STROKE

STROKE
Pathophysiology, Diagnosis, and Management

Fourth Edition

J.P. Mohr, MS, MD

Daniel Sciarra Professor of Clinical Neurology
College of Physicians and Surgeons, Columbia
    University
Stroke and Critical Care Division
Director, Doris and Stanley Tananbaum Stroke
    Campus
Neurological Institute, Columbia Campus
New York–Presbyterian Hospital
New York, New York

Dennis W. Choi, MD, PhD

Executive Vice President, Neurosciences
Merck Research Laboratories
West Point, Pennsylvania

James C. Grotta, MD

Roy M. and Phyllis Gough Huffington Distinguished
    Professor of Neurology
Director, Stroke Program
University of Texas–Houston Medical School
Houston, Texas

**Bryce Weir, OC, MD, FRCSC, FACS,
FRCSEd (Hon)**

Professor Emeritus, Departments of Surgery
University of Alberta Faculty of Medicine and
    Dentistry
Edmonton, Alberta, Canada, and
    The University of Chicago
Chicago, Illinois

Philip A. Wolf, MD

Professor of Neurology
Research Professor of Medicine (Preventive
    Medicine and Epidemiology)
Boston University School of Medicine
Professor of Public Health (Epidemiology and
    Biostatistics)
Boston University School of Public Health
Boston, Massachusetts

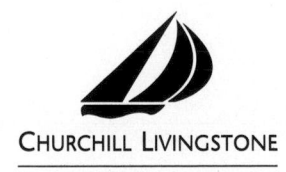

CHURCHILL LIVINGSTONE
An Imprint of Elsevier

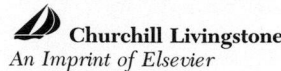 **Churchill Livingstone**
An Imprint of Elsevier

The Curtis Center
Independence Square West
Philadelphia, PA 19106

NOTICE

Neurology is an ever-changing field. Standard safety precautions must be followed, but as new research and clinical experience broaden our knowledge, changes in treatment and drug therapy may become necessary or appropriate. Readers are advised to check the most current product information provided by the manufacturer of each drug to be administered to verify the recommended dose, the method and duration of administration, and contraindications. It is the responsibility of the treating physician, relying on experience and knowledge of the patient, to determine dosages and the best treatment for each individual patient. Neither the Publisher nor the editor assumes any liability for any injury and/or damage to persons or property arising from this publication.

The Publisher

First Edition 1986. Second Edition 1992. Third Edition 1998.

Library of Congress Cataloging-in-Publication Data
Stroke : pathophysiology, diagnosis, and management / [edited by] J.P. Mohr . . . [et al.].—4th ed.
     p. ; cm.
     Includes bibliographical references and index.
     ISBN 0-443-06600-0
     1. Cerebrovascular disease.   I. Mohr, J. P.
     [DNLM: 1. Cerebrovascular Accident.   2. Cerebrovascular Disorders. WL 355 S92134 2004]
RC388.5 .S8528 2004
616.8′1—dc21

                                                                        2002031448

Acquisitions Editor: Susan Pioli
Developmental Editor: Ann Ruzycka Anderson
Project Manager: Natalie Ware
Designer: Steven Stave

Printed in the United States of America.

Last digit is the print number: 9 8 7 6 5 4 3 2

This book is dedicated to Joan Mohr, Kathryn Dreyfus, Mary Lou Weir, and Barbara Wolf, whose forbearance is herewith acknowledged with gratitude, and to our stroke patients and their families who consented to participate in the clinical research protocols that have provided us with so much of the information that is contained in this book.

Contributors

Aninda B. Acharya, MD

Instructor, Department of Neurology
Stroke Fellow
Washington University School of Medicine
St. Louis, Missouri
*Molecular Pathophysiology of White Matter Anoxic-Ischemic
Injury*

Harold P. Adams, Jr., MD

Professor of Neurology
University of Iowa Roy J. and Lucille A. Carver College
of Medicine
Attending Neurologist
University of Iowa Health Care
Iowa City, Iowa
*Aneurysmal Subarachnoid Hemorrhage
Antithrombotic Therapy for Acute Ischemic Stroke*

Lama Al-Khoury, MD

Stroke Fellow
University of California, San Diego, School of Medicine
La Jolla, California
Intravenous Thrombolysis

Adria Arboix, MD

Associate Professor
Department of Neurology, Cerebrovascular Division
University of Barcelona
Hospital Sagrat Cor
Barcelona, Catalonia, Spain
Lacunes

Roland N. Auer, MD

Professor, Departments of Pathology and Laboratory
Medicine
University of Calgary Faculty of Medicine
Neuropathologist
Foothills Hospital
Calgary, Alberta, Canada
Histopathology of Cerebral Ischemia

Issam A. Awad, MD, MSc, FACS, FAHA

Ogsbury-Kindt Professor and Chairman Department of
Neurology
University of Colorado Health Sciences Center
Denver, Colorado
Dural Arteriovenous Malformations

Alison E. Baird, MD, PhD, MPH

Chief, Stroke Neuroscience Unit
National Institute of Neurological Disorders and
Stroke
National Institutes of Health
Bethesda, Maryland
Magnetic Resonance Imaging

Henry J.M. Barnett, OC, MD, FRCP(C)

Professor Emeritus, Division of Neurology
Department of Clinical Neurological Sciences
University of Western Ontario Faculty of Medicine and
Dentistry
London, Ontario, Canada
*Cerebral Venous Thrombosis
Spinal Cord Ischemia*

Oscar Benavente, MD, FRCP(C)

Assistant Professor, Division of Neurology, Department
of Medicine
University of Texas Medical School at San Antonio
University of Texas Health Science Center at San
Antonio
San Antonio, Texas
*Secondary Prevention of Cardioembolic Stroke
Spinal Cord Ischemia*

Bernard R. Bendok, MD

Assistant Professor of Neurological Surgery and
Radiology
Co-Director, Neuroendovascular Program
Northwestern University Feinberg School of
Medicine
Chicago, Illinois
Interventional Neuroradiologic Therapy

Jeffrey R. Binder, MD

Professor of Neurology
Department of Neurology
Medical College of Wisconsin
Milwaukee, Wisconsin
Posterior Cerebral Artery Disease

Julien Bogousslavsky, MD

Professor and Chairman, Department of Neurology
Professor of Cerebrovascular Disease
University of Lausanne
Chief, Service de Neurologie
Centre Hospitalier Universitaire Vaudois
Lausanne, Switzerland
  Cervicocephalic Fibromuscular Dysplasia

Alan S. Boulos, MD

Assistant Professor of Surgery
Herman and Sunny Stall Chair of Endovascular
  Surgery
Albany Medical College
Albany, New York
  Interventional Neuroradiologic Therapy

Marie-Germaine Bousser, MD

Professor of Neurology
Director of the Neurology Department
Université Hôpital Lariboisière-Saint Louis
Paris, France
  CADASIL: Cerebral Autosomal Dominant Arteriopathy with
    Subcortical Infarcts and Leukoencephalopathy
  Cerebral Venous Thrombosis

Michael Brainin, MD

Donau-Universität Krems und Donauklinikum
Center for Postgraduate Studies in Neuroscience
Maria Gugging, Austria
  Classification of Ischemic Stroke

Robin L. Brey, PhD

Professor of Medicine, Division of Neurology
University of Texas Health Science Center at San
  Antonio
San Antonio, Texas
  Coagulation Abnormalities in Stroke

Joseph P. Broderick, MD

Professor and Chairman, Department of Neurology
University of Cincinnati College of Medicine
Staff Attending Physician
University Hospital
Cincinnati, Ohio
  Prehospital and Emergency Department Care of the Patient
    with Acute Stroke

John C.M. Brust, MD

Professor of Clinical Neurology
College of Physicians and Surgeons, Columbia University
Director, Department of Neurology
Harlem Hospital Center
New York, New York
  Anterior Cerebral Artery Disease
  Stroke and Substance Abuse

Agata Calderone

Postdoctoral Fellow
Weill Medical College of Cornell University
Department of Genetic Medicine
New York, New York
  Molecular and Cellular Mechanisms of Ischemia-Induced
    Neuronal Death

Louis R. Caplan, MD

Professor of Neurology
Harvard University Medical School
Attending Neurologist
Beth Israel Deaconess Medical Center
Boston, Massachusetts
  Intracerebral Hemorrhage
  Vertebrobasilar Disease

H. Chabriat, MD, PhD

Professor of Neurology
Department of Neurology
Université Hôpital Lariboisière-Saint Louis
Paris, France
  CADASIL: Cerebral Autosomal Dominant Arteriopathy with
    Subcortical Infarcts and Leukoencephalopathy

Angel Chamorro, MD

Neurologist
Service of Neurology
Hospital Clinic at Villarroel
Barcelona, Spain
  Anterior Cerebral Artery Disease

Sunghee Cho, PhD

Department of Neurology and Neuroscience
Cornell University Joan and Sanford I. Weill Medical
  College and Graduate School of Medical Sciences
New York, New York
  Cerebral Ischemia and Inflammation

Dennis W. Choi, MD, PhD

Executive Vice President, Neurosciences
Merck Research Laboratories
West Point, Pennsylvania
  Pathophysiology

Bruce M. Coull, MD

Professor and Chair of Neurology
Arizona Health Science Center
Tucson, Arizona
  Coagulation Abnormalities in Stroke

Edward J. Cunningham, MD

Department of Neurosurgery
St. George's Hospital Medical School
Atkinson Morley's Hospital
Wimbledon, London
United Kingdom
  Asymptomatic Carotid Occlusive Disease

Turgay Dalkara, MD, PhD

Professor, Department of Neurology
Faculty of Medicine
Hacettepe University
Ankara, Turkey
Apoptosis in Cerebral Ischemia

Patricia H. Davis, MD

Associate Professor of Neurology
University of Iowa Roy J. and Lucille A. Carver
  College of Medicine
Attending Neurologist
University of Iowa Health Care
Iowa City, Iowa
Aneurysmal Subarachnoid Hemorrhage
Antithrombotic Therapy for Acute Ischemic Stroke

Stephen M. Davis, MD, FRCP, FRACP

Department of Medicine
University of Melbourne
Director of Neurology
The Royal Melbourne Hospital
Parkville, Victoria, Australia
Single-Photon Emission Computed Tomography

Ted M. Dawson, MD, PhD

Professor of Neurology and Neuroscience
Movement Disorder Specialist
Department of Neurology
Johns Hopkins University School of Medicine
Baltimore, Maryland
Intracellular Signaling: Mediators and Protective
  Responses

Valina L. Dawson, PhD

Professor of Neurology, Neuroscience, and
  Physiology
Johns Hopkins University School of Medicine
Baltimore, Maryland
Intracellular Signaling: Mediators and Protective
  Responses

Gregory J. del Zoppo, MS, MD

Associate Professor
Department of Molecular and Experimental Medicine
The Scripps Research Institute
Member, Division of Hematology/Medical Oncology
Scripps Clinic
La Jolla, California
Mechanisms of Thrombosis and Thrombolysis
The Cerebral Microvasculature and Responses to
  Ischemia

H. C. Diener, MD

Professor and Chairman, Department of Neurology
University of Essen
Essen, Germany
Migraine and Stroke

Marco R. Di Tullio, MD

Associate Professor of Clinical Medicine
College of Physicians and Surgeons, Columbia University
Associate Attending Physician
Associate Director of the Adult Electrocardiography
  Laboratory
New York–Presbyterian Hospital
New York, New York
Atherosclerotic Disease of the Proximal Aorta

Bruce H. Dobkin, MD

Professor of Neurology
Director, Neurologic Rehabilitation and Research
  Program
David Geffen School of Medicine at UCLA
University of California, Los Angeles
Los Angeles, California
Rehabilitation and Recovery of the Patient with Stroke

Geoffrey A. Donnan, MD

Director, National Stroke Research Institute
Austin and Repatriation Medical Centre
Professor of Neurology
University of Melbourne
Heidelberg West, Victoria, Australia
Overview of Laboratory Studies

Mitchell S.V. Elkind, MS, MD

Assistant Professor of Neurology
College of Physicians and Surgeons, Columbia University
Stroke and Critical Care Division
Doris and Stanley Tananbaum Stroke Campus
Neurological Institute, Columbia Campus
New York–Presbyterian Hospital
New York, New York
Collagen Vascular and Infectious Diseases

J. Paul Elliott, MD

Assistant Clinical Professor, Department of Neurological
  Surgery
University of Colorado Health Sciences Center
Denver, Colorado
Colorado Neurological Institute
Swedish Medical Center
Englewood, Colorado
Dural Arteriovenous Malformations

Timo Erkinjuntti, MD, PhD

Chief, Memory Research Unit
Department of Neurology
University of Helsinki
Helsinki, Finland
Vascular Cognitive Impairment and Dementia

Frank M. Faraci, PhD

Professor, Department of Internal Medicine
University of Iowa Roy J. and Lucille A. Carver College
  of Medicine
Iowa City, Iowa
Vascular Biology and Atherosclerosis of Cerebral Arteries

Giora Feuerstein, MD, MSc

Merck Research Laboratories
West Point, Pennsylvania
  Cerebral Ischemia and Inflammation

J. Max Findlay, MD, PhD, FRCSC, FACS

Clinical Professor
University of Alberta Faculty of Medicine and
  Dentistry
Edmonton, Alberta, Canada
  Intraventricular Hemorrhage
  Carotid Endarterectomy

Ian G. Fleetwood, MF, FRCSC

Assistant Professor
Dalhousie University Faculty of Medicine
Director of Cerebrovascular Surgery
Co-Director of Radiosurgery
Halifax Infirmary
Halifax, Nova Scotia, Canada
  Cavernous Malformations and Venous Anomalies: Natural
    History and Surgical Management

Karen L. Furie, MD, MPH

Assistant Professor in Neurology
Harvard Medical School
Assistant in Neurology
Massachusetts General Hospital
Boston, Massachusetts
  Cardiac Diseases

Anthony J. Furlan, MD

Section Head
Stroke and Neurologic Intensive Care
Cleveland Clinic Foundation
Cleveland, Ohio
  Intra-arterial Thrombolysis in Acute Ischemic Stroke

Jean Claude Gautier, MD

Professor of Neurology (Hon)
Faculté Pitié-Salpêtrière
Médecin (Hon) de la Salpêtrière
Membre de l'Académie Nationale de Médecin
Paris, France
  Internal Carotid Artery Disease

Dimitrios Georgiadis, MD

Lecturer, Department of Neurology
University of Zurich
Zurich, Switzerland
  Critical Care of the Patient with Acute Stroke

Y. Pierre Gobin, MD

Professor of Radiology in Neurosurgery
Cornell University Joan and Sanford I. Weill Medical
  College and Graduate School of Medical Sciences
Director, Interventional Neuroradiology
Cornell Medical Center
New York, New York
  Cerebral Angiography

Mark P. Goldberg, MD

Professor, Department of Neurology
Washington University School of Medicine
St. Louis, Missouri
  Molecular Pathophysiology of White Matter Anoxic-Ischemic
    Injury

Steven Goldstein, MD*

Associate Professor, Department of Neurology
The Stroke Institute
University of Pittsburgh Medical Center
Pittsburgh, Pennsylvania
  Computed Tomography–Based Evaluation of
    Cerebrovascular Disease

Steven M. Greenberg, MD, PhD

Associate Professor of Neurology
Co-Director, Neurology Clinical Trials Unit
Massachusetts General Hospital
Boston, Massachusetts
  Cerebral Amyloid Angiopathy

James C. Grotta, MD

Roy M. and Phyllis Gough Huffington Distinguished
  Professor of Neurology
Director, Stroke Program
University of Texas–Houston Medical School
Houston, Texas
  Pharmacologic Modification of Acute Cerebral Ischemia

Robert L. Grubb, Jr., MD

Professor of Neurological Surgery
Professor of Radiation Sciences
Washington University School of Medicine
St. Louis, Missouri
Neurosurgeon
Barnes-Jewish Hospital
St. Louis, Missouri
  Extracranial-Intracranial Bypass for Cerebral Ischemia

Lee R. Guterman, MD, PhD

Assistant Professor of Neurosurgery
Co-Director, Toshiba Stroke Research Center
State University of New York at Buffalo School of
  Medicine and Biomedical Sciences
Neurosurgeon
Millard Fillmore Hospital
Buffalo, New York
  Interventional Neuroradiologic Therapy

Werner Hacke, MD

Professor and Head, Department of Neurology
University of Heidelberg
Heidelberg, Germany
  Critical Care of the Patient with Acute Stroke

---

*Deceased

John Hallenbeck, MD

Senior Investigator
Chief, Stroke Branch
National Institute of Neurological Disorders and Stroke
National Institutes of Health
Bethesda, Maryland
Cerebral Ischemia and Inflammation

Gerhard F. Hamann, MD

Professor, Department of Neurology
Ludwig-Maximilians-Universität München
Klinikum Grosshadern
Munich, Germany
The Cerebral Microvasculature and Responses to Ischemia

Andreas Hartmann, MD

Associate Professor, Department of Neurology
Freie Universität Berlin
Charite-Hochschulmedizin Berlin
Campus Benjamin Franklin
Berlin, Germany
*Arteriovenous Malformations and Other Vascular
 Anomalies*

Kazuo Hashi, MD

Professor Emeritus
Sapporo Medical University
President
Pacific Neurosurgical Consulting
Sapporo, Japan
Moyamoya Disease: Surgical Aspects

Donald D. Heistad, MD

Zahn Professor of Cardiology, Department of Internal
 Medicine
University of Iowa Roy J. and Lucille A. Carver
 College of Medicine
Iowa City, Iowa
Vascular Biology and Atherosclerosis of Cerebral Arteries

Michael Hennerici, MD

Professor and Chairman, Department of Neurology
University of Heidelberg
Mannheim Medical School
Mannheim, Germany
Ultrasonography

Juha Hernesniemi, MD

Professor and Chairman, Department of
 Neurosurgery
University Hospital of Helsinki
Helsinki, Finland
Familial Vascular Diseases of Neurosurgical Significance

Daniel B. Hier, MD

Professor and Chairman, Department of Neurology
University of Illinois at Chicago College of Medicine
Chicago, Illinois
Middle Cerebral Artery Disease

Randall T. Higashida, MD

Clinical Professor, Department of Radiology
University of California, San Francisco, School of
 Medicine
San Francisco, California
Intra-arterial Thrombolysis in Acute Ischemic Stroke

Shunichi Homma, MD

Associate Professor of Clinical Medicine
College of Physicians and Surgeons, Columbia University
Director, Echocardiography Laboratories
Columbia–Presbyterian Medical Center
New York, New York
Atherosclerotic Disease of the Proximal Aorta
Cardiac Diseases

Kazuhiro Hongo, MD

Professor and Chairman, Department of Neurosurgery
Shinshu University School of Medicine
Matsumoto, Japan
Cerebellar Infarction and Hemorrhage

L. Nelson Hopkins, MD

Professor and Chairman of Neurosurgery
Professor of Radiology
State University of New York at Buffalo School of
 Medicine and Biomedical Sciences
Chairman, Department of Neurosurgery
Kaleida Health
Buffalo, New York
Interventional Neuroradiologic Therapy

George Howard, DrPH

Professor of Biostatistics
School of Public Health
University of Alabama at Birmingham
Birmingham, Alabama
*Distribution of Stroke: Heterogeneity of Stroke by Age, Race,
 and Sex*

Virginia Howard, PhD, MSPH

Assistant Professor of Epidemiology
School of Public Health
University of Alabama at Birmingham
Birmingham, Alabama
*Distribution of Stroke: Heterogeneity of Stroke by Age, Race,
 and Sex*

Daniel Huddle, DO

Associate Professor
Interventional Neuroradiology
University of Colorado Health Sciences Center
Denver, Colorado
Dural Arteriovenous Malformations

Raymond M.M. Hupperts, MD, PhD

Neurologist, Associate Professor of Neurology
Medical Faculty, Department of Neurology
University Hospital Maastricht
Maastricht, The Netherlands
Anterior Choroidal Artery Territory Infarcts

Costantino Iadecola, MD

Department of Neurology and Neuroscience
Cornell University Joan and Sanford I. Weill
  Medical College and Graduate School of Medical
  Sciences
New York, New York
  Cerebral Ischemia and Inflammation

Bernard Infeld, MD, FRACP

Neurologist, Department of Neurology
Melbourne Neuroscience Center
Royal Melbourne Hospital
Parkville, Victoria, Australia
Director of Stroke Service
Epworth Hospital
Richmond, Victoria, Australia
  Single-Photon Emission Computed Tomography

Sriram S. Iyer, MD

Clinical Associate Professor of Medicine
New York University School of Medicine
Chief, Endovascular Services
Lenox Hill Heart and Vascular Institute
New York, New York
  Carotid Stenting

A. Joutel, MD, PhD

Senior Researcher
Faculté de Médicine Lariboisière
Laboratoire de Cytogénétique
Hôpital Lariboisière
Paris, France
  *CADASIL: Cerebral Autosomal Dominant Arteriopathy with
    Subcortical Infarcts and Leukoencephalopathy*

Teresa Jover

Research Associate
Department of Neuroscience
Albert Einstein College of Medicine of Yeshiva
  University
Bronx, New York
  *Molecular and Cellular Mechanisms of Ischemia-Induced
    Neuronal Death*

Charles A. Jungreis, MD

Professor, Department of Radiology
University of Pittsburgh Medical Center
Pittsburgh, Pennsylvania
  *Computed Tomography–Based Evaluation of
    Cerebrovascular Disease*

Mary A. Kalafut, MD

Member, Division of Neurology
Co-Director, Vascular Laboratory
Scripps Clinic and Green Hospital
La Jolla, California
  Mechanisms of Thrombosis and Thrombolysis

Carlos S. Kase, MD

Professor of Neurology
Boston University School of Medicine
Attending Neurologist
Department of Neurology
Boston Medical Center
Boston, Massachusetts
  Intracerebral Hemorrhage

Scott E. Kasner, MD

Associate Professor, Department of Neurology
Director, Comprehensive Stroke Center
University of Pennsylvania School of Medicine
Philadelphia, Pennsylvania
  Treatment of "Other" Causes of Stroke

Markku Kaste, MD, PhD FAHA

Professor of Neurology and Chairman
Department of Neurology
Helsinki University Central Hospital
University of Helsinki
Helsinki, Finland
  General Stroke Management and Stroke Units

Chelsea S. Kidwell, MD

Associate Professor, Department of Neurology
David Geffen School of Medicine at UCLA
University of California, Los Angeles
Reed Neurological Research Center
Los Angeles, California
  Magnetic Resonance Imaging

Louis J. Kim, MD

Neurosurgical Resident
Barrow Neurological Institute
Phoenix, Arizona
  Spinal Arteriovenous Malformations

Stanley H. Kim, MD

Assistant Professor of Neurosurgery
State University of New York at Buffalo School of
  Medicine and Biomedical Sciences
Buffalo, New York
Endovascular Neurosurgeon
St. David's Medical Center
Austin, Texas
  Interventional Neuroradiologic Therapy

J. Philip Kistler, MD

Professor of Neurology
Harvard Medical School
Neurologist
Massachusetts General Hospital
Boston, Massachusetts
  Cardiac Diseases

Shigeaki Kobayashi, MD

Professor and Chairman, Department of
  Neurosurgery
Shinshu University of Medicine
Matsumoto, Japan
  Cerebellar Infarction and Hemorrhage

Lise A. Labiche, MD

Neurologist
Baylor University Medical Center
Dallas, Texas
Pharmacologic Modification of Acute Cerebral Ischemia

Catherine Lamy, MD

Neurologist
University of Paris V
Hôpital Sainte-Anne
Paris, France
Hypertensive Encephalopathy

C. Geoff Lau, MD

Department of Neuroscience
Albert Einstein College of Medicine of Yeshiva
    University
Bronx, New York
*Molecular and Cellular Mechanisms of Ischemia-Induced
    Neuronal Death*

Michael T. Lawton, MD

Assistant Professor, Department of Neurological
    Surgery
University of California, San Francisco, School of
    Medicine
San Francisco, California
Intracranial Aneurysms

Ronald M. Lazar, MD

Professor of Clinical Neuropsychology in Neurology and
    Neurological Surgery
College of Physicians and Surgeons, Columbia University
Stroke and Critical Care Division
Doris and Stanley Tananbaum Stroke Campus
Neurological Institute, Columbia Campus
New York–Presbyterian Hospital
New York, New York
Middle Cerebral Artery Disease

G. Michael Lemole, Jr., MD

Assistant Professor, Department of Neurosurgery
University of Illinois Medical Center
Chicago, Illinois
Spinal Arteriovenous Malformations

Peter D. Le Roux, MD

Associate Professor and Vice Chairman, Department of
    Neurosurgery
University of Pennsylvania School of Medicine
Attending Neurosurgeon
Pennsylvania Hospital
Hospital of the University of Pennsylvania
Children's Hospital of Philadelphia
Philadelphia, Pennsylvania
*Standards for Surgical Treatment of Cerebrovascular Disease,
    Circa 2000*

Elad I. Levy, MD

Resident
Department of Neurological Surgery
University of Pittsburgh Medical Center
Pittsburgh, Pennsylvania
Interventional Neuroradiologic Therapy

Jan Lodder, MD, PhD

Associate Professor of Neurology and Neurologist,
    Department of Neurology
University Hospital Maastricht
Maastricht, The Netherlands
Anterior Choroidal Artery Territory Infarcts

Patrick D. Lyden, MD

Professor of Neuroscience
University of California, San Diego, School of
    Medicine
Staff Physician
Veterans Affairs Medical Center
La Jolla, California
Intravenous Thrombolysis

H. Ma, MD

Clinical Research Fellow
National Stroke Research Institute
Austin and Repatriation Medical Centre
Professor of Neurology
University of Melbourne
Heidelberg, West Victoria, Australia
Overview of Laboratory Studies

R. Loch Macdonald, MD, PhD

Professor of Neurosurgery, Department of Surgery
University of Chicago Pritzker School of Medicine
Chicago, Illinois
Cerebral Vasospasm

Philippe Maeder

Service de Radiodiagnostic et Radiologie
    Intervontionnelle
Centre Hospitalier Universitaire Vaudois
Lausanne, Switzerland
Cervicocephalic Fibromuscular Dysplasia

B. Elaine Marchak, MD, FRCP

Associate Clinical Professor
University of Alberta Faculty of Medicine and
    Dentistry
Head of Neuroanesthesia, University Hospital
Edmonton, Alberta, Canada
Carotid Endarterectomy

Joanne Markham, MS

Research Associate
Washington University School of Medicine
St. Louis, Missouri
*Cerebral Blood Flow and Metabolism in Cerebrovascular
    Disease*

Randolph S. Marshall, MD

Associate Professor of Clinical Neurology
College of Physicians and Surgeons, Columbia University
Stroke and Critical Care Division
Doris and Stanley Tananbaum Stroke Campus
Neurological Institute, Columbia Campus
New York–Presbyterian Hospital
New York, New York
  Middle Cerebral Artery Disease

J.L. Marti-Vilalta, MD

Professor of Neurology, Department of Neurology
Universitat Autònoma de Barcelona
Director, Cerebrovascular Unit
Hospital de la Santa Creu i Sant Pau
Barcelona, Catalonia, Spain
  Lacunes

Jean-Louis Mas, MD

Professor of Neurology
Université de Paris V
Chairman of Neurology
Hôpital Sainte-Anne
Paris, France
  Hypertensive Encephalopathy

Henning Mast, MD

Adjunct Associate Professor of Neurology
College of Physicians and Surgeons, Columbia University
Doris and Stanley Tananbaum Stroke Campus
Neurological Institute, Columbia Campus
New York–Presbyterian Hospital
New York, New York
  *Arteriovenous Malformations and Other Vascular
    Anomalies*
  Binswanger's Disease and Vascular Dementia

Junichi Masuda, MD

Professor, Department of Laboratory Medicine
Shimane Medical University
Izumo, Shimane, Japan
  Moyamoya Disease

Marc R. Mayberg, MD

Chairman, Department of Neurosurgery
Cleveland Clinic
Cleveland, Ohio
  Asymptomatic Carotid Occlusive Disease

Stephen Meairs, MD

Associate Professor of Neurology, Department of
  Neurology
University of Heidelberg
Universitätklinikum Mannheim
Mannheim, Germany
  Ultrasonography

**Alexander David Mendelow, MB, BCh, PhD,
FRCSEd (Surgical Neurology)**

Professor of Neurosurgery
University of Newcastle
Professor of Neurosurgery and Head, Department of
  Neurosurgery
Newcastle General Hospital
Newcastle upon Tyne, United Kingdom
  Intracerebral Hemorrhage

J.P. Mohr, MS, MD

Daniel Sciarra Professor of Clinical Neurology
College of Physicians and Surgeons, Columbia University
Stroke and Critical Care Division
Director, Doris and Stanley Tananbaum Stroke Campus
Neurological Institute, Columbia Campus
New York–Presbyterian Hospital
New York, New York
  Arteriovenous Malformations and Other Vascular Anomalies
  Binswanger's Disease and Vascular Dementia
  Classification of Ischemic Stroke
  Collagen Vascular and Infectious Diseases
  Internal Carotid Artery Disease
  Intracerebral Hemorrhage
  Lacunes
  Middle Cerebral Artery Disease
  Migraine and Stroke
  Overview of Laboratory Studies
  Posterior Cerebral Artery Disease
  Spinal Cord Ischemia
  Ultrasonography
  Vertebrobasilar Disease

Lewis B. Morgenstern, MD

Director of the Stroke Program
Associate Professor of Neurology, Epidemiology,
  Emergency Medicine, and Neurosurgery
University of Michigan Health System
Ann Arbor, Michigan
  *Medical Therapy of Intracerebral and Intraventricular
    Hemorrhage*

Michael A. Moskowitz, MD, MSc

Professor
Harvard–MIT Division of Health Science and
  Technology
Harvard Medical School
Massachusetts General Hospital
Boston, Massachusetts
  Apoptosis in Cerebral Ischemia

Junpei Nitta, MD

Department of Neurosurgery
Shinshu University School of Medicine
Matsumoto, Japan
  Cerebellar Infarction and Hemorrhage

Jun Ogata, MD

Advisor
Multiple Handicapped Children's Hospital
Hirakata Ryoikuen
Hirakata, Osaka, Japan
Moyamoya Disease

Adetokunbo A. Oyelese, MD, PhD

Department of Neurosurgery
Stanford University School of Medicine
Stanford, California
*Cavernous Malformations and Venous Anomalies: Natural
History and Surgical Management*

Yuko Y. Palesch, PhD

Associate Professor
Medical University of South Carolina
Department of Biometry and Epidemiology
Charleston, South Carolina
Conduct of Stroke-Related Clinical Trials

Arthur M. Pancioli, MD

Associate Professor of Emergency Medicine
Vice Chairman, Department of Emergency Medicine
University of Cincinnati College of Medicine
Cincinnati, Ohio
*Prehospital and Emergency Department Care of the Patient
with Acute Stroke*

Andrew T. Parsa, MD, PhD

Assistant Professor, Department of Neurological Surgery
University of California, San Francisco, School of
  Medicine
San Francisco, California
Vascular Malformations of the Brain

Bartlomiej Piechowski-Józwiak, MD

Assistant, Department of Neurology
Medical University of Warsaw
Warsaw, Poland
Cervicocephalic Fibromuscular Dysplasia

John Pile-Spellman, MD

Professor of Radiology and Neurosurgery
College of Physicians and Surgeons, Columbia University
Director of Research Neuroradiology
Columbia–Presbyterian Medical Center
New York, New York
Arteriovenous Malformations and Other Vascular Anomalies

William J. Powers, MD

Professor of Neurology, Neurological Surgery, and
  Radiology
Washington University School of Medicine
Attending Neurologist
Barnes-Jewish Hospital
St. Louis, Missouri
*Cerebral Blood Flow and Metabolism in Cerebrovascular
Disease*

Adnan I. Qureshi, MD

Professor, Department of Neurology and Neuroscience
UMDNJ—New Jersey Medical School
Director, Cerebrovascular Program
Endovascular Attending Physician
University Hospital
Neurological Institute of New Jersey
Newark, New Jersey
Interventional Neuroradiologic Therapy

Bruce R. Ransom, MD, PhD

Magnuson Professor and Chairman, Department of
  Neurology
Adjunct Professor, Physiology and Biophysics
University of Washington School of Medicine
Seattle, Washington
*Molecular Pathophysiology of White Matter Anoxic-Ischemic
  Injury*

Howard A. Riina, MD

Assistant Professor, Neurological Surgery, Neurology, and
  Radiology
Cornell University Joan and Sanford I. Weill Medical
  College and Graduate School of Medical Sciences
Attending Physician
New York–Presbyterian Hospital
New York, New York
Spinal Arteriovenous Malformations

Risto O. Roine, MD, PhD

Associate Professor, Department of Neurology
Chief, Acute Stroke Unit
Helsinki University Central Hospital
Helsinki, Finland
General Stroke Management and Stroke Units

Antti Ronkainen, MD, PhD

Neurosurgeon
Associate Chief Physician
Department of Neurosurgery
Kuopio University Hospital
Kuopio, Finland
Familial Vascular Diseases of Neurosurgical Significance

Gary S. Roubin, MD, PhD

Clinical Professor of Medicine
New York University School of Medicine
Lenox Hill Heart and Vascular Institute
New York, New York
Carotid Stenting

Tanja Rundek, MD, PhD

Assistant Professor of Neurology
College of Physicians and Surgeons, Columbia University
Stroke and Critical Care Division
Doris and Stanley Tananbaum Stroke Campus
Neurological Institute, Columbia Campus
New York–Presbyterian Hospital
New York, New York
Outcome following Stroke

Ralph L. Sacco, MS, MD

Professor of Neurology and Epidemiology
Associate Chair of Neurology
College of Physicians and Surgeons, Columbia University
Gertrude Sergievsky Campus, Mailman School of Public
  Health
Director, Stroke and Critical Care Division
Doris and Stanley Tananbaum Stroke Campus
Neurological Institute, Columbia Campus
New York–Presbyterian Hospital
New York, New York
  Classification of Ischemic Stroke
  Outcome following Stroke

Ronald J. Sattenberg, MD

Chief of Neuroradiology
Methodist Hospital of the New York–Presbyterian
  Hospital Center
Brooklyn, New York
  Cerebral Angiography

Jeffrey Saver, MD

Professor of Clinical Neurology
David Geffen School of Medicine at UCLA
University of California, Los Angeles
Neurology Director
UCLA Stroke Center
UCLA Center for the Health Sciences
Los Angeles, California
  Cerebral Angiography

Herrmann-Christian Schumacher, MD

Doris and Stanley Tananbaum Stroke Campus
Neurological Institute, Columbia Campus
New York–Presbyterian Hospital
New York, New York
  Arteriovenous Malformations and Other Vascular
    Anomalies

Stefan Schwab, MD

Lecturer, Department of Neurology
Director, Neurological Intensive Care
Department of Neurology
University of Heidelberg
Heidelberg, Germany
  Critical Care of the Patient with Acute Stroke

David G. Sherman, MD

Department of Medicine (Neurology)
University of Texas Health Science Center at San
  Antonio
San Antonio, Texas
  Secondary Prevention of Cardioembolic Stroke

Gerald Silverboard, MD

Clinical Associate Professor, Child Neurology
University of South Alabama College of Medicine
Mobile, Alabama
  Arterial Dissections

Monica Simionescu, MD

Resident, Department of Neurology
Loyola University Chicago Strich School of Medicine
Chicago, Illinois
  Molecular and Cellular Mechanisms of Ischemia-Induced
    Neuronal Death

Christopher G. Sobey, BSc(Hons), PhD

Research Fellow
University of Melbourne
Parkville, Victoria, Australia
  Vascular Biology and Atherosclerosis of Cerebral Arteries

Robert A. Solomon, MD

Byron Stookey Professor and Chairman
Department of Neurological Surgery
College of Physicians and Surgeons, Columbia University
Neurological Institute, Columbia Campus
New York–Presbyterian Hospital
New York, New York
  Vascular Malformations of the Brain

Robert F. Spetzler, MD

Professor, Division of Neurosurgery
University of Arizona College of Medicine
Tucson, Arizona
Director, Neurovascular Research
Barrow Neurological Institute
Phoenix, Arizona
  Intracranial Aneurysms
  Spinal Arteriovenous Malformations

Christian Stapf, MD

Assistant Professor of Neurology
Freie Universität Berlin
Berlin, Germany
  Arteriovenous Malformations and Other Vascular Anomalies

Gary K. Steinberg, MD, PhD

Lacroute-Hearst Professor and Chairman, Department
  of Neurosurgery
Stanford University School of Medicine
Chief, Neurosurgery
Stanford University Medical Center
Stanford, California
  Cavernous Malformations and Venous Anomalies: Natural
    History and Surgical Management

**Cathie Sudlow, BA, MB, BCh(Oxf),
  MMRCP(UK), MSc(London),
  DPhil(Oxf)**

Wellcome Clinician Scientist
Division of Clinical Neurosciences
University of Edinburgh
Honorary Specialist Registrar in Neurology
Western General Hospital
Edinburgh, United Kingdom
  Long-Term Medical Management of Ischemic Stroke and
    Transient Ischemic Attack Due to Arterial Disease

Barbara C. Tilley, PhD

Professor and Chair
Department of Biometry and Epidemiology
Medical University of South Carolina
Charleston, South Carolina
Conduct of Stroke-Related Clinical Trials

Danilo Toni, MD, PhD

Department of Neurological Sciences
Universitá degli Studi di Roma "la Sapienza"
Rome, Italy
Classification of Ischemic Stroke

E. Tournier-Lasserve, MD

Professor of Genetics
Université Hôpital Lariboisière-Saint Louis
Director
Laboratoire de Cytogénétique
Hôpital Lariboisière
Paris, France
*CADASIL: Cerebral Autosomal Dominant Arteriopathy with
Subcortical Infarcts and Leukoencephalopathy*

K. Vahedi, MD

Senior Clinical Neurologist, Neurology Department
Université Hôpital Lariboisière-Saint Louis
Paris, France
*CADASIL: Cerebral Autosomal Dominant Arteriopathy with
Subcortical Infarcts and Leukoencephalopathy*

G. Edward Vates, MD, PhD

Cerebrovascular and Skull Base Surgery Fellow
Department of Neurological Surgery
Brigham and Women's Hospital
Harvard Medical School
Boston, Massachusetts
Intracranial Aneurysms

Jiri J. Vitek, MD, PhD

Lenox Hill Heart and Vascular Institute
New York, New York
Carotid Stenting

Masahiko Wanibuchi, MD

Faculty
Sapporo Medical University
Sapporo, Japan
Moyamoya Disease: Surgical Aspects

Steven Warach, MD, PhD

Senior Investigator
National Institute of Neurological Disorders and
Stroke
National Institutes of Health
Bethesda, Maryland
Magnetic Resonance Imaging

**Charles P. Warlow, BA, MB BChir, FRCP,
MD, F MedSci**

Professor of Medical Neurology
University of Edinburgh
Honorary Consultant Neurologist
Western General Hospital
Edinburgh, United Kingdom
*Long-Term Medical Management of Ischemic Stroke and
Transient Ischemic Attack Due to Arterial Disease*

**Bryce Weir, OC, MD, FRCSC, FACS,
FRCSEd (Hon)**

Professor Emeritus, Departments of Surgery
University of Alberta Faculty of Medicine and Dentistry
Edmonton, Alberta, Canada, and
The University of Chicago
Chicago, Illinois
Cerebral Infarction: Surgical Treatment

Giora Weisz, MD

Lenox Hill Heart and Vascular Institute
Cardiovascular Research Foundation
New York, New York
Carotid Stenting

Babette B. Weksler, MD

Professor of Medicine
Division of Hematology/Medical Oncology
Cornell University Joan and Sanford I. Weill Medical
College and Graduate School of Medical Sciences
Attending Physician
New York–Presbyterian Hospital
New York, New York
Antiplatelet Therapy for Secondary Prevention of Stroke

K.M.A. Welch, MD

William T. Gossett Chair, Department of Neurology
Henry Ford Hospital
Detroit, Michigan
Migraine and Stroke

H. Richard Winn, MD

Professor of Neurosurgery and Neuroscience
Director of Research, Neurosurgery Department
Mount Sinai School of Medicine
New York, New York
*Standards for Surgical Treatment of Cerebrovascular Disease,
Circa 2000*

Philip A. Wolf, MD

Professor of Neurology
Research Professor of Medicine (Preventive Medicine
and Epidemiology)
Boston University School of Medicine
Professor of Public Health (Epidemiology and
Biostatistics)
Boston University School of Public Health
Boston, Massachusetts
Epidemiology of Stroke

Andrew R. Xavier, MD

Instructor, Department of Neuroscience
UMDNJ–New Jersey Medical School
Endovascular Fellow
University Hospital
Neurological Institute of New Jersey
Newark, New Jersey
  Interventional Neuroradiologic Therapy

Abutaher M. Yahia, HSC, MD

Assistant Professor, Department of Neurology and
  Neuroscience
UMDNJ–New Jersey Medical School
Neurologist/Neurointensivist
University Hospital
Neurological Institute of New Jersey
Newark, New Jersey
  Interventional Neuroradiologic Therapy

Takenori Yamaguchi, MD, PhD

President Emeritus
National Cardiovascular Center
Suita, Osaka, Japan
  Moyamoya Disease

Akira Yamaura, MD, PhD

Chairman and Professor of Neurosurgery
Graduate School of Medicine
Chiba University
Chiba, Japan
  Nontraumatic Intracranial Arterial Dissection

Hidenori Yokota, MD

Associate Professor
Jichi Medical School
Neurosurgeon
Jichi Medical School Hospital
Tochigi-Keni, Japan
  *Molecular and Cellular Mechanisms of Ischemia-Induced
    Neuronal Death*

Joseph M. Zabramski, MD

Chief, Section of Cerebrovascular Surgery
Barrow Neurological Institute
Mercy Healthcare Arizona
Phoenix, Arizona
  Intracranial Aneurysms

Allyson R. Zazulia, MD

Assistant Professor of Neurology
Washington University School of Medicine
Attending Neurologist
Barnes-Jewish Hospital
St. Louis, Missouri
  *Cerebral Blood Flow and Metabolism in Cerebrovascular
    Disease*

R. Suzanne Zukin, MD

Professor, Department of Neuroscience
Director, Neuropsychopharmacologic Center
Albert Einstein College of Medicine of Yeshiva
  University
Bronx, New York
  *Molecular and Cellular Mechanisms of Ischemia-Induced
    Neuronal Death*

Richard M. Zweifler, MD

Associate Professor of Neurology
University of South Alabama College of Medicine
Director, Stroke Center
University of South Alabama Hospitals
Mobile, Alabama
  Artertial Dissections

Preface to the Fourth Edition

The numerous contributors and editors, original and more recent, remain gratified that their efforts have justified yet another edition of this book, the first edition having begun 20 years ago. In these two decades dramatic changes have occurred in the field covered in these pages, with impacts that have changed the emphasis, chapter lengths, and even the subjects covered.

The original four editors are now down to one, the other three having given their places to new editors, and a whole new section has been created by a fifth editor. A new section for Epidemiology is now edited by Philip A. Wolf. Dennis W. Choi now heads the basic science sections formerly edited by Frank M. Yatsu. James C. Grotta has succeeded Henry J.M. Barnett for the sections on medical therapy. The chapters covering interventional and neurosurgical therapy formerly edited by Bennett M. Stein are now edited by Bryce Weir.

The scope of developments from molecular biology through clinical trials, with such a high degree of cross-fertilization between sections of this field, continues to tax the efforts by the editors to avoid redundancies in the text, so we hope readers will forgive any found as occurring in the spirit of ensuring clarity for the individual chapters. Those inclined toward page counting may notice considerable variation in chapter lengths for topics appearing in each of the editions to date, reflecting the irregular rates of advances in each subject. We hope the reader will be attracted to the more important changes in scope of the subjects covered, with the inclusion of many new ones unknown or barely in existence when the original edition was brought forth. We even hope that the information contained in this edition makes for its rapid obsolescence, so great are our aspirations for continued rapid developments in our field.

This, then, is the latest effort from a group of investigators, from bench to bedside, who look forward to the future and hope for yet another edition to be justified.

J.P. Mohr, MS, MD
Dennis W. Choi, MD, PhD
James C. Grotta, MD
Bryce Weir, MD
Philip A. Wolf, MD

Contents

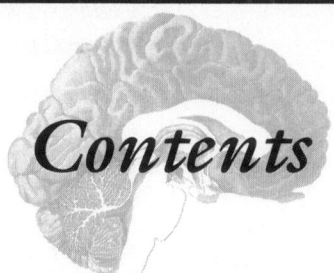

Section I

Epidemiology and Prevention

Philip A. Wolf

Epidemiology is "the study of the distribution and determinants of disease frequency" in human populations. Consideration of the *distribution* of stroke by geographic region, race-ethnicity, age, and gender is discussed comprehensively in Chapter 1. Chapter 2 focuses on risk factors for stroke and predisposing conditions, including implications for stroke prevention. An exposition of outcome following stroke, the other key determinant in stroke prevalence, morbidity, and mortality, is found in Chapter 3.

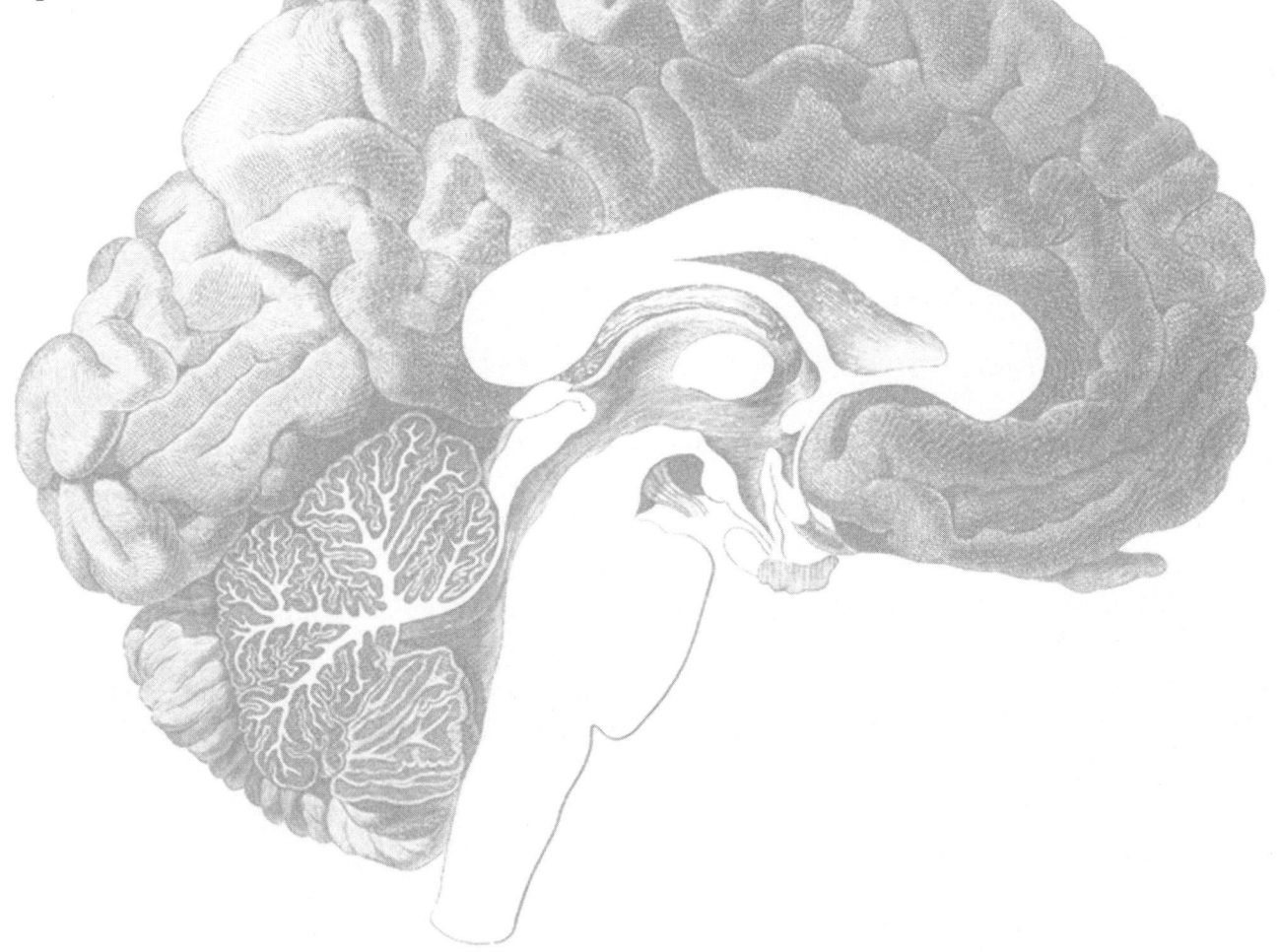

Chapter One

Distribution of Stroke: Heterogeneity of Stroke by Age, Race, and Sex

George Howard and Virginia J. Howard

INDICES OF STROKE HETEROGENEITY

Mortality, *incidence*, and *prevalence* are all indices that can be used to describe differences in the distribution or "risk" of stroke among selected populations. Each of these indices provides information that is of particular value to clinical or public health decision-makers in addressing the burden of stroke. The use of an inappropriate index, however, can lead to inappropriate conclusions and decisions. There are also striking differences between these indices in the quantity and quality of the data available. For all of these reasons, the definitions and properties of these indices should be considered.

Stroke mortality reflects deaths from stroke. In the United States, the most common source of data underlying estimates of stroke mortality rates is the vital statistics system maintained by the National Center for Health Statistics.[1] The vital statistics system requires the reporting of all death events, with information on the "underlying" (primary) and "contributing" (secondary) causes as well as demographic descriptors such as age, sex, and ethnicity. The causes of death are locally coded, generally by nonphysicians, with the use of the codes in the World Health Organization's International Classification of Diseases (ICD).[2] The ICD codes have evolved over the years, and revision 10 is currently employed.

The *stroke mortality rate* is calculated by dividing the number of deaths occurring over a fixed time (normally a year) by the estimated population at risk. Intercensus estimates are obtained by adjusting the census counts conducted each decade by regional reports of deaths and births (also part of the vital statistics reporting system). The major strength of stroke mortality rate as an index of the burden of stroke is the mandatory reporting of deaths. Because such reporting is mandatory, estimates of stroke mortality rates can be made at the national level as well as for specific regions (e.g., county level) and for specific race or sex groups.

There are, however, shortcomings in the use of stroke mortality rates as an index of the burden of stroke. Among

them is the inability to reliably report stroke death rates by stroke subtype, even at the level of distinguishing rates of death from infarction versus hemorrhage. The lack of detailed coding of causes of death requires estimates of the stroke mortality rates to be provided only for "all stroke." Specifically, Figure 1–1A shows the distribution of subtypes of 167,366 reported stroke deaths during 1999.[3] The striking feature of these data are that 91,051 (54%) were reported "stroke, not specified as hemorrhage or infarction (ICD-10: I64)." In addition, deaths from "other cerebrovascular diseases (I67)" and "sequelae of cerebrovascular disease (I69)" likely include many stroke deaths, but these codes have been shown to not be as specific as other ICD codes.[4] The ICD system also provides for coding cause of death by detailed categories within the major stroke subtypes. On the surface, this coding potentially provides the possibility of distinguishing cerebral infarctions attributable to "thrombosis of cerebral arteries (I63.3)" from those attributable to "embolism of cerebral arteries (I63.4)." However, lack of coding detail also makes this distinction problematic, as within the 14,804 deaths during 1999 from "cerebral infarction (I63)." Figure 1–1B shows that 10,101 (69%) of these deaths were reported only as "cerebral infarction, unspecified (I63.9)." For all of these reasons, use of mortality rates generally must be limited to "all stroke" comparisons.

Decision-makers must also be careful not to assume that differences among stroke mortality rates are attributable to differences in the number of stroke events, that is, incidence. Stroke mortality rates are a product of the stroke incidence and stroke case-fatality rates, and differences can be introduced from either of these sources. For example, many individuals considered the substantial 60% drop in stroke mortality occurring over the past decades to be largely attributable to a declining number of stroke events. However, because recent reports suggest that a substantial component of the declining mortality is attributable to reductions in case-fatality rates rather than the number of incident events,[5-7] clinical and public health decisions made on this assumption may be ineffective. Hence, because the emphasis of decisions is frequently on

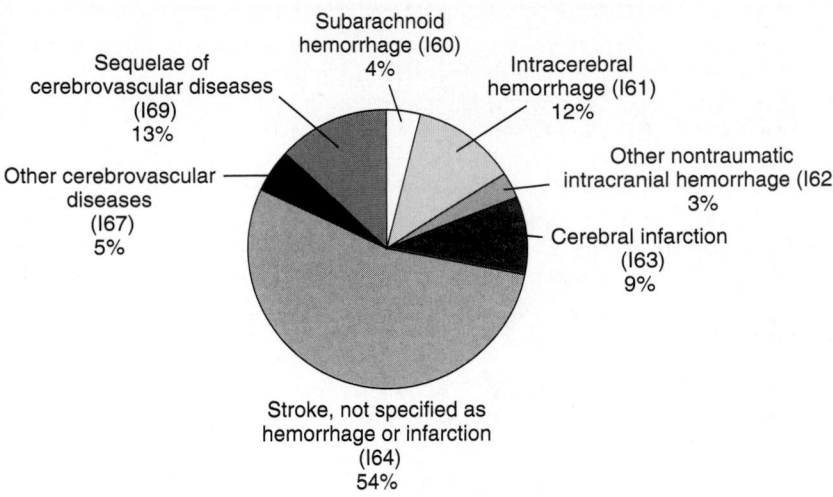

A

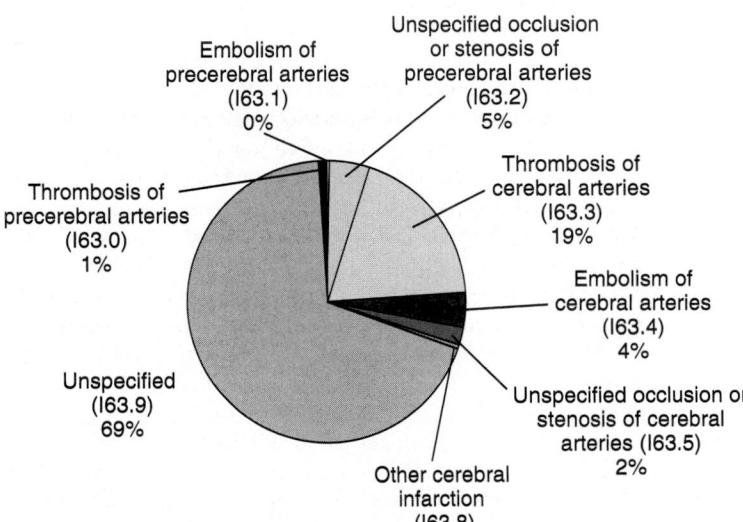

B

FIGURE 1–1 *A, Stroke subtype by International Classification of Diseases–10 (ICD-10) code (in* parentheses) *for the 167,366 stroke deaths reported for 1999. B, Detailed stroke subtype by ICD-10 code (in* parentheses) *for the 14,804 cerebral infarction deaths during 1999. (Data in* A *from the International Statistical Classification of Diseases and Health Problems, 10th revision. Geneva, World Health Organization, 2002; data in* B *from National Center for Health Statistics, Data Warehouse: Total deaths for each cause by 5-year age groups, United States, 1999. Available online at www.cdc.gov/nchs/datawh/statab/unpubd/mortabs/gmwki10.htm/; retrieved on March 10, 2002, pp 993–1008.)*

reducing the number of stroke events in a population, the use of stroke mortality rates can potentially mislead decisions by providing an index that is a function of both the number of strokes occurring and the likelihood of dying of a stroke event.

The shortcomings of stroke mortality as an index of the distribution of disease are directly addressed by the use of the stroke incidence rate. The *stroke incidence rate* is defined as the number of new stroke events per population occurring over a fixed time (normally a year). Unfortunately, there are substantial shortcomings in the use of this apparently attractive index. Most important is that, unlike for cancer and selected sexually transmitted diseases, there is no required registry of stroke events. Without such a registry, no national data are available to describe the number of incident stroke events. Current information on stroke incidence rates are based on (1) clinical reports in populations with tightly controlled referral patterns, most notably the Rochester Epidemiological Project (REP) in Olmstead County, Minnesota;[8] (2) funded stroke surveillance projects that capture admissions to

medical facilities for a fixed geographic region, such as the Greater Cincinnati/Northern Kentucky stroke project,[9] the Corpus Christi Stroke project,[10] and the Atherosclerosis Risk in Communities (ARIC) surveillance program;[11] or (3) large longitudinal epidemiologic cohort studies, such as the Framingham Study,[7] the Cardiovascular Health Study,[12] and the ARIC cohort study.[4]

In general, both surveillance and cohort studies provide stroke incidence data for specific geographic regions, but many of the regions are in northern cities with predominantly white residents (e.g., Framingham, Massachusetts, and Rochester, Minnesota). The first shortcoming of incidence data is in the assumptions required to generalize results from specific geographic and racial populations to provide either a national picture or a comparison of the disease burden between groups, such as African Americans and white persons. A second shortcoming of the use of incidence data to describe the distribution of disease is that the use or nonuse of diagnostic technologies may differentially identify milder cases of stroke. For example, it has been noted that from the 1960s through the 1990s, the number of incident strokes remained stable while the case-fatality rate fell.[7,13] One potential explanation for these patterns is the advent of neuroimaging, which made it possible to identify and diagnose previously missed strokes that were mild; its impact was to raise the incidence (by adding to the numerator of the incidence rate) and decrease the case-fatality rate (because patients with mild strokes would tend to survive). Although the potential effect of differential diagnostic evaluations is most pronounced in examination of temporal patterns, one can also argue that populations with relatively lower average socioeconomic status, such as African Americans and persons in isolated or rural communities such as those in the South, may have been less likely to have had access to these newer technologies. Such a difference would introduce a bias toward reducing the magnitude of the differences in incidence and magnifying the differences in case-fatality rate in any contrast of African Americans with whites or comparisons of residents from isolated or rural communities with residents from the rest of the nation.

Stroke is the leading cause of disability in the United States,[14] and survivors of stroke events carry this burden. The *prevalence of stroke* is defined as the proportion of the population that has survived a stroke. *Prevalence* is a proportion at a fixed point in time, distinguishing it from incidence and mortality, which are rates (number of events per population per unit of time). Although the concept is initially counterintuitive, increases in stroke prevalence are not necessarily associated with poor health outcomes. Stroke prevalence can increase not only because of the "negative"

effect of a rising stroke incidence but also because of the "positive" effect of a declining stroke case-fatality rate. Improvements in both emergency procedures and aggressive acute stroke management would be assumed to be associated with increasing stroke prevalence. Although changes in stroke prevalence are not necessarily an indication of desirable changes in the public health system, the understanding and prediction of stroke prevalence are critical to planning aspects of the health care delivery system such as the number of nursing home beds, rehabilitation services, and efforts in secondary stroke prevention.

DISTRIBUTION OF DISEASE

Stroke Mortality

In 2000, the Centers for Disease Control and Prevention (CDC) reported age-specific stroke mortality rates for 1997 for each of the major ethnic groups in the United States.[15] As shown in Figure 1–2A, there is a striking rise in stroke mortality with increasing age in all ethnic groups. However, at young ages, the stroke mortality rate for African Americans is substantially higher than the rates for other ethnic groups. For example, for the age group 35 to 44 years, the rate for African Americans is 18.2 (per 100,000), compared with 4.5 for white persons, 8.4 for Native Americans, 5.7 for Asians and Pacific Islanders, and 5.8 for Hispanic Americans. The mortality ratio for various ethnic groups, compared with white persons, is shown in Figure 1–2B. For the age group 35 to 44 years, the

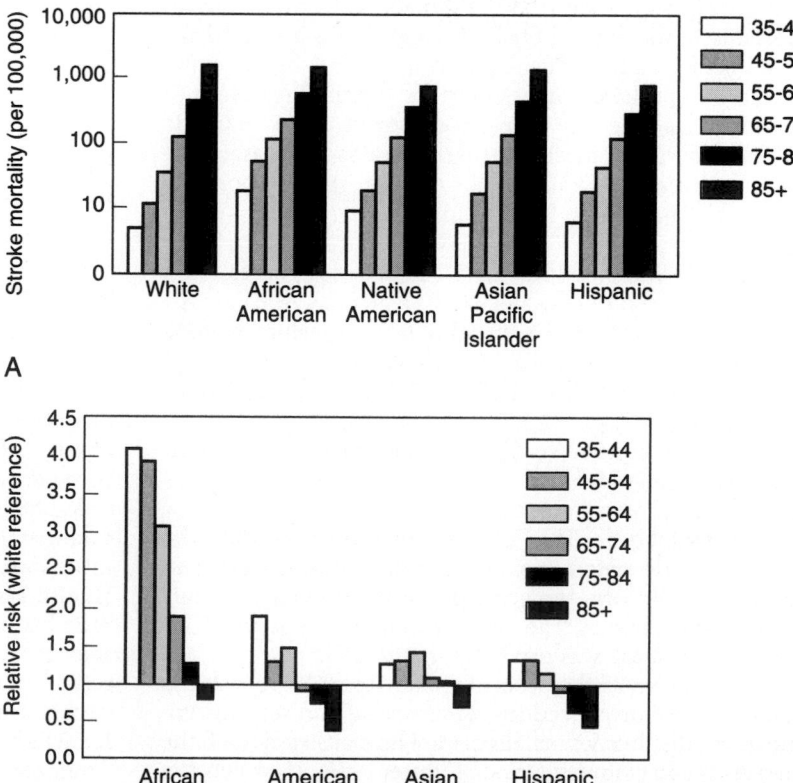

FIGURE 1–2 A, *The U.S. stroke mortality for 1997 by age and ethnic group (on a log scale). B, The age-specific relative risk for each of the ethnic groups relative to that of white persons. For example, the risk of stroke mortality is approximately three times greater for African Americans aged 35 to 44 years than for their white counterparts.*

mortality ratio for African Americans is 4.0 (18.2/4.5). Here, the mortality ratio for African Americans is strikingly different from those of other ethnic groups, for whom excess mortality rates are smaller. With increasing age, however, the ethnic disparity between African American and other ethnic groups tends to decrease, so that by age 75 years, there are no substantial differences among ethnic groups in stroke mortality. This trend continues with age; among persons older than 85 years, whites carry the highest stroke mortality rate, 1659 per 100,000; the rates for other ethnic groups range from 646 per 100,000 for American Indians to 1415 per 100,000 for African Americans.

One natural focus of this pattern of excess rates is on the extraordinarily high stroke mortality rates for young African Americans. However, equal emphasis could be placed on the striking ethnic differences in the rate of increase in stroke mortality with increasing age. For example, for both African Americans and white persons, the stroke mortality rate is 2.8 times greater for those 45 to 54 years old than for those 35 to 44 years old. Similarly, between ages 45 to 54 years and 55 to 64 years, stroke risk increases 2.9 times for whites and 2.2 times for African Americans. However, for those older than 65 years, the rate of increase in stroke mortality per decade of increasing age is strikingly higher for white persons. Specifically, stroke mortality increases 3.5 times in white persons versus 2.2 times in African Americans when one compares the age groups 55 to 64 years and 65 to 74 years. Similarly, between ages 65 to 74 years and 75 to 84 years, stroke mortality increases 3.7 times for white persons but only 2.4 times for African Americans; the increases are 3.6 and 2.5 times, respectively, for ages 75 to 84 years and 85 or more years.

Figure 1–3A shows the temporal pattern of stroke mortality in the United States between 1979 and 1997 for white persons and African Americans.[16] This figure shows both the remarkable success and the continuing failure of efforts to reduce the burden of stroke. The dramatic declines in stroke mortality that began as early as 1900[17] have continued. Figure 1–3A shows stroke mortality declines from 1979 to 1997 as follows:

- From 49.9/100,000 to 25.7/100,000 for white men (–40%)
- From 35.9/100,000 to 22.5/100,000 for white women (–37%)
- From 77.9/100,000 to 48.6/100,000 for African American men (–38%)
- From 60.9/100,000 to 37.9/100,000 for African American women (–38%)

These dramatic declines are part of the reason that the CDC recently listed the declines in heart disease and stroke as one of the ten great public health achievements of the 20th century, the only accomplishment cited for which the disease was explicitly mentioned.[17]

The similarity of the percentage declines also reveals the continuing failure to reduce ethnic-racial and sex discrepancies in the burden of disease. The consistency of the burden is explicitly shown in Figure 1–3B, in which the black-to-white stroke mortality ratio is shown for men and women, and the male-to-female stroke mortality ratio is shown for white persons and African Americans.[18] For

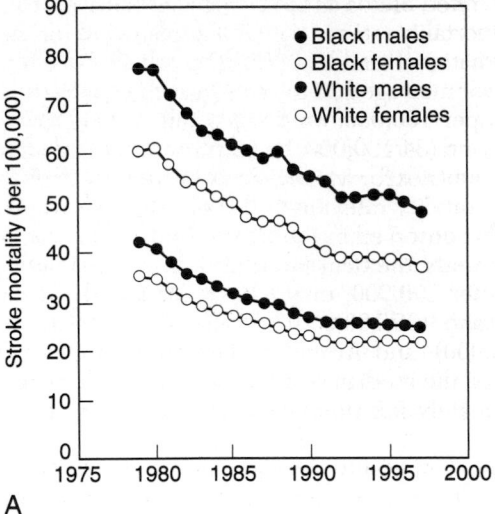

A

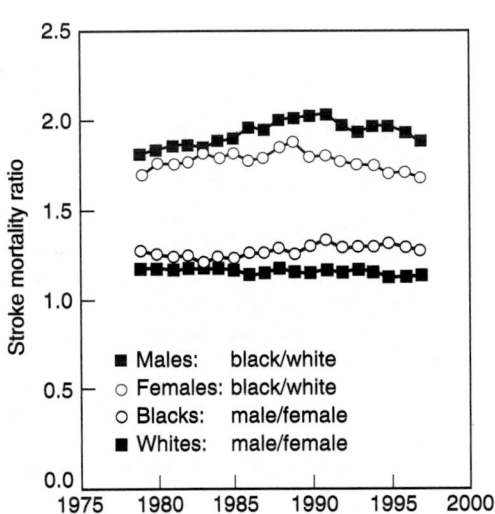

FIGURE 1–3 *A, Stroke mortality in the United States, 1979 to 1997, by race and sex. B, Stroke mortality ratios by race and sex. Black-to-white ratios are shown in black, with the ratio for men shown with squares and females shown with circles. Male-to-female ratios are shown in red, with whites shown with squares and blacks shown with circles.*

men, the black-to-white stroke mortality ratio was approximately 1.82 in 1979. This ratio rose in the 1980s and then showed a relative decline; however, the final level in 1997 was 1.89, virtually unchanged from 20 years previously. Likewise, for women, the black-to-white stroke mortality ratio was approximately 1.70 in 1979 and increased to almost 1.9 during the mid-1980s; by 1997, however, the ratio had returned to near the initial level, 1.68. As can be seen in Figure 1–3B, the male-to-female stroke mortality ratio has also proved to be remarkably stable over this period, remaining in narrow ranges between 1.14 and 1.20 for white persons and between 1.21 and 1.34 for African Americans.

There are also substantial international variations in stroke mortality, as well as variations within the United States. Although stroke is the third leading cause of death in the United States and the principal cause of disability,[14] stroke mortality rates in the United States are relatively low by international standards (Fig. 1–4).[19] The stroke mortality rate for men aged 35 to 74 years in the United States was only 42 per 100,000; only two countries had lower rates: Switzerland (34/100,000) and Canada (37/100,000). Among the 51 countries for which data were calculated, the median stroke mortality rate was 108 (Poland), approximately 2.5 times that observed in the United States. For women aged 35 to 74 years, the stroke mortality rate in the United States was 33 per 100,000; only four countries had lower rates: Switzerland (20/100,000), France (23/100,000), Canada (25/100,000), and Australia (31/100,000). Among the 51 countries, the median stroke mortality was 72 (Venezuela), approximately 2.2 times greater than that in the United States.

Although mortality rates are low for the United States, regional differences have long been recognized, with the southeastern region of the country called the "stroke belt." This *stroke belt*, first identified in 1965 as a region of high stroke mortality,[20] is commonly defined as comprising eight southern states: North Carolina, South Carolina, Georgia, Tennessee, Mississippi, Alabama, Louisiana, and Arkansas. This region of excess stroke mortality has been shown to exist since at least 1940,[21] and despite relatively minor geographic shifts,[22] it still persists today according to the latest data available.[23] Regions within the stroke belt have even higher stroke mortality, and a "buckle" region along the coastal plains of North Carolina, South Carolina, and Georgia has been identified with stroke mortality even higher than that of the rest of the stroke belt.[24]

The CDC's *Atlas of Stroke Mortality*, published in January 2003, presents a complete and extensive review of geographic variations in stroke mortality by race-ethnic group.[25] Figure 1–5, reproduced from this atlas, shows the geographic variations in stroke mortality for the nation,

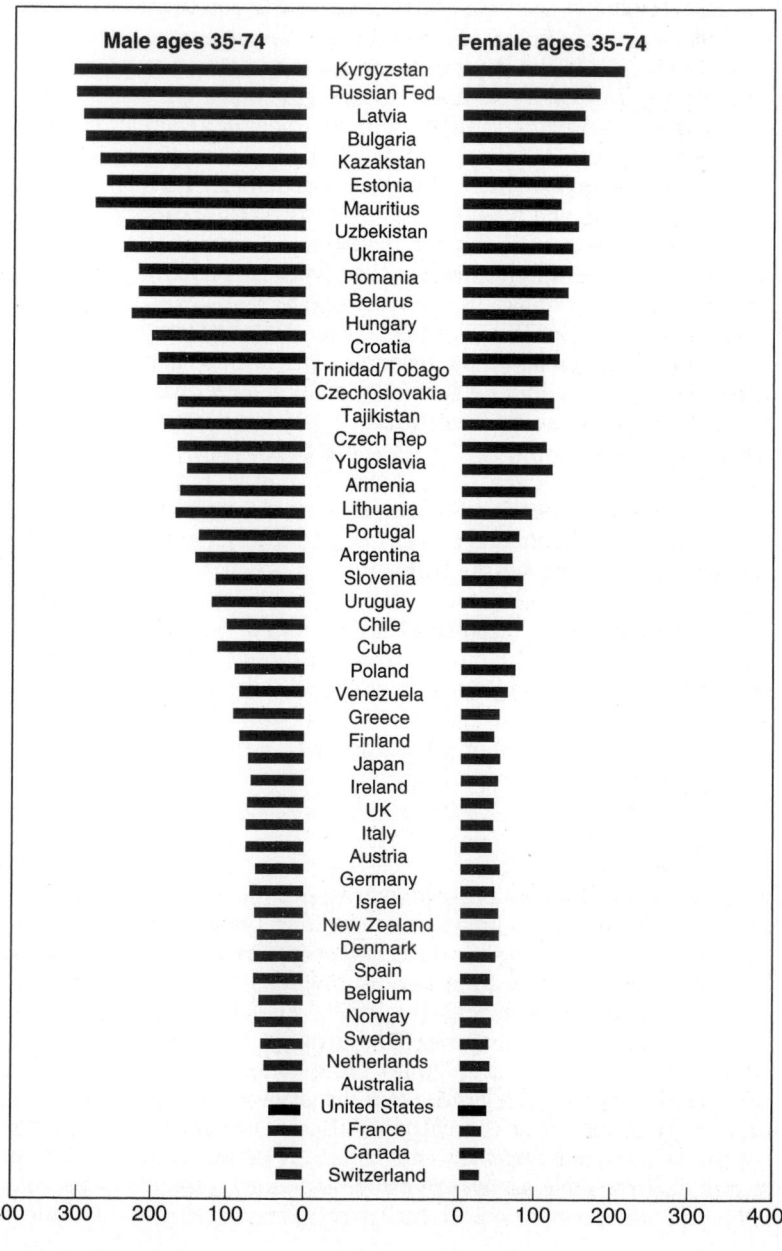

FIGURE 1–4 *Stroke mortality per 100,000 for men and women, approximately 1990. (Adapted from Sarti C, Rastenyte D, Cepaitis Z, Tuomilehto J: International trends in mortality from stroke, 1968 to 1994. Stroke 31:1588–1601, 2000.)*

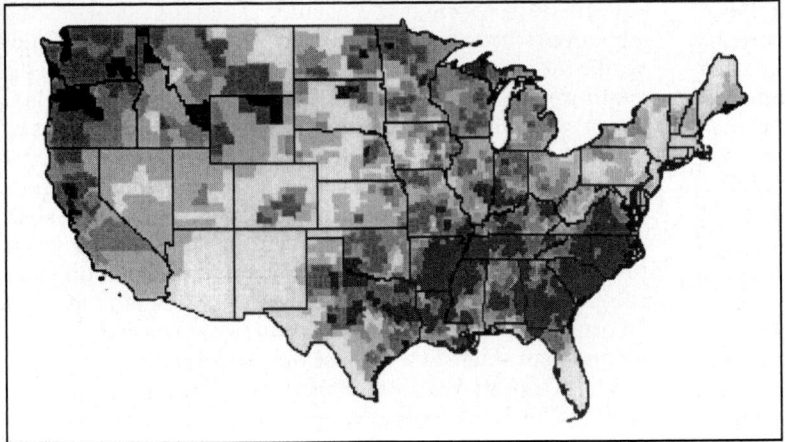

FIGURE 1–5 *Stroke mortality rates, United States, total population ages 35+ years, 1991 to 1998. Darkest colors represent areas with highest stroke mortality rates, and lightest colors represent areas with lowest rates. (Data from Casper ML, Barnett E, Williams GI, Jr, et al: Atlas of Stroke Mortality: Racial, Ethnic, and Geographic Disparities in the United States. Atlanta, US Department of Health and Human Services, Centers for Disease Control and Prevention, January 2003.)*

including the excess mortality in the southeastern United States (with particularly high rates along the coastal plains of North Carolina, South Carolina, and Georgia) and the later-occurring high stroke mortality in the northwestern United States. This atlas demonstrates a similar pattern of mortality for white persons and African Americans (i.e., higher stroke mortality rates in the Southeastern and Northwestern United States). It also reveals substantial variations for Hispanic Americans (with particularly high rates in west Texas and New Mexico), Asians (with particularly high rates in the Northwest, the Memphis area, and southern Nevada), and American Indians (with particularly high rates in the Carolinas, the Northwest, and the Northern Great Plains.) Comparisons of the total United States pattern of these racial-ethnic groups with whites and African Americans is difficult, however, because large areas of the United States lack sufficient representation of these race-ethnic groups for reliable estimates of stroke mortality.

Hence, ethnic differences in stroke mortality rates are dominated by the substantial excess risk for African Americans younger than 65 years. Although men are at higher risk of stroke death than women, the sex disparity is substantially less than the racial disparity observed between African Americans and white persons. Although stroke mortality rates have shown remarkable declines over the past several decades, there has been virtually no progress in reducing the magnitude of ethnic disparity in the risk of stroke death for African Americans.

Stroke Incidence

Several cohort studies have provided great insights into the distribution of stroke as indexed by incidence rates. For example, the ARIC study showed a clear excess risk of incident stroke among African Americans, with a black-to-white incidence rate ratio of 2.41 overall.[4] The study also revealed a greater relative risk for African Americans younger than 55 years (2.77) than those older than 55 years (2.23), reflecting the larger racial disparities observed in mortality measures at younger ages. Racial differences in stroke were only partially mediated by adjustment for risk factors such as hypertension and diabetes and by further adjustment for education as a surrogate for

socioeconomic status.[4] Several other studies have clearly documented the excess stroke incidence rate (overall and for cerebral infarctions) among African Americans, including the Northern Manhattan Stroke Study (NOMASS) (rates of 223 per 100,000 for African Americans and 93 for whites, for an incidence rate ratio of 2.4)[26] and the First National Health and Nutrition Examination Survey (NHANES I) Epidemiologic Follow-up Study (NHEFS) (age- and sex-adjusted relative risk of 2.3).[27]

A cohort study design has several advantages in providing insights into the distribution of stroke as indexed by incidence. The most notable is the ability to prospectively collect data in a manner that permits the confirmation of reported strokes as true events. For example, in the ARIC study, there were 1185 reported hospitalizations for stroke according to ICD-9 codes. Review of records found, however, that 647 (54%) of the patients showed no evidence of a residual deficit extending beyond 24 hours and as such were likely not to have experienced stroke events.[4] The rate of confirmation of stroke events varied substantially among ICD codes; record review found definite or probable evidence of stroke in only 14% of patients discharged with an ICD-9 code of 433 (occlusion and stenosis of precerebral arteries) compared with 86% of patients discharged with an ICD-9 code of 430 (subarachnoid hemorrhage). Other studies have found similar miscoding rates when careful review of records is undertaken.[4] Clearly, such a large number of miscoded discharge events raises serious concerns about the reliability of the mortality estimates discussed in the previous section.

Because incident stroke is a relatively rare event in the general population, however, the use of a cohort design to describe incidence data has the notable shortcoming of relying on relatively few incident events. For example, the ARIC study followed up 15,792 individuals for an average of 7.2 years to obtain 267 incident stroke events.[4] Likewise, over the 20-year follow-up in the Framingham Study, only 89 thromboembolic stroke events have occurred among the 1216 men.[29] Although there are a larger number of strokes among more elderly cohorts, such as the Cardiovascular Health Study (CHS), whose participants were older than 65 years at baseline,[12] much of the interest in the distribution of disease among racial groups is in younger age groups. That the number of incident events is likely to be small in cohort studies implies that the cohort design may not provide reliable subtype-specific estimates within race-sex-age strata, which are required for an understanding of the causes of racial and other differences in stroke risk. Without such information, designing clinical or public health interventions to eliminate the racial disparities is challenging. That is, substantially different approaches would be taken to reduce the difference in stroke mortality between African Americans and whites aged 45 to 64 years, depending on whether the difference is driven by largely hemorrhagic or infarction events.

The Greater Cincinnati/Northern Kentucky Stroke Study is a unique, ongoing study that has been optimally designed to provide for the assessment of racial (and sex) differences in stroke incidence in a single community.[9] Using a population-based surveillance design, the investigators in this study are obtaining a sufficient number of events to effectively describe the racial differences in the distribution of the incidence of stroke. Their approach is to identify all hospitalized patients with stroke and to obtain a sample of nonhospitalized patients with stroke managed from physician offices in a fixed geographic region. Because the basis is the total population of the region, the number of stroke events will be large enough to provide reliable estimates of incidence.

Current initial reports (available in abstract form) from the Greater Cincinnati/Northern Kentucky Stroke Study provide age-specific comparisons of racial differences in stroke incidence, but only for all stroke subtypes combined.[30] These results to date are intriguing because the patterns of incidence largely reflect the observed differences reported in mortality (Fig. 1–6A).[30] Like the age-specific racial differences in stroke mortality displayed in Figure 1–2A, the rising risk of stroke incidence with increasing age is clear, and the higher risk of incident stroke is present for African Americans in all age strata. This pattern of substantially greater risk at younger ages and declining risk with increasing age can be detected by calculating the black-to-white incidence rate ratio, as shown in Figure 1–6B. For both men and women, the risk of incident stroke among African Americans aged 35 to 44 years is approximately three times greater than that for their white counterparts; this racial disparity declines with increasing age until the risks are approximately equal for white persons and African Americans older than 75 years (see Fig. 1–6B). The Greater Cincinnati/Northern Kentucky Stroke Study is progressing, and the important information on age-specific racial differences in stroke incidence reported by stroke subtype will be available in the near future.

Unfortunately, there is no national reporting of stroke incidence rates to serve as the basis for a description of geographic variations in stroke incidence. Some geographic representation is provided by the studies already mentioned (Greater Cincinnati, ARIC). Using these studies as the basis of a description of geographic variations in stroke incidence is problematic because of (1) differences in study design and (2) the very focused geographic nature of these studies (for example, using the ARIC study data from Forsyth County to describe stroke in North Carolina). As such, there is a substantial need for studies to provide nationally comparable, generalized data

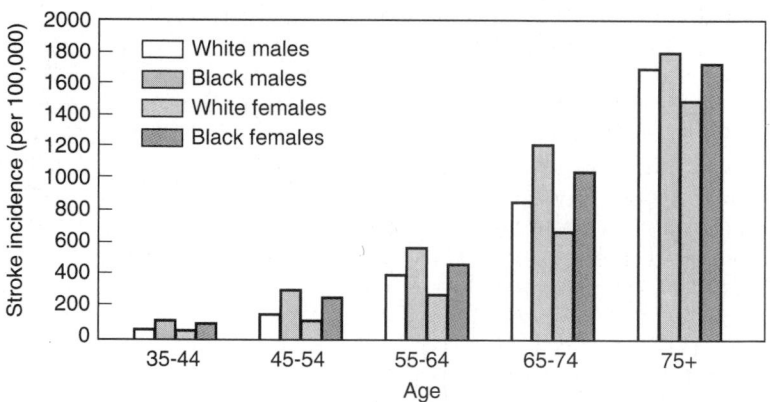

A

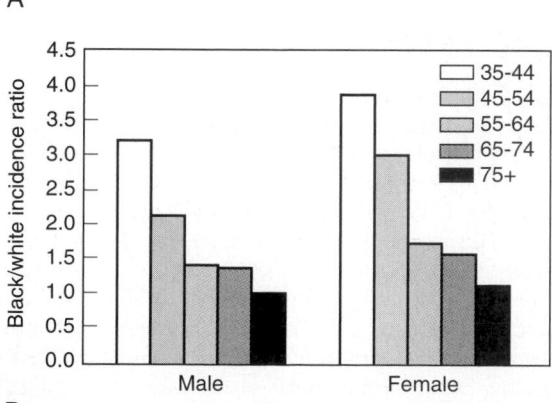

B

FIGURE 1–6 A, *Stroke incidence rates per 100,000 population from the Greater Cincinnati/Northern Kentucky Stroke Study by race and sex. B, The black-to-white stroke incidence ratio for men and women. (Data from Broderick JP, Kissela BM, Miller R, et al: Excess burden of stroke among blacks varies by age and gender [abstract]. Stroke 33:351, 2002.)*

to describe the geographic variations in stroke incidence risk.

If one assumes that stroke case-fatality rates are similar across the nation, it is tempting (and perhaps reasonable) to use stroke mortality rates to provide a description of geographic variations in incidence. Although such an approach requires the substantial assumption that there are no variations in stroke case-fatality rates, it leads to remarkable conclusions about regional differences in the public health burden of stroke. Specifically, in the eight southern states frequently regarded as being in the stroke belt, there were approximately 780,000 stroke deaths between 1968 and 1997.[16] If the stroke mortality rates in these states were similar to those of the rest of the nation, there would have been approximately 190,000 fewer stroke deaths. If one assumes the case-fatality rate for stroke to be 30%, these 190,000 "extra" stroke deaths would be the result of approximately 633,000 "extra" stroke events. The Stroke Prevention Patient Outcomes Research Team (PORT) from Duke University estimates the cost of stroke to be $104,000,[31] suggesting that over this 29-year period the higher stroke mortality in the southeastern United States was associated with an additional public health burden in excess of $65 billion (or an annual cost of more than $2 billion). These calculations require substantial assumptions, but they do underscore the potential magnitude of the geographic discrepancy in stroke.

Stroke Prevalence

Although one of the most quoted summary statistics is that stroke is the leading cause of disability among adults,[14] the focus of assessing the distribution of stroke seldom falls on the use of prevalence as an index. This is surprising because the burden of disability is borne by the survivors of stroke, which is directly indexed by measures of stroke prevalence. As important, substantial efforts in secondary stroke prevention are being made through the conduct of clinical trials, both surgical (e.g., North American Symptomatic Carotid Endarterectomy Trial [NASCET],[32] Carotid Revascularization Endarterectomy versus Stenting Trial [CREST][33]) and medical (e.g., Vitamin Intervention for Stroke Prevention [VISP],[34] Warfarin-Aspirin Recurrent Stroke Study Group [WARSS][35]). These efforts are appropriate because the risk of subsequent stroke in patients who survive a stroke is perhaps as high as 10% per year;[32] however, any potential gain in reduction of stroke risk is available only to those with prevalent stroke.

The American Heart Association estimates that there are 4,700,000 survivors of stroke alive today.[14] This estimate is based on cohort studies that reflect distinct ethnic and regional trends. For a description of differences across broad ages and by race and sex, it may be best to rely on national survey data, specifically the National Health Interview Survey.[28] The use of survey data has the strength of a substantial sample size; however, it has the weakness of dependence on self-reported conditions. With acknowledgment of this shortcoming, the prevalence rate of stroke is shown by sex and age in Figure 1–7A. In the three age strata displayed in the figure, the prevalence rates for men are 20%, 30%, and 25% higher than those observed for women—approximately the same magnitude of excess

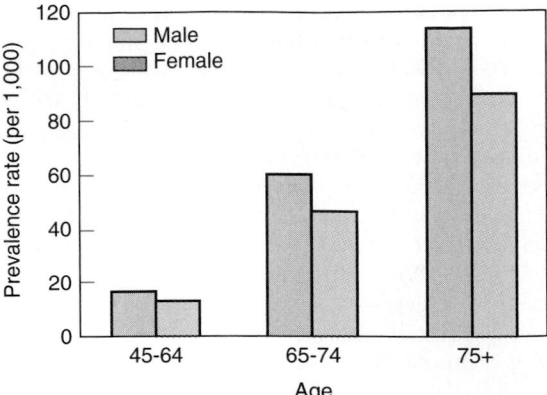

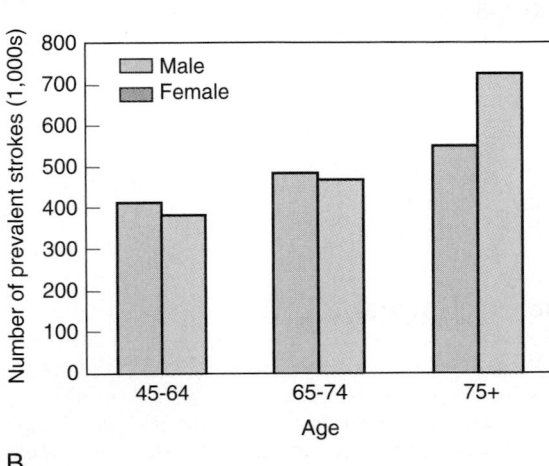

FIGURE 1–7 A, *Stroke prevalence rate per 1000 population.* B, *Number of prevalent strokes (in 1000s) as a function of age and gender.*

seen in stroke incidence rates, suggesting that case-fatality rates between the sexes are not different enough to dramatically affect the prevalence of stroke.

Because of the greater life span of women, however, focusing on the prevalence rate (number of individuals with stroke per 1000 population) fails to adequately reflect the burden of the disease as indexed by the absolute number of individuals surviving stroke. As can be seen in Figure 1–7B, although there is a slight male excess in the absolute number of stroke survivors younger than 74 years, there is a clear excess in the number of female stroke survivors older than 75 years; approximately 730,000 such women have suffered stroke, compared with "only" 555,000 men, a 31% excess. On the basis of these interview data, approximately 26% of stroke survivors are between the ages of 45 and 64 years (similar in age range to the proportion of incident strokes).

Racial differences in the prevalence rates of stroke (Fig. 1–8) largely reflect differences in incidence rates. The rate for African Americans is approximately twice as high as that for whites in those aged 45 to 64 years (27.0/1000 versus 13/1000), is 1.4 times greater in those aged 65 to 74 years (73/1000 versus 51/1000), and is approximately equal in those older than 75 years (98/1000 versus 97/1000).

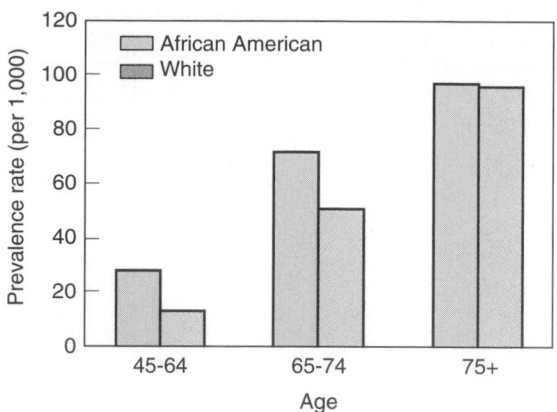

FIGURE 1–8   *Stroke prevalence rate per 1000 population by age and race.*

As with stroke incidence, there is no systematic approach for collecting data to describe geographic variations in the prevalence of stroke.

CONCLUSIONS

The measures of stroke mortality, stroke incidence, and prevalence of stroke provide important insights into the description of the distribution of the disease. Each of these indices has important strengths and weaknesses, and the measures are of particular interest to specific users of the information. Overall, several recurring patterns are clear. Perhaps the most critical is the substantially higher risk of stroke (regardless of the index of measure) among African Americans, particularly young African Americans. Other important summary observations are the greater risk for men, again particularly young men; however, the larger number of women in older age groups implies an absolutely larger number of women suffering stroke. In addition, at least by mortality measures, there is a substantial excess of stroke mortality among residents of the southeastern United States but few data to describe geographic variations in stroke incidence or prevalence.

References

1. Technical Appendix from Vital Statistics of United States: 1995: Mortality. Hyattsville, MD, US Department of Health and Human Services, Public Health Service, Centers for Disease Control and Prevention, National Center for Health Statistics, 1999.
2. The International Statistical Classification of Diseases and Health Problems, 10th revision. Geneva, World Health Organization, 2002.
3. National Center for Health Statistics: Data Warehouse GMWK I: Total deaths for each cause by 5-year age groups, United States, 1999. Available online at www.cdc.gov/nchs/datawh/statab/unpubd/mortabs/gmwki10.htm/; retrieved on March 10, 2002, pp 993–1008.
4. Rosamond WD, Folsom AR, Chambless LE, et al: Stroke incidence and survival among middle-aged adults. Stroke 30:736–743, 1999.
5. Shahar E, McGovern PG, Sprafka JM, et al: Improved survival of stroke patients during the 1980s. The Minnesota Stroke Survey. Stroke 26:1–6, 1995.
6. Howard G, Toole JF, Becker C, et al: Changes in survival following stroke in five North Carolina counties observed during two different periods. Stroke 20:345–350, 1989.
7. Wolf PA, D'Agostino RB, O'Neal MA, et al: Secular trends in stroke incidence and mortality. The Framingham Study. Stroke 23:1551–1555, 1992.
8. Petty GW, Brown RD Jr, Whisnant JP, et al: Ischemic stroke subtypes: A population-based study of incidence and risk factors. Stroke 30:2513–2516, 1999.
9. Kissela B, Broderick J, Woo D, et al: Greater Cincinnati/Northern Kentucky Stroke Study: Volume of first-ever ischemic stroke among blacks in a population-based study. Stroke 32:1285–1290, 2001.
10. Morgenstern LB, Steffen-Batey L, Smith MA, Moye LA: Barriers to acute stroke therapy and stroke prevention in Mexican Americans. Stroke 32:1360–1364, 2001.
11. White AD, Folsom AR, Chambless LE, et al: Community surveillance of coronary heart disease in the Atherosclerosis Risk in Communities (ARIC) Study: Methods and initial two years' experience. J Clin Epidemiol 49:223–233, 1996.
12. Ives DG, Fitzpatrick AL, Bild DE, et al: Surveillance and ascertainment of cardiovascular events: The Cardiovascular Health Study. Ann Epidemiol 5:278–285, 1995.
13. Howard G, Craven TE, Sanders L, Evans GW: Relationship of hospitalized stroke rate and in-hospital mortality to the decline in US stroke mortality. Neuroepidemiology 10:251–259, 1991.
14. American Heart Association: Heart Disease and Stroke Statistics—2003 Update. Dallas, American Heart Association, 2002.
15. Age-specific excess deaths associated with stroke among racial/ethnic minority populations—United States, 1997. MMWR Morb Mortal Wkly Rep 49:94–97, 2000.
16. National Center for Health Statistics: Age-adjusted death rates for 72 selected causes, United States, 1979–98. Available online at www.cdc.gov/nchs/datawh/statab/unpubd/mortabs/gmwk293.htm/; retrieved on March 22, 2002.
17. Centers for Disease Control and Prevention: Ten great public health achievements—United States, 1900–1999. MMWR Morb Mortal Wkly Rep 48:241–243, 1999.
18. National Center for Health Statistics: Age-adjusted death rates for selected causes, death registration states, 1900–1932, and United States, 1933–1998. Available online at www.cdc.gov/nchs/datawh/statab/unpubd/mortabs/hist293.htm/; retrieved on March 10, 2002.
19. Sarti C, Rastenyte D, Cepaitis Z, Tuomilehto J: International trends in mortality from stroke, 1968 to 1994. Stroke 31:1588–1601, 2000.
20. Borhani NO: Changes and geographic distribution of mortality from cerebrovascular disease. Am J Public Health 55:673–681, 1965.
21. Lanska DJ: Geographic distribution of stroke mortality in the United States: 1939–1941 to 1979–1981. Neurology 43:1839–1851, 1993.
22. Casper ML, Wing S, Anda RF, et al: The shifting stroke belt: Chances in the geographic pattern of stroke mortality in the United States, 1962 to 1988. Stroke 26:755–760, 1995.
23. Howard G, Howard VJ, Katholi C, et al: Decline in US stroke mortality: An analysis of temporal patterns by sex, race, and geographic region. Stroke 32:2213–2220, 2001.
24. Howard G, Anderson R, Johnson NJ, et al: Evaluation of social status as a contributing factor to the stroke belt of the United States. Stroke 28:936–940, 1997.
25. Casper ML, Barnett E, Williams GI Jr, et al: Atlas of Stroke Mortality: Racial, Ethnic, and Geographic Disparities in the United States. Atlanta, US Department of Health and Human Services, Centers for Disease Control and Prevention, January 2003.
26. Sacco RL, Boden-Albala B, Gan R, et al: Stroke incidence among white, black and Hispanic residents of an urban community: The Northern Manhattan Stroke Study. Am J Epidemiol 147:259–268, 1998.
27. Gillum RF: Coronary heart disease, stroke and hypertension in a U.S. national cohort: The NHANES I Epidemiologic Follow-up Study. National Health and Nutrition Examination Survey. Ann Epidemiol 6:259–262, 1996.
28. Benson V, Marano MA: Current estimates from the National Health Interview Survey, 1995. Vital Health Stat (199):101–148, 1998.
29. Rodriguez BL, D'Agostino RD, Abbott RD, et al: Risk of hospitalized stroke in men enrolled in the Honolulu Heart Program and the Framingham Study. Stroke 33:230–236, 2002.
30. Broderick JP, Kissela BM, Miller R, et al: Excess burden of stroke among blacks varies by age and gender [abstract]. Stroke 33:351, 2002.
31. Matchar DB, Duncan PW: Cost of stroke. Stroke Clin Updates 5:9–12, 1994.

32. Barnett HJ, Taylor DW, Eliasziw M, et al: Benefit of carotid endarterectomy in patients with symptomatic moderate or severe stenosis. North American Symptomatic Carotid Endarterectomy Trial Collaborators. N Engl J Med 339:1415–1425, 1998.

33. Hobson RW II: Update on the Carotid Revascularization Endarterectomy versus Stent Trial (CREST) protocol. J Am Coll Surg 194:S9–S14, 2002.

34. Spence JD, Howard VJ, Chambless LE, et al: Vitamin Intervention for Stroke Prevention (VISP) trial: Rationale and design. Neuroepidemiology 20:16–25, 2001.

35. Mohr JP, Thompson JLP, Lazar RM, et al: A comparison of warfarin and aspirin for the prevention of recurrent ischemic stroke. Warfarin-Aspirin Recurrent Stroke Study Group. N Engl J Med 345:1444–1451, 2001.

Chapter Two

Epidemiology of Stroke

Philip A. Wolf

Epidemiology is "the study of the distribution and determinants of disease frequency" in human populations.[1] Consideration of the *distribution* of stroke by geographic region, race-ethnicity, age, and gender has been dealt with comprehensively in Chapter 1. An exposition of *outcome* after stroke, the other key determinant in stroke prevalence, morbidity, and mortality is reviewed in detail in Chapter 3. This chapter focuses on determinants of stroke—risk factors and predisposing conditions—including implications for stroke prevention.

Although several medical and surgical therapies to reduce the damage from impending or recent-onset stroke have been shown to be effective in selected patients and must continue to be pursued in the future, it seems likely that *prevention* will continue to be the most effective strategy to reduce the health and economic consequences of cerebrovascular disease. Prevention is facilitated by an understanding of predisposing host and environmental factors. The relative impact of each of these factors has become clearer, chiefly through prospective epidemiologic study. Controlled clinical trials have demonstrated the effectiveness of risk factor modification in stroke prevention. In this chapter, data obtained from a number of prospective observational studies of populations are presented. In particular, assessment of risk factors measured systematically and prospectively in a variety of populations, before the appearance of disease, provides the least distorted picture of the influence of these host and environmental factors on stroke incidence.

Stroke, the most common life-threatening neurologic disease, is the third leading cause of death in the United States, after heart disease and cancer, accounting for 1 of every 15 deaths. Although stroke is more often disabling than lethal, 167,661 deaths were attributed to stroke in 2000.[2] The American Heart Association estimated that in the same year, there were 500,000 initial strokes, 200,000 stroke recurrences, and 4,700,000 stroke survivors in the United States, many of whom required long-term care.[2] Among the elderly, the segment of the population in which stroke occurs most frequently, it is a major cause of disability requiring long-term institutionalization.

INCIDENCE OF STROKE

Incidence of stroke should be ascertained by systematic evaluation of a population determined to be free of the disease at outset. Ideally, the population under study should be representative of a general population, although it is not possible to recruit and prospectively follow a large number of individuals representative of persons extant in the world, a nation, or even a smaller geographic locale such as a state or province. Nevertheless, by accumulating data derived from a number of such general population samples, one can build a more complete picture of the incidence and distribution of a condition such as stroke.

The incidence of stroke has been ascertained from prospective study over 55 years of follow-up of 5184 men and women in the Framingham Heart Study, who were 30 to 62 years old and free of stroke at entry into the Study in 1948. The population has been examined every 2 years, and follow-up has been satisfactory with approximately 85% of subjects participating in each examination. Study subjects in whom stroke was suspected have been evaluated neurologically in the hospital at the time of the stroke since 1968, and the neurologic deficit was confirmed by the Framingham study neurologist personally in more than half the cases. In the remainder, hospital records including neurologists' evaluations have usually provided confirmation. Since 1982, 91.5% of patients have had at least one computed tomography (CT) scan or magnetic resonance imaging (MRI) of the brain and arteries; many have undergone more than one study. Aside from confirming or ruling out a hemorrhage as the basis for the stroke, CT or MRI has confirmed stroke in 60.9% of cases. It has been possible, therefore, to clearly distinguish hemorrhage from infarction and to classify the ischemic stroke events into lacunar, large artery, and cardioembolic subtypes with a reasonable degree of assurance utilizing established criteria.[3] The neurologic deficit of the stroke was verified by a Framingham study neurologist. Since 1981, when surveillance was intensified, neurologic deficits have been confirmed by a Framingham study neurologist in 56.3% of cases. Follow-up of the population has been satisfactory; approximately 7% have been completely lost to follow-up by death.

After 55 years of follow-up in the Framingham study, there were 893 cases of initial completed strokes and 152 instances of isolated transient ischemic attacks (TIAs).

The average annual incidence of stroke events increased with age, approximately doubling in successive decades (Table 2.1). This pattern was true for all cerebrovascular events combined, including isolated TIAs, atherothrom-

Table 2.1 Annual Incidence of Atherothrombotic Brain Infarction (ABI) and Completed Stroke in Men and Women Aged 35 to 94 Years

Age (yrs)	Men		Women		Men and Women Combined	
	n	**Rate/1,000**	**n**	**Rate/1,000**	**n**	**Rate/1,000**
ABI						
35–44	1	0.12	1	0.1	2	0.11
45–54	15	0.97	13	0.67	28	0.81
55–64	37	1.94	35	1.4	72	1.64
65–74	80	5.14	68	3	148	3.87
75–84	79	9.06	119	7.52	198	8.07
85–94	16	8.64	72	13.79	88	12.44
Total	228	*3.60°*	308	*2.90°*	536	*3.21*
Completed stroke						
35–44	3	0.37	3	0.3	6	0.33
45–54	25	1.61	20	1.04	45	1.29
55–64	60	3.15	60	2.41	120	2.73
65–74	127	8.16	115	5.08	242	6.33
75–84	126	14.45	203	12.83	329	13.41
85–94	30	16.21	121	23.18	151	21.35
Total	371	*5.89°*	522	*4.91°*	893	*5.35*

°Age adjusted.
Data from the Framingham Heart Study: 55-Year Follow-Up.

botic brain infarctions (ABIs; see later), and *completed* strokes (ischemic strokes and hemorrhages combined) (see Table 2.1). Overall, the annual age-adjusted (ages 35 to 94 years) total initial completed stroke event rates were 5.89 per 1000 in men and 4.91 per 1000 in women, yielding a 20% excess in men (see Table 2.1). The annual age-adjusted (ages 35 to 94 years) incidence of isolated TIA also rose with age, being 1.207 per 1000 in men and 0.71 per 1000 in women.

Perspective concerning the incidence of symptomatic coronary artery disease (CHD) and stroke may be gained by comparing analogous manifestations, myocardial infarction (MI) (n = 1206) and ischemic stroke with no clear cardiac source for emboli, termed *atherothrombotic brain infarction* (n = 536) (Fig. 2–1). When these two major manifestations of atherosclerotic disease are compared, the age-adjusted average annual incidence rate of MI in men was 4.1 times that of ABI; in women, MI incidence was 1.6 times that of ABI. Comparing incidence by gender overall, MI developed 2.6 times more often in men than in women, whereas ABI was approximately 1.24 times more common in men. In both sexes, rates doubled with each decade in age. The 20-year lag in incidence of MI in women was not seen for ABI, for which age-specific rates were similar in men and women.

FREQUENCY OF STROKE BY TYPE

The in-hospital assessment of stroke in the Framingham study by a study neurologist has helped document the stroke and determine stroke subtype as well as to differentiate stroke from other neurologic diseases. Diagnosis of lacunar infarction was based on clinical and brain CT and MRI findings, although criteria for embolic infarction required a definite cardiac source for embolism. Whether cerebral infarction was due to extracranial versus intracranial

arterial disease was determined on clinical grounds as well as results of noninvasive carotid studies and magnetic resonance angiography (MRA). Contrast angiography was requested only infrequently by the study subjects' personal physicians, chiefly in subjects with extracranial carotid stenosis who were to undergo endarterectomy and those with subarachnoid hemorrhage (SAH). The occurrence of TIA was ascertained through systematic routine questioning at each biennial examination since 1971 as well as scrutiny of physician records and hospital notes. This surveillance for TIA has been comprehensive, systematic, and extended over more than 25 years. In addition to the 15.1% of ABIs preceded by TIA, there were 148 persons whose initial cerebrovascular symptom fulfilled criteria for TIA but who did not sustain a subsequent stroke. These isolated TIAs accounted for 14.8% of total cerebrovascular events in men and 12.7% of events in women.

The relative frequency of completed stroke by type was nearly identical in men and women (Table 2.2). ABI, which

Table 2.2 Frequency of Complete Stroke by Type in Men and Women Aged 35 to 94 Years

Completed Stroke	Men		Women		Total	
	n	**%**	**n**	**%**	**n**	**%**
Atherothrombotic brain infarction	228	61.5	308	59	536	60
Cerebral embolus	87	23.5	137	26.2	224	25.1
Subarachnoid hemorrhage	20	5.4	28	5.4	48	5.4
Intracerebral hemorrhage	32	8.6	42	8	74	8.3
Other	4	1.1	7	1.3	11	1.2
Total	371	*100*	522	*100*	893	*100*

Data from the Framingham Heart Study: 55-Year Follow-Up.

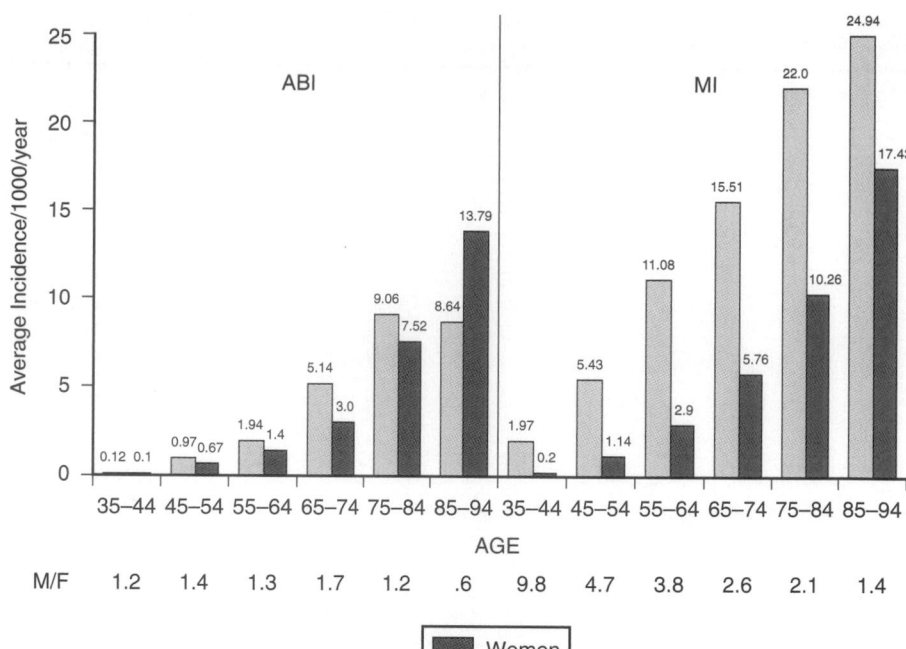

FIGURE 2–1 *Incidence of athero-thrombotic brain infarction (ABI) and myocardial infarction (MI), 50-year follow-up. (Data from the Framingham Heart Study.)*

included infarction secondary to large vessel atherothrombosis, lacunar infarction, and infarct of undetermined cause, occurred most frequently—at rates of 61.5% in men and 60.0% in women. Intracranial hemorrhage accounted for 14.0% of completed strokes in men, and 13.4% in women. Although a greater number of intracerebral hemorrhage (ICH) and SAH occurred in women than in men, age-adjusted annual incidence rates of ICH were higher in men than in women (0.52 versus 0.38 per 1000), and rates of SAH were not appreciably different (0.29 versus 0.28 per 1000). The relative frequencies of ICH and SAH varies according to the age of the population studied, with SAH predominating in persons younger than 65 years, but the frequencies being roughly equivalent in those 65 to 74 years old. At ages 75 to 84 years, ICH predominates, the annual incidence being 1.26 per 1000, compared with 0.29 per 1000 for SAH.

RISK FACTORS FOR STROKE

Identification of risk factors for stroke, awareness of the relative importance of each factor, and knowledge of their interaction should facilitate stroke prevention. Because the pathogenetic processes underlying the various types of stroke differ, it is reasonable to expect that risk factors for infarction differ from those for hemorrhage. Furthermore, precursors of intraparenchymatous bleeding are likely to differ from those for SAH. Risk factors for stroke from atherosclerosis of the carotid and vertebral arteries may well differ in impact from those for stroke from lacunar infarction. Precursors of embolic stroke are also likely to be different. Nevertheless, certain predisposing factors, particularly elevated blood pressure, are common to most stroke types.

Atherogenic Host Factors

Assessment of the importance of the major atherogenic risk factors was made utilizing data from the Framingham Heart Study and other prospective epidemiologic studies. These risk factors are hypertension, blood lipid levels, diabetes, obesity, family history, fibrinogen and other clotting factors, homocysteine levels, and cardiac disorders (coronary heart disease, CHF, atrial fibrillation, left ventricular hypertrophy, and echocardiographic abnormalities).

Hypertension

Hypertension is the principal risk factor for ischemic stroke as well as for ICH. Hypertension also predisposes to the cardiac conditions, notably MI and atrial fibrillation, promoting cerebral embolism, and elevated blood pressure also operates to increase the risk of SAH from aneurysm. Thus, hypertension serves the unique role of being a prime risk factor for stroke resulting from the most common mechanisms.

Hypertension and the Risk of Stroke

When Framingham study subjects were grouped according to the systolic blood pressure classification of JNC VI (the Sixth Report of the Joint National Committee on Prevention, Detection, Evaluation, and Treatment of High Blood Pressure),[4] the incidence of stroke generally, and of ABI in particular, was approximately three times greater in persons with stage 2 ($\geq$160 mm Hg systolic) or stage 3 ($\geq$180 mm Hg systolic) hypertension, and 50% higher in those with stage 1 hypertension (140 to 159 mm Hg systolic), than in persons with high-normal (130 to 139 mm Hg systolic) or normal (<130 mm Hg systolic) blood pressure (Fig. 2–2). This was true in both sexes and in all age categories, including 75 to 84 years. Hypertension

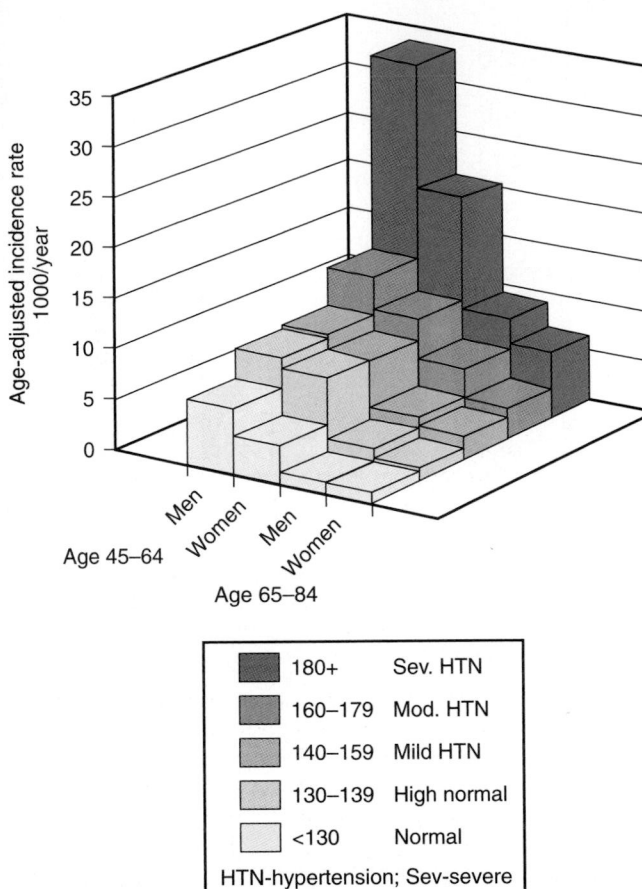

FIGURE 2–2 *Incidence of stroke and systolic blood pressure level according to the Joint National Committee VI categories. Data from 40-year Follow-up, The Framingham Study. HTN, hypertension; mod, moderate; sev, severe. (From Wolf PA: Cerebrovascular risk. In Izzo JL, Black HR [eds]: Hypertension Primer: The Essentials of High Blood Pressure, 3rd ed. [American Heart Association.] Lippincott, Williams & Wilkins, 2003, pp 239–242.)*

probably true. Systolic blood pressure continues to rise with advancing age into the eighth decade, whereas diastolic pressures decline after reaching a plateau in the early 50s. Systolic pressure level is clearly directly related to risk of stroke, particularly after age 65 years.

Isolated Systolic Hypertension

In the elderly, stage 2 (systolic ≥160 mm Hg) and stage 3 (systolic ≥180 mm Hg and diastolic <90 mm Hg) isolated systolic hypertension becomes highly prevalent, affecting approximately 25% of persons older than 80 years. Among the elderly aged 65 to 84 years in the Framingham Study, men with isolated systolic hypertension had twice the risk of stroke and women 1.5 times the risk of stroke of persons free of this condition.

Antecedent Blood Pressure and Risk of Stroke

Stroke risk predictions are generally based on measurement of current blood pressure. Clearly the duration of the blood pressure level, the height of the pressure, and other host factors contribute to cardiovascular risk. According to 50 years of blood pressure data, it is evident that for persons 60 years old, the presence of elevated midlife blood pressure during the preceding 10 years increases the relative risk of stroke by 1.68 (95% confidence interval [CI], 1.25 to 2.25) per SD increment in women and by 1.92 (95% CI, 1.39 to 2.66) per SD increment in men.[5] Similar increases in relative risk because of elevated antecedent pressures were also seen at age 70.[5] These data confirm clinical experience as well as prior prospective epidemiologic data that, at any level of blood pressure, persons with evidence of previously elevated blood pressure, such as left ventricular hypertrophy on electrocardiogram or increased

has been found to make a powerful and significant independent contribution to incidence of ABI even after age and other pertinent risk factors had been taken into account.

Although *hypertension* increases the incidence of stroke and ABI, the level of risk is clearly related to the *height* of the blood pressure. Classifying Framingham cohort subjects according to JNC VI systolic blood pressure categories makes it clear that the incidence of stroke rises with increasing blood pressure levels (see Fig. 2–2). However, more initial stroke events, hemorrhage as well as infarction, occurred in persons with mild (stage 1) hypertension than in those in any other category (see Fig. 2–1). In fact, approximately half of the initial stroke events in the Framingham study occurred in subjects with high-normal blood pressure or mild hypertension (Fig. 2–3). Traditionally, greater importance has been ascribed to the diastolic than systolic pressure level, and although most clinical trials of hypertension treatment have classified subjects according to diastolic level, evidence for the ascendancy of diastolic over systolic blood pressure is lacking. The opposite is

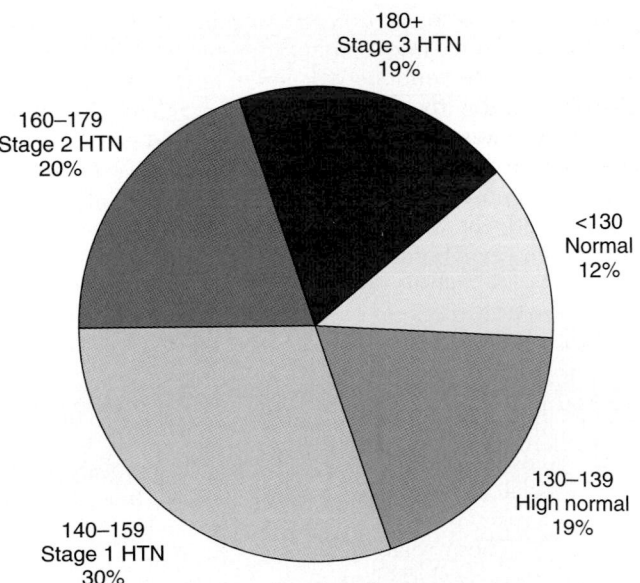

FIGURE 2–3 *Percentage of stroke by systolic blood pressure in subjects 45 to 64 years of age, from The Framingham Study. HTN, hypertension. (From Wolf PA: Cerebrovascular risk. In Izzo JL, Black HR [eds]: Hypertension Primer: The Essentials of High Blood Pressure, 3rd ed. [American Heart Association.] Lippincott, Williams & Wilkins, 2003, pp 239–242.)*

left ventricular mass on echocardiography, have a higher risk of stroke.

Blood Lipids

With rising levels of total serum cholesterol, there is a steady increase in incidence of CHD. This relationship holds in both men and women and persists after other risk factors are accounted for. The impact declines, however, with advancing age. CHD incidence is directly related to the level of low-density lipoprotein (LDL) cholesterol and inversely related to the level of high-density lipoprotein (HDL) cholesterol. The relationship of blood cholesterol to CHD incidence may best be expressed by the ratio of total serum cholesterol to HDL cholesterol, which demonstrates a significant effect on CHD incidence until age 80 years. For example, in persons age 75 to 79 years, the risk ratio for CHD with an elevated ratio of total cholesterol to HDL cholesterol is 1.6 for men and 1.8 for women.

However, stroke generally and nonembolic ischemic stroke in particular show no clear or consistent relationship with blood lipid levels. A report from the Atherosclerosis Risk in Communities (ARIC) Study found only weak and inconsistent associations between ischemic stroke and each of five lipid factors in the 305 subjects experiencing ischemic stroke after 10 years of prospective investigation.[6] The study researchers noted the absence of a relationship with these lipid factors and remarked that ischemic stroke did not demonstrate its well-known relation to coronary heart disease.[6] These findings have been corroborated by analyses utilizing the Framingham Heart Study and Cardiovascular Health Study.[7] Additionally, in a meta-analysis of 45 prospective epidemiologic studies comprising 450,000 subjects among whom 13,000 strokes occurred, no significant association between total serum cholesterol and total stroke incidence was seen.[8]

Exceptions were seen in the Honolulu Heart Study of Hawaiian men of Japanese ancestry and in the Multiple Risk Factor Intervention Trial (MRFIT) screenees.[9] In the Honolulu study, the level of total cholesterol measured years before was directly related to the incidence of thromboembolism.[10] In MRFIT, the incidence of ischemic stroke, diagnosed from death certificates, was greater in persons with the highest levels of serum total cholesterol obtained 6 years before (Fig. 2–4). A meta-analysis of the older trials of cholesterol-lowering therapies showed a definite benefit in reduction of MI but no significant impact on stroke occurrence.[11]

Although the effect of blood lipids on ischemic atherothrombotic stroke differs from the relationship of blood lipids with coronary artery atherosclerosis, serum total cholesterol and LDL cholesterol levels have been directly related to the extent of extracranial carotid artery atherosclerosis, with HDL cholesterol exerting a protective effect. These relationships also apply to extracranial carotid artery wall thickness.[12–14] Pravastatin was shown either to reduce progression or to promote regression of carotid artery plaque in an early study. These findings have been corroborated with other statins as well.[15]

In view of the lack of association of blood lipids to incidence of ischemic stroke, a significant reduction in stroke incidence was somewhat unexpected in a series of trials of

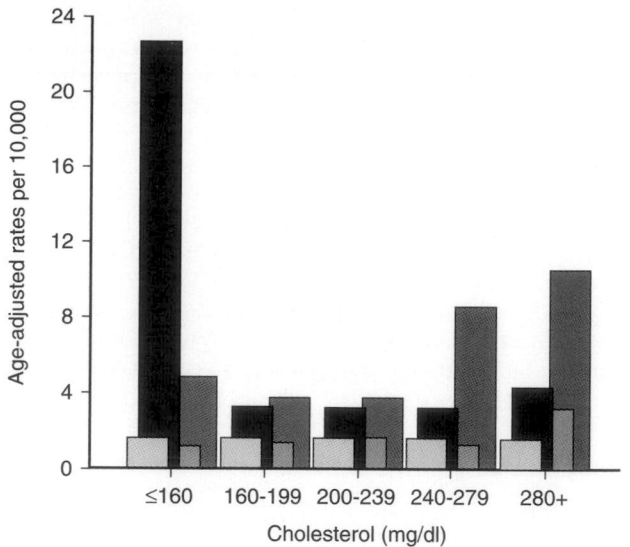

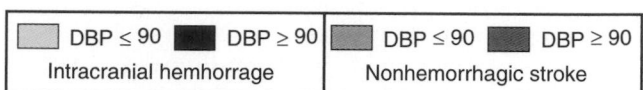

FIGURE 2–4 *Ischemic stroke and intracerebral hemorrhage death rates in men with normal and elevated diastolic blood pressure (DBP) according to screening serum cholesterol level. (From Wolf PA: Cerebrovascular risk. In Izzo JL, Black HR [eds]: Hypertension Primer: The Essentials of High Blood Pressure, 3rd ed. [American Heart Association.] Lippincott, Williams & Wilkins, 2003, pp 239–242.).*

statins in patients with clinical coronary heart disease.[16–19] The magnitude of the effect was 20% to 30% and was little different from the benefit on coronary heart disease endpoints.[16,20,21] In the Cholesterol and Recurrent Events (CARE) Trial, pravastatin and placebo were randomly allocated to 4159 survivors of a MI with total cholesterol levels below 240 mg/dL and LDL cholesterol levels of 115 to 174 mg/dL (mean 139 mg/dL).[17] The specified primary endpoint of death from CHD or nonfatal MI was reduced by 24% (95% CI, 9 to 36, $P = .003$) in the pravastatin group. Other CHD endpoints were similarly reduced during the 5 years of follow-up. Stroke occurred in 78 members (3.8%) of the placebo group and 54 members (2.6%) of the pravastatin group, a relative risk reduction of 31% (95% CI, 3 to 52, $P = .03$).[20] It was estimated that 25 strokes would be prevented by treating 1000 such patients, 60 years of age or older, with pravastatin for 5 years. This estimate compares favorably with the 27 fatal CHD events and 46 nonfatal MIs prevented in these patients, who are relatively young for stroke (mean age 59 ± 9 years).

Similar benefit in stroke prevention was seen in the Long-Term Intervention with Pravastatin in Ischaemic Disease (LIPID) trial.[18] All of these trials enrolled patients with CHD, a small percentage of whom had sustained a cerebral infarct. The later Heart Protection Study randomly assigned 20,536 high-risk individuals aged 40 to 80 years with total blood cholesterol levels of 3.5 mmol/L (135 mg/dL) to receive either simvastatin, 40 mg, or placebo daily. A 30% relative risk reduction in ischemic stroke was seen. Of the 7150 participants without diagnosed coronary disease, 1820 had prior cerebrovascular disease. The benefit in these persons was an approximate 25% relative risk reduction in overall event rate occurrence, suggesting that the simvastatin benefit occurred in the absence of prior coronary heart disease.[19]

The issue of stroke prevention with a statin was reported in the Anglo-Scandinavian Cardiac Outcomes Trial–Lipid Lowering Arm (ASCOT-LLA).[22] In ASCOT-LLA, 19,342 high-risk hypertensive patients *without* CHD were randomly assigned to receive either atorvastatin, 10 mg, or placebo. After a mean 3.3 years of follow-up, the trial was stopped; fatal and nonfatal strokes had occurred in 89 atorvastatin recipients versus 121 placebo recipients (hazard ratio 0.73 [0.56–0.96], *P* = .024).[22] This significant benefit for stroke prevention occurred in the absence of CHD in otherwise high-risk individuals, strongly suggesting an indication for statins in the primary prevention of ischemic stroke (Fig. 2–5).

The lack of benefit of statins in women in these trials may reflect the small number of women enrolled (18.8% of subjects) and the limited number of events occurring among them.

It seems likely that the significant reductions in stroke and MI in these trials did not result from the fraction of a hundredth of a millimeter reduction in plaque thickness or intimal medial thickness in the arterial wall seen in subjects in the statin arm of a number of clinical trials.[12–14,23,24] However, because extracranial large artery disease accounts for approximately 12% of stroke events and the beneficial effects in terms of plaque regression and intimal-medial thickness reduction are measured in fractions of a millimeter, it is unlikely that reversal of the atherosclerotic process alone is sufficient to account for the 20% to 30% relative risk reduction in ischemic stroke events seen in the statin trials, in which benefits occurred soon after institution of statins, often within 1 or 2 years.[19,22] It has been suggested the statin drugs acted by altering the lipid composition of the plaque, thereby reducing the tendency to rupture or fissure, by diminishing inflammation, or by improving the hemorrheologic environment.

Low Cholesterol and Hemorrhage

Low total serum cholesterol was related to an increased incidence of ICH,[25] first noted among rural Japanese after World War II who had very low serum cholesterol levels by western standards (<160 mg/dL).[26] As the subjects' nutrition improved, intake of animal fat increased, and sodium chloride intake fell, an increase in total serum cholesterol was seen in this population.[26] In men and women ages 40 to 49 years, the total serum cholesterol levels rose from 155 mg/dL in 1963 to 1966, to 175 mg/dL in 1972 to 1975, and to 181 mg/dL in 1980 to 1983. Total serum protein levels and relative weight rose significantly during these 20 years, but systolic and diastolic blood pressures declined. Accompanying these profound changes in risk factor levels were similar remarkable declines in the incidence of ICH, which fell 65% in men (*P* <.05) and 94% in women (*P* < .001) between 1964 to 1968 and 1979 to 1983.[26]

An etiologic link has been suggested by the confirmation of this relationship in other oriental populations, in Hawaiian Japanese as well as in white men in the United States. A total of 350,977 men aged 35 to 57 years were screened for entry into the MRFIT; after 6 years of follow-up, 83 deaths had occurred from ICH, and 55 from SAH.[9] In the lowest serum cholesterol category (<160 mg/dL), the risk factor–adjusted relative risk of intracranial hemorrhage was 1.0, and the relative risk at all higher levels of serum cholesterol was approximately 0.32. When data on deaths from intracranial hemorrhage were examined according to diastolic blood pressure at entry, the age-adjusted rate of death was significant only in persons with pressures of 90 mm Hg or higher (see Fig. 2–4). Death rates per 10,000 were 23.07 in the lowest serum cholesterol category (<160 mg/dL) and ranged from 3.09 to 4.83 in the four higher categories.[9]

The mechanism by which an elevated diastolic blood pressure and a very low serum cholesterol level promote ICH has been suggested to be an alteration in the cell

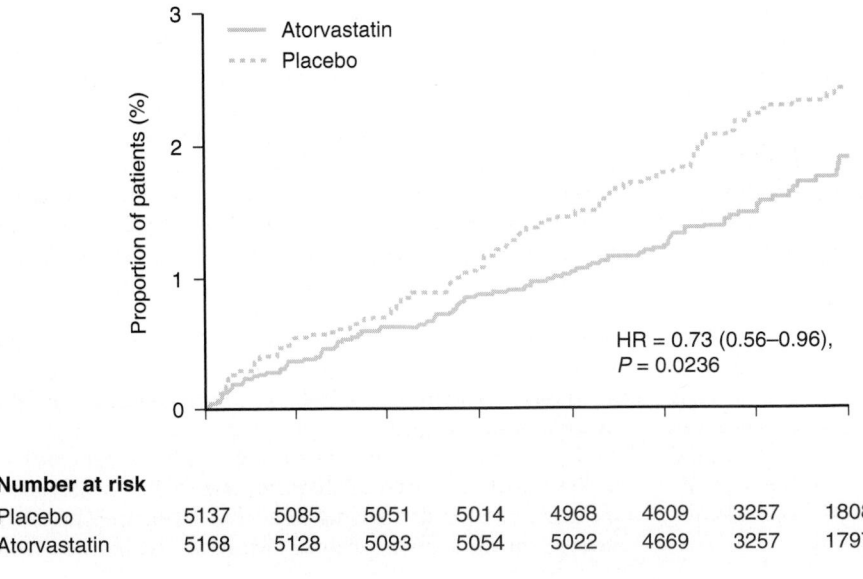

Fatal and non-fatal stroke

HR = 0.73 (0.56–0.96), *P* = 0.0236

Number at risk

Placebo	5137	5085	5051	5014	4968	4609	3257	1808
Atorvastatin	5168	5128	5093	5054	5022	4669	3257	1797

FIGURE 2–5 *Cumulative incidence for fatal and non-fatal stroke. HR, hazard ratio. (From Sever PS, Dahlof B, Poulter NR, et al: Prevention of coronary and stroke events with atorvastatin in hypertensive patients who have average or lower-than-average cholesterol concentrations, in the Anglo-Scandinavian Cardiac Outcomes Trial—Lipid Lowering Arm [ASCOT-LLA]: A multicentre randomised controlled trial. Lancet 361:1149–1158, 2003.)*

membranes that weakens the endothelium of intracerebral arteries. Despite early concerns, no significant rises in ICH rates have been noted in the many trials utilizing statins to reduce total serum and LDL cholesterol levels.

Diabetes

Diabetic persons are known to have a greater susceptibility to coronary, femoral, and cerebral artery atherosclerosis; up to 80% of those with type 2 diabetes will demonstrate or die of macrovascular disease. Hypertension is common in diabetic persons, affecting approximately 60%.[27] Surveys of patients with stroke and prospective studies have confirmed the increased risk of stroke in diabetic persons. The Honolulu Heart Study of Japanese men living in Hawaii found that rising levels of glucose intolerance conferred an increasing risk of thromboembolic stroke that was independent of other risk factors. There was no relationship with hemorrhage (Fig. 2–6).[28] Evaluation of the impact of diabetes on stroke in a population-based cohort in Rancho Bernardo, California, disclosed that relative risk of stroke was 1.8 in men and 2.2 in women even after adjustments were made for the effect of other pertinent risk factors.[29]

In the Framingham study, peripheral arterial disease with intermittent claudication occurred more than four times as often in diabetic subjects. The coronary and cerebral arteries are also affected but to a lesser extent.[30] For atherothrombotic brain infarction, the impact of glucose intolerance—physician-diagnosed diabetes, glycosuria, or a blood glucose level higher than 150 mg/l00 mL—is greater in women than men and is significant as an independent contributor to incidence only in older women. However, at all ages, in both men and women with glucose intolerance, the risk of ABI is approximately double that in nondiabetic persons.

Obesity

Obese persons have higher levels of blood pressure, blood glucose, and atherogenic serum lipids; on that account alone, they could be expected to have a higher risk of stroke. Obesity, defined as a relative weight 30% or more above average, was a significant independent contributor to incidence of ABI in younger men and older women in the Framingham original cohort. However, in all age groups and in both sexes, obesity exerts an adverse influence on health status that is probably mediated through elevated blood pressure, impaired glucose tolerance, and other mechanisms. In the Honolulu Heart Study, obesity was a risk factor for stroke that was independent of associated hypertension, glucose intolerance, and other covariates.

In the Nurses' Health Study (NHS),[30a] the incidence of stroke rose in direct relationship with body mass index in women aged 30 to 55 years after adjustment for other risk factors. No such relationship was seen, however, in the men aged 40 to 75 years participating in the Health Professionals Follow-up Study. Abdominal or central obesity seems more closely related to adverse cardiovascular outcomes, including stroke, than overall elevated body mass index. In 28,643 male health professionals, the relative risk of stroke was significantly greater (relative risk 2.33; 95% CI, 1.25 to 4.37) in men with a waist-to-hip ratio in the uppermost quintile. Obesity as reflected in the body mass index was less strongly related to stroke incidence than waist circumference, perhaps as a result of the impact of central or truncal obesity.[31]

Family History of Stroke

Although family history of stroke is perceived to be an important marker of increased stroke risk, confirmation by epidemiologic study has been lacking. Maternal history of death from stroke was significantly related to stroke incidence in a cohort of Swedish men born in 1913.[32] Other significant risk factors were hypertension, abdominal pattern of obesity, and fibrinogen level; however, maternal history of fatal stroke was independently related to stroke even after these variables were taken into account.

In a study of familial predisposition to stroke in Framingham, there was no relationship between a *history of stroke death* in parents and documented stroke in subjects. However, definite nonfatal and fatal strokes in these cohort members were related to the occurrence of stroke in their children (members of the Framingham Offspring Study cohort). In these analyses, both maternal stroke and paternal stroke were associated with approximately a 1.5-fold increased risk of stroke even after other risk factors were taken into account.[33] Thus, family history of stroke, so frequently acknowledged as risk factor for stroke, has been only recently identified and documented as such by epidemiologic study.

Fibrinogen, Clotting Factors, and Inflammation

Elevated serum fibrinogen value has been implicated in atherogenesis and in arterial thrombus formation. In a

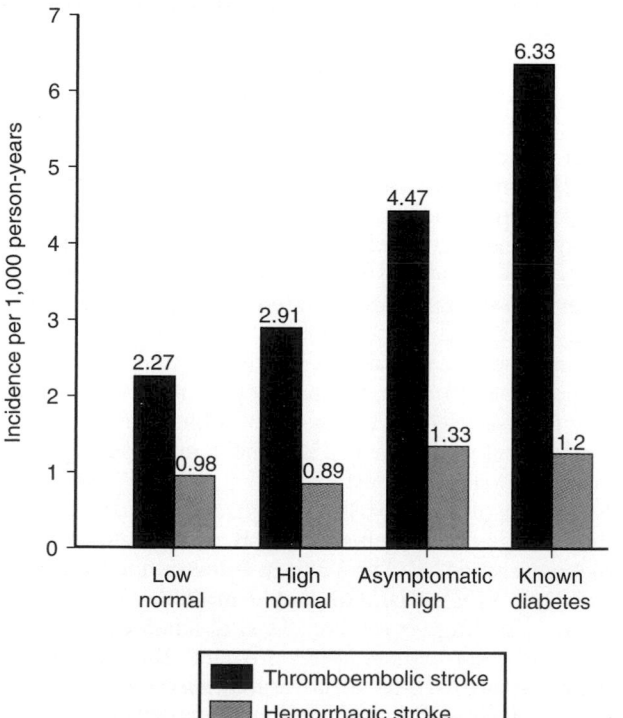

FIGURE 2–6 *Incidence of stroke and glucose intolerance in the the Honolulu Heart Study; 22-year follow-up. (From Burchfiel CM, Curb JD, Rodriquez BL, et al: Glucose intolerance and 22-year stroke incidence. The Honolulu Heart Program. Stroke 25:951–957, 1994.)*

number of epidemiologic studies, a significant independent increase in incidence of cardiovascular disease, including stroke, was related to fibrinogen level. In a prospective study of 54-year-old Swedish men, fibrinogen value in combination with elevated systolic blood pressure was found to be a potent risk factor for stroke.[34] Level of fibrinogen, measured on the tenth biennial examination in Framingham, was also significantly related to incidence of cardiovascular disease including stroke.[35]

However, fibrinogen value was associated with many other risk factors for stroke, including age, hypertensive status, hematocrit level, obesity, and diabetes.[36-38] In the Cardiovascular Health Study, fibrinogen was found to be related to the presence of subclinical atherosclerotic disease. In this study, fibrinogen and factor VIII were the only clotting factors associated with subclinical atherosclerotic disease. It seems likely the atherogenic and procoagulant effects of inflammation are related to cardiovascular disease incidence including stroke. In the Framingham original cohort, C-reactive protein (CRP) level was found to be an independent risk marker for stroke and incidence of TIA over 14 years of follow-up.[39] Men with CRP levels in the highest quartile had double the risk of stroke and TIA as men in the lowest quartile; for women, risk in the upper quintile was increased nearly three-fold[39] after other pertinent risk factors were taken into account.[39] CRP was also a potent independent risk marker for cardiovascular disease in the Women's Health Study. CRP value was said in this study to be a stronger predictor than the LDL cholesterol level and made an independent contribution to cardiovascular disease risk prediction above and beyond that provided by the Framingham risk score.[40]

Blood Homocysteine Levels

In a number of cross-sectional studies, in case-control studies, and in a meta-analysis, elevated values of plasma homocysteine (tHcy) were found to be associated with a higher incidence of CHD (odds ratio [OR], 1.6 per 5 µmol/L tHcy) and an increased incidence of stroke (OR, 1.5 per 5 µmol/L tHcy).[41] Level of tHcy is also directly related to many of the major components of the cardiovascular risk profile, which are male sex, increasing age, cigarette smoking, increased blood pressure, elevated blood cholesterol level, and lack of exercise.[42] However, even after these factors were taken into account, risk of stroke was independently related to nonfasting tHcy level in the original Framingham cohort after 9.9 years of follow-up with a relative risk in quartile 4, compared with quartile 1, of 1.82 (CI, 1.14 to 2.91) and the linear trend across the quartiles was significant (*P* < .001). A nested case-control study within the British Regional Heart Study cohort demonstrated a powerful and independent relationship between nonfasting tHcy level and stroke incidence.[43] There was a graded increase in risk with rising levels of tHcy (Fig. 2–7). Levels less than 10.3 µmol/L, repre-senting the lowest quartile, were the referent group; the risk factor-adjusted OR increased from 1.2 (10.3 to 12.49 µmol/L), to 2.6 (12.5 to 15.39 µmol/L), to 4.7 (≥15.4 µmol/L) in successive quartiles of tHcy (*P* = .03 for trend). Risk in the uppermost quartile was 4.7-fold greater than that in the lowest quartile. This was a graded response with no threshold discernible that occurred after

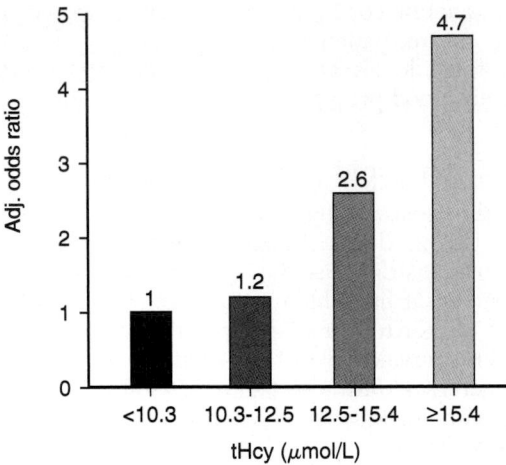

FIGURE 2–7 *Homocysteine level and stroke risk in men; data from a case-control study. (From Wolf PA: Epidemiology and Risk Factor Management. Welch M, Caplan L, Reis D, et al [eds]: Primer on Cerebrovascular Disease. San Diego, Academic Press, 1997, pp 751–757.)*

adjustment for serum creatinine level (associated with increased tHcy levels), age, social class, blood pressure, and other pertinent risk factors.[43] However, in other large population studies—the ARIC Study, Physicians' Health Study, Finnish Study, and MRFIT—no statistically significant relationship was found.[44,45]

With regard to carotid atherosclerosis, the ARIC study noted a strong independent relationship between fasting plasma tHcy concentrations and carotid artery intimal medial wall thickening.[46] Increased levels of fasting plasma homocysteine were also related to ultrasonography-assessed extracranial common carotid artery stenosis of 25% or higher in the Framingham cohort.[47] Furthermore, levels of homocysteine are inversely related to levels of dietary and plasma folic acid and vitamins B_{12} and B_6.[47,48]

The *fasting* tHcy level may miss persons with impaired homocysteine metabolism, because approximately 40% of persons who demonstrate elevated homocysteine levels in response to a methionine challenge and are thought to be at increased cardiovascular risk have normal fasting homocysteine levels. Further, the homocysteine level is similar to other physiologic measures, such as blood pressure and serum cholesterol, as a graded and continuous variable without clear threshold effect.

A number of clinical trials have used folic acid supplements, along with vitamins B_6 and B_{12}, to prevent MI and stroke recurrence.[49,50] The Vitamin Intervention for Stroke Prevention (VISP) trial, conducted in 3600 patients with mild nondisabling stroke and TIA, did not find vitamin supplementation with folic acid, B_6 and B_{12} to have any benefit in stroke, MI, or cardiovascular disease prevention. Such supplementation will reduce homocysteine levels even in persons with adequate dietary intake and normal plasma vitamin levels.[51-53] Evidence of benefit for such supplementation is currently lacking. During the VISP trial there appeared to be no risk of supplementation, and the cost of these vitamins is minimal. Adding 1 mg of cyanocobalamin should alleviate concerns about masking pernicious anemia or B_{12} deficiency. It may well be that, in the near future, patients will be expected to know their homocysteine levels as they are currently supposed to know their blood pressure and cholesterol levels.

Heart Disease and Impaired Cardiac Function

Cardiac diseases and impaired cardiac function are disease states or organ dysfunctions that predispose to stroke. Hypertension is the preeminent risk factor for strokes of all types, but at each blood pressure level, persons with impaired cardiac function have a significantly higher stroke risk.[54] The prevalence of these cardiac contributors to stroke increases with age (Fig. 2–8). After 36 years of follow-up, the prevalence of cardiovascular disease among patients with stroke in the Framingham study was high; 80.8% were hypertensive; 32.7% had prior CHD; 14.5% had prior CHF; 14.5% had atrial fibrillation (AF); and only 13.6% had none of these diseases. Cardiac disease is an important precursor of stroke; this subject is also discussed in detail in several other chapters.

Coronary Heart Disease

In the Framingham study, CHD was ascertained prospectively on biennial examination as well as through monitoring of hospitalizations. CHD predisposes to stroke by a variety of mechanisms—as a source for embolism from the heart; by virtue of shared risk factors; as an untoward effect of medical and surgical treatments for coronary atherosclerotic disease; and less commonly, as a consequence of pump failure. Stroke occurs most frequently within 2 weeks after acute MI, affecting between 0.7% and 4.7% of MI patients.[55] As expected, older age and ventricular dys-

function (chiefly, decreased ejection fraction) after MI raised stroke risk.[55] Consistent with an embolic mechanism, treatment with aspirin and particularly with warfarin anticoagulation decreased the incidence of stroke in a large group of MI survivors.[55,56]

Stroke occurs most frequently after *anterior* wall MI, in 2% to 6% of cases. The mechanism is cerebral embolism principally from left ventricular mural thrombus, which is demonstrable on echocardiographic studies in 40% of cases. Inferior wall MI is an uncommon cause of mural thrombus or stroke. Often, however, the mechanism of stroke in persons with CHD is less apparent. Persons with uncomplicated angina pectoris (AP), non–Q wave infarction, and clinically silent MI also have an increased incidence of ischemic stroke. Data from the Framingham study suggest that survivors of silent or unrecognized MI had a 10-year incidence of stroke of 17.8% for men and 17.3% for women; these figures are not that much lower than those seen after recognized MI, 19.5% for men and 29.3% for women.

Atrial Fibrillation

In association with rheumatic heart disease and mitral stenosis, AF is acknowledged to predispose to stroke. Chronic AF without valvular heart disease, previously considered to be innocuous, has been associated with approximately a five-fold increase in stroke incidence. AF is also the most prevalent persistent cardiac arrhythmia in the elderly. In the Framingham study, AF incidence more than doubled with successive decades of age, rising from 0.2 per 1000 for subjects 30 to 39 years old to 39.0 per 1000 for those 80 to 89 years old. Atrial fibrillation was particularly important in the elderly, because the proportion of total

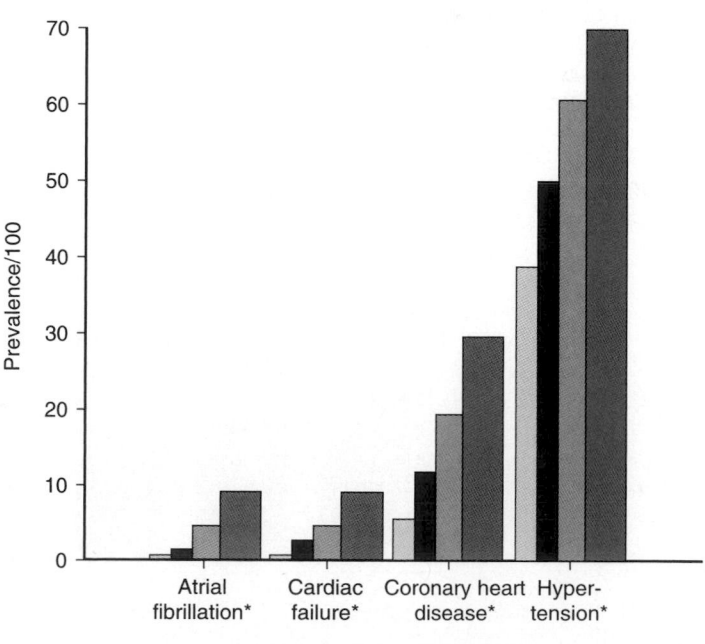

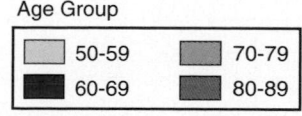

FIGURE 2–8 *Prevalence of cardiovascular abnormality with increasing age, men and women combined; 34-year follow-up. °, significant trend for age* (P < .001). *(Data from the Framingham Heart Study.)*

strokes associated with this arrhythmia rose steadily with age, reaching 36.2% for those aged 80 to 89 years.[57]

Although the prevalence of other cardiac contributors to stroke also increased with age, the greater incidence of stroke in persons with AF was more likely to be a consequence of the AF and not of the associated coronary heart disease or CHF. This pattern becomes apparent when age trends in risk of stroke are examined (Fig. 2–9). Although attributable risk of stroke increased with age for AF, that for cardiac failure, CHD, and hypertension declined with age.[57] Notably, in the oldest age group (80 to 89 years), the proportion of strokes attributable to AF was 23.5%, approaching that attributable to hypertension (33.4%), which is a far more prevalent disorder.

A dispute as to whether AF is an independent risk factor or merely a risk "marker" for other conditions predisposing to stroke raged for several years.[58,59] This issue would seem to have been settled by the remarkable concordance of results of a half-dozen randomized clinical trials demonstrating a stroke risk reduction of 68% on intention-to-treat analyses and of more than 80% on efficacy (on-treatment) analyses of warfarin for stroke prevention in AF.[60] The reduction in risk of stroke far outweighs the risk of serious and particularly intracranial bleeding. Aspirin has a far less potent effect and seems to prevent milder noncardioembolic strokes.[61] From a pooled analysis of the five primary prevention trials, the following four risk factors were shown to increase stroke risk: (1) increasing age, (2) prior stroke or transient ischemic attack, (3) history of diabetes, and (4) history of hypertension.[60] Warfarin reduced the incidence of stroke in persons with any one of these risk factors and in all three age groups— younger than 65 years, 65 to 75 years, and older than 75 years (Fig. 2–10). For all age groups, in the presence or absence of risk factors, the four-fold higher incidence of stroke was reduced to approximately 1% by warfarin anticoagulation. For subjects in the youngest age group (<65 years) who had no risk

factors, the incidence without warfarin was 1%; it is only this group for which anticoagulation is not currently indicated. These individuals, denoted as having "lone AF," may be treated with aspirin alone. This conclusion is based on relatively sparse data and will require more studies to further refine who may safely be observed without receiving warfarin therapy.

The relative lack of efficacy of aspirin was clearly demonstrated in a large secondary prevention trial, the European Atrial Fibrillation Trial, in patients who experienced a stroke or TIA within 3 months of enrollment. The annual stroke rate, 12%, was not significantly reduced by aspirin, 300 mg per day, and was the same as was seen in the placebo group.[62] Virtually identical rates occurred with aspirin, and no case of intracranial bleeding was seen in the warfarin group, although many were elderly. In this high-risk group, elderly persons with AF and a prior cerebrovascular event, 90 events (mostly strokes) would be prevented in 1 year for every 1000 patients receiving anticoagulation therapy. The study's investigators have suggested that a target international normalized ratio (INR; an index of prothrombin activity) of 3.0 would produce the lowest rates of ischemic stroke without an increase in the risk of serious hemorrhage.[63] In another study, the risk of stroke rose steeply as the INR fell below 2.0.[64] At an INR of 1.7, the adjusted OR for stroke was 2.0 (95% CI, 1.6 to 2.4); at an INR of 1.5, it was 3.3 (95% CI, 2.4 to 4.6).[64] Combinations of subtherapeutic doses of warfarin combined with aspirin provided little protection. There were no lower rates of hemorrhage, and stroke prevention was far less effective than therapeutic levels of warfarin anticoagulation.[65] Nevertheless, both physicians and patients are reluctant to use warfarin, particularly for elderly patients, in whom risk of stroke is highest.[66] Patients 80 years or older are least likely to be given warfarin. In 1992 to 1993, only 19% of eligible octogenarians were given such treatment. On the positive side, overall, use of warfarin for

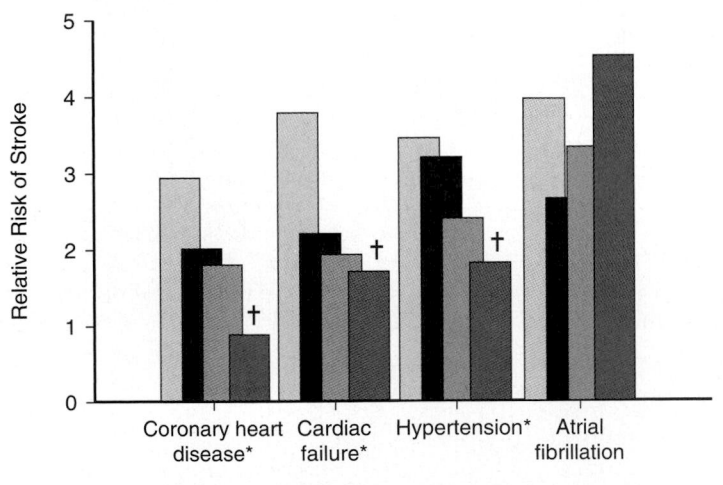

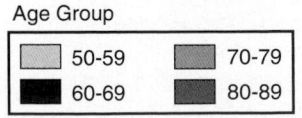

FIGURE 2–9 *Estimated relative risk of stroke with advancing age according to the presence of coronary heart disease, cardiac failure, hypertension, and atrial fibrillation; 34-year follow-up. °, significant inverse trend for age (P < .05); †, no significant excess of strokes. (Data from the Framingham Heart Study.[57])*

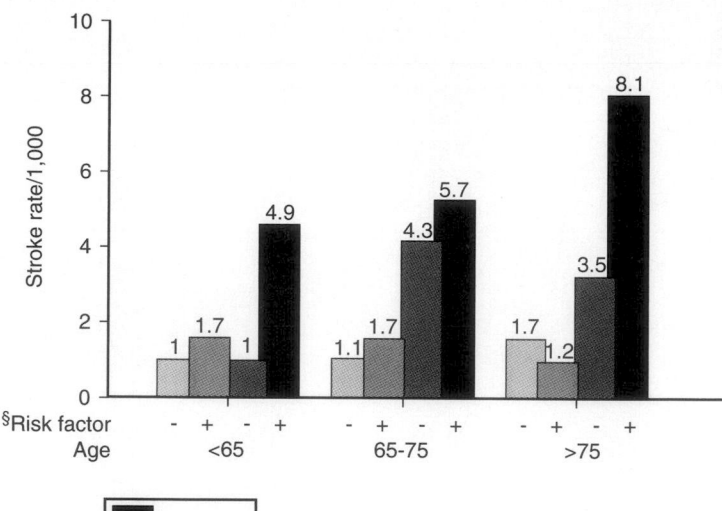

FIGURE 2–10 *Efficacy of warfarin by risk category[§] (hypertension, diabetes, prior stroke or transient ischemic attack); pooled analysis of atrial fibrillation trials. +, one or more risk factors; –, no risk factors.*

stroke prevention in AF has increased from 7% in 1980 to 1981 to 32% in 1992 to 1993.[66]

Warfarin anticoagulation requires dosage adjustment and monitoring of the INR. There is a narrow therapeutic window beyond which embolic stroke occurs on the low side, and bleeding, including intracranial bleeding, occurs with INR values above 4.5. The preliminary results of the SPORTIF III trial of the oral direct thrombin inhibitor ximelagatran, in a fixed dose at 36 mg twice daily, demonstrated noninferiority by intention-to-treat analysis with a 29% relative risk reduction of stroke and systemic embolism for the ximelagatran group.[66a] On-treatment analysis showed a 41% relative risk reduction in the ximelagatran group, which was superior to that for warfarin (P = .018).[66a] There was no significant difference in rates of major or minor bleeding and, particularly, no increase in intracranial hemorrhage with ximelagatran (0.2% per year in the ximelagatran group versus 0.5% per year for the subjects given warfarin). Clearly, if these preliminary findings are reproduced, this drug (or others in this class) offers promise for a greater likelihood of physician prescription and better patient compliance, facilitating stroke prevention in patients with atrial fibrillation.

Left Ventricular Hypertrophy by Electrocardiogram
Left ventricular hypertrophy demonstrated on electrocardiogram (LVH by ECG) increases in prevalence with age and blood pressure. Risk of ABI rose by more than fourfold in men and six-fold in women with this abnormal ECG pattern. The higher risk persisted even after the influence of age and other atherogenic precursors, including systolic blood pressure, were taken into account.

A more sensitive and precise measure of cardiac muscle hypertrophy, left ventricular mass (LVM-to-height ratio), on echocardiography is now frequently available. LVM as determined on M-mode echocardiography has been directly related to incidence of stroke.[67] The hazard ratio

for stroke and TIA, with comparison of the uppermost quartile of LVM-to-height ratio with the lowest, was 2.72 after adjustments were made for age, gender, and cardiovascular risk factors. There was a graded response with a hazard ratio of 1.45 for each quartile increment of LVM-to-height ratio. Thus, echocardiographic findings provide prognostic information beyond that available from traditional risk factors.

Other Host Factors

Race
The distribution of stroke incidence, prevalence, and mortality is dealt with in detail in Chapter 1. Clearly, these rates differ according to race, the bases of which are not dealt with here (Fig. 2–11).[68]

Migraine
As a result of clinical observations, case reports, and clinical series, the notion evolved that migraine predisposes to stroke, particularly ischemic stroke. Complicated migraine with aura and migraine with neurologic concomitants appeared most likely to be followed by stroke. Examples of the association between migraine and stroke occur in certain uncommon syndromes and instances. For instance, in CADASIL (cerebral autosomal dominant arteriopathy with subcortical infarcts and leukoencephalopathy), migraine headache is associated with white matter disease, dementia, and subcortical strokes.[69] Another syndrome of migraine and increased stroke risk is said to occur in the antiphospholipid antibody syndrome, in which migraine is associated with clearly elevated stroke risk and elevated titers of antiphospholipid antibodies.[69] Atypical migraine syndromes such as hemiplegic migraine, are also associated with stroke but are quite rare.[70]

The relationship of stroke to the common migraine syndromes encompassing migraine with aura and migraine

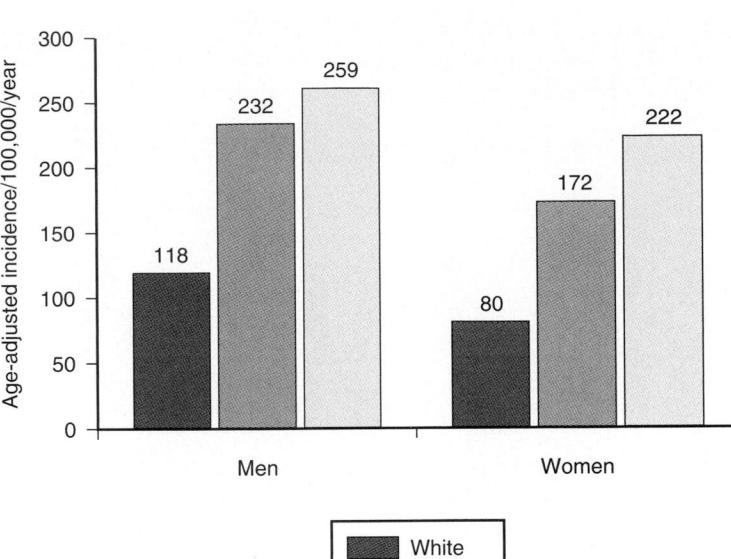

FIGURE 2–11 *Stroke incidence according to race or ethnicity in the Northern Manhattan Stroke Study (NOMASS). (From Sacco RL, Boden-Albala B, Gan R, et al: Stroke incidence among whites, blacks and Hispanics from the same community of Northern Manhattan. Am J Epidemiol 147:259–268, 1998.)*

without aura has been investigated in two large case-control studies, the Italian National Research Council Study Group on Stroke in the Young[71] and a sub-study of the World Health Organization (WHO) Collaborative Study of Cardiovascular Disease and Steroid Hormone Contraception.[85] Migraine as a predisposing factor for stroke, evaluated in the Physicians' Health Study, was associated with an increased risk of ischemic stroke in all of these aforementioned studies with relative risks or ORs ranging from 2.0 to 3.8.[72] The studies that distinguished between migraine with and migraine without aura usually detected a higher risk for migraine with aura. The contribution of migraine to stroke risk drops with increasing age. The WHO study and other case-control studies found an increase in stroke risk in women younger than 45 years who smoked and in those who used oral contraceptives.

Unruptured Intracranial Aneurysms

Detection of an unruptured intracranial aneurysm (UIA) presents a therapeutic dilemma in which risk of future rupture must be weighed against the risks of intervention. Guidance comes from data obtained from the International Study of Unruptured Intracranial Aneurysms (ISHUA), which examined two groups.[73] A retrospective cohort was assembled to permit examination of the outcome of UIAs in subjects with and without a history of SAH. Another prospective cohort was formed to examine the morbidity and mortality of surgery for UIAs. The retrospective cohort consisted of 727 subjects who had UIAs and no history of SAH, and 722 subjects who had UIAs and a history of SAH from another aneurysm.[73] For those with no history of previous SAH, aneurysm size was found to be the major predictor of rupture. The rupture rate for aneurysms smaller than 10 mm was low, 0.05% per year, compared with nearly 1% per year for aneurysms 10 mm or larger, and 6% in the first year for giant aneurysms (>25 mm). Location was another major predictor, with posterior communicating, vertebrobasilar–posterior cerebral,

and basilar tip aneurysms having a higher rate of rupture. For subjects with a history of SAH, aneurysms smaller than 10 mm had a rupture rate of 0.5% per year, 10 times higher than for subjects with aneurysms of the same size without a history of SAH. Aneurysms 10 mm or larger had a slightly higher hemorrhage rate, of 0.65% per year. The only other clear predictor in this group was basilar tip location.

For subjects without a history of SAH, the prospective component of ISHUA found the 30-day mortality rate for surgical treatment of UIAs to be 2.3%. Unlike previous studies, the ISHUA measured cognitive function as well as functional status to determine disability after surgery. Twelve percent of patients had cognitive or functional disability at 1 year after surgery. This finding suggests a high toll for surgery in these subjects, who were for the most part neurologically normal before surgery. Clearly, further study is needed, particularly with the availability and increasing utility of neurovascular interventions that promise lower rates of death and disability.

Environmental Factors

Cigarette Smoking

Cigarette smoking, a powerful risk factor for MI and sudden death, has been clearly linked to brain infarction as well as to ICH and SAH.[74,75] A similar relationship between cigarette smoking and stroke was found in Hawaiian Japanese men after 10 years of follow-up in the Honolulu Heart Study, in which cigarette smoking made a significant independent contribution to cerebral infarction and risk of intracranial hemorrhage.[76]

In the late 1970s, several studies of oral contraceptives and stroke in young women identified cigarette smoking as an important risk factor. Surprisingly, the association between cigarette smoking, oral contraceptives, and stroke was related primarily to SAH. In the Royal College of General Practitioners study of oral contraceptive use, the higher risk of SAH occurred principally in women older than 35 years who were current or former users of oral contraceptives and who smoked cigarettes.[77]

In the NHS, a cohort of nearly 120,000 women were followed prospectively for 8 years for the development of stroke. Risk of SAH as well as thrombotic stroke was increased in cigarette smokers. Relative risk of SAH showed a dose-response relationship from 4-fold in light smokers to 9.8-fold in smokers of 25 or more cigarettes daily.[77] Of note, in each smoking category, the relative risk of SAH, whether or not other associated risk factors were taken into account, was twice as great as that of thromboembolic stroke (Table 2.3).

The association between cigarette smoking and SAH from aneurysm was also found in men, in the Framingham study[78] and in a case-control analysis from New Zealand.[79] In a case-control study of 114 patients with SAH in a defined region in Finland, cigarette smokers were significantly more prevalent in patients with SAH than in controls matched for age, sex, and domicile.[80] Relative risk of SAH in smokers, compared with nonsmokers, was 2.7 in men and 3.0 in women. The investigators of this suggested that smoking promoted a temporary increase in blood pressure that, acting in concert with the "metastatic emphysema effect," was responsible for SAH from cerebral aneurysm. No more reasonable hypothesis has been promulgated to explain this powerful relationship.

That cigarette smoking raises the risk of thrombotic stroke and SAH is generally accepted; the relationship of cigarette smoking to ICH is less well established. Data from the Honolulu Heart Study firmly links cigarette smoking in Hawaiian men of Japanese ancestry to stroke both "thromboembolic and hemorrhagic."[76] Risk of "hemorrhagic" stroke was significantly greater (relative risk 2.5) in cigarette smokers than in nonsmokers; this excess risk of stroke was independent and persisted at a relative risk of 2.8 even after the other associated risk factors—age, diastolic blood pressure, serum cholesterol, alcohol consumption, hematocrit, and body mass—were accounted for.

In a meta-analysis of 32 separate studies, including those cited here, cigarette smoking was found to be a significant independent contributor to stroke incidence in both sexes and at all ages and was associated with an approximately 50% higher risk overall compared with not smoking.[81] The risk of stroke generally, and of ABI specifically, rose as number of cigarettes smoked per day increased, in both men and women.

Oral Contraceptives

In the 1970s, risk of stroke was estimated to be increased five-fold in women using oral contraceptives. This higher risk was most marked in older women—older than 35 years—and predominantly in those with other cardiovascular risk factors, particularly hypertension and cigarette smoking.[82] However, the mechanism of stroke in oral contraceptive users is unclear. Cerebral infarction is more likely to be due to thrombotic disease than to atherosclerosis; it is known that clotting is enhanced by the oral contraceptive–induced increase in platelet aggregability and by the alteration of clotting factors to favor thrombogenesis. In a young woman with unexplained ischemic stroke, use of oral contraceptives is presumed to be the "cause" of the infarct; in a series of carefully studied patients, however, stroke was attributed to oral contraceptive use in no more than 10% of cases.[83]

There was no increase in stroke or other cardiovascular disease in the NHS among former users of oral contraceptives.[84] An international ischemic stroke and oral contraceptive study assessed risk of stroke in women in Europe and in less developed countries.[85] Incidence of stroke was increased with an OR of 2.99 (95% CI, 1.65 to 5.40), and was lowest in younger women and in nonsmokers in whom blood pressure had been recently checked and found not to be elevated. Women with hypertension had an OR of 10.7 (95% CI, 2.04 to 56.6). In Europe, stroke incidence in current use of low-dose oral contraceptives (<50 mg estrogen) was 1.53 (95% CI, 0.71–3.31).[85]

In the United States, a population-based case-control study of oral contraceptive use in women with stroke, in which the oral contraceptive preparations contained the current low-dose estrogen dose, was conducted through the California Kaiser Permanente Medical Care Program.[86] Compared with former users and nonusers of oral contraceptives, the OR for ischemic stroke in current users was 1.18 (95% CI, 0.54 to 2.59) after adjustment for other risk factors for stroke.[86] Thus, risk of ischemic stroke is quite

Table 2.3 Age-Adjusted Relative Risks (RRs) of Stroke (Fatal and Nonfatal Combined), by Daily Number of Cigarettes Consumed among Current Smokers*

Event	Never Smoked	Former Smoker	Current Smoker	No. of Cigarettes Smoked per Day among Current Smokers			
				1–14	15–24	25–34	35 or More
Total stroke	1.00	1.35 (0.98–1.85)	2.73 (2.18–3.41)	2.02 (1.29–3.14)	3.34 (2.38–4.70)	3.08 (1.94–4.87)	4.48 (2.78–7.23)
Subarachnoid hemorrhage	1.00	2.26 (1.16–4.42)	4.85 (2.90–8.11)	4.28 (1.88–9.77)	4.02 (1.90–8.54)	7.95 (3.50–18.07)	10.22 (4.03–25.94)
Ischemic stroke	1.00	1.27 (0.85–1.89)	2.53 (1.91–3.35)	1.83 (1.04–3.23)	3.57 (2.36–5.42)	2.73 (1.49–5.03)	3.97 (2.09–7.53)
Cerebral hemorrhage	1.00	1.24 (0.64–2.42)	1.24 (0.64–2.42)	1.68 (0.34–5.28)	2.53 (0.71–6.05)	1.41 (0.39–5.05)	

*Numbers in parentheses are 95% confidence intervals. RR adjusted for age in 5-year intervals, follow-up period (1976–1978, 1978–1980, 1980–1982, 1982–1984,1984–1986,or 1986–1988), history of hypertension, diabetes, high cholesterol levels, body mass index, past use of oral contraceptives, postmenopausal estrogen therapy, and age at starting smoking.
Adapted from Kawachi I, Colditz GA, Stampfer MJ: Smoking cessation and decreased risk of stroke in women. JAMA 269: 223, 1993.

low in women of childbearing age and is not definitely increased in nonsmokers without hypertension. A 2000 meta-analysis involved 16 studies published from 1960 to 1999 and addressed the relationship of oral contraceptive use and stroke. The overall relative risk of ischemic stroke with all preparations and study designs was 2.75 (95% CI, 2.24 to 3.38).[87] The relative risk in population-based studies of low-estrogen preparations, after data were controlled for both smoking and hypertension, was 1.93 (95% CI, 1.35 to 2.74). If these latter results are valid, low-dose oral contraceptive pills might lead to one stroke for every 24,000 women-users, or 425 ischemic strokes in the United States each year. These results must be interpreted with caution because other studies did not find the same association between stroke and low-dose estradiol contraceptives.

With regard to SAH, the interaction between the older preparations of oral contraceptives (containing high doses of estrogens), cigarette smoking, and SAH is of particular interest. Prospective observation of more than 40,000 women, half of whom were taking oral contraceptives, showed an increased risk of fatal SAH (not cerebral infarction) in women taking these agents. Risk was increased four-fold in cigarette smokers older than 35 years, with most cases confined to this group.[77] The OR for hemorrhagic stroke in users of oral contraceptives in the California Kaiser Permanente Program study was also not significantly greater.[86] There was a positive (nonsignificant) interaction for hemorrhage in current users who smoked, with an OR of 3.64 (95% CI, 0.95 to 13.87).[86] In the WHO Collaborative Study of Cardiovascular Disease and Steroid Hormone Contraception, risk of hemorrhagic stroke was not increased in younger women and only slightly higher in older women.[88] The bulk of these hemorrhages were subarachnoid (200 of 248 in Europe), and risk was significantly greater in women aged 35 years or older. The OR for hemorrhage among current oral contraceptive users, 35 years or older, who were also current cigarette smokers was 3.91 (95% CI, 1.54 to 9.89).[88]

Hormone Replacement Therapy

Observational studies have either shown no influence of hormone replacement therapy (HRT) on stroke or a weak protective effect. The Women's Estrogen for Stroke Trial (WEST) randomly assigned 652 postmenopausal women aged 46 to 91 years to receive either placebo or estradiol within 90 days of a TIA or nondisabling stroke. After a mean 2.7-year follow-up, there was no difference between the two groups as to outcome of nonfatal stroke or death.[89] This result was consistent with previous findings of no protective impact of HRT on stroke incidence.

However, the largest trial to date examining the issue of HRT and cardiovascular disease was the Women's Health Initiative Randomized Controlled Trial, which randomly assigned 16,608 subjects to receive either conjugated estrogens plus progesterone or placebo.[90] The trial was stopped after 5.2 years because of a significant rise in rate of breast cancer in the treatment group and because a global statistic indicated that the risks of treatment exceeded the benefit. Women taking HRT had a higher risk of stroke, with a relative risk of 1.41 (1.07 to 1.8590). Despite a large body of observational evidence supporting a preventive effect of HRT on CHD, women receiving treatment also had a significantly higher risk of CHD and stroke. Pending further evidence to the contrary, HRT increases stroke and other negative outcomes and cannot be recommended as a measure to prevent cardiovascular disease.

Alcohol Consumption

As in MI, the effect of alcohol consumption on stroke risk is related to the amount of alcohol consumed. Heavy alcohol use, either habitual daily heavy alcohol consumption or binge drinking, seems to be related to higher rates of cardiovascular disease. Light or moderate alcohol consumption, on the other hand, is inversely related to incidence of CHD.[91] Light and moderate alcohol use tends to raise the HDL cholesterol, whereas high levels of alcohol intake are linked to hypertension and hypertriglyceridemia and may, in this way, predispose to fatal and nonfatal CHD.

The relationship of alcohol consumption to stroke occurrence is less clear.[92] Available evidence suggests there is a U-shaped relationship between level of alcohol consumption and ischemic stroke risk. Minimal consumption or total abstinence and heavy alcohol consumption seem to increase ischemic stroke occurrence, whereas moderate alcohol use is associated with the lowest risk. Risk of stroke due to hemorrhage rises with the amount of alcohol consumed.[93] There was a powerful dose-response relationship between alcohol consumption and incidence of ICH and SAH in the Honolulu Heart Study of men of Japanese ancestry, even after other pertinent risk factors, particularly blood pressure, were taken into account. Increases in alcohol consumption were related to rising levels of blood pressure, to cigarette smoking, and to lower serum cholesterol levels, all risk factors for ICH. However, even after these factors were taken into account, alcohol consumption was independently related to incidence of intracranial hemorrhage, both subarachnoid and intracerebral; no significant relationship was found between alcohol and thromboembolic stroke. Compared with nondrinkers, age-adjusted relative risk of ICH was 2.1 for light drinkers (1 to 14 oz per month), 2.4 for moderate drinkers (15 to 39 oz per month), and 4.0 for heavy drinkers (40 or more oz per month). After adjustment was made for the other associated risk factors, ICH was 2.0, 2.0, and 2.4 times as frequent, respectively, in these alcohol consumption categories.[93] However, there was no significant relationship between alcohol consumption and thromboembolic stroke. Data from the Framingham study also suggest a higher incidence of brain infarction and stroke with increased levels of alcohol use, but only in men.[92]

There are a number of mechanisms by which heavy alcohol consumption may predispose to, and moderate alcohol consumption protect from, stroke.[94] Cigarette smoking is more common in heavy drinkers, and contributes to the hemoconcentration accompanying heavy alcohol consumption, which increases hematocrit and viscosity.[95] In addition, rebound thrombocytosis during abstinence has been observed. Cardiac rhythm disturbances, particularly AF, occur with alcohol intoxication, producing what has been called "holiday heart."[96] Acute alcohol intoxication has been cited as a precipitating factor in stroke in young people, both in thrombotic stroke and in SAH.[95,97] Other researchers have found a relationship to acute intoxication; a case-control study failed to find an effect of alcohol consumption that was independent of other risk factors, particularly cigarette smoking.[98]

Physical Activity

Leisure-time and work-associated vigorous physical activity has been linked to lower incidence of CHD. Vigorous exercise may exert a beneficial influence on risk factors for atherosclerotic disease by lowering elevated blood pressure as a result of weight loss and by reducing the pulse rate, raising HDL cholesterol, lowering LDL cholesterol, improving glucose tolerance, and promoting a lifestyle conducive to favorably changing detrimental health habits such as cigarette smoking. However, physical activity has only recently been found to be associated with reduced stroke incidence.[99–103] In the Framingham study, physical activity in subjects with a mean age of 65 years was associated with a reduced stroke incidence.[101] In men, the relative risk was 0.41 (95% CI, 0.24 to 0.69, p = 0.0007) after analysts accounted for the effects of potential confounders, including systolic blood pressure, serum cholesterol, glucose intolerance, vital capacity, obesity, LVH on ECG, AF, valvular heart disease, CHF, coronary heart disease, and occupation. However, no evidence was found for a protective effect of physical activity on risk of stroke in women. As in coronary heart disease, *moderate* physical activity conferred no less benefit than *heavy* activity levels. In a number of other population studies and in a series of case-control studies, low levels of physical activity were associated with higher incidence of stroke. A beneficial effect has been found in women.[102]

A graded response to exercise was seen in 7735 male British civil servants, aged 40 to 59 years, with the greatest benefit in reduced stroke incidence derived from the most intense level of exercise and an intermediate protective effect from medium levels.[100] In the Honolulu Heart Program study of Hawaiian Japanese men, after adjustment for other risk factors, higher levels of physical activity was found to be associated with lower rates of both ischemic and hemorrhagic stroke.[99] Data from the First National Health and Nutrition Examination Survey (NHANES 1) Epidemiologic Follow-Up Study disclosed a consistent association of low levels of physical activity with higher risk of stroke in women as well as men and in both black and white subjects.[101,103–105] Moderate levels of activity tended to provide an intermediate level of protection.[103]

Physical activity exerts a beneficial influence on risk factors for atherosclerotic disease by reducing blood pressure and weight, reducing the pulse rate, raising HDL cholesterol, lowering LDL cholesterol, decreasing platelet aggregability, and increasing insulin sensitivity with improved glucose tolerance, and promoting a lifestyle conducive to changing diet and promoting cessation of cigarette smoking. Increased physical activity levels have now been rather convincingly associated with lower incidence of stroke. Moderate levels of recreational and nonrecreational physical activity provide substantial benefit and may be recommended as a sensible lifestyle modification to reduce the risk of cardiovascular disease including stroke.

Diet

Consumption of grains, fruits and vegetables, and fish in the diet have been related to a reduced incidence of stroke in a number of studies. In the NHS of more than 75,000 women, the relative risk of ischemic stroke was 0.69 in the uppermost quintile of grain consumption relative to the lowest quintile, after adjustment for other stroke risk factors.[106] Whole grain consumption was also associated with lower risk of stroke (relative risk 0.69; 95% CI, 0.52 to 0.92), in an analysis combining the Nurses Health Study and the Health Professionals Follow-up Study.[106] Nurses in the NHS who consumed 5 or more servings of fish per week had an adjusted relative risk for stroke of 0.38 compared with women consuming less than 1 serving per month, implying a protective effect of omega-3 fatty acids.[108]

Vitamin C and E levels have been related to stroke incidence, but the findings have been inconsistent. In the Shibata study, a prospective cohort of 880 men and 1241 women, the relative risk of stroke adjusted for all other risk factors was 0.71 in the subjects with the highest vitamin C levels relative to those with the lowest levels after 20 years of follow-up. The Health Professionals Follow-up Study also looked at this issue, administering food frequency questionnaires to 43,738 men aged 40 to 75 years. After 8 years of follow-up, there were no significant relationships between consumption of vitamins C and E and the risk of stroke.[109] Consumption of fish, once a week or more frequently, was associated with an approximate 50% reduction in stroke incidence in women and in black men.[110] Incidence was reduced by a nonstatistically significant 15% in white men who consumed fish compared with those who never ate fish.[110]

In the Heart Outcomes Prevention Evaluation (HOPE) Trial, a randomized controlled clinical trial, 9541 patients 55 years or older who had coronary heart disease, stroke, peripheral vascular disease, or diabetes mellitus and one other risk factor received (in a 2 × 2 factorial design) vitamin E, ramipril, neither, or both. There was no benefit from vitamin E intake on the composite outcome of MI, stroke, or vascular death.[124]

STROKE PREVENTION THROUGH RISK FACTOR MANAGEMENT

The rapid and remarkable 60% decline in death rates from stroke in the United States and most other industrialized nations since 1972 offers strong support that modifiable environmental influences are operating. Part of the decline may result from a reduction in the severity and maybe the incidence of stroke perhaps as a result of improved detection and treatment of hypertension as well as control of other risk factors.[111] On the basis of data from randomized clinical trials and from observational study, we can conclude that stroke may be prevented, and stroke recurrence risk reduced, by a number of risk factor interventions, as follows:

- Reduction of elevated blood pressure
- Cessation of cigarette smoking
- Use of warfarin anticoagulation in AF
- Increase in physical activity and promotion of weight reduction
- Treatment of high-risk individuals with hMG CoA (3-hydroxy-3 methylglutaryl coenzyme A) reductase inhibitors

- Use of angiotensin-converting enzyme (ACE) inhibitors and angiotensin receptor blockers (ARBs)

Lowering plasma homocysteine and achieving better control of blood sugar in diabetic patients may achieve further reductions in risk of stroke. It is likely that prevention and treatment of predisposing cardiac diseases such as CHD, CHF, AF, increased left ventricular mass, and valvular heart disease would also reduce stroke occurrence.

Control of Hypertension and Stroke Prevention

A combined analysis of 9 major prospective (observational) studies of 420,000 individuals, revealed a graded relationship between diastolic pressure and incidence of stroke and CHD.[112] There was no threshold level below which risk gradients were flat, implying a steadily rising risk with increasing diastolic pressure *even in the normal range*. This impact was also seen in another meta-analysis of drug treatment for hypertension.[112] The incidence of stroke increased 46% and CHD increased 29% from baseline with each 7.5 mm Hg increase in diastolic pressure.

These findings were validated by randomized trials of blood pressure reduction; reducing elevated blood pressure prevented stroke.[113,114] The findings of 14 treatment trials in 37,000 hypertensive subjects finally put to rest the long-standing concern that control of elevated blood pressure in hypertensive persons precipitates stroke. The average diastolic blood pressure reduction of 5.8 mm Hg resulted in a 42% lower stroke incidence. This observed reduction in stroke incidence closely approximated that expected on the basis of prospective observational studies.[113,114] In these studies, the duration of blood pressure reduction was brief, from 2 to 5 years. The dramatic impact on stroke incidence within this short period suggests that treatment removed or reduced precipitating factors as well as reducing the progression of atherosclerosis. Presumably, more prolonged blood pressure control would have both effects.

In virtually all of the older treatment trials, the diastolic pressure was been emphasized, although stroke risk clearly is directly related to systolic pressure levels.[115] In the elderly, in whom isolated elevation of the systolic pressure is common, it was thought that treatment would be ineffective in reducing pressure, hazardous in terms of side effects, and unwarranted on the basis of available epidemiologic data. The Systolic Hypertension in the Elderly Program (SHEP) trial enrolled 4736 persons older than 60 years with systolic blood pressure levels in excess of 160 mm Hg and diastolic pressure levels less than 90 mm Hg.[116] In the treated group, blood pressure reduction was associated with a 36% reduction in stroke and a 27% reduction in MI and coronary death after 4.5 years of follow-up. These findings have enormous importance because two thirds of all individuals with hypertension between the ages of 65 and 89 years have isolated systolic hypertension and the majority of strokes occur in this age group.[117]

It is clear from the SHEP trial, and from the European Working Party on Hypertension in the Elderly (EWPHE) study, that antihypertensive medication is well tolerated by the elderly.[117-119] The SHEP trial demonstrated that reduction of blood pressure can be accomplished with relative ease, approximately half of cases being controlled with the thiazide diuretic chlorthalidone alone, and that it is well tolerated, as evidenced by a 90% compliance rate in the active treatment group at 5 years. Because increased blood pressure is the most powerful risk factor for stroke and because the benefits of treatment occur so promptly, control of increased blood pressure, systolic as well as diastolic, is the cornerstone of stroke prevention. These findings were confirmed in the Syst-Eur trial, conducted in 4695 persons with isolated systolic hypertension, in which nitrendipine, a dihydropyridine calcium channel blocker, was compared with placebo.[120] A 42% reduction in stroke incidence was seen after a mean of 2 years of follow-up (95% CI, −60 to −17; P = .003). Of particular interest is that cardiovascular outcomes in the 492 diabetic subjects in the Syst-Eur Trial were compared with outcomes in the 4203 nondiabetic subjects in post hoc analyses.[121] In the treated diabetic subjects, overall mortality was reduced by 55%, mortality from cardiovascular disease by 76%, all cardiovascular events by 69%, and risk of stroke by 73%.

Consonant with the findings of this trial were the results reported by the UK Prospective Diabetes Study Group.[122] Tight control of diastolic blood pressure in the elderly diabetic subjects of this trial resulted in a 44% relative risk reduction in stroke compared with subjects in whom control was less stringent. Because increased blood pressure is the most powerful risk factor for stroke and the benefits of treatment appear so promptly, control of increased blood pressure, systolic as well as diastolic levels, is the cornerstone of stroke prevention. It would appear that diabetic patients benefit to a greater extent from antihypertensive therapy than nondiabetic patients.

The Effectiveness of Various Classes of Antihypertensive Agents

The effectiveness of the newer classes of antihypertensive agents, calcium channel blockers, and ACE inhibitors was compared with thiazide diuretics and beta-blockers in the Antihypertensive and Lipid-Lowering Treatment to Prevent Heart Attack Trial (ALLHAT).[123] The results of this and other trials suggest that all of these antihypertensive drugs have similar efficacy in the prevention of stroke, with the size of benefit proportional to the level of blood pressure control achieved. The medications also had similar safety profiles, and earlier concerns regarding the safety of calcium channel blockers did not appear to be justified. However, later trials of ACE inhibitors and angiotensin receptor blockers have raised the question of whether these newer agents have an effect on stroke prevention above and beyond their effect on blood pressure reduction.

Angiotensin-Converting Enzyme Inhibitors and Angiotensin Receptor Antagonists

In HOPE Trial, as already mentioned, 9297 subjects with cardiovascular disease (coronary artery disease, stroke, or peripheral vascular disease) or diabetes plus one other risk factor were randomly assigned to receive either 10 mg/day of the ACE inhibitor ramipril or placebo.[124,125,126] The ramipril group experienced a 26% reduction in rate of cardiovascular death, a 20% reduction in rate of MI, and a 32% reduction in rate of stroke compared with the placebo arm. Although blood pressure in the ramipril group was reduced by an average of 3 mm Hg systolic and 3 mm Hg diastolic, the researchers suggested that this level of risk reduction could not be explained by the blood pressure reduction alone. It would appear that the protective effect of ramipril is mediated by other mechanisms, such as beneficial effects on endothelial function, fibrinolysis, and smooth muscle proliferation.[126]

The Perindopril Protection Against Recurrent Stroke Study (PROGRESS) recruited 6105 subjects, both with and without hypertension, who had a history of stroke or TIA to undergo either a perindopril-based treatment protocol or placebo treatment.[127] The benefit of reduction in elevated blood pressures in patients with prior cerebrovascular disease in significantly lowering rates of recurrence was clearly demonstrated; details of this study are given in Chapter 3.

The latest trial of ACE inhibition in stroke prevention was the Losartan Intervention For Endpoint (LIFE) reduction in hypertension study.[128] The trial randomly assigned 9193 patients with hypertension and LVH treatment with either atenolol or the angiotensin II type 1 receptor antagonist losartan. After a mean follow-up of 4.8 years, mean systolic blood pressure reduction was 30.2 mm Hg in the losartan group, and 29.1 mm Hg in the atenolol group. Diastolic blood pressure reduction was 18.5 mm Hg in the losartan group and 19.2 mm Hg in the atenolol group. Compared with subjects given atenolol, subjects undergoing losartan therapy had a 13% reduction in the composite outcome of cardiovascular mortality, stroke, and MI and an impressive 25% reduction in stroke. The incremental benefit of losartan over atenolol was not likely to be due to differences in systolic or diastolic blood pressure levels, which were actually quite similar in the two treatment arms.

Treatment with ramipril or losartan produces a level of stroke risk reduction greater than that expected from the extent of blood pressure reduction alone.

Prevention of the Complications of Diabetes

Despite the increased risk of stroke in diabetic patients, tight diabetic control in type 1 and type 2 diabetes patients in the recent UK Prospective Diabetes Study and in the earlier Diabetes Control and Complications Trial was not found to reduce stroke incidence over 9 years of follow-up. Given that even tight diabetic control is not sufficient in this high-risk population to prevent cardiovascular events such as stroke, some of the focus has shifted to strategies for primary prevention of type 2 diabetes. In a trial of diet and lifestyle change utilizing the Dietary Approaches to Stop Hypertension (DASH) diet promoting weight reduction, decreases in sodium, total fat and saturated fat intake in the diet and increases in physical activity, a 58% reduction in the development of diabetes was observed.[129]

As noted, many diabetic persons have coexisting hypertension, and this combination is particularly hazardous in terms of elevated stroke risk. However, as in the Syst-Eur Trial, diabetic subjects experienced a more marked risk

reduction as a result of control of hypertension than nondiabetic subjects. Therefore, aggressive blood pressure control in diabetic patients is a proven strategy for risk reduction and, at present, is a major strategy for stroke prevention in diabetics. Only a small portion of the benefits derived from the treatment of elevated blood pressure in hypertensive persons has been achieved to date. An estimated 50 million Americans have elevated blood pressure (systolic blood pressure 140 mm Hg or greater and/or diastolic blood pressure 90 mm Hg or greater) or are taking antihypertensive medication.[130] Although 65% of these persons are aware that their blood pressures are elevated, and 49% are receiving treatment, has blood pressure control been achieved in only 21%. Thus, using the $\geq140/\geq90$ mm Hg level as normal, four-fifths of Americans are either unaware of high blood pressure, and their hypertension either is not being treated or not being controlled. If one uses the older classification of normal, $\geq160/\geq95$ mm Hg, the corresponding rates are 84% aware, 73% treated, and 55% controlled, still leaving uncontrolled the hypertension of nearly half of those with the disorder.[4]

Cessation of Cigarette Smoking

Data from Framingham and the NHS make it clear that cigarette smokers who stop smoking reduce their stroke risk by about 60%.[74,131] This reduction in risk occurs in a remarkably short time and is similar to the reduction in CHD risk, which decreases by approximately 50% within 1 year of smoking cessation and reaches the level of those who never smoked within 5 years. In the Framingham study, risk of stroke in former cigarette smokers, both men and women, did not differ from that of persons who never smoked by the end of 5 years from the time they stopped smoking.[74] There was no interaction with age, suggesting that cigarette smoking exerts a precipitating effect on stroke regardless of age or duration of smoking. Similar findings from the NHS show a sizable reduction of risk within 2 years and a reduction to a relative risk of 0.4 (same as that for women who never smoked) from a referent level for current smokers of 1.0 (Fig. 2–12).[131] Because smoking confers an increase in stroke risk of 40% in men and 60% in women, after all other pertinent risk factors have been taken into account, cessation of smoking may be expected to significantly reduce the risk of stroke.

Warfarin Anticoagulation in Atrial Fibrillation

Prophylactic anticoagulation with warfarin is indicated in all persons with AF, with the possible exception of persons younger than 65 years who have no history of hypertension, diabetes, TIA or stroke and who are free of structural heart disease. Persons in whom anticoagulants are contraindicated may take aspirin, 325 mg/day. On the basis of currently available information, anticoagulation may be safely administered to persons older than 75 years and should be continued indefinitely and at an intensity to achieve an INR greater than 2.0, with a target INR of 3.0.[63,64,132] Because there appears to be no lower risk of stroke in the presence of paroxysmal AF, warfarin is indicated in patients with this disorder as well. It is likely further refinement of treatment guidelines will be

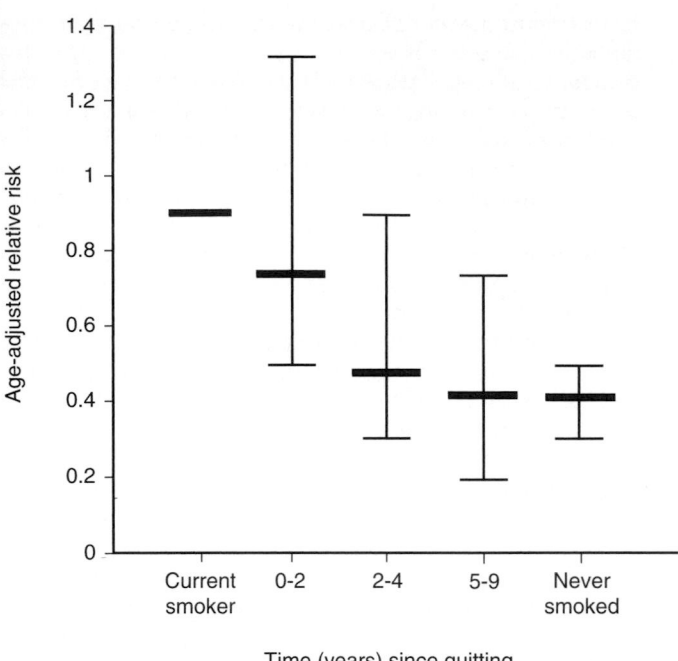

FIGURE 2–12 *Smoking cessation and risk of stroke in women. (From Kawachi I, Colditz GA, Stampfer MJ, et al: Smoking cessation and decreased risk of stroke in women. JAMA 269:232–236, 1993.*

forthcoming, and high-risk and low-risk groups better defined.

Stroke Prevention with Statins

The evidence from trials of hMG CoA reductase inhibitors in men with elevated LDL cholesterol and, usually, preexisting CHD that such treatment reduces stroke incidence opens a new area for stroke prevention.[19,22] Because the influence of cholesterol on stroke appears to be less important than for CHD, some authorities have speculated that other actions of the statins are responsible for the reduction in stroke incidence (which is equivalent to the reduction in CHD incidence in some studies).[133] It has been suggested that the statins influence hemorrheologic factors, plaque geometry, and plaque thrombogenicity as well as promote plaque regression.[133]

Prevention and Treatment of Heart Disease, Including Atrial Fibrillation

CHD, CHF, and AF predispose to stroke, so prevention of these cardiovascular conditions can be anticipated to reduce incidence of stroke.[59] On the basis of current knowledge of the epidemiology of CHF, prevention of obesity and treatment of hypertension may be beneficial. In addition to control of hypertension and cessation of smoking, reduction of CHD risk requires dietary or pharmacologic treatment to reduce elevated total and LDL cholesterol values and to increase the HDL cholesterol fraction. Prevention of AF might best be accomplished by preventing the appearance of the major precursor of AF, which is heart disease, particularly CHD.

Physical Activity

As with cigarette smoking, data from the latest observational studies strongly suggest an association of increased levels of physical activity with longer life span and reduced cardiovascular disease, including CHD and stroke. Whether benefit accrues from physical fitness and training over and above that achieved from weight reduction, blood pressure reduction, improved glucose tolerance, and other physiologic effects on clotting factors is unknown. Data on the benefit of intensive versus moderate exercise are conflicting. No randomized clinical trial findings are likely to appear to bolster these data, but better measures of physical activity, both recreational and nonrecreational, and of physical fitness may help clarify these issues. Nevertheless, the beneficial effects of greater physical activity on vigor and feeling of well-being, as well as its positive effects on cardiovascular risk factors are compelling. It is clear that regular moderate physical activity should be an integral part of a lifestyle that will help reduce the risk of stroke and other cardiovascular diseases.

Folic Acid to Lower Total Plasma Homocysteine Levels

Several clinical trials are under way to determine whether reduction of plasma homocysteine levels by vitamin supplementation will reduce recurrence of stroke or MI. It seems likely that the adverse effects of homocysteine will receive greater attention in the future.

Intensive Diabetes Therapy

Intensive therapy with insulin, three or more doses per day, to achieve tight control of hyperglycemia, in recent-onset insulin-dependent diabetes mellitus was shown to reduce microvascular complications, nephropathy, and retinopathy as well as peripheral neuropathy.[134] This demonstration that improved glycemic control reduces some complications of diabetes is the first clear evidence of what was previously thought likely but was unproven before publications by the Diabetes Control and Complications Trial (DCCT) Research Group.[134] Whether improved glycemic control will reduce the risk of stroke and other macrovascular diseases in diabetic persons remains to be demonstrated.

Identification of High-Risk Candidates for Stroke Prevention

Each physician can identify among his or her patients those who are at increased risk of stroke. Even patients with high-normal blood pressure, in addition to those with mild, moderate, and severe hypertension, will definitely require aggressive pharmacologic treatment to achieve and maintain normotension and help prevent stroke.[4] For persons with high-normal blood pressure, the following hygienic measures are recommended: weight loss, dietary modification with reduction of salt, calories and fat, and assurance of adequate amounts of fruits, vegetables, and potassium. In addition, cigarette smoking cessation, weight reduction, and moderate physical activity are all measures that should be advocated.

To help to identify persons at increased risk of stroke, a risk profile has been developed; it utilizes data from 36 years of follow-up from Framingham and allows the physician to determine a patient's probability of stroke.[135] This determination can be made on the basis of information collected from the medical history, physical examination, and an ECG. Using a table that is sex-specific, the physical determines the probability with a point system utilizing age, systolic blood pressure, use of antihypertensive therapy, presence of diabetes or cigarette smoking, history of cardiovascular disease (CHD or CHF), and EKG abnormalities (LVH or AF). Risk is distributed over a wide range and permits the physician to rapidly relate a particular patient's probability of stroke to that of an average person of the same age and sex.

The stroke risk profile helps the physician identify which borderline hypertensive patients need pharmacologic treatment by virtue of a greater probability of stroke, usually attributable to the presence of several other risk factor abnormalities. Figure 2–13 shows the risk profile for men aged 70 years with two systolic blood pressure levels, 120 mm Hg and 180 mm Hg. The probability of stroke in 10 years ranges from less than half the average level to nearly 100%, depending on the risk factor burden. The probability of stroke may be higher in a man with a normal systolic blood pressure (120 mm Hg) and multiple risk factor abnormalities than in a man with a blood pressure of 180 mm Hg who is free of diabetes and cardiovascular disease and does not smoke. This risk profile provides a quantitative assessment of the level of risk, which is particularly helpful in the patient with multiple borderline risk factor abnormalities. The graphic and percentage display gives the patient, and the physician, a concrete estimate of the patient's probability of stroke as below, at, or severalfold higher than average. It also provides an illustration of how control of certain risk factors, treatment of which has been demonstrated to reduce stroke risk, may result in a decrease in stroke probability. A patient can be shown that reduction of the systolic blood pressure from 180 mm Hg to 140 mm Hg or lower through treatment, cessation of cigarette smoking, and administration of warfarin anticoagulation if he or she has AF may reduce a significantly elevated risk of stroke to nearly normal.[135]

The risk profile may be used to identify patients at highest probability of stroke and therefore in need of antihypertensive drug treatment. For example, if one restricts drug treatment to persons with borderline systolic blood pressure level who have two or more other risk factor

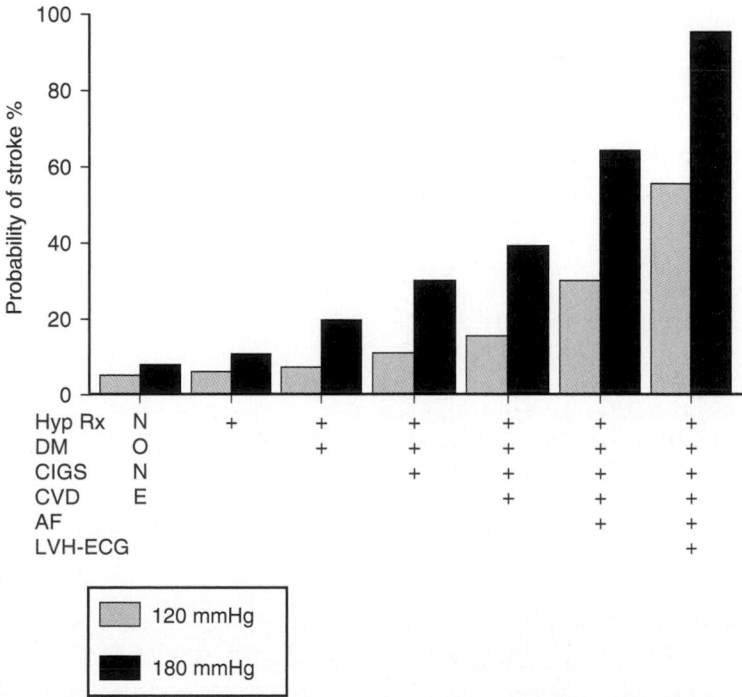

FIGURE 2–13 *Probability of stroke in 10 years at two systolic blood pressure levels. Impact of other risk factors for a 70-year old man. AF, atrial fibrillation; CIGS, cigarette smoking; CVD, previously diagnosed coronary heart disease, cardiac failure, or intermittent claudication; DM, diabetes mellitus; Hyp Rx, antihypertensive therapy; LVH-ECG, left ventricular hypertrophy revealed by electrocardiogram. Plus signs indicate presence of risk factors. (From Wolf PA, D'Agostino RB, Belanger AJ, Kannel WB: Probability of stroke: A risk profile from the Framingham Study. Stroke 22:312–318, 1991.)*

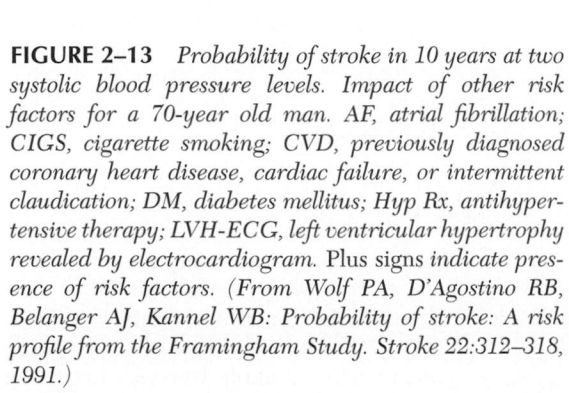

abnormalities (not including age and male sex), it is possible to identify a group consisting of 22% of the men and 14% of women at high risk. In this group, approximately 40% of stroke occur within the subsequent 10 years.[135,136]

Clearly, there are other situations not considered here in which a patient can be identified to be at substantially increased risk of stroke—recent TIA, particularly in the presence of internal carotid artery stenosis of 70% or greater; recent-onset AF; recent MI; during and immediately after cardiac surgery and cerebral angiography; and others dealt with elsewhere in this volume.

References

1. MacMahon B, Pugh TF, Ipsen J: Epidemiologic Methods. Boston, Little, Brown, 1960.
2. American Heart Association: Heart and Stroke Facts Statistics: 1997 Statistical Supplement. Dallas, American Heart Association, 1997.
3. Sacco RL, Ellenberg JH, Mohr JP, et al: Infarcts of undetermined cause: The NINCDS Stroke Data Bank. Ann Neurol 25:382–390, 1989.
4. The sixth report of the Joint National Committee on prevention, detection, evaluation, and treatment of high blood pressure [erratum appears in Arch Intern Med 158:573, 1998] [see comments]. Arch Intern Med 157:2413–2446, 1997.
5. Seshadri S, Wolf PA, Beiser A, et al: Elevated midlife blood pressure increases stroke risk in elderly persons: The Framingham Study. Arch Intern Med 161:2343–2350, 2001.
6. Shahar E, Chambless LE, Rosamond WD, et al: Plasma lipid profile and incident ischemic stroke: The Atherosclerosis Risk in Communities (ARIC) study. Stroke 34:623–631, 2003.
7. Wolf PA, D'Agostino RB, Belanger AJ, et al: Are blood lipids risk factors for stroke? Stroke 22:26, 1991.
8. Prospective Studies Collaboration: Cholesterol, diastolic blood pressure and stroke: 13,000 strokes in 450,000 people in 45 prospective cohorts. Lancet 346:1647–1653, 1995.
9. Iso H, Jacobs DR Jr, Wentworth D, et al: Serum cholesterol levels and six-year mortality from stroke in 350,977 men screened for the Multiple Risk Factor Intervention Trial. N Engl J Med 320:904–910, 1989.
10. Benfante R, Yano K, Hwang LJ, et al: Elevated serum cholesterol is a risk factor for both coronary heart disease and thromboembolic stroke in Hawaiian Japanese men: Implications for shared risk. Stroke 25:814–820, 1994.
11. Atkins D, Psaty BM, Koepsell TD, et al: Cholesterol reduction and the risk for stroke in men: A meta-analysis of randomized, controlled trials. Ann Intern Med 119:136–145, 1993.
12. Fine-Edelstein JS, Wolf PA, O'Leary DH, et al: Precursors of extracranial carotid atherosclerosis in the Framingham Study. Neurology 44:1046–1050, 1994.
13. Wilson PWF, Hoeg JM, Belanger AJ, et al: Cholesterol-years, blood pressure-years, pack-years and carotid stenosis. Circulation 92:I-519, 1995.
14. O'Leary DH, Polak JF, Kronmal RA, et al: Thickening of the carotid wall: A marker for atherosclerosis in the elderly? Stroke 27:224–231, 1996.
15. Furberg CD, Adams HP Jr, Applegate WB, et al: Effect of lovastatin on early carotid atherosclerosis and cardiovascular events: Asymptomatic Carotid Artery Progression Study (ACAPS) Research Group. Circulation 90:1679–1687, 1994.
16. Randomised trial of cholesterol lowering in 4444 patients with coronary heart disease: The Scandinavian Simvastatin Survival Study (4S). Scandinavian Simvastatin Survival Study Group. Lancet 344:1383–1389, 1994.
17. Sacks FM, Pfeffer MA, Moye LA, et al: The effect of pravastatin on coronary events after MI in patients with average cholesterol levels. Cholesterol and Recurrent Events Trial investigators. N Engl J Med 335:1001–1009, 1996.
18. Prevention of cardiovascular events and death with pravastatin in patients with coronary heart disease and a broad range of initial cholesterol levels. The Long-Term Intervention with Pravastatin in Ischaemic Disease (LIPID) Study Group [see comments]. N Engl J Med 339:1349–1357, 1998.
19. MRC/BHF Heart Protection Study of cholesterol lowering with simvastatin in 20,536 high-risk individuals: A randomised placebo-controlled trial. Heart Protection Study Collaborative Group. Lancet 360:7–22, 2002.
20. Plehn JF, Davis BR, Sacks FM, et al: Reduction of stroke incidence after MI with pravastatin: The Cholesterol and Recurrent Events (CARE) study. The Care Investigators [see comments]. Circulation 99:216–223, 1999.
21. Shepherd J, Cobbe SM, Ford I, et al: Prevention of coronary heart disease with pravastatin in men with hypercholesterolemia. West of Scotland Coronary Prevention Study Group. N Engl J Med 333:1301–1307, 1995.
22. Sever PS, Dahlof B, Poulter NR, et al: Prevention of coronary and stroke events with atorvastatin in hypertensive patients who have average or lower-than-average cholesterol concentrations, in the Anglo-Scandinavian Cardiac Outcomes Trial–Lipid Lowering Arm (ASCOT-LLA): A multicentre randomised controlled trial. Lancet 361:1149–1158, 2003.
23. Tell GS, Crouse JR, Furberg CD: Relation between blood lipids, lipoproteins, and cerebrovascular atherosclerosis: A review. Stroke 19:423–430, 1988.
24. O'Leary DH, Anderson KM, Wolf PA, et al: Cholesterol and carotid atherosclerosis in older persons: The Framingham Study. Ann Epidemiol 2:147–153, 1992.
25. Yano K, Reed DM, MacLean CJ: Serum cholesterol and hemorrhagic stroke in the Honolulu Heart Program. Stroke 20:1460–1465, 1989.
26. Shimamoto T, Komachi Y, Inada H, et al: Trends for coronary heart disease and stroke and their risk factors in Japan. Circulation 79:503–515, 1989.
27. Vijan S, Hayward R: Treatment of hypertension in type 2 diabetes mellitus: Blood pressure goals, choice of agents, and setting priorities in diabetes care. Ann Intern Med 138:593–602, 2003.
28. Burchfiel CM, Curb JD, Rodriguez BL, et al: Glucose intolerance and 22-year stroke incidence: The Honolulu Heart Program. Stroke 25:951–957, 1994.
29. Barrett Connor E, Khaw KT: Diabetes mellitus: An independent risk factor for stroke? Am J Epidemiol 128:116–123, 1988.
30. Kannel WB, McGee DL: Diabetes and cardiovascular disease: The Framingham Study. JAMA 241:2035–2038, 1979.
30a. Rexrode KM, Hennekens CH, Willett WC, et al: A prospective study of body mass index, weight change, and risk of stroke in women. JAMA 277:1539–1545, 1997.
31. Walker SP, Rimm EB, Ascherio A, et al: Body size and fat distribution as predictors of stroke among US men. Am J Epidemiol 144:1143–1150, 1996.
32. Welin L, Svardsudd K, Wilhelmsen L, et al: Analysis of risk factors for stroke in a cohort of men born in 1913. N Engl J Med 317:521–526, 1987.
33. Kiely DK, Wolf PA, Cupples LA, et al: familial aggregation of stroke: The Framingham Study. Stroke 24:1366–1371, 1993.
34. Wilhelmsen L, Svardsudd K, Korsan Bengtsen K, et al: Fibrinogen as a risk factor for stroke and MI. N Engl J Med 311:501–505, 1984.
35. Kannel WB, Wolf PA, Castelli WP, D'Agostino RB: Fibrinogen and risk of cardiovascular disease: The Framingham Study. JAMA 258:1183–1186, 1987.
36. Kannel WB, D'Agostino RB, Belanger AJ: Fibrinogen, cigarette smoking, and risk of cardiovascular disease: Insights from the Framingham Study. Am Heart J 113:1006–1010, 1987.
37. Folsom AR, Qamhieh HT, Flack JM, et al: Plasma fibrinogen: Levels and correlates in young adults. Am J Epidemiol 138:1023–1036, 1993.
38. Lee AJ, Lowe GD, Woodward M, Tunstall-Pedoe H: Fibrinogen in relation to personal history of prevalent hypertension, diabetes, stroke, intermittent claudication, coronary heart disease, and family history: The Scottish Heart Health Study. Br Heart J 69:338–342, 1993.
39. Rost NS, Kase CS, Wolf PA, et al: Plasma C-reactive protein, systolic hypertension and risk of ischemic stroke and TIA: The Framingham Study. Stroke 32:330, 2001.
40. Ridker PM, Rifai N, Rose L, et al: Comparison of C-reactive protein and low-density lipoprotein cholesterol levels in the prediction of first cardiovascular events. N Engl J Med 347:1557, 2002.
41. Boushey CJ, Beresford SAA, Omenn GS, Motulsky AG: A quantitative assessment of plasma homocysteine as a risk factor for vascular disease: Probable benefits of increasing folic acid intakes. JAMA 274:1049–1057, 1995.

42. Nygard O, Vollset SE, Refsum H, et al: Total plasma homocysteine and cardiovascular risk profile: The Hordaland Homocysteine Study. JAMA 274:1526–1533, 1995.

43. Perry IJ, Refsum H, Morris RW, et al: Prospective study of serum total homocysteine concentration and risk of stroke in middle-aged British men. Lancet 346:1395–1398, 1995.

44. Stampfer MJ, Malinow MR, Willett WC, et al: A prospective study of plasma homocyst(e)ine and risk of MI in US physicians. JAMA 268:877–881, 1992.

45. Verhoef P, Hennekens CH, Malinow MR, et al: A prospective study of plasma homocyst(e)ine and risk of ischemic stroke. Stroke 25:1924–1930, 1994.

46. Malinow MR, Nieto FJ, Szklo M, et al: Carotid artery intimal-medial wall thickening and plasma homocyst(e)ine in asymptomatic adults: The Atherosclerosis Risk in Communities Study. Circulation 87:1107–1113, 1993.

47. Selhub J, Jacques PF, Bostom AG, et al: Association between plasma homocysteine concentrations and extracranial carotid-artery stenosis [see comments]. N Engl J Med 332:286–291, 1995.

48. Selhub J, Jacques PF, Bostom AG, et al: Relationship between plasma homocysteine, vitamin status and extracranial carotid-artery stenosis in the Framingham Study population. J Nutr 126(Suppl):1258S–1265S, 1996.

49. Stampfer MJ, Malinow MR: Can lowering homocysteine levels reduce cardiovascular risk? N Engl J Med 332:328–329, 1995.

50. Stampfer MJ, Rimm EB: Folate and cardiovascular disease: Why we need a trial now [editorial; comment]. JAMA 275:1929–1930, 1996.

51. Stampfer MJ, Willett WC: Homocysteine and marginal vitamin deficiency: The importance of adequate vitamin intake. JAMA 270:2726–2727, 1993.

52. Selhub J, Jacques PF, Wilson PWF, et al: Vitamin status and intake as primary determinants of homocysteinemia in an elderly population. JAMA 270:2693–2698, 1993.

53. Robinson K, Mayer EL, Miller DP, et al: Hyperhomocysteinemia and low pyridoxal phosphate: Common and independent reversible risk factors for coronary artery disease. Circulation 92:2825–2830, 1995.

54. Wolf PA, Kannel WB, McNamara PM, Gordon T: The role of impaired cardiac function in atherothrombotic brain infarction: The Framingham Study. Am J Public Health 63:52–58, 1973.

55. Loh E, Sutton MSJ, Wun CC, et al: Ventricular dysfunction and the risk of stroke after MI. N Engl J Med 336:251–257, 1997.

56. Smith P, Arnesen H, Holme I: The effect of warfarin on mortality and reinfarction after MI. N Engl J Med 323:147–152, 1990.

57. Wolf PA, Abbott RD, Kannel WB: Atrial fibrillation: A major contributor to stroke in the elderly: The Framingham Study. Arch Intern Med 147:1561–1564, 1987.

58. Chesebro JH, Fuster V, Halperin JL: Atrial fibrillation: Risk marker for stroke. N Engl J Med 323:1556–1558, 1990.

59. Wolf PA, Abbott RD, Kannel WB: Atrial fibrillation as an independent risk factor for stroke: The Framingham Study. Stroke 22:983–988, 1991.

60. Risk factors for stroke and efficacy of antithrombotic therapy in atrial fibrillation: Analysis of pooled data from five randomized controlled trials. Atrial Fibrillation Investigators. Arch Intern Med 154:1449–1457, 1994.

61. Miller VT, Rothrock JF, Pearce LA, et al: Ischemic stroke in patients with atrial fibrillation: Effect of aspirin according to stroke mechanism. Neurology 43:32–36, 1993.

62. Secondary prevention in non-rheumatic atrial fibrillation after transient ischaemic attack or minor stroke. European Atrial Fibrillation Trial (EAFT) Study Group. Lancet 342:1255–1262, 1993.

63. Optimal oral anticoagulant therapy in patients with nonrheumatic atrial fibrillation and recent cerebral ischemia. The European Atrial Fibrillation Trial Study Group. N Engl J Med 333:5–10, 1995.

64. Hylek EM, Skates SJ, Sheehan MA, Singer DE: An analysis of the lowest effective intensity of prophylactic anticoagulation for patients with nonrheumatic atrial fibrillation. N Engl J Med 335:540–546, 1996.

65. Adjusted-dose warfarin versus low-intensity, fixed-dose warfarin plus aspirin for high-risk patients with atrial fibrillation: Stroke Prevention in Atrial Fibrillation III randomized clinical trial. Stroke Prevention in Atrial Fibrillation Investigators. Lancet 348:633–638, 1996.

66. Stafford RS, Singer DE: National patterns of warfarin use in atrial fibrillation. Arch Intern Med 156:2537–2541, 1996.

66a. Halperin JL: The Executive Steering Committee, on behalf of the SPORTIF III and V Study Investigators: Ximelagatran compared with warfarin for prevention of thromboembolism in patients with nonvalvular atrial fibrillation: rationale, objectives, and design of a pair of clinical studies and baseline patient characteristics (SPORTIF III and V) [Trial design] Am Heart J 146(3):431–438, 2003.

67. Bikkina M, Levy D, Evans JC, et al: Left ventricular mass and risk of stroke in an elderly cohort. JAMA 272:33–36, 1994.

68. Sacco RL, Boden-Albala B, Gan R, et al: Stroke incidence among white, black, and Hispanic residents of an urban community: The Northern Manhattan Stroke Study. Am J Epidemiol 147:259–268, 1998.

69. Chabriat H, Vahedi K, Iba-Zizen MT, et al: Clinical spectrum of CADASIL: A study of 7 families. Lancet 346:934–939, 1995.

70. Tanne D, Triplett DA, Levine SR: Antiphospholipid-protein antibodies and ischemic stroke: Not just cardiolipin any more [editorial; comment]. Stroke 29:1755–1758, 1998.

71. Carolei A, Marini C, De Matteis G: History of migraine and risk of cerebral ischaemia in young adults. The Italian National Research Council Study Group on Stroke in the Young. Lancet 347:1503–1506, 1996.

72. Buring JE, Hebert P, Romero J, et al: Migraine and subsequent risk of stroke in the Physicians' Health Study. Arch Neurol 52:129–134, 1995.

73. Unruptured intracranial aneurysms: Risk of rupture and risks of surgical intervention. The International Study of Unruptured Intracranial Aneurysms Investigators. N Engl J Med 339:1725, 1998.

74. Wolf PA, D'Agostino RB, Kannel WB, et al: Cigarette smoking as a risk factor for stroke: The Framingham Study. JAMA 259:1025–1029, 1988.

75. Colditz GA, Bonita R, Stampfer MJ, et al: Cigarette smoking and risk of stroke in middle-aged women. N Engl J Med 318:937–941, 1988.

76. Abbott RD, Yin Y, Reed DM, Yano K: Risk of stroke in male cigarette smokers. N Engl J Med 315:717–720, 1986.

77. Further analyses of mortality in oral contraceptive users: Royal College of General Practitioners' Oral Contraception Study. Lancet 1(8219):541–546, 1981.

78. Sacco RL, Wolf PA, Bharucha NE, et al: Subarachnoid and intracerebral hemorrhage: Natural history, prognosis, and precursive factors in the Framingham Study. Neurology 34:847–854, 1984.

79. Bonita R: Cigarette smoking, hypertension and the risk of subarachnoid hemorrhage: A population-based case-control study. Stroke 17:831–835, 1986.

80. Fogelholm R, Murros K: Cigarette smoking and subarachnoid haemorrhage: A population-based case-control study. J Neurol Neurosurg Psychiatry 50:78–80, 1987.

81. Shinton R, Beevers G: Meta-analysis of relation between cigarette smoking and stroke. BMJ 298:789–794, 1989.

82. Stadel BV: Oral contraceptives and cardiovascular disease (second of two parts). N Engl J Med 305:672–677, 1981.

83. Adams HP Jr, Butler MJ, Biller J, Toffol GJ: Nonhemorrhagic cerebral infarction in young adults. Arch Neurol 43:793–796, 1986.

84. Stampfer MJ, Willett WC, Colditz GA, et al: A prospective study of past use of oral contraceptive agents and risk of cardiovascular diseases. N Engl J Med 319:1313–1317, 1988.

85. Ischaemic stroke and combined oral contraceptives: Results of an international, multicentre, case-control study. WHO Collaborative Study of Cardiovascular Disease and Steroid Hormone Contraception. Lancet 348:498–505, 1996.

86. Petitti DB, Sidney S, Bernstein A, et al: Stroke in users of low-dose oral contraceptives [see comments]. N Engl J Med 335:8–15, 1996.

87. Gillum LA, Mamidipudi SK, Johnston SC: ischemic stroke risk with oral contraceptives: A meta-analysis. JAMA 284:72, 2000.

88. Haemorrhagic stroke, overall stroke risk, and combined oral contraceptives: Results of an international, multicentre, case-control study. WHO Collaborative Study of Cardiovascular Disease and Steroid Hormone Contraception. Lancet 348:505–510, 1996.

89. Viscoli CM, Brass LM, Kernan WN, et al: A clinical trial of estrogen-replacement therapy after ischemic stroke. N Engl J Med 345:1243, 2001.

90. Risks and benefits of estrogen plus progestin in healthy postmenopausal women: Principal results from the women's Health Initiative randomized controlled trial. Writing Group for the Women's Health Initiative Investigators. JAMA 288:321, 2002.

91. Stampfer MJ, Colditz GA, Willett WC, et al: A prospective study of moderate alcohol consumption and the risk of coronary disease and stroke in women. N Engl J Med 319:267–273, 1988.

92. Djousse L, Ellison RC, Beiser A, et al: Alcohol consumption and risk of ischemic stroke: The Framingham Study. Stroke 33:907–912, 2002.

93. Donahue RP, Abbott RD, Reed DM, Yano K: Alcohol and hemorrhagic stroke: The Honolulu Heart Program. JAMA 255:2311–2314, 1986.

94. Camargo CA Jr: Moderate alcohol consumption and stroke: The epidemiologic evidence. Stroke 20:1611–1626, 1989.

95. Hillbom M, Kaste M, Rasi V: Can ethanol intoxication affect hemocoagulation to increase the risk of brain infarction in young adults? Neurology 33:381–384, 1983.

96. Ettinger PO, Wu CF, De La Cruz C Jr, et al: Arrhythmias and the "holiday heart": Alcohol-associated cardiac rhythm disorders. Am Heart J 95:555–562, 1978.

97. Taylor JR, Combs-Orme T: Alcohol and strokes in young adults. Am J Psychiatry 142:116–118, 1985.

98. Gorelick PB: The status of alcohol as a risk factor for stroke. Stroke 20:1607–1610, 1989.

99. Abbott RD, Rodriguez BL, Burchfiel CM, Curb JD: Physical activity in older middle-aged men and reduced risk of stroke: The Honolulu Heart Program. Am J Epidemiol 139:881–893, 1994.

100 Wannamethee G, Shaper AG: Physical activity and stroke in British middle aged men. BMJ 304:597–601, 1992.

101. Kiely DK, Wolf PA, Cupples LA, et al: Physical activity and stroke risk: The Framingham Study. Am J Epidemiol 140:608–620, 1994.

102. Manson JE, Stampfer MJ, Willett WC, et al: Physical activity and incidence of coronary heart disease and stroke in women [abstract]. Circulation 91:927, 1995.

103. Gillum RF, Mussolino ME, Ingram DD: Physical activity and stroke incidence in women and men: The NHANES I Epidemiologic Follow-up Study. Am J Epidemiol 143:860–869, 1996.

104. Lee IM, Hennekens CH, Berger K, et al: Exercise and risk of stroke in male physicians. Stroke 30:1, 1999.

105. Hu FB, Stampfer MJ, Colditz GA, et al: Physical activity and risk of stroke in women. JAMA 283:2961–2967, 2000.

106. Liu S, Manson JE, Stampfer MJ, et al: Whole grain consumption and risk of ischemic stroke in women: A prospective study. JAMA 284:1534–1540, 2000.

107. Joshipura KJ, Ascherio A, Manson JE, et al: Fruit and vegetable intake in relation to risk of ischemic stroke. JAMA 282:1233–1239, 1999.

108. Iso H, Rexrode KM, Stampfer MJ, et al: Intake of fish and omega-3 fatty acids and risk of stroke in women. JAMA 285:304–312, 2001.

109. Ascherio A, Rimm EB, Hernan MA, et al: Relation of consumption of vitamin E, vitamin C, and carotenoids to risk for stroke among men in the United States. Ann Intern Med 130:963–970, 1999.

110. Gillum RF, Mussolino ME, Madans JH: The relationship between fish consumption and stroke incidence: The NHANES I Epidemiologic Follow-up Study (National Health and Nutrition Examination Survey). Arch Intern Med 156:537–542, 1996.

111. Bonita R, Beaglehole R: The enigma of the decline in stroke deaths in the United States: The search for an explanation. Stroke 27:370–372, 1996.

112. MacMahon S, Rodgers A: The epidemiological association between blood pressure and stroke: Implications for primary and secondary prevention. Hypertens Res 17(Suppl):S23–S32, 1994.

113. Collins R, Peto R, MacMahon S, et al: Blood pressure, stroke, and coronary heart disease. Part 2: Short-term reductions in blood pressure: Overview of randomised drug trials in their epidemiological context. Lancet 335:827–838, 1990.

114. MacMahon S, Peto R, Cutler J, et al: Blood pressure, stroke, and coronary heart disease. Part 1: Prolonged differences in blood pressure: Prospective observational studies corrected for the regression dilution bias. Lancet 335:765–774, 1990.

115. Kannel WB, Dawber TR, Sorlie P, Wolf PA: Components of blood pressure and risk of atherothrombotic brain infarction: The Framingham study. Stroke 7:327–331, 1976.

116. Prevention of stroke by antihypertensive drug treatment in older persons with isolated systolic hypertension: Final results of the Systolic Hypertension in the Elderly Program (SHEP). SHEP Cooperative Research Group. JAMA 265:3255–3264, 1991.

117. Wilking SV, Belanger A, Kannel WB, et al: Determinants of isolated systolic hypertension. JAMA 260:3451–3455, 1988.

118. Amery A, Birkenhager W, Brixko P, et al: Mortality and morbidity results from the European Working Party on High Blood Pressure in the Elderly trial. Lancet 1:1349–1354, 1985.

119. Staessen J, Amery A, Birkenhager W, et al: Syst-Eur: A multicenter trial on the treatment of isolated systolic hypertension in the elderly: first interim report. J Cardiovasc Pharmacol 19:120–125, 1992.

120. Staessen JA, Fagard R, Thijs L, et al: Randomised double-blind comparison of placebo and active treatment for older patients with isolated systolic hypertension. The Systolic Hypertension in Europe (Syst-Eur) Trial Investigators [see comments]. Lancet 350:757–764, 1997.

121. Curb JD, Pressel SL, Cutler JA, et al: Effect of diuretic-based antihypertensive treatment on cardiovascular disease risk in older diabetic patients with isolated systolic hypertension. Systolic Hypertension in the Elderly Program Cooperative Research Group [published erratum appears in JAMA 277:1356, 1997] [see comments]. JAMA 276:1886–1892, 1996.

122. Tight blood pressure control and risk of macrovascular and microvascular complications in type 2 diabetes: UKPDS 38. UK Prospective Diabetes Study Group [published erratum appears in BMJ 318:29, 1999] [see comments]. BMJ 317:703–713, 1998.

123. Major outcomes in high-risk hypertensive patients randomized to angiotensin-converting enzyme inhibitor or calcium channel blocker vs diuretic: The Antihypertensive and Lipid-Lowering Treatment to Prevent Heart Attack Trial (ALLHAT). The ALLHAT Officers and Coordinators for the ALLHAT Collaborative Research Group. JAMA 288:2981, 2002.

124. Yusuf S, Sleight P, Pogue J, et al: Effects of an angiotensin-converting-enzyme inhibitor, ramipril, on cardiovascular events in high-risk patients. The Heart Outcomes Prevention Evaluation Study Investigators [see comments]. N Engl J Med 342:145–153, 2000.

125. Bosch J, Yusuf S, Pogue J, et al: Use of ramipril in preventing stroke: Double blind randomised trial. BMJ 324:699, 2002.

126. Lonn E, Yusuf S, Dzavik V, et al: Effects of ramipril and vitamin E on atherosclerosis: The study to evaluate carotid ultrasound changes in patients treated with ramipril and vitamin E (SECURE). Circulation 103:919–925, 2001.

127. Randomised trial of a perindopril-based blood-pressure-lowering regimen among 6,105 individuals with previous stroke or transient ischaemic attack. PROGRESS Collaborative Group. Lancet 358:1033–1041, 2001.

128. Kjeldsen SE, Dahlof B, Devereux RB, et al: Effects of losartan on cardiovascular morbidity and mortality in patients with isolated systolic hypertension and left ventricular hypertrophy: A Losartan Intervention For Endpoint Reduction (LIFE) Substudy. JAMA 288:1491–1498, 2002.

129. Vollmer WM, Sacks FM, Ard J, et al: Effects of diet and sodium intake on blood pressure: Subgroup analysis of the DASH-sodium trial. Ann Intern Med 135:1019–1028, 2001.

130. The fifth report of the Joint National Committee on Detection, Evaluation, and Treatment of High Blood Pressure/National High Blood Pressure Education Program, National Institutes of Health, National Heart, Lung, and Blood Institute. (NIH Publication 95-1088.) Bethesda, MD, NIH, 1995.

131. Kawachi I, Colditz GA, Stampfer MJ, et al: Smoking cessation and decreased risk of stroke in women. JAMA 269:232–236, 1993.

132. Laupacis A, Albers G, Dalen J, et al: Antithrombotic therapy in atrial fibrillation. Chest 114:579S–589S, 1998. Fifth ACCP Consensus conference on Antithrombotic Therapy.

133. Vaughan CJ, Murphy MB, Buckley BM: Statins do more than just lower cholesterol. Lancet 348:1079–1082, 1996.

134. The effect of intensive diabetes therapy on the development and progression of neuropathy. The Diabetes Control and Complications Trial Research Group. Ann Intern Med 122:561–568, 1995.

135. Wolf PA, D'Agostino RB, Belanger AJ, Kannel WB: Probability of stroke: A risk profile from the Framingham Study. Stroke 22:312–318, 1991.

136. D'Agostino RB, Wolf PA, Belanger AJ, Kannel WB: Stroke risk profile: Adjustment for antihypertensive medication. The Framingham Study. Stroke 25:40–43, 1994.

Chapter Three

Outcome following Stroke

Tanja Rundek and Ralph L. Sacco

As the second most common cause of death in the world[1] and a major cause of long-term disability, stroke continues to have a great effect on public health.[2] In the United States, there are an estimated 731,000 strokes and 4 million stroke survivors annually,[3] 4% to 15% of whom suffer a recurrent stroke within a year after incident stroke and 25% by 5 years.[4] Stroke accounts for the greatest number of hospitalizations for neurologic disease.[5] The estimated lifetime cost of first strokes in the United States was approximately $40.6 billion in 1990—$5.6 billion for SAH, $6.0 billion for ICH, and $29.0 billion for ischemic stroke.[6] Costs for acute care incurred in the 2 years after a first stroke accounted for 45%, long-term ambulatory care accounted for 35%, and nursing home costs accounted for 17.5% of aggregate lifetime costs of stroke. Despite the growing knowledge about novel strategies of stroke prevention, including the results from randomized clinical trials of blood pressure–lowering drugs on the risk reduction of initial and recurrent stroke,[7–10] the real challenge still remains: to successfully implement these strategies in stroke prevention programs worldwide.

Tertiary and late secondary prevention programs require an elucidation of the outcomes after stroke, including death, stroke recurrence, worsening, functional disability, quality of life, depression, and dementia. Because the majority of strokes are cerebral infarcts, we give most attention to the prognosis for this type of stroke. We begin by addressing some important observations regarding prognosis after subarachnoid and intracerebral hemorrhage and then discuss the outcomes after ischemic strokes in more depth. We focus on results of the latest stroke outcome studies on mortality, recurrence, functional disability, quality of life, depression, and dementia after ischemic stroke.

PROGNOSIS AFTER SUBARACHNOID HEMORRHAGE

Subarachnoid hemorrhage (SAH) affects more than 25,000 people every year in the United States.[11] Patients with SAH are often younger or middle-aged adults (30 to 60 years), in the prime of life at the time of their stroke, who present with more life-threatening situations than patients with cerebral infarction.[12,13] Advances in the medical, surgical, and endovascular management of SAH have resulted in a dramatic decline in hospital mortality over the past 40 years, from more than 50% in the 1960s to approximately 10% to 20% in the late 1990s.[11,14–16] Poor neurologic status within 24 hours after ictus, advanced age, and large aneurysm have been identified as predictors of mortality and poor functional outcome after SAH.[17]

Early Mortality after Subarachnoid Hemorrhage

Thirty-day case-fatality rates for SAH range from 25% to 55% and depend on the clinical presentation at onset.[18–24] In the Northern Manhattan Stroke Study (NOMASS), the 30-day case-fatality rate for SAH was 26%, depending on severity of symptoms at presentation, patient age, and lesion location.[24] In the Framingham Study cohort, coma at onset was associated with a case-fatality rate of 83%, compared with 56% for patients with focal deficits and 13% for those with no focal deficits.[18] Other studies have also found a direct relationship between the clinical grade (i.e., Hunt and Hess grade) at presentation and mortality rate.

In Rochester, Minnesota, the 30-day case-fatality rates were 30% for patients with clinical grades 1 and 2 at presentation, 65% for those with grade 3, and 85% for those with grades 4 and 5.[17] Fatality rates are also associated with the age at presentation, the presence of intracranial hematoma, the consumption of alcohol, and the presence of hypertension.[17,18,25] Computed tomography (CT) evidence of delayed global cerebral edema after SAH was identified as an independent predictor of mortality and poor 3-month outcome after SAH.[26] Global edema on admission was present in 6% to 8% of patients with SAH.[26,27] Delayed global edema was identified in 12% of patients within 2 to 16 days (average of 6 days) after the onset of the hemorrhage. Evidence of delayed global edema was found in 20% of patients who died or were severely disabled 3 months after onset but in only 7% of survivors.[26] Besides global edema, aneurysm size, loss of consciousness, a poor National Institutes of Health Stroke Scale (NIHSS) score, and old age were independent predictors of death or severe disability 3 months after SAH (Table 3.1).

Late Mortality after Subarachnoid Hemorrhage

Only a few long-term outcome studies after SAH have been published.[27–29] It is commonly believed that patients

Table 3.1　Predictors of Mortality and Severe Disability 3 Months after Subarachnoid Hemorrhage

Predictor	Dead?			Dead or Severely Disabled?		
	Yes (n = 90), % (N)	No, (n = 284), % (N)	P	Yes (n = 137), % (N)	No (n = 237), % (N)	P
Age (years)	60 ± 16	52 ± 14	<.001	60 ± 15	51 ± 14	<.001
Loss of consciousness	62 (56)	29 (81)	<.001	56 (76)	26 (61)	<.001
National Institutes of Health Stroke Scale score	14.0	0	<.001	11.0	0	<.001
Any global edema	40 (36)	13 (37)	<.001	34 (46)	11 (27)	<.001
Aneurysm size >10 mm	31 (28)	17 (48)	<.001	31 (42)	14 (34)	<.001

who have recovered well after successful treatment of ruptured aneurysm have the same life expectancy as the general population. Long-term outcome studies after SAH have supported that observation, indicating that survival in patients who survive the early period approaches that of a general population sample but is worse in those with significant neurologic deficits.[27,28] A study from Finland involving 1714 SAH patents, however, showed that aneurysmal SAH is associated with excess long-term mortality even in patients who recovered well from initial bleeding and surgical treatment.[29] The mortality rate of patients with good recovery at 12 months after SAH was twice that of the general population. This excess tended to be higher in younger age groups.

Cerebrovascular and cardiovascular diseases were the principal causes of premature death after SAH. Nearly 20% of deaths at 12 months after SAH were caused by cerebrovascular events, and a new SAH was the cause of death in 52% of cases. More attention should be paid to the treatment of vascular risk factors in patients with SAH, and long-term follow-up is needed even for patients with SAH who have recovered well.

Recurrence of Subarachnoid Hemorrhage

Recurrence of SAH is more common than that expected among nonsurgically treated survivors, with annual rates ranging from 2.2% to 3.5%, but less common than that expected among surgically treated patients and patients treated with endovascular therapy.[28–31] Current surgical practice favors earlier intervention, because the results from the North American centers of the International Cooperative Study on the Timing of Aneurysm Surgery have shown better outcomes when surgery was performed between day 0 and day 3 after SAH.[32] There is a definite risk of rebleeding among ruptured aneurysms, which may be as high as 20% in the first 2 weeks after SAH and 50% over the first 60 days. The risk of rebleeding is greatest within the first 24 to 72 hours and persists at 3% per year after 6 months.[33] Besides rebleeding, there is a risk of delayed focal neurologic deficits from cerebral vasospasm, with the rate of occurrence of cerebral infarctions approaching 33%.[34]

In the long-term studies of SAH after surgical clipping, patients with completely obliterated ruptured aneurysms still had a relatively high risk for recurrent SAH secondary to formation of a new aneurysm or regrowth of the original aneurysm.[35,36] In the Japanese long-term follow-up angiography study, the reported annual rate of de novo

aneurysm formation was 0.89%.[36] Long-term follow-up after SAH may be indicated even 10 years after surgery because the cumulative risk of aneurysm recurrence may exceed 10%.[36]

Psychosocial Outcomes after Subarachnoid Hemorrhage

Functional dependence due to brain injury is present in 10% to 20% of survivors after SAH.[37] Many survivors suffer from significant long-term emotional and cognitive disturbances that lead to impairment of social functioning. These problems most often involve deficits in memory, psychomotor speed, executive functions, visual-spatial function, attention, mood, concentration, and depression.[38–41] Even among patients with good clinical grades, approximately 50% of those employed full time before SAH do not return to the same level of work.[27,42] Significant strains on interpersonal relationships and impairment of role functioning are also common. The improvement in survival after SAH observed in later years has probably led to an increase in the relative proportion of patients who became chronically disabled by severe cognitive deficits. Subtle cognitive impairment, increased mood disturbance, and impairment of social functioning may be present in up to 60% of patients with SAH even 12 months after onset of SAH.[43,44] In the hospital-based SAH study of 113 patients from Columbia University, impairment of global mental status as assessed by Telephone Interview of Cognitive Status (TICS) was associated with poor recovery, functional disability, and reduced quality of life after the hemorrhage.[45,46] Performance of the study population 3 months after SAH was significantly below that of published norms in the cognitive tests. Data on long-term psychosocial outcome after SAH are limited, and little is known about risk factors associated with poor quality of life after SAH.

PROGNOSIS AFTER INTRACEREBRAL HEMORRHAGE

Spontaneous intracerebral hemorrhage (ICH) constitutes 10% to 20% of all strokes but carries the highest risk of mortality and morbidity of all stroke types.[47] Approximately 37,000 persons in the United States experience ICH each year. ICH is more common in men than women and in black persons younger than 54 years and Asians than in white persons of similar age.[47]

Mortality after Intracerebral Hemorrhage

A number of studies have suggested that mortality related to ICH has fallen more rapidly than that related to the other stroke subtypes.[48] The reduction in type-specific cerebrovascular mortality rate in the United States and in Japan was largest for ICH in the 1970s (nearly a 50% decline).[49,50] Although decrements in both ICH incidence and case-fatality rate are presumably responsible for these trends, improved detection of smaller, nonlethal hemorrhages by CT may contribute to some of this decline.[51] Studies have documented lower case-fatality rates for ICH, ranging from 25% to 64%.[24,52-56] In NOMASS, the adjusted 30-day case-fatality rate was 33%, being higher with greater patient age, lobar location, and more severe stroke syndrome at onset (Fig. 3–1).[24] The 30-day case-fatality rate was similar among various race-ethnic groups, suggesting that higher mortality rates due to stroke among black and Hispanic persons are the result of higher stroke incidence rather than increased fatality rates.

Decreasing mortality for ICH is probably due to an improvement in general medical care and critical care management.[57] In the Project Impact Study, which prospectively collected data over 3 years from 42 participating intensive care units (ICUs) (medical, neurologic, and surgical) across the United States, results from 1038 acute ICH patients have shown a lower in-hospital mortality rate among those who were admitted and treated in neurologic intensive care units than those treated in general intensive care units.[58]

Predictors of Death after Intracerebral Hemorrhage

Predictors of death after ICH have included large size of the hemorrhage (ICH volume), enlargement of hemorrhage (hematoma growth), high degree of impairment of consciousness on admission, lower Glasgow Coma Scale score, presence of intraventricular hemorrhage, increased pulse pressure, older age, and infratentorial origin of ICH.[24,59-63] Early mortality in patients with *hematoma growth* after admission (defined as increase in volume on CT by 20 cm³) is extremely high, in most studies exceeding 50%.[59,62,64]

Other possible predictors of poor outcome in ICH, including early seizure and status epilepticus, which are found more frequently in ICH than in other stroke types, have not been associated with increased mortality. In NOMASS, early seizures were identified among 14% of patients with lobar ICH and 4% of those with deep ICH, in comparison with 0.6% of patients with deep infarct and 6% of those with lobar infarct.[65] Neither early seizure nor status epilepticus was associated with greater early mortality after first stroke.

Recurrence after Intracerebral Hemorrhage

Recurrence after ICH is usually low; however, the rate has not been well documented, probably because of the high early mortality of this hemorrhage.[66] In the systematic review of studies reporting recurrent stroke in survivors of primary ICH between 1982 and 2000, 10 studies were found to have published data on 1880 survivors of ICH with a mean follow-up of 3.4 patient-years.[67] The recurrence rate for any stroke was 4.3% per patient-year. About three fourths of recurrent strokes were ICHs, at a rate of 2.3% per patient-year; the recurrence rate for ischemic stroke was significantly lower, 1.1% per patient-year. Patients with a primary lobar ICH had a higher rate of recurrent ICH (4.4% per patient-year) than those with deep hemispheric ICH (2.1% per patient-year). On the contrary, in the Toronto study,[52] the recurrence rate for ICH was lower (2.4% per year) than the rate of ischemic stroke occurring after ICH (3.0% per year). Although this difference may have implications for the prevention of recurrent ICH, the use of antiplatelet therapy for patients with prior ICH is controversial.

There has been evidence that patients with lobar ICH, which often is not associated with hypertension, may represent a distinct pathogenetic subgroup with respect to etiology and prognosis.[68,69] Cerebral amyloid angiopathy is a common cause of lobar ICH.[69] Patients with cerebral amyloid angiopathy and ICH have a lower mortality rate and a greater risk of recurrence than patients with other types of ICH. Recurrence is uniformly associated with greater disability and a higher mortality rate.[69] O'Donnell and colleagues[70] have reported the importance of a genetic marker, apolipoprotein E, as a predictor of recurrent hemorrhage in patients with cerebral amyloid angiopathy. They found apolipoprotein E ε4 and ε2 alleles to be predictors of recurrent lobar hemorrhage. The risk of recurrence at 2 years was 28% for carriers of the two alleles, compared with 10% for patients with the normal variant, yielding a relative risk (RR) of 3.8. Prior symptomatic brain hemorrhage was also a strong predictor of recurrence, with a risk of 61% at 2 years and an RR of 6.4; this latter finding suggests the possibility of other risk factors, genetic or environmental, that have not yet been identified.[69,70] Gradient-echo (GRE) magnetic resonance imaging (MRI) may be useful in detecting multiple lobar hemorrhages at the patient's initial presentation.[69] Follow-up gradient-echo MRI studies can be useful for detecting subclinical signs of recurrent hemorrhage; recurrent hemorrhages are detected by MRI within 1.5 years after the first

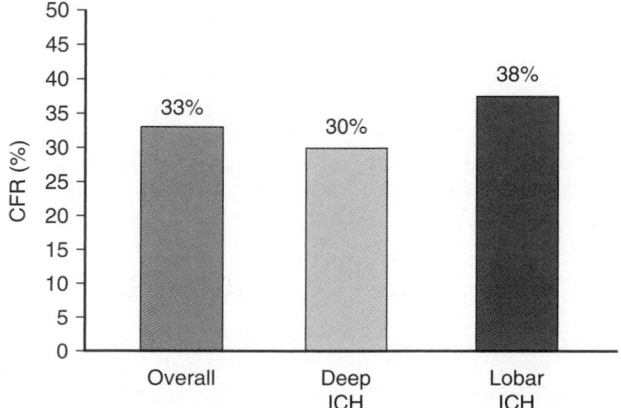

FIGURE 3–1 *Intracerebral hemorrhage (ICH) 30-day case-fatality rates overall and by ICH location in the Northern Manhattan Stroke Study.*

hemorrhage in as many as 38% of patients with ICH and cerebral amyloid angiopathy.[71]

PROGNOSIS AFTER ISCHEMIC STROKE

Mortality after Ischemic Stroke

Death rates from stroke declined throughout the last century.[72] Stroke is estimated to be responsible for 9.5% of all deaths and for 5.1 million of the 16.7 million deaths due to cardiovascular disease worldwide. Two thirds or more of stroke deaths occur in the developing world. Prevention of first and recurrent strokes is inadequate.[73,74]

Early Mortality after Ischemic Stroke

The greatest risk of death for patients with cerebral infarction occurs in the first 30 days, with case-fatality rates ranging from 8% to 20%.[75-77] In the Framingham Study, the 30-day case-fatality rate for patients with atherothrombotic infarction was 15%. The rates in men and women were similar and increased directly with age.[78] During this early period, death was more likely caused by the stroke itself or cardiopulmonary complications.[79] In Rochester, Minnesota, the 30-day case-fatality rate decreased by 50% between the periods 1945 to 1949 and 1980 to 1984.[80] Among 1111 residents of the city, the risk of death after first cerebral infarction was 7% at 7 days and 14% at 30 days.[81] In the NOMASS cohort, the 30-day mortality rate decreased from 7.7% in the 1980s (1983 to 1988) to 5.0% in the 1990s (1990 to 1997).[82] The 30-day cumulative mortality risk reported for the NOMASS cohort, 5%, was lower than that reported for other cohorts (Table 3.2), possibly because of inclusion of younger patients, exclusion of prior strokes, the higher proportion of lacunar infarcts (26%), and less severe strokes at onset in the NOMASS cohort.

In the United States, hospitalization rates for stroke grew by 18.6% between 1988 and 1997, the increase largely occurring in patients 65 years and older.[83] A decline, however, in the in-hospital case-fatality rate from stroke was observed during the same period. The decline in case-fatality rate suggested general improvements in the management of acute stroke patients, decreases in the severity of strokes, or the detection of milder cases of stroke secondary to greater use of neuroimaging technology. A decline in case-fatality rate was also observed in other countries.[84-86] "Jubilation" over the decline in stroke case-fatality rate should be tempered, however, by the recognition that part of the decline may have been due to shorter lengths of hospital stay, resulting in more out-of-hospital deaths.[85] Questions still remain as to how much of the improvement in survival after ischemic stroke is due to better management and therefore a drop in 30-day case-fatality rate, to the decreasing proportion of severe strokes, or to a reduction in mortality among 30-day survivors.

Causes of Early Death after First Ischemic Stroke

The immediate cause of death after first ischemic stroke is related to stroke itself in more than 60% of cases.[72,87,88] Death within 30 days after a first stroke due to incident stroke was found in 91% of patients in the Oxfordshire Community Stroke Project (OCSP) and 85% in the Perth Community Stroke Study.[89,90] After 1 month, cardiovascular disorders, stroke, and diseases resulting from stroke were the causes of death in up to 80% of the patients, a substantially greater percentage than that in the age- and gender-matched general population.[88] Impaired consciousness on admission, posterior circulation infarcts, and transtentorial herniation were the most important causes of death during the first week after stroke onset.[91] Thereafter, cardiac causes, pneumonia, pulmonary embolism, sepsis, and other medical complications accounted for the majority of deaths within the first month after stroke onset. The proportion of 30-day deaths after first ischemic stroke in NOMASS was 75%.[87] Incident (53%) or recurrent (4%) stroke caused early deaths in 57% of patients. Cardiac causes of early death have been reported to be higher among black persons than among other races or ethnicities.[92,93] In the Trial of ORG 10172 in Acute Stroke Therapy (TOAST), which involved 292 African-American and 801 white patients, there was a trend toward a higher rate of nonfavorable outcomes in the African-American patients at 7 days.[94] Excess mortality related to cardiovascular disease has been described among young black and Caribbean Hispanic patients in other studies.[77,87]

Late Mortality after Ischemic Stroke

Longitudinal studies among patients with ischemic stroke have demonstrated that the risk of death at 5 years ranged from 40% to 60%, including early fatalities.[80,89,95] The average annual mortality rate in the 30-day stroke survivors ranges from 8% to 9%, and a risk of death is two to three times higher for such patients than for the age- and sex-matched general population.[89,95] In the National Survey of Stroke, only 53% of stroke patients who survived the initial 6 months lived for 5 years.[96] Five-year survival was 75% in patients younger than 65 years and 23% in those 85 years or older. In the OCSP, stroke mortality was 10% at 30 days, 23% at 1 year and 51% at 5 years.[89] In Rochester, Minnesota, the risk of death after first cerebral infarction was 27% at 1 year and 53% at 5 years.[81] In the Danish MONICA (MONItoring Trends and Determinants in CArdiovascular Disease) Project, the estimated cumulative risks for death at 1 year after stroke was 41% and 60% at

Table 3.2 Stroke Mortality and Recurrence Rates

	Mortality (%)	Mortality in NOMASS (%)	Recurrence (%)	Recurrence in NOMASS (%)
30-day	8–20	5.7	1–6	2.0
1-year	20–35	16.5	5–25	8.3
5-year	38–75	38.5	15–40	15.9

NOMASS, Northern Manhattan Stroke Study.

5 years.[97] The lifetable cumulative risks of ischemic stroke mortality in NOMASS were 5% at 30 days, 16% at 1 year, and 41% at 5 years after stroke.[87] In the Framingham Study, 5-year mortality rates after atherothrombotic brain infarction were 44% for men and 36% for women, similar to the rates for the standard population.[78] In the same cohort, however, patients who survived stroke for 20 years or longer had higher mortality rates than age- and sex-matched control subjects.[98]

It is still not clear how much the long-term survival after ischemic stroke is influenced by the initial or recurrent stroke or by other associated comorbidities. Furthermore, stroke mortality declined, especially in the 1970s. Although the observed reduction in stroke mortality has been attributed to declining stroke incidence, new evidence is showing a secular trend in decline of stroke severity.[81,89,99] Stroke with severe neurologic deficit decreased in later decades, with a fall in rates of severe stroke cases in which patients were unconscious on admission to the hospital.[99]

Predictors of Death after Ischemic Stroke

Predictors of death after ischemic stroke may differ for early and late death (Table 3.3). Most of the predictors, however, affect both early and late mortality, and a clear distinction cannot be made. Early recognition of predictors of death after stroke onset is of special importance when one is accounting for relevant clinical variables available within the first 72 hours after stroke. Although the prediction of stroke outcome could probably be improved by including variables that are assessed later, the practical value would be limited, because the prediction could not be made as soon after stroke onset. In addition, development of early prediction models taking into account only variables that are evaluated within the first 6 hours after onset would be of value for designing acute stroke interventional clinical trials. Determinants of death in 30-day survivors of ischemic stroke are less well understood. Stroke risk factors that are less important during the early period may have a greater effect on long-term outcome.

Age, Gender, and Race-Ethnicity

Nonmodifiable factors, such as patient age, gender, and race-ethnicity, have been identified as potential determinants of stroke outcome.[106–113] Age is an independent prognostic factor of both early and late death due to stroke.[100–105] Elderly patients have a higher risk of subsequent complications and thereby lower probability of recovering from stroke.

The age-standardized case-fatality rates have frequently been found to be greater for women than for men.[106] The reports do not offer any explanation for the gender difference in case-fatality rate. In the Danish MONICA Project, women had a higher risk for death than men for as long as 1 year after stroke.[107] The female stroke patients were older, but the effect of age was controlled for in the analyses. In the Framingham Study, however, women had a better survival than men after stroke.[108] Further studies are needed to explore gender differences in stroke mortality.

Differences in mortality rates among various race-ethnic groups were observed in several cohorts.[87,109] In the Cardiovascular Health Study cohort of patients 65 years or older, African Americans had a greater risk of death than others after an ischemic stroke.[109] The NOMASS 5-year cumulative lifetable mortality estimates after stroke differed only slightly among the three race-ethnic groups.[87] The rates were 8% at 1 month, 26% at 1 year, and 54% at 5 years for white persons; 5%, 17%, and 39%, respectively, for black persons; and 4%, 12%, and 33%, respectively, for Caribbean Hispanic persons (Fig. 3–2). Further studies will determine how many of the possible differences in

Table 3.3 Definite and Potential Predictors of Death after Ischemic Stroke

	Definite Predictors	*Potential Predictors*
Demographics	Age	Gender Race-ethnicity
Clinical parameters	Initial severity of stroke (National Institutes of Health Stroke Scale Score) Decreased consciousness Infarct size Large hemispheral or basilar syndrome Ischemic stroke subtype Fever Hypertension Atrial fibrillation Congestive heart failure	Other cardiac disease Previous stroke Prestroke disability
Biochemical parameters	Hyperglycemia C-reactive protein	Type 2 diabetes Erythrocyte sedimentation rate Fibrinogen level White blood cell count Uric acid/creatinine levels

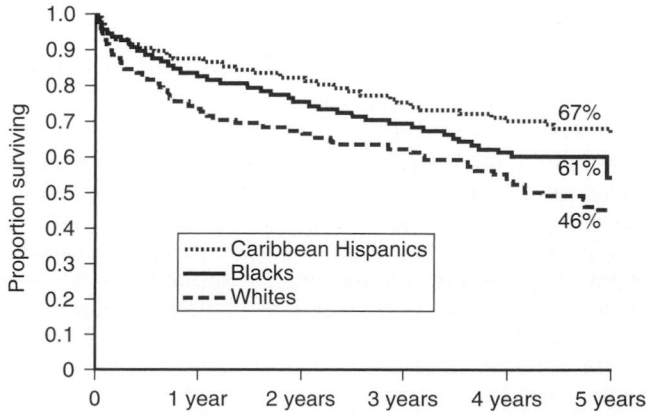

FIGURE 3–2 *Survival after first ischemic stroke in the Northern Manhattan Stroke Study.* °*5-year lifetable survival estimate in each race-ethnic group. (From Hartman A, Rundek T, Mast H, et al: Mortality and causes of death after first ischemic stroke. The Northern Manhattan Stroke Study. Neurology 57:2000–2005, 2001.)*

outcome by race-ethnicity may be explained by differences in stroke risk factors and subtype.

Initial Stroke Severity

Initial severity of stroke, often measured by the NIHSS score,[110,111] is one of the major predictors of poor outcome, including mortality, after stroke in many studies.[100–104,112] The baseline NIHSS score in the TOAST strongly predicted mortality and functional outcome; one additional point on the baseline NIHSS score decreased by 24% the likelihood of survival and excellent outcome at 7 days and by 17% at 3 months.[113] This study has shown that an NIHSS score of 16 or higher predicts a high probability of death or severe disability and that a score of 6 or lower predicts a good recovery. Four studies have shown that in patients with nonlacunar infarcts in the carotid artery territory arriving at the hospital within 6 hours, severity of the neurologic deficit was the strongest indicator of both 30-day and 6-month outcomes.[114–117]

Markers of initial stroke severity, such as depressed consciousness, infarct size, severity of the neurologic deficit, and the type of stroke syndrome on admission, have been reported as clinical predictors of early outcome.[4,118–122] In the NOMASS cohort, patients in coma had the worst prognosis with a greater likelihood of herniation from the mass effect or cerebral edema associated with the size of the infarct.[4] The German Stroke Database, consisting of 1754 prospectively collected records of patients with acute ischemic stroke, showed orientation, limb paresis, trunk ataxia, and dysphagia to be independent predictors of early death after stroke.[100]

The type of initial stroke syndrome has been found to be another important clinical determinant of mortality. In the NOMASS, patients presenting with a major hemispheric or basilar syndrome had the worst early death rate, those with minor hemispheric syndromes were associated with an intermediate survival, and those with a lacunar syndrome had the best prognosis.[4] In the OCSP cohort, patients with total anterior cerebral infarcts had the worst survival.[123]

Fever

Pyrexia after stroke onset has been associated with a marked increase in morbidity and mortality. Admission body temperature is considered a major determinant of early as well as late death after stroke.[124–126] During the first days after acute stroke, a fever or subfebrile temperature elevation develops in one fifth to almost one half of patients.[127–130] Subfebrile temperatures (37.5°C to 39°C) and fever (>39°C) after a stroke are associated with relatively large infarct volumes, high case-fatality rates, and poor functional outcome, even after adjustment of the data for initial stroke severity.[128,129–132] Hyperthermia occurring within the first 12 to 24 hours of stroke onset may have a more predictive outcome than later fever.[132] The significant stroke prognostic influence of initial body temperature was confirmed by a meta-analysis of nine studies involving 3790 patients.[133] Fever of more than 38°C within 3 days of stroke onset was among the most important predictors for death or functional dependence after stroke.[100,134–136]

In the Copenhagen Stroke Study, the mortality rate at 60 months after stroke was higher for patients with hyperthermia on admission (73%) than for those without it (59%).[126] A 1°C increase in admission body temperature independently predicted a 30% relative increase (95% confidence interval [CI], 4% to 57%) in long-term mortality risk. An association between admission body temperature and stroke mortality was noted to be independent of stroke severity. RR for 1-year mortality of hyperthermic versus normothermic patients was 3.4 (95% CI, 1.6 to 7.3).[137]

In patients with acute ischemic stroke, a pharmacologic reduction of body temperature or body cooling procedures may improve functional outcome.[138–140]

Stroke Subtypes and Stroke Mortality

Stroke subtype is an important determinant of mortality. In many prospective community stroke studies and clinical trials—including cohorts from Rochester, Minnesota; the National Institute of Neurological Diseases and Stroke (NINDS) Stroke Data Bank; Perth Community Stroke Study,; the Erlangen Stroke Project in Germany; NOMASS; OCSP; and TOAST—survival was significantly better for patients with lacunar infarcts than for those with nonlacunar infarcts.[81,113,123,141–144]

In the NOMASS cohort, presentation with a lacunar syndrome was associated with a significantly better 5-year survival (Fig. 3–3).[4] Data on long-term outcome in patients with lacunar stroke have shown that for the first few years after lacunar infarct, the risk of death is similar to that for the general population.[18,145] Later, however, a clear excess mortality was observed, indicating that the long-term prognosis with lacunar infarction appears less favorable than that previously reported.[145]

Ischemic stroke subtype classified according to the TOAST criteria[146] was a significant predictor of stroke survival after adjustment for age and sex.[143] The highest mortality was reported for cardioembolic and large atherothrombotic strokes and the lowest for lacunar strokes.[90,143,144,146] In the Rochester Epidemiology Project, the case-fatality rates for cardioembolic stroke at 1 month (30.3%), 1 year (53%), and 2 years (61.4%)[144] were higher than those reported in other cohorts, most likely because the patients in the Rochester cohort were older (mean age

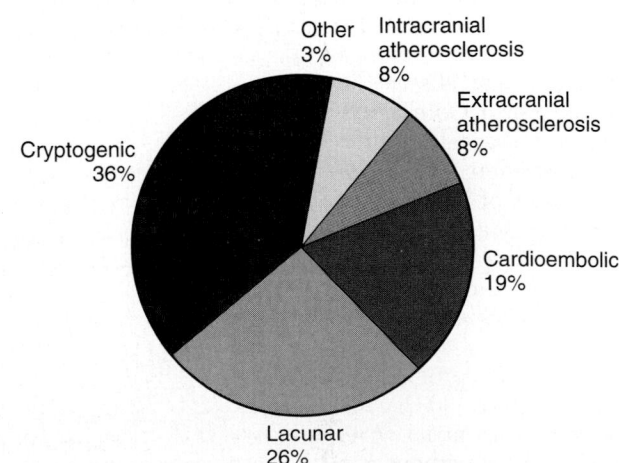

FIGURE 3–3 *Distribution of ischemic stroke subtypes among 992 patients in the Northern Manhattan Stroke Study.*

for those with cardioembolic stroke was 80 years).[147] Patients with cardioembolic stroke were nearly 4 times more likely to be dead 30 days after stroke and 2.5 times more likely to be dead 5 years after stroke than patients with stroke due to large-vessel atherosclerosis with stenosis. In the New England Medical Center Posterior Circulation Registry, a low mortality rate at 30 days after stroke onset (3.6%) was observed among patients with vertebrobasilar occlusive strokes.[148] Poor outcome was associated with basilar artery involvement, embolic stroke mechanism, and multiple posterior circulation intracranial territory strokes.

Blood Pressure, Atrial Fibrillation, and Heart Failure

Elevated *blood pressure* (BP) in stroke survivors raises the risk of death.[149,150] Blood pressure reduction after stroke recovery using diuretics, angiotensin-converting enzyme inhibitors, or both lowers stroke mortality and recurrence.[9,151,152]

Three quarters of patients with acute ischemic stroke have elevated BP at presentation.[153] Blood pressure declines spontaneously over the first week after stroke onset and returns to prestroke levels in two thirds of patients. Most studies have found that high BP in the acute phase of stroke, whether measured as casual or 24-hour ambulatory readings, is associated with a poor outcome.[149,154] Although not proven, high blood pressure in acute stroke might promote early recurrence, hemorrhagic transformation, or cerebral edema.[155]

In the International Stroke Trial (IST), which involves 17,398 patients with stroke, both high BP and low BP were independent prognostic factors for poor outcome 6 months after stroke.[149] The rate of early death increased by 3.8% for every 10 mm Hg above 150 mm Hg and by 17.9% for every 10 mm Hg below 150 mm Hg. In the Multicenter rt-PA Stroke Survey, which comprised data from 1205 patients treated in routine clinical practice with intravenous recombinant tissue-type plasminogen activator (rt-PA) within 3 hours of onset of stroke symptoms, elevated pretreatment mean BP was a main attribute associated with higher case-fatality rate and rate of ICH.[156]

Cardiac disease was a prominent predictor of survival in multiple studies. In Rochester, Minnesota, independent risk factors for death after first cerebral infarction were congestive heart failure, persistent atrial fibrillation, and ischemic heart disease.[81] Predictors of death within 1 year in the Perth Community Stroke Study included cardiac failure and atrial fibrillation.[90] In a 14-year follow-up study from Sweden, heart failure and history of diabetes were predictors of long-term mortality.[157] Stroke survivors with cardiac disease had a worse 1-year survival in the Community Hospital–based Stroke Programs and a lower rate of 10-year survival in the Framingham Study.[78,121,158]

Atrial fibrillation (AF), the most prevalent chronic cardiac arrhythmia in the elderly, also has a well-documented impact on the prognosis of first stroke.[88,159–162] In the Framingham Study, 30-day mortality and stroke severity in the subjects with atrial fibrillation was 25%, compared with 14% in those without.[160] Other studies report 30-day mortality rates of 23% to 35% for patients with and 7% to 14% for those without atrial fibrillation.[88,159,161,162] The difference

in mortality between subjects with and without atrial fibrillation was more evident in the extreme elderly. Half of the strokes in subjects 75 years or older with atrial fibrillation were either severe or fatal.

Congestive heart failure (CHF) is also a significant predictor of stroke severity and case-fatality rate.[88,162,163] Patients with dilated cardiomyopathy have a high incidence of left ventricular thrombus formation and are at increased risk of embolic complications.[164] In the Framingham Study, heart failure was the second most important factor in cardiogenic stroke risk, with a two- to threefold RR.[165,166] CHF is associated with high mortality; the 15-year mortality rate is estimated at 39% for women and 72% for men.[167] In the Helsinki Ageing Study, the presence of CHF doubled the age- and sex-adjusted risk of death from all causes, and quadrupled the risk of death from stroke and cardiovascular diseases during 4-year follow-up.[168] Among 30-day survivors in the NOMASS cohort, congestive heart failure was an independent predictor of death 5 years after stroke onset.[4]

Hyperglycemia and Diabetes

Abnormal results of admission blood tests have also been evaluated as clinical predictors of early mortality. The most frequently studied abnormality has been *hyperglycemia*, which has been associated with higher mortality after stroke in patients both with and without diabetes.[4,169–174] Hyperglycemia during acute ischemic stroke may augment brain injury, predispose to ICH, or both.[175] Alternatively, the effect of hyperglycemia may be confounded by the acute stress reaction secondary to an infarct.[169–171] The NINDS rt-PA Stroke Trial showed that higher admission glucose levels were associated with significantly lower odds of desirable clinical outcomes regardless of rt-PA treatment.[175] In the NOMASS cohort, hyperglycemia was associated with poor prognosis after stroke independent of the size or severity of the ischemic stroke.[4]

Diabetes mellitus was found to be a prognostic variable for death in several studies.[100,102,104] This finding could be due to greater preexisting comorbidity in diabetic patients as well as to greater neuronal damage of ischemic tissue in those with hyperglycemia. In a prospective observational study of 4585 patients with type 2 diabetes conducted in England, Scotland, and Northern Ireland, each 1% reduction in mean hemoglobin A_{1c} level was associated with the following reductions in risk: 21% for deaths related to diabetes, 14% for deaths related to myocardial infarction (MI), and 37% for deaths related to microvascular complications including stroke.[176] The rate of early death after stroke in patients with type 2 diabetes was 28%.

Serologic Markers and Other Biochemical Blood Parameters

Serologic abnormalities, including *C-reactive protein* (CRP) elevation, have been shown to predict poor outcome after stroke.[177–181] CRP elevation within 12 to 72 hours of stroke is associated with a higher risk of death.[180,182–185] Although elevation of serum CRP is common in acute ischemic stroke, its presence at hospital discharge is strongly related to the occurrence of subsequent vascular events or death. Data on 193 patients with ischemic stroke enrolled in the Villa Pini Stroke Data Bank suggest that elevated CRP may be a marker of increased ischemic stroke risk at 1 year.[182] Patients with serum CRP levels higher than 1.5 mg/dL had a worse prognosis. Additional well designed epidemiologic studies are needed to validate these findings.

Several studies have shown that *fibrinogen* concentration, *erythrocyte sedimentation rate*, and *leukocyte count* are elevated after ischemic stroke and that increases in these markers are independently associated with the risk of stroke death and recurrence.[182,184,186–188] Further clarification of these biochemical parameters in the prediction of stroke risk is needed.

Uric acid and other parameters of renal dysfunction have been associated with poor long-term survival after stroke. Elevation of urate has been reported to be associated with a threefold increase in RR of cardiac death within 5 years after stroke.[189] Other findings signifying renal dysfunction, even subtle dysfunction, have also been noted to be prognostic indicators of overall mortality in many patient groups.[190,191] In a Scottish 7-year follow-up study of 2042 patients with stroke, reduced *creatinine clearance*, raised *serum creatinine* and urea concentrations, and raised *ratio of urea to creatinine* on admission were significant predictors of increased mortality.[191]

Stroke Outcome Prediction Models

Discrepancies in identifying predictors of mortality have been observed among the studies. They may result from the age and stroke subtype composition of the cohorts, the definition of the predictors used in the studies, the duration of follow-up, the timing of the outcome of interest, and the relative contributions of other predictors.

The great variability in outcome seen in patients with stroke has led to an interest in identifying predictors of outcome through the use of prediction models. Combining clinical variables and imaging variables as predictors of stroke outcome in a multivariable risk adjustment model may be more powerful than using either type of variable alone. Age and severity of presenting clinical deficit are consistently found to be predictive of outcome.[4,18,19,23,102,112,144,192] Many other predictors have been reported to have a univariable relationship with outcome, but their multivariable relationship to outcome is less clear.[4,192]

A model of 1-year survival after ischemic stroke was developed from the Perth Community Stroke Study. The best model included coma, urinary incontinence, cardiac failure, severe paresis, and atrial fibrillation.[90] The sensitivity, specificity, and negative predictive value for predicting death were 90%, 83%, and 95%, respectively. In the NOMASS cohort, independent determinants of 5-year mortality among 30-day survivors were age, major hemispheric or basilar syndrome, congestive heart failure, and admission glucose greater than 140 mg/dL.[4] In the Randomized Trial of Tirilazad Mesylate in Acute Stroke (RANTTAS),[193] greater baseline NIHSS score, small-vessel infarct, history of previous stroke, history of diabetes, history of prestroke disability, and greater infarct volume at 7 to 10 days were significant predictors of survival and excellent outcome as determined by the NIHSS score of 1 at 3 months.[192] For very poor outcome including death, only infarct volume was a significant predictor of NIHSS score of 20 or death at 3 months.

Other studies have also combined clinical and imaging variables to predict stroke outcomes.[194–196] Findings of these studies suggested that because the final size of an infarct cannot be detected on CT for several days after the event, infarct volume does not improve the predictive ability of such models. New MRI techniques that identify lesion volume in the acute setting, such as diffusion-weighted imaging, may improve our ability to predict stroke outcome in the acute period.[197–200]

Recurrence after Ischemic Stroke

Recurrent stroke is a major cause of morbidity and mortality among stroke survivors. With improvements in survival after first ischemic stroke, stroke recurrence may account for a greater share of the future annual cost of stroke-related health care.[4] Despite advances in stroke prevention strategies and treatments, stroke recurrence is still the major threat to any stroke survivor.

Prospective, large, community-based studies indicate that the risk of recurrence after stroke varies from 1.7% to 4% in the first 30 days, from 6% to 13% in the first year, and from 5% to 8% per year for the next 2 to 5 years, culminating in a cumulative risk of stroke recurrence within 5 years of 19% to 42%.[4,81,192,201–204] Lower recurrent stroke rates have been observed among selected groups of patients in large clinical trials, such as TOAST,[146] IST,[149] and Warfarin-Aspirin Recurrent Stroke Study (WARSS),[205] as well as in some prospective community studies.[76,82,123,144] The reasons for the differences in recurrence rates between various studies may reflect the study design (hospital-based vs. community-based), sociodemographics of the study population, definitions of recurrent stroke, and the use of preventive medications such as antiplatelet agents. Several studies reported recurrent stroke rates for individual subtypes of ischemic stroke.[144,206–209] Higher early recurrence rates for ischemic stroke due to large-vessel atherosclerosis have been reported.[144,208–210]

In Rochester, Minnesota, the risk of recurrent stroke after first cerebral infarction was 2% at 7 days, 4% at 30 days, 12% at 1 year, and 29% at 5 years.[81,207] In the NINDS Stroke Data Bank, 3.3% of the hospitalized cohort had a stroke recurrence within 30 days, accounting for 30% of the recurrent strokes in 2 years of follow-up.[206] Cumulative recurrence rates at 5 years after an infarction in the Framingham Study were 42% for men and 24% for women.[18] Cumulative rates were lower in Rochester, Minnesota, 19.3% at 5 years and 28.8% at 10 years.[207] In the Perth Community Stroke Study, involving 343 patients with first-ever stroke, approximately 1 in 6 survivors (15%) of a first-ever stroke experienced recurrent strokes during 5 years, of which 25% were fatal within 28 days.[204] The 5-year cumulative risk of first recurrent stroke was 22.5%. In the NOMASS cohort of 992 patients with first-ever ischemic stroke, the cumulative life-table estimated risks of recurrent stroke were 2.0% at 30 days, 8.3% at 1 year, and 15.9% at 5 years (Fig. 3–4).[208]

Prognostic factors for recurrent stroke are clinically important because they help identify patients at high risk for recurrence and provide insights into ways to modify outcomes. Factors that have been associated with an increased risk of recurrent stroke in community-based and hospital-based series are as follows:

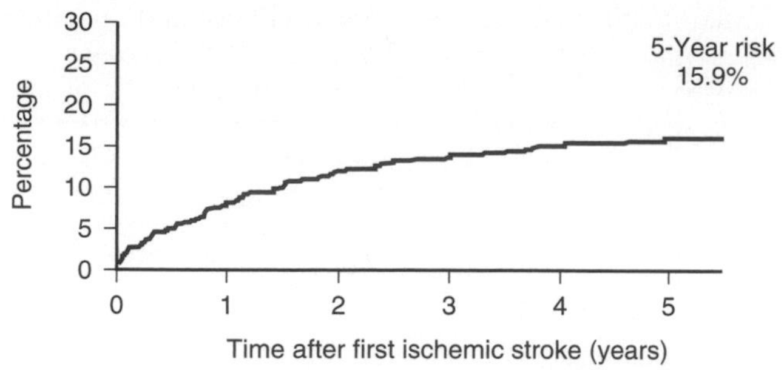

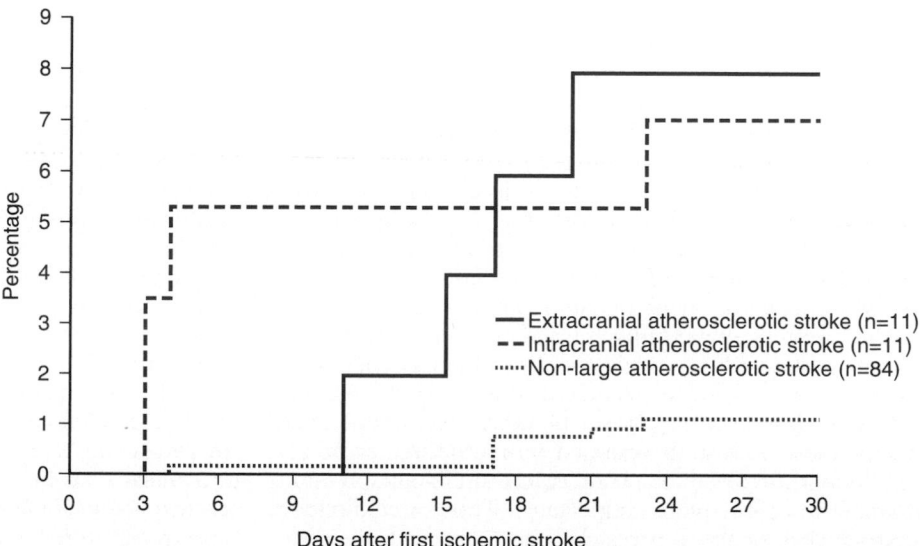

FIGURE 3–4 *Overall cumulative risk of recurrent stroke in the Northern Manhattan Stroke Study.*

- Increasing age[81,208,211–213]
- Male sex;[214,215] female sex[216]
- Clinical stroke syndrome[217]
- History of transient cerebral ischemic attack[218,219]
- Hypertension[4,111,194,214,215,218,220,239]; initially elevated blood pressure[149,194,220,240]; low blood pressure[149,195]
- Cigarette smoking[217]
- Alcohol abuse[4,221,239]
- Diabetes mellitus[4,81,194]; blood glucose elevation[4,216]
- History of coronary heart disease,[213,280] atrial fibrillation,[208,215,222,223] and other cardiac diseases (valvular heart disease, congestive heart failure, patent foramen ovale [PFO], and aortic arch atheroma)[216,224–230]
- Abnormal findings on initial brain CT[192,194]
- Dementia after stroke[209]

Predictors of Early Stroke Recurrence

Predictors of recurrent stroke may be time-specific and therefore may be different for early and late recurrences.

Ischemic stroke subtype has been shown to be a predictor of early stroke recurrence. In the Rochester Epidemiology Project, ischemic stroke due to large-vessel atherosclerosis with stenosis had a higher risk of early recurrence.[144] More than 18% of patients with this stroke subtype had a recurrent stroke within 30 days of the first

stroke, greater than the range of 8% to 14% reported in previous population and hospital-based studies.[4,208,209,231] The variations in recurrence rates may be due to demographic and clinical characteristics of the study subjects as well as to the methodologic differences among the studies. A high 30-day recurrence risk for stroke due to large-artery atherosclerotic disease was also found in the NOMASS (Table 3.4 and Fig. 3–5). Estimated rates of recurrent stroke were greater for extracranial atherosclerotic infarcts (8.8%) and intracranial atherosclerotic infarcts (9.7%) than for cardioembolic (3.7%), lacunar (2.0%), and cryptogenic (0.4%) infarcts. Patients with large atherosclerotic infarcts were seven times more likely to experience recurrent stroke 30 days after the index stroke than parents with other subtypes of ischemic stroke.

The rate of early stroke recurrence in cardioembolic stroke was reported to be low in several studies.[208,232] The frequent use of anticoagulants may prevent early cardioembolic events and therefore may reduce the risk of early recurrence. Patients with stroke due to large-artery stenotic disease are particularly prone to procedure-related cerebral ischemia, a feature that may partly account for the higher risk of early recurrent stroke for this stroke subtype.[233]

Infarct subtype has usually not been determined at admission; rather, it depends on the diagnostic in-patient

Table 3.4 Recurrence Risk by Ischemic Stroke Subtype in the Northern Manhattan Stroke Study

	30-Day Risk (%)	*1-Year Risk (%)*	*5-Year Risk (%)*
All strokes	2.0	8.3	15.9
Stroke subtype			
Extracranial atherosclerotic	8.7	11.3	23.1
Intracranial atherosclerotic	7.7	11.8	16.3
Cardioembolic	2.6	7.1	21.1
Lacunar	1.4	10.3	14.2
Cryptogenic	0.4	6.2	14.8

FIGURE 3–5 *Thirty-day cumulative risk of stroke recurrence in the Northern Manhattan Stroke Study.*

evaluation. In formulation of predictors of early recurrence, the best method would be to rely upon factors that can be classified readily upon first encounter with the patient through the clinical history, physical examination, initial neuroimaging, and laboratory testing.

In addition to ischemic stroke subtype, the most significant predictors associated with early stroke recurrence in the NOMASS were atrial fibrillation (RR 4.0; 95% CI, 1.1 to 14.6), alcohol consumption (2 to 4 drinks per day vs. none; RR 6.8; 95% CI, 1.2 to 39.9), and hypercholesterolemia (RR 0.15; 95% CI, 0.1 to 0.7).[208] Other studies have also identified atrial fibrillation and the presence of a potential cardioembolic source as predictors of early recurrent stroke.[234–236] Data from the IST for 17,398 patients with acute stroke showed that high and low systolic blood pressure values were associated with increased stroke recurrence within 14 days of stroke onset.[149] The rate of recurrent ischemic stroke within 14 days rose by 4.2% for every 10 mm Hg increase in systolic blood pressure, and this association was present in both fatal and nonfatal recurrent strokes. Also, relatively low blood pressure (systolic blood pressure < 120 mm Hg), although an uncommon clinical finding (5% of patients) was also associated with poor outcome. Both relationships appeared to be independent of age, stroke severity, level of consciousness, and atrial fibrillation. This finding may provide an explanation for the worsening of outcome after the use of calcium channel blockers in some studies of acute ischemic stroke—most likely due to a reduction of cerebral perfusion.[237,238]

Predictors of Late Stroke Recurrence

Some nonmodifiable and modifiable predictors of late recurrence after ischemic stroke have been identified.

Among *nonmodifiable predictors*, age is the most important predictor of survival after stroke but has not consistently been found to be a determinant of recurrence.

The lack of a significant association between age and stroke recurrence has been observed in several studies.[81,210–212] Most studies have found similar stroke recurrence rates for men and women. Fewer studies have evaluated stroke recurrence in different race-ethnic groups. Stroke recurrence was slightly more common among black and Hispanic persons in the NOMASS, but the differences did not reach statistical significance.[4]

In the Rochester, Minnesota, study, ischemic stroke due to atherosclerosis with stenosis was associated with fewer recurrent strokes than cardioembolic stroke,[144] and in the NOMASS, the late recurrence risks were not significantly different for the large atherosclerotic and nonlarge atherosclerotic strokes (Fig. 3–6).[4,208,239]

Modifiable predictors of late recurrence after ischemic stroke have not been uniformly established. Even the effect of *hypertension* has been debated. Some researchers have found no effect of hypertension, and others have suggested that hypertension increases the risk of recurrence after stroke.[4,5,8,11,219,240,241] The effect of hypertension on late stroke recurrence is not clearly defined and may depend on stroke subtype. Also, because hypertension is very prevalent among stroke patients, the level of blood pressure control may be more important. The recommended optimal goal for blood pressure reduction to achieve good

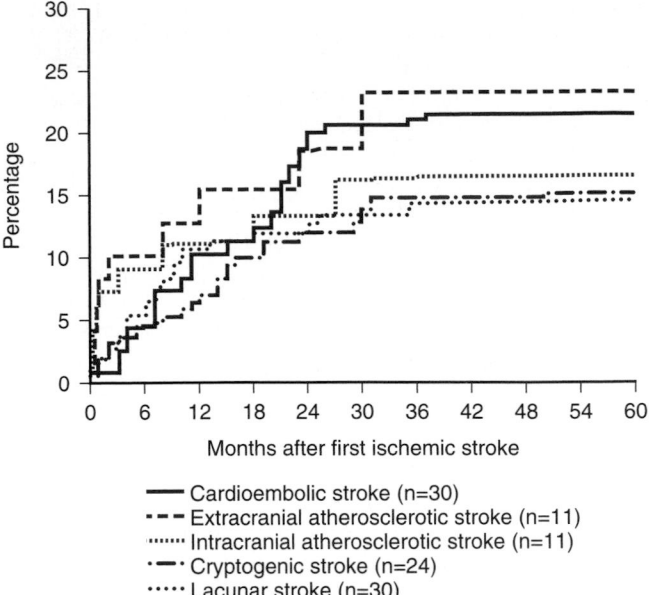

FIGURE 3–6   *Cumulative risk of recurrence by ischemic stroke subtype in the Northern Manhattan Stroke Study.*

control has been lowered to 120 mm Hg systolic/80 mm Hg diastolic.[242] A J-shaped relationship between blood pressure and stroke in treated hypertensive patients has been suggested.[243,244] In the Lehigh Valley Stroke Study, the risk of recurrent stroke was reduced when diastolic blood pressure was below 80 mmHg.[245] This finding is consistent with that of a meta-analysis of antihypertensive medication intervention trials in which BP-lowering drug interventions reduced the risk of stroke recurrence.[246] PROGRESS (Perindopril pROtection aGainst REcurrent Stroke Study), a randomized controlled trial conducted in subjects with previous stroke or TIA, showed that a BP-lowering regimen with perindopril and indapamide reduced the risk of recurrent stroke by more than a quarter.[9] Over 4 years, annual stroke recurrence in the trial was reduced from 3.8% to 2.7%. Importantly, stroke risk was also reduced among patients classified as nonhypertensive (with mean BP at entry of 136/79 mmHg).

Cardiac disease has also been found to be a determinant of recurrence after ischemic stroke. In Rochester, Minnesota, cardiac valvular disease and congestive heart failure were independent predictors of recurrent stroke.[53] The odds ratio associated with stroke recurrence in the Lehigh Valley Stroke Study was approximately 8.0 for either MI or other coronary disease.[247] In the OCSP, atrial fibrillation was not associated with a recurrent stroke within the first 30 days, and there was only a mild increase in the average annual risk of recurrent stroke, from 8.2% in patients with normal sinus rhythm to 11% in those with atrial fibrillation.[223] Atrial fibrillation markedly curtails life expectancy after stroke, but whether it has an independent effect on late recurrence needs further investigation.

Diabetes has been found to be a determinant of stroke recurrence in some studies. In Rochester, Minnesota, age and diabetes mellitus were the only significant independent predictors of recurrent stroke.[81] Patients at the lowest risk for 2-year stroke recurrence in the Stroke Data Bank had no history of diabetes.[4] Because hyperglycemia at stroke onset is more common among diabetic patients and has been found to predict stroke recurrence, some of the effect of hyperglycemia may depend on the presence of diagnosed or undiagnosed diabetes.[4] Further clarification is needed to determine whether control of diabetes after stroke is associated with a reduction in the risk of stroke recurrence.

There is a paucity of data on the effect of *smoking* and *alcohol* on stroke recurrence, particularly because these risk factors were not well established during the design of earlier epidemiologic stroke studies. Whether smoking is a risk factor for recurrent stroke is still controversial.[248] Cohort studies have suggested that cessation of smoking after MI is associated with a significant decrease in mortality.[249] Knowledge about modification of smoking habits after stroke is nevertheless scant.[250] Whether cessation of smoking after stroke reduces the risk of new major vascular events is still unknown. Despite the current lack of proof, advice on cessation of smoking is included in the strategy for secondary prevention in patients with stroke.[251]

The stroke recurrence rate was significantly higher among patients with prior heavy alcohol use in the NOMASS cohort.[4] Nearly half of subjects in this study with a history of heavy alcohol use had a recurrent stroke within 5 years, compared with 22% of those with no such history. The effect of alcohol use was observed in smokers and nonsmokers as well as in black and Hispanic persons although not in white persons. Ethanol could theoretically increase recurrent stroke risk through numerous mechanisms, including hypertension, hypercoagulable states, cardiac arrhythmias, and cerebral blood flow reduction.[252] Ethanol consumption has rarely been identified as a predictor of outcome after stroke except in patients with aneurysmal subarachnoid hemorrhage.[253-256] Because both alcohol and cigarette smoking are modifiable behaviors, it is important to determine their impact on stroke recurrence. In urban populations, these behaviors may be more prevalent and may demand greater attention in stroke recurrence prevention programs.

Some *new predictors* of recurrent stroke have been suggested, including mitral valve prolapse,[230] aortic atheromas,[228,229,257] and PFO,[224-227,258] but all require further research. In the French Study of Aortic Plaques in Stroke, atherosclerotic plaques 4mm or more in thickness in the aortic arch were significant predictors of recurrent brain infarction and other vascular events.[259] A large cohort of 360 patients with stroke enrolled in the Patent Foramen Ovale in Cryptogenic Stroke Study (PICSS)[258] had a prevalence of PFO of 33.8%, but there was no significant difference in the rates of recurrent stroke or death over 2 years between those with PFO of any size (14.8%) and those without PFO (15.4%). In a 4-year follow-up study of 267 patients with cryptogenic stroke who were younger than 55 years and had PFO, a 4.5% recurrent stroke rate was reported.[227]

The evidence for the relationship between stroke recurrence and inflammatory and hemostatic markers has been accumulating.[260-262] Possible biochemical and clinical predictors of recurrent stroke include CRP, cholesterol level, white blood cell count, fibrinogen level, hematocrit, the albumin-to-globulin ratio, protein C deficiency, free protein S deficiency, lupus anticoagulant, anticardiolipin antibodies, increased homocysteine, and obesity.[263-268] Whether these predictors are causal risk factors for recurrent stroke or markers of increased risk remains uncertain. These features have not been established as valid predictors of stroke recurrence.

Worsening after Ischemic Stroke

The term *worsening after ischemic stroke* encompasses a broad range of causes with variations in onset, duration, and course.[269] Ideally, physicians should attempt to alter a declining course of illness that begins at the time of symptom onset. Worsening during the first few hours often has quite different explanations from those for worsening that appears 12 to 48 hours after stroke. Unfortunately, it is often difficult to quantify deficits present before the patient is seen by medical personnel merely on the basis of accounts of the patient and observers. There are three main categories of worsening: (1) neurologic deterioration, consisting of gradual or stepwise progression of neurologic focal deficits while the patient usually remains alert and free of medical complications; (2) brain edema, a complication of mostly large strokes, especially hemorrhages, that is accompanied by headache and decreased alertness; and (3) medical complications, especially febrile illnesses, which affect the patient systemically and may also increase brain ischemia.

Neurologic deterioration, reported to occur in 20% to 58% of patients with acute stroke, increases both mortality and morbidity.[269-271] The frequency of clinical worsening after hospitalization varies according to stroke type and the delay between symptom onset and entry into the hospital. In the Harvard Stroke Registry, 20% of patients with stroke showed progression of neurologic deficit after stroke onset.[272] Progression was most common in patients with lacunar infarcts (37%) and large-artery occlusive disease (33%) and least common in patients with embolism (7%). In the Barcelona Stroke Registry involving more than 3500 patients, 37% experienced worsening after onset.[273] Data from the more than 3000 patients in the Lausanne Stroke Registry showed that worsening after admission occurred in 29% of all patients and in 34% of patients with noncardioembolic ischemic stroke.[274] Among the patients with noncardioembolic stroke who experienced worsening, 58% showed progression of symptoms during the first 24 hours. In a Japanese study of 350 stroke patients, 25% experienced progression after admission, 26% of whom had lacunar stroke.[275] When worsening occurred after acute ischemic stroke, it was usually due to stroke evolution. Of the 1271 patients with ischemic stroke in the NINDS Stroke Data Bank, the cause of worsening in 72% of those who experienced it during hospitalization was stroke evolution.[206]

The causes of neurologic deterioration have not been clearly identified, although several variables have been associated with deterioration. Progression of thrombosis or recurrent embolism has attracted some attention. Variables reported as predictive of neurologic deterioration include high systolic blood pressure, hyperglycemia on admission, and carotid territory involvement.[276,277] Deterioration within 4 days of stroke onset occurred mainly in cases in which arterial occlusion led to large infarctions, with secondary edema found on the brain CT studies.[270] Studies using MRI technology show that patients in whom perfusion-weighted imaging (PWI) shows a larger area of involvement than diffusion-weighted imaging (DWI) and who have persistent occlusive lesions on magnetic resonance angiography have larger infarcts and more severe clinical deficits than patients with open arteries and no PWI-DWI mismatch.[278,279] In patients with stenosis or occlusion of large arteries or penetrating artery disease, severe reduction of flow to ischemic brain areas may occur. Hypoperfusion and distal embolization are likely the most important mechanisms that lead to progressive infarction.

Severe stroke has been shown to be an important predictor of clinical worsening.[280] In a study from the University of Copenhagen, patients with neurologic deterioration had more severe strokes than nondeteriorating patients.[281] In the first European Cooperative Acute Stroke Study (ECASS I), coronary heart disease, diabetes, and early signs of infarction on CT scan were predictive of deterioration within 24 hours, whereas advanced age, severe stroke, and brain swelling were predictive of deterioration between 24 hours and 7 days after stroke.[276]

Worsening after stroke is most often related to the stroke subtype. Although hemodynamic infarction from large-artery occlusion or stenosis is associated with a greater risk of worsening, small-vessel lacunar infarcts worsen as well. A number of studies focused on progression and worsening in series of patients with lacunar strokes.[282–284] In the subpopulation with lacunar infarcts in the NINDS Stroke Data Bank, a pure motor syndrome had a better outcome in terms of improvement of motor deficits than the other lacunar syndromes.[285] In a German study, 24% of patients had worsening of motor deficits after hospitalization, predominantly in lacunar strokes.[284] Progression of deficits in patients with lacunar strokes, even evolving within days after onset, has often been noted. Mohr,[283] in a 1982 review of lacunar infarcts, commented that "this surprisingly leisurely mode of onset" characterizes many lacunar strokes.

Cardiac Events after Stroke

For people who have experienced a stroke, the risk of MI is increased by a factor of two to three compared with the stroke-free population.[286] MI and other cardiac conditions are a frequent cause of death in stroke survivors. In an older unselected series of 843 cases of cerebral thrombosis followed up for 9 to 19 years, 41% of the initial survivors died from recurrent strokes and 30% from heart disease.[154] In Rochester, Minnesota, stroke survivors died from heart disease twice as often as those from recurrent stroke.[203] The annual risk of vascular death after minor or major stroke has been estimated from various clinical trials to be 3.2% to 3.5%.[75] Forty percent of patients with a history of ischemic stroke or TIA have concomitant coronary artery disease.[287]

Observation of other abnormalities, such as depolarization and ischemia-like electrocardiographic (ECG) changes, during the acute phase of stroke is quite common. Ischemia-like ECG changes, QT prolongation, or both are present in more than 90% of unselected patients with ischemic stroke and ICH and most often represent preexisting coronary artery disease.

Functional Disability and Handicap After Stroke

Functional disability, the lack of ability to perform an activity or task in the range considered normal for an individual, is an important outcome after nonfatal stroke. Reliable and valid scales have been developed for activities of daily living (ADLs) and other indices for measuring functional dependence. One of the most commonly used is the Barthel Index.[288,289] The approximate proportion of stroke survivors who are independent at 6 months ranges from 40% to 65%, depending on the characteristics of the study population. A high Barthel Index score at hospital discharge is a good predictor of a favorable functional prognosis.[290] Functional activity measured by Barthel Index score has often been used as a primary outcome in randomized acute stroke clinical trials. In the Glycine Antagonist in Neuroprotection (GAIN) Americas trial, 38% of patients were functionally independent according to Barthel Index score (range 95–100) and 27% according to Rankin Scale score (0 or 1) at 3 months after an acute onset of ischemic stroke.[291]

The potential for recovery and the likelihood of long-term survival free of dependence on others are of concern for survivors of stroke, their families, and health care professionals. This information should be based on predictive models derived from data sets that include complete follow-up of cases of first-ever stroke from large, community-based cohorts with the standard diagnostic criteria and clinical assessments of disease severity, comorbidity, and sociodemographic factors and standardized measures of functional outcome. There are several studies of long-term functional outcome after stroke, but only a few reliable estimates of long-term functional outcome after first-ever ischemic stroke are available.[292–308] The most important are summarized in Table 3.5.

One of the largest functional outcome studies was the Auckland Stroke Study, in which information on disability and health-related quality of life (HRQOL) was available for nearly all of the 639 6-year survivors (36%) of the original cohort of 1761 patients registered in 1991 and 1992.[293] In this study, 42% of patients were dependent in at least one aspect of ADLs 6 years after stroke. Of the 30-day survivors of initial stroke in the Perth Community Stroke Study, one third remained disabled, and one in seven was in permanent institutional care.[292] The major predictors of poor long-term outcome in this group were a low level of activity before the stroke, subsequent recurrent stroke, older age, baseline disability defined by Barthel Index score, and severe stroke at onset. In the NOMASS cohort, functional outcome was assessed by Barthel Index (BI) at two time points: at 7 to 10 days and at 6 months after stroke onset.[309] Of the 359 stroke survivors, 35% were independent, 37% moderately dependent, and 28% dependent 7 to 10 days after first ischemic stroke (Fig. 3–7). Six months after stroke, 55% of patients were independent according to the BI. In the multivariate model, only greater BI assessed at 7 to 10 days was predictive of 6-month

Table 3.5 Studies of Disability or Handicap at Least 3 Months after Stroke

Study*	Strokes (No.)	Age (Mean or Range, yr)	Duration of Follow-up	Outcome(s) Measured	Survival (%)	Outcome Independence/ Survival (%)
Community-Based Studies						
Auckland Stroke Study[293,300]	1761	71	6 yr	Disability (ADLs)/SF-36	—	39
	680	70	6 mo	Disability (Katz)		76
Rochester, Minnesota[144,294]	292	72	5 yr	Disability (ADLs)/SF-36	—	39
				Disability (Katz)		76
Perth Community Stroke Study[292]	492	73	5 yr	Disability (BI)	59	38
Newcastle, UK[301]	229	82	3 yr	Disability (BI)	49	45
OSCP[296,297]	675	72	1 yr	Handicap (Rankin)		71
NEMESIS[298]	264	72	1 yr	Handicap (Rankin)	77	65
Southern England[303]	456	65	1 yr	Disability (BI)	—	71
L'Aquila Registry[304]	819	75	1 yr	Disability (BI)	64	76
Bristol, UK[299]	976	75	6 mo	Disability (BI)	63	64
Tartu, Estonia[305]	519	70	6 mo	Disability (undefined)	63	24
NOMASS[309]	395	69	6 mo	Disability (ADLs)	59	33
Hospital-Based Studies						
Iowa Registry of Stroke in Young Adults[307]	296	15–45	16 yr	Disability (BI)	79	49
Southeast London, UK[308]	291	71	5 yr	Disability (BI)	42	34
				Handicap (Rankin)		36
Hong Kong[306]	304	70	20 mo	Disability (BI)	58	57
GAIN Americas[291]	1367	70	3 mo	Disability (BI)	80	38
				Handicap (Rankin)		27

ADLs, activities of daily living; BI, Barthel Index; GAIN, Glycine Antagonist in Neuroprotection (trial); Katz, Katz Index of Independence in Activities of Daily Living; NEMESIS, North East MElbourne Stroke Incidence Study; NOMASS, NOrthern MAnhattan Stroke Study; SF-36, Medical Outcome Study's 36-item short-form health survey; OSCP, Oxfordshire Community Stroke Project.
*Superscript numbers indicate chapter references.

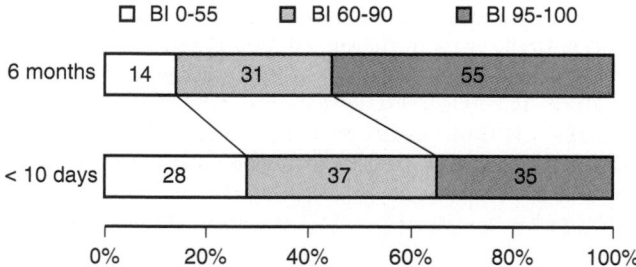

FIGURE 3–7 *Functional outcome assessed by the Barthel Index at 6 months and 7–10 days after onset of first ischemic stroke among 359 survivors from the Northern Manhattan Stroke Study.*

functional independence, indicating that long-term functional independence was strongly influenced by early functional recovery after stroke.

Handicap is the disadvantage for an individual resulting from an impairment or disability that limits or prevents the fulfillment of a role (depending on age, sex, and social and cultural factors) that is normal for that individual.[310] Although post-stroke disability has been the subject of much discussion in the literature, handicap has received little attention. Handicap is an important target of rehabilitation. Some domains of handicap are potentially modifiable, but knowledge about which aspects of handicap are

most affected in stroke survivors is limited.[311] NEMESIS (North East MElbourne Stroke Incidence Study) investigators found stroke survivors to be handicapped over a wide range of domains.[298] The most disadvantages occurred in the domains of physical independence and occupation, and handicap increased with severity of disability. A study from London reported that patients with total anterior circulatory infarcts (TACIs) were the most disabled and handicapped 3 and 12 months after stroke.[312] Using the modified Rankin Scale, researchers in both the OCSP and the Perth Community Stroke Study found that patients with total anterior circulatory infarcts (TACIs) had a low likelihood of living independently 12 months after stroke.[313,314] Patients with lacunar anterior circulatory infarcts (LACIs) were least disabled. Similarly, in the Rochester Epidemiology Project, patients with lacunar infarcts had the best functional outcomes, more than 80% having minimal or no functional impairment 1 year after stroke. Patients with cardioembolic stroke had poorer prestroke functional status, more severe neurologic deficits at the time of stroke, and poorer functional outcome than those with other subtypes.[144]

Some limitations of the BI and Rankin scales need to be noted. One of them is the "ceiling effect." Patients who are functionally independent on the BI (with the highest score) may continue to improve after stroke, and this improvement cannot be detected with the current scales of activities of daily living. The modified Rankin Scale, although easy to use and widely adopted as a measure of handicap in stroke clinical trials, is a fairly nonspecific instrument that measures a mix of impairment, disability, and handicap through assessment of natural history data and the effects of intervention on outcome.[315] Furthermore, summary scores in any of the currently available scales based on aggregated data may hide wide interindividual variations. Some patients make a rapid, early recovery; others have a more prolonged recovery. Continuing improvement may also be minimized by the effects of aging and the development of other disabilities that may or may not be stroke related. Better and more complete scales for the assessments of functional disability and handicap after stroke still need to be developed.

Quality of Life after Stroke

Quality of life (QOL) is another important outcome after stroke. Recreational and social activities are reduced for most stroke survivors after they return home, whether or not they have made a complete functional recovery.[316–318] QOL instruments have begun to be developed and applied to the evaluation of prognosis after stroke.[319] Standard multidimensional health-related QOL survey tools involve some measurement of physical status, mental and psychological status, social activity status, and functional status.[320] Numerous instruments have been developed, including the Stroke Impact Scale (SIS), Sickness Impact Profile, the Medical Outcome Study's 36-item short-form survey (SF-36), the Nottingham Profile, EuroQOL, and the Quality of Well-Being.[321–326]

The assessment of outcomes, including QOL, after stroke is important for both clinical practice and research, yet there is no consensus on the best measures of stroke outcome in either clinical practice or research. Existing measures have not been sensitive in detecting changes after mild stroke.[327] Very few studies have quantified the impact of stroke on QOL. However, no stroke-specific outcome measure has been developed that assesses other dimensions of health-related QOL: emotion, communication, memory and thinking, and social role function. The Stroke Impact Scale has been developed as a stroke-specific outcome measure, especially in patients with mild to moderate strokes.[328] The scale was developed to evaluate input from the patient and caregiver. This new, stroke-specific outcome measure seems to be reliable, valid, and sensitive to change. However, more studies are required to evaluate both the Stroke Impact Scale itself in larger and more heterogeneous populations and the feasibility and validity of proxy responses for the most severely impaired patients.

In the Northern Manhattan population–based case-control study of 207 patients older than 39 years with first cerebral infarction, the Quality of Well-Being (QWB) scale was used to assess quality of life after stroke.[329] In the comparison with the prestroke QWB score, the 6-month QWB score was 27% lower. Even among those patients who were functionally independent at 6 months (BI score ≥70), there was still a 12% decrease in QWB score.

The SF-36 is the most widely used generic instrument for measuring quality of life (QOL), although it is not specific to stroke patients.[330] The instrument has been translated into numerous languages, and the validity of its eight subscales is confirmed in general populations and in a wide variety of patient groups in more than 2000 articles. In view of the current evidence that the subscales of the SF-36 are psychometrically sound to measure QOL in a range of patient populations, SF-36 may be a useful measure of QOL in stroke.[330,331]

Stroke-specific QOL scores and patient impairments predict patient-reported overall HRQOL after stroke.[331] Disease-specific HRQOL measures are more sensitive to meaningful changes in post-stroke HRQOL and may thus aid in identifying specific aspects of post-stroke function that clinicians and "trialists" can target to improve patients' HRQOL after stroke.

Several limitations of the QOL scales must be emphasized. Most existing stroke QOL outcome measures suffer from floor effects, ceiling effects, or both, and the summary scores may inadequately reflect a patient's physical and mental health.[332–334] When traditional multi-item instruments such as the SF-36 are used, summated scores depend on the number of various items included in the different instruments; therefore, it is impossible to compare scores obtained on different instruments. Furthermore, the clinical interpretation of summated scores is not straightforward. For example, the clinical meaning of a mean score of 47.6 on the SF-36 in a patient with stroke would be unclear for most neurologists. This problem is amplified by the ordinal nature of summated scores, meaning that a given difference in scores at one point on the scale does not necessarily represent the same amount of functional change at another point on the scale.

In response to growing dissatisfaction with the traditional scales, the alternative item response theory (IRT) method has been introduced.[335] This statistical paradigm uses a logistic regression analysis to model the responses of the patients to the individual items. Therefore, the items can be placed on the same hierarchical continuous scale, a feature that helps the assessment and interpretation of the scales. In spite of interest in IRT in clinical outcome measurement, these methods must still be developed in stroke research as a useful supplement to the traditional QOL approach.[336]

Depression after Stroke

Major depression is a common occurrence after stroke.[337–339] Besides benefiting the emotional well-being of the stroke survivor, the recognition and treatment of depression are important because depression is associated with disability,[340] cognitive impairment,[341,342] suicide, and death.[343] Depression has been associated with excess stroke disability,[338,344–349] poor rehabilitation outcomes,[350,351] morbidity and mortality,[352,353] and suicidal thoughts and plans.[354]

If standard diagnostic criteria (either those of the *Diagnosis and Statistical Manual of Mental Disorders* [DSM] or *Research Diagnostic Criteria*[355]) are used to establish the presence of a major depressive episode (MDE), depression occurs, at least temporarily, in up to 30% to 40% of stroke survivors.[337] Although the term *post-stroke depression* (PSD) has already been established in the literature, standardized criteria for this diagnosis do not exist. In most cases, the DSM-IV (4th edition of the *Manual*) or the World Health Organization's International Classification of Diseases of the World (ICD) system is applied. Other investigators use various psychiatric rating scales. Although it is generally acknowledged that there is a high prevalence of depression after stroke, it is underdiagnosed and often left untreated. Also, little is known about the course of major depression after a stroke. Prevalence clearly varies over time, with an apparent peak 3 to 6 months after a stroke and a subsequent decline at 1 year to about 50% of initial rates.[356]

Treatment or prevention of depression after stroke depends greatly on understanding of the pathophysiologic mechanism linking stroke and depression. Even though the DSM-IV classification implies that strokes "cause" depression through a direct biologic mechanism, the nature of the mechanism linking stroke and depression remains debated in the literature.[337] Some researchers propose a primary biologic mechanism, according to which ischemic insults directly affect neural circuits involved in mood regulation, whereas others propose a psychosocial mechanism, according to which the social and psychological stressors associated with a stroke constitute the primary cause of depression.[357–359]

Stroke survivors in active rehabilitation programs have been shown to have lower rates of depression.[360] It has also been reported that depressed stroke survivors with cognitive impairment had a greater duration of depression for longer time periods or longer-term depression than depressed stroke survivors without significant cognitive impairment.[361] Furthermore, left anterior ischemic lesions were associated with cognitive impairment in stroke survivors with major depression; this finding indicates that ischemic lesions in the area of the striatofrontal circuit identified on brain imaging are associated with more severe cognitive impairment and longer-term depression.[362]

Depression after stroke is a common occurrence associated with higher levels of disability, cognitive impairment, and mortality. Post-stroke depression appears not to be the result of a "pure" biologic or psychological cause but instead to be multifactorial in origin and consistent with the biopsychosocial model of mental illness. Better understanding of the pathomechanism, incidence, prevalence, and factors associated with depression after stroke is needed.

Dementia after Stroke

Cerebrovascular disease, particularly stroke, is a major cause of dementia. Approximately 25% of patients with stroke meet operationalized criteria for dementia 3 months after a stroke, and a greater number have cognitive impairment without dementia.[363–368] Compared with individuals who do not have ischemic brain disease, patients who are cognitively intact 3 months after a stroke have a six- to ninefold greater risk of dementia in the first 12 months. The higher risk for dementia is still present several years later.[369]

The relationship between acute stroke and prevalent and incident dementia has been studied in several hospitalized cohorts.[365,367,368] In the longitudinal study of 334 stroke patients who did not have dementia 3 months after stroke onset and 241 stroke-free controls, the crude incidence rate

of dementia (defined according to *Diagnostic and Statistical Manual of Mental Disorders, Revised Third Edition* criteria through a comprehensive neuropsychological and clinical evaluation) was 8.49 cases per 100 person-years in the stroke group and 1.37 cases per 100 person-years among the controls.[368] The RR for incident dementia among patients with stroke was 4.4 (95% CI, 2.20 to 8.85), similar to the RR reported by other groups.[363,365,366] These incidence and RR figures highlight the magnitude of the problem of dementia after ischemic stroke.[370]

The findings of the other longitudinal studies that have been based on series of hospitalized patients with stroke also suggested that the risk of incident dementia associated with stroke is high. In one series, the incidence of dementia was 6.7% among patients 60 to 64 years old and 26.5% among patients older than 85 years after 1 year of follow-up in a sample of 610 patients who initially had no dementia after stroke.[371] In a cohort of 169 patients without dementia before stroke onset, the rate of incident dementia was 21.3% after 3 years of follow-up.[372] New dementia appeared immediately after the index stroke in most cases, however, and only 7% of patients without dementia 6 months after the index stroke experienced incident dementia during the remainder of the 3 years of follow-up. In a hospitalized cohort of 175 patients initially without dementia after stroke, 32% demonstrated incident dementia during 5 years of follow-up after first ischemic stroke.[373]

In the Rochester, Minnesota, population–based study of stroke and incident dementia in 971 patients who had been free of dementia before first stroke, the cumulative incidence of dementia, which includes prevalent cases, was 7% at 1 year, 10% at 3 years, 15% at 5 years, and 23% at 10 years.[374] In the Kungsholmen Project, Stockholm, Sweden, the RR of incident dementia associated with prior stroke was 1.7 (95% CI, 1.1 to 2.6) after adjustment for potential confounders, and prior stroke was particularly potent when it had occurred within the preceding 3 years.[375]

The clinical determinants of post-stroke dementia included (1) features of the presenting stroke, such as its size and location; (2) vascular risk factors, such as diabetes mellitus and prior stroke; and (3) host characteristics, such as older age.[363,365–367,369] The risk of dementia was found to be elevated in patients who had intercurrent illnesses that can produce hypoxia, including conditions causing transient (seizures and syncope) and prolonged (heart failure, MI) hypoxia.[368] Similarly, other studies have found that in patients with dementia, cerebral hypoperfusion was the primary cause of the dementia syndrome.[376] In an autopsy study, 28.8% of patients with vascular dementia had neuropathologic evidence of cerebral hypoperfusion, with either selective, incomplete infarction of the cerebral white matter or borderzone infarction.[377]

More research relevant to dementia after stroke needs to be conducted on (1) the qualitative features of the index stroke that are predictors of dementia, (2) quantitative brain imaging measures (e.g., the volume or number of clinically "silent" cerebral infarctions, severity of diffuse white matter disease, severity of atrophy), (3) standardized imaging of symptomatic and clinically "silent" recurrent stroke, and (4) state-of-the-art brain imaging techniques (e.g., diffusion tensor imaging to assess the integrity of subcortical pathways). Genetic factors may also be important predictors, whether as risk markers, such as the apolipoprotein E ε4 allele, or as primary independent risk factors, such as Notch3 mutations in cerebral autosomal dominant arteriopathy with subcortical infarcts and leukoencephalopathy (CADASIL).[378,379]

Finally, the results of studies of dementia after stroke are influenced by the paradigm selected for use in the diagnosis of dementia. Standardized diagnostic methods must be used to minimize systematic errors in the estimation of the incidence and prevalence of dementia after stroke.

References

1. Murray CJL, Lopez AD: Mortality by cause for 8 regions of the world: Global burden of disease study. Lancet 349:1269–1276, 1997.
2. Murray CJL, Lopez AD: Global mortality, disability and the contribution of risk factors: Global burden of disease study. Lancet 349:1436–1442, 1997.
3. Broderick J, Brott T, Kothari R, et al: The Greater Cincinnati/Northern Kentucky Stroke Study: Preliminary first-ever and total incidence rates of stroke among blacks. Stroke 29:415–421, 1998.
4. Sacco RL, Shi T, Zamanillo MC, Kargman DE: Predictors of mortality and recurrence after hospitalized cerebral infarction in an urban community: The Northern Manhattan Stroke Study. Neurology 44:626–634, 1994.
5. Wolf PA, Clagett P, Easton JD, et al: Preventing ischemic stroke in patients with prior stroke and TIA: A statement for healthcare professionals from the Stroke Council of the American Heart Association. Stroke 30:1991–1994, 1999.
6. Taylor TN, Davis PH, Torner JC, et al: Lifetime cost of stroke in the United States. Stroke 27:1459–1466, 1996.
7. Collins R, MacMahon S: Blood pressure, antihypertensive drug treatment and risk of stroke and coronary heart disease. Br Med Bull 50:272–298, 1994.
8. Neal B, MacMahon S, Chapman N, et al: Effects of ACE inhibitors, calcium antagonists and other blood pressure lowering drugs: Results of the prospectively designed overviews of randomised trials. Blood Pressure Lowering Treatment Trialists' Collaboration. Lancet 356:1955–1964, 2000.
9. Randomized trial of perindopril-based blood-pressure-lowering regimen among 6105 individuals with previous stroke or transient ischemic attack. PROGRESS Collaborative Group. Lancet 358:1033–1041, 2001.
10. Effects of an angiotensin-converting-enzyme inhibitor, ramipril, on cardiovascular events in high-risk patients. Heart Outcomes Prevention Evaluation Study Investigators. N Engl J Med 342:145–153, 2000.
11. Mayberg MR, Batjer HH, Dacey R, et al: Guidelines for the management of aneurysmal subarachnoid hemorrhage: A statement for healthcare professionals from a special writing group of the Stroke Council, American Heart Association. Circulation 90:2592–2605, 1994.
12. Measuring and improving quality of care: A report from the American Heart Association/American College of Disease and Stroke Quality of Care and Outcomes Research in CVD and Stroke Working Groups. Stroke 31:1002–1012, 2000.
13. Ogungbo B, Gregson BA, Blackburn A, Mendelow AD: Trends over time in the management of subarachnoid hemorrhage in Newcastle: Review of 1609 patients. Newcastle Subarachnoid Study Group. Br J Neurosurg 15:388–395, 2001.
14. Haley EC Jr, Kassell NF, Apperson-Hansen C, et al: A randomized double-blind vehicle-controlled trial of tirilazad mesylate in patients with aneurysmal subarachnoid hemorrhage: A cooperative study in North America. J Neurosurg 86:467–474, 1997.
15. Lanzio G, Kassell NF: Double-blind randomized vehicle-controlled study of high-dose tirilazad mesylate in women with aneurysmal subarachnoid hemorrhage. Part II: A cooperative study in North America. J Neurosurg 90:1018–1024, 1999.
16. Lanzio G, Kassell NF, Dorsch NW, et al: Double blind randomized vehicle controlled study of high dose tirilazad mesylate in women with aneurysmal subarachnoid haemorrhage. Part I: A cooperative
17. study in Europe, Australia, New Zealand, and South Africa. J Neurosurg 90:1011–1017, 1999.
18. Phillips LH, Whisnant JP, O'Fallon WM, Sundt TM: The unchanging pattern of subarachnoid hemorrhage in a community. Neurology 30:1934–1940, 1980.
19. Sacco RL, Wolf PA, Bharucha NE, et al: Subarachnoid and intracerebral hemorrhage: Natural history, prognosis, and precursive factors in the Framingham Study. Neurology 34:847–854, 1984.
20. Bonita R, Thompson S: Subarachnoid hemorrhage: Epidemiology, diagnosis, management and outcome. Stroke 16:591–594, 1985.
21. Giroud M, Milan C, Beuriat P, et al: Incidence and survival rates during a two-year period of intracerebral and subarachnoid hemorrhages, cortical infarcts, lacunes and transient ischaemic attacks. The Stroke Registry of Dijon: 1985–1989. Int J Epidemiol 120:892–899, 1991.
22. Sarti C, Tuomilehto J, Salomaa V, et al: Epidemiology of subarachnoid hemorrhage in Finland from 1983 to 1985. Stroke 22:848–853, 1991.
23. Longstreth WT Jr, Nelson LM, Koepsell TD, Van Belle G: Clinical course of spontaneous subarachnoid hemorrhage: A population-based study in Kings County, Washington. Neurology 43:712–718, 1993.
24. Broderick JP, Brott TG, Duldner JE, et al: Initial and recurrent bleeding are the major causes of death following subarachnoid hemorrhage. Stroke 25:1342–1347, 1994.
25. Labovitz DL, Rundek T, Benson R, Sacco LS: 30-Day case fatality in a multi-ethnic, population-based incident stroke cohort in Northern Manhattan. Stroke 31:2793, 2000.
26. Juvela S: Alcohol consumption as a risk factor for poor outcome after aneurysmal subarachnoid hemorrhage. BMJ 304:1663–1667, 1992.
27. Claassen J, Carhuapoma R, Kreiter KT, et al: Global cerebral edema after subarachnoid hemorrhage: Frequency, predictors and impact on outcome. Stroke 33:1225–1232, 2002.
28. Kassell NF, Torner JC. Haley EC, et al: The International Cooperative Study on the Timing of Aneurysm Surgery. I: Overall management results. J Neurosurg 73:18–36, 1990.
29. Olafsson E, Hauser WA, Gudmundsson G, et al: A population-based study of prognosis of ruptured cerebral aneurysm: Mortality and recurrence of subarachnoid hemorrhage. Neurology 48:1191–1195, 1997.
30. Ronkainen A, Niskanen N, Rinne J, Koivisto T, et al: Evidence for excess long-term mortality after treated subarachnoid hemorrhage. Stroke 32:2850–2853, 2001.
31. Winn HR, Richardson AE, Jane JA: The long term prognosis in untreated cerebral aneurysm. 1: The incidence of late hemorrhage in cerebral aneurysm: A 10 year evaluation of 364 patients. Ann Neurol 1:358–370, 1977.
32. Ogungbo B, Gregson BA, Blackburn A, Mendelow AD, Newcastle Subarachnoid Study Group: Trends over time in the management of subarachnoid haemorrhage in Newcastle: Review of 1609 patients. Br J Neurosurg 15:388–395, 2001.
33. Haley EC, Kassell NF, Torner JC: The International Cooperative Study on the Timing of Aneurysm Surgery: The North American experience. Stroke 23:205–214, 1992.
34. Kassell NF, Torner JC: Aneurysmal rebleeding: A preliminary report from the Cooperative Aneurysm Study. Neurosurgery 13:479–481, 1983.
35. Pickard JD, Murray GD, Illingworth R, et al: Effect of oral nimodipine on cerebral infarction and outcome after subarachnoid hemorrhage. British Aneurysm Nimodipine Trial. BMJ 298:636–642, 1989.
36. Tsutsumi K, Ueki K, Usui M, et al: Risk of recurrent subarachnoid hemorrhage after complete obliteration of cerebral aneurysms. Stroke 29:2511–2513, 1998.
37. Tsutsumi K, Ueki K, Morita A, et al: Risk of aneurysm recurrence in patients with clipped cerebral aneurysms. Results of long-term follow up angiography. Stroke 32:1191–1194, 2001.
38. Hop JW, Rinkel GJ, Algra A, van Gijn J: Case-fatality and functional outcome after SAH: A systematic review. Stroke 28:660–664, 1997.
39. Bornstein RA, Weir BKA, Petruk KC, et al: Neuropsychological function in patients after SAH. Neurosurgery 21:651–654, 1987.
40. Tidswell P, Dias MB, Sagar HJ, et al: Cognitive outcome after aneurysm rupture: Relationship to aneurysm site and perioperative complications. Neurology 45:875–882, 1995.
41. Vilkki J, Holst P, Ohman J, et al: Social outcome related to cognitive performance and computed tomographic findings after surgery for a ruptured intracranial aneurysm. Neurosurgery 26:579–585, 1990.

41. Ogden JA, Mee EW, Henning M: A prospective study of impairment of cognition and memory and recovery after subarachnoid hemorrhage. Neurosurgery 33:572–587, 1993.

42. Ropper AH, Zervas NT: Outcome 1 year after subarachnoid hemorrhage from cerebral aneurysm: Management morbidity, mortality, and functional status in 122 consecutive patients. J Neurosurg 60:909–915, 1984.

43. Powell J, Kitchen N, Heslin J, Greenwood R: Psychological outcomes at three and nine months after good neurological recovery from aneurysmal subarachnoid hemorrhage: Predictors and prognosis. J Neurol Neurosurg Psychiatry 72:772–781, 2002.

44. Hackett ML, Anderson CS: Health outcomes 1 year after SAH: An international population-based study. The Australian Cooperative Research on Subarachnoid Hemorrhage Study Group. Neurology 55:658–662, 2000.

45. Mayer SA, Kreiter KT, Copeland D, et al: Global and domain-specific impairment and outcome after subarachnoid hemorrhage. Neurology 59:1750–1758, 2002.

46. Kreiter KT, Copeland D, Bernardini GL, et al: Predictors of cognitive dysfunction after subarachnoid hemorrhage. Stroke 33:200–208, 2002.

47. Broderick JP, Brott T, Tomsick T, et al: Intracerebral hemorrhage more than twice as common as subarachnoid hemorrhage. J Neurosurg 78:188–191, 1993.

48. Bonita R, Stewart A, Beaglehole R: International trends in stroke mortality: 1970–1985. Stroke 21:989–992, 1990.

49. Baum HM, Goldstein M: Cerebrovascular disease type-specific mortality: 1968–1977. Stroke 13:810–817, 1982.

50. Omae T: Prevention of stroke. Jpn J Stroke 3:97–99, 1981.

51. Drury I, Whisnant JP, Garraway WM: Primary intracerebral hemorrhage: Impact of CT on incidence. Neurology 34:653–657, 1984.

52. Hill MD, Silver FL, Austin PC, Tu JV: Rate of stroke recurrence in patients with primary intracerebral hemorrhage. Stroke 31:123–127, 2000.

53. Broderick JP, Phillips SJ, Whisnant JP, et al: Incidence rates of stroke in the eighties: The end of the decline in stroke? Stroke 20:577–582, 1989.

54. Bamford J, Sandercock P, Dennis M, et al: A prospective study of acute cerebrovascular disease in the community: The Oxfordshire Community Stroke Project 1981–86. 2: Incidence, case-fatality rates and overall outcome at one year of cerebral infarction, primary intracerebral and subarachnoid hemorrhage. J Neurol Neurosurg Psychiatry 53:16–22, 1990.

55. Fogelholm R, Nuutila M, Vuorela A-L: Primary intracerebral hemorrhage in the Jyvaskyla region, Central Finland, 1985–89: Incidence, case-fatality rate, and functional outcome. J Neurol Neurosurg Psychiatry 55:546–552, 1992.

56. Broderick JP, Brott T, Tomsick T, et al: The risk of subarachnoid and intracerebral hemorrhages in blacks as compared to whites. N Engl J Med 326:733–736, 1992.

57. Broderick JP, Adams HP Jr, Barsan W, et al: Guidelines for the management of spontaneous intracerebral hemorrhage: A statement for healthcare professionals from a special writing group of the Stroke Council, American Heart Association. Stroke 30:905–915, 1999.

58. Diringer MN, Edwards DF: Admission to a neurologic/neurosurgical intensive care unit is associated with reduced mortality rate after intracerebral hemorrhage. Crit Care Med 29:635–640, 2001.

59. Mayer SA, Sacco RL, Shi T, Mohr JP: Neurologic deterioration in non-comatose patients with supratentorial intracerebral hemorrhage. Neurology 44:1379–1384, 1994.

60. Massaro AR, Sacco RL, Mohr JP, et al: Clinical discriminators between lobar and deep hemorrhage: The Stroke Data Bank. Neurology 41:1881–1885, 1991.

61. Steinke W, Sacco RL, Mohr JP, et al: Thalamic stroke: Presentation and prognosis of infarcts and hemorrhages. Arch Neurol 49:703–710, 1992.

62. Broderick JP, Brott T, Duldner JE, et al: Volume of intracerebral hemorrhage: A powerful and easy-to-use predictor of 30-day mortality. Stroke 24:987–993, 1993.

63. Hemphill JC, Bonovich DC, Besmertis L, et al: The ICH score: A simple, reliable grading scale for intracerebral hemorrhage. Stroke 32:891–897, 2001.

64. Fujii Y, Takeuchi S, Sasaki O, et al: Multivariate analysis of predictors of hematoma enlargement in spontaneous intracerebral hemorrhage. Stroke 29:1160–1166, 1998.

65. Labovitz DL, Hauser WA, Sacco RL: Prevalence and predictors of early seizure and status epilepticus after first stroke. Neurology 57:200–206, 2001.

66. Broderick JP, Brott T, Tomsick T, et al: Intracerebral hemorrhage more than twice as common as subarachnoid hemorrhage. J Neurosurg 78:188–191, 1993.

67. Bailey RD, Hart RG, Benavente O, Pearce LA: Recurrent brain hemorrhage is more frequent than ischemic stroke after intracranial hemorrhage. Neurology 56:773–777, 2001.

68. Massaro AR, Sacco RL, Mohr JP, et al: Clinical discriminators of lobar and deep hemorrhages. Neurology 41:1881–1885, 1991.

69. Sacco RL: Lobar intracerebral hemorrhage. N Engl J Med 342:276–279, 2000.

70. O'Donnell HC, Rosand J, Knudsen KA, et al: Apolipoprotein E genotype and the risk of recurrent lobar intracerebral hemorrhage. N Engl J Med 342:240–245, 2000.

71. Greenberg SM, O'Donnell HC, Schaefer PW, Kraft E: MRI detection of new hemorrhages: Potential marker of progression in cerebral amyloid angiopathy. Neurology 53:1135–1138, 1999.

72. U.S. Department of Health and Human Services. Healthy People 2010: Understanding and Improving Health, 2nd ed. Washington, DC, U.S. Government Printing Office, 2000.

73. Gorelick PB: Stroke prevention therapy beyond antithrombotics: Unifying mechanisms in ischemic stroke pathogenesis and implications for therapy, an invited review. Stroke 33:862–875, 2002.

74. Sacco RL, Wolf PA, Gorelick PB: Risk factors and their management for stroke prevention: Outlook for 1999 and beyond. Neurology 53(Suppl 4):S15–S24, 1999.

75. Wilterdink JL, Easton JD: Vascular event rates in patients with atherosclerotic cerebrovascular disease. Arch Neurol 49:857–863, 1992.

76. Sacco RL: Current epidemiology of stroke. In Fisher M, Bogousslavsky J (eds): Current Review of Cerebrovascular Disease. Philadelphia, Current Medicine, 1993.

77. Sacco RL: Prognosis of stroke. In Bogousslavsky J, Ginsberg MD (eds): Cerebrovascular Disease—Pathophysiology, Diagnosis and Management. Malden, MA: Blackwell Science, 1998, pp 879–891.

78. Sacco RL, Wolf PA, Kannel WB, McNamara PM: Survival and recurrence: The Framingham Study. Stroke 13:290–295, 1982.

79. Howard G, Evans GW, Murros KE, et al: Cause specific mortality following cerebral infarction. J Clin Epidemiol 42:45–51, 1989.

80. Garraway WM, Whisnant JP, Drury I: The changing pattern of survival following stroke. Stroke 14:699–703, 1983.

81. Petty GW, Brown RD Jr, Whisnant JP, et al: Survival and recurrence after first cerebral infarction: A population-based study in Rochester, Minnesota, 1975 through 1989. Neurology 50:208–216, 1998.

82. Sacco RL, Shi T, Zamanillo MC, Kargman D: Predictors of mortality and recurrence after hospitalized cerebral infarction in an urban community: The Northern Manhattan Stroke Study. Neurology 44:626–634, 1994.

83. Fang J, Alderman MH: Trend of stroke hospitalization, United States, 1988–1997. Stroke 32:2221–2226, 2001.

84. D'Alessandro G, Bottacchi E, Di Giovanni M, et al: Temporal trends of stroke in Valle d'Aosta, Italy: Incidence and 30-day fatality rates. Neurol Sci 21:13–18, 2000.

85. Mayo NE, Neville D, Kirkland S, et al: Hospitalization and case-fatality rates for stroke in Canada from 1982 through 1991: The Canadian collaborative study group of stroke hospitalizations. Stroke 27:1215–1220, 1996.

86. Truelsen T, Gronbaek M, Schnohr P, Boysen G: Stroke case fatality in Denmark from 1977–1992: The Copenhagen City Heart Study. Neuroepidemiology 21:22–27, 2002.

87. Hartmann A, Rundek T, Mast H, et al: Mortality and causes of death after first-ischemic stroke: The Northern Manhattan Stroke Study. Neurology 57:2000–2005, 2001.

88. Loor HI, Groenier KH, Limburg M, et al: Risks and causes of death in a community-based stroke population: 1 month and 3 years after stroke. Neuroepidemiology 18:75–84, 1999.

89. Dennis MS, Burn JPS, Sandercock PAG, et al: Long-term survival after first-ever stroke: The Oxfordshire Community Stroke Project. Stroke 24:796–800, 1993.

90. Ward G, Jamrozik K, Stewart-Wynne E: Incidence and outcome of cerebrovascular disease in Perth, Western Australia. Stroke 19:1501–1506, 1988.

91. van der Worp HB, Kappelle LJ: Complications of acute ischemic stroke. Cerebrovasc Dis 8:124–132, 1998.

92. Karter AJ, Gazzaniga JM, Cohen RD, et al: Ischemic heart disease and stroke mortality in African-American, Hispanic, and non-Hispanic white men and women, 1985 to 1991. West J Med 169:139–145, 1998.

93. Sung JF, Harris-Hooker SA, Schmid G, et al: Racial differences in mortality from cardiovascular disease in Atlanta, 1979–1985. J Natl Med Assoc 84:259–263, 1992.

94. Hassaballa H, Gorelick PB, West CP, et al: Ischemic stroke outcome: Racial differences in the trial of danaparoid in acute stroke (TOAST). Neurology 57:691–697, 2001.

95. Lai SM, Alter M, Friday G, Sobel E: Prognosis for survival after an initial stroke. Stroke 26:2011–2015, 1995.

96. National Survey of Stroke: Survival and prevalence. Stroke 12:159–168, 1981.

97. Bronnum-Hansen H, Davidsen M, Thorvaldsen P: Long-term survival and causes of death after stroke. Danish MONICA Study Group. Stroke 32:2131–2136, 2001.

98. Gresham GE, Kelly-Hayes M, Wolf PA, et al: Survival and functional status 20 or more years after first stroke: The Framingham Study. Stroke 29:793–797, 1998.

99. Wolf PA, D'Agostino RB, O'Neal MA, et al: Secular trends in stroke incidence and mortality: The Framingham Study. Stroke 23:1551–1555, 1992.

100. Weimar C, Ziegler A, König IR, Diener H-C, et al: Predicting functional outcome and survival after acute ischemic stroke. J Neurol 249:888–895, 2002.

101. Henon H, Godefroy O, Leys D, et al: Early predictors of death after acute cerebral ischemic event. Stroke 26:392–398, 1995.

102. Johnston KC, Connors AF, Wagner DP, et al: A predictive risk model for outcomes of ischemic stroke. Stroke 31:448–455, 2000.

103. Macciocchi SN, Diamond PT, Alves WM, Mertz T: Ischemic stroke: Relation of age, lesion location, and initial neurologic deficit to functional outcome. Arch Phys Med Rehabil 79:1255–1257, 1998.

104. Sankai T, Iso H, Imano H, et al: Survival and disability in stroke by stroke subtype based on computed tomographic findings in three rural Japanese communities. Nippon Koshu Eisei Zasshi 45:552–563, 1998.

105. Tanne D, Gorman MJ, Bates VE, et al: Intravenous tissue plasminogen activator for acute ischemic stroke in patients aged 80 years and older: The tPA stroke survey experience. Stroke 31:370–375, 2000.

106. Thorvaldsen P, Asplund K, Kuulasmaa K, et al: Stroke incidence, case fatality, and mortality in the WHO MONICA Project: World Health Organization Monitoring Trends and Determinants in Cardiovascular Disease. Stroke 26:361–367, 1995.

107. Bronnum-Hansen H, Davidsen M, Thorvaldsen P: Long-term survival and causes of death after stroke: The Danish MONICA Study. Stroke 32:2131–2136, 2001.

108. Gresham GE, Kelly-Hayes M, Wolf PA, et al: Survival and functional status 20 or more years after first stroke: The Framingham Study. Stroke 29:793–797, 1998.

109. Longstreth WT Jr, Bernick C, Fitzpatrick A, et al: Frequency and predictors of stroke death in 5,888 participants in the Cardiovascular Health Study. Neurology 56:368–375, 2001.

110. Lyden P, Brott T, Tilley B, et al: Improved reliability of the NIH stroke scale using video training. NINDS TPA Stroke Study Group. Stroke 25:2220–2226, 1994.

111. Tissue plasminogen activator for acute ischemic stroke. The National Institute of Neurological Disorders and Stroke rt-PA Stroke Study Group. N Engl J Med 333:1581–1587, 1995.

112. Moroney JT, Bagiella E, Paik MC, et al: Risk factors for early recurrence after ischemic stroke: The role of stroke syndrome and subtype. Stroke 29:2118–2124, 1998.

113. Adams HP Jr, Davis PH, Leira EC, et al: Baseline NIH Stroke Scale score strongly predicts outcome after stroke: A report of the Trial of Org 10172 in Acute Stroke Treatment (TOAST). Neurology 53:126–131, 1999.

114. Censori B, Camerlingo M, Casto L, et al: Prognostic factors in first-ever stroke in the carotid artery territory seen within 6 hours after onset. Stroke 24:532–535, 1993.

115. Albers GW, Bates V, Clark WM, et al: Intravenous tissue-type plasminogen activator for treatment of acute stroke: The Standard Treatment with Alteplase to Reverse Stroke (STARS) study. JAMA 283:1145–1150, 2000.

116. Jansen O, Schellinger P, Fiebach J, et al: Early recanalisation in acute ischaemic stroke saves tissue at risk defined by MRI. Lancet 353:2036–2037, 1999.

117. Adams HP Jr, Bendixen BH, Leira E, et al: Antithrombotic treatment of ischemic stroke among patients with occlusion or severe stenosis of the internal carotid artery: A report of the Trial of Org 10172 in Acute Stroke Treatment (TOAST). Neurology 53:122–125, 1999.

118. Rasmussen D, Kohler O, Worm-Petersen S, et al: Computed tomography in prognostic stroke evaluation. Stroke 23:506–510, 1992.

119. Schmidt EV, Smirnov VE, Ryabova VS: Results of the seven-year prospective study of stroke patients. Stroke 19:942–949, 1988.

120. Bonita R, Ford MA, Stewart AW: Predicting survival after stroke: A three-year follow-up. Stroke 19:669–673, 1988.

121. Howard G, Walker MD, Becker C, et al: Community hospital-based stroke programs: North Carolina, Oregon, and New York. III: Factors influencing survival after stroke: Proportional hazards analysis of 4219 patients. Stroke 17:294–299, 1986.

122. Smithard DG, O'Neill PA, Parks C, Morris J: Complications and outcome after acute stroke: Does dysphagia matter? Stroke 27:1200–1204, 1996.

123. Bamford J, Sandercock P, Dennis M, et al: Classification and natural history of clinically identifiable subtypes of cerebral infarction. Lancet 337:1521–1526, 1991.

124. Wang Y, Lim LL, Heller RF, Fisher J: Influence of admission body temperature on stroke mortality. Stroke 31:404–409, 2000.

125. Maher J, Hachinski V: Hypothermia as a potential treatment for cerebral ischemia. Cerebrovasc Brain Metab Rev 5:277–300, 1993.

126. Kammersgaard LP, Jorgensen HS, Rungby JA, et al: Admission body temperature predicts long-term mortality after acute stroke: The Copenhagen Stroke Study. Stroke 33:1759–1762, 2002.

127. Przelomski MM, Roth RM, Gleckman RA, Marcus EM: Fever in the wake of a stroke. Neurology 36:427–429, 1986.

128. Castillo J, Martinez F, Leira R, et al: Mortality and morbidity of acute cerebral infarction related to temperature and basal analytic parameters. Cerebrovasc Dis 4:66–71, 1994.

129. Azzimondi G, Bassein L, Nonino F, et al: Fever in acute stroke worsens prognosis: A prospective study. Stroke 26:2040–2043, 1995.

130. Hindfelt B: The prognostic significance of subfebrility and fever in ischaemic cerebral infarction. Acta Neurol Scand 53:72–79, 1976.

131. Castillo J, Davalos A, Marrugat J, Noya M: Timing for fever-related brain damage in acute ischemic stroke. Stroke 29:2455–2460, 1998.

132. Reith J, Jorgensen HS, Pedersen PM, et al: Body temperature in acute stroke: Relation to stroke severity, infarct size, mortality, and outcome. Lancet 347:422–425, 1996.

133. Hajat C, Hajat S, Sharma P: Effects of poststroke pyrexia on stroke outcome: A meta-analysis of studies in patients. Stroke 31:410–414, 2000.

134. Azzimondi G, Bassein L, Nonino F, et al: Fever in acute stroke worsens prognosis. Stroke 26:2040–2043, 1995.

135. Wang Y, Lim LL, Levi C, et al: Influence of admission body temperature on stroke mortality. Stroke 31:404–409, 2000.

136. Schwab S, Georgiadis D, Berrouschpt J, et al: Feasibility and safety of moderate hypothermia after massive hemispheric infarction. Stroke 32:2033–2035, 2001.

137. Wang Y, Lim LL, Heller RF, Fisher J: Influence of admission body temperature on stroke mortality. Stroke 31:404–409, 2000.

138. Dippel DW, van Breda EJ, van Gemert HM, et al: Effect of paracetamol (acetaminophen) on body temperature in acute ischemic stroke: A double-blind, randomized phase II clinical trial. Stroke 32:1607–1612, 2001.

139. Georgiadis D, Schwarz S, Aschoff A, Schwab S: Hemicraniectomy and moderate hypothermia in patients with severe ischemic stroke. Stroke 33:1584–1588, 2002.

140. Georgiadis D, Schwarz S, Kollmar R, Schwab S: Endovascular cooling for moderate hypothermia in patients with acute stroke: First results of a novel approach. Stroke 32:2550–2553, 2001.

141. Sacco SE, Whisnant JP, Broderick JP, et al: Epidemiological characteristics of lacunar infarcts in a population. Stroke 22:1236–1241, 1991.

142. Ward G, Jamrozik K, Stewart-Wynne E: Incidence and outcome of cerebrovascular disease in Perth, Western Australia. Stroke 19:1501–1506, 1988.

143. Kolominsky-Rabas PL, Weber M, Gefeller O, et al: Epidemiology of ischemic stroke subtypes according to TOAST criteria: Incidence,

recurrence, and long-term survival in ischemic stroke subtypes: A population-based study. Stroke 32:2735–2740, 2001.

144. Petty GW, Brown RD Jr, Whisnant JP, et al: Ischemic stroke subtypes: A population-based study of functional outcome, survival, and recurrence. Stroke 31:1062–1068, 2000.

145. Staaf G, Lindgren A, Norrving B: Pure motor stroke from presumed lacunar infarct: Long-term prognosis for survival and risk of recurrent stroke. Stroke 32:2592–2596, 2001.

146. Adams Jr HP, Bendixen BH, Kappelle LJ, et al: Classifications of subtype of acute ischemic stroke: Definitions for use in a multicenter clinical trial. TOAST Investigators. Stroke 24:35–41, 1993.

147. Sacco RL, Wolf PA, Gorelick PB: Risk factors and their management for stroke prevention: Outlook for 1999 and beyond. Neurology 53(Suppl 4):S15–S24, 1999.

148. Glass TA, Hennessey PM, Pazdera L, et al: Outcome at 30 days in the New England Medical Center Posterior Circulation Registry. Arch Neurol 59:369–376, 2002.

149. Leonardi-Bee J, Bath PM, Phillips SJ, et al: Blood pressure and clinical outcomes in the International Stroke Trial. IST Collaborative Group. Stroke 33:1315–1320, 2002.

150. Rodgers A, MacMahon S, Gamble G, et al: Blood pressure and risk of stroke in patients with cerebrovascular disease. The United Kingdom Transient Ischaemic Attack Collaborative Group. BMJ 313:1470, 1996.

151. Post-stroke Antihypertensive Treatment Study: A preliminary result. PATS Collaborating Group. Chin Med J 108:710–717, 1995.

152. Effects of an angiotensin-converting-enzyme inhibitor, ramipril, on cardiovascular events in high-risk patients. Heart Outcome Prevention Evaluation Study Investigators. N Engl J Med 342:145–153, 2000.

153. Britton M, Carlsson A, de Faire U: Blood pressure course in patients with acute stroke and matched controls. Stroke 17:861–864, 1986.

154. Robinson T, Waddington A, Ward-Close S, et al: The predictive role of 24-hour compared to casual blood pressure levels on outcome following acute stroke. Cerebrovasc Dis 7:264–272, 1997.

155. Bath FJ, Bath PMW: What is the correct management of blood pressure in acute stroke? The Blood Pressure in Acute Stroke Collaboration. Cerebrovasc Dis 7:205–213, 1997.

156. Tanne D, Kasner SE, Demchuk AM, et al: Markers of increased risk of intracerebral hemorrhage after intravenous recombinant tissue plasminogen activator therapy for acute ischemic stroke in clinical practice: The Multicenter rt-PA Stroke Survey. Circulation 105:1679–1685, 2002.

157. Eriksson SE, Olsson JE: Survival and recurrent strokes in patients with different subtypes of stroke: A fourteen-year follow-up study. Cerebrovasc Dis 12:171–180, 2001.

158. Sacco RL, Wolf PA, Kannel WB, McNamara PM: Survival and recurrence following stroke. The Framingham Study. Stroke 13(3):290–295, 1982.

159. Sandercock P, Bamford J, Dennis M, et al: Atrial fibrillation and stroke: Prevalence in different types of stroke and influence on early and long term prognosis (Oxfordshire Community Stroke Project). BMJ 305:1460–1465, 1992.

160. Lin HJ, Wolf PA, Kelly-Hayes M, et al: Stroke severity in atrial fibrillation: The Framingham study. Stroke 27:1760–1764, 1996.

161. Jørgensen HS, Nakayama H, Reith J, et al: Acute stroke with atrial fibrillation: The Copenhagen Stroke Study. Stroke 27:1765–1769, 1996.

162. Appelros P, Nydevik I, Seiger A, Terent A: Predictors of severe stroke: Influence of preexisting dementia and cardiac disorders. Stroke 33:2357–2362, 2002.

163. Sacco RL, Shi T, Zamanillo MC, Kargman DE: Predictors of mortality and recurrence after hospitalized cerebral infarction in an urban community: The Northern Manhattan Stroke Study. Neurology 44:626–634, 1994.

164. Gottdiener JS, Gay JA, VanVoorhees L, et al: Frequency and embolic potential of left ventricular thrombus in dilated cardiomyopathy: Assessment by 2-dimensional echocardiography. Am J Cardiol 52:1281–1285, 1983.

165. Kannel WB, Wolf PA, Verter J: Manifestations of coronary disease predisposing to stroke: The Framingham study. JAMA 250:2942–2946, 1983.

166. Al-Khadra AS, Salem DN, Rand WM, et al: Warfarin anticoagulation and survival: A cohort analysis from the Studies of Left Ventricular Dysfunction. J Am Coll Cardiol 31:749–753, 1998.

167. Pullicino PM, Halperin JL, Thompson JL: Stroke in patients with heart failure and reduced left ventricular ejection fraction. Neurology 54:288–294, 2000.

168. Kupari M, Lindroos M, Iivanainen AM, et al: Congestive heart failure in old age: Prevalence, mechanisms and 4-year prognosis in the Helsinki Ageing Study. J Intern Med 241:387–394, 1997.

169. Kiers L, Davis SM, Larkins R, Hopper J et al: Stroke topography and outcome in relation to hyperglycemia and diabetes. J Neurol Neurosurg Psychiatry 55:263–270, 1992.

170. Melamed E: Reactive hyperglycemia in patients with acute stroke. J Neurol Sci 29:267–275, 1976.

171. Oppenheimer S, Halfbraid BI, Oswald GA, Yudkin JS: Diabetes mellitus and early mortality from stroke. BMJ 291:1014–1015, 1985.

172. Pulsinelli WA, Levy DE, Sigsbee B, et al: Increased damage after ischemic stroke in patients with hyperglycemia with or without established diabetes mellitus. Am J Med 74:540–544, 1983.

173. Candelise L, Landi G, Orazio EN, Boccardi E: Prognostic significance of hyperglycemia in acute stroke. Arch Neurol 42:661–663, 1985.

174. Williams LS, Rotich J, Qi R, et al: Effects of admission hyperglycemia on mortality and costs in acute ischemic stroke. Neurology 59:67–71, 2002.

175. Bruno A, Levine SR, Frankel MR, et al: Admission glucose level and clinical outcomes in the NINDS rt-PA Stroke Trial. NINDS rt-PA Stroke Study Group. Neurology 59:669–674, 2002.

176. Stratton IM, Adler AI, Neil HA, et al: Association of glycaemia with macrovascular and microvascular complications of type 2 diabetes (UKPDS 35): Prospective observational study. BMJ 321:405–412, 2000.

177. Chamorro A, Vila N, Ascaso C, et al: Early prediction of stroke severity—role of the erythrocyte sedimentation rate. Stroke 26:573–576, 1995.

178. Di Napoli M, Papa F, Bocola V: C-reactive protein in ischemic stroke: An independent prognostic factor. Stroke 32:917–924, 2001.

179. Gorelick PB: Stroke prevention therapy beyond antithrombotics: Unifying mechanisms in ischemic stroke pathogenesis and implications for therapy: An invited review. Stroke 33:862–875, 2002.

180. Winbeck K, Poppert H, Etgen T, et al: Prognostic relevance of early serial C-reactive protein measurements after first ischemic stroke. Stroke 33:2459–2464, 2002.

181. Rost NS, Wolf PA, Kase CS, et al: Plasma concentration of C-reactive protein and risk of ischemic stroke and transient ischemic attack: The Framingham study. Stroke 32:2575–2579, 2001.

182. Di Napoli M, Papa F, Bocola V: C-reactive protein in ischemic stroke: An independent prognostic factor. Stroke 32:917–924, 2001.

183. Lagrand WK, Visser CA, Hermens WT, et al: C-reactive protein as a cardiovascular risk factor: More than an epiphenomenon? Circulation 100:96–102, 1999.

184. Ridker PM, Cushman M, Stampfer MJ, et al: Inflammation, aspirin, and risks of cardiovascular disease in apparently healthy men. N Engl J Med 336:973–979, 1997.

185. Beamer NB, Coull BM, Clark WM, et al: Persistent inflammatory response in stroke survivors. Neurology 50:1722–1728, 1998.

186. Kannel WB, Anderson K, Wilson PWF: White blood cell count and cardiovascular disease: Insights from the Framingham study. JAMA 267:1253–1256, 1992.

187. Quizilbash N: Fibrinogen and cerebrovascular disease. Eur Heart J 16(Suppl A):S45–S46, 1995.

188. Gussekloo J, Schaap MC, Frolich M, et al: C-reactive protein is a strong but nonspecific risk factor of fatal stroke in elderly persons. Arterioscler Thromb Vasc Biol 20:1047–1051, 2000.

189. Wong KYK, Macwalter RS, Fraser HW, et al: Urate predicts subsequent cardiac death in stroke survivors. Eur Heart J 23:788–793, 2002.

190. Wannamethee SG, Shaper AG, Perry IJ: Serum creatinine concentration and risk of cardiovascular disease: A possible marker for increased risk of stroke. Stroke 28:557–563, 1997.

191. MacWalter RS, Wong SY, Wong KY, et al: Does renal dysfunction predict mortality after acute stroke? A 7-year follow-up study. Stroke 33:163–165, 2002.

192. Johnston KC, Connors AF Jr, Wagner DP, et al: A predictive risk model for outcomes of ischemic stroke. Stroke 31:448–455, 2000.

193. A Randomized Trial of Tirilazad Mesylate in Patients With Acute Stroke (RANTTAS). The RANTTAS Investigators. Stroke 27:1453–1458, 1996.

194. Hénon H, Godefroy O, Leys D, et al: Early predictor of death and disability after acute cerebral ischemic event. Stroke 26:392–398, 1995.

195. Toni D, Fiorelli M, Bastianello S, et al: Acute ischemic strokes improving during the first 48 hours of onset: Predictability, outcome, and possible mechanisms: A comparison with early deteriorating strokes. Stroke 22:10–14, 1997.

196. Harrell FE, Lee KL, Mark DB: Tutorial in biostatistics: Multivariable prognostic models: Issues in developing models, evaluating assumptions and adequacy, and measuring and reducing errors. Stat Med 15:367–387, 1996.

197. Warach S, Gaa J, Siewert B, et al: Acute human stroke studied by whole brain echo planar diffusion-weighted magnetic resonance imaging. Ann Neurol 37:231–241, 1995.

198. Singer MB, Chong J, Lu D, et al: Diffusion-weighted MRI in acute subcortical infarction. Stroke 29:133–136, 1998.

199. Baird AE, Benfield A, Schlaug G, et al: Enlargement of human cerebral ischemic lesion volumes measured by diffusion-weighted magnetic resonance imaging. Ann Neurol 41:581–589, 1997.

200. Fisher M, Albers GW: Applications of diffusion-perfusion magnetic resonance imaging in acute ischemic stroke. Neurology 52:1750–1756, 1999.

201. Nadeau SE, Jordan JE, Mishra SK, Haerer AF: Stroke rates in patients with lacunar and large vessel cerebral infarctions. J Neurol Sci 114:128–137, 1993.

202. Burn J, Dennis M, Bamford J, et al: Long-term risk of recurrent stroke after a first-ever stroke: The Oxfordshire Community Stroke Project. Stroke 25:333–337, 1994.

203. Matsumoto N, Whisnant JP, Kurland LT, Okazaki H: Natural history of stroke in Rochester, Minnesota, 1955 through 1969, an extension of a previous study. Stroke 4:20–29, 1973.

204. Hankey GJ, Jamrozik K, Broadhurst RJ, et al: Long-term risk of first recurrent stroke in the Perth Community Stroke Study. Stroke 29:2491–2500, 1998.

205. Mohr JP, Thompson JLP, Lazar RM, et al: A comparison of warfarin and aspirin for the prevention of recurrent ischemic stroke. The Warfarin-Aspirin Recurrent Stroke Study Group. N Engl J Med 345:1444–1451, 2001.

206. Sacco RL, Foulkes MA, Mohr JP, et al: Determinants of early recurrence of cerebral infarction: Stroke Data Bank. Stroke 20:983–989, 1989.

207. Meissner I, Whisnant JP, Garraway WM: Hypertension management and stroke recurrence in a community (Rochester, Minnesota, 1950–79). Stroke 19:459–463, 1988.

208. Rundek T, Elkind MS, Chen X, et al: Increased early stroke recurrence among patients with extracranial and intracranial atherosclerosis: The Northern Manhattan Stroke Study. Neurology 4(50):A75:S09.001, 1998.

209. Moroney JT, Bageila E, Paik MC, et al: Risk factors for early recurrence after ischemic stroke: The role of stroke syndrome and subtype. Stroke 29:2118–2124, 1998.

210. Hier DB, Foulkes MA, Swiontoniowski M, et al: Stroke recurrence within 2 years after ischemic infarction. Stroke 22:155–161, 1991.

211. Broderick J, Brott T, Kothari R, et al: The Greater Cincinnati/Northern Kentucky Stroke Study: Preliminary first-ever and total incidence rates of stroke among blacks. Stroke 29:415–421, 1998.

212. Wade DT, Wood VA, Hewer RL: Recovery after stroke: The first 3 months. J Neurol Neurosurg Psychiatry 48:7–13, 1985.

213. Lefkovits J, Davis SM, Rossiter SC, et al: Acute stroke outcome: Effects of stroke type and risk factors. Aust N Z J Med 22:30–35, 1992.

214. Jongbloed L: Prediction of function after stroke: A critical review. Stroke 17:765–776, 1986.

215. Jorgensen HS, Nakayama H, Reith J, et al: Stroke recurrence: Predictors, severity, and prognosis. The Copenhagen Stroke Study. Neurology 48:891–895, 1997.

216. Saver JL, Johnston KC, Homer D, et al: Infarct volume as a surrogate or auxiliary outcome measure in ischemic stroke clinical trials. The RANTTAS Investigators. Stroke 30:293–298, 1999.

217. DeGraba TJ, Hallenbeck JM, Pettigrew KD, et al: Progression in acute stroke value of the initial NIH Stroke Scale score on patient stratification in future trials. Stroke 30:1208–1212, 1999.

218. Censori B, Camerlingo M, Casto L, et al: Prognostic factors in first-ever stroke in the carotid artery territory seen within 6 hours after onset. Stroke 24:532–535, 1993.

219. Hornig CR, Lammers C, Buttner T, et al: Long-term prognosis of infratentorial transient ischemic attacks and minor strokes. Stroke 23:199–204, 1992.

220. Fiorelli M, Alpérovitch A, Argentino C, et al: Prediction of long-term outcome in the early hours following acute ischemic stroke. Italian Acute Stroke Study Group. Arch Neurol 52:250–255, 1995.

221. Chambers BR, Norris JW, Shurvell BL, Hachinski VC: Prognosis of acute stroke. Neurology 37:221–225, 1987.

222. Secondary prevention in non-rheumatic atrial fibrillation after transient ischaemic attack or minor stroke. European Atrial Fibrillation Trial Study Group. Lancet 342:1255–1262, 1993.

223. Sandercock P, Bamford J, Dennis M, et al: Atrial fibrillation and stroke: Prevalence in different types of stroke and influence on early and long term prognosis (Oxfordshire Community Stroke Project). BMJ 305:1460–1465, 1992.

224. Lechat P, Mas JL, Lascault G, et al: Prevalence of patent foramen ovale in patients with stroke. N Engl J Med 318:1148–1152, 1988.

225. Webster MW, Chancellor AM, Smith HJ, et al: Patent foramen ovale in young stroke patients. Lancet 2:11–12, 1988.

226. Di Tullio MR, Sacco RL, Gopal AS, et al: Patent foramen ovale as a risk factor for cryptogenic stroke. Ann Intern Med 117:461–465, 1992.

227. Mas JL, Arquizan C, Lamy C, et al: Recurrent cerebrovascular events associated with patent foramen ovale, atrial septal aneurysm, or both. N Engl J Med 345:1740–1746, 2001.

228. Amarenco PA, Cohen A, Tzourio C, et al: Atherosclerotic disease of the aortic arch and the risk of ischemic stroke. N Engl J Med 331:1474–1479, 1994.

229. Di Tullio MR, Sacco RL, Gersony D, et al: Aortic atheromas and acute ischemic stroke: A transesophageal echocardiographic study in an ethnically mixed population. Neurology 46:1560–1566, 1996.

230. Orencia AJ, Petty GW, Khandheria BK, et al: Mitral valve prolapse and the risk of stroke after initial cerebral ischemia. Neurology 45:1083–1086, 1995.

231. Beneficial effect of carotid endarterectomy in symptomatic patients with high-grade carotid stenosis. North American Symptomatic Carotid Endarterectomy Trial Collaborators. N Engl J Med 325:445–453, 1991.

232. Grau AJ, Weimar C, Buggle F, et al: Risk factors, outcome, and treatment in subtypes of ischemic stroke: The German Stroke Data Bank. Stroke 32:2559–2566, 2001.

233. Petty GW, Brown RD, Whisnant JP, et al: Ischemic stroke subtypes: A population-based study of incidence and risk factors. Stroke 30:2513–2516, 1999.

234. Sage JI, VanUitert RL: Risk of recurrent stroke in patients with atrial fibrillation and non-valvular heart disease. Stroke 14:537–540, 1983.

235. Hart RG, Coull BM, Hart D: Early recurrent embolism associated with nonvalvular atrial fibrillation: A retrospective study. Stroke 14:688–693, 1983.

236. Sherman DG, Hart RG, Easton JD: The secondary prevention of stroke in patients with atrial fibrillation. Arch Neurol 43:68–70, 1986.

237. Ahmed N, Nasman P, Wahlgren NG: Effect of intravenous nimodipine on blood pressure and outcome after acute stroke. Stroke 31:1250–1255, 2000.

238. Squire IB, Lees KR, Pryse-Phillips W, et al: The effects of lifarizine in acute cerebral infarction: A pilot study. Cerebrovasc Dis 6:156–160, 1996.

239. Rundek T, Chen X, Steiner MM, et al: Predictors of 1-year stroke recurrence: The Northern Manhattan Stroke Study. Cerebrovasc Dis 7(4):68, epi 10, 1997.

240. Alter M, Sobel E, McCoy RL, et al: Stroke in the Lehigh Valley: Risk factors for recurrent stroke. Neurology 37:503–507, 1987.

241. Effect of antihypertensive treatment on stroke recurrence. Hypertension-Stroke Cooperative Study Group. JAMA 229:409–418, 1974.

242. The Sixth Report of the Joint National Committee on Detection, Evaluation, and Treatment of High Blood Pressure (JNC VI). Arch Intern Med 157:2413–2446, 1997.

243. Vokó Z, Bots ML, Hofman A, et al: J-shaped relation between blood pressure and stroke in treated hypertensives. Hypertension 34:1181–1185, 1999.

244. Irie K, Yagamuchi T, Minematsu K, Omae T: The J-curve phenomenon in stroke recurrence. Stroke 24:1844–1849, 1993.

245. Friday G, Alter M, Lai S-M: Control of hypertension and risk of stroke recurrence. Stroke 33:2652–2657, 2002.

246. Gueyffier F, Boissel J-P, Boutitie F, et al: Effect of antihypertensive treatment in patients having already suffered from stroke: Gathering the evidence. Stroke 28:2557–2562, 1997.

247. Sobel E, Alter M, Davanipour Z, et al: Stroke in the Lehigh Valley: Combined risk factors for recurrent ischemic stroke. Neurology 39:669–672, 1989.

248. Bak S, Sindrup SH, Alslev T, et al: Cessation of smoking after first-ever stroke: A follow-up study. Stroke 33:2263–2269, 2002.

249. Wilson K, Gibson N, Willan A, Cook D: Effect of smoking cessation on mortality after myocardial infarction. Arch Intern Med 160:939–944, 2000.

250. Redfern J, McKevitt C, Dundas R, et al: Behavioural risk factor prevalence and lifestyle change after stroke. Stroke 31:1877–1881, 2000.

251. Boysen G, Truelsen T: Prevention of recurrent stroke. Neurol Sci 21:67–72, 2000.

252. Gorelick PB: Alcohol and stroke. Stroke 18:268–271, 1987.

253. Camargo CA: Moderate alcohol consumption and stroke: The epidemiologic evidence. Stroke 20:1611–1626, 1989.

254. Gill JS, Zezulka AV, Shipley MJ, et al: Stroke and alcohol consumption. N Engl J Med 315:1041–1046, 1986.

255. Gorelick PB, Rodin MB, Langenberg P, et al: Weekly alcohol consumption, cigarette smoking, and the risk of ischemic stroke: Results of a case-control study at three urban medical centers in Chicago, Illinois. Neurology 39:339–343, 1989.

256. Klatsky AL, Armstrong MA, Friedman GD: Alcohol use and subsequent cerebrovascular disease hospitalizations. Stroke 20:741–746, 1989.

257. Di Tullio MR, Sacco RL, Homma S: Atherosclerotic disease of the aortic arch as a risk factor for recurrent ischemic stroke. N Engl J Med 335:1464–1465, 1996.

258. Homma S, Sacco RL, Di Tullio MR, et al: Effect of medical treatment in stroke patients with patent foramen ovale. Patent Foramen Ovale in Cryptogenic Stroke Study Investigators. Circulation 105:2625, 2002.

259. Atherosclerotic disease of the aortic arch as a risk factor for recurrent ischemic stroke. The French Study of Aortic Plaques in Stroke Group. N Engl J Med 334:1216–1221, 1996.

260. Di Napoli M, Papa F, Villa Pini Stroke Data Bank Investigators: Inflammation, hemostatic markers, and antithrombotic agents in relation to long-term risk of new cardiovascular events in first-ever ischemic stroke patients. Stroke 33:1763–1771, 2002.

261. Feinberg WM, Erickson LP, Bruck D, Kittelson J: Hemostatic markers in acute ischemic stroke: Association with stroke type, severity, and outcome. Stroke 27:1296–1300, 1996.

262. Tohgi H, Konno S, Takahashi S, et al: Activated coagulation/fibrinolysis system and platelet function in acute thrombotic stroke patients with increased C-reactive protein levels. Thromb Res 100:373–379, 2000.

263. Beamer N, Coull BM, Sexton G, et al: Fibrinogen and the albumin-globulin ratio in recurrent stroke. Stroke 24:1133–1139, 1993.

264. Sacco RL, Owen J, Mohr JP, Tatemichi TK: Free protein S deficiency: A possible association with intracranial vascular occlusion. Stroke 20:1657–1661, 1989.

265. Mayer SA, Sacco RL, Hurlet-Jensen A, et al: Free protein S deficiency in acute ischemic stroke: A case-control study. Stroke 24:224–227, 1993.

266. Kittner SJ, Gorelick PB: Antiphospholipid antibodies and stroke: An epidemiologic perspective. Stroke 23(Suppl 2):I19–I22, 1992.

267. Hankey GJ, Eikelboom JW: Homocysteine levels in patients with stroke: Clinical relevance and therapeutic implications. CNS Drugs 15:437–443, 2001.

268. Anticardiolipin antibodies are an independent risk factor for first ischemic stroke. Antiphospholipid Antibodies in Stroke Study Group. Neurology 43:2069–2073, 1993.

269. Caplan LR: Worsening in ischemic stroke patients: Is it time for a new strategy? Stroke 33:1443–1445, 2002.

270. Toni D, Fiorelli M, Gentile M, et al: Progressing neurological deficit secondary to acute ischemic stroke: A study on predictability, pathogenesis and prognosis. Arch Neurol 52:670–675, 1995.

271. Fisher CM: The use of anticoagulants in cerebral thrombosis. Neurology 8:311–322, 1985.

272. Mohr JP, Caplan LR, Melski JW, et al: The Harvard Cooperative Stroke Registry: A prospective registry. Neurology 28:754–762, 1978.

273. Marti-Vilalta JL, Arboix A: The Barcelona Stroke Registry. Eur Neurol 41:135–142, 1999.

274. Yamamoto H, Bogousslavsky J, van Melle G: Different predictors of neurological worsening in different causes of stroke. Arch Neurol 55:481–486, 1998.

275. Tei H, Uchiyama S, Ohara K, et al: Deteriorating ischemic stroke in 4 clinical categories classified by the Oxfordshire Community Stroke Project. Stroke 31:2049–2054, 2000.

276. Dávalos A, Cendra E, Teruel J, et al: Deteriorating ischemic stroke: Risk factors and prognosis. Neurology 40:1865–1869, 1990.

277. Jørgensen HS, Nakayama H, Raaschou HO, Olsen TS: Effect of blood pressure and diabetes on stroke in progression. Lancet 344:156–159, 1994.

278. Thijs VN, Adami A, Neumann-Haefelin T, et al: Clinical and radiological correlates of reduced cerebral blood flow measured using magnetic resonance imaging. Arch Neurol 59:233–238, 2002.

279. Parsons MW, Barber PA, Chalk J, et al: Diffusion- and perfusion-weighted MRI response to thrombolysis in stroke. Ann Neurol 51:28–37, 2002.

280. DeGraba T, Hallenbech JM, Pettigrew KD, et al: Progression in acute stroke. Stroke 30:1208–1212, 1999.

281. Christensen H, Boysen G, Johannesen HH, et al: Deteriorating ischaemic stroke: Cytokines, soluble cytokine receptors, ferritin, systemic blood pressure, body temperature, blood glucose, diabetes, stroke severity, and CT infarction-volume as predictors of deteriorating ischaemic stroke. J Neurol Sci 201:1–7, 2002.

282. Marti-Vilalta JL, Norrving B, Cronqvist S: Clinical and radiologic features of lacunar and nonlacunar stroke. Stroke 20:59–64, 1989.

283. Mohr JP: Lacunes. Stroke 13:3–13, 1982.

284. Steinke W, Ley SC: Lacunar stroke is the major cause of progressive motor deficits. Stroke 33:1510–1516, 2002.

285. Libman RB, Sacco RL, Shi T, Mohr JP: Spontaneous improvement in pure motor stroke: Implications for clinical trials. Neurology 42:1713–1716, 1992.

286. Alberts MJ: Secondary prevention of stroke and the expanding role of the neurologist. Cerebrovasc Dis 13:12–16, 2002.

287. McDermott MM, Lefevre F, Arron M, et al: ST segment depression detected by continuous electrocardiography in patients with acute ischemic stroke or transient ischemic attack. Stroke 25:1820–1824, 1994.

288. Wade DT, Collin C: The Barthel ADL Index: A standard measure of physical disability? Int Disabil Stud 10:64–67, 1988.

289. Wade DT, Hewer RL: Functional abilities after stroke: Measurement, natural history and prognosis. J Neurol Neurosurg Psychiatry 50:177–182, 1987.

290. Granger CV, Hamilton BB, Gresham GE, Kramer AA: The stroke rehabilitation outcome study. II: Relative merits of the total Barthel Index Score and a four-item subscore in predicting patient outcomes. Arch Phys Med Rehabil 70:100–103, 1989.

291. Sacco RL, DeRosa JT, Haley EC, et al: Glycine antagonist in neuroprotection for patients with acute stroke: GAIN Americas: A randomized controlled trial. GAIN Americas investigators. JAMA 285:1719–1728, 2001.

292. Hankey GJ, Jamrozik K, Broadhurst RJ, et al: Long-term disability after first-ever stroke and related prognostic factors in the Perth Community Stroke Study, 1989–1990. Stroke 33:1034–1040, 2002.

293. Hackett M, Duncan J, Anderson C, et al: Health-related quality of life among long-term survivors of stroke: Results from the Auckland Stroke Study, 1991–1992. Stroke 31:440–447, 2000.

294. Dombovy M, Basford J, Whisnant J, Bergstrahl E: Disability and use of rehabilitation services following stroke in Rochester, Minnesota, 1975–1979. Stroke 18:830–836, 1987.

295. Kojima S, Omura T, Wakamatsu W, et al: Prognosis and disability of stroke patients after 5 years in Akita, Japan. Stroke 21:72–77, 1990.

296. Dennis MS, Burn JPS, Sandercock PAG, et al: Long term survival after first-ever stroke: The Oxfordshire Community Stroke Project. Stroke 24:796–800, 1993.

297. Bamford J, Sandercock P, Dennis M, et al: A prospective study of acute cerebrovascular disease in the community: The Oxfordshire Community Stroke Project—1981–86. 2: Incidence, case fatality rates and overall outcome at one year of cerebral infarction, primary intracerebral and subarachnoid haemorrhage. J Neurol Neurosurg Psychiatry 53:16–22, 1990.

298. Sturm JW, Dewey HM, Donnan GA, et al: Handicap after stroke: How does it relate to disability, perception of recovery, and stroke

subtype? The North East Melbourne Stroke Incidence Study (NEMESIS). Stroke 33:762–768, 2002.

299. Wade DT, Hewer RL: Functional abilities after stroke: Measurement, natural history, prognosis. J Neurol Neurosurg Psychiatry 50:177–182, 1987.

300. Bonita R, Beaglehole R: Recovery of motor function after stroke. Stroke 19:1497–1500, 1988.

301. Greveson G, Gray C, French J, James OF: Long-term outcome for patients and carers following hospital admission for stroke. Age Ageing 20:337–344, 1991.

302. Taub NA, Wolfe CD, Richardson E, Burney PG: Predicting the disability of first-time stroke sufferers at 1 year: 12 month follow-up of a population-based cohort in southeast England. Stroke 25:352–357, 1994.

303. Wolfe CD, Taub NA, Bryan S, et al: Variations in the incidence, management and outcome of stroke in residents under the age of 75 in two health districts of southern England. J Pub Health Med 17:411–418, 1995.

304. Carolei A, Marini C, Di Napoli M, et al: High stroke incidence in the prospective community-based L'Aquila registry (1994–1998): First year's results. Stroke 28:2500–2506, 1997.

305. Korv J, Roose M, Haldre S, Kaasik AE: Registry of first-ever stroke in Tartu, Estonia, 1991 through 1993: Outcome of stroke. Acta Neurol Scand 99:175–181, 1999.

306. Woo J, Yuen YK, Kay R, Nicholls MG: Survival, disability, and residence 20 months after acute stroke in a Chinese population: Implications for community care. Disabil Rehabil 14:36–40, 1992.

307. Kappelle LJ, Adams HP Jr, Heffner ML, et al: Prognosis of young adults with ischemic stroke: A long-term follow-up study assessing recurrent vascular events and functional outcome in the Iowa Registry of Stroke in Young Adults. Stroke 25:1360–1365, 1994.

308. Wilkinson PR, Wolfe CD, Warburton FG, et al: A long-term follow-up of stroke patients. Stroke 28:507–512, 1997.

309. Rundek T, Boden-Alabala B, DeRosa J, et al: Functional outcome 6 months after ischemic stroke: The influence of discharge destination after acute care hospitalization. 123rd Annual Meeting of the American Neurological Association, October 18–21, 1998, Montreal, Quebec, Canada, T205:79–80, 1998.

310. World Health Organization International Classification of Impairments, Disabilities and Handicaps. Geneva, WHO, 1980.

311. Walker MF, Gladman JRF, Lincoln NB, et al: Occupational therapy for stroke patients not admitted to hospital: A randomised controlled trial. Lancet 354:278–280, 1999.

312. Jenkinson C, Mant J, Carter J, et al: The London Handicap Scale: A re-evaluation of its validity using standard scoring and simple summation. J Neurol Neurosurg Psychiatry 68:365–367, 2000.

313. Anderson CS, Taylor BV, Hankey GJ, et al: Validation of a clinical classification for subtypes of acute cerebral infarction. J Neurol Neurosurg Psychiatry 57:1173–1179, 1994.

314. Bamford J, Sandercock P, Dennis M, et al: Classification and natural history of clinically identifiable subtypes of cerebral infarction. Lancet 337:1521–1526, 1991.

315. Wolfe CD, Taub NA, Woodrow EJ, Burney PG: Assessment of scales of disability and handicap for stroke patients. Stroke 22:1242–1244, 1991.

316. Lawrence L, Christie D: Quality of life after stroke: A three year follow-up. Age Ageing 8:167–172, 1979.

317. Labi MLC, Phillips TF, Gresham GE: Psychosocial disability in physically restored long-term stroke survivors. Arch Phys Med Rehabil 61:561–565, 1980.

318. Angeleri F, Angeleri VA, Foschi N, et al: The influence of depression, social activity, and family stress on functional outcome after stroke. Stroke 24:1478–1483, 1993.

319. Kaplan RM: Health outcome models for policy analysis. Health Psychol 8:723–735, 1989.

320. Guyatt G, Feeny D, Patrick D: Measuring health-related quality of life. Ann Intern Med 118:622–629, 1993.

321. Duncan PW, Lai SM, Tyler D, et al: Evaluation of proxy responses to the Stroke Impact Scale. Stroke 33:2593–2599, 2002.

322. Bergner M, Bobbitt R, Kressel S, et al: The Sickness Impact Profile: Conceptual formulation and methodology for the development of a health status measure: Social and behavioral criteria. Int J Health Serv 6:393, 1976.

323. Ware JE, Shelbourne CD, Davies AR: The MOS 36-item short-form health survey (SPF-36). I: Conceptual framework and item selection. Med Care 30:473–483, 1992.

324. McEwen J: The Nottingham Health Profile. In Walker SR, Rosser RM (eds): Quality of Life: Assessment and Application. Lancaster, England, MTP Press, 1988, p 95.

325. EuroQOL: A new facility for the measurement of health-related quality of life. EuroQOL Group. Health Policy 16:199–208,1990.

326. Kaplan RM, Bush JW: Health-related quality of life measurement for evaluation research and policy analysis. Health Psychol 1:61–67, 1982.

327. Roberts L, Counsell C: Assessment of clinical outcomes in acute stroke trials. Stroke 29:986–991, 1998.

328. Pamela WD, Wallace D, Min Lai S, et al: The Stroke Impact Scale Version 2.0: Evaluation of reliability, validity, and sensitivity to change. Stroke 30:2131–2140, 1999.

329. Sacco RL, Boden-Albala B, Kargman DE, Gu Q: Quality of life after ischemic stroke: The Northern Manhattan Stroke Study. Ann Neurol 38:322, 1995.

330. de Haan RJ: Measuring quality of life after stroke using the SF-36. Stroke 33:1176, 2002.

331. Williams LS, Weinberger M, Harris LE, Biller J: Measuring quality of life in a way that is meaningful to stroke patients. Neurology 53:1839–1843, 1999.

332. Simon GE, Revicky DA, Grothaus L, Von Korff M: SF-36 summary scores: Are physical and mental health truly distinct? Med Care 36:567–572, 1998.

333. Wilson D, Parsons J, Tucker G: The SF-36 summary scales: Problems and solutions. Soz Praventivmed 45:239–246, 2000.

334. Taft C, Karlsson J, Sullivan M: Do SF-36 summary component scores accurately summarize subscale scores? Qual Life Res 10:395–404, 2001.

335. Van der Linden WJ, Hambleton RK: Handbook of Modern Item Response Theory. New York, Springer, 1997.

336. Fayers PM, Machin D: Quality of Life: Assessment, Analysis and Interpretation. London, John Wiley & Sons, 2000, pp 85–87.

337. Whyte EM, Mulsant BH: Post stroke depression: Epidemiology, pathophysiology, and biological treatment. Biol Psychiatry 52:253–264, 2002.

338. Burvill P, Johnson G, Jamrozik K, et al: Prevalence of depression after stroke: The Perth Community Stroke Study. Br J Psychiatry 166(3):320–327, 1995.

339. House A, Dennis M, Mogridge L, et al: Mood disorders in the year after first stroke. Br J Psychiatry 158:83–92, 1991.

340. Lenze E, Rogers J, Martire L, et al: The association of late-life depression and anxiety with physical disability: A review of the literature and prospectus for future research. Am J Geriatr Psychiatry 9:113–135, 2001.

341. Austin M, Mitchell P, Goodwin G: Cognitive deficits in depression: Possible implications for functional neuropathology. Br J Psychiatry 178:200–206, 2001.

342. Butters M, Becker J, Nebes R, et al: Changes in cognitive functioning following treatment of late-life depression. Am J Psychiatry 157:1949–1954, 2000.

343. Schulz R, Beach S, Ives D, et al: Association between depression and mortality in older adults: The Cardiovascular Health Study. Arch Intern Med 160:1761–1768, 2000.

344. Åström M, Adolfsson R, Asplund K: Major depression in stroke patients: A 3-year longitudinal study. Stroke 24:976–982, 1993.

345. Herrmann N, Black S, Lawrence J, et al: The Sunnybrook Stroke Study: A prospective study of depressive symptoms and functional outcome. Stroke 29:618–624, 1998.

346. Kauhanen M, Korpelainen J, Hiltunen P, et al: Poststroke depression correlates with cognitive impairment and neurological deficits. Stroke 30:1875–1880, 1999.

347. Pohjasvaara T, Leppavuori A, Siira I, et al: Frequency and clinical determinants of poststroke depression. Stroke 29:2311–2317, 1998.

348. Singh A, Black S, Herrmann N, et al: Functional and neuroanatomic correlations in poststroke depression: The Sunnybrook Stroke Study. Stroke 31:637–644, 2000.

349. Vataja R, Pohjasvaara T, Leppavuori A, et al: Magnetic resonance imaging correlates of depression after ischemic stroke. Arch Gen Psychiatry 58:925–931, 2001.

350. Gillen RTH, McKee TE, Gernert-Dott P, Affleck G: Depressive symptoms and history of depression predict rehabilitation efficiency in stroke patients. Arch Phys Med Rehabil 82:1645–1649, 2001.

351. Paolucci S, Antonucci G, Grasso M, et al: Post-stroke depression, antidepressant treatment and rehabilitation results: A case-control study. Cerebrovasc Dis 12:264–271, 2001.

352. Parikh R, Robinson R, Lipsey J, et al: The impact of poststroke depression on recovery in activities of daily living over a 2-year follow-up. Arch Neurol 47:785–789, 1990.

353. House A, Knapp P, Bamford J, Vial A: Mortality at 12 and 24 months after stroke may be associated with depressive symptoms at 1 month. Stroke 32:696–701, 2001.

354. Pohjasvaara T, Leppavuori A, Siira I, et al: Frequency and clinical determinants of poststroke depression. Stroke 2911:2311–2317, 1998.

355. Spitzer R, Endicott J, Robins E: Research Diagnostic Criteria (RDC) for a Group of Functional Disorders. New York, New York Psychiatric Institute, Biometrics Research Division, 1975.

356. Robinson R, Bolduc P, Price T: Two-year longitudinal study of poststroke mood disorders: Diagnosis and outcome at one and two years. Stroke 18:837–843, 1987.

357. Beblo T, Wallesch C, Herrmann M: The crucial role of frontostriatal circuits for depressive disorders in the postacute stage after stroke. Neuropsychiatry Neuropsychol Behav Neurol 12:236–246, 1999.

358. Gainotti G, Azzoni A, Marra C: Frequency, phenomenology and anatomico-clinical correlates of major post-stroke depression. Br J Psychiatry 175:163–167, 1999.

359. Katz I: Presidential address: On the inseparability of mental and physical health in aged persons: Lessons from depression and medical comorbidity. Am J Geriatr Psychiatry 4:1–16, 1996.

360. Kotila M, Numminen H, Waltimo O: Depression after stroke: Results of the FINNSTROKE study. Stroke 29:368–372, 1998.

361. Downhill J, Robinson R: Longitudinal assessment of depression and cognitive impairment following stroke. J Nerv Ment Dis 182:425–431, 1994.

362. Alexopoulos G, Meyers B, Young R: Clinically defined vascular depression. Am J Psychiatry 154:562–565, 1997.

363. de Koning I, Dippel DW, van Kooten F, Koudstaal PJ: A short screening instrument for poststroke dementia: The R-CAMCOG. Stroke 31:1502–1508, 2000.

364. Pohjasvaara T, Erkinjuntti T, Vataja R, Kaste M: Dementia three months after stroke: Baseline frequency and effect of different definitions of dementia in the Helsinki Stroke Aging Memory Study (SAM) cohort. Stroke 28:785–792, 1997.

365. Tatemichi TK, Desmond DW, Stern Y, et al: Cognitive impairment after stroke: Frequency, patterns, and relationship to functional activity. J Neurol Neurosurg Psychiatry 57:202–207, 1994.

366. Barba R, Martínez-Espinosa S, Rodríguez-García E, et al: Post stroke dementia: Clinical features and risk factors. Stroke 31:1494–1501, 2000.

367. Desmond DW, Moroney JT, Paik MC, et al: Frequency and clinical determinants of dementia after ischemic stroke. Neurology 54:1124–1131, 2000.

368. Desmond DW, Moroney JT, Sano M, Stern Y: Incidence of dementia after ischemic stroke: Results of a longitudinal study. Stroke 33:2254–2262, 2002.

369. Tatemichi TK, Paik M, Bagiella E, et al: Risk of dementia after stroke in a hospitalized cohort: Results of a longitudinal study. Neurology 44:1885–1891, 1994.

370. Merino JG: Dementia after stroke: High incidence and intriguing associations [editorial comment]. Stroke 33:2263–2264, 2002.

371. Tatemichi TK, Foulkes MA, Mohr JP, et al: Dementia in stroke survivors in the Stroke Data Bank cohort: Prevalence, incidence, risk factors, and computed tomographic findings. Stroke 21:858–866, 1990.

372. Hénon H, Durieu I, Guerouaou D, et al: Poststroke dementia: Incidence and relationship to prestroke cognitive decline. Neurology 57:1216–1222, 2001.

373. Bornstein NM, Gur AY, Treves TA, et al: Do silent brain infarctions predict the development of dementia after first ischemic stroke? Stroke 27:904–905, 1996.

374. Kokmen E, Whisnant JP, O'Fallon WM, et al: Dementia after ischemic stroke: A population-based study in Rochester, Minnesota (1960–1984). Neurology 46:154–159, 1996.

375. Zhu L, Fratiglioni L, Guo Z, et al: Incidence of dementia in relation to stroke and the apolipoprotein E ε_4 allele in the very old: Findings from a population-based longitudinal study. Stroke 31:53–60, 2000.

376. Skoog I, Nilsson L, Palmertz B, et al: A population-based study of dementia in 85-year-olds. N Engl J Med 328:153–158, 1993.

377. Brun A: Pathology and pathophysiology of cerebrovascular dementia: Pure subgroups of obstructive and hypoperfusive etiology. Dementia 5:145–147, 1994.

378. Slooter AJ, Tang MX, van Duijn C, et al: Apolipoprotein E ε_4 and the risk of dementia with stroke: a population-based investigation. JAMA 277:818–821, 1997.

379. Joutel A, Corpechot C, Ducros A, et al: Notch3 mutations in CADASIL, a hereditary adult-onset condition causing stroke and dementia. Nature 383:707–710, 1996.

Section II

Clinical Manifestations

J. P. Mohr

This section continues the attempt to cover the major syndromes of stroke, and, where possible, to point to issues of pathophysiology that bear on the diagnosis of stroke subtype, both ischemic and hemorrhagic.

The great expansion of knowledge in areas of epidemiology and risk factors has justified the subjects being treated in separate sections of the book. Despite efforts to segregate topics, there is an unavoidable degree of duplication of some of the material in the chapters on clinical manifestations by vascular territory or by mechanism and in those chapters on therapy, but, where possible, every effort has been made to keep it to a minimum.

The clinical features of many of the major stroke syndromes continue to be the foundation for the understanding of brain function, as reflected in focal small or large syndromes, so some discussion is still presented on the pathophysiologic and functional cerebral organizational insights provided by the study of these syndromes.

The advances in therapy since the last edition have also prompted a condensation of historical aspects for clinical manifestations and diagnosis. Those seeking more historical review than may be found in this edition are encouraged to seek out copies of the earlier edition of this book.

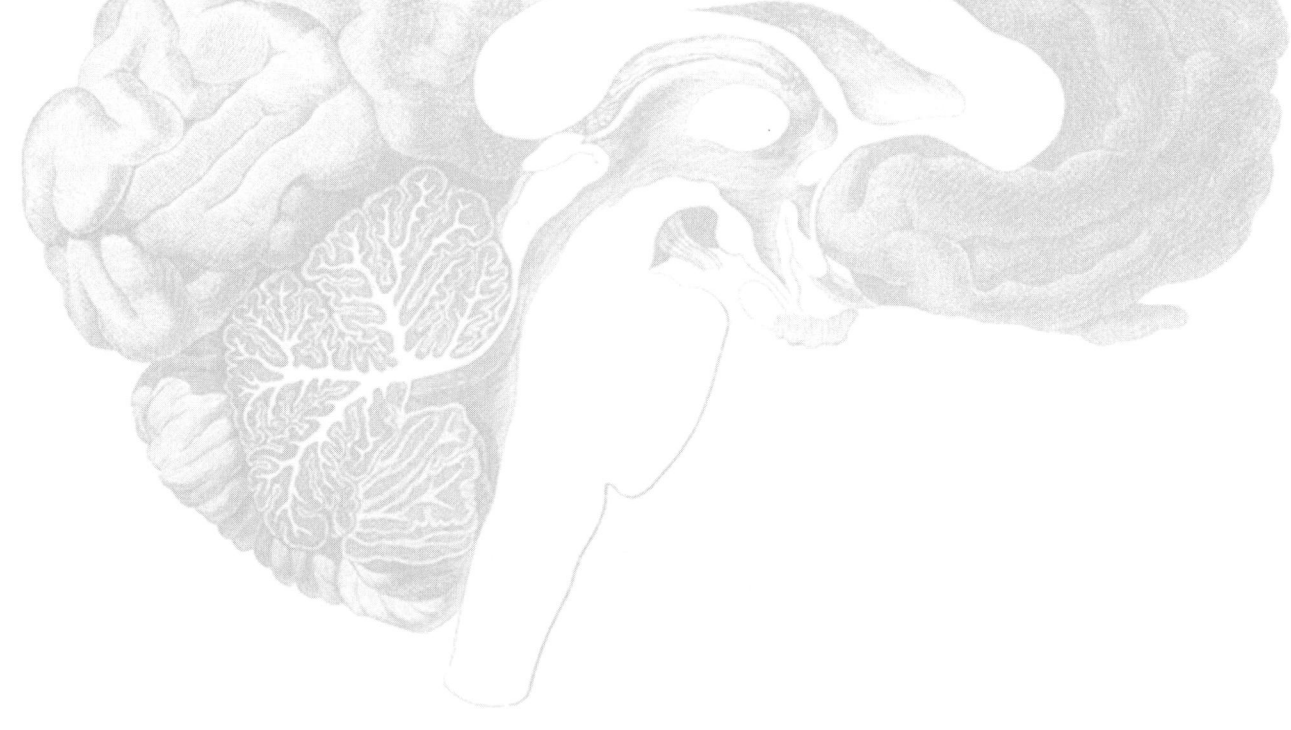

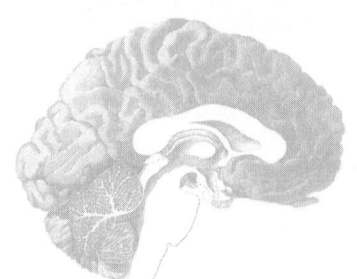

Chapter Four

Classification of Ischemic Stroke

Ralph L. Sacco, Danilo Toni, Michael Brainin, and J. P. Mohr

Since 1990, advances in imaging technologies for the brain and blood vessels have improved the diagnostic accuracy of the classification of ischemic stroke. Infarct subtype used to be determined chiefly on clinical grounds, with a heavy reliance on the clinical syndrome, neurologic findings, and coexisting risk factors. In the unfortunate patient who died, autopsy confirmation was often the basis of the classification. With the widespread application of computed tomography (CT), magnetic resonance imaging (MRI), duplex Doppler and transcranial Doppler (TCD) ultrasonography, single-photon emission computed tomography (SPECT), and other diagnostic studies, clinical impressions have been refined and supported by laboratory confirmation of the infarct subtype.

Moreover, the evolution of acute stroke therapies aimed at saving brain tissue provided the opportunity to differentiate stroke subtypes in the early hours after stroke onset, an important distinction because the treatment time window was narrow.[1] The need for early differentiation of ischemic subtypes for specific therapies is exemplified by the demonstration of the delicate balance between striking improvement and potentially disastrous hemorrhagic side effects with thrombolysis.[2-4] It has become important for the practicing physician to be able to exclude from therapy patients who have a high likelihood of spontaneous good functional recovery, such as those with some lacunar infarcts,[5-7] and to select appropriate thrombolytic approaches for patients with large artery thrombosis[8,9] and those with embolic occlusions of intracranial arteries.

FORMS OF INFARCTION: BLAND AND HEMORRHAGIC

When perfusion pressure falls to critical levels, ischemia develops, progressing to infarction if the effect persists long enough. Ischemic infarction is pathologically divided into bland infarction and hemorrhagic infarction. When the cause is thrombus, the usual occlusion persists, preventing reperfusion of the infarcted region and resulting in pale, anemic, or bland infarction.[10] In regions exposed to circulating blood, such as the edge of a bland infarct, widespread leukocyte infiltration occurs within days. For periods of up to several weeks, macrophages invade the infarct and are

active for some months until all the products of infarction are carried off. Only scattered red cells are found.

Hemorrhagic infarction, in contrast to the bland form, occurs when varying amounts of red blood cells are found among the necrotic tissues.[11,12] In some cases, the concentration of red blood cells (RBCs) is enough to make a high-density appearance consistent with blood on CT or MRI, and at autopsy, the specimen shows hemorrhagic foci ranging from a few petechiae scattered through the infarct to a mass of confluent petechial foci having almost the appearance of frank hematoma. The timing of hemorrhagic infarction varies widely, from as early as a few hours to as late as 2 weeks or more after an arterial occlusion.

The explanation for hemorrhagic infarction has long been thought to result from reperfusion of the vascular bed of the infarct after relief of the occlusion, such as would occur after fragmentation and distal migration of an embolus[13] or after early reopening of a large vessel occlusion in the setting of an established large infarction.[14,15] Presumably, the renewed pressure of arterial blood into capillaries results in a diapedesis of RBCs through their hypoxic walls. The more intense the reperfusion and the more severely damaged the capillary walls, the more confluent the hemorrhagic infarction. Assuming that hemorrhagic infarction reflects restored lumen patency, it should be a consequence of spontaneous or thrombolytic recanalization of an embolic occlusion, because the occlusion from thrombosis of an atherosclerotic stenosis would be more difficult to completely relieve. This hypothesis is supported by the greater frequency of hemorrhagic infarction found among cardioembolic infarcts.[11,16]

The simple explanation for hemorrhagic infarction previously given has been challenged by observations made by investigators using third-generation CT devices[17,18] and MRI.[19] These researchers have demonstrated that hemorrhagic infarction may frequently develop distal to the site of a persisting occlusion in the arterial bed exposed at best only to retrograde collaterals.[20,21] The severity of the hemorrhagic focus may differ from the more or less extended hematoma observed as a consequence of large artery recanalization. In these former cases, the occurrence of petechial, scattered hemorrhagic infarction may be related to surges in arterial blood pressure and the suddenness, severity, and size of the infarction.[11,18,21] It is presumed that edema initially surrounds the large infarct and compresses pial vessels. As edema subsides, retrograde reperfusion through pial collaterals ensues, leading to petechial hemorrhagic infarction.[17,18]

PROBLEMS IN THE DIAGNOSIS OF INFARCTION

Before modern neuroimaging was routinely available, many physicians persisted in believing that a definitive diagnosis as to stroke mechanism was merely a technical problem awaiting the proper laboratory procedures. In most circumstances the clinical features and CT or MRI findings suffice to differentiate acute intracerebral hemorrhage from infarction within the first hours after stroke onset. Clinical scores that have been developed to help differentiate infarct from hemorrhage rely on decreased consciousness, headache, and nausea and vomiting as predictors of hemorrhage.[22–26] The current utility of such scales would be to improve diagnoses in studies with no access to CT or to help with early mobilization of stroke teams who are alerted by emergency room personnel of a potential high-probability infarction case. Because small, deep, or lobar hematomas can manifest as circumscribed focal deficits and can easily lead those relying on the clinical syndrome alone to diagnose infarction mistakenly, these scores can never be used to make a definitive diagnosis. The advent of CT and MRI has led to the correction of these potential misdiagnoses, resulting in a greater proportion of hemorrhages in stroke series[27] and eliminating the inadvertent use of anticoagulation in the case of a "masquerading" hemorrhage.[28]

The use of CT, MRI, noninvasive vascular imaging, and angiography has greatly improved our ability to diagnose ischemic stroke but has still left large issues unresolved. Ischemic strokes can now be classified into subtype well enough to justify management decisions, but the classification is far from precise. Clinical grounds alone, with the use of age, risk factors, and so forth, have been the time-honored means of determining the subtype of infarction, such as separating embolism from thrombosis. However, it is often difficult to classify patients by different mechanism of cerebral infarction on clinical criteria alone. A thorough diagnostic evaluation is required, because the presenting clinical syndromes are usually not distinctive enough to enable one to infer the cause. This is even more apparent in the acute setting, in which the common cognitive impairment, agitation, and poor cooperation of patients may hinder a thorough assessment of neurologic functions.

Even when strenuous efforts are made to establish the exact mechanism of infarction, the problem remains difficult. Duplex Doppler ultrasonography, MR angiography (MRA), and conventional angiography often fail to show either the expected arterial stenosis or occlusion; also, when a significant carotid stenosis is found, judging whether the clinical syndrome arose from an embolic or hemodynamic mechanism is often difficult.[29] The findings of brain imaging performed during the acute stage may suggest an occlusion of the middle cerebral artery (MCA), on the basis of the detection of a high-attenuation spot along the course of the artery, a finding in 30% to 50% of

patients with angiographically proven arterial occlusion; such findings do not always settle the problem of the underlying mechanism. The identification of early signs of parenchymal damage and brain edema, proved to be useful as a prognostic index,[2,30–33] is not that helpful in the differentiation of ischemic pathogenetic mechanisms.

Few studies have collected detailed information on the clinical and radiologic characteristics of large homogeneous subsets of patients with acute cerebral infarction. The Stroke Data Bank, created by the National Institute of Neurological Diseases and Stroke (NINDS), provided a large collection of prospectively collected information on patients with different subtypes of infarction.[34] A deliberate attempt was made to classify patients into distinct categories and to create new subsets on the basis of the presumed mechanism of infarction. This effort resulted in some changes in the large categories of stroke due to infarction. In particular, the atherothrombosis category was divided into two subgroups: large artery thrombosis with no evidence of embolic infarction and a form of artery-to-artery embolism arising from an atherosclerotic source. A separate category, infarct of undetermined cause, was created to help ensure the homogeneity of the Stroke Data Bank diagnostic groups (Fig. 4–1).

Efforts to establish the diagnosis for the subtype of infarction proved remarkably difficult in a disappointingly high percentage of cases.[35] Despite efforts to arrive at the diagnosis with CT scan or angiogram, it was apparent that the basis for the diagnosis in many of the cases was still a best clinical guess. When laboratory data were available, the results indicated that large artery atherosclerotic occlusive disease was a less common cause of stroke; that small vessel or lacunar and cardioembolic infarctions were relatively common; and that the cause of most cases of infarction could not be classified into these traditional diagnostic categories. The high frequency of surface infarcts in the setting of a normal or distal branch arterial occlusion led most investigators to regard these unexplained cerebral infarcts as examples of embolism with an undetected

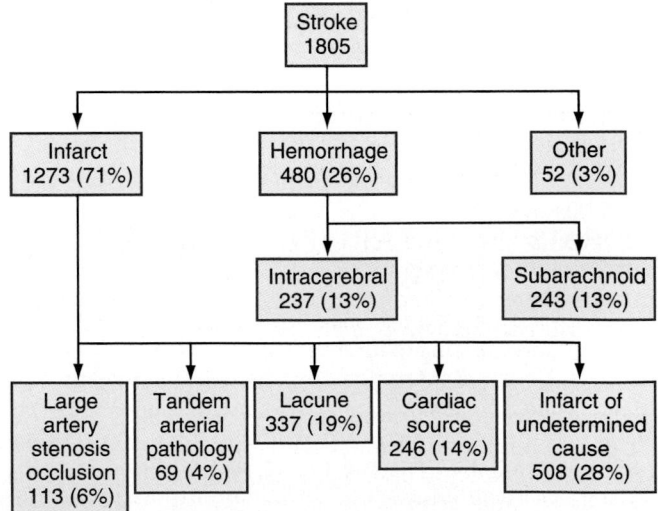

FIGURE 4–1 *Classification of stroke based on data from the NINDS Stroke Data Bank (1983–1986).*

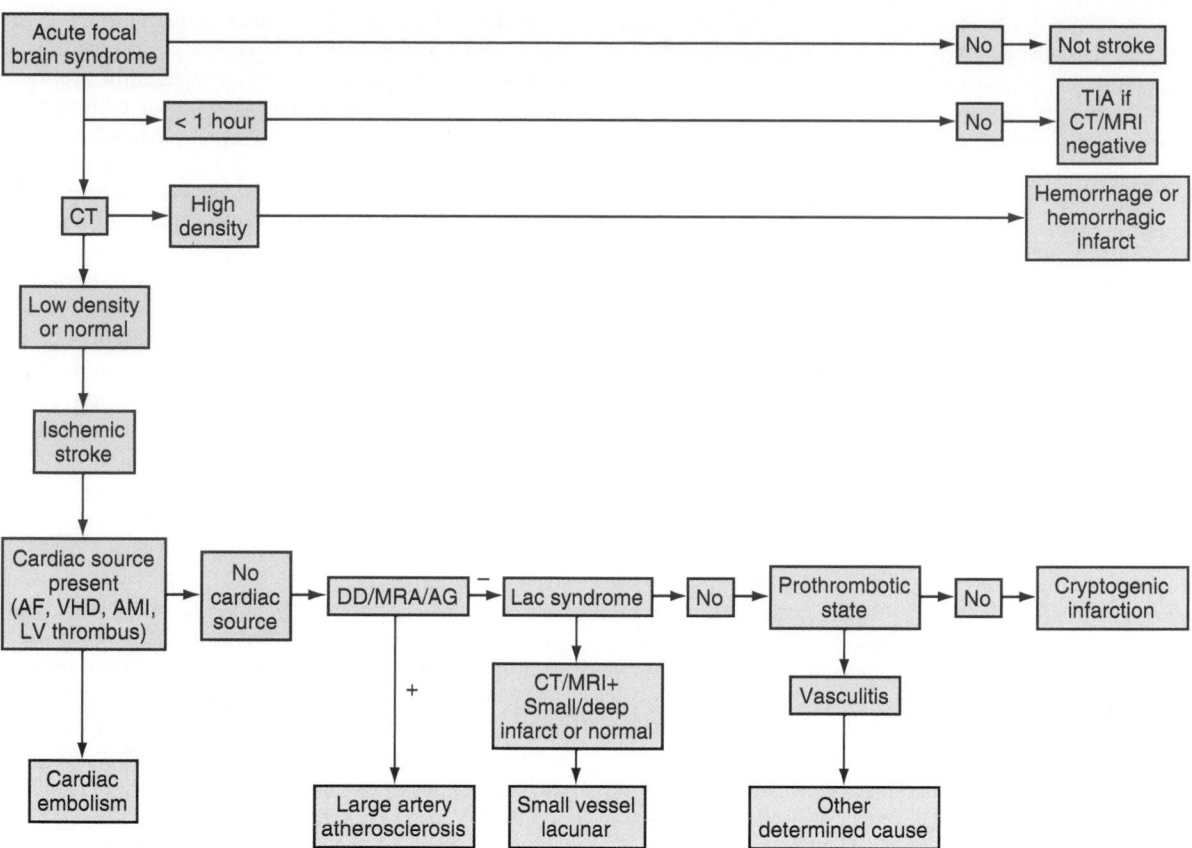

FIGURE 4–2 *Stroke diagnostic algorithm. AF, atrial fibrillation; AG, cerebral angiogram; AMI, acute myocardial infarction; DD, duplex and transcranial Doppler; lac syndrome, currently described classic lacunar syndromes, possibly including other syndromes from focal-deep infarction (e.g., cognitive changes from thalamic or caudate infarcts); LV, left ventricular; MRA, magnetic resonance angiography; TIA, transient ischemic attack; VHD, valvular heart disease.*

thrombotic source.[36] In the Stroke Data Bank, a separate diagnostic category was created for cases with unproven mechanisms of infarction: infarct of undetermined cause or cryptogenic infarction. Apart from a few common features, infarctions in this category are still poorly understood and have not yet been successfully characterized as a clinical group (Fig. 4–2).

SUBTYPES OF ISCHEMIC STROKE

Infarct with Large Artery Thrombosis

The classification of a stroke with an infarction due to large artery thrombosis was sometimes a diagnosis of exclusion in the days of less sophisticated laboratory investigations. Strokes were classified into one of three major diagnostic categories, as follows: hemorrhage if the spinal fluid was bloody, embolism if atrial fibrillation or rheumatic heart disease was present, and thrombosis if none of the foregoing was present. Syndromes previously attributed to large artery atherosclerosis, when more closely evaluated with current technology, have been reclassified. The gradual decline in large artery thrombosis as a leading diagnosis has resulted from several factors. Among the most important are the more frequent use of duplex or TCD ultrasonography in the pursuit of stroke diagnosis; the

recognition of several clinical subtypes of thrombosis, especially lacunes[5,37–39]; documentation proving that some ischemic strokes associated with large artery atherothrombosis are produced by artery-to-artery embolism (local embolism)[36,40–46]; and discontinuation of the casual classification of a stroke as atherothrombotic in favor of the additional category "undetermined."[35,47–50]

Many of the descriptions leading to the definition of this subtype stem from pathologic studies of the past.[51] Atherosclerotic lesions were found at bifurcations and curves of the larger vessels; the more proximal the location in the vascular tree, the more severe the atherosclerotic lesions.[52,53] Primary occlusion of the arteries distally located over the cerebral surface was rare.[54,55] Atherosclerotic plaque usually led to progressive stenosis, with the final large artery occlusion being due to thrombosis of the narrowed lumen. Intraplaque hemorrhage sometimes led to accelerated occlusion,[56] although the frequency of this condition is more often a matter of speculation rather than confirmed in pathologic specimens.[57,58] The possibility of achieving an in vivo characterization of the carotid plaque with MRI has been suggested[59] but needs further confirmation.

Infarct Mechanism: Perfusion Failure

Stroke in the patient with atherothrombus was initially attributed to perfusion failure distal to the site of severe stenosis or occlusion of the major vessel.[55,60,61] In some instances, the major vessel occlusion was rather proximal in the arterial tree, and some degree of collateral flow was interposed between the occlusion and the cerebral territory at risk of infarction.[62] Some cases with interposed collateral were spared infarction of any kind, whereas in others the infarct was located mainly along the most distal brain regions originally supplied by the occluded vessel.[45,55,61,63–65] In the carotid territory, these regions were the suprasylvian frontal, central, and parietal portions of the hemisphere, and in the vertebrobasilar territory, they were the bilateral occipital poles. Internal borderzone regions have also been postulated as existing in the white matter of the corona radiata supplied by both superficial MCA pial penetrators and lenticulostriate arteries.

The usually accepted mechanism of perfusion failure is more readily accepted in occlusive disease but becomes more difficult to define when, instead, the extracranial vessel is patent but highly stenotic. Some positron emission tomography–based studies have not found supportive evidence for selective hemodynamic impairment among patients with transient ischemic attacks (TIAs) and severe carotid stenosis.[29,66] The development of borderzone ischemia probably depends on multiple factors, not just on the severity of stenosis.[14,65,67]

Infarct Mechanism: Artery-to-Artery Embolism

In addition to vascular occlusion at the site of atherosclerosis, infarcts are produced by emboli arising from atheromatous lesions situated proximally to otherwise healthy branches located more distal in the arterial tree.[41] Embolic fragments may arise from extracranial arteries affected by stenosis or ulcer,[9,45,68–70] stenosis of any major cerebral artery stem,[43,71,72] or the basilar artery[73]; from the stump of the occluded internal carotid artery (ICA)[74]; and even from the intracranial tail of the anterograde thrombus atop an occluded carotid.[46,75] Nowadays embolism from a carotid source has become recognized as another, perhaps more common, cause of stroke in a setting of arterial stenosis and even occlusion.[36,40,42] In the Stroke Data Bank, this mechanism of infarction was labeled "tandem arterial pathology." In later stroke series, borderzone infarcts appear to be less common than previously thought, leading to the presumption that embolism was the actual mechanism even in the presence of ICA tight stenoses or occlusions. To add to the difficulty in distinguishing between these two mechanisms of infarction, cases of perfusion failure due to embolism have been demonstrated. Internal borderzone infarcts have been demonstrated after embolic occlusion of MCA pial branches.[76] This finding may be an example of an embolic stroke with a possible local hemodynamic effect as the final mechanism of the infarct.

Clinical Features

Focal cortical syndromes are usually found in patients with large artery thrombosis, but syndromes often attributed to lacunar disease, such as pure motor or sensorimotor stroke, can easily represent the first sign of impending flow failure.[31] Discriminating among infarct subtypes on clinical grounds alone is difficult. To determine some of these distinguishing clinical features in the Stroke Data Bank, investigators compared demographic, stroke risk,

clinical, and radiologic features for 246 cardioembolic cerebral infarcts and 113 large vessel atherosclerotic cerebral infarcts.[77] The Stroke Data Bank definitions ensured more TIAs in atherosclerotic infarcts and more cardiac disease in cardioembolic infarcts, but the diagnosis was distinguished further. Cases with fractional arm weakness (shoulder different from the hand), hypertension, diabetes, and male gender occurred more frequently with atherosclerotic than with cardioembolic infarcts. Patients with atherosclerotic infarcts were more likely to have a fractional arm weakness regardless of infarct size.

Distinguishing between the infarct mechanisms (hemodynamic versus embolism) in patients with large artery disease is quite difficult even for the most astute clinician. The sudden mode of onset may suggest, but does not confirm, a diagnosis of embolism.[78] Other clinical features may not enable such a distinction. Moreover, it is even more difficult to discriminate between emboli from a cardiac source and those from an arterial source. Comparisons in the NINDS Stroke Data Bank between the 246 patients with cardioembolic cerebral infarction and the 66 patients with arterial embolic cerebral infarction demonstrated some differences.[30] Even after the data were controlled for differences in the frequency of cardiac disease, TIAs, and carotid bruits, the probability of an artery-to-artery embolism was increased by the finding of a superficial infarct alone or by a higher hematocrit value. The probability of cardiac embolism was greater for patients who initially had decreased consciousness or for whom findings on first CT were abnormal. These findings suggested that these two embolic infarct subtypes differed as to the location and extent of the cortical infarction. Smaller and more distal infarction in embolism from an arterial source compared with cardiogenic embolism suggested a smaller embolic particle size. Clinical features observed at stroke onset can help distinguish cerebral infarction subtypes but are not reliable enough to lead to a definite determination of infarct subtype without confirmatory laboratory data.

Results of Diagnostic Tests
Brain Imaging

The only abnormalities on MRI or CT that are directly attributable to cerebral infarction from carotid artery thrombosis are those that can be interpreted to reflect the distal field effect along the borderzone between middle and anterior cerebral territories, especially on the middle cerebral side.[45,55,60,79] This topographic pattern involves the suprasylvian frontal and central regions, shading toward normal in the parieto-occipital region, sparing the region of the sylvian fissure (operculum, insula) and the penetrating territories of the lenticulostriates. The centripetal spread in more severe cases may involve so much of the hemisphere that a differentiation from embolism to the MCA stem is impossible.

CT and MRI are of help in supporting a diagnosis of embolism when (1) an infarct in the territories of large cerebral arteries or their branches is detected,[80] (2) a hyperdense spot along the course of the MCA is seen,[63] or (3) a scattered infarct pattern is seen on diffusion-weighted MRI.[81,82] However, none of the mentioned imaging techniques is of help in inferring embolism source from the neck. When occlusions involve the territories of the anterior, middle, or posterior cerebral artery or the basilar artery, brain imaging cannot distinguish between thrombosis and embolism if the scan or image shows low density only in the proximal fields of the arterial territory.

Vascular Imaging

In the clinical setting, for a diagnosis of large artery atherosclerotic occlusive disease, angiography and Doppler ultrasonography remain the most important laboratory tests. On conventional cerebral angiogram, the occlusion of the ICA at its origin or in the siphon has the appearance of a pencil point, blunt end, smooth end, or shoulder, with the intracranial portion of the internal carotid or major cerebral artery stems and branches open.[83] Spiral occlusions of the extracranial portion of the internal carotid beyond 2 cm of its origin (a finding consistent with dissection)[84] helps to indicate that the carotid lesion may be the source of the stroke, but not by means of atherosclerosis. Because of the risks of cerebral angiography,[85–87] there has been increased reliance on duplex Doppler and TCD ultrasonography techniques to show no or highly resistant flow in the extracranial carotid with dampened pulsatility in the ipsilateral MCA.[86,88–93] MRA and CT angiography are quickly becoming reliable diagnostic tools for the detection of extracranial and intracranial large artery stenosis,[94] leading to less reliance on conventional angiography.[43]

No satisfactory criteria have yet been developed to certify that a stroke is caused by extracranial arterial disease through the mechanism of embolism. The mechanism is inferred when the clinical syndrome suggests a cortical branch territory; when no obvious cardioembolic source is present and the extent of stenosis is less than 80% (which would not explain the stroke on the grounds of hemodynamic insufficiency); or when ulcerative plaque is imaged by noninvasive duplex Doppler ultrasonography, MRA, or cerebral angiogram.

On the other hand, angiographic evidence of intracranial occlusion above a carotid stenosis or ulcer is not proof of the source, but when present, it serves to classify this type of stroke into the present category.[62] The frequency of occurrence of embolism of particles large enough to cause stroke and the variety or severity of carotid lesions giving rise to such embolization remain poorly understood. In a continuous series of patients who underwent angiography within the first 6 hours of stroke onset,[36] MCA stem or branch occlusion accounted for 60% of the cases. Possible embolic sources included carotid plaque (19%), an occlusion of the ipsilateral ICA (14%), and a potential source of emboli both arterial and cardiac (27%). Conversely, 58% of patients with ICA occlusion had a tandem MCA occlusion. Despite a normal intracranial arterial tree, the remainder had a territorial infarct on CT, a finding that implied that an artery-to-artery embolism occurred with embolus fragmentation preceding angiography.

Intracranial atherosclerotic artery stem stenoses or occlusions may be due to arteriosclerotic thrombosis but are often difficult to distinguish from emboli of any extracerebral source.[95–97] If one or more appropriate TIAs occurred within the past 30 days, the diagnosis of thrombus may be correct, but the matter can be settled only if a widely patent lumen is subsequently found by serial TCD ultrasonography evaluations or a second angiogram.[98] The latter is diagnostic of embolism, whereas persistence of the occlusion leaves the mechanism unsettled.

Basilar occlusion on angiogram is usually considered the mechanism for brainstem stroke even though in many such cases the clinical syndrome fits the criteria for lacune,[73,99–101] because the territory of infarction, however small, is in the field of supply of a vessel thrombosed by the major basilar atheroma.[102] As for the carotid artery, the finding of stenosis of the basilar artery prevents a definite diagnosis as to the mechanism of infarction, because infarcts more distal in the vertebrobasilar territory might well be the result of distal embolization.[95] Atheromatous disease of the basilar artery often affects the vessel at sites where local branches directly supply brain tissue.[102,103] In the carotid artery, the atheroma involves the vessel proximal to the point where its branches supply the brain.[53] When the clinical syndrome of basilar stroke can be localized to the point of the stenosis, infarction may be caused by mural atheroma that only slightly stenoses the basilar artery but totally occludes a small penetrator departing from the basilar artery at that location. This point, established in a few instances by autopsy, can only be inferred in cases studied by angiogram; CT scanning is usually not of technically high enough quality to detect the small brainstem infarcts. However, MRI has defined the lesion and permitted better delineation of such cases.

Blood flow techniques have also helped confirm the perfusion failure mechanism in patients with atherosclerotic stenosis or occlusive disease through SPECT,[104] xenon-enhanced CT,[105] regional cerebral blood flow measurements,[21] MRI,[106–108] and positron emission tomography.[29,109,110] The more widespread use of these techniques should allow for more accurate distinction between embolism and perfusion failure in the clinical setting.

Embolism Attributed to Cardiac Sources

Embolism from any source probably accounts for between 15% and 70% of all cases of ischemic stroke,[34,36,44,49,50,111] many of which occur from embolism into the territory of the MCA. Although the subject of embolism seems clear enough, in that a particle is swept through the blood stream until it jams in an artery too small to allow it to pass, the many complexities of the embolic process make it anything but easy to account for on a case-by-case basis.

The biggest clinical problem in arriving at a diagnosis of embolism is identifying the source. Embolism was diagnosed in earlier studies mainly when a cardiac source (atrial fibrillation with valvular disease) was obvious.[51] The results of later studies have shown that emboli, diagnosed angiographically from isolated branch occlusions, may occur despite all efforts to identify the source.[36,50,112,113] Given the many possibilities and given the traditional use of the term *embolism* to refer to a cardiac source,[114–117] the following discussion is limited to that subject.

Properties of Emboli

The instability of the embolic material is a point of prime importance in clinical and angiographic analysis of cases of embolism. Mural thrombi and platelet aggregates are the materials most commonly embolized to the brain. These materials are remarkably evanescent, as has been repeatedly inferred from findings on angiogram. Embolic fragments are found in more than 75% of cases studied by angiography within 8 hours of onset of the stroke,[36,118,119] whereas embolism is demonstrated in 40% of clinically identical cases in which angiogram is delayed for up to 72 hours after clinical onset of the stroke,[120] and in only 15% of cases studied more than 72 hours after onset. These decreasing proportions imply that embolic occlusions are liable to spontaneous recanalization in a sizable number of cases. Serial studies with TCD ultrasonography demonstrated a recanalization of MCA main-stem or branch occlusions in up to 52% of cases within the first 48 hours of stroke.[121–123] Second angiographic evaluations, performed in subsets of patients in whom arterial occlusion was demonstrated by an earlier angiogram, showed recanalization in 30% to 60% of cases.[36,98]

No reliable means have been developed thus far to identify which embolic occlusions will persist and which will disappear, although it is inferred that the more friable materials will disperse more rapidly. In one of the TCD ultrasonography studies mentioned, patients with an arterial source of emboli experienced recanalization of the vessel less commonly than those with a cardiac source, suggesting a different composition or size of emboli.[122] The size of the emboli is also probably responsible, at least in part, for the highest frequency of both spontaneous[122,123] and pharmacologic[8,124–126] recanalization in cases of distal MCA occlusion.

This evanescent quality of embolic material may explain the wide variation in the frequency with which embolism is diagnosed in retrospective or prospective studies of stroke. The size of the material embolized determines the site at which it initially comes to rest in the circulation but does not determine its final point of arrest. Embolic material stops where the lumen diameter is too small to permit it to pass. Bifurcations or foci of atheroma at curves in the artery are the two sites where emboli arrest. Fibrin-platelet complexes and those also laden with bacteria vary considerably in size; some are so huge that they have obstructed the stem of the MCA,[127] and others have been so small they have lodged asymptomatically in a sensitive region such as the rolandic branch of the MCA. Calcific plaques have only rarely been described as producing large embolic strokes[69,128]; more often, they seem to produce TIAs but not persisting cerebral deficits.[68] For noncompressible objects such as shotgun pellets, the site of embolus can easily be predicted from its size.[121] For the more common fibrin-platelet complexes, however, other factors are involved, especially the poorly understood compressibility of the mass and the time required to transit a certain point of narrowing in the arterial tree. The few cases that document the passage of fibrin-platelet emboli through the arterial tree[129] show considerable alteration in the length and width of the material at different points, indicating that it possesses a remarkable elasticity and friability. What is sufficient lumen reduction to arrest the material may not be enough to keep it from changing shape or fragmenting within minutes to hours, leaving the site of the original embolic occlusion widely patent.

Embolic obstruction of an arterial lumen is most commonly cleared by recanalization with fibrinolysis. A column of blood develops between the embolus and the arterial wall, enlarges, and erodes the embolus until the lumen is finally cleared. The exact sequence of events is not fully understood in human material, but cases documented at different stages during the process make it clear that recanalization is accomplished within periods as short as hours to days.[125,128,129] The timetable for this process is also poorly understood. In some instances, the erosion takes enough time that noninvasive studies may document stenoses that create turbulences identical to those seen with atheroma. The angiographic appearance of the gradually eroding embolus is indistinguishable from that of atherostenosis. During this process, the lumen may appear stenotic.[130,131]

At the site of occlusion, opportunity exists for thrombus to develop in anterograde fashion throughout the length of the vessel, but this event seems to occur only rarely. Lack of anterograde thrombus implies either that an active flow is present proximal to the occlusion or that the occlusion was too short-lived to permit the development of the anterograde thrombus. At autopsy it is common to find the vessel distended by the embolus, yet the histologic appearance of the wall at that point usually shows no significant abnormalities. The frequent finding that the vessel wall itself is not significantly injured by the embolus argues against a role for endothelial injury, vasospasm, or necrotizing effects in the pathogenesis of the infarction from embolism.

Clinical Features

It was once taught that the sudden onset of a clinical deficit was typical of embolism and that a non-sudden onset would be more typical of thrombosis. Numerous case examples have now amply demonstrated that onset may be sudden in either condition. Non-sudden or fluctuating onset occurs in 5% to 6% of documented embolic strokes, the syndrome often requiring 36 hours or so to evolve.[55,132] A clinical diagnosis of multiple TIAs is often entertained. The reestablishment of flow, presumed further migration of embolic material, and subsequent repeat of these events are thought to be the mechanisms involved. Embolic material has even been documented to go to the same site on repeated occasions,[133] the opposite of traditional predictions.

In the past, many syndromes were considered almost specific for embolism. In each of these syndromes, it was assumed that the infarct was so focal and so far distal in the arterial tree that local atheroma was not a serious possibility. Hemianopia without hemiparesis or hemisensory disturbances, Wernicke's aphasia, ideomotor apraxia, and involvement of specific territories (the posterior division of the MCA, the anterior cerebral artery, the cerebellum, multiple territories) were more commonly associated with the presence of a potential cardiac source of embolism in the Lausanne Stroke Registry.[16] CT and MRI have shown that any of these syndromes may arise from hematoma, and modern neurologists have become wary of administering anticoagulation therapy on the basis of clinical syndrome analysis alone.

One syndrome seems to have held its own as a sign of embolism, although it is met only rarely. A spectacular shrinking deficit can occur when the embolus is introduced into the internal carotid artery, causing a profound full hemispheral syndrome, after which it passes up the artery to its final resting place in, say, the angular branch of the MCA, leaving only a mild aphasia after a few days or a week.[134] Especially characteristic of the MCA migratory embolism is the syndrome of fading hemiparesis with Wernicke's aphasia: The embolus lodges initially at the stem of the MCA, occluding the penetrating lenticulostriate branches long enough to produce scattered foci of infarction through the basal ganglia and internal capsule, the involvement of the latter producing the hemiparesis. Distal migration of the embolus then occurs, finally occluding the lower division of the MCA at the superior temporal plane and beyond. This infarct yields Wernicke's aphasia. Two separate foci of infarction occur, but they result from the same embolic event.

The cardiac history of the patient often provides important clues about a potential embolic source. In the Stroke Data Bank, besides a greater frequency of cardiac disease, patients with cardioembolic infarction more often presented with reduced consciousness.[30,77] Cardioembolic infarcts were more likely to have nonfractional arm weakness, except for those with infarctions smaller than 20 mL, in which fractional weakness was more common. In a separate Stroke Data Bank analysis, a history of systemic embolism and an abrupt onset were historical features significantly associated with cardiac sources of embolism.[135] Clinical features observed at stroke onset help distinguish the cardioembolic group from other subtypes, but the diagnosis largely depends on confirmatory laboratory findings that suggest a definite cardiac source of embolism.[136]

Results of Diagnostic Tests

The role of CT and MRI in the diagnosis of embolism is limited. Only when the infarction is confined to the cerebral surface territory of a single branch can embolism be inferred from a scan or image. Infarcts involving branches of different divisions of major cerebral arteries strongly suggest that embolism explains at least some of the clinical strokes that have occurred. A diagnosis of embolism is suggested by a large zone of low density that encompasses what amounts to the entire territory of a major cerebral artery or its main divisions and is larger than one lobe. Embolism is also the leading diagnosis when hemorrhagic infarction is seen on brain imaging.[11,16] As already mentioned, this assumption is plausible in the presence of a more or less extended hematoma, but it may not be true for other cases displaying petechial, scattered high density along the margins or in the infarct zone.[17,18] In some 30% to 50% of cases, the CT scan (or MRI) may show the occlusion itself, as the presence of the hyperdense MCA sign. Finally, as mentioned previously, a scattered infarct pattern on diffusion-weighted MRI may suggest embolism from whatever source.[81,82]

Angiography was once considered sufficient to diagnose embolism from any source if the angiogram showed branch occlusion in the absence of other occlusive disease elsewhere.[98,137,138] This rule still holds for practical purposes, but isolated branch occlusions may occur in arteritis, and growing evidence shows that intracranial atherosclerosis is common enough in some races, especially blacks, that

MCA stem occlusions may be atheromatous as well as embolic. Recanalizing embolus may mimic all the angiographic features of atherosclerosis.[130] Only when a second angiogram is performed within days of the angiogram demonstrating occlusion, and the initial occlusion is gone, can a diagnosis of embolism be made with confidence. Measures this extreme are impractical for the management of most patients.

In the presence of a cardiac source of embolism, the diagnosis is certain for all practical purposes. Establishing the cardiac source is not always a simple task. The most common sources of cardiac embolism are (1) valvular heart disease (mitral stenosis, mitral regurgitation, rheumatic heart disease); (2) intracardiac thrombus, particularly along the left ventricular wall (mural thrombus), after anterior myocardial infarction, or in the left atrial appendage in patients with atrial fibrillation; (3) ventricular or septal aneurysm; and (4) cardiomyopathies leading to stagnation of blood flow and a greater propensity for the formation of intracardiac thrombus. A paradoxical embolus occurs when a thrombus crosses from the venous circulation to the left side of the heart, most often through a patent foramen ovale. Other possible causes of cardiac embolism are atrial myxoma, atrial septal aneurysm, spontaneous echo contrast, marantic endocarditis, and prolapse of the mitral valve. Finally, aortic arch plaques, particularly when they protrude and are complicated, have been identified as potentially active sources of emboli.[139,140–142]

The cardiac diagnostic evaluation starts with an electrocardiogram to look for atrial fibrillation, acute myocardial infarction, or other arrhythmias. Holter monitoring for 24 hours is sometimes necessary to detect paroxysmal atrial fibrillation. Identification of the cardiac source depends most on transthoracic and transesophageal echocardiography, which has become more sensitive and has greatly improved the detection of sources of embolism. Bubble contrast is needed to diagnose a patent foramen ovale. Unfortunately, embolic material large enough to produce a focal stroke is so small that it may escape detection by echocardiography and all too often eludes all efforts at diagnosis. Future advances in cardiac imaging may help improve sensitivity for detecting cardiac sources of embolism.

Lacunar Infarction

Cases of lacunar infarction represent a special group that warrants description because they often occur as a common set of clinical syndromes, angiographic findings are usually normal, and the zone of ischemia is confined to the territory of a single vessel, usually quite small. Lacunar infarctions are understood to reflect arterial disease of the vessels penetrating the brain to supply the capsule, basal ganglia, thalamus, and paramedian regions of the brainstem.[143] Only a handful have been studied by autopsy, and an even smaller number have been subjected to serial section.[144] The most common lesion is a tiny focus of microatheroma or lipohyalinosis stenosing one of the deep penetrating arteries. Less frequent causes are stenosis of the MCA stem[10,145] and microembolization to penetrant arterial territories.[144]

Histopathologic studies have rarely included patients with lacunar strokes, because the in-hospital mortality of such patients is the lowest for all those with ischemic stroke. In one stroke registry, the in-hospital mortality for lacunar cases was only 2.9%.[146] A serial study of 100 autopsy cases with acute ischemic strokes has shown that hypoperfusion is an underestimated mechanism and was considered to be a definite cause of the infarct in 5 cases, whereas atheromatous causes were found in 10 cases. All infarcts were more than 10 mm in diameter, and no "classic" lacunes were seen as the corresponding infarcts, probably owing to the selection of cases reaching autopsy.[147] One single autopsied case study has shown a thrombus formation in the MCA as a convincing cause of striatocapsular infarction.[148]

Multiple infarcts in the centrum semiovale are rarely of lacunar origin, even if they do not exceed 1.5 cm in diameter. Mostly they represent consequences of hemodynamic failure, and have been described to have a rosary-like appearance. For example, in an MRI study of 16 patients, centrum semiovale infarcts were thought to be caused by occluded or highly stenosed carotid vessels on the ipsilateral side.[149] One other pathologic study of centrum semiovale infarcts showed that in 10 of 12 consecutive cases, the underlying mechanism was thought to be either cardiogenic or due to large vessel disease.[150]

Because of the lack of autopsy data demonstrating lacunes, detailed MRI investigations have been undertaken. In one such study of nine patients with lacunar syndrome, the occluded perforator was visualized together with leaks of blood and fluid in the perivascular space.[151]

Investigators have used the term *lacunar hypothesis* to refer to the clinicopathophysiologic correlation of the condition. The hypothesis consists of two parts: (1) symptomatic lacunes are usually present with a small number of distinct lacunar syndromes and (2) lacunes are caused by a characteristic disease of the penetrating artery.[37] After satisfying both parts of the hypothesis, the stroke can be classified as a lacunar infarction. Lacunes were slow to gain clinical acceptance, but they are now considered to account for between 15% and 20% of all cases of stroke.[5,34,48,49,64,152]

Clinical Features

The diagnosis of lacunar strokes has long been based on clinical characteristics alone, a practice that has contributed little to their popularity among clinical researchers in the field. The term *lacunar syndrome* refers to the constellation of clinical features that may indicate, although not invariably, a lacune. The characteristic features of all these syndromes are their relative purity and their failure to involve higher cerebral functions such as language, praxis, behavior controlled by the nondominant hemisphere, memory, and vision.[153] The classic lacunar syndromes include pure motor, pure sensory, and sensorimotor syndromes; ataxic hemiparesis; clumsy hand dysarthria; and hemichorea/hemiballism. However, other combinations of findings may be attributed to small, deep infarcts due to a lacunar mechanism. Efforts to expand the diagnosis into new formulas that account for the presence of cognitive changes have shaken the earlier purity and confounded the appealing simplicity of the initial syndromes,[154] leading some to question the separate nosologic identity of lacunar infarcts.[155,156] Some skeptics have

suggested the abolition of terms like "lacunar syndrome," "lacune," and "lacunar infarction" because of confusion. However, most of the investigations that have included analyses of clinical syndromes, results of diagnostic imaging, etiopathophysiologic correlations, and treatment implications justify the continued use of the term *lacune*.

The correspondence between lacunar syndrome and lacunar infarction depends on the timing of presentation and examination. The concordance is greatest among patients examined up to 96 hours after stroke onset[37,157] and is much less when patients are tested in the first few hours of stroke onset.[40,44,158,159]

There are clearly examples of thrombotic or embolic infarcts manifesting as pure motor hemiparesis or sensorimotor stroke, and, conversely, large lacunar infarcts in the caudate nucleus or thalamus that may initially manifest as impairment of higher cerebral functions. The latter syndromes are probably due to a reversible functional disconnection between the subcortical infarcted areas and their cortical projections.[160,161] In the acute setting, therefore, the reliance on clinical grounds alone for the identification of lacunar infarcts can be misleading for both prognostic estimates and therapeutic choices.[7]

Using data from the Northern Manhattan Stroke Study, Gan and colleagues[162] were able to evaluate the value of lacunar syndromes in predicting radiologic lacunes as well as the value of clinicoradiologic lacunes in predicting lacunar infarction as a final stroke mechanism. Lacunar syndromes were found in 225 of 591 patients, and the proportions of lacunar infarction in blacks and Hispanics were nearly twice that in white patients. The positive predictive value for finding a small, deep infarct on brain imaging after a presenting lacunar syndrome was 87% and was best for pure sensory syndrome (100%) and ataxic hemiparesis (95%), intermediate for sensorimotor syndrome (87%), and least for pure motor hemiparesis (79%). Among the 195 patients who presented with a lacunar syndrome and in whom radiologic evaluation confirmed a small deep infarct, 147 were classified with a final diagnosis of lacunar infarct mechanism (positive predictive value, 75%). Extracranial or intracranial atherosclerosis accounted for 16 cases (8%), cardioembolism for 10 (5%), cryptogenic causes for 19 (10%), and other causes for 3 (2%). These investigators concluded that lacunar syndromes, especially pure sensory syndrome and ataxic hemiparesis, were highly predictive of small deep infarcts; however, about 1 in 4 patients presenting with lacunar syndromes that are confirmed radiologically may ultimately be proved to have a nonlacunar infarct mechanism. A complete diagnostic evaluation of large vessels and potential cardiogenic sources of embolism is warranted in these patients.

Results of Diagnostic Tests

CT scanning is positive only for roughly half of cases of even the most common form of lacune, pure motor stroke.[5,38,163] Visualizing lacunes depends on their location, and MRI is clearly superior to CT in evaluating lesions, especially in the posterior fossa. Overall, MRI has improved the yield of finding a strategically placed, small, deep infarct.[164] A complex diagnostic evaluation, including MRA and diffusion-weighted MRI, has been suggested to significantly improve the differential diagnosis among stroke subtypes, when its findings are added to the Trial of Org 10172 in Acute Stroke Treatment (TOAST) or the Oxford Community Stroke Project (OCSP) clinical criteria of classification in patients seen within 24 hours of stroke onset. Particularly, the diagnosis of lacunar infarcts according to the TOAST criteria improved from 35% to 100% with addition of this evaluation, and that with the OCSP classification from 78% to 100%.[165]

In the Northern Manhattan Stroke Study, using either CT or MRI, Gan and colleagues were able to detect radiologically small deep infarcts in appropriate locations in 84% of cases of lacunar syndromes.[162] The radiologic equivalent of a lacune was defined as a small deep lesion on brain imaging usually less than 1 cm in diameter with a density or signal consistent with an infarct located in the appropriate area of the brain to explain the syndrome, or the absence of a responsible lesion despite a second evaluation. The latter definition is based on the fact that some lacunes are too small to be seen on CT or MRI despite a repeat scan.

Large deep infarcts, some of which have been called super lacunes or giant lacunes, may be seen on CT or MRI as a focal, deep site of infarction without involvement of the cerebral surface.[163] A problem arises in the interpretation of these deep lesions, because an embolus may initially be arrested in the stem of the MCA, causing a large swath of infarction scattered through the lenticulostriate territories. When accompanied by a separate cerebral surface low-density area, such large deep infarcts are easily reclassified as examples of embolism, nonthrombotic infarction, or infarction of other cause. Therefore, most of these large, deep infarcts are really not lacunes.

In cases of pure motor hemiparesis, lacunes can be most commonly found in the internal capsule and corona radiata, but they have also been imaged in the basal ganglia, pons, and thalamus. Scan findings in the capsule, adjacent corona radiata, thalamus, or pons have been reported on occasion for the ataxic-hemiparesis, dysarthria–clumsy hand syndrome and hemiballism.[38,166] Pure sensory strokes have been reported from small thalamic infarcts, some so small as to cause selective proprioceptive loss without pain or temperature deficits.[113] Reports of pure sensory stroke from low densities in the centrum semiovale are probably lacunar, although surface infarction has rarely been demonstrated.[167]

Because the vascular lesion lies in vessels some 200 to 400 μm in diameter, it is perhaps no surprise that conventional cerebral angiographic and MRA findings are normal. Incidental large vessel disease may be found in some series, but whether it is etiologically related to the site of infarction is often unclear.[38,159] A normal angiogram could also be expected if microembolism was the cause of the deep infarction. Whether the outlook for stenosis of the MCA stem or the basilar artery differs if the syndrome is lacunar or not remains unsettled. Because some of the cases of pure motor stroke have been associated with MCA stenosis, the mere presence of such a syndrome has not been an indicator of the status of the major artery in question. TCD ultrasonography of the MCA stem or basilar artery has helped to establish the patency of these large vessels. MRA or conventional angiography may be required to settle the matter in some cases, and it remains the preferred diagnostic technique when TCD ultrasonography is technically unsatisfactory and CT or MRI shows a large band of low density that spans several sections and whose abnormality is seen down to the base of the affected basal ganglia.[163] Such a large infarct is not easily accounted for by primary disease in the penetrating artery itself, justifying angiography to seek stenosis of the MCA stem. The prognosis for later hemisphere symptoms in the patient with stem stenosis manifesting as a lacunar infarct is unknown.

Cryptogenic Infarction or Infarct of Undetermined Cause

Despite efforts to arrive at a diagnosis, the cause of the infarction may remain undetermined. A number of explanations can be offered. The first of the three major reasons for the failure is easily understood: no appropriate laboratory studies are performed. Advanced age, coexisting severe disease with a poor prognosis, and patient's or physician's unwillingness are only a few of the many reasons for deferring an evaluation. One reason no longer valid for this approach is that the mechanism of stroke has been diagnosed satisfactorily on clinical grounds alone. Among the syndromes attributed to ischemia, only the Wallenberg syndrome has yet to be reported from hematoma, and causes other than stroke have been so often reported with most of the classic focal brain syndromes that this point need not be labored.

A second common cause of failure to arrive at a diagnosis is improper timing of the appropriate laboratory studies. Angiography for embolism performed more than 48 hours after the ictus has a yield as low as 15% for evidence of the responsible occlusion.[118] Brain scans performed once only within a few hours of the onset of an ischemic stroke have a similarly low yield. Findings of brain scans performed no matter how often may remain negative in some cases of small lacunar infarction, if the lesion is below the limits of resolution of the scan technique.

As many as 40% of the cases of ischemic stroke of undetermined cause are in the third category, in which normal or ambiguous findings are reached despite appropriate laboratory studies performed at the appropriate time. This last group of cases poses special problems for research in stroke diagnosis. It would be comforting if most of these cases occurred in patients with the milder deficits, perhaps accounting for the normal laboratory findings by virtue of the relative insensitivity of such tests to smaller lesions. However, the scanty data on the subject indicate that this is not true; such cases are roughly as severe as ischemic strokes for which a cause is found.

In the Stroke Data Bank, a rigorous diagnostic scheme resulted in a high frequency of infarcts that were difficult to classify into the traditional subtypes. Despite considerable effort at evaluation, there remained a large proportion, fully 40% of patients, for whom the infarct mechanism escaped explanation and who were classified as having infarcts of undetermined cause.[34,35] Not all patients in the Stroke Data Bank underwent angiography, and when the procedure was performed, it was rarely in the first 48 to 72 hours after stroke. In other series in which

Clinical Manifestations

patients underwent angiography within 6 hours of stroke onset,[36] the application of the same diagnostic scheme as that used in the Stroke Data Bank has led to a reduction in the number of cases labeled as strokes of undetermined cause to only 15%.

Clinical Features

Cases categorized as ischemic stroke of undetermined cause show no bruit or TIA ipsilateral to the hemisphere affected by stroke and have no obvious source of embolism; in short, the affected patients do not have the risk factors or prior history that help suggest a cardiac embolus or large artery thrombosis.[35,49] In the Stroke Data Bank, the mean age at stroke for infarcts of undetermined cause studied by CT and angiogram was 58 years.[35] Hemispheral syndromes predominated in 66%; basilar syndromes occurred in 15%. Very few patients have lacunar syndromes. Twenty-seven percent had worsening symptoms in the hospital, and 41% had a moderate to severe weakness score.

Results of Diagnostic Tests

Findings of CT or MRI performed within 7 days may be normal, may show an infarct limited to a surface branch territory, or may show a large zone of infarction affecting regions larger than that accounted for by a single penetrant arterial territory. In the Stroke Data Bank, among the cryptogenic infarcts fully evaluated, CT demonstrated clinically relevant infarcts in 57%; surface infarction was found in 40%.[35] Noninvasive vascular imaging fails to demonstrate an underlying large vessel occlusion or stenosis. No definite cardiac source of embolism is uncovered by echocardiography, electrocardiography, or Holter monitoring.

If angiography is performed, the findings may be normal or may show a distal branch occlusion or occlusion of a major cerebral artery stem or the top of the basilar artery. Because MCA stem or branch occlusions can have thrombotic or embolic causes, their demonstration does not settle the mechanism in all cases, particularly among black, Asian, and Hispanic patients, in whom intracranial atheroma has been more frequently detected.[152] In white patients, on the other hand, pathologic examination of MCA occlusion rarely demonstrated an organized thrombus,[116,168] so the angiographic identification of an intracranial occlusion can usually be considered typical for embolism despite the absence of a source.[36] In the most extreme case, in which angiography is repeated and the original occlusion is no longer found, a definitive diagnosis of embolism can be made.

Potential Explanations of Cryptogenic Stroke

Some examples of the forms of stroke attributed to meningitis, migraine, lupus anticoagulant, arteritis, dissection, hypercoagulable states, and the like may be represented in the cryptogenic subgroup. Efforts should be made in each case to establish the existence of these unusual causes, and all such instances should be identified and classified as cerebral infarction from *other determined cause.* Adding together all the estimated frequencies with which such unusual causes manifest without accompanying evidence of the underlying disease cannot remotely approach the high frequency of the cryptogenic subgroup of stroke documented in the Stroke Data Bank.

Emerging technologies have led to the suggestions that some of the cases of cryptogenic infarct may be explained by hematologic disorders causing hypercoagulable states from protein C, free protein S, lupus anticoagulant, or anticardiolipin antibody abnormalities and mutations of coagulation factors like factor II and factor V.[169,170]

Hyperhomocysteinemia, either acquired (environmental) or consequent to mutations of the MTHFR gene, has also received attention.[171-173] Other investigators have implicated paradoxic emboli through a patent foramen ovale[174-176] or emboli from the ascending tract of the aortic arch,[139,140] both of which have been better identified with the more widespread use of transesophageal echocardiography. The number of cases of cryptogenic infarction attributed to the lack of appropriate diagnostic examinations previously mentioned should diminish as newer and more sensitive diagnostic techniques are introduced.

One approach to dealing with this cohort of cases is their forced reclassification into the traditional categories of atherothrombosis, embolism, or lacune. The presentation of a hemispheral syndrome, a surface infarction shown by CT, and angiographic findings that either are normal or show a corresponding branch occlusion have long been considered suggestive of embolism. Nonthrombotic ischemia has been used to describe those cases with normal angiograms. Such findings could be inferred to represent emboli, even though no cardiac source for embolism is documented by clinical or laboratory criteria. There is ample evidence of many occult sources of emboli, the difficulty in proving their existence, and their role in the first or succeeding ischemic strokes. Reclassification of such cases (and others in which CT shows limited cerebral infarction) as embolism with unobvious source would add most of the cryptogenic infarct patients to the embolism category, making embolism from all sources the largest subtype of stroke.[35,36] Alternatively, maintaining a separate category of cryptogenic strokes is useful to determine whether this group of cases differs in some way from those in which the mechanism of stroke is better defined and to encourage the continued search for causes of brain infarction and precipitants of thromboembolism.

References

1. Pulsinelli W: Pathophysiology of acute ischaemic stroke. Lancet 339:533–536, 1992.
2. Hacke W, Kaste M, Fieschi C, et al: Safety and efficacy of intravenous thrombolysis with a recombinant tissue plasminogen activator in the treatment of acute hemispheric stroke. JAMA 27:1017–1025, 1995.
3. The National Institute of Neurological Disorders and Stroke rt-PA Stroke Study Group: Tissue plasminogen activator for acute ischemic stroke. N Engl J Med 333:1581–1587, 1995.
4. Wardlaw JM, del Zoppo G, Yamaguchi T: Thrombolysis for acute ischaemic stroke. Cochrane Database Syst Rev 2:CD000213, 2000.
5. Mohr JP: Lacunes. Neurol Clin North Am 1:201–221, 1983.
6. Mohr JP: Lacunes. In Barnett HJM, Stein BH, Yatsu FM (eds): Stroke: Pathophysiology, Diagnosis and Management. New York, Churchill Livingstone, 1986, pp 475–496.
7. Toni D, Fiorelli M, De Michele M, et al: Clinical and prognostic correlates of stroke subtype misdiagnosis within 12 hours from onset. Stroke 26:1837–1840, 1995.
8. del Zoppo GJ, Poeck K, Pessin MS, et al: Recombinant tissue plasminogen activator in acute thrombotic and embolic stroke. Ann Neurol 32:78–86, 1992.

9. Von Kummer R, Forsting M, Sartor K, Hacke W: Intravenous recombinant tissue plasminogen activator in acute stroke. In Hacke W, del Zoppo GJ, Hirschberg M (eds): Thrombolytic Therapy in Acute Ischemic Stroke. Berlin, Springer-Verlag, 1991, pp 161–167.

10. Araki G: Small infarctions of the basal ganglia with special reference to transient ischemic attacks. Recent Adv Gerontol 469:161, 1978.

11. Beghi E, Bogliun G, Cavaletti G, et al: Hemorrhagic infarction: Risk factors, clinical and tomographic features, and outcome: A case-control study. Acta Neurol Scand 80:226–231, 1989.

12. Gacs G, Fox AJ, Barnett HJM, Vinuela F: CT visualization of intracranial arterial thromboembolism. Stroke 14:756, 1983.

13. Fisher CM, Adams RD: Observations on brain embolism with special reference to the mechanism of hemorrhagic infarction. J Neuropathol Exp Neurol 10:92, 1951.

14. De Ley G, Weyne J, Demeester G, et al: Experimental thromboembolic stroke studied by positron emission tomography: Immediate versus delayed reperfusion by fibrinolysis. J Cereb Blood Flow Metab 8:539–545, 1988.

15. Sloan MA: Thrombolysis and stroke: Past and future. Arch Neurol 44:748–768, 1987.

16. Bogousslavsky J, Cachin C, Regli F, et al: Cardiac sources of embolism and cerebral infarction: Clinical consequences and vascular concomitants: The Lausanne Stroke Registry. Neurology 41:855–859, 1991.

17. Hornig CR, Dorndorf W, Agnoli AL: Hemorrhagic cerebral infarction—a prospective study. Stroke 17:179–185, 1986.

18. Toni D, Fiorelli M, Bastianello S, et al: Hemorrhagic transformation of brain infarct: Predictability in the first five hours from stroke onset and influence on clinical outcome. Neurology 46:341–345, 1996.

19. Hornig CR, Bauer T, Simon C, et al: Hemorrhagic transformation in cardioembolic cerebral infarction. Stroke 24:465–468, 1993.

20. Mohr JP, Duterte DI, Oliveira VR, et al: Recanalization of acute middle cerebral artery occlusion. Neurology 38(Suppl):215, 1988.

21. Ogata J, Yutani C, Imakita M, et al: Hemorrhagic infarct of the brain without a reopening of the occluded arteries in cardioembolic stroke. Stroke 20:876–883, 1989.

22. Massaro AR, Sacco RL, Scaff M, Mohr JP: Clinical discriminators between acute brain hemorrhage and infarction—a practical score for early patient identification. Arq Neuropsiquiatr 60(2-A):185–191, 2002.

23. Panzer RJ, Feibel JH, Barker WH, Griner PF: Predicting the likelihood of hemorrhage in patients with stroke. Arch Intern Med 145:1800–1803, 1985.

24. Sandercock PAG, Allen CMC, Corston RN, et al: Clinical diagnosis of intracranial haemorrhage using Guy's Hospital Score. BMJ 291:1675–1677, 1985.

25. Spitzer K, Thie A, Caplan LR, Kunze K: The MICRO-STROKE expert system for stroke type diagnosis. Stroke 20:1353–1356, 1989.

26. Von Arbin M, Britton M, de Faire U, et al: Accuracy of bedside diagnosis in stroke. Stroke 12:288–293, 1981.

27. Fieschi C, Carolei A, Fiorelli M, et al: Changing prognosis of primary intracerebral hemorrhage: Result of a clinical and computed tomographic study of 104 patients. Stroke 19:192–195, 1988.

28. Drurys I, Whisnant JP, Garraway WM: Primary intracerebral hemorrhage: Impact of CT on incidence. Neurology 34:653–657, 1984.

29. Powers WJ: Cerebral hemodynamics in ischemic cerebrovascular disease. Ann Neurol 29:231–240, 1991.

30. Timsit S, Sacco RL, Mohr JP, et al: Brain infarction severity differs according to cardiac or arterial embolic source: The NINDS Stroke Data Bank. Neurology 43:728–733, 1993.

31. Toni D, Fiorelli M, Gentile M, et al: Progressing neurological deficit secondary to acute ischemic stroke: Study on predictability, pathogenesis and prognosis. Arch Neurol 52:670–675, 1995.

32. von Kummer R, Meyding-Lamadi U, Forsting M, et al: Sensitivity and prognostic value of early CT in occlusion of the middle cerebral artery trunk. AJNR Am J Neuroradiol 15:9–15, 1994.

33. Pexman JH, Barber PA, Hill MD, et al: Use of the Alberta Stroke Program Early CT Score (ASPECTS) for assessing CT scans in patients with acute stroke. AJNR Am J Neuroradiol 22:1534–1542, 2001.

34. Foulkes MA, Wolf PA, Price TR, et al: The Stroke Data Bank: Design, methods, and baseline characteristics. Stroke 19:547–554, 1988.

35. Sacco RL, Ellenberg JA, Mohr JP, et al: Infarction of undetermined cause: The NINDS Stroke Data Bank. Ann Neurol 25:382–390, 1989.

36. Fieschi C, Argentino C, Lenzi GL, et al: Clinical and instrumental evaluation of patients with ischemic stroke within the first six hours. J Neurol Sci 91:311–321, 1989.

37. Bamford JM, Warlow CP: Evolution and testing of the lacunar hypothesis. Stroke 19:1074–1082, 1988.

38. Chamorro AM, Sacco RL, Mohr JP, et al: Lacunar infarction: Clinical-CT correlations in the Stroke Data Bank. Stroke 22:175–181, 1991.

39. Toni D, Del Duca R, Fiorelli M, et al: Pure motor hemiplegia and sensorimotor stroke: Accuracy of the very early clinical diagnosis of lacunar stroke. Stroke 25:92–96, 1994.

40. Edwards JH, Kricheff II, Riles T, Imparato A: Angiographically undetected ulceration of the carotid bifurcation as a cause of embolic stroke. Radiology 132:369, 1979.

41. Fisher CM, Karnes WE: Local embolism. J Neuropathol Exp Neurol 24:174, 1965.

42. Imparato AM, Riles TS, Gorstein F: The carotid bifurcation plaque: Pathologic findings associated with cerebral ischemia. Stroke 10:238, 1979.

43. Masuda J, Ogata J, Yutani C, et al: Artery to artery embolism from a thrombus formed in stenotic middle cerebral artery: Report of an autopsy case. Stroke 18:680–684, 1987.

44. Droste DW, Dittrich R, Kemeny V, et al: Prevalence and frequency of microembolic signals in 105 patients with extracranial carotid artery occlusive disease. J Neurol Neurosurg Psychiatry 67:525–528, 1999.

45. Tsiskaridze A, Devuyst G, de Freitas GR, et al: Stroke with internal carotid artery stenosis. Arch Neurol 58:605–609, 2001.

46. El-Mitwalli A, Saad M, Christou I, et al: Clinical and sonographic patterns of tandem internal carotid artery/middle cerebral artery occlusion in tissue plasminogen activator–treated patients. Stroke 33:99–102, 2002.

47. Bogousslavsky J, Van Melle G, Regli F: The Lausanne Stroke Registry: Analysis of 1000 consecutive patients with first stroke. Stroke 19:1083–1092, 1988.

48. Gross CR, Kase CS, Mohr JP, Cunningham SC: Stroke in south Alabama: Incidence and diagnostic features. Stroke 15:249, 1984.

49. Kunitz S, Gross CR, Heyman A, et al: The pilot stroke data bank: Definition, design, data. Stroke 15:740, 1984.

50. Mohr JP, Caplan LR, Melski JW, et al: The Harvard cooperative stroke registry: A prospective registry of cases hospitalized with stroke. Neurology 28:754, 1978.

51. Aring CD, Merritt HH: Differential diagnosis between cerebral hemorrhage and cerebral thrombosis. Arch Intern Med 56:435, 1935.

52. Fisher CM, Gore I, Okabe N, White PD: Atherosclerosis of the carotid and vertebral arteries: Extracranial and intracranial. J Neuropathol Exp Neurol 24:455, 1965.

53. Samuel KC: Atherosclerosis and occlusion of the internal carotid artery. J Pathol Bacteriol 71:391, 1956.

54. Fisher CM: Cerebral thromboangiitis obliterans. Medicine (Baltimore) 36:169, 1957.

55. Mohr JP: Neurologic complications of cardiac valvular disease and cardiac surgery. In Vinken PJ, Bruyn GW (eds): Handbook of Clinical Neurology, Vol. 34: Medical Conditions. Amsterdam, North Holland, 1979, p 143.

56. Ogata J, Masuda J, Yutani C, Yamaguchi T: Rupture of atheromatous plaque as a cause of thrombotic occlusion of stenotic internal carotid artery. Stroke 21:1740–1745, 1990.

57. Lennihan L, Kupsky WJ, Mohr JP, et al: Lack of association between carotid plaque hematoma and ipsilateral cerebral symptoms. Stroke 18:879–881, 1987.

58. Ballotta E, Da Giau G, Renon L: Carotid plaque gross morphology and clinical presentation: A prospective study of 457 carotid artery specimens. J Surg Res 89:78–84, 2000.

59. Hatsukami TS, Ross R, Polissar NL, Yuan C: Visualization of fibrous cap thickness and rupture in human atherosclerotic carotid plaque in vivo with high-resolution magnetic resonance imaging. Circulation 102:959–964, 2000.

60. Bogousslavsky J, Regli F: Borderzone infarctions distal to internal carotid artery occlusion: Prognostic implications. Ann Neurol 20:346–350, 1986.

Clinical Manifestations

61. Hultquist GT: Ueber Thrombose und Embolie der Arteria carotis und herbei vorkommende gehirnveraenderungen: Eine pathologisch-anatomische Studie. Stockholm, Gustav Fischer Verlag, 1942.

62. Pessin MS, Hinton RC, Davis KR, et al: Mechanisms of acute carotid stroke: A clinicoangiographic study. Ann Neurol 6:245, 1979.

63. Ring BA: Diagnosis of embolic occlusions of smaller branches of the intracerebral arteries. AJR Radium Ther Nucl Med 97:575, 1966.

64. Romanul FCA, Abramowicz A: Changes in brain and pial vessels in arterial borderzones. Arch Neurol (Chic) 11:40, 1964.

65. Torvick A: The pathogenesis of watershed infarcts in the brain. Stroke 15:221–223, 1984.

66. Carpenter DA, Grubb RL Jr, Powers WJ: Borderzone hemodynamics in cerebrovascular disease. Neurology 40:1587–1592, 1990.

67. Powers WJ, Tempel LW, Grubb RL Jr: Influence of cerebral hemodynamics on stroke risk: One year follow up of 30 medically treated patients. Ann Neurol 25:325–330, 1989.

68. Beal MF, Williams RS, Richardson EP, Fisher CM: Cerebral embolism as a cause of transient ischemic attacks and cerebral infarction. Neurology (NY) 31:860, 1981.

69. David NJ, Gordon KK, Friedberg SJ, et al: Fatal atheromatous cerebral embolism associated with bright plaques in the retinal arterioles. Neurology 13:708, 1963.

70. Koennecke HC, Mast H, Trocio SS, et al: Frequency and determinants of microembolic signals on transcranial Doppler in unselected patients with acute carotid territory ischemia—A prospective study. Cerebrovasc Dis 8:107–112, 1998.

71. Adams HP, Gross CE: Embolism distal to stenosis of the middle cerebral artery. Stroke 12:228, 1981.

72. Segura T, Serena J, Castellanos M, et al: Embolism in acute middle cerebral artery stenosis. Neurology 56:497–501, 2001.

73. Castaigne P, Lhermitte F, Gautier J-C, et al: Arterial occlusions in the vertebro-basilar system: A study of forty-four patients with post-mortem data. Brain 96:133, 1973.

74. Barnett HJM, Peerless SJ, Kaufmann JCE: "Stump" of internal carotid artery—a source for further cerebral embolic ischemia. Stroke 9:448, 1978.

75. Russell RW: Atheromatous retinal embolism. Lancet 2:1354, 1963.

76. Angeloni U, Bozzao L, Fantozzi L, et al: Internal border zone infarction following acute middle cerebral artery occlusion. Neurology 40:1196–1198, 1990.

77. Timsit S, Sacco RL, Mohr JP, et al: Early clinical differentiation of atherosclerotic and cardioembolic infarction: Stroke Data Bank. Stroke 23:486–491, 1992.

78. Fieschi C, Sette G, Fiorelli M, et al: Clinical presentation and frequency of potential sources of embolism in acute ischemic stroke patients: The experience of the Rome Acute Stroke Registry. Cerebrovasc Dis 5:75–78, 1995.

79. Ringelstein EB, Zeumer H, Angelou D: The pathogenesis of strokes from internal carotid artery occlusion: Diagnostic and therapeutic implications. Stroke 14:867, 1983.

80. Ringelstein EB, Koschorke S, Holling A, et al: Computed tomographic patterns of proven embolic brain infarctions. Ann Neurol 26:759–765, 1989.

81. Ay H, Oliveira-Filho J, Buonanno FS, et al: Diffusion-weighted imaging identifies a subset of lacunar infarction associated with embolic source Stroke 30:2644–2650, 1999.

82. Koennecke HC, Bernarding J, Braun J, et al: Scattered brain infarct pattern on diffusion-weighted magnetic resonance imaging in patients with acute ischemic stroke. Cerebrovasc Dis 11:157–163, 2001.

83. Pessin MS, Duncan GW, Davis KR, et al: Angiographic appearance of carotid occlusion in acute stroke. Stroke 11:485, 1980.

84. Quisling RG, Friedman WA, Rhoton AL: High cervical dissection: Spontaneous resolution. AJNR Am J Neuroradiol 1:463, 1980.

85. Dion JE, Gates PC, Fox AJ, et al: Clinical events following neuroangiography: A prospective study. Stroke 18:997–1004, 1987.

86. Hankey GJ, Warlow CP, Sellar RJ: Cerebral angiographic risk in mild cerebrovascular disease. Stroke 21:209–222, 1990.

87. Leow K, Murie JA: Cerebral angiography for cerebrovascular disease: The risks. Br J Surg 75:428–430, 1988.

88. Caplan LR, Brass LM, DeWitt LD, et al: Transcranial Doppler ultrasound: Present status. Neurology 40:696–700, 1990.

89. DeWitt LD, Wechsler LR: Transcranial Doppler. Stroke 19:915–921, 1988.

90. Grolimund P, Seiler RW, Aaslid R, et al: Evaluation of cerebrovascular disease by combined extracranial and transcranial Doppler sonography: Experience in 1,039 patients. Stroke 18:1018–1024, 1987.

91. Tatemichi TK, Chamorro A, Petty GW, et al: Hemodynamic role of ophthalmic artery collateral in internal carotid artery occlusion. Neurology 40:461–464, 1990.

92. Zanette EM, Fieschi C, Bozzao L, et al: Comparison of cerebral angiography and transcranial Doppler sonography in acute stroke. Stroke 20:899–903, 1989.

93. Zierler RE, Kohler TR, Strandness DE Jr: Duplex scanning of normal or minimally diseased carotid arteries: Correlation with arteriography and clinical outcome. J Vasc Surg 12:447–454, 1990.

94. Hirai T, Korogi Y, Ono K, et al: Prospective evaluation of suspected stenoocclusive disease of the intracranial artery: Combined MR angiography and CT angiography compared with digital subtraction angiography. AJNR Am J Neuroradiol 23:93–101, 2002.

95. Castaigne P, Lhermitte F, Gautier J-C: Role des lésions artérielles dans les accidents ischemiques cérébraux de l'athérosclerose. Rev Neurol (Paris) 113:1, 1965.

96. Castaigne P, Lhermitte F, Gautier J-C, et al: Internal carotid artery occlusion: A study of 61 instances in 50 patients with post-mortem data. Brain 93:231, 1970.

97. Torvik A, Jorgensen L: Thrombotic and embolic occlusions of the carotid arteries in an autopsy material. Part 2: Cerebral lesions and clinical course. J Neurol Sci 3:410, 1966.

98. Dalal PM, Shah PM, Aiyar RR: Arteriographic study of cerebral embolism. Lancet 2:358, 1965.

99. Caplan LR: Occlusion of the vertebral or basilar artery: Follow up analysis of some patients with benign outcome. Stroke 10:277, 1979.

100. Caplan LR: "Top of the basilar" syndrome. Neurology 30:72, 1980.

101. Castaigne P, Lhermitte F, Buge A, et al: Paramedian thalamic and midbrain infarcts: Clinical and neuropathological study. Ann Neurol 10:127, 1981.

102. Fisher CM: Bilateral occlusion of basilar artery branches. J Neurol Neurosurg Psychiatry 40:1182, 1977.

103. Caplan LR: Intracranial branch atheromatous disease: A neglected, understudied, and underused concept. Neurology 39:1246–1250, 1989.

104. Heiss WD, Herholz K, Podreka I, et al: Comparison of ^{99m}Tc HMPAO SPECT with ^{18}F fluoromethane PET in cerebrovascular disease. J Cereb Blood Flow Metab 10:687–697, 1990.

105. Johnson DW, Stringer WA, Marks MP, et al: Stable xenon CT cerebral blood flow imaging: Rationale for and role in clinical decision making. AJNR Am J Neuroradiol 12:201–213, 1991.

106. Edelman RR, Mattle HP, Atkinson DJ, et al: Cerebral blood flow: Assessment with dynamic contrast enhanced T2°-weighted MR imaging at 1.5 T. Radiology 176:211–220, 1990.

107. Apruzzese A, Silvestrini M, Floris R, et al: Cerebral hemodynamics in asymptomatic patients with internal carotid artery occlusion: A dynamic susceptibility contrast MR and transcranial Doppler study. AJNR Am J Neuroradiol 22:1062–1067, 2001.

108. Nasel C, Azizi A, Wilfort A, et al: Measurement of time-to-peak parameter by use of a new standardization method in patients with stenotic or occlusive disease of the carotid artery. AJNR Am J Neuroradiol 22:1056–1061, 2001.

109. Baron JC, Frackowiak RS, Herholz K, et al: Use of PET methods for measurement of cerebral energy metabolism and hemodynamics in cerebrovascular disease. J Cereb Blood Flow Metab 9:723–742, 1989.

110. Sette G, Baron JC, Mazoyer B, et al: Local brain haemodynamics and oxygen metabolism in cerebrovascular disease: Positron emission tomography. Brain 112:931–951, 1989.

111. Kolominsky-Rabas PL, Weber M, Gefeller O, et al: Epidemiology of ischemic stroke subtypes according to TOAST criteria: Incidence, recurrence, and long-term survival in ischemic stroke subtypes: A population-based study. Stroke 32:2735–2740, 2001.

112. Caplan LR, Hier DB, D'Cruz I: Cerebral embolism in the Michael Reese Stroke Registry. Stroke 14:30, 1983.

113. Sacco RL, Bello JA, Traub RD, Brust JCM: Selective proprioceptive sensory loss from a thalamic lacunar stroke. Stroke 18:1160–1163, 1987.

114. Cardiogenic brain embolism: The second report of the Cerebral Embolism Task Force. Arch Neurol 46:727–743, 1989.

115. Hinton RC, Kistler JP, Fallon JT, et al: Influence of etiology of atrial fibrillation on incidence of systemic embolism. Am J Cardiol 40:509, 1977.

116. Lhermitte F, Gautier JC, Derouesne C, Guiraud B: Ischemic accidents in the middle cerebral artery territory (a study of the causes in 122 cases). Arch Neurol 19:248, 1968.

117. Santamaria J, Graus F, Rubio F, et al: Cerebral infarction of the basal ganglia due to embolism from the heart. Stroke 14:911, 1983.

118. Bozzao L, Fantozzi LM, Bastianello S, et al: Ischaemic supratentorial stroke: Angiographic findings in patients examined in the very early phase. J Neurol 236:340–342, 1989.

119. del Zoppo GJ, Higashida RT, Furlan AJ, et al: PROACT: A phase II randomized trial of recombinant pro-urokinase by direct arterial delivery in acute middle cerebral artery stroke. Stroke 29:4–11, 1998.

120. Fieschi C, Bozzao L: Transient embolic occlusion of the middle cerebral and internal carotid arteries in cerebral apoplexy. J Neurol Neurosurg Psychiatry 32:236–240, 1969.

121. Kase CS, White L, Vinson L, Eichelberger P: Shotgun pellet embolus to the middle cerebral artery. Neurology 31:458, 1981.

122. Zanette EM, Roberti C, Mancini G, et al: Spontaneous middle cerebral artery reperfusion in ischemic stroke: A follow-up study with transcranial Doppler. Stroke 26:430–433, 1995.

123. Toni D, Fiorelli M, Zanette EM, et al: Early spontaneous improvement and deterioration of ischemic stroke patients: A serial study with transcranial Doppler. Stroke 29:1144–1148, 1998.

124. Mori E, Yoneda Y, Tabuchi M, et al: Intravenous recombinant tissue plasminogen activator in acute carotid artery territory stroke. Neurology 42:976–982, 1992.

125. Ringelstein EB, Biniek R, Weiller C, et al: Type and extent of hemispheric brain infarctions and clinical outcome in early and delayed middle cerebral artery recanalization. Neurology 42:289–298, 1992.

126. Von Kummer R, Hacke W: Safety and efficacy of intravenous tissue plasminogen activator and heparin in acute middle cerebral artery stroke. Stroke 23:646–652, 1992.

127. Friedlich AL, Castleman B, Mohr JP: Case records of the Massachusetts General Hospital. N Engl J Med 278:1109, 1968.

128. Sacco RL, Owen J, Mohr JP, Tatemichi TK: Free protein S deficiency: A possible association with intracranial vascular occlusion. Stroke 20:1657–1661, 1989.

128. Zatz LM, Iannone AM, Eckman PB, Hecker SP: Observations concerning intracerebral vascular occlusion. Neurology 15:390–401, 1965.

129. Liebeskind A, Chinichian A, Schechter MM: The moving embolus seen during serial cerebral angiography. Stroke 2:440, 1971.

130. Irino T, Tandea M, Minami T: Angiographic manifestations in postrecanalized cerebral infarction. Neurology 27:471, 1977.

131. Little JR, Shawhan B, Weinstein M: Pseudo-tandem stenosis of the internal carotid artery. Neurosurgery 7:574, 1980.

132. Fisher CM, Pearlman A: The non-sudden onset of cerebral embolism. Neurology (Minneap) 17:1025, 1967.

133. Whisnant JP: Multiple particles injected may all go to the same cerebral artery branch. Stroke 13:720, 1982.

134. Minematsu K, Yamaguchi T, Omae T: Spectacular shrinking deficit: Rapid recovery from a full hemispheral syndrome by migration of an embolus. Neurology 41(Suppl):329, 1991.

135. Kittner SJ, Sharkness CM, Price TR, et al: Infarcts with a cardiac source of embolism in the NINDS Stroke Data Bank: Historical features. Neurology 40:281–284, 1990.

136. Ramirez Lassepas M, Cipolle RJ, Bjok RJ, et al: Can embolic stroke be diagnosed on the basis of neurologic clinical criteria? Arch Neurol 44:87–89, 1987.

137. Bladin PF: A radiologic and pathologic study of embolism of the internal carotid–middle cerebral arterial axis. Radiology 82:614, 1964.

138. Tomsick TA, Brott TC, Olinger CP, et al: Hyperdense middle cerebral artery: Incidence and quantitative significance. Neuroradiology 31:312–315, 1989.

138. David DO, Rumbaugh CL, Gilson JM: Angiographic diagnosis of small-vessel cerebral emboli. Acta Radiol (Stockh) 9:264, 1969.

139. Amarenco P, Duyckaerts C, Tzourio C, et al: The prevalence of ulcerated plaques in the aortic arch in patients with stroke. N Engl J Med 326:221–225, 1992.

140. Amarenco P, Cohen A, Tzourio C, et al: Atherosclerotic disease of the aortic arch and the risk of ischemic stroke. N Engl J Med 331:1474–1479, 1994.

141. The French Study of Aortic Plaques in Stroke Group: Atherosclerotic disease of the aortic arch as a risk factor for recurrent ischemic stroke. N Engl J Med 334:1216–1221, 1996.

142. Tenenbaum A, Fisman EZ, Schneiderman J, et al: Disrupted mobile aortic plaques are a major risk factor for systemic embolism in the elderly. Cardiology 89:246–251, 1998.

143. Fisher CM: Lacunes: Small deep cerebral infarcts. Neurology (Minneap) 15:774, 1965.

144. Tohgi H, Kawashima M, Tamura K, Suzuki H: Coagulation fibrinolysis abnormalities in acute and chronic phases of cerebral thrombosis and embolism. Stroke 21:1663–1667, 1990.

144. Fisher CM: The arterial lesions underlying lacunes. Acta Neuropathol (Berl) 12:1, 1969.

145. Hinton RC, Mohr JP, Ackerman RA, et al: Symptomatic middle cerebral artery stem stenosis. Ann Neurol 5:152, 1979.

146. Moulin T, Tatu L, Vuillier F, et al: Role of a stroke data bank in evaluating cerebral infarction subtypes: Patterns and outcome of 1776 consecutive patients from the Besançon Stroke Registry. Cerebrovasc Dis 10:261–271, 2000.

147. MacKenzie JM: Are all cardio-embolic strokes embolic? An autopsy study of 100 consecutive acute ischemic strokes. Cerebrovasc Dis 10:289–292, 2000.

148. Nishida N, Ogata J, Yutani C, et al: Cerebral artery thrombosis as a cause of striatocapsular infarction: A histopathological case study. Cerebrovasc Dis 10:151–154, 2000.

149. Krapf H, Widder B, Skalej M: Small rosarylike infarctions in the centrum semiovale suggest hemodynamic failure. AJNR Am J Neuroradiol 19:1479–1484, 1998.

150. Lammie GA, Wardlaw JM: Small centrum ovale infarcts: A pathological study. Cerebrovasc Dis 9:82–90, 1999.

151. Wardlaw JM, Dennis MS, Warlow CP, Sandercock PA: Imaging appearance of the symptomatic perforating artery in patients with lacunar infarction: Occlusion or other vascular pathology? Ann Neurol 50:208–215, 2001.

152. Sacco RL, Kargman DE, Gu Q, Zamanillo MC: Race-ethnicity and determinants of intracranial atherosclerotic cerebral infarction: The Northern Manhattan Stroke Study. Stroke 26:14–20, 1995.

153. Nelson RF, Pullicino P, Kendall BE, Marshall J: Computed tomography on patients presenting with lacunar syndromes. Stroke 11:256, 1980.

154. Fisher CM: Lacunar strokes and infarcts: A review. Neurology (NY) 32:871, 1982.

155. Landau WM: Clinical neuromythology VI. Au clair de lacune: Holy wholly, holey logic. Neurology 39:725–730, 1989.

156. Millikan C, Futrell N: The fallacy of the lacunar hypothesis. Stroke 21:1251–1257, 1990.

157. Bamford J, Sandercock P, Dennis M, et al: Classification and natural history of clinically identifiable subtypes of cerebral infarction. Lancet 337:1521–1526, 1991.

158. Chimowitz MI, Furlan AJ, Sila CA, et al: Etiology of motor or sensory stroke: A prospective study of the predictive value of clinical and radiological features. Ann Neurol 30:519–525, 1991.

159. Toni D: Hyperacute diagnosis of subcortical infarction. In Donnan G, Norrving B, Bamford J, Bogousslavsky J (eds): Lacunar and Other Subcortical Infarctions. Oxford, UK, Oxford University Press, 2002.

160. Perani D, Vallar G, Cappa S, et al: Aphasia and neglect after subcortical stroke: A clinical/cerebral perfusion study. Brain 110:1211–1229, 1987.

161. Takano T, Kimura K, Nakamura M, et al: Effect of small deep hemispheric infarction on the ipsilateral cortical blood flow in man. Stroke 16:64–69, 1985.

162. Gan R, Sacco RL, Kargman DE, et al: Testing the validity of the lacunar hypothesis: The Northern Manhattan Stroke Study experience. Neurology 48:1204–1211, 1997.

163. Rascol A, Clanet M, Manelfe C: Pure motor hemiplegia: CT study of 30 cases. Stroke 13:11, 1982.

164. Hommel M, Besson G, Le Bas JF, et al: Prospective study of lacunar infarction using magnetic resonance imaging. Stroke 21:546–554, 1990.

165. Lee LJ, Kidwell CS, Alger J, et al: Impact on stroke subtype diagnosis of early diffusion-weighted magnetic resonance imaging and magnetic resonance angiography. Stroke 31:1081–1089, 2000.

166. Sunohara N, Mukoyama M, Mano Y, Satoyoshi E: Action-induced rhythmic dystonia: An autopsy case. Neurology (Cleveland) 34:321, 1984.

167. Derouesne C, Mas JL, Bolgert AF, Castaigne P: Pure sensory stroke caused by a small cortical infarct in the middle cerebral artery territory. Stroke 15:660, 1984.

Clinical Manifestations

168. Jorgensen L, Torvik A: Ischaemic cerebrovascular diseases in an autopsy series. Part I: Prevalence, location and predisposing factors in verified thromboembolic occlusions, and their significance in the pathogenesis of cerebral infarction. J Neurol Sci 3:490–495, 1966.
169. Longstreth WT Jr, Rosendaal FR, Siscovick DS, et al: Risk of stroke in young women and two prothrombotic mutations: Factor V Leiden and prothrombin gene variant (G20210A). Stroke 29:577–580, 1998.
170. De Stefano V, Chiusolo P, Paciaroni K, et al: Prothrombin G20210A mutant genotype is a risk factor for cerebrovascular ischemic disease in young patients. Blood 91:3562–3565, 1998.
171. Markus HS, Ali N, Swaminathan R, et al: A common polymorphism in the methylenetetrahydrofolate reductase gene, homocysteine and ischemic cerebrovascular disease. Stroke 28:1739–1743, 1997.
172. Arruda VR, von Zuben PM, Chiaparini LC, et al: The mutation Ala677Val in the methylene tetrahydrofolate reductase gene: A risk factor for arterial and venous thrombosis. Thromb Haemost 77:818–821, 1997.
173. Fletcher O, Kessling AM: MTHFR association with arteriosclerotic vascular disease? Hum Genet 103:11–21, 1998.
174. Di Tullio MR, Gopal AS, Sacco RL, et al: Prevalence of patent foramen ovale in older cryptogenic stroke patients assessed by contrast echocardiography. J Am Soc Echocardiogr 4:294, 1991.
175. Falk RH: PFO or UFO? The role of a patent foramen ovale in cryptogenic stroke [editorial]. Am Heart J 121:1264–1266, 1991.
176. Lechat P, Mas JL, Lascault G, et al: Prevalence of patent foramen ovale in patients with stroke. N Engl J Med 318:1148–1152, 1988.

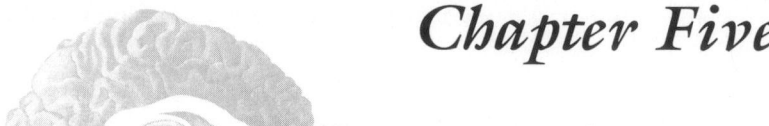

Chapter Five

Internal Carotid Artery Disease

J. P. Mohr and Jean Claude Gautier

Clinical
Manifestations

The bifurcation of the common carotid artery and the origin of the internal carotid artery (ICA) have been the focus of neurologic attention for many years. They are by far the most common sites of significant, atherosclerotic ICA lesions; the extracranial ICA is, as a rule, devoid of atherosclerosis from beyond its origin to its entry into the skull. The extracranial ICA can be examined clinically and by ultrasonography and is easy to approach surgically; even some of its less usual disorders, such as dissecting aneurysms, are to some extent amenable to conventional surgery. The intracranial ICA lends itself poorly to clinical and ultrasonographic examination, and even angiograms of the vessel are often difficult to evaluate precisely. The diseases and mechanisms to which the artery is subject cover the entire spectrum of occlusive disease.

CAROTID ANATOMY AND LESION DEVELOPMENT

The anatomy of the cerebral artery tree is presented in Figure 5–1.

Extracranial Bifurcation

The mechanisms that underlie the development of atheroma remain incompletely understood, but efforts have been directed to identifying some of the major factors. For example, the ICA more severely affected by atherosclerosis on one side appears more commonly to be the smaller,[1] the one more angulated,[2] and the one in which flow separation is more easily demonstrated.[3-6]

Hemodynamically Significant Extracranial Stenosis

Reduced cross-sectional area is the main factor in making a stenosis hemodynamically significant.[7-9] Lesser roles are played by the length of the stenosis,[7] blood flow velocity,[10] and blood viscosity.[11] Brice and colleagues[8] were among the first to define the characteristics of a hemodynamically significant stenosis in vitro, showing reduced flow in excised human ICAs when the lumen was constricted to a cross-sectional area of 4 to 5 mm^2 along a length of 3 mm (Fig. 5–2). During the days when humans underwent staged cross-clamping of the common carotid artery as a treatment for intracranial aneurysms, the point of sudden fall

in pressure distal to the stenosis occurred when the lumen reached an estimated diameter less than 2 mm. The length of the stenosis was far less significant than was the total cross-sectional area at the narrowest point. Lesions in tandem produced cumulative effects only if separated by less than 3 cm (the usual condition that applies in carotid territory stenoses in tandem). The study by Brice and colleagues[8] founded the principle that the carotid stenosis must be 2 mm or tighter to be considered hemodynamically significant. Others have used the method of percentage reduction in vascular lumen, claiming hemodynamic significance when the diameter is reduced by 50%, a figure corresponding to a cross-sectional reduction of 75% to 80%,[7,12] but Archie and Feldtman[13] demonstrated that the hemodynamic effect of stenosis is significant when 84% diameter stenosis and 96% area stenosis were achieved.

Angiography, once the "gold standard" for estimation of severity of stenosis, is fast being superseded by modern duplex Doppler methods,[14] but data from most of the larger clinical trials for endarterectomy were based on angiographic assessment, so some familiarity with the methods appears useful to review. With the use of angiography, the methods to calculate the percentage by the formula used by the North American Symptomatic Carotid Endarterectomy Trial (NASCET)—(1 − minimum residual lumen/normal distal cervical ICA diameter) × 100—differed somewhat from that for the Asymptomatic Carotid Atherosclerosis Study (ACAS). They also illustrate the problems posed by the angiogram method, leaving aside the difficulties of a biplane technique for a non-annular lesion. The method for selection of the sites in the vessel is shown in Figure 5–3.

Studies by Gagne and associates[15] indicated that the technique translates well. The percentage of stenosis from 219 consecutive angiograms was assessed by two vascular surgeons and two radiologists (neither group was aware of the results of the other group), who classified stenoses into less than or more than 60% (the break point used in the ACAS) and less than 30%, 30% to 60%, and 70% or more (as was used in the NASCET). High kappa values, 0.825 to 0.903, were found for ACAS criteria; and values of 0.729 to 0.793 for NASCET criteria. By comparison, interobserver agreement on measurements for digital subtraction angiograms and magnetic resonance angiograms has not

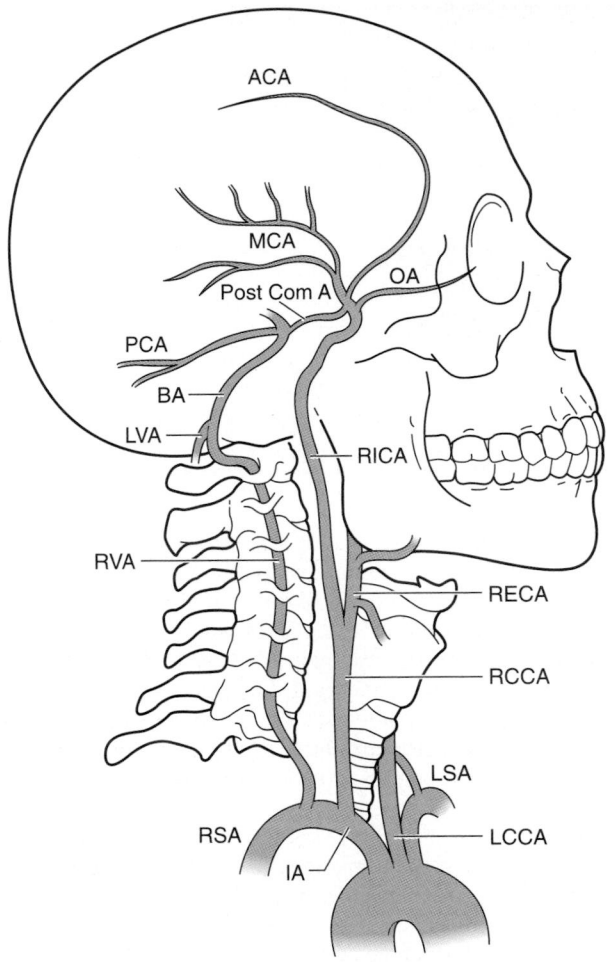

FIGURE 5–1 *Anatomy of the extracranial cerebral-bound arteries and their main intracranial supplies, lateral view from the right. ACA, anterior cerebral artery; BA, basilar artery; IA, innominate artery; LCCA, left common carotid artery; LSA, left subclavian artery; LVA, left vertebral artery; MCA, middle cerebral artery; OA, ophthalmic artery; PCA, posterior cerebral artery; Post Com A, posterior communicating artery; RCCA, right common carotid artery; RECA; right external carotid artery; RICA, right internal carotid artery; RSA, right subclavian artery; RVA, right vertebral artery. The anterior choroidal artery is not depicted. (From Gautier, JC, Mohr JP: Ischemic stroke. In Mohr JP, Gautier JC [eds]: Guide to Clinical Neurology. New York, Churchill Livingstone, 1995, p 543.)*

been high. Practices also differ between continents: in the United States, a method of measuring the angiogram may yield a diagnosis of 60% stenosis, whereas the method used in Europe may produce a diagnosis of 75% stenosis from basically the same angiographic images.[16]

Tempo of Development of Carotid Bifurcation Lesions

On the basis of studies dating from the days of digital subtraction methods[17] through those using conventional angiography[18] or noninvasive techniques, atheromatous stenoses may develop swiftly over months or slowly over years or may even remain static despite being hemodynamically significant. The 167 asymptomatic cases followed by Roederer and coworkers[19] by duplex Doppler ultrasonography found some progression in 60% of cases, which was symptomatic in 10 cases (transient ischemic attack [TIA] in 6 and stroke in 4) and accompanied by disease progression in 8. Within 6 months, 1 of 5 arteries with 80% to 90% stenosis had become occluded; occlusion in 7 of 46 increased from between 50% and 79% to between 80% and 99% stenosis; and 4 of 67 increased from between 16% and 49% to between 50% and 79% stenosis. At 24 months, of 33 arteries that were initially diagnosed with 50% to 79% stenosis, 2 were occluded and 2 had increased to 80% to 99% stenosis; of 38 that were initially diagnosed at 16% to 49%, 1 was occluded, 1 had become 80% to 99% stenosed, and 7 increased to 50% to 79% stenosis. At 3 years, of 11 arteries initially at 50% to 79% stenosis, 1 was occluded and 2 had advanced to 80% to 99% stenosis.

Hope has been held out for years first that Doppler ultrasonography (and, more recently, color-coded techniques) could distinguish features predictive of stroke from those found in patients who remained asymptomatic. To date, however, there has been no improvement in the conclusions of The Consensus Conference for Carotid Plaque Morphology and Risk (Consensus sur la Morphologie et le Risque des Plaques Carotidiennes), held in December 1996 in Paris, that it is the *degree of stenosis* that is associated with stroke risk, not the ultrasonographic features of the plaque.[20] Other investigators continue to report studies suggesting a link between subsequent TIA or stroke and appearance of ulcerative plaque on Doppler ultrasonography (see later).

Although atherosclerosis has been considered the basic disease process in the vast majority of cases, evidence is

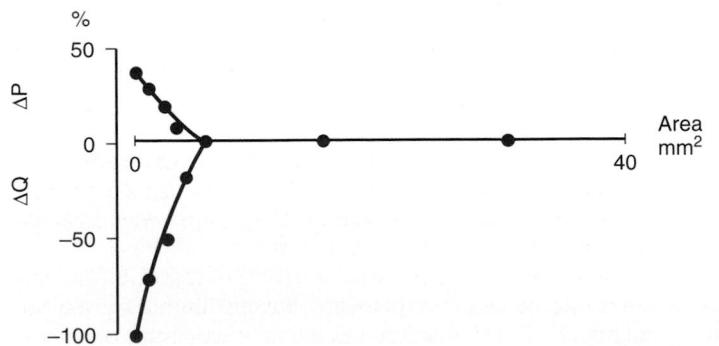

FIGURE 5–2 *Effect of cross-sectional area on pressure and flow.*

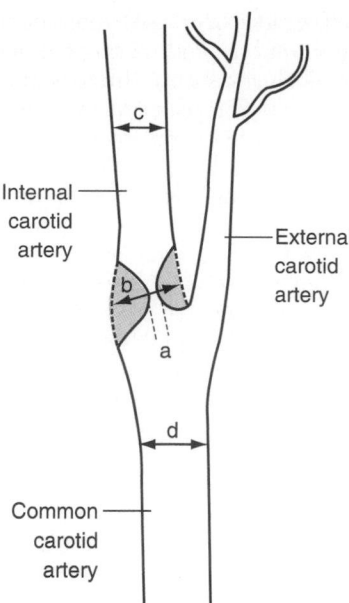

FIGURE 5–3 *Position of measurements for stenosis. a, Site of maximum stenosis (whether or not in the carotid bulb); b, original internal carotid lumen; c, internal carotid distal to the stenosis; d, common carotid lumen. (From Young GR, Humphrey PR, Nixon TE, Smith ET: Variability in measurement of extracranial internal carotid artery stenosis as displayed by both digital subtraction and magnetic resonance angiography: An assessment of three caliper techniques and visual impression of stenosis. Stroke 27:467, 1996, with permission.)*

emerging that *Chlamydia pneumoniae* may have a role as a cause of relentlessly progressing carotid stenosis. Its treatment with antibiotics has been reported in some series to be associated with a reduction in the rate of progression of the lesions.[21]

Other Causes of Extracranial Carotid Disease

Although major attention is given to atherosclerosis, there are other causes of carotid artery occlusion. Prominent among them are embolism from cardiac or arterial sources, and arterial dissection (see Chapter 23). A few additional causes are uncommon, some of them approaching the status of medical curiosities.[22]

Fibromuscular Dysplasia
A rare condition, fibromuscular dysplasia is encountered in less than 0.6% of cases of ICA disease.[23] It may account for kinks (see later), and intracranial aneurysm occurs in almost 25% of cases of fibromuscular dysplasia (see later). Its clinical importance is unclear, but the disease has been the subject of publication often enough that it is discussed in a separate chapter (see Chapter 26).

Arterial Kinks
Kinking of the ICA may achieve the same hemodynamic effects as atheromatous stenosis. Kinking of the carotid artery is an acquired condition and is not identical with coiling, which is believed to be congenital and of no clinical significance.[24,25] Kinking is thought to be caused by

atherosclerosis or to occur as a complication of fibromuscular dysplasia.

The significance of kinking arises when positional head changes produce transient cerebral ischemia, a situation in which dramatic reductions in cerebral blood flow (CBF) have been documented in some cases during intraoperative studies; as yet, the degree of stenosis observed angiographically has not proved an adequate basis to determine the need for corrective surgery without the additional studies of the effect of head position change.

Kinking caused by alteration in artery position appears to be a rare cause of TIAs. Handa and colleagues[26] described a patient who had undergone extracranial-intracranial bypass and then experienced recurrent TIAs precipitated by yawning. The stretching and kinking of the donor artery by the mouth opening during the yawning was the alleged mechanism.

Primary Tumors of the Vascular Structures
Primary tumors of vascular structures are uncommon, usually arising from mesoblastic and neural elements such as chemodectomas and paragangliomas.[27] Only 5% are bilateral. Such masses grow slowly, manifesting as dysphagia and hoarseness, although dyspnea, Horner's syndrome, and facial pain may also occur.[28] The lesions produce metastases in only about 2% of cases. Local recurrence is uncommon and is usually delayed for many years.

Complications of Head and Neck Cancer
Involvement of the extracranial carotid artery by direct extension of local tumor is distinctly uncommon.[29] However, this complication occurs often enough in hospitals with a large oncology case load to warrant consideration here. Direct tumor invasion of the arterial wall was described in 37 of 64 carotid arteries taken from patients with head or neck cancer in a study at Memorial Hospital in New York.[30] Three examples of such involvement in the siphon from parasellar tumors were reported by Spallone.[31] Two were meningiomas, and the third was a pituitary adenoma. This complication appears to be extremely rare; Spallone[31] reported having encountered it in only 3 cases among more than 10,000 examined angiographically in his institution over a period of approximately 25 years.

Surgical approaches to tumor resection that involve taking the carotid artery along with the tumor carry considerable risk. Experience at Iowa showed a stroke rate of 25% for the procedure.[32] Snyderman and D'Amico[33] reviewed the literature to 1991 for all cases of squamous cell carcinoma treated by carotid artery resection; neurologic complications occurred in 17% of patients but seemed unrelated to the method of attempted carotid reconstruction. Such methods include interposition grafting[34]; the greater saphenous vein graft is preferred, the nonreversed graft having better patency than the reversed graft.[35] Later studies have shown the value of using positron emission tomography (PET) assessment of intracranial flow to determine the outcomes expected from inclusion of the carotid artery in surgical resections for local tumor.[36]

Studies using quantitative regional CBF (rCBF) measurements by xenon inhalation during temporary carotid occlusion to predict the effects of permanent occlusion found only the reduction of rCBF less than 30 mL/ 100 g/min to be significant among the variables, including quantitative CBF values, neurologic findings, sustained-attention test results, age, sex, and side of occlusion.[37]

Radiation may induce or accelerate atherosclerosis, through means still unclear,[38] but arterial stenosis of the carotid artery is a recognized complication of irradiation of the head and neck. Huvos and associates[30] found this form of atherosclerosis in 15 of their 64 cases of head and neck tumor with carotid artery complication. Supervoltage therapy had been given to 24 of the patients, and 45 had undergone preoperative radiation therapy to the neck. Levinson and coworkers[39] described 3 patients with atypical, presumably atherosclerotic lesions that developed more than 25 years after external cervical irradiation. The syndromes occurred through a variety of inferred mechanisms, including cerebral embolization, impaired retinal perfusion, and decreased total cerebral perfusion.

Intracranial Internal Carotid Artery

Despite painstaking studies, the problem of the significance of atherosclerotic lesions of the *intracranial* ICA is still largely unsettled. Discrepancies between studies in which more occlusions occurred in the intracranial ICA than in the extracranial ICA and those in which no occlusion occurred in the intracranial ICA are obvious. Useful comparison between some of the series is difficult if not impossible because grading systems were different and occlusions were not always separated from stenoses. These studies appeared from 1956 through 1966, when the hemodynamic significance of stenoses may not have been clear to all pathologists. Today, terms such as "significant" and "severe" would probably not be applied to stenoses that reduce the lumen by about half. The intracranial ICA, especially the cavernous part, is the second site of predilection of atherosclerosis, but the extent and severity of the lesions are far behind those of the sinus; and a number (unspecified) of atherosclerotic primary occlusive thromboses occur in the intracranial ICA.

No clear evidence indicates that a siphon stenosis increases the risk of occlusive thrombosis of a stenosis at the ICA origin, and vice versa.[40–42] Likewise, tandem stenoses appear not to raise the risk of the carotid endarterectomy.[43]

Anterograde and retrograde secondary thromboses of the intracranial ICA are a subject for which only a scanty literature exists. Primary thrombotic occlusion of the sinus is in most cases followed by extensive stagnation thrombosis. However, occlusions occasionally remain segmental. Pathologically well-studied instances of intracranial ICA thrombotic occlusion are rare. In Hutchinson and Yates'[44] cases Nos. 58, 72, 78, and 93, the intracranial ICA was occluded by thrombus, but data are lacking about anterograde and retrograde thrombus. In cases Nos. 58 and 93 (the latter being a bilateral ICA occlusion), the rostral part of the plug remained proximal to the posterior communicating artery and there was no pericerebral occlusion. In both cases an ipsilateral hemispheral infarct was present. In case No. 72 there was no cerebral infarct; the occluding material was old. In Torvik and Jörgensen's[45,46] 28 intracranial ICA occlusions, 5 showed anterograde

thrombus, 6 retrograde thrombus, and 1 both anterograde and retrograde thrombus, and 16 showed none. However, these "primary" occlusions were thromboembolic, and the part played by atherosclerotic lesions cannot be estimated. Nevertheless, these researchers noted that all occlusions more than 1.5 months old were longer than 2 cm and that in 3 of 7 cases with retrograde propagation, the thrombus extended down to the extracranial division of the artery.

In the study reported by Castaigne and associates,[40] of six primary occlusions of the siphon, two had no retrograde thrombosis (one of them was a very short occlusion between the origins of the ophthalmic and posterior communicating arteries), in one a retrograde thrombus extended to the cervical part of the artery, and in three it extended down to the ICA origin. Luessenhop[47] found that when angiography was performed during the first month after the onset of symptoms, 31% of the occlusions were in the region of the siphon, but that with the passage of time, this percentage decreased, approaching zero at 30 months. He thought that this change was undoubtedly a consequence of proximal propagation of the thrombi. Most probably, in this series, not all occlusions were of atherosclerotic origin. On the basis of this literature, it seems reasonable to assume that retrograde thrombi developing down to the ICA origin are not rare. Thus, arrest of contrast medium at the sinus on angiograms does not allow firm conclusions as to where the primary occlusion started, inasmuch as the angiographic appearance of the proximal end of carotid occlusion does not predict the age of the occlusion, at least within the first 6 days from stroke onset (Fig. 5–4).[48]

Discontinuous occlusions (i.e., the presence of a patent segment of the ICA between the extracranial occluded ICA and the intracranial ICA) may be found at autopsy, and it may be difficult or impossible to decide whether the distal plug is thrombotic or embolic.[40,45,46,49] This pathologic situation should be kept in mind as a source of technical difficulties during surgical endarterectomies to remove occlusions of the ICA.

PATHOPHYSIOLOGY OF CAROTID ARTERY ISCHEMIA

The clinical syndromes that occur from disease involving the carotid artery itself result from two basic mechanisms: (1) intracranial arterial occlusion, due to either embolism or anterograde extension of thrombus across the circle of Willis into the stems of the major cerebral arteries, and (2) perfusion failure due to inadequate collateral pathways distal to hemodynamically significant stenosis or occlusion (Fig. 5–5). Both mechanisms may even be operative in the same patient.[50,51]

Collateral Pathways

When the ICA is unable to supply its usual intracranial territory, five major sources of collateral flow may develop, individually or in combination (Fig. 5–6).[52–54] As expected, but rarely documented, studies have indicated that the development and extent of such collateral pathways mirror the severity of the carotid stenosis they are intended to compensate.[55]

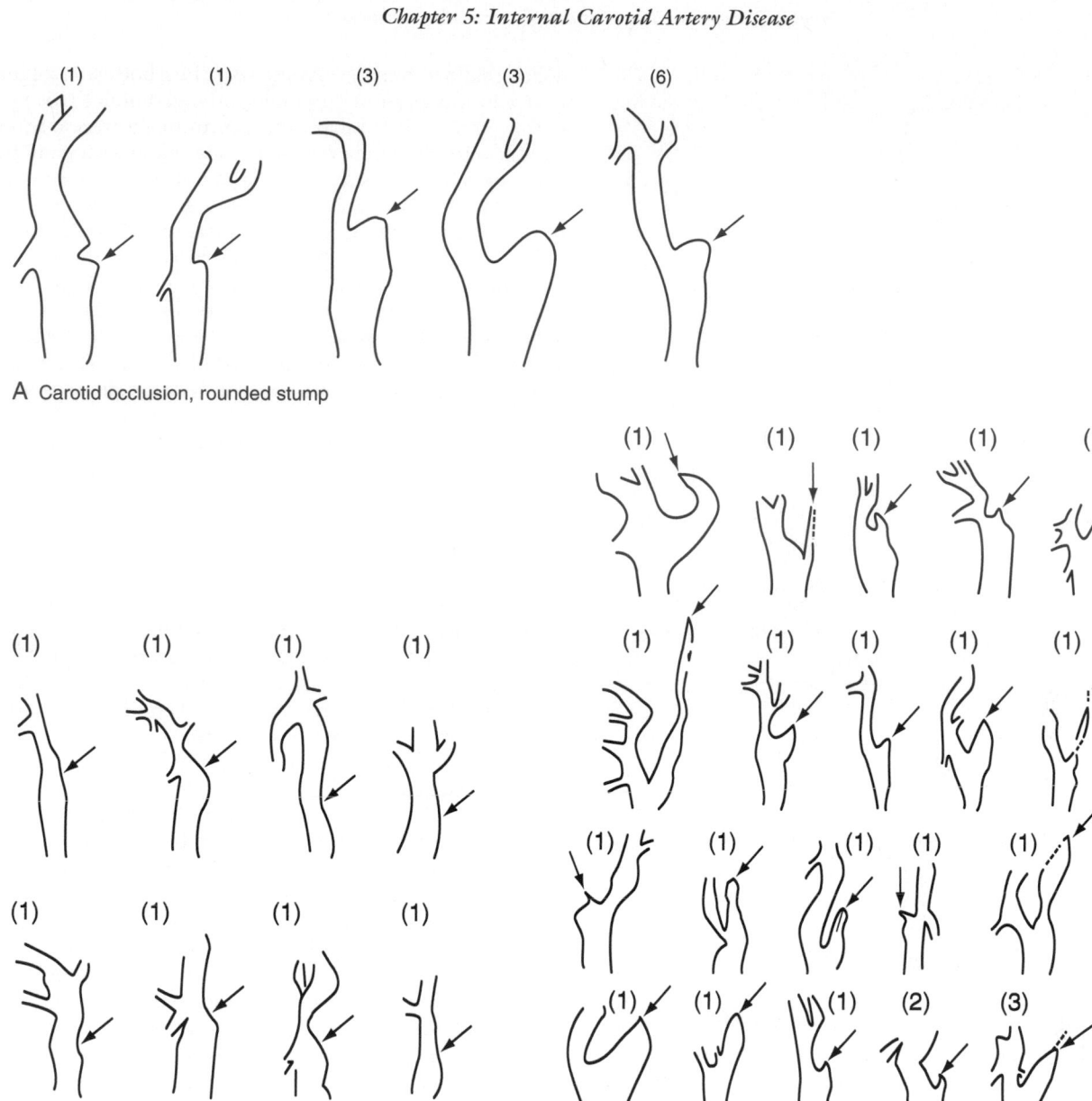

A   Carotid occlusion, rounded stump

B   Carotid occlusion, absent artery   C   Carotid occlusion, pointed stump

FIGURE 5–4 *Angiographic appearance of different types of internal carotid artery occlusion. Numbers in parentheses indicate days between stroke onset and angiography.*

The most readily recognized extracranial source is an anastomosis *via the external carotid artery (ECA) through the orbit*. Anterograde blood flow up the ECA to the orbit allows links with the ophthalmic branch of the intracranial ICA, reversing the direction of flow in the ophthalmic artery and then allowing distal anterograde flow in the supra-ophthalmic portion of the ICA. These paths of anastomoses occur mainly between the maxillary branch of the ECA and the ophthalmic artery in the floor of the orbit. Smaller anastomoses occur over the roof of the orbit between the facial and frontal branches of the ECA and the supratrochlear and supraorbital branches of the

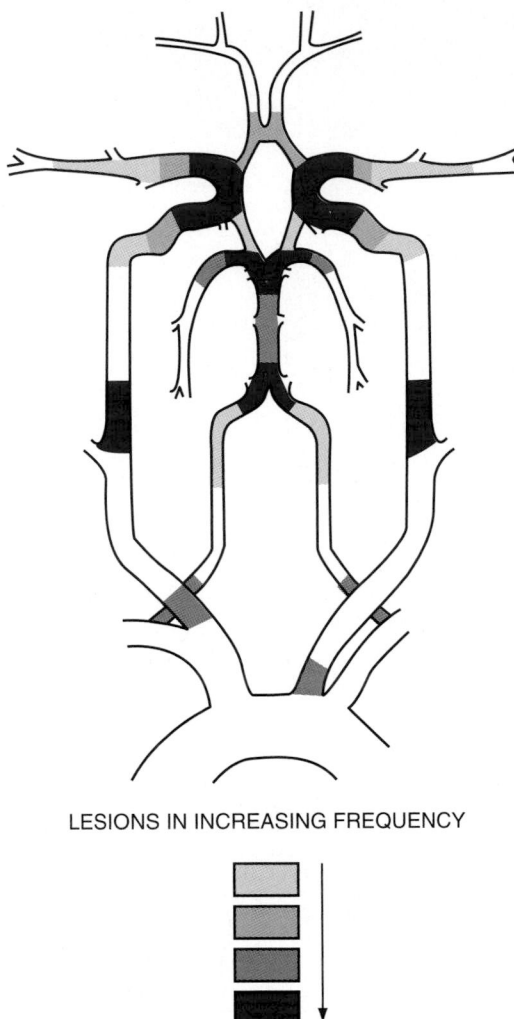

LESIONS IN INCREASING FREQUENCY

FIGURE 5–5   *Distribution of lesions in the carotid territory.*

ophthalmic artery. The blood flows from these anastomoses retrogradely in the ophthalmic artery to reach the intracranial portion of the ICA at the siphon. From there the flow continues distally toward the circle of Willis in the usual anterograde fashion. Collateral flow to the ophthalmic artery may come from meningeal branches of the ECA. Rarely, the ophthalmic artery is not a branch of the ICA, instead receiving its entire flow from the meningeal artery, a linkage that offers little intracranial supply to the circle of Willis.

The most important source of collateral circulation for a hemisphere comes from the *contralateral ICA via the circle of Willis*. In this case, blood flows anterogradely up the opposite ICA and then across the circle of Willis at the anterior communicating artery, from which it may pass anterogradely along the cortical branches of the anterior cerebral artery and on the other hand retrogradely along the stem of the anterior cerebral artery to the middle cerebral stem, and then distally into the territory of the middle cerebral artery in the usual anterograde fashion.

Because this form of collateral flow depends on an intact anterior half of the circle of Willis, the many minor variations in the circle of Willis often conspire to prevent this collateral flow from developing fully. Leading among them is an azygous anterior cerebral artery, in which the supply to the anterior cerebral artery arises from a common trunk, with no anterior cerebral stem on one side to complete the circle of Willis. In such cases, the two anterior cerebral artery territories may be involved with infarction or may be spared together, depending on the vascular anatomy.

The *vertebrobasilar system* may supply the middle and anterior cerebral artery territories by means of collateral flow through the ipsilateral posterior communicating artery. This collateral flow is the posterior equivalent of the collateral flow via the anterior half of the circle of Willis. It depends on the presence of a posterior communicating artery that is both patent and large, which is far less common than a patent, large anterior communicating artery. Rarely, the flow into the ICA territory from the basilar artery is by way of a persisting trigeminal artery, which usually reaches the ICA near the base of the skull (Fig. 5–7).

Flow retrograde from cerebral arteries *through the border zones over the brain surface* may spare some or all of the cortical surface branches of the endangered arterial territories. In this setting, the anatomy of the circle of Willis plays a vital role: If the posterior communicating artery is too small to carry much collateral flow, the distal ends of the cortical branches of the posterior cerebral artery may supply collateral flow to the anterior or middle cerebral artery territories through the borderzone anastomoses over the hemisphere surface. If the stem of the anterior cerebral artery ipsilateral to the occluded ICA is likewise too small, the anterior cerebral artery may collateralize some or all of the middle cerebral surface branches through the borderzone. In such instances, the retrograde flow into the endangered territories ranges from full collateral flow all the way to the stem of the recipient vessel to little more than feeble flow into the distal cortical surface branches.

Other paths of collateral flow may develop under special circumstances, all of them so exceptional that they could not be counted on under normal conditions. Thus, cerebral surface vessels may anastomose with an extracranial arterial source through a craniotomy site, and extremely rare instances have been described in which the deep penetrating arteries (the lenticulostriates) have linked through the deep white matter to the cerebral convexity borderzones.

It has long been obvious that the mere angiographic demonstration of collateral flow bears little relationship to its physiologic effect. Using PET measurements (CBF, blood volume, oxygen extraction fraction), Powers and colleagues[56] found that neither the percent stenosis nor the residual lumen diameter of the extracranial ICA was a reliable predictor of the hemodynamic state of the cerebral circulation in patients. Hemodynamic insufficiency of the hemisphere correlated best with angiographic patterns of meningeal and ophthalmic arterial collateral paths. Similarly, transcranial Doppler (TCD) ultrasonography has shown that ophthalmic collateral flow is an insufficient source of supply to the brain and that its presence indicates that the more common sources of collateral flow are unavailable or incompetent. Prominent ophthalmic collateral flow is probably a poor, not a favorable, prognostic sign.[57,58]

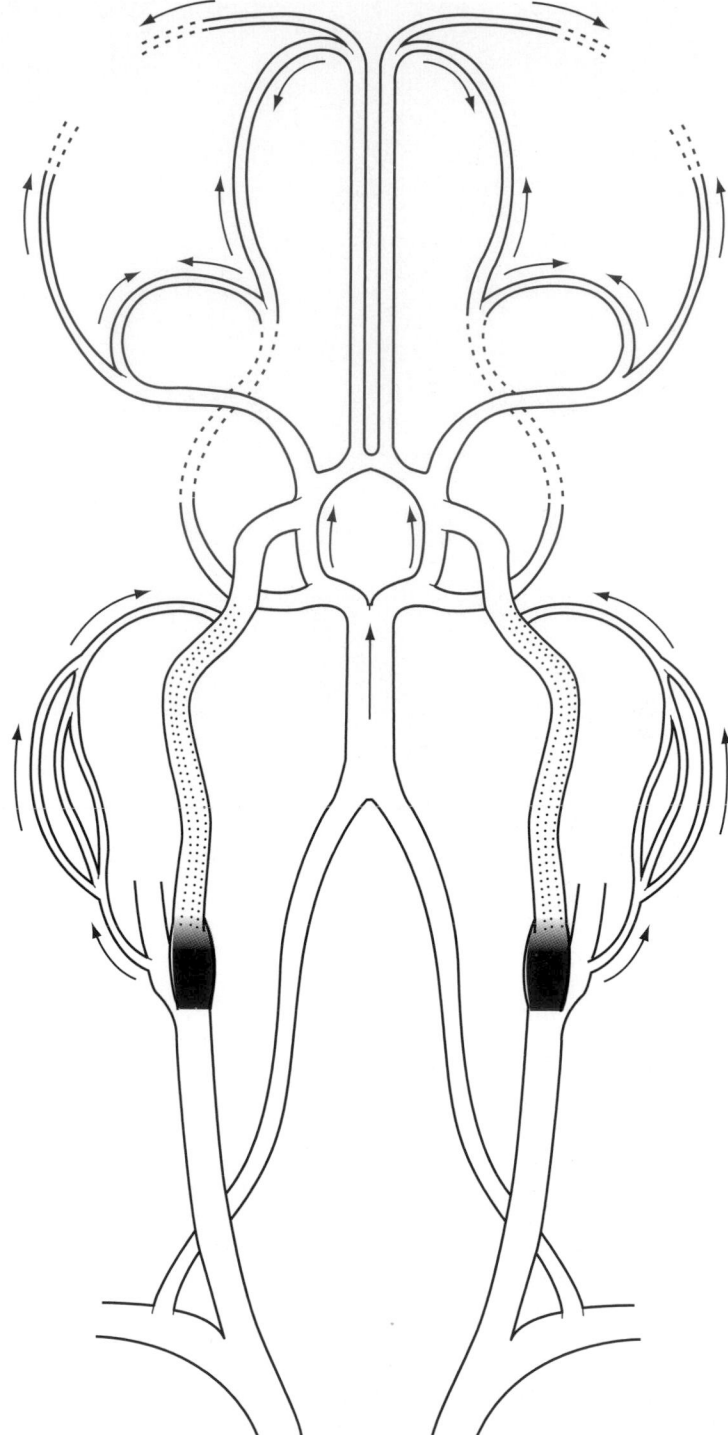

FIGURE 5–6 *Sources of collateral flow for occlusion of the internal carotid territory (red, site of occlusion; stippled, distal flow failure) showing external carotid collateral to the ophthalmic (1) and intracranial collaterals via the basilar (2) through the posterior communicating arteries (3), the borderzone vessels linking the distal branches of the anterior-middle cerebral arteries (4) and posterior cerebral to anterior (5) and middle cerebral arteries (6). (From Gautier, JC, Mohr JP: Ischemic stroke. In Mohr JP, Gautier JC [eds]: Guide to Clinical Neurology. New York, Churchill Livingstone, 1995, p 543.)*

Mechanisms of Ischemic Stroke

The problem in diagnosis and management of carotid artery disease lies mainly in (1) clarifying which one of these principles is at work in a given case, (2) identifying the source of an embolus, (3) determining the severity of the perfusion failure, and (4) predicting future events.

Most cases of carotid territory ischemia are broadly attributed to atherosclerosis, but a variety of mechanisms of infarction seem to be involved. For TIAs, these mech-

anisms could entail a temporary cessation of flow either in a distal branch artery from embolus or over the distal territories of the underperfused carotid artery during periods when systemic hypotension, bradyarrhythmia, or other causes of "low flow" exist. With restoration of blood flow, the ischemic region of the brain would quickly recover, and the clinical deficit (TIA) vanish. For infarction, the processes would presumably be the same, but the effects of the occlusion would persist. No studies have unequivocally established this mechanism.

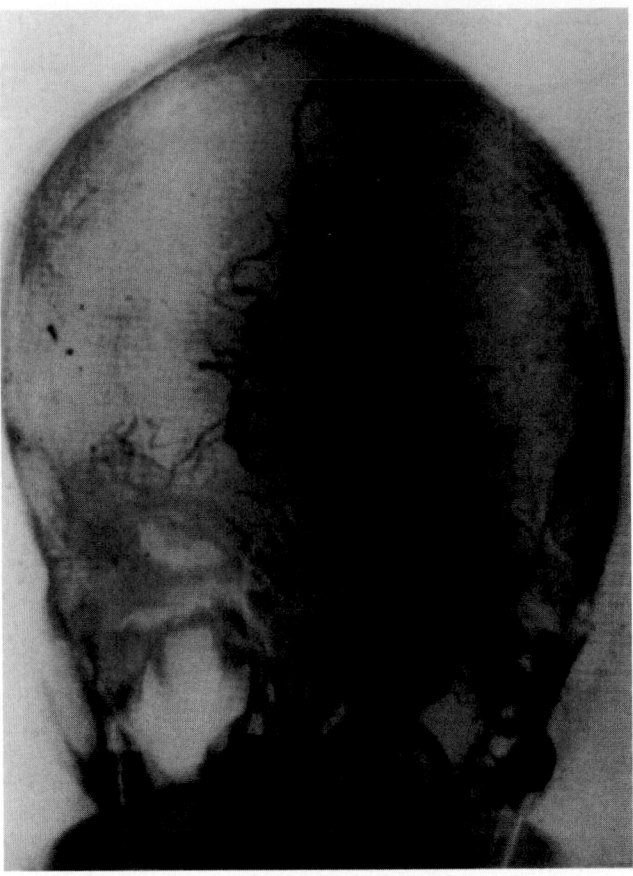

FIGURE 5–7   *Example of a persistent trigeminal artery.*

Anterograde propagation of carotid thrombosis is the easiest to understand of the effects of carotid artery occlusion. Although uncommonly documented in clinical series, extension to and beyond the circle of Willis, involving the stems of the anterior and middle cerebral arteries, usually creates devastating cerebral infarction.[51,59] One result is the rare telodiencephalic syndrome,[60] which consists of contralateral brachiofacial hemiparesis occasionally accompanied by homonymous hemianopia and aphasia but associated with ipsilateral hemihypohidrosis and an ipsilateral Horner syndrome. We believe that it is caused by an ischemic lesion of crossed pathways descending from the cerebrum and the uncrossed hypothalamic-spinal sympathetic pathways. The syndrome was attributed to occlusion of the ICA and occasionally the middle cerebral artery.

Embolism is a common cause of both TIA and stroke, whether into the carotid artery from a source proximal to the ICA (e.g., cardiac, aortic arch)[61–64] or from the carotid artery toward intracranial territories. Early autopsy studies documented intracranial embolism rising from extracranial carotid occlusive disease as a cause of hemisphere infarction. The clinical effects were usually serious and commonly occurred with no warning. Any part of the intracranial carotid circulation could be affected, but frequently the embolus impacted the middle cerebral artery stem or major branches, resulting in a sizable infarct with a serious clinical syndrome. The source of the embolus might be fragmentation and distal migration of a thrombus

at the time of, or shortly after, acute carotid occlusion, or in the setting of severe stenosis. Alternatively, anterograde propagation of thrombus into the circle of Willis, without fragmentation, may also account for intracranial obstruction.

Embolism from whatever source is a frequent cause of stroke. In the study by Pessin and associates,[51] the clinical picture for the 42 patients with angiographic evidence of embolism contrasted sharply with that for the 22 patients with no such evidence. A significantly lower proportion (40%) of those with an embolic (or suspected embolic) mechanism had preceding TIAs, compared with 73% of the 22 patients with a nonembolic mechanism. Stroke deficits were more severe in the embolic group than in the non-embolic group. The syndromes have not proved possible to differentiate from embolism of cardiac sources.[65]

Although cardiogenic embolism into the carotid artery and its branches is well established by pathology studies, embolism *from* the carotid artery itself has long been assumed but also has been difficult to prove.[66] Early success with anticoagulant therapy supported the assumption that embolism was being prevented.[63,67,68] Proof of the embolic mechanism might be difficult to find, because angiographic[69–73] and pathologic studies[61] have shown how promptly cerebral emboli fragments disappear, leaving a patent vessel supplying the clinically affected region. Fisher[74] and Ross Russell[75] observed material passing through the retinal circulation during attacks of transient monocular blindness, documenting that migrating particles could be associated with transient symptoms, but left unsettled whether the material seen was actually embolic in character or could be compared to the "cattle trucking" (i.e., spaces of clumped red cells alternating with spaces of plasma) seen in retinal vessels in a setting of hypotension associated with cardiac arrest. Evidence has also been presented for clinically asymptomatic cerebral embolization in patients suffering symptomatic transient monocular blindness.[76] Fisher and Ojemann's[77] findings in a study of 90 carotid endarterectomy specimens have challenged the embolic theory of TIAs. They found that three clinical categories—hemispheric TIAs, transient monocular blindness, and asymptomatic, severe carotid obstruction producing near occlusion—led to hemodynamic insufficiency as the cause of the transient symptoms. Mural thrombus, present in many of the specimens, contributed to the overall obstructive process but had little independent serious consequences beyond this effect (Fig. 5–8). Other case reports have been explained as embolism,[78,79] instances inferred to have passed up the ophthalmic artery, having arisen from the patent "stump" proximal ICA (Fig. 5–9).[80] Embolism has also been inferred to have reached the basilar from the carotid artery via a persistent trigeminal artery.[81]

Despite the classic literature, hopes for a clear proof of a carotid origin for embolism are often confounded: The famous case of Chiari, dating from 1905,[82] which was the index case of inferred embolism from carotid ulcer (Fig. 5–10), involved a patient whose autopsy also showed a patent cardiac foramen ovale, which is nowadays regarded as equally or possibly more suspect as a source of stroke.

The issue of source aside, that of *particle size* is obviously of great importance. The size of embolic material

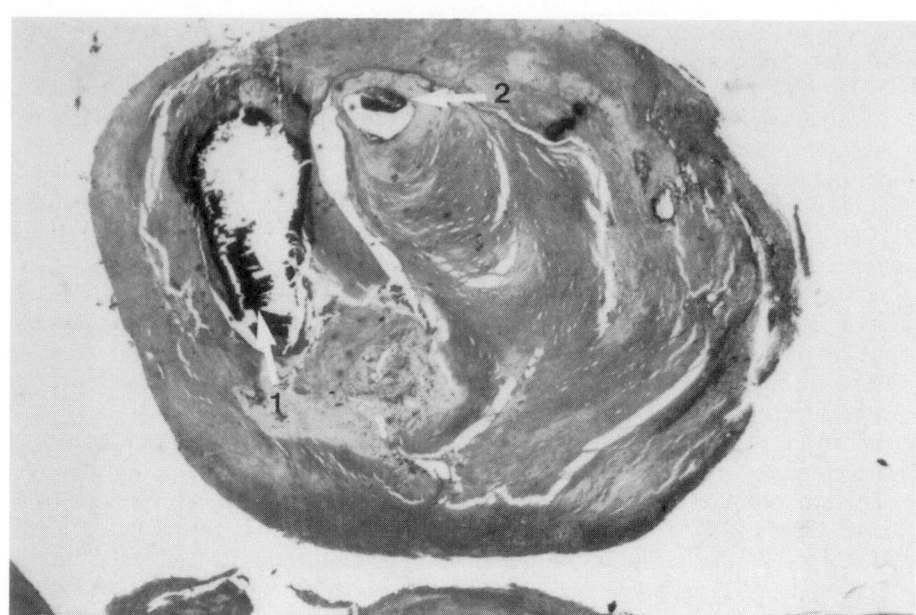

FIGURE 5–8 *Histology of severe stenosis, showing intraplaque hematoma and fibrin-platelet thrombus in lumen. (Courtesy of W. Kupsky, MD.)*

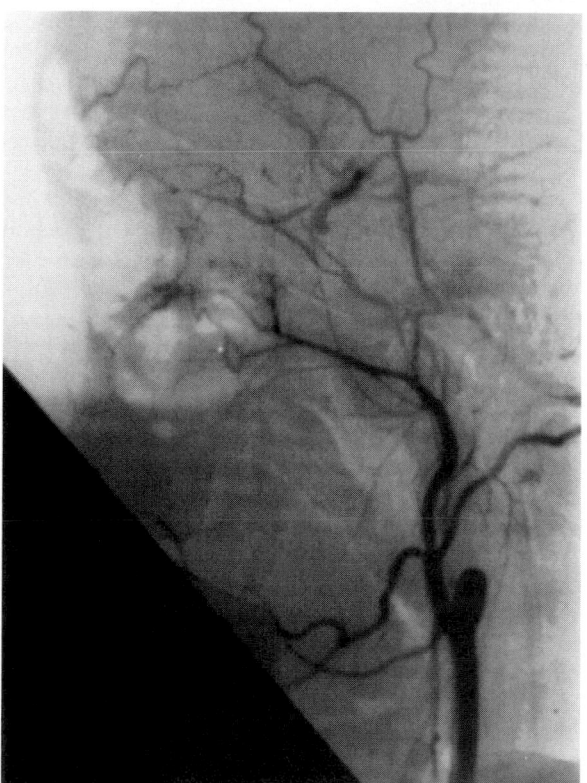

FIGURE 5–9 *Occluded internal carotid artery with a large stump.*

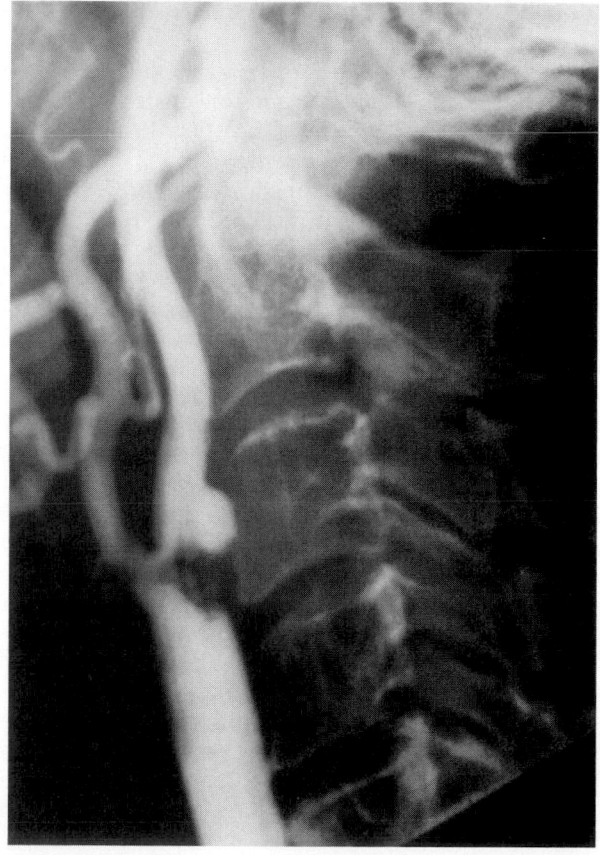

FIGURE 5–10 *Internal carotid artery with combined stenosis and large ulceration.*

sufficient to cause retinal ischemia may be too small to affect or block any but the tiny pial surface branches in the hemisphere and is unlikely to cause symptoms. This point alone may explain the usually asymptomatic state of cases in which cholesterol emboli are found in retinal vessels. However, once carotid territory embolism has occurred, no matter how small the particle size, no studies to date

permit the inference of continued small particle embolism; subsequent emboli may be quite a bit larger, as indicated by a few discouraging cases.[59,73]

The possibility of a major stroke in a setting of presumably minor carotid artery disease is the dreaded complication that continues to dictate many management decisions. The mural hemorrhage thesis of Lusby and coworkers[83] dating back several decades raised the worry that a small ulcer or modest atheroma may suffice to allow a subintimal dissection to develop, usually caused by subintimal hemorrhage. The resultant hemorrhage could thus suddenly convert a modest lesion to a severe stenosis and, fragmenting, could dislodge a "shower" of particles distally. This unsettling hypothesis, which offered endarterectomy as a way of avoiding all these risks, has had little support from observational studies or clinical trials in the years since its presentation.[77,84,85] Later studies using magnetic resonance imaging (MRI) may encourage more work in this field, because it has become possible to identify fibrous caps[86] and even rupture of the cap in the carotid lesion with this technique.[87]

The embolic theory can account for different types of carotid territory TIAs on the basis of separate embolic material occluding different intracranial branches, and probably many TIAs occur as a result of this short-lived embolic mechanism.[88] The clinical and angiographic details in many of these cases suggest that they are a variant but not the usual type of TIA. Duration of the TIA deficit in embolic cases appears to be far longer (hours or more) than the usual brief period (minutes).[89] Later assessments of syndrome duration also support the notion that longer events relate to risk factors associated with embolism, in particular atrial fibrillation.[90]

The classic, so-called stereotypic TIAs, in which attacks replicate themselves again and again, have proved difficult to document.[89] Their occurrence at any frequency is a major problem for the embolic theory, save for a single publication showing artificial emboli injected in the carotid circulation in a dog model gathered in the same vessel.[91] In the published experience with aberrant embolization from polymeric silicone (Silastic) ball therapy used for arteriovenous malformations, several cases have been reported in which a similar syndrome occurred from embolism to a variety of different middle cerebral branches; the complaints included focal weakness of the arm[92] persisting for only a few minutes and transient dysesthesia of the contralateral hand, both common symptoms of TIA. Sadly, such details are often lost on physicians from other specialties, as shown by studies indicating that many events that neurologists label as TIAs are not those of minor stroke, whereas minor stroke is often included among the conditions labeled as TIAs by non-neurologists.[93]

Perfusion failure with distal insufficiency has long been recognized as a major mechanism that may account for cerebral ischemia. This theory has proved attractive because the topography of cerebral infarcts in many cases of carotid occlusion closely mimics that found in obvious settings of hypotension such as cardiac arrest, and because the most reliable correlation with TIAs is severe stenosis.

The distal insufficiency concept for ischemia or infarction implies decreased vascular perfusion on those areas of the brain parenchyma located at the greatest distance from the site of severe stenosis or occlusion.[94] As a consequence, stagnation thrombus may develop from local circulatory failure at these distant sites,[95] and infarction follows. The areas at risk include the most distal segments of the cortical branches of the middle cerebral artery, in particular the superior parietal and posterior temporal-occipital area.[96]

A lengthy list of publications documents the existence of infarction found along the superior frontal, superior parietal, and lateral occipital regions in a setting of carotid occlusions or high-grade stenosis (Fig. 5–11).[97–105] Interest in the subject became more keen after Schneider's 1953 proposal of the thesis of infarction by the process of distal insufficiency.[106] Despite the implied mechanism of transient hypotensive theories such as that cited previously, the autopsy-documented cases with such infarct topography have been found in a high percentage of cases to be associated with a thrombus or severe stenosis of the carotid artery. The advent of modern imaging studies, ranging from computed tomography (CT)[101,105] including xenon CT and PET scanning, has confirmed the correlation of a distal field topography with high-grade carotid stenosis or occlusion.[107–112]

Current studies, led mainly by Lin and colleagues,[113] have teased out of the case material a cohort of patients whose oxygen extraction fraction is increased, as shown by PET scanning, have succeeded in correlating MRI and PET findings to assess CBF, and have found a correlation with deep white matter infarct along the ventricular wall and low rCBF as assessed by PET.[114] Known also as the "misery perfusion syndrome,"[115] this syndrome has been explained by reduced cerebral metabolism and has proved to be surgically reversible from carotid stenosis and from intracranial angioplasty.[116]

Separate from PET studies, quantitative TCD ultrasonography has also been used to assess perfusion failure in carotid occlusive disease. Low reactivity of middle cerebral blood vessels in a setting of hypercapnia, a sign of fully dilated collateral vessels, has been documented by a number of groups to have a significant relationship ($P = .04$) to high-grade carotid stenosis.[37,117,118] The demonstration of such an extreme degree of sensitivity of cerebral flow to alterations in PCO_2 may help resurrect interest in notions of cerebral claudication,[119] which is a well-recognized clinical effect in the moyamoya disorder but is less well studied in carotid stenosis and occlusion. Computer modeling is being attempted to estimate the probability of success of extracranial-intracranial bypass surgery.[120]

There is also the possibility of *multimechanism infarction*. Modern imaging has allowed some assessment of the frequencies of embolism or signs of perfusion failure. A study of 102 consecutive cases with varying degrees of carotid stenosis found distal field lesions in approximately 50% of patients with high-grade carotid stenosis or occlusion, and almost an equal number with "territorial infarctions" (i.e., inferred single-branch occlusions in those with occlusion). Of special interest was the observation that 77.8% of the cases with high-grade carotid stenosis had a perfusion-diffusion "mismatch"—that is, larger zones of impairment on perfusion-weighted MRI compared with the somewhat smaller lesions documented on diffusion-weighted MRI.[121]

CLINICAL SYNDROMES

The basic clinical features of extracranial carotid disease were described over the years of the 20th century. The

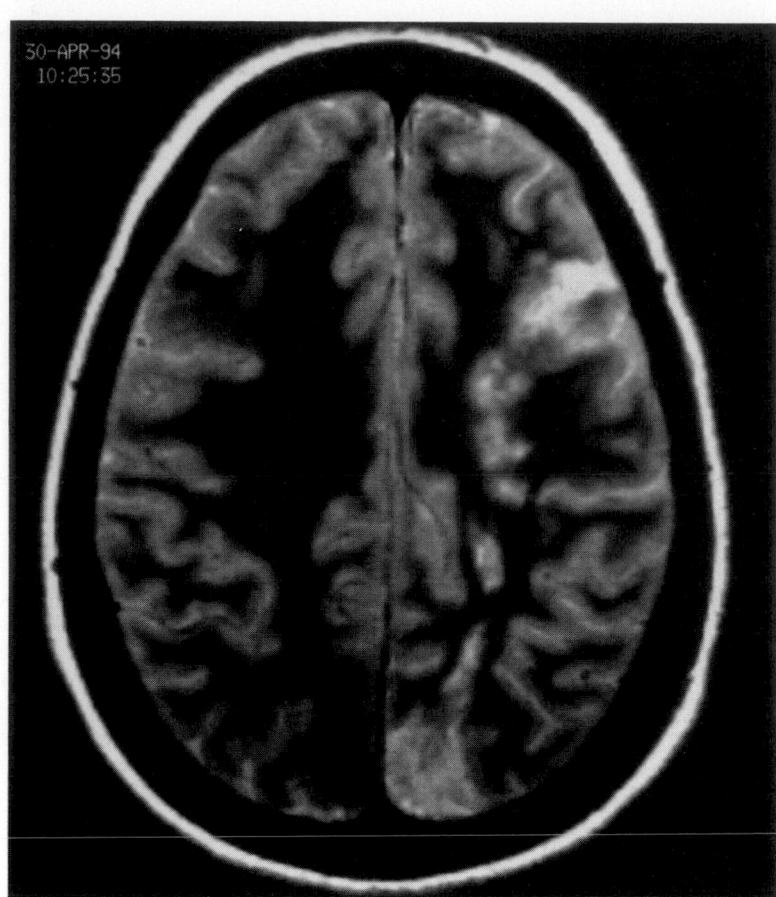

30-APR-94
10:25:35

FIGURE 5–11 *MRI scan of a distal-field (border-zone) infarction (From Gautier, JC, Mohr JP: Ischemic stroke. In Mohr JP, Gautier JC [eds]: Guide to Clinical Neurology. New York, Churchill Livingstone, 1995, p 543.)*

characteristic clinical syndrome of ICA occlusion has long been taken known to consist of "premonitory fleeting symptoms including paresthesias, paralysis, monocular blindness and aphasia," a description that preceded the concepts later to be known as TIAs.[122] It was the prospect of therapy that prompted so much interest in carotid disease. C.M. Fisher played a major role after World War II in the renewal of interest in the clinical importance of carotid disease. In his early clinicopathologic studies, he described the prodromal transient neurologic events frequently preceding stroke, discussed possible stroke mechanisms, and even predicted the surgical treatment. Eastcott and associates[123] were the first to reconstruct an extracranial ICA lesion successfully. Thus began the modern era in diagnosis and management of extracranial carotid artery disease.

Transient Ischemic Attacks

TIAs have been defined as a temporary, focal neurologic deficit presumably related to ischemia and lasting less than 24 hours.[124,125] The history of this time frame for a TIA seems to have arisen not so much from the documented time course of a typical attack as from uncertainty about to its cause. Because it has long been agreed that in a patient with a focal deficit lasting longer than 24 hours one would be expect to find a focus of ischemic infarction at autopsy, the definition of a TIA as any spell lasting less than this time can be seen as a negative definition.

It appears likely that the interest and energy of Irving Wright, a cardiologist at New York Hospital, led to the founding of the Princeton Cerebrovascular Conferences, at which issues of definitions for TIA were first discussed in detail in the Americas. The first such conference, held at the Nassau Inn in Princeton, New Jersey, in January 1954, and entitled "Cerebral Vascular Diseases," was held under the "auspices" of the American Heart Association, with Irving S. Wright as chairman and E. Hugh Luckey, a prominent New York Hospital internist, as editor. During this first session, early results of treatment of 57 patients with warfarin, 31 of whom had valvular heart disease and 29 had atrial fibrillation, were presented by E. McDevitt of Cornell. The second conference, held in 1956, was notable for having published a report, reprinted from a 1958 issue of the journal *Neurology*, featured a "Classification and Outline of Cerebrovascular Diseases," which also acknowledged among other entities the existence of a diagnosis termed "infarction of undetermined cause." At the third conference, in 1960, the subject of clinical diagnosis was defined in three stages of focal arterial disease, the last being "completed stroke." At the same conference, CM Fisher, from the Massachusetts General Hospital's Neurology Service, presented results of anticoagulant therapy from the National Cooperative study begun in 1958. Thus well under way, and before being supported by large, current clinical trials, was the notion that antithrombotics, in this case warfarin, had a role in the treatment of ischemic stroke.

How the notion of a 24-hour duration for TIAs became established has been difficult to determine. As best we can discover, far shorter durations were widely recognized during the years of the early Princeton Conferences. The first citation suggesting such a long duration was that by Marshall,[126] whose review cited only a few instances of focal events lasting longer than a few minutes; nevertheless, he proposed 24 hours as a means to ensure not including in the definition cases in which the origin was not vascular. This expanded definition became widely accepted, based as it was on clinical criteria only in the days long before modern imaging.

When the subject has been studied through the use of actual case material, the 24-hour criterion has been recognized to be excessive.[89] The typical carotid territory TIAs are brief, typically lasting only some 7 to 10 minutes, as stated by patients in retrospective interviews. (TIAs are almost always assessed by interview, but in the patients we have observed during an attack, there is often a distortion of time in a patient's memory.) These brief spells have a high correlation with angiographic evidence of tight carotid stenosis, better than that of spells lasting an hour or longer. However, the prognosis for subsequent stroke appears to be the same whether the spell is brief or long.[127,128] More important, a literature has developed demonstrating the evidence of brain infarction in patients whose syndrome lasts longer than an hour[129] with disturbed MR spectroscopy findings in the ipsilateral hemisphere.[130] Calls for a redefinition of TIA limited to an hour are thus not new.[131] An effort by a small consortium has attempted a redefinition of TIA as lasting an hour or less.[132]

Differential Diagnosis of Transient Ischemic Attacks

Interobserver agreement on the diagnosis has remained a problem.[93,133] Many types of spells similar or even partly identical to TIAs have different pathogeneses and stroke prognoses.[133,134] The concept of TIA is based on an atherothrombotic mechanism, especially that of high-grade carotid stenosis, a preventable form of subsequent stroke, making search for this cause well worth distinguishing TIAs from other types of spells.[135]

Seizures, migraine accompaniments, syncope, isolated dizziness, and transient memory disturbance are common disturbances that may be confused with TIAs. These spells, however, have no proven atheromatous basis, and their treatments and outcomes differ significantly from those of TIAs. Even spells considered to meet the definition of TIAs may have an underlying vascular mechanism other than large artery atherothrombotic disease. TIAs may be related to small, penetrating arterial disease that causes lacunar infarction. They may occur as a flurry in the hours before stroke, or as isolated events without stroke. The clinical features of lacunar TIAs may be indistinguishable from those of large artery TIAs, yet the diagnostic evaluation, treatment, and stroke risks are probably different. Also, rapidly fading cerebral embolism may give rise to a short-lived neurologic deficit consistent with the time criterion of TIA, but no atherothrombotic mechanism may exist. In one study,[89] such TIAs of a presumed embolic mechanism tended to be of longer duration, more than 1 hour, than TIAs from a carotid atheromatous cause.

All these variations should alert the clinician to the heterogeneous nature of TIAs. They are best viewed as symptoms, much like seizure and headache, and not as a homogeneous, pathogenic state. Further clarification of the underlying cerebrovascular mechanisms may lead to more rational therapy and more reliable prognostication.

Natural History

The importance of carotid TIAs is highlighted when they are viewed from the perspective of carotid stroke. Patients who suffer carotid stroke from extracranial carotid artery occlusion disease have a known prior TIA incidence of 50% to 75%.[89,136–138]

This situation contrasts sharply with the low incidence of TIAs (approximately 10%) associated with all types of stroke and reinforces the strong relationship between these transient events and underlying atherothrombotic occlusive disease. The available data, both prospective and retrospective, indicate that the TIAs may be impressive warnings of stroke in some patients, and their recognition provides the opportunity for therapeutic intervention.

Despite the large numbers of studies on TIAs, so many differences exist in definitions and methodology that all too many of the studies are disappointingly unhelpful. Few have focused on carotid territory TIAs alone, and even fewer have separated transient monocular blindness (TMB) from transient hemispheral attacks (THAs). Some studies emphasize incidence, and others describe prevalence. The TIAs have been documented by various methods, some by personal periodic examinations and others by search of clinical records; questionnaires have been tried.[139–146]

The available data show a wide range in prevalence and incidence. The prevalence varies from 1.1 to 77 per 1000 persons, and the incidence rate from 2.2 to 8 per 1000 persons per year.[139,142,143] The stroke risk associated with TIAs is significant, although no well-designed, controlled, randomized study has provided unequivocal information on the natural history of TIAs, nor is such a study likely to be done today. Past studies have assessed the stroke risk to be between 2% and 50%, results so discrepant as to be useless in an individual case.[68,126,147–153] These studies suffer from several limitations, including ambiguity of TIA definition, lumping together of carotid and vertebral basilar TIAs, and, most important, no angiographic verification of underlying vascular disease. Despite the limitations of these early studies, the view emerged that a considerable stroke risk attends TIAs, namely, in the range of 35% over 5 years, or 5% to 6% a year.[142]

Many of the important questions relating TIAs to specific carotid lesion configurations, such as irregular plaque, ulcer, severe stenosis, and occlusion, remain unanswered despite all the effort expended on the subject thus far.[154] At the least, the available evidence indicates that a serious stroke may follow a TIA in a discouraging number of patients, but the factors contributing to the risks for individuals have remained elusive.

The argument whether the outlook for TIA cases was too benign for endarterectomy to influence outcome favorably[19,155–157] has been settled by the dramatic results of the studies for symptomatic patients: Both the NASCET and the European Cooperative Study showed a clear advantage of surgery over medical (aspirin) therapy (see Chapter 65 on endarterectomy for further details). Neither trial tested surgery against anticoagulation, and the most striking of the positive findings were in those patients whose stenosis exceeded 70%. For NASCET, over a period of 18 months, in patients who were symptomatic with TIAs and were found to have stenosis of 70% to 90%, 7% of the 300 who underwent surgery suffered stroke or death, mostly in the perioperative period, whereas 24% of the 295 undergoing aspirin therapy had a stroke or died. This difference favoring surgery was highly significant ($P < .001$).[158] The risk of stroke was higher in patients with brain imaging showing "leukoariosis" than in those without such findings.[138] The outcome and best management plan for those whose stenosis is in the 30% to 70% range were less striking, with only modest or minimal benefits for surgery.

Transient Ischemic Attacks with Intracranial Internal Carotid Artery Disease

TIAs can be expected to occur in atherosclerosis of the intracranial ICA, as in extracranial ICA disease. However, precise data are lacking. One reason is that most studies of TIAs have not isolated those specifically due to intracranial ICA lesions, and the few that did so have not dealt with symptoms, only with duration or prevalence. The common association is the occurrence of TIAs with lesions elsewhere, and the common occurrence of tandem lesions makes it difficult to sort out those TIAs that could specifically result from intracranial ICA disease.[41,42] Even though the ophthalmic artery arises from the intracranial ICA, amaurosis fugax (transient monocular blindness) has been difficult to demonstrate as an association with atherosclerosis in that portion of the vessel.[89,159-164] Very few specific cases have been recorded. Gerstenfeld[165] reported on a 30-year-old man who suffered many attacks of amaurosis fugax of the right eye. White streaks were seen in the retinal arterioles. Angiography disclosed an ICA occlusion above the level of the ophthalmic artery. In addition, the ophthalmic artery had an unusually early origin from the ICA because it arose from the infraclinoid part. It should be noted that a severe right frontal headache was mentioned, a very uncommon feature of amaurosis fugax, and in such a young patient, atherosclerosis would appear unlikely. Dyll and associates[166] reported on a patient with four attacks of amaurosis fugax and roughening and narrowing of the uncoiled carotid siphon proximal to the origin of the ophthalmic artery. David[167] also described a case of amaurosis fugax with siphon lesions and a possible embolic mechanism.

Transient Monocular Blindness

TMB, also known as amaurosis fugax, has been recognized as an important manifestation of carotid artery disease since early reports.[168] TMB may be considered a brief monocular visual obscuration described by patients as a fog, blur, cloud, mist, and so forth. A shade or curtain effect occurs in only a minority of cases, approximately 15% to 20%, and is no more predictive of carotid artery disease than other variations of monocular visual loss.[134] The duration of visual impairment is brief, usually less than 15 minutes and rarely exceeding 30 minutes, with most patients affected for only 1 to 5 minutes.[75,159,163,169,170]

Flashing lights, scintillations, colors, and fortification spectra rarely occur as TIA manifestations and usually signify a migrainous event.[170] However, the presence of visual phenomena during TMB, in patients with greater than 75% stenosis, has been recorded by Goodwin and coworkers,[171] making differentiation from retinal migraine difficult, in some cases, on clinical grounds alone.

The number of TMB attacks that occur before a patient seeks medical attention varies greatly. Patients may experience a few or as many as 100 attacks of TMB over a span of several days to a year or more.[89] Vision is usually fully restored after an attack, although in long-term follow-up studies of affected patients,[162] a small number may sustain permanent visual loss from retinal infarction. TMB rarely occurs simultaneously with other neurologic deficits, and headache is not part of the disturbance. Hemisphere stroke is an infrequent sequel of TMB alone,[162,172,173] but careful studies of such cases occasionally reveal evidence of clinically unobvious cerebral embolism.[76] In most instances, clinically obvious stroke is preceded by one or more THAs. TMB tends to precede the first THA and can be documented with a careful history.

TMB poses endless diagnostic interpretation difficulties. The failure of the retinal arteries to show any abnormality during a period of TMB has been so often described that that the normal appearance of the retinal arteries has been speculated to be a sign that the inferred embolic material or low-flow state applies to the choroidal circulation, which would not be visualized by the ophthalmoscope. However, experimental occlusion of the central retinal artery for up to 98 minutes was not revealed by ophthalmoscopic change, and no significant permanent neurologic damage was observed.[174] Occlusion for 105 minutes or longer, however, produced irreversible damage, but even then no permanent injury was obvious in the retinal vascular bed. Only a transient leakage of fluorescein was observed 2.5 to 3 hours after the occlusion. These findings show that ophthalmoscopically normal vessels may be observed even in a setting of complete retinal artery occlusion.[161]

More than a century ago, Gowers[175] believed he had found intravascular material in his report on embolic material in the vessels supplying the eye. Cholesterol crystals, now known by his name (Hollenhorst plaques), were described by the Mayo ophthalmologist Hollenhorst.[176] He emphasized the association of the retinal material with systemic atherosclerosis and significant cardiovascular mortality, although he was uncertain about concomitant visual symptoms related to this particulate material.[176,177] He noted, however, that the embolic material in some cases was not necessarily associated with TMB. Reports prompted by the rare opportunity to observe a patient during an attack of TMB have described white or grayish material passing through the retinal circulation, presumably platelet complexes, perhaps mixed with fibrin.[74,75] This material is believed by many to be what is visualized by the ophthalmoscope in the rare instances of TMB studied during an attack.

Although he has been credited with the first description of such material observed during an attack, Fisher[74] was careful not to make too great a claim for how the material reached the vascular tree, and he left open the possibility that it may have been embolic or generated by local events

Clinical Manifestations

such as sludging from inadequate perfusion. Gerstenfeld[165] found similar white bodies, but the disease in his reported cases was confined to the ICA above the origin of the ophthalmic artery. In other case reports, only pallor of the disc was found, even given a source for embolic material in the proximal ICA.[166] McBrien and colleagues[178] succeeded in demonstrating a platelet origin for some of the embolic material seen in the retina in a 37-year-old man who suffered two episodes of blindness, the last one leaving him with a permanent nasal field defect. Platelet material was found in a superior nasal branch (apparently serving a portion of the visual field that was clinically unaffected). In the rare instances of calcium emboli to the retinal artery, an opportunity was provided to document the visual loss associated with focal branch occlusions. Brockmeier and associates[179] described four patients whose accompanying visual loss corresponded to the location of the retinal embolus. Transient visual loss of the type attributed to retinal branch occlusion with platelet aggregates was not encountered. These investigators suggested that the small size of the calcific emboli was sufficient to plug retinal arteries but insufficient to precipitate clinical symptoms in the cerebrum. However, Beal and coworkers[62] documented several sites of cerebral infarction in a 69-year-old man who experienced numerous brief spells of numbness and weakness consistent with hemispheral TIAs, indicating that some such particles can be large enough to precipitate symptoms. "Cattle trucking," a sign described in agonal settings, has also been seen in the vessels during some attacks.[161]

A rare case of transient vertical monocular hemianopia has also been described, the attacks being attributed to an anomalous arteriolar pattern, in that both the superior and inferior nasal quadrants were supplied by the same arterial branch.[180] Microembolization to this common arteriolar trunk may have accounted for the six episodes of monocular vertical hemianopia occurring in a 3-day period in this case.

Winterkorn and associates[181] described nine patients in whom TMB was associated with a variety of medical conditions unrelated to emboli or carotid hypoperfusion. This benign form was attributed to vasoconstriction of the retinal arterioles observed during funduscopic examination in several of their patients. The symptoms were responsive to calcium channel blockers. The clinical features show some variation from the TMB associated with carotid disease. Almost half of the patients in this report were older than 50 years and had had multiple attacks, some as many as 40, and often several a day over a brief period. Retro-orbital ache was noted in four of the nine patients. Several of the younger patients had a history of migraine or autoimmune conditions, but these features were not present in the older patients. In two older patients, temporal artery biopsy results were negative for temporal arteritis. This mechanism may partly explain the well-known clinical recognition of a benign form of TMB in younger patients.

Yet another variant of TMB has been reported by Furlan and coworkers[182]; in five patients with high-grade ICA stenosis or occlusion, exposure to bright light (often sunlight) precipitated transient unilateral visual loss. All the patients also had typical, unprovoked TMB and reduced retinal artery pressure in the affected eye; three also had hemispheric TIAs. Hemodynamic insufficiency of the retinal circulation was the probable mechanism leading to reduced photochemical resynthesis of visual pigments by the retinal rods and cones. Donnan and colleagues[183] recorded impairment of visual evoked responses in four patients with similar symptoms. Wiebers and associates[275] extended these observations to include four patients with episodic bilateral visual blurring or dimming in response to bright light; all the patients had severe bilateral carotid occlusive disease. Apart from TMB, persisting visual deficit from ocular infarction may also occur (see later).

Compared with THA (see below), TMB has a less malevolent prognosis for stroke; for the 198 cases of TMB in the nonsurgical treatment arm of the NASCET, the 3-year ipsilateral stroke rate was half that for the 417 medially treated cases of THA (adjusted hazard ratio, 0.53; 95% confidence interval [CI], 0.30 to 0.94).[184]

Transient Hemispheral Attacks

The symptoms reported for THAs have generally been weakness or numbness (or both) of part or all of the side of the body contralateral to the affected hemisphere, with presence or absence of a speech disturbance depending on whether the dominant hemisphere is affected.[67,122,126,185] An accurate history may be difficult to obtain because the episodes are brief and frightening to the patient, are not usually observed by another person, and may involve the right hemisphere, making the patient's report unreliable.

The most common constellation of symptoms involves motor and sensory dysfunction of the contralateral limbs, followed by pure motor dysfunction, pure sensory dysfunction, and lastly, isolated dysphasia.[89] The contralateral distal arm and hand are the body parts that most consistently suffer in the attack, and their symptoms may be the only manifestation. The deficit presumably reflects ischemia to a portion of the motor cortex in the distal field of the carotid circulation, by means of either embolism or perfusion failure.

Like occurrences of TMB, THAs are typically brief in duration (<15 minutes, with most lasting for 1 to 10 minutes). In one study, patients with THAs lasting for 1 hour or more tended to have wide open carotid arteries with evidence of intracranial branch occlusion, suggesting that the THAs reflected a short-lived cerebral embolus.[89] Patients may have one or many THAs before coming to medical attention; a few have 20 or more.[276] Most patients have THAs over several weeks to a few months, but some may have a history spanning months to a year, and rarely longer.

One distinctive if uncommon form of THA involves limb shaking.[122,186–192] Typically associated with severe carotid stenosis or occlusion, the attacks feature recurrent, involuntary, irregular, wavering movements of the contralateral arm or leg. The movements are described as shaking, trembling, twitching, flapping, or wavering. Limb shaking may be an initial form of THA, making distinction of THA from focal epilepsy an important differential point. In the limited number of patients reported to date, endarterectomy appears to be beneficial. The mechanism underlying the shaking TIAs is presumed to be hemodynamic insufficiency.

Nonsimultaneous Transient Monocular Blindness and Transient Hemispheral Attacks

Patients with carotid territory TIAs, depending on when they come to medical attention, may have had TMB, THA, or both types of TIA, although rarely simultaneously. There may be a stronger correlation with severe extracranial carotid artery disease in patients with a history of separate episodes of eye and hemispheral TIAs than in those with either type of spell alone.

Stroke Risk Associated with Transient Monocular Blindness and Transient Hemispheral Attacks

The NASCET provided important information on the stroke risk associated with the first clinically experienced (so-called first-ever) retinal versus hemispheral TIAs and high-grade (>70%) carotid stenosis.[193] Of the 129 medically treated patients, 59 had retinal TIAs, and 70 had hemispheral TIAs. Kaplan-Meier estimates of the risk of ipsilateral stroke at 2 years were 16.6% ± 5.6% for patients with retinal TIAs and 43.5% ± 6.7% for patients with hemisphere TIAs (P = .002). Patients with hemispheral TIAs were older and had a higher prevalence of most risk factors for stroke. In patients with TMB, duration of delay before seeking medical treatment was longer. The researchers in this study speculated that TMB may reflect an earlier stage in the development of carotid atherosclerosis, at which small thromboemboli may have a greater impact on sensitive retinal tissue, but little consequence (because of size) on cortical tissue. An important feature not presented in this report that bears on the conclusions is whether patients with TMB who had stroke had antecedent episodes of THAs.[194]

Angiographic Correlations with Transient Ischemic Attacks

A strong relationship exists between carotid territory TIAs (either TMB or THA) and extracranial carotid artery disease.[195–199] The correlation with severe stenosis is by no means a chance: It is prevalent in only 7% on autopsy in a population that is asymptomatic for carotid disease[200] and in less than 10% of patients with stroke due to another mechanism, such as hemorrhage.[136]

Apart from the degree of stenosis, no distinctive angiographic[201] or ultrasonographic[202] appearances have been found that separate symptomatic from asymptomatic patients who have the same severity of stenosis. Lesser degrees of stenosis do not have the same high correlation with TIA. However, misestimation of the stenosis is common when the imaging is based on conventional angiography. A severe stenosis found at surgery may be misread on angiogram as a lesser degree of stenosis because of minor variations in lumen display or in the judgment of individuals (Fig. 5–12).[23,203] Oblique films of the carotid bifurcation, which should be obtained in addition to the standard anteroposterior and lateral views, discloses irregular or ulcerative lesions not appreciated on the standard views.

Transient Ischemic Attacks and Nonstenosing Carotid Lesions

Despite a high correlation with severe stenosis, clinical impressions persist that any form of carotid atheromatous plaque can harbor thrombus and serve as a source of emboli causing TIAs. Early studies seemed to suggest that TIAs could be attributable to any degree of stenosis by

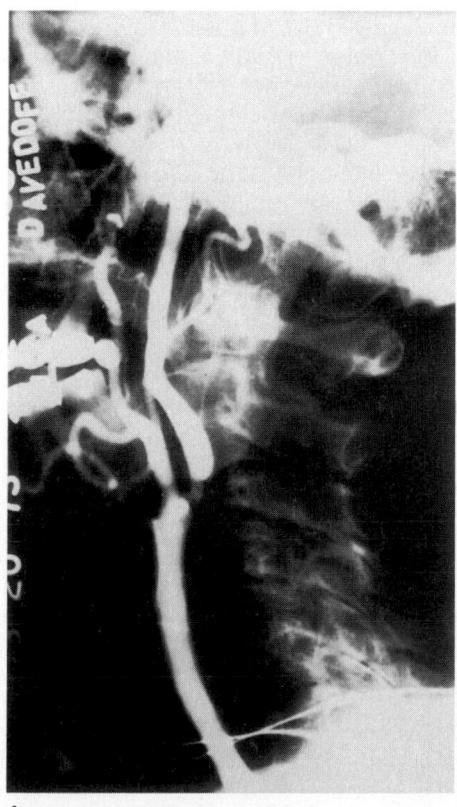 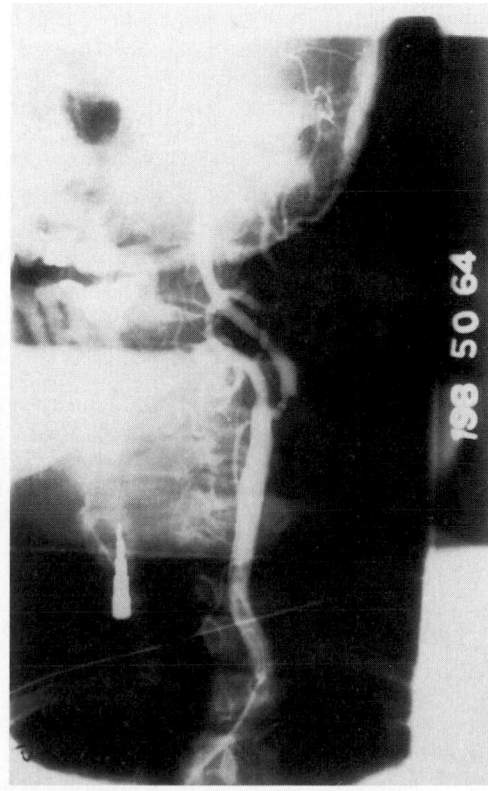

FIGURE 5–12 A *and* B, *Two views of the same stenosis.* A   B

means of microembolization.[85,88,196,199] Evidence in support of this view arose from individual case reports, to which whole series of cases were later added.[73,85,204–208] However, compared with stenosis and occlusion, ulcerations are not the common finding in patients with TIAs. With Doppler studies, it has been difficult—we would say thus far impossible—to predict the mechanism of stroke (perfusion failure or embolism) reliably from the ultrasonographic appearance of the plaque in cases of coexisting carotid stenosis.[205]

Despite the results of the NASCET and European Cooperative Study, debate continues on whether ulcers are important in stroke. Studies from individual centers continue to indicate that plaque morphology may have a predictive value in subsequent stroke risk.[209,210] It is sad to admit, however, that inter-rater reliability on the interpretation of carotid plaque morphology has not been high in any study,[211] an observation that may limit the value of single-center reports on correlations between plaque morphology and clinical event.

Ulcers are often found in surgical specimens.[204–206,212] The smaller ulcers are difficult to demonstrate angiographically, and considerable interobserver variation exists in the diagnosis of ulceration.[106] As many as 40% are missed on routine angiogram, and many ulcers are found at operation in "smooth, benign-appearing plaques. . . ."[205] Ulceration may be an erroneous angiographic diagnosis for a lesion that is actually due to subintimal hemorrhage into a shallow plaque, a finding that may even resolve spontaneously.[213]

Fisher and Ojemann's[77] pathologic study of carotid endarterectomy plaques found no important clinical correlation with ulcerations or cul-de-sacs (defined as rounded pouches of diverticula protruding from the lumen into the plaque) in 90 patients who had hemispheral TIAs or TMB or who were asymptomatic, or in a separate group of 51 patients with persistent neurologic deficit. Of 30 cases of ulceration and 7 cul-de-sacs in the patients with TIAs, no definite examples of clinical embolic events had occurred. This point is underscored by the observation that 9 ulcerations and 5 cul-de-sacs were found in 33 asymptomatic patients. Similarly, of 51 patients with persistent neurologic deficit signifying infarction, only 10 had ulcerations or cul-de-sacs, and 6 of these were associated with a severe stenosis (residual lumen < 1 mm). The remaining 4 patients, with widely patent lumens, had minor neurologic signs.

Opinions on the importance of ulceration per se have been changing over time.[214] The risk of TIA and stroke for complex, deep ulcers is still a subject of dispute, but the undeniable correlation with high-grade stenosis makes it difficult to perform a separate study of one of the two coexisting elements.

REVERSIBLE ISCHEMIC NEUROLOGIC DEFICIT

The usefulness of the older concept of reversible ischemic neurologic deficit has been questioned on the grounds that it has no prognostic value.[127,215] Arguments have now been put forward that a syndrome that clears off slowly and requires more than 24 hours to do so is a sign of infarction, as has been corroborated many times by imaging.[65]

Some carotid-related strokes begin and progress in such a way that accumulation of neurologic deficit occurs over hours to a day or more, giving rise to the term *progressive stroke* or *evolving stroke*. The brain has clearly suffered infarction in this situation, but the patient may have only a submaximal neurologic deficit for the arterial territory affected. For example, if a patient has only mild to moderate right arm and hand weakness but face, leg, speech, and visual field function are spared, the patient is considered to have a submaximal deficit for the territory involved, even though infarction may be present even on a CT scan. The mechanism responsible for this deficit might recur, leading to further disability, unless treatment is offered. This approach, which stresses submaximal deficit rather than whether or not the brain has suffered infarction, allows for the opportunity of treatment (surgical or medical) in the hopes of preventing further disability.

ISCHEMIC STROKE FROM CAROTID ARTERY DISEASE

Ocular Infarction

The ipsilateral eye and brain are the usual sites of clinical symptoms in stroke affecting a given ICA territory. Although both the eye and the brain are susceptible, it is remarkable how infrequently the eye is affected by permanent deficit compared with the brain. Even rarer is the simultaneous occurrence of eye and brain infarction from hemodynamic carotid artery disease, known as the *opticocerebral syndrome*. Bogousslavsky and colleagues[216] found this phenomenon in 3 (0.5%) of 612 consecutive patients with carotid territory stroke. In our experience, the opticocerebral syndrome is rare and gives too much emphasis to the notion that the eye and brain are involved at the same time in TIAs, a view that should be de-emphasized, not resurrected.

The relationship between retinal infarction (eye stroke) and extracranial ICA disease is complicated. Since the study of the natural history of TMB by Marshall and Meadows,[162] it has been known that associated retinal infarction may occur in a small percentage of patients monitored over the long term. The presumed mechanism is embolic occlusion of either a retinal branch or the central retinal artery. Considerable controversy, however, has centered on the relationship between the embolic material and associated carotid artery disease as a potential source (see earlier discussion). Cholesterol crystals discovered in the retinal circulation, a marker for systemic atherosclerosis known from Hollenhorst's original report,[176] are often incidentally noted on routine ophthalmologic examination in asymptomatic patients.[217,218] Hollenhorst[176] first documented that TMB was not usually associated with cholesterol emboli, an observation corroborated in clinical practice.

Even the role of cholesterol emboli in causing other types of permanent monocular visual loss is unclear. Some studies suggest a relationship to retinal branch occlusion with the carotid artery as the embolic source.[75,164] Other studies, however, identify a strong correlation between retinal infarct from branch occlusion and carotid occlusive disease, but the embolic material is usually platelet debris rather than cholesterol. When permanent visual loss related to central retinal artery occlusion is included, a condition in which the embolic obstruction may not be visualized, cardiac embolic sources, albeit occult, as well as the carotid artery, may be the underlying embolic mechanism. The simple and unitary idea that TMB and retinal stroke are all manifestations of one entity, with extracranial carotid artery disease giving rise to cholesterol emboli as the offending material, is probably incorrect. However, the possibility that moderate to severe carotid artery disease is similarly associated with different retinal embolic events has been raised by Pessin and colleagues,[219] who found 42 instances of retinal cholesterol plaques, branch retinal artery occlusion, or central retinal artery occlusion in 39 patients; the incidence of carotid disease (56% to 60%) was not different for the groups with these separate types of retinal symptoms.

Central Retinal Artery Occlusion

Several large series of patients with central retinal artery occlusion who underwent cerebral angiography have documented ipsilateral carotid artery disease (ulcerative nonstenotic, stenotic without ulceration or irregularity, or occlusive) consistent with an embolic source in 50% to 70% of cases.[219–221] Carotid territory TIAs, including TMB, had occurred in many patients before central retinal artery occlusion.

Ischemic Optic Neuropathy

A host of ocular disorders included in the term ischemic optic neuropathy may attend chronic orbital ischemia as a result of extracranial carotid occlusive disease. Remarkably, ischemic optic neuropathy is an uncommon complication of carotid occlusive disease, estimated to affect approximately 5% of patients in one of the early series.[225] Embolism may be the cause in some cases.[222] The ocular abnormalities are (1) pupillary dilatation with poor light reaction, (2) neovascularization of the iris (rubeosis iridis), (3) elevated intraocular pressure with secondary glaucoma, and (4) proliferative retinopathy (Figs. 5–13 and 5–14) with microaneurysms, scattered flame-shaped hemorrhages, and prominent venous stasis.[222–226] Significant visual loss sometimes ending in blindness with optic atrophy makes this a serious condition. The presumed pathogenesis of reduced orbital blood flow has led some investigators to claim that the chronic changes of ocular ischemia may be reversible with extracranial-intracranial arterial grafting, but others have not found this measure beneficial.[226]

Unusual Syndromes

A small series of cases have been described with symptoms and signs referable to the orbit in cases of carotid artery disease. For some, a variant of migraine, Raeder's syndrome, and the like have been described. Gelmers[227] described two cases with facial pain and ipsilateral oculosympathetic paresis, which he labeled the pericarotid syndrome. This researcher attributed the ocular disturbance to disease affecting the cervical portion of the ICA, as demonstrated angiographically.

Cerebral Infarction

The number of instances of cerebral infarction in the territory of the ICA far exceeds the instances in which the mechanism of the stroke is determined.[29] Difficulties in determining whether the ICA is occluded, severely stenosed, slightly stenosed, ulcerated, or merely the conduit for the embolic material remain a major obstacle to progress in the analysis of cases of stroke in the carotid artery territory. However, this difficulty is brushed aside when the clinical syndromes of carotid artery disease are discussed in detail, as is apparent in the material that follows.

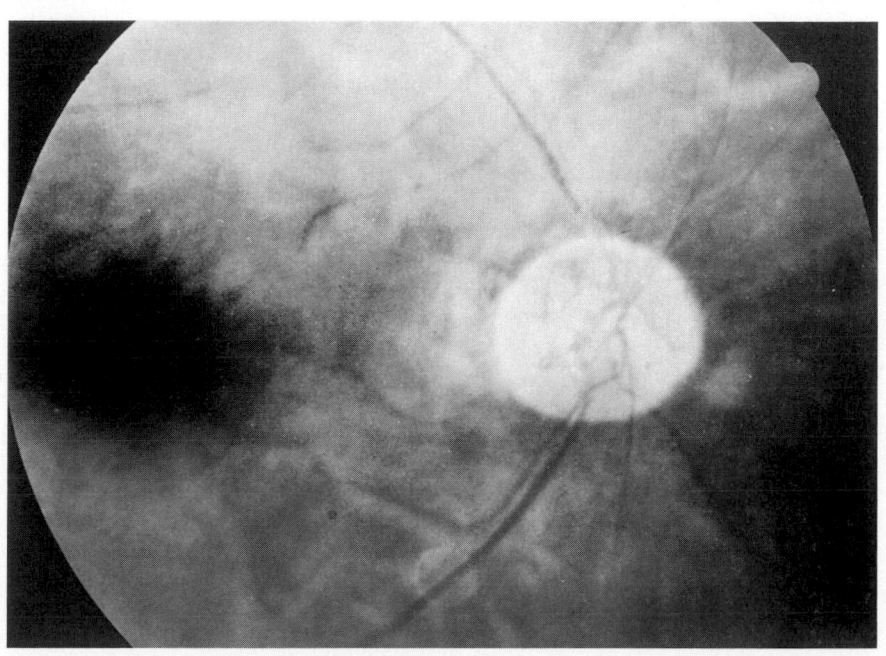

FIGURE 5–13 *Attenuated retinal vessels.*

Clinical Manifestations

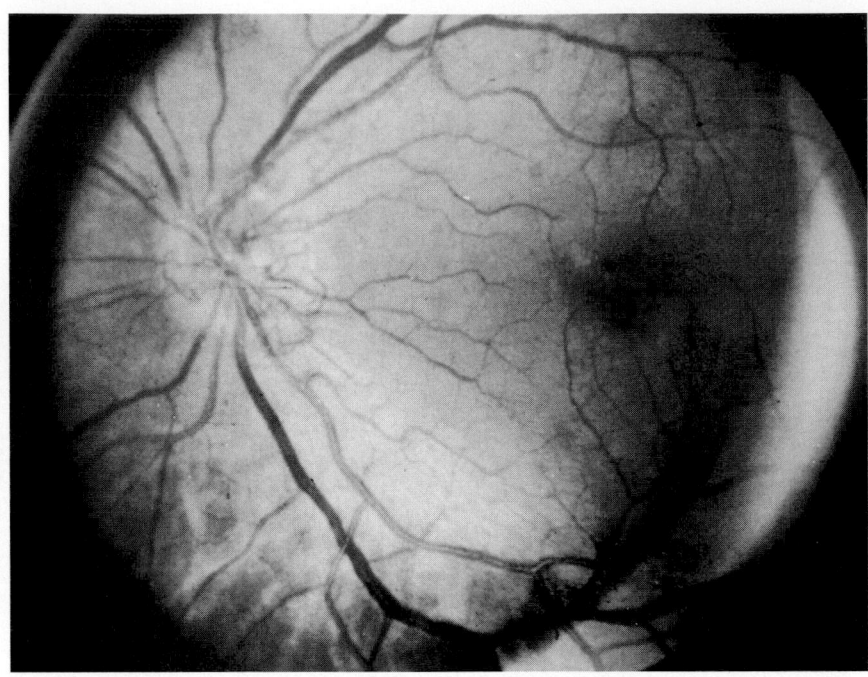

FIGURE 5–14 *Neovascular proliferation affecting the disc.*

After a variable number of TIAs, the completed stroke that results from severe stenosis or occlusion of the ICA reflects infarction from anterograde extension, embolization, or distal flow failure.[40,203] Embolism is probably most common, because it accounts for virtually two thirds of strokes with ICA occlusion.[51] Distal insufficiency appears to account for the other third. Simultaneous infarction of the eye and brain is rare.[228] The spectrum of clinical findings after carotid artery occlusion is wide, ranging from no symptoms to disastrous outcome.[229]

Anterograde Extension of Thrombus

Pathologic studies of ICA thrombosis have documented anterograde extension of thrombus intracranially for varying distances. In a number of cases, extension occurred across the circle of Willis into the stems of the anterior and middle cerebral artery, yielding devastating cerebral infarction.[40,97,98,200,230] One result of this form of extension may be the rare telodiencephalic syndrome.[277] The syndrome consists of contralateral brachiofacial hemiparesis occasionally accompanied by hemianopia and aphasia but mainly accompanied by ipsilateral hemihypohidrosis with ipsilateral Horner's syndrome. We consider it to be caused by an ischemic lesion of the crossed pathways descending from the cerebrum and the uncrossed hypothalamic-spinal sympathetic pathways. The syndrome was attributed to occlusion of the ICA and, occasionally, the middle cerebral artery.

Intracranial Internal Carotid Artery Embolism

Intracranial ICA embolism has also been commonly found in autopsy studies.[83,148,231,232] Embolism has also been the proposed mechanism in prior studies for some of the strokes that are delayed in onset after carotid artery occlusion.[40,80,200,230,233,234] This type of outlook is far more serious and seems to occur with little warning.

Apart from cardiac, transcardiac (e.g., patent cardiac foramen ovale), or aortic arch sources (discussed in other chapters) embolism from carotid artery origin may arise from several sources. Anterograde propagation of the thrombosis intracranially may result in a tail of thrombus that lies at the top of the ICA, the tail being available to be swept distally via retrograde flow through the ophthalmic artery and into the middle and anterior cerebral arteries above.[75,235] Lethal hemispheric stroke has been encountered in one patient 3 days after angiographically documented occlusion of the ipsilateral cerebral ICA. The autopsy evidence was consistent with embolism from the distal intracranial tail of the propagated carotid thrombus. An infarct this large had not previously been reported.[235] Embolization may also arise from the stump of the ICA that remains emanating from the bifurcation of the common carotid artery after ICA occlusion; the Venturi effect of blood passing up the common carotid artery to the ECA may sweep material from the stump distally to reach the intracranial arteries.[80] Other sources have not yet been defined.

Embolism, source clarified or not, may be a common cause of stroke associated with carotid artery thrombosis. In the series reported by Pessin and colleagues,[51] fully 25 of the 64 cases evaluated angiographically showed evidence of intracranial main stem or branch middle cerebral artery occlusion, and another 17 had findings consistent with or suggestive of earlier embolization. The clinical picture in these 43 cases contrasted sharply with the 22 with no signs of embolism; less than half of the patients (17 of 43) had experienced prior TIA, and 12 suffered severe strokes, which were moderately severe in 7 patients, and mild in only 6. This difference in TIA frequency and stroke severity was the reverse of the pattern in the group whose symptoms were attributed to distal insufficiency. On clinical grounds of severity and topography of cerebral infarction, there appears to be no essential difference between the type and severity of the syndromes with carotid and cardiac sources.[51,101] The clinical details of these syndromes is discussed in more detail in the chapter on middle cerebral artery disease (see Chapter 7).

Microembolism—that is, embolism inferred to be occurring in patients in whom high-intensity transient signals (HITS) found at TCD ultrasonography were interpreted as evidence of platelet or plaque material but not regarded as harbingers or causes of stroke—has been increasingly suggested as a potential cause of a dementia-like picture slowly emerging over time (see later).[236] Endarterectomy may also contribute to a cognitive decline through presumably similar mechanisms.[237]

Infarction with Distal Insufficiency

The pathophysiologic basis of distal insufficiency has already been covered in detail (see previous discussion). The clinical syndromes from cerebral infarction in this distribution should be characterized by a prominent visual field defect, aphasia or hemi-inattention features (from dominant or nondominant hemisphere involvement, respectively), and variable degrees of contralateral sensorimotor deficit. Based on now somewhat outmoded classic clinicopathologic correlations of the homunculus,[238] the latter should affect the proximal more than the distal segments of the upper limb, reflecting the location of the infarct along the upper portions of the frontal-parietal convexity.[94] Although the preceding constellation of symptoms is commonly found (bilaterally) in cases of cardiac arrest and hypotension with resulting bilateral distal field infarction, its unilateral occurrence from ICA atherothrombosis was not documented by CT scan until the mid-1980s.[96]

In the study of symptoms with carotid occlusion by Pessin and colleagues,[51] the clinical differences between the patients whose angiographic findings suggested no intracranial embolism had a higher frequency of preceding TIAs and less severe clinical deficits. Those with intracranial occlusions suggesting embolism had fewer TIAs and more severe deficits.

From these considerations, it is apparent that a distal insufficiency mechanism of reduced cerebral flow, although a possible explanation for recurrent stereotypical TIAs,[134] has proved hard to document as the source of cerebral infarction from ICA disease, a situation in which distal embolism appears to account for the great majority of events. As a result, the neurologic findings in themselves have no distinctive elements to suggest that extracranial ICA atherothrombosis is the cause of the stroke.

Numerous autopsy-documented studies have detailed the clinical picture in suprasylvian unilateral cerebral infarcts, even when the exact cause (e.g., thrombosis with perfusion failure or embolism) of the infarction has been unclear.[40,94,97,98,102,106,200,230] In many of the cases, the infarct developed in relation to carotid occlusion, under which circumstances the main bulk of the endangered territory lay between the anterior and middle cerebral arteries, causing the softening in the upper frontal lobe.

The effects most commonly reported have been unilateral infarctions. The symptoms to be expected in such cases have been described by a number of investigators.[97,51,95,98-103,239] Common symptoms are weakness, paralysis, dyspraxia, numbness and tingling, and stereodysnomia

in one or more fingers or the hand, wrist, or arm and leg. Grasp reflex has been observed. Transient impairment of ocular motility is often reported; in cases in which it is not reported, the meaning of the omission is unclear. Disturbances in higher cerebral function have included episodes of speechlessness and of change in personality[60,95,98] as well as dysgraphia of both the paretic and dyspraxic types.

A few well-known examples from the older literature indicate the long-standing recognition of the syndrome and have not yet been eclipsed by more modern case descriptions. The patient reported by Elder in 1900 was a 69-year-old messenger who developed stepwise attacks of worsening right arm and leg paresis with slight dysarthria.[240] Sensation was said to be normal, and he had no hemianopia. His left eye was frequently painful. A right grasp was noted. The attacks progressed to hemiplegia, which spared his face. The patient's speech was intact, as were auditory comprehension and repetition. His writing was clumsy, large, and confined to his own name and a few letters; he found copying difficult. He named objects presented at sight easily. He was unable to read aloud and could manage only a few letters with frequent repetitions. At autopsy, white vessel and extensive infarction was observed extending from the upper frontal region to involve almost the entire lateral parietal and occipital regions. Spatz's famous case from 1935 occurred in a 43-year-old man whose problems began with attacks of headache and shimmering in the left eye.[103] He later experience weakness in the right arm and disturbance of speech in which he often failed to find a word. A right homonymous hemianopia was observed. No tests of reading were reported. At autopsy, the suprasylvian territory of the left cerebral hemisphere from the frontal through posterior parietal regions was involved with "granular atrophy."

High-Convexity Infarction Syndrome

The predominance of high-convexity infarction in carotid syndromes of distal insufficiency has yielded some distinctive syndromes. In a study of clinical features separating embolic from carotid thrombotic syndrome, Timsit and coworkers[241] found that the cases of carotid thrombotic syndrome contained examples of fractional (different degrees of) weakness in the shoulder versus the hand, which was thought to reflect the upper convexity infarction from distal insufficiency. Examples of embolism more often showed comparable degrees of weakness of the hand and shoulder, consistent with the larger and lower-convexity infarction (Fig. 5–15). The probability of carotid artery disease rather than embolism was greater when fractional arm weakness (strength in shoulder different from that in hand) was present (odds ratio, 5.3; 95% CI interval, 3.1 to 9.0), findings confirmed by the same group in another study.[242]

A preponderance of leg weakness has also been described in two separate reports.[231,243] The 19 patients described Yanagihara and associates[243] had episodic or progressive lower extremity weakness contralateral to severe extracranial ICA occlusive disease (16 patients) or carotid siphon stenosis (3 patients). Cerebral blood measurements, using xenon-133 in some of the patients, corroborated reduced hemispheric flow on the appropriate side localized to the borderzone in the frontoparietal areas corresponding to motor function of the lower extremity.

Clinical Manifestations

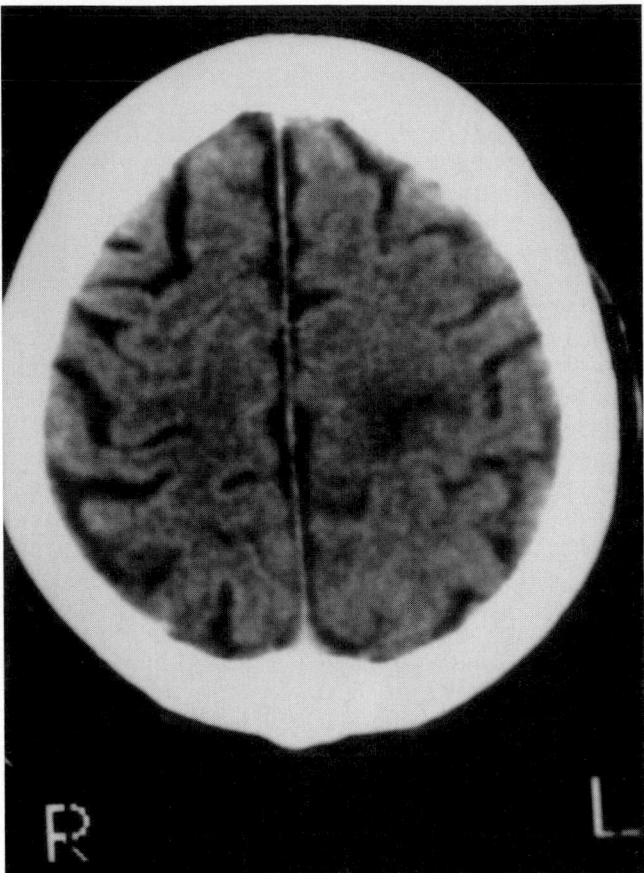

FIGURE 5–15 *High-convexity infarct in a case of fractional weakness (see text).*

Pure Dementia

Clinical syndromes of pure dementia have proved difficult to document, but case reports continue to appear describing a picture referred to as dementia in a setting of high convexity, "distal field" infarction with high-grade carotid stenosis.[244-246] Studies of mental function after carotid endarterectomy have used a battery of tests of memory and mental agility. Reports have appeared in which scores on tests conducted before and after successful endarterectomy indicate an improvement.[247] Extracranial-intracranial bypass has been reported in some small series.[247,248] Some have shown improvement after stenting[249] and some not.[250]

ASYMPTOMATIC CAROTID ARTERY DISEASE

Asymptomatic Carotid Artery Occlusion

The documentation of carotid artery occlusion by a noninvasive study or angiography is fairly common, and the literature dates back several decades.[251] A series of studies attempted to use the case-control method to estimate stroke risk, the first and still the dominant study that conducted by Furlan and Whisnant,[252] in which the annual rate of 2% was derived from 6 cases among 138 cases that were evaluated angiographically and studied retrospectively. Similar event rates have been reported in other series

from angiography.[50,253] The cohort studies reported by Sacquegna and coworkers[254] consisted of a consecutive series of 100 patients with angiographically proven ICA occlusion, 68 of whom were monitored from 17 to 69 months; 7 of the patients suffered new strokes, only 3 of which were in the territory of the occluded carotid artery, and 4 had TIAs during follow-up. The observed stroke rate was 4.7% at 1 year, 12.2% at 3 years, and 17.1% at 5 years.

Noninvasive Doppler ultrasonography provided the database for other studies. The early study by Bernstein and Norris[255] documented an annual stroke rate of 3.8%. Similar or higher rates have been published in other series, including the original extracranial-intracranial bypass study. In that study, 34 of 74 patients identified as having carotid artery occlusion were randomly assigned to undergo nonsurgical treatment and were followed up for a mean of 42 months. The annual stroke rate was 13% per patient-year; 50% of the survivors were symptom free or had minor disability.[256]

Asymptomatic Carotid Artery Stenosis

The risk of stroke in a setting of asymptomatic carotid artery stenosis, reported as case series in numerous publications,[19,155,257] was addressed in the largest study to date, the ACAS.[258] This trial randomly assigned all eligible patients with asymptomatic carotid stenosis consisting of 60% or greater lumen reduction to receive 325 mg of aspirin daily or to undergo carotid endarterectomy. All patients received appropriate counseling and treatment for risk factor reduction. The endpoints TIA and stroke in the distribution of the randomized arteries were used to assess the two treatments. Brott and colleagues[259] reviewed 1132 patients in the ACAS and discovered 126 (15%) with what was characterized as silent infarct. For fully 72% of these patients, the infarcts were small, deep lesions often considered asymptomatic, but the remainder had convexity infarctions, some as large as half a lobe. After a median follow-up of 2.7 years, the risk of ipsilateral stroke in the ACAS projected to occur over 5 years or of any perioperative stroke or death was 5.1% for surgically treated patients and 11.0% for medically treated patients. A low Mini-Mental State examination score was correlated with a higher mortality rate.[260]

The favorable outcome for surgically treated patients was predicated on a remarkably low perioperative risk of stroke or death—2.3%. The 5-year reduction in stroke risk was different for men (67%) and women (17%), this difference in part explained by a higher perioperative complication rate in women. The arteriographically related stroke rate was 1.2% for the 414 patients who underwent arteriography before endarterectomy. Despite strong clinical opinions to the contrary, the severities of increasing stenosis (60% to 69%, 70% to 79%, and 80% to 99%) were not statistically related to reduction of the 5-year risk of the primary event. These data provide the first scientifically derived information on the stroke risk and benefits of carotid endarterectomy for asymptomatic carotid artery disease and are now the new benchmark for this condition.[258]

Since these studies appeared, additional evidence has accumulated indicating the existence of intracranial perfusion impairment, as assessed by TCD ultrasonography—

an evaluation not widely used in the ACAS—adds to the risk of TIA and stroke when present. In a study of 114 patients with 80% to 99% stenosis of an extracranial ICA assessed by duplex Doppler ultrasonography, Hartmann and colleagues[261] found that evidence of intracranial waveform blunting as assessed by TCD ultrasonography had a highly significant correlation with the symptomatic patients (odds ratio, 7.5; 95% CI, 3.1–18.1; $P < .001$). In another study, "exhausted" collateral vessels (i.e., blunted intracranial waveforms ipsilateral or bilateral atop ICA stenosis, and inferred to be fully dilated because not showing further dilation after CO_2 inhalation) were the principal independent risk factor for TIA and stroke in a cohort of 153 patient studies by Blaser and coworkers.[262]

Modern data on the advance in stenosis over time was summarized by the late D. Eugene Strandness, Jr.,[263] whose career spanned the development of Doppler ultrasonography. His advice was to recheck in 6-month intervals all patients with clinically asymptomatic stenosis of 50% to 79%, but only annually for those with stenosis less than 50%. These observations are in general agreement with those of other large series.[264]

Asymptomatic Ulcerative Disease

Very few autopsy-based studies have been conducted on the stroke risk for ulcerative disease alone.[44,265] The results of the NASCET, drawn from operative specimens, have largely superseded earlier efforts. Irrespective of the degree of stenosis, a sensitivity of 45.9% and a specificity of 74.1% for ulceration were found for the first 500 specimens, yielding a somewhat disappointing positive predictive value of 71.8%.[193]

Asymptomatic Bruit

With widespread availability of Doppler studies, much of the earlier anxieties about bruits have been relieved. A bruit in the neck is commonly encountered in routine clinical examination. It occurs in 4% to 5% of the population aged 45 to 80 years.[266,267] A local cervical bruit can be detected in approximately 70% to 89% of patients with a tight (75% stenosis, or ≤ 2 mm residual lumen) stenosis of the ICA.[268,269] The site of maximal intensity of the bruit usually corresponds to the carotid bifurcation area, in front of the upper portion of the thyroid cartilage. It can radiate into the ocular region, and its intensity usually decreases with the Valsalva's maneuver. The latter point should be useful for differentiating cervical bruits from bruits originating from the ECA, which should not change with this maneuver, although the finding is disappointingly unreliable.[270] A bruit may also be absent in some patients with tight stenosis because of a slow-flow state through the patent but severely stenotic artery.[269] In some instances, the bruit can be explained by a tight, diaphragm-like lesion not easily imaged by conventional angioghaphy.[271]

Postendarterectomy Doppler Ultrasonography Findings

Despite the fervent hope that a successful endarterectomy has rid the patient of the risk of further disease at that site,

recurrence is discouragingly frequent. Estimates vary, but no less an authority than the late D. Eugene Strandness, Jr. cited an early restenosis rate of up to 20% but also noted that the recurrent lesions have a far more benign prognosis, surgery being suggested only for the patient whose recurrence advances to hemodynamically important stenosis. His advice was to undertake a study shortly after endarterectomy to confirm the success of the operation and provide a baseline.[263] The success rate for a second endarterectomy in experienced hands appears to approximate that for the first operation.[272,273]

References

1. Caplan LR, Baker R: Extracranial occlusive vascular disease: Does size matter? Stroke 11:63, 1980.
2. Schneidau A, Harrison MJ, Hurst C: Predicting the normal dimensions of the internal carotid artery. Eur J Vasc Surg 2:273–274, 1988.
3. LoGerfo FW, Crawshaw HN, Nowak M, et al: Effect of flow split on separation and stagnation in a model vascular bifurcation. Stroke 12:660, 1981.
4. LoGerfo FW, Nowak MD, Quist WC, et al: Flow studies in a model of carotid bifurcation. Arteriosclerosis 1:235, 1981.
5. Wood CPL, Smith BR, McKinney CL, Toole JF: Non-invasive detection of boundary layer separation in the normal carotid artery bifurcation. Stroke 13:120, 1982.
6. Zarins CK, Giddens DP, Balasubramanian K, et al: Carotid plaques localized in regions of low flow velocity and shear stress. Circulation 64:44, 1981.
7. Berguer R, Hwang NHC: Critical arterial stenosis: A theoretical and experimental solution. Ann Surg 180:39, 1974.
8. Brice JG, Dowsett DJ, Lowe RD: Haemodynamic effects of carotid artery stenosis. BMJ 2:1363, 1964.
9. Shipley RE, Gregg DE: The effect of external constriction of a blood vessel on blood flow. Am J Physiol 141:389, 1944.
10. Young DF, Cholvin NR, Kirkeeide RL, Roth AC: Hemodynamics of arterial stenoses at elevated flow rates. Circ Res 41:99, 1977.
11. Byar D, Fiddian RV, Quereau M, et al: The fallacy of applying the Poiseuille equation to segmental arterial stenosis. Am Heart J 70:216, 1965.
12. May AG, DeWeese JA, Rob CG: Hemodynamic effects of arterial stenosis. Surgery 53:513, 1963.
13. Archie JP, Feldtman RW: Critical stenosis of the internal carotid artery. Surgery 89:67, 1981.
14. Kuntz KM, Skillman JJ, Whittemore AD, Kent KC: Carotid endarterectomy in asymptomatic patients—is contrast angiography necessary? A morbidity analysis. J Vasc Surg 22:706, 1995.
15. Gagne PJ, Matchett J, MacFarland D, et al: Can the NASCET technique for measuring carotid stenosis be reliably applied outside the trial? J Vasc Surg 24:449, 1996.
16. Bousser MG: Faut-il opérer les sténoses carotidiennes asymptomatiques? Rev Neurol 151:363, 1995.
17. Schneidau A, Harrison MJ, Hurst C, et al: Arterial disease risk factors and angiographic evidence of atheroma of the carotid artery. Stroke 20:1466–1471, 1989.
18. Javid H, Ostermiller WE Jr, Hengesh JW, et al: Natural history of carotid bifurcation atheroma. Surgery 67:80, 1970.
19. Roederer GO, Langlois YE, Jager KA, et al: The natural history of carotid arterial disease in asymptomatic patients with cervical bruits. Stroke 15:605, 1984.
20. Mohr JP: Plaques Carotides: Diagnostic, Evaluation, Pronostic. Paris, Sauramps, 1997, p 11.
21. Sander D, Winbeck K, Klingelhofer J, et al: Reduced progression of early carotid atherosclerosis after antibiotic treatment and *Chlamydia pneumoniae* seropositivity. Circulation 106:2428–2433, 2002.
22. Fisher CM: Cerebral ischemia—less familiar types. Clin Neurosurg 18:267, 1971.
23. Croft RJ, Ellam LD, Harrison MJG: Accuracy of carotid angiography in the assessment of atheroma of the internal carotid artery. Lancet 1:997, 1980.
24. Cioffi FA, Meduri M, Tomasello F, et al: Kinking and coiling of the internal carotid artery. J Neurosurg Sci 19:15, 1975.

25. Correll JW, Quest DO, Carpenter DB: Nonatheromatous lesions of the extracranial cerebral arteries. In Smith RR (ed): Stroke and the Extracranial Vessels. Philadelphia, Lippincott-Raven, 1984, p 321.

26. Handa J, Nakasu Y, Kidooka M: Transient cerebral ischemia evoked by yawning: An experience after superficial temporal artery—middle cerebral artery bypass operation. Surg Neurol 19:46, 1983.

27. Merino MJ, Livolsi V: Malignant carotid body tumors. Cancer 47:1403, 1981.

28. Harrington HJ, Mayman CI: Carotid body tumor associated with partial Horner's syndrome and facial pain ("Raeder's syndrome"). Arch Neurol 40:564, 1983.

29. Grobe T: Diagnostik und Behandlungsmöglichkeiten extrakranieller Verschlussprozesse der Arteria carotis. Fortschr Neurol Psychiatr 49:335, 1981.

30. Huvos AG, Leaming RH, Moore OS: Clinicopathologic study of the resected carotid artery. Am J Surg 126:570, 1973.

31. Spallone A: Occlusion of the internal carotid artery by intracranial tumors. Surg Neurol 15:51, 1981.

32. Maves MD, Bruns MD, Keenan MJ: Carotid artery resection for head and neck cancer. Ann Otol Rhinol Laryngol 101:778, 1992.

33. Snyderman CH, D'Amico F: Outcome of carotid artery resection for neoplastic disease: A meta-analysis. Am J Otolaryngol 13:373, 1992.

34. Okamoto Y, Inugami A, Matsuzaki Z, et al: Carotid artery resection for head and neck cancer. Surgery 120:54, 1996.

35. Wright JG, Nicholson R, Schuller DE, Smead WL: Resection of the internal carotid artery and replacement with greater saphenous vein: A safe procedure for en bloc cancer resections with carotid involvement. J Vasc Surg 23:775, 1996.

36. Okamoto Y, Inugami A, Matsuzaki Z, et al: Carotid artery resection for head and neck cancer. Surgery 120:54–59, 1996.

37. Marshall RS, Lazar RM, Young WL, et al: Clinical utility of quantitative cerebral blood flow measurements during internal carotid artery test occlusions. Neurosurgery 50:996–1004, 2002.

38. Piedbois P, Becquemin JP, Pierquin B, et al: Les sténoses artérielles après radiothérapie. Bull Cancer Radiother 77:3, 1990.

39. Levinson SA, Close MB, Ehrenfeld WK, et al: Carotid artery of occlusive disease following external cervical irradiation. Arch Surg 107:395, 1973.

40. Castaigne P, Lhermitte F, Gautier JC, et al: Internal carotid artery occlusion: A study of 61 instances in 50 patients with post-mortem data. Brain 93:321, 1970.

41. Craig DR, Meguro K, Watridge C, et al: Intracranial internal carotid artery stenosis. Stroke 13:825, 1982.

42. Marzewski DJ, Furlan AJ, St. Louis P, et al: Intracranial internal carotid artery stenosis: Long term prognosis. Stroke 13:821, 1982.

43. Schuler JJ, Falnigan DP, Lim LT, et al: The effect of carotid siphon stenosis on stroke rate, death, and relief of symptoms following elective carotid endarterectomy. Surgery 92:1058, 1982.

44. Hutchinson EC, Yates PO: Carotico-vertebral stenosis. Lancet 1:2, 1957.

45. Torvik A, Jörgensen L: Ischemic cerebrovascular disease in an autopsy series. Part 1: Prevalence, location and predisposing factors in verified thrombo-embolic occlusion and their significance in the pathogenesis of cerebral infarction. J Neurol Sci 3:490, 1966.

46. Torvik A, Jörgensen L: Ischemic cerebrovascular disease in an autopsy series. Part 2: Prevalence, location, pathogenesis and clinical course of cerebral infarcts. J Neurol Sci 9:285, 1969.

47. Luessenhop AJ: Occlusive disease of carotid artery: Observations on the prognosis and surgical treatment. J Neurosurg 16:705, 1959.

48. Pessin MS, Duncan GW, Davis KR, et al: Angiographic appearance of carotid occlusion in acute stroke. Stroke 11:485, 1982.

49. Baud JM, De Bray JM, Delanoy P, et al: Reproductibilité ultrasonore dans la caractérisation des plaques carotidiennes. J Echograph Med Ultrason 17:377, 1996.

50. Bogousslavsky J, Regli F, Hungerbühler J-P, Chrzanowski R: Transient ischemic attacks and external carotid artery occlusion: A retrospective study of 23 patients with an occlusion of the internal carotid artery. Stroke 12:627, 1981.

51. Pessin MS, Hinton RC, Davis KR, et al: Mechanisms of acute carotid stroke. Ann Neurol 6:245, 1979.

52. Burnbaum MD, Selhorst JB, Harbison JW, Brush JJ: Amaurosis fugax from disease of the external carotid artery. Arch Neurol 34:532, 1977.

53. Krayenbühl H, Yasargil MG: Die Cerebrale Angiographie. Stuttgart, George Thieme Verlag, 1965.

54. Van der Eecken HM: Anastomoses Between the Leptomeningeal Arteries of the Brain. Springfield, IL, Charles C Thomas, 1959.

55. Henderson RD, Eliasziw M, Fox AJ, et al: Angiographically defined collateral circulation and risk of stroke in patients with severe carotid artery stenosis: North American Symptomatic Carotid Endarterectomy Trial (NASCET) Group. Stroke 31:128–132, 2000.

56. Powers WJ, Press GA, Grubb RL, et al: The effect of hemodynamically significant carotid artery disease on the hemodynamic status of the cerebral circulation. Ann Intern Med 106:27, 1987.

57. Schneider PA, Rossman ME, Bernstein EF, et al: Noninvasive assessment of cerebral collateral blood supply through the ophthalmic artery. Stroke 22:31, 1991.

58. Tatemichi TK, Chamorro A, Petty GW, et al: Hemodynamic role of ophthalmic artery collateral in internal carotid artery occlusion. Neurology 40:461, 1990.

59. David NJ, Gordon KK, Friedberg SJ, et al: Fatal atheromatous cerebral embolism associated with bright plaques in the retinal arterioles. Neurology 13:708, 1963.

60. Zülch KJ, Kleihues P: Neuropathology of Cerebral Infarction: Thule International Symposium. Stockholm, Nordiska Bokhandling Forlag, 1957, p 57.

61. Adams RD, Fisher CM: Pathology of cerebral arterial occlusion. In Fields WS (ed): Houston Symposium on Pathogenesis and Treatment of Cerebrovascular Disease. Springfield, IL, Charles C Thomas, 1961.

62. Beal MF, Williams RS, Richardson EP, Fisher CM: Cerebral embolism as a cause of transient ischemic attacks and cerebral infarction. Neurology (NY) 31:860, 1981.

63. Castaigne P, Lhermitte F, Gautier JC: Role des lésions artérielles dans les accidents ischémiques cérébraux de l'athérosclerose. Rev Neurol (Paris) 113:1, 1965.

64. Fisher CM: Clinical syndromes of cerebral thrombosis, hypertensive hemorrhage, and ruptured saccular aneurysm. Clin Neurosurg 22:117, 1975.

65. Waxman SG, Toole JF: Temporal profile resembling TIA in the setting of cerebral infarction. Stroke 14:433, 1983.

66. Gunning AJ, Pickering GW, Robb-Smith AHT, et al: Mural thrombosis of the internal carotid artery and subsequent embolism. Q J Med 33:155, 1964.

67. Millikan CH: The pathogenesis of transient focal cerebral ischemia. Circulation 32:438, 1965.

68. Olsson JE, Muller R, Berneli S: Long-term anticoagulant therapy for TIAs and minor strokes with minimum residuum. Stroke 7:444, 1976.

69. Delal PM, Shah PM, Aiyar RR: Arteriographic study of cerebral embolism. Lancet 2:358, 1965.

70. Liebeskind A, Chinichian A, Schechter MM: The moving embolus seen during serial cerebral angiography. Stroke 2:440, 1971.

71. Ring BA: Diagnosis of embolic occlusions of smaller branches of the intracerebral arteries. Am J Roentgenol Radium Ther Nucl Med 97:575, 1966.

72. Taveras JM, Wood EH: Diagnostic Neuroradiology, 2nd ed. Vol 2, Sect 4: Vascular Diseases. Baltimore, Williams & Wilkins, 1976, p 850.

73. Zatz LM, Iannone AM, Eckman PB, Hecker SP: Observations concerning intracerebral vascular occlusion. Neurology 15:390, 1965.

74. Fisher CM: Observations of the fundus oculi in transient monocular blindness. Neurology 9:337, 1959.

75. Ross Russell RW: Observations on the retinal blood vessels in monocular blindness. Lancet 2:1422, 1961.

76. Harrison MJG, Marshall J: Evidence of silent cerebral embolism in patients with amaurosis fugax. J Neurol Neurosurg Psychiatry 40:651, 1977.

77. Fisher CM, Ojemann RG: A clinico-pathologic study of carotid endarterectomy plaques. Rev Neurol (Paris) 142:573, 1986.

78. Countee RW, Sapru HN, Vijayanathan T, Wu SZ: "Other syndromes" of the carotid bifurcation. In Smith RR (ed): Stroke and the Extracranial Vessels. Philadelphia, Lippincott-Raven, 1984, p 345.

79. Ross Russell RW: Atheromatous retinal embolism. Lancet 2:1354, 1963.

80. Barnett HJM, Peerless SJ, Kaufmann JCE: The "stump" of internal carotid artery—a source for further cerebral embolic ischemia. Stroke 9:448, 1978.

81. Waller FT, Simons RL, Kerber C, et al: Trigeminal artery and microemboli to the brain stem: Report of two cases. J Neurosurg 46:104, 1977.

82. Chiari H: Ueber das Verhalten der Teilungswinkels der Carotid communis bei der Endarteritis chronica deformans. Verh Dtsch Ges Pathol 9:326, 1905.

83. Lusby RJ, Ferrell LD, Ehrenfeld WK, et al: Carotid plaque hemorrhage: Its role in production of cerebral ischemia. Arch Surg 117:1479, 1982.

84. Lennihan L, Kupsky WJ, Mohr JP, et al: Lack of association between carotid plaque hematoma and ipsilateral cerebral symptoms. Stroke 18:879, 1987.

85. Moore WS, Hall AD: Ulcerated atheroma of the carotid artery: A major cause of transient cerebral ischemia. Am J Surg 116:237, 1968.

86. Winn WB, Schmiedl UP, Reichenbach DD, et al: Detection and characterization of atherosclerotic fibrous caps with T2-weighted MRI. AJNR Am J Neuroradiol 19:129–134, 1998.

87. Yuan C, Zhang SX, Polissar NL, et al: Identification of fibrous cap rupture with magnetic resonance imaging is highly associated with recent transient ischemic attack or stroke. Circulation 105:181–185, 2002.

88. Moore WS, Hall AD: Importance of emboli from carotid bifurcation in pathogenesis of cerebral ischemic attacks. Arch Surg 101:708, 1970.

89. Pessin MS, Duncan GW, Mohr JP, Poskanzer DC: Clinical and angiographic features of carotid transient ischemic attacks. N Engl J Med 296:358, 1977.

90. Mead GE, Lewis SC, Wardlaw JM, Dennis MS: Comparison of risk factors in patients with transient and prolonged eye and brain ischemic syndromes. Stroke 33:2383–2390, 2002.

91. Whisnant JP: Multiple particles injected may all go to the same cerebral artery branch. Stroke 13:720, 1982.

92. Wolpert SM, Stein BM: Catheter embolization of arteriovenous malformations as an aid to surgical excision. Neuroradiology 10:73, 1975.

93. Ferro JM, Falcao I, Rodrigues G, et al: Diagnosis of transient ischemic attack by a nonneurologist. Stroke 27:2225, 1996.

94. Mohr JP: Neurological complications of cardiac valvular disease and cardiac surgery including systemic hypotension. In Klawans HL (ed): Neurological Manifestations of Systemic Diseases. (Handbook of Clinical Neurology, Vol 38.) Amsterdam, North Holland, 1979, p 143.

95. Fisher CM: Cerebral thromboangiitis obliterans. Medicine (Baltimore) 36:169, 1957.

96. Bogousslavsky J, Regli F: Borderzone infarctions distal to internal carotid artery occlusion: Prognostic implications. Ann Neurol 20:346, 1986.

97. Fisher CM: Occlusion of the internal carotid artery. AMA Arch Neurol Psychiatry 69:346, 1951.

98. Fisher CM: Occlusion of the carotid arteries: Further experiences. AMA Arch Neurol Psychiatry 72:187, 1954.

99. Lindenberg R, Spatz F: Ueber die Thromboendarteritis obliterans der Hirngefässe. Virchows Arch [A] 305:531, 1940.

100. Pentschew A: Die granuläre Atrophie der Grosshirnrinde. Arch Psychiatr Nervenkr 101:80, 1934.

101. Ringelstein EB, Zeumer H, Angelou D: The pathogenesis of strokes from internal carotid artery occlusion. Stroke 14:867, 1983.

102. Romanul FCA, Abramowicz A: Changes in brain and pial vessels in arterial borderzones. Arch Neurol (Chicago) 11:40, 1964.

103. Spatz A: Uber die Beteiligung des Gehirns bei v. Winiwarter-Buergerische Krankheit. Dtsch Z Nervenheilk 136:86, 1935.

104. Torvik A: The pathogenesis of watershed infarcts in the brain. Stroke 15:221, 1984.

105. Wodarz R, Ratzka M, Grosse D: Der Grenzzoneninfarkt als besondere Infarktkonstellation bei Karotisinsuffizienz. Fortschr Röntgenstr 134:128, 1981.

106. Schneider M: Durchblutung und Sauerstoffversorgung des Gehirns. Verh Dtsch Ges Kreislauf Forsch 19:3, 1953.

107. Carpenter DA, Grubb RL Jr, Powers WJ: Borderzone hemodynamics in cerebrovascular disease. Neurology 40:1587, 1990.

108. Leblanc R, Yamamoto YL, Tyler JL, et al: Borderzone ischemia. Ann Neurol 22:707, 1987.

109. Toyama H, Takeshita G, Takeuchi A, et al: SPECT measurement of cerebral hemodynamics in transient ischemic attack patients: Evaluation of pathogenesis and detection of misery perfusion. Kaku Igaku 26:1487, 1989.

110. Vorstrup S, Hemmingsen R, Henriksen L, et al: Regional cerebral blood flow in patients with transient ischemic attacks studied by xenon-133 inhalation and emission tomography. Stroke 14:903–910, 1983.

111. Raichle M: Discussion. In Reivich M, Hurtig H (eds): Cerebrovascular Disorders. XIIIth Research (Princeton) Conference. Philadelphia, Lippincott-Raven, 1983.

112. Yamauchi H, Fukuyama H, Kimura J, et al: Hemodynamics in internal carotid artery occlusion examined by positron emission tomography. Stroke 21:1400, 1990.

113. Lin W, Celik A, Derdeyn C, et al: Quantitative measurements of cerebral blood flow in patients with unilateral carotid artery occlusion: A PET and MR study. J Magn Reson Imaging 14:659–667, 2001.

114. Derdeyn CP, Khosla A, Videen TO, et al: Severe hemodynamic impairment and border zone—region infarction 1. Radiology 220:195–201, 2001.

115. Baron JC, Bousser MG, Rey A, et al: Reversal of focal "misery-perfusion syndrome" by extra-intracranial arterial bypass in hemodynamic cerebral ischemia. Stroke 12:454, 1981.

116. Derdeyn CP, Cross DT III, Moran CJ, Dacey RG Jr: Reversal of focal misery perfusion after intracranial angioplasty: Case report. Neurosurgery 48:436–439, 2001.

117. Levine RL, Dobkin JA, Rozental JM, et al: Blood flow reactivity to hypercapnia in strictly unilateral carotid disease: Preliminary results. J Neurol Neurosurg Psychiatry 54:204, 1991.

118. Markus H, Cullinane M: Severely impaired cerebrovascular reactivity predicts stroke and TIA risk in patients with carotid artery stenosis and occlusion. Brain 124:457–467, 2001.

119. Coakham HB, Duchen LW, Scaravilli F: Moyamoya disease: Clinical and pathological report of a case with associated myopathy. J Neurol Neurosurg Psychiatry 42:289, 1979.

120. Charbel FT, Guppy KH, Zhao M, Clark ME: Computerized hemodynamic evaluation of the cerebral circulation for bypass. Neurosurg Clin North Am 12:499–508, 2001.

121. Szabo K, Kern R, Gass A, et al: Acute stroke patterns in patients with internal carotid artery disease: A diffusion-weighted magnetic resonance imaging study. Stroke 32:1323–1329, 2001.

122. Fisher CM: Concerning recurrent transient cerebral ischemic attacks. Can Med Assoc J 86:1091, 1962.

123. Eastcott HG, Pickering GW, Rob CG: Reconstruction of internal carotid artery in a patient with intermittent attacks of hemiplegia. Lancet 2:994, 1954.

124. Genton E, Barnett HJM, Fields WS, et al: Cerebral ischemia: The role of thrombosis and of antithrombotic therapy. Joint Committee for Stroke Resources. Stroke 8:147, 1977.

125. Heyman A, Leviton A, Nefzger D, et al: Transient focal cerebral ischemia: Epidemiological and clinical aspects. Stroke 5:277, 1974.

126. Marshall J: The natural history of transient ischemic cerebrovascular attacks. Q J Med 33:309, 1964.

127. Loeb C, Priano A, Albano C: Clinical features and long-term follow-up of patients with reversible ischemia attacks (RIA). Acta Neurol Scand 57:471, 1978.

128. Regli F: Die flüchtigen ischämischen zerebralen Attacken. Deutsch Med Wochenschr 96:526, 1971.

129. Kidwell CS, Alger JR, Di Salle F, et al: Diffusion MRI in patients with transient ischemic attacks. Stroke 30:1174–1180, 1999.

130. Bisschops RH, Kappelle LJ, Mali WP, van der Grond J: Hemodynamic and metabolic changes in transient ischemic attack patients: A magnetic resonance angiography and (1)H-magnetic resonance spectroscopy study performed within 3 days of onset of a transient ischemic attack. Stroke 33:110–115, 2002.

131. Mohr JP: Some clinical aspects of acute stroke: Excellence in Clinical Stroke Award Lecture. Stroke 28:1835–1839, 1997.

132. Albers GW, Caplan LR, Easton JD, et al: Transient ischemic attack—proposal for a new definition. N Engl J Med 347:1713–1716, 2002.

133. Koudstaal PJ, van Gijn J, Staal A, et al: Diagnosis of transient ischemic attacks: Improvement of interobserver agreement by a check-list in ordinary language. Stroke 17:723–728, 1986.

134. Duncan GW, Pessin MS, Mohr JP, Adams RD: Transient cerebral ischemic attacks. Adv Intern Med 21:1–20, 1976.

135. Fisher CM: Perspective: Transient ischemic attacks. N Engl J Med 347:1642–1644, 2002.

136. Mohr JP, Caplan LR, Melski JW, et al: The Harvard Cooperative Stroke Registry: A prospective registry. Neurology 28:754, 1978.

137. Russo LS: Carotid system transient ischemic attacks: Clinical, racial, and angiographic correlations. Stroke 12:470, 1981.

Clinical Manifestations

138. Streifler JY, Eliasziw M, Benavente OR, et al: Prognostic importance of leukoaraiosis in patients with symptomatic internal carotid artery stenosis. Stroke 33:1651–1655, 2002.
139. Boysen G, Jensen G, Schnor P: Frequency of focal cerebral transient ischemic attacks during a 12 month period. Stroke 10:533, 1979.
140. Karp HR, Heyman A, Heyden S, et al: Transient cerebral ischemia: Prevalence and prognosis in a biracial community. JAMA 225:125, 1973.
141. Ostfeld AM, Shekelle RB, Klawans HL: Transient ischemic attacks and risk of stroke in an elderly poor population. Stroke 4:980, 1973.
142. Whisnant JP, Matsumoto N, Elveback LR: The effect of anticoagulant therapy on the prognosis of patients with transient cerebral ischemic attacks in a community: Rochester, Minnesota, 1955 through 1969. Mayo Clin Proc 48:844, 1973.
143. Wilkinson WE, Heyman A, Burch JG, et al: Use of a self-administered questionnaire for detection of transient cerebral ischemic attacks: Survey of elderly persons living in retirement facilities. Ann Neurol 6:40, 1979.
144. Wolf PA, Dawber TR, Colton T, et al: Transient cerebral ischemic attacks and risk of stroke: The Framingham Study. Cardiovascular Disease Epidemiol Newslett 22:52, 1977.
145. Fratiglioni L, Arfaioli C, Nencini P, et al: Transient ischemic attacks in the community: Occurrence and clinical characteristics: A population survey in the area of Florence, Italy. Neuroepidemiology 8:87–96, 1989.
146. Dennis MS, Bamford JM, Sandercock PA, Warlow CP: Incidence of transient ischemic attacks in Oxfordshire, England. Stroke 20:333–339, 1989.
147. Baker RN, Ramseyer JG, Schwartz WS: Prognosis in patients with cerebral ischemic attacks. Neurology 18:1157, 1968.
148. Frank G: Comparison of anticoagulation and surgical treatments of TIA: A review and consolidation of recent natural history and treatment studies. Stroke 2:369, 1971.
149. Friedman GD, Wilson WS, Mosier JM, et al: Transient ischemic attacks in a community. JAMA 210:1428, 1969.
150. Link H, Lebram G, Johansson I, Radberg C: Prognosis in patients with infarction and TIA in carotid territory during and after anticoagulant therapy. Stroke 10:529, 1979.
151. Pearce JMS, Gubbay SS, Walton JN: Longterm anticoagulant therapy in transient cerebral ischemic attacks. Lancet 1:6, 1965.
152. Siekert RG, Whisnant JP, Millikan CH: Surgical and anticoagulant therapy of occlusive cerebrovascular disease. Ann Intern Med 58:637, 1963.
153. Ziegler DK, Hassanein RS: Prognosis in patients with transient ischemic attacks. Stroke 4:666, 1973.
154. Consensus sur la morphologie et la risque des plaques carotidiennes. J Echograph Med Ultrason 17:300, 1996.
155. Durward QJ, Ferguson GG, Barr HWK: The natural history of asymptomatic carotid bifurcation plaques. Stroke 13:459, 1982.
156. Kagan A, Popper J, Rhoads GG, et al: Epidemiologic studies on coronary artery disease and stroke in Japanese men living in Japan, Hawaii, and California: Prevalence of stroke. In Scheinberg P (ed): Cerebrovascular Diseases. Philadelphia, Lippincott, 1976, p 267.
157. Shah AB, Coull BM, Howieson J, et al: Does natural history of transient ischemic attacks (TIAs) justify surgery [letter to editor]? Stroke 14:828, 1983.
158. Haynes RB, Taylor DW, Sackett DL, et al: Prevention of functional impairment by endarterectomy for symptomatic high-grade carotid stenosis: North American Symptomatic Carotid Endarterectomy Trial Collaborators. JAMA 271:1256–1259, 1994.
159. Adams HP Jr, Putnam SF, Corbett JJ, et al: Amaurosis fugax: The results of arteriography in 59 patients. Stroke 14:742, 1983.
160. DeBono DP, Warlow CP: Potential sources of emboli in patients with presumed transient cerebral or retinal ischemia. Lancet 1:343, 1981.
161. Gautier JC: Clinical presentation and differential diagnosis of amaurosis fugax. In Bernstein EF (ed): Amaurosis Fugax. New York, Springer-Verlag, 1990.
162. Marshall J, Meadows S: The natural history of amaurosis fugax. Brain 91:419, 1968.
163. Mungas JE, Baker WH: Amaurosis fugax. Stroke 8:232, 1977.
164. Wilson LA, Warlow CP, Ross Russell RW: Cardiovascular disease in patients with retinal arterial occlusion. Lancet 1:292, 1979.
165. Gerstenfeld J: The fundus oculi in amaurosis fugax. Am J Ophthalmol 58:198, 1964.
166. Dyll LM, Margolis M, David NJ: Amaurosis fugax: Funduscopic and photographic observations during an attack. Neurology (Minneap) 16:135, 1966.
167. David NJ: Amaurosis fugax and after. In Glaser JS (ed): Neuroophthalmology. St. Louis, CV Mosby, 1979.
168. Elschnig A: Ueber den Einfluss des Verschlusses der Arteria ophthalmica und der Carotis auf das Sehorgan. Graefes Arch Clin Exp Ophthalmol 39:151, 1893.
169. Fisher CM: Transient monocular blindness associated with hemiplegia. AMA Arch Ophthalmol 47:167, 1952.
170. Wagener HP: Amaurosis fugax: A specific type of transient loss of vision. Ill Med J January:21, 1957.
171. Goodwin JA, Gorelick PB, Helgason CM: Symptoms of amaurosis fugax in atherosclerotic carotid artery disease. Neurology 37:829, 1987.
172. Eisenberg RL, Mani RL: Clinical and arteriographic comparison of amaurosis fugax with hemispheric transient ischemic attacks. Stroke 9:254, 1978.
173. Hooshmand H, Vines FS, Lee HM, Grindal A: Amaurosis fugax: Diagnostic and therapeutic aspects. Stroke 5:643, 1974.
174. Hayreh SS, Weingeist TA: Experimental occlusion of the central artery of the retina. I: Ophthalmoscopic and fluorescein fundus angiographic studies. Br J Ophthalmol 64:896, 1980.
175. Gowers WR: On a case of simultaneous embolism of central retinal and middle cerebral arteries. Lancet 2:794, 1875.
176. Hollenhorst RW: Significance of bright plaques in the retinal arterioles. JAMA 178:23, 1961.
177. Praffenbach DD, Hollenhorst RW: Morbidity and survivorship of patients with embolic cholesterol crystals in the ocular fundus. Am J Ophthalmol 75:66, 1973.
178. McBrien DJ, Bradley RD, Ashton N: The nature of retinal emboli in stenosis of the internal carotid artery. Lancet 1:697, 1963.
179. Brockmeier LB, Adolph RJ, Gustin BW, et al: Calcium emboli to the retinal artery in calcific aortic stenosis. Am Heart J 101:32, 1981.
180. Wolpow ER, Lupton RG: Transient vertical monocular hemianopsia with anomalous retinal artery branching. Stroke 12:691, 1981.
181. Winterkorn JMS, Kupersmith MJ, Wirtschafter JD, Forman S: Brief report: Treatment of vasospastic amaurosis fugax with calcium-channel blockers. N Engl J Med 329:396, 1993.
182. Furlan AJ, Whisnant JP, Kearns TP: Unilateral visual loss in bright light: An unusual symptom of carotid artery occlusive disease. Arch Neurol 36:675, 1979.
183. Donnan GA, Sharbrough FW, Whisnant JP: Carotid occlusive disease: Effect of bright light on visual evoked responses. Arch Neurol 39:687, 1982.
184. Benavente O, Eliasziw M, Streifler JY, et al: Prognosis after transient monocular blindness associated with carotid-artery stenosis. N Engl J Med 345:1084–1090, 2001.
185. Barnett HJM: Delayed cerebral ischemic episodes distal to occlusion of major cerebral arteries. Neurology 28:769, 1978.
186. Baquis GD, Pessin MS, Scott RM: Limb shaking—a carotid TIA. Stroke 16:444, 1985.
187. Fisch BJ, Tatemichi TK, Prohovnik I, et al: Transient ischemic attacks resembling simple partial motor seizures, abstracted. Neurology 38(Suppl):264, 1988.
188. Ross Russell RW, Page NGR: Critical perfusion of brain and retina. Brain 106:419, 1983.
189. Tatemichi TK, Young WL, Prohovnik I, et al: Perfusion insufficiency in limb shaking transient ischemic attacks. Stroke 21:341, 1990.
190. Yanagihara T, Klass DW: Rhythmic involuntary movement as a manifestation of transient ischemic attacks. Trans Am Neurol Assoc 106:46, 1981.
191. Klempen NL, Janardhan V, Schwartz RB, Stieg PE: Shaking limb transient ischemic attacks: Unusual presentation of carotid artery occlusive disease: Report of two cases. Neurosurgery 51:483–487, 2002.
192. Radberg J, Sanner J, Bojo L, et al: [Limb-shaking—a rare manifestation of hemodynamic-related TIA]. Lakartidningen 97:4313–4316, 2000.
193. Streifler JY, Eliasziw M, Fox AJ, et al: Angiographic detection of carotid plaque ulceration: Comparison with surgical observations in a multicenter study: North American Symptomatic Carotid Endarterectomy Trial. Stroke 25:1130, 1994.

Clinical Manifestations

194. Streifler JY, Eliasziw M, Bonavente OR, et al: The risk of stroke in patients with first-ever retinal vs. hemispheric transient ischemic attacks and high-grade carotid stenosis. Arch Neurol 52:246, 1995.

195. Eisenberg RL, Nemzek WR, Moore WS, Mani RL: Relationship of transient ischemic attacks and angiographically demonstrable lesions of carotid artery. Stroke 8:483, 1977.

196. Horenstein S, Hambrook G, Roat GW, et al: Arteriographic correlates of transient ischemic attacks. Trans Am Neurol Assoc 97:132, 1972.

197. Janeway R, Toole JF: Vascular anatomic status of patients with transient ischemic attacks. Trans Am Neurol Assoc 97:137, 1971.

198. Ramirez-Lassepas M, Sandok BA, Burton RC: Clinical indicators of extracranial carotid artery disease in patients with transient symptoms. Stroke 4:537, 1973.

199. Toole JF, Janeway R, Choi K, et al: Transient ischemic attacks due to atherosclerosis: A prospective study of 160 patients. Arch Neurol 32:5, 1975.

200. Fisher CM, Gore I, Okabe N, White PD: Atherosclerosis of the carotid and vertebral arteries—extracranial and intracranial. J Neuropathol Exp Neurol 24:455, 1965.

201. Rothwell PM, Salinas R, Ferrando LA, et al: Does the angiographic appearance of a carotid stenosis predict the risk of stroke independently of the degree of stenosis? Clin Radiol 50:830, 1955.

202. Hennerici M, Steinke W, Rautenberg W, Mohr JP: Symptomatic and asymptomatic high-grade carotid stenosis in Doppler color flow imaging. Neurology 42:131, 1992.

203. Chikos PM, Fisher LD, Hirsch JH, et al: Observer variability in evaluating extracranial carotid artery stenosis. Stroke 14:885, 1983.

204. Blaisdell FW, Glickman M, Trunkey DD: Ulcerated atheroma of the carotid artery. Arch Surg 108:491, 1974.

205. Edwards JH, Kricheff II, Riles T, Imparato A: Angiographically undetected ulceration of the carotid bifurcation as a cause of embolic stroke. Radiology 132:369, 1979.

206. Kishore PRS, Chase NE, Kricheff II: Carotid stenosis and intracranial emboli. Radiology 100:351, 1971.

207. Meyer WW: Cholesterinkrystall embolic kleiner Organarterien und ihre Folgen. Virchows Arch [A] 314:616, 1947.

208. Wood EH, Correll JW: Atheromatous ulceration in major neck vessels as a cause of cerebral embolism. Acta Radiol Diagn (Stockh) 9:520, 1969.

209. Aburahma AF, Thiele SP, Wulu JT Jr: Prospective controlled study of the natural history of asymptomatic 60% to 69% carotid stenosis according to ultrasonic plaque morphology. J Vasc Surg 36:437–442, 2002.

210. Tegos TJ, Sohail M, Sabetai MM, et al: Echomorphologic and histopathologic characteristics of unstable carotid plaques. AJNR Am J Neuroradiol 21:1937–1944, 2000.

211. Hartmann A, Mohr JP, Thompson JL, et al: Interrater reliability of plaque morphology classification in patients with severe carotid artery stenosis. Acta Neurol Scand 99:61–64, 1999.

212. Imparato AM, Riles TS, Gorstein F: The carotid bifurcation plaque: Pathologic findings associated with cerebral ischemia. Stroke 10:238, 1979.

213. Kishore PRS, Dick AR: Spontaneous disappearance of carotid stenosis. Radiology 129:721, 1978.

214. Kroener JM, Dorn PL, Shoor PM, et al: Prognosis of asymptomatic ulcerating carotid lesions. Arch Surg 115:1387, 1980.

215. Caplan LR: Are terms such as completed stroke or RIND of continued usefulness? Stroke 14:431, 1983.

216. Bogousslavsky J, Regli F, Zografos L, Uske A: Optico-cerebral syndrome: Simultaneous hemodynamic infarction of optic nerve and brain. Neurology 37:263, 1987.

217. Bunt TJ: The clinical significance of the asymptomatic Hollenhorst plaque. J Vasc Surg 4:559, 1986.

218. Schwarcz TH, Eton D, Ellenby MI, et al: Hollenhorst plaques: Retinal manifestations and the role of carotid endarterectomy. J Vasc Surg 11:635, 1990.

219. Pessin MS, Estol CJ, DeWitt LD, et al: Retinal emboli and carotid disease [abstract]. Neurology 40(Suppl 1):249, 1990.

220. Douglas DJ, Schuler JJ, Buchbinder D, et al: The association of central retinal artery occlusion and extracranial carotid artery disease. Ann Surg 208:85, 1988.

221. Sheng FC, Quinones-Baldrich W, Machleder HI, et al: Relationship of extracranial carotid occlusive disease and central retinal artery occlusion. Am J Surg 152:175, 1986.

222. Magargal LE, Sanborn GE, Zimmerman A: Venous stasis retinopathy associated with embolic obstruction of the central retinal artery. J Clin Neuroophthalmol 2:113, 1982.

223. Fisher CM: Some neuro-opthalmological observations. J Neurol Neurosurg Psychiatry 30:383, 1967.

224. Hedges TR: Ophthalmoscopic findings in internal carotid artery occlusions. Bull Johns Hopkins Hosp 111:89, 1962.

225. Kearns TP, Hollenhorst RW: Venous-stasis retinopathy of occlusive disease of the carotid artery. Staff Meet Mayo Clin 38:304, 1963.

226. Young LHY, Appen RE: Ischemic oculopathy: A manifestation of carotid artery disease. Arch Neurol 38:358, 1981.

227. Gelmers HJ: The pericarotid syndrome. Acta Neurochir (Wien) 57:37, 1981.

228. Bogousslavsky J, Regli F: Cerebral infarction with transient signs (CITS): Do TIAs correspond to small deep infarcts in internal carotid artery occlusion? Stroke 15:536, 1984.

229. Macchi C, Molino LR, Miniati B, et al: Collateral circulation in internal carotid artery occlusion: A study by duplex scan and magnetic resonance angiography. Minerva Cardioangiol 50:695–700, 2002.

230. Lhermitte F, Gautier JC, Derouesne C: Anatomie et physiopathologie des sténoses carotidiennes. Rev Neurol (Paris) 115:641, 1966.

231. Chimowitz MI, Lafranchise EF, Furlan AJ, Awad IA: Ipsilateral leg weakness associated with carotid stenosis. Stroke 21:1362, 1990.

232. Karis R: Asymptomatic carotid artery disease [letter to the editors]. Stroke 14:443, 1983.

233. Dandy WE: Results following ligation of the internal carotid artery. Arch Surg 45:521, 1942.

234. Fleming JFR, Petrie D: Traumatic thrombosis of the internal carotid artery with delayed hemiplegia. Can J Surg 11:166, 1968.

235. Finklestein S, Kleinman GM, Cuneo R, Baringer JR: Delayed stroke following carotid occlusion. Neurology (Minneapolis) 30:84, 1980.

236. Russell D: Cerebral microemboli and cognitive impairment. J Neurol Sci 203–204(C):211–214, 2002.

237. Heyer EJ, Sharma R, Rampersad A, et al: A controlled prospective study of neuropsychological dysfunction following carotid endarterectomy. Arch Neurol 59:217–222, 2002.

238. Mohr JP, Foulkes MA, Polis AB, et al: Infarct topography and hemiparesis profiles with cerebral convexity infarction: The Stroke Data Bank. J Neurol Neurosurg Psychiatry 56:344, 1993.

239. Liebers M: Alzheimerische Krankheit bei schwerer Gehirnarteriosklose. Z Ges Neurol Psychiatr 124:639, 1932.

240. Elder W: The clinical varieties of visual aphasia (case 1). Edinb Med J 49:433, 1900.

241. Timsit SG, Sacco RL, Mohr JP, et al: Early clinical differentiation of atherosclerotic and cardioembolic infarction: The Stroke Data Bank (SDB). In: 1st European Stroke Conference, Duesseldorf, May 10–11, 1990.

242. Timsit S, Logak M, Manai R, Rancurel G: Evolving isolated hand palsy: A parietal lobe syndrome associated with carotid artery disease. Brain 120:2251–2257, 1997.

243. Yanagihara T, Sundt TM Jr, Piepgras DG: Weakness of the lower extremity in carotid occlusive disease. Arch Neurol 45:297, 1988.

244. Rao R: The role of carotid stenosis in vascular cognitive impairment. J Neurol Sci 203–204(C):103–107, 2002.

245. Maeshima S, Terada T, Yoshida N, et al: Cerebral angioplasty in a patient with vascular dementia. Arch Phys Med Rehabil 78:666–669, 1997.

246. Hashiguchi S, Mine H, Ide M, Kawachi Y: Watershed infarction associated with dementia and cerebral atrophy. Psychiatry Clin Neurosci 54:163–168, 2000.

247. Jacobs LA, Ganji S, Shirley JG, et al: Cognitive improvement after extracranial reconstruction for the low flow-endangered brain. Surgery 93:683, 1983.

248. Tatemichi TK, Desmond DW, Prohovnik I, Eidelberg D: Dementia associated with bilateral carotid occlusions: Neuropsychological and haemodynamic course after extracranial to intracranial bypass surgery. J Neurol Neurosurg Psychiatry 58:633–636, 1995.

249. Sakoh M, Ueda T, Kumon Y, et al: [Bilateral carotid stenting for bilateral carotid artery stenosis improved vascular dementia]. No Shinkei Geka 30:759–765, 2002.

250. Rabee HM, Saadani MK, Iqbal KM, Al Salman MM: Neurobehavioral effects of carotid endarterectomy. Saudi Med J 22:433–437, 2001.

Clinical Manifestations

251. Dyken ML, Doepker JF, Kiovsky R, et al: Asymptomatic occlusion of an internal carotid artery in a hospital population: Determined by directional Doppler ophthalmosonometry. Stroke 5:714, 1974.

252. Furlan AJ, Whisnant JP: Long-term prognosis after carotid artery occlusion. Neurology (Minneapolis) 30:986, 1980.

253. Grillo P, Paterson RH: Occlusion of the carotid artery: Prognosis (natural history) and the possibilities of surgical revascularization. Stroke 6:17, 1975.

254. Sacquegna T, DeCarolis P, Pazzaglia P, et al: The clinical course and prognosis of carotid artery occlusion. J Neurol Neurosurg Psychiatry 45:1037, 1982.

255. Bernstein NM, Norris JW: Benign outcome of carotid occlusion. Neurology 39:6, 1989.

256. Wade JPH, Wong W, Barnett HJM, Vandervoort P: Bilateral occlusion of the internal carotid arteries: Presenting symptoms in 74 patients and a prospective study of 34 medically treated patients. Brain 110:667, 1987.

257. Hennerici M, Rautenberg W: Stroke risk from symptomless extracranial arterial disease. Lancet 2:1180, 1982.

258. Endarterectomy for asymptomatic carotid artery stenosis. Executive Committee for the Asymptomatic Carotid Atherosclerosis Study. JAMA 273:1421–28, 1995.

259. Brott T, Tomsick T, Feinberg W, et al: Baseline silent cerebral infarction in the Asymptomatic Carotid Atherosclerosis Study. Stroke 25:1122, 1994.

260. Pettigrew LC, Thomas N, Howard VJ, et al: Low mini-mental status predicts mortality in asymptomatic carotid arterial stenosis: Asymptomatic Carotid Atherosclerosis Study investigators. Neurology 55:30–34, 2000.

261. Hartmann A, Mast H, Thompson JL, et al: Transcranial Doppler waveform blunting in severe extracranial carotid artery stenosis. Cerebrovasc Dis 10:33–38, 2000.

262. Blaser T, Hofmann K, Buerger T, et al: Risk of stroke, transient ischemic attack, and vessel occlusion before endarterectomy in patients with symptomatic severe carotid stenosis. Stroke 33:1057–1062, 2002.

263. Strandness DE Jr: Screening for carotid disease and surveillance for carotid restenosis. Semin Vasc Surg 14:200–205, 2001.

264. Lovelace TD, Moneta GL, Abou-Zamzam AM Jr, et al: Optimizing duplex follow-up in patients with an asymptomatic internal carotid artery stenosis of less than 60%. J Vasc Surg 33:56–61, 2001.

265. Mohr JP: Asymptomatic carotid artery disease. Stroke 13:431, 1982.

266. Heyman A, Wilkinson WE, Heyden S, et al: Risk of stroke in asymptomatic persons with cervical arterial bruits. N Engl J Med 302:838, 1980.

267. Wolf PA, Kannel WB, Sorlie P, McNamara P: Asymptomatic carotid bruit and the risk of stroke. JAMA 245:1442, 1981.

268. Gautier JC, Rosa A, L'hermitte F: Auscultation carotidienne: Correlations chez 200 patients avec 332 angiographies. Rev Neurol (Paris) 131:175, 1975.

269. Pessin MS, Panis W, Prager RJ, et al: Auscultation of cervical and ocular bruits in extracranial carotid occlusive disease: A clinical and angiographic study. Stroke 14:246, 1983.

270. Lees RS, Kistler JP: Carotid phonoangiography. In Bernstein E (ed): Noninvasive Diagnostic Techniques in Vascular Disease. St. Louis, CV Mosby, 1978, p 187.

271. Lipchik EO, DeWeese JA, Schenk EA, et al: Diaphragm-like obstructions of the human arterial tree. Radiology 113:43, 1974.

272. Archie JP Jr: Reoperations for carotid artery stenosis: Role of primary and secondary reconstructions. J Vasc Surg 33:495–503, 2001.

273. O'Hara PJ, Hertzer NR, Karafa MT, et al: Reoperation for recurrent carotid stenosis: Early results and late outcome in 199 patients. J Vasc Surg 34:5–12, 2001.

Clinical Manifestations

Chapter Six

Anterior Cerebral Artery Disease

John C. M. Brust and Angel Chamorro

ETIOLOGY

Infarction in the territory of one or both anterior cerebral arteries (ACAs) is commonly secondary to vasospasm after rupture of saccular aneurysms of the ACA or the anterior communicating artery (ACoA). When such cases are excluded, ACA infarcts have been reported to represent 0.6% to 3% of acute ischemic strokes.[1–4] As with infarcts in the middle cerebral artery territory, those involving the ACA are more often associated with internal carotid artery (ICA) atherosclerosis than with primary stenosis or thrombosis of the ACA itself.[5] In a clinical series of 27 patients, 17 (63%) had probable emboli from the ICA or the heart; other causes were isolated proximal ACA occlusion, paraneoplastic disseminated intravascular coagulation, ICA dissection with embolic occlusion of the opposite ACA, acute ethanol intoxication, and hypertensive occlusion of a small penetrating branch of the ACA. Six patients with no obvious cause were older than 50 years, five of whom had risk factors for atherosclerotic stroke.[1] In an autopsy series of 55 patients with ACA infarcts, 10 had probable cardiac emboli and only 5 had atherosclerosis primarily involving the ACA itself.[6] ACA territory infarction has resulted from vessel compression during transfalcial herniation.[7]

Dissecting aneurysms of the ACA have affected either proximal or distal segments, have produced both infarction and subarachnoid hemorrhage, and have occurred either spontaneously or after head trauma.[8–12] Intracranial carotid artery dissection is nearly always associated with ACA occlusion.[13] A few case reports suggest embolic occlusion from small aneurysms of the distal ICA.[14]

A patient with transient ischemic attacks had fibromuscular dysplasia of both pericallosal arteries.[15] In another report, bilateral ACA infarction occurred in a patient with sickle cell trait during acute ethanol intoxication and withdrawal.[16] Bilateral ACA infarction has also followed intracranial extension of Wegener's granulomatosis.[17] ACA occlusion has resulted from arteritis secondary to subarachnoid neurocysticercosis[18,19] and tuberculous meningitis[20] as well as from radiation vasculitis 19 years after cranial irradiation for acute lymphoblastic leukemia.[21] Dolichoectasia is rarely reported, including an unusual example involving the anterior and middle cerebral arteries.[22] Dissecting aneurysm has been described so rarely that only scattered individual case reports exist.[23]

Symptoms and signs, including weakness, sensory loss, and behavioral disturbance, vary widely among patients with ACA infarcts. To understand this variety one must be familiar with the relevant anatomy.

ANATOMY

The ACA can be divided into a proximal or A1 segment, from its origin as the medial component of the internal carotid bifurcation to its junction with the ACoA, and a distal or postcommunicating artery segment (Fig. 6–1).[24–28] The distal segment has been variably subdivided by different authorities,[25,26,28–41] for example, into an A2 segment beginning at the ACoA and passing in front of the lamina terminalis as far as the junction of the rostrum and genu of the corpus callosum, an A3 segment passing around the genu of the corpus callosum, an A4 segment from above the corpus callosum to just beyond the coronal suture, and an A5 segment extending to the artery's termination.[32] The A2 and A3 segments have together been referred to as the "ascending segment" and the A4 and A5 segments as the "horizontal segment."[27]

The A1 segment passes over the optic chiasm (in 70% of cases) or optic nerve (30%), varying in length from 7.2 to 18 mm (average 12.7 mm).[26] Its diameter ranges from 0.9 to 4.0 mm (average 2.6 mm) and is greater than 1.5 mm in 90% of brains. In 74% of brains, both A1 segments are larger than the ACoA, the diameter of which ranges from 0.2 to 3.4 mm (average 1.5 mm).[26]

The ACAs pass over the corpus callosum side by side in only a minority of cases, so the ACoA is most often directed obliquely or even anteroposteriorly; thus, it is often best seen with angiography on oblique projections.[26]

The recurrent artery of Heubner[42] arises either at the level of the ACoA or just proximal or distal to it;[43] in different series, it was described as arising most often from the A1 segment,[44] from the A2 segment,[26] or at the level of the ACoA.[45–58] Usually the largest branch of the A1 or proximal A2 segment, Heubner's artery doubles back on the ACA for a variable distance and then, either as a single trunk or with

Clinical Manifestations

101

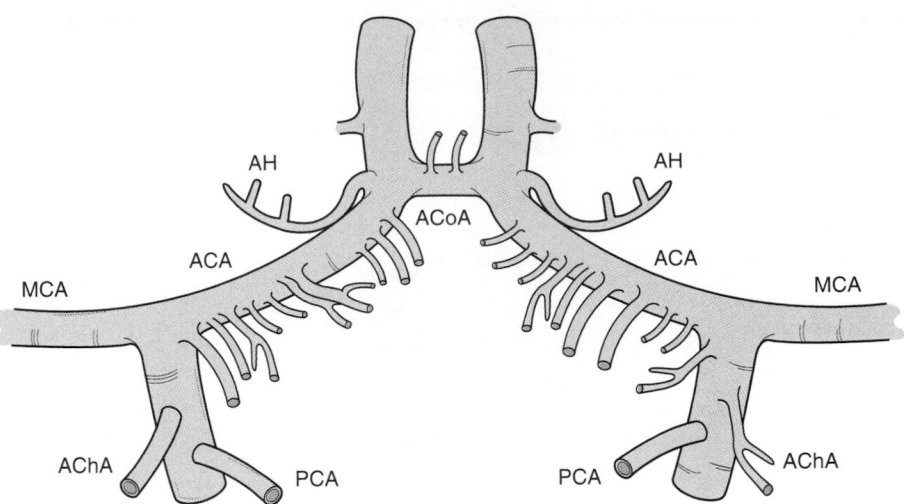

FIGURE 6–1 *Diagram of the dorsal surface of the anterior circle of Willis, showing branches from the A1 segment of the anterior cerebral artery and from the anterior communicating artery. ACA, anterior cerebral artery; AChA, anterior choroidal artery; ACoA, anterior communicating artery; AH, Heubner's artery; MCA, middle cerebral artery; PCA, posterior communicating artery. (From Dunker RO, Harris AB: Surgical anatomy of the proximal anterior cerebral artery. J Neurosurg 44:359, 1976.)*

as many as 12 branches, penetrates the anterior perforated substance above the ICA bifurcation or lateral to it in the sylvian fissure; some branches enter the olfactory sulcus, the gyrus rectus, or more lateral inferior frontal areas.[26,49] Of obvious importance to the neurosurgeon[50–52] is the fact the Heubner's artery most consistently supplies the head of the caudate, the anterior inferior part of the internal capsule's anterior limb, the anterior globus pallidus, and parts of the uncinate fasciculus, olfactory regions, and anterior putamen and hypothalamus.[26,31,43,44,46,49,53–55]

In addition to Heubner's artery, the A1 and A2 segments give off smaller basal perforating branches, up to 15 from each A1 segment[26,46] and up to 10 from each A2 segment.[26–28,50] One of these, called the short central artery, is considered more consistent than others, in some people supplying part of the caudate nucleus and anterior limb of the internal capsule.[57,58] Other proximal branches penetrate the anterior perforated substance and the optic tract and supply, variably, parolfactory structures, the medial anterior commissure, globus pallidus, caudate, and putamen, and the anterior limb of the internal capsule; these vessels also commonly supply the genu and contiguous posterior limb of the internal capsule, part of the anterior nucleus of the thalamus, and most of the anterior hypothalamus.[46] More distal A1 penetrating branches are smaller and supply the optic nerve, chiasm, and tract;[46,59] gyrus rectus and inferior frontal lobe; anterior perforated substance; and suprachiasmatic area.[26] Additional supply to the anterior inferior striatum and anterior hypothalamus comes from A2 segment branches, which can arise either separately or from a larger common trunk (the precallosal artery).[27] Similar penetrating branches from the ACoA,[46,60] 13 or fewer in number,[46,60] supply the suprachiasmatic and parolfactory areas, dorsal optic chiasm, anterior perforated substance, inferior frontal lobe, septum pellucidum, columns of the fornix, corpus callosum, septal region, and anterior hypothalamus and cingulum.[24,26,59,60]

Vascular anastomoses are less functional in the diencephalon and basal ganglia than elsewhere in the cerebral hemispheres, and the territories supplied by these

ACA penetrating end-zone arteries are no exception. Capillary anastomoses, which are difficult to demonstrate by standard perfusion techniques, exceed arterial anastomoses.[30,61–65]

The distal ACAs, deep in the interhemispheric fissure, are the only example of major cerebral arteries running side by side, although as noted, one (usually the left) is often posterior to the other, and because of crossover of branches to the other hemisphere, occlusion of either artery can cause contralateral or bilateral infarction.[27] Beyond the lamina terminalis, the main trunk of the ACA—the pericallosal artery—runs above the corpus callosum in the pericallosal cistern (or, less often, over the cingulate gyrus or in the cingulate sulcus[29]), passes around the splenium of the corpus callosum, and terminates in the choroid plexus of the third ventricle; its posterior extent depends on the anterior extent of the posterior cerebral artery (PCA).[27,66] Except most posteriorly, the pericallosal artery lies below the free edge of the falx cerebri and can therefore shift across the midline.

The pericallosal artery has been variably defined as beginning at the ACoA[28,40] or at the point where the ACA gives off the callosomarginal artery; however, the callosomarginal artery is absent in 18% to 60% of brains.[27,37,38] The callosomarginal artery has been defined as that branch of the ACA traveling in or near the cingulate sulcus and giving off at least two major cortical branches.[37] It originates from just beyond the ACoA to the genu of the corpus callosum, most often from the A3 segment,[27] and can be of the same diameter, larger, or smaller than the pericallosal artery.[25,27] Any or all of the callosomarginal artery's usual branches can arise from the pericallosal artery[27]; these branches supply the inferior frontal lobe (including the gyrus rectus, the orbital part of the superior frontal gyrus, the medial part of the orbital gyri, and the olfactory bulb and tract), the medial surface of the hemisphere (including the cingulate gyrus, the superior frontal gyrus, the paracentral lobule, and the precuneus), and the superior 2 cm of the lateral convexity (including the superior frontal, precentral, central, and postcentral gyri), anastomosing there with branches of the middle cerebral artery (MCA).[29] (These borderzones of shared arterial territory are of clinical importance: In a radionuclide study of 365 consecutive patients with stroke, infarction occurred in the "watershed" between the ACA and the MCA in 5% of patients, compared with the MCA territory in 28% and the ACA territory in 1%.)[67-69] The band of lateral convexity supplied by the ACA is wider anteriorly than posteriorly and may extend into the middle frontal gyrus.

Although variable in number and in whether they arise directly from the pericallosal artery or from its callosomarginal branch, eight major cortical branches of the distal ACA can usually be defined.[27] The orbitofrontal artery arises from the A2 segment except, infrequently, when it shares a common trunk with the frontopolar artery[28] or arises just proximal to the ACoA.[26] Running forward in the floor of the anterior fossa as far as the planum sphenoidale, the orbitofrontal artery supplies the gyrus rectus, olfactory bulb and tract, and orbital surface of the frontal lobe. The frontopolar artery arises from the A2 segment (or, uncommonly, from the callosomarginal artery), passes to the frontal pole along the medial hemispheric surface, and supplies parts of the medial and lateral surfaces of the frontal pole.

The anterior, middle, and posterior frontal arteries arise separately from the A2, A3, and A4 segments of the pericallosal artery or from the callosomarginal artery; infrequently they arise from a common stem.[27,38] They supply the anterior, middle, and posterior parts of the superior frontal gyrus and the cingulate gyrus. The paracentral artery, arising from A4 or the callosomarginal artery, supplies premotor, motor, and sensory areas of the paracentral lobule.

The superior parietal artery, arising anterior to the splenium of the corpus callosum from A4, A5, or the callosomarginal artery, passes through the marginal limb of the cingulate sulcus and supplies the superior part of the precuneus. The inferior parietal artery, subdivided by some authorities into the precuneal and parieto-occipital arteries,[29,31] is the most commonly absent cortical branch of the ACA (36% of brains in one series[27]); it arises from the A5 segment (or rarely from the callosomarginal artery) just above the splenium of the corpus callosum and supplies

the posterior inferior part of the precuneus and portions of the cuneus.

The rostrum, genu, body, and splenium of the corpus callosum are supplied by short callosal arteries, pericallosal artery branches that pass through the callosum to supply, additionally, the septum pellucidum, anterior pillars of the fornix, and anterior commissure.[27,29] Posteriorly, the pericallosal artery extends around the splenium of the corpus callosum (the posterior pericallosal artery[28]) and then passes forward, ending on the inferior surface of the splenium[70] or extending all the way to the foramen of Monro.[28]

Of obvious importance in interpreting symptoms and signs is the normal variability of the boundaries (or borderzones) between the anterior, middle, and posterior cerebral arteries. Figure 6–2, which is based on postmortem injection studies of 25 normal brains, illustrates the range of cortical distribution of the ACA.[71] In those with the most extensive ACA distribution, the primary motor and sensory cortices were supplied by the ACA not only medially but also over the convexity as far as the inferior frontal sulcus. In those with the least extensive ACA distribution, the ACA supplied little or none of the primary motor cortex, even medially.

Anomalies and Species Differences

The anatomy of the anterior circle of Willis is so varied among otherwise normal people that whether a variation should be called an anomaly is sometimes difficult to define. Especially common are hypoplastic A1 segments, from mildly narrow to nonfunctionally threadlike, with both distal ACAs filling from the larger A1 segment.[50,72-75] In one study, 7% of brains had a stringlike A1 segment, and 6% had a hypoplastic ACoA.[76] In another study, 22% of brains had A1 segment hypoplasia, which was severe in 8% of cases and was associated with additional anomalies of the ACA or the posterior cerebral, posterior communicating, or basilar arteries in 82%.[77] Such anomalies are associated with a greater frequency of saccular aneurysms, and ACA occlusion secondary to cardiac embolism is often accompanied by proximal hypoplasia of the contralateral ACA.[75,78-80]

FIGURE 6–2 *Cortical distribution of the anterior cerebral artery. A, Area of variation on the cerebral convexity. B, Area of variation on the cerebral medial surface. Horizontal or vertical lines represent a composite of maximal extent. Crosshatched lines represent a composite of minimal extent. CS, central sulcus; IFS, inferior frontal sulcus; PCS, precentral sulcus; POS, parieto-occipital sulcus; SFS, superior frontal sulcus. (From Van der Zwan A, Hillen B, Tulleken CAF, et al: Variability of the territories of the major cerebral arteries. J Neurosurg 77:927, 1992.)*

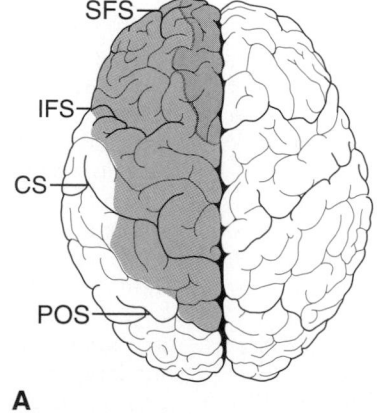

A

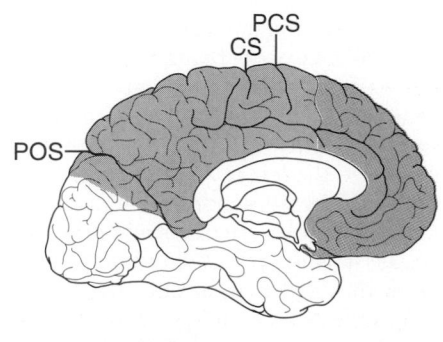

B

A smaller ACA often occurs on the same side as a smaller ICA,[81] and a hypoplastic A1 segment tends to be associated with an ACoA of larger diameter than usual.[26,82] Small A1 segments are several times more common among patients with symptomatic cerebrovascular disease than in the general population.[55] Cerebral angiography in one young man with episodic vertigo, loss of consciousness, and left leg weakness showed absence of the ACAs; the MCAs and one intracavernous carotid artery provided collateral vessels to the patient's medial cerebral hemispheres.[83]

In 50 adult autopsy specimens, 60% had one ACoA, 30% two, and 10% three[26]; other investigators have also found doubling and tripling of this vessel, and some have found absence of the ACoA.[31,84] A1 segment duplication also occurs,[26] as well as a third or median ACA arising from the ACoA (arteria termatica), which is sometimes as large as the two other ACAs and may be the major supplier to the posterior medial hemispheres.[28,31,46,85]

The recurrent artery of Heubner rarely arises from the ICA at its bifurcation, from the MCA, or from the ACoA itself.[26] Absence or doubling of Heubner's artery has occurred.[49] Embryologically, this artery is a remnant of the primitive olfactory artery, and so a patient with a persistent primitive olfactory artery has no Heubner's artery.[86]

Another well-recognized anomaly is a supernumerary vessel arising from the ICA at the level of the ophthalmic artery, coursing below the optic nerve, ascending in front of the optic chiasm, and terminating on the ipsilateral ACA near the ACoA. The A1 segment may be normal, hypoplastic, or absent[87–91]; in one instance both ACAs were absent.[92] Such an anomaly, which may be bilateral,[93] is commonly associated with ACA saccular aneurysm[43,88,90,92,94] and with other anomalies, such as duplication of the MCA,[95] median corpus callosum artery, distal moyamoya, aortic coarctation,[96] facial congenital defects, cerebral lipoma,[44] and absence of the ICA (with the remaining carotid artery giving off a branch that passes beneath the optic nerve and divides into two ACAs and the other MCA arising from the PCA).[97] The anomalous vessel itself can cause visual symptoms from compression of the optic nerve or chiasm.[98]

The infraoptic ACA has been considered a remnant of the embryonic primitive maxillary artery, present in 3- to 4-mm embryos as an ICA branch and normally becoming a cavernous carotid branch, the inferior hypophyseal artery.[87,88,98,99] (The ACA normally arises from the primitive olfactory artery, eventually becoming the dominant vessel.)

Other anomalies, reported in an autopsied infant, include unilateral absence of the proximal MCA, ACA, and anterior choroidal artery, with much of the ipsilateral inferior frontal lobe being supplied by branches from the opposite ACA, and secondary porencephaly of the orbital frontal lobe.[100] Autopsy of a neurologically normal man showed a plexiform anterior communicating system connected to the left ICA by an anomalous vessel arising from the ICA near the ophthalmic artery, a single distal ACA, marked right A1 segment hypoplasia, and right plexiform vessels in the area of Heubner's artery, along with other anomalies of the posterior circulation.[101] Such anomalies, rare in combination, are not unusual individually. For example, in a series of 1250 consecutive autopsies, a plexiform anterior communicating system was found in 15% of subjects, hypoplastic ACAs in 4%, and fused distal ACAs in 4%; a plexiform Heubner artery was much less common.[101] An ophthalmic artery arising from the ACA has also been reported,[70,102,103] as has an accessory MCA arising from the A2 segment of the ACA.[104]

In a study of 381 brains, distal ACA anomalies were found in 25%,[29] including pericallosal artery triplication, absence of ACA pairing, branches from one ACA to the other hemisphere, and bihemispheric branches (Fig. 6–3).[27,31,72,84,85,105,106] Triplicate ACAs with a variably developed midline accessory artery arising from the ACoA and supplying little, much, or most of either or both hemispheres have been observed in up to 22% of autopsy specimens.[29,58,84,107–111] Also, a long callosal artery (medial artery of the corpus callosum, anterior MCA) can arise from the pericallosal artery and pass parallel to it, giving off callosal perforating branches.[27,28] At angiography, these anomalies, like a hypoplastic A1 segment, produce apparent bilateral ACA filling after unilateral injection of a carotid artery.[29,36,112–114] Bihemispheric ACAs, with either ACA taking over the supply of part or all of the other hemisphere, have been reported in up to 64% of brains.[27,29,105,111] (The highest value comes from a study in which any contralateral supply, however small, was included; brains in which most of both hemispheres are supplied by one of two ACAs are less common.)[27,105]

In the fetus, there is gradual embryonic transition from one to two ACAs.[107,115] An unpaired or azygous ACA, arising through proximal union of the ACAs without an ACoA, occurs in 5% or less of adult brains.[29,84,85,107–110,116,117] Sometimes, the ACAs fuse for up to 3.9 cm and an ACoA is absent.[83] Azygous ACAs are associated with a variety of other anomalies, including hydranencephaly, septum pellucidum defects, meningomyelocele, hydroencephalodysplasia, and vascular malformations,[118] and, like other ACA anomalies, with a higher frequency of saccular aneurysm.[119,120] In holoprosencephaly (fusion of the frontal neocortex and absence of the interhemispheric fissure), an azygous ACA courses just beneath the inner table of the skull.[96]

As noted, ACA anomalies are associated with an increased frequency of saccular aneurysms, especially at the ACoA, but also on distal or anomalous branches.[49,86,121–130] The embryonic prominence of the interhemispheric arterial plexus that develops into the ACoA is the most common site for the development of intracranial aneurysms.[131] Of 206 patients with ACoA aneurysms in one study, 44 (21.4%) had ACA anomalies, especially a median artery of the corpus callosum and duplication of the ACoA.[126] Ruptured fusiform aneurysm of the A1 segment of the ACA has been reported.[132] Giant aneurysms have been found on azygous ACAs.[133,134] After subarachnoid hemorrhage, a congenitally narrow A1 segment may be mistaken for vasospasm. Furthermore, proximal ACA ligation in patients with surgically unclippable ACoA aneurysms is not a valid option if one A1 segment fills both distal ACAs or if, in the absence of cross-compression, the aneurysms fill well from either side.[43,73,135–138]

A common anomaly, ACA fenestration has no clinical significance except when it is mistaken for an aneurysm on angiography.[139] Vestibulocochlear symptoms developed in a 22-year-old patient with fenestration and ectasia of the left ACA and persistence of the right trigeminal artery.[140]

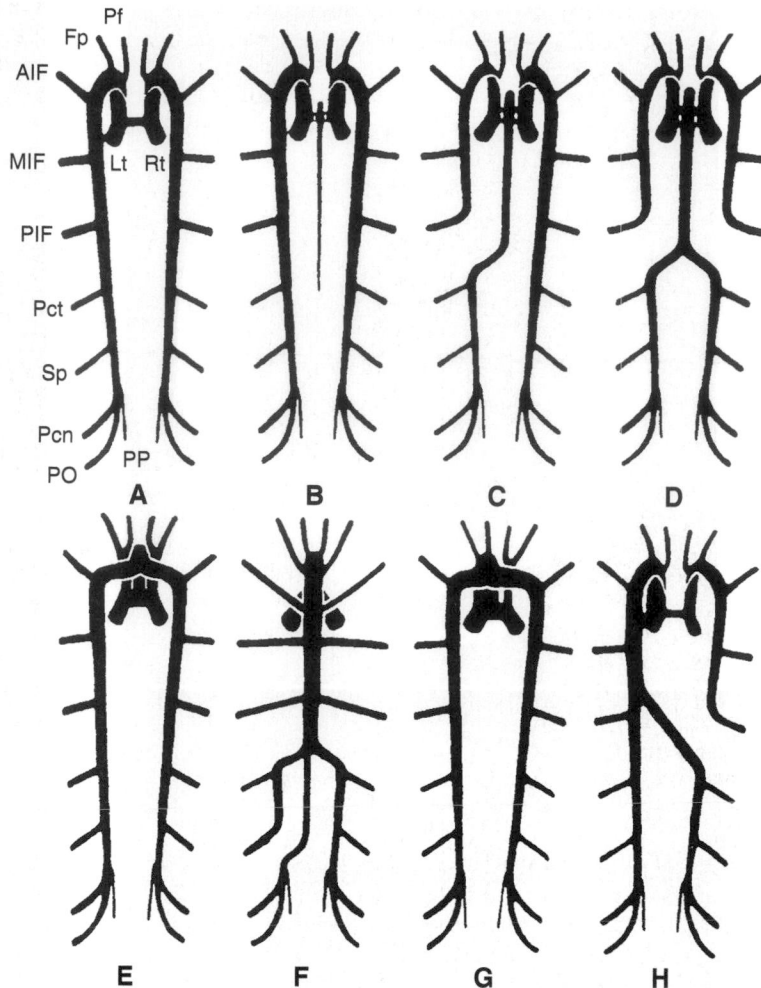

FIGURE 6–3 *Variations in the distal anterior cerebral artery including patterns without (A) and with (B) a medial artery of the corpus callosum and variously developed accessory (C to E), unpaired (F), and bihemispheric lateral arteries (G and H). AIF, anterior internal frontal; Fp, frontopolar; MIF, middle internal frontal; Pcn, precuneal; Pct, paracentral; Pf, prefrontal (orbitofrontal); PIF, posterior internal frontal; PO, parieto-occipital; pp, posterior pericallosal; Sp, superior parietal. (From Baptista AG: Studies on the arteries of the brain. II: The anterior cerebral artery: Some anatomic features and their clinical implications. Neurology [NY] 13:825, 1963.)*

Species differences in the anatomy of the ACA (and other cerebral vessels) must be kept in mind when one is interpreting animal studies of cerebral ischemia and stroke. For example, birds, amphibians, and anteaters have paired arteries without an ACoA or other left-to-right anastomoses.[31] In most mammals, the two ACAs join to form a single pericallosal (azygous) artery, which may or may not bifurcate distally, and there is no ACoA.[31] In subhuman primates, several recurrent medial striate arteries (the equivalent of Heubner's artery in humans) supplying the anterior caudate, putamen, and globus pallidus have rich preparenchymal anastomoses with lateral lenticulostriate arteries from the MCA; the orbitofrontal artery, supplying most of the orbital surface of the frontal lobe, arises from the MCA and anastomoses with branches of the ACA, and extensive anastomoses exist between the ACA and the proximal MCA in the sylvian fissure.[54,141–144] In cats, the presence of an ACoA has been both claimed[145,146] and denied.[147] The feline ACA supplies the medial hemispheric cortex containing hind limb motor representation, but cerebral arterial occlusion tends to cause smaller and deeper infarcts than in higher primates.[148] In rats the rostral caudatoputamen is supplied by penetrating ACA branches and a vessel running alongside the lateral olfactory tract, and this area accounts for

25% of strokes in stroke-prone, spontaneously hypertensive rats.[149,150]

SYMPTOMS AND SIGNS

Weakness and Sensory Loss

ACA occlusion causes infarction of the paracentral lobule and, as a result, weakness and sensory loss in the contralateral leg (Fig. 6–4).[151–156] The deficit is usually greatest distally for the following two reasons: (1) the proximal leg is represented on the primary sensorimotor cortex either superiorly on the medial hemisphere or on the high convexity with, therefore, richer collateral vessels from the MCA and (2) proximal muscles have substantial representation in the ipsilateral hemisphere.[157] If infarction extends to the upper convexity, there may be proximal arm weakness or, as is usual with cortical lesions, clumsiness or slowness out of proportion to the actual loss of strength.

Paretic muscles are initially most often flaccid, becoming spastic over days or weeks; at the outset, tendon reflexes may be decreased, normal, or increased.[159] (This common early dissociation between tone and tendon reflexes has been attributed to the loss of supraspinal influence on

A woman with left ACA territory infarction had difficulty naming her left fingers and moving her named left fingers; she also had difficulty pointing to her own body parts with her left hand.[222] It was suggested that the patient's "body schema" was organized principally in her left cerebral hemisphere and was therefore as a consequence of callosal infarction, disconnected from her right hemisphere.

Occlusion of an ACA that extends around the splenium of the corpus callosum can produce pure alexia in the left visual field or other visual anomic or agnostic problems.[27,212]

A problem in evaluating these patients is the extent to which they differ from those who have undergone surgical callosectomy. Left-sided apraxia to verbal commands occurs immediately after complete section of the corpus callosum and anterior commissure, usually with preserved ability to carry out the act in imitation of the examiner.[223,224] Right-sided movements, when governed by the right hemisphere (e.g., drawing an object seen only in the left visual field), are also impaired.[225] Such deficits tend to improve over days, however,[224] unless severe extracallosal brain damage is present.[223] Lasting deficit after callosal and commissural section is most likely to affect homolateral control of fingers (e.g., moving the left fingers to identify areas corresponding to regions stimulated on the right fingers or mimicking with the left hand postures shown pictorially to the right visual field). When left hemispheric damage occurs early in life, the minor hemisphere can comprehend spoken or written names of familiar objects[226–229] but, except in the setting of prolonged stimulus exposure[230] or in rare instances of unusual plasticity in speech organization,[231,232] usually cannot comprehend verbs or action nouns.[227,233,234] Such lack of comprehension accounts for the inability of a patient who has callosectomy to follow verbal commands with either hand when the information is given to the minor hemisphere. Recovery of all but the most distal and subtle apraxia when commands are given to the language hemisphere is explained by each hemisphere's control over homolateral as well as contralateral limbs.

A patient with anterior callosal hemorrhage and bilateral ACA vasospasm had alexia in the left hemifield, anomia for objects held in the left hand, and left-handed agraphia and apraxia (including imitation and object use).[235] She also had bilateral pseudoneglect: Visual or tactile line bisection produced left hemineglect with the right hand in the left hemispace and right hemineglect with the left hand in the right hemispace. A proposed explanation was disconnection of "the hemisphere important for directing attention-intention into the contralateral hemispace" from "the hemisphere important for controlling sensory motor processing of the limb" as an explanation.[235] By contrast, left hemispatial neglect "confined to right-hand and verbal responses" occurred in a patient with infarction of the posterior genu and whole trunk of the corpus callosum plus the left medial frontal and temporo-occipital lobes.[236] These findings were consistent with the hypothesis that "the left hemisphere is only concerned with attending to the contralateral hemispace," whereas "the right hemisphere is specialized for attending to both sides of space." Also consistent with previous reports, hemineglect does not seem to occur with lesions restricted to the corpus callosum but requires additional destruction (e.g., medial frontal lobe) that blocks transmission through extracallosal commissures.[216,237]

In a right-handed patient who had undergone callosectomy but displayed unusually rich right hemispheric verbal comprehension, there was no left-sided apraxia to verbal information presented to the right hemisphere.[234] This finding argues against the notion that motor engrams reside solely in one hemisphere, language-dominant or not.[207,238–244] In other patients undergoing callosectomy, visual nonverbal stimulation has also produced normally coordinated contralateral motor acts.[244]

Consistent with the view that extracallosal damage is probably crucial to the appearance of anterior callosal disconnection syndrome after ACA occlusion is the finding that left tactile anomia, apraxia for verbal commands, and agraphia did not occur in two patients who underwent sectioning of the anterior commissure and only the anterior two thirds of the corpus callosum.[224] These patients, moreover, performed a variety of nonverbal cross-integration tasks, matching visual or tactile stimuli directed separately to each hemisphere.[245] Conversely, selective sectioning of the splenium, sparing the genu and body, does produce verbal deficits for left visual field and tactile stimuli[208,246] as well as for tactile-motor tasks requiring interhemispheric integration.[243,244] It appears that "the anterior commissure and the rostral callosum do not transfer either lateralized visual images that elicit motor activity or the specific motor program needed to carry out the appropriate movement."[244] An isolated 3-cm midcallosal section impairs interhemispheric transfer of tactile data but not of information obtained visually.[247] Section of the posterior-most 1.5 cm of the callosum disrupts naming of visual stimuli in the left visual field,[246,248–250] and an additional 1.5 cm section further impairs sensorimotor integration and tactile naming.[244,251] What information is transferred across the rostral callosum, that part most often damaged after ACA occlusion, is unclear; it has been suggested that the anterior callosum transfers information after processing it into higher-order abstraction.[244,252] Tomaiuolo and colleagues[253] performed simple reaction times for interhemispheric transfer tasks in a patient with callosal lesions sparing the splenium and rostrum. They measured unimanual responses to simple lateralized visual displays presented tachistoscopically. The impaired responses, when compared with those of a patient with complete callosal section, led Tomaiuolo and colleagues[253] to conclude that "specific callosal channels mediate the basic visuomotor interhemispheric transfer times (ITTs), and these do not include the rostrum and/or the splenium of the corpus callosum." (After posterior callosal section, interhemispheric transfer of sensory information from the right hemisphere is lost, but transfer of semantic information is still possible; after complete section, neither sensory nor semantic information can be transferred.)[252]

Akinetic Mutism (Abulia)

Coma can probably occur after bilateral proximal ACA occlusion, but when aneurysm surgery[254] or vasospasm after subarachnoid hemorrhage[255] is the cause of coma, interpretation is difficult. Dandy[256] believed that left ACA occlusion (i.e., surgical ligation) caused permanent coma, and this view was promulgated by Poppen,[257] who nevertheless considered hypotension during surgery to be a critical factor. Subsequent writers have perpetuated the idea that coma can follow unilateral ACA occlusion.[29,258] However, Dandy's[256] attribution of coma to striatal damage was soon discredited,[259,260] and it is now recognized that coma requires either bihemispheric or ascending reticular activating system lesions.[261] Probably those patients in whom coma seemed to follow ACA occlusion either had brain damage not restricted to one hemisphere, as a result of one of the several vascular anomalies described previously, or were akinetic, mute, and more alert than they seemed.

Akinetic mutism is "a state of limited responsiveness to the environment in the absence of gross alteration of sensorimotor mechanisms operating at a more peripheral level."[262] Neither paralysis nor coma accounts for the symptoms. Patients may open their eyes and seem alert, and brief movement, speech, or even agitation may follow powerful stimuli, but patients are otherwise "indifferent, detached, frozen, and apathetic."[262] The term akinetic mutism was used by Cairns and associates[263] to describe such a state in association with a tumor of the third ventricle. Patients with such lesions often have ophthalmoparesis and fluctuating or continuous somnolence.[264–270]

Akinetic mutism also occurs with lesions of the anteromedial frontal lobes, including infarction.[252,271–274] Ophthalmoparesis (except for early gaze preference) is then not present, and the patient, whose open eyes may follow objects, is more obviously alert than the patient with mesencephalic or thalamic lesions; the patient may make brief, monosyllabic, but appropriate responses to questions. Striking dissociation occurs between spontaneous verbal communication, which is often totally absent, and solicited communication, which is often retained although restricted.[271] *Abulia* refers to a continuum of such abnormalities, from mild to severe, having in common decreased spontaneous movement and speech, latency in responding to verbal and other stimuli, and impersistence in responses and tasks.[96,275] Although verbal responses are "late, terse, incomplete, and emotionally flat," the patient who is sufficiently prodded sometimes reveals a cognitive capacity much more normal than expected.[57] When the patient is literally akinetic and mute, however, the condition must be differentiated from true stupor or coma, a locked-in state, extrapyramidal akinesia, catatonia, hysteria, and a persistent vegetative state. The two structures most often implicated in the production of abulia are the cingulate gyrus and the supplementary motor area (SMA).

Abulia has occurred after bilateral cingulate gyrus lesions. A woman had a sudden headache and then "lay staring at the ceiling, not asking for water or food, and never speaking spontaneously."[276] She was incontinent of urine, ate and drank when food or water was brought, comprehended spoken speech, answered questions monosyllabically, and did not display any emotional reaction. Right-sided hyperreflexia and bilateral Babinski signs were present. At autopsy, embolic hemorrhagic infarction of the cingulate gyri bilaterally and of the corpus callosum was seen. A clinically and pathologically similar patient showed Babinski signs but no hypertonus, and there were

"no visible reactions to pain."[277] Inability to walk despite normal strength has been specifically mentioned in other reports.[278] In another report, however, unilateral cingulate infarction in two patients was followed by seizures in one and personality change in another, with no reduction in motor activity.[278] Akinetic mutism occurred in one patient with presumed unilateral cingulate (and pontine) damage, but autopsy findings were incomplete.[279] A patient with hemorrhage into the right medial frontal lobe had marked bradykinesia of the left limbs that improved when the limbs were placed in his right hemispace.[280] This disturbance was considered motor neglect ("a failure of the intentional systems that lead to preparation and activation of movement"), possibly secondary to SMA damage.[280] It is not unusual for patients with unilateral ACA territory infarction (or medial frontal lobe surgical ablation) to have several days of abulia followed by return of verbal and ipsilateral motor responses, persistence of weakness in the contralateral leg, and a disinclination to move the contralateral arm. Motor neglect thus might be viewed as unilateral abulia.[31,165,281–284] Chamorro and associates[158] demonstrated that motor neglect explains some of the apparent hemiparesis affecting the face, arm, and leg in infarction in the ACA territory, as revealed by computed tomography (CT) or magnetic resonance imaging (MRI) and, in one case, by autopsy correlation (Fig. 6–6). Before the report of these cases, the usual explanation for such face-arm-leg hemiparesis had been involvement of the primary motor cortex or the deeper pathways, neither of which was involved in this series of eight patients. Instead, defective supramotor planning, unilateral hypokinesia, and motor neglect were due to damage of medial premotor areas. Five of the patients had a total lack of voluntary movement in the contralateral limbs that prevented adequate testing of motor praxis and performance of bimanual tasks. Movement could not be elicited by the examiner despite strong verbal and gestural commands. Pain reaction was also defective or absent in the limbs contralateral to the lesion. Transcranial motor stimulation demonstrated absence of responses to cortical stimulation in the lower limbs of the affected side, interpreted as a sign of functional interruption of the corticospinal tract. In the upper limbs, the response to transcranial motor stimulation was normal; this finding indicated that the impaired voluntary function reflected impairment of circuits involved in motor planning or in the initiation of motor action.

With further improvement, signs can become increasingly subtle, for example, difficulty with sequential movements involving different joints or coordinating the movements of both arms.[284,285] In one report there was inability to reproduce rhythms from memory,[286] and in another, in patients with bilateral SMA lesions, there was inability to perceive as separate two successive tactile stimuli applied to the body.[287] Observations such as these have led to the hypotheses that the SMA (and perhaps other premotor structures) is responsible for generating "sequences from memory that fit into a precise timing plan."[286]

Patients with abulia or motor neglect often display relative preservation of reflexic (externally stimulated) movements, in contrast to anticipated or willed movements.

Clinical Manifestations

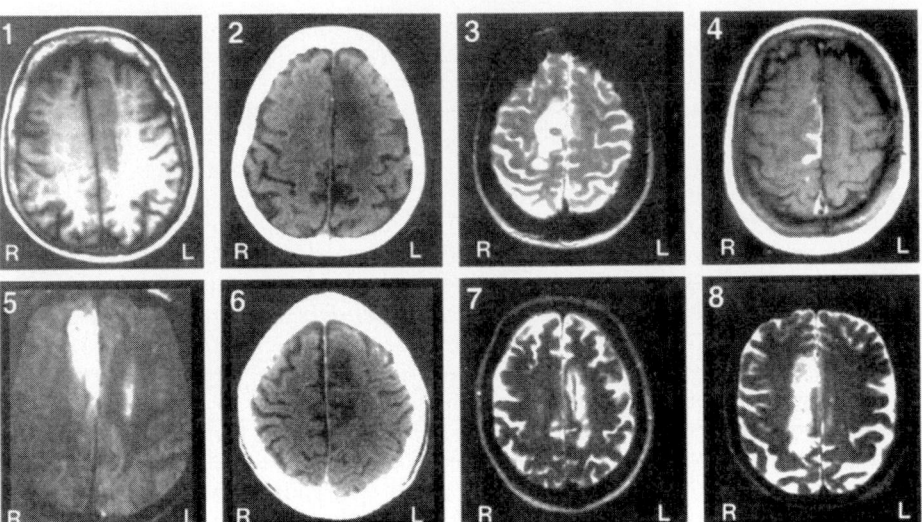

FIGURE 6–6 *Representative axial magnetic resonance (MR) images and computed tomography (CT) scans of the brains of eight patients with anterior cerebral artery (ACA) infarctions. 1, T1-weighted axial MR image. 2, CT scan. 3, T2-weighted MR image. 4, T1-weighted MR image. 5, Proton-density MR image. 6, CT scan. 7, T2-weighted MR image. 8, T2-weighted MR image. (From Chamorro A, Marshall RS, Valls-Sole J, et al: Motor behavior in stroke patients with isolated medial frontal ischemic infarction. Stroke 28:1755, 1997.)*

(A comparable dissociation is seen in parkinsonism.) Disinhibition of unanticipated complex motor movements as a result of SMA damage has been invoked to explain such phenomena as alien hand syndrome, diagonistic apraxia, and utilization behavior.[288]

Cingulectomy in monkeys caused reduction of motor activity and "loss of social conscience"; the animals treated their fellows as inanimate objects not to be feared.[144] Monkeys in which the medial temporal lobes were removed and with Klüver-Bucy syndrome (quietness, no fear, and increased curiosity with compulsive nosing and smelling of all objects) showed gradual clearing of symptoms, which returned after bilateral cingulectomy.[289] In cingulectomized cats, motor signs suggested catatonia.[289] The consequences of surgical cingulate ablation for psychiatric disturbance in humans are difficult to interpret, because the amount of cingulate removed is usually small,[127,290] and the importance of cingulothalamic disconnection in frontal lobotomy has never been defined.[278,291]

The full syndrome of akinetic mutism or abulia has thus not been produced in animals by experimental cingulectomy or in humans by surgical cingulectomy, and even bilateral ACA ligation in humans has on occasion failed to cause the syndrome.[257,272] In an autopsy report of eight patients with akinetic mutism and bilateral cingulate destruction, no difference was seen in the clinical picture whether or not additional lesions existed in the medial orbital cortex or septal region.[278] Most reports, however, have emphasized additional lesions or diffuse compressive cerebral injury,[261,271,272] and electroencephalograms usually show bilateral cerebral slowing.[261,272] An angiographic study of patients with subarachnoid hemorrhage showed correlation of unilateral or bilateral ACA vasospasm with akinetic mutism, but it was unclear whether brain damage was limited to one hemisphere in the patients with unilateral vasospasm.[292]

Abulia has also followed unilateral or bilateral caudate infarction (most likely from occlusion of the recurrent artery of Heubner). In one series of unilateral caudate infarction in 17 patients, abulia was the most prominent feature in 10 patients (6 left, 4 right).[57] In 4 patients, CT showed the lesions to be restricted to the caudate; in others, the anterior limb of the internal capsule was involved. Three abulic patients had alternating restlessness and hyperactivity, and in 4 others, hyperactivity was present without abulia. In another report it was proposed that abulia resulted from damage to the dorsolateral caudate (which connects to the dorsolateral frontal lobe) and disinhibition from damage to the ventromedial caudate (which connects to orbitofrontal areas).[293]

After surgical partial section of the anterior corpus callosum, acute akinetic mutism is often seen that tends to recover over days.[294,295] Positron emission tomography studies in baboons have shown that the procedure causes transient depression of cortical metabolism in widespread areas of both frontal lobes (diaschisis).[296]

Language Disturbance

Unilateral ACA occlusion can produce language disturbance, but whether the disturbance is aphasic is uncertain.[297,298] Details are often lacking in case reports.[43] In some patients, "reduction of spontaneous verbal expression"[281] or muteness, often in association with more global psychomotor bradykinesia,[281,299] seems to be a manifestation of abulia; in such patients, comprehension of spoken speech may be untestable.[300] Some investigators have described true impairment of speech comprehension,[301] word-finding difficulty, alexia,[34] and phonemic or verbal paraphasias on spontaneous speech, reading aloud, or writing.[301,302] Others, however, have emphasized the absence of paraphasias[260,299,303,304] or have considered the difficulty "partly defects of an aphasic order and partly those of a dysarthria."[31] A number of reports have described impairment of spontaneous speech with normal repetition and sometimes echolalia (transcortical aphasia),[260,261,300,303,305–307] and in one instance, echolalia and palilalia occurred without other evidence of aphasia.[164] A man with transcortical motor aphasia, although lacking echolalia and echopraxia, could not refrain from completing the sentences of others.[260] Some patients have had transcortical aphasia (or, as Luria[308,309] calls it, dynamic aphasia), with a strikingly greater impairment of list naming than of naming to confrontation,[303] or particularly impaired speech initiative, as in attempts to narrate stories or describe complex pictures.[260]

In one report, a patient with transcortical mixed aphasia had infarction of both the medial frontal and the medial parietal lobes, whereas two other patients with transcortical motor aphasia had infarction of only the medial frontal lobe.[310] After a large left ACA infarction, one patient had transcortical motor aphasia and mirror writing.[151] Another, who was right-handed, had left-handed mirror writing after infarction of the right medial frontal cortex sparing the corpus callosum, leading to the conjecture that the SMA is "responsible for nonmirror transformation of motor programs originating in the left hemisphere before execution by the primary motor area in the right hemisphere."[311] A woman with aphasia that included impairment of comprehension, repetition, reading, and writing had medial frontal infarction plus an old infarct over the rolandic convexity.[312]

In some patients, speech disturbance was transient, whereas paucity of other movements, including writing, persisted.[301] *Strategic infarct dementia* is a term also used to describe the paucity of speech and motor behavior, accompanied by long delays in response and poor scores on tests involving narrative and naming response. Deep infarcts, in the anterior limb of the internal capsule or anterior thalamus, have been inferred to have interrupted frontal lobe–bound neurotransmitter pathways to create this syndrome, some of them caused by infarcts in the ACA territory.[313,314] Lack of standard testing may have created some overlap in the syndrome names discussed here, leaving unclear exactly how different the eponymic and descriptive syndromes actually are.

Reports of severe language impairment after pathologically documented ACA occlusion have involved left-sided lesions[151] with one exception,[315] a right-handed woman with left hemiparesis, diffuse bradykinesia, speech limited to short replies to questions, and a tendency to echolalia; naming and comprehension of spoken or written language seemed impaired in this patient but were difficult to test. At autopsy, infarction was found in the territory of the right ACA, including the head of the caudate, the anterior limb of the internal capsule, the anterior putamen, the anterior cingulate and superior frontal gyri, and the entire SMA (Fig. 6–7). Several reports describe language disturbance after bilateral ACA occlusion,[300,316,317] including stuttering[318]; in one report with neither postmortem examination nor disclosure of the patient's handedness, the patient had occlusion of the right ACA.[281]

Most investigators, whether or not they consider these abnormalities to be truly aphasic, attribute them to damage to the SMA on the medial surface of the frontal lobe, anterior to the paracentral lobule, and between the cingulate and superior frontal gyri (i.e., the medial hemispheric part of Brodmann's area 6).[297,319–322] Of 10 right-handed patients with left ACA territory infarcts described in one report, 4 had transcortical motor aphasia, and in each, the SMA was involved. Three other patients with sparing of the SMA but involvement of the cingulate had only "alterations of verbal memory."[323] In monkeys, stimulation of this area causes arm and leg movements and head turning,[324] and

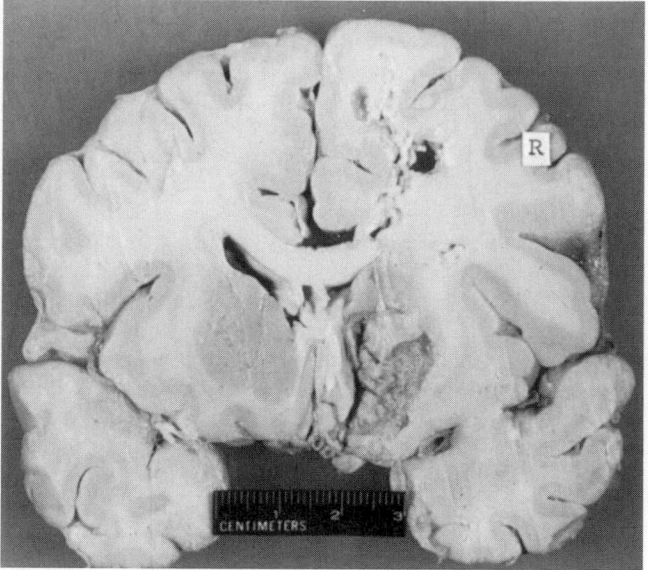

FIGURE 6–7 *Autopsy specimen showing a coronal section of the anterior frontal and temporal lobes. There is infarction in the territories of both the proximal and distal portions of the right anterior cerebral artery. Affected areas include the caudate, putamen, internal capsule's anterior limb, cingulate gyrus, and supplementary motor area. (From Brust JCM, Plank C, Burke A, et al: Language disorder in a right-hander after occlusion of the right anterior cerebral artery. Neurology [NY] 32:492, 1982.)*

there seems to be rostral-caudal forelimb–hind limb somatotopy.[325–331] Unilateral ablation of the SMA in monkeys produces a deficit in tasks of bimanual coordination.[332] In humans, SMA stimulation induces bodily postures (e.g., turning of the head and eyes toward a contralaterally uplifted arm) or repetitive movements (e.g., stepping or hand-waving).[321] Such responses are often bilateral and can occur after ablation of area 4 (the primary motor cortex). SMA stimulation can also cause speech and movement arrest or vocalization.

Whereas stimulation of the face region of area 4 causes vocalization of continuous vowel sounds,[333,334] SMA stimulation on either hemisphere[157] produces intermittently repeated words, syllables, or meaningless combinations of syllables (saccadic vocalization).[321,322] The repeated word might be a palilalia of what was being said at the onset of stimulation. Rhythmic mouth and jaw movements sometimes accompany the vocalization. Speech arrest, hesitation, or slowing also occurs, sometimes with mouth movements suggesting attempted speech or with arrest of other voluntary movement. Speech comprehension is usually preserved, but anomia and paraphasias have occurred.[157]

Such symptoms, with or without other motor, sensory, or autonomic phenomena, may be the manifestation of seizures caused by structural lesions affecting the SMA, especially meningiomas.[116,311,322,335–341] Although experimental stimulation of either the right or left SMA can cause speech arrest or repetition, seizures causing altered speech have only rarely occurred in right-handed persons with lesions of the right SMA.[342,343] Both stimulation and seizure phenomena raise the question of whether true aphasia is occurring and which brain structures are in fact responsible.

Destructive lesions, including infarction, are similarly problematic. Medial hemispheric structural lesions such as neoplasm,[242,306,338,339,344-347] vascular malformation,[211,340] subdural empyema,[348] surgical ablation,[339,349-351] and trauma[309] not only can directly affect more regions than the SMA but also can produce distant effects from edema or brain distortion. SMA excision for the treatment of epilepsy has led to language disturbance, but interpretation of such cases has varied. One group found that excision of the language hemisphere's SMA back to area 4 caused muteness, whereas excision of the language hemisphere's anterior SMA or the nonlanguage hemisphere's entire SMA produced "no specific deficit."[352] Others found, after excision of either SMA, more lasting speech disturbances, although they seemed nonaphasic and secondary to bradykinesia.[349] Transcortical motor aphasia was reported to occur after excision of the left SMA.[351] Bilateral ideomotor apraxia without aphasia affected two patients with ACA infarction involving both the left SMA and the corpus callosum.[353]

The SMA receives afferents from the ipsilateral primary and secondary somatosensory cortex and has reciprocal connections to ipsilateral area 4, posterior parietal cortex, upper convexity premotor cortex (area 6), several thalamic nuclei, and, across the corpus callosum, the contralateral SMA and convexity area 6.[322,354-356] It has been suggested, therefore, that the SMA is "an area of sensory convergence."[325] Efferents project bilaterally to the cingulate gyrus and striatum;[247,299,357,358] ipsilaterally to the red nucleus, pontine nuclei, and dorsal column nuclei;[325] and contralaterally to area 4 and the midconvexity premotor region (area 8).[299] There are also SMA neurons that project to the spinal cord.[326,359,360] Regional cerebral blood flow (rCBF) increases in the SMA during automatic speech and during repetitive finger movement but not during isometric hand muscle contraction.[43,261-263,265] Cerebral blood flow also increases in the SMA during planning of sequential movements.[364-366] (By contrast, the cerebral blood flow of area 4 increases only during execution of such movements.[365]) In monkeys, medullary pyramidal section did not affect movements produced by SMA stimulation,[367] increased discharge of SMA neurons preceded stereotyped learned motor tasks of either the ipsilateral or contralateral extremities, and SMA neurons fired in response to sensory signals "only when the signal called for a motor response."[329] Neurons in the SMA are, however, less responsive to peripheral stimuli than those in area 4,[325,330] suggesting that part of the SMA's function may be "to 'gate' or suppress the afferent influences on area 4"[163] (perhaps accounting for the transient contralateral grasp reflex commonly seen after SMA ablation).[157,303,321,330,368-370] Such suppression would convert area 4's activity from a closed loop to an open loop mode,[330,371] consistent with the further notion that the SMA develops "a preparatory state" for impending movement[329,372] or that it elaborates "programs for motor subroutines necessary in skilled voluntary motion,"[373] including, with its "sequences of fast isolated muscular contraction," human speech.[365] ACA occlusion and SMA damage may therefore affect "an elementary part of language, very primitive, and lacking . . . symbols and

intellectual features"[340]; the resulting disturbances would not, strictly speaking, be aphasic.

The often cited case described by Bonhoeffer[173] in 1914 may represent ACA occlusion causing language disturbance by a different mechanism. The patient experienced right hemiplegia, with the leg weaker than the arm, plus reduction of speech to one or two words, relatively preserved comprehension of spoken speech, alexia, agraphia, and apraxia (difficulty following commands, imitating, and handling objects) that was greater on the left than the right. Abnormalities at autopsy included infarction of the posterior left middle and superior frontal gyri, the anterior four fifths of the corpus callosum, the anterior limb of the left internal capsule, and a small part of the left posterior inferior parietal lobule. Bonhoeffer[173] (and Geschwind,[207] reviewing the case 50 years later) explained the left apraxia as that resulting from the callosal lesion and the aphasia from the combined callosal and capsular lesions, which in effect isolated Broca's area; the posterior parietal lesion probably contributed to the alexia, agraphia, and right apraxia. Neither writer discussed the possible contribution of SMA destruction to the language disturbance, which theoretically could have occurred without it.

Other Mental Abnormalities

Besides abulia, apraxia, and language impairment, patients with ACA occlusion can have a variety of other emotional or intellectual disturbances, usually attributed to involvement of structures supplied by branches of the proximal ACA (A1 segment or ACoA).[52,336,374] Anxiety, fear, insomnia, talkativeness, or agitation has occurred with or without weakness, bradykinesia, or grasp and suck reflexes.[31,164,278,336] A young woman, awakening from a coma after ACoA aneurysm rupture, had severe withdrawal with unprovoked agitation and screaming; autopsy demonstrated bilateral infarction of the orbital gyri, gyri recti, septal nuclei, cingulate gyri, hippocampal formations, and right amygdala.[375] Damage to hypothalamic or other limbic structures has also been considered responsible for these symptoms,[46] which, when they predominate, can suggest nonstructural neurotic or psychotic illness.[29,258] In any event, the notion that apathy and poor motivation predictably follow dorsolateral frontal lesions, whereas orbitofrontal damage causes disinhibited behavior, appears to be an oversimplification.[180,376]

Confusion, disorientation, and memory loss, sometimes severe, also occur.[27,74,147,254,316,377-383] Retrograde and anterograde amnesia after ACoA aneurysm rupture may be subtle or severe,[384-387] with variable denial or confabulation.[169,309,388-390] In one report, a patient with bilateral infarction of both medial frontal lobes as well as the right inferior temporal lobe and pole had severely impaired recognition of previously presented words or pictures yet could spontaneously recall them.[154] In another report, five patients with lesions restricted to basal forebrain structures (sparing the hippocampus and temporal lobes) were able to recall particular stimuli (e.g., someone's name or face) but could not bring such differently learned components together as an integrated memory.[391] Structures that have been implicated in these amnestic syndromes include the hypothalamus, medial forebrain bundle, septum, nucleus of Meynert, nucleus accumbens, and fornix, with possible secondary dysfunction of medial temporal regions.[391–393]

Of 251 patients examined 3 months after acute ischemic stroke, 66 had dementia. Infarction in the territory of the left ACA was more predictive of dementia than infarction in the MCA or PCA territory.[394]

Visuospatial disturbance with difficulty dressing, drawing, or copying or with left hemineglect has occurred after infarction of the caudate and anterior limb of the internal capsule. Primary dyscalculia was also reported after infarction in the territory of the left ACA.[395] Depression has been associated with left caudate lesions.[396]

Incontinence and Other Autonomic Changes

Urinary (and, less often, fecal) incontinence can occur with either unilateral or bilateral ACA occlusion.[29,31,55,343] Involvement of the paracentral lobule (presuming homuncular representation of motor and sensory components of micturition) has been offered as an explanation,[27,93,397] even though paracentral stimulation was found to produce only contralateral sensation without motor response in the penis.[398] Damage to the superior medial frontal lobe, especially the midportion of the superior frontal gyrus, the cingulate, and the white matter in between, is a more likely cause, because such damage (e.g., from frontal leukotomy) causes transient or permanent disturbance of urination and defecation, including urgency and incontinence.[192,399–401]

Cardiorespiratory alterations are common after stroke, whether or not limbic structures are specifically damaged.[402,403] Such changes seen after ACA occlusion are therefore open to interpretation, but it is not unreasonable to incriminate damage to the hypothalamus, cingulate gyrus, or other limbic areas. Fever not always related to infection, tachycardia, and unexpected death have followed cingulate infarction in humans.[254,277,278] Human and animal cingulate stimulation can produce altered respiration, bradycardia, temporary respiratory or cardiac arrest, hypertension or hypotension, pupillary dilatation, and piloerection.[277,404–408] Diabetes insipidus, perhaps from anterior hypothalamic infarction, has occurred after surgical occlusion of a proximal ACA for ACoA aneurysm.[31,52] Gastrointestinal bleeding after ACoA aneurysm rupture has also been blamed on hypothalamic damage.[409]

Periventricular Leukomalacia of Infancy

Brains of infants dying within hours or months of birth may have necrotic foci along the lateral ventricles, considered by some investigators to be infarcts at borderzones between the territories of the ACA, MCA, and PCA.[410–412] Others have stressed that the periventricular areas are more properly called end zones and are not in anastomotic areas but rather within a few millimeters of the ventricular wall "between the terminal distributions of ventriculopetal and ventriculofugal branches of small arteries that penetrate deeply into the brain,"[413] including those from the ACA passing through the cingulate gyrus.[414] Such lesions usually spare the cerebral cortex, because the fetus has rich meningeal anastomoses between pial vessels and the white matter in newborns has a relatively higher metabolic rate.[413,415] Hypotensive newborn dogs develop decreased white matter blood flow and lesions resembling those of periventricular leukomalacia.[416] Autopsy in infants with periventricular leukomalacia and no apparent perinatal asphyxia has shown poorly developed ventriculofugal branches.[414,417] Affected infants display lethargy, hypotonia, difficulty feeding, and seizures; survivors are usually mentally retarded, with spastic quadriparesis.

Because cerebral autoregulation is impaired in neonates with asphyxia, periventricular hemorrhage in the newborn may be the result of capillary dilatation and rupture in these same deep end zones.[412]

References

1. Bogousslavsky J, Regli F: Anterior cerebral artery territory infarction in the Lausanne Stroke Registry: Clinical and etiological patterns. Arch Neurol 47:144, 1990.
2. Gacs G, Fox AJ, Barnett HJM, Vinuela F: Occurrence and mechanism of occlusion of the anterior cerebral artery. Stroke 14:952, 1983.
3. Kazui S, Sawada T, Kuriyama Y, et al: A clinical study of patients with cerebral infarction localized in the territory of anterior cerebral artery. Jpn J Stroke 9:317, 1987.
4. Hollander M, Bots ML, Del Sol AI, et al: Carotid plaques increase the risk of stroke and subtypes of cerebral infarction in asymptomatic elderly: The Rotterdam study. Circulation 105:2872, 2002.
5. Rodda RA: The arterial patterns associated with internal carotid disease and cerebral infarcts. Stroke 17:69, 1986.
6. Castaigne P, Lhermitte F, Escourelle R, et al: Étude anatomopathologique de 74 infarcts de l'artère cérébrale antérieure (55 observations). Rev Med Toulouse Suppl. 339, 1975.
7. Rothfus WE, Goldberg AL, Tabas JH, Deeb ZL: Callosomarginal infarction secondary to transfalcial herniation. AJNR Am J Neuroradiol 8:1073, 1987.
8. Amagasa M, Sato S, Otabe K: Posttraumatic dissecting aneurysm of the anterior cerebral artery: Case report. Neurosurgery 23:221, 1988.
9. Araki T, Ouchi M, Ikeda Y: A case of anterior cerebral artery dissecting aneurysm. No Shinkei Geka 24:87, 1996.
10. Ishibashi A, Kubota Y, Yokokura Y, et al: Traumatic occlusion of the anterior cerebral artery—case report. Neurol Med Chir (Tokyo) 35:882, 1995.
11. Kidooka M, Okada T, Sonabe M, et al: Dissecting aneurysm of the anterior cerebral artery: Report of two cases. Surg Neurol 39:53, 1993.
12. Yano H, Sawada M, Shinoda J, Funakoshi T: Ruptured dissecting aneurysm of the peripheral anterior cerebral artery—case report. Neurol Med Chir (Tokyo) 35:450, 1995.
13. Wada M, Kajikawa H, Fujii S, et al: Ruptured distal anterior cerebral artery aneurysm and diagionistic dyspraxia: A case report. No Shinkei Geka 23:355, 1995.
14. Smrcka M, Ogilvy C, Koroshetz W: Small aneurysms as a cause of thromboembolic stroke. Bratisl Lek Listy 103:250, 2002.
15. Shimauchi M, Kaji Y, Goya T, Kinoshita K: A case report of fibromuscular dysplasia presenting symptoms like moyamoya disease: "String of beads" appearance of the pericallosal artery. No Shinkei Geka 17:981, 1989.
16. Swanson TH, Zinkel JL, Peterson PL: Bilateral anterior cerebral artery occlusion in an alcohol abuser with sickle cell trait. Henry Ford Hosp Med J 35:67, 1987.
17. Satoh J, Miyasaka N, Yamada T, et al: Extensive cerebral infarction due to involvement of both anterior cerebral arteries by Wegener's granulomatosis. Ann Rheum Dis 47:606, 1988.
18. Levy AS, Lillehei KO, Rubinstein D, Stears JC: Subarachnoid neurocysticercosis with occlusion of the major intracranial arteries: Case report. Neurosurgery 36:183, 1995.
19. Katayama W, Enomoto T, Yanaka K, Nose T: Moyamoya disease associated with persistent primitive hypoglossal artery: Report of a case. Pediatr Neurosurg 35:262, 2001.
20. Kashiwagi S, Abiko S, Harada K, et al: [Ischemic cerebrovascular complication in tuberculous meningitis: A case of Fröhlich syndrome and hemiparesis]. No Shinkei Geka 18:1141, 1990.

21. Foreman NK, Laitt RD, Chambers EJ, et al: Intracranial large vessel vasculopathy and anaplastic meningioma 19 years after cranial irradiation for acute lymphoblastic leukaemia. Med Pediatr Oncol 24:265, 1995.

22. Starkstein SE, Bryer JB, Berthier ML, et al: Depression after stroke: The importance of cerebral hemisphere asymmetries. J Neuropsychiatry Clin Neurosci 3:276, 1991.

23. Wakabayashi Y, Nakano T, Isono M, et al: Dissecting aneurysm of the anterior cerebral artery requiring surgical treatment—case report 5. Neurol Med Chir (Tokyo) 40:624, 2000.

24. Czochra M, Kozniewska H, Muszynski A, Trojanowski T: Surgical treatment of aneurysms of the anterior communicating artery using Yasargil's approach. Neurol Neurochir Pol 13:71, 1979.

25. Krayenbuhl HA, Yasargil MS: Cerebral Angiography, 2nd ed. Philadelphia, Lippincott-Raven, 1968.

26. Perlmutter D, Rhoton AL: Microsurgical anatomy of the anterior cerebral–anterior communicating–recurrent artery complex. J Neurosurg 45:259, 1976.

27. Perlmutter D, Rhoton AL: Microsurgical anatomy of the distal anterior cerebral artery. J Neurosurg 49:204, 1978.

28. Stephens RB, Stilwell DL: Arteries and Veins of the Human Brain. Springfield, IL, Charles C Thomas, 1969.

29. Baptista AG: Studies on the arteries of the brain. II: The anterior cerebral artery: Some anatomic features and their clinical implications. Neurology (NY) 13:825, 1963.

30. Beevor CE: The cerebral arterial supply. Brain 30:403, 1907.

31. Critchley M: The anterior cerebral artery and its syndromes. Brain 53:120, 1930.

32. Fischer E: Die Lageabweichungen der vorderen Hirnarterie im Gefässbild. Zentralbl Neurochir 3:300, 1938.

33. Lazorthes G, Bastide G, Gomes FA: Les variations du trajet de la carotide interne d'après une étude artériographe. Arch Anat Pathol 9:129, 1961.

34. Liepmann H, Maas O: Fall von linksseitiger Agraphie und Apraxie bei rechtsseitiger Lähmung. J Psychol Neurol 10:214, 1907.

35. Marino R: The anterior cerebral artery. I: Anatomico-radiological study of its cortical territories. Surg Neurol 5:81, 1976.

36. Morris AA, Peck CM: Roentgenographic study of variation in normal anterior cerebral artery: One hundred cases studied in the lateral plane. AJR Am J Roentgenol 74:818, 1955.

37. Moscow N, Michotey P, Salamon G: Anatomy of the cortical branches of the anterior cerebral artery. In Newton TH, Potts DG (eds): Radiology of the Skull and Brain, Vol 2, Book 2. St Louis, CV Mosby, 1974, p 1411.

38. Ring BA, Waddington MM: Roentgenographic anatomy of the pericallosal arteries. AJR Am J Roentgenol 104:109, 1968.

39. Salamon G, Huang YP: Radiologic Anatomy of the Brain. Berlin, Springer-Verlag, 1976.

40. Snyckers FD, Drake CG: Aneurysms of the distal anterior cerebral artery: A report on 24 verified cases. S Afr Med J 47:1787, 1973.

41. Waddington MM: Atlas of Cerebral Angiography with Anatomic Correlations. Boston, Little, Brown, 1974.

42. Heubner O: Zur Topographie der Ernährungsgebiete der einzelnen Hirnarterien. Zentralbl Med Wissenschaften 10:817, 1872.

43. Ryding E, Bradvik B, Ingvar DH: Changes of regional cerebral blood flow measured simultaneously in the right and left hemispheres during automatic speech and humming. Brain 110:1345, 1987.

44. Ostrowski AZ, Webster JE, Gurdjian ES: The proximal anterior cerebral artery: An anatomic study. Arch Neurol 3:661, 1960.

45. Aydin IH, Onder A, Takei E, et al: Heubner's artery variations in anterior communicating artery aneurysms. Acta Neurochir 127:17, 1994.

46. Dunker RO, Harris AB: Surgical anatomy of the proximal anterior cerebral artery. J Neurosurg 44:359, 1976.

47. Gomes F, Dujouny M, Umansky F, et al: Microsurgical anatomy of the recurrent artery of Heubner. J Neurosurg 60:130, 1984.

48. Gorczyca W, Mohr G: Microvascular anatomy of Heubner's recurrent artery. Neurol Res 9:254, 1987.

49. Ahmed DS, Ahmed RH: The recurrent branch of the anterior cerebral artery. Anat Rec 157:699, 1967.

50. Falconer MA: The surgical treatment of bleeding intracranial aneurysms. J Neurol Neurosurg Psychiatry 14:153, 1951.

51. Gillingham FJ: The management of ruptured intracranial aneurysms. Ann R Coll Surg Engl 23:89, 1958.

52. Hegenholtz H, Morley TP: The results of proximal anterior cerebral artery occlusion for anterior communicating aneurysms. J Neurosurg 37:65, 1972.

53. Alexander MP, Freedman M: Amnesia after anterior communicating artery aneurysm rupture. Neurology (NY) 33(Suppl 2):104, 1983.

54. Gillilan LA: The arterial and venous blood supplies to the forebrain (including the internal capsule) of primates. Neurology (NY) 18:653, 1968.

55. Webster JE, Gurdjian ES, Lindner DW, Hardy WG: Proximal occlusion of the anterior cerebral artery. Arch Neurol 2:19, 1960.

56. Ghika JA, Bogousslavsky J, Regli F: Deep perforators from the carotid system: Template of the vascular territories. Arch Neurol 47:1097, 1990.

57. Caplan LR, Schmahmann JD, Kase CS, et al: Caudate infarcts. Arch Neurol 47:133, 1990.

58. Berman SA, Hayman LA, Hinck VC: Correlation of CT cerebral vascular territories with function. 1: Anterior cerebral artery. AJR Am J Roentgenol 135:253, 1980.

59. Dawson BH: The blood vessels of the human optic chiasma and their relation to those of the hypophysis and thalamus. Brain 81:207, 1958.

60. Crowell RM, Morawetz RB: The anterior communicating artery has significant branches. Stroke 8:272, 1977.

61. Abbie AA: The morphology of the forebrain arteries, with especial reference to the evolution of the basal ganglia. J Anat 68:433, 1934.

62. Alexander L: The vascular supply of the striopallidum. Res Publ Assoc Res Nerv Ment Dis 21:77, 1942.

63. Cobb S: The cerebral circulation. 13: The question of "end-arteries" of the brain and the mechanism of infarction. Arch Neurol Psychiatry 25:273, 1931.

64. Shellshear JC: The basal arteries of the forebrain and their functional significance. J Anat 55:27, 1920.

65. Van den Bergh R, Vander Eecken H: Anatomy and embryology of cerebral circulation. Prog Brain Res 30:1, 1968.

66. Zeal AA, Rhoton AL: Microsurgical anatomy of the posterior cerebral artery. J Neurosurg 48:534, 1978.

67. Booker J, Morris N, Huang C-Y: Cerebral radionuclide scintigraphy in the stroke syndrome. Med J Aust 1:625, 1978.

68. Waltz AG, Sundt TM: The microvascular and microcirculation of the cerebral cortex after arterial occlusion. Brain 90:681, 1967.

69. Watanabe O, Bremer AM, West CR: Experimental regional cerebral ischemia in the middle cerebral artery territory in primates. 1: Angioanatomy and description of an experimental model with selective embolization of the internal carotid artery bifurcation. Stroke 8:61, 1977.

70. Lasjaunias P, Vignaud J, Clay C: Radioanatomie de la vascularisation artérielle de l'orbite, à l'exception du tronc de l'artère ophtalmique. Ann Radiol 18:181, 1975.

71. Van der Zwan A, Hillen B, Tulleken CAF, et al: Variability of the territories of the major cerebral arteries. J Neurosurg 77:927, 1992.

72. Alpers BJ, Berry RG, Paddison RM: Anatomical studies of the circle of Willis in normal brain. Arch Neurol Psychiatry 81:409, 1959.

73. Pool JL: Aneurysms of the anterior communicating artery: Bifrontal craniotomy and routine use of temporary clips. J Neurosurg 18:98, 1961.

74. Tindall GT: The treatment of anterior communicating aneurysms by proximal anterior cerebral artery ligation. Clin Neurosurg 21:134, 1974.

75. Wilson G, Riggs HE, Rupp C: The pathologic anatomy of ruptured cerebral aneurysms. J Neurosurg 11:128, 1954.

76. Riggs HE, Rupp C: Variation in form of circle of Willis. Arch Neurol 8:8, 1963.

77. Marinkovic S, Kovacevic M, Milisavljevic M: Hypoplasia of the proximal segment of the anterior cerebral artery. Anat Anz 168:145, 1989.

78. Kirgis HD, Fisher WL, Llewellyn RC, Peebles EM: Aneurysms of the anterior communicating artery and gross anomalies of the circle of Willis. J Neurosurg 25:73, 1966.

79. Stebbens WE: Aneurysms and anatomic variation of cerebral arteries. Arch Pathol 75:45, 1963.

80. VanderArk GD, Kempe LC: Classification of anterior communicating aneurysms as a basis for surgical approach. J Neurosurg 32:300, 1970.

81. Lehrer HZ: Relative calibre of the cervical internal carotid artery: Normal variation with the circle of Willis. Brain 91:339, 1968.

82. Tindall GT, Kapp J, Odom GL, Robinson SC: A combined technique for treating certain aneurysms of the anterior communicating artery. J Neurosurg 33:41, 1970.

83. Kruyt RC: Aplasia of the anterior cerebral arteries: Angiographic study of a case. Neurochirurgia 14:172, 1971.

84. Windle BCA: On the arteries forming the circle of Willis. J Anat Physiol 22:289, 1888.

85. Blackburn IW: Anomalies of the encephalic arteries among the insane. J Comp Neurol Psychol 17:493, 1907.

86. Tsuji T, Abe M, Tabuchi K: Aneurysm of a persistent primitive olfactory artery. J Neurosurg 83:138, 1995.

87. Brismar J, Ackerman R, Roberson G: Anomaly of anterior cerebral artery: A case report and embryologic considerations. Acta Radiol [Diagn] (Stockh) 18:154, 1977.

88. Isherwood I, Dutton J: Unusual anomaly of anterior cerebral artery. Acta Radiol [Diagn] (Stockh) 9:345, 1969.

89. Mercier P, Velvt S, Fournier D, et al: A rare embryologic variation: Carotid–anterior cerebral artery anastomosis or infraoptic course of the anterior cerebral artery. Surg Radiol Anat 11:73, 1989.

90. Nutic S, Dilence D: Carotid–anterior cerebral artery anastomosis: Case report. J Neurosurg 44:378, 1976.

91. Robinson LR: An unusual human anterior cerebral artery. J Anat 93:131, 1959.

92. Senter HJ, Miller DJ: Interoptic course of the anterior cerebral artery associated with anterior cerebral artery aneurysm: Case report. J Neurosurg 56:302, 1982.

93. Besson G, Leguyader J, Mimassi N, et al: Anomalie rare du polygone de Willis: Trajet sous-optique des deux artères cérébrales antérieures. Aneurysme associé de la bifurcation due tronc basilaire. Neurochirurgie 26:71, 1980.

94. Padget DH: The circle of Willis: Its embryology and anatomy. In Dandy WE (ed): Intracranial Arterial Aneurysms. Ithaca, NY, Comstock, 1945, p 67.

95. Milenkovic Z: Anastomosis between internal carotid artery and anterior cerebral artery with other anomalies of the circle of Willis in a fetal brain. J Neurosurg 55:701, 1981.

96. Lehmann G, Vincentelli F, Ebagosti A: Anomalies rares du polygone de Willis: Le trajet infraoptique des artères cérébrales antérieures. Neurochirurgie 26:243, 1980.

97. Turnbull I: Agenesis of the internal carotid artery. Neurology (NY) 12:588, 1962.

98. Bosma NJ: Infra-optic course of anterior cerebral artery and low bifurcation of internal carotid artery. Acta Neurochir 38:305, 1977.

99. Padget DH: The development of the cranial arteries in the human embryo. Contrib Embryol 32:205, 1948.

100. Stewart RM, Williams RS, Luhl P, Schoenen J: Ventral porencephaly: A cerebral defect associated with multiple congenital anomalies. Acta Neuropathol 42:231, 1978.

101. McCormick WF: A unique anomaly of the intracranial arteries of man. Neurology (NY) 10:77, 1969.

102. Hassler W, Zentner J, Voigt K: Abnormal origin of the ophthalmic artery from the anterior cerebral artery: Neuroradiological and intraoperative findings. Neuroradiology 31:85, 1989.

103. Islak C, Ogut G, Numan F, et al: Persistent nonmigrated ventral primitive ophthalmic artery. J Neuroradiol 21:46, 1994.

104. Tacconi L, Johnston FG, Symon L: Accessory middle cerebral artery: Case report. J Neurosurg 83:916, 1995.

105. Moniz E: Die Cerebral Arteriographie und Phlebographie. Berlin, Springer-Verlag, 1940.

106. Van der Eecken HM: Anastomosis Between the Leptomeningeal Arteries of the Brain: Their Morphological, Pathological and Clinical Significance. Springfield, IL, Charles C Thomas, 1959.

107. De Vriese B: Sur la signification morphologique des artères cérébrales. Arch Biol 21:357, 1904/05.

108. Fawcett E, Blachford JV: The circle of Willis: An examination of 700 specimens. J Anat Physiol 40:63a, 1905/06.

109. Kleiss E: Die verschiedenen Formen des circulus arteriosus cerebralis Willisi. Anat Anz 92:216, 1942.

110. Lazorthes G, Gaubert J, Poulhes J: La distribution centrale et corticale de L'artère cérébrale antérieure: Étude anatomique et incidences neuro-chirurgicales. Neurochirurgie 2:237, 1956.

111. Van der Eecken H: Discussion of "collateral circulation of the brain." Neurology (NY) 11:16, 1961.

112. Curry RW, Culbreth GC: The normal cerebral angiogram. AJR Am J Roentgenol 65:345, 1951.

113. Ruggiero G: Factors influencing the filling of the anterior cerebral artery in angiography. Acta Radiol 37:87, 1952.

114. Saita I, Shigeno T, Aritake K, et al: Vasospasm assessed by angiography and computerized tomography. J Neurosurg 51:466, 1979.

115. Lesem WW: The comparative anatomy of the anterior cerebral artery. Postgrad Med 20:445, 1905.

116. LeMay M, Gooding CA: The clinical significance of the azygous anterior cerebral artery (ACA). AJR Am J Roentgenol 98:602, 1966.

117. Szdzuy D, Lehmann R, Nickel B: Common trunk of the anterior cerebral arteries. Neuroradiology 4:51, 1972.

118. Niizuma H, Kwak R, Uchida K, Susuki J: Aneurysms of the azygous anterior cerebral artery. Surg Neurol 15:225, 1980.

119. Fujimoto K, Waga S, Kojima T, Shimosaka S: Aneurysm of distal anterior cerebral artery associated with azygous anterior cerebral artery. Acta Neurochir 59:79, 1981.

120. Katz RS, Horoupian DS, Zingesser L: Aneurysm of azygous anterior cerebral artery: A case report. J Neurosurg 48:804, 1978.

121. Friedlander RM, Oglivy CS: Aneurysmal subarachnoid hemorrhage in a patient with bilateral A1 fenestrations associated with an azygous anterior cerebral artery: Case report and literature review. J Neurosurg 84:681, 1996.

122. Hanakita J, Nagayasu S, Nishi S, Suzuki T: An aneurysm of the distal anterior cerebral artery with a remarkably anomalous configuration. No Shinkei Geka 16:781, 1988.

123. Klein SI, Gahbauer H, Goodrich I: Bilateral anomalous anterior cerebral artery and infraoptic aneurysm. AJNR Am J Neuroradiol 8:1142, 1987.

124. Mishima H, Kim YK, Shiomi K, et al: Ruptured anterior communicating artery aneurysm associated with inter-optic course of anterior cerebral artery: Report of a case and review of the literature. No Shinkei Geka 22:495, 1994.

125. Ogasawara H, Inagawa T, Yamamoto M, Kamiya K: Aneurysm in a fenestrated anterior cerebral artery—case report. Neurol Med Chir 28:575, 1988.

126. Ogawa A, Suzuki M, Sakurai Y, Yashimoto T: Vascular anomalies associated with aneurysms of the anterior communicating artery: Microsurgical observations. J Neurosurg 72:706, 1990.

127. Sakai K, Asari S, Fujisawa M, Katagi R: Ruptured aneurysm arising from the anomalous anterior cerebral artery—case report. Neurol Med Chir (Tokyo) 32:846, 1992.

128. Schick RM, Rumbaugh CL: Saccular aneurysm of the azygous anterior cerebral artery. AJNR Am J Neuroradiol 10(Suppl):S73, 1989.

129. Suzuki M, Onuma T, Sakurai Y, et al: Aneurysms arising from the proximal (A1) segment of the anterior cerebral artery: A study of 38 cases. J Neurosurg 76:55, 1992.

130. Tracy PT: Unusual intracarotid anastomosis associated with anterior communicating artery aneurysm: Case report. J Neurosurg 67:765, 1987.

131. Truwit CL: Embryology of the cerebral vasculature. Neuroimaging Clin North Am 4:663, 1994.

132. Oba M, Suzuki M, Onuma T: Two cases of ruptured fusiform aneurysm of the proximal anterior cerebral artery (A1 segment). No Shinkei Geka 17:365, 1989.

133. Hashizume K, Nukui H, Horikoshi T, et al: Giant aneurysm of the azygous anterior cerebral artery associated with acute subdural hematoma: Case report. Neurol Med Chir (Tokyo) 32:693, 1992.

134. Shiokawa K, Tanikawa T, Satoh K, et al: Two cases of giant aneurysms arising from the distal segment of the anterior cerebral circulation. No Shinkei Geka 21:467, 1993.

135. Choudhury AR: Proximal occlusion of the dominant anterior cerebral artery for anterior communicating aneurysms. J Neurosurg 45:484, 1976.

136. Cuatico W: The phenomenon of ipsilateral innervation: One case report. J Neurosurg Sci 23:81, 1979.

137. Durity F, Logue V: The effect of proximal anterior cerebral occlusion on anterior communicating artery aneurysms: Postoperative radiological survey of 43 cases. J Neurosurg 35:16, 1971.

138. Nornes H, Wikeby P: Cerebral arterial blood flow and aneurysm surgery. 1: Local arterial flow dynamics. J Neurosurg 47:810, 1977.

139. Ito J, Washiyama K, Kim CH, Ibuchi Y: Fenestration of the anterior cerebral artery. Neuroradiology 21:277, 1981.

140. Tran-Dinh HD, Dorsch NW, Soo YS: Ectasia and fenestration of the anterior cerebral artery associated with persistent trigeminal artery: Case report. Neurosurgery 31:125, 1992.

141. Campbell JB, Forster FM: The anterior cerebral artery in the macaque monkey (*Macaca mulatta*). J Nerv Ment Dis 99:229, 1944.

142. Kaplan HA: Vascular supply of the base of the brain. In Fields WS (ed): Pathogenesis and Treatment of Parkinsonism. Springfield, IL, Charles C Thomas, 1958, p 138.

Clinical Manifestations

Clinical Manifestations

143. Molinari GF, Moseley JI, Laurent JP: Segmental middle cerebral artery occlusion in primates: An experimental method requiring minimal surgery and anesthesia. Stroke 5:334, 1974.

144. Ward AA: The anterior cingulate gyrus and personality. Res Publ Assoc Nerv Ment Dis 27:438, 1948.

145. Hayakawa T, Waltz AG: Immediate effects of cerebral ischemia: Evolution and resolution of neurological deficits after experimental occlusion of one middle cerebral artery in conscious cats. Stroke 6:321, 1975.

146. Hayakawa T, Waltz AG: On the importance of the anterior cerebral artery. Stroke 7:523, 1976.

147. Kamijyo Y, Garcia JH: Carotid arterial supply of the feline brain: Applications to the study of regional cerebral ischemia. Stroke 6:361, 1975.

148. Thompson FJ, Campbell ML: Arterial supply of the feline motor cortex. Stroke 12:233, 1981.

149. Rieke GK, Bowers DE, Penn P: Vascular supply pattern to rat caudatoputamen and globus pallidus: Scanning electronmicroscopic study of vascular endocasts of stroke-prone vessels. Stroke 12:840, 1981.

150. Yamori Y, Horie R, Akiguchi I, et al: Pathogenic mechanisms and prevention of stroke in stroke-prone spontaneously hypertensive rats. Prog Brain Res 47:219, 1977.

151. Bogousslavsky J, Assal G, Regli F: Infarctus du territoire de l'artère cérébrale antérieure gauche. 2: Troubles du langage. Rev Neurol 143:121, 1987.

152. Brust JCM: Circulation of the brain. In Kandel ER, Schwartz JH, Jessel TM (eds): Principles of Neural Science, 4th ed. New York, McGraw-Hill, 2000, p 1302.

153. Brust JCM: Cerebral infarction. In Rowland LP (ed): Merritt's Textbook of Neurology, 10th ed. Philadelphia, Lippincott Williams & Wilkins, 2000, p 232.

154. Delbecq-Derouesné J, Beauvois MF, Shallice T: Preserved recall versus impaired recognition: A case study. Brain 113:1045, 1990.

155. Reivich M: Embryology, anatomy, and pathophysiology of the cerebral circulation. In Goldensohn ES, Appel SH (eds): Scientific Approaches to Clinical Neurology. Philadelphia, Lea & Febiger, 1977, p 749.

156. Tichy F: The syndromes of the cerebral arteries. Arch Pathol 48:475, 1949.

157. Penfield W, Jasper H: Epilepsy and the Functional Anatomy of the Human Brain. Boston, Little, Brown, 1954.

158. Chamorro A, Marshall RS, Valls-Sole J, et al: Motor behavior in stroke patients with isolated medial frontal ischemic infarction. Stroke 28:1755, 1997.

159. Brodal A: Neurological Anatomy in Relation to Clinical Medicine, 3rd ed. New York, Oxford University Press, 1981.

160. Long E: Contributions à l'étude des fonctions de la zone motrice du cerveau. Rev Neurol 15:1218, 1907.

161. Long E: Monoplegia crurale, par lésion du lobule paracentrale. Nouv Icon Salpetr 21:37, 1908.

162. Wilson G: Crural monoplegia. Arch Neurol Psychiatr 10:699, 1923.

163. Winkelman NW: Two brains showing the lesions producing cerebral monoplegia. Arch Neurol Psychiatry 12:241, 1924.

164. Baldy R: Les Syndromes de l'Artère Cérébrale Antérieure. Paris, Jouve, 1927.

165. Foix C, Hillemand P: Les syndromes de l'artère cérébrale antérieure. Encephale 20:209, 1925.

166. Lhermitte J, Schiff P, Curtois A: Le phénomène de la préhension forcée, expression d'un ramollissement complet de la première convolution frontale. Rev Neurol 15:1218, 1907.

167. Schuster P, Pinéas M: Weitere Beobachtungen über Zwangsgreifen u. Nachgreifen u. deren Beziehungen zu ähnlichen Bewegungsstörungen. Dtsch Z Nervenheilkd 91:16, 1926.

168. Seyffarth H, Denny-Brown D: The grasp reflex and the instinctive grasp reaction. Brain 71:9, 1948.

169. DeLuca J, Cicerone KD: Cognitive impairments following anterior communicating artery aneurysm. J Clin Exp Neuropsychol 11:47, 1989.

170. Landau WM, Clare MH: Pathophysiology of the tonic innervation phenomenon of the foot. Arch Neurol 15:252, 1966.

171. Goldstein K: Zur Lehre von der motorischen Apraxie. J Psychol Neurol 11:169, 270, 1908.

172. Goldstein K: Der makroskopische Befund in meinem Fall v. Linksseiter motorischen Apraxie. Zentralbl Neurol 28:898, 1909.

173. Bonhoeffer K: Klischer u. anatomischer Befund zur Lehre von der Apraxie und der motorischen Sprachbahn. Monatsschr Psychiatr Neurol 35:113, 1914.

174. Ghika J, Bogousslavsky J, van Melle, Regli F: Hyperkinetic motor behaviors contralateral to hemiplegia in acute stroke. Eur Neurol 35:27, 1995.

175. Bogousslavsky J, Regli F: Capsular genu syndrome. Neurology (NY) 40:1499, 1990.

176. Schneider R, Gautier J-C: Leg weakness due to stroke: Site of lesions, weakness patterns and causes. Brain 117:347, 1994.

177. Moulin T, Bogousslavsky J, Chopard JL, et al: Vascular ataxic hemiparesis: A reevaluation. J Neurol Neurosurg Psychiatry 58:422, 1995.

178. Bogousslavsky J, Martin R, Moulin T: Homolateral ataxia and crural paresis: A syndrome of anterior cerebral artery territory infarction. J Neurol Neurosurg Psychiatry 55:1146, 1992.

179. Giroud M, Creisson E, Fayolle H, et al: Homolateral ataxia and crural paresis: A crossed cerebral-cerebellar diaschisis. J Neurol Neurosurg Psychiatry 57:221, 1994.

180. Stuss DT, Benson DF: Neuropsychological studies of the frontal lobes. Psychol Bull 95:3, 1984.

181. Greene KA, Marciano FF, Dickman CA, et al: Anterior communicating artery aneurysm paraparesis syndrome: Clinical manifestations and pathologic correlates. Neurology 45:45, 1995.

182. Borggreve F, DeDeyn PP, Marien P, et al: Bilateral infarction in the anterior cerebral artery vascular territory due to an unusual anomaly of the circle of Willis. Stroke 25:1279, 1994.

183. Chimowitz MI, Lafranchise EF, Furlan AJ, Awad IA: Ipsilateral leg weakness with carotid stenosis. Stroke 9:1362, 1990.

184. Schuster P: Zwangsgreifen u. Nachgreifen, zweipost-hemisplegische Bewegungsstörungen. Z Ges Neurol Psychiatr 83:586, 1923.

185. Schuster P: Autoptische Befunde bei Zwangsgreifen u. Nachgreifen. Z Ges Neurol Psychiatr 108:751, 1927.

186. Marie P, Foix C: Paraplégie en flexion d'origine cérébrale par nécrose sous épendymaire progressive. Rev Neurol 27:1, 1920.

187. Van Bogaert L, Ley R: Contribution à la connaissance de la paraplegie en flexion, type Babinski, d'origine cérébrale. J Neurol Psychiatry 26:547, 1926.

188. Meyer JS, Barron DW: Apraxia of gait: A clinicophysiological study. Brain 83:261, 1960.

189. Ueno E: Clinical and physiological study of apraxia of gait and frozen gait. Rinsho Shinkeigaku 29:275, 1989.

190. Denny-Brown D: The nature of apraxia. J Nerv Ment Dis 126:9, 1958.

191. Ferbert A, Thron A: Bilateral anterior cerebral artery territory infarction in the differential diagnosis of basilar artery occlusion. J Neurol 239:162, 1992.

192. Bradley WE, Timm GW, Scott FB: Innervation of the detrusor muscle and urethra. Urol Clin North Am 1:3, 1974.

193. Fisher CM: Hydrocephalus as a cause of disturbances of gait in the elderly. Neurology (NY) 32:1358, 1982.

194. Yakovlov PI: Paraplegias of hydrocephalics (clinical note and interpretation). Am J Ment Defic 51:561, 1947.

195. Yakovlev PI: Paraplegia in flexion of cerebral origin. J Neuropathol Exp Neurol 13:267, 1954.

196. Hill A, Volpe J: Decrease in pulsatile flow in the anterior cerebral arteries in infantile hydrocephalus. Pediatrics 69:4, 1982.

197. Mathew NT, Hartmann A, Meyer JS, et al: The importance of "CSF pressure-regulated cerebral blood flow dysregulation" in the pathogenesis of normal pressure hydrocephalus. In Lundberg N, Panton V, Brock M (eds): Intracranial Pressure Two: Proceedings. New York, Springer-Verlag, 1975, p 145.

198. Levin HS, Goldstein FC, Ghostine SY, et al: Hemispheric disconnection syndrome persisting after anterior cerebral artery aneurysm rupture. Neurosurgery 21:831, 1987.

199. Maas O: Ein Fall von linksseitiger Apraxie und Agraphie. Zentralbl Neurol 26:789, 1907.

200. Van Vleuten CF: Linksseitige motorische Apraxie. Z Psychiatr 64:203, 1907.

201. Yamadori A, Osumi Y, Ikeda H, Kanazawa Y: Left unilateral agraphia and tactile anomia: Disturbances after occlusion of the anterior cerebral artery. Arch Neurol 37:88, 1980.

202. Geschwind N, Kaplan E: A human cerebral disconnection syndrome: A preliminary report. Neurology (NY) 12:675, 1962.

203. Hecaen H, Gimeno-Alava A: L'apraxie idéomotrice unilatérale gauche. Rev Neurol 102:648, 1960.

204. Bouman L, Grunbaum AA: Über motorische Momente der Agraphie. Monatsschr Psychiatr Neurol 77:223, 1930.

205. Geschwind N: The apraxias: Neural mechanisms of disorders of learned movement. Am Sci 63:188, 1975.

206. Schott B, Michel F, Michel D, Dumas R: Apraxie idéomotrice unilatérale gauche avec main gauche anomique: Syndrome de déconnection calleuse? Rev Neurol 120:359, 1969.

207. Geschwind N: Disconnection syndromes in animals and man. Brain 88:237, 1965.

208. Trescher JH, Ford FR: Colloid cyst of the third ventricle. Arch Neurol 37:959, 1937.

209. Nielsen JM: Agnosia, Apraxia, Aphasia, 2nd ed. New York, Hoeber, 1946.

210. Pitres A: Considerations sur l'agraphie. Rev Med 4:855, 1884.

211. Luria AR, Tsvetkova LS: Towards the mechanism of "dynamic aphasia." Acta Neurol Belg 67:1045, 1967.

212. Watson RT, Heilman KM: Callosal apraxia. Brain 106:391, 1983.

213. Goldberg G, Mayer NH, Toglia JU: Medial frontal cortex infarction and the alien hand sign. Arch Neurol 38:683, 1981.

214. Feinberg TE, Schindler RJ, Flanagan NG, Haber LD: Two alien hand syndromes. Neurology 42:19, 1992.

215. Gasquoine PG: Alien hand sign. J Clin Exp Neuropsychol 15:653, 1993.

216. Goldenberg G: Neglect in a patient with partial callosal disconnection. Neuropsychologia 24:397, 1986.

217. Trojano L, Crisci C, Lanzillo B, et al: How many alien hand syndromes? Follow-up of a case. Neurology 43:2710, 1993.

218. Tanaka Y, Iwasa H, Yoshida M: Diagonistic dyspraxia: Case report and movement-related potentials. Neurology 40:657, 1990.

219. Chan JL, Liu AB: Anatomical correlates of alien hand syndromes 4. Neuropsychiatry Neuropsychol Behav Neurol 12:149, 1999.

220. Fukui T, Hasegawa Y, Sugita K, Tsukagoshi H: Utilization behavior and concomitant motor neglect by bilateral frontal lobe damage. Eur Neurol 33:325, 1993.

221. Lhermitte F, Pillon B, Serdaru M: Human anatomy and the frontal lobes. Part I: Imitation and utilization behavior: A neuropsychological study of 75 patients. Ann Neurol 19:326, 1986.

222. Nagumo T, Yamadori A: Callosal disconnection syndrome and knowledge of the body: A case of left hand isolation from the body schema with names. J Neurol Neurosurg Psychiatry 59:548, 1995.

223. Gazzaniga MS, Bogen JE, Sperry RW: Some functional effects of sectioning the cerebral commissures in man. Proc Natl Acad Sci U S A 48:1765, 1962.

224. Gazzaniga MS, Bogen JE, Sperry RW: Dyspraxia following division of the cerebral commissures. Arch Neurol 16:606, 1967.

225. Bogen JE, Gazzaniga MS: Cerebral commissurotomy in man: Minor hemisphere dominance for certain visuo-spacial functions. J Neurosurg 23:394, 1965.

226. Gazzaniga MS, Bogen JE, Sperry RW: Observations on visual perception after disconnection of the cerebral hemispheres in man. Brain 88:221, 1965.

227. Gazzaniga MS, Sperry RW: Language after section of the cerebral commissures. Brain 90:131, 1967.

228. Sperry RW, Gazzaniga MS: Language following surgical disconnection of the hemispheres. In Millikan CH (ed): Brain Mechanisms Underlying Speech and Language. New York, Grune & Stratton, 1966.

229. Sperry RW, Gazzaniga MS, Bogen JE: Interhemispheric relationships: The neocortical commissures: Syndromes of hemispheric disconnection. In Vinken PJ, Bruyn GW (eds): Handbook of Clinical Neurology, Vol. 4: Disorders of Speech, Perception, and Symbolic Behaviour. Holland Publishing, Amsterdam, 1969, pp 273–290.

230. Zaidel E: Unilateral auditory language comprehension on the Token Test following cerebral commissurotomy and hemispherectomy. Neuropsychologia 15:1, 1977.

231. Gazzaniga MS, Volpe BT, Smylie CS, et al: Plasticity in speech organization following commissurotomy. Brain 102:805, 1979.

232. Sidtis JJ, Volpe BT, Wilson DH, et al: Variability in right hemisphere language function after callosal section: Evidence for a continuum of generative capacity. J Neurosci 1:323, 1981.

233. Gazzaniga MS, Hillyard SA: Language and speech capacity of the right hemisphere. Neuropsychologia 9:273, 1971.

234. Gazzaniga MS, LeDoux JE, Wilson DH: Language, praxis, and the right hemisphere: Clues to some mechanisms of consciousness. Neurology (NY) 27:1144, 1977.

235. Heilman KM, Bowers D, Watson RT: Pseudoneglect in a patient with partial callosal disconnection. Brain 107:519, 1984.

236. Kashiwagi A, Kashiwagi T, Nishikawa T, et al: Hemi-spacial neglect in a patient with callosal infarction. Brain 113:1005, 1990.

237. Sine RD, Soufi A, Shah M: Callosal syndrome: Implications for understanding the neuropsychology of stroke. Arch Phys Med Rehab 65:606, 1984.

238. Heliman KM, Coyle JM, Gonyea EF, Geschwind N: Apraxia and agraphia in a left-hander. Brain 96:21, 1973.

239. Kimura D: Neuromotor mechanisms in the evolution of human communication. In Steklin HD, Raleigh MJ (eds): Neurobiology of Social Communication in Primates. San Diego, CA, Academic Press, 1979, p 197.

240. Kimura D, Archibald Y: Motor functions of the left hemisphere. Brain 97:337, 1974.

241. Kimura D, Archibald Y: Acquisition of a motor skill after left hemisphere damage. Brain 100:527, 1977.

242. Sabouraud O, Pecker J: Suspension de langage non-aphasique après intervention sur la region interhémisphérique. Rev Otoneuroophtalmol 1:42, 1960.

243. Volpe BT: Observation of motor control in patients with partial and complete callosal section: Implications for current theories of apraxia. In Reeves A (ed): Epilepsy and the Corpus Callosum. New York, Plenum Press, 1983.

244. Volpe BT, Sidtis JJ, Holzman JD, et al: Cortical mechanisms involved in praxis: Observations following partial and complete section of the corpus callosum in man. Neurology (NY) 32:645, 1982.

245. Gordon HW, Bogen JE, Sperry RW: Absence of disconnection syndrome in two patients with partial section of the neocommissures. Brain 94:327, 1971.

246. Maspes PE: Le syndrome expérimental chez l'homme de la section du splenium du corps calleus: Alexie visuelle pure hémianopique. Rev Neurol 80:100, 1948.

247. Jeeves MA, Simpson DA, Geffen G: Functional consequences of the transcollosal removal of intraventricular tumours. J Neurol Neurosurg Psychiatry 42:134, 1979.

248. Gazzaniga MS, Freedman H: Observations on visual processes after posterior callosal section. Neurology (NY) 23:1126, 1973.

249. Iwata M, Sugishita M, Toyokura Y, et al: Étude sur le syndrome de disconnection visuo-lingual après le transéction du splenium du corps calleux. J Neurol Sci 23:421, 1974.

250. Sugishita M, Iwata M, Toyokura Y, et al: Reading ideograms and phonograms in Japanese patients after partial commissurotomy. Neuropsychologia 16:417, 1978.

251. Damasio AR, Chui HC, Corbett J, Kassel N: Posterior callosal section in a non-epileptic patient. J Neurol Neurosurg Psychiatry 43:351, 1980.

252. Sidtis JJ, Volpe BT, Holtzman JD, et al: Cognitive interaction after staged callosal section: Evidence for transfer of semantic activation. Science 212:344, 1981.

253. Tomaiuolo F, Nocentini U, Grammaldo L, Caltagirone C: Interhemispheric transfer time in a patient with a partial lesion of the corpus callosum. Neuroreport 12:1469, 2001.

254. Patricolo A, Chiappetta F, Esposito S, Gazzeri G: Complicanze ipotalamiche nel trattamento chirurgio degli aneurismi della comunicante anteriore. Minerva Neurochir 15:146, 1971.

255. Takeuchi K, Hara M, Yokata M, et al: Factors influencing the development of moyamoya phenomenon. Acta Neurochir 59:79, 1981.

256. Dandy WE: Surgery of the brain. In Lewis D (ed): Practice of Surgery, vol 12. Hagerstown, MD, WF Prior, 1932, p 51.

257. Poppen JL: Ligation of the left anterior cerebral artery: Its hazards and means of avoidance of its complications. Arch Neurol Psychiatry 41:495, 1939.

258. Chavany JA, Messimy R, Pertuiset B, Hagenmuller D: Les fonctions du territoire cortical de l'artère cérébrale antérieure: Parentés séméiologiques des syndromes vasculaires traumatiques et tumoraux. Nouv Presse Med 63:512, 1955.

259. Myers R: Dandy's striatal theory of "the center of consciousness:" Surgical evidence and logical analysis indicating its improbability. Arch Neurol Psychiatry 65:659, 1951.

260. Rubens AB: Aphasia with infarction in the territory of the anterior cerebral artery. Cortex 11:239, 1975.

261. Plum P, Posner J: The Diagnosis of Stupor and Coma, 3rd ed. Philadelphia, FA Davis, 1980.

262. Segarra JM: Cerebral vascular disease and behavior. I: The syndrome of the mesencephalic artery (basilar artery bifurcation). Arch Neurol 22:408, 1970.

Clinical Manifestations

263. Cairns H, Oldfield RC, Pennybacker JB: Akinetic mutism with an epidermoid cyst of III ventricle. Brain 64:273, 1941.

264. Brage D, Morea R, Copello AR: Syndrome nécrotique tegmento-thalamique avec mutisme akinétique. Rev Neurol 104:126, 1961.

265. Castaigne P, Buge A, Cambier J, et al: Démence thalamique d'origine vasculaire par ramollissement bilateral, limité au territoire du pedicule retromammiliare. Rev Neurol 114:89, 1966.

266. Castaigne P, Buge A, Escourelle R, Masson M: Ramollissement pedonculaire median, tegmento-thalamique avec ophthalmoplegie et hypersomnie. (Étude anatomo-clinique.) Rev Neurol 106:357, 1962.

267. Facon E, Steriade M, Werthein N: Hypersomnie prolongée engendrée par des lesions bilaterales du système activateur médial: Le syndrome thrombotique de la bifurcation du tronc basilaire. Rev Neurol 98:117, 1958.

268. French JD: Brain lesions associated with prolonged unconsciousness. Arch Neurol Psychiatry 68:727, 1952.

269. Lechi A, Marchi G: Nécrose méso-diencephalique au cours d'une méningo-encephalite subaiguë: Observation anatomoclinique. Acta Neurol Belg 67:475, 1967.

270. Lhermitte F, Gautier JC, Marteau R, Chain F: Troubles de la conscience et mutisme akinetique: Étude anatomoclinique d'un ramollissement paramedian bilateral du pedoncule cérébral et du thalamus. Rev Neurol 109:115, 1963.

271. Buge A, Escourelle R, Rancurel G: "Mutisme akinétique" et ramollissement bilingulaire: Trois observations anatomo-clinique. Rev Neurol 131:121, 1975.

272. Freeman FR: Akinetic mutism and bilateral anterior cerebral artery occlusion. J Neurol Neurosurg Psychiatry 34:693, 1971.

273. Gugliotta MA, Silvestri R, DeDomenico P, Galatioto S: Spontaneous bilateral anterior cerebral artery occlusion resulting in akinetic mutism: A case report. Acta Neurol (Napoli) 11:252, 1989.

274. Wolff V, Saint Maurice JP, Ducros A, et al: [Akinetic mutism and anterior bicerebral infarction due to abnormal distribution of the anterior cerebral artery]. Rev Neurol (Paris) 158:377, 2002.

275. Fisher CM: Abulia minor versus agitated behavior. Clin Neurosurg 31:9, 1983.

276. Nielsen JM, Jacobs LL: Bilateral lesions of the anterior cingulate gyri. Bull Los Angeles Neurol Soc 16:231, 1951.

277. Barris RW, Schuman HR: Bilateral anterior cingulate gyrus lesions. Syndrome of the anterior cingulate gyri. Neurology (NY) 3:44, 1953

278. Amyes EW, Nielsen JM: Clinicopathologic study of vascular lesions of the anterior cingulate region. Bull Los Angeles Neurol Soc 20:112, 1955.

279. Skultety FM: Clinical and experimental aspects of akinetic mutism: Report of a case. Arch Neurol 19:1, 1968.

280. Meador KJ, Watson RT, Bowers D, Heilman KM: Hypometria with hemispacial and limb motor neglect. Brain 109:293, 1986.

281. Cambier J, Dehen H: Les syndromes de l'artère cérébrale antérieure. Nouv Presse Med 28:1137–1141, 1973.

282. Castaigne P, LaPlane D, Degos JD: Trois cas de negligence motrice par lesion frontal prerolandique. Rev Neurol 126:5, 1972.

283. Paillard J: À propos de la négligence motrice: Issues et perspectives. Rev Neurol 146:600, 1990.

284. Schell G, Hodge CJ, Cacayorin E: Transient neurological deficit after therapeutic embolization of the arteries supplying the medial wall of the hemisphere, including the supplementary motor area. Neurosurgery 18:353, 1986.

285. Dick JPR, Benecke R, Rothwell JC, et al: Simple and complex movements in a patient with infarction of the right supplementary area. Mov Disord 1:255, 1986.

286. Halsband U, Ito N, Tanji J, Freund H-J: The role of premotor cortex and the supplementary motor area in the temporal control of movement in man. Brain 116:243, 1993.

287. Lacruz F, Artieda J, Pastor MA, Obeso JA: The anatomical basis of somatesthetic temporal discrimination in humans. J Neurol Neurosurg Psychiatry 54:1077, 1991.

288. Paus T, Kalina M, Patockova L, et al: Medial vs lateral frontal lobe lesions and differential impairment of central-gaze fixation in man. Brain 114:2051, 1991.

289. Kennard M: The cingulate gyrus in relation to consciousness. J Nerv Ment Dis 121:34, 1955.

290. Whitty CWM, Duffield JE, Tow PM, Cairns H: Anterior cingulectomy in the treatment of mental disease. Lancet 1:475, 1952.

291. Denny-Brown D: The frontal lobes and their function. In Feiling A (ed): Modern Trends in Neurology. New York, Hoeber, 1951, p 13.

292. Fisher CM, Kistler JP, David JM: Relation of cerebral vasospasm to subarachnoid hemorrhage by computerized tomographic scanning. Neurosurgery 6:1, 1980.

293. Mendez MF, Adams NL, Lewandowski KS: Neurobehavioral changes associated with caudate lesions. Neurology (NY) 39:349, 1989.

294. Spencer SS: Corpus callosum section and other disconnection procedures for medically intractable epilepsy. Epilepsia 29(Suppl 2):S85, 1988.

295. Sussman NM, Gur RC, Gur RE, O'Connor MJ: Mutism as a consequence of callosectomy. J Neurosurg 59:514, 1983.

296. Yamaguchi T, Kunimoto M, Pappata S, et al: Effects of anterior corpus callosum section on cortical glucose utilization in baboons: A sequential positron emission tomography study. Brain 113:937, 1990.

297. Gelmers HJ: Non-paralytic motor disturbances and speech disorders: The role of the supplementary motor area. J Neurol Neurosurg Psychiatry 46:1052, 1983.

298. Jonas S: The supplementary motor region and speech emission. J Commun Disord 14:349, 1981.

299. Damasio AR, Van Hoesen GW: Structure and function of the supplementary motor area. Neurology (NY) 30:359, 1980.

300. Kornyey É: Aphasie transcorticale et écholalie: Le problème de l'initiative de la parole. Rev Neurol 131:347, 1975.

301. Masdeu JC, Schoene WC, Funkenstein H: Aphasia following infarction of the left supplementary motor area: A clinical pathological study. Neurology (NY) 28:1220, 1978.

302. Van Stockert TR: Aphasia sine aphasia. Brain Lang 1:277, 1974.

303. Alexander MP, Schmitt MA: The aphasia syndrome of stroke in the left anterior cerebral artery territory. Arch Neurol 37:97, 1980.

304. Lhermitte J, Schiff P: Le phénomène de la préhension forcée, expression d'un ramollissement complet de la première circonvolution frontale. Rev Neurol 35:175, 1928.

305. Atkinson MS: Transcortical motor aphasia associated with left frontal lobe infarction. Trans Am Neurol Assoc 96:136, 1971.

306. Damasio AR, Kassel NF: Transcortical motor aphasia in relation to lesions of the supplementary motor area. Neurology (NY) 28:396, 1978.

307. Kertesz A, Lesk D, McCabe P: Isotope localization of infarcts in aphasia. Arch Neurol 34:590, 1977.

308. Luria AR: Traumatic Aphasia. The Hague, Mouton, 1970.

309. Luria AR: Disturbances of memory and consciousness after rupture of an aneurysm of the anterior communicating artery. In Luria AR (ed): The Neuropsychology of Memory. New York, Wiley, 1976, p 255.

310. Ross ED: Left medial parietal lobe and receptive language functions: Mixed transcortical aphasia after left anterior cerebral artery infarction. Neurology (NY) 30:144, 1980.

311. Carrieri G: Sindrome da sofferenza dell'area supplementaria motoria sinistra nel corso di un meningioma parasaggitale. Riv Patol Nerv Ment 84:29, 1963.

312. Racy A, Jannotta FS, Lehner LH: Aphasia resulting from occlusion of the left anterior cerebral artery: Report of a case with an old infarct in the left rolandic region. Arch Neurol 36:221, 1979.

313. Tatemichi TK, Desmond DW, Prohovnik I: Strategic infarcts in vascular dementia: A clinical and brain imaging experience. Arzneimittelforschung 45:371, 1995.

314. Auchus AP, Chen CP, Sodagar SN, et al: Single stroke dementia: Insights from 12 cases in Singapore. J Neurol Sci 203–204:85, 2002.

315. Brust JCM, Plank C, Burke A, et al: Language disorder in a right-hander after occlusion of the right anterior cerebral artery. Neurology (NY) 32:492, 1982.

316. Hyland HH: Thrombosis of intracranial arteries: Report of three cases involving, respectively, the anterior cerebral, basilar and internal carotid arteries. Arch Neurol Psychiatry 30:342, 1933.

317. Masdeu JC: Language disturbance after mesial frontal infarction. Neurology (NY), suppl. 2, 33:243, 1983.

318. Tsumoto T, Nishioka K, Nakakita K, et al: [Acquired stuttering associated with callosal infarction: A case report.] No Shinkei Geka 27:79, 1999.

319. Iragui VJ: Ataxic hemiparesis associated with transcortical motor aphasia. Eur Neurol 30:162, 1990.

320. Penfield W, Welch K: The supplementary motor area in the cerebral cortex of man. Trans Am Neurol Assoc 74:179, 1949.

321. Penfield W, Welch K: The supplementary motor area of the cerebral cortex: A clinical and experimental study. Arch Neurol Psychiatry 66:289, 1951.

322. Wiesendanger M: Organization of secondary motor areas of cerebral cortex. In Brookhart JM, Mountcastle VB, Brooks VB, Geiger SR (eds): Handbook of Physiology, Section 1: The Nervous System, Volume II: Motor Control, Part 2. Bethesda, MD, American Physiological Society, 1981, p 1121.

323. Bogousslavsky J, Regli F: Infarctus du territoire de l'artère cérébrale antérieure gauche. 1: Correlations clinico-tomodensitometriques. Rev Neurol 143:21, 1987.

324. Munk H: Über die Functionen der Grosshirnrinde: Gesammelte Mitteilungen aus den Jahren 1877-80, mit Einleitung und Anmerkungen. Berlin, Hirschwald, 1881.

325. Brinkman C, Porter R: Supplementary motor area in the monkey: Activity of neurons during performance of a learned motor task. J Neurophysiol 42:681, 1979.

326. Macpherson JM, Marangoz C, Miles TS, Wiesendanger M: Microstimulation of the supplementary motor area (SMA) in the awake monkey. Exp Brain Res 45:410, 1982.

327. Smith AM: The activity of supplementary motor area neurons during a maintained precision grip. Brain Res 172:315, 1979.

328. Tanji J, Kurata K: Neuronal activity in the cortical supplementary motor area related with distal and proximal forelimb movements. Neurosci Lett 12:201, 1979.

329. Tanji J, Kurata K: Comparison of movement-related activity in two cortical motor areas of primates. J Neurophysiol 48:633, 1982.

330. Wise SP, Tanji J: Supplementary and pre-central motor cortex: Contrast in responsiveness to peripheral input in the hindlimb area of the unanesthetized monkey. J Comp Neurol 195:433, 1981.

331. Woolsey CN, Settlage PH, Meyer DR, et al: Patterns of localization in precentral and "supplementary" motor areas. Res Publ Assoc Res Nerv Ment Dis 30:238, 1952.

332. Brinkman C: Lesions in supplementary motor area interfere with a monkey's performance of a bimanual coordination task. Neurosci Lett 27:267, 1981.

333. Penfield W: The cerebral cortex in man. I: The cerebral cortex and consciousness. Arch Neurol Psychiatry 40:417, 1938.

334. Penfield W, Rasmussen T: Vocalization and arrest of speech. Arch Neurol Psychiatry 61:21, 1949.

335. Arseni C, Botez MI: Speech disturbances caused by tumours of the supplementary motor area. Acta Psychiatr Scand 36:279, 1961.

336. Boudouresques J, Bonnal J: Les troubles psychiques des tumeurs frontales. Rev Prat 7:1375, 1957.

337. Castaigne P: Vocalisations itératives et crises palilaliques dans les lésions prérolandiques de la face interne du lobe frontal. Neurologia 9:39, 1964.

338. Erickson TC, Woolsey CN: Observations on the supplementary motor area of man. Trans Am Neurol Assoc 76:50, 1951.

339. Guidetti B: Désordres de la parole associés à des lésions de la surface interhémisphérique frontale postérieure. Rev Neurol 97:121, 1957.

340. Petit-Dutaillis D, Guiot G, Messimy R, Bourdillon C: À propos d'une aphémie par atteinte de la zone motrice supplémentaire de Penfield, au cours de l'évolution d'un aneurisme artérioveineux: Guérison de l'aphémie par l'ablation de la lesion. Rev Neurol 90:95, 1954.

341. Talairach J, Bancaud J: The supplementary motor area in man. Int J Neurol 5:330, 1966.

342. Botez MI, Wertheim N: Expressive aphasia and amusia following right frontal lesions in a righthanded man. Brain 82:186, 1959.

343. Caplan LR, Zervas NT: Speech arrest in a dextral with a right mesial frontal astrocytoma. Arch Neurol 35:252, 1978.

344. Chusid JG, de Gutiérrez-Mahoney CG, Margules-Lavergne MP: Speech disturbances in association with parasagittal frontal lesions. J Neurosurg 11:193, 1954.

345. Cushing H, Eisenhardt L: Meningiomas: Their Classification, Regional Behavior, Life History, and Surgical End Results. Springfield, IL, Charles C Thomas, 1938.

346. Elsberg CA: The parasagittal meningeal fibroblastomas. Bull Neurol Inst N Y 1:389, 1931.

347. Magnan: On simple aphasia, and aphasia with incoherence. Brain 2:112, 1879/1880.

348. Lazorthes G, Anduze-Acher H, Coll J: Empyème sous-dural intérhemisphérique (considérations sur les centres inhibiteurs de la face interne des hémisphères). Rev Otoneuroophtalmol 26:149, 1954.

349. Laplane D, Talairach J, Meininger J, et al: Clinical consequences of corticectomies involving the supplementary motor area in man. J Neurol Sci 34:301, 1977.

350. Penfield W, Roberts L: Speech and Brain Mechanisms. Princeton, NJ, Princeton University Press, 1969.

251. Schwab O: Über vorübergehende aphasische Störungen nach Rindenexzision aus dem linken Stirnhirn bei Epileptikern. Dtsch Z Nervenheilkd 94:177, 1926.

352. Penfield W, Rasmussen T: The Cerebral Cortex of Man: A Clinical Study of Localization of Function. New York, Macmillan, 1950.

353. Watson RT, Fleet S, Gonzolez-Rothi L, Heilman KM: Apraxia and the supplementary motor area. Arch Neurol 43:787, 1986.

354. Jones EG, Coulter JD, Burton H, Porter R: Cells of origin and terminal distribution of corticostriatal fibers arising in the sensory-motor cortex of monkeys. J Comp Neurol 173:53, 1977.

355. Jones EG, Coulter JD, Hendry SHC: Intracortical connectivity of architectonic fields in the somatic sensory, motor, and parietal cortex of monkeys. J Comp Neurol 181:291, 1978.

356. Jones EG, Powell TPS: Connections of the somatic sensory cortex of the rhesus monkey. I: Ipsilateral cortical connections. Brain 92:477, 1969.

357. De Vito JL, Smith OA: Projections from the mesial frontal cortex (supplementary motor area) to the cerebral hemispheres and brain stem of the *Macaca mulatta*. J Comp Neurol 11:261, 1959.

358. Kunzle H: Bilateral projections from precentral motor cortex to the putamen and other parts of the basal ganglia: An autoradiographic study in *Macaca fascicularis*. Brain Res 88:195, 1975.

359. Biber MP, Kneisley LW, LaVail JH: Cortical neurons projecting to the cervical and lumbar enlargements of the spinal cord in young and adult rhesus monkeys. Exp Neurol 59:492, 1978.

360. Murray EA, Coulter JD: Organization of corticospinal neurons in the monkey. J Comp Neurol 195:339, 1981.

361. Ingvar DH, Schwartz MS: Blood flow patterns induced in the dominant hemisphere by speech and reading. Brain 97:273, 1974.

362. Larson B, Skinhoj E, Larsen NA: Variations in regional cortical blood flow in the right and left hemispheres during automatic speech. Brain 101:193, 1978.

363. Lassen NA, Roland PE, Larsen B, et al: Mapping of human cerebral functions: A study of the regional cerebral blood flow pattern during rest, its reproducibility and the activation seen during basic sensory and motor functions. Acta Neurol Scand Suppl 64:262, 1977.

364. Orgogozo JM, Larsen B: Activation of the supplementary motor area during voluntary movement in man suggests it works as a supramotor area. Science 206:847, 1979.

365. Roland PE, Larsen B, Lassen NA, Skinhoj E: Supplementary motor areas in organization of voluntary movements in man. J Neurophysiol 43:118, 1980.

366. Roland PE, Meyer E, Shibasaki T, et al: Regional cerebral blood flow changes in cortex and basal ganglia during voluntary movements in normal human volunteers. J Neurophysiol 48:467, 1982.

367. Woolsey CN: Cortical motor map of *Macaca mulatta* after chronic section of the medullary pyramid. In Zulch KJ, Creutzfeldt O, Galbraith GC (eds): Cerebral Localisation: An Otto Foerster Symposium. Berlin, Springer-Verlag, 1975, p 19.

368. Richter CP, Hines M: Experimental production of the grasp reflex in adult monkeys by lesions of the frontal lobes. Am J Physiol 101:87, 1932.

369. Smith AM, Bourbonnais D, Blanchette G: Interaction between forced grasping and learned precision grip after ablation of the supplementary motor area. Brain Res 222:395, 1981.

370. Travis AM: Neurological deficiencies following supplementary motor area lesions in *Macaca mulatta*. Brain 78:155, 1955.

371. Wiesendanger M, Ruegg DG, Lucier GE: Why transcortical reflexes? Can J Neurol Sci 2:295, 1975.

372. Tanji J, Taniguchi K, Saga T: Supplementary motor area: Neuronal responses to motor instructions. J Neurophysiol 43:60, 1980.

373. Roland PE, Skinhoj E, Lassen NA, Larsen B: Different cortical areas in man in organization of voluntary movements in extrapersonal space. J Neurophysiol 43:137, 1980.

374. Sengupta RP: Direct surgery of anterior communicating aneurysms and its effect on intellect and personality. J Neurol Neurosurg Psychiatry 38:406, 1975.

375. Faris AA: Limbic system infarction. J Neuropathol Exp Neurol 26:174, 1967.

376. Grafman J, Vance SC, Weingartner H, et al: The effects of lateralized frontal lesions on mood regulation. Brain 109:1127, 1986.

Clinical Manifestations

377. Davison C, Goodhart SP, Needles W: Cerebral localization in cerebrovascular disease. Res Publ Assoc Res Nerv Ment Dis 13:435, 1934.

378. Dimitri V, Victoria M: Sindrome de la arteria cerebral anterior. Rev Neurol Buenos Aires 1:81, 1936.

379. Larsson C, Forssell A, Ronnberg J, et al: Subarachnoid blood on CT and memory dysfunction in aneurysmal subarachnoid hemorrhage. Acta Neurol Scand 90:331, 1994.

380. Löhr W: Erkrankungen des Hirngefässe in arteriographischer Darstellung. Arch Klin Chir 186:298, 1936.

381. Löhr W, Jacobi W: Gefässkrankheiten des Gehirns in arteriographischer Darstellung. Arch Klin Chir 177:510, 1933.

382. Reichert T: Die Arteriographie der Hirngefässe. Berlin, JF Lehmann, 1943.

383. Scott M: Ligation of an anterior cerebral artery for aneurysms of the anterior communicating artery complex. J Neurosurg 38:481, 1973.

384. Janowsky JS, Shimamura AP, Kritchevsky M, Squire LR: Cognitive impairment following frontal lobe damage and its relevance to human amnesia. Behav Neurosci 103:548, 1989.

385. Parkin AJ, Leng NRC, Stanhope N, Smith AP: Memory impairment following ruptured aneurysm of the anterior communicating artery. Brain Cogn 7:231, 1988.

386. Stuss DT, Alexander MP, Lieberman A, Levine H: An extraordinary form of confabulation. Neurology (NY) 28:1166, 1978.

387. Vilkki J: Amnestic syndromes after surgery of anterior communicating artery aneurysms. Cortex 21:431, 1985.

388. Talland GA, Sweet WH, Ballantine HT: Amnestic syndrome with anterior communicating artery aneurysm. J Nerv Ment Dis 145:179, 1967.

389. Volpe BT, Hirst W: Amnesia following rupture and repair of an anterior communicating artery aneurysm. J Neurol Neurosurg Psychiatry 46:704, 1983.

390. Youngjohn JR, Altman IM, Van Doren J: Amnesia following anterior communicating aneurysm surgery. J Clin Exp Neuropsychol 11:61, 1989.

391. Damasio AR, Graff-Radford NR, Eslinger PJ, et al: Amnesia following basal forebrain lesions. Arch Neurol 42:263, 1985.

392. Phillips S, Sangalang V, Sterns G: Basal forebrain infarction: A clinicopathologic correlation. Arch Neurol 44:1134, 1987.

393. Wolfe N, Linn R, Babikian VL, et al: Frontal system impairment following multiple lacunar infarcts. Arch Neurol 47:129, 1990.

394. Tatemichi TK, Desmond DW, Patik M, et al: Clinical determinants of dementia related to stroke. Ann Neurol 33:568, 1993.

395. Lucchelli F, DeRenzi E: Primary dyscalculia after a medial frontal lesion of the left hemisphere. J Neurol Neurosurg Psychiatry 56:304, 1993.

396. Starkstein SE, Robinson RG, Berthier ML, et al: Differential mood changes following basal ganglia vs thalamic lesions. Arch Neurol 45:725, 1988.

397. Chusid JG: Correlative Neuroanatomy and Functional Neurology, 16th ed. Los Altos, CA, Lange Medical, 1976.

398. Penfield W, Boldrey E: Somatic motor and sensory representation in cerebral cortex of man as studied by electrical stimulation. Brain 60:384, 1937.

399. Andrew J, Nathan PW: Lesions of the anterior frontal lobes and disturbances of micturition and defecation. Brain 87:233, 1964.

400. Andrew J, Nathan PW: The cerebral control of micturition. Proc R Soc Med 58:553, 1965.

401. Risso M, Poeck K, Creutzfeld O, Pilleri G: Katamnestische Untersuchungen nach frontaler Leukotomie. I: Klinische Beobachtungen. II. Anatomischklinische Korrelationen. Bibl Psychiatr Neurol 116:1, 1962.

402. Lloyd T Jr: Effect of stroke on lung function and the pulmonary circulation. In Price TR, Nelson E (eds): Cerebrovascular Diseases: Proceedings of the Eleventh Research Conference. Philadelphia, Lippincott-Raven, 1979, p 371.

403. Vincent GM: Cardiac electrophysiologic abnormalities in the stroke syndrome. In Price TR, Nelson E (eds): Cerebrovascular Diseases: Proceedings of the Eleventh Research Conference. Philadelphia, Lippincott-Raven, 1979, p 365.

404. Dunsmore RH, Lennox MA: Stimulation and strychninization of supracallosal anterior cingulate gyrus. J Neurophysiol 13:207, 1950.

405. Kaada BR, Pribram K, Epstein JA: Respiratory and vascular responses in monkeys from temporal pole, insular, orbital surface, and cingulate gyrus. J Neurophysiol 12:347, 1949.

406. Segundo JP, Naquet R, Buser P: Cortical stimulation in monkeys. J Neurophysiol 18:236, 1955.

407. Smith WK: The functional significance of the rostral cingular cortex as revealed by its responses to electrical excitation. J Neurophysiol 8:241, 1945.

408. Ward AA: The cingular gyrus: Area 24. J Neurophysiol 11:13, 1948.

409. Tanaka S, Mori T, Ohara H, et al: Gastrointestinal bleeding in cases of ruptured cerebral aneurysms. Acta Neurochir 48:223, 1979.

410. Banker BQ, Larroche JC: Periventricular leukomalacia of infancy: A form of neonatal anoxic encephalopathy. Arch Neurol 7:386, 1962.

411. Lindenberg R: Patterns of CNS vulnerability in acute hypoxemia including anesthesia accidents. In Shade JP, McMenemey WH (eds): Selective Vulnerability of the Brain in Hypoxemia. Philadelphia, FA Davis, 1963, p 189.

412. Volpe JJ: Cerebral blood flow in the newborn infant: Relations to hypoxic-ischemic brain injury and periventricular hemorrhage. J Pediatr 94:170, 1979.

413. De Reuck J, Chatta AS, Richardson EP: Pathogenesis and evolution of periventricular leukomalacia in infancy. Arch Neurol 27:229, 1972.

414. Takashima S, Tanaka K: Development of cerebrovascular architecture and its relationship to periventricular leukomalacia. Arch Neurol 35:11, 1978.

415. Davison AN, Dobbing J: Applied Neurochemistry. Philadelphia, FA Davis, 1968.

416. Young RSK, Hernandez MJ, Yagel SK: Selective reduction of blood flow to white matter during hypotension in newborn dogs: A possible mechanism of periventricular leukomalacia. Ann Neurol 12:445, 1982.

417. Armstrong D, Norman MG: Periventricular leukomalacia in neonates: Complications and sequelae. Arch Dis Child 49:367, 1974.

Chapter Seven

Middle Cerebral Artery Disease

J. P. Mohr, Ronald M. Lazar, Randolph S. Marshall, and Daniel B. Hier

ANATOMY

The middle cerebral artery (MCA), the most commonly affected artery in stroke syndromes, is the largest of the major branches of the internal carotid artery. Its anatomy has been studied in detail over the past century.[1-6] The MCA supplies most of the convex surface of the brain. Only the frontal pole and the superior and extreme posterior rim of the convex surface have other sources of supply. Within the brain, this artery irrigates almost all of the basal ganglia and capsules, including the extreme capsule, claustrum, putamen, the upper parts of the globus pallidus, parts of the substantia innominata of Reichert, the posterior portion of the head and all of the body of the caudate nucleus, and all but the very lowest portions of the anterior and posterior limbs of the internal capsule. The thalamus is supplied almost entirely by the posterior cerebral artery, but infarcts arising in the thalamus may produce slight ischemia in the adjacent internal capsule.[7]

The internal capsule has a complex arterial supply: Its anterior limb has some supply from a large branch of the anterior cerebral artery known as Heubner's artery, although the MCA supplies the anterior limb in one third of cases; most of the posterior limb of the internal capsule and the corona radiata are fed by the deep, lenticulostriate branches of the MCA, whereas the lowest portion of the posterior limb is supplied by the anterior choroidal artery, which usually arises from the internal carotid artery.[8]

Classification

The anatomy of the MCA tree has been classified according to two major criteria, one based on the branching of the artery itself and the other based on the relationship between the vessel and the anatomic landmarks of the cerebral surface.

Stem, Divisions, and Branches

The traditional terminology analogizes the vessel as a tree with a trunk and branches (Fig. 7–1), a clinically useful descriptive method that we use throughout this chapter.

The MCA regularly begins as a single trunk or stem. Its length varies from 18 to 26 mm. The diameter at its origin is roughly 3 mm, varying from 2.5 to 4.9 mm.[9,10] The stem gives rise to most of the lenticulostriate branches, so named because they penetrate the brain to supply the lentiform nucleus (putamen and pallidum), body of the caudate nucleus (together with the putamen known as the striatum), and the internal capsule.[9] (The claustrum and extreme capsule are supplied by vessels from the surface penetrating through the insula.)[11] Typically the lenticulostriate arteries number from 5 to 17 branches, each of them end arteries. A few of the smaller lenticulostriate arteries may arise from the distal internal carotid artery, but the larger penetrating vessels do not.[10]

No clear correlations exist between the length of the MCA stem and the pattern or number of the lenticulostriate arteries, nor does the pattern on one side predict that on the other.[10] The lenticulostriate arteries arising more medially on the MCA stem are the smaller vessels, whereas those arising more laterally are larger. Three patterns of origin of the lenticulostriate arteries from the MCA have been described.[10] In the most common variant (49%), one or more of the larger lenticulostriate branches arise just beyond the major bifurcation. In the next most common permutation (39%), all the larger lenticulostriate arteries arise from the stem just proximal to its bifurcation. In the least commonly encountered pattern, some of the larger penetrators arise from the medial portion of the stem. One important anatomic feature these arteries all share is the lack of anastomoses among themselves and only rare anastomotic links to the cerebral surface vessels (see Chapter 5).

The cerebral surface, claustrum, extreme capsule, the hemispheral cortex, and white matter are supplied by those MCA branches that originate beyond (distal to) the lenticulostriate arteries. These cortical surface branches usually number 12 to 15. They arise from the MCA stem in a variety of patterns, by far the most common one (78%)[9] being two large divisions, the number of branches of which varies considerably. Less often (12%) the 12 branches arise from three major trunks (trifurcation pattern). The least differentiated and least common (10% of cases) is the continuation of the stem with no major divisions, each of the

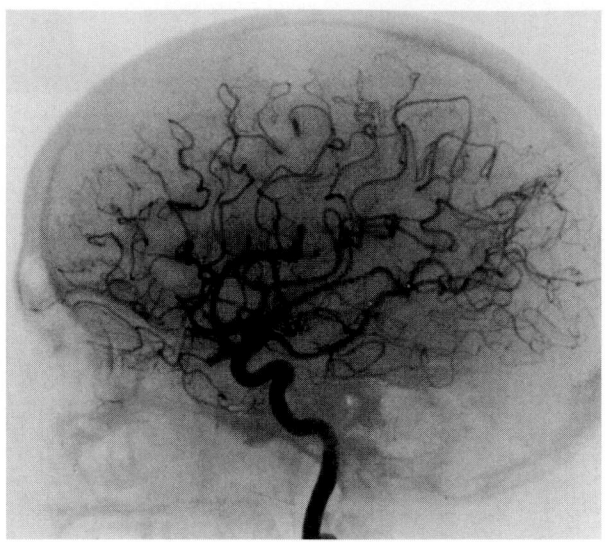

FIGURE 7–1 *Lateral view of the middle cerebral artery anatomy.*

surface branches arising in turn from the common trunk until the primary vessel has given off 11 of the usual 12 branches, after which it terminates as the angular artery.[6]

In the bifurcation patterns, the superior division, supplying the frontal lobe and rolandic regions, always contains the orbitofrontal and prefrontal branches; the inferior division, supplying the temporal, lateral occipital, and, usually, parietal lobes, always contains the temporal polar, anterior temporal, and middle temporal branches. The distribution of the remaining branches in a given division varies widely. The central (rolandic) branch is almost always in the upper division, and the posterior temporal branch is almost always in the lower division. In like manner, the anterior parietal branch is usually in the upper division and the temporo-occipital branch is usually in the lower division. The posterior parietal and angular branches, which arise in the middle of this fanlike array of vessels, have an almost equal chance of being in either division.

In the trifurcation pattern, the orbitofrontal, prefrontal, and precentral branches supplying the frontal lobe are regularly represented in the upper division. The middle division is made up of the central (rolandic), the anterior parietal, and the angular branches. Less often, the precentral branch is a member of this trunk on the frontal side, and in a few other instances, the temporo-occipital and superior temporal branches are added on the inferior side. The inferior division regularly contains the temporal polar, anterior, and middle temporal branches, to which the posterior temporal and temporo-occipital branches are less often added.

Although the frequency with which a given branch occurs in a given division may vary, the branches provide a fairly reliable supply to certain brain regions and do not appear to cross one another. No branch arising from the upper division irrigates brain regions that would be expected to be supplied from a branch of the lower division, or vice versa. That point aside, remarkable variations have been found in the exact position over gyri and sulci of individual branches within their section of the convexity. The

smallest and the shortest branches supply the frontal lobe.[12]

Only 27% of the orbital frontal branches are as large as 1 mm in diameter.[9] The largest artery is usually the artery of the central (rolandic) sulcus. The more posterior regions of the brain are supplied by fewer arteries, which are larger in diameter, give off fewer major branches, and have the longest course from the circle of Willis to their termination in a borderzone (Fig. 7–2). The temporo-occipital artery is 1 mm in diameter in 90% of cases and more than 1.5 mm in up to 63% of cases. This large diameter and the ease with which it can be followed on the surface for long distances led surgeons to prefer to use this branch when the extracranial-intracranial anastomosis operation was in its heyday. The three vessels with the longest course on the cortical surface are the angular, posterior parietal, and temporo-occipital arteries. Intraluminal diameters greater than 1 mm have been encountered in up to 86% of angular arteries, 68% of temporo-occipital arteries, and 52% of posterior parietal arteries but only 14% of central sulcus arteries.[13]

Arterial Segments in Relation to Anatomic Landmarks

Another method of classifying the branches of the MCA is based on the relationship of the artery with the major landmarks on the brain, especially the sylvian fissure, the operculum, and the convex surface. This scheme, which has found its greatest use in angiographic descriptions of the MCA and its branches, divides the MCA into four major segments (Fig. 7–3).[14] The first, or M1, segment occupies the space from the origin of the MCA to the limen insulae. The second, or M2, segment encompasses the portions of the MCA that overlie the insula. The M3 segments are those portions that curve along the surface of the operculum, and the fourth, or M4, segments describe those portions of the branches of the MCA over the convex surface of the brain.

The *M1 or sphenoidal* segment has two components.[9] The first is an undivided MCA stem from which the

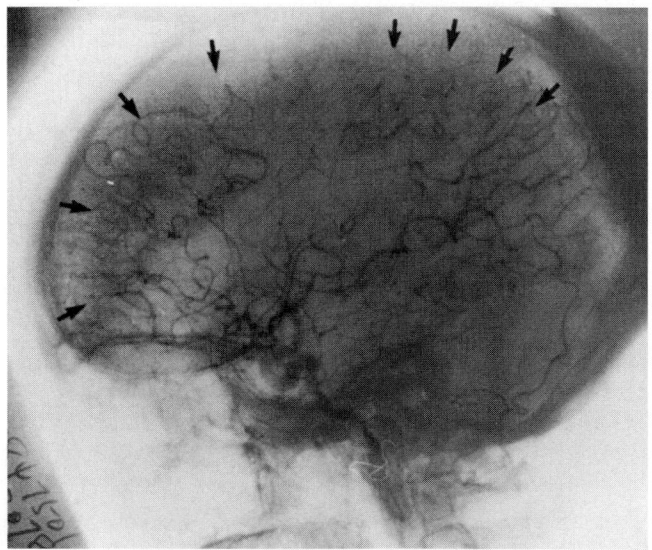

FIGURE 7–2 *Anatomy of the borderzone anastomoses (individual anastomoses shown by* arrows).

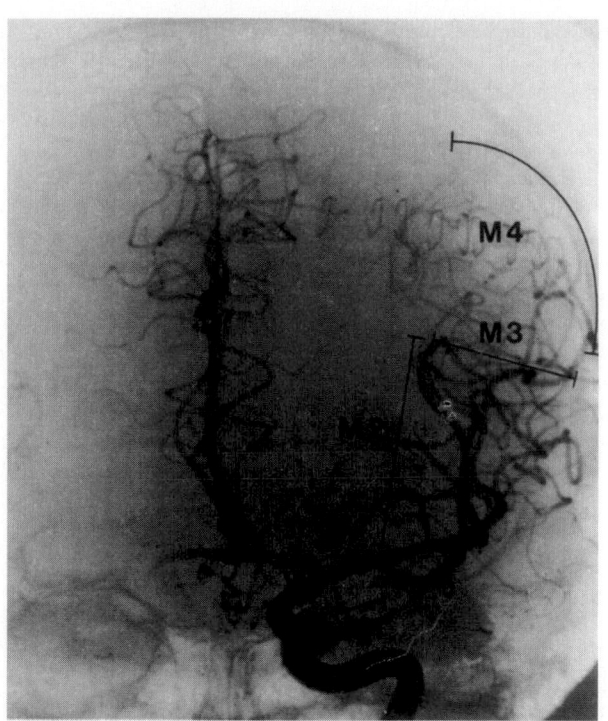

FIGURE 7–3 *Classification of the middle cerebral artery by segments.*

lenticulostriate branches arise; the second is composed of the short segments from the bifurcation of the MCA into its major divisions to their entry into the sylvian fissure. The *M2 or insular* segment gives rise to most of the cerebral surface branches. Most of them develop over the anterior portion of the insula. Branches supplying the frontal and central regions of the convexity ascend sharply upward over the course of the insula, and those supplying the posterior temporal and parietal regions course more or less parallel to the long axis of the insula.

The MCA branches that constitute the *M3 or opercular* segment follow the curve of the operculum back over the surface of the insula. Some of these branches reverse course over as much as 180 degrees,[6] especially those ascending over the frontal and central operculum to gain access to the frontal half of the cerebral convexity. The branches passing over the parietal and temporal operculum make less striking reversals of direction, some turning only a few degrees before reaching the convex surface of the temporal and parietal regions. Finally, the *M4 or cortical* segments are those portions of the branches of the MCA after they emerge from the sylvian fissure beyond the operculum and course along the sulci and gyri of the cerebral convexity. Considerable variation in their path is found from brain to brain. Some of them follow a path mainly along the depths of a given sulcus, whereas others pass long distances over the surface of a gyrus.

Anomalies

The few anomalies of the MCA described appear to occur in no more than 3% of cases.[9,15,16] Some writers even dispute their occurrence.[10] Duplication of the MCA is the more common, usually arising from the internal carotid artery and supplying the same regions that would otherwise have been supplied by the original MCA. An accessory MCA has also been described,[17] arising from the anterior cerebral artery, usually supplying frontal polar areas.

Borderzone Anastomoses

For each cerebral surface branch of the major cerebral arteries, the terminal twigs end in a narrow network of vessels that form the borderzone (see Fig. 7–2) between the major arterial territories.[18–20] Within the borderzone, the anastomoses formed are end-to-end, end-to-side, and side-to-side linkages occurring in remarkable permutations. The actual size of the anastomosis at any given point is usually quite small, on the order of 300 to 400 μm.[21] More often, the available anastomotic vessels are 200 to 400 μm, too small to provide adequate collateral supply to an endangered arterial territory. Only occasionally are the borderzone anastomoses larger than 500 μm. There are wide individual variations in the anastomotic artery-to-artery network. Direct, end-to-end anastomoses as large as 1 mm are rare. Although these tiny vessels scarcely seem of the size that could sustain collateral flow, it has proved remarkable how useful, but unpredictable, a role they play in limiting the size of a given infarct. Anastomoses between contiguous branches of the MCA are either scanty or quite small and play little or no useful role as collateral supply for occlusion of adjacent branches, compared with the value of end-to-end anastomoses via the borderzones.[3,22]

Histology

The MCA contains the same intima, media, and adventitia as other arteries, but the relative thicknesses of these component parts differ from those in peripheral arteries of comparable size.[23] The differences begin even within the intracranial internal carotid artery, which changes the histologic character of the MCA in such a way that the two blend in a smooth continuum. Compared with extracranial vessels of similar size, the MCA has a narrower adventitia with little elastic tissue and few perivascular supporting structures; the media is also thinner, with some 20 circular muscle layers.[24,25] The internal elastic lamina is thicker[26] and finely fenestrated. The intima, although somewhat thin, seems essentially the same as that of comparably sized vessels elsewhere.[25] No evidence of vasa vasorum has been demonstrated to date.[25–27]

The pathologic implications of these differences from extracranial vessels are still unclear. The thinner adventitia of intracranial vessels may be a sign of the lower exposure to stretch and trauma than that in the environment in which the extracranial vessels live.[28] Elastic tissue is concentrated in the internal elastic lamina instead of being scattered through the vessel as in other artery beds, perhaps making intracranial arteries more prone to dampen pulse waves.[26]

PATHOLOGY

Embolism

Although atherosclerosis is a major cause of disease of the extracranial carotid and intracranial basilar arteries, embolism is the more common cause of occlusion for the major cerebral arteries beyond the circle of Willis. It accounts for between 15% and 30% of strokes,[29–31] most of which occur in the territory of the MCA.

Particle Size and Composition

A size of a few millimeters is needed for embolic material to arrest in the stem of the MCA. Rigid materials such as shotgun pellets[32] (first described by Leceve and Lhermitte in 1920), catheter tips, and the like may be this large. Far smaller sources, such as calcific plaques, are too small to block the stem.[33] Calcific plaques that are large enough occur in unusual circumstances, such as direct-puncture carotid arteriography, but may arise from carotid atheroma itself. Rare causes include one case of fibrocartilaginous material.[34]

Most of the embolic material is a fragment of a thrombus. These complexes occur alone or mixed with bacteria.[4] Quite compressible,[35] such embolic fragments may alter their length and width as they pass through the arterial tree. The important issue of how large an embolic particle may arise from angiographically unobvious carotid ulceration or from thrombosis of the aortic arch remains unresolved.[36,37]

Distribution in the Middle Cerebral Artery Territory

The paths followed by embolic particles through the MCA territory are decidedly nonrandom.[31,38] Beyond the stem, flow seems equally directed to the two divisions, but the lower division receives the larger share of the emboli. In the upper division, the four posterior branches are arranged in series, providing an orderly set of opportunities for emboli to lodge.[31,38–40] The orbital frontal branch, acutely angulated from the path of flow, is rarely embolized. The lower division remains a single vessel as it passes over the insula until it reaches the superior temporal plane, where it gives off its three main branches within the space of 1 cm or less. As a result, embolization into the lower division often results in the simultaneous occlusion of more than one, or even all, of the branches of the division.

Persistence of Material

It is common to find autopsy evidence of infarction with no occlusion at the site. From the scant data available, persistence of embolic occlusion seems to be the exception rather than the rule. Some branches originally affected, however, may be found to be occluded well after 48 hours, and the occlusion observed in others has disappeared.[41] Persistence of the occlusion seems to carry a worse functional prognosis.[42] When persistent, the material has proved difficult to differentiate from an in situ thrombus at autopsy.[43]

In studies based on angiographic findings, branch occlusions have been found in the first 24 hours in more than 75% of cases, but for those found after 48 hours, the intracranial branches are often widely patent.[44,45] Although it is inferred that the more friable materials disperse rapidly, no reliable means have been developed thus far to predict which embolic occlusions persist and which disappear. Transcranial Doppler ultrasonographic studies have documented a few instances in which the occlusion has become recanalized within 40 minutes,[46] but with what frequency and how quickly emboli are dissipated past their points of initial lodgment remain unknown.[47]

Effects of Collateral Flow on Embolic Infarct Patterns

Unless adequate collateral flow is present, embolic occlusion of the MCA stem yields a gigantic infarct affecting both the superficial and deep territories of supply. When collateral flow is readily available, the resultant infarct may be remarkably circumscribed, sometimes confined to little more than those branches of the lenticulostriate arteries that were caught by the occluding embolus.[48] Little knowledge is available on what allows collateral flow to be so generous and readily available in some cases and so trivial in others, depending on the variations in the congenitally determined vascular pattern.

Etiology

Since the time of Chiari,[49] it has been appreciated that embolic occlusion may affect the MCA *stem* across the circle of Willis, but particles large enough to lodge in the MCA stem alone are less easily documented. They include such carious sources as "paradoxical" embolus from a leg vein source,[50,51] atrial fibrillation,[52] mitral valve prolapse,[53,54] marantic embolus,[55,56] fragmented thrombus complexes from a nonobstructing internal carotid artery plaque,[57,58] shotgun pellet,[32] metal fragment from a penetrating neck wound,[59] traumatic dissection of the internal carotid artery,[47] internal carotid occlusion of various causes,[45] and automobile accident with angiographically normal ipsilateral internal carotid artery.[31,47]

Embolism to the *surface branches* affecting one or more branches of the MCA may occur from almost any source of embolism.[60,61] Sources include calcific material from the ipsilateral internal carotid (although the patient in Chiari's famous case also had a patent cardiac foramen ovale),[49] spontaneous dissection of the internal carotid artery from fibromuscular hyperplasia,[62] traumatic internal carotid dissection,[63] mucin and emulsified fat from breast metastasis,[64] endocarditis due to candida,[65] mitral valve prolapse,[53] cardiac myxoma,[66] marantic embolus,[55] arterial wall fragments after resuscitation,[67] giant fusiform MCA aneurysm,[68] internal carotid occlusion from various causes, and various sources of transcardiac emboli via a patent cardiac foramen ovale.

Clinical Syndromes of Embolism

A variety of temporal profiles occur in embolism to *branches* of the MCA (Fig. 7–4). In some instances, the deficits are only transient, even with angiographic evidence of persisting occlusion or brain image evidence of focal infarction that confounds traditional clinical definitions of transient ischemic attack (TIA), raising the possibility that the nature of the material may play a role in the severity of the infarct.[69,70] In the days of polymeric silicone (Silastic) pellet therapy for arteriovenous malformations (AVMs), aberrant embolism was a well-recognized risk,[71] usually occurring near the end of the embolization procedure, when conditions initially favoring the entry of the pellets directly into the AVM vessels changed as the fistula became clogged with pellets.[71,72] In our personal series,

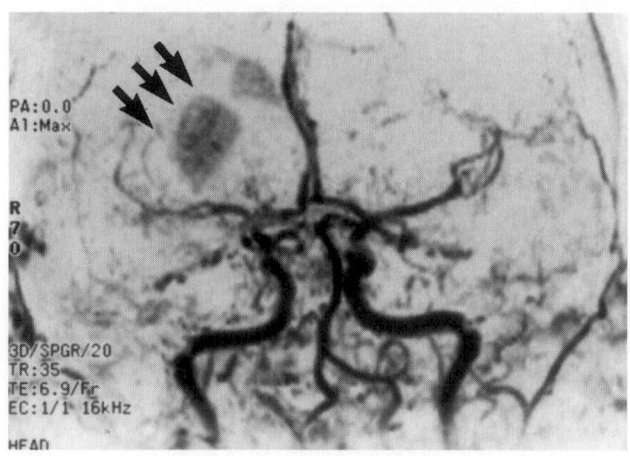

FIGURE 7–4 *Hemorrhagic infarction (arrows) shown in the deep (lenticulostriate) territories of the middle cerebral artery on coronal MR image. (From Gautier, JC, Mohr JP: Ischemic stroke. In Mohr JP, Gautier JC [eds]: Guide to Clinical Neurology. New York, Churchill Livingstone, 1995, p 543.)*

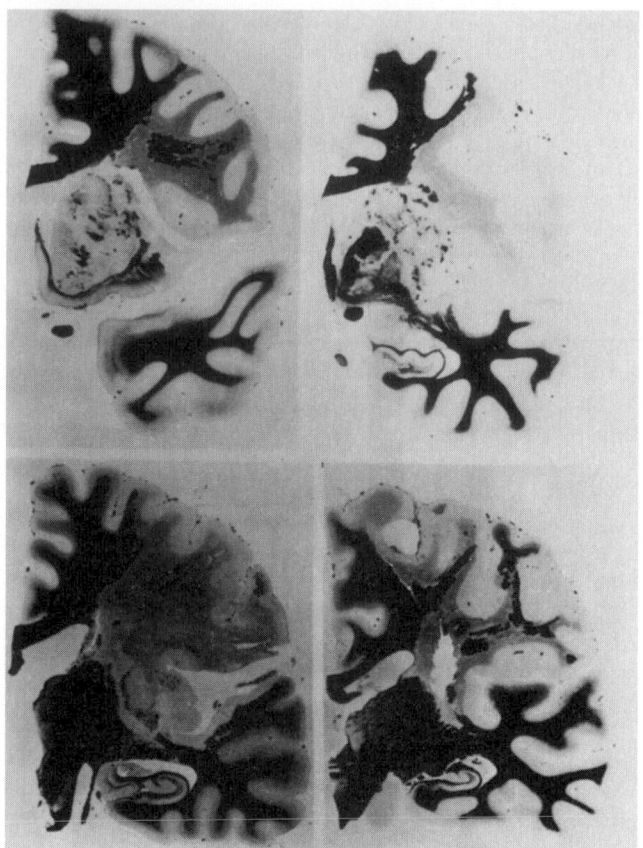

FIGURE 7–5 *Deep and superficial infarction from the same embolic occlusion (myelin stain of celloidin section). (From Friedlich AL, Castleman B, Mohr JP: Case records of the Massachusetts General Hospital. N Engl J Med 278:1109, 1968.)*

one patient in whom two beads traveled into an angular branch of the MCA experienced 15 minutes of contralateral arm numbness—a complaint not entirely predicted by classic clinicopathologic correlation—and also showed immediate distal retrograde collateral flow; the pellet remained in place. Single beads occluded parietal branches of the MCA in two other patients and an ascending frontal branch in a third, none of whom experienced any deficits; in all patients, immediate collateral flow occurred retrogradely into the embolized branch.

Emboli initially occluding the MCA stem and then later migrating to the convexity branches may leave lesions in the deep and superficial territories as *discontinuous multifocal infarction*. The lack of collateral branches to the lenticulostriates makes this territory especially vulnerable to ischemia. The distally placed embolic fragment in a cortical branch is usually considerably smaller than the mass of which it was part that initially blocked the MCA stem. The clinical picture may be predominantly that of the deep infarction affecting the penetrating vessels of the MCA stem. This clinical picture, dubbed "spectacular shrinking deficit" in earlier versions of this book and given the acronym SSS by Minematsu and colleagues,[48] can occur when the embolus occludes the internal carotid artery, causing a profound full hemisphere syndrome, after which it passes up the internal carotid to its final resting place in, for example, the angular branch of the MCA, leaving only a mild aphasia after a few days to a week. Especially characteristic of this type of migratory embolism is a syndrome of fading hemiparesis with persisting Wernicke's aphasia: The embolus presumably lodges initially at the stem of the MCA, occluding the penetrating lenticulostriate branches long enough to produce scattered foci of infarction through the basal ganglia and internal capsule, involvement of the latter producing the hemiparesis. The embolus then migrates distally, usually finally occluding the lower division of the MCA at the superior temporal plane and beyond, yielding Wernicke's aphasia. There are two separate foci of infarction, but they result from the same embolic event (Fig. 7–5).

Syndromes of nonsudden or fluctuating onset may also occur, reported in a small series in 5% to 6% of documented embolic strokes, the syndrome often requiring 36 hours or so to evolve.[31,73] A clinical diagnosis of multiple TIAs is often entertained.

Atherosclerosis

Primary arteriosclerotic occlusive thrombosis is an uncommon cause of symptomatic disease of the MCA[74] even though this diagnosis has been made clinically for years. As long ago as 1951, Fisher[75] noted that "in case after case neuropathologic examination failed to confirm the clinical impression of disease of the middle cerebral artery." Blackwood and associates[76] searched back through the records at the National Hospital and found great difficulty uncovering many convincing examples of thrombosis of the MCA, attesting to its rarity. Likewise, in a clinical and autopsy study of 122 cases of infarction in the territory of the MCA, Lhermitte and coworkers[31] diagnosed atherosclerosis in 8 of 94 cases on clinical and angiographic grounds, but in a companion series studied by autopsy, only 2 (one occlusion, one stenosis) were attributed to atherosclerosis. Resurveying the scene almost 20 years after his initial observation, Fisher[77] diagnosed arteriosclerotic thrombosis in only 7% of 68 cases of MCA occlusion according to clinical, angiographic, or pathologic criteria.

These findings lend support to the diagnosis of embolism for angiographically documented occlusions of the MCA and its branches unless shown to be otherwise at autopsy. Angiographically demonstrated middle cerebral artery stenosis found above a normal internal carotid artery suggests recanalizing embolism. When lysis and disappearance of the initial occlusion occur, a diagnosis of embolism seems acceptable[44,78,79] and is being seen repeatedly in follow-up studies using magnetic resonance angiography (MRA). The hazards of conventional angiography discouraged further studies. In those cases with persisting occlusion, the diagnostic problem remains unsettled, defeating the diagnostic efforts of even the best clinicians.

Thrombotic Occlusion

Autopsy studies indicate that thrombotic occlusion accounts for only 2% of cases of ischemic events in the MCA territory.[31] Although the distinction between thrombus and embolus on clinical grounds is difficult, the syndrome of occlusion, irrespective of cause, is worthy of mention in its own right. Asymptomatic occlusion of the MCA stem must be rare, if it occurs at all.[80,81]

Stenosis

Stenosis, although a familiar problem in the extracranial carotid artery, is uncommon anywhere in the MCA and, when found, is almost always in the stem (Fig. 7–6). Thus far, no reliable means have been developed to determine what the lesion represents when seen the first time. Atheroma not fully developed, a recent embolus undergoing recanalization, the stenosis of moyamoya disease, dissection, postradiation effects, and other causes, including infection, are all possibilities. Case series are uncommon, but the clinical course has been surprisingly mild. Five of the nine cases reported by Lascelles and Burrows[81] made an almost complete recovery. Kawase and associates[82] described only examples of TIA. Hinton and colleagues[78] reported on 17 patients, only 3 of whom were left with focal neurologic deficits, although all were treated with warfarin (Coumadin). Minor deficit characterized 8 of the 13 cases described by Feldmeyer and coworkers.[83] A progressive course was described in 5, in which deficit evolved over 12 hours. The gradual mode of onset even led to a clinical diagnosis of tumor in three instances. Day[84] mentioned TIAs alone or with mild stroke in 12 of 18 cases of stenosis. The experience reported by Corston and associates[85] was less fortunate: 14 of their 21 patients presented with stroke, yet even in this series, only 3 had a severe disability, and 7 patients presented with TIA alone.

Clinical syndromes of stenosis remain poorly described. Judging from the handful of studies available, stenosis can cause lenticulostriate or hemispheral syndromes by at least three mechanisms. Local lacunar-type syndromes affecting the lenticulostriate branches may occur if they become trapped in the atheroma, affecting the MCA itself. Ischemic events in the hemisphere distal to the stenosis may occur because of hemodynamic insufficiency[78] or because of embolism.[86] Kawase and associates[82] found four examples of capsular low density on computed tomography (CT) ipsilateral to angiographically documented

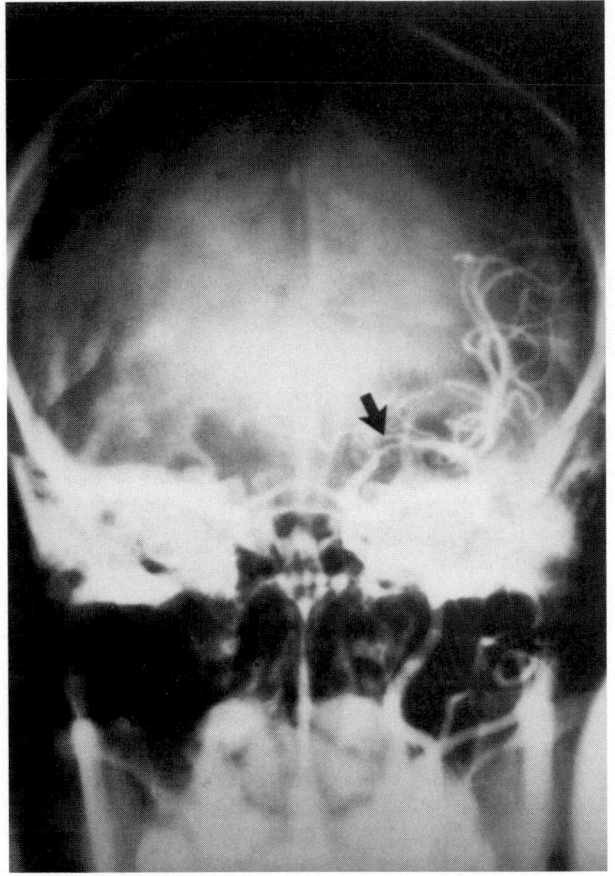

FIGURE 7–6 *Angiogram showing middle cerebral artery stem stenosis* (arrow).

stenosis of the M1 segment of the MCA in 52 Japanese patients with TIAs affecting the carotid territory.[5] They attributed the clinical syndrome and CT abnormality to the MCA stem stenosis. However, in one of the four cases, the stenosis was so far distal in the stem that it was beyond the usual point of departure of even the lateral lenticulostriate branches; in two others, the stenosis lay at the origin of the stem, and in the last, it lay in its midportion. Several of the patients (cases 2, 3, and 4) reported by Hinton and colleagues[78] had similar syndromes, limited to pure motor weakness. In each instance, however, considerable shift of the borderzone was seen on angiography, with anterior cerebral branches supplying collateral flow for the MCA. The pure motor character of the attacks and the obvious borderzone shift posed a problem in interpretation of the mechanism involved. Corston and associates[85] may have had similar experiences because they described three of their patients as having severe hemiplegia, but they did not give details of the remainder of the clinical syndrome in these patients. A shift of the borderzone was encountered in some of these cases. Other examples of lacunar syndromes in a setting of MCA stem stenosis may be found scattered through the literature.[87]

Hemispheral hemodynamic insufficiency was suggested by the clinical syndromes of 13 of the 16 cases reported by Hinton and colleagues.[78] The TIAs or minor permanent deficits were accompanied by mutism, dysarthria, or numbness. In each case, an obvious shift had occurred in the borderzone, with striking collateral flow into the MCA territory. Even given the occurrence of ischemic stroke, the syndromes were quite mild. Less encouraging results were reported by Corston and associates,[85] who described nine patients with some disturbance in higher cerebral function, one with no accompanying hemiparesis. In only one patient was shift of the borderzone described. These cases leave no doubt that some patients are left with a severe disability.

Dissection

Autopsy diagnosis of MCA dissection has been rare. A wide variety of settings are recognized—trauma,[88] strenuous physical exertion,[89] surgery,[90] fibromuscular hyperplasia,[91] atherosclerosis,[87] mucoid degeneration of the media,[88] moyamoya disease,[92] split or frayed internal elastic lamina,[93] congenital defect of the media,[94] syphilis,[95] and even migraine.[96] The disorder has been most often reported in younger patients, many of them children. The usual site is a short section of the stem, although adjacent branches may also be affected.[97]

When a precipitating factor, such as trauma, has been documented, symptoms have developed immediately or have been delayed for minutes,[97] hours,[94] or up to 4 days.[98] Once set in motion, events proceed rapidly, but in a few cases the clinical syndrome has evolved over a day or more. Because the dissections occur most often in the stem of the MCA, severe clinical deficits usually occur.

Other Diseases

The MCA, like other vessels, may fall victim to arteritis, fibromuscular hyperplasia, altered coagulation states, delayed effects of radiation, and the like. Reports in the literature remain too scant to enable determination of whether unique syndromes occur, and the reader is referred to the chapters in this book that deal with these topics individually.

CLINICAL SYNDROMES OF MIDDLE CEREBRAL ARTERY TERRITORY INFARCTION

Little has been added to the description of the major syndromes of MCA disease offered by Foix and Levy[4] and cited repeatedly in textbooks.[99] Such accounts are biased by the assumption that occlusion of a trunk, division, or branch will affect its entire territory. The effects of an arterial occlusion may be greatly mitigated by the collateral flow via borderzone vessels shared with the anterior or posterior cerebral arteries. Effective formation of collateral flow may rescue the endangered territory, resulting in the striking diminution of symptoms and signs and reducing the value of much of the clinical literature based on angiographic documentation alone.[100,101] More modern work, relying on CT, positron emission transverse tomography, and magnetic resonance imaging (MRI), has greatly expanded the scope of syndromes, both acute and chronic, that are occasioned by a given arterial occlusion.

Standard Syndromes

The textbook accounts, briefly reviewed here, assume total infarction in the territory at risk.[307,312,349] Uncollateralized occlusion of the *main trunk* of the MCA artery causes softening of the basal ganglia and internal capsule within the substance of the hemisphere as well as a large portion of the cerebral surface and subcortical white matter. The large infarct produces contralateral hemiplegia, deviation of the head and eyes toward the side of the infarct, hemianesthesia, and hemianopia. Major disturbances also occur in behavior: Global aphasia occurs when the hemisphere dominant for speech and language is involved, whereas impaired awareness of the stroke is expected when the nondominant hemisphere is affected. When the infarct is large, the hemianopia may be due to involvement of the visual radiations deep in the brain. More often, the hemianopia is part of a syndrome of hemineglect for the opposite side of the space and is accompanied by failure to turn toward the side of the hemiplegia in response to sounds from that side, a problem separate from the head and eye deviation toward the side of the infarct.

A variant of the syndrome of MCA stem occlusion, colorfully named "malignant infarction" by Hacke and associates,[102] applies in those patients experiencing subsequent herniation. Only 12 of the 55 patients studied survived. The mean Scandinavian Stroke Scale score on admission was 20. The time to severe decline was brief, between 2 and 5 days. The rapid development of a space-occupying mass effect as shown on brain imaging was a particularly predictive sign of poor outcome. Fully 43 patients suffered herniation as the terminating event. Advances in treatment have been reviewed by this group.[103] Some patients survive (see Fig. 7–7).

When the occlusion is restricted to the *upper division*, the initial deficit mimics that from occlusion of the main trunk: contralateral hemiparesis and hemisensory syndromes are the rule, accompanied by hemineglect for the other side of the space, aphasia when the dominant hemisphere is involved, or impaired awareness of the deficit when the other hemisphere is affected. However, the hemiparesis usually affects the face and arm more heavily than the leg, a picture opposite that in anterior cerebral artery disease. Because the occlusions usually affect the anterior branches of the upper division, the aphasia from dominant hemisphere infarction is usually of the motor (Broca's) type, whereas the disturbance in behavior from nondominant hemisphere infarction may be mild.

In the *lower division* syndromes, infarction typically spares the rolandic region, hemiparesis does not usually occur, head and eye deviations are rarely encountered, and even disorders of sensation are infrequent. When the infarct affects the dominant hemisphere, pure aphasia (Wernicke's type) is the rule, whereas in nondominant hemisphere infarction, the behavior disturbances may appear in relative isolation. Hemianopia may be a prominent sign.

When the involvement is limited to the territory of a small *penetrating artery* branch of the main stem, a small, deep infarct (lacune) occurs, affecting part or all of the internal capsule and producing a syndrome of pure hemiparesis unaccompanied by sensory, visual, language, or behavior disturbances.

CLINICAL SYNDROMES FROM INFARCTION OF EITHER HEMISPHERE

Loss of Consciousness

Transient loss of consciousness is uncommon in all forms of ischemic stroke and is rare in MCA territory infarction. It occurs at onset in only 8.4% of carotid ischemic strokes[104] and in 5.7% of vertebrobasilar territory strokes. Diaschisis[105] might be considered a possible explanation if one assumes it to be secondary to sudden embolization of the stem of the carotid artery with temporary global ischemia. Delayed loss of consciousness is more common, often occurring 36 hours to 4 days after hemispheral infarcts ranging in size from the entire MCA territory to only the frontotemporal region.[106] The decline in consciousness is usually part of a larger clinical picture of impending cerebral herniation and not due to an injury to a specific brain region in the MCA territory controlling consciousness (Fig. 7–7).

Hemiplegia and Hemiparesis

The terms *hemiplegia* and *hemiparesis* have been used rather loosely in many case reports, making difficult a clear correlation between the severity of weakness and a given site of infarction. Weakness of some degree and type has been encountered most often with infarcts of the branches of the upper division, but it is not regularly reported for infarcts affecting the territory of the lower division.

With more than 150 years of reports, the number of cases that correlate the hemiparesis formula and imaging or autopsy findings remains disappointingly small, and some of them, despite an autopsy study, are lacking credibility.[107] Henschen's[108] massive review of the published autopsy literature on higher cerebral function before 1920 was typical of most writers: The occurrence of hemiparesis on a case-by-case basis was mentioned only in passing, and details of the syndrome were rarely given. This literature is frustrating because many surprising instances can be found of apparent amelioration of motor deficit after infarction affecting the MCA territory on either side.

MCA stem occlusions affecting either side of the brain appear to produce the same basic motor deficit and can be described under the same heading. Such were the findings in the 488 cases of MCA territory infarction published in the pilot phase of the National Institute of Neurological and Communicative Disorders and Stroke (NINCDS) Stroke Data Bank project.[109] However, De Renzi and colleagues[110] found that the frequency of conjugate eye deviation from right hemisphere stroke greatly exceeded that from left, a finding not subsequently pursued.

Hemiplegia

The most reliable occurrence of hemiplegia follows complete occlusion of the MCA at its stem (Figs. 7–8 and 7–9). The effect of the occlusion may produce infarction involving both the deep and superficial territories of the MCA, the deep only, or the superficial only. The syndrome of hemiplegia varies enough to warrant separate descriptions.

Hemiplegia from combined deep and superficial infarction was described in detail by Foix and Levy.[4] The typical picture consists of dense contralateral hemiplegia, hemianesthesia, homonymous hemianopia, and conjugate gaze deviation to the contralateral side. The severity of the syndrome is more severe when the stem is affected.[4,81,111,112] Among the patients who die within days, contralateral hemiplegia is usually accompanied by hemianesthesia and hemianopia, which is the rule.[113]

Cases of MCA territory infarction with brain swelling massive enough to promote hemicraniectomy serve to indicate the expected course of hemiplegia in the most extensive strokes.[114] Deterioration with massive brain edema may occur in these cases as early as 36 hours, but often it is more evident by the fourth day. After reversal of the incipient herniation, the persistent neurologic deficit is usually severe hemiplegia with little clinical improvement. The syndrome among survivors without hemicraniectomy seems similar.[79] The deficit after hemispherectomy in cases of chronic infarction contains some features unusual for acute hemispheric infarct: In 1964, Obrador[115] reported on the results of hemispherectomy performed in 10 patients ranging in age from 3 to 29 years. He noted in particular that three patients showed only slight facial paresis. Another seven had only moderate lower facial paresis, and four were able to move facial muscles on each side easily. The distal functions of the limbs were very much impaired. Complete paralysis of hand and finger movements was seen in six, and the foot was completely paralyzed in nine. By contrast, the upper limbs moved well at the shoulder and elbow in seven patients, and motility of the muscles of the hip and knee was fairly well preserved, enough for walking, in all cases. Later reports have shifted the emphasis to scores from outcome scales, with limited information on the details of the hemiparesis, whether acute or chronic.[116]

Hemiplegia from deep infarction alone features several different syndromes. Foix and Levy[4] described two types: In the first, massive hemiplegia occurred, and the appearance was the same as that observed when the infarct involved both the superficial and deep territories. Initial hemiplegia gave way to marked contracture. These investigators observed no instances of involuntary movements, choreoathetosis, parkinsonism, or disturbances in balance. The second type involved a more marked hemiplegia in the leg than in the arm, rendering the patient unable to walk. Contracture in this syndrome was more common in the leg and was often associated with a permanently flaccid hemiplegia. The prognosis for recovery was poor in the second type, but the outlook for life appeared to be good in both types. Subsequent researchers have expanded these initial syndromes with autopsy studies.[117–119] CT findings also support evidence for a syndrome of hemiplegia from deep infarction described as "giant lacunes"[120] that featured a profound hemiplegia in some and incomplete in others. In a few, the course of the hemiparesis was surprisingly mild, with striking improvement despite persistence of the deep infarct.[121,122]

Other reports describing the syndromes of striatocapsular infarction have emphasized the difficulty of separating the syndrome of large, deep infarction from superficial cortical infarction on clinical grounds alone and have cited numerous instances of dysphasia, dyspraxia, and hemineglect among the prominent clinical features.[62,69] Stenosis of the MCA is a common explanation, at least in Korean subjects.[123]

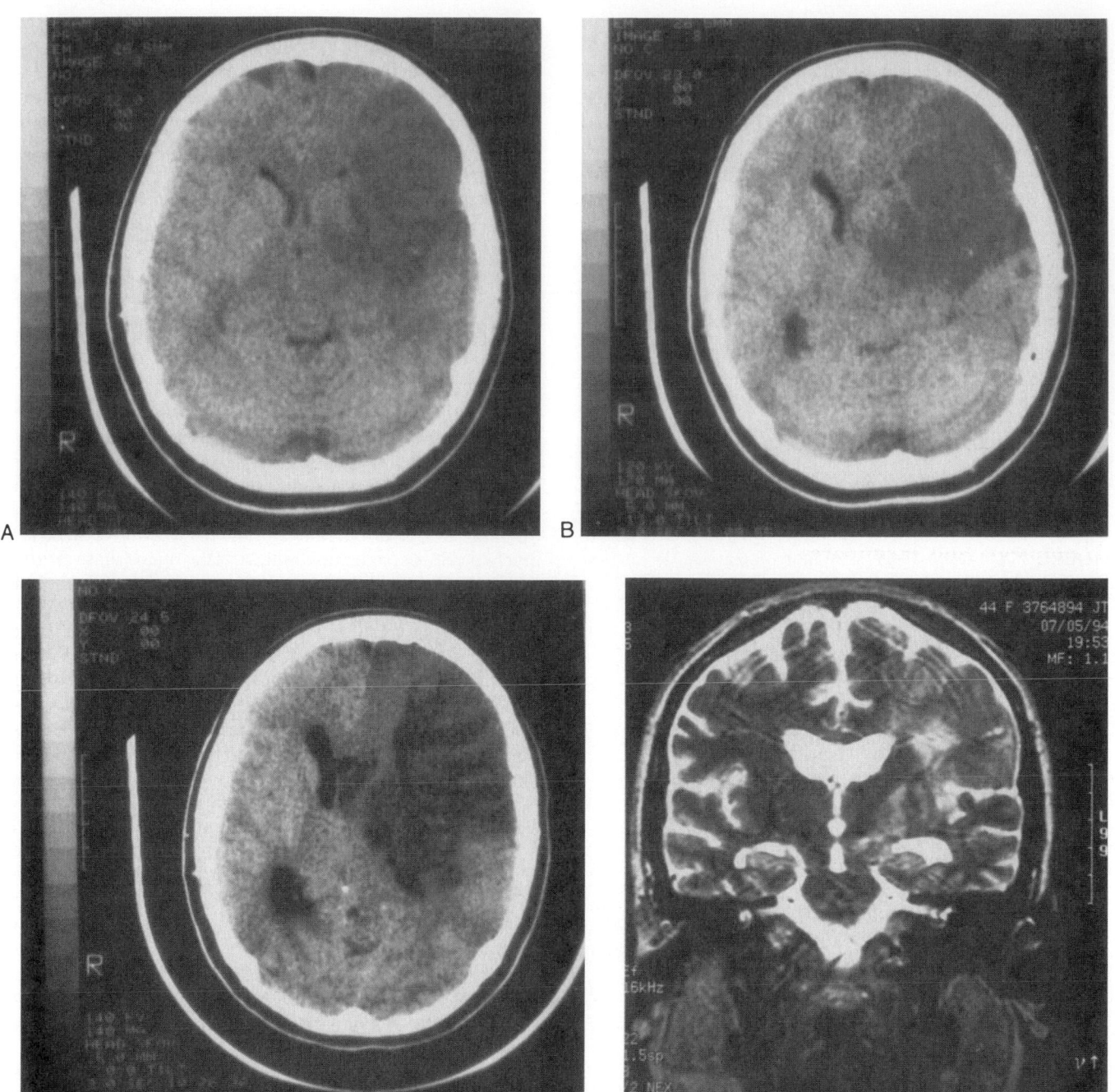

FIGURE 7–7 *Four stages of midbrain compression. A, Viewed from an axial CT scan, the large middle cerebral artery (MCA) terri-tory infarction has just begun to produce slight displacement a few hours after the acute stroke. B, By the second day, edema and "mass effect" have displaced the midbrain and thalamic structures slightly across the midline. C, By the fourth day, at the height of com-pression, the midline structures have been rotated and displaced considerably, during which time the patient appeared in a state of uncal herniation. D, A week later, a coronal T2-weighted MR image shows the midline structures back at their normal positions, and no lasting damage is evident from the displacement. (From Gautier JC, Mohr JP: Ischemic stroke. In Mohr JP, Gautier JC [eds]: Guide to Clinical Neurology. New York, Churchill Livingstone, 1995, p 543.)*

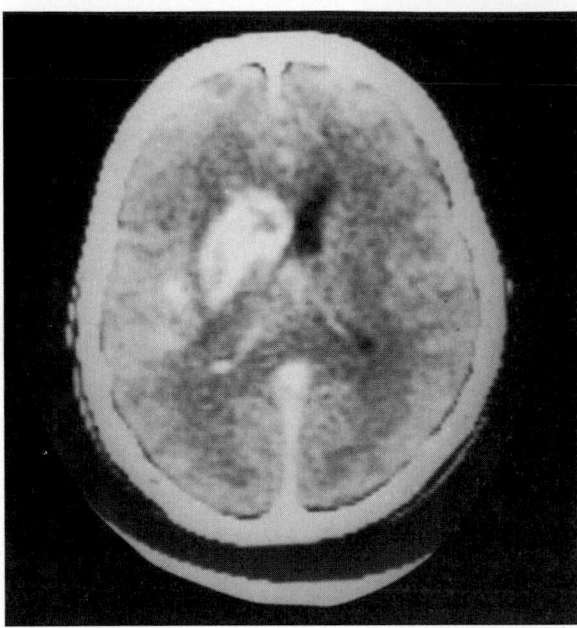

FIGURE 7–8 *Large deep infarction of the middle cerebral artery lenticulostriate territories shown by CT scan.*

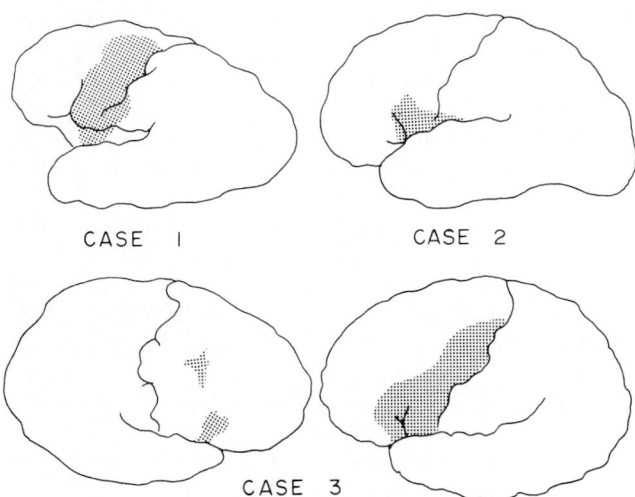

CASE 1   CASE 2

CASE 3

FIGURE 7–9 *Three examples of embolic infarction of Broca's area and surrounding cerebrum. (From Mohr JP: Broca's area and Broca's aphasia. In Whitaker H [ed]: Studies in Neurolinguistics. New York, Academic Press, 1976, p 201.)*

Hemiplegia from surface infarction is the third type. Infarction of the entire surface territory of the MCA produces a syndrome essentially identical to that found when the deep territory is also affected. A few instances of surface infarcts confined to the cortical surface of the insula and operculum have been described,[124] the syndrome involving hemiplegia with faciobrachial predominance that soon faded to a facioplegia with mild, predominantly distal paresis of the arm.

Individual branch occlusions seem only uncommonly to produce hemiplegia.[4] In most cases, either hemiparesis occurs or the syndrome of paralysis is incomplete and is confined to one or more body parts. The most reliable deficit is encountered among patients suffering occlusion of the ascending frontal branch.[65] However, Barnett and colleagues[53] described a patient with sylvian branch occlusion and contralateral hemiplegia who recovered substantially in 1 week. Two years later, only minimal right-sided weakness was found on examination. A second patient had total hemiplegia with aphasia, which remitted within 1 week. Subsequently-described cases are mixed into larger series and have proved difficult to isolate from the group case reports.[125]

Syndromes of Partial Hemiparesis

The most commonly encountered pattern of hemiparesis seems to be one with equivalent weakness of the hand, shoulder, foot, and hip. This type occurred in 71.2% of the 488 unilateral hemisphere strokes studied during the pilot phase of the NINCDS Stroke Data Bank project.[109] A few other types of hemiparesis are also well known. Among them are the classic syndromes of distal predominance to the hemiparesis (often attributed to Broadbent,[126] although we have found no source among his writings), a faciobrachial paresis, and monoplegia. The main phase of the NINCDS Stroke Data Bank study provided data for 183 of 1276 patients with convexity infarction in the MCA territory, still the largest cohort reported to date. Infarct size did not differ according to side, but the location of the main site of the infarct did: On the left side, the infarct was centered in the inferior parietal region, but on the right, it was midfrontal. There was a good correlation between infarct size and level of weakness as estimated by overall motor function on one side, the arm, or the hand alone. There was a poor correlation, however, for lesion location (lower third, middle third, or upper third on either side of the rolandic fissure) and any of the specific syndromes of focal weakness, no two cases sharing the same lesion for the same syndrome and several cases sharing the same lesion with a different syndrome. The findings indicated a difference in weakness syndromes between the two hemispheres and great individual variation of the acute syndrome caused by a given site of focal infarction along the rolandic convexity. These findings provide a framework for the smaller case studies of incomplete hemiparesis discussed later.[109]

Hemiparesis with distal predominance affects the lower face, fingers and forearm, and toes and lower leg, with relative sparing of the forehead, shoulder and upper arm, hip and thigh, neck, and trunk. This lower facial and distal predominance of hemiparesis has been taken to represent the density of the homuncular representation over the hemispheral surface.[127,129] Although widely accepted as typical of MCA territory infarction, it was encountered in the Stroke Data Bank series in only 23.5% of the 488 patients with unilateral weakness affecting the cerebrum.[109] Furthermore, this predominance pattern occurred with approximately the same frequency whether the infarct was confined to a single lobe or was as large as several lobes and whether the area involved was frontal, parietal, temporal, or opercular. As expected, hemiparesis of any kind did not occur in infarcts of the occipital region.

The syndrome of faciobrachial paresis also has a widely varying frequency, depending on the study. In an angiographic study of MCA occlusion conducted in the days before CT and with no autopsy data, Lascelles and Burrows[81] found that the lower face was affected in 51 of 59 MCA infarcts; among the patients who could be assessed, the deficit was greater in the upper than in the lower limb.[81] In patients with involvement of the insula and operculum, the weakness of the face and oropharynx may be profound; in addition to the expected lower facial plegia, the upper face may fail to wrinkle for some days or weeks.[124,128] Obvious weaknesses are present in the muscles of the jaw. Movements of the tongue and oropharynx show impairment of swallowing and occasionally of vocalization. These lower face and oral pharyngeal disturbances may persist long after the forehead movement has been restored. The initial appearance is sometimes similar to that of Bell's palsy, but the upper deviation of the eyes characteristic of peripheral facial palsy (Bell's phenomenon) is typically not present even in the earliest stages. The involvement of the upper extremity is usually more obvious in the impaired movement of the fingers and hand. A faciobrachial predominance to the hemiparesis may occur in cases of small surface infarcts of the anterior rolandic and opercular areas.[129]

In this series,[129] one patient had severe right central facial weakness with only moderate right hemiparesis (see Fig. 7–9, Case 1). Within a week, although the face and hand remained plegic, the arm strength improved to the point that the patient could lift the arm off the bed, the leg had full power, and the eyes moved freely. Within 1 month, the face and hand remained unchanged, but the arm moved freely and the patient walked easily. At 5 months, the face and fingers remained unchanged, but the wrist was now capable of making moderate movements, and the leg remained essentially free of trouble. Another patient, with more extensive spread of the infarct up the rolandic cortex, had a severe right facial and distal arm paralysis (including the hand) that persisted unchanged for 90 days before death (see Fig. 7–9, Case 2). A patient whose focal inferior frontal infarct was documented by angiography and CT was struck mute while talking but did not lose balance. Examination within an hour revealed dense right lower facial plegia during attempts to talk, grimace, or smile; preserved wrinkling of the forehead; deviation of the tongue to the right; slight weakness of the grip; and barely detectable weakness of the shoulder but full movement of the trunk and leg. The right plantar response was extensor. Within 3 weeks, the tongue moved freely and the face showed only slight weakness, but the weakness of the hand persisted. By 3 months, the facial asymmetry was barely detectable under any conditions, and the grip was improved but still noticeably weak.

Another, similar case (JPM) demonstrates that the deficit may follow a similar course when the infarct affects the right hemisphere. Over a 2-hour period, in stuttering fashion, a 54-year-old man developed dysarthria and left facial plegia, with mild weakness of grip, but retained full movement of the shoulder, trunk, and leg. Angiography revealed occlusion of the MCA at the origin of the upper division, with collateral flow retrograde from the anterior cerebral territory to the point of the occlusion. CT findings were normal. The focal deficit persisted for more than a week unchanged and then faded steadily within weeks to a barely detectable lower facial weakness upon forced grimace.

Faciobrachial paresis may even occur as an isolated sign. One of the authors' (JPM) patients had a mild faciobrachial paresis of sudden onset unaccompanied by other findings, which was correlated with a contrast enhancement on CT scan and branch occlusion on angiogram. Even the possibility of facial weakness as an isolated sign has been mentioned in the literature.[130]

Monoplegia

Monoplegia as a circumscribed disturbance is described in standard texts on the subject but is not easily found in the literature. Von Monakow[105] made reference to the possibility of an isolated brachial plegia arising from a lesion confined to the middle of the second frontal gyrus, provided that the lesion is acute and does not extend too deeply into the white matter ("wenn sie akut einsetzt und nicht zu tief in das subcorticale Mark übergrieft"). Dejerine and Regnard[131] found a case with weakness limited to the muscles of the thenar, hypothenar, and interosseous muscles; they did not mention confirmation of the presumed vascular nature of the lesion. Garcin[132] described a monoparesis with weakness predominating in the flexor movements, mimicking a median nerve palsy; the locus of the lesion was inferred in the absence of autopsy data. The only case of focal upper rolandic infarction known by the authors with autopsy documentation (Fig. 7–10) was an elderly woman, whose examination within hours of onset revealed normal power in the upper extremity including the hands and fingers, sparing the limb entirely. The only clinical signs were slight right facial weakness with initial mutism. She was monitored for months, during which time the initial deficit improved, but no disturbance of limb power occurred at any time.

Isolated brachial monoplegia has often been described as a clinical sign in carotid territory TIAs. It has also been encountered as a transient syndrome in aberrant emboli during pellet embolization in the treatment of AVMs, regardless of the MCA branch being embolized. These findings are of great interest but must be interpreted with caution, because the setting (an angiogram suite with the patient under a drape) does not lend itself to detailed evaluation of the leg and axial structures during the frantic period when the physicians are striving to reverse the acute deficit.

Schneider and Gautier,[133] in an extensive review of 1575 patients with acute stroke and predominance of leg weakness, found that only 63 had predominance of leg weakness. Although 41 patients had hemispheric convexity lesions, the MCA territory was affected in only 1.

Data from the pilot phase of the NINCDS Stroke Data Bank project contained a mere 31 cases of monoplegia involving the arm among the 488 patients with cerebral stroke,[109] yet even this small number showed a significant correlation with infarct of a single lobe rather than multiple lobes (P < .002). Although monoplegia seems to be uncommon, it has some value as a sign of circumscribed infarction. Monoplegia was encountered in infarcts involving the frontal, temporal, or parietal lobes.

Infarcts Without Hemiparesis

Infarction confined to the *lower division* of the MCA is not expected to produce hemiparesis in any form, since the site of the infarct lies so far posterior to the rolandic sulcus.

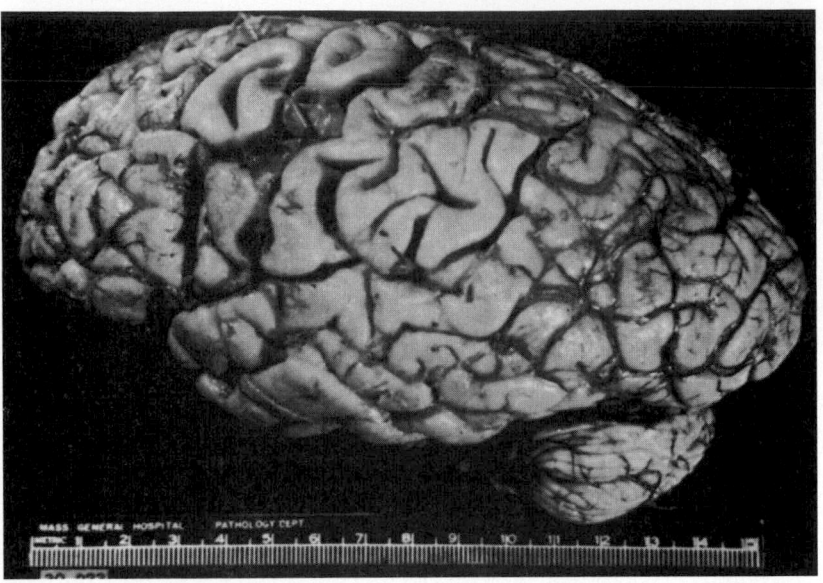

FIGURE 7–10　*Small upper rolandic infarction. The pia-arachnoid has been stripped away to show the infarct. (Courtesy of J. M. C. Pearce.)*

This point also seems to apply to the *postrolandic branches of the upper division*. Occlusion of the ascending parietal branch is uncommonly reported, but the few cases documented have been remarkably free of focal motor deficit.[135] The pilot phase of the NINCDS Stroke Data Bank study[109] documented a handful of instances of hemiparesis after *opercular infarction*. Several notable cases exist with autopsy correlation in which weakness did not occur in either the face or the limbs at any time during an acute infarction affecting the inferior frontal region's anterior operculum.[134] Reports of infarction confined to the *orbital frontal branch* of the upper division are exceedingly rare. Waddington and Ring described a 62-year-old man with a grasp reflex, inappropriate laughing *witzelsucht*, inappropriate advances toward his employees, and poor business judgment.[13] His only motor deficit consisted of the grasp reflex and contralateral extensive planar response. The case was studied by angiogram only. Rare reports of occlusion may be a result of the low frequency of embolism into this particular branch of the MCA.

Contraversive Eye and Head Deviation

Prevost[135] first described deviation of the head and eyes after unilateral lesion in 1896. Review articles nowadays rarely cite the documentation for the correlation[136–138] even though the lesions responsible and the setting for persistence of the deviation are not well understood.[139] It has long been held that the deviation of the eyes represents disruption of the frontal eye fields in and around area 8 alpha, located in the premotor region of the superior frontal lobe.[136,137,140–142] Yet few cases have been so reported,[143,144] and most cases with deviation of the head or eyes have been associated with lesions more centrally located in the MCA territory near the operculum or insula.

Types of Deviation

De Renzi and colleagues[110] encountered three types of deviations in their 120 patients with ocular motility disorders. In the first group, the head and eyes were in the midline and moved spontaneously to either side in response to stimulus, but eye movements were less complete to the side of the space served by the damaged hemisphere. In the second group, the head and eyes were found completely to one side with absence of spontaneous movements to the contralateral side and only fleeting voluntary deviation of the eyes into the side of the space served by the damaged hemisphere. In the most severely affected group, the head or eyes, or both, were completely deviated away from the side of the space served by the damaged hemisphere and failed to turn in response to verbal or sensory stimuli, with no spontaneous or voluntary movements observed to the midline or beyond. Hemi-inattention or neglect of the contralateral side of the space usually accompanied cases with head and eye deviation.

Eye Deviation and Infarct Topography

Eye deviation is the expected finding after massive infarction of the *entire* MCA territory.[81] For *upper division* syndromes encountered in studies of Broca's aphasia, one of the chapter authors (JPM) reported uncovering 10 autopsy cases from the Massachusetts General Hospital files[145]; all of the patients had experienced head and eye deviation to the site of the lesion that persisted for days and cleared within a week. Less frequent eye deviation has been found in opercular infarction. Ocular deviation with *deep infarction* has been reported in individual cases with autopsy correlation,[119] and Tijssen's[139] study of 133 consecutive patients with "acute supratentorial lesions" included 5 who showed ipsilateral eye deviation. In 4, the deviation was from hemorrhage (thalamus, frontal or frontotemporal location), and in 1, from a subdural hematoma; none were from infarction. De Renzi and colleagues[110] found a higher frequency of ocular motor deviation in *right* than in left hemisphere infarcts.

In the NINCDS Stroke Data Bank study,[146] 86 cases (16%) of supratentorial-type conjugate ocular deviation occurred among the 531 cases of hemispheral stroke diagnosed according to clinical or radiologic criteria. The occurrence of ocular deviation was significantly correlated with the larger infarcts, but among the infarcts confined to single lobes, those involving the right side were more commonly associated with ocular deviation. A frontal predominance over parietal infarcts was not found, and a parietal location was not the explanation for the effect of the right-sided stroke. The prevalence of frontal or parietal lobe location did not differ significantly in single-lobe infarcts. Ocular deviation occurred from infarction as low on the surface as the operculum. Gaze deviation of less than 5 days' duration did not correlate with lesion side, size, site, cause, or positive initial CT findings. However, the larger lesions predominated among the nine patients whose ocular deviation persisted beyond 20 days.

Duration of the Deviation and Severity of Infarct

The severity of the initial ocular motility deficit seemed greater in right hemisphere cases than in left for the first 6 to 9 days in the series by De Renzi and colleagues,[110] but at the end of 2 to 3 weeks, most of the patients showed only mild or no disturbance. Contralateral hemineglect often outlasted the disturbance in ocular motility in these cases. Patients with infarction affecting the *operculum and insula* showed what has been labeled pseudo-ophthalmoplegia for the first few days of the stroke.[124] Conjugate deviation of the head and eyes lasts for several days and then disappears. The lesion causing this condition is far away from area 8 alpha and is considered a reliable feature of infarcts of the insula and operculum.

The duration of ocular deviation following *branch occlusion* in the upper division is less well documented. In one of the chapter authors' (JPM) patients, the head and eyes were deviated to the left for several weeks.[129] The branch occlusion affected the anterior ascending branch of the MCA as high as the borderzone with the anterior cerebral artery.

Infarction with No Eye Movement Disturbances

De Renzi and colleagues[110] reported one patient who was completely free of any gaze disturbance and had a cortical-subcortical lesion (a frontal hematoma) on the left involving the areas of the rolandic fissure. The few cases with focal infarction confined to the superior frontal region, near area 8 alpha, have not confirmed the thesis that this region is vital for ocular motility.

Dizziness and Vertigo

Hemispheral infarcts have long been assumed to have a vertiginous component. A unique case reported by Brandt and associates[147] provides a contrasting view. The patient suffered "well-demarcated infarction" in the right posterior insular region and had a rotational vertigo, among other signs, for almost a week.

Sensory Disturbances

Because the most attention has been paid to the more obvious deficits in language and motor function, surprisingly few data have described sensory disturbances outside the usual claims in the textbooks. The presence of a disturbance in sensation carries an important indication of a large lesion when it accompanies hemiparesis: In the pilot data from the NINCDS Stroke Data Bank project, this correlation was highly significant for infarcts greater than a single lobe in size ($P < .001$).[109]

Hemispherectomies and Sensory Disturbances

Because the sensory disturbance from hemispheric disease may improve with time, it is worth emphasizing that the anatomic substrate may not be the surviving portion of the damaged hemisphere. The data from hemispherectomy cases permit assessment of the sensory disturbance expected under extreme conditions of tissue removal.[115] A relative preservation of sensory function in the face seems common, whereas more blunted sensation to several modalities occurs the more distally the test is performed in the arm. Complete astereognosia was common in Obrador's[115] patients. Vibration and position sense were heavily affected. No patients showed definite alteration of the body scheme. The sensory disturbances in the massive "malignant" infarcts treated with hemicraniectomy should be reported in an ongoing study in the near future for comparison with this older series.

Pure Sensory Deficits

Focal sensory deficits have been described in detail in only a handful of cases with autopsy correlation, most of which were noted because the patients seemed to show an unusual variant of the expected deficit. One syndrome described has shown a pseudoradicular pattern of sensory loss, with impairment of joint position sense, stereognosis, graphesthesia, and two-point discrimination.[130] In the few cases studied, the hand is the most severely affected, but two have been described with both hand and foot disturbances. Hemianesthesia has also been described in a few other cases.[4,13,148] The persistence of the deficit outlasts the complaints of sensory disturbances.

Hemisensory Deficits and Lesion Topography

Foix and coworkers[149] are credited with demonstrating that an infarct affecting the anterior parietal region may produce a profound hemisensory loss (pseudothalamic syndrome) with little or no accompanying hemiparesis. Their patient had a large anterior parietal infarct that was so deep it created almost a cleft in the hemisphere to the ventricular wall. Lhermitte and associates[148] had a similar patient who was studied with CT. Remarkably few other cases have been described. Derouesne and colleagues[150] reported on a 50-year-old man with sudden numbness of the left thumb and index and middle fingers, which felt frozen or asleep. Normal power was found on physical examination, but the patient dropped small objects held in the hand. A hypodense cortical and subcortical lesion was found on CT 17 days after the onset of symptoms, consistent with an infarction affecting the parietal region. The symptoms disappeared in 3 weeks, but the sensory deficit persisted unchanged at reexamination 2 months later.

Paillard and associates[151] described a woman with left MCA lower division occlusion with a large infarct including the posterior parietal region and part of the superior parietal lobule. Very little motor deficit was noted, but a right hemianesthesia persisted for several years. The disturbance affected the right cheek and gums, manifested as frequent failure of the patient to notice that food had gone to the right side of her mouth. The hand was so anesthetic that she experienced cuts and burns without noticing them. The foot was anesthetic enough that several times the patient stumbled when climbing stairs. Specific testing of the hand disclosed no joint position sense to point discrimination or ability to report pressure. However, touch could be discriminated as to both direction and general speed (whether fast or slow), and the patient proved capable of discriminating the gross size of an object (large or small) and was also capable of rough location of points of touch along the surface of the limb.

Correlations with Motor Deficits

The correlation of the sensory disturbance with motor disturbance is infrequently reported. A few unusual cases exist, suggesting that a sensory disturbance may affect an area far smaller than that of the accompanying motor disturbance. Gacs and coworkers[152] described a 50-year-old woman with a large low-density area in the right frontal region whose clinical deficit consisted of a dense left hemiplegia including the face with left hemianopia. The sensory disturbance was described only as diminution and pinpricking vibration in the left arm.

Visual Field Disturbances

Hemianopia

Standard textbook accounts of MCA territory infarction regularly refer to hemianopia accompanying hemiparesis, hemisensory disturbance, and alterations in behavior, but little clarification is provided for the value of this sign as an index of infarct site and size, and even less for the pathoanatomic correlate. There is little doubt that hemianopia to confrontation clinical testing accompanies the huge infarcts.[4] Before modern imaging provided ample contradictory evidence, the hemianopia was ascribed to involvement of the visual radiation, even though the MCA supplies only the upper half of the radiation.[153]

For less global infarcts, hemianopia has been described with infarcts involving the frontal region, some as low as the sylvian fissure.[129] However, hemianopia has been absent in some instances of focal infarction even when impaired opticokinetic nystagmus (OKN) was found. It is difficult to sustain the notion that edema involving the radiations explains hemianopia when the infarct is far away from these structures. Instead, it seems more likely that the hemianopia as described is actually a disturbance in hemispatial response that is part of a hemineglect syndrome.[154] In such cases, other faulty responses to spatial stimuli are noted, such as the patient who is suffering a left hemispheral infarction, turning toward the left in response to a voice from the right and also showing failure to blink in response to threat stimuli from the right.

Quadrantanopia

Parietal infarction deep enough to affect the fibers of the upper half of the visual radiation is presumably responsible for the infrequently described inferior quadrantanopia of MCA territory infarction (Fig. 7–11). Bounds et al[155] described a 45-year-old woman who experienced left inferior quadrantanopia attributed to embolism of the MCA 8 days after aortocoronary bypass surgery. Clinical worsening occurred 5 days later, with hemiplegia, coma, and death

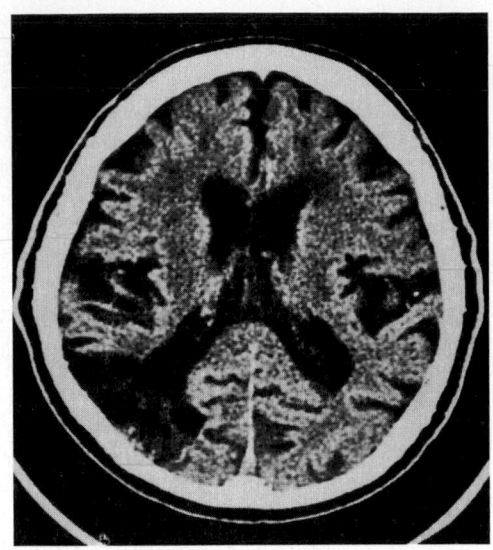

FIGURE 7–11   *Axial CT scan showing a left parietal infarct in a patient with right inferior quadrantanopia.*

from herniation. The autopsy report showed softening of most of the right hemisphere, and a specific focus of infarction correlating with the earlier quadrantanopia was not described. Remarkably enough, it is difficult to find the clinical setting in which lower quadrantanopia is found; it is even more difficult to determine whether the quadrantanopia indicates a deep cleft of infarction reaching the visual radiation or whether it may occur in a more superficial infarct.

Impairment of Opticokinetic Nystagmus

A test for OKN is assumed to detect disorders of the gaze mechanism mild enough that conjugate ocular gaze is not present at rest. Considering the number of patients tested for OKN, it is remarkable that there is still considerable controversy over the usual locus of the lesion, the pathways injured, and even the nature of the disturbance. The early view[156,157] was that OKN was a reflex activity of the cerebral cortex, that the slow component was initiated from the occipital region and the fast corrective phase from the frontal region, and that the OKN response was blunted by lesions at any point in the pathway. However, the higher prevalence of abnormal OKN in parietal lesions supported another view, namely that the slow component from the occipital region passed directly to the brainstem through a pathway adjacent to the visual radiations organized in ipsilateral pathways.[158,159] Still another approach argued that the pathway runs deep through the parietal region to the frontal lobe, crosses the posterior limb of the corpus callosum, and controls fast-phase components generated in the opposite frontal lobe.[156] Other arguments have been put forward for separate mechanisms controlling foveal and full-field pursuit.[160] These studies showed the main disturbance to be in the slow component when targets were moved into vision from the side of space served by the damaged hemisphere.

The actual documented sites vary considerably (not all in the parietal lobe), and hemianopia need not occur. Impairment of OKN has been encountered in a patient

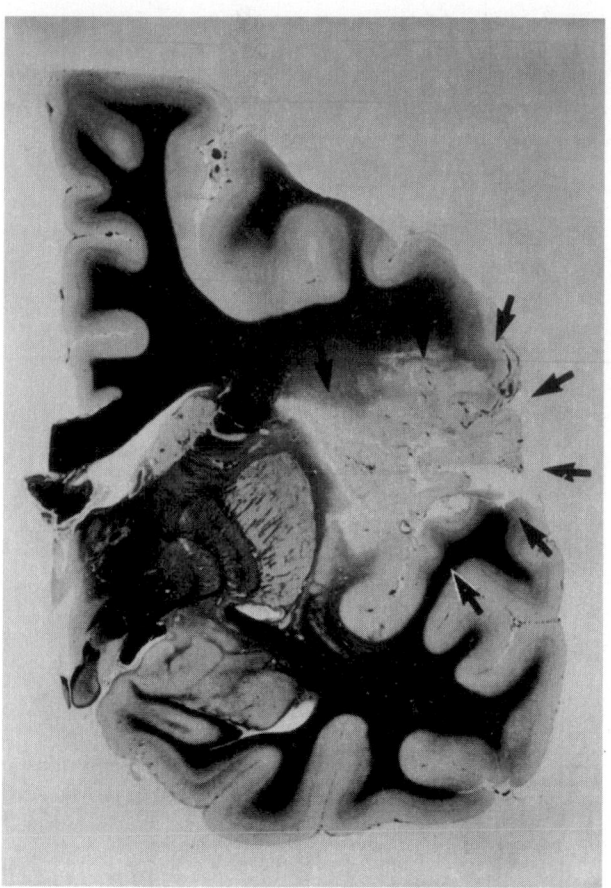

FIGURE 7–12 *Coronal view of insular and upper opercular infarction from embolism to the upper division of the middle cerebral artery. (Myelin stain of celloidin section.)*

with a small, high rolandic infarct whose visual fields were intact (see Fig. 7–10). On initial examination, a patient of the senior author (JPM), who reported the autopsy results,[129] had superficial infarction confined to the inferior frontal region and showed a brisk response by blinking from visual threat to the right side but absence of OKN for targets moving from right to left (Fig. 7–12). The patient reported by Baloh and colleagues[160] had a large infarct apparently involving the posterior cerebral artery territory, accompanied by right hemianopia and alexia but no language disturbance.

Neglect

The term *neglect* indicates disturbances shown by patients in their responses to stimuli from the right side of space, including impairment of OKN, turning to the left in response to auditory stimuli from the right, and faulty performance in reading aloud or naming objects in the right side of space.[161,162]

Neglect from Frontal Lesion

It has long been appreciated that a parietal lesion (from infarct or hemorrhage or even other causes) may be associated with an impaired response to stimuli from the opposite side of space, whether from a visual, auditory, or even somatosensory source.[163,164] These deficits are thought to reflect impaired input from sensory to motor regions. However, a similar disturbance occurs from frontal lesions as well,[165,166] whether cortical or subcortical.[167] Using positron emission transverse tomograph scanning, Deuel and Collins[168] found widespread metabolic suppression in the basal ganglia and thalamus after a unilateral frontal lesion, with little evidence of cortical hypometabolism beyond the immediate confines of the lesion. Their findings suggest that part of the syndrome might result from impaired activation of subcortical structures involved in planning motor movements. In the human, the signs of neglect from frontal lesions are remarkably transient, usually fading within a week in all but the largest infarcts.[169] (This subject is treated more fully in the section on right hemisphere disease; the following discussion applies mainly to left hemisphere disease.)

Motor Neglect

Motor neglect, said to be characterized by underutilization of one side without defects in strength reflex or sensibility, has been described by LaPlane and Degos.[170] Of the 20 cases reported, one ischemic type (located only by radionuclide scan in a prerolandic area) manifested as abnormal placement, lack of withdrawal of pain, reduced amplitude of movements, and visual hemineglect of the opposite side of space. This condition has a long history in clinical neurology. Under most circumstances of clinical examination, the patient with this syndrome appears to have a hemiparesis; with special efforts on examination, however, normal strength and dexterity can be demonstrated. The usual features are (1) a lack of spontaneous placing reaction, such as failure to place the hand in the lap or on the arm of a chair when sitting, letting it instead drag down beside the body; (2) delayed or insufficient assumption of correct postures, resulting in heavy falls to the affected side with no attempts to minimize the effect of the fall by reaching out or correcting the balance; (3) impairment of automatic withdrawal reaction to pain; and (4) excursions of the limb necessary to achieve a movement such as touching the nose, the patient instead leaning the head forward to compensate for failure to bring the finger far enough up. This disturbance may occur in the absence of a sensory disturbance or demonstrable hemiparesis. Hartmann[171] described an autopsy case with similar disturbances secondary to an infarct affecting the second frontal gyrus of the right frontal lobe. Animal studies in the monkey have demonstrated a similar transitory disturbance observed high over the prefrontal region after selective research.[172]

Neglect for Verbal Material

Leicester and associates[173] described a form of visual neglect in which the occurrence and frequency of errors were determined by the verbal content of the test materials. When the patient was required to select from an array of choices displayed directly in front, errors were seen with those materials that the patient found the most difficult to name or write; in such instances, responses were made less frequently to choices on the right-hand side of the display. When the test materials were easily named, little or no evidence of neglect for the right side of space was noted. This form of neglect, which is commonly encountered in testing of patients with aphasia, was shown not to be obligatory but to depend highly on the verbal material in the test itself. It was explained neither by defective spatial responding nor by defective sensory function, and it occurred with left-sided but not right-sided lesions.

Movement Disorders

Temporary or permanent movement disorders, including hemichorea, athetosis, and dystonia, are uncommon sequelae of MCA territory infarcts. Despite a large body of literature on the subject in children, few reports have appeared on adults.[174] Only one adult has been described with chorea: A 68-year-old woman reported by Austregesilo and Borges-Forte[175] experienced immediate torsion spasms with choreiform movements from what was presumed to have been a stroke affecting the head of the caudate nucleus, putamen, and pallidum.

Dystonia has been the subject of the other reports. The one adult described in the series reported by Demierre and Rondot[121] was a 17-year-old with left hemiplegia that improved slightly within 4 weeks, by which time signs of dystonia had appeared. A large hypodensity affecting the putamen, anterior capsule, and caudate was seen on CT. Grimes and colleagues[174] encountered two patients with CT-documented stroke in adulthood. The first was a 32-year-old woman who suffered dense hemiplegia and "cortical" sensory loss from a large deep infarct affecting the caudate and putamen that regressed considerably by 5 months. A month later, she began to experience involuntary abduction and extension of the affected fingers with ulnar deviation of the wrist; the arm flexed behind the back as she walked; and she had coarse tremor of the outstretched hand. The deficit progressed for 2 months and then stabilized. Medical therapy was ineffective. The second patient, a 50-year-old man, had a similar course with the addition of orofacial dyskinesia and dystonia that developed in the fingers and arm, with flexion of the limb behind the back during walking. The syndrome worsened for 3 months before stabilizing and was unaffected by medical therapy.

Autonomic Disturbances

Excess of sweating contralateral to an MCA territory infarction is encountered only rarely. In the small series of cases reported, all patients had major syndromes of hemiparesis, hemisensory problems, hemianopia, and altered behavior states, indicating a large lesion affecting both the superficial and deep territories of the MCA.[176] Sweating in these few cases affected the face, neck, axilla, and upper trunk contralateral to the infarct and faded to normal within days. Appenzeller[177] published an autopsy case for which the patient was described clinically as showing hyperhidrosis on the contralateral side of the body. No further details were mentioned, not even the extent of the other clinical deficits. The published photographs show a site of small hemorrhagic infarction in the upper bank of the insula and adjacent orbital surface of the operculum.

An MRI series describes hypertensive episodes in patients with infarcts restricted to the right insular cortex.[178] Contralateral rubbery edema of the affected hands and feet may occur from large MCA territory

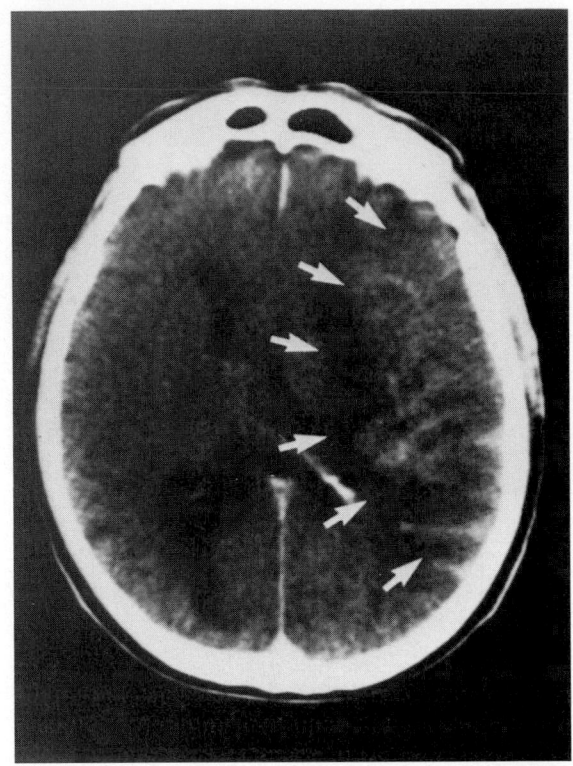

FIGURE 7–13   *Non–contrast-enhanced CT scan showing hemorrhagic infarction of the entire middle cerebral artery territory (arrows). Hemihyperhidrosis and distal arm edema were part of the clinical picture.*

infarction (Fig. 7–13). The syndrome usually becomes evident within a few hours and persists for up to 2 weeks. The exact anatomic correlates are unknown.

SYNDROMES REFERABLE TO LEFT HEMISPHERE INFARCTION

Aphasia

The cerebrum irrigated by the left MCA is of prime importance in language function. This function can be defined operationally for clinical purposes as a symbolic system in which the relations between meaningful elements (sounds, print, gestural signs, and so forth) are purely arbitrary. Aphasia (or its more commonly less severe variant known as dysphasia) is thus regarded as a disorder caused by acquired brain injury that results in dysfunctional use of rule-governed, symbolic behavior.[179,180] The sylvian fissure of the hemisphere dominant for speech and language is the region most likely to cause symptoms of dysphasia after a focal brain lesion. More than 95% of right-handed people and even most left-handed people have dominance for speech and language in the left hemisphere. Right hemisphere dominance for speech and language in a right-handed person is distinctly uncommon.

Many of the traditional clinicopathologic correlations of brain and language function have undergone revisions in the last few decades under the influence of modern imaging.[181,182] Among them has been that smaller focal brain lesions once thought to produce the major syndromes of aphasia are now known to cause less severe, minor, or even transient disturbances in production or comprehension of speech, sounds, and shapes. Much larger lesions are necessary to produce the lasting major disruptions in language function. Later work has also made it apparent that deeper structures, especially the thalamus, play vital roles in speech and language.[183] Nevertheless, there have been few additional gains over the past few years regarding the clinical characteristics of acute aphasia, with most new studies showing that lesion location is still the main determinant of the language syndrome. Rather, the contributions of new work have centered on insights achieved with functional imaging during the course of stroke recovery and with pharmacologic challenge targeted toward restitution of function.

Global or Total Aphasia

Few studies have indicated the different types of aphasia expected in a setting of acute stroke. In a survey of 850 patients, Brust and associates[184] found that 177 (21%) had acute aphasia. Fifty-seven (32%) had "fluent" aphasia and 120 (68%) "nonfluent" (see later for definitions). Nonfluency was significantly correlated ($P < .01$) with a poor prognosis for mortality. Even highly significant mortality was found for patients with fluent and nonfluent aphasia who showed hemiparesis or a visual field disturbance. Similarly, Marquardson[185] reported 769 acute patients with stroke, 133 (33%) of whom showed aphasia in the acute state; hemiplegia was less likely to improve if accompanied by aphasia, and aphasia had a better outlook when unaccompanied by hemiplegia.

Clinical Features

Occlusion of the trunk of the MCA or its upper division produces a global disruption of language function. Its effect puts out of action virtually all the brain regions mainly responsible for language. The initial disturbance is so profound that it goes by the term *total aphasia*. After the acute period, clinicians and family sometimes observe some improvement in the patient's capacity to understand context-related information (e.g., "Are you feeling better?") and to participate in the give and take of simple communication. Within weeks or months, comprehension improves, especially for nongrammatical forms, and the patient shows more disturbances in speaking and writing than in listening and reading.[186] This emphasis on dysphasia more in speaking and writing is known as *Broca's aphasia* or *major motor aphasia*.

Lesion Size

With the advent of CT and MRI, a volumetric measure of the lesion became possible during life, permitting inquiry into the issues not only of the usual lesion size associated with the syndrome but also of the minimal and maximal dimensions.[59,187] Naeser and Hayward,[188] relying on CT data, documented the lesion volume in two groups of patients, those labeled as having *mixed aphasia*, a term that broadly encompasses the clinical picture of total aphasia, and those labeled as having *global aphasia*, usually equated with total aphasia. The site of the lesion in seven cases of mixed aphasia reflected a large infarct affecting the sylvian region and beyond, but in a few instances, Broca's or Wernicke's areas proper were not mapped in the scanned lesion. The lesion size in these cases was approximately 3.9 by 3.9 cm, and such a lesion was usually seen on five CT slices. The lesion volume in five cases of global aphasia was considerably larger, on the order of 5.8 by 5.8 cm. As with the mixed aphasia cases, the site of the minimal lesion lay in the sylvian region, and the major contribution to the larger volume was its centrifugal spread into the adjacent frontal, parietal, and temporal regions. An example of such a case is shown in Figure 7–14A. With time, such lesions may evolve, leaving a major syndrome associated with considerable postinfarction atrophy (Fig. 7–14B).

Motor Aphasia

For more than 100 years, a syndrome has been recognized in which the ability to communicate by speaking or writing seems far more impaired than the comprehension of words heard or seen.[40] Although Boulliaud[189] deserves credit for popularizing the notion that a lesion of both frontal lobes disrupts the power of spoken speech, the surgeon Paul Broca, the friend of Boulliaud's son-in-law, has received most of the credit for the documentation that a left-sided sylvian infarct more reliably causes the syndrome. Broca described two patients who appeared to have lost their memory of how to speak. Considerable controversy has persisted concerning whether this characterization is suitable for the findings and for the locus of the minimal lesion to precipitate the major syndrome and whether the effects are the same when the lesion is confined to the third frontal convolution, which Broca took to be the site causing the syndrome that bears his name. The actual lesion sizes were far larger, encompassing most of the sylvian region and adjacent superior temporal lobe, lesions nowadays expected to be associated with a syndrome of total aphasia (Fig. 7–15).

Major Motor Aphasia

In its usual form, major motor aphasia appears to be an improvement of a syndrome of total aphasia and is a late sign in the course of the major sylvian cerebral infarct. In such patients, there is a sharp contrast between the hesitant, agrammatical speech and the relatively better comprehension evident in conversational tests as long as the examiner keeps the sentences and questions simple.

In the initial period after the acute infarction, the speech and language disturbances are too severe to allow a distinction between speech and language production and comprehension.[129,130,145,190–192] With the passage of a few months and some improvements in testability, the syndrome of Broca's aphasia begins to appear.

Whether the motor aphasia that emerges is a disturbance confined to speaking and writing or contains a global disturbance in the brain's capacity to deal with grammatical functions has been argued for almost 150 years. Part of the argument stems from the terms used to substitute for Broca's aphasia—expressive dysphasia, efferent motor dysphasia,[193] motor dysphasia,[194] verbal dysphasia,[195] and simply nonfluency,[191] to name but some. Despite the semantics, most investigators echo the impression of Liepmann[196] that symptoms of motor aphasia predominate and the limited capacity for spoken expression conceals the

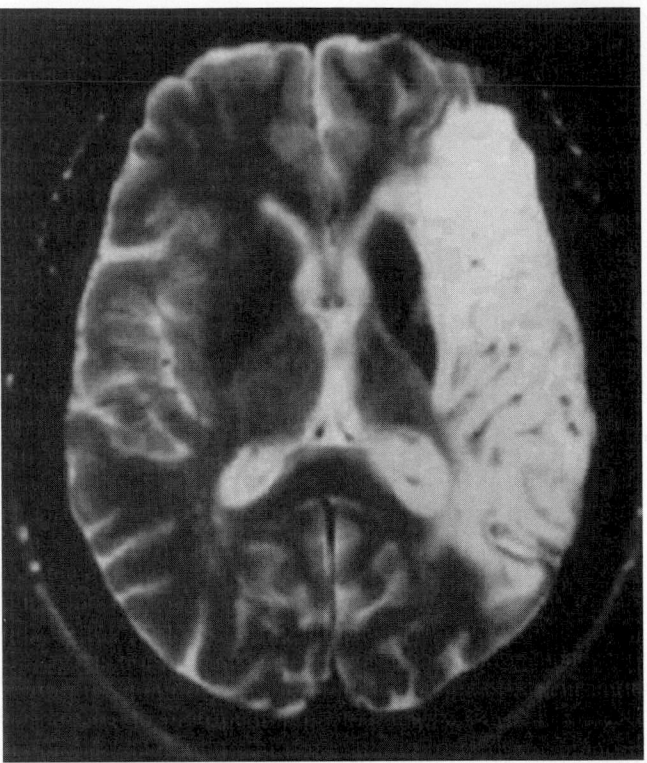

A

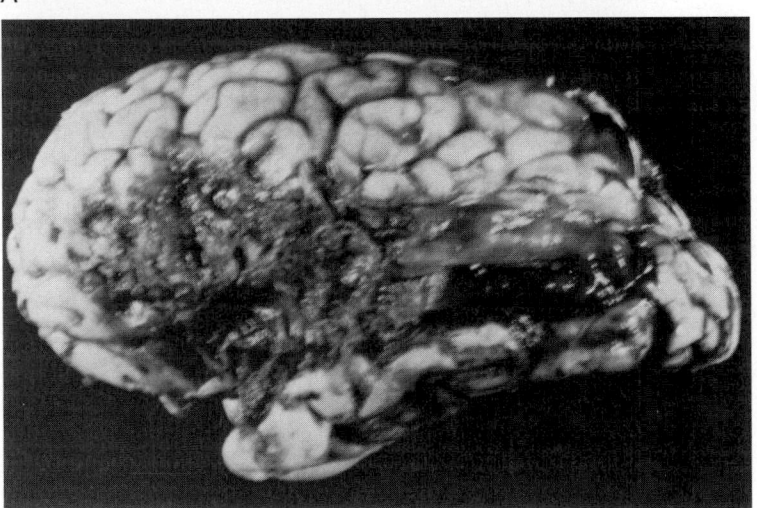

B

FIGURE 7–14   A, *Complete infarction of the surface territory of the middle cerebral artery following occlusion of the middle cerebral artery.* B, *Appearance of another similar case at a later stage.*

deeper language disturbances that persist but are less obvious.

The *speech disturbance* is evident to a similar degree whether the utterances are produced in spontaneous conversation or during efforts to repeat aloud or read aloud; that is, they are obligatory. The spoken responses are hesitant, demonstrating impairment of skilled interaction (dyspraxia) between the settings of the oropharynx and the respiratory elements that permit smooth vocalization.[197] In the production of individual words, the transitions from sound to sound are accomplished only with difficulty,[193] which is especially obvious with polysyllabic words. The disturbance disrupts the usual clustering of words to form phrases, interfering with the normal melodic intonation

that serves to indicate differences among exclamations, questions, and declarative statements. There is a high correlation between the degree of buccolingual dyspraxia and the extent of speech loss in patients with Broca's aphasia.[198]

Apart from these signs of *speech dyspraxia*, the structure of the spoken phrases may show a simplification of grammar, the language content consisting largely of single words that function as predicative elements, a performance formerly known as *telegraphic speech*, a term coined in the days when telegrams were an expensive form of communication charged by the word(s) sent. These grossly condensed utterances, lacking as they do normal sentence structure, have also been labeled *agrammatism*. In some cases, the utterances have been limited to a single word or

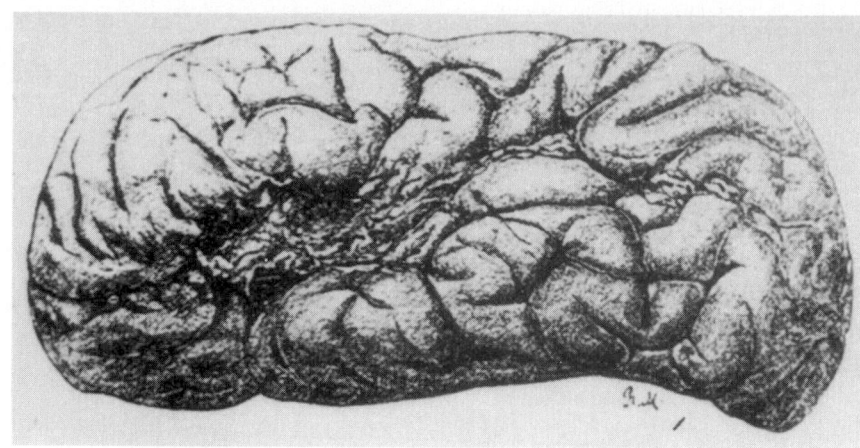

FIGURE 7–15 *One of Broca's original cases.*

phrase,[199] characterized as verbal stereotypes. The more limited the range of utterances, the more discouraging the prognosis for improvement.

Other disorders of language usage are part of the syndrome and seem independent of the difficulty in speaking aloud. They include difficulties responding to spoken or written material that features small grammatical words such as "the," "are," and "then" or involve spelling.[257] The poorest performance occurs when the meaning is highly dependent on grammatical features, especially when subject-object relations are based less on simple nouns (e.g., "John saw Jane") than on pronouns (e.g., "He saw it"), or when the passive voice is used (e.g., "He was seen by her"). The disturbances observed extend beyond the acts of speaking or writing to comprehension of the material itself. Silent reading comprehension, which requires no overt vocalization, is usually only a little disturbed for single words that are picturable nouns, but difficulties are encountered when the material to be read contains a particularly high density of such grammatical words. When it does, the comprehension may be strikingly abnormal. This condition has been termed *deep dyslexia* and has been described as a third form of dyslexia.[199] Similar disturbances can be documented in tests requiring the patient to point to visual displays containing single letters or grammatical words in response to hearing the names of the letters. Some have even shown faulty selection of a single letter among a visually presented display of letters when the test stimulus was a printed word whose pronounced sound (homophone) is identical to that of a given letter (i.e., "eye" to "i").[186] These examples are indicative of the global disturbances in language that occur and persist in patients with the major syndrome of Broca's aphasia.

The *clinicopathologic correlation* for the syndrome has evolved over the last century. Major motor or Broca's aphasia is not a syndrome expected from infarction restricted to Broca's area. It usually reflects a major infarction involving most of the territory of supply of the upper division of the left MCA, which was actually shown in Broca's original cases.[145] Accompanying disturbances in motor, sensory, and visual function usually make the diagnosis easy. The usually large size of the sylvian infarct sets the stage for contralateral hemiplegia.[200] At times, however, the main weight of the lesion may fall on the sylvian region alone, producing a surprisingly slight hemiparesis,

considering the major effect on language function (Fig. 7–16).[201] In these cases, the hemiparesis may be limited to the face and hand. Ideomotor dyspraxia of the unaffected left upper extremity is the rule, as is bilateral buccofacial dyspraxia, which has been reported in 90% of patients.[198,202] Contralateral hemineglect is the rule in the acute stage.

Autopsy documentation of the major syndrome of Broca's aphasia comes largely from the older literature;[145] living patients with the syndrome have been studied extensively by CT[203–205] and less frequently by MRI, given the extensive work already done earlier. The imaged lesions in patients with persistent Broca's aphasia were largely opercular and insular[206] and frontosylvian, sparing the temporal lobe. The larger sylvian lesions were associated with persistent nonfluency.[191] In cases with smaller lesions, destruction of the region taken to represent Broca's area was more often associated with transient deficits.

A few notable exceptions to the usual clinical picture accompanying Broca's aphasia may occur when the lesion is confined to the insula and adjacent operculum. Moutier's[207] patient Chissadon had a hemiplegia in the acute period but in the chronic state had only the slightest motor deficit. A remarkably circumscribed infarct was found along the lip of the upper bank of the sylvian fissure, which may have sufficed to interfere with language function and not with sensory motor function. A few cases of this type have been described with the use of Benson's term the "sylvian lip syndrome."[199] One of Broca's patients was also described as having no detectable motor disturbance but was examined several years after the onset of his original deficit. The issue of the smallest lesion sufficient to produce the persisting syndrome of Broca's aphasia remains unresolved. To date, no known case of an infarct confined to Broca's area alone has produced lasting, severe Broca's aphasia,[208] save for the tersely described case cited by van Gehuchten.[209]

The means by which clinical improvement occurs remains unclear. Work with metabolic imaging points to activation of tissue adjacent to the lesion site, providing supporting evidence for the process inferred from autopsy studies.

Minor Motor Aphasia

Focal infarcts affecting the operculum produce a rather circumscribed syndrome lacking the full elements of

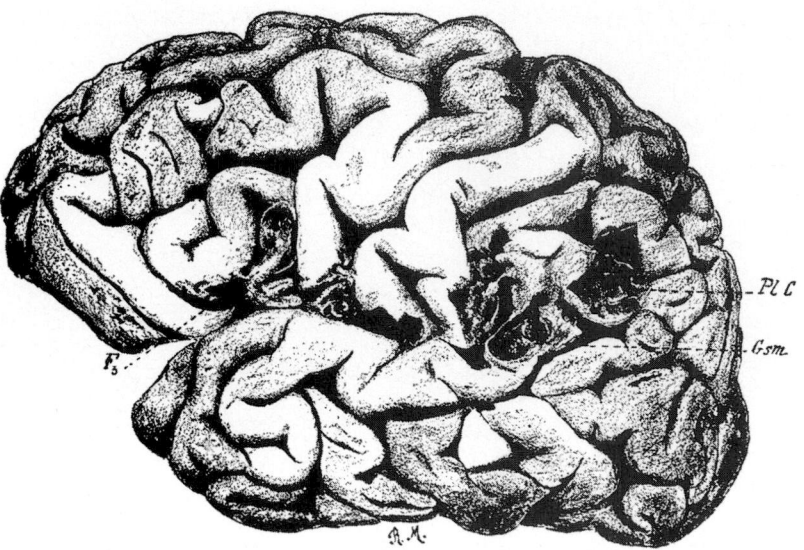

FIGURE 7–16 *Lithograph of an example of infarction limited to the sylvian lip. (From Moutier F: L'Aphasie de Broca. Paris, Thèse Médicine, 1908.)*

Broca's aphasia.[129,145,187,208,210] In the acute stages, complete mutism with ideomotor and buccofacial dyspraxia is commonly encountered. Auditory and visual comprehension for language is virtually intact, and some patients are capable of writing properly with the unaffected left hand. Improvement from the initial mutism begins within hours or at the least days and, rarely, weeks later.[205,211] Any language deficit evident in speaking and writing is extremely transitory and often disappears before it can be tested in full detail. The accompanying buccolinguofacial and ideomotor limb dyspraxia likewise disappears quickly. The dyspraxia appears to contribute to most of the disturbances in speaking. The oral cavity positions closely approximate those desired to generate given sounds, but the slight inaccuracies strike the listener's ears as mispronunciations. Also, the dyspractic disturbance in respiration interferes with the smooth flow of sounds and transition from syllable to syllable in running speech; this pattern has variously been called aphemia, oral-verbal apraxia, and apraxia of speech.[212] The disorder is not result of weakness of the muscle serving articulation.

The initial mutism is usually accompanied by contralateral hemiparesis, but limitation of the weakness to the lower face and hand is not uncommon. Head and eye deviation have been documented but not often.[129] A few cases of Broca's infarction have manifested with no hint of motor paresis.[134,213] In those reports using the term "nonfluency,"[191] a similarly transient disturbance has been seen in the smaller lesions found on CT (Fig. 7–17).

The clinicopathologic correlation has shown few exceptions to the rule that Broca's area infarction does not precipitate either the acute or the chronic forms of Broca's aphasia, an observation made from the earliest days after Broca's original publication[214] and confirmed many times

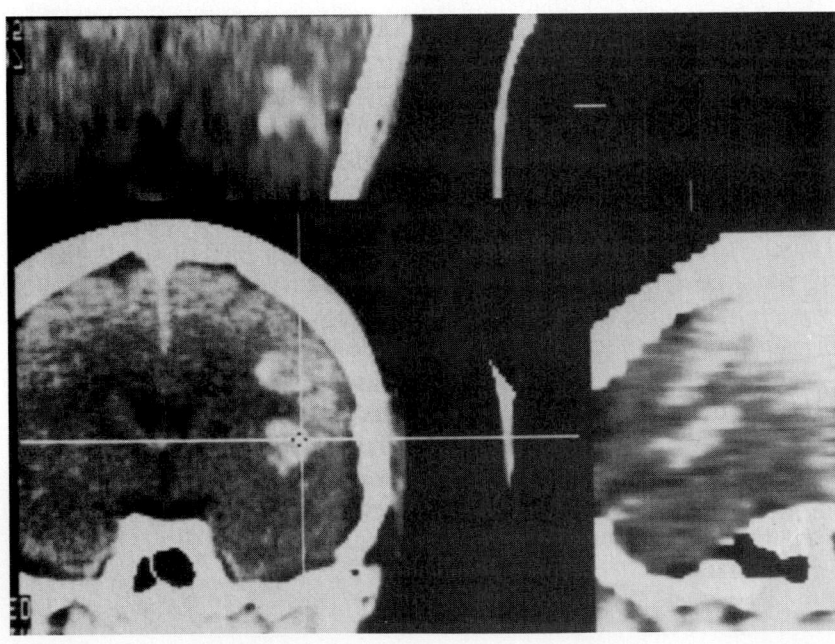

FIGURE 7–17 *CT scan showing three views of an inferior frontal infarct, presenting as minor motor aphasia.*

since.[145,205,215,216] The exceptions to this rule appear infrequent enough to warrant special comment. Van Gehuchten[209] described a 60-year-old man with sudden total loss of speech accompanied by paresis of the right upper limb and a small amount of facial involvement. The paresis diminished progressively, but the speech disturbance persisted unchanged until the man's death 1 year later. Van Gehuchten described the clinical picture as "pure motor aphasia with agraphia with no word blindness or deafness."[209] The patient was incapable of speaking. He uttered only a few sounds and sometimes a word or two. However, he could express himself adequately by gestures and wrote some letters or ordinary words from dictation but was unable to write spontaneously or from dictation under more demanding circumstances. Autopsy revealed an infarct affecting the inferior half of the middle frontal gyrus from the top to the bottom of what was described as Broca's area. The accompanying photograph disclosed the infarct but did not indicate the involvement or sparing of the insula nor whether the lesion extended deep into the brain.

Kleist[217] believed that the rare instances of a persistent and severe deficit associated with Broca's area infarction could be explained by an extension of the infarct deep into the hemisphere, disrupting the white matter fibers that serve as projection and association pathways for Broca's area. Foix[218] made a similar inference earlier, referring to infarcts affecting the deeper branches of the MCA. Goldstein[194] also made similar suggestions but did not specify the vascular territory involved in these larger lesions.

Speech Disturbances with Lower Rolandic Infarction

Few cases of lower rolandic infarction have been reported since the days of Moutier,[207] whose studies suggested that infarcts in the region did not cause motor aphasia. Three autopsied cases have appeared in the literature. Tonkonogy and Goodglass[211] described a 63-year-old man with moderate right central facial paresis, deviation of the tongue to the right, and slight right hemiparesis predominantly in the right arm with normal sensory function and visual fields. His speech was slow and dysprosodic, involving both stuttering and poor control of pitch. Articulations were deformed to the point of approximating literal paraphasias. He had a very slight disturbance in word finding. Dysprosody and articulatory disturbances remained, and moderate brachial facial dyspraxia was present. Comprehension for reading and writing was practically intact. By 3 weeks, the speech function had recovered fully or almost entirely, with just mild dysprosody; the right hand had only slight weakness. Autopsy showed an infarct of superficial size approximately 1.0 by 1.5 cm linked to an infarct in the anterior limb of the internal capsule affecting the lower cortex of the rolandic sulcus.

LaCours and Lhermitte[210] described a patient with an infarct limited to the rolandic operculum who lacked any disturbance in language but suffered a syndrome of "phonetic disintegration." Levine and Sweet[219] added a third case of rolandic infarction involving most of the precentral gyrus. The patient was only able to vocalize grunting or moaning sounds for the 10 days she was testable before her death. Autopsy disclosed a highly focal hemorrhage involving the midportion of the precentral gyrus and sparing the frontal region in Broca's area.

The overlap of this syndrome with cases producing predominantly literal paraphasias has been noted by Luria[193] under the term *afferent motor aphasia*, attributed to faulty sensory feedback from a postrolandic lesion leading to inaccurate anatomic settings of the oropharynx, with resultant mispronunciations.

Speech Disturbances from Deep Infarcts

Infarcts affecting the motor outflow of both sides have produced mutism as part of a syndrome of paralysis of both sides of the face, oropharynx, and tongue. However, a more interesting syndrome is that from a single deep infarct that has produced enough disturbance in speech and language to be described as an aphasic disorder. Bonhoeffer's[67] classic patient, unable to speak anything more than a few poorly formed vowels, had a large, deep infarct of the type described as a "giant lacune."[120] However, given its large size and the second infarct in the cortical surface territory of the anterior cerebral artery, it seems more likely that the cause of the deep infarct in this patient was embolism to the MCA stem: The infarct spread from the corner of the lateral ventricle through the caudate and internal capsule, even reaching the external capsule. The speech deficit was formulated as a double disconnection from Broca's area: The giant lacune prevented innervation of the bulbar apparatus from ipsilateral pathways, and the anterior cerebral territory infarct cut off transcallosal projections. A handful of other similar descriptions have been reported by Kleist from autopsy data[217] in the patient Bühlmeir. To date, the neuropathologic nature of the lesions remains unclarified. The six cases reported by Damasio and colleagues[220] were diagnosed from CT (with no angiographic or autopsy data), as were the seven cases of ischemic mechanism reported by Naeser and associates,[221] at least three of which had accompanying surface infarcts. These uncertainties aside, the CT abnormalities encountered in the cases with wholly deep lesion were predominantly in the anterior limb of the internal capsule, putamen, and caudate, and all were among the larger sizes consistent with the type 1 "giant lacunes" of Rascol and coworkers.[120] Remarkable dysprosody was seen, at times accompanied by dysarthria, little or no dyspraxia of limbs on either side, and a mixture of deficits in syntactic and semantic functions not typical of any of the classic syndromes of dysphasia. Other studies showing impairment of frontal reactivity in studies of cerebral blood flow suggest that the disorder may be explained by damage to thalamofrontal pathways, the diminished verbal behavior forming part of a syndrome of abulia.[222,223]

Sensory Aphasia

The syndrome known as Wernicke's aphasia is most commonly explained by occlusion of the lower division of the MCA and its branches, usually due to embolism. Because the lower division gives off its branches over an extremely short distance, the occlusion at or near the point of takeoff of these branches may give rise to several distinct variants in the size and topography of the infarction. There is a rough correlation between the extent of the language deficit and its intensity as a function of the lesion size, which is reflected in the text that follows.

Major Sensory Aphasia

When the embolus blocks the trunk of the lower division or occludes all the branches with no retrograde collateral flow from the posterior cerebral artery, a large infarct occurs, encompassing the whole posterior temporal, inferior parietal, and lateral temporo-occipital regions (Fig. 7–18). Infarcts of such huge size generate a profound deficit in language function, classically known as *Wernicke's aphasia* but here described as *major sensory aphasia*.

In contrast to motor aphasia, patients with any degree of sensory aphasia show little or no disturbance in the ability to vocalize, make smooth transitions between syllables, assemble utterances in the form of phrases, and achieve intonations of utterances that sound like questions, replies, and declarative statements, regardless of the severity of the language disturbance reflected in the content of their speech.[190]

In the acute stage of the major infarcts, the disturbance in language content manifests as such gross disturbance in the content of *spoken speech* as to contain no understandable words, a condition known as *jargon paraphasia*. The specific words expected to be uttered—the target words—are often distorted (but recognizable) in their phonetic structure (*literal paraphasia*) both in vowels and consonants, or other words in the same class are substituted (*verbal paraphasias*); these are occasionally distorted by the addition of unwanted suffixes (less often prefixes) or at times even omitted and are often contaminated by the recurrence (perseverations) of previously uttered words or word fragments. The effects on language behavior are almost the reverse of those in the insular-opercular syndromes: Speech is filled with small grammatical words but is missing the key words (the predicative elements) that contain the essence of the message. The extent of the language disturbance is often revealed only in prolonged conversation. The casual or hurried examiner may find that the patient speaks easily, engages in simple conversational exchanges, and even appears to be making an effort at communication. Because the utterances often flow in a manner suggesting attempts at declarative statements, questions, or explanations and are accompanied by gestures of the face and limbs, the patient seems to be making efforts to communicate. However, attempts to engage the patient in testing often fail to yield much evidence that the patient has understood the task and is attempting to respond. When the patient does not respond properly, the examiner is faced with the difficulty of deciding whether the fault lies in comprehension, in praxis, or in his or her own failure to make clear to the patient what is required.[224]

Writing is usually disturbed much like spoken speech. The cursive script is usually legible, but the language content reflected in the written letters and words has little communicative value. In some cases, writing and oral naming show striking differences in the severity of the language disorder, which some researchers have argued means that the two forms of expression are not under the same control.[225,226] The disturbance in *comprehension* of language for words heard or seen has long been assumed to be of the same type as that observed in spoken and written speech, a sign of the essentially unitary nature of the disorder.[202] However, despite the assumption that the brain lesion on the superior temporal plane interferes with auditory comprehension, it has been difficult to demonstrate any such disturbance in phonemic processing.[211] Instead of a disturbance in elemental phonemic processing, the problem seems to lie at the level of determining the linguistic significance of the adequately discriminated auditory stimuli.[227] It has likewise proved difficult to determine the extent to which disturbances in reading comprehension parallel those of auditory comprehension. A few patients with rather large lesions have shown a relative superiority in reading for comprehension compared with auditory comprehension.[225]

The phenomenology of major sensory aphasia has always been of interest to students of language abnormality ("What was it like?"), but the severe comprehension deficits during the acute syndrome usually preclude study. We had the rare opportunity to query a patient with a left frontal AVM about his perceptions immediately after we deliberately induced a transient Wernicke's aphasia via superselective injection of anesthetics into the lower division of the left MCA.[228] From his viewpoint, his speech was fluent and intelligible; he recalled later, "In general my mind seemed to work except that words could not be found or had turned into other words." He was unable to follow any dictated commands and had no recollection of the task after the anesthetic had dissipated. On oral naming of pictures, as he stated, "I told (the doctor) that I had just bought a tennis racket. But this was not true. What I explicitly meant to say was that I owned a tennis racket. . . . I think that no less than three times I stated that I had just bought a racket and kept repeating it." He was unable to repeat any phrases, saying afterward that "it appeared to be an issue of retention." On reading aloud, he noted that the words appeared to be a random group of letters: "I tried my best to pronounce them but it was clear even to me that I was speaking gibberish. . . . I would see a word, pronounce it, but another word would emit from my mouth." From these

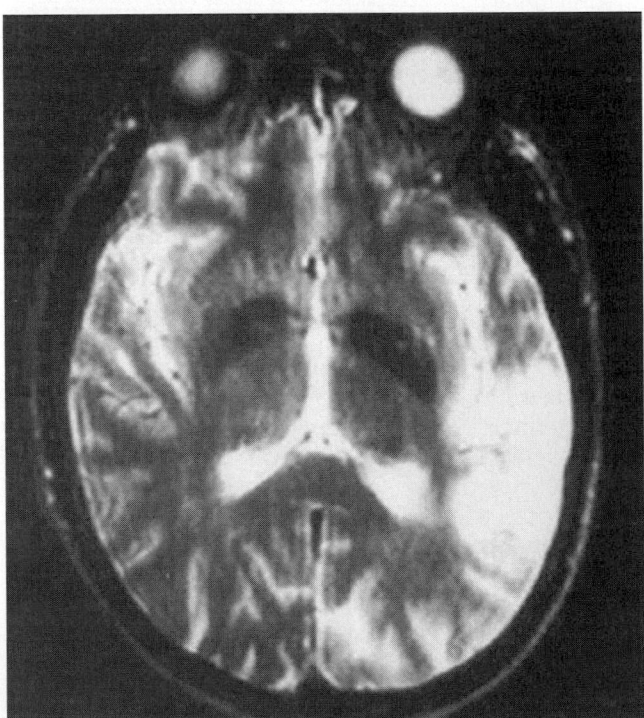

FIGURE 7–18 *Large posterior hemispheral infarct with syndrome of major sensory (Wernicke's) aphasia.*

self-reflections, it appeared that he was actually deriving more from the environment than his overt responses would have led us to infer. His recollections therefore question the long-held assumption that such profound comprehension deficits preclude the ability to analyze one's own behavior.[190] This appears to be another instance of blaming the subject for the insensitivity of the observer's measurement tools.[229]

The *clinicopathologic correlation* in Wernicke's aphasia, as in Broca's aphasia, has been with a rather large lesion. In most of the later literature, the full syndrome of Wernicke's aphasia has been correlated mainly with the larger posterior hemispheral extent of the lesions.[188,230] In the four cases clinically diagnosed as Wernicke's aphasia in Naeser's study,[188] the lesions were relatively large, on the order of 2.5 to 3.1 × 3.1 cm on the slices showing low-density lesions, and the findings were seen on three slices around the level of Wernicke's area. Although the lesion in the reported literature seems to be large in cases labeled clinically as Wernicke's aphasia, little is known about the exact correlation of the lesion site and size and the features of the syndrome. In our case material, some correlation seems to exist between lesion size and performance in special language studies comparing the spoken and written response to auditory and visual presentation of words, pictures, and sounds: Patients with small lesions were no better at language response to words, sounds, or pictures of the same items (i.e., the disturbance was just as severe for words heard as words seen or for sounds heard as pictures seen). Other patients with smaller lesions have shown more limited disturbance in either auditory or visual comprehension but not both to the same degree.[225] Patients with protracted and exaggerated spontaneous speaking (logorrhea) have been those with the larger infarcts, and those with the smaller infarcts rarely show this sign, a point that could be studied in more detail.

It has now been recognized that some of the patients with a fairly large lesion across the lower division may not show a full clinical picture of Wernicke's aphasia at all. In some, it has been suggestive of the syndrome of conduction aphasia (see later).[231,232] In these cases, comprehension is so satisfactory that the main finding is difficulty in repeating aloud. The implications are discussed in detail later.

Further, few cases have been reported in which either no detectable initial deficit in language occurred or the deficit was at most only slight and transient[233-235] even though the patient had an infarct affecting the posterior superior temporal region that was large enough to have been expected to produce Wernicke's aphasia. A chapter author (JPM) has had a similar case, an elderly right-handed woman whose cerebral embolism occurred while she was walking in her garden in the company of her internist son. She was immediately tested: She could read aloud and write correctly and could repeat and converse normally, but she experienced signs of a right hemianopia. Examination within days also failed to disclose language disturbance (Fig. 7–19). Cases of this sort serve to indicate the limitations of our present understanding of language organization in the brain.

Minor Sensory Aphasia and Variants

When collateral flow is established retrogradely from the branches of the posterior cerebral artery after an embolus

occluding at the origin of the lower division of the MCA, some reduction in total infarct size occurs, the infarction zone shrinking backward toward the site of occlusion. How often such cases occur is only now being appreciated with the widespread use of CT and MRI. Before the availability of these techniques, the mere angiographic demonstration of an occluded lower division at its origin left the physician unable to be certain how large an infarction was present distal to the occlusion. However, these cases provide an opportunity to determine how small a lesion is sufficient to precipitate the full syndrome of Wernicke's aphasia. Little is known about the spectrum of syndromes that occur as a function of differences in lesion size.

At issue is the vital question of the precise location and size of Wernicke's area. The thorough review by Bogen and Bogen[236] amply demonstrated that scarcely anyone agrees. Over the decades, the region attributed to Wernicke's area seems to have shrunk steadily from Wernicke's original notion that it was the posterior end of the sylvian fissure and adjacent parietotemporo-occipital region. From the initially large zone suggested by 19th century writers, actually encompassing much of the arterial supply of the lower division, the area critical for the syndrome has been considered to be smaller and smaller, the most shrunken being the small size of the posterior superior temporal plane in Geschwind's[237] diagrams. As previously suggested, the tendency to focus attention on this smaller zone may arise in part from the currently popular means of mapping a lesion by CT or MRI for several cases in the same cohort, seeking the site where the lesions overlap.[238] The approach has the advantage of targeting the focal lesion site common to all the cases. Because the site common to all cases is the posterior superior temporal plane, it would be easy to assume that this site represents the critical zone. However, this site may simply be an artifact of the diagrammatic method, because it is along the posterior superior temporal plane that the lower division bifurcates and where most of the embolic infarcts begin. If so, this location may merely be the essential focus of the infarct, not the site of the lesion producing Wernicke's aphasia. The precise relationship must be established in patients whose lesions are confined to this small site.

Cases of Wernicke's aphasia with a lesion confined to the superior temporal plane appear to be remarkably rare. A 20-year effort in three large hospital-based populations that we and our colleagues have reviewed has failed to reveal any examples. No less an authority than Charles Foix,[218] writing on vascular causes of Wernicke's aphasia in 1928, admitted he had seen none. In 1946, Nielsen[239] found 12 patients with Wernicke's aphasia in the literature whose deficits included reading disturbances with lesions that spared the angular gyrus. These were the same cases that Benson and Geschwind[240] later used to support their claim that severe alexia (part of the full Wernicke aphasia syndrome) can arise from a lesion confined to the superior temporal plane. However, of these 12 patients, three had been reported by the original writers (and also so noted in 1920 by Henschen[108] in his long review) to have had no alexia. Six others had large posterior sylvian lesions of which the superior temporal plane portion was rarely a part. According to the detailed description, two of the lesions appear to have been old residual subcortical

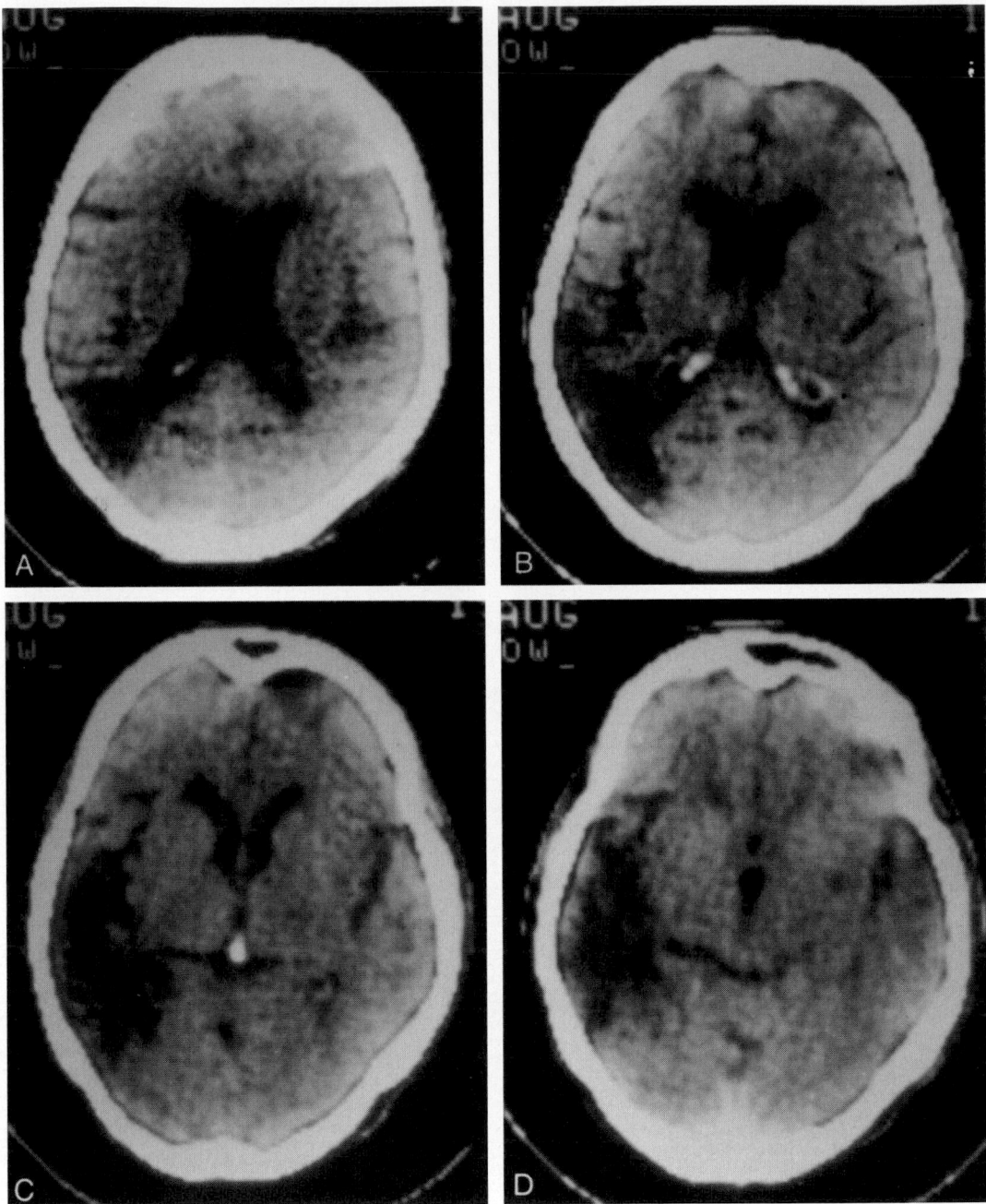

FIGURE 7–19   *A* to D, *CT evidence of large infarct involving the lower division of the middle cerebral artery in a right-handed woman who had no aphasia.*

hematomas, lesions that are arguably much larger when initially symptomatic than when observed later at autopsy.

Luria[193] considered the superior temporal plane to be Wernicke's area, but his cases were of traumatic origin from World War II, a notoriously inadequate source of material for precise localization. Kertesz and Benson[241] reported on four autopsied cases with lesions involving the superior temporal plane, but the lesions in these cases also spread into the insula and supramarginal gyri, even into the angular gyri. Naeser[206] described lesions larger than the superior temporal plane in a study of four cases documented by CT.

Our personal literature search showed that only three superior temporal plane lesions have been found with Wernicke's aphasia among 89 published cases with autopsy correlation. Two of the cases are subject to criticisms that minimize their utility, and the third is described too briefly to permit much analysis. The first, Gilbert Ballet's case,[108] was actually reported as an example of pure word deafness, a more restricted syndrome. Examined in March 1900 shortly after the stroke, the patient had pure word deafness, paraphasic speech both spontaneously and on repeating aloud, word blindness, and agraphia. Description of the autopsy performed in October 1901, 19 months later, fits that of a residue of an old subcortical (so-called slit) hemorrhage, which one can presume was larger at the time of the evaluation of the original clinical deficit (Fig. 25 in Henschen[108]). In any case, it is certainly not an isolated lesion of the superior temporal plane.

The second patient, described by Souques,[108] was followed up clinically for 14 years. The deficit faded from an initial picture of Wernicke's aphasia to almost normal within 2 years. Unfortunately, the patient was illiterate, so reading and writing were not tested. At autopsy, he appeared to have had an old hematoma, a lesion presumably large enough in the acute stage to have caused the full syndrome of Wernicke's aphasia.

The third case involved Kleist's[217] patient Papp, who was said to have sensory aphasia for 2 months until another stroke altered the clinical picture. No details of reading tests were described. The lesion was, however, confined to the temporal plane.

Henschen,[108] in a review of the literature up to the mid-1920s, concluded that a superior temporal plane lesion does not cause the full picture of Wernicke's aphasia (i.e., both "pure word deafness" and "alexia"). He based this opinion on a review of 35 patients with temporal lobe lesions, 20 of whom had "pure word deafness." In none was alexia present. Earlier, Bastian[243] had found alexia and sensory (Wernicke's) aphasia in only 5 of 16 cases of temporal lobe lesions and in most of which the lesion was large. Studies based on imaging add no qualitatively new cases: The study conducted by Naeser and colleagues[221] contained cases with medium to large lesions, whereas that reported by Mazzocchi and Vignolo[187] contained only one case with a smallish lesion, which the researchers described as an exception to the other cases in that "anomias were in the foreground."

These data provide little support for the view that a superior temporal plane lesion alone accounts for the full syndrome of Wernicke's aphasia. The infarction needed to precipitate the full syndrome in the reported cases has been much larger, well beyond the confines of the superior temporal plane. A unique case from our clinical experience further demonstrates this point.

A 20-year old right-handed man with only a very mild defect in spontaneous word retrieval underwent deliberate embolization of the left angular artery for treatment of a fusiform aneurysm–dysplastic segment. He was asymptomatic for about 4 hours, after which he began to demonstrate mild defects in auditory comprehension; otherwise, reading aloud, reading comprehension, and oral naming of pictures were normal. MRI demonstrated an infarct restricted to the territory of the angular artery, presumably Wernicke's area. The patient's language returned to baseline within a week.

There is no lack of superior temporal plane lesion cases, but simply a lack of such cases showing the full syndrome of Wernicke's aphasia. Many of the cases involving an infarct limited to less than the whole lower division territory appear to have been labeled conduction aphasia, pure word deafness, or alexia with agraphia.

Pure Word Deafness. More than 40 cases with CT or autopsy correlation are reported. According to the classic formulations, the only deficit should be auditory; spontaneous speech should be normal, as should reading comprehension and writing.[244] Eight well-known cases exist in which a unilateral lesion is confined to the superior temporal plane in the dominant hemisphere. In seven of these cases, paraphasic speaking was prominent, a clinical picture not permitted in the formulation of pure word deafness, which, by definition, should be free of a disturbance in speaking. In many cases, the elements of paraphasic speech cleared later.

The case reported by Schuster and Taterka[245] has been repeatedly cited but is a disappointment: In the acute phase, the patient had paraphasias for well over a month, in addition to the word deafness. More disappointing, at 7-month examination, no tests of reading were performed. Finally, autopsy showed the residue of an old slit hemorrhage, scarcely the stuff of precise correlation. Although this case is famous, the early phase of the illness makes it difficult to maintain the "purity" of a syndrome of pure word deafness. In Nielsen's[246] patient Sult, a left superior temporal plane lesion was demonstrated, said to be associated with pure word deafness, but there are few satisfying details in the clinical text.

Many of the patients with bilateral lesions also experienced paraphasic speaking with poor comprehension during the acute phase of the stroke.[231,247] In the famous case reported by Pick,[248] bilateral lesions including a large left temporal plane lesion left the patient paraphasic for 4 years. The deficit was only slight when Pick examined the patient 10 years later. The latest reported patient described as having pure word deafness had only a few paraphasic errors in spoken speech and in tests indicating comprehension of printed words.[231] He suffered bilateral temporal lobe infarction, documented by CT, which was inferred to have affected the primary auditory cortex. The largest lesion was on the right side.

From the foregoing discussion, one must conclude that examples of the pure word deafness syndrome occur only rarely. There is not even much current evidence that unilateral infarcts of the left temporal lobe create a state of impaired auditory discrimination.[190] Instead, small temporal lobe infarcts or parenchyma residue of an old slit hemorrhage (see Chapter 13) usually seems to set the stage for a transient form of Wernicke's aphasia, the major clinical feature of which is a disturbance in auditory comprehension, such as the aneurysm case we described earlier. The spontaneous speech contains many paraphasic errors, especially in the acute stages, enough that the listener may make a preliminary diagnosis of Wernicke's aphasia. Also, when taxed in reading aloud or comprehension tasks, patients with such lesions make enough errors that the notion of a pure disorder in auditory comprehension is not easily maintained.

Cortical Deafness. The issue of cortical deafness is another matter. At least one case report exists of an autopsied patient who was well studied clinically and found to have deafness occasioned by an infarct confined to Heschl's transverse gyrus.[249] This case supports Henschen's[108] claim that such an event can occur. Examples are rare enough that the unilateral lesion is difficult to predict on clinical grounds alone. Bilateral infarcts affecting the temporal plane are a well-recognized cause of deafness, although only a few reports have appeared. The 24-year-old man reported by Khurana and associates[250] is a typical example:

After the second cerebral embolus, he became completely deaf to all sounds, speech and nonspeech in character, and could not be startled by loud noise. The brainstem auditory evoked response studies showed normal waveforms through wave V. The patient's spontaneous speech contained the expected paraphasias, which were of the phonetic type; communication was achieved by writing, and occasional paragraphic errors were observed. The bilateral superior temporal plane infarcts were rather circumscribed.

Alexia with Agraphia. Alexia with agraphia has proved remarkably difficult to find in case descriptions in the literature. Henschen,[108] who found five "pure" cases among the more than 250 patients who had dyslexia and dysgraphia as part of larger clinical syndromes, noted that paraphasia in speaking was a common accompaniment to the syndrome.

Its general characteristics have been repeatedly described by a number of authorities as a disturbance in reading comprehension and in the morphology and language content of writing that far exceeds the disturbance in auditory comprehension or in spontaneous speech.[240] The original patient reported by Dejerine[130,251] suffered a lateral parietal infarct that penetrated as far as the ventricular wall. The disturbance in writing and reading was out of proportion to the modest dysphasia in conversation, but Dejerine did not see the patient in the acute phase. Touche[230] described a similar case, whose remarkably focal cerebral infarct involved the right posterolateral parietal region in a left-handed man; he also showed mild paraphasia in spoken speech but not to the same degree as the disturbance in reading and writing.

Among the many accounts, mention is usually made that "almost all patients suffering alexia with agraphia have some degree of aphasia which ranges from a minimal degree of word-finding difficulty to a more marked sensory aphasia with paraphasia and comprehension disturbance." [240] This observation raises the possibility that the syndrome may be another variant of Wernicke's aphasia. DeMassary[252] suggested that Dejerine himself considered this type of alexia a form of the sensory aphasia syndrome, which is more evident when the patient is seen in the early phase of the stroke. Sidman and colleagues[253,254] studied such a patient for many years; autopsy eventually showed a large lesion affecting much of the posterior left hemisphere (Fig. 7–20). His deficit began as sensory aphasia, affecting all forms of language and all conditions of testing. As time passed, the spoken response to auditory language stimuli improved, but the written response to any tests and the response to printed words remained impaired, a disturbance that could be classified grossly as dyslexia with dysgraphia.

The clinical problem posed by the syndrome is not whether it exists but whether it is only a transient, acute disorder or occurs mainly in the chronic state of an initially more severe Wernicke's aphasia. The anatomy of the lesion requires a circumscribed infarction beyond the superior temporal plane. Embolism is the only reliable source of such an infarct, apart from the focal form of vasculitis. In the unusual case in which the posterior cerebral artery takes its origin from the carotid artery, the main weight of the distal infarction could fall on the parieto-occipital lobe, which happened in the case reported by Sidman and colleagues,[254] but such an event would be most unusual. The available clinical data do not permit the determination of how acutely this syndrome can occur. The cases in the literature suggest it is a late development from an earlier syndrome of more extensive deficits. The few cases of the syndrome from nonvascular causes do not bear on this problem and are beyond the scope of this discussion.

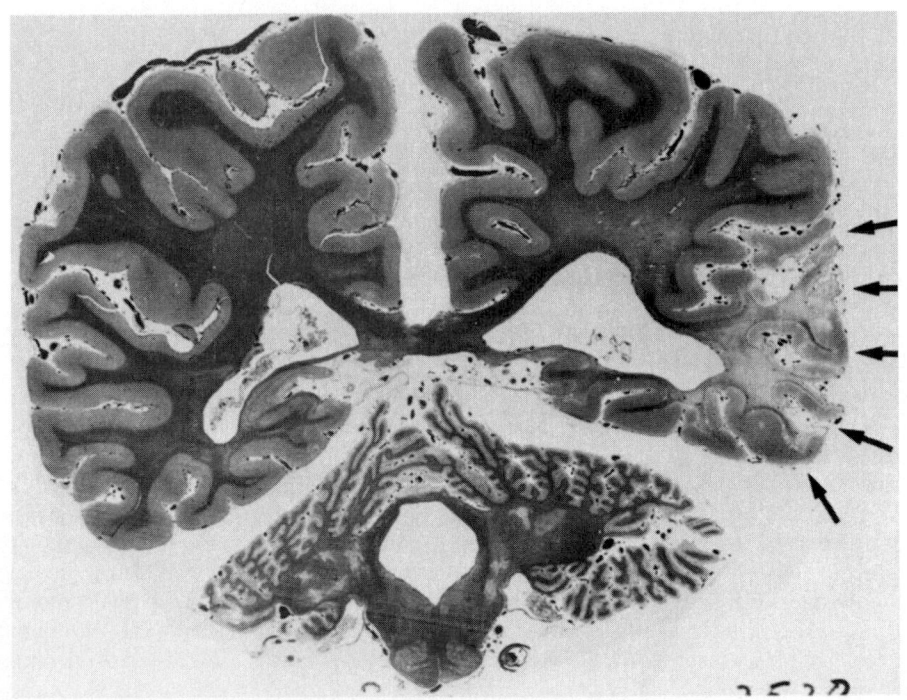

FIGURE 7–20 *Coronal section from posterior half of brain in a patient with Wernicke's aphasia that evolved over years toward a syndrome of dyslexia with dysgraphia.*

Conduction Aphasia

Conduction aphasia occupies a special position in aphasiology, mainly because of its theoretical prediction rather than its isolated occurrence as a clinical entity. Wernicke,[255] who first defined the syndrome, offered the opinion that it represented the interruption of fiber pathways connecting the sensory language zone of the posterior half of the brain with the motor language zone in the frontal lobe. For Goldstein,[194] the disorder represented disruption of a brain region located between the major sensory and motor centers, mediating the interaction of both functions simultaneously. As has been well documented by Levine and Calvanio,[256] its clinical features are not accounted for by either of the two major theories.

The term *conduction aphasia* has become accepted in clinical circles to apply to patients with poor repetition, especially for unfamiliar material, and far better auditory and visual comprehension of language than that evident in their spontaneous spoken and written efforts. That spontaneous speech is often contaminated by paraphasic utterances is not emphasized. Although auditory and visual language comprehension is relatively preserved, neither function is normal at any stage of the disorder.[221] The ease with which disturbances in comprehension and the language content of speech are demonstrated has proved to be a major stumbling block to the satisfactory application of the label *conduction aphasia* when the physician encounters such a patient at the bedside. The disturbance in repeating aloud, on which great stress has been laid,[257,258] is not as useful a distinguishing point in the acute stage of the syndrome, because it also occurs in Wernicke's aphasia. In assessing the deficits in conversation, Burns and Canter[259] found a higher incidence of unwanted phonemes and intrusion of semantically related words among those patients classified as having Wernicke's aphasia than among those with conduction aphasia, but careful testing was required to make this distinction. Patients with conduction aphasia are also said to have a greater tendency to attempt self-correction than those with Wernicke's aphasia;[240] in the authors' own experience, this point has applied only to cases of Wernicke's aphasia with the major syndrome. For ordinary clinical purposes, the distinction between the error patterns in speaking in the two types is not an easy one, except that semantic word substitutions are rare in conduction aphasia.[260,261]

Because the site of the infarct lies behind the rolandic region, there is usually no contralateral hemiparesis. Disturbances in eye movements and visual fields are also minor or not present. Buccolinguofacial dyspraxia is a common accompaniment, as is bimanual ideomotor dyspraxia. The dyspraxia of the latter state is different in the two limbs, the disorder in the limb served by the infarcted hemisphere taking the form of a deafferentation[150] and that in the other limb conforming more to the picture expected in ideomotor dyspraxia.

Conduction aphasia often proves surprisingly evanescent when seen in an acute setting. More often, the initial syndrome is a Wernicke-type aphasia, evolving later into the picture of conduction aphasia.[232] The syndrome in its late stages may prove difficult to demonstrate. Testing with difficult words that the patient repeats aloud is often required.

The clinicopathologic correlation is also at odds with the theory. The most popular current thesis envisions interruption of the arcuate fasciculus as the mechanism for the errors.[257,258] The interruption presumably prevents adequate control by the auditory system over the speech apparatus. Because this thesis hinges on a lesion interrupting the arcuate fasciculus, the findings expected on brain imaging or autopsy would be mainly subcortical. However, autopsy evidence in support of this thesis is surprisingly slight. The documented lesions have all been superficial infarcts, whose penetration into the subcortical white matter has varied considerably.[199] In some instances, the infarction was completely superficial; in only a few has it been profound enough to produce a cleft deep enough to injure the arcuate fasciculus. Damasio and Damasio[231] offered the suggestion that two projecting systems may exist and may follow pathways susceptible to injury even by superficial lesions. The cases used for their analysis were not "pure," however, because some disturbance in auditory and reading comprehension was present, although no more than that in the usual cases classified as conduction aphasia. More than 20 cases with CT, MRI, or autopsy correlation are reported with this syndrome, and many show the lesion located in the same area usually attributed to Wernicke's aphasia. Naeser[206] found no difference in the lesion size per CT slice in cases with conduction or Wernicke's aphasia, but the mean percentage of left hemispheral tissue damage was larger in patients with Wernicke's aphasia than in those with conduction aphasia ($P < .01$).

Another major thesis of the conduction aphasia theory considers the deficit to represent a disturbance in kinesthetic feedback. Luria[193] coined the term *afferent motor aphasia* to characterize this behavior. He assumed that the lesion lay in the sylvian operculum posterior to the rolandic fissure, yielding a disturbance in pronunciation resulting from faulty anatomic oropharyngeal positionings. The words pronounced would contain sounds different from those intended. These errors, analogous to the typing errors of a novice typist, require considerable listener training for their detection, rather like the recognition of typing errors by those familiar with the typewriter keyboard. The novice listener may easily mistake them for language errors (paraphasias) and may assume that the speaker has a language disorder. Such an interpretation may be inaccurate, but it remains common medical practice to refer to errors of this type as "literal paraphasias." The doubting examiner may well wonder how the patient's language comprehension can be so intact if the speech utterances are so distorted, in some cases to the point of meaningless jargon. This thesis assumes a surface lesion, such as would be expected from the embolic infarction that is almost invariably the responsible lesion. It matches with studies suggesting that the major difficulty experienced by affected patients in repeating aloud can be considered to represent a disturbance in encoding accompanied by a disturbance in short-term memory.[262] A patient with this syndrome showed CT evidence of an anterior parietal infarct.

The question of whether the impairment in conduction aphasia represents mere phonologic mistargeting or is truly language based was raised for us again when we encountered a patient with a dilated cardiomyopathy who

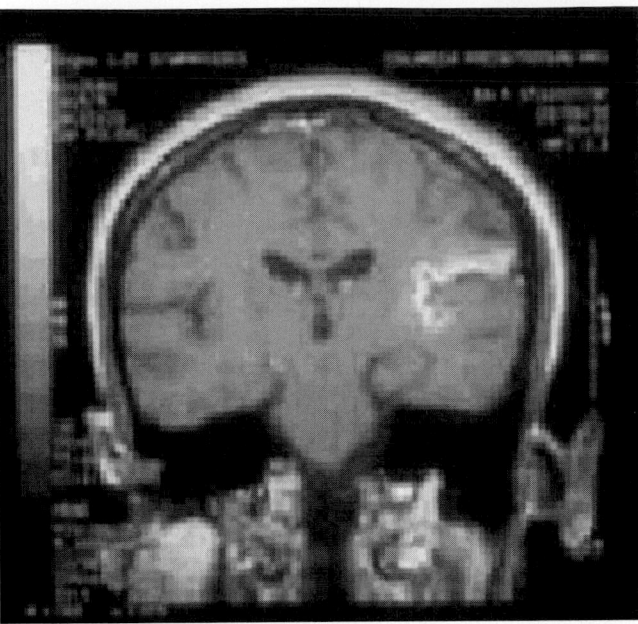

FIGURE 7–21 *Coronal T1-weighted MR image with contrast enhancement showing a posterior insular cortex infarct in a patient with conduction aphasia featuring semantic errors.*

experienced a syndrome of fluent conversational speech, normal auditory and reading comprehension, and repetition that was halting and effortful.[263] Nearly all of this patient's paraphasic errors—on naming, on repetition, on reading aloud, and on writing—were semantic substitutions. For example, "The quarterback threw the football down the field on Saturday" became "The quarterback through the baseball into the field." High-resolution MRI identified an infarct restricted to the posterior left insular cortex and intrasylvian parietal operculum (Fig. 7–21).

As a result of the more modern studies using brain imaging, it has been recognized for some time that the syndrome may occur from a lower division infarct, a point that should further trouble the thesis that Wernicke's aphasia results from superior temporal plane disease. Kleist[217] suggested that some form of mixed hemisphere dominance accounts for the patients with conduction aphasia instead of Wernicke's aphasia from an infarction of the superior temporal plane. We and others have considered the disturbance merely a mild form of sensory aphasia.[264] Many affected patients show some level of decreased auditory comprehension when tested, but their ability to read aloud and for comprehension is so much superior that they do not easily qualify as having the full syndrome of Wernicke's aphasia as traditionally defined. However, they would easily be described as having the mild form of Wernicke's aphasia.

Transcortical Aphasia

The observation of an aphasic syndrome with relatively intact ability to repeat dictated material aloud is attributed to Wernicke,[255,265] but Goldstein[194,266] has been recognized for his attempt to establish a separate entity characterized by an "isolation of the speech area." The traditional inference has been that the sylvian region is preserved, as demonstrated by intact repetition skills, and that the responsible lesion for the aphasic disorder is elsewhere. The exact anatomic basis is less well established than the term *transcortical* suggests, but three syndrome subsets have been described—motor, sensory, and mixed—corresponding to the major motor, major sensory, and global aphasias, respectively, except for the presence of otherwise preserved repetition.[267,268]

Transcortical motor aphasia (TCMA) resembles major motor aphasia (limited spontaneous speech, good comprehension) with relatively intact repetition,[256] although significant variations have made any single underlying explanation of the behavioral and anatomic mechanisms problematic. The language of some patients matches the classic behavioral description, but lesions have been found in the white matter anterolateral to the left frontal horn. They have been caused by infarction or hemorrhage in the upper division of the MCA. They demonstrated that the expected lesion location for TCMA produces varying degrees of impaired articulation, mild deficits in auditory comprehension, and stuttering. TCMA has also been described as a phase during the evolution of Broca's syndrome. It has also been observed that motor language syndromes with good repetition occur during the recovery process after infarction in the territory of the anterior cerebral artery, usually involving the supplementary motor area in the paramedian region of the frontal lobe.

Transcortical sensory aphasia (TCSA) resembles a major sensory syndrome consisting of fluent speech, impaired comprehension, alexia with agraphia, and paraphasic errors, but relatively preserved repetition ability.[269] Patients often display compulsive repetition (echolalia), suggesting more linguistic competence than is actually the case. The responsible lesion is usually large, occurring in the territory of the posterior cerebral artery and involving the temporoparieto-occipital junction[270]; occasionally an isolated thalamic infarct is present. The broad range of cognitive deficits often seen in conjunction with TCSA, including amnestic and attentional disturbances,[271] has clouded its status as a separable aphasic disorder.

Mixed transcortical aphasia is the entity to which Goldstein[266] made reference in 1917 as "isolation of the speech." These patients have a global aphasia except for retention of good repetition and virtually no other capacity for receptive or expressive propositional language. This is a very unusual syndrome. Only a small number of cases have been reported, mostly in patients with stroke, with the study of patients during the evolution of global aphasia or instances of recurrent stroke.[258] In the setting of acute stroke with no prior language disturbance, mixed transcortical aphasia has been said to occur from occlusion of the left internal carotid artery, resulting in simultaneous embolism in the anterior pial territory and perfusion failure in the terminal branches of the middle and posterior cerebral arteries.[272]

Functional Imaging in Aphasia

Following infarction, regional changes in cerebral blood flow and metabolism can be identified by single-photon emission CT (SPECT), positron emission tomography (PET), or ultrafast MRI. Hypoperfusion and hypometabolism may extend into the peri-infarct area or may be seen at a site distant from the lesion itself.[273] With the ability to evaluate physiologic effects of structural lesions in regions adjacent to or remote from the territory of infarction has come a reexamination of some clinicopathologic correlations.

Patients with moderate to severe aphasia often show regions of hypometabolism encompassing large frontoparietal or temporoparietal areas, even in the presence of modest cortical or subcortical structural lesions.[228,267,274,298] Larger metabolic defects in the acute phase of hemispheral stroke that extend beyond the borders of infarction[275,276] correlate with worse initial clinical state and appear to predict poorer recovery from aphasia.[277,278] Reversal of cortical hypometabolism may correlate with clinical improvement when lesions are deep,[231,279] although in some cases of subcortical stroke, cortical hypometabolism may persist for at least 3 months despite good clinical recovery.[280]

A PET study by Metter and colleagues[275] suggests that different aphasias may share common regions of hypometabolism regardless of lesion site. These researchers studied 44 aphasic patients with fluorodeoxyglucose (F 18) PET. Nineteen patients had "anomic," 10 had "Broca's," 8 had "conduction," 5 had "Wernicke's," 1 had "global," and 1 had "transcortical" aphasia. The researchers found that 97% of patients had metabolic decreases in the left angular gyrus, 87% in the left supramarginal gyrus, and 85% in the left posterior superior temporal gyrus. Taken all together, 100% of the patients had PET abnormalities in the left parietotemporal region. A greater degree of hypometabolism in the prefrontal region was the only imaging feature that distinguished patients with Broca's aphasia from those with Wernicke's aphasia. In functional imaging studies of normal controls performing language tasks, hyperperfusion or hypermetabolism has been demonstrated in certain brain regions. The superior temporal gyrus has been implicated both in the early acoustic processing of words and nonwords[281–283] and in the word-retrieval process required to generate verbs from noun stimuli.[284] The prefrontal region and supplementary motor area may also play a role in word selection and output.[283]

Functional imaging has also been used to explore the pathophysiology of atypical aphasias. Cappa and associates[285] showed that in two right-handed aphasics with right-sided lesions (periventricular corona radiata and lentiform nucleus), there was not only widespread hypometabolism in right cortical and subcortical structures but also decreased metabolism in the left frontal and parietal cortex, suggesting that the left hemisphere played a role in the aphasia even though the structural lesion was restricted to the right. Contralateral hemispheral contributions have also been evoked in cases of transcortical aphasias. When structural damage has unexpectedly included the left perisylvian region, SPECT and ^{133}Xe regional cerebral blood flow studies have revealed extensive hypoperfusion throughout the left hemisphere but increased blood flow in the contralateral right temporal lobe.[267] Finally, in a patient with a conduction aphasia in which the paraphasic errors were nearly all semantic substitutions, MRI showed an infarct restricted to the posterior left insular cortex and intrasylvian parietal operculum, but SPECT revealed hypometabolism in the inferomedial and lateral left temporal lobe, suggesting a physiologic but nonischemic role for these regions in the syndrome.[286]

Important functional information can also be obtained by imaging aphasic patients while they are actively engaged in a language task. Such functional imaging studies have begun to elucidate the functional reorganization that is associated with recovery of stroke-induced deficits. Although some investigators have reported that contrahemispheral mirror locations correlate with the recovery process in mildly affected aphasics, others claim that peri-infarct and other ipsilateral regions are crucial for recovery and that activation in the contralateral hemisphere may correlate with persistence of aphasia.[287] Most of the evidence to date suggests that the right hemisphere contributes to recovery from aphasia, particularly in the early phase, with ultimate recovery depending on return of function in the left hemisphere.

In a PET study of 12 aphasic patients with strokes in the left MCA territory, Heiss and coworkers[288] observed unique activation during a word-repetition task 3 to 4 weeks after the patients had experienced stroke in the right supplementary motor area (SMA); this activation was not seen in 10 roughly age-matched controls. Then, in follow-up PET performed 18 months after stroke, return of left superior temporal (Wernicke's area) activity was shown to be associated with good performance on an auditory comprehension task, suggesting that it was the return of left hemisphere function over time that was important in good recovery. Additional evidence that right hemisphere involvement in language was only the second-best mediator of recovery was demonstrated by the findings that (1) persistence of the right SMA activity was *inversely* correlated with performance on the language comprehension task and (2) persistence of right temporal activation was inversely correlated with recovery of left temporal activity. In a follow-up study, the same investigators performed PET imaging at 1 week and 8 weeks after cortical or subcortical stroke in 23 aphasic patients. They observed unique activation in the right inferior frontal region at 1 week. Good recovery of language correlated with activity in the left superior temporal region at 1 week, 8 weeks, or both and also with a disappearance of the right hemisphere activation. Patients with stroke whose original infarcts destroyed the left superior temporal region were not able to incorporate Wernicke's area back into a language network, and this was the reason, the investigators argued, that these patients had a worse prognosis for language recovery.[288]

Further evidence to support the functional significance of brain reorganization after stroke can be gained by performing functional imaging before and after a specific rehabilitative intervention. Only a few studies of this type have been done to date. The right superior temporal gyrus and left precuneus were reported to be associated with improvements in language comprehension after brief, intense language therapy in a group of four patients with post-stroke Wernicke's aphasia.[289,290] The study did not contain a comparison group who did not receive the therapy, however. Ipsihemispheral translocation of language function has also been demonstrated in patients with AVMs in the posterior, dominant hemisphere,[291] but contralesional extension of function has been seen in right frontal AVM.[228] Whatever the mechanism, it seems clear that the brain is capable of reorganization. The patho-physiology of this process remains to be elucidated.

Pharmacologic Intervention in Aphasia Treatment

Although imaging has given us descriptions of new regions assuming control of language after stroke, little is known about the means by which such areas come to acquire these functions. An approach that might ultimately shed light on recovery mechanisms is the systematic delivery of pharmacologic agents. Early animal studies by Feeney and colleagues,[292] for example, showed that administration of D-amphetamines given to rats 24 hours after surgical resection of the motor cortex produced acceleration of function. Later studies have shown these same facilitating effects in rats after experimenter-induced stroke.[293,294] After several investigations in patients with post-stroke weakness had positive results,[295–297] Walker-Batson and associates[296] showed, in a double-blind, placebo-controlled study of 21 patients with aphasia, that dextroamphetamine produced greater improvement in language scores at 1 week, but the differences were not significant when corrected for multiple comparisons.

How this class of stimulants promotes recovery remains unclear, however, so others have sought to administer pharmacologic agents that target specific transmitter systems. For example, there is good evidence that cholinergic transmission mediates cognitive processes.[298] Jacobs and colleagues[299] were among the earliest groups to demonstrate that physostigmine could ameliorate anomia in aphasic patients. Tanaka and coworkers[300] found that open-label administration of the cholinergic agonist bifemelane in 2 of 4 patients who had fluent aphasia with temporal lesions produced improvement in naming and comprehension; the 2 untreated patients showed no changes on follow-up testing. Similarly, Hughes and coworkers[301] successfully treated a patient with aphasia arising from subcortical infarction with the acetylcholinesterase inhibitor donepezil, chosen because of the presumed selective action of acetylcholine (ACh) in behaviorally relevant cortex.

The efficiency of naming seems especially vulnerable to the volume of disease in the hippocampus,[302] especially the CA1 region, which depends heavily on ACh, is believed to be important for both memory storage and retrieval systems, and projects to multiple regions in the cerebral cortex.[303] Although ACh appears to induce plasticity as a facilitator of other mechanisms, such as N-methyl-D-aspartate (NMDA) receptor–dependent long-term potentiation, it has also been shown to be an independent initiator of plasticity in rats.[304] The administration of dopaminergic agents after stroke apparently has a role that combines controlling functions for both motor performance and cognition.[305] Studies in animals and humans report that the dopamine agonist bromocriptine has improved aphasia (left hemisphere function) and left hemineglect (right hemisphere function). With regard to restoration of language after stroke, bromocriptine has been most extensively studied for treatment of motor (nonfluent) aphasias. Positive results in post-stroke patients in the initial study[306] were followed by negative findings in a second study,[307] although the patients in the latter study were described only as "brain-injured." Later work with a higher dose of bromocriptine in the first double-blind study involving patients whose strokes had occurred more than 1 year previously showed statistically significant improvement in verbal latency, repetition, reading comprehension, dictation, and free speech.[308,309] Bragoni and associates[309] propose that these findings result from dopamine's active role in neuronal projections from the midbrain to frontal brain regions, including supplementary motor areas (SMAs) and the cingulate gyrus. Speech impairment and motor planning deficits of the articulatory apparatus have been associated with the cingulate and SMA projections to the basal ganglia. Naeser and colleagues,[310,311] who reviewed CT scans of patients with severe nonfluent aphasia, judged that extensive white matter lesions in the frontal lobe were necessary for significant impairment of spontaneous speech.

We (RML, RSM) have sought to determine the importance of a transmitter system in stroke recovery through the demonstration that once a function has significantly improved after infarction, former stroke or TIA deficits can be transiently reinduced with a targeted sedating agent. For example, we administered the short-acting gamma-aminobutyric acid A (GABA$_A$) agonist midazolam to eight post-stroke patients.[312] Those with left cerebral injury demonstrated reemergence of aphasia, right-sided weakness, or both, but never left-sided weakness or left hemineglect. Conversely, patients who had suffered a right cerebral stroke demonstrated left-sided weakness, hemineglect, or both, but no aphasia or right-sided paresis. More work is needed with larger numbers of patients to clarify the relationships among the extent of deficit at stroke onset, the course of stroke recovery, and the severity of deficits later elicited by GABAergic and other agents.

Apraxias

Apraxias are acquired disorders of execution. They represent an inability to perform a previously learned, skilled act that is unexplained by weakness, visual loss, incoordination, dementia, sensory loss, or aphasia. Liepmann[313,314] described apraxia as the "incapacity for purposive movement despite retained mobility." Apraxic patients are unable to perform skilled acts because they either have lost or cannot access the motor engrams (programs) that guide skilled acts. Because these deficits in skilled movement are rarely complete, the term *dyspraxia* is often used. Apraxic deficits may affect movements of the body, face, or limbs. Liepmann proposed that the left hemisphere possesses the motor engrams necessary for skilled movements, just as it possesses the linguistic engrams necessary for speech. Kimura and Archibald[315] have also postulated left hemisphere dominance for skilled motor activity. The overwhelming proportion of right-handed patients with motor apraxia have left hemisphere lesions.[316] Ajuriaguerra and colleagues[317] noted 47 cases of ideomotor apraxia and 11 cases of ideational apraxia among 206 patients with left retrorolandic lesions and 55 patients with bilateral hemisphere lesions; motor apraxia was absent in the 151 patients with right retrorolandic lesions.

Ideomotor Apraxia

The most common type of motor apraxia is ideomotor apraxia. Liepmann[313,314] believed that dissociation occurs between the brain areas that contain the "ideas" for move-

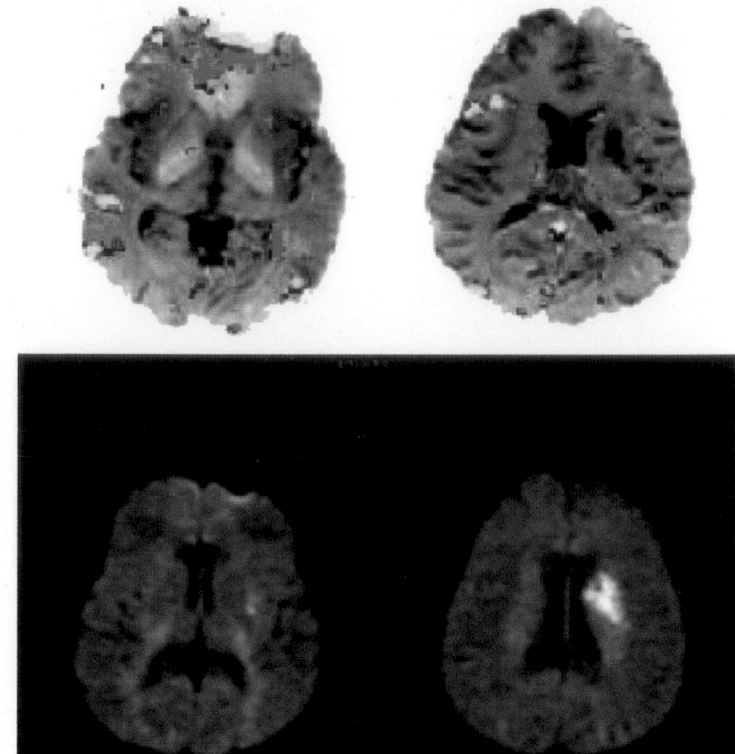

PLATE 7–1 *Aphasia recovery. Activation seen in the right frontal and temporal lobes in regions homologous to Broca's and Wernicke's areas. Infarct in left basal ganglia and periventricular white matter seen on diffusion-weighted MR image.*

ments and the "motor" areas responsible for execution. As a result, skilled movements involving the limbs are not executed accurately. Ideomotor apraxia may be elicited by asking patients to show how they would salute, wave goodbye, hammer a nail, saw wood, and so forth. In the most severe cases, the action cannot be performed at all. In moderately severe cases, the actions are vague and confused. In milder cases, the actions are clumsy and lack precision. In general, the worst performance is elicited on verbal command. Performance may improve on imitation but still remains abnormal.[318] The best performance is elicited on actual use of the object.[202] Ideomotor apraxia can take two forms—bilateral ideomotor apraxia, in which both extremities are affected, and sympathetic apraxia (callosal apraxia), in which the apraxia is limited to the nondominant left arm. Although the left hemisphere is dominant in most right-handed persons for both language and skilled motor activity, apraxia does not depend on the presence of dysphasia. Furthermore, although aphasia commonly accompanies ideomotor apraxia, there is no close relationship between ideomotor apraxia and either the severity or the type of aphasia.[319–321] Geschwind[258] has suggested cerebral disconnection between the language area and the premotor area in the frontal lobe as an explanation for ideomotor apraxia. Lesions in the vicinity of the left supramarginal gyrus with deep extension into the subjacent white matter could interrupt impulses originating in Wernicke's area that were directed toward the premotor area.

Heilman[322] has suggested an alternative explanation. He believes that the motor programs for skilled motor movements are stored in the left superior parietal lobe. Skilled motor activity depends on the transmission of these programs to the premotor area in the left frontal lobe. Ideomotor apraxia may then arise from either (1) direct destruction of motor programs in the left superior parietal lobe or (2) destruction of the pathways from the left superior parietal lobe to the premotor area of the left frontal lobe (i.e., disconnection).[323] Typically, bilateral ideomotor apraxia is associated with retrorolandic lesions in the vicinity of the parietal lobe.[318] These lesions are usually superficial cortical infarcts in the distribution of the posterior division of the left MCA. Although ideomotor apraxia is more common with superficial than with deep lesions, large, deep lesions may produce ideomotor apraxia.[215] Ideomotor apraxia does not occur with smaller lacune-type infarctions. Little is known about recovery from ideomotor apraxia.[202] However, recovery may be surprisingly rapid in certain cases. Anterior lesions have a better prognosis for recovery than posterior lesions.[319]

Ideational Apraxia

Ideational apraxia, a disorder of the sequencing and planning of complex motor acts,[324] bears an uncertain relation to ideomotor apraxia. It can be elicited by asking the patient to demonstrate complex motor tasks, such as lighting a candle or mailing a letter. Hecaen and Gimeno[318] reported 8 cases of ideational apraxia among 47 cases of ideomotor apraxia. Sittig[325] believed that ideational apraxia is only a severe form of ideomotor apraxia, but others hold that they are distinct entities.[326,327]

Ideational apraxia is generally observed after dominant hemisphere parietal lobe lesions. Associated findings may include a fluent aphasia (anomic, semantic, or Wernicke's), constructional apraxia, and elements of Gerstmann's syndrome. Dementia and confusion are noted in some cases. The localization is the same as what might be expected to produce ideomotor apraxia. Bilateral parietal lesions are present in some cases,[317,328] but isolated right parietal lesions seem to produce ideational apraxia only in individuals with anomalous cerebral dominance.[329] Little is known about the improvement over time and whether there is "recovery" or simply a new strategy in responding.

Limb-Kinetic Apraxia

Limb-kinetic (also innervational or melokinetic) apraxia is manifested as a lack of rapidity, skill, and delicacy in the performance of learned motor movements.[316] Liepmann held that in limb-kinetic apraxia "the virtuosity which practice lends to movement is lost. Therefore the movements are . . . clumsy, without precision" (quoted by Kertesz[330]). The patient is clumsy in the execution of common motor acts, such as the manipulation of objects (eating utensils, combs, brushes, saws, hammers, playing cards, and so forth). Limb-kinetic apraxia is unilateral and affects the limb contralateral to the cerebral lesion.

It may be difficult to distinguish between limb-kinetic apraxia and paresis in some cases. Commonly associated neurologic signs are ataxia, choreoathetosis, grasping, spasticity, weakness, and dystonic posturing. However, the clumsiness in using objects is out of proportion to these other deficits. The perseverative and conceptual disturbances that characterize ideational apraxia are not prominent. Patients with limb-kinetic apraxia respond poorly to commands or imitations. Performance may improve slightly with use of the object, but patients often act as if they were somewhat unfamiliar with its use.

Limb-kinetic apraxia may occur after injury to either the right or left premotor cortex or subjacent white matter.[239] Slight weakness is usually present, suggesting that injury to the pyramidal pathways is an essential feature of limb-kinetic apraxia. However, injury limited solely to the pyramidal pathways does not produce limb-kinetic apraxia. Patients with pure motor hemiplegia due to lacunar infarction in the internal capsule do not manifest limb-kinetic apraxia. Thus, the elicitation of this sign is a useful indicator that the surface cortex or subjacent white matter has been injured. The diagnosis of limb-kinetic apraxia is rarely made, reflecting the doubts of some as to its validity as an apraxic entity discrete from either pyramidal weakness or ideomotor apraxia.

Callosal Apraxia

Callosal apraxia (sympathetic apraxia) represents a restricted form of ideomotor apraxia in which the apraxia is limited to the nondominant arm. Liepmann and Maas[264] first described a patient with a right hemiplegia who was unable to perform skilled movements with his nonparetic left arm. Similar patients have been described by Geschwind and Kaplan[331] and by Watson and Heilman.[332] Critical to the syndrome is disruption of the anterior portions of the corpus callosum. Infarction of the medial or anterior left frontal lobe with Broca's aphasia and right hemiplegia is often present, but these elements are not critical to the genesis of the apraxia.

The apraxia is unilateral and limited to the nondominant arm. If the right arm is not paretic, it can be demonstrated to be free of apraxia. The apraxia of the left arm is similar to the bilateral apraxia that characterizes ideomotor apraxia. Two somewhat similar hypotheses have been offered to explain callosal apraxia. Geschwind[258] has suggested that callosal apraxia is due to a disconnection of the right premotor region from the speech area in the left temporal lobe. Verbal instructions are unable to traverse the anterior corpus callosum and reach the right premotor cortex. Hence, the left arm is deprived of verbal instructions to guide its motor activity. The patient described by Geschwind and Kaplan[331] was able to perform skilled movements with his left arm on imitation but not on verbal command; however, this has not been the general experience. Thus, this hypothesis does not explain why patients with callosal apraxia continue to be apraxic upon use of an object or on imitation of the examiner. Heilman[322] suggested that the left arm is apraxic because it is disconnected from the motor engram centers in the left hemisphere.

The lesion producing callosal apraxia may be a rare, isolated lesion of the corpus callosum. More commonly, the crossing callosal fibers are disrupted in the mesial left hemisphere by an infarction either in the left anterior cerebral artery territory or in the distribution of the anterior division of the left MCA. These anterior division left MCA territory infarctions are associated with right hemiplegia and Broca's aphasia. Injury to the corpus callosum rather than to the left supplementary motor cortex is critical to the syndrome.[333]

Oral-Buccal-Lingual Apraxia

Orofacial or oral-buccal-lingual apraxia is the inability to perform skilled movements with the oral and facial musculature on command. Hughlings-Jackson[200] had noted that some patients are unable to protrude their tongues on command. In addition, these patients may be unable to pucker their lips, cough, lick their lips, puff up their cheeks, or whistle on verbal command. They may, however, be able to perform the same acts well spontaneously. De Renzi and colleagues[324] found oral apraxia in 90% of patients with Broca's aphasia and 33% of those with conduction aphasia in one study. Oral apraxia is unusual in cases of anomic or Wernicke's aphasia. Although oral apraxia is common in global aphasia, testing for oral apraxia may be difficult because of comprehension disturbances. Hecaen and Albert[334] have emphasized that oral-buccal-lingual apraxia is not synonymous with Broca's aphasia, because some patients with Broca's aphasia are not dyspraxic and some subjects with oral-buccal-lingual apraxia are not aphasic.

Oral-buccal-lingual apraxia generally results from an inferior frontal lesion in the premotor cortex adjacent to the face area on the motor strip. Most lesions are cortical and superficial.[386] Occasionally, oral-buccal-lingual apraxia may result from large, deep lesions.[7]

SYNDROMES OF RIGHT HEMISPHERAL INFARCTION

A wide variety of behavioral abnormalities may follow stroke in the right MCA territory. These deficits are governed in general by several unifying observations.

1. Despite some rudimentary capacity to comprehend language, language plays no important role in the activities subserved by the right hemisphere.
2. The commitment of the cerebral cortex to a specific higher cortical function is less precise in the right hemisphere than in the left hemisphere. Although higher cortical functions in the left hemisphere appear to be governed by identifiable "centers" of function, higher cortical functions of the right hemisphere appear to be governed by far-flung "networks."
3. The right hemisphere is dominant for certain aspects of attention,[303] including directed attention, focused attention, and vigilance. This specialization for attention may be reflected in a variety of right hemisphere deficits, such as neglect, extinction, and impersistence.
4. Many spatial and quasispatial operations are performed by the right hemisphere. This specialization for spatial operations may be reflected in such right hemisphere deficits as prosopagnosia,[335] topographic disorientation, constructional apraxia, and dressing apraxia.
5. Confabulatory behaviors are more common after right than left hemisphere injury.[258] Both reduplicative paramnesia and anosognosia may be considered forms of confabulation that occur after right hemisphere stroke.

Patients without the many neurologic deficits from right hemispheral infarction do much better in rehabilitation than patients with these deficits. Although some patients show a steady recovery from these deficits (Plate 7–1 following page 152), others are left with persistent and disabling behavioral abnormalities, including constructional and dressing apraxias, left neglect, and motor impersistence. The size of the lesion, rather than its exact location, is a better predictor of behavioral deficits after right hemisphere damage (Fig. 7–22).

Neglect and Extinction

Extinction and neglect are two forms of hemi-inattention that may occur after right hemisphere stroke. *Extinction* implies that a "stimulus is not perceived only when a second stimulus is presented simultaneously—usually but not necessarily on the opposite side of the body."[336] Unilateral spatial neglect (USN) is a restricted syndrome in which patients fail to copy one side (usually the left) of a figure, fail to read one side of words or sentences, and bisect lines far to the right of center. The term *neglect* implies a more flagrant syndrome characterized by a failure of the patient to attend to new stimuli coming from one side (usually the left).

Neglect is often trimodal (auditory, visual, and tactile). In left-sided neglect, the patient may not explore the left side of space; the eyes and body may be turned tonically to the right.[158] Neglect is characterized by "a lack of responsivity to stimuli on one side of the body, in the absence of any sensory or motor deficit severe enough to account for the imperception."[337] Battersby and associates[338] found USN in 29% of their right brain–damaged patients and 12% of their left brain–damaged patients. Most subjects with USN had lesions involving either the parieto-occipital or temporo-occipital regions. Using a

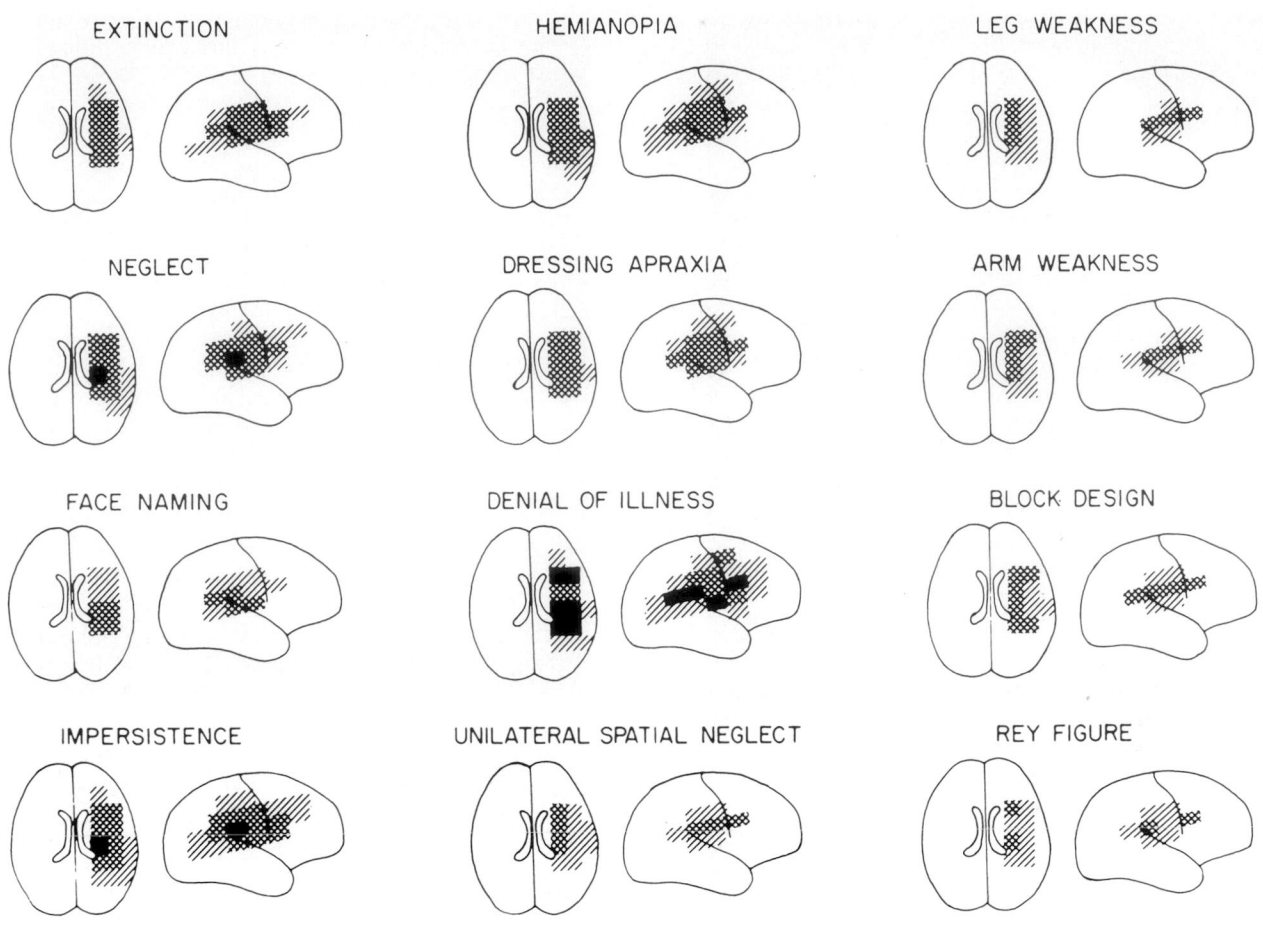

FIGURE 7–22   *Topography of infarction as documented by CT scan for patients with nondominant hemisphere deficits. (From Hier DB, Mondlock J, Caplan LR: Behavioral abnormalities after right hemisphere stroke. Neurology [NY] 33:337, 1983.)*

line-bisection test, Schenkenberg and colleagues[339] found USN to be more common after right than left brain damage.

The mechanism underlying USN is uncertain. Hemianopia, oculomotor disorders, or dementia cannot account for the phenomenon. Heilman and Valenstein[340] suggested that hemispatial hypokinesia due to hypoarousal explains USN on drawing tasks. Related to the syndrome of USN is more gross ignorance of the neglect. Affected patients behave as if they have completely lost the left side of space and the left side of their bodies. They may ignore visitors on their left side or fail to attend to sounds coming from the left. Marked left neglect tends to occur in conjunction with other markers of severe right hemisphere damage, including anosognosia (i.e., implicit unawareness of illness and its clinical manifestations)[154] and motor impersistence. By contrast, USN may occur with smaller right hemisphere strokes, which usually have a good prognosis (Fig. 7–23).

Neglect has been traditionally attributed to injury in the vicinity of the right parietal lobe. However, neglect may follow injury to the right frontal lobe,[165] right cingulum,[341] right lenticular nucleus, or right thalamus.[342] Because injury to a variety of cortical and subcortical structures produces left neglect, a cortical network in the right hemisphere underlying directed attention has been proposed.[343]

Mesulam[344] posited a "network" model for attention that consists of a reticular element (providing arousal and vigilance), a parietal element (providing sensory and spatial mapping), a frontal element (providing the motor programs for exploration), and a limbic element. Data from the series of 34 patients reported by Binder and coworkers[345] support the notion that the nature of the neglect syndrome may vary according to whether the lesion lies in the upper or lower division of the right MCA. In a sensory-motor dichotomy analogous to that found in aphasia syndromes, 11 patients with infarction in the lower division of the right MCA demonstrated rightward deviation on line bisection with an otherwise minimal or no defect on letter cancellation, suggesting abnormality in perceptual function. By contrast, 10 patients with lesions in the upper division showed neglect on letter cancellation but performed normally on line bisection, suggesting a defect in motor search behavior. In a later study, one of the authors (DBH) has also described a seemingly obligatory intrusion of other stimuli into the performance of spatial judgment in patients with right hemisphere injury.

Anosognosia (i.e., unawareness of illness or its clinical manifestations) is more likely to be associated with severe as opposed to mild hemiparesis.[346–348] Williams and associates[347] also noted an association between anosognosia and severity of hemiparesis. Nonetheless, Bisiach and

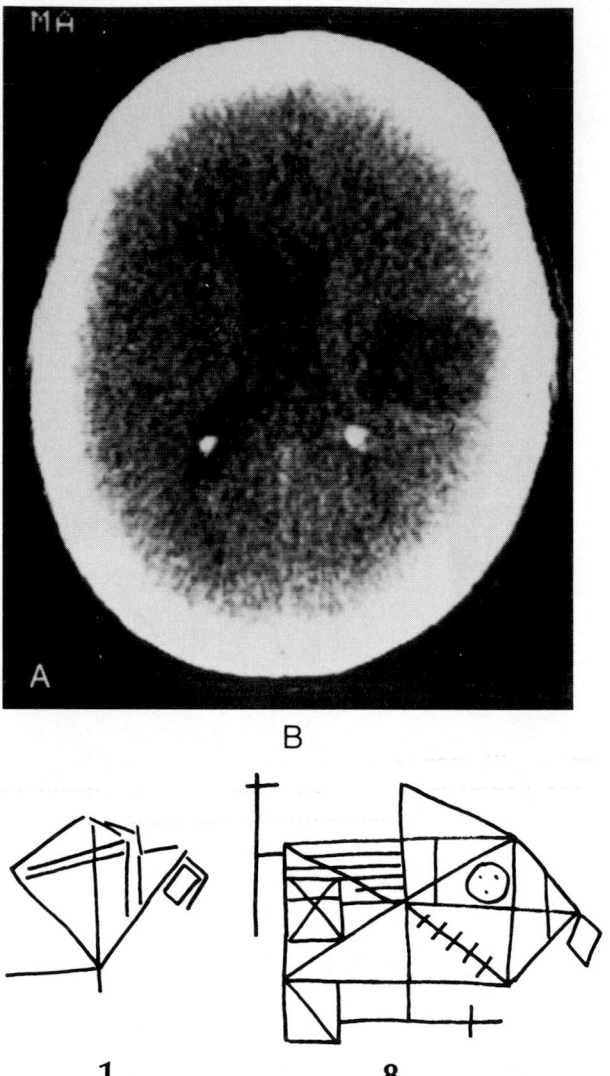

FIGURE 7–23   A, *CT scan of small right middle cerebral artery territory infarct.* B, *Drawings made by the patient with the infarct shown in A at 1 and 8 weeks after stroke.*

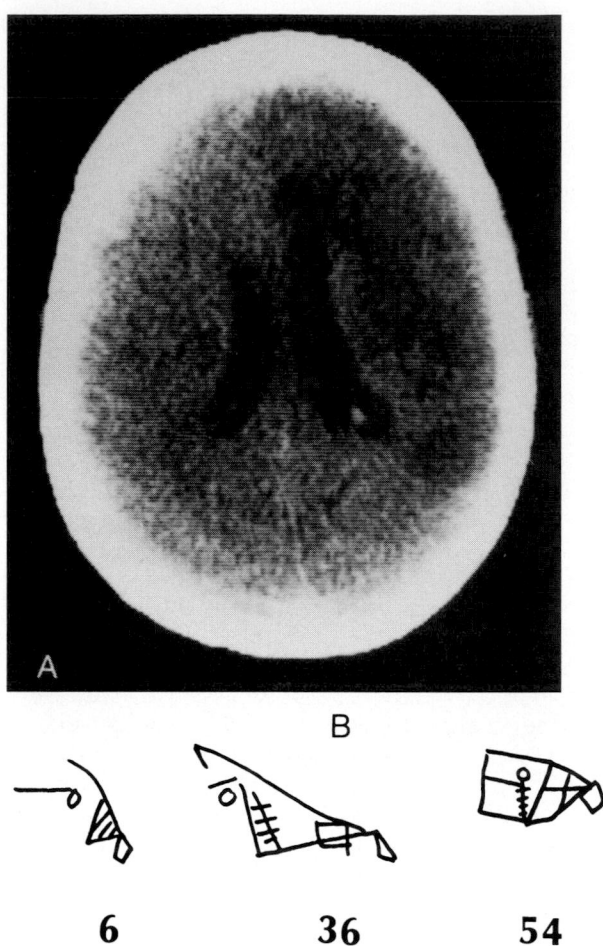

FIGURE 7–24   A, *CT scan of large right middle cerebral artery territory infarct.* B, *Drawings done by the patient with the infarct shown in A at 6, 36, and 54 weeks after stroke.*

coworkers[349] have shown that anosognosia for either hemianopia or hemiparesis can be dissociated from elementary[349] neurologic deficits or neglect. Hier and colleagues[346,350] found, in 15 patients with acute right hemisphere stroke followed up longitudinally, that all recovered from anosognosia within 22 weeks.

The lesion producing anosognosia is usually large. Hier and colleagues[346] found that the responsible lesion is often extended beyond the parietal lobe to the frontal and temporal lobes (Fig. 7–24). Extension of the lesion to the deep white matter and basal ganglia was common. It is probably incorrect to call anosognosia a "right parietal" phenomenon, because many of the lesions are massive and involve much of the right MCA territory (both deep and superficial structures). Involvement of the occipital lobe does not appear to be essential to development of anosognosia. On occasion, small, deep lesions (often basal ganglionic hemorrhages) may produce anosognosia, presumably by undercutting and isolating the cortex of the right hemisphere.

Sensory loss, confusion, or dementia cannot adequately account for anosognosia. Gerstmann[351] has viewed anosognosia as a disorder of a hypothetical "body image." Although he believed that this body image is "mapped" into the left parietal lobe, input from the right parietal lobe is essential in updating the left parietal lobe as to the condition of the left side of the body. Injury to the right parietal lobe, or to connecting pathways between the right and left parietal lobes, could lead to anosognosia. Geschwind[237] suggested that anosognosia may be due to a disconnection syndrome that prevents sensory impressions from reaching the central language zone in the left hemisphere. Another explanation for anosognosia is that structures essential for the recognition of hemiplegia or other body defects are localized to the right hemisphere. Injury to the right hemisphere could produce an agnosia for illness by disrupting structures essential for the recognition of illness. Finally, anosognosia may be viewed as a variation of "neglect" or "inattention" in that the patient with anosognosia fails to "attend" to the hemiplegia.

Impersistence

In 1956, Fisher[352] described 10 patients with left hemiplegia who were unable to persist at a variety of willed acts, including eye closure, breath-holding, conjugate gaze deviation, tongue protrusion, and hand gripping. Fisher introduced the new term *impersistence* to describe "this failure to persist in a motor act." He noted that "mental impairment of some degree was always present" and that impersistence was "encountered almost exclusively in association with left hemiplegia." Many of the patients had accompanying left neglect, constructional apraxia, and anosognosia.

Joynt and colleagues[353] documented impersistence in 19% of 48 patients with left hemisphere damage and 26% of 34 patients with right hemisphere damage. These investigators found impersistence to be more common in patients with mental impairment, especially visuospatial deficits. However, Levin[354] could not demonstrate a higher incidence of impersistence after right than after left hemisphere damage. Ben-Yishay and associates[355] found a correlation between impersistence and visuomotor and visuospatial deficits. In addition, impersistence proved to bode poorly for rehabilitation efforts. Later studies have confirmed a right hemisphere localization for motor impersistence,[356] and Hier and coworkers[346] found impersistence in 46% of 41 subjects with acute right hemisphere strokes.

Impersistence correlated with a variety of other deficits, including severity of hemiparesis, prosopagnosia, dressing apraxia, constructional apraxia, left neglect, and anosognosia.[346] Motor impersistence occurred only after the largest lesions. Injury generally extended to the frontal, parietal, temporal, and deep structures. No specific locus of injury for "impersistence" was found within the right hemisphere. Rather, impersistence reflected diffuse and widespread dysfunction. Hier and coworkers[357] found recovery from motor impersistence to be quite indolent.

The mechanism underlying impersistence is unknown. Motor impersistence may reflect a depletion of vigilance or of sustained attention after widespread injury to the right hemisphere. The anatomic locus of the structures involved in sustained attention and vigilance is unknown. Widespread networks in the right hemisphere may underlie focused attention.

Dressing Apraxia

Brain[358] described "apraxia for dressing" in 1941. *Dressing apraxia* refers to confusions in the orientation of clothing during dressing. As McFie and colleagues[359] commented, these "difficulties appeared to be due to confusions regarding top and bottom, back and front, and right and left with reference to the garments." Roth[360] noted the close association between constructional apraxia (see later) and dressing apraxia. Dressing apraxia occurs almost exclusively with lesions of the right hemisphere.

Although constructional apraxia occurs with either right or left hemisphere lesions, the constructional apraxia that occurs with left hemisphere lesions is rarely associated with dressing apraxia. After right hemisphere damage, strokes large enough to produce both dressing apraxia and constructional apraxia are larger than strokes producing only constructional apraxia. Unilateral spatial neglect contributes to difficulties in dressing as well. Dressing apraxia should not be diagnosed in the presence of disabling hemiplegia that interferes with dressing.

Loss of Topographic Memory and Disorientation for Place

Loss of topographic memory is the inability of some patients to find their way in familiar surroundings, to recognize familiar surroundings, and to learn new routes in unfamiliar surroundings. Loss of topographic memory is somewhat different from *disorientation to place*, which refers to confusion about current location.[361]

Critchley[362] described several patients who were constantly getting lost in familiar surroundings. Many of his subjects had biparietal injury. A few had lesions limited to the posterior right hemisphere. He described one patient with a right MCA territory infarction who "will often pass his home without knowing that it is his, and will wander around for many minutes trying to decide where he does live." In milder cases, patients recognize surroundings as familiar; in more severe cases, even very familiar surroundings may seem strange. Critchley described another patient with a right MCA occlusion who could not recognize "the countryside he should have known so well. His home and surroundings are no longer familiar." Loss of topographic memory is uncommon. Hecaen and Angelergues[363] reported 40 cases of loss of topographic memory, 29 in association with right hemisphere lesions and 3 with bilateral lesions. Many patients have bilateral parietal lesions, although some have unilateral right parietal lesions. Landis and coworkers[364] described 16 patients with loss of topographic familiarity; all had right medial temporoparietal lesions. Alsaadi and colleagues,[365] however, have shown that topographic disorientation can occur with unilateral stroke in either hemisphere.

The mechanism underlying loss of topographic memory is uncertain. The failure to recognize familiar surroundings suggests an agnostic defect similar to that underlying prosopagnosia.[366] The inability to follow familiar routes and the inability to orient oneself in space suggest a failure to create an internal spatial representation of the external world. Ross[367] has suggested that visual modality–specific memory defects may underlie both loss of topographic memory deficits and prosopagnosia.

Disorders of Spatial Localization

The right hemisphere plays a special role in the spatial localization of stimuli. This effect has been demonstrated for both visual and auditory stimuli. With regard to determination of spatial orientation of objects in space, the most severe deficits have been noted after posterior right hemisphere damage.[368,369] Short-term spatial memory (a skill analogous to the auditory short-term memory task of digit span) is a dominant function of the posterior right hemisphere.[368] Auditory localization of sounds in space also depends on an intact posterior right hemisphere.[349]

Confusion and Delirium

Acute confusion and delirium are states characterized by impaired orientation, diminished attention, and aberrant perception. Alertness is usually well maintained, clarity and speed of thinking are diminished, and memories are poorly formed. Inattentiveness, poor concentration, and alerting to irrelevant stimuli are present. There is overlap between confusional and delirious states, and some investigators regard delirium as a subset of confusion. Delirium is characterized by disturbed perception with terrifying hallucinations, vivid dreams, fantasies, insomnia, and overactivity.

Acute confusional states have been reported after right MCA infarctions.[370,371] Mesulam and colleagues[372] reported three cases of sudden onset of acute confusion accompanied by retropulsion, unsteady gait, incontinence, difficulty in using common objects, and lack of concern for the illness. Mental agitation evolved into a state of irritable sluggishness, inattention, and memory disorder. Mullalley and associates[373] reported acute confusion in 13 patients with right parietal lobe lesions and in 4 with right temporal lobe lesions. Levine and Finkelstein[374] added 8 patients with a behavioral disorder, characterized by hallucinations, delusions, agitation, and confusion, that was remotely related (by 1 month to 11 years) to right temporoparietal stroke or trauma. Dunne and coworkers[375] found that 3% (19) of 661 patients with stroke presented with delirium, confusion, dementia, or psychosis. Nearly all had right hemisphere lesions. Elementary neurologic findings were either absent or subtle. In 41 patients with right MCA territory infarctions, Mori and Yamadori[336] found acute confusion in 25 and acute delirium in 6.

Caplan and associates[376] found that posterior right temporal lesions were more likely to produce acute confusion than posterior right parietal lesions. The propensity of temporal lesions to produce confusional states may be explained by the proximity of these lesions to the underlying limbic system. Confusional states that follow brain infarction may result from one of two processes: disrupted modulation of affective responses in the limbic system or disruption of right hemisphere networks subserving attention.

Confabulation and Reduplicative Paramnesia

Confabulation, the unintentional production of inappropriate and fabricated information, is often associated with a failure to inhibit incorrect responses, poor error awareness, and poor self-correction abilities. Impaired memory, poor motivation, and anosognosia are often present. Because many of these associated behaviors are characteristics of frontal lobe disease, confabulation is often linked to frontal lobe damage. Although impairment of memory is often associated with confabulation, the two behaviors vary independently in severity.[377,378]

Reduplication is a special form of confabulation. It appears to reflect an attempt of the brain-injured patient to fuse experiences from two disparate periods in his or her life. In instances of reduplication for place, patients hold an inaccurate belief that two versions of a geographic location exist. They wrongly believe that they are residing in a second version of a familiar setting. Hospitalized patients may persist in believing that they are at home or at another hospital despite repeated attempts to orient them to current location. Luria,[379] describing several patients with right hemisphere lesions and reduplication for place, says he will "never forget a group of patients with deep lesions ... of the right hemisphere. ... They firmly believed that at one and the same time they were in

Moscow and also in another town. They suggested that they had left Moscow and gone to the other town. They suggested that they were still in Moscow where an operation had been performed on their brain. Yet they found nothing contradictory about these conclusions."

Environmental reduplication occurs most commonly after right frontoparietal lobe injury. Reduplication of person (a false belief that two versions of an individual exist) may also occur after right hemisphere injury. Like reduplication of place, reduplication of person is a restricted form of confabulation.

Constructional Apraxia

In 1934, Kleist[217] defined *constructional apraxia* as "a disturbance which appears in formative activities (arranging, building, drawing) and in which a spatial part of the task is missed, although there is no apraxia of single movements." Kleist's definition includes the key aspects of constructional apraxia: Patients fail at tasks that require the manipulation of objects in space. A variety of tests have been utilized to identify constructional apraxia, including the copying of block designs, the copying of simple and complex figures, puzzle constructions, mental rotations, and three-dimensional model building. Constructional apraxia is synonymous with other terms, including apractagnosia, constructional disability, and visual-spatial agnosia.

Constructional apraxia occurs after injury to either cerebral hemisphere. Among 67 patients with constructional apraxia, Piercy and colleagues[380] reported 42 with right-sided lesions and 25 with left-sided lesions. Arrigoni and De Renzi[381] found constructional apraxia to be more prevalent in subjects with damage to the right brain than to the left brain. Most lesions are in the vicinity of the parietal lobe. The nature of constructional apraxia differs according to the hemisphere injured. Patients with left-sided lesions improve their drawings when aided by visual cues, whereas patients with right-sided lesions do not. Warrington and colleagues[382] suggested that the constructional apraxia following right hemisphere damage is a visuospatial disorder, whereas that following left hemisphere damage is an executive disorder. The drawings of patients with left hemisphere damage are oversimplified, with reduced detail, whereas left unilateral neglect characterizes the drawings of patients with right hemisphere damage. However, Gainotti and coworkers[383,384] were not able to distinguish right-sided from left-sided constructional apraxia.

Critchley[362] regards constructional apraxia as "an executive defect within a visuospatial domain." Constructional apraxia may also be viewed as a spatial agnosia, that is, a defect in the comprehension of spatial relationships.[385] Similarly, Whitty and Newcombe[386] argued that "the nature of the visual spatial difficulty appears to be of an agnostic rather than simple perceptual type. The term constructional apraxia is not entirely satisfactory." Data from 37 patients in the Neurological Institute Cerebral Localization Laboratory suggest further that abnormal drawing may arise from different behavioral abnormalities correlating with different lesion sites.[286] The patients with marked drawing hemineglect had infarcts in the dorsal posterior parietal region. The patients whose drawings were unrecognizable and who performed poorly on line bisection had lesions in the temporoparieto-occipital junction. Unrecognizable drawings by patients with normal line bisection were produced by lesions in anterior subcortical locations. Similarly, Lazar and colleagues[387] reported the case of a 66-year-old woman with CT-verified infarction in the region of the right caudate nucleus and putamen who was tested with traditional clinical measures of perception, attention, and constructional apraxia, followed by the presentation of matching-to-sample procedures. The clinical measures first showed severe constructional apraxia without hemineglect; the matching procedures then provided demonstrable evidence that she could not copy Greek letter forms that she could otherwise match with perfect accuracy, thereby eliminating perceptual dysfunction as a cause of her deficit.

Allesthesia

Allesthesia (also "allochiria") is the referral of a sensory stimulus (visual, tactile, or auditory) from one side of the body to the other.[17,164] It is most often seen in the setting of right hemisphere damage with left-sided neglect. When the left side is touched, the sensation may be reported by the patient as occurring on the right side. Allesthesia may also occur in the setting of spinal cord injury or conversion hysteria.

Amusia

Amusia (loss of musical ability secondary to brain disease) has been an elusive deficit to study.[388–390] Brust[391] concluded that no simple relationship exists between the location of a lesion and extent of musical disability. Case reports of expressive amusia after right hemisphere lesions are numerous. Affected patients are unable to sing or whistle but their language function and melody recognition are preserved. Receptive amusia may also occur with right hemisphere lesions.

Because of its complexity, the neural basis of music remains obscure. Amusia is an isolated phenomenon that may occur after right hemisphere lesions of varying location, size, and etiology. A remarkable case of a blind organist who suffered left hemispheral infarction with aphasia but without amusia (some of his post-stroke compositions were published) suggests that a clear separation between the two entities is possible.[392]

Aprosody and Affective Agnosia

Monrad-Krohn[393] defined *prosody* as the musical quality of speech produced by "variations in pitch, rhythm, and stress of pronunciation." Buck and Duffy[394] reported that after right hemisphere damage, some patients are unable to intone affect into their speech; this deficit is known as *aprosody*. On the basis of their work and that of Heilman and colleagues,[395] Ross and Mesulam[396] proposed that the right hemisphere was dominant for the modulation of affective language and that this modulation was organized in a fashion analogous to left hemisphere organization for propositional language. In a subsequent study, Ross[385]

provided additional confirmatory evidence of the functional-anatomic organization of the affective components of language in the right hemisphere. By utilizing a combination of a bedside examination strategy analogous to a routine aphasia examination and CT mappings, he observed that the organization of affective language in the right hemisphere mirrored that of propositional language in the left hemisphere. The resulting disturbances of affective modulation were coined the *aprosodias*.

In analogy with the aphasias, Ross[385] proposed the existence of motor, sensory, global, conduction, and transcortical aprosodias. In *motor aprosody*, the patient is unable to utilize prosody to inject affect into speech, nor is the patient able to repeat the affect-laden prosody of others. However, the patient can comprehend the affect conveyed by the prosody of other speakers. The patient with *sensory aprosody* shows poor comprehension of affective prosody and cannot repeat affective prosody but has normal spontaneous affective prosody in speech. *Global aprosody* is reflected in the drawing errors of apraxies. Hecaen and Albert[334] suggest that "constructional apraxia may result from a breakdown in different underlying neuropsychological mechanisms, depending on the hemisphere damaged."

Heilman and Van Den Abell,[397] noting that right temporoparietal lesions cause defects in the comprehension of affective speech, term this disorder *affective agnosia*. Tucker and colleagues[398] observed that right temporoparietal lesions caused deficits both in affective comprehension and in evoking emotional intonation in a speech repetition task.

References

1. Abbie AA: The morphology of the forebrain arteries with especial reference to the evolution of the basal ganglia. J Anat 68:432, 1934.
2. Abbie AA: The vascular supply of the internal capsule. Med J Aust 1934.
3. Beevor CE: On the distribution of the different arteries supplying the human brain. Philos Trans R Soc (Biol) 1908.
4. Foix C, Levy M: Les ramollissements sylviens. Rev Neurol (Paris) 11:51, 1927.
5. Shellshear JC: A contribution to our knowledge of the arterial supply of the cerebral cortex in man. Brain 50:236, 1927.
6. Lazorthes G, Gouaze A, Salomon G: Vascularisation et Circulation de l'Encéphale. Paris, Masson, 1976.
7. Mohr JP, Kase CS, Meckler RJ, Fisher CM: Sensorimotor stroke due to thalamocapsular ischemia. Arch Neurol 34:739, 1977.
8. Alexander L: The vascular supply of the striato-pallidum. Res Publ Assoc Nerv Ment Dis 21:77, 1941.
9. Gibo H, Carver CP, Rhoton AL, et al: Microsurgical anatomy of the middle cerebral artery. J Neurosurg 54:151, 1981.
10. Grand W: Microsurgical anatomy of the proximal middle cerebral artery and the internal carotid artery bifurcation. Neurosurgery 7:151, 1980.
11. Marinkovic R, Markovic L: The role of the middle cerebral artery in the vascularization of the claustrum. Med Pregl 43:361, 1990.
12. Amyes EW, Nielsen JM: Clinicopathologic study of vascular lesions of the anterior cingulate region. Bull Los Angeles Neurol Soc 20:112, 1955.
13. Waddington MM, Ring BA: Syndromes of occlusions of middle cerebral artery branches. Brain 91:685, 1968.
14. Fischer E: Die Lageabweichungen der vorden Hirnarterie im Gefaessbild. Zentralbl Neurochir 3:300, 1938.
15. Teal JS, Rumbaugh CL, Bergeron RT, et al: Anomalies of the middle cerebral artery: Accessory artery, duplication, and early bifurcation. AJR Radium Ther Nucl Med 118:567, 1973.

Clinical Manifestations

56

16. Umansky F, Dujovny M, Ausman JI, et al: Anomalies and variations of the middle cerebral artery: A microanatomical study. Neurosurgery 22:1023, 1988.
17. Jain KK: Some observations on the anatomy of the middle cerebral artery. Can J Surg 7:134, 1964.
18. Akelatis AJ: Symmetrical bilateral granular atrophy of the cerebral cortex of vascular origin: A clinico-pathologic study. Am J Psychiatry 99:447, 1942.
19. Brierley JB, Adams JH, Connor RCR, Triep CS: The effects of systemic hypotension upon the human brain. Brain 89:235, 1966.
20. Romanul FCA, Abramowicz A: Changes in brain and pial vessels in arterial borderzones. Arch Neurol 11:40, 1964.
21. Mohr JP: Neurological complications of cardiac valvular disease and cardiac surgery including systemic hypotension. In Klawans HL (ed): Neurological Manifestations of Systemic Diseases. (Vinken PJ, Bruyn GW [eds]: Handbook of Clinical Neurology, Vol 38.) New York, North-Holland, 1979, p 143.
22. van der Eecken HM: Anastomoses Between the Leptomeningeal Arteries of the Brain. Springfield, IL, Charles C Thomas, 1959.
23. Strong KC: A study of the structure of the media of the distributing arteries by the method of microdissection. Anat Rec 72:151, 1938.
24. Baker AB: Structure of the small cerebral arteries and their changes with age. Am J Pathol 13:453, 1937.
25. Stehbens WE: Focal intimal proliferation in the cerebral arteries. Am J Pathol 36:289, 1960.
26. Wolff HG: The cerebral blood vessels—anatomical principles. Assoc Res Nerv Ment Dis 18:39, 1938.
27. Clower BR, Sullivan DM, Smith RR: Intracranial vessels lack vasa vasorum. J Neurosurg 61:44, 1984.
28. Maksimow AA, Bloom W: A Textbook of Histology, 4th ed. Philadelphia, WB Saunders, 1942.
29. Gross CR, Kase CS, Mohr JP, et al: Stroke in south Alabama: Incidence and diagnostic features—a population based study. Stroke 15:249, 1984.
30. Kunitz S, Gross CR, Heyman A, et al: The pilot stroke data bank: Definition, design, data. Stroke 15:740, 1984.
31. Lhermitte F, Gautier JC, Derouesne C: Nature of occlusions of the middle cerebral artery. Neurology (Minneap) 20:82, 1970.
32. Kase CS, White L, Vinson L, Eichelberger P: Shotgun pellet embolus to the middle cerebral artery. Neurology 31:458, 1981.
33. Steiner TJ, Rail DL, Rose FC: Cholesterol crystal embolization in rat brain—a model for atherosclerotic cerebral infarction. Stroke 11:184, 1980.
34. Toro-Gonzalez G, Navarro-Roman L, Roman GC, et al: Acute ischemic stroke from fibrocartilaginous embolism to the middle cerebral artery. Stroke 24:738, 1993.
35. Liebeskind A, Chinichian A, Schechter MM: The moving embolus seen during serial cerebral angiography. Stroke 2:440, 1971.
36. Edwards JH, Kricheff II, Riles T, Imparato A: Angiographically undetected ulceration of the carotid bifurcation as a cause of embolic stroke. Radiology 132:369, 1979.
37. Imparato AM, Riles TS, Gorstein F: The carotid bifurcation plaque: Pathologic findings associated with cerebral ischemia. Stroke 10:238, 1979.
38. Gacs G, Merei F, Bodosi M: Balloon catheter as a model of cerebral emboli in humans. Stroke 13:39, 1982.
39. Bladin PF: A radiologic and pathologic study of embolism of the internal carotid–middle cerebral arterial axis. Radiology 82:614, 1964.
40. Broca P: Remarques sur le siège de la faculté du langage articule, suivies d'une observation d'aphémie (perte de la parole). Bull Soc Anat Paris 6:330, 1861.
41. Zatz LM, Iannone AM, Eckman PB, Hecker SP: Observations concerning intracerebral vascular occlusion. Neurology 15:390, 1965.
42. Lhermitte F, Gautier JC, Derouesne C, Guiraud B: Ischemic accidents in the middle cerebral artery territory (a study of the causes in 122 cases). Arch Neurol 19:248, 1968.
43. Fisher CM, Gore I, Okabe N, White PD: Atherosclerosis of the carotid and vertebral arteries—extracranial and intracranial. J Neuropathol Exp Neurol 24:455, 1965.
44. Delal PM, Shah PM, Aiyar RR: Arteriographic study of cerebral embolism. Lancet 2:358, 1965.
45. Pessin MS, Duncan GW, Mohr JP, Poskanzer DC: Clinical and angiographic features of carotid transient ischemic attacks. N Engl J Med 296:358, 1977.

46. Mohr JP, Duterte DI, Oliveira VR, et al: Recanalization of acute middle cerebral artery occlusion. Neurology 38:215, 1988.
47. Hollin SA, Silverstein A: Transient occlusion of the middle cerebral artery. JAMA 194:243, 1965.
48. Minematsu K, Yamaguchi T, Omae T: "Spectacular shrinking deficit": Rapid recovery from a full hemispheral syndrome by migration of an embolus. Neurology 41(Suppl):329, 1991.
49. Chiari H: Ueber das Verhalten des Teilungswinkels der Carotis communis bei der Endarteritis chronic deformans. Verh Dtsch Ges Pathol 9:326, 1905.
50. Friedlich AL, Castleman B, Mohr JP: Case records of the Massachusetts General Hospital. N Engl J Med 278:1109, 1968.
51. Gleysteen JJ, Silver D: Paradoxical arterial embolism: Collective review. Am J Surg 36:47, 1970.
52. Fairfax AJ, Lambert CD, Leatham A: Systemic embolism in chronic sinoatrial disorder. N Engl J Med 275:190, 1976.
53. Barnett HJM, Jones MW, Boughner DR, Kostuk WJ: Cerebral ischemic events associated with prolapsing mitral valve. Arch Neurol 33:777, 1976.
54. Bluschke V, Hennerici M, Scharf RE, et al: Mitralklappenprolaps-Syndrom und Thrombozytenaktivität bei jungen Patienten mit zerebralen Ischämien. Dtsch Med Wochenschr 107:410, 1982.
55. Kooiker JC, MacLean JM, Sumi SM: Cerebral embolism, marantic endocarditis, and cancer. Arch Neurol 33:260, 1976.
56. Neufield HN, Cadman NL, Miller AW, Edwards JE: Embolism from marantic endocarditis as a manifestation of occult carcinoma. Proc Mayo Clin 35:292, 1960.
57. David NJ, Gordon KK, Friedberg SJ, et al: Fatal atheromatous cerebral embolism associated with bright plaques in the retinal arterioles. Neurology 13:708, 1963.
58. Wood EH, Correll JW: Atheromatous ulceration in major neck vessels as a cause of cerebral embolism. Acta Radiol Diag 9:520, 1969.
59. Kerbler S, Schober PH, Steiner H: Traumatische Embolisierung der Arteria cerebri media. Z Kinderchir 45:301, 1990.
60. Caplan LR, Hier DB, D'Cruz I: Cerebral embolism in the Michael Reese Stroke Registry. Stroke 14:30, 1983.
61. Davis DO, Rumbaugh CL, Gilson JM: Angiographic diagnosis of small-vessel cerebral emboli. Acta Radiol (Stockh) 9:264, 1969.
62. Weiller C, Ringelstein EB, Reiche W, et al: The large striatocapsular infarct: A clinical and pathophysiological entity. Arch Neurol 47:1085, 1990.
63. Stringer WL, Kelly DL: Traumatic dissection of the extracranial internal carotid artery. Neurosurgery 6:123, 1980.
64. Deck JHN, Lee MA: Mucin embolism to cerebral arteritis: A fatal complication of carcinoma of the breast. J Can Sci Neurol 5:327, 1978.
65. Glew RH: Case records of the Massachusetts General Hospital. N Engl J Med 301:36, 1979.
66. Yufe R, Karpati G, Carpenter S: Cardiac myxoma: A diagnostic challenge for the neurologist. Neurology 26:1060, 1976.
67. Bonhoeffer K: Klinischer und anatomischer Befund zur Lehre von der Apraxie und der "motorische Sprachbahn." Monatsschr Psychiatr Neurol 35:113, 1914.
68. Cohen MM, Hemalatha CP, D'Addario RT, Goldman HW: Embolism from a fusiform middle cerebral artery aneurysm. Stroke 11:58, 1980.
69. Donnan GA, Bladin PF, Berkovic SF, et al: The stroke syndrome of striatocapsular infarction. Brain 114:51, 1991.
70. Pessin MS, Hinton RC, Davis KR, et al: Mechanisms of acute carotid stroke. Ann Neurol 6:245, 1979.
71. Wolpert SM, Stein BM: Catheter embolization of intracranial arteriovenous malformations as an aid to surgical excision. Neuroradiology 10:73, 1975.
72. Kusske JA, Kelly WA: Embolization and reduction of the "steal" syndrome in cerebral AVMs. J Neurosurg 40:313, 1974.
73. Fisher CM, Pearlman A: The non-sudden onset of cerebral embolism. Neurology (Minneap) 17:1025, 1967.
74. Aring CD, Merritt HH: Differential diagnosis between cerebral hemorrhage and cerebral thrombosis. Arch Intern Med 56:435, 1935.
75. Fisher CM: Occlusion of the internal carotid artery. AMA Arch Neurol Psychiatry 69:346, 1951.
76. Blackwood W, Bratty P, Mair WGP: In Jakob H (ed): Observations on Occlusive Vascular Disease of the Brain, vol 3. Stuttgart, Thieme Verlag, 1963, p 146.
77. Fisher CM: Cerebral ischemia—less familiar types. Clin Neurosurg 18:267, 1971.

Clinical Manifestations

78. Hinton RC, Mohr JP, Ackerman RA, et al: Symptomatic middle cerebral artery stenosis. Ann Neurol 5:152, 1979.
79. Irino T, Tandea M, Minami T: Angiographic manifestations in postrecanalized cerebral infarction. Neurology 27:471, 1977.
80. Fisher CM: Capsular infarcts. Arch Neurol 36:65, 1979.
81. Lascelles RG, Burrows EH: Occlusion of the middle cerebral artery. Brain 88:85, 1966.
82. Kawase T, Mizukami M, Tazawa T, Araki G: The significance of lenticulostriate arteries in transient ischemic attack: Neuroradiological and regional cerebral blood flow studies. Brain Nerve 31:1033, 1979.
83. Feldmeyer JJ, Merendaz C, Regli F: Sténoses symptomatiques de l'artère cérébrale moyenne. Rev Neurol (Paris) 139:725, 1983.
84. Day AL: Anatomy of the extracranial vessels. In Smith RR (ed): Stroke and the Extracranial Vessels. New York, Raven Press, 1984, p 9.
85. Corston RN, Kendall BE, Marshall J: Prognosis in middle cerebral artery stenosis. Stroke 15:237, 1984.
86. Adams HP, Gross CE: Embolism distal to stenosis of the middle cerebral artery. Stroke 12:228, 1981.
87. Araki G: Small infarctions of the basal ganglia with special reference to transient ischemic attacks. Recent Adv Gerontol 469:161, 1978.
88. Hyland HH: Thrombosis of intracranial arteries. Arch Neurol Psychiatry 30:342, 1933.
89. Wolman L: Cerebral dissecting aneurysms. Brain 82:276, 1959.
90. Bigelow NH: Intracranial dissecting aneurysms: An analysis of their significance. Arch Pathol 60:271, 1955.
91. Hirsch CS, Roessmann U: Arterial dysplasia with ruptured basilar artery aneurysm: Report of a case. Hum Pathol 6:749, 1975.
92. Yamashita M, Tanaka K, Matsuo T, et al: Cerebral dissecting aneurysms in patients with moyamoya disease. J Neurosurg 58:120, 1983.
93. Dratz HM, Woodhall B: Traumatic dissecting aneurysm of left internal carotid, anterior cerebral and middle cerebral arteries. J Neuropathol Exp Neurol 6:286, 1947.
94. Yonas H, Agamanolis D, Takaoka Y, et al: Dissecting intracranial aneurysms. Surg Neurol 8:407, 1977.
95. Turnbull HM: Alterations in arterial structures, and their relation to syphilis. Q J Med 8:201, 1915.
96. Sinclair W Jr: Dissecting aneurysm of the middle cerebral artery associated with migraine syndrome. Am J Pathol 29:1083, 1953.
97. Johnson AC, Graves VB, Pfaff JP Jr: Dissecting aneurysm of intracranial arteries. Surg Neurol 7:49, 1977.
98. Duman S, Stephans JW: Post-traumatic middle cerebral artery occlusion. Neurology 13:613, 1963.
99. Adams RD, Victor M: Principles of Neurology. New York, McGraw-Hill, 1984.
100. Rosegay H, Welch KJ: Peripheral collateral circulation between cerebral arteries. J Neurosurg 11:363, 1954.
101. Rovira M, Jacas R, Lay A: The collateral circulation in thrombosis of the internal carotid and its branches. Acta Radiol Stockh 50:101, 1958.
102. Hacke W, Schwab S, Horn M, et al: 'Malignant' middle cerebral artery territory infarction: clinical course and prognostic signs. Arch Neurol 53:309, 1996.
103. Steiner T, Ringleb P, Hacke W: Treatment options for large hemispheric stroke. Neurology 57(Suppl 2):S61, 2001.
104. Bousser MG, Dubois B, Castaigne P: Pertes de connaissance brèves au cours des accidents ischemiques cérébraux. Ann Med Interne 132:300, 1981.
105. von Monakow K: Die Lokalisation im Grosshirn und der Abbau der Funktion durch Kortikale Herde. Wiesbaden, JF Begman, 1914.
106. Rengachary SS, Batnitzky S, Morantz RA, et al: Hemicraniectomy for acute mass of cerebral infarction. Neurosurgery 8:321, 1981.
107. Davison C, Goodhart SP, Needles W: Cerebral localization and cerebral vascular disease. Arch Neurol Psychiatry (Chicago) 30:749, 1933.
108. Henschen SE: Klinische und Anatomische Beitrage zur Pathologie des Gehirns. Stockholm, Nordiska, 1920.
109. Mohr JP, Foulkes MA, Polis AT, et al: Infarct topography and hemiparesis profiles with cerebral convexity infarction: The Stroke Data Bank. J Neurol Neurosurg Psychiatry 56:344, 1993.
110. De Renzi E, Colombo A, Faglioni P, Gilbertoni N: Conjugate gaze paresis in stroke patients with unilateral damage. Arch Neurol 39:42, 1982.

111. Barat M, Constant P, Mazaux JM, et al: Corrélations anatomo-cliniques dans l'aphasie: Apport de la tomodensitometrie. Rev Neurol (Paris) 134:611, 1978.
112. Rondot P: Syndromes of central motor disorder. In Vinken PJ, Bruyn GW (eds): Handbook of Clinical Neurology, vol 1: Disturbances of Nervous Function. Amsterdam, North-Holland, 1969, p 169.
113. Gazengel JGL: Etude de 276 emboles cérébrales d'origine cardiaque: Thèse Faculté de Médécine de Paris. Paris, Editions AGEMP, 1966, p 123.
114. Hacke W, Schwab S, Horn M, et al: 'Malignant' middle cerebral artery territory infarction: Clinical course and prognostic signs. Arch Neurol 53:309, 1996.
115. Obrador S: Nervous integration after hemispherectomy in man. In Schaltenbrand G, Woolsey CN (eds): Cerebral Localization and Organization. Madison, WI, University of Wisconsin Press, 1964, p 133.
116. Walz B, Zimmermann C, Bottger S, Haberl RL: Prognosis of patients after hemicraniectomy in malignant middle cerebral artery infarction. J Neurol 249:1183, 2002.
117. Fisher CM, Curry HB: Pure motor hemiplegia of vascular origin. Arch Neurol 13:30, 1965.
118. Hanaway J, Torack R, Fletcher AP, Landau WM: Intracranial bleeding associated with urokinase therapy for acute ischemic hemispheral stroke. Stroke 7:143, 1976.
119. Healton EB, Navarro C, Bressman S, Brust JCM: Subcortical neglect. Neurology (NY) 32:776, 1982.
120. Rascol A, Clanet M, Manelfe C: Pure motor hemiplegia: CT study of 30 cases. Stroke 13:11, 1982.
121. Demierre B, Rondot P: Dystonia caused by putamino-capsulo-caudate vascular lesions. J Neurol Neurosurg Psychiatry 46:404, 1983.
122. Santamaria J, Graus F, Rubio F, et al: Cerebral infarction of the basal ganglia due to embolism from the heart. Stroke 14:911, 1983.
123. Bang OY, Heo JH, Kim JY, et al: Middle cerebral artery stenosis is a major clinical determinant in striatocapsular small, deep infarction. Arch Neurol 59:259, 2002.
124. Bruyn GW, Gathier JC: The operculum syndrome. In Vinken PJ, Bruyn GW (eds): Handbook of Clinical Neurology, vol 2. Amsterdam, North Holland Publishing, 1976, p 776.
125. Irino T, Watanabe M, Nishide M, et al: Angiographical analysis of acute cerebral infarction followed by "cascade"-like deterioration of minor neurological deficits: What is progressing stroke? Stroke 14:363, 1983.
126. Broadbent WH: On the cerebral mechanism of speech and thought. Trans R Med Chir Soc (Lond) 55:145, 1872.
127. Phillips CG: Some thoughts on the organization of the motor cortex. In Eccles JC (ed): The Brain and Conscious Experience. New York, Springer-Verlag, 1966.
128. Alajouanine T, Boudin G, Pertuiset B, Pepin B: Le syndrome operculaire unilatéral avec atteinte contralatérale du territoire des V, VII, IX, XI, XIIème nerfs craniens. Rev Neurol (Paris) 101:167, 1959.
129. Mohr JP: Rapid amelioration of motor aphasia. Arch Neurol 28:77, 1973.
130. Dejerine J: Séméiologie des Affections du Système Nerveux. Paris, Masson, 1914.
131. Dejerine J, Regnard M: Monoplegie brachiale gauche limitée aux muscles des eminences thenar, hypothenar et aux interosseux: Astereognosie, épilepsie jacksonienne. Rev Neurol 1:285, 1912.
132. Garcin R: Paralysie dissociée du median d'origine corticale (sur le caractère durement familial de certains accidents vasculaires cérébraux). Médecine 137, 1932.
133. Schneider R, Gautier JC: Leg weakness due to stroke: Site of lesions, weakness patterns and causes. Brain 117:347, 1994.
134. Bramwell B: A remarkable case of aphasia. Brain 21:343, 1898.
135. Prevost JL: De la Déviation Conjuguée des Yeux et de la Rotation de la Tête. Paris, Thèse, 1896.
136. Bizzi E: Discharge of frontal eye field neurons during saccadic and following eye movements in unanesthetized monkeys. Exp Brain Res 6:69, 1968.
137. Pederson RA, Troost BT: Abnormalities of gaze in cerebrovascular disease. Stroke 12:251, 1981.
138. Pierrot-Deseilligny C: Saccade and smooth-pursuit impairment after cerebral hemispheric lesions. Eur Neurol 34:121, 1994.
139. Tijssen CC: Contralateral conjugate eye deviation in acute supratentorial lesions. Stroke 25:1516, 1994.

Clinical Manifestations

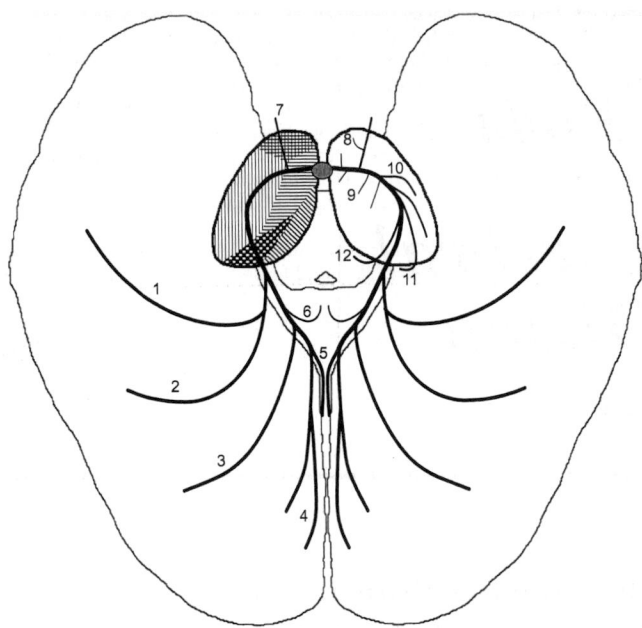

gives the vessel the appearance of the number 3 on an angiogram.[3] Proximally, it supplies part of the upper midbrain and the peduncle. After entering the choroidal fissure, it supplies the choroid plexus of the third ventricle, the anterior aspect of the pulvinar, and the medial thalamus. The terminal branches of the posteromedial choroidal artery supply the anterior nucleus of the thalamus. The last branch of the arteries supplying the deep territory is the posterior pericallosal or splenial artery.[3] Rarely, the thalamotuberal artery takes its origin from the middle cerebral artery instead of its more common origination from the posterior communicating artery.[7]

Cortical Territory

Although the cortical branches of the PCA are well known, there has been considerable disagreement as to their names (Fig. 8–3). Salamon and Huang[3] label the three major ventral temporal branches as the inferior temporal and occipitotemporal arteries, and the vessel supplying the calcarine region, as the calcarine artery. Kaul and associates[8] refer to the former group as the anterior, middle, and posterior temporal arteries. The term *parieto-occipital artery* describes the trunk from which branches arise that supply the calcarine cortex, cuneus, and precuneus.

Whatever their names, three vessels usually supply the entire ventral surface of the temporal and occipital lobes (see Fig. 8–2).[9] The anterior inferior temporal and the posterior inferior temporal arteries may arise from a single trunk, separate from the occipitotemporal, or the three may arise from a common trunk. The two anterior arteries supply the entire undersurface of the temporal lobe. The undersurface of the occipital lobe, including the posterior portion of the fusiform and lingual gyri, is supplied by the occipitotemporal branch.

The calcarine artery may be single or double.[8] Although the calcarine artery has been claimed to be the exclusive

FIGURE 8–1 *Schematic diagram of the posterior cerebral artery and its branches: 1, anterior inferior temporal artery; 2, posterior inferior temporal artery; 3, occipitotemporal artery; 4, calcarine arteries; 5, occipitoparietal artery; 6, splenial artery; 7 posterior communicating artery; 8, tuberothalamic arteries; 9, thalamoperforating arteries; 10, thalamogeniculate and posterior thalamic arteries; 11, posterolateral choroidal artery; 12, posteromedial choroidal artery. Arterial territories of the thalamus are indicated as follows: horizontal hatching, thalamoperforator territory; vertical hatching, thalamogeniculate territory; crosshatching, tuberothalamic territory; checkerboard pattern, posterolateral choroidal territory; diagonal hatching, posteromedial choroidal territory.*

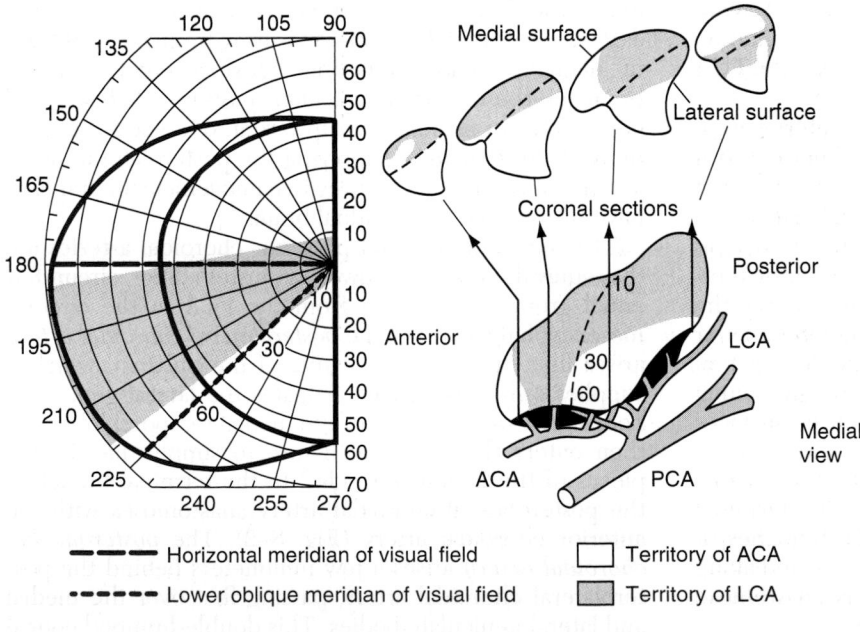

FIGURE 8–2 *Arterial supply to the lateral geniculate body showing the course of the arteries. ACA, anterior choroidal artery; LCA, posterolateral choroidal artery. (From Frisen L, Holmegaard L, Rosencrantz M: Sectorial optic atrophy and homonymous horizontal sector anopia: A lateral choroidal artery syndrome? J Neurol Neurosurg Psychiatry 41:374, 1978.)*

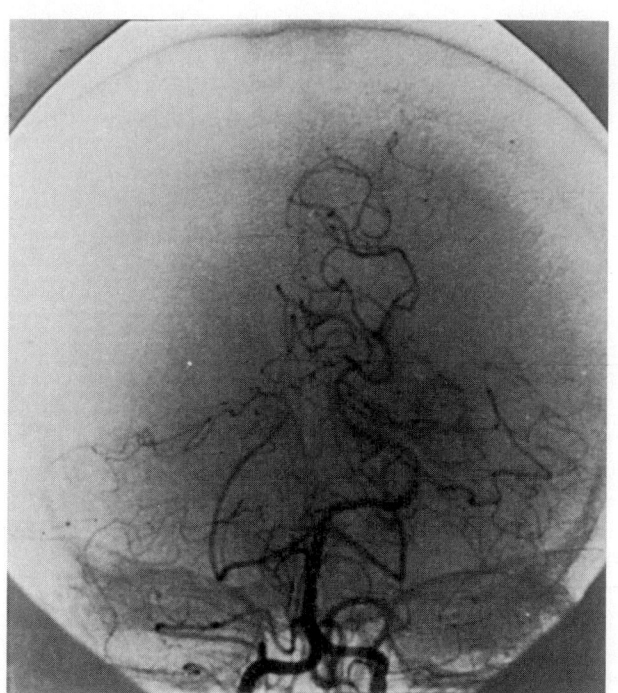

FIGURE 8–3 *Anteroposterior view of the posterior cerebral artery territory showing the cerebral surface branches supplying the inferior surface branches, which in turn supply the inferior surface of the temporal lobe and the medial occipital region.*

supply to the visual cortex in the calcarine fissure,[10] the striate area may at times be supplied in part by the occipitotemporal or occipitoparietal arteries.[11] The termination of the supply of the calcarine artery and its branches is far posterior along the occipital pole.[12] The supply commonly passes around the edge of the occipital pole and as far forward as 1 cm on the convex surface of the hemisphere, where anastomoses are formed with terminal branches of the middle cerebral artery.

Collateral Vessels

The PCA has abundant collateral connections with the middle and anterior cerebral arteries.[13] The collaterals occur in the borderzone, a narrow (usually 1-cm) strip separating two major arterial territories. Within this zone, anastomoses between end arteries occur freely in a variety of forms—end-to-end, side-to-side, and end-to-side. The actual size of the anastomosing vessels varies considerably, but most are on the order of 300 to 600 μm, only rarely as large as 1 mm. As a result, although a potential collateral vessel exists at any point along a borderzone, it is all but impossible to anticipate that a given terminal branch will receive the immediate flow through the borderzone that it may need to prevent infarction when its territory is suddenly compromised.

The anastomoses with the anterior cerebral artery usually take place along a narrow borderzone of vessels on the precuneus between the transverse parietal sulcus and the parieto-occipital fissure, from the isthmus of the gyrus fornicati inferiorly to the margin of the hemisphere superiorly. Three or four branches enter the borderzone.

With the middle cerebral artery, anastomoses occur from the orbital surface of the anterior tip of the temporal lobe inferolaterally along the margin of the hemisphere as far back as the occipital pole.[14] Between five and eight such branches can be traced into the borderzones in most hemispheres.

PATHOGENESIS

Occlusion of the PCA or its branches is less common than that of the middle cerebral artery, and reports of their relative occurrences seem constant over the decades.[15–17] Bilateral involvement was observed in 25% of the cases reported by Kleihues and Hizawa,[16] but in 6% to 13% of cases in later series.[17–21] Bilateral infarction of the entire deep and superficial territory of the PCA appears to be quite rare.[22,23] Infarction of individual branches, alone or in combination, is more common (Table 8.1), with the calcarine artery leading the list.[21,22] Isolated occlusion of the anterior temporal artery is the most rare, and clinical details for such cases are lacking. Three series based on computed tomography (CT) findings reported thalamic involvement in 19% of 221 patients,[18,22,24] and three series using magnetic resonance imaging (MRI) found thalamic infarction in 30% of 235 patients.[17,20,21] Infarction of the midbrain is much less common.[17,18,20,21]

Embolism

Embolism leads all other causes of PCA occlusion.[17–21,23,25,26] Embolic material may reach the artery via the vertebral or basilar arteries or the internal carotid artery. Castaigne and associates[15] attributed only one case to cardiac source embolism in their series of 44 autopsy studies, while finding evidence for emboli arising from plaques in the vertebrals or the basilar in 50% of cases. In vivo series, however, suggest that embolism from a cardiac source accounts for roughly 25% to 40% of all cases of PCA

Table 8.1 Regional Distribution of Infarcts

Site(s)	Number
PCA	6
CA	7
PTA	7
ATA	1
POA	2
PTA + ATA	7
CA + POA	6
CA + PTA	10
CA + PTA + ATA	11
CA + PTA + POA	1
CA + PTA + POA + PPA	2

ATA, anterior temporal artery; CA, calcarine artery; PCA, posterior cerebral artery; POA, parieto-occipital artery; PPA, posterior pericallosal artery; PTA, posterior temporal artery.
Adapted from Kinkel WR, Newman RP, Jacobs L: Posterior cerebral artery branch occlusions: CT and anatomic considerations. In Berguer R, Bauer RB (eds): Vertebrobasilar Arterial Occlusive Disease: Medical and Surgical Management. Philadelphia, Lippincott-Raven, 1984, p 117.

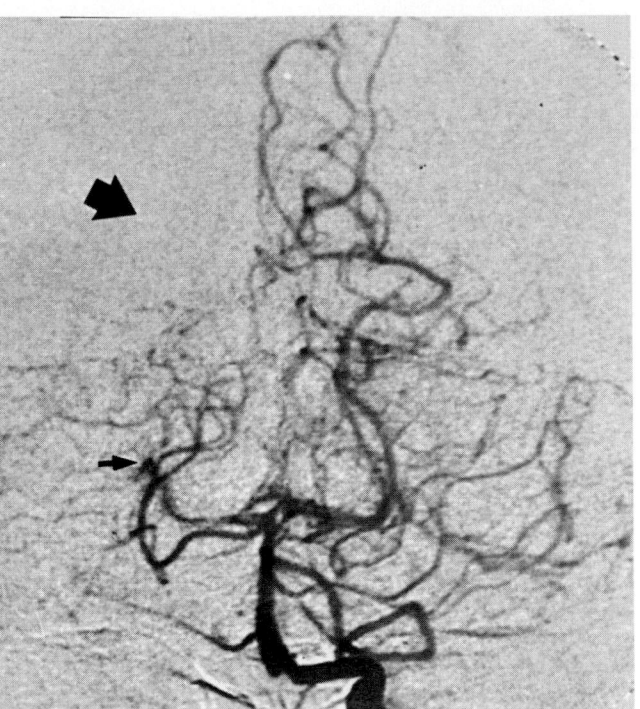

FIGURE 8–4 *Anteroposterior view of a selective left vertebral angiogram. The ambient segment of the right posterior cerebral artery is occluded (small arrow). There is no opacification of the terminal branches of this artery (large arrow).*

percutaneous transluminal angioplasty.[36] The atheroma usually affects the posterior cerebral along its course around the brain stem,[37] at approximately the same sites where embolic materials stop (Fig. 8–5). Thrombus atop preexisting stenosis is rare.[15] No clinical features specifically distinguish thrombosis from embolic occlusion in the proximal posterior cerebral artery. Occlusion from anterograde extension of thrombus from an occlusion of the upper basilar artery appears to account for half of the cases of bilateral PCA territory infarction.[38,39] The occipital lobes may suffer ischemia as a distal field effect from occlusion of the vertebral arteries bilaterally or the basilar itself,[40–43] but autopsy reports indicate embolism is the usual cause.[38]

Few studies have been made of stenosis of the posterior cerebral stem.[18,26,35,37] Duncan and Weidling's[35] patient had diplopia, ipsilateral ptosis, and contralateral hemiataxia, the syndrome reported as a mixture of Benedikt's syndrome with pupil-sparing oculomotor palsy. Pessin and coworkers[37] found six examples in a 7-year period. From

occlusion and is somewhat more common than arterial source embolism.[17–21,23] Rarely, the initial presentation of extracranial carotid occlusive disease may be a hemianopia from embolism to the PCA through a fetal origin of the PCA from the internal carotid artery.[20,27]

Emboli that travel up the posterior circulation are often arrested at the top of the basilar artery,[28] where they may produce bilateral posterior cerebral occlusions, fragment into branches bilaterally, or arrest in one PCA at any point along its course (Fig. 8–4). Common sites of arrest are the stem of the PCA where it winds around the brain stem, at the origin of the cortical surface branches, and along the course of the branches serving the occipital lobe. Although embolic occlusions confined to the anterior cortical branches serving the undersurface of the temporal lobe are theoretically possible, we found no case when searching the literature in preparation of this chapter.

Embolic occlusions often produce incomplete infarction of the territory distal to the occluded site.[6,29–33] Complete infarction affecting the gray matter and subcortical white matter to the depths of the ventricular wall is rarely reported,[3] the lesions more typically being patchy.[32]

Thrombosis

Atheromatous thrombosis of the PCA seems infrequent, accounting for roughly 5% to 15% of cases in most series.[15,17–21,23,26] PCA stenosis is uncommon enough to warrant individual case reports even in current times, given the unusual syndromes that may occur, such as Benedikt's oculomotor palsy,[35] and uncertainty about indications for

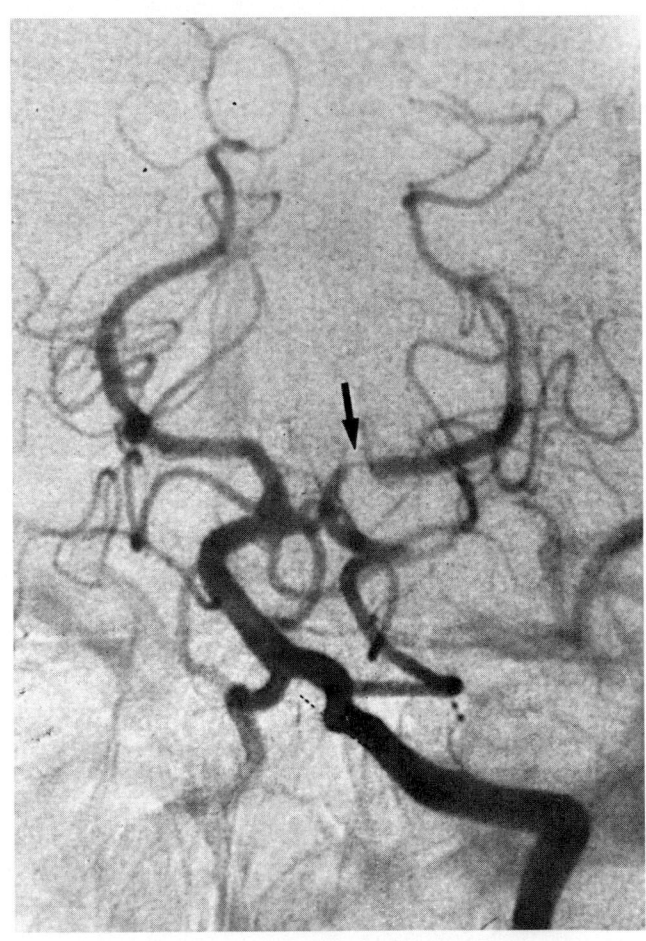

FIGURE 8–5 *Anteroposterior view of a selective left vertebral angiogram with simultaneous compression of the left carotid artery. A high-grade stenosis (arrow) can be seen in the proximal left posterior cerebral artery just distal to its junction with the left posterior communicating artery. Compression of the left carotid artery eliminated the possibility of flow artifact created by nonopacified blood from the anterior circulation. (From Pessin MS, Kwan ES, DeWitt LD, et al: Posterior cerebral artery stenosis. Ann Neurol 21:85, 1987.)*

this slender database, they found that in five patients, transient ischemic attacks (TIAs) were the major presenting complaint, and two patients had homonymous visual field defects. The TIAs were predominantly visual disturbances in the contralateral half-field, or sensory complaints in the form of paresthesias involving the arm and hand or, occasionally, the face and leg. Three patients had visual and sensory spells together.

Other Causes

Other reported causes of infarcts in the PCA territory are migraine, hypercoagulopathy, and brain herniation. Although the concept of vasoconstriction-induced ischemia in patients with migraine is accepted by many researchers,[17,21,23,44,45] other evidence suggests that in at least some patients, ischemia may induce migraine as a secondary phenomenon.[46,47] Reports of PCA territory infarction include a few patients with hypercoagulopathic states induced by neoplasm, dehydration, hyperosmolarity, systemic illness, collagen vascular disease, cryoglobulinemia, cardiolipin antibodies, or other conditions.[20,21,23,48] Transtentorial brain herniation is a well-recognized cause of PCA occlusion. The artery can be compressed in its course around the midbrain between the herniated temporal lobe medially and the tentorium laterally.[49–52] Compression may also occur contralateral to the herniation because of lateral displacement of the brainstem against the contralateral tentorium.[52]

CLINICAL SYNDROMES

Distal Basilar and Posterior Cerebral Artery Stem Occlusion

Occlusions affecting the top of the basilar artery are discussed in detail in Chapter 10. In this section, the discussion is confined to those syndromes in which the PCA is affected as part of the basilar occlusion. Castaigne and associates[38] described 4 cases with pathologically proven occlusion of the PCA: the infarct affected the red nucleus and the intralamellary, parafascicular, central, and median nuclei of the thalamus. Profound deficits occurred, featuring obtundation, stupor or coma, disturbance in memory, hemiplegia, varying degrees of hemihypesthesia, and isolated instances of hemianopia or partial third nerve paresis. Similar syndromes have been documented by others.[53–55] From the limited literature available, it is apparent that occlusion of the PCA stem between the basilar artery and the junction with the posterior communicating artery is sufficient to precipitate a hemiparesis from peduncular infarct, ocular motility disorder from deeper infarction of the midbrain, and complex disturbances in consciousness, memory, and even language for patients in whom infarcts penetrate deeper into medial thalamic structures. In some cases, hypersexuality and changes in appetite occur as well.

Unilateral occlusion of the PCA stem has caused syndromes mimicking those from middle cerebral artery territory infarction (Fig. 8–6). Involvement of both the deep and superficial territories of the PCA (right side) has produced not only contralateral plegia, hemisensory syndrome, hemianopia, and behavioral effects but also

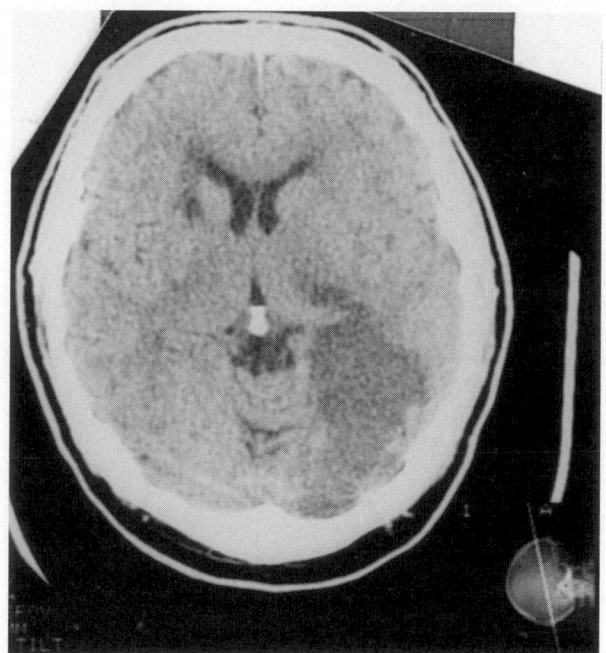

FIGURE 8–6 *Deep thalamic and occipital infarction from occlusion of the posterior cerebral artery in a patient with severe sensory loss and dense hemianopia.*

Horner's syndrome and contralateral hyperhydrosis; these last two effects are explained by involvement of the thalamus and hypothalamus.[56] Four reports have described small case series with occlusion of the proximal PCA.[18,57–59] Brain imaging (CT or MRI) was needed for accurate diagnosis, suggesting that the specific clinical features do not distinguish the syndromes clearly. Argentino and coworkers[60] reported similar frustrations during attempts to characterize patients clinically in the hyperacute stage of ischemic stroke.

Sensory Syndromes

Hypesthesia or Anesthesia
Hypesthesia or anesthesia might be an expected consequence of PCA occlusion near the stem, because the vascular supply to the ventral tier nuclei of the thalamus is in the territory of its penetrating branches.[54] Most of the literature on this subject is discussed in more detail in Chapter 10. Individual reports describing hypesthesia, and even "considerable anesthesia,"[33] can be found, including one with a large, autopsy-documented, dominant hemisphere occipital infarction but no lesions described in the thalamus (on gross inspection); the patient was described as complaining that "the whole right side of the body [felt] cold and heavy . . . the difference of sensation in the two sides being so marked he felt as if a plumb line down the middle of the head and trunk had divided him into two halves."[33]

The branches suppling the ventral tier nuclei of the thalamus come most regularly from the thalamogeniculate branch of the PCA and the posterolateral choroidal artery (Fig. 8–7), whose main target is the lateral geniculate nucleus. Frisen and coworkers[61] speculated that occlusion

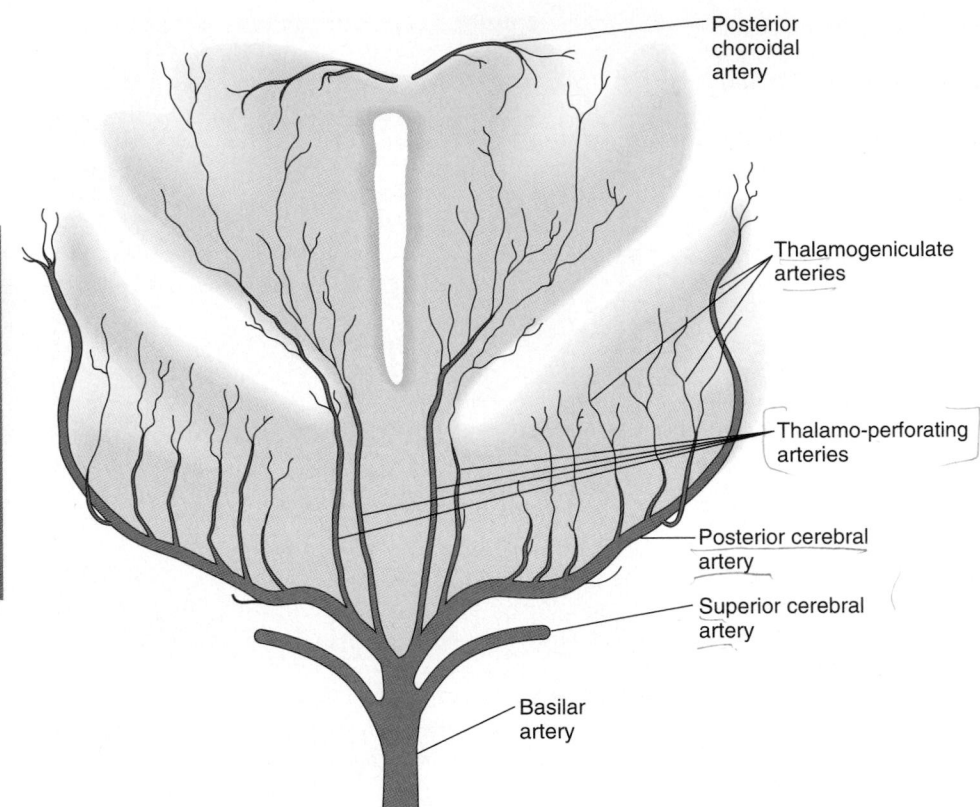

Posterior choroidal artery

Thalamogeniculate arteries

Thalamo-perforating arteries

Posterior cerebral artery

Superior cerebral artery

Basilar artery

FIGURE 8–7 *Thalamus with the usual arterial distribution. Note the multiple thalamogeniculate arteries.*

of the posterolateral choroidal artery could produce not only a somatosensory defect but also a hemianopia from involvement of the lateral geniculate body. A case studied by one of the authors (JPM) had hemianopia but no abnormality of sensation.[6]

Déjerine-Roussy Syndrome

A special form of sensory disorder occasioned by occlusion of the thalamogeniculate branch of the PCA is the source of the thalamic pain syndrome described by Déjerine and Roussy.[62] These researchers reviewed the literature up to 1906 and showed that the occlusion of this artery produced a syndrome consisting of rapidly improving hemiparesis with choreic movements and ataxia, persisting hypesthesia, and severe paroxysmal pain in the hypesthetic side. Their pathologic correlation has been reconfirmed by others over the years[57,63–65] and is described in more detail in Chapter 11.

Motor Syndromes

Although not expected from class descriptions, hemiparesis and even hemiplegia are increasingly recognized as part of the PCA syndrome.[18,59,60,66] The cause has been ascribed to involvement of the upper brainstem[26] or ischemia on the edge of the internal capsule.[18,67,68] Hyperkinetic and dystonic syndromes involving limbs contralateral to the lesion have also been described, including "jerky dystonic unsteady hand" (three cases attributed to occlusion of the posterior choroidal arteries),[63] hemichorea-hemiballism,[62,69,70] "hyperkinesie volitionnelle,"[71] asterixis, and hemidystonia.[62,69,72,73] Lesions in these cases were

most often in posterior or ventral thalamus, in the territory of thalamoperforating and thalamogeniculate penetrators.

Visual Field Disturbances

The lower portions of the visual radiations, throughout their entire course, lie in the territory of the PCA. Most of the upper portion is supplied by branches of the middle cerebral artery, especially the angular and posterior temporal branches. Disruption of the pathway may occur from infarction involving the lateral geniculate body, the radiations along their course in the temporal lobe, or at the calcarine cortex itself. Damage near the calcarine cortex may cause amblyopic disturbances featuring relative rather than absolute loss of vision.

Bilateral Infarction
Complete
Complete destruction of both the visual cortices has only rarely been reported.[16,43,74–76] Brindley and Janota's[34] patient typifies the striking clinical picture. In this patient the infarcts extended bilaterally along the entire undersurface of the temporal and occipital lobes. In the inferior temporal region, the hippocampus, parahippocampal gyrus, and fusiform gyrus were destroyed. The medial surface of the occipital lobes was affected, including both fusiform gyri, lingual gyrus and cunei, and both banks of each calcarine sulcus; the infarction affected the posterior portions of the corpus callosum and the pillars of the fornix and extended as high as the parieto-occipital fissure. Both occipital poles were spared. Throughout her life after the

stroke, this patient remained blind, with no response to optikokinetic nystagmus and no visual evoked potentials. She was unable to distinguish steady darkness from steady light, nor could she detect a light moving in front of her, although she consistently distinguished sudden darkening of a lighted room and sudden lighting of a darkened room. In another patient, visual evoked potentials to pattern stimulation were found despite a complete lack of vision on testing by clinical methods.[77] A patient described by Goldenberg,[75] in whom MRI showed all but complete bilateral destruction of the calcarine regions, denied blindness but was able to describe by recall the shapes of letters and colors typical of certain objects named by the examiners. This last case addresses the issue whether preservation of the primary visual cortex is necessary to generate conversationally tested recall of images.

The huge infarcts are often associated with severe amnestic states, amnestic aphasia, amnestic color dysnomia, topographic disorientation, and implicit unawareness of the extent of the deficit and perhaps even its existence.[78] This last point suggests that the preservation or loss of awareness of the blindness is of little value in differentiating middle from posterior cerebral territory infarction.[28]

Incomplete

Incomplete bilateral infarction is better known and produces a remarkable variety of syndromes.[17,18] Some cases have begun as complete blindness only to evolve within hours or days to less striking deficits.[41] During the time of complete blindness, the patient commonly volunteers no complaints and is unaware of the deficit.[75] In a series of 25 patients with incomplete bilateral infarction of the visual cortices, detection of movement of objects in visual space was present and sufficient for localization, but no discrimination of size or shape was possible.[79]

Superficial infarction may involve almost the whole of the calcarine cortex, but if it spares the occipital pole and the subcortical visual radiations, visual function for complex activities such as reading may be spared even if only a tiny portion of the central field remains.[42,43,74,80] Holmes[81] described a patient with a narrow wedge of preserved vision extending from the fixation point upward on either side of the vertical meridian, with its apex at the fixation point and its base at the periphery. Serial sections of the autopsy specimen from this patient showed total calcarine infarction except for a small region, nearly symmetric bilaterally, that extended along the inferior lip of the striate cortex from the anterior end to the pole.

Bilateral altitudinal hemianopia is an expected consequence of incomplete bilateral occipital infarction but has rarely been reported in detail. The onset in several cases was preceded by hallucinations of lights, prismatic or geometric forms, and other phenomena suggestive of migrainous scintillations. After the hemianopias developed, associated visual disturbances included color dysnomias, difficulties with visual form discrimination, spatial disorientation, and disordered visual search behavior of the type encountered in Balint's syndrome. However, other patients have had little such disturbance.[32] In a personal case of one of the present authors (JPM), a construction foreman was annoyed most by his inferior altitudinal hemianopia because it prevented his easy scanning of blueprints and caused difficulty in reaching for the floor-mounted gear shift in his pickup truck. Few autopsy-documented cases have been published; all of the patients had experienced inferior altitudinal hemianopia.[32,43,82] In each case, however, the superior quadrants were slightly affected as well. Autopsy showed foci of infarction scattered through the calcarine cortex with varying subcortical involvement. The visual field disturbances seemed more homogeneous than indicated by the discontinuous foci of infarction. Altitudinal hemianopia with such infarcts has also been documented on CT.[83]

For most of the patients with cortical blindness from bilateral infarction, the deficits are described by the patients as persisting and unchanging.[34] Scattered reports and our personal experience, however, indicate that some patients with bilateral cortical blindness may experience considerable remission of the deficit. Presumably, the infarction is incomplete, and the acute syndrome is misleading in its failure to predict the subsequent improvement. Although Bergman[78] addressed the issue of remission in 12 patients with cortical blindness, only one of the five whose blindness was due to infarction showed any improvement. Vision returned within a month but was confined to the macular region, suggesting sparing of the radiations and the occipital pole. The description of the autopsy specimen in this case does not settle this point.

Clinical events that herald cortical blindness are not often reported. A scattering of cases began with a unilateral hemianopia that was followed by cortical blindness. Bogousslavsky and colleagues[84] monitored 58 patients with unilateral infarction in the superficial area supplied by the PCA for up to 39 months. Thirteen of the patients experienced cortical blindness associated with a delayed contralateral occipital infarction. The investigators noted that lack of visual field improvement most accurately predicated a high risk of cortical blindness.

Unilateral Infarction

Temporal crescent sparing has been described in a few instances of unilateral infarction with sparing of the anterior end of the calcarine cortex.[85,86] This pattern, which cannot be detected with standard automated perimetry, may nonetheless be prognostically important because of the usefulness of peripheral vision in daily activites.[86]

Macular sparing is frequently encountered in unilateral (and also in bilateral) infarction of the PCA territory. The most common explanation is that the collateral flow available from the middle cerebral artery territory spares the pole.[32,74,87] For macular vision to remain, the infarct must be superficial enough to spare the visual radiations; when they are involved, anatomic integrity of the occipital pole does not suffice to preserve central vision.[34] Infarcts limited to the middle fields of supply of the PCA involve the anterior portions of the calcarine cortex and lingual gyrus.[8,13,16] The most common finding in such instances is a homonymous hemianopia with macular sparing, the most consistent deficit involving visual field adjacent to the horizontal meridian.[8] Isolated macular hemianopia, the inverse of hemianopia with macular sparing, is less common and occurs when infarction is relatively confined to the occipital pole.[32,43,88] Isa and colleagues[88] found six cases among 54 patients with PCA infarction who underwent Goldmann's perimetry testing.

Isolated infarction of the visual radiation seems rare. In contrast to middle cerebral artery territory disease, infarctions of the PCA territory have often been reported in which the subcortical component was more evident than the infarction involving the cortical surface.[6,29,43] In most instances, the damage found subcortically affected the white matter of the lingual or fusiform gyrus, often sparing the visual radiations, which pass deeper and are adjacent to the ventricular wall. Infarcts in this deep territory are rare unless they are the result of a full-thickness infarct, one that forms a schizencephalic cleft extending from the pial surface of the cortex all the way to the ependyma of the ventricle.

Lateral geniculate infarcts account for but a small fraction of the literature (see Fig. 8–2).[6,61,89,90] The anterior choroidal artery supplies the anterior hilum and the anterior and lateral aspects of the nucleus. The lateral posterior choroidal artery supplies the remainder, including the crown. The two sources of supply do not anastomose before or in the nucleus and appear to be end arteries with no collaterals. The visual field is represented in the following three parts in the nucleus: the anteromedial, which subserves inferior quadrant vision; the crown, serving macular vision; and the lateral, which serves upper quadrantic vision. The only pathologically documented infarcts produced a congruous, complete upper quadrantanopia involving the macula, with some involvement of the upper portion of the lower quadrant.[6,91] Brain imaging has shown patients with inferred infarcts of the lateral geniculate to have wedge-shaped homonymous sectoranopia, congruent upper quadrantanopia, and a quadruple sectoranopia (one case).[61,89,92] Upper and lower homonymous sectoranopias have also been reported after ligation of the anterior choroidal artery but were documented only by CT.[93]

Although such attention to detail might seem excessive, occlusion of the posterior choroidal artery yields a rather unusual syndrome: The artery supplies the lateral geniculate body, the fornix, the dorsomedial nucleus, and the posterior pulvinar. Infarction of these structures in one autopsied case studied by serial sections caused hemianopia, color dysnomia, and disturbance of memory.[6] In some cases studied with brain imaging, such infarction caused homonymous quadrantanopia or sectoranopia, with or without sensory disturbances, and a variety of behavioral disturbances, including memory disturbance and "transcortical aphasia."[92] That so complex a syndrome can arise from an occlusion very difficult to visualize on angiography and almost as difficult to document with the best CT and MRI equipment keeps this diagnosis at the forefront of clinical concerns.

Hemiamblyopias are partial visual impairments without complete loss of vision. The defect may be a complete or relative loss of color perception, referred to as *dyschromatopsia* (see later), or a reduction in the perception of light or form. In mild cases, the field defect is detected only by testing with small targets. With more severe impairments, there may be no perception of stationary targets of any size, but detection of moving stimuli may be preserved ("Riddoch phenomenon").[79,94] The pattern of loss of color perception with preserved motion perception is particularly well documented in patients with medial occipitotemporal lesions in the PCA territory.[95-97] Merigan

and coworkers[95] described a typical patient, with MRI-documented infarction of the right fusiform gyrus, who they studied using discrimination tasks with retinotopically presented stimuli. The patient was unable to discriminate colors, name objects, or discriminate grating orientations in the left upper quadrant, but showed normal perception of coherently moving dots in the same location. Such partial defects attest to the complexity of visual perception, which depends on parallel and largely independent processing pathways for color, motion, and form.[98] Lesions in most of the cases involve extrastriate regions, most notably lingual and fusiform gyri, and spare the calcarine cortex. Rare patients have had calcarine cortex lesions and what appeared to be typical dense, scotomatous field defects with no detection of moving stimuli, but they could localize in space stimuli they claimed not to see. The physiologic basis for this so-called blindsight phenomenon remains controversial, with some researchers proposing a separate geniculocortical pathway that bypasses calcarine cortex, and others favoring a mechanism based on small remnants of spared striate cortex.[99,100]

Clinical Course

The clinical course of visual field abnormalities has received insufficient attention. The majority of patients with optic radiation or calcarine cortex lesions do not show significant recovery, owing to the strictly unilateral representation of the primary visual pathway.[101] A general clinical impression is that recovery of vision is most common in paracentral regions and during the first months after onset.[102] Defects persisting beyond the first year are generally permanent.[101,103] Some investigators have observed modest improvement of target detection, color discrimination, and form discrimination in the impaired field as well as shift of the scotoma border by a few degrees with daily computerized visual training,[101,104] although others could not replicate these results.[105] Few patients have been observed long enough for the possibility that the initial deficit may undergo more gradual shrinkage to be excluded. The case of a famous pathologist who was under observation for a long period is of interest because he initially experienced a large visual field defect that later "cleared up."[32] The clinical course was not better characterized historically. As late as 1 year after onset, he was examined by an ophthalmologist, who described a large hemianopic scotoma in the left upper fields "too far from the macula to cause him any disturbances in microscopic work." Twenty-four years later, this patient's formal visual fields were plotted on a tangent screen and showed only a dense but highly circumscribed upper quadrantanopia confined to the macular region and extending some 20 degrees in the horizontal plane and 10 degrees in the vertical plane (Fig. 8–8). No comments were made on the disparity between the patient's comment that his vision had cleared up and the persisting visual field deficit. At autopsy years later, the only site of infarction affecting the calcarine cortex was a small wedge of the lower bank near the pole. However, a larger area of infarction had undermined much of the lingual gyrus and adjacent inferior bank of the calcarine cortex, within which the cellular elements were much reduced in number. The findings were interpreted by Polyak[32] as indicating that the surviving cells sufficed to

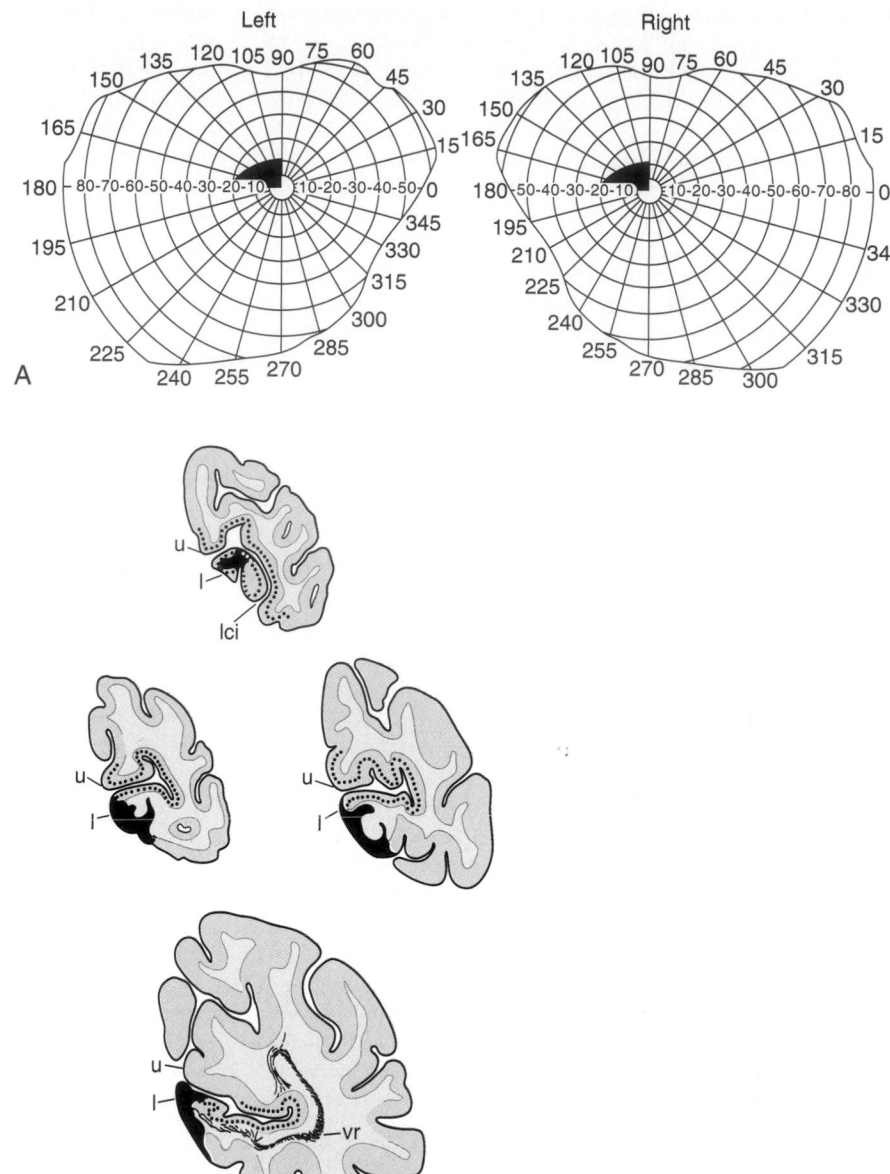

FIGURE 8–8 *(A and B) Case Mallory. The visual field examination years after the stroke showed a circumscribed upper quadrantanopia. (From Polyak SL: The Vertebrate Visual System. Chicago, University of Chicago, 1957.)*

Clinical Manifestations

permit the initial visual field defect to undergo functional resolution, a speculation that appears not to have been challenged in Polyak's lifetime.

Visual Agnosia

Extensive occipital infarction is the usual cause of visual agnosia, a rare disorder featuring an inability to recognize objects. Some of the cases occurred in a setting of cardiac arrest. Many have resulted from bilateral or unilateral PCA territory infarction.

A great deal of effort has been expended in asserting[106,107] or denying[108–110] that such syndromes exist. Opponents of the notion argue that the deficits are a combination of a "primary" visual field defect, a secondary perceptual disorder, and some degree of dementia. Those in support of the notion admit that few cases have been

fully described but that in those cases, the strict criteria have been met—intact primary visual function and no language disturbance. Two forms are said to exist: an apperceptive form, caused by "interference with the processing of primary visual sensory data,"[107] and an associative form, "caused by disorders affecting associative cortex where visual percepts are matched with previously processed sensory data for recognition."[107] Other, more detailed taxonomies based on modern studies of normal visual recognition have also been proposed.[111]

Apperceptive visual agnosia refers to a recognition defect due to imperfect visual perception. Integrity of visual perception has been assessed in a variety of ways, such as having patients discriminate lines of differing length or orientation, discriminate similar shapes, copy shapes, or match objects viewed from different angles. Given the complexity of visual object recognition, which requires integration of orientation, contour, luminance, texture, color, motion, and shape information, it is easy to imagine many subtle deficits that could result in a less than perfect perceptual representation, thus impairing recognition. Patients said to have apperceptive visual agnosia vary in their deficit patterns; typical patients are able to perform simple discriminations but are impaired in performance of more complex tasks such as discriminating and copying shapes.[111–114] Some patients are able to discriminate shapes but unable to match shapes viewed from different angles, suggesting an inability to form a three-dimensional percept.[115–117] Such patients may show better recognition of real three-dimensional objects than of photographs of the same objects.[112,118]

Associative visual agnosia refers to a failure to provide a name or other information about an object when visual perception is normal. Some patients are unable to name visually presented objects but otherwise show relatively intact knowledge by answering questions about the objects, categorizing them, or demonstrating their use through pantomime. This syndrome, which has been called "optic aphasia,"[119–121] differs from a more general amnestic (anomic) aphasia in that with optic aphasia, the same objects that cannot be named from visual input are readily named after tactile presentation or after a verbal description of the object is provided. Other patients show a more severe impairment that involves both deficient naming and an inability to retrieve knowledge about the object from visual input, but with intact knowledge retrieval with tactile input or giving of the object's name.[107,122–125] These syndromes have similar lesion localization and may simply represent ends of a continuum with varying deficit in knowledge retrieval.[126–130] The restriction of impairments to the visual modality has suggested to many investigators a functional disconnection between an intact visual perceptual system and an intact language system.[121,125,131] This formulation is supported by the frequent co-occurrence of associative visual agnosia with right homonymous hemianopia, which deprives the left hemisphere of direct visual input, and splenial damage, which interrupts the transfer of information from the intact right visual cortex to the left hemisphere.[119,121,123–125,130,132–135] Many patients with this profile have also had alexia (without writing impairment) and color dysnomia, both of which have also been attributed to visual-verbal disconnection.[136]

Bilateral PCA territory infarction has explained some instances of visual agnosia. A patient described by Rubens and Benson[107] was later the subject of an autopsy report.[29] The visual agnosia was accompanied by right hemianopia, dyslexia with preserved ability to write, color "agnosia," "impaired verbal learning," and prosopagnosia. The visual agnosia was demonstrated by the patient's ability to produce approximate drawn copies of the picture stimuli he was unable to name or point to after hearing the item named by the examiner. By comparison, he was able to name the same object immediately after palpation or when hearing its characteristic sound. At autopsy, the left PCA was found to be firmly occluded from its junction with the posterior communicating artery to its first temporal branch. On cut section, a predominantly subcortical infarct was found that undermined the left parahippocampal gyrus, undermined the entire lingual gyrus, and reached

the surface at its distal end. A smaller subcortical infarct undermined most of the right lingual gyrus. The researchers speculated that the combination of lesions prevented visual stimuli discriminated by the right hemisphere from arousing associations in the left, analogous to the dyslexia and color-associative defect also found.[29]

A similar case of associative visual agnosia was reported by Albert and colleagues;[122,137] this patient's deficit was somewhat more circumscribed. He was initially blind but regained some sight within 2 days. Vision improved by day 8 to a right upper quadrantic defect. Although able to read aloud, describe pictures, copy by drawing, and match words heard to pictures seen, the patient had difficulty naming pictures shown to him. Aller and colleagues[137] reported results of the autopsy of this patient. On the right, an infarct was found over the entire parahippocampal and lingual gyrus; on the left, a similar infarct affected the parahippocampal gyrus, and another affected part of the lingual and fusiform gyri. A small infarct was found in the left pulvinar.

In one unusual case reported by Cambier and associates,[138] the patient had bilateral infarctions, quite large on the right, but the infarct affecting the left side was confined to the fusiform gyrus. Hemianopia was confined to the left side. The patient had alexia without agraphia, but no "agnosia for colors."

Unilateral left PCA territory infarction has been documented by neuroimaging or autopsy in many cases of associative visual agnosia.[106,123,124,127,130,132,133–135,139–143] In one typical patient, a large hemorrhagic infarction resulted in right homonymous hemianopia, right visual spatial neglect, difficulty naming visual stimuli, and alexia with spared writing.[143] The patient was able to copy by drawing, and he could match a picture to another view of the same object from among six choices. However, he had great difficulty showing the use of a pictured object and could not reliably group objects together according to their functional class. Another typical patient, documented by MRI, had right homonymous hemianopia without macular sparing, difficulty naming visual stimuli including colors, and alexia with spared writing.[123] He showed normal visual perception on tests of size discrimination, shape matching, pattern matching, line orientation matching, and line length discrimination. He could match pictured objects seen from different views, indicating accurate formation of a three-dimensional percept, and he could discriminate line drawings of real objects from unreal objects with similar features, indicating a sense of familiarity. However, he could not demonstrate the use of pictured objects and was imperfect at grouping objects by semantic category. In contrast, naming and describing use of objects were normal when he was allowed to touch them. The lesion involved most of the left PCA territory, including portions of the splenium.

Such cases seem to represent an extreme form of disconnection between an intact right hemisphere visual system, which enables normal performance on visual perceptual tasks, and the left hemisphere language system, which produces the naming and categorization responses. Further evidence of this interhemispheric disconnection is seen in the actual responses given by the patients, which often have a markedly perseverative character.[121,123,124,130]

One patient, after producing a name for the first object shown, subsequently gave responses from the same semantic category as the first name regardless of what the objects actually were, as if the visual input exerted no control over the spoken responses.[123] Pantomime responses tend to be consistent with whatever name is given, whether correct or incorrect, suggesting that the pantomime is based on the name retrieved rather than the visual input.[121,130,135,144] Several patients showed better performance on pantomime and categorization tasks when prior naming was prevented than when naming was allowed, suggesting interference between the hemispheres.[124,130,135]

Yet other patients with similarly large left PCA territory lesions and right hemianopic deficits were able to categorize and pantomime the use of objects they could not name.[119,125,130,133,145] Such cases of "optic aphasia" have been explained in two ways. One explanation presupposes that the isolated right hemisphere possesses semantic capabilities and can perform pantomime and categorization tasks, as long as there is no transcallosal interference by the damaged left hemisphere.[119,130,131] Schnider and coworkers[130] argued this point on anatomical grounds, opining that the patients with optic aphasia have more damage to the corpus callosum than those with visual agnosia.[130] There are, however, several clear counterexamples, such as patients with visual agnosia and extensive splenial damage.[123,124,132] An alternative account assumes that the semantic system lies principally in the left hemisphere and that all patients with visual agnosia or optic aphasia have difficulty accessing this system from visual input.[126,146–148] What might account for individual variability in performing pantomime and categorization tasks, therefore, is individual variability in the semantic capabilities of the right hemisphere.[126,128] Functional neuroimaging studies amply demonstrate the existence of such variability.[149–151] Alternatively (or additionally), patients with visual agnosia may have greater damage to the left hemisphere semantic system than those with optic aphasia.[148]

An unexplained but repeatedly observed feature of this syndrome is relatively preserved naming and recognition of actions compared with objects.[124,130,140–142,147] Objects whose use is demonstrated through action are also better named than stationary objects.[124,130,132,140]

Prosopagnosia

Prosopagnosia is said to be present when the sufferer fails to recognize known faces at sight. This intriguing syndrome may in some cases be but a component of the larger problem currently labeled "visual agnosia." In the published literature on the subject, reviewed by several investigators,[111,152–155] prosopagnosia has usually been associated with unilateral or bilateral visual field defects, particularly involving the upper quadrants of vision. Achromatopsia, dyslexia, and topographic disorientation are also often present, as are, in a few instances, more striking disturbances of visual neglect or Balint's syndrome. As with visual agnosia, there are apperceptive forms and associative forms, though many cases appear to have been a mixture of both. Patients with apperceptive prosopagnosia have deficits in matching different views of unfamiliar faces, suggesting a high-level perceptual problem.[156–158] There may be associated difficulty in determining the age and gender of the unknown face.[159,160] This deficit of face perception has been attributed to a number of more specific impairments, such as deficiency in processing configurations[161,162] or curved surfaces.[163,164] Patients with associative prosopagnosia, in contrast, can match unfamiliar faces but are unable to recognize familiar faces, presumably because the normal percept cannot be connected to information about the identity of the individual.[156,158–160] In neither apperceptive nor associative prosopagnosia can patients discriminate familiar from unfamiliar faces.

Almost all cases of prosopagnosia have resulted from damage to ventral temporal or ventral temporo-occipital areas. More precise anatomical formulations have been difficult to derive. One point of ongoing dispute is whether prosopagnosia requires bilateral lesions, as suggested in several early reviews,[152,154] or can result from unilateral right hemisphere damage. The patient reported by Cambier and associates[138] had a large right occipital infarct and a small infarct on the left limited to the fusiform gyrus. These researchers argued for bilateral medial occipital lesions in such cases, that affect the inferior visual radiations and are not necessarily caused by large infarcts. They marshaled evidence against the traditional claim that prosopagnosia is a sign of right hemisphere dysfunction.[29,165] Their review also indicated that the larger of the bilateral lesions could be on the left, not the right, side.

Landis and coworkers[39] described a patient who died 10 days after onset of prosopagnosia and was found at autopsy to have a large unilateral right occipitotemporal infarct, indicating that unilateral involvement is sufficient for the syndrome to occur. De Renzi and colleagues[153] found 27 cases in the literature and reported on three patients of their own, all with large, unilateral right hemisphere lesions. In contrast, prosopagnosia from unilateral left hemisphere damage appears to be very rare. Nevertheless, it is doubtful that even large right PCA territory infarcts always cause prosopagnosia. One counter-example we have encountered was a young man with a very large right ventral temporal and occipital infarct accompanied by left upper quadrantanopia (Fig. 8–9). At no time did he experience difficulty recognizing familiar faces, and he performed normally on a recognition test using 20 photographs of famous people and on a test requiring matching of unfamiliar faces viewed from different angles.[166]

Much debate has centered on whether the impairment can be confined to faces or always involves other classes of visual stimuli as well. Some authorities point to particular difficulties with faces as evidence of a "face-specific" perceptual system,[167–169] and others have argued for more general perceptual problems that happen to be particularly important for discriminating faces.[170–172] When object agnosia is also present, the stimulus classes most affected are those with many perceptually similar members, such as cars, flowers, and buildings.[152,171,173,174] Some authors have argued that such deficient discrimination between similar members within a category, whether at a perceptual level or a semantic level, is the crucial deficit in prosopagnosia.[152,171]

Several functional imaging studies in normal subjects demonstrated a posterior temporal region on the fusiform

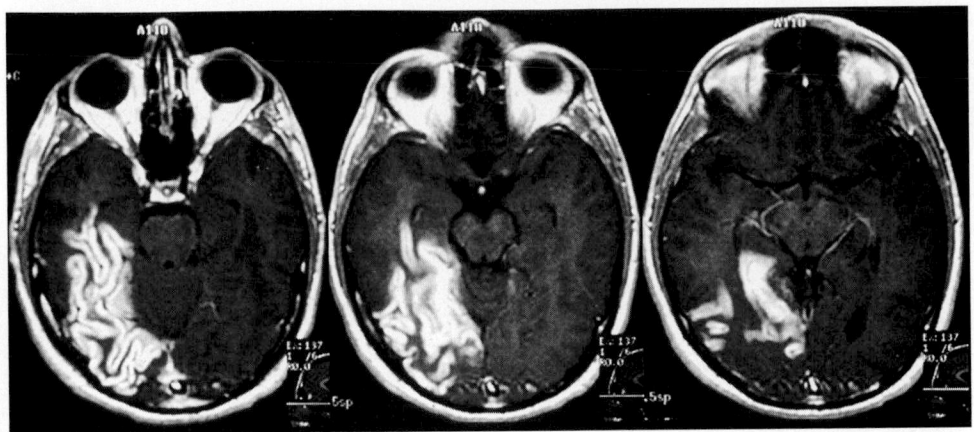

FIGURE 8–9 *Contrast-enhanced T1-weighted MR image of a 32-year-old man with infarction affecting nearly the entire ventral occipitotemporal territory of the right posterior cerebral artery. The patient had mild topographical disorientation but no prosopagnosia.*

gyrus in both hemispheres that responds more strongly to faces than to other visual stimuli.[175–179] Other studies showed stronger activation by familiar faces than by unfamiliar faces in more anterior areas of the ventral temporal lobe.[178–180] These results suggest a hierarchical processing stream progressing posteriorly to anteriorly along much of the ventral temporal lobe, which may explain why prosopagnosia can occur from ventral temporal lobe lesions in a wide variety of locations.[173]

Palinopsia

Palinopsia has been regarded as a bit of a curiosity and is not commonly a result of vascular disease.[181] The syndrome usually occurs in a patient who has an impaired visual field but is not entirely blind.[182] Many investigators have grouped together the two variants and their frequently associated experiences.[183] In one form of palinopsia, there is a persistence of some or all of a visual image immediately after it has disappeared from the environment. In the other form, the image reappears only some time later and persists for varying periods. This form is quite striking, as the time between the disappearance of the original stimulus and its reappearance may be hours or days, and the image may persist into the following day. A peculiar feature of the palinopic images is their tendency to be incorporated in the appropriate position into visual stimuli in the present environment, such as a cigar and beard appearing on the faces of all the people at a party. Frank hallucinations and illusions of visual movement are common accompaniments of both types.[184] Meadows and Munro[183] described three patients, one of whom underwent autopsy. This last patient experienced a severe headache lasting only a few hours and then suffered palinopic images beginning the next day and recurring for the remaining 7 days of her life, unaccompanied by any other obvious complaints. A congruous, left upper quadrantanopia was documented. The autopsy showed a predominantly subcortical infarct undermining the right lingual and fusiform gyri, that seemed to be at least several months old. Michel and Troost,[181] using CT only, studied three patients whose palinopic images also occurred in the affected visual field after presumed unilateral occipital infarction, affecting the right side in two and the left in one. The lesions were all large. Whether the palinopic effect represents a form of seizure is unknown, although treating such patients with anticonvulsants remains common practice.

Micropsia

An unusual complaint, *micropsia* is a visual disorder in which objects appear smaller than expected. Yamada and associates[185] reported a 63-year-old man whose micropsia occurred suddenly and was associated with an acute amnestic state (as expected from large left PCA territory infarction), but his visual field disturbance was limited to a right upper quadrantanopia. CT and MRI showed an infarct in the left occipital lobe and hippocampus. All the clinical features improved within a month, save for the persistence of the quadrantanopia. Another patient with a migraine history and postmortem right cerebral infarction has been reported.[186] The infarct was found in the inferolateral occipital region near the inferred borderzone shared by the middle and posterior cerebral arteries. The syndrome started as left homonymous hemianopia with prominent prosopagnosia. As these complaints faded over a week's time, the patient noted that objects seemed somewhat shrunken and compressed in his left visual field, making the plotting of visual fields difficult and producing an awareness that pictures seemed asymmetric. He drew the left-hand side of a pattern larger than the right so it would look symmetrical to him.

Topographical Disorientation

Patients with topographical disorientation, an infrequently described syndrome, have a striking inability to find their way around.[187,188] Infarction in the right hemisphere, left visual field defects, and, occasionally, a disorder in recognition of faces are among the usual accompanying signs. There are at least three distinct syndromes. In the first, patients have difficulty recognizing familiar environmental landmarks such as buildings and street corners.[189–193] This syndrome resembles and is often accompanied by prosopagnosia, and some investigators prefer the label *topographical agnosia* or *landmark agnosia*. In the second syndrome, landmarks are recognized but do not evoke a sense of direction; the patient is unable to retrieve the routes previously learned in going from one landmark to another.[188,194-197] Alternative terms for this type are *topographical amnesia*, *directional disorientation*, and *heading disorientation*.[187] In the third syndrome, the patient is able to recognize landmarks and follow familiar routes but is impaired in learning *new* routes.[188,198-200]

Though sometimes appearing in the setting of more global disorientation, dementia, or spatial neglect, topographical disorientation from stroke often occurs in relative isolation. In three cases we have studied, no other disturbance was discovered except for homonymous left inferior quadrantanopia in one case.[194] Although suffering a topographical directional disorientation so severe that he could not find the bathroom in the apartment he had lived in for more than 40 years, one of our patients successfully conducted a high-level law practice, with no errors in language, memory, or judgment noted by any of his many colleagues.

All variants of topographical disorientation are associated with lesions in the PCA territory, most often in the right hemisphere. Deficits of landmark recognition (landmark agnosia) typically follow bilateral or large right-sided lesions of the inferomedial occipital lobe centered on the lingual gyrus.[190,192] Most of the reported patients with preserved landmark recognition and impaired sense of direction (directional disorientation) had unilateral infarction in the right retrosplenial, posterior cingulate, or posterior parahippocampal cortex.[188,194-197] Impaired learning of new routes is strongly associated with right parahippocampal damage.[188,198-200] These localizations are supported by functional imaging studies in normal subjects that show activation of the medial occipital lobe during landmark recognition, of the posterior cingulate cortex during recall of directions, and of the parahippocampus during learning of routes and visual scenes.[178,201-205] Still, topographical disorientation has resulted from lesions in a variety of other locations, including the right parietal lobe,[206,207] right internal capsule,[208] and left splenium.[194,209]

Disorders of Reading

Ischemic lesions in the territory of the PCA produce a variety of disorders labeled *alexia* or *dyslexia*. Although some writers have characterized these disorders as rare,[210] they probably occur to varying degrees in the majority of patients with dominant hemisphere PCA infarcts.[118,211] Writing and other language functions are completely or almost completely spared in these syndromes, which have proved of interest for the opportunity they provide to test mechanisms of cerebral function as well as for the different forms of disturbance encountered. At the present time, all of these forms are casually classified as alexia or dyslexia without agraphia, yet the nature of the disorders and the extent of the underlying lesions differ enough that they each deserve a different descriptive term. Unfortunately, no such terms have yet come into standard use.

Global Alexia

Global alexia is the most severe form. The patient with this syndrome can read no words and is markedly inaccurate in naming even single letters. Characteristically, when presented with lexical stimuli, the patient responds with little hesitation and often displays no awareness that the

responses are well off the mark. For example, Wyllie's[33] patient III (Fig. 8–10) named the word "Dugald" as a series of single letters "k-a-n-i-o-i," similarly responded to the digit set "123456" as "i-r-e-i-u-e," and even named the mathematical symbols "+ − =" as "n-e-a." It makes little difference whether the letters and words are presented in typed, printed, or handwritten form; patients cannot read their own handwriting. Some words ordinarily presented in a distinctive form (e.g., the script form in which the word Coca-Cola appears in advertisements) may be read aloud easily, but the meaning of the words is derived from the unique shape of the stimuli, not from the letters themselves. Despite this marked inability to name letters, letters and digits are accurately discriminated from unfamiliar characters. For example, the patient does not distinguish between languages sharing the same characters as his own (e.g., English and Italian) but usually rejects truly novel lexical stimuli such as the alphabet of a foreign language having no characters in common (e.g., Arabic compared with English). The patient readily and spontaneously reorients letters presented in upside-down or rotated orientation. Musical notes and digits are classifiable separately from letters, but the items themselves do not convey meaning. The first reported patient with global alexia was an accomplished musician who, in addition to losing the ability to name letters, lost the power to read musical scores after his stroke, although he retained the ability to play and sing from memory.[212] In some cases, the patient can name letters and digits when his or her hand is passively traced over the shapes (Willbrand's sign), indicating that the problem is with the visual forms. Writing, spelling aloud, and naming words heard in spelled form are usually spared.

This clinical picture is often accompanied by many other disorders indicative of a major left PCA territory infarction.[118] A dense right homonymous hemianopia is nearly always present. There may also be optic aphasia or visual agnosia, color dysnomia, amnestic aphasia, transcortical sensory aphasia, or memory disturbance.[119,125,134,136,143,213-215] In other patients, the deficits accompanying the alexia have been less spectacular.[216]

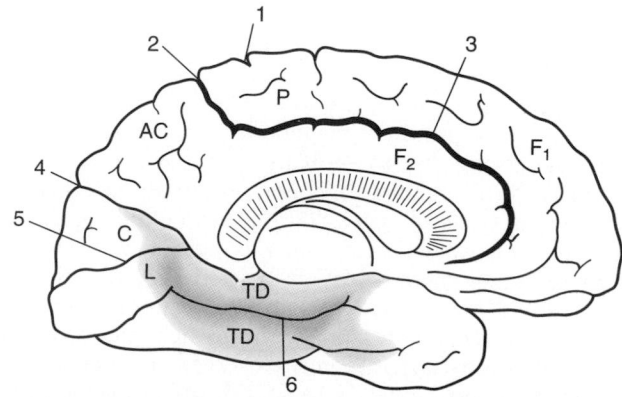

FIGURE 8–10 *Drawing of the brain in Wyllie's Case III, showing the mesial left occipital infarction that produced global alexia. (From Wyllie J: The Disorders of Speech. Edinburgh, Oliver, Boyd, 1894.)*

Clinical Manifestations

Verbal Dyslexia

Verbal dyslexia is a less severe impairment in which individual letter naming is preserved. The patient cannot read whole words but adopts a strategy of recognizing words by naming the letters one by one. This is the most common form of alexia without agraphia and has been by far the most studied, almost to the point of obscuring the existence of global alexia.[217] Many writers use the term *letter-by-letter reading* to denote the syndrome,[218–222] which has also been called *word-form dyslexia*[223] and *spelling dyslexia*.[211] Because the patient depends on sequential identification of letters, the time needed to read a word increases with word length.[219,222–224] Patients with this syndrome may initially show global alexia but, within days to weeks after onset, begin to read words by laboriously naming individual letters. Letter naming typically becomes fluent after weeks to months. We monitored five such patients and documented continued improvement in both reading accuracy and reading speed throughout the first year after stroke.[211] Some patients with verbal dyslexia have right upper quadrantanopia rather than a complete hemianopia.[211,216,225]

The phenomenon of letter-by-letter reading suggests the existence of somewhat different mechanisms serving recognition of single letters and whole words.[223] Experimental evidence in normal readers indicates that the orthographic structure of a written language, such as the frequency with which particular letter combinations occur, is coded in the brain and influences reading speed.[226,227] Damage to this "visual word-form" system may underlie verbal dyslexia. Other evidence shows that fluent reading involves a whole-word process in which the constituent letters of a word are processed in parallel rather then sequentially.[228] In some patients with verbal dyslexia, the defect may be a specific deficit of this parallel processing system, resulting in simultanognosia for letter strings.[229]

Dyslexia with No Visual Field Defect

Pure dyslexia without a visual field defect has been reported only rarely. Leff and associates,[230] reviewing 107 cases of pure dyslexia published over the past 40 years, found only 4 with quantitative visual testing that confirmed intact visual fields. The first description of the syndrome was made without autopsy or imaging data; the patient, a 20-year-old woman, walking in the street, suddenly noticed she could not read the letters on a sign or the names of the subway stations.[10] Her alexia was described as complete for all varieties of reading tasks, including musical notes. The handful of autopsied or imaged cases, the first of which were described by Greenblatt,[231,232] have been from tumors, arteriovenous malformations, hematomas, and the like, but not from infarction.[230,233–238] Most of these patients had relatively mild deficits, such as slowing or hesitation during reading, or transient dyslexia that rapidly cleared. Patients with severe deficits had large lesions of the left ventrolateral occipitotemporal cortex and lateral occipitotemporal convexity, the residue of lobar hemorrhages involving fusiform, inferior temporal, and lateral occipital gyri.[230,237] The patients read very slowly and inaccurately and showed a marked drop in word recognition with increasing word length, suggesting a letter-by-letter reading strategy.

Lesions Associated with Reading Disorders

Lesions associated with reading disorders have been subject to many interpretations.[6,136,211,216,231,239–241] *Major infarction in the PCA territory of the hemisphere dominant for speech and language, usually the left, appears necessary to precipitate the striking disorder of global or absolute alexia.*[119,125,134,136,143,211,213–215,217,239] In Déjerine's[30] frequently discussed case, the lesion, an old infarct, had damaged the inferior edge of the posterior portion of the corpus callosum as well as the cortex of the cuneus and adjacent calcarine region and had completely penetrated the underlying white matter to the wall of the ventricle (Fig. 8–11). Although this patient is commonly considered to have had hemianopia, the right visual field function was intact enough that Landolt's[242] original examination demonstrated only a hemiachromatopsia (see later discussion on color); the patient had full, albeit dim, vision in the right visual field to white targets. Déjerine proposed that the subcortical component of the infarct served to disrupt the projections to the angular gyrus (which he considered to be the site where the lexical information gained access to the language system) from both the ipsilateral calcarine cortex and the opposite side, this latter pathway via the corpus callosum. He made little mention of the callosal

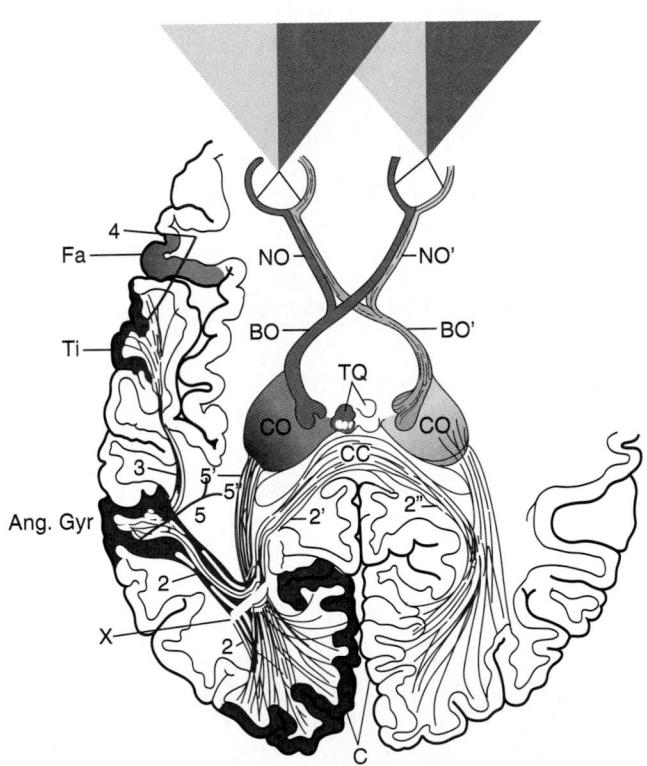

FIGURE 8–11 *Diagram of the possible site (X) of interruption of the visual pathways linking the calcarine cortices (C) with the angular gyrus (Ang. Gyr.). BO, left optic tract; BO', right optic tract; CC, corpus callosum; CO, left lateral geniculate body; CO', right lateral geniculate body; Fa, frontal operculum; NO, left optic nerve; NO', right optic nerve; Ti, superior temporal gyrus. (Adapted from Déjerine J, Vialet N: Contribution a l'étude de la localisation anatomique de la cécité verbale pure. C R Seances Soc Biol 45:790, 1893.)*

lesion, as did Vialet[241] in a thorough review of the case. In both instances, emphasis was placed on the deep paraventricular lesion. Damasio and Damasio[216] resurrected these observations and drew attention to the likelihood that the inferior fibers of the forceps major, which cross in the inferior portion of the corpus callosum and terminate in the inferior visual association cortices, were the fibers of relevance for the conveyance of lexical information from the right to the left hemisphere. The anatomical course of these fibers places them in the position to be caught in a deep infarct that penetrates to the wall of the ventricle.

We had somewhat different findings in our five patients with global alexia, whose lesions were compared with those of seven control patients with left PCA infarction in whom reading was unaffected.[211] Normal readers had damage in the medial and ventral occipital lobe, which affected the ventral occipital white matter but spared dorsal white matter pathways and the ventral temporal lobe. Global alexia was invariably accompanied by dense right homonymous hemianopia and occurred only with additional injury to the splenium, forceps major, or white matter above the occipital horn of the lateral ventricle (Fig. 8–12). Many other reports of severe alexia have also documented right hemianopia together with damage to the splenium or forceps major.[119,125,134,136,213–215,217,239,243] On the basis of these observations, we proposed that the pathway from the right visual cortex to left language areas involved in reading is most vulnerable at the splenium and forceps major, before it fans out laterally over the top of the occipital horn to synapse in ventrolateral and anterior visual association areas.[211] This formulation is different from the more inferomedial location favored by several other writers.[216,238]

Déjerine did not specify whether he believed visual information was conveyed from the right hemisphere via transcallosal pathways directly to the language zone without interruption or by an indirect route through the left visual cortex. The lesion shown in his often-reproduced diagram (see Fig. 8–11) can be interpreted either way but is placed laterally enough to emphasize his original point that it served to interrupt the pathway from both calcarine

Clinical Manifestations

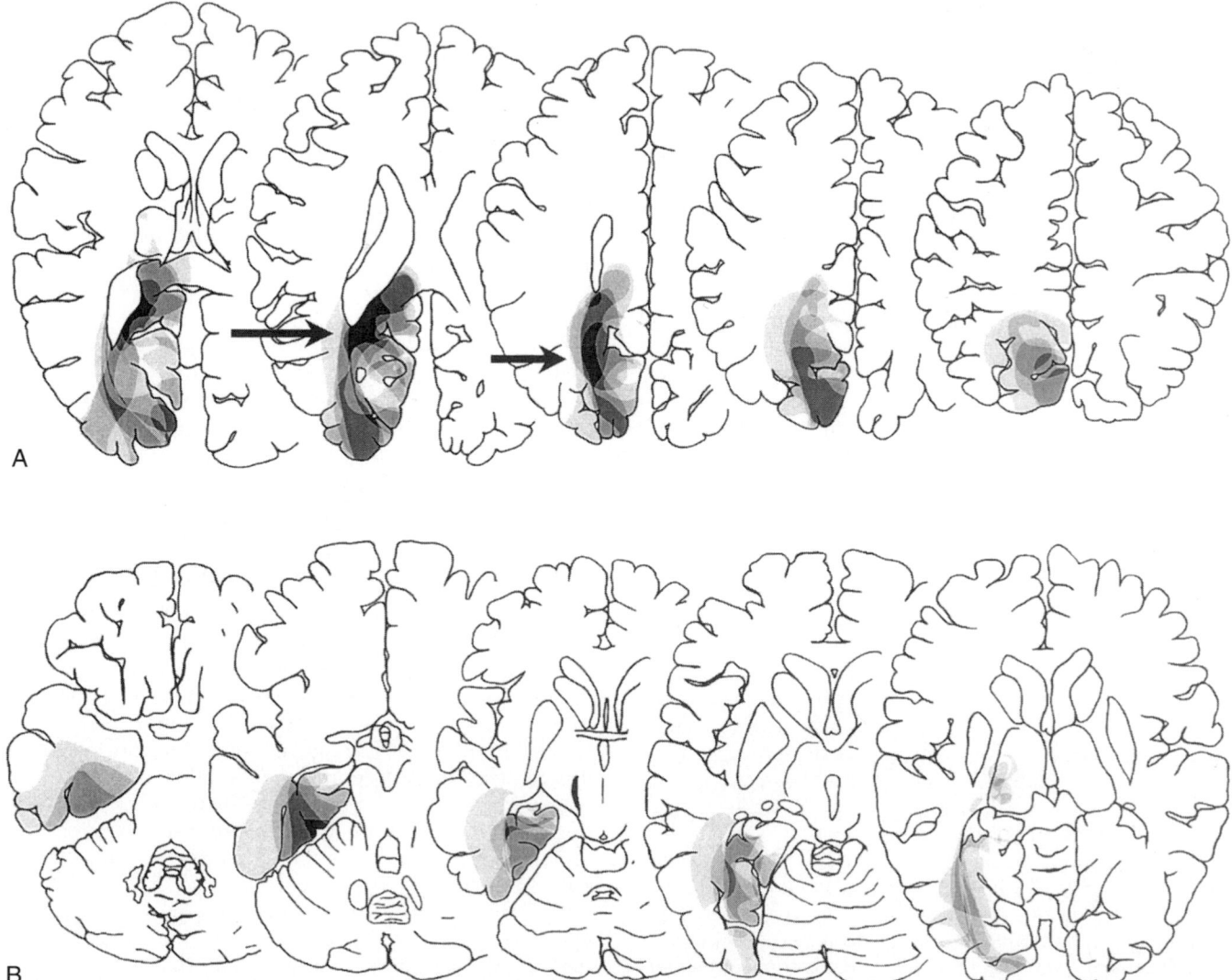

FIGURE 8–12 *Lesion overlap analyses.* A, *Common areas of damage, in patients with global alexia, that were not damaged in normal readers with left posterior cerebral artery infarcts.* B, *Common areas of damage, in patients with verbal dyslexia (letter-by-letter reading), that were not damaged in normal readers with left posterior cerebral artery infarcts.*

regions. Given that calcarine infarction alone does not cause alexia,[211,241] it is very unlikely that the transcallosal pathway passes through primary visual cortex in the left calcarine area. This inference, and the observation that some patients with mild forms of pure dyslexia have "subangular" parietal lesions that appear to completely spare the left visual system,[232,233,244] led to the idea of a direct white matter pathway from the splenium to the angular gyrus.

Arguing against this theory, however, are many cases of pure dyslexia with lesions confined to the left visual association cortex. For example, lesions in the five patients with verbal dyslexia that we studied show greater involvement of the anterior visual association cortex, primarily in the left fusiform gyrus, than the lesions in normal readers (see Fig. 8–12).[211] Other patients have had lesions involving the ventrolateral or lateral occipital cortex.[218,231,234–237,245] Patient 1 of Sakurai and colleagues,[245] for example, had an initial infarct affecting the left calcarine cortex and lingual gyrus, followed a year later by lateral extension of the lesion to the fusiform, lateral occipital, and inferior temporal gyri. The first stroke produced no reading disturbance, but the second caused abrupt dyslexia, affecting whole-word pictograms (kanji) more than phonograms (kana). These cases suggest that left visual association areas, particularly those lateral and anterior to the lingual gyrus, are critical components of the reading pathway and receive input from early visual systems in both hemispheres. This account is further supported by functional imaging studies in normal subjects showing a "visual word-form" area in the left ventrolateral visual cortex (particularly fusiform gyrus), which responds more to letters, words, and wordlike letter strings than to nonsense shapes.[246] Unlike the calcarine cortex and lingual gyrus, which are activated only by stimuli from the contralateral hemifield, this left-hemisphere visual word-form area responds to graphemic stimuli presented to either hemifield, indicating that it receives transcallosal projections from the right visual cortex.[230,246] Leff and associates[230] showed that this area is activated by graphemic stimuli not only in normal control subjects but also in good readers with macula-splitting right hemianopia from calcarine infarcts. In the same report, these investigators described a patient with verbal dyslexia but no hemianopia who had a large lesion centered in the same ventrolateral occipitotemporal area that was activated in the normal readers. These data argue strongly that (1) left medial occipital infarcts cause visual field defects but do not impair reading, (2) left lateral occipital and occipitotemporal (fusiform gyrus, inferior temporal gyrus) lesions impair reading but do not produce visual field defects, and (3) transcallosal pathways from the right visual system subserving reading project to the left lateral occipitotemporal cortex.

Hemidyslexia

Hemidyslexia was described by Wilbrand[247] as a macular hemianopic disturbance of reading (makulähemianopische Lesestörung). In our experience, it is a frequent accompaniment of a homonymous hemianopia contralateral to infarction affecting the PCA territory of the hemisphere dominant for speech and language. In some instances, the hemianopia is limited to the macular region, as demonstrated by Polyak's[32] patient Harry Kraft, or to the right upper quadrant.

For most patients with such lesions, reading of connected text is more disturbed than reading of single words, owing to a disruption of the visuomotor coordination of saccadic eye movements during text reading.[248,249] Reading speed directly depends on the amount of spared macular vision in the right hemifield.[249,250] Reading of single words is often disturbed as well, manifested as both slowed recognition and misreading of the right-hand end of longer words. The time needed to read a word increases with word length, though not nearly as dramatically as in verbal dyslexia.[230] Errors occur whether the task is reading aloud or for comprehension and whether the words are printed or written, large or small, and isolated or embedded in text, as long as the words are lengthy (four letters or more). Errors occur less often when the right-hand end of the word is easily predicted by the left-hand end (e.g., "eight") and more often when the right-hand end has many possibilities not predicted by the left-hand end (e.g., "predator"). The term *hemidyslexia* is not quite accurate, because the errors do not occur beginning at the midpoint of the stimulus but instead only at some point beyond the midline of the word.

Hemidyslexia affecting the left side of words occurs after sectioning of the corpus callosum.[234,251,252] The surgical section does no damage to the primary visual pathways but interrupts transmission of information from the right hemisphere to the left. Because the initial letters of a word fall within the left visual field during word fixation, they are transmitted first to the right hemisphere and are then misperceived because of the interhemispheric disconnection. Binder and coworkers[251] reported two patients with left hemidyslexia who also had macula-splitting *right* hemianopia. Both patients had left calcarine and splenial infarcts that occurred after treatment (embolization or resection) of left-sided retrosplenial arteriovenous malformations. Because visual input in these patients came only from the left visual field, the left-sided errors were taken as evidence that callosal transfer was weaker for letters presented farther to the left from the visual midline. This theory was confirmed by presentation of words in vertical orientation, which improved single-word reading accuracy from 55% to 93%.

Color Dysnomia and Dyschromatopsia

Some degree of faulty color discrimination may occur with dysfunction at any level along the visual pathway.[253–255] The lateral geniculate body is considered to play a role in color discrimination,[256] but deficits in color discrimination would be expected to occur only when the lesion is bilateral. However, when infarction is the cause of dyschromatopsia, it usually lies in the occipital lobe inferior to the calcarine cortex in the fusiform or lingual gyri, either with full-thickness infarction or with subcortical infarction that undermines the gyri. The lesion may be unilateral on either side[32,95,212,242,257–262] or bilateral.[31,96,97,253,257,263–267] In human functional imaging studies, the posterior fusiform gyrus responds more strongly to color stimuli than to luminance-matched grays,[263,268] suggesting that it may be the homologue of visual area V4 in the monkey, which is specialized for perception of color.[96,269]

Patients with bilateral color blindness from cerebral disease show impaired performance on tests of color discrimination (e.g., Ishihara color plates, Farnsworth-Munsell 100-hue test), though performance is usually far better than chance. Total absence of color perception (*achromatopsia*) appears to be rather rare.[265] Unilateral cases (*hemidyschromatopsia*) are best detected with color perimetry, because vision in the unimpaired hemifield is sufficient for normal performance on free-field tests such as the Ishihara plates. When the defect is quadrantic, the upper quadrants are affected, never the lower.[258,270] In typical cases, the colors in the affected field(s) are described as gray, pale, or washed out. At times, a given color is misnamed for another having a similar hue or brightness. This last finding is of little clinical value because it also occurs in patients whose color discrimination is intact (see later). Recall is normal for the color name characteristically associated with a given object (e.g., green with grass). Some improvement over time has been reported, even though an upper quadrantanopia might remain.[263,271,258] Prosopagnosia and spatial and topographical disorientation have been reported as associated findings in many patients, particularly those with bilateral lesions.[31,96,97,253,257,264,270] Dyslexia often accompanies right hemidyschromatopsia. One among these cases[30,212,242] was explained by subsequent reviewers as a disconnection syndrome,[272] which would be expected to impair color naming but not color discrimination. Unfortunately, no details were provided about whether the color recognition impairment involved one or both fields, or whether the patient was asked to name colors or simply discriminate between them.

Color and color-name disconnection describes a bidirectional impairment in relating a color to its name in the absence of deficits in color discrimination. The term *color agnosia* has also been used. The absence of deficits in color discrimination is revealed by normal performance on tests such as the Ishihara color plates. The bidirectional impairment in relating a color to its name is shown by errors in naming colors at sight and in matching color names heard or color names seen with color choices, and vice versa. Geschwind and Fusillo[136] applied the term *disconnection syndrome* to this type of case to stress the point that the lesion may have separated the adequately discriminated visual input in the right hemisphere from access to the language region of the left hemisphere. As a result, the patient presumably could not associate visual stimuli with their names, causing alexia (letters and words), defective naming of colors, and defective matching of color names to colors. In support of the disconnection notion, Geschwind and Fusillo[136] stressed that their patient "would answer at random" when shown an object and asked whether it was a certain color. This random quality of color naming has not been a feature of other reported patients, however, even in some other patients with a bidirectional failure in relating colors to their names.

The infarct in the best-known case was in the distribution of the left PCA, destroying most of the gray matter and deep white matter of the medial occipital lobe, including the visual radiation, the inferior longitudinal fasciculus, and the crossing fibers through the splenium of the corpus callosum in the tapetum.[136] A subsequent case reported by Rubens and Benson[107] showed more circumscribed subcortical infarction underlying the left lingual gyrus. Another case used by these researchers in support of their thesis[30,212,242] appears to have had right hemidyschromatopsia; it is not clear from the details of the clinical case report that a disturbance as thoroughly documented as that by Geschwind and Fusillo[136] was present. Unfortunately, for most of the other reported patients whose deficits might represent bidirectional disconnection, precise documentation of a disconnection state was lacking.[191,260,264,273–276] In only a few was complete testing performed for color discrimination, impaired color naming, and impaired matching of colors with color names.[106,136,277] Clinically, these patients also showed a right homonymous hemianopia and dyslexia. The patient described by Zihl and von Cramon[278] exhibited intact color discrimination but impaired color naming restricted to the left visual field after splenial damage, consistent with a disconnection mechanism.

Color dysnomia is often considered synonymous with the bidirectional disconnection syndrome. In the initial days after onset, a patient encountered by one of the authors (JPM) (Fig. 8–13) showed errors both in naming colors and in selecting the correct color from among an array of color choices when a color name was dictated aloud to him.[6] However, within several days, he became able to select a color from among several choices when its name was provided. He was easily able to recall the name of a color commonly associated with a given item and items commonly associated with a given color, yet he persisted in having difficulties in naming a color shown to him. His naming errors were not random or of the confabulatory type. He often named a given color using the name of another color close to it on the spectrum of hue or brightness, such as green for blue, or yellow for orange. The errors were mild enough to be overlooked on casual testing and might have been attributed to dim light in less rigorous test settings. Casual explanations such as these probably account for the infrequency with which the dysnomia is reported in patients with an infarct in a similar locale. When sought in such cases, the deficit is often easily demonstrated. The infarct is often quite modest and may be confined to the subcortical structures of the lingual gyrus.

The syndrome of color dysnomia is also of interest because it may be present without dyslexia (i.e., with preserved reading). Although the two deficits frequently coexist, color dysnomia and alexia do not reflect a common mechanism, rather, they show that spatially proximate regions of the cerebrum serving different functions are susceptible to simultaneous involvement by the same lesion if it is large enough.[279]

Amnestic color dysnomia, a syndrome so rare that it is almost nonexistent, is a disturbance in the recall of the names of the colors that are characteristic of a given object (e.g., green for grass) and vice versa. Tests of color discrimination and cross-matching of color with color names are said to be performed well.[280] No definite neuropathologic basis for this disorder has been established.

Other unusual disturbances in color naming or discrimination occur in cerebral disease.[281] However, none of them has as yet been related to a focal lesion. The delineation of most such disturbances requires the examiner to depend on the patient's subjective description of the altered appearance of color and of its relationship to the environment. The syndromes include illusory spread of color.

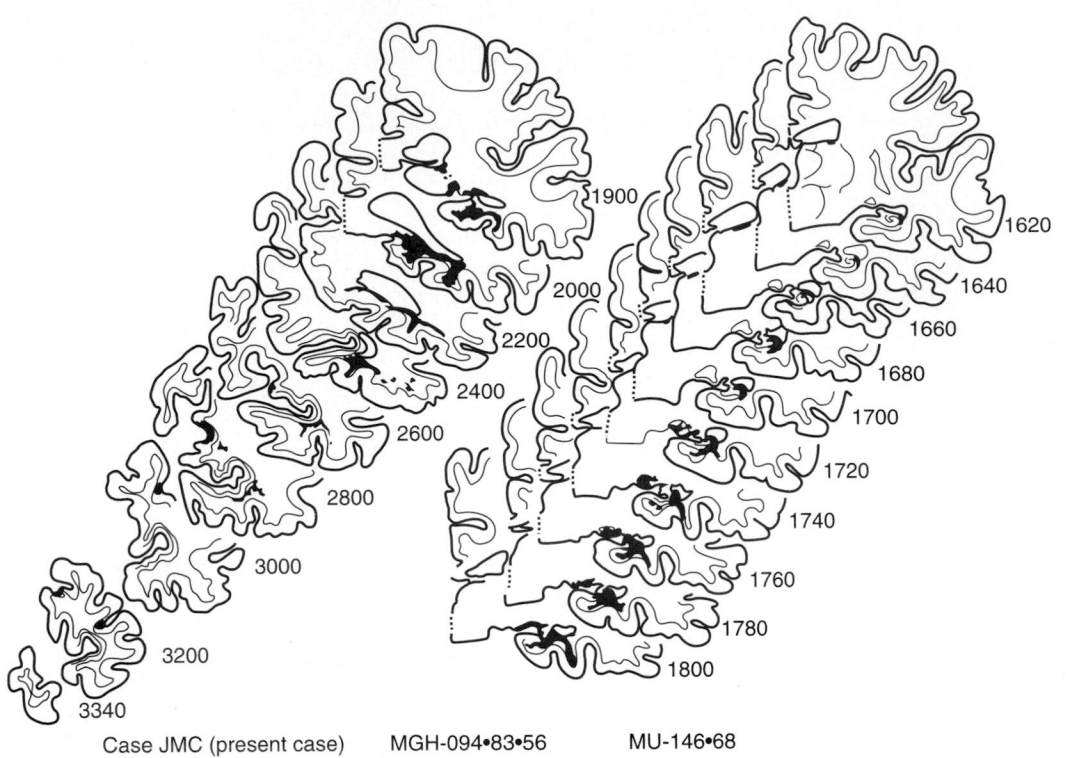

Case JMC (present case)   MGH-094•83•56   MU-146•68

FIGURE 8–13 *Traced serial sections of a posterior cerebral artery territory infarct with involvement of the lateral geniculate body, hippocampus, and subcortical portions of the calcarine region. (From Mohr JP, Leicester J, Stoddard LT, Sidman M: Right hemianopia with memory and color deficits in circumscribed left posterior cerebral artery territory infarction. Neurology 21:1104, 1971.)*

Transcortical Sensory Aphasia

That aphasia may occur with PCA territory lesions is well documented.[58,118,282] Transcortical sensory aphasia is an uncommon disturbance featuring fluent speech, accurate repetition sometimes accompanied by echolalia, and impaired comprehension of both speech and text. Data on neuroanatomical correlation is somewhat lacking. There are clear-cut cases due to infarction in the middle cerebral artery territory or arterial borderzones.[283–287] Whether to place this syndrome among the consequences of PCA territory infarction is subject to argument, but it is discussed here because of the high frequency of accompanying hemianopia, visual object agnosia, and occipitotemporal low density seen on CT or MRI.

Kertesz and associates[288] collected 15 patients with transcortical sensory aphasia diagnosed using the Western Aphasia Battery. The lesion was imaged by isotope brain scan in 12 patients and by CT in 6. A contralateral hemianopia occurred in 11, and 1 had an inferior quadrantanopia. In another 5 patients, the disturbance of higher cerebral function was accompanied by "visual agnosia." The unusual speech pattern was described by the investigators as fluent and circumlocutory, with the content mainly semantic jargon. The lesion locations were equally unusual, as practically all the patients had massive involvement of the posterior half of the brain, spreading from the occipital pole forward on both the ventral and lateral surfaces, and in many, the abnormality reached far forward along the mesial occipital lobe, well within the territory of the PCA. Kertesz and associates[288] suggested that the sites

of infarction were "in the posterior cerebral artery territory or in the watershed area . . . between posterior cerebral and middle cerebral arteries." The mechanism of these infarctions is unclear. Some could be the result of combined middle cerebral and posterior cerebral occlusion, or an internal carotid occlusion with distal field infarction affecting the parieto-occipital region in the unusual instances in which the PCA is a branch of the internal carotid artery. At least one of their patients had an arteriovenous malformation—a lesion suitable for such an unusual location, crossing as it does between two major arterial territories.

Alexander and coworkers[289] found three cases of transcortical sensory aphasia among a group of 12 patients with left PCA infarcts encountered consecutively in a rehabilitation ward. These patients had severely impaired auditory comprehension, semantically empty but fluent jargon speech, and impaired object recognition (agnosia) in both visual and tactile modalities. Eight other patients had varying degrees of visual and tactile anomia with preserved auditory comprehension (amnestic aphasia). The lesion in those with transcortical sensory aphasia was large, involving superficial and deep occipital and temporal lobes as well as the posterolateral thalamus. The feature distinguishing these lesions from those in patients with amnestic aphasia, according to the researchers, was an additional extension of the infarct into deep temporal-occipital white matter and the temporal isthmus. Alexander and coworkers[289] speculated that this lesion disrupted a distributed cortical and subcortical semantic processing network including sensory association areas, areas 37 and 39 of Brodmann, and the thalamus. The remaining patient in the series had an isolated, though large, infarct of the anterolateral and paramedian thalamus. The deficits included impaired auditory comprehension and preserved repetition, but with sparse output and spared object recognition, similar to those in several other reported patients with large thalamic infarcts.[290,291]

Servan and colleagues[282] retrospectively reviewed 76 patients with cortical PCA territory infarcts. Of these, 3 met criteria for transcortical sensory aphasia and had infarction only in the PCA territory (all on the left) without accompanying middle cerebral infarct. All had involvement of the ventromedial temporal lobe, calcarine cortex, and thalamus. Five other patients with anomia but preserved speech content and comprehension (amnestic aphasia) had similar lesions but without thalamic involvement, prompting the investigators to propose that additional damage to the thalamus provokes the deficits seen in transcortical sensory aphasia.

Amnestic Aphasia

Amnestic (or anomic) aphasia is characterized by a failure to recall the names of people as well as many other individual nouns when the stimuli are presented in visual, tactile, or auditory form. The independence of the deficit from modality of sensory input distinguishes it from *optic aphasia*, in which anomia occurs only with visual presentation. Commonly, the expected response fails to occur, with the patient often falling silent or hesitating as if the name is about to be produced momentarily ("tip of the tongue" phenomenon). When the name fails to be given, it is rare for the patient to produce a neologism or other substitutive error. Instead, attributes of the item are described, indicating the patient's familiarity with the item in question. The failures in naming are often associated with circumlocutions, lame excuses for failure, and a general acceptance of the correct name when offered.[280]

Amnestic aphasia has been associated with lesions throughout the language-dominant hemisphere, but severe and isolated anomia has classically been considered a sign of deep temporal lobe[280] or lateral temporo-occipital[292,293] damage. The syndrome has been reported, often incidentally, in patients showing infarction limited to the territory of the dominant PCA.[33,118,125,264] De Renzi and associates[118] documented multimodal anomia in 10 of 16 consecutively encountered cases of left PCA infarct. Compared with controls, naming in affected patients was most impaired for colored photograph stimuli, less for real objects presented in tactile or visual modalities, and least for verbal descriptions. Some writers have emphasized a correlation between the severity of anomia and the severity of dyslexia in such patients.[118,125] The exact pathologic correlation for naming deficits remains unclear, but one possibility is that amnestic aphasia appears when the temporal lobe component of the infarct extends sufficiently laterally (into fusiform and inferior temporal gyri) or deeply to involve lexical systems critical for name retrieval.

Memory Disorder Syndromes

PCA territory infarction may profoundly disrupt memory function,[118,294–296] through damage to the hippocampus, parahippocampus, or efferents and afferents of these structures. As with surgical lesions of the medial temporal lobe, medial temporal infarcts produce impaired acquisition of new memories (*anterograde amnesia*), with relatively little effect on retrieval of memories encoded prior to onset of the lesion (*retrograde amnesia*). Amnestic disorders have also been reported from occlusion of thalamoperforant arteries, but in these cases, the possibility of simultaneous infarction of structures supplied by larger PCA branches is not easily ruled out. On the basis of available literature, the occurrence of an amnestic state is no guide to whether the infarct is of thrombotic or embolic origin.

Bilateral infarction has been the usual setting for severe memory disorders.[34,43,295,297–301] Both embolism and thrombus have been found to be responsible.[43] The occlusions have usually been found proximally in the PCA stem and precortical segment. The infarcts frequently spread along most of the undersurface of the cerebrum, involving the parahippocampus, lingual and fusiform gyri, some as far posteriorly as the cuneus[34]; others have been extensive enough to include the fornices and fimbria of the hippocampus.[299] The hippocampus is sometimes affected in amnestic cases, though PCA infarcts always involve other structures surrounding the hippocampus as well. The best-documented case of isolated bilateral hippocampal infarction was reported by Zola-Morgan and associates.[300] The patient suffered a cardiac arrest with prolonged hypotension, from which he recovered with residual anterograde amnesia. He had severe impairments in learning word lists, learning arbitrary word pairings, recalling a story after a brief delay, and reproducing a nonsense drawing after a brief delay, indicating both verbal and nonverbal anterograde amnesia. In contrast, he performed normally on recognition of famous faces and news events from previous decades and showed no other signs of cognitive impairment. The deficits persisted until death 5 years after onset; autopsy showed complete and bilateral cell loss throughout the CA1 region of hippocampus with little abnormality elsewhere in the brain.

A large literature has accumulated indicating that bilateral hippocampal involvement is a necessary condition for amnesia to occur and to persist.[302] Numerous reports suggest that a bilateral disruption of the fornix though surgical section,[303–305] penetrating wounds,[306] or tumors[307] may achieve the same effect. In other similar cases, however, either no such deficits occurred,[308,309] or memory impairments were transient.[310,311] The exact role of fornix damage in the occurrence and persistence of anterograde memory deficits has been difficult to determine because instances of isolated bilateral fornix interruption are rare.[307] Bilateral infarction of the fornix and the anterior cingulate gyri were described by Laplane and associates[312] in a 70-year-old woman who exhibited a confabulatory-amnestic syndrome as well as complex behavioral changes. Two patients with amnesia due to fornix infarction have also been described,[313,314] but in both, the lesion involved additional regions surrounding the fornix. Gaffan and colleagues[303,304,315] offered perhaps the most persuasive argument for a critical role of the fornix in memory, citing evidence that amnesia after surgical resection of colloid cysts in the third ventricle depends primarily on bilateral damage to the fornix.

The rare case of bilateral PCA territory infarction with unilateral hippocampal or limbic infarction exists to confound efforts to settle the role of the bilateral lesion in memory disorder. Benson and colleagues[29] described a 47-year-old physician with right hemianopia, alexia, visual agnosia, color agnosia, prosopagnosia, and "impaired verbal learning." This disturbance was manifested by an "inability to learn the names of ward personnel, considerable difficulty in learning the Babcock sentence, and ability to remember only one or two of four unrelated words after five minutes." The patient was noted to have made some improvements in the first few months after onset but remained disabled. Although bilateral fusiform gyrus and posterior callosal infarcts were found, the hippocampal infarct was confined to the left side. The autopsy findings were described only in cut section.

Some cases of transient global amnesia (TGA) may represent bilateral medial temporal lobe ischemia. Single-photon emission CT (SPECT) scans performed during the amnestic ictus in TGA frequently show bitemporal hypoperfusion.[316–319] TGA is only rarely associated with embolism or thrombosis, however, and many such cases are probably caused by posterior circulation migraine.[319]

Unilateral infarcts in the left PCA territory have also produced anterograde impairments of memory.[6,115,125,136,213,295,296,298,320,321] Geschwind and Fusillo's[136] case involved a man with thrombosis of the left PCA whose infarct was detailed in serial sections. On admission, he was able to recall his name yet stated his age incorrectly and was unable to recall his address. He failed to recall any of four objects after 1 minute. In addition, prominent deficits were encountered in reading aloud and in naming of colors and simple objects. Severe disturbances in topographical orientation were also noted. No further description was given concerning his memory disorder, but when he was seen 7 weeks after onset, the recent memory deficits were said to have "cleared completely." The topographical disorientation "cleared to normal in the next few weeks." He died 15 months after the stroke occurred. On serial sections obtained at autopsy, the left hippocampus was infarcted and the left fornix had undergone complete degeneration.

A patient described by one of the authors (JPM) showed a severe memory disorder from onset that persisted unchanged until his death on day 82.[6] On initial examination within 12 hours of onset, this patient also stated his name, failed to recall his exact age, and was unable to state his address or where he had been the evening of his stroke. He repeatedly asked many questions, such as "Where is my wife?" He accepted the examiner's answer but within seconds asked the question again. When his wife arrived hours after onset of the stroke and mentioned her brother by name, the patient asked, "Ed who?" He repeatedly attempted to learn the examiner's name, often wrote it on a note pad, and when the examiner reappeared, did not recall the name or consult the note pad. Weeks after discharge, when returning to the laboratory for reexamination, the patient regularly introduced himself to the staff whom he had met on every previous occasion, and only rarely walked spontaneously in the correct direction toward the examining room. He showed a retrograde and anterograde amnesia for the events surrounding his admission, faulty retention of verbal material, impaired retension on a form discrimination test, and an amnestic dysnomia. Whether his deficit would have persisted over a longer period remains an open question. The pathologic findings indicated only unilateral infarction of the left hippocampus, with secondary degeneration of the left fornix and the precommissural bed nuclei of the septum (see Fig. 8–13).

Escourolle and Gray[321] reported an important autopsied patient with memory disturbance whose infarct affected the left occipital and temporal lobe with atrophy of the fimbria of the hippocampus, the fornix, and the anterior nucleus of the thalamus. Several similar autopsied patients with unilateral left PCA infarcts, typically quite large and accompanied by severe alexia, were documented to have anterograde amnestic syndromes persisting to the time of death.[125,214,298]

Despite this evidence, some writers, citing evidence that amnesia from unilateral temporal lobe lesions often improves with time, have proposed that bilateral lesions are necessary for memory deficits to persist.[300,320] Trillet and coworkers[298] presented preliminary evidence to the contrary. They reported 18 patients with PCA occlusion and amnestic syndrome that persisted beyond the first few months. In 3 of these patients, the lesion was probably unilateral, though no definitive anatomical evidence was provided. The systematic investigation reported by von Cramon and associates[296] included 30 patients with unilateral PCA infarction documented by CT, 12 of whom (all with left-sided lesions) had marked verbal memory and learning impairment. Although the patients were not followed longitudinally, 3 were impaired when tested at 1 year after onset, suggesting a relatively permanent deficit. Compared with patients with normal memory functions, the patients with amnestic deficits in this study had farther anterior temporal extension of the infarct into the parahippocampus, collateral sulcus, and underlying white matter (called the "collateral isthmus" by the researchers). Lesion studies in primates show that most of the structures in this region surrounding the hippocampus—posterior parahippocampus, entorhinal cortex, perirhinal cortex, fornix, and cingulum bundle—contribute to normal memory function.[322] It is likely that the larger the medial temporal component of the lesion in cases of left PCA infarct, the greater is the damage to these structures and the greater the severity and persistence of the resulting amnestic syndrome.

Cases in which details were provided have shown patients to have profound disturbances in memory, especially for recent events when tested by conversational methods. The characteristics of the memory impairments and the performance on special laboratory tests are essentially identical to those reported in patients with bilateral medial temporal surgical lesions that include the hippocampus[323,324] and with unilateral temporal lobe removal.[325–327] An acute confusional state has also been described in patients with left PCA territory infarction.[328–330] An isolated amnestic state, that is, without any additional clinical features, has yet to be reported from infarction in the PCA territory. To date, all such cases known to us have produced other deficits accompanying the amnestic state.

Thalamic lesions have also been documented to produce anterograde amnestic syndromes, whether from Wernicke-Korsakoff syndrome[331,332] trauma,[333] or infarction.[38,334,335]

Lesions in the infarct cases are usually bilateral, lie in the territory of the tuberothalamic or anterior paramedian perforators, and involve anterior nuclei and the mamillothalamic tract.

Klüver-Bucy Syndrome

Klüver-Bucy syndrome is described here because its cause is usually bilateral lesions in the territory of the PCAs. In the small number of reports, some not using this eponym,[336] the lesions have been very large, affecting most of the undersurface of the temporal lobes,[329,330,337–340] including the fusiform and lingual gyri, parahippocampal gyri, and the hippocampal structures. In addition to the fearless exploration of environment, the syndromes precipitated by these infarctions frequently include a prominent state of exaggerated motor activity; restlessness, agitation, delirium, crying out, and unwarranted excessive reaction to visual, auditory, or cutaneous stimuli may be the most striking features noted in the acute phase.[341] Within hours to days, these states usually subside.

References

1. Lazorthes G, Salamon G: Étude anatomique et radio-anatomique de la vascularisation arterielle du thalamus. Ann Radiol 14:905, 1971.
2. Abbie AA: The blood supply of the visual pathways. Med J Aust 2:199, 1938.
3. Salamon G, Huang YP: Radiologic Anatomy of the Brain. Berlin, Springer-Verlag, 1976.
4. Milisavljevic MM, Marinkovic SV, Gibo H, Puskas LF: The thalamogeniculate perforators of the posterior cerebral artery: The microsurgical anatomy. Neurosurgery 28:523, 1991.
5. Galloway JR, Greitz T: The medial and lateral choroidal arteries: An anatomic and roentgenographic study. Acta Radiol (Stockh) 53:353, 1960.
6. Mohr JP, Leicester J, Stoddard LT, Sidman M: Right hemianopia with memory and color deficits in circumscribed left posterior cerebral artery territory infarction. Neurology 21:1104, 1971.
7. Ghika JA, Bogousslavsky J, Regli F: Deep perforators from the carotid system: Template of the vascular territories. Arch Neurol 47:1097, 1990.
8. Kaul SN, DuBoulay GH, Kendall BE, Ross Russell RW: Relationship between visual field defects and arterial occlusion in the posterior cerebral circulation. J Neurol Neurosurg Psychiatry 37:1033, 1974.
9. Margolis MT, Newton TH, Hoyt WF: Cortical branches of the posterior cerebral artery anatomic-radiologic correlation. Neuroradiology 2:127, 1971.
10. Peron N, Goutner V: Alexie pure sans hemianopsie. Rev Neurol 76:81, 1944.
11. Smith CG, Richardson WFG: The course and distribution of the arteries supplying the visual striate cortex. Am J Ophthalmol 61:1391, 1966.
12. Margolis MT, Smith CG, Richardson WF: The course and distribution of the arteries supplying the visual (striate) cortex. Am J Ophthalmol 61:1391, 1966.
13. Beevor CE: On the distribution of the different arteries supplying the human brain. Philos Trans R Soc [Biol] 200:1, 1909.
14. Shellshear JL: A contribution to our knowledge of the arterial supply of the cerebral cortex in man. Brain 50:236, 1927.
15. Castaigne P, Lhermitte F, Gautier JC, et al: Arterial occlusions in the vertebro-basilar system: A study of forty-four patients with post-mortem data. Brain 96:133, 1973.
16. Kleihues P, Hizawa K: Die Infarkte der A Cerebri posterior. Arch Psychiatr Z Ges Neurol 208:263, 1966.
17. Milandre L, Brosset C, Botti G, Khalil R: Étude de 82 infarctus du territoire des artères cérébrales postérieures. Rev Neurol 150:133, 1994.
18. Brandt T, Thie A, Caplan LR, Hacke W: Infarkte im Versorgungsgebiet der A cerebri posterior: Klinik, Pathogenese und Prognose. Nervenarzt 66:267, 1995.
19. Cals N, Devuyst G, Afsar N, et al: Pure superficial posterior cerebral artery territory infarction in The Lausanne Stroke Registry. J Neurol 249:855, 2002.
20. Steinke W, Mangold J, Schwartz A, Hennerici M: Mechanisms of infarction in the superficial posterior cerebral artery territory. J Neurol 244: 571, 1997.
21. Yamamoto Y, Georgiadis AL, Chang H-M, Caplan LR: Posterior cerebral artery territory infarcts in the New England Medical Center Posterior Circulation Registry. Arch Neurol 56:824, 1999.
22. Kinkel WR, Newman RP, Jacobs L: Posterior cerebral artery branch occlusions: CT and anatomic considerations. In Berguer R, Bauer RB (eds): Vertebrobasilar Arterial Occlusive Disease: Medical and Surgical Management. Philadelphia, Lippincott-Raven, 1984, p 117.
23. Pessin MS, Lathi ES, Cohen MB, et al: Clinical features and mechanism of occipital infarction. Ann Neurol 21:290, 1987.
24. Goto K, Takagawa K, Uemura K, et al: Posterior cerebral artery occlusion: Clinical computed tomographic and angiographic correlation. Radiology 132:357, 1979.
25. Moriyasu H, Yasaka M, Minematsu K, et al: The pathogenesis of brain infarction in the posterior cerebral artery territory. Clin Neurol 35:344, 1995.
26. North K, Kan A, de Silva M, Ouvrier R: Hemiplegia due to posterior cerebral artery occlusion. Stroke 24:1757, 1993.
27. Pessin MS, Kwan ES, Scott RM, Hedges TR: Occipital infarction with hemianopsia from carotid occlusive disease. Stroke 20:409, 1989.
28. Caplan LR: "Top of the basilar" syndrome. Neurology 30:72, 1980.
29. Benson DF, Segarra J, Albert ML: Visual agnosia-prosopagnosia. Arch Neurol 30:307, 1974.
30. Déjerine J: Contribution à l'étude anatomo-pathologique et clinique des différentes variétés de cécité verbale. C R Séances Soc Biol 44:61, 1892.
31. Lenz G: Zwei Sektionsfalle doppelseitigen zentraler Farbenhemianopsie. Z Ges Neurol Psychiatr 71:135, 1921.
32. Polyak SL: The Vertebrate Visual System. Chicago, University of Chicago Press, 1957.
33. Wyllie J: The Disorders of Speech. Edinburgh, Oliver, Boyd, 1894.
34. Brindley GS, Janota I: Observations on cortical blindness and on vascular lesions that cause loss of recent memory. J Neurol Neurosurg Psychiatry 38:459, 1975.
35. Duncan GW, Weidling SM: Posterior cerebral artery stenosis with midbrain infarction. Stroke 26:900, 1995.
36. Touho H, Takaoka M, Ohnishi H, et al: Percutaneous transluminal angioplasty for severe stenosis of the posterior cerebral artery: Case report. Surg Neurol 43:42, 1995.
37. Pessin MS, Kwan ES, DeWitt LD, et al: Posterior cerebral artery stenosis. Ann Neurol 21:85, 1987.
38. Castaigne P, Lhermitte F, Buge A, et al: Paramedian thalamic and midbrain infarcts: Clinical and neuropathological study. Ann Neurol 10:127, 1981.
39. Landis T, Regard M, Bliestle A, Kleihues P: Prosopagnosia and agnosia for noncanonical views: An autopsied case. Brain 111:1287, 1988.
40. Bohdiewicz P, Juni JE: Watershed ischemia demonstrated with acetazolamide enhanced Tc-99m HMPAO SPECT. Clin Nucl Med 19:452, 1994.
41. Melamed E, Abraham FA, Lavy S: Cortical blindness as a manifestation of basilar artery occlusion. Eur Neurol 11:22, 1974.
42. Riley HA, Yaskin JC, Riggs ME, Torney AS: Bilateral blindness due to lesions in both occipital lobes. N Y J Med 43:1619, 1943.
43. Symonds C, Mackenzie I: Bilateral loss of vision from cerebral infarction. Brain 80:415, 1957.
44. Bogousslavsky J, Regli F, van Melle G, et al: Migraine stroke. Neurology 38:223, 1988.
45. Fisher CM: The posterior cerebral artery syndrome. Can J Neurol Sci 13:232, 1986.
46. Lauritzen M: Pathophysiology of the migraine aura. Brain 117:199, 1994.
47. Olesen J, Friberg L, Olsen TS, et al: Ischaemia-induced (symptomatic) migraine attacks may be more frequent than migraine-induced ischaemic insults. Brain 116:187, 1993.

48. Bruno A, LaKind E: Occipital infarction: Carotid artery and cardiac findings. J Stroke Cerebrovasc Dis 2:70, 1992.

49. Meyer A: Herniation of the brain. Arch Neurol Psychiatry 4:387, 1920.

50. Moore MT, Stern K: Vascular lesions in the brainstem and occipital lobe occurring in association with brain tumors. Brain 61:70, 1938.

51. Ropper AH: Syndrome of transtentorial herniation: Is vertical displacement necessary? J Neurol Neurosurg Psychiatry 56:932, 1993.

52. Sato M, Tanaka S, Kohama A, Fujii C: Occipital lobe infarction caused by tentorial herniation. Neurosurgery 18:300, 1986.

53. Gacs G, Fox AJ, Barnett HJM, Vinuela F: CT visualization of intracranial arterial thromboembolism. Stroke 14:756, 1983.

54. Sieben G, De Reuck J, Eecken HV: Thrombosis of the mesencephalic artery: A clinico-pathological study of two cases and its correlation with the arterial vascularization. Acta Neurol Belg 77:151, 1977.

55. Waterston JA, Stark RJ, Gilligan BS: Paramedian thalamic and midbrain infarction: The 'mesencephalothalamic syndrome.' J Clin Exp Neurol 24:45, 1987.

56. Bassetti C, Staikov IN: Hemiplegia vegetativa alterna (ipsilateral Horner's syndrome and contralateral hemihyperhidrosis) following proximal posterior cerebral artery occlusion. Stroke 26:702, 1995.

57. Caplan LR, DeWitt LD, Pessin MS, et al: Lateral thalamic infarcts. Arch Neurol 45:959, 1988.

58. Chambers BR, Brooder RJ, Donnan GA: Proximal posterior cerebral artery occlusion simulating middle cerebral artery occlusion. Neurology 41:385, 1991.

59. Hommel M, Besson G, Pollak P, et al: Hemiplegia in posterior cerebral artery occlusion. Neurology 40:1496, 1990.

60. Argentino C, De Michele M, Fiorelli M, et al: Posterior circulation infarcts simulating anterior circulation stroke: Perspective of the acute phase. Stroke 27:1306, 1996.

61. Frisen L, Holmegaard L, Rosencrantz M: Sectorial optic atrophy and homonymous horizontal sector anopia: A lateral choroidal artery syndrome? J Neurol Neurosurg Psychiatry 41:374, 1978.

62. Déjerine J, Roussy G: La syndrome thalamique. Rev Neurol (Paris) 14:521, 1906.

63. Ghika J, Bogousslavsky J, Henderson J, et al: The "jerky dystonic unsteady hand": A delayed motor syndrome in posterior thalamic infarctions. J Neurol 241:537, 1994.

64. Hayman LA, Berman SA, Hinck VC: Correlation of CT cerebral vascular territories with function. II: Posterior cerebral artery. Am J Neuroradiol 2:219, 1981.

65. Manfredi M, Curccu G: Thalamic pain revisited. In Loeb C (ed): Studies in Cerebrovascular-Disease. Milan, Masson Italia Editori, 1981, p 73.

66. Bogousslavsky J, Maeder P, Regli F, Meuli R: Pure midbrain infarction: Clinical syndromes, MRI, and etiologic patterns. Neurology 44:2032, 1994.

67. Mohr JP, Case CS, Meckler RJ, Fisher CM: Sensorimotor stroke due to thalamocapsular ischemia. Arch Neurol 34:739, 1977.

68. Ortiz N, Barraquer Bordas L, Dourado M, et al: La hemiplejia en los infartos de la arteria cerebral posterior: Un analisis de los diversos mecanismos responsables. Neurologia 8:188, 1993.

69. Ghika-Schmid F, Ghika J, Regli F, Bogousslavsky J: Hyperkinetic movement disorders during and after acute stroke: The Lausanne Stroke Registry. J Neurol Sci 146:109, 1997.

70. Lee MS, Marsden CD: Movement disorder following lesions of the thalamus or subthalamic region. Mov Disord 9:493, 1994.

71. Ferroir JP, Feve A, Khalil A, et al: Hyperkinesie volitionnelle et d'attitude d'un membre supérieur: Manifestation d'un accident ischemique dans le territoire de l'artère cérébrale postérieure. Presse Med 21:2104, 1992.

72. Gille M, Van den Bergh P, Ghariani S, et al: Delayed-onset hemidystonia and chorea following contralateral infarction of the posterolateral thalamus: A case report. Acta Neurol Belg 96:307, 1996.

73. Lazzarino LG, Nicolai A: Late onset unilateral asterixis secondary to posterior cerebral artery infarction. Ital J Neurol Sci 13:361, 1992.

74. Förster O: Ueber Rindenblindheit. Graefes Arch Ophthalmol 36:94, 1890.

75. Goldenberg G: Loss of visual imagery and loss of visual knowledge: A case study. Neuropsychologia 30:1081, 1992.

76. Spector RH, Glaser JS, David NJ, Vining DQ: Occipital lobe infarctions: Perimetry and computed tomography. Neurology (NY) 31:1198, 1981.

77. Celesia GG, Archer CR, Kuriowa Y: Visual function of the extrageniculo-calcarine system in man. Arch Neurol 37:704, 1980.

78. Bergman PS: Cerebral blindness. Arch Psychiatry Neurol 78:568, 1957.

79. Blythe IM, Kennard C, Ruddock KH: Residual vision in patients with retrogeniculate lesions of the visual pathways. Brain 110:887, 1987.

80. Meyer O: Ein- und doppleseitige homonyme Hemianopsia mit Orientirungsstörungen. Monatsschr Psychiatr Neurol 8:440, 1900.

81. Holmes G: Selected Papers of Sir Gordon Holmes. London, Blackwell, 1956, p 195.

82. Heller-Bettinger I, Kepes JJ, Preskorn SH, et al: Bilateral altitudinal anopia caused by infarction of the calcarine cortex. Neurology 26:1176, 1976.

83. Newman RP, Kinkel WR, Jacobs L: Altitudinal hemi-anopia caused by occipital infarctions. Arch Neurol 41:413, 1984.

84. Bogousslavsky J, Regli F, van Melle G: Unilateral occipital infarction: Evaluating the risks of developing bilateral loss of vision. J Neurol Neurosurg Psychiatry 46:78, 1983.

85. Benton S, Levy I, Swash M: Vision in the temporal crescent in occipital infarction. Brain 103:83, 1980.

86. Lepore FE: The preserved temporal crescent: The clinical implications of an "endangered" finding. Neurology 57:1918, 2001.

87. Holmes G, Lister WT: Disturbances of vision from cerebral lesions, with special reference to the cortical representation of the macula. Brain 39:34, 1916.

88. Isa K, Miyashita K, Yanagimoto S, et al: Homonymous defect of macular vision in ischemic stroke. Eur Neurol 46:126, 2001

89. Luco C, Hoppe A, Schweitzer M, et al: Visual field defects in vascular lesions of the lateral geniculate body. J Neurol Neurosurg Psychiatry 55:12, 1992.

90. Miller NR: Walsh and Hoyt's Clinical Neuro-Ophthalmology, 4th ed, vol 1. Baltimore, Williams & Wilkins, 1982.

91. Mackenzie I, Meighan S, Pollock EN: On the projection of the retinal quadrants on the lateral geniculate bodies and the relationship of the quadrants to the optic radiations. Trans Ophthalmol Soc U K 53:142, 1933.

92. Neau J-P, Bogousslavsky J: The syndrome of posterior choroidal artery territory infarction. Ann Neurol 39:779, 1996.

93. Frisen L: Quadruple sector anopia and sectorial optic atrophy: A syndrome of the distal anterior choroidal artery. J Neurol Neurosurg Psychiatry 42:590, 1979.

94. Riddoch G: Dissociation of visual perceptions due to occipital injuries, with especial reference to appreciation of movement. Brain 40:15, 1917.

95. Merigan W, Freeman A, Meyers SP: Parallel processing streams in human visual cortex. Neuroreport 8:3985, 1997.

96. Rizzo M, Nawrot M, Blake R, Damasio AR: A human visual disorder resembling area V4 dysfunction in the monkey. Neurology 42:1175, 1992.

97. Vaina L: Functional segregation of color and motion processing in the human visual cortex: Clinical evidence. Cereb Cortex 5:555, 1994.

98. Van Essen DC, Felleman DJ, DeYoe EA, et al: Modular and hierarchical organization of extrastriate visual cortex in the macaque monkey. Cold Spring Harb Symp Quant Biol 55:679, 1990.

99. Weiskrantz L: Blindsight: A Case Study and Implications. Oxford, Clarendon, 1986.

100. Wessinger CM, Fendrich R, Gazzaniga MS: Islands of residual vision in hemianopic patients. J Cogn Neurosci 9:203, 1997.

101. Zihl J, von Cramon D: Visual field recovery from scotoma in patients with postgeniculate damage: A review of 55 cases. Brain 108:335, 1985.

102. Walsh FB: Clinical Neuro-Ophthalmology, 2nd ed. Baltimore, William & Wilkins, 1957.

103. Nelles G, Esser J, Eckstein A, et al: Compensatory visual field training for stroke patients with hemianopia after stroke. Neurosci Lett 306:189, 2001.

104. Kasten E, Wust S, Behrens-Baumann W, Sabel BA: Computer-based training for the treatment of partial blindness. Nature Med 4:1083, 1998.

105. Balliet R, Blood KM, Bach-y-Rita P: Visual field rehabilitation in the cortically blind? J Neurol Neurosurg Psychiatry 48:1113, 1985.

106. Lissauer H: Ein fall von Seelenblindheit nebst einem Beitrage zur Theorie derselben. Arch Psychiatr Nervenkr 21:2, 1889.

107. Rubens AB, Benson DF: Associative visual agnosia. Arch Neurol 24:305, 1971.

108. Bay E: Agnose und Funktionswandel: Eine Hirnpathologische Studie. Berlin, Springer-Verlag, 1950.

109. Bender MB, Feldman M: The so-called visual agnosias. Brain 95:173, 1972.

110. Head H: Aphasia: An historical review. Brain 43:340, 1920.

111. Farah MJ: Visual Agnosia: Disorders of Object Recognition and What They Tell Us About Normal Vision. Cambridge, MA, MIT Press, 1990.

112. Davidoff J, Warrington EK: A dissociation of shape discrimination and figure-ground perception in a patient with normal visual acuity. Neuropsychologia 31:83, 1993.

113. Humphrey KG, Symons LA, Herbert AM, Goodale MA: A neurological dissociation between shape from shading and shape from edges. Behav Brain Res 76:117, 1996.

114. Riddoch MJ, Humphreys GW: A case of integrative visual agnosia. Brain 92:847, 1987.

115. De Renzi E, Lucchelli F: The fuzzy boundaries of apperceptive agnosia. Cortex 29:187, 1993.

116. Marr D: Vision. San Francisco, Freeman, 1982.

117. Warrington EK, James M: Visual object recognition in patients with right hemisphere lesions: Axes or features. Perception 15:355, 1986.

118. De Renzi E, Zambolin A, Crisi G: The pattern of neuropsychological impairment associated with left posterior cerebral infarcts. Brain 110:1099, 1987.

119. Coslett HB, Saffran EM: Preserved object recognition and reading comprehension in optic aphasia. Brain 112:1091, 1989.

120. Freund CS: Ueber optische Aphasie und Seelenblindheit. Archiv für Psychiatrie und Nervenkrankheiten 20:276, 1889.

121. Lhermitte F, Beauvois MF: A visual speech disconnection syndrome: Report of a case with optic aphasia, agnosic alexia and colour agnosia. Brain 96:695, 1973.

122. Albert ML, Reches A, Silverberg R: Associative visual agnosia without alexia. Neurology 25:322, 1975.

123. Carlesimo GA, Casadio P, Sabbadini M, Caltagirone C: Associative visual agnosia resulting from a disconnection between intact visual memory and semantic systems. Cortex 34:563, 1998.

124. Goldenberg G, Karlbauer F: The more you know the less you can tell: Inhibitory effects of visuo-semantic activation on modality specific visual misnaming. Cortex 34:471, 1998.

125. Michel F, Schott B, Boucher M, Kopp N: Alexie sans agraphie chez un malade ayant un hémisphére gauche déafférenté. Rev Neurol 135:347, 1979.

126. De Renzi E, Saetti MC: Associative agnosia and optic aphasia: Qualitative or quantitative difference? Cortex 33:115, 1997.

127. Iorio L, Faranga A, Fragassi NA, Grossi D: Visual associative agnosia and optic aphasia: A single case study and a review of the syndromes. Cortex 28:23, 1992.

128. Luzzatti C, Rumiati RI, Ghirardi GA: A functional model of visuo-verbal disconnection and the neuroanatomical constraints of optic aphasia. Neurocase 4:71, 1998.

129. Matsuda M, Nakamura K, Fujimoto N, et al: Visual agnosia evolving to optic aphasia: A case study. Clin Neurol 32:1179, 1992.

130. Schnider A, Benson DF, Scharre DW: Visual agnosia and optic aphasia: Are they anatomically distinct? Cortex 30:445, 1994.

131. Poeck K: Neuropsychological demonstration of splenial interhemispheric disconnection in a case of "optic anomia." Neuropsychologia 22:707, 1984.

132. Feinberg TE, Gonzalez Rothi LJ, Heilman KM: Multimodal agnosia after unilateral left hemisphere lesion. Neurology 36:864, 1986.

132. Greenblatt SH: Subangular alexia without agraphia or hemianopsia. Brain Lang 3:229, 1976.

133. Larrabee GJ, Levin HS, Huff FJ, et al: Visual agnosia contrasted with visual-verbal disconnection. Neuropsychologia 23:1, 1985.

134. Lindeboom J, Swinkels JA: Interhemispheric communication in a case of total visuo-verbal disconnection. Neuropsychologia 24:781, 1986.

135. Ohtake H, Fujii T, Yamadori A, et al: The influence of misnaming on object recognition: A case of multimodal agnosia. Cortex 37:175, 2001.

136. Geschwind N, Fusillo M: Color-naming defects in association with alexia. Arch Neurol 15:137, 1966.

137. Albert NL, Soffer D, Silverberg R, Raches A: The anatomic basis of visual agnosia. Neurology 29: 876, 1979

138. Cambier J, Masson M, Elghozi D, et al: Agnosie visuelle sans hemianopsie droite chez un sujet droitier. Rev Neurol (Paris) 136:727, 1980.

139. Feinberg TE, Schindler RJ, Ochoa E, et al: Associative visual agnosia and alexia without prosopagnosia. Cortex 30:395, 1994.

140. Ferreira CT, Guisiano B, Ceccaldi M, Poncet M: Optic aphasia: Evidence of the contribution of different neural systems to object and action naming. Cortex 33:499, 1997.

141. Ferro JM, Santos ME: Associative visual agnosia: A case study. Cortex 20:121, 1984.

142. McCarthy R, Warrington EK: Visual associative agnosia: A clinico-anatomical study of a single case. J Neurol Neurosurg Psychiatry 49:1233, 1986.

143. Pillon B, Signoret J-L, Lhermitte F: Agnosie visuelle associative: Rôle de l'hémisphere gauche dans la perception visuelle. Rev Neurol (Paris) 137:831, 1981.

144. Oxbury JM, Oxbury SM, Humphrey NK: Varieties of colour anomia. Brain 92:847, 1969.

145. McCormick GF, Levine DA: Visual anomia: A unidirectional disconnection. Neurology 33:664, 1983.

146. Feinberg TE, Dyckes-Berke D, Miner CR, Roane DM: Knowledge, implicit knowledge, and metaknowledge in visual agnosia and pure alexia. Brain 118:789, 1995.

147. Hillis AE, Caramazza A: Cognitive and neural mechanisms underlying visual and semantic processing: Implications from "optic aphasia." J Cogn Neurosci 7:457, 1995.

148. Warrington EK: Agnosia: The impairment of object recognition. In Frederiks JAM (ed): Handbook of Clinical Neurology, vol 1. New York, Elsevier, 1985, p 333.

149. Pujol J, Deus J, Losilla JM, Capdevila A: Cerebral lateralization of language in normal right-handed people studied by functional MRI. Neurology 52:1038, 1999.

150. Springer JA, Binder JR, Hammeke TA, et al: Language dominance in neurologically normal and epilepsy subjects: A functional MRI study. Brain 122:2033, 1999.

151. Szaflarski JP, Binder JR, Possing ET, et al: Language lateralization in left-handed and ambidextrous people: fMRI data. Neurology 59:238, 2002.

152. Damasio A, Damasio H, Van Hoesen GW: Prosopagnosia: Anatomic basis and behavioral mechanisms. Neurology (NY) 323:331, 1982.

153. De Renzi E, Perani D, Carlesimo GA, et al: Prosopagnosia can be associated with damage confined to the right hemisphere: An MRI and PET study and a review of the literature. Neuropsychologia 32:893, 1994.

154. Meadows JC: The anatomical basis of prosopagnosia. J Neurol Neurosurg Psychiatry 37:489, 1974.

155. Michel F, Poncet M, Signoret JL: Les lésions responsables de la prosopagnosie sont-elles toujours bilatérales? Rev Neurol 146:764, 1989.

156. Benton AL, Van Allen MW: Prosopagnosia and facial discrimination. J Neurol Sci 15:167, 1972.

157. De Renzi E, Faglioni P, Grossi D, Nichelli P: Apperceptive and associative forms of prosopagnosia. Cortex 27:213, 1991.

158. Schweich M, Bruyer R: Heterogeneity in the cognitive manifestations of prosopagnosia: The study of a group of single cases. Cogn Neuropsychol 10:529, 1993.

159. Carlesimo GA, Caltagirone C: Components in the visual processing of known and unknown faces. J Clin Exp Neuropsychol 17:691, 1995.

160. De Renzi E, Bonacini MG, Faglioni P: Right posterior brain-damaged patients are poor at assessing the age of a face. Neuropsychologia 27:839, 1989.

161. Levine DN, Calvanio R: Prosopagnosia: A defect in visual configural processing. Brain Cogn 10:149, 1989.

162. Saumier D, Arguin M, Lassonde M: Prosopagnosia: A case study involving problems in processing configural information. Brain Cogn 46:255, 2001.

163. Kosslyn SM, Hamilton SE, Bernstein JH: The perception of curvature can be selectively disrupted in prosopagnosia. Brain Cogn 27:36, 1995.

164. Laeng B, Caviness VS: Propagnosia as a deficit in encoding curved surface. J Cogn Neurosci 13:556, 2001.

165. Whiteley AM, Warrington EK: Prosopagnosia: A clinical, psychological and anatomical study of three patients. J Neurol Neurosurg Psychiatry 40:395, 1977.

166. Benton AL, Hamsher Kd, Varney NR, Spreen O: Contributions to Neuropsychological Assessment: A Clinical Manual. New York, Oxford University Press, 1983.

Clinical Manifestations

167. Farah MJ, Wilson KD, Drain HM, Tanaka JR: The inverted face inversion effect in prosopagnosia: Evidence for mandatory, face-specific perceptual mechanisms. Vision Res 35:2089, 1995.

168. McNeil JE, Warrington EK: Prosopagnosia: A face-specific disorder. Q J Exp Psychol 46:1, 1993.

169. Nachson I: On the modularity of face recognition: The riddle of domain specificity. J Clin Exp Neuropsychol 17:256, 1995.

170. de Gelder B, Bachoud-Lévi A-C, Degos J-D: Inversion superiority in visual agnosia may be common to a variety of orientation polarised objects besides faces. Vision Research 38:2855, 1998.

171. Dixon MJ, Bub DN, Arguin M: Semantic and visual determinants of face recognition in a prosopagnosic patient. J Cogn Neurosci 10:362, 1998.

172. Gauthier I, Behrmann M, Tarr MJ: Can face recognition really be dissociated from object recognition? J Cogn Neurosci 11:349, 1999.

173. Clark S, Lindemann A, Maeder P, et al: Face recognition and postero-inferior hemispheric lesions. Neuropsychologia 35:1555, 1997.

174. De Haan EHF, Young AW, Newcombe F: Covert and overt recognition in prosopagnosia. Brain 114:2575, 1991.

175. Allison T, Puce A, Spencer DD, McCarthy G: Electrophysiological studies of human face perception. 1: Potentials generated in occipitotemporal cortex by face and non-face stimuli. Cereb Cortex 9:415, 1999.

176. Haxby JV, Horwitz B, Ungerleider LG, et al: The functional organization of human extrastriate cortex: A PET-rCBF study of selective attention to faces and locations. J Neurosci 14:6336, 1994.

177. Kanwisher N, McDermott J, Chun MM: The fusiform face area: A module in human extrastriate cortex specialized for face perception. J Neurosci 17:4302, 1997.

178. Nakamura K, Kawashima R, Sato N, et al: Functional delineation of the human occipitotemporal areas related to face and scene processing. Brain 123:1903, 2000.

179. Sergent J, Ohta S, MacDonald B: Functional neuroanatomy of face and object processing: A positron emission tomography study. Brain 115:15, 1992.

180. Leveroni C, Seidenberg M, Mayer AR, et al: Neural systems underlying the recognition of familiar and newly learned faces. J Neurosci 20:878, 2000.

181. Michel EM, Troost BT: Palinopsia: Cerebral localization with computed tomography. Neurology 30:887, 1980.

182. Bender MB, Feldman M, Sobin AJ: Palinopsia. Brain 91:321, 1968.

183. Meadows JC, Munro SS: Palinopsia. J Neurol Neurosurg Psychiatry 40:5, 1977.

184. Critchley M: Types of visual perseveration: 'Palinopsia' and 'illusory visual spread.' Brain 74:267, 1951.

185. Yamada A, Miki H, Nishioka M: A case of posterior cerebral artery territory infarction with micropsia as the chief complaint. Rinsho Shinkeigaku 30:894, 1990.

186. Cohen L, Gray F, Meyrignac C, et al: Selective deficit of visual size perception: Two cases of hemimicropsia. J Neurol Neurosurg Psychiatry 57:73, 1994.

187. Aguirre GK, D'Esposito M: Topographical disorientation: A synthesis and taxonomy. Brain 122:1613, 1999.

188. Habib M, Sirigu A: Pure topographical disorientation: A definition and anatomical basis. Cortex 23:73, 1987.

189. Cogan DG: Visuospatial dysgnosia. Am J Ophthalmol 88:361, 1979.

190. Landis T, Cummings JL, Benson DF, Palmer E: Loss of topographic familiarity. Arch Neurol 43:132, 1986.

191. Pallis CA: Impaired identification of faces and places with agnosia for colors. J Neurol Neurosurg Psychiatry 18:218, 1955.

192. Takahashi N, Kawamura M: Pure topographical disorientation: The anatomical basis of landmark agnosia. Cortex 38:717, 2002.

193. Whiteley AM, Warrington EK: Selective impairment of topographical memory: A single case study. J Neurol Neurosurg Psychiatry 41:575, 1978.

194. Alsaadi T, Binder JR, Lazar RM, et al: Pure topographic disorientation: A distinctive syndrome with varied localization. Neurology 54:1864, 2000.

195. Cammalleri R, Gangitano M, D'Amelio M, et al: Transient topographical amnesia and cingulate cortex damage: A case report. Neuropsychologia 34:321, 1996.

196. Luzzi S, Pucci E, Di Bella P, Piccirilli M: Topographical disorientation consequent to amnesia of spatial location in a patient with right parahippocampal damage. Cortex 36:427, 2000.

197. Takahashi N, Kawamura M, Shiota J, et al: Pure topographical disorientation due to right retrosplenial lesion. Neurology 49:464, 1997.

198. Barrash J, Damasio H, Adolphs R, Tranel D: The neuroanatomical correlates of route learning impairment. Neuropsychologia 38:820, 2000.

199. Bohbot VD, Kalina M, Stepankova K, et al: Spatial memory deficits in patients with lesions to the right hippocampus and to the right parahippocampus. Neuropsychologia 36:1217, 1998.

200. Epstein R, DeYoe EA, Press DZ, et al: Neuropsychological evidence for a topographical learning mechanism in parahippocampal cortex. Cogn Neuropsychol 18:481, 2001.

201. Aguirre GK, Detre JA, Alsop DC, D'Esposito M: The parahippocampus subserves topographical learning in man. Cereb Cortex 6:823, 1996.

202. Aguirre GK, D'Esposito M: Environmental knowledge is subserved by separable dorsal/ventral neural areas. J Neurosci 17:2512, 1997.

203. Aguirre GK, Zarahn E, D'Esposito M: An area within human ventral cortex sensitive to "building" stimuli: Evidence and implications. Neuron 21:373, 1998.

204. Epstein R, Kanwisher N: A cortical representation of the local visual environment. Nature 392:598, 1998.

205. Maguire EA, Frith CD, Burgess N, et al: Knowing where things are: Parahippocampal involvement in encoding object locations in virtual large-scale space. J Cogn Neurosci 10:61, 1998.

206. De Renzi E, Faglioni P, Villa P: Topographical amnesia. J Neurol Neurosurg Psychiatry 40:498, 1977.

207. Suzuki K, Yamadori A, Hayakawa Y, Fujii T: Pure topographical disorientation related to dysfunction of the viewpoint-independent visual system. Cortex 34:589, 1998.

208. Hublet C, Demeurisse G: Pure topographical disorientation due to a deep-seated lesion with cortical remote effects. Cortex 28:123, 1992.

209. Obi T, Bando M, Takeda K, Sakuta M: A case of topographical disturbance following a left medial parieto-occipital lobe infarction. Rinsho Shinkeigaku 32:426, 1992.

210. Benson DF, Geschwind N: The alexias. In Vinken PJ, Bruyn GW (eds): Handbook of Clinical Neurology, vol 4. Amsterdam, North Holland Publishing, 1969, p 112.

211. Binder JR, Mohr JP: The topography of transcallosal reading pathways: A case-control analysis. Brain 115:1807, 1992.

212. Déjerine J, Vialet N: Contribution a l'étude de la localisation anatomique de la cécité verbale pure. C R Séances Soc Biol 45:790, 1893.

213. Beauvois MF, Saillant B: Optic aphasia for colours and colour agnosia: A distinction between visual and visuo-verbal impairments in the processing of colours. Cogn Neuropsychol 2:1, 1985.

214. Caplan LR, Hedley-White T: Cuing and memory dysfunction in alexia without agraphia: A case report. Brain 97:251, 1974.

215. Mori E, Yokoyama K, Matsuo T, Yamadori A: A clinicopathological study of vision specific anomia seen in alexia without agraphia. No To Shinkei 34:673, 1982.

216. Damasio AR, Damasio H: The anatomic basis of pure alexia. Neurology 33:1573, 1983.

217. Dalmás JF, Dansilo S: Visuographemic alexia: A new form of a peripheral acquired dyslexia. Brain Lang 75:1, 2000.

218. Buxbaum LJ, Coslett HB: Deep dyslexic phenomena in a letter-by-letter reader. Brain Lang 54:136, 1996.

219. Patterson KE, Kay J: Letter-by-letter reading: Psychological descriptions of a neurological syndrome. Q J Exp Psychol 34A:411, 1982.

220. Price CJ, Humphreys GW: Letter by letter reading? Functional deficits and compensatory strategies. Cogn Neuropsychol 9:427, 1992.

221. Rapcsak SZ, Rubens AB, Laguna JF: From letters to words: Procedures for word recognition in letter by letter reading. Brain Lang 38:504, 1990.

222. Shallice T, Saffran E: Lexical processing in the absence of explicit word identification: Evidence from a letter-by-letter reader. Cogn Neuropsychol 3:429, 1986.

223. Warrington EK, Shallice T: Word-form dyslexia. Brain 103:99, 1980.

224. Staller J, Buchanan D, Singer M, et al: Alexia without agraphia: An experimental case study. Brain Lang 5:378, 1978.

225. Orgogozo JM, Pere JJ, Strube E: Alexie sans agraphie "agnose" des couleurs et atteinte de l'hémichamp visuel droite: Un syndrome de l'artère cérébrale postérieure. Sem Hop 55:1389, 1979.

226. Andrews S: The effect of orthographic similarity on lexical retrieval: Resolving neighborhood conflicts. Psychonom Bull Rev 4:439, 1997.

227. Reicher GM: Perceptual recognition as a function of meaningfulness of stimulus material. J Exp Psychol 81:274, 1969.

228. Samuels SJ, LaBerge D, Bremer CD: Units of word recognition: Evidence for developmental changes. J of Verbal Learning and Verbal Behavior 17:715, 1978.

229. Levine DN, Calvanio R: A study of the visual defect in verbal alexia: Simultanagnosia. Brain 101:65, 1978.

230. Leff AP, Crewes H, Plant GT, et al: The functional anatomy of single-word reading in patients with hemianopic and pure alexia. Brain 124:510, 2001.

231. Greenblatt SH: Alexia without agraphia or hemianopsia: Anatomical analysis of an autopsied case. Brain 96:307, 1973.

233. Assal G, Hadj-Djilani M: Une nouvelle observation d'alexie pure sans hémianopsie. Cortex 12:169, 1976.

234. Benito-Leon J, Sanchez-Suarez C, Diaz-Guzman J, Martinez-Salio A: Pure alexia could not be a disconnection syndrome. Neurology 49:305, 1997.

235. Beversdorf DQ, Ratcliffe NR, Rhodes CH, Reeves AG: Pure alexia: Clinical-pathological evidence for a lateralized visual language association cortex. Clin Neuropathol 16:328, 1997.

236. Caffarra P: Alexia without agraphia or hemianopia. Eur Neurol 27:65, 1987.

237. Henderson VW, Friedman RB, Teng EL, Weiner JM: Left hemisphere pathways in reading: Inferences from pure alexia without hemianopia. Neurology 35:962, 1985.

238. Vincent FM, Sadowsky CH, Saunders RL, Reeves AG: Alexia without agraphia, hemianopia, or color-naming defect: A disconnection syndrome. Neurology 27:689, 1977.

239. Foix C, Hillemand P: Role vraisemblable du splenium dans la pathogénie de l'alexie pure par lésion de la cérébrale postérieure. Bull Mem Soc Med Hop Paris 49:393, 1925.

240. Henderson VW: Anatomy of posterior pathways in reading: A reassessment. Brain Lang 29:119, 1986.

241. Vialet N: Les Centres Cérébraux de la Vision et l'Appareil Nerveux Visuel Intra-Cérébral. Paris, Faculté de Medecine de Paris, 1893

242. Landolt E: De la cécité verbale. Neurol Cbl 7:605, 1888.

243. Stommel EW, Friedman RJ, Reeves AG: Alexia without agraphia associated with spleniogeniculate infarction. Neurology 41:587, 1991.

244. Iragui VJ, Kritchevsky M: Alexia without agraphia or hemianopia in parietal infarction. J Neurol Neurosurg Psychiatry 54:841, 1991.

245. Sakurai Y, Takeuchi S, Takada T, et al: Alexia caused by a fusiform or posterior inferior temporal lesion. J Neurol Sci 178:42, 2000.

246. Cohen L, Lehéricy S, Chochon F, et al: Language-specific tuning of visual cortex? Functional properties of the visual word form area. Brain 125:1054, 2002.

247. Wilbrand H: Ueber die makulär-hemianopische Lesestörung und die v Monakowsche Projektion der Makula auf die Sehspäre. Klin Monatsbl Augenheilkd 45:1, 1907.

248. Gassel MM, Williams D: Visual function in patients with homonymous hemianopia. Part II: Oculomotor mechanisms. Brain 86:1, 1963.

249. Zihl J: Eye movement patterns in hemianopic dyslexia. Brain 118:891, 1995.

250. McConkie G, Rayner K: Asymmetry of the perceptual span in reading. Bull Psychonom Soc 8:365, 1976.

251. Binder JR, Lazar RM, Tatemichi TK, et al: Left hemiparalexia. Neurology 42:562, 1992.

252. Levine DN, Calvanio R: Visual discrimination after lesion of the posterior corpus callosum. Neurology 30:21, 1980.

253. Green GJ, Lessell S: Acquired cerebral dyschromatopsia. Arch Ophthalmol 95:121, 1977.

254. Sheppard JJ: Human Color Perception. New York, Elsevier, 1968

255. Urechia CI, Cremene V, Popescu P: Hémianopsie avec chromoagnosie. Rev Neurol (Paris) 80:70, 1948.

256. LeGros Clark WE: The laminar pattern of the lateral geniculate nucleus considered in relation to color vision. Doc Ophthalmol 3:57, 1949.

257. Damasio A, Yamada T, Damasio H: Central achromatopsia: Behavioral and anatomic and physiologic aspects. Neurology 30:1064, 1980.

258. Kolmel HW: Pure homonymous hemiachromatopsia: Findings with neuro-ophthalmologic examination and imaging procedures. Eur Arch Psychiatry Neurol Sci 237:237, 1988.

259. Merle P: Aphasie et hemiachromatopsie. Rev Neurol (Paris) 21:1129, 1908.

260. Pötzl O: Ueber einige zentrale Probleme des Farbensehens. Wien Klin Wochenschr 61:706, 1949.

261. Verrey D: Hémiachromatopsie droite absolue. Arch d'Ophthalmol Paris 8:289, 1888.

262. Ziehl-Lübeck: Ueber einem Fall von Alexia and Farbenhemiagnosie. Verh Ges Dtsch Natur Aertze 67:184, 1895.

263. Beauchamp MS, Haxby JV, Rosen AC, et al: A functional MRI case study of acquired cerebral dyschromatopsia. Neuropsychologia 38:1170, 2000.

264. Heidenhain A: Beitrag zur Kenntnis der Seelenblindheit. Monatsschr Psychiatr Neurol 66:61, 1927.

265. Heywood CA, Wilson B, Cowey A: A case study of cortical colour "blindness" with relatively intact achromatic discrimination. J Neurol Neurosurg Psychiatry 50:22, 1987.

266. Kennard C, Lawden M, Morland AB, Ruddock KH: Colour identification and colour constancy are impaired in a patient with incomplete achromatopsia associated with prestriate cortical lesions. Proc R Soc Lond B Biol Sci 260:169, 1995.

267. Pearlman AL, Birch J, Meadows JC: Cerebral color blindness: An acquired defect in hue discrimination. Ann Neurol 5:253, 1979.

268. Sakurai Y, Takeuchi S, Takada T, et al: Alexia caused by a fusiform or posterior inferior temporal lesion. J Neurol Sci 178:42, 2000.

268. Zeki S, Watson JDG, Lueck CJ, et al: A direct demonstration of functional specialisation in human visual cortex. J Neurosci 11:641, 1991.

269. Zeki S: A century of cerebral achromatopsia. Brain 113:1721, 1990.

270. Meadows JC: Disturbed perception of colours associated with localized cerebral lesions. Brain 97:615, 1974.

271. Albert NL, Reches A, Silverberg R: Hemianopic colour blindness. J Neurol Neurosurg Psychiatry 38:546, 1975.

272. Geschwind N: Disconnection syndromes in animals and man. Brain 88:237, 1965.

273. Schober H: Erworbene Farbenblindheit nach Schadeltrauma. Graefes Arch Ophthalmol 148:93, 1948.

274. Siemerling: Ein Fall sogenannte Seelenblindheit nebst anderweitigen cerebralen Symptomen. Arch Psychiatr Nervenkr 21:284, 1889.

275. Sittig O: Stoerungen in Verhalten gegenuber Farben bei Aphasischen. Monatsschr Psychiatr Neurol 49:63, 1921.

276. Stengel E: The syndrome of visual alexia without colour agnosia. J Mental Sci 94:46, 1948.

277. Lewandowsky M: Ueber Abspaltung des Farbensinnes. Monatsschr Psychiatr Neurol 23:488, 1908.

278. Zihl J, von Cramon D: Color anomia restricted to the left visual hemifield after splenial disconnection. J Neurol Neurosurg Psychiatry 43:719, 1980.

279. Pötzl O: Die zweite Gruppe der optischen Agnosien. In Aschaffenburg G (ed): Handbuch der Psychiatrie die Aphasielehre I Optische-agnostischen Storungen. Wien, Franz Deuticke, 1928, p 80.

280. Goldstein K: Language and Language Disturbances. New York, Grune & Stratton, 1948.

281. Critchley M: Acquired disturbances of color perception of central origin. Brain 88:711, 1965.

282. Servan J, Verstichel P, Catala M, et al: Aphasia and infarction of the posterior cerebral artery territory. J Neurol 242:87, 1995.

283. Berthier ML, Starkstein SE, Leiguarda R, et al: Transcortical aphasia: Importance of the non speech dominant hemisphere in language repetition. Brain 114:1409, 1991.

284. Damasio H: Cerebral localization of the aphasias. In Sarno MT (ed): Acquired aphasia. Orlando, FL, Academic Press, 1981, p 27.

285. Geschwind N, Quadfasel FA, Segarra JM: Isolation of the speech area. Neuropsychologia 6:327, 1968.

286. Heubner: Über Aphasie; cited in Goldstein K (ed): Language and Language Disturbances. New York, Grune & Stratton, 1948, p 303.

287. Otsuki M, Soma Y, Koyama A, et al: Transcortical sensory aphasia following left frontal infarction. J Neurol 245:69, 1998.

288. Kertesz A, Sheppard A, MacKenzie R: Localization in transcortical sensory aphasia. Arch Neurol 39:475, 1982.

289. Alexander MP, Hiltbrunner B, Fischer RS: Distributed anatomy of transcortical sensory aphasia. Arch Neurol 46:885, 1989.

290. Graff-Radford NR, Damasio H, Yamada T, et al: Nonhemorrhagic thalamic infarction. Brain 108:485, 1985.

Clinical Manifestations

291. McFarling D, Rothi W, Heilman KM: Transcortical aphasia from ischemic infarcts of the thalamus: A report of two cases. J Neurol Neurosurg Psychiatry 45:107, 1982.

292. Foundas A, Daniels SK, Vasterling JJ: Anomia: Case studies with lesion localisation. Neurocase 4:35, 1998.

293. Mills CK, McConnell JW: The naming centre, with the report of a case indicating its location in the temporal lobe. J Nerv Ment Dis 22:1, 1895.

294. Nicolai A, Lazzarino LG: Acute confusional states secondary to infarctions in the territory of the posterior cerebral artery in elderly patients. Ital J Neurol Sci 15:91, 1994.

295. Servan J, Verstichel P, Catala M, Rancurel G: Syndromes amnesiques et fabulations au cours d'infarctus du territoire de l'artère cérébrale postérieure. Rev Neurol 150:201, 1994.

296. von Cramon DY, Hebel N, Schuri U: Verbal memory and learning in unilateral posterior cerebral infarction. Brain 111:1061, 1988.

297. Dide M, Botcazo: Amnesie continue, cécité verbale pure, perte du sens topographique, ramollisement double du lobe lingual. Rev Neurol 10:676, 1902.

298. Trillet M, Fischer C, Serclerat D, Schott B: Le syndrome amnésique des ischémies cérébrales postérieures. Cortex 16:421, 1980.

299. Victor M, Angevine JB, Mancall EL: Memory loss with lesions of the hippocampal formation. Arch Neurol (Chicago) 5:244, 1961.

300. Woods BT, Schoene W, Kneisley L: Are hippocampal lesions sufficient to cause lasting amnesia? J Neurol Neurosurg Psychiatry 45:243, 1982.

301. Zola-Morgan S, Squire LR, Amaral DG: Human amnesia and the medial temporal region: Enduring memory impairment following a bilateral lesion limited to field CA1 of the hippocampus. J Neurosci 6:2950, 1986.

302. Milner B: Amnesia following operations on the temporal lobes. In Whitty CMW, Zangwill OL (eds): Amnesia. London, Butterworth, 1966, p 109.

303. Aggleton JP, McMackin D, Carpenter K, et al: Differential cognitive effects of colloid cysts in the third ventricle that spare or compromise the fornix. Brain 123:800, 2000.

304. Gaffan EA, Gaffan D, Hodges JR: Amnesia following damage to the left fornix and to other sites: A comparative study. Brain 114:1297, 1991.

305. Sweet WH, Talland GA, Ervin FR: Loss of recent memory following section of fornix. Trans Am Neurol Assoc 84:76, 1959.

306. D'Esposito M, Verfaellie M, Alexander MP, Katz DI: Amnesia following traumatic bilateral fornix transection. Neurology 45:1546, 1995.

307. Heilman KN, Sypert GW: Korsakoff's syndrome resulting from bilateral fornix lesions. Neurology 27:490, 1977.

308. Akelaitis AJ: Study of language functions unilaterally following section of the corpus callosum. J Neuropathol Exp Neurol 2:226, 1943.

309. Woolsey RM, Nelson JS: Asymptomatic destruction of the fornix in man. Arch Neurol 32:566, 1975.

310. Milner B: In Discussion of Sweet WH, Talland GA, Ervin FR (refernce 305). Trans Am Neurol Assoc 84:78, 1959.

311. Zola-Morgan S, Squire LR, Amaral DG: Lesions of the hippocampal formation but not lesions of the fornix or mammillary nuclei produce long-lasting memory impairment in monkeys. J Neurosci 9:898, 1989.

312. Laplane D, Degos JD, Baulac M, Gray F: Bilateral infarction of the anterior cingulate gyri and of the fornices. J Neurol Sci 51:289, 1981.

313. Moudgil SS, Azzouz M, Abkulkader AA, et al: Amnesia due to fornix infarction. Stroke 31:1418, 2000.

314. Park SA, Hahn JH, Kim JI, et al: Memory deficits after bilateral anterior fornix infarction. Neurology 54:1379, 2000.

315. Gaffan D, Gaffan EA: Amnesia in man following transection of the fornix. Brain 114:2611, 1991.

316. Lin KN, Liu RS, Yeh TP, et al: Posterior ischemia during an attack of transient global amnesia. Stroke 24:1093, 1993.

317. Schmidtke K, Reinhardt M, Krause T: Cerebral perfusion during transient global amnesia: Findings with HMPAO SPECT. J Nucl Med 39:155, 1998.

318. Stillhard G, Landis T, Schiess R, et al: Bitemporal hypoperfusion in transient global amnesia: 99m-Tc-HM-PAO SPECT and neuropsychological findings during and after an attack. J Neurol Neurosurg Psychiatry 53:339, 1990.

319. Hodges JR, Warlow CP: The aetiology of transient global amnesia. Brain 113:639, 1990.

320. Benson DF, Marsden CD, Meadows JC: The amnesic syndrome of posterior cerebral artery occlusion. Acta Neurol Scand 50:133, 1974.

321. Escourolle R, Gray F: Les accidents vasculaires du système limbique. In Proceedings of the VIIth International Congress of Neuropathology. Amsterdam, Excerpta Medica, 1975, p 195.

322. Squire LR: Memory and the hippocampus: A synthesis from findings with rats, monkeys, and humans. Psychol Rev 99:195, 1992.

323. Scoville WB, Milner B: Loss of recent memory after bilateral hippocampal lesions. J Neurol Neurosurg Psychiatry 20:11, 1957.

324. Sidman M, Stoddard LT, Mohr JP: Some additional quantitative observations of immediate memory in a patient with bilateral hippocampal lesions. Neuropsychologia 6:245, 1968.

325. Dimsdale H, Logue V, Piercy M: A case of persisting impairment of recent memory following right temporal lobectomy. Neuropsychologia 1:287, 1964.

326. Milner B: Psychological aspects of focal epilepsy and its neurosurgical management. Adv Neurol 8:299, 1975.

327. Walker AE: Recent memory impairment in unilateral temporal lesions. Arch Neurol Psychiatry (Chicago) 78:543, 1957.

328. Devinsky O, Bear D, Volpe BT: Confusional states following posterior cerebral artery infarction. Arch Neurol 45:160, 1988.

329. Horenstein S, Chamberlin W, Conomy J: Infarction of the fusiform and calcarine regions: Agitated delirium and hemianopia. Trans Am Neurol Assoc 92:85, 1967.

330. Medina JL, Chokroverty S, Rubino FA: Syndrome of agitated delirium and visual impairment: A manifestation of medial temporooccipital infarction. J Neurol Neurosurg Psychiatry 40:861, 1977.

331. Mair WGP, Warrington EK, Weiskrantz L: Memory disorder in Korsakoff's psychosis: A neuropathological and neuropsychological investigation of two cases. Brain 102:749, 1979.

332. Victor M, Adams RD, Collins GH: The Wernicke-Korsakoff Syndrome. Philadelphia, FA Davis, 1971.

333. Squire LR, Amaral DG, Zola-Morgan S, et al: Description of brain injury in the amnesia patient N.A. based on magnetic resonance imaging. Exp Neurol 105:23, 1989.

334. Graff-Radford NR, Tranel D, Van Hoesen GW, Brandt JP: Diencephalic amnesia. Brain 113:1, 1990.

335. von Cramon DY, Hebel N, Schuri U: A contribution to the anatomical basis of thalamic amnesia. Brain 108:993, 1985.

336. Suzuki T, Iwakuma A, Tanaka Y, et al: Changes in personality and emotion following bilateral infarction of the posterior cerebral arteries. Jpn J Psychiatr Neurol 46:897, 1992.

337. Conomy JP, Laureno R, Massarweh W: Transient behavioral syndrome associated with reversible vascular lesions of the fusiform-calcarine region in humans, abstracted. Ann Neurol 12:83, 1982.

338. Levine DN, Finklestein S: Delayed psychosis after right temporoparietal stroke or trauma: Relation to epilepsy. Neurology 32:267, 1982.

339. Lilly R, Cummings JL, Benson DF, Frankel M: The human Klüver-Bucy syndrome. Neurology (Cleve) 33:1141, 1983.

340. Shraberg D, Weisberg L: The Klüver-Bucy syndrome in man. J Nerv Ment Dis 166:130, 1978.

341. Medina JL, Rubino FA, Ross E: Agitated delirium caused by infarctions of the hippocampal formation and fusiform and lingual gyri: A case report. Neurology 24:1181, 1974.

Chapter Nine

Anterior Choroidal Artery Territory Infarcts

Raymond M. M. Hupperts and Jan Lodder

Distinctions among different subtypes of brain infarction may be relevant for treatment and for prevention of recurrences.[1] Characteristics of brain infarcts can be studied from different points of entry, such as the clinical syndrome and the involved vascular territory. After the introduction of computed tomography (CT) scanning of the brain, infarcts in the territory of the anterior choroidal artery (AChA) have received renewed interest.[2–11] Symptomatology, risk factors and presumed pathophysiology, vascular supply areas, and prognosis differ among studies, probably because of differences in patient selection.

A clinical syndrome resulting from AChA territory infarction was first published by Foix and colleagues[12] in 1930. In the older literature, two more cases were described.[13,14] These cases featured a typical syndrome that included the triad of hemiparesis, hemianopia, and hemianesthesia. However, the clinical spectrum of AChA infarcts has been extended widely since the introduction of CT, as reviewed by several groups.[2,5,15] With respect to the later literature, the typical triad was found less often, and whether hemiparesis, hemianopia, and hemianesthesia should be regarded as "typical" signs of AChA territory infarction is disputable.

The pathophysiology of AChA territory infarcts may be related to infarct size; small infarcts may result from obstruction of small vessels, whereas larger infarcts may be caused by large artery thromboembolism or cardiac embolism. However, views on the cause of AChA territory infarcts vary in the literature, because of opposing ideas about the precise areas receiving vascular supply from the AChA. Most contentious in this respect is the posterior paraventricular corona radiata; the lateral thalamic border and the medial part of the lentiform nucleus are subjects of less debate. Although the supply areas of this artery may vary from patient to patient, the optic tract, the posterior leg of the internal capsule, the cerebral peduncle, and the choroid plexus are consistently supplied by the AChA.[13,16,17]

Little is known about the prognosis in AChA infarcts, because case histories rather than larger series have been published.

THE SYNDROME OF ANTERIOR CHOROIDAL ARTERY TERRITORY INFARCTS

Most AChA territory infarct syndromes are caused by small infarcts, which are no more than 15 to 20 mm in diameter on CT or magnetic resonance imaging (MRI) (Fig. 9–1). Large or total AChA territory infarcts are uncommon in stroke studies. AChA infarct syndromes may be caused by surgical ligation of the AChA (Parkinson's surgery), tumors, aneurysms, or arteriovenous malformations (Fig. 9–2). Patients who underwent clipping for an AChA aneurysm may be at especially high risk for postoperative ischemia.[18] Hemorrhages (mostly hypertensive) may cause AChA territory infarct syndromes but are rarely restricted to the AChA territory. In discussions of AChA territory infarct syndromes, it is important to differentiate between those due purely to AChA territory infarction and those resulting from combined infarction of the AChA and other vascular territories, and to distinguish between small (lacunar) and large AChA territory infarcts. Most small infarcts do not cause hemianopia, whereas in larger infarcts, "cortical" signs are often present (Table 9.1).[2,11,15,19]

Lacunar Syndromes

Although lacunar syndromes are very common in small deep infarcts, they are infrequently mentioned in studies on the AChA.[20] Fisher and Curry[21] were probably the first to describe a pure motor stroke in the AChA territory. Derouesné and colleagues[22] were the first to describe pure sensory stroke "in relation to an infarct in the territory of the anterior choroidal artery." Although most of the 16 patients described by these investigators had lacunar infarcts on CT, only three had lacunar syndromes (one pure motor, two pure sensory).[2] Mohr and associates[9] found pure motor strokes in 2 of 16 patients with presumed AChA territory infarcts. Some of the patients with small infarcts studied by Leys and coworkers[10] and Takahashi and colleagues[23,24] may have had pure motor syndromes. One of the 5 patients described by Helgason and associates[3] probably had a pure motor syndrome.

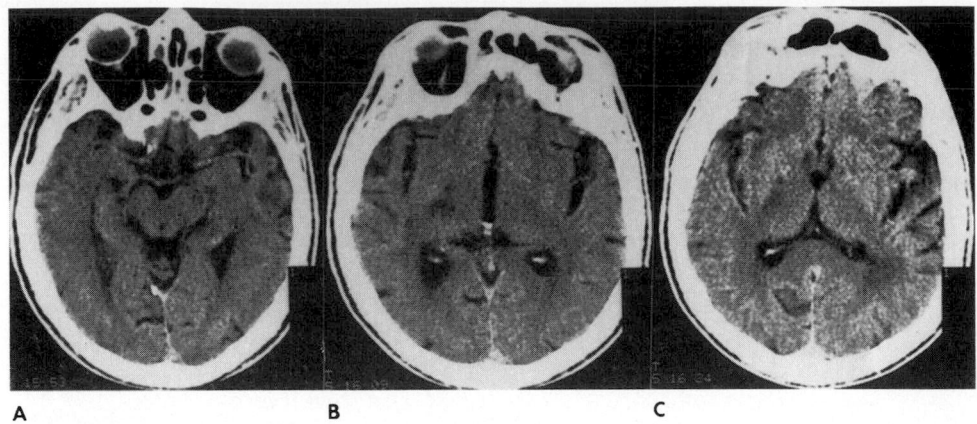

FIGURE 9–1   *CT scan taken within 1 week after admission of a patient with severe pure motor syndrome, showing involvement of the hippocampal gyrus (A), lowest level of the internal capsule and medical aspect of the pallidum (B), and posterior limb of the internal capsule, sparing the thalamus and putamen (C). (From Mohr JP, Steinke W, Timsit SG: The anterior choroidal artery does not supply the corona radiata and lateral ventricular wall. Stroke 22:1502–1507, 1991.)*

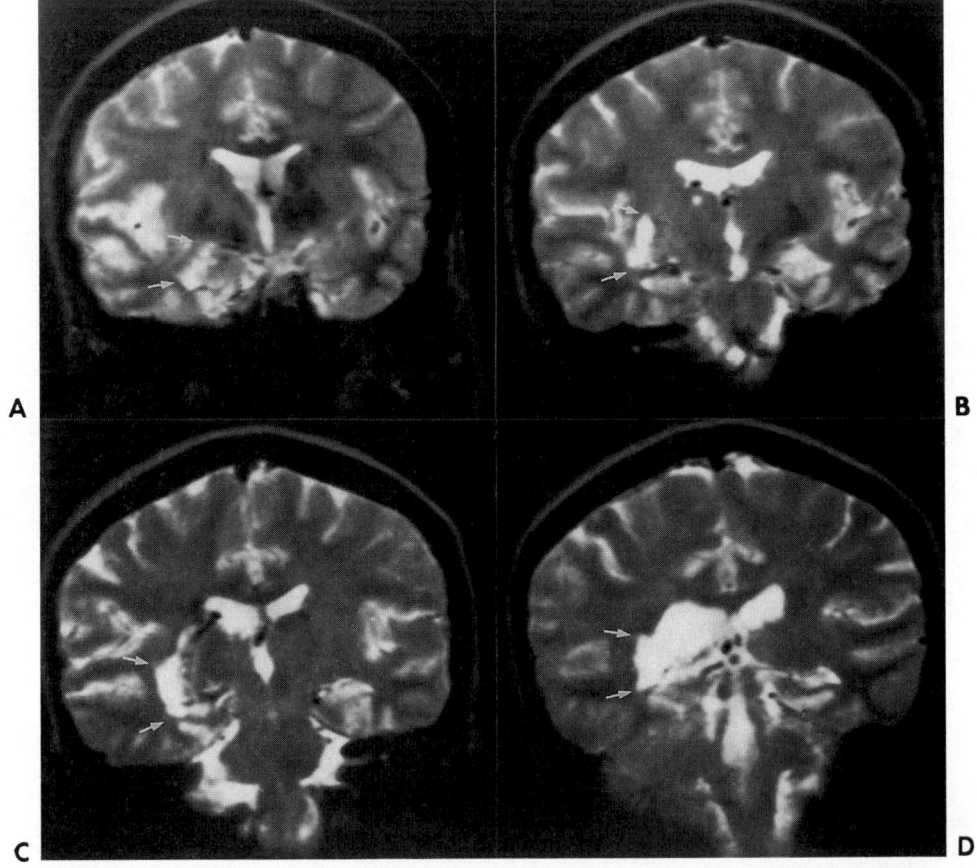

FIGURE 9–2   *MR images in the coronal plane (A through D) showing right thalamic arteriovenous malformation fed by lenticulostriate, thalamoperforating, and choroidal arteries and an associated anterior choroidal infarct (arrows) (A) after embolization therapy, the infarct affecting the posterior limb of the internal capsule (B), lateral geniculate body (C), retrolenticular fibers (D), and upper portion of the medial temporal lobe (B). (From Mohr JP, Steinke W, Timsit SG: The anterior choroidal artery does not supply the corona radiata and lateral ventricular wall. Stroke 1991; 22:1502–1507.)*

Table 9.1 Clinical Features in CT- or MRI-Documented, Presumed Unilateral Anterior Choroidal Artery Territory Infarcts

Study (Year)[°]	No. of AChA Infarcts	Lacunar Syndrome	Visual Field Deficit	Neuropsychological Higher Cortical Dysfunction	Hemiplegia Deficit	Hemisensory Dysarthria	Dysphasia/
De Bleecker et al (1988)[15]	27	PMS	HH: 4 Quadrantanopia: 1	Constructive apraxia: 18 Neglect: 11	23	21	Speech/language disturbances/ thalamic aphasia: 14
Bruno et al (1989)[6]	31	—	2	NI	31	15	Dysarthria: 22 Dysphasia NI?
Cambier et al (1983)[34]	4	—	HH: 2	Visual neglect/ constructive apraxia/alexia/ anosognosia: 3	4	Severe: 3 Moderate: 1	Aphasia paraphasia/ perseveration: 1
Decroix et al (1986)[2]	16	PMS: 1 PSS: 1	HH: 3; visual extinction	Neglect: 3	Severe: 6 Moderate: 8	Severe: 5 Moderate: 8	Dysphasia: 2 Dysarthria: 6
Helgason et al (1986)[3]	5	PMS: 1	HH: 2	Visual neglect: 2	Severe: 4	Severe: 2 Moderate: 1	Dysphasia: 1?
Helgason and Wilbur (1990)[8]	23[†]	—	—	—	—	—	—
Hupperts et al (1994)[19]	77	[‡]	HH: 3	NI	[‡]	[‡]	[‡]
Hupperts et al (1994)[19]	6	—	—	NI	—	—	—
Leys et al (1994)[10]	16	PMS: 2(?)	3	Visual neglect: 3	Severe: 12 Moderate: 4	Severe: 7 Moderate: 8	Dysphasia: 6
Mohr et al (1991)[9]	16	Ataxia: 2	HH: 5 Quadrantanopia: 1 Superior sector anopia: 1	NI	Severe: 14 Moderate: 2	Moderate: 8	Dysarthria: 6 Aphasia: 1
Takahashi et al (1994)[24]	12	PMS: 2(?)	HH: 4 Quadrantanopia: 1	Visuospatial agnosia: 1 Visual hallucinations: 1	Severe: 2 Moderate: 9	Severe: 7 Moderate: 1	Dysarthria: 4 Speech/language disturbances/ inclusive thalamic aphasia: 6

[°]Superscript numbers indicate chapter refereces.
[†]Patients with hypestetic ataxic hemiparesis.
[‡]See Table 9.2.
AChA, anterior choroidal artery; AH, ataxic hemiparesis; NI, not investigated in detail; HH, homonymous hemianopia; PMS, pure motor syndrome; PSS, pure sensory syndrome; SMS, sensorimotor syndrome.

In the prospective registry of first-ever supratentorial brain infarcts my colleagues and I[19] created, 67 of 77 small AChA territory infarcts had caused lacunar syndromes—a frequency almost the same as that for small deep infarcts in other vascular territories (Table 9.2). The frequency of lacunar syndromes in that study far exceeded the frequency reported in other CT scan studies on small AChA infarcts. However, in contrast to patients in several other studies, our patients had not undergone detailed neuropsychological analysis, and therefore, less evident cortical signs may have gone undetected. Moreover, in some of the earlier (CT) studies, no special attention was given to lacunar syndromes, a lack that may have biased the numbers of lacunar syndromes toward lower figures.

(Hypesthetic) Ataxic Hemiparesis

The syndrome of ataxic hemiparesis, first described by Fisher,[25,26] is based on the presence of pyramidal and cerebellar signs on the same side.[27] Ataxic hemiparesis seems to be common in lacunar stroke series.[28,29] A variant of this syndrome is hypesthetic ataxic hemiparesis, which was first described in association with an infarct (detected on CT) in the AChA territory by Bogousslavsky and colleagues.[30]

Table 9.2 Clinical Syndromes in Small Anterior Choroidal Artery (AChA) Infarcts Compared with Non–AChA Small Deep Infarcts

Syndrome	AChA (n = 77)	Non–AChA Small Deep Infarcts (n = 83)	AChA vs. Non–AChA Small Deep Infarcts* OR	AChA vs. Non–AChA Small Deep Infarcts* 95% CI
Cortical	10 (13%)	21 (25%)	0.44	0.18–1.09
Pure motor	35 (45%)	26 (31%)	1.83	0.90–3.70
Sensorimotor	21 (27%)	12 (14%)	2.22	0.93–5.27
Pure sensory	0 —	3 (4%)	—	—
DCHS/AH	11 (14%)	18 (22%)	0.60	0.22–1.61
Unknown	0 3	(4%) —	—	—

*OR < 1: less frequent in AChA.
AChA, anterior choroidal artery; CI, confidence interval; DCHS/AH, dysarthria clumsy hand syndrome/ataxic hemiparesis; OR, odds ratio.
Adapted from Hupperts RMM, Lodder J, Heuts-van Raak EPM, Kessels F: Infarcts in the anterior choroidal artery territory: Anatomical distribution, clinical syndromes, presumed pathogenesis and early outcome. Brain 117: 825–834, 1994.

Boiten and Lodder also found that the lesion in ataxic hemiparesis (with or without associated hypesthesia) was frequently located in the posterior internal capsule.[20] Moulin and associates[31] investigated 100 patients with ataxic hemiparesis and first-ever stroke. Thirty of the 77 infarcts documented by CT or MRI in this study were located in the posterior limb of the internal capsule, 21 involving the lower part and 9 extending into the posterior part of the corona radiata near the ventricular body. Inclusion of the corona radiata lesions in patients with ataxic symptoms was previously also described by Huang and Lui[32] and Gutmann and Scherer.[33]

Some investigators have suggested that the finding of ataxia in patients with small AChA infarcts results from inappropriate inclusion of patients with corona radiata lesions in AChA series.[9] We found no differences in frequency of ataxia between 22 AChA infarcts that were restricted to the posterior part of the internal capsule and 26 that were restricted to the posterior corona radiata. Of our patients with AChA infarcts, 14% had ataxia, as either dysarthria–clumsy hand syndrome or ataxic hemiparesis, a rate similar to the 13% reported by Ghika and associates.[7] Helgason and Wilbur[8] described a selective series of 23 patients with hypesthetic ataxic hemiparesis, 22 of whom had lacunar infarcts in the contralateral internal capsule. Fifteen of the infarcts extended into the superior paraventricular corona radiata. In our series, none of the 29 patients with infarcts located in the posterior internal capsule with upward extension had ataxia, a finding that contradicts the view of others. Only 5 of our 26 patients whose infarcts were confined to the paraventricular corona radiata had ataxia. In general, the frequency of ataxic hemiparesis is not higher in patients with small AChA territory infarcts than in those with small deep infarcts in general (see Table 9.2).

Visual Field Disturbances

A homonymous hemianopia can result from separate lesions of any three structures of the visual pathway supplied by the AChA—the optic tract, the lateral geniculate body, and the optic radiation. Generally, the optic radiation is most commonly affected.[2]

Variable visual field deficits have been described in unilateral AChA infarcts.[2,3,34] In addition to homonymous hemianopia, which is the most common, upper quadrant anopia and upper and lower sector anopia with sparing of the horizontal meridian occur.[35] A homonymous visual field defect can occasionally be the only sign of an AChA territory infarct. Abbie[13,36] described a patient with bilateral occlusion of the AChA and the complete triad of symptoms on one side but only a homonymous superior quadrant anopia on the other. Han and colleagues[37] described two patients with pure homonymous hemianopia due to small AChA territory infarcts. However, visual field disturbances are rare in small AChA infarcts but common in large ones.

In a series reported by Takahashi and associates[23] all of 4 patients with extensive AChA territory lesions had hemianopia with or without other cortical signs, but none of 4 patients with small AChA infarcts had hemianopia. Levy and associates[11] found hemianopia in 11 of 35 patients with infarcts at least involving the AChA territory.[11] De Bleecker and colleagues[15] described hemianopia in 9 of 27 patients with (probably small) AChA territory infarcts, a finding similar to the results of Mohr and associates,[9] who found hemianopia in 5 of 16 patients with (large) AChA infarcts. Decroix and coworkers[2] mentioned hemianopia in only 3 of 16 patients.[2] In our series of 77 small AChA territory infarcts, my colleagues and I[19] found only 3 patients (4%) with hemianopia.

These low rates of hemianopia may be attributable primarily to the small size of the infarcts as well as to the fact that the lesions often are located mostly in the posterior limb of the internal capsule, with consequent sparing of the visual system. Furthermore, the optic tract and lateral geniculate body may receive anastomoses from the PChA, the posterior communicating artery, or the leptomeningeal arteries.[17,38–40] This latter possibility could also explain why visual field disturbances accompanying AChA infarcts are often transient. In any case, the absence of hemianopia should not be considered to argue against AChA territory location for an infarct.

Neuropsychological or Cortical Signs

Cambier,[34] conducting extensive neuropsychological investigations in four patients with infarcts in the AChA territory, described marked cognitive dysfunctions in all four.[34] Three patients had visual neglect, constructive apraxia, anosognosia, visuospatial disorders, and motor impersistence. The patient with a left-sided hemispheric lesion had aphasia and semantic paraphasia. The extension of the infarcts in Cambier's series was not clear. De Bleecker and associates[15] studied 27 patients with small infarcts of undefined size in the posterior leg of the internal capsule and found signs of left or right hemispheric neglect in 10 patients, constructive apraxia in 18, and disturbed speech performance in 14. Decroix and coworkers[2] performed extensive neuropsychological evaluations of 16 patients with small AChA territory infarcts and found signs of visual neglect in 3. Other researchers have found signs of right hemispheric neglect in patients with small infarcts.[3,10,41] Ten of 77 patients small AChA infarcts had cortical syndromes on clinical examination in our series, but the neuropsychological study of these patients was not extensive.[19]

Rare Clinical Features

Bilateral AChA infarcts are rare. Buge and associates[42] described a case of pseudobulbar palsy with sparing of limbs resulting from anatomic-pathologically proven incomplete bilateral AChA infarcts. Fisher[43] mentioned bilateral pure motor hemiparesis with faciobuccolingual palsy. Helgason and coworkers[5,35] described nine patients with acute pseudobulbar mutism and variable bilateral hemimotor, hemiataxic, and hemisensory findings; all nine patients experienced the sequential appearance of initially unilateral, but subsequently bilateral, AChA syndromes resulting in a locked-in state. Mohr and colleagues[9] described a patient with unilateral AChA infarct and transient contralateral gaze preference, ptosis, and a Horner's syndrome ipsilateral to the infarct, and transient hemiballism.[9] The anatomic or functional relationships of some of these rare symptoms to the AChA territory were not always evident.

RISK FACTORS AND PRESUMED PATHOPHYSIOLOGY IN ANTERIOR CHOROIDAL ARTERY INFARCTS

The underlying cause of small deep and larger AChA infarcts has not been fully clarified.[6,9,44,45] In addition to clear causes, such as arterial ligation, larger AChA infarcts may result from large artery thromboembolism and cardiac embolism. Small deep AChA infarcts may occur from cerebral small vessel disease, of which small vessel atherosclerosis may be more common than lipohyalinosis.[20] Although larger AChA infarcts are rare, their underlying pathophysiology has been studied. The higher incidence of small deep AChA infarcts allowed better study of their presumed pathogenesis, but pathologic evaluation of small infarcts is hardly feasible because of the low early case-fatality rate in small deep infarcts.[1,20]

Small Deep Infarcts

Concerning small deep AChA infarcts, Mohr and associates[9] suggested that inclusion of cases of posterior corona radiata infarction would result in a "disproportionate increase in the frequency of typical small vessel disease" in AChA infarct studies. However, most symptomatic small deep infarcts are not located in this area, and the size of an infarct does not necessarily imply a certain vascular pathology.

Pathologic studies of small deep infarcts are scarce, but it might be possible to infer the cause of such infarcts from the study of risk factors for them (Table 9.3). Sterbini and associates[4] studied 28 patients with AChA infarcts of various sizes and found 41% with hypertension, 26% with diabetes mellitus, and 30% with possible cardiac or carotid embolic sources. Six of 16 cases described by Decroix and colleagues[2] had either cardiac or carotid embolic causes, and Mayer and coworkers[45] reported two cases of smaller AChA infarcts that probably resulted from carotid artery disease.

Out Of 31 patients with AChA infarct studied by Bruno and colleagues,[6] 65% had hypertension, 33% had diabetes mellitus, and only 6% had cardioembolic sources.[6] All of the patients underwent carotid studies, results of which were normal in 27. Fifteen of the 16 patients who underwent angiography had patent AChAs. The researchers concluded that "small-vessel disease" was the most common underlying vasculopathy, with hypertension as the single most important risk factor. A similar conclusion was drawn by Helgason and Wilbur,[8] who also cited diabetes mellitus as an important risk factor. Ghika and associates[7] found small artery disease the most likely cause in 42% of their 32 patients with AChA infarcts, possible embolism from carotid sources in 27%, and cardiac sources in 17%. Leys and coworkers[10] concluded, from a clinical study of 16 AChA territory infarcts, that these infarcts were probably not attributable to small vessel occlusion. However, only five of their patients had small infarcts (less than 15 mm in diameter), of whom only one had signs of carotid artery disease and none had a cardioembolic source, whereas all five had hypertension.[10]

The heterogeneity of series studied so far makes general conclusions regarding the cause of small AChA infarcts difficult. My colleagues and I[19] compared patients with AChA infarcts and those with other subtypes of infarct. Many patients had hypertension, but this did not differentiate the AChA infarcts from the non–AChA small deep or superficial infarcts (Table 9.4). Hypertension can be regarded as a nonspecific risk factor for AChA infarct, as it is for small deep infarcts in general.[20,46,47] Furthermore, cardiac and carotid embolisms are unlikely causes of small AChA infarcts. Therefore, the cause of small AChA infarction is most likely small vessel obstruction, as it is of most small deep (lacunar) infarcts in general.[20,46] However, cardiac or carotid embolism may be a more common cause in AChA infarct than in other small deep infarcts. Moreover, a series of patients with acute AChA territory infarct syndromes were successfully treated with early administration of recombinant tissue-type plasminogen activator (r-tPA), a result that may suggest a thromboembolic cause for their infarcts.[48] Diagnostic procedures and eventual carotid surgery should be considered in this subgroup of patients with small infarcts according to the same criteria as used for patients with large infarcts.[49]

Table 9.3 Vascular Risk Factors and/or Etiologic Factors in CT/MRI Documented Anterior Choroidal Artery Territory Infarcts

Study (Year)[*]	AChA Infarcts	Size	Cardiac Embolism	Carotid Embolism	Diabetes Mellitus	Hypertension	Ischemic Heart Disease	TIA
Bruno et al (1989)[6]	31	Unknown	2 (6%)	2 (6%) moderate; 3 (10%) mild	10 (32%)	20 (65%)	NM	NM
Decroix et al (1986)[2]	16	Small	2 (13%)	4 (25%)	3 (19%)	2 (13%)	1 (6%)	NM
Helgason et al (1986)[3]	5[†]	Unknown	1 (20%)	f	1 (20%)	3 (60%)	NM	NM
Helgason and Wilbur (1990)[8]	23[‡]	22 small	1 (4%)	5/12 (42%)[‖]	8 (35%)	23 (100%)	6 (26%)	NM
Hupperts et al (1994)[19]	77	Small	7 (9%)	9 (12%)	13 (17%)[¶]	37 (48%)	13 (17%)	NM
Hupperts et al (1994)[19]	6	Large	2 (33%)	1 (17%)	1 (17%)	4 (66%)	1 (17%)	NM
Mohr et al (1991)[9]	16	Unknown	2 (13%)	3 (19%)	3 (19%)	4 (25%)	2 (13%)	NM
Leys et al (1994)[10]	16	5 small, 11 large	4 (25%)	2 (13%)	4 (25%)	10 (63%)	NM	2 (17%)
Sterbini et al (1987)[4]	28	6 or more small	5 (18%)	3 (11%)	7 (25%)	11 (41%)	NM	2 (7%)
Takahashi et al (1994)[24]	12[§]	4 small 4 moderate, 4 large	NM	2 (17%)[¶]	NM	NM	NM	NM

[*]Superscript numbers indicate chapter references.
[†]Three patients with intracranial small vessel disease related to hypertension; two patients with intraoperative manipulation near the AChA.
[‡]Patients selected with stroke and ataxic hemiparesis.
[‖]Five out of 12 patients with angiography had carotid plaques.
[§]Patients selected with presumed AChA territory infarct and angiographic evidence of AChA obstruction.
[¶]Next to seven with AChA occlusion and three with AChA stenosis.
AChA, anterior choroidal artery; NM, not mentioned in this study; TIA; transient ischemic attack.

Table 9.4 Vascular Risk Factors in 77 Small Deep Anterior Choroidal Artery (AChA) Infarcts, 83 Non–AChA Small Deep Infarcts, and 384 Superficial Infarcts

Risk Factor	Small Deep AChA Infarcts (n = 77)	Non–AChA Small Deep Infarcts (n = 83)	Superficial Infarcts (n = 384)
Male	46 (60%)	46 (55%)	198 (52%)
Diabetes mellitus	13 (17%)	13 (16%)	61 (16%)
Hypertension	37 (48%)	35 (42%)	166 (43%)
Ischemic heart disease	13 (17%)	12 (14%)	110 (29%)
Carotid ultrasonography	65 (84%)	58 (70%)	249 (65%)
Carotid stenosis	9 (14%)	2 (2%)	74 (19%)
Cardioembolism	7 (9%)	16 (19%)	132 (34%)

From Hupperts RMM, Lodder J, Heuts-van Raak EPM, Kessels F: Infarcts in the anterior choroidal artery territory: Anatomical distribution, clinical syndromes, presumed pathogenesis and early outcome. Brain 117: 825–834, 1994.

Table 9.5 Clinical Features in Six Large Anterior Choroidal Artery (AChA) Infarcts and 378 Non–AChA Superficial Infarcts

Feature	AChA Infarcts (n = 6)	Superficial Infarcts (n = 378)	P Value[*]
Male patient	2 (33%)	196 (52%)	0.43
Diabetes mellitus	1 (17%)	60 (16%)	1.00
Hypertension	4 (67%)	162 (43%)	0.41
Ischemic heart disease	1 (17%)	109 (29%)	0.68
Carotid ultrasonography	6 (100%)	243 (64%)	0.09
Carotid stenosis	1 (17%)	73 (19%)	0.67
Rankin Scale score 4/5	4 (67%)	236 (62%)	1.00
Cardioembolism	2 (33%)	130 (34%)	1.00

[*]Fisher exact test.
From Hupperts RMM, Lodder J, Heuts-van Raak EPM, Kessels F: Infarcts in the anterior choroidal artery territory: Anatomical distribution, clinical syndromes, presumed pathogenesis and early outcome. Brain 117: 825–834, 1994.

Large Infarcts

In our study, the larger AChA infarcts resembled superficial infarcts with respect to vascular risk factors and potential underlying cause of stroke, although the numbers were small (Table 9.5). Several series on large AChA territory infarcts have now been reported. Leys and coworkers[10] presented 16 AChA territory infarcts documented by CT or MRI, 11 of which were more than 15 mm in diameter.[10] In 7 of the 11 large infarcts, the mesiotemporal territory was involved. Four of the seven patients with these infarcts had presumed cardioembolic causes of stroke, but none of the five patients with small AChA infarcts did. One patient with a large AChA infarct had large vessel atherosclerosis, suggesting carotid emboli, and in two patients, the infarcts were caused by carotid dissection.

Levy and associates[11] described 35 patients with neuropathologically confirmed massive infarcts involving at least the AChA territory; in none of the patients was the AChA infarct recognized clinically, nor did any of them

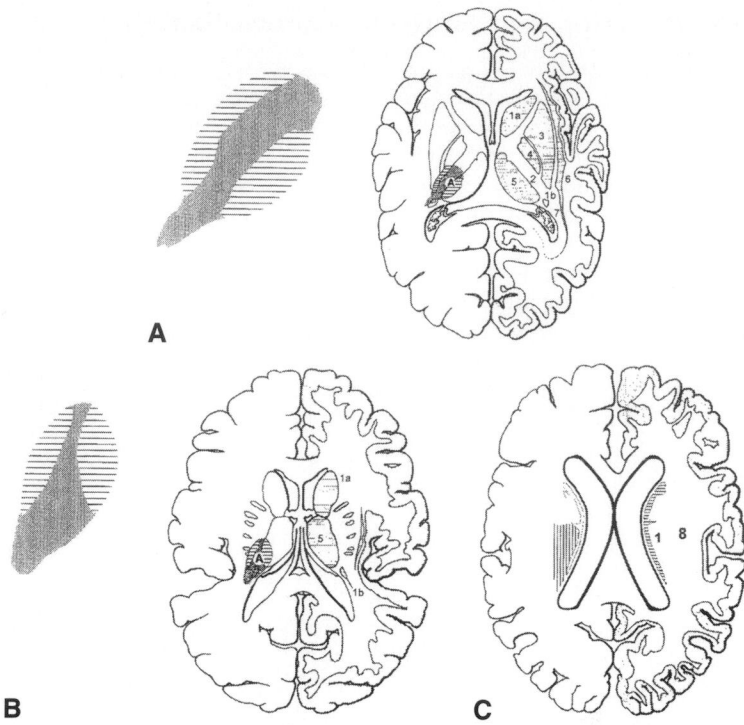

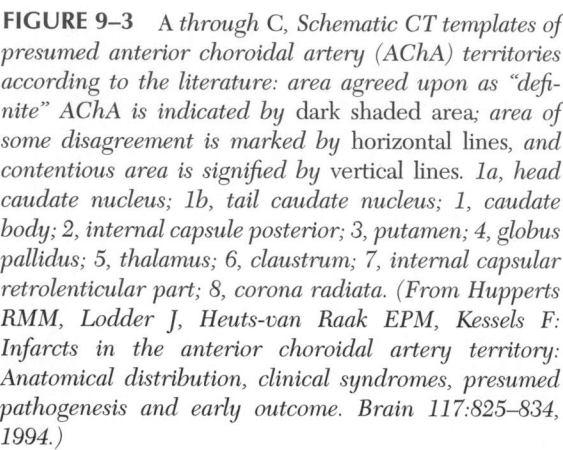

FIGURE 9–3 A *through* C, *Schematic CT templates of presumed anterior choroidal artery (AChA) territories according to the literature: area agreed upon as "definite" AChA is indicated by* dark shaded area; *area of some disagreement is marked by* horizontal lines, *and contentious area is signified by* vertical lines. *1a, head caudate nucleus; 1b, tail caudate nucleus; 1, caudate body; 2, internal capsule posterior; 3, putamen; 4, globus pallidus; 5, thalamus; 6, claustrum; 7, internal capsular retrolenticular part; 8, corona radiata. (From Hupperts RMM, Lodder J, Heuts-van Raak EPM, Kessels F: Infarcts in the anterior choroidal artery territory: Anatomical distribution, clinical syndromes, presumed pathogenesis and early outcome. Brain 117:825–834, 1994.)*

have the clinical triad hemiplegia, hemianesthesia, and hemianopia. Embolic occlusions were found in 74%, most of which were due to cardiac embolism (54%). In contrast, small artery disease (3%) and artery-to-artery embolism (17%) were rarely found. These findings may suggest a carotid or cardioembolic cause for large AChA territory infarcts, but none of the infarcts was restricted to the AChA territory. The studies by Leys and Levy and their colleagues suggest that large artery thromboembolism and cardiac embolism are the most common causes of large AChA infarcts,[10,11] as has been found for striatocapsular and superficial infarcts.[50–52]

VASCULAR SUPPLY AREAS

The AChA, with an average diameter of about 1 mm, arises most often from the stem of the internal carotid artery but sometimes from the bifurcation of the internal carotid artery, from the middle cerebral artery, or from the posterior communicating artery.[13,16,17,36,53–56] Rarely, the AChA is absent; plural (duplicate or multiple) anterior choroidal arteries have also been described.[17,57,58]

The artery courses along the lateral border of the optic tract, which it crosses from lateral to medial, and runs posteriorly along the medial border of the optic tract against the cerebral peduncle.[13,53] At the anterior pole of the lateral geniculate body, the AChA divides into many branches, most of which recross the optic tract to enter the inferior temporal horn of the lateral ventricle and the choroid plexus of the lateral ventricle.[13,16,17] The average distance for which the artery followed the optic tract in one study was 12 mm.[55]

Throughout its course, the AChA has many branches to neighboring structures. The *superficial branches* supply the optic tract, the optic radiation, the anterolateral half

and hilum of the lateral geniculate body and of the medial temporal lobe, the anterior parts of the hippocampus, the uncus, the posterior part of the amygdaloid nucleus, and the middle third of the peduncle.[13,17,55,58,59] AChA branches supply the most rostral third of the temporomedial region.[60] The *perforating branches* supply the posterior two thirds of the posterior limb of the internal capsule, the retrolenticular part of the internal capsule, the optic radiation, the medial globus pallidus, and the superficial part of the ventrolateral thalamus. Other AChA branches supply the substantia nigra, part of the red nucleus, a portion of the subthalamus, and the superficial part of the (ventro-)lateral thalamus.[5,24,54,58,59]

Variability in Supply

The number and distribution of the AChA branches are to some extent variable.[13,17,36,55] Branches of the AChA anastomose with those of the posterior communicating, posterior cerebral, internal carotid, middle cerebral, and lateral posterior choroidal arteries.[13,17,23,24,36,55] Therefore, the area supplied by the AChA may depend on differences in number of anastomoses.[5,13,16,17,36,58,61] The most consistent supply area of the AChA contains the optic tract, the posterior limb of the internal capsule, the cerebral peduncle, and the choroid plexus. Most writers agree that the posterior two thirds of the posterior leg of the internal capsule and the pars retrolenticularis are supplied by the AChA.* In clinical studies, however, supply of the lateral thalamus, the medial part of the lentiform nucleus, and especially the posterior paraventricular corona radiata by the AChA is in dispute (Fig. 9–3).[4,5,9,30,62,63]

---

*See references 2, 4, 5, 9, 13, 16, 20, 36, 56, 58, 61.

The Posterior Paraventricular Corona Radiata

Autopsy Studies

From autopsy cases, pathologic injection studies, and their own clinical series, Mohr and associates[9] (Fig. 9–4) opposed the view of Helgason and Wilbur[8] who, among others,[2,5,62] found extension of AChA infarcts into the posterior corona radiata. According to some investigators, results of several pathologic injection studies do not lend support to the view that the posterior paraventricular corona radiata should be regarded as AChA territory.[64] Takahashi and coworkers,[23] in particular, mapped the territory of the AChA in their series with a combination of angiographic evidence of AChA occlusion and CT or MRI evidence of infarction. Their maps correlate well with those from the clinical series of Mohr and associates[9] but were created independently, and Takahashi and coworkers[23] do not cite or list the Mohr series.

Issues of ambiguity remain. In his pathologic study, Beevor[16,53] did not exclude the area next to the lateral ventricle from AChA territory. Abbie's[13] India ink perfusion study allowed him to follow AChA branches as high as the upper level of the lentiform nucleus, but one may wonder whether this injection technique was able to reveal very small penetrating branches possibly continuing more rostrally. Percheron[63] studied the AChA territory in only four patients and restricted the study to AChA branches possibly supplying parts of the thalamus. He aimed to study the vasculature of the thalamus and not that of the paraventricular corona radiata. Thus, several pathologic studies do not reject the posterior paraventricular corona radiata region from AChA territory.

Clinical Studies

Clinical studies have not settled this issue. From investigations that merely used current vascular CT templates, no conclusions can be drawn as to which vessel supplies this region, because the templates were not derived from series that were actually studied.[9,65,66] If "definite" AChA infarcts that in large part are located in the posterior leg of the internal capsule extend upward into the paraventricular corona radiata, this region is probably being supplied by the AChA.

In a prospective stroke series, we found 51 such "definite" small AChA infarcts, mapped from CT scan images and inferred to have been AChA infarcts (Fig. 9–5).[19] Twenty-nine of these infarcts extended upward into the posterior paraventricular corona radiata. It is unlikely that the lower parts of these infarcts resulted from AChA obstruction and the upper parts were caused by obstruction of a separate vessel in a different vascular territory at the same time. Not only would simultaneous obstructions in two separate vascular territories producing adjacent small infarcts be unlikely; the small size of the infarcts in our series may also suggest obstruction of a single, small perforating artery (Fig. 9–6).[67] Furthermore, a composite topographic projection figure of the upwardly extending AChA infarcts overlapped with that of 26 other small deep infarcts restricted to the posterior paraventricular area, suggesting AChA branches as supplying vessels for this area. Because small deep infarcts occur frequently in the paraventricular corona radiata, this region is, in any case, most likely being supplied by small deep penetrators.[55,59,68–70]

Thus, as an alternative to the AChA, the lenticulostriate arteries would be the next most likely vessels supplying this area.[71] Pullicino[64] suggested that infarcts located in the posterior limb of the internal capsule, which is definitely AChA territory, and extending rostrally into the lateral ventricular margin are in fact in the territory of a posteriorly located lateral lenticulostriate artery. However, we found only one small deep infarct located in the lenticulostriate territory at the level of the internal capsule–basal ganglia

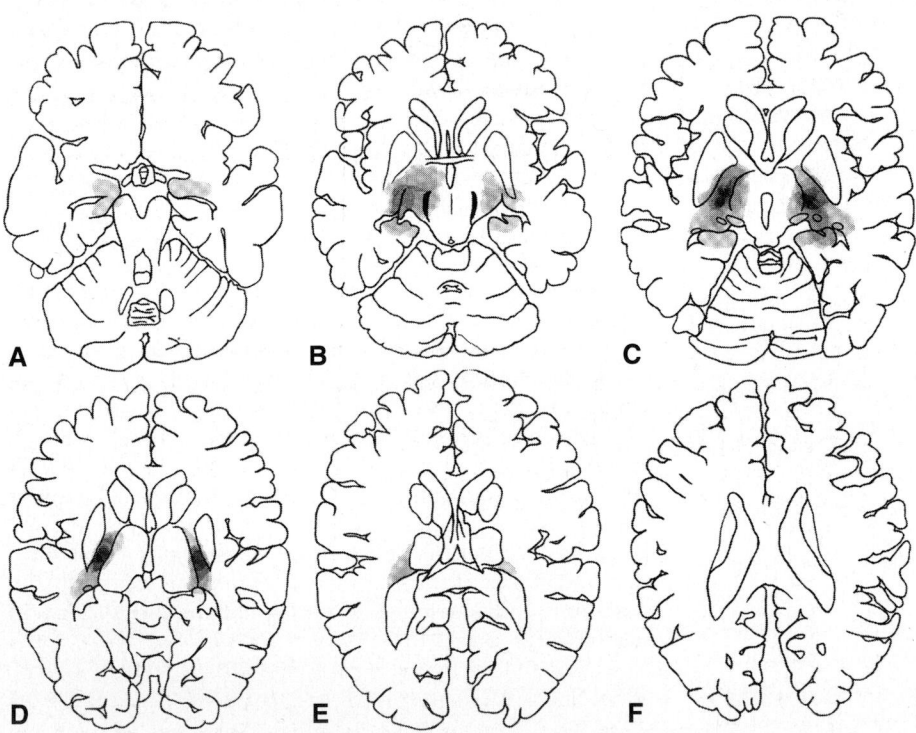

FIGURE 9–4 *A through F, Mapping of infarction as inferred from MRI or CT and attributed to occlusion of the anterior choroidal artery (AChA) by angiography or selective injection of the AChA during CT. (From Mohr JP, Timsit S: Choroidal artery disease. In Barnett HJM, Mohr JP, Stein BM, Yatsu FM [eds]: Stroke: Diagnosis, Pathophysiology, and Management, 3rd ed. New York, Churchill Livingstone, 1998, pp 503–512.)*

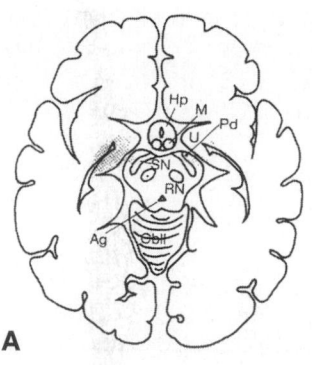 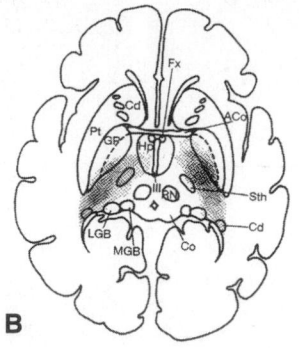 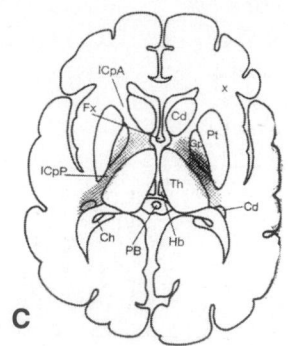

A   B   C

FIGURE 9–5 *Diagram of the distribution of lesions in the 12 cases reported by Takahashi and colleagues,[24] on axial sections through the midbrain (A), the junction of midbrain and diencephalon (B), and thalamus (C). Lightly stippled areas represent individual infarcts, and denser portions represent overlapping lesions. Although variable, the lesions are generally distributed in an arcuate zone between the striatum anterolaterally and the thalamus posteromedially. Aco, anterior commissure; Aq, aqueduct of Sylvius; Cll, cerebellum; Cd, caudate nucleus; Co, colliculi; Ch, choroid plexus; Fx, fornix; Hb, habenula; Hp, hypothalamus; IcpA and IcpC, anterior and posterior limb, respectively, of internal capsule; M, mammillary body; MGB and LGB, medial and lateral geniculate body, respectively; PB, pineal body; Pd, cerebral peduncle; RN, red nucleus; SN, substantia nigra; Sth, subthalamus; Th, thalamus, U, uncus; III, third ventricle. (From Takahashi S, Fukasawa H, Ishii K, Sakamoto K: The anterior choroidal artery syndrome I: Microangiography of the anterior choroidal artery. Neuroradiology 36:337–339, 1994.)*

that extended upward and was continuous with the posterior part of this region, whereas we found seven that extended into the anterior part.[19,72] Therefore, it is unlikely that the posterior paraventricular corona radiata is being supplied by the lenticulostriate arteries.

Infarcts extending into the paraventricular corona radiata could be "watershed infarcts" between (1) the territories of AChA and posterolateral choroidal arteries or (2) the territories of the terminal branches of the anterior-posterolateral choroidal artery and the terminal branches of the lateral lenticulostriate arteries.[64,73] However, the concept of lacunar "watershed" infarcts questionable, and the sizes of the infarcts we studied were compatible with the occlusion of a single penetrator. This latter finding argues against the idea that lacunar infarcts could be located in separate but coincidentally adjacent areas of two different vascular territories, even if some distally located small deep infarcts may be caused by low-flow state.[74] The body of the caudate nucleus and the adjacent ventricular wall superolateral to the thalamus are occasionally supplied by the PChA.[63] Therefore, anastomosis of the lateral PChA with the AChA may account for small infarcts in the posterior paraventricular corona radiata when the lateral PChA is small or stenosed.[13,17,64] However, this theoretical possibility has never been substantiated. Therefore, except for the area immediately adjacent to the ventricular wall, the posterior paraventricular corona radiata is most likely being supplied by AChA penetrating branches. Whether this region is supplied by the AChA in an individual case may depend on the diameter of the supplying penetrator; in a microdissection study, Marinkovic and associates[75] showed that the diameter of the most distal AChA penetrator, which is the capsular thalamic perforator, varied from 200 to 600 μm.

The Lateral Thalamic Border

A less controversial question is whether the lateral thalamic border and the medial part of the lentiform nucleus

are supplied by the AChA. We found, in a series of 51 "definite" AChA infarcts with the largest part of the infarct in the posterior leg of the internal capsule, that 4 infarcts involved the lateral thalamic border; this finding concurs with the conclusion by Mohr and associates[9] that a superficial involvement of the lateral thalamus may occur. Takahashi and colleagues[24] demonstrated common involvement of the lateral border of the thalamus in a microangiographic analysis of the AChA territory of 55 brains (see Fig. 9–5). In a series of 12 angiographically verified AChA territory infarcts of varying size, these researchers found that most infarcts extended into the posteromedial part of the thalamus.[23,24] Fujii and coworkers[59] described involvement of the thalamus in 10% of the patients they studied.[59] Other workers have reported similar findings.[8,55,63] CT-demonstrated thalamic involvement may be attributable merely to surrounding edema rather than to ischemic necrosis caused by obstruction of presumed AChA thalamic branches.

The Medial Part of the Lentiform Nucleus

A region more consistently involved in AChA infarcts is the medial part of the lentiform nucleus, which was involved in 12 of 16 cases described by Mohr and associates[9] and 6 of 23 cases studies by Helgason and Wilbur.[8] Both groups concluded from the available literature that the medial part of the lentiform nucleus is regularly supplied by the AChA. In our series, 22 (43%) of the 51 "definite" AChA infarcts involved the medial part of the lentiform nucleus.[19]

PROGNOSIS

Few studies have reported on prognosis in AChA infarcts, and those that have done so have been case studies. The first-described patient with bilateral AChA infarcts died of pulmonary complications.[42] Helgason and colleagues[35] described nine patients with pseudobulbar mutism and

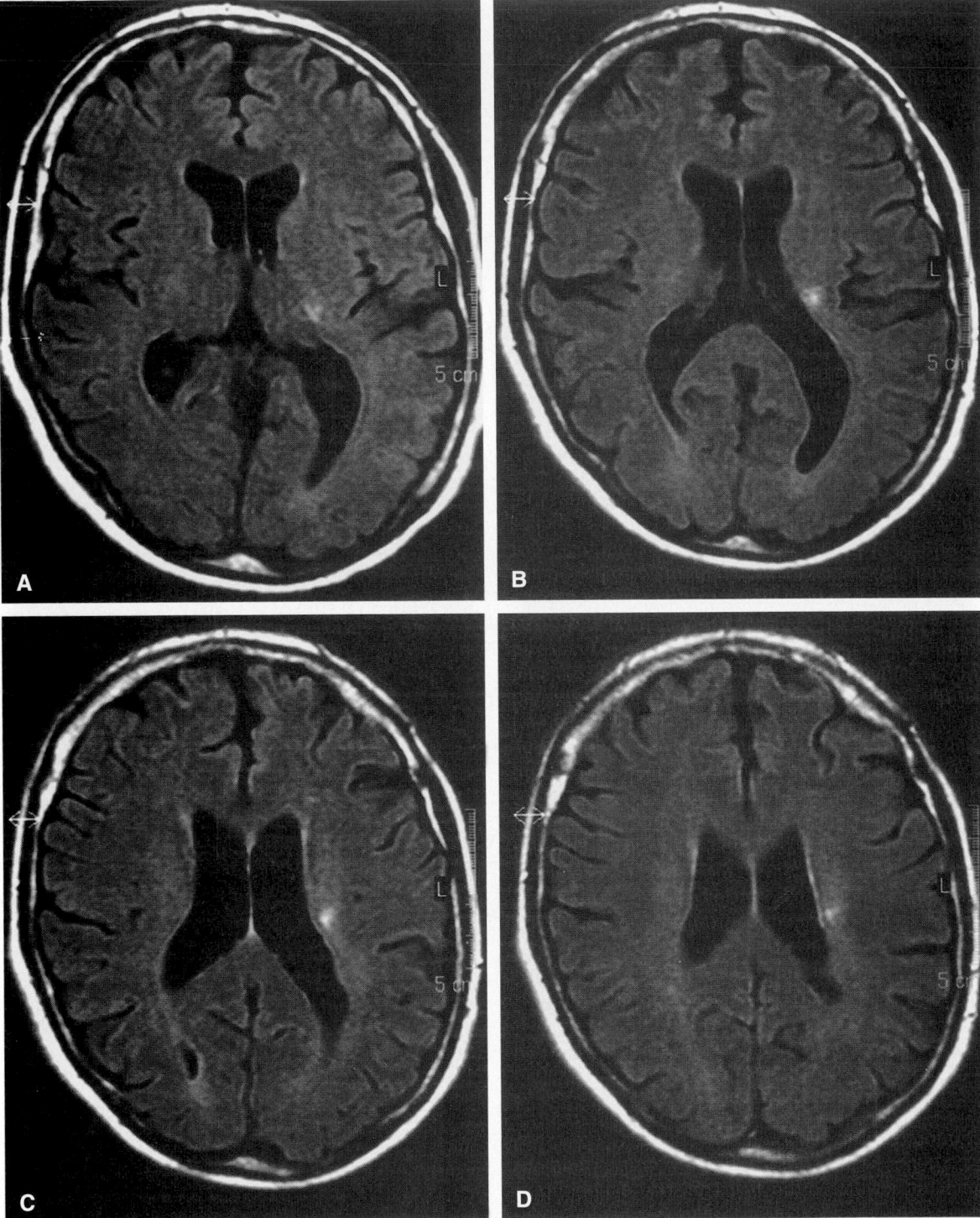

FIGURE 9–6   *A 47-year-old man suffered acute numbness of the right side of the body, choreic movements of the right arm, and slight right-sided hemiparesis. A through D, T2-weighted fluid-attenuated inversion recovery (FLAIR) MR images show a small signal-intense area compatible with a lacunar infarct extending from the posterior part of the posterior internal capsule leg upwards into the paraventricular corona radiata area.*

bilateral AChA infarct, of whom five remained severely impaired up to 1 year after stroke, and four died either of aspiration pneumonia or cardiopulmonary arrest.[35] These researchers described good prognosis in AChA infarcts that occurred after seizure focus resection, whereas

unilateral AChA infarcts occurring after aneurysm clipping were associated with moderate to severe clinical deficit. Some patients with unilateral AChA infarcts associated with small vessel disease remained moderately to severely impaired. Helgason and colleagues[35] mentioned that visual

Table 9.6 Thirty-day Case Fatality Rate, 1-year Mortality, and Rate of Functional Independence After 1 Year in Small Deep Anterior Choroidal Artery Territory Infarcts Compared with Non–AChA Small Deep Infarcts and Superficial Infarcts

	AChA Infarcts (n = 77)	Small Deep Infarcts (n = 83)					Superficial Infarcts (n = 384)				
		No.	(%)	OR°	95% CI	P value	No.	(%)	OR°	95% CI	P Value
30-day case-fatality rate	0	3	(4)			0.25[†]	49	(13)			<0.01[†]
1-year mortality	7 (9%)	18	(22)	0.36	0.13–0.99	<0.04	107	(28)	0.26	0.12–0.57	<0.0008
Functional independence at 1 year	62 (81%)	54	(65)	2.22	1.02–4.03	<0.05	196	(51)	3.96	2.21–7.10	<0.001

°OR < 1: less frequent in AChA.
[†]Fisher exact test.
AChA, anterior choroidal artery; CI, confidence interval; OR, odds ratio.
From Hupperts RMM, Lodder J, Heuts-van Raak EPM, Kessels F: Infarcts in the anterior choroidal artery territory: Anatomical distribution, clinical syndromes, presumed pathogenesis and early outcome. Brain 117: 825–834, 1994.

field deficits and sensory loss improved, whereas patients with hemiparesis recovered little. They suggested that discrepant prognosis of postoperative and spontaneous-onset AChA infarcts may be explained by poor collateral circulation and anastomoses resulting from diffuse disease of the cardiac and cerebral vascular system in the older, nonsurgical group.

In our series, the rate of functional independence after 1 year was higher, and the 30-day case-fatality rate and 1-year mortality lower, for patients with small deep infarcts than for those with superficial infarcts. The rates were even more favorable for patients with small deep AChA infarcts than for those with non–AChA small deep infarcts, a difference that probably was related to the younger age of the patients with AChA infarcts (Table 9.6).

CONCLUSION

The areas supplied by the AChA have been studied extensively. The areas most consistently supplied by this artery contain the optic tract, posterior limb of the internal capsule, cerebral peduncle, and choroid plexus. After the introduction of CT scanning, some presumed "AChA territories" became controversial. The posterior part of the paraventricular corona radiata is the area in most dispute, but in our view, it is most likely supplied by the AChA.

Although the AChA territory infarct syndrome consists of a classic triad—hemiparesis, hemianesthesia, and hemianopia—the syndrome often is incomplete or is accompanied by other signs commonly related to higher cortical dysfunction, even in larger infarcts. Most, but not all, AChA infarcts give rise to one of the lacunar syndromes.

The cause of small AChA infarcts is most likely small vessel obstruction, as it is for most small deep infarcts in general. Carotid stenosis, although less common in small AChA infarcts than in cortical infarcts, may be more common in small AChA infarcts than in small infarcts in general. Large artery thromboembolism, cardiac embolism, or both is the most probable cause of large AChA infarcts.

Clinical symptoms, vascular risk factor profiles, presumed underlying causes, and prognoses, in terms of rate

of functional independence, 30-day case-fatality rate, and 1-year mortality, have all failed to lend support to the idea that small deep infarcts in the AChA territory should be regarded as a clinical entity separate from other small deep infarcts. Similar conclusions can be drawn with regard to large AChA infarcts compared with superficial infarcts. Consequently, the small and large infarcts in the territory of the AChA should, in general, be investigated and treated as small deep and superficial infarct subtypes, respectively. Future development in imaging techniques such as MRI, MR angiography, and physiologic measurements may shed further light on causes and proposed treatment of AChA territory infarcts.[76,77]

References

1. Bamford J, Sandercock P, Dennis M, et al: Classification and natural history of clinically identifiable subtypes of cerebral infarction. Lancet 337:1521–1526, 1991.
2. Decroix JP, Graveleau Ph, Masson M, Cambier J: Infarction in the territory of the anterior choroidal artery: A clinical and computerized tomographic study of 16 cases. Brain 109:1071–1085, 1986.
3. Helgason C, Caplan LR, Goodwin J, Hedges T: Anterior choroidal artery-territory infarction: Report of cases and review. Arch Neurol 43:681–686, 1986.
4. Sterbini GLP, Agatiello LM, Stocchi A, Solivetti FM: CT of ischemic infarctions in the territory of the anterior choroidal artery: A review of 28 cases. Am J Neuroradiol 8:229–232, 1987.
5. Helgason CM: A new view of anterior choroidal artery territory infarction. J Neurol 235:387–391, 1988.
6. Bruno A, Graff-Radford NR, Biller J, Adams HP: Anterior choroidal artery territory infarction: Small vessel disease. Stroke 20:616–619, 1989.
7. Ghika J, Bogousslavsky J, Regli F: Infarcts in the territory of the deep perforators from the carotid system. Neurology 39:507–512, 1989.
8. Helgason CM, Wilbur AC: Capsular hypesthetic ataxic hemiparesis. Stroke 21:24–33, 1990.
9. Mohr JP, Steinke W, Timsit SG: The anterior choroidal artery does not supply the corona radiata and lateral ventricular wall. Stroke 22:1502–1507, 1991.
10. Leys D, Mounier-Vehier F, Lavenu I, et al: Anterior choroidal artery territory infarcts: Study of presumed mechanisms. Stroke 25:837–842, 1994.
11. Levy R, Duyckaerts C, Hauw JJ: Massive infarcts involving the territory of the anterior choroidal artery and cardioembolism. Stroke 26:609–613, 1995.
12. Foix Ch, Chavany JA, Hillemand P, Schiff Wertheimer S: Oblitération de l'artère choroidienne antérieure: Ramollissement de son

territoire cérébral, hemiplégie, hémianesthésie, hemianopsie. Bull Soc Ophthalmol (Paris) 27:221–223, 1925.

13. Abbie AA: The blood supply of the lateral geniculate body, with a note of the morphology of the choroidal arteries. J Anat 67:491–527, 1933.

14. Steegman A, Roberts D: The syndrome of the anterior choroidal artery: Report of a case. JAMA 104:1695–1697, 1935.

15. De Bleecker J, De Reuck J, Vingergoets G, et al: Het arteria choroidea anterior syndroom. Tÿdschrift voor Geneeskunde 44:259–262, 1988.

16. Beevor CE: The cerebral arterial supply. Brain 30:403–425, 1907.

17. Carpenter MB, Noback CR, Moss ML: The anterior choroidal artery: Its origins, course, distribution, and variations. Arch Neurol Psychiatry (Chicago) 71:714–722, 1954.

18. Friedman JA, Pichelmann MA, Piepgras DG, et al: Ischemic complications of surgery for anterior choroidal artery aneurysms. J Neurosurg 94:565–572, 2001.

19. Hupperts RMM, Lodder J, Heuts-van Raak EPM, Kessels F: Infarcts in the anterior choroidal artery territory: Anatomical distribution, clinical syndromes, presumed pathogenesis and early outcome. Brain 117:825–834, 1994.

20. Boiten J, Lodder J: Lacunar infarcts: Pathogenesis and validity of the clinical syndromes. Stroke 22:1374–1378, 1991.

21. Fisher CM, Curry HB: Pure motor hemiplegia of vascular origin. Arch Neurol 13:13–44, 1965.

22. Derouesné C, Yelnik A, Castaigne P: Déficit sensitif isolé par infarctus dans le territoire de l'artère choroidienne antérieure. Rev Neurol 141:311–314, 1985.

23. Takahashi S, Ishii K, Matsumoto K, et al: The anterior choroidal artery syndrome II: CT and/or MR in angiographically verified cases. Neuroradiology 36:340–345, 1994.

24. Takahashi S, Fukasawa H, Ishii K, Sakamoto K: The anterior choroidal artery syndrome I: Microangiography of the anterior choroidal artery. Neuroradiology 36:337–339, 1994.

25. Fisher CM, Cole M: Homolateral ataxia and crural paresis: A vascular syndrome. J Neurol Neurosurg Psychiatry 28:48–55, 1965.

26. Fisher CM: Ataxic hemiparesis: A pathologic study. Arch Neurol 35:126–128, 1978.

27. Hommel M, Besson G: Advances in neurology. In Pullicino PM, Caplan LR, Hommel M (eds): Cerebral Small Artery Disease, vol 62. New York, Raven, 1993, pp 141–180.

28. Boiten J, Lodder J: Discrete lesions in the sensorimotor control system: A clinical-topographical study of lacunar infarcts. J Neurol Sci 105:150–154, 1991.

29. Chamorro A, Sacco RL, Mohr JP, et al: Clinical-computed tomographic correlations of lacunar infarction in the Stroke Data Bank. Stroke 22:175–181, 1991.

30. Bogousslavsky J, Regli F, Delaloye B, et al: Hémiataxie et déficit sensitif ipsilateral: Infarctus du territoire de l'artère choroïdienne antérieure: Diaschisis cérébelleux croisé. Rev Neurol 142:671–676, 1986.

31. Moulin T, Bogousslavsky J, Chopard J, et al: Vascular ataxic hemiparesis: A re-evaluation. J Neurol Neurosurg Psychiatry 58:422–427, 1995.

32. Huang CY, Lui FS: Ataxic hemiparesis, localization and clinical features. Stroke 15:363–366, 1984.

33. Gutmann DH, Scherer S: Magnetic resonance imaging of ataxic hemiparesis localized in the corona radiata. Stroke 20:1571–1573, 1989.

34. Cambier J, Graveleau Ph, Decroix JP, et al: Le syndrome de l'artère choroidienne antérieure étude neuropsychologique de 4 cas. Rev Neurol (Paris) 131:553–559, 1983.

35. Helgason C, Wilbur A, Weiss A, et al: Acute pseudobulbar mutism due to discrete capsular infarction in the territory of the anterior choroidal artery. Brain 11:507–524, 1988.

36. Abbie AA: The clinical significance of the anterior choroidal artery. Brain 56:233–246, 1933.

37. Han SW, Sohn YH, Lee PH, et al: Pure homonymous hemianopia due to anterior choroidal artery territory infarction. Eur Neurol 43:35–8, 2000.

38. Rand RW, Brown WJ, Stern WE: Surgical occlusion of anterior choroidal arteries in parkinsonism. Neurology (Minn) 6:390–401, 1956.

39. Ueda M, Morinaga K, Matsumoto Y, et al: Infarction in the territory of the anterior choroidal artery due to embolic occlusion of the internal carotid artery: Report of two cases. No To Shinkei 42:655–660, 1990.

40. Zwan van der A, Hillen B, Tulleken CAF, et al: Variability of the territories of the major cerebral arteries. J Neurosurg 77:927–940, 1992.

41. Bogousslavsky J, Miklossy J, Regli F, et al: Subcortical neglect: Neuropsychological, SPECT and neuropathological correlations with anterior choroidal artery territory infarction. Ann Neurol 23:448–452, 1988.

42. Buge A, Escourolle R, Hauw J, et al: Syndrome pseudobulbaire aigu par infarctus bilateral limité du territoire des artères choroidiennes antérieures. Rev Neurol (Paris) 135:313–318, 1979.

43. Fisher CM: Capsular infarcts: The underlying vascular lesions. Arch Neurol 36:65–73, 1979.

44. Fisher M, Lingley JF, Blumenfield A, Felice K: Anterior choroidal artery territory infarction and small-vessel disease [letter comment in Stroke 20:616–619, 1989]. Stroke 20:1591–1592, 1989.

45. Mayer JM, Lanoë Y, Pedetti L, Fabry B: Anterior choroidal artery territory infarction and carotid occlusion. Cerebrovasc Dis 2:315–316, 1992.

46. Lodder J, Bamford J, Sandercock PAG, et al: Are hypertension or cardiac embolism likely causes of lacunar infarction? Stroke 21:375–381, 1990.

47. Lodder J, Boiten J: Incidence, natural history, and risk factors in lacunar infarction: Review. Adv Neurol 62:213–227, 1993.

48. Trouillas P, Derex L, Nighoghossian N, et al: RtPA intravenous thrombolysis in anterior choroidal artery territory stroke. Neurology 54:666–673, 2000.

49. Rothwell PM, Mayberg MR, Warlow CP, et al: Meta-analysis of individual patient data from randomised controlled trials of carotid endarterectomy for symptomatic stenosis: The efficacy of surgery in important pre-defined subgroups. Carotid Endarterectomy Trialists' Collaboration. Cerebrovasc Dis 10(Suppl 2):108, 2000.

50. Weiller C, Ringelstein B, Reiche W, et al: The large striatocapsular infarct: A clinical and pathophysiological entity. Arch Neurol 47:1085–1091, 1990.

51. Boiten J, Lodder J: Large striatocapsular infarcts: Clinical presentation and pathogenesis in comparison with lacunar and cortical infarcts. Acta Neurol Scand 86:298–303, 1992.

52. Weiller C, Willmes K, Reiche W, et al: The case of aphasia or neglect after striatocapsular infarction. Brain 116:1509–1525, 1993.

53. Beevor CE: On the distribution of the different arteries supplying the human brain. Philos Trans R Soc London (Biol), 200:1–55, 1909.

54. Herman LH, Fernando OU, Gurdjian ES: The anterior choroidal artery: An anatomical study of its area of distribution. Anat Rec 154:95–102, 1966.

55. Rhoton AL Jr, Fujii K, Fradd B: Microsurgical anatomy of the anterior choroidal artery. Surg Neurol 12:171–187, 1979.

56. Saeki N, Rhoton AL Jr: Microsurgical anatomy of the upper basilar artery and the posterior circle of Willis. J Neurosurg 46:563–578, 1977.

57. Hussein S, Renella RR, Dietz H: Microsurgical anatomy of the anterior choroidal artery. Acta Neurochir 92:19–28, 1988.

58. Pullicino PM: The course and territories of cerebral small arteries. Adv Neurol 62:11–41, 1993.

59. Fujii K, Lenkey C, Rhoton AL: Microsurgical anatomy of the choroidal arteries: Lateral and third ventricles. J Neurosurg 52:165–188, 1980.

60. Ludemann W, Schneekloth C, Samii M, Hussein S: Arterial supply of the temporo-medial region of the brain: Significance for preoperative vascular occlusion testing. Surg Radiol Anat 23:39–43, 2001.

61. Pullicino PM: Diagnosis of perforating artery territories in axial, coronal and sagittal planes. Adv Neurol 62:41–72, 1993.

62. Graff-Radford N, Damasio H, Yamada T, et al: Nonhemorrhagic thalamic infarction. Brain 108:485–516, 1985.

63. Percheron G: Les artères du thalamus humain: Les artères choroidiennes. Rev Neurol 133:547–558, 1977.

64. Pullicino PM: Infarcts in the anterior artery territory [letter to the editor]. Brain 118:1353–1355, 1995.

65. Damasio H: A computed tomographic guide to the identification of cerebral vascular territories. Arch Neurol 40:138–142, 1983.

66. Ghika JA, Bogousslavsky J, Regli F: Deep perforators from the carotid system: Template of the vascular territories. Arch Neurol 47:1097–1100, 1990.

67. Bamford JM, Warlow CP: Evolution and testing of the lacunar hypothesis. Stroke 19:1074–1082, 1988.

68. van den Bergh R: Centrifugal elements in the vascular pattern of the deep intracerebral blood supply. Angiology 20:88–94, 1969.

69. De Reuck J, Van der Eecken HM: The arterial angioarchitecture in lacunar state. Acta Neurol Belg 76:142–149, 1976.

Clinical Manifestations

70. Bogousslavsky J, Regli F: Centrum ovale infarcts: Subcortical infarction in the superficial territory of the middle cerebral artery. Neurology 42:1992–1998, 1992.

71. De Reuck J: The human periventricular arterial blood supply and the anatomy of cerebral infarctions. Eur Neurol 5:321–334, 1971.

72. Hupperts RMM, Lodder J, Heuts-van Raak EPM, Kessels F: Infarcts in the anterior choroidal artery territory [letter to the editor]. Brain 118:1355–1356, 1995.

73. Leys D, Lejeune JP, Bourgeois P, et al: Syndrome pseudo-bulbaire aigue. Rev Neurol 141:814–818, 1985.

74. Bladin CF, Chambers BR: Clinical features, pathogenesis, and computed tomographic characteristics of internal watershed infarction. Stroke 24:1925–1932, 1993.

75. Marinkovic S, Hirohiko G, Brigante L, et al: The surgical anatomy of the perforating branches of the anterior choroidal artery. Surg Neurol 52:30–36, 1999.

76. Wiesmann M, Yousry I, Seelos KC, Yousry TA: Identification and anatomic description of the anterior choroidal artery by use of 3D-TOF source and 3D-CISS MR imaging. AJNR Am J Neuroradiol 22:305–310, 2001.

77. Rousseaux M, Froger J, Kozlowski O, Steinling M: Cerebral blood flow disturbances after anterior choroidal artery infarcts: Anatomical and functional correlates. Rev Neurol 157:187–197, 2001.

Clinical Manifestations

Chapter Ten

Vertebrobasilar Disease

J. P. Mohr and Louis R. Caplan

Clinicians of the 19th century described in detail the clinical and pathologic findings in patients with softening or hemorrhage limited to portions of the brainstem. Interest lay primarily in defining the anatomy and function of the various brainstem nuclei and tracts. The nature and location of the responsible vascular lesion and the mechanism of the parenchymatous damage were given little attention, because they were at that time of no practical concern.

In the late 19th century and the early years of the 20th century, attention turned to the pathology and anatomy of the intracranial vessels. Interest in the anatomy of the intracranial vessels started with the landmark descriptions by Henri Duret[1,2] in 1873 and 1874. Isolated cases of basilar artery (BA) occlusion, usually attributed to syphilitic endarteritis, had been described in the later 19th century,[3,4] but in 1911, Marburg[5] first reviewed the topic of brainstem infarction and described clinical examples of basilar territory syndromes. In 1932, Pines and Gilinsky[6] published a detailed report that included serial sections of the brainstem in a patient with thrombosis of the rostral BA. Meanwhile, Stopford[7,8] in England and Foix and colleagues[9–11] in France had defined the anatomy of branches of BA and described syndromes caused by paramedian and lateral ischemia. By 1934, Lhermitte and Trelles,[12] in their review of BA arteriosclerosis and its clinicoanatomic consequences, showed that pathologists at that time knew that arteriosclerosis (as well as syphilis) affected the intracranial arteries and led to softening and that the BA and its branches were especially vulnerable to atheroma formation.

In 1946, Kubik and Adams[13] published a meticulous analysis of 18 cases, studied both clinically and at postmortem, of patients with occlusion of the BA. These researchers emphasized the severity of the disorder and expressed the belief that it was diagnosable during life. In their series, the onset was usually abrupt, and death invariably ensued from extensive brainstem infarction. The possibility that patients occasionally survived was also entertained, and clinical details of four living patients in whom BA occlusion was suspected were offered. This landmark report brought the subject of BA occlusion to the full attention of the neurologic community. With the advent of arteriography, and careful pathologic studies of the entire vascular tree, the 1950s saw an awakening of interest in the extracranial vessels. Fisher[14] showed that severe atherosclerotic occlusive vascular disease in the internal carotid artery in the neck was a common cause of hemispheral

softening. Hutchinson and Yates[15] carefully dissected the cervical vertebral arteries and demonstrated that severe occlusive disease also occurs frequently in these vessels. Meyer and colleagues[16] used arteriography to corroborate the frequency of occlusive disease in the basilar and nuchal vertebral arteries during life. In his seminal article on carotid artery disease, Fisher[14] emphasized that warning spells (transient ischemic attacks [TIAs]) frequently occurred before cerebral hemisphere infarctions. Other writers called these attacks "carotid insufficiency."

As the clinical findings associated with posterior circulation infarction became more widely recognized, Williams and Wilson,[17,18] Denny-Brown,[19] Fang and Palmer,[20] Millikan and Siekert,[21] and others called attention to transient episodes of dysfunction within the posterior circulation territory.[22] The term *vertebrobasilar insufficiency* was born, and interest in the 1960s shifted away from the pathology and clinical symptoms to an attempt to understand the pathophysiology of these vascular lesions. Microembolization, intermittent obstruction of the vertebral arteries by bony osteophytes, and clotting and viscosity factors within the blood were identified as important factors. Intense physiologic studies by Denny-Brown[23] added emphasis to the nature and capability of the collateral circulation with its dependence on systemic factors such as blood pressure, blood volume, cardiac output, body position and activity, and pharmacologic agents.

During the 1970s and 1980s, emphasis shifted from diagnosis to treatment. As a result of a number of uncontrolled observations, enthusiasm for the use of warfarin anticoagulation grew in the 1960s.[24,25] In a review in 1969, Browne and Poskanzer[26] stated, "If anticoagulation has value, it may be more useful in the patient with vertebrobasilar disease, with its high morbidity, than in other forms of cerebral vascular thrombosis." Aspirin and other agents that affect platelet agglutination, such as dipyridamole, sulfinpyrazone, and ticlopidine, have also been used in an attempt to modify coagulation factors in patients with posterior circulation disease. Surgically created shunts from the occipital artery to long circumferential cerebellar artery branches of the vertebral and basilar arteries and to the posterior cerebellar artery have been devised to improve circulation to the brainstem and posterior hemispheral regions.[27–29] Vertebral[30] and carotid endarterectomy[31] and bypass and transluminal dilatation of the BA[32] involve more direct surgical correction of occlusive disease in the posterior circulation.

Advances in interventional neuroradiology now make it possible to introduce catheters and therapeutic agents into the vertebral artery (VA) and the larger intracranial arteries within the posterior circulation. Intravenous and intra-arterial thrombolytic agents, such as streptokinase, urokinase, and recombinant tissue plasminogen activator, have been infused to lyse thrombi in patients with VA and BA occlusions.[33–36] During the 1980s, there were also dramatic improvements in diagnostic technology. Brain imaging became possible in the 1970s after the introduction of computed tomography (CT). This imaging modality proved useful for posterior circulation hemorrhages but was less helpful in occlusive disease, because the brainstem was difficult to image. Magnetic resonance imaging (MRI), introduced in the 1980s, permitted far superior imaging of brainstem and cerebellar infarcts.[37–39] Axial, sagittal, and coronal sections allow localization of brainstem lesions in rostrocaudal, tegmentobasal, and medial-lateral directions. Flow voids on MRI give information about aneurysms and occlusions in the plane of the section.

Technology for the study of the posterior circulation arteries has also improved greatly. Duplex scanning, color-coded Doppler ultrasonography, and continuous-wave Doppler ultrasonography allow detection of lesions in the extracranial vertebral arteries,[40–46] and transcranial Doppler (TCD) ultrasonography has improved detection of intracranial lesions.[46–49] Magnetic resonance angiography (MRA) offers promise for allowing safe imaging of the vertebrobasilar vessels without risk to patients.[50–52] Transesophageal echocardiography, cardiac imaging, and sophisticated rhythm monitoring now also allow detection of cardiac sources of embolism to the posterior circulation.[53] Angiography using standard arterial catheterization and dye opacification has also become safer because of improvements in catheters, dyes, and filming as well as greater experience of the personnel performing the procedure.

Clearly, physicians practicing in the 1990s have much greater capabilities for defining the brain and vascular lesions in patients with vertebrobasilar arterial occlusive disease than were possible a decade ago. The physicians in the 19th and early 20th centuries had virtually no therapy that could influence the course of serious cerebrovascular disease. Now in the 21st century, clinicians have a variety of potent treatments and an increasing awareness of the range of syndromes and levels of severity associated with vertebrobasilar disease.[54] Despite such advances, basic questions remain, such as how disease within vessels produces TIAs[55] or stroke and why, in some patients with severe occlusive disease, many regions escape damage. Individual case reports continue to remind us that even the most experienced clinicians can be misled by diagnoses other than vascular disease, which can mimic brainstem symptoms.[56] Whatever else is being learned, it is increasingly clear that posterior circulation disease is not a homogeneous entity.[54]

ANATOMY

Embryology

The vertebrobasilar arterial system has several unique features. For a period in the embryologic life of the fetus,

most of the blood to the hindbrain structures comes from the carotid circulation. Because of its paired systems and the many changes that it undergoes during fetal development, the vertebrobasilar system has a high incidence of variations, anomalies, and persistent fetal vessels. It is one of the only regions in the body where two large arteries merge into a single larger trunk. The posterior circulation also supplies the anterior spinal artery, which usually forms from smaller arterial branches of each vertebral artery. In addition, because the vertebral arteries course through and around many bony structures and ligaments and are fixed in a part of their course, they are especially vulnerable to traumatic injury.

Vascular Anatomy

Vertebral Artery

The vertebral artery is divided into segments (Fig. 10–1).[57–59] In the first segment, the artery courses directly cephalad from its origin as the first branch of the subclavian artery (SA) to enter the costotransverse foramen of C6 or C5. The second segment is entirely within the transverse foramina from C6 to C2. The third segment is highly tortuous: The VA emerges from the transverse foramen of C2 and courses posteriorly and laterally toward the costotransverse foramen of the atlas. It circles the posterior arch of C1 and passes between the atlas and occiput within the suboccipital triangle. During its course, the third segment of the VA is covered by muscles and nerves and is pressed against bone while being covered by the atlanto-occipital membrane. The fourth segment of the VA is its intracranial portion after the vessel pierces the dura mater to enter

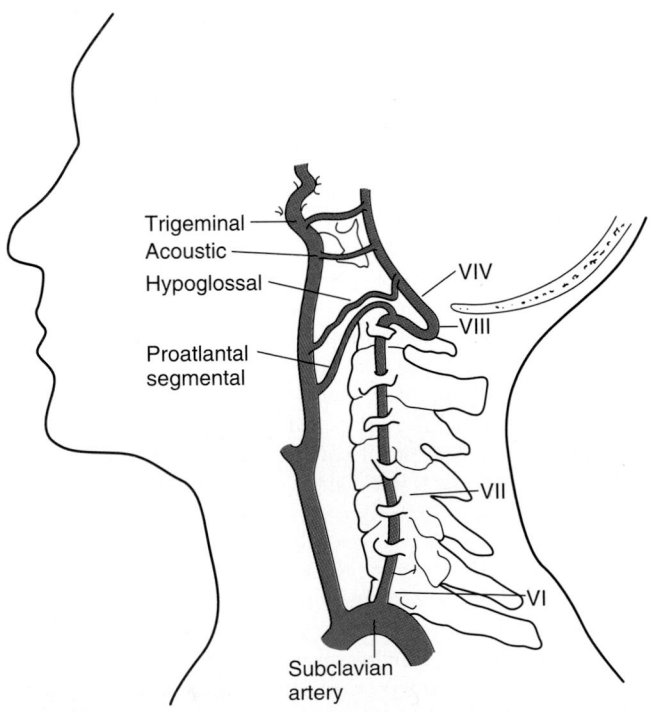

FIGURE 10–1 *Vertebral artery segments and persisting primitive anastomotic connections within the carotid arterial tree (VI to VIV denote vertebral artery segments 1 to 4).*

the foramen magnum. As the VA pierces the dura, its adventitial and medial coats are less thick, and there is a gross reduction in elastic lamina.[60]

Usually at the level of the pontomedullary junction, the two VAs merge to form the BA. The junction is sometimes higher, in which case the VA supplies the middle and lower pons; occasionally the BA has a low origin. The BA becomes somewhat smaller as it travels distally, and frequently it curves slightly in the direction away from the larger VA. It divides near the pontomesencephalic junction to form the two posterior cerebral arteries (PCAs).

Variations are relatively common. In approximately 8% of humans, the left VA originates directly from the aortic arch and not from the SA (in which case the left VA would not fill from a left brachial injection). Rarely, the right VA arises as a separate branch from the innominate artery and not from the SA. The VAs are commonly asymmetric (in 45% of people the left VA is larger, in 21% the right VA is larger, and in 24% the arteries are of equal size).

Cerebellar Arteries

The *posterior inferior cerebellar artery* (PICA), usually the largest branch of the VA, arises from its intradural segment approximately 1.5 cm from the origin of the BA. The PICA usually arises from the VA an average of 8.6 mm above the foramen magnum but sometimes originates from the VA as low as 24 mm below the foramen magnum.[11,61] Occasionally, the PICA arises extracranially and courses cephalad within the spinal canal[62] or originates from the ascending pharyngeal artery.[63]

The VA may terminate in the PICA, in which case the distal segment (which usually communicates with the BA) is hypoplastic or nonexistent, and the VA is smaller than the contralateral VA.[64] The medial branch of the PICA may also arise directly from the VA, with the lateral branch arising from the BA or, more commonly, from the anterior inferior cerebellar artery (AICA).[2] One PICA is entirely lacking in 15% of individuals and is hypoplastic in 5%.[65] The posterior spinal arteries may arise from the PICA rather than from their usual VA origin.[66] The PICA and AICA are often reciprocally related in size; for example, a large PICA may supply most of the inferior surface of the cerebellum, and the AICA on the same side is quite small with little cerebellar supply. When the AICA on one side is large, the ipsilateral PICA is frequently small. The lateral medulla is rarely fed primarily from the PICA; in most cases, the major blood supply is from direct lateral medullary branches of the VA.[67–69] The only part of the medulla that the PICA constantly supplies is the dorsal tegmental area, and this it supplies together with the posterior spinal arteries.[2,11,67] This region is supplied by rami from the medial PICA.[70]

Anterior Inferior Cerebellar Artery

The AICA arises from the caudal third of the BA in 75% of people, sometimes from the middle third, and occasionally from its inferior limit; the AICA is lacking in only 4% of individuals.[8,71] However, it can arise from the VA or the BA by a common trunk together with the PICA. Rarely, several small vessels arising directly from the BA or from the internal auditory artery replace the AICA. Because of its small size, the AICA supplies a small area of the anterior and medial cerebellum (i.e., the middle cerebellar peduncle and the flocculus).[71] Proximal branches of the AICA usually supply the lateral portion of the pons, including the facial, trigeminal, vestibular, and cochlear nuclei, the root of the seventh and eighth cranial nerves, and the spinothalamic tract (Fig. 10–2).[67,72]

Superior Cerebellar Artery

The superior cerebellar artery (SCA) arises from the rostral BA just before its bifurcation into the posterior cerebral arteries. Each SCA has a short trunk that divides into two main branches, a medial (mSCA) branch and a lateral (lSCA) branch. These two branches sometimes arise separately from the BA, follow the pontomesencephalic sulcus, and pass around the superior cerebellar peduncle to ramify onto the rostral cerebellum (Fig. 10–3). The SCA courses along the anterosuperior margin of the cerebellum. The mSCA starts with a course parallel to that of the lSCA but soon turns medially to reach the lateral surface of the mesencephalon and the inferior colliculus; from there, the mSCA makes a rostral loop along the superior margin of the colliculus and then courses over the superior vermis (see Fig. 10–3). The SCA supplies the rostral half of the cerebellar hemispheres as well as the dentate nucleus.[73] Along its course, branches of the SCA supply the laterotegmental portion of the rostral pons (see Fig. 10–2).

Cerebellum and its Arterial Supply

The cerebellum is supplied by the long circumferential vessels (see Fig. 10–3)[11]; the PICA encircles the medulla and supplies the suboccipital surface in the caudal part of the cerebellum, whereas the AICA encircles the lower pons and relates to a usually small ventral surface in the anteromedial part of the cerebellum, while the SCA supplies the tentorial surface (the rostral part of the cerebellum) after encircling the upper pons. When a large AICA is present on one side, the ipsilateral PICA is often hypoplastic, and the AICA territory encompasses the whole anterior inferior aspect of the cerebellum.

The PICA has a sinuous course with several loops (see Fig. 10–3). It travels dorsally, lateral to the medulla, below the roots of the ninth and tenth cranial nerves. From there, it courses inferiorly, makes the first (caudal) loop at a variable level, and goes up onto the posterior surface of the medulla in the sulcus separating the medulla and the tonsil. At the top of the tonsil, the PICA makes a second (cranial) loop around the tonsil and then goes downward to the inferior part of the vermis. Sometimes the second loop occurs at the midpoint of the tonsil. Thus, the PICA has lateral medullary, dorsal medullary (ventral tonsillar), superior tonsillar, and dorsal tonsillar segments.

The PICA divides into two main branches, the medial (mPICA) and the lateral (lPICA).[74] The mPICA climbs along the inferior and dorsal surface of the vermis and the internal part of the hemispheres, making a third loop. The lPICA most often arises from the upper part of the dorsal medullary segment of the parent trunk, between the first and second loops, and then gives rise to several terminal branches to the caudal hemisphere.[75] Sometimes it arises from the first loop. The caudal loop is usually found at the level of the foramen magnum. It can be found below this level, but rami from the lPICA that supply the tonsil are

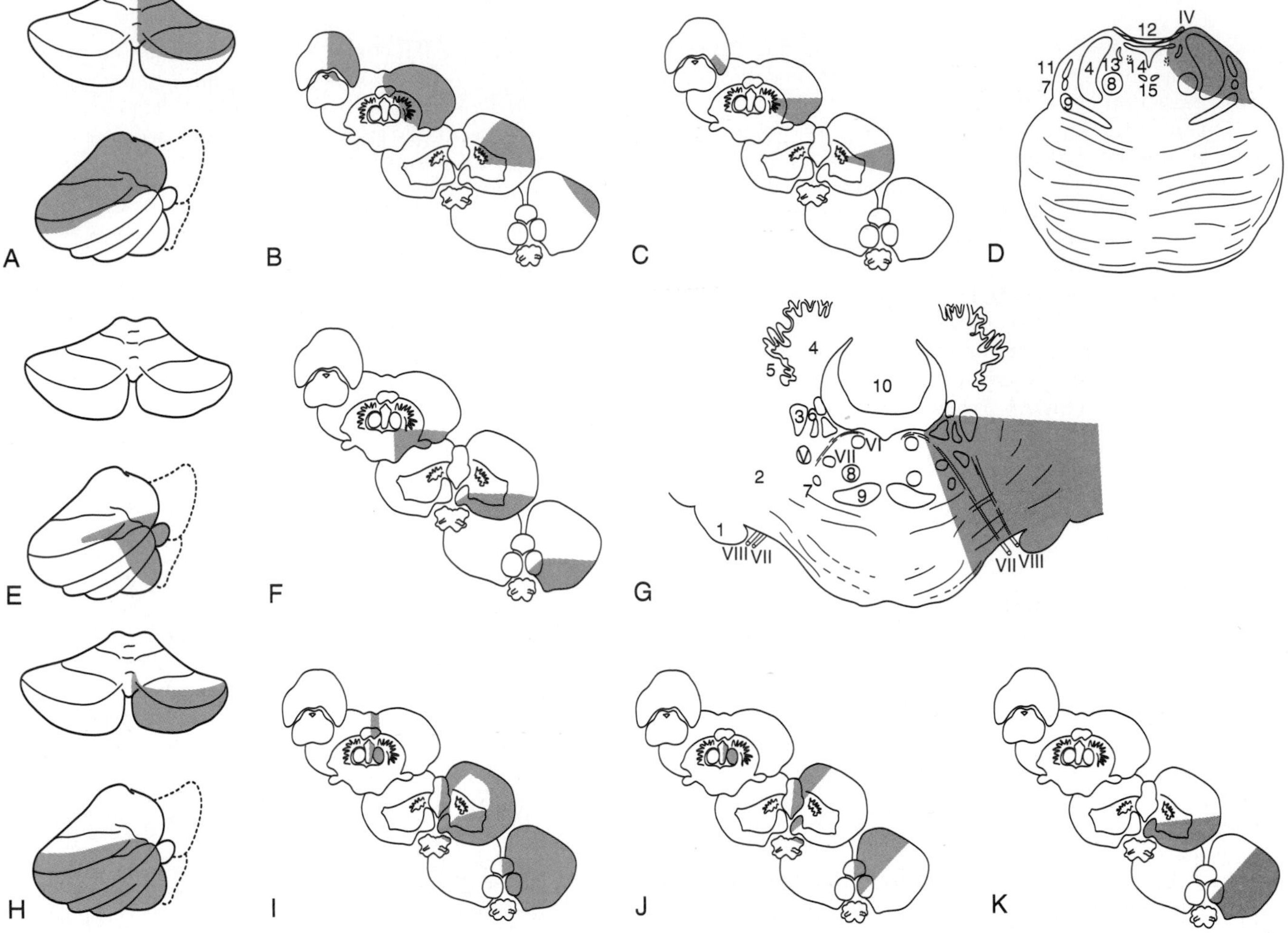

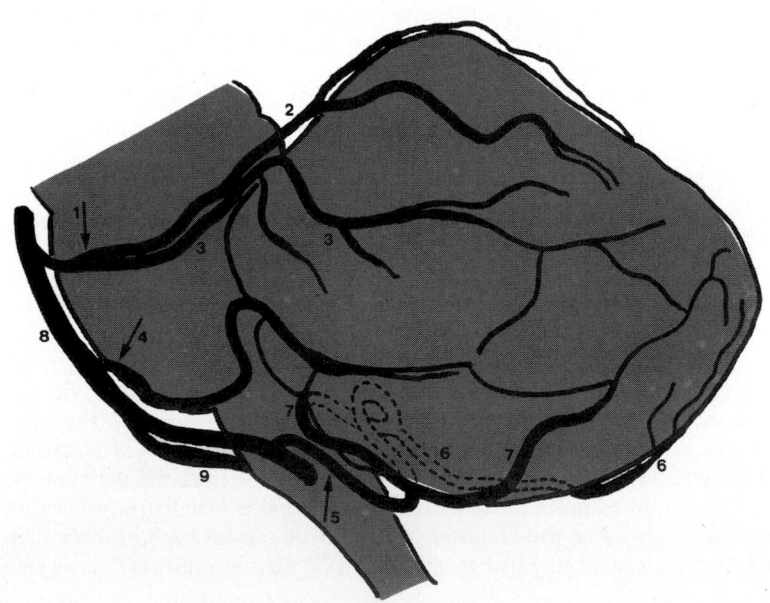

FIGURE 10–2 *Anatomic drawings of the territory of cerebellar arteries and their branches at autopsy. A, Superior cerebellar artery (SCA) territory (superior, dorsal view; inferior, lateral view). B, SCA territory (sections from the rostral to the caudal cerebellum). C, Lateral SCA territory. D, Brainstem territory of SCA. E, Anterior inferior cerebellar artery (AICA) territory (dorsal and lateral views). F, AICA territory. G, Brainstem territory of AICA. H, Posterior inferior cerebellar artery territory (dorsal and lateral views). I, PICA territory. J, Medial PICA territory. K, Lateral PICA territory. 1, Flocculus; 2, middle cerebellar peduncle; 3, inferior cerebellar peduncle; 4, superior cerebellar peduncle; 5, dentate nucleus; 6, vestibular nuclei; 7, spinothalamic tract; 8, central tegmental tract; 9, medial lemniscus; 10, nodulus; 11, lateral lemniscus; 12, decussation of trochlear nerve; 13, mesencephalic trigeminal tract; 14, locus ceruleus; 15, medial longitudinal fasciculus. (Data from references 72, 76, and 440.)*

FIGURE 10–3 *Lateral view of cerebellar arteries. 1, Superior cerebellar artery (SCA); 2, medial branch of the SCA; 3, lateral branch of the SCA; 4, anterior inferior cerebellar artery; 5, posterior inferior cerebellar artery (PICA); 6, medial branch of the PICA; 7, lateral branch of the PICA; 8, basilar artery; 9, vertebral artery.*

always above the foramen magnum except for instances of tonsillar herniation.[74] Rami from the cranial loop supply the choroid plexus of the fourth ventricle.

Two main areas of supply can be distinguished within the PICA territory.[76] The dorsomedial area is supplied by the mPICA, whose territory includes the dorsolateral portion of the medulla. The anterolateral area is supplied by the lPICA, which never supplies the medulla (see Fig. 10–2).

These three major arteries (the PICA, AICA, and SCA) and their branches are connected by numerous free anastomoses, which limit infarct size in patients who have cerebellar, vertebral, or basilar artery occlusions. Drawings of the territory of each cerebellar artery and their branches conform to the CT and MRI horizontal axial sections (Fig. 10–4).

Basilar Artery and Its Main Branches

The major branches of the BA are generally uniform, the most common variation being that the internal auditory artery, usually an AICA branch, may arise directly from the BA. The SCAs occasionally are duplicated or arise from the PCA. Even more uniform are the smaller penetrating branches of the vertebral and basilar arteries.[67,68,77–79] The three groups of arterial penetrators are (Fig. 10–5): (1) median arteries, which usually take a slightly caudal course and then penetrate the brainstem and supply the paramedian basal and tegmental regions, (2) short lateral circumferential arteries, which give rise to branches that penetrate the brainstem and supply the intermediate tegmental and basal regions, and (3) long lateral circumferential arteries, which course around the brainstem and supply the lateral basal and tegmental regions. Stephens and Stilwell,[58] using elegant injection techniques, have shown that many lateral circumferential vessels arise from the vertebral and basilar arteries directly as well as from the long cerebellar vessels. In the medulla and midbrain, there are also posterior branches, which arise from the long lateral circumferential cerebellar vessels (the SCA, PICA, and AICA), course in a horizontal and dorsoventral direction, and supply the lateral tegmentum (see Fig. 10–5). Penetrating vessels are usually less than 100 μm in diameter, their size being roughly proportional to their length.[80] The medial penetrating vessels arise from the anterior spinal, vertebral, and basilar arteries as well as from the AICA and PCA; lateral penetrators frequently enter the brainstem along the laterally emerging nerve roots and arise from the vertebral, PICA, AICA, basilar, SCA, and posterior choroidal arteries. The medial tegmental region has a prominent rich collateral supply, making it more resistant to ischemia than the base or lateral tegmentum.

The distal basilar segments are also the source of occasional variations. During early fetal life, the internal carotid artery (ICA) supplies the posterior hemispheres and brainstem via posterior communicating arteries. In one third of humans, this primitive vascular pattern persists, and the connecting segment from the BA to the PCA (variously called the basilar communicating artery or mesencephalic artery or P1 segment of the PCA) remains vestigial.[79–81] In these patients, the PCA may fill from carotid injection, and not after VA opacification. In 2% of humans, this primitive

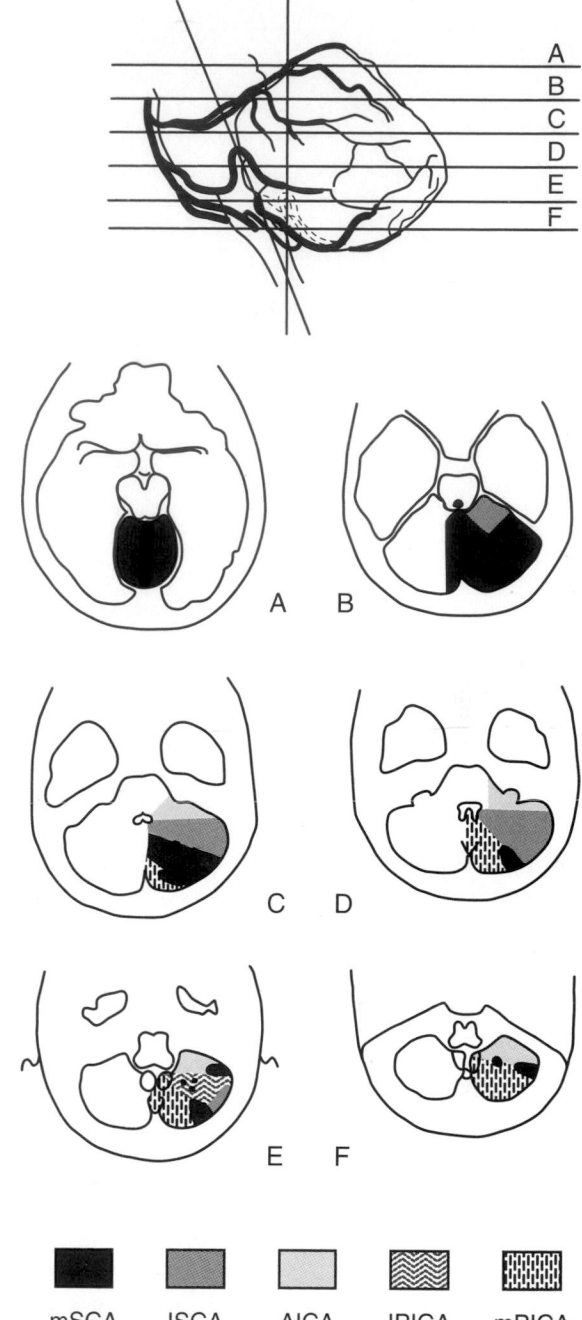

mSCA   lSCA   AICA   lPICA   mPICA

FIGURE 10–4 *Anatomic drawings (A to F) of the territory of branches of the cerebellar arteries as they appear on CT and MRI. (Data from Amarenco P, Kase CS, Rosengart A, et al: Very small [border zone] cerebellar infarcts: Distribution, mechanisms, causes and clinical features. Brain 116:161, 1993.)*

circulatory pattern is bilateral; even more rarely, the BA may be hypoplastic in its distal segment and end in the SCAs.[81] Penetrating branches from the distal basilar communicating artery, SCA, and proximal PCA pass through the posterior perforating substance and supply the paramedian midbrain and diencephalon.

The paramedian mesencephalic arteries arise from the proximal portion of the basilar communicating artery to

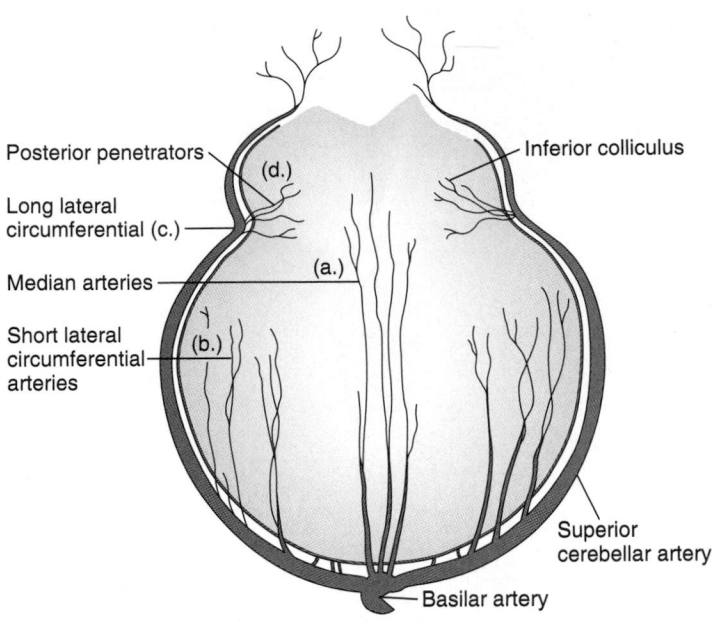

FIGURE 10–5 *Rostral pons with the usual arterial distribution. A, Median penetrating arteries. B, Short lateral circumferential arteries. C, Long lateral circumferential artery. D, Posterior penetrating arteries.*

supply the cerebral peduncle and red nucleus.[6,7,11,74,82] The lateral midbrain is supplied by peduncular perforating branches arising from the proximal portion of the PCA and from its earliest main branches, the posterior choroidal arteries.[67,82] There are usually two separate paramedian thalamoperforating arteries,[59,83–87] (1) the polar artery (also called tuberothalamic artery) and the preliminary pedicles[11,84,88] and (2) the thalamic-subthalamic arteries (also called the paramedian thalamic,[89] deep interpeduncular profunda,[84] and the thalamoperforating pedicle[11,88]). The polar artery arises from the posterior communicating artery and supplies the anterolateral thalamus, including the mamillothalamic tract, the paraventricular region, and a part of the reticular nucleus.[84,90,91] Occasionally, the right and left thalamoperforating arteries arise from a common single trunk that originates from the P1 segment of the PCA on one side (Percheron's artery).[89] The lateral portions of the thalamus are supplied by a series of thalamogeniculate arteries, often called the thalamogeniculate pedicle, and not a large vessel as was formerly believed (Fig. 10–6).[1,11,58,91] The thalamogeniculate pedicle arises from the ambient segment of the PCAs and penetrates the thalamus between the geniculate bodies.[92] These arteries supply the posterolateral and posteromedial ventral somatosensory nuclei, part of the ventralis lateralis, part of the centromedian nucleus, and the rostrolateral portion of the pulvinar. The posterior choroidal arteries arise from the PCAs more laterally and supply portions of the medial nuclei, the habenular nucleus, and the rostromedial pulvinar.

Anastomotic Links

Occasionally, primitive connections from the ICA to the posterior circulation vessels persist into adult life.[12,58,59] The most common persisting channel is the trigeminal artery, which remains in 0.1% to 0.2% of adults.[93] The trigeminal artery arises from the ICA, as it enters the cavernous sinus proximal to the carotid siphon, and penetrates the sella turcica or the dura near the clivus to join the BA between the AICA and SCA branches. The VAs and proximal BA are commonly small or hypoplastic, as is true in many patients with other persistent anastomoses. Persistence of the hypoglossal artery is the next most common variant.[93–95] This vessel originates from the ICA in the neck, usually between C1 and C3, and courses posteriorly to enter the hypoglossal canal, from which it joins the BA.[95] A persistent otic artery is a rarer anomaly; this vessel leaves the ICA within the petrous bone and enters the posterior fossa with the seventh and eighth cranial nerves at the internal acoustic meatus, later to join the mid-BA. The rarest fetal communicating channels are the persistent proatlantal intersegmental arteries, which originate from the nuchal internal or external carotid artery at C2 and C3 and join the horizontal (third) segment of the VA suboccipitally.[96] Isolated reports have documented communications between the common or proximal ICA and the lower VAs.[97]

PATHOLOGY

Atherosclerosis

Atherosclerosis is by far the most common vascular condition responsible for posterior circulation ischemia. Fatty streaks, fibrous plaques, calcified lesions, and complicated lesions (fibrous plaques on which hemorrhage, ulceration, or thrombosis has developed) have all been frequently identified within the larger vessels of the vertebrobasilar system and do not differ qualitatively from atherosclerosis of other vessels.[98–104]

Ulceration in plaques is less common in the posterior circulation.[104,105] However, when ulceration occurs, it usually involves the SA at the origin of the VA or in the most proximal portion of the VA in the neck.[104,106] As in the anterior circulation, thrombosis may occur in the absence of severe preexisting atherosclerosis of the vessel wall.[107]

Ulcerated atherosclerotic plaques in the aortic arch have been found in association with posterior circulation ischemia at necropsy.[108–110] However, the most common

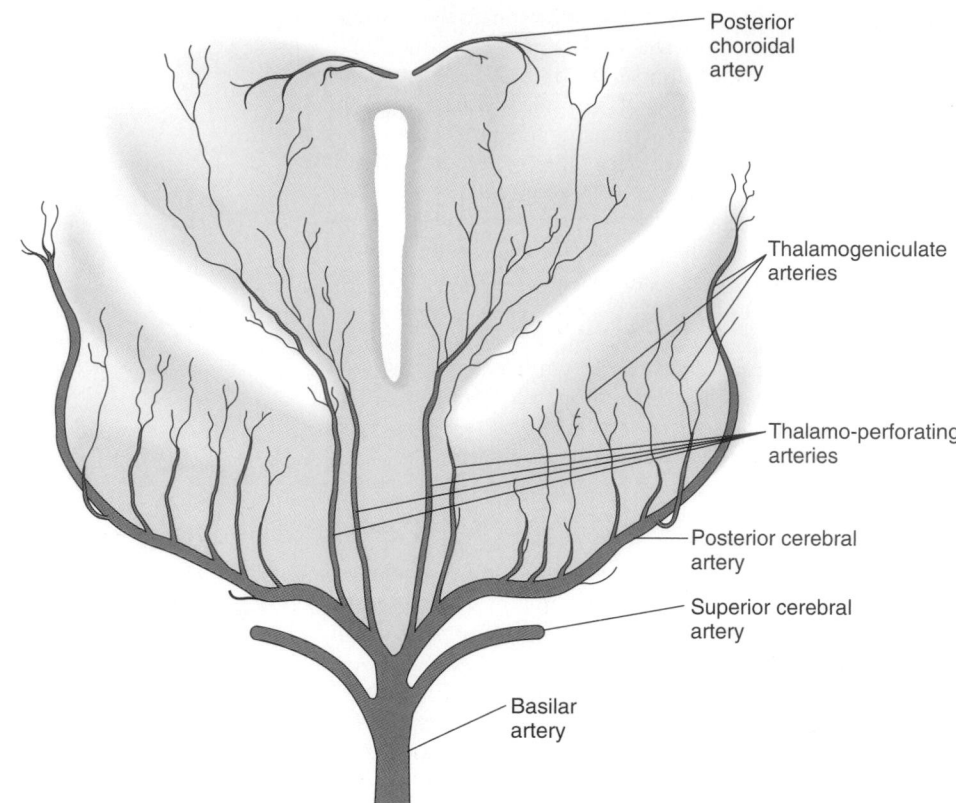

Posterior
choroidal
artery

Thalamogeniculate
arteries

Thalamo-perforating
arteries

Posterior cerebral
artery

Superior cerebral
artery

Basilar
artery

FIGURE 10–6 *Diagram of the thalamic arteries.*

site of atherosclerotic stenosis is at the origin of the VAs.[15,77,104,111–113] Plaque forms and may assume a ringlike extension from the SA to encircle the VA orifice.[111] The left and right VAs are approximately equally affected by atherosclerosis, but there is some indication that when the two vessels are unequal in diameter, the smaller vessel is more frequently occluded.[104,114] The intracranial VA, after it pierces the dura, is another common site of occlusive disease.[77,111,112] Aside from these sites, fibrous plaques and fatty streaks are distributed along the VA without any single site of predilection.[15,77,111,112] Often in the second segment of the VA, during its course through the transverse foramina, a ladder-like arrangement of fibrous plaques, seemingly related to the anatomy of the adjacent cervical spine structures, is found.[112]

When thrombosis occurs within the extracranial vertebral artery (ECVA), the clot usually develops at a site of atherosclerotic stenosis and seldom forms a long anterograde or retrograde extension.[77,115] By contrast, a thrombus within the extracranial ICA often extends the length of the vessel up to the first branch, the ophthalmic artery. The limited length of the VA thrombus may be related to this vessel's more extensive branching and the possibility that extensive collateral channels keep blood circulating above and below the clot.[116] Thrombus formed within the intracranial VA (ICVA), however, frequently extends into the proximal BA.[77]

Within the BA, fatty sudanophilic plaques are more prevalent on the ventral surface, and stenosis or occlusion is common in the proximal 2 cm of the vessel.[34,77,101,117] Atherosclerotic stenosis of the distal portion of the BA may be

common in persons of African origin.[118] *Thrombi* within the BA also tend to have limited propagation,[88] frequently extending only to the orifice of the next long circumferential cerebellar artery (the AICA or SCA). At the distal end of the BA, the proximal PCAs are also sites of atherosclerotic lesions, such lesions being less common here than in the middle cerebral artery (MCA).[77,112] *Embolic material* is most often found within the distal basilar tributaries, especially the PCA branches; less often, an embolus lodges in the more proximal vertebral or basilar arteries, especially at sites of luminal encroachment by preexisting atherosclerotic lesions.[13,53,77]

Angiographic studies[16,119–121] have corroborated that the origins of the VA, the intradural VA,[122] the BA,[16] and the SA proximal to the VA origin are the most common sites of occlusive disease. Atherosclerotic stenosis of the extracranial ICA occurs approximately twice as often as stenosis of the ECVA,[104,105,111,112] but often, both vessels are severely compromised.[123] The location and severity of occlusive disease in these two vessels are extremely variable; Castaigne and associates[77] reported that 60% of their patients with occlusions in the vertebrobasilar system had no serious occlusive disease within the anterior circulation. Atherothrombosis in the aortic arch causing artery-to-artery embolism in the posterior circulation has probably been neglected until now because of the lack of clinical diagnostic tools.[124]

The frequency of atherosclerotic lesions in the subclavian and proximal VAs is different in men and women and in persons of different racial backgrounds.[118,125,126] People with atheromatous lesions of the VAs, however, have the same epidemiologic and demographic features as those with carotid artery bifurcation lesion in the neck.[15,127] There is a strong association between lesions in the vertebral and carotid arteries and coronary and peripheral vascular occlusive disease, smoking, hypertension, and hypercholesterolemia.[127] Men are more often affected than women.[127] White persons have a relatively higher incidence of severe extracranial occlusive disease, whereas black persons and persons of Japanese and Chinese ancestry have a preponderance of intracranial occlusive disease, especially of medium-sized branches (the PICA, AICA, SCA, and PCA).[118,125,126,128,129] Black, Japanese, and Chinese persons and women with predominantly intracranial branch disease have a high incidence of hypertension but a relatively low frequency of coronary and peripheral vascular occlusive disease and hypercholesterolemia. Occlusive lesions of the intracranial vertebral and basilar arteries have less clear sex and racial preponderance.[126]

Atherosclerosis may also affect the branches of the vertebral and basilar arteries.[130] Whereas AICA occlusions are atherothrombotic in most cases,[72,109,131] situated in the basilar wall as situ occlusions, PICA occlusions are equally divided between in situ atherothrombosis and cardioembolism; SCA occlusions are most commonly cardioembolic.[109,132,133] Most infarctions in the vascular territories of these vessels are due to narrowing or occlusion of the parent vessel that blocks or diminishes blood flow into the major tributaries.[109,134] The smaller penetrating branches (approximately 0.5 mm in diameter) are vulnerable to occlusive disease. Fisher and Caplan[135] found four such small basilar branch occlusions in a serial section (Fig. 10–7). Two branches were blocked as they traversed the intramural portion of the parent BA, one by a foamy macrophage plaque causing blockage of the orifice of the branch. In the other two vessels, a junctional plaque extended from the parent BA into the proximal branch and occluded the branch lumen. Microatheromas as the cause of infarction in regions of the pons and diencephalon supplied by paramedian penetrating branches are found three or four times more commonly in patients with diabetes than in nondiabetics.[136] The morphology of the presumed branch disease in these patients has not been studied but could represent similar microatheromata.[130] Figure 10–7 depicts mechanisms of branch occlusion.

Lipohyalinosis

The pathology of smaller penetrating arteries (<200 µm) within the brainstem parenchyma is qualitatively quite different from atherosclerosis of larger vessels.[100,137–140] a distinctive process that Fisher[139,140] labeled *lipohyalinosis*, can lead to disorganization and disruption of the lumen of the vessel. The hyaline material readily stains for fat, accumulates subintimally, and may weaken the wall, allowing aneurysmal dilations. Red blood cells may become extravasated through the disintegrating wall.

Lipohyalinosis leads to functional occlusion of the vessel by a subintimal process that obliterates the lumen and leads to ischemia distal to the lesion. Because the ischemic lesions are generally small and somewhat round, the term *lacune* (hole) has been applied. In addition, the same vascular process can lead to a break in the vessel wall and

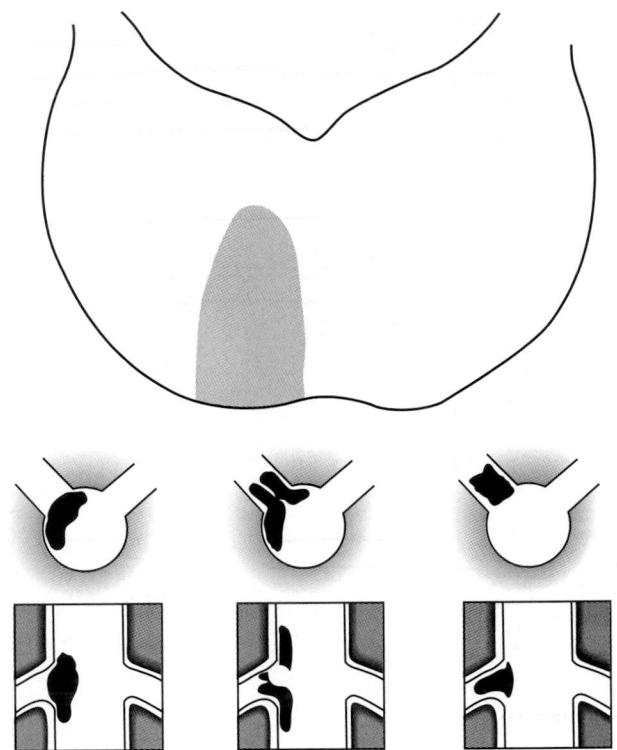

FIGURE 10–7 *Diagrammatic representation of types of branch occlusion.* Left to right, *Luminal plaque blocking the orifice of a branch, junctional plaque spreading into a branch, and a clot in the proximal part of a branch.*

parenchymatous hemorrhage.[141] Most patients with lipohyalinosis and lacunar infarctions are or have been hypertensive, although lipohyalinosis is not limited to patients with hypertension. The incidence of lipohyalinosis increases with the age of the patient but is not correlated with atheroma of larger vessels.

Aneurysms

Saccular Aneurysms

Saccular aneurysms are usually discovered during evaluation of subarachnoid hemorrhage. Ischemic stroke has been reported from blockage of the orifice of tributary vessels due to embolization from clot within the aneurysm.[142] Saccular aneurysms accounted for only 3.6% (64 of 1769) of those analyzed in Bull's large series.[143] The most common site of saccular aneurysms in the posterior circulation is the basilar apex (60%); less often, they occur in the vertebral-PICA junction (20%) and the basilar-SCA junction (11%), and occasionally, aneurysms involve the junction of the vertebral and basilar arteries (3%).[59,143,144] Basilar apex aneurysms may grow quite large, splaying the cerebral peduncle (Fig. 10–8)[145]; when these apex aneurysms leak, blood in the interpeduncular fossa may lead to spasm and infarction in the territory of vessels within the posterior perforated substance, producing a complex clinical picture of rostral brainstem ischemia.

Despite their frequency, it is unusual for basilar apex aneurysms to manifest as isolated third nerve palsy.[146] Only

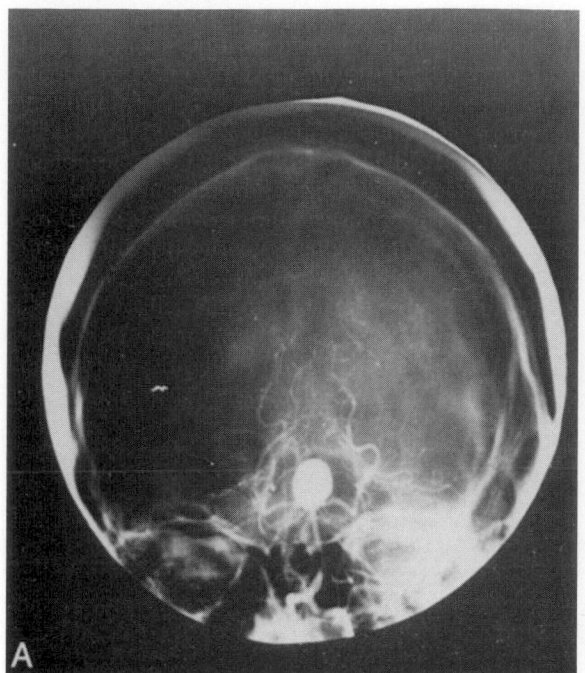
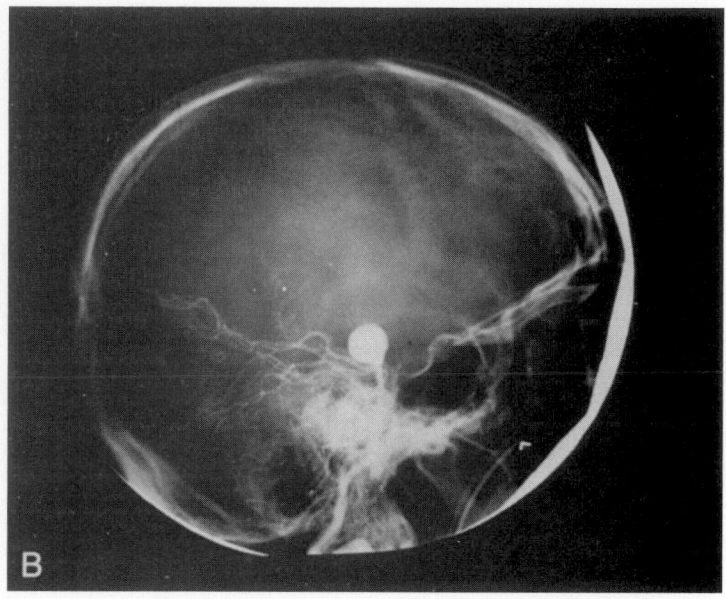

FIGURE 10–8 *Basilar apex aneurysm.* A, *Anteroposterior view.* B, *Lateral view.*

4% of aneurysms causing a third nerve palsy arise from the vertebrobasilar system.[146] In a case report of a large aneurysm at the junction of the BA and left PCA, paroxysmal hypertension occurred, closely simulating a pheochromocytoma[147]; blood pressure normalized after clipping of the aneurysm. Partially thrombosed giant basilar aneurysms are seen on CT scan as calcified, partially enhancing lesions, often near the cerebellopontine angle (Fig. 10–9).[148] However, MRI, MRA, and CT angiography undoubtedly improve their detection.[149,150]

Fusiform (Dolichoectatic) Aneurysms

Fusiform aneurysms are often different in embryology from saccular aneurysms. As suggested by their name, they are tortuous, elongated, ectatic variations of the normal arterial anatomy (see Fig. 10–9).[151] They are now increasingly identified by CT scanning or MRI and MRA, on which they appear as dilated enhancing channels crossing the cerebellopontine angle. Symptoms occur either by compression and traction on posterior fossa structures[152,153] or by ischemia[154] from several mechanisms, including obstruction of blood flow related to atherosclerotic stenosis of the vertebrobasilar arteries, local embolism from in situ thrombus within the aneurysm, and compromise of the orifice of tributary vessels.[155–157] Occipital-nuchal headache is common. Cranial nerve compression and traction may result in neuropathies, usually affecting the seventh and eighth cranial nerves, some manifesting as hemifacial spasm, tinnitus, deafness, vertigo,[158–161] glossopharyngeal and trigeminal–like pain, hiccups, and even hypoglossal paralysis.[158] The larger BA aneurysms can even compress the basis points or cerebral peduncle (leading to spastic paraparesis[162]), may cause hydrocephalus,[157] or may manifest as cerebellopontine angle masses.[163,164] VA aneurysms have compressed the medulla[165] or upper brainstem.[157]

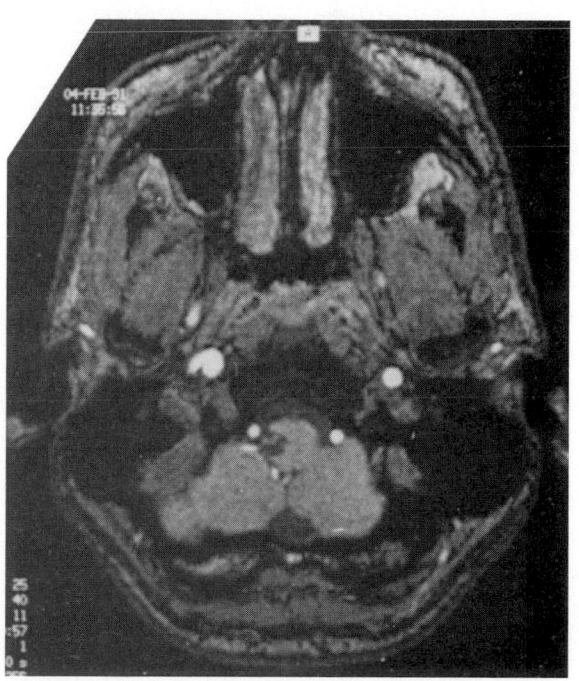

FIGURE 10–9 *T1-weighted MR image showing a lateral medullary infarct sparing the cerebellum.*

The pathogenesis of these aneurysms involves congenital, degenerative, and genetic influences—underlying structural arterial defects, including connective tissue replacement and deficient elastin,[166] fibrous dysplasia and degeneration of internal elastic lamina,[167] and fibrous and collagen replacement of the media. In adults, atherosclerotic changes in the vessels may interact with congenital structural defects to result in fusiform aneurysm formation. A genetic deficiency in α-glucosidase was found in three adolescent brothers with fusiform basilar aneurysms, two of whom had ruptures of the aneurysms; the third had cerebellar infarction.[168] In some patients with structural defects, the arterial abnormalities are widespread, affecting other vessels.[159,169] An association with aneurysms of the abdominal aorta occurs in up to 45% of patients with dolichoectatic basilar arteries.[170] Fusiform aneurysms therefore appear to represent a heterogeneous mixture of vascular causes. Atherosclerosis may be a prominent factor in many adult patients, and other cardiopathies play a role in some patients, especially children. One patient has been described as having a fusiform aneurysm in association with ulcerative colitis.[171]

Dolichoectatic VA and BA aneurysms are also readily visualized on MRI and MRA. The heterogeneity of echo densities and morphology of flow voids usually allows detection of thrombus within the aneurysm. MRA accurately detects the vast majority of sizable saccular and fusiform aneurysms.[51,52,102] Angiography or metrizamide CT cisternography can confirm the diagnosis but is not usually needed if high-quality plain and contrast-enhanced CT or MRI has been performed with special attention to the posterior fossa, or if MRA is available.[172] The pons appears to be the most common site,[173] and lacunar presentation predominates,[174] but a wide range of syndromes can occur, including hydrocephalus, pseudotumor, cranial nerve dysfunction (all from compression), ischemic stroke, and even subarachnoid hemorrhage.[175]

Arterial Dissection

Dissection of the vertebral and basilar arteries has been increasingly recognized since the clinical and angiographic descriptions of ICA dissection.[176–182] The artery most commonly affected in the posterior circulation is the ECVA; dissection usually occurs well above the origin from the subclavian and below the intradural intracranial penetration of the vessel. The initial reports of ECVA dissection featured chiropractic or other neck manipulations, but minor trauma and even spontaneous dissection are now recognized.[183–189] Minor trauma causes of dissection include riding on a rollercoaster,[190] heavy coughing, falling on the back (not the neck) from a handstand, turning the head to back a car, and falling while water-skiing.

VA dissections have been associated with conditions such as Marfan's syndrome, Ehlers-Danlos syndrome, pseudoxanthoma elasticum, lentiginosis, systemic lupus erythematosus, fibromuscular dysplasia, congenital bicuspid aortic valves,[191–194] and arterial redundancy.[195,196] Simultaneous dissection of the carotid and vertebral arteries is a common angiographic finding, and simultaneous dissection of both cervical and renal arteries in a setting of fibromuscular dysplasia suggests an underlying morbid systemic process.[191] Genetic factors may also predispose to dissection. Whereas the risk of recurrent dissection is 1% a year, it is as high as 50% in patients with a familial history of dissection.[197,198]

The most common symptom of VA dissection is pain in the head or neck. Usually, the pain is in the posterior neck with radiation to the occiput, sometimes to the shoulder.[182]

Headache and neck pain may be the only complaints. Ischemic symptoms and signs may develop at the same time as the pain or after a delay of hours to a few days. The lateral medulla and cerebellum are the brainstem regions most susceptible to ischemia from ECVA dissection.[179–181] The clinical features usually correspond to a partial lateral medullary syndrome. Vertigo and isolated face dysesthesia are common symptoms. Visual blurring, diplopia, and oscillopsia also occur. Ipsilateral cerebellar dysfunction and gait ataxia occur frequently. Horner's syndrome is usually present. If isolated cerebellar infarction occurs, dizziness and ataxia predominate. Unilateral symptomatic VA dissection may be associated with asymptomatic dissection of the other VA or even the ICA.

ICVA dissection is less common than ECVA dissection. Two major clinical presentations have been described: subarachnoid hemorrhage (SAH) and brainstem infarction.[199] Less commonly, the dissection may act as a mass lesion compressing posterior fossa structures.[199] SAH as a complication of ICVA dissection reflects, in part, the differences in vessel morphology of intracranial and extracranial arteries. The intracranial arteries have thinner media and adventitial layers, and only an internal elastic lamina; extracranial arteries have thicker media and adventitial layers, and an external as well as an internal elastic lamina. If an intracranial dissection involves the media and spreads to the outer layers, rupture and SAH may occur. When the dissection occurs in the media and subintimal layers, obstruction to blood flow from a narrowing of the lumen or local embolism may lead to brainstem infarction. When SAH is present, it is no different from SAH due to saccular aneurysm rupture.

Headache, often chronic, is common in all presentations of ICVA dissection. Acute headaches associated with prodromal leaks have also been suspected as explained by dissection. As with SAH from saccular aneurysms, the outcome is poor. When brainstem infarction occurs, it is usually severe and is often fatal. Initially unilateral signs frequently become bilateral, with coma and quadriparesis. Deficits limited to the lateral medulla, as in ECVA dissection, are unusual when the dissection involves the ICVA. Dissecting aneurysms of the ICVA may manifest as mass lesions without SAH or stroke. Headache, neck pain, and signs of progressive lower cranial nerve compression have been the hallmarks.[200–202]

Dissection of the BA and its major branches is very uncommon compared with VA dissection. Most descriptions are isolated case reports diagnosed at postmortem examination.[177,203–207] The most common clinical presentation is sudden coma with no history of preceding events. Major brainstem infarction correlates with the clinical findings. SAH as the initial presentation of basilar dissection has also been documented. Rare reports have described dissection beginning in the right ICVA and extending into the BA,[147] some of the cases with remarkably mild initial syndromes.[208]

Watson[206] described a 32-year-old man who experienced headache, confusion, blindness, and pontine dysfunction. The cerebrospinal fluid contained no blood. Postmortem examination showed a dissection of the BA between the media and internal elastic lamina that had narrowed the basilar lumen to a small slit. Unusual loose connective tissue was identified in the media and may have contributed to the dissection. Wolman[209] described a similar case in a 33-year-old man who suddenly became comatose and died of brainstem and cerebellar infarction. The BA dissection had begun at the distal end and spread into the PCA and SCA. The lumen of the BA may have predisposed this patient to the dissection. Alexander and colleagues[203] also reported two patients with basilar dissection. One had a month-long chronic course characterized by altered mental state and paraparesis; the basilar dissection had enlarged the vessel, resulting in considerable mass effect. In the other patient, who had long-standing migraine, sudden brainstem infarction developed secondary to dissection of the BA. Premonitory symptoms were not noted in any of these cases of basilar dissection. However, Escourolle and associates[204] described a patient who tested positive for syphilis in whom severe headache and episodes of left hemiplegia developed before a fixed quadriplegic deficit. Postmortem examination revealed a dissection beginning in the right ICVA and extending up the BA to the SCA.

The principal features thought to distinguish carotid artery dissection from atherosclerotic occlusion are (1) local neck or jaw pain, (2) migrainous spells of scintillation, (3) relatively rapid onset with multiple spells (carotid allegro), and (4) Horner's syndrome.[177] We have seen several patients in whom VA occlusion was heralded by severe headache, local posterior occipital and nuchal discomfort, and caudal brainstem dysfunction. In some of these cases, angiography has shown a VA occlusion, but the extent of the vascular lesion could not be clarified angiographically, and so the presence of dissection could not be verified. Migraine has been found to be significantly associated with dissection.[210] Some investigators have proposed that migraine may predispose to dissection by producing edema of the media of vessels.[206,211] Are we failing to diagnose most examples of VA dissection? Is dissection a more common cause of posterior circulation stroke than currently appreciated?

VA dissections can be imaged at the C2 and C3 levels by means of high-quality color-flow ultrasonography.[212] MRA is also a useful screening test, but the sensitivity and specificity of this method is not yet as good for VA dissection as it is for carotid artery dissection.[213,214] Standard angiography combined with axial MR images of the arteries is still the best way to diagnose VA dissections.

Cervical Spondylosis

In 1960 Sheehan and coworkers[215] popularized the idea that compression of the VA by osteophytes was a common cause of vertebrobasilar insufficiency. Spondylitic osteophytes project from the vertebral joints adjacent to the transverse foramina through which the VAs course. In cadavers, extreme neck turning can cut off VA flow, especially at C5 to C6.[216] Angiographic studies have shown stenosis to be common but occlusion rare at the point of maximal concavity.[216] Clinical examples are decidedly uncommon: Only two patients in one series experienced symptoms on neck turning (dizziness, blurred vision, and confusion), and in only two other patients (not the symptomatic patients) was angiographically measured stenosis worsened by turning. In 6 of 26 patients studied by

angiogram, the only symptom was drop attacks, dubiously attributable to vascular disease. However, ECVAs can occasionally be intermittently occluded by spondylitic spurs.[217-219] In many cases, either the ECVA contralateral to the compressed VA is hypoplastic or previously occluded, or the ICVA ends in the PICA; thus, the compressed ECVA could be the major supply to the posterior circulation.

Chin[217] reported a well-documented example of a patient who experienced a left PICA cerebellar and right PCA territory infarct in relation to a high-grade stenosis of the left ECVA at the V4 level. A large vertebral osteophyte projected into the narrowed transverse foramen at this level. Rosengart and associates[219] reported a similar case of a patient with intermittent vertigo and downbeat nystagmus provoked by head turning. His ECVA was compressed by a large osteophyte, and symptoms disappeared after removal of the osteophytic obstruction. Similarly, fibrous tissue bands and muscles have occasionally been found to compress the ECVAs, usually in the distal portion of the V1 portions of the arteries before they enter the intravertebral foramina.[220-223] Symptoms are often intermittent and may be precipitated by turning or rotation of the neck during which the ECVA can become occluded. These cases are rare. Although turning or sudden motion may further compromise kinks or smaller atherosclerotic vessels and can lead to vascular occlusion or dissection, the mechanism only rarely involves spondylosis.

Several cogent arguments challenge the theory that spondylosis is a common cause of symptomatic vascular compression: First, in postmortem studies, although slight ridging or streaks are frequently seen in the midcervical area,[112] this region is infrequently a site of severe stenosis or occlusion[77,104,111]; in large radiographic series, severe lateral displacement by osteophytes is rare (2 of 203 cases reported by Radner[224]). Second, most reported patients with intermittent posterior circulation ischemia and spondylosis have coexistent atherosclerosis, and some spondylosis is ubiquitous in patients older than 40 years.[215,225] Finally, In some patients, spondylosis itself may cause transient rostral spinal cord signs—for example, drop attacks. In other supposed examples of spondylosis–vascular disease, the only symptom is vertigo on neck motion, a common phenomenon in the elderly and one frequently produced by labyrinthine and other nonvascular mechanisms.[226] Until a clearer relationship between spondylosis and vascular disease can be demonstrated, surgery of spondylitic lesions should not be performed for the sole purpose of treating vertebrobasilar insufficiency.

Neck Rotation or Trauma

Although earlier reports have described individual case histories of posterior circulation infarction that occurred after neck manipulation, the mechanism has now been further elucidated. In 1947, Pratt-Thomas and Berger[227] provided an account of two previously healthy individuals, a 32-year-old man and a 35-year-old woman, who became unconscious during chiropractic manipulation and died in less than 24 hours without regaining consciousness. Occlusion of the BA, left AICA, and right PICA with brainstem and bilateral cerebellar hemisphere softenings were found in one patient, and occlusion of the right vertebral and basilar arteries and left PICA in the other. Since this original report, more than 50 additional patients have been described in whom posterior circulation stroke followed neck rotation or injury.[184,188,228–236] Most cases occur after chiropractic manipulation, but manipulation of the neck by a patient's wife,[184] neck turning while driving a car, wrestling,[233] and practicing archery and yoga[228] have also been implicated. Most of the patients have been young (average age, 37 years)[234] and have had no evidence of preexisting vascular disease or cervical fractures or dislocations.

In most patients, the syndrome is unilateral, and ischemia is limited to the lateral medulla or pons and the ipsilateral cerebellum.[183,228,230–233] Arteriography in those with predominantly unilateral findings has documented narrowing or occlusion of the VA in its third segment, usually in the region of C2 or C1 before the vessel penetrates the dura. One report documented the occlusive process in the intracranial VA[183]; in another, the VA was occluded at C6 because of neck trauma and paraplegia.[58] Only one patient had a lesion at the level of the VA origin, but this patient, who suffered an acute traumatic injury, was studied 7 weeks after the initial injury, a period that would allow retrograde extension of clot.[230] Pseudoaneurysm formation has been seen in 5 patients, also at the C2 to C1 region. Unilateral lesions tend to develop at the time of neck rotation and often (14 of 21 cases) do not progress.[188] Only 1 of the 21 patients in one series died of the unilateral stroke.[188] Cerebellar softening with subsequent edema and increased posterior fossa pressure may occur and may require surgical decompression.[237]

When initial findings indicate bilateral brainstem lesions, the course is often progressive (9 of 13 cases) and fatal (6 of 13 cases). Symptoms appear at the time of neck rotation or injury in approximately one third of cases, symptoms develop minutes or days later in one third, and symptoms progress after the onset in one third.[234] Autopsy usually confirms extensive brainstem and cerebellar infarctions and thrombosis in the basilar or vertebral artery. In one report, the right VA was perforated, with disruption of the media and internal elastic membrane, and hemorrhage surrounded the VA and vein[234]; in one other (of an 8-year-old boy who fell from a tree), a true traumatic aneurysm of the right VA ruptured, leading to death from SAH.[237] In some cases, dissection of the VA is suggested by the radiographic appearance of pseudoaneurysm but is not found on postmortem examination. Mas and colleagues[238] reported the case of a 35-year-old woman with 3 weeks of cervical pain who experienced ischemia in the BA territory after cervical manipulation and died less than 24 hours later. At postmortem examination, a dissecting aneurysm was found within the third segment of the right VA. Pathologic changes in the lower and upper parts of the dissecting aneurysm were different, indicating recurrent bleeding. These investigators hypothesized that spontaneous dissection had led to the original neck pain, which prompted neck manipulation, which in turn precipitated the stroke by inducing bleeding within the dissecting aneurysm.[238]

Especially susceptible to injury during neck rotation is the third segment of the VA, which lies in relation to the atlas, axis, and atlanto-occipital membrane. Injury to the intima activates clotting mechanisms and leads to the formation of thrombus in the VA, usually at the C2 to C1 region. Thrombus may propagate distally or may embolize to more rostral portions of the basilar arterial tree. Filling defects in the distal vascular bed are occasionally verified angiographically.[178,234] In unusual instances, the VA may be perforated or a dissection may be initiated at the injured segment. Anticoagulation has been occasionally used in an attempt to stop clot propagation and embolization.[234] The variability of the natural course and the scarcity of treated patients make it impossible at present to estimate the utility of anticoagulation in patients with vertebrobasilar artery injury due to neck manipulation or trauma.

Fibromuscular Dysplasia

Fibromuscular dysplasia (FMD) is characterized by hyperplasia of the intima and media of arteries with adventitial sclerosis and breakdown of normal elastic tissue. Thickened septa and ridges protrude into the lumen. At postmortem examination, basilar occlusion with brainstem infarction has been documented; the BA has been severely ectatic and atherosclerotic with focal variations in wall thickness and aneurysm formation. Homonymous hemianopia has been reported with FMD of the PCA,[239,240] and cephalic FMD is strongly associated with an accompanying intracranial aneurysm.[239,241–244] A relationship between cephalic FMD and dissection has also been noted.[205] The angiographic changes of pseudoaneurysm formation seen in FMD are also commonly described in dissection of cervical vessels.[177] The mechanisms of ischemia distal to lesions of FMD are unclear, as are the need for and types of treatment.

Temporal Arteritis

Headache and visual loss, the most common clinical manifestations of temporal arteritis, are caused by giant cell granulomatous disease of the ophthalmic branches to the optic nerve and central retinal arteries and the superficial temporal and occipital branches of the external carotid artery (see Chapter 5). The most frequently described intracranial vessel disease in temporal arteritis is thrombus formation without local arteritis; it is probably due to embolization from the extracranial arteritic occlusive disease.[245] Rarely, smaller intracranial vessels, including posterior circulation branches, may demonstrate granulomatous arteritis.[245] The related clinical findings are headache, cerebrospinal fluid pleocytosis, and multifocal cranial nerve and parenchymatous dysfunction, including some typically distinctive basilar branch syndromes such as one-and-a-half ocular palsies (see later)[246]; many such cases do not have clear histories of stroke.[245]

Other Diseases

Less common diseases affecting vascular structures of the posterior fossa are mentioned only briefly here because of their rarity and the lack of data on their special features within the posterior circulation.

Aspergillosis seems to have a special tropism for the posterior circulation vessels.[247] It involves the brain by infarction due to occlusion of distal branches in the cerebellum or occipital lobes. Infarctions are commonly small and hemorrhagic. Later, abscesses may develop at the borderzone of the infarcted area. Aspergillosis is a usually nosocomial fungal infection that disseminates via the blood route and develops in the presence of oxygen, a feature that explains why the borderzone area of infarcted tissue is the best site for development of an abscess. Unlike cryptococcosis, another fungal infection, aspergillosis rarely occurs together with meningitis.[248] Mechanisms of arterial occlusion are (1) thromboangiitis with presence of aspergillosis in the arterial wall and in the thrombus and (2) embolic occlusion from an endocarditis due to *Aspergillus*.[247] Endocarditis is most difficult to diagnose even with transesophageal echocardiography but is found in as many as 50% of patients with aspergillosis at autopsy.[249] Diagnosis of aspergillosis in the presence of brain infarctions is usually very difficult and is based on repeated serology, biopsy, and culture of an associated arthritis or spondylitis infection,[250] culture of a catheter of perfusion, or presence of pneumonia due to *Aspergillus*, especially in severely ill patients in intensive care units, patients with chronic polyinfection, and drug users.[248,251]

Meningitis due to other fungal infections or tuberculosis commonly produces changes within vessels, most often in branches of the MCA and in arteries that traverse the interpeduncular fossa to penetrate the rostral brainstem. The exudate somehow produces a reaction in the media of these vessels, usually referred to as Heubner's arteritis. Sudden stupor may be due to infarctions of the brainstem, often with third cranial nerve palsies and bilateral pyramidal tract dysfunction. Headache, fever, cranial nerve palsies, and confusion dominate the clinical picture, and examination of the cerebrospinal fluid usually confirms the diagnosis.

Fibrous bands crossing the proximal VA before it enters the transverse foramina may constrict the vessel when the neck is turned.[223]

Sickle cell disease is associated with occlusion of small and larger vessels[252]; the larger vessels frequently show extensive intimal proliferation of fibrodysplasia, possibly related to abnormal flow mechanisms.[253] Stroke often occurs during a sickle cell crisis and is heralded by seizures. Few data are available concerning the findings related to posterior circulation occlusion in this group of patients; pseudobulbar signs are more common than bulbar paralysis.

Young women taking oral contraceptives may suffer occlusion of the ECVA, and for unclear reasons, BA occlusion occasionally occurs in the first two decades of life.

Syphilis can also produce an arteritis and can be associated with brainstem infarcts, usually in branch distribution.

Systemic lupus erythematosus and granulomatous angiitis do affect cerebral blood vessels, but a strokelike picture is rarely found. CT or MRI shows very small infarcts often in borderzone areas of the cerebellum or occipital lobes.[254]

Homocystinuria, Marfan's syndrome, Ehlers-Danlos syndrome, pseudoxanthoma elasticum, polyarteritis nodosa, Kohl-Meyer-Degos disease, and Fabry's disease are associated with ischemic strokes, but little is known of the incidence and site of involvement in the vertebrobasilar system in these diseases.

Takayasu's pulseless disease often involves the SA and VA orifices as well as the aorta.[255,256] Occasionally, the intracranial arteries also show intensive inflammation typical of Takayasu's arteritis.[257] Brainstem lesions are especially common in Behçet's syndrome.[258]

Behçet's disease was first described by a Turkish ophthalmologist; although rare, this disorder is less uncommon in the Middle East and Mediterranean countries. Clinical findings include aphthous stomatitis and genital ulcers, uveitis, cells in the cerebrospinal fluid, and multifocal neurologic signs.[259,260] The neurologic symptoms often relate to the brainstem and develop quickly or gradually. CT usually shows a low-density abnormality, and T2-weighted MRI shows an area of hypersignal in the brainstem, cerebellum, or cerebral white matter that enhances acutely.[259] Mass effect may be seen. With time, enhancement is lost, and the patient stabilizes or improves. Angiography usually does not show arterial occlusions, but dural sinus occlusions are common. At necropsy, inflammatory lesions are seen with perivascular lymphocytic cuffing around capillaries and ventricles, especially in the brainstem.[259]

Neurofibromatosis has been rarely reported as a cause of basilar compression with stroke.[261]

PATHOPHYSIOLOGY

Luminal Obstruction

Many factors determine whether or not an ischemic tissue becomes infarcted. Blockage of the lumina of blood vessels by atheroma, by clot, or by swollen vessel wall, embolization of intraluminal material distally, or by activation of clotting factors with propagation of clot all act to increase luminal obstruction and diminish blood flow to a given region. Concomitantly, however, reduction of flow to a region leads to accumulation of metabolites, especially lactate, and an increase in collateral circulation. Fibrinolysis and other enzymatic processes act to lyse and solidify the local clot. Embolic fragments pass through the vascular bed, allowing resumption of flow. In addition, systemic factors such as blood pressure, cardiac output, blood viscosity, red blood cell count, and pulmonary function all affect the rheology and oxygen-carrying capacity of the blood reaching a given ischemic region. The sum of these factors determines the survival of a given ischemic zone. The process can be viewed schematically (Table 10.1) as the summation of vectors, those tending to increase ischemia and those promoting additional blood flow to reduce the ischemic deficit.

Within the posterior circulation, there are multiple collateral channels for augmenting flow. Reduction of flow through one VA can often be compensated for by

Table 10.1 Pathophysiology of Tenuous Equilibrium after Occlusion of an Artery

Factors Promoting Deficit	Factors Defending Against Deficit
Blood flow to lesion diminished by stenosis of occlusion	Collateral circulation and autoregulation
Embolization from plaque or clot	Passing of emboli
Activation of clotting factors	Thrombolysis (?)

collateral vessels from the other VA, the thyrocervical trunk, and occipital artery branches of the external carotid artery, which direct flow toward the nuchal vertebral artery. Intracranially, the long circumferential cerebellar arteries (the AICA, PICA, and SCA) form an active collateral system. For example, in a lesion blocking flow in the proximal BA, blood can course from the VA to the PICA, and into hemispheral branches of the AICA and SCA, and back to the BA beyond the region of blockage. Similarly, blood may pass from the SCA to AICA or PICA branches. The ICA may serve as a major source of collateral circulation, with blood flowing via the posterior communicating artery to the PCA and down the BA and SCAs, the latter supplying collaterals to the lower brainstem through the cerebellar hemispheral branches. Collateral circulation is especially rich in the brainstem tegmentum, making this region more resistant to ischemia.

The time course of development and progression of symptoms are well correlated with prognosis and give information about the sum of pathophysiologic factors operative in the individual patient. Symptoms develop in one of the following temporal patterns: (1) TIAs, either as an isolated finding or preceding a stroke, (2) sudden-onset deficits that are maximal at onset, (3) fluctuating clinical deficits punctuated by improvements and deteriorations, and (4) gradually progressive stroke.[262,263] Clinical fluctuations during a period of 2 to 3 weeks may be sensitive to blood pressure and postural changes.[262,264] Simply sitting up or raising the head of the bed to eat could cause temporary aggravation of a deficit, which may be quickly relieved by lowering the head.

The presence of preceding TIAs indicates some chronicity in the occlusive process, allowing more time for collateral circulation to develop. Improvement in function indicates that collateral circulation has developed or the occlusive process is less operant (e.g., lysis of embolic clot). Perhaps for these reasons patients with TIAs and a fluctuating course have a better prognosis. Other patients had sudden-onset deficits sometimes heralded by TIAs or progressive accumulation of deficit without significant temporary improvement in function. Sudden-onset deficits are usually embolic. Prognosis depends on the length of time the embolus blocks the vessel as well as on clot lysis or passage. Steady progression of symptoms without stabilization or improvement indicates poor formation of collateral vessels and has a bad prognosis.

Few reports have considered the temporal course. Jones and colleagues[265] analyzed the course of 37 patients with vertebrobasilar territory infarction; 12 had had at least one preceding TIA, and in 30 patients, the onset of stroke was precipitous. Fluctuations commonly occurred during the first week but were unusual thereafter. Progressive deterioration in function was common (16 of 37 cases), usually reached its maximum within the first 4 days, and had a bad prognosis. Similarly, Patrick and associates[266] reviewed 39 patients with vertebrobasilar territory infarction and commented on the instability of the early clinical course but rarity of late (over 3 weeks) progression. In neither series was there frequent corroboration of the nature and locus of the vascular lesion during life.

TIAs are caused by either diminished blood flow (with temporarily insufficient collateral circulation) or embolization of clot or plaque material. The fixed deficit is often noticed in the morning, having accumulated at night during a time of more sluggish flow. Once the VA or BA is occluded, propagation of clot, embolization, and diminished blood flow may result. The critical period for development of neurologic deficit is at the time of occlusion and during the next few weeks. Denny-Brown[19] emphasized a contributory role of systemic factors in compounding the clinical deficit and called these fluctuations *reversible hemodynamic crises*. These factors seemed most operant in the first 2 weeks after vascular occlusion and were less clinically important thereafter. Sundt and Piepgras[267] also emphasized the effect of postural changes on flow during the early critical period. Naritomi and coworkers[268] showed that reduction in regional blood flow to the posterior circulation, as measured by xenon inhalation, rarely persisted 3 weeks after transient ischemic symptoms, but that defective autoregulation (i.e., change in flow after induced postural hypotension) was more widespread and long-lasting after vertebrobasilar insufficiency than after carotid attacks. Careful scrutiny of blood pressure, maintenance of blood volume with optimal oxygenation, and careful surveillance of patients when they assume sitting or upright postures are very important during the first few weeks after a vertebrobasilar territory stroke, because collateral circulation is still developing. This is especially true in occlusive disease of larger vessels (VA or BA), but extension of deficit after reduced blood pressure may also occur in basilar branch occlusion.[269]

Intra-Arterial Embolism

Although embolic occlusion is considered by some to be unusual in patients with vertebrobasilar infarction,[270] Castaigne and associates[77] have documented the frequency of emboli within the PCAs, and syndromes related to the rostral BA are likely to be more frequently embolic.[271] Other common recipient sites for embolism are the SCA, PICA, and distal VAs.[108,109,134] Initial syndromes are often severe, but reports now indicate that some affected patients may experience benign outcomes,[272] presumably through rapid recanalization without major infarction. Artery-to-artery embolisms do occur within the posterior circulation, but their frequency has not been documented. Emboli probably account for the sudden-onset deficits.

The most important donor sites for intra-arterial emboli are the aortic arch, SA, VA origin, and distal VA.[273] The most common donor sites are the VA origin (either recent thrombosis[274] or ulcerated plaques[106]) and the ICVA. In a series of 67 patients with brainstem and cerebellar ischemia, intra-arterial embolism was the mechanism of stroke in 9 (13%).[53] Among these 9 patients, the donor site was the proximal ECVA in 5, distal ECVA dissection in 3, and a thrombus within the ICVA in 1. Emboli went to the ICVA-PICA in 3, the BA in 3, and the BA-SCA region in another 3.[53] Embolism from VA origin occlusive disease was recognized in a series of 10 patients with distal intra-arterial embolism. The VA lesions were complete occlusion in 7 patients and severe atherosclerotic stenosis in 3. Recipient sites were the intracranial VA-PICA in 8 cases and the distal BA and its SCA and PCA branches in 7 patients.[274] Cardiac cavities are other important donor sites of embolism, probably the most prevalent sites in posterior circulation infarction, especially cerebellar and occipital lobe infarctions.[109,133,275,276]

Worsening

Generally, progressive neurologic deficits imply propagation of clot or failure of collateral circulation to compensate for reduced flow. Involvement of a larger vessel usually implies a poor prognosis.[262,277] Another cause of worsening of symptoms within the posterior circulation is infarction of the cerebellum with progressive swelling and pressure on the brainstem and ventricular pathways.[278] This problem has a high mortality rate, but it is amenable to surgical decompression. The deficit can also progress within the territory of a basilar branch, but this situation usually occurs over a shorter period (from hours to a week), and the deficit is limited to the territory supplied by the single branch or its previously occluded neighboring branches.[279]

Worsening can also be caused by alterations in cardiovascular and respiratory function resulting from ischemic brainstem dysfunction. Lability of blood pressure and blood flow can result from lesions of the medulla and pons.[280] Reis and colleagues[281] documented the importance of the fastigial nucleus of the cerebellum in altering vertebral blood flow. Stimulation of regions within the brainstem tegmentum can alter heart rate and rhythm.[282,283] Khurana[280] described persistent tachycardia, orthostatic hypotension without cardiac acceleration, episodic bradycardia, and even cardiorespiratory arrest in four patients with bilateral pontomedullary lesions. Even unilateral lesions can be accompanied by tachycardia and lability of blood pressure. Bogousslavsky and associates[284] reported two patients studied clinically and at necropsy who had severe hypoventilation related to lateral tegmental pontomedullary infarcts. Intermittent apnea, especially during sleep, and failure to respond during CO_2 retention were prominent features, and each patient died of the complications of respiratory failure.

Activation of clotting factors, polycythemia, or thrombocytosis can exaggerate occlusive disease and in some situations may alone be responsible for sluggish posterior circulation flow and clinical attacks. One patient with elevations of hemoglobin content, platelet count, and platelet agglutination experienced frequent spells of vertebrobasilar ischemia and claudication of the legs; no lesion could be detected angiographically, and the spells disappeared after aspirin therapy. This experience prompts the suggestion that a hematologic survey be part of the evaluation of all patients with transient or persistent ischemic symptoms. In the individual patient, the anatomic location of the lesion producing the neurologic signs and the time course of development of the deficit help the physician predict the affected vessel, the nature of the pathologic process in the vessel, and the adequacy of collateral circulation. Laboratory investigations, especially angiography, confirm the location of the responsible vascular lesion, give additional information concerning previous disease or maldevelopment in other extracranial and intracranial vessels, and help define the source and adequacy of collateral circulation.

CLINICAL FINDINGS IN PATIENTS WITH VASCULAR LESIONS IN VARIOUS LOCATIONS

Occlusion or Severe Stenosis of the Basilar Artery

Historical Aspects

Kubik and Adams,[13] in their landmark description of occlusion of the BA, summarized the findings as follows:

The onset is sudden and is not preceded by tangible causal factors. The first symptom is usually headache, dizziness, confusion, or coma. Difficulty in speaking and unilateral paresthesias occur in a large proportion of the cases. Common findings are pupillary abnormalities, disorders of ocular movement, facial palsy, hemiplegia, quadriplegia, or both, and bilateral extensor plantar reflexes. Cranial nerve palsies and contralateral hemiplegia may be combined. It is common for temporary improvement, lasting hours or days, to occur during the course of the illness. In the majority of cases, death takes place between 2 days and 5 weeks from onset. Rare cases have been reported in which the first symptom was deafness.[285]

In an early angiography study, Archer and Horenstein[286] also found severe deficits in 20 patients with angiographically confirmed BA occlusion: 15 patients died, and the other 5 were left severely disabled. By contrast, Caplan[262] described 4 patients among 6 with verified basilar occlusion who survived the associated acute ischemic event with little (1 patient) or no (3 patients) deficit. Other investigators have also noted examples of survival without crippling deficit after BA occlusion[21,98,287–289]; in fact, Kubik and Adams,[13] in their original paper, mentioned 4 patients with clinical findings identical to those with documented basilar occlusion who survived the stroke and were alive months later.

Patterns of Infarction

The regions of infarction in patients with confirmed BA occlusion vary considerably, depending on the portion of the BA occluded. At times the occlusion is quite limited and segmental, whereas at others, thrombosis can affect multiple segments or can even occlude the entire BA and extend into the VA and PCA.[77,290]

Kubik and Adams[13] studied 18 patients with BA occlusion, including six examples of presumed embolic occlusion: eight involved the rostral BA, five the proximal third, two the middle third, and three the entire artery. In their material, the patterns of infarction and vascular occlusion are neatly diagrammed. In the patients with sparing of the rostral tip of the BA, the infarcts were predominantly pontine, usually centering on the midpons. In these cases, the most lateral margins of the basis pontis were often spared, and the basis pontis was affected to a far greater degree than the tegmentum. When the basilar tip was occluded, the lesions were predominantly in the midbrain, diencephalon, and rostral pons, and the tegmentum of the pons and midbrain were more often involved than in occlusion of the caudal BA. In one third of cases, the infarcts were symmetric, and in many cases, the softenings were patchy. The cerebellum was also spared in most cases; the extensive brainstem softening contrasted strikingly with the normal or minimally damaged cerebellum.

Silverstein[291] reported 11 examples of verified BA occlusion in his series; in 8 patients, the lesion affected the distal third, in 1 patient the proximal third, and in 2 patients the middle third of the artery. He remarked, "Embolism was not recorded clinically or pathologically in our series," but 3 patients had minimal atherosclerosis of the BA, brainstem infarcts, and emboli in various viscera. The infarctions centered on the midpons (again predominantly in a paramedian distribution), were occasionally patchy, and were almost invariably anemic rather than hemorrhagic.

Loeb and Meyer[292] reviewed and tabulated previous reports of BA occlusion and the pattern of brainstem infarction. They found that pontine infarcts always favored median and paramedian zones, with relative sparing of the lateral margins. Biemond[293] noted frequent tegmental sparing and sought to explain it by emphasizing that the tegmentum is supplied mainly by the SCA and its branches. The SCA is the most anatomically constant long circumferential branch vessel and often has a prominent anastomosis with the PCA. Biemond[293] followed small branches of the SCA and found that they formed a corona around the cranial part of the pontine tegmentum and anastomosed with the SCA branches of the other side. When a lateral branch of the SCA was injected, the tegmentum was stained bilaterally; when the BA was injected from the VA, the basis pontis was deeply stained but the tegmentum remained entirely clear. Biemond[293] also obtained little tegmental staining from injection of the AICA.

According to the study by Kubik and Adams,[13] the tegmentum is involved most commonly when the occlusive lesions extend to the basilar tip, thus obstructing the SCA orifices. Angiographic material in patients with BA occlusion reported by Caplan and Rosenbaum[263] also demonstrated retrograde filling of the PCA and SCA from carotid injection and the prominence of cerebellar artery anastomotic vessels that fill other lateral circumferential cerebellar artery branches. Tegmental involvement thus depends on the involvement of the distal BA and the adequacy of collateral vessels. Collateral circulation through the PICA is poor when the VA and BA are both obstructed. Archer and Horenstein[286] wondered whether hypertension, by reducing the number and adequacy of collateral vessels, might considerably affect prognosis.

Angiographic and MRI Diagnosis

Angiography performed with the standard Seldinger technique and intra-arterial digital subtraction angiography have been the principal methods of corroborating the clinical impression of BA occlusive disease. Now, absence of a signal void in the artery in various MRI slices can often suggest occlusion.[37] MRA shows great promise for allowing corroboration of BA occlusion without invasive catheterization or dye injection.[51,52] TCD ultrasonography is probably accurate in lesions of the proximal BA but to date has not been sensitive to lesions of the middle and distal BA.[49]

Diagnosis of BA occlusion hinges on angiographic demonstration of blocked cephalad flow (not simply poor filling or ending of the VA in the PICA) and collateral filling of rostral structures. Carotid artery injection frequently leads to flow through the posterior communicating artery to the PCA, basilar tip, and SCA. Figure 10–10

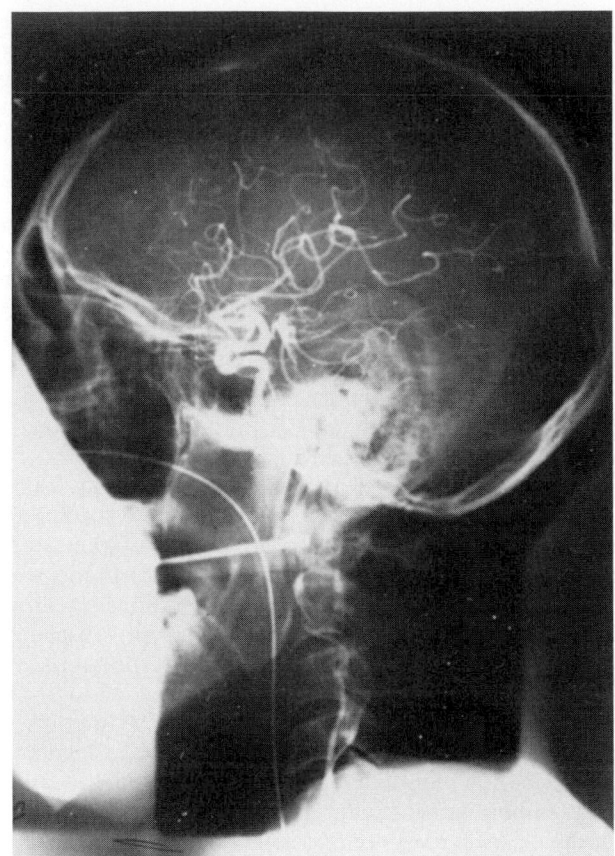

FIGURE 10–10   *Carotid arteriogram demonstrating retrograde filling of the basilar artery and the posterior cerebral and superior cerebellar arteries. Note the midbasilar occlusion.*

is an example of such a retrograde filling. Even in the presence of a tiny incompetent posterior communicating artery, the PCA may be opacified via anastomoses between posterior branches of the MCA and the branches of the PCA, with subsequent filling of the distal BA. In addition to the anastomoses between the vermian and hemispheric branches of the PICA, AICA, and SCA, there is also filling via the posterior meningeal branches of the VA and the meningohypophyseal branch of the ICA.[288]

Angiographic definition of the disease in the BA can help determine whether long-term warfarin anticoagulation therapy should be used in a patient with slight deficits. Angiography must be performed if surgery to create shunts that would increase posterior circulation flow is under consideration. The risk of angiography in posterior circulation disease has been surprisingly low when the procedure is performed in large centers by trained neuroradiologists and a large number of cases. CT is helpful in documenting cerebellar infarction but to date has been disappointing in defining acute brainstem softenings.

MRI has been a great advance in mapping and defining infarcts in the brainstem and cerebellum. The pattern of brainstem infarction—that is, whether unilateral or bilateral, tegmental or basal and medial or lateral, as well as rostrocaudal level—can indicate whether the lesion involves the territory of the unilateral or bilateral intracranial VAs, the BA, or single penetrating or circumferential branches. The pattern of cerebellar infarction, most readily seen on T2-weighted sagittal sections for the vermis and coronal sections for the hemispheres, also helps define the likely arterial territory and pathology.[134]

General Clinical Features

Atherosclerotic disease of the BA has been recognized at the preocclusive stage of severe stenosis (see Fig. 10–10). It is relatively uncommon compared with occlusion of the BA. In the Joint Study of Extracranial Arterial Occlusion, BA stenosis was identified in 7.7% of 3778 patients undergoing four-vessel angiography.[294]

Pessin and colleagues[295] identified nine patients with angiographically proven middle or distal segment basilar stenosis and, in reviewing their other angiographic and pathologic cases, found that occlusion affected all three BA segments (proximal, middle, and distal) with relatively equal frequency. These investigators also found that TIAs were a common feature of the clinical presentation in patients with BA stenosis, occurring in six of the nine cases. The TIAs usually preceded brainstem stroke, but in two patients, they were the sole clinical manifestation. Features of TIA consisted of the brief duration of two or more of the following symptoms: dizziness, slurred speech, double vision, dysphagia, and unilateral or bilateral weakness. The TIAs occurred during a period of 1 day to 6 months before stroke. Stroke severity and infarct location varied, but the pons was a common locus of injury. The short-term prognosis was good; most patients remained free of symptoms for periods of 1 month to 2 years, usually with anticoagulation or on antiplatelet treatment. Three patients died, one from the original stroke, another from a new basilar territory infarct, and the third from unrelated causes.[295]

No uniform syndrome or outcome is applicable to all patients with BA occlusion. Should this come as a surprise? The situation in the carotid artery is clearly comparable. Sometimes when the ICA is occluded, patients complain of amaurosis fugax followed by symptoms and signs of total ischemia of the anterior and MCA branches of the ICA. Such patients are readily diagnosed. Other patients with ICA occlusion have transient or partial deficits, and diagnosis can be made only with laboratory confirmation, usually angiography. There is a wide spectrum of symptomatology, severity of signs, and outcome.[296]

The situation in the BA is not very different. Because confirmation of BA occlusion requires angiography, the frequency of this angiographic diagnosis depends at present on the indications for angiography in a given institution. TCD ultrasonography has documented at least one example of high-grade basilar stenosis manifesting clinically in the early stage as "herald hemiparesis."[297] Archer and Horenstein[286] studied severely ill patients with angiography; Meyer and colleagues[16] excluded patients with severe brainstem infarction from angiography, but nevertheless identified two patients with unusual BA occlusion. Prognosis depends on the rate and extent of occlusion, presence of collateral circulation, systemic factors (see earlier discussion of pathophysiology), and, possibly, treatment.

Patients with documented severe stenotic lesions of the BA or the ICVAs have a relatively poor prognosis for subsequent brainstem infarction or death.[298] In the New England Medical Center Registry, the mortality rate for brainstem infarcts was low overall (3.6%) at 30 days, but the group with the poor outcome were those with BA involvement, embolic mechanism, and multiple intracranial posterior circulation infarcts.[299] For patients in the Lausanne Registry, dysarthria, pupillary disorders, lower cranial nerve involvement, and disorders of consciousness on admission had the worst prognostic value compared with other syndromic elements ($P < .001$).[300] In one series, the stroke rate for such patients was 17 times the expected rate for a matched normal population.

Because there is no absolutely uniform syndrome of BA occlusion, the remainder of this discussion describes common neurologic findings not previously commented on that occur with BA occlusion, characterizes the common patterns of infarction documented at postmortem, and covers angiographic diagnosis and clinical tempo.

Clinical Tempo and Course

Information correlating the usual tempo of neurologic deficit acquisition and the location of vascular occlusion is very scanty. Subjects in many studies are chosen solely because of the availability of necropsy material, a factor that eliminates the less severely affected patients.[13,291] The clinical studies often lack angiographic or pathologic confirmation.[22,301] Angiographic studies commonly do not detail temporal profiles.[287] Larger series of patients with BA occlusion antedated the widespread use of angiography.

Caplan[262] analyzed the clinical course of surviving patients with BA occlusions that have been verified angiographically, but the series was quite small (six cases). TIAs were quite common before the stroke (four of the six cases). The last TIA occurred within 1 month of the stroke in all these patients (within 1 week in three cases). The initial TIA preceded the stroke by a wide range (1 week to 1 year). After onset of a prolonged deficit, five of the six patients had either progression of the deficit over 2 to 3 days or fluctuations. Fluctuations occurred over 2 weeks and were sensitive to position in bed.[264] Two patients had sudden-onset deficits; in one, the deficit subsequently fluctuated for less than 2 weeks. Only one patient had a progressive course without stabilization or fluctuation over the first 3 days.

In another clinical series, Jones and colleagues[265] noted that a temporal profile consisting of an unstable course characterized by progression or remission and relapses was more common in patients who had vertebrobasilar system infarction (54%) compared with patients who had carotid system disease (26%). In this series, the neurologic deficit in patients with vertebrobasilar disease rarely progressed after 4 days, and most changes occurred within the first 48 hours. Declining consciousness was an ominous sign. Patrick and colleagues[266] also analyzed the temporal profile in their series of 39 cases of clinical vertebrobasilar infarction (7 with angiography). Sudden onset followed by stabilization (12 patients) and gradual onset with later progression (9 patients) were common patterns. Only 2 patients' deficits progressed after 24 hours, one over 48 hours and the other over 1 week. Deficits in a total of 13 patients progressed after being stable for 24 hours or more; 8 patients experienced progression on day 2, 2 on day 3, and one each on days 4, 6, and 7. As in other series, coma

Clinical Manifestations

was a poor prognostic sign. These studies indicate that sudden-onset deficits are common, a point also emphasized by Kubik and Adams.[13]

Ferbert and colleagues[302] analyzed the early symptoms and course in their 85 patients with angiographically proven BA occlusion. More than half had some premonitory symptoms, usually in the 2 weeks before stroke onset. Vertigo and headache were especially common symptoms. Acute onset of stroke was noted in 31 patients, 11 of whom had TIAs or other prodromal symptoms. In 54 of the 85 patients (64%), the course was progressive with or without prodromal symptoms.

Sudden onset might point to an embolic mechanism (thrombus breaking loose from a more proximal arterial site within the ICVA or the lower BA). Fluctuations and progressions are common but are almost invariably documented only within the first 2 weeks after stroke onset, usually within the first 48 hours; few occur between 1 and 2 weeks. Gradual progression without improvement, especially if stupor develops, is a grave prognostic sign. This evidence, in our view, favors treatment before the stroke in patients with TIAs and emphasizes the importance of treatment during the first 1 to 2 weeks after stroke onset. Vigorous treatment after the deficit is stable, especially after 2 weeks, would not seem to be warranted in patients with BA occlusion, because late deficits are rare.

The introduction of thrombolytic treatment in patients with BA occlusion has brought new therapeutic promise for treatment of a potentially devastating illness. After angiography has confirmed a BA occlusion, patients have been treated with local catheter infusion of streptokinase or urokinase[33,36] or recombinant tissue plasminogen activator,[303] and with intravenously administered doses of the last.[304] The optimum route of administration, the optimum dose, and the need for and dangers of the concurrent or postinfusion use of platelet anti-aggregants, heparin, or warfarin have still to be defined. Endovascular techniques for treatment of BA disease also have untested promise for the future.

Common Clinical Phenomena

Ischemic disease of the BA and its branches can generate a wide variety of disturbances in ocular motility.[305] The more distinctive syndromes are described here.

Coma

Unresponsiveness to external stimuli occurs in some patients with BA occlusion. Chase and coworkers[91] analyzed eight of their own cases (7 basilar occlusions, 1 pontine hemorrhage) and 12 prior reports in an attempt to correlate the state of consciousness and electroencephalographic changes with the necropsy findings. Bilateral damage to the medial pontine tegmentum was present in all the comatose patients, whereas of the 11 patients with no more than unilateral tegmental damage, 8 were either alert or only "slightly obtunded." No patient with bilateral tegmental damage was fully alert. There was no reliable relationship between the resting electroencephalogram and the size or localization of the lesions, but attempts to activate the electroencephalography by voice or painful cutaneous stimuli were unsuccessful in the unresponsive patient. Lesions of the mesencephalic reticular formation

can produce prolonged coma.[306–308] In animals, damage to the central tegmental region in the rostral pons, midbrain, and dorsal hypothalamus is associated with unresponsiveness.[308] Lesions below the trigeminal nerve entry zone of the pons usually do not interrupt alertness in the experimental animal.[308]

Motor Signs

Paresis. Some paresis, either transient or persistent, accompanies nearly all cases of BA occlusion. Fisher[269] emphasized that the initial motor weakness can be quite lateralized, referring to this phenomenon as "herald hemiparesis of BA occlusion." Fisher[269] described five patients, in four of whom quadriparesis soon developed, and one of whom exhibited jerking of the limbs contralateral to the hemiparesis. Although hemiparesis may occur, the spared side invariably demonstrates some slight paresis, hyperreflexia, and Babinski's sign.[13]

It is of practical importance to separate clinically the paramedian penetrating branch lesions with hemiplegia from more serious BA occlusion with bilateral involvement. When basilar artery occlusion begins with a hemiplegia, the other limbs are generally affected within 24 hours. In one such case with angiographic verification of BA occlusion, which one of the chapter authors (LRC) personally examined, the patient was hemiplegic when first seen, but the contralateral limbs had episodic shivering movements; the next day he was quadriplegic. At times, the hemiplegia alternates from one side to the other. Biemond[293] described a patient who initially experienced a right hemiplegia; later, after the right limb weakness had cleared, she became dysarthric and had a left hemiplegia. Right hemiplegia, bilateral tongue and face weakness, and bilateral extensor plantar responses then developed. Postmortem examination showed the left VA to be occluded and the thrombus extended into the caudal BA.

Asymmetries probably depend on VA involvement, adequacy of collaterals on each side, and presence of distal emboli. In the 18 cases carefully studied by Kubik and Adams,[13] one side of the body was generally more affected than the other. Stupor often made precise motor examination difficult. Crossed motor paralysis, ipsilateral facial or conjugate gaze paralysis, and contralateral hemiparesis were found in 4 of the 18 cases studied by Kubik and Adams.[13] Among the 85 patients of Ferbert and colleagues[302] with angiographically proven BA occlusion, 31 patients had tetraparesis, 15 had tetraplegia, and 21 had hemiparesis at presentation. In France, a society has been founded to seek better treatment and outcome for patients with the locked-in syndrome.[309]

Decerebrate Responses. Decerebrate responses are common in patients with extensive BA infarction, although at times, the inferior extremity flexes as the arms extend, a response correlated with lesions at the level of the vestibular nuclei in the pontine tegmentum.[308] Some of the findings have the appearance of seizures in the opinion of some observers; in some patients, the responses take the form of tonic-clonic movements, in others they appear to be myoclonic jerks, and in still others they are fasciculation, shivering, and generalized nonclonic shaking movements.[310]

Locked-in Syndrome. Kemper and Romanul[307] described a patient who, although paralyzed and speechless, could move his eyes horizontally and raise his eyebrows. Postmortem examination of this case showed extensive destruction of the pontine base and only slight encroachment on the ventral part of the pontine tegmentum unilaterally. These researchers sought to differentiate this paralytic state from akinetic mutism, a condition in which the patient could, under certain circumstances, speak and move. Plum and Posner[308] coined the term *locked-in syndrome* to describe a state in which severe paralysis prevents the usual means of gestural or vocal communication. Usually the patient can communicate by way of vertical eye movements or blinking and can demonstrate full comprehension of his plight and the environment. In some locked-in patients, oral automatisms in the form of chewing and sucking movements can be reflex-induced by oral and perioral stimulation, indicating loss of voluntary control over bulbar masticatory function.[311] These patients have been likened to the character M. Noirtier de Villefort, in the Dumas novel *The Count of Monte Cristo*, who while encased in armor could not communicate except with his eyes.

The most common vascular lesion underlying the locked-in syndrome is BA occlusion with extensive destruction of the pontine base. Vertical eye movements are usually spared. Midbrain lesions may also produce a locked-in state. In one affected patient, the lesions were confined to the ventral mesencephalon, and eye and lid movement was preserved.[312] In another patient, studied only clinically, bilateral third cranial nerve paralysis, mutism, and quadriplegia were present, but the patient could signal with one hand.[313] Caplan and Zervas[314] described two similar patients with presumed Duret hemorrhages who could communicate by hand signals despite bilateral third cranial nerve paralysis and mutism. The necessary substrate for the locked-in syndrome is bilateral paralysis despite preserved consciousness.

Ataxia. Ataxia is frequently hidden by weakness and has been difficult to analyze, although the location of necropsy findings would predict its presence. Nystagmus is common in patients with tegmental ischemia but may be overshadowed by nuclear, internuclear, or gaze paresis. Vertical nystagmus commonly accompanies internuclear ophthalmoplegia and pontine infarction. Dysarthria, dysphagia, and facile laughing and crying can be due to pseudobulbar paralysis and are present to some degree in most patients with moderate to severe limb paresis.

Palatal Myoclonus. *Palatal myoclonus* is a rhythmic involuntary jerking movement of the soft palate and pharyngopalatine arch, often involving the diaphragm and laryngeal muscles.[315] It usually appears some time after the acute brainstem process, which is most often an infarction. The locus and nature of the responsible vascular lesion have not been analyzed, but the parenchymatous lesion involves the dentate nucleus of the cerebellum, the red nucleus, the inferior olivary nucleus, or their connections (the Guillain-Mollaret triangle). The dentate nucleus and contralateral inferior olive are somatotopically related. Fibers from the dentate nuclei travel in the superior cerebellar peduncle and decussate in the midbrain to the region of the contralateral red nucleus, from which the central tegmental tract descends to the inferior olivary nucleus of the same side.[316] The pathologic lesion most often seen in patients with palatal myoclonus is hypertrophic degeneration of the inferior olive, often associated with a lesion of the ipsilateral central tegmental tract or the contralateral dentate nucleus. The olivary lesion consists of enlarged neurons, loss of the other neurons, and gliosis, usually with enlargement of the olive; these changes are thought to be trans-synaptic and secondary to lesions of the neuronal system afferent to the inferior olivary nucleus.

The brachial movements may vary in rate (40 to 200 motions per min).[315] The patient may complain of an audible clicking noise due to movement of the eustachian tube, or the noise may be heard by the examiner applying a stethoscope to the lateral neck. The movements of the pharynx can be readily seen and are often accompanied by a fluttering of the diaphragm, which is usually obvious on chest fluoroscopy. Palatal myoclonus has surprisingly little effect on swallowing.

Neuro-ophthalmologic Observations

Ocular Bobbing. Fisher[317] introduced the term *ocular bobbing* to describe an unusual vertical movement of the eyes: "The eyeballs intermittently dip briskly downward through an arc of a few millimeters and then return to the primary position in a kind of bobbing action." He believed that this was a sign of "advanced pontine disease" and of little diagnostic importance because "the site of the disease process is usually obvious from the other ocular abnormalities" and clinical findings.

Fisher described three examples of ocular bobbing in pontine disease; two patients with pathologic documentation of BA occlusion and extensive infarction of the pontine base and tegmentum, and one with a pontine hemorrhage. In the patients with pontine lesions, voluntary and reflex horizontal gaze was lost. The eyes moved conjugately, but the vertical excursion of the bob was only one fourth to one third of the normal full voluntary vertical movement. Downward movement was quicker than upward; between downward jerks, the eyes rested quietly. Fisher also noted atypical bobbing, either dysconjugate, as in one case of cerebellar hemorrhage, or unilateral. Unilateral ocular bobbing occurred in a patient with a left sixth cranial nerve palsy and consisted of a downward bob of the left eye on attempted left lateral gaze. Nelson and Johnston[318] added four cases of bilateral ocular bobbing, all in patients with pontine hemorrhage, one of whom had a hemorrhage to the tegmentum and fourth ventricle.

The mechanism of ocular bobbing in pontine lesions proposed by Fisher[317] and supported by Nelson and Johnston[318] relates the bobbing to roving eye movements. In patients with coma due to bilateral supratentorial lesions, the eyes rove from side to side freely. In pontine lesions, horizontal gaze is lost but vertical gaze is preserved because the midbrain tegmentum is spared; therefore, the vertical vector of gaze is accentuated so that the eyes "bob" down. In addition, caloric irrigation increases the bobbing, acting as an afferent stimulus to gaze. Similarly, a unilateral bob (downward dip), when the affected eye is pointed toward the direction of paralytic lateral gaze, could evoke a downward movement.

Yap and colleagues[211] described two clinical cases of ocular bobbing (one vascular and one probably demyelinative) in which the ocular bobbing occurred synchronously with palatal myoclonus, raising the possibility that an unusual tremor or movement disorder affecting brainstem structures is a mechanism of bobbing. Bosch and colleagues[319] questioned the value of bobbing as a reliable sign of intrapontine disease; they presented a case of "typical ocular bobbing" (referring to bilateral conjugate downward movements) in a patient with a large cerebellar hemorrhage who had no extensive pontine lesion. However, that patient was in a deep coma and had distortion of the pons and a small unilateral Duret-type hemorrhage in the adjacent pontine tegmentum. Surely, distortion with physiologic disruption of pontine function was the basis of the bobbing, absence of horizontal gaze, and decerebration state.

Others have described ocular bobbing in cerebellar hemorrhage[317,320] and cerebellar infarction.[321] Newman and associates[322] described a patient in a coma after cranial gunshot wounds. The necrotic temporal lobe was removed, at which time the patient had no spontaneous or reflex oculocephalic eye movements. He became alert after surgery; ocular bobbing appeared and was accentuated during voluntary eye movements, especially when he attempted to gaze into fields of gaze with limitation of horizontal eye movements. We have also noted, in patients with pontine lesions (hemorrhage or infarction) and preserved consciousness, the tendency for bobbing to occur, bilaterally or unilaterally, on attempted voluntary gaze into a field of limited gaze. Newman and colleagues[322] raised the possibility that the vertical vectors could originate inferior to the lesion, for example, in the medulla or vestibular nuclei; they emphasized the possibility of recovery.

Ocular bobbing occurs in a variety of situations in which horizontal gaze is affected despite sparing of vertical gaze capabilities. It usually indicates pontine dysfunction due to an intrinsic pontine lesion, external pressure, or toxic or metabolic disruption of function.[323]

Skew Deviation. *Skew deviation* refers to an altered vertical position of the eyes, with one eye situated above the other and the vertical displacement remaining nearly constant in all planes of gaze. Skew is quite common in patients with brainstem infarction, especially those whose lesions are asymmetric. When skew deviation is associated with a unilateral internuclear ophthalmoplegia, the elevated eye is usually ipsilateral to the lesion.[324] Asymmetric lesions in the region of the vestibular nuclei, dorsolateral medulla, brachium pontis, cerebellum, and rostral midbrain may all produce skewing.

Internuclear Ophthalmoplegia. In the 1950s, Cogan and associates[325–327] revised the nomenclature and described the usual findings in patients with internuclear ophthalmoplegia. Earlier investigators had originally designated two types of internuclear ophthalmoplegia: an anterior type, in which the medial rectus muscle is paralyzed for conjugate movements toward the side of the lesion but functions normally in convergence and the lateral rectus muscle operates normally on lateral gaze, and a posterior type, in which both internal recti function normally on convergence and lateral gaze movements but the extremus on the side of the lesion is paralyzed for voluntary conjugate movements even though it can function on labyrinthine stimulation.

Smith and Cogan,[327] stating that posterior internuclear ophthalmoplegia was merely a partial sixth cranial nerve palsy, proposed a new designation that is now in common usage. In their terminology, internuclear ophthalmoplegia always involves paralysis of the adducting eye; the posterior type designates cases in which the medial rectus works normally during convergence, and the anterior type consists of absence of medial rectus function in either convergence or conjugate lateral gaze. In either type, nystagmus of the abducting eye occurs, a phenomenon that had led other writers to designate internuclear ophthalmoplegia as "ataxic nystagmus," a term still used in some regions.[328] Furthermore, analysis of 58 cases (29 unilateral and 29 bilateral) led Smith and Cogan[327] to assert that bilateral internuclear ophthalmoplegia was "invariably indicative of multiple sclerosis" and unilateral internuclear ophthalmoplegia was most commonly vascular in etiology.

Christoff and colleagues,[329] among others, reviewed previous examples of clinicopathologic correlation in patients with internuclear ophthalmoplegia and added three of their own; they implicated the ipsilateral medial longitudinal fasciculus (MLF) in the production of internuclear ophthalmoplegia. Damage to the right MLF would result in absence of adduction of the right medial rectus on leftward gaze and abducting nystagmus of the left eye. Vertical nystagmus and skew deviation were frequent concomitant findings. Gonyea[330] later described a number of patients with bilateral internuclear ophthalmoplegia due to vascular disease (only one had documented BA occlusion) and reviewed previous examples from the literature; as a result, he took exception to the dictum of Smith and Cogan[327] that bilateral involvement is invariably due to multiple sclerosis. In BA occlusion with extensive pontine infarction, tegmental infarcts are frequently patchy and asymmetric, so unilateral internuclear ophthalmoplegia is more common than the bilateral type. Absence of associated convergence does not necessarily implicate the more rostral midbrain MLF, as Cogan and associates[325,331] initially believed.

Although the eyes are generally conjugate at rest in patients with internuclear ophthalmoplegia, some patients have bilateral exotropia; this situation has been referred to as *wall-eyed bilateral internuclear ophthalmoplegia.*[332] Outward deviation of the eyes has been used as evidence of medial rectus nuclear involvement, but Gonyea[330] and Cogan and associates[325,331] emphasize that exotropia is to be anticipated with dysconjugate impairment of medial rectus function at any level, including the MLF.

MRI studies of patients with internuclear ophthalmoplegia showed damage of the MLF and adjacent structures.[333] When internuclear ophthalmoplegia was associated with loss of convergence or abnormality of abduction of the contralateral eye, the medial tegmental lesions were usually more extensive than when the only defect was an internuclear ophthalmoplegia.

Conjugate Horizontal Gaze Palsy. Fibers from the frontal eye fields affecting conjugate lateral gaze cross at or near the level of the abducens nucleus in the pons[296] and end in the reticular gray region in the neighborhood of the contralateral abducens nucleus.[334] This region is usually referred to as the *paramedian pontine reticular formation* (PPRF) or, by some, as the pontine lateral gaze center. Damage to the abducens nucleus can probably produce an ipsilateral gaze palsy for all lateral eye movements, voluntary and reflex (caloric or vestibulo-ocular).[335]

MRI shows that in patients with a unilateral abduction weakness (sixth cranial nerve palsy), the lesion invariably involves the intrapontine nerve fascicles and not the abducens nucleus.[99] Involvement of the PPRF leads to absence of voluntary lateral gaze to the side of the lesion with preservation of reflex movements.[335] The PPRF also mediates ipsilaterally directed saccades within the contralateral hemifield of movement. Bilateral lesions in the pontine tegmentum involving the abducens nucleus and PPRF produce paralysis of all horizontal eye movements, with sparing of vertical gaze because it is mediated at a more rostral level. Halsey and coworkers[336] described a patient with subsequently documented BA occlusion and infarction restricted to the basis pontis ventral to the PPRF who had absence of voluntary lateral gaze. Voluntary vertical gaze was preserved, and labyrinthine stimuli produced full conjugate lateral gaze except for absence of adduction of one eye (due to a more rostral MLF lesion). These investigators postulated that the descending fibers for voluntary conjugate gaze travel with the corticobulbar and aberrant corticobulbar fibers in the base of the pons in the region of the medial lemniscus. The senior author of this chapter (JPM) has observed one patient with pontine hemorrhage who was conscious but could not look voluntarily to either side; reflex lateral gaze could be readily evoked by doll's-eye maneuver. In unilateral lesions of the PPRF there is often some conjugate deviation of the eyes toward the contralateral side, but the deviation is less than is usually found with supratentorial lesions.

MRI studies of patients with unilateral conjugate gaze palsy show lesions in the paramedian pons, including the abducens nucleus, the nucleus reticularis pontis oralis, and the lateral portion of the nucleus reticularis pontis caudalis. These latter two structures are identified in animals as responsible for lateral gaze and contain burst neurons of the PPRF. Patients with bilateral horizontal gaze palsies usually have bilateral medial pontine lesions, but some have unilateral lesions that include the pontine tegmental raphe.[99] Patients with bilateral horizontal gaze palsies often also have slowness of vertical gaze saccades or limitation of upgaze. Horizontal gaze palsies are common in patients with BA occlusive disease. In one series of 85 patients with proven BA occlusion, 22 had a horizontal gaze palsy.[302]

One-and-a-Half Syndrome. Fisher[115] introduced the term *one-and-a-half syndrome* to refer to "a paralysis of eye movements in which one eye lies centrally and fails completely to move horizontally while the other eye lies in an abducted position and cannot be adducted past the midline." A unilateral pontine lesion involving the PPRF produces an ipsilateral conjugate gaze palsy and also affects the MLF on the same side, leading to paralysis of adduction of the ipsilateral eye on conjugate gaze to the opposite side.[115,335] MRI has disclosed infarcts affecting the superior, inferior, or widely scattered in the pons of patients with one-and-a-half syndrome.[337] If normal conjugate gaze to either side is rated 1, full horizontal gaze would score 2. Patients with combined PPRF and MLF lesions on one side only move a single eye in abduction to one side; they are therefore lacking one and one-half components of normal gaze. Others have called this deficit "paralytic pontine exotropia" because of the deviation of the eye at rest.[338]

Ptosis. Common in patients with BA occlusion, ptosis is usually attributed to involvement of the descending sympathetic fibers in the lateral pontine tegmentum. However, even with severe bilateral ptosis, the pupils may not be miotic.[115] Pontine ptosis is often more severe than the ptosis that usually accompanies peripheral Horner's syndrome or Horner's syndrome found in patients with lateral medullary syndrome. Pontine ptosis is often modified by involvement of the seventh cranial nerve or a hemiparesis.[339] In patients with hemiparesis, whether brainstem or supratentorial, ptosis is often more severe on the hemiparetic side. A peripheral type of facial weakness diminishes the ptosis by paralyzing the orbicularis oculi muscle, widening the palpebral fissure. If BA occlusion produces infarction of a third nerve nucleus, complete bilateral ptosis is the rule.

Pontine Pupils. Pupillary disturbances from pontine infarction are frequently pinpoint,[115] but reaction can be seen if a bright light and magnification are used.[308] When pontine and midbrain infarctions coexist, the pupils are often at midposition but poorly reactive. Lesions in the midbrain alone, with sparing of the pons, produce fixed dilated pupils. Pupillary constriction is more severe with pontine infarction or hemorrhage than with peripheral Horner's syndrome; some investigators have postulated parasympathetic irritation as well as a destructive sympathetic process to explain the pinpoint pupils.

Nystagmus. Common in patients with basilar occlusion, nystagmus varies in frequency of occurrence and severity of clinical presentation according to the locus of infarction and the severity of paresis of eye movements. Vertical nystagmus is an important sign of pontine infarction; rhythmic vertical nystagmus does not occur with higher brainstem lesions, although other disorders of vertical gaze are hallmarks of mesencephalic and diencephalic damage.[308]

Sensory Findings

Sensory findings are quite variable in BA occlusion and clearly depend on the locus of infarction. Stupor or altered capability of communication often makes determination of sensory abnormalities imprecise. Usually the motor dysfunction far outweighs the sensory signs. Perhaps this situation is explained by the predominantly medial location of infarction; the more lateral regions, which contain the spinothalamic tracts, and, more rostrally, the main somatosensory lemniscus are supplied by lateral circumferential collaterals and are relatively spared. Eleven of the 85 patients reported on by Ferbert and associates[302] were said to have a hemihypoesthesia. In our experience, hemisensory signs usually indicate additional involvement of the medulla (VA) or spread of infarction to the thalamus or PCA territory. Occasional patients with BA disease have bilateral, severe, unusual pain sensations in the face. Some patients have likened the feeling to having salt and pepper thrown on the face.[340] This symptom could be due to involvement of fibers crossing the midline from the trigeminal nuclei to join the medial border of the spinothalamic tracts. Alternatively, the symptoms could be explained by involvement of the nucleus raphe magnus in the periaqueductal gray matter. This nucleus has serotonergic projections to the spinal tracts of the fifth cranial nerve and their nuclei.

Clinical Manifestations

Abnormalities of Respiration

Abnormalities of respiration are also common, but their mechanism is difficult to determine because of the extensiveness of the infarction and the presence of general medical factors (aspiration, fever, hypoventilation). Apneustic breathing with a hang-up of the inspiratory phase and grossly regular breathing (ataxic respirations) occasionally occur terminally in patients with BA occlusion and carry an ominous prognosis. Fisher[323] and Plum and Posner[308] have summarized other respiratory irregularities and discussed their clinicoanatomic significances. Silverstein[291,341] has described the frequency of symptoms and signs in 83 patients with infarction within the "distribution of the BA."

Top of the Basilar Artery Occlusion

Occlusive lesions of the rostral tip of the BA lead to bilateral infarction of midbrain, thalamus, and occipital and medial temporal lobes. In this area, in addition to the major tributary branches of the basilar apex, the SCA, posterior communicating artery, and PCA, numerous smaller perforating midbrain arteries and vessels course through the posterior perforating substance to feed the hypothalamus and paramedian diencephalic structures (Fig. 10–11). Atherosclerosis is generally most severe in the proximal BA; in the more cephalad portion, atherosclerotic stenosis is less common, and the vessel gradually tapers in size. Occlusions of the basilar apex are generally embolic, arising from thrombi originating from the heart or proximal vertebrobasilar system.[109,221] Included in the list is Chagas' disease.[342] The extent of infarction depends on the size of the thrombus, the length of time it obstructs the main BA, its eventual destination in tributary vessels, and the adequacy of collateral circulation. In some cases, the ischemic damage is limited to one or both PCA hemispheric territories, and in others, the brunt of the damage is to the rostral brainstem structures.

At times the syndrome of rostral basilar territory ischemia occurs after posterior circulation angiography, usually in patients in whom the posterior circulation

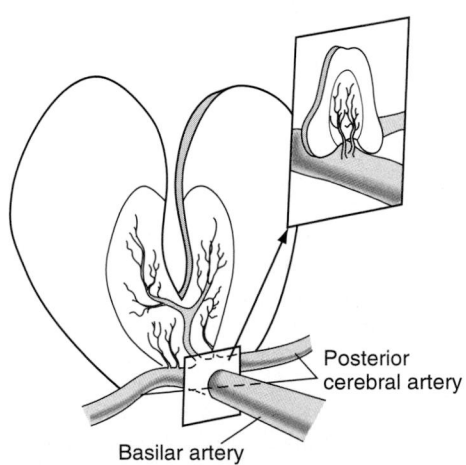

FIGURE 10–11 *Diagrammatic representations of blood supply from the distal basilar artery. Note the single midline vessel supplying the thalamus bilaterally. The area of infarction is the zone within the ellipse. Inset, Midbrain with shaded area of infarction.*

Posterior
cerebral artery

Basilar artery

vessels have been found to be widely patent and to have no important occlusive disease. Cortical blindness, agitated delirium, and an amnesic state are the cardinal features, usually with accompanying headache. The symptoms and signs reverse within 24 hours, leaving a permanent amnesia for the period of the angiography and its sequelae. Mehler[343,344] studied 61 patients with ischemia in the rostral BA territory. Fourteen of the patients (23%) had vascular stroke risk factors and previous episodes of vertebrobasilar ischemia and presented with severe bilateral vessel, oculomotor, and behavioral abnormalities; thrombosis engrafted on atherosclerotic stenosis and artery-to-artery emboli from the proximal system were common mechanisms of stroke in this group. The remaining 47 patients had less severe syndromes that were often reversible. Cardiac embolism was more prominent in this second group. Among the total series of 61 cases, 28 (46%) were considered to have an embolic cause (8 intra-arterial, 14 of cardiac origin, and 6 of unknown source). In situ thrombosis was believed to be responsible in 11 patients (18%), and 7 patients (11%) had symptoms after angiography, some of whom had documented transient contrast extravasation.

In the following section, we discuss findings only in patients with embolism or atherosclerotic occlusions of the BA apex in whom ischemia involves multiple tributaries of the BA. Similar findings, although of more limited extent, can occur in branch occlusions of these basilar apex branches; they are reviewed later (see discussions of midbrain, thalamic, and SCA territory infarcts in the section on basilar branch occlusion).

Major Clinical Syndromes

Abnormalities of Alertness, Attention, and Behavior. The medial mesencephalon and diencephalon contain the most rostral portions of the reticular activating system. Infarcts in these regions frequently affect consciousness, sleep, and behavior. Facon and colleagues[345] and Castaigne and associates[117] described patients with basilar apex occlusions in whom prolonged sleep and third cranial nerve palsies were the most prominent features. Segarra[346] later outlined the distribution of the infarction that causes this syndrome, which he believed was due to occlusion of the perforating branches of the mesencephalic artery (the first portion of the PCA as it courses around the midbrain). These vessels, which have been studied by Foix and Hillemand,[11] Lazorthes,[71] Percheron,[86] and Castaigne and associates,[88] are called the *paramedian mesencephalic arteries* and the *anterior and posterior thalamosubthalamic paramedian arteries.* They form the most rostral group of vessels in the posterior perforated substance and supply the paramedian midbrain and diencephalon. There is some evidence that a single midline vessel may branch to supply both banks of the third ventricle (Fig. 10–12).[88] Because the reticular gray matter is adjacent to the third cranial nerve nuclei and the vertical gaze regions near the posterior commissure, somnolence is invariably associated with pupillary abnormalities, third cranial nerve palsies, and defects of vertical gaze, although lateralized motor or sensory signs are often absent. A similar syndrome can occur after herniation, presumably as a result of extension pressure on these same vascular structures, caused by

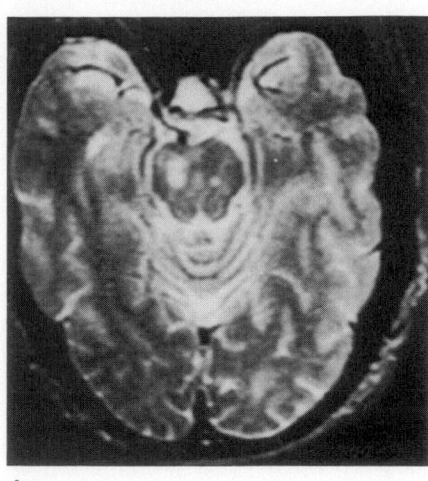
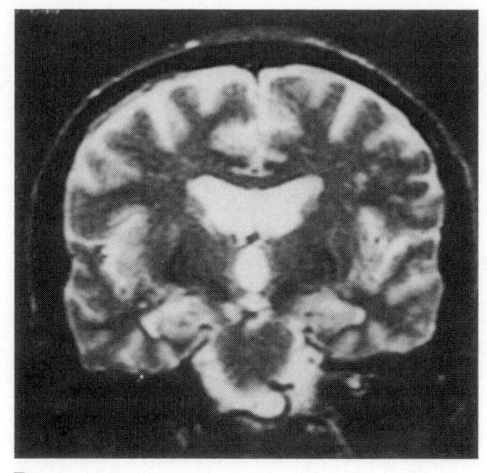

A   B

FIGURE 10–12   *T2-weighted MR images of pontomesencephalic infarct. (A) Axial plane. (B) Coronal plane.*

wedging of the mammillary bodies into the interpeduncular fossa, a situation that causes either median brainstem infarction[347] or Duret hemorrhages.[314] Among our own patients, one with a large putaminal hemorrhage survived the acute stroke but was left with third cranial nerve palsies and slept nearly continuously for 2 years in a nursing home. Postmortem examination showed an old slit cavity in the putamen and that butterfly distribution infarctions in the medial midbrain and thalamus had developed, probably during the period of herniation. Of 28 patients with rostral brainstem infarcts studied by Castaigne and associates,[88] 15 had hypersomnia caused by paramedian tegmental lesions, usually bilateral.

Pupillary Abnormalities. When ischemia affects the medial midbrain tegmentum or medial diencephalon, pupillary reactivity is usually abnormal, because the afferent limb of the pupillary reflex arc is interrupted in its course from the optic tract of the Edinger-Westphal nucleus. Midbrain pupils are frequently eccentric (corectopia iridis) and may acutely shift position.[348,349] If the lesion affects only the Edinger-Westphal nucleus, the pupils are generally fixed and dilated, but if rostral extension of the lesion occurs with resultant sympathetic paralysis, the deficit involves a midposition, fixed pupil. In some cases the pupil is oval, a phenomenon that is usually transient and most often found in patients with supratentorial vascular catastrophes that lead to tentorial herniation.[350] Occasionally a pupil becomes oval in a patient with midbrain infarction when a third cranial nerve paralysis is developing or recovering.[350] Thalamic infarcts are associated with small, poorly reactive pupils.

Among 61 patients with rostral BA territory infarction, Mehler[344] found that 18 (30%) had abnormal pupillary size, shape, or function. Six patients had discrepancies in pupillary reaction between accommodation and light stimuli. Despite abnormal light reactivity, 4 patients with dorsal midbrain infarcts had constriction on forced lid closure, normal dilatation with psychosensory stimuli, normal-sized pupils, and normal dilatation in response to drugs applied locally. Two other patients had normal pupillary light reactions but impaired response to convergence accommodation.

Oculomotor Dysfunction. Vertical gaze–vertical plane eye movements are voluntarily generated by bilaterally simultaneous activation of the frontal and parietal occipital conjugate gaze centers. Vertical gaze pathways then converge on the periaqueductal region beneath the collicular plate, near the interstitial nucleus of Cajal and the posterior commissure.[351–353] In this region in the monkey, there is a cluster of neurons important in vertical gaze; it is situated among fibers of the medial longitudinal fasciculus and is generally referred to as the *rostral interstitial nucleus* of the MLF[354] or the *nucleus of the prerubral field.*[353] Clinically, there is often a disparity between paralysis of voluntary vertical gaze and vertical eye movements reflex-induced by vertical doll's-eyes maneuver, bilateral simultaneous caloric stimulation, or Bell's phenomenon, although the anatomic basis for the disparity is not clear. Most commonly, upgazes and downgazes are affected together. Debate still centers on the question whether such dysfunctions occur only with bilateral lesions, because unilateral stereotactic placed lesions[355] or unilateral vascular[356] and metastatic[145] lesions have on occasion produced upward gaze paralysis. In monkeys and humans, lesions of the pretectum in the posterior commissure region are necessary to produce paralysis of upward gaze.[357,358] Selective paralysis of downward gaze is much rarer; when it occurs, the lesions usually border the red nucleus and lie more ventral and caudal, producing paralysis of upward gaze.[353,359,360]

In one patient with selective downgaze palsy, the lesions were situated bilaterally in the dorsolateral periaqueductal gray matter, involving the crossing fibers of the commissure of the superior colliculus.[361] The eyes may rest down and are often skewed in asymmetric lesions of the mesodiencephalic junction.[271] Some patients with unilateral lesions of the paramedian midbrain and caudal diencephalon have abnormal control of head and eye posture in the roll plane.[362] Halmagyi and colleagues[362] reported four patients and Mehler[344] two patients with ocular tilt reactions. All of these patients had a head tilt, conjugate eye torsion, and skewing with hypotropia to the side ipsilateral or contralateral to the mesodiencephalic lesion. All patients with ocular tilt reactions also had vertical, predominantly upward gaze, palsies. Some patients with mesodiencephalic infarcts have had vertical one-and-a-half syndrome.[363,364] Deleu and coworkers[364] reported a patient in whom all downward saccadic and smooth pursuit eye movements were lost bilaterally, but only a monocular paresis of upgaze was present. MRI showed the lesion to be confined to the rostral interstitial nucleus of the MLF bilaterally. These investigators hypothesized that the lesion affected upgaze premotor fibers in the tracts from these nuclei before or after their decussation in the posterior commissure. Bogousslavsky and Regli[363] reported a patient with a unilateral mesodiencephalic lesion with bilateral upgaze palsy but only monocular paresis of downgaze. Unilateral lesions, by affecting the crossing or commissural fibers, can produce bilateral defects in vertical gaze. Among Mehler's[344] series of 61 patients with top of the basilar territory infarction, 47 (77%) had some abnormality of vertical eye position or gaze.

Abnormalities of Convergence. Ocular convergence is probably controlled in the medial midbrain tegmentum, although there is considerable debate as to whether a formal nuclear structure, such as the nucleus of Perlia, subserves this function. One or both eyes may rest in, and convergence vectors are frequently evident on attempted upward gaze. Rhythmic convergence nystagmus may be elicited by having the eyes follow a downgoing opticokinetic target. Convergence vectors may also modify lateral gaze. Voluntary lateral movements of the lateral rectus are balanced against convergence vectors, thus limiting abduction and giving the superficial appearance of a sixth cranial nerve palsy (pseudo–sixth nerve palsy).[271] Lid abnormalities are also a common sign of rostral brainstem disease. Unilateral infarction of a third cranial nerve nucleus can lead to complete bilateral ptosis.[339] Retraction of the upper lid, giving the eye a prominent stare (Collier's sign), is also common in tectal lesions.[365]

Hallucinations. Complaints of hallucination are also made by patients with rostral brainstem infarction, leading to application of the term *peduncular hallucinosis*, first used by Lhermitte[366] in 1922 and then by Van Bogaert.[367,368] All of the patients who have been described with this phenomenon have experienced hallucinations at twilight or during the night, and all have sleep disorders (nocturnal insomnia or daytime hypersomnolence).[271] The hallucinations are usually vivid, are most commonly visual, and contain multiple colors, objects, and scenes. Blood and red hair, horses and green serpents against a red background, and brightly plumed parrots are examples. Occasionally, auditory or tactile hallucinations are associated. Similar hallucinations also accompany sleep deprivation or drug intoxication and may relate to dysfunction of the reticular activating system.

In addition to hallucinations, impulsive reports, which have been called *extraordinary confabulation*, are often made by patients with rostral brainstem infarcts.[369] They consist of descriptions of behavior or present whereabouts that are totally unrealistic. The reports have no approximation to reality and are influenced by surrounding stimuli. For example, a 60-year-old woman was questioned while a newscast of a school incident was on an adjacent television set. She said that she was in school at a lunch bar ready to order English muffins and, if the examiners did not get out of the way, she would be late for her next

seventh grade class. When asked why she was wearing a nightgown and seemed to be in a hospital bed, she said that she was too lazy that day to get fully dressed and simply came to school in her nightgown in bed. Similarly, other patients have incorporated into their replies reality items provided by the questioner. Many such patients "dream a lot," and they may be reporting their imaginings as reality.

In most patients with peduncular hallucinations, the lesions have been large, making it difficult to relate the abnormality to any particular anatomic structure. McKee and associates[370] reported a single patient with peduncular hallucinations who had very discrete small bilateral lesions in the medial portions of the substantia nigra pars reticulata. This patient was a diabetic man with previous third cranial nerve palsies that developed 2 years apart, each recovering within 2 months. After a seizure, the patient reported visual hallucinations of animals and people with obscured faces walking across his field of vision. Often these visual hallucinations were preceded by the sensation of being touched on the shoulder or face. The lesions were limited entirely to the pars reticulata and may have affected adjacent fibers of the third cranial nerve just medial to the infarcts, but tegmental structures were completely spared. The pars reticulata has connections with the pedunculopontine nucleus and shows increased discharge during rapid eye movement sleep.

Hemiballism and Abnormal Movements. It has long been known that involuntary movements occur from deep upper brainstem lesions. In 1927, Martin[371] described a hypertensive man who suddenly developed violent movements of the right limbs associated with facial grimacing, dysarthria, agitation, and finally death. Necropsy revealed a small hemorrhage located in the left subthalamus in the region of the subthalamic nucleus (corpus Luysii). Martin[371] reviewed 12 earlier cases of hemichorea associated with lesions in this region that were verified postmortem; the lesions were small hemorrhages in 8 cases and metastases in 3, and in 1 case the lesion was unspecified.

Whittier[372] later reviewed the subject and attempted to differentiate *ballism*—that is, incessant violent, limb flinging proximal movements—from other types of adventitious movements such as chorea. Lesions in 30 of the cases he reviewed involved the subthalamic region or "the connections of this region." The most common etiology was hemorrhage, but infarctions in this region were also described. Moersch and Kernohan[373] noted a single patient with hemiballism due to two small adjacent softenings in the subthalamic nucleus but unfortunately did not comment on the offending vascular lesion.

It has become clear from CT correlation that lesions in other sites, especially the striatum and thalamus, can produce a movement disorder difficult to distinguish from that caused by lesions in the subthalamic nucleus.[301] Infarction of the subthalamus can result in a severe movement disorder that is unilateral and characterized by nearly constant flinging and often rotatory proximal arm and leg movements on one side of the body. Frequently, a hemiparesis precedes or follows the movement disorder, the movement disappearing as the limbs are paralyzed and returning when the paralysis clears. Unfortunately, the offending vascular lesion in the subthalamus, which is fed by branches of the posterior communicating and posterior choroidal arteries and the PCA, has seldom if ever been characterized.[373] One of the authors (LRC) has seen a patient in whom unilateral hemiballism was associated with stupor and eye signs typical of basilar apex brainstem infarction (no hemorrhage on CT), but unfortunately, the patient's vascular lesion was not verified.

Abnormal movements other than ballistic were present in 7 of 28 patients with rostral brainstem infarcts studied by Castaigne and associates.[88] The movements were frequently delayed in onset and had a predilection for the face, arm, and thumb. Clonic, athetoid, and myoclonic movements were described in patients with bilateral paramedian thalamic infarcts that at times extended to the upper pole of the red nucleus and affected Meynert's tract and the decussation of the brachium conjunctivum. When emboli block the penetrating vessels of the basilar apex, limb paralysis is usually transient or absent. When the most proximal portion of the PCA is affected, a contralateral hemiplegia may occur, at times accompanied by a contralateral third nerve palsy.[82] Often, however, the clinical findings are dominated by unilateral or bilateral PCA territory hemispheral infarction.

Basilar Branch Disease

A heterogeneous group of disorders, *basilar branch disease* involves all occlusive disease arising in small or larger branches of the basilar arteries. Convenient subdivisions, which are used in this discussion, are (1) intraparenchymatous occlusions resulting in lacunar infarctions due to hypertensive arteriolopathy, usually within the tiny penetrating parenchymatous vessels, (2) extraparenchymatous occlusion of small branches, such as median pontine or thalamogeniculate arteries, usually by miniature atherosclerotic plaques or junctional lesions involving the BA wall,[135,279] and (3) stenosis or occlusion of larger circumferential branches, such as the AICA and SCA.

Lacunar Infarctions

Lacunes are the single most common lesion found in the brainstem at postmortem examination. These small deep infarcts are caused by disruption of vessels less than 200 μm in diameter by lipohyalinosis or, less commonly, by blockage of arteries 0.1 to 1 mm in diameter by miniature atherosclerotic plaques.[139] Precise clinicopathologic correlation has been infrequent, because the prognosis for recovery from the individual strokes is good, leaving less opportunity for pathologic confirmation. At postmortem examination, lacunes tend to be multiple, providing a dilemma as to which ones were responsible for which symptoms or signs. A lacunar infarct can vary from a pinpoint hole to a larger cavitated lesion 1.5 cm in diameter. Lacunes are most common in the pons and thalamus but do occur in the medulla and midbrain. In the medulla, pons, and midbrain, the lesions usually occupy the basal portion,[374] especially medially, seldom extend far into the tegmentum, and are never limited solely to the tegmentum.

Fisher's[375] intent in describing specific lacunar syndromes was to call attention to combinations of clinical findings that had an extremely high probability of being caused by lacunar infarctions; many lacunes, however, manifest as slight deficits impossible to distinguish from incomplete stroke due to large vessel disease or embolism. The risk factors for the well-defined syndromes help make them a homogeneous group, separable from other small deep infarcts not associated with the most commonly defined syndrome.[376] Several syndromes known to be caused by brainstem lacunes are reviewed in the following sections.

The tempo of lacunar infarctions in the posterior circulation has been similar to that of infarctions in a supratentorial location.[377] TIAs occur but are less common than with larger vessel disease. The neurologic deficit usually develops over a period of hours to a few days and rarely evolves over more than 7 days. There is no accompanying headache. The patients generally remain alert. Hypertension, either previous or current, is the nearly invariable requirement for the development of lacunes; the diagnosis should not be made in its absence. Other syndromes also occur, including pure dysarthria and toppling to the side whenever the erect position is attained but an absence of symptoms and signs when the patient is examined supine or seated, and pure sensory stroke of just half the face and head. The pathologic basis for these lesions is unknown, but the etiology, tempo of onset, clinical course, and negative radiologic findings all suggest lacunar infarction as the most probable cause. The main lacunar syndromes are briefly described here and more thoroughly described in Chapter 11.

Pure Motor Hemiplegia. Weakness of the face, arm, and leg is not accompanied by visual or sensory signs or deficits of higher cortical function in pure motor hemiplegia. Of the nine original patients studied by Fisher,[378] three had lesions in the basis pontis. One of these patients also had a conjugate gaze paresis to the ipsilateral side, identifying the pontine locus of the stroke. Transient tegmental symptoms or signs (diplopia, dizziness, nystagmus, or internuclear ophthalmoplegia), prominent dysarthria, an ataxic quality to the movements of the hemiparetic side, and bilateral extensor plantar reflexes sometimes give a clue to the brainstem origin. To date, CT has not been effective in predictably verifying these lesions, although one of us (LRC) has seen one patient with a previous pure motor hemiparesis in whom, months after the stroke, a definite pontine lacune was seen on CT. MRI is the best imaging technique to show lacunar infarcts.[379, 380] A lacune in the medial medullary pyramid[381–383] or cerebral peduncle[384] can also produce a pure motor hemiparesis, usually with sparing of the face in medullary lesions. A progressing pure motor syndrome in eight cases with infarction extending to the ventral pontine surface has been described.[385]

Dysarthria–Clumsy Hand Syndrome. The cardinal features of dysarthria–clumsy hand syndrome are moderate to severe dysarthria, corticobulbar weakness of the lower face and tongue, and slowness of fine movements of one hand. In some cases there is slight ataxia, hyperreflexia, or Babinski's sign on the side of the clumsy hand. The lesion is a small infarct in the dorsal basis pontis just below the medial lemniscus, disrupting the corticobulbar fibers in this location.[386] The limb findings are due to dysfunction of extrapyramidal or pyramidal fibers within the basis pontis.

Ataxic Hemiparesis. A syndrome in which motor hemiparesis (usually of slight degree) occurs with incoordination of the cerebellar type is termed *ataxic hemiparesis*.[137] Occasionally, the pyramidal and cerebellar dysfunction is limited to the lower extremity; this variant is then called homolateral ataxia and crural hemiparesis.[387] The lesion responsible for ataxic hemiparesis is usually in the more rostral pons, interrupting crossing fibers as well as the pyramidal fibers in the pontine base. We have also seen a patient with this syndrome whose postmortem lesion involved the brachium conjunctivum and cerebral peduncle at the midbrain level. Slight ataxia of the other (normal) leg has been a clue to the pontine location of this syndrome. At times, horizontal or vertical nystagmus and dysarthria accompany the limb ataxia and hemiparesis.[137]

Pure Sensory Stroke. A lacune in the somatosensory nuclei of the thalamus and ventral posterolateral and ventral posteromedial nuclei produces sensory symptoms on the opposite side of the body and face without motor, cerebellar, or higher cortical function abnormalities.[375,388–390] Paresthesias are usually characterized as tingling, prickling, or a sleepy, cold, hard, numb, or dead feeling. Usually at least two parts, such as face and arm or arm and leg, are involved.[388] The limbs are involved more than the face, but often the whole hemicorpus is affected, including the abdomen, chest, and face (as well as the eye, ear, and inside of the mouth). Cortical representation in the postcentral gyrus for the ear, eye, and trunk is quite small. Involvement of these structures usually signifies a lesion in a tract or a thalamic nucleus rather than a parietal cortical lesion. When the hand is affected, usually all digits are affected. The symptoms of sensory dysfunction commonly far exceed the objective signs; in fact, objective parameters of sensory function may be completely normal. In one reported patient with a right lateral thalamic lacune, the sensory loss consisted only of proprioceptive loss, the temperature and pain sensations both being intact.[391]

Helgason and Wilbur[392] described 10 patients with pontine infarcts identified on MRI in whom sensory symptoms and signs were the most prominent clinical findings. In 4 of the patients, infarcts were localized to the lateral pontine tegmentum at various levels.

Sensorimotor Stroke. A lacune may involve both the thalamic sensory nuclei and the adjacent posterior limb of the internal capsule. This picture leads to a combination of hemiparesis, pyramidal signs, and hemisensory loss, all on the contralateral side, unaccompanied by visual or intellectual dysfunction.[393] This syndrome is nearly impossible to differentiate from larger vessel ischemic disease or deep hemorrhage except with CT and angiography.

Basilar Branch Arteries in Their Extraparenchymatous Course

Occlusion of medium-sized penetrating vessels is probably quite common, but the disease within these vessels has been verified in detail in only three cases.[135,279] All of these patients were hypertensive and, in addition, two had known diabetes. Atherosclerotic basilar branch disease is probably more common than is currently realized.[130] Diagnosis rests on a clinical syndrome limited to dysfunction in a unilateral branch[8,10,12,79] and CT or MRI[379,394] findings of

infarction in the territory of a single branch. The infarct may extend to the pontine basal surface, confirming that the occlusive process must have involved the branch before penetration of the parenchyma (Fig. 10–13). MRA or standard arterial opacification through catheters shows the patency of the parent BA. Kumral and associates[395] studied 150 cases of consecutive pontine brainstem infarcts and found that they could be sorted into five syndromic clusters—anteromedial (58%), anterolateral (17%), tegmental (56%), bilateral (11%), and unilateral multiple (4%). The cause of stroke was most often BA branch disease and far less often large artery basilar disease. Few reports have documented syndromic change with recurrent pontine infarction. Kim and colleagues[396] found five such cases; the recurrent event added to the initial syndrome quadriparesis, dysarthria, and dysphagia, features not present in a matched group of five patients with pontine infarcts who did not suffer recurrence.

Basilar Branch Occlusion with Pontine Infarcts. The two patients with unilateral basilar branch occlusion had transient tegmental signs: ipsilateral small pupil in one patient, and lateral gaze palsy, internuclear ophthalmoplegia, and horizontal and vertical nystagmus in the other.[135]

One patient with bilateral branch occlusion was a hypertensive diabetic man who, 2 months previously, had had a minor stroke characterized by right hemiparesis, dysarthria, and transient diplopia.[130] This lesion was later

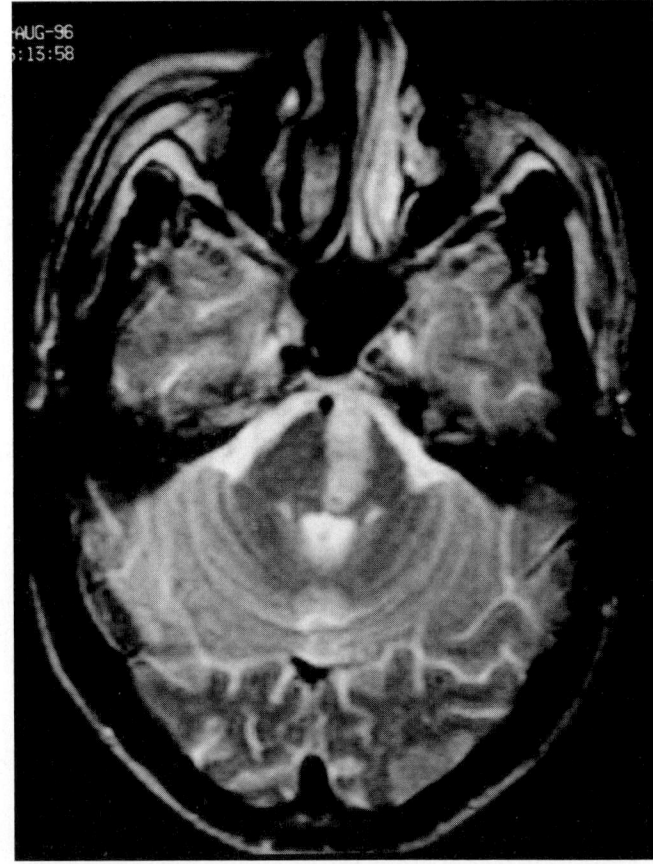

FIGURE 10–13 *Paramedian infarct in the pons on a T2-weighted MR image. Note that the basilar artery is patent.*

traced to a bead of atheroma blocking a left pontine paramedian branch. He then demonstrated dysarthria and a severe left hemiparesis. After his blood pressure was lowered precipitously and heparin was given, the patient became quadriplegic and lost all lateral gaze. Those caring for the patient (LRC) thought he had an occlusion of the main BA with extensive pontine infarction. To everyone's surprise, postmortem examination showed the BA to be widely patent and the vascular lesions to be limited to two adjacent paramedian branches. There was an old infarct in the left pons, and fresh infarctions were superimposed in both the left and right paramedian zones of the pontine base. In this case, prior branch occlusion and rapid reduction in blood pressure led to a large zone of ischemia much wider than would be expected in disease of a single branch. The pathology of the branch lesions in this case was described earlier in this chapter.

The distribution and size of pontine infarcts depends heavily on the anatomy of the penetrating artery branches. Figure 10–14 shows the distribution within the pons of the arterial territories; the drawings were modeled after those of Foix and Hillemand,[11] Gillian,[79] and Duvernoy.[67] The four major arterial territories are anteromedial, anterolateral, lateral tegmental, and posterior.[67] Foix and Hillemand[10] in 1926 and Lhermitte and Trelles[12] in 1934 first focused attention on small unilateral pontine infarcts, either paramedian infarcts or small lacunes, as infarcts *en chapelet* (Fig. 10–15). These investigators summarized

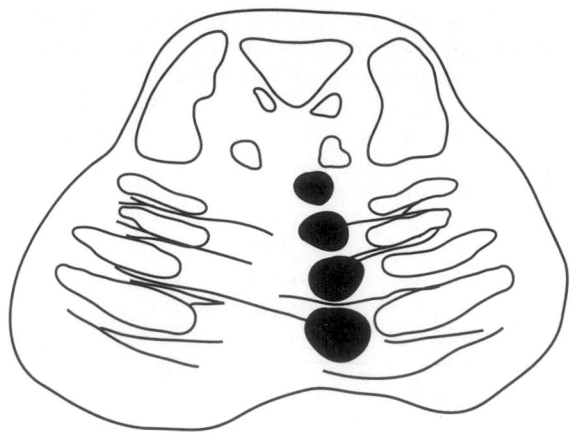

FIGURE 10–15 *Infarcts en chapelet by Foix and Hillemand. (From Foix C, Hillemand P: Contribution à l'étude des ramollissements protubérantiels. Rev Med 43:287, 1926.)*

their experience without describing their case material in detail. They realized that these ventral pontine infarcts may have a different clinical presentation from that of pontine tumors or hemorrhages, in which tegmental signs (i.e., cranial nerve involvement) are common, giving rise to complex syndromes (Millard-Gübler, Foville's, and other alternating syndromes). They called attention to a few patients presenting with clinical symptoms and signs of these paramedian pontine infarcts, described as pure motor hemiparesis, hemiparesis with crural predominance at times associated with some ataxia of cerebellar type (forme fruste of cerebellar signs), or some clumsiness of a limb.[10] Bilateral infarcts in the ventromedial area of the pons were responsible for pseudobulbar signs due to bilateral lacunes[10] and for pontine paraplegia in cases of larger infarcts.[12]

In their initial description, Foix and Hillemand[10] noted that these pontine infarcts are due to involvement of one of the paramedian pontine arteries (i.e., penetrator branches) and that larger paramedian infarcts were due to BA disease that blocks the origin of one or several paramedian arteries.[254] Lhermitte and Trelles[12] established a parallel between small paramedian and short circumferential arteries and lenticulostriate arteries; both arise at right angles from a very large parent artery (the BA for the former and the MCA for the latter), and their ostia may frequently be blocked by atherosclerotic plaques within the BA.[397] Landmark demonstration of BA branch occlusions was brought forth in 1971 by Fisher and Caplan,[135] as reported previously.[76] Foix and Hillemand[10] also reported on pontine infarcts in the lateral territory of the short circumferential arteries with isolated ipsilateral cerebellar signs involving the arm and leg described as cerebellar hemiplegia.

Infarcts in these territories have been reevaluated with MRI.[379,394,398,399] The most common site of infarction is medial along the base in the territory of the large anteromedial penetrating arteries. Bassetti and colleagues[379] reported the MRI lesions in their patients with infarcts in the pons to be in anteromedial territory. Of their 36 patients with isolated pontine infarcts, 12 (33%) had

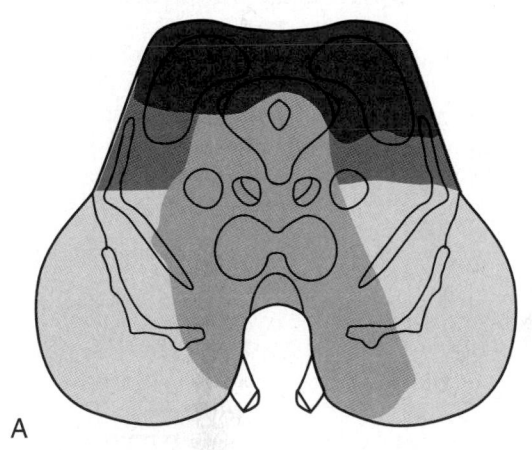

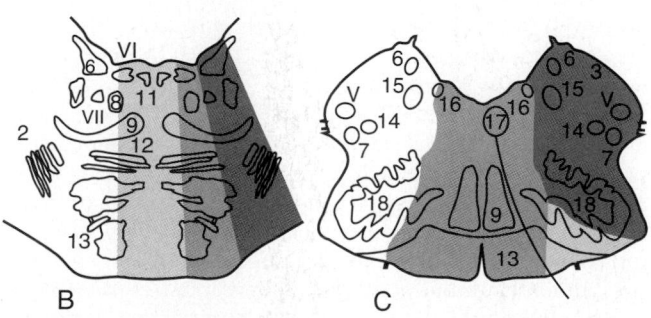

FIGURE 10–14 *Drawing of the arterial territories in the (A) medulla, (B) pons, and (C) mesencephalon.*

lesions in this distribution. Anterolateral infarcts are probably the next most common distribution. These infarcts are located in the basis pontis but more lateral than the medial basal infarcts. Infarcts in this anterolateral distribution tend to be smaller than medial lesions, probably because the penetrating arteries are smaller. Hematomas in this location are also smaller than medial pontine hemorrhages. Anterolateral infarcts were found in 9 of the 36 patients (25%) in the series reported by Bassetti and colleagues.[379] The lateral territory of the caudal pons, including the lateral tegmental area, is usually supplied by branches arising from the AICA. The lateral portion of the tegmentum in the rostral portion of the pons is fed by penetrating artery branches of the long circumferential arteries (usually the SCAs). Lateral tegmental infarcts are less common than basis pontis infarcts. The posterior (dorsomedial) territories are supplied by a variety of circumferential arteries and are not known to be supplied by penetrating artery branches. Infarcts in the distribution of these circumferential vessels are usually accompanied by cerebellar infarcts or more widespread brainstem infarction due to BA occlusion. The most difficult infarcts to classify according to territory are those lesions that are purely tegmental but are not in the midline. This region is probably fed by anteromedial, anterolateral, and lateral tegmental branches varying in individual patients.

Basilar Branch Occlusion with Midbrain Infarcts. Lipohyalinosis and atheromatous branch occlusions also occur frequently in arterial penetrating branches of the BA apex and the adjacent basilar communicating, posterior communicating, and proximal posterior cerebral arteries. MRI is now able to identify infarcts limited to the territory of individual penetrating branches.[394,400] However, the only pathologic studies of lesions in penetrating arteries have been Fisher's[388,389,401] studies of patients with pure sensory stroke due to lateral thalamic infarction.

Paramedian arteries originate from the proximal basilar communicating artery (also called the P1 segment of the PCA by some) and supply the cerebral peduncles, medial portions of the substantia nigra, fascicles of the third cranial nerve, and the red nuclei.[82,402] Peduncular perforating arteries originate from the distal end of the basilar communicating arteries and the proximal portions (P2a) of the PCAs as they course around the peduncles.[11,67,79,82] These arteries supply the more lateral portions of the ventral midbrain, including the lateral portions of the cerebral peduncles and substantia nigra.

Clinical studies have demonstrated a spectrum of syndromes based on medial, lateral, posterior, and combined mesencephalic infarcts.[403] Infarctions in the territory of the paramedian penetrating mesencephalic arteries are probably responsible for some examples of Weber's syndrome (ipsilateral third cranial nerve palsy and contralateral hemiplegia), Claude's syndrome (ipsilateral third cranial nerve palsy and contralateral limb dysmetria due to involvement of the lower part of the red nucleus), and Benedikt's syndrome (ipsilateral third cranial nerve palsy and contralateral movement disorders due to involvement of the upper part of the red nucleus). Some diabetic third cranial nerve palsies probably involve the parenchymatous portions of the third cranial nerve before the fascicle exit from the midbrain.[404] Unilateral nuclear involvement of the third

cranial nerve by a small infarct results in vertical gaze paresis[405] and bilateral ptosis.[127] Pure motor hemiplegia could also result from infarction limited to the cerebral peduncle. In the case of peduncular hallucinosis related to bilateral infarcts in the substantia nigra pars reticulata cited earlier, infarction was probably due to bilateral small paramedian artery disease.[370] An organized occlusion with recanalization was identified in one small penetrating artery within the substantia nigra. Some patients with caudal midbrain infarcts have predominant sensory abnormalities.[400]

In the series reported by Bogousslavsky and coworkers,[400] 12 patients, all with infarcts in the middle midbrain group, had third nerve dysfunction. Five patients with paramedian tegmental infarcts showed evidence of involvement of the third nerve nucleus, which usually caused bilateral ptosis and bilateral superior rectus weakness. Some also had bilateral mydriasis. Two of these patients also had contralateral limb motor weakness or ataxia. The 7 patients with infarcts that were more ventral and lateral had peripheral-type unilateral third nerve paralysis without other major signs. In one of these patients, the palsy was only partial, involving just elevation and adduction of the ipsilateral eye. The other 6 patients had weakness of all third nerve–innervated muscles, severe ptosis, and mydriasis.[400] In a report from Tatemichi and colleagues,[394] 2 patients had nuclear third nerve palsies with a complete third nerve palsy on one side and ptosis and elevation palsy on the other side. Contralateral weakness or ataxia was often associated.

Basilar Branch Occlusion with Thalamic Infarcts. The four main groups of arteries penetrate the thalamus, arising from the region of the BA bifurcation, are two groups of thalamoperforating arteries, the polar (tuberothalamic) arteries and the thalamic-subthalamic (thalamoperforating) arteries, and the thalamogeniculate and the posterior choroidal arteries.

Polar Artery. The polar artery (also called the anterior internal optic artery by Duret,[1] the premammillary pedicle by Foix and Hillemand,[11,86,89] and the tuberothalamic artery[83,84]) usually arises from the middle portion of the posterior communicating artery to supply the anterolateral portion of the thalamus. In about a third of cases this artery is absent, and the thalamic-subthalamic artery also supplies this territory. The polar artery supply includes the lateral portion of the anterior thalamic pole but not the anterior nucleus. Portions of the ventral lateral, dorsomedial, and reticular nuclei are supplied as well as part of the mammillothalamic tract.[83,84,90] Supply is said to be always unilateral by single branches. Infarcts can result from penetrating branch disease or clipping of an ICA or posterior communicating artery aneurysm.

Unilateral infarcts cause minor or negligible contralateral motor signs, for example, slight often transient hemiparesis, asymmetric facial expression, slight asymmetry of arm swing, and spontaneous or automatic use of the contralateral limbs. Sensory and oculomotor findings are generally absent.[83,84,90] Cognitive and behavioral abnormalities predominate. Initially, patients may appear confused and disoriented. Later, the predominant findings are lack of initiation and spontaneity, long latency in responding, and inability to persevere with protracted tasks. Fisher[406] has called these deficits *abulia*. They are identical to the dysfunction found in patients with disease of the frontal lobes and caudate nuclei[407] and probably indicate loss of function of corticostriatothalamic projections from the anterior thalamic nuclei.[88]

Patients with left anterolateral thalamic infarcts may also have slight aphasic abnormalities with paraphasic errors and verbal perseverations, but they retain the ability to repeat spoken language.[83] With right anterolateral thalamic infarction, constructional praxis and visual-spatial abnormalities may also be found.[83,90] Verbal memory is affected in left-sided lesions, and visual memory in right-sided infarcts.[84,408] The abulia and cognitive and behavioral abnormalities are often transient and usually regress and substantially recover during the 3 to 6 months after the stroke. Kotila and colleagues[409] studied cognitive functions during the acute phase and after 1 year in seven patients with left polar artery territory infarcts. The most severe impairments in these patients were in memory functions. The memory performance of all the patients was far below average, and five fulfilled criteria for having amnesic syndromes. The most severe deficits were in memorizing verbal material. Intellectual performances generally improved to normal, including orientation and visual memory. Verbal memory also improved, but difficulties remained in the learning and recall of verbal material and names of individuals.[409] The memory deficits prevented three of the four patients who attempted to return to work from retaining their previous jobs.

The abulia and apathy often improve dramatically in patients with unilateral lesions. Occasional patients have been reported with bilateral, nearly symmetric polar artery territory infarcts.[410] One patient suddenly became abulic and unconcerned after cardiac catheterization and has remained abnormal—very apathetic and unmotivated in the years since. Memory loss and abulia are more severe and more persistent in patients with bilateral lesions. The occurrence of bilateral isolated polar artery territory infarcts suggests that, in some patients, the polar artery, like the thalamic-subthalamic arteries, may emerge from a single artery or an arcade of vessels.[86,410] Polar territory infarcts are responsible for what has been referred to as "acute thalamic dementia."

Thalamic-Subthalamic Arteries. The thalamic-subthalamic arteries (also called interpeduncular profunda arteries, the paramedian thalamic arteries by Percheron,[86,89] the posterior internal optic arteries by Duret,[1] and the thalamoperforating pedicle by Foix and Hillemand[11]) arise from the basilar communicating artery segment of the PCA. The arterial pattern is quite homogeneous. Single arteries to each side can arise, or bilateral branches may arise from a unilateral single artery, or arteries to both sides may arise from a pedicle.[83,88,89,351] These arteries may also supply territory usually supplied by the polar arteries. Medial thalamic infarcts in the territories of the thalamic-subthalamic arteries usually involve the subthalamus, the rostral interstitial nucleus of the medial longitudinal fasciculus, the nucleus parafascicularis, and the medial part of the centromedian nucleus.[83,84,88,411] Ischemia in the territory of these arteries can be caused by atheromatous branch disease, emboli to the basilar apex, or aneurysms at the basilar bifurcation.

Reported patients with unilateral paramedian left thalamic infarcts all have had upgaze pulses and loss of convergent eye movement.[84,88,412–414] Temporary downgaze paresis may also be present. The vertical gaze abnormality affects voluntary saccades, smooth pursuit, and vestibulo-ocular reflex motions.[83] Disorientation and severe amnesic deficits have also been noted.[84,88,412,413] Some patients have also had aphasic abnormalities characterized by occasional paraphasic errors and loss of naming abilities. A minor right hemiparesis, consisting of decreased spontaneous and associated movements of the right limbs, may be present.[84,88,412] One patient had reduced pain and touch sensation in the right face.[83,412] Insufficient examples of unilateral right-sided paramedian infarction limited to the territory of the thalamic-subthalamic artery are reported to permit clinicopathologic correlation. Bilateral paramedian infarcts cause hypersomnolence, vertical gaze palsies predominantly of upgaze, loss of ocular convergence, and amnesic syndrome.[83,87,88,117,351,415] Elements of third cranial nerve palsies may also be present. The deficits in patients with bilateral lesions have been qualitatively similar to but more severe and more persistent than those found in patients with unilateral posteromedial infarcts. Patients with bilateral paramedian thalamic infarcts usually have persistent severe amnesia and vertical gaze palsies.[416] Malamut and colleagues[416] found that explicit memory (i.e., ability of patients to repeat, on confrontation after a delay, items that were previously told to them) was very defective but that implicit memory (i.e., unconscious learning as shown from action) was relatively preserved. A permanent Korsakoff-like syndrome often develops in patients with bilateral posteromedial infarcts.

Apathy, disinterest, flattening of emotions, lack of insight, and indifference to people and the environment may be severe. Affective responses to the environment are usually reduced, and patients appear changed in their interpersonal relations: They are described as being less warm and caring and more stoic and introverted. Bogousslavsky and colleagues[90,417] used the term coined by Laplane, "lack of psychic self-activation," to describe aspects of this behavior. One of their patients would "sit at the table to eat only when asked by nurses or family and would stop eating after a few seconds unless repeatedly stimulated. During the day, he would stay in bed or in an armchair unless asked to go for a walk. He did not react to unusual stimuli in the room such as grand mal seizures in another patient. He did not read newspapers and did not watch television."[417] In this patient and some others, single-photon emission computed tomography or positron emission tomography has shown medial frontal lobe hypometabolism.[417,418]

So-called utilization behavior, in which patients automatically and inappropriately handle and use objects placed before them even though told not to use them, has also been described in patients with posteromedial bilateral thalamic infarcts.[419] This phenomenon, described and named by Lhermitte,[420] has usually been described in patients with frontal lobe disease. In a report by Hashimoto and coworkers,[421] a patient with a large right thalamic infarct that probably included some of the territory of both the polar and thalamic-subthalamic arteries was noted to have utilization behavior; she had diffuse decrease in uptake on single-photon emission computed tomography scans in the entire right hemisphere, especially frontally. Hypersomnolence may be more prolonged and severe in patients with bilateral disease. One patient had a compulsive tendency to lie in a sleeping position with her eyes closed throughout the day.[422] She was also apathetic, disinterested, and inactive. It is of great interest that administration of bromocriptine in large doses ($\leq$120 mg/day) to this patient resulted in an increase in spontaneous activities and lessening of the sleeplike behavior.[422]

Thalamogeniculate Arteries. The thalamogeniculate arteries arise as a pedicle or group of arteries from the ambient segment of the PCA. The pedicle usually consists of six to eight arteries that vary widely in diameter and penetrate the ventral lateral thalamus between the geniculate bodies.[11,59,92] These arteries supply the somatosensory nuclei, the ventral posterolateral and posteromedial nuclei, the inferior and posterior portions of the ventral lateral nucleus, the lateral portion of the centromedial nucleus, and the rostrolateral portion of the pulvinar.[92] In most cases, the thalamogeniculate arteries probably also supply a portion of the posterior limb of the internal capsule,[92] as can be seen from the lesions in the original cases of Dejerine and Roussy.[423]

Three somewhat distinct syndromes result from infarction in the territory supply of the thalamogeniculate arteries and their branches. These vessels are the posterior circulation counterpart of the lenticulostriate branches of the MCAs. Lesions of small branches can produce infarction restricted to the somatosensory nuclei, causing the clinical syndromes of pure sensory stroke or sensory loss limited to the face.[388,401] Occlusion of branches supplying the lateral thalamus and posterior limb of the internal capsule can give rise to a sensorimotor stroke in which the deficits are restricted to paresis, decreased pin and touch perception, and pyramidal signs without cognitive or behavioral abnormalities.[92,393] Larger lateral thalamic infarcts cause a syndrome originally described by Dejerine and Roussy,[423] which consisted of hemiataxia, hemichorea, transient hemiparesis, and hemisensory symptoms and signs.[92]

Choroidal Arteries. The anterior choroidal artery is also inferred to supply a small portion of the thalamus,[1] although this is still debated.[11,86,89] However, infarction restricted to the thalamus after occlusion of this artery has not been documented.[424]

Lateral geniculate body infarction can occur secondary to occlusive lesions of either the anterior or posterior choroidal arteries and produce characteristic visual field deficits. Infarcts in the territory of the medial and lateral posterior choroidal arteries are the least well known and most rarely reported of all thalamic infarcts.[425,426] The lateral arteries supply mostly the pulvinar, a portion of the lateral geniculate body, and the anterior nucleus. The medial arteries supply the habenula, anterior pulvinar part of the center median nucleus, and the paramedial nuclei.[11] There have been very few clinicopathologic[427–429] and clinicoradiographic reports of patients with posterior choroidal territory infarcts.[127,430–433] This syndrome is summarized by Neau and Bogousslavsky.[432]

The first reported necropsy case was in a 52-year-old man who became confused and aphasic and was found at postmortem examination to have an infarct in the thalamus in the distribution of the posterior choroidal arteries.[427,429]

The second case involved a 67-year-old woman who had abnormalities of vertical eye movements, including retraction nystagmus, and later a hemiparesis.[427,428] Although a number of different phenomena may occur in patients with posterior choroidal territory infarction, the most specific abnormality relates to the visual fields. The posterior choroidal arteries and their lateral choroidal artery branches supply a portion of the lateral geniculate body reciprocal to that supplied by the anterior choroidal arteries. The characteristic visual field defect in patients with posterior choroidal artery territory infarcts is a sectoranopia involving a wedge defect on each side of the horizontal meridian.[432,434] By contrast, the visual field defect in patients with anterior choroidal artery territory infarcts can include loss of the upper and lower quadrants with sparing of vision in a line along the median horizontal meridian. Patients with posterior choroidal territory infarcts can also have either an upper or lower quadrantanopia.

Other clinical deficits are less well established. Pulvinar ischemia can cause aphasia, visual hallucinations, and abnormal limb movements and postures. The anterior nucleus of the thalamus with its frontal lobe projections can also be involved. In the Stroke Data Bank series of patients with thalamic infarcts, the most common restricted focal infarcts were in the territory of the posterior choroidal arteries.[435] Two of the patients with posterior choroidal territory infarcts had prominent contralateral neglect. Little is known about infarcts limited to the pulvinar or the anterior nucleus of the thalamus. Ghika and associates[436] reported on a patient with an infarct in the left posterior thalamus involving the internal medullary lamina and the pulvinar in the territory of the left lateral posterior choroidal artery. This patient, who was severely hypertensive, had burning paresthesia in his right hand and foot at the onset of the stroke but later experienced restlessness, akathisia, and an irrepressible urge to move the right limbs, symptoms that improved after he was given clonazepam.[436] Lateral posterior choroidal territory infarcts can involve fibers synapsing in the thalamic sensory nuclei, possibly resulting in hemisensory syndromes.[127]

Occlusion of Long Circumferential Branches of the Basilar Artery

The most common mechanism of occlusion of the circumferential (cerebellar) branches of the BA is embolism, atheroma, or thrombus in the parent BA that blocks the orifices of these branches. The nomenclature is a bit misleading, the three vessels more easily being described as superior, midline and inferior, but because the brainstem and cerebellum lie in a forward angle, they have traditionally been broken into two groups, superior and inferior (anterior inferior and posterior inferior). Despite objections, it seems unlikely that any change will be achieved in this nomenclature. Because of the intimate association of the PICA with the lateral medullary syndrome and vertebral artery occlusion, the discussion that follows reviews the cerebellar arterial occlusion in reverse order—superior, anterior inferior, and then posterior inferior.

Superior Cerebellar Artery Occlusions

SCA infarctions are among the most common of the cerebellar stroke syndromes. Fifty percent to 65% of all cerebellar infarctions appear in the distribution of this artery.[132,133,275,437–439] SCA territory infarctions are characterized by the rarity of clinical involvement of the brainstem territory of the SCA and do not frequently manifest as the classic SCA syndrome.[132,133,276,277,439] They typically have partial cerebellar involvement, a cardioembolic origin, and a relatively benign prognosis.[133,275,437,440–442] The SCA supplies the rostral surface of the cerebellum down to the great horizontal sulcus (see Fig. 10–3), including the lobulus centralis, culmen, clivus, folium, and tuber of the vermis; the anterior, simplex, and superior semilunar lobules of the cerebellar hemispheres; and, rarely, the upper part of the inferior semilunar lobules.[76] Hemispheric branches can be classified as *medial, intermediate* (both arising from mSCA), and *lateral* (arising from lSCA) groups.[443]

Causes. Arterial occlusions leading to strokes in the SCA distribution usually involve the distal tip of the BA, the ICVA, the ECVA at its origin, and, less frequently, the SCA itself.[109,132,275,277,439,442] However, in most patients with SCA strokes, no arterial occlusion is found. Presumably, the thromboembolus has moved on or has been lysed by the time of angiography or postmortem examination. Thus, the frequency of SCA occlusion is probably underestimated.

Every autopsy and clinical series concerned with SCA infarctions emphasizes cardiogenic embolism as the most common cause of SCA territory infarction, whatever the extent of the stroke.[109,132,133,275,439,440,442,444] Cardiac sources of emboli have been observed variously in 35%,[442] 40%,[133] 61%,[439] and 70% of cases.[132] Sometimes the responsible stroke mechanism is artery-to-artery embolism from atherosclerotic occlusion of the VA artery or from ulcerated plaques in the aortic arch,[109,132–134,439,442] or VA dissection.[133,199,439,442,445] Atherosclerotic occlusion occurs in 30% of patients.[132,439] Rare causes of SCA territory stroke in the young include SCA dissection and fibromuscular dysplasia,[446,447] migraine,[448,449] and transcardiac embolism a patent foramen ovale during Valsalva's maneuver.[440]

Anatomical Aspects. The *medial group* of hemispheric branches of the SCA supplies the vermis and gives rise to two branches. A paramedian branch on the vermal surface anastomoses with the contralateral mSCA; the other branch runs parallel to the first paramedian branch but more laterally on the medial surface of the hemisphere (Fig. 10–16). Sometimes it is replaced by an artery from the intermediate group.

The *intermediate group* contains one to four arteries running obliquely, dorsally, and laterally, giving rise to numerous rami, some of which anastomose with branches from the PICA. One of the arteries from the intermediate group often runs directly down, giving few rami to the rostral cortex and anastomosing directly with one of the PICA branches. The *lateral group*, arising from the lSCA, runs anteriorly on the anterosuperior margin dividing the superior and anterior aspects of the cerebellum (see Fig. 10–16). The territory of the lSCA includes the anterior rostral cerebellar cortex and adjacent white matter (the anterior part of the anterior simplex, and superior semilunar lobules) and the ventral aspect of the dentate nucleus.[440] The lSCA probably never supplies the flocculus. Anastomoses exist between the lateral group of the lSCA and branches of the AICA. The boundary zone between SCA and PICA territories usually lies just above the great horizontal sulcus. The SCA rarely supplies the upper part of the inferior semilunar lobule and never the cerebellar tonsil.[443] As far as the vermis is concerned, the SCA and PICA territories usually overlap on the tuber or the clivus.

The *deep territory* of the SCA is larger than that of the other two cerebellar arteries. It supplies the dentate, intermediate (the embolus and globulus), and fastigial nuclei and most of the cerebellar white matter.[443,450] The white matter is supplied by branches arising from the cortex that penetrate the cortex perpendicularly and extend toward the dentate nucleus. These branches anastomose in the dentate nucleus with early branches of the parent trunk that follow the superior cerebellar peduncle, giving rise to an internal anastomotic network between deep and superficial branches of the SCA.[443]

In the *brainstem*, the SCA supplies the dorsolaterotegmental area of the upper pons (see Fig. 10–2), which includes the superior cerebellar peduncle, lateral lemniscus, spinothalamic tract, corticotegmental tract, descending sympathetic tracts, mesencephalic trigeminal tract, locus ceruleus, and, more dorsally, the root of the contralateral fourth cranial nerve.[11,67,79,450–452] The SCA participates in the supply of the inferior colliculus[11,79,453] and,

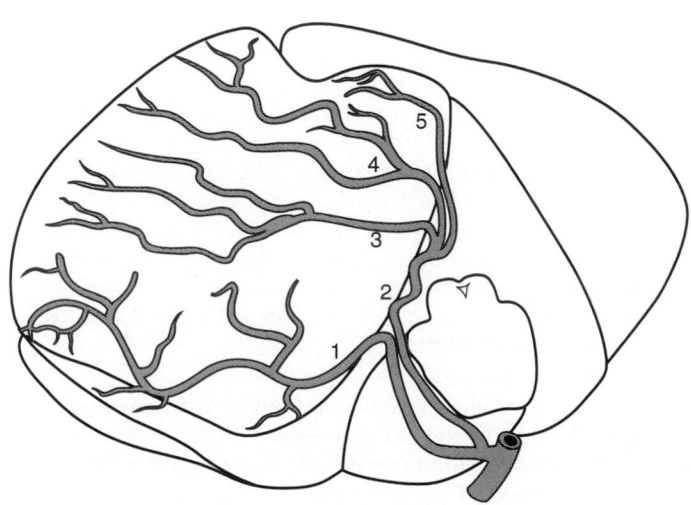

FIGURE 10–16 *Superior cerebellar artery branches (three-quarter view). The lateral branch of the SCA and medial branch of the SCA and its vermal branches, paravermal branches, and hemispheric branches.*

at times, of the superior colliculus as well.[11,79,450] The SCA also supplies the choroid plexus of the fourth ventricle.[450]

The largest early description of SCA occlusion concerned seven patients with SCA territory infarcts reported by Davison and colleagues[450] in 1935. Then Thompson[444] described five cases of SCA infarction emphasizing cardioembolic causes. Many of the patients in this series had infarction in the brainstem and cerebellar territory of the SCA. During the first half of the 20th century, neurologists and neuroanatomists became very interested in clinicoanatomic correlations and would posit likely symptoms that might result from lesions at various sites. The so-called classic syndrome of the SCA was mostly a product of hypotheses, because actual patients with this syndrome are extremely rare. The classic SCA syndrome is said to consist of ipsilateral limb ataxia, ipsilateral Horner's syndrome, contralateral loss of pain and temperature sensibility of the face, arm, leg, and trunk, and contralateral fourth nerve palsy.[132] Abnormal spontaneous involuntary movements on the same side of the body were also known to occur.[132,277,454]

In 1985, Kase and associates[277] reported on three patients with infarcts that included the SCA. All three patients had partial infarcts, each identified on CT scan. In 1987, Savoiardo and coworkers[455] published templates of the territories of the PICA, AICA, and SCA on axial, coronal, and sagittal sections of CT. On the basis of the complete necropsy analysis of 64 cases of cerebellar infarctions, the territories of the cerebellar arteries and their main branches (mSCA, lSCA, mPICA, and lPICA) have been identified both on axial pathologic sections of the cerebellum and brainstem[76] (see Fig. 10–2) and on CT and MRI axial sections (see Fig. 10–4).[73,456]

Five years after the report by Kase and associates,[277] Amarenco and Hauw[132] described the largest single clinicopathologic analysis of SCA territory infarcts. They reported on findings in specimens from 33 patients who had 41 cerebellar infarcts in the territory of the SCA and its main medial and lateral branches; the patients were selected from among all neuropathologic specimens studied at the Salpêtrière hospital during a 20-year period.[132] The same group of researchers then identified the territory and the clinical syndrome of infarction of the lateral branch of the SCA at necropsy and on CT and MRI.[440] Several large series—including the landmark study by Kase and colleagues[439] and those of Chaves and coworkers[275] and the experience of others,[133,437,441,442,457,458]—noted the frequency and locations of cerebellar infarcts identified on CT, MRI, or both; such series have commonly tabulated the underlying vascular lesions, stroke mechanisms, and clinical findings.

Clinical Aspects. Infarctions in the full territory of the SCA are usually accompanied by other infarctions in the rostral territory of the BA. In 73% of autopsy cases the involved territory includes the occipitotemporal lobes unilaterally or bilaterally, the thalamic and subthalamic areas, and the mesencephalon.[132] Some infarctions involve the ventral aspect of the pons or occur together with PICA and AICA infarcts (one third of autopsy cases).[132] Infarctions of the SCA are frequently edematous, sometimes giving rise to brainstem compression and tonsillar herniation.[132,459] Some SCA infarctions occur together with embolic occlusion of the MCA.

Although partial territory SCA infarctions may be associated with rostral BA infarctions,[132] they more commonly involve the rostral cerebellum alone.[133,275,439,440,442] The brainstem territory of the SCA supplied by branches arising early from the parent trunk is usually unaffected in patients with partial territory SCA infarctions. Partial territory infarctions are the most common type of SCA infarction[133,275,437,439] and differ from full territory infarctions in having routinely benign outcomes.[133,439,440]

Six distinct clinical patterns arise with SCA occlusion (Table 10.2). The previously described *classic SCA syndrome*, first described by Mills[460,461] and Guillain and associates,[454] is rarely seen[132,277,439] being found in only 3% of autopsy specimens from patients with SCA occlusions.[132] This syndrome develops with involvement of the brainstem territory of the SCA (see Fig. 10–2). Signs characteristic of the syndrome are ipsilateral limb dysmetria, ipsilateral Horner's syndrome,[462] contralateral pain and temperature sensory loss,[450,452,454,462–465] and contralateral fourth nerve palsy.[452] Other signs less commonly reported are ipsilateral loss of emotional expression in the face,[282] unilateral or bilateral hearing loss (possibly due to involvement of the lateral lemniscus), and sleep disorders (due to locus ceruleus damage).[461] Ipsilateral abnormal limb movements are more unusual.[277,450,452,454,464,465] Movement disorders occurring with classic SCA syndrome, described as choreiform[277] or athetotic,[450,452,465] consist of slow, undulatory movements[454,464] of large amplitude.[277,452,465] They appear with effort or emotion,[464] at rest, on assumption of certain postures, or continuously. Guillain and associates[454] noted some unsteadiness of the head in their patient with SCA occlusion and the classic syndrome. Some patients have coarse tremors.[450,462] Movement disorders are presumed to arise from involvement of the dentate nucleus or damage to the superior cerebellar peduncle. A few weeks after ischemic injury, palatal myoclonus and contralateral hypertrophy of the inferior olivary nucleus may occur with dentate nucleus damage.[462] Palatal myoclonus is occasionally accompanied by synchronous myoclonic movements of the jaw, face,[462] tongue, and ipsilateral vocal cord, producing voice disorders.[465] Davison and colleagues[450] described a patient with SCA infarction without palatal myoclonus who had myoclonus of the jaw and a coarse tremor of the hand.

The *rostral BA syndrome* is one of the most striking clinical presentations of SCA occlusion in the autopsy series described by Amarenco and Hauw.[132] This syndrome occurs in 25% of patients with SCA territory infarction.[132] The presenting signs are visual field defects, vomiting, dizziness, diplopia, paresthesia, clumsiness of limbs, weakness, and drowsiness. These signs and symptoms suggest occipitotemporal lobe damage. Some patients clearly have cortical blindness or hemianopia, memory loss or confusion, or paralysis of visual fixation (Balint's syndrome).

Thalamomesencephalic involvement is manifest in other patients as multimodal sensory loss, contralateral Horner's syndrome, ipsilateral hemianopia, appendicular ataxia or pendular reflexes, behavioral changes, abulia, unilateral spatial neglect, memory loss, transcortical motor aphasia, and vertical gaze palsy. Subthalamic damage may produce hemiballism. Mesencephalic damage usually manifests as one of several syndromes—Benedikt's syndrome of third

Table 10.2 Cerebellar Stroke Syndromes

Location of Cerebellar Infarct	Associated Infarcts	Clinical Syndrome
Rostral (SCA)	Mesencephalon, subthalamic area, thalamus, occipitotemporal lobes	Rostral basilar artery syndrome or coma from onset ± tetraplegia
	Laterotegmental area of the upper pons	Dysmetria and Horner's syndrome (ipsilateral), temperature and pain sensory loss, and CN IV palsy (contralateral)
	—	Dysarthria, headache, dizziness, vomiting, ataxia, and delayed coma (pseudotumoral form)
Dorsomedial (mSCA)	—	Dysarthria
		Ataxia
Ventrolateral (lSCA)	—	Dysmetria, axial lateropulsion (ipsilateral) ataxia, and dysarthria
Medial (AICA)	Lateral area of the lower pons	CN V, VII, and VIII, Horner's syndrome, dysmetria (ipsilateral), temperature and pain sensory loss (contralateral)
	—	Pure vestibular syndrome
Caudal (PICA)	—	Vertigo, headache, vomiting, ataxia, and delayed coma (pseudotumoral form)
Dorsomedial (mPICA)	Dorsolateromedullary area	Wallenberg's syndrome
	—	Isolated vertigo or vertigo with dysmetria and axial lateropulsion (ipsilateral) and ataxia
Ventrolateral (lPICA)	—	Vertigo, ipsilateral limb dysmetria
Caudal and medial	Lateral area of the lower pons or lateromedullary area, or both	AICA syndrome ± delayed coma (pseudotumoral form)
Rostrocaudal	—	Vertigo, vomiting, headache, ataxia, dysarthria, and delayed coma (pseudotumoral form)
	Brainstem, thalamus, occipitotemporal lobes	Coma from onset ± tetraplegia

AICA, anterior inferior cerebellar artery; CN, cranial nerve; lPICA, lateral branch of the PICA; lSCA, lateral branch of the SCA; mPIVA, medial branch of the PICA; mSCA, medial branch of the SCA; PICA, posterior inferior cerebellar artery; SCA, superior cerebellar artery.

nerve palsy with contralateral limb movement disorders, Claude's syndrome with third nerve palsy and contralateral limb dysmetria, Weber's syndrome with contralateral limb weakness, or Parinaud's syndrome with vertical gaze paresis. Some individuals with mesencephalic damage have also had pseudo–sixth nerve palsy, tonic deviation of gaze, palpebral retraction, pupillary disturbances, drowsiness, hallucinosis, and confusion.[132,271,343] Additional signs are ipsilateral Horner's syndrome, limb dysmetria, hemiplegia, contralateral pain and temperature sensory loss, and internuclear ophthalmoplegia. Usually only two or three of these signs of rostral BA occlusion are present; in such circumstances, the SCA involvement is commonly difficult to recognize or is unexpectedly discovered on CT.[132,466]

Coma from onset, together with tetraplegia and oculomotor palsy, is another common clinical finding in patients in whom autopsy identifies SCA occlusion. Patients with this presentation represent about 33% of cases of SCA infarctions that come to autopsy. These clinical findings arise with embolic obstruction of the rostral end of the BA.[132]

SCA occlusion may be *clinically inapparent* if there is simultaneous embolic infarction in the distribution of the ICA with a resultant brachiofacial sensorimotor deficit and aphasia. This second infarction, identified in 9% of patients with SCA occlusion who came to autopsy in one series, was associated with a cardiac source of embolism.[132] Occasionally this infarction also occurs along with occlusion of the

innominate artery with intra-arterial embolism to the right MCA and embolism through the VA to the SCA.

Cerebellar and vestibular signs are the prominent presenting features in many clinical series.[133,276,437,439,440,442] They are due to partial involvement of the SCA territory (see Fig. 10–4). Symptoms are headache, gait abnormalities, and, in about 35% of patients, dizziness and vomiting.[133,275,439,442] In a series of 30 patients with unilateral, isolated infarctions of the SCA territory as documented on CT,[286] patients most often presented with appendicular ataxia (73%), gait ataxia (67%), nystagmus (50%), and brainstem signs (30%).[439] Nystagmus was horizontal and ipsilateral in 20% of patients, horizontal and contralateral in 3%, horizontal and bilateral in 20%, and vertical in 7%.[439] In an unselected CT series of 17 SCA infarctions, 15 patients had limb ataxia and 12 had truncal ataxia and dysarthria.[442] Dysarthria, one of the main symptoms of SCA infarction, seems to be the counterpart of the vertigo that typically develops with PICA infarctions.[440] Hemiparesis occurs in nearly one fourth of patients.[442]

The *lSCA syndrome* has been described by Amarenco and colleagues.[440] Occlusions of the lateral branch of the SCA involve the anterior rostral cerebellum (see Fig. 10–4). The same investigators first described the typical territory of these infarctions in one pathologic case and in nine additional patients examined with CT and MRI.[132,440] Since then, large series of cerebellar infarctions from prospective registries have shown that infarction in the lSCA territory is the most common of SCA infarctions, accounting for about half the cases.[127,133] The lSCA syndrome consists of dysmetria of the ipsilateral limbs, ipsilateral axial lateropulsion, dysarthria, and gait unsteadiness.[440] The findings can mimic the dysarthria–clumsy hand lacunar syndrome,[467] may manifest as isolated axial lateropulsion,[468] and may be associated with prominent dysmetria, nystagmus, or contrapulsion of saccades.[277,469] Occasionally, lSCA infarctions may manifest as transient symptoms (transient blurring of vision, unsteadiness of gait, and tinnitus lasting a few seconds) and no clinical neurologic signs.[73]

Clinical syndromes due to *dorsomedial infarction* of the rostral cerebellum in the territory of the mSCA have not been fully characterized, although some individual patients have been reported.[277,457,470] In large registries of cerebellar infarctions, mSCA infarcts represent 10% to 20% of all SCA infarctions,[132] but no specific clinical syndrome has been reported.[127,133] Among the individual patients who have been described, those in whom the most medial branches were involved have shown isolated unsteadiness of gait.[277] In those in whom the anterior cerebellar lobe (i.e., the lingula, central, culmen lobules of the vermis, and the anterior lobule of the hemisphere) was involved, some appendicular ataxia and spontaneous posturing of the neck, trunk, and limbs occurred.[470] With involvement of more lateral branches the paravermal territory, isolated dysarthria was found.[457] Lechtenberg and Gilman[471] showed that the paravermal zone of the lateral rostral cerebellum was the most commonly damaged in 31 patients with cerebellar dysarthria and nondegenerative cerebellar disease. However, no patient with pure dysarthria and cerebellar infarction was found. The report of an isolated infarction of this paravermal area demonstrates that this zone is involved in the control of the voice and that dysarthria should be considered one of the main features of mSCA infarctions.[457]

Prognosis. SCA territory infarctions can have a pseudotumoral presentation, a characteristic observed in 21% of autopsy cases.[132] However, the course and outcome of SCA infarctions are best evaluated in CT and MRI series of patients.[133,275,437,439,458] Ninety-three percent of patients in whom CT demonstrates the lesion to be limited to the SCA territory have partial SCA involvement. They have benign outcomes and are left minimally disabled or neurologically intact.[439] Only 7% of patients have a pseudotumoral pattern leading to coma and, occasionally, death.[439] This relatively benign course is seen with both lSCA and mSCA infarctions.

Anterior Inferior Cerebellar Artery Occlusions

AICA infarctions are exceedingly rare, although probably many go undiagnosed.[72] MRI reveals a higher incidence of strokes due to AICA infarction than was previously suspected (see Fig. 10–4).[131] This type of pontocerebellar infarction differs strikingly from SCA and PICA infarctions in terms of brainstem signs associated with the clinical presentation.

The cerebellar territory of the AICA (see Fig. 10–2) varies as a function of its caliber. The arteries on the two sides usually have different calibers. The artery nearly always supplies the flocculus, the only territory of the cerebellum usually vascularized solely by the AICA.[71] The flocculus is supplied by the PICA rather than the AICA in only 3% to 5% of individuals. In 40% of subjects, the AICA ends on the flocculus.[71] In others, it follows the sulcus separating the anterior lobule and the semilunar lobule and gives rise to terminal branches that supply the neighboring lobules: anterior, simplex, superior semilunar, inferior semilunar, gracilis, and lobulus biventer in 18% to 50% of individuals.[71,472] The AICA can replace a hypoplastic PICA, taking over the supply to most of the inferior surface of the cerebellum, including the anterolateral part of the tonsil but not the vermis. According to Stopford,[8] Foix and Hillemand,[11] Atkinson,[472] Takahashi and associates,[411] and Perneczky and colleagues,[473] a balance in size exists between the AICA and the PICA, the artery giving rise to the lateral branch of the PICA being able to arise from AICA. The terminal branches of the AICA anastomose with the ipsilateral SCA and the PICA at the borderzone areas of these arteries.

The pontine distribution of the AICA (see Fig. 10–2) has been precisely described by Duvernoy.[67] The AICA always supplies the middle cerebellar peduncle, in most cases the lower third of the lateral pontine territory, frequently its middle third, and in a few individuals the superior part of the lateral region of the medulla.

Few reports on AICA infarctions have been published to date, and series of patients studied pathologically[72] and with MRI[131] did not appear until 1990. The first full report of the AICA syndrome was made by Adams[474] in 1983 in a clinicopathologic study of one patient. Goodhart and Davison[70] briefly described a patient 7 years earlier who had an infarct limited to the AICA territory of the cerebellum and whose only symptom was vertigo. The most extensive clinical necropsy study of 20 patients with AICA territory infarcts was reported by Amarenco and Hauw[72] in 1990.

With the advent of MRI, precise localization of brainstem and cerebellar infarcts became possible during life. In 1993, Amarenco and associates[131] reported on nine patients with AICA territory infarcts identified by CT and MRI. Matsushita and colleagues[475] also reported on five patients whose AICA territory infarcts were diagnosed with MRI. Fisher[476] described one patient whose AICA infarct was diagnosed with MRI.

Most AICA infarcts involve a small territory restricted to the lateral region of the caudal pons and, in the cerebellum, to the middle cerebellar peduncle (100% of cases) and flocculus (69% of cases). Involvement of this region accounts for most of the clinical signs described for AICA occlusions.[72] Infarctions often also affect other cerebellar lobules (75% of cases) but usually remain limited in size.

Infarcts commonly involve a small part of the cerebellum comprising the central white matter, the flocculus, and a thin rim of cerebellar cortex located at the junction of the territories of the three major cerebellar arteries, as illustrated in Figure 10–3, but this involvement does not modify the clinical presentation. When the AICA is large (and the PICA is hypoplastic), the AICA territory encompasses the whole anterior inferior cerebellum. There is no significant clinical difference between the signs and symptoms initially observed after infarctions arising with relatively limited AICA involvement and those observed after infarctions arising in vascular systems in which both the

AICA and the PICA arise from a common trunk from the vertebral or basilar artery.[72]

In most AICA infarctions, the inferolateral pontine territory is involved, the infarction sometimes extending up to the middle third of the lateral pons and down to the superior part of the lateral medulla. It involves neither the upper third of the lateral pons, which is supplied by the superior lateral pontine artery, a branch of the BA or of the medial branch of the SCA, nor the ventral aspect of the pons. AICA territory infarctions are associated with PICA and SCA infarcts in 35% of autopsy cases, and this association frequently occurs with ventromedian pontine infarction and tonsillar herniation.[72] Other partial AICA infarctions involve at least the middle cerebellar peduncle, the core of the vessel's territory.

Cause. The arterial occlusion usually seen postmortem involves the lower BA and, less frequently, the end of the VA above the PICA ostium.[72] In many cases, there have been associated anomalies of the vertebrobasilar system, such as a hypoplastic VA, dolichoectatic BA, or patent trigeminal artery. The mechanism is mostly atherosclerotic occlusion.[72] In studies reported by Amarenco and colleagues,[72,109] one patient with an isolated AICA territory infarction and one with AICA-SCA-PICA infarctions had no arterial occlusion at necropsy, but each had high-risk cardiac sources of emboli—mitral stenosis with atrial fibrillation and an acute myocardial infarction with a mural thrombus. These two cases provide additional evidence that emboli of cardiac origin can occasionally cause a unilateral AICA territory infarct.

In a series of 9 patients with AICA infarction studied during life who were diagnosed with MRI and contrast angiography, Amarenco and associates[131] could clearly identify two groups of patients. Four diabetic patients had isolated unilateral AICA infarction, patent BAs, and probably basilar branch occlusion due to BA plaques that extended into the AICA or microatheroma that blocked the AICA origin. The other 5 patients had AICA infarction together with other pontine, midbrain, occipital, PICA, or SCA infarction. They all had BA occlusion including the AICA level and reconstitution of the distal BA by collaterals through hemispheric anastomoses from the PICAs and posterior communicating arteries.[131] Among 79 consecutive patients with territorial cerebellar infarcts, Amarenco and coworkers[133] included 9 patients with AICA territory infarcts. Seven of the 9 likely had occlusive branch disease, and the others had ICVA or BA occlusion, or both. Intracranial giant cell arteritis was shown to have caused an occlusion of AICA in one patient studied at necropsy.[477] Cases associated with migraine have also been reported.[448]

Clinical Aspects. Four distinct clinical pictures can be distinguished in patients with AICA occlusions (see Table 10.2).

The classic syndrome of the AICA, first described by Adams[474] in one patient, is the most common clinical picture described with AICA occlusions.[72] Symptoms are vertigo, vomiting, tinnitus, and dysarthria. Signs comprise ipsilateral facial palsy, hearing loss, trigeminal sensory loss, Horner's syndrome, appendicular dysmetria, and contralateral temperature and pain sensory loss over the limbs and trunk.[72,474] The AICA syndrome may also include ipsilateral conjugate lateral gaze palsy due to involvement of the flocculus rather than damage to the abducens nucleus, dysphagia due to extension of the infarction to the superior part of the lateral medulla, and ipsilateral limb weakness due to contralateral involvement of the corticospinal tract in the pons or mesencephalon.[72] Because some signs are crossed and otherwise some are similar to signs observed in Wallenberg's syndrome, an AICA occlusion is often misdiagnosed as lateral medullary infarction. However, signs unusual in Wallenberg's syndrome, such as severe facial palsy, deafness, tinnitus, and multimodal sensory impairment over the face, allow accurate clinico-topographic diagnosis.[72]

A complete AICA syndrome was observed in 30% of autopsy cases in individuals with AICA occlusion in one series, an almost complete syndrome in 35%, and an incomplete syndrome in 10%.[72] Limb weakness was found in half these patients.

Coma with tetraplegia from onset occurred in 20% of cases of AICA that came to autopsy in the same series.[72] It was due to massive ventromedial involvement of the basis pontis together with cerebellar infarction in the territory of all three cerebellar arteries.

Isolated vertigo, mimicking labyrinthitis, occurs in partial AICA territory infarcts. This was suspected for a long time,[70,474] initially posited in case 1 described by Rubenstein and coworkers,[478] in which the CT findings were not convincing, and finally demonstrated with MRI by Amarenco and colleagues.[73,479,480] Oas and Baloh[481] reported on two patients with unilateral AICA territory infarcts in whom attacks of vertigo preceded the strokes by 12 months or 3 months. Each patient also had unilateral hearing loss. However, owing to the extent of the territory usually supplied by the AICA, isolated vertigo as the sole clinical presentation is likely to be exceptional.

In the case reported by Amarenco and associates in which vertigo was the sole clinical presentation without cranial nerve involvement, mimicking a labyrinthitis,[73,480] MRI showed involvement of only the vestibular nuclei, middle cerebellar peduncle, and flocculus areas. Surprisingly, the angiogram showed two AICAs on the same side. The one of large caliber arose from the mid-BA; the other was hypoplastic and arose from the proximal part of the BA, then reached the flocculus area, where it ended and ramified.[480] This small AICA corresponded to the lower supplementary cerebellar artery described by Jakob.[482] No occlusion was seen on angiography, but this small AICA was thought likely to be responsible for the lesion. Only this very unusual arterial disposition in this patient made possible the small extent of the AICA infarction and its unique clinical presentation. Another explanation for isolated vertigo in patients with AICA occlusion is occlusion of the internal auditory artery, which supplies the labyrinth and cochlea and arises from the AICA in 80% of individuals. However, good clinicopathologic reports of such cases are lacking. AICA territory infarctions can also cause *isolated cerebellar signs,* as demonstrated in a clinical MRI report of an infarction in a child.[483]

Prognosis. Although most cases reported in the literature have been based on autopsies, AICA infarctions may have a better outcome than would be predicted from the published reports. Most of the reported patients died from remote complications, such as pulmonary embolism and infections. Clinical MRI reports that have been published depict patients with benign outcomes and minimal neurologic residua.[131,476,480] Descriptions of banal, isolated vertigo with benign outcome suggest that partial AICA territory infarctions may be more frequent than has been recognized.[480,481] Alternatively, AICA occlusion may be a very rare cause of isolated vertigo, as in the patient with an unusual supplementary AICA described by Amarenco and associates.[480] In some cases, AICA territory infarctions may herald massive BA thrombosis.[73,131]

Posterior Inferior Cerebellar Artery Infarctions

PICA infarcts are due to PICA occlusion. Occlusion involves the ICVA facing the PICA ostium or (directly) the main stem of the PICA. However, the two sites of occlusion have the same causes.[484] Symptoms of cerebellar infarction are nonspecific, including vertigo, headache, vomiting, dysarthria, and gait unsteadiness. The major sign is gait and trunk ataxia, ipsilateral axial lateropulsion, or both, which usually prevent standing in an upright position. Usually, patients able to walk or stand in tandem position are unlikely to have important cerebellar infarction.[456] Other signs are nystagmus, ipsilateral limb dysmetria, and dysarthria. Impairment of consciousness, ranging from drowsiness to deep coma, occurs in half the patients either at onset or later. More than half the patients have signs of associated brainstem infarction (facial palsy, trigeminal involvement, ocular motor abnormalities, motor weakness, and sensory loss) or occipitotemporal infarction (visual field defects, cortical blindness, memory loss).

The clinical presentation is similar to that of cerebellar hemorrhage, but unenhanced CT allows distinction between the two conditions.[320,485] In cerebellar infarcts, CT usually shows focal hypodensity in the cerebellum, mass effect on the fourth ventricle, or compression of adjacent posterior fossa cisterns. However, CT findings can be normal or difficult to interpret because of bone artifacts. MRI, now the "gold standard" for the early and accurate visualization of cerebellar infarctions, shows an area of increased signal on T2-weighted axial, coronal, and sagittal sections (Fig. 10–17). Outcome of cerebellar infarctions is usually benign, with relatively good recovery, but cerebellar infarctions can sometimes take a pseudotumoral form because of edema, cerebellar swelling, brainstem compression, obstruction of the fourth ventricle, and hydrocephalus (see later). In that case, life-saving surgery is needed if deterioration of consciousness appears.

PICA infarcts were formerly the most studied and were presumed to be the most common of all cerebellar infarctions. Most often the pseudotumoral form and the form associated with Wallenberg's syndrome have been emphasized. MRI has shown that these forms are not common. Awareness of both presentations is very important, because a patient with the pseudotumoral form may need life-saving surgical treatment and a patient with Wallenberg's syndrome may require gastrostomy. Other more common presentations have a benign course.

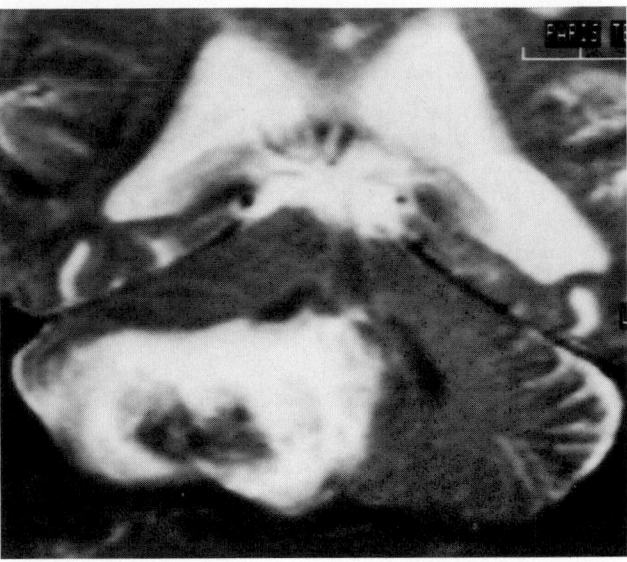

FIGURE 10–17 *Posterior inferior cerebellar artery territory infarction on T2-weighted MR image.*

Clinicopathologic and clinicoradiologic series show that PICA infarcts are actually about as common as SCA infarcts.[133,275,437–439,484] In 64 autopsy cases with cerebellar infarctions, 10 of which involved both PICA and SCA territories, there were 28 PICA infarcts and 33 SCA infarcts.[484] In 66 isolated unilateral cerebellar infarcts, there were 36 PICA infarcts and 30 SCA infarcts.[439] Macdonell and colleagues[441] found 7 PICA infarcts among 19 autopsy cases of cerebellar infarcts, and Hinshaw and coworkers[438] found that 29% of 42 radiologically demonstrated instances of cerebellar infarction were PICA infarcts. In the series reported by Kase and associates,[439] PICA infarcts accounted for half of the cerebellar infarctions; and in another large, consecutive series of 115 patients with cerebellar infarcts, 35 had PICA infarcts, 30 had SCA infarcts, 9 had AICA infarcts, and 36 had small nonterritorial infarcts not localizable to a given arterial territory.[133]

PICA infarcts were historically, but partly erroneously, associated closely with lateral medullary infarctions (i.e., Wallenberg's syndrome; see later). After the anatomic descriptions by Duret in 1873,[1] in which only the PICA was posited to supply the lateral region of the medulla, and Wallenberg's description[486,487] of a case of lateral medullary infarction due to PICA occlusion, every lateral medullary infarction was assumed to be due to a PICA occlusion[488–493] even when no occlusion could be found.[489–491,493,494] In fact, necropsy showed that Wallenberg's original patient also had an ipsilateral ICVA occlusive lesion.

Subsequently, the lateral medullary syndrome was confused with the PICA syndrome. Further studies revealed that the lateral region of the medulla is supplied most often by three or four small branches arising from the distal ICVA between the PICA ostium and the origin of the BA, and less commonly by small branches arising from the PICA.[68,110,495–497] Krayenbühl and Yasargil[498] estimated that the PICA participated in the supply to this region in 22%

or fewer persons. Consequently, PICA infarctions sparing the lateral medullary territory are the most common, and paradoxically, syndromes featuring occlusion of the PICA were not described until Duncan and coworkers[499] emphasized the frequency of vertigo as the prominent presenting symptom. In summary, the PICA (1) sometimes participates in the supply of the lateral medullary area, usually together with branches from the VA but alone in 22% of individuals and (2) usually participates in the supply of the dorsal medullary area together with the posterior spinal arteries.[498]

Clinical Aspects. The arterial occlusion primarily involves the intracranial portion of the VA facing the PICA ostium and the origin of the PICA. The mechanisms of occlusion are equally divided into cardioembolic and atherosclerotic causes.[439,484] Other mechanisms are VA dissection,[133,439] ulcerated plaques in the aortic arch,[109] and occlusion of the mPICA by tonsillar herniation due to raised posterior fossa pressure.[459]

Two different clinical situations occur, depending on whether the medulla is involved. In the autopsy series reported by Amarenco and colleagues[484] from the Salpêtrière Hospital, the medulla was involved in its dorsolateral aspects in one third of patients. No lateral medullary infarction was seen without associated infarction in the dorsal medullary territory. PICA infarctions were much less frequently associated with other vertebrobasilar (pontine, mesencephalic, thalamic, or occipitotemporal) infarctions than AICA or SCA infarctions. The full PICA territory was involved in isolation in only 7% of autopsy cases and was more routinely associated with SCA infarction, AICA infarction, or both (46%). These combined infarctions were frequently edematous and produced brainstem compression.

Partial PICA territory infarctions were very common (46%) in the autopsy cases reported by Amarenco and colleagues.[484] They usually involved the dorsomedial area of the caudal cerebellum—that is, the territory of the mPICA (32%)—and less frequently the lateral area, the territory of the lPICA (18%).[484] Partial infarctions represented 75% of PICA infarctions in one clinical series[439] and two thirds in another series.[133] Such infarctions are never edematous. Thus, when restricted to branch PICA territory, they are often small and benign.[439] In the clinical series reported by Kase and associates,[439] 9 of 36 patients had signs of brainstem compression, and all 9 had full PICA territory infarction. Seven of these patients had obstructive hydrocephalus, and four died from cerebellar swelling. No clinically significant differences exist between full PICA and mPICA territory lesions.[500]

Clinical Pictures. PICA territory cerebellar infarcts are undoubtedly underrecognized and underdiagnosed. Norrving and colleagues[501] studied 24 patients aged 50 to 75 years who came to the hospital in Lund, Sweden, with isolated severe vertigo. Six of the patients had PICA territory cerebellar infarcts (two mPICA, two adjacent parts of mPICA and lPICA, and two full PICA). Among the 6 patients with cerebellar infarcts, 3 had embolisms of cardiac origin, and three had VA occlusions. These investigators estimated that perhaps one fourth of elderly patients presenting with severe vertigo and nystagmus may have PICA territory cerebellar infarcts. Several clinical syndromes can be distinguished.

The *dorsal lateral medullary syndrome*[68,70,486,487,502] occurred in 25% of autopsy cases of PICA territory infarcts in one series[457] and in one third of 36 patients in a clinical series of 36 PICA infarctions.[439] Conversely, because dorsal medullary infarctions are almost constantly associated with PICA infarctions and 13% of cases of lateral medullary infarctions occur together with dorsal medullary infarctions,[69] a PICA territory cerebellar infarction is estimated to exist in 13% of cases of lateromedullary infarction.[484] Wallenberg's syndrome can be complete or partial, with vertigo, nystagmus, loss of pain and temperature on the ipsilateral face, ninth and tenth cranial nerve palsies, ipsilateral Horner's syndrome, appendicular ataxia, and contralateral temperature and pain sensory loss.

Patients with *PICA territory infarctions sparing the medulla* usually present with vertigo, headache, gait ataxia, limb ataxia, and horizontal nystagmus.[439,503–506] Headache is cervical, occipital, or both, occasionally with periauricular or hemifacial-ocular radiation. Unilateral headaches are ipsilateral to the cerebellar infarction.[439] Nystagmus is the most common sign (75%), being either horizontal (ipsilateral in 47% of patients, contralateral in 5%, bilateral in 11%) or vertical (11% of patients).[439] In addition to vertigo, one of the most striking findings in patients with PICA infarctions is ipsilateral axial lateropulsion, a phenomenon suggestive of a lateral displacement of the central representation of the center of gravity.[456] This sign is distinct from lateral deviation of the limbs (i.e., past-pointing) and gait veering. Kase and associates[439] also frequently noted that a patient's attempts to stand or walk led to falling toward the side of the cerebellar infarction. In one of four patients with this type of PICA infarction, there are signs of brainstem compression, such as drowsiness and lateral gaze palsy, followed by progressive coma.[439]

The *isolated acute vertigo* form of PICA infarction, mimicking labyrinthitis, was first described clinicopathologically by Duncan and coworkers[499] in a patient who died of acute myocardial infarction 3 weeks after the onset of vertigo. The autopsy showed a recent medial and caudal cerebellar infarction with no other brain lesions. Subsequently, several convincing clinical cases were reported.[478,507–509] Amarenco and associates[73,484] reported a second typical case with necropsy confirmation of an old dorsomedial infarction of the right caudal cerebellum in the territory of mPICA with normal brainstem (Fig. 10–18). It was due to an embolic occlusion of the ipsilateral VA involving the V2, V3, and V4 portions due to atrial fibrillation. MRI will probably establish the actual frequency of PICA infarctions causing isolated vertigo.

PICA infarctions should be sought in any vertiginous patient older than 50 years who has vascular risk factors, and in circumstances supporting a vascular mechanism in the young. Normal caloric responses and direction-changing nystagmus on gaze to each side or after a patient changes head position or lies down, are additional signs suggesting a pure vestibular syndrome with a PICA territory infarction.[499,505] Vertigo is explained by involvement of the uvulonodular complex of the vermis, which is part of the vestibular portion of the cerebellum. Because the

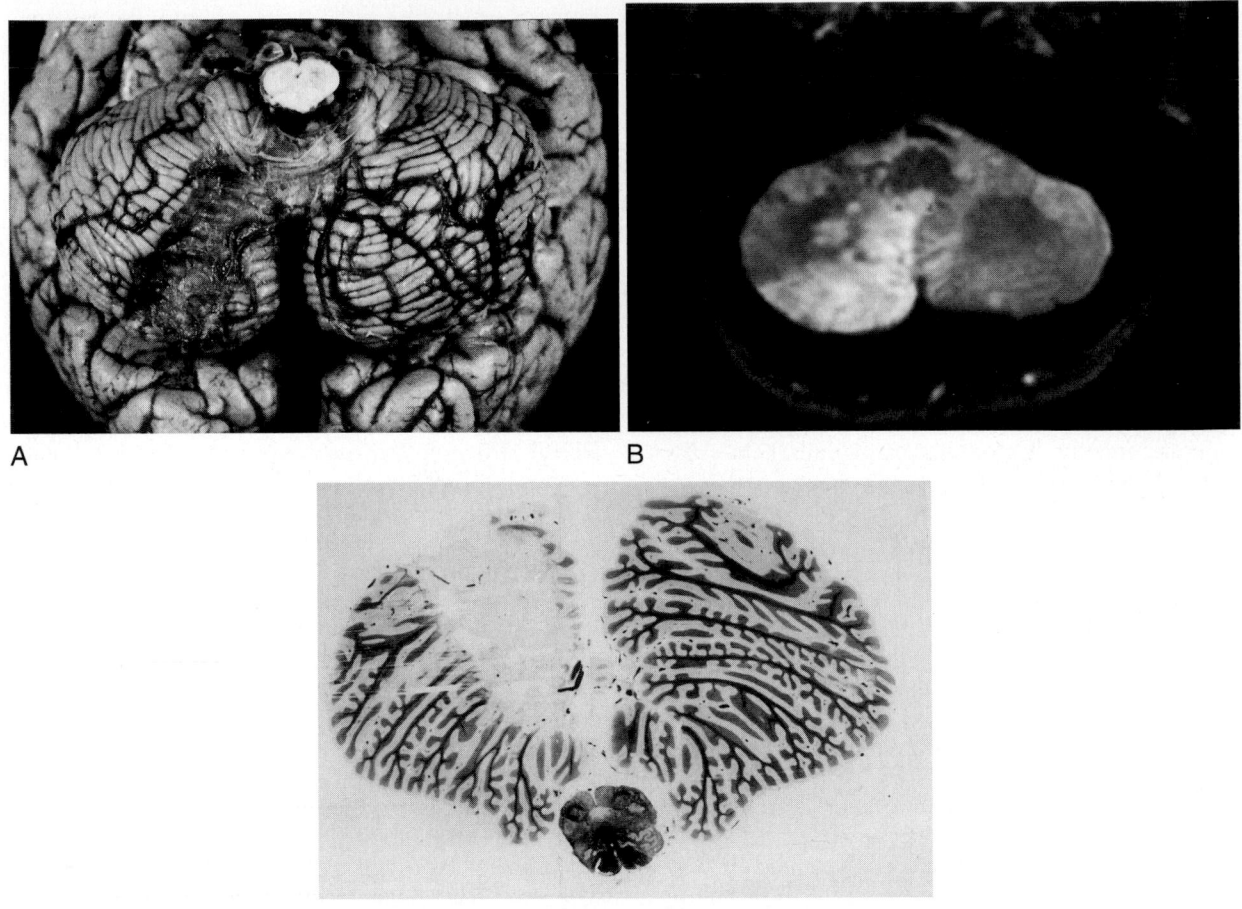

FIGURE 10–18 *Infarctions in the territory of the medial branch of the posterior inferior cerebellar artery (mPICA) (A) at autopsy, (B) on a T2-weighted MR image, and (C) in a drawing.*

nodulus is supplied by the PICA and the flocculus by the AICA, these infarctions should not be labeled "flocculonodular."

Infarcts of the *lateral branch of the PICA* have been reported as chance autopsy findings with no available clinical information.[70,484] Amarenco and colleagues[73] reported one patient who presented with isolated dysmetria (Fig. 10–19). Then Barth, and colleagues[510] described a series of 10 patients with cerebellar infarction in the territory of the lateral branch of the PICA. All patients presented with cerebellar dysmetria ipsilateral to the infarct without dysarthria, nystagmus, or rotatory vertigo.

PICA territory infarctions associated with AICA or SCA infarctions are much more severe in clinical presentation than isolated PICA territory infarctions.[484] They often manifest a pseudotumoral pattern or with deep coma and tetraplegia. *Syndromes of the mPICA* are now common MRI findings.[133,437,456,500,511] The first documentation of the territory of the mPICA was reported in 1989 (Fig. 10–18).[484] Amarenco and coworkers[500] then described the typical territory of mPICA infarctions on T2-weighted MRI axial sections as areas of increased signal in a triangular zone, dorsomedially directed with the dorsal base and the ventral point directed toward the fourth ventricle,

consistent with the appearance on pathologic sections of the cerebellum at necropsy (see Fig. 10–18). Infarctions with occlusion of the medial branch may be clinically silent[484,500] or may manifest in one of three principal patterns[500]: (1) isolated vertigo, often misdiagnosed as labyrinthitis, (2) vertigo together with ipsilateral axial lateropulsion of the trunk and gaze,[512] and dysmetria or unsteadiness, and (3) Wallenberg's syndrome in patients in whom the medulla is also involved. By contrast with PICA, only the mPICA gives rise to rami to the dorsolateral aspect of the medulla.

Prognosis. Clinical series have shown that PICA infarctions have a much more benign outcome than usually thought.[439] Sypert and Alvord's[513] autopsy series emphasized the high incidence of brainstem compression and tonsillar herniation in acute PICA infarctions, but most acute cases were detected only at necropsy, thus biasing the series to fatal cases with large infarcts. Cerebellar swelling should always be the major concern of clinicians caring for patients with large cerebellar infarcts (see later). However, Sypert and Alvord[513] excluded from their analysis 46% of their patients in whom cerebellar infarction was not seen acutely but was diagnosed at autopsy. Kase and

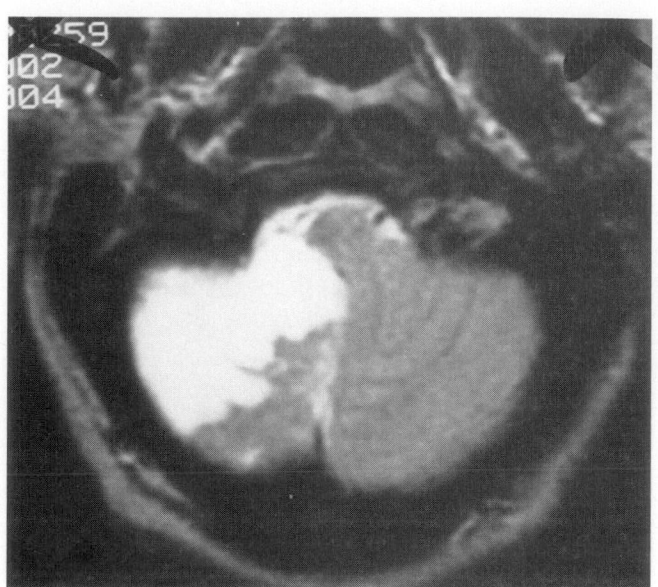

FIGURE 10–19 *Infarction in the territory of the lateral branch of the PICA (lPICA) on T2-weighted MR image.*

associates[439] found signs of brainstem compression in one fourth of their 36 patients (all of whom had full PICA territory infarcts) and acute hydrocephalus in 7 patients; only 4 patients died from cerebellar swelling. Most full and partial PICA territory infarctions have a relatively benign course.[133,439,500]

Intracranial Vertebral Artery Occlusive Disease

Occlusive disease of the intracranial portion of the VA is much more serious than extracranial disease and is commonly associated with infarction of posterior circulation structures. When the one VA that is responsible for supplying the major source of the blood flow is occluded (the contralateral VA being tiny, previously occluded, severely narrowed, or ending in the PICA), the resulting syndrome is indistinguishable from that caused by occlusion of the BA. Fisher[514] used the term *basilarization* of the VA to describe the situation of dependence on one VA for maintenance of the posterior circulation. Clot formed within the distal VA may propagate into the proximal BA, again producing a syndrome indistinguishable from that seen with BA occlusion.

In the more common situation of bilaterally competent VAs, occlusion of a single VA may be asymptomatic or may be associated with one of the following clinical pictures: (1) lateral medullary infarction, (2) PICA infarction due to obstruction of the ostium of the PICA by an occlusive thrombus in the intracranial VA, (3) ischemia of the ipsilateral hemimedulla through obstruction of the ostia of the anterior spinal artery arising from the intracranial portion of the VA, (4) embolic occlusion in vessels of the distal basilar arterial tree, the embolus originating from the VA clot, and (5) transient spells without infarction. Because these syndromes are common, quite distinct, and

clinically important, they are considered separately in detail here.

Lateral Medullary Infarction
Anatomic Vascular Aspects

The issue of vascular supply from the vertebral or posterior inferior cerebellar artery in lateral medullary infarction has a long history. In the comprehensive anatomic description of the brain supply by Duret[1] in 1873, the PICA was described as supplying the lateral region of the medulla. Then Dumenil[502] in 1875, in a clinical and pathologic report, expressed the realization that unilateral palsy of the palate can be attributed to lateral medullary infarction and PICA occlusion. In 1895, Wallenberg[486] reasoned, from the clinical findings in a single case and what he knew of brainstem anatomy and physiology, that the responsible lesion should be in the lateral medulla.[515] Furthermore, he injected the vessels of seven other autopsied human brains to define the arterial supply to the medulla and concluded that the PICA should be occluded in patients with infarcts in the lateral medulla. In fact, postmortem examination of the single case studied clinically did verify infarction of the cerebellum and medulla and occlusion of the PICA. However, when Fisher and colleagues[68] examined the pattern of vascular occlusion in 17 of their own cases of lateral medullary infarction, the occlusive lesion was located solely within the PICA in only 2 cases. In 13 cases, the vertebral artery was occluded, and in 1 case, severely stenosed. In 20 earlier reports in which the responsible vascular lesion had been documented, 15 patients had VA occlusion; only 4 had occlusion within the PICA itself. In about half the cases, the thrombus in the VA extended to block the PICA orifice.

Fisher and colleagues[68] and Escourolle and associates[110] demonstrated that not one (Foix's artery or the PICA as stated by Wallenberg) but several small arteries from the VA usually supply the lateral medullary area. Foix and coworkers probably described an infrequent arterial anomaly, and Wallenberg an unusual lateral medullary supply, because the PICA participates in the supply of the lateral medulla in less than one third of cases. However, the mPICA always participates in the supply of the dorsal medulla along with branches from the posterior spinal arteries.[67] If indeed the intrinsic arterial distribution is usually fixed and divided into medial, lateral, and dorsal areas, the extrinsic arterial supply is extremely variable from one individual to the next.[11]

The series reported by Norrving and Cronqvist[516] from Lund, Sweden, was the first to report the vascular lesions as determined in vivo by either angiography or ultrasonography in 43 patients with lateral medullary infarcts. The most common vascular lesions involved the VAs.[516] Among the 12 patients with angiographically documented VA occlusions, 9 patients had no proximal VA opacification, one VA filled for 4 to 5 cm, and two occlusions involved the distal ECVA. These researchers made no comments about the mechanism by which the ECVA occlusive lesions caused the medullary infarcts, but either propagation or embolism of clot into the ICVA must have occurred. In 2 patients with distal ECVA stenosis and 1 patient with PICA stenosis, dissection was the cause of the vascular narrowing.

Clinical Manifestations

Disease in the contralateral subclavian-vertebral arteries was rare. An angiogram of one patient showed contralateral SA stenosis, and one patient was found at necropsy to have contralateral VA stenosis. Five patients had coexisting carotid artery disease with greater than 50% stenosis in the neck.[516]

In the series described by Sacco and colleagues[517] from Columbia University, vascular studies were performed in 33 patients, and the ipsilateral VA was abnormal in 24 (73%). In 18 patients, duplex Doppler ultrasonography of the VA showed either high-resistance flow or no flow in an imaged artery. Fifteen patients underwent angiography, which showed that 5 had VA stenoses, 3 had VA occlusions, and 5 had VA dissections. In 2 patients with VA dissection or stenosis, the PICA was also occluded, but in no patient was PICA disease the only finding. In 2 patients, angiographic findings were normal.[517] In another clinical MRI study, ICVA disease was the most common etiology.[518] Among patients with large dorsolateral infarcts, 75% had severe stenosis or occlusion of the ICVA. Dissections of the VAs and cardioembolism were each thought to account for one seventh of the cases.[518]

Infarct Topography

The infarct usually involves a wedge of the medulla extending from the lateral edge (see Fig. 10–9). It usually affects a portion of the olive ventrally and in some cases extends dorsally to involve the restiform body. Currier and associates[519] divided the pattern of infarction into ventral, superficial, and dorsal lesions, indicating that the extent of infarction was quite variable. When the dorsal medulla is infarcted, the lesion is almost always accompanied by cerebellar infarction.[69] Because the lesion extends dorsally to the olive, the older terminology referred to the lesion as the "retro-olivary syndrome."[520] The zone of infarction usually extends 7 to 10 mm in a rostrocaudal dimension, occurring most commonly in the middle part of the olive but frequently extending into its upper or lower third.[68] In 9 of 24 lateral medullary infarcts studied by Hauw and colleagues,[69] the lesion extended to the pontomedullary junction. Vuilleumier and coworkers[518] published data from the Lausanne registry on MRI-clinical correlations in 28 patients with medullary infarcts.[518] They showed that the distribution of infarcts suggested earlier by Currier and associates[519] could be confirmed by MRI. The most common locations of medullary infarcts in the Lausanne series were small midlateral, dorsolateral, inferolateral, and inferodorsolateral. Dorsal infarcts were always accompanied by medial PICA territory cerebellar infarcts.[518]

In the series reported by Sacco and associates,[517] the selection of cases was predominantly clinical—all patients with lateral medullary syndrome were included.[517] Although all 33 patients underwent CT (none showed a brainstem infarct but 3 showed cerebellar infarcts), MRI was performed in only 22 (66%); a typical lateral medullary infarct was present in only 12 patients (37% of the total number), and 8 had other brainstem infarcts with or without lateral medullary infarction.[517] All 33 patients in the series reported by Kim and colleagues[521] were selected because MRI in these patients showed unilateral lesions involving mainly the dorsolateral medulla.[521] The infarcts involved the rostral medulla in 8 patients, the middle

medulla in 8, and the caudal medulla in 9; among the remaining 8 patients, 4 had rostral and middle infarcts, and 4 had middle and caudal involvement.[521] Accompanying cerebellar infarction was uncommon on neuroimaging scans, occurring in 3 patients (9%) in the Columbia series,[517] in 7 patients (21%) in Kim's series,[521] and in 6 of 30 (20%) patients in the Swedish study.[516] As with thrombosis elsewhere, TIAs commonly precede the stroke by days or weeks, more rarely months, and are noted in about half the patients with lateral medullary infarction.

Vascular Pathology

Vascular pathology also plays a role. Among the patients studied at necropsy by Fisher and assoicates,[68] 14 were thought to have *atherostenotic thrombotic occlusions*, and 3 were thought to represent *embolic occlusions*. Two patients with embolism had cardiac sources in the form of congenital heart disease and bacterial endocarditis; the other patient with presumed embolism had multiple scattered brain infarcts and no occlusion of the VA or PICA at necropsy, suggesting an embolism that fragmented and passed. This group also reviewed previous reports of embolism causing lateral medullary infarcts. In the first reported case, described by Hallopeau, a patient studied at necropsy by Charcot was thought to have a distal VA embolus that arose from ulcerated atheromatous plaques in the aorta. A patient described by Breuer and Marburg had a cardiac mural thrombus and nonadherent gray embolic thrombus in the ICVA leading to a lateral medullary infarct.[53,68] A patient studied by Richter[522] had a PICA embolus from a bicuspid aortic valve.

Escourolle and colleagues[110] found 14 VA occlusions and 3 occlusions of the PICA among 23 examples of lateral medullary infarction. When the infarction was located in the dorsal medulla, the occlusion was more likely to be in the stem of the PICA (four of five patients). Foix and colleagues[496] found in an autopsy case that the lateral medulla was supplied by a single lateral medullary artery that arose from the very proximal portion of the BA; they postulated that the syndrome was caused by occlusion of "the artery of the lateral sulcus of the medulla." Subsequently, however, Goodhart and Davison[70] found such an artery only once and Escourolle and colleagues[110] twice.

In cases of PICA infarctions due to VA occlusion, autopsy-documented multiple vascular occlusions including the VA has been reported by a number of workers.[484] McCusker and colleagues[523] described a patient with a locked-in syndrome that was likely due to an embolus to the BA arising from a previously occluded VA. Fisher and Karnes[524] noted 18 examples of local artery-to-artery embolism within the posterior circulation, 5 in relation to a unilateral VA occlusion. Castaigne and associates[77] also described examples of artery-to-artery emboli within the posterior circulation, and Caplan[262] reported a patient (case 5) with spells of transient dizziness who experienced a stroke when embolic material originating in a unilateral VA occlusion embolized to the SCA. George and Laurian[66] described two patients with unilateral VA stenosis, and in whom angiography subsequently verified occlusion, who suffered embolism arising from the diseased VAs. George and Laurian[66] found that 80% of patients with a lateral medullary or cerebellar infarct and 65% of patients with basilar trunk territory infarcts had greater than 50% stenosis of a VA, leading the researchers to suspect that the stenotic VA was a common source of embolism.

Koroshetz and Ropper[525] systematically studied patients with PCA territory strokes who also had brainstem symptoms. Six patients had occlusive lesions of the ICVA (combined with extracranial lesions in three); these investigators judged that these lesions had served as donor sites for intra-arterial emboli to the PCA. Pessin and coworkers[526] reported on a patient with a major BA territory infarct in whom angiography showed occlusion of one intracranial VA and an intraluminal filling defect embolus in the distal BA. Among a series of 85 patients with recent BA thrombi who underwent acute thrombolytic treatment, 16 had stenotic or occlusive lesions of the ICVAs that likely served as sources of artery-to-artery emboli to the BA.

Figure 10–20 shows an example of VA intracranial occlusion with an embolus to the distal BA. In patients with distal BA territory infarction, scant data are available concerning the incidence of coincidentally discovered VA occlusion that might have provided an embolic source. Within the anterior circulation, occlusion of the ICA is commonly heralded by a distal embolus.

Symptoms

The symptoms of lateral medullary infarction are explained by the distinctive anatomy of the lesion (Fig. 10–21).

Vertigo. The most common symptom is dizziness or vertigo, often accompanied by staggering and double

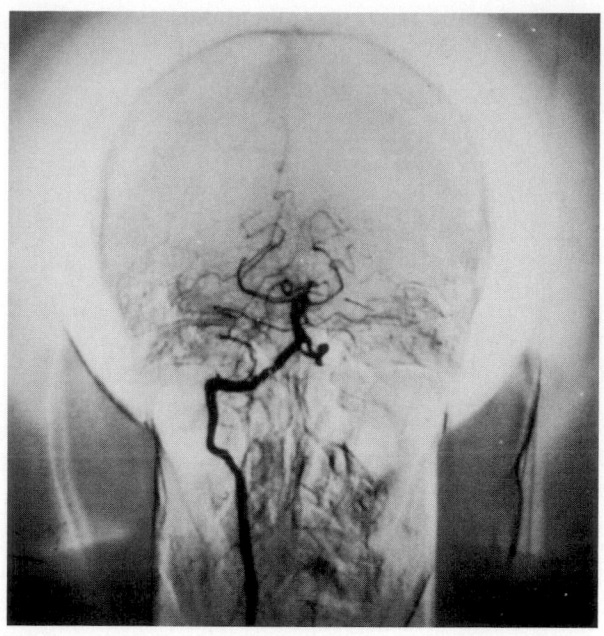

FIGURE 10–20 *Vertebral angiogram showing right vertebral artery intracranial occlusion. The top of the basilar artery and posterior cerebral arteries are not opacified, probably owing to embolus from the vertebral artery clot.*

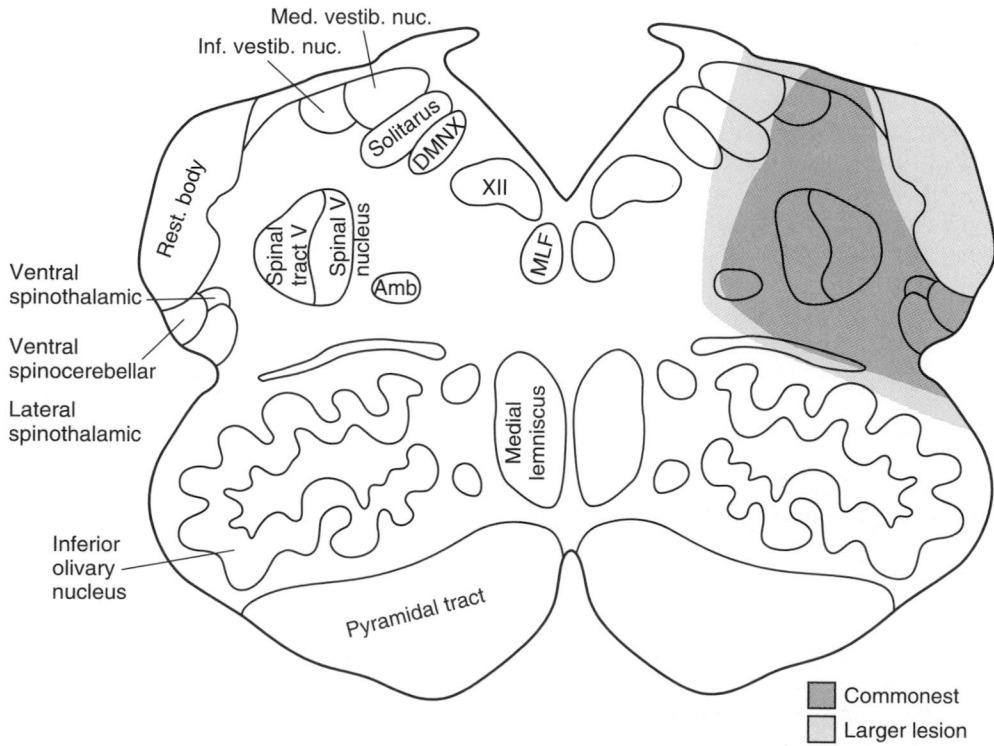

FIGURE 10–21 *Lateral medullary infarction. The most common involvement and largest extent of the lesion are designated by the shaded areas, as described in the key. (Based on a figure in Currier R, Giles C, Dejong R: Some comments on Wallenberg's lateral medullary syndrome. Neurology [NY] 11:778, 1961.)*

vision. Difficulty in focusing and numbness of the face are other common components of the TIAs. Headache, especially in the occipital region, may accompany other symptoms or may occur alone. The deficit may develop suddenly, but more commonly it progresses gradually over 24 to 48 hours. Fluctuations or stepwise deterioration frequently characterizes the first week after stroke onset, but is less common thereafter and distinctly unusual after 2 weeks.

Facial Pain. Facial pain is more diagnostic and is a cardinal feature of the syndrome. Of 39 patients studied in one large series, 27 had persisting (18 patients) or transient face pain ipsilateral to the lesion.[519] Sharp, single stabs or jolts of pain are felt in the eye or face. Occasionally, these may occur in flurries like a machine gun. Sticking, burning, stinging, tingling, and numbness are other commonly used descriptive terms. The eye is the most commonly affected region, but the pain may be limited to the ear or isolated spots on the forehead or cheeks. Pain frequently affects the entire face, including the lips and inside the mouth, but is rarely if ever limited to the mandibular division of the trigeminal nerve.

Unpleasant facial sensations, when present, usually appear at the very onset of the stroke and are often the first symptom perceived by the patient. The coexistent contralateral hemianalgesia of the body is seldom mentioned but is usually evident to the patient only after pain or temperature testing. The striking contrast between the spontaneous sudden facial pain due to involvement, presumably, of the nucleus of the descending tract of the fifth cranial nerve and the lack of perception of the hemianalgesia related to ischemia of the spinothalamic tract led Fisher[527] to postulate that dysfunction of sensory neurons (either within the dorsal root ganglia or buried within the central nervous system, as in the nucleus of the tract of the fifth cranial nerve or in its main sensory nucleus) produces spontaneous pain, but lesions of white matter or nerves do not generally evoke pain as an early finding. Occasionally, burning facial pain, likened by one patient to having salt and pepper thrown on the face, may be seen transiently in tegmental ischemia other than in a lateral medullary location.[340] The presence of facial pain or dysesthetic feelings may not be mentioned spontaneously by the patient because of their bizarre or unusual nature. Because they are so diagnostic of brainstem involvement, the presence of such sensations should be diligently sought by the examiner.

Feelings of Disequilibrium. Vertigo or other feelings of disequilibrium are nearly always present. Although frank whirling or rotational turning may be described, feelings of swaying or falling, feeling seasick, or being off balance are the most common terms used. These perceptions are probably due to involvement of the vestibular nuclei or their connections. Alteration of vision, another common complaint, may even be described as diplopia (18 of 39 cases) or, less commonly, as the illusion that objects are oscillating or moving.[519] The visual deficit is not monocular, and decreased visual acuity, visual field defects, and extraocular muscle palsies are not found to explain the visual symptoms. In the patient complaining of altered vision, the most common neuro-ophthalmologic finding is nystagmus; the visual complaints are probably due to

sudden alteration in the vestibulo-ocular system, sometimes resulting in skew deviation or even in conjugate ipsilateral horizontal gaze palsy. Occasionally, patients with lateral medullary infarction complain of tilting of the visual world with a 90- to 180-degree inversion of the visual images.[110] Even with persisting nystagmus, the patient's visual symptoms are usually transient, indicating the nervous system's compensatory ability to adapt to chronic nystagmus and vestibular dysfunction.

Nausea and Vomiting. Nausea and vomiting are also common symptoms (affecting 18 of the 35 patients reported by Peterman and Siekert,[528] and 27 of those studied by Currier and associates[519]) and are due to vestibular dysfunction or to involvement of the dorsal tegmentum—the *vomiting centers* identified by Borison and Wang[529] in the floor of the fourth ventricle. The nucleus ambiguus is near the vomiting centers; some writers have therefore argued that because signs of ninth and tenth cranial nerve dysfunction frequently occur in patients with vomiting, the floor of the fourth ventricle is incriminated as the site of origin of the vomiting.[519] We have not seen a patient with nausea and vomiting without accompanying dizziness or nystagmus, and we wonder whether vomiting is simply a reflection of disease of the vestibular nuclei and their connections.

Ataxia. Ataxia is the rule rather than the exception. Virtually no patient with documented lateral medullary infarction walks normally, and all patients complain of altered gait. Walking is usually characterized by veering to the side, leaning, or stumbling. The patient is also aware of the ipsilateral cerebellar dysfunction and describes the arm as clumsy, unreliable, or weak.

Hiccups. Hiccups (affecting 19 of the 74 patients reported by Currier and associates[519]) are a common complaint, usually developing some time after the onset. In most patients with hiccups, the lateral medullary infarct is typically complete and is usually not ventral or superficial. The origin of the hiccups is uncertain but could relate to dysfunction of "respiratory centers" or to involvement of tenth cranial nerve fibers.[519,530] Difficulty in swallowing is common (55 of the 74 total patients reported by Currier and associates[19] and Peterman and Siekert[528]).

Food or secretions may have unusually free influx into the air passages, a phenomenon unusual in patients with peripheral ninth and tenth cranial nerve involvement at the jugular foramen. Disturbances of the coordination of epiglottic closure and palatal and pharyngeal function may be more likely with a central lesion of the nucleus ambiguus. Food gets stuck in the piriform recess of the pharynx adjacent to the larynx; patients attempt to extricate the material by an unusual cough-like maneuver. This crowing-like cough is characteristic, and its presence in a patient with stroke is virtually diagnostic of lateral medullary infarction.

Hoarseness is also common but may be absent in ventral or more superficial lesions. Some patients with involvement of the spinothalamic tract mention numbness, burning, or perverted sensations in the contralateral limbs or trunk, but these symptoms most commonly occur later in the course, sometimes weeks or months after the stroke.[531] Ipsilateral stuffy nose, altered taste, and dysarthria are less common.

Headache. Moderate or severe headache is common in lateral medullary infarction and is related either to involvement of the descending spinal tract of the fifth cranial nerve and its nucleus or to vascular distension produced by the occlusive process within the vertebral artery. In 1836, Bright[532] called attention to posterior headache in vascular disease. He described a "gentleman past the meridian of life" who had apoplectic attacks and complained, "I feel completely knocked up and have much pain in the back of the head, like a rheumatic pain, generally at the same spot the right side of the back part of the head." Bright commented, "This pain would itself chiefly direct our suspicions to disease of the vertebral arteries."

Steady or, less commonly, pulsatile headache is located most often in the occipital region and is unilateral in about half of cases.[514] Headache is usually centered just below the external occipital protuberance and extends into the suboccipital and nuchal regions, usually nearer the midline than the ear. Frequently it extends into the frontal region, and occasionally, the headache may be dull and only frontal in location.

Signs

The signs accompanying lateral medullary infarction have been extensively reviewed.[519,528,530,531,533,536] This discussion is confined to a review of the seven main signs.

Diminished Sensation in the Ipsilateral Face. Involvement of the descending tract of the fifth cranial nerve and its nucleus usually produces decreased pain and temperature sensation of the ipsilateral face. Almost invariably, the corneal reflex is lost or severely reduced. The forehead and rest of the ophthalmic division are more analgesic than the lower face. Pain and cold sensitivities are generally affected equally. At times, although single pinpricks feel less sharp and less discrete, there may be a dysesthetic quality, with spread and persistence of the perceived stimulus. When the ipsilateral face is severely analgesic, the lower border does not usually conform to the limits of the peripheral mandibular division of the fifth cranial nerve, but can be portrayed as a gentle curve sloping downward and medially from the tragus to the mandible, where the facial artery lies.[528] Touch may also be diminished in the analgesic face.[531] The sensory defect in the face usually clears more quickly than that on the contralateral body, although the loss of corneal reflex usually persists.[531]

Diminished Pain and Temperature Sensation on the Contralateral Body. Ischemia of the lateral spinothalamic tract is responsible for diminished pain and temperature sensation on the side of the body contralateral to the infarct. As previously noted, patients infrequently report contralateral hemianalgesia, but some described a numbness or cold feeling. The sensory loss may affect the entire hemicorpus, but often the cervical region is spared. At onset, a level of pain and temperature sensation may be delimited either near the nipple line or on the trunk or abdomen, in which case the arm frequently has normal sensibility.

Pain and temperature should always be checked in the lower extremity; some examiners "retire" their pins to abbreviate the examination of a patient who has perceived pain normally in the arm. The fibers within the spinothalamic tract are laminated, with the sacral fibers most lateral and the arm more medial. The arm and upper neck and trunk are spared in more superficial lesions. When the lesion extends far medially, it may even involve the quintothalamic fibers, which have already crossed to join the medial border of the spinothalamic tract, producing a complete contralateral hemianalgesia including the contralateral face.

In patients with bilateral facial analgesia, the pin feels different on the two sides of the face, the loss being more severe on the side of the infarction. Without very careful testing, the contralateral face could be assessed as normal unless the pin sensibility here is compared with that in the normal ipsilateral arm or trunk.

With time, the hemianalgesia frequently improves, and a pain-numbness level may become apparent over the trunk.[534] Less often the analgesia clears both rostrally and caudally, leaving a band of altered sensibility on the trunk.[530] Although at onset the loss of pain and temperature sensibility tends to be homogeneous over affected areas, greater degrees of sensibility appear later, leaving patches of perverted sensation. The analgesia usually extends to the midline at onset, but the paramedian region of the body often clears more in the front than in the back.[531]

At times, the loss of pain and temperature can be entirely crossed, occurring in the face, arm, trunk, and leg contralateral to the infarct. The lesions that cause this unilateral pattern of sensory loss are located more medially and involve the crossing fibers in the ventral trigeminal thalamic tract and the fibers in the crossed lateral spinothalamic tract. At times, the discomfort is severe and is comparable to thalamic pain, with which it probably shares a common mechanism. Rubbing of the involved part, the pressure of tight clothing, or excessive heat or cold may aggravate the discomfort. When pain makes a delayed appearance on the contralateral side of the body, the pain generally persists and is relatively resistant to pharmacologic treatments.[531]

Horner's Syndrome. Sympathetic nervous system fibers course through the lateral reticular substance and are involved in most cases of lateral medullary infarction (affecting 25 of 35 patients in the series reported by Hauw and colleagues[69]), resulting in ipsilateral Horner's syndrome. Usually, the syndrome is incomplete; ptosis is the most common element and leads to drooping of the upper eyelid and some elevation of the lower lid, narrowing the palpebral fissure. Miosis is also very common, the pupil usually retaining its reactivity to light. Anhydrosis is the least common element of the Horner's syndrome in lateral medullary infarction.

Ataxia. Gait ataxia and limb ataxia are very important signs of lateral brainstem infarction and are due to ischemia of the restiform body or to associated infarction of the inferior cerebellum in the territory of the PICA. The gait ataxia seen in the lateral medullary syndrome is different from that seen with the vermal degeneration of alcoholism. Leaning, veering, falling, or toppling to the side when the patient is placed in an erect or sitting position is characteristic of medullary infarction and can be contrasted with the wide-based gait with truncal titubation

cerebrovascular disease, lesions of the SA were avidly sought and surgically repaired. More importantly, the concept of blood flowing from one vessel to rescue a more distant circulation gave rise to the concept that the cerebrovascular bed was an open net in which decreased input at any point of entry could conceivably lead to decreased flow in any distant site. To determine *ischemia at a distance*, clinicians would fully opacify the entire vascular bed, including the aortic arch and the four major extracranial vessels. Any obstructive lesion, even if it did not directly supply the ischemic region, might then be subjected to surgical repair.

In the 40 years since the original report, a clearer definition of the clinical findings has been accomplished, and with it, a lessening of the role of surgery. Patients with subsequently verified subclavian steal may present with one of several types of symptoms, (1) headache, (2) intermittent episodes of cerebral ischemia, or (3) claudication or pain in the ischemic arm. However, many are entirely asymptomatic from the subclavian lesion, as was the case in fully 74% of the 155 lesions evaluated by Hennerici and colleagues.[603] The lesion is often discovered only when angiographic or noninvasive evaluation of pulse or blood pressure changes in the arm, peripheral vascular disease in the legs, or abnormalities in the carotid circulation reveal the subclavian lesion.

Headache is common and is usually located in the mastoid, occiput, or neck. The major symptom of the first patient encountered by Reivich and colleagues[595] was recurrent throbbing pain in the left mastoid area, which radiated to the left parietal and occipital regions. The headache may be more generalized, may be isolated, or may accompany symptoms of cerebral ischemia. The headache may be precipitated by exercise. Surprisingly, symptoms of severe ischemia in the involved arm are rare. Patients may complain of fatigue, claudication with exercise, paresthesia, sensitivity to cold, and sensations of heaviness or coolness in the arm; symptoms are often exercise-related.

The usual slow development of the occlusion and the richness of collateral supply tend to make upper extremity ischemia a relatively minor problem unless the patient exercises the arm frequently, as has been the case in some noted golfers and baseball pitchers.[369,604,605] Sudden downward arm motions can cause angulation of the SA over the first rib or a cervical rib, where the artery courses over the flat surface of the first rib on its way out of the thorax. Pitchers and cricket bowlers may subject the SAs of their throwing arms to chance trauma with subsequent thrombosis. Fatigue, arm pain, loss of pitching velocity and accuracy, and lack of stamina in the throwing arm result.[603]

Cerebral symptoms are common but usually transient, lasting seconds to minutes but often recurring over months or even years.[600,602] In many patients, subclavian stenosis occurs as one of many vessels affected by severe atherosclerotic disease; coexistent significant atherosclerotic lesions in the carotid artery and other extracranial and intracranial vessels are quite common and might even be considered the rule rather than the exception. The source of the transient ischemic cerebral symptoms is thus often difficult to discover.[595,600] In the series of Hennerici and colleagues,[603] lateralized hemispheric symptoms of cerebral ischemia were about twice as frequent in patients with uni-

lateral subclavian steal and associated carotid disease as in those without carotid lesions. Hemispheric brain symptoms occurred more often (29 patients [62%]) in patients with severe carotid artery stenosis than in those with less severe obstruction (18 patients [38%]).

Other symptoms and signs may reflect peripheral arterial effects. The arm may show more cyanosis when held above heart level. A bruit may be heard in the supraclavicular region and may radiate into the axilla or along the posterior neck to the mastoid region. Sometimes one can distinguish the subclavian or vertebral origin of a bruit by pumping a blood pressure cuff above systolic pressure. This maneuver decreases distal subclavian flow but may increase cephalad flow in the VA, because blood goes into the proximal branches rather than the arm. In disease of the proximal SA, the bruit usually decreases because of less flow through the stenotic segment and less retrograde vertebral flow; in VA stenosis, the bruit is usually augmented. Focal neurologic deficits caused by subclavian-vertebral siphonage are rare and are usually explained by coexistent carotid artery disease, which should be sought on examination.

The most common cause of subclavian occlusive disease is atherosclerosis, although congenital lesions such as preductal coarctation of the aorta with patent ductus arteriosus,[262] atresia of the left SA,[606] and a pseudocoarctation of the aorta with kinked left SA[144] occasionally produce the syndrome. Sometimes, subclavian steal follows surgical manipulation of the SA, as in the Blalock-Taussig procedure for tetralogy of Fallot, in which the SA is anastomosed to the pulmonary artery. Traumatic injury, embolism, and arteritis (temporal arteritis and Takayasu's arteritis) may also cause subclavian steal. In the large series reported by North and coworkers,[600] the left SA was affected alone in 33 cases and the right subclavian or innominate artery in 13 cases, and 13 cases were bilateral.

The frequency with which the arteries are affected varies. The left SA is involved approximately three times more frequently than the right innominate or subclavian artery. Among 155 patients with a unilateral subclavian steal in one series, 71% of the cases were left-sided, and 29% of the patients had Raynaud's phenomenon. In the SA, occlusive disease does not always cause retrograde vertebral flow. Of 20 cases of SA stenosis evaluated by Berguer and associates,[607] only half showed evidence of reversed VA flow. There are many other possible collateral channels to augment distal subclavian flow, including the inferior and external thyroid, internal mammary, intercostal, and ascending cervical arteries.[608] At times, the VA ipsilateral to the SA stenosis originates from the aortic arch, ends distally in the PICA, or is tiny or occluded, and so is unavailable as a source of collateral supply.[62]

The anatomy of the right side of the aortic arch differs from that of the left. The innominate artery is larger and usually rises higher in the supraclavicular fossa than its left counterpart. The right SA has a more intimate relationship with the right common carotid artery. Clot in the right axillary or subclavian artery may propagate into the innominate artery and extend or embolize to the carotid system. Although this phenomenon is rare, most of the patients affected have been young and have presented a striking clinical picture. Symonds[609] described two patients with diminished arterial pulsation in the right arm, probably due to a cervical rib in which sudden left hemiplegia developed. Yates and Guest[236] reported a patient with progressive pain and weakness in the right arm who had an non-united fracture of the right clavicle. This patient suddenly experienced visual loss, went into a coma, had left hemiplegia, and subsequently died. At postmortem, the right SA was found to be displaced by the fractured bone and occluded. Clot extended into the innominate artery and had embolized to the BA bifurcation. Hoobler[610] reported a similar patient with a cervical rib, weak right arm pulses, and sudden left hemiparesis. Damage to the SA may be caused by cervical ribs, trauma, or the use of crutches. Clot or aneurysm forms at the site of compression and leads to symptoms of ischemia or Raynaud's phenomenon in the arm; the clot embolizes on the right, into the distal carotid or vertebral arterial tree. Although a similar lesion could occur on the left, it would involve only the left VA and might be difficult to recognize.

Stenosis or occlusion of the innominate artery is less common than SA disease. Brewster and colleagues[611] collected data on 71 patients operated on in one hospital for innominate artery lesions during a 20-year period. Thirty-six of the patients had atherosclerotic occlusive disease involving the origin of the innominate artery from the aortic arch or the heart.

The diagnosis of subclavian steal in the early series was usually confirmed by angiography, which is best accomplished through selective transfemoral or transaxillary catheterization of the normal VA with delayed films to show retrograde flow down the contralateral VA. Arch angiography provides suboptimal detail of the involved vessels. In addition, more dye is required for arch angiography, and complications are more common. Digital subtraction angiography is used less often nowadays,[612,613] having largely been replaced by MRA.[50–52]

Noninvasive testing now accurately documents severe innominate and SA occlusive disease with a high degree of reliability.[42,43,46,48] Liljequist and coworkers[44] demonstrated that directional Doppler ultrasonography of flow in the VA located just below the transverse process of the atlas reliably detects the presence of retrograde VA blood flow in patients with angiographically verified subclavian steal. Berguer and colleagues[607] measured the relative velocity of pulsed-wave propagation in both arms of subjects and concluded that a delay in propagation was well correlated with angiographically verified reversal of VA flow in the innominate and subclavian arteries. Provocative tests such as decreasing peripheral resistance in the upper arm could cause temporary BA flow reversal, which can be insonated by TCD ultrasonography.[47,87]

Surgical treatment for subclavian steal, at one time popular, has received less application in the last decade. Among the procedures are endarterectomy of the subclavian lesion, which usually requires a thoracotomy, and cervical or thoracic prosthetic or venous bypass grafts and ligation of the ipsilateral VA.[608] VA ligation can cause thrombosis of the artery with later propagation of clot into the cranium or distal embolization.[85,614] A physician or surgeon who is deciding whether surgery is indicated in a particular patient with subclavian steel should keep the following three points in mind:

1. Subclavian steal is a relatively benign phenomenon. Although transient spells are common, brainstem infarction is rare. Cerebellar infarction has been observed, but only after hypotension. In other words, there is usually more smoke than fire.
2. Coexistent serious extracranial and intracranial vascular disease is the rule. It is easy to be seduced by the intriguing collateral pathways and the clearly demonstrable physical signs of subclavian disease and thereby to miss the more important, more relevant vascular lesion in the individual patient.
3. Subclavian or innominate artery surgery is somewhat more complex and is associated with higher morbidity rates than other extracranial vascular surgery if a thoracotomy is needed. Patients who could tolerate a local neck procedure, such as carotid endarterectomy or venous bypass grafting, may not be able to survive a thoracotomy satisfactorily. Unfortunately, the open net theory of cerebral circulation has given license to surgical repair of an angiographic stenosis whether or not it is directly related to the symptomatology.

Mobile Thrombus in the Aortic Arch

See Chapter 30 for a full discussion of this disorder.

Edematous Cerebellar Infarction Manifesting as a Space-Occupying Mass

Although benign forms of cerebellar infarcts are much more common than lethal infarctions, the possibility of rapidly progressive cerebellar swelling with acute hydrocephalus and death must be kept in mind, because surgery in this situation may be life saving. This form was first described by Menzies[615] in 1893. However, Fairburn and Oliver[616] and Lindgren[283] deserve considerable credit because they showed, 50 years ago, that total recovery could be obtained with surgical treatment. They emphasized the clinical findings in patients with these infarcts. Edema causes cerebellar swelling, raised pressure in the posterior fossa, and brainstem compression. Aqueductal or fourth ventricle displacement or occlusion leads to obstructive hydrocephalus and acute intracranial hypertension. Cerebellar swelling may cause downward tonsillar herniation through the foramen magnum and transtentorial upward herniation of the culmen of the vermis.

Involved Artery Territories and Mechanisms in Patients with Pseudotumoral Cerebellar Infarcts

In autopsy series, pseudotumoral infarctions involved the PICA territory,[513] SCA territory, or both.[459] In clinical series, the PICA territory is more frequently involved than the SCA territory.[439] Swelling of the cerebellum seems to be related to at least four factors, as follows: (1) mainly the large size of the infarction with involvement of more than one third of the cerebellar hemisphere volume,[513] (2) the site of the embolic occlusion, with disease at the rostral end of the BA affecting the SCA ostia or with bilateral VA occlusions affecting the PICA ostia, as well as the failure of collateral supply,[459] (3) the increase in vasogenic edema with reperfusion after the migration of an embolus,[459] and (4) the presence of a massive SCA infarction, the

Clinical Manifestations

However, only MRI revealed a high frequency of very small cerebellar infarcts (<2 cm in extent) and located in borderzone areas.

Two studies summarize the main findings.[133,254] Among a consecutive series of 115 patients with cerebellar infarcts (diagnosed with MRI in 85% of patients), 36 (31%) had only small borderzone infarcts.[133] These infarcts were usually small and deep or cortical, involving the borderzones between territories of cerebellar arteries or their branches. Both reports sought to identify the stroke mechanisms and clinical findings in patients with small cerebellar infarcts. Were these lesions the posterior circulation counterparts of cerebral borderzone lesions attributable in some patients to systemic hypoperfusion? Could some infarcts represent cerebellar lacunes due to lipohyalinosis, or intracranial branch atheromatous disease, or both? Instead, were the causes of small infarcts identical to those of larger cerebellar infarcts, but the small size explained by the rapid development of adequate collateral circulation or by the passage and fragmenting of emboli with fragments blocking small distal arterial branches?

Amarenco and colleagues[254] analyzed a series of very small cerebellar infarcts. The series consisted of 47 patients with small infarcts that were found by extensive review of CT and MRI findings in patients with cerebellar infarcts studied at the New England Medical Center (29 patients) and Boston University Medical Center (8 patients) in Boston and at the Hôpital Saint-Antoine in Paris (10 patients). These small cerebellar infarcts accounted for 43%, 26%, and 28% of cerebellar infarcts at these hospitals, respectively.[254]

Patterns of Infarction

Amarenco and colleagues[254] observed that the infarcts seemed to fit five different anatomic patterns (Fig. 10–24). Group I infarcts (29 patients) were cortical and linear and were directed toward the subcortical cerebellar white matter, perpendicular to the cortex and parallel to the penetrating branches. Group II infarcts (15 patients) were very small and were located in the deep white matter. Group III infarcts (5 patients) were located in the rostral and medial cerebellum. Group IV (2 patients) infarcts were

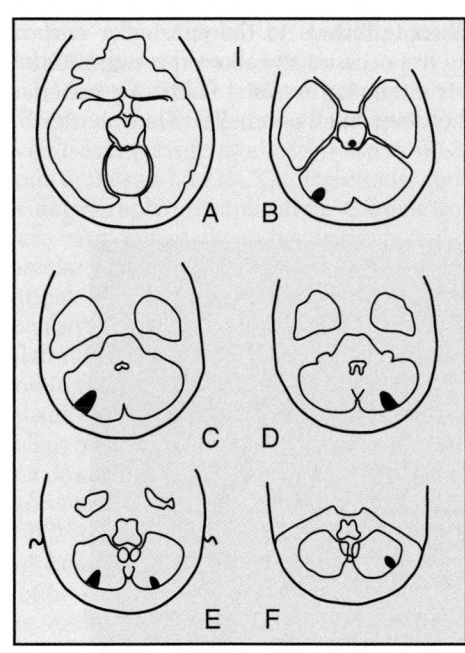
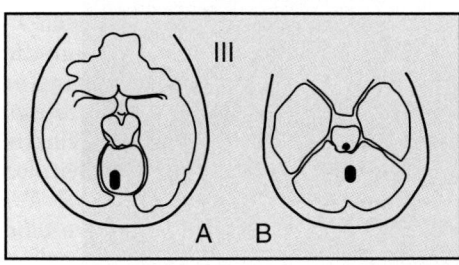
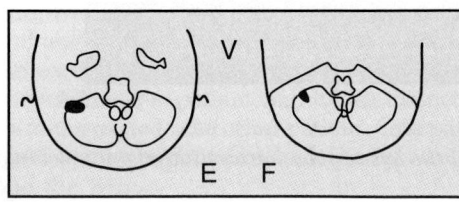
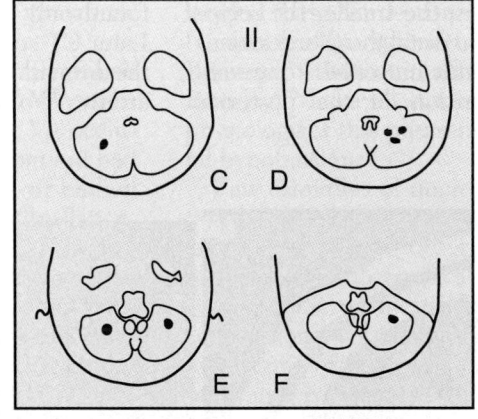
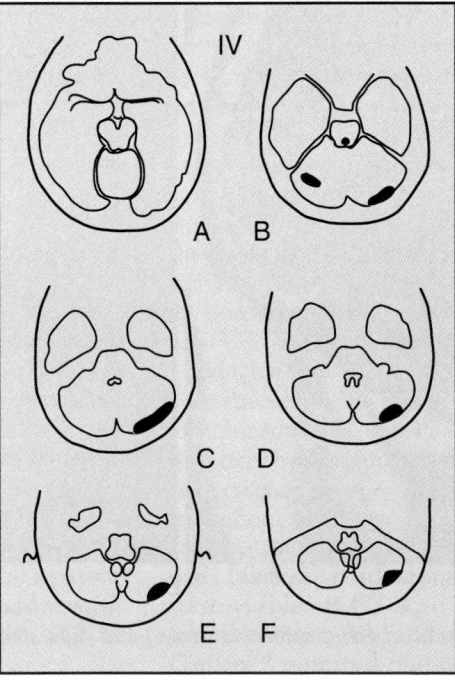

FIGURE 10–24 *Pattern of distribution of cerebellar borderzone infarcts.*

cortical superficial infarcts. Group V (1 patient) infarcts were cortical and ventral and were aligned parallel to penetrating branches.

Some patients had more than one type of infarct.[254] The researchers divided the causes of these infarcts into four groups: In group A (2 patients), cardiac arrest or systemic hypoperfusion was the cause of infarction. Group B (9 patients) were considered to have occlusive disease of small penetrating or pial arteries caused by various conditions. In this group, 1 patient had Wegener's granulomatosis; 4 had hypercoagulability (2 disseminated intravascular coagulation, 1 thrombocytosis, 1 polycythemia); in 3 patients, the absence of large artery lesions and the presence of diabetes and lacunes suggested disease of small arteries as the cause; and in 1 patient, cholesterol crystal embolism was proven by muscle biopsy. Group C, the largest group, consisted of 27 patients in whom large artery occlusive disease or brain embolism was the likely cause of stroke. Sixteen had occlusive lesions, most often involving the VAO, ICVA, and BA. Eleven had embolism, 9 of cardiac origin and 2 intra-arterial. In group D, which consisted of 9 patients, the cause of the small cerebellar infarcts was unknown, mostly because of incomplete evaluation.[254] In this study, systemic hypoperfusion was a very rare cause of small infarcts, and in very few patients was intrinsic atherostenotic disease of small penetrating or pial arteries the cause of the small infarcts.[254]

Amarenco and colleagues[133] later prospectively collected patients with territorial and small nonterritorial infarcts studied at the Hôpital Saint-Antoine in Paris during a 6-year period. Thirty-six of the 115 cerebellar infarcts (31%) were small and not readily localizable to one of the cerebellar artery territories. The causes of territorial and small, nonterritorial infarcts were very similar. About one third of the patients in each group had cardiac sources of embolism; one fourth had large artery occlusive disease; and in about one fourth, no definite cause could be established. Small artery inflammatory disease and hypercoagulable states were more common in patients with small nonterritorial infarcts than in patients with territorial infarcts.[133] Systemic hypoperfusion and penetrating and pial artery branch disease were not important causes of small infarcts in either series.[133] Infarcts distal to unilateral occlusive lesion of one VA occurred in 18% of patients with territorial cerebellar infarcts and in 5% of patients with small nonterritorial (borderzone) infarcts, but this difference was not statistically significant. However, infarcts distal to bilateral vertebral or BA occlusions occurred with a low-flow state at angiography in 14% of patients with nonterritorial (borderzone) cerebellar infarcts but in none of the patients with territorial infarcts. These investigators concluded that small nonterritorial infarcts have the same high rate of embolic mechanism (about 50% of cases) as territorial infarcts, more commonly are associated with hypercoagulable states and small artery inflammatory disease than territorial infarcts, and sometimes have a hemodynamic mechanism.[133]

One other study reported eight borderzone infarcts among a series of 34 patients diagnosed with MRI, which were attributed to "severe vertebrobasilar atherosclerosis."[437] Mounier-Vehier and coworkers[644] reported a series of 14 consecutive patients with borderzone infarcts and confirmed that most (9 patients) had a cardioembolic mechanism; 3 of the 14 had VA dissections.

Distal Field Ischemia in the Brainstem

Brainstem lesions due to hypotension have been hypothesized but seldom documented. Romanul[637] identified the medial zone at the tegmentobasal junction of the mid-pons (the area damaged in central pontine myelinolysis) as a possible zone of vulnerability between medial penetrating branches and tegmental supply from the circumferential cerebellar vessels supplying the tegmentum, but did not refer to necropsy specimens supporting this idea. Jurgensen and colleagues[645] described a 44-year-old epileptic woman who was found to be hypotensive, hypothermic, and comatose after presumed multiple-drug injection. Necropsy revealed bilateral, symmetric, round, hemorrhagic infarcts distributed in a columnar fashion in the lateral brainstem tegmentum extending the length of the lower pons and medulla. They were between the short lateral circumferential penetrators and the lateral edge. There were also bilateral hemorrhagic lesions in the lateral putamen. Gilles[646] described isolated necrosis of brainstem nuclei in children after hypotension.

The authors have seen two adult patients with a clinical picture after hypotension that closely mimicked pontine hemorrhage: small pupils, absence of horizontal gaze, and deep coma. In one of these patients, no gross lesion was visible at postmortem, but extensive necrosis of brainstem nuclei was seen microscopically, especially in the pons. Postmortem examination was not performed in the other patient. Lance and Adams[647] described patients with hypotension who made fine or coarse muscular jerks, especially on conscious attempts at precise movement. These researchers called this phenomenon "intention and action myoclonus." Myoclonus was related to probable cerebellum system damage but was not precisely localized. Keane[648] wondered whether the sustained upward gaze found in 15 patients who had suffered a cardiorespiratory arrest could be due to a "symmetrical cerebellar hypoxic change" that was found at postmortem in the 6 autopsied patients. Downward nystagmus and severe truncal and extremity cerebellar dysfunction were also noted in several patients, leading Keane[648] to suggest a posterior circulation locus for the pathogenic mechanism.

Migraine

In 1961, Bickerstaff[649] reported a distinct symptom complex occurring in adolescent girls that consisted of repeated episodes of altered vision, vertigo, ataxia, dysarthria, and numbness and tingling of the limbs and sometimes face, followed by headache. The common family history of migraine and clearing of ischemic symptoms by the time the headache began stamped the disorder as migrainous for Bickerstaff, who called this disorder *basilar artery migraine*. Swanson and Vick[650] have corroborated the existence of this syndrome, noted its occasional onset in adult life, and described an occasional familial tendency.[651]

Although traditionally considered a disorder beginning in the first two or three decades of life, migraine occurring late in life is more common than is generally realized.

Clinical Manifestations

Fisher[652] analyzed the nature of migraine accompaniments in a group of patients and contrasted their clinical features with those in a comparable group of patients in whom ischemia was due to verified atherosclerotic occlusive disease. Migrainous deficits developed over a period of 15 to 30 minutes. "Positive" phenomena (for example, scintillations or brightness in the visual sphere or tingling in the tactile sphere) were perceived first and gradually spread within each sensory modality; for example, scintillations traveled gradually across the visual field and paresthesias spread from one digit to the next and slowly up the limbs. The "positive" phenomena left in their wake "negative" phenomena, for example, blackness or numbness. As positive and later negative phenomena spread within the sensory modality, the regions affected earliest would clear, and finally all symptoms related to that modality would return to normal before a second modality would be affected. Headache would usually, but not always, appear after the deficits had disappeared. Using these clinical criteria and the absence of appropriate angiographic atherosclerotic lesions that might explain the clinical phenomenon, Fisher[653] defined a group of patients whom he believed had transient migrainous spells beginning after the age of 50 years. Our experience (LRC) with such patients includes those with (1) a clinical tempo matching that described by Fisher,[652] (2) multiple attacks in a variety of regions, (3) absence of angiographic disease or a source of cerebral emboli, and (4) response to commonly used prophylactic anti-migraine agents such as propranolol, phenytoin, and methysergide. In many such patients, attacks are within the distribution of the posterior circulation.

The term basilar artery migraine is perhaps redundant, because it has long been known, but not understood, that migraine tends to involve the BA and its branches. Visual scintillations are the most common accompaniments of migraine and are occipital (PCA) in origin. Examples of transient global amnesia are known in migraine, and the pathologic anatomy and physiology of memory suggest a dominant PCA localization.[654] Physiologic studies using xenon-133 have documented oligemia as an early finding or as occurring subsequent to focal hyperemia.[655,656] Blood flow changes are maximal in the occipitoparietal regions.[657] Also, angiography performed during the prodromal phase of migraine has demonstrated filling of the PCA from carotid injection, suggesting low pressure in the basilar system. Any of these patients might fall within the usually accepted nosology of migraine.[654]

Caplan[448] reviewed his experience with patients who had migraine (classic or common) and posterior circulation ischemic attacks and strokes and underwent angiography. Nine patients were presented. Men and women of widely varying ages were included. The clinical patterns involved just TIAs, single strokes, single stroke followed by attacks, and multiple strokes. In some patients, classic migraine developed only months or years later. CT and MRI confirmed infarctions in patients who had strokes with persistent neurologic deficits (seven of nine patients).[448] Angiography showed BA occlusions, severe diffuse narrowing of vertebrobasilar arteries (rather persistent in one patient), or normal posterior circulation vessels. The mechanism of infarction was not elucidated, but clearly, vasoconstriction, which was often protracted, and BA occlusion did occur. Caplan[448] posited that ischemia was due to protracted vasoconstriction or to vascular thrombosis precipitated by activation of platelet adhesion and agglutination and activation of the intrinsic and extrinsic coagulation pathways.

References

1. Duret H: Recherches anatomiques sur la circulation de l'encéphale. Arch Physiol Norm Pathol 3:60, 1874.
2. Duret H: Sur la distribution des artères nourricières du bulbe rachidien. Arch Physiol Norm Pathol 2:97, 1873.
3. Hayem G: Sur la thrombose par artérite du tronc basilaire comme cause de mort rapide. Arch Physiol Norm Pathol 1:270, 1868.
4. Leyden E: Uber die Thrombose der basilar Arterie. Z Klin Med 5:165, 1882.
5. Marburg O: Uber die neuren Fortschritte in der topischen Diagnostic du Pons und Oblongata. Dtsch Z Nervenheilkd 41:41, 1911.
6. Pines L, Gilinsky E: Uber die Thrombose der Arteria basilaris und uber die Vascularization de Brucke. Arch Psychiatr 26:380, 1932.
7. Stopford J: The arteries of the pons and medulla oblongata. I. J Anat Physiol 50:131, 1915.
8. Stopford J: The arteries of the pons and medulla oblongata. II. J Anat Physiol 50:255, 1916.
9. Caplan LR: Charles Foix: The first modern stroke neurologist. Stroke 21:348, 1990.
10. Foix C, Hillemand P: Contribution à l'étude des ramollissements protubérantiels. Rev Med 43:287, 1926.
11. Foix C, Hillemand P: Les artères de l'axe encéphalique jusqu'au diencéphale inclusivement. Rev Neurol 32:705, 1925.
12. Lhermitte J, Trelles JO: L'artério-sclérose du tronc basilaire et ses conséquences anatomo-cliniques. Jahrbücher Psychiatr Neurol 51:91, 1934.
13. Kubik C, Adams R: Occlusion of the basilar artery: A clinical and pathologic study. Brain 69:73, 1946.
14. Fisher CM: Occlusion of the internal carotid artery. Arch Neurol Psychiatry 65:345, 1951.
15. Hutchinson E, Yates P: Carotico-vertebral stenosis. Lancet 1:2, 1957.
16. Meyer JS, Sheehan S, Bauer R: An arteriographic study of cerebrovascular disease in man: Stenosis and occlusion of the vertebral basilar arterial system. Arch Neurol 2:27, 1960.
17. Williams D: The syndromes of basilar insufficiency. In Garland H (ed): Scientific Aspects of Neurology. Baltimore, Williams & Wilkins, 1961, p 202.
18. Williams D, Wilson T: The diagnosis of the major and minor syndromes of basilar insufficiency. Brain 85:741, 1962.
19. Denny-Brown D: Basilar artery syndromes. Bull N Engl Med Cent 15:53, 1953.
20. Fang H, Palmer J: Vascular phenomena involving brainstem structures. Neurology (NY) 6:402, 1956.
21. Millikan C, Siekert R: Studies in cerebrovascular disease: The syndrome of intermittent insufficiency of the basilar arterial system. Proc Staff Meet Mayo Clin 30:61, 1955.
22. Wolf J: The Classical Brainstem Syndromes. Springfield, IL, Charles C Thomas, 1971.
23. Denny-Brown D: Recurrent cerebrovascular episodes. Arch Neurol 2:194, 1960.
24. Millikan C, Siekert R, Shick R: Studies in cerebrovascular disease: The use of anticoagulant drugs in the treatment of insufficiency or thrombosis within the basilar arterial system. Proc Staff Meet Mayo Clin 30:116, 1955.
25. Millikan C, Siekert R, Whisnant J: Anticoagulant therapy in cerebrovascular disease: Current status. JAMA 166:587, 1958.
26. Browne T, Poskanzer D: Treatment of strokes. N Engl J Med 281:594, 1969.
27. Ausman JI, Diaz FG, Pearce JE, et al: Endarterectomy of the vertebral artery from C-2 to posterior inferior cerebellar artery intracranially. Surg Neurol 18:400, 1982.
28. Khodadad G, Singh R, Olinger C: Possible prevention of brainstem stroke by microvascular anastomosis in the vertebrobasilar system. Stroke 8:316, 1977.

29. Sundt T, Whisnant J, Piepgras D, et al: Intracranial bypass grafts for vertebral basilar ischemia. Mayo Clin Proc 53:12, 1978.

30. Imparato A, Riles T, Kim G: Cervical vertebral artery angioplasty for brainstem ischemia. Surgery 90:842, 1981.

31. McNamara J, Heyman A, Silver D, et al: The value of carotid endarterectomy in treating transient cerebral ischemia of the posterior circulation. Neurology (NY) 27:682, 1977.

32. Sundt T, Smith H, Campbell J, et al: Transluminal angioplasty for basilar artery stenosis. Mayo Clin Proc 55:673, 1980.

33. Hacke W, Zeumer H, Ferbert A, et al: Intra-arterial thrombolytic therapy improves outcome in patients with acute vertebrobasilar occlusive disease. Stroke 19:1216, 1988.

34. Pessin MS, del Zoppo GJ, Estol C: Thrombolytic agents in the treatment of stroke. Clin Neuropharmacol 13:271, 1990.

35. Zeumer H: Vascular recanalizing technique in interventional neuroradiology. J Neurol 231:287, 1985.

36. Zeumer H, Hacke W, Ringelstein EB: Local intraarterial thrombolysis in vertebrobasilar thromboembolic disease. AJNR Am J Neuroradiol 4:401, 1983.

37.. Biller J, Yuh W, Mitchell GW: Early diagnosis of basilar artery occlusion using magnetic resonance imaging. Stroke 19:297, 1988.

38. Kistler JP, Buonnano FS, DeWitt LD, et al: Vertebral-basilar posterior cerebral territory stroke: Delineation by proton nuclear magnetic resonance imaging. Stroke 15:417, 1984.

39. Simmons Z, Biller J, Adams HP, et al: Cerebellar infarction: Comparison of computed tomography and magnetic resonance imaging. Ann Neurol 19:291, 1986.

40. Ackerstaff RG, Hoenefeld H, Slowikowski JM, et al: Ultrasonic duplex scanning in atherosclerotic disease of the innominate, subclavian and vertebral arteries: A comparative study with angiography. Ultrasound Med Biol 10:409, 1984.

31. Bluth EL, Merritt CR, Sullivan MA, et al: Usefulness of duplex ultrasound in evaluating vertebral arteries. J Ultrasound Med 8:229, 1989.

42. Ekestrom S, Eklund B, Liljequist L, et al: Noninvasive methods in the evaluation of obliterative disease of the subclavian or innominate artery. Acta Med Scand 206:467, 1979.

43. Hennerici M, Rautenberg W, Schwartz A: Transcranial Doppler ultrasound for the assessment of intracranial arterial flow velocity. II: Evaluation of intracranial arterial disease. Surg Neurol 27:523, 1987.

44. Liljequist L, Ekerstrom S, Nordhus O: Monitoring direction of vertebral artery blood flow by Doppler shift ultrasound in patients with suspected subclavian steal. Acta Chir Scand 147:421, 1981.

45. Touboul PJ, Bousser MG, Laplane D, et al: Duplex scanning of normal vertebral arteries. Stroke 17:97, 1986.

46. von Reutern GM, Budingen JH: Ultraschalldiagnostik der Hirnversorgenden Arterien. Stuttgart, Thieme, 1989.

47. Caplan LR, Brass LM, DeWitt LD, et al: Transcranial Doppler ultrasound: Present status. Neurology (NY) 40:696, 1990.

48. Hennerici M, Rautenberg W, Sitzer G, et al: Transcranial Doppler ultrasound for the assessment of intracranial arterial flow velocity. I: Examination of technique and normal values. Surg Neurol 27:439, 1987.

49. Tettenborn B, Estol C, DeWitt LD, et al: Accuracy of transcranial Doppler in the vertebrobasilar circulation. J Neurol 237:159, 1990.

50. Dumoulin CL, Hart HR: MR angiography. Radiology 161:717, 1986.

51. Edelman RR, Mattle HP, Atkinson DJ, et al: MR angiography. AJR Am J Roentgenol 154:937, 1990.

52. Zuccoli G, Guidetti D, Nicola F, et al: Carotid and vertebral artery dissection: Magnetic resonance findings in 15 cases. Radiol Med (Torino) 104:466–471, 2002.

53. Caplan LR, Tettenborn B: Embolism in the Posterior Circulation in Vertebrobasilar Disease. St. Louis, Quality Medical Publishing, 1991, p 52.

54. Prognosis of patients with symptomatic vertebral or basilar artery stenosis. The Warfarin-Aspirin Symptomatic Intracranial Disease (WASID) Study Group. Stroke 29:1389, 1998.

55. Alajouanine T, Lhermitte F, Gautier J: Transient cerebral ischemia in atherosclerosis. Neurology (NY) 10:906, 1960.

56. Libman R, Benson R, Einberg K: Myasthenia mimicking vertebrobasilar stroke. J Neurol 249:1512, 2002.

57. Krayenbüll H, Yasargil M: Radiological anatomy and tomography of the cerebral arteries. In Vinken P, Bruyn G (eds): Handbook of Clinical Neurology, vol 2. Amsterdam, North-Holland, 1972, p 65.

58. Stephens R, Stilwell D: Arteries and Veins of the Human Brain. Springfield, IL, Charles C Thomas, 1969.

59. Takahashi S: Atlas of Vertebral Angiography. Baltimore, University Park Press, 1974.

60. Wilkinson I: The vertebral artery. Arch Neurol 27:392, 1972.

61. Lister J, Rhoton A, Matsushima T, et al: Microsurgical anatomy of the posterior inferior cerebellar artery. Neurosurgery 10:170, 1982.

62. Fankhauser H, Kamano S, Hanamura T, et al: Abnormal origin of the posterior inferior cerebellar artery. J Neurosurg 51:569, 1979.

63. Lasjaunias P, Guibert-Tranier F, Braun JP: The pharyngo-cerebellar artery or ascending pharyngeal artery origin of the posterior inferior cerebellar artery. J Neuroradiol 8:317, 1981.

64. Guillard A: Pathologie ischemique cérébrale et anomalie de terminaison intracranienne de l'artère vertébrale. Semin Hop Paris 62:2755, 1986.

65. Margolis MT, Newton TH: The posterior inferior cerebellar artery. In Newton TH, Potts G (eds): Radiology of the Skull and Brain: Angiography, vol 68. St. Louis, CV Mosby, 1974, p 1710.

66. George B, Laurian C: Vertebro-basilar ischemia with thrombosis of the vertebral artery: Report of two cases with embolism. J Neurol Neurosurg Psychiatry 45:91, 1982.

67. Duvernoy HM: Human Brainstem Vessels. Heidelberg, Springer-Verlag, 1978.

68. Fisher CM, Karnes W, Kubik C: Lateral medullary infarction: The pattern of vascular occlusion. J Neuropathol Exp Neurol 20:323, 1961.

69. Hauw J-J, Der Agopian P, Trelles L, et al: Les infarctus bulbaires. J Neurol Sci 28:83, 1976.

70. Goodhart S, Davison C: Syndrome of the posterior inferior and anterior inferior cerebellar arteries and their branches. Arch Neurol Psychiatry 35:501, 1936.

71. Lazorthes G: Vascularisation et Circulation Cérébrales. Paris, Masson, 1961

72. Amarenco P, Hauw J-J: Cerebellar infarction in the territory of the anterior and inferior cerebellar artery: A clinicopathological study of 20 cases. Brain 113:139, 1990.

73. Amarenco P, Hauw J-J, Caplan LR: Cerebellar infarctions. In Lechtenberg R (ed): Handbook of Cerebellar Diseases. New York, Marcel Dekker, 1993, p 251.

74. Taveras JM, Wood EH: Diagnostic Neuroradiology, vol II. Baltimore, Williams & Wilkins, 1976, p 783.

75. Greitz T, Sjögren S: The posterior inferior cerebellar artery. Acta Radiol 1:284, 1963,

76. Amarenco P, Hauw J-J: Anatomie des artères cérébel-leuses. Rev Neurol 145:267, 1989.

77. Castaigne P, Lhermitte F, Gautier J-C, et al: Arterial occlusions in the vertebral-basilar system. Brain 96:133, 1973.

78. Foix C, Hillemand P: Irrigation de la protubérance. C R Soc Biol Paris 42:35, 1925.

79. Gillian L: The correlation of the blood supply to the human brainstem with brainstem lesions. J Neuropathol Exp Neurol 23:78, 1964.

80. Gillian L: Anatomy and embryology of the arterial system of the brainstem and cerebellum. In Vinken P, Bruyn G (eds): Handbook of Clinical Neurology, vol 2. Amsterdam, North-Holland, 1972, p 24.

81. Szdzuy D, Lehman R: Hypoplastic distal part of the basilar artery. Neuroradiology 4:118, 1972.

82. Hommel M, Besson G, Pollak P, et al: Hemiplegia in posterior cerebral artery occlusion. Neurology (NY) 40:1496, 1990.

83. Caplan LR: Vertebrobasilar system syndromes. In Vinken PJ, Bruyn GW, Klawans HL (eds): Handbook of Clinical Neurology. Amsterdam, North-Holland, 1988, p 371.

84. Graff-Radford NR, Damasio H, Yamada T, et al: Non-haemorrhagic thalamic infarction. Brain 108:495, 1985.

85. Hopkins LN, Martin NA, Hadley MN, et al: Vertebrobasilar insufficiency. II: Microsurgical treatment of intracranial vertebrobasilar disease. J Neurosurg 66:662, 1987.

86. Percheron GMJ: Etude anatomique du thalamus de l'homme adulte et de sa vascularisation artérielle. Paris, Thesis, 1966

87. von Cramm D, Hebel N, Schieri U: A contribution to the anatomical basis of thalamic amnesia. Brain 108:993, 1985.

88. Castaigne P, Lhermitte F, Buge A, et al: Paramedian thalamic and midbrain infarcts: clinical and neuropatho-logical study. Ann Neurol 10:127, 1981.

89. Percheron G: Les artères du thalamus humain. Rev Neurol (Paris) 132:297, 1976.

Clinical Manifestations

90. Bogousslavsky J, Regli F, Assal G: The syndrome of unilateral tuberothalamic artery territory infarction. Stroke 17:434, 1986.

91. Chase T, Moretti L, Prensky A: Clinical and electro-encephalographic manifestations of vascular lesions of the pons. Neurology (NY) 18:357, 1968.

92. Caplan LR, DeWitt LD, Pessin MS, et al: Lateral thalamic infarcts. Arch Neurol 45:959, 1988.

93. Lie T: Congenital malformations of the carotid and vertebral arterial systems, including the persistent anastomoses. In Vinken P, Bruyn G (eds): Handbook of Clinical Neurology, vol 2. Amsterdam, North-Holland, 1972, p 289.

94. Kingsley D, Radue E, DuBoulay E: Evaluation of computed tomography in vascular lesions of the vertebrobasilar territory. J Neurol Neurosurg Psychiatry 43:193, 1980.

95. Pinkerton J, Davidson K, Hibbard B: Primitive hypoglossal artery and carotid endarterectomy. Stroke 6:658, 1980.

96. Obayashi T, Furuse M: The proatlantal intersegmental artery. Arch Neurol 37:387, 1980.

97. Parkinson D, Reddy V, Ross R: Congenital anastomosis between the vertebral artery and internal carotid artery in the neck. J Neurosurg 51:697, 1979.

98. Asplund K, Wester P, Fodstad H, et al: Long time survival after vertebral/basilar occlusion. Stroke 11:304, 1980.

99. Bronstein AM, Morris J, DuBoulay G, et al: Abnormalities of horizontal gaze: Clinical, oculographic and magnetic resonance imaging findings. I: Abducens palsy. J Neurol Neurosurg Psychiatry 53:194, 1990.

100. Caplan LR: Lacunar infarction: A neglected concept. Geriatrics 3:71, 1976.

101. Cornhill J, Akins D, Hutson M, et al: Localization of atherosclerotic lesions in the human basilar artery. Atherosclerosis 35:77, 1980.

102. Echiverri HC, Rubino FA, Gupta SR, et al: Fusiform aneurysm of the vertebrobasilar arterial system. Stroke 20:1741, 1989.

103. Feigin I, Budzilovich G: The general pathology of cerebrovascular disease. In Vinken P, Bruyn G (eds): Handbook of Clinical Neurology, vol 2. Amsterdam, North-Holland, 1972, p 128.

104. Schwartz C, Mitchell J: Atheroma of the carotid and vertebral arterial systems. BMJ 2:1057, 1961.

105. Fisher CM, Ojemann RG: A clinico-pathologic study of carotid endarterectomy plaques. Rev Neurol (Paris) 142:573, 1986

106. Pelouze GA: Plaque ulcérée de l'ostium de l'artère vertébrale. Rev Neurol 145:478, 1989.

107. Reznik M: Le ramollissement du tronc cérébral. Acta Neurol Belg 81:257, 1981.

108. Amarenco P, Duyckarets C, Tzourio C, et al: The prevalence of ulcerated plaques in the aortic arch in patients with stroke. N Engl J Med 326:221, 1992.

109. Amarenco P, Hauw J-J, Gautier J-C: Arterial pathology in cerebellar infarction. Stroke 21:1299, 1990.

110. Escourolle R, Hauw J-J, Der Agopian P, et al: Les infarctus bulbaires. J Neurol Sci 28:103, 1976.

111. Fisher C, Gore I, Okabe N, et al: Atherosclerosis of the carotid and vertebral arteries: Extracranial and intracranial. J Neuropathol Exp Neurol 24:455, 1965.

112. Moosy J: Morphology, sites and epidemiology of cerebral atherosclerosis. Proc Assoc Res Nerv Ment Dis 51:1, 1966.

113. Whisnant J, Martin M, Sayre G: Atherosclerotic stenosis of cervical arteries. Arch Neurol 5:429, 1961.

114. Caplan L, Baker R: Extracranial occlusive disease: Does size matter? Stroke 11:63, 1980.

115. Fisher C: Some neuro-ophthalmological observations. J Neurol Neurosurg Psychiatry 30:383, 1967.

116. Fields WS: Collateral circulation in cerebrovascular disease. In Vinken P, Bruyn G (eds): Handbook of Clinical Neurology, vol 2. Amsterdam, North-Holland, 1972, p 168.

117. Castaigne P, Buge A, Escourolle R, et al: Ramollissement pédonculaire médian, tégmentothalamique avec ophtalmoplégie et hypersomnie. Rev Neurol 106:357, 1962.

118. Caplan LR, Gorelick PB, Hier DB: Race, sex and occlusive cerebrovascular disease: A review. Stroke 17:648, 1986.

119. Bauer R, Sheehan S, Wechsler N, et al: Arteriographic study of sites, incidence and treatment of arteriosclerotic cerebrovascular lesions. Neurology (NY) 12:698, 1962.

120. Stein B, McCormick W, Rodriques J, et al: Incidence and significance of occlusive vascular disease of the extracranial arteries as documented by post-mortem angiography. Trans Am Neurol Assoc 86:60, 1961.

121. Ueda K, Toole J, McHenry L: Carotid and vertebrobasilar transient ischemia attacks: Clinical and angiographic correlation. Neurology (NY) 29:1094, 1979.

122. Thompson JR, Simmons C, Hasso A, et al: Occlusion of the intradural vertebrobasilar artery. Neuroradiology 14:219, 1978.

123. Hutchinson E, Yates P: The cervical portion of the vertebral artery: A clinico-pathological study. Brain 79:319, 1956.

124. Tunick PA, Kronzon I: Protruding atherosclerotic plaque in the aortic arch of patients with systemic embolization: A new finding seen by transesophageal echocardiography. Am Heart J 120:658, 1990.

125. Feldmann E, Daneault N, Kwan E, et al: Chinese-white differences in the distribution of occlusive cerebrovascular disease. Neurology (NY) 40:1541, 1990.

126. Gorelick PB, Caplan LR, Hier DB, et al: Racial differences in the distribution of posterior circulation occlusive disease. Stroke 16:785, 1985.

127. Caplan LR (ed): Posterior Circulation Disease. Cambridge, UK, Blackwell Science, 1996.

128. Kieffer SA, Takeya Y, Resch JA, et al: Racial differences in cerebrovascular disease: Angiographic evaluation of Japanese and American populations. AJR Am J Roentgenol 101:94, 1967.

129. Resch JA, Okabe N, Loewenson RB, et al: Patterns of vessel involvement in cerebral atherosclerosis: A comparative study between a Japanese and Minnesota population. J Atherosclerosis Res 9:239, 1969.

130. Caplan LR: Intracranial branch atheromatous disease: A neglected, understudied and underused concept. Neurology (NY) 39:1246, 1989.

131. Amarenco P, Rosengart A, DeWitt LD, et al: Anterior inferior cerebellar artery territory infarcts: Mechanisms and clinical features. Arch Neurol 50:154, 1993.

132. Amarenco P, Hauw J-J: Cerebellar infarction in the territory of the superior cerebellar artery. Neurology (NY) 40:1383, 1990.

133. Amarenco P, Lévy C, Cohen A, et al: Causes and mechanisms of territorial and nonterritorial cerebellar infarcts in 115 consecutive cases. Stroke 25:105, 1994.

134. Amarenco P, Caplan LR: Vertebrobasilar occlusive disease: Review of selected aspects. 3: Mechanisms of cerebellar infarctions. Cerebrovasc Dis 3:66, 1993.

135. Fisher CM, Caplan L: Basilar artery branch occlusion: A cause of pontine infarction. Neurology (NY) 21:900, 1971.

136. Peress N, Kane WC, Aronson SM: Central nervous system findings in a tenth decade autopsy population. Prog Brain Res 40:473, 1973.

137. Fisher CM: Ataxic hemiparesis: A pathologic study. Arch Neurol 35:126, 1978.

138. Fisher CM: Cerebral ischemia: Less familiar types. Clin Neurosurg 18:267, 1971.

139. Fisher CM: The arterial lesions underlying lacunes. Acta Neuropathol 12:1, 1967.

140. Fisher CM: The vascular lesion in lacunae. Trans Am Neurol Assoc 90:243, 1965.

141. Fisher CM: Pathological observations in hypertensive cerebral hemorrhage. J Neuropathol Exp Neurol 30:536, 1971.

142. Barrows L, Kubik C, Richardson E: Aneurysms of the basilar and vertebral arteries: A clinicopathologic study. Trans Am Neurol Assoc 81:181, 1956.

143. Bull J: Contribution of radiology to the study of intracranial aneurysms. BMJ 2:1701, 1962.

144. Lochaya S, Kaplan B, Shaffer AB: Pseudocoarctation of the aorta with bicuspid aortic valve and kinked left subclavian artery, a possible cause of subclavian steal. Am Heart J 73:369, 1967.

145. Auerbach S, De Piero T, Romanul F: Sylvian aqueduct syndrome caused by unilateral midbrain lesion. Ann Neurol 11:91, 1982.

146. Barnes KL, Ferrario CM: Role of the central nervous system in cardiovascular regulation. In Furlan A (ed): The Heart and Stroke. Heidelberg, Springer Verlag, 1987.

147. Emanuele M, Dorsch T, Scarff T, et al: BA aneurysm simulating pheochromocytoma. Neurology (NY) 31:1560, 1981.

148. Naheedy M, Tyler H, Wolf M, et al: Diagnosis of thrombotic giant basilar artery aneurysm on computed tomographic scan. Arch Neurol 39:64, 1982.

149. Aichner FT, Felber SR, Birhamer GG, Posch A: Magnetic resonance imaging and magnetic resonance angiography of vertebrobasilar dolichoectasia. Cerebrovasc Dis 3:280, 1993.

150. Schwartz A, Rautenberg W, Hennerici M: Dolichoectatic intracranial arteries: Review of selected aspects. Cerebrovasc Dis 3:273, 1993.

151. Yu Y, Moseley I, Pullicino P, et al: The clinical pictures of ectasia of the intracerebral arteries. J Neurol Neurosurg Psychiatry 45:29, 1982.
152. Moseley I, Holland I: Ectasia of the basilar artery: The breadth of the clinical spectrum and the diagnostic value of computed tomography. Neuroradiology 18:83, 1979.
153. Pessin MS, Chimowitz MI, Levine SR, et al: Stroke in patients with fusiform vertebrobasilar aneurysms. Neurology (NY) 39:16, 1989.
154. Hirsh L, Gonzalez C: Fusiform basilar aneurysm simulating carotid transient ischemic attacks. Stroke 10:598, 1979.
155. DeBosscher J: Anévrysme de l'artère vertébrale gauche chez un homme 45 ans. Acta Neurol Psychiatr Belg 52:1, 1952.
156. Denny-Brown D, Foley J: The syndrome of basilar aneurysm. Trans Am Neurol Assoc 77:30, 1952.
157. Ekbom K, Grietz T, Kugelberg E: Hydrocephalus due to ectasia of the basilar artery. J Neurol Sci 8:465, 1969.
158. Kerber C, Margolis M, Newton T: Tortuous vertebrobasilar system: A cause of cranial nerve signs. Neurocardiology 4:74, 1972.
159. Nishizaki T, Tamikl N, Takeda N: Dolichoectatic basilar artery: A review of 23 cases. Stroke 17:1277, 1986.
160. Passerini A, Tagliabue G: Aneurysms of the vertebrobasilar system. Radiol Clin Biol 35:257, 1966.
161. Paulson G, Nashold B, Margolis G: Aneurysms of the vertebral artery. Neurology (NY) 9:590, 1959.
162. Milandre L, Bonnefoi B, Pestre P, et al: Dolichoectasies artérielles vertébrobasilaires: Complications et pronostique. Rev Neurol (Paris) 147:714, 1991.
163. Pollock M, Blennerhassett J, Clarke A: Giant cell arteritis and the subclavian steal syndrome. Neurology 23:653, 1973.
164. Rao K, Woodlief C: Stimulation of cerebellopontine tumor by tortuous vertebrobasilar artery. AJR Am J Roentgenol 132:602, 1979.
165. Maruyama K, Tanaka M, Ikeda S, et al: A case report of quadriparesis due to compression of the medulla oblongata by the elongated left vertebral artery. Rinsho Shinkeigaku 29:108, 1989.
166. Paulson G, Boesel C, Evans W: Fibromuscular dysplasia. Arch Neurol 35:287, 1978.
167. Hirsch CS, Roessmann U: Arterial dysplasia with ruptured basilar artery aneurysm: Report of a case. Hum Pathol 6:749, 1975.
168. Makos MM, McComb RD, Hart MN, et al: Alphaglucosidase deficiency and basilar artery aneurysm: Report of a sibship. Ann Neurol 22:629, 1987.
169. Little JR, St. Louis P, Weinstein M, et al: Giant fusiform aneurysm of the cerebral arteries. Stroke 12:183, 1981.
170. Gautier JC, Hauw JJ, Awada A, et al: Artères cérébrales dolichoectasiques: Association aux anévrysmes de l'aorte abdominales. Rev Neurol (Paris) 144:437, 1988.
171. Monge-Argiles J, et al: [Megadolicobasilar, ulcerative colitis and ischemic stroke]. Neurologia 18:221, 2003.
172. del Zoppo GJ, Zeumer H, Harker LA: Thrombolytic therapy in stroke: Possibilities and hazards. Stroke 17:595, 1986.
173. Passero S, Filosomi G: Posterior circulation infarcts in patients with vertebrobasilar dolichoectasia. Stroke 29:653, 1998.
174. Ince B, et al: Dolichoectasia of the intracranial arteries in patients with first ischemic stroke: A population-based study. Neurology 50:1694, 1998.
175. de Oliveira R de M, Cardeal JO, Lima JG: [Basilar ectasia and stroke: Clinical aspects of 21 cases]. Arq Neuropsiquiatr 55:558, 1997.
176. Alpert J, Gerson L, Hall R, et al: Reversible angiopathy. Stroke 13:100, 1982.
177. Fisher CM, Ojemann R, Roberson G: Spontaneous dissection of cervico-cerebral arteries. J Can Sci Neurol 5:9, 1978.
178. Caplan L, Young RR: EEG findings in certain lacunar stroke syndromes. Neurology (NY) 22:403, 1972.
179. Chiras J, Marciano S, Vega Molina J, et al: Spontaneous dissecting aneurysm of the extracranial vertebral artery (20 cases). Neuroradiology 27:327, 1985.
180. Mas JL, Bousser MG, Hasboun D, et al: Extracranial vertebral artery dissection: A review of 13 cases. Stroke 18:1037, 1987.
181. Mokri B, Houser OW, Sandok BA, Piepgras DG: Spontaneous dissections of the vertebral arteries. Neurology 38:880, 1988.
182. Silbert PL, Mokri B, Schievink W: Headache and neck pain in spontaneous internal carotid and vertebral artery dissections. Neurology 45:1517, 1995.
183. Easton JD, Sherman DG: Cervical manipulation and stroke. Stroke 8:594, 1977.
184. Ford F, Clark D: Thrombosis of the basilar artery with softenings in the cerebellum and brainstem due to manipulation of the neck. Bull Johns Hopkins Hosp 98:37, 1956.
185. Frumkin L, Baloh R: Wallenberg's syndrome following neck manipulation. Neurology 40:611, 1990.
186. Goldstein S: Dissecting hematoma of the cervical vertebral artery. J Neurosurg 56:451, 1982.
187. Houser OW, Baker H, Sandok B, et al: Cephalic arterial fibromuscular dysplasia. Radiology 101:605, 1971.
188. Kreuger B, Okazaki H: Vertebral-basilar distribution infarction following chiropractic cervical manipulation. Mayo Clin Proc 55:322, 1980.
189. Norris JW, Beletsky V, Nadareishvili ZG: Sudden neck movement and cervical artery dissection. The Canadian Stroke Consortium. CMAJ 163:38, 2000.
190. Biousse V, Chabriat H, Amarenco P, Bousser M-G: Roller-coaster-induced vertebral artery dissection. Lancet 346:767, 1995.
191. Amarenco P, Seux-Levieil M-L, Lévy C, et al: Carotid artery dissection with renal infarcts: Two cases. Stroke 25:2488, 1994.
192. Schievink WI, Michels VV, Mokri B, et al: A familial syndrome of arterial dissections with lentiginosis. N Engl J Med 332:576, 1995.
193. Schievink WI, Mokri B, Piepgras DG, Kuiper JD: Recurrent spontaneous arterial dissections: Risk in familial versus nonfamilial disease. Stroke 27:622, 1996.
194. Youl BD, Coutellier A, Dubois B, et al: Three cases of spontaneous extracranial vertebral artery dissection. Stroke 21:618, 1990.
195. Barbour PJ, Castaldo JE, Rae-Grant AD, et al: Internal carotid artery redundancy is significantly associated with dissection. Stroke 25:1201, 1994.
196. Ben Hamouda-M'Rad I, Biousse V, Bousser M-G, et al: Internal carotid artery redundancy is significantly associated with dissection. Stroke 26:1962, 1995.
197. Schievink WI, Mokri B: Familial aorto-cervicocephalic arterial dissections and congenitally bicuspid aortic valve. Stroke 26:1935, 1995.
198. Schievink WI, Mokri B, O'Fallon WM: Spontaneous recurrent cervical-artery dissection. N Engl J Med 330:393, 1994.
199. Caplan LR, Baquis G, Pessin MS, et al: Dissection of the intracranial vertebral artery. Neurology (NY) 38:868, 1988.
200. Alom J, Matias-Gurer J, Padeo L, et al: Spontaneous dissection of intracranial vertebral artery: Clinical recovery with conservative treatment. J Neurol Neurosurg Psychiatry 49:599, 1986.
201. Caplan L, Goodwin J: Hypertensive lateral tegmental brainstem hemorrhage. Neurology (NY) 32:252, 1982.
202. Deeb Z, Janetta P, Rosenbaum A, et al: Tortuous vertebrobasilar arteries causing cranial nerve syndromes: Screening by computed tomography. J Comput Assist Tomogr 3:774, 1965.
203. Alexander C, Burger P, Goree J: Dissecting aneurysms of the basilar artery. Stroke 10:294, 1979.
204. Escourolle R, Gautier J-C, Rosa A, et al: Anévrysme dissequant vertébrobasilaire. Rev Neurol 128:95, 1972.
205. Ringel S, Harrison S, Norenberg M, et al: Fibromuscular dysplasia: Multiple "spontaneous" dissecting aneurysms of the major cranial arteries. Ann Neurol 1:301, 1977.
206. Watson AJ: Dissecting aneurysm of arteries other than the aorta. J Pathol Bacteriol 72:439, 1956.
207. Lacour JC, et al: [Isolated dissection of the basilar artery]. Rev Neurol (Paris) 156:654, 2000.
208. Endoh H, et al: [A case of vertebrobasilar dissection which was associated with progressing stroke and was successfully treated by intravascular surgery in the acute stage]. No Shinkei Geka 26:1001, 1998.
209. Wolman L: Cerebral dissecting aneurysms. Brain 82:276, 1959.
210. D'Anglejan-Chatillon J, Ribeiro V, Mas J-L, et al: Migraine-risk factor for dissection of cervical arteries. Headache 29:560, 1989.
211. Yap C, Mayo C, Barron K: "Ocular bobbing" in palata: Myoclonus. Arch Neurol 18:304, 1968.
212. Touboul P-J, Mas J-L, Bousser M-G, Laplane D: Duplex scanning in extracranial vertebral artery dissection. Stroke 18:116, 1987.
213. Lévy C, Laissy J-P, Raveau V, et al: 3D-time-of-flight MR angiography and MR imaging versus angiography in carotid and vertebral artery dissections: A prospective study in 18 patients. Radiology 190:97, 1994.
214. Rother J, Schwartz A, Rautenberg W, Hennerici M: Magnetic resonance angiography of spontaneous vertebral artery dissection suspected on Doppler ultrasonography. J Neurol (Germany) 242:430, 1995.

Clinical
Manifestations

215. Sheehan S, Bauer R, Meyer J: Vertebral artery compression in cervical spondylosis. Neurology (NY) 10:968, 1960.

216. Tatlow W, Bammer H: Syndrome of vertebral artery compression. Neurology (NY) 7:331, 1957.

217. Chin JH: Recurrent stroke caused by spondylitic compression of the vertebral artery. Ann Neurol 33:558, 1993.

218. Powers SR, Drislane TM, Nevins S: Intermittent vertebral artery compression: A new syndrome. Surgery 49:257, 1961.

219. Rosengart A, Hedges TR III, Teal PA, et al: Intermittent downbeat nystagmus due to vertebral artery compression. Neurology 43:216, 1993.

220. Dadsetan MR, Skeihut HEI: Rotational vertebrobasilar insufficiency secondary to vertebral artery occlusion from fibrous band of the longus coli muscle. Neuroradiology 32:514, 1990.

221. George B, Laurian C: Impairment of vertebral artery flow caused by extrinsic lesions. Neurosurgery 24:206, 1989.

222. Hardin CA, Poser CA: Rotational obstruction of the vertebral artery due to redundancy and extraluminal cervical fascial bands. Ann Surg 158:133, 1963.

223. Mapstone T, Spetzler R: Vertebrobasilar insufficiency secondary to vertebral artery occlusion from a fibrous band. J Neurosurg 56:581, 1982.

224. Radner S: Vertebral angiography by catheterization. Acta Radiol [Suppl] (Stockh) 87:1–133, 1951.

225. Hardin C, Williamson W, Steegman T: Vertebral artery insufficiency produced by cervical osteoarthritic spurs. Neurology (NY) 10:855, 1960.

226. Fisher CM: Vertigo in cerebrovascular disease. Arch Otolaryngol 85:529, 1967.

227. Pratt-Thomas H, Berger K: Cerebellar and spinal injuries after chiropractic manipulation. JAMA 133:600, 1947.

228. Hanus S, Homer T, Harter D: Vertebral artery occlusion complicating yoga exercises. Arch Neurol 34:547, 1977.

229. Heros R: Cerebellar infarction resulting from traumatic occlusion of a vertebral artery. J Neurosurg 51:111, 1979.

230. Levy R, Dugan T, Bernat J, et al: Lateral medullary syndrome after neck injury. Neurology (NY) 30:788, 1980.

231. Mueller S, Sahs A: Brainstem dysfunction related to cervical manipulation. Neurology (NY) 26:547, 1976.

232. Robertson J: Neck manipulation as a cause of stroke. Stroke 12:1, 1981.

233. Rogers L, Sweeney P: Stroke: A neurological complication of wrestling. Am J Sports Med 7:352, 1979.

234. Sherman D, Hart R, Easton JD: Abrupt change in head position and cerebral infarction. Stroke 12:2, 1981.

235. Woolsey R, Chang H: Fatal basilar artery occlusion following cervical spine injury. Paraplegia 17:280, 1979.

236. Yates A, Guest D: Cerebral embolism due to an ununited fracture of the clavicle and subclavian thrombosis. Lancet 2:25, 1928.

237. Pawl G, Shaw C, Wray L: True traumatic aneurysms of the vertebral artery. J Neurosurg 53:101, 1980.

238. Mas JL, Hénin D, Bousser MG, et al: Dissecting aneurysm of the vertebral artery and cervical manipulation: A case report with autopsy. Neurology 39:512, 1989.

239. Frens D, Petajan J, Anderson R, et al: Fibromuscular dysplasia of the posterior cerebral artery: Report of a case and review of the literature. Stroke 5:161, 1974.

240. Osborn A, Anderson R: Angiography spectrum of cervical and intracranial fibromuscular dysplasia. Stroke 8:617, 1977.

241. Corrin LS, Sandok BA, Houser W: Cerebral ischemic events in patients with carotid artery fibromuscular disease. Arch Neurol 38:616, 1981.

242. Handa J, Kamijo Y, Handa H: Intracranial aneurysms associated with fibromuscular hyperplasia of the renal and internal carotid arteries. Br J Radiol 43:483, 1970.

243. Mettinger K: Fibromuscular dysplasia and the brain. II: Current concepts of the disease. Stroke 13:53, 1982.

244. So EL, Toole JF, Dalal P, et al: Cephalic fibromuscular dysplasia in 32 patients: Clinical findings and radiologic features. Arch Neurol 38:619, 1981.

245. Goodwill J: Temporal arteritis. In Vinken P, Bruyn G (eds): Handbook of Clinical Neurology, vol 39. Amsterdam, North-Holland, 1980, p 313.

246. Zamarbide ID, Maxit MJ: [Fisher's one and half syndrome with facial palsy as clinical presentation of giant cell temporal arteritis]. Medicina (B Aires) 60:245, 2000.

247. Walsh TJ, Hier DB, Caplan LR: Aspergillosis of the central nervous system: Clinicopathological analysis of 17 patients. Ann Neurol 18:574, 1985.

248. Young RC, Bennett JE, Vogel CL, et al: Aspergillosis: The spectrum of the disease in 98 patients. Medicine (Baltimore) 49:147, 1970.

249. Walsh TJ, Hutchins GM, Bukley BH, Mendelsohn G: Fungal infections of the heart: Analysis of 51 autopsy cases. Am J Cardiol 45:357, 1980.

250. Tack KJ, Rhame FS, Brown B, Thompson RC: Aspergillus osteomyelitis: Report of four cases and review of the literature. Am J Med 83:295, 1982.

251. Caplan LR, Thomas C, Banks G: Central nervous system complications of addiction to "T's and Blues." Neurology 32:623, 1982.

252. Wood D: Cerebrovascular complications of sickle cell anemia. Stroke 9:73, 1978.

253. Merkel K, Grinsberg P, Parker J, et al: Cerebrovascular disease in sickle cell anemia: A clinical, pathological, and radiological correlation. Stroke 9:45, 1978.

254. Amarenco P, Kase CS, Rosengart A, et al: Very small (border zone) cerebellar infarcts: Distribution, mechanisms, causes and clinical features. Brain 116:161, 1993.

255. Ishikawa K: Natural history and classification of occlusive thromboarteriopathy (Takayasu disease). Circulation 57:27, 1978.

256. Lupi-Herrera E, Sanchez-Torres G, Marcushamer J, et al: Takayasu's arteritis: Clinical study of 27 cases. Am Heart J 93:94, 1977.

257. Molnar P, Hegedus K: Direct involvement of intracerebral arteries in Takayasu's arteritis. Acta Neuropathol (Berl) 63:83, 1984.

258. McMenemy WH, Lawrence BJ: Encephalomyelopathy in Behçet's syndrome. Lancet 2:353, 1957.

259. Herskovitz S, Lipton RB, Lantos G: Neuro-Behçet's disease. Neurology (NY) 38:1714, 1988.

260. Seldarogiu P, Yazici H, Ozdemir C, et al: Neurologic involvement in Behçet's syndrome: A prospective study. Arch Neurol 46:265, 1989.

261. Piovesan EJ, et al: Neurofibromatosis, stroke and basilar impression: Case report. Arq Neuropsiquatr 57:484, 1999.

262. Caplan L: Occlusion of the vertebral or basilar artery. Stroke 10:277, 1979.

263. Caplan LR, Rosenbaum A: Role of cerebral angiography in vertebrobasilar occlusive disease. J Neurol Neurosurg Psychiatry 38:601, 1975.

264. Caplan L, Sergay S: Positional cerebral ischemia. J Neurol Neurosurg Psychiatry 39:385, 1976.

265. Jones HE, Millikan C, Sandok B: Temporal profile (clinical course) of acute vertebrobasilar system cerebral infarction. Stroke 11:173, 1980.

266. Patrick B, Ramirez-Lassepas M, Snyder B: Temporal profile of vertebrobasilar territory infarction. Stroke 11:643, 1980.

267. Sundt TM, Piepgras D: Occipital to posterior inferior cerebellar artery bypass surgery. J Neurosurg 49:916, 1978.

268. Naritomi H, Sakai F, Meyer J: Pathogenesis of transient ischemic attacks within the vertebrobasilar arterial system. Arch Neurol 36:121, 1979.

269. Fisher CM: The "herald hemiparesis" of basilar artery occlusion. Arch Neurol 45:1301, 1988.

270. Babinski J, Nageotte J: Hémiasynergie, lateropulsion et myosis bulbaires avec hémianesthésie et croisées. Rev Neurol 10:358, 1902.

271. Caplan L: "Top of the basilar" syndrome: Selected clinical aspects. Neurology (NY) 30:72, 1980.

272. Schwarz S, et al: Basilar artery embolism: Clinical syndrome and neuroradiologic patterns in patients without permanent occlusion of the basilar artery. Neurology 49:1346, 1997.

273. Caplan LR: Brain embolism, revisited. Neurology 43:1281, 1993.

274. Caplan LR, Amarenco P, Rosengart A, et al: Embolism from vertebral artery origin occlusive disease. Neurology 42:1505, 1992.

275. Chaves CJ, Caplan LR, Chung CS, et al: Cerebellar infarcts in the New England Medical Center Posterior Circulation Stroke Registry. Neurology 44:1385, 1994.

276. Chaves CJ, Pessin MS, Caplan LR, et al: Cerebellar hemorrhagic infarction. Neurology 46:346, 1996.

277. Kase CS, White JL, Joslyn N, et al: Cerebellar infarction in the superior cerebellar artery distribution. Neurology (NY) 35:705, 1985.

278. Lehrich J, Winkler G, Ojemann R: Cerebellar infarction with brainstem compression: Diagnosis and surgical treatment. Arch Neurol 22:490, 1970.

279. Fisher CM: Bilateral occlusion of basilar artery branches. J Neurol Neurosurg Psychiatry 40:1182, 1977.

280. Khurana R: Autonomic dysfunction in pontomedullary stroke. Ann Neurol 12:86, 1982.

281. Reis DJ, Iadecola C, Nakai M: Control of cerebral blood flow and metabolism by intrinsic neural systems in brain. In Plum P, Pulsinelli W (eds): Cerebrovascular Diseases: Proceedings of the Fourteenth (Princeton) Conference. Philadelphia, Lippincott-Raven, 1985, p 1.

282. Barnes M, Hunt B, Williams I: The role of vertebral angiography in the investigation of third nerve palsy. J Neurol Neurosurg Psychiatry 44:1153, 1981.

283. Lindgren SO: Infarctions simulating brain tumors in the posterior fossa. J Neurosurg 13:575, 1956.

284. Bogousslavsky J, Khurana R, Deruaz JP, et al: Respiratory failure and unilateral caudal brainstem infarction. Ann Neurol 28:668, 1990.

285. Toyoda K, et al: Bilateral deafness as a prodromal symptom of basilar artery occlusion. J Neurol Sci 193:147, 2002.

286. Archer C, Horenstein S: Basilar artery occlusion: Clinical and radiological correlation. Stroke 8:383, 1977.

287. Fields W, Ratinov G, Weibel J, et al: Survival following basilar artery occlusion. Arch Neurol 15:463, 1966.

288. Moscow N, Newton T: Angiographic implications in diagnosis and prognosis of basilar artery occlusion. AJR Am J Roentgenol 119:597, 1973.

289. Pochaczevsky R, Uygur Z, Berman A: Basilar artery occlusion. J Can Assoc Radiol 22:261, 1971.

290. Labauge R, Pages M, Marty-Double C, et al: Occlusion du tronc basilaire. Rev Neurol 137:545, 1981.

291. Silverstein A: Acute infarctions of the brainstem in the distribution of the basilar artery. Conf Neurol 24:37, 1964.

292. Loeb C, Meyer JS: Strokes Due to Vertebro-Basilar Disease. Springfield, IL, Charles C Thomas, 1965.

293. Biemond A: Thrombosis of the basilar artery and the vascularization of the brainstem. Brain 74:300, 1951.

294. Hass WK, Fields WS, North RR, et al: Joint study of extracranial arterial occlusion. II: Arteriography, technique, sites, and complications. JAMA 203:159, 1986.

295. Pessin MS, Gorelick PB, Kwan ES, et al: Basilar artery stenosis: Middle and distal segments. Neurology (NY) 37:1742, 1987.

296. Ackerman E, Levinsohn M, Richards D, et al: Basilar artery occlusion in a 10-year-old boy. Ann Neurol 1:204, 1977.

297. Montaner J, et al: 'Herald hemiparesis' of basilar artery occlusion: Early recognition by transcranial Doppler ultrasound. Eur J Neurol 7:91, 2000.

298. Moufarrij NA, Little JR, Furlan AJ, et al: Basilar and distal vertebral artery stenosis: Long-term follow-up. Stroke 17:938, 1986.

299. Glass TA, et al: Outcome at 30 days in the New England Medical Center Posterior Circulation Registry. Arch Neurol 59:369, 2002.

300. Devuyst G, et al: Stroke or transient ischemic attacks with basilar artery stenosis or occlusion: Clinical patterns and outcome. Arch Neurol 59:567, 2002.

301. Kase C, Maulsby G, De Juan C, et al: Hemichorea-hemiballism and lacunar infarction in the basal ganglia. Neurology (NY) 31:452, 1981.

302. Ferbert A, Bruckmann H, Drummen R: Clinical features of proven basilar artery occlusion. Stroke 21:1135, 1990.

303. Henze T, Boeer A, Tebbe U, et al: Lysis of basilar artery occlusion with tissue plasminogen activator. Lancet 2:1391, 1987.

304. Wildemann B, Hutschenreuter M, Kriegtl D, et al: Infusion of recombinant tissue plasminogen activator for basilar artery occlusion. Stroke 21:1513, 1990.

305. Moncayo J, Bogousslavsky J: Vertebro-basilar syndromes causing oculo-motor disorders. Curr Opin Neurol 16:45, 2003.

306. Ingvar D, Sourander P: Destruction of the reticular core of the brainstem. Arch Neurol 23:1, 1970.

307. Kemper T, Romanul F: State resembling akinetic mutism in basilar artery occlusion. Neurology (NY) 17:74, 1967.

308. Plum F, Posner J: The Diagnosis of Stupor and Coma, 3rd ed. Philadelphia, FA Davis, 1980.

309. Leon-Carrion J, et al: The locked-in syndrome: A syndrome looking for a therapy. Brain Inj 16:571, 2002.

310. Saposnik G, Caplan LR: Convulsive-like movements in brainstem stroke. Arch Neurol 58:654, 2001.

311. Bauer G, Prugger M, Rumpl E: Stimulus evoked oral automatisms in the locked-in syndrome. Arch Neurol 39:435, 1982.

312. Karp J, Hurtig H: "Locked-in" state with bilateral midbrain infarcts. Arch Neurol 30:176, 1974.

313. Meienberg O, Mumenthaler M, Karbowski K: Quadriparesis and nuclear oculomotor palsy with total bilateral ptosis mimicking coma. Arch Neurol 36:708, 1979.

314. Caplan L, Zervas N: Survival with permanent midbrain dysfunction after surgical treatment of traumatic sub-dural hematoma: The clinical picture of a Duret hemorrhage. Ann Neurol 1:587, 1977.

315. Tahmoush A, Brooks J, Keltner J: Palatal myoclonus associated with abnormal ocular and extremity movements. Arch Neurol 27:431, 1972.

316. Lapresle J, Ben Hamida M: The dentato-olivary pathway. Arch Neurol 22:135, 1970.

317. Fisher CM: Ocular bobbing. Arch Neurol 11:543, 1964.

318. Nelson J, Johnston C: Ocular bobbing. Arch Neurol 22:348, 1970.

319. Bosch E, Kennedy S, Aschenbrenner C: Ocular bobbing: The myth of its localizing value. Neurology (NY) 25:949, 1975.

320. Ott K, Kase C, Ojemann R, et al: Cerebellar hemorrhage: Diagnosis and treatment. Arch Neurol 31:160, 1974.

321. Susac J, Hoyt W, Daroff R, et al: Clinical spectrum of ocular bobbing. J Neurol Neurosurg Psychiatry 33:771, 1970.

322. Newman N, Gay A, Heilbrun M: Disconjugate ocular bobbing: Its relation to midbrain, pontine and medullary function in a surviving patient. Neurology (NY) 21:633, 1971.

323. Fisher CM: The neurological examination of the comatose patient. Acta Neurol Scand 45(Suppl 36):1, 1969.

324. Smith M, Lauria J: Upward gaze paralysis following unilateral pretectal infarction. Arch Neurol 38:127, 1981.

325. Cogan D, Kubik C, Smith WL: Unilateral internuclear ophthalmoplegia. Arch Ophthalmol 44:783, 1950.

326. Cogan DG: Supranuclear connections of the ocular motor system. In Neurology of the Ocular Muscles, 2nd ed. Springfield, IL, Charles C Thomas, 1956, p 84.

327. Smith JL, Cogan D: Internuclear ophthalmoplegia. Arch Ophthalmol 61:687, 1959.

328. Harris W: Ataxic nystagmus: A pathognomonic sign in disseminated sclerosis. Br J Ophthalmol 28:40, 1944.

329. Christoff N, Anderson P, Nathanson M, et al: Problems in anatomical analysis of lesions of the medial longitudinal fasciculus. Arch Neurol 2:293, 1960.

330. Gonyea E: Bilateral internuclear ophthalmoplegia: Association with occlusive cerebrovascular disease. Arch Neurol 31:168, 1974.

331. Cogan D: Internuclear ophthalmoplegia, typical and atypical. Arch Ophthalmol 84:583, 1970.

332. Daroff R, Hoyt W: Supranuclear disorders of ocular control systems in man. In Bach Y, Rita P, Collins C (eds): The Control of Eye Movements. Orlando, FL, Academic Press, 1977, p 175.

333. Bronstein AM, Rudge P, Gresty MA, et al: Abnormalities of horizontal gaze: Clinical, oculographic and magnetic resonance imaging findings. II: Gaze palsy and internuclear ophthalmoplegia. J Neurol Neurosurg Psychiatry 53:200, 1990.

334. Crosby E, Yoss R, Henderson J: The mammalian midbrain and isthmus regions. II: The fiber connections. D: The pattern for eye movement in the frontal eye fields and the discharge of specific portions of this field to and through midbrain levels. J Comp Neurol 97:357, 1952.

335. Pierrot-Deseilligny C, Chain F, Serdaru M, et al: The one and a half syndrome. Brain 104:665, 1981.

336. Halsey J, Ceballos R, Crosby E: The supranuclear control of voluntary lateral gaze. Neurology (NY) 17:928, 1967.

337. de Seze J, et al: One-and-a-half syndrome in pontine infarcts: MRI correlates. Neuroradiology 41:666, 1999.

338. Sharpe J, Rosenberg M, Hoyt W, et al: Paralytic pontine exotropia. Neurology (NY) 24:1076, 1974.

339. Caplan L: Ptosis. J Neurol Neurosurg Psychiatry 37:1, 1974.

340. Caplan L, Gorelick P: Salt and pepper in the face pain in acute brainstem ischemia. Ann Neurol 13:344, 1983.

341. Silverstein A: Pontine infarction. In Vinken P, Bruyn G (eds): Handbook of Clinical Neurology, vol 12. Amsterdam, North-Holland, 1972, p 13.

342. Carod-Artal FJ, et al: ["Top-of-the-basilar" syndrome and Chagas' disease]. Rev Neurol 35:337, 2002.

343. Mehler MF: The rostral basilar artery syndrome: Diagnosis, etiology, prognosis. Neurology 39:9, 1989.

344. Mehler MF: The neuro-ophthalmologic spectrum of the rostral basilar artery syndrome. Arch Neurol 45:966, 1988.

Clinical Manifestations

345. Facon E, Steriade M, Werthein N: Hypersomnie prolongée engendrée par des lésions bilatérales du système activateur médial: Le syndrome thrombotique de la bifurcation du tronc basilaire. Rev Neurol 98:117, 1958.

346. Segarra J: Cerebral vascular disease and behavior. I: The syndrome of the mesencephalic artery (basilar artery bifurcation). Arch Neurol 22:408, 1970.

347. Lindenberg R: Compression of brain arteries as a pathogenetic factor for tissue necrosis and their areas of predilection. J Neuropathol Exp Neurol 14:223, 1955.

348. Selhorst J, Hoyt W, Feinsod M, et al: Midbrain corectopia. Arch Neurol 33:193, 1976.

349. Wilson SAK: Ectopia pupillae in certain mesencephalic lesions. Brain 29:524, 1906.

350. Fisher CM: Oval pupils. Arch Neurol 37:502, 1980.

351. Meissner I, Sapir S, Kokmen E, et al: The paramedian diencephalic syndrome: A dynamic phenomenon. Stroke 18:380, 1987.

352. Pedersen R, Troost BT: Abnormalities of gaze in cerebrovascular disease. Stroke 12:251, 1981.

353. Trojanowski J, Wray S: Vertical gaze ophthalmoplegia: Selective paralysis of downgaze. Neurology (NY) 30:605, 1980.

354. Buttner-Ennever J, Buttner U, Cohen B, et al: Vertical gaze paralysis and the rostral interstitial nucleus of the medial longitudinal fasciculus. Brain 105:125, 1982.

355. Nashold B, Seaber J: Defects of ocular mobility after stereotactic midbrain lesions in man. Arch Ophthalmol 88:245, 1972.

356. White DN, Ketelaars EJ, Cledgett PR: Non-invasive techniques for the recording of vertebral artery flow and their limitations. Ultrasound Med Biol 6:315, 1980.

357. Christoff N: A clinicopathological study of vertical eye movements. Arch Neurol 31:1, 1974.

358. Pasik P, Pasik T, Bender M: The pretectal syndrome in monkeys. I: Disturbance of gaze and body posture. Brain 92:521, 1969.

359. Halmagyi G, Evans W, Hallinan J: Failure of downward gaze. Arch Neurol 35:22, 1978.

360. Jacobs L, Anderson P, Bender M: The lesion producing paralysis of downward but not upward gaze. Arch Neurol 28:319, 1973.

361. Jacobs L, Heffner RR, Newman RP: Selective paralysis of downward gaze caused by bilateral lesions of the mesencephalic periaqueductal gray matter. Neurology (NY) 35:516, 1985.

362. Halmagyi MB, Brandt T, Dieterich M, et al: Tonic contraversive ocular tilt reaction due to unilateral mesodiencephalic lesion. Neurology (NY) 40:1503, 1990.

363. Bogousslavsky J, Regli F: Upgaze palsy and monocular paresis of downgaze from ipsilateral thalamo-mesencephalic infarction: A vertical one-and-a-half syndrome. J Neurol 231:43, 1984.

364. Deleu D, Buisseret T, Ebinger G: Vertical one-and-a-half syndrome: Supranuclear downgaze paralysis with monocular elevation palsy. Arch Neurol 46:1361, 1989.

365. Collier J: Nuclear ophthalmoplegia with especial reference to retraction of the lids and ptosis and to lesions of the posterior commissure. Brain 50:488, 1927.

366. Lhermitte J: Syndrome de la calotte du pédoncule cérébral: Les troubles psycho-sensoriels dans les lesions du mésocephale. Rev Neurol (Paris) 38:1359, 1922.

367. Van Bogaert L: L'hallucinose pedonculaire. Rev Neurol (Paris) 43:608, 1927.

368. Van Bogaert L: Syndrome inferieure du noyau rouge, troubles psycho-sensoriels d'origine mésocephalique. Rev Neurol (Paris) 40:416, 1924.

369. Strukel RJ, Garrick JG: Thoracic outlet compression in athletes: A report of four cases. Am J Sports Med 6:35, 1978.

370. McKee AC, Levine DN, Kowall NW, et al: Peduncular hallucinosis associated with isolated infarction of the substantia nigra pars reticulata. Ann Neurol 27:500, 1990.

371. Martin JP: Hemichorea resulting from a local lesion of the brain (the syndrome of the body of Luys). Brain 50:637, 1927.

372. Whittier J: Ballism and the subthalamic nucleus. Arch Neurol Psychiatry 58:672, 1947.

373. Moersch F, Kernohan J: Hemiballismus, a clinicopathological study. Arch Neurol Psychiatry 41:365, 1939.

374. Kataoka S, et al: Paramedian pontine infarction. Neurological/topographical correlation. Stroke 28:809, 1997.

375. Fisher CM: Lacunar strokes and infarcts: A review. Neurology (NY) 32:871, 1982.

376. Besson G, Hommel M, Perret J: Risk factors for lacunar infarcts. Cerebrovasc Dis 10:387, 2000.

377. Mohr JP, Caplan L, Melski JW, et al: Harvard Cooperative Stroke Registry: A prospective registry. Neurology (NY) 28:754, 1978.

378. Fisher CM: Pure motor hemiplegia of vascular origin. Arch Neurol 13:30, 1965.

379. Bassetti C, Bogousslavsky J, Barth A, Regli F: Isolated infarcts of the pons. Neurology 46:165, 1996.

380. Hommel M, Besson G, Le Bas JF, et al: Prospective study of lacunar infarction using magnetic resonance imaging. Stroke 21:546, 1990.

381. Ho K, Meyer K: The medial medullary syndrome. Arch Neurol 38:385, 1981.

382. Paulson GW, Yates AJ, Paltan-Ortiz JD: Does infarction of the medullary pyramid lead to spasticity? Arch Neurol 43:93, 1986.

383. Ropper A, Fisher CM, Kleinman G: Pyramidal infarction in the medulla: A cause of pure motor hemiplegia sparing the face. Neurology (NY) 29:91, 1979.

384. Ho K: Pure motor hemiplegia due to infarction of the cerebral peduncle. Arch Neurol 39:524, 1982.

385. Kaps M, et al: Basilar branch disease presenting with progressive pure motor stroke. Acta Neurol Scand 96:324, 1997.

386. Fisher CM: A lacunar stroke: The dysarthria clumsy hand syndrome. Neurology (NY) 17:614, 1967.

387. Fisher CM, Cole M: Homolateral ataxia and crural paresis: A vascular syndrome. J Neurol Neurosurg Psychiatry 28:48, 1965.

388. Fisher CM: Pure sensory stroke and allied conditions. Stroke 13:434, 1982.

389. Fisher CM: Pure sensory stroke involving face, arm, and leg. Neurology (NY) 15:76, 1965.

390. Kim J: Pure sensory stroke: Clinical-radiological correlates of 21 cases. Stroke 23:983, 1992.

391. Sacco RL, Bello JA, Traub R, et al: Selective proprioceptive loss from a thalamic lacunar stroke. Stroke 18:1160, 1987.

392. Helgason CM, Wilbur AC: Basilar branch pontine infarction with prominent sensory signs. Stroke 22:1129, 1991.

393. Mohr JP, Kase C, Meckler R, et al: Sensorimotor stroke due to thalamocapsular ischemia. Arch Neurol 34:739, 1977.

394. Tatemichi T, Steinke W, Duncan C, et al: Paramedian thalamopeduncular infarction: Clinical syndromes and magnetic resonance imaging. Ann Neurol 32:162, 1992.

395. Kumral E, Bayulkem G, Evyapan D: Clinical spectrum of pontine infarction: Clinical-MRI correlations. J Neurol 249:1659, 2002.

396. Kim JS: Recurrent pontine base infarction: A controlled study. Cerebrovasc Dis 13:257, 2002.

397. Babinski J, Nageotte J: Hémiasynergie, latéropulsion et myosis bulbaire. Nouv Iconog Salpetriere 15:492, 1902.

398. Kim JS, Lee JH, Im JH, Lee MC: Syndromes of pontine base infarction: A clinical-radiological correlation study. Stroke 26:950, 1995.

399. Toyoda K, Saku Y, Ibayashi S, et al: Pontine infarction extending to the basal surface. Stroke 25:2171, 1994.

400. Bogousslavsky J, Maeder P, Regli F, et al: Pure midbrain infarction: Clinical syndromes, MRI, and etiologic patterns. Neurology 44:2032, 1994.

401. Fisher CM: Thalamic pure sensory stroke: A pathologic study. Neurology (NY) 28:1141, 1978.

402. Zeal AA, Rhoton AL: Microsurgical anatomy of the posterior cerebral artery. J Neurosurg 48:534, 1978.

403. Kumral E, et al: Mesencephalic and associated posterior circulation infarcts. Stroke 33:2224, 2002.

404. Hopf HC, Gutmann L: Diabetic 3rd nerve palsy: Evidence for a mesencephalic lesion. Neurology 40:1041–1045, 1990.

405. Hommel M, Bogousslavsky J: The spectrum of vertical gaze palsy following unilateral brainstem stroke. Neurology 41:1229–1234, 1991.

406. Fisher CM: Honored guest lecture: Abulia minor vs agitation behavior. Clin Neurosurg 31:9, 1983.

407. Caplan LR, Schmahmann JD, Kase CS, et al: Caudate infarcts. Arch Neurol 47:133, 1990.

408. Caplan L: Bilateral distal vertebral artery occlusion. Neurology (NY) 33:552, 1983.

409. Kotila M, Hokkainen L, Laaksonen R, Valanne L: Long-term prognosis after left tuberothalamic infarction: A study of 7 cases. Cerebrovasc Dis 4:44, 1994.

410. Kaplan RF, Estol CJ, Damasio H, et al: Bilateral polar territory infarcts. Neurology 41:329, 1991.

411. Takahashi S, Goto K, Fukasawa H, et al: Computed tomography of cerebral infarction along the distribution of the basal perforating arteries. II: Thalamic arterial group. Radiology 155:119, 1985.

412. Bogousslavsky J, Miklossy J, Deruaz JP, et al: Unilateral left paramedian infarction of the thalamus and midbrain: A clinicopathological study. J Neurol Neurosurg Psychiatry 49:686, 1986.

413. Mori E, Yamadori A, Mitani Y: Left thalamic infarction and disturbance of verbal memory: A clinicoanatomical study with a new method of computed tomographic stereotaxic lesion localization. Ann Neurol 20:671, 1986.

414. Wall M, Slamovits T, Weisberg LA, et al: Vertical gaze ophthalmoplegia from infarction in the area of the posterior thalamosubthalamic paramedian artery. Stroke 17:546, 1986.

415. Swanson R, Schmidley J: Amnestic syndrome and vertical gaze palsy: Early detection of bilateral thalamic infarction by CT and MRI. Stroke 16:823, 1985.

416. Malamut BL, Graff-Radford N, Chawluk J, et al: Memory in a case of bilateral thalamic infarction. Neurology 42:163, 1992.

417. Bogousslavsky J, Regli F, Delaloye B, et al: Loss of psychic self-activation with bithalamic infarction: Neurobehavioural, CT, MRI, and SPECT correlates. Acta Neurol Scand 83:309, 1991.

418. Bewermeyer H, Dreesbach HA, Rackl A, et al: Presentation of bilateral thalamic infarction on CT, MRI, and PET. Neuroradiology 27:414, 1985.

419. Eslinger PJ, Warner GC, Grattan LM, Easton JD: "Frontal lobe" utilization behavior associated with paramedian thalamic infarction. Neurology 41:450, 1991.

420. Lhermitte F: "Utilization behavior" and its relation to lesions of the frontal lobes. Brain 106:237, 1983.

421. Hashimoto R, Yoshida M, Tanaka Y: Utilization behavior after right thalamic infarction. Eur Neurol 35:58, 1995.

422. Catsman-Berrevoets CE, Harskamp F: Compulsive pre-sleep behavior and apathy due to bilateral thalamic stroke: Response to bromocriptine. Neurology 38:647, 1988.

423. Dejerine J, Roussy G: Le syndrome thalamique. Rev Neurol 14:521, 1906.

424. Helgason C, Caplan LR, Goodwin J, et al: Anterior choroidal artery territory infarction: Case reports and review. Arch Neurol 3:681, 1986.

425. Bogousslavsky J, Caplan LR: Vertebrobasilar occlusive disease: Review of selected aspects. III: Thalamic infarcts. Cerebrovasc Dis 3:193–205, 1993.

426. Bogousslavsky J, Regli F, Uske A: Thalamic infarcts: Clinical syndromes, etiology, prognosis. Neurology 38:837, 1988.

427. Bogousslavsky J: Thalamic infarcts in lacunar and other subcortical infarcts. In Donnan G, Bamford J, Norrving B, Bogousslavsky J (eds): Lacunar Strokes. Oxford, Oxford University Press, 1995, pp 149–170.

428. Devic M, Michel F, Lenglet JP: Nystagmus retractorius, paralysie de la verticalité, aréflexie pupillaire et anomalie de la posture du regard par ramollissement dans le térritoire de la choroidienne postérieure. Rev Neurol 10:399–404, 1964.

429. Besson G, Bogousslavsky J, Regli F: Posterior choroidal artery infarct with homonymous horizontal sectoranopia. Cerebrovasc Dis 1:117, 1991.

430. Luco C, Hoppe A, Schweitzer M, et al: Visual field defects in vascular lesions of the lateral geniculate body. J Neurol Neurosurg Psychiatry 55:12, 1992.

431. Neau J-P, Bogousslavsky J: The syndrome of posterior choroidal artery territory infarction. Ann Neurol 39:779, 1996.

432. Serra Catafan J, Rubio F, Peres Serra J: Peduncular hallucinosis associated with posterior thalamic infarction. J Neurol 239:89, 1992.

433. Waither H: Uber einen Dammerzustand mit triebhafter Erregung nach Thalamusschadigung. Monatsschr Psychiatr Neurol 111:1, 1945–46.

434. Frisen L, Holmegaard L, Rosencrantz M: Sectorial optic atrophy and homonymous horizontal sectoranopia: A lateral choroidal artery syndrome? J Neurol Neurosurg Psychiatry 41:374, 1978.

435. Steinke W, Sacco RL, Mohr JP, et al: Thalamic stroke: Presentation and prognosis of infarcts and hemorrhages. Arch Neurol 49:703, 1992.

436. Ghika J, Bogousslavsky J, Regli F: Delayed unilateral akathisia with posterior thalamic infarct. Cerebrovasc Dis 5:55, 1995.

437. Barth A, Bogousslavsky J, Regli F: The clinical and topographic spectrum of cerebellar infarcts: A clinical-magnetic resonance imaging correlation study. Ann Neurol 33:451, 1993.

438. Hinshaw D, Thompson J, Hasso A, et al: Infarction of the brainstem and cerebellum: A correlation of computed tomography and angiography. Radiology 137:105, 1980.

439. Kase CS, Norrving B, Levine SR, et al: Cerebellar infarction: Clinico-anatomic correlations. Stroke 24:76, 1993.

440. Amarenco P, Roullet E, Goujon C, et al: Infarction in the anterior rostral cerebellum (the territory of the lateral branch of the superior cerebellar artery). Neurology 41:253, 1991,

441. Macdonell RAL, Kalnins RM, Donnan GA: Cerebellar infarction: Natural history, prognosis, and pathology. Stroke 18:849, 1987.

442. Struck LK, Biller J, Bruno A, et al: Superior cerebellar artery territory infarction. Cerebrovasc Dis 1:71, 1991.

443. Lazorthes G, Gouazé A, Salamon G, et al: La vascularisation artérielle du cervelet. In Lazorthes G, Gouazé A, Salamon G (eds): La Vascularisation Cérébrale. Paris, Masson, 1978, pp 205–219.

444. Thompson GN: Cerebellar embolism. Bull Los Angeles Neurol Soc 9:140, 1944.

445. Levine SR, Welch KMA: Superior cerebellar artery infarction and vertebral artery dissection. Stroke 19:1431, 1988.

446. Kalyan-Raman UP, Kowalski RV, Lee RH, Fierer JA: Dissecting aneurysm of superior cerebellar artery. Arch Neurol 40:120, 1983.

447. Perez-Higueras A, Alvarez-Ruiz F, Martinez-Bermejo A, et al: Cerebellar infarction from fibromuscular dysplasia and dissecting aneurysm of the vertebral artery: Report of a child. Stroke 19:521, 1988.

448. Caplan LR: Migraine and vertebrobasilar ischemia. Neurology (NY) 41:55, 1991.

449. Titus F, Montalban J, Molins A, et al: Migraine-related stroke: Brain infarction in superior cerebellar artery territory demonstrated by nuclear magnetic resonance. Acta Neurol Scand 79:357, 1989.

450. Davison C, Goodhart S, Savitsky N: The syndrome of the superior cerebellar artery and its branches. Arch Neurol Psychiatry 33:1143, 1935.

451. Gillian LA: The arterial blood supply of the human brainstem correlated with vascular lesions. J Neuropathol Exp Neurol 21:303, 1962,

452. Girard PF, Bonamour Garde, Etienne: Les syndromes de l'oblitération de l'artère cérébelleuse supérieure et du ramollissement global de la calotte protubérantielle dans son tiers supérieur: Participation du pathétique. Rev Neurol (Paris) 83:199, 1950.

453. Alezais D'Astros L: La circulation artérielle du pédoncule cérébral. J Anat Physiol 28:519, 1892.

454. Guillain G, Bertrand L, Péron N: Le syndrome de l'artère cérébelleuse supérieure. Rev Neurol 2:835, 1928.

455. Savoiardo M, Bracchi M, Passerini A, et al: The vascular territories in the cerebellum and brainstem: CT and MR study. AJNR Am J Neuroradiol 8:199, 1987.

456. Amarenco P: The spectrum of cerebellar infarctions. Neurology 41:973, 1991.

457. Amarenco P, Chevrie-Muller C, Roullet E, Bousser M-G: Paravermal infarct and isolated cerebellar dysarthria. Ann Neurol 30:211, 1991.

458. Tohgi H, Takahashi S, Chibra K, et al: Cerebellar infarction: Clinical and neuroimaging analysis in 293 patients. Stroke 24:1697, 1993.

459. Amarenco P, Hauw J-J: Infarctus cérébelleux œdémateux: Etude clinico-pathologique de 16 cas. Neurochirurgie 36:234, 1990.

460. Mills CK: Hemianesthesia to pain and temperature and loss of emotional expression on the right side with ataxia of the upper limb on the left. J Nerv Ment Dis 35:331, 1908.

461. Mills CK: Preliminary note on a new symptom complex due to lesion of the cerebellum and cerebello-rubro-thalamic system, the main symptoms being ataxia of the upper and lower extremities of one side, and the other side deafness, paralysis of emotional expression in the face, and loss of the senses of pain, heat, and cold over the entire half of the body. J Nerv Ment Dis 39:73, 1912.

462. Freeman W, Jaffe D: Occlusion of the superior cerebellar artery. Arch Neurol Psychiatry 46:115, 1941.

463. Russel CK: The syndrome of brachium conjunctivum and the tractus spinothalamicus. Arch Neurol Psychiatry 25:1003, 1931.

464. Worster-Drought C, Allen I: Thrombosis of the superior cerebellar artery. Lancet 2:1137, 1929.

465. Cossa P, Richard S: Sur deux cas de syndrome de l'artère cérébelleuse supérieure (ou de ses branches). Rev Neurol (Paris) 633, 1955.

466. Levine SR, Welch KMA: Superior cerebellar artery territory stroke [abstract]. Neurology 38(Suppl 1):344, 1988.

Clinical Manifestations

467. Tougeron A, Samson Y, Schaison M, et al: Syndrome dysarthrie-main malhabile par infarctus cérébelleux. Rev Neurol (Paris) 144:596, 1988.

468. Bogousslavsky J, Régli F: Latéro-pulsion axiale isolée lors d'un infarctus cérébelleux flocculo-nodulaire. Rev Neurol (Paris) 140:140, 1984.

469. Ranalli PJ, Sharpe JA: Contrapulsion of saccades and ipsilateral ataxia: A unilateral disorder of the rostral cerebellum. Ann Neurol 20:311, 1986.

470. Ringer RA, Culberson JL: Extensor tone disinhibition from an infarction within the midline anterior cerebellar lobe. J Neurol Neurosurg Psychiatry 52:1597, 1989.

471. Lechtenberg R, Gilman S: Speech disorders in cerebellar diseases. Ann Neurol 3:285, 1978.

472. Atkinson WJ: The anterior inferior cerebellar artery. J Neurol Neurosurg Psychiatry 12:137, 1949.

473. Perneczky A, Perneczky G, Tschabitscher M, et al: The relationship between the caudolateral pontine syndrome and the anterior inferior cerebellar artery. Acta Neurochir 58:245, 1981.

474. Adams R: Occlusion of the anterior inferior cerebellar artery. Arch Neurol Psychiatry 49:765, 1983.

475. Matsushita K, Naritomi H, Kazui S, et al: Infarction in the anterior inferior cerebellar artery territory: Magnetic resonance imaging and auditory brainstem responses. Cerebrovasc Dis 3:206, 1993.

476. Fisher CM: Lacunar infarct of the tegmentum of the lower lateral pons. Arch Neurol 46:566, 1989.

477. McLean CA, Gonzales MF, Dowling JP: Systemic giant cell arteritis and cerebellar infarction. Stroke 24:899, 1993.

478. Rubenstein RL, Norman D, Schindler R, et al: Cerebellar infarction: A presentation of vertigo. Laryngoscope 90:505, 1980.

479. Amarenco P, Debroucker T, Cambier J: Dysarthrie et instabilité révélant d'un infarctus distal de l'artère cérébelleuse supérieure gauche. Rev Neurol (Paris) 144:459, 1988.

480. Amarenco P, Roullet E, Chemouilli P, Marteau R: Infarctus pontin inféro-latéral: Deux aspects cliniques. Rev Neurol (Paris) 146:433, 1990.

481. Oas JG, Baloh RW: Vertigo and the anterior inferior cerebellar artery syndrome. Neurology 42:2274, 1992.

482. Jakob A: Das Kleinhirn. In Von Möllendorff W (ed): Handbuch der mikroskopischen Anatomie des Menschen, vol 4. Berlin, Julius Springer, 1928.

483. Philips PC, Lorentsten KJ, Shropshire LC, Ahn HS: Congenital odontoid aplasia and posterior circulation stroke in childhood. Ann Neurol 23:410, 1988,

484. Amarenco P, Hauw J-J, Henin D, et al: Les infarctus du territoire de l'artère cérébelleuse postéro-inférieure: étude clinico-pathologique de 28 cas. Rev Neurol 145:277, 1989.

485. Heros R: Cerebellar hemorrhage and infarction. Stroke 13:106, 1982.

486. Wallenberg A: Acute bulbar affection. Arch Psychiatr Nervenheilkd 27:504, 1895.

487. Wallenberg A: Anatomischer Befund in einem als "Acute Bulbäraffection (Embolie der art. cerebellar. post. inf. sinistr.?)." Beschriebenem falle. Arch F Psychiatr 34:923, 1901.

488. Diggle FH, Stopford JSB: PICA and vertebral artery thrombosis. Lancet 1:1214, 1935.

489. Hall AJ, Eaves EC: Posterior inferior cerebellar thrombosis (autopsy). Lancet 2:975, 1934.

490. Hun H: Analgesia, thermic anesthesia, and ataxia, resulting from foci of softening in the medulla oblongata and cerebellum due to occlusion of the left PICA. N Y Med J 65:513, 1897.

491. Spiller WG: The symptom-complex of occlusion of PICA. J Nerv Ment Dis 35:365, 1908.

492. Thomas HM: Symptoms following the occlusion of the PICA. J Nerv Ment Dis 34:48, 1907.

493. Wilson G, Winkelman NW: Occlusion of the PICA. J Nerv Ment Dis 65:125, 1927.

494. Harris TH, Hauser A: Occlusion of the right posterior inferior cerebellar artery and right vertebral artery. Arch Neurol Psychiatry 26:396, 1931.

495. Breuer R, Marburg O: Zur Klinik und Pathologie der apoplektiformen Bulbärparalyse. Arb Neurol Inst Wien Univ 9:181, 1902.

496. Foix C, Hillemand P, Schalit I: Sur le syndrome latéral due bulbe et l'irrigation du bulbe supérieur: L'artère de la fossette latérale du bulbe, le syndrome de la cérébelleuse inférieure, territoire de ces artères. Rev Neurol 32:160, 1925.

497. Ramsbottom A, Stopford JSB: Occlusion of the PICA. BMJ 1:364, 1924.

498. Krayenbüll H, Yasargil MG: Die vaskulären Erkrankungen im Gebiet der Arteria vertebralis und Arteria basilaris. Stuttgart, George Thieme, 1957.

499. Duncan G, Parker S, Fisher CM: Acute cerebellar infarction in the PICA territory. Arch Neurol 32:364, 1975.

500. Anson JA, Spetzler RF: Endarterectomy of the intradural vertebral artery via the far lateral approach. Neurosurgery 33:804, 1993.

501. Norrving B, Magnusson M, Holtas S: Isolated acute vertigo in the elderly: Vestibular or vascular disease? Acta Neurol Scand 91:43, 1995,

502. Dumenil L: De la paralysie unilatérale du voile du palais d'origine centrale. Arch Gen Med 25:385, 1875.

503. Ho SU, Kim KS, Berenberg RA, Ho HT: Cerebellar infarction: A clinical and CT study. Surg Neurol 16:350, 1981.

504. Samson M, Milhout B, Onnient Y, et al: Les ramollissements cérébelleux: Données diagnostiques et pronostiques. Semin Hop Paris 62:2766, 1986.

505. Samson M, Milhout B, Thiebot J, et al: Forme bénigne des infarctus cérébelleux. Rev Neurol 137:373, 1981.

506. Tomaszek DE, Rosner MJ: Cerebellar infarction: Analysis of twenty-one cases. Surg Neurol 24:223, 1985.

507. Feely MP: Cerebellar infarction. Neurosurgery 4:7, 1979.

508. Guiang RL, Ellington OB: Acute pure vertiginous disequilibrium in cerebellar infarction. Eur Neurol 16:11, 1977.

509. Huang CY, Yu YL: Small cerebellar strokes may mimic labyrinthine lesions. J Neurol Neurosurg Psychiatry 48:263, 1985.

510. Barth A, Bogousslavsky J, Régli F: Infarcts in the territory of the lateral branch of the posterior inferior cerebellar artery. J Neurol Neurosurg Psychiatry 57:1073, 1994.

511. Amarenco P, Roullet E, Hommel M, et al: Infarction in the territory of the medial branch of the posterior inferior cerebellar artery. J Neurol Neurosurg Psychiatry 53:731, 1990.

512. Caplan LR, Flamm ES, Mohr JP, et al: Lumbar puncture in stroke. Stroke 18:540A, 1987.

513. Pierrot-Deseilligny C, Amarenco P, Roullet E, et al: Vermal infarct with pursuit eye movement disorders. J Neurol Neurosurg Psychiatry 53:519, 1990.

514. Sypert G, Alvord E: Cerebellar infarction: A clinicopathological study. Arch Neurol 32:357, 1975.

515. Fisher CM: Headache in cerebrovascular disease. In Vinken P, Bruyn G (eds): Handbook of Clinical Neurology, vol 5. Amsterdam, North-Holland, 1968, p 124.

516. Wilkins R, Brody I: Wallenberg's syndrome. Arch Neurol 22:379, 1970.

517. Norrving B, Cronqvist S: Lateral medullary infarction: Prognosis in an unselected series. Neurology 41:244, 1991.

518. Sacco RL, Freddo L, Bello JA, et al: Wallenberg's lateral medullary syndrome: Clinical-magnetic resonance imaging correlation. Arch Neurol 50:609, 1993,

519. Vuilleumier P, Bogousslavsky J, Regli F: Infarction of the lower brainstem: Clinical, aetiological and MR-topographical correlations. Brain 118:1013, 1995.

520. Currier R, Giles C, Dejong R: Some comments on Wallenberg's lateral medullary syndrome. Neurology (NY) 11:778, 1961.

521. Sheehan D, Smith G: A study of the anatomy of vertebral thrombosis. Lancet 2:614, 1937.

522. Kim JS, Lee JH, Suh DC, Lee MC: Spectrum of lateral medullary syndrome: Correlation between clinical findings and magnetic resonance imaging in 33 subjects. Stroke 25:1405, 1994.

523. Richter R: Collaterals between the external carotid artery and the vertebral artery in cases of thrombosis of the internal carotid artery. Acta Radiol [Diagn] (Stockh) 40:108, 1953.

524. McCusker E, Rudick R, Honch G, et al: Recovery from the locked-in syndrome. Arch Neurol 39:145, 1982.

525. Fisher CM, Karnes WE: Local embolism. J Neuropathol Exp Neurol 24:174, 1965.

526. Koroshetz WJ, Ropper AH: Artery-to-artery embolism causing stroke in the posterior circulation. Neurology (NY) 37:292, 1987.

527. Pessin MS, Daneault N, Kwan E, et al: Local embolism from vertebral artery occlusion. Stroke 19:112, 1988.

528. Fisher CM: Is pressure on nerves and roots a common cause of pain? Trans Am Neurol Assoc 97:282, 1972.

529. Peterman A, Siekert R: The lateral medullary (Wallenberg) syndrome: Clinical features and prognosis. Med Clin North Am 44:887, 1960.

530. Borison H, Wang S: Physiology and pharmacology of vomiting. Pharmacol Rev 5:193, 1953.

531. Louis-Bar D: Sur le syndrome vasculaire de l'hémibulbe (Wallenberg). Monatsschr Psychiatr Neurol 112:53, 1946.

532. Soffin G, Feldman M, Bender M: Alterations of sensory levels in vascular lesions of lateral medulla. Arch Neurol 18:178, 1968.

533. Bright R: Cases illustrative of the effects produced when the arteries and brain are diseased. Guys Hosp Rep 1:9, 1836.

534. Merritt H, Finland M: Vascular lesions of the hindbrain (lateral medullary syndrome). Brain 53:290, 1930.

535. Matsumoto S, Okuda B, Imai T, et al: A sensory level on the trunk in lower lateral brainstem lesions. Neurology (NY) 38:1515, 1988.

536. Morrow MJ, Sharpe JA: Torsional nystagmus in the lateral medullary syndrome. Ann Neurol 24:390, 1988.

537. Estanol B, Lopez-Rios G: Neuro-otology of the lateral medullary infarct syndrome. Arch Neurol 39:176, 1982.

538. Bjewer K, Silkerskjold BP: Lateropulsion and imbalance in Wallenberg's syndrome. Acta Neurol Scand 44:91, 1968.

539. Kommerell G, Hoyt W: Lateropulsion of saccadic eye movements. Arch Neurol 28:313, 1973.

540. Meyer K, Baloh R, Krohel G, et al: Ocular lateropulsion: A sign of lateral medullary disease. Arch Ophthalmol 98:1614, 1980.

541. Keane JR: Ocular tilt reaction following lateral pontomedullary infarction. Neurology 42:259, 1992.

542. Brandt T, Dieterich M: Skew deviation with ocular torsion: A vestibular brainstem sign of topographic diagnostic value. Ann Neurol 33:528, 1993.

543. Dieterich M, Brandt T: Ocular torsion and tilt of subjective visual vertical are sensitive brainstem signs. Ann Neurol 33:292, 1993.

544. Dieterich M, Brandt T: Wallenberg's syndrome: Lateropulsion, cyclorotation, and subjective visual vertical in thirty-six patients. Ann Neurol 31:399, 1992.

545. Currier R, Giles C, Westerberg M: The prognosis of some brainstem vascular syndromes. Neurology (NY) 8:664, 1958.

546. Levin B, Margolis G: Acute failure of automatic respirations secondary to a unilateral brainstem infarct. Ann Neurol 1:583, 1977.

547. Devereaux M, Keane J, Davis R: Automatic respiratory failure associated with infarction of the medulla: Report of two cases with pathologic study of one. Arch Neurol 29:46, 1973.

548. Levine SR, Patel VM, Welch KMA, et al: Are heart attacks really brain attacks? In Furlan A (ed): The Heart in Stroke. Heidelberg, Springer-Verlag, 1987.

549. Ross MA, Biller J, Adams HP, et al: Magnetic resonance imaging in Wallenberg's lateral medullary syndrome. Stroke 17:542, 1986.

550. Duffy P, Jacobs G: Clinical and pathologic findings in vertebral artery thrombosis. Neurology (NY) 8:862, 1958.

551. Marinesco G, Draganesco S: Hémisyndrome bulbaire relevant d'un ramollissement de l'étage moyen du bulbe, suite de thrombus de l'artère vertébrale droite. Ann Med 13:1, 1923.

552. Dhamoon SK, Igbal J, Collins GH: Ipsilateral hemiplegia and the Wallenberg syndrome. Arch Neurol 41:179, 1984.

553. Davison C: Syndrome of the anterior spinal artery of the medulla oblongata. J Neuropathol Exp Neurol 3:73, 1944.

554. Kumral E, et al: Spectrum of medial medullary infarction: Clinical and magnetic resonance imaging findings. J Neurol 249:85, 2002.

555. Sawada H, Seriu N, Udaka F, Kameyama M: Magnetic resonance imaging of medial medullary infarction. Stroke 21:963, 1990.

556. Kleineri G, Fazekas F, Kleinert R, et al: Bilateral medial medullary infarction: Magnetic resonance imaging and correlative histopathologic findings. Eur Neurol 33:74, 1993.

557. Toyoda K, Hasegawa Y, Yonehara T, et al: Bilateral medial medullary infarction with oculomotor disorders. Stroke 23:1657, 1992.

558. Kase C, Varakis J, Stafford J, et al: Medial medullary infarction from fibrocartilaginous embolism to the anterior spinal artery. Stroke 14:413, 1983.

559. Jagiella WM, Sung JH: Bilateral infarction of the medullary pyramids in humans. Neurology 39:21, 1989.

560. Milandre L, Habib M, Hassoun J, Khalil R: Bilateral infarction of the medullary pyramids. Neurology 40:556, 1990.

561. Mizutani T, Lewis R, Gonatas N: Medial medullary syndrome in a drug abuser. Arch Neurol 37:425, 1980.

562. Trelles J, Trelles L, Urquraga C: Le ramollissement médian du bulbe. Rev Neurol 129:91, 1973.

563. Tatemichi TK, Oropeza LA, Sacco RL, et al: Doppler diagnosis of vertebral artery occlusion: Role of runoff into the posterior inferior cerebellar artery. Ann Neurol 26:158, 1989.

564. Tatsumi T, Shenkin H: Occlusion of the vertebral artery. J Neurol Neurosurg Psychiatry 28:235, 1965.

565. Allen G, Cohen R, Preziosi T: Microsurgical endarterectomy of the intracranial vertebral artery for vertebrobasilar transient ischemic attacks. Neurosurgery 81:56, 1981.

566. Ausman J, Lee M, Chater N, et al: Superficial artery to superior cerebellar artery anastomosis for distal basilar artery stenosis. Surg Neurol 12:277, 1979.

567. Imparato A, Riles T, Kim G, et al: Vertebral artery reconstruction. Stroke 12:125, 1981.

568. Higashida RT, Tsai FY, Halbach VV, et al: Transluminal angioplasty for atherosclerotic disease of the vertebral and basilar arteries. J Neurosurg 78:192, 1993.

569. Alexander A: The treatment of epilepsy by ligature of the vertebral arteries. Brain 5:170, 1882.

570. Fisher CM: Occlusion of the vertebral arteries. Arch Neurol 22:13, 1970.

571. Maruyama M, Asai T, Kuriyama Y, et al: Positive platelet scintigram of a vertebral aneurysm presenting thromboembolic transient ischemic attacks. Stroke 20:687, 1989.

572. Keane JR: Locked-in syndrome after head and neck trauma. Neurology (NY) 36:80, 1986.

573. Labauge R, Boukobza M, Pages M, et al: Occlusion de l'artère vertébrale. Rev Neurol 143:490, 1987.

574. Moufarrij NA, Little JR, Furlan AJ, et al: Vertebral artery stenosis: Long-term follow-up. Stroke 15:260, 1984.

575. Hennerici M, Aulich A, Sandmann W, et al: Incidence of asymptomatic extracranial arterial disease. Stroke 12:750, 1981.

576. Martin PJ, Evans DH, Naylor AR: Transcranial color-coded sonography of the basal cerebral circulation: Reference data from 115 volunteers. Stroke 25:390, 1994.

577. Kimura K, Yasaka M, Moriyasu H, et al: Ultrasonographic evaluation of vertebral artery to detect vertebrobasilar axis occlusion. Stroke 25:1006, 1994.

578. Trattnig S, Hubsch P, Schuster H, et al: Color-coded Doppler imaging of normal vertebral arteries. Stroke 21:1222, 1990.

579. Hesselink JR, Teresi L, Davis K, et al: Intravenous digital subtraction angiography of arteriosclerotic vertebrobasilar disease. AJR Am J Roentgenol 142:255, 1984.

580. Berguer R, Feldman AJ: Surgical reconstruction of the vertebral artery. Surgery 93:670, 1983.

581. Edwards WH, Mulherin JL: The surgical reconstruction of the proximal subclavian and vertebral artery. In Berguer R, Bauer R (eds): Vertebrobasilar Arterial Occlusive Disease. Philadelphia, Lippincott-Raven, 1984.

582. Imparato A: Vertebral artery reconstruction: A nineteen year experience. J Vasc Surg 2:626, 1985.

583. Lee RE: Reconstruction of the proximal vertebral artery. In Berguer R, Caplan LR (eds): Vertebrobasilar Arterial Disease. St. Louis, Quality Medical, 1992, pp 211–223.

584. Reul GJ, Cooley DA, Olson SK, et al: Long-term results of direct vertebral artery operations. Surgery 96:854, 1984.

585. Roski R, Spetzler R, Hopkins L: Occipital artery to posterior inferior cerebellar artery bypass for vertebrobasilar ischemia. Neurosurgery 10:44, 1982.

586. Spetzler RF, Hadley MN, Martin NA, et al: Vertebrobasilar insufficiency. I: Microsurgical treatment of extracranial vertebrobasilar disease. J Neurosurg 66:648, 1987.

587. Albuquerque FC, Fiorella D, Han P, et al: A reappraisal of angioplasty and stenting for the treatment of vertebral origin stenosis. Neurosurgery 53:607–614, 2003.

588. Jensen ME, Mathis JM, DeNardo AJ, Dion JE: Angioplasty of brachiocephalic and cerebral vessels in atherosclerotic disease. Stroke 25:155, 1994.

589. Schutz H, Yeung H, Chiu M, et al: Dilatation of vertebral artery stenosis. N Engl J Med 304:732, 1981.

590. Shin HK, et al: Bilateral intracranial vertebral artery disease in the New England Medical Center, Posterior Circulation Registry. Arch Neurol 56:1353, 1999.

591. Bogousslavsky J, Gates PC, Fox AJ, et al: Bilateral occlusion of vertebral artery. Neurology (NY) 36:1309, 1986.

592. Desmet Y, Brucher JM: L'infarctus bilatéral du territoire latéral du bulbe. Acta Neurol Belg 85:137, 1985.

593. Ausman J, Nicoloff D, Chou S: Posterior fossa revascularization anastomosis of vertebral artery to PICA with interposed radial artery graft. Surg Neurol 9:281, 1978.

Clinical Manifestations

594. Ausman J, Diaz F, de los Reyes RA, et al: Occipital artery to anterior inferior cerebellar artery anastomosis for vertebrobasilar junction stenosis. Surg Neurol 16:99, 1981.

595. Sundt T, Piepgras D, Houser O, et al: Interposition saphenous vein grafts for advanced occlusive disease and large aneurysms in the posterior circulation. J Neurosurg 56:205, 1982.

596. Reivich M, Holling E, Roberts B, et al: Reversal of blood flow through the vertebral artery and its effect on cerebral circulation. N Engl J Med 265:88, 1961.

597. Fisher CM: A new vascular syndrome: "The subclavian steal" [editorial]. N Engl J Med 265:912, 1961.

598. Daves J, Treger A: Vertebral grand larceny. Circulation 29:911, 1964.

599. Fields WS, Lemak N: Joint study of extracranial arterial occlusion. VII: Subclavian steal. JAMA 222:1139, 1972.

600. Heyman A, Young W, Dillon M, et al: Cerebral ischemia caused by occlusive lesions of the subclavian or innominate arteries. Arch Neurol 10:581, 1964.

601. North R, Fields W, DeBakey M, et al: Brachial-basilar insufficiency syndrome. Neurology (NY) 12:810, 1962.

602. Patel A, Toole J: Subclavian steal syndrome: Reversal of cephalic blood flow. Medicine (Baltimore) 44:289, 1965.

603. Siekert R, Millikan C, Whisnant J: Reversal of blood flow in the vertebral arteries. Ann Intern Med 61:64, 1964.

604. Hennerici M, Klemm C, Rautenberg W: The subclavian steal phenomenon: A common vascular disorder with rare neurologic deficits. Neurology (NY) 38:669, 1988.

605. Fields WS: Neurovascular syndromes of the neck and shoulders. Semin Neurol 1:301, 1981.

606. Fields WS, Lemak NA, Ben-Menachem Y: Thoracic outlet syndrome: Review and reference to a stroke in a major league pitcher. AJNR Am J Roentgenol 7:73, 1986.

607. Gerber N: Congenital atresia of the subclavian artery producing subclavian steal syndrome. Am J Dis Child 113:709, 1967.

608. Berguer R, Higgins R, Nelson R: Non-invasive diagnosis of reversal of vertebral artery blood flow. N Engl J Med 302:1349, 1980.

609. Baker R, Rosenbaum A, Caplan L: Subclavian steal syndrome. Contemp Surg 4:96, 1974.

610. Symonds C: Two cases of thrombosis of subclavian artery with contralateral hemiplegia of sudden onset, probably embolic. Brain 50:259, 1927.

611. Hoobler S: The syndrome of cervical rib with subclavian arterial thrombosis and hemiplegia due to cerebral embolism. N Engl J Med 226:942, 1942.

612. Brewster DC, Moncure AC, Darling C, et al: Innominate artery lesions: Problems encountered and lessons learned. J Vasc Surg 2:99, 1985.

613. Lahitte M, Marc-Vergnes J, Rascol A, et al: Intravenous angiography of the extracranial arteries. Radiology 137:705, 1980.

614. Weibel J, Fields W: Angiography of the posterior cervicocranial circulation. AJR Am J Roentgenol 98:660, 1966.

615. French LA, Haines GL: Unilateral vertebral artery ligation. J Neurosurg 7:156, 1950.

616. Menzies WF: Thrombosis of inferior cerebellar artery. Brain 15:436–439, 1893.

617. Fairburn B, Oliver LC: Cerebellar softening: A surgical emergency. BMJ 1:1335, 1956.

618. Cuneo R, Caronna J, Pitts L, et al: Upward transtentorial herniation. Arch Neurol 36:618, 1989.

619. Fisher CM, Picard E, Polak A, et al: Acute hypertensive cerebellar hemorrhage: Diagnosis and surgical treatment. J Nerv Ment Dis 140:38, 1965.

620. Ludwig B, Swerdlow ML: Lethal cerebellar infarction with normal EMI scan: Two cases [abstract]. Neurology 27:402, 1977.

621. Hornig CR, Rust DS, Busse O, et al: Space-occupying cerebellar infarction: Clinical course and prognosis. Stroke 25:372, 1994.

622. Kanis KB, Ropper AH, Adelman LS: Homolateral hemiparesis as an early sign of cerebellar mass effect. Neurology 44:2194, 1994.

623. Momose KJ, Lehrich JR: Acute cerebellar infarction presenting as a posterior fossa mass. Radiology 109:343, 1973.

624. Shenkin HA, Zavala M: Cerebellar strokes: Mortality, surgical indications, and results of ventricular drainage. Lancet 11:429, 1982.

625. De Reuck J, Vander Eecken H: Cerebellar infarction and internal hydrocephalus. Acta Neurol Belg 78:129, 1978.

626. Géraud G, Guillaume J, Lagarrigue J, et al: Les ramollissements pseudo-tumoraux du cervelet. Rev Neurol (Paris) 134:183, 1978.

627. Norris JW, Eisen AA, Branch CL: Problems in cerebellar hemorrhage and infarction. Neurology 19:1043, 1969.

628. Taneda M, Ozaki K, Wakayama A, et al: Cerebellar infarction with obstructive hydrocephalus. J Neurosurg 57:83, 1982.

629. Wood MW, Murphey F: Obstructive hydrocephalus due to infarction of a cerebellar hemisphere. J Neurosurg 30:260, 1969.

630. Khan M, Polyzoidis KS, Adegbite ABO, McQueen JD: Massive cerebellar infarction: Conservative management. Stroke 14:745, 1983.

631. Cioffi FA, Bernini FP, Punzo A, D'Avanzo R: Surgical management of acute cerebellar infarction. Acta Neurochir 74:105, 1985.

632. Kase CS, Wolf PA: Cerebellar infarction: Upward transtentorial herniation after ventriculostomy. Stroke 24:1096, 1993.

633. Chen H-J, Lee T-C, Wei C-P: Treatment of cerebellar infarction by decompressive suboccipital craniectomy. Stroke 23:957, 1992.

634. No reference cited.

635. Schneider M: Durchblutung und Sausrstoffversorgung des Gehirns. Verh Dtsch Geskreislauf Forsch 19:3, 1953.

636. Zülch KJ: On circulatory disturbances in borderline zones of cerebral and spinal vessels. In Proceedings of the Second International Congress of Neurology. London, Excerpta Medica, 1955.

637. Zülch KJ, Behrend R: The pathogenesis and topography of anoxia, hypoxia, and ischemia of the brain in man. In Meyer J, Gastaut H (eds): Cerebral Anoxia and the EEG. Springfield, IL, Charles C Thomas, 1961, p 144.

638. Romanul F: Examination of the brain and spinal cord. In Tedeschi CG (ed): Neuropathology: Methods and Diagnosis. Boston, Little, Brown, 1970, p 131.

639. Romanul F, Abramowicz A: Changes in brain and pial vessels in arterial boundary zones. Arch Neurol 11:40, 1964.

640. Mohr JP: Neurological complications of cardiac valvular disease and cardiac surgery including systemic hypotension. In Vinken P, Bruyn G (eds): Handbook of Clinical Neurology, vol 38. Amsterdam, North-Holland, 1979, p 143.

641. Brierley JB: The neuropathology of brain hypoxia. In Critchley M, O'Leary J, Jennett B (eds): Scientific Foundations of Neurology. Philadelphia, FA Davis, 1972, p 243.

642. Zülch KJ: The Cerebral Infarct. Berlin, Springer-Verlag, 1986.

643. Rodda R: The vascular lesions associated with cerebellar infarcts. Proc Aust Assoc Neurol 8:101, 1971.

644. Sevestre H, Vercken JB, Hénin D, et al: Encéphalopathie anoxique après incompétence cardio-circulatoire: Etude neuropathologique à propos de 16 cas. Ann Med Intern 139:245, 1988.

645. Mounier-Vehier F, Gedaey I, Leclerc X, Leys D: Cerebellar border zone infarcts are often associated with presumed cardiac sources of ischemic stroke. J Neurol Neurosurg Psychiatry 59:87, 1995.

646. Jurgensen J, Brennan R, Towfighi J: Brainstem arterial end-zone infarction following hypotension in man. Neurology (NY) 31:92, 1981.

647. Gilles F: Hypotensive brainstem necrosis. Arch Pathol 88:32, 1969.

648. Lance J, Adams R: The syndrome of intention and action myoclonus as a sequel of hypoxic encephalopathy. Brain 86:111, 1963.

649. Keane J: Sustained upgaze in coma. Ann Neurol 9:409, 1981.

650. Bickerstaff E: Basilar artery migraine. Lancet 1:15, 1961.

651. Swanson J, Vick N: Basilar artery migraine. Neurology (NY) 28:782, 1978.

652. Caplan L: A tale of two brothers. Headache 17:49, 1977.

653. Fisher CM: Migrainous accompaniments versus arteriosclerotic ischemia. Trans Am Neurol Assoc 93:211, 1968.

654. Fisher CM: Transient migrainous accompaniments of late onset. Stroke 10:96, 1979.

655. Caplan L, Chedru F, Lhermitte F, et al: Transient global amnesia and migraine. Neurology (NY) 31:1167, 1981.

656. Simard D: Cerebral vasomotor paralysis during migraine attack. Arch Neurol 29:207, 1973.

657. Skinhoj E: Hemodynamic studies within the brain during migraine. Arch Neurol 29:95, 1973.

658. Olesen J, Larsen B, Lauritzen M: Focal hyperemia followed by spreading oligemia and impaired activation of CBF in classic migraine. Ann Neurol 9:344, 1981.

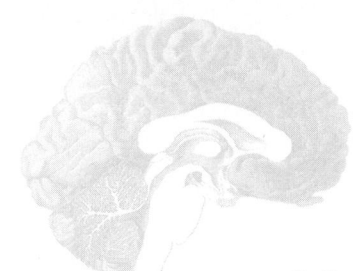

Chapter Eleven

Lacunes

J. L. Marti-Vilalta, Adria Arboix, and J. P. Mohr

HISTORICAL ASPECTS

In 1838, Dechambre[1] used the term *lacune* for the first time with pathologic criteria. From its initial description until the end of the nineteenth century, *lacune* was frequently misused in descriptions of cerebral specimens, and the entity was confused with other cavitary lesions in the brain such as état criblé (small bilateral, multiple lesions in the white matter described by Durand-Fardel[2] in 1842; Fig. 11–1), residual necrotic tissue of small infarcts or hemorrhages, enlarged perivascular spaces (Fig. 11–2), and porosis due to postmortem bacterial autolysis.

In 1901, Pierre Marie[3] used *lacune* as his descriptive term for 50 cases of capsular infarction and clearly established the concept and classification of different small cavities in the brain, ending the period of morphologic confusion. He formulated a syndrome featuring sudden onset of incomplete hemiplegia unaccompanied by persisting sensory loss, homonymous hemianopia, or permanent aphasia. Considerable improvement in the paralysis occurred within hours to days, but complete recovery was unusual. Walking was disturbed in a special fashion, the patients taking small steps described as marche à petits pas de Dejerine. In modern times this latter state has been attributed to patients with many foci of lacunar infarction, the so-called lacunar state. Marie emphasized a capsular and lenticular location for the syndrome. Ferrand[4] claimed, the next year, that the same syndrome occurred whether the lesion was capsular or pontine in location. More than 20 years later, Foix and Levy[5] reiterated these principles, adding the claim that a deep lesion produced a hemiparesis without visual or sensory disturbance and the formulation that the hemiparesis affected the arm and leg equally. In another publication, Foix and Hillemand[6] described the effects of a pontine infarction as a "simple" hemiplegia affecting the arm more than the leg, with an associated mild dysarthria.

During the first quarter of the twentieth century, doubts persisted about the etiology and pathogenesis of lacunes—whether they were ischemic, hemorrhagic, or inflammatory. The German pathologists Cecil and Oscar Vogt[7] firmly established the ischemic etiology. Only passing references to a capsular lesion producing a pure hemiplegia can be found in most standard textbooks of neurology published from the 1930s to the 1960s.[8,9]

Lacunes began their modern comeback almost entirely through the efforts of C.M. Fisher. Largely alone but in a few instances accompanied by or in support of younger colleagues, Fisher described pure motor hemiplegia,[10] pure sensory stroke,[11] homolateral ataxia and crural paresis (known mainly thereafter as ataxic hemiparesis),[12] dysarthria–clumsy hand syndrome,[13] sensorimotor stroke,[14] basilar branch syndromes,[15] and the vascular pathology underlying lacunes.[16] The position was so thoroughly developed that it triggered companion studies, many corroborating[14,17] and others enlarging on the clinical entities, vascular pathology, and clinicoradiologic correlations.[18–20] Other researchers attacked the basic principles,[21–23] some arguing for other causes including embolism[24] and others recommending that the concepts be abandoned altogether.[25] However, the high frequency of publications worldwide[26] indicates that the subject has become firmly established among the syndromes of stroke. In some countries, notably China, the high frequency of deep infarcts has even been proposed to have a racial or ethnic basis.[27,28]

The initial concept of lacunes as a set of clinical syndromes with pathologic criteria was soon diluted by new findings. Although none of the findings has fundamentally altered the basic concepts, so many exceptions to the basic concepts have appeared that some investigators have challenged their utility. Numerous studies have claimed that the syndromes may have causes other than hypertensive arteriopathy.[12,29–32] Although the individual reports often contained one or more clinical elements that deviated from the original syndromes, the effect was to blunt the impact of a causal relation of the syndromes with hypertension. Not long after the introduction of high-quality brain imaging, a wider range of locations of small, deep infarcts was found, together with an expansion of the syndromes associated with such lesions, now including the brainstem, parts of the thalamus, and other nuclei in the basal ganglia, corona radiata, centrum semiovale, and even some straddling of the thalamus and internal capsule; the concept was thus expanded to include syndromes overlapping with those caused by Binswanger's disease.[22,23,29,33,34] The earlier insistence on autopsy studies has largely been lost under the weight of publications based entirely on computed tomography (CT) or magnetic resonance imaging (MRI) findings. In recent years, it has been the exception, not the rule, to find a case report with autopsy correlation. Lamentably, *lacune* has passed into common use to refer

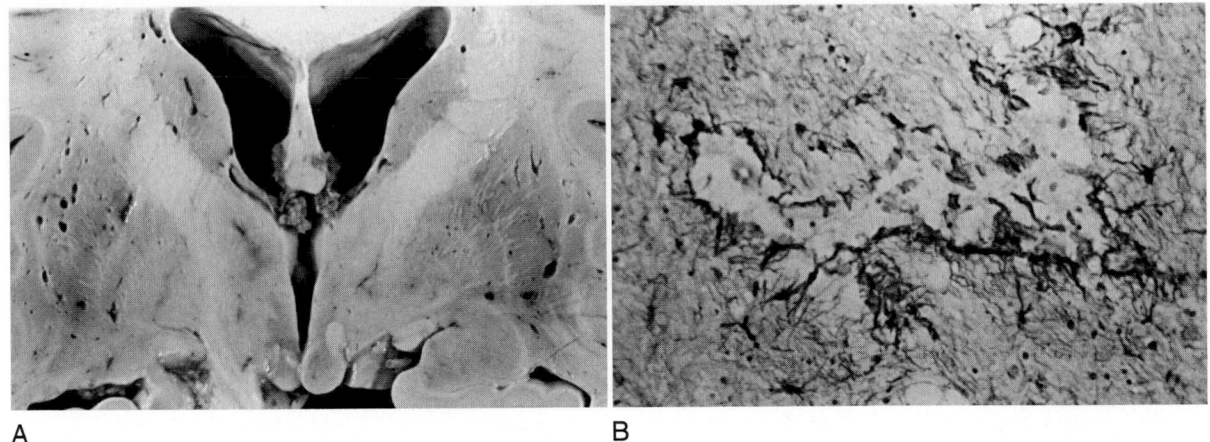

FIGURE 11–1   *État criblé. A, Macroscopic coronal section. B, Microscopic pathologic specimen. (GFAP stain.)*

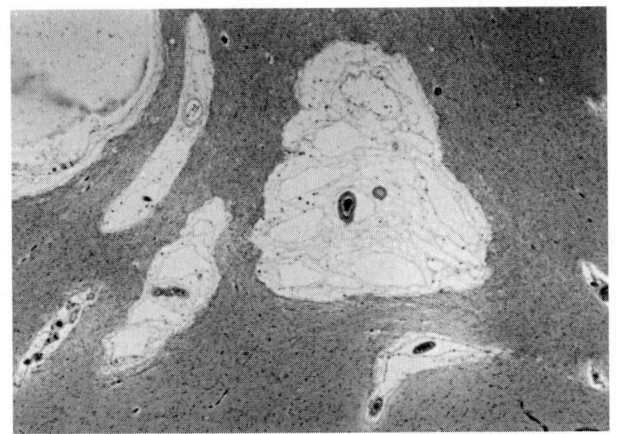

FIGURE 11–2   *Multiple enlarged perivascular spaces in the putamen of a patient with marked small blood vessel disease. (H&E, ×40.) (From Garcia JH, Ho KL: Pathology of hypertensive arteriopathy. Neurosurg Clin North Am 3:487, 1992.)*

to any small, deep lesion. Many researchers at least attempt to show that the cause is ischemic, but some have exercised no such caution, and the notion has even been introduced that lacunes may come from small hemorrhages. Despite these shortcomings, *lacune* has become firmly established among the syndromes of stroke and is a useful term when it refers to a lacunar syndrome implying a variety of causes, topographies, and clinical features that need careful study by the clinician and not a simple diagnosis at the bedside.

DEFINITIONS

As a term based on neuropathologic findings, *lacune* refers to a small, deep infarct attributable to a primary arterial disease that involves a penetrating branch of a large cerebral artery (Fig. 11–3). It should not be used to describe lesions of nonvascular origin, nor does it apply to deep infarction that is simply part of a larger stroke affecting the

cerebral surface in continuity or separately, such as that which occurs in embolism affecting the middle cerebral artery. It is also inapplicable to describe deep infarction from disease involving the stems of the large cerebral arteries (such as the middle or anterior cerebral vessels) that affects the penetrating branches.

The low frequency of autopsy studies has forced modification of the definitions to include small, deep lesions found by brain imaging, whether CT or MRI. Numerous attempts at definitions have been made, but the most widely seen is the attempt to distinguish among a small, deep infarct, the residue of a small hemorrhage, and dilated Virchow-Robin spaces; for those readers inclined to use numbers, these are types I, II, and III lacunes, respectively. In an attempt to keep this presentation orderly, we discuss first the autopsy-based material, then the studies based only on brain imaging, and finally the clinical studies.

PATHOANATOMY

Table 11.1 summarizes the findings of pathologic series of lacunar infarcts.

Size

Most autopsy-documented lacunar infarcts are small, ranging from 0.2 to 15 mm³ in size.[35] They vary according to the territory supplied by the occluded vessel feeding the infarct. In general, vessels are 100 to 400 μm[11] in size and serve territories varying from little more than a cylinder the size of the vessel itself to wedges as large as 15 mm on a side. Although the smallest infarcts are unresolved by CT scanners, and occasionally even escape detection at autopsy,[19] the largest, the so-called super lacunes, are as large as 15 mm³.[35] They are seen as obvious abnormalities at several levels on a CT scan. Thus, far fewer of these super lacunes have been examined at autopsy, and in some that were examined, no detailed search for the underlying vascular disorder was made. Embolism into the stem of the middle cerebral artery with occlusion of several of the lenticulostriate branches is a possible cause of such

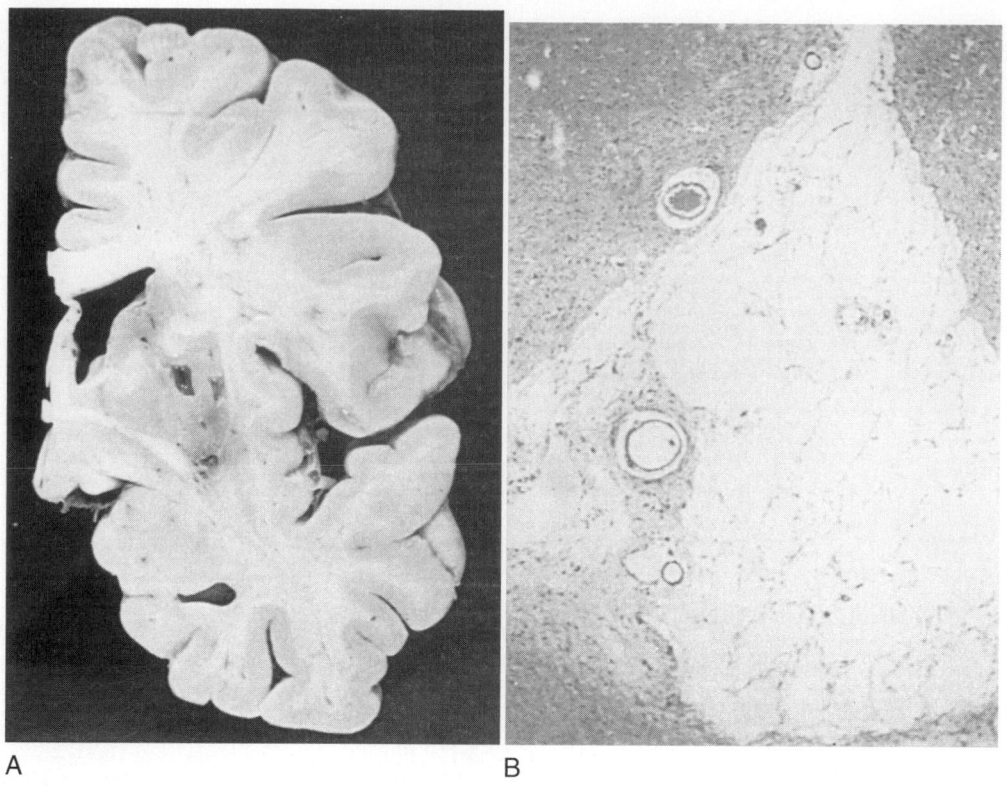

FIGURE 11–3   *Lacunes in the basal ganglia.* A, *Macroscopic coronal section.* B, *Microscopic pathologic specimen.* (H&E stain.)

Table 11.1   Lacunar Infarcts: Pathologic Series

Series (Year)°	Number of Cases	Number of Lacunar Infarcts per case	Topography	Risk Factors	Clinical Data	Causes of Death
Marie (1901)[3]	50	—	Lenticular nucleus	—	Pseudobulbar palsy Hemiparesis	—
Ferrand (1902)[4]	88	2.4	Lenticular nucleus	—	Pseudobulbar palsy	—
Hughes and Dodgson (1954)[237]	15	—	Lenticular nucleus (putamen/caudate)	—	Pseudobulbar palsy	—
Fisher (1965)[29]	114	3	Putamen/pons/ thalamus	Hypertension (>90%)	Silent ischemic stroke	—
Fang (1972)[238]	51	—	Basal ganglia	—	—	—
De Reuck and van der Eecken (1976)[102]	75	4.4	Putamen/thalamus	—	—	—
Ishii et al (1986)[239]	30	12	Frontal white matter	Hypertension (86%)	Pseudobulbar palsy/ dementia	—
Mancardi et al (1988)[240]	51	2.02	Putamen/thalamus/ frontal white matter/ caudate	—	Pseudobulbar palsy	—
Tuszynski et al (1989)[88]	169	1.9	Basal ganglia/ internal capsule/ putamen/thalamus	Hypertension (59%)	Pure motor hemiparesis (31%)	Ischemic heart disease/acute stroke
Dozono et al (1991)[241]	532	2.36	Frontal white matter/ putamen/pons	Hypertension (58%)	—	—
Arboix et al (1996)[242]	25	4.2	Putamen/pons/ frontal white matter	Hypertension (84%)	Silent ischemic stroke/ pseudobulbar palsy/pure motor stroke	Respiratory events (pulmonary thromboembolism/ lower respiratory tract infection)

°Superscript numbers indicate chapter references.

infarcts, which do not deserve the name lacune except for their location in the depths of the brain.[36]

Location

Lacunes predominate in the basal ganglia, especially the putamen, the thalamus, and the white matter of the internal capsule and pons, and they occur occasionally in the white matter of the cerebral gyri. They are rare in the gray matter of the cerebral surface as well as in the corpus callosum, visual radiations, centrum semiovale of the cerebral hemispheres, medulla, cerebellum, and spinal cord.[37] In general, the larger the series, the more widespread the lesions.[38] In the largest autopsy series thus far reported (169 found among 2859 patients), 81% of the lacunes seem to have been asymptomatic in life, arguing that many lacunes seen nowadays on brain imaging are of uncertain clinical significance.

Attempts to include the centrum semiovale and white matter of the temporal lobes in the regions subject to lacunes involves a challenge (thus far not justified by available data) to a principle long thought important in the production of lacunes: the lack of gradual step-down in vascular size between the major cerebral artery trunks and the penetrating vessels involved in lacunes. The medullary arteries of the white matter arise from the cortical branches and not directly from the large trunks. If their disease is the same as that of the lenticulostriate and thalamoperforating vessels, the similarity has not yet been demonstrated.

Vascular Territories Involved

Most lacunes occur in the territories of the lenticulostriate branches of the anterior and middle cerebral arteries, the thalamoperforating branches of the posterior cerebral arteries, and the paramedian branches of the basilar artery. Their occurrence is rare in the territories of the cerebral surface branches.

The lenticulostriate vessels arise from the circle of Willis and the stems of the anterior and middle cerebral arteries to supply the putamen, globus pallidus, caudate nucleus, and internal capsule. They are composed of two main groups: those more medial whose diameters are 100 to 200 μm and those more lateral whose diameters are 200 to 400 μm.[35] The thalamoperforating vessels arise from the posterior half of the circle of Willis and the stems of the posterior cerebral arteries to supply the midbrain and thalamus.[39] Their size varies from 100 to 400 μm. The paramedian branches of the basilar artery mainly supply the pons. Few branches have been measured, but sizes ranging from 40 to as large as 500 μm have been observed.[16,40] These arteries have in common both a tendency to arise directly from much larger arteries and an unbranching end-artery anatomy. The penetrators are all less than 500 μm in size and arise directly from the larger, 6- to 8-mm, internal carotid or basilar artery. Their small size and their points of origin rather proximal in the arterial network are thought to expose these vessels to forces that scarcely reach other arteries of similar size in the cerebral cortex.[41] These latter arteries are apparently protected by a gradual step-down in size from the 8-mm internal

carotid, to the 3- to 4-mm middle cerebral, to the 1- to 2-mm surface branches, from which the intracortical vessels whose diameters are less than 500 μm arise. Perhaps this difference explains the low frequency of lacunes in the cerebral surface vessels.[42,43]

The lack of collateral circulation for the penetrators results in an infarct that spreads distally from the point of occlusion through the entire territory of the vessel affected. The exact volume of tissue supplied by each penetrating artery varies enormously.[16] Some arteries supply little more than a territory of the same diameter as the vessels,[35] whereas others arborize widely and leave an infarct shaped like a wedge or cone.[16] Most capsular infarcts arise from arteries 200 to 400 μm in size and produce infarcts of about 2 to 3 mm³. These small infarcts are found regularly only on MRI with 1.5 tesla, are commonly missed on CT scanning, and are easily overlooked at autopsy.[19]

The arterial occlusion usually occurs in the first half of the course of the penetrating vessel, a location ensuring that most such occlusions are quite small. These sites are not usually detected on angiography because the course of the individual vessels is difficult to plot to show that one is missing. However, in disease involving the stem of the cerebral artery from which the penetrator arises, or from one of the small number of large penetrators, a bigger infarction results. Occlusions at the ostium of a penetrator where it departs from the parent major cerebral artery may yield a swath of infarction some 15 mm large.[3] These so-called super lacunes[35] are large enough to produce a striking abnormality at several levels on the CT scan. In most instances, however, super lacunes result from occlusions of larger vessels and are not a sign of primary arteriopathy of the penetrating vessels.

ARTERIOPATHIES UNDERLYING LACUNES

Microatheroma

Several distinct but related arteriopathies cause lacunes. Microatheroma is believed to be the most common mechanism of arterial stenosis underlying symptomatic lacunes (Fig. 11–4).[16,35,44] The artery is usually involved in the first half of its course. Microatheroma stenosing or occluding a penetrating artery was found in 6 of 11 capsular infarcts in the only published pathologic study on the cause of capsular infarcts,[35] and it was the cause of the only published case of a thalamic lacune.[11] The histologic characteristics of the microatheroma are identical to those affecting the larger arteries.

These tiny foci of atheromatous deposits are commonly encountered in chronic hypertension. In the usual non-hypertensive case, atheroma appears mostly in the extracranial internal carotid and basilar arteries but only rarely in the stems of the major cerebral arteries.[45,46] In hypertension, however, the lesions not only are more advanced for the patient's age but also are spread more distally in the arterial system, at times involving even some of the cerebral surface arteries. In patients with advanced hypertension, miniature foci of typical atherosclerotic plaques are found even in arteries as small as 100 to 400 μm in diameter, resulting in a stenosis or occlusion that sets the

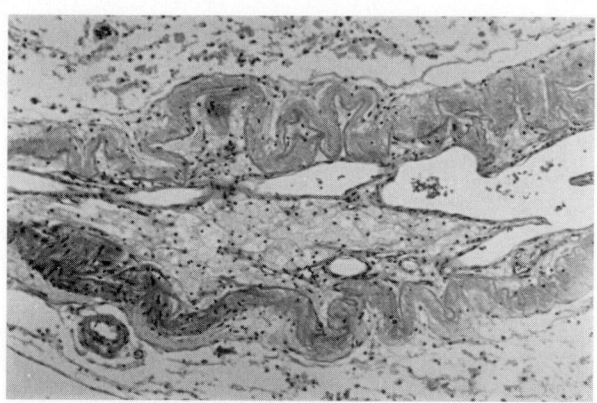

FIGURE 11–4 *Intimal deposit of lipid-laden macrophages in a penetrating intracerebral artery that shows partial occlusion of the lumen. (H&E, ×100.) (Courtesy of J.H. Garcia, MD.)*

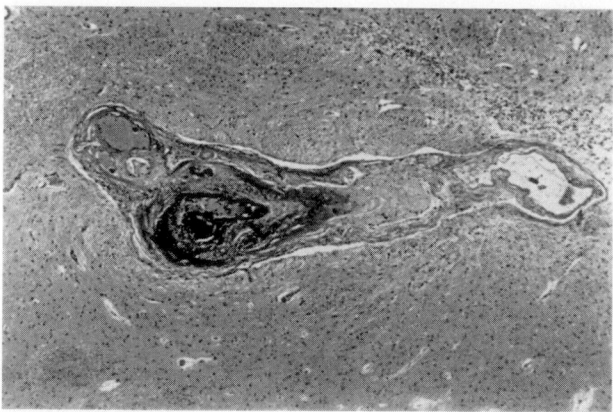

FIGURE 11–5 *Terminal segment of a lenticulostriate artery showing marked mural changes (hyalinization and fibrinoid change) as well as occlusion of the lumen. (H&E, ×60.) (From Garcia JH, Ho KL: Pathology of hypertensive arteriopathy. Neurosurg Clin North Am 3:487, 1992.)*

stage for a lacune. In a retrospective autopsy study of 70 brains with microscopic evidence of small vessel disease, the morphology of the vessel disease, the arteriolosclerosis, was similar in normotensive and hypertensive subjects. Lacunes were as prevalent in normotensive subjects(36%) as in hypertensive patients (40%), suggesting that the control of hypertension has modified the pathology of small vessel disease.[47]

Lipohyalinosis and Fibrinoid Necrosis

Other arterial disorders seem less common. Lipohyalinosis, formerly considered the most frequent cause of lacunes, affects penetrating arteries in a segmental fashion in chronic hypertension.[41] It was the cause attributed to 40 of 50 lacunes studied in serial section by Fisher[16] in four cases of stroke. It seems to occur most often in the smaller penetrating arteries, those less than $200\,\mu m$ in diameter, and accounts for many of the smaller lacunes, especially those that are clinically asymptomatic. Lipohyalinosis has been thought to be an intermediate stage between the fibrinoid necrosis of severe hypertension and the microatheroma associated with more long-standing hypertension.[16,40,43]

Fibrinoid necrosis is a related condition found in arterioles and capillaries of the brain (Fig. 11–5), retina, and kidneys in a setting of extremely high blood pressure.[48] It appears histopathologically as a brightly eosinophilic, finely granular, or homogeneous deposit involving the connective tissue of blood vessels.[49] The mechanism is believed to involve disordered cerebrovascular autoregulation[50,51] with a necrotizing consequence.[38] This thesis envisions that the thickened arterial walls are unable to constrict, resulting in a resetting of cerebrovascular autoregulation at higher blood pressure levels. Continued high pressure produces increased capillary hydrostatic pressure and capillary damage. The overdistension[30,52] of these small arteries occurs in segmental fashion,[53] leading to vascular necrosis,[38,42,54] which allows red blood cells, plasma, and protein ultrafiltrates into the stretched segments of the wall.[53]

That other vessels are spared such injury is not easily explained. However, the arteriolar and capillary necrosis

encountered in severe hypertension does not occur in renal arteries, which are protected from hypertension distal to an experimental arterial clamp or to renal arterial stenosis. Larger vessels seem able to absorb enough in the subintima and in their thicker muscularis layer to resist such change, and the tiny cerebral cortical arteries of a size similar to the deep branches of the circle of Willis are protected by their more distal location.[30,38,43]

Fibrinoid necrosis shares some of the histochemical, electron-microscopic,[30,55] and immunofluorescent[56] characteristics of lipohyalinosis,[57] another cause of lacunes. Both occur in the brain[16,35] in a setting of hypertension, and both occur in a segmental location along the course of the arteries.[16] The two conditions have also been labeled hyalinosis, hyaline fatty change, hyaline arterionecrosis, angionecrosis, fibrinoid arteritis, plasmatic vascular destruction, atherosclerosis of small arteries, and segmental arterial disorganization. Although often considered identical,[16,35] segmental fibrinoid necrosis and lipohyalinosis differ histochemically in that fibrinoid necrosis is said to stain strongly for phosphotungstic acid hematoxylin, whereas lipohyalinosis does not.[48,53] Also, lipohyalinosis is found most commonly in a setting of chronic, nonmalignant hypertension,[16,40] whereas fibrinoid necrosis is said to be found only with extreme blood pressure elevations[43,48] such as those that occur in hypertensive encephalopathy[43] and eclampsia.

Charcot-Bouchard Aneurysms

A long-standing, little noted controversy concerns whether lipohyalinosis or microatheroma is the precursor, is the result, or is even related to another commonly encountered arteriopathy in chronic hypertensives, Charcot-Bouchard aneurysms (Fig. 11–6).[16,32,59,60] The controversy also involves the following questions:

- Does the Charcot-Bouchard arteriopathy represent a true aneurysm formation, merely a dissection into the wall of a microatheroma, or twists, coils, and loops that are misdiagnosed as aneurysms?[61]

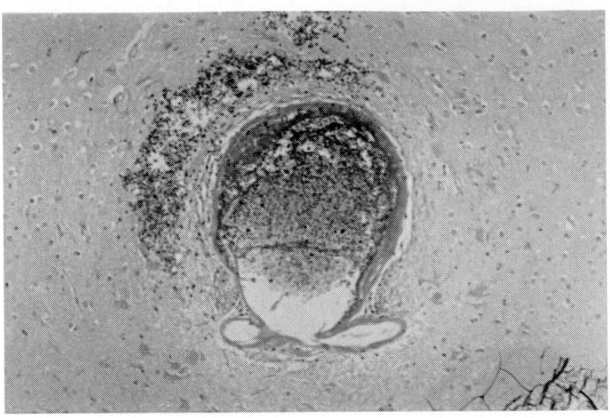

FIGURE 11–6 *A saccular microaneurysm (Charcot-Bouchard aneurysm) with extravasated erythrocytes and reactive astrocytes. The longitudinally sectioned vessel is seen at the bottom. (H&E, ×33.) (From Garcia JH, Ho KL: Pathology of hypertensive arteriopathy. Neurosurg Clin North Am 3:487, 1992.)*

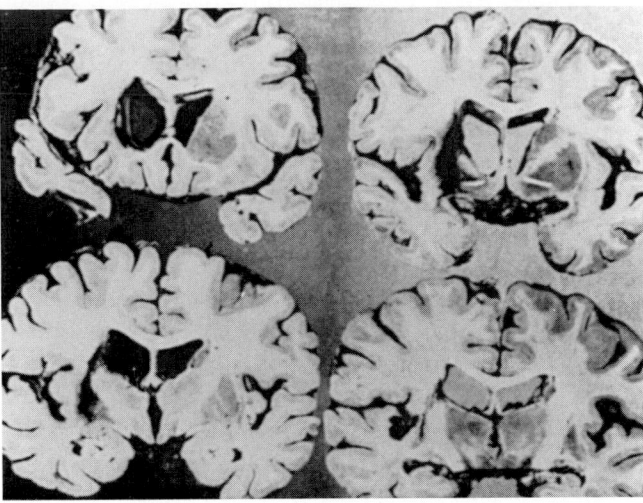

FIGURE 11–7 *Large, deep infarct reported in the original series of pure motor stroke syndrome. (From Fisher CM, Curry HB: Pure motor hemiplegia of vascular origin. Arch Neurol (Chic) 13:30, 1965.*

- Do both lipohyalinosis and Charcot-Bouchard aneurysms deserve consideration as pathologic processes separate from microatheroma of the penetrating arteries?
- Are these lesions simply variants along a spectrum of vascular effects of hypertension?

The available evidence suggests that lipohyalinosis is more significant than Charcot-Bouchard aneurysms in the development of lacunes.[16,60] No evidence has appeared to support an earlier suggestion that lipohyalinosis is the end stage of a preceding Charcot-Bouchard aneurysm.[32]

Other Causes

Microembolism has been inferred in a few serially sectioned lacunes shown to have normal arteries leading to the infarct.[35] Macroembolism is considered elsewhere, but one such case (case 10) is to be found among Fisher and Curry's[10] original descriptions of pure motor stroke (Fig. 11–7). Cholesterol emboli from atheromatous changes in the aortic arch have been shown in pathologic examination, occluding small arteries around multiple lacunar infarcts.[62] Even polycythemia has been thought to be a cause of lacunes,[63] the small vessels being obstructed by the sludged blood. Small, deep infarcts have been found in patients with antiphospholipid antibodies.[64] Dissection of a tiny artery may occur in the process leading to Charcot-Bouchard aneurysms.[65] Attempts have been made[66] to relate severe extracranial carotid stenosis to deep infarcts on a hemodynamic basis, the lacunar infarct being imaged on brain scan. Although the mechanism has been presumed to be perfusion failure in the symptomatic deep territory, the lack of autopsy data leaves unsettled the question whether such infarction is from embolism from the carotid disease or is associated with severe stenosis of a penetrating artery.[67] Amyloid angiopathy related to aging can narrow the lumen of small arteries through deposition of amyloid in the adventitia and media and can produce small infarcts.[68] Varying forms of arteritis may also occur, especially due to chronic meningitis (so-called Heubner's

arteritis),[69,70] chronic neurosyphilis,[71,72] any severe granulomatous meningitis, and chronic fibrosing meningitis. Neurocysticercosis,[73] neuroborreliosis,[74] and acquired immunodeficiency syndrome (AIDS)[75] affecting small arteries can produce lacunar infarcts. Arteritides of unknown cause, such as polyarteritis nodosa and granulomatous angiitis, autoimmune disorders like lupus erythematosus,[76] and drug abuse, particularly of cocaine,[77] may produce small, deep infarcts. Lacunar strokes due to thrombotic microangiopathy, not vasculitis, in deep, small or penetrating arteries is the main cause of early ischemia in patients with polyarteritis nodosa.[78]

Arteritis may have been a major cause of small, deep infarcts[79] when chronic neurosyphilis was in its heyday. However, two major works[70,80] on the subject contain no specific cases, even though the authors of one opined that "they undoubtedly occur."[70] This opinion was not shared by Pentschew,[72] who doubted whether "syphilitic endarteritis" was actually of syphilitic origin. In patients with first-ever stroke, chronic *Helicobacter pylori* infection detected by immunoglobulin (Ig) G antibodies was associated with risk of small artery occlusion.[81]

GENERAL CLINICAL FEATURES

Lacunar infarctions share many risk factors, the most common being hypertension and diabetes mellitus. These two common accompaniments of lacunar disease have been present with comparable frequencies in those clinical series exceeding 100 patients collected over the last 20 years: 75% and 29%, respectively, of lacunar cases diagnosed in the Harvard Cooperative Stroke Registry;[34] 74% and 27%, respectively, of cases in the south Alabama population study[11]; and 72% and 28%, respectively, of the Barcelona series reported by Arboix and colleagues,[82] in which only 26% of patients had cardiac disease. A high frequency (93%) of hypertension or left ventricular hypertrophy was found by Reimers and associates,[83] whereas no clear correlation with blood pressure or hypertension was found in some of the smaller series.[84] In a prospective epidemiologic study of 3660 elderly people examined with cranial MRI, 23% had one or more lacunes; the lacunes were single in 66% of subjects and silent in 89%. Risk factors associated independently with lacunar infarcts were age, diastolic blood pressure, creatinine level, smoking, and carotid artery stenosis of more than 50%.[85] In other studies, the risk factors for silent lacunar infarcts were age, systolic blood pressure,[86] and plasma homocysteine level.[87]

The largest currently reported autopsy-based study was that of Tuszynski and coworkers[88] (2859 patients), who found lacunar infarctions in 169 patients (6%). Hypertension was present in 64%, diabetes in 34%, and smoking in 46% of patients, and there were no known risk factors for cerebrovascular disease in 18%. A correlation was found between high hematocrit value and hypertension in the patients with lacunar syndromes in a population-based study.[89] In the Barcelona Stroke Registry, 399 (11%) of the 3577 patients with acute stroke had a lacunar infarct.[90] In the Stroke Data Bank project of the National Institute of Neurological and Communicable Diseases and Stroke (NINCDS), 337 (27%) of the 1273 patients diagnosed as having infarction had typical lacunar syndromes. In this large cohort, no striking differences were found among the risk factors for each of the lacunar subtypes, but differences were found between lacunar syndrome stroke as a group and other types of infarcts.[91] Lacunar syndrome strokes shared risk factors with large vessel infarction except for fewer transient ischemic attacks (TIAs) (13% versus 40%, respectively) and prior stroke (19% versus 39%). Compared with cardioembolism, lacunar syndrome strokes were more strongly associated with hypertension (75% for lacunar syndrome strokes versus 60% for cardioembolism) and diabetes (26% versus 17%) and less with cardiac disease (24% versus 77%).[92] Lacunar syndrome strokes may be more common among black patients.[71] Diabetes and hyperlipidemia are associated independently with lacunes in patients with carotid artery stenosis.[93]

Atrial fibrillation, one of the hallmarks of embolism, has a low frequency of small, deep infarcts (5%),[94] similar to the frequency in the general population older than 60 years. In very elderly patients (older than 85 years), there is a high frequency of atrial fibrillation (28%) as a consequence of age.[95] In a series comparing patients with atrial fibrillation with control subjects, in which neither group was known to have symptomatic stroke, Kempster and associates[96] found that all infarcts with atrial fibrillation were peripheral and consistent with embolism. In the control group, three asymptomatic infarcts were lacunes.

Prior TIAs are documented in approximately 20% of cases of lacunar infarcts, a frequency intermediate between embolism (5%) and large artery atherostenosis (40%). No correlation has yet been documented among the type of lacune, severity of the clinical deficit, and occurrence of TIAs. Compared with TIAs in large vessel infarcts, TIAs in lacunar infarcts have a higher number of episodes, a longer duration of neurologic deficit in each TIA, and a shorter latency between the first and last TIA and the definitive infarction. Stepwise or stuttering onset is more common in lacunar infarcts with TIA than in those without. There is a positive correlation between the number of prior TIAs and the volume of the lacunar infarct.[97]

Compared with the sudden onset more typical of infarction in other territories, a leisurely mode of onset has occurred in many lacunar strokes, delayed over enough time that an opportunity often exists to determine the effects of intervention. In contrast to major atheromatous or embolic stroke, in which a gradual onset is encountered in less than 5% of cases, as many as 30% of lacunes develop over a period of up to 36 hours.[11,35,98,99] During this time, a mild weakness may evolve into total paralysis, usually by intensifying the initial deficit but occasionally by spreading into limbs not affected initially.[11] This smooth onset occurs with equal frequency in all types of lacunar syndromes. Sudden onset occurs in only 40% of cases.[99] The progression of initial motor deficit is associated with poor functional outcome.[100] The rate of evolution of the stroke appears not to predict the severity of the eventual defect, but this matter has not yet received much detailed study. With respect to the circadian rhythm, the pattern of onset is uniform throughout the 24 hours.[101]

Lacunes typically manifest as the highly focal symptoms described later, but a few nonfocal symptoms have been reported in clinical series of patients with the typical motor or sensory syndromes. Lability of mood was once taken as a sign of multiple lacunes. This sign occurs in 26% of patients, with equal frequency whether single or multiple lacunes are visible on CT scan.[102] It may simply be that multiple lacunes are present pathologically but are too small to be seen on CT scan. To date, headache (9% to 15%),[103,104] lightheadedness, hiccup, and asterixis do not occur in a predictable manner with a high frequency, nor has any symptom been correlated with the presence of a CT scan abnormality or with the size or location of the lacunes shown on CT scan. Also, none appears to predict the clinical outcome.

CLINICAL SYNDROMES

Lacunar State

For many years, lacunar state was what most clinicians understood was meant by the term *lacunes*. It was part of the original description by Marie.[3] His syndrome included a progressive decline in neurologic function punctuated by a few episodes of mild hemiparesis and followed by the appearance of dysarthria, imbalance, incontinence, pseudobulbar signs, and a short-step gait (marche à petits pas). It was easy to envision that the small infarcts, widely scattered throughout the deep white matter, might accumulate gradually, each infarct inconspicuous but the cumulative effect devastating. Despite a few dissenting voices, matters have remained thus over the years.

Whether because of the effects of antihypertensive treatment or from some other undefined cause, the lacunar state is a rarity in modern times. One reason might be that the syndrome had been due to other causes. Fisher[65] pointed out that symptomatic occult hydrocephalus may have been the more common cause and that Marie's own published cases show such findings. He further noted that most lacunar infarcts are symptomatic and that the number of infarcts is small compared with the greatly deteriorated state of the patients. Earnest and colleagues[105] and Koto and associates[106] have observed a correlation between lacunar infarcts and hydrocephalus, suggesting that the infarcts may arise from the pressure on the white matter.

Pure Motor Stroke

Pure motor stroke is undoubtedly the most common of any lacunar form, accounting for between one half and two thirds of cases, depending on the series.[82,83,88,107] It was the first lacunar syndrome recognized clinically,[3,10] and its features have been the most thoroughly explored.

Clinicoanatomic Correlations

Pure motor stroke, also known as pure motor hemiparesis, has been reported from autopsied cases with focal infarction involving the corona radiata (Fig. 11–8),[102] internal capsule,[10,35] pons,[15] and medullary pyramid.[10,21,26] The most common correlations have been with capsular locations. Of the two ends of the capsule, the greater number of lacunes has been reported in the posterior limb (Fig. 11–9). Posterior limb capsular lacunes usually involve the globus pallidus and posterior limb of the capsule,[108] which are supplied by the lenticulostriate branches of the middle cerebral artery. The vessels occluded vary in size from small, medially placed penetrators to the larger lateral lenticulostriate vessels. The infarcts range in location from the genu to the back of the posterior limb. It is in this group that most of the data referable to the classic views of a homunculus in the internal capsule are to be found. Lesions in this region, especially those affecting the corona radiata, have also produced the syndrome of ataxic hemiparesis.

Anterior limb capsular lacunes constitute a smaller number of cases and are smaller infarcts that may affect the caudate in addition to the anterior limb of the

capsule.[19] Some of them are in the territory of supply of the anterior cerebral artery, including the largest of the penetrating vessels, the recurrent artery of Heubner. Syndromes of hemiparesis constitute only one of the many permutations of anterior capsular infarcts,[108,109] which also include ataxic hemiparesis[110] and some unusual speech and language disorders.[111,112]

Compared with the small number of cases with autopsy correlation, a steadily growing group of cases of pure motor stroke have been documented by CT scan alone. In the NINCDS Pilot Stroke Data Bank project, fully 45 of the 100 cases of lacunes were diagnosed on CT scan, most often as instances of pure motor stroke.[14] The pathology in such cases is rarely defined.

Other Causes of Pure Motor Syndromes

Nonlacunar pure motor syndromes have also been described, indicating that the clinical picture alone is not invariably due to deep infarction. Less than a year after Marie's description of lacunes, protests against his definitions were lodged. In an earlier thesis Abadie[113] contrasted the great frequency with which a capsular lesion was diagnosed clinically and the rarity with which such a lesion was found without other complaints accompanying the hemiparesis. His objection set the stage for the many others down through the years.

After Fisher and Curry's 1965 report[10] of pure motor stroke, several articles appeared challenging the lacunar origin by detailing a similar syndrome due to a variety of other causes, including nocardial abscess of the motor cortex,[23] ischemia-edema after craniotomy for postoperative bleeding,[114] internal carotid artery occlusion in the neck,[115] and cerebral cortical surface infarction or ventromedial pontine infarction due to a propagating thrombosis of the basilar branch.[116] Lesions rostral to the capsule have been described in cases studied only by CT,[20] and the syndrome has also been encountered with both deep and

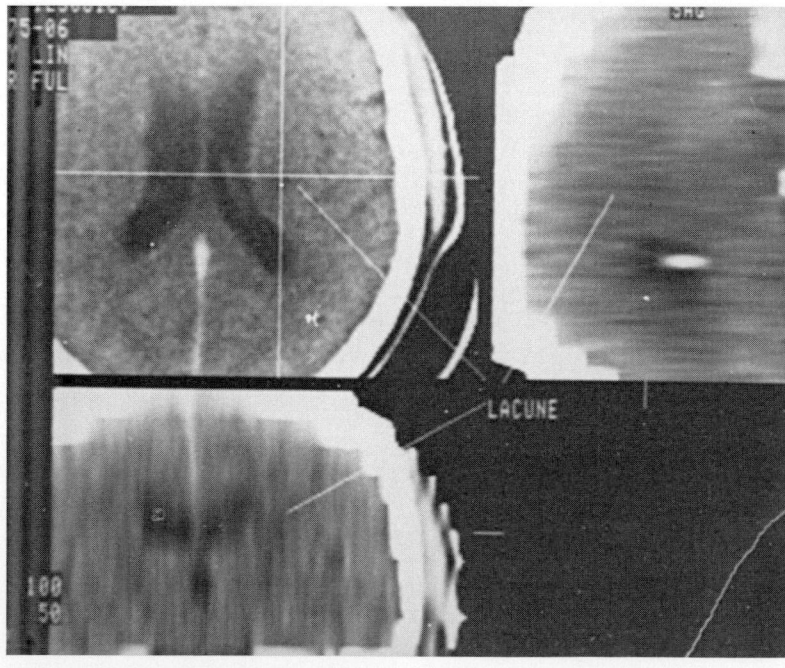

FIGURE 11–8 *Lacune affecting the corona radiata.*

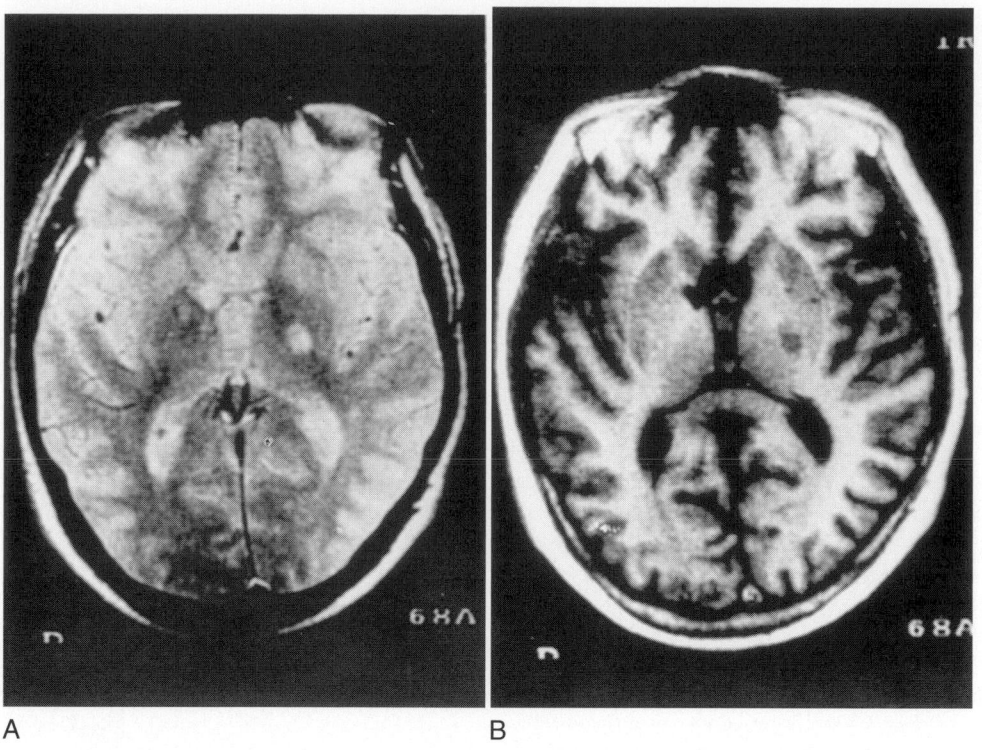

A   B

FIGURE 11–9 *Axial (A) T2-weighted and (B) T1-weighted magnetic resonance images showing a lacunar infarct in the posterior limb of the internal capsule.*

superficial low-density lesions on CT that were inferred to be from infarction.[19] A few such cases have even been reported from hemorrhage.[108,117–120]

The clinical picture itself has also come under criticism. Richter and associates[121] studied all cases of stroke that occurred in a single hospital and found that pure motor stroke occurred rarely, was not more prevalent among hypertensives, and did not usually have a good clinical outlook.

Even the most careful studies exploring the limits of the syndrome and its causes, however, have found a remarkably high percentage of cases with a clinical and radiologic picture conforming to the original syndrome described by Fisher and Curry[10]; Pullicino and coworkers[19] studied 297 consecutive patients whose CT scans showed one or more foci of low density and found among them 42 single, small, deep lesions. Hypertension was more prevalent in this group than in the 122 patients with large lesions. Nine of the 42 (21%) with small lesions had a pure motor deficit, in contrast to only 3 of 122 (2%) with large lesions, a highly significant difference ($P < .0005$). Furthermore, in another 13 cases with isolated deep lesions, either the clinical deficit could not be related to the lesion or there was no clinical deficit at all, a point consistent with the observation that deep infarcts may spare the capsule.

Clinical Features

Pure motor stroke is most easily diagnosed when the stroke affects the face, arm, and leg equally on the same side, sparing sensation, vision, language, and behavior.[10] The complete syndrome is somewhat uncommon, however. As a clinical rule, as long as the syndrome is purely motor, the diagnosis applies when the affected side involves one part more than the other. Some cases have been described in which the face is essentially spared, the best known being from pyramid infarction.[122] In a series of 22 patients with a brachiofacial pure motor stroke, four had a cortical infarct in the superficial middle cerebral artery.[123] Pure motor monoparesis is almost never due to a lacunar infarct.[124] The term *pure motor stroke* was initially used to draw attention to the lack of expected accompanying sensory, visual, or behavior disturbances, especially considering the severity of the weakness. In this sense only is it "pure."

Pure motor stroke has been described in both capsular and pontine locations, producing a clinical picture essentially identical to that first suggested by Ferrand.[4] Some reports suggested that a case with capsular infarct might have an associated conjugate eye movement disturbance that would follow the hemispheral pattern (i.e., deviation of the eyes toward the side of the lesion) and that those involving the pons would have the opposite effect, the so-called wrong way eyes.[10,125] However, this finding occurs too infrequently to serve a useful function.[34]

Despite earlier opinions expressed by Ferrand[4] and by Foix and Levy,[5] it has become clear that pure motor stroke may be associated with considerable variations among the syndromes involving the face, arm, and leg. Fisher and Curry[10] found the arm severely affected in all 50 of their cases of pure motor stroke, but the lower the lesion occurred in the neuraxis, the less the face was involved.

When the lacune affects the internal capsule and corona radiata, the motor deficits encountered have shown considerable variety in both severity and formula. Despite the many CT correlations with capsular lesions, only a handful of cases exists with a capsular infarct for which the syndrome was fully studied in life. Among this small group, there are remarkable variations. The most compact lesion with a hemiplegia was an autopsied case with an infarct confined to the third quarter of the posterior limb of the internal capsule.[126] This location corresponds to the approximate pathway of the motor fibers as inferred from whole brain anatomic dissections.[127] The clinical deficit had persisted for years, affecting the face, arm, and leg equally. In another autopsied case involving the same site in the posterior limb of the internal capsule, the deficit was less severe. Spastic hemiparesis developed over many hours and lasted for the remaining 9 months of the patient's life, paralyzing the tongue, palate, face, arm, and hand but only slightly affecting the leg.[48] In still another case, ischemia involving the posterior quarter of the internal capsule was associated with a hemiparesis that only slightly affected the face.[34]

Most of the initial imaging studies were based on CT scan. Donnan and colleagues[18] found a hemiplegia involving the face, arm, and leg in equivalent fashion in all 36 patients with infarction involving the capsule, but 22 other patients in the same series had incomplete syndromes, the most common being paresis of the arm and leg that spared the face. The inferred lacune in these latter cases occurred more often in the fibers of the corona radiata or at the extreme ends of the capsule. One lacune with pure facial weakness was located at the genu, whereas another associated with pure leg weakness lay at the extreme posterior end of the capsule. Rascol and associates[108] also found a spectrum of syndromes of hemiparesis that varied at one end from equal involvement of the face, arm, and leg to partial syndromes of faciobrachial weakness, in a few cases purely crural[108]; similar incomplete formulas of hemiparesis occurred in the smaller capsulopallidal cases and also in the anterior capsulocaudate infarcts. In both the NINCDS Pilot Stroke Data Bank project[107] and the population-based study of stroke conducted in southern Alabama,[128] lacunes located more posteriorly in the capsule produced a deficit greater in the leg than in the arm, but several varieties were encountered, including some in which the arm was worse than the leg. Lesions affecting the anterior limb and genu have also been a source of syndromes of partial hemiparesis, in a few cases featuring greater weakness of the face than of the leg.[18] In cases studied in the Stroke Data Bank, lesions seen in the corona radiata were associated with a hemiparesis that took highly variable forms, whereas those located lower in the capsule produced a wide variety of syndromes (Fig. 11–10).[92] Taken together, the CT scan correlations with the syndromes of hemiparesis showed only slight support for the classic view of a homunculus in the internal capsule with the face, arm, and leg displayed in an anteroposterior distribution.

When these findings are taken together, it is no longer possible to infer the exact site and size of the lesion in the motor pathway using the clinical formulation based on the older dogma[129] that the motor fibers occupy a certain functionally reliable position in the posterior limb of the internal capsule. The case material only vaguely supports the traditional impression of a homunculus whose face is

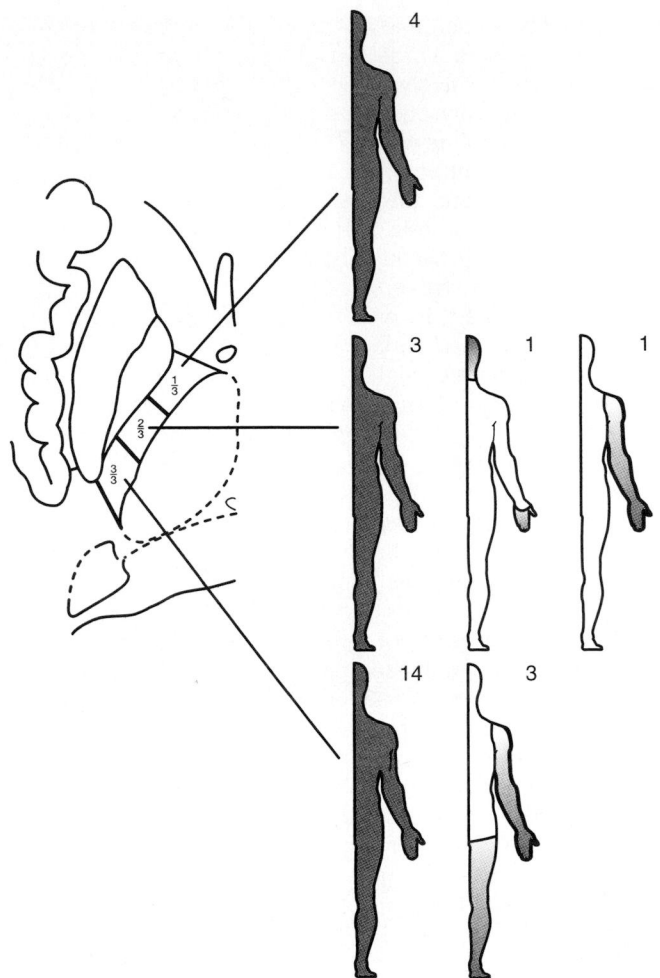

FIGURE 11–10 *Hemiparesis formulas for capsular lesions of the anterior, middle, and posterior thirds of the posterior limb of the internal capsule. (From Chamorro AM, Saco RL, Mohr JP, et al: Lacunar infarction: Clinical-CT correlations in the Stroke Data Bank. Stroke 22:175, 1991.)*

forward and whose leg is located posteriorly. These findings suggest that even more careful attention to the clinical details in future cases might permit a clearer understanding of the variability and reliability of the pathways that make up the capsule.[22,82,109,127] At the least, the findings thus far indicate that partial syndromes of hemiparesis are common manifestations of lacunar infarction affecting the internal capsule and adjacent territory.

Associated Complaints

Although the main elements of the pure motor stroke syndromes are motor, other complaints are not rare, especially sensory disturbances, which occur initially in as many as 42% of cases.[18] These complaints usually present as numbness, heaviness, and loss of feeling. Only scant abnormalities are found on clinical examination. Given their vague character, they are all too easily brushed aside or ignored. However, complaints of undue coldness, at times confined to the distal arm, are less easily ignored, and in a few cases personally observed by one of the authors, they have lasted for years.[34] The anatomic disorder of these complaints has not been resolved. These sensory complaints are thought to reflect slight involvement of the projections to the sensory cortex from occlusion of the larger lateral striate vessels, although few such cases have actually been documented by autopsy. When the perception threshold for temperature and thermal pain is measured, a significant thermal hypesthesia on the affected side is found. This semiologic finding has also been reported in pure motor and sensorimotor stroke.[130]

No disturbance in visual field function has been described from such infarcts. Dysphasia, dyspraxia, and other disturbances of higher cerebral function have rarely been described.

Clinical Course

Improvement is seen in a high percentage of cases. It is usually more rapid and more complete than that following cerebral surface infarction with a similar initial motor deficit.[19] The syndromes of partial hemiparesis show the best prognosis, as do those with the smaller infarct size on CT scan, but cases of complete plegia with virtually total recovery have been encountered. Rascol and associates[108] found that all their patients regained the ability to walk. Fully 19 of the 30 patients experienced a favorable outcome, whereas another 6 were left with functional incapacity of the upper extremity. Thirty-five of the 42 patients documented in the pilot phase of the NINCDS Stroke Data Bank improved to a functionally useful level within a few months.[14] The improvement occurred regularly in the patients whose initial syndrome was incomplete. Unfortunately, of the 7 patients initially paralyzed, only 2 experienced much improvement in the first few months, and both of them improved almost to normal. In 5 patients with pure motor hemiparesis, pontine (3) and capsular (2) functional MRI in the acute phase showed activation in the ipsilateral sensorimotor cortex and contralateral supplementary motor area and reduction in the contralateral sensorimotor cortex. After recovery, the activity normalized in the contralateral cortex.[131]

Pure Sensory Stroke

Pure sensory stroke is assumed to be due to infarction of the sensory pathway of the brainstem, thalamus, or thalamocortical projections. The thalamus is supplied by very small arteries susceptible to the effects of chronic hypertension.[39] Few autopsy-documented cases have been reported, and the syndrome was not noted in one large autopsy-based series.[58] In this small group, the most common location was the thalamus,[11,14,132] mostly in the ventral posterior tier nuclei, the main sensory relay nuclei to the cerebrum.[132] The only autopsied case with pure sensory stroke from a lesion outside the thalamus[133] consisted of a small hemorrhage that involved the corona radiata of the posterior limb of the internal capsule.

CT has been the basis of identification of the other sites associated with pure sensory stroke (Fig. 11–11). One case, inferred to be due to a lacune because of the small size of the lesion, affected the centrum semiovale, presumably with involvement of the thalamocortical projection area.[134] Caution is necessary in this interpretation, because lacunes

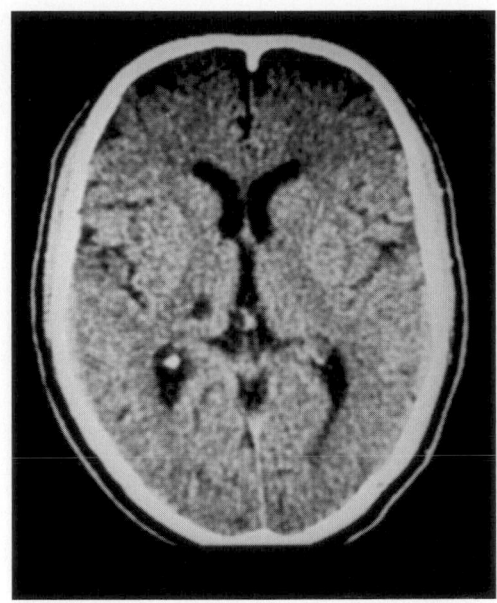

FIGURE 11–11 *Computed tomography scan showing thalamic lacunar infarct.*

in the centrum semiovale are distinctly uncommon in series based on autopsy data.[29,102] Involvement of subthalamic brainstem pathways has not yet been reported to be associated with pure sensory stroke. Pure sensory stroke due to a pontine tegmentum lesion can cause ipsilateral impairment of the smooth pursuit eye movements, which can be differentiated to thalamic topography.[135]

Observations of the arterial disease are confined to two cases. In one, a microatheroma was found narrowing the lumen of a small artery to the posterior thalamus,[16] which led to a lacunar infarct. The report did not mention whether the lacune was symptomatic. In the other case, a pure sensory syndrome was described clinically.[11] The 54-year-old patient was recovering from a right-sided pure motor hemiplegia when a feeling of pins and needles developed in the left lower lip, the left side of the mouth, and the fingers of the left hand; the sole of the left foot tingled and felt numb, dull, and swollen many hours later. No sensory deficit was evident on examination. Unpleasant paresthesias affected the left side of the face and the left foot. CT scan was normal on the fourth day. At autopsy 6 months later, a lacune measuring $2 \times 2 \times 3.7$ mm was found in the right ventral posterior nucleus, fed by four tiny arteries that arose from a single artery destroyed by lipohyalinosis.

The lacunes in both of the reported autopsied cases were quite small. If they are typical, it is easy to understand why many thalamic lacunes have thus far escaped detection by CT and require the higher-grade image provided by MRI. Larger lesions may be seen with both techniques (Fig. 11–12).

Complete Hemisensory Syndromes

Typically, the disturbance in sensation extends over the entire side of the body, involving the face, proximal as well as distal limbs, and axial structures including the scalp, neck, trunk, and genitalia right to the midline, even

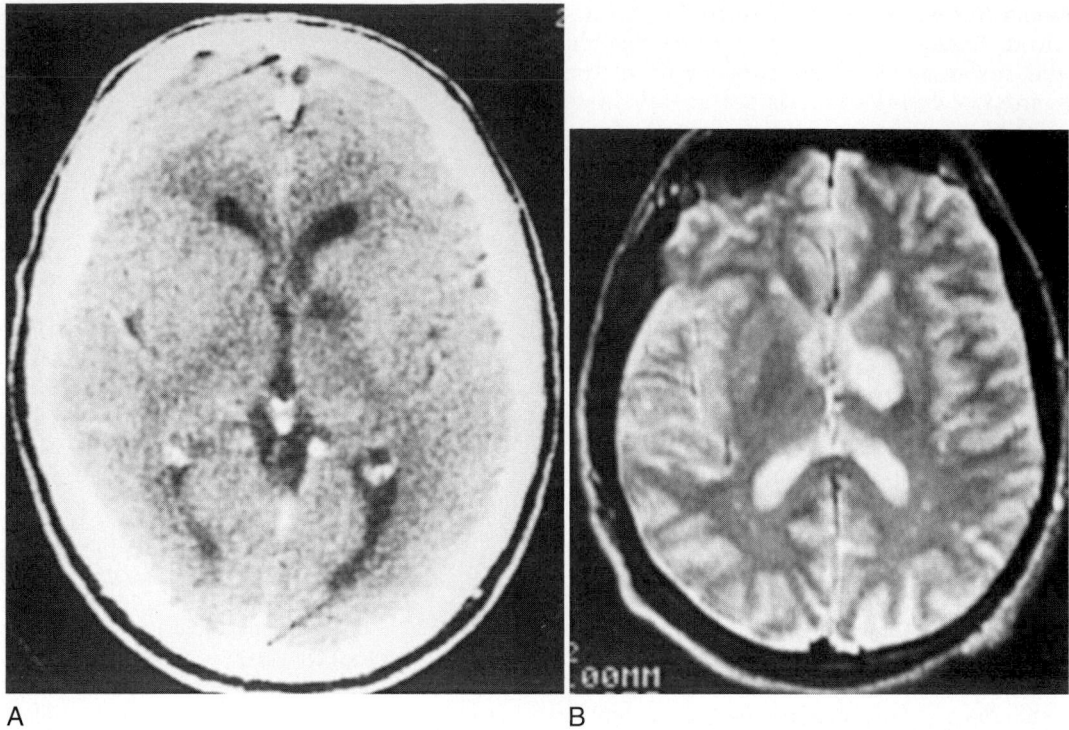

FIGURE 11–12 *Anterior thalamic infarct seen on (A) computed tomography scan and (B) magnetic resonance image of the same patient.*

splitting the two sides of the nose, tongue, penis, and anus.[34,132] This remarkable midline split, especially when the trunk or abdomen is involved, may be unique to thalamic or thalamocortical pathway lesions. This type of hemisensory syndrome affected one patient with a thalamic infarction measuring $4 \times 4 \times 2$ mm.

In the earliest report of a patient with a complete hemisensory syndrome, which was not attributed to a lacune, Wyllie[136] described the clinical picture as if a plumb had been dropped down the exact center of the patient's body so that exactly one half only was affected. In this case, the responsible thalamic infarct was not reported: Wyllie's main interest was the associated disturbances in higher cerebral function from the remainder of the large left posterior cerebral artery territory infarction. This complaint of total hemisensory loss has also been part of the syndrome in the small number of patients with the syndrome of sensorimotor stroke.

Incomplete Hemisensory Syndromes

Variants in the topography of pure sensory stroke have been reported that involve less than the entire side of the body. One patient, reported with autopsy correlation (case 9 in Fisher's original collection of pure sensory stroke[132]), suffered only TIAs affecting at one time the right fingers and at another time the right upper and lower lips, right side of the tongue, and the two medial toes of the right foot. At autopsy, a lacune 7 mm in diameter was found in the left ventral posterior nucleus. The complaints in other cases without autopsy documentation have involved the face, arm, and leg; head, cheek, lips, and hand; unilateral intraoral and perioral sites and fingers, the so-called

cheiro-oral syndrome; face, fingers, and foot; shoulder tip and lower jaw; distal forearm alone; fingers alone; and leg alone.[37,132] How many permutations exist is a subject of some interest, because establishing them might serve to determine the organization of a sensory homunculus in the ventral tier nuclei.

Lapresle and Haguenau[137] found partial sensory syndromes involving the face, the arms, the leg, the oral cavity, the peribuccal area and forearm, and the peribuccal area and radial edge of the forearm, all from focal thalamic softening of lacunar size. As already mentioned, the patient in Fisher's case 9 suffered only TIAs affecting the right fingers at one time and the right upper and lower lips, the right side of the tongue, and the two medial toes of the right foot at another time.[11] A lacune 7 mm in diameter affecting the left ventral posterior nucleus was found at autopsy. In another autopsied case also previously described, a 54-year-old patient recovering from a right pure motor hemiplegia experienced a feeling of pins and needles in the left lower lip, the left side of the mouth, and the fingers of the left hand; the sole of the left foot tingled and felt numb, dull, and swollen many hours later. No sensory deficit was evident on examination. Unpleasant paresthesias affected the left side of the face and the left foot. CT scan was normal on the fourth day. At autopsy 6 months later, a $2 \times 2 \times 3$-mm lacune was found in the right ventral posterior thalamus.[11] The complaints in other cases without autopsy documentation have involved the face, arm, and leg; head, cheek, lips, and hand; face, fingers, and foot; shoulder tip and lower jaw; distal forearm alone; fingers alone; and leg alone. The full array of permutations has been subject to considerable study.[138]

Electrophysiologic studies have found a well-organized topographic arrangement of the ventroposterolateral nucleus of the thalamus in animals, which has been confirmed in humans by single-unit studies of thalamic neurons. The location and size of the receptive field have been mapped, showing a high number of cells concentrated on perioral and digital sensation and only a few for the forearm and upper arm.[139] The organization of the cells is in the sagittal plane with cutaneous and deep stimuli aligned toward each other. The failure of the clinical syndromes from infarction to reflect this type of organization may be explained by the vascular anatomy. The small vessels, individually occluded, may cause an infarct that cuts across the functional anatomic fields of somatosensory projections, causing clusters of symptoms and signs from lesions that are at variance with the normal organization.

Nature of the Sensory Complaints

The patients complain of striking alterations in spontaneous sensations.[132,140] The parts feel stretched, hot, and sunburned, as if being stuck by pins, larger, smaller, or heavier. Contacts with the skin from eyeglasses, bedclothes, rings, watches, and sheets feel heavier on the affected side and may transiently aggravate the sensory disturbance. The stimulus seems to persist for a few seconds after its removal. In the patients with severe disturbances, the occurrence of a stimulus is better reported than its exact location. In a series of 21 cases, impairment of all sensory types (touch, pinprick, vibration, and position sense) was usually associated with large lacunes in the lateral thalamus; restricted sensory complaints suggest small lacunes at any level of the sensory pathway.[141]

The Dejerine-Roussy syndrome[142] is an uncommon accompaniment of lacunar infarction of the thalamus, although dysesthetic accompaniments are common in pure sensory stroke, as described previously. The full Dejerine-Roussy syndrome was originally described as the effect of occlusion of the thalamogeniculate branch of the posterior cerebral artery, with infarction of the ventral posterolateral and ventral posteromedial nuclei, largely sparing the remaining nuclei of the thalamus. Cases documented only by CT have shown a lesion small enough to qualify for a clinical diagnosis of lacunar infarction.[143] Suffice it to say here that the initial deficit usually consists of a hemiparesis and a hemisensory syndrome. The pain, which is an inconstant feature in cases with such infarcts, may begin at the onset of the syndrome or appear only later; delays of up to several months are common. The pains are intermittent or constant, appear spontaneously, or at other times are provoked by contact with the affected parts. They are usually accompanied by many other disturbances in sensation, including tingling, feelings of excessive weight, and feelings of cold, although a few cases exist in which the sensory function is normal on clinical testing. The special disturbance known as *hyperpathia* is particularly characteristic but not common: After a sensory stimulus, a disagreeable response occurs that is usually delayed in onset, may spread over a large area, persists after removal of the stimulus, and may even increase in intensity over several seconds. The syndrome may outlast other features of the original stroke syndrome and may even become permanent. Amitriptyline has been used with some success;

treatment begins with doses of 10 mg at bedtime and increases to 25 mg after a week in most patients who tolerate the dry mouth and to even higher levels in some cases. A month or more may be required for benefit to appear in patients who show response to the therapy.

Associated Disturbances

Disturbances in motor function, language, and vision might be expected in a setting of thalamic infarction but have thus far been unreported except for a single example of sensorimotor stroke due to a thalamic lacune (see later).[144] Given the anatomy of the thalamus and its widely varying projections to the cerebrum, such syndromes should be encountered but have thus far eluded the most careful diagnostic efforts of vascular neurologists.

Clinical Course

Improvement appears to be the rule, often to normal within weeks.[138] The topography of the shrinking deficit may be rather unusual. Improvement in the trunk with persistence of deficit in the distal extremities, a pattern common in hemispheral disease, is only occasionally encountered. In one case, the deficit shrank to a vertical band from the axilla down the lateral trunk to the thigh,[98] a finding encountered by one of the authors (JPM) in several cases studied in southern Alabama.

Sensorimotor Stroke

Three autopsied cases of sensorimotor stroke have been reported to date,[14,118,136] only one being published with "sensorimotor stroke" in the title.[14] Such cases, although rare, are important because they attest to the occurrence of a combined motor and sensory deficit from a small, deep infarct. Their vascular anatomy also helps clarify the vascular supply to the thalamus and adjacent internal capsule. The rarity of these cases should obviate any casual assumption that small, deep infarcts cause most cases of sensorimotor stroke.

The first case report that we found was published by Garcin and Lapresle[145] as part of a review of sensory disorders from thalamic infarction. The patient was a 65-year-old woman who suddenly developed left hemiparesis and a combination of hypesthesia and dysesthesia in the left peribuccal area and forearm. At autopsy, a small infarct was found straddling the intersection of the ventral posterior lateral and medial nucleus of the right thalamus. Involvement of the internal capsule was not mentioned.

The patient reported by Mohr and colleagues[14] was a 61-year-old man. The sensory component preceded the motor component by several hours. The syndrome evolved smoothly and steadily over approximately a day and then stabilized for many days before beginning to improve. The sensory component involved the entire half of the body, including the neck, ear, and genitalia. The sensory and motor deficits each followed a temporal course and clinical profile typical of pure sensory stroke and pure motor stroke, respectively. Neither deficit faded completely with time, but both underwent considerable improvement. The hemihypalgesia shrank to a vertical band from the axilla down the lateral trunk to the thigh. At autopsy, a

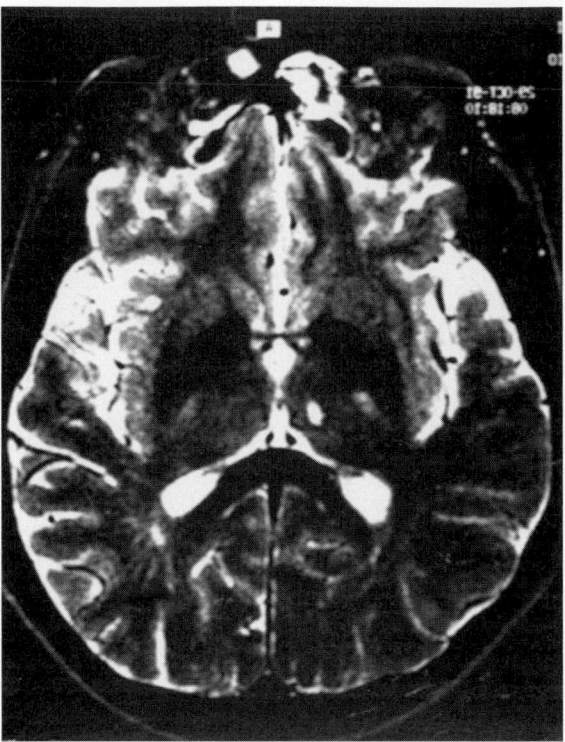

FIGURE 11–13 *Magnetic resonance image showing a small thalamic lacune.*

well-developed lacune 4 × 4 × 2 mm was found in the ventral lateral nucleus of the thalamus, and the adjacent internal capsule showed a slight pallor (Fig. 11–13). Efforts to track down the vascular supply to the infarct by means of serial sections were frustrated by the gross horizontal section made before embedding. The small artery found in the infarct was tracked downward toward its expected source from the posterior cerebral artery. Instead of gradually enlarging, however, the vessel gradually became smaller and vanished, leaving the investigators to infer that its origin was from above the infarct. Efforts to trace the artery upward also proved futile when the serial sections crossed the plane of the original gross section. Here the discontinuity was too great to permit matching of sections to map the course of the artery.

The third patient attracted more interest because of his action-induced rhythmic dystonia than because of the sensorimotor stroke.[146] The stroke occurred when the patient was 61 years old and had been known to be diabetic for 4 years. He fell suddenly, with left leg weakness. On examination, he was found to have a left hemiparesis "with loss of all sensory modalities." He improved within a week and was able to walk with support within a month. Involuntary movements began in the left leg by the fourth month. When examined by the investigators 4 years after the stroke, the patient had slight lower facial weakness and slightly exaggerated left-sided reflexes but normal strength and sensation. Autopsy revealed an infarct 3 × 3 × 10 mm involving the ventral posterolateral nucleus of the right thalamus and adjacent internal capsule. No mention was made of the arterial anatomy of the lesion.

The neurovascular issues raised by the case are also of importance. Before such cases were documented, the vascular supply to the internal capsule was believed to be wholly separate from that to the thalamus. The lenticulostriate branches of the middle cerebral artery presumably supplied the capsule, and the thalamus was artery presumed to receive its supply from the perforating branches of the posterior cerebral artery.[144] The extreme posterior nuclei of the thalamus received a few branches from the choroidal arteries.[39] However, three cases now exist showing that a single infarct may involve both the thalamus and the adjacent internal capsule. These cases suffice to overturn earlier claims and to reopen the issues of the boundary line between the middle and posterior cerebral artery territories.

At least 13 clinical examples of sensorimotor stroke have been documented by CT.[18,107,109,147] In these cases, the lesions were fairly large. Donnan and coworkers[18] described one extending from the left putamen to the corona radiata, not obviously involving the thalamus. One of the chapter authors (JPM) encountered two other examples in southern Alabama. The first case began as an incomplete pure motor stroke to which the hemisensory component was added within hours. This pattern was the reverse of the author's autopsy-documented case of sensorimotor stroke. In the series reported by Weisberg,[109] eight cases were described with "weakness and sensory disturbance and were found to have a hemiparesis and a decreased appreciation of pinprick, light-touch, vibration, and position sense involving the face, arm, and leg."[109] Large caudatoputaminal infarcts were seen on CT scan. It is presumed that these CT-documented cases affected the thalamocortical projections. However, apart from the cases reported by Groothius and associates,[133] no autopsy-documented material has appeared to clarify the course followed by the thalamocortical fibers.

Ataxic Hemiparesis

The syndrome of ataxic hemiparesis has both cerebellar and pyramidal elements.[45] It was initially described as homolateral ataxia with crural paresis, its most familiar form.[12,148] The investigators of the original report speculated that the lesion might lie either in the anterior limb of the internal capsule or in the adjacent corona radiata. However, the first autopsied cases showed a pontine lesion of the small size typical of lacunar infarction.[45]

Since these early observations, numerous case reports have shown a low-density CT lesion lying in the corona radiata[149] or the posterior limb of the internal capsule, thalamus, lentiform nucleus, cerebellum, and frontal cortex.[45,99,102,109,150,151] These lesions have not been in the same site in each case and have been encountered as far forward as the head of the caudate and as far posterior as the posterior limb of the internal capsule.[102] As the lesions in all these cases have been documented by CT scan alone, their exact correlation with the syndrome has been called into question by the disturbing case reported by Kistler and associates.[152] The CT scan showed a corona radiata lesion; a nuclear MR scan revealed a recent pontine lesion that better explained the deficit. The pontine lesion was not seen on CT scan owing to the difficulty in averaging the bone densities adjacent to the brainstem. Because this effect prevents all but the largest pontine infarcts from being seen on CT scan, other cases may have had a similar second lesion as well. In the series reported by Gorman and colleagues,[153] 3% of patients with stroke fulfilled criteria for a diagnosis of ataxic hemiparesis. Although the syndrome is best known to occur from infarction, it has also been reported from tumor,[154] although not in as pure a form, or as intracerebral hemorrhage in the parasagittal part of the precentral area.[155]

The clinical features have been rather similar from case to case. The usual form manifests as a mild to moderate weakness of the leg, especially the ankle, with little or no weakness of the upper limb and face, accompanied by an ataxia of the arm and leg on the same side. In a few cases, a mild and transient hemisensory deficit may initially accompany the motor findings.[65,149] In one series of 100 patients with ataxic hemiparesis, sensory disturbances were frequently associated in the capsular location.[150] The syndrome commonly develops only gradually, requiring from hours to a day or more to reach its peak.[149] There are a few instances of a chronic state, but some degree of improvement within days or months is usual. In some cases, the syndrome changes, the hemiparesis clearing and the ataxia remaining.[149]

Efforts to separate a hemispheral location from a brainstem location have met with only limited success:[12,149] Patients with the former are said to have paresthesias when the lesion is in the thalamus and those with the latter to have a slightly higher frequency of dysarthria and trigeminal weakness. In most instances, however, no distinctive features separate the cases of capsular or radiation origin from those involving the pons. The extent of weakness accompanying the ataxia is no guide to the location. In both the capsular and pontine cases, weakness may involve more structures than the leg, at times affecting the face and arm to almost the same extent. In all cases, the severity of ataxia is more striking than the weakness and exceeds that attributable to weakness alone.

Dysarthria–Clumsy Hand Syndrome

The dysarthria–clumsy hand syndrome has the advantage of emphasizing the distinctive elements of the stroke: In patients presenting with the syndrome, the dysarthria and the ataxia of the upper limb appear to be the prominent components of the clinical deficit, but they do not occur in isolation. The syndrome usually also includes facial weakness, which at times may be profound; dysphagia; and some weakness of the hand and even of the leg. The reflexes on the affected side are usually exaggerated, and the plantar response is extensor. The clinical picture usually develops suddenly. The cases with autopsy correlation have shown no sensory deficit. In one case, the facial weakness was accompanied by impaired strength in opening the jaw.[156] In the case of pontine hemorrhage, several features differed from those reported with infarction: Vomiting and lethargy occurred at onset; balance was impaired enough that the patient was unable to stand; and the facial weakness was mild. It was only after a week that the persisting deficit was reduced to dysarthria and a clumsy hand.

Some researchers have equated the dysarthria–clumsy hand syndrome with ataxic hemiparesis,[157] whereas Fisher,[65] the originator, has come to the view that it is a variant. The best-recognized association has been with lacunes of the anterior limb of the internal capsule.[29] Other sites have been reported less often: Spertell and Ransom[158] described a case with a low-density lesion near the genu, and two of Fisher's patients with anterior capsular infarcts had combinations of mild ataxia and dysarthria. In a few other cases, the lesion has been in the basis pontis.[159] The syndrome has also been reported from hemorrhage of the pons.[155] The outlook for functional recovery is good.

Movement Disorders

Several types of movement disorders have been described with small, deep infarcts. Although the exact vascular occlusion has not been demonstrated in many of these cases, the small size of the infarct and its occurrence in territories fed by small penetrating arteries justify its possible inclusion among the lacunar syndromes. The disorder may appear as the only sign of the infarct or may develop later, after an initial syndrome, different in character, has resolved.

Hemichorea-Hemiballismus

Hemichorea-hemiballismus is the most commonly documented form of movement disorder, accounting for 68% in a series of 22 patients with movement disorders of vascular origin, lacunar infarcts being the most frequent cause.[160] The infarcts found in different parts of the striatum have been of lacunar size,[161,162] including those in the head of the caudate nucleus and adjacent corona radiata,[163] the subthalamic nucleus,[17,164] and the thalamus.[98,162,165] The onset is typically abrupt and is usually unaccompanied by other complaints. The chorea usually involves the forearm, hand, and fingers. In one case, it was accompanied by hemiparesis that faded within 3 months even though the chorea persisted unchanged.[163] In some cases, chorea has been delayed by some weeks or months after the initial occurrence of hemiparesis. One patient familiar to one of the authors (JPM), whose putaminal lesion was documented only by CT scan,[166] suffered choreic movements of the distal parts of the arm and leg that interfered with normal activity and prevented easy walking for more than 4 weeks. In this case the chorea improved, only to relapse a few weeks later. Rare ballistic movements were superimposed. The examination revealed normal strength, sensation, and reflexes.

Treatment with haloperidol is a common approach but has not been uniformly effective.[163] Doses as high as 5 mg three times daily have been required to suppress the chorea.[166]

Dystonia

Two types of dystonia have been described in cases of lacunes. Action-induced rhythmic dystonia has been documented by an autopsy study. In the case reported, the syndrome began as a sensorimotor stroke.[146] Both of the deficits improved within a month. By 3 months, the movement disorder began in the left leg, which had been the most severely affected part in the initial stroke. The disorder spread to involve the patient's entire left side. The fingers of the affected hand became flexed into the palm, leaving only the thumb free. When the patient was examined 4 years later, the hand was unchanged, but strength was otherwise normal. Voluntary movements of any parts of the body, including even eye closure, precipitated rhythmic dystonic extension and rotation of the left arm and leg (sparing the trunk) that subsided a few seconds after the voluntary movements ceased. Clonazepam and 5-hydroxytryptophan were successful in suppressing the involuntary movement disorder. At autopsy, an infarct $5 \times 1 \times 2$ mm was found straddling the ventral posterolateral nucleus and the adjacent posterior limb of the internal capsule.

The other type is a focal dystonia. One patient has been described whose CT scan showed a low density in the right lenticular nucleus.[167] As with the cases of hemichorea and hemiballismus, the deficit appeared abruptly, unaccompanied by weakness or sensory disturbances. Only the distal end of the upper extremity was affected. Although it was described as dystonic, the disorder featured changing postures: "The movements were slow and caused the patient's fingers to assume unusual positions. Activity exacerbated the movements ... the left hand and forearm showed involuntary movements that produced an unusual posture, with hyperpronation and flexion at the wrist, extension of the fingers, and opposition of the thumb." Haloperidol, 1 mg three times daily, relieved much of the movement and posture disorder. Attempts to remove the medication more than 8 months later produced relapse, requiring reinstitution of therapy to suppress the disorder.

Pseudochoreoathetosis

The syndrome pseudochoreoathetosis, consisting of piano-playing movements of the fingers contralateral to the lesion and due to a loss of proprioception, has been described during the acute phase in three patients with lacunar thalamic infarcts.[168]

Asterixis and Tremor

The unilateral flapping tremor or asterixis affecting an upper extremity may be produced by a lacunar infarct in the basal ganglia, thalamus, internal capsule, or midbrain, although no cases with pathologic images have been published.[169,170] Unilateral tremor can appear several months after the initial lacunar infarction in the caudate nucleus or the thalamus.[171,172]

Speech and Language Disorders

Mutism, Aphonia, and Anarthria

Bilateral capsular lacunar infarctions have been a cause of mutism in the absence of any disturbance in language or praxis. One patient reported by Fisher,[35] in whom infarction was documented by microscopic vascular pathology, had no difficulty with speech after his first infarct but became mute with the second infarct, which involved the left internal capsule. The left capsular lacune was $4 \times 4 \times 5$ mm and lay at the genu. Marie[3] had earlier reported a case of unilateral stroke with "anarthria" and no aphasic symptoms, but the cause of the small, deep lesion was a putaminal hemorrhage.

In subsequent years, several such cases, in which the lesions were documented on brain imaging, have been reported. None of these patients with bilateral capsular infarcts have had aphasia apart from the disturbance in articulation. One of the author's (JPM) collection includes a case of an infarct affecting the posterior limb of the right internal capsule followed by an infarct affecting the left internal capsule at the genu.[107] This last infarct was so small that it was barely visible on CT scan, yet it yielded virtual anarthria, severe dysphonia, and dysphagia but only a mild right arm weakness. Three others have been reported, each with bilateral capsular infarcts involving the genu or anterior limb of the capsule.[88,173,174]

Disorders of Language

Considerable doubt still remains as to whether aphasic disturbances per se occur from lacunes. At least one case indicates that they may.[65] In most instances, the cause is not the primary arteriopathy but instead is embolism into the stem of the middle cerebral artery with involvement of many lenticulostriate vessels together. Fisher's patient is the only autopsy-verified patient to date reported with a language disorder from an infarct involving the territory of a lenticulostriate. The syndrome included a modified pure motor hemiparesis with "motor aphasia." It was attributed to a large infarct involving the genu and anterior limb of the internal capsule and adjacent white matter of the corona radiata. Speech initially was dysarthric, progressed later to mispronunciation of words and then to a state of utterance of single-syllable unintelligible sounds, and ended in mutism. Comprehension was reportedly intact. The accompanying weakness severely affected the right side of the face and moderately involved the right hand. This case is important not because of the large size of the infarct but because the underlying lesion was a thrombosis of a lenticulostriate artery.

One case diagnosed on CT scan only has also been associated with a small lesion.[175] It was but one among eight large, deep infarcts attributed to cardiac embolism; the patient presented with an "expressive dysphasia." The disturbance was characterized by "nonfluent conversational speech, naming and reading difficulties, dysgraphia, and normal auditory comprehension." This case is of special interest, given the small size of the lesion demonstrated on the CT scan, because a lacunar cause is in the differential diagnosis.

That unilateral, large, deep infarcts may disrupt language function to some extent has never been the subject of serious dispute (Fig. 11–14). Several well-known cases attest to the correlation. However, except for the case noted previously, in each case the infarct was quite large, of the super lacune category, well beyond the usual limits of the infarcts caused by primary disease of the penetrating arteries. Although it is described in more detail elsewhere in this volume, the subject is touched on here to settle the point of the larger size of the infarcts.

Two famous cases are on record with large infarctions documented by autopsy. Bonhoeffer's[176] classic case was associated with a large, deep lesion typical of the type 1 lacuna described by Rascol and associates,[108] involving the caudate nucleus, internal capsule, and putamen as far laterally as the external capsule. The patient was unable to speak

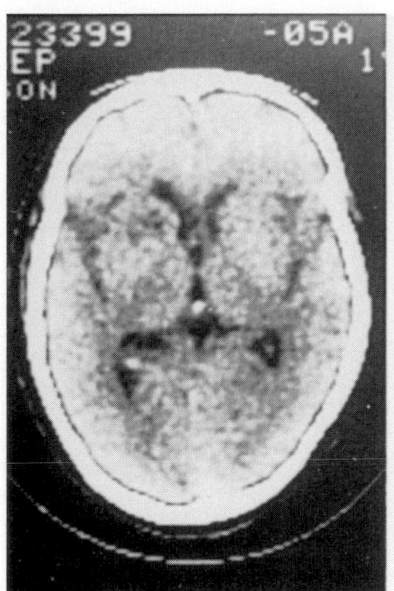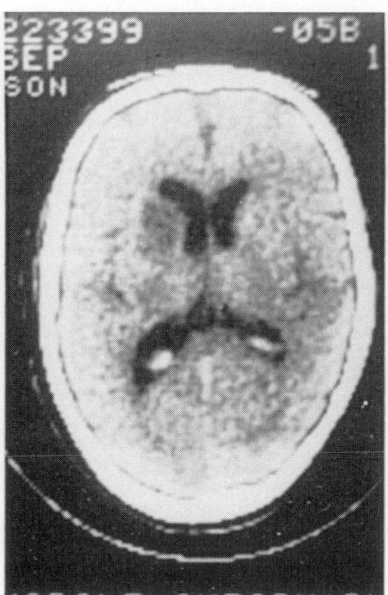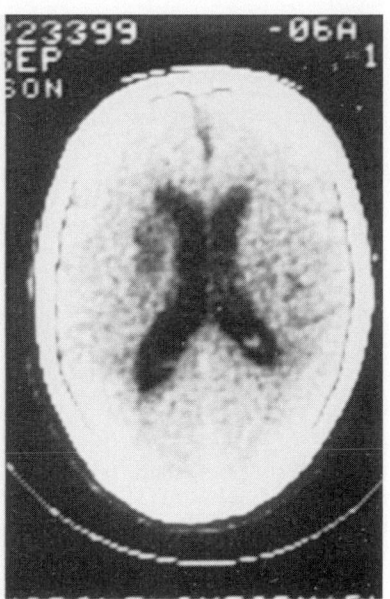

FIGURE 11–14 *Large anterior capsular infarct with dysnomia.*

anything more than a few poorly formed vowels. The cause of the lesion was undetermined, but its large size suggested occlusion of the middle cerebral artery stem. An embolic mechanism was suggested by the second infarct, of fairly large size, affecting almost the entire anterior cerebral artery territory. Kleist[177] reported a case with an infarct of similar size and location (Bühlmeir case) featuring severe dysarthria, rare paraphasias, and only slight disturbance in comprehension. No mention was made of the vascular pathology.

Thirteen other patients to date have been documented by CT scan, all of whom had large, deep infarcts.[111,112,175] In the series reported by Naeser and colleagues,[112] at least three had accompanying surface infarcts. That an accompanying surface infarct that is not obvious on CT scan might be the cause keeps the value of the reports based entirely on CT scan well below that of reports with autopsy documentation. These cases have been characterized by dysprosody, at times accompanied by dysarthria and a mixture of deficits in syntactic and semantic functions not typical of any of the classic syndromes of dysphasia.

Other Disorders of Higher Cerebral Function

A single instance of pure motor stroke with "confusion" has been reported, in which a 1.2-cm lacune affecting the anterior limb and the anterior portion of the posterior limb of the right internal capsule has been documented.[35] The behavior disorder was characterized as "acute onset of confusion and impairment of attention and memory." Later studies using brain imaging to document the lesion have found a few instances of deep infarction, usually affecting the genu or anterior limb of the internal capsule with a greatly reduced level of activity. In a study comparing 11 patients who had multiple lacunes with 11 controls, Wolfe and colleagues[178] found that patients with lacunar infarcts showed neuropsychological signs of frontal system disturbance, although only 27% met clinical criteria for a diagnosis of dementia. The disturbances were described as

"shifting mental set, response inhibition, and executive function," and the patients with these disturbances "were more often rated apathetic on a behavior-rating scale."

Symptomatic supratentorial lacunar infarction, even single, can determine neuropsychological impairment, decreased performance for mental capacities, and, more often than in controls, emotional disturbances.[179]

Some insight into the underlying mechanisms was provided in the study of one patient by Satomi and coworkers,[180] who performed a single-photon emission computed tomogram (SPECT) study with ^{123}I iodoamphetamine; this study showed decreased vasoreactivity, predominantly to the frontal lobes. Tatemichi and associates[181] studied a right-handed man whose infarct was limited to the genu of the capsule in the left hemisphere; they suggested that the impaired SPECT reactivity could be from interruption of thalamofrontal projections passing below the genu, producing a syndrome of frontal lobe dysfunction without a direct lesion to the frontal lobe. This patient became the index case for a series subsequently reported with similar clinical features.

The literature continues to document disorders of language, memory, orientation, and activity after infarction of the paramedian thalamic nuclei. Except for two reports,[58,182] CT has been the basis for lesion localization. In many of these cases, including some of the autopsied material collected by Castaigne and associates,[58] embolism to the top of the basilar artery or to the posterior cerebral artery stem or thrombosis of the basilar artery may have been the cause, rather than vascular disease of the lacunar type. Given the origin of these cases, CT might not reveal all the foci of infarction, making the correlation of clinical features with CT findings a bit unreliable.[24,183–185] In the few cases with autopsy documentation, the arterial disease has been rather unusual. Poirer and colleagues,[182] for example, encountered a picture of thalamic dementia. Autopsy showed many small, deep infarcts of lacunar size.

Clinical Manifestations

These researchers formed the impression that the lesion was an angitis hitherto undefined. Among the cases documented only by CT, hypertension, a normal angiogram, several spells typical of TIAs before the final stroke, and then the emergence of a CT-positive low-density lesion have been documented in a few instances; this pattern seems consistent with the course expected of lacunar disease. The patient reported by Michel and associates[24] is such an example, described as having a thalamic lacune. The initial deficit consisted of right hemiparesis with agitation, disorientation, and language disturbances. The language disorder was of the expressive type, with reduction in language, slowness in response, and some verbal paraphasias. Verbal memory was greatly disturbed and was the subject of a special investigation. The presence of the hemiparesis might mean that the scope of the lesion exceeded that seen on CT scan, but this issue was not settled.

A single case of dysphasia with a small thalamic infarction documented by CT scan has been reported.[60] The infarct was large enough to include the ventral anterior and rostral ventral lateral nucleus, which might be too large for an infarct from primary disease of the thalamoperforating vessels. No cause of the infarct was found. In the other cases in the literature, the infarcts were bilateral or large enough to make it unlikely that they were due to primary arteriopathy of the penetrating vessels. These cases are detailed elsewhere in this book. The last word has not been written on the syndromes of deep infarction with disturbances in speech and language.

LABORATORY STUDIES

Computed Tomography

Technical limitations of the most modern CT scanners prevent the resolution of most lacunes smaller than 2 mm in the internal capsule and almost all of those in the thalamus and brainstem[23,186] because of an obscuring artifact. For the lacunar syndromes documented in the NINCDS Stroke Data Bank, a lesion was found in 39% of cases on the first CT scan; most lesions were located in the posterior limb of the internal capsule and corona radiata.[92] Repeat CT scan increased the yield to 35%. Brainstem lesions were not often visualized. The mean infarct volume in this cohort was greater in pure motor and sensorimotor stroke syndromes than in ataxic hemiparesis, dysarthria–clumsy hand, and pure sensory stroke syndromes. In those patients with pure motor stroke and posterior capsule infarction, there was a correlation between lesion size and severity of hemiparesis, except for the small number of patients whose infarcts involved the lowest portion of the capsule, supplied by the anterior choroidal artery, where severe deficits occurred without regard for lesion size. Enhancement of small, deep infarcts on CT with intravenous contrast is seen in 13% to 40% of patients, mainly during the second and third weeks after onset.[186,187]

Magnetic Resonance Imaging

MRI has greatly changed the frequency with which small infarcts are demonstrated.[188] Although CT is still used,

MRI has now surpassed it in sensitivity for detection of lacunes.[73,189]

In their study of 227 patients with lacunar infarcts, Arboix and colleagues[82] found that CT findings were positive in 100 patients (44%), whereas MRI findings were positive in 35 of 45 (78%). MRI was significantly better ($P < .001$) than CT for imaging lacunes, especially those located in either the pons ($P < .005$) or the internal capsule ($P < .001$). Motor stroke, pure or sensorimotor, has the highest positive rate on MRI and pure sensory stroke the lowest. This finding corresponds to the main volumes of the classic lacunar syndromes on MRI: sensorimotor, 1.7 mL; pure motor, 1.2 mL; ataxic hemiparesis, 0.6 mL; and pure sensory, 0.2 mL. Hommel and coworkers[189] used MRI for 100 patients hospitalized with a lacunar infarct syndrome and also found it more sensitive. MRI detected at least one lacune appropriate to the symptoms in 89 patients in whom 135 lacunes were found on imaging. MRI was more effective when it was performed a few days after the stroke.

The superiority of MRI over CT for detection of small lesions now seems generally accepted. Enhancement of small, deep infarcts on MRI with use of an intravenous contrast agent (gadolinium) is seen in 67% of cases during the first week and in 100% by the second week; this finding is useful in differentiating the present lacune from old ones.[119,190] The hyperintense signals on T2-weighted images in MRI may be lacunar infarcts, état criblé, or dilated perivascular spaces, wallerian degeneration, later stages of small hemorrhages, small artery ectasia, myelin loss, and other incidental white matter lesions, and they must be differentiated. In a pathologic study of small hyperintense foci in the basal ganglia on MRI, lesions with smooth margins and putaminal locations were mainly dilated perivascular spaces, whereas lesions with irregular margins and thalamic locations were mainly lacunes.[191] Echoplanar gradient-echo T2-weighted MRI is effective for the detection of small hypointense lesions due to lacunar hemorrhages; these lesions were found in 68% of patients with multiple lacunar infarcts.[192]

MRI may have a higher yield, as inferred from the experiences of Kistler and colleagues[152] and the authors. To date, only a few lesions seen on MRI have been confirmed by autopsy. Autopsy correlations with CT findings indicate that CT overestimates lacunar size by as much as 100%.[18] The yield on scans performed within 2 days of the stroke is very low, but by 10 days, more than 50% of the lacunes that eventually show on CT can be detected.[18-20,107,109] The high yield in the study reported by Rascol and associates[108] may have been an artifact of selection, but fully 29 of their 30 cases of hemiparesis were documented by CT. The population-based study conducted in southern Alabama noted that 13% of the strokes were due to lacunes; 40% of these were documented by fourth-generation CT.[128] Some of the lesions seen on MRI have been judged to be incidental.[193]

Diffusion-Weighted Magnetic Resonance Imaging

Diffusion-weighted (DW) MRI is the most sensitive and specific imaging method for detection of acute subcortical ischemic lesions and can differentiate acute from nonacute lesions. Acute lacunar infarcts show a high value on DW MRI, appearing as a bright area of decreased apparent diffusion coefficient (ADC); a subacute lacunar infarct is shown as an area of decreased or normal ADC and a chronic infarct as normal or increased ADC.[194] In all or nearly all patients with the clinical acute subcortical infarction, focal areas of high intensity appeared on DW MRI that correlated with all or part of the patients' clinical syndromes.[195,196]

DW MRI performed in 62 patients with well-defined lacunar syndrome during the first 3 days after onset showed the clinically relevant lesion in 68% of cases and additional simultaneous lesions in 16%. These data confirm the need to investigate the etiology and possible embolic mechanism in every patient with a classic clinical picture of lacunar infarction.[197]

Magnetic Resonance Angiography

Magnetic resonance angiography (MRA) can detect intracranial large artery diseases, stenoses, or occlusions in 21% of patients meeting clinical and radiologic criteria for lacunar infarcts, but only in 10% is the artery disease related to the affected penetrating vessel.[198] In 4 of 11 patients with paramedian pontine infarction of lacunar type and a clinical lacunar syndrome in one study (10 with pure motor hemiparesis and 1 with ataxic hemiparesis), MRA disclosed a basilar artery stenosis.[199]

Angiography

Similar technical limitations apply to arteriography. Because the artery affected is usually in the range of 100 to 500 μm, conventional angiography does not often demonstrate abnormalities.[60] However, in the case of giant lacunes, stenosis of the middle cerebral artery stem or, occasionally, one of the larger lateral lenticulostriate arteries may be documented.[108] In a series of young patients with lacunar infarcts (≤50 years old), conventional angiography was performed in 19 to search for unusual vascular disorders such as vasculitis and extracranial artery dissection; findings were normal in all cases.[67] Ipsilateral extracranial carotid stenosis has a low incidence in patients with lacunar infarcts (89%)[93] and an uncertain relationship.[200] Insufficient cases have been studied to determine how often angiography shows major extracranial or intracranial atheroma in classic lacunar syndromes (Fig. 11–15) and what prognostic interaction exists between such findings and the lacunar syndromes. Nowadays, angiography by MRA can help in providing the true incidence of abnormalities in large extracranial or intracranial vessels in lacunar stroke patients.

Transcranial Doppler Ultrasonography

In patients with lacunes, transcranial Doppler ultrasonography (TCD) can be used to determine whether the lacunar infarct is associated with stenosis of the middle cerebral artery or basilar artery. In these cases, if the origin of lenticulostriate or paramedian branches corresponds to the stenotic segment, the perfusion pressure could be reduced in the vessel's territories and a hemodynamic mechanism could be involved. One study has shown that the pulsatility indices measured by TCD can be elevated, reflecting increased vascular resistance.[201] In another

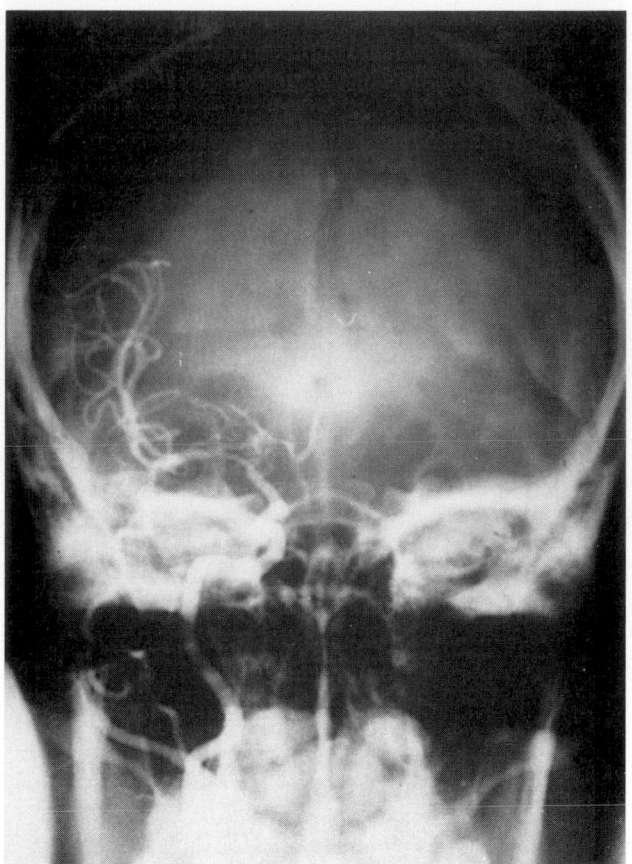

FIGURE 11–15 *Angiographic evidence of middle cerebral artery stem stenosis in a patient with dysnomia. The computed tomography scan of this patient is shown in Figure 11–14.*

study, the vascular resistance was higher in patients with silent lacunar infarcts.[202]

Echocardiography

Transesophageal echocardiography demonstrated atheromatous aortic plaques greater than 5 mm in 20% of patients with lacunar stroke and in 4% of control cases in one study.[203] In a prospective series, the main significant risk factor for recurrence was the cardioembolic source detected by transesophageal echocardiography.[204]

Neurophysiologic Studies

Electroencephalography

Their small size prevents most individual lacunes from disrupting enough of the general brain function to produce changes in the conventional electroencephalogram (EEG).[205] In the data from the NINCDS Pilot Stroke Data Bank, no significant EEG abnormalities were encountered even in patients with positive CT findings.[107] EEG abnormalities were so uncommon in their 56 patients with lacunes that Falcone and colleagues[206] considered a normal EEG a helpful sign suggesting a lacune. Quantitative analysis of the different frequencies of the α- and μ-rhythms with the EEG has not been useful in the diagnosis and prognosis of lacunar infarcts.[107,205–207]

Evoked Cerebral Responses

A few studies of the somatosensory response have shown alterations in the waveform suggesting a subclinical sensory impairment in clinically pure motor strokes. Efforts to find an abnormality in the sensory evoked potential were disappointing in a study by Mohr and associates[122]; only patients with a large CT lesion and an accompanying motor deficit showed such abnormalities. Other even larger series have also failed to show the usefulness of evoked potentials, except in patients with the largest lesions and sensorimotor deficits.[208] As a test for brain image–negative lacunes, the evoked potential seems thus far to have little use.

Cerebral Blood Flow Measurement

The cerebral blood flow measured in the cortex of patients with lacunar infarcts after stroke is lower in those with multiple lacunes than in those with single lacunar infarcts. The changes induced in cerebral blood flow by intravenous injection of acetazolamide are also lower in multiple than in single lacunar infarctions. These data suggest that atherosclerosis is more advanced and widespread in patients with multiple lacunar infarctions.[209]

PROGNOSIS

In general, the patient with a lacunar infarction has a good prognosis, a finding that Pierre Marie and Miller Fisher noted as one of the characteristics of lacunes. In comparison with other vascular processes (ischemic or hemorrhagic, hemispheric or in brainstem), lacunes have the best prognosis (not always as good as we expect, however). The prognosis of lacunes is influenced by several factors. The presence of TIAs before the infarct indicates a poor prognosis, more recurrences, and coronary artery disease in the clinical evolution.[8] Generally, when the motor or sensory deficit is complete (affecting the face, arm, and leg), the prognosis is worse than with an incomplete deficit. The size of the lacunar infarction on CT or MRI is usually correlated with prognosis, being better for smaller lesions. Hyperglycemia, which is associated with poor outcome in acute ischemic strokes due to large vessel atherothrombotic or cardioembolic disease, does not affect the prognosis in lacunar cerebral infarction.[210,211]

Prognosis in such vascular processes as lacunes implies four aspects: survival, recovery of deficits, general or neurologic complications in the acute phase, and recurrences. Survival is the rule during the acute phase. The possibility of death in this phase is related to other complications rather than the lacunar infarct. The risk of death after the acute phase is no different from that in the general population.[212,213] Recovery of deficits is generally good in the first few weeks after onset. Related functional outcome at 6 months[112] to 94% of patients is independent.[214] Complications in the acute phase occur in 18% of patients, urinary infections being the most common.[215] The prognosis for recurrence of stroke in lacunar infarcts at 1 year in hospital studies or community series is about 10%. The rate of recurrence in following years is similar[213,216]; the rate is 23.5%, however, with a follow-up of 10 years, as shown in one series of pure motor stroke from presumed lacunar infarction.[217] The proportion of lacunar infarction has been reported in about one fourth of recurrences and is especially related to hypertension[213,218] and a cardioembolic source of embolus detected by transesophageal echocardiography.[204]

TREATMENT

The use of thrombolytic therapy in patients in whom lacunar infarct is clinically suspected can be controversial, but the results of the NINDS study[100] as well as those of others,[219] in which three of every four patients with lacunar infarction had a favorable outcome, can support its indication.

The patient with a lacunar infarction may have had prior TIAs (20%) close to the infarct onset or a leisurely mode of onset (30%). In both cases anticoagulant therapy did not prove its efficacy. No specific treatment exists for the necrotic tissue of a small, deep infarct, but we can act on its causes and consequences. Atherosclerosis is the most important cause, usually affecting small vessels and less frequently affecting main intracranial or extracranial trunks; the current treatment is directed at correcting vascular risk factors such as hypertension, diabetes mellitus, and cigarette smoking. Specific drugs acting against platelet aggregation, such as aspirin, ticlopidine, and clopidogrel, can be used, but their efficacy has not been proven. Mohr and colleagues[220] found that after the first ever lacunar infarction, aspirin and warfarin do not show a difference in the prevention of recurrence during a 2-year period. Extracranial carotid stenosis must be regarded as asymptomatic, except in cases in which stenosis is the sole etiologic factor, which could produce lacunes by embolism or hemodynamically.

Hypertension must be treated as in other types of cerebral infarction—that is, not in the first days of the acute phase, when values are greater than 190 to 200 mm Hg systolic and 110 to 115 mm Hg diastolic. After the acute phase, hypertension must be accurately controlled.[67] The continuous control of blood pressure levels, during the day and night, can avoid the development of new silent lacunes.[221] Heart diseases (ischemia, atrial fibrillation, or valvulopathy) are regarded and treated as risk factors. Similarly, diabetes mellitus must be treated in all patients as a risk factor and occasionally as the cause of a lacune.

When elevated hematocrit value (>45%) is the sole cause, phlebotomy may be indicated.[89] When arteritis is the cause of lacunes, as in chronic neurosyphilis, granulomatosis, cysticercosis, or tuberculosis, treatment with penicillin, steroids, praziquantel, or antituberculous drugs, respectively, is indicated. In relation to the symptoms of lacunar infarct, the treatment can be specific. In all patients with motor deficit, prevention of deep venous thrombosis with low-molecular-weight heparin (0.2 mL/day subcutaneously) is the rule. In a double-blind, crossover placebo study, the motor performance in patients with pure motor stroke was modulated by a single dose of fluoxetine, with hyperactivation in the primary motor cortex ipsilateral to the lesion as evaluated by functional MRI; this treatment enhanced motor performance.[222] Motor rehabilitation must be started as soon as possible. When hyperpathia is present in sensory stroke, amitriptyline, carbamazepine, gabapentin, or clonazepam has been used with an inconsistent response. Movement disorders such as hemichorea-hemiballismus or dystonia can be relieved with haloperidol, 1 to 5 mg tid,[30] but this treatment has not always been effective. Pallidotomy can be useful to reduce hemichorea.[223] When motor aphasia is present, speech therapy is started.

Although primary prevention of lacunes has not been investigated, the treatment of hypertension and the other established risk factors (such as diabetes mellitus and cigarette smoking) is probably the best way to avoid lacunes in the symptomatic and asymptomatic forms.

Practical Approach

An acute or stuttering unilateral or focal deficit referable to the brain with motor, sensory, ataxic, or dysarthric deficits in the form of one of the five lacunar syndromes (pure motor, pure sensory, sensorimotor, ataxic hemiparesis, or dysarthria–clumsy hand) suggests the probability of a lacunar infarction. However, this diagnosis is only a possibility that must be confirmed. A patient with a motor deficit must be admitted to the hospital. All cases must be investigated with the aim of confirming the presumed diagnosis, establishing its cause, and starting the best treatment. The clinical picture can never be regarded as synonymous with a lacunar infarction.

The diagnosis of a lacunar syndrome has a 20% possibility of being explained by other processes, vascular or not. The clinical diagnosis of lacunar infarction has a sensitivity—that is, the proportion of patients with the same diagnosis at the initial examination and at the end of the study—between 81% and 95%. Specificity—or the proportion of patients with different final diagnoses who also had other initial diagnoses—is between 81% and 93%.[224–226]

The first step in the study of a patient is to confirm the lacunar infarction and differentiate it from other possible diagnoses. CT scan excludes such other possibilities as intracerebral hemorrhage, tumor, metastasis, subdural hematoma, and abscess, with a positive rate in lacunes of between 15% and 58%,[227,228] but MRI is the best and most useful exploration, confirming lacunar infarction in 74% to 98% of cases.[229,230] MRI can also establish the topography (68%), diagnose silent infarcts (13%) in neurologically normal adults,[231] and differentiate a lacune from other small, deep hyperintensive signals.

Once the lacunar infarct is confirmed by MRI or is suspected because the clinical picture is appropriate and MRI findings are normal, the next step is the etiologic investigation. This is the most important work in the management of a patient with lacunar infarct, and hypertension can never be considered the sole cause of the infarct. Although carotid and other vascular lesions, cardioembolic disease, and hematologic alterations have a low etiologic incidence in patients with lacunar infarct, they must be investigated.[94,232–235] Etiologic study consists of looking for vascular risk factors (mainly hypertension and diabetes mellitus) and trying to find a vascular abnormality on TCD ultrasonography or MRA, a cardioembolic disease on electroencephalogram and echocardiogram, and a hematologic process. Patients with lacunes have a risk of developing dementia in the next 4 years of 23%[236]; because of this it is important to perform a neuropsychological study as a reference point for the follow-up. Treatment of vascular risk factors, other possible causes, and the consequences of stroke is the next step.

Evidence shows that one in every five patients with ischemic stroke has a lacune; such evidence has good sensitivity and specificity in clinical diagnosis and good correlation with lacunar syndromes and with pathologic studies. Thus, small vessel disease producing lacunes is a well-established subtype of ischemic stroke; in one study at 28 medical centers, small vessel disease was the most common initial diagnosis (38%) in 479 patients with ischemic stroke.[226] In spite of this evidence, complete investigations must be performed in all patients presenting with a lacunar syndrome due to this stroke subtype, because the others have many problematic aspects in terms of etiology, pathology, topography, and treatment that deserve careful and exhaustive clinical study and research.[243]

References

1. Dechambre A: Mémoire sur la curabilité du ramollissement cérébral. Gaz Med Paris 6:305, 1838.
2. Durand-Fardel M: Mémoire sur une alteration particulière de la substance cérébrale. Gaz Med Paris 10:23, 1842.
3. Marie P: Des foyers lacunaire de désintegration et de différents autres états cavitaires du cerveau. Rev Med 21:281, 1901.
4. Ferrand J: Essai sur l'hémiplegie des vieillards, les lacunes de désintegrations cérébrale. Thesis, Rousset, Paris, 1902.
5. Foix C, Levy M: Les ramollissements sylviens. Rev Neurol 11:1, 1927.
6. Foix C, Hillemand P: Contribution à l'étude des ramollissements protruberantiels. Rev Med 43:287, 1926.
7. Vogt C, Vogt O: Zur Lehre der Erkrankungen des striaren Systems. J Psychol Neurol 25:627, 1920.
8. Alpers BJ: Clinical Neurology. Philadelphia, FA Davis, 1958.
9. Weschler IS: Textbook of Clinical Neurology. Philadelphia, WB Saunders, 1943.
10. Fisher CM, Curry HB: Pure motor hemiplegia of vascular origin. Arch Neurol (Chic) 13:30, 1965.
11. Fisher CM: Thalamic pure sensory stroke: A pathologic study. Neurology (NY) 28:1141, 1978.
12. Fisher CM, Cole M: Homolateral ataxia and crural paresis: A vascular syndrome. J Neurol Neurosurg Psychiatry 28:48, 1965.
13. Fisher CM: A lacunar stroke: The dysarthria–clumsy hand syndrome. Neurology (Minneap) 17:614, 1967.
14. Mohr JP, Kase CS, Meckler RJ, Fisher CM: Sensorimotor stroke. Arch Neurol 34:739, 1977.
15. Fisher CM, Caplan LR: Basilar artery branch occlusion: A cause of pontine infarction. Neurology (Minneap) 21:900, 1971.
16. Fisher CM: The arterial lesions underlying lacunes. Acta Neuropathol (Berl) 12:1, 1969.
17. Melamed E, Korn Lubetzki I, Reches A, et al: Hemiballismus: Detection of focal hemorrhage in subthalamic nucleus by CT scan. Ann Neurol 4:582, 1978.
18. Donnan GA, Tress BM, Bladin PF: A prospective study of lacunar infarction using computerized tomography. Neurology 32:49, 1982.
19. Pullicino P, Nelson RF, Kendall BE, Marshall J: Small deep infarcts diagnosed on computed tomography. Neurology 30:1090, 1980.
20. Weisberg LA: Computed tomography and pure motor hemiparesis. Neurology (NY) 29:490, 1979.
21. Chokroverty S, Rubino FA, Haller C: Pure motor hemiplegia due to pyramidal infarction. Arch Neurol 2:647, 1975.
22. Rottenberg, DA, Talman W, Chernik NL: Location of pyramidal tract questioned. Neurology (Minneap) 26:291, 1976.
23. Weintraub MI, Glaser GH: Nocardial brain abscess and pure motor hemiplegia. N Y J Med 70:2717, 1970.
24. Michel D, Laurent B, Foyatier N, et al: Infarctus thalamique paramedian gauche. Rev Neurol (Paris) 138:6, 1982.

Clinical Manifestations

25. Landau WM: Clinical neuromythology VI: Au clair de lacune: Holy, wholly, holey logic. Neurology 39:725, 1989.

26. Leestma JE, Noronha A: Pure motor hemiplegia, medullary pyramid lesion, and olivary hypertrophy. Arch Neurol 39:877, 1976.

27. Davis LE, Xie JG, Zou AH, et al: Deep cerebral infarcts in the People's Republic of China. Stroke 21:394, 1990.

28. Huang CY, Chan FL, Yu YL, et al: Cerebrovascular disease in Hong Kong Chinese. Stroke 21:230, 1990.

29. Fisher CM: Lacunes: small deep cerebral infarcts. Neurology (Minneap) 15:774, 1965.

30. Goldblatt H: Studies on experimental hypertension. VII: The production of the malignant phase of hypertension. J Exp Med 67:809, 1938.

31. Nelson RF, Pullicino P, Kendall BE, Marshall J: Computed tomography on patients presenting with lacunar syndromes. Stroke 11:256, 1980.

32. Ross Russell RW: Observations on intracerebral aneurysms. Brain 86:425, 1963.

33. Loeb C: The lacunar syndromes. Eur Neurol 29:2, 1989.

34. Mohr JP, Caplan LR, Melski JW, et al: The Harvard Cooperative Stroke Registry. Neurology 28:754, 1978.

35. Fisher CM: Capsular infarcts. Arch Neurol 36:65, 1979.

36. Bokura H, Kobayashi S, Yamaguchi S: Distinguishing silent lacunar infarction from enlarged Virchow-Robin spaces: A magnetic resonance imaging and pathological study. J Neurol 245:116, 1998.

37. Combarros O, Polo JM, Pascual J, et al: Evidence of somatotopic organization of the sensory thalamus based on infarction in the nucleus ventralis posterior. Stroke 22:1445, 1991.

38. Byrom FB, Dodson LF: The causation of acute arterial necrosis in hypertensive disease. J Pathol Bacteriol 60:357, 1948.

39. Percheron SMJ: Les artères du thalamus humain. Rev Neurol 132:297, 1976.

40. Heptinstall RH: Pathology of the Kidney, 2nd ed, vol 1. Boston, Little, Brown, 1974, p 121.

41. Gautier JC: Cerebral ischemia in hypertension. In Ross Russell RW (ed): Cerebral Arterial Disease. London, Churchill Livingstone, 1978, p 181.

42. Byrom FB: The pathogenesis of hypertensive encephalopathy and its relation to the malignant phase of hypertension. Lancet 2:201, 1954.

43. Chester EM, Agamanolis DP, Banker Q, Victor M: Hypertensive encephalopathy: A clinicopathologic study of 20 cases. Neurology 28:928, 1978.

44. Fisher CM: Bilateral occlusion of basilar artery branches. J Neurol Neurosurg Psychiatry 40:1182, 1977.

45. Fisher CM: Ataxic hemiparesis. Arch Neurol 35:126, 1978.

46. Fisher CM, Gore I, Okabe N, White PD: Atherosclerosis of the carotid and vertebral arteries: Extracranial and intracranial. J Neuropathol Exp Neurol 24:455, 1965.

47. Lammie GA, Brannan F, Slattery J, Warlow CH: Nonhypertensive cerebral small-vessel disease: An autopsy study. Stroke 28:2222, 1997.

48. Hanaway J, Young RR: Localization of the pyramidal tract in the internal capsule of man. J Neurol Sci 34:63, 1977.

49. Rosenberg EF: The brain in malignant hypertension: A clinicopathological study. Arch Intern Med 65:545, 1940.

50. Ekstrom Jodal B, Haggendal E, Linder LE, et al: Cerebral blood flow autoregulation at high arterial pressures and different levels of carbon dioxide tension in dogs. Eur Neurol 6:6, 1972.

51. Skinhoj E, Strandgaard S: Pathogenesis of hypertensive encephalopathy. Lancet 1(7801):461, 1973.

52. Hill GS: Studies on the pathogenesis of hypertensive vascular disease: Effect of high pressure intraarterial injections in rats. Circ Res 27:657, 1970.

53. Giese J: The pathogenesis of hypertensive vascular disease. Dan Med Bull 14:259, 1967.

54. Byrom FB: The Hypertensive Vascular Crisis. New York, Grune & Stratton, 1969.

55. Wiener J, Spiro D, Lattes RG: The cellular pathology of experimental hypertension. II: Arteriolar hyalinosis and fibrinoid change. Am J Pathol 47:457, 1965.

56. Paronetto F: Immunocytochemical observations on the vascular necrosis and renal glomerular lesions of malignant nephrosclerosis. Am J Pathol 46:901, 1965.

57. Feigin I, Prose P: Hypertensive fibrinoid arteritis of the brain and gross cerebral hemorrhage: A form of "hyalinosis." Arch Neurol 1:98, 1959.

58. Castaigne P, Lhermitte F, Buge A, et al: Paramedian thalamic and midbrain infarcts: Clinical and neuropathologic study. Ann Neurol 10:127, 1981.

59. Cole FM, Yates PO: Pseudo-aneurysms in relationship to massive cerebral haemorrhage. J Neurol Neurosurg Psychiatry 30:61, 1967.

60. Fisher CM: Cerebral ischemia: Less familiar types. Clin Neurosurg 18:267, 1971.

61. Challa VR, Moody DM, Bell MA: The Charcot-Bouchard aneurysm controversy: Impact of a new histologic technique. J Neuropathol Exp Neurol 51:264, 1992.

62. Laloux P, Broucher JM: Lacunar infarctions due to cholesterol emboli. Stroke 22:1440, 1991.

63. Pearce JMS, Chandrasekera CP, Ladusans EJ: Lacunar infarcts in polycythemia with raised packer cell volumes. BMJ 287:935, 1983.

64. Levine SR, Deegan MJ, Futrell N, et al: Cerebrovascular and neurologic disease associated with antiphospholipid antibodies: 48 cases. Neurology 40:1181, 1990.

65. Fisher CM: Lacunar strokes and infarcts: A review. Neurology (NY) 32:871, 1982.

66. Waterston JA, Brown MM, Butler P, Swash M: Small deep cerebral infarcts associated with occlusive internal carotid artery disease: A hemodynamic phenomenon? Arch Neurol 47:953, 1990.

67. Luijckx GJ, Boiten J, Lodder J, et al: Cardiac and carotid embolism, and other rare definite disorders are unlikely causes of lacunar ischaemic stroke in young patients. Cerebrovasc Dis 6:28, 1996.

68. Loeb DJ, Biller J, Yuh WTC, et al: Leukoencephalopathy in cerebral amyloid angiopathy: MR imaging in four cases. AJNR Am J Neuroradiol 11:485, 1990.

69. Kribs M, Kleihues J: The recurrent artery of Heubner. In Zulch KJ (ed): Cerebral Circulation and Stroke. New York, Springer-Verlag, 1971, p 40.

70. Merritt HH, Adams RD, Solomon HC: Neurosyphilis. New York, Oxford University Press, 1946.

71. Gorelick PB, Caplan LR: Racial differences in the distribution of anterior circulation occlusive disease. Neurology 34:54, 1984.

72. Pentschew A: Gibt es eine Endarteritis luica der kleinen Hirnrindengefässe (Nissl Alzheimer)? Nervenartz 8:393, 1935.

73. Barinagarrementeria F, Del Brutto OH: Lacunar syndrome due to neurocysticercosis. Arch Neurol 46:415, 1989.

74. Kohler J, Kern U, Kasper J, et al: Chronic central nervous system involvement in Lyme borreliosis. Neurology 38:863, 1988.

75. Park YD, Belman AL, Kim TS, et al: Stroke in pediatric acquired immunodeficiency syndrome. Ann Neurol 28:303, 1990.

76. Devinsky O, Petito CK, Alonso DR: Clinical and neuropathological findings in systemic lupus erythematosus: The role of vasculitis, heart emboli, and thrombotic thrombocytopenic purpura. Ann Neurol 23:380, 1988.

77. Fredericks RK, Leflowitz DS, Challa VR, et al: Cerebral vasculitis associated with cocaine abuse. Stroke 22:1437, 1991.

78. Reichart MD, Bogousslavsky J, Janzer RC: Early lacunar strokes complicating polyarteritis nodosa. Neurology 54:883, 2000.

79. Ho KL: Pure motor hemiplegia due to infarction of the cerebral peduncle. Arch Neurol 39:524, 1982.

80. Dattner B, Thomas EW, Wexler G: The Management of Neurosyphilis. New York, Grune & Stratton, 1944.

81. Heuschemann PU, Neureiter D, Gesslein M, et al: Association between infection with *Helicobacter pylori* and *Chlamydia pneumoniae* and risk of ischemic stroke subtypes: Results from a population-based case-control study. Stroke 32:2253, 2001.

82. Arboix A, Marti-Vilalta JL, Garcia JH: Clinical study of 227 patients with lacunar infarcts. Stroke 21:842, 1990.

83. Reimers J, de Wytt C, Seneviratne B: Lacunar infarction: A 12 month study. Clin Exp Neurol 24:28, 1987.

84. Lazzarino LG, Nicolai A, Poldelmengo P, et al: Risk factors in lacunar strokes: A retrospective study of 52 patients. Acta Neurol (Napoli) 11:265, 1989.

85. Longstreth WT, Bernick CH, Manolio TA, et al: Lacunar infarcts defined by magnetic resonance imaging of 3660 elderly people. Arch Neurol 55:1217, 1998.

86. Shintani S, Shiigai T, Arinami T: Silent lacunar infarction on magnetic resonance imaging (MRI): Risk factors. J Neurol Sci 160:82, 1998.

87. Toshifumi M, Arai H, Yuzuriha T, et al: Elevated plasma homocysteine levels and risk of silent brain infarction in elderly people. Stroke 32:1116, 2001.

88. Tuszynski MH, Petito CK, Levy DE: Risk factors and clinical manifestations of pathologically verified lacunar infarctions. Stroke 20:990, 1989.

89. LaRue L, Alter M, Lai SM, et al: Acute stroke, hematocrit, and blood pressure. Stroke 18:565, 1987.

90. Marti-Vilalta JL, Arboix A: The Barcelona Stroke Registry. Eur Neurol 41:135, 1999.

91. Mast H, Thompson JL, Lee SH, et al: Hypertension and diabetes mellitus as determinants of multiple lacunar infarcts. Stroke 26:30, 1995.

92. Chamorro AM, Sacco RL, Mohr JP, et al: Lacunar infarction: Clinical-CT correlations in the Stroke Data Bank. Stroke 22:175, 1991.

93. Inzitari D, Eliasziw M, Sharpe BL, et al: Risk factors and outcome of patients with carotid artery stenosis presenting with lacunar stroke. Neurology 54:660, 2000.

94. Arboix A, Marti-Vilalta JL: Presumed cardioembolic lacunar infarcts. Stroke 23:1841, 1992.

95. Arboix A, Garcia-Eroles L, Massons J, et al: Lacunar infarcts in patients aged 85 years and older. Acta Neurol Scand 101:25, 2000.

96. Kempster PA, Gerraty RP, Gates PC: Asymptomatic cerebral infarction in patients with chronic atrial fibrillation. Stroke 19:955, 1988.

97. Arboix A, Marti-Vilalta JL: Transient ischemic attacks in lacunar infarct. Cerebrovasc Dis 1:20, 1991.

98. Hyland HH, Forman DM: Prognosis in hemiballismus. Neurology (Minneap) 7:381, 1957.

99. Ichikawa K, Tsutsumishita A, Fujioka A: Capsular ataxic hemiparesis: A case report. Arch Neurol 39:585, 1982.

100. Nakamura K, Saku Y, Ibayashi S, Fujishima M: Progressive motor deficits in lacunar infarction. Neurology 52:29, 1999.

101. Arboix A, Marti-Vilalta JL: Acute stroke and circadian rhythm. Stroke 21:826, 1990.

102. De Reuck J, van der Eecken H: The topography of infarcts in the lacunar state. In Meyer JS, Lechner H, Reivich M (eds): Cerebral Vascular Disease: 7th International Conference, Salzburg. New York, Thieme Edition/Publishing Sciences Group, 1976, p 162.

103. Kumral E, Bogousslavsky J, Van Melle G, et al: Headache at stroke onset: The Lausanne Stroke Registry. J Neurol Neurosurg Psychiatry 58:490, 1995.

104. Vestergaard K, Andersen G, Nielsen MI, et al: Headache in stroke. Stroke 24:1621, 1993.

105. Earnest MP, Fahn S, Karp JH, Rowland LP: Normal pressure hydrocephalus and hypertensive cerebrovascular disease. Arch Neurol 31:262, 1974.

106. Koto A, Rosenberg G, Zingesser LH, et al: Syndrome of normal pressure hydrocephalus: Possible relation to hypertensive and arteriosclerotic vasculopathy. J Neurol Neurosurg Psychiatry 40:73, 1977.

107. Mohr JP, Kase CS, Wolf PA, et al: Lacunes in the NINCDS Pilot Stroke Data Bank [abstract]. Ann Neurol 12:84, 1982.

108. Rascol A, Clanet M, Manelfe C, et al: Pure motor hemiplegia: CT study of 30 cases. Stroke 13:11, 1982.

109. Weisberg LA: Lacunar infarcts. Arch Neurol 39:37, 1982.

110. Iragui VJ, McCutchen CB: Capsular ataxic hemiparesis. Arch Neurol 39:528, 1982.

111. Damasio AR, Damasio H, Rizzo M, et al: Aphasia with nonhemorrhagic lesions of the basal ganglia and internal capsule. Arch Neurol 39:15, 1982.

112. Naeser MA, Alexander MP, Helm Estabrooks N, et al: Aphasia with predominantly subcortical lesion sites. Arch Neurol 39:2, 1982.

113. Abadie JL: Les localisations functionelles de la capsule interne. Thesis, Bordeaux, 1900.

114. Igapashi S, Mori K, Ishijima Y: Pure motor hemiplegia after recraniotomy for postoperative bleeding. Arch Jpn Chir 41:32, 1965.

115. Aleksie SN, George AE: Pure motor hemiplegia with occlusion of the extracranial carotid artery. J Neurol Sci 19:331, 1973.

116. Kaps M, Klostermann W, Wessel K, et al: Basilar branch diseases presenting with progressive pure motor stroke. Acta Neurol Scand 96:324, 1997.

117. Arboix A, García-Eroles L, Massons J, et al: Hemorrhagic lacunar stroke. Cerebrovasc Dis 10:229, 2000.

118. Misra UK, Kalita J: Putaminal haemorrhage leading to pure motor hemiplegia. Acta Neurol Scand 91:283, 1995.

119. Miyashita K, Naritomi H, Sawada T, et al: Identification of recent lacunar lesions in cases of multiple small infarctions by magnetic resonance imaging. Stroke 19:834, 1988.

120. Tapia JF, Kase CS, Sawyer RH, Mohr JP: Hypertensive putaminal hemorrhage presenting as pure motor hemiparesis. Stroke 14:505, 1983.

121. Richter RW, Brust JCM, Bruun B, Shafer SQ: Frequency and course of pure motor hemiparesis: A clinical study. Stroke 8:58, 1977.

122. Robinson RK, Richey ET, Kase CS, Mohr JP: Somatosensory evoked potentials in pure sensory stroke and allied conditions [abstract]. Neurology 34:231, 1984.

123. Fraix V, Besson G, Hommel M, Perret J: Brachiofacial pure motor stroke. Cerebrovasc Dis 12:34, 2001.

124. Melo TP, Bogousslavsky J, Van Melle G, et al: Pure motor stroke: A reappraisal. Neurology 42:789, 1992.

125. Fisher CM: Some neuroophthalmologic observations. J Neurol Neurosurg Psychiatry 30:383, 1967.

126. Englander RN, Netsky MG, Adelman LS: Location of human pyramidal tract in the internal capsule: Anatomic evidence. Neurology 25:823, 1975.

127. Ross ED: Localization of the pyramidal tract in the internal capsule by whole brain dissection. Neurology (NY) 30:59, 1980.

128. Gross CR, Kase CS, Mohr JP, Cunningham SC: Stroke in south Alabama: Incidence and diagnostic features. Stroke 15:249, 1984.

129. Dejerine J, Dejerine Klumpke H: Anatomie des Centres Nerveux, Vol 2. Paris, Rueff, 1901.

130. Samuelsson M, Samuelsson L, Lindell D: Sensory symptoms and signs and results of quantitative sensory thermal testing in patients with lacunar infarct syndromes. Stroke 25:2165, 1994.

131. Lazar RM, Perera GM, Marshall RS, et al: The evolution of fMRI activation following pure motor stroke. Neurology 50:402, 1998.

132. Fisher CM: Pure sensory stroke involving face, arm and leg. Neurology (Minneap) 15:76, 1965.

133. Groothius DR, Duncan GW, Fisher CM: The human thalamocortical sensory path in the internal capsule: Evidence from a capsular hemorrhage causing a pure sensory stroke. Ann Neurol 2:328, 1977.

134. Rosenberg NL, Koller R: Computerized tomography and pure sensory stroke. Neurology (NY) 31:217, 1981.

135. Jokura H, Matsumoto S, Komiyama A, et al: Unilateral saccadic pursuit in patients with sensory stroke: Sign of pontine tegmentum lesion. Stroke 29:2377, 1998.

136. Wyllie J: The Disorders of Speech. Edinburgh, Oliver & Boyd, 1894, p 340.

137. Lapresle J, Haguenau S: Anatomico-clinical correlation in focal thalamic lesions. Z Neurol 205:29, 1973.

138. Fisher CM: Pure sensory stroke and allied conditions. Stroke 13:434, 1982.

139. Lenz FA, Dostrovsky JO, Tasker RR, et al: Single unit analysis of the human ventral thalamic nuclear group: Somatosensory responses. J Neurophysiol 59:299, 1988.

140. Mohr JP: Lacunes. Neurol Clin North Am 1:201, 1983.

141. Kim JS: Pure sensory stroke: Clinical-radiological correlates of 21 cases. Stroke 23:983, 1992.

142. Dejerine J, Roussy G: La syndrome thalamique. Rev Neurol (Paris) 14:521, 1906.

143. Manfredi M, Cruccu G: Thalamic pain revisited. In Loeb C (ed): Studies in Cerebrovascular Disease. Milano, Masson Italiano, 1981, p 73.

144. Plets C, De Reuck J, Vander Eecken H, et al: The vascularization of the human thalamus. Acta Neurol Belg 70:685, 1970.

145. Garcin R, Lapresle J: Syndrome sensitif de type thalamique et etopographie cheiro orale par lesion localisée du thalamus. Rev Neurol 90:124, 1954.

146. Sunohara N, Mukoyama M, Mano Y, Satoyoshi E: Action-induced rhythmic dystonia: An autopsy case. Neurology (Cleve) 34:321, 1984.

147. Gursahani RD, Khadilkar SV, Surya N, Singhal BS: Capsular involvement and sensorimotor stroke with posterior cerebral artery territory infarction. J Assoc Physicians India 38:939, 1990.

148. Perman GP, Racey A: Homolateral ataxic and crural paresis: Case report. Neurology 30:1013, 1980.

149. Huang CY, Lui FS: Ataxic hemiparesis: Localization and clinical features. Stroke 15:363, 1984.

150. Moulin T, Bogousslavsky J, Chopard JL, et al: Vascular ataxic hemiparesis: A re-evaluation. J Neurol Neurosurg Psychiatry 58:422, 1995.
151. Sage JI: Ataxic hemiparesis from lesions of the corona radiata. Arch Neurol 40:449, 1983.
152. Kistler JP, Buonanno FS, DeWitt LD, et al: Vertebral basilar posterior cerebral territory stroke delineation by proton nuclear magnetic resonance imaging. Stroke 15:417, 1984.
153. Gorman MJ, Dafer R, Levine SR: Ataxic hemiparesis: Critical appraisal of a lacunar syndrome. Stroke 29:2549, 1998.
154. Bendheim PE, Berg BO: Ataxic hemiparesis from a midbrain mass. Ann Neurol 9:405, 1981.
155. Tjeerdsma HC, Rinkel GJE, van Gijn J: Ataxic hemiparesis from a primary intracerebral haematoma in the precentral area. Cerebrovasc Dis 6:45, 1996.
156. Sakai T, Murakami S, Ito K: Ataxic hemiparesis with trigeminal weakness. Neurology (NY) 31:635, 1981.
157. Tuhrim S, Yang WC, Rubinowitz H, Weinberger J: Primary pontine hemorrhage and the dysarthria–clumsy hand syndrome. Neurology (NY) 31:635, 1982.
158. Spertell RB, Ransom BR: Dysarthria–clumsy hand syndrome produced by capsular infarct. Ann Neurol 6:268, 1979.
159. Glass JD, Levey AI, Rothstein JD: The dysarthria–clumsy hand syndrome: A distinct clinical entity related to pontine infarction. Ann Neurol 27:487, 1990.
160. D'Olhaberriague L, Arboix A, Marti-Vilalta JL, et al: Movement disorders in ischemic stroke: Clinical study of 22 patients. Eur J Neurol 2:553, 1995.
161. Goldblatt D, Markesbery W, Reeves AG: Recurrent hemichorea following striatal lesions. Arch Neurol 31:51, 1974.
162. Martin JP: Hemichorea (hemiballismus) without lesions in the corpus Luysii. Brain 80:1, 1957.
163. Saris S: Chorea caused by caudate infarction. Arch Neurol 40:590, 1983.
164. Meyers R: Ballismus. In Vinken PJ, Bruyn GW (eds): Handbook of Clinical Neurology, vol 6. Amsterdam, North Holland, 1968, p 476.
165. Antin SP, Prockop LD, Cohen SM: Transient hemiballismus. Neurology (Minneap) 17:1068, 1967.
166. Kase CS, Maulsby GO, de Juan E, Mohr JP: Hemichorea hemiballism and lacunar infarction in the basal ganglia. Neurology 31:454, 1981.
167. Russo LS: Focal dystonia and lacunar infarction of the basal ganglia. Neurology (NY) 40:61, 1983.
168. Kim JW, Kim SH, Cha JK: Pseudochoreoathetosis in four patients with hypesthetic ataxic hemiparesis in a thalamic lesion. J Neurol 246:1075, 1999.
169. Massey EW, Goodman JC, Stewart C, et al: Unilateral asterixis: Motor integrative dysfunction in focal vascular disease. Neurology 29:1188, 1979.
170. Yagnik P, Dhopesh V: Unilateral asterixis. Arch Neurol 38:601, 1981.
171. Dethy S, Luxen A, Bidaut LM, et al: Hemibody tremor related to stroke. Stroke 24:2094, 1993.
172. Kim JS: Delayed onset hand tremor caused by cerebral infarction. Stroke 23:292, 1992.
173. Croisile B, Henry E, Trillet M, Aimard G: Loss of motivation for speaking with bilateral lacunes in the anterior limb of the internal capsule. Clin Neurol Neurosurg 91:325, 1989.
174. Laitinen LV: Loss of motivation for speaking with bilateral lacunes in the anterior limb of the internal capsule. Clin Neurol Neurosurg 92:177, 1990.
175. Santamaria J, Graus F, Rubio F, et al: Cerebral infarction of the basal ganglia due to embolism from the heart. Stroke 14:911, 1983.
176. Bonhoeffer K: Klinischer und anatomischer Befund zur Lehre von der Apraxie und der "motorischen Sprachbahn." Monatsschr Psychiatr Neurol 35:113, 1914.
177. Kleist K: Gehirnpathologie. Leipzig, Barth, 1934, p 930.
178. Wolfe N, Linn R, Babikian VL, et al: Frontal systems impairment following multiple lacunar infarcts. Arch Neurol 47:129, 1990.
179. Van Zandvoort MJE, Kappelle LJ, Algra A, et al: Decreased capacity for mental effort after single supratentorial lacunar infarct may affect performance in everyday life. J Neurol Neurosurg Psychiatry 56:697, 1998.
180. Satomi K, Terashima Y, Goto K, et al: Capsular pseudobulbar mutism in a patient of lacunar state. Rinsho Shinkeigaku 30:299, 1990.
181. Tatemichi TK, Desmond DW, Prohovnik I, et al: Confusion and memory loss from capsular genu infarction: A thalamocortical disconnection syndrome? Neurology 42:1966, 1992.
182. Poirer J, Barbizet J, Gaston A, Meyrignac C: Démence thalamique. Rev Neurol (Paris) 139:5, 1983.
183. Guberman A, Stuss D: The syndrome of bilateral paramedian thalamic infarction. Neurology (Cleve) 33:540, 1983.
184. Schott B, Maugiere F, Laurent B, et al: L'amnésie thalamique. Rev Neurol (Paris) 136:117, 1980.
185. Wallesch CW, Kornhuber HH, Kunz T, Brunner RJ: Neuropsychological deficits associated with small unilateral thalamic lesions. Brain 106:141, 1983.
186. Pullicino P, Kendall BE: Contrast enhancement in ischaemic lesions. I: Relationship to prognosis. Neuroradiology 19:235, 1980.
187. Launay M, N'Diaye M, Bories J: X-ray computed tomography (CT) study of small, deep and recent infarcts (SDRIs) of the cerebral hemispheres in adults. Neuroradiology 27:494, 1985.
188. Arboix A, Marti-Vilalta JL, Pujol J, et al: Lacunar infarct and nuclear magnetic resonance: A review of sixty cases. Eur Neurol 30:47, 1990.
189. Hommel M, Besson G, Le Bas JF, et al: Prospective study of lacunar infarction using magnetic resonance imaging. Stroke 21:546, 1990.
190. Elster AD: MR contrast enhancement in brainstem and deep cerebral infarction. AJNR Am J Neuroradiol 12:1127, 1991.
191. Takao M, Koto A, Tanahashi N, et al: Pathologic findings of silent, small hyperintense foci in the basal ganglia and thalamus on MRI. Neurology 52:666, 1999.
192. Kinoshita T, Okudera T, Tamura H, et al: Assessment of lacunar hemorrhage associated with hypertensive stroke by echo-planar gradient-echo T2-weighted MRI. Stroke 31:1646, 2000.
193. Awad IA, Johnson PC, Spetzler RF, Hodak JA: Incidental subcortical lesions identified on magnetic resonance imaging in the elderly. II: Postmortem pathological correlations. Stroke 17:1090, 1986.
194. Noguchi K, Nagayoshi T, Watanabe N, et al: Diffusion-weighted echo-planar MRI of lacunar infarcts. Neuroradiology 40:448, 1998.
195. Schonewille WJ, Tuhrim S, Singer MB, et al: Diffusion-weighted MRI in acute lacunar syndromes: A clinical-radiological correlation study. Stroke 30:2066, 1999.
196. Singer MB, Chong J, Dongfeng L, et al: Diffusion-weighted MRI in acute subcortical infarction. Stroke 29:133, 1998.
197. Ay H, Oliveira-Filho J, Buonanno FS, et al: Diffusion-weighted imaging identifies a subset of lacunar infarction associated with embolic stroke. Stroke 30:2644, 1999.
198. Sweeny R, Cheng EM, Kidwell CHS, et al: Incidence of intracranial large vessel disease in patients with radiologic lacunar stroke. Neurology 52(suppl 2):557, 1999.
199. Thompson DW, Cruz S, Eichholz KM: Magnetic resonance angiography in patients with paramedian pontine infarcts and a lacunar syndrome. Neurology 50:A-215, 1998.
200. Kapelle LJ, van Gijn J: Carotid angiography in patients with subcortical ischaemia. In Donnan GA, Norrving B, Bamford JM, Bogousslavsky J (eds): Lacunar and Other Subcortical Infarctions. Oxford, Oxford University Press, 1995, p 80.
201. Kidwell CS, El-Saden S, Livshits Z, et al: Transcranial Doppler pulsatility indices as a measure of diffuse small-vessel disease. J Neuroimag 11:229, 2001.
202. Chamorro A, Saiz A, Vila N, et al: Contribution of arterial blood pressure to the clinical expression of lacunar infarction. Stroke 27:388, 1996.
203. Donnan GA, Kazui S, Levi CR, et al: Risk factors for lacunar stroke: A case-control transesophageal echocardiographic study. Stroke 31:284, 2000.
204. Kazui S, Levi CR, Jones EF, et al: Lacunar stroke: Transoesophageal echocardiographic factors influencing long-term prognosis. Cerebrovasc Dis 12:325, 2001.
205. Caplan LR, Young RR: EEG findings in certain lacunar stroke syndromes. Neurology 22:403, 1972.
206. Falcone N, Fensore C, Lanzetti A, et al: Clinical considerations and EEG-CT correlations in lacunar infarcts. Rev Neurol 56:396, 1986.
207. Kapelle LJ, van Huffelen AC: Electroencephalography in patients with small, deep infarcts. In Donnan GA, Norrving B, Bamford JM, Bogousslavsky J (eds): Lacunar and Other Subcortical Infarctions. Oxford, Oxford University Press, 1995, p 87.

208. Labar DR, Petty GW, Emerson RG, Mohr JP, Pedley TA: Abnormal somatosensory evoked potentials in patients with motor deficits due to lacunar strokes. Electroencephalogr Clin Neurophysiol 67:74, 1987.
209. Mochizuki Y, Oishi M, Takasu T: Cerebral blood flow in single and multiple lacunar infarctions. Stroke 28:1458, 1997.
210. Bruno A, Biller J, Adams HP Jr, et al: Acute blood glucose level and outcome from ischemic stroke. Neurology 52:280, 1999.
211. Chan RKT, Chong PN: Hyperglycemia is not associated with adverse outcome in patients with lacunar infarcts. Neurology 52(suppl 2):301, 1999.
212. Millikan C, Futrell N: The fallacy of the lacune hypothesis. Stroke 21:1251, 1990.
213. Sacco SE, Whisnant JP, Broderick J, et al: Epidemiological characteristics of lacunar infarcts in a population. Stroke 22:1236, 1991.
214. Boiten J: Lacunar stroke: A prospective clinical and radiological study. Thesis, Maastricht, 1991.
215. Arboix A, Marti-Vilalta JL: Lacunar syndromes not due to lacunar infarcts. Cerebrovasc Dis 2:287, 1992.
216. Hier DB, Foulkes MA, Swiontoniowski M, et al: Stroke recurrence within 2 years after ischaemic infarction. Stroke 22:155, 1991.
217. Staaf G, Lindgren A, Norrving B: Pure motor stroke from presumed lacunar infarct: Long-term prognosis for survival and risk of recurrent stroke. Stroke 32:2592, 2001.
218. Clavier I, Hommel M, Besson G, et al: Long-term prognosis of symptomatic lacunar infarcts: A hospital-based study. Stroke 25:2005, 1995.
219. Frey JL, Snider RM, Jahnke H, et al: rt-PA in lacunar infarction. Neurology 50:A-406, 1998.
220. Mohr JP, Thompson JLP, Lazar RM, et al: A comparison of warfarin and aspirin for the prevention of recurrent ischemic stroke. N Engl J Med 345:1444, 2001.
221. Yamamoto Y, Akiguchi I, Oiwa K, et al: Adverse effect of nighttime blood pressure on the outcome of lacunar infarct patients. Stroke 29:570, 1998.
222. Pariente J, Loubinoux I, Carel C, et al: Fluoxetine modulates motor performance and cerebral activation of patients recovering from stroke. Ann Neurol 50:718, 2001.
223. Hashimoto T, Morita H, Tada T, et al: Neuronal activity in the globus pallidus in chorea caused by striatal lacunar infarction. Ann Neurol 50:528, 2001.
224. Boiten J, Lodder J: Lacunar infarcts: Pathogenesis and validity of the clinical syndromes. Stroke 22:1374, 1991.
225. Gan R, Sacco RL, Kargman DE, et al: Testing the validity of the lacunar hypothesis: The Northern Manhattan Stroke Study experience. Neurology 48:1204, 1997.
226. Madden KP, Karanjia PN, Adams HP, et al: Accuracy of initial stroke subtype diagnosis in the TOAST study. Neurology 45:1975, 1995.
227. Rothrock JF, Lyden PD, Yee J, et al: "Crescendo" transient ischemic attacks: Clinical and angiographic correlations. Neurology 38:198, 1988.
228. Salgado ED, Weinstein M, Furlan AF, et al: Proton magnetic resonance imaging in ischaemic cerebrovascular disease. Ann Neurol 20:502, 1986.
229. Brown MM, Hesselink JR, Rothrock JF: MR and CT of lacunar infarcts. AJNR Am J Neuroradiol 9:477, 1988.
230. Rothrock JF, Lyden PD, Hesselink JR, et al: Brain magnetic resonance imaging in the evaluation of lacunar infarcts. Stroke 18:781, 1987.
231. Kobayashi S, Okada K, Yamashita K: Incidence of silent lacunar lesion in normal adults and its relation to cerebral blood flow and risk factors. Stroke 22:1379, 1991.
232. Horwitz DR, Tuhrim S, Weinberger JM: Mechanism in lacunar infarction. Stroke 23:325, 1992.
233. Kilpatrick TJ, Matkovic Z, Davis SM, et al: Hematologic abnormalities occur in both cortical and lacunar infarction. Stroke 24:1945, 1993.
234. Mast H, Thompson JL, Voller H, et al: Cardiac sources of embolism in patients with pial artery infarcts and lacunar lesions. Stroke 25:776, 1994.
235. Tegeler CH, Shi F, Morgan T: Carotid stenosis in lacunar stroke. Stroke 22:1124, 1991.
236. Loeb C, Gandolfo C, Croce R, et al: Dementia associated with lacunar infarction. Stroke 23:1225, 1992.
237. Hughes M, Dodgson MCH: Chronic cerebral hypertensive disease. Lancet 2:770, 1954.
238. Fang HCH: Lacunar infarction: Clinico-pathologic correlation study [abstract]. J Neuropathol Exp Neurol 31:212, 1972.
239. Ishii N, Nishihara Y, Imamura T: Why do frontal lobe symptoms predominate in vascular dementia with lacunes? Neurology 36:340, 1986.
240. Mancardi GL, Romagnoli P, Tassinari T, et al: Lacunes and cribriform cavities of the brain: Correlations with pseudobulbar palsy and parkinsonism. Eur Neurol 28:11, 1988.
241. Dozono K, Ishii N, Nishihara Y, Horie A: An autopsy study of the incidence of lacunes in relation to age, hypertension, and arteriosclerosis. Stroke 22:993, 1991.
242. Arboix A, Ferrer I, Marti-Vilalta JL: Análisis clinico-anatomo-patológico de 25 pacientes con infartos lacunares. Rev Clin Esp 196:370, 1996.
243. The National Institute of Neurological Disorders and Stroke. Rt-PA Stroke Study Group. Tissue plasminogen activator for acute ischemic stroke. N Engl J Med 333:1581, 1995.

Clinical Manifestations

Chapter Twelve

Cerebral Venous Thrombosis

Marie-Germaine Bousser and Henry J. M. Barnett

In 1825, Ribes[1] described the clinical history of a 45-year-old man who died after a 6-month history of severe headache, epilepsy, and delirium. Postmortem examination showed thrombosis of the superior sagittal sinus (SSS), the left lateral sinus (LS), and a cortical vein in the parietal region. This was probably the first detailed description of cerebral venous thrombosis (CVT) in a human. Since then, numerous case reports and series have been published, most of them from autopsy material.[2–10] They led to the classic description of a rare and severe disease characterized clinically by headache, papilledema, seizures, focal deficits, progressive coma, and death and pathologically by hemorrhagic infarction that was thought to contraindicate the use of anticoagulants.

This early literature and the history of CVT have been extensively covered in two old excellent French[5] and English[6] monographs. However, angiography, magnetic resonance imaging (MRI),[11–30] and magnetic resonance angiography (MRA) have made intra vitam diagnosis possible, and evidence has accumulated that many cases do not fit this classic description. The later literature[30] has convincingly shown that

- CVT is far more common than previously assumed.
- The spectrum of its clinical presentation is extremely wide.
- Its mode of onset is highly variable.
- Its outcome is usually favorable.
- The treatment of choice is heparin.

Because of its frequently misleading presentation, its wide variety of causes, its unpredictable course, and its occasional treatment problems, CVT remains a challenge for the clinician.

RELEVANT VENOUS ANATOMY

Blood from the brain is drained by cerebral veins that empty into dural sinuses, themselves mostly drained by the internal jugular veins.[5,6,30–33]

Dural Sinuses

The dural sinuses most commonly affected by thrombosis are the SSS, the LSs, and the cavernous sinuses (Figs. 12–1 and 12–2).

Superior Sagittal Sinus

The SSS lies in the attached border of the falx cerebri. It starts at the foramen cecum and runs back toward the occipital protuberance, where it joins with the straight sinus (SS) and the LS to form the torcular herophili. The anterior part of the SSS is narrow but is sometimes absent, replaced by two superior cerebral veins that join behind the coronal suture.[7,16,30] Consequently, the anterior part of the sinus is often poorly visualized on angiography, and its isolated lack of filling is not sufficient to indicate thrombosis.[7,16]

The SSS receives superficial cerebral veins and drains the major part of the cortex. It also receives the diploic veins, which are themselves connected to scalp veins by emissary veins, an arrangement that explains some cases of SSS thrombosis after cutaneous infections or contusions. The SSS and other sinuses play a major role in cerebrospinal fluid (CSF) circulation, because they contain most of the arachnoid villi and granulations (pacchionian bodies) in which much of the CSF absorption takes place. Thus, CSF pressure depends directly on the intracranial venous pressure, accounting for the frequency of raised intracranial pressure in SSS or LS thrombosis.

Lateral Sinuses

Each LS extends from the torcular herophili to the jugular bulbs and consists of two portions: the transverse portion, which lies in the attached border of the tentorium, and the sigmoid portion, which runs on the inner aspect of the mastoid process and is thereby susceptible to infectious thrombosis in patients with mastoiditis or otitis media. The LSs drain blood from the cerebellum, brainstem, and posterior part of the cerebral hemispheres. They also receive some of the diploic veins and some small veins from the middle ear, yet another possible source of septic thrombosis.

Numerous anatomic variations of the LSs may be misinterpreted as sinus occlusion on angiography. In particular, the right LS, which is often a direct continuation of the SSS, is commonly larger than the left, which receives most of its supply from the SS. In Hacker's[31] study, the transverse portions were not visualized on ipsilateral carotid angiograms in 14% of cases on the left side and in 3.3% on the right side; in contrast, the sigmoid portions, which may be directly injected via cerebral veins, did not fill in 4% of cases on the left side but were always demonstrated on the

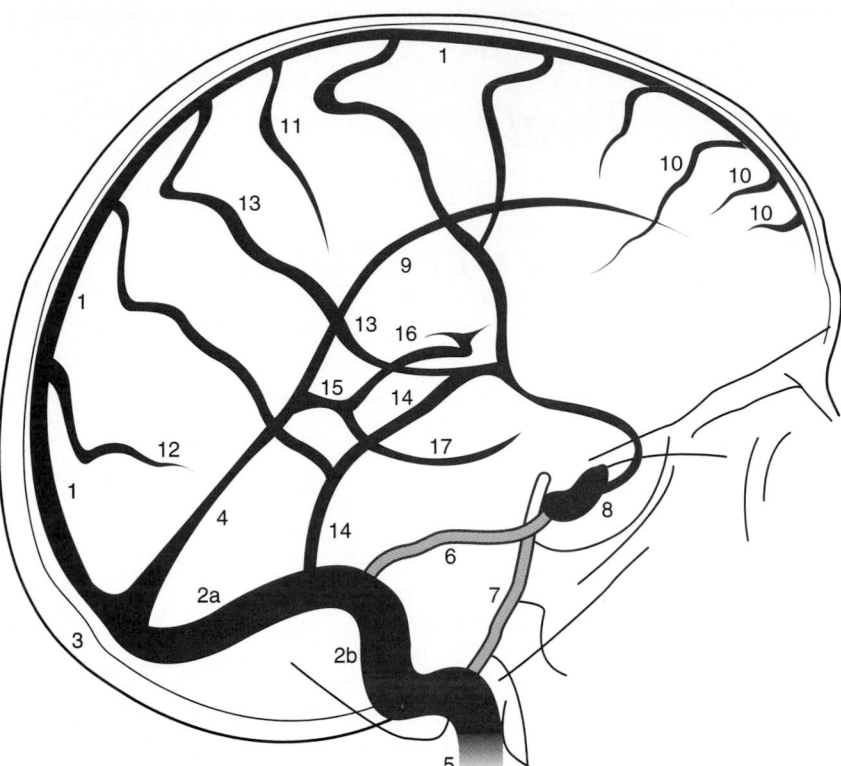

FIGURE 12–1 *Superficial and deep cerebral veins and dural sinuses: 1, superior sagittal sinus; 2a, transverse portion of lateral sinus; 2b, sigmoid portion of lateral sinus; 3, torcular herophili; 4, straight sinus; 5, internal jugular vein; 6, superior petrosal sinus; 7, inferior petrosal sinus; 8, cavernous sinus; 9, inferior sagittal sinus; 10, frontal veins; 11, parietal vein; 12, occipital vein; 13, Trolard's vein; 14, Labbé's vein; 15, great vein of Galen; 16, internal cerebral vein; 17, basal vein.*

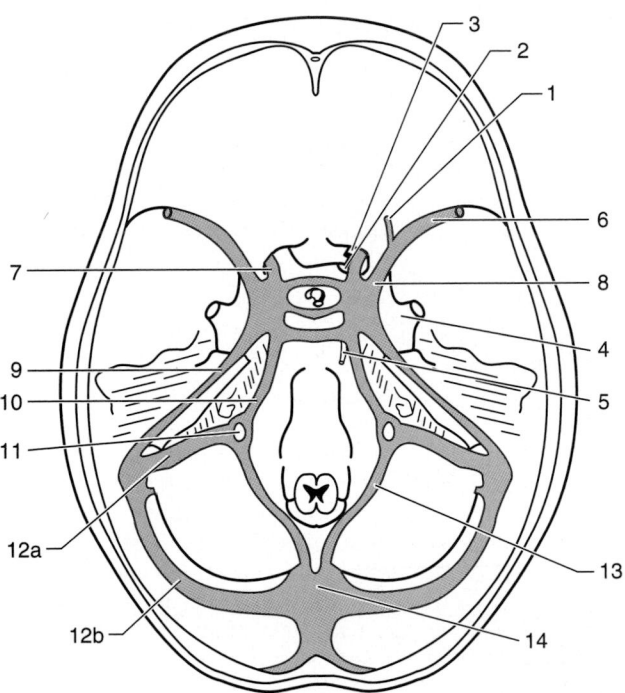

FIGURE 12–2 *Cavernous sinus and dural sinuses: 1, trochlear cranial nerve; 2, carotid artery; 3, optic nerve; 4, trigeminal nerve; 5, oculomotor nerve; 6, sphenoparietal sinus; 7, ophthalmic vein; 8, cavernous sinus; 9, superior petrosal sinus; 10, inferior petrosal sinus; 11, internal jugular vein; 12a, sigmoid portion of lateral sinus; 12b, transverse portion of lateral sinus; 13, posterior occipital sinus; 14, torcular herophili.*

right. An isolated lack of filling of a left transverse sinus is thus suggestive more of hypoplasia than of thrombosis.

Cavernous Sinuses

The cavernous sinuses consist of trabeculated cavities formed by the separation of the layers of the dura and located on either side of the sella turcica, superolaterally to the sphenoid air sinuses. The oculomotor and trochlear cranial nerves, along with the ophthalmic and maxillary branches of the trigeminal nerve, course along the lateral wall of the cavernous sinuses, whereas the abducens nerve and the carotid artery with its surrounding sympathetic plexus are located within the center of the sinus itself.

Cavernous sinuses drain the blood from the orbits through the ophthalmic veins and from the anterior part of the base of the brain by the sphenoparietal sinus and the middle cerebral veins. They empty into both the superior and inferior petrosal sinuses and ultimately into the internal jugular veins. Because of their situation, cavernous sinuses are often thrombosed in relation to infections of the face or sphenoid sinusitis and, in contrast to other varieties of sinus thrombosis, infection is still the leading cause of thrombosis.[34]

Rarely injected on carotid angiograms, cavernous sinuses are now well visualized on computed tomography (CT) and MRI.

Cerebral Veins

The three groups of veins that drain the blood supply from the brain are the superficial cerebral (or cortical) veins, the deep cerebral veins, and the veins of the posterior fossa (see Fig. 12–1).[6,30,32,33]

Superficial Cerebral Veins

Some of the cortical veins—the frontal, parietal, and occipital superior cerebral veins—drain the cortex up into the SSS, whereas others, mainly the middle cerebral veins, drain down into the cavernous sinuses. These veins are linked by Trolard's great anastomotic vein, which connects the SSS to the middle cerebral veins, which are themselves connected to the LS by Labbé's vein.

These cortical veins present some peculiarities[6,30] that are important to understanding some of the clinical features of CVT. They have thin walls, no muscle fibers, and no valves, thereby permitting both their dilatation and reversal of the direction of blood flow when the sinus into which they drain is occluded. They are linked by numerous anastomoses, allowing the development of a collateral circulation (angiographically visible as corkscrew vessels), that probably explains the good prognosis of some cases of CVT. The number and location of cortical veins are inconsistent, making the angiographic diagnosis of isolated cortical vein thrombosis extremely difficult. This anatomic variability, together with the possibility of flow reversal and the development of collateral circulation, accounts for the absence of well-delineated venous territories and consequently of well-defined clinical syndromes of cortical vein thrombosis.

Deep Cerebral Veins

Blood from the deep white matter of the cerebral hemispheres and from the basal ganglia is drained by internal cerebral and basal veins that join to form the great vein of Galen, which drains into the straight sinus. In contrast to the superficial veins, the deep system is consistent and is always visualized at angiography, so any thrombosis in this system is easily recognized.

Veins of the Posterior Fossa

Posterior fossa veins may be divided into the following three groups[32,33]: superior veins draining into the galenic system, anterior veins draining into the petrosal sinuses, and posterior veins draining into the torcular and neighboring SS and LS. They are variable in course, and angiographic diagnosis of their occlusion is extremely difficult.

PATHOLOGY

Pathologic findings have been extensively described.[3,5,6,8,9,30] They vary according to the site of thrombosis and the interval between the onset of symptoms and death.

The *thrombus* itself is like other venous thrombi elsewhere in the body: When it is fresh, it is rich in red blood cells and fibrin and poor in platelets; when it is old, it is replaced by fibrous tissue (Fig. 12–3), sometimes showing recanalization. Its formation is due to the usual pathogenetic factors—mostly venous stasis, increased clotting tendency, and changes in the vessel wall. Its location and extension are variable. In autopsy series,[3,4,6] extensive thrombosis of the SSS and tributary veins is the most common finding, but this pattern of involvement no longer reflects the common expression of clinically diagnosable CVT.

The consequences of CVT in the brain are also highly variable; some thromboses, particularly of the lateral sinus, may have no consequence for the brain and may be completely latent[30]. Brain edema can be the only consequence in thrombosis restricted to the SSS,[6,30] whereas occlusion of cerebral veins usually leads to what is usually called a "venous infarct." Such infarcts affect the cortex and adjacent white matter and are often hemorrhagic, explaining the possibility of associated subarachnoid hemorrhage and subdural or intracerebral hematomas. The classic anatomic presentation is that of extensive bilateral hemorrhagic infarcts, located in the superior and internal parts of both hemispheres, due to thrombosis of the SSS and its tributary cortical veins (Fig. 12–4). However, studies with magnetic resonance diffusion have shown that these "venous

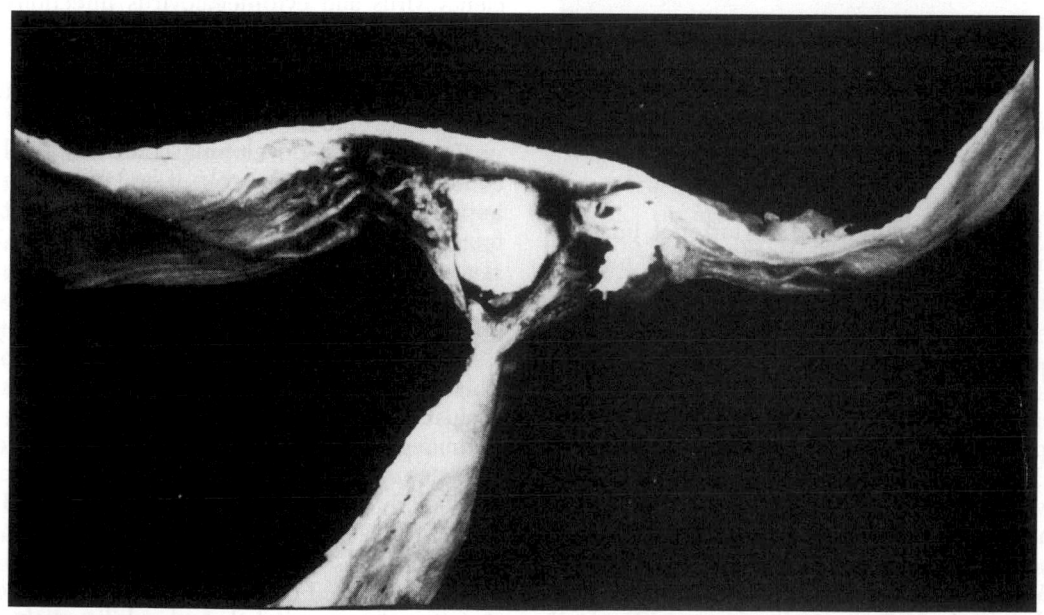

FIGURE 12–3   *Old superior sagittal sinus thrombosis.*

Clinical Manifestations

Table 12.2 Percentages of Appearance of Main Clinical Signs in Series of Patients with Cerebral Venous Thrombosis

Sign	Einhäupl et al (1990)[49] (n = 71)	Cantu and Barrinagarrementeria (1993)[51] Puerperal (n = 67)	Nonpuerperal (n = 46)	Daif et al (1995)[46] (n = 40)	Ferro et al (2001)[53] (n = 142)	Bousser[3] (2001)* (n = 200)
Headache	91	88	70	82	92	85
Papilledema	27	40	52	80	45	47
Focal deficits	66	79	76	27	42	42
Seizures	48	60	63	10	37	41
Altered consciousness	56	63	59	10	13	29

*Personal series.

symptom in two thirds of cases.[30] The headache has no specific features. It is mostly diffuse, progressive, and permanent, but it can be misleading, mimicking migraine or the typical headache of subarachnoid hemorrhage.

Headache is almost invariably associated with other neurologic signs, such as papilledema, focal deficits, and seizures. The frequency of papilledema is highly variable, from 7%[25] to 80%.[46] It can be associated with transient visual obscurations, indicating a high-grade papilledema and threatened vision. Focal deficits are inaugural in 15% of cases and are present at some time during the course of the disease in about 50% of patients (see Table 12.2). The type of deficit varies with the site and extent of thrombosis; the most common are motor and sensory deficits, usually unilateral and often predominating in the leg.

Other symptoms of CVT are aphasia, cranial nerve palsies, and, more rarely, hemianopia. Seizures are inaugural in 12% to 15% of cases and are present at some time during the course of CVT in about 40% of cases (see Table 12.2). Seizures are about equally divided between focal and generalized types, and the association of both types is very common. Seizures are uncommon and usually generalized in patients who present with isolated intracranial hypertension; by contrast, seizures are common and often partial in patients who have focal deficits. Status epilepticus may occur and can be difficult to control. Seizures are particularly common in children (58%), especially neonates (71%).[58]

Alteration of consciousness is present in about half of patients with CVT (see Table 12.2). Rarely inaugural, this sign is usually a late one. Other signs, such as cerebellar incoordination and psychiatric disturbances, may occur. It should be noted that the classic picture of SSS thrombosis with its bilateral or alternating deficits, seizures, or both is a very late pattern of presentation that is now rarely encountered (3% in our series of 200 patients).

Unlike in arterial stroke, the mode of onset of symptoms in CVT is highly variable. Onset is subacute (>48 hours but <30 days) in 50% to 80% of cases, acute (<48 hours) in 20% to 30% of cases, and chronic (>30 days) in 10% to 20% of cases, particularly in patients presenting with isolated intracranial hypertension.[30]

With such a wide spectrum of neurologic signs and modes of onset, the clinical presentation of CVT is extremely variable. It can be separated into the following five patterns: isolated intracranial hypertension, focal cerebral signs, cavernous sinus syndrome, a subacute encephalopathy, and unusual presentations.

Isolated Intracranial Hypertension

Isolated intracranial hypertension with headache, papilledema, and sixth nerve palsy, mimicking benign intracranial hypertension (pseudotumor cerebri), is the most homogeneous pattern, occurring in up to 40% of our patients.[30] It can evolve over days, months,[45] or even years.[30] Even though SSS and LS thromboses have long been recognized as two of the leading causes of "benign" intracranial hypertension,[5,6,10,45,99–102] this syndrome is still often subjected only to clinical, CSF, and CT investigation. Because CVT can mimic all the features of idiopathic intracranial hypertension,[30,45,100,101] normal four-vessel angiography or normal MRI and MRA should be added to the classic diagnostic evaluation of this syndrome.[100,101]

Focal Cerebral Signs

Focal signs characterize the presentation in the largest group of patients, accounting for roughly 75% of published cases. The clinical picture is heterogeneous, however, depending on the mode of onset of focal signs, their nature (deficits and/or seizures), and their possible association with altered consciousness. Acute cases with, for instance, a sudden hemiplegia, simulate an arterial stroke, but the unusual severity or isolated occurrence of leg involvement, the presence of seizures, and the absence of a well-defined arterial syndrome should alert the clinician to the possibility of CVT, particularly if the patient's condition deteriorates steadily. Chronic cases simulate tumors, whereas subacute cases mimic brain abscesses, particularly in patients with fever, increased erythrocyte sedimentation rate, and CSF pleocytosis.[30]

Cavernous Sinus Thrombosis

Cavernous sinus thrombosis has a distinctive clinical picture that includes, in classic acute cases, chemosis, proptosis, and painful ophthalmoplegia, initially unilateral but frequently becoming bilateral.[5,6,30,34,103,104] Dramatic complications can occur such as extension to other sinuses[34] and stenosis (with a mycotic aneurysm in one case) of the intracavernous portion of the internal carotid arteries.[103] Cavernous sinus thrombosis is not always acute, however. It can also take a more indolent form (either spontaneously or because of the masking effect of an inadequate antibiotic regimen), with an isolated abducens nerve palsy and only mild chemosis and proptosis leading to great diagnostic difficulties.[34]

Subacute Encephalopathy

Subacute encephalopathy is the fourth pattern of presentation[30] (i.e., a generalized encephalopathic illness without localizing signs or recognizable features of raised intracranial pressure). The patients are often either very old or very young and are suffering from cachexia or malignant or cardiac diseases; the cerebral thrombosis is often a terminal event.[3] A depressed level of consciousness is the most constant finding, varying from drowsiness to deep coma. This type of presentation is extremely misleading. The differential diagnosis includes encephalitis, disseminated intravascular coagulation, marasmic endocarditis, and cerebral vasculitis.

Unusual Presentations

The grouping of signs of CVT into the foregoing four main patterns (isolated intracranial hypertension, focal signs, cavernous sinus syndrome, and subacute encephalopathy) does not account for every case. Some rare cases initially manifest as isolated intracranial hypertension and later demonstrate focal neurologic signs.[30] Some patients may initially present with isolated headache, which can, for instance, be mistaken for a post–dural puncture headache[105] after delivery or for migraine in the presence of aura-like phenomena.[30] After dural puncture of any cause, CVT should be suspected when the headache loses its postural component and becomes permanent.[105] Other patients present with transient ischemic attacks[30,45,106] or with grand mal seizures and headache, a presentation mimicking eclampsia.

Psychiatric disturbances (irritability, lack of interest, anxiety, depression) are sometimes the prevailing symptoms. They are particularly misleading during the postpartum period, when they raise the possibility of postpartum psychosis. Other cases manifest as thunderclap headache with or without evidence of subarachnoid hemorrhage, simulating a ruptured intracranial aneurysm.[30,42,45,107] Yet others cause more or less isolated cranial nerve involvement.[108–110] Finally, CVT may be so insidious that it is totally asymptomatic[30,111] or is discovered at postmortem, particularly in elderly patients dying of congestive heart failure.[3]

It is clear from the preceding description that signs and symptoms of CVT are extremely variable and often misleading. One must consider CVT in all the clinical presentations just described and must make the appropriate investigations to reach the diagnosis. Another important general diagnostic principle is to consider CVT as a possibility in any condition that raises the suspicion of the more common phenomenon, crural and pelvic vein thromboses (e.g., puerperium, postoperative and post-traumatic conditions, cardiac failure, and wasting conditions).

Neonates

In neonates, the most common presentation of CVT is that of an acute illness with seizures (71% of cases) and diffuse neurologic signs (58%).[58] Focal neurologic signs are less common (29%). It has been suggested that CVT is an important and under-recognized cause of seizures and diffuse encephalopathy in the first 2 weeks of life in term infants.[98] In older children, the presentation resembles that of CVT in adults.

TOPOGRAPHIC DIAGNOSIS

Table 12.3 lists the relative distribution of sites of CVT. This distribution should be regarded as a rough estimate, particularly for cortical vein involvement, which is often missed at angiography. Furthermore, it is uncommon for thrombosis to be confined to a single vessel. Thus, in about 75% of cases, multiple veins or sinuses are involved.[30] The

Table 12.3   Disposition of Venous Thrombosis in Series of Patients with Cerebral Venous Thrombosis*

Veins	Milandre et al (1988)[54] (n = 20)	Cantu and Barinagarrementeria (1993)[51] Puerperal (n = 67)	Nonpuerperal (n = 46)	Tsai et al (1995)[25] (n = 29)	Daif et al (1995)[46] (n = 40)	Ferro et al (2001)[53] (n = 142)	Bousser (2001)[‡] (n = 200)
Superior sagittal sinus	13 (4)	60 (22)	45 (11)	19 (11)	34 (22)	94	128 (25)
Lateral sinus	2	23 (1)	20 (1)	15 (9)	14 (4)	92	148 (47)
Straight sinus	5	0	0	3	3	12	28 (1)
Cavernous sinus	1	0	0	0		0	4 (0)
Cortical or cerebellar veins	10 (2)	13	14	1	4	5	39 (5)
Deep venous system	1 (1)	17 (4)	10			9	15 (1)
Association[†]	12	39	34	9	26	74	121

Data represent numbers of patients. Numbers in parentheses indicate cases in which the venous structure alone was involved.
[†]*More than one structure involved.*
[‡]*Personal series.*

frequent multiple vein involvement, the variability of the cortical venous system, and the rapid development of collateral circulation explain the lack of well-defined topographic clinical syndromes that are described in arterial occlusion. There are broad patterns according to the site of venous occlusion, but at present, topographic diagnosis is usually not important for the management of CVT; the crucial step is to recognize CVT itself.

The sinus most commonly affected is the SSS: 72% in Ameri and Bousser's series,[42] 64% in our current series, 85% in Daif and colleagues' series,[46] and 92% in Cantu and Barinagarrementeria's series.[51] The SSS was involved alone in a minority of cases (13%, 55%, 15%, and 29%, respectively, in the four series listed). The LS is more often affected than the SSS in our current series (74%) but far less commonly in the other series (38%).[51] Isolated involvement of the LS is rare, occurring in 9% of patients in our series and in 2% in the other series. Cerebral veins are affected in about 40% of cases, but this figure is probably an underestimation, given the much higher frequency of focal clinical signs. Thrombosis of the galenic system is rare, occurring in some 80 reported cases. Only a few cases of petrosal sinus, isolated cortical, or cerebellar vein thrombosis have been described but these conditions are also likely to be underdiagnosed because of the extreme difficulty of their diagnosis.

Superior Sagittal Sinus Thrombosis

When thrombosis is restricted to the SSS, the clinical presentation is that of isolated intracranial hypertension, as previously described. In Ameri and Bousser's series,[42] 33% of 79 cases of SSS thrombosis manifested as idiopathic intracranial hypertension. Grand mal seizures and psychiatric disturbances occasionally occur in pure SSS thrombosis. In most cases, thrombosis also involves one or both LSs, with intracranial hypertension as the main clinical presentation. Extension to cortical veins, particularly those of the rolandic and parietal lobes, is common and is characterized by the acute or progressive onset of a focal motor or sensory deficit, classically more marked in the leg and associated with focal or generalized seizures.

Lateral Sinus Thrombosis

Like SSS thrombosis, LS thrombosis has a variable presentation. Although it can be asymptomatic, isolated LS thrombosis usually manifests as raised intracranial pressure; hence the term *otitic hydrocephalus* coined by Symonds[10] to describe the effects of LS thrombosis secondary to an active or latent ear infection. LS thrombosis commonly extends to other sinuses and veins, especially to the SSS, manifesting as isolated intracranial hypertension. Focal signs occur when thrombosis extends to (1) the superior or inferior petrosal sinuses with involvement of the 5th and 6th cranial nerves, respectively, (2) the straight sinus and deep venous system (see later), (3) adjacent cortical veins with aphasia in left LS thrombosis (see later), and (4) the jugular bulb with involvement of the 9th, 10th, and 11th cranial nerves. Cases have been reported of isolated involvement of the cranial nerves (III to VIII) in LS thrombosis.[108–110]

Cortical Vein Thrombosis

Any cortical vein can be the seat of thrombosis, but the most often involved are the superior cerebral veins (rolandic, parieto-occipital, and posterior temporal), which drain into the SSS. The consequences of a cortical vein thrombosis are variable; in an unknown proportion of cases, collateral circulation develops rapidly, and there is no parenchymal lesion. In other cases, an area of localized edema appears that can still be asymptomatic. At a further stage, neurons become edematous or partially ischemic, but this injury is mostly reversible, as judged from the frequency of totally regressive focal deficits. Remarkably, even when an infarct occurs and is confirmed by neuroimaging, clinical recovery can be complete in some cases.

Isolated cortical vein thrombosis is extremely rare, with an overall frequency of about 2%.[30,42,45,48,112] It may be overlooked, however, because of its difficult diagnosis, even with MRI. This disorder manifests as focal deficits or seizures of sudden or progressive onset (or both), mimicking a stroke or a space-occupying lesion. In most cases, thrombosis extends to the SSS with signs of raised intracranial pressure and, occasionally, to cortical veins on the opposite side, leading to the classic picture of a bilateral parasagittal infarct.

Thrombosis of the Deep Venous System

The clinical presentation of thrombosis of the galenic system is highly variable. The classic picture is that of a child with an acute coma associated with decerebration, decortication, extrapyramidal hypertonia, signs of raised intracranial pressure, pupillary changes, and rise in blood pressure leading to death in a few hours or days.[4,113,114] Similar cases have been reported in adults. When patients survive, severe sequelae, such as akinetic mutism, mental retardation, dementia, bilateral athetoid movements, hemiparesis, vertical gaze palsy, and dystonia, are common.[4,6,8,30,115] Some reports have illustrated the possibility of benign forms of galenic system thrombosis. The most common symptoms are headache, nausea and vomiting, gait ataxia, neuropsychological deficits, and drowsiness of a variable degree.[42,113,116–119] Other signs are unusual, including impaired upward conjugate gaze, vertical nystagmus, trismus, hemiparesis that may be bilateral or alternating, limb or axial rigidity, tremor, seizures, and signs of raised intracranial pressure.[120] Neuropsychological disturbances with impaired anterograde memory are sometimes severe, resembling Korsakoff's psychosis,[117] but they are usually mild or moderate.[30,116,121] A case has been reported in which acute micrographia and hypophonia were the sole manifestations of extensive deep venous system thrombosis.[119]

Cerebellar Vein Thrombosis

Cerebellar venous infarction is extremely rare and had not been recognized during life until 1965.[8] Cerebellar vein thrombosis is nearly always associated with LS thrombosis.[30,42,45,122–124]

The clinical presentation is variable. The most common signs are headache, vomiting, ataxia, and unilateral dysmetria.[30,42,45,122–124] They are usually of acute onset, but subacute and even chronic cases have been reported.[45] An early decrease in conscious level and, commonly, papilledema occur, indicating obstructive hydrocephalus.[124] Cranial nerve palsies can occur,[45] and the involvement of the 9th and 10th nerves may suggest propagation of thrombosis to the internal jugular vein.

Thrombosis of the Superior and Inferior Petrosal Sinuses

Thrombosis of the superior and inferior petrosal sinuses is usually a sequela of cavernous sinus thrombosis or infection in the temporal bone with LS thrombosis. Mainly described in the older literature, it is characterized by cranial nerve palsies—CN V palsy in thrombosis of the superior sinus and CN VI palsy in thrombosis of the inferior sinus.[5,9,10]

Internal Jugular Vein Thrombosis

Internal jugular vein thrombosis may be initiated by cannulae used for long-term venous access or, more commonly, may spread there from the sigmoid sinus.[30,125] In most cases, this extension of thrombosis from the LS to the jugular vein is totally asymptomatic. Rarely, there are signs of local infection with pain and swelling in the mastoid region and a palpable, tender thrombosed vein. A jugular foramen syndrome is seen if the infection involves the skull base. There is a risk of venous thromboembolism to the lungs, and in rare instances, there may be widespread propagation of thrombus to the superior vena cava and subclavian veins.

INVESTIGATIONS

Computed Tomography

CT scanning with and without injection of contrast material is usually the first neuroimaging examination carried out in patients with headache, focal deficits, or seizures, particularly on an emergency basis. CT scanning is extremely useful for ruling out the many conditions that CVT can mimic. The modality occasionally detects lesions that can themselves cause CVT, such as meningiomas, abscesses, sinusitis, and mastoiditis. CT scanning is also useful in showing brain or sinus changes suggestive of CVT.

CT findings have been described in detail in numerous reports and are now well established.[111,118,126–139] They can be divided into direct signs and indirect signs.

Direct Signs of Cerebral Venous Thrombosis

Three abnormalities are considered direct signs of CVT: the cord sign, the dense triangle, and the delta or empty triangle sign.

The *cord sign*, visible on unenhanced CT scans, represents the spontaneous visualization of a thrombosed cortical vein; it is very rare,[129,133,134] and its diagnostic value is debated. The cord sign can also be seen in thrombosis of the internal cerebral veins and of the vein of Galen.[137]

The *dense triangle sign* also reflects spontaneous SSS opacification by freshly congealed blood[30] (Fig. 12–5A). It

is a very early sign but an extremely rare one, being present in less than 2% of cases. The dense triangle is difficult to assess, particularly in other sinuses (LS and SS), which can be spontaneously hyperdense in normal children or in patients with hemoconcentration.

The *empty delta sign*, described by Buonanno and colleagues,[130] appears after injection of contrast material. It reflects the contrast between the opacified collateral veins in the SSS wall and the nonopacification of the clot inside the sinus (see Fig. 12–5B). It is the most common direct sign, present in approximately 35% of published cases.[126,130,134,139] The empty delta sign is absent, however, when (1) thrombosis does not affect the posterior third of the SSS or (2) CT scanning is performed either in the first 5 days or more than 2 months after onset of symptoms.[136]

The sensitivity and specificity of the empty delta sign are enhanced with some technical refinements, such as orthogonal sectioning, different window and level settings, and multiplanar reformations.[111,127,133–135] These factors probably explain why this sign is found in only 10% to 20% of CT scans performed routinely to rule out other conditions in patients suspected to have CVT.[131] Furthermore, it is not pathognomonic, because early division of the SSS can be responsible for a false delta sign.

Indirect Signs of Cerebral Venous Thrombosis

Indirect and nonspecific abnormalities are more common in CVT. Intense contrast enhancement of the falx and tentorium is present in some 20% of cases (Fig. 12–6).[129,130,131,134] Intense enhancement is easily recognized in the tentorium but can be difficult to assess in the falx, particularly in aged patients. It indicates venous stasis or hyperemia of the dura mater. Tentorial enhancement is usually thought to suggest SS thrombosis,[134] but it is not rare in SSS thrombosis.[45,131] It can be associated with dilated transcerebral medullary veins, indicating a major venous stasis, usually in relation to an extensive SSS thrombosis.[126]

A common finding is the presence of small ventricles with swelling and sometimes diffuse low density suggestive of edema.[30,45,129,131,133,134] Although reported in 20% to 50% of cases, this finding is not a useful sign because it is nonspecific and is frequently difficult to differentiate from normal brain, particularly in the young. In some cases, the cerebral swelling can be confirmed by the later increase in size of ventricles, which were initially small. However, the opposite finding (i.e., enlarged ventricles) may occur, particularly in cerebellar vein thrombosis, and therefore does not exclude the diagnosis.

White matter hypodensity without contrast enhancement suggestive of cerebral edema is present in up to 75% of cases.[133] It can be diffuse or localized and is sometimes associated with a mass effect. This finding is usually associated with abnormalities suggestive of a venous infarct, but it can occasionally be the only sign of CVT.

Usually described by pathologists as hemorrhagic, venous infarcts on CT scan manifest as a spontaneous hyperdensity in 10% to 50% of cases.[30,42,45,128,130,131,134] Two main aspects are encountered: large subcortical often multifocal hematomas and petechial hemorrhages within large hypodensities (Fig. 12–7). In rare instances, there is an associated subarachnoid hemorrhage or a subdural

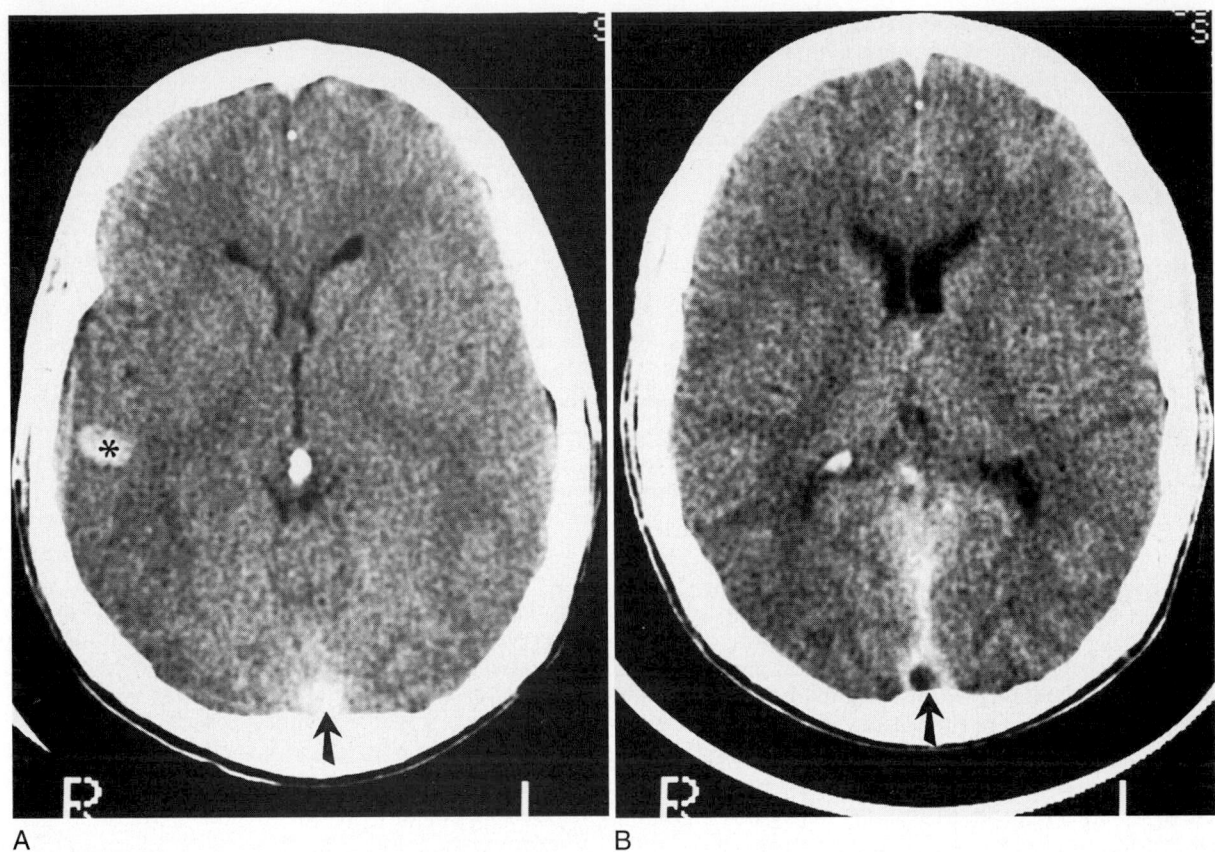

FIGURE 12–5   A, *Unenhanced CT scan. Dense triangle in a recent SSS thrombosis* (arrow) *with a small cortical hemorrhage* (asterisk). B, *Enhanced CT scan in the same patient 10 days later. Empty delta sign* (arrow).

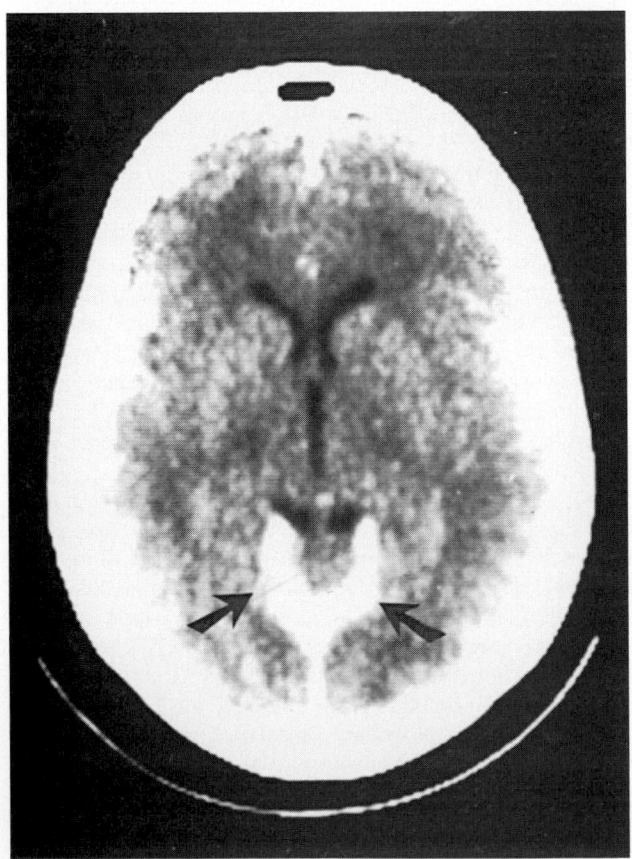

FIGURE 12–6   *Enhanced CT scan. Intense tentorial enhancement in a patient with superior sagittal sinus and thrombosis of both lateral sinuses* (arrows).

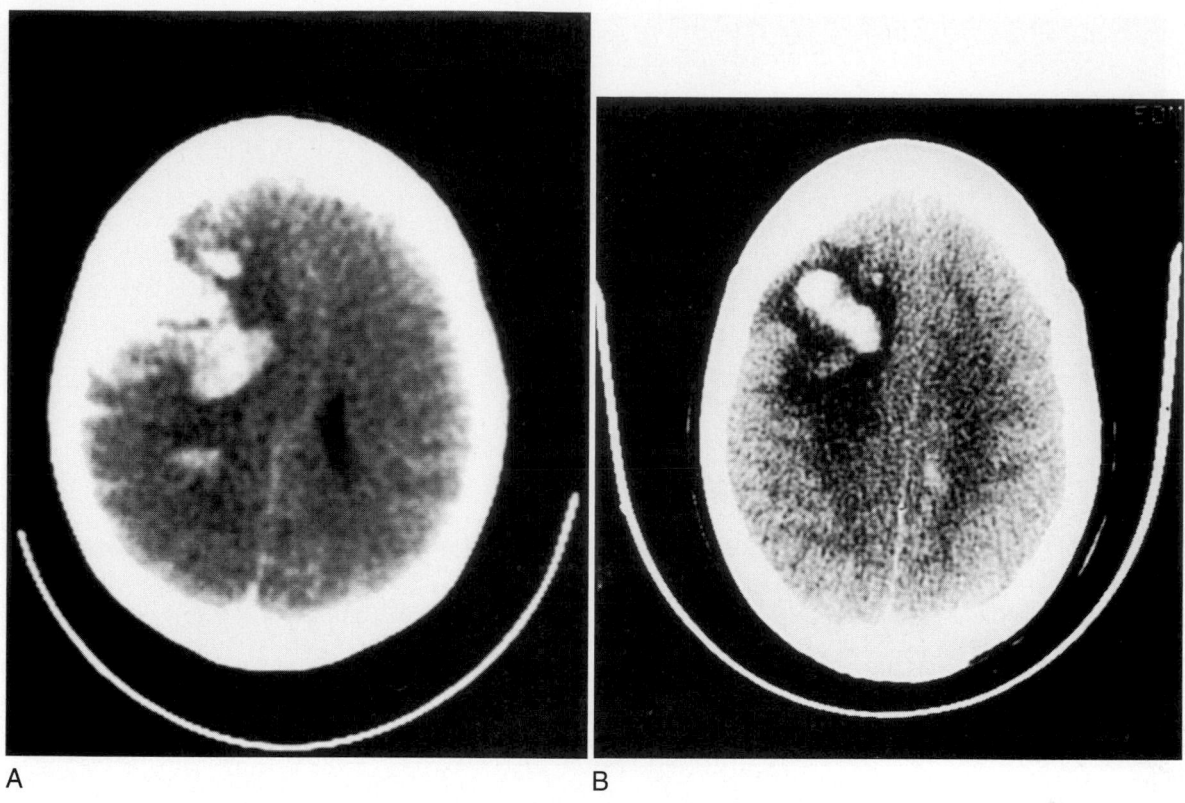

FIGURE 12–7　*Unenhanced CT scans in two patients with superior sagittal sinus thrombosis. A, Spontaneous hyperdensity with severe mass effect suggestive of a hemorrhagic infarct. B, Bilateral hemorrhagic infarct.*

hematoma, which can sometimes be the only signs of CVT.[131] Nonhemorrhagic venous infarcts are almost as common. They are protean in appearance,[131] taking the form of focal hypodensity with gyral enhancement, areas of hypodensity without enhancement, or isolated gyral enhancement (Fig. 12–8). Hemorrhagic or nonhemorrhagic infarcts can be unilateral or bilateral, single or multiple.[30,42,131] They are seen superficially in the hemispheres in SSS thrombosis and within the basal ganglia in deep venous system thrombosis.

Cavernous Sinus Thrombosis
The CT scan can sometimes be useful in demonstrating cavernous sinus thrombosis,[103,132] showing on post-contrast CT scans as multiple irregular filling defects with bulging cavernous sinuses and enlarged orbital veins.[132] The presence of air, seen on coronal sections, has been reported in septic thrombosis.[103]

Normal CT Scan
In 10% to 20% of cases, CT scanning is normal in patients with proven CVT, more commonly (up to 50%) in patients presenting with isolated intracranial hypertension than in those with focal signs (<10%).[30,131]

Summary
The place of CT scanning in the diagnostic strategy of CVT is mainly to rule out other conditions, such as arterial stroke, abscess, tumors, and subarachnoid hemorrhage on an emergency basis. It should be performed at first without contrast enhancement, and then, in the absence of

hemorrhagic infarct, with contrast enhancement. In a minority of cases, CT scanning shows the direct pathognomonic signs of CVT; more frequently, however, only indirect signs are present, and MRI or angiographic confirmation must be obtained.

Angiography

Intra-arterial Angiography
Angiography has been the key procedure in the diagnosis of CVT for many years and remains the method of reference in some difficult cases. It requires a perfect technique; four-vessel angiography (conventional or digitized intra-arterial) with visualization of the entire venous phase on at least two projections (frontal and lateral) and three, if possible, oblique views are the best combination for visualization of the entire SSS.[30,42,45,140]

The partial or complete lack of filling of veins or sinuses is the best angiographic sign of CVT. Easily recognized when it affects the posterior or whole SSS (Fig. 12–9), both LSs (Fig. 12–10), or the deep venous system (Fig. 12–11), lack of filling may be more difficult to interpret in other locations, such as the anterior third of the SSS or the left LS, where it can be confused with hypoplasia.[114] For occlusion of the anterior part of the SSS to be established, either involvement of another sinus or unequivocal indirect signs of CVT, such as delayed emptying and dilated collateral veins, must be present. For LS thrombosis, the main evidence is the absence of filling of the whole sinus or of its sigmoid portion, contrasting with the presence of the sinus

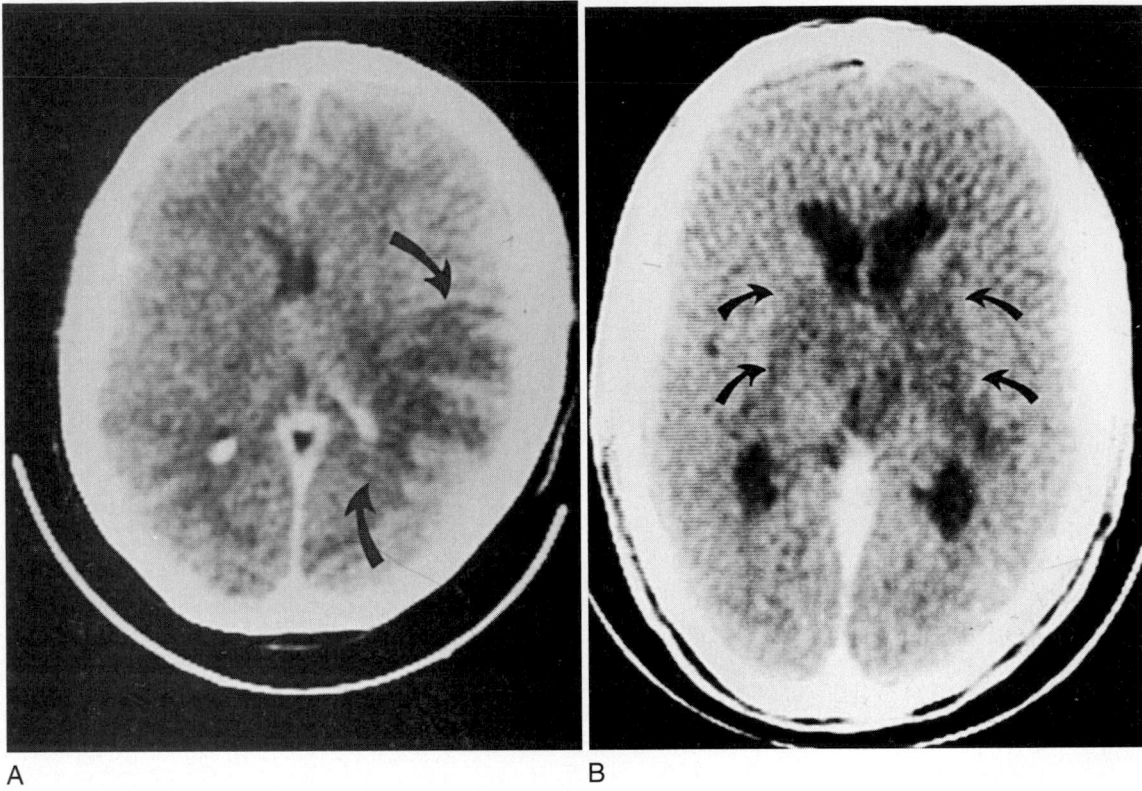

FIGURE 12–8 *Enhanced CT scans. A, Large area (arrows) of cortico-subcortical hypodensity with mass effect on the lateral ventricle in a patient with superior sagittal sinus thrombosis. B, Bilateral basal ganglia hypodensity (arrows) in a patient with deep cerebral vein thrombosis.*

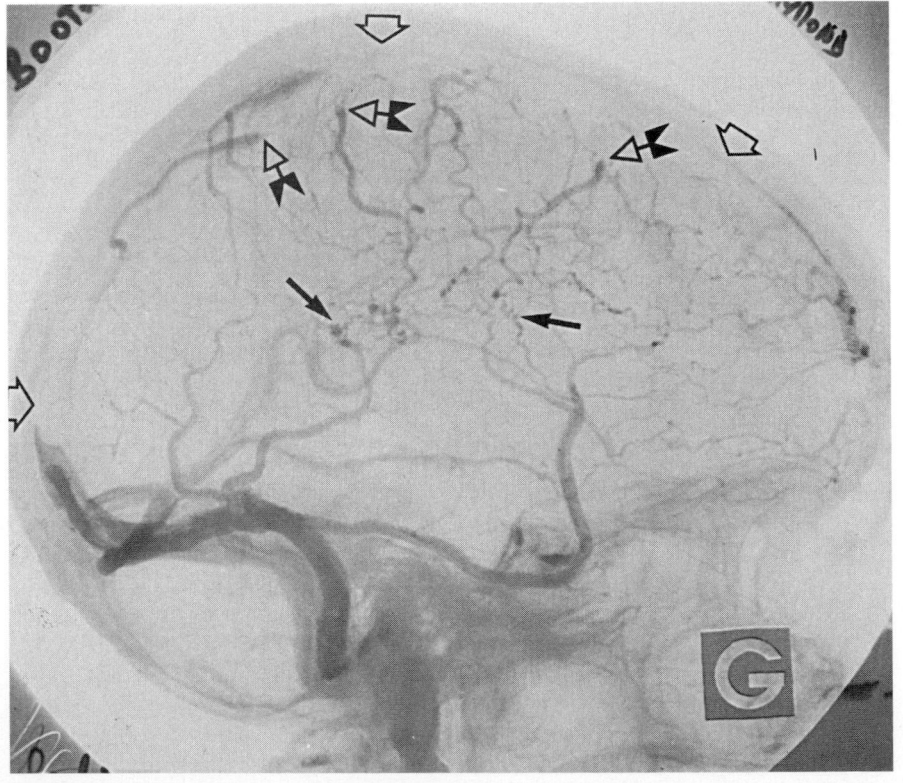

FIGURE 12–9 *Left carotid angiogram. Total occlusion of the superior sagittal sinus (white arrows) with occlusion of the frontoparietal veins (tailed arrows) and anastomotic cortical veins with a corkscrew appearance (straight arrows).*

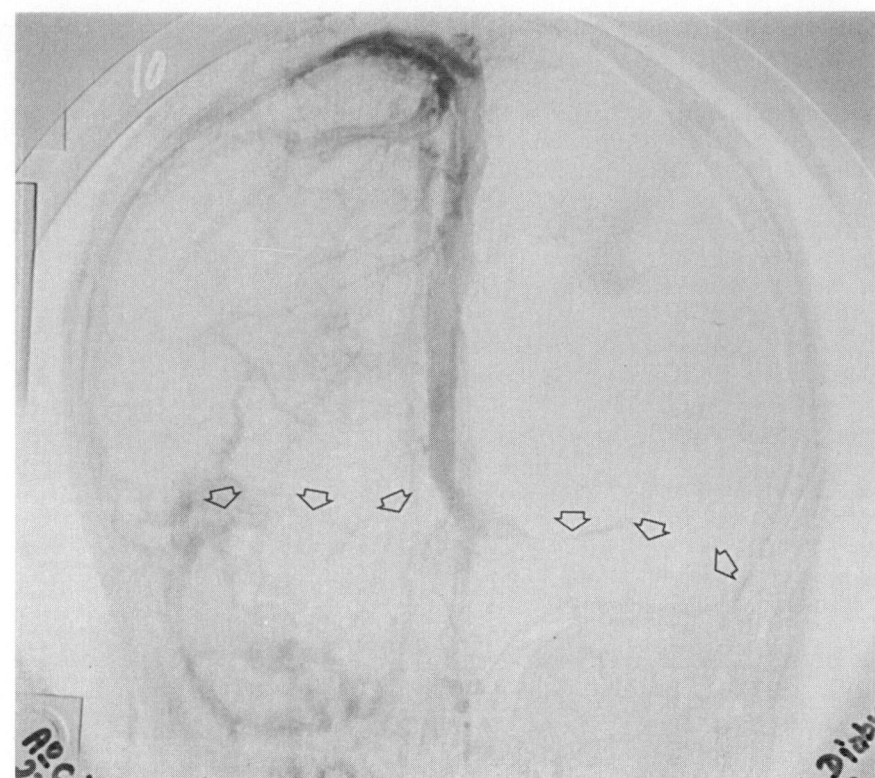

FIGURE 12–10 *Right carotid angiogram. Lack of filling of both lateral sinuses (white arrows). (From Bousser MG, Chiras J, Sauron B, et al: Cerebral venous thrombosis: A review of 38 cases. Stroke 16:199, 1985.)*

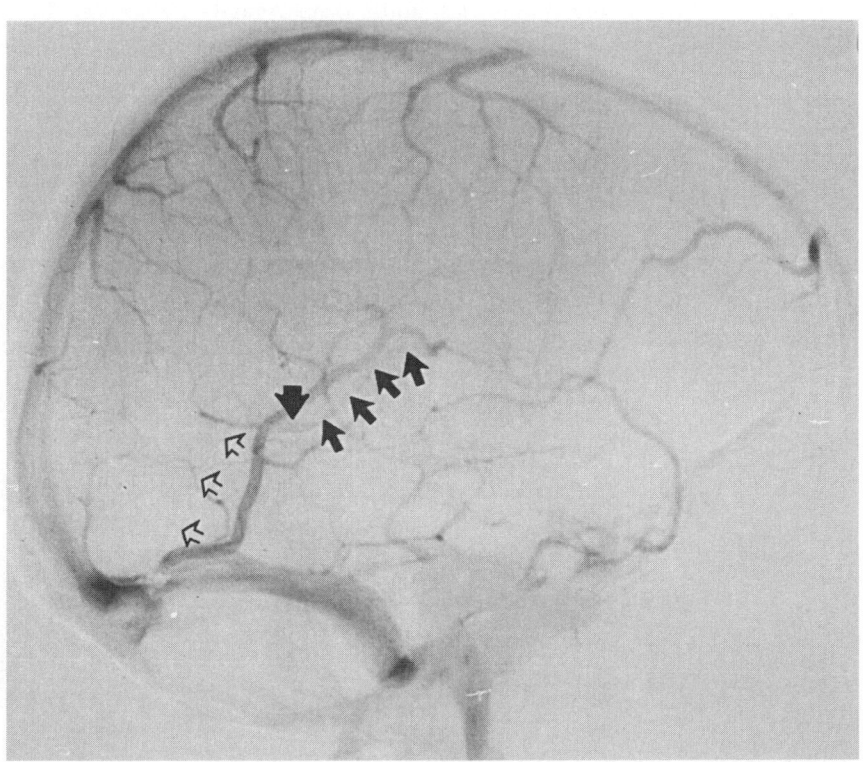

FIGURE 12–11 *Right carotid angiogram. Poor filling of internal cerebral vein (narrow black arrows) and vein of Galen (wide black arrow) and lack of filling of straight sinus (white arrows).*

groove and normality of the jugular foramen on plain radiographs of the skull. However, in some cases, such signs are lacking, and MRI is required to differentiate between thrombosis and hypoplasia (Fig. 12–12).[17]

The absence of a cortical vein is difficult and sometimes impossible to detect except when the vein is partly visualized but stops suddenly and is surrounded by dilated collateral veins (see Fig. 12–9). Another angiographic finding is delayed emptying; collateral venous pathways, found in about 50% of cases, almost invariably indicate SSS thrombosis. Dilated and tortuous cortical collateral veins with a corkscrew appearance are much more common (see Fig. 12–9) than transcerebral or intradural collateral vessels.[30,31,45,138,140] An important mass effect is extremely rare and has been reported in only a few cases.[30,138]

Magnetic Resonance Angiography

The tendency now is to use MRA instead of intra-arterial angiography for the diagnosis of CVT. Several methods can be used: two-dimensional time-of-flight (TOF), three-dimensional TOF, and phase contrast.[11,21,25,26,141–143] Two-dimensional TOF is the most commonly used, with 1.5- and 3-mm-thick slices in the coronal and axial planes. As with intra-arterial angiography, the typical appearance of CVT on MRA is the absence of flow, indicating a complete thrombosis (see Fig. 12–12). Specific limitations exist for each of the MRA techniques as well as the limitations common to all varieties of angiography in CVT: the difficulty in diagnosing partial thrombosis, the inability to differentiate hypoplasia and thrombosis, and the poor yield for detection of cortical vein and cavernous sinus thromboses. However, MRA has the advantages of being easily repeatable and noninvasive. In most cases, it is combined with MRI, this association now being the best diagnostic tool in CVT.

CT Angiography (Helical CT Venography)

Helical cerebral CT venography has been developed to study the venous circulation.[30,48] Excellent images of sinus thrombosis have been obtained; filling defects, sinus wall enhancement, abnormal collateral venous drainage, and tentorial enhancement are common abnormalities.[144] It has been suggested that CT venograms are easier to interpret and have fewer artifacts than magnetic resonance venography (MRV). CT venography is particularly interesting in the acute setting because it can easily be performed immediately after non–contrast-enhanced CT, which is usually the first procedure performed in emergencies.

Magnetic Resonance Imaging

Thrombosis Imaging

MRI offers the following major advantages for the evaluation of possible CVT: sensitivity to blood flow, ability to visualize the thrombus itself, and noninvasiveness. A variety of MRI findings have been described, mainly relating to the evaluation of thrombosis.[14,17,18,24,141,145–147] At a very early stage, flow void is absent, and the occluded vessel appears isointense on T1-weighted images and hypointense on T2-weighted images. The diagnosis at that stage is often impossible on MRI alone. Angiography (or MRA) is required to demonstrate the absence of flow in the thrombosed vessel.

A few days later, the absence of flow void persists, but the thrombus becomes hyperintense, initially on T1- and then on T2-weighted images (Fig. 12–13).[145] In large vessels, these changes start in the periphery and proceed toward the center. They represent the aging of the thrombus with biochemical conversion of oxyhemoglobin to methemoglobin rather than extension of thrombosis. This intermediate pattern (increased signal on T1- and

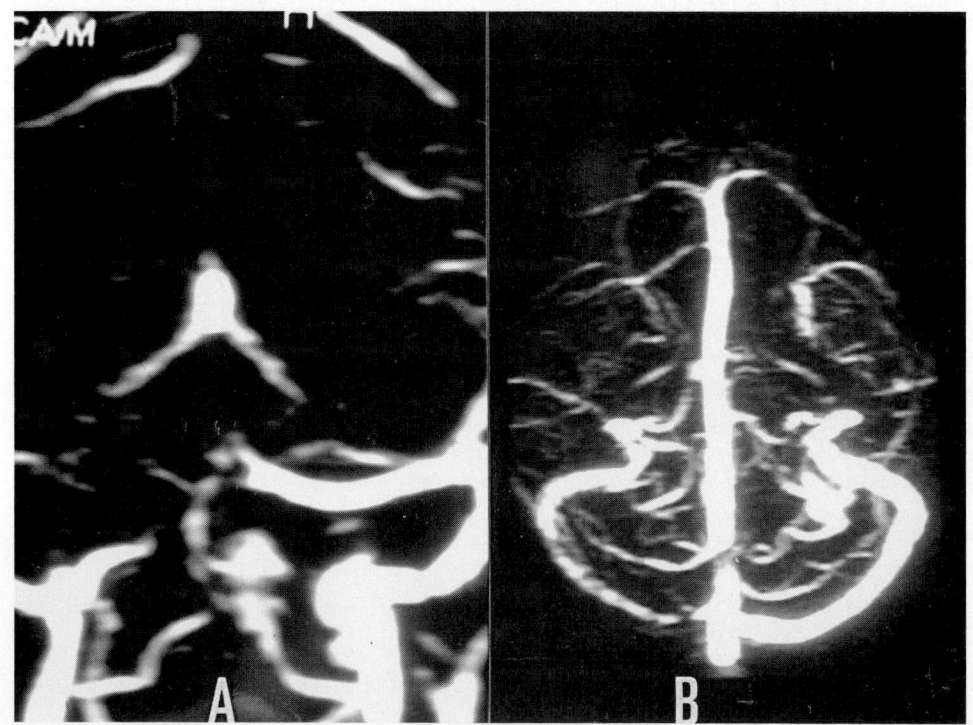

FIGURE 12–12 *Magnetic resonance angiography (phase contrast). Superior sagittal sinus thrombosis before (A) and 7 days after (B) heparin treatment (recanalization). (Courtesy of Dr. Beyssac, Toulon, France.)*

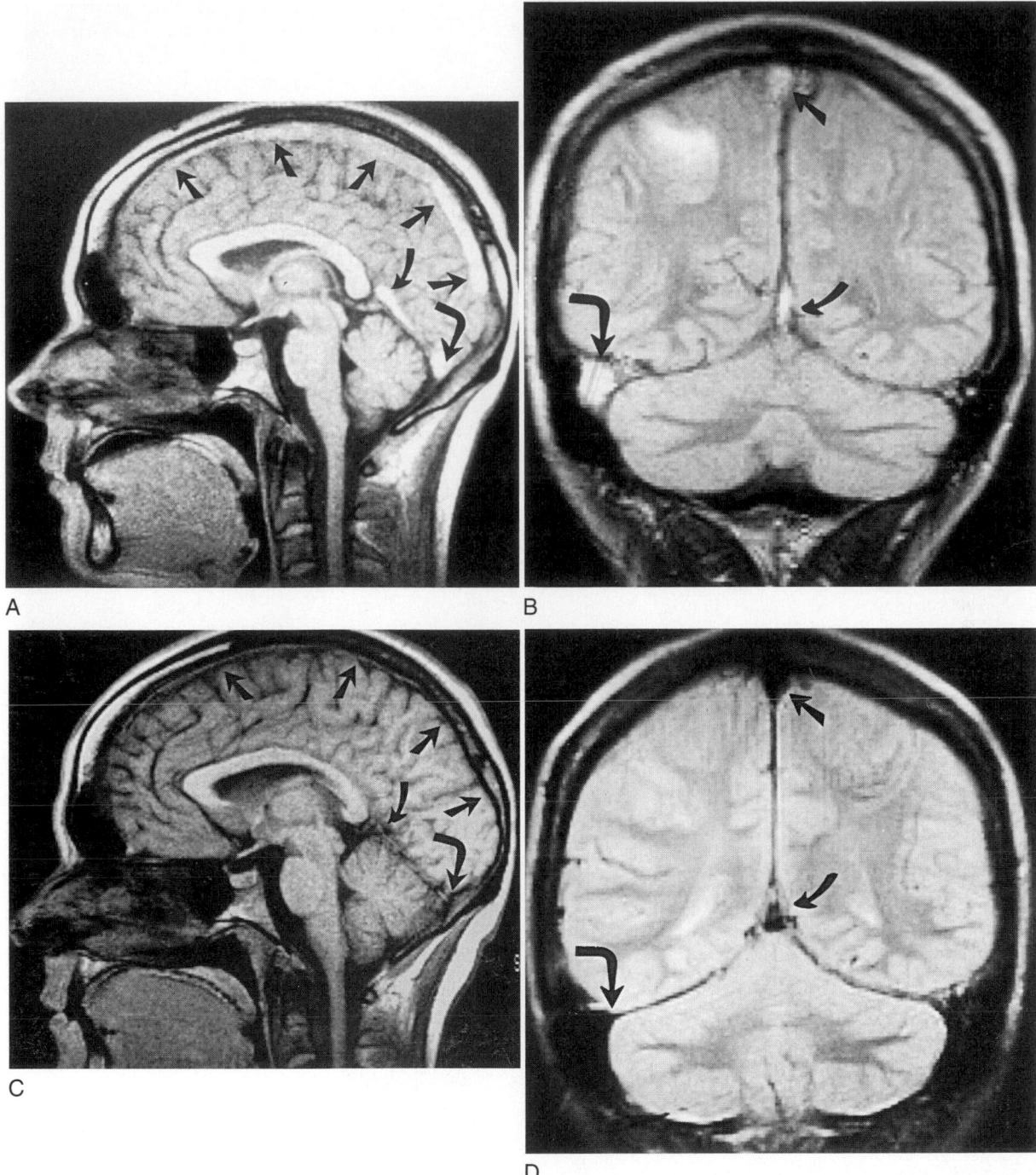

FIGURE 12–13   *MRI, T1-weighted images. A and B, Hyperintense signal indicating thrombosis of the superior sagittal sinus (straight arrows), lateral sinuses (angled arrows), and straight sinus (curved arrows). C and D, Same patient 3 months later. Normal flow void in previously thrombosed sinuses.*

T2-weighted images) is diagnostic of CVT and is by far the most common. It is usually found between 4 or 5 and 30 to 35 days after the onset of symptoms.[30,145]

Late changes (approximately 2 to 4 weeks after onset) can reveal the beginning of vascular recanalization with the resumption of flow void in the previously thrombosed vessel. However, at 6 months, more than two thirds of cases still show some heterogeneous localized signal abnormalities, which can persist for years and should not be

mistaken for a recurrent acute CVT.[141,145] MRI thus can reveal not only venous thrombosis but also the natural history of the thrombotic process (see Fig. 12–13). MRI diagnosis is particularly easy in SSS thrombosis,[22,24,30,145,147] but convincing images have also been obtained in cases of thrombosis involving the LS (Fig. 12–14), the SS (Fig. 12–15), the internal cerebral veins and vein of Galen (see Fig. 12–15), the cavernous sinus, and the cortical veins.[19,22,42,145,147,148]

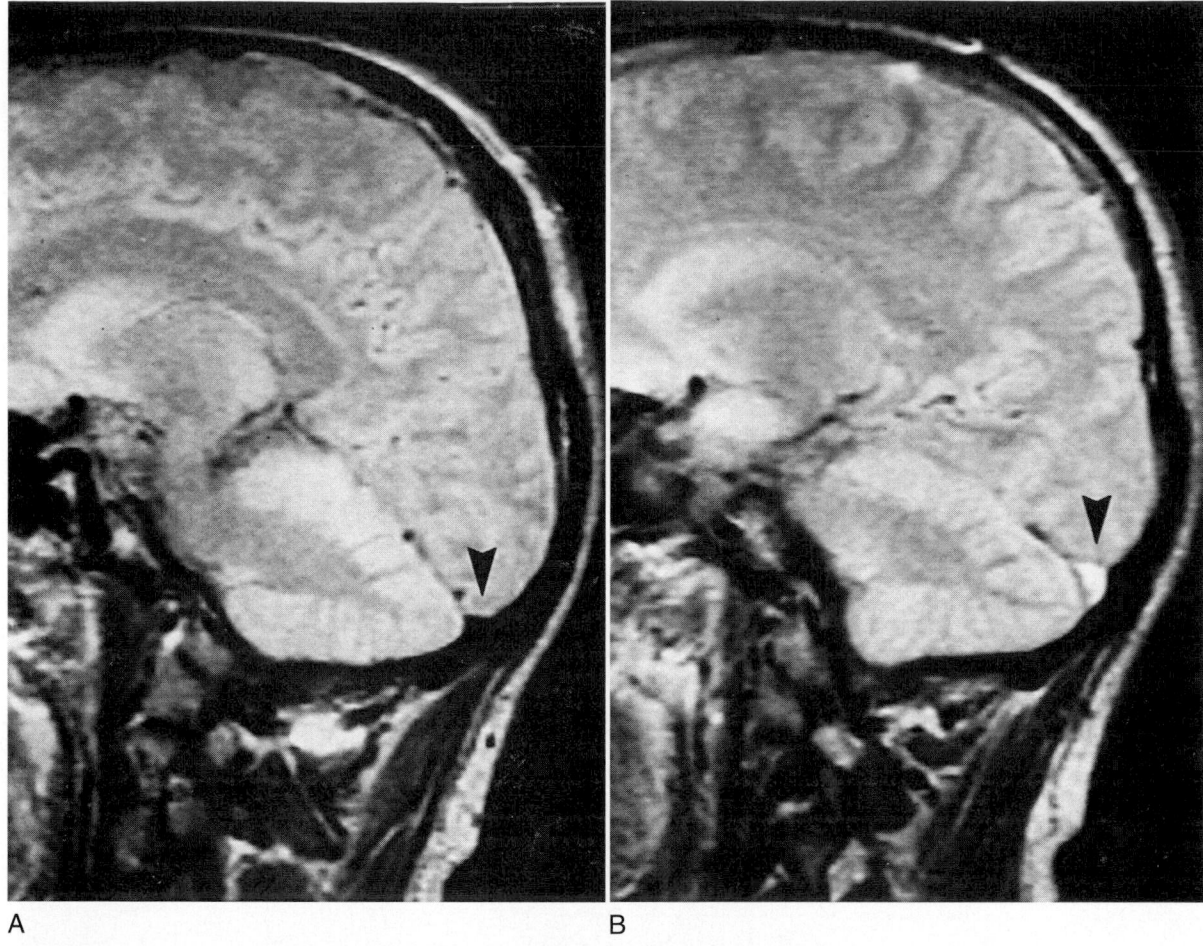

FIGURE 12–14 *MRI, T2-weighted images.* A, *Lateral sinus hypoplasia* (arrowhead). B, *Lateral sinus thrombosis* (arrowhead).

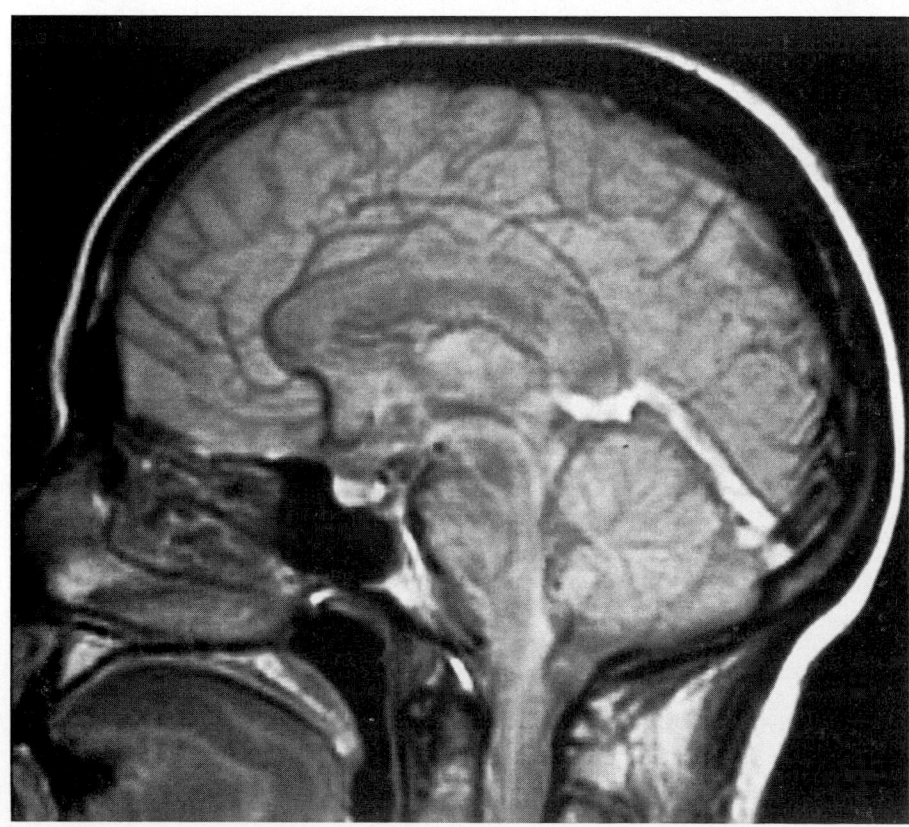

FIGURE 12–15 *MRI, T2-weighted image (first echo; TR = 2000 msec, TE = 40 msec) hyperintense signal indicating thrombosis of the vein of Galen and superior sagittal sinus.*

In some cases, however, interpretation of MRI findings is not easy because of false-negative and false-positive appearances. False-negative appearances are rare and mostly correspond to a very early or very late stage or to isolated cortical vein thrombosis. Most false-positive appearances are created by slowly flowing blood. Repositioning the patient, repeating the sequence in a different plane, using at least two sequences, and, sometimes, obtaining specialized acquisitions are helpful in eliminating these artifacts.[19,22–24,30,145-148]

Parenchymal Lesions

Besides visualizing the thrombus itself, MRI detects its parenchymal consequences: brain swelling with mass effect and cortical sulcal effacement; increased signal on T2-weighted images with isointense or hypointense signal on T1-weighted images suggestive of edema; and increased signal on both T1- and T2-weighted images, indicating a hemorrhagic component.[145] These findings are nonspecific, but their diagnosis is easy because of the associated MRI signs of sinus thrombosis. The main difficulty is with isolated cortical vein thrombosis, which can be mistaken for a tumor unless angiography demonstrates typical stop sign with corkscrew collateral veins.

Diffusion-weighted imaging (DWI), which has also been studied in patients with CVT, seems to have several advantages.[13,15,36–39,151] First, the clot can be directly visualized as a high signal intensity in the affected sinus. Whether this abnormality will result in a greater diagnostic yield for DWI compared with conventional MRI and MRV remains unknown, however.

Second, the main interest of DWI is to show, in the so-called venous infarcts, a diffusion pattern highly different from that in arterial infarcts. The most common pattern is an heterogeneous signal intensity with a normal or increased apparent diffusion coefficient (ADC) corresponding mostly with vasogenic edema combined with some areas of cytotoxic edema.[13,15,36–39,149] Another pattern consists of a multifocal increased signal with moderately decreased ADC; unlike in arterial infarcts, however, areas of reduced ADC values may not be predictive of ultimate venous infarction.[37] In a third pattern, there is no abnormality in diffusion. Thus the DWI-ADC pattern of brain lesions in CVT is highly heterogeneous, mostly suggestive of vasogenic edema, and markedly different from that of arterial infarcts. This accounts for the much better recovery observed in venous brain lesions than in arterial infarcts.

The vast difference between venous and arterial ischemia is also illustrated by a case of deep venous system thrombosis with large bilateral thalamic lesions, reported by Hsu and Lirng.[150] Hydrogen 1 magnetic resonance spectroscopy (MRS) showed a normal N-acetyl aspartate (NAA) peak and only a small lactate peak. These findings contrast with the marked loss of NAA and increase in lactates observed in arterial infarction and they suggest that the neurons, though functionally impaired, were still viable.[150]

Summary

The combination of non–contrast-enhanced MRI plus MRA is currently the best method for the diagnosis and follow-up of CVT. It should be performed as a first-line investigation in patients in whom clinical suspicion of CTS is high. Its use is limited in certain situations, such as deeply comatose subjects requiring artificial ventilation. In such patients as well as in dubious cases—such as isolated cortical vein thrombosis—intra-arterial angiography may still be required.

Other Neurologic Investigations

Other investigations were most useful in the pre-CT era. *Electroencephalographic* changes are constantly found in SSS thrombosis with extension to cortical veins; they are present in roughly 75% of all CVT cases.[30,42,48] These changes are nonspecific; the most common pattern is a severe generalized slowing more marked on one side, with frequent superimposed epileptic activity. In some patients with focal symptoms, a generalized slowing indicates a more diffuse lesion than clinically suspected.

Isotope brain scanning with technetium Tc 99m– or indium In 111–labeled platelets has been used to detect sinus thrombosis,[151,152] but the technique has now been supplanted by MRI.

CSF examination is still a useful diagnostic tool because the CSF is very rarely (10%) entirely normal in CVT, in either composition or pressure.[6,30,42,59,101] Abnormalities in composition include raised protein content as well as the presence of red blood cells (in two thirds of cases) and pleocytosis (in one third). Mainly seen when focal signs are present, pleocytosis and the presence of red blood cells can also be found in patients presenting with benign intracranial hypertension; the presence of these abnormalities should therefore suggest sinus thrombosis as the possible cause of this syndrome. CSF examination is crucial to ruling out meningitis, which is extremely difficult to exclude on clinical grounds alone. With the advent of CT scanning and MRI, CSF study has become obsolete in most cases of nonseptic CVT manifesting as focal signs. The examination remains crucial, however, in patients with isolated intracranial hypertension, to rule out meningitis, to measure CSF pressure, and to remove CSF when the patient's vision is threatened.

Transcranial Doppler ultrasonography (TCD) has a very limited role in the diagnosis of CVT. In the past few years, however, attempts have been made to assess the venous circulation by means of conventional TCD and transcranial color-coded duplex sonography.[153–157] SSS thrombosis has been associated with elevated venous blood velocities in the deep venous system and with microembolic signals in the internal jugular vein. TCD has thus been used to detect massive SSS thrombosis and to provide day-to-day monitoring of severe cases that cannot be studied by MRI.

General Investigations

After CVT has been established, investigations should be directed toward demonstrating the underlying cause. Because of the multiplicity of causes, this task is long and difficult whenever the cause is not clinically evident. Fever, increased erythrocyte sedimentation rate, or raised polymorphonuclear white blood cell count points to infective, inflammatory, or malignant causes. However, even with such underlying diseases, these abnormalities are

Clinical Manifestations

sometimes lacking; by contrast, they are occasionally found in idiopathic cases.[30] Their presence is particularly useful as an indication of CVT in patients presenting with benign intracranial hypertension.

Detailed coagulation studies have only rarely been performed in series of CVT, and their results have been conflicting. Some investigators have found hypercoagulability state,[71] an increase in platelet adhesiveness and aggregability,[43] and a decrease in fibrinolytic activity,[43] but these findings were obtained during pregnancy or the puerperium or in women taking oral contraceptives. Other studies did not confirm these results[64] or found an increased platelet aggregation with the lowest dose of epinephrine as the only abnormality.[45] On the whole, there is no consistent abnormality indicating the presence of a thrombotic process except, as in other varieties of venous thrombosis, a significant increase (although not constant) in D-dimer levels. The main interest of coagulation studies is to detect possible causative conditions such as congenital thrombophilia. Such conditions should be systematically sought in patients with CVT, whether or not other potential causes are present, because they (1) imply a systematic family study and (2) modify the long-term management of the patients (see discussion of etiology).

OUTCOME

Short-Term Outcome

Mortality

Before the introduction of angiography, CVT was diagnosed mainly at autopsy and was therefore thought to be usually lethal.[3,5,6,8] In early angiographic series, mortality still ranked between 30% and 50%,[7] but in later series, it was lower, ranging from 6% to 38% (Table 12.4). In the ISCVT,[57] the mortality rate at hospital discharge for the 450 patients recruited worldwide was only 3.6% (95% CI, 1.7–5.4).

The three main causes of death in CVT are (1) the brain lesion itself, particularly when a massive hemorrhagic infarct is present; (2) intercurrent complications such as sepsis, uncontrolled seizures, and pulmonary embolism, present in 11% of 203 published cases reviewed by Diaz and colleagues,[158] with a mortality rate of 94%, and (3) underlying conditions, such as carcinomas, septicemias, leukemias, and paroxysmal nocturnal hemoglobinuria.[30,42,44,45,55]

Factors classically considered to suggest a bad prognosis are as follows:

- Rate of evolution of thrombosis[6]
- Age of the patient (mortality rate is high in infants and the aged)
- An infectious cause[34,44,48]
- Focal symptoms and coma[5,6,30,34,44]
- Presence of a hemorrhagic infarct
- Empty delta sign on CT scan[139]

The topography of the cerebral veins involved is also an important prognostic factor, deep cerebral vein thrombosis and cerebellar vein thrombosis carrying much higher risks than cortical vein thrombosis.[4,30,113,115] Among the underlying conditions, the postpartum state is a favorable one, with a survival of 90% in most later series.[30]

Functional Recovery

It has long been recognized that if the patient with CVT survives, the prognosis for recovery of function is much better than for patients with arterial thrombosis.[30,45,48,49,159] A minority (15% to 25%) of patients are left with disabling sequelae, such as optic atrophy and focal deficits.[24,30,45,48,159] Any combination of neurologic signs can persist, according to the site, extent, and severity of the parenchymal lesion and to the severity of raised intracranial pressure. In neonates, the functional outcome is usually normal in the absence of associated asphyxia but is frequently abnormal in preterm neonates who have suffered asphyxia.[58,98,160]

It is thus apparent that although CVT is less severe than classically thought, its natural history and prognosis are highly variable. Some patients with acute cases can have a fulminating course leading to death in a few days, whereas others recover rapidly and completely, and still others are left with sequelae. Some patients with chronic disease show progressive worsening and sequelae, whereas others recover spontaneously. In extremely benign forms, symptoms are limited to transient ischemic attacks, headache, or epilepsy; the patients recover spontaneously and are probably still under-recognized. On the whole, isolated sinus thrombosis carries a good prognosis, provided that intracranial hypertension is controlled; however, sinus thrombosis can extend to cerebral veins at any moment, leading to death or sequelae, although in a minority of cases.

Table 12.4   Outcome (Percentage) in a Series of Patients with Cerebral Venous Thrombosis

Outcome	Einhäupl et al (1990)[49] (n = 71)	Cantu and Barinagarrementeria (1993)[51] Puerperal (n = 67)	Cantu and Barinagarrementeria (1993)[51] Nonpuerperal (n = 46)	Tsai et al (1995)[25] (n = 29)	Daif et al (1995)[46] (n = 40)	De Bruijn et al (2001)[52] (n = 59)	Ferro et al (2001)[53] (n = 142)	Bousser (2001)° (n = 200)
Total recovery	59	53.7	52	71	72	24	68	76.5
Minor sequelae	18.5	28.3	6.5	0	8	59	22	11
Major sequelae	8.5	9	9	3.5	10	7	4	9
Death	14	9	33	21	10	10	6	3.5

°Personal series.

Long-Term Outcome

Little is known about the long-term outcome of patients with CVT. Only two studies have so far addressed this issue.[159,161] In the earliest study, which was retrospective,[161] the prognosis was essentially good, 86% of patients being without neurologic symptoms during a mean follow-up of 6.5 years. In the second study,[161] which was prospective, the outcome was far less favorable; 44% of the patients had some degree of handicap or significant cognitive impairment after 1 to 4 years. A few reports suggest that LS thrombosis can later induce arteriovenous malformations affecting the transverse sinus.[30,45,141,162,163] Residual epilepsy has been reported in 10% to 30% of patients who had seizures during the acute stage of CVT.[54,161] Seizures usually occur in the first year and are easily controlled with antiepileptic drugs. In a 1996 study, no seizures were observed during long-term follow-up in patients who did not have focal signs and did not suffer seizures during the acute stage.[161] The frequency of long-term epilepsy is also low in neonates who suffer CVT without associated asphyxia.[98]

Recurrence of CVT seems infrequent, the rate being 11.7% in one series of 77 patients who were monitored for a mean of 77.8 months.[161] Recurrences have been reported in cases with known prothrombotic conditions but also in idiopathic cases. The risk of recurrence during a later pregnancy is poorly known but seems low; recurrence was seen in none of 16 pregnancies in a series reported by Preter and associates.[161]

TREATMENT

Because CVT is an uncommon disease with a great variability in natural history, treatment is still controversial. It is based on a combination of symptomatic, etiologic, and antithrombotic medications on a case-by-case basis.

Symptomatic Treatment

Some investigators favor the systematic use of anticonvulsant treatment,[6,48,164] whereas others restrict it to patients who present with seizures.[30,42,59] Any of the major antiepileptic drugs can be used. The duration of treatment remains an open question. In our series, anticonvulsants were progressively discontinued 1 year after CVT in patients with a normal electroencephalogram and no recurrent seizures.[161]

Opinions on reducing intracranial pressure are more divergent, and various approaches have been used— steroids, mannitol, glycerol, dextran, acetazolamide, lumbar punctures, shunting, barbiturate-induced coma, LS venous bypass, or even surgical decompression.[30,59,164,165] The choice among these methods depends on the individual clinical situation. Minor brain swelling often needs no specific treatment. In a patient who has isolated intracranial hypertension, particularly whose vision is threatened, we favor performance of one lumbar puncture before starting heparin. If vision continues to deteriorate or if consciousness becomes abnormal, mannitol is usually added.[164] In the very rare cases of life-threatening raised intracranial pressure, drastic methods such as shunting or barbiturate-induced coma might be required.[166,167]

Etiologic Treatment

Whenever possible, the cause of the CVT should be treated. This statement applies particularly to septic thrombosis, which requires wide-spectrum combination antibiotics, along with surgical treatment of the primary site of infection in some cases. It also applies to all the general conditions that can promote CVT and must be specifically treated, such as malignancies, connective tissue diseases, and hematologic disorders.

Antithrombotic Treatment

Although jugular vein ligation and surgical thrombectomy have been performed in the past for CVT,[6,102] these surgical methods have been abandoned. Antithrombotic treatment is based primarily on anticoagulants and secondarily on antiplatelet drugs and thrombolytics.

Anticoagulants

Although the use of heparin has been advocated for more than 50 years,[66,168] some investigators have been skeptical about its value for two main alleged reasons, the risk of intracerebral bleeding, particularly in an already hemorrhagic infarct, and the lack of enough evidence of its efficacy.[165,169] It is remarkable that the risk of intracerebral bleeding with heparin therapy has been emphasized again and again[3,56,165,169] even though hardly any undisputable cases have been reported. The two cases most often cited are those reported by Gettelfinger and Kokmen[170]; in one of these cases, however, the patient's condition worsened after heparin *and* urokinase therapy, and the other patient suffered paroxysmal nocturnal hemoglobinuria, a notoriously severe underlying condition with an increased hemorrhagic risk.

It is clear that the risk of hemorrhage has been overestimated, an impression confirmed by the large number of cases and case series in which heparin has been given without deleterious effects.* There is now ample evidence that heparin is safe even when CT or MRI demonstrates a hemorrhagic lesion.[30,68,172–175] Evidence of the efficacy of heparin in CVT is based on illustrative cases, on retrospective and prospective series, and on two randomized trials. A number of well-documented cases have been reported in which a dramatic improvement occurred shortly after the initiation of heparin in patients who had previously been deteriorating steadily.[24,30,45,69,171] Moreover, the condition of some of these patients worsened when heparin was changed to oral anticoagulants and rapidly improved again after heparin was resumed.[24,30,69]

Heparin has been used in many cases and series with apparently good results.† Thus, in German and French series combined,[60] 143 patients received heparin, and only 4 of them died. This figure could be difficult to interpret, because (1) patients with CVT can recover spontaneously and (2) it could be argued that the most severe cases were excluded.[165] However, the latter argument does not hold because the German and the French groups have used heparin in all their CVT patients during the last 20 years. An important contribution has been made by Diaz and col-

---

*6,7,24,30,45,48,49,60,69,164,171,173
†24,30,42,45,48–60,69,164,171,174,176

leagues,[158] who reviewed 203 cases of CVT reported between 1942 and 1990 and compared the outcomes of patients who were treated (n = 56) with those who were not treated (n = 226) with heparin; 91% survived in the first group, compared with 36% in the second.

The best evidence of the efficacy of heparin was obtained by the randomized study performed by Einhäupl and coworkers[174] in Germany; high-dose intravenous heparin was compared with placebo in patients with angiographically proven CVT. The study had to be stopped after the first 20 patients because of a statistically significant difference in favor of heparin ($P < .05$). After 3 months, all 10 heparin-treated patients either had completely recovered or were left with a slight neurologic deficit, whereas in the control group, 4 patients died or had severe sequelae.

This trial has been criticized because of the use of an unvalidated scale and of the long delay (30 days) before the patients were randomly assigned to treatment groups. In a new trial, 60 patients were randomized between low-molecular-weight heparin (nadroparin) and matching placebo.[169] A poor outcome, defined as death or a Barthel index score of ≤15 was observed at 12 weeks in 13% of the patients treated with low-molecular-weight heparin and in 21% of the patients receiving placebo. The difference was not statistically significant, but it is interesting to note that no worsening attributable to new or enlarged cerebral hemorrhage was observed in patients undergoing anticoagulant therapy, even among the 15 in whom hemorrhagic lesions were demonstrated by CT. Therefore, this study confirmed the following important facts about CVT: (1) the mortality rate is lower than historically thought, (2) full recovery is possible without antithrombotic treatment, (3) the prognosis of CVT is more severe with hemorrhage, and (4) heparin is safe, even in patients with CT evidence of hemorrhagic lesions on CT. However, the study raised more questions about the efficacy of heparin in CVT.[177]

The authors of the European trial[169] have performed a meta-analysis of the two available trials that shows that with heparin, there is an absolute risk reduction in mortality of 14% and in death or dependency of 15%, with relative risk reductions of 70% and 56%, respectively. Although the sample size is small and confidence intervals are large (explaining why differences do not reach statistical significance), these results are highly meaningful from a clinical standpoint.[177] Thus, when one considers the safety of heparin and the unpredictability of the outcome of patients with CVT, these results reinforce the use of heparin as first-line treatment for CVT.[177] Another argument in favor of heparin treatment is the risk of pulmonary embolism during the acute phase of CVT.[158]

There is no consensus as to the best modality of heparin treatment. Some investigators use low-molecular-weight heparin because of its better pharmacokinetics and lower associated incidence of thrombocytopenia. We favor the use of intravenous heparin, consisting of a bolus of 80 UI/kg followed by a continuous infusion of 18 UI/kg/hr with control APTT 2.5 times the control.[60,174,177]

The optimal duration of heparin is not established. For deep vein thrombosis of the leg, oral anticoagulants are started after a few days of heparin, to reduce the risk of heparin-induced thrombocytopenia. Warfarin is usually adjusted to obtain an international normalized ratio between 2 and 3. There are no controlled data on the required duration of oral anticoagulation, but 6 months is usually recommended,[30,177] particularly when there is a known acute cause of CVT, such as minor head trauma, postpartum state, or local infection. In contrast, prolonged treatment is warranted in any patient with a continuing risk of thrombosis, such as lengthy immobilization, malignant disease, inflammatory disease (Behçet's disease or systemic lupus erythematosus), inherited thrombophilia, or recurrent venous thrombosis.[30]

Very few data have been reported on the use of anticoagulant treatment during later pregnancies in women with previous CVT.[65,161] Our approach is to use preventive low-molecular-weight heparin treatment when the initial CVT occurred during pregnancy and in patients who have a history of venous thrombosis. In other cases, we recommend close monitoring with appropriate investigations and treatment at the earliest suspicion of CVT. For women who had postpartum CVT, we favor the use of preventive low-molecular-weight heparin immediately after delivery and then for 1 month.

Thrombolytics

The use of heparin is now challenged by the advocates of direct endovascular thrombolytic therapy.[178–196] Intravenous urokinase was used for CVT first by Vines and David[138] in 1971, and then 10 years later by Di Rocco and colleagues.[180] In 1988, Scott and associates[191] reported a patient with extensive SSS thrombosis who was successfully treated with urokinase administered directly into the SSS through a frontal bur hole. Since then, approximately 200 reported cases[197] have been treated by local infusion of urokinase via the internal jugular or, more commonly, the femoral route. Also, local recombinant tissue-type plasminogen activator (rt-PA) has been used in combination with heparin.[181,185,189]

Both local urokinase and rt-PA , however, carry an indisputable risk of hemorrhagic complications. Indeed, there have been some reports, in patients with CVT who underwent local thrombolysis, of bleeding at the femoral puncture site,[185] pelvic bleeding,[185] or worsening of pretreatment intracranial bleeding.[181] These reports contrast with the absence of deterioration in the patients with hemorrhagic lesions who were treated with heparin in both the German[174] and European[169] trials. In patients without pretreatment hemorrhage, local thrombolysis appears safe, but the numbers are still small compared with the large number of patients treated with heparin. The best method of thrombolytic administration, whether urokinase or rt-PA should be used, and the optimal dosage remain to be determined. Thus, although more and more patients are treated by local endovascular urokinase or rt-PA therapy, it is still extremely difficult to assess the risk-benefit ratio of this treatment precisely.[173,197] Local thrombolysis appears to restore flow more often and more rapidly than heparin alone[196]; this treatment has been claimed to be more effective than heparin alone,[196] but there is no good evidence so far that the clinical outcome is better. This statement applies equally to other local intravascular techniques, such as rheolytic thrombectomy, which has been advocated in heparin-resistant, extensive CVT.[198,199] Therefore, there is reason to recommend local thrombolysis as the first-line treatment for CVT.[199,202] The question of local thrombolysis arises only if the condition of the patient worsens despite adequate anticoagulation and symptomatic treatment, provided that other causes of worsening, such as uncontrolled seizures, concomitant pulmonary embolism, and aggravation of an underlying condition, have been excluded.[197,200]

Summary

Treatment of CVT should be started as early as possible. It is based primarily on heparin, followed by warfarin. The efficacy of other modalities of antithrombotic treatment is at present anecdotal. Heparin therapy should be associated, whenever necessary, with symptomatic treatment (anticonvulsants and reduction of raised intracranial pressure) and, whenever possible, with etiologic treatment, such as antibiotics in septic cases.

CONCLUSION

Over the past 20 years, the better recognition of CVT has greatly modified our knowledge of this condition, and the range of underlying causes has also expanded. Studies have shown that treatment with heparin or even thrombolytics is safe in CVT. Because of its large variety of presentations, its highly variable mode of onset, its numerous causes, and its unpredictable outcome, however, CVT remains a diagnostic and therapeutic challenge.

References

1. Ribes MF: Des recherches faites sur la phlébite. Revue Médicale Française et Etrangère et Journal de Clinique de l'Hôtel-Dieu et de la Charité de Paris 3:5, 1825.
2. Bailey OT, Hass GM: Dural sinus thrombosis in early life, clinical manifestations and extent of brain injury in acute sinus thrombosis. J Pediatr 11:755, 1937.
3. Barnett HJM, Hyland HH: Noninfective intracranial venous thrombosis. Brain 76:36, 1953.
4. Ehlers H, Courville CB: Thrombosis of internal cerebral veins in infancy and childhood: Review of literature and report of five cases. J Pediatr 8:600, 1936.
5. Garcin R, Pestel M: Thrombophlébites Cérébrales. Paris, Masson, 1949.
6. Kalbag RM, Woolf AL: Cerebral Venous Thrombosis, vol 1. Oxford, Oxford University Press, 1967.
7. Krayenbühl H: Cerebral venous and sinus thrombosis. Clin Neurosurg 14:1, 1967.
8. Noetzel H, Jerusalem F: Die Hirnvenen und sinusthrombosen. Monographien aus dem Gesamtgebiete der Neurologie und Psychiatrie 106:1, 1965.
9. Symonds CP: Cerebral thrombophlebitis. BMJ 2:348, 1940.
10. Symonds CP: Hydrocephalic and focal cerebral symptoms in relation to thrombophlebitis of the dural sinuses and cerebral veins. Brain 60:531, 1937.
11. Anderson CM, Edelman RR, Turski PA: Magnetic resonance venography and cerebral venous thrombosis. Anderon CM, Edelman RR, Turski PA (eds): In Clinical Magnetic Resonance Angiography, Vol. 1. Philadelphia, Lippincott-Raven, 1993, p 289.
12. Ayanzen RH, Bird CR, Keller PJ: Cerebral MR venography: Normal anatomy and potential diagnostic pitfalls. Am J Neuroradiol 21:74, 2000.
13. Chu K, Kang DW, Yvon BW, et al: Diffusion-weighted magnetic resonance in cerebral venous thrombosis. Arch Neurol 58:1569, 2001.
14. Isensee CH, Reul J, Thron A: Magnetic resonance imaging of thrombosed dural sinuses. Stroke 25:29, 1994.
15. Keller E, Flacke S, Urbach H, et al: Diffusion and perfusion-weighted magnetic resonance imaging in deep cerebral venous thrombosis. Stroke 30:1144, 1999.
16. Krayenbühl H: Cerebral venous thrombosis: The diagnostic value of cerebral angiography. Schweiz Arch Neurol Neurochir Psychiatr 74:261, 1954.
17. Mas JL, Meder JF, Meary E, Bousser MG: Magnetic resonance imaging in lateral sinus hypoplasia and thrombosis. Stroke 21:1350, 1990.
18. Mattle HP, Wentz KU, Edelman RR, et al: Cerebral venography with MR. Radiology 178:453, 1991.
19. McMurdo SK, Brant-Zawadzki M, Bradley WG, et al: Dural sinus thrombosis study using intermediate field strength MR imaging. Radiology 161:83, 1986.
20. Medlock MD, Olivero WC, Hanigan WC, et al: Children with cerebral venous thrombosis diagnosed with magnetic resonance imaging and magnetic resonance angiography. Neurosurgery 31:870, 1992.
21. Padayachee TS, Bingham JB, Grave MJ, et al: Dural sinus thrombosis: Diagnosis and follow-up by magnetic resonance angiography and imaging. Neuroradiology 33:165, 1991.
22. Snyder TC, Sachdev HS: MR imaging of cerebral dural sinus thrombosis. J Comput Assist Tomogr 10:889, 1986.
23. Sze G, Simmons B, Krol G, et al: Dural sinus thrombosis: Verification with spin echo techniques. AJNR 9:679, 1988.
24. Thron A, Wessel K, Linden D, et al: Superior sagittal sinus thrombosis: Neuroradiological evaluation and clinical findings. J Neurol 233:283, 1986.
25. Tsai FY, Wang AM, Matovich V, et al: MR staging of acute dural sinus thrombosis: Correlation with venous pressure measurements and implications for treatment and prognosis. AJNR 16:1021, 1995.
26. Tsuruda JS, Shimakawa A, Pecl NJ, et al: Dural sinus occlusions: Evaluation with phase sensitive gradient echo MR imaging. AJNR 12:481, 1991.
27. Vogl TJ, Bergman C, Villringer A, et al: Dural sinus thrombosis: Value of venous MR angiography for diagnosis and follow-up. Am J Roentgenol 162:1191, 1994.
28. Vogl TJ, Hoffmann Y, Muhler A, et al: Contrast medium enhanced MR angiography. Radiologe 34:423, 1994.
29. Wang AM: MRA of venous sinus thrombosis. Clin Neurosci 4:158, 1997.
30. Bousser MG, Russell RR: Cerebral Venous Thrombosis. London, WB Saunders, 1997.
31. Hacker H: Normal supratentorial veins and dural sinuses. In Newton TH, Potts DG (eds): Radiology of the Skull and Brain. St. Louis, CV Mosby, 1974.
32. Huang YP, Wolf BS: Veins of posterior fossa—superior or galenic draining group. Am J Roentgenol Radiat Ther Nucl Med 95:808, 1965.
33. Huang YP, Wolf BS, Antin SP, Okudera T: The veins of the posterior fossa-anterior or petrosal draining group. Am J Roentgenol Radiat Ther Nucl Med 104:36, 1968.
34. Dinubile MJ: Septic thrombosis of the cavernous sinuses: Neurological review. Arch Neurol 45:567, 1988.
35. Bernstein R, Albers GW: Potential utility of diffusion-weighted imaging in venous infarction. Arch Neurol 58:1538, 2001.
36. Doege CA, Tavakolian R, Kerskens CM, et al: Perfusion and diffusion magnetic resonance imaging in human cerebral venous thrombosis. J Neurol 248:564, 2001.
37. Ducreux D, Oppenheim C, Vandamme W, et al: Diffusion-weighted imaging patterns of brain damage associated with cerebral venous thrombosis. AJNR 22:261, 2001.
38. Forbes KPN, Pipe JG, Heiserman JE. Evidence for cytotoxic edema in the pathogenesis of cerebral venous infarction. AJNR 22:450, 2001.
39. Lövblad KO, Bassetti C, Schneider J, et al: Diffusion-weighted MR in cerebral venous thrombosis. Cerebrovasc Dis 11:169, 2001.
40. Towbin A: The syndrome of latent cerebral venous thrombosis: Its frequency and relation to age and congestive heart failure. Stroke 4:419, 1973.
41. Averback P: Primary cerebral venous thrombosis in young adults: The diverse manifestations of an underrecognized disease. Ann Neurol 3:81, 1978.
42. Ameri A, Bousser MG: Cerebral venous thrombosis. Neurol Clin 10:876, 1992.
43. Bansal BC, Gupta RR, Prakash C: Stroke during pregnancy and puerperium in young females below the age of 40 years as a result of cerebral venous/sinus thrombosis. Jpn Heart J 21:171, 1980.

44. Barinagarrementeria F, Cantu C, Arredondo H: Aseptic cerebral venous thrombosis: Proposed prognostic scale. J Stroke Cerebrovasc Dis 2:34, 1992.

45. Bousser MG, Chiras J, Sauron B, et al: Cerebral venous thrombosis: A review of 38 cases. Stroke 16:199, 1985.

46. Daif A, Awada A, Al-Rajeh S, et al: Cerebral venous thrombosis in adult: A study of 40 cases from Saudi Arabia. Stroke 26:1193, 1995.

47. De Bruijn SF, Stam J, Vandenbroucke JP: Increased risk of cerebral venous sinus thrombosis with third-generation oral contraceptive. Cerebral Venous Sinus Thrombosis Study Group. Lancet 351:1404, 1998.

48. Einhäupl KM, Masuhr F: Cerebral venous and sinus thrombosis: An update. Eur J Neurol 1:109, 1994.

49. Einhäupl KM, Villringer A, Habert RL, et al: Clinical spectrum of sinus venous thrombosis. In Einhäupl KM, Kempski O, Baethmann A (eds): Cerebral Sinus Thrombosis: Experimental and Clinical Aspects. New York, Plenum Press, 1990, p 149.

50. Enevoldson TP, Russell RW: Cerebral venous thrombosis: New causes for an old syndrome. Q J Med 77:1255, 1990.

51. Cantu C, Barinagarrementeria F: Cerebral venous thrombosis associated with pregnancy and puerperium: Review of 67 cases. Stroke 24:1880, 1993.

52. De Bruijn SFTM, de Haan RJ, Stam J: Clinical features and prognostic factors of cerebral venous sinus thrombosis in a prospective series of 59 patients. J Neurol Neurosurg Psychiatry 70:105, 2001.

53. Ferro JM, Correia M, Pontes C, et al: Cerebral vein and dural sinus thrombosis in Portugal: 1980–1988. Cerebrovasc Dis 11:177, 2001.

54. Milandre L, Gueriot C, Girard N, et al: Les thromboses veineuses cérébrales de l'adulte. Ann Med Intern 139:544, 1988.

55. Rondepierre P, Hamon M, Leys D, et al: Thromboses veineuses cérébrales: étude de l'évolution. Rev Neurol (Paris) 151:100, 1995.

56. Rousseaux P, Bernard MH, Scherpereel B, et al: Thrombose des sinus veineux intra-crâniens (à propos de 22 cas). Neurochirurgie 24:197, 1978.

57. Canhao P, Barinagarrementeria F, Bousser MG, et al: International study on cerebral vein thrombosis. Cerebrovasc Dis 11(suppl 4):31, 2001.

58. DeVeber G, Andrew M, Adams C, et al: Cerebral sinovenous thrombosis in children. N Engl J Med 345:417, 2001.

59. Bousser MG: Cerebral venous thrombosis: diagnosis and management. J Neurol 247:252, 2000.

60. Villringer A, Bousser MG, Einhäupl KM: Cerebral sinus venous thrombosis. In Hacke W (ed): Neurocritical Care, vol 1. Berlin, Springer-Verlag, 1994, p 654.

61. Sekhar LN, Dujovny M, Rao GR: Carotid cavernous sinus thrombosis caused by *Aspergillus fumigatus*. J Neurosurg 52:120, 1980.

62. Evans RW, Patten BM: Trichinosis associated with superior sagittal sinus thrombosis. Ann Neurol 11:216, 1982.

63. Meyohas MC, Roullet E: Cerebral venous thrombosis and dural primary infection with human immunodeficiency virus and cytomegalovirus. J Neurol Neurosurg Psychiatry 52:1010, 1989.

64. Estanol B, Rodriguez A, Conte G, et al: Intracranial venous thrombosis in young women. Stroke 10:680, 1979.

65. Lamy C, Hamon JB, Coste J, et al: Ischemic stroke in young women: Risk of recurrence during subsequent pregnancies. French Study Group on Stroke in Pregnancy. Neurology 55:269, 2000.

66. Martin JP, Sheenan HL: Primary thrombosis of cerebral veins (following childbirth). BMJ 1:349, 1941.

67. Buchanan DS, Brazinsky JH: Dural sinus and cerebral venous thrombosis: Incidence in young women receiving oral contraceptives. Arch Neurol 22:440, 1970.

68. De Bruijn SF, Stam J, Koopman MMW, et al: Case-control study of risk of cerebral sinus thrombosis in oral contraceptive users who are carriers of hereditary prothrombotic conditions. Cerebral Venous Sinus Thrombosis Study Group. BMJ 316:589, 1998.

69. Fairburn B: Intracranial venous thrombosis complicating oral contraception: Treatment by anticoagulant drugs. BMJ 2:647, 1973.

70. Martinelli I, Sacchi E, Landi G, et al: High risk of cerebral vein thrombosis in carriers of prothrombin-gene mutation and in users of oral conraceptives. N Engl J Med 338:1793, 1998.

71. Poltera AA: The pathology of intracranial venous thrombosis in oral contraception. J Pathol 106:209, 1972.

72. Biousse V, Conard J, Brouzes C, et al: Frequency of the 20210 G→A mutation in the 3'-untranslated region of the prothrombin gene in 35 cases of cerebral venous thrombosis. Stroke 29:1398, 1998

73. Deschiens MA, Conard J, Horellou MH, et al: Coagulation studies, factor V Leiden, and antiphospholipid antibodies in 40 cases of cerebral venous thrombosis. Stroke 27:1724, 1996.

74. Wechsler B, Vidailhet M, Piette JC, et al: Cerebral venous thrombosis in Behçet's disease: Clinical study and long-term follow-up of 25 cases. Neurology 42:614, 1992.

75. Bertina RM, Koeleman BPLC, Koiser T, et al: Mutation in blood coagulation factor V associated with resistance to activated protein C. Nature 369:64, 1994.

76. Brey RL, Coull BM: Cerebral venous thrombosis: Role of activated protein C resistance and factor V gene mutation. Stroke 27:1719, 1996.

77. Dahlback B, Carlsson M, Svensson PJ: Familial thrombophilia due to a previously unrecognized mechanism characterized by poor anticoagulant response to activated protein C. Proc Natl Acad Sci U S A 90:1004, 1993.

78. Engesser L, Broekmans AW, Briet E, et al: Hereditary protein S deficiency: Clinical manifestations. Ann Intern Med 106:31, 1987.

79. Huberfeld G, Kubis N, Lot G, et al: G20210A prothrombin gene mutation in two siblings with cerebral venous thrombosis. Neurology 51:316, 1998.

80. Ludeman P, Nabavi DG, Junker R, et al: Factor V Leiden mutation is a risk factor for cerebral venous thrombosis: A case-control study of 55 patients Stroke 29:2507, 1998.

81. Martinelli I, Landi G, Merati G, et al: Factor V gene mutation is a risk factor for cerebral venous thrombosis. Thromb Haemost 75:393, 1996.

82. Reuner KH, Ruf A, Grau A, et al: Prothrombin gene G 20210→A transition is a risk factor for cerebral venous thrombosis Stroke 29:1765, 1998.

83. Vielhaber N, Ehrenforth S, Koch HC, et al: Cerebral venous sinus thrombosis in infancy and childhood: Role of genetic and acquired risk factors of thrombophilia. Eur J Pediatr 157:555, 1998.

84. Weih M, Vetter B, Ziemer S, et al: Increased rate of factor V Leiden mutation in patients with cerebral venous thrombosis. J Neurol 245:149, 1998.

85. Weih M, Mehraein S, Valdueza JM, et al: Coincidence of factor V Leiden mutation and a mutation in the prothrombin gene at position 20210 in a patient with puerperal cerebral venous thrombosis. Stroke 29:1739, 1998.

86. Zuber M, Toulon P, Marnet L, et al: Factor V Leiden mutation in cerebral venous thrombosis. Stroke 27:1721, 1996.

87. Sauron B, Chiras J, Chain G, et al: Thrombophlébite cérébelleuse chez un homme porteur d'un déficit familial en antithrombine III. Rev Neurol (Paris) 138:685, 1982.

88. Tarras S, Gadia C, Mester L, et al: Homozygous protein C deficiency in a newborn: Clinicopathologic correlation. Arch Neurol 45:214, 1988.

89. Azzarelli B, Itani AL, Catanzaro PT: Cerebral phlebothrombosis: A complication of lymphoma. Arch Neurol 37:126, 1980.

90. Feinberg WM, Swenson MR: Cerebrovascular complications of L-asparaginase therapy. Neurology 38:127, 1988.

91. Hickey WF, Garnick MB, Henderson JC, Dawson DM: Primary cerebral venous thrombosis in patients with cancer—a rarely diagnosed paraneoplastic syndrome. Am J Med 73:740, 1982.

92. Meininger V, James JM, Rio B, Zittoun R: Occlusions des sinus veineux de la dure-mère au cours des hémopathies. Rev Neurol (Paris) 141:228, 1985.

93. Smith WDF, Sinar J, Carey M: Sagittal sinus thrombosis and occult malignancy. J Neurol Neurosurg Psychiatry 46:187, 1983.

94. Bousser MG, Bletry O, Launay M, et al: Thrombose veineuse cérébrale au cours de la maladie de Behçet: A propos de deux cas. Revue Neurol (Paris) 136:753, 1980.

95. Levine SR, Kieran S, Puzio K, et al: Cerebral venous thrombosis with lupus anticoagulants: Report of 2 cases. Stroke 18:801, 1987.

96. Vidailhet M, Piette JC, Wechsler B, et al: Cerebral venous thrombosis in systemic lupus erythematosus: Report of 6 cases and review. Stroke 21:1226, 1990.

97. Rivkin MJ, Anderson ML, Kaye EM: Neonatal idiopathic cerebral venous thrombosis: An unrecognized cause of transient seizures or lethargy. Ann Neurol 32:51, 1992.

98. Shevell MI, Silver K, O'Gorman AM, et al: Neonatal dural sinus thrombosis. Pediatr Neurol 5:161, 1989.

99. Barthelemy M, Bousser MG, Jacobs C: Thrombose veineuse cérébrale au cours d'un syndrome néphrotique. Nouv Presse Med 9:367, 1980.

100. Biousse V, Ameri A, Bousser MG: Isolated intracranial hypertension as the only sign of cerebral venous thrombosis. Neurology 53:1537, 1999.

101. Tehindrazanarivelo AD, Evrard S, Schaison M, et al: Prospective study of cerebral sinus venous thrombosis in patients presenting with benign intracranial hypertension. Cerebrovasc Dis 2:22, 1992.

102. Ray BS, Dunbar HS: Thrombosis of dural venous sinuses as cause of "pseudotumor cerebri." Ann Surg 134:376, 1951.

103. Curnes JT, Creasy JL, Whaley RL, Scatliff JH: Air in the cavernous sinus thrombosis [letter]. AJNR 8:176, 1987.

104. Levine SR, Twyman RE, Gilman S: The role of anticoagulation in cavernous sinus thrombosis. Neurology 38:517, 1988.

105. Aidi S, Chaunu MP, Biousse V, et al: Changing pattern of headache pointing to cerebral venous thrombosis after lumbar puncture and intravenous high-dose corticosteroids. Headache 39:559, 1999.

106. Ferro JM, Falcao F, Melo TP et al: Dural sinus thrombosis mimicking "capsular warning syndrome." J Neurol 247:802, 2000

107. De Bruijn SF, Stam J, Kappelle LJ: Thunderclap headache as first symptom of cerebral venous thrombosis. Lancet 348:1623, 1996.

108. Crassard I, Biousse V, Meyer B, et al: Hearing loss revealing lateral sinus thrombosis in a patient with factor V Leiden mutation. Stroke 28:876, 1997.

109. Kuehnen J, Schwartz A, Neff W, et al: Cranial nerve syndrome in thrombosis of the transverse/sigmoid sinuses. Brain 121:381, 1998.

110. Straub J, Magistris MR, Delavelle J, et al: Facial palsy in cerebral venous thrombosis transcranial stimulation and pathophysiological considerations. Stroke 31:1766, 2000.

111. Goldberg AL, Rosenbaum AE, Wang H, et al: Computed tomography of dural sinus thrombosis. J Comput Assist Tomogr 10:16, 1986.

112. Jacobs K, Moulin T, Bogousslavsky J, et al: The stroke syndrome of cortical vein thrombosis. Neurology 47:376, 1996.

113. Eick JJ, Miller KD, Bell KA, et al: Computed tomography of deep cerebral venous thrombosis in children. Radiology 140:399, 1981.

114. Johnsen S, Greenwood R, Fischman MA: Internal cerebral vein thrombosis. Arch Neurol 28:205, 1973.

115. Bots GAM: Thrombosis of the galenic system veins in the adult. Acta Neuropathol 17:227, 1971.

116. Baumgartner RW, Landi T: Venous thalamic infarction. Cerebrovasc Dis 2:353, 1992.

117. Haley EC, Brasmear HR, Barth JT, et al: Deep cerebral venous thrombosis: Clinical, neuroradiological and neuropsychological correlates. Arch Neurol 46:337, 1989.

118. Kim KS, Walczak TS: Computed tomography of deep cerebral venous thrombosis. J Comput Assist Tomogr 10:386, 1986.

119. Murray BJ, Llinas R, Caplan LR, et al: Cerebral deep venous thrombosis presenting as acute micrographia and hypophonia. Neurology 54:751, 2000.

120. Alecu C, de Bray JM, Penisson-Besnier I, et al: Trismus, syndrome pseudobulbaire et thrombose veineuse profonde cérébrale. Rev Neurol 157:309, 2001.

121. Lacour JC, Ducrocq X, Anxionnat R, et al: Les thromboses veineuses profondes de l'encéphale de l'adulte: Aspects cliniques et approche diagnostique. Rev Neurol (Paris) 156:739, 2000.

122. Eng LJ, Longstreth WT, Shaw CM, et al: Cerebellar venous infarction: Case report with clinicopathologic correlation. Neurology 40:837, 1990.

123. Nayak AK, Karnad D, Mahajan MV, et al: Cerebellar venous infarction in chronic suppurative otitis media: A case report with review of four other cases. Stroke 25:1958, 1994.

124. Rousseaux M, Lesoin F, Barbaste P, et al: Infarctus cérébelleux pseudo-tumoral d'origine veineuse. Rev Neurol (Paris) 144:209, 1988.

125. Girard DE, Reuler JB, Mayer BS, et al: Cerebral venous sinus thrombosis due to indwelling transvenous pacemaker catheter. Arch Neurol 37:113, 1980.

126. Anderson SC, Shah CP, Murtagh FR: Congested deep subcortical veins as a sign of dural venous thrombosis: MR and CT correlations. J Comput Assist Tomogr 11:1059, 1987.

127. Brant-Zawadzki M, Chang GY, McCarty GE: Computed tomography in dural sinus thrombosis. Arch Neurol 39:446, 1982.

128. Brismar J: Computed tomography in superior sagittal sinus thrombosis. Acta Radiol (Stockh) 21:321, 1980.

129. Buonanno F, Moody DM, Ball MR, Laster DW: Computed cranial tomographic findings in cerebral sino-venous occlusion. J Comput Assist Tomogr 2:281, 1978.

130. Buonanno FS, Moody DM, Ball RM: CT scan findings in cerebral sinovenous occlusion. Neurology 12:288, 1982.

131. Chiras J, Bousser MG, Meder JF, et al: CT in cerebral thrombophlebitis. Neuroradiology 27:145, 1985.

132. De Slegte RGM, Kaiser MC, van der Baan S, Smit L: Computed tomographic diagnosis of septic sinus thrombosis and their complications. Neuroradiology 30:160, 1988.

133. Ford K, Sarwar M: Computed tomography of dural sinus thrombosis. AJNR 2:539, 1981.

133. Kingsley DPE, Kendall BE, Moseley LF: Superior sagittal sinus thrombosis, an evaluation of the changes demonstrated on computed tomography. J Neurol Neurosurg Psychiatry 41:1065, 1978.

134. Rao KCVG, Knipp HC, Wagner EJ: CT findings in cerebral sinus and venous thrombosis. Radiology 140:391, 1981.

135. Segall HD, Ahmadi J, McComb JG, et al: Computed tomographic observations pertinent to intracranial venous thrombotic and occlusive disease in childhood. Radiology 143:441, 1982.

136. Kinal ME: Traumatic thrombosis of dural venous sinuses in closed head injuries. J Neurosurg 27:142, 1967.

136. Shinohara Y, Yositomoshi M, Yoshii F: Appearance and disappearance of empty delta sign in superior sagittal sinus thrombosis. Stroke 17:1282, 1986.

137. Ur Rahman N, Al-Tahan AR: Computed tomographic evidence of an extensive thrombosis and infarction of the deep venous system. Stroke 24:744, 1993.

138. Vines FS, Davis DO: Clinical radiological correlation in cerebral venous occlusive disease. Radiology 98:9,1971.

139. Virapongse C, Cazenave C, Quisling R, et al: The empty delta sign: Frequency and significance in 76 cases of dural sinus thrombosis. Radiology 162:779, 1987.

140. Yasargil MG, Damur M: Thrombosis of the cerebral veins and dural sinuses. In Newton TH, and Potts DG (eds): Radiology of the Skull and Brain. St. Louis, CV Mosby, 1974.

141. Mas JL, Meder JF, Meary E: Dural sinus thrombosis: Long term follow-up by magnetic resonance imaging. Cerebrovasc Dis 2:137, 1992.

142. Mattle H, Edelkman RR, Reis MA, Atkinson DJ: Flow quantification in the superior sagittal sinus using magnetic resonance. Neurology 40:813, 1990.

143. Rippe DJ, Boyko OB, Spritzer CE, et al: Demonstration of dural sinus occlusion by the use of MR angiography. AJNR 11:199, 1990.

144. Casey SO, Alberico RA, Patel M: Cerebral CT venography. Radiology 198:163, 1996.

145. Dormont D, Anxionnat R, Evrard S, et al: MRI in cerebral venous thrombosis. J Neuroradiol 21:81, 1994.

146. Dormont D, Sag K, Biondi A, et al: Gadolinium-enhanced MR of chronic dural sinus thrombosis. AJNR 16:1347, 1995.

147. Macchi PJ, Grossman RI, Gomori JM, et al: High field MR imaging of cerebral venous thrombosis. J Comput Assist Tomogr 10:10, 1986.

148. Savino PJ, Grossman RI, Schatz NJ, et al: High field magnetic resonance imaging in the diagnosis of cavernous sinus thrombosis. Arch Neurol 43:1081, 1986.

149. Manzione J, Newman GC, Shapiro A, et al: Diffusion and perfusion weighted MR imaging of dural sinus thrombosis. AJNR 21:68, 2000.

150. Hsu LC, Lirng JF, Fuh JL, et al: Proton magnetic resonance spectroscopy in deep cerebral venous thrombosis. Clin Neurol Neurosurg 100:27, 1998.

151. Barnes BD, Winestock DP: Dynamic radionuclide scanning in the diagnosis of thrombosis of the superior sagittal sinus thrombosis. Neurology 27:656, 1977.

152. Bridgers SL, Strauss E, Smith EO, et al: Demonstration of superior sagittal sinus thrombosis by indium 111 platelet scintigraphy. Arch Neurol 43:1079, 1986.

153. Valdueza JM, Schultz M, Harms L, et al: Venous transcranial Doppler ultrasound monitoring in acute dural sinus thrombosis: Report of two cases. Stroke 26:1196, 1995.

154. Valdueza JM, Harms L, Doepp F, et al: Venous microembolic signals detected in patients with cerebral sinus thrombosis. Stroke 28:1607, 1997.

155. Valdueza JM, Hoffmann O, Weih M, et al: Monitoring of venous hemodynamics in patients with cerebral venous thrombosis by transcranial Doppler. Arch Neurol 25:229, 1999.

156. Wardlaw JM, Vaughan GT, Steers AJW, et al: Transcranial Doppler ultrasound findings in venous sinus thrombosis. J Neurosurg 80:332, 1994.

Clinical Manifestations

157. Canhao P, Batista P, Ferro JM: Venous transcranial Doppler in acute dural sinus thrombosis. J Neurol 245:276, 1998.

158. Diaz JM, Schiffman JS, Urban ES, Maccario M: Superior sagittal sinus thrombosis and pulmonary embolism: A syndrome rediscovered. Acta Neurol Scand 86:390, 1992.

159. de Bruijn SFTM, Budde M, Teunisse S, et al: Long-term outcome of cognition and functional health after cerebral venous thrombosis. Neurology 54:1687, 2000.

160. Barron TF, Gusnard DA, Simmermann RA, Clancy RR: Cerebral venous thrombosis in neonates and children. Pediatr Neurol 8:112, 1992.

161. Preter M, Tzourio C, Ameri A, et al: Long term prognosis in cerebral venous thrombosis: A follow up of 77 patients. Stroke 27:243, 1996.

162. Houser OW, Campbell JK, Campbell RJ, et al: Arteriovenous malformation affecting the transverse dural venous sinus: An acquired lesion. Mayo Clin Proc 54:651, 1979.

163. Kutluk K, Schumacher M, Mironov A: The role of sinus thrombosis in occipital dural arteriovenous malformations: Development and spontaneous closure. Neurochirurgia 34:144, 1991.

164. Villringer A, Meraein S, Einhäupl KM: Treatment of sinus venous thrombosis—beyond the recommendation of anticoagulation. J Neuroradiol 21:72, 1994.

165. Stam J: Treatment of cerebral venous thrombosis. Cerebrovasc Dis 3:329, 1993.

166. Feldenzer JA, Bueche MJ, Venes JL, Gebarski SS: Superior sagittal sinus thrombosis with infarction in sickle cell trait. Stroke 18:656, 1987.

167. Hanley DF, Feldman E, Borel CO, et al: Treatment of sagittal sinus thrombosis associated with cerebral hemorrhage and intracranial hypertension. Stroke 19:903, 1988.

168. Stansfield FR: Puerperal cerebral thrombophlebitis treated by heparin. BMJ 1:436, 1942.

169. De Bruijn SF, Stam J, for the Cerebral Venous Sinus Thrombosis Study Group: Randomized placebo controlled trial of anticoagulant treatment with low molecular weight heparin for cerebral sinus thrombosis. Stroke 30:484, 1999.

170. Gettelfinger DM, Kokmen E: Superior sagittal sinus thrombosis. Arch Neurol 34:2, 1977.

171. Halpern JP, Morris JGL, Driscoll GL: Anticoagulants and cerebral venous thrombosis. Aust N Z J Med 14:643, 1984.

172. Brucker AB, Vollert-Rogenhofer H, Wagner M, et al: Heparin treatment in acute cerebral sinus venous thrombosis: A retrospective clinical and MR analysis of 42 cases. Cerebrovasc Dis 8:331, 1998.

173. DeVeber G, Chan A, Monagle P, et al: Anticoagulation therapy in pediatric patients with sinovenous thrombosis: A cohort study. Arch Neurol 55:1533, 1998.

174. Einhäupl KM, Villringer A, Meister W, et al: Heparin treatment in sinus venous thrombosis. Lancet 338:597, 1991.

175. Fink JN, McAuley DL: Safety of anticoagulation for cerebral venous thrombosis associated with intracerebral hematoma. Neurology 57:1138, 2001.

176. Greitz T, Link H: Aseptic thrombosis of intracranial sinuses. Radiol Clin Biol 35:111, 1966.

177. Bousser MG: Cerebral venous thrombosis: Nothing, heparin, or local thrombosis ? Stroke 30:481, 1999.

178. Barnwell SL, Higashida RT, Halbach VV, et al: Direct endovascular thrombolytic therapy for dural sinus thrombosis. Neurosurgery 28:135, 1991.

179. D'Alise MD, Fichtel F, Horowitz M, et al: Sagittal sinus thrombosis following minor head injury treated with continuous urokinase infusion. Surg Neurol 49:430,1998.

180. DiRocco C, Lanelli A, Leone G, et al: Heparin-urokinase treatment in a septic dural sinus thrombosis. Arch Neurol 38:431, 1981.

181. Frey JL, Muro GJ, McDougall CG, et al: Cerebral venous thrombosis: Combined intrathrombus rTPA and intravenous heparin. Stroke 30:489, 1999.

182. Gerszten PC, Welch WC, Spearman MP, et al: Isolated deep cerebral venous thrombosis treated by direct endovascular thrombolysis. Surg Neurol 48:261, 1997.

183. Holder CA, Bell DA, Lundell AL, et al: Isolated straight sinus and deep cerebral venous thrombosis: Successful treatment with local infusion of urokinase. Case report. J Neurosurg 86:704; 1997.

184. Horowitz M, Purdy P, Unwin H, et al: Treatment of dural sinus thrombosis using elective catheterization and urokinase. Ann Neurol 38:58, 1995.

185. Kim SY, Suh JH: Direct endovascular thrombolytic therapy for dural sinus thrombosis: Infusion of alteplase. AJNR Am J Neuroradiol 18:639, 1997.

186. Kuether TA, O'Neill O, Nesbit GM, Barnwell SL: Endovascular treatment of traumatic dural sinus thrombosis: Case report. Neurosurgery 42:1163, 1998.

187. Niwa J, Ohyama H, Matumura S, et al: Treatment of acute superior sagittal sinus thrombosis by rt-PA infusion via venography—direct thrombolytic therapy in the acute phase. Surg Neurol 49:425, 1998.

188. Philips MF, Bagley LJ, Sinson GP, et al: Endovascular thrombolysis for symptomatic cerebral venous thrombosis. J Neurosurg 90:65, 1999.

189. Rael JR, Orrison WW Jr, Baldwin N, et al: Direct thrombolysis of superior sagittal sinus thrombosis with coexisting intracranial hemorrhage. AJNR Am J Neuroradiol 18:1238, 1997.

190. Renowden SA, Oxbury J, Molyneux AJ: Case report: Venous sinus thrombosis: The use of thrombolysis. Clin Radiol 52:396, 1997.

191. Scott JA, Pascuzzi RM, Hall PV, et al: Treatment of dural sinus thrombosis with local urokinase infusion. J Neurosurg 68:284, 1988.

192. Smith AG, Cornblath WT, Deveikis JP: Local thrombolytic therapy in deep cerebral venous thrombosis. Neurology 48:1613, 1997.

193. Smith TP, Higashida R, Barnwell S, et al: Treatment of dural sinus thrombosis by urokinase infusion. AJNR 15:801, 1994.

194. Tsai FY, Higashida RT, Matovich V, et al: Acute thrombosis of the intracranial dural sinus: direct thrombolytic treatment. AJNR 13:1137, 1992.

195. Wasay M, Bakshi R, Kojan S, et al: Superior sagittal sinus thrombosis due to lithium: Local urokinase thrombolysis treatment. Neurology 54:532, 2000.

196. Wasay M, Bakshi R, Kojan S, et al: Nonrandomised comparison of local urokinase thrombolysis versus systemic heparin anticoagulation for superior sagittal sinus thrombosis. Stroke 32:2310, 2001.

197. Canhao P, Ferro J: Thrombolytics for cerebral sinus thrombosis: A systematic review. Cerebrovasc Dis 11(suppl 4):122, 2001.

298. Chow K, Gobin P, Saver J, et al: Endovascular treatment of dural sinus thrombosis with rheolytic thrombectomy and intra-arterial thrombolysis. Stroke 31:1420, 2000.

299. Dowd CF, Malek AM, Phatouros CC, et al: Application of a rheolytic thrombectomy device in the treatment of dural sinus thrombosis: A new technique. AJNR Am J Neuroradiol 20:568, 1999.

200. Benamer HTS, Bone I: Cerebral venous thrombosis: Anticoagulants or thrombolytic therapy? J Neurol Neurosurg Psychiatry 69:427, 2000.

201. Pfister HW, Borasio GD, Dirnagl V, et al: Cerebrovascular complications of bacterial meningitis in adults. Neurology 42:1497, 1992.

202. El Alaoui Faris M, Birouk N, Slassi I, et al: Thrombose du sinus longitudinal supérieur et ostéite cranienne syphilitique. Rev Neurol 148:783, 1992.

203. van Dyke DC, Eldalah MK, Bale JF, et al: *Mycoplasma pneumoniae*-induced cerebral venous thrombosis treated with urokinase. Clin Pediatr (Phila) 31:501, 1992.

204. Ergan M, Hansen von Bunau F, Courtheoux P, et al: Cerebral vein thrombosis after an intrathecal glucocorticoid injection. Rev Rhum Engl Ed 64:513, 1997.

205. Brown MT, Friedeman HS, Oakes WJ, et al: Sagittal sinus thrombosis and leptomeningeal medulloblastoma. Neurology 41:455, 1991.

206. Nadel L, Braun IF, Muizelaar JP, et al: Tumoral thrombosis of cerebral venous sinuses: Preoperative diagnosis using magnetic resonance phase imaging. Surg Neurol 35:189, 1991.

207. Souter RG, Mitchell A: Spreading venous cortical thrombosis due to infusion of hyperosmolar solution into the internal jugular vein. BMJ 285:935, 1982.

208. Patel A, Lo R: Electric injury with cerebral venous thrombosis: Case report and review of the literature. Stroke 24:903, 1993.

209. Patchell RA, Posner JB: Neurologic complications of carcinoid. Neurology 36:745, 1986.

210. Al Hakim M, Katirji MB, Osorio I, Weisman R: Cerebral venous thrombosis in paroxysmal nocturnal hemoglobinuria: Report of two cases. Neurology 43:742, 1993.

211. Van Vleymen B, de Haenne I, van Hoof A, et al: Cerebral venous thrombosis in paroxysmal nocturnal haemoglobinuria. Acta Neurol Belg 87:80, 1987.

212. Jacquin V, Salama J, Le Roux G, Delaporte P: Thromboses veineuses cérébrales et des membres supérieurs associées à une thrombopénie, induites par le polysulfate de pentosane. Ann Med Intern 139:194, 1988.

213. Meyer-Lindenberg A: Fatal cerebral venous sinus thrombosis in heparin induced thrombotic thrombocytopenia. Eur Neurol 37:191, 1997.

214. Schutta HS, Williams EC, Baranski BG, et al: Cerebral venous thrombosis with plasminogen deficiency. Stroke 22:401, 1991.

215. Achiron A, Gornish M, Melamed E: Cerebral sinus thrombosis as a potential hazard of antifibrinolytic treatment in menorrhagia. Stroke 21:817, 1990.

216. Norlund L, Zoller B, Ohlin AK: A novel thrombomodulin gene mutation in a patient suffering from sagittal sinus thrombosis. Thromb Haemost 78:1164, 1997.

217. Carhuapoma JR, Mitsias P, Levine SR: Cerebral venous thrombosis and anticardiolipin antibodies. Stroke 28:2163, 1997.

218. Yerby MS, Bailey GM: Superior sagittal sinus thrombosis 10 years after surgery for ulcerative colitis. Stroke 11:294, 1980.

219. Mickle JP, McLennan JE, Lidden CW: Cortical vein thrombosis in Wegener's granulomatosis. J Neurosurg 46:248, 1977.

220. Urban E, Jabbari B, Robles H: Concurrent cerebral venous sinus thrombosis and myeloradiculopathy in Sjögren syndrome. Neurology 44:554, 1994.

221. Hughes JP, Stovin PG: Segmental pulmonary artery aneurysms with peripheral venous thrombosis. Br J Dis Chest 53:19, 1959.

222. Byrne JV, Lawton CA: Meningeal sarcoidosis causing intracranial hypertension secondary to dural sinus thrombosis. Br J Radiol 56:755, 1983.

223. Eikmeier G, Kuhlmann R, Gastpar M, et al: Thrombosis of cerebral veins following intravenous application of clomipramine. J Neurol Neurosurg Psychiatry 52:1461, 1989.

224. Shiozawa Z, Yamada H, Mabuchi C, et al: Superior sagittal sinus thrombosis associated with androgen therapy for hypoplastic anaemia. Ann Neurol 12:578, 1982.

225. Rothwell PM, Grant R: Cerebral venous sinus thrombosis induced by "ecstasy." J Neurol Neurochir Psychiatry 56:1035, 1993.

226. Cochran FB, Packman S: Homocystinuria presenting as sagittal sinus thrombosis. Eur Neurol 32:1, 1992.

227. Siegert CEH, Smelt AHM, De Bruin TWA: Superior sagittal sinus thrombosis and thyrotoxicosis. Possible association in two cases. Stroke 26:496, 1995.

228. Finelli PF, Carley MD: Cerebral venous thrombosis associated with epoetin alfa therapy. Arch Neurol 57:260, 2000.

Clinical Manifestations

Chapter Thirteen

Intracerebral Hemorrhage

Carlos S. Kase, J. P. Mohr, and Louis R. Caplan

EPIDEMIOLOGY

Intracerebral hemorrhage (ICH) occurs as a result of bleeding from an arterial source directly into the brain substance. Although its relative frequency in patients with stroke is subject to geographic and racial variations, values between 5% and 10% are most commonly quoted.[1–3] In a consecutive series of 938 patients with stroke entered into the National Institute of Neurological and Communicative Diseases and Stroke (NINCDS) Data Bank, primary ICH accounted for 10.7% of the cases.[4] Similar figures were obtained in population or community studies from Denmark (10.4%),[5] Holland (9%),[6] Oxfordshire, England (10%),[7] and southern Alabama (8%).[8] The incidence of ICH increases with advancing age,[3,9] a feature that applies to all types of stroke, both ischemic and hemorrhagic.

The incidence rates are relatively constant in predominantly white populations, with rates between 7 and 11 cases per 100,000 (Table 13.1).[9–13] The figures were higher in a U.S. population (southern Alabama) with a mixture of white and black people, because the former had an incidence rate of 12 per 100,000, whereas in blacks the rate was 32 per 100,000.[8] Similar comparisons between white and black people in Cincinnati, Ohio, yielded an overall age- and sex-adjusted incidence of ICH that was 1.4-fold higher in black people.[9] The difference in ICH incidence was even higher (2.3-fold) for black persons who were younger than 75 years. Also, a Hispanic population in New Mexico had a high incidence of ICH (34.9/100,000), whereas non-Hispanic whites from the same population had an incidence rate (16.6/100,000) comparable to that of whites in other geographic locations.[14] Some series from Asian countries, such as that from Shibata, Japan,[15] report severalfold higher incidence rates of ICH (61/100,000).

Along with these differing incidence rates from various geographic locations, a general trend toward declining rates of ICH has been detected, starting in the 1960s with the initial observation in Göteborg, Sweden,[16] and subsequently confirmed in the United States in the population of Rochester, Minnesota.[10,17] From analysis of data encompassing a 32-year period (1945 to 1976), Furlan and associates[10] showed a significant decrease in incidence between the first and second parts of this period: 13.3 per 100,000 for 1945 to 1960 and 6.7 per 100,000 for 1961 to 1976. These figures correlated with a similar decline in the frequency and severity of hypertension in the population studied. A similarly declining trend in the incidence of ICH has been reported from Hisayama, Japan,[18] where it was also related to a decrease in the frequency of hypertension.

The role of *hypertension* as a leading risk factor is well established, and its frequency has been estimated to be between 72%[2,10,19] and 81%.[2,10,19] The causative role of hypertension is supported by the high frequency of left ventricular hypertrophy in autopsy cases of ICH[20–22] and the significantly higher admission blood pressure readings in patients with ICH than in those with other forms of stroke.[23] The autopsy study by McCormick and Rosenfield[24] challenged the view that hypertension represents the main causative factor in ICH. Their series included a large number of cases of ICH due to blood dyscrasias, vascular malformations, and tumors, and hypertension was regarded as the sole basis for the bleeding in only 25% of the total. This difference from most reported series of ICH may reflect a referral pattern bias in this series as well as more stringent criteria for establishing a causal relationship between hypertension and ICH. However, clinical series have also questioned the validity of the concept of ICH as a condition most commonly related to hypertension. Brott and colleagues[12] found a history of hypertension in only 45% of 154 patients, a figure that rose to only 56% when electrocardiographic or chest radiographic evidence of cardiomegaly were added to criteria for the diagnosis of hypertension. Similarly, Schütz and associates[13] labeled only 59% of their cases of ICH as due to hypertension. Certain subgroups of hypertensive patients, however, appear to be at particularly high risk for ICH. They include subjects who are 55 years or younger, smokers, and those who have stopped taking their antihypertensive medications.[25] Finally, the beneficial effects of antihypertensive treatment with regard to risk of ICH have been documented in the PROGRESS (Perindopril Protection Against Recurrent Stroke Study) trial[26]: The combination of the ACE inhibitor perindopril and the diuretic indapamide resulted in a 76% relative risk reduction of ICH in comparison with the placebo-treated group after 4 years of follow-up.

A number of other risk factors in addition to advancing age, hypertension, and race have been evaluated, including cigarette smoking, alcohol consumption, and serum cholesterol levels. Abbott and coworkers[27] showed a higher

Table 13.1 Incidence of Intracerebral Hemorrhage in Studies from Various Geographic Locations

Location	Chapter Reference	No. of Cases	Rate*
Rochester, Minnesota	11	81	7
Framingham, Massachusetts	3	58	10
Southern Alabama	8	13	12
Cincinnati, Ohio	12	154	11
Giessen, Germany	13	100	11
Shibata, Japan	15	97	61
Bernalillo Co., New Mexico	14		
Non-Hispanic whites		47	17
Hispanics		39	35

*Per 100,000 population.

risk of intracranial hemorrhage (both ICH and subarachnoid hemorrhage [SAH]) in *cigarette-smoking* Hawaiian men of Japanese ancestry. The risk of "hemorrhagic stroke" was 2.5 times higher in smokers, an effect that was independent of other risk factors. However, the diagnosis of ICH was often made on clinical grounds, without verification by imaging or autopsy findings. In a study based on computed tomography (CT) diagnosis of ICH in Finland, Juvela and colleagues[28] found that smoking was not an independent risk factor for ICH. However, recent data from the Physicians' Health Study and the Women's Health Study[29a] documented a significant association[29a] between cigarette smoking and both SAH and ICH risk in men and women.[29,29a] After the analysis was controlled for a number of vascular risk factors, smoking 20 or more cigarettes per day emerged as an independent risk factor for SAH (relative risk [RR] 3.22; 95% confidence interval [CI], 1.26–8.18) and ICH (RR 2.06; 95% CI, 1.08–3.96) in a cohort of predominantly white male physicians.[29] Corresponding figures for women who smoked 15 or more cigarettes per day were RR of 4.02 (95% CI, 1.63–9.89) for SAH and 2.67 (95% CI, 1.04–6.90) for ICH in the Women's Health Study.[29a]

The series reported by Donahue and associates[30] and Juvela and colleagues[28] also documented an increased risk of ICH in relation to *alcohol ingestion*, an effect that operated independently of other risk factors. Both studies showed a strong dose-response relationship between alcohol use and ICH. Juvela and colleagues[28] documented a similar effect for alcohol ingestion within 24 hours and within 1 week before onset of ICH. *Low serum cholesterol* level, defined as serum cholesterol less than 160 mg/dL, has been shown to be associated with a higher risk of ICH in Japanese men[15] as well as in Hawaiian men of Japanese origin.[31] Other risk factors have been suggested in some studies. *Cirrhosis* was highly represented (15.5%) in the autopsy series of Boudouresques and associates,[32] but its significance could not be assessed, because comparison with a control autopsy series of the general population was not available. The occasional association of ICH with cirrhosis has been linked to thrombocytopenia and other abnormalities in coagulation.[33] The role of *aspirin use* in the risk of ICH is controversial. The Physicians' Health Study, which evaluated the effect of low-dose aspirin (325 mg every other day) in comparison with placebo in the primary prevention of coronary events, documented a bor-

derline-significant increase in relative risk of hemorrhagic stroke (ICH and SAH) in the aspirin group.[34] Similarly, the SALT (Swedish Aspirin Low-Dose Trial) secondary stroke prevention trial documented a significantly higher frequency of hemorrhagic stroke in the group assigned to aspirin (75 mg/day) than in the group given placebo.[35] These data contrast with those from other secondary stroke prevention trials, in which various doses of aspirin did not lead to a higher risk of ICH.[36–41]

GENETICS

The study of the genetics of cerebrovascular disease has focused mainly on ischemic stroke, but some researchers have addressed ICH as well.[42] Alberts and coworkers[43] addressed the issue of familial aggregation of cases of ICH. Their prospective study in North Carolina found that 10% of probands had a history of ICH. No significant clinical or demographic differences separated those with and without family history of ICH. Data reported by Woo and colleagues[44] indicated that the presence of a first-degree relative is a risk for ICH of the lobar variety. These investigators also documented that the occurrence of lobar ICH is associated with the e2 and e4 alleles of the apolipoprotein E gene. These alleles, particularly e4, have been identified as factors related to an increased risk of lobar ICH, presumably due to the presence of cerebral amyloid angiopathy (CAA).[45] In addition, the presence of the e4 allele was found to determine an earlier age of onset of ICH in its carriers compared with the age of presentation of CAA-related ICH in those without the allele.[45]

A potential novel association between a point mutation in codon 34 of exon 2 for factor XIII Val34Leu and ICH was suggested by Catto and associates.[46] The suggested association was based on the known protective effect of this mutation for myocardial infarction (MI), as a result of its interfering with the formation of cross-linked fibrin. This last feature suggested the hypothesis that the mutation may result in an increased risk of ICH via the formation of weak fibrin structures. The study, which involved a large cohort of patients with stroke of both ischemic and hemorrhagic varieties, suggested that the mutation was significantly more common in subjects with ICH than in controls and in those with cerebral infarction.[46] However, a similar study from Korea did not show an association between factor XIII Val34Leu polymorphism and ICH.[47] These inconsistent observations may simply reflect the differences in the cohorts studied, and further data from other population samples will be required before a definitive statement can be made about the potential role of this mutation in the risk of ICH.

Further advances in the area of the genetics of stroke—such as the identification of genetic defects that result in an increased risk of specific stroke subtypes, including ICH—are likely in the near future.

PATHOLOGIC FEATURES AND PATHOGENESIS

Spontaneous ICH occurs predominantly in the deep portions of the cerebral hemispheres. Its most common location is the putamen; this site accounts for 35% to 50%

Table 13.2 Distribution by Site of 100 Cases of Intracerebral Hemorrhage at the University of South Alabama Medical Center

Type	No. of Cases
Putaminal	34
Lobar	24
Thalamic	20
Cerebellar	7
Pontine	6
Miscellaneous	
Caudate	5
Putaminothalamic	4

of the cases.[2,4,10,48-50] The second site of preference varies in different series; in most, it is the subcortical white matter,[2,10,21,49] with a frequency of 30%. The thalamus follows, with a uniform frequency of 10% to 15%.[2,4,10,49-53] Pontine hemorrhage accounts for 5% to 12% of cases of ICH.[2,4,10,49,51] The distribution figures in a series of 100 unselected cases of ICH are shown in Table 13.2.

The hemorrhages of putaminal, thalamic, and pontine location occur in the vascular distribution of small, perforating intracerebral arteries, the lenticulostriate, thalamoperforating, and basilar paramedian groups, respectively. Cerebellar hemorrhage occurs in the area of the dentate nucleus,[54,55] which is supplied by small branches of both the superior and the posterior-inferior cerebellar arteries.[54] Thus, most ICHs originate from the rupture of small, deep arteries[56] with diameters between 50 and 200 µm. The same arteries are recognized to be those occluded in cases of lacunar infarcts,[57] a form of stroke correlated primarily with chronic hypertension and diabetes.[58,59] Thus, it is apparent that these various groups of small arteries, located in well-defined anatomic areas, become the targets of chronic hypertension, and the result can be either occlusion or rupture, leading to lacunar infarcts or ICH, respectively.

Vascular Rupture

The actual mechanism of vascular rupture leading to ICH has been the subject of considerable interest, and several detailed pathologic studies[60-62] have addressed this point. Because hypertension is one of its main causative factors,[63] arterial changes associated with it have been commonly implicated in its pathogenesis. Since Charcot and Bouchard[64] described "miliary aneurysms" in brain specimens from patients with hypertensive ICH in 1868, these lesions have been the subject of extensive interest. Initially, they were thought to represent true dilatations of the arterial wall, and their preferential location deep in the hemispheres lent support to their pathogenic role. In the early 20th century, however, with the use of a more precise histologic technique, Ellis[65] was able to show that miliary aneurysms represent "false aneurysms" and are actually made of blood collected outside the vessel wall, as "masses of blood" surrounded by either "remains of the vessel wall" or fibrin. His view of the pathogenesis of ICH implied a primary intimal lesion, with or without secondary involvement of the media and adventitia, the former often leading to passage of blood into the vessel wall, with formation of a dissecting aneurysm. Either form of vascular abnormality (dissecting aneurysm or simple "weakening" of the vessel wall by extension of the primary intimal lesion into the media and adventitia) would then be responsible for rupture and hemorrhage.

Over the following years, miliary aneurysms in the brain of hypertensive patients were shown through the use of thick frozen sections[66] and x-ray imaging of brain specimens injected with radiopaque media.[67] Green[66] demonstrated three such lesions, two of which were associated with a fresh hemorrhage in the pons and frontal lobe. His view was that these lesions were mainly related to atherosclerosis and that they "may be responsible for some cases of cerebral hemorrhage." However, the definitive work that established the relationship between hypertension and miliary aneurysms was performed by Ross Russell,[67] who combined postmortem angiography with routine histologic study of brain specimens. He found miliary aneurysms in 15 of 16 brains of hypertensive patients and in 10 of 38 normotensive patients. The aneurysms were found mostly in the basal ganglia, internal capsule, and thalamus and less commonly in the centrum semiovale and cortical gray matter. Ross Russell[67] regarded these lesions as most likely acquired, strongly related to hypertension, and possibly causally related to ICH. He rejected the notion that aneurysms may be consequences rather than causes of ICH, as they were present in brains of hypertensive patients without ICH.

This study was followed by a series of observations reported by Cole and Yates[60,61,68] in a systematic analysis of 100 brains from hypertensive patients and an equal number of brains from normotensive persons. Miliary aneurysms were found in 46% of hypertensive brains, but only in 7% of normotensive brains; furthermore, they occurred in 85% of the hypertensive patients with massive ICH, and in all of those with small "slit" hemorrhages, suggesting that small hemorrhages probably result from microaneurysmal "leaks."[60] These researchers did not, however, establish a relationship between microaneurysms and bleeding sites, thereby failing to prove that these "leaks" had a causal role in ICH.

In 1971, Fisher[56] reported the study of two brains containing three ICHs, one pontine and two putaminal, by serial sections of blocks of tissue containing the hemorrhage. In both putaminal hemorrhages, the primary arterial bleeding sites were identified along with multiple sites of secondary bleeding. The latter was thought to result from mechanical disruption and tearing of smaller vessels at the periphery of the enlarging hematoma. In the pontine ICH, only the secondary bleeding sites were recognized. No instances of microaneurysm formation were found in immediate relationship to the hematomas, whereas "lipohyalinosis" was a common abnormality of the walls of small arteries harboring the bleeding sites. Miliary aneurysms were identified in both hemorrhages, although not in relation to the bleeding points. Fisher[56] thought the aneurysms were unlikely to be sources of major hemorrhage and more probably the end result of old small sites of arterial rupture ("the end stage of a limited extravasation"). A year later, Fisher[69] reported a detail of the types of microaneurysms found in brains of hypertensive patients. He described "saccular," "lipohyalinotic," and "fusiform" varieties of microaneurysms and suggested that the lipohyalinotic form may be the process underlying ICH (as well as

Clinical Manifestations

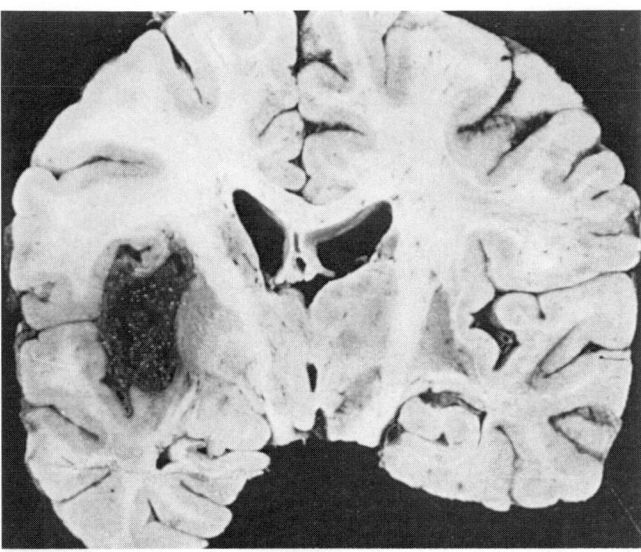

FIGURE 13–10 *A 2-month-old right putaminal-insular hemorrhage, with partial cavitation, good demarcation from the adjacent parenchyma, and lack of signs of mass effect.*

arterial rupture leads to local accumulation of blood, which in part destroys the parenchyma locally, displaces nervous structures in the vicinities, and dissects at some distance from the initial focus. The bleeding sites are at times difficult to locate, and serial sections are needed to show them.[56] The bleeding sites appear as round collections of platelets admixed with and surrounded by concentric lamellae of fibrin, so-called bleeding globes or fibrin globes.[56] These fibrin or bleeding globes at the

primary and secondary sites are histologically identical, except that the fibrin globes are larger. The bulk of the hematoma is formed by a compact mass of red blood cells, and the bleeding sites are characteristically found at its periphery.

García and colleagues[92] have described in detail the sequential histologic changes that take place in the hematoma. After hours or days, extracellular edema develops at the periphery of the hematoma, resulting in pallor and vacuolation of myelin sheaths. After 4 to 10 days, the red blood cells begin to lyse, eventually turning into an amorphous mass of methemoglobin. Cellular infiltration by polymorphonuclear leukocytes appears at the periphery of the hematoma as early as 2 days after onset, and the number of leukocytes peaks at 4 days.[93] This event is followed by the arrival of microglial cells, which become foamy macrophages after the ingestion of cellular debris, including products of disintegration of myelin as well as blood-derived pigments, especially hemosiderin. The final stages of this process consist of the proliferation of astrocytes at the periphery of the hematoma, where these cells become enlarged and display prominent eosinophilic cytoplasm (gemistocytes), which at times contains hemosiderin granules. Once the chronic stage of hematoma reabsorption and repair has been reached, the astrocytes are replaced by abundant glial fibrils.

This histologic process is correlated with macroscopic changes in the hematoma, which initially becomes a soft, spongy mass of brick-red, altered blood (Fig. 13–10). After many months of slowly progressing phagocytosis, the residua of the hematoma is confined to a flat, collapsed cavity lined by reddish orange discoloration resulting from the accumulation of hemosiderin-laden macrophages (Fig. 13–11).[22]

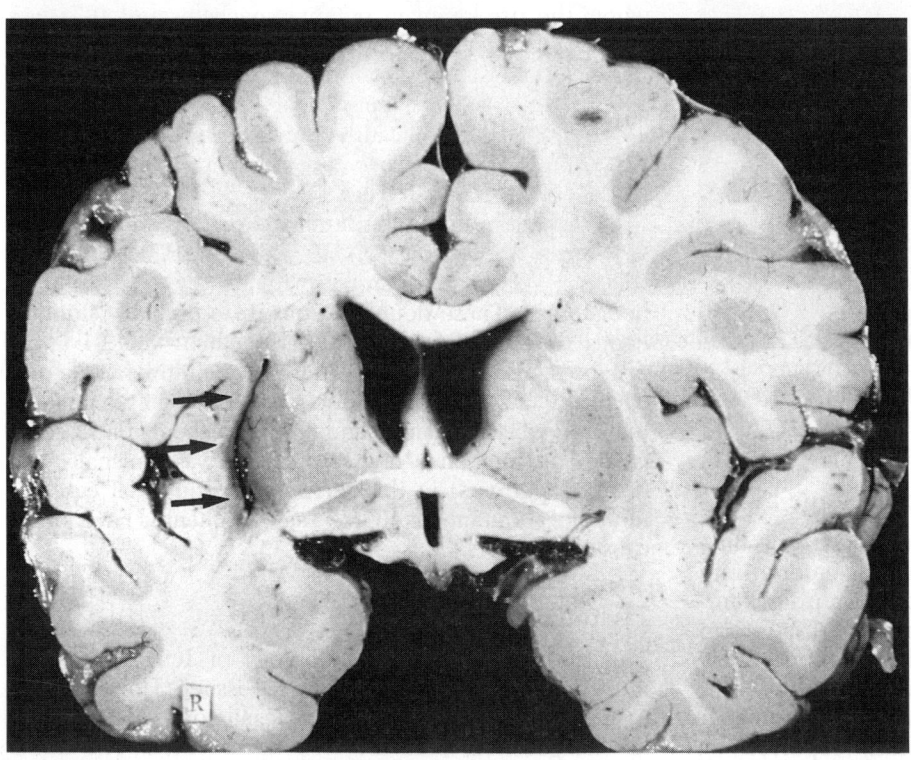

FIGURE 13–11 *Old right putaminal hemorrhage reduced to a slit with hemosiderin-stained edges (arrows). (From García JH, Ho KL, Caccamo DV: Intracerebral hemorrhage: Pathology of Selected Topics. In Kase CS, Caplan LR [eds]: Intracerebral Hemorrhage. Boston, Butterworth-Heinemann, 1994, p 45.)*

Nonhypertensive Causes of Intracerebral Hemorrhage

There are a number of instances in which ICH occurs in the absence of a history of long-standing hypertension. These mechanisms of ICH are (1) small vascular malformations, (2) sympathomimetic drugs, (3) brain tumors, (4) anticoagulants, (5) fibrinolytic agents, and (6) vasculitis. CAA, another mechanism of nonhypertensive ICH, is discussed in Chapter 33.

Small Vascular Malformations

Small vascular malformations, also referred to as angiomas, are commonly implicated in cases of ICH, especially lobar ICH.[94] Margolis and associates[95] first called attention to these lesions in 1951, when they reported four cases of fatal ICH in young patients, in whom pathologic examination disclosed small vascular malformations—one arteriovenous, two venous, and one probably cavernous. These researchers add two other cases in which malformations were incidentally found (not associated with ICH), a cavernous angioma and a telangiectasis. Margolis and associates[95] stressed the need to consider such lesions in cases of nonhypertensive ICH, especially in the young.

Since that report, several researchers have shared this point of view.[96–98] Fisher[51] recorded 17 such lesions in his series of ICH and suggested that the hemorrhages they produce are less massive or slower to develop than most hypertensive ones.

Crawford and Russell[96,98] reported 21 examples of ICH due to small vascular malformations, 20 of which were arteriovenous, and only 1 a cavernous angioma. The 20 arteriovenous lesions were located in the cerebral convexity (10 cases), deep portions of the hemispheres (4 cases), and cerebellum (6 cases). Because of their small size and the difficulties in diagnosing them in life, the term *cryptic* was proposed for these malformations. However, the term has become obsolete since the introduction of CT and especially of magnetic resonance imaging (MRI); the latter

technique routinely demonstrates these small lesions, which were previously undetectable on cerebral angiography. Multiple series have now documented instances of ICH due to rupture of small vascular malformations that occur either sporadically[97,99–101] or on a familial basis.[102–106]

In the series of 18 cases reported by Becker and colleagues,[99] the hemorrhages were predominantly lobar, reflecting the usually cortical location of the malformations. These investigators found a mean age at diagnosis of 23 years in their series and documented a female preponderance of 2.5:1, similar to the sex distribution of 42 cases previously reported in the literature.

Cavernous angiomas are thought to have a generally lower bleeding potential than the arteriovenous variety (Fig. 13–12). However, they occasionally lead to progressive, subacute deficits that result from protracted bleeding or recurrent small hemorrhages, mimicking brainstem tumors[101] or even multiple sclerosis.[107] Natural history data suggest that bleeding from cavernous angiomas may be more common than previously recognized. Bleeding rates of 0.7%[108] and 1.1%[109] per year were recorded in two reports with follow-up periods of 2.2 years. In a third series, Kondziolka and associates[110] found the bleeding risk on follow-up to differ according to the initial presentation. They documented bleeding rates of 0.6% per year for patients without a history of ICH and 4.5% per year for patients with prior ICH (Table 13.3).

The availability of MRI has greatly facilitated the diagnosis of cavernous angiomas (Fig. 13–13). They characteristically appear, on T2-weighted sequences, as irregular lesions with a central core of mixed (high and low) signal, surrounded by a halo of hypodensity corresponding to hemosiderin deposits, which represent previous episodes of bleeding around the malformation.[111–113] Although these lesions generally occur in isolation and with a preference for the cortical and subcortical regions of the cerebral hemispheres and the pons,[111,114] occasional examples are multiple,[112] in which case a familial occurrence is likely.[115] The latter appears to be particularly common among

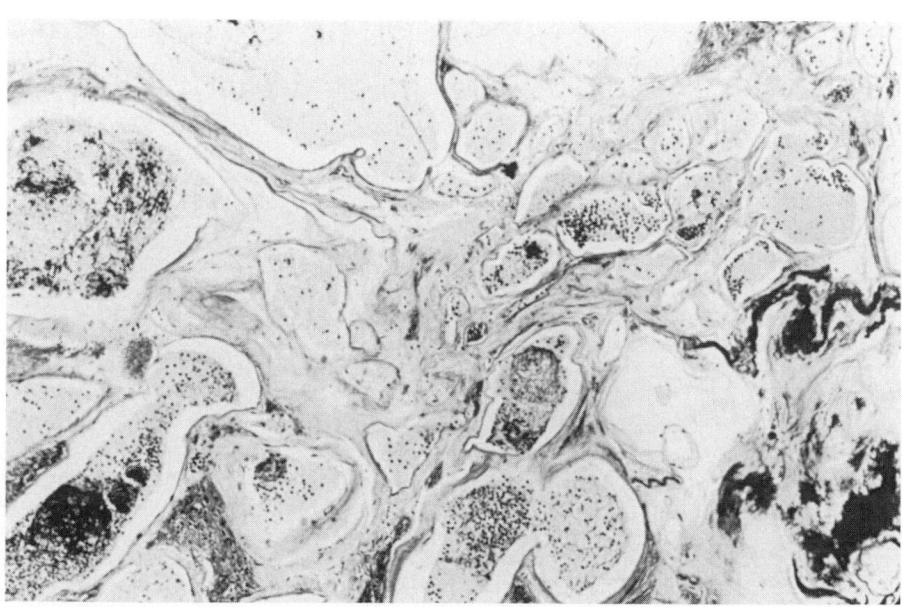

FIGURE 13–12 *Incidentally found cavernous angioma in the subcortical white matter of the left frontal lobe, showing widely separated vascular channels with primitive walls and without intervening brain parenchyma. Areas of calcification are shown in the right lower corner. (Hematoxylin and eosin, × 48.)*

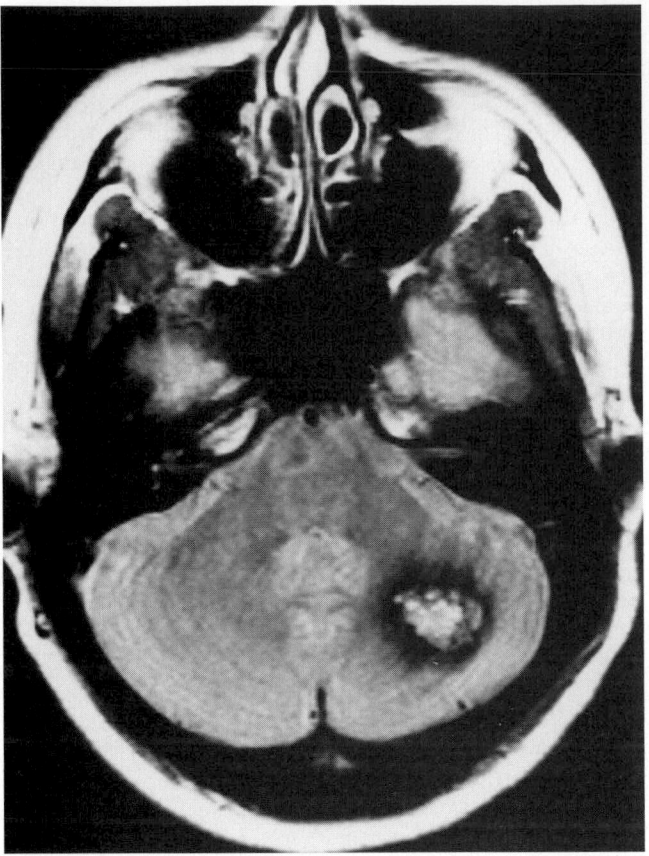

FIGURE 13–13 *MR image (T2-weighted) of left cerebellar cavernous angioma, with mixed-signal central core and peripheral low-signal hemosiderin ring.*

individuals of Mexican-American descent,[115] in whom cavernous angiomas are inherited as an autosomal dominant pattern linked to a mutation that has been mapped to the short arm of chromosome 7.[116,117]

On the basis of the preceding reports, it now seems well established that small vascular malformations, both arteriovenous and cavernous, are likely to bleed and may be responsible for cases of nonhypertensive ICH. The frequency of this occurrence is difficult to establish, but one figure is available from the autopsy study by Russell,[98] who obtained 21 cases with vascular formations from a total of 461 cases of ICH, a frequency of 4.5%.

Sympathomimetic Drugs

ICH related to the use of *amphetamines* has been documented in several publications.[118–121] The preparation most

Table 13.3   Natural History of Cavernous Angiomas

Study	No. of Patients	Bleeding Rate per Year (%)
Robinson et al[108]	57	0.7
Zabramski et al[109]	31	1.1
Kondziolka et al[110]	122	2.63
Without prior intracerebral hemorrhage	61	0.6
With prior intracerebral hemorrhage	61	4.5

commonly implicated has been intravenous methamphetamine,[118] but cases related to intranasal[120] or oral[119] use of this drug and amphetamine have also been reported. Another sympathomimetic drug, *pseudoephedrine*, has been associated with one reported instance of ICH.[121] In these cases, ICHs have developed usually within minutes (20 to 40) to a few hours (4 to 6) after the use of the drug; frequently, the ICH represents an established pattern of drug abuse for months beforehand, but at times it has followed a first-time use.[119] An association with transiently elevated blood pressure has been noticed in about 50% of cases, and most of the hematomas have been of lobar location.[120,121] Their pathogenesis has been related to either transient drug-induced elevation in blood pressure[119] or an arteritis-like vascular change histologically similar to periarteritis nodosa.[122] The latter is considered either a direct "toxic" effect of the drug on cerebral blood vessels or a hypersensitivity reaction to the drug or its vehicle.

The cerebral "arteritis" related to use of these drugs is characterized angiographically by beading (multiple areas of focal arterial stenosis or constriction) of medium-sized and large intracranial arteries,[120,121,123–125] an effect that has been shown to be reversible after use of steroids and discontinuation of drug abuse.[125] However, it is likely that these reversible vascular changes correspond not to a true vasculitis but rather to a nonspecific phenomenon of multifocal spasm related to the effects of the sympathomimetic drug on the vessel wall. In isolated instances, intravenous use of methamphetamine precipitated an ICH from a sylvian-region AVM,[126] and oral use of dextroamphetamine was associated with SAH in the presence of a small middle cerebral artery aneurysm.[127] Most other reports of amphetamine-related ICH and SAH have not documented preexisting vascular malformations or mycotic aneurysms.

Other sympathomimetic agents have been related to episodes of ICH. *Phenylpropanolamine* (PPA) has been associated with instances of ICH and SAH. Most affected patients have been young (median age in the 30s), have been women more often than men, and generally have lacked other risk factors for ICH.[128] Results of a case-control study reported by Kernan and associates[129] have suggested the potential association between PPA and ICH. These investigators found that women who used appetite suppressants containing PPA had a significantly higher risk of intracranial hemorrhage (odds ratio [OR] = 16.58; 95% CI, 1.51–182.21; P = .02). The hemorrhages occur shortly after PPA ingestion, most between 1 and 8 hours.[128–134] The ICHs are most commonly of lobar location, and about two thirds of the cases that have undergone angiography have showed widespread beading of intracranial arteries (Fig. 13–14), without documentation of other vascular lesions responsible for bleeding, such as AVM and aneurysm. Histologic examination of blood vessels from biopsy material has been nondiagnostic except for one instance in which changes consistent with vasculitis were found.[135]

The pathogenesis of these PPA-related hemorrhages is obscure. Although rare patients have been previously hypertensive, transient hypertension was noted at presentation in about 50% of the reported cases.[128] This finding suggests that a possible mechanism of vascular rupture is drug-induced transient hypertension associated with

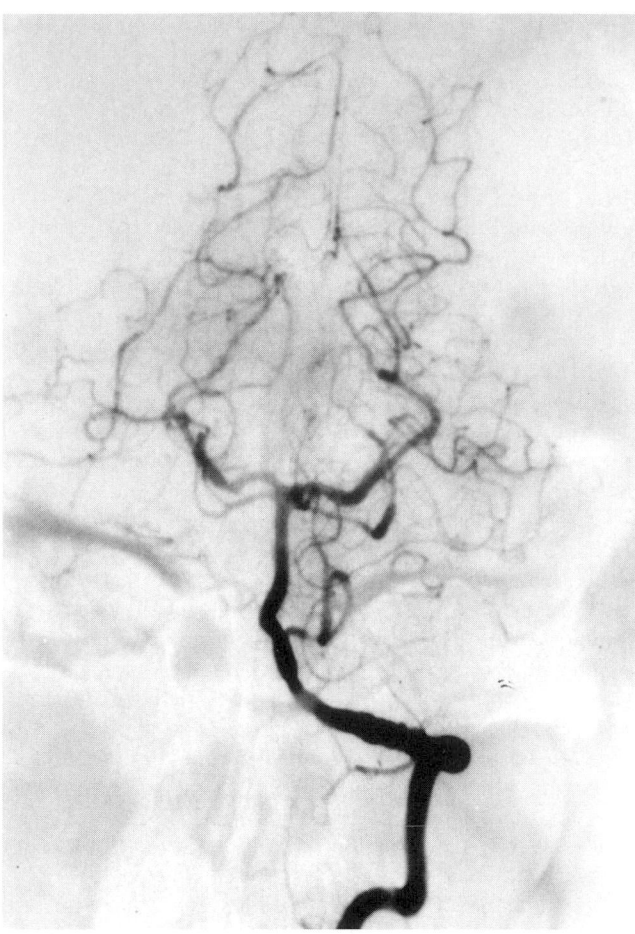

FIGURE 13–14 *Multifocal areas of arterial constriction and dilatation ("beading") in the vertebrobasilar system after an episode of severe headache and transient hypertension (200/110 mm Hg), shortly after the ingestion of a phenylpropanolamine-containing nasal decongestant. (From Kase CS, Foster TE, Reed JE, et al: Intracerebral hemorrhage and phenylpropanolamine use. Neurology [NY] 37:399, 1987.)*

ICHs, which in turn have shown a stronger association with AVMs or aneurysms as the bleeding mechanism.[137] This association suggests that the hypertensive response that commonly follows cocaine use may act in some instances as a precipitant of ICH in preexisting vascular malformations. In one case, ICH after cocaine use was related to pathologically documented vasculitis of a small intraparenchymal artery.[139]

Intracranial Tumors

Intracranial tumors are a well-recognized but uncommon cause of ICH. Underlying tumors have accounted for 1% to 2% of cases of ICH in autopsy series,[21] whereas rates of 6% to 10% have been found in clinical-radiologic series.[140,141] The great majority of the underlying neoplasms have been malignant, either primary or metastatic, but rarely, meningiomas[142] or oligodendrogliomas[140] have manifested as ICH. An example of a generally benign tumor with relatively high tendency to bleed is pituitary adenoma, which was associated with bleeding in 15% of the cases in one large series of brain tumors.[143] Among the primary malignant brain tumors causing ICH, glioblastoma multiforme predominates[140]; the metastatic tumors have been melanoma, choriocarcinoma, renal cell, and bronchogenic carcinoma.[141,144–147] The frequency of hemorrhagic metastases was estimated at 60% for germ cell tumors, 40% for melanoma, and 9% for bronchogenic carcinoma.[148]

multifocal arterial changes due to vasospasm or, less commonly, vasculitis. However, transient hypertension alone is an unlikely explanation for these hemorrhages, because the hypertension has generally been modest, even in comparison with blood pressure rises documented under physiologic conditions.[136] These observations suggest that mechanisms other than transient hypertension must be present in order for intracranial hemorrhage to occur under these circumstances.

Cocaine is being increasingly reported as a cause of cerebral hemorrhage in young individuals, especially in its precipitate form, known as "crack." Instances of ICH and SAH have occurred within minutes to 1 hour from use of crack cocaine.[137] The ICHs are either lobar or deep ganglionic (Fig. 13–15); occasionally there are multiple hemorrhages in both locations.[138] The mechanism of these ICHs is unclear, although these lesions are in many respects similar to those related to use of amphetamine or PPA; the angiographic beading that characterizes ICHs due to amphetamine or PPA use is relatively uncommon in cocaine-related

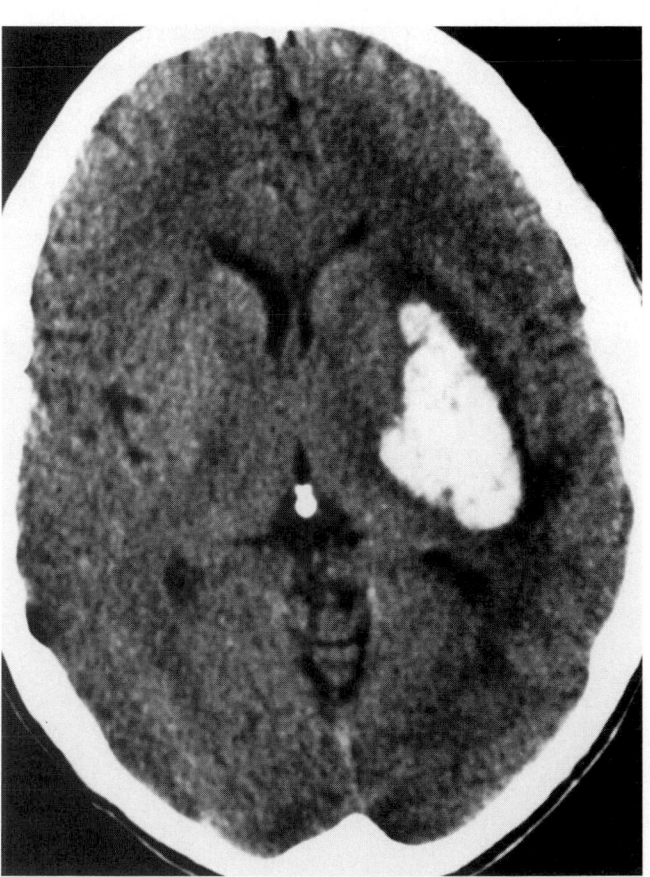

FIGURE 13–15 *Left putaminal hemorrhage secondary to use of crack cocaine.*

The bleeding tendency in neoplasms is thought to be directly related to the richness of their vascular components and their pathologic, neoplastic character.[149] In the case of metastatic choriocarcinoma, these features are enhanced by the normal biologic tendency of trophoblastic tissue to invade the walls of blood vessels.[145,150] The location of the hemorrhage relates to some extent to the type of neoplasm involved: Hemorrhages occurring in glioblastoma multiforme are frequently deep into the hemispheres, basal ganglia, or corpus callosum.[140] Hemorrhages due to metastatic tumors occur more often in the subcortical white matter[144] (Fig. 13–16), because metastatic nodules commonly deposit at the gray-white matter junction.

In approximately half of the reported instances of ICH within an intracerebral tumor, the hemorrhage was the first clinical manifestation of the neoplasm. The radiologic diagnosis by CT can be established easily in instances of multiple metastatic lesions,[144] but cases of ICH into a single tumor can be more difficult to diagnose. Such a diagnosis should be suspected with the finding of large areas of low-density edema surrounding the hematoma (Fig. 13–17) or of an area of contrast enhancement at the periphery of the hematoma, frequently forming a ring pattern on initial presentation with ICH.[140,144] Because ring enhancement is not expected on presentation of spontaneous, hypertensive ICH,[150–153] its presence should strongly suggest the possibility of an underlying, previously asymptomatic primary or metastatic brain tumor. Other features suggesting ICH into a brain tumor are (1) finding of papilledema at presentation with acute ICH; (2) atypical location of the ICH, in areas such as the corpus callosum, which is rarely the site of "spontaneous" ICH and is commonly involved by malignant gliomas (Fig. 13–18); and (3) a ringlike high-density area corresponding to blood around a low-density center, resulting from bleeding by tumor vessels at the junction of tumor and adjacent brain parenchyma.[154] In addition, Iwama and colleagues[155] have suggested that a low-density indentation of the periphery of an ICH on CT should raise the suspicion of an underlying tumor nodule. These clinical and radiologic features should prompt a search for a primary or metastatic brain tumor with MRI and cerebral angiography. If the results of these studies are inconclusive, biopsy of the hematoma cavity should be considered to establish the diagnosis of an underlying brain tumor, because the therapeutic options and prognosis are radically different from those for spontaneous or hypertensive ICH.

Anticoagulant Therapy
Warfarin

Long-term oral anticoagulation with warfarin is often listed among the causes of ICH. In a consecutive series of 100 cases of ICH that Kase and associates[156] observed over a 3-year period, warfarin anticoagulation was a factor in 9% of the cases. Boudouresques and colleagues[32] reported that in their autopsy series of 500 cases of ICH, anticoagulation was implicated in 11%. After excluding cases due to trauma, ruptured aneurysm, or concomitant brain tumor, Rådberg and coworkers[157] documented an anticoagulant-related mechanism in 14% of 200 consecutive patients with ICH. Furthermore, anticoagulation is second only to hypertension as a causative factor in series of cerebellar[158] and lobar[84] locations. The risk of ICH in patients undergoing long-term oral anticoagulation has been shown to be 8 to 11 times that in patients of similar age who are not receiving anticoagulants.[159–162]

The incidence of ICH in patients receiving warfarin after MI is approximately 1% a year.[160] A number of factors are known to contribute to a higher risk of ICH in these patients, including advanced age (>70 years),[163,164] hypertension,[156,162,163,165–167] and concomitant use of aspirin, which has been estimated to double the rate of ICH in comparison with individuals on oral anticoagulants alone.[160,168]

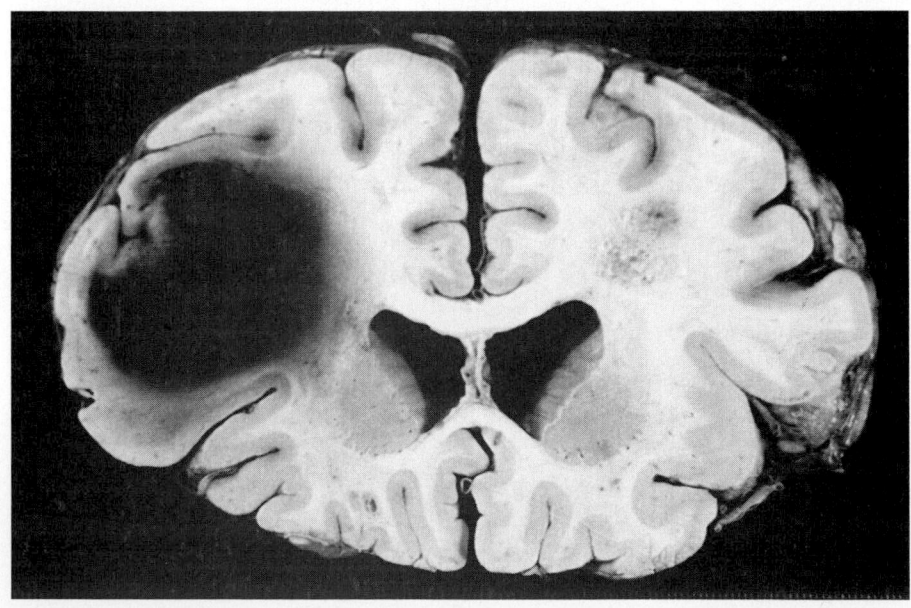

FIGURE 13–16 *Large hemorrhage into a metastatic lesion (from bronchogenic carcinoma) in the right frontal subcortical white matter. A second, nonhemorrhagic metastasis is present in the white matter of the left frontal lobe.*

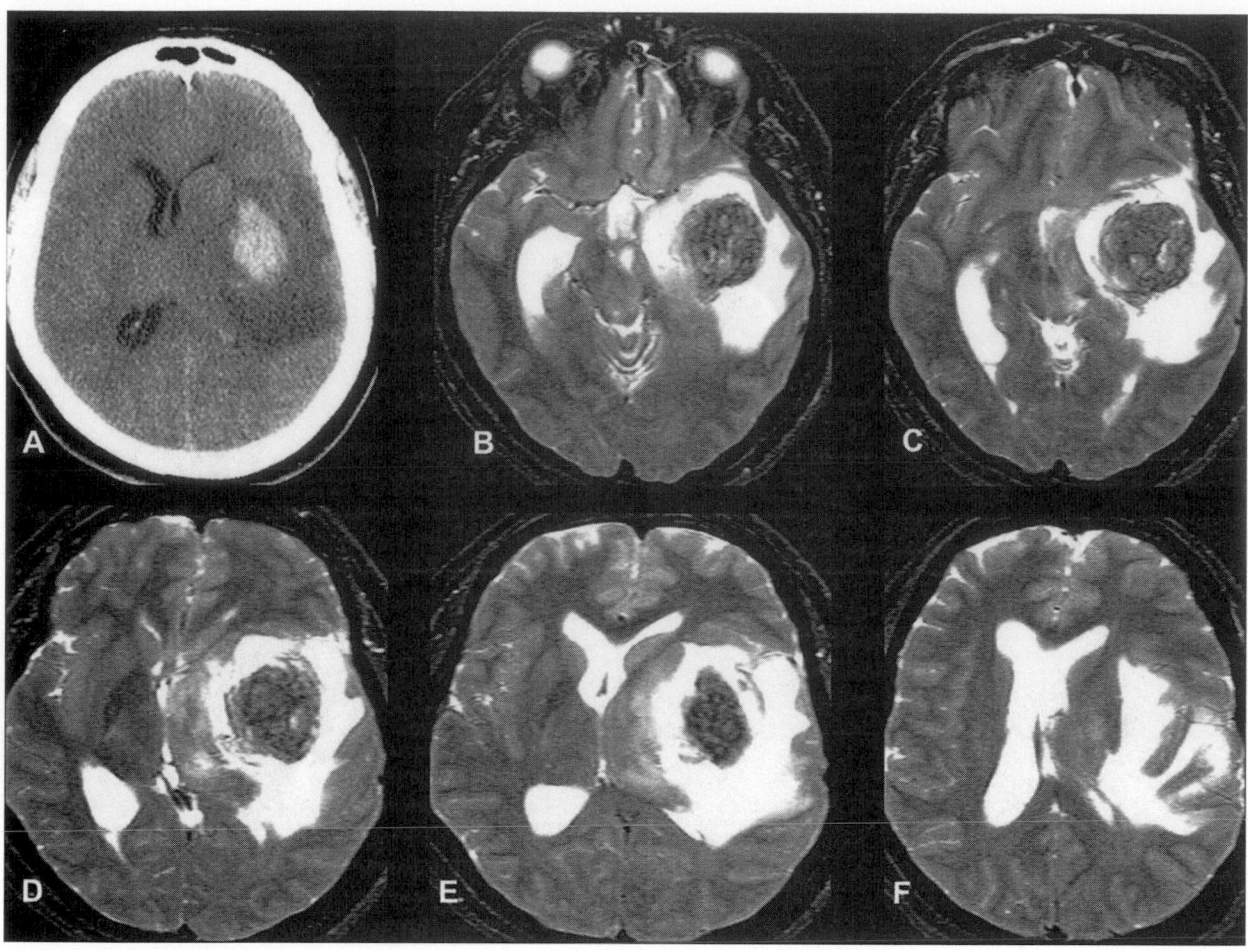

FIGURE 13–17 *CT scan (A) and T2-weighted MR images (B to F) of acute hemorrhage into a glioblastoma multiforme, showing the acute hematoma with marked edema extending well beyond the immediate vicinity of the acute hemorrhage.*

Other features related to ICH in patients receiving anticoagulants are as follows:

Duration of Anticoagulation Therapy before Onset of ICH. In two series, most ICHs (70%,[156] 54%[157]) occurred during the first year after start of treatment. In another report, only one third of ICHs occurred after that period of time,[159] the other two thirds appearing between 2 and 18 years after start of treatment.

Relationship between Intensity of Anticoagulant Effect and Risk of ICH. Excessive anticoagulant effect is now well established as a powerful risk factor for ICH.[156,162–165,167,169] Hylek and Singer,[163] reporting data from an anticoagulant therapy unit, showed that the risk of ICH doubled with each 0.5-point increase in the prothrombin time ratio above the recommended limit of 2.0. Data from the Stroke Prevention in Reversible Ischemia Trial,[170] a secondary stroke prevention trial in which patients with TIA or minor ischemic stroke were randomly assigned to receive either aspirin (30 mg/day) or warfarin (to achieve an international normalized ratio [INR] of 3.0 to 4.5), add further evidence of the effect of excessive anticoagulation and frequency of ICH: The trial was stopped early, after the occurrence of 24 ICHs (14 fatal) in the warfarin group

in comparison with only 3 ICHs (1 fatal) in the aspirin group; there was a strong relationship between bleeding complications and rise in INR values.

Presence of Leukoaraiosis. Severe and confluent areas of leukoaraiosis were associated with a higher risk of ICH in warfarin-anticoagulated subjects in the Stroke Prevention in Reversible Ischemia Trial.[170] Similarly, data reported by Smith and colleagues[167] documented CT-detected leukoaraiosis as an independent risk factor (OR = 12.9; 95% CI, 28–59.8) for ICH in subjects receiving anticoagulation therapy with warfarin after an episode of ischemic stroke.

Location of ICH. A high frequency of cerebellar location was found in some studies,[156,157,171] whereas others found no differences in location of ICH between patients who were and were not receiving anticoagulation therapy.[159,160,162]

Characteristics. Characteristics of these hemorrhages include a tendency to occur in the absence of signs of systemic bleeding, lack of relationship between the ICH and preceding cerebral infarction, frequent leisurely progression of the focal neurologic deficits (at times over periods as long as 48 to 72 hours), and high mortality (46%

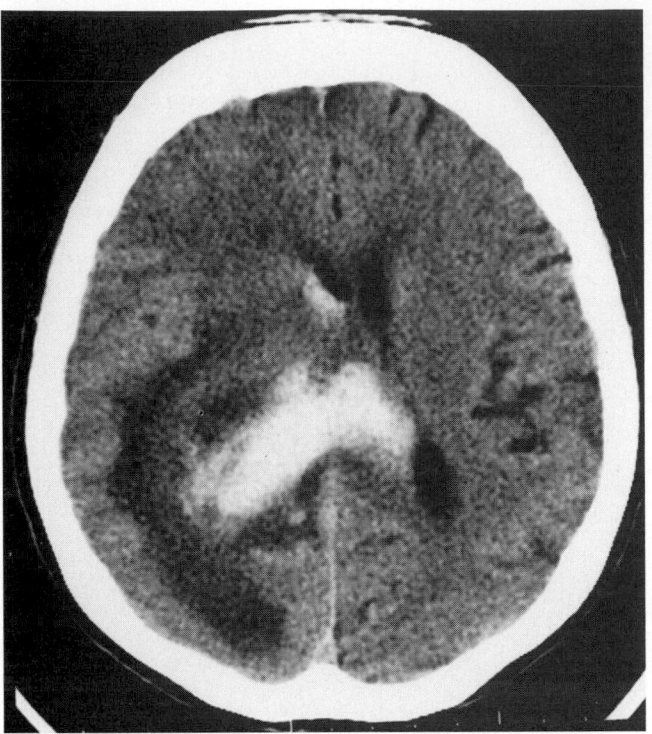

FIGURE 13–18   *CT scan of hemorrhage into glioblastoma multiforme, with bleeding into the corpus callosum and adjacent thalamus and deep parietal lobe as well as extensive surrounding low-density edema.*

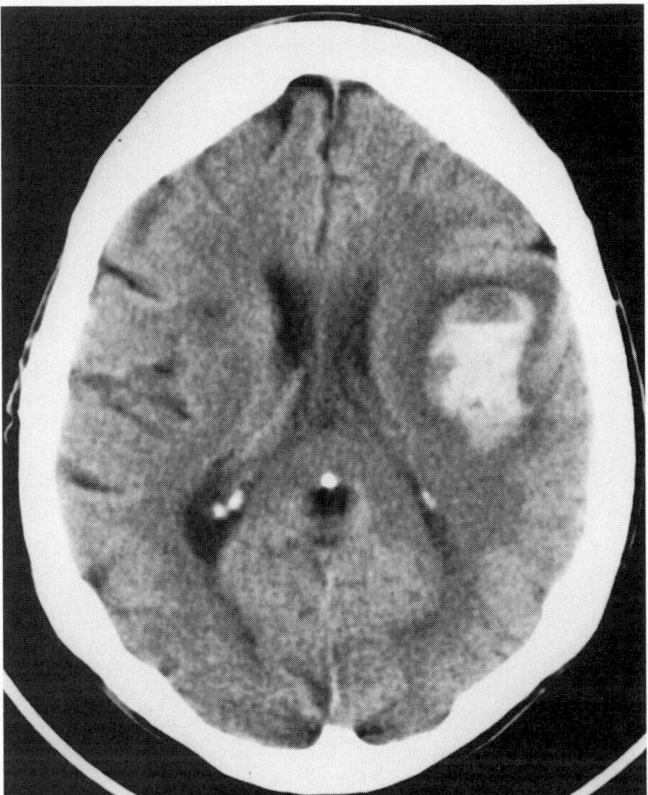

FIGURE 13–19   *CT of acute intracerebral hemorrhage in left frontal white matter, with blood-fluid level.*

to 68%) related to hematoma size (the hematoma is generally larger than in hypertensive ICH).[157,159,160] On CT scan, the hemorrhages often show blood-fluid levels, which result from "sedimentation" of red blood cells in a hematoma that does not clot because of the anticoagulation effect (Fig. 13–19).

The actual mechanism of ICH in patients undergoing anticoagulation is unknown, in part owing to the lack of adequate pathologic studies with serial histologic sections aimed at identifying the type of bleeding vessel and the histopathologic abnormality at the bleeding site. Such studies should determine whether anticoagulant-related ICHs have a different microscopic pathology from that of spontaneous ICH, in terms of the type of affected vessel as well as the eventual presence of local vascular disease (microaneurysm, fibrinoid necrosis, lipohyalinosis, CAA) at the rupture site as a possible substrate for this complication of warfarin anticoagulation. Hart and colleagues[160] have hypothesized that ICH in patients undergoing anticoagulation could result from enlargement of small, spontaneous hemorrhages that would otherwise occur without clinical consequence in individuals with normal coagulation function. The contributing role of local vascular disease, such as CAA, is favored by observation of a high frequency of this angiopathy in individuals with warfarin-related ICH. Rosand and associates[172] documented CAA in brain tissue samples from 7 of 11 patients with warfarin-related ICH. In addition, these investigators found an over-representation of the apoE-e2 allele, a marker of

CAA, in patients with warfarin-related ICH in comparison with a control group.

Heparin

The occurrence of ICH during intravenous heparin anticoagulation represents a different situation, because this complication generally occurs in the setting of preceding acute cerebral infarction (because ICH is extremely uncommon in patients receiving intravenous heparin for noncerebrovascular indications, such as deep vein thrombosis and MI[173,174]). Thus, a recent cerebral infarction with local ischemic blood vessels is a likely site for the occurrence of secondary ICH, especially in embolic infarcts, which tend to become hemorrhagic as part of their natural history.[175] ICH in this setting occurs within 24 to 48 hours of the start of heparin treatment,[176] and excessive prolongation of the activated partial thromboplastin time (aPTT) is common.[177,178] Other risk factors for ICH in the setting of intravenous heparin therapy for acute cerebral infarction are infarcts of large size and uncontrolled hypertension (blood pressure exceeding 180 mm Hg systolic/ 100 mm Hg diastolic).[179]

These findings have led to recommendations that the immediate use of intravenous heparin anticoagulation in acute nonseptic cerebral infarction be limited to those patients with subtotal infarcts in a given vascular territory but without uncontrolled hypertension (i.e., blood pressure <180/100 mm Hg) and that it be accompanied by close adherence to a prolongation of the aPTT value within the recommended therapeutic range (1.5 times the control value).[178] However, the immediate use of intravenous heparin after cerebral infarction has been questioned in view of the lack of data supporting the value of any parenteral antithrombotic agents in this setting.[180] Because intravenous heparin has not been properly tested in patients with acute ischemic stroke of nonlacunar type, a prospective, randomized clinical trial investigating this use (the RAPID trial) is currently under way in Europe.[181]

Fibrinolytic Agents

Fibrinolytic agents, especially tissue-type plasminogen activator (t-PA) are increasingly being used in the treatment of coronary and arterial and venous thrombosis in the limbs and pulmonary circulation. The ability of these agents to produce clot lysis and a relatively low level of systemic hypofibrinogenemia makes them ideal choices for the treatment of acute thrombosis. However, the major complication, although it is relatively infrequent, continues to be hemorrhage, in particular ICH. ICH has been reported in 0.4% to 1.3% of patients with acute MI treated with the single-chain t-PA alteplase.[182] The clinical and CT features of ICHs related to coronary thrombolysis with t-PA have been extensively reviewed.[183–187] The hemorrhages tend to occur early after start of t-PA treatment: In one study, 40% of the hemorrhages started during the infusion, and another 25% occurred within 24 hours of the start of treatment.[183] In 70% to 90% of cases, the hemorrhages are lobar. In about 30% of cases the hemorrhages are multiple[184]; and the mortality for multiple hemorrhages is high (44% to 66%).[183–186]

The mechanism of bleeding in this setting is unknown. On several occasions, patients have had excessively prolonged aPTT values at the time of onset of intracranial hemorrhage, as a result of the use of intravenous heparin (aimed at preventing reocclusion of reperfused coronary arteries).[184–186] Other factors suggested as significant in raising the risk of ICH after the use of t-PA in acute MI are advanced age (>65 years), history of hypertension, and use of aspirin before t-PA therapy[186]; in one study, however, none of these factors was found to be significantly different in patients with and without ICH.[185] A possible role for local cerebral vascular disease has been considered, because examples of pretreatment head trauma[185] and concomitant CAA[187–189] have been documented in association with ICH after use of t-PA. Other coagulation defects related to this treatment, such as hypofibrinogenemia and thrombocytopenia, have not been found to correlate with this complication.

In addition to their established role in the treatment of acute MI, thrombolytic agents have been extensively tested in the management of acute ischemic stroke. Initial pilot studies with the use of intra-arterial agents, mainly urokinase and t-PA, yielded encouraging rates of reperfusion, on the order of 55% of patients treated, with hemorrhagic complications (hemorrhagic infarction, ICH) and neurologic deterioration occurring in about 11% of patients.[190] Attention has also been directed at the less invasive administration of intravenous t-PA and streptokinase. The initial experience with intravenous t-PA administered within 8 hours of stroke onset, reported by del Zoppo and colleagues,[191] yielded angiographically documented rates of reperfusion at a disappointingly low level, in the range of 26% to 38%. Despite this low level of recanalization, hemorrhagic changes with neurologic deterioration occurred in 9% of patients. In addition, the study showed that the rate of hemorrhagic complications was significantly higher in patients to whom t-PA was administered more than 6 hours after stroke onset, in comparison with patients treated within 6 hours.[192] Other potential risk factors for intracranial hemorrhage after use of t-PA in acute ischemic stroke are less clearly defined. In an exploratory analysis of their pilot experience with intravenous t-PA given within 3 hours of stroke onset, Levy and colleagues[193] found diastolic hypertension and a t-PA dose of 0.95 mg/kg or higher to be associated with an increased risk of ICH.

Nonangiographic studies of intravenous t-PA in acute stroke, the European Cooperative Acute Stroke Study[194] and the National Institute of Neurological Diseases and Stroke (NINDS) rt-PA Stroke Study,[195] used entry windows (time after onset during which patient could be entered into the study) of 6 hours and 3 hours, respectively, and doses of alteplase of 1.1 mg/kg (to a maximum of 100 mg) and 0.9 mg/kg (to a maximum of 90 mg), respectively. Results of both studies were positive, especially those of the NINDS study, which showed an improved functional outcome at 3 months in the group treated with t-PA without a higher mortality due to hemorrhagic complications. Despite a 10-fold increase in symptomatic ICH during the first 36 hours in patients treated with t-PA (6.4% versus 0.6% for the placebo group), a net benefit accrued for the t-PA–treated group as measured by three functional scales 3 months after treatment. The intracranial hemorrhages in the t-PA group occurred in both the lobar white matter and the deep gray nuclei (Fig. 13–20), and they carried a high mortality (45%).[196]

Three clinical trials of intravenous streptokinase in acute ischemic stroke have found an alarmingly high rate of ICH and mortality.[197–199] The use of 1.5 million IU of streptokinase within 4[197] or 6[198,199] hours from stroke onset resulted in rates of symptomatic ICH between 6%[198] and 21.2%,[197] with mortality rates of 19%[198] and 34%[199] at 10 days, and 43.4%[197] at 90 days, resulting in the termination of the trials. It is possible that the higher rates of ICH after streptokinase therapy than after t-PA therapy in acute ischemic stroke may reflect a dose of streptokinase that is too high for this indication (as opposed to its safer profile in the treatment of patients with acute MI[200]). Additional possible reasons for such observation include a more pronounced and longer-lasting systemic fibrinolytic effect with streptokinase than with t-PA.[201]

The use of intra-arterial recombinant pro-urokinase (proUK) was tested in the PROACT (PROlyse in Acute Cerebral Thromboembolism) I[202] and II trials.[203] When given directly into an MCA clot, proUK was associated with a recanalization rate of 66% (compared with 18% for the control group) in the PROACT II study.[203] This rate correlated with a significantly better functional outcome at 3 months for the treated group, without differences in mortality even though the rate of symptomatic ICH was 10% in treated patients, and only 2% in the controls. Virtually all proUK-related ICHs were massive (Fig. 13–21), and all occurred in the area of the qualifying

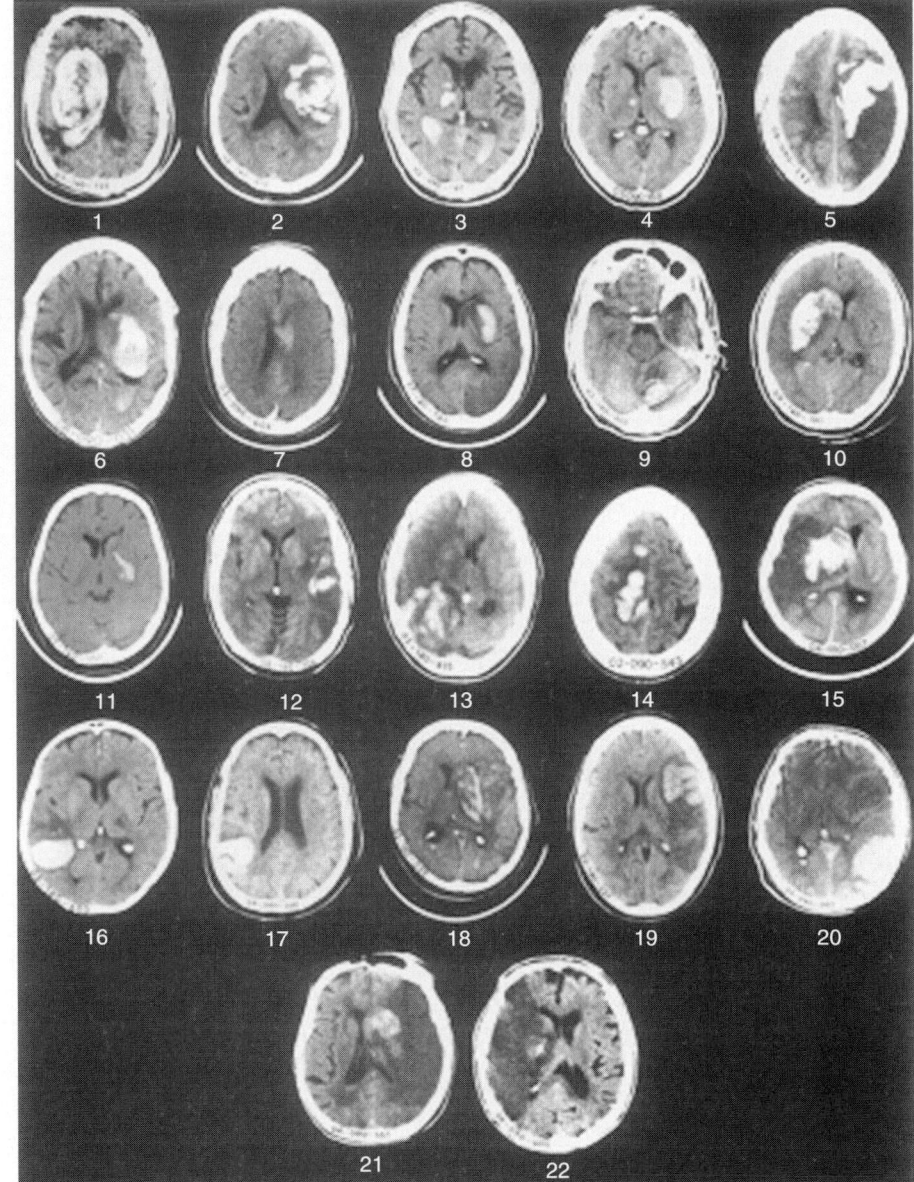

FIGURE 13–20 *CT scans of hemorrhages from the National Institutes of Neurological Diseases and Stroke (NINDS) trial of tissue-type plasminogen activator (t-PA). Cases 1 through 20 are from the t-PA–treated group; cases 21 and 22 are from the control group. (From Intracerebral hemorrhage after intravenous t-PA therapy for ischemic stroke. The NINDS t-PA Stroke Study Group. Stroke 28:2109, 1997.)*

acute infarct in the middle cerebral artery distribution.[204] Among a number of possible risk factors for post-proUK symptomatic ICH, only hyperglycemia at baseline was identified as being potentially associated with a higher risk.[204] Data on ICH after IV t-PA have also suggested that hyperglycemia at baseline increases the risk of symptomatic ICH.[205]

Vasculitis

The cerebral vasculitides generally result in arterial occlusion and cerebral infarction, only rarely being responsible for ICH. Most of these unusual examples of ICH secondary to cerebral arteritis have been secondary to *granulomatous angiitis of the nervous system* (GANS).[206] This primary cerebral vasculitis occurs in the absence of systemic involvement. Histologically, it is characterized by mononuclear inflammatory exudates with giant cells in the media and adventitia of small and medium-sized arteries and veins. This vascular inflammation is occasionally associated with the formation of microaneurysms. The cerebral disease evolves with chronic headache, progressive cognitive decline, seizures, and recurrent episodes of cerebral infarction.[207] Owing to its primary cerebral location, systemic features such as malaise, fever, weight loss, arthralgias, myalgias, anemia, and elevated sedimentation rate are absent.[207,208] The diagnosis is favored by the finding of lymphocytic cerebrospinal fluid (CSF) pleocytosis with elevated protein, and angiography may show a beading pattern in multiple medium-sized and small intracranial arteries. The instances of ICH reported in patients with GANS have occurred in the setting of progressive encephalopathy or myelopathy,[209,210] although ICH has occasionally been the first manifestation of the condition.[211] The hemorrhages have been predominantly lobar in location, and in rare instances, histologic examination of cerebral vessels has shown the association of GANS with CAA,[212,213] suggesting that either vascular lesion could have been responsible for the episode of ICH.

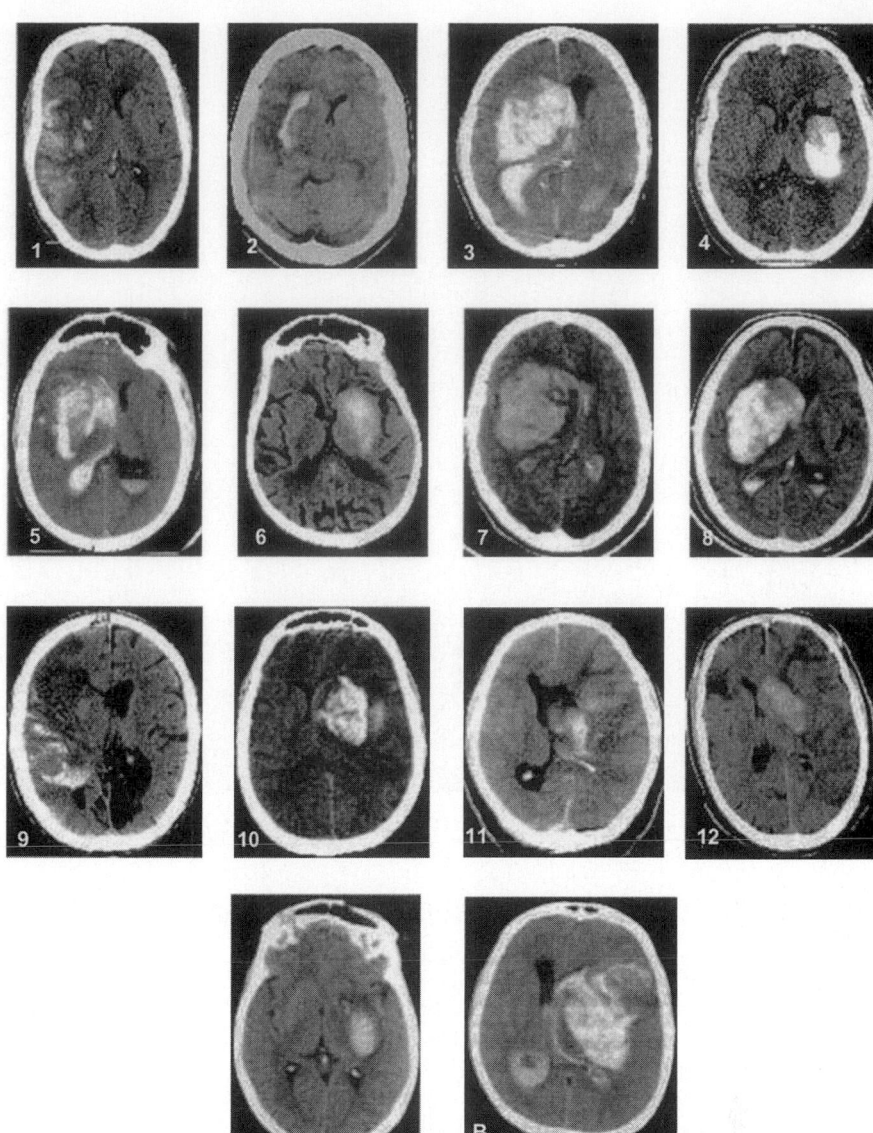

FIGURE 13–21 *CT scans of hemorrhages from the PROlyse in Acute Cerebral Thromboembolism (PROACT) II trial. Cases 1 through 12 are from the recombinant pro-urokinase (r-proUK) group, and cases A and B from the control group. (From Kase CS, Furlan AJ, Wechsler LR, et al: Symptomatic intracerebral hemorrhage after intra-arterial thrombolysis with prourokinase in acute ischemic stroke: The PROACT II trial. Neurology 57:1603, 2001.)*

BRAIN IMAGING

The imaging aspects of ICH are discussed in Chapters 18, 19, and 20. This section only briefly highlights developments in this area.

The view that CT is superior to MRI for the diagnosis of acute ICH has been challenged by new observations. With the use of susceptibility-weighted (also known as gradient-echo) MRI sequences, Linfante and coworkers[214] were able to document acute ICHs within periods as short as 30 minutes after symptom onset. Their observations, along with those of others,[215,216] suggest that in the acute phase of ICH, MRI protocols that include susceptibility-weighted sequences are as reliable as CT for diagnosis.

An additional value of these MRI sequences is their ability to document areas of "micro-hemorrhage," detected as areas of low signal of up to 5 mm in diameter (Fig. 13–22) that result from the presence of deposits of hemosiderin as a sequela from past episodes of minor bleeding.[217–219] The importance of these lesions stems from their potential role in instances of major hemorrhage in subjects receiving anticoagulants or after treatment with thrombolysis.[220] In addition, they may be markers of arteriopathies with potential for bleeding,[221] such as CAA.[222] Finally, their high prevalence in the aging population, estimated to be in the order of 16% for patients older than 75 years,[223] makes them a likely substrate for bleeding, either by reflecting the presence of CAA or by leading to major ICH in the setting of antithrombotic, anticoagulant, or thrombolytic therapy.

GENERAL CLINICAL AND LABORATORY FEATURES

The different forms of ICH share a number of clinical features that result from the progressive accumulation of a mass of blood in the parenchyma. These features include mode of onset as well as clinical manifestations reflecting increased intracranial pressure. ICH occurs characteristically during activity,[55,56] and its onset during sleep is extremely rare.[224] It occurred in only one instance in the

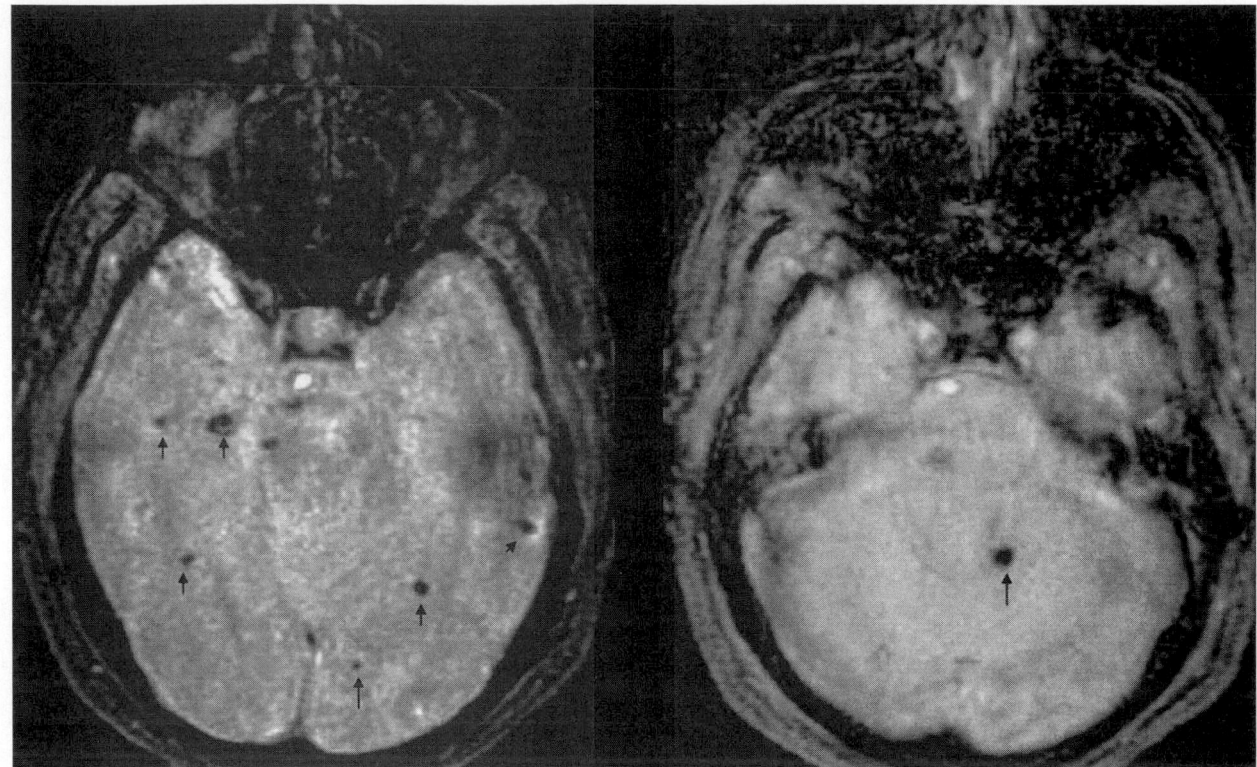

FIGURE 13–22   *MRI, using gradient-echo sequences, showing multiple microhemorrhages* (arrows) *as small black round images corresponding to hemosiderin deposits.*

series reported by Fisher,[224] and in only 3% of ICH cases included in the NINDS Data Bank.[4] The type of onset, studied in 70 cases of ICH prospectively included in the Harvard Cooperative Stroke Registry, was found to be one of gradual and smooth progression in two thirds of the cases, the deficit being maximal at onset in the remainder.[2] No cases showed a regressive course in the acute phase, supporting the clinical dictum that a definite improvement in the early hours of a stroke syndrome rules out ICH.[225] Along with a gradual onset over periods of 5 to 30 minutes, patients with ICH frequently show some decrease in alertness at the time of admission. The frequency and severity of this sign vary to some extent according to the location of the hemorrhage, but when all forms are considered, a decrease in alertness is present in at least 60% of cases,[2,82] in two-thirds of them to a level of coma.[2,50] Coma has been correlated with ventricular extension of the hemorrhage,[50,217] large hematoma,[82] and poor vital prognosis.[50,82,226,227]

The clinical features of ICH associated with increased intracranial pressure are headache and vomiting. Although these features also vary widely in frequency with the location of hemorrhage, their overall diagnostic value at the onset of ICH is limited.[2] Of 54 patients alert enough to report the symptom, only 36% reported headache in the study by Mohr and colleagues[2]; in Aring's[228] series, the frequency of headache was 23%. The reporting of vomiting at onset follows similar frequencies, being 44%[2] and 22%[228] in these two series. These findings stress the important clinical point that absence of headache or vomiting does

not rule out ICH. On the other hand, when present, these signs suggest ICH (or SAH) as the most likely diagnosis, because they are present in less than 10% of occlusive strokes.[2]

Seizures at the onset of ICH are uncommon. They have been reported at rates as low as 7%,[2] 11%,[10] and 14%[228] when all forms of ICH are considered together. In some groups, such as in patients with lobar hemorrhages, seizures have been reported in as many as 32%.[49]

In the general physical examination, a common abnormality is hypertension, found in as many as 91% of the cases in some series.[2] The high frequency of elevated blood pressure on admission in all forms of ICH correlates with other physical signs indicative of hypertension, such as left ventricular hypertrophy[229] and hypertensive retinopathy.[224] The examination of the ocular fundi in a case of suspected ICH serves the dual purpose of detecting signs of hypertensive retinopathy and allowing careful search for subhyaloid hemorrhages. The latter represent blood collections in the preretinal space, and their presence is virtually diagnostic of SAH,[225] because they rarely occur in primary ICH.[84,158,225] Although an occasional case of massive primary ICH does show this sign,[230] its presence has a high correlation with ruptured aneurysm as the cause of the intracranial hemorrhage. The neurologic findings permit the differentiation of the different topographic varieties of ICH (see later).

Communication of the hematoma with the ventricular space accounts for the presence of bloody or xanthochromic CSF in 70% to 90% of cases.[2,10,50,158,224,228,231] **A** somewhat lower frequency of bloody CSF (63%) has been reported in hematomas of lobar location,[84] probably reflecting the less frequent communication with the ventricular system[49] due to the subcortical location of the hematoma. The small percentages of cases with clear CSF in all series of ICH reflect hematomas of small size that do not reach the ventricular system even though located close to it. Furthermore, on account of the smaller size of such hematomas, the clinical presentation may not clearly indicate ICH; signs of increased intracranial pressure may be lacking in such cases, so differentiating them from ischemic strokes is difficult. It is in this particular group of strokes that CT scan has had its most dramatic impact.

In addition to simple inspection of the CSF for bloody or xanthochromic content, spectrophotometric CSF analysis can disclose blood products in virtually 100% of cases.[232] However, this technique is not currently used, because the two widely available anatomic means of diagnosis (CT and MRI) have made CSF examination unnecessary in establishing the presence of an ICH. Moreover, the uncommon but well-recognized precipitation of uncal or tonsillar herniation by lumbar puncture in supratentorial ICH[51,225,233] has contributed to the abandonment of this test for the diagnosis of ICH.

The value of angiography in the evaluation of cases of ICH has similarly declined since the introduction of CT and MRI. Angiography most commonly shows the non-specific signs of mass effect at the site of the hematoma[234] and occasionally has detected extravasation of contrast medium.[235,236] The study by Mizukami and associates[237] correlated the angiographic pattern of displacement of the lenticulostriate arteries with functional prognosis in putaminal hemorrhage. Because of the obvious advantages of CT and MRI in disclosing most of the anatomic features of ICH, angiography is now used only in selected instances. Its main role at present is in the evaluation of nonhypertensive forms of ICH, multiple ICHs, and ICHs located in atypical sites (hemispheral white matter, head of the caudate nucleus), to look for AVM, aneurysm, or tumor as the possible cause of the hemorrhage. Even this role for angiography is steadily diminishing with improvement in noninvasive brain imaging.

SUPRATENTORIAL INTRACEREBRAL HEMORRHAGE

Most cases of intracerebral hemorrhage occur in the supratentorial compartment, usually involving the deep structures of the cerebral hemispheres, the basal ganglia, and the thalamus.[2,10,23,48–50] In addition, a substantial number of hemispheral ICHs occur at the level of the subcortical white matter of the cerebral lobes, the so-called lobar hemorrhages.[49,84] These various forms of ICH have distinctive features in terms of clinical presentation, CT aspects, course, and therapy.

Putaminal Hemorrhage

The several clinical subtypes of putaminal hemorrhage, which is the most common form of ICH, are determined by the size and pattern of extension of the hematoma. Each of these variables independently determines the prognosis.

Overall, a mortality of 37% is expected,[82] a value that is far lower than those quoted in the pre-CT literature,[238] which did not include the undiagnosed smaller cases.

The classic presentation of putaminal hemorrhage comprises massive hemorrhages (Fig. 13–23), with rapidly evolving unilateral weakness accompanied by sensory, visual, and behavioral abnormalities. Headache is common, as is vomiting, within a few hours of onset.[2] Although the onset is abrupt, there is often a gradual worsening of both the focal deficit and the level of consciousness in the following minutes or hours.[224,225] A "maximal from the onset" deficit is uncommon. Whether with sudden or gradual onset, medium-sized or large hematomas are invariably accompanied by a decreased level of alertness correlated with hematoma size. Once the syndrome is well developed, neurologic examination shows a dense flaccid hemiplegia with a hemisensory syndrome and homonymous hemianopia, with global aphasia if the hematoma is in the dominant hemisphere, and hemi-inattention if it is in the nondominant hemisphere.[224,225] A horizontal gaze palsy, with the eyes conjugately deviated toward the side of the lesion, is usually found, which can be reversed momentarily by doll's head maneuver or ice-water caloric testing.[227] The pupillary size and reactivity are normal unless uncal herniation has occurred; if it has, signs of an ipsilateral third cranial nerve palsy are present.[224] These abnormalities in oculomotor function have a poor

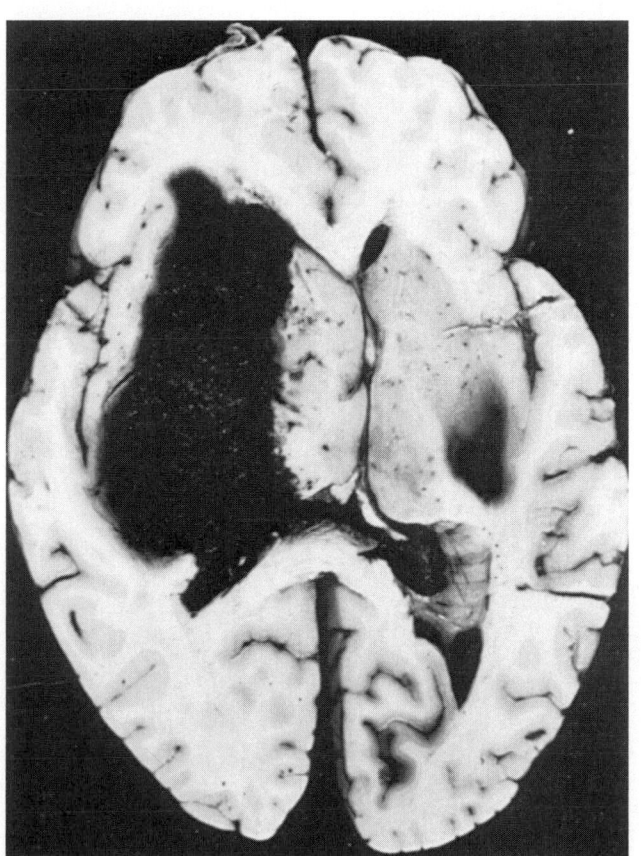

FIGURE 13–23 *Massive right putaminal hemorrhage with ventricular extension. Incidental finding of a small hemorrhage on the posterior corner of the contralateral (left) putamen.*

prognosis.[82] Total unilateral motor deficit, coma, and clinical progression after admission all correlate with large hematoma size and poor functional and vital prognosis, as does ventricular extension of the hematoma by CT scan.[82]

The presence of two hypertensive putaminal hemorrhages, one recent and one old, has been described in pathologic material.[21,33,52,56] The occurrence of simultaneous fresh bilateral putaminal hemorrhages (Fig. 13–24), although occasionally reported,[239] is distinctly uncommon: It was observed in only 2 of 86 cases in Fisher's series,[48] and in none of 42 hypertensive ICH cases from the series reported by McCormick and Schochet.[33] Multiple ICHs are rare unless due to bleeding diathesis associated with thrombocytopenia,[48,240] metastatic tumor,[144] or CAA.[241]

Syndromes Due to Small Hemorrhages

The availability of CT and MRI allows the diagnosis of a number of variations in the presentation of small putaminal ICHs, which in the pre-CT era would have been clinically diagnosed as small infarcts. They are as follows:

Pure Motor Stroke. Instances of pure motor stroke due to small putaminal-capsular hemorrhages have been rarely documented.[242,243] The clinical presentation in such cases has consisted of a mild and transient pure motor syndrome affecting the face and limbs, and the small hematomas originated from the posterior angle of the putamen, with impingement of the posterior limb of the

internal capsule. At times, a small capsular hemorrhage has manifested as pure motor stroke and dysarthria,[244] although the clinical syndrome has been more properly that of a "pure sensory-motor" stroke, related to a component of lateral thalamic compression accompanying the capsular lesion.

Pure Sensory Stroke. The syndrome of pure sensory stroke, related to thalamic lacunar infarction, has rarely been due to a small putaminal ICH. Three such cases were reported among a group of 152 patients with putaminal ICH.[245] All 3 patients had posteriorly located putaminal hemorrhages that were adjacent to the posterior limb of the internal capsule and the adjacent thalamus. The clinical syndrome was a contralateral hemisensory syndrome involving both superficial and deep sensory modalities, with more severe involvement of the leg than of the arm and face. The imaging studies demonstrated involvement of the dorsolateral thalamus or the ascending thalamocortical projections located in the posterior ("retrolenticular") portion of the posterior limb of the internal capsule.

Hemichorea-Hemiballism. A unilateral dyskinetic syndrome, hemichorea-hemiballism is most commonly due to lacunar infarction in the basal ganglia, thalamus, or subthalamic nucleus but can rarely result from a small putaminal hemorrhage.[246,247] In both series reporting such cases, a right, laterally placed putaminal hemorrhage manifested as contralateral chorea and ballism in the absence of hemiparesis, hemisensory loss, gaze paresis, and hemineglect. The prognosis was excellent in both cases.

Clinical Syndromes in Relationship to the Location of Putaminal Hemorrhage

In a study 100 patients with putaminal hemorrhage, Weisberg and colleagues[248] established the following clinicoanatomic correlations:

1. *Medial hemorrhages* extended medially from the putamen and involved the genu and posterior limb of the internal capsule. This finding correlated with a contralateral hemisensory syndrome but there were no abnormalities of ocular motility, visual fields, or level of consciousness. Affected patients generally had full clinical recovery.

2. *Lateral hemorrhages* originated from the lateral putamen and extended anteriorly along the external capsule. They produced a contralateral hemiplegia and sensory deficits. More than half the patients showed delayed neurologic deterioration, and persistent deficits were more common than full recovery.

3. *Putaminal hemorrhages with extension to the internal capsule and subcortical white matter* extended medially through the internal capsule and superiorly into the corona radiata, causing a more severe syndrome of hemiplegia and hemianesthesia, often but not always with homonymous hemianopia and conjugate ocular deviation. Most patients were left with persistent neurologic sequelae.

4. *Putaminal hemorrhages with subcortical and hemispheric extension* were large hematomas that extended into the white matter of adjacent cerebral lobes, causing mass effect on the lateral ventricle and frequently extending into the ventricular system. They were clinically similar to those of the preceding group, except for

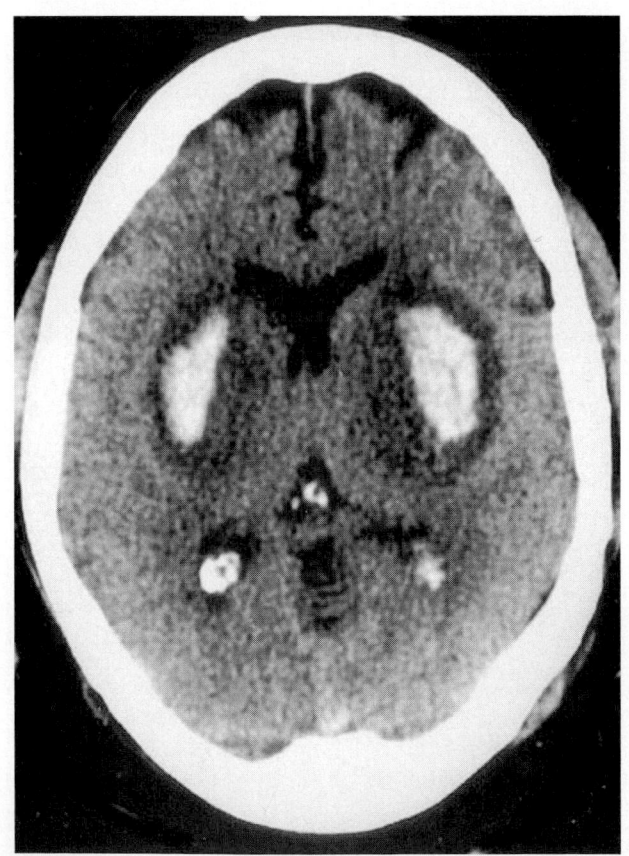

FIGURE 13–24 *CT scan of bilateral, symmetric putaminal hemorrhages in a hypertensive subject. (From Silliman S, McGill J, Booth R: Simultaneous bilateral hypertensive putaminal hemorrhages. J Stroke Cerebrovasc Dis 12:44, 2003.)*

having more prominent aphasia or parietal lobe findings and impaired consciousness. Mortality in this group was 16%, and the majority of the survivors had deficits that interfered with independent living.

5. *Putaminal-thalamic hematomas*, the largest, extended from the putamen into the thalamus (through the internal capsule) and into the subcortical white matter. They all were accompanied by intraventricular hemorrhage. The clinical picture included impaired consciousness in all patients, frequently associated with hemiplegia, abnormalities of horizontal more than vertical gaze, and homonymous hemianopia. Mortality in this group was 79%.

These clinical-CT correlations allowed Weisberg and colleagues[248] to characterize a number of clinically useful patterns, as follows: (1) intraventricular hemorrhage was seen with large hematomas, and both features were associated with high mortality; (2) all patients had combined motor and sensory deficits; (3) the best functional outcome was seen in patients with medial or lateral putaminal hematomas that did not involve the internal capsule or the corona radiata; and (4) delayed neurologic deterioration occurred only in patients with hematomas that extended into the cerebral hemisphere or the thalamus.

Chung and associates[244] analyzed the clinicoanatomic correlations in 192 patients with putaminal hemorrhage. They divided their cases into five anatomic types—middle, posteromedial, posterolateral, lateral, and massive—and related the outcomes to the presumed ruptured arterial branches leading to hematoma formation. The *middle* type (Fig. 13–25) was caused by rupture of medial lenticulostriate arteries, with bleeding into the medial putamen and globus pallidus; the result was a benign syndrome of mild contralateral hemiparesis and hemisensory loss, with a low frequency of impairment of consciousness and with transient conjugate ocular deviation toward the side of the hematoma. Intraventricular extension of the hemorrhage did not occur, and all patients survived. This group of lesions was equivalent to the medial putaminal hemorrhages described by Weisberg and colleagues.[248]

The *posteromedial* type (Fig. 13–26) corresponded to small hematomas confined to the posterior limb of the internal capsule ("capsular" hemorrhages) and were associated with contralateral hemiparesis, hemisensory loss, and dysarthria. The small hematomas, which did not reach the ventricular system, were associated with excellent functional outcome and no mortality. The bleeding vessel in this type of hemorrhage is a branch of the anterior choroidal artery, which supplies a portion of the posterior limb of the internal capsule.[249]

The *posterolateral* type (Fig. 13–27) was a putaminocapsular hemorrhage, caused by rupture of posterior branches of the lateral lenticulostriate arteries. These larger hematomas occasionally ruptured into the lateral ventricle and produced a more severe syndrome consisting of impaired consciousness, frequent conjugate ocular deviation toward the affected hemisphere, and constant and generally severe contralateral hemiparesis and hemisensory loss, along with aphasia or hemineglect, depending on hematoma location in the dominant or nondominant hemisphere, respectively.

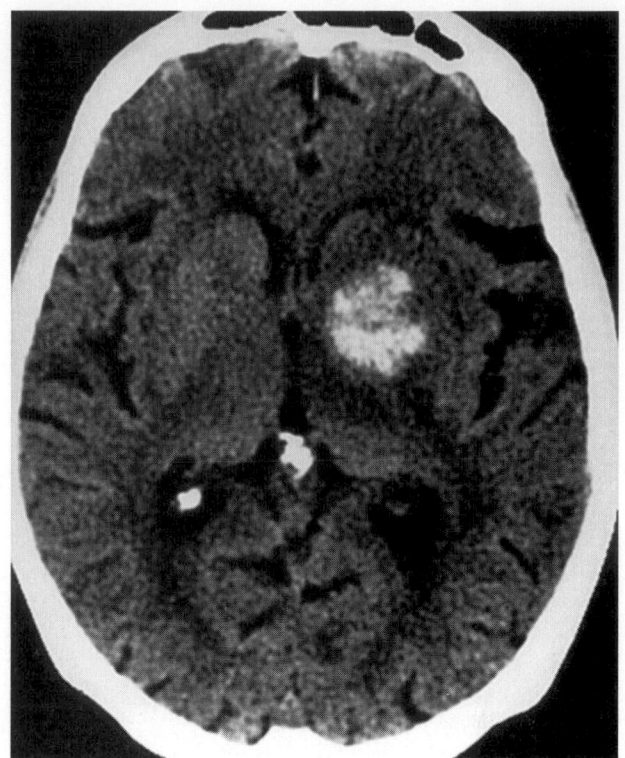

FIGURE 13–25 *CT scan of the medial variety of striatocapsular (putaminal) hemorrhage with minimal mass effect on the frontal horn of the lateral ventricle. (From Chung C, Caplan LR, Yamamoto Y, et al: Striatocapsular haemorrhage. Brain 123:1850, 2000.)*

The *lateral* type of hematoma (Fig. 13–28) originated from rupture of the most lateral branches of the lenticulostriate arteries. It remained confined to an elliptical hematoma collected between the putamen and the insular cortex, producing contralateral hemiparesis, often without an associated hemisensory loss but frequently with either aphasia or hemineglect, depending on the side of the brain involved. The outcome was generally excellent, except in cases of large hematomas, which frequently ruptured into the ventricular system and often required surgical treatment, which in turn was generally associated with good outcome. This "lateral" type of putaminal ICH in the dominant hemisphere has rarely been associated with the syndrome of conduction aphasia.[250]

The *massive* type (Fig. 13–29) involved the entire striatocapsular area and probably resulted from rupture of the same branches (posteromedial branches of the lateral lenticulostriate arteries) that cause the posterolateral type of putaminal ICH. Affected patients had a depressed level of consciousness and hemiparesis, frequently associated with ipsilateral conjugate eye deviation, and often progressed to coma with brainstem involvement and death despite treatment with surgical drainage of the hematoma. This group corresponds to the "putaminal-thalamic" group described by Weisberg and colleagues.[248]

In a separate study, Weisberg and colleagues[251] analyzed 14 cases of massive putaminal-thalamic hemorrhage. All of their patients were young African-Americans with

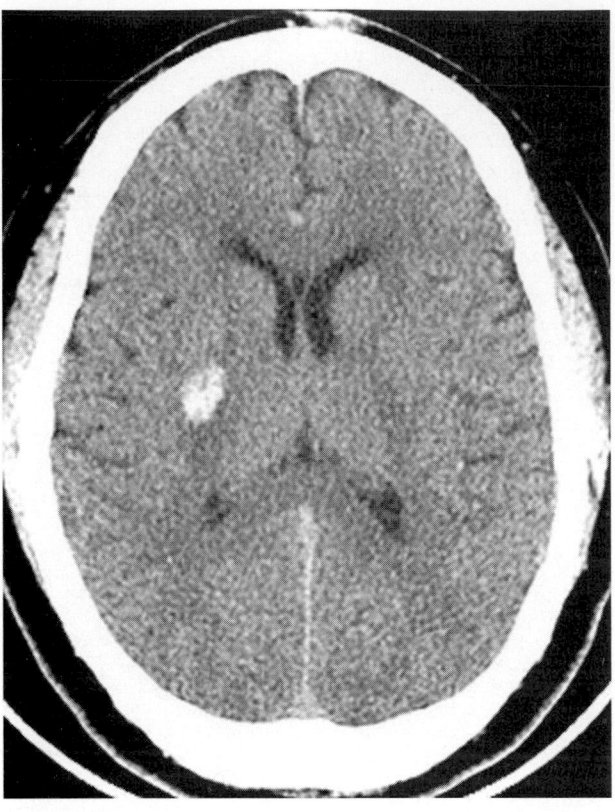

FIGURE 13–26 *CT scan of posteromedial ("capsular") form of putaminal hemorrhage. This small hemorrhage is limited to the posterior limb of the internal capsule.*

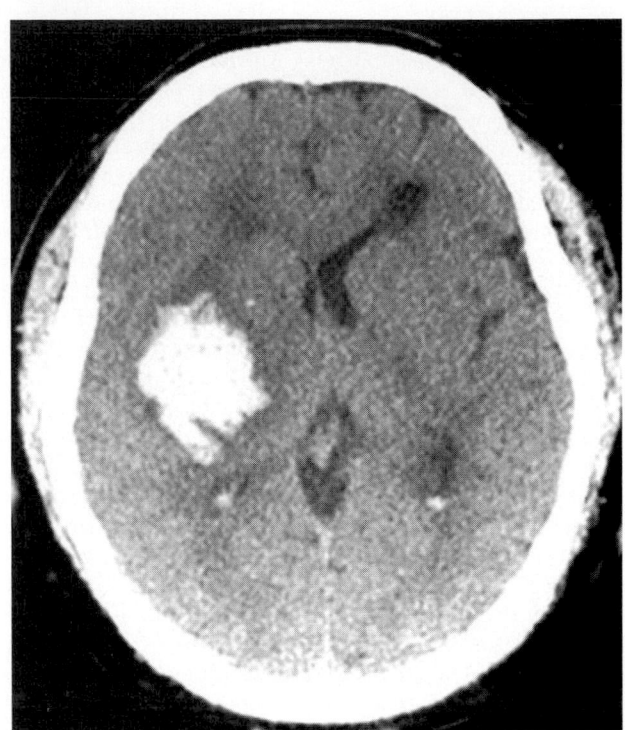

FIGURE 13–27 *CT scan of posterolateral putaminal hemorrhage. Moderate-size hematoma originating in the posterior putamen, with compression and medial displacement of the posterior limb of the internal capsule but without ventricular extension.*

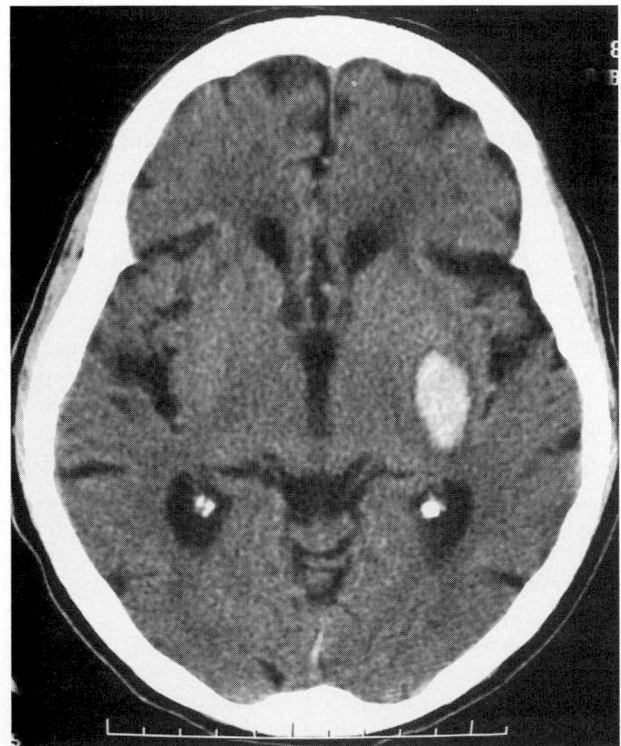

FIGURE 13–28 *CT scan of lateral variety of putaminal hemorrhage. The small lens-shaped hematoma has collected between the insula and the posterior putamen without ventricular extension.*

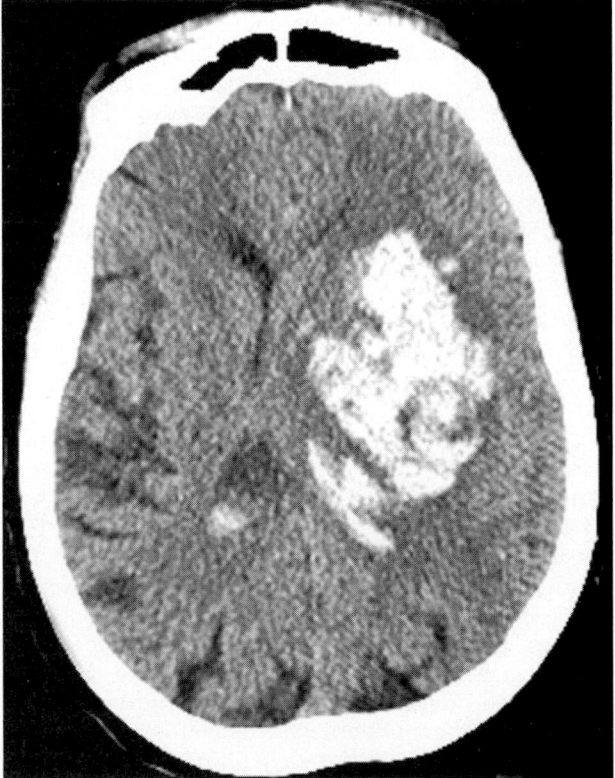

FIGURE 13–29 *CT scan of massive type of putaminal hemorrhage, showing marked mass effect with midline shift and effacement of the lateral ventricle as well as intraventricular extension.*

hypertension who presented with headache several hours before the onset of the focal deficit, and all became hemiplegic and comatose over periods of 4 to 12 hours. The hematomas were large, with marked mass effect and intraventricular extension. All patients died within 72 hours of onset of symptoms despite treatment of hypertension and increased intracranial pressure.

Caudate Hemorrhage

Caudate hemorrhage represents approximately 5% to 7% of cases of ICH (see Table 13.2).[81] Most of the published series on caudate ICH have identified hypertension as its leading cause.[81,252,253] However, other causes not generally associated with deep spontaneous ICH are frequently identified, including cerebral aneurysms,[254] arteriovenous malformations,[99,255] and the basal vascular abnormalities associated with moyamoya disease.[252,256] The last mechanism is thought to lead to ICH through rupture of the anastomotic channels that develop in the area of the basal ganglia, including the head of the caudate, as a result of the progressive occlusion of trunks of the circle of Willis.[257]

The bleeding vessels correspond to deep penetrating branches of the anterior and middle cerebral arteries, vessels similar in diameter to those that supply the putamen and thalamus.[258] Because of its paraventricular location, the caudate also receives blood supply from ependymal arteries that flow outward from the ventricular surface into the parenchyma. These arteries originate beneath the ependymal surface as terminal branches of the anterior choroidal artery, posterior choroidal artery, and striatal rami of the middle cerebral artery.[259]

A number of reported cases of spontaneous hemorrhage in the caudate nucleus have delineated a relatively consistent clinical picture.[81,252–254,260,261] The onset has generally been abrupt, with headache and vomiting commonly followed by variably decreased level of consciousness, resembling the onset of SAH from aneurysmal rupture. Seizures at onset have been reported rarely[99] and were not encountered in the series of 12 patients reported by Stein and coworkers.[81] Consistent physical findings have included neck stiffness and various types of behavioral abnormalities, the latter most commonly being abulia, impairment of memory (both short-term and long-term), and abnormalities of speech, especially verbal fluency.[81,252] These deficits are thought to occur as a result of interruption of cortical-subcortical tracts between the caudate nucleus and the frontal cortex.[252]

The neuropsychologic abnormalities of caudate hemorrhage have been described in detail by Fuh and Wang[252] and by Kumral and associates.[253] A common pattern is that of presentation with abulia, confusion, and disorientation at onset, followed by the development of a prominent amnestic syndrome, at times accompanied by language disturbances. The latter have most often included a nonfluent aphasia,[253] and occasional examples of transcortical motor aphasia have been recorded as well.[249] Hematomas in the nondominant hemisphere generally do not produce unilateral disturbances of attention,[81,249] although one patient reported by Kumral and associates[253] developed visuospatial neglect.

In approximately 50% of cases, the common clinical features are accompanied by others, which most often take the form of transient gaze paresis and contralateral hemiparesis, and rarely elements of an ipsilateral Horner's syndrome.[81] The abnormalities described in gaze mechanisms have most often been horizontal gaze palsies with conjugate deviation or preference toward the side of the hemorrhage, with full correction by oculocephalic maneuvers. Less commonly, vertical gaze palsy has been described, either combined with a horizontal gaze palsy or, more commonly, as an isolated phenomenon. Occasionally, the motor deficit is accompanied by a transient hemisensory syndrome. In those cases in which hemiparesis is a feature, the weakness tends to be slight (never to the point of hemiplegia) and transient, resolving within days of the onset.[81,260] The generally small size and localized character of caudate hemorrhage are the reason that focal neurologic deficits such as transient hemiparesis are relatively uncommon (in 30% of the 23 cases studied by Chung and associates[244]). The virtually consistent extension into the ventricular system accounts for the high frequency of headache and meningeal signs, which resemble those in the onset of SAH. Rare instances of bilateral caudate ICH[262] or hemorrhage associated with intraventricular extension with acute hydrocephalus[81] can have a more dramatic presentation, with coma and ophthalmoplegia, the latter presumably due to oculomotor nuclei involvement as a result of aqueductal dilatation.[263]

In typical cases, CT scan shows a hematoma located in the area of the head of the caudate nucleus (Fig. 13–30). Ventricular extension into the frontal horn of the ipsilateral ventricle is an invariable feature.[81] In approximately 75% of cases, mild to moderate hydrocephalus of the body and temporal horns of the lateral ventricles has been present.

Hemorrhages that are medium or large are frequently accompanied by transient gaze palsies and hemiparesis, and those accompanied by an ipsilateral Horner's syndrome extend more inferiorly and laterally. Occasionally, the hematomas extend from the region of the head of the caudate nucleus into the anterior portions of the thalamus (Fig. 13–31). In those instances, the clinical syndrome has featured a prominent but transient short-term memory defect.[81] Before the introduction of CT, these cases of caudate ICH with consistent extension into the ventricular system may have been diagnosed as "subarachnoid hemorrhage with negative arteriography," or even as "primary intraventricular hemorrhage."[259] The latter is probably a rare condition,[23] in most instances reflecting a lack of documentation of the parenchymal or meningeal (in cases of ruptured aneurysm) site of origin of the hemorrhage rather than a hemorrhage truly confined to the ventricular space.

Caudate hemorrhage can be separated from putaminal and thalamic hemorrhage clinically and radiographically. Headache, nausea, vomiting, and stiff neck regularly accompany caudate hemorrhage[81] but are less common manifestations in putaminal hemorrhage.[82] Disorders of language are regular features of putaminal and thalamic hemorrhage in the dominant hemisphere,[53,82,264] whereas hemorrhages that remain confined to the caudate nucleus are only rarely associated with aphasia.[253] Furthermore, caudate hemorrhages in the nondominant hemisphere do not cause hemi-inattention and anosognosia, the

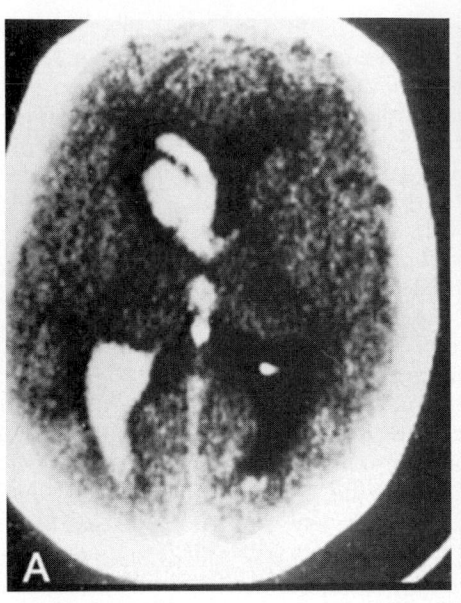
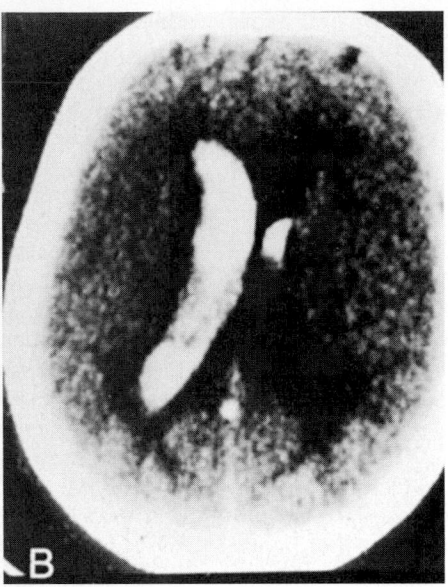

FIGURE 13–30 *A, Hemorrhage originating in the head of the right caudate nucleus with extension into the anterior limb of the internal capsule and into the lateral ventricle and third ventricle. B, Extensive amount of intraventricular blood in the body of the lateral ventricles, primarily on the right side, associated with moderate hydrocephalus.*

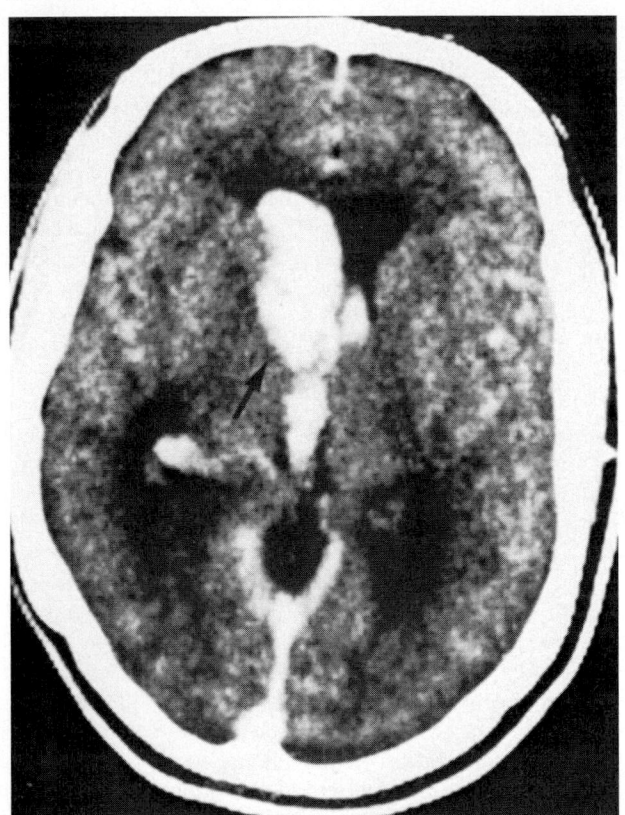

FIGURE 13–31 *Hemorrhage originating from the head of the left caudate nucleus with extension into the anterior-dorsal aspect of the thalamus (arrow), lateral ventricle, and third ventricle.*

behavioral abnormalities associated with thalamic[265–267] and putaminal[82] hemorrhages in that hemisphere.

Caudate hemorrhage also must be distinguished from anterior communicating artery aneurysms that bleed into the brain parenchyma. In primary caudate hemorrhage, there is no accumulation of blood in the interhemispheric fissure, and most of the blood is located in the lateral ventricle adjacent to the involved caudate nucleus. In addition, extension of the hemorrhage into the basal frontal region, a feature invariably seen when hemorrhage into the parenchyma results from ruptured anterior communicating aneurysm, is rarely present in caudate ICH.[81]

The outcome in caudate hemorrhage is usually benign, and most patients recover fully, without permanent neurologic deficits.[81] The accompanying hydrocephalus characteristically tends to disappear as the hemorrhage resolves, and ventriculoperitoneal shunting for persistent hydrocephalus is rarely required.[81] This generally benign outcome in caudate ICH occurs despite the virtually consistent ventricular extension of the hemorrhage, stressing the fact that the latter in itself is not necessarily a bad prognostic sign in hemorrhages that originate in the vicinity of the ventricular system, as in caudate and thalamic ICHs.

Thalamic Hemorrhage

The thalamic form of ICH accounts for 10% to 15% of parenchymatous hemorrhage.[2,4,48–50,52,53] Its clinical and pathologic characteristics are well recognized, and the spectrum of clinical variations reflects the size and pattern of extension of the hematoma. The mass originates in the thalamus and, if it enlarges, extends laterally (into the internal capsule), medially (into the third ventricle), inferiorly (into the subthalamus and dorsal midbrain), upward, and into the parietal white matter.[225,266,268]

The main cause of thalamic hemorrhage is hypertension, which accounts for 74% to 83% of cases.[268–270] Other reported mechanisms are the use of anticoagulant and thrombolytic agents,[271] use of cocaine,[268] rupture of posterior cerebral artery aneurysm,[272] and cavernous malformations.[273] The hemorrhages due to these mechanisms are not clinically different from those caused by hypertension, except for (1) the tendency toward recurrent bleeding in those due to cavernous angioma[273] and (2) the potential for multiple ICHs after use of cocaine[138] and after thrombolysis.[271]

Table 13.4 Clinical Features of Thalamic Hemorrhage

	Walshe et al[53] (N = 18)	Barraquer-Bordas et al[274] (N = 23)
History		
Age (yr) (mean)	64	68
Headache	22%	30%
Vomiting	77%	48%
Physical findings		
Level of consciousness		
Alert	6%	21%
Drowsy	33%	40%
Stuporous	33%	18%
Comatose	28%	21%
Hemiplegia-hemiparesis	100%	100%
Hemisensory deficit	100%	100%
Homonymous hemianopia	—	18%
Aphasia	4/7°	4
Mutism	1	1
Anosognosia	2/3°	2
Upward gaze palsy	94%	35%
Horizontal ocular deviation		
Toward side of lesion	6	3
Opposite side of lesion	3	6
Pupillary abnormalities		
Miosis	100%	70%
Absence of light reflex	62%	13%
Mortality	50%	39%

°Number of patients with deficit/number of patients tested.

The clinical picture has several distinctive features. They are listed in Table 13.4, which summarizes data from a total of 41 patients in two series.[53,274] A typical mode of presentation features a rapid onset of unilateral sensorimotor deficit, frequent occurrence of vomiting (about half the cases), but a low frequency of headache (less than one third of cases). In some, the onset was signaled by coma.[53] A slowly progressive initial course with headache preceding the focal deficits is distinctly uncommon,[225] and only 4 of 13 patients in the series reported by Walshe and associates[53] experienced symptoms for 1 to 2 hours before hemiparesis occurred. In a few cases, unilateral sensory symptoms (numbness) precede the onset of hemiparesis and stupor.[53,275]

The physical findings include hemiparesis or hemiplegia in 95% of cases,[53,264,265,274] virtually all of which have an associated severe hemisensory syndrome (see Table 13.4). This syndrome usually appears as a decrease or loss of all sensory modalities over the contralateral limbs, face, and trunk.[270] The severity and distribution of the motor and sensory symptoms are similar to those of putaminal hemorrhage and therefore are not useful differentiating points. Homonymous hemianopia is an uncommon finding and tends to be transient,[51,224] probably reflecting the location of the lateral geniculate body below and lateral to the hematoma. This sign would be expected in large hemorrhages with extrathalamic extension, but these lesions also affect consciousness severely, precluding detection of the visual field defect.

The clinical presentation of thalamic hemorrhage has distinctive oculomotor findings. The most characteristic combination is one of upward gaze palsy with miotic unreactive pupils,[51,53,224,275] elements of Parinaud's syndrome caused when the enlarging mass exerts effects on the upper midbrain. The upward gaze palsy determines the ocular position at rest of conjugate downward deviation, sometimes associated with convergence, as if the eyes were peering at the tip of the nose.[51] In addition, nystagmus retractorius on attempted upward gaze, and skew deviation are commonly present.[51,224] Other, less common oculomotor abnormalities reported in thalamic hemorrhage are downward gaze palsy[51,224]; anisocoria with ipsilateral miosis, sometimes associated with palpebral ptosis[224]; transient opsoclonus[276]; and ipsilateral[53,274] or contralateral[274,277] horizontal ocular deviation.

The classic combination of upward gaze palsy with miotic unreactive pupils has high diagnostic value, and it is due to compressive or destructive effects of the thalamic hematoma on the underlying midbrain tectum.[51,224,230,274] The precise anatomic structures involved in these oculomotor abnormalities have been delineated by experimental studies in monkeys[278,279] and a number of observations in humans.[280,282] The experimental observations of Pasik and colleagues[279] established that involvement of the posterior commissure and the "nucleus interstitialis of the posterior commissure" were consistently associated with upward gaze palsy. Areas that were not essential for the development of the gaze palsy included the superior colliculi, the nucleus of Darkschewitsch and the interstitial nucleus of Cajal, and the medial thalamus. Christoff and associates,[280,281] from their observations in human clinicopathologic material, concluded that most lesions producing upward gaze palsy required bilateral or midline involvement of the midbrain tectum, particularly when loss of pupillary light reflex was also present.[280] Denny-Brown and Fischer,[278] however, performed unilateral midbrain tegmental lesions in monkeys, which resulted in upward gaze palsy, skew deviation (with the ipsilateral eye in a higher position than the contralateral eye), and head tilt. Also after performing unilateral stereotactic lesions of the dorsolateral midbrain tegmentum in humans for the treatment of pain syndromes, Nashold and Seaber[282] recorded symmetric upward gaze palsy in 13 of 16 subjects. In 10 subjects, downward gaze was impaired as well, but never without upward gaze palsy. Of their 16 patients, 15 had miotic nonreactive pupils, 11 had convergence paralysis, and 10 showed skew deviation, with the ipsilateral eye in a lower position in two thirds.

In summary, virtually all the oculomotor findings observed in thalamic hemorrhage have been described after unilateral tegmental midbrain lesions in humans. This fact supports the view that the oculomotor findings in this condition are due to compression or extension of the hemorrhage into the midbrain tegmentum. However, other observations suggest that CSF hypertension and hydrocephalus associated with the hemorrhage may play an additional role in the production of the oculomotor findings, because ventricular shunting has been shown to reverse these manifestations.[275,283,284] In conclusion, a compressive effect upon the tegmental-tectal portion of the midbrain, either directly from unilateral compression by the hematoma or indirectly through hydrocephalus, results in the classic oculomotor and pupillary abnormalities of thalamic hemorrhage.

Clinical Manifestations

types of ICH have been noted.[49,84,304,308] The circumstances at onset are listed in Table 13.7, which compares series of lobar ICH with those involving all forms of ICH.[2,49,84,304,308–310] The distinguishing features of lobar ICH are lower frequency of hypertension and coma on admission and higher frequency of headache and seizures. The higher frequency of headache at onset may reflect the larger number of patients with lobar ICH who are awake and can give a history. Ropper and Davis[84] described the headaches as located in and around the ipsilateral eye in occipital hematomas, around the ear in temporal hemorrhages, bilateral anteriorly in frontal hemorrhage, and anterior temporal (temple) in parietal lobe hematomas. The low incidence of coma on admission in lobar ICH is probably related to the peripheral location of the hematoma, at a distance from midline structures.[84]

Seizure as a common event at the onset of lobar ICH has been well documented.[49,304,308,311–315] The mechanism of seizures in lobar hematomas may reflect the location of the hemorrhage in the gray matter–white matter interface, which creates a situation similar to the surgical isolation of cortex by subcortical injury that results in sustained paroxysmal activity from the isolated cortex.[316]

The neurologic deficits seen with lobar ICH depend on the location and size of the hematoma.[84] They include (1) sudden hemiparesis, worse in the arm, with retained ability to walk, in frontal hematoma; (2) combined sensory and motor deficits, the former predominating, and visual field defects in parietal hemorrhage; (3) fluent paraphasic speech with poor comprehension and relative sparing of repetition in left temporal lobe hematomas; and (4) homonymous hemianopia, occasionally accompanied by mild sensory changes (extinction to double simultaneous stimulation), in occipital lobe hemorrhages. In the group of 24 patients described by Kase and associates,[49] hemiparesis and visual field defects were the most common abnormality, found in 60% and 30% of patients who were not comatose on admission, respectively. Those patients in whom the two signs coexisted had larger and more anteriorly placed hematomas, whereas those with hemianopia and no hemiparesis had posterior hemorrhages. From these data, the clinical presentation in a lobar parieto-occipital hematoma emerges as sudden onset of headache, sometimes associated with vomiting, not uncommonly associated with seizure activity, with state of consciousness in the alert or obtunded level, associated with mild contralateral hemiparesis and visual field defect. Specific deficits in speech or spatial function are seen when the hematomas are of dominant frontotemporal or nondominant parietal location, respectively, mimicking the deficits seen with infarction.[317,318]

Prognosis

The prognosis in lobar hematomas is usually less grave than in other forms of ICH. The mortality rates reported have been between 11.5% and 29%,[49,84,152,319] all lower than the rates for the other varieties of ICH. A low frequency (6%) has been reported in an autopsy series,[52] whereas in clinical series, the frequency is between 10% and 32%.[49,84,152] In addition, the functional outcome for survivors is generally better than in those of deep hemispheric ICHs, with good outcome reported in 57% to 85% of patients.[319–321]

Computed Tomography Aspects

After the acute phase of the ICH, lobar hematomas can adopt a number of residual patterns, as analyzed by Sung and Chu.[322] Frequently (27%), the ICH leaves no CT-demonstrated residual, although a slit and a round cavity (34%) are the most common CT sequelae; rarely (3%), only calcification at the ICH site remains.

Ropper and Davis[84] provided two-dimensional measurements of 26 hematomas and commented on the tendency of these lesions to enlarge mostly in the transverse and anteroposterior planes of the CT section. In Weisberg's[152] series of 45 patients with lobar ICH, 10 were found to have intraventricular extension, a factor that did not affect the mortality rates in this group.

The CT features of the 22 cases reported by Kase and associates[49] are shown in Table 13.8. The hematomas could be divided by volume into three main groups, which in turn correlated with the presence and severity of mass effect. Ventricular extension was a factor that correlated with location (proximity to ventricular system) rather than size of the hematoma. The outcome was in part a function of hematoma size; no patient with a hematoma larger than 60 mL survived, whereas all those with small hematomas (<20 mL) did. In the group with moderate-size

Table 13.7 Comparison of Clinical Features of Lobar Intracerebral Hemorrhage (ICH) with All Forms of ICH

	All Forms of ICH (%)[*]		Lobar ICH (%)[*]			
Feature	HCSR[2]	Lausanne[309]	Kase et al[49]	Ropper and Davis[84]	Weisberg[308]	SDB[304]
Hypertension						
History	72		22	31	30	55
On admission	91	55[†]	66	46	56	?
Headache	33	40	61	46	72	60
Vomiting	51	?	33	61	32	29
Seizures	6	7	33	0	28	16
Coma	24	22	18	0.4	?	19

HCSR, Harvard Cooperative Stroke Registry; SDB, Stroke Data Bank; ?, information not provided.
[*]Percentages rounded to the closest whole number (decimals from the original omitted).
[†]Not specified whether hypertension was diagnosed by history or at entry examination.
From Kase CS: Lobar hemorrhage. In Kase CS, Caplan LR (eds): Intracerebral Hemorrhage. Boston, Butterworth-Heinemann, 1994, p 363.

Table 13.8 Computed Tomography Features and Outcome of Lobar Intracerebral Hematomas

Hematoma Size	No. of Cases	Midline Shift	Ventricular Extension	Outcome/Operated
Small (<20 mL)	5	1	0	5 improved/0
Moderate (20–40 mL)	7	6	1	6 improved/3 1 died/0
Massive (>40 mL)	10	10	7	4 improved/2 6 died/1
Total	22	17	8	

From Kase CS, Williams JP, Wyatt DA, Mohr JP: Lobar intracerebral hematomas: Clinical and CT analysis of 22 cases. Neurology (NY) 32:1146, 1982.

hematomas, 75% survived, and the functional level was in general poorer than in the group with small hematomas. These figures, in addition, give some indication of the possible role of surgical drainage as a therapeutic option in lobar ICH. Writers of some studies of lobar ICH have stated that surgery offers no advantage over medical therapy,[84,323] whereas results of the uncontrolled study reported by Kase and associates[49] suggested a trend toward better outcome after surgery. Surgery as a possible option for lobar hematomas is further encouraged by the superficial location of the hemorrhage, which makes it more easily accessible.[324] This form of therapy is particularly indicated in patients with medium-sized or large hematomas who show signs of progressive neurologic deterioration after diagnosis.[23,49,325]

Flemming and coworkers[326] have further analyzed the surgical management of lobar ICH. In a review of 61 patients, these researchers found neurologic deterioration after admission in 16 patients (26%) and predictors of a deteriorating course to be a decreased level of consciousness, ICH volume greater than 60 mL, and CT signs of mass effect. The main cause of neurologic decline was hematoma enlargement. These data further strengthen the view that early aggressive management, including hematoma evacuation, should be considered in patients with lobar ICH who meet the preceding criteria. In a subsequent analysis of Mayo Clinic data, Flemming and colleagues[327] reported observations on 81 patients with lobar ICH. Volume larger than 40 mL on CT was associated with poor outcome; in patients with hemorrhage smaller than 40 mL, interval from symptom onset to hospital presentation of less than 17 hours and a Glasgow Coma Scale GCS (score) of 13 or less were predictive of a poor outcome. These data stressed the importance of hematoma enlargement as a factor in the deterioration of patients who present early after onset of lobar ICH.

HEMORRHAGE AFFECTING THE BRAINSTEM AND CEREBELLUM

Cerebellar Hemorrhage

In a landmark paper in 1959, Fisher and colleagues[55] described the main clinical features of cerebellar hemorrhage. Especially important diagnostic features were the inability to walk, gaze palsy without hemiplegia, and the absence of unilateral limb paresis. These investigators found that surgical decompression could be lifesaving, occasionally even in patients in deep coma before surgery.

More important, patients who had been treated surgically were often able to return to active lives without the overwhelming disability often retained by survivors of basal ganglionic hemorrhage. Although these diagnostic formulations were initially subject to dispute, CT scanning and MRI have made the detection of smaller cerebellar hematomas possible,[328,329] essentially confirming the report by Fisher and colleagues.[55]

Cerebellar hemorrhage appears at a rate variously quoted as between 5% and 15%.[48,54,330–333] The average rate is about 10%, which is also approximately the percentage of brain in weight accounted for by the cerebellum. Although 10% is a relatively low frequency, the importance of establishing the diagnosis resides in the good prognosis after prompt surgical treatment.[48,158,334] Cerebellar hemorrhage usually occurs in one of the hemispheres, generally originating in the region of the dentate nucleus, probably from distal branches of the superior cerebellar artery[55] or occasionally the posterior-inferior cerebellar artery.[126] In the study by Fisher and colleagues,[55] the left hemisphere was affected twice as often as the right. McKissock and associates[335] also commented on a left hemisphere preponderance in cerebellar hemorrhage. Most other series do not report hemorrhage laterality.

The hematoma collects around the dentate and spreads into the hemispheral white matter, commonly extending into the cavity of the fourth ventricle as well (Fig. 13–37). The adjacent brain stem (pontine tegmentum) is rarely involved directly by the hematoma but is often compressed by it, at times leading to pontine necrosis. The midline variant of cerebellar hemorrhage originates from the vermis and represents only about 5% of the cases.[55] It virtually always communicates directly with the fourth ventricle through its roof and frequently extends into the pontine tegmentum bilaterally (Fig. 13–38). The bleeding vessel in this variety usually corresponds to distal branches of the superior or the posterior-inferior cerebellar artery. These two forms of cerebellar hemorrhage have distinctive clinical and prognostic features.

Distribution of etiologic factors in cerebellar hemorrhage is similar to that in other forms of ICH, hypertension being the leading cause.[55,158] AVMs are said to be common in the cerebellum.[332,335] AVMs accounted for 5 of 15 cerebellar hematomas in the autopsy series reported by McCormick and Rosenfield[24]; in other series,[158] lower rates of AVMs (4%), similar to those for ICH at other sites, have been reported.[84] Anticoagulation is an important etiologic factor in cerebellar hemorrhage and was the second most common cause reported by Ott and coworkers.[158] Among

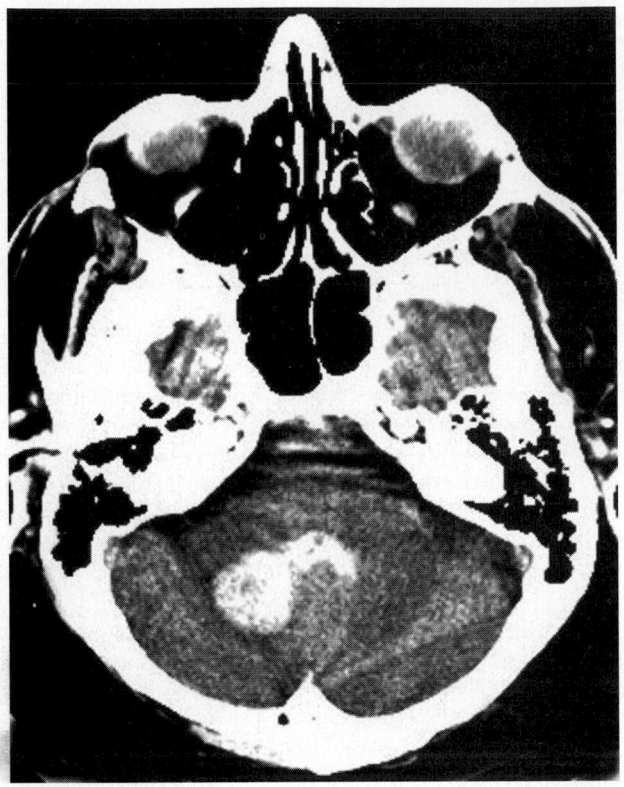

FIGURE 13–37   *CT scan of right cerebellar hemorrhage originating in the area of the dentate nucleus, with extension into the adjacent fourth ventricle.*

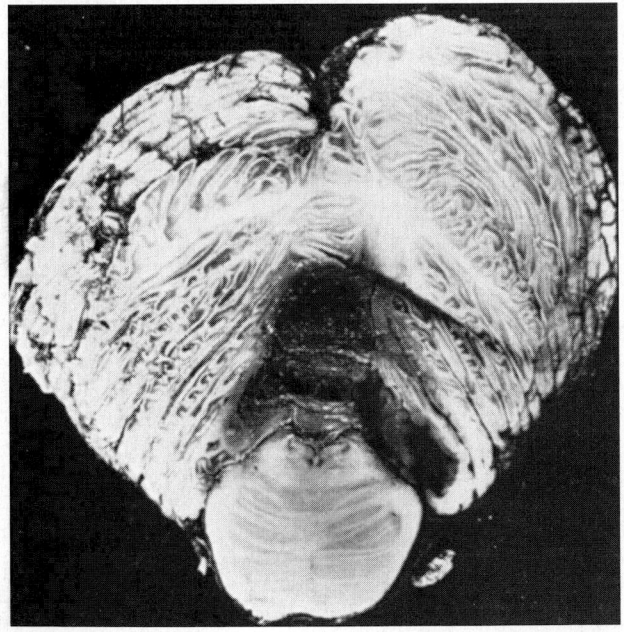

FIGURE 13–38   *Vermian cerebellar hemorrhage with pressure on the pontine tegmentum.*

24 ICHs in patients undergoing oral anticoagulant therapy,[156] 9 occurred in the cerebellum. Three of these were of the less common vermian or midline variety. Fisher and colleagues[55] commented on a relative female preponderance in their series (13:8); in other series, the female-to-male ratio was reported as 26:30,[335] 6:6,[54] 5:14,[336] and 17:17.[335]

Symptoms usually develop while the patient is active. Occasionally a single prodromal episode of dizziness or facial numbness may precede the hemorrhage. The most common symptom is *an inability to stand or walk*, which in many patients has been dramatic in onset. One man leaned against a fence while painting and could not right himself; another bumped downstairs on his bottom to call for help. Crawling or propelling oneself prone on the floor to get to the bathroom to vomit has been mentioned. Rare patients maintain their ability to walk a few steps, but scarcely any patient with a sizable hemorrhage (>2 cm) walks into the emergency room or physician's office.

Vomiting is also very common, being present in 42 of 44 patients,[158] 12 of 12 patients,[334] and 14 of 18 patients[55] in various series. Vomiting usually occurs soon after the onset in cerebellar and subarachnoid hemorrhage but often develops later, after other symptoms, in putaminal hemorrhage. *Dizziness* is also common, occurring in 24 of 44 patients,[158] 8 of 21 patients,[55] and 4 of 12 patients[334] in various series. More often the feeling is one of insecurity, a "drunken feeling," or wavering rather than true rotational vertigo.

Headache is also very common, occurring in 32 of 44 patients,[158] 10 of 21 patients,[55] and 12 of 12 patients[54] in various series. Most often the pain is occipital, but occasionally it can occur on the side of the head or frontally. At times the headache is abrupt and excruciating, closely mimicking SAH. In other patients the pain is located primarily in the neck or shoulder. Dysarthria, tinnitus, and hiccups occur but are less common. Loss of consciousness at onset is unusual,[158,337] and only one third of patients are obtunded by the time they reach the hospital.[158] Most patients show gradual worsening over 1 to 3 hours, as in other forms of ICH.[2]

The classic physical findings are a combination of a unilateral cerebellar deficit with variable signs of ipsilateral tegmental pontine involvement. These are detailed in Table 13.9, from an analysis of 38 noncomatose patients in the series reported by Ott and coworkers.[158] Appendicular and gait ataxias occurred in 65% and 78%, respectively, of patients who were alert enough to cooperate for cerebellar function testing. Other patients lean to the side when placed upright. On the side of the hemorrhage, there usually is overshoot or inability to brake the limb quickly; this sign is more common than finger-to-nose or finger-to-object ataxia. Signs of involvement of the ipsilateral pontine tegmentum include peripheral facial palsy, ipsilateral horizontal gaze palsy, sixth cranial nerve palsy, depressed corneal reflex, and miosis. In some patients the hemorrhage presses laterally in the area of the cerebellopontine angle, producing peripheral facial palsy, deafness, and diminished corneal response.

From analysis of the relative frequency of signs in noncomatose patients reported by Ott and coworkers,[158] a characteristic triad consisting of appendicular ataxia,

Table 13.9 Neurologic Findings in Cerebellar Hemorrhage for Noncomatose Patients

Neurologic Finding	No.	%
Appendicular ataxia	17/26	65
Truncal ataxia	11/17	65
Gait ataxia	11/14	78
Dysarthria	20/32	62
Gaze palsy	20/37	54
Cranial nerve findings		
Peripheral facial palsy	22/36	61
Nystagmus	18/35	51
Miosis	11/37	30
Decreased corneal reflex	10/33	30
Abducens palsy	10/36	28
Loss of gag reflex	6/30	20
Skew deviation	4/33	12
Trochlear palsy	0/36	—
Hemiparesis	4/35	11
Extensor plantar response	23/36	64
Respiratory irregularity	6/28	21
Nuchal rigidity	14/35	40
Subhyaloid hemorrhage	0/34	—

From Ott KH, Kase CS, Ojemann RJ, Mohr JP: Cerebellar hemorrhage: Diagnosis and treatment. Arch Neurol 31:160, 1974.

ipsilateral gaze palsy, and peripheral facial palsy was suggested; at least two of the three signs were present in 73% of the patients tested for all three. Skew ocular deviation is also common.[330] Additional findings useful in differential diagnosis are hemiplegia and subhyaloid hemorrhages, both of which are uncommon enough in cerebellar hemorrhage that their presence essentially rules out the diagnosis.[158] The frequency of unilateral limb weakness in cerebellar hemorrhage has been a matter of controversy. In the study by Fisher and colleagues,[55] hemiplegia was observed only in the setting of a prior stroke; and similar findings were recorded by Ott and coworkers.[158] In two autopsy series, however, hemiplegia was reported in 50% and 20% of the cases,[332,334] and Richardson[333] noted contralateral hemiplegia in more than 50% of cases in his clinical series. Although in some instances reports of ipsilateral hemiplegia may have corresponded to decreased mobility of grossly ataxic limbs or decreased spontaneous movement, a contralateral hemiplegia cannot be explained on those bases, so one must assume involvement of the corticospinal tract in the ipsilateral basis pontis.

Other neurologic findings add little specific diagnostic data: The pupils are commonly small and reactive to light, dysarthria is present in two thirds of cases, and the respiratory rhythm is usually unaffected.[158] Unilateral involuntary eye closure has been occasionally observed,[285,338] the involved eye usually being contralateral to the hematoma. This sign has been interpreted as eye closure for avoidance of diplopia, but this interpretation is probably not always correct, because the sign occurs in the absence of diplopia, in both infratentorial and supratentorial strokes.[285] Other less common oculomotor abnormalities, such as ocular bobbing, have occasionally been reported in cerebellar hemorrhage,[158,339,340] but with a lower frequency than in pontine hemorrhage and infarction. Some patients have a head tilt. Neck stiffness and unwillingness to move the head or neck either actively or passively probably signify increased pressure in the posterior fossa.

Along with these focal neurologic manifestations, patients with cerebellar hemorrhage may present with variable levels of decreased alertness. Of the 56 cases reported by Ott and coworkers,[158] 14 (25%) were alert, 22 (40%) drowsy, 5 (9%) stuporous, and 15 (26%) comatose. That two thirds of the patients are responsive (alert or drowsy) on admission justifies the intensive efforts to diagnose this condition early, because the surgical prognosis largely depends on the preoperative level of consciousness.

The clinical course in cerebellar hemorrhage is notoriously unpredictable: Some patients who are alert or drowsy on admission can deteriorate suddenly to coma and death without warning,[55,158,341] whereas others with similar clinical status have an uneventful course with complete recovery of function. Of those patients who were not comatose on admission, only 20% had a smooth, uneventful recovery in the series reported by Ott and coworkers[158]; 80% deteriorated to coma, one fourth of them within 3 hours of onset (Fig. 13–39). A similar frequency was observed in the study by Fisher and colleagues,[55] in which only 2 of 18 patients had a benign course, the other 16 deteriorating to coma at variable intervals, mostly within a few hours after onset. Most patients deteriorate early in the course, but occasional patients have shown fatal decompensation at a later stage, even a month later, after being stable in the interim.[342]

Because prediction of the clinical course cannot be made on the basis of clinical parameters on admission, Ott and coworkers[158] recommended that surgical evacuation of the hematoma should be undertaken whenever the diagnosis is made within 48 hours of onset.[158] They justified the need for prompt diagnosis and emergency surgery by pointing to poor surgical outcome with worsening preoperative mental status, the surgical mortality being 17% for responsive and 75% for unresponsive patients.[158] These figures have proved generally accurate, despite occasional reports of good surgical results in comatose patients.[343]

The use of CT and MRI in cerebellar hemorrhage has permitted the recognition of many different aspects of these lesions, some of which are useful early predictors of clinical course.[328,329,344] Little and coworkers[328] reported two groups of patients with cerebellar hemorrhage; one group had abrupt onset, a more severely depressed level of consciousness, and a tendency toward progressive deterioration, and the other had a more benign, stable course. The first group required surgical treatment, whereas the second group did well with a medical program. CT scans of the first group showed hematomas 3 cm or more in diameter, obstructive hydrocephalus, and ventricular extension of the hemorrhage; in the second group of patients, all of whom had hematomas less than 3 cm in diameter, the other two features were absent. These observations, along with those of others,[345] have identified a group of cerebellar hemorrhages with a benign course. It may be possible to make accurate predictions from the combined analysis of clinical and CT data at the time of onset. Especially important is careful monitoring of the status of the patient. The development of obtundation and extensor plantar responses is ominous and is virtually

Clinical Manifestations

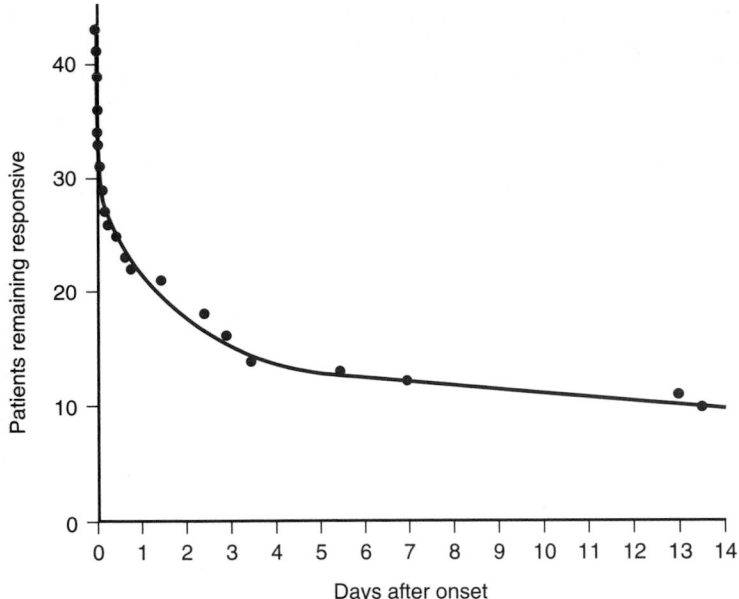

FIGURE 13–39   *Coma in patients with cerebellar hemorrhage as a function of time after onset. (From Ott KH, Kase CS, Ojemann RG, Mohr JP: Cerebellar hemorrhage: Diagnosis and treatment. Arch Neurol 31:160, 1974.)*

always followed by a fatal outcome unless surgery is performed.

In an attempt to identify predictors of neurologic deterioration, St. Louis and associates[341] analyzed a series of 72 patients with cerebellar hemorrhage. For the 33 patients (46%) with deterioration, independent predictors of such a course were a vermian location of the hemorrhage and hydrocephalus. On the basis of these data, St. Louis and associates[341] suggested that patients with these features are likely to require neurosurgical treatment. The same group analyzed clinical factors predictive of poor outcome in a group of 94 patients. Poor outcome was predicted by admission systolic blood pressure higher than 200 mm Hg, hematoma diameter more than 3 cm, brainstem distortion, and acute hydrocephalus, and death was predicted by abnormal brainstem reflexes (corneal and oculocephalic), Glasgow Coma Scale score less than 8, acute hydrocephalus, and intraventricular hemorrhage.[346]

Kirollos and associates[347] have made further refinements in the approach to the treatment of cerebellar hemorrhage. They evaluated 50 consecutive patients and used level of mass effect in the fourth ventricle (graded as absent, compression, or complete obliteration), size of hematoma, Glasgow Coma Scale score, and hydrocephalus as the parameters correlated with type of management and outcome. Their findings indicated that patients with obliterated fourth ventricle, even if conscious on admission, had a high rate (43%) of subsequent neurologic deterioration and that surgical treatment with posterior fossa craniectomy for clot evacuation was recommended before these patients experienced neurologic deterioration. Of interest, 60% of subjects in whom hematoma diameter was more than 3 cm but who had only moderate compression or normal size of the fourth ventricle did not require surgery for clot evacuation.

The uncommon midline (vermian) cerebellar hematoma still represents a serious diagnostic challenge, and its outcome is generally poor. Its frequency in autopsy series has been 6% of all cerebellar hemorrhages.[54] Our experience has documented syndromes featuring relatively acute onset of coma, ophthalmoplegia, and respiratory abnormalities, with variable severity of bilateral limb weakness. Early extension of the vermian hematoma into the midline pontine tegmentum is probably responsible for the abrupt onset of coma and bilateral oculomotor signs (Fig. 13–40). This variant of cerebellar hematoma carries a poor prognosis, similar to that of primary pontine hemorrhage. At times, a relatively small hematoma in this location results in fatal brainstem compression.

Midbrain Hemorrhage

Spontaneous, nontraumatic mesencephalic hemorrhage is rare. In most instances the hemorrhage has dissected down from the thalamus or putamen, is part of a lesion originating in the cerebellum or pons, or arises from blood dyscrasias or AVMs.

Mesencephalic AVMs generally produce a stepwise progressive deterioration. Ataxia and ophthalmoplegia (especially third cranial nerve palsy and paralysis of upward gaze) are common. Aqueductal or third ventricular blockage or distention often leads to hydrocephalus. Bleeding diathesis can lead to isolated midbrain hemorrhage, as shown in Figure 13–41, a brain tissue specimen from an elderly woman with leukemia in whom a third cranial nerve palsy and contralateral intention tremor developed shortly before death. Hypertensive primary mesencephalic hemorrhage is very rare but does occur. One might predict that the hemorrhage would be in the tegmentum in the territory supplied by branches of the superior cerebellar arteries, as in the hypertensive patients reported by several groups.[348–350] The details of these cases follow.

Durward and colleagues[349] described two patients with mesencephalic hematomas. Their first patient was a 71-year-old hypertensive man (blood pressure 230/130 mm Hg) who suddenly could not stand or open his eyes. Signs included bilateral third cranial nerve paralysis, bulbar weakness, and extensor plantar responses. CT scan

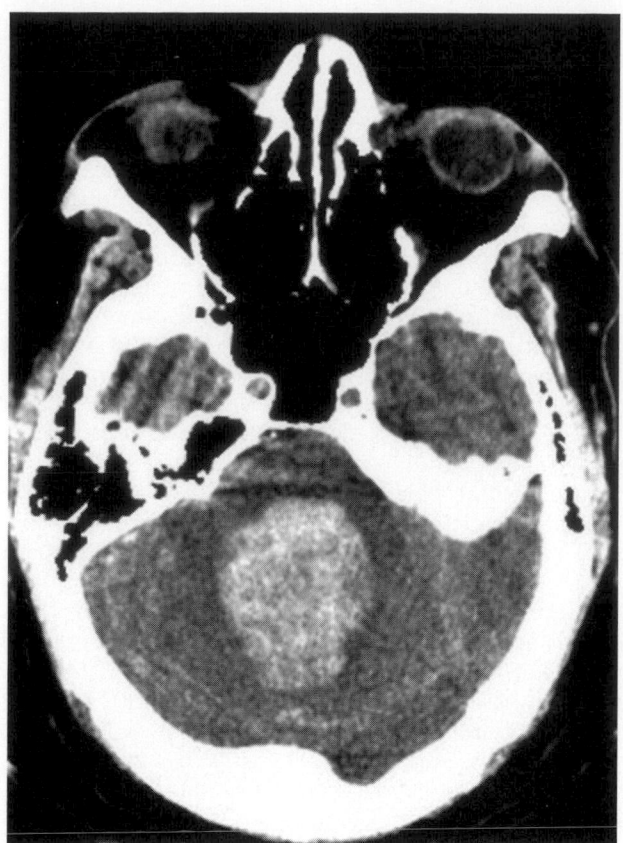

FIGURE 13–40 *CT scan of large midline (vermian) cerebellar hemorrhage with extension into the fourth ventricle and compression of the tegmentum of the pons.*

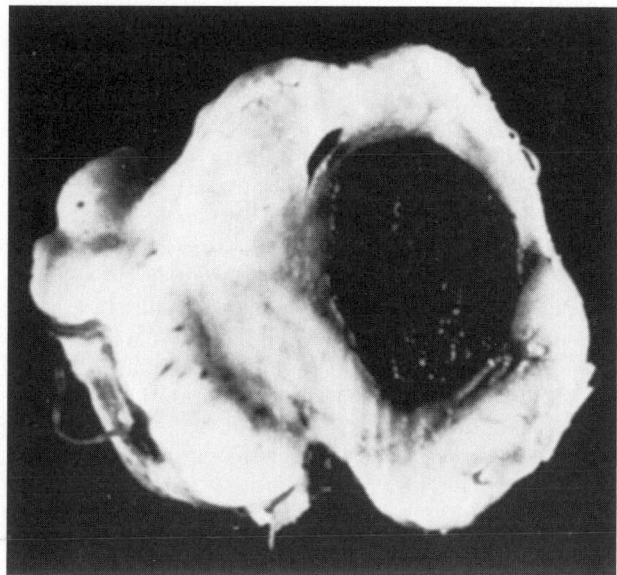

FIGURE 13–41 *Midbrain hemorrhage in a patient with bleeding diathesis.*

revealed a 1-cm hematoma in the ventral tegmentum of the midbrain with rupture into the third ventricle. He experienced obstructive hydrocephalus, which was treated with a ventriculoperitoneal shunt, and survived with bilateral third cranial nerve palsies and poor balance with a tendency to fall backward. Arteriographic findings were normal. Although there was no pathologic confirmation, this case may represent a primary hypertensive mesencephalic tegmental hematoma. The second patient was a normotensive young man who experienced Weber's syndrome (crossed third cranial nerve palsy and hemiparesis) after a week of prodromal headache. The CT scan showed a right midbrain hematoma. After further deterioration, the hematoma was surgically decompressed, and microscopic examination of the wall of the hematoma revealed an AVM. The patient survived but was grossly ataxic.

A 71-year-old patient reported by Morel-Maroger and associates[350] had midbrain hemorrhage due to hypertension. After being treated for hypertension for 5 years, he suddenly lost consciousness and awakened confused and dizzy. He had a diffuse headache and vomited. Clinical findings included a right third cranial nerve palsy, left hemiparesis, and a cerebellar-type ataxia of the right limbs. Blood pressure was 290/110 mm Hg. CT scan documented a 12 × 16-mm hematoma in the right superior cerebellar peduncle. The patient recovered after antihypertensive therapy without surgical intervention.

Roig and coworkers[48] described two patients with hypertensive mesencephalic hematomas detected on CT. One patient had an ipsilateral third cranial nerve paralysis with contralateral hemihypesthesia and limb ataxia. The hyperdense lesion was high in the right mesencephalic tegmentum near the midline, probably draining into the third ventricle. Vertebral angiographic findings were normal. A second patient had a right third cranial nerve palsy and left hemiparesis. The lesion was high in the right side of the midbrain. Both patients survived.

A 10-year-old boy reported by Humphreys[351] suddenly demonstrated right hemiparesis and confusion. Neuro-ophthalmologic findings were not given in detail. A CT scan showed a large hematoma in the basis pedunculi extending into the interpeduncular fossa. The lesion was drained surgically and was found to contain nuclear debris. The nature of the lesion is unknown, but it was likely a hemorrhage into an AVM or a benign tumor.

LaTorre and associates[352] described a 38-year-old woman who, after complaining of headache and intermittent diplopia for 2 years, vomited and demonstrated bilateral sixth cranial nerve palsies and paralysis of upward gaze. Cerebrospinal fluid was found to contain blood, and ventriculography visualized a beaded aqueduct and hydrocephalus. Surgical exploration of the midbrain discovered an AVM of the quadrigeminal plate with a blood clot embedded in the sylvian aqueduct.

A single patient was reported by Scoville and Poppen.[353] The 44-year-old woman experienced an ataxic right hemiparesis in stepwise fashion over 1.5 years. Vomiting, bilateral third cranial nerve paralysis, stupor, and pinpoint pupils suddenly supervened. After a blood clot was drained from her left cerebral peduncle, the patient awakened. Normal blood pressure and coagulation values and the gradual onset favored an AVM in this patient.

Clinical Manifestations

A number of further observations have stressed the presentation of small midbrain hemorrhages with features of isolated forms of ophthalmoplegia.[354-356] These have included isolated fourth[354] and third[355,356] nerve palsies as well as various combinations of a dorsal midbrain syndrome.[357,358] Most of these cases were remarkable for the absence or paucity of signs of long-tract involvement, stressing the fact that small midbrain ICHs can present with isolated ophthalmoplegia.

Pontine Hemorrhage

The early clinicopathologic observations in pontine hemorrhage correspond to those made by Fang and Foley[359] and later by Dinsdale,[54] who reviewed the necropsies at Boston City Hospital and found 511 ICHs among 19,093 autopsies, of which 30 were pontine (6%). Two thirds of the patients in this autopsy series had been comatose when first seen, 13% vomited, and 78% were dead within 48 hours. One patient who survived for 23 days had a small hemorrhage in the right pontine tegmentum. All of the remainder had massive hemorrhage, usually in the midpons at the junction of the basis pontis and tegmentum, that frequently spread rostrally into the midbrain; the hemorrhages almost never spread caudally to the medulla but frequently ruptured into the fourth ventricle.

In 1971 Fisher,[56] using serial sections from a patient with a massive fatal pontine hemorrhage, identified numerous small vessels with "fibrin globes," which he thought were related to the vascular rupture causing the hemorrhage. "From the gaping end of each of these torn vessels there protruded a large mass of platelets partially encircled by thin concentric layers of fibrin." He suggested that the primary hemorrhage led to pressure on surrounding vessels, which subsequently ruptured, causing a cascade or avalanche effect and producing gradual enlargement of the hematoma. Ross Russell[67] had demonstrated large asymptomatic fusiform enlargements on the penetrating vessels of the pons in patients with "atherosclerosis" and hypertensive vascular disease. Cole and Yates,[60] Rosenblum,[62] Fisher,[56] and Caplan[360] all explained bleeding in hypertensive patients as leakage from tiny penetrating vessels damaged by lipohyalinosis and containing small microaneurysms.

Kornyey[361] reported a patient whose pontine hemorrhage occurred during clinical observation; the slow march of signs was similar to the pattern of development seen in ganglionic and thalamic hemorrhages, providing support for Fisher's postulation of the slowly evolving avalanche. Kornyey's patient was a 39-year-old man referred for admission because of malignant hypertension. While his admission history was being taken, he complained of numb hands, weakness, and dizziness. His blood pressure was 245/170 mm Hg. He became restless and apprehensive and complained that he could not hear and had difficulty swallowing and breathing. A bilateral sixth cranial nerve palsy and dilated pupils developed, and his corneal reflexes disappeared. Speech became "bulbar," he was deaf, and he could not move his left leg. Within 15 minutes the patient was comatose; the pupils were small, and the eyes were converged. Bilateral bulbar palsy, stiff limbs with exaggerated reflexes, and extensor plantar responses were observed. Two hours after onset, the patient died. A large hemorrhage in the tegmentum of the pons, with some spread into the right basis pontis, was found at necropsy.[361] In other patients observed during the onset of pontine hemorrhage, development of the deficit usually evolved gradually over minutes (1 to 30 minutes) and was not as instantaneous as aneurysmal subarachnoid hemorrhage.

In the pons, the largest penetrating arteries enter medially, arise perpendicular to the basilar artery, and course from the base to the tegmentum. Other small penetrating arteries originate from the short and long circumferential vessels and enter more laterally, also coursing from base to tegmentum. Some arteries enter the tegmentum laterally and course horizontally across it.[56] Because vessels in all of these sites are potentially susceptible to hypertensive damage and lipohyalinosis, they could theoretically also be sites for pontine bleeding. Silverstein,[362,363] reviewed the pathologic material from Philadelphia General Hospital and confirmed that these sites (Fig. 13-42) were the usual regions of pontine hemorrhage. Of 50 cases, 28 were massive central hemorrhages presumably arising from large paramedian penetrators; 11 were more lateralized, usually spreading from base to tegmentum; and 11 had a tegmental location, 4 remaining unilateral and 7 involving the tegmentum bilaterally.

Not until the mid-1970s, when CT became available, was it possible to diagnose smaller nonfatal pontine hemorrhages accurately and to separate them positively from pontine infarction during life. MRI data, acquired through the use of gradient-echo sequences, indicate that pontine microhemorrhages tend to adopt a distribution similar to that of the large, symptomatic hemorrhages,[364] favoring the dorsal aspect of the basis pontis.

Large Paramedian Pontine Hemorrhage

Massive pontine hemorrhage results from rupture of parenchymal midpontine branches originating from the basilar artery. The bleeding vessel is thought to be a paramedian perforator in its distal portion,[54] causing initial hematoma formation at the junction of tegmentum and basis pontis,[54,363] from which the mass grows into its final round or oval shape and replaces most of both subdivisions of the pons (Fig. 13-43). The lesion usually begins in the middle of the pons and extends along the longitudinal axis of the brainstem into the lower midbrain. The hematoma may track into the middle cerebellar peduncles but usually does not extend caudally beyond the pontomedullary junction.[54] In the process of rapid hematoma expansion, destruction of tegmental and ventral pontine structures results, with the classic combination of signs caused by involvement of cranial nerve nuclei, long tracts, autonomic centers, and structures responsible for maintenance of consciousness. Large pontine hematomas also regularly rupture into the fourth ventricle.[54,362,363]

The classic form of pontine hemorrhage, bilateral and massive, is almost exclusively of hypertensive origin. Other etiologies, such as cryptic vascular malformation, account for 10% or less of the cases in most series.[54,363] Russell[98] regarded pontine hemorrhage as a form of ICH most likely to occur in patients with malignant hypertension or hypertension associated with chronic nephropathy. Clinical presentation is characteristically one of rapid development of

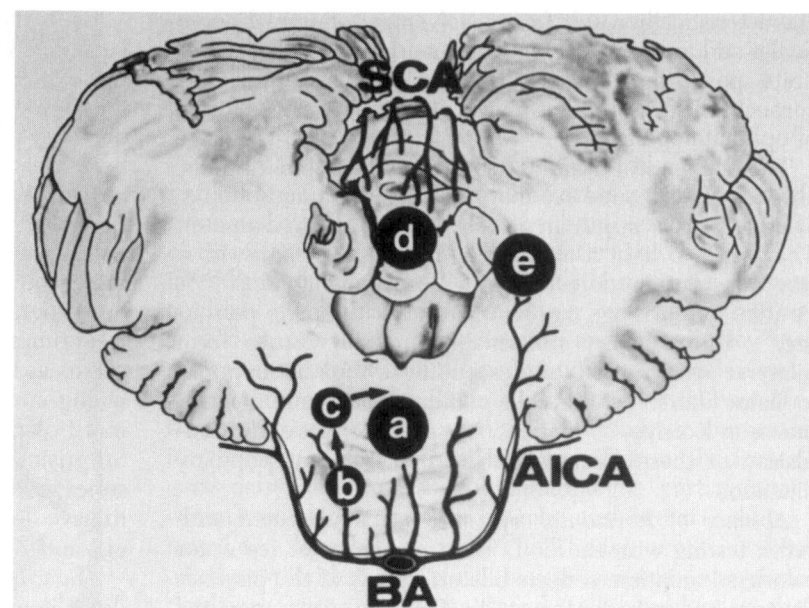

FIGURE 13–42 *Schematic representation of common sites of hypertensive pontine and cerebellar hemorrhages: a, massive, paramedian pontine; b, basal pontine; c, lateral tegmental pontine; d, cerebellar vermian; e, cerebellar hemispheral. AICA, anterior-inferior cerebellar artery; BA, basilar artery; SCA, superior cerebellar artery.*

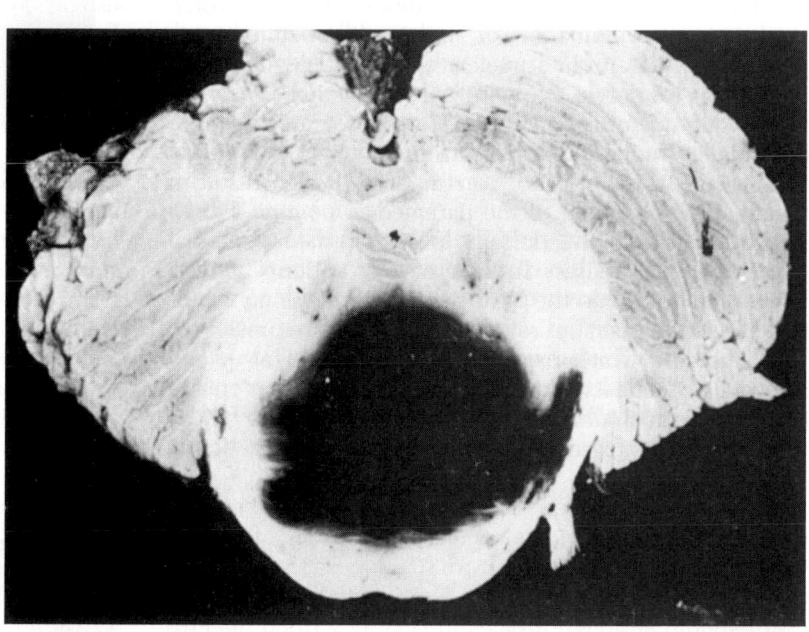

FIGURE 13–43 *Massive pontine hemorrhage with dissection into brachium pontis and fourth ventricle.*

coma (80% of cases) without warning signs. Dana[365] recognized that some patients were conscious when first examined; in three different series, 4 of 19 patients (22%),[359] 10 of 30 patients (33.3%),[54] and 5 of 50 patients (10%)[362,363] were alert when initially seen. By 48 hours, approximately 80% were dead.[54,359] In some patients (30%), a complaint of severe occipital headache preceded by minutes the catastrophic onset of coma.[362,366] Vomiting was noted in 4 of 30 (13%)[54] and 4 of 19 (22%)[359] patients in two series, occasionally being a prominent early symptom.

The frequency of seizures at onset, estimated to be as high as 22%,[362] probably represents a combination of true convulsive phenomena in rare instances, along with episodes of spasmodic decerebrate posturing and even the sometimes violent shivering associated with autonomic dysfunction and rapidly evolving hyperthermia. Some patients present before the development of coma with focal pontine signs, such as facial or limb numbness, deafness, diplopia, bilateral leg weakness, or progressive hemiparesis. Physical examination often reveals an abnormal respiratory rhythm or apnea.[54,363,367] Steegmann[367] analyzed these respiratory abnormalities in detail and reported a variety of abnormal respiratory patterns, including "inspiratory gasps of apneustic respiration," Cheyne-Stokes rhythm, slow and labored respirations, "gasping" respiration, and apnea. Two thirds of his 17 patients exhibited either apnea or severely abnormal patterns of hypoventilation. Hyperthermia frequently coexisted, with temperatures above 39°C in more than 80% of the patients,[366] in one fourth of whom it reached levels of 42°C to 43°C,[362] usually in the preterminal stages. Neurologic findings

Table 13.10   Tegmental Pontine Hemorrhages

Study	Extraocular Movements	Motor	Sensory	Other Cranial Nerves	Cerebellar
Computed tomography diagnosis					
Caplan and Goodwin[86]	No vertical, R gaze, R 6th, bilat. INO	L ↑ toe	L ↓ pin	R 7th, dysarthria, ptosis	Ataxia R > L
Caplan and Goodwin[86]	"1½", vertical nystagmus	L hemip, ↑↑ toes	L ↓ pin	R 7th, 8th, ptosis, dysarthria	Ataxia L > R
Müller et al[329]	R INO	L hemip, ↑↑ toes	L ↓ pin	R 5th, 7th	—
Kase et al[85]	"1½", No ↑ gaze,	R hemip	R ↓ pin and joint position sense	Dysarthria, L 7th	Ataxia L
Kase et al[85]	L INO and 6th, R 4th, bobbing	R hemip	R ↓ pin	Dysphagia, L 7th	Ataxia R & L
Autopsy cases					
Caplan and Goodwin[86]	"1½", bobbing, OD ↓ & inward	L hemip, Babinski	L ↓ pin	Dysarthria	Ataxia R > L
Tyler and Johnson[382]	No horizontal or ↑ gaze, bobbing, skew	L hemip, ↑↑ toes	L ↓ pin	R 5th, 7th, dysarthria, dysphagia, ptosis	R tremor
Dinsdale[54]	R gaze palsy	L hemip	L ↓ pin	R 7th, 8th	—
Silverstein[363]	R gaze palsy	L hemip, ↑↑ toes	L ↓ pin	R 7th, ptosis, dysphagia	—
Pierrott-Deseilligny et al[370]	"1½"	L hemip, ↑↑ toes	L hemis	R 5th, 7th, 8th	Ataxia R arm

Hemip, hemiparesis; hemis, hemisensory syndrome; INO, internuclear ophthalmoplegia; OD, right eye; "1½," the "one-and-one-half" syndrome; R, right; L, left.

"palatal myoclonus" as a sequela of lateral tegmental hematomas.

Medullary Hemorrhage

Hemorrhage into the medulla oblongata (Fig. 13–46) is even more rare than hemorrhage into the midbrain.

Arseni and Stanciu[385] described a 40-year-old woman with dizziness, vomiting, and headache with diplopia and right limb paresthesias. She suddenly became somnolent and ataxic, with a stiff neck, left hemiparesis, diminished pain and temperature sensation on the left side of the face, left limb ataxia, nystagmus, dysphonia, and dysphagia. Surgical exploration found a hematoma on the floor of the fourth ventricle laterally. After drainage of the clot, the patient was said to do well.

Kempe[386] reported on a similar patient who had a lateral medullary hematoma. The 25-year-old woman noted diminished hearing on the left and then suddenly became ill with headache, vomiting, vertigo, and hiccups. She was ataxic and fell to the left. Findings included left nystagmus, diminished pain and temperature sensation on the left side of the face, and left facial weakness; the left ear was deaf and unreactive to caloric stimuli. Pneumoencephalography documented a defect in the rhomboid fossa of the fourth ventricle, which at surgical exploration was found to be a clot bulging through the floor of the fourth ventricle medial to the restiform body. Both this patient and the one described by Arseni and Stanciu[386] had findings similar to those in patients with lateral medullary infarcts, and each had a stepwise course. Arteriography was not performed, and CT and MRI were not available. We suspect that the underlying process in both patients was a cavernous angioma.

In another patient,[227] the explanation was an AVM. At age 37, the woman experienced weakness and decreased position sense in her left arm and leg. Right vocal cord and hypoglossal paralysis developed at age 60, and 2 years later, she became gradually and then abruptly worse and was hypertensive. Necropsy revealed a hemorrhage in the medial medullary tegmentum with spread into the dorsal medulla and right lateral medulla.

Mastaglia and associates[387] reported two cases of medullary hemorrhage with quite different clinical features. In one case, an 87-year-old hypertensive woman was found unconscious with a right gaze palsy, right facial weakness, and left hemiplegia. The hemorrhage was largest in the lateral pons and descended into the medullary pyramid. The cause seems to have been a pontine basal-tegmental hemorrhage with unusual caudal dissection, but its clinical picture did not differ from that already described in unilateral pontine hemorrhage. The other patient was hypertensive and had been undergoing anticoagulation with warfarin. She demonstrated an unusual clinical picture consisting of markedly decreased postural sensation and incoordination of her left arm and leg, diminished left arm reflexes, numbness over the right eye, and subjective numbness of the right limbs. Autopsy showed a hemorrhage into the rostral spinal cord with rostral dissection into the left medullary pyramid. The most likely etiologic factor in this patient was anticoagulation, perhaps compounded by hypertension.

There is one well-documented case of medullary hemorrhage due to hypertension, but whether the hemorrhage

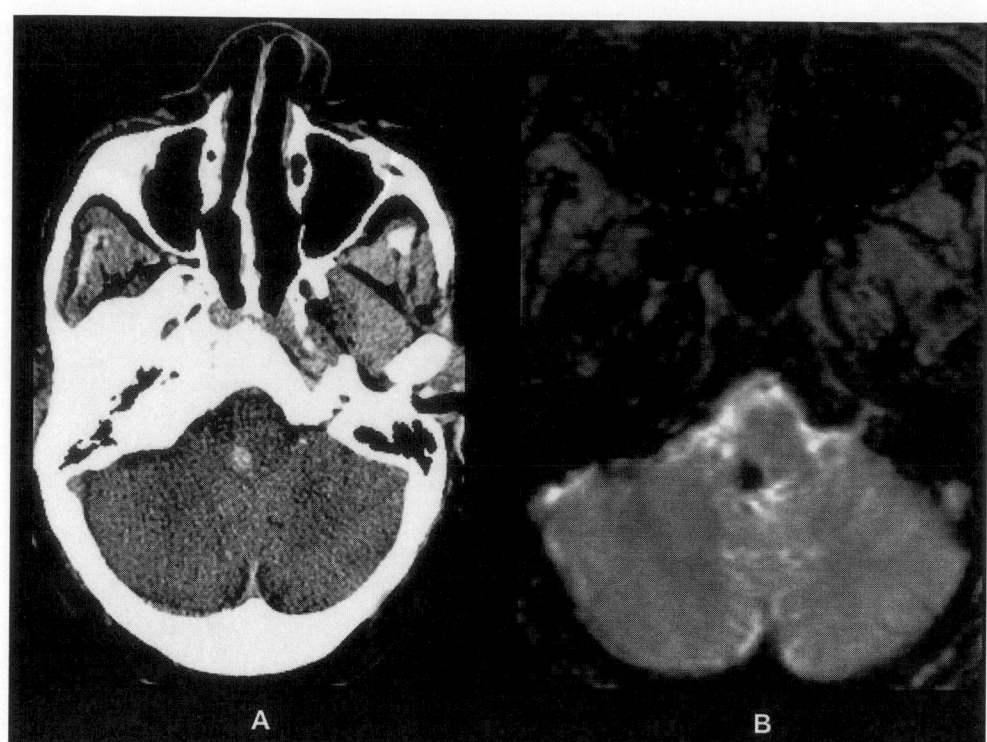

FIGURE 13–46 *Right dorsolateral medullary hemorrhage on CT scan (A) and gradient-echo MR image (B).*

arose in the medulla or arose in the caudal pontine tegmentum and dissected into the medulla is not certain.[345] The patient, 56-year-old, previously hypertensive man, experienced difficulty swallowing, and examination found paralysis of the left side of the face, soft palate, vocal cord, and tongue. A left Horner's syndrome, deafness in the left ear, and paresthesias of the right limbs were also found. CT scan showed a left medullary tegmental hematoma, but the signs of deafness and facial palsy might indicate some pontine involvement.

Barinagarrementeria and Cantú[388] described four cases of their own and reviewed 12 others from the literature. The characteristic profile was one of sudden onset of headache, vertigo, dysphagia, dysphonia or dysarthria, and limb incoordination. Common findings on examination were palatal weakness (88%), nystagmus, cerebellar ataxia, or both (75%), limb weakness (68%), and hypoglossal nerve palsy (56%). Less common signs were facial palsy and Horner's syndrome. The mechanism of the medullary hemorrhage could be determined in only 7 of the 16 patients, corresponding to ruptured vascular malformation (3), hypertension (3), and anticoagulant treatment (1). The mortality rate for the group was 19% (3 of 16), and in most of the survivors, residual neurologic deficits were either mild (56%) or absent (19%).

Unusual presentations of medullary hemorrhage have included a patient with isolated hiccups from a small dorsal ICH,[389] and a second patient with dorsolateral hemorrhage into an area of infarction[390] who presented initially with features of Wallenberg's syndrome.

References

1. Kurtzke JF: Epidemiology of Cerebrovascular Disease. Berlin, Springer-Verlag, 1969.
2. Mohr JP, Caplan LR, Melski JW, et al: The Harvard Cooperative Stroke Registry: A prospective registry. Neurology (NY) 28:754, 1978.
3. Sacco RL, Wolf PA, Bharucha NE, et al: Subarachnoid and intracerebral hemorrhage: Natural history, prognosis, and precursive factors in the Framingham Study. Neurology (NY) 34:847, 1984.
4. Kunitz SC, Gross CR, Heyman A, et al: The Pilot Stroke Data Bank: Definition, design and data. Stroke 15:740, 1984.
5. Hansen BS, Marquardsen J: Incidence of stroke in Frederiksberg, Denmark. Stroke 8:663, 1977.
6. Herman B, Schulte BPM, Van Luijk JH, et al: Epidemiology of stroke in Tilburg, The Netherlands: The population-based stroke incidence register. 1: Introduction and preliminary results. Stroke 11:162, 1980.
7. Bamford J, Sandercock P, Dennis M, et al: A prospective study of acute cerebrovascular disease in the community: The Oxfordshire Community Stroke Project, 1981–86. 2: Incidence, case fatality rates and overall outcome at one year of cerebral infarction, primary intracerebral and subarachnoid haemorrhage. J Neurol Neurosurg Psychiatry 53:16, 1990.
8. Gross CR, Kase CS, Mohr JP, et al: Stroke in south Alabama: Incidence and diagnostic features—a population based study. Stroke 15:249, 1984.
9. Broderick J, Brott T, Tomsick T, et al: The risk of subarachnoid and intracerebral hemorrhages in blacks as compared with whites. N Engl J Med 326:733, 1992.
10. Furlan AJ, Whisnant JP, Elveback LR: The decreasing incidence of primary intracerebral hemorrhage: A population study. Ann Neurol 5:367, 1979.
11. Drury I, Whisnant JP, Garraway WM: Primary intracerebral hemorrhage: Impact of CT on incidence. Neurology (NY) 34:653, 1984.
12. Brott T, Thalinger K, Hertzberg V: Hypertension as a risk factor for spontaneous intracerebral hemorrhage. Stroke 17:1078, 1986.
13. Schütz H, Bödeker R-H, Damian M, et al: Age-related spontaneous intracerebral hematoma in a German community. Stroke 21:1412, 1990.
14. Bruno A, Carter S, Qualls C, et al: Incidence of spontaneous intracerebral hemorrhage among Hispanics and non-Hispanic whites in New Mexico. Neurology 47:405, 1996.
15. Tanaka H, Ueda Y, Date C, et al: Incidence of stroke in Shibata, Japan, 1976–1978. Stroke 12:460, 1981.

Clinical Manifestations

16. Aurell M, Head B: Cerebral hemorrhage in a population after a decade of active anti-hypertensive treatment. Acta Med Scand 176:377, 1964.

17. Garraway WM, Whisnant JP, Drury I: The continuing decline in the incidence of stroke. Mayo Clin Proc 58:520, 1983.

18. Ueda K, Omae T, Hirota Y, et al: Decreasing trend in incidence and mortality from stroke in Hisayama residents, Japan. Stroke 12:154, 1981.

19. Qureshi AI, Suri MAK, Safdar K, et al: Intracerebral hemorrhage in blacks: Risk factors, subtypes, and outcomes. Stroke 28:961, 1997.

20. Brewer DB, Fawcett FJ, Horsfield GI: A necropsy series of non-traumatic cerebral haemorrhages and softenings, with particular reference to heart weight. J Pathol Bacteriol 96:311, 1968.

21. Mutlu N, Berry RG, Alpers BJ: Massive cerebral hemorrhage: Clinical and pathological correlations. Arch Neurol 8:74, 1963.

22. Stehbens WE: Pathology of the Cerebral Blood Vessels. St. Louis, CV Mosby, 1972.

23. Ojemann RG, Heros RC: Spontaneous brain hemorrhage. Stroke 14:468, 1983.

24. McCormick WF, Rosenfield DB: Massive brain hemorrhage: A review of 144 cases and an examination of their causes. Stroke 4:946, 1973.

25. Thrift AG, McNeil JJ, Forbes A, et al: Three important subgroups of hypertensive persons at greater risk of intracerebral hemorrhage. Hypertension 31:1223, 1998.

26. Randomised trial of a perindopril-based blood-pressure-lowering regimen among 6105 individuals with previous stroke or transient ischaemic attack. PROGRESS Collaboration Group. Lancet 358:1033, 2001.

27. Abbott RD, Yin Y, Reed DH, Yano K: Risk of stroke in male cigarette smokers. N Engl J Med 315:717, 1986.

28. Juvela S, Hillbom M, Palomaki H: Risk factors for spontaneous intracerebral hemorrhage. Stroke 26:1558, 1995.

29. Kurth T, Kase CS, Berger K, et al: Smoking and the risk of hemorrhagic stroke in men. Stroke 34:1151, 2003.

29a. Kurth T, Kase CS, Berger K, et al: Smoking and risk of hemorrhagic stroke in women. Stroke 34:2792, 2003.

30. Donahue RP, Abbott RD, Reed DM, Yanko K: Alcohol and hemorrhagic stroke: The Honolulu Heart Program. JAMA 255:2311, 1986.

31. Ueshima H, Iida M, Shimamoto T, et al: Multivariate analysis of risk factors for stroke: Eight-year follow-up of farming villages in Akita, Japan. Prevent Med 9:722, 1980.

32. Boudouresques G, Hauw JJ, Meininger V, et al: Étude neuropathologique des hémorragies intracraniennes de l'adulte. Rev Neurol 135:197, 1979.

33. McCormick WF, Schochet SS: Atlas of Cerebrovascular Disease. Philadelphia, WB Saunders, 1976, p 328.

34. Final report on the aspirin component of the ongoing Physicians' Health Study. Steering Committee of the Physicians' Health Study Research Group. N Engl J Med 321:129, 1989.

35. Swedish Aspirin Low-dose Trial (SALT) of 75 mg aspirin as secondary prophylaxis after cerebrovascular ischaemic events. The SALT Collaborative Group. Lancet 338:1345, 1991

36. Bousser MG, Eschwege E, Haguenau M, et al: "AICLA" controlled trial of aspirin and dipyridamole in the secondary prevention of atherothrombotic cerebral ischemia. Stroke 14:5, 1983.

37. A randomized trial of aspirin and sulfinpyrazone in threatened stroke. Canadian Cooperative Study Group. N Engl J Med 299:53, 1978.

38. Persantine aspirin trial in cerebral ischemia. Part II: Endpoint results. The American-Canadian Co-Operative Study Group. Stroke 16:406, 1985.

39. The European Stroke Prevention Study (ESPS): Principal endpoints. The ESPS Group. Lancet 2:1351, 1987.

40. United Kingdom Transient Ischaemic Attack (UK-TIA) aspirin trial: Interim results. UK-TIA Study Group. BMJ 296:316, 1988.

41. Diener HC, Cunha L, Forbes C, et al: European Stroke Prevention Study. 2: Dipyridamole and acetylsalicylic acid in the secondary prevention of stroke. J Neurol Sci 143:1, 1996.

42. Alberts MJ: Stroke genetics update. Stroke 34:342, 2003.

43. Alberts MJ, McCarron MO, Hoffman KL, et al: Familial clustering of intracerebral hemorrhage: A prospective study in North Carolina. Neuroepidemiology 21:18, 2002.

44. Woo D, Sauerbeck LR, Kissela BM, et al: Genetic and environmental risk factors for intracerebral hemorrhage: Preliminary results of a population-based study. Stroke 33:1190, 2002.

45. Greenberg SM, Briggs ME, Hyman BT, et al: Apolipoprotein E e4 is associated with the presence and earlier onset of hemorrhage in cerebral amyloid angiopathy. Stroke 27:1333, 1996.

46. Catto AJ, Kohler HP, Bannan S, et al: Factor XIII Val 34 Leu: A novel association with primary intracerebral hemorrhage. Stroke 29:813, 1998.

47. Cho KH, Kim BC, Kim MK, et al: No association of factor XIII Val34Leu polymorphism with primary intracerebral hemorrhage and healthy controls in Korean population. J Korean Med Sci 17:249, 2002.

48. Fisher CM: The pathology and pathogenesis of intracerebral hemorrhage. In Fields WS (ed): Pathogenesis and Treatment of Cerebrovascular Disease. Springfield, IL, Charles C Thomas, 1961, p 295.

49. Kase CS, Williams JP, Wyatt DA, Mohr JP: Lobar intracerebral hematomas: Clinical and CT analysis of 22 cases. Neurology (NY) 32:1146, 1982.

50. Wiggins WS, Moody DM, Toole JF, et al: Clinical and computerized tomographic study of hypertensive intracerebral hemorrhage. Arch Neurol 35:832, 1978.

51. Fisher CM: The pathologic and clinical aspects of thalamic hemorrhage. Trans Am Neurol Assoc 84:56, 1959.

52. Freytag E: Fatal hypertensive intracerebral haematomas: A survey of the pathological anatomy of 393 cases. J Neurol Neurosurg Psychiatry 31:616, 1968.

53. Walshe TM, Davis KR, Fisher CM: Thalamic hemorrhage: A computed tomographic-clinical correlation. Neurology (NY) 27:217, 1977.

54. Dinsdale HB: Spontaneous hemorrhage in the posterior fossa: A study of primary cerebellar and pontine hemorrhage with observations on the pathogenesis. Arch Neurol 10:200, 1964.

55. Fisher CM, Picard EH, Polak A, et al: Acute hypertensive cerebellar hemorrhage: Diagnosis and surgical treatment. J Nerv Ment Dis 140:38, 1965.

56. Fisher CM: Pathological observations in hypertensive cerebral hemorrhage. J Neuropathol Exp Neurol 30:536, 1971.

57. Fisher CM: The arterial lesions underlying lacunes. Acta Neuropathol 12:1, 1969.

58. Fisher CM: Lacunes: Small, deep cerebral infarcts. Neurology (Minneap) 15:774, 1965.

59. Fisher CM: Cerebral ischemia: Less familiar types. Clin Neurosurg 18:267, 1971.

60. Cole FM, Yates PO: Intracranial microaneurysms and small cerebrovascular lesions. Brain 90:759, 1967.

61. Cole FM, Yates PO: Pseudo-aneurysms in relationship to massive cerebral hemorrhage. J Neurol Neurosurg Psychiatry 30:61, 1967.

62. Rosenblum WI: Miliary aneurysms and "fibrinoid" degeneration of cerebral blood vessels. Hum Pathol 8:133, 1977.

63. Cole FM, Yates PO: Comparative incidence of cerebrovascular lesions in normotensive and hypertensive patients. Neurology (NY) 18:255, 1968.

64. Charcot JM, Bouchard C: Nouvelles recherches sur la pathogénie de l'hémorragie cérébrale. Arch Physiol Norm Pathol 1:110, 1868.

65. Ellis AG: The pathogenesis of spontaneous cerebral hemorrhage. Proc Pathol Soc (Phila) 12:197, 1909.

66. Green FHK: Miliary aneurysms in the brain. J Pathol Bacteriol 33:71, 1930.

67. Ross Russell RW: Observations on intracerebral aneurysms. Brain 86:425, 1963.

68. Cole FM, Yates PO: The occurrence and significance of intracerebral microaneurysms. J Pathol Bacteriol 93:393, 1967.

69. Fisher CM: Cerebral miliary aneurysms in hypertension. Am J Pathol 66:313, 1972.

70. Herbstein DJ, Schaumburg HH: Hypertensive intracerebral hematoma: An investigation of the initial hemorrhage and rebleeding using chromium Cr 51-labeled erythrocytes. Arch Neurol 30:412, 1974.

71. Kelley RE, Berger JR, Scheinberg P, Stokes N: Active bleeding in hypertensive intracerebral hemorrhage: Computed tomography. Neurology (NY) 32:852, 1982.

72. Broderick JP, Brott TG, Tomsick T, et al: Ultra-early evaluation of intracerebral hemorrhage. J Neurosurg 72:195, 1990.

73. Fehr MA, Anderson DC: Incidence of progression or rebleeding in hypertensive intracerebral hemorrhage. J Stroke Cerebrovasc Dis 1:111, 1991.

74. Fujii Y, Tanaka R, Takeuchi S, et al: Hematoma enlargement in spontaneous intracerebral hemorrhage. J Neurosurg 80:51, 1994.

75. Kazui S, Naritomi H, Yamamoto H, et al: Enlargement of spontaneous intracerebral hemorrhage: Incidence and time course. Stroke 27:1783, 1996.

76. Brott T, Broderick J, Kothari R, et al: Early hemorrhage growth in patients with intracerebral hemorrhage. Stroke 28:1, 1997.

77. Tatu L, Moulin T, El Mohamad R, et al: Primary intracerebral hemorrhage in the Besançon stroke registry: Initial clinical and CT findings, early course and 30-day outcome in 350 patients. Eur Neurol 43:209, 2000.

78. Broderick J, Brott TG, Duldner JE, et al: Volume of intracerebral hemorrhage: A powerful and easy-to-use predictor of 30-day mortality. Stroke 24:987, 1993.

79. Kothari RU, Brott T, Broderick JP, et al: The ABCs of measuring intracerebral hemorrhage volumes. Stroke 27:1304, 1996.

80. Lisk DR, Pasteur W, Rhoades H, et al: Early presentation of hemispheric intracerebral hemorrhage: Prediction of outcome and guidelines for treatment allocation. Neurology 44:133, 1994.

81. Stein RW, Kase CS, Hier DB, et al: Caudate hemorrhage. Neurology (NY) 34:1549, 1984.

82. Hier DB, Davis KR, Richardson EP, Mohr JP: Hypertensive putaminal hemorrhage. Ann Neurol 1:152, 1977.

83. Fisher CM: Capsular infarcts. Arch Neurol 36:65, 1979.

84. Ropper AH, Davis KR: Lobar cerebral hemorrhages: Acute clinical syndromes in 26 cases. Ann Neurol 8:141, 1980.

85. Kase CS, Maulsby GO, Mohr JP: Partial pontine hematomas. Neurology (NY) 30:652, 1980.

86. Kaplan LR, Goodwin JA: Lateral tegmental brainstem hemorrhages. Neurology (NY) 32:252, 1982.

87. Fieschi C, Carolei A, Fiorelli M, et al: Changing prognosis of primary intracerebral hemorrhage: Results of a clinical and computed tomographic follow-up study of 104 patients. Stroke 19:192, 1988.

88. González-Duarte A, Cantú C, Ruiz-Sandoval JL, Barinagarrementeria F: Recurrent primary cerebral hemorrhage: Frequency, mechanisms, and prognosis. Stroke 29:1802, 1998.

89. Bae H, Jeong D, Doh J, et al: Recurrence of bleeding in patients with hypertensive intracerebral hemorrhage. Cerebrovasc Dis 9:102, 1999.

90. Hickey WF, King RB, Wang A-M, Samuels MA: Multiple simultaneous intracerebral hematomas: Clinical, radiologic, and pathologic findings in two patients. Arch Neurol 40:519, 1983.

91. Weisberg L: Multiple spontaneous intracerebral hematomas: Clinical and computed tomographic correlations. Neurology (NY) 31:897, 1981.

92. García JH, Ho KL, Caccamo DV: Intracerebral hemorrhage: Pathology of selected topics. In Kase CS, Caplan LR (eds): Intracerebral Hemorrhage. Boston, Butterworth-Heinemann, 1994, p 45.

93. Jenkins A, Maxwell W, Graham D: Experimental intracerebral hematoma in the rat: Sequential light microscopic changes. Neuropathol Appl Neurobiol 15:477, 1989.

94. Ruiz-Sandoval JL, Cantú C, Barinagarrementeria F: Intracerebral hemorrhage in young people: Analysis of risk factors, location, causes, and prognosis. Stroke 30:537, 1999.

95. Margolis G, Odom GL, Woodhall B, Bloor BM: The role of small angiomatous malformations in the production of intracerebral hematomas. J Neurosurg 8:564, 1951.

96. Crawford JV, Russell DS: Cryptic arteriovenous and venous hamartomas of the brain. J Neurol Neurosurg Psychiatry 19:1, 1956.

97. Krayenbühl H, Siebenmann R: Small vascular malformations as a cause of primary intracerebral hemorrhage. J Neurosurg 22:7, 1965.

98. Russell DS: The pathology of spontaneous intracranial haemorrhage. Proc Soc Med 47:689, 1954.

99. Becker DH, Townsend JJ, Kramer RA, Newton TH: Occult cerebrovascular malformations: A series of 18 histologically verified cases with negative angiography. Brain 70:530, 1979.

100. Roberson GH, Kase CS, Wolpow ER: Telangiectases and cavernous angiomas of the brainstem: "Cryptic" vascular malformations. Neuroradiology 8:83, 1974.

101. Wakai S, Ueda Y, Inoh S, et al: Angiographically occult angiomas: A report of thirteen cases with analysis of the cases documented in the literature. Neurosurgery 17:549, 1985.

102. Bicknell JM, Carlow TJ, Kornfeld M, et al: Familial cavernous angiomas. Arch Neurol 35:746, 1978.

103. Clark JV: Familial occurrence of cavernous angiomata of the brain. J Neurol Neurosurg Psychiatry 33:871, 1970.

104. Kattapong VJ, Hart BL, Davis LE: Familial cerebral cavernous angiomas: Clinical and radiologic studies. Neurology 45:492, 1995.

105. Labauge P, Brunereau L, Levy C, et al: The natural history of familial cerebral cavernomas: A retrospective MRI study of 40 patients. Neuroradiology 42:327, 2000.

106. Labauge P, Brunereau L, Laberge S, Houtteville JP: Prospective follow-up of 33 asymptomatic patients with familial cerebral cavernous malformations. Neurology 57:1825, 2001.

107. Stahl SM, Johnson KP, Malamud N: The clinical and pathological spectrum of brainstem vascular malformations: Long-term course simulates multiple sclerosis. Arch Neurol 37:25, 1980.

108. Robinson JR, Awad IA, Little JR: Natural history of the cavernous angioma. J Neurosurg 75:709, 1991.

109. Zabramski JM, Wascher TM, Spetzler RF, et al: The natural history of familial cavernous malformations: Results of an ongoing study. J Neurosurg 80:422, 1994.

110. Kondziolka D, Lunsford LD, Kestle JR: The natural history of cerebral cavernous malformations. J Neurosurg 83:820, 1995.

111. Requena I, Arias M, Lopez-Ibor L, et al: Cavernomas of the central nervous system: Clinical and neuroimaging manifestations in 47 patients. J Neurol Neurosurg Psychiatry 54:590, 1991.

112. Rigamonti D, Drayer BP, Johnson PC, et al: The MRI appearance of cavernous malformations (angiomas). J Neurosurg 67:518, 1987.

113. Zimmerman RS, Spetzler RF, Lee KS, et al: Cavernous malformations of the brain stem. J Neurosurg 75:32, 1991.

114. Simard JM, Garcia-Bengochea F, Ballinger WE, et al: Cavernous angioma: A review of 126 collected and 12 new clinical cases. Neurosurgery 18:162, 1986.

115. Rigamonti D, Hadley MN, Drayer BP, et al: Cerebral cavernous malformations: Incidence and familial occurrence. N Engl J Med 319:343, 1988.

116. Gil-Nagel A, Dubovsky J, Wilcox KJ, et al: Familial cerebral cavernous angioma: A gene localized to a 15-cM interval on chromosome 7q. Ann Neurol 39:807, 1996.

117. Günel M, Awad IA, Finberg K, et al: A founder mutation as a cause of cerebral cavernous malformation in Hispanic Americans. N Engl J Med 334:946, 1996.

118. Delaney P, Estes M: Intracranial hemorrhage with amphetamine abuse. Neurology (NY) 30:1125, 1980.

119. D'Souza T, Shraberg D: Intracranial hemorrhage associated with amphetamine use [letter]. Neurology (NY) 31:922, 1981.

120. Harrington H, Heller HA, Dawson D, et al: Intracerebral hemorrhage and oral amphetamine. Arch Neurol 40:503, 1983.

121. Loizou LA, Hamilton JG, Tsementzis SA: Intracranial hemorrhage in association with pseudoephedrine overdose. J Neurol Neurosurg Psychiatry 45:471, 1982.

122. Citron BP, Halpern M, McCarron M, et al: Necrotizing angiitis associated with drug abuse. N Engl J Med 283:1003, 1970.

123. Margolis MT, Newton TH: Methamphetamine ("speed") arteritis. Neuroradiology 2:179, 1971.

124. Rumbaugh CL, Bergeron RT, Fang HCH, McCormick R: Cerebral angiographic changes in the drug abuse patient. Radiology 101:335, 1971.

125. Yu YJ, Cooper DR, Wellenstein DE, Block B: Cerebral angiitis and intracerebral hemorrhage associated with methamphetamine abuse. J Neurosurg 58:109, 1983.

126. Lukes SA: Intracerebral hemorrhage from an arteriovenous malformation after amphetamine injection. Arch Neurol 40:60, 1983.

127. Matick H, Anderson D, Brumlik J: Cerebral vasculitis associated with oral amphetamine overdose. Arch Neurol 40:253, 1983.

128. Kase CS, Foster TE, Reed JE, et al: Intracerebral hemorrhage and phenylpropanolamine use. Neurology (NY) 37:399, 1987.

129. Kernan WN, Viscoli CM, Brass LM, et al: Phenylpropanolamine and the risk of hemorrhagic stroke. N Engl J Med 343:1826, 2000.

130. Barinagarrementeria F, Méndez A, Vega F: Hemorragia cerebral asociada al uso de fenilpropanolamina. Neurología 5:292, 1990.

131. Bernstein E, Diskant BM: Phenylpropanolamine: A potentially hazardous drug. Ann Emerg Med 11:311, 1982.

132. Fallis RJ, Fisher M: Cerebral vasculitis and hemorrhage associated with phenylpropanolamine. Neurology (NY) 35:405, 1985.

133. Kikta DG, Devereaux MX, Chandar K: Intracranial hemorrhages due to phenylpropanolamine. Stroke 16:510, 1985.

134. Stoessl AJ, Young GB, Feasby TE: Intracerebral haemorrhage and angiographic beading following ingestion of catecholaminergics. Stroke 16:734, 1985.

Clinical Manifestations

135. Glick R, Hoying J, Cerullo L, Perlman S: Phenylpropanolamine: An over-the-counter drug causing central nervous system vasculitis and intracerebral hemorrhage. Neurosurgery (NY) 20:969, 1987.

136. MacDougall JD, Tuxen D, Sale DG, et al: Arterial blood pressure response to heavy exercise. J Appl Physiol 58:785, 1985.

137. Levine SR, Brust JCM, Futrell N, et al: Cerebrovascular complications of the use of the "crack" form of alkaloid cocaine. N Engl J Med 323:699, 1990.

138. Green RM, Kelly KM, Gabrielsen T, et al: Multiple intracranial hemorrhages after smoking "crack" cocaine. Stroke 21:957, 1990.

139. Tapia JF, Golden JA: Case records of the Massachusetts General Hospital (Case 27-1993). N Engl J Med 329:117, 1993.

140. Little JR, Dial B, Bellanger G, Carpenter S: Brain hemorrhage from intracranial tumor. Stroke 10:283, 1979.

141. Scott M: Spontaneous intracerebral hematoma caused by cerebral neoplasms: Report of eight verified cases. J Neurosurg 42:338, 1975.

142. Modesti LM, Binet EF, Collins GH: Meningiomas causing spontaneous intracranial hematomas. J Neurosurg 45:437, 1976.

143. Wakai S, Yamakawa K, Manaka S, Takakura K: Spontaneous intracranial hemorrhage caused by brain tumors: Its incidence and clinical significance. Neurosurgery 10:437, 1982.

144. Gildersleve N, Koo AH, McDonald CJ: Metastatic tumor presenting as intracerebral hemorrhage. Radiology 124:109, 1977.

145. Gurwitt LJ, Long JM, Clark RE: Cerebral metastatic choriocarcinoma: A postpartum cause of "stroke." Obstet Gynecol 45:583, 1975.

146. Mandybur TI: Intracranial hemorrhage caused by metastatic tumors. Neurology (NY) 27:650, 1977.

147. Vaughan HG, Howard RG: Intracranial hemorrhage due to metastatic chorionepithelioma. Neurology (NY) 12:771, 1962.

148. Graus F, Rogers LR, Posner JB: Cerebrovascular complications in patients with cancer. Medicine 64:16, 1985.

149. Zülch KJ: Neuropathology of intracranial haemorrhage. Prog Brain Res 30:151, 1968.

150. Shuangshoti S, Panyathanya R, Wichienkur P: Intracranial metastases from unsuspected choriocarcinoma: Onset suggestive of cerebrovascular disease. Neurology (NY) 24:649, 1974.

151. Herold S, von Kumer R, Jaeger CH: Follow-up of spontaneous intracerebral haemorrhage by computed tomography. J Neurol 228:267, 1982.

152. Weisberg LA: Computerized tomography in intracranial hemorrhage. Arch Neurol 36:422, 1979.

153. Zimmerman RD, Leeds NE, Naidich TP: Ring blush associated with intracerebral hematoma. Radiology 122:707, 1977.

154. Kase CS: Intracerebral hemorrhage: Non-hypertensive causes. Stroke 17:590, 1986.

155. Iwama T, Ohkuma A, Miwa Y, et al: Brain tumors manifesting as intracranial hemorrhage. Neurol Med Chir 32:130, 1992.

156. Kase CS, Robinson RK, Stein RW, et al: Anticoagulant-related intracerebral hemorrhage. Neurology (NY) 35:943, 1985.

157. Rådberg JA, Olsson JE, Rådberg CT: Prognostic parameters in spontaneous intracranial hematomas with special reference to anticoagulant treatment. Stroke 22:571, 1991.

158. Ott KH, Kase CS, Ojemann RG, Mohr JP: Cerebellar hemorrhage: Diagnosis and treatment. Arch Neurol 31:160, 1974.

159. Franke CL, deJonge J, van Swieten JC, et al: Intracerebral hematomas during anticoagulant treatment. Stroke 21:726, 1990.

160. Hart RG, Boop BS, Anderson DC: Oral anticoagulants and intracranial hemorrhage. Stroke 26:1471, 1995.

161. Whisnant JP, Cartlidge NEF, Elveback LR: Carotid and vertebral-basilar transient ischemic attacks: Effect of anticoagulants, hypertension, and cardiac disorders on survival and stroke occurrence in a population study. Ann Neurol 3:107, 1978.

162. Wintzen AR, de Jonge H, Loeliger EA, Bots GTAM: The risk of intracerebral hemorrhage during oral anticoagulant treatment: A population study. Ann Neurol 16:553, 1984.

163. Hylek EM, Singer DE: Risk factors for intracranial hemorrhage in outpatients taking warfarin. Ann Intern Med 120:897, 1994.

164. Landefeld CS, Goldman L: Major bleeding in outpatients treated with warfarin: Incidence and prediction by factors known at the start of outpatient therapy. Am J Med 87:144, 1989.

165. Barron KD, Fergusson G: Intracranial hemorrhage as a complication of anticoagulant therapy. Neurology (NY) 9:447, 1959.

166. Dawson I, van Bockel JH, Ferrari MD, et al: Ischemic and hemorrhagic stroke in patients on oral anticoagulants after reconstruction for chronic lower limb ischemia. Stroke 24:1655, 1993.

167. Smith EE, Rosand J, Knudsen KA, et al: Leukoaraiosis is associated with warfarin-related hemorrhage following ischemic stroke. Neurology 59:193, 2002.

168. Hart RG, Pearce LA: In vivo antithrombotic effect of aspirin: Dose versus nongastrointestinal bleeding. Stroke 24:138, 1993.

169. Snyder M, Renaudin J: Intracranial hemorrhage associated with anticoagulation therapy. Surg Neurol 7:31, 1977.

170. A randomized trial of anticoagulants versus aspirin after cerebral ischemia of presumed arterial origin. The Stroke Prevention In Reversible Ischemia Trial (SPIRIT) Study Group. Ann Neurol 42:857, 1997.

171. Warfarin versus aspirin for prevention of thromboembolism in atrial fibrillation. Stroke Prevention in Atrial Fibrillation Investigators. Lancet 343:687, 1994.

172. Rosand J, Hylek EM, O'Donnell HC, Greenberg SM: Warfarin-associated hemorrhage and cerebral amyloid angiopathy: A genetic and pathologic study. Neurology 55:947, 2000.

173. Drapkin A, Merskey C: Anticoagulant therapy after acute myocardial infarction: Relation of therapeutic benefit to patient's age, sex, and severity of infarction. JAMA 222:541, 1972.

174. Handley AJ, Emerson PA, Fleming PR: Heparin in the prevention of deep vein thrombosis after myocardial infarction. BMJ 2:436, 1972.

175. Fisher CM, Adams RD: Observations on brain embolism with special reference to the mechanism of hemorrhagic infarction. J Neuropathol Exp Neurol 10:92, 1951.

176. Camerlingo M, Casto L, Censori B, et al: Immediate anticoagulation with heparin for first-ever ischemic stroke in the carotid artery territories observed within 5 hours of onset. Arch Neurol 51:462, 1994.

177. Babikian VL, Kase CS, Pessin MS, et al: Intracerebral hemorrhage in stroke patients anticoagulated with heparin. Stroke 20:1500, 1989.

178. Chamorro A, Villa N, Saiz A, et al: Early anticoagulation after large cerebral embolic infarction: A safety study. Neurology 45:861, 1995.

179. Immediate anticoagulation of embolic stroke: Brain hemorrhage and management options. Cerebral Embolism Study Group. Stroke 15:779, 1984.

180. Adams HP: Emergent use of anticoagulation for treatment of patients with ischemic stroke. Stroke 33:856, 2002.

181. Chamorro A: Immediate anticoagulation in acute focal brain ischemia revisited: Gathering the evidence. Stroke 32:577, 2001.

182. Comparison of invasive and conservative strategies after treatment with intravenous tissue plasminogen activator in acute myocardial infarction: Results of the Thrombolysis in Myocardial Infarction (TIMI) phase II trial. TIMI Study Group. N Engl J Med 320:618, 1989.

183. Gore JM, Sloan M, Price TR, et al: Intracerebral hemorrhage, cerebral infarction, and subdural hematoma after acute myocardial infarction and thrombolytic therapy in the Thrombolysis in Myocardial Infarction Study: Thrombolysis in myocardial infarction, phase II, pilot and clinical data. Circulation 83:448, 1991.

184. Kase CS, O'Neal AM, Fisher M, et al: Intracranial hemorrhage after use of tissue plasminogen activator for coronary thrombolysis. Ann Intern Med 112:17, 1990.

185. Kase CS, Pessin MS, Zivin JA, et al: Intracranial hemorrhage following coronary thrombolysis with tissue plasminogen activator. Am J Med 92:384, 1992.

186. O'Connor CM, Aldrich H, Massey EW, et al: Intracranial hemorrhage after thrombolytic therapy for acute myocardial infarction: Clinical characteristics and in-hospital outcome [abstract]. J Am Coll Cardiol 15:213A, 1990.

187. Sloan MA, Price TR, Petito CK, et al: Clinical features and pathogenesis of intracerebral hemorrhage after rt-PA and heparin therapy for acute myocardial infarction: The Thrombolysis in Myocardial Infarction (TIMI) II pilot and randomized clinical trial combined experience. Neurology 45:649, 1995.

188. Pendlebury WW, Iole ED, Tracy RP, Dill BA: Intracerebral hemorrhage related to cerebral amyloid angiopathy and t-PA treatment. Ann Neurol 29:210, 1991.

189. Wijdicks EFM, Jack CR: Intracerebral hemorrhage after fibrinolytic therapy for acute myocardial infarction. Stroke 24:554, 1993.

190. Pessin MS, del Zoppo GJ, Estol CJ: Thrombolytic agents in the treatment of stroke. Clin Neuropharmacol 13:271, 1990.

191. del Zoppo GJ, Poeck K, Pessin MS, et al: Recombinant tissue plasminogen activator in acute thrombotic and embolic stroke. Ann Neurol 32:78, 1992.

Clinical Manifestations

192. Wolpert SM, Bruckmann H, Greenlee R, et al: Neuroradiologic evaluation of patients with acute stroke treated with recombinant tissue plasminogen activator: The rt-PA Acute Stroke Study Group. AJNR Am J Neuroradiol 14:3, 1993.

193. Levy DE, Brott TG, Haley EC Jr, et al: Factors related to intracranial hematoma formation in patients receiving tissue-type plasminogen activator for acute ischemic stroke. Stroke 25:291, 1994.

194. Hacke W, Kaste M, Fieschi C, et al: Intravenous thrombolysis with recombinant tissue plasminogen activator for acute hemispheric stroke: The European Cooperative Acute Stroke Study (ECASS). JAMA 274:1017, 1995.

195. Tissue plasminogen activator for acute ischemic stroke. The National Institute of Neurological Disorders and Stroke rt-PA Stroke Study Group. N Engl J Med 333:1581, 1995.

196. Intracerebral hemorrhage after intravenous t-PA therapy for ischemic stroke. The NINDS t-PA Stroke Study Group. Stroke 28:2109, 1997.

197. Donnan GA, Davis SM, Chambers BR, et al: Trials of streptokinase in severe acute ischaemic stroke [letter]. Lancet 345:578, 1995.

198. Randomised controlled trial of streptokinase, aspirin, and combination of both in treatment of acute ischaemic stroke. Multicentre Acute Stroke Trial–Italy (MAST-I) Group. Lancet 346:1509, 1995.

199. Thrombolytic therapy with streptokinase in acute ischemic stroke. The Multicenter Acute Stroke Trial–Europe Study Group. N Engl J Med 335:145, 1996.

200. GISSI-2: A factorial randomised trial of alteplase versus streptokinase and heparin versus no heparin among 12,490 patients with acute myocardial infarction. Gruppo Italiano per lo Studio della Sopravvivenza nell' Infarto Miocardico. Lancet 336:65, 1990.

201. Clark WM, Lyden PD, Madden KP, et al: Thrombolytic therapy in acute ischemic stroke [letter]. N Engl J Med 336:65, 1997.

202. Del Zoppo GJ, Higashida RT, Furlan AJ, et al: PROACT: A phase II randomized trial of recombinant pro-urokinase by direct arterial delivery in acute middle cerebral artery stroke. Stroke 29:4, 1998.

203. Furlan A, Higashida R, Wechsler L, et al: Intra-arterial prourokinase for acute ischemic stroke: The PROACT II Study: A randomized controlled trial. JAMA 282:2003, 1999.

204. Kase CS, Furlan AJ, Wechsler LR, et al: Symptomatic intracerebral hemorrhage after intra-arterial thrombolysis with prourokinase in acute ischemic stroke: The PROACT II trial. Neurology 57:1603, 2001.

205. Bruno A, Levine SR, Frankel MR, et al: Admission glucose level and clinical outcomes in the NINDS rt-PA stroke trial. Neurology 59:669, 2002.

206. Kolodny EH, Rebeiz JJ, Caviness VS, Richardson EP: Granulomatous angiitis of the central nervous system. Arch Neurol 19:510, 1968.

207. Moore PM, Cupps TR: Neurological complications of vasculitis. Ann Neurol 14:155, 1983.

208. Hankey GJ: Isolated angiitis/angiopathy of the central nervous system. Cerebrovasc Dis 1:2, 1991.

209. Clifford-Jones RE, Love S, Gurusinghe N: Granulomatous angiitis of the central nervous system: A case with recurrent intracerebral hemorrhage. J Neurol Neurosurg Psychiatry 48:1054, 1985.

210. De Reuck J, Crevits L, Sieben G, DeCoster W: Granulomatous angiitis of the nervous system: A clinicopathological study of one case. J Neurol 227:49, 1982.

211. Biller J, Loftus CM, Moore SA, et al: Isolated central nervous system angiitis first presenting as spontaneous intracranial hemorrhage. Neurosurgery 20:310, 1987.

212. Probst A, Ulrich J: Amyloid angiopathy combined with granulomatous angiitis of the central nervous system: Report on two patients. Clin Neuropathol 4:250, 1985.

213. Shintaku M, Osawa K, Toki J, et al: A case of granulomatous angiitis of the central nervous system associated with amyloid angiopathy. Acta Neuropathol 70:340, 1986.

214. Linfante I, Llinas RH, Caplan LR, et al: MRI features of intracerebral hemorrhage within two hours from symptom onset. Stroke 30:2263, 1999.

215. Schellinger PD, Jansen O, Fiebach JB, et al: A standardized MRI stroke protocol: Comparison with CT in hyperacute intracerebral hemorrhage. Stroke 30:765, 1999.

216. Patel MR, Edelman RR, Warach S: Detection of hyperacute primary intraparenchymal hemorrhage by magnetic resonance imaging. Stroke 27:2321, 1996.

217. Tanaka A, Ueno Y, Nakayama Y, et al: Small chronic hemorrhages and ischemic lesions in association with spontaneous intracerebral hematomas. Stroke 30:1637, 1999.

218. Roob G, Schmidt R, Kapeller P, et al: MRI evidence of past cerebral microbleeds in a healthy elderly population. Neurology 52:991, 1999.

219. Atlas SW, Thulborn KR: MR detection of hyperacute parenchymal hemorrhage of the brain. Am J Neuroradiol 19:1471, 1998.

220. Kidwell CS, Saver JL, Villablanca JP, et al: Magnetic resonance imaging detection of microbleeds before thrombolysis: An emerging application. Stroke 33:95, 2002.

221. Tsushima Y, Aoki J, Endo K: Brain microhemorrhages detected on T2-weighted gradient-echo MR images. AJNR Am J Neuroradiol 24:88, 2003.

222. Greenberg SM, Finklestein SP, Schaefer PW: Petechial hemorrhages accompanying lobar hemorrhage: Detection by gradient-echo MRI. Neurology 46:1751, 1996.

223. Jeerakathil TJ, Wolf PA, Beiser AB, et al: Gradient-echo cerebral microbleeds predict diminished cognitive function in a community-based sample: The Framingham Study [abstract]. Stroke 33:345, 2002.

224. Fisher CM: Clinical syndromes in cerebral hemorrhage. In Fields WS (ed): Pathogenesis and Treatment of Cerebrovascular Disease. Springfield, IL, Charles C Thomas, 1961, p 318.

225. Ojemann RG, Mohr JP: Hypertensive brain hemorrhage. Clin Neurosurg 23:220, 1976.

226. Portenoy RK, Lipton RB, Berger AR, et al: Intracerebral hemorrhage: A model for the prediction of outcome. J Neurol Neurosurg Psychiatry 50:976, 1987.

227. Tuhrim S, Dambrosia JM, Price TR, et al: Prediction of intracerebral hemorrhage survival. Ann Neurol 24:258, 1988.

228. Aring CD: Differential diagnosis of cerebrovascular stroke. Arch Intern Med 113:195, 1964.

229. Abu-Zeid HAH, Choi NW, Maini KK, et al: Relative role of factors associated with cerebral infarction and cerebral hemorrhage. Stroke 8:106, 1977.

230. Walsh FB, Hoyt WK: Clinical Neuro-ophthalmology, 3rd ed. Baltimore, Williams & Wilkins, 1969, p 1786.

231. Myoung CL, Heany LM, Jacobson RL, Klassen AC: Cerebrospinal fluid in cerebral hemorrhage and infarction. Stroke 6:638, 1975.

232. Kjellin KG, Soderstrom CE: Cerebral haemorrhages with atypical clinical patterns: A study of cerebral hematomas using CSF spectrophotometry and computerized transverse axial tomography ("EMI scanning"). J Neurol Sci 25:211, 1975.

233. Plum F, Posner JB: The Diagnosis of Stupor and Coma, 3rd ed. Philadelphia, FA Davis, 1980.

234. Taveras JM, Wood EH: Diagnostic Neuroradiology, 2nd ed, Vol 2. Baltimore, Williams & Wilkins, 1976, p 1018.

235. Kowada M, Yamaguchi K, Matsuoka S, Ito Z: Extravasation of angiographic contrast material in hypertensive intracerebral hemorrhage. J Neurosurg 36:471, 1972.

236. Mizukami M, Araki G, Mihara H, et al: Arteriographically visualized extravasation in hypertensive intracerebral hemorrhage: Report of seven cases. Stroke 3:527, 1972.

237. Mizukami M, Araki G, Mihara H: Angiographic sign of good prognosis for hemiplegia in hypertensive intracerebral hemorrhage. Neurology (NY) 24:120, 1974.

238. Merritt HH: A Textbook of Neurology, 6th ed. Philadelphia, Lea & Febiger, 1979, p 160.

239. Silliman S, McGill J, Booth R: Simultaneous bilateral hypertensive putaminal hemorrhages. J Stroke Cerebrovasc Dis 12:44, 2003.

240. Silverstein A: Intracranial hemorrhage in patients with bleeding tendencies. Neurology (NY) 11:310, 1961.

241. Gilles C, Brucher JM, Khoubesserian P, Vanderhaeghn JJ: Cerebral amyloid angiopathy as a cause of multiple intracerebral hemorrhages. Neurology (NY) 34:730, 1984.

242. Tapia JF, Kase CS, Sawyer RH, Mohr JP: Hypertensive putaminal hemorrhage presenting as pure motor hemiparesis. Stroke 14:505, 1983.

243. Kim JS, Lee JH, Lee MC: Small primary intracerebral hemorrhage: Clinical presentation of 28 cases. Stroke 25:1500, 1994.

244. Chung C, Caplan LR, Yamamoto Y, et al: Striatocapsular haemorrhage. Brain 123:1850, 2000.

245. Kim JS: Lenticulocapsular hemorrhages presenting as pure sensory stroke. Eur Neurol 42:128, 1999.

246. Jones HR, Baker RA, Kott HS: Hypertensive putaminal hemorrhage presenting with hemichorea. Stroke 16:130, 1985.

Clinical Manifestations

247. Altafullah I, Pascual-Leone A, Duvall K, et al: Putaminal hemorrhage accompanied by hemichorea-hemiballism. Stroke 27:1093, 1990.

248. Weisberg LA, Stazio A, Elliott D, Shamsnia M: Putaminal hemorrhage: Clinical-computed tomographic correlations. Neuroradiology 32:200, 1990.

249. Mohr JP, Steinke W, Timsit SG, et al: The anterior choroidal artery does not supply the corona radiata and lateral ventricular wall. Stroke 22:1502, 1991.

250. D'Esposito M, Alexander MP: Subcortical aphasia: Distinct profiles following left putaminal hemorrhage. Neurology 45:38, 1995.

251. Weisberg LA, Elliott D, Shamsnia M: Massive putaminal-thalamic nontraumatic hemorrhage. Comput Med Imaging Graph 16:353, 1992.

252. Fuh JL, Wang SJ: Caudate hemorrhage: Clinical features, neuropsychological assessments and radiological findings. Clin Neurol Neurosurg 97:296, 1995.

253. Kumral E, Evyapan D, Balkir K: Acute caudate vascular lesions. Stroke 30:100, 1999.

254. Weisberg LA: Caudate hemorrhage. Arch Neurol 41:971, 1984.

255. Waga S, Fujimoto K, Okada M, et al: Caudate hemorrhage. Neurosurgery 18:445, 1986.

256. Steinke W, Tatemichi TK, Mohr JP, et al: Caudate hemorrhage with moyamoya-like vasculopathy from atherosclerotic disease. Stroke 23:1360, 1992.

257. Suzuki J, Kodama N: Moyamoya disease: A review. Stroke 14:104, 1983.

258. Stephen R, Stillwell D: Arteries and Veins of the Human Brain. Springfield, IL, Charles C Thomas, 1969.

259. Butler AB, Partian RA, Netsky MG: Primary intraventricular hemorrhage: A mild and remediable form. Neurology (NY) 22:675, 1972.

260. Beck DW, Menezes AH: Intracerebral hemorrhage in a patient with eclampsia. JAMA 246:1442, 1981.

261. Cambier J, Elghozi D, Strube E: Hémorragie de la tête du noyau caudé gauche. Rev Neurol (Paris) 135:763, 1979.

262. Bertol V, Gracia-Naya M, Oliveros A, Gros B: Bilateral symmetric caudate hemorrhage. Neurology 41:1157, 1991.

263. Caplan LR: Caudate hemorrhage. In Kase CS, Caplan LR (eds): Intracerebral Hemorrhage. Boston, Butterworth-Heinemann, 1994, p 329.

264. Mohr JP, Watters WC, Duncan GW: Thalamic hemorrhage and aphasia. Brain Lang 2:3, 1975.

265. Watson RT, Heilman KM: Thalamic neglect. Neurology (NY) 29:690, 1979.

266. Cambier J, Elghozi D, Strube E: Trois observations de lésions vasculaires du thalamus droit avec syndrome de l'hémisphère mineur: Discussion du concept de négligence thalamique. Rev Neurol (Paris) 136:105, 1980.

267. Schott B, Laurent B, Mauguiere F, Chazot G: Négligence motrice par hématome thalamique droit. Rev Neurol (Paris) 137:447, 1981.

268. Chung CS, Caplan LR, Han W, et al: Thalamic haemorrhage. Brain 119:1973, 1996.

269. Kumral E, Kocaer T, Ertubey NO, Kumral K: Thalamic hemorrhage: A prospective study of 100 patients. Stroke 26:964, 1995.

270. Steinke W, Sacco R, Mohr JP, et al: Thalamic stroke: Presentation and prognosis of infarcts and hemorrhages. Arch Neurol 49:703, 1992.

271. Dromerick AX, Meschia JF, Kumar A, Hanton RE: Simultaneous bilateral thalamic hemorrhages following the administration of intravenous tissue plasminogen activator. Arch Phys Med Rehab 78:92, 1997.

272. Crum BA, Wijdicks EF: Thalamic hematoma from a ruptured posterior cerebral artery aneurysm. Cerebrovasc Dis 10:475, 2000.

273. Pozzati E: Thalamic cavernous malformations. Surg Neurol 53:30, 2000.

274. Barraquer-Bordas L, Illa I, Escartin A, et al: Thalamic hemorrhage: A study of 23 patients with a diagnosis by computed tomography. Stroke 12:524, 1981.

275. Waga S, Okada M, Yamamoto Y: Reversibility of Parinaud syndrome in thalamic hemorrhage. Neurology (NY) 29:407, 1979.

276. Keane JR: Transient opsoclonus with thalamic hemorrhage. Arch Neurol 37:423, 1980.

277. Keane JR: Contralateral gaze deviation with supratentorial hemorrhage: Three pathologically verified cases. Arch Neurol 32:119, 1975.

278. Denny-Brown D, Fischer EG: Physiological aspects of visual perception. II: The subcortical visual direction of behavior. Arch Neurol 33:228, 1976.

279. Pasik P, Pasik T, Bender MB: The pretectal syndrome in monkeys. I: Disturbances of gaze and body posture. Brain 92:521, 1969.

280. Christoff N: A clinicopathologic study of vertical eye movements. Arch Neurol 31:1, 1974.

281. Christoff N, Anderson PJ, Bender MB: A clinicopathologic study of associated vertical eye movements. Trans Am Neurol Assoc 87:184, 1962.

282. Nashold BS, Seaber JH: Defects of ocular motility after stereotactic midbrain lesions in man. Arch Ophthalmol 88:245, 1972.

283. Gilner LI, Avin B: A reversible ocular manifestation of thalamic hemorrhage: A case report. Arch Neurol 34:715, 1977.

284. Reynolds AF, Harris AB, Ojemann GA, Turner PT: Aphasia and left thalamic hemorrhage. J Neurosurg 48:570, 1978.

285. Fisher CM: Some neuro-ophthalmological observations. J Neurol Neurosurg Psychiatry 30:383, 1967.

286. Pessin MS, Adelman LS, Prager RJ, et al: "Wrong-way eyes" in supratentorial hemorrhage. Ann Neurol 9:79, 1981.

287. Tijssen CC: Contralateral conjugate eye deviation in acute supratentorial lesions. Stroke 25:1516, 1994.

288. Alexander MP, LoVerme SR: Aphasia after left hemispheric intracerebral hemorrhage. Neurology (NY) 30:1193, 1980.

289. Heilman JM, Valenstein E: Frontal lobe neglect in man. Neurology (Minneap) 22:660, 1972.

290. Karussis D, Leker RR, Abramsky O: Cognitive dysfunction following thalamic stroke: A study of 16 cases and review of the literature. J Neurol Sci 172:25, 2000.

291. Liebson E: Anosognosia and mania associated with right thalamic haemorrhage. J Neurol Neurosurg Psychiatry 68:107, 2000.

292. Manabe Y, Kashibara K, Ota T, et al: Motor neglect following left thalamic hemorrhage: A case report. J Neurol Sci 171:69, 1999.

293. Dejerine J, Roussy G: Le syndrome thalamique. Rev Neurol (Paris) 12:521, 1906.

294. Percheron SMJ: Les artères du thalamus humain. Rev Neurol (Paris) 132:297, 1976.

295. Wilkins RH, Brody IA: The thalamic syndrome (Neurological Classics 18). Arch Neurol 20:559, 1969.

296. Fisher CM: Pure sensory stroke involving face, arm and leg. Neurology (Minneap) 15:76, 1965.

297. Abe K, Yorifuji S, Nishikawa Y: Pure sensory stroke resulting from thalamic haemorrhage. Neuroradiology 34:205, 1992.

298. Paciaroni M, Bogousslavsky J: Pure sensory syndromes in thalamic stroke. Eur Neurol 39:211, 1998.

299. Shintani S, Tsuruoka S, Shiigai T: Pure sensory stroke caused by a cerebral hemorrhage: Clinical-radiologic correlations in seven patients. AJNR Am J Neuroradiol 21:515, 2000.

300. Dobato JL, Villanueva JA, Gimenez-Roldan S: Sensory ataxic hemiparesis in thalamic hemorrhage. Stroke 21:1749, 1990.

301. Fisher CM: Ataxic hemiparesis: A pathologic study. Arch Neurol 35:126, 1978.

302. Mori S, Sadoshina S, Ibayashi S, et al: Impact of thalamic hematoma on six-month mortality and motor and cognitive functional outcome. Stroke 26:620, 2000.

303. Maeshima S, Truman G, Smith DS, et al: Functional outcome following thalamic haemorrhage: Relationship between motor and cognitive functions and ADL. Disabil Rehabil 11:459, 1997.

304. Massaro AR, Sacco RL, Mohr JP, et al: Clinical discriminators separate lobar and subcortical hemorrhage: The Stroke Data Bank. Neurology (NY) 41:1881, 1991.

305. Masdeu JC, Rubino FA: Management of lobar intracerebral hemorrhage, medical or surgical. Neurology (Cleve) 34:381, 1984.

306. Broderick J, Brott T, Tomsick T, Leach A: Lobar hemorrhage in the elderly: The undiminishing importance of hypertension. Stroke 24:49, 1993.

307. O'Donnell HC, Rosand J, Knudsen K, et al: Apolipoprotein E genotype and the risk of recurrent lobar intracerebral hemorrhage. N Engl J Med 342:240, 2000.

308. Weisberg LA: Subcortical lobar intracerebral hemorrhage: Clinical-computed tomographic correlations. J Neurol Neurosurg Psychiatry 48:1078, 1985.

309. Bogousslavsky J, Van Melle G, Regli F: The Lausanne Stroke Registry: Analysis of 1,000 consecutive patients with first stroke. Stroke 19:1083, 1988.

310. Kase CS: Lobar hemorrhage. In Kase CS, Caplan LR (eds): Intracerebral Hemorrhage. Boston, Butterworth-Heinemann, 1994, p 363.

311. Faught E, Peters D, Bartolucci A, et al: Seizures after primary intracerebral hemorrhage. Neurology 39:1089, 1989.

312. Lipton RB, Berger AR, Lesser ML, et al: Lobar vs thalamic and basal ganglion hemorrhage: Clinical and radiographic features. J Neurol 234:86, 1987.

313. Sung C-Y, Chu N-S: Epileptic seizures in intracerebral hemorrhage. J Neurol Neurosurg Psychiatry 52:1273, 1989.

314. Arboix A, Comes E, Garcia-Eroles L, et al: Site of bleeding and early outcome in primary intracerebral hemorrhage. Acta Neurol Scand 105:282, 2002.

315. Passero S, Rocchi R, Rossi S, et al: Seizures after spontaneous supratentorial intracerebral hemorrhage. Epilepsia 43:1175, 2002.

316. Echlin FA, Arnett V, Zoll J: Paroxysmal high voltage discharges from isolated and partially isolated human and animal cerebral cortex. EEG Clin Neurophysiol 4:147, 1952.

317. Mohr JP, Pessin MS, Finkelstein S, et al: Broca aphasia: Pathologic and clinical aspects. Neurology (Minneap) 28:311, 1978.

318. Naeser MA, Hayward RW: The resolving stroke and aphasia: A case study with computerized tomography. Arch Neurol 36:233, 1979.

319. Helweg-Larsen S, Sommer W, Strange P, et al: Prognosis for patients treated conservatively for spontaneous intracerebral hematomas. Stroke 15:1045, 1984.

320. Richardson A: Spontaneous intracerebral and cerebellar hemorrhage. In Russell RWR (ed): Cerebral Arterial Disease. New York, Churchill-Livingstone, 1976, p 210.

321. Steiner I, Gomori JM, and Melded E: The prognostic value of the CT scan in conservatively treated patients with intracerebral hematoma. Stroke 15:279, 1984.

322. Sung CY, Chu NS: Late CT manifestations in spontaneous lobar hematoma. Compat Assist Tomogram 25:938, 2001.

323. McKusick W, Richardson A, Taylor J: Primary intracerebral hemorrhage: A controlled trial of surgical and conservative treatment in 180 unsolicited cases. Lancet 2:221, 1961.

324. Crowell RM, Ojemann RG: Surgery for brain hemorrhage. In Moossy J, Reinmuth OM (eds): Cerebrovascular Diseases: Twelfth Research Conference. Philadelphia, Lippincott-Raven, 1981, p 233.

335. Broderick JP, Adams HP, Barsan W, et al: Guidelines for the management of spontaneous intracerebral hemorrhage: A statement for healthcare professionals from a special writing group of the Stroke Council, American Heart Association. Stroke 30:905, 1999.

326. Flemming K, Wijdicks EFM, St. Louis EK, Li H: Predicting deterioration in patients with lobar haemorrhages. J Neurol Neurosurg Psychiatry 66:600, 1999.

327. Flemming KD, Wijdicks EF, Li H: Can we predict poor outcome at presentation in patients with lobar hemorrhage? Cerebrovasc Dis 11:183, 2001.

328. Little JR, Tubman DE, Ethier R: Cerebellar hemorrhage in adults: Diagnosis by computerized tomography. J Neurosurg 48:575, 1978.

329. Müller HR, Wüthrich R, Wiggli U, et al: The contribution of computerized axial tomography to the diagnosis of cerebellar and pontine hematomas. Stroke 6:467, 1975.

330. Freeman RE, Onofrio BM, Okazaki H, Dinapoli RP: Spontaneous intracerebellar hemorrhage. Neurology (NY) 23:84, 1973.

331. Hyland HH, Levy D: Spontaneous cerebellar hemorrhage. Can Med Assoc J 71:315, 1954.

332. Rey-Bellet J: Cerebellar hemorrhage: A clinicopathologic study. Neurology 10:217, 1960.

333. Richardson AE: Spontaneous cerebellar hemorrhage. In Vinken PJ, Bruyn GW (eds): Handbook of Clinical Neurology, Vol. 12. Amsterdam, North-Holland Publishing, 1972, p 54.

334. Brennan RW, Bergland RM: Acute cerebellar hemorrhage: Analysis of clinical findings and outcome in 12 cases. Neurology (NY) 27:527, 1977.

335. McKissock W, Richardson A, Walsh L: Spontaneous cerebellar hemorrhage: A study of 34 consecutive cases treated surgically. Brain 83:1, 1960.

336. Norris JW, Eisen AA, Branch CL: Problems in cerebellar hemorrhage and infarction. Neurology (NY) 19:1043, 1969.

337. Fisher CM: The neurological examination of the comatose patient. Acta Neurol Scand Suppl 45:44, 1969.

338. Messert B, Leppik IE, Sato Y: Diplopia and involuntary eye closure in spontaneous cerebellar hemorrhage. Stroke 7:305, 1976.

339. Bosch EP, Kennedy SS, Aschenbrener CA: Ocular bobbing: The myth of its localizing value. Neurology (NY) 25:949, 1975.

340. Fisher CM: Ocular bobbing. Arch Neurol 11:543, 1964.

341. St. Louis EK, Wijdicks EF, Li H: Predicting neurologic deterioration in patients with cerebellar hematomas. Neurology 51:1364, 1998.

342. Brillman J: Acute hydrocephalus and death one month after nonsurgical treatment for acute cerebellar hemorrhage. J Neurosurg 50:374, 1979.

343. Yoshida S, Sasaki M, Oka H, et al: Acute hypertensive cerebellar hemorrhage with signs of lower brainstem compression. Surg Neurol 10:79, 1978.

344. Greenberg J, Skubick D, Shenkin H: Acute hydrocephalus in cerebellar infarct and hemorrhage. Neurology (NY) 29:409, 1979.

345. Heiman TD, Satya-Murti S: Benign cerebellar hemorrhages. Ann Neurol 3:366, 1978.

346. St. Louis EK, Wijdicks EF, Li H, Atkinson JD: Predictors of poor outcome in patients with a spontaneous cerebellar hematoma. Can J Neurol Sci 27:32, 2000.

347. Kirollos RW, Tyagi AK, Ross SA, et al: Management of spontaneous cerebellar hematomas: A prospective treatment protocol. Neurosurgery 49:1378, 2001.

348. Roig C, Carvajal A, Illa I, et al: Hémorragies mésencephaliques isolées. Rev Neurol (Paris) 138:53, 1982.

349. Durward QJ, Barnett HJM, Barr HWK: Presentation and management of mesencephalic hematoma. J Neurosurg 56:123, 1982.

350. Morel-Maroger A, Metzger J, Bories J, et al: Les hématomes benins du tronc cérébral chez les hypertendus artériels. Rev Neurol (Paris) 138:437, 1982.

351. Humphreys RP: Computerized tomographic definition of mesencephalic hematoma with evacuation through pedunculotomy. J Neurosurg 49:749, 1978.

352. LaTorre E, Delitala A, Sorano V: Hematoma of the quadrigeminal plate. J Neurosurg 49:610, 1978.

353. Scoville WB, Poppen JL: Intrapeduncular hemorrhage of the brain. Arch Neurol Psychiatry 61:688, 1949.

354. Galetta SL, Balcer LJ: Isolated fourth nerve palsy from midbrain hemorrhage. J Neuroophthalmol 18:204, 1998.

355. Isikay CT, Yucesan C, Yucemen N, et al: Isolated nuclear oculomotor nerve syndrome due to mesencephalic hematoma. Acta Neurol Belg 100:248, 2000.

356. Mizushima H, Seki T: Midbrain hemorrhage presenting with oculomotor nerve palsy: Case report. Surg Neurol 58:417, 2002.

357. Lee AG, Brown DG, Diaz PJ: Dorsal midbrain syndrome due to mesencephalic hemorrhage: Case report with serial imaging. J Neuroophthalmol 16:281, 1996.

358. Pego R, Martinez-Vazquez F, Branas F, et al: Hemorragia espontánea en la lámina cuadrigémina: Presentación de dos casos. Rev Neurol (Spain) 25:1414, 1997.

359. Fang HCM, Foley JM: Hypertensive hemorrhages of the pons and cerebellum. Arch Neurol Psychiatry 72:638, 1954.

360. Caplan LR: Intracerebral hemorrhage. In Tyler HR, Dawson DM (eds): Current Neurology, Vol II. Boston, Houghton Mifflin, 1979, p 185.

361. Kornyey S: Rapidly fatal pontile hemorrhage: Clinical and anatomic report. Arch Neurol Psychiatry 41:793, 1939.

362. Silverstein A: Primary pontile hemorrhage. Conf Neurol 29:33, 1967.

363. Silverstein A: Primary pontine hemorrhage. In Vinken PJ, Bruyn GW (eds): Handbook of Clinical Neurology, Vol 12, Part II. Amsterdam, North-Holland Publishing, 1972, p 37.

364. Jeong JH, Yoon SJ, Kang SJ, et al: Hypertensive pontine microhemorrhage. Stroke 33:925, 2002.

365. Dana C: Acute bulbar paralysis due to hemorrhage and softening of the pons and medulla. Med Rec 64:361, 1903.

366. Okudera T, Uemura K, Nakajima K, et al: Primary pontine hemorrhage: Correlations of pathologic features with postmortem microangiographic and vertebral angiography studies. Mt Sinai J Med 45:305, 1978.

367. Steegmann AT: Primary pontile hemorrhage. J Nerv Ment Dis 114:35, 1951.

368. Sharpe JA, Rosenberg MA, Hoyt WF, Daroff RB: Paralytic pontine exotropia: A sign of acute unilateral pontine gaze palsy and internuclear ophthalmoplegia. Neurology (NY) 24:1076, 1974.

369. Becker DH, Silverberg GD: Successful evacuation of an acute pontine hematoma. Surg Neurol 10:263, 1978.

Clinical Manifestations

370. Pierrott-Deseilligny C, Chain F, Serdaru M, et al: The "one-and-a-half" syndrome: Electro-oculographic analysis of five cases with deductions about the physiological mechanisms of lateral gaze. Brain 104:665, 1981.

371. Halsey JH, Ceballos R, Crosby EC: The supranuclear control of voluntary lateral gaze. Neurology (NY) 17:928, 1967.

372. Susac JO, Hoyt WF, Daroff RB, Lawrence W: Clinical spectrum of ocular bobbing. J Neurol Neurosurg Psychiatry 33:771, 1970.

373. Goto N, Kaneko M, Hosaka Y, Koga H: Primary pontine hemorrhage: Clinicopathologic correlations. Stroke 11:84, 1980.

374. Payne HA, Maravilla KR, Levinstone A, et al: Recovery from primary pontine hemorrhage. Ann Neurol 4:557, 1978.

375. Wijdicks EF, St. Louis E: Clinical profiles predictive of outcome in pontine hemorrhage. Neurology 49:1342, 1997.

376. O'Laoire SA, Crockard HA, Thomas DGT, Gordon DS: Brain-stem hematoma. J Neurosurg 56:222, 1982.

377. Zuccarello M, Iavicoli R, Pardatscher K, et al: Primary brain stem hematomas. Diagnosis and treatment. Acta Neurochir 54:45, 1980.

378. Gobernado JM, Fernandez de Molina AR, Gimeno A: Pure motor hemiplegia due to hemorrhage in the lower pons. Arch Neurol 37:393, 1980.

379. Schnapper RA: Pontine hemorrhage presenting as ataxic hemiparesis. Stroke 13:518, 1982.

380. Tuhrim S, Yang WC, Rubinowitz H, Weinberger J: Primary pontine hemorrhage and the dysarthria clumsy hand syndrome. Neurology (NY) 32:1027, 1982.

381. Freeman W, Ammerman HH, Stanley M: Syndromes of the pontile tegmentum, Foville's syndrome: Report of 3 cases. Arch Neurol Psychiatry 50:462, 1943.

382. Tyler HR, Johnson PC: Case records of the Massachusetts General Hospital (Case 36-1972). N Engl J Med 287:506, 1972.

383. Pullicino PM, Wong EH: Tonic downward and inward ocular deviation ipsilateral to pontine tegmental hemorrhage. Cerebrovasc Dis 10:327, 2000.

384. Lawrence WH, Lightfoote WE: Continuous vertical pendular eye movements after brainstem hemorrhage. Neurology (NY) 25:896, 1975.

385. Arseni C, Stanciu M: Primary hematomas of the brain stem. Acta Neurochir 28:323, 1973.

386. Kempe LG: Surgical removal of an intramedullary hematoma simulating Wallenberg's syndrome. J Neurol Neurosurg Psychiatry 27:78, 1964.

387. Mastaglia FL, Edis B, Kakulas BA: Medullary hemorrhage: A report of two cases. J Neurol Neurosurg Psychiatry 32:221, 1969.

388. Barinagarrementeria F, Cantú C: Primary medullary hemorrhage: Report of four cases and review of the literature. Stroke 25:1684, 1994.

389. Kumral E, Acarer A: Primary medullary hemorrhage with intractable hiccup. J Neurol 245:620, 1998.

390. Jung HH, Baumgartner RW, Hess K: Symptomatic secondary hemorrhagic transformation of ischemic Wallenberg's syndrome. J Neurol 247:463, 2000.

Chapter Fourteen

Aneurysmal Subarachnoid Hemorrhage

Harold P. Adams, Jr. and Patricia H. Davis

Subarachnoid hemorrhage (SAH) accounts for 5% to 10% of all strokes and, unlike most other types of stroke, has not declined in incidence during the last 30 years. The leading cause of SAH, accounting for approximately 80% of cases, is rupture of an intracranial saccular aneurysm. This distinction is important, because patients with bleeding secondary to ruptured saccular aneurysms have a poorer prognosis and present more complicated management problems than patients with SAH of other causes.

Outcomes among patients who do not have aneurysms are also better. Such patients, including those with a perimesencephalic pattern of bleeding found on computed tomography (CT), often are not seriously ill and uncommonly experience either rebleeding or delayed cerebral ischemia.[1,2] As a result, the treatment of patients with nonaneurysmal SAH differs from that of patients with aneurysmal SAH. We restrict discussion in this chapter to management of patients with aneurysmal SAH and emphasize medical measures to treat these seriously affected patients.

Despite early diagnosis and better medical and surgical treatment that probably are reducing the mortality, SAH remains a common cause of death and disability. The 30-day mortality rate of SAH approaches 50%. Most deaths occur within 1 week of the ictus; 10% of patients die before reaching medical attention, and 25% die within 24 hours.[3–5] Causes of sudden death include a large intraparenchymal hematoma, destruction of brain tissue, acute hydrocephalus, increased intracranial pressure, myocardial ischemia, cardiac arrhythmias, pulmonary edema, and respiratory failure. These critically ill patients, who are moribund, often have ataxic or periodic respirations, suggesting brainstem failure. In these cases, CT usually shows massive intracerebral, intraventricular, or subarachnoid hemorrhage. Survival in these instances is unlikely even with prompt and aggressive medical care.

Even if terminally ill patients are excluded from consideration, the natural history of SAH is grim. The 3-month mortality rate among patients who reach a major medical center is approximately 25%.[6] The leading causes of death are sequelae of the initial hemorrhage, recurrent aneurysmal rupture, and vasospasm leading to ischemic stroke. In addition, severe medical complications may add

significantly to mortality rates after SAH.[7] Another 20% to 40% of hospitalized patients have major neurologic impairments.[8–10] Because SAH affects a relatively young group of otherwise healthy patients, the economic and social effects of the disease are great.[11] The chief reasons for neurologic residual effects are the consequences of the initial rupture, vasospasm and ischemia, recurrent hemorrhage, hydrocephalus, complications of surgery, and complications of medical management.[12] Sequelae include cranial nerve palsies, paralysis, aphasia, cognitive impairments, behavioral disorders, and psychiatric disturbances that could hamper return to gainful employment or independence. Nevertheless, improvements in care are leading to reductions in mortality and disability after SAH.[11,13,14]

The two most important factors that influence prognosis after SAH are the interval from the ictus and the person's level of consciousness.[10] Most deaths and complications occur within 2 weeks of SAH; patients surviving this period without major complications generally have a favorable prognosis. When examining the possible usefulness of any intervention, one should consider the interval from the onset of SAH to initiation of treatment. The key test of any medical or surgical therapy is whether it improves outcome among acutely ill patients treated within the first few days after SAH. The admitting level of consciousness is the most predictive clinical factor (Table 14.1). In one study, the 6-month mortality rate among comatose patients was 71%, whereas only 11% of initially alert patients died during the same period.[15]

The size of the aneurysm was a major determinant of prognosis in one study,[16] but not in another study.[9] Although data conflict, aneurysms located on the basilar artery or its branches appear to be associated with a poorer prognosis.[5,10] Patients older than 65 years have a poorer prognosis than younger patients.[16,17] Favorable outcomes are less common among women than among men.[9,18] Fever, presumably of central origin, occurs commonly with SAH, and patients with fever often have poor outcomes.[19] Preexisting medical conditions, such as hypertension and diabetes mellitus, do not have major effects on prognosis. In one study, smoking had a protective effect on mortality[17]; the reason for this effect is not clear, and the

Table 14.1 Factors Predicting Less Favorable Outcome after Subarachnoid Hemorrhage

Clinical factors	Admitting level of consciousness (coma)
	Interval from subarachnoid hemorrhage (<3 days)
	Age (>65 years)
	Prior unrecognized hemorrhage or warning leak
	Presence of focal neurologic signs on admission
	Presence of severe comorbid disease or extraneural organ involvement
Diagnostic test results	Hyponatremia or hypovolemia
	Abnormal CT scan
	Local, thick, or diffuse collection of subarachnoid blood
	Intracerebral or intraventricular blood
	Mass effect
	Hydrocephalus
	Evidence of rebleeding detected by sequential CT scans
	Vasospasm detected by arteriography or by transcranial Doppler ultrasonography
	Aneurysm located on anterior cerebral or vertebrobasilar arteries
	Size of aneurysm (≥10 mm)

Table 14.2 Complications of Aneurysmal Subarachnoid Hemorrhage

Neurologic (intraparenchymal hematoma)
Intraventricular hemorrhage
Brain edema
Hydrocephalus (acute, subacute, chronic)
Recurrent hemorrhage
Vasospasm-induced ischemic stroke
Seizures
Systemic
   Arterial hypotension or hypertension
   Electrolyte disturbances (hyponatremia, hypernatremia, hypokalemia)
   Cardiac (myocardial infarction, arrhythmia, congestive heart failure)
Pulmonary (neurogenic pulmonary edema, adult respiratory distress syndrome, atelectasis, pneumonia)
Gastrointestinal bleeding
Sepsis
Renal or hepatic dysfunction
Venous thromboembolism
Bleeding disorders, including thrombocytopenia

observation needs further study. Patients who do not reach medical attention until after a second rupture of the aneurysm have a worse prognosis than patients who have a single hemorrhage.[6] Evidence of extracerebral organ dysfunction and acute systemic inflammatory response syndrome also predict higher mortality and morbidity in patients with SAH.[20,21]

The results of the initial CT examination also provide prognostic clues (see Table 14.1).[10,15] In general, CT and clinical findings are parallel and correlate with the time lag from SAH.[15] Patients with CT evidence of hydrocephalus, mass effect, intracerebral hematoma, intraventricular evidence, or diffuse subarachnoid blood have a poorer prognosis than those with normal CT findings or a minimal amount of subarachnoid blood. Early elevations in thrombin–antithrombin III complex, plasmin α_2–plasmin inhibitor complex, and D dimer are more common among patients with severe hemorrhages and poor outcomes.[22] Mack and colleagues[23] noted that elevations of serum intercellular adhesion molecule-1 (ICAM-1) levels were associated with poorer outcomes after SAH.

The complications of SAH that can lead to death or disability are summarized in Table 14.2. Neurologic injuries secondary to a number of complications lead to greater morbidity or mortality from SAH, especially among the most seriously ill patients.[24] Because rebleeding and ischemic complications from cerebral vasospasm account for approximately 60% of unfavorable outcomes, considerable attention is directed toward their prevention or treatment. Still, approximately one third of patients who die or are disabled from SAH are injured primarily by the consequences of the initial hemorrhage.[4,12] The goals of medical management are (1) to stabilize an acutely ill patient and to prevent early complications, (2) to forestall recurrent hemorrhage, and (3) to avoid the ischemic complications of vasospasm. Treatment is multifactorial and complex; therapies aimed at prevention of one complication might interfere with management of another complication. In addition, successful treatment of one complication can leave the patient at risk for another. For example, prevention of early rebleeding means that cerebral ischemia from vasospasm might develop. Considerable research has focused on individual components of management. Still, much of the treatment of SAH is empirical or is based on anecdotal evidence; several components of care have not been tested in clinical trials. Thus, some recommendations for management are based on weak or conflicting scientific evidence. In the future, considerable research will focus on refining the utility of several elements of acute management after SAH.

DIAGNOSIS

The key to successful management of SAH is early treatment, which, in turn, is based on prompt recognition and accurate diagnosis.[6] The drive to popularize the concept of stroke as a "brain attack" is stimulated, in part, by the successful early treatment of patients with ruptured aneurysms.[25] Therapies of proven utility are available, and the goal is to offer these interventions to patients with SAH, who are acutely ill. Approximately 10% of patients or their families do not recognize the serious nature of the symptoms and do not seek medical attention quickly. More disconcerting is that physicians initially diagnose disorders other than SAH in 25% to 50% of cases.[26–28] Such misdiagnoses can delay treatment for days.[27–29] Even more bothersome is that the chance of misdiagnosis is greatest among the least seriously ill patients—who are most likely to be helped by early medical or surgical interventions.

ACUTE MANAGEMENT

The patient with recent SAH is critically ill and should be evaluated and treated urgently.[30,31] He or she should be transported rapidly to a medical center that has the expertise to treat a patient with a ruptured aneurysm. Acute, potentially life-threatening complications should be anticipated (see Table 14.2). Personnel should assess the patient quickly and should measure vital signs and assess neurologic status frequently. The heart rate and rhythm should be monitored. The airway, breathing, and circulation should be supported, and if necessary, supplemental oxygen, endotracheal intubation, or ventilatory assistance should be given.[31] Intravenous access is established to expedite emergency administration of medications. Normal saline can be given at a slow rate to maintain patency of the intravenous line. Unfortunately, the urgent approach to acute management of SAH is often suboptimal in emergency departments.[32] Each institution should develop a protocol for the management of SAH in the emergency department, including plans for both acute treatment and urgent evaluation.

The initial evaluation should include CT scan, chest radiograph, electrocardiogram, and blood studies (Table 14.3). CT can demonstrate subarachnoid blood and a number of other acute intracranial complications (Table 14.4 and Fig. 14–1). When CT shows intracranial bleeding, a lumbar puncture can be avoided. The findings of CT that is performed within 24 hours after onset of symptoms with the use of third-generation scanners are normal in approximately 2% to 7% of cases.[27] If the CT findings are normal, a cerebrospinal fluid (CSF) specimen should be obtained.

Magnetic resonance imaging (MRI) may not be as sensitive as CT in detecting subarachnoid blood in the acute setting but may be more sensitive than CT in patients presenting in the subacute phase. The most sensitive MRI sequences for detecting SAH are gradient-echo T2 images

Table 14.4 Abnormalities Found by Unenhanced Cranial CT in Patients with Recent Subarachnoid Hemorrhage

Abnormality	%
Subarachnoid blood	93–98 (<24 hours)
Focal, thin collection	
Focal, thick collection	
Diffuse, thin collection	
Diffuse, thick collection	
Intraventricular blood	15–20
Intraparenchymal blood	15–20
Subdural blood	1–2
Hydrocephalus	10–20
Mass effect	5–8
Ischemic lesion	1–2
Aneurysm	5

followed by fluid attenuation inversion recovery (FLAIR) images (Fig. 14–2).[33] Once the diagnosis of SAH is confirmed, arteriography is needed to demonstrate the presence and location of the aneurysm (Fig. 14–3).[29] Both carotid circulations and the entire vertebrobasilar system should be examined, although the sequence of the arterial studies is influenced by the findings on CT.

Magnetic resonance angiography can be used to screen for larger aneurysms, but it is probably not as effective as arteriography in the evaluation of patients with SAH. CT angiography is becoming a useful alternative to conventional arteriography to detect aneurysms[34,35] and in some cases may detect aneurysms missed by angiography.[36] A potential advantage of CT angiography is its ability to demonstrate the topographic anatomy of the cerebral aneurysms and surrounding structures.[37] If results of the first arteriographic study are normal, a second study is usually performed approximately 10 to 14 days after SAH among patients whose bleeding is not in a perimesencephalic pattern. The second arteriogram obtained 1 week later can detect an aneurysm in an additional 1% to 2% of patients.

Patients should be admitted to a unit that has monitoring equipment and is staffed by neurologically trained nurses. Acute care can be divided into general supportive efforts and therapies aimed at preventing or controlling specific complications (Table 14.5).[30,31] For the first 24 hours, blood pressure, vital signs, and neurologic status should be assessed hourly. Thereafter, examinations can be spaced further apart in stable patients. Cardiac monitoring and, if necessary, continuous intra-arterial or noninvasive blood pressure monitoring are extended for at least 24 to 48 hours after admission.

Forced bed rest is a traditional part of management. Visitors and external stimuli are restricted. Passive range-of-motion exercises and frequent turning are performed. A water mattress or an alternating-pressure pneumatic bed can reduce the risk of pressure sores and atelectasis. Patients are assisted with self-care activities, such as bathing and eating. Black and associates[38] showed that external pneumatic calf compression stockings and devices reduce the incidence of deep vein thrombosis. The use of heparin as a prophylaxis against deep venous thrombosis is generally avoided until the ruptured aneurysm is treated.

Table 14.3 Initial Diagnostic Evaluation of a Patient with a Suspected Subarachnoid Hemorrhage

Laboratory tests
  Complete blood count and platelet count
  International Normalized Ratio, activated partial thromboplastin time
  Serum electrolytes, glucose, calcium
  Blood urea nitrogen and serum creatinine
  Urinalysis
  Electrocardiogram
Imaging studies
  Non–contrast-enhanced cranial CT
  Chest radiograph
  Cerebral angiogram (4-vessel)
Cerebrospinal fluid exam (if CT results are negative)
Optional tests
  CT angiography
  Cervical spine radiography (if patient is comatose with a possible spine injury)
  MRI of brain or cervical spine (if angiogram results are negative)
  Arterial blood gas measurements
  Liver function tests
  Electroencephalogram
  Cerebral blood flow study
  Transcranial Doppler ultrasonography

Clinical Manifestations

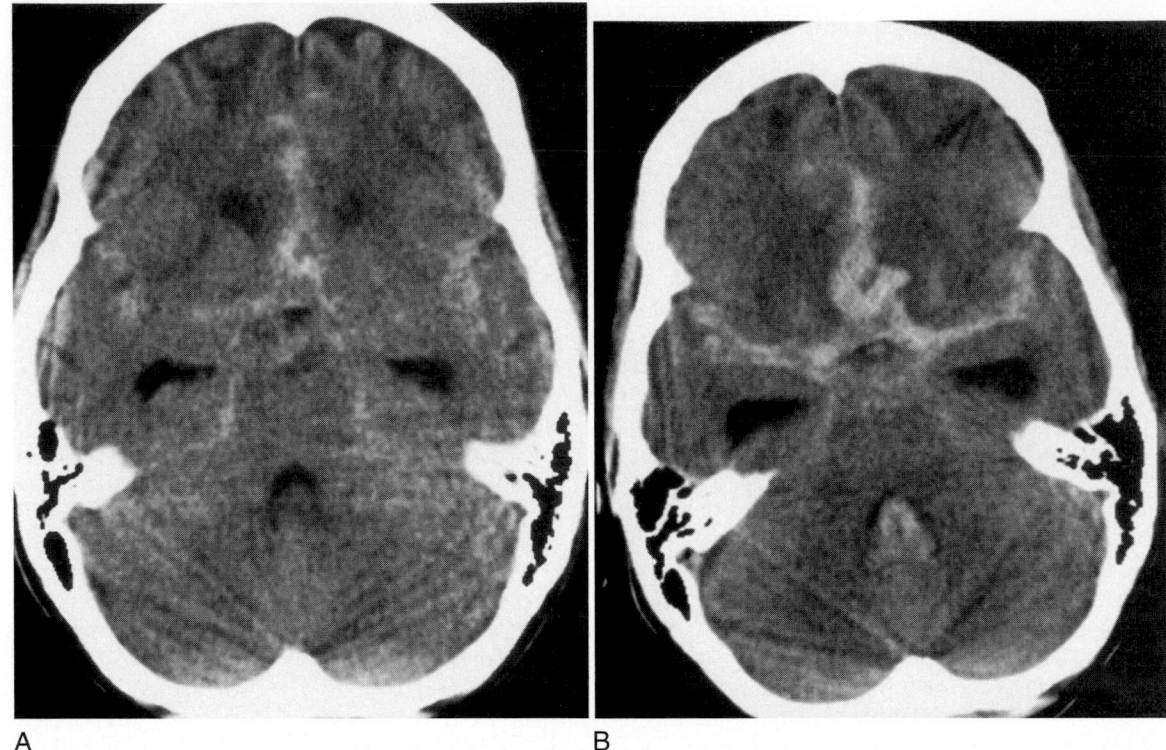

A   B

FIGURE 14–1 *Two CT scans obtained approximately 4 hours apart in a patient who had a recurrent hemorrhage. A, Subarachnoid blood can be seen in interhemispheric fissure and basal cisterns. The patient's condition suddenly deteriorated. B, The second study shows additional subarachnoid blood and intraventricular hemorrhage. Hydrocephalus (enlargement of the temporal horns) is also present.*

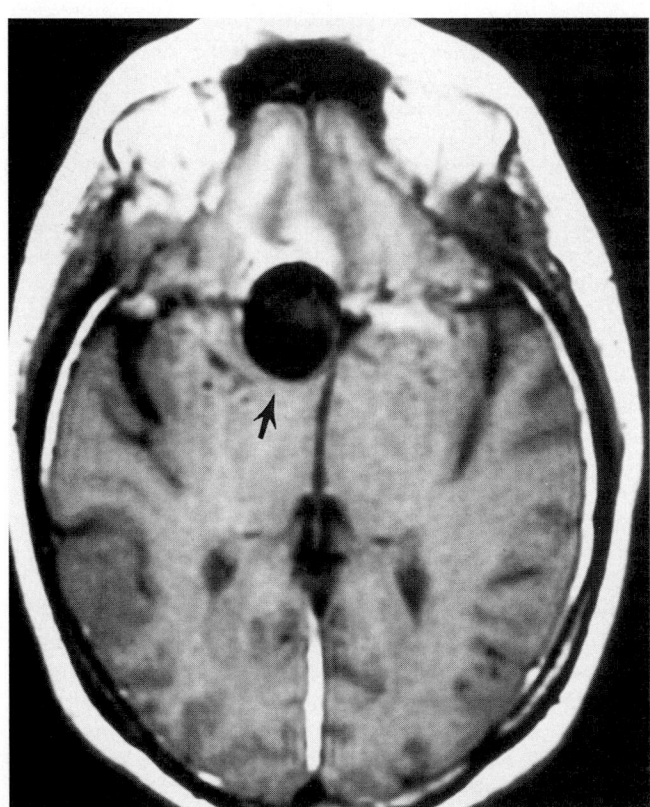

FIGURE 14–2 *T1-weighted MRI scan demonstrates a large aneurysm (arrow) arising from the right internal carotid artery.*

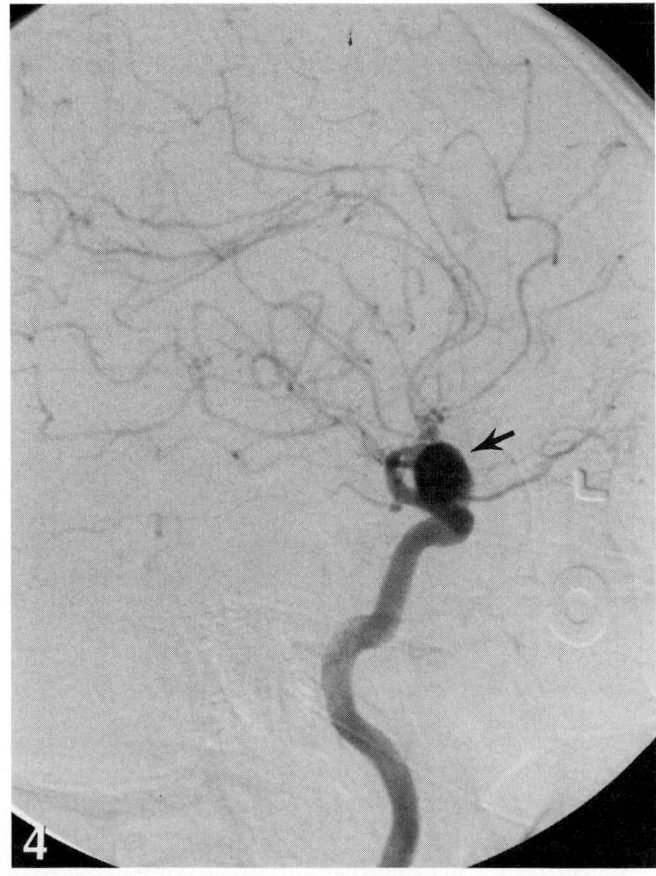

FIGURE 14–3 *Left lateral carotid arteriogram obtained with the use of subtraction technique shows an aneurysm of the internal carotid artery (arrow) in the region of the carotid siphon.*

Table 14.5 Medical Management of Persons with Aneurysmal Subarachnoid Hemorrhage

Emergency treatment
  Support airway
  Supplemental oxygen
  Ventilatory assistance
  Intravenous access—normal saline
Other immediate treatment
  Close observation
    Cardiac monitoring
    Arterial pressure monitoring
  Bed rest
    Passive/active range of movement
    Water/alternating-pressure mattress
    Assistance with self-care
    Gentle pulmonary toilet
    Avoidance of indwelling bladder catheter, if possible
    Pneumatic compression stockings
  Intravenous saline with multiple vitamins—2.5–3.5 L per day
  Stool softeners
  Stress ulcer prophylaxis
  Diet—soft, high-fiber if patient is alert; nasogastric feeding if patient is obtunded
Symptomatic treatment
  Pain or discomfort—codeine, meperidine, morphine, acetaminophen
  Nausea and vomiting—prochlorperazine, promethazine, trimethobenzamide, ondansetron
  Seizures—anticonvulsants
  Cardiac arrhythmias—correct electrolytes, β-blocker, calcium channel blocker
  Arterial hypertension
    Moderate—labetalol, enalaprilat, hydralazine
    Severe—nicardipine, esmolol, nitroprusside, fenoldopam
  Hyponatremia—isotonic or hypertonic fluids, fludrocortisone, no diuretics, fluid restriction only if patient is euvolemic or hypervolemic
  Increased intracranial pressure
    Elevate head of bed
    Intracranial pressure monitoring
    Correct metabolic disturbances
    Hyperventilation
    Mannitol, furosemide, hypertonic saline
    Cerebrospinal fluid drainage—multiple lumbar punctures or intraventricular catheter placement
    Surgical decompression
  Rebleeding
    Aminocaproic acid/tranexamic acid
    Secure aneurysm—surgical clipping or endovascular obliteration
  Neurogenic pulmonary edema
    Dobutamine
    Positive end-expiratory pressure, gentle diuresis

Gentle pulmonary suctioning and nursing care are important for avoiding pneumonia. The value of absolute bed rest in preventing rebleeding was tested by the Cooperative Study of Intracranial Aneurysms and Subarachnoid Hemorrhage; the cumulative rate of rebleeding was 25% during the first 14 days after SAH.[39] In general, the prognosis of patients treated only with absolute bed rest now represents the natural history of SAH.

Because intravenously administered medications are often needed, a slow infusion of saline is continued. Alert patients are usually given a soft, high-fiber diet supplemented by stool softeners.[31] Caffeinated beverages are avoided. Stuporous and comatose patients are not fed during the acute treatment period. If a seriously ill person is stable several days after SAH and the airway is secured, nasogastric feedings can be instituted.

SYMPTOMATIC TREATMENT

Patients with SAH are often confused or agitated as a result of brain injury, hydrocephalus, or increased intracranial pressure. Pain or nausea can also lead to irritability. Agitation raises the risk of rebleeding and aggravates increased intracranial pressure. Control of pain or nausea can calm an upset patient. Regular administration of diazepam or phenobarbital may be useful in providing sedation for agitated patients.

The headache of SAH is intense, and patients should receive ample doses of analgesics.[30,31] Most alert patients require a medication such as codeine, meperidine, or morphine. The agent is usually administered parenterally. These medications can be combined with acetaminophen, hydroxyzine hydrochloride, or promethazine. Some patients have photophobia and phonophobia; a quiet, dark environment can help relieve some of these conditions, which otherwise might worsen the head pain. Sedation and sleep might also help control pain. Aspirin affects platelet aggregation and prolongs the bleeding time; there is concern that aspirin might potentiate rebleeding.

Severe nausea and vomiting are common and important complaints, particularly during the first 24 hours after SAH. Nauseated patients should receive an antiemetic, such as ondansetron, trimethobenzamide, or prochlorperazine, to control these complaints.

ANTICONVULSANTS

Approximately 25% of patients have seizures, most of which occur within the first 24 hours.[40–42] Rhoney and colleagues[41] reported that seizures were most common among patients with thick cisternal clots. Most seizures happen before the patient reaches the hospital.[41] Hart and associates[40] noted that 63% of the seizures happened at the time of aneurysmal rupture. However, some of these "seizures" may not be truly epileptic phenomena but may represent transient decerebrate posturing secondary to increased intracranial pressure.[40,43] There is no correlation between epileptic seizures at the time of aneurysmal rupture and the risk of rebleeding, early mortality, or major morbidity.[40,42]

Although seizures occurring after hospitalization are uncommon, they can be associated with recurrent hemorrhage. Physicians prescribe anticonvulsants to patients who have experienced a seizure as part of SAH, but the prophylactic use of these agents in treatment of patients who have not had a seizure is controversial. The rationale for prophylactic administration of anticonvulsants is that a seizure is a dangerous event in a person with a recent SAH. Because of the low rate of seizures after admission, however, Hart and associates[40] and Sundaram and Chow[42] question the necessity for routine prescription of anticonvulsants to patients with recent SAH. However, regular use of phenytoin or another parenterally administered anti-convulsant is recommended to reduce the likelihood of seizures. No trial has tested the value of anticonvulsants in management of patients with recent SAH. Pending such a trial, the decision to prescribe these medications is individualized. The benefit of prophylaxis against seizures must be weighed against potential adverse reactions, which occurred in 4.1% of patients in one series.[41] If a patient has had or is having convulsions, intravenous doses of anticonvulsants are given.

TREATMENT OF MYOCARDIAL ISCHEMIA AND CARDIAC ARRHYTHMIAS

Cardiac arrhythmias can be detected in almost all patients during the first few hours after SAH; in approximately 20% of cases, the arrhythmias can be severe or life-threatening (Table 14.6).[44–48] Ventricular arrhythmias are a potential cause of sudden death after SAH. Di Pasquale and coworkers[45] noted torsades de pointes in 3.8% of 132 patients with SAH who underwent Holter monitoring. Machado and colleagues[49] correlated the development of torsades de pointes with hypokalemia rather than the direct effects of the SAH. Increased QT dispersion is a common electrocardiographic finding after SAH.[48]

Changes resembling those seen in acute myocardial ischemia can be noted in 25% to 80% of patients.[35,50] In fact, many people with SAH have secondary myocardial ischemia and left ventricular dysfunction.[51,52] An elevation of the cardiac isoenzyme creatine kinase can be detected. Subendocardial areas of focal ischemic necrosis are found among patients who died of SAH even those without prior history of coronary artery disease. Abnormal left ventricular function is seen most commonly among patients with elevated creatine kinase levels.[53] Severe left ventricular dysfunction after SAH may necessitate a delay in aneurysm surgery.[51] In addition, the reduction of cardiac output after severe SAH might increase the risk of cerebral ischemia secondary to vasospasm.[53]

The frequency of electrocardiographic changes can be predicted from (1) the severity of bleeding detected on CT and (2) the patient's neurologic status. The changes are most common among seriously ill patients with diffuse subarachnoid blood, intraventricular hemorrhage, or a large intracerebral hematoma.[46,54] The presence of a large clot in the right sylvian cistern and fissure is associated with electrocardiographic changes. Although Brouwers and associates[55] correlated elevated plasma levels of norepinephrine with a poor outcome after SAH, they could not find a relationship between norepinephrine and cardiac ischemia. Still, it is assumed that the release of catecholamines by the posterior hypothalamus is key to the development of the cardiovascular complications of SAH. Presumably, the markedly elevated levels of norepinephrine lead to hypokalemia, systemic hypertensive effects, left ventricular strain, coronary artery vasospasm, a "stunned" myocardium, or cardiac toxicity.[47,52,56] Administration of a β-blocking medication might reduce the number and severity of cardiac sequelae.[57,58]

Further study on the potential value of cardioprotective agents in reducing the cardiac complications of SAH is needed. The risk of cardiac causes of death seems to be low.[54] There may be a group of patients who are particularly vulnerable to such complications. Pending more definitive data, β-blockers can be given on a case-by-case basis. The first 24 to 48 hours are the period of highest risk for cardiac complications, so there is little reason to start treatment with cardioprotective medications after that time.

Neurogenic pulmonary edema is a rare, but often fatal complication that occurs in critically ill patients. Markedly increased extravascular lung water and an intrapulmonary shunt lead to hypoxia. This complication is frequently ascribed to greater sympathetic activity resulting in acute cardiac changes.[31] Treatment is difficult but consists of oxygen and positive-pressure ventilatory assistance.[31] Dobutamine (5 to 10 μg/kg/hr) increases both the cardiac index and left ventricular stroke work index and decreases the total peripheral vascular resistance, leading to diuresis and a reduction in pulmonary congestion; this agent is now recommended for the treatment of neurogenic pulmonary edema after SAH.[31,59]

ANTIHYPERTENSIVE TREATMENT

Arterial hypertension is common in SAH, resulting from elevations of catecholamines and renin produced by hypothalamic disturbances (see Table 14.5).[60,61] Additionally, increased intracranial pressure can induce arterial hypertension as a means to maintain adequate cerebral perfusion pressure. Arterial hypertension also can be secondary to seizures, vomiting, agitation, or pain. In addition, the patient may have preexisting hypertension.

Hypertension after SAH has been found to correlate with increases in the risk of vasospasm and mortality.[61] Arterial hypertension also puts patients at high risk for recurrent hemorrhage. Administration of antihypertensive agents is a traditional component of early medical management of SAH.[30,31] However, rapid or steep reductions in blood pressure might be dangerous. Patients with vasospasm or increased intracranial pressure may experience a drop in cerebral perfusion in conjunction with a decline in blood pressure; neurologic deterioration can result. Some antihypertensive agents (nitroglycerin, sodium nitroprusside, fenoldopam) are potent cerebral vasodilators, and enlargement of the cerebrovascular bed secondary to their administration could further increase intracranial pressure.

Table 14.6 Electrocardiographic Abnormalities after Subarachnoid Hemorrhage

Prominent P waves
Prolonged/shortened PR interval
Broad/inverted/flattened T waves
Prolonged/shortened QT interval
Elevation/depression ST segment
Prominent/inverted U waves
Pathologic Q waves
S in V_1 and R in V_5 combined >35 mm
Rhythm disturbances

The blood pressure often returns to normal after the patient with SAH is admitted to the hospital or when symptoms such as headache are treated; thus, aggressive antihypertensive therapy might be avoided in some cases. The level of arterial hypertension that mandates treatment is not known. Patients with moderate hypertension (mean arterial blood pressure lower than 120 mm Hg) probably do not need to be treated. On the other hand, patients whose mean blood pressure is 120 mm Hg or higher or whose systolic blood pressure is higher than 180 mm Hg should receive medication. The goal should be to cautiously lower the blood pressure to levels normal for the patient and to avoid inducing hypotension.

Although alert patients with elevated blood pressures can receive oral medications, parenteral agents have the advantage of a prompt response. Antihypertensive agents that were used before SAH are usually continued, and they should not be stopped abruptly. Short-acting antihypertensive agents are desirable because of the rapid resolution of the unwanted effects of an excessive decline in blood pressure. Because patients are often dehydrated or hyponatremic, diuretics are avoided. β-blockers, calcium channel blockers, and angiotensin-converting enzyme inhibitors are the oral agents most commonly prescribed. Nimodipine or nicardipine may be useful antihypertensive agents in the patient with SAH.

The patient with a markedly elevated or unstable arterial blood pressure reading may require a continuous intravenous infusion of labetalol, sodium nitroprusside, or fenoldopam. The rate of infusion is adjusted in response to blood pressure values. Intravenous infusions of antihypertensive agents should be given only if intra-arterial or frequent noninvasive blood pressure monitoring can be achieved. The dosage must be individualized, because a patient may be very sensitive to a medication, and the resulting drop in blood pressure may exceed expectations. Doses required in patients with SAH can be lower than those required for other hypertensive emergencies.

Drug-induced hypotension might help prevent early rebleeding in SAH. This regimen was compared with absolute bed rest in a randomized trial.[62] Mortality and rebleeding rates were similar in the two groups. Although the study was performed more than 25 years ago and older antihypertensive medications were prescribed, there is no evidence that induced hypotension should be part of the acute management of patients with SAH. The potential for low arterial blood pressure to aggravate the ischemic effects of vasospasm is another reason to avoid vigorous lowering of blood pressure. If a patient does experience ischemic symptoms secondary to vasospasm, antihypertensive agents are usually discontinued to help efforts to increase cerebral perfusion pressure.

MANAGEMENT OF ELECTROLYTE AND FLUID BALANCE

Disturbances in water and sodium balance occur in approximately one third of patients with SAH.[63] These complications are most likely to develop in critically ill patients with large hemorrhages. Hyponatremia and volume depletion correlate with a poor prognosis and the subsequent development of hydrocephalus, vasospasm, and ischemic stroke.[64] Severe hyponatremia can cause convulsions and is a potential cause of coma.

The primary indication for rapid correction of hyponatremia is the development of seizures in a patient without neurologic disease; however, this indication becomes blurred in patients with recent SAH. In the past, hyponatremia after SAH was attributed to the syndrome of inappropriate secretion of antidiuretic hormone (SIADH) and was treated with fluid restriction. It is now recognized, however, that a more common cause of hyponatremia in patients with SAH is cerebral salt wasting (CSW). The mechanism of water and sodium loss in CSW has been correlated with disturbances in levels of atrial natriuretic peptide, brain natriuretic peptide, and c-type natriuretic peptide as well as with direct neural effects on renal function.[65-67] The key to diagnosis of this syndrome is the urinary excretion of large amounts of sodium and chloride at a time when the extracellular fluid volume is contracted. Declines in plasma volume, red blood cell mass, and total blood volume occur;[63,68] these findings are unlike those in SIADH, in which the patient is euvolemic or hypervolemic. In contrast to therapy for SIADH, the appropriate therapy for CSW is replacement of salt and water rather than fluid restriction. Assessment of volume status by means of careful recording of inputs and outputs to calculate sodium and chloride balance, daily body weights, or laboratory test results suggesting dehydration, such as elevated hematocrit or blood urea nitrogen–creatinine ratio, can be useful in choosing therapy.[65,69]

Fluid restriction to control hyponatremia or to reduce the course of brain edema was tested in a randomized study, but no improvement in outcomes was noted.[70] Fluid restriction is dangerous in CSW because it leads to a contracted blood volume, increased blood viscosity, and hemoconcentration—effects that might increase the risk of ischemia among patients with vasospasm.[64] The best strategy is to give at least maintenance volumes of colloid and crystalloid solutions. The usually daily administration of liquids, including dietary and intravenous fluids, should be approximately 2.5 to 3.5 L.[31,71] Adjustments may be required, depending on urinary or insensible water losses. Central venous pressure or pulmonary artery wedge pressure monitoring might be needed to monitor the cardiac status of patients given large volumes of fluids. Increased volumes of sodium-containing fluids will overcome the volume contraction but may not reverse the hyponatremia.[72]

If the serum sodium concentration does not normalize despite a euvolemic status, modest fluid restriction or an infusion of a hyperosmolar solution containing sodium can be started. The serum sodium concentration should be corrected no more rapidly than 0.7 mEq/hour to avoid central pontine myelinolysis.[65] In 39 patients with recent SAH, Wijdicks and associates[73] administered 0.2 mg of fludrocortisone twice a day, combined with daily fluid intake of at least 3 L, and noted improvements in plasma volume and sodium balance. As a result, these investigators recommend that fludrocortisone be added to the fluid management regimen if the serum concentration of sodium is less than 125 mmol/L. Hypokalemia after SAH probably results from vomiting but can be secondary to elevated

Clinical Manifestations

levels of corticosteroids, renin, or catecholamines. Because cardiac arrhythmias can be associated with hypokalemia, this imbalance should be corrected promptly.

TREATMENT OF OTHER MEDICAL COMPLICATIONS

Gastrointestinal bleeding can result from hemorrhagic gastritis, stress gastric ulcers, or an esophageal tear secondary to vomiting. Because of the risk of bleeding, patients are often given intravenous histamine$_2$-receptor antagonists or proton pump inhibitors via nasogastric tube.[30] Sucralfate does not have central nervous system side effects, so it has potential advantages in preventing gastrointestinal side effects among critically ill patients prone to depression in consciousness.[73]

Obtunded patients are at high risk for adult respiratory distress syndrome, atelectasis, pulmonary hypoventilation, and aspiration pneumonia. Gruber and colleagues,[20] evaluating pulmonary function among 207 patients with SAH, noted that severe lung dysfunction was uncommon but that its presence was correlated with a greater likelihood of poor outcome. Securing of the airway, careful bronchopulmonary management, and ventilatory assistance may be required. Events such as renal failure, hepatic dysfunction, and urinary tract infections as well as other illnesses should be treated. Measures to avoid pressure sores or orthopedic complications also are important.

Using data from a large multicenter randomized trial, Solenski and associates[7] found a frequency of 40% for life-threatening medical complications in patients with SAH. Careful monitoring to avoid systemic complications is important in these critically ill patients. Patients with SAH who have evidence of an acute systemic inflammatory response with elevations in temperature, heart rate, respiratory rate, and white cell count have worse outcomes.[20,21] The central nervous system injury may predispose such patients to systemic inflammation, so therapies to modulate cytokine-induced inflammation may have potential to reduce these systemic complications.

TREATMENT OF INCREASED INTRACRANIAL PRESSURE

A decline in consciousness is the hallmark of increased intracranial pressure, which, in turn, can result from a large intracerebral or intraventricular hematoma, the mass effect of a secondary ischemic lesion, cerebral edema, or hydrocephalus. SAH also causes vasoparalysis and loss of autoregulation; secondary dilation of intracranial vessels might aggravate intracranial pressure by expanding the vascular compartment. Intracranial pressure is markedly elevated within a few minutes of aneurysmal rupture; the sudden increase in pressure may help halt the bleeding. In addition, the elevated intracranial pressure may transiently equal mean arterial blood pressure. A massive rise in intracranial pressure is probably one of the causes of sudden death after SAH. High intracranial pressure may also lead to hypoperfusion, which induces brain ischemia. Prompt aggressive treatment of increased intracranial pressure is one of the keys to successful management of SAH.[31]

Several medical and surgical measures are available to treat brain edema or increased intracranial pressure. Continuous monitoring of intracranial pressure is indicated for many patients; the results might guide the timing of surgical or medical interventions. Continuous intraventricular drainage combined with monitoring is an option if the patient has intraventricular hemorrhage or acute hydrocephalus. Treatment of increased intracranial pressure consists of (1) elevation of the head of the bed to promote venous drainage, (2) fluid restriction, (3) correction of hyponatremia, (4) treatment of fever or agitation, and (5) prevention of hypoventilation and secondary hypercarbia.

Intubation and hyperventilation are indicated if a patient's condition is deteriorating. There is no evidence that dexamethasone is useful in managing brain edema after intracranial hemorrhage. Furosemide, which can reduce intracranial pressure by limiting the production of CSF, can be given in an emergency. However, the diuretic effects of furosemide can lead to electrolyte disturbances and hypovolemia. Mannitol is an osmotic agent that can be given to control increased intracranial pressure. A response is noted within minutes, and the duration of effect is approximately 4 to 6 hours. The dosage can be repeated as needed. Secondary dehydration, hyperosmolarity, and a rebound increase in brain edema are possible complications. Measurements of serum osmolality and serum electrolytes should be performed often, especially if repeated doses of mannitol are prescribed. Measurement of central venous or pulmonary artery wedge pressure might be needed. Hypertonic saline has also been used in refractory cases to lower intracranial pressure and has the advantage of expanding intravascular volume.[74] In a small retrospective study, hypertonic saline did not produce adverse effects in patients with SAH and vasospasm.[75]

Increased intracranial pressure may be caused by large intracerebral hematomas, which are usually located in the basal ganglia and adjacent white matter and are most commonly seen with ruptured aneurysms of the internal carotid or middle cerebral arteries. Surgical evacuation of the hematoma can be lifesaving in a rapidly deteriorating patient. Some patients can recover and return to independent activity.[31,76,77] Stereotactic aspiration combined with the thrombolysis has also been performed successfully.[78] This approach might be better than direct surgical exploration if the hematoma is located deep within the hemisphere. Patients with CT evidence of very large hematomas, extensive intraventricular bleeding, or shifts of midline structures have the poorest postoperative outcomes. In general, patients who are in better clinical condition and those who have a ruptured aneurysm of the middle cerebral artery are most likely to benefit.

Patients with intraventricular extension of bleeding might benefit from the combination of ventricular drainage and instillation of fibrinolytic agents.[79] However, no randomized trials have tested this approach. Shimoda and coworkers[80] reported that direct surgical evacuation of major intraventricular hemorrhages is not successful. Unfortunately, patients who are in poor condition are the ones most commonly referred for operation. Although data are lacking to support a recommendation for surgical removal of a large hematoma associated with a ruptured aneurysm, operation is an option for a patient showing no response to medical measures. Still, both the physician and the family must be aware that the patient's life might be saved but the neurologic sequelae might be considerable.

MANAGEMENT OF HYDROCEPHALUS

Hydrocephalus is a common complication of SAH, resulting from the massive collections of blood that fill the ventricles, block the aqueduct of Sylvius, or obstruct the fourth ventricle. Blood can fill the subarachnoid cisterns or coat the arachnoid villi. The prolonged presence of extensive subarachnoid clots is strongly associated with the appearance of hydrocephalus; thus, an intervention that extends the presence of these clots might promote development of hydrocephalus. Conversely, therapies that stimulate clot lysis might lessen the risk of hydrocephalus.

Sheehan and associates[81] reported that hydrocephalus developed in approximately one fourth of their patients during the acute treatment period. Hydrocephalus is more common among patients who, upon admission, have severe neurologic impairments or CT evidence of ventricular dilation or intraventricular hemorrhage. In addition, women, patients with preexisting hypertension, and patients with a history of alcohol abuse have higher rates of hydrocephalus.[81]

The hydrocephalus after SAH may be classified according to its time of appearance as (1) acute—appearing within 12 hours after aneurysmal rupture, (2) subacute—developing a few days after the ictus, or (3) delayed—noted as ventricular dilation weeks to years later.[82,83] Acute hydrocephalus is an important cause of increased intracranial pressure and coma. Subacute hydrocephalus is a cause of a gradual decline in consciousness that can occur approximately 7 to 10 days after SAH. In this situation, intracranial pressure may be modestly elevated. Delayed hydrocephalus often manifests as a subacute dementia, gait apraxia, and bladder incontinence. In this setting, intracranial pressure often fluctuates and may not be consistently elevated.

Approximately 16% to 34% of patients have CT findings consistent with acute hydrocephalus. Some patients with ventricular enlargement may be asymptomatic, but most have decreased consciousness. Symptoms of acute hydrocephalus in addition to decline in alertness are bilateral motor signs, miosis, and downward deviation of the eyes. Acute hydrocephalus predicts increased mortality and morbidity and is correlated with subsequent development of vasospasm and ischemic stroke. A patient with acute hydrocephalus can be observed, medically managed, monitored with sequential CT studies, and treated with serial lumbar punctures. Although acute hydrocephalus may resolve spontaneously, most cases require placement of a temporary ventriculocaval or ventriculoperitoneal catheter.[82,83] Insertion of a ventricular catheter may be difficult in a patient with an intraventricular clot, because blood can occlude the catheter. Continuous cisternal drainage might relieve intracranial pressure and expedite lavage of blood from the subarachnoid space.

Placement of a shunt is recommended for any patient with depressed consciousness and enlarging ventricles.

Some patients require only temporary shunting. If necessary, the shunt can be made permanent later. Shunting is not always effective, however. Hasen and colleagues[84] reported a high rate of shunt-related complications, including intracranial infections, among their patients with SAH and acute hydrocephalus.

PREVENTION OF RECURRENT HEMORRHAGE

Recurrent hemorrhage is a feared complication of SAH because it is a leading cause of death or neurologic morbidity during the first 2 weeks after SAH.[12,85] In the series reported by Broderick and associates,[4] rebleeding accounted for half of the deaths that occurred more than 2 days after SAH. Mortality rates among patients who have rebleeding are approximately twice those of patients who have a single hemorrhage. Even in centers performing early surgery, rebleeding remains a major cause of poor outcome after SAH.[86]

Preventing recurrent hemorrhage is a major goal of the medical management of SAH. Torner and colleagues[87] found that the period of greatest risk for rebleeding is the first 24 hours after the ictus; the risk peaked at approximately 4% during that time. These results are supported by other studies. In a Swedish series, 9.6% of all patients admitted within 24 hours of SAH had very early rebleeding; most of these patients died.[85] Fujii and coworkers[88] found that rebleeding occurred within 24 hours of admission in 31 of 174 patients (17.3%)—most of whom were waiting for surgery. Steiger and associates[89] found a low rate of recurrent hemorrhage between 5 and 13 days after SAH. The cumulative rate of rebleeding during the first 2 weeks after SAH is approximately 15% to 20%.[87] The high rate of early recurrent hemorrhage has implications for the choice of treatment. Bleeding might recur even before a surgical team can be mobilized or before a medication can reach "therapeutic" levels in the blood and CSF.

Several clinical features identify those patients at the highest risk for early rebleeding. The most important is the level of consciousness at admission; patients admitted in coma are at the greatest risk. Rebleeding is also more common among older people, women, and people whose systolic blood pressure exceeds 170 mm Hg. The results of the baseline CT do not predict recurrent hemorrhage.

Recurrent hemorrhage usually causes a sudden headache and a rapid change in neurologic condition, including a drop in consciousness. Extensor spasms and posturing are important early signs. A "convulsion" that occurs immediately after SAH also can mark a recurrent hemorrhage.[40] However, rebleeding in a comatose patient may be overlooked. It may be manifested only by a sudden change in respiratory pattern or vital signs. Recurrent hemorrhage should be sought whenever a patient experiences a new headache or worsens neurologically.

The differential diagnosis of rebleeding is listed in Table 14.7. The clinical diagnosis of rebleeding can be incorrect in as many as a third of cases. Other causes of the worsening are seizures, ischemia, and medical complications. The diagnosis of rebleeding should not be made solely on clinical features, because this approach leads to

catheterization in small- to medium-sized arteries at the base of the brain. Angioplasty does stretch and disrupt the arterial wall.[182] Bejjani and associates[183] performed angioplasty at approximately 7 days after SAH in 31 patients, treating a total of 81 vessels. These investigators noted major clinical improvements in 12 cases and moderate improvements in another 11. They encountered no major neurologic complications and concluded that angioplasty is a potentially useful treatment for patients who show no response to other therapies. Polin and coworkers[184] found that angioplasty is effective in reversing angiographically confirmed vasospasm, but they did not observe clinical improvements with treatment. At present, angioplasty is usually reserved for treatment of SAH that does not respond to medical measures.

CONCLUSION

Considerable progress is being made in the management of SAH. Medical and surgical therapies that effectively prevent rebleeding and vasospasm are reflected by declines in mortality and morbidity. Still, there is considerable room for improvement. Several promising therapies are being tested; one or more of these interventions likely will be shown to further improve outcomes after SAH. However, most successful therapies are based on early treatment. Thus, the medical community must give greater attention to the early diagnosis of SAH and the acute care of patients with SAH who are critically ill.

References

1. Rinkel GJE, Wijdicks EF, Vermeulen M: The clinical course of perimesencephalic non-aneurysmal subarachnoid haemorrhage. Ann Neurol 29:463, 1991.
2. Velthuis BK, Rinkel GJ, Ramos LM, et al: Perimesencephalic hemorrhage: Exclusion of vertebrobasilar aneurysms with CT angiography. Stroke 30:1103–1109, 1999.
3. Arboix A, Marti-Vilalta JL: Predictive clinical factors of very early in-hospital mortality in subarachnoid hemorrhage. Clin Neurol Neurosurg 101:100–105, 1999.
4. Broderick JP, Adam SA, Mann JI: Initial and recurrent bleeding are the major causes of death following subarachnoid hemorrhage. Stroke 25:1342–1347, 1994.
5. Schievink WI, Wijdicks EFM, Parisi JE: Sudden death from aneurysmal subarachnoid hemorrhage. Neurology 45:871–874, 1995.
6. Edner G, Ronne-Engstrom E: Can early admission reduce aneurysmal rebleeds? A prospective study on the aneurysmal incidence, aneurysmal rebleeds, admission and treatment delays in a defined region. Br J Neurosurg 5:601, 1991.
7. Solenski NJ, Haley EC Jr, Kassell NF: Medical complication of aneurysmal subarachnoid hemorrhage: A report of the multicenter, cooperative aneurysm study. Participants of the Multicenter Cooperative Aneurysm Study. Crit Care Med 23:1007–1017, 1995.
8. Proust F, Hannequin D, Langlois O: Causes of morbidity and mortality after ruptured aneurysm surgery in a series of 230 patients: The importance of control angiography. Stroke 26:1553, 1995.
9. Rosenorn J, Eskesen V, Schmidt K: Clinical features and outcome in females and males with ruptured intracranial saccular aneurysms. Br J Neurosurg 7:287, 1993.
10. Saveland H, Brandt L: Which are the major determinants for outcome in aneurysmal subarachnoid hemorrhage? Acta Neurol Scand 90:245, 1994.
11. Johnston SC, Selvin S, Gress DR: The burden, trends, and demographics of mortality from subarachnoid hemorrhage. Neurology 50:1413–1418, 1998.
12. Roos YB, de Haan RJ, Beenen LF, et al: Complications and outcome in patients with aneurysmal subarachnoid haemorrhage: A prospective hospital based cohort study in the Netherlands. J Neurol Neurosurg Psychiatry 68:337–341, 2000.
13. Cesarini KG, Hardemark H-G, Persson L: Improved survival after aneurysmal subarachnoid hemorrhage: Review of case management during a 12-year period. J Neurosurg 90:664–672, 1999.
14. Johansson M, Giuliana K, Contant CF, et al: Changes in intervention and outcome in elderly patients with subarachnoid hemorrhage. Stroke 32:2845–2849, 2001.
15. Adams HP Jr, Kassell NF, Torner JC: Usefulness of computed tomography in predicting outcome after aneurysmal subarachnoid hemorrhage. Neurology 35:1263–1267, 1985.
16. Roos EJ, Rinkel GJ, Velthuis BK, Algra A: The relation between aneurysm size and outcome in patients with subarachnoid hemorrhage. Neurology 54:2334–2336, 2000.
17. Pobereskin LH: Influence of premorbid factors on survival following subarachnoid hemorrhage. J Neurosurg 95:555–559, 2001.
18. Kongable GL, Lazino G, Germanson TP: Gender-related differences in aneurysmal subarachnoid hemorrhage. J Neurosurg 84:43–48, 1996.
19. Oliveira-Filho J, Ezzeddine MA, Segal AZ, et al: Fever in subarachnoid hemorrhage: Relationship to vasospasm and outcome. Neurology 56:1299–1304, 2001.
20. Gruber A, Reinprecht A, Gorzer H, et al: Pulmonary function and radiographic abnormalities related to neurological outcome after aneurysmal subarachnoid hemorrhage. J Neurosurg 88:28–37, 1998.
21. Yoshimoto Y, Tanaka Y, Hoya K: Acute systemic inflammatory response syndrome in subarachnoid hemorrhage. Stroke 32:1989–1993, 2001.
22. Fujii Y, Takeuchi S, Sasaki O, et al: Serial changes of hemostasis in aneurysmal subarachnoid hemorrhage with special reference to delayed ischemic neurological deficits. J Neurosurg 86:594–602, 1997.
23. Mack WJ, Mocco J, Hoh DJ, et al: Outcome prediction with serum intercellular adhesion molecule-1 levels after aneurysmal subarachnoid hemorrhage. J Neurosurg 96:71–75, 2002.
24. Enblad P, Persson L: Impact on clinical outcome of secondary brain insults during the neurointensive care of patients with subarachnoid haemorrhage: A pilot study. J Neurol Neurosurg Psychiatry 62:512–516, 1997.
25. Camarata PJ, Heros PC, Latchaw RE: "Brain attack": The rationale for treating stroke as a medical emergency. Neurosurgery 34:144–158, 1994.
26. Adams HP Jr, Jergenson DD, Kassell NF: Pitfalls in the recognition of subarachnoid hemorrhage. JAMA 244:794–796, 1980.
27. Edlow JA, Caplan LR: Avoiding pitfalls in the diagnosis of subarachnoid hemorrhage. N Engl J Med 342:29–36, 2000.
28. Neil-Dwyer G, Lang D: 'Brain attack'—aneurysmal subarachnoid haemorrhage: Death due to delayed diagnosis. J R Coll Physicians Lond 31:49–52, 1997.
29. Findlay JM: Current management of aneurysmal subarachnoid hemorrhage: Guidelines from the Canadian Neurosurgical Society. Can J Neurol Sci 24:161–170, 1997.
30. Mayberg MR, Batjer HH, Dacey R: Guidelines for the management of aneurysmal subarachnoid hemorrhage. Circulation 90:2592–2605, 1994.
31. Wijdicks EFM: Worst case scenario: Management in poor-grade aneurysmal subarachnoid hemorrhage. Cerebrovasc Dis 5:163–169, 1995.
32. Thomson S, Ryan JM, Lyndon J: Brain attack:—how good is the early management of subarachnoid haemorrhage in accident and emergency departments? South Thames A&E Specialty Sub Committee Audit Group. Emerg Med J 17:176–179, 2000.
33. Mitchell P, Wilkinson ID, Hoggard N, et al: Detection of subarachnoid haemorrhage with magnetic resonance imaging. J Neurol Neurosurg Psychiatry 70:205–211, 2001.
34. Velthuis BK, Rinkel GJ, Ramos LM, et al: Subarachnoid hemorrhage: Aneurysm detection and preoperative evaluation with CT angiography. Radiology 208:423–430, 1998.
35. Zouaoui A, Sahel M, Marro B, et al: Three-dimensional computed tomographic angiography in detection of cerebral aneurysms in acute subarachnoid hemorrhage. Neurosurgery 41:125–130, 1997.
36. Hashimoto H, Jun-Ichi I, Hironaka Y, et al: Use of spiral computerized tomography angiography in patients with subarachnoid

hemorrhage in whom subtraction angiography did not reveal cerebral aneurysms. J Neurosurg 92:278–283, 2000.

37. Lenhart M, Bretschneider T, Gmeinwieser J, et al: Cerebral CT angiography in the diagnosis of acute subarachnoid hemorrhage. Acta Radiol 38:791–796, 1997.

38. Black PM, Crowell RM, Abbott WM: External pneumatic calf compression reduces deep vein thrombosis in patients with ruptured intracranial aneurysms. Neurosurgery 18:25–28, 1986.

39. Nishioka H: Report of the Cooperative Study of Intracranial Aneurysms and Subarachnoid Hemorrhage. Section VII, Part I: Evaluation of conservative measurement of ruptured aneurysms. J Neurosurg 25:574, 1966.

40. Hart RG, Byer JA, Slaughter JR: Occurrence and implications of seizures in subarachnoid hemorrhage due to ruptured intracranial aneurysms. Neurosurgery 8:417, 1981.

41. Rhoney DH, Tipps LB, Murry KR, et al: Anticonvulsant prophylaxis and timing of seizures after aneurysmal subarachnoid hemorrhage. Neurology 55:258–265, 2000.

42. Sundaram MBM, Chow F: Seizures associated with spontaneous subarachnoid hemorrhage. Can J Neurol Sci 13:229–231, 1986.

43. Fisher CM: Clinical syndromes in cerebral thrombosis, hypertensive hemorrhage and ruptured saccular aneurysm. Clin Neurosurg 22:117, 1975.

44. Di Pasquale G, Andreoli A, Lusa AM, et al: Cardiologic complications of subarachnoid hemorrhage. J Neurosurg Sci 42:33–36, 1998.

45. Di Pasquale G, Pinelli G, Andreoli A: Torsades de pointes and ventricular flutter-fibrillation following spontaneous cerebral subarachnoid hemorrhage. Int J Cardiol 18:163, 1988.

46. Manninen PH, Ayra B, Gelb AW: Association between electrocardiographic abnormalities and intracranial blood in patient with acute subarachnoid hemorrhage. J Neurosurg Anesthesiol 7:12–16, 1995.

47. Oppenheimer SM, Hachinski V: Neurogenic cardiac effects of cerebrovascular disease. Curr Opin Neurol 7:20–24, 1994.

48. Randell T, Tanskanen P, Scheinin M, et al: QT dispersion after subarachnoid hemorrhage. J Neurosurg Anesthesiol 11:163–166, 1999.

49. Machado C, Baga JJ, Kawasaki R, et al: Torsades de pointes as a complication of subarachnoid hemorrhage: A critical reappraisal. J Electrocardiol 30:31–37, 1997.

50. Gascon P, Ley TJ, Toltzis RJ, Bonow RO: Spontaneous subarachnoid hemorrhage simulating acute transmural myocardial infarction. Am Heart J 105:511, 1983.

51. Sakka SG, Huettemann E, Reinhart K: Acute left ventricular dysfunction and subarachnoid hemorrhage. J Neurosurg Anesthesiol 11:209–213, 1999.

52. Yuki K, Kodama Y, Onda J: Coronary vasospasm following subarachnoid hemorrhage as a cause of stunned myocardium. J Neurosurg 75:308–311, 1991.

53. Mayer SA, Lin J, Homma S, et al: Myocardial injury and left ventricular performance after subarachnoid hemorrhage. Stroke 30:780–786, 1999.

54. Zaroff JG, Rordorf GA, Newell JB, et al: Cardiac outcome in patients with subarachnoid hemorrhage and electrocardiographic abnormalities. Neurosurgery 44:34–39, 1999.

55. Brouwers PJAM, Westenberg HGM, van Gijn J: Noradrenaline concentration and electrocardiographic abnormalities after aneurysmal subarachnoid hemorrhage. J Neurol Neurosurg Psychiatry 58:614, 1995.

56. Donaldson JW, Pritz MB: Myocardial stunning secondary to aneurysmal subarachnoid hemorrhage. Surg Neurol 55:12–16, 2001.

57. Hamann G, Haass A, Schimrigk K: Beta blockade in acute aneurysmal subarachnoid hemorrhage. Acta Neurochir (Wien) 121:119, 1993.

58. Neil-Dwyer G, Walter P, Cruikshank JM: Effect of propranolol and phentolamine on myocardial necrosis after subarachnoid hemorrhage. Br Med J 2:990, 1978.

59. Levy ML, Rabb CH, Zelman V, Giannotta SL: Cardiac performance enhancement from dobutamine in patients refractory to hypervolemic therapy for cerebral vasospasm. J Neurosurg 79:494, 1993.

60. Neil-Dwyer G, Walter P, Shaw HJH: Plasma renin activity in patients after a subarachnoid hemorrhage: A possible predictor of outcome. Neurosurgery 7:578, 1980.

61. Toftdahl DB, Torp-Pedersen C, Engel UH: Hypertension and left ventricular hypertrophy in patients with spontaneous subarachnoid hemorrhage. Neurosurgery 37:235, 1995.

62. Nibbelink DW: Considerations in the treatment of stroke: Cooperative Aneurysm Study: Antihypertensive and antifibrinolytic therapy following subarachnoid hemorrhage from ruptured intracranial aneurysm. In Whisnant JP, Sandok BA (eds): Cerebral Vascular Diseases. Orlando, Grune & Stratton, 1975, p 155.

63. Wijdicks EFM, Vermeulen M, Ten Haaf JA: Volume depletion and natriuresis in patients with ruptured intracranial aneurysm. Ann Neurol 18:211–216, 1985.

64. Wijdicks EFM, Vermeulen M, Hijdra A: Hyponatremia and cerebral infarction in patients with ruptured intracranial aneurysms: Is fluid restriction harmful? Ann Neurol 17:137–140, 1985.

65. Harrigan MR: Cerebral salt wasting syndrome. Crit Care Clin 17:125–138, 2001.

66. Sviri GE, Feinsod M, Soustiel JF: Brain natriuretic peptide and cerebral vasospasm in subarachnoid hemorrhage: Clinical and TCD correlations. Stroke 31:118–122, 2000.

67. Wijdicks EF, Schievink WI, Burnett JC Jr: Natriuretic peptide system and endothelin in aneurysmal subarachnoid hemorrhage. J Neurosurg 87:275–280, 1997.

68. Sato K, Karibe H, Yoshimoto T: Circulating blood volume in patients with subarachnoid haemorrhage. Acta Neurochir 141:1069–1073, 1999.

69. Carlotti APCP, Bohn D, Rutka JT, et al: A method to estimate urinary electrolyte excretion in patients at risk for developing cerebral salt wasting. J Neurosurg 95:420–424, 2001.

70. Nibbelink DW, Torner JC, Burmeister LF: Fluid restriction in combination with antifibrinolytic therapy. In Sahs AL, Nibbelink DW, Torner JC (eds): Aneurysmal Subarachnoid Hemorrhage. Baltimore, Urban & Schwarzenberg, 1981, p 307.

71. van Gijn J, Rinkel GJE: Subarachnoid haemorrhage: Diagnosis, causes and management. Brain 124:249–278, 2001.

72. Diringer MN, Wu KC, Verbalis VG: Hypervolemic therapy prevents volume contraction but not hyponatremia following subarachnoid hemorrhage. Ann Neurol 31:543–550, 1992.

73. Wijdicks EFM, Vermeulen M, Van Brummelen P: The effect of fludrocortisone acetate on plasma volume and natriuresis in patients with aneurysmal subarachnoid hemorrhage. Clin Neurol Neurosurg 90:209–214, 1988.

74. Qureshi AI, Suarez JI: Use of hypertonic saline solutions in treatment of cerebral edema and intracranial hypertension. Crit Care Med 28:3301–3313, 2000.

75. Suarez JI, Qureshi AI, Parekh PD, et al: Administration of hypertonic (3%) sodium chloride/acetate in hyponatremic patients with symptomatic vasospasm following subarachnoid hemorrhage. J Neurosurg Anesthesiol 11:178–184, 1999.

76. Nowak G, Schwachenwald R, Arnold H: Early management in poor grade aneurysm patients. Acta Neurochir (Wien) 126:33, 1994.

77. Stachnick JB, Layon AJ, Day AL, Gallagher J: Craniotomy for intracranial aneurysm and subarachnoid hemorrhage: Is course, cost or outcome affected by age? Stroke 27:276, 1996.

78. Montes J, Wong J, Fayad P, Awad IA: Stereotactic computed tomographic-guided aspiration and thrombolysis of intracerebral hematoma: Protocol and preliminary experience. Stroke 31:834–840, 2000.

79. Nieuwkamp DJ, de Gans K, Rinkel GJ, Algra A: Treatment and outcome of severe intraventricular extension in patients with subarachnoid or intracerebral hemorrhage: A systematic review of the literature. J Neurol 247:117–121, 2000.

80. Shimoda M, Oda S, Shibata M, et al: Results of early surgical evacuation of packed intraventricular hemorrhage from aneurysm rupture in patients with poor-grade subarachnoid hemorrhage. J Neurosurg 91:408–414, 1999.

81. Sheehan JP, Polin RS, Sheehan JM, et al: Factors associated with hydrocephalus after aneurysmal subarachnoid hemorrhage. Neurosurgery 45:1120–1127, 1999.

82. Graff-Radford NR, Torner J, Adams HP Jr: Factors associated with hydrocephalus after subarachnoid hemorrhage: A report of the Cooperative Aneurysm Study. Arch Neurol 46:744–752, 1989.

83. Heros RC: Acute hydrocephalus after subarachnoid hemorrhage. Stroke 20:715, 1989.

84. Hasen D, Vermeulen M, Wijdicks EFM: Management problems in acute hydrocephalus after subarachnoid hemorrhage. Stroke 20:747, 1989.

85. Hillman J, von Essen C, Leszniewski W, Johansson I: Significance of "ultra-early" rebleeding in subarachnoid hemorrhage. J Neurosurg 68:901, 1988.

Clinical Manifestations

86. Roos YB, Beenen LF, Groen RJ, et al: Timing of surgery in patients with aneurysmal subarachnoid haemorrhage: Rebleeding is still the major cause of poor outcome in neurosurgical units that aim at early surgery. J Neurol Neurosurg Psychiatry 63:490–493, 1997.
87. Torner JC, Kassell NF, Wallace RB: Preoperative prognostic factors for rebleeding and survival in aneurysm patients receiving fibrinolytic therapy: Report of the Cooperative Aneurysm Study. Neurosurgery 9:506–513, 1981.
88. Fujii Y, Takeuchi S, Sasaki O: Ultra-early rebleeding in spontaneous subarachnoid hemorrhage. Neurosurgery 84:35–42, 1996.
89. Steiger HJ, Fritschi J, Seiler RW: Current pattern of in-hospital aneurysmal rebleeds. Acta Neurochir (Wien) 127:21, 1994.
90. Perret GE, Nibbelink DW: Randomized treatment study: Carotid ligation. In Sahs AL, Nibbelink DW, Torner JC (eds): Aneurysmal Subarachnoid Hemorrhage. Baltimore, Urban & Schwarzenberg, 1981, p 121.
91. Brown JA, Wollmann RL, Mullan S: Myopathy induced by epsilon-aminocaproic acid. J Neurosurg 57:130, 1983.
92. Kassell NF, Torner JC, Adams HP Jr: Antifibrinolytic therapy in the acute period following aneurysmal subarachnoid hemorrhage: Preliminary observations from the Cooperative Aneurysm Study. J Neurosurg 61:225–230, 1984.
93. Vermuelen M, Lindsay KW, Murray GD: Antifibrinolytic treatment in subarachnoid hemorrhage. N Engl J Med 311:432–437, 1984.
94. Stroobandt G, Lambert O, Menard E: The association of tranexamic acid and nimodipine in the pre-operative treatment of ruptured intracranial aneurysms. Acta Neurochir 140:148–160, 1998.
95. Roos Y: Antifibrinolytic treatment in subarachnoid hemorrhage: A randomized placebo-controlled trial. STAR Study Group. Neurology 54:77–82, 2000.
96. Roos YB, Rinkel GJ, Vermeulen M, et al. Antifibrinolytic therapy for aneurysmal subarachnoid haemorrhage. Cochrane Database Syst Rev CD00124, 2000.
97. Roos YB, Vermeulen M, Rinkel GJ, et al: Systematic review of antifibrinolytic treatment in aneurysmal subarachnoid haemorrhage. J Neurol Neurosurg Psychiatry 65:942–943, 1998.
98. Maurice-Williams RS, Wadley JP: Delayed surgery for ruptured intracranial aneurysms: A reappraisal. Br J Neurosurg 11:104–109, 1997.
99. Juvela S, Kaste M, Hillbom M: The effects of earlier surgery and shorter bedrest on the outcome in patients with subarachnoid haemorrhage. J Neurol Neurosurg Psychiatry 52:776, 1989.
100. LeRoux PD, Elliott JP, Downey L: Improved outcomes after rupture of anterior circulation aneurysms: A retrospective 10-year review of 224 good-grade patients. J Neurosurg 83:394, 1995.
101. Nishimoto A, Veta K, Onbe H: Nationwide cooperative study of intracranial aneurysm surgery in Japan. Stroke 16:48, 1985.
102. Ohman J, Heiskanen O: Timing of operation for ruptured supratentorial aneurysms: A prospective randomized study. J Neurosurg 70:55, 1989.
103. Miyaoka M, Sato K, Ishii S: A clinical study of the relationship of timing to outcome of surgery for ruptured cerebral aneurysms: A retrospective analysis of 1,622 cases. J Neurosurg 79:373–378, 1993.
104. Kassell NF, Torner JC, Haley EC: The International Cooperative Study on the Timing of Aneurysm Surgery. II: Surgical results. J Neurosurg 73:34–36, 1990.
105. Kassell NF, Torner JC, Haley EC: The International Cooperative Study on the Timing of Aneurysm Surgery. I: Overall management results. J Neurosurg 73:18–33, 1990.
106. Deruty R, Mottolese C, Pecisson-Guyotat I, Soustiec JF: Management of the ruptured intracranial aneurysm: Early surgery, late surgery, or modulated surgery. Acta Neurochir (Wien) 113:1, 1991.
107. Larson JJ, Tew JM Jr, Tomsick T: Treatment of aneurysms of the internal carotid artery by intravascular balloon occlusion: Long-term follow-up of 58 patients. Neurosurgery 36:23–30, 1995.
108. Kinugasa K, Mandai S, Kamata I: Prophylactic thrombosis to prevent new bleeding and to delay aneurysm surgery. Neurosurgery 36:661, 1995.
109. McDougall CG, Halbach VV, Dowd CF: Endovascular treatment of basilar tip aneurysms using electrolytically detachable coils. J Neurosurg 84:393, 1996.
110. Casasco AE, Aymard A, Gobin P: Selective endovascular treatment of 71 intracranial aneurysms with platinum coils. J Neurosurg 79:3, 1993.
111. Sinson G, Philips MF, Flamm ES: Intraoperative endovascular surgery for cerebral aneurysm. J Neurosurg 84:63, 1996.
112. Birchall D, Khangure M, McAuliffe W, et al: Endovascular treatment of posterior circulation aneurysms. Br J Neurosurg 15:39–43, 2001.
113. Eskridge J, Song J: Endovascular embolization of 150 basilar tip aneurysms with Guglielmi detachable coils: Results of the Food and Drug Administration multicenter clinical trial. J Neurosurg 89:81–86, 1998.
114. Cognard C, Weill A, Castaings L, et al: Intracranial berry aneurysms: Angiographic and clinical results after endovascular treatment. Radiology 206:499–510, 1998.
115. Raymond J, Roy D: Safety and efficacy of endovascular treatment of acutely ruptured aneurysms. Neurosurgery 41:1235–1245, 1997.
116. Lefkowitz MA, Gobin YP, Akiba Y, et al: Balloon-assisted Guglielmi detachable coiling of wide-necked aneurysms: Part II—clinical results. Neurosurgery 45:531–537, 1999.
117. Treggiari-Venzi MM, Suter PM, Romand JA: Review of medical prevention of vasospasm after aneurysmal subarachnoid hemorrhage: A problem of neurointensive care. Neurosurgery 48:249–261, 2001.
118. Smith RR, Clower BR, Grotendorst GM: Arterial wall changes in early human vasospasm. Neurosurgery 16:171, 1985.
119. Dietrich HH, Dacey RG Jr: Molecular keys to the problems of cerebral vasospasm. Neurosurgery 46:517–530, 2000.
120. Nagatani K, Masciopinto J, Letarte PB: The effect of hemoglobin and its metabolites on energy metabolism in cultured cerebrovascular smooth-muscle cells. J Neurosurg 82:244, 1995.
121. Pasqualin A: Epidemiology and pathophysiology of cerebral vasospasm following subarachnoid hemorrhage. J Neurosurg Sci 42:15–21, 1998.
122. Hirashima Y, Endo S, Ohmori T: Platelet-activating factor (PAF) concentration and PAF acetylhydrolase activity on cerebrospinal fluid of patients with subarachnoid hemorrhage. J Neurosurg 80:31, 1994.
123. Gaetani P, Rodriguez Y, Baena R: Endothelin and aneurysmal subarachnoid hemorrhage: A study of subarachnoid cisternal cerebrospinal fluid. J Neurol Neurosurg Psychiatry 66:57, 1994.
124. Pickard JD, Walker V, Brandt L: Effect of intraventricular haemorrhage and rebleeding following subarachnoid haemorrhage on CSF eicosanoids. Acta Neurochir (Wien) 129:152, 1994.
125. Seifert V, Loffler BM, Zimmerman M, et al: Endothelin concentrations in patients with aneurysmal subarachnoid hemorrhage: Correlation with cerebral vasospasm, delayed ischemic neurologic defects and volume of hematoma. J Neurosurg 82:55, 1995.
126. Yundt KD, Grubb RL Jr, Diringer MN, Powers WJ: Autoregulatory vasodilation of parenchymal vessels is impaired during cerebral vasospasm. J Cereb Blood Flow Metab 18:419–424, 1998.
127. Shimoda M, Oda S, Tsugane R, Sato O: Prognostic factors in delayed ischaemic deficit with vasospasm in patients undergoing early aneurysm surgery. Br J Neurosurg 11:210–215, 1997.
128. Charpentier C, Audibert G, Guillemin F, et al: Multivariate analysis of predictors of cerebral vasospasm occurrence after aneurysmal subarachnoid hemorrhage. Stroke 30:1402–1408, 1999.
129. Hop JW, Rinkel GJ, Algra A, van Gijn J: Initial loss of consciousness and risk of delayed cerebral ischemia after aneurysmal subarachnoid hemorrhage. Stroke 30:2268–2271, 1999.
130. Qureshi AI, Sung GY, Razumovsky AY, et al: Early identification of patients at risk for symptomatic vasospasm after aneurysmal subarachnoid hemorrhage. Crit Care Med 28:984–990, 2000.
131. Juvela S: Aspirin and delayed cerebral ischemia after aneurysmal subarachnoid hemorrhage. J Neurosurg 82:945, 1995.
132. Hop JW, Rinkel GJ, Algra A, et al: Randomized pilot trial of postoperative aspirin in subarachnoid hemorrhage. Neurology 54:872–878, 2000.
133. Claassen J, Bernardini GL, Kreiter K, et al: Effect of cisternal and ventricular blood on risk of delayed cerebral ischemia after subarachnoid hemorrhage: The Fisher Scale revisited. Stroke 32:2012–2020, 2001.
134. Fisher CM, Kistler JP, Davis JM: Relation of cerebral vasospasm to subarachnoid hemorrhage visualized by computerized tomographic scanning. Neurosurgery 6:1–9, 1982.
135. Conway JE, Tamargo RJ: Cocaine use is an independent risk factor for cerebral vasospasm after aneurysmal subarachnoid hemorrhage. Stroke 32:2338–2343, 2001.
136. Fisher CM, Roberson GH, Ojemann RG: Cerebral vasospasm with ruptured saccular aneurysm: The clinical manifestations. Neurosurgery 1:245, 1977.

137. Rajendran JG, Lewis DH, Newell DW, Winn HR: Brain SPECT used to evaluate vasospasm after subarachnoid hemorrhage: Correlation with angiography and transcranial Doppler. Clin Nucl Med 26:125–130, 2001.

138. Grosset DG, Straiton J, McDonald I: Angiographic and Doppler diagnosis or cerebral artery vasospasm following subarachnoid hemorrhage. Br J Neurosurg 7:291–298, 1993.

139. Laumer R, Steinmeier R, Gonner F: Cerebral hemodynamics in subarachnoid hemorrhage evaluated by transcranial Doppler sonography. Neurosurgery 33:11–18, 1993.

140. Boecher-Schwarz HG, Ungersboeck K, Ulrich P, et al: Transcranial Doppler diagnosis of cerebral vasospasm following subarachnoid haemorrhage: Correlation and analysis of results in relation to the age of patients. Acta Neurochir (Wien) 127:32, 1994.

141. Ekelund A, Saveland H, Romner B: Transcranial Doppler ultrasound in hypertensive versus normotensive patients after aneurysmal subarachnoid hemorrhage. Stroke 26:2071–2074, 1995.

142. Giller CA, Purdy P, Giller A: Elevated transcranial Doppler ultrasound velocities following therapeutic arterial dilation. Stroke 26:123–127, 1995.

143. Steinmeier R, Laumer R, Bondar I: Cerebral hemodynamics in subarachnoid hemorrhage evaluated by transcranial Doppler sonography. Part 2: Pulsatility indices: Normal reference values and characteristics in subarachnoid hemorrhage. Neurosurgery 33:10, 1993.

144. Brinker T, Seifert V, Dietz H: Subacute hydrocephalus after experimental subarachnoid hemorrhage: Its prevention by intrathecal fibrinolysis with recombinant tissue plasminogen activator. Neurosurgery 31:306, 1992.

145. Mizoi K, Yoshimoto T, Takahashi A: Prospective study on the prevention of cerebral vasospasm by intrathecal fibrinolytic therapy with tissue type plasminogen activator. J Neurosurg 78:430, 1993.

146. Sasaki T, Ohta T, Kikuchi H: A phase II clinical trial of recombinant human tissue-type plasminogen activator against cerebral vasospasm after aneurysmal subarachnoid hemorrhage. Neurosurgery 35:597–605, 1994.

147. Usui M, Saito N, Hoya K, Todo T: Vasospasm prevention with postoperative intrathecal thrombolytic therapy: A retrospective comparison of urokinase, tissue plasminogen activator, and cisternal drainage alone. Neurosurgery 34:235, 1994.

148. Kodama N, Sasaki T, Kawakami M, et al: Cisternal irrigation therapy with urokinase and ascorbic acid for prevention of vasospasm after aneurysmal subarachnoid hemorrhage: Outcome in 217 patients. Surg Neurol 53:110–117, 2000.

149. Allen AS, Ahn HS, Preziosi TJ: Cerebral arterial spasm—a controlled trial of nimodipine in patients with subarachnoid hemorrhage. N Engl J Med 308:619, 1983.

150. Ohman J, Servo A, Heiskanen O: Long-term effects of nimodipine on cerebral infarcts and outcome effects after aneurysmal subarachnoid hemorrhage and surgery. J Neurosurg 74:8, 1991.

151. Pickard JD, Murray GD, Illingworth R: Effect of oral nimodipine on cerebral infarction and outcome after subarachnoid haemorrhage: British Aneurysm Nimodipine Trial. Br Med J 298:636–642, 1989.

152. Barker FGI, Ogilvy CS: Efficacy of prophylactic nimodipine for delayed ischemic deficit after subarachnoid hemorrhage: A meta-analysis. J Neurosurg 84:405–414, 1996.

153. Feigin VL, Rinkel GJ, Algra A, et al: Calcium antagonists for aneurysmal subarachnoid haemorrhage. Cochrane Database Syst Rev CD000277, 2000.

154. Tettenborn D, Dycka J: Prevention and treatment of delayed ischemic dysfunction in patients with aneurysmal subarachnoid hemorrhage. Stroke 21(Suppl):IV85, 1990.

155. Haley EC Jr, Kassell NF, Torner JC: A randomized trial of nicardipine in subarachnoid hemorrhage: Angiographic and transcranial Doppler ultrasound results. A report of the Cooperative Aneurysm Study. J Neurosurg 78:548–553, 1993.

156. Haley EC Jr, Kassell NF, Torner JC, et al: A randomized, controlled trial of high-dose intravenous nicardipine in aneurysmal subarachnoid hemorrhage: A report of the Cooperative Aneurysm Study. J Neurosurg 78:537–547, 1993.

157. Haley EC Jr, Kassell NF, Torner JC, and the participants: A randomized trial of two doses of nicardipine in aneurysmal subarachnoid hemorrhage: A report of the Cooperative Aneurysm Study. J Neurosurg 80:788, 1994.

158. Shibuya M, Suzuki Y, Enomoto H: Effects of prophylactic intrathecal administration of nicardipine on vasospasm in patients with severe aneurysmal subarachnoid haemorrhage. Acta Neurochir (Wien) 131:19, 1994.

159. Effect of calcitonin-gene-related peptide in patients with delayed postoperative cerebral ischaemia after aneurysmal subarachnoid haemorrhage. European CGRP in Subarachnoid Hemorrhage Study Group. Lancet 339:831–834, 1992.

160. Clouston JE, Numaguchi Y, Zoarski GH: Intraarterial papaverine infusion for cerebral vasospasm after subarachnoid hemorrhage. Am J Neuroradiol 16:2, 1995.

161. Firlik KS, Kaufmann AM, Firlik AD, et al: Intra-arterial papaverine for the treatment of cerebral vasospasm following aneurysmal subarachnoid hemorrhage. Surg Neurol 51:66–74, 1999.

162. Kaku Y, Yonekawa Y, Tsukahara T, Kazekawa K: Superselective intra-arterial infusion of papaverine for the treatment of cerebral vasospasm after subarachnoid hemorrhage. J Neurosurg 77:842, 1992.

163. Carhuapoma JR, Qureshi AI, Tamargo RJ, et al: Intra-arterial papaverine-induced seizures: Case report and review of the literature. Surg Neurol 56:159–163, 2001.

164. Arakawa Y, Kikuta K, Hojo M, et al: Milrinone for the treatment of cerebral vasospasm after subarachnoid hemorrhage: Report of seven cases. Neurosurgery 48:713–728, 2001.

165. Finfer SR, Ferch R, Morgan MK: Barbiturate coma for severe, refractory vasospasm following subarachnoid haemorrhage. Intensive Care Med 25:406–409, 1999.

166. Haley ECJ, Kassell NF, Apperson-Hansen C, et al: A randomized, double-blind, vehicle-controlled trial of tirilazad mesylate in patients with aneurysmal subarachnoid hemorrhage: A cooperative study in North America. J Neurosurg 86:467–474, 1997.

167. Kassell NF, Haley EC Jr, Apperson-Hansen C: Randomized, double-blind, vehicle-controlled trial of tirilazad mesylate in patients with aneurysmal subarachnoid hemorrhage: A cooperative study in Europe, Australia, and New Zealand. J Neurosurg 84:221–221, 1996.

168. Lanzino G, Kassell NF: Double-blind, randomized, vehicle-controlled study of high-dose tirilazad mesylate in women with aneurysmal subarachnoid hemorrhage. Part II: A cooperative study in North America. J Neurosurg 90:1018–1024, 1999.

169. Kassell NF, Peerless SJ, Durward QJ, et al: Treatment of ischemic deficits from vasospasm with intravascular volume expansion and induced arterial hypertension. Neurosurgery 11:337–343, 1982.

170. Mori K, Arai H, Nakajima K: Hemorrheological and hemodynamic analysis of hypervolemic hemodilution therapy for cerebral vasospasm after aneurysmal subarachnoid hemorrhage. Stroke 26:1620–1626, 1995.

171. Egge A, Waterloo K, Sjoholm H, et al: Prophylactic hyperdynamic postoperative fluid therapy after aneurysmal subarachnoid hemorrhage: A clinical, prospective, randomized, controlled study. Neurosurgery 49:593–606, 2001.

172. Qureshi AI, Suarez JI, Bhardwaj A, et al: Early predictors of outcome in patients receiving hypervolemic and hypertensive therapy for symptomatic vasospasm after subarachnoid hemorrhage. Crit Care Med 28:824–829, 2000.

173. Lennihan L, Mayer SA, Fink ME, et al: Effect of hypervolemic therapy on cerebral blood flow after subarachnoid hemorrhage: A randomized controlled trial. Stroke 31:383–391, 2000.

174. Feigin VL, Rinkel GJ, Algra A, van Gijn J: Circulatory volume expansion for aneurysmal subarachnoid hemorrhage. Cochrane Database Syst Rev CD000483, 2000.

175. Darby JM, Yonas H, Marks EC: Acute cerebral blood flow response to dopamine-induced hypertension after subarachnoid hemorrhage. J Neurosurg 80:857, 1994.

176. Oropello JM, Weiner L, Benjamin E: Hypertensive, hypervolemic, hemodilutional therapy for aneurysmal subarachnoid hemorrhage: Is it efficacious? No! Crit Care Clin 12:709–730, 1996.

177. Ullman JS, Bedersom JB: Hypertensive hypervolemic, hemodilutional therapy for aneurysmal subarachnoid hemorrhage. Is it efficacious? Yes. Crit Care Clin 12:697–707, 1996.

178. Terada T, Komai N, Hayashi S: Hemorrhagic infarction after vasospasm due to ruptured cerebral aneurysm. Neurosurgery 18:415, 1986.

179. Shimoda M, Oda S, Tsugane R, Sato O: Intracranial complication of hypervolemic therapy in patients with a delayed ischemic deficit attributed to vasospasm. J Neurosurg 78:423, 1993.

Clinical Manifestations

180. Trumble ER, Muizelaar JP, Myseros JS: Coagulopathy with the use of hetastarch in the treatment of vasospasm. J Neurosurg 82:44, 1995.

181. Coyne TJ, Montanera WJ, Macdonald RL: Percutaneous transluminal angioplasty for cerebral vasospasm after subarachnoid hemorrhage. Can J Surg 37:391–396, 1994.

182. Honma Y, Fujiwara T, Irie K: Morphological changes in human cerebral arteries after percutaneous transluminal angioplasty for vasospasm caused by subarachnoid hemorrhage. Neurosurgery 36:1073, 1995.

183. Bejjani GK, Bank WO, Olan WJ, Sekhar LN: The efficacy and safety of angioplasty for cerebral vasospasm after subarachnoid hemorrhage. Neurosurgery 42:979–986, 1998.

184. Polin RS, Coenen VA, Hansen CA, et al: Efficacy of transluminal angioplasty for the management of symptomatic cerebral vasospasm following aneurysmal subarachnoid hemorrhage. J Neurosurg 92:284–290, 2000.

Clinical Manifestations

Chapter Fifteen

Arteriovenous Malformations and Other Vascular Anomalies

J. P. Mohr, Andreas Hartmann, Henning Mast, John Pile-Spellman,
Herrmann-Christian Schumacher, and Christian Stapf

HISTORY

The pathologic case material provides the earliest examples of what we call today a brain arteriovenous malformation (AVM). The 1846 publication by Viennese pathologist Rokitansky[1] may be the first to mention the existence of such lesions. He did not provide a detailed morphologic description of what he called "vascular brain tumors in pial tissue," but he was puzzled by the structural analogy between their "cavernous textures" and the "gaps, windows or canals in certain blastemas of the vascular system" that he had noted in embryonic tissue. This observation led him to the idea that a developmental derangement was the most likely underlying cause for this type of lesion. Half a century later Carl Emanuel, a pathologist working at Heidelberg University, published one of the first detailed histopathologic case studies.[2] He had already described "substantial enlargement of the microcirculatory pathways" reflecting the lack of a capillary bed in the angioma arteriale racemosum. Emanuel's report is noteworthy because he appears to be the first researcher considering three possible causes of such lesions: congenital, secondary development from an innate telangiectasia, or a sequel to trauma. His landmark proposal drafted the three major etiologic concepts—embryologic derangement, dynamic development, and vascular trauma—upon which most future theories were built and further elaborated.[3]

ETIOLOGY

Growing insight into the embryology of the human cerebrovascular system during the first half of the 20th century fostered theories on the developmental basis of persistent cerebral arteriovenous (AV) shunts.[3–6] The introduction of cerebral angiography into clinical practice[7] offered the first in vivo opportunities for a better understanding of AVM angioarchitecture and its inherent flow pattern. Among the different types of intracerebral AV fistulas, vein of Galen aneurysmal malformations may actually constitute the only embryonic disorder (Table 15.1). The fistula links the choroidal artery system to a persistent ectatic median vein of the prosencephalon, which represents the embryonic precursor of the vein of Galen.[8,9]

Thanks to now routinely applied fetal ultrasound screening, an increasing number of vein of Galen aneurysmal malformations has been detected during gestation, and a few patients have been studied by prenatal magnetic resonance imaging (MRI).[10,11] Information on comparable cases with an intrauterine diagnosis of a brain AVM, however, are lacking; none has as yet been reported from studies on routine fetal ultrasound evaluations, which are commonly performed between the 20th and 22nd gestational week.[12,13] Probably the youngest individual so far reported may be a preterm neonate (born at 32 weeks' gestation) who died during the second postnatal day from acute hemorrhage of an infratentorial AVM that was fed by the superior cerebellar artery.[14] The lack of observed cases in which a brain AVM was detected at earlier fetal stages hence challenges the widespread assumption that these lesions also arise from an embryonic disturbance at the time of the vessel formation.[15]

The vascular topography in many AVMs also argues against a genuine embryonic disorder. Brain AVMs commonly affect distal arterial branches, and in roughly half the cases, the malformation is found in the borderzone region shared by the distal anterior, middle, and posterior cerebral arteries.[16] These "watershed areas" constitute anatomic remnants of the manifold artery-to-artery links that once covered the brain surface at its lissencephalic state. With the onset of cortical gyration (29th gestational week), the original arterial mesh regresses, giving rise eventually to the defined arterial territories of the leptomeningeal arteries. In the distal fields of these arterial territories, pial anastomoses between otherwise separated brain arteries persist, even though the number, size, and exact location of the leptomeningeal anastomoses show numerous interindividual variations.[17–19] Their persistence may depend on the local composition of the extracellular matrix,[20] the formation of capillary basement membranes,[21,22] and the influence of angiogenetic factors on the

Table 15.1   Differential Diagnosis of Arteriovenous (AV) Malformations of the Brain: Other Intracranial AV Fistulas

Entity*	Pathogenesis	Clinical Characteristics
Vein of Galen malformation[9, 233]	Persistent dilated embryonic vein of the prosencephalon; posterior choroidal artery affected	Hemorrhage, congestive heart failure in neonates
Dural AV fistula[9]	Different types (congenital, traumatic, secondary to venous occlusion, etc.)	Arterial supply through meningeal arterial branches; high recurrence rate
Hereditary hemorrhagic telangiectasia (Rendu-Osler-Weber syndrome)[234]	Capillary regression leads to multiple small AV shunts in various tissues	Vascular abnormalities in nose, skin, lung, brain, and gastrointestinal tract
Encephalotrigeminal (Sturge-Weber syndrome)[235]	Phakomatosis	Neurocutaneous syndrome
Cerebro-retinal angiomatosis (von Hippel–Lindau disease)[235]	Phakomatosis	Neurocutaneous syndrome
Wyburn-Mason syndrome[236, 237]	Phakomatosis	Neurocutaneous syndrome
Neovascular collateral vessels	Venous thrombosis or arterial occlusion may lead to focal angioneogenesis with false AV connections	Post-thrombotic syndrome, moyamoya disease, etc.
Traumatic AV fistulas	Traumatic disruption of adjacent arterial and venous vessel walls	Cavernous sinus fistula, etc.

*Superscript numbers indicate chapter references.

Clinical Manifestations

course of the regression process.[23,24] This possibility suggests that the initial lesion may actually arise with a timely link to the formation of the arterial borderzones, that is, at some point after the 29th gestational week.[19,25] In one case report in which the interplay between cortical gyration and borderzone formation was disturbed by a primary migration disorder such as schizencephaly, an AVM had developed at the site where the neural defect straddled the arterial borderzone territory.[26]

The relatively high rate of arterial aneurysms associated with AVMs (up to 58% in two series)[27,28] has led to the notion of a similar underlying pathogenesis in AVMs and aneurysms,[29–31] thereby suggesting a structural or functional smooth muscle disorder in the context of AVM development. The formation of the arterial smooth muscle layer shows a spatiotemporal sequence, slowly progressing from proximal to distal arterial segments. In the human fetus, the first smooth muscle layer detected at proximal levels of the leptomeningeal arteries appears in the 16th gestational week, subsequently followed by the striatal (20th to 22nd gestational week), extrastriatal medullary (term to first postnatal month), and cortical arteries (6th to 9th month).[25] The time frame for this histologic maturation process coincides with the arterial borderzone development (29th gestational week to end of the first year of life). The idea of a primary smooth muscle defect at the level of the distal arterial branches may therefore provide a testable hypothesis for AVM development, especially in patients in whom the malformation is located in the arterial borderzone territory. On the basis of theoretical vascular modeling, data from a study using the modeling now support the notion that a lack of local flow control at the distal arterial level may be the cause, rather than the result, of an AVM.[32]

The pathogenetic mechanisms leading to the lack of capillaries in the AVM nidus remain as yet unclear. The capillary density—that is, the number of capillaries in a given volume of brain tissue—remains stable after the fourth month of gestation, whereas the relative capillary volume in the cortex increases in a linear fashion from the end of

the first trimester throughout infancy.[33,25] Any presumed capillary disease has as yet not found its morphologic correlate, and the morphology of endothelial cells in vessels within or adjacent to an AVM has been described as being normal.[34–40] A higher endothelial turnover in the AVM vasculature, however, may suggest the presence of active angiogenesis or ongoing vascular remodeling.[41]

Much effort is currently being devoted to defining the predisposing factors at the molecular level of the developing brain vasculature. Possible germline mutations affecting distinct angiogenetic pathways have been proposed to be the underlying cause of a variety of vascular malformations in the brain. As to AVMs, several candidate proteins are currently under investigation, including endothelial angiopoietin receptor Tie-2,[42–44] basic fibroblast growth factor (FGF-2),[45] nitric oxide synthase (NOS),[46] transforming growth factor beta (TGF-β),[47,48] vascular endothelial growth factor (VEGF),[49] and endoglin.[50] Many of these proteins show mutual interactions,[43,47,51] commonly affect the signal pathways between the vascular endothelium and the smooth muscle layer of the arterial wall, but do not seem to affect the physiologic maturation process in the vessels involved. In fact, the basement membranes of AVM vessels have been shown to predominantly express laminin, a glycoprotein that is typically seen in mature (i.e., postembryonic) vessels.[22] Fibronectin, a histochemical marker for embryonic vessels, is barely detectable in AVMs, suggesting that an AVM nidus consists of abnormal but not immature vessels.

Once the initial lesion has emerged, the permanent intraluminal stress arising from abnormal flow and pressure may lead to so-called secondary angiopathy, a nonreversible abnormal remodeling process in otherwise normal neighboring vessels.[9] Whether any of the suggested molecular factors may also play a role amid the biologic mechanisms that eventually lead to AVM growth, to secondary vascular changes, and to phenomena like spontaneous obliteration[52] and recurrence after successful therapy[53,54] has yet to be determined.

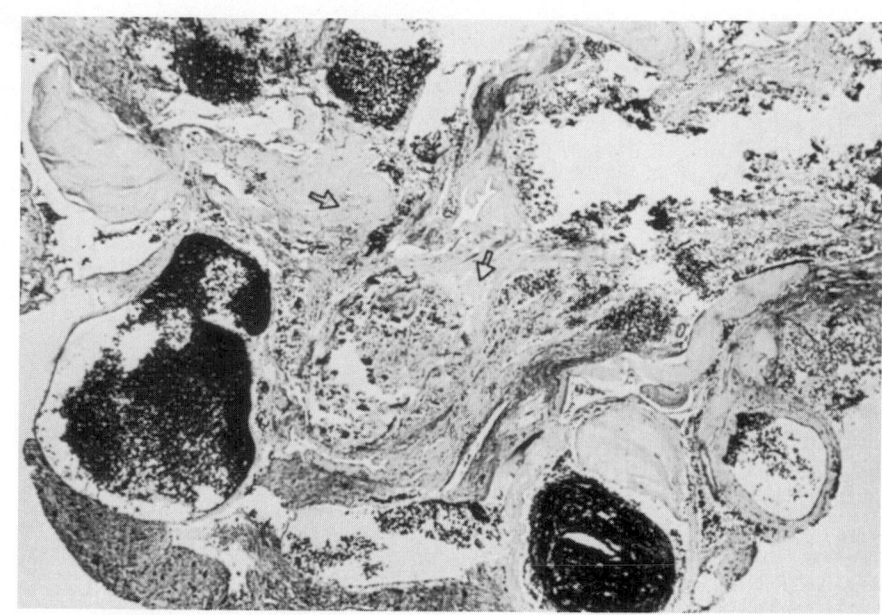

FIGURE 15–1 *Photomicrograph of an arteriovenous malformation at low power, demonstrating areas of gliosis (arrows) between large thin-walled cavernous sinuses.*

Clinical
Manifestations

MORPHOLOGY

An AVM resembles a tortuous agglomeration of abnormally dilated arteries and veins in the brain, commonly supplied through branches of one or more leptomeningeal arteries, and with drainage into deep veins, superficial veins, or both. In its core region or nidus, the AVM lacks a capillary bed, thereby allowing high-flow AV shunting through one or more fistulas.

Histologic evaluation of AVMs demonstrates that the walls of the large vascular components of the malformation are mostly devoid of elastic and significant muscular components (Fig. 15–1).[37,55] Within the malformation, the arteries show subendothelial thickening, medial hypertrophy, and, occasionally, thrombosis; the veins are thin walled and vary in size, with poorly developed muscular and elastic components. Corrosion preparation of AVMs injected with inert substances after removal of the brain at autopsy have shown that there is no normal cerebral tissue within the confines of an AVM (Fig. 15–2). The intense gliosis suggests that the neurons captivated within the margins of a malformation are probably nonfunctional (see Fig. 15–1). Presumably, cerebral function that should be located in the brain occupied by the malformation is displaced to the malformation's margins or even remote from it.[56,57]

Feeding arteries may supply the malformation directly via terminal branches or may continue "en passage," thereby supplying normal brain tissue distal to the AVM (Fig. 15–3). Arterial supply may arise from single arterial

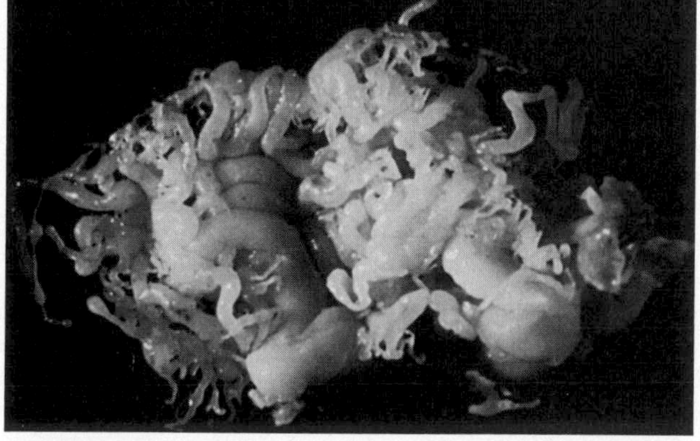

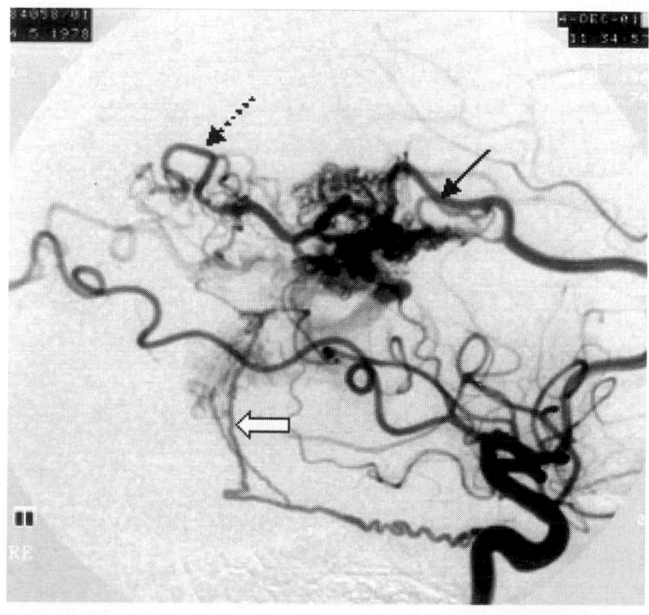

FIGURE 15–2 *Corrosion specimen of an arteriovenous malformation obtained after the injection of acrylate into the malformation and dissolution of the soft tissue by potassium hydroxide. The specimen reveals the three-dimensional anatomy of the malformation and the configuration of the large venous sinusoids.*

FIGURE 15–3 *An "en passage" feeder vessel (black arrow) supplies the nidus, then continues to healthy brain tissue (dotted arrow). Note the meningeal supply to a second nidus (white arrow).*

territories or may straddle the arterial borderzones, thereby recruiting feeding vessels from two or more adjacent arterial territories.[58] Deep arterial feeders originating from branches or main trunks of the major cerebral arteries in the lenticulostriate, choroidal, or thalamoperforating arteries may reach the AVM after passing through healthy brain tissue. In a few cases, feeding arteries may stenose or even occlude over time; in these instances, so-called moyamoya-type changes refer to any pattern of collateral small vessel recruitment due to proximal feeding artery stenosis or occlusion.

Concurrent arterial aneurysms are commonly defined as saccular dilatations of the lumen two or more times the width of the arterial vessel that carry the dilatation. Such arterial aneurysms may be located either on feeding arteries (so-called flow-related arterial aneurysms; Fig. 15–4), within the margins of the AVM nidus ("intranidal aneurysms"; Fig. 15–5), or on vessels unrelated to blood flow to the AVM.[59] The reported rates of concurrent aneurysms in patients with AVMs show large variations, ranging from 3%[60] to 58%.[61] Some of this variation may result from low interrater agreement.[62] Referral bias toward tertiary treatment centers may also influence the rate of detected aneurysms in the study cohort.[63] Finally, different study definitions of the term concurrent aneurysm may further contribute to variations in reported aneurysm rates. Therefore, there is now common agreement that infundibula, arterial ectasias (i.e., dilated feeding vessels), and intranidal aneurysmal dilatations seen during the venous phase of angiography are not to be diagnosed as arterial aneurysms.

The most common route of *venous AVM drainage* is toward the superficial veins of the brain directly or via collaterals to the major sinuses (Fig. 15–6). An alternative

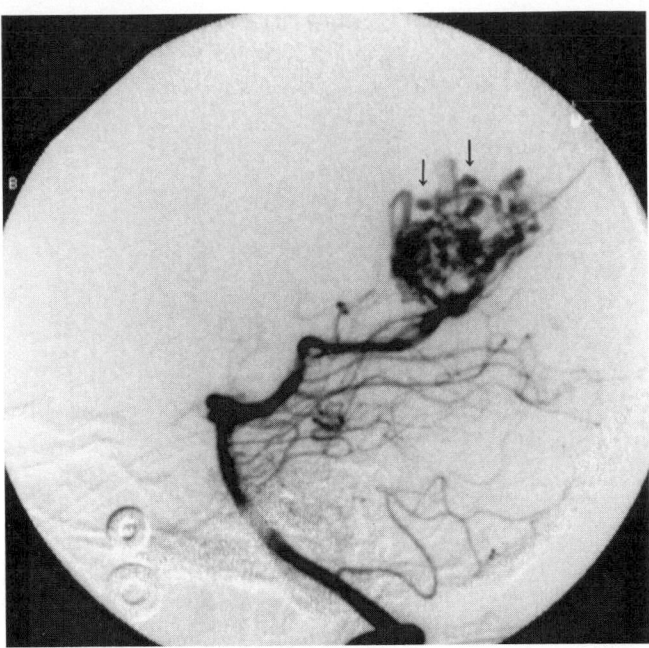

FIGURE 15–5   *Multiple intranidal arterial aneurysms* (arrows) *in a right occipital arteriovenous malformation with feeders from the posterior cerebral artery.*

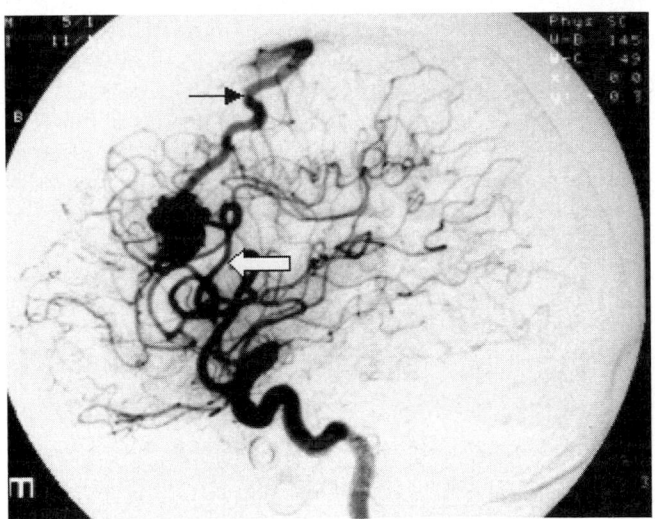

FIGURE 15–6   *Angiogram of a compact arteriovenous malformation fed by branches of the middle cerebral artery* (white arrow) *and draining into a single superficial vein* (black arrow).

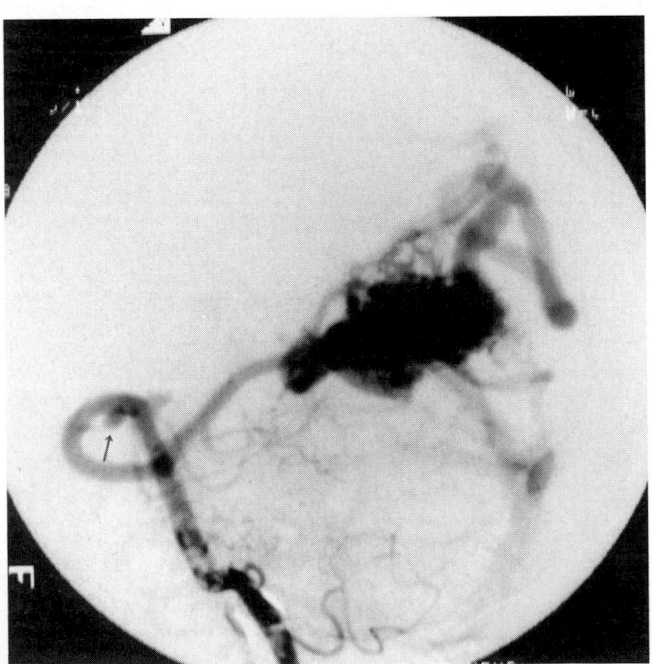

FIGURE 15–4   *Flow-related arterial aneurysm* (arrow) *in a right occipital arteriovenous malformation fed by the ipsilateral posterior cerebral artery.*

route is through deep venous channels that may reach the ependymal surface of the ventricular system and drain via the deep venous system. Variations of normal venous drainage anatomy may be found in up to 30% of all patients with AVM,[64,65] and adaptations of the venous system to compensate for the large blood volume leads to sometimes extensive collateral veins. In clinical AVM research, the overall venous drainage pattern is usually categorized as angiographically demonstrated drainage into the superficial cortical veins ("superficial venous drainage"), drainage into the deep venous system ("deep venous drainage")

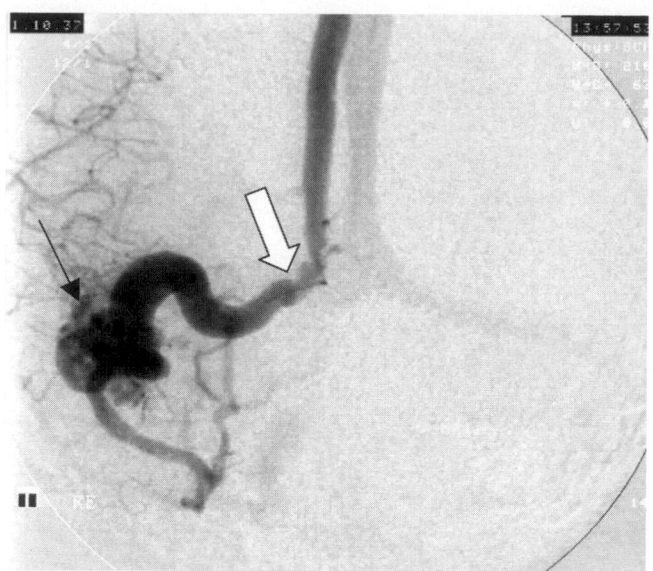

FIGURE 15–7 *Arteriovenous malformation* (black arrow) *with a single large draining vein. Note the venous stenosis* (white arrow).

such as the internal cerebral veins, basal veins, and vein of Galen, and combined superficial and deep drainage. It is generally agreed that "in the posterior fossa, only cerebellar hemispheric veins that drain directly into the straight sinus, torcula Herophili, or transverse sinus are considered to be superficial."[66] Stenosis and thrombosis of venous drainage pathways have been described in prior observations.[67-69] For research purposes, "venous stenosis" is usually defined as a greater than two-fold caliber narrowing of any draining vein outflow pathway seen in two angiographic views. Correspondingly, "venous ectasia" is usually recorded in cases with a greater than two-fold caliber increase in any draining venous channel (Fig. 15–7).

EPIDEMIOLOGY

No population-based prevalence data on AVMs are currently available. In the Cooperative Study of Subarachnoid Hemorrhage, still the largest such series to date, symptomatic AVMs were found in 549 of 6,368 cases, representing an incidence of 8.6% of subarachnoid hemorrhages (SAHs).[70,71] Because SAH accounts for roughly 10% of strokes, AVMs make up approximately 1% of all strokes.

Calculated estimates from hospital-based autopsy data may be unreliable, showing a wide range from 5 to as many as 613 AVMs per 100,000 persons.[72-75] The early studies suggested a very low prevalence; their figures were contradicted by McCormick and Rosenfield,[76] who uncovered 196 AVMs among 4530 consecutive autopsies, an incidence of 4.3%. Although not derived from a population-based study, these data are of special interest because they represent a careful autopsy-based effort to document the prevalence of AVMs, both symptomatic and asymptomatic. Only 24 of the 196 (12.2%) patients in this study had experienced symptoms of an AVM. This figure yields a symptomatic stroke incidence of 0.52% in this autopsied

population, which is in the range of the 1% incidence found in purely clinical studies. Among the 24 patients with symptomatic AVMs, 21 had suffered hemorrhage, which was massive in 16 patients, and the remainder had epilepsy or steal phenomena. The distribution of AVMs 118 (60%) in cerebral hemispheres, 28 (14%) affecting the brainstem, and 5 (3%) in the spinal cord. This distribution closely approximates those from series of clinically symptomatic patients. Given the patterns of case referral, it is no surprise that the larger series of cases of AVMs come mainly from surgical clinics. The low frequency of the disorder prevents all but a few interested physicians and surgeons from having any but a passing encounter with such cases. In one report of 100 patients evaluated angiographically for tandem lesions in a setting of high-grade carotid stenosis, two AVMs were found.[77]

Prior data from a large series in which more than 4000 volunteers were screened with brain MRI did not lead to the detection of any brain AVMs.[78,79] Assuming a hypothetical prevalence of 10 patients with AVMs per 100,000, brain MRI screening of 1 million people would be necessary to yield estimates with sufficiently narrow confidence intervals (CIs).[80]

Figure 15–8 summarizes available incidence rates for both AVM detection and associated intracranial hemorrhage (ICH). The age- and gender-adjusted incidence of ICH due to any type of intracranial vascular malformation is 0.82 per 100,000 (95% CI, 0.46–1.19) in a retrospective, population-based study conducted over 27 years in Olmsted County, Minnesota.[81,82] Of the 20 patients recorded, 17 (85%) had an underlying brain AVM. No separate incidence for AVM hemorrhage was calculated. In the Netherlands Antilles between 1980 and 1990, an annual incidence of 1.1 symptomatic AVMs per 100,000 people was described.[83] Of the 17 patients identified as having an AVM, 16 presented with ICH. In this fairly isolated and homogeneous population, however, an unusually high proportion of the patients with AVM (35%) had hereditary hemorrhagic telangiectasia (Rendu–Osler–Weber disease). Further, 25% of the patient cohort showed multiple brain AVMs, making it difficult to compare the findings with those in other populations. Finally, a mixed prospective and retrospective series from Linköping University, Sweden, estimated an AVM detection rate of 1.24 per 100,000 person-years (95% CI, 0.75–1.56).[84] The relatively high estimated incidence of AVM hemorrhage (0.87 per 100,000 person-years; 95% CI, 0.57–1.19) may have been biased by patient referrals from outside the geographic study area. Incidence data derived from non–population-based studies have been shown to be highly variable, likely because of referral bias and underascertainment of AVM hemorrhage.

The New York Islands Study

The New York Islands AVM Hemorrhage Study is an ongoing prospective population-based survey determining the incidence of AVM hemorrhage and associated morbidity and mortality rates in a population defined by U.S. Post Office Zip Code boundaries. The New York islands—Manhattan Island, Staten Island, and Long Island (the latter including the New York City boroughs of Brooklyn

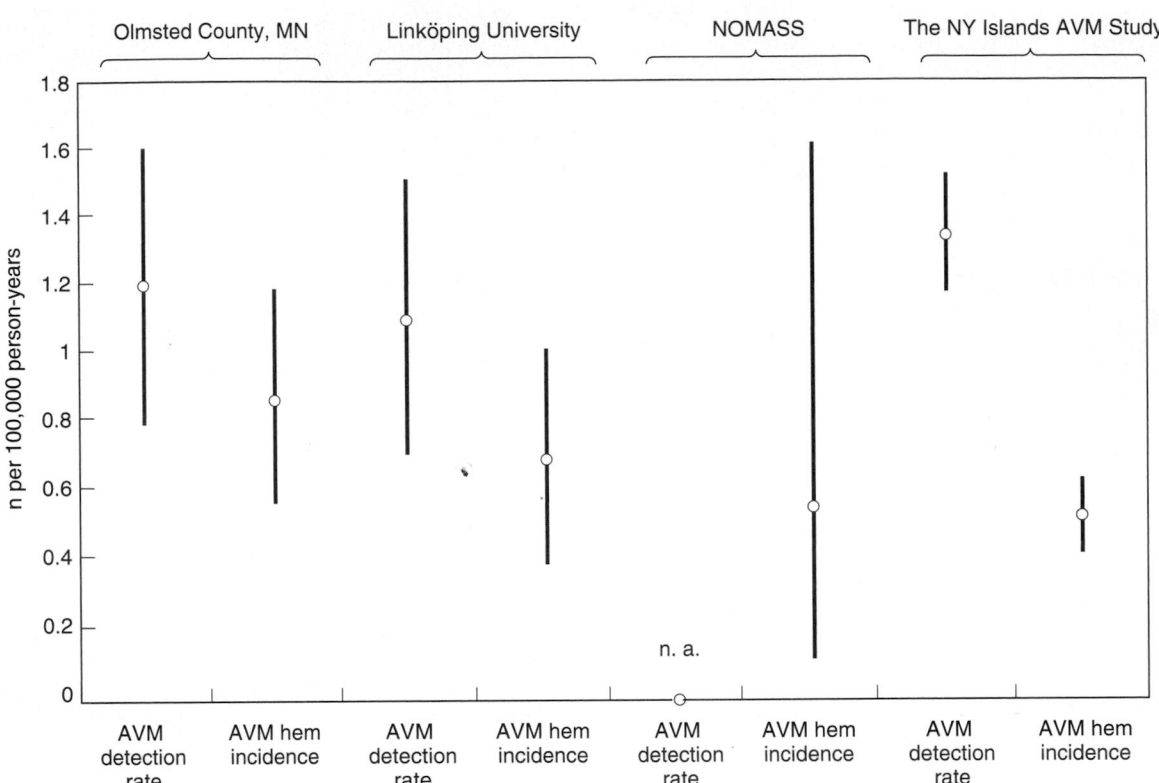

FIGURE 15–8 *Synopsis of population-based arteriovenous malformation (AVM) detection rates and incidence of AVM hemorrhage. Average annual rates per 100,000 and 95% confidence limits are given on the basis of data from references 81, 82, 84, 86, and 166. hem, hemorrhage; n.a., not available.*

and Queens and the counties of Nassau and Suffolk)—contain a population of 9,429,541 persons according to the 2000 U.S. Census. Since March 15, 2000, all major New York Islands hospitals and their related hospital networks have cooperated prospectively to report weekly data on consecutive patients living in the study area with a diagnosis of brain AVM, and have included in their reports whether or not the patients had suffered AVM hemorrhage. Patients who are referred to these hospitals but live outside the ZIP code–defined study area are excluded from the study population.

As of June 14, 2002, 284 prospective patients with AVM were encountered, leading to a calculated prospective AVM detection rate of 1.34 per 100,000 person-years (95% CI, 1.18–1.49). Mean age among identified patients was 35 years (± 18 SD), and 49% were women. Overall, 108 patients presented with a first-ever acute AVM hemorrhage; the currently estimated incidence of AVM hemorrhage in the New York Islands population is thus 0.51 per 100,000 person-years (95% CI, 0.41–0.61). The prevalence of AVM hemorrhage among detected cases (n = 144) was 0.68 per 100,000 person-years (95% CI, 0.57–0.79).[85]

Northern Manhattan Stroke Study

The Northern Manhattan Stroke Study (NOMASS) was a prospective, population-based, stroke incidence survey collecting data in a ZIP code–defined area in New York City that contains 136,623 white, black, and Hispanic

residents older than 20 years, according to the 1990 U.S. Census. An active surveillance program was used to identify all hospitalized and nonhospitalized patients with first-ever (incident) stroke older than 20 years. All patients underwent computed tomography (CT), MRI, or both of the brain, and clinical data were systematically collected from their medical records.[86,87]

Data on all patients with incident ICH (i.e., any ICH or SAH, with or without intraventricular blood) occurring between July 1, 1993, and June 30, 1997, were analyzed. Those suspected to have underlying AVMs underwent further studies, including cerebral angiography at the discretion of the treating physicians. The investigators did not include patients whose AVMs were identified before their strokes, nor those with ICH due to trauma, tumor, or any other type of intracranial vascular malformation (e.g., dural AV fistula, vein of Galen type malformation).

Overall, first-ever ICH occurred in 207 patients during 546,492 person-years of observation, including 3 patients (1.4%) with an underlying brain AVM. The crude incidence rate for first-ever AVM hemorrhage in the adult population was 0.55 per 100,000 person-years (95% CI, 0.11–1.61).[88]

GENETICS

The presumably congenital nature of AVMs might be expected to yield many cases with a family history, but the familial incidence appears to be quite rare.[89–93] Only seven families had been reported through 1990, involving 15 people in all. The mode of inheritance is uncertain. In contrast to the general male preponderance for AVMs reported in clinical surgical services, the sexes are equally represented in the scanty family history data, a feature that has been confirmed in the ongoing New York Islands Study. With a greater awareness of the successes in surgery, greater effort is being made to diagnose the condition in the older population. In large modern centers, this effort at diagnosis has shifted the age of onset upward. Therefore, AVM is no longer to be considered a diagnosis mainly involving the young, even though most hemorrhages occur in younger patients. Dural and extracerebral AVMs are the only types thought to be usually acquired from trauma.

AVMs usually occur in isolation, unrelated to other disease states, but a few have been associated with the Rendu-Osler-Weber disease, most of them small.[94,95] In one large study,[95] 31 of 136 patients from a hereditary hemorrhagic telangiectasia clinic were inferred from MRI findings to have cerebral AVMs. Eighteen of these patients underwent angiogram; findings in all 18 were positive, and 7 had multiple (three or more) AVMs. The AVMs varied in size from 3 to 25 mm in maximal dimension. AVMs have also been described in the Wyburn-Mason syndrome.[96]

DIAGNOSIS AND CLASSIFICATION

Cerebral angiography represents the key imaging technique for adequate diagnosis, morphologic characterization (vascular supply and drainage, related aneurysms), and treatment planning for AVMs.[61,97] A meta-analysis has demonstrated that the risk of diagnostic angiography is significantly lower in patients with AVM (0.3%–0.8%) than in those evaluated for TIA or stroke (3.0%–3.7%).[98] Noninvasive conventional and functional MRI techniques are playing an increasing role in the interventional management because they facilitate localization of the nidus in relation to the brain (Fig. 15–9) and further identify functionally important brain areas adjacent to the nidus (Plate 15–1 following page 408).[99–101] Finally, based on flow velocity and resistance pattern, transcranial Doppler (TCD) ultrasonography (conventional B-mode, echo-enhanced, or color-coded TCD) has been demonstrated to be a noninvasive and cost-effective screening tool for both detection and follow-up evaluation of brain AVMs (Plate 15–2).[102–104]

Despite proposals for a uniform terminology in clinical AVM research,[105] common international standards for diagnosing brain AVMs have not as yet been established.[62] Brain AVMs must be separated from other intracranial AV fistulas, which at times have similar morphologic features, because these lesions differ in terms of pathogenesis, natural course, and treatment strategies (Table 15.2). This nosologic heterogeneity in reported AVM series still confounds the literature and makes it difficult to compare different AVM study populations.[63,106] The ninth revision of the International Classification of Diseases (ICD-9)—still widely used in clinical and administrative practice—does not offer a separate code for brain AVMs, clustering them together with any other "congenital anomalies of cerebral vessels" such as cavernous malformations and unruptured

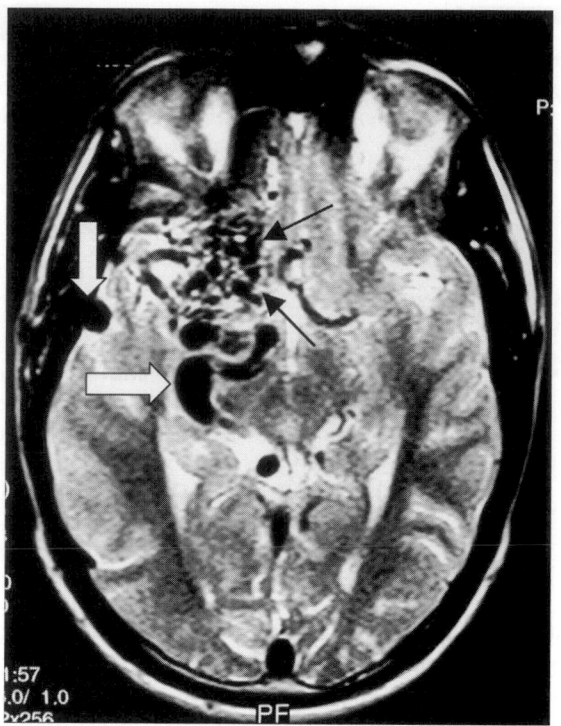

FIGURE 15–9 *Large frontotemporal arteriovenous malformation* (black arrows) *with superficial and deep venous drainage* (white arrows) *and mass effect leading to midbrain compression.*

arterial aneurysms.[107] The current ICD-10 codes provide an individual code for unruptured "arteriovenous malformations of cerebral vessels." Hemorrhage from the AVM, however, regardless of the bleeding location, is still classified among "other causes of SAH."[108]

Size

AVMs vary in size from tiny, so-called cryptic malformations (Fig. 15–10) to massive anomalies that encompass a number of cerebral lobes (Fig. 15–11). The arterial supply also varies enormously, from the extremes of all major cerebral, brainstem, or cerebellar arterial systems, to a single artery, to a single vein draining a fistula. The feeding arteries in the larger malformations frequently are abnormally enlarged and ectatic, reflecting the large loads they carry. Deep arterial feeders often feed the malformation as well. These deep vessels usually arise from branches or main trunks of the major cerebral arteries in the lenticulostriate, choroidal, or thalamoperforating arteries (Fig. 15–12) and reach the AVM after passing through healthy tissues. The venous drainage of AVMs eventually reaches recognizable venous channels, usually appearing abnormally distended because of the large volumes of blood flow through the shunt. The veins follow two basic routes, the more common being superficial drainage coursing over the cortex directly to the major sinuses or collateral venous channels that lead to the major sinuses. The other route is through deep venous channels that reach the ependymal surface of the ventricular system and drain via the deep venous system. In the larger lesions, there is often a dual

Clinical Manifestations

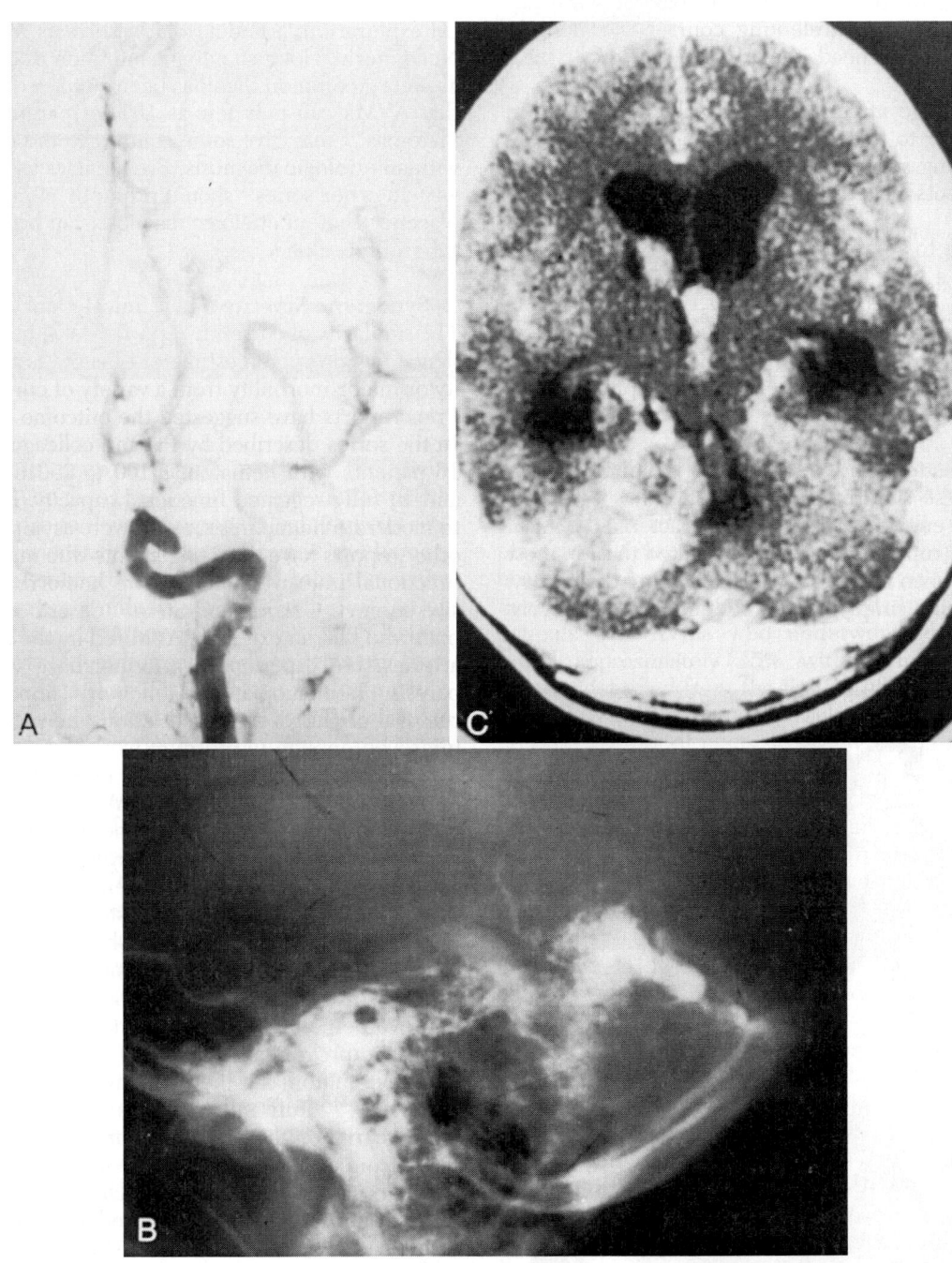

FIGURE 15–17   *Intense vasospasm (A) observed after (B) the rupture of a posterior fossa arteriovenous malformation (C) with massive outpouring of blood into the basal cisterns and ventricles.*

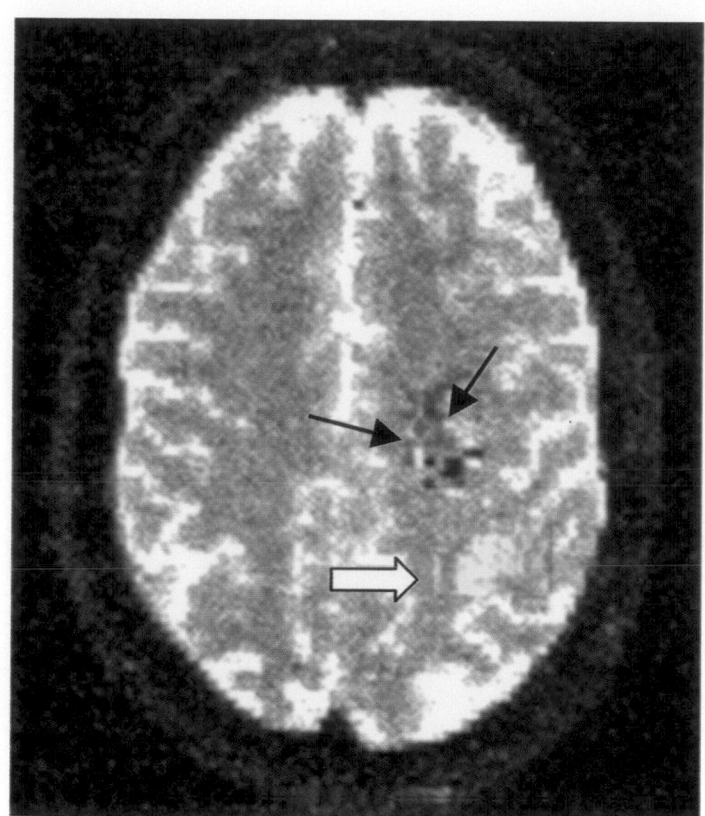

PLATE 15–1 *Functional magnetic resonance imaging study obtained as the patient performed finger-tapping shows brain activation (white arrow) in the vicinity of an arteriovenous malformation (black arrows) in slightly more posterior location than expected.*

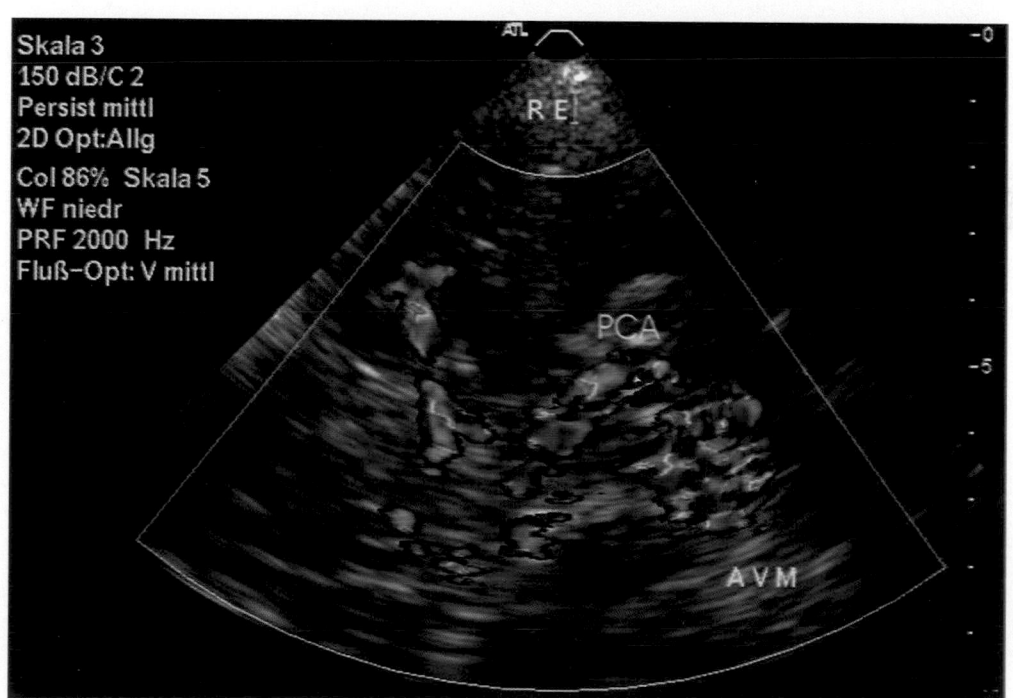

Skala 3
150 dB/C 2
Persist mittl
2D Opt:Allg
Col 86% Skala 5
WF niedr
PRF 2000 Hz
Fluß–Opt: V mittl

R E

PCA

AVM

PLATE 15–2 *Transcranial color-coded duplex sonogram of a small midbrain arteriovenous malformation mainly fed by the posterior cerebral artery (PCA).*

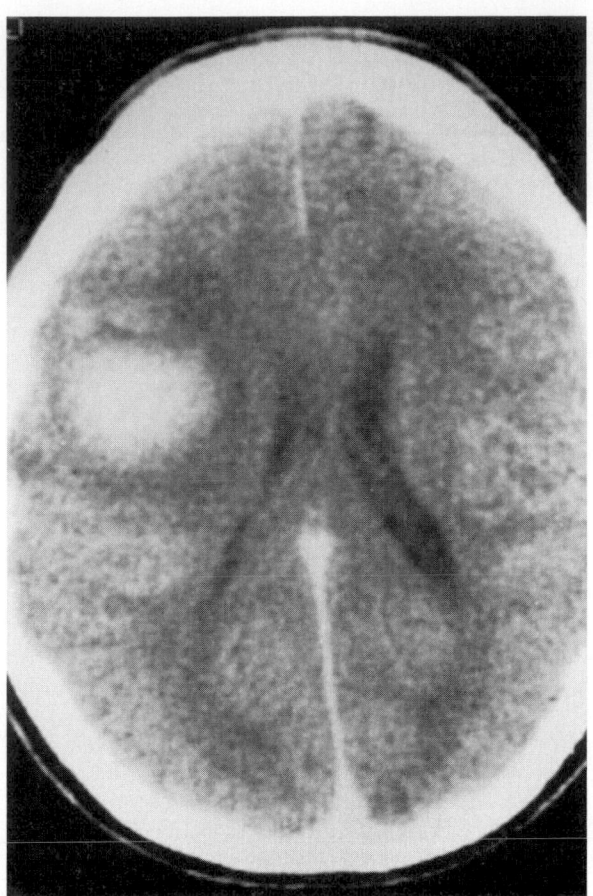

FIGURE 15–18 *Computed tomography scan demonstrating parenchymatous hemorrhage after the rupture of a previously unsuspected arteriovenous malformation.*

The location of the incident bleeds was supratentorial in 99 (86%) patients. Of the 16 (14%) cases with infratentorial lesions, 4 (4%) were located in the brainstem, and 12 (10%) in the cerebellum. The type of initial and follow-up hemorrhage was identical in 23/27 patients (85%). Follow-up hemorrhages were similarly distributed: 29 (94%) supratentorial, and 2 (7%) infratentorial.

In 54 (47%, CI 38%-56%) patients the incident hemorrhage resulted in no neurologic deficit, an additional 43 (37%, CI 28%-46%) patients were independent in their daily activities (Rankin 1). Fifteen (13%, CI 7%-19%) patients were moderately disabled (Rankin 2 or 3), and 3 (3%, CI 0%-6%) were severely disabled (Rankin 4). The mean Rankin score for the cases with incident hemorrhage was 0.76 (0.91), and for the cases with incident and follow-up hemorrhage the mean was 0.89 (1.09). The difference between the means of the two groups was not significant (0.13, 95% CI -0.31 to 0.57). No patient had died during the observation period.

Parenchymal hemorrhages were most likely to result in a neurologic deficit (52%). Type and morbidity of hemorrhage during follow-up were similar to incident events. Twenty (74%) of 27 patients with both incident and follow-up hemorrhages were normal or independent (Rankin 0 or 1). None of the patients with a hemorrhage during follow-up died during the observation period.

Based on these observations, hemorrhage from cerebral AVMs appears to have a lower morbidity rate than currently assumed. However, if AVMs have a better clinical outlook, more effort to deal aggressively with such hematomas than is routinely the case in many institutions might be appropriate.

Risk of Rehemorrhage

Once hemorrhage has occurred, the risk of rehemorrhage is known to rise, but the extent and the timing of rehemorrhage are uncertain. In our own studies, an 18% annual rehemorrhage rate has been found in patients who already had bled.[150] Other studies report a wide variety of rates.[70,151] Graf and colleagues[152] reviewed the records of 191 patients with AVMs, but the mean period of follow-up was relatively short (2 to 5 years). Nevertheless, they found a high rate of initial hemorrhage in age group 11 to 35 years old, and the rate of rebleeding was about 2% a year. Smaller lesions were more prone to hemorrhage, and approximately 13% of the patients died as a result of the hemorrhage. It is generally accepted that approximately 15% of operated AVMs show evidence of prior but asymptomatic hemorrhage.[133]

Vasospasm

The rarity of vasospasm, symptomatic or merely an angiographic finding, has been a source of special commentary.[153,154] Although AVMs are generally said to be associated with a lower incidence of cerebral vasospasm than cerebral aneurysms, this statement may be based on artifact, because AVMs (1) hemorrhage with less frequency into the large basal cisterns than aneurysms, (2) are less common than cerebral aneurysms, and (3) may be evaluated in the acute stage by arteriography, whereas spasm is generally seen on follow-up arteriography performed a few days after the SAH to evaluate the progress of a cerebral aneurysm or its readiness for surgery. The approach just described for vasospasm is not commonly the course of action taken with AVMs once they are identified. Anecdotal cases have certainly been observed in which delayed cerebral vasospasm has been intense after the rupture of an AVM; this spasm may go on to produce death or severe neurologic abnormalities (see Fig. 15–17). It is our impression that the incidence of cerebral vasospasm, in which the quantity of blood is sufficient within the entire subarachnoid space, is probably the same after rupture of a cerebral AVM as that after rupture of a cerebral aneurysm, but most AVMs do not rupture in ways that bring large amounts of blood into the basal cisterns. If present, vasospasm should be treated vigorously by whatever techniques are in current practice.

Aneurysms

Several retrospective studies suggested a higher risk of hemorrhage in patients with AVM and concurrent arterial aneurysms.[29,155-160] The retrospective actuarial analysis by Brown and colleagues[161] demonstrated an increased annual risk of 7.0% for ICH in the setting of unruptured AVMs

Clinical Manifestations

with a concurrent arterial aneurysm (any coexisting saccular aneurysm seen on brain angiography) compared with a 1.7% per year risk for patients who have AVM without concurrent aneurysm. A few retrospective[162,163] and prospective[164,165] studies have found no independent effect of concurrent arterial aneurysms on the risk of ICH. The presence of such aneurysms, however, influences treatment decisions (i.e., surgical, endovascular, or radiation therapy) and acute patient management (i.e., invasive versus conservative care).

We undertook an analysis of our data to address these points. In a cross-sectional study, the 463 consecutive, prospectively enrolled patients from the Columbia AVM Databank were analyzed. Concurrent arterial aneurysms demonstrated on brain angiography were classified as (1) feeding artery aneurysms, (2) intranidal aneurysms, or (3) aneurysms unrelated to blood flow to the AVM. Clinical presentation (diagnostic event) was categorized as (1) ICH proven by imaging or (2) nonhemorrhagic presentation. Univariate and multivariate statistical models were applied to test the effect of age, gender, AVM size, venous drainage pattern, and the three different types of aneurysms on the risk of AVM hemorrhage at initial presentation.

ICH was the presenting symptom in 204 (44%) patients with AVM; 132 of them presented with ICH, 34 with intraventricular hemorrhage, and 29 with SAH. Because of missing data, the hemorrhage type was undefined in 9 patients. Of the 117 (25%) patients with concurrent arterial aneurysms, 93 had a single aneurysm type (54 had feeding artery aneurysms, 21 had intranidal aneurysms, and 18 had aneurysms unrelated to flow to the AVM). The remaining 24 patients showed more than one aneurysm type (10 with feeding artery and intranidal aneurysms, 10 with feeding artery and unrelated aneurysms, 1 with intranidal and unrelated aneurysms, and 3 with all three types of aneurysm).

Concurrent arterial aneurysms were significantly more common in patients presenting with AVM hemorrhage than in those with nonhemorrhagic AVM presentation ($P < .0001$). The difference remained significant ($P < .0001$) in a multivariate model controlling for age, gender, AVM size, and deep venous drainage (odds ratio 3.17; 95% CI, 1.91–5.28).

Feeding artery aneurysms were detected in 77 (17%) patients with AVM and were found significantly more often in those presenting with ICH than in those with nonhemorrhagic presentation (see Fig. 15–4). The difference remained significant in the multivariate model controlling for age, gender, AVM size, venous drainage pattern, and other concurrent aneurysm types (Table 15.2). On the basis of these findings, the attributable risk of incident hemorrhage in feeding artery aneurysms for patients with AVM was estimated to be 6% (95% CI, 1%–11%). Feeding artery aneurysms were significantly more common among the 29 patients presenting with SAH (52%; n = 15) than in the 132 cases with intracerebral hemorrhage (17%; n = 23) or in the 34 patients with intraventricular hemorrhage (15%; n = 5; $P < .001$).

Intranidal aneurysms occurred in 35 (8%) patients with AVM. By univariate comparison, intranidal aneurysms were detected significantly more often in patients who presented with ICH (11%; n = 22) than in those without

Table 15.2 Multivariate Logistic Regression Model Testing the Effect of Different Aneurysm Types on Incident Hemorrhage in 463 Patients with Arteriovenous Malformation (AVM)

	Odds Ratio	95% Confidence Interval	P Value
Feeding artery aneurysm	2.11	1.18–3.78	.012
Intranidal aneurysm	1.83	0.79–4.21	.158
Unrelated aneurysms	1.69	0.72–3.95	.228
Patient age	1.00	0.99–1.01	.923
Female gender	0.65	0.43–0.98	.042
AVM size°	0.94	0.93–0.96	<.0001
Deep venous drainage component	2.42	1.58–3.69	<.0001

°Maximum diameter in mm increments.

hemorrhagic presentation (5%; n = 13) ($P = .023$) (see Fig. 15–5). The effect of intranidal aneurysms on AVM hemorrhage, however, was not significant in the multivariate model controlling for age, gender, AVM size, venous drainage pattern, and the two other aneurysm types (Table 15.2). No significant association was found for intranidal aneurysms with intracerebral (12%), intraventricular hemorrhage (15%), or SAH (3%) ($P = .3$) (see Table 15.2).

Thirty-two (7%) patients were found to have *arterial aneurysms unrelated to blood-flow to the AVM.* No significant associations were found between unrelated arterial aneurysms and AVM hemorrhage at initial presentation or with either ICH (7%), intraventricular hemorrhage (3%), or SAH (18%) ($P = .2$).

Our findings suggest that feeding artery aneurysms constitute an independent risk factor for hemorrhagic AVM presentation and may therefore be considered for surgical or endovascular treatment. However, a number of limitations should caution against final conclusions about treatment recommendations: Currently, population-based rates of death after AVM hemorrhage are unknown, and data from referral center patient cohorts may underestimate the overall frequency of AVM hemorrhage,[166] thereby leading to the possibility of a systematic error in this single-center analysis. Second, only 22% of our patients with incident ICH demonstrated aneurysms on an AVM feeding vessel, and only 52% of all patients presenting with SAH had a feeding artery aneurysm. Given the prevalence of feeding artery aneurysms in our sample, the attributable risk calculation suggests that only 6% of hemorrhages would have been prevented if all feeding artery aneurysms in the study sample had been eliminated.

Seizures

Seizures—not caused by hemorrhage—are the initial symptom in 16% to 53% of patients,[167] often alerting the physician to the presence of an AVM before it ruptures. Although seizure frequency has rarely been reported, the treatment response to antiepileptic medication is good.[168]

The available literature documents a remarkable variation in incidence of seizure (Table 15.3). The rate of seizure as a presenting feature of AVM varies from 28% (Cooperative Study) to 67%.[71] Reports vary too widely for one to consider that the severity,[169,170] ease of control with

Table 15.3 Seizure as the First Sign of Arteriovenous Malformation

Study (Year)[°]	No. of Cases	Cases with Seizure Presentation (%)				
		Total	Seizures Alone	Seizures plus Hemorrhage	Generalized Seizures	Focal Seizures
Stein and Wolpert (1980)[119,238]	121	43.8	36.8	7.4	—	—
Parkinson and Bachers (1980)[239]	100	67	—	—	—	—
Pertuiset et al (1979)[240]	162	37.6	25.3	12.3	41	59
Morello and Borhi[118]	154	35.0	20.1	14.9	—	—
Troupp et al (1970)[241]	138	26	—	—	—	—
Cooperative Study (1966)[71]	406	28	—	—	—	—
Paterson and McKissock (1956)[60]	110	46.4	—	—	—	—
Moody and Poppen (1970)[242]	105	50.5	40	10.5	55	45
Tönnis (1967)[243]	215	48.3	—	—	—	—
Krayenbühl and Yasargil (1959)[151]	608	41.2	—	—	—	—

[°]Superscript numbers indicate chapter references.

medication, and prognosis for hemorrhage are fully understood. The frequency of seizures correlates so poorly with AVM location that at present no specific relationships can be claimed. None was found in our series.

The *type of seizure* is often unreported. Several types of attacks labeled as seizures occur. The majority are partial or partial complex seizures, and the grand mal type is encountered in 27% to 35% of all seizures.[63,168] Some are typical focal epileptic seizures not associated with loss of consciousness. Others have been of the jacksonian type, with or without the loss of consciousness. Finally, several patients have experienced only a sudden loss of function, without tonic-clonic activity and without headache or loss of consciousness. Whether this latter group has epilepsy per se is difficult to determine.[70] Ozer and colleagues[171] were unable to distinguish focal AVM seizures from those of other causes in their 14 cases of seizure among 65 AVMs. Earlier opinions continue to influence clinical thinking but have been superseded by modern data. The most persistent opinion currently unsupported by data is the notion that there is more variation in type and frequency of attacks in AVM seizures than in cryptogenic or traumatic epilepsy.[116,172]

A small but separate literature exists for occipital AVMs, in which the seizures appear to have migrainous features,[173] including such complaints as "sudden dimming of everything in the right side of vision," "dimming of vision," and seeing "swirling spots of brightly colored lights," "red spots," or "frosted glass." In several cases, the visual complaints were followed by generalized seizure.

The *role of anatomic location* in seizure occurrence has received limited study, but suggestions have been made of a correlation of seizure with AVMs at the cortical surface. Turjman and associates[71,140,174,175] found seizures associated with AVMs of the cerebral surface but not with deep AVMs. We did find an independent association of seizures at initial AVM presentation and a vascular borderzone location (odds ratio 2.2; 95% CI, 1.3–3.7).[176]

The incidence of seizures alone compared with *seizures in association with hemorrhage* varies widely. Hemorrhage occurred within 1 year in only 15% of 90 cases of seizure in the Cooperative Study.[71] Turjman and colleagues[177] postulated a relationship between seizures and cortical AVMs

and a history of hemorrhage.[178] Whether the character of the seizure differs when it is associated with hematoma is not certain.

Headache

Headache is the presenting symptom in 7% to 48% of patients with AVM.[167] In contrast to early assumptions,[179] the headache in AVM is of no distinctive type, frequency, persistence, or severity. Speculations about a pattern that distinguishes AVM headache from classic or common migraine or that recurrent unilateral headache reflects an underlying AVM have proved unfounded.[180] The former idea appears to have originated with Mackenzie,[116] who emphasized the tendency of the headaches to occur before the aura and for the aura to persist beyond the few minutes that typifies migraine, a finding not confirmed by others. Because headache is a common complaint in the population at large, it has been difficult to determine whether the headache associated with AVM is unique to the condition. That the character of the headache can by migrainous and have the classic aura is amply documented.[181,182]

Nevertheless, the notion that recurrent unilateral headache should arouse suspicion of an ipsilateral AVM is outmoded. It may have started with Northfield,[183] whose 1940 report stated that the headache "may affect only one side of the head, usually the side on which the angioma is situated." Very little evidence supports this claim. The yield for AVMs in evaluation for headache is low; in one study, only 0.2% of patients with normal neurologic findings who underwent neuroimaging for headache were diagnosed with an AVM.[184] Rates of response to pharmacologic headache treatment in patients with AVM have not been studied so far.

The postoperative disappearance of migraine headaches is not unusual and may occur after any type of operation. Disappearance of migraine after operation was a common feature of the early literature, which comprised mostly single case reports. The question raised now is whether all patients with migraine should be evaluated for an AVM. At the very least, CT with administration of a large bolus of contrast agent should be carried out in such patients. If anything suspicious is noted, then MRI should be performed.

Clinical Manifestations

Neurologic Deficits

Focal neurologic deficits without signs of underlying hemorrhage have been reported in 1% to 40% of patients with AVMs.[185] This large range most likely reflects nonuniformity of definitions.[63] Slowly progressing neurologic deficits, which were once considered common,[186] are part of the presentation in only a few patients (4% to 8%). Progressing syndromes were thought to be due to "steal"—that is, cerebral artery hypotension leading to ischemia in brain tissue adjacent to the lesion caused by shunting of large blood volumes through the fistulas.[187,188] AVMs sometimes induce remarkable levels of arterial hypotension, but evidence for a causal link with symptoms is lacking.[185,189] Venous hypertension and mass effect of the nidus offer alternative explanations for progressing focal neurologic deficits.[190] Although AVMs occupy space, they do not act like tumors with invasive growth or perifocal edema, and their bulk effect is usually recognized only in terms of massive, distended draining veins. They may even hinder the circulation of cerebrospinal fluid, leading to hydrocephalus. Displacement of healthy brain tissue by the AVM sufficient to cause neurologic symptoms is rare.

PHYSIOLOGIC STUDIES

Physiologic evaluation of vascular malformations has centered on the study of AVMs.[191–195] Cerebral blood flow recordings indicate a varying degree of AV blood shunting within an AVM. The amount of shunting depends on the ratio of the feeding arteries to draining veins, the size of the lesion, and the number of shunts within the lesion. When shunting is great enough, left ventricular cardiac failure can occur, as has been seen in children with larger AVMs. Early intraoperative studies by Nornes and Grip[196]

underscore the dynamic changes that occur in blood flow through these malformations during occlusion of the various nutrient arteries and with systemic changes of blood pressure and flow. The fall in pressures proceeds in an orderly manner from the parent artery through branches, leading finally to the AVM, where pressures may be quite low; by inference, pressures are also low in normal adjacent brain supplied by these branches.[197] Remarkably little difference is found between the shear forces in vessels involved by an AVM and those in healthy vessels.

Evidence is now clear that the large feeding arteries lack autoregulation.[198] Angiographic signs of disordered autoregulation after surgery include enlargement of an artery proximal to an AVM in the days after the malformation is occluded by either embolization or surgical ligation (Fig. 15–19). This postocclusion ectasia remains for days to weeks. Persistent ectasia leads to decreased flow and stasis in the arterial system proximal to the AVM,[131] indicating that obliteration of the shunt results in a global increase in blood flow.

In the postoperative state, arterial stasis, even vein thrombosis and venous infarction in the normal brain, has been described.[119,199] The pressure in the feeding arteries is initially high after surgery and may lead to hemorrhagic complications described by Spetzler and associates[200] as "perfusion pressure breakthrough." The pressure and flow that drive the nutrient blood to an AVM are thought to be redirected to the normal circulation after the obliteration of an AVM. This rerouted blood pressures the local arteries beyond their capacities, resulting in edema and then hemorrhage in the area. Postoperative stasis, high arterial pressures, hemorrhagic complications, or a combination of these findings have been described by others as well.[110,131,201–204] Studies from our institution have indicated a shift of the autoregulation limits toward lower pressures,

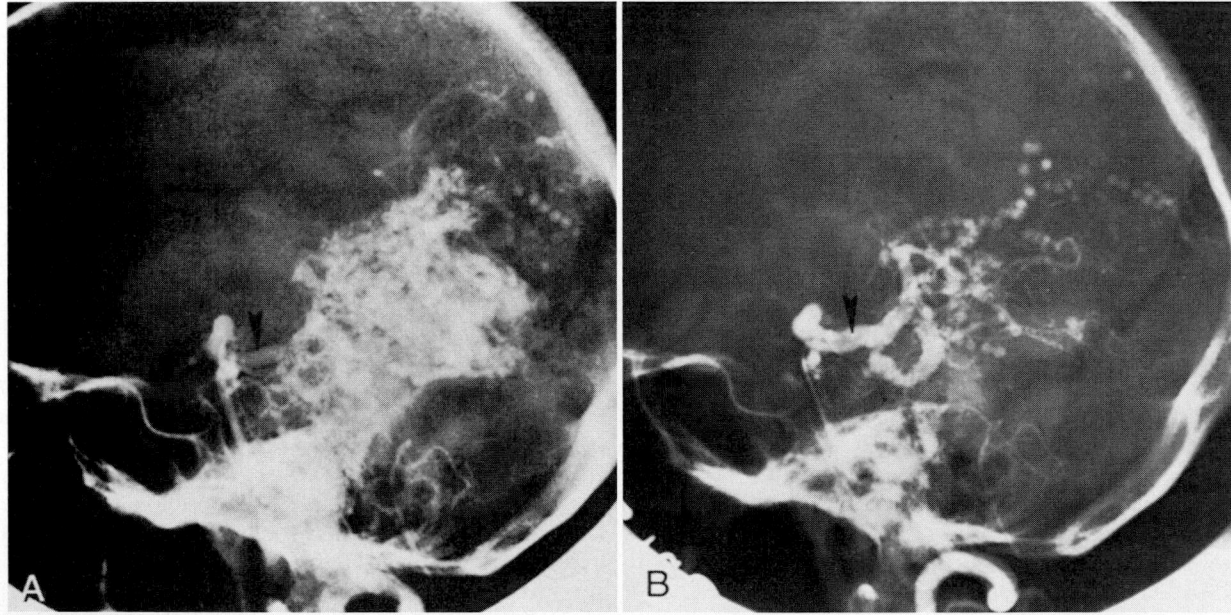

FIGURE 15–19   A, *Large arteriovenous malformation (AVM) fed by a posterior cerebral artery* (arrowhead). *B, Enlargement of the posterior cerebral artery* (arrowhead) *after successful embolic occlusion of portions of the AVM and feeding artery, with marked reduction of flow through the AVM but with enlargement of the feeding artery.*

preserved responsiveness to CO_2, and pharmacologically induced vasodilatation in arteries adjacent to AVMs.[197,205]

Former assumptions of perfusion defects in the brain adjacent to an AVM have proved difficult to certify. In a study of 11 cases of hemispheral AVM, single-photon emission computed tomography (SPECT) was used to compare the regions of the AVM with a matching contralateral site before and after administration of acetazolamide. The defects in flow surrounding the AVM lesions were found to be related to the size of the AVM, not to any effects explained by local arterial pressure.[206] Preservation of cerebrovascular reserve was also evident, arguing against a specific defect in perfusion around an AVM such as that postulated for steal.

OTHER VASCULAR MALFORMATIONS

Distinction from Other Vascular Malformations

Once grouped together with other intracranial vascular malformations and abnormalities, AVMs have become better defined in the past few decades, distinguishing them from other entities. Lesions mislabeled as "AVM" are included in older data sets, often rendering long-term studies on the natural history and outcome of AVMs fruitless. The heterogeneity continues to confound current studies. Clearly, international common standards relying on modern imaging techniques and consensus agreements for diagnosing brain AVMs are needed. Among the lesions historically and currently contributing to the uncertainty in nomenclature are AV fistulas caused by trauma, occlusion of the venous sinus or sinuses with the subsequent formation of new collaterals, occlusion of branch arteries with the compensatory formation of pial-to-pial arterial collaterals, and a group of currently rather well-defined malformations and abnormalities. In order to better delineate the population in this present study, such lesions warrant more detailed descriptions, because they are so similar to AVMs in clinical presentation, detection with diagnostic techniques, and treatment options. For the current study, patients with any of these malformations and abnormalities have been excluded from the study population unless the lesions were found as concurrent conditions.

Acquired Arteriovenous Fistulas

Some AV fistulas that appear on angiography to be AVMs arise from trauma and thrombosis of large veins or sinuses. Two major causes have been identified, trauma and venous thrombosis.

Trauma

Trauma to the brain surface from closed-head injury presumably may join or enlarge the existing AV shunts roughly 90 μm near the superior sagittal sinus and possibly in other sites. Once linked or enlarged, such fistulas would presumably lose their autoregulation and be subject to the same enlargement typical of any AV link. Patients with such lesions should have a history or should show evidence of prior head injury, and the injury should be confined to

the brain surface. To date, no ready classification for these lesions has been developed.

Venous Thrombosis

Thrombosis of a large vein or sinus may create a high enough resistance to normal arterial flow to force creation of new pathways.[175,207,208] Angiography usually shows delayed filling of the carotid or vertebrobasilar arteries and those branches having access to a patent vein or sinus, such as the meningeal and other dural arteries, which dilate and convolute in a manner seen in congenital AVMs. These shunts can develop in a fairly short time, possibly months. If sinus thrombosis occurs, a major hemorrhagic lesion may follow. There is still uncertainty about (1) whether the hypertrophied channels become independent of autoregulation or can be expected to subside if the venous obstruction is relieved is still unknown; (2) whether they have certain theoretical limits in size and extent or continue to develop until they hemorrhage; and (3) whether their proper treatment is ligation or neglect.

Dural Arteriovenous Fistulas

The majority of dural AV fistulas are supplied by branches of the external carotid artery or muscular branches of the vertebral artery (Fig. 15–20). Their venous channels usually empty into the major sinus, depending on the location of the AV shunt. They may be congenital, but posttraumatic occurrence or manifestation of an AV fistula in the setting of a sinus thrombosis is also known. Often the

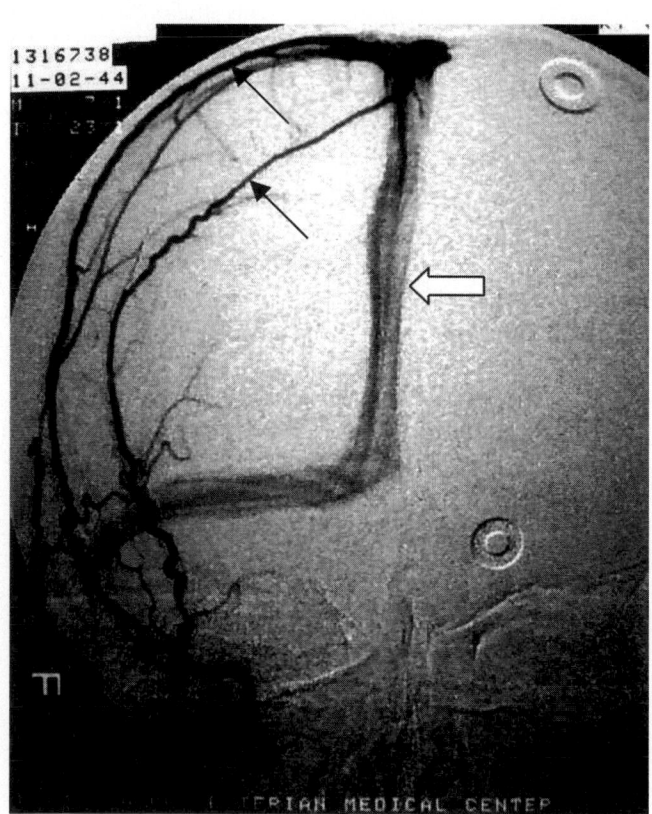

FIGURE 15–20 *Dural fistula connecting branches of the external carotid artery* (black arrows) *with the superior sagittal sinus* (white arrow).

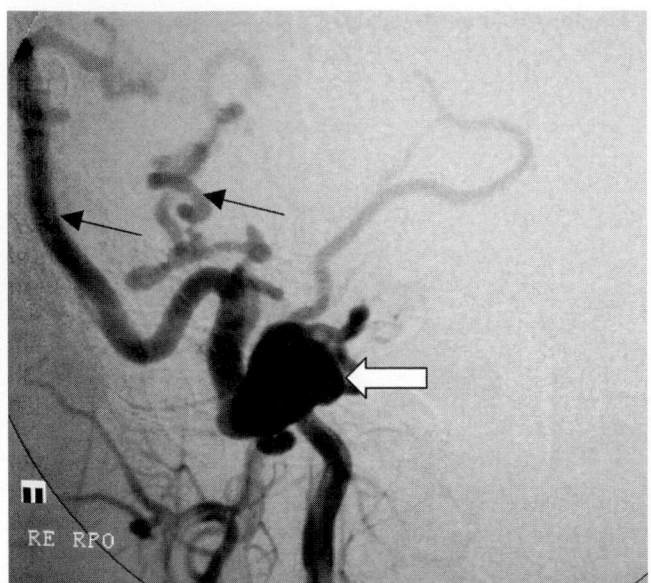

FIGURE 15–21 *Carotid-cavernous fistula filling the cavernous sinus* (white arrow) *and draining through the intracranial venous system* (black arrows).

lesions manifest as bruits, headaches, and signs of increased intracranial pressure, but they may also cause hemorrhage.

A common presentation in a dural AV shunt is the carotid-cavernous fistula (Fig. 15–21). This subtype consists mainly of a single shunt that links the internal carotid artery during its passage through the cavernous sinus with a portion of the cavernous sinus. Although they often arise after trauma, dural AV shunts are also known to occur spontaneously. The classic symptom complex features an injected sclera of the affected eye, chemosis, ophthalmoplegia, a bruit, and, in severe cases, even loss of vision.

Other Anomalies with Fistulae

Vein of Galen Malformations

Vascular malformations that involve the vein of Galen region and that are characterized by venous dilatation of the great cerebral vein or its precursors have long been grouped together, regardless of vastly differing pathology. It was only in 1986 that Raybaud and Strother[8] described the dilated midline vein as the embryologic precursor of the vein of Galen, the median vein of the prosencephalon. The vein of Galen and the straight sinus form after the stage of the 50-mm embryo. Because the pallium is beginning to grow without established intrinsic vascularization between 21 to 23 mm (6 weeks' gestation) and 50 mm (11 weeks' gestation), the event leading to the defect must occur at the stage of the 21- to 23-mm embryo. There are fundamental differences between lesions in which the vein of Galen is absent (the malformation per se) and a situation in which a deep-seated AVM drains into a dilated vein of Galen. Prenatal diagnoses of the latter confirmed true vein of Galen malformations further support their distinction from AVMs, for which in utero findings are yet missing.[10,11] Consequently, vein of Galen malformations become clinically manifest in neonates with cardiac failure due to high intracranial shunt flow, whereas infants present with macrocephaly or neurologic symptoms.[9] Vein of Galen malformations are usually not detected at later stages of life.

Developmental Venous Anomalies

Developmental venous anomalies (DVAs) represent extreme variations of hemispheric white matter and tectal venous drainage. These lesions have come under scrutiny because of the use of MRI (Fig. 15–22) and sophisticated angiography. They are represented by a deep prominent vein that appears late on the venous phase of an arteriogram and is associated with a finger-like projection from the main vein. This appearance is characteristic on angiography, the lack of an arterial component in DVAs distinguishing them from AVMs. They are associated with cavernous malformations in more than 30% of cases[209] and often remain clinically asymptomatic. Their role in ischemic or hemorrhagic events may best be explained by secondary failure of efficient drainage of brain tissue due to insufficient autoregulation mechanisms or by undetected associated lesions.

Cavernous Malformations (Cavernomas)

Cavernous malformations (cavernomas) represent the only true venous malformation of the brain. Studies from the pre-MRI era estimate an incidence of 0.5%.[210] Because of their characteristic appearance on MRI (less so on CT), cavernous malformations are becoming more and more the subject of reports in the literature.[143,211–213] These lesions rarely occupy a clinically significant amount of space in the brain but may be located in clinically important cortical or subcortical regions and are occasionally multiple. Although they are masses, they do not produce displacements commensurable with those of neoplasms. Cavernous malformations are composed of cavernous channels with multiple areas of thrombosis. Because the flow through these lesions

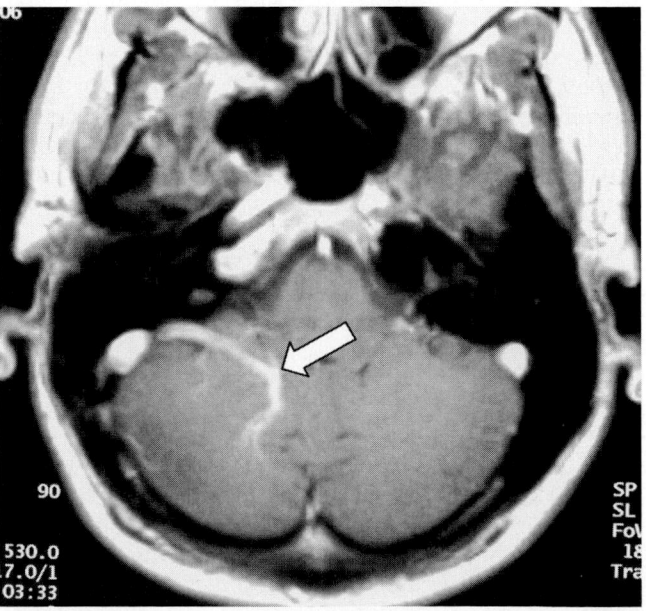

FIGURE 15–22 *Developmental venous anomaly (DVA) of the cerebellum* (arrow).

is minimal, they are rarely seen on angiograms. They are identified by contrast enhancement on CT scans and their characteristic configuration. They are frequently associated with headache and seizures, and occasionally with hemorrhage. Although cavernous malformations are not readily identified on CT, the distinctive cat's-eye appearance on MRI has made their diagnosis more common since the introduction of this modality. The cat's-eye appearance is no longer considered pathognomonic for cavernous angiomas.

The clinical importance of cavernous malformations is unclear except in a differential diagnosis from tumor and other contrast-enhancing masses. They usually manifest as a seizure disorder, like venous malformation.[121,183,214–216] Cavernous malformations may also be seen in patients with headaches, which may or may not be related to the lesions. It is very often difficult to determine a one-to-one relationship between lesion and symptoms. The lesions may occur anywhere, including the cortical surface and deep in the brainstem. MRI has allowed study of family members, which in a small series of cases has suggested a hereditary basis for some instances of multiple cavernous malformations.[91,217] A predominance among Hispanic people has been suggested.[218]

Clinically, hemorrhage from cavernous and venous malformations is not as common as hemorrhage from AVMs.[193,213,215,219] However, as these heretofore obscure conditions are recognized with increasing frequency on CT, we have come to realize that they can be the source of parenchymal and ventricular hemorrhage. Hemorrhages from telangiectasis are rarely recognized by the clinician, although some of these cases may actually be hemorrhage from cryptic malformations.[143] On the other hand, pathologists have recognized a high incidence of microscopic hemorrhages associated with cavernous, venous, and telangiectatic malformations.

Cavernomas are occasionally multiple,[220] and familial forms with autosomal dominant transmission have been found. Simultaneous occurrence of cavernomas with AVMs has been seen in a few patients (Fig. 15–23). In some cases, an anomaly of endothelial growth factor has been identified.[221] Alterations on chromosomes 3 and 7 have been detected as genetic correlates.[222]

Telangiectasis

Telangiectases are uncommon anomalies composed of small clusters of capillary-like vessels located in the brainstem or cerebellum.[223] They are often deep and multiple. Their clinical significance is dubious. Telangiectases may rarely be the source of a large hemorrhage, which may cause death if located in a critical area. Mostly, these lesions are curiosities noted postmortem. Although they frequently demonstrate small microhemorrhages on histologic examination, the hemorrhage does not appear to be large enough to create a clinical syndrome. When associated with Rendu-Osler-Weber disease, telangiectasia is recognized elsewhere in the body. Rapid advances in genetics are shedding light on the chromosomal aberrations that underlie these anomalies. For the autosomal dominant disorder that is hereditary hemorrhagic telangiectasia, linkage studies have implicated chromosome 12.[224]

The telangiectases have long been considered curiosities for the pathologist to describe, with only rare clinical significance,[225] but findings now suggest otherwise.[95] Before

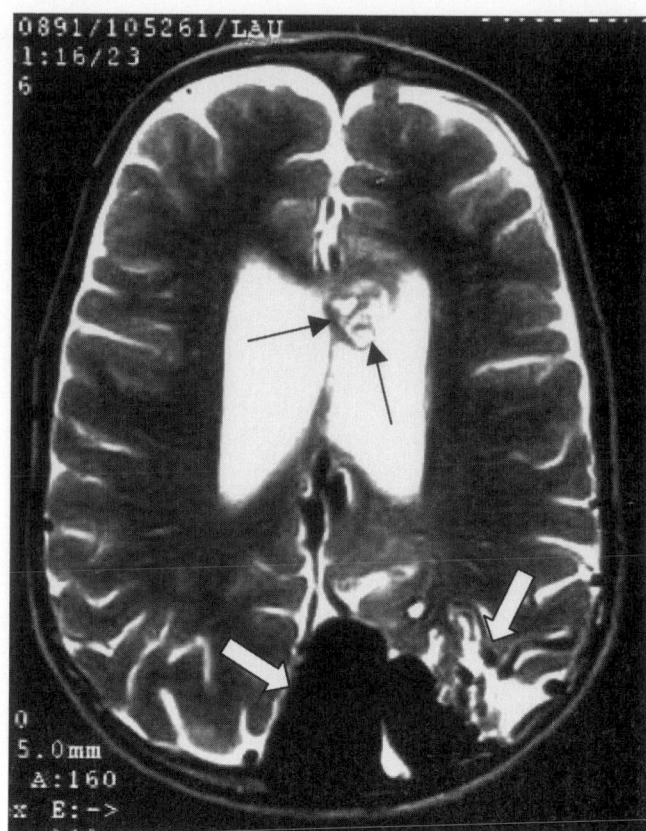

FIGURE 15–23 *Cavernous malformation* (black arrows) *and large posterior arteriovenous malformation with ectatic draining veins* (white arrows).

the availability of high-field MRI, they were most commonly found only at postmortem examinations.

In telangiectasia that manifests clinically, hemorrhage is the common syndrome, most often in the white matter of the brainstem, cerebellum, and diencephalic regions, their usual sites of occurrence. Rarely, the hemorrhages may be incapacitating or fatal, and postmortem examination may uncover the lesion as a thrombosed telangiectasia.

Moyamoya Disease

Moyamoya is an unusual form of chronic cerebrovascular occlusive disease with angiographic findings of bilateral stenosis or occlusion of the terminal portion of the internal carotid artery together with a vascular network at the base of the brain.[229] The Japanese word *moyamoya* has been translated as "hazy puff of smoke." The description arose from the initial angiographic appearance of this pathologic vascularization: The tiny size and large number of vessels imaged made the combination look like a cloud or a puff of smoke instead of single arteries. The numerous, dilated small vessels have also been termed "rete mirabile."[230] Formerly described only in Japanese patients, moyamoya disease has now been found in other populations, although rarely. The disease shows a female preponderance (female-to-male ratio 1.8); age distribution peaks at 10 to 14 years, with another, smaller increase at 25 to 49 years (adult-type moyamoya).[229]

None of the proposed hypotheses for the pathogenesis of this disease—congenital or acquired—has been confirmed, and the etiology remains unknown. Hereditary factors may play a role in the occurrence of or susceptibility to the disease, as suggested by the occasional familial occurrence and association with other congenital diseases, such as sickle cell anemia, von Recklinghausen's disease, and Down's syndrome. However, the clinical manifestation and disease progression are not congenital, and proposed disease mechanisms include vasculitis, infection, thrombosis, juvenile atherosclerosis, cranial trauma, and abnormalities of sympathetic nerve endings.

In the vascular network of perforating arteries (the so-called moyamoya vessels), the following histologic changes can be observed: dilated vessels with a relatively thin wall, this type being more prominent in children, and thick-walled arteries showing luminal stenosis. With hemodynamic stress or aging, the dilated arteries with attenuated walls may predispose to the formation of microaneurysms, the rupture of which is considered one of the mechanisms leading to parenchymatous hemorrhages in patients with moyamoya disease. Clinically, ischemic and hemorrhagic symptoms are encountered. The ischemic type dominates in childhood, and transient ischemic attacks occur more often than infarctions, manifesting a variety of symptoms. The hemorrhagic type is more common in adult patients. Bleeding occurs, commonly in multiple and repetitive intervals, and massive bleeding, although infrequent, often leads to death.

Typical angiographic findings were considered indispensable to the diagnosis of moyamoya disease. As the quality of MRI and magnetic resonance angiography improved, however, the diagnosis was also made if either modality clearly demonstrated all the findings indicative of moyamoya. Moyamoya-type vascular changes have been observed in patients with AVMs (Fig. 15–24).[231] Whether

the two entities are linked biologically or genetically, or whether the moyamoya-type vascular pathology observed in patients with AVMs merely results from hemodynamic changes associated with the AVM, remains unclear.

Moyamoya Disease and "High-Flow Angiopathy"
Growing awareness of a relationship between AVMs and high-grade intracranial stenoses has left unsettled which of the two processes begins first. Some investigators envision a so-called high-flow angiopathy with the development of lesions to the intima in vessels feeding an AVM, the lesions building to the point of causing severe stenosis and occlusion of feeding arteries.[232] Another thesis is that the underlying process of severe stenosis known as moyamoya triggers sufficient vasodilatation in distal vessels as to cause AV links, which take on a life of their own and have the angiographic appearance of AVMs. Further work is needed to clarify these issues.

References

1. Rokitansky C: Handbuch der allgemeinen pathologischen Anatomie. Wien, Austria, Braumüller & Seidel, 1846, pp 276–277.
2. Emmanuel C: Ein Fall von Angioma arteriale racemosum des Gehirns. Deutsche Zeitschr Nervenheilk 14:288–318, 1899.
3. Stapf C, Mohr JP, Mast H: History of concepts on the etiology of brain arteriovenous malformations. Neurology 58(Suppl 3):A342, 2002.
4. Mall FP: On the development of the blood-vessels of the brain in the human embryo. Am J Anat 4:1, 1905.
5. Evans HM: On the development of the aortae, cardinal and umbilical veins, and the other blood vessels of vertebrate embryos from capillaries. Anat Rec 3:498–519, 1909.
6. Streeter GL: The developmental alterations in the vascular system of the brain of the human embryo. (Carnegie Inst Wash Pub 271.) Contrib Embryol 8:5–38, 1918.
7. Moniz E: L'encéphalographie artérielle, son importance dans la localisation des tumeurs cérébrales. Rev Neurol 2:72–90, 1927.
8. Raybaud CA, Strother CM: Persisting abnormal embryonic vessels in intracranial arteriovenous malformations. Acta Radiol Suppl 369:136–138, 1986.
9. Lasjaunias P: Vascular Diseases in Neonates, Infants and Children: Interventional Neuroradiology Management. Berlin, Springer-Verlag, 1997.
10. Yuval Y, Lerner A, Lipitz S, et al: Prenatal diagnosis of vein of Galen aneurysmal malformation: Report of two cases with proposal for prognostic indices. Prenat Diagn 17:972–977, 1997.
11. Campi A, Scotti G, Filippi M, et al: Antenatal diagnosis of vein of Galen aneurysmal malformation: MR study of fetal brain and postnatal follow-up. Neuroradiology 38:87–90, 1996.
12. Pschyrembel W, Dudenhausen JW: Praktische Geburtshilfe mit geburtshilflichen Operationen, 17th ed. Berlin, Walter de Gruyter, 1991.
13. Weaver DD, Brandt IK. Catalog of Prenatally Diagnosed Conditions, 3rd ed. Baltimore, Johns Hopkins University Press, 1999.
14. Baird WF, Stitt DG: Arteriovenous aneurysm of the cerebellum in a premature infant. Pediatrics 24:455–457, 1959.
15. Padget DH: The development of the cranial arteries in the human embryo. (Carnegie Inst Wash Pub. 575.) Contrib Embryol 32:205, 1948.
16. Stapf C, Mohr JP, Sciacca RR, et al: Incident hemorrhage risk of brain arteriovenous malformations located in the arterial border-zones. Stroke 31:2365–1268, 2000.
17. van den Bergh R, van der Eecken H: Anatomy and embryology of the cerebral circulation. Prog Brain Res 30:1, 1968.
18. Van den Bergh R, van der Eecken H: Anatomy and embryology of cerebral circulation. Prog Brain Res 30:1–25, 1968.
19. Van der Eecken HM, Fisher CM, Adams RD: The anatomy and functional significance of the meningeal arterial anastomoses of the human brain. J Neuropathol Exp Neurol 12:132–157, 1953.

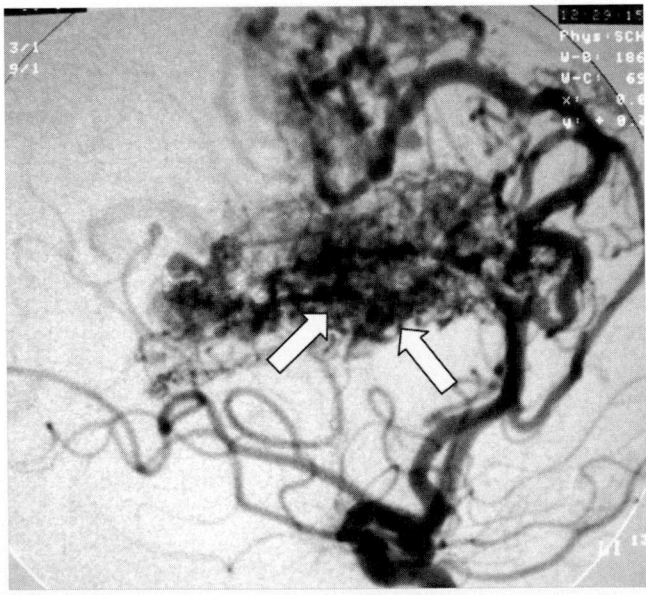

FIGURE 15–24 *Angioproliferative changes (arrows) in an arteriovenous malformation resembling those found in moyamoya disease.*

20. Risau W, Lemmon V: Changes in the vascular extracellular matrix during embryonic vasculogenesis and angiogenesis. Dev Biol 125:441–450, 1988.
21. Bär T, Wolff JR: The formation of capillary basement membranes during internal vascularization of the rat's cerebral cortex. Z Zellforsch 133:231–248, 1972.
22. Krum JM, More NS, Rosenstein JM: Brain angiogenesis: Variations in vascular basement membrane glycoprotein immunoreactivity. Exp Neurol 111:152–165, 1991.
23. Bobik A, Campbell JH: Vascular derived growth factors: Cell biology, pathophysiology, and pharmacology. Pharm Rev 45:1–42, 1993.
24. Risau W: Angiogenetic factors. Progr Growth Factor Res 2:71–79, 1990.
25. Nelson MD, Gonzalez-Gomez I, Gilles FH: The search for human telencephalic ventriculofugal arteries. AJNR Am J Neuroradiol 12:215–222, 1991.
26. Hung PC, Wang HS, Yeh YS, et al: Coexistence of schizencephaly and intracranial arteriovenous malformation in an infant. AJNR Am J Neuroradiol 17:1921–1922, 1996.
27. Turjman F, Massoud TF, Viñuela F, et al: Correlation of the angioarchitectural features of cerebral arteriovenous malformations with clinical presentation of hemorrhage. Neurosurgery 37:856–862, 1995.
28. Meisel HJ, Mansmann U, Alvarez H, et al: Cerebral arteriovenous malformations and associated aneurysms: Analysis of 305 cases from a series of 662 patients. Neurosurgery 46:793–802, 2000.
29. Anderson RMcD, Blackwood W: The association of arteriovenous angioma and saccular aneurysm of arteries of the brain. J Pathol Bacteriol 77:101–110, 1959.
30. Voigt K, Beck U, Reinshagen G: A complex cerebral vascular malformation studied by angiography: Multiple aneurysms, angiomas and arterial ectasia. Neuroradiology 5:117–123, 1973.
31. Miyasaka K, Wolpert SM, Prager RJ: The association of cerebral aneurysms, infundibula, and intracranial arteriovenous malformations. Stroke 13:196–203, 1982.
32. Quick CM, Hashimoto T, Young WL: Lack of flow regulation may explain the development of arteriovenous malformations. Neurol Res 23:641–644, 2001.
33. Otto KB, Lierse W: Die Kappilarisierung verschiedener Teile des menschlichen Gehirns in der Fetalperiode und in der ersten Lebensjahren. Acta Anat (Basel) 77:25–36, 1970.
34. Laves W: Ein Fall von Angioma arteriali racemosum des Gehirnes im Bereiche der rechten Arter: Cerebri media, nebst einem Beitrag zur Frage der Entwicklung von Rankenangiomen im Gehirn. Jahrb Psychiatr Neurol 44:55, 1925.
35. Müller G: Zur Pathologie der arterio-venösen Rankenangiome des Gehirns. Dtsch Z Nervenheilk 172:361–376, 1954.
36. Kaplan HA, Aronson SM, Browder EJ: Vascular malformations of the brain: An anatomical study. J Neurosurg 18:830–635, 1961.
37. McCormick WF: The pathology of vascular ("arteriovenous") malformations. J Neurosurg 24:807–816, 1966.
38. Isoda K, Fukuda H, Takamura N, Hamamoto Y: Arteriovenous malformation of the brain: Histological study and micrometric measurement of abnormal vessels. Acta Pathol Jpn 31:883–893, 1981.
39. Challa VR, Moody DM, Brown WR: Vascular malformations of the central nervous system. J Neuropathol Exp Neurol 54:609–621, 1995.
40. Lamszus K, Schmidt NO, Ergün S, Westphal M: Isolation and culture of human neuromicrovascular endothelial cells for the study of angiogenesis in vitro. J Neurosci Res 55:370–381, 1999.
41. Hashimoto T, Mesa-Tejada R, Quick CM, et al: Evidence of increased endothelial cell turnover in brain arteriovenous malformations. Neurosurgery 49:124–131, 2001.
42. Gallione CJ, Pasyk KA, Boon LM, et al: A gene for familial venous malformations maps to chromosome 9p in a second large kindred. J Med Genet 32:197–199, 1995.
43. Hashimoto T, Lam T, Boudreau NJ, et al: Abnormal balance in the angiopoietin-Tie2 system in human brain arteriovenous malformations. Circ Res 89:111–113, 2001.
44. Vikkula M, Boon LM, Carraway KL, et al: Vascular dysmorphogenesis caused by an activating mutation in the receptor tyrosine kinase TIE2. Cell 87:1181–1190, 1996.
45. Rothbart D, Awad IA, Lee J, et al: Expression of angiogenic factors and structural proteins in central nervous system vascular malformations. Neurosurgery 38:915–924, 1996.
46. Hashimoto T, Emala CW, Joshi S, et al: Abnormal pattern of Tie-2 and vascular endothelial growth factor receptor expression in human cerebral arteriovenous malformations. Neurosurgery 47:910–918, 2000.
47. Hirschi KK, Rohovski SA, D'Amore PA: PDGF, TGF-beta, and heterotypic cell-cell interactions mediate endothelial cell-induced recruitment of 10T1/2 cells and their differentiation to a smooth muscle fate. J Cell Biol 141:805–814, 1998.
48. Malik G, Abdulrauf S, Yang XY, et al: Expression of transforming growth factor-beta complex in arteriovenous malformations. Neurol Med Chir (Tokyo) 38(Suppl):161–164, 1998.
49. Sonstein WJ, Kader A, Michelsen WJ, et al: Expression of vascular endothelial growth factor in pediatric and adult cerebral arteriovenous malformations: An immunocytochemical study. J Neurosurg 85:838–845, 1996.
50. Bourdeau A, Cymerman U, Paquet ME, et al: Endoglin expression is reduced in normal vessels but still detectable in arteriovenous malformations of patients with hereditary hemorrhagic telangiectasia type 1. Am J Pathol 156:911–923, 2000.
51. Blottner D: Nitric oxide and fibroblast growth factor in autonomic nervous system: Short- and long-term messengers in autonomic pathway and target organ control. Prog Neurobiol 51:423–438, 1997.
52. Abdulrauf SI, Malik GM, Awad IA: Spontaneous angiographic obliteration of cerebral arteriovenous malformations. Neurosurgery 44:280–287, 1999.
53. Kader A, Goodrich JT, Sonstein WJ, et al: Recurrent cerebral arteriovenous malformations after negative postoperative angiograms. J Neurosurg 85:14–18, 1996.
54. Robinson JR, Awad IA, Zhou P, et al: Expression of basement membrane and endothelial cell adhesion molecules in vascular malformations of the brain: Preliminary observations and working hypothesis. Neurol Res 17:49–58, 1995.
55. Yamada S, Liwnicz B, Lonser RR, Knierim D: Scanning electron microscopy of arteriovenous malformations. Neurol Res 21:541–544, 1999.
56. Burchiel KJ, Clarke H, Ojemann GA, et al: Use of stimulation mapping and corticography in the excision of arteriovenous malformations in sensorimotor and language-related neocortex. Neurosurgery 24:322–327, 1989.
57. Lazar RM, Marshall RS, Pile-Spellman J, et al: Interhemispheric transfer of language in patients with left frontal cerebral arteriovenous malformation 1. Neuropsychologia 38:1325–1332, 2000.
58. Stapf C, Mohr JP, Sciacca RR, et al: Incident hemorrhage risk of brain arteriovenous malformations located in the arterial borderzones. Stroke 31:2365–2368, 2000.
59. Stapf C, Mohr JP, Pile-Spellman J, et al: Concurrent arterial aneurysms in brain arteriovenous malformations with hemorrhagic presentation. J Neurol Neurosurg Psychiatry 73:294–298, 2002.
60. Paterson JH, McKissock W: A clinical survey of intracranial angiomas with special reference to their mode of progression and surgical treatment: A report of 110 cases. Brain 79:233, 1956.
61. Turjman F, Massoud TF, Vinuela F, et al: Aneurysms related to cerebral arteriovenous malformations: Superselective angiographic assessment in 58 patients. AJNR Am J Neuroradiol 15:1601–1605, 1994.
62. Stapf C, Hofmeister C, Mast H, et al: The feasibility of an Internet web-based, international study on brain arteriovenous malformations (The AVM World Study) [abstract]. Stroke 31:322, 2000.
63. Hofmeister C, Stapf C, Hartmann A, et al: Demographic, morphological, and clinical characteristics of 1289 patients with brain arteriovenous malformation. Stroke 31:1307–1310, 2000.
64. Yasargil MG (ed): Microneurosurgery. New York, Thieme Medical, 1987.
65. Willinsky R, Lasjaunias P, terBrugge K, Pruvost P: Brain arteriovenous malformations: Analysis of the angio-architecture in relationship to hemorrhage (based on 152 patients explored and/or treated at the hopital de Bicetre between 1981 and 1986). J Neuroradiol 15:225–237, 1988.
66. Spetzler RF Martin NA: A proposed grading system for arteriovenous malformations. J Neurosurg 65:476–483, 1986.
67. Nehls DG, Pittman HW: Spontaneous regression of arteriovenous malformations. Neurosurgery 11:776–780, 1982.
68. Willinsky R, Lasjaunias P, terBrugge K, Pruvost P: Brain arteriovenous malformations: Analysis of the angio-architecture in relationship to hemorrhage (based on 152 patients explored and/or treated

at the hopital de Bicetre between 1981 and 1986). J Neuroradiol 15:225–237, 1988.

69. Morgan MK, Sekhon LH, Finfer S, Grinnell V: Delayed neurological deterioration following resection of arteriovenous malformations of the brain. J Neurosurg 90:695–701, 1999.

70. Perret G: The epidemiology and clinical course of arteriovenous malformations. In Pia HW, Gleave JRW, Grote E, Zierski J (eds): Cerebral Angiomas: Advances in Diagnosis and Therapy. New York, Springer-Verlag, 1975, p 21.

71. Perret G, Nishioka H: Report on the cooperative study of intracranial aneurysms and subarachnoid hemorrhage. Section VI: Arteriovenous malformations. An analysis of 545 cases of cranio-cerebral arteriovenous malformations and fistulae reported to the cooperative study. J Neurosurg 25:467–490, 1966.

72. Courville CB: Intracranial tumors: Notes upon a series of three thousand verified cases with some current observations pertaining to their mortality. Bull Los Angeles Neurol Soc 32(Suppl 2):1–80, 1967.

73. Jellinger K: The morphology of centrally-situated angiomas. In Pia HW, Gleave JRW, Grote E, Zierski J (eds): Cerebral Angiomas: Advances in Diagnosis and Therapy. New York, Springer-Verlag, 1975, pp 9–20.

74. Jellinger K: Vascular malformations of the central nervous system: A morphological overview. Neurosurg Rev 9:177–216, 1986.

75. Sarwar M, McCormick WF: Intracerebral venous angioma: Case report and review. Arch Neurol 35:323–325, 1978.

76. McCormick WF, Rosenfield DB: Massive brain hemorrhage: A review of 144 cases and an examination of their causes. Stroke 4:946–954, 1973.

77. Griffiths PD, Worthy S, Gholkar A: Incidental intracranial pathology in patients investigated for carotid stenosis. Neuroradiology 38:25, 1996.

78. Yue NC, Longstreth WT Jr, Elster AD, et al: Clinically serious abnormalities found incidentally at MR imaging of the brain: Data from the Cardiovascular Health Study. Radiology 202:41–46, 1997.

79. Katzman GL, Dagher AP, Patronas NJ: Incidental findings on brain magnetic resonance imaging from 1000 asymptomatic volunteers. JAMA 282:36–39, 1999.

80. Berman MF, Sciacca RR, Pile-Spellman J, et al: The epidemiology of brain arteriovenous malformations. Neurosurgery 47:389–396, 2000.

81. Brown RD Jr, Wiebers DO, Torner JC, O'Fallon WM: Incidence and prevalence of intracranial vascular malformations in Olmsted County, Minnesota, 1965 to 1992. Neurology 46:949–952, 1996.

82. Brown RD Jr, Wiebers DO, Torner JC, O'Fallon WM: Frequency of intracranial hemorrhage as a presenting symptom and subtype analysis: A population-based study of intracranial vascular malformations in Olmsted Country, Minnesota. J Neurosurg 85:29–32, 1996.

83. Jessurun GA, Kamphuis DJ, van der Zande FH, Nossent JC: Cerebral arteriovenous malformations in The Netherlands Antilles: High prevalence of hereditary hemorrhagic telangiectasia-related single and multiple cerebral arteriovenous malformations. Clin Neurol Neurosurg 95:193–198, 1993.

84. Hillman J: Population-based analysis of arteriovenous malformation treatment. J Neurosurg 95:633–637, 2001.

85. Stapf C, Mast H, Sciacca RR, et al: The New York Islands AVM Study: Design, study progress, and initial results. Stroke 34:e29–e33, 2003.

86. Stapf C, Labovitz DL, Sciacca RR, et al: Incidence of adult brain arteriovenous malformation hemorrhage in a prospective population-based stroke survey. Cerebrovasc Dis 13:43–46, 2002.

87. Sacco RL, Boden-Albala B, Gan R, et al: Stroke incidence among white, black, and Hispanic residents of an urban community. Am J Epidemiol 147:259–268, 1998.

88. Stapf C, Labovitz DL, Sciacca RR, et al: Incidence of adult brain arteriovenous malformation hemorrhage in a prospective population-based stroke survey. Cerebrovasc Dis 13:43–46, 2002.

89. Barre RG, Suter CG, Rosenblum WI: Familial vascular malformation or chance occurrence? Case report of two affected family members. Neurology 28:98–100, 1978.

90. Boyd MC, Steinbok P, Paty DW: Familial arteriovenous malformations: Report of four cases in one family. J Neurosurg 62:597–599, 1985.

91. Dobyns WB, Michels VV, Groover RV, et al: Familial cavernous malformations of the central nervous system and retina. Ann Neurol 21:578–583, 1987.

92. Gerosa MA, Cappellotto P, Licata C, et al: Cerebral arteriovenous malformations in children (56 cases). Childs Brain 8:356–371, 1981.

93. Snead OC III, Acker JD, Morawetz R: Familial arteriovenous malformation. Ann Neurol 5:585–587, 1979.

94. Kadoya C, Momota Y, Ikegami Y, et al: Central nervous system arteriovenous malformations with hereditary hemorrhagic telangiectasia: Report of a family with three cases. Surg Neurol 42:234–239, 1994.

95. Putman CM, Chaloupka JC, Fulbright RK, et al: Exceptional multiplicity of cerebral arteriovenous malformations associated with hereditary hemorrhagic telangiectasia (Osler-Weber-Rendu syndrome). AJNR Am J Neuroradiol 17:1733–1742, 1996.

96. Willinsky RA, Lasjaunias P, terBrugge K, Burrows P: Multiple cerebral arteriovenous malformations (AVMs): Review of our experience from 203 patients with cerebral vascular lesions. Neuroradiology 32:207–210, 1990.

97. Meder JF, Nataf F, Delvat D, et al: [Radioanatomy of cerebral arteriovenous malformations]. Cancer Radiother 2:173–179, 1998.

98. Cloft HJ, Joseph GJ, Dion JE: Risk of cerebral angiography in patients with subarachnoid hemorrhage, cerebral aneurysm, and arteriovenous malformation: a meta-analysis. Stroke 30:317–320, 1999.

99. Latchaw RE, Hu X, Ugurbil K, et al: Functional magnetic resonance imaging as a management tool for cerebral arteriovenous malformations. Neurosurgery 37:619–625, 1995.

100. Schlosser MJ, McCarthy G, Fulbright RK, et al: Cerebral vascular malformations adjacent to sensorimotor and visual cortex: Functional magnetic resonance imaging studies before and after therapeutic intervention. Stroke 28:1130–1137, 1997.

101. Zimmerman RS, Spetzler RF, Lee KS, et al: Cavernous malformations of the brain stem. J Neurosurg 75:32–39, 1991.

102. Mast H, Mohr JP, Thompson JL, et al: Transcranial Doppler ultrasonography in cerebral arteriovenous malformations: Diagnostic sensitivity and association of flow velocity with spontaneous hemorrhage and focal neurological deficit. Stroke 26:1024–1027, 1995.

103. Uggowitzer MM, Kugler C, Riccabona M, et al: Cerebral arteriovenous malformations: Diagnostic value of echo-enhanced transcranial Doppler sonography compared with angiography. AJNR Am J Neuroradiol 20:101–106, 1999.

104. Kilic T, Pamir MN, Budd S, et al: Grading and hemodynamic follow-up study of arteriovenous malformations with transcranial Doppler ultrasonography. J Ultrasound Med 17:729–738, 1998.

105. Reporting terminology for brain arteriovenous malformation clinical and radiographic features for use in clinical trials. Stroke 32:1430–1442, 2001.

106. Willinsky RA, Lasjaunias P, terBrugge K, Burrows P: Multiple cerebral arteriovenous malformations (AVMs): Review of our experience from 203 patients with cerebral vascular lesions. Neuroradiology 32:207–210, 1990.

107. U.S. Dept. of Health and Human Services, Public Health Service, Health Care Financing Administration. The International Classification of Diseases, 9th Revision, Clinical Modification: ICD-9. (Dept. of Health and Human Service Publication 91–1260.) 1991.

108. ICD-10: International Statistical Classification of Diseases and Related Health Problems. Geneva, World Health Organization, 1992.

109. Andoh T, Sakai N, Yamada H, et al: [Cerebellar AVM—clinical analysis of 14 cases]. No To Shinkei 42:913–921, 1990.

110. Batjer HH, Devous MD Sr, Meyer YJ, et al: Cerebrovascular hemodynamics in arteriovenous malformation complicated by normal perfusion pressure breakthrough. Neurosurgery 22:503–509, 1988.

111. Kupersmith MJ, Vargas ME, Yashar A, et al: Occipital arteriovenous malformations: Visual disturbances and presentation. Neurology 46:953–957, 1996.

112. Symon L, Tacconi L, Mendoza N, Nakaji P: Arteriovenous malformations of the posterior fossa: A report on 28 cases and review of the literature. Br J Neurosurg 9:721–732, 1995.

113. Santoreneos S, Blumbergs PC, Jones NR: Choroid plexus arteriovenous malformations: A report of four pathologically proven cases and review of the literature. Br J Neurosurg 10:385–390, 1996.

114. Picard L, Miyachi S, Braun M, et al: Arteriovenous malformations of the corpus callosum: Radioanatomic study and effectiveness of intranidus embolization. Neurol Med Chir (Tokyo) 36:851–859, 1996.

115. Schlachter LB, Fleischer AS, Faria MA Jr, Tindall GT: Multifocal intracranial arteriovenous malformations. Neurosurgery 7:440–444, 1980.

Clinical Manifestations

116. Mackenzie I: The clinical presentation of cerebral angioma: A review of 50 cases. Brain 76:184, 1953,

117. Maspes PE, Marini G: Results of the surgical treatment of intracranial arteriovenous malformations. Vasc Surg 4:164–170, 1970.

118. Morello G, Borghi GP: Cerebral angiomas: A report of 154 personal cases and a comparison between the results of surgical excision and conservative management. Acta Neurochir (Wien) 28:135–155, 1973.

119. Stein BM, Wolpert SM: Arteriovenous malformations of the brain. I: Current concepts and treatment. Arch Neurol 37:1–5, 1980.

120. Trumpy JH, Eldevik P: Intracranial arteriovenous malformations: Conservative or surgical treatment? Surg Neurol 8:171–175, 1977.

121. Walter W: The influence of the type and localization of the angioma on the clinical syndrome. In Pia HW, Gleave JRW, Grote E, Zierski J (eds): Cerebral Angiomas: Advances in Diagnosis and Therapy. New York, Springer-Verlag, 1975, p 271.

122. Stapf C, Mast H, Sciacca RR, et al: The New York Islands AVM Study: Detection rates for brain AVM and incident AVM hemorrhage. Stroke 32:368, 2001.

123. Marks MP, Lane B, Steinberg GK, Chang PJ: Hemorrhage in intracerebral arteriovenous malformations: angiographic determinants. Radiology 176:807–813, 1990.

124. Duong DH, Young WL, Vang MC, et al: Feeding artery pressure and venous drainage pattern are primary determinants of hemorrhage from cerebral arteriovenous malformations. Stroke 29:1167–1176, 1998.

125. Crawford JV Russell DS: Cryptic arteriovenous and venous hamartomas of the brain. J Neurol Neurosurg Psychiatry 19:1, 1956.

126. Dandy WE: Arteriovenous aneurysm of the brain. Arch Surg (Chicago) 17:190, 1928.

127. Forster DM, Steiner L, Hakanson S: Arteriovenous malformations of the brain: A long-term clinical study. J Neurosurg 37:562–570, 1972.

128. Fox JL AMO: Embolization of an arteriovenous malformation of the brain stem. Surg Neurol 8:7, 1977.

129. Henderson WR, Gomez RD: Natural history of cerebral angiomas. Br Med J 4:571–574, 1967.

130. Kusske JA, Kelly WA: Embolization and reduction of the "steal" syndrome in cerebral arteriovenous malformations. J Neurosurg 40:313–321, 1974.

131. Young WL, Prohovnik I, Ornstein E, et al: The effect of arteriovenous malformation resection on cerebrovascular reactivity to carbon dioxide. Neurosurgery 27:257–266, 1990.

132. Höök OJ: Intracranial arteriovenous aneurysms: A follow-up study with particular attention to their growth. Arch Neurol Psychiatry 80:39, 1958.

133. Krayenbühl H, Siebenmann R: Small vascular malformations as a cause of primary intracerebral hemorrhage. J Neurosurg 22:7, 1965.

134. Mohr JP, Caplan LR, Melski JW, et al: The Harvard Cooperative Stroke Registry: A prospective registry. Neurology 28:754–762, 1978.

135. Paterson JH, McKissock W: A clinical survey of intracranial angiomas with special reference to their mode of progression and surgical treatment: A report of 110 cases. Brain 79:233, 1956.

136. Lanzino G, Jensen ME, Cappelletto B, Kassell NF: Arteriovenous malformations that rupture during pregnancy: A management dilemma. Acta Neurochir (Wien) 126:102–106, 1994.

137. Horton JC, Chambers WA, Lyons SL, et al: Pregnancy and the risk of hemorrhage from cerebral arteriovenous malformations. Neurosurgery 27:867–871, 1990.

138. Kelly DL Jr, Alexander E Jr, Davis CH Jr, Maynard DC: Intracranial arteriovenous malformations: Clinical review and evaluation of brain scans. J Neurosurg 31:422–428, 1969.

139. Guidetti B, Delitala A: Intracranial arteriovenous malformations: Conservative and surgical treatment. J Neurosurg 53:149–152, 1980.

140. Garrido E, Stein B: Removal of an arteriovenous malformation from the basal ganglion. J Neurol Neurosurg Psychiatry 41:992–995, 1978.

141. Hier DB, Davis KR, Richardson EP Jr, Mohr JP: Hypertensive putaminal hemorrhage. Ann Neurol 1:152–159, 1977.

142. Wilson CDJ: Microsurgical treatment of intracranial vascular malformations. J Neurosurg 51:446, 1979.

143. McCormick WF, Nofzinger JD: "Cryptic" vascular malformations of the central nervous system. J Neurosurg 24:865–875, 1966.

144. Pia HW, Gleave JRW, Grote E, et al: Cerebral Angiomas: Advances in Diagnosis and Therapy. New York, Springer-Verlag, 1975, p 285.

145. Hosobuchi Y, Fabricant J, Lyman J: Stereotactic heavy-particle irradiation of intracranial arteriovenous malformations. Appl Neurophysiol 50:248–252, 1987.

146. Massoud TF, Ji C, Guglielmi G, Vinuela F: Endovascular treatment of arteriovenous malformations with selective intranidal occlusion by detachable platinum electrodes: Technical feasibility in a swine model. AJNR Am J Neuroradiol 17:1459–1466, 1996.

147. Ruff RM, Arbit E: Aphemia resulting from a left frontal hematoma. Neurology 31:353, 1981.

148. Kase CS, Williams JP, Wyatt DA, Mohr JP: Lobar intracerebral hematomas: Clinical and CT analysis of 22 cases. Neurology 32:1146–1150, 1982.

149. Stein R, Kase CS, Heir DB, et al: Caudate hemorrhage. Neurology 34:1549, 1984.

149a. Hartmann A, Mast H, Mohr JP, et al: Morbidity of intracranial hemorrhage in patients with cerebral arteriovenous malformation. Stroke 29:931-934, 1998.

150. Mast H, Young WL, Koennecke HC, et al: Risk of spontaneous haemorrhage after diagnosis of cerebral arteriovenous malformation. Lancet 350:1065–1068, 1997.

151. Krayenbühl H, Yasargil G: L'Aneurismo Cerebral. (Documenta Geigy, Series Chirurgica 4.) Basel, Geigy, 1959.

152. Graf CJ, Perret GE, Torner JC: Bleeding from cerebral arteriovenous malformations as part of their natural history. J Neurosurg 58:331–337, 1983.

153. Hayashi S, Arimoto T, Itakura T, et al: The association of intracranial aneurysms and arteriovenous malformation of the brain: Case report. J Neurosurg 55:971–975, 1981.

154. Lazar ML, Watts CC, Kilgore B, Clark K: Cerebral angiography during operation for intracranial aneurysms and arteriovenous malformations: Technical note. J Neurosurg 34:706–708, 1971.

155. Marks MP, Lane B, Steinberg GK, Chang PJ: Hemorrhage in intracerebral arteriovenous malformations: Angiographic determinants. Radiology 176:807–813, 1990.

156. Batjer HH, Devous MD Sr, Seibert GB, et al: Intracranial arteriovenous malformation: Relationships between clinical and radiographic factors and ipsilateral steal severity. Neurosurgery 23:322–328, 1988.

157. Lasjaunias P, Piske R, terBrugge K, Willinsky R: Cerebral arteriovenous malformations (C. AVM) and associated arterial aneurysms (AA). Analysis of 101 C. AVM cases, with 37 AA in 23 patients. Acta Neurochir (Wien) 91:29–36, 1988.

158. Turjman F, Massoud TF, Vinuela F, et al: Correlation of the angioarchitectural features of cerebral arteriovenous malformations with clinical presentation of hemorrhage. Neurosurgery 37:856–860, 1995.

159. Westphal M, Grzyska U: Clinical significance of pedicle aneurysms on feeding vessels, especially those located in infratentorial arteriovenous malformations. J Neurosurg 92:995–1001, 2000.

160. Redekop G, terBrugge K, Montanera W, Willinsky R: Arterial aneurysms associated with cerebral arteriovenous malformations: Classification, incidence, and risk of hemorrhage. J Neurosurg 89:539–546, 1998.

161. Brown RD Jr, Wiebers DO, Forbes GS: Unruptured intracranial aneurysms and arteriovenous malformations: Frequency of intracranial hemorrhage and relationship of lesions. J Neurosurg 73:859–863, 1990.

162. Langer DJ, Lasner TM, Hurst RW, et al: Hypertension, small size, and deep venous drainage are associated with risk of hemorrhagic presentation of cerebral arteriovenous malformations. Neurosurgery 42:481–486, 1998.

163. Nataf F, Meder JF, Roux FX, et al: Angioarchitecture associated with haemorrhage in cerebral arteriovenous malformations: A prognostic statistical model. Neuroradiology 39:52–58, 1997.

164. Mansmann U, Meisel J, Brock M, et al: Factors associated with intracranial hemorrhage in cases of cerebral arteriovenous malformation. Neurosurgery 46:272–279, 2000.

165. Stefani MA, Porter PJ, terBrugge KG, et al: Angioarchitectural factors present in brain arteriovenous malformations associated with hemorrhagic presentation. Stroke 33:920–924, 2002.

166. Brown RD Jr, Wiebers DO, Torner JC, O'Fallon WM: Incidence and prevalence of intracranial vascular malformations in Olmsted County, Minnesota, 1965 to 1992. Neurology 46:949–952, 1996.

167. Mast H, Mohr JP, Osipov A, et al: 'Steal' is an unestablished mechanism for the clinical presentation of cerebral arteriovenous malformations. Stroke 26:1215–1220, 1995.

Clinical Manifestations

168. Osipov A, Koennecke HC, Hartmann A, et al: Seizures in cerebral arteriovenous malformations: Type, clinical course, and medical management. Interv Neuroradiol 3:37–41, 1997.

169. Leblanc R, Feindel W, Ethier R: Epilepsy from cerebral arteriovenous malformations. Can J Neurol Sci 10:91–95, 1983.

170. Leblanc E, Meyer E, Zatorre R, et al: Functional PET scanning in the preoperative assessment of cerebral arteriovenous malformations. Stereotact Funct Neurosurg 65:60–64, 1995.

171. Ozer MN, Sencer W, Block J: A clinical study of cerebral vascular malformations: The significance of migraine. J Mt Sinai Hosp 31: 403, 1964.

172. Olivecrona H, Ladenheim J: Congenital Arteriovenous Aneurysms of the Carotid and Vertebral Systems. Berlin, Springer-Verlag, 1957.

173. Troost BT, Newton TH: Occipital lobe arteriovenous malformations: Clinical and radiologic features in 26 cases with comments on differentiation from migraine. Arch Ophthalmol 93:250–256, 1975.

174. Turjman F, Massoud TF, Sayre JW, et al: Epilepsy associated with cerebral arteriovenous malformations: A multivariate analysis of angioarchitectural characteristics. AJNR Am J Neuroradiol 16:345–350, 1995.

175. Graeb DA, Dolman CL: Radiological and pathological aspects of dural arteriovenous fistulas: Case report. J Neurosurg 64:962–967, 1986.

176. Stapf C, Mohr JP, Sciacca RR, et al: Incident hemorrhage risk of brain arteriovenous malformations located in the arterial borderzones. Stroke 31:2365–2368, 2000.

177. Turjman F, Massoud TF, Sayre JW, et al: Epilepsy associated with cerebral arteriovenous malformations: A multivariate analysis of angioarchitectural characteristics. AJNR Am J Neuroradiol 16:345–350, 1995.

178. Kilpatrick CJ, Davis SM, Tress BM, et al: Epileptic seizures in acute stroke. Arch Neurol 47:157–160, 1990.

179. Mackenzie I: The clinical presentation of cerebral angioma: A review of 50 cases. Brain 76:184, 1953.

180. Frishberg BM: Neuroimaging in presumed primary headache disorders. Semin Neurol 17:373–382, 1997.

181. Ennoksson P, Bynke H: Visual field defects in arteriovenous aneurysms of the brain. Acta Ophthalmol 36:586, 1958.

182. Lees F: The migrainous symptoms of cerebral angiomata. J Neurol Neurosurg Psychiatry 25:45, 1962.

183. Northfield DWC: Angiomatous malformations of the brain. Guys Hosp Rep 90:149, 1940.

184. Evans RW: Diagnostic testing for the evaluation of headaches. Neurol Clin 14:1, 1996.

185. Mast H, Mohr JP, Osipov A, et al: 'Steal' is an unestablished mechanism for the clinical presentation of cerebral arteriovenous malformations. Stroke 26:1215–1220, 1995.

186. Carter LP, Gumerlock MK: Steal and cerebral arteriovenous malformations. Stroke 26:2371–2372, 1995.

187. Carter LP, Gumerlock MK: Steal and cerebral arteriovenous malformations. Stroke 26:2371–2372, 1995.

188. Nornes H, Grip A: Hemodynamic aspects of cerebral arteriovenous malformations. J Neurosurg 53:456–464, 1980.

189. Young WL, Pile-Spellman J, Prohovnik I, et al: Evidence for adaptive autoregulatory displacement in hypotensive cortical territories adjacent to arteriovenous malformations. Columbia University AVM Study Project. Neurosurgery 34:601–610, 1994.

190. Miyasaka Y, Kurata A, Tanaka R, et al: Mass effect caused by clinically unruptured cerebral arteriovenous malformations. Neurosurgery 41:1060–1063, 1997.

191. Feindel W, Yamamoto YL, Hodge CP: Red cerebral veins as an index of cerebral steal. Scand J Clin Lab Invest Suppl 102:X:C, 1968.

192. Norlen G: Arteriovenous aneurysms of the brain: Report of ten cases of total removal of the lesion. J Neurosurg 6:475, 1949.

193. Numaguchi Y, Kitamura K, Fukui M, et al: Intracranial venous angiomas. Surg Neurol 18:193–202, 1982.

194. Shenkin HA, Spitz EB, Grant FC, Kety SS: Physiologic studies of arteriovenous anomalies of the brain. J Neurosurg 6:165, 21948.

195. Waltimo O: The relationship of size, density and localization of intracranial arteriovenous malformations to the type of initial symptom. J Neurol Sci 19:13–19, 1973.

196. Nornes H, Grip A: Hemodynamic aspects of cerebral arteriovenous malformations. J Neurosurg 53:456–464, 1980.

197. Fogarty-Mack P, Pile-Spellman J, Hacein-Bey L, et al: The effect of arteriovenous malformations on the distribution of intracerebral arterial pressures. AJNR Am J Neuroradiol 17:1443–1449, 1996.

198. Tarr RW, Johnson DW, Rutigliano M, et al: Use of acetazolamide-challenge xenon CT in the assessment of cerebral blood flow dynamics in patients with arteriovenous malformations. AJNR Am J Neuroradiol 11:441–448, 1990.

199. Spetzler RF, Wilson CB: Enlargement of an AVM documented by angiography: Case report. J Neurosurg 43:767, 1975.

200. Spetzler RF, Wilson CB, Weinstein P: Normal perfusion pressure breakthrough theory. Clin Neurosurg 25:651, 1978.

201. Kvam DA, Michelsen WJ, Quest DO: Intracerebral hemorrhage as a complication of artificial embolization. Neurosurgery 7:491–494, 1980.

202. Morgan MK, Johnston I, Besser M, Baines D: Cerebral arteriovenous malformations, steal, and the hypertensive breakthrough threshold: An experimental study in rats. J Neurosurg 66:563–567, 1987.

203. Mullan S, Brown FD, Patronas NJ: Hyperemic and ischemic problems of surgical treatment of arteriovenous malformations. J Neurosurg 51:757–764, 1979.

204. Muraszko K, Wang HH, Pelton G, Stein BM: A study of the reactivity of feeding vessels to arteriovenous malformations: Correlation with clinical outcome. Neurosurgery 26:190–199, 1990.

205. Young WL, Pile-Spellman J, Prohovnik I, et al: Evidence for adaptive autoregulatory displacement in hypotensive cortical territories adjacent to arteriovenous malformations. Columbia University AVM Study Project. Neurosurgery 34:601–610, 1994.

206. Hacein-Bey L, Nour R, Pile-Spellman J, et al: Adaptive changes of autoregulation in chronic cerebral hypotension with arteriovenous malformations: An acetazolamide-enhanced single-photon emission CT study. AJNR Am J Neuroradiol 16:1865–1874, 1995.

207. Lasjaunias P, Chiu M, ter Brugge K, et al: Neurological manifestations of intracranial dural arteriovenous malformations. J Neurosurg 64:724–730, 1986.

208. Svien HJ, McRae JA: Arteriovenous anomalies of the brain: Fate of patients not having definitive surgery. J Neurosurg 23:23–28, 1965.

209. Rabinov JD: Diagnostic imaging of angiographically occult vascular malformations 1. Neurosurg Clin North Am 10:419–432, 1999.

210. Otten P, Pizzolato GP, Rilliet B, Berney J: [131 cases of cavernous angioma (cavernomas) of the CNS, discovered by retrospective analysis of 24,535 autopsies] 1. Neurochirurgie 35:82–31, 1989.

211. Hashim AS, Asakura T, Koichi U, et al: Angiographically occult arteriovenous malformations. Surg Neurol 23:431–439, 1985.

212. Tsitsopoulos P, Andrew J, Harrison MJ: Occult cerebral arteriovenous malformations. J Neurol Neurosurg Psychiatry 50:218–220, 1987.

213. Voigt K, Yasargil MG: Cerebral cavernous haemangiomas or cavernomas: Incidence, pathology, localization, diagnosis, clinical features and treatment. Review of the literature and report of an unusual case. Neurochirurgia (Stuttg) 19:59–68, 1976.

214. Fierstien SB, Pribram HW, Hieshima G: Angiography and computed tomography in the evaluation of cerebral venous malformations. Neuroradiology 17:137–148, 1979.

215. Giombini S, Morello G: Cavernous angiomas of the brain: Account of fourteen personal cases and review of the literature. Acta Neurochir (Wien) 40:61–82, 1978.

216. Pool JL Potts DG: Aneurysms and Arteriovenous Anomalies of the Brain: Diagnosis and Treatment. New York, Harper & Row, 1965, p 463.

217. Rigamonti D, Spetzler RF, Medina M, et al: Cerebral venous malformations. J Neurosurg 73:560–564, 1990.

218. Kattapong VJ, Hart BL, Davis LE: Familial cerebral cavernous angiomas: Clinical and radiologic studies. Neurology 45:492–497, 1995.

219. Saito Y, Kobayashi N: Cerebral venous angiomas: Clinical evaluation and possible etiology. Radiology 139:87–94, 1981.

220. Steiger HJ, Tew JM Jr: Hemorrhage and epilepsy in cryptic cerebrovascular malformations. Arch Neurol 41:722–724, 1984.

221. Humphreys RP, Hoffman HJ, Drake JM, Rutka JT: Choices in the 1990s for the management of pediatric cerebral arteriovenous malformations. Pediatr Neurosurg 25:277–285, 1996.

222. Craig HD, Gunel M, Cepeda O, et al: Multilocus linkage identifies two new loci for a mendelian form of stroke, cerebral cavernous malformation, at 7p15–13 and 3q25.2-27. Hum Mol Genet 7:1851–1858, 1998.

223. McCormick WF, Hardman JM, Boulter TR: Vascular malformations ("angiomas") of the brain, with special reference to those occurring in the posterior fossa. J Neurosurg 28:241–251, 1968.

Clinical Manifestations

224. Johnson DW, Berg JN, Gallione CJ, et al: A second locus for hereditary hemorrhagic telangiectasia maps to chromosome 12. Genome Res 5:21–28, 1995.
225. Farrell DF, Forno LS: Symptomatic capillary telangiectasis of the brainstem without hemorrhage: Report of an unusual case. Neurology 20:341–346, 1970.
226. Moritake K, Handa H, Mori K, et al: Venous angiomas of the brain. Surg Neurol 14:95–105, 1980.
227. Wendling LR, Moore JS Jr, Kieffer SA, et al: Intracerebral venous angioma. Radiology 119:141–147, 1976.
228. Mullan S, Mojtahedi S, Johnson DL, Macdonald RL: Cerebral venous malformation-arteriovenous malformation transition forms. J Neurosurg 85:9–13, 1996.
229. Masuda J, Ogata J, Yutani C: Smooth muscle cell proliferation and localization of macrophages and T cells in the occlusive intracranial major arteries in moyamoya disease. Stroke 24:1960–1967, 1993.
230. Nishimoto A, Takeuchi S: Abnormal cerebrovascular network related to the internal carotid arteries. J Neurosurg 29:255, 1968.
231. Enam SA, Malik GM: Association of cerebral arteriovenous malformations and spontaneous occlusion of major feeding arteries: Clinical and therapeutic implications. Neurosurgery 45:1105–1111, 1999.
232. Pile-Spellman JM, Baker KF, Liszczak TM, et al: High-flow angiopathy: Cerebral blood vessel changes in experimental chronic arteriovenous fistula. AJNR Am J Neuroradiol 7:811–815, 1986.
233. Raybaud CA, Strother CM, Hald JK: Aneurysms of the vein of Galen: Embryonic considerations and anatomical features relating to the pathogenesis of the malformation. Neuroradiology 31:109–128, 1989.
234. Guttmacher AE, Marchuk DA, White RI: Hereditary hemorrhagic telangiectasia. N Engl J Med 333:918–224, 1995.
235. Alberts ML: Intracerebral hemorrhage and vascular malformations. In Alberts MJ (ed): Genetics of Cerebrovascular Disease. Armonk, NY, Future Publishing, 1999, pp 209–236.
236. Patel U, Gupta SC: Wyburn-Mason syndrome: A case report and review of the literature. Neuroradiology 31:544–546, 1990.
237. Ponce FA, Han PP, Spetzler RF, et al: Associated arteriovenous malformation of the orbit and brain: A case of Wyburn-Mason syndrome without retinal involvement. Case report. J Neurosurg 95:346–349, 2001.
238. Stein BM, Wolpert SM: Arteriovenous malformations of the brain I: Current concepts and treatment. Arch Neurol 37:1-5, 1980.
239. Parkinson D, Bachers G: Arteriovenous malformations. Summary of 100 consecutive supratentorial cases. J Neurosurg 53:285-299, 1980.
240. Pertuiset B, Sichez JP, Philippon J: Mortalité et morbidité après exerèse chirurgicale totale de 162 malformations artérioveneuses intracraniennes. Rev Neurol 135:319-329, 1979.
241. Troupp H, Marttila I, Halonen V: Arteriovenous malformations of the brain: Prognosis without operation. Acta Neurochir 22:125-128, 1970.
242. Moody RA, Poppen JL: Arteriovenous malformations. J Neurosurg 32:503-511, 1970.
243. Tönnis W, Walter W: On the differential diagnosis of apoplexy in neurosurgery. Dtsch Med J 18:162-176, 1967.

Clinical Manifestations

Chapter Sixteen

Spinal Cord Ischemia

J. P. Mohr, Oscar Benavente, and Henry J. M. Barnett

Spinal cord infarction, although rare, remains incompletely studied. Its incidence is unknown, and no large epidemiologic study has been conducted. The increase in accidental production of cord infarct by modern cardiovascular surgery and the advances in imaging techniques, including computed tomography (CT) and magnetic resonance imaging (MRI), have led to more documentation.[1-3] One hopes that the better visualization of the spinal cord and improvements in the accurate localization, diagnosis, and management of vascular lesions may eventually improve its management.[4-6]

HISTORICAL ASPECTS

Blackwood,[7] reviewing the records of 3737 autopsies conducted over 50 years, found only five cases of spinal cord infarction. Surprisingly, no cases were due to atherosclerosis or hypertensive vascular disease. Slager and Webb,[8] however, found microinfarcts of the spinal cord in 3% of 200 consecutive autopsies performed in asymptomatic patients. Sandson and Friedman[9] described eight cases of spinal cord infarction, representing roughly 1.2% of all admissions for stroke in their center. Despite numerous well-documented case reports of spinal cord infarction, misconceptions still exist regarding its pathogenesis and clinical course.

Studies in animals reported in the distant past showed that aortic clamping led to paralysis. Clinically, paraparesis as a result of aortic obstruction was recognized at the end of the 19th century.[10] Bastian[11] in 1882 suggested that spinal cord softening may be the result of vascular occlusion; however, it was not until 1904 that Preobrashenski[12] described the syndrome of anterior spinal artery infarct.

BLOOD SUPPLY TO THE SPINAL CORD

The basic pattern of the arterial blood supply to the spinal cord consists of three longitudinal vessels that arise rostrally from the cervical region and descend as far as the conus medullaris, plus numerous feeder arteries and radicular vessels. Anastomoses between the descending and segmentally oriented vessels occur on the surface of the spinal cord, leading to the formation of a rich vascular plexus from which medullary vessels penetrate both white and gray matter. These vessels are end arteries and do not anastomose further.[2]

Longitudinal Arteries

There are three longitudinal arteries, the anterior spinal artery and the two posterior spinal arteries.

The *anterior spinal artery* forms rostrally from the union of the two anterior spinal branches of each vertebral artery at the level of the foramen magnum. From this site, it descends up to the tip of the conus medullaris. It lies in relation to the anterior median sulcus (Fig. 16–1).[13,14] The caliber of the artery is largest in the lumbosacral region and smallest in the thoracic region, which has been considered a vulnerable zone for ischemia. The anterior spinal artery is reinforced by successive contributions of feeder arterial branches, which enter the artery in a caudal direction and supply the spinal cord below the point of entry. At the conus medullaris and along the filum terminale, the anterior spinal artery communicates through anastomotic branches with the posterior spinal arteries.[13,14]

The two *posterior spinal arteries* originate directly from the vertebral arteries (Fig. 16–2). Each vessel descends on the posterior surface of the spinal cord along the posterolateral sulcus. The arteries are commonly found to be discontinuous, and sometimes one artery moves across to supply the other side.[14] Throughout its course, each posterior spinal artery gives off branches that penetrate the cord to supply the posterior columns, dorsal gray matter, and superficial dorsal aspect of the lateral columns.

Radicular Tributary Arteries

Thirty-one pairs of radicular arteries penetrate the spinal canal through the intervertebral foramina. Usually 7 or 8 of these 62 radicular branches contribute to the vascularization of the spinal cord and define three major spinal arterial territories—cervicothoracic, midthoracic, and thoracolumbar.[5,15]

The *cervicothoracic* territory consists of the cervical spinal cord, its brachial plexus enlargement, and the first two or three thoracic segments. This territory is richly supplied by the anterior spinal artery arising from the intracranial vertebral arteries, the midcervical radicular branches of the vertebral artery, and the branches of the costocervical trunk.

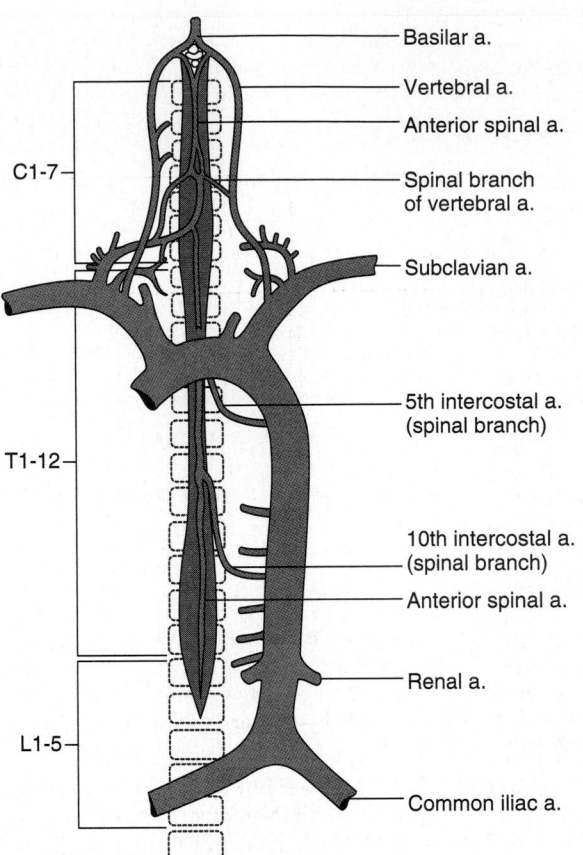

FIGURE 16–1 *Extrinsic vascular supply of the spinal cord. Schematic representation of the anterior spinal artery. (Adapted from Gray H: Development and gross anatomy of the human body. In Clemente CD [eds]: Anatomy of the Human Body, 30th ed. {American Ed.} Philadelphia, Lea & Febiger, 1984; from Benavente OR, Barnett HJM: Spinal cord infarction. In Carter LP, Spetzler RF [eds]: Neurovascular Surgery. New York, McGraw-Hill, 1995, p 1229.)*

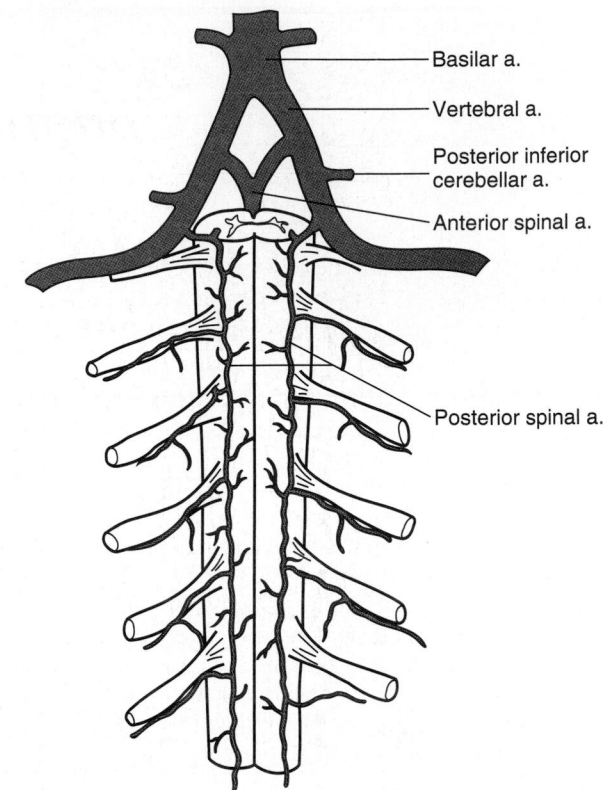

FIGURE 16–2 *Extrinsic vascular supply of the spinal cord. Schematic representation of the posterior spinal arteries. (Adapted from Gray H: Development and gross anatomy of the human body. In Clemente CD [eds]: Anatomy of the Human Body, 30th ed. {American Ed.} Philadelphia, Lea & Febiger, 1984; from Benavente OR, Barnett HJM: Spinal cord infarction. In Carter LP, Spetzler RF [eds]: Neurovascular Surgery. New York, McGraw-Hill, 1995, p 1229.)*

In the *midthoracic* territory, the radicular arteries supplying the middle and lower thoracic cord are less prominent.[16] This territory is usually supplied by a radicular branch arising at about the T7 level; it comprises the fourth to eighth segments of the thoracic cord.

In addition to the lower thoracic segments, the *thoracolumbar* territory contains the lumbar enlargement, which relates to the lumbosacral plexus. This segment receives its blood supply from a single artery, called the artery of Adamkiewicz. Although the artery of Adamkiewicz is well-known by name, the site of origin varies widely from the left 9th, 10th, 11th, or 12th intercostal artery, and the artery itself varies considerably in size.[15] This irregular augmentation of the anterior spinal artery system results in watershed areas that may be vulnerable to hypoperfusion, most marked in the thoracic area.[16] These radicular tributaries may be subdivided into two groups according to their origin. The first group consists of those derived from the subclavian artery; the second group is supplied directly from the aorta. At the level of the second thoracic spinal cord segment, the arterial supply changes, from a subclavian supply to a direct aortic supply.[17]

Intrinsic Blood Supply of the Cord

When the radicular arteries reach the surface of the spinal cord, they form two distinct systems of intrinsic blood supply (Figs. 16–3 and 16–4). The first is the posterolateral and peripheral plexus formed by the two posterior spinal arteries, which are interconnected by anastomotic channels.[18] This plexus, a centripetal vascular territory, is formed by radial arteries directed inward as branches from the coronal arterial plexus surrounding the spinal cord. It supplies from one third to one half of the outer rim of the cord, including the lateral and ventral spinothalamic tracts. These radial arteries are longer in the posterior white columns than in the anterior and lateral columns. This difference in length could explain the size and localization of pathologic changes related to vascular disorders.[14]

The second arterial system to the spinal cord is a centrifugal system formed by the sulcal arteries, which arise from the anterior spinal artery and pass backward in the anterior medial sulcus. These arteries enter the gray commissure and, turning left or right, supply the gray matter and adjacent white matter. The corticospinal tract is nourished by both arterial systems.[14]

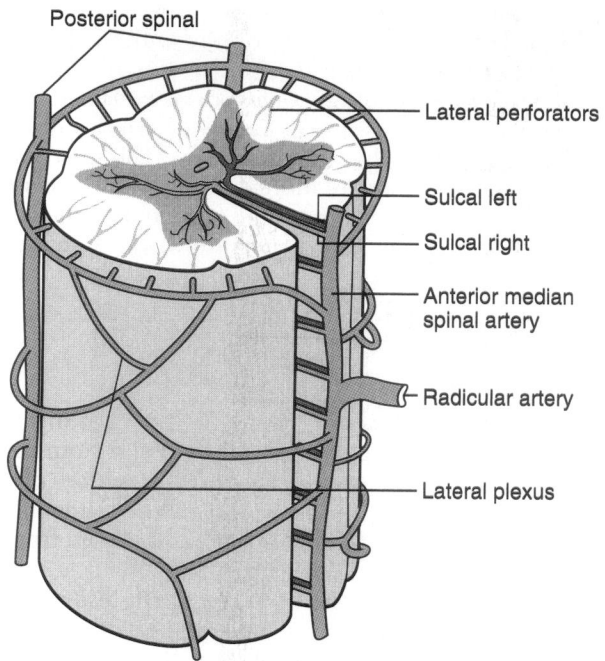

FIGURE 16–3 *Intrinsic vascular supply of the cord. The central sulcal artery is supplied from the anterior median artery, and the lateral artery from the anterior and posterior spinal arteries, forming the vasa corona. (From Buchan AM, Barnett HJM: Infarction of the spinal cord. J Neurosurg 35:253, 1971.)*

Both arterial systems are interconnected by a capillary anastomosis in the spinal cord. The number of sulcal arteries supplying each segment of the spinal cord varies with the region of the cord. They are most numerous in the thoracolumbar segment and least numerous in the upper thoracic segment.[19]

Venous System

Two *intrinsic venous systems* and one *extrinsic venous system* drain the spinal cord.[15,18–21]

Intrinsic Venous System

The anterior median group (central veins) collects blood from both halves of the medial aspects of the anterior horns, anterior gray commissure, and white matter of the anterior funiculus. The central veins also drain adjacent levels above and below through intersegmental anastomoses. They commonly anastomose with other veins within the fissure. Finally, the central veins empty into the anterior median spinal vein.

The other group consists of radial veins that arise from capillaries near the periphery of the gray matter or from the white matter. They are radially oriented and directed outward toward the surface of the spinal cord, where they join the superficial plexus of veins surrounding the cord and form a venous vasa corona or corona plexus. These veins are more numerous in the white matter of the posterior and lateral funiculi, but they are also found in the anterior funiculus. The radial veins are more prominent at certain cervical and thoracic levels; they drain laterally from the gray matter of the lateral horns as well as posteriorly from the dorsal nucleus of Clark.

Extrinsic Venous System

The extrinsic venous system is very conspicuous on the posterior aspect of the spinal cord and is especially prominent in the lumbosacral region. There is a rich anastomosis between the large venous trunks. The median posterior spinal vein descends in the region of the posterior median septum. This vessel drains blood from the posterior white columns and the end of the posterior horns.

The anterior spinal vein accompanies the anterior spinal artery and receives the sulcal veins. Both the anterior spinal veins and the median posterior spinal vein empty into the radicular veins, which accompany the anterior or posterior spinal roots. These radicular veins drain into the paravertebral and intervertebral plexuses, and then into the azygos and pelvic venous systems.[14] The absence of venous valves may allow infections in the abdominal cavity to spread to the spinal cord. Their absence also renders the spinal veins susceptible to Valsalva maneuvers, increasing the intra-abdominal pressure.

PHYSIOLOGY OF SPINAL CORD BLOOD FLOW

The regulation of spinal cord blood flow is similar to that of brain blood flow. The spinal cord blood vessels are affected by changes in PCO_2 and hypoxia. Hypercapnia

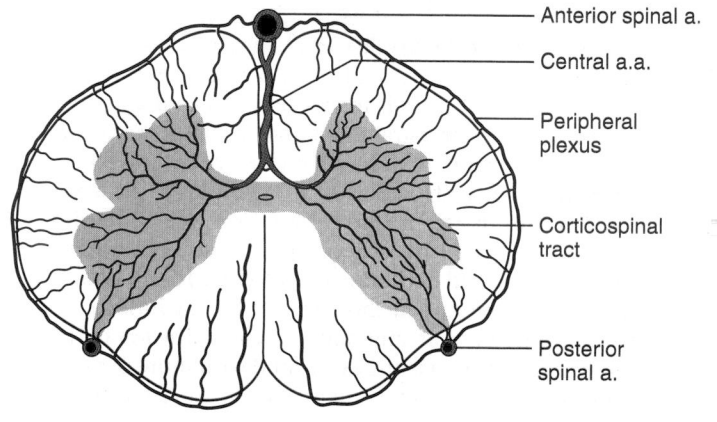

FIGURE 16–4 *Cross-sectional diagrammatic representation of the territories of the anterior and posterior spinal arteries. (From Mawad ME, Rivera V, Crawford S, et al: Spinal cord ischemia after resection of the thoracoabdominal aortic aneurysms: MR findings in 24 patients. AJNR Am J Neuroradiol 155:987, 1990.)*

Chapter Seventeen

Overview of Laboratory Studies

Geoffrey A. Donnan, H. Ma, and J. P. Mohr

ACUTE STROKE

Faced with an acute stroke, the physician must determine the cause, estimate the severity, consider the possibility of progression or recurrence, and seek ways of stabilizing or provide appropriate treatment, especially thrombolytic therapy, which is proven to decrease the chance of significant disability. Investigations should be designed to assist clinicians in subcategorizing cases at the following four specific levels: (1) separating strokes from nonstrokes such as cerebral tumors and subdural hematoma, (2) distinguishing hemorrhage from infarction, (3) identifying specific pathophysiologic subtypes of cerebral infarction, and (4) determining eligibility for thrombolytic therapy.[1] Because the possibility of worsening or recurrence is paramount, speedy efforts should be made to arrive at a diagnosis of stroke mechanism using this approach. The ideal test should be inexpensive, noninvasive, accessible, accurate, and informative. If investigations are used in a logical sequence and are related to the clinical syndrome, unnecessary tests can be avoided, and more cost-effective approaches adopted. An example of a suggested sequence of investigations, with these points taken into consideration, is given in Table 17.1.[1]

Brain Imaging

In most hospitals, the first testing step is an attempt to image the injured site by computed tomography (CT) or magnetic resonance imaging (MRI).[2,3] If neither modality is available, estimates of risk factor and clinical assessments of the syndrome help greatly but cannot substitute for brain imaging. Rapid acquisition of images with spiral CT (seconds only) is available in many centers.

Computed Tomography

The initial scan should separate hemorrhage from ischemia or infarction. For the CT scan, high-density signal attenuation (about 80 Hounsfield units [HU]) points to hemorrhage and low density to ischemia; on MRI, common method, long T2 sequence, the reverse is true: high-intensity signal indicates ischemia, and low-intensity signal hemorrhage. On CT, the high-density abnormality from parenchyma-

tous hemorrhage is usually rather circumscribed in the acute stage, gradually losing its density over 1 week in the smaller hemorrhages but persisting as long as months for the larger or more intense hemorrhage. Infarction followed by hemorrhagic transformation is more easily recognized when it is confined to the cerebral surface,[4] but it may mimic the findings in hematoma, making a certain differential diagnosis difficult.[5] One exception, a finding that seems specific for hemorrhage, is the pooling of blood found in some lobar hemorrhages.[6]

Hemorrhagic infarction is uncommon in the first hours after stroke, although this pattern is not universal. Hemorrhagic infarction can be inferred when the lesion lies in the ribbon-like fashion, but even these findings have been mimicked in lobar hemorrhage. MRI shows the same uniform density as does CT for hematomas but suffers the same problem as CT in showing minor examples of hemorrhagic infarction. In some instances, autopsy-documented hemorrhagic infarction has appeared isodense or even hypodense on CT and has been seen as scattered flecks of very low signal peppered through the infarct site. T2-weighted gradient spin-echo sequences[7] and multimodal protocol[8] have improved the sensitivity of MRI in the diagnoses of acute intracerebral hemorrhage. Multimodal stroke MRI has been reported to be as reliable as CT for the assessment of hyperacute intracranial hemorrhage.[8]

On CT, infarction appears as a low-density focus as early as 3 hours but more often not before 6 hours.[9] After 12 hours, CT findings are positive in almost half the cases,[10] and certainly after 48 hours,[11] reaching a plateau within 3 days in more than 60% of cases. Later studies suggest that both CT and MRI (with diffusion-weighted imaging [DWI]) are comparable for detecting the lesion in the earliest hours, and neither has much success before 3 to 4 hours from onset.[10] One study using advanced equipment reported detection of abnormality on CT within 6 hours in 94% of patients.[12] On CT, the low-density abnormality is seen early more often with embolic infarction, in which the infarcts have more complete tissue necrosis and edema, and is seen later with perfusion failure from thrombosis of large arteries, in which the necrosis may be more patchy and the edema less obvious.[13]

Table 17.1   Investigation of TIA and Stroke

	Clinical Presentation				
	TIA or Minor Stroke			**Severe Stroke**	
Investigation Sequence	**Lacunar**	**Hemispheric**	**Brainstem**		*Reason for Investigation*
CT at presentation (not enhanced)°	Yes	Yes	Yes	Yes	Distinguish hemorrhage from infarction, tumor, subdural hematoma
Ultrasonography of carotid arteries, MRI/MRA, or both	No[†]	Yes if good recovery	No[†]	No	Assess patency of carotid vessels
Echocardiography	No	Yes if carotid ultrasonography/MRA normal	Yes if clinical evidence of cardiac disease	No	Cardiac source of embolism
Intra-arterial digital subtraction angiography	No	Yes if ultrasonography/MRA shows significant stenosis[§]	Usually no[†]	No	More precise evaluation of extracranial and intracranial vessels
Repeat CT at day 7–10 (not enhanced) or MRI even earlier	Yes if early CT normal	Yes if early CT normal	Yes if early CT normal	Yes if early CT normal	Topography for infarct mechanism and prognosis

°Standard investigations may also be arranged at this time (see text).
[†]May be performed as risk factor assessment or MRA to detect basilar stenosis in brainstem ischemia.
[‡]Sometimes if patient is younger than 55 years or events are repeated.
[§]Definition may vary from center to center, but usually > 50% stenosis or evidence of ulceration or both.
CT, computed tomography; MRA, magnetic resonance angiography; MRI, magnetic resonance imaging; TIA, transient ischemic attack.
Modified from Donnan G: Investigation of patients with stroke and transient ischaemic attacks. Lancet 339:473, 1992.

Diagnostic Studies

Hyperacute CT scanning with advanced equipment provides important information for decision-making in applying thrombolytic therapy within 3 to 6 hours of the onset of the stroke symptoms. Loss of delineation between gray matter and white matter can be detected as early as 1 hour.[14] Early parenchymatous signs—attenuation of the lentiform nucleus, loss of the insular ribbon, and hemispheric sulcus effacement—are associated with subsequent infarct location and extension. The presence of these signs is associated with extended middle cerebral artery (MCA) infarct and poor outcome.[12] Evaluation of the CT findings in the first European Cooperative Acute Stroke Study (ECASS-1) showed that in patients with small (< 33%) parenchymal hypoattenuation of the MCA, treatment with tissue-type plasminogen activator (t-PA) increased the chance of good outcome.[15] It has been suggested that patients with significant parenchymal changes (> 33% of the MCA territory) are at risk of intracerebral hemorrhage, but this issue is still controversial. A large prospective study showed the specificity and positive predictive value of hypoattenuation (ischemic edema) on baseline CT (performed within 6 hours) for brain infarcts to be 85% and 96%, respectively.[16] The infarct volume is related to stroke outcome.[17,18] However, in the XXX (RANTTAS) trial, the infarct volume on CT scan at 1 week did not provide any additional clinical benefit for the prediction of 3-month outcome.[19]

Neuroradiologists have proved to be most reliable and consistent in the detection of early ischemic changes on CT scans.[20,21] In an acute situation, an expert neuroradiologist may not be available in some institutions to evaluate a patient's eligibility for thrombolytic therapy. One study showed a variable level of sensitivity, averaging 67%, for the correct diagnosis of intracerebral hemorrhage and early CT changes for emergency physicians evaluating CT scans.[22] A post hoc review by the ECASS investigators revealed that early infarction was missed in 11% of the initial assessments.[23]

Hyperdense MCA sign (HMCAS) is an early CT sign of MCA occlusion and indirectly indicates ischemia.[24–26] It has a relatively low sensitivity (47%)[26] and high specificity (85% to 100%) for cerebral ischemia.[27] The value of HMCAS as an isolated predictor of stroke outcome is unclear,[12,26,28] although some studies have found that HMCAS is associated with poor clinical outcome.[29,30] Heavily calcified intracranial arteries may appear as HMCAS, but this finding is often bilateral.

In the cerebrum, the topography of the CT abnormality may assist in differentiating distal infarction due to larger artery thrombosis from infarction attributed to embolism: The former is higher over the convexity and usually spares the sylvian region, whereas the latter conforms more to the territory supplied by one or more cerebral surface branches. Small surface infarcts are not always easily visualized on CT, because they may be hidden in the gyral pattern of the convexity; MRI is a better tool. On CT scans acquired late after onset of stroke, some low-density lesions are the late effect of parenchymatous hematoma; this diagnosis is more easily made from MRI, in which the residual methemoglobin leaves a permanent signal change.

The development of spiral CT, multidetector rows, and subsecond scanning time in CT angiography (CTA) technology allows accurate study of the extracranial carotid arteries and MCA.[27] The combination of CT, CTA, and xenon-enhanced CT (XeCT) can provide information about which vessel or vessels are occluded and the extent of blood flow compromise in the affected vascular territory.[31]

Magnetic Resonance Imaging and Novel Techniques

Over the last decade the progress in MRI technology has contributed significantly to the understanding of the pathophysiology of acute stroke and its management.

DWI relies on the cytotoxic edema (intracellular) in ischemic tissue.[32] This edema causes hyperintense signal on DWI, which is achieved by two diffusion-sensitizing gradients placed symmetrically around the 180-degree radiofrequency pulse of a spin-echo sequence. The apparent diffusion coefficient (ADC) map that quantifies the degree of water proton mobility from one magnetic field to another appears hypointense in the region of restricted diffusion (hyperintense on DWI).[33] It is important to realize that there are two situations in which false-positive results can occur: (1) transient global amnesia, epilepsy, tumors, migraine, and multiple sclerosis can cause hyperintense DWI, and (2) "T2 shine-through," whereby in subacute or chronic infarcts, the T2 signal may become dominant and appears hyperintense on DWI despite normal diffusion.[34] Interpretation in these situations can be helped by the realization that ADC values are not reduced and are often increased in vasogenic edema in tumors and abscesses. After 7 to 14 days, the abnormalities on DWI begin to resolve.[35]

As mentioned earlier, thrombolytic therapy may be contraindicated in patients in whom CT indicates that more than 33% of the MCA is involved. MRI with DWI is more sensitive than CT in the identification of acute ischemia (within 6 hours of the onset of symptoms)[36] and achieved a 100% predictive value in an Australian study compared with CT.[37] MRI with DWI also was superior to T2-weighted MRI for the detection of ischemia.[36,38]

Perfusion-weighted imaging (PWI) relies on the dynamic magnetic susceptibility effects (T2 images) within the brain tissue during the first pass of an intravenously injected gadolinium-based contrast agent.[39–41] There are two types of PWI techniques, bolus tracking (BT-PWI) and arterial spin labeling (ASL-PWI). Multiple-slice imaging of the whole brain is possible with single-shot echoplanar imaging (EPI), giving it an advantage over the single-slice technique of CT perfusion imaging. Various hemodynamic parameters can be derived from the time–signal intensity curve. They include the time to peak (TTP), the mean transit time (MTT), and the relative cerebral blood flow (rCBF) and volume (rCBV). It is important to realize that these are only semi-quantitative data and may be underestimated by bolus-delay effect.[42] MTT is the earliest and most consistent sign of perfusion impairment,[43] and the rCBV map correlates reasonably with the final infarct volume.[44,45] One study has shown that first moment method and deconvolution method are the two most sensitive calculation methods in this setting.[46]

In regard to the clinical application, the acute clinical severity scale for stroke based on National Institutes of Health Stroke Scale (NIHSS) was correlated with acute lesion volumes, in particular hypoperfusion and tissue at risk volumes, and the difference between the volume at risk on images acquired in acute stroke and the infarct volume correlated with the change in clinical severity.[38,47–50] A similar correlation was seen at 7 days.[51] PWI and DWI mismatch (TTP delays of ≥ 6 seconds) in acute stroke indicates a high risk of lesion enlargement and presence of salvageable ischemic tissue.[52,53] Calculation of the absolute ADC value may further identify the tissue at risk,[54] although doubts have been raised about the validity of this observation.[55] Compared with CT, DWI is more accurate and sensitive for the identification of acute infarction and greater than 33% involvement of the MCA. The lesion volume on acutely obtained DWI correlates with the final infarct volume,[56] which is often smaller.[50] Reduction of lesion volumes on DWI and PWI has been demonstrated after successful thrombolytic therapy, a finding that goes at least some way in validating these measures as possible surrogate outcomes in clinical trials.[57]

Further, in hyperacute stroke, the defect on PWI is often larger than that on DWI, and patients with such mismatch have the greatest potential to benefit from thrombolytic therapy.[58,59]

MRI is the preferred method for detecting hemorrhagic transformation and microbleeds. In the early stage, the extent of contrast enhancement correlates with the occurrence and severity of the transformation.[60] This information may become important for risk stratification before thrombolytic treatment is begun.[61]

Magnetic resonance spectroscopy (MRS) measures the relative concentration of major cerebral biochemical substances. Proton [^{1}H]-MRS demonstrates a relative increase in lactate level and a reduction in *N*-acetyl aspartate (NAA) level in the ischemic tissue in comparison with the contralateral hemisphere.[62,63] The application of this technique in the clinical setting is unclear. Knowledge of the infarct volume makes possible a better prediction of morbidity in patients with stroke.[64,65]

MRI offers a clear advantage over CT for imaging of flowing blood, which appears black on the MR image, allowing a diagnosis with a high degree of accuracy.[66] This physiologic effect enables the diagnosis of arteriovenous malformations (AVMs) in ways difficult for CT scan, which relies on hemorrhage, calcification, or contrast enhancement to suggest the diagnosis even though the findings are positive in up to 80% cases.[67] MRI has also become the tool of choice for demonstration of cavernous angiomas, which have a low-signal center and a high-signal rim, commonly called a "tiger eye." These small angiographically occult lesions may cause brain hemorrhage. MRI may also demonstrate the thrombosed dome of a recently ruptured aneurysm, a difficult imaging feat rarely achieved by CT scan.

Both CT and MRI can document deep infarcts,[68] with MRI showing smaller lesions than those seen on CT, especially in the basal ganglia and thalamus.[69] MRI is preferred over CT for the smaller infarcts deep in the brain and for those in the brainstem, especially if a fluid-attenuated inversion-recovery (FLAIR) sequence is used.[70,71] However, the mere imaging of these smaller lesions does not elucidate whether the mechanism in a particular case is thrombotic or embolic.[72] When a core of very low signal is seen on MRI, the uncommon deep lesions from old hemorrhage can be differentiated from those of infarction. The sensitivity of detection of old hemorrhage can be improved

Diagnostic Studies

by EPI sequences.[41] Coexisting surface infarcts often confound attempts to attribute physiologic abnormalities to deep infarcts on CT scan.[73-76] Many of the larger deep infarcts are not due to microatheroma in the lenticulostriate arteries but have had an associated cerebral surface component that reflects their embolic origin. No findings on CT or MRI reliably separate a deep lesion due to thrombosis of a small feeding artery from one caused by occlusion from embolism.

Duplex and Transcranial Doppler Ultrasonography

In experienced hands, duplex and transcranial Doppler (TCD) methods of ultrasonography may provide useful information within minutes, adding to the assessment of acute stroke.[77,78] In a setting of occlusion in the early hours after stroke, before brain imaging can demonstrate the changes of infarction, duplex Doppler ultrasonography may disclose high-grade stenosis of a carotid or vertebral artery. The internal carotid artery peak systolic velocity (ICAPSV) and the ratio of ICAPSV to common carotid artery peak systolic velocity (CCAPSV) add accuracy to the diagnosis of crucial 60% to 70% stenosis.[79,80] Severe stenosis can often be difficult to distinguish from an occlusion; color Doppler ultrasonography and the use of an intravenous contrast medium can improve the accuracy.[81] The morphology,[82] echogenicity,[83,84] and surface ulceration[85] provide further information on the risk of cerebral infarction.

From TCD ultrasonography findings, one may infer extracranial carotid occlusion[86] or high-grade stenosis by a collateral across the circle of Willis to the affected side, signaled by reversal of flow in the ipsilateral anterior cerebral vessels (particularly the A1 segment) ipsilateral to a hemodynamically significant lesion.[87,88] Very few patients with lacunar infarction have significant artery abnormalities.[87]

Intracranial disease may also be documented as stenosis of the basilar artery or a major cerebral artery. When the MCA velocity signal is missing ipsilateral to symptomatic hemisphere dysfunction, the sensitivity and specificity of TCD ultrasonography in the detection of stenosis or occlusion are 87.5% and 88.6% respectively, in comparison with angiography.[89,90] Proof of occlusion of a major cerebral artery is difficult to demonstrate directly, but increased velocity in an adjacent cerebral artery may indicate an augmentation flow-bearing collateral vessel.[91] The sensitivity and specificity of TCD ultrasonography in the detection of the site of arterial occlusion are 80% and 94%, respectively.[92] The degree of arterial occlusion demonstrated by this modality within 4 hours of admission is significantly associated with clinical outcome.[93] The rate of recanalization or recovery of flow in the MCA coincides with angiographic resolution and clinical recovery.[94,95] When the Doppler waveforms indicate greatly reduced resistance to flow, an arteriovenous shunt may be suspected, helping to suggest AVM in some instances of brain hemorrhage. Although vasospasm after acute rupture of an aneurysm is not usually found in the first day or so, TCD ultrasonography has proved to be a useful tool for the early detection of vasospasm and a means of following its course.[96]

Technical difficulty with poor signal quality is encountered in 5% to 15% of patients.[97] Echocontrast-enhanced TCD ultrasonography studies can improve the quality and diagnostic confidence but come with a price of increase in rate of false-positive results.[98]

TCD ultrasonography has also been shown to be of potential benefit in detecting embolic (high-intensity) signals in the middle cerebral and carotid arteries, but the practical uses of this information are still being determined.[99] Specifically, it remains to be shown whether these signals translate into increased stroke risk in various clinical settings, such as symptomatic or asymptomatic carotid stenosis.[100] In one study, the inferred detection of microembolism over 20 minutes was associated with early relapse in patients with infarctions or transient ischemic attacks.[101] Findings of TCD ultrasonography are similar in the setting of symptomatic carotid stenosis[102] and carotid artery dissection with stenosis.[103] The use of anticoagulation may decrease the microembolic signals, but its clinical value is unclear (see Chapter 21).[104]

Doppler ultrasonography can quickly provide information about carotid or vertebral artery dissection, but MRA (see later) or digital subtraction angiography (DSA) may provide more complete information.

Echocardiography

Transesophageal echocardiography (TEE), which is being used increasingly to identify cardiac or aortic arch sources of embolism not previously realized, is superior to transthoracic echocardiography (TTE) for this use.[105] Although the procedure is modestly invasive, in that it usually requires the patient to be sedated during the passage of the probe down the esophagus, the information provided may help determine subsequent stroke risk and possibly assist in therapy. A major issue is now the finding that aortic arch atheroma may be a more common cause of ischemic stroke than previously realized, although which form of therapy is most effective is as yet unclear.[106] Through the use of TEE, cardiac causes of emboli have also been detected that could not be visualized with TTE. Of these, stasis within the atrium, which causes a swirling pattern of left atrial spontaneous echocontrast, is the most notable and is usually present in association with atrial fibrillation. This information is applicable to all stroke subtypes, including lacunar stroke.[107]

Patent foramen ovale (PFO) is frequently associated with embolic stroke, particularly in patients younger than 55 years.[108,109] TEE is the preferred investigation for the detection of PFO.[110] For patients who are not suitable candidates for TEE, contrast-enhanced TCD ultrasonography is the alternative investigation modality.[111] Intrapulmonary shunts may produce false-positive results for contrast-enhanced TCD ultrasonography.[112]

Lumbar Puncture

Long the mainstay of diagnosis, lumbar puncture has been relegated to a minor role now that high-quality brain imaging is available. Widespread subarachnoid hemorrhage or local subarachnoid collections can usually be detected by CT, and MRI can demonstrate most of the larger aneurysms and all the AVMs and cavernous angiomas, obviating the purpose of lumbar puncture, which simply proves the existence of subarachnoid hemorrhage but not the cause. When imaging is not available, lumbar puncture is distinctive for identification of subarachnoid hemorrhage; analysis of the cerebrospinal fluid (CSF) usually detects blood, high protein level, and xanthochromia in the major syndrome caused by parenchymatous brain hemorrhage but findings may be normal in small brain hemorrhage. In this last setting, differentiating hemorrhage from infarction is important; whether or not to treat with anticoagulants must be decided. Therefore in this case, lumbar puncture alone is not sufficient to rule out hemorrhage if the CSF is clear. In the rare instance of arteritis, lumbar puncture may show elevated white blood cell counts and high protein level in CSF, findings also encountered in large infarcts.

Angiography and Magnetic Resonance Angiography

Angiography remains the preferred tool for demonstrating aneurysm and vasospasm and for easy diagnosis of AVM.[113] There has been a steady decline in the use of this technique in the management of ischemic cerebrovascular disease since the introduction of the noninvasive approaches discussed earlier. Many embolic occlusions are quite transient, so that there must be a plan for prompt angiography, if it is to be performed to confirm a diagnosis of occlusion due to embolism.[114,115] Thrombosis is expected to persist. The search for a source of embolism is a separate issue from documenting the occurrence of brain embolism. In the case of the former, conventional monitoring of arrhythmia, blood cultures, echocardiography, and the like usually takes days. If delayed until the results of these tests are complete, angiography could have a negative result.

DSA is fast being eclipsed in some centers by MRA,[116] which has almost matched conventional angiography in estimation of disease at the carotid bifurcation[117] and demonstration of vascular occlusion before and recanalization after thrombolytic treatment.[118–120] However, MRA tends to overestimate the degree of stenosis compared with conventional angiography, a difference that may have the effect of falsely identifying patients as candidates for carotid endarterectomy, given the current trial evidence for symptomatic disease (70% stenosis or greater).[121] MRA has been reported to have 100% sensitivity and specificity in differentiating carotid occlusion from a greater than 95% stenosis.[122] Gadolinium-enhanced MRA has a 92% compatibility with DSA in the grading of carotid stenosis and a 100% detection rate for occlusion.[123] For the detection of vertebral artery stenosis, MRA has more than 98% sensitivity and specificity.[122]

In both DSA and MRA, the circle of Willis and the basilar artery, their main branches, and many of the large surface vessels can be imaged well enough for one to determine whether some are occluded.[124] CTA is sometimes used to complement other studies, but the extra computer time required to construct the images can be a disadvantage.[125]

Fat-suppression T1- and T2-weighted MRI is superior to MRA in the demonstration of carotid dissection. Both DSA and MRA show AVMs, but neither method is as yet the equal of cut-film angiography in showing vasospasm and the widespread stenoses found in arteritis. MRA has been found to have only moderate sensitivity and specificity for the detection of aneurysm in subarachnoid hemorrhage.[126]

Studies of Blood Flow and Metabolism

Xenon-Enhanced Computed Tomography
XeCT blood flow imaging is occasionally used[127] but has now been supplemented by single-photon emission CT (SPECT).[128] Both methods demonstrate both local and distant functional effects after stroke, and some investigators have used the methods to show effects on resting flows remote from the site of infarction. If either method is applied quickly after infarction, the deficit in local flow may be evident before the tissue signal changes appear on CT or MRI, and reasonable sensitivities and specificities for subsequent infarction have been shown.[7] An XeCT CBF study allows for the rapid and quantitative assessment of CBF. Critical values less than $6 cm^3/100g/min$ in the ischemic region may presage future infarction.[129] A small study showed patients with no infarction on initial CT and normal XeCT CBF findings within 24 hours of onset of stroke symptoms had significantly fewer new infarctions than those with compromised CBF on initial study.[31]

Neither technique separates hemorrhage from infarction. It remains uncertain whether SPECT and XeCT will predict the potential for clinical recovery.[130] A combination of TCD ultrasonography and CBF evaluation has been helpful in tracking the course of vasospasm in subarachnoid hemorrhage.[131]

Perfusion-Weighted Computed Tomography
Perfusion-weighted CT (PWCT) imaging is a new technique that reflects low CBV within a collapsed vascular bed, allowing better delineation of the injured tissue from the normal. The modality is relatively rapid in acquisition and low in cost.[132] Its clinical application and correlation with outcome measures are unclear.[133] One study has shown that PWCT enables the accurate prediction of final infarct size at the time of emergency evaluation.[134]

Positron Emission Tomography
Positron emission tomography (PET) has demonstrated its power in documenting the functional metabolic response of the brain to focal infarction, but its availability is still limited.[135] PET remains the best method for demonstrating viable tissue in cerebral ischemia,[5,136] the time window for which may be longer than previously realized.[137] The method has been able to demonstrate the remote effects of infarctions, some spread over wide areas[138] and some explained as trans-synaptic depression or dischesis.[139] Tissue cubes, as small as 10 to 15 mm on a side, are being imaged by these techniques.[140]

TRANSIENT ISCHEMIC ATTACKS

Transient ischemic attacks (TIAs) are defined as neurologic symptoms of vascular etiology that resolve within 24 hours. Traditionally one would not expect to see the corresponding lesion on a CT scan in acute stroke. MRI with DWI

Diagnostic Studies

demonstrated ischemic changes in 48% of patients in one study, half of whom progressed to infarction.[141] The percentage of patients with a DWI lesion increases with the duration of the symptoms. It is of interest that about half of these DWI lesions are reversible.[39,141,142] ADC maps of these patients typically show less severe lesions than those of patients with acute stroke. This information is useful in the localization of the event and its etiology, especially in patients with atypical symptoms. Its effect on morbidity is not yet proved.[141]

Only after the symptoms have faded is a diagnosis of TIA justified. In the acute symptomatic phase, the approach is the same as that for an acute stroke. Symptoms may fade or may entirely disappear, yet brain imaging demonstrates recent ischemic lesions. The old definition of TIA as any neurologic deficit resolving in 24 hours is out of date. The actual duration of a brief ischemic event is typically measured in minutes, not hours. In patients whose symptoms have lasted longer than 1 hour, a higher frequency of brain lesions has been found than in patients whose symptoms have lasted for minutes.

After it is certain that all symptoms have disappeared, investigation of a TIA is directed at underlying disease, which may predict the risk of recurrence in the same or a different vascular territory.

By habit and because there is a surgical option for therapy, TIAs are often equated with the surgically correctable disease in the neck at the carotid bifurcation. However, TIAs may occur in territories remote from this site. For those affecting the carotid territory, duplex and TCD ultrasonography should suffice to determine whether high-grade stenosis or occlusion exists and to detect indications of the development of collateral vessels. Embolism may account for many TIAs, yet some may be explained by distal insufficiency in the far fields of the MCA or in the borderzone between the middle and anterior cerebral arteries.[143] This suprasylvian location would be expected to produce a clinical deficit involving the forearm and hand.

A high frequency of stereotypic neurologic deficits has been reported in patients suffering repeated TIAs.[144] Even in single attacks, distal brachial sensorimotor syndromes lead all other syndromes in frequency. PET and SPECT can determine whether the brain being supplied through the stenosis or by collateral vessels around the stenosis or occlusion suffers from inadequate flow[139] (i.e. misery perfusion syndrome),[145] which has been shown to be surgically reversible in some instances. In the even more severe state of distal intracranial internal carotid artery stenosis with abundant collateral vessels associated with moyamoya disease, hyperventilation has been shown to precipitate focal symptoms.[146] The demonstration of such an extreme degree of sensitivity of cerebral flow to alteration in PCO_2 suggests that cerebral claudication may even occur.[69]

Angiography, DSA,[147] CTA,[124] and MRA have all become popular for demonstrating stenosis or occlusion of the carotid. Venous bolus angiography has become less popular because of poor resolution and the high dose of intravenous contrast agent required.[148] In experienced centers, the combination of Doppler ultrasonography to demonstrate high-grade stenosis and the extent of collateral circulation with MRA to show anatomy may replace all invasive angiography in the evaluation of extracranial occlusive disease. Even though the risks are small, angiographic complications in direct injection studies remain a risk to be avoided when possible.[149] However, conventional angiography is still the tool of choice to show ulceration, a component of carotid disease that may still explain many forms of stroke. When Doppler ultrasonography or MRA fails to indicate high-grade stenosis, DSA may not be fully justified.

ASYMPTOMATIC DISEASE

Asymptomatic disease manifests usually as a bruit discovered on routine office evaluation or stenosis on Doppler ultrasonography performed as a screening test.[150] The bruit of carotid stenosis and from radiated heart murmurs is difficult to distinguish clinically. The improvement in Doppler technology has been so great that a bruit is no longer regarded as a sign of stenosis of the carotid artery but only as an indication for evaluation by Doppler ultrasonography.[151]

Doppler ultrasonographic evaluation of the flow velocities through arteries has been available for years.[152] Some of the devices using Doppler signals display the different velocities encountered along an artery in different colors according to velocity, allowing the clinician to see the stenosis in one color and the normal flow in another. Like spectral analysis, Doppler studies can be useful to follow the course of a stenosis.[153] Although impressive, the information from conventional continuous-wave Doppler analysis adds little to that available from other methods and has its own sources of error.[152] Pulse-wave, range-gated Doppler ultrasonographic techniques have been developed that can scan the lumen from wall to wall in tiny steps.[147] Newer devices that allow color-coded displays permit better characterization of the flow patterns. Despite such improved characterizations, it has not yet become evident that the extra information obtained relates to stroke risk.[154] To date, the role of progression of the extracranial carotid stenosis, not the specific characteristics of the velocity profiles, has predicted subsequent symptoms.

Brain imaging may demonstrate prior stroke. In roughly 20% of patients with high-grade stenosis, and in a similar number of patients seen for their first symptomatic stroke, CT scan shows evidence of prior brain infarction. Most of the lesions are small and are in brain region not likely to cause major symptoms, but a small percentage have been as large as a portion of a cerebral lobe, a finding not easily dismissed although not in any way explained.

Asymptomatic aneurysms, AVMs, cavernous angiomas, and dural fistulas have also been shown by brain imaging. Little is known of the prognostic significance of such findings, except for aneurysms: A few studies have indicated a higher risk of hemorrhage from aneurysms measuring 8 to 15 mm.

References

1. Donnan GA: Investigation of patients with stroke and transient ischaemic attacks. Lancet 339:473, 1992.
2. Kistler JP, Nuonanno FS, Dewitt LD, et al: Vertebral basilar posterior cerebral territory stroke delineation by proton nuclear magnetic resonance imaging. Stroke 15:417, 1984.

3. McCullough EC, Baker HL Jr: Nuclear magnetic resonance. Radiol Clin North Am 20:3, 1982.

4. Brahme FJ: CT diagnosis of cerebrovascular disorders: A review. Comput Tomogr 2:173, 1978.

5. Yamauchi H, Fukuyama H, Kimura J, et al: Hemodynamics in internal carotid artery occlusion examined by positron emission tomography. Stroke 21:1400, 1990.

6. Zilkha A: Intraparenchymal fluid-blood level: A CT sign of recent intracerebral hemorrhage. J Comput Assist Tomogr 7:301, 1983.

7. Brass LM, Walovitch RC, Joseph JL, et al: The role of single photon emission computed tomography brain imaging with ^{99m}Tc-bicisate in the localization and definition of mechanism of ischemic stroke. J Cereb Blood Flow Metab 14(Suppl 1):S91–S98, 1994.

8. Schellinger PD, Jansen O, Fiebach JB, et al: A standard MRI stroke protocol: Comparison with CT in hyperacute intracerebral hemorrhage. Stroke 30:765, 1999.

9. Inoue Y, Takemoto K, Miyamoto T, et al: Sequential computed tomography scans in acute cerebral infarction. Radiology 135:655, 1980.

10. Mohr JP, Biller J, Hilal SK, et al: MR vs CT imaging in acute stroke. Stroke 26:807, 1995.

11. Tatemichi TK, Mohr JP, Rubinstein LV, et al: CT findings and clinical course in acute stroke: The NINCDS stroke data bank. Presented at the Tenth International Joint Conference on Stroke and Cerebral Circulation, New Orleans, February 22, 1985.

12. Moulin T, Cattin F, Crepin-Leblond T, et al: Early CT signs in acute middle cerebral artery infarction: Predictive value for subsequent infarct locations and outcome. Neurology 47:366, 1996.

13. Schuknecht B, Ratzka M, Hofmann E: The "dense artery sign": Major cerebral artery thromboembolism demonstrated by computed tomography. Neuroradiology 32:98, 1990.

14. Tomura N, Uemura K, Inugami A, et al: Early CT finding in cerebral infarction: Obscuration of the lentiform nucleus. Radiology 1168:463, 1988.

15. Von Kummer R, Allen KL, Holle R, et al: Acute stroke: Usefulness of early CT findings before thrombolytic therapy. Radiology 205:327, 1997.

16. Von Kummer R, Bourquain H, Bastianello S, et al: Early prediction of irreversible brain damage after ischaemic stroke at CT. European Cooperative Acute Stroke Study II Group. Radiology 219:95, 2001.

17. Saver JL, Johnston KC, Homer D, et al: Infarct volume as a surrogate or auxiliary outcome measure in ischaemic stroke clinical trial. Stroke 30:293, 1999.

18. Brott T, Marler JR, Olinger CP, et al: Measurement of acute cerebral infarction: Lesion size by computed tomography. Stroke 20:871, 1989.

19. Johnston KC, Wagner DP, Haley EC, et al: Combined clinical and imaging information as an early stroke outcome measure. RANTTAS Investigators. Stroke 33:466, 2002.

20. Kalafut MA, Schriger DL, Saver JL, Starkman S: Detection of early CT signs of > 1/3 middle cerebral artery infarctions: Interrater reliability and sensitivity of CT interpretation by physicians involved in acute stroke care. Stroke 31:1667, 2000.

21. Von Kummer R, Holle R, Grzyska U, et al: Interobserver agreement in assessing early CT signs of middle cerebral artery infarction. Am J Neuroradiol 17:1743, 1996.

22. Schrifer D, Kalafut M, Starkman S, et al: Cranial computed tomography interpretation in acute stroke. JAMA 279:1293, 1998.

23. Hacke W, Kaste M, Fieschi C, et al: Intravenous thrombolysis with recombinant tissue plasminogen activator for acute hemisphere stroke. The European Cooperative Acute Stroke Study (ECASS). JAMA 274:1017, 1995.

24. Bastianello S, Pierallini A, Colonnese C: Hyperdense middle cerebral artery CT sign: Comparison with angiography in the acute phase of ischaemic supratentorial infarction. Neuroradiology 33:207, 1991.

25. Tomsick TA, Brott TG, Olinger CP: Hyperdense middle cerebral artery: Incidence and quantitative significance. Neuroradiology 31:312, 1989.

26. Von Kummer R, Meyding-Lamade U, Forsting M, et al: Sensitivity and prognostic value of early CT in occlusion of the middle cerebral artery trunk. Am J Neuroradiol 15:9, 1994.

27. Leys D, Pruvo JP, Godefroy O, et al: Prevalence and significance of hyperdense middle cerebral artery in acute stroke. Stroke 23:317, 1992.

28. Manelfe C, Larrue V, von Kummer R, et al: Association of hyperdense middle cerebral artery sign with clinical outcome in patients treated with tissue plasminogen activator. Stroke 30:769, 1999.

29. Launes J, Ketonen L: Dense middle cerebral artery infarction. J Neurol Neurosurg Psychiatry 50:1550, 1987.

30. Tomsick TA, Brott TG, Barsan W, et al: Prognostic value of the hyperdense middle cerebral artery sign and stroke scale score before ultraearly thrombolytic treatment. Am J Neuroradiol 17:79, 1996.

31. Kilpatrick MM, Yonas H, Goldstein S, et al: CT-based assessment of acute stroke: CT, CT angiography, and xenon-enhanced CT cerebral blood flow. Stroke 32:2543, 2001.

32. Provenzale J, Sorensen G: Diffusion-weighted MR imaging in acute stroke: Theoretic considerations and clinical applications. AJR Am J Roentgenol 173:1459, 1999.

33. Fisher M, Albers GW: Applications of diffusion-perfusion magnetic resonance imaging in acute ischaemic stroke. Neurology 52:1750, 1999.

34. Burdette JH, Elster AD, Ricci PE: Acute cerebral infarction: Quantification of spin-density and T2 shine-through phenomena on diffusion-weighted MR images. Radiology 212:333, 1999.

35. Schlaug G, Siewert B, Benfield A, et al: Time course of the apparent diffusion coefficient (ADC) abnormality in human stroke. Neurology 49:113, 1997.

36. Gonzalez RG, Schaefer PW, Buonanno FS, et al: Diffusion-weighted MR imaging: Diagnostic accuracy in patients imaged within 6 hours of stroke symptom onset. Radiology 210:155, 1999.

37. Barber PA, Darby DG, Desmond PM, et al: Identification of major ischaemic change: Diffusion-weighted imaging versus computed tomography. Stroke 30:2059, 1999.

38. Van Everdingen KJ, Van der Grond J, Kappelle LJ, et al: Diffusion-weighted magnetic resonance imaging in acute stroke. Stroke 29:1783, 1998.

39. Baird AE, Warach S: Magnetic resonance imaging of acute stroke. J Cereb Blood Flow Metab 18:583, 1998.

40. Calamante F, Thomas DL, Pell GS, et al: Measuring cerebral blood flow using magnetic resonance imaging techniques. J Cereb Blood Flow Metab 19:701, 1999.

41. Jager HR: Diagnosis of stroke with advanced CT and MR imaging. Br Med Bull 56:318, 2000.

42. Ostergarrd L, Chesler DA, Weisskoff RM, et al: Modeling cerebral blood flow and flow heterogeneity from magnetic resonance residue data. J Cereb Blood Flow 18:1143, 1999.

43. Beauchamp N, Barker P, Wang P, van Zijl P: Imaging of acute cerebral ischemia. Radiology 212:307, 1999.

44. Sorensen AG, Copen WA, Ostergaard L, et al: Hyperacute stroke: Simultaneous measurement of relative cerebral blood volume, relative cerebral blood flow, and mean tissue transit time. Radiology 210:519, 1999.

45. Ueda T, Yuh W, Maley J, et al: Outcome of acute ischaemic lesions evaluated by diffusion and perfusion MR imaging. AJNR Am J Neuroradiol 20:983, 1999.

46. Yamada K, Wu O, Gonzalez G, et al: Magnetic resonance perfusion-weighted imaging of acute cerebral infarction: Effect of the calculation methods and underlying vasculopathy. Stroke 33:87, 2002.

47. Baird AE, Lovblad KO, Dashe JF, et al: Clinical correlations of diffusion and perfusion lesion volumes in acute ischaemic stroke. Cerebrovasc Dis 10:441, 2000.

48. Beaulieu C, de Crespigny A, Tong DC, et al: Longitudinal magnetic resonance imaging study of perfusion and diffusion in stroke: Evolution of lesion volume and correlation with clinical outcome. Ann Neurol 46:568, 1999.

49. Lev MH, Segal AZ, Farkas J, et al: Utility of perfusion-weighted CT imaging in acute middle cerebral artery stroke treated with intra-arterial thrombolysis: Prediction of final infarct volume and clinical outcome. Stroke 32:2021, 2001.

50. Schwamm LH, Koroshetz WJ, Sorensen G, et al: Time course of lesion development in patients with acute stroke: Serial diffusion- and hemodynamic-weighted magnetic resonance imaging. Stroke 29:2268, 1998.

51. Tong DC, Yenari MA, Albers GW, et al: Correlation of perfusion- and diffusion-weighted MRI with NIHSS score in acute (<6.5 hours) ischaemic stroke. Neurology 50:864, 1998.

Diagnostic Studies

52. Barber PA, Darby DG, Desmond PM, et al: Prediction of stroke outcome with echoplanar perfusion- and diffusion-weighted MRI. Neurology 51:418, 1998.

53. Neumann-Hadfelin T, Wittsack H-J, Wenserski F, et al: Diffusion- and perfusion-weighted MRI: The DWI/PWI mismatch region in acute stroke. Stroke 30:1591, 1999.

54. Oppenheim C, Grandin C, Samson Y, et al: Is there an apparent diffusion coefficient threshold in predicting tissue viability in hyperacute stroke? Stroke 32:2486, 2001.

55. Fiehler J, Foth M, Kucinski T, et al: Severe ADC decreases do not predict irreversible tissue damage in humans. Stroke 33:79, 2002.

56. Lansberg MG, Albers GW, Beaulieu C, Marks MP: Comparison of diffusion-weighted MRI and CT in acute stroke. Neurology 54:1557, 2000.

57. Kidwell CS, Saver JL, Mattiello J, et al: Thrombolytic reversal of acute human cerebral ischaemic injury shown by diffusion/perfusion magnetic resonance imaging. Ann Neurol 47:462, 2000.

58. Marks MP, Tong DC, Beaulieu C, et al: Evaluation of early reperfusion and i.v. tPA therapy using diffusion and perfusion-weighted MRI. Neurology 52:1792, 1999.

59. Schellinger PD, Jansen O, Fiebach JB, et al: Monitoring intravenous recombinant tissue plasminogen activator thrombolysis for acute ischaemic stroke with diffusion and perfusion MRI. Stroke 31:1318, 2000.

60. Mayer TE, Schuffe-Altedorneburg G, Droste DW, Bruchmann H: Serial CT and MRI of ischaemic cerebral infarcts: Frequency and clinical impact of haemorrhagic transformation. Neuroradiology 42:233, 2000.

61. Kidwell CS, Saver JL, Villablanca P, et al: Magnetic resonance imaging detection of microbleeds before thrombolysis: An emerging application. Stroke 33:95, 2002.

62. Gillard JH, Barker PB, van Zijl PCM, et al: Proton MR spectroscopy in acute middle cerebral artery stroke. AJNR Am J Neuroradiol 17:873, 1996.

63. Saunders D, Howe FA, van den Boogaart A, et al: Continuing ischaemic damage after acute middle cerebral artery infarction in humans demonstrated by short-echo proton spectroscopy. Stroke 26:1007, 1995.

64. Pereira AC, Saunders DE, Doyle VL, et al: Measurement of initial N-acetyl aspartate using magnetic resonance spectroscopy and initial infarct volume using MRI predicts outcome in patients with middle cerebral artery territory infarction. Stroke 30:1577, 1999.

65. Wardlaw JM, Marshall I, Wild J, et al: Studies of acute stroke with proton magnetic resonance spectroscopy: Relation between time from onset, neurological deficit, metabolite abnormalities in the infarct, blood flow, and clinical outcome. Stroke 29:1618, 1998.

66. Nussel F, Wegmuller H, Huber P: Comparison of magnetic resonance angiography, magnetic resonance imaging and conventional angiography in cerebral arteriovenous malformation. Neuroradiology 33: 56, 1991.

67. Leblanc R, Ethier R, Litter JR: Computerized tomography findings in arteriovenous malformations of the brain. J Neurosurg 51:765, 1979.

68. Sipponen JT, Kaste M, Sepponen RE, et al: Nuclear magnetic resonance imaging in reversible cerebral ischaemia. Lancet 1:294, 1983.

69. Mohr JP: Discussion. In Reivich M (ed): Cerebrovascular Disease: Proceedings of the Thirteenth Princeton Conference in Cerebrovascular Disease. Philadelphia, Lippincott-Raven, 1983.

70. Alexander JA, Sheppard D, Davies PC, Salverda P: Adult cerebrovascular disease: Role of modified rapid fluid-attenuated inversion-recovery sequences. AJNR Am J Neuroradiol 17:1507, 1996.

71. Savoiardo M, Bracchi M, Passerini A, Visciani A: The vascular territories in the cerebellum and brainstem: CT and MR study. AJNR Am J Neuroradiol 8:199, 1987.

72. Mohr JP: Lacunes. Neurol Clin North Am 1:201, 1983.

73. Castaigne P, Lhermitte F, Buge A, et al: Paramedian thalamic and midbrain infarcts: Clinical and neuropathological study. Ann Neurol 10:127, 1981.

74. Rascol A, Clanet M, Manelfe C: Pure motor hemiplegia: CT study of 30 cases. Stroke 13:11, 1982.

75. Wallesch CW, Kornhuber HH, Kunz T, Brunner RJ: Neuropsychological deficits associated with small unilateral thalamic lesions. Brain 106:141, 1983.

76. Weaver RG Jr, Howard G, McKinney WM, et al: Comparison of Doppler ultrasonography with arteriography of the carotid bifurcation. Stroke 4:402, 1980.

77. Comerota AJ, Crabley JJ, Cook SE: Real-time B-mode carotid imaging in diagnosis of cerebrovascular disease. Surgery 6:718, 1981.

78. Tatemichi TK, Oropeza LA, Saco RL, et al: Doppler diagnosis of vertebral artery occlusion: Role of run off into the posterior inferior cerebellar artery. Ann Neurol 26:58, 1989.

79. Hunink MGM, Polak JF, Barlan MM, O'Leary DH: Detection and quantification of carotid artery stenosis: Efficacy of various Doppler velocity parameters. Am J Roentgenol 160:619, 1993.

80. Moneta GL, Edwards JM, Chitwood RW, et al: Correlation of North American Symptomatic Carotid Endarterectomy Trial (NASCET) angiographic definition of 70% to 99% internal carotid artery stenosis with duplex scanning. J Vasc Surg 17:152, 1993.

81. Sitzer M, Furst G, Siebler M, Steinmetz H: Usefulness of an intravenous contrast medium in the characterization of high-grade internal carotid stenosis with color Doppler-assisted duplex imaging. Stroke 25:385, 1994.

82. Hatsukami TS, Ferguson MS, Beach KW, et al: Carotid plaque morphology and clinical events. Stroke 28:95, 1997.

83. Geroulakos G, Ramaswami G, Nicholaides A, et al: Characterisation of symptomatic and asymptomatic carotid plaques using high-resolution real-time ultrasonography. Br J Surg 80:1274, 1993.

84. Sterpetti AV, Schultz RD, Feldhaus RJ, et al: Ultrasonographic features of carotid plaque and the risk of subsequent neurologic deficits. Surgery 104:652, 1988.

85. Zukowski AJ, Nicolaides AAN, Lewis RT, et al: The correlation between carotid plaque ulceration and cerebral infarction seen on CT scan. J Vasc Surg 1:782, 1984.

86. Kaps M, Damian MS, Reschendorf U, Dorndorf W: Transcranial Doppler ultrasound findings in middle cerebral artery occlusion. Stroke 21:532, 1990.

87. Mead GE, Wardlaw JM, Dennis MS, et al: Relationship between pattern of intracranial artery abnormalities on transcranial Doppler and Oxfordshire Community Stroke Project clinical classification of ischaemic stroke. Stroke 31:714, 2000.

88. Taemichi TK, Chamorro A, Petty GW, et al: Hemodynamic role of ophthalmic artery collateral in internal carotid artery occlusion. Neurology (NY) 40:461, 1990.

89. Alexandrov AV, Demchuk AM, Wein TH, Grotta JC: Yield of transcranial Doppler in acute cerebral ischemia. Stroke 30:1604, 1999.

90. Kushner MJ, Zaenette EM, Bastianello S, et al: Transcranial Doppler in acute hemispheric brain infarction. Neurology (NY) 41:109, 1990.

91. Mohr JP, Caplan LR, Melski JW, et al: The Harvard Cooperative Stroke Registry: A prospective registry of cases hospitalized with stroke. Neurology (NY) 28:754, 1978.

92. Nabavi DG, Droste DW, Kemeny V, et al: Potential and limitations of echocontrast-enhanced ultrasonography in acute stroke patients. Stroke 29:949, 1998.

93. Alexandrov AV, Bladin CF, Norris JW: Intracranial blood flow velocities in acute ischaemic stroke. Stroke 25:1378, 1994.

94. Burgin WS, Malkoff M, Felberg RA, et al: Transcranial Doppler ultrasound criteria for recanalization after thrombolysis for middle cerebral artery stroke. Stroke 31:1128, 2000.

95. Mohr JP, Duterte DI, Oliveira VR, et al: Recanalization of acute middle cerebral artery occlusion. Neurology (NY) 38:215, 1988.

96. Lennihan L, Petty GW, Mohr JP, et al: Transcranial Doppler detection of anterior cerebral artery vasospasm. Stroke 20:151, 1989.

97. Egido JA, Sanchez C: Neurosonology in cerebral ischemia: Future application of transcranial Doppler in acute stroke. Cerebrovasc Dis 11(Suppl 1):15, 2001.

98. Baumgartner RW, Mattle HP, Aaslid R: Transcranial color-coded duplex sonography, magnetic resonance angiography, and computed tomography angiography: Methods, applications, advantages and limitations. J Clin Ultrasound 23:89, 1995.

99. Delcker A, Schnell A, Wilhelm H: Microembolic signals and clinical outcome in patients with acute stroke: A prospective study. Eur Arch Psychiatry Clin Neurosci 250:1, 2000.

100. Siebler M, Kleinschmidt A, Sitzer M, et al: Cerebral microembolism in symptomatic high grade internal carotid artery stenosis. Neurology 44:615, 1994.

101. Valton L, Larrue V, Pavy le Traon A, et al: Microembolic signals and risk of early stroke recurrence in patients with stroke or transient ischaemic attack. Stroke 29:2125, 1998.

Diagnostic Studies

102. Markus HS, Harrison MJ: Microembolic signal detection using ultrasound. Stroke 26:1517, 1995.

103. Droste DW, Junker K, Stogbauer F, et al: Clinically silent circulating microemboli in 20 patients with carotid or vertebral artery dissection. Cerebrovasc Dis 12:181, 2001.

104. Batista P, Oliveira V, Ferro JM: The detection of microembolic signals in patients at risk of recurrent cardioembolic stroke: Possible therapeutic relevance. Cerebrovasc Dis 9:314, 1999.

105. Donaldson RM, Emanuel RW, Earl CJ: The role of two dimensional echocardiography in the detection of potentially embolic intracardiac masses in patients with cerebral ischemia. J Neurol Neurosurg Psychiatry 44:803, 1981.

106. Amarenco P, Cohen A, Tzourio C, et al: Atherosclerotic disease of the aortic arch and the risk of ischemic stroke. N Engl J Med 331:1474, 1994.

107. Kazui S, Levi CR, Jones EF, et al: Lacunar stroke: Transesophageal echocardiographic factors influencing long-term prognosis. Cerebrovasc Dis 12:325, 2001.

108. Hausmann D, Mugge A, Becht I, Daniel WG: Diagnosis of patent foramen ovale by transesophageal echocardiography and association with cerebral and peripheral embolic events. Am J Cardiol 70:668, 1992.

109. Teague SM, Sharma MK: Detection of paradoxical cerebral echo contrast embolization by transcranial Doppler ultrasound. Stroke 22:740, 1991.

110. Baguet JP, Besson G, Tremel F, et al: Should one use echocardiography or contrast transcranial Doppler ultrasound for the detection of a patent ovale after an ischaemic cerebrovascular accident? Cerebrovasc Dis 12:318, 2001.

111. Jauss M, Zanette E: Detection of right-to-left shunt with ultrasound contrast agent and transcranial Doppler sonography. Cerebrovasc Dis 10:490, 2000.

112. Devuyst G, Despland PA, Bogousslavsky J, Jeanrenaud X: Complementary of contrast transcranial Doppler and contrast transesophageal echocardiography for the detection of patent foramen ovale in stroke patients. Eur Neurol 38:21, 1997.

113. Liliequist B, Lindqvist M, Valdimarsson E: Computed tomography and subarachnoid haemorrhage. Neuroradiology 14:21, 1977.

114. Delal PM, Shah PM, Aiyar RR: Arteriographic study of cerebral embolism. Lancet 2:358, 1961.

115. Irino T, Tandea M, Minami T: Angiographic manifestations in postrecanalized cerebral infarction. Neurology 27:471, 1977.

116. Ludwig JW, Verhoeven LHJ, Engels PHC: Digital video subtraction angiography (DVSA) equipment: Angiographic technique in comparison with conventional angiography in different vascular areas. Br J Radiol 55:54, 1982.

117. Mattle HP, Kent KC, Edelman RR, et al: Evaluation of the extracranial carotid arteries: Correlation of magnetic resonance angiography, duplex ultrasonography, and conventional angiography. J Vasc Surg 13:838, 1991.

118. Ohue S, Kohno K, Kusunoki K, et al: Magnetic resonance angiography in patients with acute stroke treated by local thrombolysis. Neuroradiology 40:536, 1998.

119. Phan T, Huston J, Bernstein MA, et al: Contrast-enhanced magnetic resonance angiography of the cervical vessels. Experience with 422 patients. Stroke 32:2282, 2001.

120. Tarnawski M, Padayavhee S, Graves MJ, et al: Measurement of time-average flow in the middle cerebral artery by magnetic resonance imaging. Br J Radiol 64:178, 1991.

121. Levi CR, Donnan GA, Fitt G: Magnetic resonance angiography. Cerebrovasc Dis (in press).

122. Clifton AG: MR angiography. Br Med Bull 56:367, 2000.

123. Remonda L, Head O, Silroth G: Carotid artery stenosis, occlusion and pseudo-occlusion: First-pass gadolinium-enhanced, three dimensional MR angiography—preliminary study. Radiology 209:95, 1998.

124. Cline HE, Lorensen WE, Souza SP, et al: 3D surface rendered MR images of the brain and its vasculature. J Comput Assist Tomogr 15:344, 1991.

125. Frisen L, Kjallman L, Lindberg B, Svenden P: Detection of extracranial carotid stenosis by computed tomography. Lancet 1:1319, 1979.

126. Wardlaw JM, White PM: The detection and management of unruptured intracranial aneurysm. Brain 123:205, 2000.

127. Lassen N, Ingva DH, Skinhoj E: Brain function and blood flow: Changes in the amount of blood flowing in areas of the human cerebral cortex, reflecting changes in the activity of those areas, are graphically revealed with the aid of radioactive isotope. Sci Am 239:62, 1978.

128. Hanyu H, Arai H, Kobayashi Y, et al: Remote effects in cerebral infarction—123I-IMP SPECT study. Kaku Igaku 27:629, 1990.

129. Kaufmann A, Firlik A, Fukui M, et al: Ischaemic core and penumbra in human stroke. Stroke 30:93, 1999.

130. Demeurisse M, Verhas M, Capon A, Paternot J: Lack of evolution of the cerebral blood flow during clinical recovery of a stroke. Stroke 14:77, 1983.

131. Jakobsen M, Enevoldsen E, Dalager T: Spasm index in subarachnoid haemorrhage: Consequences of vasospasm upon cerebral blood flow and oxygen extraction. Acta Neurol Scand 82:331, 1990.

132. Koroshetz W, Gonzales R: Imaging stroke in progress: Magnetic resonance advances but computed tomography is poised for counterattack. Ann Neurol 46:556, 1999.

133. Furlan AJ: Perfusion-weighted CT in acute MCA stroke: Teaching old dogs new tricks. Stroke 32:2027, 2001.

134. Wintermark M, Reichhart M, Thiran J-P, et al: Prognostic accuracy of cerebral blood flow measurement by perfusion computed tomography, at the time of emergency room admission, in acute stroke patients. Ann Neurol 51:417, 2002.

135. Frackowiak RSJ, Wise RJS: Positron tomography in ischemic cerebrovascular disease. Neurol Clin North Am 1:183, 1983.

136. Powers WJ, Martin ERW, Herscovitch P, et al: Extracranial-intracranial bypass surgery: Hemodynamic and metabolic effects. Neurology (NY) 34:1168, 1984.

137. Marchal G, Beaudouin V, Rioux P, et al: Prolonged persistence of substantial volumes of potentially viable brain tissue after stroke: A correlative PET-CT study with voxelbased data analysis. Stroke 27:599, 1996.

138. Kiyosawa M, Bosley TM, Kushner M, et al: Middle cerebral artery strokes causing homonymous hemianopia: positron emission tomography. Ann Neurol 28:180, 1990.

139. Baron JC, Bousser MG, Comar D, Castaigne P: "Crossed cerebellar diaschisis": A remote functional depression secondary to supratentorial infarction of man. J Cereb Blood Flow Metab 1 (Suppl 1):500, 1981.

140. Phelps ME, Mazziotta JC, Kuhl DE, et al: Tomographic mapping of human cerebral metabolism: Visual stimulation and deprivation. Neurology (NY) 31:517, 1981.

141. Kidwell CS, Alger JR, Di Salle F, et al: Diffusion MRI in patients with transient ischaemic attacks. Stroke 30:1174, 1999.

142. Hasegawa Y, Fisher M, Latour LL, et al: MRI diffusion mapping of reversible and irreversible ischemic injury in focal brain ischemia. Neurology 44:1484, 1994.

143. Pessin MS, Hinton RC, Davis KR, et al: Mechanisms of acute carotid stroke: A clinicoangiographic study. Ann Neurol 6:245, 1979.

144. Pessin MS, Duncan GW, Mohr JP, Poskanzer DC: Carotid artery territory transient ischemic attacks. N Engl J Med 296:358, 1977.

145. Baron JC, Bousser MG, Rey A, et al: Reversal of focal "misery-perfusion syndrome" by extra-intracranial arterial bypass in haemodynamic cerebral ischemia. Stroke 12:454, 1981.

146. Suzuki J, Kodama N: Moyamoya disease—a review. Stroke 14:104, 1983.

147. Furlan AJ, Weinstein MA, Little JR, Modic MT: Digital subtraction angiography in the evaluation of cerebrovascular disease. Neurol Clin North Am 1:55, 1983.

148. Ducos de Lahitte M, Marc-Vergnes JP, Rascol A, et al: Intravenous angiography of the external cerebral arteries. Radiology 137:705, 1980.

149. Hankey GJ, Warlow CP, Sellar RJ: Cerebral angiographic risk in mild cerebrovascular disease. Stroke 21:209, 1990.

150. Mohr JP: Asymptomatic carotid artery disease. Stroke 13:431, 1982.

151. Gautier JC, Rosa A, Lhermitte F: [Carotid auscultations: Correlation in 200 patients with 332 angiograms.] Rev Neurol 131:175, 1975.

152. Zwiebel WJ, Crummy AB: Sources of error in Doppler diagnosis of carotid occlusive disease. AJNR Am J Neuroradiol 2:231, 1982.

153. Norrving B, Nilsson B, Olsson J: Progression of carotid disease after endarterectomy: A Doppler ultrasound study. Ann Neurol 12:548, 1982.

154. Hennerici M, Steinke W, Rautenberg W, Mohr JP: Symptomatic and asymptomatic high-grade carotid stenosis in Doppler color flow imaging. Neurology (NY) 42:131, 1992.

Diagnostic Studies

Chapter Eighteen

Computed Tomography–Based Evaluation of Cerebrovascular Disease

*Charles A. Jungreis and Steven Goldstein**

Computed tomography (CT) of the brain has been the mainstay of imaging in patients with cerebrovascular disease. When a patient presents with an acute neurologic deficit, the differential diagnosis includes ischemic stroke, hemorrhagic stroke, and transient ischemic attack (TIA) as well as mass lesions of traumatic, neoplastic, and infectious causes. Conventional CT has been revolutionary in the examination of brain parenchymal and extra-axial anatomy. Technologic advances have given us the ability to examine vascular anatomy through the use of CT angiography (CTA) and brain physiology through the investigation of cerebral blood flow (CBF) using the techniques of xenon-enhanced CT (XeCT) and dynamic CT perfusion (CTP). When these techniques are combined, CT-based imaging constitutes a powerful tool in both the diagnosis and the treatment of patients with cerebrovascular disease.

IMMEDIATE COMPUTED TOMOGRAPHY EVALUATION OF ISCHEMIC STROKE

CT represents the "gold standard" for the detection of intracranial hemorrhage. However, with the use of thrombolytic agents in acute ischemic stroke, concern has been raised about the ability of standard CT imaging to detect acute ischemic change. Such early ischemic changes have been associated with a higher risk of intracranial hemorrhage and aggressive edema with poorer outcomes after thrombolytic therapy.[1–3]

A number of acute ischemic signs are well visualized on conventional CT. They include the finding of a hyperdense middle cerebral artery (MCA) (Fig. 18–1), cortical effacement, edema, hypodensity, and loss of the insular ribbon (Fig. 18–2). The sensitivity and specificity of even experienced stroke clinicians to detect these changes remains

variable. Barber and colleagues,[4] in an effort to develop a standardized quantitative method of detecting early ischemic changes on CT, proposed a CT grading system for acute anterior circulation ischemic stroke. Using this grading system, they detected ischemic changes in 75% of the 156 patients in their study who had anterior circulation ischemia and who had been treated within 3 hours of symptom onset with intravenous tissue-type plasminogen activator (t-PA). In addition, baseline CT score predicted functional outcome as indicated by the modified Rankin scale score at 3 months (sensitivity 0.78 and specificity 0.96) as well as symptomatic intracerebral hemorrhage (sensitivity 0.90 and specificity 0.62). Combining such a quantitative grading scale of high-resolution helical CT images with CT-based cerebral blood flow techniques (see later discussion) may act to give the treating clinician better information on the risks of acute stroke treatment and may predict functional outcome.

COMPUTED TOMOGRAPHY ANGIOGRAPHY

The technologic advances in CT have enabled scanners to acquire data very quickly. In fact, during injection of a contrast agent, CT scanners can acquire data during the vascular phase. The primary innovation enabling such rapid data acquisition has been the advent of "helical" or "spiral" acquisitions. With this technique, data acquisition occurs continuously while the gantry table moves the patient through the gantry, so a volume of interest can be scanned in a relatively short time. The acquired data is then divided into packets of information sufficient to reconstruct cross-sectional images. The technical factors, such as the rate at which the table moves, the current (milliamperes), the kilovoltage, the tube heating capacity, and the algorithm for reconstruction, can be varied and so can have the usual impact on image quality. Such technical factors are beyond the scope of this discussion; it is

*Deceased

CASE 1 - PRE RX

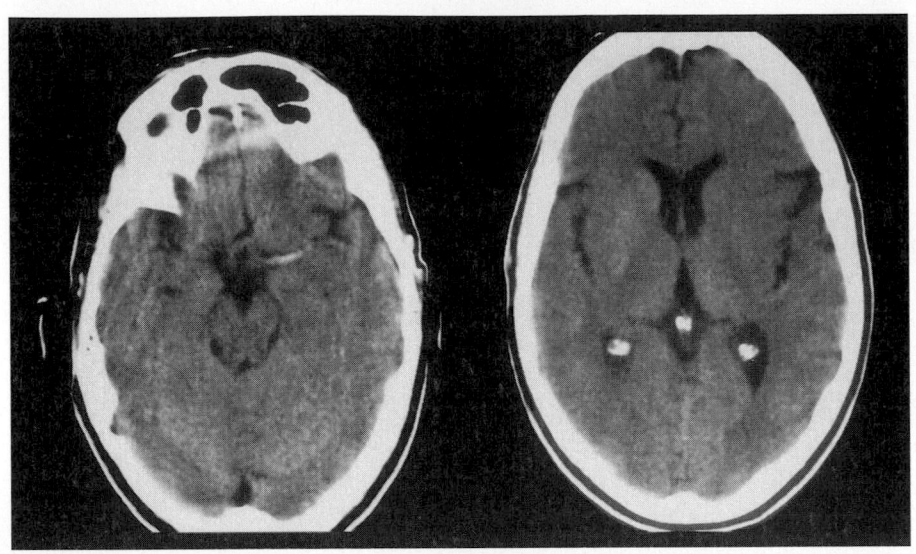

FIGURE 18–1 *Hyperdense middle cerebral artery sign demonstrated on a non–contrast-enhanced CT in a patient with an acute ischemic infarct.*

CASE 4 - PRE TREATMENT

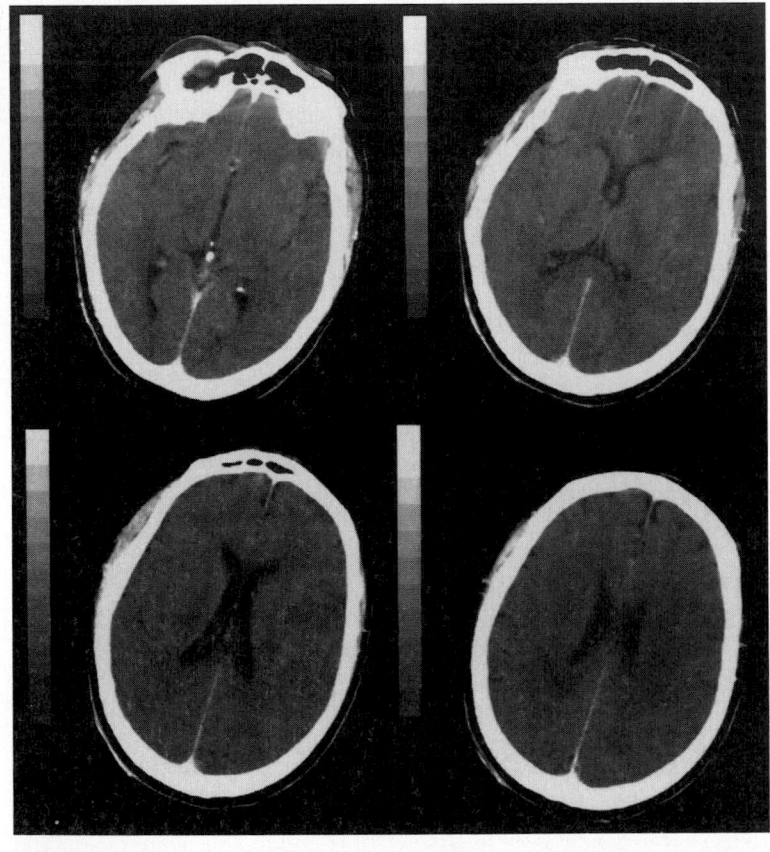

FIGURE 18–2 *Cortical effacement, edema, hypodensity, and loss of insular ribbon on a non–contrast-enhanced CT in a patient with an acute ischemic stroke.*

sufficient to say that diagnostic quality images are obtainable of large volumes of tissue in much shorter times than were possible with previous generations of scanners. Hence, CTA has gained credibility and popularity.

Some limitations remain. As in many imaging examinations, motion artifact and the usual CT artifacts, such as those often seen near the petrous bones, can be problematic. Sometimes the course of a vessel is such that a cross-sectional image is difficult to interpret, and contrast volumes are not inconsequential on a typical CT angiogram.

However, because the data are digital, images in alternate planes and three-dimensional renderings are easy to reconstruct on commercially available work stations. Although much of the diagnostic information is gleaned from the baseline cross-sectional images, the three-dimensional reconstructions are particularly helpful when vessels are tortuous. The utility of CTA is tremendous, and it has already replaced conventional catheter angiography in many situations.

Clinical Applications

Extracranial Carotid Artery Disease

Cerebral angiography has been the diagnostic procedure of choice for the quantification of extracranial carotid arterial stenosis. Although generally safe, angiography is still associated with a 0.5% to 5% rate of stroke as a complication when used in routine clinical practice.[5-12] With the advent of ultrafast helical CT imaging, the complication is avoided and CTA is being used with increasing frequency in the diagnosis of extracranial carotid artery stenosis. An example of severe right internal carotid stenosis is depicted in Figure 18–3, on conventional arteriography, and Figure 18–4, on CTA (axial cuts).

Several studies to date have reported excellent agreement between conventional catheter cerebral angiography and CTA. In a comparative study of CTA, conventional angiography, and magnetic resonance angiography (MRA), a strong correlation was found between CTA and angiography ($r = 0.987$; $P < .0001$) in 128 carotid bifurcations in 64 patients.[13] CTA has the additional benefit of providing precise information regarding the surrounding vascular and bony anatomy that cannot be evaluated on standard cerebral angiography or MRA. Another group of investigators compared CTA with conventional angiography in 20 patients and found agreement between the two techniques in 95% of arteries studied.[14]

In a prospective study, 40 patients (80 carotid arteries) underwent evaluation by CTA, digital subtraction angiography (DSA), and Doppler ultrasonography.[15] The overall correlation between Doppler ultrasonography and DSA was less robust ($r = 0.808$) than that between CTA and DSA ($r = 0.099$; axial source images). CTA provided superb correlation in the detection of mild stenosis (0–29%), stenosis greater than 50%, and carotid occlusion, with sensitivities and specificities exceeding 0.90. CTA performed less well in the detection of 70% to 99% stenosis, with a sensitivity of 0.73 (axial source images) and a positive predictive value of only 0.62 (negative predictive value of 0.95). The relatively poorer degree of discrimina-

Diagnostic Studies

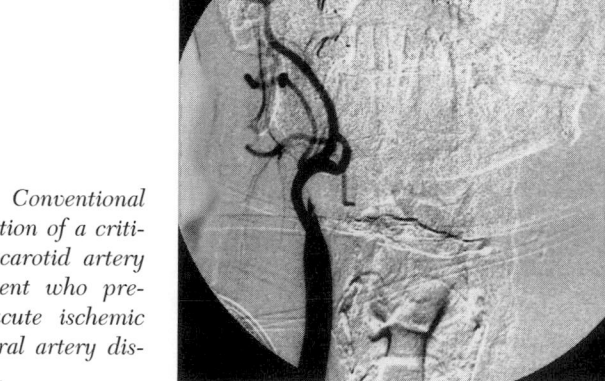
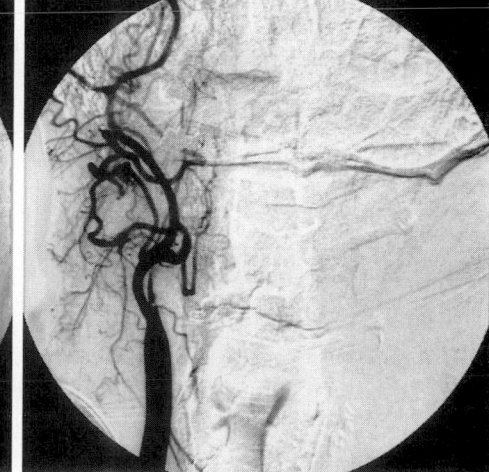

FIGURE 18–3 *Conventional angiographic depiction of a critical right internal carotid artery stenosis in a patient who presented with an acute ischemic right middle cerebral artery distribution infarction.*

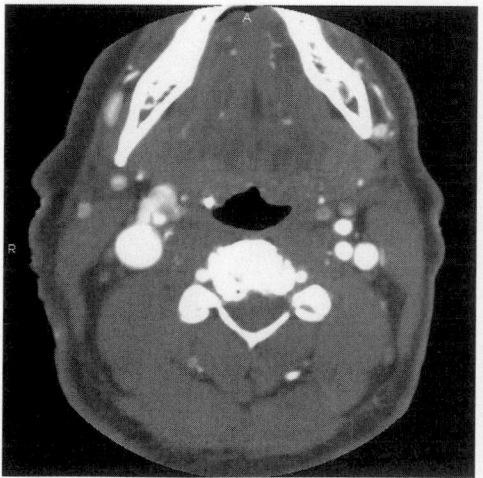
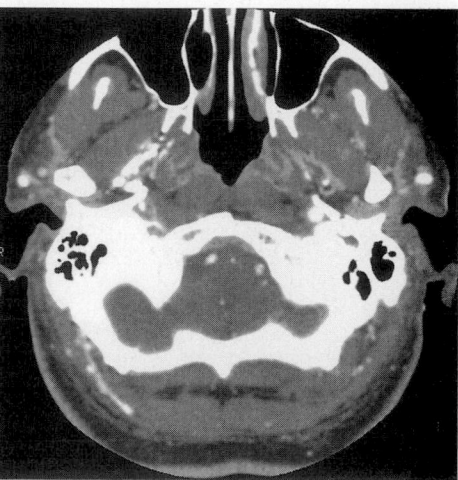

FIGURE 18–4 *CT angiography (axial cuts) of the same critical right internal carotid artery stenosis demonstrated in Figure 18–3.*

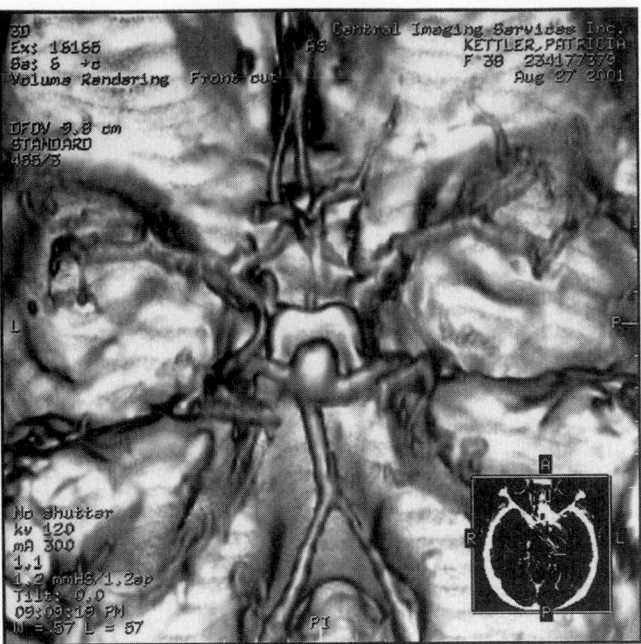

FIGURE 18–5 *Reconstructed CT angiographic image of a large basilar aneurysm.*

tion on CTA in this study between moderate (50%–69%) and severe (70%–99%) stenosis is an important limiting factor to consider in the use of this technology. It is hoped that further prospective data acquisition with simultaneous 16-slice technology will shed additional light on this issue.

Intracranial Disease

CTA has been used with growing frequency in the detection of intracranial aneurysms (Fig. 18–5) and intracranial stenosis (Fig. 18–6). One of the most exciting applications of intracranial CTA is in the rapid triage of patients with acute stroke due to intracranial stenosis. Both combined

intravenous–intra-arterial (IV/IA) thrombolysis[16] and IA thrombolysis[17] (time from symptom onset <6 hours) have demonstrated promise in improving outcome after acute stroke due to occlusion of major vessels. The need for rapid decision-making makes CTA an ideal technique in the detection of large vessel intracranial arterial stenosis. Lev and associates[18] studied 44 consecutive patients presenting with acute stroke within 6 hours or less of onset, who underwent non–contrast-enhanced CT followed immediately by CTA. A total of 572 vessels in the circle of Willis were visually evaluated with these techniques, and angiographic correlation was available for 224 of the vessels. Sensitivity and specificity for CTA were both 98%, and accuracy as calculated by receiver operating characteristic analysis was 99%. Mean time for CTA reconstruction was 15 minutes. CTA represents an ideal tool for the rapid and accurate detection of intracranial stenosis of the major vessels of the circle of Willis.

COMPUTED TOMOGRAPHY–BASED EVALUATION OF CEREBRAL BLOOD FLOW

The use of functional neuroimaging in the form of CBF measurement is rapidly expanding in the care of patients with cerebrovascular disease, head trauma, seizure disorders, and many other disease states involving the central nervous system. CT-based assessment of CBF offers many advantages in the care of patients with disorders of the central nervous system. CT-based technology capable of evaluating CBF can be readily combined with routine CT scanning equipment, thus both improving the availability and reducing the costs of this technology. Monitoring of patients with respiratory and hemodynamic instability is also more easily accomplished with CT-based technology. In addition, patients with mechanical heart valves, permanent cardiac pacemakers, and other ferromagnetic devices can be safely studied. Most patients with stroke undergo CT scanning for detection of hemorrhage; the addition of CT-based CBF measurements to the evaluation avoids

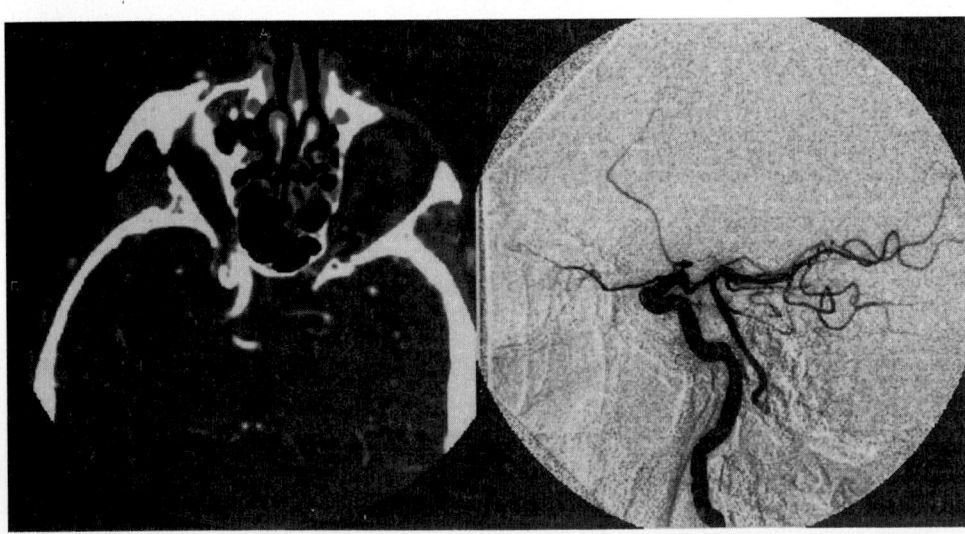

FIGURE 18–6 *CT angiographic demonstration of a distal intracranial internal carotid artery occlusion and its corresponding conventional angiographic image.*

moving the patient to a magnetic resonance imaging (MRI) or positron emission tomography (PET) unit for another evaluation, reducing the overall time needed to acquire physiologic data. This point is particularly important in the treatment of patients with acute stroke.

Two primary CT-based imaging techniques are clinically available to evaluate CBF, XeCT and CTP. These techniques are based on two entirely different mathematical models. XeCT is based on the well-established diffusible tracer model, whereas CTP is based on a nondiffusible tracer kinetic model that can be applied to both CTP and magnetic resonance perfusion (MRP).

Xenon-Enhanced Computed Tomography

Theory

Xenon (Xe), a naturally occurring element, is an inert gas at room temperatures. With an atomic number of 54, close to that of iodine, Xe is radiodense and can therefore be employed as a contrast agent. Unlike iodine, Xe is not reactive and is freely diffusible throughout most tissues in the body, including the blood-brain barrier. These properties, which do not depend on radioactivity, have led to a commercially available product that can be used with most modern CT scanners and is capable of measuring blood flow quantitatively.[19,20]

The technique of stable XeCT quantitative CBF measurement is based on the same principle as the nitrous oxide method of Kety and Schmidt,[21] namely, that the rate of uptake and clearance of a diffusible tracer in a tissue is proportional to the CBF in that tissue. XeCT is a quantitative method of high-resolution tomographic cerebral blood flow (qCBF) measurement that uses stable xenon gas as a contrast agent in association with conventional CT scanning. The arterial concentration of xenon over time, $C_a(t)$, is assumed to be equal to the end-tidal alveolar concentration of xenon directly measured by a thermoconductivity analyzer in the exhaled gas. The brain concentration of xenon over time, $C_b(t)$, is calculated from the density changes detected by the CT scanner (directly measured from the scanner) and knowledge of the partition coefficient (λ), which is defined as the equilibrium ratio of the concentration of Xe in tissue and in blood. κ is a rate constant for the uptake of Xe. These variables are combined to solve the Kety-Schmidt equation.

A quantitative CBF value is calculated for each voxel per CT level and displayed in a color-coded flow map. A confidence image is presented that is derived as a normalized sum of the square of the differences between the actual enhancement data and the fitted data. A simple pictorial representation of data reliability is generated. Regions of interest may be placed over the image for perfusion analysis in different vascular distributions or anatomic locations.

The accuracy for measurement has been cross-correlated with other quantitative CBF techniques, such as radiolabeled microspheres, xenon 133 inhalation, and iodoantipyrine CBF techniques.[22–25] Patients inhale a 28% to 33% xenon, 40% oxygen mixture for 4.3 minutes. CT images with 10-mm slice thickness are obtained at up to six levels through the brain. Acquisition of qCBF data is available for clinical review within 5 minutes of study completion. An inhalation time of 4 minutes allows us to maximize the gray and white matter data while minimizing the side effects associated with inhalation times longer than 5 minutes.[26]

Xe is an inert noble gas that does not cause allergic reactions. Side effects are minimal (mild sensory and cognitive symptoms) and always transient, and the technique is well tolerated. Even brief, mild sensorial side effects have been significantly reduced as the concentration of xenon has been brought to less than 30% through improvements in CT technology.

Although several concerns about the safety and validity of the XeCT method have been raised in the literature, nearly all have been resolved as of 1998. One concern is that Xe may cause apnea. Although it has been reported that breathing 100% Xe can produce apnea,[27] apnea is an extremely rare event with an Xe inhalation concentration of 28%, and it is easily reversed by having the patient breathe, either by giving instructions or through sensory stimulation. Another concern has been the effect of Xe on intracranial pressure (ICP); however, no changes in ICP have been observed as long as carbon dioxide retention is prevented.[28,29] The ability of XeCT to yield quantitative CBF information has been the subject of criticism because of the concern that Xe inhalation may alter CBF. The effect of flow activation on XeCT-derived CBF values has proved to be insignificant, however, because of the robustness of the Kety-Schmidt equation[3] and because early, frequent scanning allows for characterization of CBF before significant flow activation occurs.[30] Activation of CBF with Xe inhalation becomes significant only after 2.5 minutes[31]; using only wash-in data with a heavy dependence on these earlier data provides an error of less than 5%.[32,33]

XeCT has a few technical pitfalls. The major problem encountered is related to patient motion. Because the technique requires a series of sections to be obtained at precisely the same locations, any movement between slice acquisitions can be a source of error. If a patient moves between image acquisitions, the pixels are misaligned, and the accuracy of the calculations is reduced. With attention to gaining the trust of the patient, careful positioning and securing of the head, and occasional intravenous sedation, more than 90% of studies performed with patients awake yield useful information. For studies performed with patients who are paralyzed and intubated, this figure approaches 100%. A second problem is gas leak in the administration set or in the mouthpiece; the monitoring systems usually detect these quickly. The third pitfall is that, in theory, pulmonary disease sufficient to cause poor diffusion of the Xe gas across the capillary membranes from the alveoli to the blood stream might impair the uptake and alter the apparent equilibrium. In more than 9000 studies at my institution, however, this has rarely been a problem. The one issue related to pulmonary disease that occasionally has been problematic occurs in patients for whom high percentages of oxygen are needed in a ventilator to maintain oxygenation. The addition of Xe gas may require a decrease in the percentage of oxygen during the blood flow examination and, in some clinical situations, this decrease may be intolerable for the patient.

Diagnostic Studies

Clinical Applications
Determinants of Irreversible Cerebral Ischemia in Acute Stroke

The primary goal of thrombolytic therapy in acute stroke is to reestablish tissue perfusion before the onset of irreversible ischemia. The two major determinants of irreversible cerebral ischemia leading to tissue infarction are the duration and the severity of reduced CBF.[34] In a review of thresholds of ischemia in different animal models, Hossmann[35] demonstrated a distinct rank order of susceptibilities to eventual infarction. The sodium-potassium ratio of brain tissue, an important marker of anoxic depolarization, increases at CBF values below 10 to 15 mL/100 g/min,[36] and extracellular ion changes occur at CBF values between 6 and 15 mL/100 g/min.[37-39] In the baboon, Yonas and coworkers[40] showed that selective occlusion of the lenticulostriate arteries caused reduction of CBF to less than 8 mL/100 g/min. At this level of CBF, tissue infarction was consistently produced after 60 minutes.[40,41]

In a study of the ischemic *core* (tissue destined to go on to irreversible cell death and necrosis) and *penumbra* (salvageable tissue) in human stroke by means of XeCT, Kaufmann and colleagues[42] found that the area of most severe ipsilateral ischemia, with a CBF of 6 mL/100 g/min or less, best corresponded to the final area of infarction on follow-up CT scans. These investigators demonstrated a tight correlation between the final infarct volume measured on follow-up CT scan and the volume of qCBF that was less than 6 mL/100 g/min on the initial XeCT qCBF scan in 20 patients presenting with acute MCA occlusion (Pearson correlation coefficient of 0.90; $P < .01$). This statistically significant correlation held independent of whether the patient was treated with thrombolytic agents, suggesting that the early extent of severe ischemia defines the final extent of infarction.

It has been reported that the ischemic core follows a predictable course in acute MCA infarction.[43] Jovin and colleagues[43] used a reproducible experimental primate model to study the time course of ischemic core qCBF

values (0–10 mL/100 g/min) over the first 6 hours after reproducible experimental MCA infarction. They observed little variation in qCBF over time. For each primate, the probability that an MCA qCBF value would remain within the range of 0 to 10 mL/100 g/min at any time during the 6 hours was 95% (Fig. 18–7). The clinical ramification of this finding might be that qCBF determination in ischemic stroke demonstrating the presence of an ischemic core measured within the first 6 hours after symptom onset is unlikely to be significantly different if measured before or after the clinical study upon which treatment decisions may potentially be based.

Acute Stroke

In patients with acute stroke, direct measurement of CBF is potentially helpful in maximizing the benefit of immediate therapy and reducing the complications. To accomplish these goals, an imaging method must distinguish brain already infarcted or destined to become infarcted from reversibly ischemic brain capable of returning to normal functioning with reperfusion. In addition, some vessels become recanalized in the first few hours after stroke despite persistent neurologic deficits. In such cases, the presence of normal CBF values suggests that reperfusion has already occurred and that interventional therapy is not necessary, possibly avoiding angiography or thrombolytic therapy.

XeCT provides quantitative CBF values that can potentially be used for triage of patients with acute stroke. In one study, CBF values less than 6 mL/100 g/min measured in the setting of acute stroke correlated with subsequent infarction on follow-up CT, whether or not reperfusion had occurred after thrombolytic therapy.[42] Patients with occlusion of the M1 segment of the MCA had significantly lower mean CBF values in the MCA territory than those without MCA occlusion.[44] In all patients with M1 occlusions, mean MCA CBF values were less than 20 mL/100 g/min. Thus, within the first few hours after stroke, XeCT may identify areas of brain already infarcted and may predict the presence of proximal arterial occlusion. Reperfusion of

Diagnostic Studies

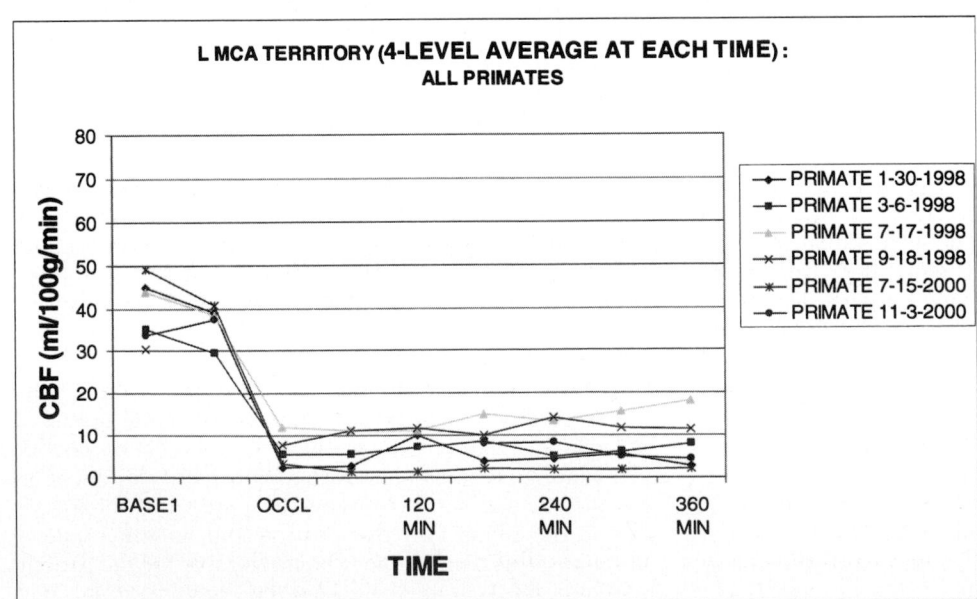

FIGURE 18–7 *Graph showing left middle cerebral artery (L MCA) qCBF over time after MCA occlusion in a primate model of MCA infarction. Note that when qCBF approaches 10 mL/100 g/min, there is little variation of flow over time.*

infarcted brain does little to improve neurologic function but may cause neurologic worsening because of hemorrhage or cerebral edema with herniation. Mean CBF values for the whole MCA territory that were less than 15 mL/100 g/min were associated with a greater risk of hemorrhage or herniation in patients treated with thrombolytic therapy after acute stroke.[45]

CBF can act as a predictor for the identification of patients at high risk for symptomatic hemorrhagic conversion (SHC) or clinical herniation (CH) after treatment with thrombolytic therapy for acute ischemic stroke. My colleagues and I[46] compared the ability of CBF with that of admission National Institutes of Health Stroke Scale Score (A-NIHSS) to correctly identify patients destined to suffer the complication of SHC or CH after treatment for acute ischemic stroke. We studied 32 patients with acute cerebral infarction in whom CBF measurements in the affected vascular distribution had been determined by XeCT before or during thrombolytic therapy. Of these patients, 9 suffered SHC or CH after thrombolytic therapy. The median CBF in these 9 patients with SHC or CH after thrombolysis was 13.6 mL/100 g/min. In the 23 patients without SHC or CH, the median CBF was 27.6 mL/100 g/min (Wilcoxon Rank Sum test; $P = .0003$). The median core CBF (core CBF representing the two regions of interest that have the lowest blood flow values within the entire affected cortical territory) in patients with SHC or CH after thrombolysis was 7.5 mL/100 g/min. In patients without SHC or CH, the core CBF was 17.2 mL/100 g/min (Wilcoxon Rank Sum test; $P = .0006$). The median A-NIHSS in patients with SHC or CH was 19, and that in patients without SHC or CH was 12 ($P = 0.008$). After adjustment for time to treatment and age of the patient, the overall number of patients correctly classified by XeCT as having or not having SHC or CH (29/32) was also greater than the number of patients classified according to A-NIHSS (23/32) ($P = 0.07$).

Plate 18–1 (following page 460) shows a severe perfusion defect with a CBF less than 10 mL/100 g/min (suggesting irreversible ischemic necrosis) in the MCA territory. Plate 18–2 demonstrates a mild perfusion defect treated with thrombolytic therapy.

Initial CBF values may also predict long-term outcome in patients with acute stroke.[47] Mean CBF in the affected vascular distribution measured within 6 hours of stroke onset in patients treated with intra-arterial urokinase were found to predict long-term outcome better than time to treatment, which correlated poorly with long-term deficits.[48] Similarly, CBF measured by XeCT in the first few hours after stroke was more predictive of subsequent infarction on CT than time from onset of symptoms to CBF measurement.[49]

In some patients, despite significant neurologic deficits, CBF in the affected vascular territory is normal. This finding suggests that reperfusion has already occurred and that there is little to gain from an attempt at thrombolysis. In many such patients, neurologic deficits resolve over the ensuing 24 hours without acute stroke interventions.[50] The ability to avoid therapy that has the potential to cause intracerebral hemorrhage in patients destined to improve may be a valuable contribution of quantitative CBF measurements in the setting of acute stroke.

Intermediate levels of CBF measured by XeCT may predict brain regions that can be salvaged with acute stroke therapy. Ultimately, the optimal CBF technique in acute stroke will be able to consistently identify areas of brain that are potentially recoverable by reperfusion or other acute stroke therapies. CBF values less than 20 mL/100 g/min (indicating ischemia) but more than 6 mL/100 g/min (the level at which irreversible ischemia occurs even within the first few hours after stroke) hold the promise of identifying such reversibly ischemic areas.

Chronic Ischemia

The role of hemodynamic factors in the risk of recurrent stroke in patients with extracranial carotid occlusive disease remains controversial. From 1977 to 1985, The International Cooperative Study of Extracranial-Intracranial Arterial Anastomosis compared the efficacy of the superficial temporal artery to middle cerebral artery (STA–MCA) bypass procedure with medical management using aspirin therapy in a group of patients who experienced minor strokes or TIAs 3 months or less before surgery.[51] Despite this study's negative results, many investigators have continued to demonstrate that patients with compromised hemodynamics may benefit from revascularization procedures.

Later data suggest that patients in whom compromised cerebrovascular reserve is demonstrated may constitute a subgroup at high risk for recurrent stroke. Increased oxygen extraction fraction (OEF) as measured by PET has been reported to be associated with a statistically higher incidence of prior ischemic events (42%) than normal OEF (16%) in patients with carotid occlusive disease.[52] In a prospective study of 419 patients with symptomatic carotid occlusion monitored over an average of 31.5 months and studied by PET, stroke occurred in 11 of 39 patients with increased OEF but in only 2 of 42 patients without a significant increase in OEF ($P = .004$).[53] Using XeCT before and after a intravenous acetazolamide challenge, both Yonas and colleagues[54] and Webster and associates[55] identified a group of patients with carotid occlusive disease and evidence of hemodynamic compromise or "steal," defined as a 5% decrease in qCBF measured after acetazolamide challenge. These patients went on to have a stroke rate of 36% within 6 months. These findings demonstrate that measurement of cerebrovascular reserve after vasodilatory challenge as well as increased OEF as measured by PET can potentially identify patients at high risk of recurrent cerebral ischemia after symptomatic carotid occlusive disease. Planning of prospective trials is under way to reassess the utility of intracranial bypass in patients with carotid occlusion and compromised hemodynamic profile as defined by increased OEF and cerebrovascular reserve.

Intracerebral Hemorrhage

Parenchymal intracerebral hemorrhage (ICH), commonly associated with hypertension, remains the most common form of hemorrhagic stroke and is an important cause of morbidity and mortality.[56] Substantial growth in the overall volume of ICH has been reported to occur in 26% of patients from baseline examination to a 1-hour CT scan, and an additional 12% of all patients experience further growth in the volume of ICH during the interval between

1-hour and 20-hour CT scans.[57] Thus, early volume expansion is common.[58] Such volume expansion is a potentially important contributor to overall patient morbidity and mortality. Efforts at acute blood pressure reduction may offer an important treatment option to lower this rate of early volume expansion.[59] Alternatively, such blood pressure reduction may lead to regional or global cerebral ischemia by decreasing CBF.[60]

In an attempt to address this issue, investigators have begun to monitor global and regional CBF during attempts at aggressive blood pressure reduction in ICH. Powers and colleagues[61] studied CBF changes with PET after blood pressure reduction in 9 patients with hypertensive ICH. Intravenous labetalol or nicardipine was used to achieve a 15% reduction in mean arterial pressure (MAP). These 9 patients did not demonstrate a significant change in mean hemispheric or regional CBF at the lower blood pressure. My colleagues and I[62] reported on the effect of aggressive blood pressure reduction on CBF in a retrospective series of 6 hypertensive patients with ICH studied by XeCT. Five of the 6 patients tolerated reduction to normotensive blood pressure levels without a significant decline in global or regional quantitative CBF. Further studies designed to demonstrate the utility of CBF monitoring during blood pressure reduction in ICH and the efficacy of this strategy in improving outcome in these critically ill patients are under way.

Subarachnoid Hemorrhage and Vasospasm

The rupture of an intracranial aneurysm is the most common cause of nontraumatic subarachnoid hemorrhage (SAH), the incidence of which is estimated to be 10 in 100,000 per year.[63] It is a devastating disease with a 30-day mortality rate of 45%, and half the survivors are disabled because of irreversible brain injury.[64] Symptomatic cerebral vasospasm is a major cause of delayed morbidity and mortality, occurring in approximately 30% of all patients. Early detection of vasospasm allows for more timely intervention with both medical and endovascular treatment strategies. Angiography has been held to be the "gold standard" for diagnostic measurement of vasospasm; because of its invasive nature, however, routine monitoring with angiography is not practical.

Transcranial Doppler (TCD) ultrasonography has been used to diagnose and monitor the course of vasospasm in patients with SAH for the better part of two decades. In 1990, the American Academy of Neurology formally endorsed the utility of TCD in diagnosis and monitoring of SAH due to rupture of an aneurysm.[65] Two parameters, the time course of vasospasm and the residual lumen diameter, have demonstrated a significant correlation between TCD and angiography. In general, mean velocities of 120 to 200 cm/sec as measured in the MCA by TCD correlate with moderate vasospasm on angiography, whereas mean velocities higher than 200 cm/sec have correlated with severe vasospasm.[66]

Ultimately, symptomatic vasospasm can result in decreased cerebral perfusion at the parenchymal level, leading to tissue ischemia and, in some cases, irreversible necrosis. Although reduced TCD velocities measured in large conductance vessels have at times correlated with a reduction in blood flow, this has not always been the case.

In a study of 50 patients with SAH undergoing a total of 94 paired TCD and XeCT studies, Clyde and associates[67] found that elevated TCD velocities in the affected MCA territory were correlated with increased qCBF as measured by XeCT. TCD is also insensitive to second- and third-order vessel spasm, which can occur without significant involvement of the more proximal vessels examined by TCD. Not infrequently, this insensitivity has led a treating physician to the false conclusion that there was no problem with blood delivery, although the patient could have been suffering an ischemic infarction. In addition, focal neurologic deficits correlated only with decreased qCBF and not with the TCD velocity. In another study, the association of high TCD velocities with hyperemic CBF, as measured by single photon emission computed tomography (SPECT) 15 to 20 days after SAH, was also demonstrated.[68]

In conclusion, although TCD generally correlates well with angiographic vasospasm, it is likely that measurement of regional qCBF yields the most important evidence of clinically significant vasospasm—that is, significant tissue hypoperfusion.

Traumatic Brain Injury

A primary goal in the treatment of patients with severe traumatic brain injury is the detection and prevention of secondary brain injury. Such secondary injury results from edema, increased ICP, hypotension, and hypocapnia and eventually results in tissue ischemia and infarction. Some data clearly demonstrate a correlation between poorer outcome and reduced regional qCBF and reduced vasoreactivity to CO_2 after acetazolamide administration, as measured by XeCT, in patients with traumatic brain injury.[69-71] Current treatment strategies for this group of patients involve manipulation of PCO_2, blood pressure management, and control of increased ICP. XeCT is a potentially useful guide to such management strategies.

Computed Tomography Perfusion

Theory

With the development of helical CT scanning technology, it is now possible to track a bolus of intravenous contrast material as it passes through the brain. The measurement technique for CBF has its theoretical basis in the central volume principle,[72,73] which relates CBF (mL/100 g/min), cerebral blood volume (CBV; mL/100 g), and mean transit time (MTT; sec) by the following equation:

$$CBF = \frac{CBV}{MTT}$$

It is assumed that a linear relationship exists between the CT enhancement and the concentration of contrast material within brain tissue and arteries. After intravenous administration of a bolus of iodinated contrast agent, measurements are made of the arterial enhancement curve, $C_a(t)$, of the supplying artery and the tissue enhancement curve, $Q(t)$, for a region of the central parenchyma. For the calculation of MTT, a mathematical process of deconvolution is applied to the functions $C_a(t)$ and $Q(t)$ to determine an impulse function, $R(t)$, which would be the theoretical tissue enhancement curve obtained from a rapidly injected bolus of contrast material. The MTT is calculated from the following formula:

$$MTT = \frac{\text{area underneath R(t)}}{\text{height of R(t) plateau}}$$

CBV is calculated from Q(t) and C_a(t) the two parameters measured directly during the CTP study:

$$CBV = \frac{\text{area underneath Q(t)}}{\text{area underneath } C_a(t)}$$

Although this technique is rapidly evolving, difficulties remain, involving partial averaging effects, effects of drawing regions of interest (ROIs) directly over arterial vessels, and the proper selection of the arterial input vessel to yield the most accurate results. Attempts at quantitative validation of this technology in humans through comparison with other techniques, such as XeCT, are ongoing.[74]

Technical Limitations of CTP in Quantitative Cerebral Blood Flow Measurement

My colleagues and I[75] have correlated the qCBF obtained by CTP with the "gold-standard," XeCT, in a patient with a right MCA occlusion. XeCT was performed first, followed by CTP (10-minute delay between studies). Two co-registered levels were analyzed, and 24 identical ROIs were overlaid per slice. Spearman correlation coefficients (SCCs) were determined in order to correlate the qCBF determined from XeCT and CTP using the right and left MCAs as arterial inputs.

In the right MCA vascular distribution, the mean CBF measured by XeCT was 12.7 mL/100 g/min (level 2); a cor-

responding CTP image of level 2 is demonstrated in Plate 18–3. In the ROIs excluding the right MCA, there was no significant correlation between qCBF obtained by XeCT and CTP images (Fig. 18–8). Efforts to improve the measurement of qCBF by CTP are under way.

In a study correlating the measurement of qCBF by CTP and XeCT, Wintermark and colleagues[74] found that in pixels that include cerebral parenchyma and arterial branches qCBF values obtained by CTP consistently exceed those obtained by XeCT.[51] In addition, these investigators commented on the fact that the vessel used as the arterial input function can strongly influence the final qCBF map obtained by CTP. Research groups are currently collecting data in patients with ischemic vascular disease.

Clinical Application in Cerebrovascular Disease

CTP is a fairly new technique, and only a few clinical studies assessing its utility have been published. Because of the ease of the technique, interest in the utility of CTP in patients with acute stroke has been growing. However, owing to the technical limitations of CTP, absolute measurement of CBV, MTT, and CBF do not provide accurate results.[76] Alternative parameters relying on ratios or qualitative analysis have therefore been employed.

For example, in 1998, Hunter and colleagues[77] described their assessment of CTP in nine patients with no history of stroke, eight patients with a history of established stroke, and five patients with acute stroke at less than 3 hours from onset. In theory, regions of cerebral ischemia due to major vessel occlusion are associated with an increase in CBV as a result of greater capillary recruitment. Along with this increase in CBV, MTT rises, resulting in a decrease in CBF. These investigators described the parameter "percent perfused cerebral blood volume (%PBV)," which is reported to reflect the delivery of contrast mate-

Diagnostic Studies

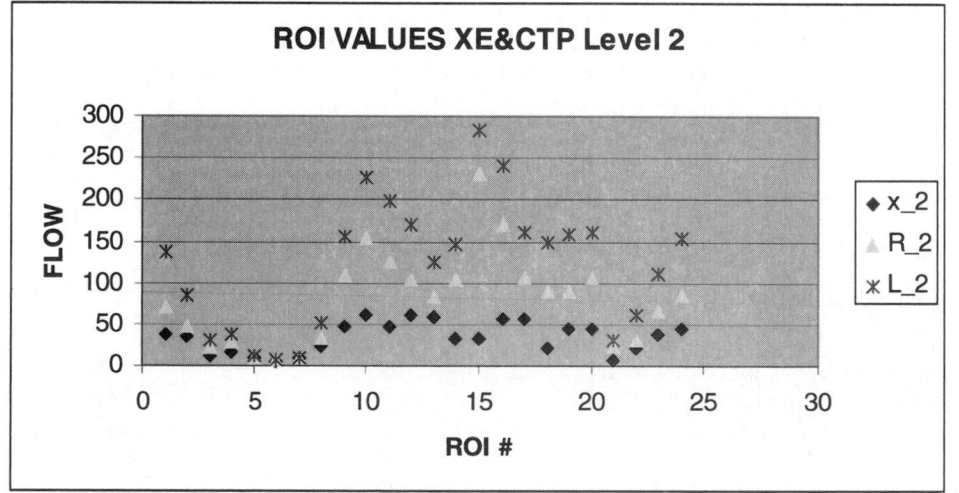

FIGURE 18–8 *Correlation of qCBF values in selected regions of interest (ROIs), comparing xenon-enhanced CT (XeCT) level 2 (diamonds), dynamic CT perfusion (CTP)–left middle cerebral artery (MCA) arterial input, level 2 (stars), and CTP–right MCA (RMCA) arterial input, level 2 (triangles) in the patient with RMCA occlusion whose XeCT and CTP images are depicted in Plate 18–3. Spearman correlation coefficient was significant in the region of severe hypoperfusion but was without significance on the other ROIs.*

ROI 3-8; 21-22 (RMCA); Spearman Correlation 0.833 (L) & 0.881(R) p=0.02

ROI Excluding above; Spearman Correlation 0.297 (L) & 0.362(R) p=NS

rial to those vessels that still receive blood. It is claimed that %PBV is proportional to CBF. Using this variable, Hunter and colleagues[77] demonstrated that %PBV decreases in regions of ischemia, the volume of which is a function of collateral flow as measured by CTA. Although %PBV may have the potential to yield useful quantitative perfusion information that would allow the distinction between penumbra and core, threshold levels for this variable have not been defined to date.

Lee and associates[78] reported a qualitative volumetric study using CTP in eight patients with acute stroke who were evaluated within 3 hours of stroke onset. These researchers found a correlation between the volume of hypoperfusion noted on CTP and angiographic data. The study was limited by the lack of quantitative data as well as the lack of specific information as to which variable was measured by the technique. Koenig and colleagues[79] reported on the quantitative assessment of cerebral ischemia by perfusion-related parameters measured by CTP. They studied 34 patients with acute ischemic stroke within 6 hours of onset by means of conventional CT and CTP. The CTP study was performed with a single-slice dynamic CT scan at the level of the basal ganglia. Because of the inaccuracies inherent in calculation of CBV, these investigators used MTT and CBF ratios to calculate relative values. A value of 0.60 for relative CBV ($P = .02$) and 0.48 for relative CBF ($P = 0.21$; not significant) discriminated between tissue that went on to infarction on follow-up CT and non-infarcted tissue.

A potential caution should be noted in the interpretation of results that rely on ratios involving contralateral ROIs. Our group has demonstrated, using XeCT, that CBF in the contralateral hemisphere after acute stroke is indeed not normal and is consistently 10 to 15 mL/100 g/min below normal CBF; in addition, the flow values in the contralateral hemisphere are also quite variable.[80,81] Thus, reliance on the contralateral hemisphere as a benchmark for CBF may be faulty.

Preliminary assessment of CBF by CTP in intracerebral hemorrhage has also been reported. Eskey and coworkers[82] studied three patients with acute ICH by CTP within 12 hours of onset. Relative CBF values, based on a ratio analysis using the contralateral hemisphere, were reported. A thin rim of decreased perfusion was seen surrounding the hematoma, but global flows were not reduced.

CONCLUSION

The need for quantitative physiologic information continues to expand as more emphasis is placed on immediate therapeutic intervention in a host of disease states affecting the central nervous system. These techniques offer the possibility of improved patient selection and lower rate of complications from aggressive interventional techniques. However, in order to be of clinical usefulness, these techniques must be capable of being rapidly performed with minimal delay in time to treatment. Also, to have a true clinical impact, they must be widely available. CT-based systems now offer exquisite visualization of tissue and vascular anatomy using conventional CT and CT angiography. In addition, CT-based perfusion techniques provide physiologic information that is becoming increasingly important in clinical decision-making. All this information (CT, CTA, and XeCT and/or CTP CBF) may be obtained in less than 20 minutes with current technology.

Given the current state of CT perfusion imaging, XeCT remains the "gold standard" for the measurement of CBF.[83] CTP is a promising technique for future development but is currently limited by technical difficulties. These difficulties include, but are not limited to, the appropriate selection of an arterial input function, ROIs containing blood vessels yielding inappropriately high perfusion values, and assumptions in the mathematical model on which the technique is based. Given the current state of affairs, absolute measurement of CBV, MTT, and CBF has not been standardized. However, it is expected that these difficulties will be resolved as interest in CTP continues to grow.

References

1. Hacke W, Kaste M, Fieschi C, et al: Intravenous thrombolysis with recombinant tissue plasminogen activator for acute hemispheric stroke: The European Cooperative Acute Stroke Study (ECASS). JAMA 274:1017–1225, 1995.
2. Hacke W, Kaste M, Fieschi C, et al: Randomised double-blind placebo-controlled trial of thrombolytic therapy with intravenous alteplase in acute ischaemic stroke (ECASS II). Lancet 352:1245–1250, 1998.
3. Tissue plasminogen activator for acute ischemic stroke: The National Institute of Neurological Disorders and Stroke rt-PA Stroke Study Group. N Engl J Med 333:1581–1587, 1995.
4. Barber PA, Demchuk AM, Zhang J, Buchan AM: Validity and reliability of a quantitative computed tomography score in predicting outcome of hyperacute stroke before thrombolytic therapy. Lancet 355(9216):1670–1674, 2000.
5. Johnston DCC, Chapman KM, Goldstein L: Low rate of complications of cerebral angiography in routine clinical practice. Neurology 57:2012–2014, 2001.
6. Kerber CW, Cromwell LD, Drayer BP, Bank WO: Cerebral ischemia. I: Current angiographic techniques, complication and safety. Am J Roentgenol 130:1097–1103, 1978.
7. Mani RL, Eisenberg RL, McDonald EJ, et al: Complications of catheter cerebral arteriography; analysis of 5000 procedures. I: Criteria and incidence. Am J Roentgenol 131:861–865, 1978.
8. Mani RL, Eisenberg RL, McDonald EJ, et al: Complications of catheter cerebral arteriography; analysis of 5000 procedures. II: Relation of complication rates to clinical and arteriographic diagnoses. Am J Roentgenol 131:867–869, 1978.
9. Mani RL, Eisenberg RL, McDonald EJ, et al: Complications of catheter cerebral arteriography; analysis of 5000 procedures. III: Assessment of arteries injected, contrast medium used, duration of procedure, and age of patient. Am J Roentgenol 131:871–874, 1978.
10. Dion JE, Gates PC, Fox AJ, et al: Clinical events following neuroangiography: A prospective study. Stroke 18:997–1004, 1987.
11. Grzyska U, Freitag J, Zeumer H: Selective cerebral intra-arterial DSA: Complication rate and control of risk factors. Neuroradiology 32:296–299, 1990.
12. Mamourian A, Drayer BP: Clinically silent infarcts shown by MR after cerebral angiography. AJNR Am J Neuroradiol 11:1084, 1990.
13. Shameshima T, Futami S, Morita Y, et al: Clinical usefulness of and problems with three-dimensional CT angiography for the evaluation of arteriosclerotic stenosis of the carotid artery: Comparison with conventional angiography, MRA, and ultrasound sonography. Surg Neurol 51:301–308, 1999.
14. Leclerc X, Godefroy O, Pruvo JP, Leys D: Computed tomographic angiography for the evaluation of carotid artery stenosis. Stroke 26:1577–1581, 1995.
15. Anderson GB, Ashforth R, Steinke DE, et al: CT angiography for the detection and characterization of carotid artery bifurcation disease. Stroke 31:2168–2174, 2000.
16. Ernst R, Pancioli A, Tomsick T, et al: Combined intravenous and intra-arterial recombinant tissue plasminogen activator in acute ischemic stroke. Stroke 31:2552–2557, 2000.

17. Furlan A, Higashida R, Wechsler L, et al: Intra-arterial prourokinase for acute ischemic stroke. The PROACT II study: A randomized controlled trial. Prolyse in Acute Cerebral Thromboembolism. JAMA 282:1–9, 1999.

18. Lev MH, Farkas J, Rodriguez VR, et al: CT angiography in the rapid triage of patients with hyperacute stroke to intra-arterial thrombolysis: Accuracy in the detection of large vessel thrombus. J Comput Assist Tomogr 25:520–528, 2001.

19. Good WF, Gur D: Xenon-enhanced CT of the brain: Effect of flow activation on desired cerebral blood flow measurements. Am J Neuroradiol 12:83–85, 1991.

20. Gur D, Yonas H, Wolfson SK Jr, et al: Xenon and iodine enhanced cerebral CT: A closer look. Stroke 12:573–578, 1981.

21. Ketty SS, Schmidt CF: The nitrous oxide method for the quantitative determination of cerebral blood flow in man: Theory, procedure and normal values. J Clin Invest 27:476–483, 1948.

22. Yonas H, Johnson DW, Pindzola RR: Xenon-enhanced CT of cerebral blood flow. Sci Am 2:58–67, 1995.

23. Wolfson SKJ, Clark J, Greenberg JH, et al: Xenon-enhanced computed tomography compared with [^{14}C]iodoantipyrine for normal and low cerebral blood flow states in baboons. Stroke 21:751–757, 1990.

24. DeWitt DS, Fatouros PP, Wist AO, et al: Stable xenon versus radiolabeled microsphere cerebral blood flow measurements in baboons. Stroke 20:1716–1723, 1989.

25. Fatouros PP, Wist AO, Kishore PR, et al: Xenon/computed tomography cerebral blood flow measurements: Methods and accuracy. Invest Radiol 22:705–712, 1987.

26. Yonas H, Darby JM, Marks EC, et al: CBF measured by XeCT: Approach to analysis and normal values. J Cereb Blood Flow Metab 11:716–725, 1991.

27. Winkler S, Turski P, Holden J, et al: Xenon effects on CNS control of respiratory rate and tidal volume: The danger of apnea. In Hartmen A, Hoyer S (eds): Cerebral Blood Flow and Metabolism Measurement. Berlin, Springer Verlag, 1985, pp 356–360.

28. Darby JM, Yonas H, Pentheny S, Marion D: Intracranial pressure response to stable Xe inhalation in patients with head injury. Surg Neurol 32:343–345, 1989.

29. Marion DW, Crosby K: The effect of stable Xe on ICP. J Cereb Blood Flow Metab 11:347–350, 1991.

30. Good WF, Gur D: Xenon enhanced CT of the brain: Effect of flow activation on derived cerebral blood flow measurements. AJNR Am J Neuroradiol 12:83–85, 1991.

31. Marks EC, Yonas H, Sander MH, et al: Physiologic implications of adding small amounts of carbon dioxide to the gas mixture during inhalation of Xe. Neuroradiology 34:297–300, 1992.

32. Obrist WD, Zhang Z, Yonas H: Effect of xenon induced flow activation on XeCT CBF calculations. J Cereb Blood Flow Metab 18:1192–1195, 1998.

33. Witt JP, Holl K, Heissler HE, Dietz H: Stable Xe CT CBF: Effects of blood flow alterations on CBF calculation during inhalation of 33% stable Xe. AJNR Am J Neuroradiol 12:973–975, 1991.

34. Jones TH, Morawetz RB, Crowell RM, et al: Thresholds of focal cerebral ischemia in awake monkeys. J Neurosurg 54:773–782, 1981.

35. Hossmann K-A: Viability thresholds and the penumbra of focal ischemia. Ann Neurol 36:557–564, 1994.

36. Hossman K-A, Schuier FJ: Experimental brain infarcts in cats: Pathophysiological observations. Stroke 11:583–592, 1980.

37. Astrup J, Symon L, Branston NM: Cortical evoked potential and extracellular K$^+$ and H$^+$ at critical levels of brain ischemia. Stroke 8:51–57, 1977.

38. Branston NM, Strong AJ, Symon L: Extracellular potassium activity, evoked potential and tissue blood flow: Relationships during progressive ischaemia in baboon cerebral cortex. J Neurol Sci 32:305–321, 1977.

39. Morawetz RB, Crowell RH, DeGirolami U: Regional cerebral blood flow thresholds during cerebral ischemia. Fed Proc 38:2493–2494, 1979.

40. Yonas H, Gur D, Claassen D, et al: Stable xenon enhanced computed tomography in the study of clinical and pathologic correlates of focal ischemia in baboons. Stroke 19:228–238, 1988.

41. Yonas H, Gur D, Claassen D, et al: Stable xenon-enhanced CT measurement of cerebral blood flow in reversible focal ischemia in baboons. J Neurosurg 73:266–273, 1990.

42. Kaufmann AM, Firlik AD, Fukui MB, et al: Ischemic core and penumbra in human stroke. Stroke 30:93–99, 1999.

43. Jovin TG, Goldstein S, Gebel J, et al: Patterns of core and penumbra in acute M1 occlusion and their clinical correlates. Abstract accepted as a poster presentation to the 26th American Heart Association International Stroke Conference, February 14–16, 2001. Stroke 32:348, 2001.

44. Firlik AD, Kaufmann AM, Wechsler LR, et al: Quantitative cerebral blood flow determinations in acute ischemic stroke: Relationship to computed tomography and angiography. Stroke 28:2208–2213, 1997.

45. Firlik AD, Yonas H, Kaufmann AM, et al: Relationship between cerebral blood flow and the development of swelling and life-threatening herniation in acute ischemic stroke. J Neurosurg 89:67–73, 1998.

46. Goldstein S, Yonas H, Gebel JM, et al: Acute cerebral blood flow as a predictive physiologic marker for symptomatic hemorrhagic conversion and clinical herniation after thrombolytic therapy. Abstract accepted as an oral presentation to the 25th AHA International Stroke Conference, 2000. Stroke 31:275, 2000.

47. Goldstein S, Yonas H, Gebel JM, et al: Cerebral blood flow as a predictor of clinical outcome after thrombolytic therapy for acute ischemic stroke. Stroke 31:327, 2000.

48. Goldstein S, Jungreis CA, Wechsler LR, et al: Time to Treatment and Cerebral Blood Flow as Predictive Measures of Clinical Outcome in Patients Treated with Intra-arterial Thrombolytic Therapy. Accepted as an oral presentation to the American Society of Neuroradiology (ASNR) 39th Annual Meeting, April 26, 2001.

49. Kilpatrick MM, Goldstein S, Yonas H, et al: Sensitivity and specificity of quantitative cerebral blood flow vs. time from symptom onset as a predictor of cerebral infarction. Abstract accepted to the 26th American Heart Association International Stroke Conference, February 14–16, 2001. Stroke 32:348, 2001.

50. Firlik AD, Rubin G, Yoans H, Wechsler LR: Relation between cerebral blood flow and neurologic deficit resolution in acute ischemic stroke. Neurology 51:177–182, 1998.

51. Failure of extracranial-intracranial arterial bypass to reduce the risk of ischemic stroke. The EC/IC Bypass Study Group. N Engl J Med 313:1191–1200, 1985.

52. Derdeyn CP, Yundt KD, Videen TO, et al: Increased oxygen extraction fraction is associated with prior ischemic events in patients with carotid occlusion. Stroke 29:754–758, 1998.

53. Grubb RL, Derdeyn CP, Fritsch SM, et al: Importance of hemodynamic factors in the prognosis of symptomatic carotid occlusion. JAMA 280:1055–1060, 1998.

54. Yonas H, Smith H, Durham S, et al: Increased stroke risk predicted by compromised cerebral blood flow reactivity. J Neurosurg 79:483–489, 1993.

55. Webster MW, Makaroun MS, Steed DL, et al: Compromised cerebral blood flow reactivity is a predictor of stroke in patients with symptomatic carotid artery occlusive disease. J Vasc Surg 21:338–345, 1995.

56. Broderick JP, Brott T, Tomsick BT, et al: Intracerebral hemorrhage is more than twice as common as subarachnoid hemorrhage. J Neurosurg 78:188–191, 1993.

57. Brott T, Broderick J, Kothari R, et al: Early hemorrhage growth in patients with intracerebral hemorrhage. Stroke 28:1–5, 1997.

58. Kazui S, Naritomi H, Yamamoto H, et al: Enlargement of spontaneous intracerebral hemorrhage. Stroke 27:1783–1787, 1996.

59. Dandapani BK, Suzuki S, Kelley RE, et al: Relation between blood pressure and outcome in intracerebral hemorrhage. Stroke 26:21–24, 1995.

60. Powers WJ: Acute hypertension after stroke: The scientific basis for treatment decisions. Neurology 43:461–467, 1993.

61. Powers WJ, Adams RE, Yundt KD, et al: Acute pharmacological hypotension after intracerebral hemorrhage does not change cerebral blood flow [abstract]. Stroke 30:242, 1999.

62. Gebel JM, Kassam AB, Snyder JV, et al: Effects of aggressive blood pressure reduction on cerebral blood flow in patients with acute intracerebral hemorrhage. Stroke 31:283, 2000.

63. Wiebers DO, Whisnant JP, Sundt TM Jr, O'Fallon WM: The significance of unruptured intracranial aneurysms. N Engl J Med 304:696–698, 1981.

64. Graves EJ: Detailed diagnoses and procedures: National Hospital Discharge Survey, 1990. Vital Health Stat 13:1–225, 1992.

65. Assessment: Transcranial Doppler. Report of the American Academy of Neurology, Therapeutics and Technology Assessment Subcommittee. Neurology 40:680–681, 1990.

66. Sloan MA, Wozniak MA, Macko RF: Monitoring of vasospasm after subarachnoid hemorrhage. In Babikian VL, Wechsler LR (eds):

Diagnostic Studies

Transcranial Doppler Ultrasonography, 2nd ed. Boston: Butterworth-Heinemann, 1999, pp 109–127.

67. Clyde BL, Resnick DK, Yonas H et al: The relationship of blood velocity as measured by transcranial Doppler ultrasonography to cerebral blood flow as determined by stable xenon computed tomographic studies after aneurysmal subarachnoid hemorrhage. Neurosurgery 38:896, 2001.

68. Iacopino DG, Todaro C, Alafaci C, et al: Transorbital Doppler: An approach that increases transcranial Doppler sensitivity in the detection of SAH vasospasm. Stroke 24:519, 1993.

69. Marion DW, Darby J, Yonas H: Acute regional cerebral blood flow changes caused by severe head injuries. J Neurosurg 74:407–414, 1991.

70. Marion DW, Bouma GJ: The use of stable xenon-enhanced computed tomographic studies of cerebral blood flow to define changes in cerebral carbon dioxide vasoresponsivity caused by a severe head injury. Neurosurgery 29:869–873, 1991.

71. Adelson PD, Clyde B, Kochanek PM, et al: Cerebrovascular response in infants and young children following severe traumatic brain injury: A preliminary report. Pediatr Neurosurg 26:200–207, 1997.

72. Meier P, Zierler KL: On the theory of the indicator-dilution method for measurement of blood flow and volume. J Appl Physiol 6:731–744, 1954.

73. Roberts GW, Larson KB: The interpretation of mean transit time measurements for multi-phase tissue systems. J Theor Biol 39:447–475, 1973.

74. Wintermark M, Thiran J, Maeder P, et al: Simultaneous measurement of regional cerebral blood flow by perfusion CT and stable xenon CT: A validation study. AJNR Am J Neuroradiol 22:905–914, 2001.

75. Goldstein S, Herron J, Wintermark M, et al: Comparison of quantitative cerebral blood flow measured by CT perfusion v. xenon enhanced computerized tomography in cerebral infarction. IRB approved study funded by GE.

76. Koenig M, Kraus M, Theek C, et al: Quantitative assessment of the ischemic brain by means of perfusion-related parameters derived from perfusion CT. Stroke 32:431–437, 2001.

77. Hunter GJ, Hamberg LM, Ponzo JA, et al: Assessment of cerebral perfusion and arterial anatomy in hyperacute stroke with three-dimensional functional CT: Early clinical results. AJNR Am J Neuroradiol 19:29–37, 1998.

78. Lee KH, Cho S, Byun HS, et al: Triphasic perfusion computed tomography in acute middle cerebral artery stroke. Arch Neurol 57:990–999, 2000.

79. Koenig M, Kraus M, Theek C, et al: Quantitative assessment of the ischemic brain by means of perfusion-related parameters derived from perfusion CT. Stroke 32:431–437, 2001.

80. Firlik AD, Kaufmann AM, Wechsler LR, et al: Quantitative cerebral blood flow determinations in acute ischemic stroke: Relationship to computed tomography and angiography. Stroke 28:2208–2213, 1997.

81. Rubin G, Firlik AD, Pindzola RR, et al: The effect of reperfusion therapy on cerebral blood flow in acute stroke. J Stroke Cerebrovasc Dis 8:9–16, 1999.

82. Eskey CJ, Rosand J, Greenberg S, et al: Dynamic CT perfusion assessment of cerebral blood flow in acute intracerebral hemorrhage. Boston, ASNR Proceedings, 2001, p 239.

83. Dillon WP: CT techniques for detecting acute stroke and collateral circulation: In search of the Holy Grail. AJNR Am J Neuroradiol 19:191–192, 1998.

Diagnostic Studies

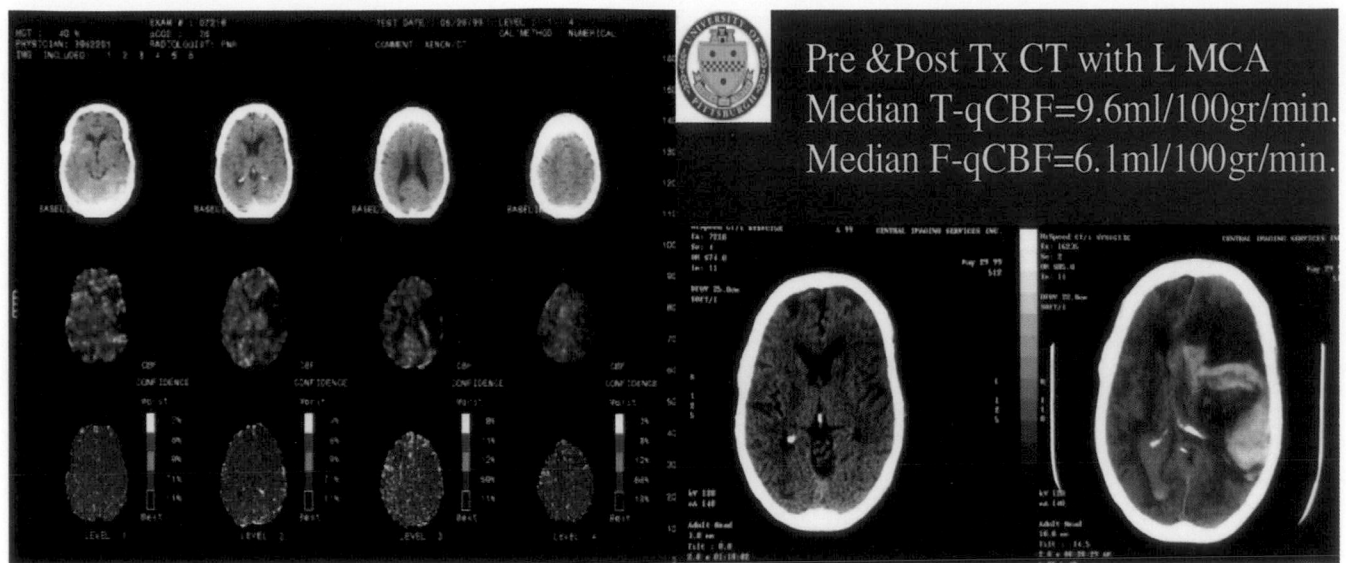

PLATE 18–1 *The pre-treatment xenon-enhanced CT (XeCT) cerebral blood flow (CBF) study (left side of picture) with the pre-treatment and post-treatment CT scans (paired CT images in right side of picture) in a case of severe hypoperfusion with a median T-qCBF in the left middle cerebral artery (L MCA) territory of 9.6 mL/100 g/min and an F-qCBF of 6.1 mL/100 g/min treated with combined intravenous and intra-arterial administration of tissue-type plasminogen activator (t-PA), which resulted in symptomatic hemorrhagic conversion and death.*

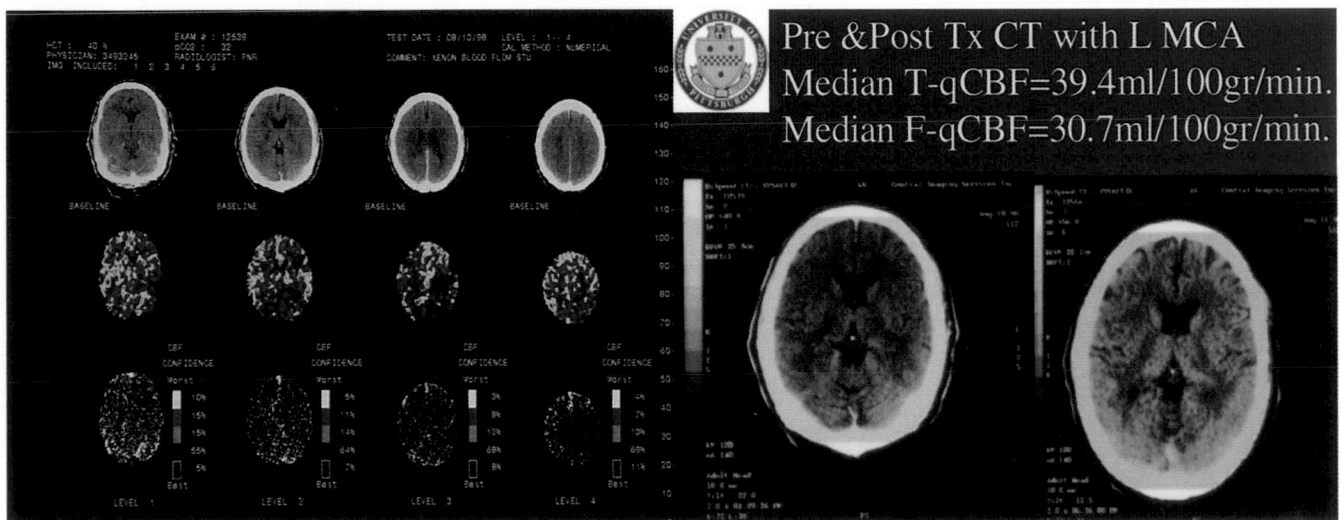

PLATE 18–2 *The pre-treatment xenon-enhanced CT (XeCT) cerebral blood flow (CBF) study (left) with pre-treatment and post-treatment paired CT scans (right) in a case of mild hypoperfusion with a median T-qCBF in the left middle cerebral artery (L MCA) territory of 39.4 mL/100 g/min and a F-qCBF of 30.7 mL/100 g/min treated with intravenous tissue-type plasminogen activator (t-PA). (Modified Rankin scale score at discharge equaled 0-1; no or minimal disability).*

XeCT and CTP Level 2

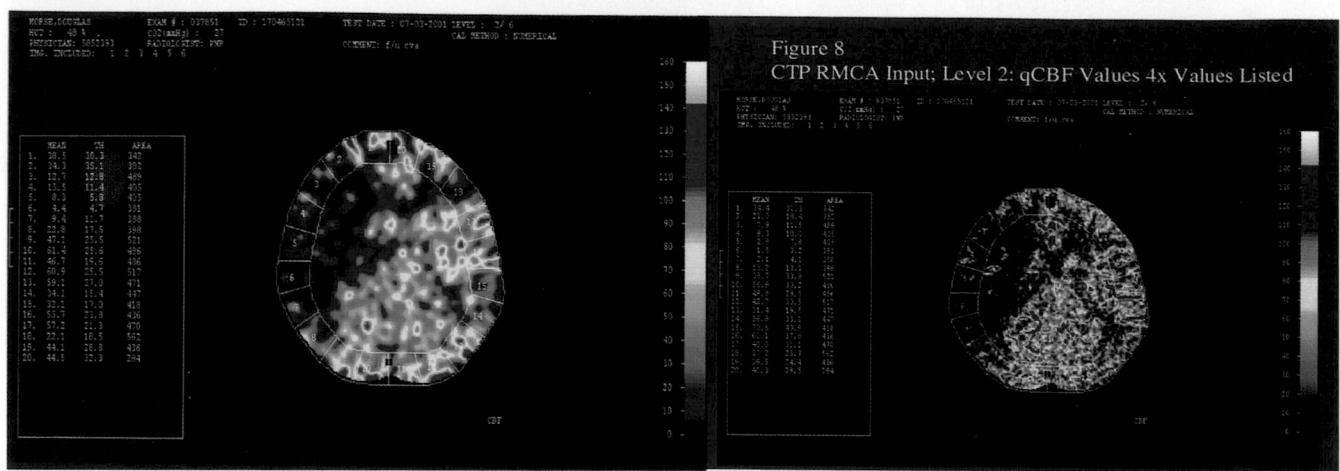

Figure 8
CTP RMCA Input; Level 2: qCBF Values 4x Values Listed

PLATE 18–3 *In the right middle cerebral artery (RMCA) vascular distribution* (left), *the mean cerebral blood flow CBF measured by xenon-enhanced CT (XeCT) was 12.7 mL/100 g/min (level 2), and a corresponding CT perfusion (CTP) image of level 2* (right) *is demonstrated.*

DWI
ADC
PWI
Pretreatment
Post-treatment

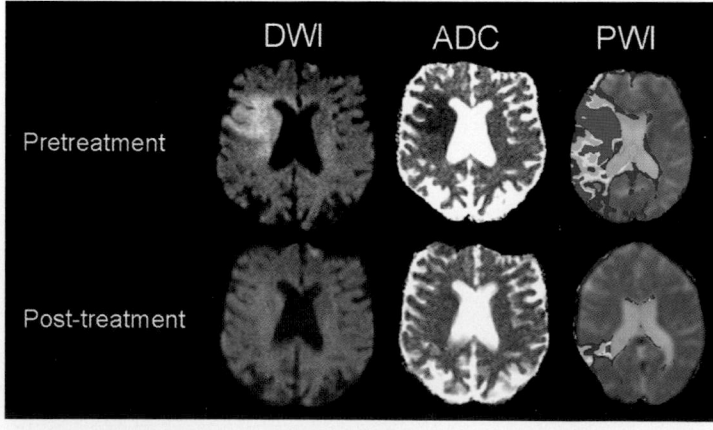

PLATE 19–1 *Examples of diffusion-weighted (DWI) and perfusion-weighted (PWI) images from a patient treated with intra-arterial thrombolytic therapy for a right middle cerebral artery occlusion.* Top row, *Pretreatment images;* bottom row, *early posttreatment images. Perfusion images are in the form of color-coded maps of the time to peak of the residue function (Tmax), with red indicating greatest delay. After vessel recanalization, there is complete reversal of initial DWI and apparent diffusion coefficient (ADC) abnormalities and almost complete reversal of the initial perfusion lesion.*

Chapter Nineteen

Magnetic Resonance Imaging

Steven Warach, Chelsea S. Kidwell, and Alison E. Baird

Nuclear magnetic resonance techniques were first employed in the 1940s, and the first images were obtained in the 1970s. In the 1980s structural nuclear magnetic resonance imaging (MRI) emerged as a clinically useful diagnostic modality for stroke and other neurologic disorders.[1-5] In the detection of ischemic stroke lesions, structural MRI is more sensitive than computed tomography (CT), particularly for small infarcts and in sites such as the cerebellum, brainstem, and deep white matter.[6-8] In the investigation of ischemic stroke, conventional structural MRI techniques, such as T1-weighted imaging (T1WI), T2-weighted imaging (T2WI), and fluid-attenuated inversion recovery (FLAIR) imaging, are valuable for the assessment of infarct extent and location after the first 12 to 24 hours from onset. These methods can be combined with MR angiography (MRA) to noninvasively assess the intracranial and extracranial vasculature.

During the critical first 3 to 6 hours, however, the probable period of greatest therapeutic opportunity, these methods do not adequately assess the extent and severity of ischemia. The 1990s witnessed the development of reliable imaging of ischemic events within the first 6 hours from onset: cerebral perfusion and early, potentially reversible parenchymal injury. Diffusion-weighted imaging (DWI) sequences have been developed that are sensitive to the self-diffusion of water and early ischemic changes,[9,10] as have contrast-based, perfusion-sensitive techniques that delineate hemodynamic changes.[11,12] These techniques were recognized for their potential clinical utility in the early detection and investigation of patients with stroke.[13,14] That initial optimism is now bearing fruit as further technical developments, most notably echo planar imaging,[15] have made routine clinical diffusion and perfusion MRI feasible in clinical practice. The detection of hyperacute intraparenchymal hemorrhagic stroke by susceptibility-weighted MRI also shows much promise. In combination with MRA, these methods allow the detection of the site, age, extent, mechanism, and tissue viability of acute stroke lesions in one imaging study.

A number of potential clinical applications have emerged that could allow therapeutic and clinical decisions to be based on the physiologic state of the tissue in addition to clinical assessment. At the beginning of the 21st century,

MRI is typically applied as a multimodal examination to evaluate the patient with stroke for arterial disease, hemodynamic changes, hyperacute parenchymal injury, subacute and chronic infarction, and evidence of acute or chronic hemorrhage. However, even where multimodal MRI is available, the information now obtainable is not always being utilized to its fullest potential, and clinical applications are yet to be standardized. The emerging and most promising applications of current MRI methodology are as a patient selection tool for experimental and interventional therapies and as a biomarker of therapeutic response in clinical trials.

In this review, we describe the applications of structural and functional MR techniques in cerebrovascular disease. First we describe the relevant technological and methodological aspects, then the pathophysiologic considerations and background, and last the potential clinical applications. A fuller treatment of the technical and clinical topics discussed in this chapter may be found elsewhere.[16,17]

GENERAL PRINCIPLES AND BASIC PULSE SEQUENCES

Routine MRI is based on the interaction of radio waves with nuclei (most commonly protons or hydrogen nuclei) in tissue. Hydrogen is present in nearly all of the organs of the body. Water and fat protons are the most extensively imaged nuclei. Other nuclei that can be imaged are those of sodium and phosphorus, but they are much less abundant than hydrogen. Protons have a net magnetic moment such that when they are placed in a magnetic field, they align with it. They also can be excited by intermittent radiofrequency (RF) pulses.

In MRI the patient is placed in a strong magnetic field. The strength of the magnetic field depends on the specific scanner. In practice, most of the current clinical MRI is performed at 1.0 tesla (T) and 1.5 T, but scanners with lower and higher field strengths are also in use. Over the next decade, clinical 3.0 T MRI will become commonplace. In general, for brain and cerebrovascular imaging, higher field strengths give greater signal to noise, which is advantageous for reducing scanning time and increasing spatial resolution. For the acquisition of images, RF pulses are applied at the Lamour frequency for hydrogen, the proton's resonant spin frequency. The energy from the RF pulses is absorbed and then released until the tissue being scanned has completely reemitted the energy absorbed and undergone complete relaxation. The echo time (TE) is the time the machine waits after the applied RF pulse to receive the RF echo from the patient. The repetition time (TR) is the time between RF pulses. The energy released occurs over a short time according to two relaxation constants, known as T1 (longitudinal relaxation constant) and T2 (transverse relaxation constant). Varying the TE and the TR enables images of different contrast to be obtained, depending on which of the constants is dominant.

Conventional Pulse Sequences

Conventional MRI pulse sequences are T2-weighted imaging, T1 weighted imaging, proton density imaging, and fluid attenuated inversion recovery imaging. These are of most value in the evaluation of subacute and chronic stroke. The conventional sequences are based on two families of sequences, termed *spin echo* (or fast spin echo) and *gradient echo*. In the former, the energy is refocused through the use of a series of RF pulses, whereas the latter uses a reversal of the magnetic field gradient to refocus the energy. The gradient echo sequences are most useful for MR angiography and hemorrhage detection.

T1-Weighted Images

T1-weighted images are based on the longitudinal relaxation of spins. They are generated primarily from sequences of short TE and short TR; the shorter the TE and TR, the more T1-weighted the image is. On T1WI, the cerebrospinal fluid (CSF) has a low signal intensity, whereas fat has a high signal intensity. Gray matter appears less intense (darker) than white matter. Ischemic infarcts appear hypointense on T1WI.

T2-Weighted Images

T2-weighted images are based on the transverse relaxation of spins. They are generated from sequences of long TE and long TR. On T2WI, the CSF signal is hyperintense, whereas fat has almost no signal. Gray matter appears less intense (darker) than white matter. Ischemic lesions also appear hyperintense and may be difficult to distinguish from normal CSF spaces, a problem with smaller lesions.

Proton Density Images

Proton density images are generated with long TR and short TE, and the CSF and fat are of similar signal intensity. One advantage of PDI is that lesions appear hyperintense relative to CSF.

Fluid-Attenuated Inversion Recovery Images

On FLAIR images, an additional RF pulse (inversion pulse) is applied with the purpose of nulling signal from the CSF. When the technique is applied in routine practice, the CSF signal is nearly fully suppressed and appears dark as in T1WI, but the lesions appear bright, as in T2WI, allowing better visualization of cortical and periventricular lesions. In practice, FLAIR may be used in place of PDI

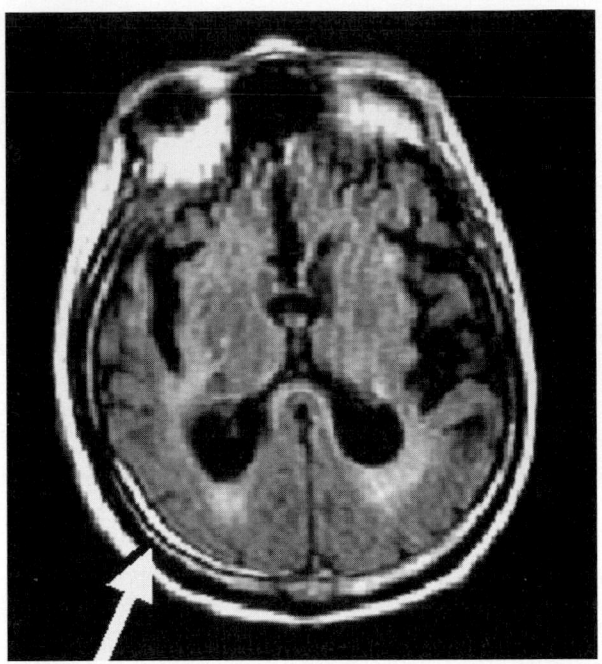

FIGURE 19–1   *An example of a subdural hematoma seen on fluid-attenuated inversion recovery (FLAIR) imaging (arrow), with clear contrast between the hyperintensity of the blood and the background tissue. This small subdural was not seen on computed tomography.*

and is often used in preference to T2WI, although FLAIR acquisition times are somewhat longer. Unique features of FLAIR for acute stroke imaging include hyperintensity of extra-axial blood (e.g., subarachnoid hemorrhage,[18] subdural hematoma, Fig. 19–1) and hyperintense arterial signal indicative of very slow flow associated with acute occlusions or severe stenosis (Fig. 19–2).[19,20]

Functional Magnetic Resonance Imaging Sequences

The advances in functional or physiologic MRI that have occurred over the past 10 to 12 years provide valuable information in the emergency evaluation of acute stroke, supplementing the anatomic information obtained from conventional sequences. These protocols are diffusion-weighted imaging, perfusion imaging, MR angiography, and gradient-recalled echo (GRE) imaging. Echo planar imaging (EPI) became a clinical application essential to diffusion and perfusion imaging, because its short acquisition time minimizes the effects of motion due either to head movement or to physiologic pulsations of the brain. These sequences allow a multimodal evaluation of the patient with acute stroke through imaging of tissue injury, perfusion, and the vasculature.

Diffusion-Weighted Imaging

DWI allows the detection of ischemic stroke lesions within minutes after the onset of symptoms, well before changes are detectable on CT and T2WI (Fig. 19–3). DWI detects the self-diffusion of water, which is the mobility of water molecules among other water molecules (brownian

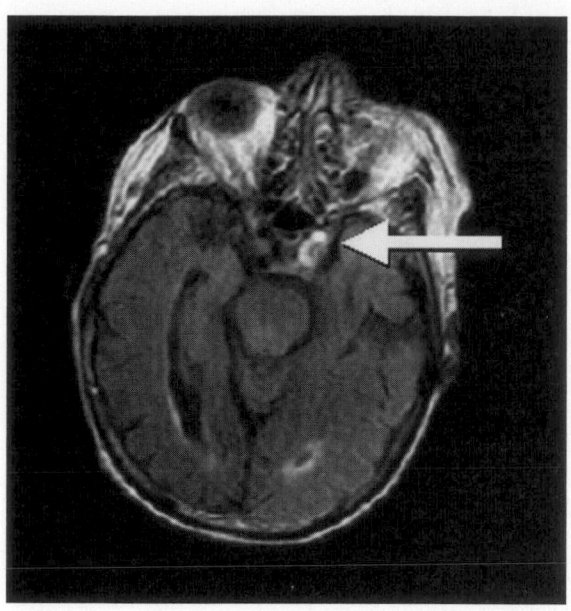

FIGURE 19–2 *Hyperintense acute occlusion sign on fluid-attenuated inversion recovery (FLAIR) imaging in a patient with a 2-hour-old occlusion of the left internal carotid artery (arrow). Note the normal flow void (hypointensity) of the contralateral carotid artery.*

motion).[9,10] With the use of EPI, whole-brain DWI of stroke can be obtained in a scanning time of 2 seconds.[21] The diffusion-sensitive MRI pulse sequence involves the addition of a bipolar pair of diffusion-sensitizing magnetic field gradient pulses to a pulse sequence (typically a T2WI) to cause a dephasing and then rephasing of the spinning protons in water molecules.[10] Where there has been net movement of a water molecule (i.e., protons) between application of the two diffusion gradient pulses (approximately 40 milliseconds for an echo planar image), there is a net dephasing and subsequent signal loss in the resulting image. The more the water has moved, the greater the signal loss, so that signal intensity is reduced everywhere but relatively less where water movement is restricted. CSF appears very dark, normal brain appears intermediate, and ischemic brain, where parenchymal diffusion is reduced, appears relatively bright.

DWI is quantitative in that it both measures a physiologic parameter—the apparent diffusion coefficient (ADC) of water in tissue—and permits volumetric analysis of lesions that can be used to study ischemic pathophysiology in vivo. Diffusion measurements also contain geometric information, primarily axonal orientation, because DWI acquisitions acquire their information in one direction at a time. For routine stroke imaging, it is preferable to minimize this anisotropy by effectively averaging the diffusion measurements in three orthogonal directions, eliminating hyperintensity not due to ischemia. However, diffusion tensor imaging has emerged as a technique for applications in which axonal direction and integrity are the questions of interest.[22,23]

In acute cerebral ischemia, the ischemic lesion appears hyperintense (bright) on DWI and hypointense (dark) on an ADC map. This reflects cytotoxic edema and a reduction in the volume and an increase in the tortuosity of the extracellular space. As the ischemic lesion evolves through the phases of cytotoxic edema, vasogenic edema, tissue necrosis, and cavitation, the ADC normalizes and then becomes elevated in the chronic phase of stroke. This feature makes it possible to distinguish old ischemic lesions from new through calculation of the ADC value. As a rule of thumb, DWI hyperintensity without T2WI or FLAIR changes implies reduced ADC and can be taken as evidence of acute ischemic injury. A combination of DWI with FLAIR in a single pulse sequence eliminates partial volume effects of CSF in the brain parenchyma and increases lesion contrast.[24,25] In addition to acute ischemia, signal hyperintensity on DWI can also be due to prior stroke (the T2 shine through effect), to susceptibility artifacts, or rarely, to nonischemic diseases.[26] For these reasons, in patients with suspected ischemic stroke, DWI should always be interpreted with T2WI, FLAIR, or a calculation of the ADC.

Perfusion Imaging

Brain perfusion, defined in the broadest sense as some aspect of cerebral circulation, may be studied by various MRI strategies. Two MRI methods, one requiring the injection of contrast material and the other not, have been used to study abnormal perfusion in human stroke (mainly ischemic). The first strategy, dynamic contrast-enhancing blood volume imaging, involves a bolus injection of gadolinium and the rapid acquisition of a series of susceptibility-weighted gradient echo images.[11,12] The intravascular passage of gadolinium in sufficiently high concentration distorts the local magnetic field because of magnetic susceptibility effects, causing dephasing of spins in brain tissue adjacent to the blood vessels, and therefore results in signal loss. The amount of signal loss over time in a series of rapidly acquired images has been shown to be proportional to cerebral blood volume (CBV) in healthy brain tissue. The time it takes for the change in signal intensity to reach a maximum is related to the mean transit time (MTT) of an idealized bolus of contrast agent. Because cerebral blood flow (CBF) in these intravascular models equals the ratio CBV/MTT, information about cerebral blood flow can potentially be inferred with this technique. In patients with acute stroke, qualitative perfusion maps of the relative MTT (rMTT), relative CBF, and relative CBV have been generated and have permitted visualization of perfusion defects in acute infarcts, tissue reperfusion occurring after recanalization of blood vessels, and hyperperfusion of subacute infarcts. Postprocessing of these images has been time consuming in the past, but qualitative perfusion maps of transit time and blood volume can now be generated within 10 minutes of image acquisition and so are rapidly available to the treating physician. Absolute quantification of CBF parameters with bolus tracking MRI perfusion may be possible[27–31] but are not routinely applied in clinical practice, and questions persist about the accuracy of the quantification algorithms.

The second MR perfusion strategy involves arterial spin labeling (ASL) methods that use RF inversion pulses to magnetically label spins in the arterial supply to brain regions, using arterial water as an endogenous diffusible tracer.[32] This can be applied as either pulsed[33,34] or continuous[35] labeling. In ischemic stroke, ASL appears to give

Diagnostic Studies

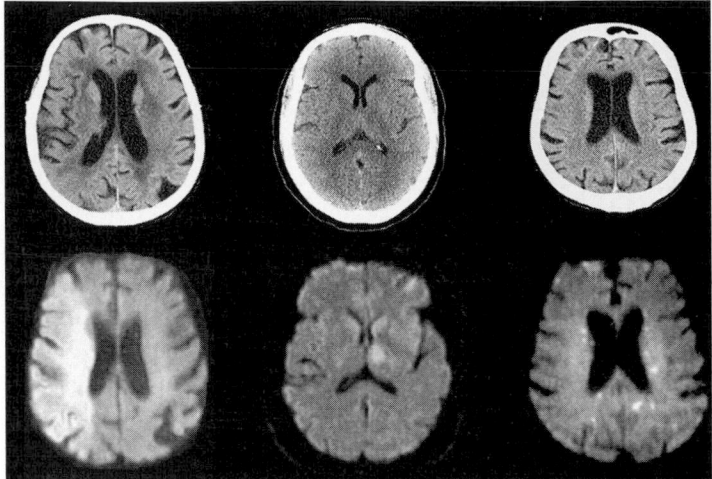

A

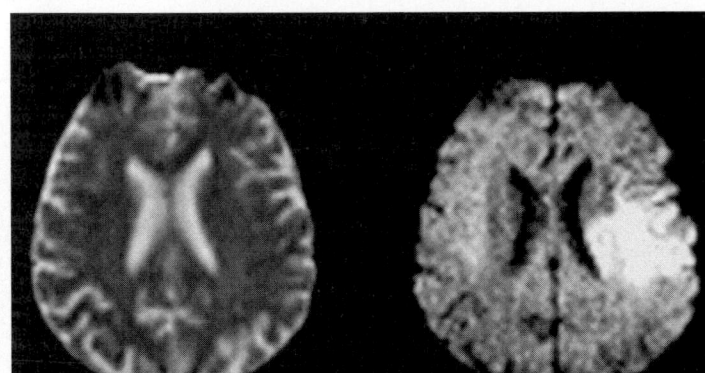

B

FIGURE 19–3 *Detection of hyperacute ischemic stroke with diffusion-weighted imaging (DWI). A, Traditional brain imaging methods such as computed tomography (CT) (top row) and conventional magnetic resonance imaging (MRI) do not at present show ischemic lesions reliably for up to 12 to 24 hours after onset. Diffusion-weighted images (bottom row) clearly show the acute strokes in these three patients. B, At 2 hours after onset of symptoms, DWI (left) shows a hyperintense lesion in the left cerebral hemisphere, but the corresponding T2-weighted image (right) is normal.*

diagnostic information comparable to that provided by the gadolinium bolus tracking methods,[36] but longer acquisition times and limited slice coverage have limited its routine clinical use. However, the more straightforward quantitative measurement of tissue perfusion with ASL[37] is a significant advantage of this methodology compared with the bolus tracking method, even though the reduced signal-to-noise ratio requires averaging of multiple acquisitions and thus significantly longer acquisition times and greater vulnerability to motion artifacts. Innovations have permitted multiple brain slices to be imaged with ASL.[38]

Magnetic Resonance Angiography

Three types of MRA are in clinical use, two-dimensional and three dimensional time-of-flight MRA, and phase-contrast MRA.

Time-of-flight (TOF) MRA depends on the movement of blood into the imaging field. The magnetization of protons in stationary tissue are saturated by repeated low-flip-angle RF pulses, whereas protons in the vessels flowing into the tissue remain unsaturated and appear relatively bright. The data are then postprocessed using a maximum intensity projection (MIP) algorithm for angiographic reconstruction. In practice, inspection of the source images is often necessary to evaluate subtle or ambiguous findings. Three-dimensional rather than two-dimensional

TOF MRA is the most common implementation of MRA in clinical practice, because it gives superior spatial resolution and is less prone to signal loss from turbulent flow at sites of stenoses, although two-dimensional TOF MRA may be more sensitive to slower flow.

Phase-contrast MRA is another technique of generating angiographic type images based on the velocity and direction of flow. Phase-contrast MRA is based on the principle that moving spins develop a phase shift relative to stationary spins when they move in the presence of a pair of opposing magnetic field gradients. There is superior background suppression with phase-contrast MRA, but acquisition times tend to be longer and more prone to artifacts.

Susceptibility-Weighted Imaging

Magnetic susceptibility is the property of matter that distorts an applied magnetic field. Although often a source of artifacts at the interface of differing tissue types, this principle can be used to make pulse sequences sensitive to hemorrhage, to functional changes in blood oxygenation, and to hemodynamic parameters. The GRE pulse sequences (also called T2*-weighted images or susceptibility-weighted images) can be made sensitive to the susceptibility effects of paramagnetic molecules such as gadolinium containing contrast agents, deoxyhemoglobin and other hemoglobin breakdown products that are

Table 19.1 Magnetic Resonance Imaging Sequences in Acute Ischemic Stroke*

Sequence	Detection
DWI	Acute ischemic lesions as early as 39 minutes from onset
	Distinguish old lesions from new by quantitative measurement of the apparent diffusion coefficient
	Lesions as small as 2 mm detected
	High sensitivity (much higher than T2WI, FLAIR, and CT) but patient can have perfusion defects without DWI lesions
	Lesions in the posterior fossa may be less easy to detect because of susceptibility artifacts and small size
T2WI	Subacute and chronic ischemic lesions
FLAIR	Subacute and chronic ischemic lesions
Susceptibility-weighted imaging	Intracranial hemorrhage as early as 2 to 3 hours after onset
	Sensitivity and specificity being evaluated
MRA	Arterial lesions (intracranial)
	With the use of a head-and-neck coil and gadolinium injection, MRA can image from the aortic arch to the circle of Willis in 2 minutes
Perfusion Imaging	Tissue perfusion—semiquantitative measurements of relative mean transit time (rMTT), relative cerebral blood volume (rCBV), and relative cerebral blood flow (rCBF)
	In combination with DWI and MRA patterns of mismatch

*First obtain MRI checklist to exclude patients with metallic implants.
CT, computed tomography; DWI, diffusion-weighted imaging; FLAIR, fluid-attenuated inversion recovery; MRA; magnetic resonance angiography; T2WI, T2-weighted imaging.

present during all stages of intracranial hemorrhage. Single-shot echo planar imaging (EPI) has intrinsic susceptibility weighting, and EPI using a GRE technique is the most sensitive of all to susceptibility effects.

Multimodality Magnetic Resonance Imaging

The objective of multimodal MRI of acute stroke is to obtain diagnostic information about the acute parenchymal injury, chronic infarct, arterial disease, tissue perfusion, and presence of hemorrhage. The multimodal MR sequences listed in Table 19.1 can be acquired on the latest generation of 1.5 T MRI scanners in a 20-minute scanning period. More time is required for moving the patient on and off the scanning table and confirming that the patient is free of metallic implants.

TRANSIENT ISCHEMIC ATTACKS

Conventional MRI is more sensitive than standard CT at identifying both new and preexisting ischemic lesions in patients with transient ischemic attacks (TIAs). Among various studies, MRI has shown evidence of at least one infarct somewhere in the cerebrum in 46% to 81% of patients with TIA.[39,40] Some of these infarcts are in locations that could have accounted for the deficits observed during the TIA. Among patients meeting clinical criteria for TIA, 31% to 39% demonstrate neuroanatomically relevant infarcts on conventional MRI.[39,41] It is difficult with both conventional MRI and CT to determine what proportion of these appropriately localized infarcts occurred at the time of the index TIA and what proportion existed before the presenting event.

The earliest report of MRI findings in patients with TIA came from Awad and colleagues.[42] This group studied 22 patients with both MRI and CT. They found that MRI showed focal ischemic changes in 77% of patients but that CT showed such changes in only 32%. However, the majority of lesions did not correlate with symptomatology. Fazekas and associates[39] reported the results of conventional MRI in 62 patients with hemispheric TIAs. Forty-five of the patients also underwent contrast-enhanced studies. These investigators found that 81% of the cohort had MRI evidence of focal ischemic injury, and that 31% demonstrated evidence of an acute TIA-associated infarct.

Additional insight regarding lesion location and clinical characteristics of patients with TIA-associated lesions with conventional MRI comes from two additional studies. In their study of 64 patients with carotid territory TIAs studied with MRI, Kimura and coworkers[41] found that lesions in 16 of 41 patients demonstrated contrast enhancement; the majority of contrast-enhancing lesions were cortical (81%).

Bhadelia and associates[40] studied 100 patients with and without a history of TIA from the Cardiovascular Health Study, who were evaluated with standard MRI sequences.[40] Brain infarcts were shown in 46% of the patients with TIA compared with 28% of patients without a history of TIA. In stepwise logistic regression analysis, diastolic blood pressure and internal carotid intima-media thickness were shown to be predictive of infarction on MRI. These investigators also found a higher frequency of cortical infarcts and multiple infarcts in the patients with TIA.

Preliminary data regarding neuroimaging prognosis in TIA patients are now available. Walters and colleagues[42a] performed serial MRI studies over a 2-year period in 125 patients with TIA and compared the results with those in 75 controls. Follow-up MRI in 47% of the patients with TIA showed evidence of new asymptomatic lesions compared with 12% of controls. Thirteen patients with TIA had new transient cerebral symptoms, of whom two had new relevant MRI lesions. In addition, four patients with TIA experienced a clinical stroke during the follow-up period (3 ischemic events, 1 intracerebral hemorrhage). Factors that correlated with a greater risk of a new ischemic lesion were elevated diastolic blood pressure, male sex, increasing age, and initial severity of MRI ischemic lesions. Also of note, these researchers found that patients with TIA had an accelerated rate of cerebral atrophy.

Kidwell and colleagues[43] provided the first systematic report of DWI in TIA, demonstrating that DWI abnormalities could be visualized in 48% of patients. Five of the 20 patients with a DWI lesion (25%) did not show a lesion correlate on initial T2-weighted (T2W) sequences (Fig. 19–4). The remaining 15 patients did exhibit abnormalities

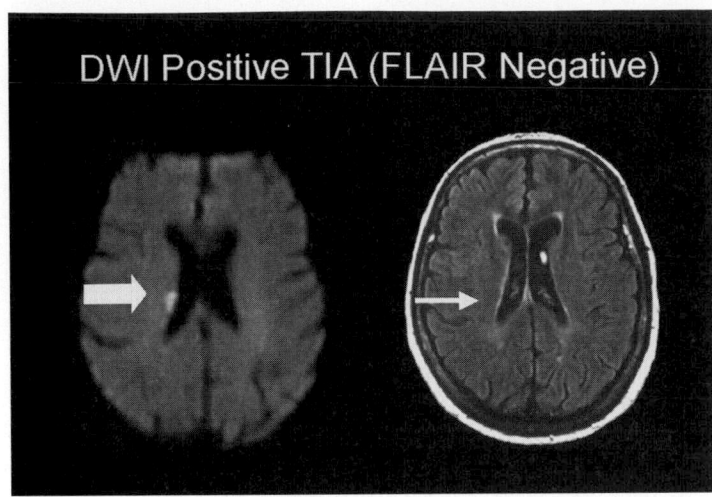

FIGURE 19–4 *Diffusion-weighted imaging (DWI) of a transient ischemic attack. A 63-year-old man with a 30-minute episode of left arm weakness underwent magnetic resonance imaging 4 hours after resolution of the symptoms. The DWI sequence (left) shows a right periventricular white matter lesion (thick arrow) that is not apparent on the fluid-attenuated inversion recovery (FLAIR) sequence (right, thin arrow).*

on T2-weighted sequences in the same regions as the DWI alterations.

Studies from five groups have now confirmed DWI provides a more precise evaluation of ischemic insult in patients with TIA than standard CT and MRI studies.[43–47] These studies show convergent results regarding the frequency of DWI positivity among patients with TIA; in the five studies encompassing 202 patients, the aggregate rate of DWI positivity was 44%, ranging from 35% to 48% (Table 19.2).

One noteworthy finding that has evolved from DWI studies in patients with TIA is that DWI-positive TIA lesions do not consistently evolve to completed infarctions on follow-up imaging studies. In the series reported from the University of California at Los Angeles,[43] only 5 of 9 patients (56%) undergoing follow-up imaging demonstrated a subsequent infarct in the region corresponding to the original DWI abnormality. In addition, there are two case reports in the literature of DWI lesions associated with TIA in which reversibility of the DWI abnormalities was seen on follow-up imaging.[48,49] Of note, however, in the series of 19 TIA patients reported by Takayama and associates,[47] all of the DWI-positive lesions (7 patients) evolved to persistent T2W lesions. This discrepancy may be related to patient characteristics and timing of the imaging studies.

Data regarding perfusion imaging findings in patients with clinical TIAs are scarce. However, two case reports in the literature provide some insight into the potential role of perfusion imaging in the evaluation of TIA. In one report, the initial DWI study was negative but the perfusion study demonstrated a perfusion deficit in a region compatible with the focal symptoms.[50] Despite resolution of the clinical symptoms, the follow-up DWI study showed a small lesion in the initially hypoperfused area. In the second report, a patient with a prolonged reversible ischemic neurologic deficit underwent acute and follow-up diffusion-weighted and perfusion imaging.[49] The initial perfusion scan showed a large lesion with a smaller, relatively less conspicuous DWI abnormality. At the time of follow-up imaging, both the clinical and imaging abnormalities had completely resolved.

These two cases suggest that perfusion imaging is likely to be even more sensitive than DWI in detecting acute ischemic changes in some TIA patients. Because perfusion imaging is able to detect regions of relative hypoperfusion that remain above the threshold of tissue bioenergetic compromise required to cause a lesion on DWI, a greater number of patients with modest degrees of ischemia may be identified with this technique. The anticipated utility of perfusion MR imaging is supported by perfusion studies employing other imaging modalities that have demonstrated detectable blood flow abnormalities in a substantial proportion of patients with TIA.[51,52]

Taken as a whole, these neuroimaging studies suggest a need to reexamine the utility and accuracy of the current time-based definition of TIA. Accumulating evidence suggests that any time cutoff for TIA is inaccurate in reflecting end-organ injury. Accordingly, efforts are under way to redefine TIAs using a tissue-based definition that takes into account the fundamental physiologic processes indexed by imaging or other laboratory measures, rather than a strict time limit.[53,54]

Table 19.2　Time Intervals and Yield of Diffusion Magnetic Resonance Imaging (MRI) in Patients with Transient Ischemia Attack (TIA): Five Series

Series[°]	TIA Duration (mean)	Time from TIA Onset to MRI (mean)	Frequency of Positive DWI Findings on MRI (%)
UCLA (n = 42)[43]	3.2 hr[†]	17 hr	48
Duke (n = 40)[44]	4.8 hr	37 hr	35
MGH (n = 57)[45]	1.9 hr	39 hr	46
Takayama (n = 19)[46]	—	—	37
Bisschops (n = 44)[42]	—	—	47
Total (n = 202)	—	—	44

[°]Superscript numbers indicate chapter references.
[†]Median duration was 2.0 hours.

ACUTE STROKE

Within the first few hours of ischemia, standard MRI sequences (T1WI, T2WI, and proton-density sequences) are relatively insensitive to ischemia, showing abnormalities in less than 50% of cases.[55] The earliest changes, seen as increased signal on T2WI and FLAIR sequences, are due to a net increase in overall tissue water content, a process that takes several hours to develop to levels visible on MRI. These changes are rarely seen earlier than 6 hours from onset but are readily appreciated by 12 to 24 hours. Although the majority of ischemic lesions are evident on both CT and conventional MRI by 24 hours, standard MRI is superior to CT in identifying lesions at an earlier point, smaller lesions, and lesions in the posterior fossa.[6,7] Conventional MRI sequences are sensitive to patient motion, degrading image quality. Although ischemic parenchymal changes are not apparent on conventional sequences in the first few hours, intravascular signs of acute stroke may be apparent: absence of arterial flow void on T2WI, intravascular hyperintensity on FLAIR sequences,[19,56,57] and the hypointense intravascular sign due to acute thrombus on GRE sequences.[58,59]

DWI allows visualization of regions of ischemia within minutes of symptom onset.[60] Decreased water diffusion associated with cytotoxic edema leads causes an increased (bright) signal on DWI sequences, which can be quantitatively measured on the apparent diffusion coefficient (ADC) maps, where darker areas represent decreased diffusion. The increase in signal on DWI may persist for several weeks or longer partially due to a T2 effect. The average ADC, however, remains reduced for only 4 to 7 days, then returns to normal or supranormal levels within 7 to 10 days from onset of ischemia.[61–63] Although the average ADC generally follows this pattern, studies have now clearly demonstrated that marked heterogeneity of the ADC value can occur within the ischemic lesion, even in the hyperacute time window.[64]

DWI has a high degree of sensitivity (88% to 100%) and specificity (95% to 100%) for acute ischemia, even very early in the process.[65–68] In the study by Ay and colleagues,[65] of 782 consecutive patients presenting with strokelike deficits, DWI findings were positive in 765 and negative in 27, including 10 patients whose deficits had non-stroke causes and 10 patients whose deficits were reversible. Studies performed in the acute stroke setting have consistently demonstrated marked superiority in accuracy of the diagnosis of ischemic change for DWI (95% to 100%) compared with CT (42% to 75%) and standard MRI sequences such as FLAIR (46%).[69–72] A study comparing DWI lesions with pathologically confirmed infarction at autopsy also demonstrated an overall accuracy of 95%.[73] Occasionally, DWI hyperintensities may be seen in a number of other cerebral disorders, including status epilepticus, tumors, and Jakob-Creutzfeldt disease.

Information on the natural history of the growth of DWI-demonstrable lesions comes from several clinical trials and case series. Warach and colleagues,[74] analyzing serial imaging studies from patients enrolled in the placebo arm of a neuroprotective trial, demonstrated that the natural history of diffusion lesions is to grow over time during acute and subacute periods.[74] Ischemic lesions follow a relatively consistent pattern of growth during the first 3 days, followed by subsequent decrease in size to day 5 through 7.[75–78]

Numerous studies have shown that initial DWI lesion volume correlates well both with final infarct volume as well as neurologic and functional outcomes in patients with stroke, suggesting that DWI can provide important early prognostic information.[77,79–85] Building on this data, Baird and colleagues[86] showed that the combination of clinical and DWI factors provided better prediction of stroke recovery than any factor alone.

Although these correlations have been repeatedly demonstrated in anterior circulation ischemia, several small case series have suggested that acute DWI lesion volumes correlate poorly with clinical measures in the posterior circulation, because small strategic brainstem infarcts can lead to devastating clinical syndromes but large cerebellar infarcts may cause minimal symptoms.[87]

A growing number of studies have provided data demonstrating the clinical utility of DWI in current practice.[88,89] Diffusion imaging allows early identification of lesion size, neuroanatomic site, and vascular territory involved. A distinctive advantage of DWI is its ability to distinguish acute from chronic ischemia, allowing new lesions to be identified in patients even those near or within areas of prior ischemic injury.[90,91] Another important insight into stroke pathophysiology offered by DWI is the frequent visualization of multiple acute lesions in different vascular territories in patients who have only one clinically symptomatic acute insult, providing evidence of an embolic stroke mechanism.

Perfusion imaging employing the bolus contrast passage method is playing an ever more important role in the initial evaluation and treatment of the patient with acute stroke. Perfusion measures that can be derived from this technique include mean transit time (MTT), relative cerebral blood volume (rCBV), time to peak measures, and relative cerebral blood flow (rCBF). Quantitative measures of cerebral tissue perfusion may be calculated using an arterial input function.[92–95] Controversy persists regarding the best perfusion measure and the ability to obtain reliable quantitative perfusion measures in the acute stroke setting.

Both DWI and T2WI have allowed the detection of many silent or previously undetected small cortical and cerebellar infarcts. Further, DWI has shown that there are commonly multiple acute infarcts and that new ischemic lesions can occur over time. In the study by Baird and colleagues,[86] multiple acute lesions were seen in 17% of patients. These were attributed to multiple emboli. The lesions occurred in both anterior and posterior circulations or in both cerebral hemispheres in 3% to 5% of patients, suggesting a proximal source of embolism. Otherwise, the lesions were seen in the vascular territories of one hemisphere and were attributed to multiple emboli or to the breakup of an embolus.

SUBACUTE STROKE

Subacute infarcts are characterized by varying amounts of vasogenic edema and, frequently, hemorrhagic transformation of the infarct. Vasogenic edema is maximum between 1 and 6 days but persists to varying degrees for 3 or 4 weeks. T2WI and FLAIR sequences show signal hyperintensity in the area of infarction. There may be a variable amount of edema. On T1WI, the area of infarction appears hypointense. After the administration of gadolinium, there is usually enhancement of the lesion on T1WI or of the blood vessels within the ischemic lesion, indicating slow flow in the area of infarction. In acute and subacute stroke, gadolinium enhancement occurs in regions of blood-brain barrier breakdown. The typical sequence of enhancement of the infarct is that enhancement is uncommon in the first 6 days, is most common between 7 and 30 days, and disappears after 30 days but can persist for up to 6 weeks.[97] Two patterns of enhancement have been seen, a slowly progressive form that follows the T2WI changes and then an early form of enhancement that may be associated with better outcome. Occasionally, a fogging effect may be seen in this phase or in the acute phase that is postulated to be due to developing hemorrhagic infarction.

On DWI, the ischemic lesion may be isointense (phase of pseudonormalization) or, less commonly, hyperintense as in the acute phase. Over time, as the ischemic lesion evolves through the phases of cytotoxic edema, vasogenic edema, and tissue necrosis and cavitation, the ADC normalizes (termed "pseudonormalization"); it then becomes elevated in the chronic phase of stroke. This feature makes it possible to distinguish old from new ischemic lesions through calculation of the ADC.

CHRONIC STROKE (OLDER THAN 30 DAYS)

In the chronic stage of stroke, the edema that was present in the subacute phase has resolved. Very late, there may be atrophy and cavity formation. On T2WI and FLAIR sequences, infarcts appear hyperintense. On T1WI, infarcts are hypointense and no longer have contrast enhancement. On DWI they are usually hypointense, except with the "T2 shine through pattern" or if the ADC is elevated.

Wallerian degeneration may be seen as a secondary phenomenon in the white matter tracts. Kuhn and associates[98] used sequential MRI to show wallerian degeneration after cerebral infarction.

Incidental focal hyperintensities in the subcortical white matter on T2WI or FLAIR sequences, a common feature in patients undergoing brain MRI for cerebrovascular or other indications, signify chronic microvascular disease. Pathologic correlations performed by Awad and colleagues[99–102] found these hyperintensities to be associated with advanced age, history of hypertension, and a variety of antopsy findings, including the pathologic changes of arteriosclerosis, dilated perivascular spaces, vascular ectasia, and chronic cerebrovascular disease. These incidental or silent white matter hyperintensities have also been studied extensively by Fazekas and coworkers,[103–108] who confirmed their association with risk factors for cerebrovascular disease. The associations were strongest for age but were strong also for reduced white matter cerebral blood flow, history of hypertension, diabetes, cardiac disease, elevated fibrinogen levels, and reduced levels of total cholesterol and alpha-tocopherol. Such white matter lesions may progress in number and frequency, but their clinical significance in an asymptomatic patient for cognitive decline or risk of stroke, independent of the other coexisting stroke risk factors, is uncertain.

HEMORRHAGE

Intraparenchymal Hemorrhage

The appearance of blood on various MRI sequences depends on the stage of breakdown of the blood products (Table 19.3). The hemoglobin that is present in freshly extravasated blood exists primarily in the form of oxyhemoglobin, which is nonparamagnetic. However, conversion of oxyhemoglobin to deoxyhemoglobin likely begins at the outer rim of the hematoma almost immediately. Deoxyhemoglobin contains four unpaired electrons making it highly paramagnetic. Around day 2 or 3, deoxyhemoglobin is converted to methemoglobin, which initially is formed intracellularly then becomes extracellular as the red blood cells lyse. Around day 7, macrophages and phagocytes begin transforming the methemoglobin to hemosiderin and ferritin.

Although conventional T1WI and T2WI are highly sensitive for the detection of subacute and chronic blood, they are less sensitive to parenchymal hemorrhage less than 6 hours old. Studies now suggest that hyperacute parenchymal blood can be accurately detected using GRE (T2*-weighted) MRI or echo planar imaging (EPI). As already mentioned, EPI has intrinsic susceptibility weighting, so that even an EPI T2WI, such as is used for the b0 images of the diffusion-weighted sequence, is sufficiently susceptibility

Table 19.3   Signal Features of Hyperacute Intracerebral Hemorrhage on Magnetic Resonance Imaging

	Center	Periphery	Surrounding Rim	Acute Evolution
Susceptibility-weighted imaging	Iso/hyperintense, heterogeneous	Hypointense	Hyperintense Hypointense later	Progressive enlargement of hypointense periphery toward the center
T2-weighted imaging	Iso/hyperintense, heterogeneous, larger than on SWI	Hypointense, smaller than on SWI	Hyperintense	Hypointense periphery and outer rim enlarges toward the center
T1-weighted imaging	Iso/hypointense heterogeneous	None	Hypointense	Hypointense rim enlarges
Interpretation	Oxyhemoglobin dominant	Deoxyhemoglobin dominant	Vasogenic edema	Progressive increase in the concentration of deoxyhemoglobin from the periphery toward the center

weighted to have a high sensitivity to blood products. These sequences detect the paramagnetic effects of deoxy-hemoglobin and methemoglobin, which lead to a loss of signal in regions of both acute and chronic blood.

Hyperacute (in the first few hours) hemorrhage has a characteristic appearance on gradient echo (GRE) sequences.[109–112] Typically, the rim of tissue outside the hematoma appears hyperintense, indicative of edema surrounding the mass; the peripheral part of the hematoma is hypointense, signifying deoxyhemoglobin, and the hematoma center is hetergenous with a mixture of hyperintense, hypointense, and isointense signals in the initial hours (Fig. 19–5; see Table 19.3). With time, more of the central hematoma becomes deoxygenated and hypointense. It should be noted that the sequences used to diagnose acute intracerebral hemorrhage would appear normal if the stroke were ischemic; thus the distinction of ischemic stroke from hemorrhage in the setting of a hyperacute stroke syndrome is easily made.

Several case series and now two large multicenter prospective studies suggest that these MRI sequences may, in fact, be as reliable as CT in the identification of acute blood.[109,111,113,114] These findings may now allow MRI to be employed as the sole imaging modality to evaluate patients with acute stroke, including candidates for thrombolytic treatment.

Microbleeds

In addition, GRE sequences have the ability to detect clinically silent prior microbleeds not visualized on CT (Fig. 19–6). MRI evidence of microbleeds is seen in 38% to 66% of patients with primary intracerebral hemorrhages, in 21% to 26% of patients with ischemic stroke, and in 5% to 6% of asymptomatic or healthy elderly individuals.[115–117] In their study of patients with a history of atherosclerosis, Kwa and colleagues[117] found that hemosiderin deposits visualized with MRI were significantly associated with cerebral white matter lesions. Fazekas and associates,[118] performing a histopathologic analysis of small regions of signal loss visualized on GRE MRI sequences, confirmed that these regions signify previous extravasation of blood and are related to bleeding-prone microangiopathy, usually due to hypertension, prior ischemic injury, or amyloid angiopathy.[118,119]

A growing body of data suggests that microbleeds visualized on GRE MRI represent markers of bleeding-prone angiopathy and increased risk of hemorrhagic transformation after antithrombotic and thrombolytic therapy.[115,120–122] If these findings are confirmed, GRE MRI and EPI-SWI sequences may be useful in pretreatment screening of candidates for thrombolytic therapy and in providing information for antithrombotic treatment decisions in all patients with stroke.

Hemorrhagic Transformation

Hemorrhagic transformation of an ischemic infarction is a common occurrence, visualized in 42% or more of patients in pathologic series. Numerous studies have demonstrated that hemorrhagic transformation is much more common in cardioembolic strokes, with estimates ranging from 30% to 74% in CT studies. The frequency of hemorrhagic transformation is also significantly higher in patients treated with thrombolytic trials; rates of asymptomatic transformation ranged from 10.6% to 67.8% in trials of intravenous thrombolytic therapy and 57% in the PROACT II trial of intra-arterial pro-urokinase. Generally, a distinction is

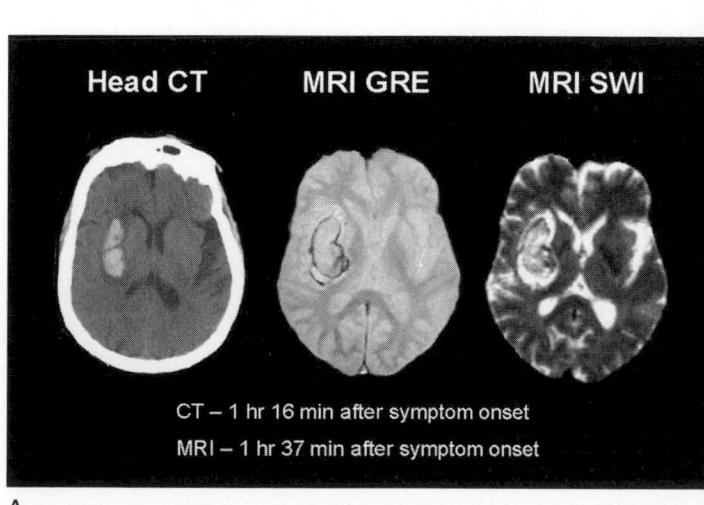

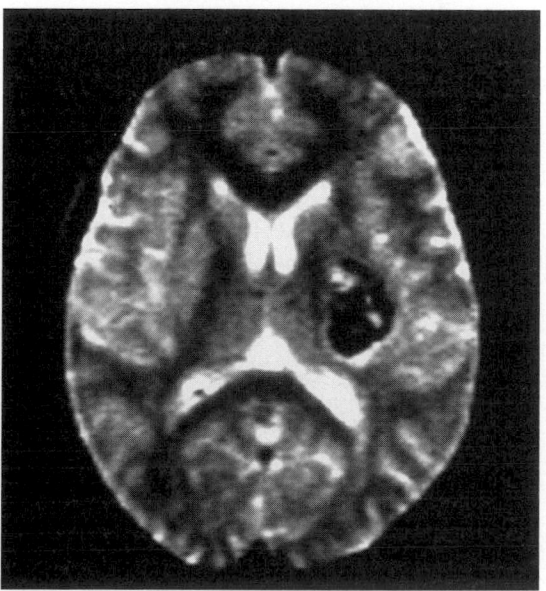

A   B

FIGURE 19–5 *A, An example of an acute intraparenchymal hematoma, less than 2 hours after onset, on computed tomography (CT) as well as gradient-recalled echo (or T2°-weighted) magnetic resonance imaging (GRE MRI) and echo planar, susceptibility MRI (SWI MRI). Note on MRI the appearance of a heterogenous central hypointense periphery of the hematoma, surrounded by the hyperintense rim of edema. B, In a hematoma at a later time, approximately 3 hours from onset in this figure, hypointensity predominates.*

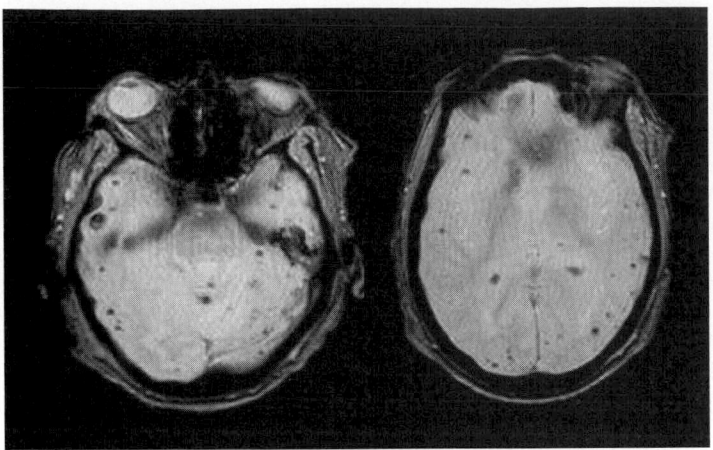

FIGURE 19–6   *Gradient echo magnetic resonance imaging sequence demonstrating multiple scattered old microbleeds (punctate hypointensities) in a patient with cerebral amyloid angiopathy.*

made between parenchymatous hematomas, which are frequently symptomatic, and petechial hemorrhagic transformation, which is generally asymptomatic.

The MR appearance of hemorrhagic transformation of an ischemic infarct is similar to that seen with primary intracerebral hemorrhage. Commonly, gradient echo sequences may demonstrate regions of petechial hemorrhage not visualized with CT or standard MR sequences. Prospective studies employing serial MRI with gradient echo sequences are required to clarify the frequency of these findings in various subtypes of stroke and their role in antithrombotic treatment decisions.

Subarachnoid Hemorrhage

Several studies have explored the clinical utility of MR sequences in patients with subarachnoid hemorrhage. Although standard spin-echo sequences are relatively insensitive to subarachnoid blood, newer sequences, including FLAIR and gradient echo T2°-weighted imaging, have been shown to have high sensitivity, particularly in the subacute phase, when CT findings are often negative.[123–126] Subarachnoid blood appears as a region of high signal intensity relative to normal cerebrospinal fluid on FLAIR sequences (see Fig. 19–1), and as a region of hypointensity on gradient echo images, similar in characteristic to intraparenchymal blood. In one study, gradient echo sequences were shown to be superior to FLAIR sequences, with sensitivities of 94% in the acute phase and 100% in the subacute phase, compared with 81% and 87%, respectively, for FLAIR sequences.[125]

Evaluation of patients with vasospasm is an emerging role for multimodal MRI. Several reports have demonstrated that patients with vasospasm secondary to aneurysmal subarachnoid hemorrhage have a high rate of DWI lesions, often indicative of silent ischemia.[127,128] In studies employing perfusion imaging, these ischemic lesions were associated with regions of hemodynamic compromise associated with angiographic evidence of vessel vasospasm.[129–131]

Subdural and Epidural Hematomas

Subdural hematomas appear as crescent-shaped lesions and epidural hematomas as lentiform lesions adjacent to the brain parenchyma. The MR appearance depends on the age of the hematoma and the sequences acquired. FLAIR sequences may be particularly sensitive for the detection of small subacute subdural hemorrhages that may be difficult to diagnose with CT (see Fig. 19–1). In epidural hematomas, the displaced dura appears as a thin line of low signal intensity between the brain and hematoma. The MR appearance of chronic subdural hematomas may be quite variable.

VASCULAR DISEASE

MRA rivals conventional angiography for the detection of arterial stenoses and occlusions,[132] although there is a tendency on MRA to overestimation of the severity of stenosis because of dephasing of protons caused by turbulent flow or calcifications at the site of the stenosis, and the smaller intracranial vessels are not well visualized. A normal screening MRA is reliable to exclude hemodynamically significant stenoses. False-positive results can occur (1) when the degree of carotid stenosis is overestimated, (2) when the carotid artery is kinked or changes direction abruptly, (3) in the distal carotid artery as it enters the carotid canal because of a susceptibility artifact between vessel and bone, and (4) in the presence of surgical clips. A false-positive occlusion on MRA is usually deducible from the reconstitution of flow distal to the point of signal loss. Sensitivity and specificity of MRA for carotid occlusion have been reported as 100% for most studies.

In general, if MRA shows no stenosis or a stenosis of less than 70%, no further evaluation is necessary. If MRA shows a stenosis of 70% or more, duplex ultrasonography should be done. If findings of the two studies agree, no further evaluation is suggested,[133,134] and appropriate management can be provided. If MRA and duplex ultrasonography findings do not agree, further evaluation with conventional angiography is recommended.

The most promising new approach is contrast-enhanced MRA of the carotid arteries, in which a more rapid MR acquisition (<1 minute) is timed to a bolus injection of contrast agent over a larger field of view. This modality compares favorably with conventional angiography for the diagnosis of carotid stenosis.[135–138] The accuracy of the contrast-enhanced MRA technique for the detection of vascular disease of vertebral artery origins and the aortic arch is being investigated.

The diagnosis of dissection of the internal carotid artery or the vertebral artery can be made with MRI and MRA.[139–142] Findings suggestive of dissection on MRI are (1) increased signal from parts of or the entire vessel wall on axial T1WI (with fat suppression) consistent with hematoma (Fig. 19–7), (2) a border of increased signal surrounding the lumen with luminal narrowing, (3) poor or absence of visualization of the vessel, and (4) significant compromise of the vessel lumen by adjacent abnormal increased signal tissue. If a false lumen with an intimal flap is present, it is best appreciated on T2WI. Vessel abnormalities such as narrowing, aneurysmal dilatation, and a second lumen may be demonstrable by MRA. When a TOF technique is used, MRA may show a normal or simply widened vessel at the site of dissection. This is due to the addition of a signal from the vessel wall because of methemoglobin in the hematoma, and from the high-flow lumen. Contrast-enhanced MRA techniques demonstrate the intimal flap as a linear enhancing structure similar to the vessel wall. False-negative MRI or MRA assessments for dissection occur, and conventional angiography is recommended if there is a high degree of clinical suspicion in a patient with normal MRI or MRA findings.

MRA has a sensitivity of 92% to 95% for the detection of intracranial aneurysms.[143,144] Lesions as small as 2 to 3 mm in diameter have been shown by MRA, and the technique has occasionally demonstrated small aneurysms missed on conventional x-ray angiography.[145] However, aneurysms smaller than 5 mm may be missed on MRA. Slow flow and turbulence within small aneurysms may interfere with their detection in up to 27% of cases, leading to limitation in study interpretation.[146] These problems can be partially overcome through the use of intravenous contrast media. Small aneurysms may be difficult to differentiate from vessel loops because, unlike on x-ray angiography, there is no increase in signal at the point of vessel overlap with a maximal intensity projection algorithm. The use of

MRA as a screen for aneurysms is still controversial.[147,148] If aneurysmal size is the only risk factor for hemorrhage, the insensitivity of MRA to small aneurysms may not be of clinical importance. The accuracy of MRA in detecting small aneurysms is likely to improve as techniques are further refined.

A newer application of vascular imaging with MRI is high spatial resolution multimodal imaging of the carotid plaque to identify the various components, such as lipid deposits, fibrous caps, calcium, and thrombus.[149–151] Although not yet a routine practice, high-resolution carotid plaque imaging appears promising as a way to document decreased lipid content and plaque stabilization after lipid-lowering therapy[152] and to identify a ruptured fibrous cap associated with a recent history of TIA or stroke.[151]

CEREBRAL VENOUS THROMBOSIS

Although diagnosis of cerebral venous thrombosis remains a diagnostically challenging entity, advances in MRI have substantially improved the ability of physicians to perform a rapid, noninvasive, and comprehensive neuroimaging evaluation. Moreover, MRI has provided further insight into the underlying differences in the pathophysiologic processes involved in venous versus arterial infarction. In cerebral venous thrombosis, breakdown of the blood-brain barrier combined with venous congestion leads to a unique combination of coexistent vasogenic and cytotoxic edema that in turn often leads to frank infarction, hemorrhage, or both. Imaging studies are able to visualize venous congestion, venous infarction, and hemorrhage.

Venous hypertension may produce cytotoxic edema, vasogenic edema, or both. These changes may be visualized as hyperintensity on T2WI or FLAIR sequences. If venous hypertension is mild, no signal abnormalities may occur. In patients with superior sagittal sinus thromboses, parasagittal lesions are common and may be bilateral. Transverse sinus thrombosis frequently causes posterior temporal lobe lesions, whereas thrombosis of the deep sinus system often causes bithalamic or subcortical lesions. With administration of a contrast agent, lesion enhancement may appear in a tumor-like pattern. Hemorrhagic transformation of venous infarction occurs frequently and has the typical MR appearance of hemorrhage based on the stage of the blood breakdown product (see earlier discussion of hemorrhage). Vessel occlusion is usually well-demonstrated by MR venography (MRV), making angiography unnecessary in the majority of cases. Thrombosed veins or sinuses may also be visualized on axial gradient echo T2*-weighted sequences with greater conspicuity than on standard T1WI and T2WI.[153] Some studies suggest that the majority of cases can be initially diagnosed by a combination of MRI and MRA or MRV and that MR studies are useful for follow-up.[154]

Reports have begun to elucidate the diffusion-perfusion MR characteristics of venous sinus thrombosis. Abnormal DWI signal intensity may be associated with low ADC values indicative of cytotoxic edema, high ADC values indicative of vasogenic edema, or mixed values indicative of a combination of both vasogenic and cytotoxic edema.[155–157] Consequently, MR lesions caused by venous thrombosis

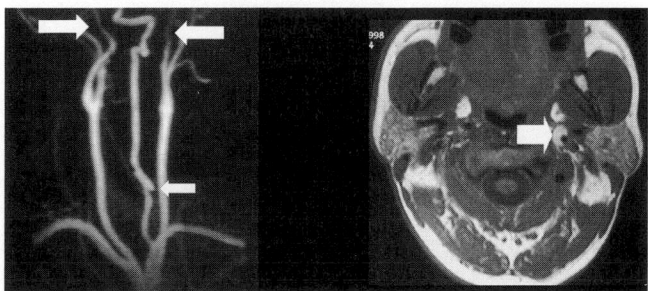

FIGURE 19–7 *Magnetic resonance images from a 48-year-old man with dissections of bilateral carotid and vertebral arteries. Left, Power-injector contrast-enhanced neck magnetic resonance angiogram shows an intimal flap in the left vertebral artery as well as progressive tapering of the distal internal carotid arteries. Right, A T1-weighted axial image through the internal carotid artery illustrates the pathognomonic crescent sign of dissection. In this image, the blood within the vessel wall of the right internal carotid artery appears hyperintense.*

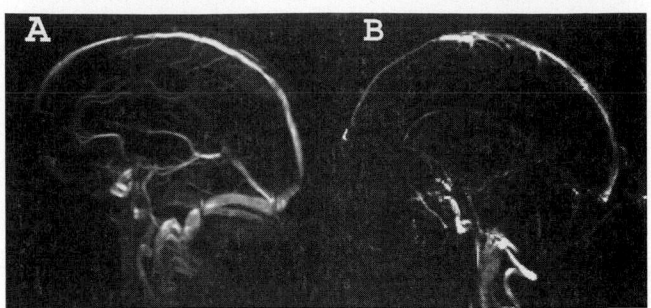

FIGURE 19–8 A, *Normal magnetic resonance venogram of the brain. B, Straight sinus thrombosis. Note the lack of flow signal in the straight sinus, lateral sinus, vein of Galen, and internal cerebral veins.*

Diagnostic Studies

are more frequently reversible than those due to arterial ischemia, likely reflecting the reversibility of vasogenic edema. Several groups have also demonstrated perfusion imaging abnormalities, including increased mean transit time[158] and increased CBV.[159]

MRV has been accepted as the procedure of choice in the diagnosis of sagittal sinus thrombosis.[156,160,161] It is particularly valuable because the clinical diagnosis of sinus venous thrombosis is often occult owing to a wide spectrum of clinical presentations and a highly variable clinical presentation. Direct findings of cerebral thrombosis on MRV include lack of typical high flow signal from a sinus and direct visualization of thrombus on individual frames of the two-dimensional slices (Fig. 19–8). These must be distinguished from an aplastic or hypoplastic sinus and from the appearance of a sinus after recanalization. Signs of infarct, hemorrhage, and intravascular thrombus on other MR pulse sequences may also raise the suspicion of sinus or venous thrombosis.[153]

Problems in interpreting MRV are largely related to slow flow or in-plane flow causing signal loss and therefore mimicking thrombosis. These obstacles can be overcome by using thinner slices on two-dimensional TOF sequences to detect slow flow or choosing a different imaging plane (for example, switching from a coronal to an axial imaging plane). Another potential pitfall is a high signal intensity thrombus resembling flow signal, especially on two-dimensional and three-dimensional TOF sequences. Phase contrast techniques may help distinguish high signal intensity thrombus from flow.

FUNCTIONAL MAGNETIC RESONANCE IMAGING AND RECOVERY

Functional MRI (fMRI) has an important application in the study of the mechanisms of recovery after stroke and has been used predominantly to study motor recovery[162] with the blood oxygenation level dependent (BOLD) technique. The results have largely complemented and confirmed the earlier work using positron emission tomography.[163] In several studies, a hand movement task paradigm has been used. In normal controls, a hand movement task results in contralateral activation of the sensorimotor cortex (SMC) and the supplementary motor area (SMA)

on fMRI. In patients with stroke not only the contralateral SMC and SMA are activated, often to a larger extent than control, but also the SMC ipsilateral to the hand movement (i.e., unaffected hemisphere). These functional changes suggest that plasticity or reorganization of the cortical network for motor control may contribute to adaptations leading to functional recovery of post-stroke hemiparesis and that there is recruitment of preexisting uncrossed motor pathways (normally around 10% to 15%). Near-infrared spectroscopy (NIRS) confirmation of the fMRI findings has been reported.[164]

Using fMRI, Feydy and colleagues[165] have characterized two patterns of cortical reorganization after stroke and its relation to the site of the stroke-induced lesion and the extent of motor recovery. These researchers studied 14 patients with stroke and an affected upper limb longitudinally. Three fMRI sessions were performed over a period of 1 to 6 months after stroke. Upper limb recovery, wallerian degeneration of the pyramidal tract, and responses to transcranial magnetic stimulation were assessed. Feydy and colleagues[165] found two main patterns of cortical reorganization. Pattern 1, identified in 9 patients, was focusing, in which, after initial recruitment of additional ipsilateral and contralateral areas, activation gradually developed toward a pattern of activation restricted to the contralateral sensorimotor cortex. Five patients were found to have pattern 2, persistent recruitment, in which there was an initial and sustained recruitment of ipsilateral activity. Occurrence of recruitment or focusing seemed to depend mainly on whether the primary motor cortex (M1) was lesioned; persistent recruitment was observed in 3 of 4 patients with M1 injury, and focusing was seen in 8 of 10 patients with spared M1. These patterns had no relation to the extent of recovery; in particular, focusing did not imply recovery. However, there was a clear relation between the extent of recovery and the severity of wallerian degeneration. These results suggested that (1) ipsilateral recruitment after stroke corresponds to a compensatory corticocortical process related to the lesion of the contralateral M1 and (2) the process of compensatory recruitment persists if M1 is lesioned but otherwise is transient.[165]

Sensory recovery has also been reported. Carey and associates[166] demonstrated the potential for post-stroke return of activation in regions normally involved in touch discrimination in a serial, whole-brain fMRI study of a patient with marked sensory loss followed by good recovery. They observed a return of activation in ipsilesional primary and bilateral secondary somatosensory cortices at 3 months after stroke that was maintained at 6 months, indicating a reemergence of activation after the interval of somatosensory recovery. There was little evidence of neural plastic changes early after stroke (2 weeks), when sensory loss was severe.

DWI has been used to study wallerian degeneration after stroke, both early[167] and late.[98] Diffusion tensor imaging has the potential to provide additional new insights into white matter tract reorganization after stroke.

SPINAL CORD

When a patient has acute spinal cord symptoms in an emergency setting, structural MRI has an established role in the exclusion of space-occupying lesions, which would require neurosurgical intervention. The high spatial resolution of MRI means that it also allows the detection of many spinal cord infarcts. These lesions are generally rare and have various causes. Weidauer and coworkers[168] have reported on the utility of DWI in spinal cord infarction. Two of their patients presented with anterior spinal artery syndrome caused by infarction of the thoracolumbar spinal cord including the conus medullaris. Although T2-weighted images obtained 4 hours and 28 hours after onset of clinical symptoms showed only slight, unspecific signal changes, DWI showed clear infarction and detected spinal cord ischemia in an early stage, showing signal intensity conversion comparable to that in acute cerebral stroke. Also, Stepper and Lovblad[169] have reported the utility of DWI in the clinical setting of spinal cord infarction.

PREDICTION OF TISSUE AND CLINICAL OUTCOME

Prediction of Tissue Outcome

Multimodality MRI may have a valuable role in the prediction of tissue outcome, which could help identify the tissue destined to become infarcted soonest after stroke onset. The combination of DWI and perfusion imaging allows the identification of four ischemic patterns. In approximately 70% of patients studied within 24 hours of symptom onset, there is a "perfusion-diffusion mismatch," in which the area of DWI abnormality is surrounded by a larger area of hypoperfusion, most commonly measured by the relative MTT perfusion map.[170–177] It has been proposed that tissue that is hypoperfused but has a normal DWI signal may be the tissue that is ischemic but not yet irreversibly injured and is at risk for infarct progression. In other patients, the DWI lesion is larger than the perfusion lesion in approximately 10% (presumed partial or total reperfusion), and the DWI and perfusion lesions are of equivalent size (likely little viable tissue, operationally defined as a completed infarct) in 10% to 15%.

Several studies have demonstrated that baseline MR perfusion lesion volumes correlate well with final infarct volume as well as neurologic and functional outcome—that in fact, they correlate somewhat better than baseline diffusion lesion volumes.[80–82,85] It is speculated that the stronger association is explained by the fact that the perfusion lesion volume identifies all tissue at risk of infarction if vessel recanalization does not occur. Several groups have reported that CBV measures provide the greatest accuracy in predicting final infarct size and clinical outcome.[170–173]

Diffusion-perfusion MR studies have begun to elucidate the evolution of ischemic lesions in humans. It has been suggested that early MR can characterize the ischemic penumbra as regions of perfusion but not diffusion abnormality (diffusion-perfusion mismatch, Plate 19–1, facing page 461). These are regions in which blood flow is reduced but tissue bioenergetic failure, as evidenced by cytotoxic edema, has not yet developed. This hypothesis is supported by studies demonstrating that the natural history of diffusion MR abnormalities is to grow over time as noted previously, particularly in patients studied early after symptom onset.[74,75,78,174] An important finding that

arose from combined diffusion-perfusion studies was that a substantial number of patients still have regions of mismatch up to 24 hours or longer, even though the likelihood of mismatch decreases with time after stroke.[174,175]

Serial MRI studies performed in patients with diffusion-perfusion mismatch have confirmed that infarct growth occurs primarily in patients with large regions of mismatch,[77,82,171,176,177] suggesting gradual failure of the ischemic penumbra within the region of mismatch as it is incorporated into the infarct core. Schellinger and colleagues,[178] studying patients with mismatch and evidence of a vessel occlusion at baseline, found that patients with subsequent early recanalization had substantially smaller final infarct lesions than those without recanalization and the former had a better clinical outcome.

Although mismatch may provide a simple and practical means of identifying the penumbra in acute stroke, it is important to note that prior animal studies and case series in humans undergoing thrombolytic therapy have shown that diffusion abnormalities can be partially reversed with early reperfusion.[179–181] These data suggest that early after ischemia onset, the penumbra likely includes not only regions of diffusion-perfusion mismatch but also portions of the region of diffusion abnormality (see Fig. 19–9).

Efforts are under way to identify thresholds that will distinguish tissue that will proceed to infarction from salvageable, penumbral tissue. Several groups have found that relative ADC values could reliably differentiate regions that would proceed to infarction from those that would not within the initial hypoperfused region.[182] These findings are in accord with those of Schlaug and colleagues,[197] who found ADC values 56.4% of normal in the core, and values 91.3% of normal in the penumbra. However, these findings apply generally to untreated patients or to patients in whom early recanalization does not occur. In patients with early vessel recanalization, ADC decreases may not reliably indicate tissue infarction independent of the duration and severity of ischemia.[183] Thresholds for infarct progression, malignant middle cerebral artery infarct, and risk of hemorrhagic transformation may be identified by quantitative diffusion or perfusion MRI,[184–193] but these thresholds are not absolute thresholds; rather, they depend on the technique of measurement and analysis, the time from onset, the therapeutic intervention, and interactions with other physiologic and clinical variables.[194]

Several prior studies have delineated perfusion thresholds that distinguish benign oligemia from ischemic penumbral tissue by determining values that predict final infarct size in patients not being treated with thrombolysis, in whom the infarct grows to consume the entire penumbra to the benign oligemia border.[187,190,195,196]

A large number of studies have analyzed early MR characteristics in untreated patients with stroke to identify predictors of final infarct volume. These natural history studies generally provide predictive models of tissue outcome, under the assumption that early recanalization does not occur in most patients. Schlaug and colleagues[197] used a logistic regression model to differentiate regions of ultimate infarction from noninfarction on the basis of baseline perfusion measures to operationally define the ischemic penumbra. Other groups have employed gener-

Diagnostic Studies

alized linear model algorithms, multiparametric techniques, and other automated strategies to predict final tissue status. All of these approaches have demonstrated good overall accuracy.[195,198,199]

Several groups have reported that an altered evolution of infarction can be visualized on serial diffusion and perfusion imaging studies in patients undergoing intravenous thrombolytic therapy. Inhibition of lesion growth has been clearly demonstrated in patients experiencing reperfusion compared with those who have persistent perfusion deficits or vessel occlusions.[200,201] In addition, several groups have found regions of higher ADC within the initial ischemic field on follow-up imaging in patients undergoing reperfusion within 36 hours of onset compared with those who did not experience reperfusion, suggesting tissue salvage.[202,203] Further compelling data come from Parsons and colleagues,[203a] who compared MRI signatures in patients treated with intravenous tissue-type plasminogen activator (tPA) within 6 hours of onset and in a group of matched controls. These researchers found a significant decrease in the amount of mismatch tissue proceeding to infarction as well as less infarct expansion in the group undergoing thrombolysis.

These studies suggest that it is feasible and potentially advantageous to use diffusion-perfusion MR to identify patients who would benefit from thrombolytic therapy, employing MRI to characterize the extent of perfusion impairment and the amount of remaining salvageable tissue. Efforts are under way to identify specific MR signatures and criteria to distinguish regions of reversible and irreversible infarction. Kidwell and colleagues[204] used automated image registration techniques to analyze diffusion-perfusion MR data in patients treated with intraarterial thrombolytic therapy.[204] They performed stepwise discriminant analysis using baseline ADC, MTT, rCBV, and rCBF values to identify tissue that was labeled as infarction or normal at day 7. In this preliminary model, baseline diffusion-perfusion MR variables differentiated ultimate tissue infarction from noninfarction to a high degree. There is also a growing body of data suggesting that baseline MRI characteristics may be used to predict risk of hemorrhagic transformation.[193,205] Further characterization of the MR signatures of penumbra, core infarction, and hemorrhage risk may allow extension of the time window for treatment beyond current standards and improve safety, because treatment decisions could be based on individual patient pathophysiology rather than rigid time windows.

In addition to demonstrating lesion evolution through infarct growth in patients with mismatch and a persistent vessel occlusion, serial multimodal MRI studies have provided important additional insights into the evolving pathophysiology of human ischemia, particularly in patients undergoing vessel recanalization. The phenomenon of postischemic hyperperfusion has been demonstrated in approximately half of patients undergoing successful vessel recanalization with intra-arterial thrombolysis.[206] In addition, late secondary ischemic injury, visualized on DWI and ADC maps, has now been demonstrated in humans, as in animal models, after vessel recanalization.[207] These findings may become important targets for neuroprotective therapy in the future.

Table 19.4   Three-Item Scale for the Early Prediction of Stroke Recovery*

Factor		Assigned Points
Volume of lesion on diffusion-weighted imaging (DWI) (mL)	≤14.1	1
	>14.1	0
National Institutes of Health Stroke Scale (NIHSS) score	≤3	4
	4–15	2
	>15	0
Time from onset (hr)	≤3	0
	3 < time ≤ 6	1
	>6	2
Total score (sum of assigned points)		0–7

*The physician should identify the NIHSS score for the patient, the time in hours from onset to magnetic resonance imaging (MRI) and the DWI lesion volume. These values should be matched with the assigned points in each category. The three sets of points should then be added to give a total score. A total score of 0–2 is associated with a low (7%) probability of stroke recovery (defined as a Barthel score ≥90 at 3 months); a total score of 3–4 with an intermediate (53%) probability of recovery; and a total score of 5–7 with a high (87%) probability of recovery at 3 months.

Early Prediction of Stroke Recovery

DWI lesion volume correlates with acute stroke severity as measured by the National Institutes of Health Stroke Scale (NIHSS) score.[80] Further, DWI lesion size, clinical stroke severity, and a number of other clinical factors each provides prognostic information in ischemic stroke. Baird and coworkers[86] have reported that the combination of clinical factors (NIHSS score and time in hours from onset to MRI evaluation) and DWI factors (DWI lesion volume) allowed improved prediction of stroke recovery as early as 3 to 6 hours after onset. The findings were externally validated in an independent series of patients with high sensitivity and specificity. These investigators developed a three-item scale for the early prediction of stroke recovery, in which a total score of 5 to 7 indicates a high likelihood of recovery (Table 19.4).[86]

References

1. Bydder GM, Steiner RE, Young IR, et al: Clinical NMR imaging of the brain: 140 cases. AJR Am J Roentgenol 139:215–236, 1982.
2. Brant-Zawadzki M, Davis PL, Crooks LE, et al: NMR demonstration of cerebral abnormalities: Comparison with CT. AJR Am J Roentgenol 140:847–854, 1983.
3. Buonanno FS, Kistler JP, DeWitt LD, et al: Proton (1H) nuclear magnetic resonance (NMR) imaging in stroke syndromes. Neurol Clin 1:243–262, 1983.
4. Bydder GM, Steiner RE, Thomas DJ, et al. Nuclear magnetic resonance imaging of the posterior fossa: 50 cases. Clin Radiol 34:173–188, 1983.
5. Ramadan NM, Deveshwar R, Levine SR: Magnetic resonance and clinical cerebrovascular disease: An update. Stroke 20:1279–1283, 1989.
6. Bryan RN, Levy LM, Whitlow WD, et al: Diagnosis of acute cerebral infarction: Comparison of CT and MR imaging. AJNR Am J Neuroradiol 12:611–620, 1991.
7. Yuh WT, Crain MR, Loes DJ, et al: MR imaging of cerebral ischemia: Findings in the first 24 hours. AJNR Am J Neuroradiol 12:621–629, 1991.

8. Amarenco P, Kase CS, Rosengart A, et al: Very small (border zone) cerebellar infarcts: Distribution, causes, mechanisms and clinical features. Brain 116:161–186, 1993.
9. Le Bihan D, Breton E, Lallemand D, et al: MR imaging of intravoxel incoherent motions: Application to diffusion and perfusion in neurologic disorders. Radiology 161:401–417, 1986.
10. Moseley ME, Kucharczyk J, Mintorovitch J, et al: Diffusion-weighted MR imaging of acute stroke: Correlation with T2-weighted and magnetic susceptibility-enhanced MR imaging in cats. AJNR Am J Neuroradiol 11:423–429, 1990.
11. Belliveau JW, Rosen BR, Kantor HL, et al: Functional cerebral imaging by susceptibility-contrast NMR. Magn Reson Med 14:538–546, 1990.
12. Rosen BR, Belliveau JW, Buchbinder BR, et al: Contrast agents and cerebral hemodynamics. Magn Reson Med 19:285–292, 1991.
13. Warach S, Chien D, Li W, et al: Fast magnetic resonance diffusion-weighted imaging of acute human stroke. Neurology 42:1717–1723, 1992.
14. Warach S, Li W, Ronthal M, Edelman RR: Acute cerebral ischemia: Evaluation with dynamic contrast-enhanced MR imaging and MR angiography. Radiology 182:41–47, 1992.
15. Stehling MK, Turner R, Mansfield P: Echo-planar imaging: Magnetic resonance imaging in a fraction of a second. Science 254:43–50, 1991.
16. Davis S, Fisher M, Warach S (eds): Magnetic Resonance Imaging in Stroke. Cambridge, UK, Cambridge University Press, 2003.
17. Edelman RR, Hesselink JR, Zlatkin MB (eds): Clinical Magnetic Resonance Imaging, 2nd ed. Philadelphia, WB Saunders, 1996.
18. Noguchi K, Ogawa T, Inugami A, et al: MR of acute subarachnoid hemorrhage: A preliminary report of fluid-attenuated inversion-recovery pulse sequences. AJNR Am J Neuroradiol 15:1940–1943, 1994.
19. Toyoda K, Ida M, Fukuda K: Fluid-attenuated inversion recovery intraarterial signal: An early sign of hyperacute cerebral ischemia. AJNR Am J Neuroradiol 22:1021–1209, 2001.
20. Kamran S, Bates V, Bakshi R, et al: Significance of hyperintense vessels on FLAIR MRI in acute stroke. Neurology 55:265–269, 2000.
21. Warach S, Gaa J, Siewert B, et al: Acute human stroke studied by whole brain echo planar diffusion-weighted magnetic resonance imaging. Ann Neurol 37:231–241, 1995.
22. Basser PJ, Mattiello J, LeBihan D: Estimation of the effective self-diffusion tensor from the NMR spin echo. J Magn Reson B 103:247–254, 1994.
23. Pierpaoli C, Jezzard P, Basser PJ, et al: Diffusion tensor MR imaging of the human brain. Radiology 201:637–648, 1996.
24. Lansberg MG, Thijs VN, O'Brien MW, et al: Evolution of apparent diffusion coefficient, diffusion-weighted, and T2-weighted signal intensity of acute stroke. AJNR Am J Neuroradiol 22:637–644, 2001.
25. Latour LL, Warach S: Cerebral spinal fluid contamination of the measurement of the apparent diffusion coefficient of water in acute stroke. Magn Reson Med 48:478–486, 2002.
26. Schaefer PW: Diffusion-weighted imaging as a problem-solving tool in the evaluation of patients with acute strokelike syndromes. Top Magn Reson Imaging 11:300–309, 2000.
27. Rempp KA, Brix G, Wenz F, et al: Quantification of regional cerebral blood flow and volume with dynamic susceptibility contrast-enhanced MR imaging. Radiology 193:637–641, 1994.
28. Smith AM, Grandin CB, Duprez T, et al: Whole brain quantitative CBF, CBV, and MTT measurements using MRI bolus tracking: Implementation and application to data acquired from hyperacute stroke patients. J Magn Reson Imaging 12:400–410, 2000.
29. Smith AM, Grandin CB, Duprez T, et al: Whole brain quantitative CBF and CBV measurements using MRI bolus tracking: Comparison of methodologies. Magn Reson Med 43:559–564, 2000.
30. Ostergaard L, Sorensen AG, Kwong KK, et al: High resolution measurement of cerebral blood flow using intravascular tracer bolus passages. Part II: Experimental comparison and preliminary results. Magn Reson Med 36:726–736, 1996.
31. Ostergaard L, Johannsen P, Host-Poulsen P, et al: Cerebral blood flow measurements by magnetic resonance imaging bolus tracking: Comparison with [(15)O]H2O positron emission tomography in humans. J Cereb Blood Flow Metab 18:935–940, 1998.
32. Roberts DA, Detre JA, Bolinger L, et al: Quantitative magnetic resonance imaging of human brain perfusion at 1.5 T using steady-state inversion of arterial water. Proc Natl Acad Sci U S A 91:33–37, 1994.
33. Kim SG, Tsekos NV, Ashe J: Multi-slice perfusion-based functional MRI using the FLAIR technique: Comparison of CBF and BOLD effects. NMR Biomed 10:191–196, 1997.
34. Edelman RR, Siewert B, Darby DG, et al: Qualitative mapping of cerebral blood flow and functional localization with echo-planar MR imaging and signal targeting with alternating radio frequency. Radiology 192:513–520, 1994.
35. Detre JA, Alsop DC: Perfusion magnetic resonance imaging with continuous arterial spin labeling: Methods and clinical applications in the central nervous system. Eur J Radiol 30:115–124, 1999.
36. Siewert B, Schlaug G, Edelman RR, Warach S: Comparison of EPISTAR and T2*-weighted gadolinium-enhanced perfusion imaging in patients with acute cerebral ischemia. Neurology 48:673–679, 1997.
37. Wong EC, Buxton RB, Frank LR: Quantitative perfusion imaging using arterial spin labeling. Neuroimaging Clin North Am 9:333–342, 1999.
38. Alsop DC, Detre JA: Multisection cerebral blood flow: MR imaging with continuous arterial spin labeling. Radiology 208:410–416, 1998.
39. Fazekas F, Fazekas G, Schmidt R, et al: Magnetic resonance imaging correlates of transient cerebral ischemic attacks. Stroke 27:607–611, 1996.
40. Bhadelia RA, Anderson M, Polak JF, et al: Prevalence and associations of MRI-demonstrated brain infarcts in elderly subjects with a history of transient ischemic attack. The Cardiovascular Health Study. Stroke 30:383–388, 1999.
41. Kimura K, Minematsu K, Wada K, et al: Lesions visualized by contrast-enhanced magnetic resonance imaging in transient ischemic attacks. J Neurol Sci 173:103–108, 2000.
42. Awad I, Modic M, Little JR, et al: Focal parenchymal lesions in transient ischemic attacks: Correlation of computed tomography and magnetic resonance imaging. Stroke 17:399–403, 1986.
42a. Walters RJ, Holmes PA, Thomas PJ: Silent cerebral ischemic lesions and atrophy in patients with apparently transient cerebral ischemic attacks. Cerebrovasc Dis 10(Suppl 4):12–13, 2000.
43. Kidwell CS, Alger JR, Di Salle F, et al: Diffusion MRI in patients with transient ischemic attacks. Stroke 30:1174–1180, 1999.
44. Engelter ST, Provenzale JM, Petrella JR, Alberts MJ: Diffusion MR imaging and transient ischemic attacks. Stroke 30:2762–2763, 1999.
45. Ay H, Buonanno FS, Schaefer PW, et al: Clinical and diffusion-weighted imaging characteristics of an identifiable subset of TIA patients with acute infarction [abstract]. Stroke 30:235A, 1999.
46. Takayama H, Mihara B, Kobayashi M, et al: [Usefulness of diffusion-weighted MRI in the diagnosis of transient ischemic attacks]. No To Shinkei 52:919–923, 2000.
47. Bisschops RHC, Kappelle LJ, Mali W, van der Grond J: Hemodynamic and metabolic changes in transient ischemic attack patients. Stroke 33:110–115, 2001.
48. Lecouvet FE, Duprez TP, Raymackers JM, et al: Resolution of early diffusion-weighted and FLAIR MRI abnormalities in a patient with TIA. Neurology 52:1085–1087, 1999.
49. Neumann-Haefelin T, Wittsack HJ, Wenserski F, et al: Diffusion- and perfusion-weighted MRI in a patient with a prolonged reversible ischaemic neurological deficit. Neuroradiology 42:444–447, 2000.
50. Ide C, De Coene B, Trigaux JP, et al: Discrepancy between diffusion and perfusion imaging in a patient with transient ischaemic attack. J Neuroradiol 28:118–122, 2001.
51. Laloux P, Jamart J, Meurisse H, et al: Persisting perfusion defect in transient ischemic attacks: A new clinically useful subgroup? Stroke 27:425–430, 1996.
52. You DL, Shieh FY, Tzen KY, et al: Cerebral perfusion SPECT in transient ischemic attack. Eur J Radiol 34:48–51, 2000.
53. Kidwell CS, Saver JL: Head CT and MRI findings in patients with transient ischemic attacks. In Chaturvedi S, Levine S (eds): Transient Ischemic Attacks. Armonk, NY, Futura Publishing, In Press.
54. Saver JL, Kidwell CS: Magnetic resonance imaging in transient ischemic attacks: Clinical utility and insights into pathophysiology. In Davis SA, Fisher M, Warach S (eds): Magnetic Resonance Imaging in Cerebrovascular Disease. New York, Cambridge University Press, In Press.
55. Mohr JP, Biller J, Hilal SK, et al: Magnetic resonance versus computed tomographic imaging in acute stroke. Stroke 26:807–812, 1995.

56. Maeda M, Yamamoto T, Daimon S, et al: Arterial hyperintensity on fast fluid-attenuated inversion recovery images: A subtle finding for hyperacute stroke undetected by diffusion-weighted MR imaging. AJNR Am J Neuroradiol 22:632–636, 2001.

57. Koga M, Kimura K, Minematsu K, Yamaguchi T: Hyperintense MCA branch sign on FLAIR-MRI. J Clin Neurosci 9:187–189, 2002.

58. Flacke S, Urbach H, Keller E, et al: Middle cerebral artery (MCA) susceptibility sign at susceptibility-based perfusion MR imaging: Clinical importance and comparison with hyperdense MCA sign at CT. Radiology 215:476–482, 2000.

59. Chalela JA, Haymore JB, Ezzeddine MA, et al: The hypointense MCA sign. Neurology 58:1470, 2002.

60. Baird AE, Warach S: Magnetic resonance imaging of acute stroke. J Cereb Blood Flow Metab 18:583–609, 1998.

61. Schlaug G, Siewert B, Benfield A, et al: Time course of the apparent diffusion coefficient (ADC) abnormality in human stroke. Neurology 49:113–119, 1997.

62. Fiebach JB, Jansen O, Schellinger PD, et al: Serial analysis of the apparent diffusion coefficient time course in human stroke. Neuroradiology 44:294–298, 2002.

63. Lansberg MG, Thijs VN, O'Brien MW, et al: Evolution of apparent diffusion coefficient, diffusion-weighted, and T2-weighted signal intensity of acute stroke. AJNR Am J Neuroradiol 22:637–644, 2001.

64. Nagesh V, Welch KM, Windham JP, et al: Time course of ADC changes in ischemic stroke: Beyond the human eye! Stroke 29:1778–1782, 1998.

65. Ay H, Buonanno FS, Rordorf G, et al: Normal diffusion-weighted MRI during stroke-like deficits. Neurology 52:1784–1792, 1999.

66. Lövblad KO, Laubach HJ, Baird AE, et al: Clinical experience with diffusion-weighted MR in patients with acute stroke. AJNR Am J Neuroradiol 19:1061–1066, 1998.

67. van Everdingen KJ, van der Grond J, Kappelle LJ, et al: Diffusion-weighted magnetic resonance imaging in acute stroke. Stroke 29:1783–1790, 1998.

68. Gonzalez RG, Schaefer PW, Buonanno FS, et al: Diffusion-weighted MR imaging: Diagnostic accuracy in patients imaged within 6 hours of stroke symptom onset. Radiology 210:155–162, 1999.

69. Mullins ME, Schaefer PW, Sorensen AG, et al: CT and conventional and diffusion-weighted MR imaging in acute stroke: Study in 691 patients at presentation to the emergency department. Radiology 224:353–360, 2002.

70. Perkins CJ, Kahya E, Roque CT, et al: Fluid-attenuated inversion recovery and diffusion- and perfusion-weighted MRI abnormalities in 117 consecutive patients with stroke symptoms. Stroke 32:2774–2781, 2001.

71. Lansberg MG, Albers GW, Beaulieu C, Marks MP: Comparison of diffusion-weighted MRI and CT in acute stroke. Neurology 54:1557–1561, 2000.

72. Barber PA, Darby DG, Desmond PM, et al: Identification of major ischemic change: Diffusion-weighted imaging versus computed tomography. Stroke 30:2059–2065, 1999.

73. Kelly PJ, Hedley-Whyte ET, Primavera J, et al: Diffusion MRI in ischemic stroke compared to pathologically verified infarction. Neurology 56:914–920, 2001.

74. Warach S, Pettigrew LC, Dashe JF, et al: Effect of citicoline on ischemic lesions as measured by diffusion- weighted magnetic resonance imaging: Citicoline 010 Investigators. Ann Neurol 48: 713-7-22, 2000.

75. Baird AE, Benfield A, Schlaug G, et al: Enlargement of human cerebral ischemic lesion volumes measured by diffusion-weighted magnetic resonance imaging [see comments]. Ann Neurol 41:581–589, 1997.

76. Lansberg MG, O'Brien MW, Tong DC, et al: Evolution of cerebral infarct volume assessed by diffusion-weighted magnetic resonance imaging. Arch Neurol 58:613–617, 2001.

77. Beaulieu C, de Crespigny A, Tong DC, et al: Longitudinal magnetic resonance imaging study of perfusion and diffusion in stroke: Evolution of lesion volume and correlation with clinical outcome. Ann Neurol 46:568–578, 1999.

78. Schwamm LH, Koroshetz WJ, Sorensen AG, et al: Time course of lesion development in patients with acute stroke: Serial diffusion- and hemodynamic-weighted magnetic resonance imaging. Stroke 29:2268–2276, 1998.

79. Warach S, Dashe JF, Edelman RR: Clinical outcome in ischemic stroke predicted by early diffusion-weighted and perfusion magnetic resonance imaging: A preliminary analysis. J Cereb Blood Flow Metab 16:53–59, 1996.

80. Lovblad KO, Baird AE, Schlaug G, et al: Ischemic lesion volumes in acute stroke by diffusion-weighted magnetic resonance imaging correlate with clinical outcome. Ann Neurol 42:164–170, 1997.

81. Tong DC, Yenari MA, Albers GW, et al: Correlation of perfusion- and diffusion-weighted MRI with NIHSS score in acute (<6.5 hour) ischemic stroke. Neurology 50:864–870, 1998.

82. Barber PA, Darby DG, Desmond PM, et al: Prediction of stroke outcome with echoplanar perfusion- and diffusion-weighted MRI. Neurology 51:418–426, 1998.

83. Thijs VN, Adami A, Neumann-Haefelin T, et al: Clinical and radiological correlates of reduced cerebral blood flow measured using magnetic resonance imaging.PG 233–8. Arch Neurol. 59:233–238, 2002.

84. Thijs VN, Lansberg MG, Beaulieu C, et al: Is early ischemic lesion volume on diffusion-weighted imaging an independent predictor of stroke outcome? A multivariable analysis. Stroke 31:2596–2602, 2000.

85. Baird AE, Lovblad KO, Dashe JF, et al: Clinical correlations of diffusion and perfusion lesion volumes in acute ischemic stroke. Cerebrovasc Dis 10:441–448, 2000.

86. Baird AE, Dambrosia J, Janket S, et al: A three-item scale for the early prediction of stroke recovery. Lancet 357:2095–2099, 2001.

87. Linfante I, Llinas RH, Schlaug G, et al: Diffusion-weighted imaging and National Institutes of Health Stroke Scale in the acute phase of posterior-circulation stroke. Arch Neurol 58:621–628, 2001.

88. Lutsep HL, Albers GW, DeCrespigny A, et al: Clinical utility of diffusion-weighted magnetic resonance imaging in the assessment of ischemic stroke. Ann Neurol 41:574–580, 1997.

89. Lee LJ, Kidwell CS, Alger J, et al: Impact on stroke subtype diagnosis of early diffusion-weighted magnetic resonance imaging and magnetic resonance angiography. Stroke 31:1081–1089, 2000.

90. Fitzek C, Tintera J, Müller-Forell W, et al: Differentiation of recent and old cerebral infarcts by diffusion-weighted MRI. Neuroradiology 40:778–782, 1998.

91. Schonewille WJ, Tuhrim S, Singer MB, Atlas SW: Diffusion-weighted MRI in acute lacunar syndromes: A clinical-radiological correlation study. Stroke 30:2066–2069, 1999.

92. Ostergaard L, Johannsen P, Høst-Poulsen P, et al: Cerebral blood flow measurements by magnetic resonance imaging bolus tracking: Comparison with [(15)O]H2O positron emission tomography in humans. J Cereb Blood Flow Metab 18:935–940, 1998.

93. Ostergaard L, Sorensen AG, Kwong KK, et al: High resolution measurement of cerebral blood flow using intravascular tracer bolus passages. Part II: Experimental comparison and preliminary results. Magn Res Med 36:726–736, 1996.

94. Ostergaard L, Weisskoff RM, Chesler DA, et al: High resolution measurement of cerebral blood flow using intravascular tracer bolus passages. Part I: Mathematical approach and statistical analysis. Magn Res Med 36:715–725, 1996.

95. Smith AM, Grandin CB, Duprez T, et al: Whole brain quantitative CBF, CBV, and MTT measurements using MRI bolus tracking: Implementation and application to data acquired from hyperacute stroke patients. J Magn Reson Imaging 12:400–410, 2000.

96. Baird AE, Lovblad KO, Schlaug G, et al: Multiple acute stroke syndrome: Marker of embolic disease? Neurology 54:674–678, 2000.

97. Crain MR, Yuh WT, Greene GM, et al: Cerebral ischemia: Evaluation with contrast-enhanced MR imaging. AJNR Am J Neuroradiol 12:631–639, 1991.

98. Kuhn MJ, Mikulis DJ, Ayoub DM, et al: Wallerian degeneration after cerebral infarction: Evaluation with sequential MR imaging. Radiology 172:179–182, 1989.

99. Awad IA, Johnson PC, Spetzler RF, Hodak JA: Incidental subcortical lesions identified on magnetic resonance imaging in the elderly. II: Postmortem pathological correlations. Stroke 17:1090–1097, 1986.

100. Awad IA, Spetzler RF, Hodak JA, et al: Incidental subcortical lesions identified on magnetic resonance imaging in the elderly. I: Correlation with age and cerebrovascular risk factors. Stroke 17:1084–1089, 1986.

101. Awad IA, Spetzler RF, Hodak JA, et al: Incidental lesions noted on magnetic resonance imaging of the brain: Prevalence and clinical significance in various age groups. Neurosurgery 20:222–227, 1987.

Diagnostic Studies

102. Awad IA, Masaryk T, Magdinec M: Pathogenesis of subcortical hyperintense lesions on magnetic resonance imaging of the brain: Observations in patients undergoing controlled therapeutic internal carotid artery occlusion. Stroke 24:1339–1346, 1993.

103. Fazekas F, Kleinert R, Offenbacher H, et al: The morphologic correlate of incidental punctate white matter hyperintensities on MR images. AJNR Am J Neuroradiol 12:915–921, 1991.

104. Schmidt R, Fazekas F, Kleinert G, et al: Magnetic resonance imaging signal hyperintensities in the deep and subcortical white matter: A comparative study between stroke patients and normal volunteers. Arch Neurol 49:825–827, 1992.

105. Schmidt R, Fazekas F, Hayn M, et al: Risk factors for microangiopathy-related cerebral damage in the Austrian stroke prevention study. J Neurol Sci 152:15–21, 1997.

106. Schmidt R, Schmidt H, Fazekas F, et al: Apolipoprotein E polymorphism and silent microangiopathy-related cerebral damage: Results of the Austrian Stroke Prevention Study. Stroke 28:951–956, 1997.

107. Schmidt R, Fazekas F, Kapeller P, et al: MRI white matter hyperintensities: Three-year follow-up of the Austrian Stroke Prevention Study. Neurology 53:132–139, 1999.

108. Fazekas F, Niederkorn K, Schmidt R, et al: White matter signal abnormalities in normal individuals: Correlation with carotid ultrasonography, cerebral blood flow measurements, and cerebrovascular risk factors. Stroke 19:1285–1288, 1988.

109. Patel MR, Edelman RR, Warach S: Detection of hyperacute primary intraparenchymal hemorrhage by magnetic resonance imaging. Stroke 27:2321–2324, 1996.

110. Schellinger PD, Jansen O, Fiebach JB, et al: A standardized MRI stroke protocol: Comparison with CT in hyperacute intracerebral hemorrhage. Stroke 30:765–768, 1999.

111. Linfante I, Llinas RH, Caplan LR, Warach S: MRI features of intracerebral hemorrhage within 2 hours from symptom onset. Stroke 30:2263–2267, 1999.

112. Kidwell CS, Saver JL, Mattiello J, et al: Diffusion-perfusion MR evaluation of perihematomal injury in hyperacute intracerebral hemorrhage. Neurology 57:1611–1617, 2001.

113. Kidwell CS, Chalela JA, Saver JL, et al: Hemorrhage early MRI evaluation (HEME) study: Preliminary results of a multicenter trial of neuroimaging in patients with acute stroke symptoms within 6 hours of onset. Stroke 34:239(Abstract), 2003.

114. Schellinger PD, Fiebach JB, Gass A, et al: Accuracy of stroke MRI in hyperacute intracerebral hemorrhage < 6 hours: A prospective standardized blinded multicenter study. Stroke In Press.

115. Roob G, Lechner A, Schmidt R, et al: Frequency and location of microbleeds in patients with primary intracerebral hemorrhage. Stroke 31:2665–2669, 2000.

116. Roob G, Schmidt R, Kapeller P, et al: MRI evidence of past cerebral microbleeds in a healthy elderly population. Neurology 52:991–994, 1999.

117. Kwa VI, Franke CL, Verbeeten B Jr, Stam J: Silent intracerebral microhemorrhages in patients with ischemic stroke. Amsterdam Vascular Medicine Group. Ann Neurol 44:372–377, 1998.

118. Fazekas F, Kleinert R, Roob G, et al: Histopathologic analysis of foci of signal loss on gradient-echo T2°-weighted MR images in patients with spontaneous intracerebral hemorrhage: Evidence of microangiopathy-related microbleeds. AJNR Am J Neuroradiol 20:637–642, 1999.

119. Greenberg SM, O'Donnell HC, Schaefer PW, Kraft E: MRI detection of new hemorrhages: Potential marker of progression in cerebral amyloid angiopathy. Neurology 53:1135–1138, 1999.

120. Kidwell CS, Saver JL, Villablanca JP, et al: Magnetic resonance imaging detection of microbleeds before thrombolysis: An emerging application. Stroke 33:95–98, 2002.

121. Coutts S, Frayne R, Sevick R, Demchuk A: Microbleeding on MRI as a marker for hemorrhage after stroke thrombolysis. Stroke 33:1457–1458, 2002.

122. Nighoghossian N, Hermier M, Adeleine P, et al: Old microbleeds are a potential risk factor for cerebral bleeding after ischemic stroke: A gradient-echo T2°-weighted brain MRI study. Stroke 33:735–742, 2002.

123. Noguchi K, Ogawa T, Inugami A, et al: MRI of acute cerebral infarction: A comparison of FLAIR and T2-weighted fast spin-echo imaging. Neuroradiology 39:406–410, 1997.

124. Singer MB, Atlas SW, Drayer BP: Subarachnoid space disease: Diagnosis with fluid-attenuated inversion-recovery MR imaging and comparison with gadolinium-enhanced spin-echo MR imaging—blinded reader study. Radiology 208:417–422, 1998.

125. Mitchell P, Wilkinson ID, Hoggard N, et al: Detection of subarachnoid haemorrhage with magnetic resonance imaging. J Neurol Neurosurg Psychiatry 70:205–211, 2001.

126. Wiesmann M, Mayer TE, Yousry I, et al: Detection of hyperacute subarachnoid hemorrhage of the brain by using magnetic resonance imaging. J Neurosurg 96:684–689, 2002.

127. Condette-Auliac S, Bracard S, Anxionnat R, et al: Vasospasm after subarachnoid hemorrhage: Interest in diffusion-weighted MR imaging. Stroke 32:1818–1824, 2001.

128. Hadeishi H, Suzuki A, Yasui N, et al: Diffusion-weighted magnetic resonance imaging in patients with subarachnoid hemorrhage. Neurosurgery 50:741–774; discussion 747–748, 2002.

129. Rordorf G, Koroshetz WJ, Copen WA, et al: Diffusion- and perfusion-weighted imaging in vasospasm after subarachnoid hemorrhage. Stroke 30:599–605, 1999.

130. Shimoda M, Takeuchi M, Tominaga J, et al: Asymptomatic versus symptomatic infarcts from vasospasm in patients with subarachnoid hemorrhage: Serial magnetic resonance imaging. Neurosurgery 49:1341–1348; discussion 1348–1450, 2001.

131. Griffiths PD, Wilkinson ID, Mitchell P, et al: Multimodality MR imaging depiction of hemodynamic changes and cerebral ischemia in subarachnoid hemorrhage. AJNR Am J Neuroradiol 22:1690–1697, 2001.

132. Siewert B, Patel MR, Warach S: Magnetic resonance angiography. Neurologist 1:167–184, 1995.

133. Anderson CM, Saloner D, Lee RE, et al: Assessment of carotid artery stenosis by MR angiography: Comparison with x-ray angiography and color-coded Doppler ultrasound. AJNR Am J Neuroradiol 13:989–1003; discussion 1005–1008, 1992.

134. Long A, Lepoutre A, Corbillon E, Branchereau A: Critical review of non- or minimally invasive methods (duplex ultrasonography, MR- and CT-angiography) for evaluating stenosis of the proximal internal carotid artery. Eur J Vasc Endovasc Surg 24:43–52, 2002.

135. Huston J 3rd, Fain SB, Wald JT, et al: Carotid artery: Elliptic centric contrast-enhanced MR angiography compared with conventional angiography. Radiology 218:138–143, 2001.

136. Sundgren PC, Sunden P, Lindgren A, et al: Carotid artery stenosis: Contrast-enhanced MR angiography with two different scan times compared with digital subtraction angiography. Neuroradiology 44:592–599, 2002.

137. Remonda L, Senn P, Barth A, et al: Contrast-enhanced 3D MR angiography of the carotid artery: Comparison with conventional digital subtraction angiography. AJNR Am J Neuroradiol 23:213–219, 2002.

138. Randoux B, Marro B, Koskas F, et al: Carotid artery stenosis: Prospective comparison of CT, three-dimensional gadolinium-enhanced MR, and conventional angiography. Radiology 220:179–185, 2001.

139. Sue DE, Brant-Zawadzki MN, Chance J: Dissection of cranial arteries in the neck: Correlation of MRI and arteriography. Neuroradiology 34:273–278, 1992.

140. Provenzale JM, Barboriak DP, Taveras JM: Exercise-related dissection of craniocervical arteries: CT, MR, and angiographic findings. J Comput Assist Tomogr 19:268–276, 1995.

141. Rother J, Schwartz A, Rautenberg W, Hennerici M: Magnetic resonance angiography of spontaneous vertebral artery dissection suspected on Doppler ultrasonography. J Neurol 242:430–436, 1995.

142. Stringaris K, Liberopoulos K, Giaka E, et al: Three-dimensional time-of-flight MR angiography and MR imaging versus conventional angiography in carotid artery dissections. Int Angiol 15:20–25, 1996.

143. Ross JS, Masaryk TJ, Modic MT, et al: Intracranial aneurysms: Evaluation by MR angiography. AJNR Am J Neuroradiol 11:449–455, 1990.

144. Huston J 3rd, Nichols DA, Luetmer PH, et al: Blinded prospective evaluation of sensitivity of MR angiography to known intracranial aneurysms: Importance of aneurysm size. AJNR Am J Neuroradiol 15:1607–1614, 1994.

145. Curnes JT, Shogry ME, Clark DC, Elsner HJ: MR angiographic demonstration of an intracranial aneurysm not seen on conventional angiography. AJNR Am J Neuroradiol 14:971–973, 1993.

146. Schuierer G, Huk WJ, Laub G: Magnetic resonance angiography of intracranial aneurysms: Comparison with intra-arterial digital subtraction angiography. Neuroradiology 35:50–54, 1992.

147. Ronkainen A, Puranen MI, Hernesniemi JA, et al: Intracranial aneurysms: MR angiographic screening in 400 asymptomatic individuals with increased familial risk. Radiology 195:35–40, 1995.

Diagnostic Studies

148. Raaymakers TW, Buys PC, Verbeeten B Jr, et al: MR angiography as a screening tool for intracranial aneurysms: Feasibility, test characteristics, and interobserver agreement. AJR Am J Roentgenol 173:1469–1475, 1999.

149. Fayad ZA, Fuster V: Clinical imaging of the high-risk or vulnerable atherosclerotic plaque. Circ Res 89:305–316, 2001.

150. Yuan C, Mitsumori LM, Beach KW, Maravilla KR: Carotid atherosclerotic plaque: Noninvasive MR characterization and identification of vulnerable lesions. Radiology 221:285–299, 2001.

151. Yuan C, Zhang SX, Polissar NL, et al: Identification of fibrous cap rupture with magnetic resonance imaging is highly associated with recent transient ischemic attack or stroke. Circulation 105:181–185, 2002.

152. Zhao XQ, Yuan C, Hatsukami TS, et al: Effects of prolonged intensive lipid-lowering therapy on the characteristics of carotid atherosclerotic plaques in vivo by MRI: A case-control study. Arterioscler Thromb Vasc Biol 21:1623–1629, 2001.

153. Selim M, Fink J, Linfante I, et al: Diagnosis of cerebral venous thrombosis with echo-planar T2*-weighted magnetic resonance imaging. Arch Neurol 59:1021–1026, 2002.

154. Lafitte F, Boukobza M, Guichard JP, et al: MRI and MRA for diagnosis and follow-up of cerebral venous thrombosis (CVT). Clin Radiol 52:672–679, 1997.

155. Lovblad KO, Bassetti C, Schneider J, et al: Diffusion-weighted MR in cerebral venous thrombosis. Cerebrovasc Dis 11:169–176, 2001.

156. Chu K, Kang DW, Yoon BW, Roh JK: Diffusion-weighted magnetic resonance in cerebral venous thrombosis. Arch Neurol 58:1569–1576, 2001.

157. Ducreux D, Oppenheim C, Vandamme X, et al: Diffusion-weighted imaging patterns of brain damage associated with cerebral venous thrombosis. AJNR Am J Neuroradiol 22:261–268, 2001.

158. Doege CA, Tavakolian R, Kerskens CM, et al: Perfusion and diffusion magnetic resonance imaging in human cerebral venous thrombosis. J Neurol 248:564–571, 2001.

159. Keller E, Flacke S, Urbach H, Schild HH: Diffusion- and perfusion-weighted magnetic resonance imaging in deep cerebral venous thrombosis. Stroke 30:1144–1146, 1999.

160. Yuh WT, Simonson TM, Wang AM, et al: Venous sinus occlusive disease: MR findings. AJNR Am J Neuroradiol 15:309–316, 1994.

161. Vogl TJ, Bergman C, Villringer A, et al: Dural sinus thrombosis: Value of venous MR angiography for diagnosis and follow-up. AJR Am J Roentgenol 162:1191–1198, 1994.

162. Cramer SC, Nelles G, Benson RR, et al: A functional MRI study of subjects recovered from hemiparetic stroke. Stroke 28:2518–2527, 1997.

163. Chollet F, DiPiero V, Wise RJ, et al: The functional anatomy of motor recovery after stroke in humans: A study with positron emission tomography. Ann Neurol 29:63–71, 1991.

164. Kato H, Izumiyama M, Koizumi H, et al: Near-infrared spectroscopic topography as a tool to monitor motor reorganization after hemiparetic stroke: A comparison with functional MRI. Stroke 33:2032–2036, 2002.

165. Feydy A, Carlier R, Roby-Brami A, et al: Longitudinal study of motor recovery after stroke: Recruitment and focusing of brain activation. Stroke 33:1610–1617, 2002.

166. Carey LM, Abbott DF, Puce A, et al: Reemergence of activation with poststroke somatosensory recovery: A serial fMRI case study. Neurology 59:749–752, 2002.

167. Castillo M, Mukherji SK: Early abnormalities related to postinfarction Wallerian degeneration: Evaluation with MR diffusion-weighted imaging. J Comput Assist Tomogr 23:1004–1007, 1999.

168. Weidauer S, Dettmann E, Krakow K, Lanfermann H: [Diffusion-weighted MRI of spinal cord infarction—description of two cases and review of the literature]. Nervenarzt 73:999–1003, 2002.

169. Stepper F, Lovblad KO: Anterior spinal artery stroke demonstrated by echo-planar DWI. Eur Radiol 11:2607–610, 2001.

170. Kluytmans M, van Everdingen KJ, Kappelle LJ, et al: Prognostic value of perfusion- and diffusion-weighted MR imaging in first 3 days of stroke. Eur Radiol 10:1434–1441, 2000.

171. Sorensen AG, Copen WA, Ostergaard L, et al: Hyperacute stroke: Simultaneous measurement of relative cerebral blood volume, relative cerebral blood flow, and mean tissue transit time. Radiology 210:519–527, 1999.

172. Ueda T, Yuh WT, Maley JE, et al: Outcome of acute ischemic lesions evaluated by diffusion and perfusion MR imaging. AJNR Am J Neuroradiol 20:983–989, 1999.

173. Karonen JO, Liu Y, Vanninen RL, et al: Combined perfusion- and diffusion-weighted MR imaging in acute ischemic stroke during the 1st week: A longitudinal study. Radiology 217:886–894, 2000.

174. Neumann-Haefelin T, Wittsack HJ, Wenserski F, et al: Diffusion- and perfusion-weighted MRI: The DWI/PWI mismatch region in acute stroke. Stroke 30:1591–1597, 1999.

175. Darby DG, Barber PA, Gerraty RP, et al: Pathophysiological topography of acute ischemia by combined diffusion- weighted and perfusion MRI. Stroke. 30:2043–2052, 1999.

176. Baird AE, Benfield A, Schlaug G, et al: Enlargement of human cerebral ischemic lesion volumes measured by diffusion-weighted magnetic resonance imaging. Ann Neurol 41:581–589, 1997.

177. Karonen JO, Vanninen RL, Liu Y, et al: Combined diffusion and perfusion MRI with correlation to single-photon emission CT in acute ischemic stroke: Ischemic penumbra predicts infarct growth. Stroke 30:1583–1590, 1999.

178. Schellinger PD, Fiebach JB, Jansen O, et al: Stroke magnetic resonance imaging within 6 hours after onset of hyperacute cerebral ischemia. Ann Neurol 49:460–469, 2001.

179. Kidwell CS, Saver JL, Mattiello J, et al: Thrombolytic reversal of acute human cerebral ischemic injury shown by diffusion/perfusion magnetic resonance imaging. Ann Neurol 47:462–469, 2000.

180. Lutsep HL, Nesbit GM, Berger RM, Coshow WR: Does reversal of ischemia on diffusion-weighted imaging reflect higher apparent diffusion coefficient values? J Neuroimaging 11:313–316, 2001.

181. Uno M, Harada M, Okada T, Nagahiro S: Diffusion-weighted and perfusion-weighted magnetic resonance imaging to monitor acute intra-arterial thrombolysis. J Stroke Cerebrovasc Dis 9:113–120, 2000.

182. Desmond PM, Lovell AC, Rawlinson AA, et al: The value of apparent diffusion coefficient maps in early cerebral ischemia. AJNR Am J Neuroradiol 22:1260–1267, 2001.

183. Fiehler J, Foth M, Kucinski T, et al: Severe ADC decreases do not predict irreversible tissue damage in humans. Stroke 33:79–86, 2002.

184. Oppenheim C, Samson Y, Manai R, et al: Prediction of malignant middle cerebral artery infarction by diffusion-weighted imaging. Stroke 31:2175–2181, 2000.

185. Oppenheim C, Grandin C, Samson Y, et al: Is there an apparent diffusion coefficient threshold in predicting tissue viability in hyperacute stroke? Stroke 32:2486–2491, 2001.

186. Oppenheim C, Samson Y, Dormont D, et al: DWI prediction of symptomatic hemorrhagic transformation in acute MCA infarct. J Neuroradiol 29:6–13, 2002.

187. Grandin CB, Duprez TP, Smith AM, et al: Which MR-derived perfusion parameters are the best predictors of infarct growth in hyperacute stroke? Comparative study between relative and quantitative measurements. Radiology 223:361–370, 2002.

188. Rohl L, Sakoh M, Simonsen CZ, et al: Time evolution of cerebral perfusion and apparent diffusion coefficient measured by magnetic resonance imaging in a porcine stroke model. J Magn Reson Imaging 15:123–129, 2002.

189. Wu O, Koroshetz WJ, Ostergaard L, et al: Predicting tissue outcome in acute human cerebral ischemia using combined diffusion- and perfusion-weighted MR imaging. Stroke 32:933–942, 2001.

190. Thijs VN, Adami A, Neumann-Haefelin T, et al: Relationship between severity of MR perfusion deficit and DWI lesion evolution. Neurology 57:1205–1211, 2001.

191. Fiehler J, Knab R, Reichenbach JR, et al: Apparent diffusion coefficient decreases and magnetic resonance imaging perfusion parameters are associated in ischemic tissue of acute stroke patients. J Cereb Blood Flow Metab 21:577–584, 2001.

192. Tong DC, Adami A, Moseley ME, Marks MP: Prediction of hemorrhagic transformation following acute stroke: Role of diffusion- and perfusion-weighted magnetic resonance imaging. Arch Neurol 58:587–593, 2001.

193. Kidwell CS, Saver JL, Carneado J, et al: Predictors of hemorrhagic transformation in patients receiving intra- arterial thrombolysis. Stroke 33:717–724, 2002.

194. Warach S: Tissue viability thresholds in acute stroke: The 4-factor model. Stroke 32:2460–461, 2001.

195. Rose SE, Chalk JB, Griffin MP, et al: MRI based diffusion and perfusion predictive model to estimate stroke evolution. Magn Reson Imaging 19:1043–1053, 2001.

196. Liu Y, Karonen JO, Vanninen RL, et al: Cerebral hemodynamics in human acute ischemic stroke: A study with diffusion- and perfusion-

weighted magnetic resonance imaging and SPECT. J Cereb Blood Flow Metab 20:910–920, 2000.

197. Schlaug G, Benfield A, Baird AE, et al: The ischemic penumbra: Operationally defined by diffusion and perfusion MRI. Neurology 53:1528–1537, 1999.

198. Wu O, Koroshetz WJ, Ostergaard L, et al: Predicting tissue outcome in acute human cerebral ischemia using combined diffusion- and perfusion-weighted MR imaging. Stroke 32:933–942, 2001.

199. Jacobs MA, Mitsias P, Soltanian-Zadeh H, et al: Multiparametric MRI tissue characterization in clinical stroke with correlation to clinical outcome: Part 2. Stroke 32:950–957, 2001.

200. Jansen O, Schellinger P, Fiebach J, et al: Early recanalisation in acute ischaemic stroke saves tissue at risk defined by MRI [letter]. Lancet 353:2036–2037, 1999.

201. Schellinger PD, Jansen O, Fiebach JB, et al: Monitoring intravenous recombinant tissue plasminogen activator thrombolysis for acute ischemic stroke with diffusion and perfusion MRI. Stroke 31:1318–1328, 2000.

202. Marks MP, Tong DC, Beaulieu C, et al: Evaluation of early reperfusion and i.v. tPA therapy using diffusion- and perfusion-weighted MRI [see comments]. Neurology 52:1792–1798, 1999.

203. Taleb M, Lovblad KO, El-Koussy M, et al: Reperfusion demonstrated by apparent diffusion coefficient mapping after local intra-arterial thrombolysis for ischaemic stroke. Neuroradiology 43:591–594, 2001.

203a. Parsons MW, Barber PA, Chalk J, et al: Diffusion-and perfusion-weighted MRI response to thrombolysis in stroke. Ann Neurol 51:28–37, 2002.

204. Kidwell CS, Alger JR, Saver JL, et al: MR signatures of infarction vs. salvageable penumbra in acute human stroke: A preliminary model. Stroke 31:285, 2000.

205. Tong DC, Adami A, Moseley ME, Marks MP: Prediction of hemorrhagic transformation following acute stroke: Role of diffusion- and perfusion-weighted magnetic resonance imaging. Arch Neurol 58:587–593, 2001.

206. Kidwell CS, Saver JL, Mattiello J, et al: Diffusion-perfusion MRI characterization of post-recanalization hyperperfusion. Neurology 57:2015–2021, 2001.

207. Kidwell CS, Saver JL, Starkman S, et al: Late secondary ischemic injury in patients receiving intraarterial thrombolysis. Ann Neurol 52:698–703, 2002.

Diagnostic Studies

Chapter Twenty

Cerebral Angiography

Ronald J. Sattenberg, Jeffrey Saver, and Y. Pierre Gobin

After Egas Moniz invented cerebral angiography in 1927, it became the method of choice for the diagnosis of brain lesions,[1,2] until the development of computed tomography (CT) and later magnetic resonance imaging (MRI) limited the indication for catheter angiography to visualization of cerebral vessels. CT angiography (CTA) and magnetic resonance angiography (MRA) have demonstrated excellent performance in noninvasively imaging large cervicocerebral vessels, further reducing the need for invasive angiography. Other noninvasive imaging techniques, such as duplex ultrasonography and transcranial Doppler ultrasonography, provide hemodynamic information that further limits the indications for cerebral angiography. Because of its ability to show the smallest vascular lesions, however, cerebral angiography is still the "gold standard" for imaging the cervicocerebral vasculature. Moreover, the dramatic expansion of percutaneous treatments for ischemic and hemorrhagic cerebrovascular disease has brought a resurgence in catheter angiography as a necessary prelude and guide to endovascular interventions.

TECHNIQUE

With miniaturization and other advances in catheter technology and the development of non-ionic contrast agents, a cerebral angiogram now is usually a straightforward procedure that takes 30 to 60 minutes to complete. Cerebral angiography is painless and can generally be performed with the use of local anesthesia administered at the groin and no or mild sedation. General anesthesia is required only in patients unable to cooperate or in children. With the use of a closure device such as a collagen plug or percutaneous arterial suture for hemostasis, patients may be ambulatory within 1 hour after the procedure is completed, and anticoagulation need not be halted before the procedure. However, closure devices are only used in a select population of patients. Without closure devices, the patient can usually ambulate within 6 to 8 hours.

Vascular access is most often obtained via the common femoral artery, and rarely via the brachial or axillary artery. After arterial puncture, an arterial sheath is placed into the artery. A *sheath* is a short catheter with a diaphragm at its exterior end that allows the passage and manipulation of additional smaller catheters without damaging the femoral artery. Catheterization of the aortic arch and further selective catheterizations are performed with the combined use of a catheter and a guidewire. Many catheters and guidewires are available. Selection of the catheters and guidewires used in a particular patient is based on the patient's vascular anatomy, the diagnostic question to be answered by the procedure, and the preferences of the operator. We routinely use a hockeystick-shaped catheter and a guidewire with a simple 45-degree curve, both with hydrophilic coating. For difficult anatomy, other catheter shapes are available. The catheter is continuously flushed with heparinized saline to prevent thrombus formation.

The precise vessels catheterized depend on the indication for the procedure. Sometimes catheterizing only one vessel is all that is required—for instance, for immediate follow-up evaluation after aneurysm clipping. At other times, the bilateral vertebral arteries, bilateral external and internal carotid arteries, and bilateral common carotid arteries all must be catheterized. In many instances, catheterization and angiography of the aortic arch and three to four vessels are necessary.

At the very end of the procedure, the common femoral artery sheath is removed, and manual compression is applied at the access site until hemostasis is obtained. Multiple arteriotomy closing devices have now gained popularity. These are essentially tools that percutaneously place a suture into or a plug at the puncture site to obtain immediate hemostasis. The indications for the use of a percutaneous closure device vary among institutions. One common approach is not to use these devices for routine angiograms, but to reserve their application in patients who are undergoing anticoagulation, who are being treated with fibrinolytics, or have coagulation deficits from other causes.

RISKS

The risk of cerebral angiography has declined over the years. Increasing procedural safety is due to many factors, including non-ionic contrast agents, new catheters and guidewires that have safer designs and are made of less thrombogenic materials, and digital subtraction angiography.[3,4]

The risks of cerebral angiography are related to patient age and medical condition, the number of catheter exchanges, the total time for the procedure, and the load of contrast agent.[4,5] Cerebral angiography is more risky in the elderly, and in patients with particular conditions that predispose to thrombus formation on the catheter (hypercoagulable states) and to vessel dissection and rupture (e.g., Marfan's disease).

Many studies have been performed to quantify the risks of cerebral angiography. Hankey and associates[6] reviewed several series and found the general risk for permanent neurologic sequelae after cerebral angiography to be 1%. The mortality rate was less than 0.1%. The overall risk for a neurologic complication was about 4%.[6] In a prospective study by Dion and colleagues,[4] of 1002 cerebral angiography procedures, the rate of permanent neurologic deficit was 0.1%, and that of transient deficits 1.2%. Other studies cite a persistent neurologic deficit rate of 0.3% to 0.5% and a total neurologic complication rate of 0.5% to 2%.[3]

Among the potential neurologic complications of cerebral angiography are embolic events and vascular dissections. Transcranial Doppler ultrasonography studies monitoring for microembolic events during diagnostic angiography have shown that although nonpathogenic air emboli introduced at the time of contrast injection are common, formed element emboli are uncommon.[7] Carotid or vertebral artery dissections secondary to catheterization depend on operator experience and are less frequent (0.4%) with the newer, safer catheter designs.[8] Although neurologically symptomatic complications from a cerebral angiogram are rare, clinically silent "complications," diagnosed on diffusion-weighted MRI, are more common, being found in 26% of diagnostic angiography procedures.[10] Covert MRI diffusion lesions are associated with the presence of multiple vascular risk factors, greater difficulty in probing vessels, amount of contrast medium needed, longer fluoroscopy time, and the use of multiple catheters.[10]

One particular concern of cerebral angiography in the setting of recently ruptured cerebral aneurysms is the risk of precipitating rebleeding by injecting contrast agent with an increased pressure head. This risk is extremely low. In the meta-analysis of 415 patients with acute subarachnoid hemorrhage, Cloft and associates[9] found no cases of rebleeding during angiography.

Non-neurologic complications consist of local complications (i.e., hematoma, pseudoaneurysm, and infection), renal failure, contrast agent allergies, and arterial occlusions. In a cooperative study among leading interventional radiologic societies, non-neurologic major complications rates were as follows: renal failure, 0% to 0.15%; arterial occlusion requiring surgical intervention, 0% to 0.4%; arteriovenous fistula or pseudoaneurysm, 0.01% to 0.22%; and hematoma requiring transfusion or evacuation, 0.26% to 1.5%.[5]

When allergy to iodine contrast medium is known before procedure initiation, premedication with steroids and antihistamines is usually sufficient to prevent any adverse reactions. In patients with previous severe allergy such as shock, in whom iodine is contraindicated even with premedication, gadolinium-based contrast agents, which are radiopaque as well as paramagnetic, may be employed.

ANGIOGRAPHIC CEREBRAL VASCULATURE: NORMAL ANATOMY

In order to recognize and understand vascular disease, one must first be acquainted with the normal angioarchitecture of the cerebrovascular system and its variants. The three phases of an angiographic imaging sequence—the arterial, capillary, and venous—are shown in Figures 20–1 to 20–3. Each phase has its particular sensitivity for the different pathologic entities. One should be able to recognized common variants, such as persistent fetal anomalies and vascular fenestrations (Fig. 20–4).

INDICATIONS

Intracranial Hemorrhage

Intracranial hemorrhage may be epidural, subdural, subarachnoid, or intraparenchymal.

Epidural hemorrhage is usually secondary to head trauma. The vessels coursing in the epidural space, most notably the middle meningeal artery, are torn, with resultant arterial bleeding. These hemorrhages are often associated with skull fractures. Because epidural hemorrhages are usually of traumatic origin, correlation with the clinical history as well as noninvasive imaging almost invariably identifies the cause, obviating the need for angiographic evaluation.

Subdural hemorrhage (SDH) is secondary to bleeding from the cortical bridging veins that drain into the superior sagittal sinus or other dural sinuses. The characteristic angiographic appearance is a lentiform avascular collection outlined by displaced cortical vessels. The cortical bridging veins are vulnerable to venous hypertension or tearing in the subdural space secondary to trauma. Venous hypertension can be caused by a variety of reasons, including sinus thrombosis and dural arteriovenous fistulas (Fig. 20–5). Uncommonly, a subdural hematoma may result when an intracerebral aneurysm that previously hemorrhaged creates adhesions that direct subsequent hemorrhage into the subdural compartment. In this situation, an intraparenchymal focus of hemorrhage is often present as

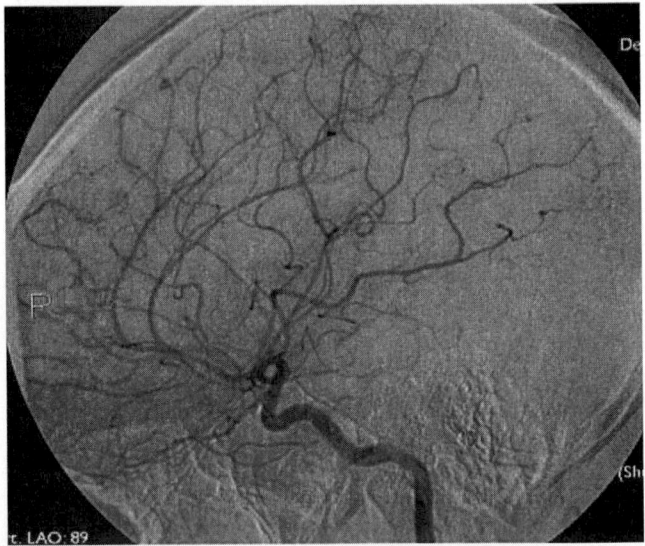

FIGURE 20–1 *Internal carotid artery injection, lateral projection, arterial phase. The arteries are primarily opacified during this phase.*

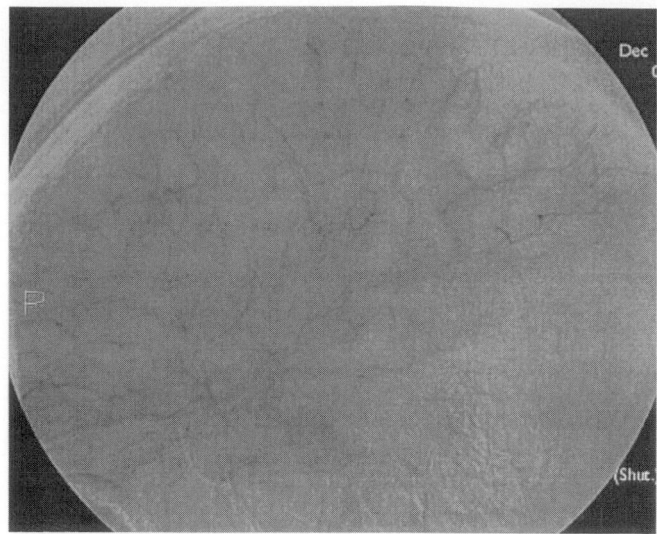

FIGURE 20–2 *Internal carotid artery injection, lateral projection, capillary phase. No significant arterial or venous opacification is noted during this phase.*

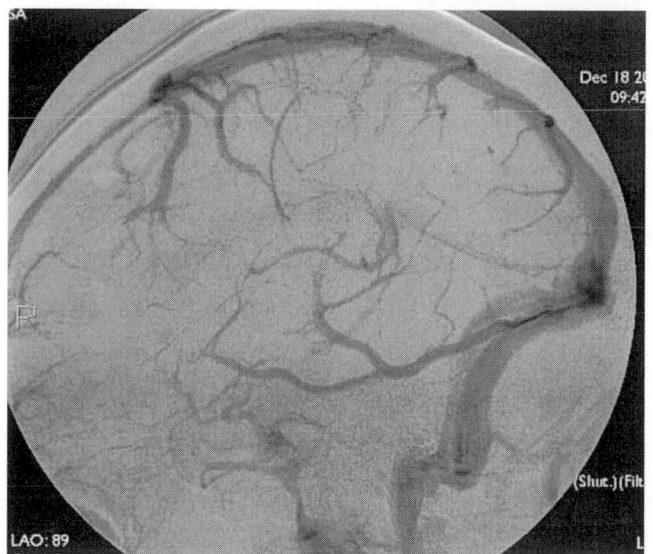

FIGURE 20–3 *Internal carotid artery injection, lateral projection, venous phase. The veins are primarily opacified during this phase.*

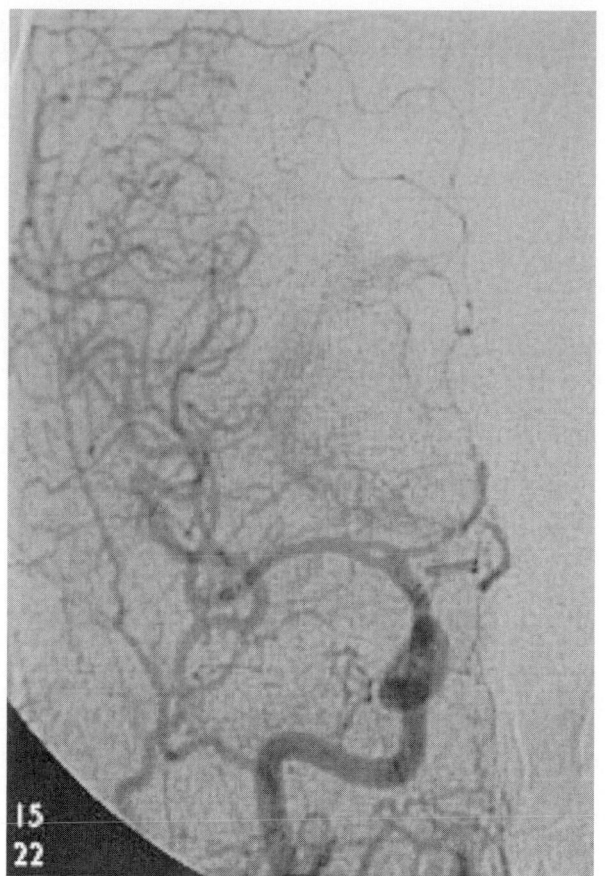

FIGURE 20–4 *Common carotid artery injection, anteroposterior projection. Note the "filling defect" in the M1 segment, just at the carotid bifurcation. This is a fenestration.*

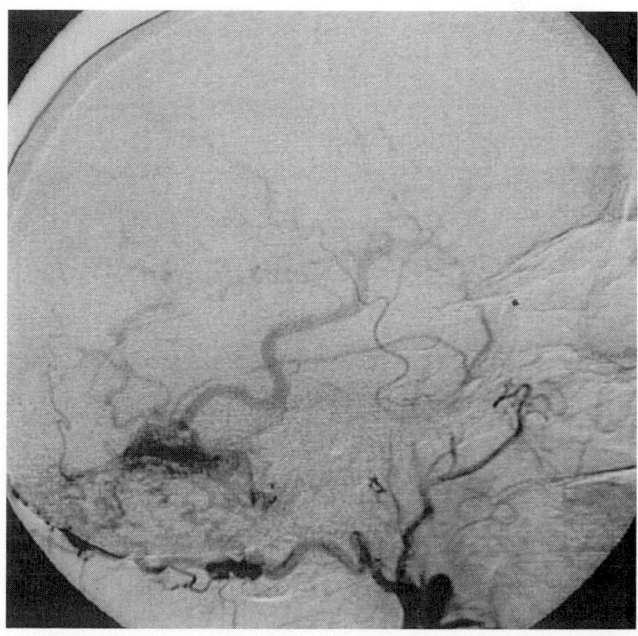

FIGURE 20–5 *External carotid artery injection, lateral projection. There is arterial and early venous opacification with contrast simultaneously. The dural fistula is opacified as well.*

well, detection of which should raise the suspicion for an aneurysmal bleed. In a subdural hemorrhage, if a dural arteriovenous fistula or aneurysm is suspected, a cerebral angiogram should be performed. Otherwise, if trauma or significant brain parenchyma atrophy is present in an older patient, angiography should be reserved.

Subarachnoid hemorrhage (SAH) has an incidence of 6 to 8 per 100,000 person-years, and studies suggest that 2% to 6% of the population have an intracranial aneurysm.[11] In 85% of SAHs, the cause is a ruptured aneurysm, usually a berry aneurysm. Among the other causes of SAH are trauma (in which case a parenchyma focus of contusion or hemorrhage is often seen on imaging), intraparenchymal hemorrhage extending into the ventricular system, cerebral or cervical arteriovenous malformation or fistula, mycotic aneurysm, nonaneurysmal perimesencephalic hemorrhage, vasculitis, and dissections; some SAHs are cryptogenic.[12]

In less than 5% of arteriovenous malformations (AVMs) that bleed, the hemorrhage is confined to the subarachnoid space with no intraparenchymal blood. Generally, if the findings of angiography performed in the acute phase of a nontraumatic SAH are normal, the procedure should be repeated after 1 week. There are several explanations why an aneurysm may not be detected on angiography; among these are parenchymal hematoma compressing the aneurysm, thrombus in the aneurysm, its neck, or both, perianeurysmal vasospasm, and suboptimal views of the region harboring the aneurysm. The diagnostic yield of a second cerebral angiogram in eight different series was 17%.[12] If findings on the second angiogram are also normal, a third angiogram performed several months later can be of benefit. In one series, aneurysm was detected by a third angiogram in 1 out of 14 patients.[12] For a patient in whom a CT scan shows a truly perimesencephalic hemorrhage pattern, the probability that cerebral angiography will reveal a vertebrobasilar aneurysm is 4%.[13] Thus, the diagnosis of perimesencephalic hemorrhage requires a normal cerebral angiogram. In a truly perimesencephalic pattern of SAH, a second angiogram is not necessary if findings of the first angiogram are normal.

Berry or sacciform aneurysms are the most prevalent intracranial aneurysms. They are localized mostly in the anterior circulation (90%) as follows: anterior communicating artery, 40%; middle cerebral artery bifurcation, 30%; intracranial internal carotid artery, 20%; and posterior circulation, 10%.[10] Other cerebral aneurysms are fusiform, traumatic (pseudoaneurysm), mycotic, or dissecting. A selection of aneurysms is illustrated in Figures 20–6 to 20–18. Associations of cerebral aneurysm with autosomal dominant polycystic kidney disease and Marfan's syndrome have been discussed.[14–16]

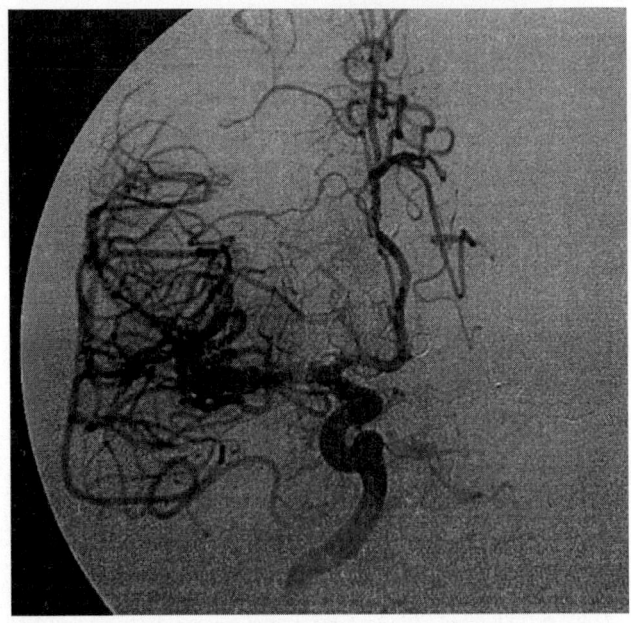

FIGURE 20–7 *Right internal carotid artery injection, anteroposterior projection, after embolization. The previously anterior communicating artery aneurysm seen is no longer opacifying.*

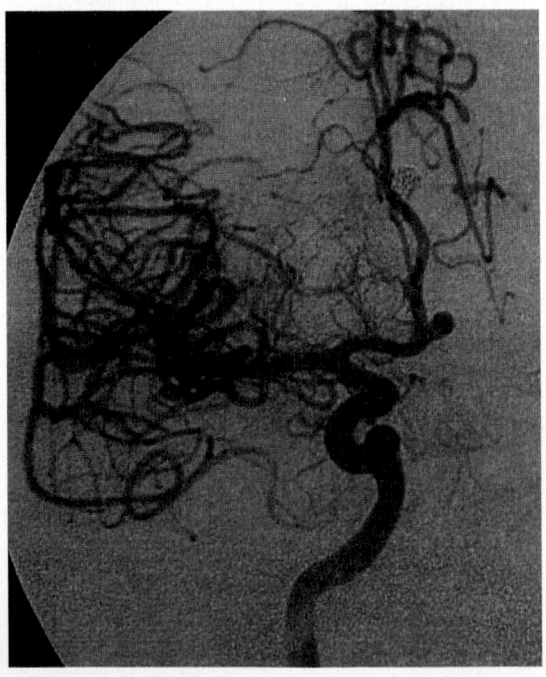

FIGURE 20–6 *Right internal carotid artery injection, frontal projection, demonstrates an anterior communicating artery aneurysm. The aneurysm dome points superomedially.*

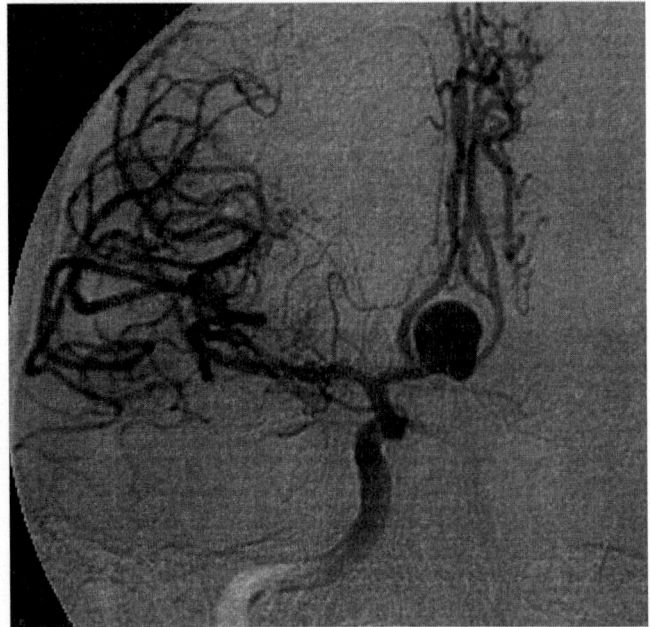

FIGURE 20–8 *Right internal carotid artery injection, frontal view, arterial phase, demonstrating a large anterior communicating artery aneurysm. Notice how the A2 segments of the anterior cerebral artery are splayed by the aneurysm.*

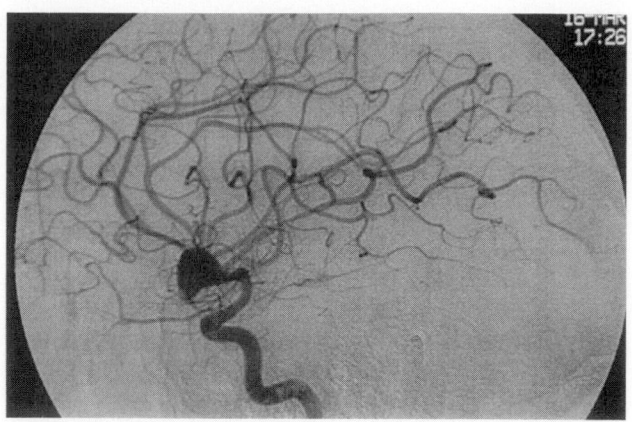

FIGURE 20–9 *Internal carotid artery injection, lateral projection, arterial phase, demonstrating a large anterior communicating artery aneurysm.*

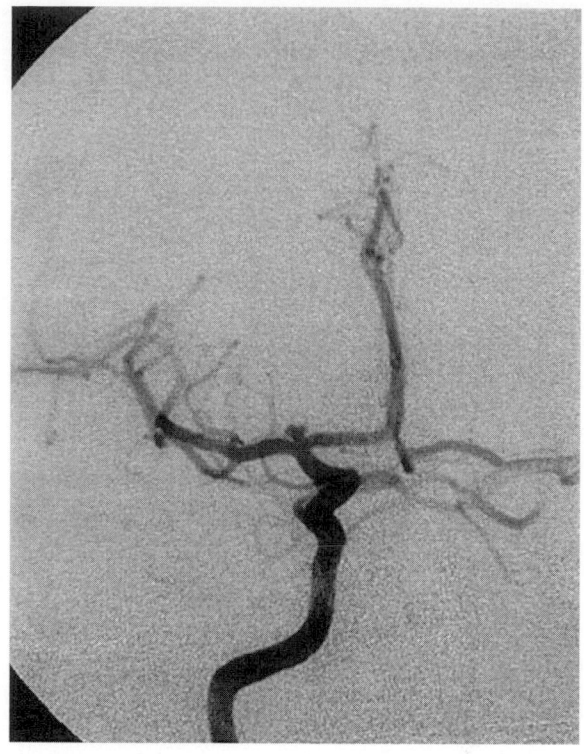

FIGURE 20–10 *Right internal carotid artery injection, anteroposterior projection, arterial phase, demonstrating a carotid bifurcation aneurysm. The aneurysm is bilobed and irregular in contour.*

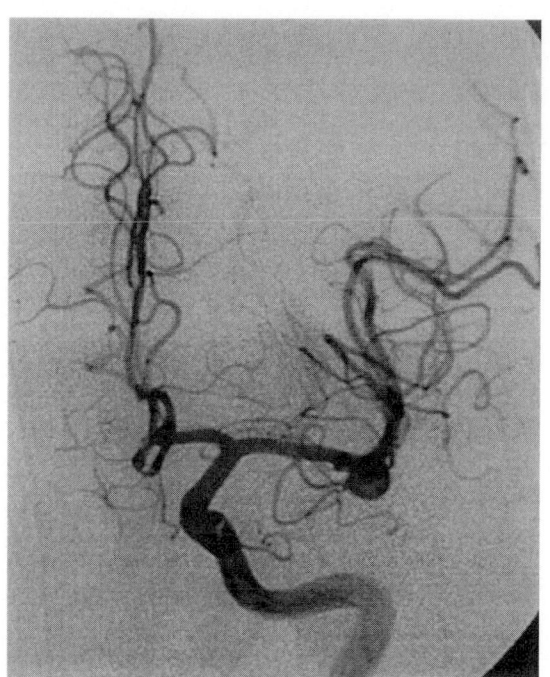

FIGURE 20–11 *Left internal carotid artery injection, frontal projection, arterial phase, demonstrating a middle cerebral artery aneurysm. The aneurysm dome is pointing inferiorly.*

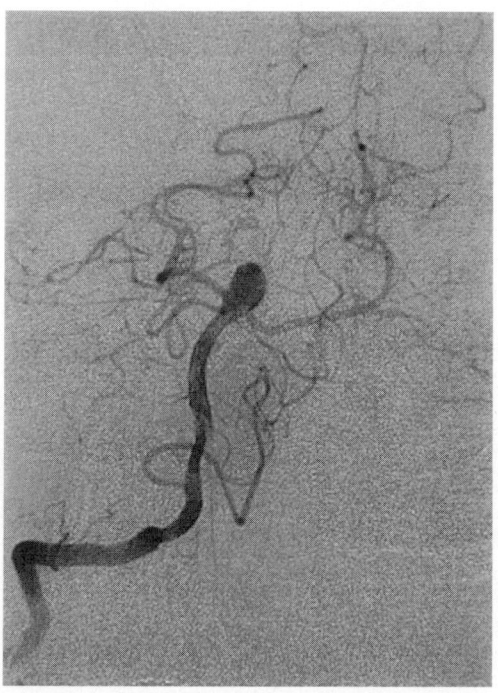

FIGURE 20–12 *Right vertebral artery injection, frontal projection, arterial phase, demonstrating a basilar tip aneurysm.*

Diagnostic Studies

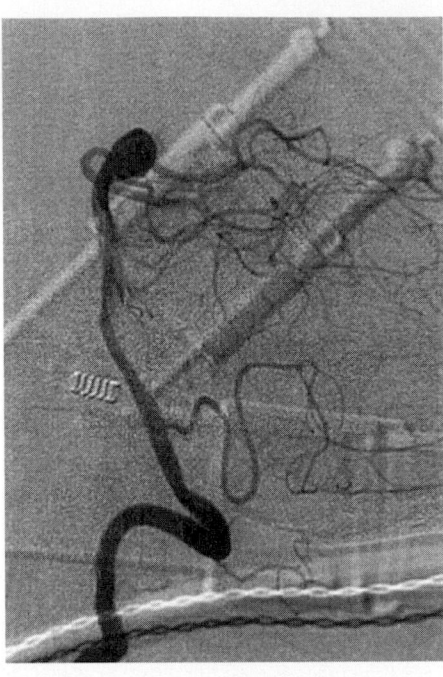

FIGURE 20–13 *Vertebral artery injection, lateral projection, arterial phase, demonstrating a basilar tip aneurysm.*

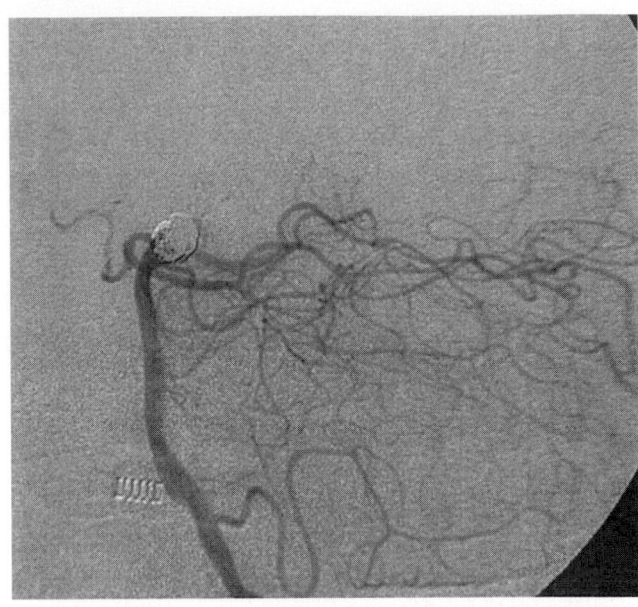

FIGURE 20–14 *Lateral projection, posterior circulation, arterial phase. Status post embolization, the basilar tip aneurysm is no longer opacifying.*

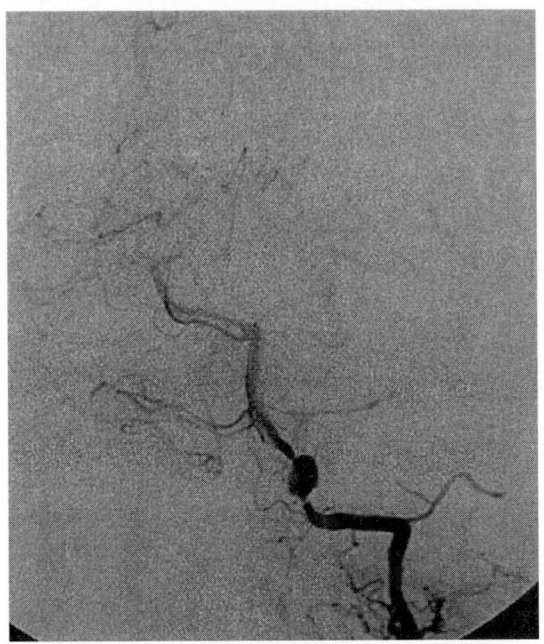

FIGURE 20–15 *Vertebral artery injection, frontal projection, demonstrating a vertebrobasilar aneurysm. Notice how the contrast column rapidly narrows and there is significantly decreased opacification of the vasculature distal to the aneurysm. This is consistent with a dissecting aneurysm.*

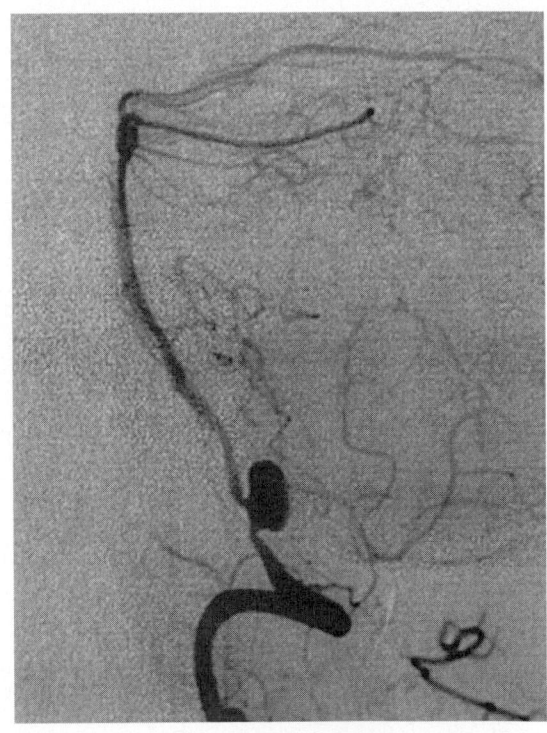

FIGURE 20–16 *Vertebral artery injection, lateral projection, arterial phase, demonstrating a dissecting vertebrobasilar aneurysm.*

Diagnostic Studies

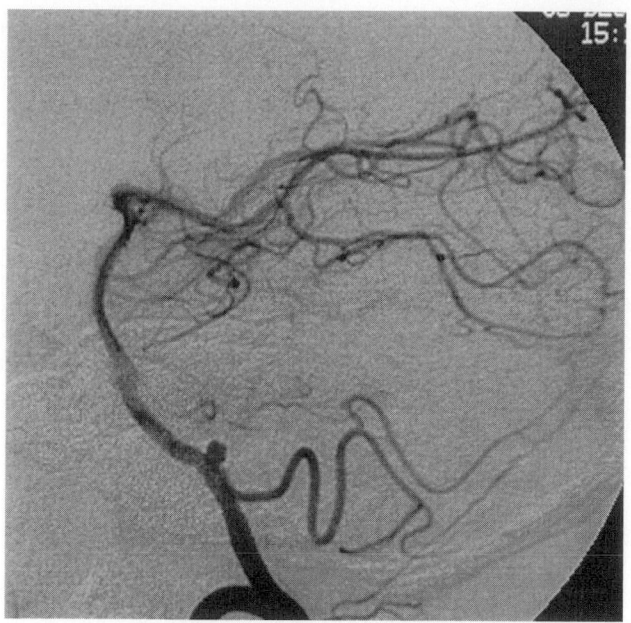

FIGURE 20–17 *Vertebral artery injection, lateral projection, arterial phase, demonstrating a posterior inferior cerebellar artery (PICA) aneurysm.*

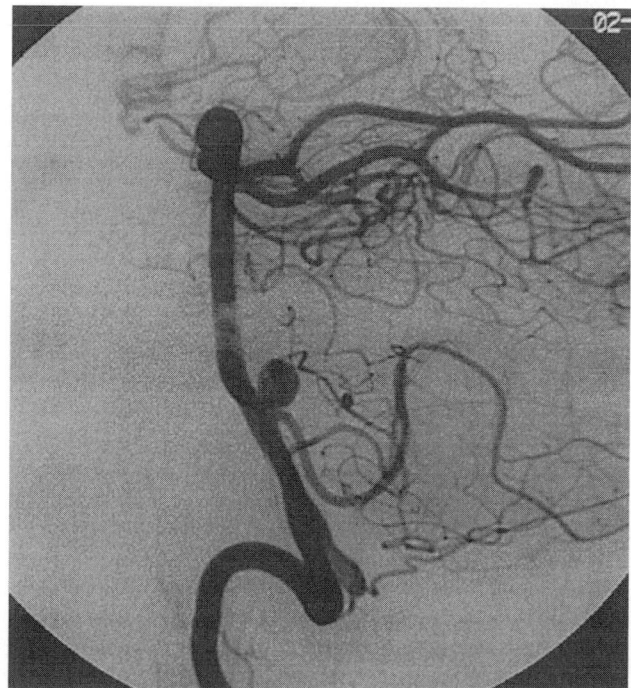

FIGURE 20–18 *Vertebral artery injection, lateral projection, arterial phase, demonstrating both a basilar tip aneurysm, as well as a posterior inferior cerebellar artery aneurysm.*

The angiogram should evaluate location of the aneurysm, size of the neck and dome (dome to neck ratio), morphology, and relationship to the parent vessel and should show whether the aneurysm incorporates the origin of other vessels. Multiple aneurysms are found in 20% of aneurysmal SAHs, and it may be difficult to identify which

aneurysm bled and should be treated first. Three important features indicating the causative aneurysm are (1) the location of the aneurysm in relation to the SAH, (2) the aneurysm shape, because a ruptured aneurysm may be lobulated or have a teat, and (3) the aneurysm size. Active extravasation of contrast material from an aneurysm at the time of angiography is exceptional and indicates intraprocedural rupture.

Intraparenchymal hemorrhage can be secondary to a variety of pathologic entities, including hypertension (80%),[10] amyloid angiopathy, trauma, hemorrhagic conversion of ischemic stroke, arterial dissection, tumor, sinus thrombosis, AVM, cavernous hemangioma, and saccular aneurysm. About 20% of hemorrhages due to intracranial aneurysms have an intraparenchymal component, especially if a mycotic aneurysm is the cause. If an AVM is suspected on MRI or CT, an angiogram is required to characterize the lesion, its venous drainage, arterial feeding arteries (feeders), and nidus. The characteristic angiographic appearance of an AVM consists of enlarged arterial feeders, a nidus, and early draining veins (Figs. 20–19 to 20–22).

The association of AVMs and aneurysms on the arterial feeders is well known and is secondary to the high-flow state through the AVM (Figs. 20–21 and 20–22). Furthermore, selection of optimal treatment modalities for AVMs requires knowledge of the detailed angioarchitecture of the lesion. For example, the presence of a lenticulostriate arterial supply to the nidus makes surgery more difficult (see Fig. 20–22).

In general, angiography is indicated in the evaluation of intracranial hemorrhage (ICH) in (1) any patient younger than 70 years with a lobar hemorrhage and (2) any patient of any age with a deep hemorrhage who does not have a history of hypertension or CT or MRI evidence of small vessel arteriopathy.

Ischemia

Cerebral Infarction and Transient Ischemic Attack
Cerebral angiography remains a mainstay in the evaluation of cerebral ischemia in the young (e.g., <45 years), in

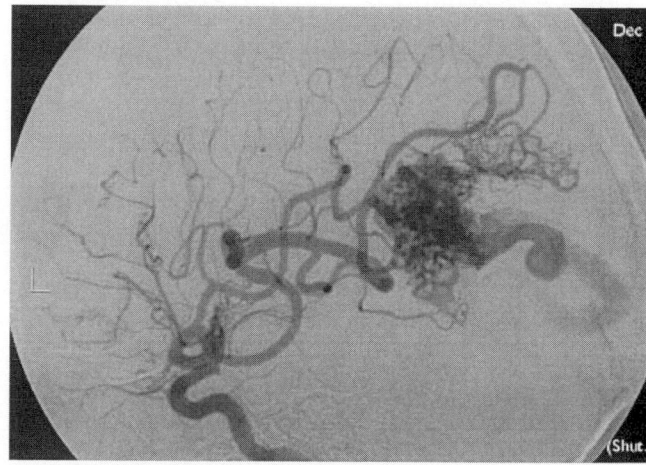

FIGURE 20–19 *Internal carotid artery injection, lateral projection, arterial phase, demonstrating early venous opacification, as well as a nidus, consistent with an arteriovenous malformation.*

Diagnostic Studies

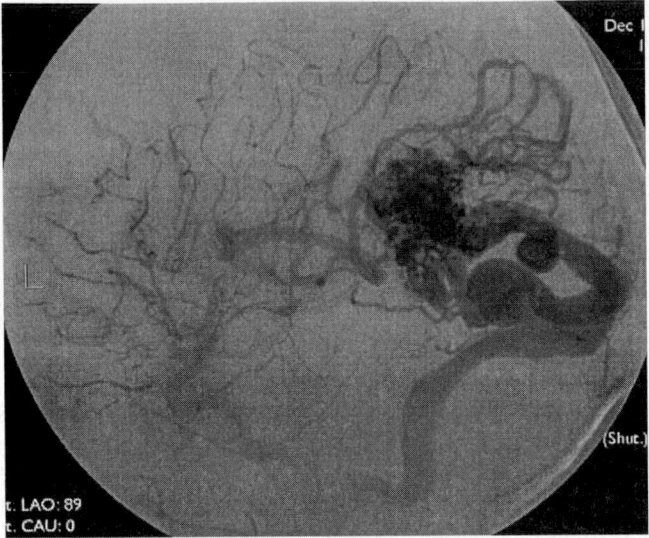

FIGURE 20–20 *Internal carotid artery injection, lateral projection, venous phase, demonstrating the venous phase of an arteriovenous malformation. Note the enlarged vein draining the arteriovenous malformation nidus.*

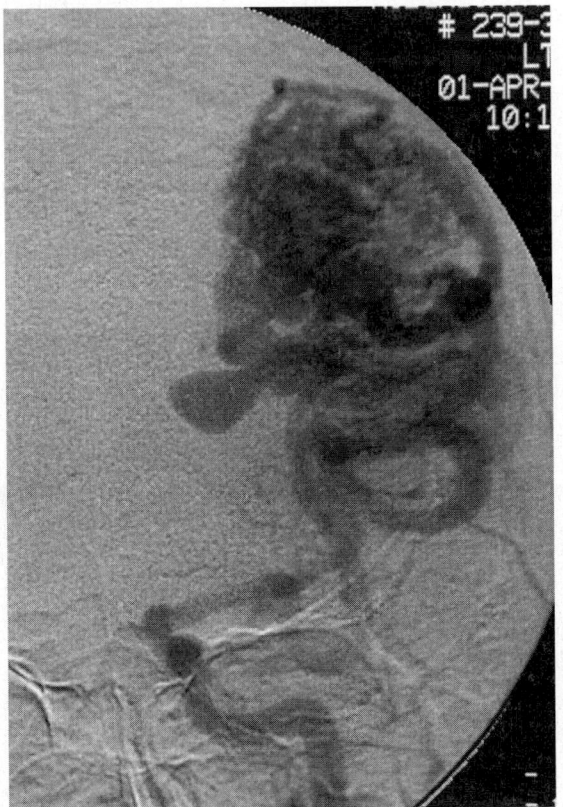

FIGURE 20–21 *Left internal carotid artery injection, anteroposterior projection, arterial phase, demonstrating an enlarged middle cerebral artery vasculature feeding an arteriovenous malformation with an aneurysm whose dome points inferomedially.*

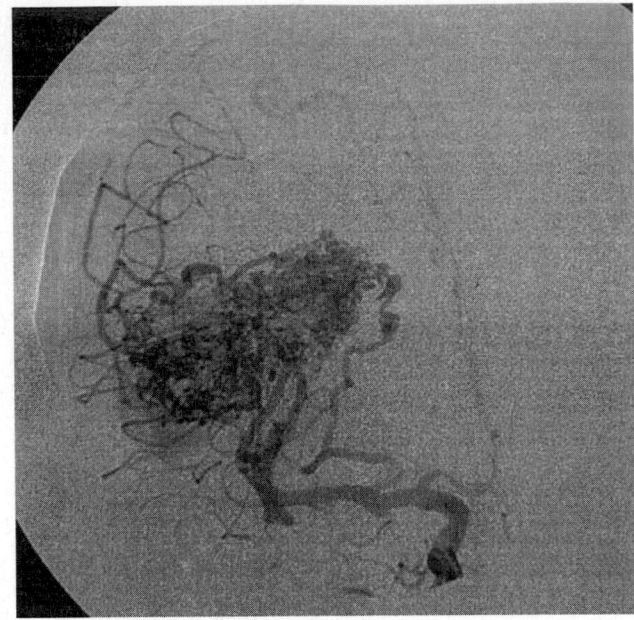

FIGURE 20–22 *Right internal carotid artery injection, frontal projection, arterial phase, demonstrating an arteriovenous malformation being opacified by middle cerebral arterial vessels, as well as a lenticulostriate artery originating from the M1 segment of the middle cerebral artery.*

whom the potential causes are diverse and include entities often best characterized on angiographic studies, including vasculitis and dissection.

Angiography remains fundamentally important in the evaluation of cervical carotid atherosclerosis. The decision whether to proceed with carotid endarterectomy or carotid stenting depends on the extent of stenosis at the carotid bifurcation. In general, patients with symptomatic carotid disease benefit from surgical intervention if the severity of stenosis on angiography is 50% to 99%, whereas those with asymptomatic stenosis derive a modest benefit from surgery if severity of stenosis is 60% to 99%. The common noninvasive imaging modalities, carotid duplex ultrasonography, CT angiography, and MRA, are generally quite good, but each has intrinsic as well as operator- and reader-dependent limitations. When two noninvasive tests provide congruent results regarding the severity of stenosis, a decision for or against surgery may be made with confidence. If noninvasive test results disagree, however, catheter angiography is desirable to definitively characterize the lesion.[17]

Another important advantage of cerebral angiography over standard carotid duplex ultrasonography is that although both modalities can assess the severity of an internal carotid artery stenosis well, evaluation of the morphology of a plaque is best accomplished by catheter angiography (Figs. 20–23 and 20–24). Plaque morphology can be very important, because even if stenosis is not severe, an ulcerated plaque can be the cause of transient ischemic attacks (TIAs) and similarly may be the harbinger of a stroke.

Also among the causes of cerebral infarction and transient ischemic attacks is intracranial atherosclerotic

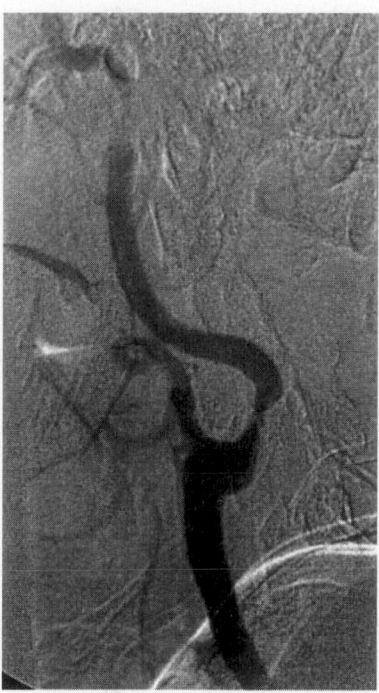

FIGURE 20–23 *Common carotid artery injection, lateral projection, arterial phase, demonstrates an internal carotid artery stenosis just distal to the bifurcation.*

stenosis (Figs. 20–25 and 20–26). For middle cerebral artery atherosclerotic stenosis, a stroke rate of 7.8% annually is reported.[21-24] The intracranial vasculature can be assessed with CT angiography, MRA, and transcranial Doppler ultrasonography to some extent; however, these intracranial vessels are smaller in diameter than the internal carotid artery, and the sensitivity and specificity of noninvasive studies for detecting and characterizing intracranial stenoses are not yet as well documented as for cervical stenoses. Quantifying the severity of intracranial stenosis at angiography requires a different measurement technique from that used for extracranial stenosis—that established by the North American Symptomatic Carotid Endarterectomy Trial (NASCET). Intracranial vessels tend to taper distal to stenoses, leading to possible underestimation of the extent of narrowing if the NASCET method were employed.

Acute Ischemia

In approximately 80% of acute ischemic strokes, early angiography demonstrates a large artery occlusion, either embolic (from arterial origin or cardioembolic) or due to in situ atherothrombosis.[18-20] Cerebral angiography is indicated as an emergency procedure if intra-arterial thrombolysis or mechanical embolectomy is being considered.

The cerebral angiographic findings in acute ischemic stroke are varied. One finding is the abrupt cutoff of a vessel (Figs. 20–27 to 20–33). If an embolus is the

Diagnostic Studies

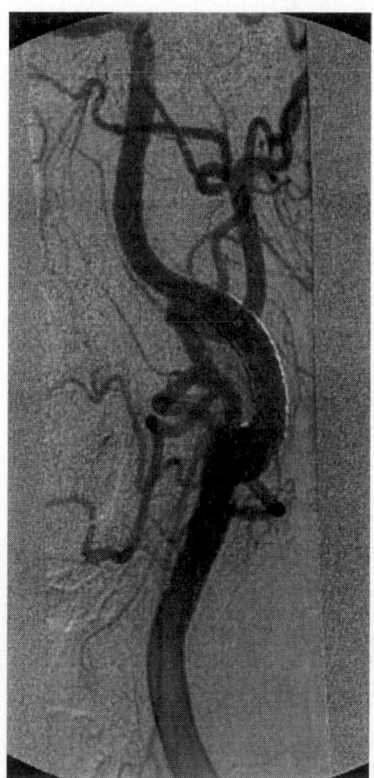

FIGURE 20–24 *Common carotid artery injection, lateral projection, arterial phase, demonstrating an internal carotid artery status post angioplasty and stent placement. The stenotic segment is no longer present.*

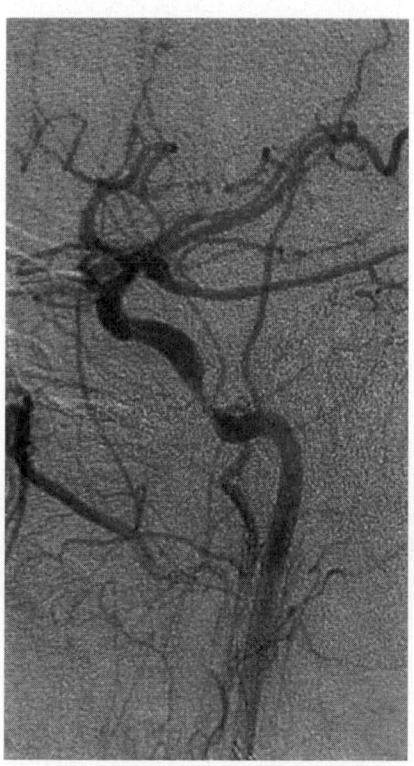

FIGURE 20–25 *Common carotid artery injection, lateral projection, arterial phase, demonstrating a stenosis in the petrous segment of the internal carotid artery. Note that there is opacification of some of the external carotid artery vasculature as well.*

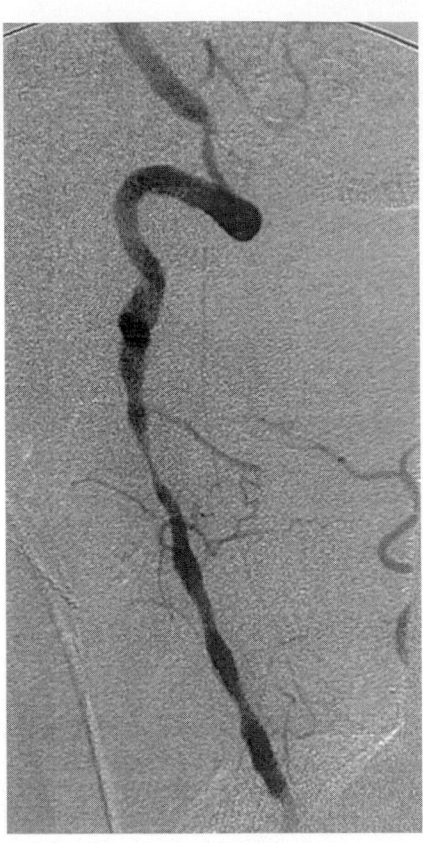

FIGURE 20–26   *Vertebral artery injection, lateral projection, arterial phase. Note the tandem stenoses.*

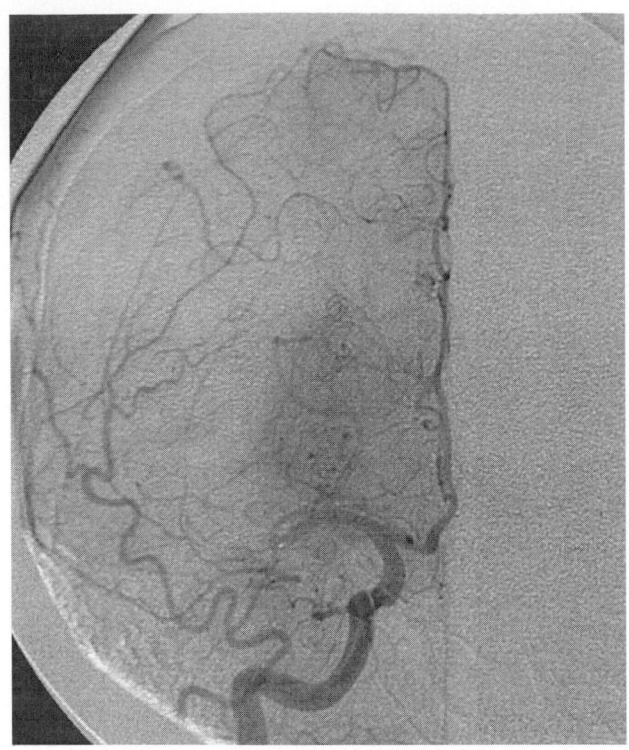

FIGURE 20–27   *Right internal carotid artery injection, frontal projection, demonstrating an abrupt M1 segment "cutoff."*

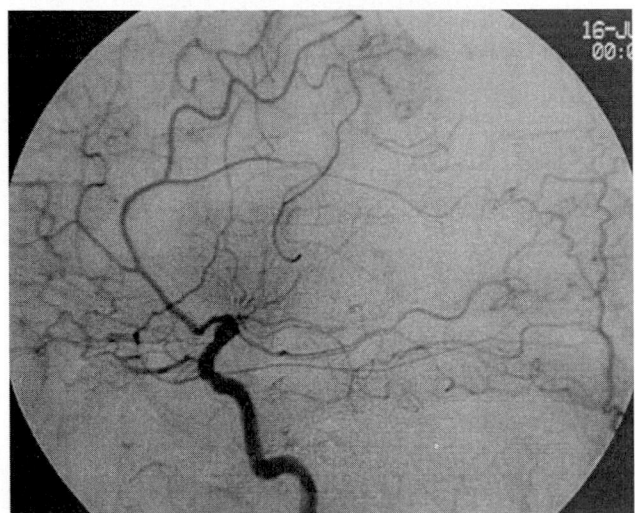

FIGURE 20–28   *Internal carotid artery injection, lateral projection, demonstrating the absence of opacification of the middle cerebral artery vasculature.*

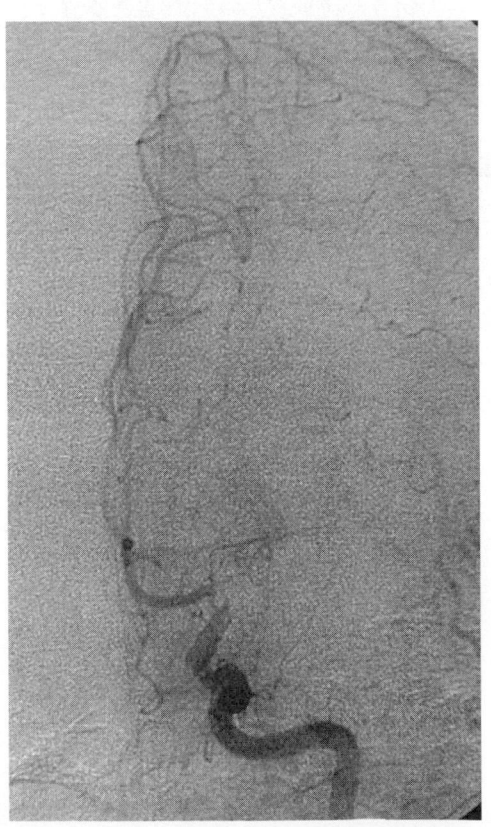

FIGURE 20–29   *Left internal carotid artery injection, frontal projection, demonstrates significant occlusion at the top of the internal carotid artery at its bifurcation. Note that some opacification of the left anterior cerebral artery vasculature is seen.*

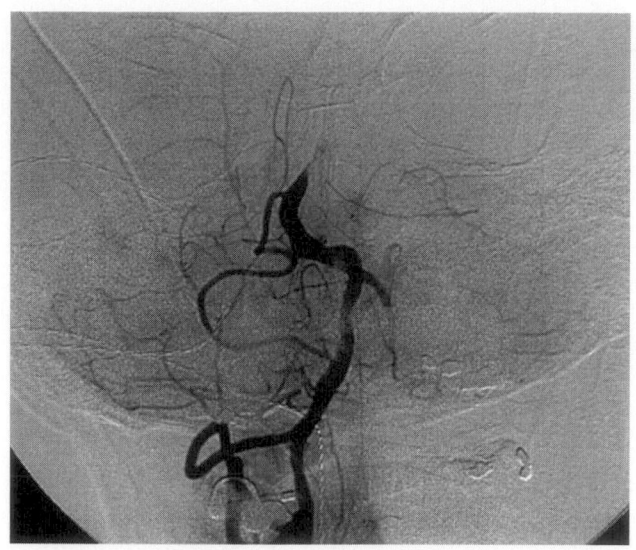

FIGURE 20–30 *This anteroposterior projection of the vertebrobasilar artery demonstrates occlusion of the basilar artery. Notice the parenchymal blush.*

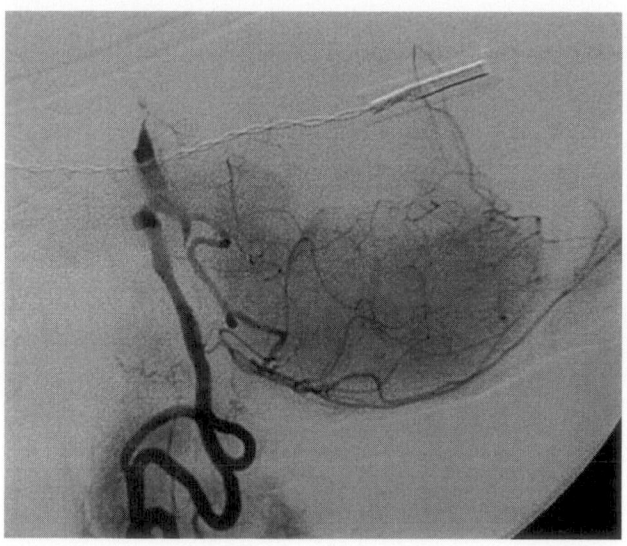

FIGURE 20–31 *Vertebral artery injection, lateral projection, demonstrating an abrupt "cutoff" of the basilar artery opacification.*

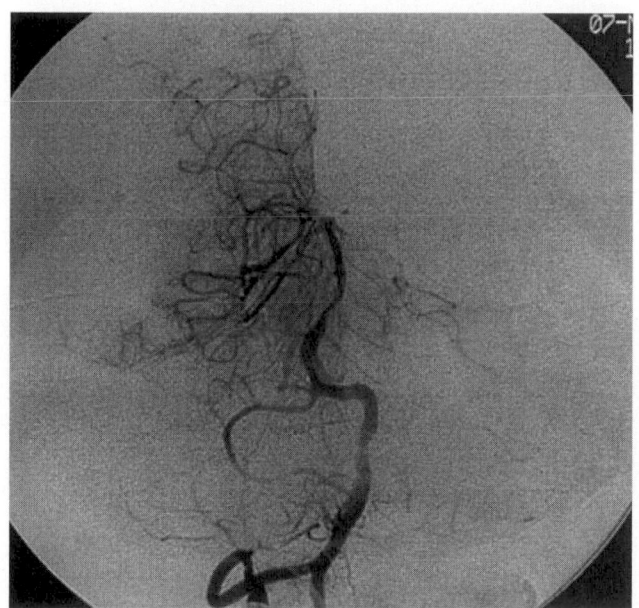

FIGURE 20–32 *Vertebral artery injection, anteroposterior projection, status post thrombolysis, demonstrates opacification of the entire basilar artery and the posterior cerebral artery vasculature.*

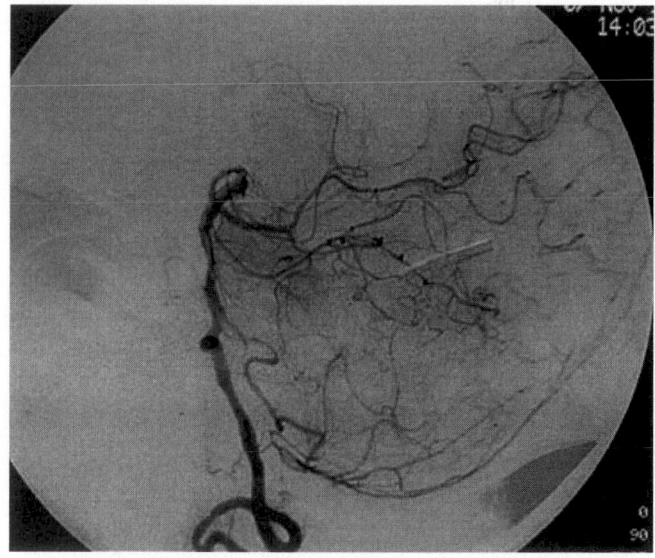

FIGURE 20–33 *Vertebral artery injection, lateral projection, demonstrating basilar artery status post thrombolysis with opacification of the entire basilar artery as well as posterior cerebral artery opacification.*

Diagnostic Studies

cause, a meniscus sign is often seen. Another finding is a relatively bare area seen in the capillary phase of the examination (this is perhaps the most sensitive angiographic sign of ischemia). Collateralization should be assessed in acute strokes, because the presence of collateral vessels indicates that the hypoperfused region has some blood supply, so irreversible injury may not occur for some time. Collateralization can take the following forms: (1) flow through the circle of Willis (i.e., anterior communicating artery and posterior communicating artery); (2) flow from the external carotid artery through the ophthalmic artery and then to the internal carotid artery, and (3) pial-to-pial flow. In the subacute phase, hours to weeks after ischemic strokes, "luxury perfusion" (hyperperfusion visualized as increased contrast radiodensity) may be seen.

Arteriovenous Malformations

An *arteriovenous malformation* is an abnormal connection between arteries and veins without an intervening capillary, producing a high-flow state with arteriovenous shunting of blood (see Figs. 20–19 to 20–22). These lesions can be associated with headaches, seizures, and other neurologic symptoms. Hemorrhages may be due to nidus vessel rupture or to rupture of an associated aneurysm. Associated aneurysms may be in the nidus or on a feeding artery, so-called flow-related aneurysms (see Figs. 20–21 and 20–22). This diagnosis is often made or at least suspected on MRI, MRA, or CT. Cerebral angiography is necessary to adequately characterize the arterial feeders and venous drainage as well as to search for associated aneurysms.

Treatment is based on the characteristics of the AVM and whether it involves neurologically eloquent territory. Among the treatment modalities are endovascular embolization, surgery, and stereotactic radiation surgery. Often, a combination of two or three therapies is required.[25]

Cervicocephalic Artery Dissection

Cervicocephalic arterial dissection has many possible causes, including trauma, fibromuscular dysplasia, and other vasculopathies. Dissection can manifest as ischemic stroke, and less often, SAH. The diagnosis of dissection can often be made on MRI, MRA, or CT angiography. In particular, nonenhanced axial T1-weighted, fat-saturated, MR images are sensitive for subacute dissection, because the blood in the vessel wall appears as high-signal intensity, contrasting with the flow void in the vessel lumen. Characteristic of dissection on angiography is tapering or narrowing of the vessel, in some cases to a string, or even total occlusion; in other cases, a flap may be visualized. Dissecting aneurysms may also be seen (see Figs. 20–15 and 20–16). Affected patients are most often managed medically.[26-28] However, in case of progressing ischemia, an endovascular procedure involving angioplasty and stenting may be beneficial.

Vasculitis

Intracranial vasculitis is suspected when multiple cerebral infarcts are detected in different vascular territories. There are many causes of intracranial vasculitis, both autoim-

mune and infectious. CT and especially MRI can strongly suggest the diagnosis in conjunction with the clinical history, but a cerebral angiogram is generally required for confirmation. The angiographic findings in intracranial vasculitis range from normal to demonstration of focal concentric narrowings, most prominent in the more distal vasculature. This appearance may mimic the vasospasm of SAH, but the clinical history distinguishes the two entities. Cerebral angiography is important to confirming the diagnosis of vasculitis before a patient is subjected to long-term corticosteroid and cytotoxic therapies with their potential side effects.

Another benefit of the cerebral angiogram in suspected vasculitis is that the external carotid artery can be injected as part of the procedure, to help plan for a superficial temporal artery biopsy if it is indicated to aid in diagnosis.

Takayasu's arteritis involves the proximal segments of the supra-aortic arteries. Its angiographic appearance is shown in Figure 20–34.

Fibromuscular Dysplasia

Fibromuscular dysplasia (FMD) is a vasculopathy of medium-sized arteries, with a prevalence of 0.5% to 0.7%.[29,31] This entity affects the cervical and intracranial vasculature. Most lesions occur at the C1–C2 level and spare the proximal aspect of the supra-aortic arteries.[29] The diagnosis is often made incidentally on a cerebral angiogram performed for diagnosis of intracranial aneurysm or dissection, both of which are often associated with fibromuscular dysplasia. The characteristic angiographic finding is alternation of dilated and stenosed regions to give a "string

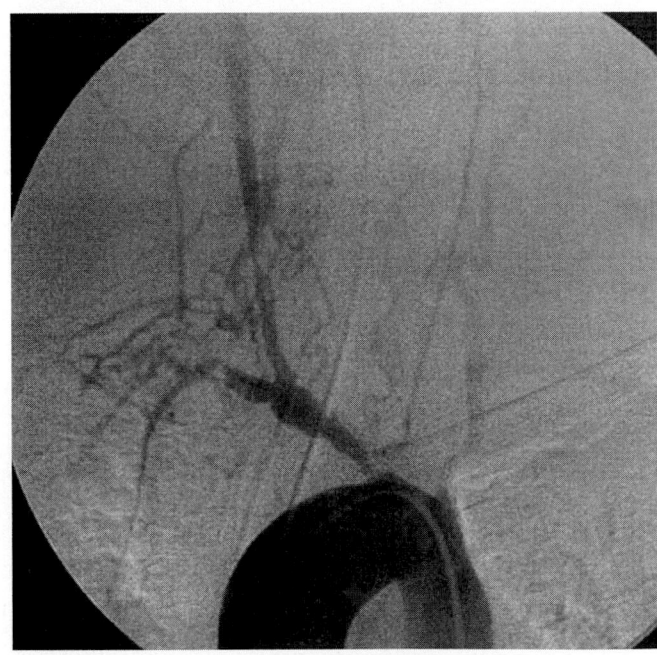

FIGURE 20–34 *Aortic arch injection demonstrating multiple large vessel tandem stenoses in Takayasu's arteritis. Notice how poorly the arch vessels are opacifying secondary to stenoses at vessel origins.*

of beads" appearance or, alternatively, a long tubular stenosis.[29–31]

Moyamoya Disease

Moyamoya disease is a condition named for its cerebral angiographic appearance—*moya moya* is the Japanese word for "puff of smoke." The cloudlike collateral networks of vessels in moyamoya disease are multiple small channels formed in response to the chronic occlusive vasculopathy affecting large arteries at the base of the brain.[32] Moyamoya disease can produce both ischemic and hemorrhagic strokes, with cerebral infarcts predominating in children and hemorrhagic and ischemic events relatively equally common in adults. Among the pathologic concomitants of this disease are aneurysms and AVMs, which were detected in 11% of patients reported by Chiu and coworkers.[32]

The diagnosis of moyamoya disease may be suspected from MRI or MRA findings. Cerebral angiography is required, however, for confirmation, precise anatomic depiction, and study of the external carotid circulation to guide revascularization therapy. The angiographic findings consist of bilateral stenotic occlusive disease in the intracranial internal carotid artery with thin multiple collateral vessels (Fig. 20–35).[33–35] The angiographic changes of moyamoya occur idiopathically in moyamoya disease but also in response to stenosing vasculopathy from diverse identified causes (moyamoya syndrome), including radiation vasculopathy, Down's syndrome, and early-onset intracranial atherosclerosis.

Cerebral Arterial Vasospasm

Arterial vasospasm of the intracranial arteries after SAH has an associated 15% to 20% risk of mortality.[36] Vasospasm is most common between 3 and 10 days after SAH. It is the principal cause of death and disability once the aneurysm has been secured by clipping or coiling. The diagnosis of vasospasm is generally suspected from clinical findings as well as transcranial Doppler ultrasonography, but confirmation usually requires a cerebral angiogram. Patients with symptomatic vasospasm despite adequate medical management, including hypertensive-hypervolemic therapy, are usually candidates for urgent cerebral angiography and angioplasty (balloon and/or chemical). In a patient with vasospasm, angiography shows narrowing of the vessels in a single or multiple regions. Spasm in the proximal intracranial arteries may be amenable to balloon angioplasty, and more distal spasm may be treated with intra-arterial injection of papaverine.

Cerebral Venous Thrombosis

Cerebral venous thrombosis refers to the occlusion of the cerebral veins or sinuses by thrombus. The superior sagittal sinus is affected in 72% of cases, and the lateral sinuses in 70%.[37] Multiple predisposing factors are associated with cerebral venous thrombosis, and a predisposing factor is identified in as much as 80% of cases.[37] Among these factors are intracranial infection, sepsis, brain surgery, tumor, hormonal causes, puerperium,[38] oral contraceptives,[39] hypercoagulable states, and dehydration. The clinical scenario is often one of slow progression of symptoms. Initial symptoms are generally nonspecific. Headache is the most common presenting symptom. Additional common symptoms are papilledema, vomiting, seizures, and focal neurologic deficits.[40] The diagnosis is often suggested by CT or MRI findings.

The angiographic appearance of cerebral venous thrombosis is characteristically seen in the venous phase of the imaging sequence. There is no (or little) opacification of the thrombosed sinus. A long arterial injection as well as a long imaging time must be used so as to give the venous system an adequate chance to opacify. Anteroposterior (AP), lateral, and oblique views should be obtained. Oblique imaging is very valuable, because often the entire sinus cannot be shown on the lateral view, and the anterior and posterior aspects of the sinus overlap on a true AP view. Imaging of superior sagittal sinus thrombosis is shown in Figure 20–36.

Anticoagulation is usually the first treatment attempted for cerebral venous thrombosis. If the patient's symptoms progress or there is no improvement over time, local catheter-guided pharmacologic or mechanical thrombolysis can be considered.[41–43]

Brain Death

The diagnosis of brain death rarely requires a cerebral angiogram. If confirmatory laboratory tests are needed to supplement clinical findings, a diagnosis can be established with the use of nuclear medicine, electrophysiology, transcranial Doppler ultrasonography, and other noninvasive methods. For brain death to be diagnosed on cerebral angiography, there should be no contrast opacification of intracranial vessels after injection of contrast agent into the brachiocephalic vasculature. The shutdown of the entire cerebral circulation reflects increased intracranial pressure due to brain swelling.

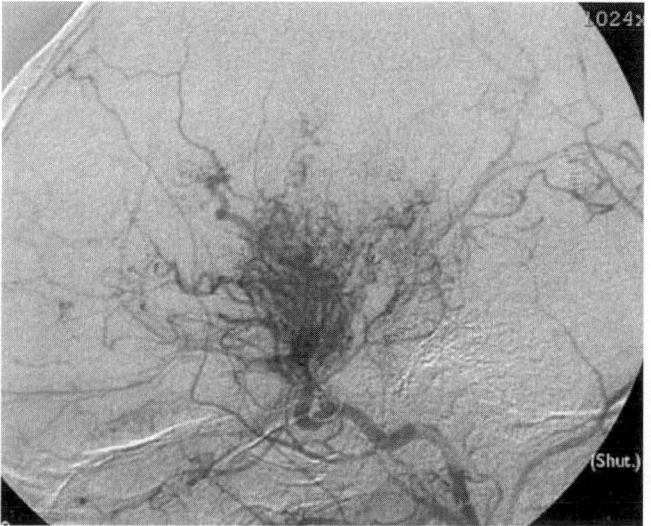

FIGURE 20–35 *Internal carotid artery injection, lateral projection, demonstrating absence of the normal vasculature and a "puff of smoke" appearance to the distribution of opacification.*

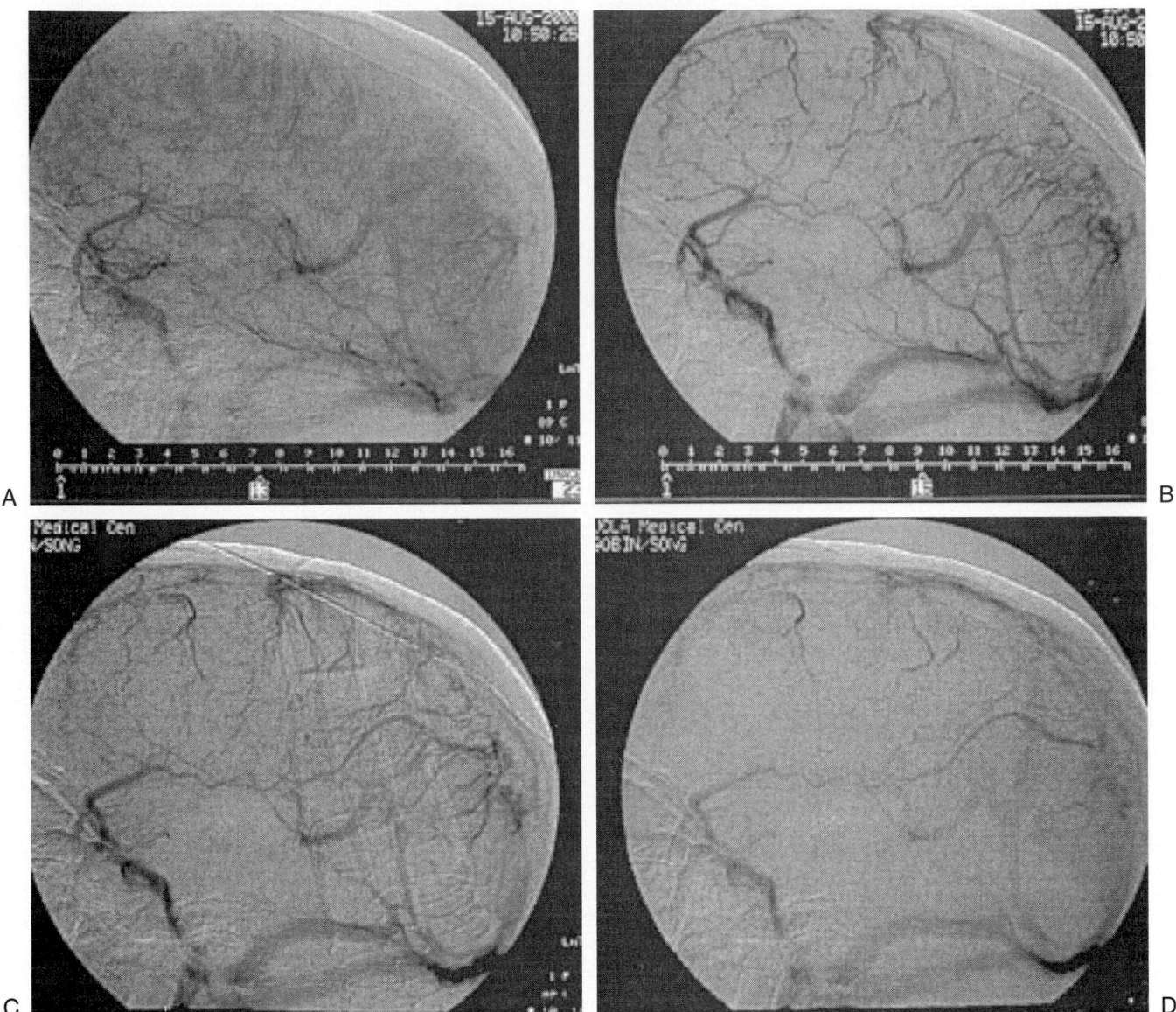

FIGURE 20–36   A–D. *Lateral view of entire venous phase demonstrating no significant opacification of the superior saggital sinus. (Images are a sequence of the "verous phase"—A being earlier than D.)*

References

1. Wolpert SM: Neuroradiology classics. AJNR Am J Neuroradiol 20:1752–1753, 1999.
2. Rosenbaum AE, Eldevik OP, Mani JR, et al: In re: Amundsen P. Cerebral angiography via the femoral artery with particular reference to cerebrovascular disease, Acta Neurol Scand Suppl, 31:115, 1967. AJNR Am J Neuroradiol 22:584–589, 2001.
3. Leffers AM, Wagner A: Neurologic complications of cerebral angiography: A retrospective study of complication rate and patient risk factors. Acta Radiol 41:204–210, 2000.
4. Dion JE, Gates PC, Fox AJ, et al: Clinical events following neuroangiography: A prospective study. Stroke 18:997–1004, 1987.
5. Quality improvement guidelines for adult diagnostic neuroangiography: Cooperative study between ASITN, ASNR and SCVIR. American Society of Interventional and Therapeutic Neuroradiology. American Society of Neuroradiology. Society of Cardiovascular and Interventional Radiology. J Vasc Interv Radiol 11:129–234, 2000.
6. Hankey GJ, Warlow CP, Sellar RJ: Cerebral angiographic risk in mild cerebrovascular disease. Stroke 21:209–222, 1990.
7. Gerraty RP, Bowser DN, Infeld B, et al: Microemboli during carotid angiography: Association with stroke risk factors or subsequent magnetic resonance imaging changes? Stroke 27:1543–1547, 1996.
8. Cloft HJ, Jensen ME, Kallmes DF, Dion JE: Arterial dissections complicating cerebral angiography and cerebrovascular interventions. AJNR Am J Neuroradiol 21:541–545, 2000.
9. Cloft HJ, Joseph GJ, Dion JE: Risk of cerebral angiography in patients with subarachnoid hemorrhage, cerebral aneurysm, and arteriovenous malformation: A meta-analysis. Stroke 30:317–320, 1999.
10. Bendszus M, Koltzenberg M, Burger R, et al: Silent embolism in diagnostic cerebral angiography and neurointerventional procedures: A prospective study. Lancet 354:1594–1597, 1999.
11. Wardlaw JM, White PM: The detection and management of unruptured intracranial aneurysms [review]. Brain 123:205–221, 2000.
12. van Gijn J, Rinkel GJ: Subarachnoid haemorrhage: Diagnosis, causes and management. Brain 124:249–278, 2001.
13. Ruigrok YM, Rinkel GJ, Buskens E, et al: Perimesencephalic hemorrhage and CT angiography: A decision analysis. Stroke 31:2976–2983, 2000.

Diagnostic Studies

14. Mariani L, Bianchetti MG, Schroth G, Seiler RW: Cerebral aneurysms in patients with autosomal dominant polycystic kidney disease—to screen, to clip, to coil? Nephrol Dial Transplant 14:2319–2322, 1999.

15. Pirson Y, Chauveau D, Torres V: Management of cerebral aneurysms in autosomal dominant polycystic kidney disease. J Am Soc Nephrol 13:269–276, 2002.

16. van den Berg JS, Limburg M, Hennekam RC: Is Marfan syndrome associated with symptomatic intracranial aneurysms? Stroke 27:10–12, 1996.

17. Culebras A, Kase CS, Masdeu JC, et al: Practice guidelines for the use of imaging in transient ischemic attacks and acute stroke: A report of the Stroke Council, American Heart Association. Stroke 28:1480–1497, 1997.

18. Gonner F, Remonda L, Mattle H, Sturzenegger M, et al: Local intra-arterial thrombolysis in acute ischemic stroke. Stroke 29:1894–1900, 1998.

19. Keris V, Rudnicka S, Vorona V, et al: Combined intraarterial/intravenous thrombolysis for acute ischemic stroke. AJNR Am J Neuroradiol 22:352–358, 2001.

20. Tissue plasminogen activator for acute ischemic stroke: The National Institute of Neurological Disorders and Stroke rt-PA Stroke Study Group. N Engl J Med 333:1581–1587, 1995.

21. Sliwka U, Klotzsch C, Popescu O, et al: Do chronic middle cerebral artery stenoses represent an embolic focus? A multirange transcranial Doppler study. Stroke 28:1324–1327, 1997.

22. Lyrer PA, Engelter S, Radu EW, Steck AJ: Cerebral infarcts related to isolated middle cerebral artery stenosis. Stroke 28:1022–1027, 1997.

23. Segura T, Serena J, Castellanos M, et al: Embolism in acute middle cerebral artery stenosis. Neurology 56:497–501, 2001.

24. Thijs VN, Albers GW: Symptomatic intracranial atherosclerosis: Outcome of patients who fail antithrombotic therapy. Neurology 55:490–497, 2000.

25. Al-Shahi R, Warlow C: A systematic review of the frequency and prognosis of arteriovenous malformations of the brain in adults [review]. Brain 124:1900–1926, 2001.

26. Bassetti C, Carruzzo A, Sturzenegger M, Tuncdogan E: Recurrence of cervical artery dissection: A prospective study of 81 patients. Stroke 27:1804–1807, 1996.

27. Brandt T, Orberk E, Weber R, et al: Pathogenesis of cervical artery dissections: Association with connective tissue abnormalities. Neurology 57:24–30, 2001.

28. Schievink WI, Mokri B, O'Fallon WM: Recurrent spontaneous cervical-artery dissection. N Engl J Med 330:393–397, 1994.

29. Kubis N, Von Langsdorff D, Petitjean C, et al: Thrombotic carotid megabulb: Fibromuscular dysplasia, septae, and ischemic stroke. Neurology 52:883–886, 1999.

30. Osborn AG, Anderson RE: Angiographic spectrum of cervical and intracranial fibromuscular dysplasia. Stroke 8:617–626, 1977.

31. Finsterer J, Strassegger J, Haymerle A, Hagmuller G: Bilateral stenting of symptomatic and asymptomatic internal carotid artery stenosis due to fibromuscular dysplasia. J Neurol Neurosurg Psychiatry 69:683–686, 2000.

32. Chiu D, Shedden P, Bratina P, Grotta JC: Clinical features of moyamoya disease in the United States. Stroke 29:1347–1351, 1998.

33. de Veber G:: Vascular occlusion in moyamoya: A multitude of mechanisms [editorial comment]? Stroke 32:1791–1792, 2001.

34. Bonduel M, Hepner M, Sciuccati G, et al: Prothrombotic disorders in children with moyamoya syndrome. Stroke 32:1786–1792, 2001.

35. Bitzer M, Topka H: Progressive cerebral occlusive disease after radiation therapy. Stroke 26:131–136, 1995.

36. Lysakowski C, Walder B, Costanza MC, Tramer MR: Transcranial Doppler versus angiography in patients with vasospasm due to a ruptured cerebral aneurysm: A systematic review. Stroke 32:2292–2298, 2001.

37. Allroggen H, Abbott RJ: Cerebral venous sinus thrombosis. Postgrad Med J 76:12–15, 2000.

38. Lanska DJ, Kryscio RJ: Risk factors for peripartum and postpartum stroke and intracranial venous thrombosis. Stroke 31:1274–1282, 2000.

39. Vandenbroucke JP: Cerebral sinus thrombosis and oral contraceptives: There are limits to predictability. BMJ 317(7157):483–484, 1998.

40. Daif A, Awada A, al-Rajeh S, et al: Cerebral venous thrombosis in adults: A study of 40 cases from Saudi Arabia. Stroke 26:1193–1195, 1995.

41. Chow K, Gobin YP, Saver J, et al: Endovascular treatment of dural sinus thrombosis with rheolytic thrombectomy and intra-arterial thrombolysis. Stroke 31:1420–1425, 2000.

42. Frey JL, Muro GJ, McDougall CG, et al: Cerebral venous thrombosis: Combined intrathrombus rtPA and intravenous heparin. Stroke 30:489–494, 1999.

43. Benamer HT, Bone I: Cerebral venous thrombosis: Anticoagulants or thrombolytic therapy? J Neurol Neurosurg Psychiatry 69:427–430, 2000.

Diagnostic Studies

Chapter Twenty-One

Ultrasonography

Stephen Meairs, Michael Hennerici, and J. P. Mohr

More than three decades ago, continuous-wave (CW) Doppler ultrasonography was introduced as the first neurosonologic method for evaluation of cerebrovascular disease. Since that time, the continuous development of noninvasive ultrasound techniques has resulted in many clinical applications for assessment of extracranial and intracranial arterial diseases. In this chapter, we discuss the clinical merits and limitations of ultrasonographic techniques for evaluation of both early and advanced cerebrovascular disease. We outline approaches for identification of stroke etiology and summarize how neurosonology is used for monitoring of patients with stroke. We also address recent developments in both qualitative and quantitative assessment of cerebral perfusion as well as advances in ultrasonographic techniques for molecular imaging, acceleration of thrombolysis, and gene therapy.

ULTRASOUND TECHNOLOGY

Doppler Ultrasonography

Ultrasonographic Doppler techniques are commonly used for examining the intracranial and extracranial arteries supplying the brain. Interpretation of Doppler signals is based on analysis of the audio signals and of the frequency spectrum. The *Doppler effect* is named after Christian Doppler, who in 1842 described the change in frequency of light emitted by moving objects. This effect is familiar to anyone who has stood in one place and listened to a source of sound passing by. The sound rises in pitch as the source approaches the listener and then equally drops off as the source moves away after passing. In clinical applications, this effect is known as the *Doppler frequency shift*, which is the difference between emitted and received ultrasonography frequency, and is proportional to the velocity of moving blood cells.

CW Doppler systems use two transducers, one of which emits while the other receives ultrasound continuously (Fig. 21–1). Although this simple system is easily applicable for the detection of a broad range of alterations in flow velocity, including the high blood flow velocities associated with severe stenosis, it provides only limited information about the topographic origin of the ultrasound-reflecting source. In contrast, pulsed-wave (PW) Doppler systems, in which ultrasound is both emitted from and received by a single piezoelectric crystal in the transducer, can provide

a depth estimate of the site being insonated (Fig. 21–2). This feature, along with information on the direction of the Doppler frequency shift, is used in transcranial PW Doppler ultrasonography to locate and differentiate intracranial cerebral arteries. Although CW and PW Doppler techniques are simple, inexpensive screening procedures for detection of stenoses and occlusions in the extracranial arteries, they have been largely replaced by more sophisticated ultrasonographic techniques offering real-time display of the vessel walls and lumen combined with color-coded visualization of blood flow (Fig. 21–3). PW Doppler transcranial, however, still plays a significant role in transcranial investigation of cerebrovascular disease.

Imaging Techniques

A number of complementary ultrasonographic techniques are available for evaluation of the intracranial and extracranial arteries and for visualization of the brain parenchyma. They are summarized here.

B-mode scanning displays the morphologic features of normal and diseased vessels.[1-4] Because the extracranial carotid and vertebral arteries lie near the skin, linear-array transducers are commonly used at ultrasound frequencies of 7.0 to 12.0 MHz. A number of transcranial imaging applications for assessment of structural alterations in the brain have emerged. The brain must be imaged through the transtemporal bone window, so these applications usually employ 2.0 MHz phased or curved-array transducers.

Duplex ultrasonography combines integrated PW Doppler spectrum analysis and B-mode scanning. In addition to providing information about the presence and morphology of arterial lesions, the B-mode image serves as a guide for the placement of the PW Doppler sample volume (Fig. 21–4). Distinct criteria of the Doppler spectrum analysis (see later) are then used to evaluate hemodynamics and to categorize carotid artery stenoses. The common carotid artery (CCA), internal carotid artery (ICA), and external carotid artery (ECA) are usually characterized by a relatively distinct Doppler frequency spectrum, allowing their identification upon insonation with a PW Doppler system. The emission frequency of the integrated PW Doppler system ranges between 4 and 7 MHz.

Color Doppler flow imaging (CDFI) preserves the advantages of duplex ultrasonography and also demonstrates

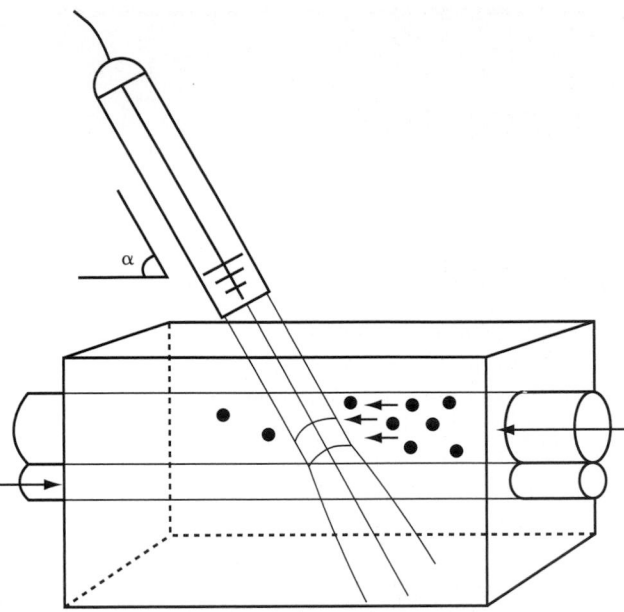

FIGURE 21–1 *Continuous-wave Doppler ultrasonography uses a single piezo crystal for both transmitting and receiving ultrasound signals. (From Hennerici M, Rautenberg W, Steinke W: Ultrasonography. In Mohr JP, Gautier J-C [eds]: Guide to Clinical Neurology. St. Louis, Churchill Livingstone, 1995, p 185.)*

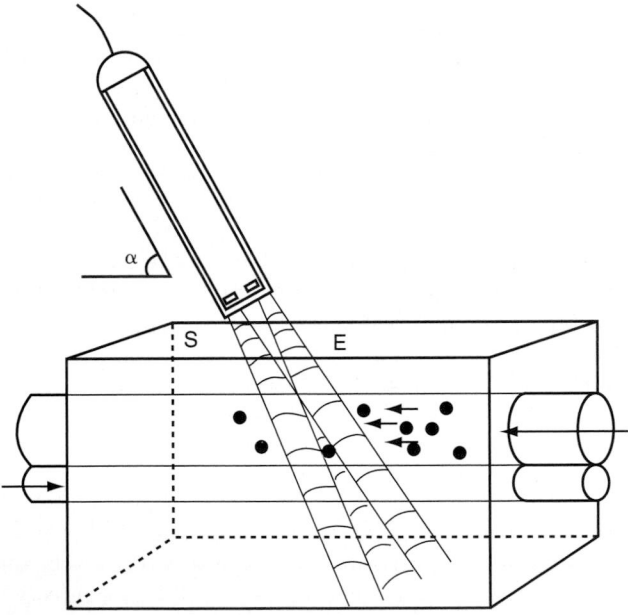

FIGURE 21–2 *Pulsed-wave Doppler ultrasonography uses separate piezo crystals, one emitting (E) and one receiving (S) ultrasound waves. This allows location of the sample volume. (From Hennerici M, Rautenberg W, Steinke W: Ultrasonography. In Mohr JP, Gautier J-C [eds]: Guide to Clinical Neurology. St. Louis, Churchill Livingstone, 1995, p 185.)*

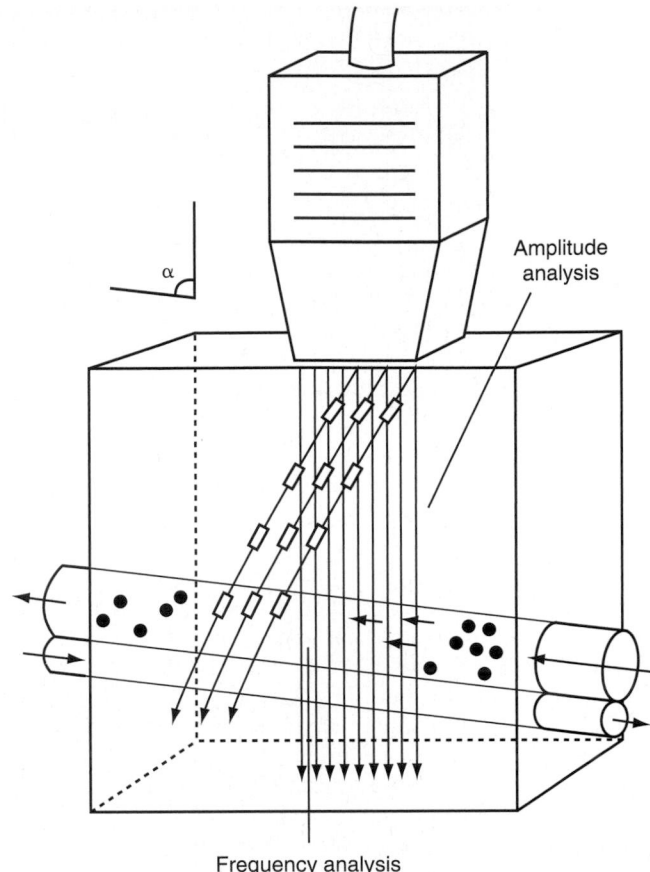

FIGURE 21–3 *Color-coded duplex ultrasonography combines B-mode echotomography and flow velocity signals for structural and hemodynamic analysis. (From Hennerici M, Rautenberg W, Steinke W: Ultrasonography. In Mohr JP, Gautier J-C [eds]: Guide to Clinical Neurology. St. Louis, Churchill Livingstone, 1995, p 185.)*

color-coded blood flow patterns superimposed on the grayscale B-mode image.[5–7] With use of a defined color scale, the direction and the average mean velocity of moving blood cells within the sample volume at a given point in time are encoded. Generation of color signals is based on the detection of frequency and phase shifts by means of a multigate transducer. The technique of autocorrelation is used to obtain a real-time visualization of color-coded hemodynamics.

Power Doppler imaging (PDI) displays the amplitude of Doppler signals. Color and brightness of the signals are related to the number of blood cells producing the Doppler shift. PDI is more sensitive for detection of blood flow than CDFI (Table 21.1). The reason is that PDI is less angle-dependent than CDFI, thus allowing better display of curving or tortuous vessels. Reliance upon Doppler amplitude means that there is no aliasing, which appears when an analog signal is sampled at a frequency that is lower than the half of its maximum frequency. The lack of aliasing of signal improves the display of vessel wall disease in areas of turbulent flow. Moreover, more of the dynamic range of the Doppler signal can be used in PDI to improve

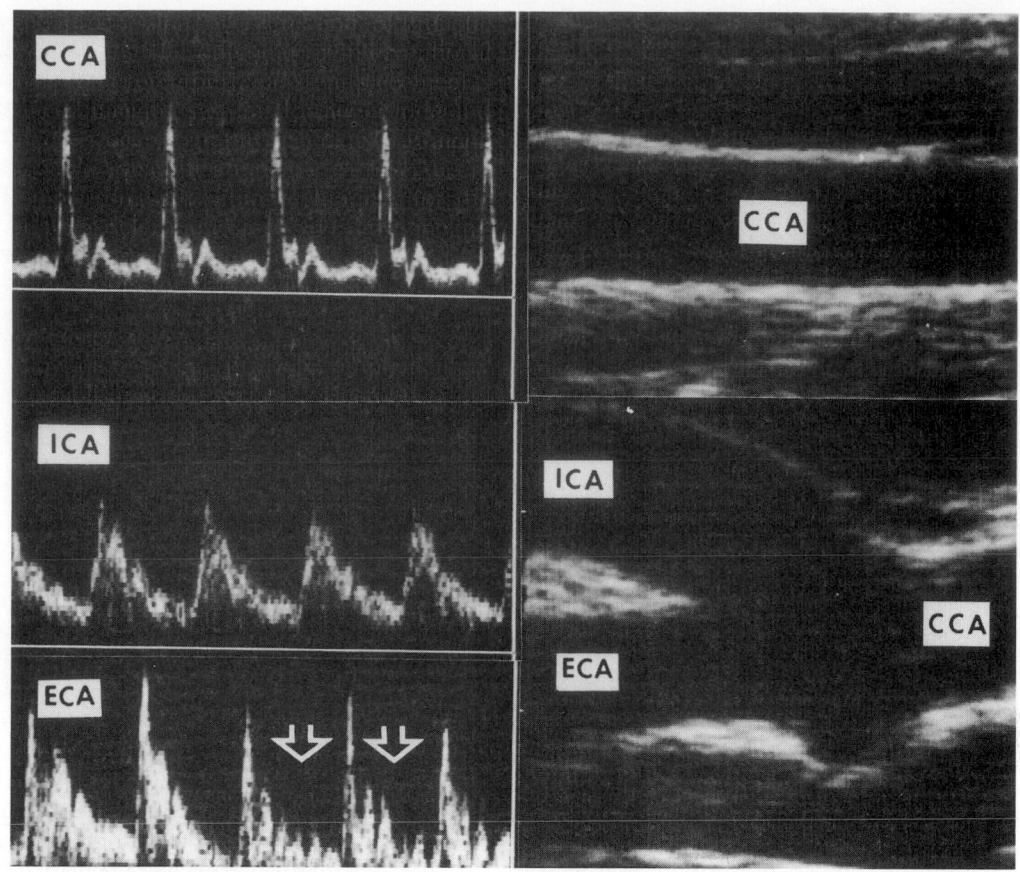

FIGURE 21–4 *Duplex system analysis of a normal carotid artery. Doppler frequency spectra* (left) *and B-mode echotomograms* (right) *of the common carotid artery* (CCA) *and the bifurcation with internal carotid artery* (ICA) *and external carotid artery* (ECA). *High systolic flow and low diastolic flow and transmitted oscillation* (open arrows) *in the ECA from tapping of the superficial temporal artery. Flow in the ICA is high in diastole, reflecting a low-resistance pattern. The Doppler waveform in the CCA reflects the two vascular beds it supplies, but it is dominated by the low-resistance flow to the brain.*

Table 21.1   Technical Differences between Color Doppler Flow Imaging (CDFI) and Power Doppler Imaging (PDI)

	CDFI	PDI
Physical principle	Frequency and phase shift	Echo amplitude
Color-coded information	Mean velocity and direction	Density of blood cells
Hemodynamic information	Display in real time	None
Angle dependence of color display	Present	Absent
Aliasing phenomenon	Above Nyqist limit	Absent
	Good definition of plaque surface	Improved display of high-grade stenoses
Intravascular color contrast		Improved visualization in calcified plaques
Motion artifacts	Rare	Frequent

sensitivity. PDI is a valuable technique for displaying plaque surface structure (Plate 21–1 following page 504).[8,9]

Real-time compound imaging is a new modality that enhances ultrasonographic visualization and characterization of carotid artery plaques.[10,11] This technique acquires ultrasound beams, which are steered off-axis from the orthogonal beams used in conventional ultrasonography. The number of frames and steering angles varies, depending on the transducer characteristics. Frames acquired from sufficiently different angles contain independent random speckle patterns, which are averaged to reduce speckle and improve tissue differentiation.

Three-dimensional (3D) ultrasonography can be used for both qualitative and quantitative analysis of plaques in the carotid artery. Surface features of carotid plaques, which are not readily appreciated in conventional two-dimensional B-mode scanning, can be clearly demonstrated by 3D ultrasonography. In some cases, use of this modality may lead to a diagnosis not obtainable with other imaging techniques.[12] New developments in 3D ultra-

Diagnostic Studies

sonography image acquisition involve the use of position and orientation measurement (POM) devices capable of tracking scanheads in six degrees of freedom (6-DOF).[13–16] This approach allows "freehand" scanning to collect image data from different perspectives and potentially offers the ability to maximize tissue information that is not readily available from one imaging plane alone (Plate 21–2). Methods for enhanced reconstruction and visualization of 6-DOF ultrasonography data are now available.[17]

Contrast harmonic imaging (CHI) is based on the non-linear emission of harmonics by resonant microbubbles pulsating in an ultrasound field. The emission at twice the driving frequency, termed the *second harmonic*, can be detected and separated from the fundamental frequency. The advantage of the harmonic over the fundamental frequency is that microbubbles of contrast agent resonate with harmonic frequencies, whereas adjacent tissues do so very little. In this way, CHI may enhance the signal-to-noise ratio and the ability of B-mode scanners to differentiate bubbles in the tissue vascular space from the echogenic surrounding avascular tissue (Fig. 21–5).

MONITORING ATHEROSCLEROSIS

Intima-Media Thickness

Pignoli and coworkers were the first to characterize a "double-line" pattern of the normal carotid artery wall with B-mode ultrasonography.[18] They described the first echogenic line on the far wall to represent the lumen-intima interface and the second line to correspond to the media-adventitia interface. Significantly, they demonstrated that the distance between these two echogenic lines correlated highly with measurements of intima-media thickness (IMT) in tissue specimens from common carotid arteries. This initial report on measurement of IMT with B-mode scanning was later validated in vitro[19] and was shown to enable good intraobserver and interobserver reproducibility.[20]

Many studies have used high-resolution ultrasonography to establish associations between common carotid IMT, cardiovascular risk factors,[21,22] and the prevalence of cardiovascular disease.[23] The Cardiovascular Health Study Collaborative Research Group has identified carotid artery IMT as a risk factor for both myocardial infarction and stroke in older adults.[24] The growing importance of common carotid IMT is reflected by its use as a surrogate endpoint for determining the success of interventions that lower the levels of low-density lipoprotein cholesterol. Likewise, IMT measurements have been used to assess the effect of supplementary vitamin E intake in reducing the progression of atherosclerosis while the process is still confined to the arterial wall.[25] Another study demonstrated the positive impact of antibiotic treatment on the progression of IMT in patients with stroke who were seropositive for *Chlamydia pneumoniae*.[26] IMT evaluation has also been utilized to assess the anti-atherosclerotic action of the calcium antagonist lacidipine.[27]

Sampling

Because of the focal location of sites of reactive intimal thickening and initial plaque development in the carotid arteries is related to geometric transitions, the selection of precise regions for measurement of IMT is important (Plate 21–3). Any single examination by ultrasonography may not identify the site of maximal intimal thickening. Therefore, IMT examinations over a range of incident angles and axial locations are necessary. Several IMT sampling protocols have been introduced. Some use IMT measurements of the CCA, where the double-line pattern is easier to visualize. Others include IMT at the carotid bifurcation and at the ICA. Some studies have calculated IMT means obtained from both normal and abnormal walls.[20,28,29] Use of these aggregate measurements has been shown to improve reliability.[20] The type of IMT sampling used—combined measurements at different sites, measurements only at the CCA, mean or maximum wall thickness—may largely depend on the research question and on the relative emphasis accorded to confirmed atherosclerotic lesions.[30]

Serial Measurements

A major source of error in the longitudinal assessment of IMT is the difficulty of retrieving the same echographic view of the vessel. Although the mean IMT might be regarded as a reproducible parameter by which to evaluate differences between populations exposed to diverse risk factors, evolutionary or therapy-induced changes in the individual may be better monitored in defined carotid

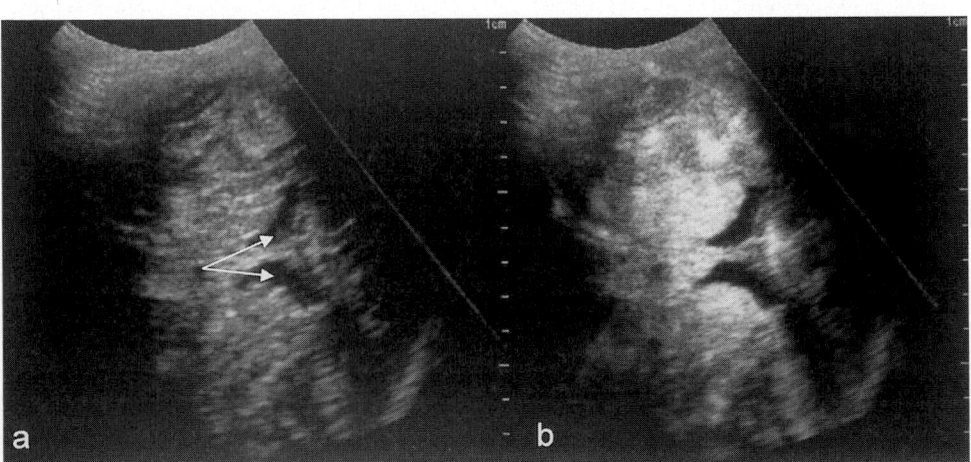

FIGURE 21–5 *Pulse-inversion contrast harmonic imaging of the brain using a 2- to 5-MHz dynamic range, curved-array transducer on an HDI 5000 platform (Philips Ultrasound). The images from a transverse section through the brain at the level of the frontal horns of the lateral ventricles* (arrows) *illustrate tissue contrast enhancement before* (**A**) *and after* (**B**) *an intravenous bolus injection of galactose and palmitic acid (Levovist).*

sectors. External reference points have been proposed to improve reproducibility.[31] Another approach uses matching of baseline ultrasonographic images with a corresponding view that minimizes the vessel contour by means of the discrete Fourier transform.[32] Although the feasibility of these methods has been demonstrated, there are no data supporting their use in larger clinical trials of serial IMT measurements.

Quality Control

Sources of potential variability in IMT measurements associated with both image acquisition (sonographers) and interpretation (readers) have led to development of quality control procedures in many laboratories. These procedures include periodical expert review by trained neurologists or neuroradiologists, replicate baseline readings to identify outliers, standard films to check against reader variability and drift, second readings for data verification, use of standardized ultrasound equipment, and appropriate blinding of sonographers and technicians to clinical status or treatment assignment.

Pathophysiologic Correlates

Although an increased IMT is generally considered to reflect early atherosclerotic plaque formation, this consideration may not always be true. Intimal hyperplasia and intimal fibrocellular hypertrophy are two types of nonatherosclerotic intimal reactions associated with local modifications of flow and mural tension that are likely to represent adaptive or self-limiting compensatory changes. Intimal fibrocellular hypertrophy, a layered widening of both smooth muscle cells and matrix fibers, can be quite extensive in a particular arterial segment and is not necessarily of uniform width. Early atherosclerotic lesions, on the other hand, are characterized by a focal eccentric accumulation of lipid in the intima, in the extracellular matrix interstices as well as in smooth muscle cells and macrophages. These early lesions do not project into the vessel lumen or modify the surface contour, and endothelial cells are anatomically intact. Superimpositions of intimal fibrocellular hypertrophy, intimal hyperplasia, and atherosclerosis are common. IMT, as measured by B-mode scanning, is a heterogeneous entity reflecting normal ageing and atherosclerosis, the differentiation of which is limited and possible only from subsequent follow-up studies to some extent.

Intima-Media Thickness and Future Stroke Research

As a marker integrating endogenous and exogenous risk factors of atherosclerosis, IMT measurements may be used to screen populations exposed to vascular disease. However, several problems pertaining to the standardization of these measurements must be solved. The differentiation among atherosclerosis, remodeling, inflammatory processes, and unknown mechanisms that can lead to thickening of the arterial wall requires further elucidation. Prospective studies on large populations will be necessary to define the predictive values of a normal or thickened arterial wall for ischemic stroke. This definition may allow the introduction of IMT measurements into clinical practice for improved assessment of stroke risk in individual patients. Likewise, because many studies have demonstrated stabilization or regression of IMT with hypolipidemic drug therapy, IMT monitoring may provide new parameters for evaluation of therapeutic interventions in patients with both early and advanced atherosclerotic disease.

Endothelium-Dependent Flow-Mediated Vasodilation

The endothelium synthesizes and releases nitric oxide (NO) to regulate homeostatic function. Endothelium-derived NO maintains a nonthrombogenic surface, prohibits leukocyte attachment, and promotes vascular relaxation. In situations associated with atherothrombosis, the bioavailability of NO is decreased because of diminished synthesis and release as well as increased generation of reactive oxygen species. This decrease alters vascular homeostatic mechanisms and promotes platelet aggregation, inflammatory cell diapedesis, and vasoconstriction.

Endothelial dysfunction may be evaluated with high-frequency ultrasonographic imaging of the brachial artery to assess endothelium-dependent flow-mediated dilation (FMD) of blood vessels.[33] The technique provokes the release of NO, resulting in vasodilation, which serves as an index of vasomotor function. Ischemia-induced hyperemia in the distal forearm is usually used as a stimulus to produce a two- to five-fold increase in brachial blood flow.[34,35] High-resolution B-mode scanning measures the diameter of the artery before and after the flow stimulus. A detailed description of ultrasonographic assessment of FMD with guidelines for research application of this technique has been published by the International Brachial Artery Reactivity Task Force.[36]

Ultrasonographic studies of FMD have demonstrated an abnormal endothelium-dependent vasodilation in subjects with coronary artery disease (CAD).[37] Patients with CAD had lower FMD than controls, and this difference was statistically significant after smokers were excluded. In addition, not only is brachial artery reactivity impaired in patients with CAD but also the impairment is related to the extent and severity of CAD.[38] Hypercholesterolemia is associated with abnormal FMD in children and in adults with significant correlations between levels of low-density lipoprotein (LDL) and Lp(a) lipoprotein and endothelium-dependent vasodilation.[33,39] The mechanism by which hypercholesterolemia impairs endothelial function is not completely understood, but evidence suggests that oxidative stress has an important role in mediating the effects of hypercholesterolemia. Likewise, significantly reduced FMD has been found in insulin-dependent diabetes,[40] the magnitude of which correlates with duration of disease and levels of LDL cholesterol.[41] Impairment of nitric oxide–mediated vasodilation has also been shown in patients with non–insulin-dependent diabetes mellitus.[42] One study has found correlations between levels of circulating endothelial progenitor cells and FMD.[43] This is a particularly interesting finding, because endothelial progenitor cells derived from bone marrow may have a role in ongoing endothelial repair, and impaired mobilization or depletion of these cells may contribute to endothelial dysfunction and cardiovascular disease progression.

Diagnostic Studies

Although the assessment of endothelial function with FMD is a promising technique that may reflect an independent measure of cardiovascular disease (CVD) risk, additional prospective research is needed to demonstrate that this technique can truly add to standard CVD risk prediction. Standardization and improvement of the measurement technique are needed before this modality can become a part of routine clinical assessment of CVD risk.[44]

Assessment of Advanced Atherosclerotic Disease

In the initial period of the development of methods of cerebrovascular ultrasonographic studies, insonation of the ophthalmic artery was used as an indirect test for detection of significant carotid artery stenosis.[45–48] This periorbital technique rapidly provides information about the existence of collateral pathways. In the presence of severe stenosis or occlusion of the ICA, retrograde blood supply from the ECA via the ophthalmic anastomosis can be easily detected with CW Doppler ultrasonography. However, with sufficient collateralization from the contralateral carotid artery or the vertebrobasilar systems, orthograde perfusion of the ophthalmic artery may occur. Accordingly, this indirect test fails to detect even hemodynamically significant ipsilateral carotid obstruction in up to 20% of patients. Thus, although detection of retrograde perfusion in the ophthalmic artery is a strong indicator of severe disease within the ipsilateral extracranial carotid system, finding normal perfusion of the ophthalmic branches cannot exclude severe carotid stenosis or occlusion.

Doppler ultrasonography can be used directly over the extracranial carotid artery to detect various degrees of carotid obstruction. According to the distribution of abnormal blood flow patterns measured within, proximal to, or distal to a narrowed arterial segment, this technique provides data on the extent, site, and severity of lesions of more than 40% lumen narrowing. In such lesions, the sensitivity (92% to 100%) and specificity (93% to 100%) of various Doppler techniques have been shown to be similar to those of arteriography.[49,50] Special transducers can be used to assess distal extracranial lesions of the ICA, such as carotid dissections,[51] fibromuscular dysplasia, and atypically located atherosclerosis.

Grading Carotid Artery Stenosis

An international consensus meeting has established criteria for the quantification of ICA stenosis.[52] Recommendations for interpretation of maximum Doppler shift velocities (Table 21.2), systolic velocity ratios, and residual area are summarized here.

Mild stenosis (40% to 60% of lumen diameter) is characterized by a local increase of peak and mean flow velocities. Systolic peak velocities range above 120 cm/sec (4-MHz probe).

Moderate stenosis (60% to 80%) shows a distortion of normal pulsatile flow in addition to a local increase of peak and mean frequencies. Typically, systolic flow decelerations are found in the post-stenotic segment. The systolic peak velocity ranges from 120 to 240 cm/sec.

Severe stenosis (more than 80% as estimated by Doppler studies) produces markedly increased peak flow velocities exceeding 240 cm/sec and occasionally reaching over 600 cm/sec (Plate 21–4). In addition, pre- and post-stenotic blood flow velocities are significantly lower than those in the contralateral, unaffected carotid artery. Retrograde flow in the ophthalmic artery may occur.

Subtotal stenosis (more than 95%) is characterized by variable, usually low peak flow velocities, which decrease once a stenosis becomes pseudo-occlusive. This condition is difficult to separate from complete occlusion and may be misdiagnosed.

ICA occlusion is characterized by the absence of any signal along the cervical course of the ICA. Frequently, a low-velocity Doppler signal with predominant reversed signal component and absence of diastolic flow can be recorded at the presumed origin of the ICA (stump flow). Blood flow velocity in the CCA is reduced, and frequently, retrograde perfusion of the ophthalmic artery occurs. The diagnosis of carotid occlusion by B-mode echotomography alone without Doppler ultrasonography is not reliable, because the residual vascular lumen frequently cannot be visualized adequately in complicated, heterogeneous, partially calcified high-grade obstructions. In acute thrombotic occlusion, echolucent material fills the vascular lumen, which can hardly be differentiated on gray scale from blood flow in a patent ICA. CW Doppler and duplex ultrasonography techniques have a significantly higher accuracy for the diagnosis of ICA occlusion; however, differentiation of this entity from a subtotal stenosis is sometimes difficult. The PW Doppler spectrum and color signals in ICA occlusion typically demonstrate a marked reduction of the systolic and diastolic blood flow velocity in the CCA and an internalized ECA with high diastolic flow velocity, indicating collateral supply via the ophthalmic artery. Color-coded intravascular Doppler signals are absent in the occluded ICA; however, blue-coded flow reversal in the residual stump at the bifurcation (stump flow) may occur. The capacity of modern CDFI and PDI instruments to detect very slow blood flow velocities has markedly improved the sensitivity for the diagnosis of a subtotal ICA stenosis and pseudo-occlusion.

CCA occlusion is a relatively rare condition that can be diagnosed reliably by conventional duplex ultrasonography and CDFI.[53,54] It is important to assess whether the ICA distal to the CCA occlusion is patent, because patency of this area is a prerequisite for surgical intervention.[55–58] CDFI typically displays blue-coded signals in the ECA because of reversed flow direction and orthograde filling of the ICA in the absence of Doppler signals in the CCA.

Severe intracranial obstructions within the carotid siphon or the middle cerebral artery (MCA) may lead to dampened spectra in the ipsilateral extracranial carotid

Table 21.2   **Criteria for the Classification of Internal Carotid Artery Stenosis by Pulsed-Wave Doppler Sonography**

Diameter Stenosis (%)	Peak Systolic Frequency (kHz)	Peak Systolic Velocity (cm/s)	End Diastolic Frequency (kHz)	End Diastolic Velocity (cm/s)
40–60	>4.0	>120	<1.3	<40
61–80	>4.0	>120	>1.3	>40
81–90	>8.0	>240	>3.3	>100

artery. In addition, alterations of flow direction and signal frequency may occur in the ophthalmic artery, depending on the site and severity of the lesion. Intracranial arteriovenous malformations (AVMs) and shunts may lead to increased flow velocities in the ipsilateral proximal vessel segments. Such findings on extracranial Doppler examination should therefore prompt an appropriate evaluation for suspected intracranial AVM.

The combination of B-mode imaging and PW Doppler ultrasonography in duplex instruments considerably improves the accuracy of the noninvasive diagnosis and grading of carotid stenosis. The degree of stenosis can be estimated from distinct parameters of the Doppler frequency spectrum. However, instead of Doppler shift frequencies, equivalent flow-velocity values can be obtained after correction of the Doppler insonation angle according to the flow direction in the vessel segment. In CDFI, three sources of information are available for the classification of carotid stenosis: the Doppler frequency spectrum, measurement of the residual vessel lumen, and characteristic color-flow patterns.

Doppler Frequency Spectrum
Assessment of the Doppler spectrum is important because it can often be recorded even when plaque calcification prevents adequate visualization of color-flow patterns and of the residual vessel lumen. Parameters from the Doppler spectrum such as the peak systolic frequency or velocity[59–61] (see Table 21.1) agree well with angiography for grading of carotid stenosis.

Measurement of Residual Vessel Lumen
The methodologic limitations of measurements of residual vessel lumen with B-mode imaging are well documented.[62–64] With the use of sequential longitudinal and transverse sections, both CDFI and PDI allow more reliable assessment of plaque configuration and relative obstruction by contrasting the intravascular surface.[65–69] Assuming a concentric stenosis, the percentage area reduction in cross-sections is higher than the relative diameter. There is a good correlation between transverse lumen reduction on CDFI and diameter reduction on corresponding angiograms of carotid stenosis.[69,70] Measurement of local diameter and area reduction in carotid stenosis can be performed more reliably by PDI than by CDFI because of better visualization of the residual stenotic lumen by the former technique.[8,9]

The volumetric potential of 3D ultrasonography has important clinical implications in serial follow-up studies for observing the progression or regression of stenotic lesions and for evaluating the outcome of interventional procedures such as endarterectomy and stent placement.[71] The use of advanced imaging systems for acquisition and offline analysis of electrocardiography-gated, axial B-mode scans allows reliable quantification of carotid artery plaques.[72] In comparison with other techniques for the quantification of atherosclerotic lesions, 3D ultrasonography angiography offers a precise quantitative method for prospective, clinical studies of atherosclerosis.[73]

Color Doppler Flow Patterns
Color Doppler flow patterns can provide complementary information for establishing the severity of carotid artery stenosis. Mild stenosis is associated with a relatively long segment of decreased color saturation with absence of or minimal poststenotic turbulence.[7] In moderate obstructions, the decreased color saturation is more circumscribed, and flow velocity remains high during diastole. Post-stenotic flow is turbulent, and flow reversal occurs frequently (Plate 21–5). Severe stenosis is characterized by a mosaic pattern indicating high flow velocity and mixed turbulence.[74] A short segment of maximal color fading or aliasing with severe post-stenotic turbulence and flow reversal provides further evidence for severe stenosis.[7]

Plaque Morphology
Because of its noninvasive nature, real-time capabilities and general availability, ultrasonography has been the most extensively utilized imaging technique for the study of carotid plaque morphology. High-resolution B-mode imaging alone, and in conjunction with color Doppler flow and PDI techniques, has been used to define parameters for identification of symptomatic or vulnerable plaques. The parameters have included echogenicity, surface structure, and ulcerations of the plaques.

Carotid artery plaques of homogeneous, moderate-intensity echogenicity consist mainly of fibrotic tissue.[1,3] Such plaques rarely show ulceration, perhaps accounting for the lack of a significant correlation between homogeneous echogenicity and the occurrence of focal cerebral ischemia. Heterogeneous plaques, by comparison, represent matrix deposition, cholesterol accumulation, necrosis, calcification, and intraplaque hemorrhage.[1,3,4] Several studies have demonstrated that high-resolution B-mode scanning can characterize echomorphologic features of carotid plaques (Fig. 21–6) that correlate with histopathologic criteria.[75] Although echolucent areas within the plaque may represent thrombotic material or hemorrhage, lipid accumulation may have similar echogenicity.[76] Plaque calcification causes acoustic shadowing. Depending on the location of the plaque and on the extent of calcification, acoustic shadowing can be a major obstacle to adequate

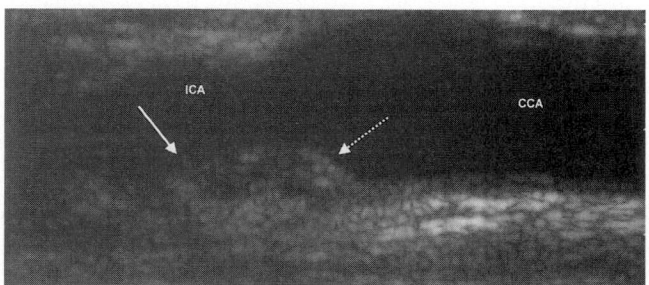

FIGURE 21–6 *B-mode scan (using a 8- to 13-MHz, dynamic-range, linear transducer) of heterogeneous plaque (arrows) of the internal carotid artery (ICA) at the level of the carotid bifurcation. The fibrous cap displays stronger echoes on the proximal plaque surface (broken arrow) than on its more distal surface (solid arrow), where thinning of the cap is evident. The plaque displays a relatively smooth surface structure protruding into the lumen of the ICA. Beneath the plaque surface is an area of weaker echoes, corresponding to lipid accumulation. CCA, common carotid artery.*

ultrasonographic visualization. Initial studies of plaque echogenicity with B-mode ultrasonography reported an association between heterogeneous plaques and the occurrence of cerebrovascular events.[77–81] Support for this association was provided by several investigations of endarterectomy specimens that suggested a correlation between intraplaque hemorrhage and transient ischemic attacks (TIAs) and stroke.[82–85] Later studies, however, were unable to confirm these observations.[86–88]

Whether differences in plaque echogenicity can distinguish between symptomatic and asymptomatic plaques continues to be a debatable subject. Later ultrasonographic studies have renewed the notion that heterogeneous carotid plaques are more often associated with intraplaque hemorrhage and neurologic events, and conclude that evaluation of plaque morphology may be helpful in selecting patients for carotid endarterectomy.[89–91] Other researchers argue that lipid-rich plaques are more prone to rupture and suggest that an association between intraplaque hemorrhage and a high lipid content as revealed by B-mode scanning may support this theory.[92] These newer findings have been negated by yet other research groups who find little correlation between plaque morphology and histologic specimens.[93] A definitive study on the significance of heterogeneous plaque structure found no differences in volume of intraplaque hemorrhage, lipid core, necrotic core, or plaque calcification in patients with highly stenotic carotid lesions undergoing endarterectomy, regardless of preoperative symptom status.[94]

Attempts to characterize plaque surface structure with B-mode scanning have been disappointing. Although a relatively good differentiation between smooth, irregular and ulcerative plaque surfaces has been obtained for postmortem carotid artery specimens,[3] the accuracy of in vivo findings in comparison with findings at carotid endarterectomy has been considerably poorer.[59,75,93,95] Commonly used parameters for identification of plaque ulceration have been surface defects showing a depth and length of 2 mm or more with a well-defined base in the recess.[50] B-mode imaging using these criteria has failed to provide a satisfactory diagnostic yield for ulcerative plaques, with a sensitivity of only 47%.[75] Other groups have been unable to distinguish between the presence and absence of intimal ulcerations with B-mode scans.[96] Diagnostic sensitivity for detection of plaque ulceration with ultrasonography is affected by the severity of carotid stenosis, increasing to 77% in plaques associated with 50% or less stenosis.[75]

Whether plaque surface irregularities or ulcerations are useful parameters for defining patients at risk for carotid embolism remains unclear. Advocates of a pathophysiologic relationship maintain that ulcerations represent fertile ground for potential thrombosis and consequent embolic events. This contention is supported by studies demonstrating an association between angiographically defined ulcerations and an increased risk of stroke in medically treated symptomatic patients.[97] In spite of the poor sensitivity and specificity of arteriography for detection of plaque ulceration,[75] it should be remembered that many ulcers are smooth and thick, containing no thrombus at all[98] for putative plaque embolism. Moreover, pathologic studies have shown that in asymptomatic carotid plaques with stenosis exceeding 60%, there is a higher frequency

of plaque hemorrhages, ulcerations, and mural thrombi as well as of numerous healed ulcerations and organized thrombi.[99] Likewise, comparisons of symptomatic with asymptomatic large and stenotic carotid endarterectomy plaques have revealed a high incidence of complex plaque structure and complications in each.[86,100] There appears, therefore, to be little difference in plaque constituents or plaque surface structure between specimens from symptomatic and asymptomatic patients. These findings suggest that a simple description of plaque structure or an identification of plaque ulceration as depicted in current clinical imaging techniques—ultrasonography, magnetic resonance imaging (MRI) and angiography—may be of doubtful significance for predicting the vulnerability of carotid plaques.

Plaque Motion

Experimental work has suggested that analysis of plaque motion—that is, translational plaque movements coincident with those of arterial walls, plaque rotations, and local, plaque-specific deformations—may provide new insights into plaque modeling as well as into mechanisms of plaque rupture with subsequent embolism. Plaque surface movement may be attributable to deformations resulting from propagation of multiple local internal tears in the plaque. Theoretically, identification of local variations in surface deformability might provide information on the relative vulnerability of a plaque to fissuring or rupture.

Four-dimensional (4D) ultrasonography was used to acquire temporal three-dimensional ultrasonography data on carotid artery plaques.[101] The ultrasonography data was analyzed with motion detection algorithms to determine apparent velocity fields, also known as optical flow, of the plaque surface. This technique allowed characterization of plaque motion patterns in patients with symptomatic and asymptomatic carotid artery disease.[101] Asymptomatic plaques showed a homogenous orientation and magnitude of computed surface velocity vectors, coincident with arterial wall movement. Symptomatic plaques, however, demonstrated evidence of plaque deformation, irrespective of arterial wall movements. Further data are required to substantiate these initial findings.

Vertebral Artery Stenosis

Examination of the extracranial vertebral artery with ultrasonography is limited to its origin from the subclavian artery, its proximal pretransverse segment, short intertransverse segments between the third and sixth cervical vertebrae, and the atlas loop. Although PW Doppler criteria for vertebral artery stenosis are similar to those used for diagnosis of carotid artery stenosis and have been defined by several duplex studies, classification and detection of stenosis or occlusion in the vertebral arteries are more difficult than in the carotid arteries.[102–104] One reason for this difficulty is that variations in arterial caliber are common in vertebral arteries. In addition, numerous collateral pathways of the vertebral system can permit orthograde flow to the basilar artery even in the presence of vertebral occlusion. These features make examination of the vertebral artery at several locations mandatory. CDFI allows noninvasive quantification of flow in the vertebral artery system in more than 95% of all patients[105] and facilitates

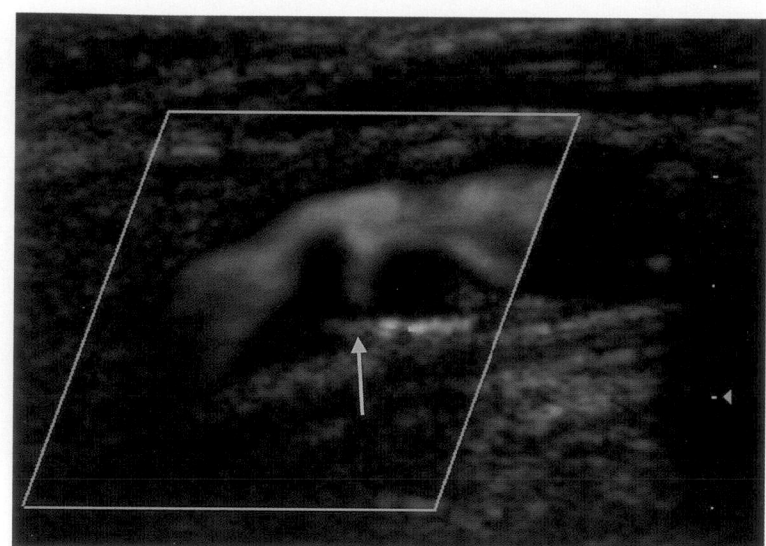

PLATE 21–1 *Deep plaque ulceration (arrow) in the left internal carotid artery as depicted by power Doppler imaging. The plaque is practically anechoic, typical of lipid-filled plaques.*

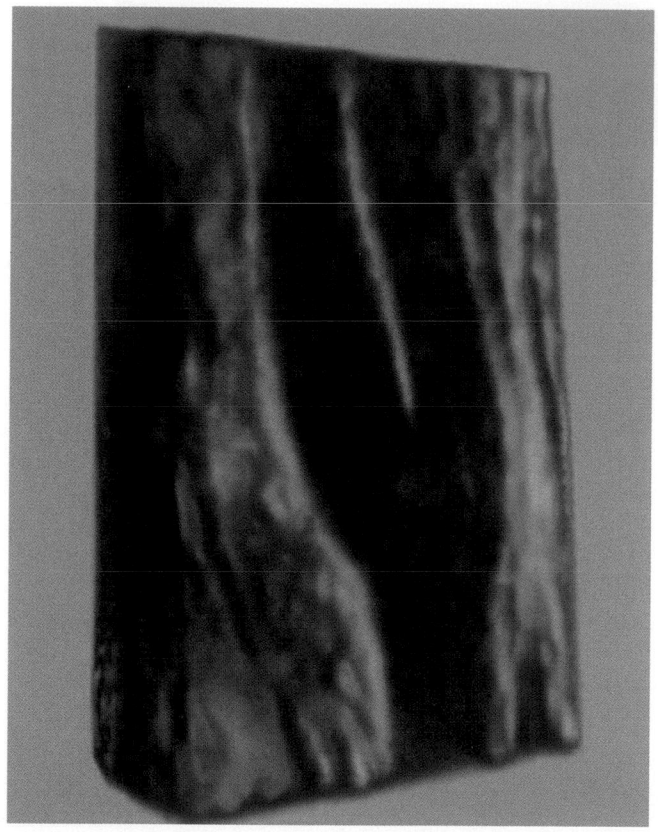

PLATE 21–2 *Volume rendering of the three-dimensional ultrasound reconstruction of the carotid artery. Data were acquired with a position and orientation device that tracks the transducer during freehand scanning.*

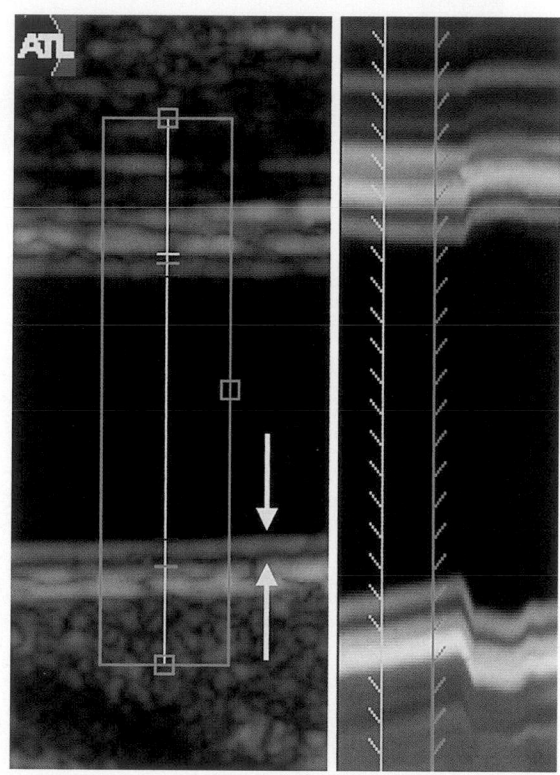

PLATE 21–3 *Intima-medial thickness (IMT) measurements can be performed for a defined segment of the cardiac cycle using automated systems. Right, The green region of interest specifies the area in which IMT (as shown with white arrows) is measured. Right, A user-defined specification of the segment of the cardiac cycle (diastole) in the M-mode display of arterial diameter over time.*

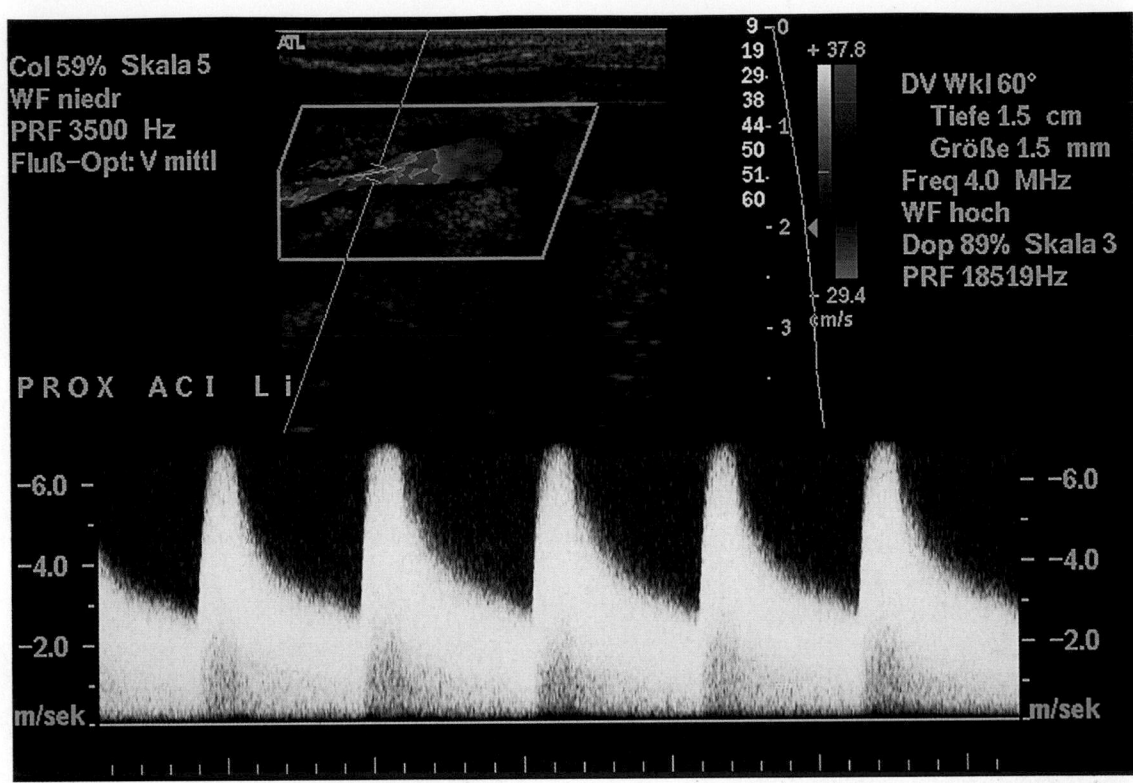

PLATE 21–4 *The Doppler spectrum identifies a high-grade stenosis of the carotid artery with maximum peak velocity exceeding 600 cm/sec, causing left hemispheric stroke. Color Doppler flow imaging demonstrates a mosaic pattern indicating high-flow velocity and mixed turbulence.*

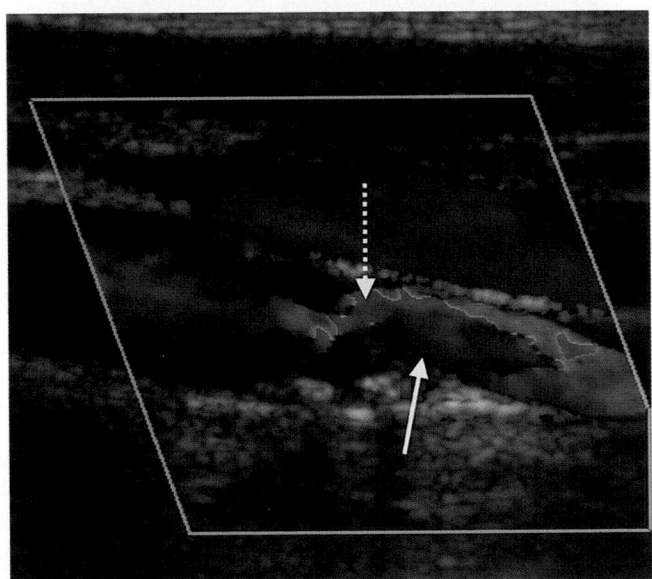

PLATE 21–5 *High-resolution B-mode scan of a heterogeneous, asymptomatic plaque in the right internal carotid artery. The display is facilitated with color Doppler flow imaging, showing a 70% stenosis with turbulent flow (dotted arrow). The plaque is weakly echogenic at the surface with calcifications near the arterial wall. The blue area represents flow reversal (white arrow).*

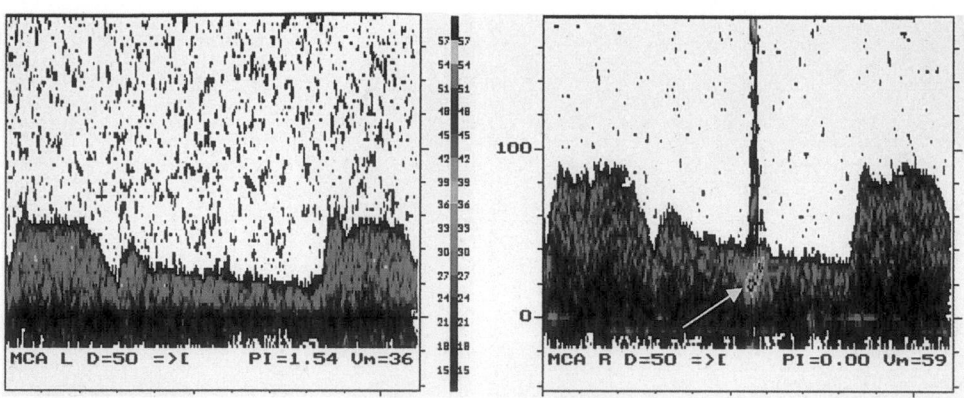

PLATE 21–6 *Two images showing simultaneous transcranial Doppler monitoring of high-intensity transient signals (HITS) in the left and right middle cerebral arteries (MCAs). Note the HITS (arrow) occurring in the right MCA, presumably of microembolic origin.*

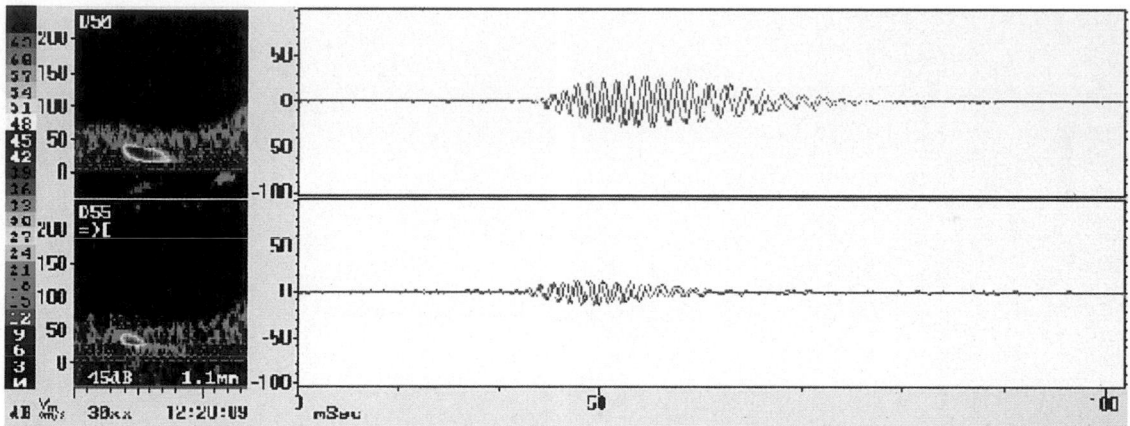

PLATE 21–7 *Multigate Doppler technique for improved identification of microemboli. Here the middle cerebral artery is insonated simultaneously at two locations. The delay in time between the appearance of high-intensity signals at the two gates is strong evidence for a microembolic particle (an artifact would appear simultaneously at both gates).*

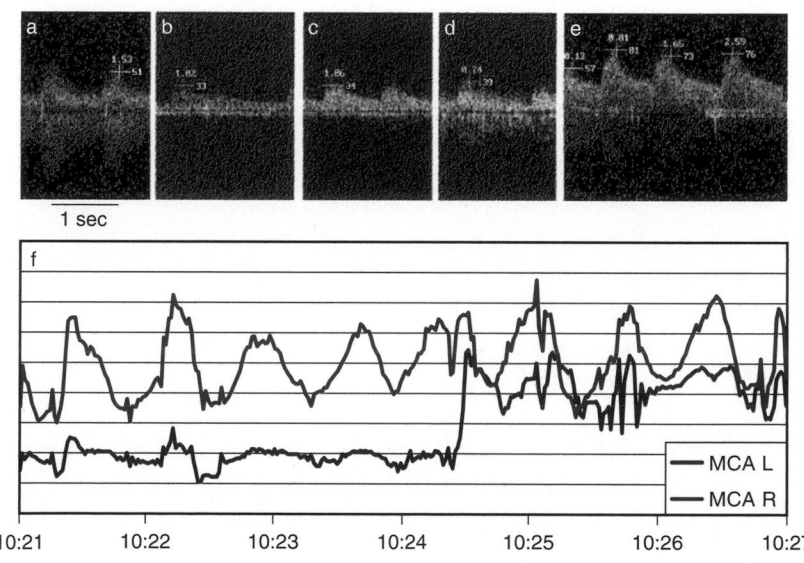

PLATE 21–8 *A 63-year-old man with sudden onset of right-sided sensorimotor hemiparesis and aphasia at 8:30 AM. A, Transcranial Doppler ultrasonography shows a minimal signal in the left middle cerebral artery (MCA). B and C, Cerebral blood flow velocity decreases further. D, An improvement in signal intensity is detected at 10:24 AM, signifying the onset of recanalization. E, The signal abruptly changes to a normal waveform in less than 1 second. F, Recanalization starts within minutes of administration of a bolus of tissue-type plasminogen activator and is complete within seconds, leading to complete recanalization of the distal M1 segment of the MCA.*

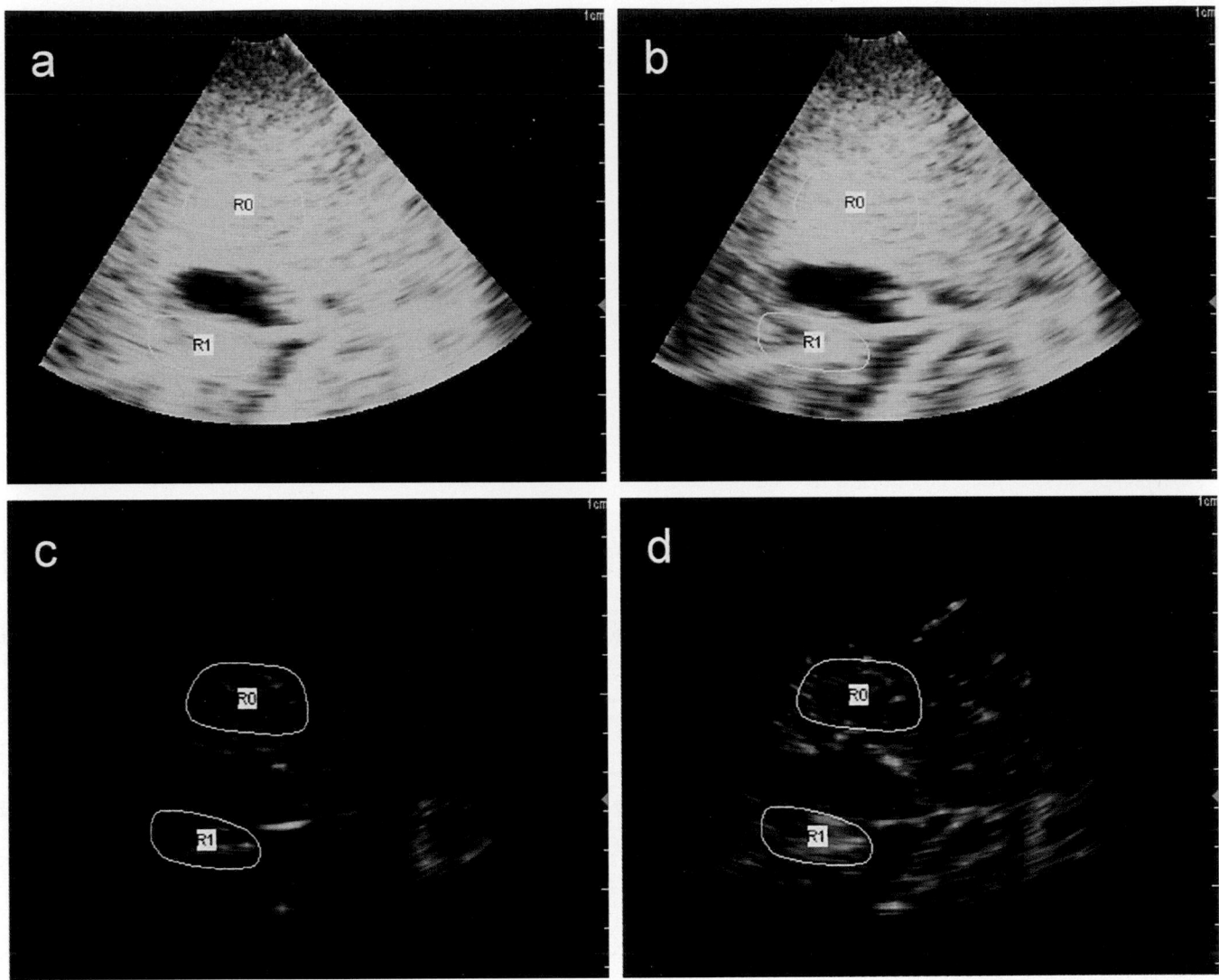

PLATE 21–9 *Real-time power pulse inversion contrast imaging of ipsilateral middle cerebral artery (MCA) infarction with recanalization of the MCA. A and B, Real-time destruction of the contrast agent Sonovic using an high mechanical index (pulse interval 60 ms). B demonstrates color desaturation after bubble destruction. In C and D, a low mechanical index is used that does not destroy microbubbles, thus allowing contrast replenishment to be monitored in real time; C was acquired directly after bubble destruction, and D approximately 5 seconds later. Two regions of interest (R0 and R1 in A through D) have been set to allow evaluation of bubble destruction and replenishment kinetics in both hemispheres.*

identification of the proximal segment and ostium, the predominant location of extracranial vertebral stenosis, as well as of the atlas loop.[106,107] Using this technique, investigators have documented normal flow velocities of the vertebral artery origin (V0 segment), the pretransverse segment (V1 segment), and the intertransverse (V2 segment).[108]

Correct interpretation of Doppler results in a vertebral artery requires knowledge of Doppler parameters from both the contralateral vertebral artery and from the carotid system. For example, an increase in the systolic or diastolic velocity profile of the proximal vertebral artery, although suggestive of stenosis, can also occur as a compensatory response to a variety of conditions of the contralateral vertebral artery, such as hypoplasia, aplasia, stenosis, and occlusion, as well as to severe obstruction of the carotid system.

The predominant site of extracranial vertebral artery stenosis is the ostium of the subclavian artery (Fig. 21–7). The atlas loop (V3) and intracranial (V4) segment are involved less commonly, and stenoses in the intertransverse segments are rare. A peak systolic frequency exceeding 4 kHz assessed by means of the integrated PW Doppler system indicates a relevant vertebral stenosis. Features of color-coded Doppler signals correspond to those of carotid stenosis. As luminal narrowing is greater, decreased color saturation becomes more circumscribed, and turbulence as well as post-stenotic flow reversal more severe. Hemodynamically significant obstruction of the intracranial vertebral artery produces a high-resistance Doppler waveform with a resistivity index exceeding 0.80.[107] However, the Doppler spectrum may be normal if flow to the ipsilateral posterior inferior cerebellar artery is preserved. In acute proximal vertebral artery occlusion, PW Doppler spectra cannot be recorded, and color Doppler signals are absent in the pretransverse and intertransverse segments. However, demonstration of the vascular lumen differentiates this condition from vertebral hypoplasia, which is defined in pathoanatomical studies as a decrease in vascular lumen diameter to less than 2 mm.[109]

NONATHEROSCLEROTIC VASCULAR DISEASE

Carotid Artery Dissection

Ultrasonography is useful for diagnosis of carotid artery dissection, a cause of transient or permanent neurologic deficits, particularly in young patients. ICA dissection usually occurs spontaneously and results in a typical syndrome of focal cerebral deficits, headache, neck pain, and ipsilateral Horner's syndrome.

Various patterns can be observed in carotid dissection. CDFI can show marked flow reversal at the origin of the ICA in systole and absence of or minimal blood flow in diastole, a pattern that corresponds to a high-resistance bidirectional Doppler signal.[110] B-mode scans can demonstrate a tapered lumen and occasionally a floating intimal flap.[111] Narrowing of the true lumen by the false lumen thrombus can be associated with a low-velocity Doppler waveform. The direction of flow in a patent false lumen can vary from being forward to being reversed or bidirectional. The flow dynamics in carotid dissections are

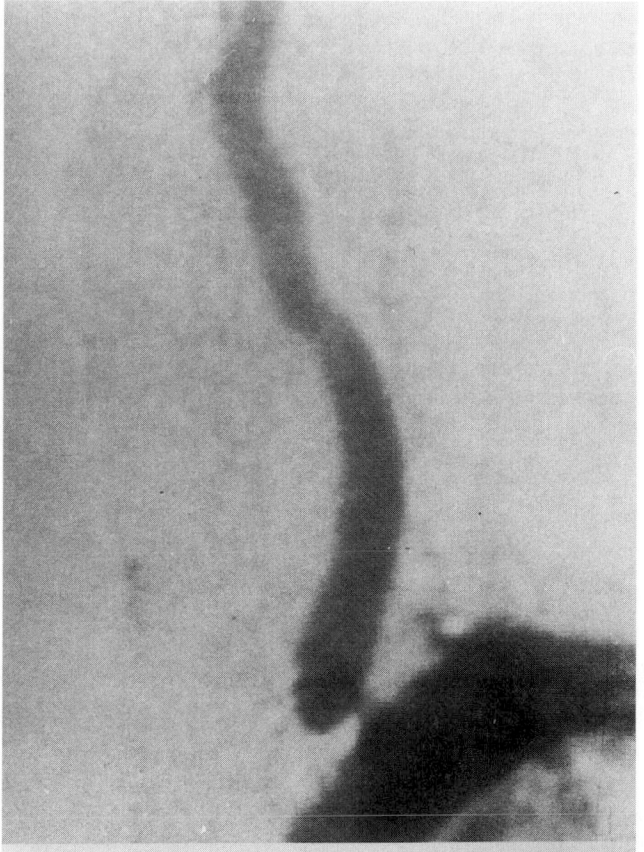
A

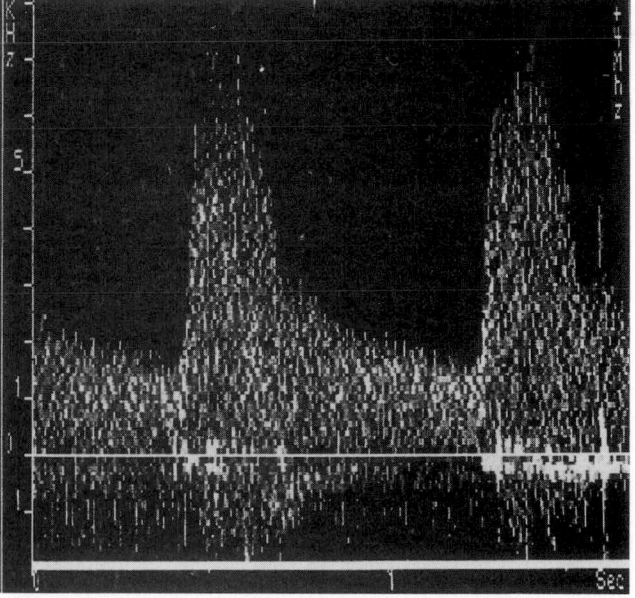
B

FIGURE 21–7 *Tight stenosis at the origin of the vertebral artery. A, angiogram; B, Doppler spectra.*

complex and depend primarily on the presence of thrombus within the false lumen, the entry and exit flaps if the false lumen is patent, the motion of the flap wall, and the extent of the dissection.[112] In some patients, the only finding may be a retromandibular high-velocity signal associated with a distal stenosis of the cervical carotid artery.[113]

Diagnostic Studies

Follow-up examinations of carotid dissections demonstrate gradual normalization of the Doppler spectrum, indicating recanalization of the ICA within a few weeks to months in more than two thirds of patients.[114] Carotid aneurysms can occur as complications of ICA dissections. Their follow-up with angiography and MR angiography (MRA) or MRI can be complemented with ultrasonography because of development of broad-band transducers with improved axial resolution and depth penetration.[51]

Vertebral Artery Dissection

Vertebral artery dissection is one of the most common causes of brainstem strokes in young patients.[115,116] It manifests as neck pain, occipital headache, and signs and symptoms of brainstem or cerebellar ischemia in about 90% of patients and commonly leaves a permanent deficit.[117–119] The role of ultrasonography in diagnosis of this condition remains uncertain. There is no pathognomonic ultrasonographic finding for vertebral artery dissection if the lesion affects the V2 through V4 segments. Examination of the atlas loop can reveal absence of flow signals, low bidirectional flow signals, or low poststenotic flow signals.[120] In dissections of the V1 segment, the stenotic segment can be visualized, whereas absence of flow in the intertransverse segments should similarly raise the question of vertebral dissection. Further findings can include a localized increase in the diameter of the artery with hemodynamic signs of stenosis or occlusion at the same level, decreased pulsatility, and the presence of intravascular echogenicity in the enlarged segment.[121,122] Occasionally, the specific finding of an intramural hematoma is found.[123]

Transcranial Doppler (TCD) can be helpful in determining the length of dissection.[124] In one study, combined use of extracranial and TCD and duplex ultrasonography methods has been found to improve the diagnostic yield to detect vertebral artery dissection. Consideration of any abnormal ultrasonographic finding resulted in a diagnostic yield of 86%, whereas reliance upon definite abnormal findings (absence of flow signal, severely reduced flow velocities, absence of diastolic flow, bidirectional flow, or stenosis signal) resulted in a diagnostic yield of only 64%.[120] Similar results were obtained in another study, in which ultrasonography abnormalities (high-resistance signal, occlusion, and bilateral retrograde flow) were found in eight of ten vertebral artery dissections.[125] Detection of abnormal flow patterns in the vertebral artery in cases of suspected dissection may guide further diagnostic imaging procedures and therapeutic measures. However, because unremarkable ultrasound findings do not exclude the diagnosis of vertebral dissection, further workup in these cases is mandatory.

TRANSCRANIAL DOPPLER IN THE EVALUATION OF STROKE

TCD uses high-energy bidirectional pulsed Doppler, typically at a low frequency of 2 MHz, for intracranial vascular examination via transtemporal, transorbital, and transnuchal bone windows (Fig. 21–8). Applications for TCD in stroke imaging include detection of intracranial stenosis and occlusion, evaluation of intracranial collateral circulations, detection of vasospasm in subarachnoid hemorrhage (SAH), and assessment of cerebral autoregulation. TCD monitoring techniques are available for detection of high-intensity transient signals suggestive of microembolism and for surveillance of intracranial hemodynamics during

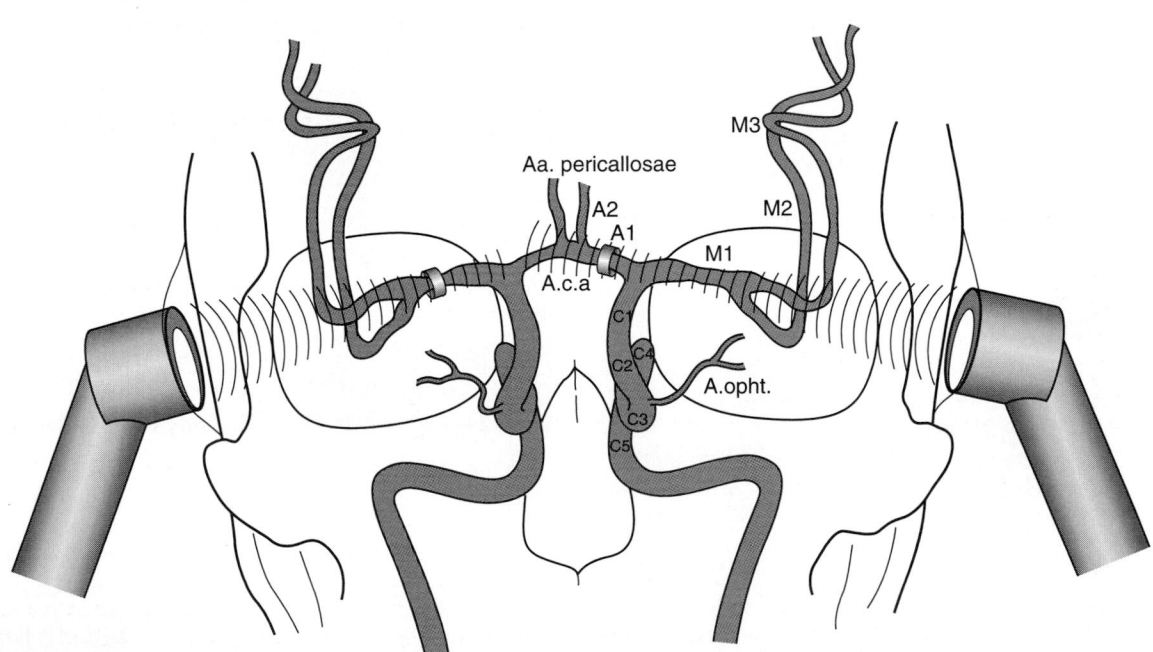

FIGURE 21–8   *Schematic illustration of the position of the sample volume inside the skull, using the transtemporal approach. Aa. pericallosae, pericallosal arteries; A.c.a., anterior communicating artery; A. opht., ophthalmic artery; C1 through C5, segments of the internal carotid artery; M1, M2, and M3, segments of the middle cerebral artery.*

stroke therapy. The introduction of transcranial CDFI has led to greater accuracy in vessel identification. Reports on the merits of transcranial CDFI for detection of cerebral aneurysms, evaluation of AVMs, and characterization of vessel morphology are now available.

Technologic advances have enhanced the capabilities of TCD. They include transcranial PDI, contrast-enhanced CDFI, 3D transcranial PDI, and contrast harmonic perfusion imaging.

With conventional TCD, intracranial basal arteries are identified from flow direction, depth of the Doppler sample volume, and probe position (Table 21.3). Because flow velocities of intracranial vessels are known to vary with age and sex,[126] hematocrit value,[127] and end-tidal partial pressure of carbon dioxide, a standardized TCD examination procedure is mandatory.[128] Normal values for flow velocities in the basal cerebral arteries have been determined in several studies (Table 21.4).[49,129–134] Optimal performance and correct interpretation of TCD studies require knowledge of both the clinical setting and the results of extracranial ultrasonography examinations.

Transcranial CDFI facilitates identification of basal cerebral arteries.[135] Although conventional TCD ultrasonography assumes a 0-degree Doppler angle for the calculation of flow velocities, transcranial CDFI allows correction for the Doppler insonation angle. The magnitude of the angle of insonation and the effect on flow velocity estimates in intracranial vessels have been determined through visually controlled measurements of the Doppler insonation angle of made by color-flow imaging; angle-corrected peak systolic flow velocities were 3% to 30% higher than uncorrected velocity readings obtained with conventional Doppler ultrasonography.[136] Similar findings were reported in another study; in 14.5% of subjects, the angle-corrected velocity was 25% to 50% higher, and in 10.8%, it was more than 50% higher than the uncorrected velocity readings.[137] Although transcranial CDFI is con-

Table 21.4 Normal Values of Transcranial Doppler Examination

Vessel	Age Group (yr)	Systolic Peak Velocity (cm/s)	Mean Velocity (cm/s)	Diastolic Velocity (cm/s)
MCA (50 mm)	<40	94.5 ± 13.6	58.4 ± 8.4	45.6 ± 6.6
	40–60	91.0 ± 16.9°	57.7 ± 11.5°	44.3 ± 9.5°
	>60	78.1 ± 15.0†	44.7 ± 11.1†	31.9 ± 9.1°
ACA (70 mm)	<40	76.4 ± 16.9	47.3 ± 13.6	36.0 ± 9.0
	40–60	86.4 ± 20.1	53.1 ± 10.5	41.1 ± 7.4†
	>60	73.3 ± 20.3	45.3 ± 13.5	34.2 ± 8.8†
PCA (60 mm)	<40	53.2 ± 11.3	34.3 ± 7.8	25.9 ± 6.5
	40–60	60.1 ± 20.6	36.6 ± 9.8	28.7 ± 7.5†
	>60	51.0 ± 11.9	29.9 ± 9.3	22.0 ± 6.9†
VA/BA (75 mm)	<40	56.3 ± 7.8	34.9 ± 7.8	27.0 ± 5.3
	40–60	59.5 ± 17.0	36.4 ± 11.7	29.2 ± 8.4†
	>60	50.9 ± 18.7	30.5 ± 12.4	21.2 ± 9.2†

Pulsatility Index (all age groups)	
MCA	0.92 ± 0.25
ACA	0.8 ± 0.16
PCA	0.88 ± 0.21

ACA, anterior cerebral artery; BA, basilar artery; MCA, middle cerebral artery; PCA, posterior cerebral artery; VA, vertebral artery.
°p <.02.
†p <.05.

sidered by many to be the ultrasonic method of choice for evaluation of the intracranial circulation, there are no data on the failure rate of transcranial CDFI in a large group of patients. There are no prospective data on the ability of transcranial CDFI to detect intracranial stenosis in a large group of patients.

Intracranial Stenosis and Occlusion

Significant narrowing of intracranial arteries results in localized increases in mean and peak flow velocities, turbulence and reversed flow phenomena, and reduction of pre- or post-stenotic flow velocities.[138–140] Stenosis that narrows the lumen by more than 50% can be reliably detected in arterial segments with anatomically favorable insonation angles such as the M1 segment of the MCA and the P1 segment of the posterior cerebral artery (PCA).

A reliable diagnosis of occlusion in the M1 segment can be made only when unequivocal evidence of blood flow in the ipsilateral anterior cerebral artery (ACA) or PCA can be obtained, thus differentiating this condition from high ultrasound attenuation and poor echo window insonation. Further findings supporting MCA occlusion are dampened spectra in segments proximal to the occlusion, reversed flow direction in distal MCA branches, and abnormally elevated flow velocities in the ipsilateral ACA.[141] In one series of 467 patients, the sensitivity for the detection of MCA occlusion by TCD ultrasonography was 79% with a specificity of 100%.[142] Contrast-enhanced transcranial CDFI may be more accurate than TCD ultrasonography in

Table 21.3 Transcranial Doppler Criteria for the Identification of Basal Intracranial Vessels Using the Transtemporal, Transorbital, and Nuchal Approaches

Vessel	Probe	Depth (mm)	Flow Direction
Transtemporal approach			
MCA	Medial	30–65	Toward probe
ACA	Medial	55–80	Away from probe
ICA	Caudal	55–75	Toward probe
PCA, P1	Posterior	55–80	Toward probe
PCA, P2	Posterior	55–75	Away from probe
Transorbital approach			
Ophthalmic artery		30–60	Toward probe
ICA, C4, C5		60–80	Toward probe
ICA, C2, C3		60–80	Away from probe
Nuchal approach			
VA		50–100	Away from probe
BA		75–120	Away from probe

ACA, anterior cerebral artery; BA, basilar artery; ICA, internal carotid artery; MCA, middle cerebral artery; PCA, posterior cerebral artery; VA, vertebral artery.

Diagnostic Studies

demonstrating occlusions of the MCA[143] and is particularly useful in cases of inadequate bone windows.[144] A multicenter has demonstrated that transcranial CFDI is a feasible, fast, and valid noninvasive bedside method for evaluating the MCA in an acute stroke setting, particularly when contrast enhancement is applied.[145]

TCD ultrasonography examinations of the vertebrobasilar arteries are less reliable than those of the anterior circulation. The junction of the basilar artery is difficult to define by TCD criteria alone, and investigation of the entire course of the basilar artery, which is usually limited by excessive insonation depth with poor signal-to-noise ratio,[146] can be achieved in only 30% of patients. As in the anterior circulation, partial obstructions are easier to detect than total occlusion. Using intra-arterial digital subtraction angiography (DSA) as a standard reference, two groups of investigators have found that TCD ultrasonography demonstrated sensitivities of 74% to 87% and specificities of 80% to 86% for detection of large vessel occlusive disease of the intracranial vertebrobasilar system.[147,148] Best results, however, are obtained when TCD ultrasonography is used in combination with cerebral angiography[146] or MR angiography.[149] Unfortunately, TCD ultrasonography detection of basilar artery occlusion is poor, with a sensitivity of only 36%.[150] This fact is of major clinical importance in the evaluation of patients suspected of suffering from acute basilar artery thrombosis.

3D ultrasonographic imaging of the intracranial vessels allows a comprehensive visualization of the basal arteries and circle of Willis. Details not appreciated on 2D images alone are well shown with this technique. In particular, the origin of small arteries perpendicular or diagonal to the scanning plane can be easily identified with 3D ultrasonography. Contrast-enhanced 3D power Doppler imaging (PDI) may allow superior demonstration of intracerebral vascular disease and increase operator diagnostic confidence.[151] Measurement of 3D transcranial images can be a difficult task, because the appearance of surface reconstructions of intracranial arteries can be significantly affected by the quality of the acquired images, the accuracy of the spatial registration, the reconstruction algorithm used, and the selection of isosurface parameters. Moreover, there can be significant distortion of the ultrasound beam when it transverses the temporal bone window, leading to unpredictable results in some cases.[152] Nevertheless, first reports on the characterization of intracranial stenosis with 3D PDI have been encouraging.[153] Further work is needed to validate the ability of 3D ultrasonography to provide accurate data for quantitative assessment of the intracranial arteries and to establish parameters for standardization of this technique.

Assessment of Intracranial Collateralization

The presence of intracranial collateralization in patients with stenosis or occlusion of the extracranial carotid arteries can be investigated with conventional TCD ultrasonography. Findings compatible with the presence of collateral flow over the anterior communicating artery include retrograde flow in the ipsilateral ACA, increased peak and mean velocities in both ACAs, increased velocities and low-frequency signals in the midline indicating functional stenosis of the anterior communicating artery, and decreased MCA velocity during compression of the contralateral CCA. Collateralization from the posterior circulation is suggested by increased velocities in the ipsilateral P1 segment of the PCA or in the basilar artery as well as by low-frequency signals in the posterior communicating artery. Leptomeningeal anastomosis, although more difficult to assess, may be associated with increased velocities in proximal and distal segments of the PCA and with retrograde flow signals in distal MCA branches. TCD ultrasonography can also detect retrograde flow in the ophthalmic artery, another avenue for collateralization.

Flow velocities in the MCA distal to significant stenosis and occlusion vary with regard to the efficacy of intracranial collateralization. Although reduced MCA velocities and pulsatility indexes have been found ipsilateral to symptomatic carotid occlusion,[154,155] normal peak and mean velocities indicating adequate collateralization have been reported in asymptomatic patients.[156]

Microembolic Signal Detection

TCD ultrasonography is used by a number of specialized centers to detect microembolic signals (MES) entering the cerebral circulation. This technique, first reported almost two decades ago,[157] may benefit patients who are at increased risk for stroke during interventional investigations and carotid surgery.[158] The methodology of MES detection consists of fixing a Doppler probe with a frequency of approximately 2 MHz over the temporal bone and adjusting its position, orientation, and the Doppler sample volume depth to obtain a good signal from blood flow within the ipsilateral MCA. Because a microembolus has different acoustic properties from those of the blood in which it is traveling, there is a transient increase in the back-scattered ultrasonic power as it passes through the Doppler sample volume (high-intensity transient signal, or HITS); therefore, careful monitoring of the Doppler signal provides a means of classification and artifact rejection (Plate 21–6). HITSs corresponding to both gaseous and solid microembolic materials have been detected during angiography,[159,160] carotid angioplasty,[161] open heart surgery,[162,163] and carotid endarterectomy[164,165] as well as in patients with TIAs or stroke,[166–169] asymptomatic carotid stenosis,[170] heart valve prosthesis,[171,172] and intracranial arterial disease.[173]

Definition of High-Intensity Transient Signals

HITS are usually visualized in the fast Fourier transform (FFT). In 1995, using this signal analysis approach, consensus committee[174] proposed the following three criteria for defining a HITS: (1) duration is less than 300 msec, (2) exceeds the background by at least 3 dB, and (3) is unidirectional within the Doppler velocity spectrum. HITS detection can be performed by insonating any of the three major vessels of the circle of Willis, although monitoring of the carotid arteries[175] and the jugular veins[176] has also been reported. In most cases, the main stem of the middle cerebral artery is insonated with a 2-MHz probe using the temporal bone window. Sophisticated multigate techniques have been developed that interrogate two sample volumes along a vessel to enable better differentiation between artifacts and moving particles (Plate 21–7).

Differentiation

To date most, studies of embolic signals have relied on trained human observers to identify candidate events and to distinguish between true embolic signals and signals due to other mechanisms. Indeed, the detection of HITS shows a high interobserver agreement,[177,178,179] with kappa values in the range of 0.95. The technique is very time consuming, however, and there are a number of drawbacks associated with HITS monitoring, in terms of both cost and reliability.

If the technique is to become widely accepted in clinical practice, some form of automatic recognition will become mandatory. A number of attempts have been made to provide commercial automated systems, but none has been independently shown to be able to discriminate artifacts from signals due to microemboli.[180] Such systems must also be capable of distinguishing between signals from emboli of different types, because the clinical consequences of microemboli, although currently unclear, are expected to vary greatly; for example, patients with prosthetic heart valves can show more than 40,000 HITS per day or more than 1 million HITS per month without any neurologic or neuropsychological sequelae. New signal analysis techniques, such as simultaneous insonation with two frequencies (e.g., 1 and 2 MHz),[181] nonlinear forecasting,[182] recognition of specific postembolic spectral patterns,[183] and the application of the narrow band hypothesis[184] have been introduced to illuminate specific properties of HITS. Recent applications for automatic online microembolic signal detection using a multifrequency Doppler instrument[185,186] and a rule-based expert system[187] have given favorable results, suggesting that such approaches may well provide the necessary basis for automatic MES detection systems in the future.

Localizing the Source of Embolism in Patients with Stroke

Data on the frequency of HITS suggestive of microemboli from the heart or from the proximal arteries of the intracranial circulation have been variable.[188,189] In patients with heart valve prosthesis, thousands of clinically silent events can be recorded, whereas in patients with symptomatic carotid stenoses, HITS are relatively rare events. It appears that emboli of cardiac and carotid origin may have different ultrasonic characteristics, which are probably related to composition and size.[190] The clinical relevance of these features, however, is unclear.

After the report of HITS detection during carotid endarterectomy,[191] similar signals that occurred spontaneously were recognized in patients with symptomatic carotid artery disease.[166,168,170] Because the MES disappeared after carotid endarterectomy,[167,192,193] it was assumed that the atherosclerotic carotid plaque had been the source of the signals. In an unselected group of patients with stroke examined within 1 month of cerebral infarction, however, the prevalence of ipsilateral MES in the largest series published was approximately 10%.[194] If the interval after the acute event is shorter, the prevalence of MES may increase. In another study, monitoring with TCD ultrasonography within 2 days after admission showed that approximately 25% of an unselected group of patients had MES.[195] Patients with a carotid stenosis of at least 40%

have been reported to have significantly more MES (39%) than those without a carotid stenosis (18%). Similarly, the prevalence of MES in a comparable group of patients was reported to approach 50% when monitoring was performed immediately after admission and 1 and 2 days thereafter.[196] Of the studied group, 44% of patients had a carotid stenosis or occlusion, and 62% of these patients were MES positive.

Apart from the role of the timing of examination in determining the likelihood of MES detection in symptomatic carotid artery disease,[192,197,198] the severity of carotid stenosis may correlate with the number of measured MES; that is, the more severe the narrowing, the more MES are detected.[196,199,200] Interestingly, complete carotid occlusion has been found to be associated with a high MES count.[200] Contrary to the preceding discussion on the doubtful relevance of plaque ulcerations in pathoanatomical studies, other studies maintain that there is a relationship between preoperative MES count and carotid plaque ulceration.[201] Similarly, HITS monitored in the MCAs of patients with carotid stenosis have been reported to correlate with the appearance of ipsilateral plaque ulceration.[202]

There is some evidence that HITS detected during the dissection phase of carotid endarterectomy may correlate with clinically silent infarctions demonstrated with MRI.[164] Moreover, in a few cases, a relationship between persistent particulate embolization in the immediate postoperative period and both incipient carotid artery thrombosis and the development of major neurologic deficits has been observed.[165] In carotid angioplasty, embolization at the time of intervention is very common but usually asymptomatic. Late embolization, occurring in a minority of patients, may account for the small but significant risk of delayed stroke.[161]

Carotid dissections can cause neurologic deficits by either hemodynamic or embolic mechanisms. Because anticoagulants are often used in this setting to prevent neurologic deterioration and stroke recurrence, it would be valuable to differentiate between the two mechanisms. HITS detection would seem an ideal technique for this purpose. Reports on the relationship between MES and the clinical or imaging features of carotid dissection have been conflicting, however. One study of patients with carotid dissections reported that the detection of HITS had no clinical significance,[203] but another investigation found that MES occurrence on serial TCD ultrasonography monitoring sessions was associated with an increased risk of early ischemic recurrence.[204] Further studies are necessary to settle this issue.

HITS occur predominantly in patients with large vessel territory stroke patterns and persisting deficits, most likely due to artery-to-artery or cardiogenic embolism.[194] In contrast, patients with small vessel disease only occasionally present with HITS. Thus, the detection of HITS may support the classification of the individual pathogenesis of cerebral ischemia, particularly when multiple risk constellations for stroke coexist. Moreover, detection of recurrent microembolic events by TCD ultrasonography monitoring can provide useful guidance for pathophysiologically oriented treatment of patients with stroke.[205] Microembolism can also occur in giant cell arteritis[206] and may be related to disease activity in systemic lupus erythematosus with antiphospholipid syndrome.[207] HITS are also significantly associated with large aortic arch atheromas in elderly patients with stroke, an observation supporting the causal role of aortic atheromas in ischemic stroke.[208]

Predicting Early Recurrence of Ischemia

Microemboli detected by TCD ultrasonography in patients with stroke may be associated with a higher prevalence of prior cerebrovascular ischemia,[197,200] thus suggesting a role of MES as a risk factor for cerebral ischemia. Asymptomatic carotid stenoses are associated with MES, but to a much lesser extent than symptomatic stenoses.[193,199,209,210] Studies addressing early recurrent ischemic events after stroke or TIA in patients with a carotid stenosis[211,212] have found the presence of MES to be a predictor for early ischemic recurrence.

Future Aspects of Microembolic Signal Detection

In the majority of cases in which HITS are detected, whether these phenomena are associated with an increased risk of functional or morphologic brain damage remains unclear.[213] This problem has been compounded by the wide variety of parameters used by different investigators for MES detection. The International Consensus Group on Microembolus Detection reported guidelines for the proper use of microembolism detection by TCD ultrasonography in clinical practice and scientific investigations.[180] They suggested that technical instruments (ultrasound device, transducer size and type, FFT size, FFT length, FFT overlap, and high-pass filter settings), methodology (identification of arteries insonated, insonation depth, detection threshold, scale settings, axial extension of sample volume, recording time) and methods for analysis and interpretation (algorithms for signal intensity measurement, standardization of interobserver and intraobserver variability, and comparison of semiautomatic embolus detection algorithms) should be reported and validated in each laboratory to establish the required sensitivity and specificity for clinical use and scientific application.

If embolus detection is to realize its full potential, both in clinical trials and in routine monitoring situations, it is necessary to derive automatic methods of processing Doppler data so that vast amounts of information can be speedily and accurately evaluated. As novel applications for dynamic quantitative evaluation of cerebral perfusion with second-generation ultrasonography contrast agents emerge,[214,215] new approaches using systems that can automatically analyze multiple gaseous particles may prove beneficial. Such techniques could be applied, for example, to discriminate embolus material through the use of targeted microbubbles that attach to solid emboli and hence establish their characteristics from the bubble signatures. Moreover, exciting new applications for site-specific monitoring of microbubbles in ultrasonography-mediated gene therapy are also conceivable. Indeed, such extended applications of this monitoring technique, originally designed for embolus detection, may significantly increase its therapeutic relevance and serve to promote further advances in this important field of ultrasonography.

Dolichoectatic Arteries and Intracranial Vasculopathies

Noninvasive diagnosis of intracranial dolichoectatic arteries,[216] a cause of TIAs or stroke,[217] can be achieved with TCD ultrasonography in combination with CT or MRI. The dramatic reduction in peak and mean flow velocities that are often observed in these patients suggests a thromboembolic mechanism of ischemia in slow flow territories. TCA is also sensitive and specific for the detection of arterial vasculopathy in sickle cell disease[218,219] and has been used for assessment of reversible multisegmental narrowing of cerebral arteries in postpartum cerebral angiopathy.[220]

Detection of Right-to-Left Cardiac Shunts

Paradoxical embolism through a patent foramen ovale (PFO) is a known cause of embolic strokes and TIAs in patients with stroke of uncertain etiology. TCD ultrasonography monitoring of the basal intracranial vessels during intravenous injection of contrast media can be used for the detection of right-to-left shunts through documentation that microbubbles reach the brain.[221-223] TCD ultrasonography findings correlate well with those of transesophageal echocardiography when a standardized procedure including the Valsalva maneuver is used.[224] In some patients, TCD ultrasonography studies can identify microbubbles in the absence of PFO, thus suggesting pulmonary shunting. Careful CT assessment of the thorax can identify such abnormal pathways, which sometimes require interventional treatment.

Contrast TCD ultrasonography performed with galactose suspension (Echovist), but not with saline, has 100% sensitivity for identification of cardiac right-to-left shunt that has been proven by transesophageal echocardiography (TEE).[225] The sensitivity of diagnosing PFO with both TCD ultrasonography and TEE may be higher with injection of contrast media into the femoral vein than into the antecubital vein.[226] This difference may be related to different inflow patterns to the right atrium, because inferior vena caval flow is directed to the right atrial septum and superior vena caval flow to the tricuspid valve. The timing of the Valsalva maneuver, the dose of the contrast medium, and the patient's posture during the examination are further factors influencing detection of PFO.[227,228]

ECHOCONTRAST STUDIES IN STROKE DIAGNOSIS

The ability of intravenous contrast media to increase the echogenicity of flowing blood has been known for some time.[229] Only in the last several years, however, has there been a growing demand for use of echo-enhancing agents in assessment of cerebrovascular disease. Common applications employing contrast agents are TCD ultrasonography studies in patients with severe hyperostosis of the skull, quantification of internal carotid stenosis in the presence of calcification, differentiation between internal carotid occlusion and pseudo-occlusion, assessment of intracranial aneurysms and AVMs, and investigation of the basilar and intracranial vertebral arteries.

Commercially available contrast agents consist of microbubbles with average diameters from $3\,\mu m$ to $6\,\mu m$ in concentrations typically on the order of 10^8 microbubbles per mL. The microbubbles are normally stabilized against dissolution by surfactants, phospholipids, or a surface layer of partially denatured albumin. Current contrast agents can enhance the ultrasound signal by 10 dB to 30 dB,[230] thus enabling the detection of flow in deeper and smaller vessels.

The first generation of ultrasonography contrast agents consisted of air-filled microbubbles. Examples of such agents are Albunex (Molecular Biosystems Inc., San Diego, CA), which is produced by controlled sonication of a 5% human serum albumin solution, and Levovist (Schering AG, Berlin), a galactose-based agent stabilized by 0.01% palmitic acid. Albunex is approved by the U.S. Food and Drug Administration (FDA) for use in the United States, and Levovist is approved for use in Europe. However, because of the low concentration of air gases in the systemic circulation, the air contained inside these agents quickly diffuses out of the microbubbles after injection into the body.[231] The type of gas inside the bubble determines the dwell time in the circulation[232] and can also affect the back-scattered signal in both linear and nonlinear regimens.[233] Thus, a second generation of ultrasonic agents was developed, which consists of microbubbles containing less soluble gases, such as perfluorocarbons and sulfur hexafluoride.

Carotid Artery Stenosis

Clinical studies with echo contrast agents have claimed to be effective in improving diagnostic confidence in patients with carotid artery stenosis. Contrast enhancement reduces operator variability, improves ultrasonographic image quality, and aids in distinguishing between pseudo and true occlusions.[234] Although first reports on the use of ultrasonic contrast media to investigate carotid arteries suggested a significant improvement in characterization and quantification of severe internal carotid stenosis,[235,236] further studies demonstrated that unenhanced PDI provides the same diagnostic yield as the combined approach for assessment of carotid artery pseudo-occlusion.[237] Now that new analysis of the data from the European Carotid Surgery Trial study has shown that patients with subtotal ICA stenosis do not benefit from carotid endarterectomy,[238] the importance of distinguishing between pseudo-occlusions and true occlusions with ultrasonography has diminished. In this context, the use of echo contrast agents for detection of carotid artery pseudo-occlusion is not justified.

Insufficient Transcranial Bone Windows

In TCD ultrasonography, insonation through the transtemporal bone window is often impaired by an insufficient signal-to-noise ratio, especially in elderly patients. Echo contrast agents have been shown to yield conclusive TCD ultrasonography findings in most patients in whom ultrasonography penetration is insufficient. Most studies have been performed with the galactose-based microbubble agent Levovist. Depending on the concentration of Levo-

vist, the average maximal TCD signal enhancement is approximately 12.0 ± 5.4 dB for 300 mg/mL.[239] Albunex has likewise been shown to improve the quality of TCD ultrasonography examinations through better visualization of the ICA, the MCA, and the circle of Willis,[240] although the relatively short duration of the contrast enhancement is a limiting factor.

Contrast agents have also been shown to enhance diagnoses by transcranial CDFI in patients with poor tissue penetration in whom imaging of vessels would otherwise be inadequate.[241] Other studies have confirmed these initial findings in patients whose basal arteries could not be assessed adequately with transcranial CDFI. After administration of Levovist, more than 85% of examinations of the MCA, the ACA, the P1 and P2 segments of the PCA, and the supraclinoid portion of the ICA siphon were satisfactory.[242] Moreover, use of intravenous contrast material often enables the entire circle of Willis to be evaluated from a single temporal-bone acoustic window in both PDI and CDFI.[243] Contrast agents have also been used to enable intracranial insonation through lateral and paramedian frontal bone windows, thus offering a new approach to study the circle of Willis, the venous midline vasculature, and the frontal parenchyma.[244] The technical success rate of 3D transcranial PDI investigations has also been improved with contrast agents.[245]

There is good evidence that echo contrast agents are valuable in TCD ultrasonography examinations of patients with acute cerebrovascular disease. In an investigation of patients presenting with ischemic strokes and TIAs who had insufficient temporal bone windows, results of contrast-enhanced transcranial CDFI studies in 66% of patients were conclusive.[246] These findings have been confirmed by a similar study of patients with acute stroke in whom investigations performed without contrast enhancement were inadequate.[247]

The quality of transtemporal pre–contrast enhancement scans is strongly predictive of the potential diagnostic benefit that is to be expected from application of an intravenous contrast agent. In patients whose intracranial structures are not visible in B-mode imaging and whose vessel segments are not depicted with CDFI, there is little chance that the use of a contrast agent will provide diagnostic confidence.[248] This has also been shown in patients with acute cerebral ischemia. In one study b identification of any cerebral artery before contrast enhancement provided an overall accuracy of 97% in predicting that an investigation with contrast agent would be conclusive, whereas in patients in whom vessel identification was not possible before the use of contrast enhancement, there were no conclusive contrast studies.[246]

Vertebral and Basilar Arteries

Examinations of the intracranial vertebral arteries and the basilar artery are also facilitated with echo contrast agents. Use of an echo contrast agent for insonation through the foramen magnum during color-coded duplex ultrasonography can increase the depth at which vessels can be identified[249] and improve the number of pathologic findings not seen in unenhanced scans by about 20%.[250] Moreover,

Diagnostic Studies

echo-contrast enhancement of the vertebral and basilar arteries may significantly improve diagnostic confidence. This is particularly true in cases of acute basilar artery occlusion, because the detection rate of basilar artery flow for contrast-enhanced transcranial CDFI is more than 98%, as opposed to 76% without contrast agent.[251] Some evidence suggests that PDI may be just as effective as contrast-enhanced transcranial CDFI in visualizing the vertebrobasilar system.[252]

Intracranial Aneurysms

Contrast-enhanced transcranial CDFI and contrast-enhanced PDI (CE PDI) employing Levovist have been used to detect and measure the size of intracranial aneurysms.[253] Although CE PDI missed 4 of 36 angiographically verified aneurysms in one study, measurements of aneurysm size correlated well with angiographic findings. Other ultrasonography studies have suggested that aneurysm dimensions may vary with intracranial pressure (ICP), being larger and less pulsatile at low ICP and smaller but more pulsatile at high ICP.[254] Intraoperative transcranial CDFI allows characterization and localization of aneurysms[255] as well as identification of vessels potentially threatened by clipping,[256] whereas intraoperative microvascular Doppler ultrasonography has been shown to be an effective alternative to intraoperative angiography for assessment of vessel patency in aneurysm surgery.[257] An important remaining question is whether, in cases of acute SAH, TCD ultrasonography is capable of detecting not only the bleeding aneurysm but also other asymptomatic aneurysms that may require neurosurgical intervention.

Arteriovenous Malformations

Transcranial CE PDI with Levovist has also been used to evaluate AVMs.[258] In one study, CE PDI identified all angiographically confirmed AVMs in patients with adequate temporal bone windows. Although this technique slightly underestimated AVM size, it consistently showed feeding arteries. Coincidental blood supply from another intracranial or extracranial vessel, however, was missed by CE PDI in all cases. These results are encouraging and demonstrate the potential of CE PDI for evaluation and follow-up of AVMs.

Venous Thrombosis

TCD methods can also be used to evaluate the basal cerebral veins, which can be identified on the basis of their anatomic relation to specific arteries.[259] As in other applications, power- and frequency-based color-coded duplex ultrasonography aids in the assessment of cerebral veins and sinuses.[260] Standardized protocols for intracranial venous examinations and reference data for clinical applications have been described.[261]

Evidence suggests that TCD ultrasonography can detect and monitor intracranial venous hemodynamics and collateral pathways in patients with confirmed cerebral venous thrombosis (CVT).[262,263] Transcranial CDFI evaluation of venous drainage patterns in acute CVT have shown that both initially normal venous flow and normalization of initially diseased venous flow within 90 days of CVT are related to a favorable outcome.[264] Transcranial CDFI appears to enable a more reliable evaluation of the major deep cerebral veins and posterior fossa sinuses in cases of sinus thrombosis. The anterior and middle portions of the superior sagittal sinus and cortical veins, however, cannot be assessed by this means.[265] Here, increased venous blood flow velocity can be used as indirect evidence of a cerebral venous thrombosis. Superior evaluation of transverse sinus thrombosis can be obtained by with the use of echo contrast agents[266] (see later). Further prospective studies are needed to establish the sensitivity and specificity of neurosonologic techniques for diagnosis and monitoring of intracranial venous thrombosis.

MONITORING IN ACUTE STROKE

Monitoring of Thrombolysis

Recanalization time as determined in vitro is an important measure of thrombolysis when clot is exposed to tissue-type plasminogen activator (t-PA) (Plate 21–8). This time is usually given as the time of complete clot dissolution with washout to the distal vasculature and the veins. In human stroke, complete recanalization correlates with clinical recovery, as predicted from animal models. Recanalization, however, is a process that often begins many minutes before restoration of cerebral blood flow (CBF), because t-PA binding and activity on the clot surface are proportional to the area exposed to blood flow. Once recanalization starts, the clot softens and partially dissolves. As a result, residual flow improves, allowing more t-PA to bind with fibrinogen sites. This process facilitates clot lysis and continually improves residual flow until the clot breaks up under the pressure of arterial blood pulsations.

Recanalization time may be an important clinical parameter of thrombolysis. Although prolonged clot dissolution delays complete recanalization and may be associated with a longer duration of cerebral ischemia, a sudden increase in blood flow may disrupt the blood-brain barrier and lead to edema or hemorrhage. Alexandrov and coworkers[267] have addressed this issue using real-time ultrasonography monitoring of residual flow signals during thrombolysis with t-PA in patients with occlusion of the MCA or basilar artery. These researchers classified recanalization as sudden (abrupt appearance of a normal or stenotic low-resistance signal), stepwise (flow improvement over 1 to 29 minutes), or slow (≥30 minutes to improvement). The results showed that recanalization began at a median of 17 minutes and was completed at 35 minutes after bolus administration of t-PA, with a mean duration of recanalization of 23 ± 16 minutes. Complete recanalization occurred considerably faster (median 10 minutes) than partial recanalization (median 30 minutes). Importantly, rapid arterial recanalization was associated with better short-term improvement, whereas slow flow improvement and dampened flow signals were less favorable prognostic signs. These findings, by providing valuable information on temporal patterns of recanalization, may assist in identification of patients who need additional pharmacologic or interventional treatment.

Detection of MES by TCD at the site of arterial obstruction can indicate clot dissolution. Alexandrov and coworkers[268] detected clusters of MES distal to a high-grade M1 stenosis before spontaneous clinical recovery; they also documented minimal MCA flow signals followed by MES, increased velocities, and normal flow signals over a period of 2 minutes preceding complete recanalization.[268] Further studies are needed to establish the role of MES detection in monitoring of thrombolytic therapy.

Monitoring of Midline Shift

Transcranial color-coded duplex ultrasonography is a non-invasive, easily reproducible, and reliable method for monitoring midline dislocation of the third ventricle in patients with stroke.[269] It is well suited for monitoring the space-occupying effect of both supratentorial and infratentorial strokes during treatment in critical care and stroke units.[270] The technique can also be used to facilitate the identification of patients who are unlikely to survive without decompressive craniectomy.[271]

Assessment of Vasospasm

TCD has become a standard examination procedure for detection, quantification, and follow-up of vasospasms after SAH.[132,272,273] Vasospasms generally occur on the fourth day after SAH, and peak flow velocities can be observed between the 11th and 18th days. Normalization of flow velocities occurs within the third or fourth week after SAH. Rapid increase of velocities 4 to 8 days after SAH is associated with a higher risk of ischemic stroke.

Although early reports claimed that TCD results mirror the extent of obstruction commonly demonstrated in angiograms of stroke-prone patients after SAH, other observations have questioned a simple focal narrowing of the arterial lumen, analogous to that in atherosclerotic disease, as the cause of altered Doppler flow patterns after SAH. The pathophysiology of subarachnoid vasospasm is complex. Elevated ICP may lead to an increase in vasomotor resistance of capillary and arteriolar vessels with consequent dampening of the Doppler flow velocity in major proximal arteries. This may result in false-negative Doppler results despite angiographically demonstrable vasospasm. Moreover, local flow turbulences may be found despite normal angiographic findings if peripheral vasomotor dysregulation and large vessel vasoconstriction occur subsequent to SAH.

Importantly, TCD findings in patients with SAH are greatly influenced by changing therapeutic concepts. Only 28% of patients treated with calcium channel blockers have a significant increase in flow velocities before the onset of delayed ischemic stroke, suggesting that vasospasm may occur in more distal arterial segments inaccessible to TCD insonation.[274] TCD is further limited in patients with SAH by its relatively poor diagnostic accuracy in the ACA territory, a common site of aneurysms.[275]

Increased Intracranial Pressure

TCD can be useful in monitoring ICP in patients with bleeding diatheses and other contraindications to invasive ICP monitoring. Simultaneous recordings of Doppler signals from the basal cerebral arteries, systemic blood pressure, and ICP with epidural devices have shown that a progressive reduction in diastolic and systolic velocities can occur with increasing ICP. Moreover, various patterns of flow alterations have been demonstrated in different regions of the brain, indicating the existence of varying pressure gradients inside the skull.[276] When the ICP rises above diastolic blood pressure, Doppler signals from the basal cerebral arteries are severely altered. Mild or moderate increases in ICP, however, can be compensated by an increase in the systemic blood pressure, thus resulting in normal TCD findings. Measurements of the absolute ICP value cannot be performed with this method, but changes in TCD findings parallel changes in ICP value, assuming a constant arterial CO_2 content and a constant level of distal vasoconstriction. Thus, at least under certain conditions, a quantitative estimation of the ICP could be made on the basis of consistent relationships between flow velocity parameters recorded from intracranial arteries and continuous but noninvasive arterial blood pressure measurement. Schmidt and colleagues[277] supported this concept and showed that a mathematical model could predict ICP modulations from shapes of arterial blood flow and pulse noninvasively. These preliminary findings suggest that TCD may prove useful in evaluating strategies to improve cerebral autoregulation as well as in the optimal management of ICP control.

Functional Studies

The introduction of bilateral continuous TCD monitoring has resulted in the development of a variety of new sophisticated applications as supplementary tools to positron emission tomography (PET) and functional MRI studies. They include evaluation of functional recovery after stroke.

Changes in cerebral perfusion during motor activity in patients with stroke who have early recovery of motor function may be monitored with TCD ultrasonography.[278,279] Increased flow velocities in both the contralateral and ipsilateral MCAs during motor tasks have been demonstrated, suggesting that areas of the healthy hemisphere can be activated soon after a focal ischemic injury and can contribute to the positive evolution of a functional deficit. This phenomenon of contralateral recovery from activation is not transient, because it is evident months after stroke onset. In patients with Broca aphasia after ischemic stroke, a similar increase in MCA flow velocities has been detected after successful speech therapy, providing additional support for contralateral hemispheric involvement in functional recovery after stroke.[280]

Ultrasonographic Brain Perfusion Imaging

Because perfusion imaging may detect ischemic lesions earlier than CT and may distinguish the stroke subtype and severity of cerebral ischemia, there is growing interest in the use of perfusion imaging to predict recovery, differentiate stroke pathogenesis, and monitor therapy. Validated proportional indicators of CBF and potential diagnostic tools in stroke are single-photon emission CT using technetium ^{99m}Tc–hexamethyl-propyleneamineoxime (HMPAO), positron emission tomography, xenon-enhanced CT, and perfusion-weighted MRI. The main disadvantages of

Diagnostic Studies

these methods are that they are time consuming, require the use of radioactive tracers, are expensive, or cannot be tolerated by critically ill or restless patients. Noninvasive and easily available perfusion studies are clearly needed. In this regard, contrast harmonic imaging (CHI) may represent a useful bedside tool for a reliable measurement of brain perfusion.

Contrast Harmonic Imaging

Physiologic and pathologic myocardial perfusion has been assessed with CHI.[281,282] Several studies of this modality have shown that it may enable identification of physiologic parenchymal cerebral echo-contrast enhancement in different brain areas.[283–288] First applications of CHI in patients with CVD have demonstrated its potential to detect perfusion deficits.[289]

Although CHI is capable of imaging brain tissue perfusion, it has some drawbacks. Energy loss, signal reverberations, and aberrations occur during insonation through the transtemporal bone window. Moreover, in dual-frequency harmonic imaging, the bandwidths have to be narrow to avoid overlap between the fundamental and second harmonic frequencies. This requirement leads to an inherent tradeoff in image resolution, thus accentuating the problem of the transtemporal bone window.

Stimulated Acoustic Emission

Stimulated acoustic emission, also called "contrast burst imaging," involves CDFI or PDI with the transmitting power set high enough to ensure disruption of contrast agent bubbles on the first pulse. Certain ultrasonography contrast agents, such as those with thin polymer coatings, are durable linear scatterers at low acoustic pressures but undergo destruction, fusion, or splitting at higher acoustic pressures that are within the range of diagnostic ultrasonography.[290] causing a transient high-amplitude broadband response.[291] Because Doppler ultrasonography systems correlate the signals back-scattered from a target within a number of successive pulses, the loss of signal correlation caused by the transient bubble collapse is interpreted by the machine as a random Doppler shift, resulting in a mosaic of colors at the location of the microbubbles, even without flow. This technique has been shown to be useful in detecting bleeding sites[292] and liver tumors.[293,294] The ability of stimulated acoustic emission to visualize brain perfusion has been demonstrated.[290]

Pulse Inversion Contrast Harmonic Imaging

Pulse-inversion CHI (PICHI) is an ultrasonography technique that minimizes some of the shortcomings of CHI. It uses a two-pulse sequence with an 180-degree phase difference to cancel the effect of transmitted second harmonics on the received signal.[295] By preserving axial resolution and avoiding harmonic frequency overlaps, PICHI offers new possibilities for both qualitative and quantitative evaluation of the cerebral circulation.

Early results with PICHI demonstrated excellent ultrasonographic visualization of adult brain tissue.[215] Exceptional depth penetration allows simultaneous measurement of harmonic microbubble contrast enhancement in both ipsilateral and contralateral temporal lobes, providing a basis for qualitative comparison of perfusion char-

acteristics with a single bolus injection of contrast agent. Although preliminary, the results provide evidence that PICHI may be very sensitive in the characterization of brain perfusion.

Quantitative Perfusion Studies

Comparison of echo-contrast washout curves has shown a significant decrease in signal intensity in investigations of similar brain structures at different insonation depths.[296] Because of this depth dependence of measured contrast enhancement, it is unlikely that a classical approach using indicator dilution modeling can provide a valid measurement of CBF in different regions of the brain.

A promising new method for determination of tissue blood flow with CHI has been developed.[214] This approach is based on measurement of the reappearance rate of microbubbles after their destruction by ultrasound. Under steady-state conditions, measurement of the microbubble reappearance rate provides a measure of mean microbubble velocity, thus allowing blood flow to be calculated as a product of the reappearance rate and of the cross-sectional volume of the region of interest being measured according to the following equation:

$$\gamma = A(1 - e^{-\beta t})$$

where γ is the measured acoustic intensity at a pulse interval t, A is the plateau of acoustic intensity, and β is the rate constant that determines the rate of rise of acoustic intensity.

The technique using microbubble refill kinetics has been used to measure blood flow to various tissues, including the myocardium,[214] skeletal muscle,[297] and kidney.[298] It has also been shown to be applicable for assessment of CBF in animal experiments.[299] Rim and coworkers[300] have demonstrated that measurement of CBF can be obtained using real-time PICHI in dog brains. Real-time power PICHI, a hybrid method using power Doppler and pulse inversion technology, is a promising new technique that may give rise to significant advances in both ultrasonographic visualization of brain infarctions and in assessment of CBF (Fig. 21–9 and Plate 21–9).

NEW HORIZONS IN CEREBROVASCULAR ULTRASONOGRAPHY

Thrombolysis with Ultrasound

Deficiencies of current thrombolytic stroke therapy include slow and incomplete thrombolysis and frequent bleeding complications. Growing evidence from in vitro and animal studies indicates that application of ultrasound as an adjunct to thrombolytic therapy offers a unique approach to improve effectiveness and decrease bleeding complications. The potential for high-frequency ultrasound to dissolve intra-arterial thrombi was first reported by Trubestein and associates[301] in 1976. In these experiments, a 26.5-kHz ultrasound transducer was used to recanalize thrombosed iliofemoral arteries in dogs with minimal complications. In the ensuing 25 years, further

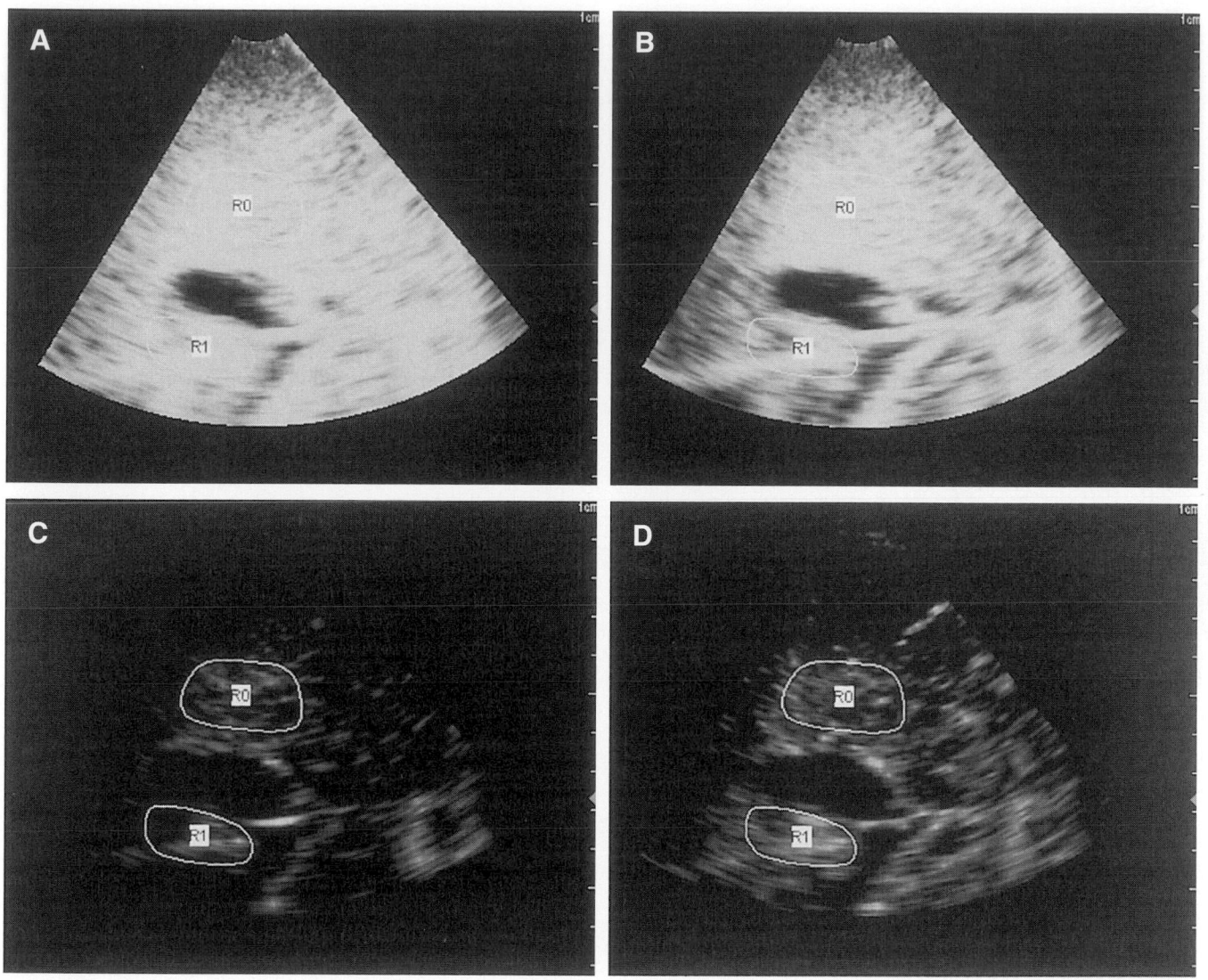

FIGURE 21–9 *Real-time power pulse inversion contrast imaging of ipsilateral middle cerebral artery (MCA) infarction with recanalization of the MCA. A and B, Real-time destruction of the contrast agent Sonovue using an high mechanical index (pulse interval 60 ms). B demonstrates color desaturation after bubble destruction. In C and D, a low mechanical index is used that does not destroy microbubbles, thus allowing contrast replenishment to be monitored in real time; C was acquired directly after bubble destruction, and D approximately 5 seconds later. Two regions of interest (R0 and R1 in A through D; ROI in E and F) have been set to allow evaluation of bubble destruction*

Continued

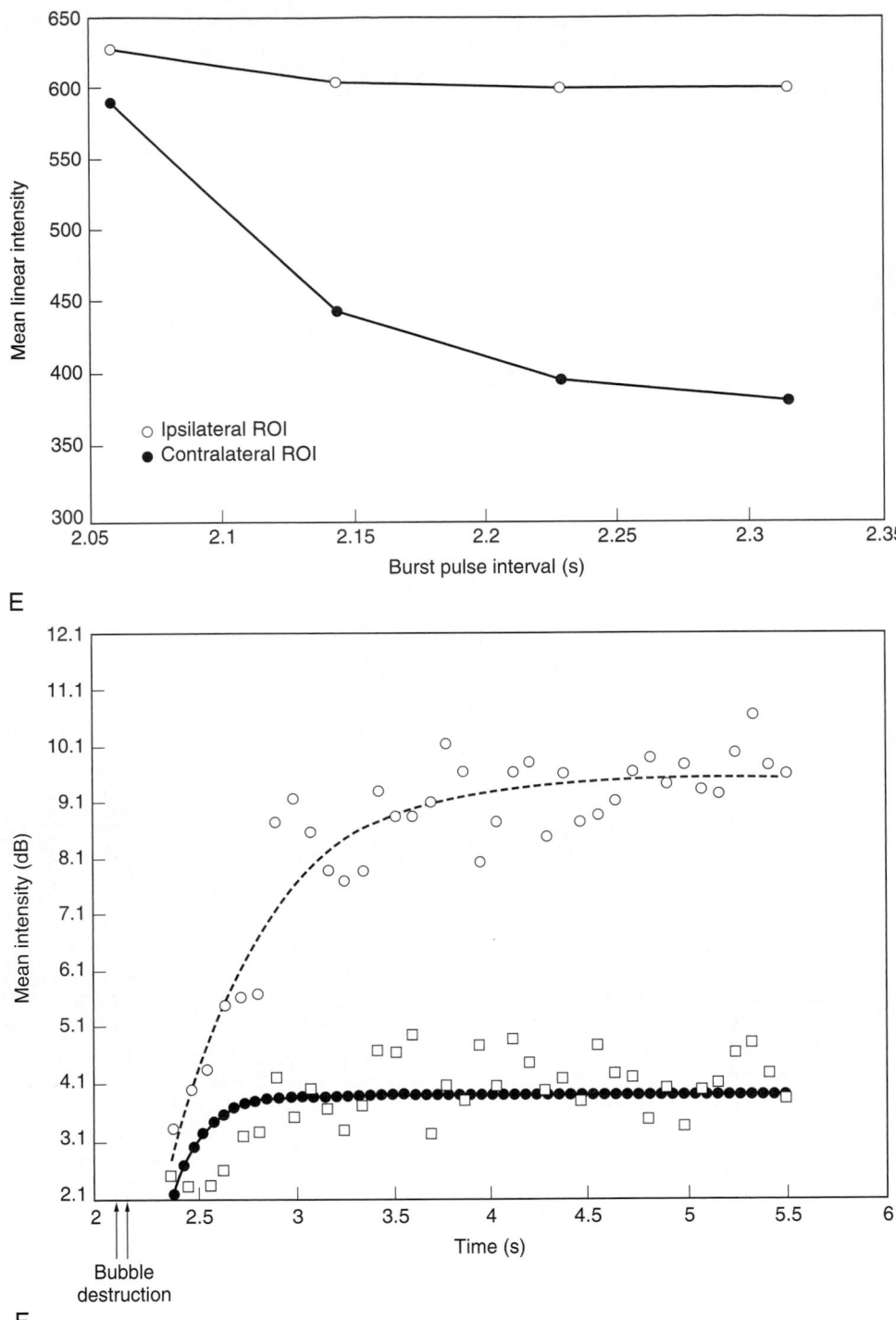

FIGURE 21–9, cont'd. (E) *and replenishment kinetics* (F) *in both hemispheres. In* F, *the* squares *depict mean intensities overtime in ROI of ipsilateral infarction, and the* circles *denote mean intensities in contralateral tissue.*

studies using catheter-based or transcutaneous ultrasound focused mainly on the ability of ultrasound to enhance the effect of fibrinolytic agents in recanalizing acutely thrombosed arteries.[302,303–308] Later animal studies have suggested that intravenously injected microbubbles may enhance the effects of ultrasound and may even produce recanalization of acutely thrombosed arteries in the presence of ultrasound without the need for fibrinolytic agents.[309,310]

Although in vitro studies have observed microfragmentation of thrombi in the presence of microbubbles and ultrasound, the precise mechanism by which ultrasound and microbubbles induce thrombus dissolution remains unknown.

In vitro studies have shown that very-low-frequency ultrasound transducers (33 to 71 kHz) can significantly potentiate the effect of t-PA–mediated thrombolysis when delivered through the temporal bone.[311,312] There is some evidence that TCD, even at diagnostic frequencies, can accelerate thrombolysis. In one study, dramatic recovery during t-PA therapy occurred in 20% of all patients when infusion was continuously monitored with TCD.[313] Clinical studies are under way to assess the value of both diagnostic and low-frequency ultrasound in enhancing thrombolysis in acute ischemic stroke.

Molecular Imaging

Molecular imaging can be defined as the characterization and measurement of biologic processes at the cellular and molecular level by means of remote imaging detectors. Goals of molecular imaging include noninvasive detection of disease using disease-associated molecular signatures, in vivo delineation of complex molecular mechanisms of disease, and detection of gene expression. Targeted ultrasound techniques combine ultrasound imaging technology with specific contrast agents for the assessment of molecular or genetic signatures for disease. Because of the high echogenicity of ultrasonographic contrast agents in comparison with tissue or plasma, the echo from a single microbubble can be detected with ultrasonographic imaging techniques. This means that the system is sensitive to a volume in the order of 0.004 pico liters,[314] thus offering a high level of resolution that is not currently achieved with other imaging modalities.

Addition of targeted ligands to microbubbles opens new avenues for the identification of vascular occlusion or areas of vascular injury. Adhesion molecules such as the integrin $\alpha_v\beta_3$, intercellular adhesion molecule-1 (ICAM-1), and fibrinogen receptor GPIIb/IIIa are overexpressed in regions of angiogenesis, inflammation, and thrombus, respectively. These molecular signatures can be used to localize ultrasonographic contrast agents through the use of complementary receptor ligands. This approach has been demonstrated for imaging of angiogenesis using microbubbles targeted to α_v-integrins.[315] Likewise, lipid-based perfluorobutane-filled microbubbles have been synthesized with various densities of anti–ICAM-1 monoclonal antibodies conjugated to the bubble shell to investigate early stages of atherosclerosis.[316] Targeted microbubbles directed to the GPIIb/IIIa receptor of activated platelets have also been developed for visualization of thrombus,[317,318] and leukocyte-targeted microbubbles can be used to characterize the severity of postischemic myocardial inflammation[319] and to identify inflamed plaques.[320]

Although application of targeted contrast-enhanced ultrasonography for molecular imaging is in the early stages of development, it is potentially easily translatable to routine clinical practice, because the technique is relatively inexpensive, is portable, and employs technology that is already widely used to evaluate vascular disease.

Gene Delivery

The promise of gene therapy in acute stroke lies in the potential to increase the brain's resistance to ischemic damage by upregulating genes known to improve cell survival. This goal may be accomplished by incorporating transfected genes into neurons already suffering from an ischemic insult or into those in which such an event is anticipated. Ultrasound may be a valuable tool in gene therapy by virtue of its ability to enhance transgene expression. Simple exposure to ultrasound has been shown to enhance transgene expression in vascular cells by up to 10-fold after naked DNA transfection. Likewise, transfection studies performed using marker genes that do not exert a therapeutic effect—that is, *p*-chloramphenicolacetyltransferase, β-galactosidase, and green fluorescent protein—demonstrated that ultrasound consistently increased gene expression in cell lines such as HeLa, NIH t-3, and COS-1 cells.[321] The enhancement of transfection occurred at levels of ultrasound of about 0.5 W/cm^2 and duration of exposure of only about 15 seconds and did not appreciably heat the cells or adversely affect their survival. Similar results on the effect of ultrasound on gene expression have been obtained in cell cultures during liposomal transfection experiments.[322] Ultrasound enhances transfection mostly likely through cavitation,[323] which in turn increases microvascular permeability. This effect can be dramatically enhanced in the presence of ultrasonographic contrast agents.[324] Microbubble cavitation by ultrasound produces local shock waves. This process increases transcapillary passage of macromolecules or nanospheres codelivered with the microbubbles.[325,326] Cavitation probably opens micropores in small blood vessel walls, making the vessels more permeable to molecules and nanoparticles. Microvascular permeability due to cavitation of microbubbles may therefore be exploited therapeutically to increase local delivery of therapeutic materials such as genes.

Not only can microbubbles be used to enhance the effects of ultrasound on gene expression. They may also be employed as carriers of gene therapeutic agents.[321,327] There are a number of ways to entrap different drugs with microbubbles. One technique is to incorporate them into the membrane- or wall-forming materials that stabilize microbubbles. Charged drugs can be stabilized in or onto the surfaces of microbubbles by virtue of electrostatic interactions. In this way, cationic lipid–coated microbubbles can bind DNA, which is a polyanion and binds avidly to cationic (positively charged) microbubbles. Drugs can also be incorporated into the interior of microbubbles (gas-filled microspheres). Another way to entrap drugs in microbubbles is to create a layer of oil (e.g., triacetin) to stabilize the outer surface of the bubble. Hydrophobic drugs can then be incorporated into the oil layer. Regardless of the technique used to incorporate the drugs, they are released when ultrasound energy cavitates the microbubble. These methods for making drug-carrying microbubbles are most applicable to drugs that are highly active. This is the case for gene-based drugs, in which the amount of gene injected is usually on the order of micrograms or milligrams. Therefore, large volumes of bubbles are not required to deliver highly active drugs such as genes.

In summary, ultrasound may be used to enhance gene expression. In the presence of microbubbles, a synergistic effect is attained, and cavitation is a likely mechanism. Acoustically active materials that bind or entrap genetic materials have a potential role for gene delivery. These materials can be injected intravenously, and targeted gene delivery is attained within the tissue exposed to ultrasound.

Diagnostic Studies

This new technology holds the promise of delivering genes more selectively than other methods and less invasively than direct injection. The ability to focus ultrasound and cause local cavitation with these new gene carriers may provide a powerful new tool for gene delivery in patients with stroke.

References

1. Goes E, Janssens W, Maillet B, et al: Tissue characterization of atheromatous plaques: Correlation between ultrasound image and histological findings. J Clin Ultrasound 18:611–617, 1990.
2. Hennerici M, Steinke W: Carotid plaque developments: Aspects of hemodynamic and vessel wall-platelet interaction. Cerebrovasc Dis 1:142–148, 1991.
3. Hennerici M, Reifschneider G, Trockel U, et al: Detection of early atherosclerotic lesions by duplex scanning of the carotid artery. J Clin Ultrasound 12:455–464, 1984.
4. Wolverson MK, Bashiti HM, Peterson GJ: Ultrasonic tissue characterisation of atheromatous plaques using high resolution real time scanner. Ultrasound Med Biol 9:599–609, 1983.
5. Merritt CR: Doppler color flow imaging. J Clin Ultrasound 15:591–597, 1987.
6. Middleton WD, Foley WD, Lawson TL: Color Doppler flow imaging of carotid artery abnormalities. Am J Roentgenol 150:419–425, 1988.
7. Steinke W, Kloetzsch C, Hennerici M: Carotid artery disease assessed by color Doppler flow imaging: Correlation with standard Doppler sonography and angiography. Am J Neuroradiol 11:259–266, 1990.
8. Steinke W, Meairs S, Ries S, et al: Sonographic assessment of carotid artery stenosis: Comparison of power Doppler imaging and color Doppler flow imaging. Stroke 27:91–94, 1996.
9. Griewing B, Morgenstern C, Driesner F, et al: Cerebrovascular disease assessed by color-flow and power Doppler ultrasonography: Comparison with digital subtraction angiography in internal carotid artery stenosis. Stroke 27:95–100, 1996.
10. Jespersen SK, Wilhjelm JE, Sillesen H: In vitro spatial compound scanning for improved visualization of atherosclerosis. Ultrasound Med Biol 26:1357–1362, 2000.
11. Kofoed SC, Gronholdt ML, Wilhjelm JE, et al: Real-time spatial compound imaging improves reproducibility in the evaluation of atherosclerotic carotid plaques. Ultrasound Med Biol 27:1311–1317, 2001.
12. Meairs S, Timpe L, Beyer J, et al: Acute aphasia and hemiplegia during karate training. Lancet 356:40, 2000.
13. Detmer PR, Bashein G, Hodges T, et al: 3D ultrasonic image feature localization based on magnetic scanhead tracking: In vitro calibration and validation. Ultrasound Med Biol 20:923–936, 1994.
14. Hodges TC, Detmer PR, Burns DH, et al: Ultrasonic three-dimensional reconstruction: In vitro and in vivo volume and area measurement. Ultrasound Med Biol 20:719–729, 1994.
15. Leotta DF, Detmer PR, Martin RW: Performance of a miniature magnetic position sensor for three-dimensional ultrasound imaging. Ultrasound Med Biol 23:597–609, 1997.
16. Barry CD, Allott CP, John NW, et al: Three-dimensional freehand ultrasound: Image reconstruction and volume analysis. Ultrasound Med Biol 23:1209–1224, 1997.
17. Meairs S, Beyer J, Hennerici M: Reconstruction and visualization of irregularly sampled three- and four-dimensional ultrasound data for cerebrovascular applications. Ultrasound Med Biol 26:263–272, 2000.
18. Pignoli P, Tremoli E, Poli A, et al: Intimal plus medial thickness of the arterial wall: A direct measurement with ultrasound imaging. Circulation 74:1399–1406, 1986.
19. Wong M, Edelstein J, Wollman J, et al: Ultrasonic-pathological comparison of the human arterial wall: Verification of intima-media thickness. Arterioscler Thromb 13:482–486, 1993.
20. Riley WA, Barnes RW, Applegate WB, et al: Reproducibility of non-invasive ultrasonic measurement of carotid atherosclerosis: The Asymptomatic Carotid Artery Plaque Study. Stroke 23:1062–1068, 1992.
21. Poli A, Tremoli E, Colombo A, et al: Ultrasonographic measurement of the common carotid artery wall thickness in hypercholesterolemic patients: A new model for the quantitation and follow-up of preclinical atherosclerosis in living human subjects. Atherosclerosis 70:253–261, 1988.
22. O'Leary DH, Polak JF, Kronmal RA, et al: Thickening of the carotid wall: A marker for atherosclerosis in the elderly? Cardiovascular Health Study Collaborative Research Group. Stroke 27:224–231, 1996.
23. Bots ML, Hoes AW, Koudstaal PJ, et al: Common carotid intima-media thickness and risk of stroke and myocardial infarction: The Rotterdam Study. Circulation 96:1432–1437, 1997.
24. O'Leary DH, Polak JF, Kronmal RA, et al: Carotid-artery intima and media thickness as a risk factor for myocardial infarction and stroke in older adults. Cardiovascular Health Study Collaborative Research Group. N Engl J Med 340:14–22, 1999.
25. Azen SP, Qian D, Mack WJ, et al: Effect of supplementary antioxidant vitamin intake on carotid arterial wall intima-media thickness in a controlled clinical trial of cholesterol lowering. Circulation 94:2369–2372, 1996.
26. Sander D, Winbeck K, Klingelhofer J, et al: Reduced progression of early carotid atherosclerosis after antibiotic treatment and *Chlamydia pneumoniae* seropositivity. Circulation 106:2428–2433, 2002.
27. Zanchetti A, Bond MG, Hennig M, et al: Calcium antagonist lacidipine slows down progression of asymptomatic carotid atherosclerosis: Principal results of the European Lacidipine Study on Atherosclerosis (ELSA), a randomized, double-blind, long-term trial. Circulation 106:2422–2427, 2002.
28. Folsom AR, Eckfeldt JH, Weitzman S, et al: Relation of carotid artery wall thickness to diabetes mellitus, fasting glucose and insulin, body size, and physical activity. Atherosclerosis Risk in Communities (ARIC) Study Investigators. Stroke 25:66–73, 1994.
29. Furberg CD, Borhani NO, Byington RP, et al: Calcium antagonists and atherosclerosis: The Multicenter Isradipine/Diuretic Atherosclerosis Study. Am J Hypertens 6:24S–29S, 1993.
30. Crouse JR: Sources of arterial wall thickness measurement variability. In Touboul PJ (ed): Intima Media Thickness and Atherosclerosis: Predicting the Risk? New York, Parthenon, 1997, pp 59–68.
31. Baldassarre D, Werba JP, Tremoli E, et al: Common carotid intima-media thickness measurement: A method to improve accuracy and precision. Stroke 25:1588–1592, 1994.
32. Bruschi G, Cabassi A, Orlandini G, et al: Use of Fourier shape descriptors to improve the reproducibility of echographic measurements of arterial intima-media thickness. J Hypertens 15:467–474, 1997.
33. Celermajer DS, Sorensen KE, Gooch VM, et al: Non-invasive detection of endothelial dysfunction in children and adults at risk of atherosclerosis. Lancet 340:1111–1115, 1992.
34. Corretti MC, Plotnick GD, Vogel RA: Technical aspects of evaluating brachial artery vasodilatation using high-frequency ultrasound. Am J Physiol 268:H1397–H1404, 1995.
35. Uehata A, Lieberman EH, Gerhard MD, et al: Noninvasive assessment of endothelium-dependent flow-mediated dilation of the brachial artery. Vasc Med 2:87–92, 1997.
36. Corretti MC, Anderson TJ, Benjamin EJ, et al: Guidelines for the ultrasound assessment of endothelial-dependent flow-mediated vasodilation of the brachial artery: A report of the International Brachial Artery Reactivity Task Force. J Am Coll Cardiol 39:257–265, 2002.
37. Corretti MC, Plotnick GD, Vogel RA: Correlation of cold pressor and flow-mediated brachial artery diameter responses with the presence of coronary artery disease. Am J Cardiol 75:783–787, 1995.
38. Neunteufl T, Katzenschlager R, Hassan A, et al: Systemic endothelial dysfunction is related to the extent and severity of coronary artery disease. Atherosclerosis 129:111–118, 1997.
39. Arcaro G, Zenere BM, Travia D, et al: Non-invasive detection of early endothelial dysfunction in hypercholesterolaemic subjects. Atherosclerosis 114:247–254, 1995.
40. Johnstone MT, Creager SJ, Scales KM, et al: Impaired endothelium-dependent vasodilation in patients with insulin-dependent diabetes mellitus. Circulation 88:2510–2516, 1993.
41. Clarkson P, Celermajer DS, Donald AE, et al: Impaired vascular reactivity in insulin-dependent diabetes mellitus is related to disease duration and low density lipoprotein cholesterol levels. J Am Coll Cardiol 28:573–579, 1996.

Diagnostic Studies

42. Williams SB, Cusco JA, Roddy MA, et al: Impaired nitric oxide-mediated vasodilation in patients with non-insulin-dependent diabetes mellitus. J Am Coll Cardiol 27:567–574, 1996.

43. Hill JM, Zalos G, Halcox JP, et al: Circulating endothelial progenitor cells, vascular function, and cardiovascular risk. N Engl J Med 348:593–600, 2003.

44. Greenland P, Abrams J, Aurigemma GP, et al: Prevention Conference V: Beyond secondary prevention: Identifying the high-risk patient for primary prevention: Noninvasive tests of atherosclerotic burden: Writing Group III. Circulation 101:E16–E22, 2000.

45. Maroon JC, Pieroni DW, Campbell RL: Ophthalmosonometry: An ultrasonic method for assessing carotid blood flow. J Neurosurg 30:238–246, 1969.

46. Melis-Kisman E, Mol JMF: L'application de l'effet Doppler à l'exploration cérébrovasculaire: Rapport préliminaire. Rev Neur 122:470–472, 1970.

47. Müller HR: Direktionelle Dopplersonographie der A. frontalis medialis. EEG EMG Z Elektroenzephalogr Elektromyogragr Verwandte Geb 2:816–823, 1971.

48. LoGerfo FW, Mason GR: Directional Doppler studies of supraorbital artery flow in internal carotid stenosis and occlusion. Surgery 76:723–728, 1974.

49. Büdingen HJ, von Reutern GM: Ultraschalldiagnostik der hirnversorgenden Arterien. Stuttgart, Thieme, 1994.

50. Hennerici M, Neuerburg-Heusler D: Vascular Diagnosis with Ultrasound. New York, Thieme, 1998.

51. Meairs S, Hennerici M: Long-term follow-up of aneurysms developed during extracranial internal carotid artery dissection. Neurology 54:2190, 2000.

52. De Bray JM, Glatt B: Quantification of atheromatous stenosis in the extracranial internal carotid artery. Cerebrovasc Dis 5:414–426, 1995.

53. Levine SR, Welch KM: Common carotid artery occlusion. Neurology 39:178–186, 1989.

54. Zbornikova V, Lassvik C: Common carotid artery occlusion: Haemodynamic features. Cerebrovasc Dis 1:136–141, 1991.

55. Belkin M, Mackey WC, Pessin MS, et al: Common carotid artery occlusion with patent internal and external carotid arteries: Diagnosis and surgical management. J Vasc Surg 17:1019–1028, 1993.

56. Dashefsky SM, Cooperberg PL, Harrison PB, et al: Total occlusion of the common carotid artery with patent internal carotid artery: Identification with color Doppler flow imaging. J Ultrasound Med 10:417–421, 1991.

57. Riles TS, Imparato AM, Posner MP, et al: Common carotid occlusion. Ann Surg 199:363–366, 1984.

58. Steinke W, Rautenberg W, Sliwka U, et al: Common carotid artery occlusion: Clinical significance of a patent internal carotid artery. Neurol Sci 20:140, 1993.

59. Robinson ML, Sacks D, Perlmutter GS, et al: Diagnostic criteria for carotid duplex sonography. AJR Am J Roentgenol 151:1045–1049, 1988.

60. Taylor DC, Strandness DE Jr: Carotid artery duplex scanning. J Clin Ultrasound 15:635–644, 1987.

61. Zwiebel WJ, Knighton R: Duplex examination of the carotid arteries. Semin Ultrasound CT MRI 11:97–135, 1990.

62. Comerota AJ, Cranley A, Cook S: Real-time B-mode imaging in diagnosis of cerebrovascular disease. Surgery 89:718–729, 1981.

63. Ricotta JJ, Bryan FA, Bond MG, et al: Multicenter validation study of real-time (B-mode) ultrasound, arteriography, and pathologic examination. J Vasc Surg 6:512–520, 1987.

64. Zwiebel WJ, Austin CW, Sackett JF, et al: Correlation of high-resolution, B-mode and continuous-wave Doppler sonography with arteriography in the diagnosis of carotid stenosis. Radiology 149:523–532, 1983.

65. Sliwka U, Rother J, Steinke W, et al: [The value of duplex sonography in cerebral ischemia] Die Bedeutung der Duplexsonographie bei zerebralen Ischämien. Bildgebung 58:182–191, 1991.

66. Erickson SJ, Mewissen MW, Foley WD, et al: Stenosis of the internal carotid artery: Assessment using color Doppler imaging compared with angiography. Am J Roentgenol 152:1299–1305, 1989.

67. Middleton WD, Foley WD, Lawson TL: Flow reversal in the normal carotid bifurcation: Color Doppler flow imaging analysis. Radiology 167:207–210, 1988.

68. Steinke W, Kloetzsch C, Hennerici M: Variability of flow patterns in the normal carotid bifurcation. Atherosclerosis 84:121–127, 1990.

69. Steinke W, Hennerici M, Rautenberg W, et al: Symptomatic and asymptomatic high-grade carotid stenoses in Doppler color-flow imaging. Neurology 42:131–138, 1992.

70. Sitzer M, Fuerst G, Fischer H, et al: Between-method correlations in quantifying internal carotid stenosis. Stroke 24:1513–1518, 1993.

71. Yao J, van Sambeek MR, Dall'Agata A, et al: Three-dimensional ultrasound study of carotid arteries before and after endarterectomy: Analysis of stenotic lesions and surgical impact on the vessel. Stroke 29:2026–2031, 1998.

72. Delcker A, Diener HC: Quantification of atherosclerotic plaques in carotid arteries by three-dimensional ultrasound. Br J Radiol 67:672–678, 1994.

73. Griewing B, Schminke U, Morgenstern C, et al: Three-dimensional ultrasound angiography (power mode) for the quantification of carotid artery atherosclerosis. J Neuroimaging 7:40–45, 1997.

74. Hallam MJ, Reid JM, Cooperberg PL: Color-flow Doppler and conventional duplex scanning of the carotid bifurcation: Prospective, double-blind, correlative study. Am J Roentgenol 152:1101–1105, 1989.

75. Comerota AJ, Katz ML, White JV, et al: The preoperative diagnosis of the ulcerated carotid atheroma. J Vasc Surg 11:505–510, 1990.

76. Bock RW, Lusby RJ: Carotid plaque morphology and interpretation of the echolucent lesion. In Labs KH, Jäger KA, Fitzgerald DE, et al (eds): Diagnostic Vascular Imaging. London, Arnold, 1992, pp 225–236.

77. Bluth EI, Kay D, Merritt CRB, et al: Sonographic characterization of carotid plaque: detection of hemorrhage. Am J Roentgenol 146:1061–1065, 1986.

78. Langsfeld M, Gray Weale AC, Lusby RJ: The role of plaque morphology and diameter reduction in the development of new symptoms in asymptomatic carotid arteries. J Vasc Surg 9:548–557, 1989.

79. O'Donnell TF, Erdoes L, Mackay WC, et al: Correlation of B-mode ultrasound imaging and arteriography with pathologic findings at carotid endarterectomy. Arch Surg 120:443–449, 1985.

80. Sterpetti AV, Schultz RD, Feldhaus RJ, et al: Ultrasonographic features of carotid plaque and the risk of subsequent neurologic deficits. Surgery 104:652–660, 1988.

81. Aldoori MI, Baird R: Duplex scanning and plaque histology in cerebral ischaemia. Eur J Vasc Surg 1:159–164, 1987.

82. Imparato AM, Riles TS, Gostein F: The carotid bifurcation plaque: Pathologic findings associated with cerebral ischemia. Stroke 10:238–245, 1979.

83. Fisher M, Blumenfeld AM, Smith TW: The importance of carotid artery plaque disruption and hemorrhage. Arch Neurol 44:1086–1089, 1987.

84. Imparato AM, Riles TS, Mintzer R, et al: The importance of hemorrhage in the relationship between gross morphologic characteristics and cerebral symptoms in 376 carotid artery plaques. Ann Surg 197:195–203, 1983.

85. Lusby RJ, Ferrell LD, Ehrenfeld WK, et al: Carotid plaque hemorrhage: Its role in production of cerebral ischemia. Arch Surg 117:1479–1488, 1982.

86. Bassiouny HS, Davis H, Massawa N, et al: Critical carotid stenoses: Morphologic and chemical similarity between symptomatic and asymptomatic plaques. J Vasc Surg 9:202–212, 1989.

87. Leen EJ, Feeley TM, Colgan MP, et al: "Haemorrhagic" carotid plaque does not contain haemorrhage. Eur J Vasc Surg 4:123–128, 1990.

88. Lennihan L, Kupsky WJ, Mohr JP, et al: Lack of association between carotid plaque hematoma and ischemic cerebral symptoms. Stroke 18:879–881, 1987.

89. AbuRahma AF, Kyer PD, Robinson PA, et al: The correlation of ultrasonic carotid plaque morphology and carotid plaque hemorrhage: Clinical implications. Surgery 124:721–726, 1998.

90. Park AE, McCarthy WJ, Pearce WH, et al: Carotid plaque morphology correlates with presenting symptomatology. J Vasc Surg 27:872–878, 1998.

91. Golledge J, Cuming R, Ellis M, et al: Carotid plaque characteristics and presenting symptom. Br J Surg 84:1697–1701, 1997.

92. Gronholdt ML, Wiebe BM, Laursen H, et al: Lipid-rich carotid artery plaques appear echolucent on ultrasound B-mode images and may be associated with intraplaque haemorrhage. Eur J Vasc Endovasc Surg 14:439–445, 1997.

93. Droste DW, Karl M, Bohle RM, et al: Comparison of ultrasonic and histopathological features of carotid artery stenosis. Neurol Res 19:380–384, 1997.

Diagnostic Studies

94. Hatsukami TS, Ferguson MS, Beach KW, et al: Carotid plaque morphology and clinical events. Stroke 28:95–100, 1997.
95. Widder B, Paulat K, Hackspacher J, et al: Morphological characterization of carotid artery stenoses by ultrasound duplex scanning. Ultrasound Med Biol 16:349–354, 1990.
96. Bluth EI, McVay LVI, Merritt CR, et al: The identification of ulcerative plaque with high resolution duplex carotid scanning. J Ultrasound Med 7:73–76, 1988.
97. Eliasziw M, Strifler JY, Fox AJ, et al: Significance of plaque ulceration in symptomatic patients with high-grade carotid stenosis. Stroke 25:304–308, 1994.
98. Fischer CM, Ojemann RJ: A clinico-pathologic study of carotid endarterectomy plaques. Rev Neurol 142:573, 1986.
99. Svindland A, Torvik A: Atherosclerotic carotid disease in asymptomatic individuals: An histological study of 53 cases. Acta Neurol Scand 78:506–517, 1988.
100. Glagov S, Bassiouny HS, Giddens DP, et al: Intimal thickening: Morphogenesis, functional significance and detection. J Vasc Invest 1:1–14, 1995.
101. Meairs S, Hennerici M: Four-dimensional ultrasonographic characterization of plaque surface motion in patients with symptomatic and asymptomatic carotid artery stenosis. Stroke 30:1807–1813, 1999.
102. Ackerstaff RG, Hoeneveld H, Slowikowski JM, et al: Ultrasonic duplex scanning in atherosclerotic disease of the innominate, subclavian and vertebral arteries: A comparative study with angiography. Ultrasound Med Biol 10:409–418, 1984.
103. Bendick PJ, Jackson VP: Evaluation of the vertebral arteries with duplex sonography. J Vasc Surg 3:523–530, 1986.
104. Davis PC, Nilsen B, Braun IF, et al: A prospective comparison of duplex sonography vs angiography of the vertebral arteries. Am J Neuroradiol 7:1059–1064, 1986.
105. Bendick PJ, Glover JL: Hemodynamic evaluation of vertebral arteries by duplex ultrasound. Surg Clin North Am 70:235–244, 1990.
106. Bartels E: [Color-coded Doppler sonography of the vertebral arteries: Comparison with conventional duplex sonography] Farbkodierte Dopplersonographie der Vertebralarterien: Vergleich mit der konventionellen Duplexsonographie. Ultraschall Med 13:59–66, 1992.
107. Trattnig S, Schwaighofer B, Hubsch P, et al: Color-coded Doppler sonography of vertebral arteries. J Ultrasound Med 10:221–226, 1991.
108. Kuhl V, Tettenborn B, Eicke BM, et al: Color-coded duplex ultrasonography of the origin of the vertebral artery: Normal values of flow velocities. J Neuroimaging 10:17–21, 2000.
109. Fisher CM, Gore I, Okabe N, et al: Atherosclerosis of the carotid and vertebral arteries—extracranial and intracranial. Neuropathol Exp Neurol 24:455–476, 1965.
110. Hennerici M, Steinke W, Rautenberg W: High-resistance Doppler flow pattern in extracranial carotid dissection. Arch Neurol 46:670–672, 1989.
111. Steinke W, Rautenberg W, Schwartz A, et al: Ultrasonographic diagnosis and monitoring of cervicocephalic arterial dissection. Cerebrovasc Dis 2:195, 1992.
112. Sidhu PS, Jonker ND, Khaw KT, et al: Spontaneous dissections of the internal carotid artery: Appearances on colour Doppler ultrasound. Br J Radiol 70:50–57, 1997.
113. Sturzenegger M, Mattle HP, Rivoir A, et al: Ultrasound findings in carotid artery dissection: Analysis of 43 patients. Neurology 45:691–698, 1995.
114. Steinke W, Rautenberg W, Schwartz A, et al: Noninvasive monitoring of internal carotid artery dissection. Stroke 25:998–1005, 1994.
115. Caplan LR, Zarins CK, Hemmatti M: Spontaneous dissection of the extracranial vertebral arteries. Stroke 16:1030–1038, 1985.
116. Hart RG: Vertebral artery dissection. Neurology 38:987–989, 1988.
117. Greselle JF, Zenteno M, Kien P, et al: Spontaneous dissection of the vertebro-basilar system: A study of 18 cases (15 patients). J Neuroradiol 14:115–123, 1987.
118. Josien E: Extracranial vertebral artery dissection: Nine cases. J Neurol 239:327–330, 1992.
119. Mokri B, Houser OW, Sandok BA, et al: Spontaneous dissections of the vertebral arteries. Neurology 38:880–885, 1988.
120. Sturzenegger M, Mattle HP, Rivoir A, et al: Ultrasound findings in spontaneous extracranial vertebral artery dissection. Stroke 24:1910–1921, 1993.
121. Touboul PJ, Mas JL, Bousser MG, et al: Duplex scanning in extracranial vertebral artery dissection. Stroke 19:116–121, 1988.
122. Bartels E, Flügel KA: Evaluation of extracranial vertebral artery dissection with duplex color-flow imaging. Stroke 27:290–295, 1996.
123. Lu CJ, Sun Y, Jeng JS, et al: Imaging in the diagnosis and follow-up evaluation of vertebral artery dissection. J Ultrasound Med 19:263–270, 2000.
124. De Bray JM, Missoum A, Dubas F, et al: [Doppler transcranial ultrasonography in carotid and vertebral dissections: 36 cases involving angiography] Le Doppler transcranien dans les dissections carotidiennes et vertebrales: Étude de 36 cas arteriographies. J Mal Vasc 19:35–40, 1994.
125. Hoffmann M, Sacco RL, Chan S, et al: Noninvasive detection of vertebral artery dissection. Stroke 24:815–819, 1993.
126. Ackerstaff RG, Keunen RW, van Pelt W, et al: Influence of biological factors on changes in mean cerebral blood flow velocity in normal ageing: A transcranial Doppler study. Neurol Res 12:187–191, 1990.
127. Brass LM, Pavlakis SG, DeVivo D, et al: Transcranial Doppler measurements of the middle cerebral artery: Effect of hematocrit. Stroke 19:1466–1469, 1988.
128. Gomez CR, Brass LM, Tegeler CH, et al: The transcranial Doppler standardization project. J Neuroimaging 3:190–192, 1993.
129. Aaslid R, Markwalder TM, Nornes H: Noninvasive transcranial Doppler ultrasound recording of flow velocity in basal arteries. J Neurosurg 57:769–774, 1982.
130. Arnolds BJ, von Reutern GM: Transcranial Doppler sonography: Examination technique and normal reference values. Ultraschall Med 12:115–123, 1987.
131. Büdingen HJ, Staudacher T: Die Identifizierung der Arteria basilaris mit der transkraniellen Dopplersonographie. Ultraschall 8:95–101, 1987.
132. Harders A: Neurosurgical Applications of Transcranial Doppler Sonography. New York, Springer-Verlag, 1986.
133. Hennerici M, Rautenberg W, Sitzer G, et al: Transcranial Doppler ultrasound for the assessment of intracranial arterial flow velocity. Part 1: Examination technique and normal values. Surg Neurol 27:439–448, 1987.
134. Lindegaard KF, Bakke SJ, Grolimund P, et al: Assessment of intracranial hemodynamics in carotid artery disease by transcranial Doppler ultrasound. J Neurosurg 63:890–898, 1985.
135. Bogdahn U, Becker G, Winkler J, et al: Transcranial color-coded real-time sonography in adults. Stroke 21:1680–1688, 1990.
136. Bartels E, Flugel KA: Quantitative measurements of blood flow velocity in basal cerebral arteries with transcranial duplex color-flow imaging: A comparative study with conventional transcranial Doppler sonography. J Neuroimaging 4:77–81, 1994.
137. Eicke BM, Tegeler CH, Dalley G, et al: Angle correction in transcranial Doppler sonography. J Neuroimaging 4:29–33, 1994.
138. Hennerici M, Rautenberg W, Schwartz A: Transcranial Doppler ultrasound for the assessment of intracranial arterial flow velocity. Part 2: Evaluation of intracranial arterial disease. Surg Neurol 27:523–532, 1987.
139. Lindegaard KF, Bakke SJ, Aaslid R, et al: Doppler diagnosis of intracranial artery occlusive disorders. J Neurol Neurosurg Psychiatry 49:510–518, 1986.
140. Spencer MP, Whisler D: Transorbital Doppler diagnosis of intracranial arterial stenosis. Stroke 17:916–921, 1986.
141. Mattle H, Grolimund P, Huber P, et al: Transcranial Doppler sonographic findings in middle cerebral artery disease. Arch Neurol 45:289–295, 1988.
142. Rautenberg W, Schwartz A, Mull M, et al: Noninvasive detection of intracranial stenoses and occlusions. Stroke 21:149, 1990.
143. Goertler M, Kross R, Baeumer M, et al: Diagnostic impact and prognostic relevance of early contrast-enhanced transcranial color-coded duplex sonography in acute stroke. Stroke 29:955–962, 1998.
144. Postert T, Braun B, Federlein J, et al: Diagnosis and monitoring of middle cerebral artery occlusion with contrast-enhanced transcranial color-coded real-time sonography in patients with inadequate acoustic bone windows. Ultrasound Med Biol 24:333–340, 1998.
145. Gerriets T, Goertler M, Stolz E, et al: Feasibility and validity of transcranial duplex sonography in patients with acute stroke. J Neurol Neurosurg Psychiatry 73:17–20, 2002.
146. Mull M, Aulich A, Hennerici M: Transcranial Doppler ultrasonography versus arteriography for assessment of the vertebrobasilar circulation. J Clin Ultrasound 18:539–549, 1990.

147. Cher LM, Chambers BR, Smidt V: Comparison of transcranial Doppler with DSA in vertebrobasilar ischaemia. Clin Exp Neurol 29:143–148, 1992.

148. Tettenborn B, Estol C, DeWitt LD, et al: Accuracy of transcranial Doppler in the vertebrobasilar circulation [abstract]. J Neurol 237:159, 1990.

149. Röther J, Wentz KU, Rautenberg W, et al: Magnetic resonance angiography in vertebrobasilar ischemia. Stroke 24:1310–1315, 1993.

150. Meairs S, Steinke W, Mohr JP, Hennerici M: Ultrasound imaging and Doppler sonography. In Barnett HJM, Mohr JP, Stein BM, Yatsu F (eds): Stroke: Pathophysiology, Diagnosis and Management, 3rd ed. New York, Churchill Livingstone, 1998, pp 207–326.

151. Postert T, Braun B, Pfundtner N, et al: Echo contrast-enhanced three-dimensional power Doppler of intracranial arteries. Ultrasound Med Biol 24:953–962, 1998.

152. Deverson S, Evans DH, Bouch DC: The effects of temporal bone on transcranial Doppler ultrasound beam shape. Ultrasound Med Biol 26:239–244, 2000.

153. Klotzsch C, Bozzato A, Lammers G, et al: Contrast-enhanced three-dimensional transcranial color-coded sonography of intracranial stenoses. AJNR Am J Neuroradiol 23:208–212, 2002.

154. Schneider PA, Rossman ME, Bernstein EF, et al: Effect of internal carotid artery occlusion on intracranial hemodynamics: Transcranial Doppler evaluation and clinical correlation. Stroke 19:589–593, 1988.

155. Schneider PA, Rossman ME, Torem S, et al: Transcranial Doppler in the management of extracranial cerebrovascular disease: Implications in diagnosis and monitoring. J Vasc Surg 7:223–231, 1988.

156. Rautenberg W, Hennerici M: Intracranial hemodynamic measurements in patients with severe asymptomatic extracranial carotid disease. Cerebrovasc Dis 1:216–222, 1991.

157. Padayachee TS, Gosling RG, Bishop CC, et al: Monitoring middle cerebral artery blood velocity during carotid endarterectomy. Br J Surg 73:98–100, 1986.

158. Naylor AR: Transcranial Doppler monitoring during carotid endarterectomy. In Hennerici M, Meairs S (eds): Cerebrovascular Ultrasound—Theory, Practice and Future Developments. Cambridge, UK Cambridge University Press, 2001, pp 317–323.

159. Rautenberg W, Schwartz A, Hennerici M: Transkranielle Dopplersonographic während der zerebralen Angiographie. In Widder B (ed): Transkranielle Dopplersonographie bei zerebrovaskulären Erkrankungen. Berlin, Springer-Verlag, 1987, pp 144–148.

160. Markus HS, Loh A, Isrrael D, et al: Microscopic air embolism during cerebral angiography and strategies for avoidance. Lancet 341:784–787, 1993.

161. Markus HS, Clifton A, Buckenham T, et al: Carotid angioplasty: Detection of embolic signals during and after the procedure. Stroke 25:2403–2406, 1994.

162. Ries F, Eicke M: Auswirkungen der extrakorporalen Zirkulation auf die intrazerebrale Hämodynamik—Erklärung postoperativer neuropsychiatrischer Komplikationen. In Widder B (ed): Transkranielle Doppler-Sonographie bei zerebrovaskulären Erkrankungen. New York, Springer-Verlag, 1987, pp 100–103.

163. Bunegin L, Wahl D, Albin MS: Detection and volume estimation of embolic air in the middle cerebral artery using transcranial Doppler sonography. Stroke 25:593–600, 1994.

164. Jansen C, Ramos LM, van Heeswijk JP, et al: Impact of microembolism and hemodynamic changes in the brain during carotid endarterectomy. Stroke 25:992–997, 1994.

165. Gaunt ME, Martin PJ, Smith JL, et al: Clinical relevance of intraoperative embolization detected by transcranial Doppler ultrasonography during carotid endarterectomy: A prospective study of 100 patients. Br J Surg 81:1435–1439, 1994.

166. Siebler M, Sitzer M, Steinmetz H: Detection of intracranial emboli in patients with symptomatic extracranial carotid artery disease. Stroke 23:1652–1654, 1992.

167. Siebler M, Sitzer M, Rose G, et al: Silent cerebral embolism caused by neurologically symptomatic high-grade carotid stenosis: Event rates before and after carotid endarterectomy. Brain 116:1005–1015, 1993.

168. Grosset DG, Georgiadis D, Abdullah I, et al: Doppler emboli signals vary according to stroke subtype. Stroke 25:382–384, 1994.

169. Georgiadis D, Grosset DG, Quin RO, et al: Detection of intracranial emboli in patients with carotid disease. Eur J Vasc Surg 8:309–314, 1994.

170. Markus HS, Droste DW, Brown MM: Detection of asymptomatic cerebral embolic signals with Doppler ultrasound. Lancet 343:1011–1012, 1994.

171. Grosset DG, Cowburn P, Georgiadis D, et al: Ultrasound detection of cerebral emboli in patients with prosthetic heart valves. J Heart Valve Dis 3:128–132, 1994.

172. Georgiadis D, Mallinson A, Grosset DG, et al: Coagulation activity and emboli counts in patients with prosthetic cardiac valves. Stroke 25:1211–1214, 1994.

173. Diehl RR, Sliwka U, Rautenberg W, et al: Evidence for embolization from a posterior cerebral artery thrombus by transcranial Doppler monitoring. Stroke 24:606–608, 1993.

174. Basic identification criteria of Doppler microembolic signals. Consensus Committee of the Ninth International Cerebral Hemodynamics Symposium. Stroke 26:1123, 1995.

175. Georgiadis D, Baumgartner RW, Karatschai R, et al: Further evidence of gaseous embolic material in patients with artificial heart valves. J Thorac Cardiovasc Surg 115:808–810, 1998.

176. Valdueza JM, Harms L, Doepp F, et al: Venous microembolic signals detected in patients with cerebral sinus thrombosis. Stroke 28:1607–1609, 1997.

177. Georgiadis D, Kaps M, Siebler M, et al: Variability of Doppler microembolic signal counts in patients with prosthetic cardiac valves. Stroke 26:439–443, 1995.

178. Markus H, Bland JM, Rose G, et al: How good is intercenter agreement in the identification of embolic signals in carotid artery disease? Stroke 27:1249–1252, 1996.

179. Van Zuilen EV, Mess WH, Jansen C, et al: Automatic embolus detection compared with human experts: A Doppler ultrasound study. Stroke 27:1840–1843, 1996.

180. Ringelstein EB, Droste DW, Babikian VL, et al: Consensus on microembolus detection by TCD. International Consensus Group on Microembolus Detection. Stroke 29:725–729, 1998.

181. Georgiadis D, Wenzel A, Zerkowski HR, et al: Influence of transducer frequency on Doppler microemboli signals in an in vivo model. Neurol Res 20:198–200, 1998.

182. Keunen RW, Stam CJ, Tavy DL, et al: Preliminary report of detecting microembolic signals in transcranial Doppler time series with nonlinear forecasting. Stroke 29:1638–1643, 1998.

183. Ries F, Tiemann K, Pohl C, et al: High-resolution emboli detection and differentiation by characteristic postembolic spectral patterns. Stroke 29:668–672, 1998.

184. Roy E, Abraham P, Montresor S, et al: The narrow band hypothesis: An interesting approach for high-intensity transient signals (HITS) detection. Ultrasound Med Biol 24:375–382, 1998.

185. Russell D, Brucher R: Online automatic discrimination between solid and gaseous cerebral microemboli with the first multifrequency transcranial Doppler. Stroke 33:1975–1980, 2002.

186. Brucher R, Russell D: Automatic online embolus detection and artifact rejection with the first multifrequency transcranial Doppler. Stroke 33:1969–1974, 2002.

187. Fan L, Evans DH, Naylor AR: Automated embolus identification using a rule-based expert system. Ultrasound Med Biol 27:1065–1077, 2001.

188. International Workshop on Cerebral Embolism. Cerebrovasc Dis 5:67–158, 1995.

189. Rautenberg W, Ries S, Bäzner H, et al: Emboli detection by TCD monitoring. Can J Neurol Sci 20:138–139, 1993

190. Grosset DG, Georgiadis D, Kelman AW, et al: Quantification of ultrasound emboli signals in patients with cardiac and carotid disease. Stroke 24:1922–1924, 1993.

191. Spencer MP, Thomas GI, Nicholls SC, et al: Detection of middle cerebral artery emboli during carotid endarterectomy using transcranial Doppler ultrasonography. Stroke 21:415–423, 1990.

192. van Zuilen EV, Moll FL, Vermeulen FE, et al: Detection of cerebral microemboli by means of transcranial Doppler monitoring before and after carotid endarterectomy. Stroke 26:210–213, 1995.

193. Markus HS, Thomson N, Brown MM: Asymptomatic cerebral embolic signals in symptomatic and asymptomatic carotid artery disease. Brain 118:1005–1011, 1995.

194. Daffertshofer M, Ries S, Schminke U, et al: High-intensity transient signals in patients with cerebral ischemia. Stroke 27:1844–1849, 1996.

195. Koennecke HC, Mast H, Trocio SHJ, et al: Frequency and determinants of microembolic signals on transcranial Doppler in unselected patients with acute carotid territory ischemia: A prospective study. Cerebrovasc Dis 8:107–112, 1998.

Diagnostic Studies

196. Sliwka U, Lingnau A, Stohlmann WD, et al: Prevalence and time course of microembolic signals in patients with acute stroke: A prospective study. Stroke 28:358–363, 1997.

197. Tong DC, Albers GW: Transcranial Doppler-detected microemboli in patients with acute stroke. Stroke 26:1588–1592, 1995.

198. Forteza AM, Babikian VL, Hyde C, et al: Effect of time and cerebrovascular symptoms on the prevalence of microembolic signals in patients with cervical carotid stenosis. Stroke 27:687–690, 1996.

199. Wijman CA, Babikian VL, Matjucha IC, et al: Cerebral microembolism in patients with retinal ischemia. Stroke 29:1139–1143, 1998.

200. Eicke BM, von Lorentz J, Paulus W: Embolus detection in different degrees of carotid disease. Neurol Res 17:181–184, 1995.

201. Sitzer M, Muller W, Siebler M, et al: Plaque ulceration and lumen thrombus are the main sources of cerebral microemboli in high-grade internal carotid artery stenosis. Stroke 26:1231–1233, 1995.

202. Valton L, Larrue V, Arrué P, et al: Asymptomatic cerebral embolic signals in patients with carotid stenosis: Correlation with appearance of plaque ulceration on angiography. Stroke 26:813–815, 1995.

203. Oliveira V, Batista P, Soares F, et al: HITS in internal carotid dissections. Cerebrovasc Dis 11:330–334, 2001.

204. Molina CA, Alvarez-Sabin J, Schonewille W, et al: Cerebral microembolism in acute spontaneous internal carotid artery dissection. Neurology 55:1738–1740, 2000.

205. Behrens S, Daffertshofer M, Hennerici MG: Stroke treatment guided by transcranial Doppler monitoring in a patient unresponsive to standard regimens. Cerebrovasc Dis 9:175–177, 1999.

206. Schauble B, Wijman CA, Koleini B, et al: Ophthalmic artery microembolism in giant cell arteritis. J Neuroophthalmol 20:273–275, 2000.

207. Fukuchi K, Kusuoka H, Watanabe Y, et al: Correlation of sequential MR images of microsphere-induced cerebral ischemia with histologic changes in rats. Invest Radiol 34:698–703, 1999.

208. Rundek T, Di Tullio MR, Sciacca RR, et al: Association between large aortic arch atheromas and high-intensity transient signals in elderly stroke patients. Stroke 30:2683–2686, 1999.

209. Siebler M, Kleinschmidt A, Sitzer M, et al: Cerebral microembolism in symptomatic and asymptomatic high-grade internal carotid artery stenosis. Neurology 44:615–618, 1994.

210. Babikian VL, Hyde C, Pochay V, et al: Clinical correlates of high-intensity transient signals detected on transcranial Doppler sonography in patients with cerebrovascular disease. Stroke 25:1570–1573, 1994.

211. Valton L, Larrue V, le Traon AP, et al: Microembolic signals and risk of early recurrence in patients with stroke or transient ischemic attack. Stroke 29:2125–2128, 1998.

212. Babikian VL, Wijman CA, Hyde C, et al: Cerebral microembolism and early recurrent cerebral or retinal ischemic events. Stroke 28:1314–1318, 1997.

213. Hennerici M. High intensity transcranial signals (HITS): A questionable "jackpot" for the prediction of stroke risk. J Heart Valve Dis 3:124–125, 1994.

214. Wei K, Jayaweera AR, Firoozan S, et al: Quantification of myocardial blood flow with ultrasound-induced destruction of microbubbles administered as a constant venous infusion. Circulation 97:473–483, 1998.

215. Meairs S, Daffertshofer M, Neff W, et al: Pulse-inversion contrast harmonic imaging: Ultrasonographic assessment of cerebral perfusion. Lancet 355:550–551, 2000.

216. Schwartz A, Rautenberg W, Hennerici M: Dolichoectatic intracranial arteries: Review of selected aspects. Cerebrovasc Dis 3:273–279, 1993.

217. Rautenberg W, Aulich A, Röther J, et al: Stroke and dolichoectatic intracranial arteries. Neurol Res 14:201–203, 1992.

218. Adams RJ, Nichols FT, Aaslid R, et al: Cerebral vessel stenosis in sickle cell disease: Criteria for detection by transcranial Doppler. Am J Pediatr Hematol Oncol 12:277–282, 1990.

219. Adams RJ, Nichols FT, Figueroa R, et al: Transcranial Doppler correlation with cerebral angiography in sickle cell disease. Stroke 23:1073–1077, 1992.

220. Bogousslavsky J, Despland PA, Regli F, et al: Postpartum cerebral angiopathy: Reversible vasoconstriction assessed by transcranial Doppler ultrasounds. Eur Neurol 29, 1989.

221. Chimowitz MI, Nemec JJ, Marwick TH, et al: Transcranial Doppler ultrasound identifies patients with right-to-left cardiac or pulmonary shunts. Neurology 41:1902–1904, 1991.

222. Di Tullio M, Sacco RL, Venketasubramanian N, et al: Comparison of diagnostic techniques for the detection of a patent foramen ovale in stroke patients. Stroke 24:1020–1024, 1993.

223. Itoh T, Matsumoto M, Handa N, et al: Paradoxical embolism as a cause of ischemic stroke of uncertain etiology: A transcranial Doppler sonographic study. Stroke 25:771–775, 1994.

224. Jauss M, Kaps M, Keberle M, et al: A comparison of transesophageal echocardiography and transcranial Doppler sonography with contrast medium for detection of patent foramen ovale. Stroke 25:1265–1267, 1994.

225. Droste DW, Lakemeier S, Wichter T, et al: Optimizing the technique of contrast transcranial Doppler ultrasound in the detection of right-to-left shunts. Stroke 33:2211–2216, 2002.

226. Hamann GF, Schatzer KD, Frohlig G, et al: Femoral injection of echo contrast medium may increase the sensitivity of testing for a patent foramen ovale. Neurology 50:1423–1428, 1998.

227. Schwarze JJ, Sander D, Kukla C, et al: Methodological parameters influence the detection of right-to-left shunts by contrast transcranial Doppler ultrasonography. Stroke 30:1234–1239, 1999.

228. Droste DW, Jekentaite R, Stypmann J, et al: Contrast transcranial Doppler ultrasound in the detection of right-to-left shunts: Comparison of Echovist-200 and Echovist-300, timing of the Valsalva maneuver, and general recommendations for the performance of the test. Cerebrovasc Dis 13:235–241, 2002.

229. Ophir J, Parker KJ: Contrast agents in diagnostic ultrasound. Ultrasound Med Biol 15:319–333, 1989.

230. Burns PN: Overview of echo-enhanced vascular ultrasound imaging for clinical diagnosis in neurosonology. J Neuroimaging 7(Suppl 1):S2–S14, 1997.

231. Van Liew HD, Burkard ME: Bubbles in circulating blood: Stabilization and simulations of cyclic changes of size and content. J Appl Physiol 79:1379–1385, 1995.

232. Kabalnov A, Bradley J, Flaim S, et al: Dissolution of multicomponent microbubbles in the bloodstream. 2: Experiment. Ultrasound Med Biol 24:751–760, 1998.

233. Chang PH, Shung KK, Levene HB: Quantitative measurements of second harmonic Doppler using ultrasound contrast agents. Ultrasound Med Biol 22:1205–1214, 1996.

234. Strandness DE, Eikelboom BC: Carotid artery stenosis: Where do we go from here? Eur J Ultrasound 7(Suppl 3):S17–S26, 1998.

235. Sitzer M, Furst G, Siebler M, et al: Usefulness of an intravenous contrast medium in the characterization of high-grade internal carotid stenosis with color Doppler-assisted duplex imaging. Stroke 25:385–389, 1994.

236. Sitzer M, Rose G, Furst G, et al: Characteristics and clinical value of an intravenous echo-enhancement agent in evaluation of high-grade internal carotid stenosis. J Neuroimaging 7(Suppl 1):S22–S25, 1997.

237. Furst G, Saleh A, Wenserski F, et al: Reliability and validity of non-invasive imaging of internal carotid artery pseudo-occlusion. Stroke 30:1444–1449, 1999.

238. Rothwell PM, Gutnikov SA, Warlow CP: Reanalysis of the final results of the European Carotid Surgery Trial. Stroke 34:514–523, 2003.

239. Ries F, Honisch C, Lambertz M, et al: A transpulmonary contrast medium enhances the transcranial Doppler signal in humans. Stroke 24:1903–1909, 1993.

240. Haggag KJ, Russell D, Brucher R, et al: Contrast enhanced pulsed Doppler and colour-coded duplex studies of the cranial vasculature. Eur J Neurol 6:443–448, 1999.

241. Otis S, Rush M, Boyajian R: Contrast-enhanced transcranial imaging: Results of an American phase-two study. Stroke 26:203–209, 1995.

242. Gerriets T, Seidel G, Fiss I, et al: Contrast-enhanced transcranial color-coded duplex sonography: Efficiency and validity. Neurology 52:1133–1137, 1999.

243. Murphy KJ, Bude RO, Dickinson LD, et al: Use of intravenous contrast material in transcranial sonography. Acad Radiol 4:577–582, 1997.

244. Stolz E, Kaps M, Kern A, et al: Frontal bone windows for transcranial color-coded duplex sonography. Stroke 30:814–820, 1999.

245. Delcker A, Turowski B: Diagnostic value of three-dimensional transcranial contrast duplex sonography. J Neuroimaging 7:139–144, 1997.

246. Baumgartner RW, Arnold M, Gonner F, et al: Contrast-enhanced transcranial color-coded duplex sonography in ischemic cerebrovascular disease. Stroke 28:2473–2478, 1997.

247. Nabavi DG, Droste DW, Kemeny V, et al: Potential and limitations of echocontrast-enhanced ultrasonography in acute stroke patients: A pilot study. Stroke 29:949–954, 1998.

248. Nabavi DG, Droste DW, Schulte-Altedorneburg G, et al: Diagnostic benefit of echocontrast enhancement for the insufficient transtemporal bone window. J Neuroimaging 9:102–107, 1999.

249. Iglseder B, Huemer M, Staffen W, et al: Imaging the basilar artery by contrast-enhanced color-coded ultrasound. J Neuroimaging 10:195–199, 2000.

250. Droste DW, Nabavi DG, Kemeny V, et al: Echocontrast enhanced transcranial colour-coded duplex offers improved visualization of the vertebrobasilar system. Acta Neurol Scand 98:193–199, 1998.

251. Koga M, Kimura K, Minematsu K, et al: Relationship between findings of conventional and contrast-enhanced transcranial color-coded real-time sonography and angiography in patients with basilar artery occlusion. AJNR Am J Neuroradiol 23:568–571, 2002.

252. Postert T, Meves S, Bornke C, et al: Power Doppler compared to color-coded duplex sonography in the assessment of the basal cerebral circulation. J Neuroimaging 7:221–226, 1997.

253. Griewing B, Motsch L, Piek J, et al: Transcranial power mode Doppler duplex sonography of intracranial aneurysms. J Neuroimaging 8:155–158, 1998.

254. Wardlaw JM, Cannon J, Statham PF, et al: Does the size of intracranial aneurysms change with intracranial pressure? Observations based on color "power" transcranial Doppler ultrasound. J Neurosurg 88:846–850, 1998.

255. Woydt M, Greiner K, Perez J, et al: Intraoperative color duplex sonography of basal arteries during aneurysm surgery. J Neuroimaging 7:203–207, 1997.

256. Mursch K, Schaake T, Markakis E: Using transcranial duplex sonography for monitoring vessel patency during surgery for intracranial aneurysms. J Neuroimaging 7:164–170, 1997.

257. Bailes JE, Tantuwaya LS, Fukushima T, et al: Intraoperative microvascular Doppler sonography in aneurysm surgery. Neurosurgery 40:965–970, 1997.

258. Uggowitzer MM, Kugler C, Riccabona M, et al: Cerebral arteriovenous malformations: Diagnostic value of echo-enhanced transcranial Doppler sonography compared with angiography. Am J Neuroradiol 20:101–106, 1999.

259. Valdueza JM, Schmierer K, Mehraein S, et al: Assessment of normal flow velocity in basal cerebral veins. A transcranial Doppler ultrasound study. Stroke 27:1221–1225, 1996.

260. Baumgartner RW, Gonner F, Arnold M, et al: Transtemporal power- and frequency-based color-coded duplex sonography of cerebral veins and sinuses. AJNR Am J Neuroradiol 18:1771–1781, 1997.

261. Stolz E, Kaps M, Kern A, et al: Transcranial color-coded duplex sonography of intracranial veins and sinuses in adults: Reference data from 130 volunteers. Stroke 30:1070–1075, 1999.

262. Valdueza JM, Hoffmann O, Weih M, et al: Monitoring of venous hemodynamics in patients with cerebral venous thrombosis by transcranial Doppler ultrasound. Arch Neurol 56:229–234, 1999.

263. Canhao P, Batista P, Ferro JM: Venous transcranial Doppler in acute dural sinus thrombosis. J Neurol 245:276–279, 1998.

264. Stolz E, Gerriets T, Bodeker RH, et al: Intracranial venous hemodynamics is a factor related to a favorable outcome in cerebral venous thrombosis. Stroke 33:1645–1650, 2002.

265. Stolz E, Kaps M, Dorndorf W: Assessment of intracranial venous hemodynamics in normal individuals and patients with cerebral venous thrombosis. Stroke 30:70–75, 1999.

266. Ries S, Steinke W, Neff KW, et al: Echocontrast-enhanced transcranial color-coded sonography for the diagnosis of transverse sinus venous thrombosis. Stroke 28:696–700, 1997.

267. Alexandrov AV, Burgin WS, Demchuk AM, et al: Speed of intracranial clot lysis with intravenous tissue plasminogen activator therapy: Sonographic classification and short-term improvement. Circulation 103:2897–2902, 2001.

268. Alexandrov AV, Demchuk AM, Felberg RA, et al: Intracranial clot dissolution is associated with embolic signals on transcranial Doppler. J Neuroimaging 10:27–32, 2000.

269. Stolz E, Gerriets T, Fiss I, et al: Comparison of transcranial color-coded duplex sonography and cranial CT measurements for determining third ventricle midline shift in space-occupying stroke. AJNR Am J Neuroradiol 20:1567–1571, 1999.

270. Bertram M, Khoja W, Ringleb P, et al: Transcranial colour-coded sonography for the bedside evaluation of mass effect after stroke. Eur J Neurol 7:639–646, 2000.

271. Gerriets T, Stolz E, Konig S, et al: Sonographic monitoring of midline shift in space-occupying stroke: An early outcome predictor. Stroke 32:442–447, 2001.

272. Aaslid R, Huber P, Nornes H: Evaluation of cerebrovascular spasm with transcranial Doppler ultrasound. J Neurosurg 60:37–41, 1984.

273. Seiler RW, Grolimund P, Aaslid R, et al: Cerebral vasospasm evaluated by transcranial ultrasound correlated with clinical grade and CT-visualized subarachnoid hemorrhage. J Neurosurg 64:594–600, 1986.

274. Laumer R, Steinmeier R, Gönner R, et al: Cerebral hemodynamics in subarachnoid hemorrhage evaluated by transcranial Doppler sonography. Neurosurgery 31:1–9, 1993.

275. Lennihan L, Petty GW, Fink E, et al: Transcranial Doppler detection of anterior cerebral vasospasm. J Neurol Neurosurg Psychiatry 56:906–909, 1993.

276. Hassler W, Steinmetz H, Gawlowski J: Transcranial Doppler ultrasonography in raised intracranial pressure and in intracranial circulatory arrest. J Neurosurg 68:745–751, 1988.

277. Schmidt B, Klingelhofer J, Schwarze JJ, et al: Noninvasive prediction of intracranial pressure curves using transcranial Doppler ultrasonography and blood pressure curves. Stroke 28:2465–2472, 1997.

278. Silvestrini M, Cupini LM, Placidi F, et al: Bilateral hemispheric activation in the early recovery of motor function after stroke. Stroke 29:1305–1310, 1998.

279. Caramia MD, Palmieri MG, Giacomini P, et al: Ipsilateral activation of the unaffected motor cortex in patients with hemiparetic stroke. Clin Neurophysiol 111:1990–1996, 2000.

280. Silvestrini M, Troisi E, Matteis M, et al: Correlations of flow velocity changes during mental activity and recovery from aphasia in ischemic stroke. Neurology 50:191–195, 1998.

281. Porter TR, Xie F, Kricsfeld D, et al: Improved myocardial contrast with second harmonic transient ultrasound response imaging in humans using intravenous perfluorocarbon-exposed sonicated dextrose albumin. J Am Coll Cardiol 27:1497–1501, 1996.

282. Linka AZ, Sklenar J, Wei K, et al: Assessment of transmural distribution of myocardial perfusion with contrast echocardiography. Circulation 98:1912–1920, 1998.

283. Postert T, Federlein J, Rose J, et al: Ultrasonic assessment of physiological echo-contrast agent distribution in brain parenchyma with transient response second harmonic imaging. J Neuroimaging 11:18–24, 2001.

284. Postert T, Hoppe P, Federlein J, et al: Ultrasonic assessment of brain perfusion. Stroke 31:1460–1462, 2000.

285. Postert T, Muhs A, Meves S, et al: Transient response harmonic imaging: An ultrasound technique related to brain perfusion. Stroke 29:1901–1907, 1998.

286. Wiesmann M, Seidel G: Ultrasound perfusion imaging of the human brain. Stroke 31:2421–2425, 2000.

287. Seidel G, Algermissen C, Christoph A, et al: Harmonic imaging of the human brain: Visualization of brain perfusion with ultrasound. Stroke 31:151–154, 2000.

288. Seidel G, Greis C, Sonne J, et al: Harmonic grey scale imaging of the human brain. J Neuroimaging 9:171–174, 1999.

289. Federlein J, Postert T, Meves S, et al: Ultrasonic evaluation of pathological brain perfusion in acute stroke using second harmonic imaging. J Neurol Neurosurg Psychiatry 69:616–622, 2000.

290. Postert T, Hoppe P, Federlein J, et al: Contrast agent specific imaging modes for the ultrasonic assessment of parenchymal cerebral echo contrast enhancement. J Cereb Blood Flow Metab 20:1709–1716, 2000.

291. Uhlendorf V, Hoffmann C: Nonlinear acoustical response of coated microbubbles in diagnostic ultrasound. In Ultrasonics Symposium Proceedings 1994. New York, Institute of Electrical and Electronics Engineers, 1994, pp 1559–1562.

292. Goldberg BB, Merton DA, Liu JB, et al: Evaluation of bleeding sites with a tissue-specific sonographic contrast agent. J Ultrasound Med 17:609–616, 1998.

293. Moriyasu F, Kono Y, Kamiyama N, et al: Flash echo imaging of liver tumors using ultrasound contrast agent and intermittent color Doppler scanning. J Ultrasound Med 17:S63, 1998.

294. Forsberg F, Goldberg BB, Liu JB, et al: Tissue-specific US contrast agent for evaluation of hepatic and splenic parenchyma. Radiology 210:125–132, 1999.

295. Krishnan S, O'Donnell M. Transmit aperture processing for nonlinear contrast agent imaging. Ultrason Imaging 18:77–105, 1996.

Diagnostic Studies

296. Postert T, Muhs A, Meves S, et al: Transient response harmonic imaging: An ultrasound technique related to brain perfusion. Stroke 29:1901–1907, 1998.

297. Vincent MA, Dawson D, Clark AD, et al: Skeletal muscle microvascular recruitment by physiological hyperinsulinemia precedes increases in total blood flow. Diabetes 51:42–48, 2002.

298. Wei K, Le E, Bin JP, et al: Quantification of renal blood flow with contrast-enhanced ultrasound. J Am Coll Cardiol 37:1135–1140, 2001.

299. Seidel G, Claassen L, Meyer K, et al: Evaluation of blood flow in the cerebral microcirculation: Analysis of the refill kinetics during ultrasound contrast agent infusion. Ultrasound Med Biol 27:1059–1064, 2001.

300. Rim SJ, Leong-Poi H, Lindner JR, et al: Quantification of cerebral perfusion with "real-time" contrast-enhanced ultrasound. Circulation 104:2582–2587, 2001.

301. Trubestein G, Engel C, Etzel F, et al: Thrombolysis by ultrasound. Clin Sci Mol Med Suppl 3:697s–698s, 1976.

302. Harpaz D, Chen X, Francis CW, et al: Ultrasound accelerates urokinase-induced thrombolysis and reperfusion. Am Heart J 127:1211–1219, 1994.

303. Rosenschein U, Gaul G, Erbel R, et al: Percutaneous transluminal therapy of occluded saphenous vein grafts: Can the challenge be met with ultrasound thrombolysis? Circulation 99:26–29, 1999.

304. Luo H, Birnbaum Y, Fishbein MC, et al: Enhancement of thrombolysis in vivo without skin and soft tissue damage by transcutaneous ultrasound. Thromb Res 89:171–177, 1998.

305. Riggs PN, Francis CW, Bartos SR, et al: Ultrasound enhancement of rabbit femoral artery thrombolysis. Cardiovasc Surg 5:201–207, 1997.

306. Hamm CW, Steffen W, Terres W, et al: Intravascular therapeutic ultrasound thrombolysis in acute myocardial infarctions. Am J Cardiol 80:200–204, 1997.

307. Rosenschein U, Roth A, Rassin T, et al: Analysis of coronary ultrasound thrombolysis endpoints in acute myocardial infarction (ACUTE trial): Results of the feasibility phase. Circulation 95:1411–1416, 1997.

308. Yock PG, Fitzgerald PJ: Catheter-based ultrasound thrombolysis. Circulation 95:1360–1362, 1997.

309. Birnbaum Y, Luo H, Nagai T, et al: Noninvasive in vivo clot dissolution without a thrombolytic drug: Recanalization of thrombosed iliofemoral arteries by transcutaneous ultrasound combined with intravenous infusion of microbubbles. Circulation 97:130–134, 1998.

310. Nishioka T, Luo H, Fishbein MC, et al: Dissolution of thrombotic arterial occlusion by high intensity, low frequency ultrasound and dodecafluoropentane emulsion: An in vitro and in vivo study. J Am Coll Cardiol 30:561–568, 1997.

311. Behrens S, Daffertshofer M, Spiegel D, et al: Low-frequency, low-intensity ultrasound accelerates thrombolysis through the skull. Ultrasound Med Biol 25:269–273, 1999.

312. Spengos K, Behrens S, Daffertshofer M, et al: Acceleration of thrombolysis with ultrasound through the cranium in a flow model. Ultrasound Med Biol 26:889–895, 2000.

313. Alexandrov AV, Demchuk AM, Felberg RA, et al: High rate of complete recanalization and dramatic clinical recovery during tPA infusion when continuously monitored with 2-MHz transcranial Doppler monitoring. Stroke 31:610–614, 2000.

314. Dayton PA, Ferrara KW: Targeted imaging using ultrasound. J Magn Reson Imaging 16:362–377, 2002.

315. Leong-Poi H, Christiansen J, Klibanov AL, et al: Noninvasive assessment of angiogenesis by ultrasound and microbubbles targeted to alpha(v)-integrins. Circulation 107:455–460, 2003.

316. Weller GE, Villanueva FS, Klibanov AL, et al: Modulating targeted adhesion of an ultrasound contrast agent to dysfunctional endothelium. Ann Biomed Eng 30:1012–1019, 2002.

317. Schumann PA, Christiansen JP, Quigley RM, et al: Targeted-microbubble binding selectively to GPIIb-IIIa receptors of platelet thrombi. Invest Radiol 37:587–593, 2002.

318. Tardy I, Pochon S, Theraulaz M, et al: In vivo ultrasound imaging of thrombi using a target-specific contrast agent. Acad Radiol 9(Suppl 2):S294–S296, 2002.

319. Christiansen JP, Leong-Poi H, Klibanov AL, et al: Noninvasive imaging of myocardial reperfusion injury using leukocyte-targeted contrast echocardiography. Circulation 105:1764–1767, 2002.

320. Lindner JR: Detection of inflamed plaques with contrast ultrasound. Am J Cardiol 90:32L–35L, 2002.

321. Unger EC, Hersh E, Vannan M, et al: Local drug and gene delivery through microbubbles. Prog Cardiovasc Dis 44:45–54, 2001.

322. Unger EC, McCreery TP, Sweitzer RH: Ultrasound enhances gene expression of liposomal transfection. Invest Radiol 32:723–727, 1997.

323. Koch S, Pohl P, Cobet U, et al: Ultrasound enhancement of liposome-mediated cell transfection is caused by cavitation effects. Ultrasound Med Biol 26:897–903, 2000.

324. Lawrie A, Brisken AF, Francis SE, et al: Microbubble-enhanced ultrasound for vascular gene delivery. Gene Ther 7:2023–2027, 2000.

325. Price RJ, Skyba DM, Kaul S, et al: Delivery of colloidal particles and red blood cells to tissue through microvessel ruptures created by targeted microbubble destruction with ultrasound. Circulation 98:1264–1267, 1998.

326. Skyba DM, Price RJ, Linka AZ, et al: Direct in vivo visualization of intravascular destruction of microbubbles by ultrasound and its local effects on tissue. Circulation 98:290–293, 1998.

327. Shohet RV, Chen S, Zhou YT, et al: Echocardiographic destruction of albumin microbubbles directs gene delivery to the myocardium. Circulation 101:2554–2556, 2000.

Diagnostic Studies

Chapter Twenty-Two

Single-Photon Emission Computed Tomography

Bernard Infeld and Stephen M. Davis

Single-photon emission computed tomography (SPECT) has become a widely available functional neuroimaging technique, with an expanding role in the investigation and management of a wide range of neurologic disorders. This functional neuroimaging modality complements conventional computed tomography (CT) and magnetic resonance imaging (MRI) techniques, which image brain structure. The most common form of SPECT images cerebral perfusion and is therefore well suited to the study of cerebrovascular disease.

Through the use of SPECT technology, a three-dimensional dataset representing aspects of cerebral function, mainly regional perfusion and neuroreceptor distribution, is generated. After intravenous injection of a radioisotope, images of radionuclide activity in the brain are acquired with one of several different types of camera systems—rotating gamma camera, multiple head cameras, or ring-type imaging systems. After computer-generated reconstruction, these data can be presented three-dimensionally or as a series of two-dimensional slices in the axial, coronal, and sagittal planes.

Perfusion SPECT provides images of the relative distribution of blood flow in the brain. Because regional cerebral blood flow (rCBF) and metabolism are normally matched, except in certain pathologic conditions such as acute ischemia, it is generally assumed that the information obtained with SPECT corresponds to brain function. However, these parameters may be discordant in various disease states, particularly acute ischemia. Although cortical and subcortical structures are well delineated, the resolution of SPECT is less than that achieved with CT, MRI, or positron emission tomography (PET). SPECT systems are now available in most nuclear medicine departments with rotating gamma cameras and commercially marketed radionuclides (Table 22.1).

In the assessment of cerebral perfusion, SPECT imaging has largely replaced the earlier planar xenon-133 (^{133}Xe) technique, in which the radiotracer was administered intravenously, inhalationally, or intra-arterially and extracranial detecting probes were placed over each hemisphere. SPECT is logistically far simpler and less expensive, but with currently available radiotracers, SPECT cannot image regional metabolism. The nonradioactive xenon CT technique has also been used to image rCBF with excellent spatial resolution, but the advantage of perfusion SPECT, particularly in the acute stroke setting, is that the mildly anesthetic effects of the xenon gas are avoided. The newer echoplanar MRI techniques, which are able to rapidly provide information about cerebral perfusion and water diffusion, are being increasingly used in the study of cerebrovascular disease, but SPECT still has much to offer as an investigative modality in this field.[1–3]

The radionuclides used in SPECT imaging emit a single photon. In contrast, the positron emitters used in PET scanning that generate two photons in coincidence, after the annihilation reaction between the positron and a tissue electron. Rotating gamma camera or fixed ring detector systems are used to measure these cerebral emissions in SPECT, and the regional counts correlate with functional activity in different brain regions. As in PET, counts are normally much higher in the gray matter of the cortex, basal ganglia, and cerebellum than in the white matter of the centrum semiovale.

Radionuclide SPECT technology can be categorized into perfusion SPECT and neuroreceptor SPECT methods. Virtually all studies in cerebrovascular disease have involved perfusion SPECT. The four principal techniques developed are the ^{133}Xe clearance method and three techniques in which brain retention of a radioligand generates cerebral images representing regional perfusion.

PERFUSION TECHNIQUES

Table 22.1 summarizes the perfusion techniques of SPECT.

Xenon-133 Clearance SPECT

The xenon-133 clearance method was a development of the earlier, nontomographic (planar) ^{133}Xe method, relating the cerebral clearance of ^{133}Xe to rCBF. This method has the advantage of providing quantification of rCBF in mL/100 g/min. Furthermore, because ^{133}Xe is rapidly cleared, multiple studies can be performed on the same day. However, image quality is inferior to that of the later retention SPECT techniques; the poorer spatial resolution is explained by both the low photon energy of the ^{133}Xe radiotracer and its rapid cerebral clearance. In addition,

Table 22.1 Perfusion Techniques of Single-Photon Emission Computed Tomography

	^{133}Xe	^{123}I-IMP	^{99m}Tc-HMPAO	^{99m}Tc-ECD
Advantages	Quantification of rCBF Multiple studies can be performed on the same day	Validated rCBF technique	Steady state for several hours Good spatial resolution Readily available radioligand Extensive published experience	Superior to 99mTc-HMPAO in subacute stroke Good spatial resolution Greater stability in vitro than 99mTc-HMPAO
Disadvantages	Inferior spatial resolution Requires specialized detection instruments	Inferior Imaging quality inferior to that of technetium-based methods Cerebral imaging must be performed <1 hour after injection May underestimate rCBF in cerebral acidosis	Quantification of rCBF extremely difficult Hyperfixation artifact in subacute stroke	May not detect luxury perfusion

^{123}I-IMP, iodine-123 *N*-isopropyl-*p*-iodoamphetamine; rCBF, regional cerebral blood flow; ^{99m}Tc-ECD, technetium-99m-ethyl cysteinate dimer; ^{99m}Tc-HMPAO, technetium-99m-hexamethylpropyleneamine oxime; ^{133}Xe, xenon-133 clearance.

this method requires specialized instrumentation.[4] For these reasons, the ^{133}Xe SPECT clearance method is rarely used in clinical practice.

Brain Radiopharmaceutical Perfusion (Retention) Techniques

Developments in perfusion SPECT over the past two decades have used radiotracers that cross the blood-brain barrier, distribute in the brain in proportion to perfusion, and remain fixed for a sufficient time to allow extracranial tomographic imaging of the gamma emissions. Three techniques have now come into clinical practice.[5]

Iodine-123-IMP SPECT

Because iodine-123 (^{123}I) requires cyclotron generation, the ^{123}I-IMP (iodine-133 *N*-isopropyl-*p*-iodoamphetamine) technique has more limited availability than the technetium-based methods (see later). It has been validated as a reliable rCBF technique.[6,7] Redistribution of this substance in the body is fairly rapid, so cerebral imaging must be performed within 1 hour of injection. The ^{123}I-IMP technique may underestimate rCBF in acidotic brain, a feature that is pertinent in acute cerebral ischemia.[4,8] Because of lower dosimetry and lower photon flux, the imaging quality of ^{123}I-IMP is somewhat inferior to that of the technetium-based methods.[5]

^{99m}Tc-HMPAO SPECT

Of the perfusion tracers currently available for SPECT imaging, that using the technetium Tc99m (^{99m}Tc) ligand d,l-hexamethylpropyleneamine oxime (HMPAO; exametazime [Ceretec, Amersham International]), developed in the mid-1980s,[9,10] has been the method most commonly used for research in cerebrovascular disease. ^{99m}Tc-HMPAO has several advantages over the earlier perfusion SPECT tracers ^{133}Xe and ^{123}I-IMP. Being a ^{99m}Tc ligand, it benefits from the optimal physical characteristics of the radionuclide, such as a 140-keV monoenergetic photon, 6-hour half-life, and potential for on-site labeling.[4] Also, ^{99m}Tc-HMPAO has the most stable in vivo binding, lasting

several hours, offers better spatial resolution, and is readily available commercially at a lower cost.[11]

A lipophilic agent, ^{99m}Tc-HMPAO is rapidly taken up across the blood-brain barrier in proportion to rCBF.[9,12–15] The first-pass extraction fraction is moderately high, around 80%.[14,16] There is little brain washout, which lasts only 2 to 3 minutes, after which steady-state conditions are reached.[9,12] The radiopharmaceutical then remains fixed in the brain for several hours after being converted to a hydrophilic form in the presence of intracellular glutathione.[13] It is not redistributed between gray matter and white matter. Subsequent loss of activity is due to physical decay of the isotope.[17] Imaging can then be performed from 2 minutes to several hours after injection and is limited only by decay of the isotope.

^{99m}Tc-HMPAO SPECT is a validated tracer of rCBF, comparing favorably with other techniques, such as ^{133}Xe washout[6,18] and PET[19,20] in both normal and pathologic conditions. Also, autoradiographic studies comparing rCBF values derived with ^{99m}Tc-HMPAO and the ^{14}C-iodoantipyrine method have found a good correlation.[21] ^{99m}Tc-HMPAO and ^{133}Xe rCBF values have also been demonstrated to correlate closely in clinical situations in which blood flow and metabolism are no longer coupled. During the luxury perfusion phenomenon seen in subacute stroke (see later discussion), the uptake of ^{99m}Tc-HMPAO follows the high flow that occurs,[22,23] validating it as an accurate tracer of blood flow. ^{123}I-IMP SPECT, on the other hand, tends to underestimate blood flow when plasma pH is low, as in cerebral ischemia.[4] It could be said that the ^{123}I-IMP method of SPECT is more sensitive to cerebral infarction than the ^{99m}Tc-HMPAO method during the subacute stages, indicating a profound perfusion defect,[23] but ^{99m}Tc-HMPAO follows blood flow more reliably and therefore reflects brain pathophysiology more closely.

^{99m}Tc-ECD SPECT

A newer technetium ligand, ^{99m}Tc-ethyl cysteinate dimer (^{99m}Tc-ECD), has high cerebral uptake with slow clearance and optimal characteristics for SPECT imaging.[24] An additional advantage is the stability of the ^{99m}Tc-ECD ligand in vitro for about 6 hours.[4,5] Its uptake by brain tissue depends on cellular viability in addition to perfusion and has been shown to correlate better with cerebral oxygen metabolism (on PET) than with rCBF in subacute stroke.[25–27] The intracerebral distribution of ^{99m}Tc-ECD has been shown to be similar to rCBF as measured by ^{133}Xe imaging.[28,29] With ^{99m}Tc-HMPAO SPECT, focal hyperfixation of the radionuclide in subacute stroke can give spuriously high, artifactual estimates of rCBF in some patients, with poor clinical correlations at these times between regional perfusion changes and neurologic parameters.[30,31] Because this hyperfixation artifact does not occur with ^{99m}Tc-ECD SPECT, the method appears to be preferable in the assessment of rCBF in subacute stroke.[32]

NEURORECEPTOR SPECT

Various neuroreceptor ligands have been developed for muscarinic and cholinergic receptors, dopamine D_2 receptors, and the serotonin 2 and benzodiazepine receptors.[4,33,34] Few studies of these ligands have been conducted in cerebrovascular disease, and they are not used in routine clinical practice.[5]

IMAGING SYSTEMS

Instrumentation for SPECT imaging relies on the use of rotating gamma cameras or ring-type dedicated imaging systems. The tomographic gamma camera systems can be used for body as well as dedicated head scanning.[4] The spatial resolution of current SPECT systems is between 7 mm and 10 mm,[4] but that of state-of-the-art triple- or four-head systems reaches only 6 to 7 mm.

When interpreting brain SPECT studies, one must appreciate that the thickness of the cerebral cortex, which is the main area of interest, is less than 5 mm,[35] below the resolution of current SPECT systems.[4] The effects of image degradation resulting from the combination of photon scatter and partial voluming lessen the intensity of the cortical image, so its margins are widened and blurred.

Quantification of Hypoperfusion Using SPECT

Unlike the ^{133}Xe clearance and PET methods, which allow direct quantification of rCBF in mL/100 g/min, ^{99m}Tc-HMPAO SPECT is a semiquantitative method that routinely measures only regional counts of activity that correlate with rCBF. Quantification of rCBF cannot be performed easily with this method because of its complex blood-brain kinetics.[14] Through the use of arterial sampling with ^{99m}Tc-HMPAO SPECT, quantitative estimates of rCBF can be obtained that correlate with values achieved by other quantitative rCBF methods.[20,36,37] Arterial sampling, however, is not in widespread use.

A variety of semiquantitative methods have been proposed for obtaining a measure of rCBF with SPECT.[16,38–61] These methods principally measure the number of counts within a region of interest (ROI) and express it as a mathematical fraction, normalized with respect to either global brain activity[49,50,53,54,59,60] or the activity within a reference region that is believed to be unaffected by the disease under study.[16,38–48,51,53,55–58,60,61] These techniques differ either by the number of slices analyzed, the method of defining ROIs, or the normalization algorithm. There is no standardized or validated method of semiquantitative analysis, and this disparity makes comparison of studies difficult.

In our laboratory at the Royal Melbourne Hospital (RMH), we have developed a method of volumetric analysis of regional hypoperfusion with SPECT.[62] This analysis integrates both the size and severity of perfusion reduction, yielding an equivalent volume of cortical tissue (in mL) having zero blood flow. This method of volume measurement has been validated in vitro through the use of a Hoffman brain phantom[63,64] fitted with simulated lesions of different sizes, demonstrating that the method is robust, accurate, and reproducible with two different camera systems. We have also shown that this method has negligible interobserver variability.[62]

A few other methods for volumetric analysis of cerebral hypoperfusion that take both the size and severity of perfusion reduction into account have been proposed,[38,65] but none has been validated in vitro. Image degradation and distortion due to photon attenuation and scatter, inadequate spatial resolution, and partial volume effects are the major limitations to accurate quantification. Quantitative volumetric measurement is useful for statistical comparisons with clinical parameters in cerebrovascular research, but qualitative image analysis is generally used in clinical practice.

SPECT IN CEREBROVASCULAR DISEASE

In the 1980s, SPECT was shown to demonstrate regional hypoperfusion in acute stroke. It was found to demonstrate brain ischemia more sensitively than early CT, and the hypoperfusion deficits correlated with clinical measures of neurologic severity.[11] A wide range of SPECT studies in various cerebrovascular conditions over subsequent years included the analysis of serial perfusion changes in acute and evolving stroke through to brain recovery, the use of perfusion SPECT in stroke prognosis, measurement of perfusion abnormalities in patients with clinically transient cerebral ischemia, evaluation of perfusion changes after pharmacologic interventions in acute stroke, analysis of functional perfusion reserve in patients with carotid occlusive disease, and measurement of perfusion abnormalities in patients with subarachnoid hemorrhage and arteriovenous malformations. Other related SPECT studies have focused on the diagnosis of vascular dementia and focal epileptic disorders. Interest has also focused on the role of SPECT in the identification of patients to be treated with new interventional stroke therapies such as thrombolysis. Table 22.2 summarizes the SPECT abnormalities observed in cerebrovascular disease along with their clinical usefulness.

Acute Ischemic Stroke: Diagnosis and Clinical Correlations

Many studies have demonstrated that the diagnostic sensitivity of perfusion SPECT in acute ischemic stroke is

Diagnostic Studies

Table 22.2   Abnormalities Found by Single-Photon Emission Computed Tomography (SPECT) in Cerebrovascular Disease and Their Clinical Usefulness

Disease or Category	SPECT Abnormalities	Clinical Usefulness
Acute Stroke		
Early diagnosis	Regional hypoperfusion	Accurate diagnosis of acute cerebral ischemia
Stroke prognosis	Regional acute hypoperfusion predicts functional outcome	Adds little to clinical prognostic determinants
Diagnosis of stroke subtype	Regional hypoperfusion useful in predicting cortical, borderzone, and lacunar infarcts	Limited
Interventional therapy	Reperfusion correlated with clinical benefits; conflicting results from studies	Potentially useful in selection of patients for reperfusion therapies
Diaschisis	Crossed cerebellar diaschisis correlates with acute stroke severity	Not evaluated
	May give insight into metabolism at infarct site	
Transient ischemic attacks	Regional hypoperfusion in patients with clinical recovery	May identify subset of high-risk patients
	Impaired perfusion reserve in some patients	
Subarachnoid hemorrhage	Regional hypoperfusion correlates with site of vasospasm producing tissue ischemia	Role in monitoring tissue ischemia due to vasospasm
	Correlates with delayed neurologic deficits	Template for therapy such as angioplasty
Arteriovenous malformations	Preoperative and postoperative hypoperfusion linked to clinical deficits and prognosis	Limited
Stroke-related epilepsy	Interictal hypoperfusion	Very useful in temporal lobe epilepsy.
	Ictal hyperperfusion	Not specifically evaluated in post-stroke epilepsy
Vascular dementia	Multifocal hypoperfusion deficits	Useful in distinction between multi-infarct and Alzheimer's-type dementias
	Distinctly different pattern from Alzheimer's disease	

superior to that of CT scanning or conventional MRI (Plate 22–1, following page 536).[16,39,66–77] The reason is that hypoperfusion, the hallmark of acute ischemia, occurs instantly after stroke, whereas the structural alterations imaged by CT and the increases in tissue water content detected by T2-weighted MRI take much longer to develop (see Plate 22–1). Findings of only 20% of CT scans are positive within 8 hours of cortical infarction,[4,11,78,79] but nearly 90% of SPECT scans demonstrate hypoperfusion by that point,[16,72] with a diagnostic specificity of 98%.[32]

This difference in sensitivity between structural and functional modalities disappears within 72 hours and is partly due to development of *luxury perfusion*, in which the rCBF becomes inappropriately elevated relative to the tissue's metabolic needs (see later discussion).[4,11,23] Acute cerebral hypoperfusion has also been found to correlate well with both the topographic site of the stroke and the severity of neurologic deficits, particularly after cortical infarction.[11,32,39–42,80,81]

In contrast, the diagnostic sensitivity of SPECT in lacunar infarction is significantly lower than that of the structural modalities CT and MRI, around 58%, because of the inferior spatial resolution of SPECT.[32,72,75,76] Therefore, false-negative results in subcortical lacunar strokes are a well-recognized problem with SPECT. Brass and colleagues,[32] using ^{99m}Tc-ECD SPECT, showed nonetheless that a normal image or small subcortical hypoperfusion defect on SPECT was highly predictive of lacunar infarction, whereas the method was both highly sensitive and specific in the diagnosis and localization of cortical infarction. The technique is also clinically useful as an aid in the

pathogenetic differentiation between embolic and borderzone infarcts.[75]

Stroke Prognosis

Given the early diagnostic sensitivity of SPECT in acute ischemic stroke, several investigators have focused on its prognostic potential. Early published reports suggested a poor correlation between acute hypoperfusion deficits and stroke outcome.[40,43,71,82–84] Most of these studies were, however, flawed by inclusion of patients evaluated after the acute stage of stroke.[40,71,82–84] It subsequently became clear that measurements of perfusion in the subacute stage after stroke displayed a poor correlation with neurologic parameters and outcome because of the presence of luxury perfusion shown to be prevalent on SPECT scans at these times.[85,86]

Later investigators analyzed cerebral hypoperfusion with SPECT during the acute stage of stroke and established a good correlation of findings with clinical outcome.[44,81,87–89] Bushnell and associates,[87] using ^{99m}Tc-IMP SPECT, found that the defect volume predicted language and neurologic recovery even though they evaluated only two patients within 7 days of stroke. Similarly, Launes and coworkers[81] found that the perfusion defect volume measured with either ^{99m}Tc-IMP or ^{99m}Tc-HMPAO SPECT correlated with performance of activities of daily living at outcome. In a study conducted by Giubilei and colleagues,[44] severe hypoperfusion within 6 hours of stroke onset predicted poor outcome at 1 month. Limburg and associates[88,89] reported that large acute flow deficits detected within 24 hours of stroke onset predicted early death from transtentorial herniation and that acute flow deficits correlated with neurologic and functional outcomes at 6 months.

Studies at the RMH stroke research laboratory have shown that acute hypoperfusion on ^{99m}Tc-HMPAO SPECT performed within 72 hours of stroke onset is a strong predictor of both neurologic impairment and functional disability after 3 months.[80] Large acute hypoperfusion deficits were typically seen in patients at high risk for death or poor functional outcome. The predictive value of acute hypoperfusion on SPECT was compared in this study with two clinical prognostic scores, the Canadian Neurological Scale (CNS)[90] and Allen's prognostic score.[91] Functional status and neurologic severity were measured at least 3 months after stroke with the Barthel Index (BI)[92] and CNS, respectively. Although acute hypoperfusion measurements strengthened the clinical scores in the prediction of neurologic outcome, they added little independent prognostic power to the acute clinical scores in the prediction of functional outcome. In addition, the acute hypoperfusion deficit has been shown to correlate with outcome tissue loss as measured on CT scan at 3 months.[44,93-95]

Subsequent studies have confirmed the prognostic value of acute hypoperfusion measured early after stroke onset using ^{99m}Tc-HMPAO SPECT.[42,45,96-98] Hanson and colleagues[42] reported that acute hypoperfusion assessed within 6 hours of stroke onset, corresponding with the likely time window for the use of acute interventional therapies, correlated with long-term functional outcome. Shimosegawa and associates[45] used the same method within 6 hours of stroke onset to distinguish morphologically viable brain tissue from infarcted tissue. Laloux and coworkers[98] found that the level of acute hypoperfusion predicted functional outcome at 1 month. Similarly, Bowler and associates[97] reported that measurement of acute infarct volume with ^{99m}Tc-HMPAO SPECT predicted both neurologic and functional outcomes at 3 months. Like the RMH researchers,[80] however, both of the latter two groups[97,98] found that SPECT was no better at predicting final outcome than clinical assessment using the CNS score.[90]

Conversely, in a larger study of 458 consecutive patients by Alexandrov and colleagues,[96] ^{99m}Tc-HMPAO SPECT not only was of prognostic value independent of clinical grading but also statistically improved the predictive power of the CNS score if performed within the first 72 hours after stroke onset. In a novel study, Hirano and associates[99] assessed a small group of patients with ^{99m}Tc-HMPAO SPECT within 6 hours of stroke onset and coregistered the SPECT images with CT scans obtained 7 to 10 days later that showed the final infarct volume. They found that identifying tissue with cerebral blood flow below a threshold value of 63.7% (of the contralateral mean hemispheric CBF) reliably predicted the final infarct volume. Hence, under conditions of stable CBF, tissues with CBF values above this threshold are likely to survive, and those with values below the threshold are destined for infarction.

Barthel and colleagues[100] have found that ^{99m}Tc-ECD SPECT performed within 6 hours of stroke onset had prognostic values for both death and disability. They also found the method could predict evolution of middle cerebral artery (MCA) infarction more reliably than

conventional CT.[100] Other researchers have also argued that ^{99m}Tc-ECD SPECT is probably superior to ^{99m}Tc-HMPAO SPECT in assessing prognosis because it reflects regional metabolism and cellular viability more accurately than perfusion.[25-27,101] Hence, ^{99m}Tc-ECD SPECT might be well suited to identifying candidates for therapeutic intervention.

Because acute hypoperfusion has prognostic value for both clinical outcome and tissue survival, early measurements of rCBF with SPECT can serve as a template for the investigation of experimental acute stroke therapies, particularly those aimed at improving brain perfusion. The ^{99m}Tc-HMPAO SPECT method provides a practical technique for evaluating reperfusion after acute interventional therapies. The properties of ^{99m}Tc-HMPAO allow injection of the radionuclide 2 to 3 minutes before administration of therapy. It is rapidly fixed in the brain in proportion to regional perfusion, and images can then be acquired in the nuclear medicine department up to 4 hours later. Thus, the method provides a pretherapy snapshot of CBF without significantly delaying initiation of therapy. A second SPECT study can be performed 24 hours later to determine the level of reperfusion after therapy.

The Confounding Problem of Luxury Perfusion

An understanding of the natural history of evolving perfusion changes imaged by ^{99m}Tc-HMPAO SPECT after acute stroke is important to the interpretation of findings of reperfusion after experimental stroke therapies. One must also appreciate that the ischemic penumbra and regions of luxury perfusion cannot be prospectively detected with SPECT; unlike PET, current SPECT methods are not able to visualize regional metabolism. Several previous investigators have made serial assessments of CBF in patients with acute cerebral infarction using SPECT and a variety of radiotracers.[39,44,70,89] They have identified three discrete stages of perfusion as visualized by SPECT in the course of cortical cerebral infarction (Plates 22–2 and 22–3). The acute stage, consisting of the first 3 days, is characterized by regional hypoperfusion at the infarct site that correlates with the severity of neurologic deficits and predicts late functional outcome. This early hypoperfusion typically exceeds the focal deficit demonstrated by either CT scanning or MRI performed in the acute stage of stroke.

During the subacute stage, between 3 days and 2 weeks after stroke onset, rCBF at the infarct site tends to spontaneously improve, so that SPECT may show either reduced, normal, or increased (hyperemia) regional blood flow. The increase in rCBF during the subacute stage can be on the order of 59% to 108%, even in patients in whom CT shows large infarcts.[70] Subacute perfusion deficits usually do not correlate with concurrent clinical severity or with functional outcome.[39,44,89] These subacute perfusion changes are consistent with the phase of luxury perfusion (see Plate 22–3).

A phenomenon originally described by Lassen,[102] luxury perfusion is thought to be due to a combination of impairment of local cerebral autoregulation and vasodilatation produced by localized metabolic acidosis. Luxury perfusion is readily appreciated on oxygen-15 PET during the subacute stage after stroke; it is characterized by a mismatch between rCBF and regional oxygen metabolism such that rCBF becomes elevated relative to metabolism, thereby reducing the regional oxygen extraction fraction.[103–106] Raynaud and associates,[86] in a cross-sectional analysis of patients with stroke during the subacute stage and again at 3 months, found that luxury perfusion progressively increased with time, peaking at day 15, and then gradually decreased, stabilizing at day 50. Other studies have shown that luxury perfusion may follow spontaneous recanalization of the MCA or may even be present with persistent MCA occlusion.[107–109] Cordes and associates[85] reported that luxury perfusion was associated with increases in regional cerebral blood volume and gadolinium enhancement on MRI, indicating regional vasodilatation accompanied by disruption of the blood-brain barrier.

An advantage of ^{99m}Tc-ECD over other SPECT tracers is that it is more reliable in identifying subacute infarction, as it is unaffected by luxury perfusion. Conversely, ^{99m}Tc-ECD SPECT may fail to demonstrate luxury perfusion.[110] In a study comparing ^{99m}Tc-ECD and ^{133}Xe as SPECT tracers of CBF in patients with a variety of neurologic conditions including different stages of stroke, Lassen and Sperling[110] found good agreement between the two radiotracers in all subjects except the patients with subacute stroke. In those with subacute stroke, the ^{99m}Tc-ECD technique showed low count rates in the infarct region, but the ^{133}Xe SPECT technique showed normal or elevated flow at the infarct site, consistent with reperfusion or luxury perfusion. Hence, the usefulness of the ^{99m}Tc-ECD method is to detect the true extent of cerebral ischemia during the subacute stage after stroke, when reperfusion may mask the true extent and severity as measured by other methods.

Studies using ^{99m}Tc-HMPAO may exaggerate hyperemia during the subacute stage, in part reflecting a hyperfixation artifact peculiar to this tracer in addition to the presence of luxury perfusion.[30] Artifactually elevated rCBF due to hyperfixation of ^{99m}Tc-HMPAO is most commonly seen in strokes evaluated between 1 and 4 weeks after onset but is not likely to account for hyperemia or reperfusion before this time.

In the chronic stage, beyond 2 to 3 months, rCBF at the infarct site decreases again, and regional hypoperfusion may resemble that seen in the acute stage (see Plate 22–3).[70] Perfusion deficits on SPECT at the chronic stage again correlate with clinical severity of stroke.[89] Some investigators have identified a region of depressed perfusion surrounding the anatomic area of tissue loss, which indicates that the extent of hypoperfusion may exceed the size of the infarct on correlative CT.[70,111,112] This depressed rCBF in apparently histologically normal tissue may reflect functionally depressed cerebral activity, termed *diaschisis*, which is consequent on neuronal deafferentation or deefferentation.

At the RMH stroke research laboratory, Davis and colleagues[80] studied a cohort of 38 patients with MCA cortical infarction using ^{99m}Tc-HMPAO SPECT within 72 hours of stroke onset, and 18 of them again after 3 months. These researchers found that mean infarct hypoperfusion volume paradoxically increased between the acute and outcome stages, despite clinical improvement over the same period. They concluded that the increase in mean hypoperfusion volume between acute and outcome CBF studies was due to luxury perfusion during the first 72 hours that was no longer present at 3 months. This conclusion was supported by the finding of a weak correlation between acute hypoperfusion volume and acute neurologic deficit and a stronger correlation between hypoperfusion volume and neurologic deficit at the outcome stage. Another possible explanation is the presence of hypoperfusion in excess of tissue loss during the chronic stage because of either peri-infarct diaschisis, as previously suggested,[70,111,112] or a persisting penumbra (ischemic but morphologically intact tissue).

In later studies at the RMH stroke research laboratory, mean chronic infarct hypoperfusion on SPECT and tissue loss on CT were in close agreement.[93,95] Also, mean chronic infarct hypoperfusion volume did not alter after vasodilatory challenge with acetazolamide. Similarly, Vorstrup[112] found no significant change in side-to-side asymmetry in the peri-infarct areas when evaluating vasodilatory capacity using acetazolamide in five of six patients with chronic infarction. These results argue against the presence of chronic peri-infarct diaschisis and in favor of early luxury perfusion as the cause of the paradoxic increase in infarct hypoperfusion with brain recovery.

In a later report, Bowler and coworkers[113] evaluated 50 patients with acute ischemic stroke using serial ^{99m}Tc-HMPAO SPECT studies at 1 day, 1 week, and 3 months after stroke onset. They found that the median SPECT perfusion defect decreased between the first and second scans, indicating early reperfusion, then increased between the second and third examinations. These investigators concluded that the observed early spontaneous reperfusion was mainly transient and non-nutritional. Their findings confirm the conclusions reached by Davis and colleagues.[80]

In yet another study performed in the RMH stroke laboratory, Barber and associates[114] examined the natural history of serial perfusion changes after acute ischemic stroke by combining SPECT data from patients enrolled in the placebo arm of the Australian Streptokinase Trial[115] and the nimodipine study[116] as well as a cohort of other, untreated patients.[117] All of the patients underwent serial HMPAO SPECT within 4[115] or 12[116] hours of stroke onset, 24 hours later, and at 3 months. Barber and associates[114] found that spontaneous, partial early reperfusion occurred in 61% of patients, which was followed by expanding hypoperfusion between the subacute and outcome stages. These results extend previous RMH work and confirm that spontaneous reperfusion is common after stroke but is also incomplete and has both nutritional and non-nutritional components.

These serial changes in imaged rCBF explain the paradoxic increase in hypoperfusion found by RMH investigators between SPECT studies performed within 3 days of stroke onset and those performed at 3 months—it is caused by early luxury perfusion on the acute SPECT scans.[80,115,117] Vorstrup and associates[70] had documented similar changes in an earlier study using the ^{133}Xe technique. Therefore, for assessment of reperfusion after stroke, outcome SPECT studies must be performed to retrospectively discriminate between the proportion of early flow that is retained at 3 months and is hence nutritional from the proportion that is not apparent at 3 months and so was not supplying viable tissue in the acute stage of stroke. One SPECT study indicated that postinfarction hyperemia could occur with some infarcts as early as 6 hours after onset.[45]

Comparison of SPECT Imaging with Echoplanar Magnetic Resonance Imaging

Few comparisons have been made between SPECT perfusion techniques and perfusion-weighted imaging (PWI) and diffusion-weighted (DWI) modalities of MRI. Kim and associates[118] compared ^{99m}Tc-ECD SPECT with T2-weighted MRI, PWI, and DWI during the acute and subacute stages after stroke in ten patients.[118] They found that the sensitivity of ^{99m}Tc-ECD SPECT in detecting new lesions during the hyperacute stage was equal to that of PWI and superior to those of both DWI and T2-weighted MRI. During the subacute stage, ^{99m}Tc-ECD SPECT was more sensitive than PWI because of pseudonormalization of the PWI images. These investigators concluded that ^{99m}Tc-ECD SPECT is comparable to PWI in detecting acute stroke and is more useful than PWI for subacute stroke.[118]

Similarly, CBF measured with ^{99m}Tc-HMPAO SPECT has also been found to correlate closely with PWI, but this comparison was made in patients assessed only within 6 hours of stroke onset.[119] Close correlation between CBF measurements on ^{99m}Tc-HMPAO SPECT and PWI has also been demonstrated in chronic stroke.[120]

The Relationship between Early Reperfusion and Clinical Gains after Stroke

A number of SPECT studies have addressed the relationship between early perfusion changes and clinical gains in untreated patients[107,113,121] and in patients undergoing acute interventional therapy with either thrombolytic agents[38,42,122,123] or calcium channel antagonists.[124,125]

Untreated Patients
Uemura and colleagues[107] used the ^{133}Xe intra-arterial injection technique to study 50 patients between 1 day and 2 months after stroke onset. Second rCBF examinations were carried out in 15 patients. These investigators noted the frequent appearance of regional hyperemia consistent with luxury perfusion and found that the presence of luxury perfusion was associated with a poorer prognosis than its absence, despite the presence of arterial recanalization. In a study by Jorgensen and coworkers,[121] the incidence of "hyperperfusion" (which we assume to mean spontaneous reperfusion) was 77% in patients with cortical infarcts. Marked clinical improvement was observed in patients with hyperperfusion, but no improvement in those without hyperperfusion. However, both of these studies suffer from several methodologic flaws.

Other investigators have sequentially evaluated rCBF at various stages after stroke along with neurologic recovery.[39,41,44,83,89,97] Vallar and coworkers[41] found that almost complete spontaneous clinical recovery occurred in association with significant improvement of cortical perfusion between the subacute and chronic stages. In contrast, Demeurisse and colleagues[83] found progressive clinical improvement that was not accompanied by improvement

of rCBF. Several other studies, however, have demonstrated early reperfusion that was not associated with clinical gains or with functional outcome.[39,44,89,97]

In the serial perfusion study reported by Bowler and coworkers,[113] in which sequential SPECT scans were performed 1 day, 1 week, and 3 months after stroke, reperfusion was defined on visual inspection as either an absolute increase in ^{99m}Tc-HMPAO uptake in the affected infarct area on any scan, termed "absolute hyperemia," or a relative increase in ^{99m}Tc-HMPAO uptake between two consecutive SPECT studies, termed "relative reperfusion." Lesser levels of reperfusion were interpreted as being present when the apparent perfusion defect determined by volume measurement was smaller in the second SPECT scan than in either the first or third scan. Reperfusion, as defined by any of these criteria, was observed in 42% of patients studied and was never seen on the 3-month scan. Absolute hyperemia and relative reperfusion occurred in 28% of patients at a mean time of 5.8 days from onset. Reperfusion was, however, associated with clinical improvement in only 2% of cases. Overall, there was no difference in CT infarct volume or in neurologic or functional outcome between those patients with and without reperfusion. These findings are not surprising, as it would be unlikely for reperfusion occurring as late as 1 week after onset to be clinically beneficial. This study emphasizes the need for early serial SPECT studies to be performed no more than 24 hours apart, and beginning within the first few hours after stroke onset.

In the natural history study by Barber and associates,[114] the majority of patients were from the placebo arms in trials of either streptokinase or nimodipine and therefore underwent SPECT within 4 to 12 hours of stroke onset and again 24 hours later. Patients with early reperfusion had better neurologic outcome and greater neurologic improvement than those without early reperfusion. Early reperfusion also tended to be associated with better functional outcome and smaller degrees of tissue loss. This study demonstrates that the spontaneous but incomplete early reperfusion occurring in the majority of patients with stroke is probably of some nutritional benefit.

SPECT and Interventional Therapy: Thrombolysis
A number of SPECT studies have addressed the relationship between acute changes in perfusion and the clinical gains seen after intravenous thrombolytic therapy.[38,42,122,123,126,127] Most studies have used the ^{99m}Tc-HMPAO SPECT technique, imaging perfusion before and after treatment. This technique readily provides images of cerebral perfusion and is therefore ideal for evaluation of reperfusion after acute thrombolysis. It also allows imaging of pretherapy cerebral perfusion without delaying treatment. The rapid brain uptake of ^{99m}Tc-HMPAO in proportion to regional perfusion and its stable binding allow injection of radiotracer 2 to 3 minutes before administration of thrombolytics. Image acquisition can be delayed up to 4 hours and provides an estimate of pretherapy rCBF.[9,12–14] A second SPECT scan can then be performed 24 hours later to determine the extent of reperfusion after therapy.

This group of studies has yielded conflicting results concerning the relation between reperfusion after therapy and

Diagnostic Studies

clinical gains. Overgaard and associates[123] reported that reperfusion after open treatment with recombinant tissue-type plasminogen activator (rt-PA) correlated with angiographic patency, clinical improvement, and smaller infarcts on outcome CT in a study that lacked controls. Baird and colleagues[38] found that open administration of streptokinase by either the intravenous or intra-arterial route tended to be associated with more frequent and greater reperfusion than that seen in controls and that reperfusion was of significant prognostic value. Grotta and Alexandrov[126] reported the results of SPECT studies in a small number of patients who were entered into the National Institute of Neurological Diseases and Stroke (NINDS) rt-PA study. These investigators found that reperfusion was greater in patients receiving rt-PA than in those receiving placebo and was often complete. This improved reperfusion was associated with greater clinical improvement over the first 24 hours. However, this study did not include data on clinical outcome at 3 months.

Yasaka and associates[127] studied 37 patients in the Australian Streptokinase Trial (ASK) using ^{99m}Tc-HMPAO SPECT, transcranial Doppler ultrasonography (TCD), or both, and found that streptokinase improved the hemodynamic parameters of reperfusion and recanalization but that these changes were neither sufficiently early nor extensive enough to have a positive effect on clinical outcome. No patient showed early recanalization within 3 hours, but only 3 patients in this study were treated within 3 hours. Discordance was observed between SPECT and TCD findings. At baseline, the findings of a perfusion defect on SPECT and MCA occlusion on TCD did not always match; some patients without MCA occlusion had a perfusion defect. In addition, there was a poor correlation between reperfusion and recanalization after therapy. In determining prognosis, however, reperfusion was found to be more important than restoration of vessel patency alone. These observations indicate the greater importance at the tissue level of reperfusion than of recanalization.

In the study by Herderscheê and coworkers,[122] there was no relation between reperfusion and clinical change after open treatment with rt-PA, although one patient with complete reperfusion had complete clinical recovery. This was, however, a small open study without controls. Hanson and colleagues[42] combined data from patients treated in either a thrombolysis or glutamate antagonist trial and evaluated results that were blinded as to treatment. They found no relation between perfusion changes and clinical changes over the first 24 hours. They did, however, find a threshold of perfusion on initial SPECT below which either poor outcome or the complications of hemorrhagic conversion or cerebral edema were reliably predicted.

It is likely that the disparity between these reports regarding the relation between reperfusion and clinical outcome after thrombolysis reflects the variable contributions of nutritional and non-nutritional flow in the reperfusion phase after acute stroke. Although the level of luxury perfusion (or non-nutritional reperfusion—marked by depression of the oxygen extraction fraction[103,106]) can be prospectively analyzed by means of PET, the components of reperfusion measured by SPECT that are nutritional or non-nutritional can be distinguished only retrospectively with an outcome SPECT study at the chronic (3-month) stage. Non-nutritional reperfusion may be estimated as that proportion that does not persist at the chronic stage, when regional perfusion is matched to both metabolism and anatomic infarct size.[93,95,103,104] Nutritional reperfusion, on the other hand, would be equivalent to the remaining proportion of early reperfusion that is maintained at the outcome stage and would be associated with clinical improvement. Because none of the previous studies of reperfusion after thrombolysis has analyzed cerebral perfusion during the chronic stage, the contribution of luxury perfusion has not yet been examined.

We studied 24 patients in the Australian Streptokinase Trial with ^{99m}Tc-HMPAO SPECT before therapy, 24 hours after therapy, and at 3 months and found no differences in acute reperfusion between those receiving intravenous streptokinase and those receiving placebo.[115] However, streptokinase was associated with a significantly larger amount of non-nutritional reperfusion than placebo. This luxury perfusion was associated with poor functional outcome. We also found an association between non-nutritional flow and hemorrhagic transformation; this finding suggests that luxury perfusion may be an important determinant of reperfusion injury. Luxury perfusion was more prominent in the patients with larger acute hypoperfusion regions; this finding correlated with results of another trial suggesting that established or large infarcts have a worse outcome after thrombolysis.[128] Finally, nutritional reperfusion was more likely with earlier treatment. This observation underlies the reason two other trials found that efficacy of therapy is critically related to the timing of thrombolysis.[129,130]

A small number of studies have used ^{99m}Tc-ECD SPECT to evaluate thrombolysis. This technique has the advantage of more accurately reflecting nutritional reperfusion than ^{99m}Tc-HMPAO SPECT during the subacute stage and is therefore well suited to the evaluation of reperfusion after therapy.[25,131] Berrouschot and colleagues[133] assessed patients enrolled in the second European Cooperative Acute Stroke Study (ECASS II)[132] with ^{99m}Tc-ECD SPECT before treatment, 6 to 8 hours after treatment, and again at 7 days.[133] They found that reperfusion after therapy or at 7 days was associated with both improved clinical outcome and smaller infarcts on outcome CT. Parenchymal hemorrhage occurred in patients without reperfusion. However, there was no association between treatment and reperfusion.[133] These findings reflect those of ECASS II[132] and are in agreement with our study using ^{99m}Tc-HMPAO SPECT to evaluate streptokinase,[115] in that they show a relation between nutritional reperfusion and outcome.

Iseda and coworkers[134] have evaluated a cohort of patients with acute MCA occlusion treated with a protocol consisting of percutaneous transluminal angioplasty and intra-arterial t-PA. These researchers used ^{99m}Tc-ECD SPECT to evaluate rCBF before treatment and coregistered the results with 3-month outcome CT scans. They found that tissue salvage depended critically on timing of therapy within the first 3 hours but was related to the rCBF derangement after the first 3 hours.[134] These observations add further evidence that timing of therapy and extent of reduction in perfusion are but two of the many complex factors that influence the outcome of therapeutic reperfusion after stroke.

Calcium Channel Antagonists

Two studies have used ^{133}Xe SPECT to evaluate the efficacy of calcium channel antagonists after stroke,[124,125] but neither included outcome evaluations, and both lacked control subjects. Pozzilli and associates[125] used the ^{133}Xe inhalation technique to measure the effect of intravenous nimodipine on rCBF, administering treatment within 6 hours of stroke onset, in seven patients. They found a significant improvement after nimodipine in rCBF in the ischemic borderzone but not in the infarct core. There was no associated clinical benefit. Gelmers and coworkers[124] reported that nimodipine produced a dose-dependent increase in CBF throughout both hemispheres, but reperfusion in the infarct region over and above this general increase was seen in only three out of 10 patients studied. The associated clinical effects were not described. Also, their report furnished no information about the interval between stroke onset and nimodipine administration, except those patients were studied electively; one patient was treated 3 days after onset.

We have previously reported the largest study to date of the effects of (oral) nimodipine on reperfusion after acute ischemic stroke and the only study to include outcome CBF data.[116] In a blinded, randomized trial, we used ^{99m}Tc-HMPAO SPECT to evaluate perfusion changes and their relation to outcome in 46 patients in whom either oral nimodipine, 120 mg daily, or placebo was started within 12 hours of stroke onset and continued for 14 days. SPECT was performed before therapy, 24 hours after therapy, and at 3 months. We demonstrated that nimodipine improved early reperfusion compared with placebo but to only a modest degree compared with thrombolysis (another reperfusion strategy).[115] The early reperfusion associated with nimodipine was not maintained at outcome, however, and was therefore non-nutritional in nature. The presence of non-nutritional reperfusion after nimodipine correlated with poor clinical outcome and greater tissue loss. On the other hand, spontaneous reperfusion in the patients receiving placebo had a positive effect on outcome. There was a tendency for earlier treatment to be associated with greater reperfusion.

The results of this study suggest either that the lack of efficacy of nimodipine in acute ischemic stroke might relate to its potency as a reperfusion agent or that the benefit of reperfusion was outweighed by reperfusion injury. These findings may have related to the relatively late timing of therapy. The Dutch Very Early Nimodipine Use in Stroke (VENUS) Trial, a larger, randomized, placebo-controlled trial of oral nimodipine published subsequent to our SPECT study, used a shorter treatment time window, 6 hours.[135] The trial was terminated early after 439 of the planned 1500 patients had been assigned for therapy. No beneficial effect of early nimodipine administration was found, but this trial is believed to have had several pertinent design flaws. Patients were entered into the trial by general practitioners, and CT scans were not performed in approximately one third of patients.

Blood Pressure Reduction

SPECT has been used to study the effect of antihypertensive agents on CBF after acute ischemic stroke. Lisk and coworkers[136] used the modality to evaluate the effect of acute pharmacologic (with nicardipine, captopril, or clonidine versus placebo) reduction of blood pressure after ischemic stroke in hypertensive patients. They demonstrated a negative relationship between the extent of blood pressure reduction and the improvement in cerebral blood flow, a finding that suggests the presence of impaired cerebrovascular autoregulation and cautions against aggressive treatment of hypertension in the acute stroke setting. Similarly, Waldemar and associates[137] used ^{133}Xe-inhalation SPECT to study the effect of captopril on blood flow after stroke and did not demonstrate any improvement.

The Role of SPECT in Acute Ischemic Stroke

Stroke Subtype

SPECT is a useful tool in the diagnosis of acute ischemic stroke and in predicting prognosis, particularly early on in the course, when CT findings may be normal or may not reveal the complete extent of infarction. SPECT may also be clinically useful to delineate stroke pathogenesis and subtype, and therefore, influence stroke management. In light of the difference in sensitivity of SPECT to evaluate cortical versus lacunar infarctions at the acute stage, patients with acute hemispheric stroke and normal SPECT findings are likely to have lacunar infarcts.[32,66,72,75,76] Also, lacunar strokes may demonstrate reduced radiopharmaceutical uptake at the site of the lesion or in the overlying cortex that resolves concurrently with clinical improvement.[138]

Transient Ischemic Attack

Various SPECT techniques have been used to show prolonged disturbances in regional cerebral hemodynamics in patients with clinically defined transient cerebral ischemic attacks (TIAs). Hartmann and colleagues[139] detected rCBF abnormalities in 60% of patients on the day of a TIA, but in only 40% on the day after a TIA. Bogousslavsky and coworkers[140] found that persistent perfusion abnormalities identified a high-risk group of patients who were predisposed to early infarction.[140] Laloux and colleagues[141] reported that the sensitivity of SPECT was higher than that of CT in patients with TIA, although SPECT did not necessarily provide additional clinical information about etiology.

SPECT may be able to differentiate acute stroke from a TIA within the first 6 hours of symptom onset, a period during which acute intervention may be considered. In one series of patients who underwent ^{99m}Tc-ECD SPECT within 6 hours of symptom onset, those with TIAs tended to have perfusion defects that either were less apparent on visual analysis or were less severe with regional activity count rates of at least 70% of the homologous contralateral region.[142] This difference would be potentially useful in identifying patients with TIA so as to avoid the risks of interventional therapy at a time when the natural history may not be clinically predictable and conventional CT findings may be normal and therefore unable to discriminate between stroke and TIA.

Watershed Infarction

In patients with watershed infarction, SPECT performed in the acute stage may be more sensitive than conventional

CT, showing perfusion defects in the appropriate watershed distribution.[143,144] The sensitivity of SPECT in detecting watershed ischemia is improved with the use of acetazolamide (see later).[145]

Possible Role in Selecting Patients for Thrombolysis

The results of the trials using intravenous t-PA[128,129] have led to optimism that a group of patients with acute ischemic stroke will benefit from early interventional thrombolytic therapy. The ECASS trial showed benefits of using intravenous rt-PA within 6 hours of stroke onset, but only in those patients in whom CT scans did not show signs of major early ischemia and who therefore were not at a high risk for hemorrhagic transformation.[128] The NINDS Stroke Study showed overall benefits for patients treated within 3 hours of stroke onset, when acute CT changes are unusual; nevertheless, the rate of symptomatic hemorrhagic transformation was at least ten times greater with rt-PA than with placebo.[129]

Alexandrov and colleagues[146,147] have suggested that ^{99m}Tc-HMPAO SPECT may have a clinical role in patient selection for thrombolysis during the early hours of stroke. The feasibility of performing SPECT studies in the short time available before the start of urgent thrombolytic therapy in acute stroke has been demonstrated by several studies.[38,42,115,122,123,126] The excellent retention properties of ^{99m}Tc-HMPAO allow scanning to be delayed for several hours after its injection and initiation of therapy.[13,14] SPECT can determine the depth, extent, and location of ischemia during the "therapeutic window," when CT findings may be normal or inconclusive.[4] Patients with normal perfusion associated with minor or resolving stroke or lacunar syndromes who have a favorable prognosis[96] can be identified and spared the hazards of thrombolysis. Patients with severe, extensive reduction in perfusion, who are at high risk of hemorrhagic transformation or reperfusion injury and therefore are less likely to benefit from treatment, can be distinguished from those with moderate perfusion defects, who might be more likely to benefit from thrombolysis without an appreciable risk of suffering adverse effects. SPECT will be useful in selecting patients for thrombolysis, however, only if scans can be obtained and interpreted before the initiation of therapy. This goal necessitates the development of rapid image acquisition protocols as well as standardized, validated methods of simple visual or semiquantitative image analysis.

Cerebrovascular Reserve

The concept of cerebrovascular or perfusion "reserve" refers to the ability of regional cerebral tissue to increase its perfusion in response to a vasodilatory stimulus such as intravenous acetazolamide or inhaled carbon dioxide. Intravenous acetazolamide is currently more commonly used, but the two techniques have similar mechanisms.

Acetazolamide is a cerebral vasodilator that has been used to evaluate vasodilatory capacity in patients with cerebrovascular disease.[112] Although the exact mechanism of action of acetazolamide remains to be elucidated, vasodilatation is believed to be mediated by the drug's potent inhibition of carbonic anhydrase. The inhibition produces a drop in pH in brain tissue and extracellular fluid, similar to the effect of breathing carbon dioxide. The resulting carbonic acidosis leads to an increase in CBF that is dose-dependent and can be as high as 66% after a single 1-g IV dose of acetazolamide.[112]

With any of the perfusion SPECT techniques, perfusion reserve can be calculated after a vasodilatory challenge with either 1 g of intravenously injected acetazolamide or 5% CO_2 administered by inhalation.[112,148] These vasodilatory agents increase rCBF in normal brain. In ischemic brain regions, which may appear to be normal on evaluation by structural brain techniques, cerebral arterioles are already vasodilated to optimize microvascular perfusion (rCBF). After the vasodilatory challenge, the response to acetazolamide is attenuated or abolished in the regions of affected perfusion, in contrast to increased rCBF in surrounding normal brain, reflecting a degree of "vasoparalysis."[149-151] These regions of relative vasoparalysis are identified through comparison of the baseline with post-challenge scans.

These focal changes in functional vasoreactivity, which can be correlated with other structural parameters indicating hemodynamic compromise—occlusive lesions on angiography, arterial flow changes shown by TCD, and borderzone infarction on CT scans—indicate the adequacy of cerebral hemispheric collateral supply in patients with severe arterial occlusive lesions.[152,153] A clinical application of this approach could be to enhance angiographic information in patients with intracranial occlusive arterial disease so as to identify high-risk patients who should undergo intervention with angioplasty rather than medical therapy.[153]

Carotid Stenosis

The role of SPECT in evaluating patients with extracranial carotid stenosis has been examined in several reports. Post-acetazolamide SPECT scans demonstrate perfusion deficits that are not present on resting (pre-acetardamide) scans, thereby providing objective evidence of hemodynamic significance.[149] Several investigators have demonstrated impairment hemispheric perfusion using the pre- and post-acetazolamide SPECT algorithm in both symptomatic and asymptomatic patients with extracranial carotid stenoses of more than 70% in severity.[154-160] They also found that the cerebral perfusion reserve returned to normal after carotid endarterectomy.[155-159] Although it is already accepted that patients with symptomatic carotid stenosis greater than 70% benefit from carotid endarterectomy,[161-164] this technique might be useful in excluding from carotid endarterectomy patients who have carotid stenosis but are at low risk of stroke or selecting for the procedure high-risk asymptomatic patients or patients with orthostatic symptoms.[155,157,165]

Carotid and Cerebral Artery Occlusion

It has also been suggested that post-acetazolamide SPECT can identify patients with internal carotid occlusion who would be at high risk of stroke if treated medically. Two groups have demonstrated a higher risk of subsequent major stroke associated with either symptomatic internal carotid or middle cerebral artery occlusion but with minimal neurologic deficit, in the presence of significant ipsilateral impairment of cerebrovascular reactivity.[166] However, whether this finding can be used to select such patients for extracranial-intracranial bypass is hypothetical and yet to be tested. Furthermore, other therapeutic implications remain unclear.[166–168]

Transient Ischemic Attacks

Studies in patients who have experienced carotid territory TIAs have shown impairment of cerebrovascular perfusion reserve after acetazolamide in the relevant vascular territory, even a month after the event.[150] Abnormalities are demonstrated in patients who do not have associated internal carotid artery stenosis, although these abnormalities are smaller than in patients with internal carotid artery lesions. This finding suggests a persistent vasoparalysis from the ischemic event itself, which may be useful to confirm a clinical diagnosis in unusual or difficult cases. There has also been a report of the diagnostic usefulness of this technique in a patient with vertebrobasilar territory ischemia, presumably due to vertebrobasilar arterial disease.[169]

Watershed Infarcts

Given that the pathophysiology of watershed, or borderzone, infarcts is thought to have a hemodynamic basis, there may be a role for post-acetazolamide SPECT in the evaluation of patients with such infarcts. Moriwaki and associates[170] divided 29 patients with watershed cerebral infarction and major cerebral arterial obstruction into two groups according to whether they had internal or cortical watershed infarction.[170] When evaluated with acetazolamide and SPECT, patients with internal watershed infarction showed evidence of severely impaired perfusion reserve, whereas those with cortical watershed infarcts had normal perfusion reserve. This finding suggested that watershed infarcts might be multifactorial in nature but that internal watershed infarcts are more likely to be due to hemodynamic impairment whereas external watershed infarcts might have an embolic basis.

Diaschisis and Stroke

Diaschisis refers to functional deactivation of morphologically intact brain regions remote from but connected to an area of primary structural damage.[171–173] The term, coined by von Monakow[171] in 1914, is derived from the Greek *schizein* meaning "to split."[174] The three general types of diaschisis that have been recognized are (1) contralateral effects on the opposite hemisphere in the mirror regions to the injury (interhemispheric, transhemispheric, or transcallosal diaschisis); (2) ipsilateral effects on the injured cerebral hemisphere but separate from the injury; and (3) effects on the cerebellum contralateral to the affected cerebral hemisphere (crossed cerebellar diaschisis [CCD]).

Interhemispheric Diaschisis

Depression of rCBF, metabolism in the contralateral hemisphere, or both after cerebral infarction has been recognized in numerous studies.[46,70,72,83,86,104,175–185] It has been attributed to transhemispheric diaschisis, and the mechanism is thought to be transcallosal neuronal depression. Transhemispheric diaschisis usually occurs in association with large cerebral infarcts, and the extent of rCBF or metabolic reduction is proportional to but less than that occurring in the infarct region.[70,182] The effect is usually maximal between 7 and 10 days after stroke onset, and it gradually returns to normal, in contrast to the ipsilateral rCBF and metabolic changes, which generally persist.[46,70,104,176,178] Other confounding factors that may contribute to the rCBF and metabolic changes contralateral to infarction are chronic hypertension, previous cerebral infarction, and large vessel occlusion with a "steal" phenomenon.[173] The effects of raised intracranial pressure or transtentorial herniation also must be considered, given the time course and association with large infarcts. Wise and associates[181] have suggested that the depression of contralateral metabolism may have preceded infarction because they found no difference between regional cerebral metabolic rate of oxygen (rCMRO$_2$) value contralateral to infarction and that found in patients who had extracranial vascular disease but no evidence of infarction.[181] We have not observed interhemispheric diaschisis in our published studies, but none of our patients was studied during the 7- to 10-day window, when this phenomenon is maximal.[80,114–117]

Subcortical-Cortical Diaschisis

In patients with lesions of subcortical white matter, basal ganglia, or thalamus, depression of rCBF and metabolism has been found in the ipsilateral overlying cortex.[41,47,61,70,72,179,180,183,186–197] The depression is thought to be due to interruption of neural connections between subcortical structures and cortex and, therefore, to represent diaschisis. This form of diaschisis has been found to correlate with the presence of cortical deficits such as aphasia, neglect, visual field defects, visuospatial abnormalities, and other neuropsychological deficits associated with subcortical lesions.[41,186–188,193,195] One specific and well-recognized example is the aphasia seen with thalamic lesions that is associated with thalamocortical diaschisis. The relationship between clinical recovery and resolution of this diaschisis is, however, variable.[41,195]

Chu and associates[198] used both ^{99m}Tc-HMPAO SPECT and magnetic resonance spectroscopy to study cerebral diaschisis associated with internal capsule infarction. They evaluated cortical diaschisis with SPECT and compared it with the severity of white matter diaschisis as determined with spectroscopy. The measures of diaschisis in the cortex and white matter were found to be proportional, such that larger reductions in cortical rCBF were associated with greater levels of white matter metabolic derangement.[198] These findings would be consistent with the proposition that diaschisis is related to functional deactivation transmitted by existing neuronal connections.

Cortical-Subcortical Diaschisis

The reverse process of the preceding condition has also been reported. In patients with hemispheric cortical infarction, remote effects have been observed in the structurally intact ipsilateral thalamus.[179,180,183,191] Although this finding might be due to decreased excitation of thalamic neurones secondary to loss of afferent input from the region of cortical infarction, other explanations must be considered. They include direct ischemia due to involvement of small penetrating arteries and compression of the thalamic circulation by postinfarction edema of perithalamic tissue. The effects of limited resolution and photon scatter from neighboring structures that produce blurred lesion margins, making lesions on functional modalities appear larger than with structural imaging, also must be taken into account.

Intrahemispheric Diaschisis

Depression of rCBF and regional glucose metabolism have been observed in the frontal and parietal cortices adjacent to hemispheric lesions.[61,179,199] Although this depression might be related to interruption of afferent input to these regions as a result of undercutting of associative fibers, several other factors might also play a role. They include direct extension of the ischemic processes including tissue edema, raised intracranial pressure, diffusion of toxic waste products from the necrotic core, and selective neuronal cell death without necrosis.[173] The existence of this "intracortical" or "intrahemispheric diaschisis" is therefore controversial. The finding of depressed rCBF adjacent to cerebral infarction has also been proposed to reflect a persistent ischemic penumbra in collaterally perfused tissue.[200] The effects of margin blurring due to limited spatial resolution, as mentioned previously, also warrant consideration.

Crossed Cerebellar Diaschisis

Crossed cerebellar diaschisis (CCD) is a matched depression of blood flow and metabolism in the cerebellar hemisphere contralateral to a focal, supratentorial lesion, and is a well-recognized phenomenon after cerebral infarction. Because the initial description in patients with supratentorial infarction by Baron and colleagues[201–203] in the early 1980s using the ^{15}O steady-state PET technique, CCD has been studied with numerous tomographic modalities, including ^{15}O PET[194,204–210]; fluorodeoxyglucose (FDG) PET[179,194,211–215]; ^{18}F-fluoromethane PET[180]; ^{133}Xe inhalation SPECT[216–218]; ^{123}I-IMP SPECT[183,219–221]; ^{123}I-labeled hydroxyiodobenzyl propanediamine (HIPDM) SPECT[46,47,68,222,223]; thallium-201-labeled diethyldithiocarbamate (^{201}Tl-DDC) SPECT[73]; and ^{99m}Tc-HMPAO SPECT.[61,190,196,199,224–226] As well as being seen after cerebral infarction (Plate 22–4),[*] CCD has been reported in patients with cerebral hemorrhage,[47,61,194,206,210,218] tumors,[196,209,211–215,221] TIAs,[46,224] arteriovenous malformations,[221,227] and pure white matter lesions such as progressive multifocal leukoencephalopathy.[228] The incidence of CCD in patients with supratentorial lesions varies between 41% and 89%, depending on the individual series and the method of patient selection.[†] This proportion does not appear to depend on the nature of the disorder. In regard to lesion topography, CCD has been observed in association with isolated lesions of the frontal cortex,[73,204,214] parietal cortex,[104,211,214] and multilobar lesions[207,221] but not with pure temporal lobe lesions.[207,221] It has also been observed in association with deep MCA or capsular infarctions,[194,201,207,223] nonlacunar subcortical strokes,[47,229] and basal ganglia and putaminal lesions[218,223]

but not with pure thalamic lesions.[218] Less commonly, lacunar infarctions involving the corona radiata or internal capsule have been observed to produce CCD.[190] Unilateral brainstem and pontine lesions have also been associated with CCD.[209,214,219,222] CCD does not have any neurologic manifestations.

Mechanism

The most likely mechanism underlying CCD is thought to be interruption of the corticopontocerebellar connections by the lesion causing deafferentation and transneural metabolic depression of the contralateral cerebellar hemisphere.[179,203,204,207,211,216] The corticopontocerebellar pathway provides the major excitatory input from the cerebral cortex to the cerebellar cortex.[173,212] The corticopontine portion arises from the frontal and parietal cortices and forms excitatory synapses on the ipsilateral pontine nuclei.[231,232] Second-order neurones then cross to the opposite cerebellar hemisphere via the middle cerebellar peduncle and synapse in the granule cell layer of the cerebellar cortex. It follows, then, that interruption of the corticopontine pathway at any point along its course decreases the excitatory activity in its projections in the ipsilateral pons and also in the contralateral cerebellar hemisphere.

This proposed mechanism is supported by the finding, reported by Fulham and associates,[212] that cerebral lesions producing CCD were associated with decreased glucose metabolism in the structurally intact ipsilateral pons. These investigators also found that glucose metabolism in the dentate nucleus of the affected cerebellar hemisphere was relatively preserved, suggesting that afferent input to the deep cerebellar nuclei from the Purkinje cells in the cerebellar cortex was preserved. Also, Yamauchi and colleagues[210] described a correlation between cerebellar metabolic asymmetry and the extent of hypometabolism in the pons. This mechanism is also supported by the topographic distribution of cerebral lesions associated with CCD as well as the observation by several investigators that upper pontine lesions, but not lower pontine lesions, produce CCD.[209,214,219,222]

Functional Nature

Structural Abnormalities in the Affected Cerebellar Hemisphere. Baron and colleagues[201,203] originally proposed that CCD is the early metabolic correlate of crossed cerebellar atrophy seen in long-standing unilateral brain lesions acquired in early life. Only a small number of studies, however, have attempted to determine whether chronic CCD associated with long-standing cerebral lesions progresses to crossed cerebellar atrophy. Three studies used MRI to study cerebellar morphology in patients with long-standing supratentorial lesions and crossed cerebellar hypometabolism due to infarct, hemorrhage, or tumor.[194,212,215] All found no structural abnormalities in the affected cerebellar hemisphere for lesions acquired during adulthood or late childhood despite duration of clinical signs and symptoms of up to 30 years. Cerebellar atrophy was, however, found with lesions acquired in early childhood and was associated with contralateral supratentorial hemispheric atrophy and intractable seizures.[215] These results suggest that CCD does not usually produce antegrade transneuronal degeneration

---

[*]See references 46, 47, 68, 73, 179, 180, 183, 194, 201–204, 206, 207, 210, 211, 216, 221.
[†]See references 46, 47, 61, 68, 73, 104, 199, 207, 210, 211, 213, 216, 223, 229, 230.

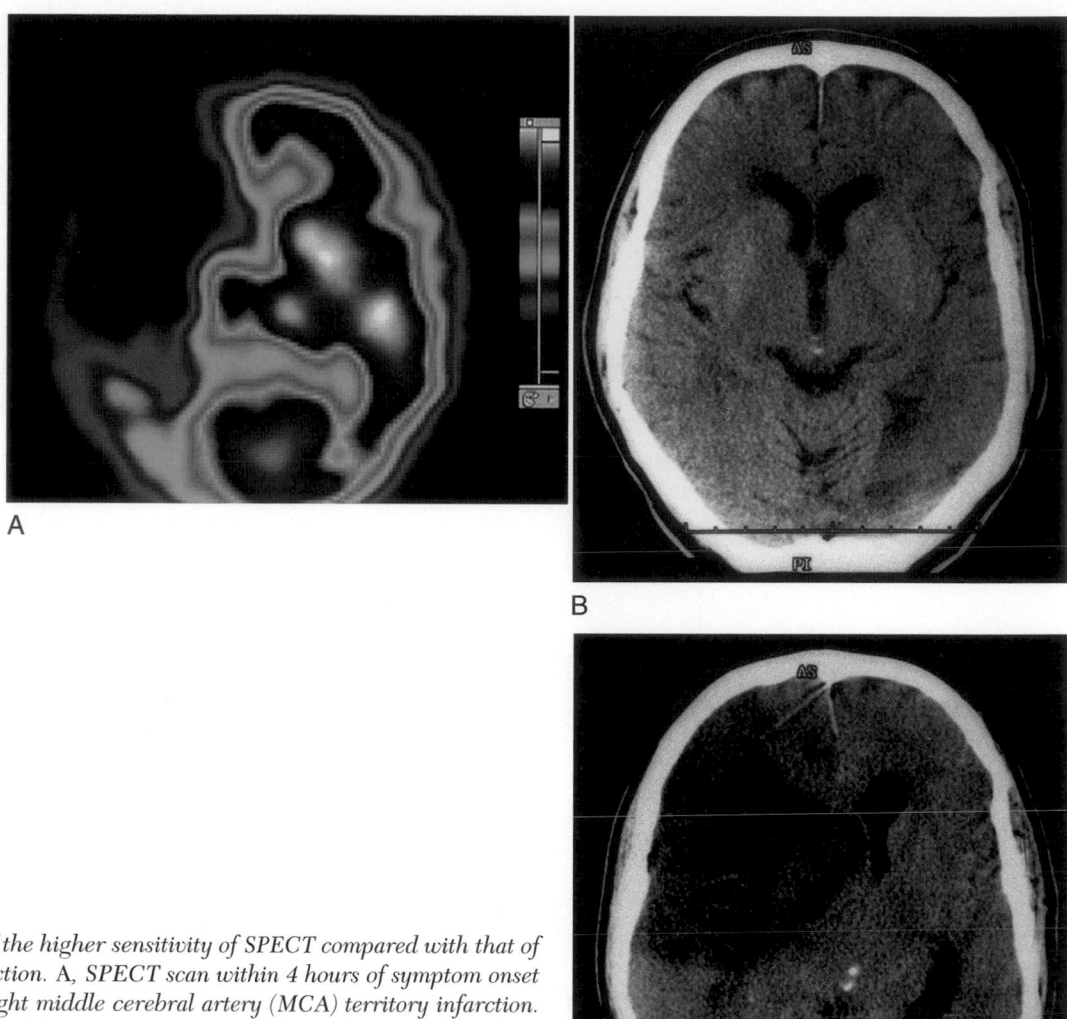

PLATE 22–1 *Example of the higher sensitivity of SPECT compared with that of CT in early cerebral infarction. A, SPECT scan within 4 hours of symptom onset in a patient with severe right middle cerebral artery (MCA) territory infarction. The clinical features were left hemiplegia and gaze palsy with visual and sensory neglect. The SPECT scan demonstrates severe perfusion reduction involving the entire right MCA territory. B, CT scan obtained within 4 hours of stroke onset in the same patient, showing minor early infarct changes, in contrast to the striking hypoperfusion seen on the SPECT scan. C, CT scan obtained 2 days later showing extensive right MCA territory infarction and associated cerebral edema with mass effect and transtentorial herniation. The patient died 3 days after the stroke as a result of cerebral edema and transtentorial herniation.*

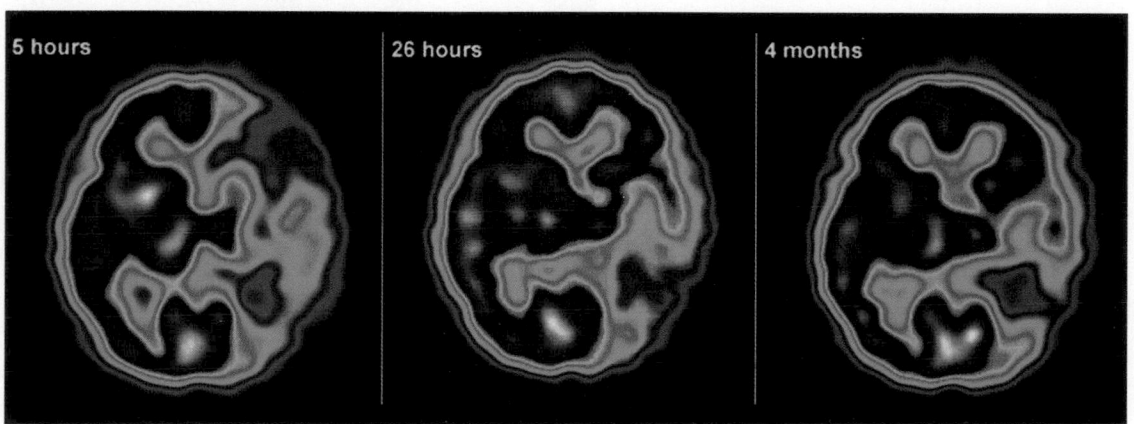

PLATE 22–2 *Example of nutritional reperfusion. Serial SPECT scans of a patient with left middle cerebral artery cortical infarction at 5 hours, 26 hours, and 4 months after stroke onset. Reperfusion has occurred between the first and second scans, which was accompanied by clinical improvement. This reperfusion is maintained at the chronic stage and is therefore nutritional in nature.*

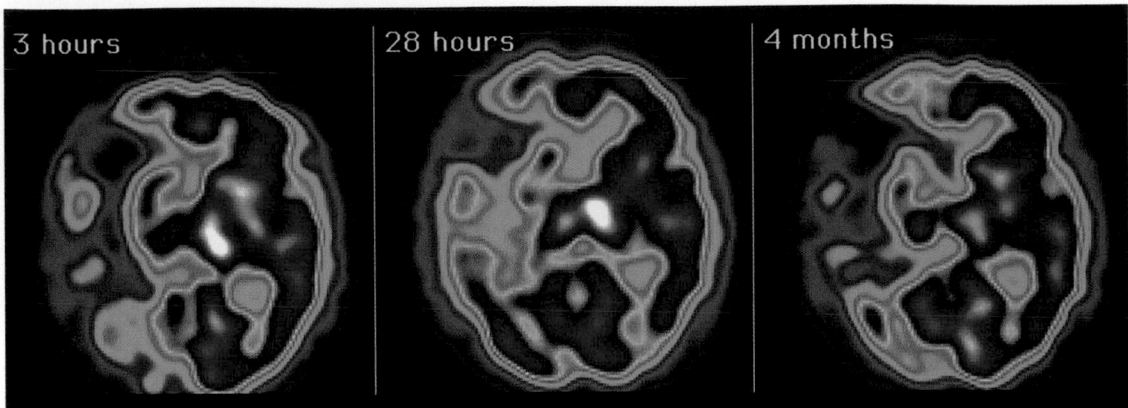

PLATE 22–3 *Example of non-nutritional reperfusion. Serial SPECT scans of a patient with right middle cerebral artery cortical infarction at 3 hours, 28 hours, and 4 months after stroke onset. Although there is reperfusion between the first and second scans, it was not accompanied by clinical improvement. Furthermore, hypoperfusion is increased at the chronic stage and is similar in severity to that on the initial scan. The reperfusion was therefore non-nutritional.*

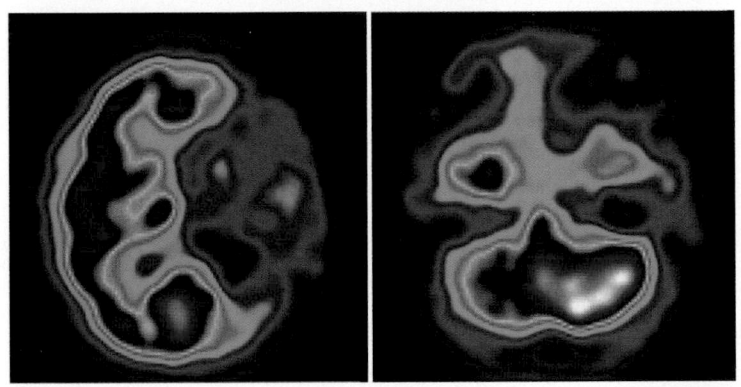

PLATE 22–4 *Example of crossed cerebellar diaschisis. SPECT scan of a patient with acute left middle cerebral artery cortical infarction. Left cerebral hypoperfusion (top) is associated with right cerebellar hypoperfusion (bottom). The cerebellum was structurally normal on a correlative CT scan.*

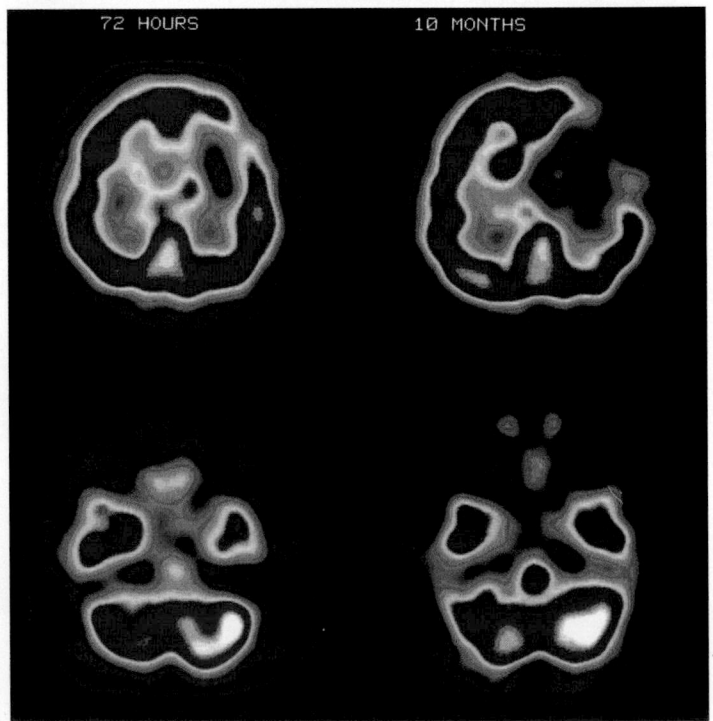

PLATE 22–5 *Changes in crossed cerebellar diaschisis (CCD) and infarct hypoperfusion with recovery. SPECT scans of a patient with left middle cerebral artery territory infarction at 72 hours (left images) and at 10 months (right images). The transverse slices through the cerebral hemispheres (upper images) show increasing hypoperfusion despite clinical recovery. The cerebellar images (lower images) show persistent, unchanged right-sided CCD.*

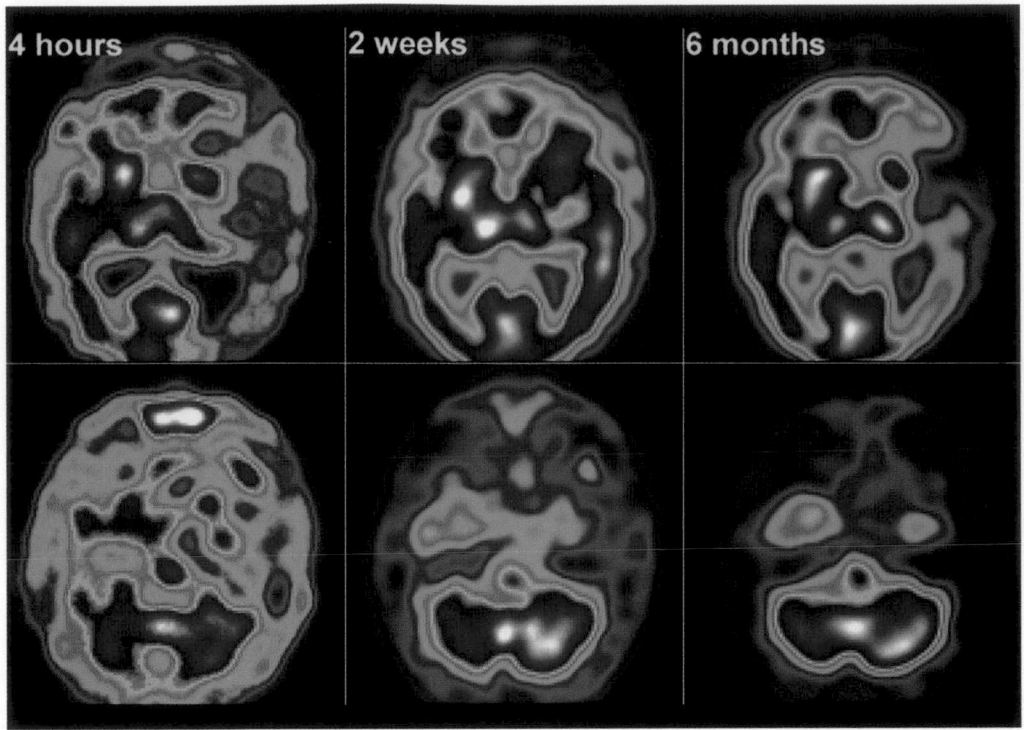

PLATE 22–6 *Crossed cerebellar diaschisis (CCD) and non-nutritional reperfusion. Serial SPECT scans of a patient with left middle cerebral artery territory cortical infarction. The scans were performed 4 hours, 2 weeks, and 6 months after stroke onset. The transaxial slices through the cerebral hemispheres* (upper images) *show non-nutritional reperfusion at 2 weeks that is not maintained at 6 months. The cerebellar images* (lower images) *show persistent CCD. (The 24-hour study was technically unsatisfactory.)*

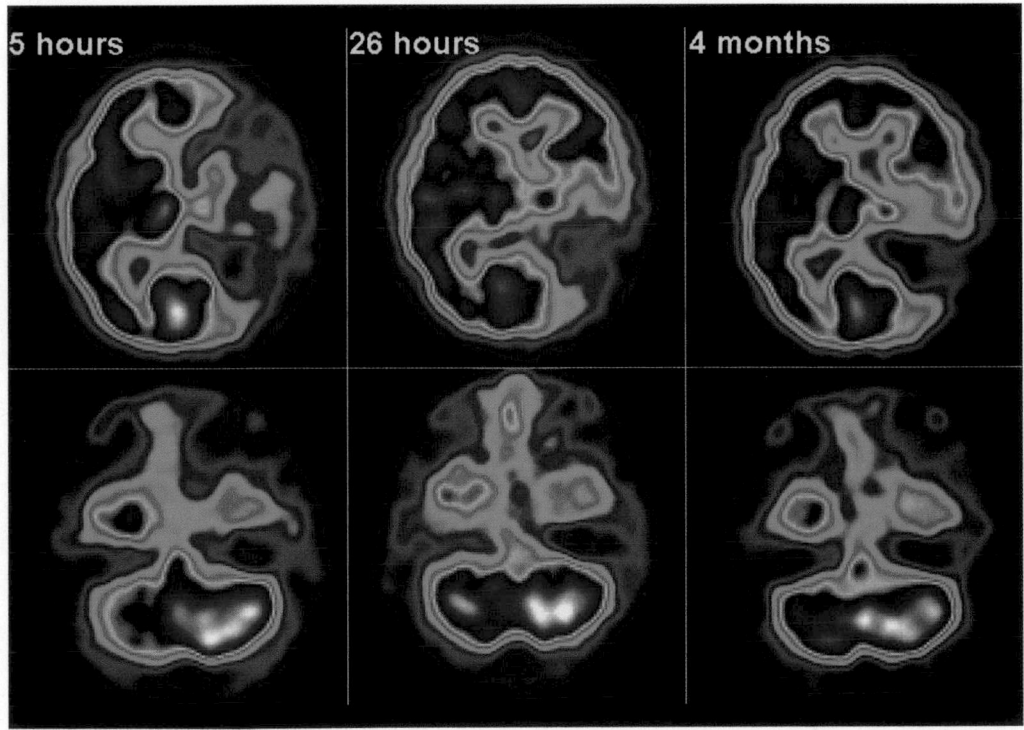

PLATE 22–7 *Crossed cerebellar diaschisis (CCD) and nutritional reperfusion. Serial SPECT scans of a patient with left middle cerebral artery territory cortical infarction. The scans were performed 5 hours, 26 hours, and 4 months after stroke onset. The transaxial slices through the cerebral hemispheres* (upper images) *show nutritional reperfusion at 26 hours that is maintained at 4 months. The cerebellar images* (lower images) *show concurrently improving CCD.*

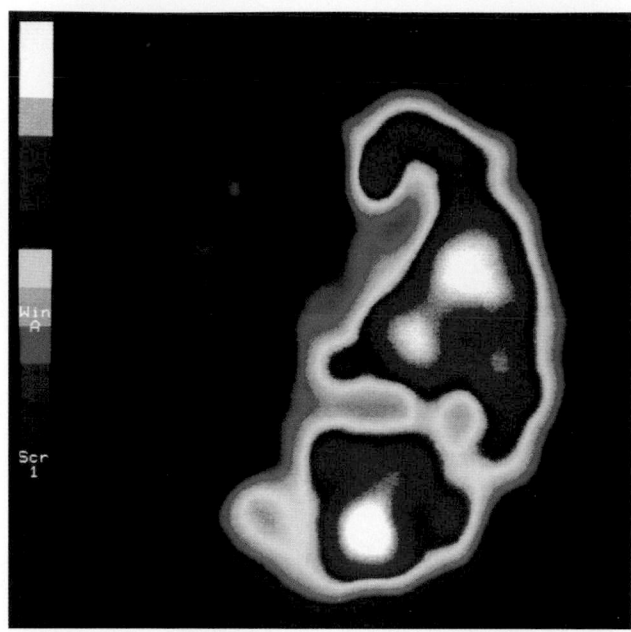

PLATE 22–8 *Right cerebral hypoperfusion due to severe symptomatic cerebral vasospasm after subarachnoid hemorrhage.*

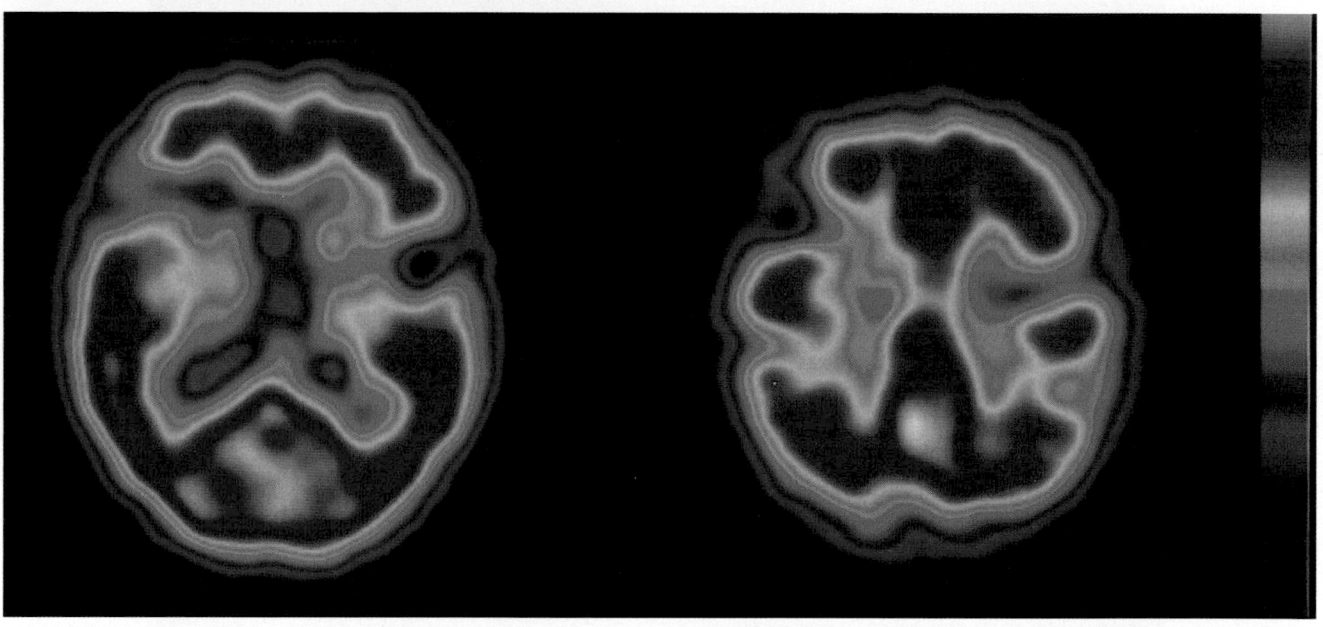

PLATE 22–9 *Multifocal perfusion defects in a patient with dementia, indicating a multi-infarct cause.*

unless the lesion is acquired in early childhood, before significant growth.

Effect of Acetazolamide. Intravenous injection of acetazolamide increases both cerebral and cerebellar blood flow within minutes in normal subjects.[112] In patients with impaired cerebrovascular hemodynamic reserve, the response to acetazolamide is attenuated or abolished in the regions of affected perfusion, reflecting a level of vasoparalysis.[149,150] Three studies have evaluated the effect of acetazolamide on cerebellar blood flow (CbBF) using SPECT in patients with unilateral cerebral infarction.[217,220,225] All studies found that cerebellar vasoreactivity was preserved in the affected cerebellar hemispheres, in contrast to that in the cerebral infarct region.

Takano and associates[197] assessed vasoreactivity to changes in carbon dioxide levels in cerebral regions with diaschisis in patients with capsular infarction, although they did not specifically study CCD. They found that in areas with diaschisis, hypercapnia after carbon dioxide inhalation produced a greater increase in rCBF, whereas hypocapnia after hyperventilation was associated with an attenuated decrease in rCBF compared with areas without diaschisis. We have also found that vasoreactivity in the affected cerebellar hemisphere is preserved in CCD.[117] These results lend further support to the concept that CCD is associated with vasoconstriction in the resting state due to decreased tissue production of carbon dioxide, which is in turn secondary to metabolic depression by loss of normal excitatory afferent input. Further evidence that CCD is associated with local vasoconstriction produced by metabolic suppression is the observation on PET by Yamauchi and coworkers[210] of raised regional cerebellar oxygen extraction in association with decreased cerebellar blood volume (CbBV) without an alteration in the ratio of CbBF to CbBV in the affected cerebellar hemisphere.

Other Evidence. Several other studies have provided evidence that CCD is a phenomenon secondary to functional deactivation rather than to direct vascular or structural alterations. The observation of transient CCD after hemispheric TIA[224] and after balloon test occlusion of the carotid artery[233–235] are suggestive of transient ischemic loss of corticocerebellar excitation. Similarly, the appearance of reversible CCD accompanying ipsilateral cerebral hypoperfusion after performance of the Wada test,[236–238] which involves intracarotid injection of a short-acting barbiturate, indicates an indirect pharmacologic effect on the contralateral cerebellar hemisphere mediated through the corticocerebellar connections.

Activation studies using PET have also shed light on CCD. Di Piero and colleagues[208] studied a patient 1 month after recovery from a cerebral hemorrhage. Both the reduced rCBF and rCMRO$_2$ in the frontotemporoparietal cortex ipsilateral to the anatomic lesion and the associated CCD, present on an early study, had resolved. After motor activation with a fine finger motor task of the contralateral hand, rCBF increased significantly in the sensorimotor and supplementary motor areas but decreased in the contralateral cerebellar hemisphere. This finding suggests persisting functional incompetence of the cerebral projections to the contralateral cerebellar hemisphere.

Barker and associates[239] studied the effect of verbal memory and somatosensory tasks on cerebral and cere-

bellar glucose metabolism in healthy normal volunteers. They found that both tasks produced coupled metabolic activation in the appropriate cerebral hemisphere and the other cerebellar hemisphere. The level of metabolic activation in the cerebellar hemisphere was proportional to that in the contralateral sensorimotor area. This coupled metabolic activation probably represents the inverse phenomenon of CCD but further supports its functional nature mediated via anatomic connections.

Whether chronic cerebellar hypometabolism associated with cerebral infarction leads to transneural degeneration and morphologic changes has been addressed in only two small MRI studies,[194,215] which found no evidence of cerebellar atrophy. In contrast, crossed cerebellar atrophy on MRI has been noted in patients with long-standing cerebral hemispheric atrophy associated with intractable seizures and onset at birth or in childhood.[215]

Crossed Cerebellocerebral Diaschisis
The opposite effect of CCD, crossed cerebellocerebral diaschisis, was reported in the 1990s. Depression of rCBF in the structurally normal frontal cortex and basal ganglia has been observed contralateral to unilateral cerebellar lesions (infarct, hemorrhage, or tumor).[240–243]

Several possible mechanisms have been proposed. The most favored mechanism is antegrade transneuronal depression via the cerebellodentatothalamocortical pathway.[240–243] This pathway originates in the cerebellar dentate nuclei, passes through the superior cerebellar peduncle, and ends on the ventrolateral and ventroanterior nuclei of the thalamus. Neurones from these nuclei then project to the frontal cortex. Another possible anatomic pathway is the nigrostriatal dopaminergic projections that pass from the dentate nucleus to the neostriatum.[240,243] This pathway would account for the decreased rCBF observed in the basal ganglia. A third possibility is retrograde transneuronal depression via the corticopontocerebellar pathway.[241,242] It has been suggested that crossed cerebellocerebral diaschisis might account for neuropsychological deficits that are often found in patients with chronic cerebellar lesions, but this issue remains to be clarified.[240,241,244]

Crossed Cerebellar Diaschisis and Brain Recovery after Acute Stroke
In the RMH laboratory, we studied a cohort of patients with acute middle cerebral cortical infarction and ^{99m}Tc-HMPAO SPECT within 72 hours of onset, followed up after 3 months.[117] Our study showed that CCD is a functional phenomenon that correlates with both severity of stroke and volume of infarct hypoperfusion and persists despite neurologic recovery (Plate 22–5). The extent of CCD could be correlated with the severity of the acute neurologic deficit and was also prognostic of functional outcome and tissue loss at 3 months, although it was not independently predictive after the prognostic value of the volume of the acute hypoperfusion deficit was considered. In a later study, Takasawa and associates[245] reported that CCD during the subacute stage of stroke indicates a worse functional outcome but also that acute CCD did not have any predictive ability.

We also found that CCD is unaffected by nonnutritional reperfusion, in contrast to the infarct site which

Diagnostic Studies

is affected by non-nutritional reperfusion (Plate 22–6). Meneghetti and associates[216] reported that CCD was less variable than the relative supratentorial infarct-related hyperemia. Lin and coworkers[246] used ^{99m}Tc-HMPAO SPECT to sequentially study rCBF in patients with acute MCA territory infarction at 1 day and at weekly intervals for 3 weeks.[246] They found that the incidence of luxury perfusion at the infarct site progressively increased while the incidence of CCD remained relatively stable.

Because CCD in the acute stage is not affected by luxury perfusion, it might reflect the extent of metabolic derangement at the infarct site, which cannot be measured with current SPECT methods. For example, relatively preserved rCBF at the infarct site associated with marked CCD might suggest a significant level of luxury perfusion. A few previous studies of CCD using PET have advanced a similar hypothesis.[205,229,247] On the other hand, CCD in the acute stage of stroke that decreases or resolves in association with early reperfusion might indicate nutritional reperfusion (Plate 22–7). Whether evaluation of early serial changes in acute CCD in tandem with early reperfusion after therapeutic intervention might permit prospective distinction between nutritional reperfusion and non-nutritional reperfusion has yet to be explored.

Subarachnoid Hemorrhage

The most important cause of morbidity after subarachnoid hemorrhage (SAH) is cerebral ischemia due to vasospasm, producing delayed neurologic deterioration in approximately 30% of patients. Davis and colleagues[248] reported that in patients with aneurysmal SAH, regional hypoperfusion on ^{99m}Tc-HMPAO SPECT (Plate 22–8) could be correlated with the presence and severity of delayed neurologic deficits, providing more information than CT scans. Regional hypoperfusion deficits correlated with clinical evidence of focal neurologic abnormalities and were most severe in the patients who later died. In contrast, asymptomatic patients usually had normal rCBF.[248] Similar findings were reported by other groups.[249–251] One study correlated hypoperfusion on SPECT with the site of ruptured aneurysms.[252] Localized hypoperfusion has also been shown after aneurysm clipping without clinical deterioration, possibly reflecting local edema.[253]

Because of the established value of TCD in the diagnosis of large vessel vasospasm,[254] Davis and colleagues[255] compared serial MCA velocities with TCD and rCBF changes with ^{99m}Tc-HMPAO SPECT after SAH and correlated the hemodynamic data with clinical evidence of delayed ischemia.[255] Of the patients who did not exhibit clinical signs of delayed neurologic deterioration, 50% had vasospasm according to TCD criteria, but regional hypoperfusion as shown on SPECT was rare. Concordant MCA vasospasm and regional cortical hypoperfusion were typically present in patients with delayed ischemia and a lateralizing neurologic deficit, such as hemiplegia, dysphasia, and neglect. These researchers concluded that regional hypoperfusion was a more specific indicator of cerebral ischemia after SAH than the demonstration of vasospasm on TCD. Grosset and coworkers[256] also used ^{99m}Tc-HMPAO SPECT to study rCBF changes in patients exhibiting rapid increases in arterial velocities after SAH.

They found that correlative focal hypoperfusion occurred in most patients before the onset of any focal neurologic deficit.

These studies highlight the complementary nature of the information provided by these two hemodynamic techniques and show that SPECT is more specific to tissue ischemia. On the basis of the detection of focal abnormalities in SAH, SPECT imaging has been used to select the type and intensity of therapy for vasospasm. For example, Lewis and coworkers[257] used ^{99m}Tc-HMPAO SPECT to select patients for angioplasty.

Arteriovenous Malformations

The SPECT technique has also been used to study patients with arteriovenous malformations (AVMs). Cerebrovascular steal in such patients can be evaluated with SPECT. Abnormally enhanced reactivity has been linked to postoperative hyperemia and poor outcomes.[258] SPECT evidence of postoperative hypoperfusion has been correlated with cognitive and behavioral abnormalities.[259] Awad and colleagues[260] correlated intractable postoperative intracranial hypertension in lesions 6 cm or greater with preoperative hypoperfusion.

Epileptic Seizures in Acute and Chronic Stroke

Epileptic seizures are a well-recognized complication of acute ischemic stroke. Our group reported a 4.4% incidence of seizures in 1000 consecutive patients with stroke and TIAs; seizures occurred only in those with cortical ischemia or lobar hemorrhage.[261] In addition, seizures as a late manifestation of cerebral infarction are observed in about 10% of patients.[262,263] The use of SPECT has found increasing application in the investigation and management of patients with intractable seizure disorders, particularly those with complex partial seizures of temporal lobe origin. In this disorder, interictal SPECT demonstrates regional hypoperfusion with a sensitivity of 50% to 90%.[264–266] At the time of an epileptic discharge, there is a marked focal increase in rCBF. A number of studies have shown that perfusion SPECT is very valuable in the localization of a seizure focus at the time of the ictus or in the immediate postictal phase.[267–269] Although post-stroke epilepsy is rarely an intractable problem, the successful application of SPECT in comprehensive epilepsy programs incorporating surgery for selected patients with refractory temporal lobe epilepsy may in the future assist in the management of other medically refractory seizure disorders. In patients with vascular malformations and epilepsy, SPECT has been used to evaluate focal perfusion abnormalities.[270]

Multi-infarct Dementia

Functional neuroimaging with SPECT is useful in the evaluation of dementia, because there are specific differences in the pattern between multi-infarct dementia and the more common Alzheimer's disease. In Alzheimer's disease, SPECT characteristically shows diffuse bilateral and symmetrical hypoperfusion in the temporal and parietal lobes, correlating with the clinical manifestations and severity of the dementia progress.[4,271–273] In contrast, the characteristic pattern on SPECT in multi-infarct dementia consists of multiple asymmetrical perfusion deficits that involve both the cortex and deep structures (Plate 22–9).[274,275] In addition, unlike patients with Alzheimer's disease, patients with multi-infarct dementia typically show frontal lobe perfusion abnormalities on SPECT.[276] The use of the vasodilator acetazolamide, which detects vasoparalysis or impaired perfusion reserve in patients with focal regions of brain ischemia, can also be useful in the distinction between a multi-infarct state and Alzheimer's disease.[277]

CONCLUSIONS

A variety of SPECT techniques have now been available for more than a decade, but the use of this technology in cerebrovascular disease is still chiefly confined to centers with a special interest in brain perfusion rather than finding widespread application in routine clinical practice. This situation is likely to alter if knowledge of cerebral perfusion changes proves to be relevant to clinical decision-making in cerebrovascular disease. The most important role of this technique may well be to facilitate selection of interventional therapies in acute ischemic stroke, particularly thrombolysis, in which a rapid analysis of regional hypoperfusion may be valuable for the identification of patients whose disease is likely to respond to a potentially dangerous therapy.[146] The clinical application of SPECT in cerebrovascular disease, which often depends on the interpretation of complex imaging data, should involve a close collaboration between neurologists and nuclear medicine physicians.[5]

References

1. Fisher M, Prichard JW, Warach S: New magnetic resonance techniques for acute ischemic stroke. JAMA 274:908–911, 1995.
2. Warach S, Dashe JF, Edelman RR: Clinical outcome in ischemic stroke predicted by early diffusion-weighted and perfusion magnetic resonance imaging: A preliminary analysis. J Cereb Blood Flow Metab 16:53–59, 1996.
3. Barber PA, Darby DG, Desmond PM, et al: Prediction of stroke outcome with echoplanar perfusion- and diffusion-weighted MRI. Neurology 51:418–426, 1998.
4. Holman BL, Devous MD Sr: Functional brain SPECT: The emergence of a powerful clinical method. J Nucl Med 33:1888–1904, 1992.
5. Assessment of brain SPECT. Report of the Therapeutics and Technology Assessment Subcommittee of the American Academy of Neurology. Neurology 46:278–285, 1996.
6. Nakano S, Kinoshita K, Jinnouchi S, et al: Comparative study of regional cerebral blood flow images by SPECT using xenon-133, iodine-123 IMP, and technetium-99m HM-PAO. J Nucl Med 30:157–164, 1989.
7. Podreka I, Baumgartner C, Suess E, et al: Quantification of regional cerebral blood flow with IMP-SPECT: Reproducibility and clinical relevance of flow values. Stroke 20:183–191, 1989.
8. Kuhl DE, Barrco JR, Huang SC, et al: Quantifying local cerebral blood flow by N-isopropyl-p-I-123 iodoamphetamine (IMP) tomography. J Nucl Med 23:196–203, 1982.
9. Ell PJ, Hocknell JM, Jarritt PH, et al: A 99Tcm-labelled radiotracer for the investigation of cerebral vascular disease. Nucl Med Commun 6:437–441, 1985.
10. Neirinckx RD, Canning LR, Piper IM, et al: Technetium-99m d,l-HM-PAO: A new radiopharmaceutical for SPECT imaging of regional cerebral blood perfusion. J Nucl Med 28:191–202, 1987.
11. Fayad PB, Brass LM: Single photon emission computed tomography in cerebrovascular disease. Stroke 22:950–954, 1991.
12. Andersen AR, Friberg H, Knudsen KB, et al: Extraction of [99mTc]-d,l-HM-PAO across the blood-brain barrier. J Cereb Blood Flow Metab 8(Suppl 1):S44–S51, 1988.
13. Neirinckx RD, Burke JF, Harrison RC, et al: The retention mechanism of technetium-99m-HM-PAO: Intracellular reaction with glutathione. J Cereb Blood Flow Metab 8(Suppl 1):S4–S12, 1988.
14. Andersen AR: 99mTc-D,L-hexamethylene-propyleneamine oxime (99mTc-HMPAO): Basic kinetic studies of a tracer of cerebral blood flow. Cerebrovasc Brain Metab Rev 1:288–318, 1989.
15. Holmes RA, Chaplin SB, Royston KG, et al: Cerebral uptake and retention of 99Tcm-hexamethylpropyleneamine oxime (99Tcm-HM-PAO). Nucl Med Commun 6:443–447, 1985.
16. Podreka I, Suess E, Goldenberg G, et al: Initial experience with technetium-99m HM-PAO brain SPECT. J Nucl Med 28:1657–1666, 1987.
17. Costa DC, Ell PJ, Cullum ID, et al: The in vivo distribution of 99Tcm-HM-PAO in normal man. Nucl Med Commun 7:647–658, 1986.
18. Andersen AR, Friberg H, Lassen NA, et al: Serial studies of cerebral blood flow using 99Tcm-HMPAO: A comparison with 133Xe. Nucl Med Commun 8:549–557, 1987.
19. Yonekura Y, Nishizawa S, Mukai T, et al: SPECT with [99mTc]-d,l-hexamethyl-propylene amine oxime (HM-PAO) compared with regional cerebral blood flow measured by PET: Effects of linearization. J Cereb Blood Flow Metab 8(Suppl 1):S82–S89, 1988.
20. Inugami A, Kanno I, Uemura K, et al: Linearization correction of 99mTc-labeled hexamethyl-propylene amine oxime (HM-PAO) image in terms of regional CBF distribution: Comparison to C15O2 inhalation steady-state method measured by positron emission tomography. J Cereb Blood Flow Metab 8(Suppl 1):S52–S60, 1988.
21. Lear JL: Quantitative local cerebral blood flow measurements with technetium-99m HM-PAO: Evaluation using multiple radionuclide digital quantitative autoradiography. J Nucl Med 29:1387–1392, 1988.
22. Spreafico G, Cammelli F, Gadola G, et al: Luxury perfusion syndrome in cerebral vascular disease evaluated with technetium-99m HM-PAO. Clin Nucl Med 12:217–218, 1987.
23. Moretti JL, Defer G, Cinotti L, et al: "Luxury perfusion" with 99mTc-HMPAO and 123I-IMP SPECT imaging during the subacute phase of stroke. Eur J Nucl Med 16:17–22, 1990.
24. Holman BL, Hellman RS, Goldsmith SJ, et al: Biodistribution, dosimetry, and clinical evaluation of technetium-99m ethyl cysteinate dimer in normal subjects and in patients with chronic cerebral infarction. J Nucl Med 30:1018–1024, 1989.
25. Shishido F, Uemura K, Inugami A, et al: Discrepant 99mTc-ECD images of CBF in patients with subacute cerebral infarction: A comparison of CBF, CMRO2 and 99mTc-HMPAO imaging. Ann Nucl Med 9:161–166, 1995.
26. Shishido F, Uemura K, Murakami M, et al: Cerebral uptake of 99mTc-bicisate in patients with cerebrovascular disease in comparison with CBF and CMRO2 measured by positron emission tomography. J Cereb Blood Flow Metab 14(Suppl 1):S66–S75, 1994.
27. Tsuchida T, Nishizawa S, Yonekura Y, et al: SPECT images of technetium-99m-ethyl cysteinate dimer in cerebrovascular diseases: Comparison with other cerebral perfusion tracers and PET. J Nucl Med 35:27–31, 1994.
28. Garrett K, Villanueva J, Kuperus J, et al: A comparison of regional cerebral blood flow with Xe133 to SPECT Tc99mECD. J Nucl Med 29:913, 1988.
29. Devous MD Sr, Payne JK, Lowe JL, et al: Comparison of technetium-99m-ECD to xenon-133 SPECT in normal controls and in patients with mild to moderate regional cerebral blood flow abnormalities. J Nucl Med 34:754–761, 1993.
30. Sperling B, Lassen NA: Hyperfixation of HMPAO in subacute ischemic stroke leading to spuriously high estimates of cerebral blood flow by SPECT. Stroke 24:193–194, 1993.
31. Lassen NA: Imaging brain infarcts by single-photon emission tomography with new tracers. Eur J Nucl Med 21:189–190, 1994.
32. Brass LM, Walovitch RC, Joseph JL, et al: The role of single photon emission computed tomography brain imaging with 99mTc-bicisate in the localization and definition of mechanism of ischemic stroke. J Cereb Blood Flow Metab 14(Suppl 1):S91–S98, 1994.
33. Eckelman WC, Reba RC, Rzeszotarski WJ, et al: External imaging of cerebral muscarinic acetylcholine receptors. Science 223:291–293, 1984.

34. Savic I, Persson A, Roland P, et al: In-vivo demonstration of reduced benzodiazepine receptor binding in human epileptic foci. Lancet 2:863–866, 1988.

35. Gray's Anatomy, 36th edition. Edinburgh, Churchill Livingstone, 1980.

36. Isaka Y, Itoi Y, Imaizumi M, et al: Quantitation of rCBF by ^{99m}Tc-hexamethylpropyleneamine oxime single photon emission computed tomography combined with ^{133}Xe CBF. J Cereb Blood Flow Metab 14:353–357, 1994.

37. Pupi A, De Cristofaro MT, Bacciottini L, et al: An analysis of the arterial input curve for technetium-99m-HMPAO: Quantification of rCBF using single-photon emission computed tomography. J Nucl Med 32:1501–1506, 1991.

38. Baird AE, Donnan GA, Austin MC, et al: Reperfusion after thrombolytic therapy in ischemic stroke measured by single-photon emission computed tomography. Stroke 25:79–85, 1994.

39. Rango M, Candelise L, Perani D, et al: Cortical pathophysiology and clinical neurologic abnormalities in acute cerebral ischemia: A serial study with single photon emission computed tomography. Arch Neurol 46:1318–1322, 1989.

40. Lee RG, Hill TC, Holman BL, et al: Predictive value of perfusion defect size using N-isopropyl-(I-123)-p-iodoamphetamine emission tomography in acute stroke. J Neurosurg 61:449–452, 1984.

41. Vallar G, Perani D, Cappa SF, et al: Recovery from aphasia and neglect after subcortical stroke: Neuropsychological and cerebral perfusion study. J Neurol Neurosurg Psychiatry 51:1269–1276, 1988.

42. Hanson SK, Grotta JC, Rhoades H, et al: Value of single-photon emission-computed tomography in acute stroke therapeutic trials. Stroke 24:1322–1329, 1993.

43. Defer G, Moretti JL, Cesaro P, et al: Early and delayed SPECT using N-isopropyl p-iodoamphetamine iodine 123 in cerebral ischemia: A prognostic index for clinical recovery. Arch Neurol 44:715–718, 1987.

44. Giubilei F, Lenzi GL, Di Piero V, et al: Predictive value of brain perfusion single-photon emission computed tomography in acute ischemic stroke. Stroke 21:895–900, 1990.

45. Shimosegawa E, Hatazawa J, Inugami A, et al: Cerebral infarction within six hours of onset: Prediction of completed infarction with technetium-99m-HMPAO SPECT. J Nucl Med 35:1097–1103, 1994.

46. Pantano P, Lenzi GL, Guidetti B, et al: Crossed cerebellar diaschisis in patients with cerebral ischemia assessed by SPECT and ^{123}I-HIPDM. Eur Neurol 27:142–148, 1987.

47. Perani D, Di Piero V, Lucignani G, et al: Remote effects of subcortical cerebrovascular lesions: A SPECT cerebral perfusion study. J Cereb Blood Flow Metab 8:560–567, 1988.

48. Goulding P, Burjan A, Smith R, et al: Semi-automatic quantification of regional cerebral perfusion in primary degenerative dementia using 99m technetium-hexamethylpropylene amine oxime and single photon emission tomography. Eur J Nucl Med 17:77–82, 1990.

49. Hellman RS, Tikofsky RS, Collier BD, et al: Alzheimer disease: Quantitative analysis of I-123-iodoamphetamine SPECT brain imaging. Radiology 172:183–188, 1989.

50. Hooper HR, McEwan AJ, Lentle BC, et al: Interactive three-dimensional region of interest analysis of HMPAO SPECT brain studies. J Nucl Med 31:2046–2051, 1990.

51. Jagust WJ, Reed BR, Seab JP, et al: Alzheimer's disease: Age at onset and single-photon emission computed tomographic patterns of regional cerebral blood flow. Arch Neurol 47:628–633, 1990.

52. Johnson KA, Holman BL, Mueller SP, et al: Single photon emission computed tomography in Alzheimer's disease: Abnormal iofetamine I-123 uptake reflects dementia severity. Arch Neurol 45:392–396, 1988.

53. Karbe H, Kertesz A, Davis J, et al: Quantification of functional deficit in Alzheimer's disease using a computer-assisted mapping program for ^{99m}Tc-HMPAO SPECT. Neuroradiology 36:1–6, 1994.

54. Maurer AH, Siegel JA, Comerota AJ, et al: SPECT quantification of cerebral ischemia before and after carotid endarterectomy. J Nucl Med 31:1412–1420, 1990.

55. Montaldi D, Brooks DN, McColl JH, et al: Measurements of regional cerebral blood flow and cognitive performance in Alzheimer's disease. J Neurol Neurosurg Psychiatry 53:33–38, 1990.

56. O'Mahony D, Coffey J, Murphy J, et al: The discriminant value of semiquantitative SPECT data in mild Alzheimer's disease. J Nucl Med 35:1450–1455, 1994.

57. Perani D, Di Piero V, Vallar G, et al: Technetium-99m HM-PAO-SPECT study of regional cerebral perfusion in early Alzheimer's disease. J Nucl Med 29:1507–1514, 1988.

58. Rowe CC, Berkovic SF, Austin MC, et al: Visual and quantitative analysis of interictal SPECT with technetium-99m-HMPAO in temporal lobe epilepsy. J Nucl Med 32:1688–1694, 1991.

59. Spreafico G, Gadola G, Cammelli F, et al: Semiquantitative assessment of regional cerebral perfusion using ^{99m}Tc HM-PAO and emission tomography. Eur J Nucl Med 14:565–568, 1988.

60. Waldemar G, Hasselbalch SG, Andersen AR, et al: ^{99m}Tc-d,l-HMPAO and SPECT of the brain in normal aging. J Cereb Blood Flow Metab 11:508–521, 1991.

61. Rousseaux M, Steinling M, Huglo D, et al: Perfusion mapping with Tc-HMPAO in cerebral haematomas. J Neurol Neurosurg Psychiatry 54:1040–1043, 1991.

62. Infeld B, Binns D, Lichtenstein M, et al: Volumetric analysis of cerebral hypoperfusion on SPECT: Validation and reliability. J Nucl Med 38:1447–1453, 1997.

63. Hoffman EJ, Cutler PD, Digby WM, et al: 3-D phantom to simulate cerebral blood flow and metabolic images for PET. IEEE Trans Nucl Sci 37:616–620, 1990.

64. Hoffman EJ, Cutler PD, Guerrero TM, et al: Assessment of accuracy of PET utilizing a 3-D phantom to simulate the activity distribution of [^{18}F]fluorodeoxyglucose uptake in the human brain. J Cereb Blood Flow Metab 11(Suppl 1):A17–A25, 1991.

65. Mountz JM: A method of analysis of SPECT blood flow image data for comparison with computed tomography. Clin Nucl Med 14:192–196, 1989.

66. Hill TC, Magistretti PL, Holman BL, et al: Assessment of regional cerebral blood flow (rCBF) in stroke using SPECT and N-isopropyl-(I-123)-p-iodoamphetamine (IMP). Stroke 15:40–45, 1984.

67. Hill TC, Holman BL, Lovett R, et al: Initial experience with SPECT (single-photon computerized tomography) of the brain using N-isopropyl I-123 p-iodoamphetamine: Concise communication. J Nucl Med 23:191–195, 1982.

68. Brott TG, Gelfand MJ, Williams CC, et al: Frequency and patterns of abnormality detected by iodine-123 amine emission CT after cerebral infarction. Radiology 158:729–734, 1986.

69. de Bruine JF, van Royen EA, van Weeren F, et al: Functional brain imaging with I-123-amphetamine: First experience in the Netherlands. Clin Neurol Neurosurg 88:253–261, 1986.

70. Vorstrup S, Paulson OB, Lassen NA: Cerebral blood flow in acute and chronic ischemic stroke using xenon-133 inhalation tomography. Acta Neurol Scand 74:439–451, 1986.

71. Hayman LA, Taber KH, Jhingran SG, et al: Cerebral infarction: Diagnosis and assessment of prognosis by using ^{123}IMP-SPECT and CT. AJNR Am J Neuroradiol 10:557–562, 1989.

72. De Roo M, Mortelmans L, Devos P, et al: Clinical experience with Tc-99m HM-PAO high resolution SPECT of the brain in patients with cerebrovascular accidents. Eur J Nucl Med 15:9–15, 1989.

73. de Bruine JF, Limburg M, van Royen EA, et al: SPET brain imaging with 201 diethyldithiocarbamate in acute ischemic stroke. Eur J Nucl Med 17:248–251, 1990.

74. Feldmann M, Voth E, Dressler D, et al: ^{99m}Tc-hexamethylpropylene amine oxime SPECT and X-ray CT in acute cerebral ischemia. J Neurol 237:475–479, 1990.

75. Baird AE, Donnan GA, Austin M, et al: Preliminary experience with 99mTc-HMPAO SPECT in cerebral ischemia. Clin Exp Neurol 28:43–49, 1991.

76. Laloux P, Doat M, Brichant C, et al: Clinical usefulness of technetium-99m HMPAO SPECT imaging to map the ischemic lesion in acute stroke: A reevaluation. Cerebrovasc Dis 4:280–286, 1994.

77. Spreafico G, Cammelli F, Gadola G, et al: Initial experience with SPECT of the brain using ^{99m}Tc-hexamethyl-propyleneamine oxime (^{99m}Tc-HM-PAO). Eur J Nucl Med 12:557–559, 1987.

78. Fieschi C, Argentino C, Lenzi GL, et al: Clinical and instrumental evaluation of patients with ischemic stroke within the first six hours. J Neurol Sci 91:311–321, 1989.

79. Bose A, Pacia SB, Fayad P, et al: Cerebral blood flow imaging compared to CT during the initial 24 hours of cerebral infarction. Neurology 40:190, 1990.

80. Davis SM, Chua MG, Lichtenstein M, et al: Cerebral hypoperfusion in stroke prognosis and brain recovery. Stroke 24:1691–1696, 1993.

81. Launes J, Nikkinen P, Lindroth L, et al: Brain perfusion defect size in SPECT predicts outcome in cerebral infarction. Nucl Med Commun 10:891–900, 1989.

Diagnostic Studies

82. Burke AM, Younkin D, Gordon J, et al: Changes in cerebral blood flow and recovery from acute stroke. Stroke 17:173–178, 1986.

83. Demeurisse G, Verhas M, Capon A, et al: Lack of evolution of the cerebral blood flow during clinical recovery of a stroke. Stroke 14:77–81, 1983.

84. Nagata K, Yunoki K, Kabe S, et al: Regional cerebral blood flow correlates of aphasia outcome in cerebral hemorrhage and cerebral infarction. Stroke 17:417–423, 1986.

85. Cordes M, Henkes H, Roll D, et al: Subacute and chronic cerebral infarctions: SPECT and gadolinium-DTPA enhanced MR imaging. J Comput Assist Tomogr 13:567–571, 1989.

86. Raynaud C, Rancurel G, Tzourio N, et al: SPECT analysis of recent cerebral infarction. Stroke 20:192–204, 1989.

87. Bushnell DL, Gupta S, Mlcoch AG, et al: Prediction of language and neurologic recovery after cerebral infarction with SPECT imaging using N-isopropyl-p-(I 123) iodoamphetamine. Arch Neurol 46:665–669, 1989.

88. Limburg M, van Royen EA, Hijdra A, et al: Single-photon emission computed tomography and early death in acute ischemic stroke. Stroke 21:1150–1155, 1990.

89. Limburg M, van Royen EA, Hijdra A, et al: rCBF-SPECT in brain infarction: When does it predict outcome? J Nucl Med 32:382–387, 1991.

90. Côté R, Battista RN, Wolfson C, et al: The Canadian Neurological Scale: Validation and reliability assessment. Neurology 39:638–643, 1989.

91. Allen CM: Predicting the outcome of acute stroke: A prognostic score. J Neurol Neurosurg Psychiatry 47:475–480, 1984.

92. Collin C, Wade DT, Davies S, et al: The Barthel ADL Index: A reliability study. Int Disabil Stud 10:61–63, 1988.

93. Davis SM, Chua MG, Lichtenstein M, et al: Perfusion changes with recovery after stroke. Aust N Z J Med 23:568, 1993.

94. Davis SM, Chua MG, Lichtenstein M, et al: Perfusion changes with recovery after stroke. In 2nd International Conference on Stroke, May 12–15, 1993, Geneva, Switzerland.

95. Davis SM, Infeld B, Chua MG, et al: Reperfusion after stroke and non-nutritional flow. In 1994 Annual Scientific Meeting of the Stroke Society of Australasia, October 6–7, 1994, Sydney, Australia.

96. Alexandrov AV, Black SE, Ehrlich LE, et al: Simple visual analysis of brain perfusion on HMPAO SPECT predicts early outcome in acute stroke. Stroke 27:1537–1542, 1996.

97. Bowler JV, Wade JP, Jones BE, et al: Single-photon emission computed tomography using hexamethylpropyleneamine oxime in the prognosis of acute cerebral infarction. Stroke 27:82–86, 1996.

98. Laloux P, Richelle F, Jamart J, et al: Comparative correlations of HMPAO SPECT indices, neurological score, and stroke subtypes with clinical outcome in acute carotid infarcts. Stroke 26:816–821, 1995.

99. Hirano T, Read SJ, Abbott DF, et al: Prediction of the final infarct volume within 6 h of stroke using single photon emission computed tomography with technetium-99m hexamethylpropylene amine oxime. Cerebrovasc Dis 11:119–127, 2001.

100. Barthel H, Hesse S, Dannenberg C, et al: Prospective value of perfusion and x-ray attenuation imaging with single-photon emission and transmission computed tomography in acute cerebral ischemia. Stroke 32:1588–1597, 2001.

101. Mahagne MH, Darcourt J, Migneco O, et al: Early (99m)Tc-ethylcysteinate dimer brain SPECT patterns in the acute phase of stroke as predictors of neurological recovery. Cerebrovasc Dis 10:364–373, 2000.

102. Lassen NA: The luxury-perfusion syndrome and its possible relation to acute metabolic acidosis localised within the brain. Lancet 2:1113–1115, 1966.

103. Baron JC, Bousser MG, Comar D, et al: Noninvasive tomographic study of cerebral blood flow and oxygen metabolism in vivo: Potentials, limitations, and clinical applications in cerebral ischemic disorders. Eur Neurol 20:273–284, 1981.

104. Lenzi GL, Frackowiak RS, Jones T: Cerebral oxygen metabolism and blood flow in human cerebral ischemic infarction. J Cereb Blood Flow Metab 2:321–335, 1982.

105. Wise RJ, Bernardi S, Frackowiak RS, et al: Serial observations on the pathophysiology of acute stroke: The transition from ischemia to infarction as reflected in regional oxygen extraction. Brain 106:197–222, 1983.

106. Ackerman RH, Alpert NM, Correia JA, et al: Positron imaging in ischemic stroke disease. Ann Neurol 15(Suppl):S126–S130, 1984.

107. Uemura K, Goto K, Ishii K, et al: Sequential changes of regional circulation in cerebral infarction. Neuroradiology 16:228–232, 1978.

108. Companioni JM, Lassen NA, Tfelt-Hansen P, et al: Delayed reflow of an ischemic infarct after spontaneous thrombolysis studied by CBF tomography using SPECT and Tc-99m HMPAO. Am J Physiol Imaging 6:167–171, 1991.

109. Sugiyama H, Christensen J, Skyhoj Olsen T, et al: Monitoring CBF in clinical routine by dynamic single photon emission tomography (SPECT) of inhaled xenon-133. Stroke 17:1179–1182, 1986.

110. Lassen NA, Sperling B: 99mTc-bicisate reliably images CBF in chronic brain diseases but fails to show reflow hyperemia in subacute stroke: Report of a multicenter trial of 105 cases comparing 133Xe and 99mTc-bicisate (ECD, Neurolite) measured by SPECT on same day. J Cereb Blood Flow Metab 14(Suppl 1):S44–S48, 1994.

111. Raynaud C, Rancurel G, Samson Y, et al: Pathophysiologic study of chronic infarcts with I-123 isopropyl iodo-amphetamine (IMP): The importance of periinfarct area. Stroke 18:21–29, 1987.

112. Vorstrup S: Tomographic cerebral blood flow measurements in patients with ischemic cerebrovascular disease and evaluation of the vasodilatory capacity by the acetazolamide test. Acta Neurol Scand 114:1–48, 1988.

113. Bowler JV, Wade JP, Jones BE, et al: Natural history of the spontaneous reperfusion of human cerebral infarcts as assessed by 99mTc HMPAO SPECT. J Neurol Neurosurg Psychiatry 64:90–97, 1998.

114. Barber PA, Davis SM, Infeld B, et al: Spontaneous reperfusion after ischemic stroke is associated with improved outcome. Stroke 29:2522–2528, 1998.

115. Infeld B, Davis SM, Donnan GA, et al: Streptokinase increases luxury perfusion after stroke. Stroke 27:1524–1529, 1996.

116. Infeld B, Davis SM, Donnan GA, et al: Nimodipine and perfusion changes after stroke. Stroke 30:1417–1423, 1999.

117. Infeld B, Davis SM, Lichtenstein M, et al: Crossed cerebellar diaschisis and brain recovery after stroke. Stroke 26:90–95, 1995.

118. Kim HS, Kim DI, Lee JD, et al: Significance of 99mTc-ECD SPECT in acute and subacute ischemic stroke: Comparison with MR images including diffusion and perfusion weighted images. Yonsei Med J 43:211–222, 2002.

119. Kim JH, Lee EJ, Lee SJ, et al: Comparative evaluation of cerebral blood volume and cerebral blood flow in acute ischemic stroke by using perfusion-weighted MR imaging and SPECT. Acta Radiol 43:365–370, 2002.

120. Barber PA, Consolo HK, Yang Q, et al: Comparison of MRI perfusion imaging and single photon emission computed tomography in chronic stroke. Cerebrovasc Dis 11:128–136, 2001.

121. Jorgensen HS, Sperling B, Nakayama H, et al: Spontaneous reperfusion of cerebral infarcts in patients with acute stroke: Incidence, time course, and clinical outcome in the Copenhagen Stroke Study. Arch Neurol 51:865–873, 1994.

122. Herderscheê D, Limburg M, van Royen EA, et al: Thrombolysis with recombinant tissue plasminogen activator in acute ischemic stroke: Evaluation with rCBF-SPECT. Acta Neurol Scand 83:317–322, 1991.

123. Overgaard K, Sperling B, Boysen G, et al: Thrombolytic therapy in acute ischemic stroke: A Danish pilot study. Stroke 24:1439–1446, 1993.

124. Gelmers HJ: Effect of nimodipine (Bay e 9736) on postischaemic cerebrovascular reactivity, as revealed by measuring regional cerebral blood flow (rCBF). Acta Neurochir (Wien) 63:283–290, 1982.

125. Pozzilli C, Di Piero V, Pantano P, et al: Influence of nimodipine on cerebral blood flow in human cerebral ischemia. J Neurol 236:199–202, 1989.

126. Grotta JC, Alexandrov AV: tPA-associated reperfusion after acute stroke demonstrated by SPECT. Stroke 29:429–432, 1998.

127. Yasaka M, O'Keefe GJ, Chambers BR, et al: Streptokinase in acute stroke: Effect on reperfusion and recanalization. Australian Streptokinase Trial Study Group. Neurology 50:626–632, 1998.

128. Hacke W, Kaste M, Fieschi C, et al: Intravenous thrombolysis with recombinant tissue plasminogen activator for acute hemispheric stroke: The European Cooperative Acute Stroke Study (ECASS). ECASS Study Group. JAMA 274:1017–1025, 1995.

129. Tissue plasminogen activator for acute ischemic stroke. The National Institute of Neurological Disorders and Stroke rt-PA Stroke Study Group. N Engl J Med 333:1581–1587, 1995.

Diagnostic Studies

130. Donnan GA, Davis SM, Chambers BR, et al: Streptokinase for acute ischemic stroke with relationship to time of administration: Australian Streptokinase (ASK) Trial Study Group. JAMA 276:961–966, 1996.

131. Ishizu K, Yonekura Y, Magata Y, et al: Extraction and retention of technetium-99m-ECD in human brain: Dynamic SPECT and oxygen-15-water PET studies. J Nucl Med 37:1600–1604, 1996.

132. Hacke W, Kaste M, Fieschi C, et al: Randomised double-blind placebo-controlled trial of thrombolytic therapy with intravenous alteplase in acute ischemic stroke (ECASS II): Second European-Australasian Acute Stroke Study Investigators. Lancet 352:1245–1251, 1998.

133. Berrouschot J, Barthel H, Hesse S, et al: Reperfusion and metabolic recovery of brain tissue and clinical outcome after ischemic stroke and thrombolytic therapy. Stroke 31:1545–1551, 2000.

134. Iseda T, Nakano S, Yano T, et al: Time-threshold curve determined by single photon emission CT in patients with acute middle cerebral artery occlusion. AJNR Am J Neuroradiol 23:572–576, 2002.

135. Horn J, de Haan RJ, Vermeulen M, et al: Very Early Nimodipine Use in Stroke (VENUS): A randomized, double-blind, placebo-controlled trial. Stroke 32:461–465, 2001..

136. Lisk DR, Grotta JC, Lamki LM, et al: Should hypertension be treated after acute stroke? A randomized controlled trial using single photon emission computed tomography. Arch Neurol 50:855–862, 1993.

137. Waldemar G, Vorstrup S, Andersen AR, et al: Angiotensin-converting enzyme inhibition and regional cerebral blood flow in acute stroke. J Cardiovasc Pharmacol 14:722–729, 1989.

138. Toso V: Single photon emission tomography findings in lacunar lesions. Eur Neurol 29 Suppl 2:36–38, 1989.

139. Hartmann A: Prolonged disturbances of regional cerebral blood flow in transient ischemic attacks. Stroke 16:932–939, 1985.

140. Bogousslavsky J, Delaloye-Bischof A, Regli F, et al: Prolonged hypoperfusion and early stroke after transient ischemic attack. Stroke 21:40–46, 1990.

141. Laloux P, Jamart J, Meurisse H, et al: Persisting perfusion defect in transient ischemic attacks: A new clinically useful subgroup? Stroke 27:425–430, 1996.

142. Berrouschot J, Barthel H, Hesse S, et al: Differentiation between transient ischemic attack and ischemic stroke within the first six hours after onset of symptoms by using 99mTc-ECD-SPECT. J Cereb Blood Flow Metab 18:921–929, 1998.

143. Sullivan T, Villanueva-Meyer J, Liu CK, et al: Watershed infarcts, Tc-99m HMPAO SPECT and CT correlation: Case reports. Clin Nucl Med 16:170–173, 1991.

144. Baird AE, Donnan GA, Saling M: Mechanisms and clinical features of internal watershed infarction. Clin Exp Neurol 28:50–55, 1991.

145. Bohdiewicz P, Juni JE: Watershed ischemia demonstrated with acetazolamide enhanced Tc-99m HMPAO SPECT. Clin Nucl Med 19:452–454, 1994.

146. Alexandrov AV, Grotta JC, Davis SM, et al: Brain SPECT and thrombolysis in acute ischemic stroke: Time for a clinical trial. J Nucl Med 37:1259–1262, 1996.

147. Alexandrov AV, Masdeu JC, Devous MD Sr, et al: Brain single-photon emission CT with HMPAO and safety of thrombolytic therapy in acute ischemic stroke. Proceedings of the meeting of the SPECT Safe Thrombolysis Study Collaborators and the members of the Brain Imaging Council of the Society of Nuclear Medicine. Stroke 28:1830–1834, 1997.

148. Leinsinger G, Piepgras A, Einhaupl K, et al: Normal values of cerebrovascular reserve capacity after stimulation with acetazolamide measured by xenon 133 single-photon emission CT. AJNR Am J Neuroradiol 15:1327–1332, 1994.

149. Burt RW, Witt RM, Cikrit DF, et al: Carotid artery disease: Evaluation with acetazolamide-enhanced Tc-99m HMPAO SPECT. Radiology 182:461–466, 1992.

150. Chollet F, Celsis P, Clanet M, et al: SPECT study of cerebral blood flow reactivity after acetazolamide in patients with transient ischemic attacks. Stroke 20:458–464, 1989.

151. Matsuda H, Higashi S, Kinuya K, et al: SPECT evaluation of brain perfusion reserve by the acetazolamide test using Tc-99m HMPAO. Clin Nucl Med 16:572–579, 1991.

152. Knop J, Thie A, Fuchs C, et al: 99mTc-HMPAO-SPECT with acetazolamide challenge to detect hemodynamic compromise in occlusive cerebrovascular disease. Stroke 23:1733–1742, 1992.

153. Ozgur HT, Kent Walsh T, Masaryk A, et al: Correlation of cerebrovascular reserve as measured by acetazolamide-challenged SPECT with angiographic flow patterns and intra- or extracranial arterial stenosis. AJNR Am J Neuroradiol 22:928–936, 2001.

154. Asenbaum S, Reinprecht A, Brucke T, et al: A study of acetazolamide-induced changes in cerebral blood flow using 99mTc HMPAO SPECT in patients with cerebrovascular disease. Neuroradiology 37:13–19, 1995.

155. Cikrit DF, Burt RW, Dalsing MC, et al: Acetazolamide enhanced single photon emission computed tomography (SPECT) evaluation of cerebral perfusion before and after carotid endarterectomy. J Vasc Surg 15:747–753, 1992.

156. Lord RS, Yeates M, Fernandes V, et al: Cerebral perfusion defects, dysautoregulation and carotid stenosis. J Cardiovasc Surg (Torino) 29:670–675, 1988.

157. Ramsay SC, Yeates MG, Lord RS, et al: Use of technetium-HMPAO to demonstrate changes in cerebral blood flow reserve following carotid endarterectomy. J Nucl Med 32:1382–1386, 1991.

158. Russell D, Dybevold S, Kjartansson O, et al: Cerebral vasoreactivity and blood flow before and 3 months after carotid endarterectomy. Stroke 21:1029–1032, 1990.

159. Vorstrup S, Engell HC, Lindewald H, et al: Hemodynamically significant stenosis of the internal carotid artery treated with endarterectomy: Case report. J Neurosurg 60:1070–1075, 1984.

160. Imaizumi M, Kitagawa K, Hashikawa K, et al: Detection of misery perfusion with split-dose 123I-iodoamphetamine single-photon emission computed tomography in patients with carotid occlusive diseases. Stroke 33:2217–2223, 2002.

161. Beneficial effect of carotid endarterectomy in symptomatic patients with high-grade carotid stenosis. North American Symptomatic Carotid Endarterectomy Trial Collaborators. N Engl J Med 325:445–453, 1991.

162. Barnett HJ, Taylor DW, Eliasziw M, et al: Benefit of carotid endarterectomy in patients with symptomatic moderate or severe stenosis. N Engl J Med 339:1415–1425, 1998.

163. MRC European Carotid Surgery Trial: Interim results for symptomatic patients with severe (70–99%) or with mild (0–29%) carotid stenosis. European Carotid Surgery Trialists' Collaborative Group. Lancet 337:1235–1243, 1991.

164. Randomised trial of endarterectomy for recently symptomatic carotid stenosis: Final results of the MRC European Carotid Surgery Trial (ECST). Lancet 351:1379–1387, 1998.

165. Yonas H, Smith HA, Durham SR, et al: Increased stroke risk predicted by compromised cerebral blood flow reactivity. J Neurosurg 79:483–489, 1993.

166. Kuroda S, Houkin K, Kamiyama H, et al: Long-term prognosis of medically treated patients with internal carotid or middle cerebral artery occlusion: Can acetazolamide test predict it? Stroke 32:2110–2116, 2001.

167. Ogasawara K, Ogawa A, Terasaki K, et al: Use of cerebrovascular reactivity in patients with symptomatic major cerebral artery occlusion to predict 5-year outcome: Comparison of xenon-133 and iodine-123-IMP single-photon emission computed tomography. J Cereb Blood Flow Metab 22:1142–1148, 2002.

168. Ogasawara K, Ogawa A, Yoshimoto T: Cerebrovascular reactivity to acetazolamide and outcome in patients with symptomatic internal carotid or middle cerebral artery occlusion: A xenon-133 single-photon emission computed tomography study. Stroke 33:1857–1862, 2002.

169. Delecluse F, Voordecker P, Raftopoulos C: Vertebrobasilar insufficiency revealed by xenon-133 inhalation SPECT. Stroke 20:952–956, 1989.

170. Moriwaki H, Matsumoto M, Hashikawa K, et al: Hemodynamic aspect of cerebral watershed infarction: Assessment of perfusion reserve using iodine-123-iodoamphetamine SPECT. J Nucl Med 38:1556–1562, 1997.

171. von Monakow C: Diaschisis [1914 article translated by G. Harris]. *In* Pribram KH (ed): Brain and Behaviour I: Mood States and Mind. Baltimore, Penguin Books, 1969, pp 27–36.

172. Kempinsky WH: Experimental study of distant effects of acute focal brain injury: A study of diaschisis. Arch Neurol Psychiatry 79:376–389, 1958.

173. Feeney DM, Baron JC: Diaschisis. Stroke 17:817–830, 1986.

174. Dorland's Illustrated Medical Dictionary, 26th ed. Philadelphia, WB Saunders, 1981.

Diagnostic Studies

175. Hoedt-Rasmussen K, Skinhoj E: Transneural depression of the cerebral hemispheric metabolism in man. Acta Neurol Scand 40:41–46, 1964.

176. Meyer JS, Shinohara Y, Kanda T, et al: Diaschisis resulting from acute unilateral cerebral infarction: Quantitative evidence for man. Arch Neurol 23:241–247, 1970.

177. Lavy S, Melamed E, Portnoy Z: The effect of cerebral infarction on the regional cerebral blood flow of the contralateral hemisphere. Stroke 6:160–163, 1975.

178. Slater R, Reivich M, Goldberg H, et al: Diaschisis with cerebral infarction. Stroke 8:684–690, 1977.

179. Heiss WD, Pawlik G, Wagner R, et al: Functional hypometabolism of noninfarcted brain regions in ischemic stroke. J Cereb Blood Flow Metab 3(Suppl 1):S582–S583, 1983.

180. Celesia GG, Polcyn RE, Holden JE, et al: Determination of regional cerebral blood flow in patients with cerebral infarction: Use of fluoromethane labeled with fluorine 18 and positron emission tomography. Arch Neurol 41:262–267, 1984.

181. Wise R, Gibbs J, Frackowiak R, et al: No evidence for transhemispheric diaschisis after human cerebral infarction. Stroke 17:853–861, 1986.

182. Lagreze HL, Levine RL, Pedula KL, et al: Contralateral flow reduction in unilateral stroke: Evidence for transhemispheric diaschisis. Stroke 18:882–886, 1987.

183. Johansson T, Soderborg B, Virgin J: Cerebral infarctions studied by [^{123}I]iodoamphetamine: Clinical aspects of the findings on single photon emission computed tomography and transmission computed tomography. Eur Neurol 28:18–23, 1988.

184. Dobkin JA, Levine RL, Lagreze HL, et al: Evidence for transhemispheric diaschisis in unilateral stroke. Arch Neurol 46:1333–1336, 1989.

185. Andrews RJ: Transhemispheric diaschisis: A review and comment. Stroke 22:943–949, 1991.

186. Baron JC, D'Antona R, Pantano P, et al: Effects of thalamic stroke on energy metabolism of the cerebral cortex: A positron tomography study in man. Brain 109:1243–1259, 1986.

187. Baron JC, Levasseur M, Mazoyer B, et al: Thalamocortical diaschisis: Positron emission tomography in humans. J Neurol Neurosurg Psychiatry 55:935–942, 1992.

188. Bogousslavsky J, Miklossy J, Regli F, et al: Subcortical neglect: Neuropsychological, SPECT, and neuropathological correlations with anterior choroidal artery territory infarction. Ann Neurol 23:448–452, 1988.

189. Bosley TM, Rosenquist AC, Kushner M, et al: Ischemic lesions of the occipital cortex and optic radiations: Positron emission tomography. Neurology 35:470–484, 1985.

190. Bowler JV, Costa DC, Jones BE, et al: High resolution SPECT, small deep infarcts and diaschisis. J R Soc Med 85:142–146, 1992.

191. Kuhl DE, Phelps ME, Kowell AP, et al: Effects of stroke on local cerebral metabolism and perfusion: Mapping by emission computed tomography of ^{18}FDG and ^{13}NH$_3$. Ann Neurol 8:47–60, 1980.

192. Pappata S, Mazoyer B, Tran Dinh S, et al: Effects of capsular or thalamic stroke on metabolism in the cortex and cerebellum: A positron tomography study. Stroke 21:519–524, 1990.

193. Perani D, Vallar G, Cappa S, et al: Aphasia and neglect after subcortical stroke: A clinical/cerebral perfusion correlation study. Brain 110:1211–1229, 1987.

194. Pappata S, Tran Dinh S, Baron JC, et al: Remote metabolic effects of cerebrovascular lesions: Magnetic resonance and positron tomography imaging. Neuroradiology 29:1–6, 1987.

195. Demeurisse G, Capon A, Verhas M, et al: Pathogenesis of aphasia in deep-seated lesions: Likely role of cortical diaschisis. Eur Neurol 30:67–74, 1990.

196. Lindegaard MW, Skretting A, Hager B, et al: Cerebral and cerebellar uptake of ^{99m}Tc-(d,1)-hexamethyl-propyleneamine oxime (HMPAO) in patients with brain tumor studied by single photon emission computerized tomography. Eur J Nucl Med 12:417–420, 1986.

197. Takano T, Nagatsuka K, Ohnishi Y, et al: Vascular response to carbon dioxide in areas with and without diaschisis in patients with small, deep hemispheric infarction. Stroke 19:840–845, 1988.

198. Chu WJ, Mason GF, Pan JW, et al: Regional cerebral blood flow and magnetic resonance spectroscopic imaging findings in diaschisis from stroke. Stroke 33:1243–1248, 2002.

199. Bowler JV, Wade JP, Jones BE, et al: Contribution of diaschisis to the clinical deficit in human cerebral infarction. Stroke 26:1000–1006, 1995.

200. Olsen TS, Larsen B, Herning M, et al: Blood flow and vascular reactivity in collaterally perfused brain tissue: Evidence of an ischemic penumbra in patients with acute stroke. Stroke 14:332–341, 1983.

201. Baron JC, Bousser MG, Comar D, et al: "Crossed cerebellar diaschisis" in human supratentorial brain infarction. Ann Neurol 8:128, 1980.

202. Baron JC, Bousser MG, Comar D, et al: "Crossed cerebellar diaschisis": A remote functional depression secondary to supratentorial infarction of man. J Cereb Blood Flow Metab 1(Suppl 1):S500–S501, 1981.

203. Baron JC, Bousser MG, Comar D, et al: "Crossed cerebellar diaschisis" in human supratentorial brain infarction: Trans Am Neurol Assoc 105:459–461, 1980.

204. Martin WR, Raichle ME: Cerebellar blood flow and metabolism in cerebral hemisphere infarction. Ann Neurol 14:168–176, 1983.

205. Serrati C, Marchal G, Rioux P, et al: Contralateral cerebellar hypometabolism: A predictor for stroke outcome? J Neurol Neurosurg Psychiatry 57:174–179, 1994.

206. Tanaka M, Kondo S, Hirai S, et al: Crossed cerebellar diaschisis accompanied by hemiataxia: A PET study. J Neurol Neurosurg Psychiatry 55:121–125, 1992.

207. Pantano P, Baron JC, Samson Y, et al: Crossed cerebellar diaschisis: Further studies. Brain 109:677–694, 1986.

208. Di Piero V, Chollet F, Dolan RJ, et al: The functional nature of cerebellar diaschisis. Stroke 21:1365–1369, 1990.

209. Fukuyama H, Kameyama M, Harada K, et al: Thalamic tumours invading the brain stem produce crossed cerebellar diaschisis demonstrated by PET. J Neurol Neurosurg Psychiatry 49:524–528, 1986.

210. Yamauchi H, Fukuyama H, Kimura J: Hemodynamic and metabolic changes in crossed cerebellar hypoperfusion. Stroke 23:855–860, 1992.

211. Kushner M, Alavi A, Reivich M, et al: Contralateral cerebellar hypometabolism following cerebral insult: A positron emission tomographic study. Ann Neurol 15:425–434, 1984.

212. Fulham MJ, Brooks RA, Hallett M, et al: Cerebellar diaschisis revisited: Pontine hypometabolism and dentate sparing. Neurology 42:2267–2273, 1992.

213. Patronas NJ, Di Chiro G, Smith BH, et al: Depressed cerebellar glucose metabolism in supratentorial tumors. Brain Research 291:93–101, 1984.

214. Rozental JM, Levine RL, Nickles RJ, et al: Cerebral diaschisis in patients with malignant glioma. J Neuro-Oncol 8:153–161, 1990.

215. Tien RD, Ashdown BC: Crossed cerebellar diaschisis and crossed cerebellar atrophy: Correlation of MR findings, clinical symptoms, and supratentorial diseases in 26 patients. AJR Am J Roentgenol 158:1155–1159, 1992.

216. Meneghetti G, Vorstrup S, Mickey B, et al: Crossed cerebellar diaschisis in ischemic stroke: A study of regional cerebral blood flow by ^{133}Xe inhalation and single photon emission computerized tomography. J Cereb Blood Flow Metab 4:235–240, 1984.

217. Bogsrud TV, Rootwelt K, Russell D, et al: Acetazolamide effect on cerebellar blood flow in crossed cerebral-cerebellar diaschisis. Stroke 21:52–55, 1990.

218. Kanaya H, Endo H, Sugiyama T, et al: "Crossed cerebellar diaschisis" in patients with putaminal hemorrhage. J Cereb Blood Flow Metab 3(Suppl 1):S27–S28, 1983.

219. Fazekas F, Payer F, Valetitsch H, et al: Brain stem infarction and diaschisis: A SPECT cerebral perfusion study. Stroke 24:1162–1166, 1993.

220. Sakashita Y, Matsuda H, Kakuda K, et al: Hypoperfusion and vasoreactivity in the thalamus and cerebellum after stroke. Stroke 24:84–87, 1993.

221. Flores LG II, Futami S, Hoshi H, et al: Crossed cerebellar diaschisis: Analysis of iodine-123-IMP SPECT imaging. J Nucl Med 36:399–402, 1995.

222. Perani D, Lucignani G, Pantano P, et al: Cerebellar diaschisis in pontine ischemia: A case report with single-photon emission computerized tomography. J Cereb Blood Flow Metab 7:127–131, 1987.

223. Shih WJ, Dekosky ST, Coupal JJ, et al: I-123 hydroxyiodobenzyl propanediamine (HIPDM) cerebral blood flow imaging demonstrating transtentorial diaschisis. Clin Nucl Med 15:623–629, 1990.

224. Perani D, Gerundini P, Lenzi GL: Cerebral hemispheric and contralateral cerebellar hypoperfusion during a transient ischemic attack. J Cereb Blood Flow Metab 7:507–509, 1987.

Diagnostic Studies

225. Matsuda H, Tsuji S, Sumiya H, et al: Acetazolamide effect on vascular response in areas with diaschisis as measured by Tc-99m HMPAO brain SPECT. Clin Nucl Med 17:581–586, 1992.

226. Pantano P, Formisano R, Ricci M, et al: Prolonged muscular flaccidity in stroke patients is associated with crossed cerebellar diaschisis. Cerebrovasc Dis 3:80–85, 1993.

227. Tanaka K, Yonekawa Y, Kaku Y, et al: Arteriovenous malformation and diaschisis. Acta Neurochir (Wien) 120:26–32, 1993.

228. Kiyosawa M, Bosley TM, Alavi A, et al: Positron emission tomography in a patient with progressive multifocal leukoencephalopathy. Neurology 38:1864–1867, 1988.

229. Yamauchi H, Fukuyama H, Yamaguchi S, et al: Crossed cerebellar hypoperfusion in unilateral major cerebral artery occlusive disorders. J Nucl Med 33:1637–1641, 1992.

230. Miura H, Nagata K, Hirata Y, et al: Evolution of crossed cerebellar diaschisis in middle cerebral artery infarction. J Neuroimaging 4:91–96, 1994.

231. Brodal P: The corticopontine projection in the rhesus monkey: origin and principles of organization. Brain 101:251–283, 1978.

232. Brodal A: Neurological Anatomy in Relation to Clinical Medicine. New York, Oxford University Press, 1981.

233. Brunberg JA, Frey KA, Horton JA, et al: Crossed cerebellar diaschisis: Occurrence and resolution demonstrated with PET during carotid temporary balloon occlusion. AJNR Am J Neuroradiol 13:58–61, 1992.

234. Eckard DA, Purdy PD, Bonte F: Crossed cerebellar diaschisis and loss of consciousness during temporary balloon occlusion of the internal carotid artery. AJNR Am J Neuroradiol 13:55–57, 1992.

235. Nathan MA, Bushnell DL, Kahn D, et al: Crossed cerebellar diaschisis associated with balloon test occlusion of the carotid artery. Nucl Med Commun 15:448–454, 1994.

236. Biersack HJ, Linke D, Brassel F, et al: Technetium-99m HM-PAO brain SPECT in epileptic patients before and during unilateral hemispheric anesthesia (Wada test): Report of three cases. J Nucl Med 28:1763–1767, 1987.

237. Ryding E, Sjoholm H, Skeidsvoll H, et al: Delayed decrease in hemispheric cerebral blood flow during Wada test demonstrated by 99mTc-HMPAO single photon emission computed tomography. Acta Neurol Scand 80:248–254, 1989.

238. Kurthen M, Reichmann K, Linke DB, et al: Crossed cerebellar diaschisis in intracarotid sodium Amytal procedures: A SPECT study. Acta Neurol Scand 81:416–422, 1990.

239. Barker WW, Yoshii F, Loewenstein DA, et al: Cerebrocerebellar relationship during behavioral activation: A PET study. J Cereb Blood Flow Metab 11:48–54, 1991.

240. Botez MI, Leveille J, Lambert R, et al: Single photon emission computed tomography (SPECT) in cerebellar disease: Cerebellocerebral diaschisis. Eur Neurol 31:405–412, 1991.

241. Boni S, Valle G, Cioffi RP, et al: Crossed cerebello-cerebral diaschisis: A SPECT study. Nucl Med Commun 13:824–831, 1992.

242. Rousseaux M, Steinling M: Crossed hemispheric diaschisis in unilateral cerebellar lesions. Stroke 23:511–514, 1992.

243. Sonmezoglu K, Sperling B, Henriksen T, et al: Reduced contralateral hemispheric flow measured by SPECT in cerebellar lesions: Crossed cerebral diaschisis. Acta Neurol Scand 87:275–280, 1993.

244. Gomez BM, Garcia-Monco JC, Quintana JM, et al: Diaschisis and neuropsychological performance after cerebellar stroke. Eur Neurol 37:82–89, 1997.

245. Takasawa M, Watanabe M, Yamamoto S, et al: Prognostic value of subacute crossed cerebellar diaschisis: Single-photon emission CT study in patients with middle cerebral artery territory infarct. AJNR Am J Neuroradiol 23:189–193, 2002.

246. Lin WY, Kao CH, Wang PY, et al: Serial changes in regional blood flow in the cerebrum and cerebellum of stroke patients imaged by $^{99}Tc^m$-HMPAO SPET. Nucl Med Commun 17:208–211, 1996.

247. Yamauchi H, Fukuyama H, Kimura J, et al: Crossed cerebellar hypoperfusion indicates the degree of uncoupling between blood flow and metabolism in major cerebral arterial occlusion. Stroke 25:1945–1951, 1994.

248. Davis S, Andrews J, Lichtenstein M, et al: A single-photon emission computed tomography study of hypoperfusion after subarachnoid hemorrhage. Stroke 21:252–259, 1990.

249. Hasan D, van Peski J, Loeve I, et al: Single photon emission computed tomography in patients with acute hydrocephalus or with cerebral ischemia after subarachnoid hemorrhage. J Neurol Neurosurg Psychiatry 54:490–493, 1991.

250. Naderi S, Ozguven MA, Bayhan H, et al: Evaluation of cerebral vasospasm in patients with subarachnoid hemorrhage using single photon emission computed tomography. Neurosurg Rev 17:261–265, 1994.

251. Kimura T, Shinoda J, Funakoshi T: Prediction of cerebral infarction due to vasospasm following aneurysmal subarachnoid hemorrhage using acetazolamide-activated 123I-IMP SPECT. Acta Neurochir (Wien) 123:125–128, 1993.

252. Rawluk D, Smith FW, Deans HE, et al: Technetium 99m HMPAO scanning in patients with subarachnoid hemorrhage: A preliminary study. Br J Radiol 61:26–29, 1988.

253. Rosen JM, Butala AV, Oropello JM, et al: Postoperative changes on brain SPECT imaging after aneurysmal subarachnoid hemorrhage: A potential pitfall in the evaluation of vasospasm. Clin Nucl Med 19:595–597, 1994.

254. Aaslid R, Huber P, Nornes H: Evaluation of cerebrovascular spasm with transcranial Doppler ultrasound. J Neurosurg 60:37–41, 1984.

255. Davis SM, Andrews JT, Lichtenstein M, et al: Correlations between cerebral arterial velocities, blood flow, and delayed ischemia after subarachnoid hemorrhage. Stroke 23:492–497, 1992.

256. Grosset DG, Straiton J, du Trevou M, et al: Prediction of symptomatic vasospasm after subarachnoid hemorrhage by rapidly increasing transcranial Doppler velocity and cerebral blood flow changes. Stroke 23:674–679, 1992.

257. Lewis DH, Eskridge JM, Newell DW, et al: Brain SPECT and the effect of cerebral angioplasty in delayed ischemia due to vasospasm. J Nucl Med 33:1789–1796, 1992.

258. Batjer HH, Devous MD Sr: The use of acetazolamide-enhanced regional cerebral blood flow measurement to predict risk to arteriovenous malformation patients. Neurosurgery 31:213–217, 1992.

259. Gomez-Tortosa E, Sychra JJ, Martin EM, et al: Postoperative cognitive and single photon emission computed tomography assessment of patients with resection of perioperative high-risk arteriovenous malformations. Neurosurgery 36:447–457, 1995.

260. Awad IA, Magdinec M, Schubert A: Intracranial hypertension after resection of cerebral arteriovenous malformations: Predisposing factors and management strategy. Stroke 25:611–620, 1994.

261. Kilpatrick CJ, Davis SM, Tress BM, et al: Epileptic seizures in acute stroke. Arch Neurol 47:157–160, 1990.

262. Kilpatrick CJ, Davis SM, Hopper JL, et al: Early seizures after acute stroke: Risk of late seizures. Arch Neurol 49:509–511, 1992.

263. Burn J, Dennis M, Bamford J, et al: Epileptic seizures after a first stroke: The Oxfordshire community stroke project. Br Med J 315:1582–1587, 1997.

264. Duncan R, Patterson J, Hadley DM, et al: CT, MR and SPECT imaging in temporal lobe epilepsy. J Neurol Neurosurg Psychiatry 53:11–15, 1990.

265. Jibiki I, Kubota T, Fujimoto K, et al: Regional relationships between focal hypofixation images in 123I-IMP single photon emission computed tomography and epileptic EEG foci in interictal periods in patients with partial epilepsy. Eur Neurol 31:360–365, 1991.

266. Pantano P, Matteucci C, di Piero V, et al: Quantitative assessment of cerebral blood flow in partial epilepsy using Xe-133 inhalation and SPECT. Clin Nucl Med 16:898–903, 1991.

267. Rowe CC, Berkovic SF, Austin M, et al: Postictal SPET in epilepsy. Lancet 1:389–390, 1989.

268. Newton MR, Berkovic SF, Austin MC, et al: Dystonia, clinical lateralization, and regional blood flow changes in temporal lobe seizures. Neurology 42:371–377, 1992.

269. Rowe CC, Berkovic SF, Austin MC, et al: Patterns of postictal cerebral blood flow in temporal lobe epilepsy: Qualitative and quantitative analysis. Neurology 41:1096–1103, 1991.

270. Kraemer DL, Awad IA: Vascular malformations and epilepsy: Clinical considerations and basic mechanisms. Epilepsia 35(Suppl 6):S30–43, 1994

271. Jagust WJ, Budinger TF, Reed BR: The diagnosis of dementia with single photon emission computed tomography. Arch Neurol 44:258–262, 1987.

272. Jobst KA, Smith AD, Barker CS, et al: Association of atrophy of the medial temporal lobe with reduced blood flow in the posterior parietotemporal cortex in patients with a clinical and pathological diagnosis of Alzheimer's disease. J Neurol Neurosurg Psychiatry 55:190–194, 1992.

273. O'Brien JT, Eagger S, Syed GM, et al: A study of regional cerebral blood flow and cognitive performance in Alzheimer's disease. J Neurol Neurosurg Psychiatry 55:1182–1187, 1992.

274. Buell U, Costa DC, Kirsch G, et al: The investigation of dementia with single photon emission tomography. Nucl Med Commun 11:823–841, 1990.

275. Gemmell HG, Sharp PF, Besson JA, et al: Differential diagnosis in dementia using the cerebral blood flow agent 99mTc HM-PAO: A SPECT study. J Comput Assist Tomogr 11:398–402, 1987.

276. Starkstein SE, Sabe L, Vazquez S, et al: Neuropsychological, psychiatric, and cerebral blood flow findings in vascular dementia and Alzheimer's disease. Stroke 27:408–414, 1996.

277. Bonte FJ, Devous MD Sr, Reisch JS, et al: The effect of acetazolamide on regional cerebral blood flow in patients with Alzheimer's disease or stroke as measured by single-photon emission computed tomography. Invest Radiol 24:99–103, 1989.

Diagnostic Studies

Section IV

Specific Medical Diseases and Stroke

J. P. Mohr

The authors of the individual chapters in this section have focused on those aspects of a given disease as it relates to stroke. Their wider, non-neurological, clinical manifestations have been presented in summary form at most, the reader being referred to standard texts for the specialities represented.

The topics chosen represent the major disease processes which cause stroke as part of the clinical picture. Others also exist, but the list chosen was considered to be the most important. Because the book is organized into sections on laboratory science, diagnostic studies, clinical sciences, and therapy, specific comments on the management of the diseases in this section are deferred where possible to the more general discussion of therapy in the last section of the book.

Although all topics from the prior edition are included again, new topics also appear. The authors of some of the chapters in earlier editions have graciously given way to new authors, whose emphases and writing styles differ.

For some subjects, radical changes in chapter structure have been required and a spill-over into the therapy section has occurred.

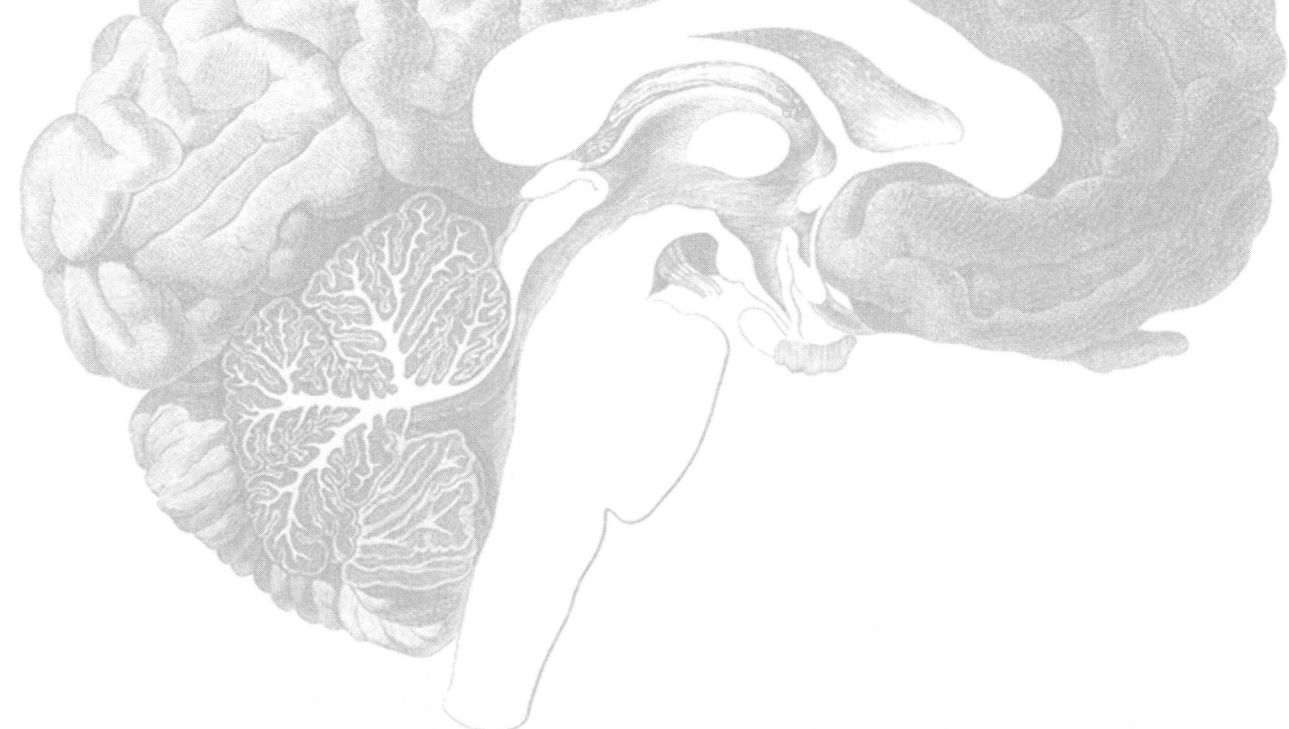

Chapter Twenty-Three

Arterial Dissections

Richard M. Zweifler and Gerald Silverboard

EPIDEMIOLOGY

Cervicocerebral arterial dissections account for approximately 2% of all ischemic strokes, but they are among the most important causes of stroke in young and middle-aged patients.[1-6] Most patients with dissection are between 30 and 50 years of age, with the mean age approximately 40 years.[3,4] In patients younger than 45 years, arterial dissection is the second leading cause of stroke, accounting for 10% to 25% of ischemic strokes.[6-9] Although there is no overall gender predilection in adults, females with arterial dissection are approximately 5 years younger at the time of dissection.[3] Childhood arterial dissections are unique in that they occur more commonly in boys.[10,11]

Population-based studies have reported the incidence of dissection as ranging from 2.6 to 2.9 cases per 100,000 per year.[2,3] The true incidence of cervicocerebral arterial dissection is likely higher than these estimates, however, because asymptomatic patients and patients with pain but no neurologic symptoms are underdiagnosed.[12] The annual incidence of cervical internal carotid artery (ICA) dissection was 3.5 per 100,000 in those older than 20 years in a Mayo Clinic series.[3] Seventy percent of cervical internal carotid dissections occur in patients between 35 and 50 years of age, with a mean age at presentation of 44 years; there is no sex predilection.[13] Patients with intracranial carotid dissection tend to be younger than those with cervical dissections. In a review of 59 reported cases of intracranial carotid dissection, the mean age at onset was 30 years and there was a slight male predominance.[14] The annual incidence of spontaneous vertebral artery dissection is one third that of ICA dissection[5,15-17] with estimates of 1 to 1.5 per 100,000.[18] Extracranial vertebral artery dissection is more common, accounting for up to 15% of the reported cases of cervicocerebral dissection, whereas dissection of the intracranial vertebral artery is uncommon, accounting for approximately 5%.[19] The mean age at onset of intracranial vertebral dissection is the late 40s for isolated dissection and the late 30s for dissection with extension to the basilar artery.[20-23] In contrast to extracranial carotid and vertebral artery dissections, intracranial vertebral artery dissections are more common in men than in women.[20,24]

PATHOLOGY

Arterial dissections usually arise from an intimal tear that allows the development of an intramural hematoma (false lumen) (Figs. 23–1 and 23–2). In some patients, no communication between the true and false lumens can be demonstrated, suggesting that some dissections are the result of a primary intramedial hematoma. Furthermore, intimal disruption could occur as a result of rupture of a primary intramural hematoma into the intima. Although it is likely that the former mechanism is more common, both could occur.

The intramural hematoma is located within the layers of the tunica media but may be eccentric toward the intima (subintimal dissection) or adventitia (subadventitial dissection). Subintimal dissections are more likely to cause luminal stenosis, whereas subadventitial dissections may cause arterial dilatation (aneurysm). The aneurysms are often referred to as "false aneurysms" or "pseudoaneurysms," but they are true aneurysms because their walls contain blood vessel elements (i.e., media and adventitia)[18]; they are better termed "dissecting" aneurysms.[25,26] The absence of an external elastic lamina and a thin adventitia makes intracranial arteries prone to subadventitial dissection and subsequent subarachnoid hemorrhage. Subarachnoid hemorrhage is reported in about one fifth of intracranial ICA dissections and in more than half of intracranial vertebral artery dissections.[10,20,22,23,27-31]

Pathogenesis

The pathogenesis of most spontaneous arterial dissections is unknown. Dissections can be iatrogenic or due to severe trauma, in which cases the causes are obvious, but most occur spontaneously or are associated with antecedent trivial trauma. Precipitating events reported to antedate dissection include sudden head movement, coughing, vomiting, sneezing, chiropractic manipulation, performing yoga, painting a ceiling, vigorous nose blowing, sexual activity, anesthesia administration, resuscitation, and many types of sports activity.[32-48] Such activities may cause arterial injury from mechanical stretching. A prospective study found that 81% of dissections were associated with some form of sudden neck movement.[35] Estimates of dissection

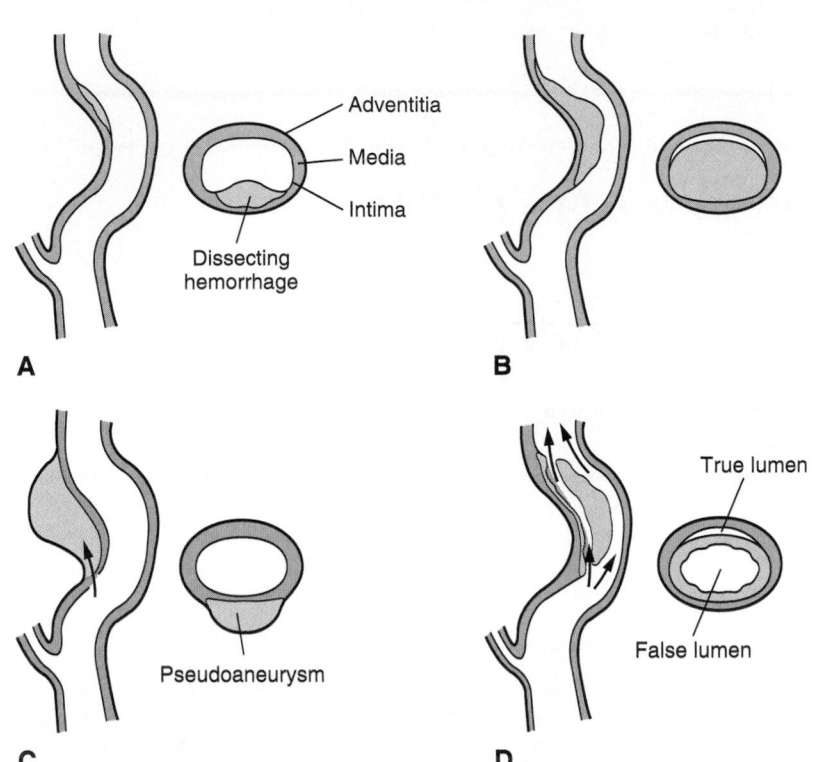

FIGURE 23–1 *Anatomy of dissections. A, Lateral (left) and cross-sectional (right) schematic views of internal carotid artery demonstrate initial phase of intramedial and subintimal dissecting aneurysm; the three basic arterial layers (intima, media, and adventitia) are delineated. B, Comparable views of the progression of intramedial hemorrhage; the arterial lumen is reduced in size. C, Comparable views of an intramedial hemorrhage that dissects into the subadventitial, rather than the subintimal plane, as in A and B; a large pseudoaneurysm results. D, Dissecting hemorrhage ruptures through the intima, establishing communication with the true lumen; recanalization may occur, enlarging the true or false lumen. (From Friedman AH, Day AL, Quisling RGJ, et al: Cervical carotid dissecting aneurysms. Neurosurgery 7:207, 1980.)*

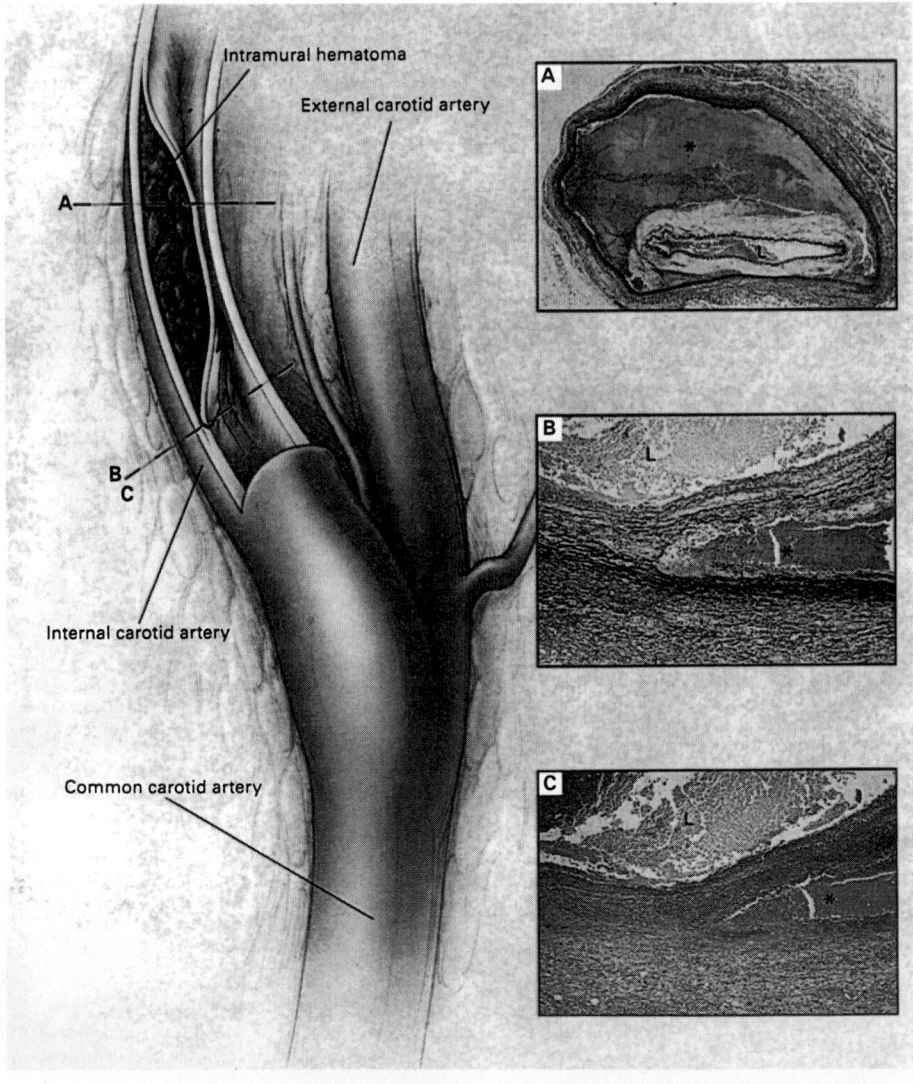

FIGURE 23–2 *Pathologic findings in a 37-year-old woman with a dissection of the internal carotid artery. Photomicrographs of the right extracranial internal carotid artery (A through C) show a dissection within the outer layers of the tunica media, resulting in stenosis of the arterial lumen (L). The blue dashed lines on the left indicate the sites of the photomicrographs. A, The intramural hemorrhage (°) extends almost entirely around the artery (van Gieson stain, ×4). B and C, Higher-power views of the internal carotid artery at the point of dissection show fragmentation of elastic tissue (B; van Gieson stain, ×25), with the accumulation of pale ground-glass substance in the tunica media, indicated by the blue-staining mucopolysaccharides (C; Alcian blue, ×25). These changes are consistent with a diagnosis of cystic medial necrosis. (From Schievink WI: Spontaneous dissection of the carotid and vertebral arteries. N Engl J Med 344:898, 2001.)*

risk after chiropractic manipulation vary widely with the study methodology but range from 1 in 5.85 million manipulations[36] to as many as 1 in 20,000 manipulations.[49] One study found connective tissue disorders in one fourth of patients with cervical artery dissection after chiropractic manipulation.[50]

An underlying arteriopathy has been postulated to lead to structural instability of the arterial wall. Fibromuscular dysplasia is found in approximately 15% to 20% of all patients with cervicocephalic dissection and is seen in more than half of those with bilateral carotid involvement.[3,19,51-56] One percent to 5% of patients have an identifiable heritable connective tissue disorder,[57] such as Ehlers-Danlos syndrome type IV[58,59] Marfan's syndrome,[53,54,60,61] autosomal dominant polycystic kidney disease,[54] osteogenesis imperfecta type I,[54] pseudoxanthoma elasticum,[54,62] type I collagen point mutation,[63] or α_1-antitrypsin deficiency.[64] Dissection has also been associated with other arteriopathies, such as cystic medial necrosis[3,65] and moyamoya disease.[66-68] The association with arterial redundancies (e.g., coils, kinks, and loops),[69,70] increased arterial distensibility,[71] widened aortic root,[72] and intracranial aneurysms[73,74] provides indirect evidence of an underlying arteriopathy.

Five percent of patients with spontaneous cervicocephalic dissection have at least one family member with a spontaneous dissection of the aorta or its main branches, including the vertebral and carotid arteries.[75] Atherosclerosis does not appear to be a risk factor.[26] Other reported risk factors for dissection are migraine,[76,77] recent infection,[78-80] pregnancy,[81,82] hyperhomocyst(e)inemia,[83,84] smoking,[26,85] hypertension,[26,86] and oral contraceptive use.[26] The possibility of an infectious etiology is supported by the reported seasonal variation of cervical artery dissection, with a 58% increase in frequency in the autumn.[55] Schievink and colleagues[87,88] have reported familial associations between dissection and multiple cutaneous lentigines and bicuspid aortic valves, suggesting an underlying neural crest defect.

Ultrastructural aberrations of dermal collagen fibrils and elastic fibers have been reported in 54% to 68% of patients with spontaneous cervical artery dissection in whom there is no clinical evidence of a known connective tissue disorder,[89-91] suggesting a molecular defect in the biosynthesis of the extracellular matrix.[92] A study of skin biopsy specimens from healthy relatives of patients with dissection indicates a familial occurrence of connective tissue abnormalities.[93] No genetic mutation responsible for the majority of patients with cervical artery dissection has been identified.[90] Screening for mutations in the genes for type V procollagen (*COL5A1*),[94] type III collagen (*COL3A1*),[95,96] and tropoelastin (*ELN*)[97] has been negative.

Despite an association with many disorders (Table 23.1), the precise cause of cervicocephalic dissection remains unknown in most cases. The pathogenesis is likely multifactorial with mechanical factors and underlying arteriopathy, possibly genetic or infectious, playing roles.

Sites of Dissection

Dissection of the extracranial carotid and vertebral arteries accounts for approximately 80% to 90% of all cervico-

Table 23.1 Predisposing Factors for Cervicocephalic Dissection

Trauma
  Mild or trivial
  Major
  Iatrogenic
Arteriopathies
  Fibromuscular dysplasia
  Cystic medial necrosis
  Ehlers-Danlos syndrome type IV
  Marfan syndrome
  Type I collagen point mutation
  α-Antitrypsin deficiency
  Osteogenesis imperfecta type I
  Pseudoxanthoma elasticum
  Autosomal dominant polycystic kidney disease
  Moyamoya disease
  Redundancies (e.g., coils, kinks, and loops)
  Intracranial aneurysms
Migraine
Family history
Recent infection
Hyperhomocyst(e)inemia
Less well-established factors:
  Hypertension
  Pregnancy
  Smoking
  Oral contraceptives

cephalic dissections.[98,99] This disparity may be explained by the greater mobility of the extracranial segments and the potential for injury by contact with bony structures such as the transverse processes of the upper cervical vertebrae and the styloid process (Fig. 23–3).[13] Extracranial ICA dissection typically occurs at least 2 cm distal to the bifurcation, near the C2-C3 vertebral level, and extends superiorly for a variable distance. It usually terminates before the artery enters the petrous bone, where mechanical support appears to limit further dissection in the majority of cases.[13] This location is distinct from that of atherosclerosis, which most commonly affects the ICA origin or the siphon. The vertebral artery is most mobile, and most susceptible to mechanical injury, at the C1-C2 level, as it leaves the transverse foramen of the axis and abruptly turns to enter the intracranial cavity (the V3 segment) (Fig. 23–4). The C1-C2 site is involved in one half to two thirds of all vertebral artery dissections and in 80% to 90% of rotation-related dissections.[16,100-102]

Intracranial arterial dissection is more common in children and adolescents than in adults, although intracranial dissection in children usually affects the anterior circulation, and intracranial posterior circulation dissection is more common in adults.[10] The most commonly involved intracranial sites are the supraclinoid segment of the ICA and the middle cerebral artery stem.[103,104] The most common site of intracranial vertebral artery dissection is the V4 segment at or near the origin of the posterior inferior cerebellar artery. At this level, the artery may be compressed during head maneuvers, the media and adventitia diminish in size and elastic components, and the external elastic lamina terminates. Approximately 20% of vertebral

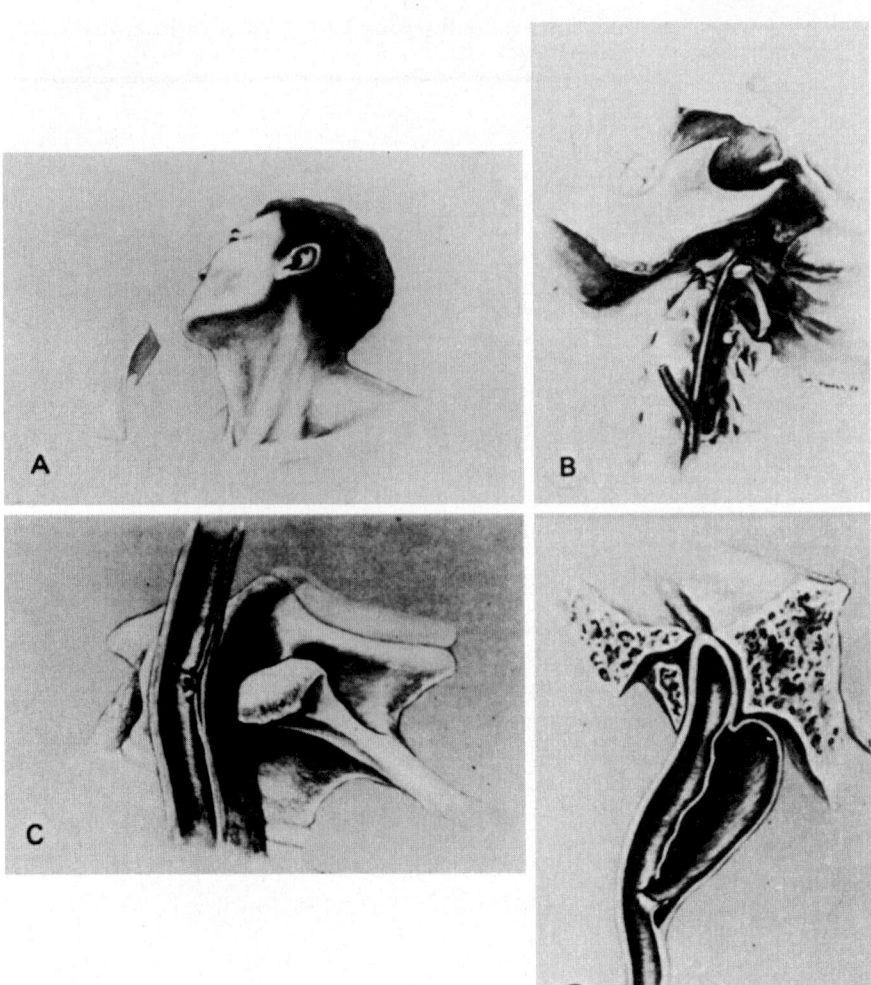

FIGURE 23–3 *Presumed mechanism of carotid injury induced by neck rotation. A, Direction of hyperextension. B, Impingement of artery on the process of the vertebra. C, Intimal tear caused by impingement. D, Progression of intimal tear to dissection. (From Stringer WL, Kelly DLJ: Traumatic dissection of the extracranial internal carotid artery. Neurosurgery 6:123, 1980.)*

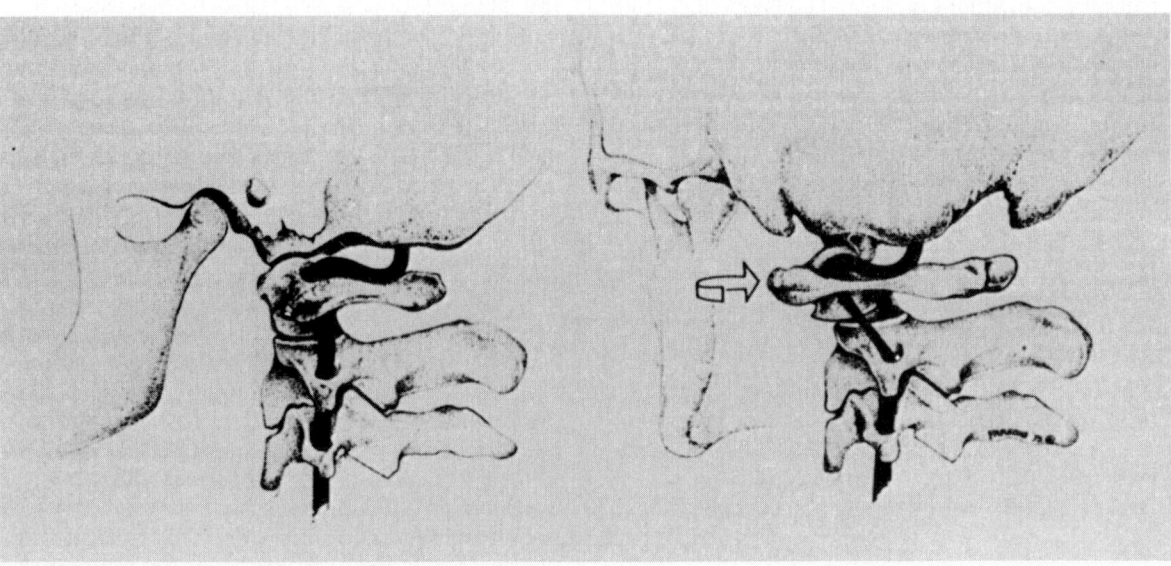

FIGURE 23–4 *Vertebral artery injury with abrupt cervical rotation. The vertebral artery is subject to stretch and mechanical trauma between C1 and C2 when the neck is vigorously rotated and extended. (From Barnett HJM: Progress towards stroke prevention. Neurology [NY] 30:1212, 1980.)*

artery dissections involve both the extracranial and intracranial segments.[105]

Mechanism of Ischemia

Cervicocephalic dissection can cause ischemic symptoms due to hemodynamic compromise secondary to luminal narrowing or occlusion, thromboembolism, or both. Several reports investigating the pattern of infarction in patients with carotid dissection indicate that most strokes are the result of distal embolization.[106–110] A high incidence of middle cerebral artery microemboli correlating with stroke symptoms has been found in patients with carotid artery dissection, further supporting a thromboembolic mechanism.[111]

CLINICAL MANIFESTATIONS

Extracranial Carotid Artery Dissection

Local Signs and Symptoms

The major presenting features of extracranial carotid dissection are pain in the ipsilateral head, face, or neck associated with focal ischemic symptoms (cerebral or retinal). In about one third of cases, partial Horner's syndrome is present. Saver and Easton[19] summarized the clinical, radiologic, and prognostic features of 635 patients reported in the literature (Table 23.2).

Pain (in head, face, or neck) is the most common overall symptom, present in more than 80% of symptomatic cases, and is the initial presenting symptom in one half to two thirds of patients.[10,19,51,77,106,108,110,112–120]

Headache, present in 60% to 75% of patients, may precede other signs or symptoms by hours or weeks.[106,110,113,116,119,121] The pain is typically ipsilateral over the anterior head but may be more diffuse or bilateral, even with unilateral dissection.[77,119,122] Onset of headache is usually gradual, although sudden "thunderclap" headache has been reported.[119,122] The headache is usually nonthrobbing and severe, and ipsilateral scalp tenderness may occur.[77,119,122] Unilateral neck pain is present in 20% to 30% of patients and may involve the anterior neck with radiation toward the ear, scalp, jaw, face, or pharynx.[106,110,119] Facial or orbital pain has been reported in more than 50%.[119]

Ipsilateral partial oculosympathetic paresis (Horner's syndrome), present in approximately one third of patients, results from involvement of sympathetic fibers of the internal carotid plexus.[110,116,119] Ptosis and miosis are seen, but facial sweating remains intact (except for a focal area of the ipsilateral forehead) because the majority of sympathetic fibers supplying the face travel with the external carotid artery.[26]

Cranial nerve palsies have been reported in 12% of patients with spontaneous ICA dissection.[123] Lower cranial nerve palsies are most common and are found in approximately 5% to 10% of patients.[110,119,123] Figure 23–5 displays the anatomic relationship of the lower cranial nerves and the carotid artery. The most commonly affected cranial nerve is CN XII, followed in frequency by nerves IX, X, XI, and V.[119,123–129] The facial, oculomotor, abducens, and trochlear nerves may also be involved.[119,123,130] Dysgeusia is reported in about 10%.[119] Pulsatile tinnitus or a subjective

Table 23.2 Clinical Features of Extracranial Carotid Dissection

No. of cases	635
Patient age	Mean 44.4 yr; range 4–74 yr
Patient sex	
Male	53%
Female	47%
Laterality	
Unilateral	86%
Left	60%
Right	40%
Bilateral	14%
Major presenting complaint°	
Cerebral infarction	46%
Transient ischemic attack	30%
Neck or head pain	21%
Pulsatile tinnitus only	2%
Asymptomatic bruit only	2%
Associated features at diagnosis	
Symptoms	
Neck pain	20%
Headache	64%
Neck or head pain	67%
Tinnitus or subjective bruit	3%
Signs	
Partial Horner's syndrome	32%
Cervical bruit	18%
Linguinal paresis	6%
Early outcome	
Angiographic	
Normal or mildly stenotic vessels on follow-up imaging	70%
Clinical	
Neurologically normal	50%
Mild deficits only	21%
Moderate to severe deficits	25%
Death	4%

°*Major presenting complaint leading to evaluation, not necessarily the initial symptom.*

bruit is reported in up to one fourth of patients, and an objective bruit may be heard in nearly one fifth.[51,62,119]

Ischemic Signs and Symptoms

Ischemic manifestations have been reported in 50% to 95% of patients,[110,113,119] although the highest rates were reported in older studies. At the time of the earlier reports, the diagnosis of dissection was typically suspected only in the presence of ischemic signs, and noninvasive diagnostic techniques were not available.[113] Most ischemic symptoms occur within 1 week of the onset of pain[113,119,121]; one study reported a median delay in the appearance of other symptoms of 4 days.[119] A 1998 case report describes a disabling stroke occurring 5 months after traumatic ICA dissection, although the patient did suffer a silent stroke at the time of the dissection.[131] Most infarctions are territorial (as opposed to borderzone), supporting an embologenic etiology.[106–110] Transient ischemic attacks are common, being reported in about 50% of patients, and they are recurrent in half of the cases.[113] Of patients with stroke, approximately 75% report at least one preceding transient

Specific Medical Diseases and Stroke

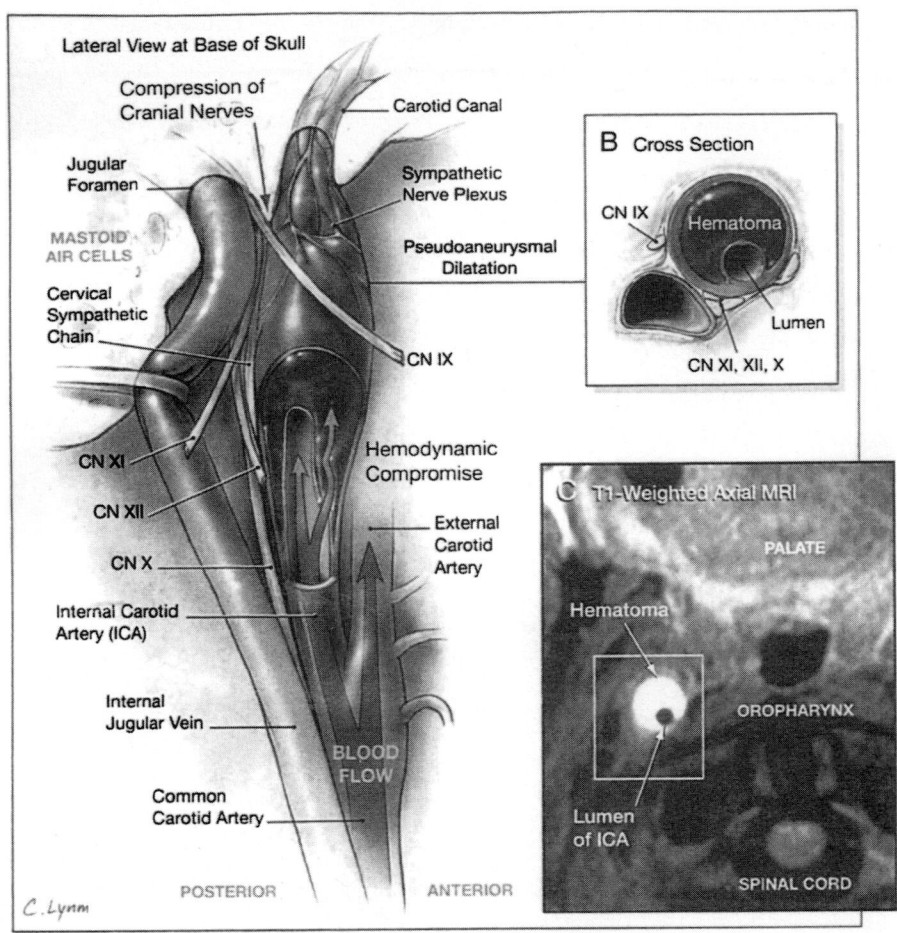

FIGURE 23–5 *Anatomy of carotid artery dissection. A, Diagram demonstrating hematoma tracking into the vessel wall, resulting in a long segment of narrowing distal to the carotid artery bifurcation. B, Pseudoaneurysmal dilatation of the carotid artery at the base of the skull due to dissection may injure adjacent lower cranial nerves. C, T1-weighted axial magnetic resonance image of the upper neck. The hematoma in the wall of the internal carotid artery appears as a bright crescent around the residual vessel lumen (appearing as a dark flow void in the center of the vessel). (From Wityk RJ: Stroke in a healthy 46-year-old man. JAMA 285:2757, 2001.)*

ischemic attack.[113] Transient monocular blindness occurs in one fourth of cases.[119] Other ischemic ocular syndromes, such as central retinal artery occlusion and anterior ischemic optic neuropathy, are rare.[98,132,133]

Baumgartner and associates[110] have reported that dissections causing ischemic events are more often associated with occlusions and stenosis greater than 80%, and that dissections that do not cause ischemic events are more often associated with Horner's syndrome and lower cranial nerve palsies.

Intracranial Carotid and Middle Cerebral Artery Dissection

As noted previously, dissection of the intracranial ICA and its branches occurs in younger patients than does extracranial dissection. A male preponderance has been reported.[14] Severe unilateral headache is almost universally present, and ischemic symptoms typically occur with a much shorter delay (within minutes or hours) compared with extracranial dissection. Seizures or syncope can be the presenting symptom, and half the patients have altered levels of consciousness.[19] Three quarters of cases involve the supraclinoid ICA or the middle cerebral artery stem; the anterior cerebral artery is infrequently involved.[10,135] Although reported, bilateral dissections occur less commonly in the intracranial circulation than in the

extracranial circulation.[68,104,136,137] Subarachnoid hemorrhage, resulting from subadventitial hematoma rupture through the external vessel wall, occurs in approximately 20% of cases.[14,104,138]

Extracranial Vertebral Artery Dissection

Saver and Easton[19] have previously summarized the clinical features and course of 174 cases of extracranial vertebral dissection from the literature (Table 23.3).

Local Signs and Symptoms

Headache occurs in one half to two thirds of patients with extracranial vertebral dissection and is typically ipsilateral and occipital.[19,102,105,119,139–141] The pain can be either throbbing or pressure-like.[119] Neck pain occurs in approximately half of patients and is typically gradual in onset.[19,102,105,119,139–142] The pain is usually unilateral but is bilateral in one third of cases.[119]

Ischemic Signs and Symptoms

The majority of patients with vertebral artery dissection have ischemic symptoms, although this observation may reflect an underdiagnosis of cases without ischemic manifestations. The median interval between onsets of neck pain and headache and the development of ischemic symptoms is 2 weeks and 15 hours, respectively.[119] Lateral

Table 23.3 Clinical Features of Extracranial Vertebral Dissection

No. of cases	174
Patient age	Mean 38.9 yr; range 3–67 yr
Patient sex	
Male	43%
Female	57%
Laterality	
Unilateral	69%
Left	56%
Right	44%
Bilateral	31%
Clinical features at presentation	
Cerebral infarction	75%
At onset	17%
Delayed	83%
Transient ischemic attack	25%
Neck pain	55%
Headache	53%
Head or neck pain	75%
Lateral medullary symptoms	33%
Associated conditions	
Hypertension	25%
Migraine	13%
Oral contraceptives (among women)	24%
Fibromuscular dysplasia	17%
Early outcome	
Angiographic	
Normal or mildly stenotic vessel on follow-up imaging	78%
Clinical	
Neurologically normal or mild deficits only	83%
Moderate to severe deficits	11%
Death	6%

Major presenting complaint leading to evaluation, not necessarily the initial symptom.
Data from references 19, 139–141.

medullary signs and symptoms may be seen in isolation or in combination with other brainstem, posterior cerebral artery distribution, or upper cervical spinal cord findings.[13,51,119,143–147] Cervical radiculopathy (most commonly at C5-C6) has been reported, although it is unclear whether the etiology is ischemic or mechanical.[144,145]

Intracranial Vertebral and Basilar Artery Dissections

Intracranial vertebral artery dissection is distinguished clinically from extracranial dissection by the association with subarachnoid hemorrhage. Coexistent subarachnoid hemorrhage has been reported to occur in as many as one half to two thirds of adult cases,[20,22,23,27–31] but the association has not been reported in children.[10] Basilar artery dissections are rare. They may be isolated (primary) or associated with concomitant vertebral artery dissection. Clinical manifestations vary according to the extent of involvement. Primary basilar dissection typically manifests as rapidly progressive brainstem signs, although it can manifest as headache and more slowly developing focal signs or as a mass

lesion due to intravascular hematoma.[24,28,104,105,138,148–173] Like other intracranial dissections, basilar dissections can manifest as subarachnoid hemorrhage and dissecting aneurysm if the dissection plane is subadventitial or transmural.[28,104,138,149,150,154,158,159,167]

DIAGNOSIS

When clinical presentation suggests cerebrovascular arterial dissection, whether spontaneous or traumatic in occurrence, an aggressive diagnostic approach is immediately warranted. The combination of magnetic resonance imaging (MRI) and magnetic resonance angiography (MRA) are at present the most direct noninvasive modalities for confirmation of arterial dissection.[18,18,174–181] In the traumatized patient for whom transport to an MRI unit may be an issue, carotid ultrasonography (US) transcranial Doppler ultrasonography (TCD), or both, can provide direct or indirect evidence of dissection.[182–188] Helical computerized tomographic angiography (CTA) is also noninvasive and may be particularly advantageous in the traumatized patient with suspected arterial dissection.[189,190] Conventional angiography remains a mainstay in accurately defining the exact level and arterial territory of dissection and for imaging complications associated with dissection, such as pseudoaneurysm, double lumen, and presence of intraluminal or distal clot.[9,30,99,178,191] Neuroendovascular therapy, including balloon angioplasty and placement of stents and coils, is an option that may be performed in tandem with conventional angiography.

Ultrasonography

The combination of extracranial carotid B-mode imaging and carotid color-flow Doppler ultrasonography combined with TCD offers the most reliable systematic US investigation.[111,117,121,182–188,192] Extracranial vertebral artery dissection may also be diagnosed using a multimodal US approach.[192] Indirect rather than direct evidence of extracranial carotid artery dissection is often more prominent on US, because extracranial carotid artery dissection typically occurs 2 cm or more distal to the carotid bulb, the latter being the more common site of atherosclerotic abnormalities.[19,183] Decrease or absence of flow velocities in the affected vessel, retrograde flow in supraorbital vessels, or bidirectional ICA flow suggests more distal obstruction or moderate to high-grade stenosis resulting from dissection. Direct US visualization of tapering of the ICA lumen may be achieved, as well as presence of a true and false lumen with an intraluminal flap in 15% of cases (Figs. 23–6 and 23–7).[183,186]

Extracranial color-flow duplex ultrasonography has been effective in detecting abnormalities in extracranial vertebral artery dissection, similarly demonstrating indirect evidence of absence, reduction, or reversal of flow in the vertebral artery or, rarely, direct evidence of intimal hemorrhage.[184,185,192] The severity of stenosis and the presence of occlusion and site of dissection significantly affect the sensitivity and specificity of US in extracranial carotid and vertebral artery dissection.[183] Insonating the high cervical (retromandibular) region in extracranial carotid artery

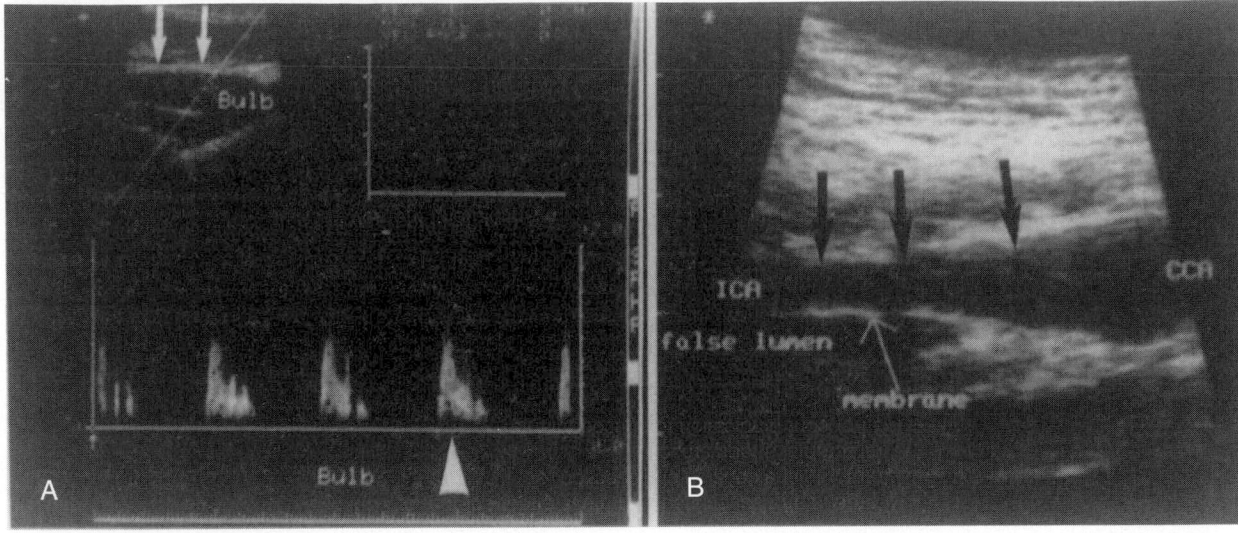

FIGURE 23–6   A, *Duplex ultrasonography demonstrates a patent bulb without atherosclerotic wall changes* (arrows). *Doppler sample in the bulb demonstrates only short systolic flow signal without diastolic flow (stump flow)* (arrowhead). B, *B-mode imaging of bulb and proximal internal carotid artery shows tapering luminal narrowing* (black arrows) *and a membrane* (white arrow) *separating true from false lumen. (From Sturzenegger M: Spontaneous internal carotid artery dissection: Early diagnosis and management in 44 patients. J Neurol 242:231, 1995.)*

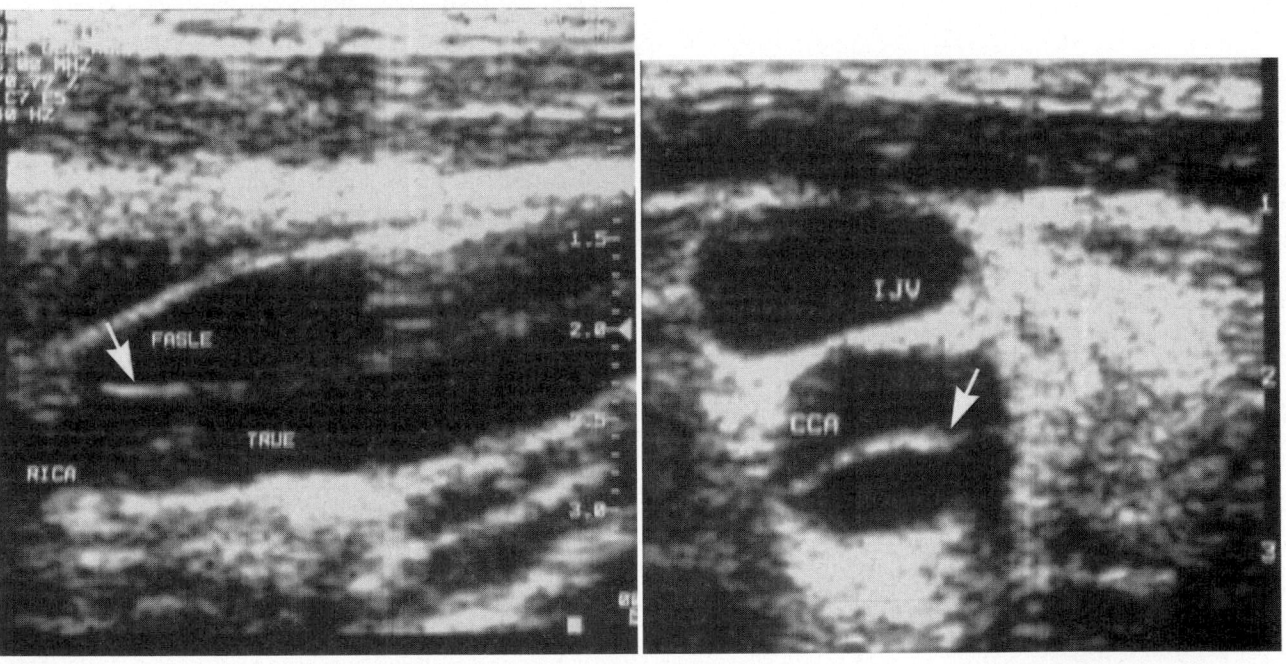

FIGURE 23–7   *B-mode ultrasonography images of a carotid artery dissection demonstrating the true and false lumen separated by a membrane* (white arrows). *(Courtesy of Christine Miles, RVT.)*

dissection and stepwise segmental insonation of the vertebral artery in extracranial vertebral artery dissection improve detection of suspected dissection.[19,183] TCD delineates flow abnormalities distal to vascular luminal narrowing or occlusion by dissection, including signs of carotid-carotid collateral cross-flow; artery-to-artery embolic middle cerebral artery stem occlusion is suggested when the middle cerebral artery signal is absent and the ipsilateral anterior cerebral and posterior cerebral artery velocities are increased.[19,188] Serial examination of extracranial carotid and vertebral artery dissection for spontaneous or therapy-based recanalization with these US techniques allows outpatient monitoring and the use of clinical decision algorithms.[183–186,192,193]

Magnetic Resonance Imaging

MRI coupled with MRA currently offers sophisticated noninvasive imaging of cerebrovascular arterial dissection. Simultaneous definitions of the brain and the major cervical and intracranial arteries are achieved with conventional T1- and T2-weighted and fluid attenuation inversion recovery (FLAIR) axial MRI with three-dimensional time-of-flight (TOF) MRA (Fig. 23–8). The typical abnormalities associated with dissection are most easily defined in extracranial carotid (Fig. 23–9) and vertebral artery dissection, whereas intracranial arterial dissection imaging often shows less specific abnormalities.[19] Characteristic imaging findings on MRI in extracranial carotid artery dissection include diminution or absence of signal flow void and a crescent sign, due to narrowing of the vessel by intramural dissection of blood appearing in a semilunar fashion as a spiraling periarterial rim of intramural hematoma in cross-section on T1-weighted and FLAIR axial views (see Figs. 23–8 and 23–9; see Fig. 23-5C).[18,19,174–181,194–197]

The intensity of the hematoma on T1- and T2-weighted images depends on the age of the dissection, because the hyperintense signal corresponds to intramural hematoma with methemoglobin signal intensity; in some dissections, all or part of the intramural hematoma appears hypointense on T2-weighted images as a result of acute clot deoxyhemoglobin or hemosiderin in the chronic type.[111] Subtle abnormalities also include (1) high signal intensity from the entire vessel, (2) significant compromise of the vessel lumen by adjoining abnormal increased signal tissue, (3) enlargement of the vessel diameter, and (4) poor or no visualization of the vessel. Fat suppression techniques are important to differentiate small intramural hematomas from surrounding soft tissues.[18] In the absence

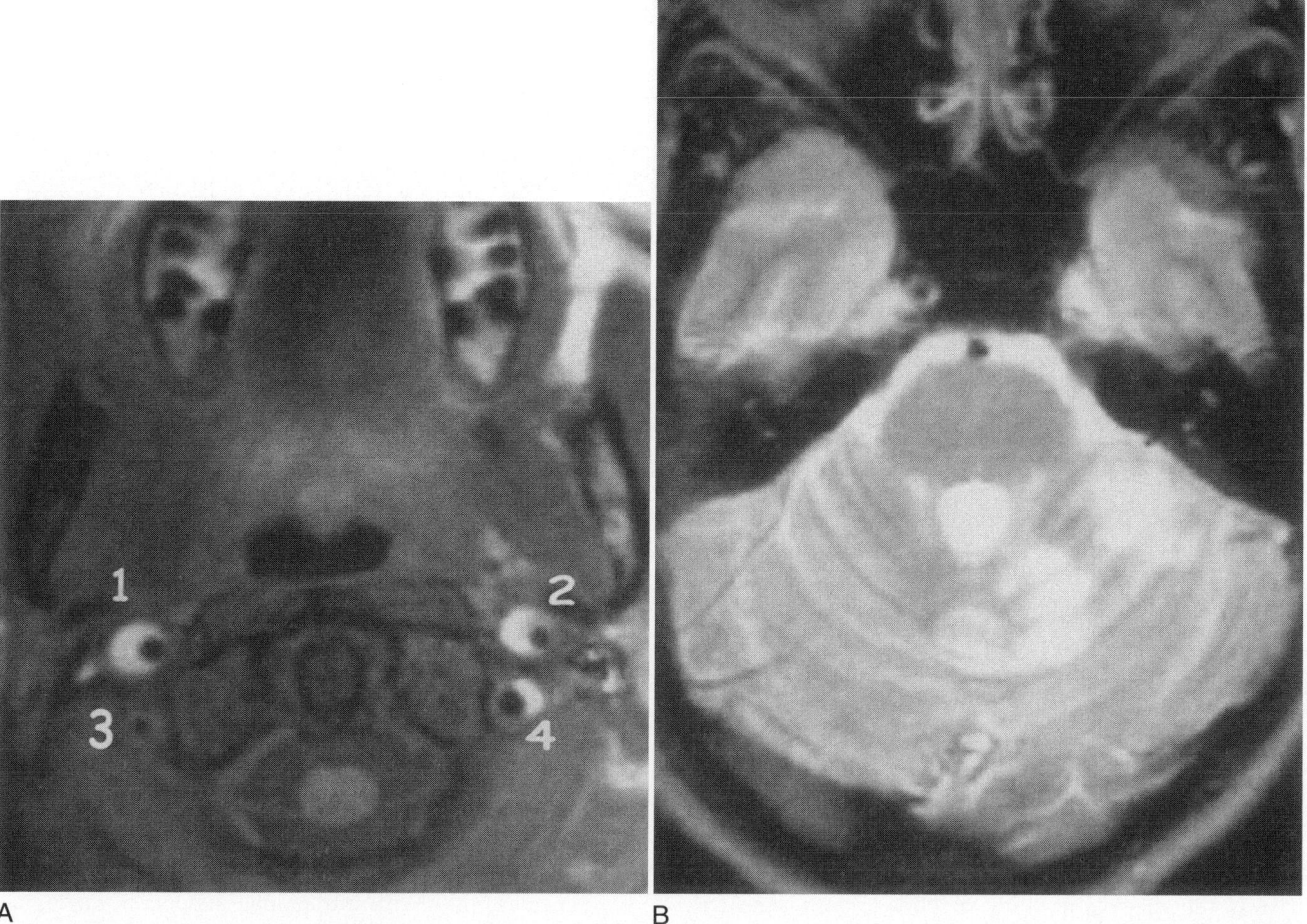

A   B

FIGURE 23–8 *T1-weighted (A) and T2-weighted (B) axial magnetic resonance images from a patient with vertigo and ataxia who was found to have a spontaneous four-vessel dissection. Note the crescent of methemoglobin in the wall of all the cerebral vessels. A, Dissection in the right internal carotid artery (1), left internal carotid artery (2), right vertebral artery (3), and left vertebral artery (4). The findings in the right vertebral artery (3) are subtle. B, Multiple cerebellar infarcts (arrows). (From Silverboard G, Tart R: Cerebrovascular arterial dissection in children and young adults. Semin Pediatr Neurol 7:278, 2000.)*

Specific Medical Diseases and Stroke

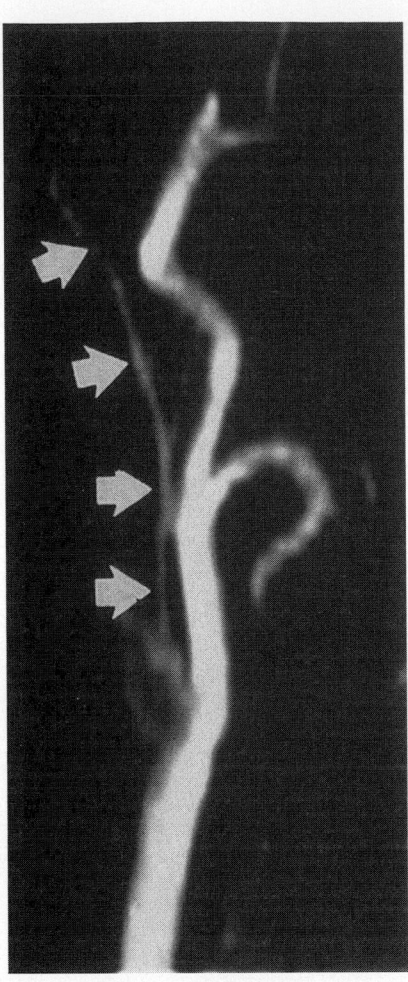

FIGURE 23–9 *Lateral projection from a segmented cervical carotid magnetic resonance angiogram demonstrating complete occlusion of the high cervical portion of the internal carotid artery (arrows). This spontaneous dissection manifested as a minor stroke. The patient made a near-complete recovery with anticoagulation therapy. (From Silverboard G, Tart R: Cerebrovascular arterial dissection in children and young adults. Semin Pediatr Neurol 7:278, 2000.)*

of significant luminal stenosis or compromise, MRI may detect carotid dissection missed by conventional angiography; however, MRI may fail to demonstrate mural hematoma even though associated vessel wall thickening is present. The pattern of stroke associated with extracranial carotid artery dissection is predominantly cortical (83%) and subcortical (60%) with the middle cerebral artery territory affected in 99%, the anterior cerebral artery territory in 4%, and the posterior cerebral artery territory in 3%, with borderzone infarcts in 5% of cases.[109,110] In extracranial carotid artery dissection, MRA in tandem with MRI is the diagnostic study of choice, with sensitivity and specificity of 95% and 99%, respectively, for MRA and 84% and 99%, respectively, for MRI.[19,179] Dissecting aneurysms may be missed in the acute stage by three-dimensional TOF MRA if the hematoma is isointense.[178] Intracranial carotid arterial dissection produces less specific abnormalities on noninvasive studies, although MRI

may demonstrate intramural hematoma.[19,198,199] The presence of subarachnoid hemorrhage, occurring in one fifth of cases, is notable and may clinically suggest dissection; however, cerebral angiography rather than MRI-MRA is the standard for diagnosis of intracranial carotid artery dissection.[19,30,99,105]

Extracranial vertebral artery dissection is the second most common site of dissection and typically occurs at the C1-C2 site. Although unilateral extracranial vertebral artery dissection may go unrecognized because of collateral flow by the uninvolved vertebral artery, bilateral vertebral artery dissection is well recognized. It may be associated with cerebellar, brainstem, or hemispheric infarction noted on routine MRI; concurrent carotid artery dissections may also occur.[19,105,200,201] The entire spectrum of MRI-MRA findings seen in extracranial carotid artery dissection may occur in extracranial vertebral artery dissection, although these two modalities are not as sensitive in extracranial vertebral artery dissection; one study reported sensitivity and specificity of 60% and 98%, respectively, for MRI and 20% and 100%, respectively, for MRA.[179] Conventional angiography is warranted if MRI-MRA findings are nondiagnostic in spite of a high clinical index of suspicion for extracranial vertebral artery dissection.

Intracranial vertebral artery dissection occurs at or near the origin of the posterior inferior cerebellar artery. Although the presentation is similar to that of extracranial vertebral artery dissection, with brainstem, cerebellar, or hemispheric infarction, intracranial vertebral artery dissection may be distinguished on the basis of its association with subarachnoid hemorrhage.[19,20,22,23,27,28] MRI-MRA may demonstrate a crescent sign or suggestion of dissecting aneurysm, but angiography is warranted in most instances of intracranial vertebral or basilar artery dissection or suspected basilar artery embolization associated with vertebral artery dissection.

Angiography

Although the complementary use of MRI, MRA, and US is usually sufficient for the diagnosis of extracranial carotid artery dissection and some instances of extracranial vertebral artery dissection, angiography is the most definitive test for investigation of intracranial dissection as well as extracranial vertebral artery dissection. Angiography, although invasive, yields excellent delineation of abnormalities associated with dissection (Fig. 23–10), including intimal flaps, intraluminal clots, flame-shaped tapering occlusion, double lumen, vessel stenosis with string sign, and dissecting aneurysm formation. Double lumen and intimal flaps are the most specific angiographic findings in dissection. More often, angiographic features of intracranial dissection are not definitive but suggest dissection by demonstrating irregular or scalloped stenoses, a "string of beads," or complete vessel occlusion.[178] With intracranial dissection, angiography may delineate cerebral aneurysm from dissection causing subarachnoid hemorrhage (Fig. 23–11). The finding at angiography of aneurysmal formation at a non-bifurcation location suggests dissection. Irregular narrowing of the affected artery may give a wavy ribbon appearance. The presence of fibromuscular dysplasia

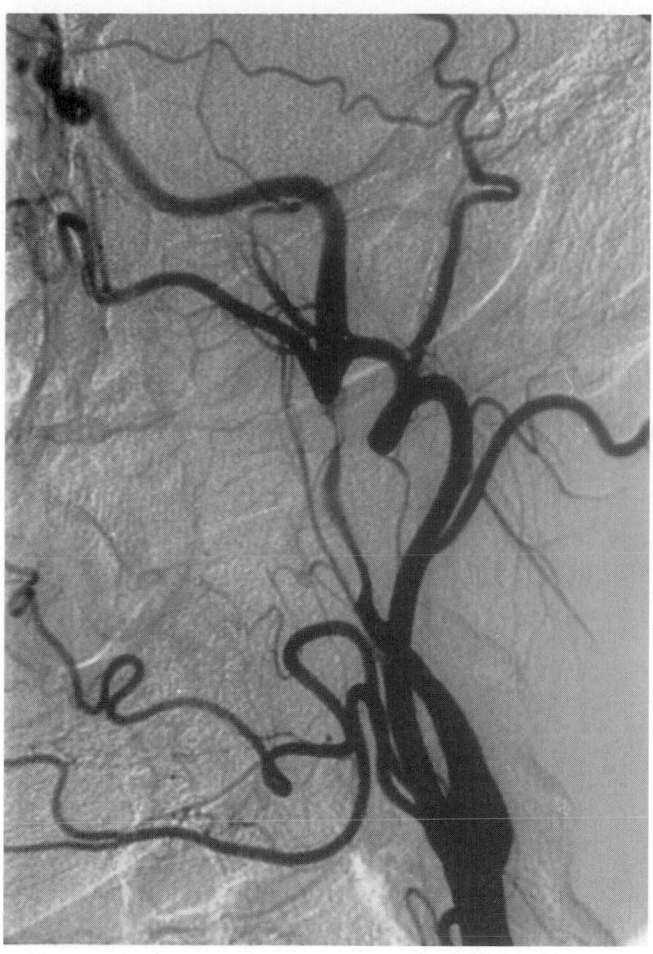

FIGURE 23–10 *Digital subtraction angiogram (lateral view) showing irregular narrowing of the left internal carotid artery beginning approximately 3 cm distal to the bifurcation in a 38-year-old woman who presented with expressive aphasia and right hemiparesis. Note that the dissection terminates at the skull base, with a normal-appearing intracranial internal carotid artery.*

(Fig. 23–12) in 15% of cases may be associated with multi-vessel dissections.[202–204] Atherosclerotic disease should be suspected in lesions seen proximal to and within 2 cm of the carotid bifurcation.

Computed Tomography

Advanced CT applications such as helical CTA may be particularly suited for investigation of dissection in traumatized patients (Fig. 23–13).[190] Traumatic effects depend on the extent and location of damage to the vessel wall. Dissection occurs more often in blunt rather than penetrating trauma. CTA is rapid, allowing unstable patients to be imaged without compromising patient monitoring. Experience with CTA is limited, but in preliminary studies, this modality appears to provide high sensitivity and specificity while revealing findings similar to those of conventional angiography, although small dissections may escape detection.[190]

TREATMENT

Medical Therapy

Although treatment of extracranial cerebrovascular dissection is controversial and large controlled clinical trials are lacking, treatment is based both on empiric and clinical observations that most cerebral injuries, at least acutely, result from secondary thrombotic events, particularly artery-to-artery embolism.[19] Medical intervention, consisting of anticoagulation with heparin given as acute therapy in the symptomatic patient and subsequent warfarin therapy, is the most commonly suggested therapy; therapy is reassessed in the stable patient at 3 months by means of multimodal US studies or MRI-MRA.[18,19,106,111,205] If imaging studies show that dissection has resolved, antiplatelet therapy may be warranted after discontinuation of warfarin; some investigators, however, would discontinue all therapies. If at 3 months reconstitution has not occurred and severe luminal irregularity or stenosis is

Specific Medical Diseases and Stroke

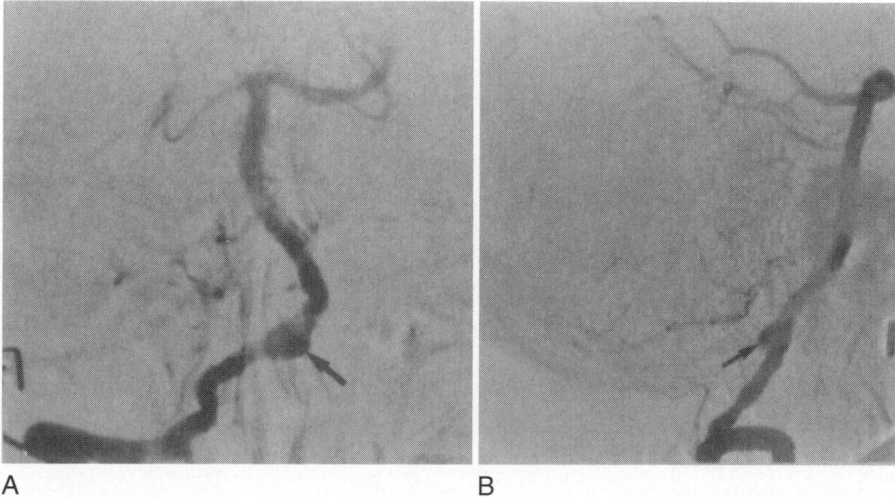

FIGURE 23–11 *Vertebral angiography.* A, *Anteroposterior view showing right irregular aneurysm* (arrow) *with proximal narrowing.* B, *Lateral view. Aneurysm is more obvious* (arrow). *(From Caplan LR, Baquis GD, Pessin MS, et al: Dissection of the intracranial vertebral artery.* Neurology 38:868, 1988.)

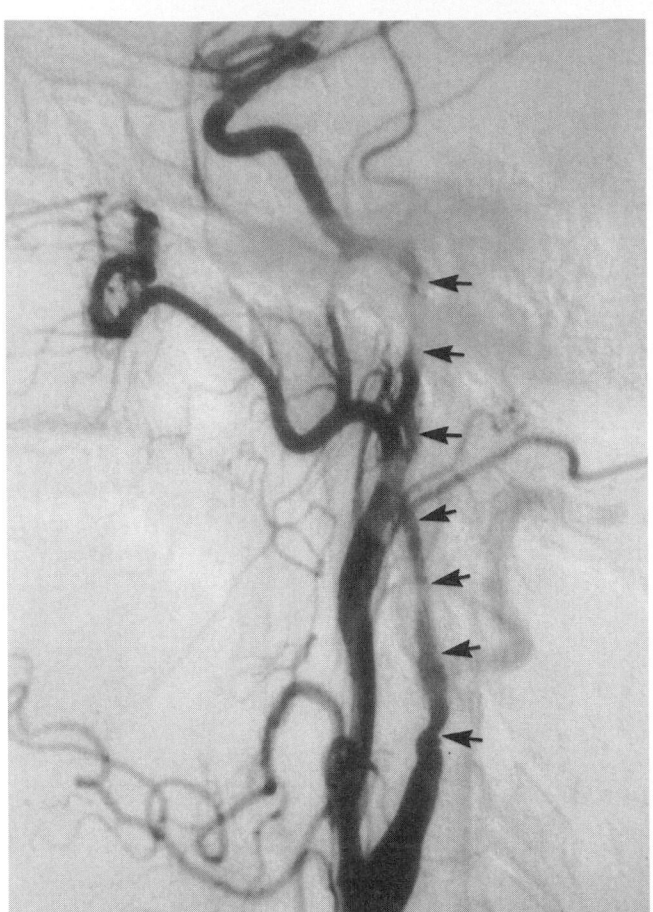

FIGURE 23–12 *Lateral view from a digital subtraction angiogram showing the high cervical internal carotid artery. In this patient with fibromuscular dysplasia (more prominently seen on the opposite side, not shown), there is a long, irregular narrowing of the internal carotid artery. The dissection involves nearly the entire cervical portion of the internal carotid artery (black arrows), starting just beyond the cervical bifurcation and ending in the petrous portion of the internal carotid artery with a normal carotid siphon. (From Silverboard G, Tart R: Cerebrovascular arterial dissection in children and young adults. Semin Pediatr Neurol 7:278, 2000.)*

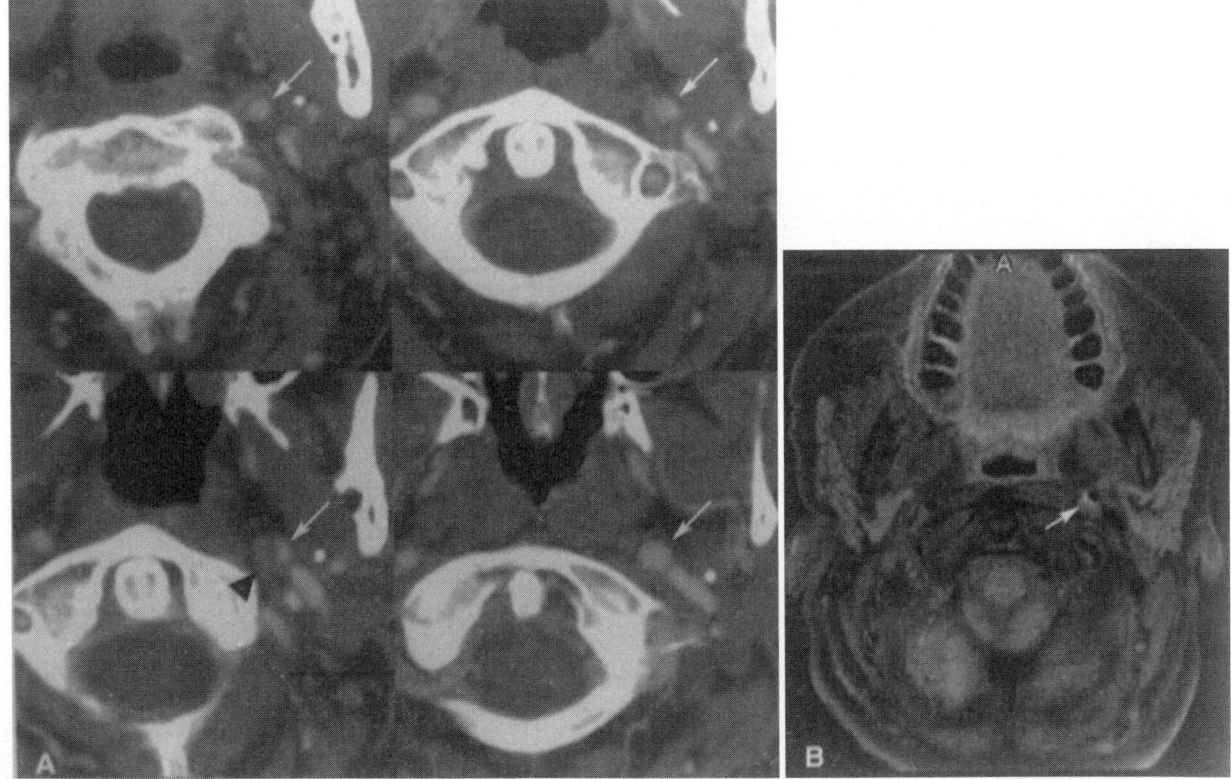

FIGURE 23–13 (A, upper left to lower right) *Axial mutliplanar volume reconstruction computed tomographic angiograms obtained because of the possibility of acute carotid dissection shows that the caudal configuration of the internal carotid artery (ICA) is normal (upper left, arrow). Moving rostrally in the neck (upper right, lower left), the caliber of the ICA narrows (arrows). A crescent-shaped intraluminal thrombus is visible (lower left, arrowhead). Superior to the lesion (lower right), the ICA is enlarged abnormally, suggesting a postdissection pseudoaneurysm (arrow). B, The next day, a fat-saturated, T1-weighted axial magnetic resonance image through the lesion shows a crescent-shaped area of abnormally high signal intensity (arrow) consistent with intramural thrombus related to the acute dissection. (From Fredenberg P, Forbes K, Toye L, et al: Assessment of cervical vascular injury with CT angiography. BNI Q 17:44, 2001.)*

noted or there is persistence of dissecting aneurysm, warfarin is continued for 3 months longer.[19] Rupture of dissecting aneurysms is not commonly described; rather, thromboembolism from the dissecting aneurysm or expansion of the aneurysm compressing adjacent structures merits continued monitoring.[206]

Anticoagulation is typically avoided (albeit on empiric grounds) in the presence of intracranial dissection because of the increased risk of subarachnoid hemorrhage. This precaution is particularly true for vertebrobasilar dissection, for which the risk of subarachnoid hemorrhage, either early or late, may be 50% or greater. Other relative contraindications to anticoagulation are the presence of a large infarct with mass effect, hemorrhagic transformation of the infarcted arterial territory, and presence of an intracranial aneurysm.[25] In a 2003 *Cochrane Review* on the use of antithrombotic drugs for carotid artery dissection, no evidence was found to support the routine use of anticoagulant or antiplatelet drugs for the treatment of extracranial carotid artery dissection.[238] Schievink and associates[206] have proposed a treatment algorithm for the medical management of cervicocephalic dissection that reflects our practice (Fig. 23–14).

Acute thrombolysis with tissue plasminogen activator (tPA), given both intravenously and intra-arterially through superselective arterial catheterization, has been administered safely after dissection-related stroke.[207-212] Increased intramural hemorrhage with exacerbation of

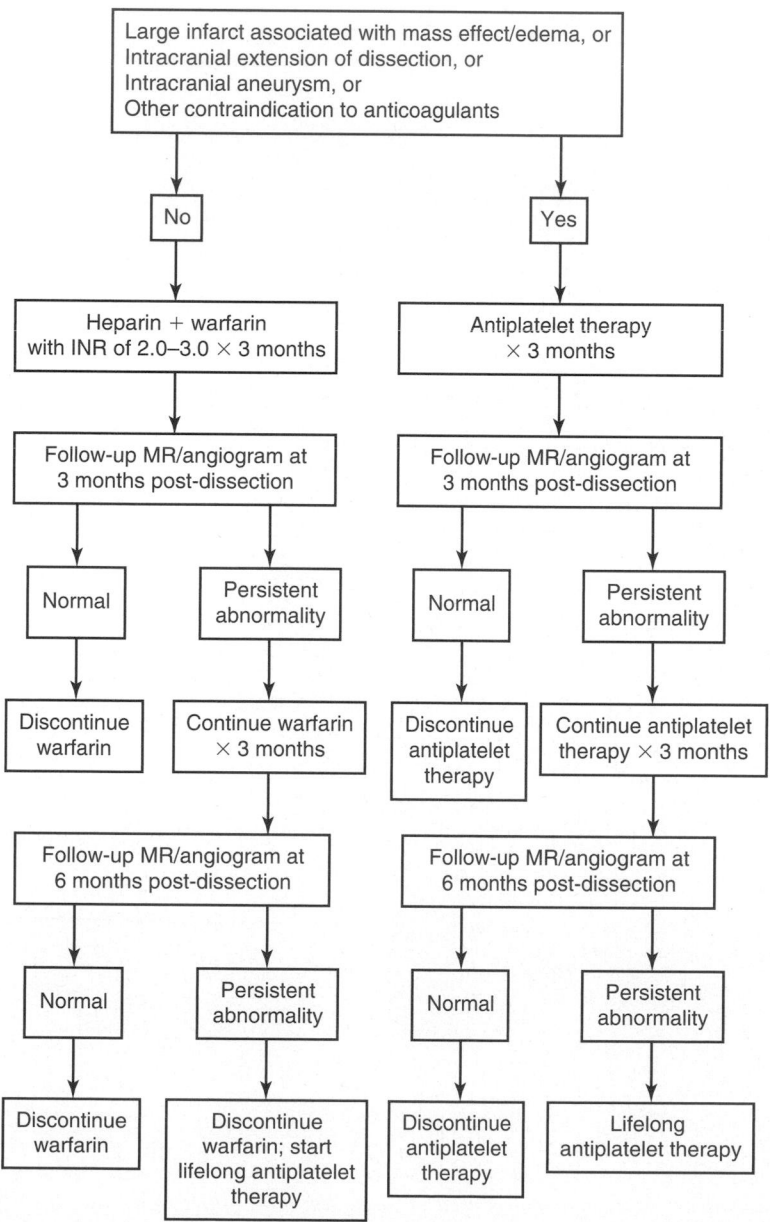

FIGURE 23–14 *Algorithmic approach to the medical treatment of spontaneous carotid and vertebral artery dissections. INR, international normalized ratio; MR, magnetic resonance. (From Schievink WI: Spontaneous dissection of the carotid and vertebral arteries. N Engl J Med 344:898, 2001.)*

Specific Medical Diseases and Stroke

dissection-related stenosis has not been reported. Experience with thrombolytic therapy after dissection is limited, however, with only 30 reported cases in the literature.

Neuroendovascular Interventional Therapy

Neuroendovascular intervention is increasingly being employed in patients for whom medical therapy has failed and who have (1) persistent ischemic symptoms, (2) contraindications to anticoagulation, (3) surgically inaccessible lesions, (4) limited reserve due to involvement of other vessels, or (5) persistent or expanding dissecting aneurysm.[213] For both spontaneous and traumatic dissections, endovascular therapy in appropriate circumstances allows reestablishment of the true lumen by means of balloon angioplasty and stenting with either balloon-expandable or metallic self-expanding stents, resulting in the obliteration of the false lumen and restoration of hemodynamic flow in the true lumen and thereby reducing the risk of artery-to-artery embolism (Fig. 23–15).[25,29,165,213–232] Through the use of a covered stent or coil embolization placed through the interstices of the stent when necessary, obliteration of dissecting aneurysms

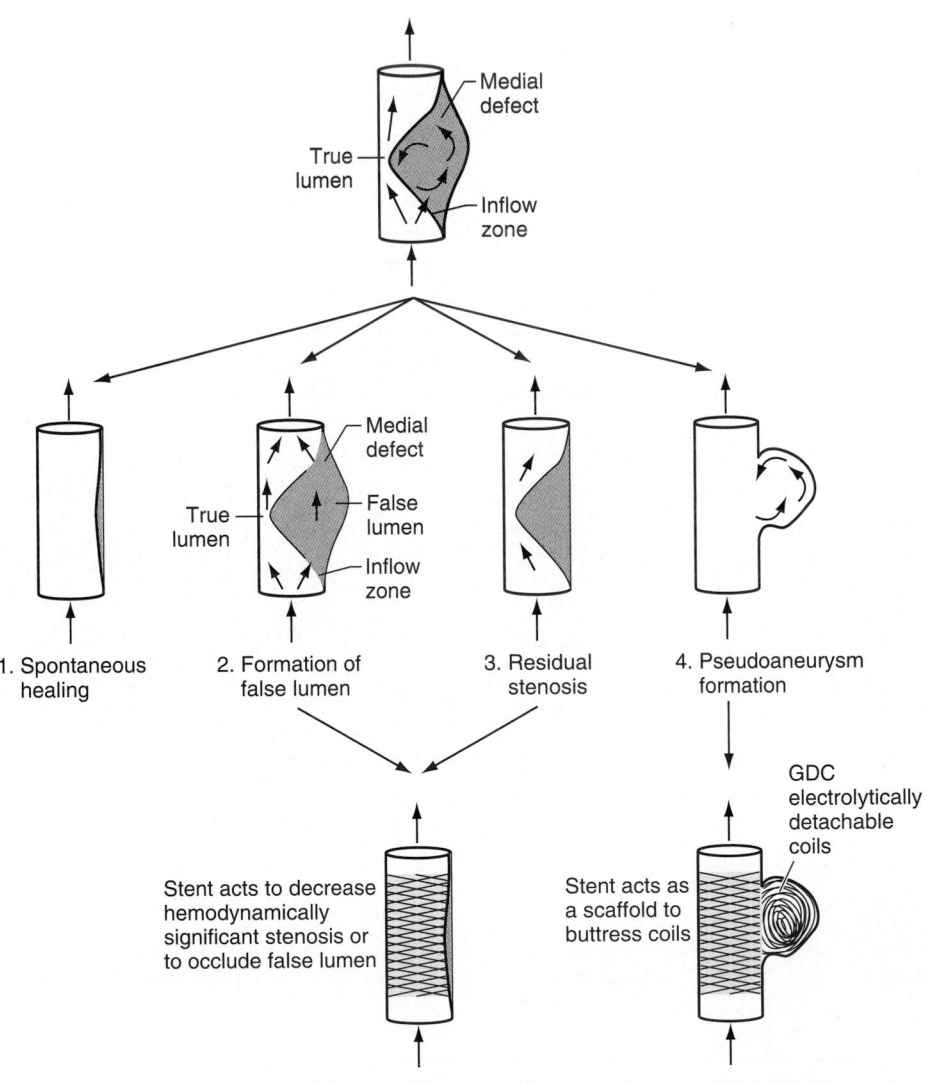

ACUTE CAROTID ARTERY DISSECTION

FIGURE 23–15 *Simplified schematic illustration of the pathophysiologic process of carotid artery dissection proceeding from the acute stage to either spontaneous healing (1), formation of false lumen (2), residual stenosis of varying degree or complete occlusion (3), and formation of a pseudoaneurysm (4). A stent is used in cases that have not responded to medical therapy either to relieve a hemodynamically significant stenosis, to occlude a false lumen, or to serve as a scaffold to enable coil embolization of a wide-necked pseudoaneurysm. (From Malek AM, Higashida RT, Phatouros CC, et al: Endovascular management of extracranial carotid artery dissection achieved using stent angiography. Am J Neuroradiol 21:1380, 2000.)*

in both the extracranial carotid and vertebral arteries may be accomplished (Fig. 23–16).[29,218,220,221,223,227,229,230,233] Endovascular therapy can reestablish hemodynamic flow in severely stenotic or totally occluded true lumens in selected cases (Figs. 23–17 and 23–18); sequential reconstruction of the true lumen is accomplished by means of stents that provide gradual radial force, permitting apposition of the dissected segment to the vessel wall and thereby obliterating the false lumen and resolving the consequent loss of vascular continuity.[206,223] Extracranial and intracranial components of dissection can be addressed simultaneously if necessary.

When intracranial extension has occurred, endovascular techniques are also applicable and may be of particular benefit for balloon occlusion of intracranial dissection of the vertebral artery if temporary occlusion studies suggest adequate collateral blood flow. Long-term efficacy and endovascular therapy-related complications are still being assessed, although results of limited published series are promising.[207,233–237] Complications of endovascular intervention include retroperitoneal hemorrhage, vasospasm, which may be treated with angioplasty during the endovascular procedure, and the possibility of recurrent stenosis and distal embolism if there is large thrombus burden.[206] Because the risk of recurrent embolization is low and dissecting aneurysms do not usually rupture, stenting as an initial therapy is not warranted and should be reserved in most cases for cases in which medical therapy has failed.[25,206,238] When stenting is performed, antiplatelet agents are administered for at least 4 weeks to prevent stent occlusion.[206]

Surgical Therapy

With the advent of endovascular techniques, the need for surgical intervention as the treatment for symptomatic dissecting aneurysm or post-dissection stenosis has decreased. Formerly, aneurysms accounted for 0.3% of extracranial ICA operations performed at the Cleveland Clinic[239] and 0.2% of those performed by the neurovascular surgical service at the Mayo Clinic.[206,240] Surgery is now reserved for patients who are symptomatic despite optimal medical therapy and who are not candidates for endovascular intervention.[25,206,241] Patients with impaired cerebral vasoreactivity who are at increased risk for stroke may need surgical revascularization.[25,242]

Surgical treatment consists of carotid ligation, aneurysmal resection with carotid reconstruction, and cervical-to-intracranial ICA bypass (supraclinoid or petrous ICA). Aneurysmal clipping is usually not an option because of the fusiform configuration usually found at surgery. Extracranial dissecting aneurysms rarely need surgery; they often resolve spontaneously, particularly those that are not traumatic in origin.[206,243] Surgical excision of the symptomatic dissecting aneurysm with reconstruction of the ICA to eliminate the aneurysm and maintain the artery's hemodynamic flow may be accomplished with interposition of a saphenous vein graft or primary

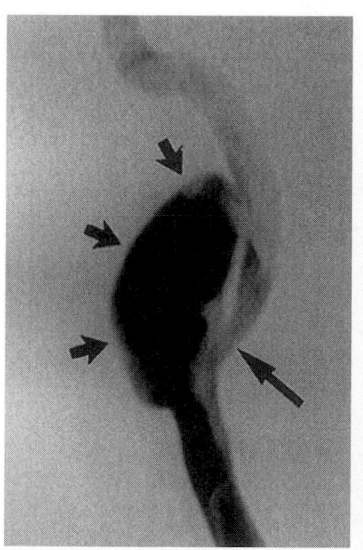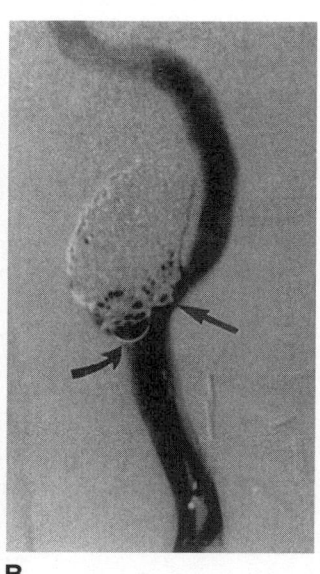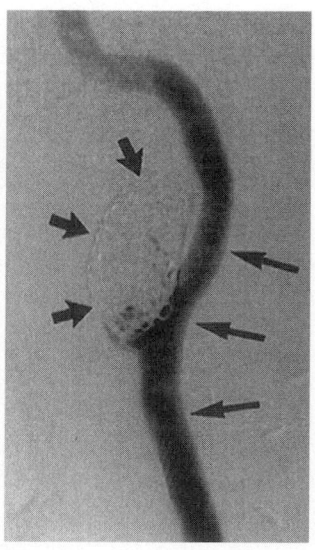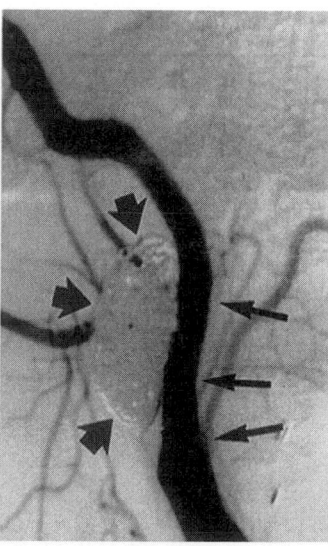

A   **B**   **C**   **D**

FIGURE 23–16 *A 30-year-old woman with a left cervical internal carotid artery (ICA) pseudoaneurysm. A, Left internal carotid injection, lateral view, shows pseudoaneurysm (short arrows) and narrowed ICA (long arrow). B, Left ICA angiogram after embolization with Guglielmi detachable coils shows the coils protruding into the parent artery (arrows). C, Left ICA angiogram after embolization and stent placement shows the occluded pseudoaneurysm (short arrows) and the remodeled, stented carotid artery (long arrows). D, At 6-month follow-up, left common carotid angiogram shows total occlusion of the pseudoaneurysm (short arrows) and normal width and patency of the stented segment of the ICA (long arrows). (From Klein GE, Szolar DH, Raith J, et al: Post-traumatic extracranial aneurysm of the internal carotid artery: Combined endovascular treatment with coils and stents. AJNR Am J Neuroradiol 18:1261, 1997.)*

Specific Medical Diseases and Stroke

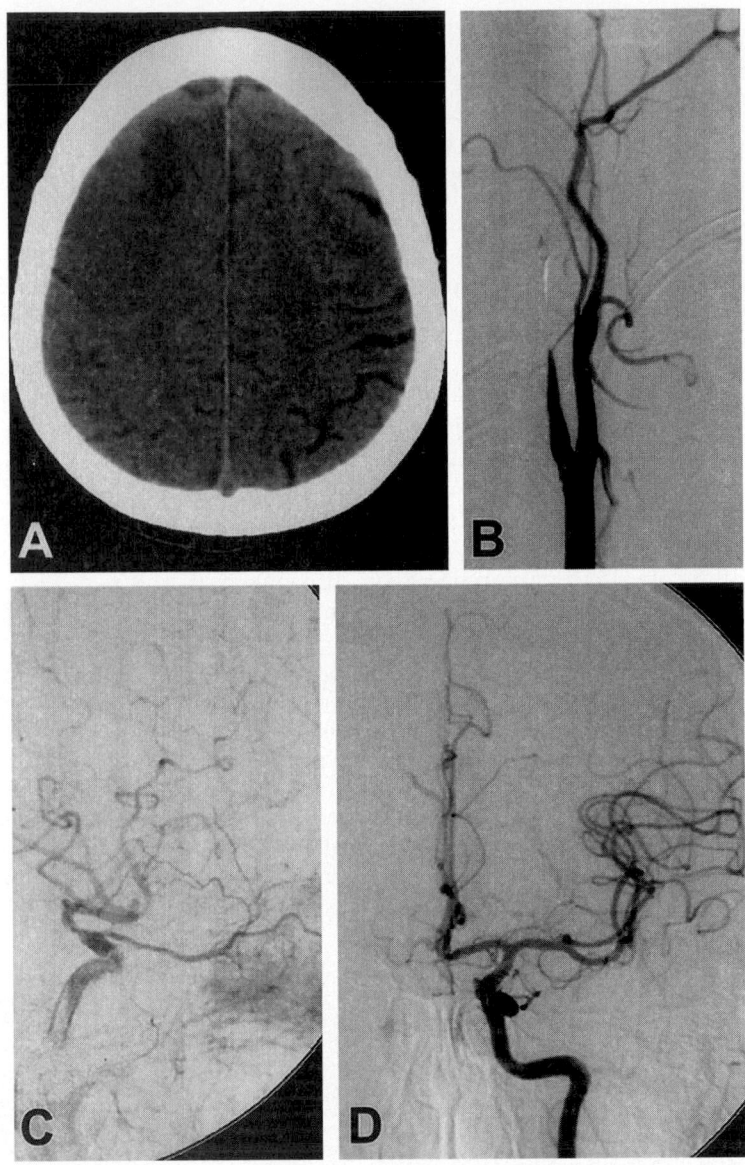

FIGURE 23–17   *A 45-year-old woman noted to have left hemiparesis after diagnostic angiography. A, Head computed tomography scan shows evidence of a previous focal infarct as well as diffuse edema in the right posterior frontal lobe. B, Digital subtraction angiogram of the right common carotid artery reveals tapering of the right internal carotid artery, to a complete occlusion, with appearance consistent with dissection. C, Injection of the right external carotid artery shows retrograde collateral flow through the right ophthalmic artery, with filling of the cavernous segment of the right internal carotid artery. D, Injection of the left internal carotid artery shows no significant flow across the anterior communicating artery.*

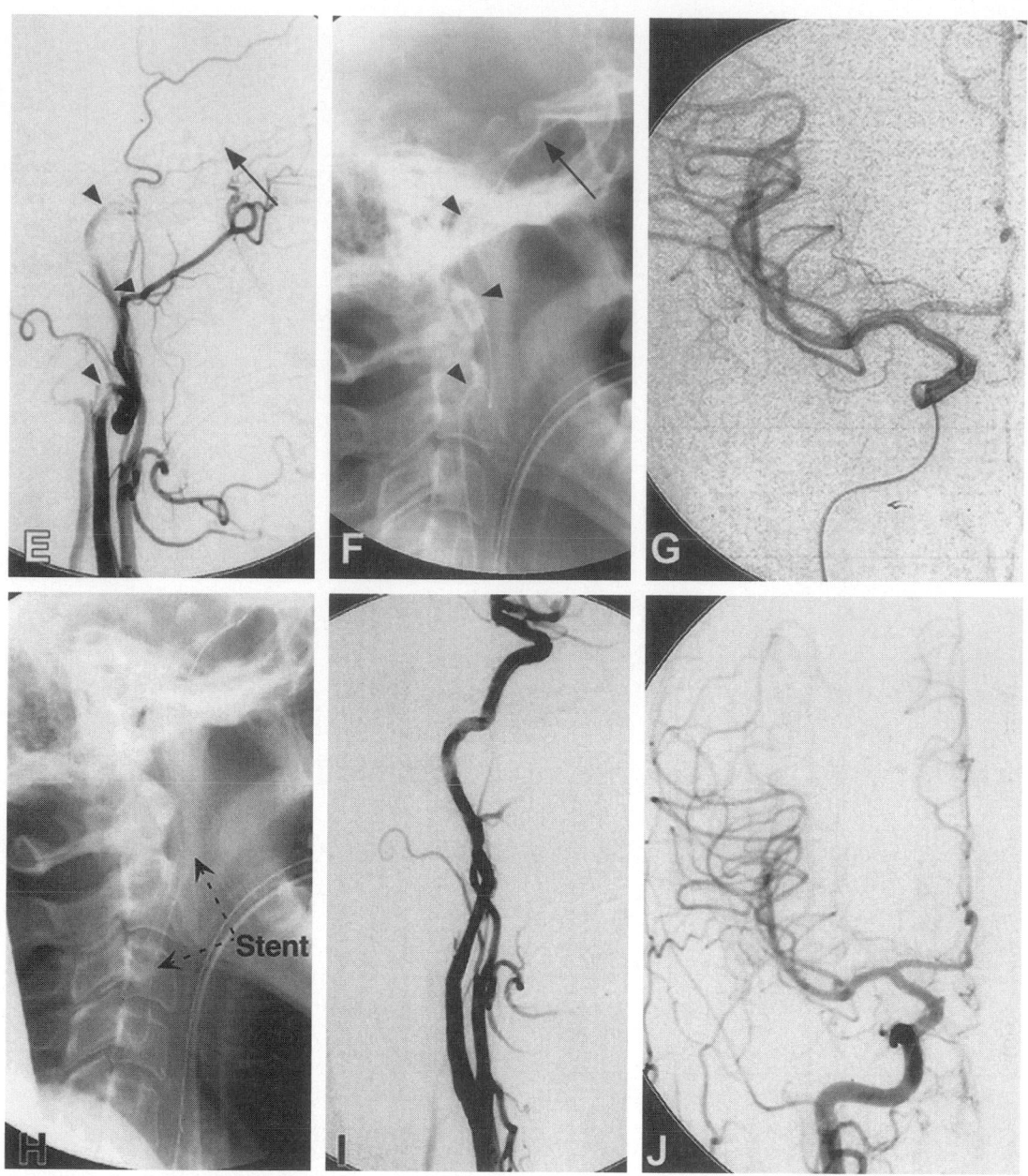

FIGURE 23–17—cont'd *Treatment approach consisted of initial recanalization of the dissected right internal carotid artery achieved by entering the true lumen with the use of a Rapid Transit microcatheter and Instinct-10 microguidewire (E; arrowheads), advancing them up to the cavernous portion of the right internal carotid artery (F; arrow). G, Superselective injection shows a patent right middle and anterior cerebral artery. H, An 8 mm × 2 cm Wallstent was then deployed at the dissection site over a Stabilizer exchange microguidewire at the C2 level. The reconstitution of the lumen of the right internal carotid artery is shown by injection of the right common carotid artery (I), with resumption of intracranial perfusion (J). (From Malek AM, Higashida RT, Phatouros CC, et al: Endovascular management of extracranial carotid artery dissection achieved using stent angiography. Am J Neuroradiol 21:1380, 2000.)*

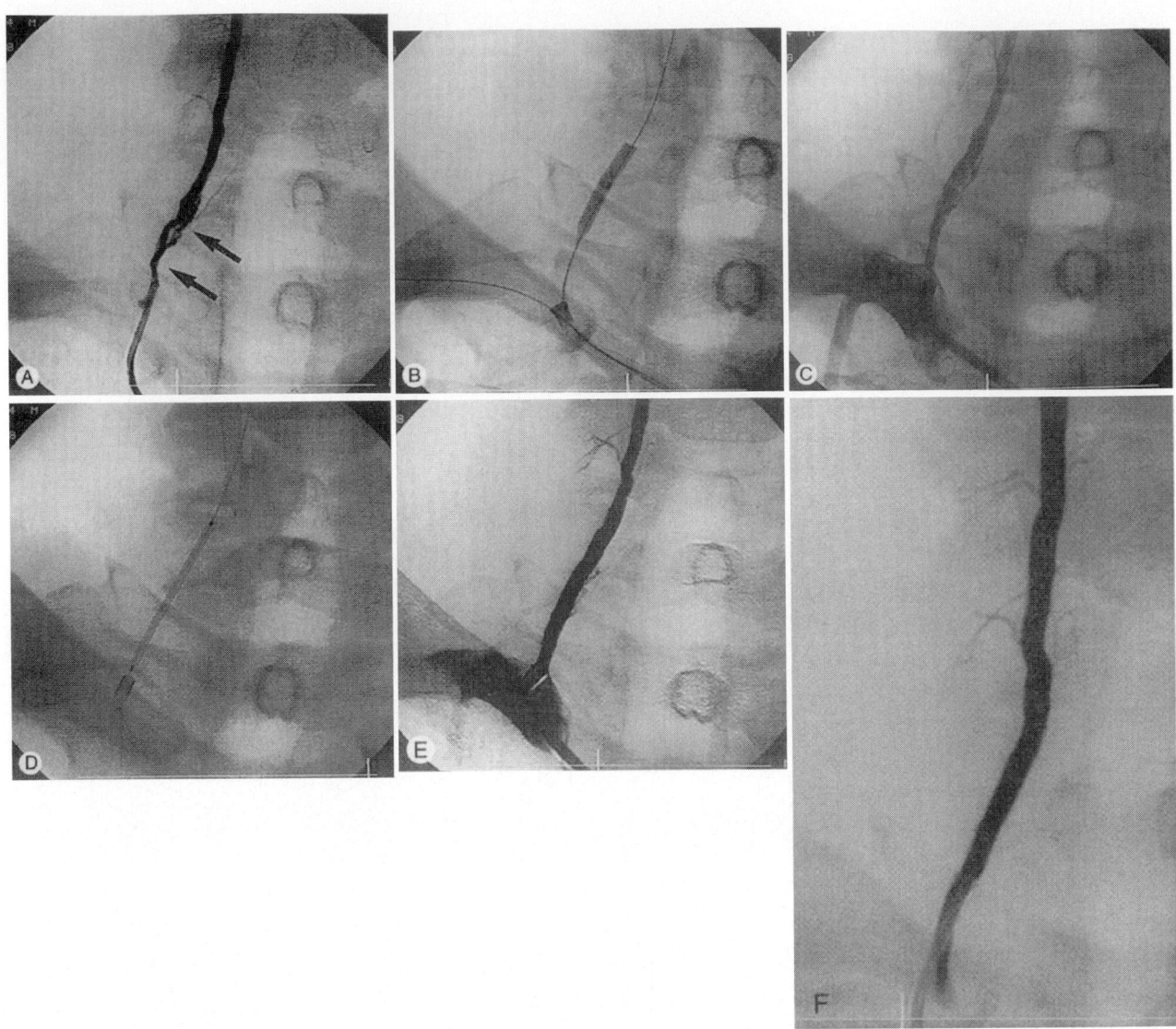

FIGURE 23–18   A, *Traumatic dissection of proximal right vertebral artery in a 36-year-old man who suffered a brainstem infarction. After conservative treatment for 1 year, the vessel still appeared damaged, so endovascular therapy was offered. Note the multiple lumens (arrows) that force the interventionist to find the true lumen before inflating balloons and using stents. B, Once the true lumen is found, balloon angioplasty allows enlargement of this lumen in order to properly fit and deploy the stents. C, After predilation, note improvement of the true lumen, although further reconstruction of the vessel seems to be required. D, Balloon-expandable stent is properly positioned and deployed. E, Final result shows normalization of the true lumen of vessel with obliteration of false lumens. F, Six-month control follow-up angiogram shows preservation of the architecture of the vessel. (From Gomez CR, May AK, Terry JB, et al: Endovascular therapy of traumatic injuries of the extracranial cerebral arteries. Crit Care Clin 15:789, 1999.)*

reanastomosis (Fig. 23–19).[25] Because the majority of carotid dissecting aneurysms occur in the distal carotid artery near the skull base, surgery may cause pharyngeal and superior laryngeal branch injuries of the vagus nerve and resultant, although usually transient, dysphonia or dysphagia.[25]

Carotid artery ligation, provided that adequate collateral flow is documented, has been performed. Complications include delayed ischemia due to embolization in the immediate postoperative period and long-term potential occurrence of cerebral ischemia or cerebral aneurysms.[25] Because of the risk of recurrent dissection in another vessel, preservation of vessel integrity is a practical and

potentially critical consideration. Schievink[25] favors cervical-to-intracranial ICA bypass using a saphenous vein graft between the cervical carotid artery and the petrous or supraclinoid portion of the ICA or, less often, the proximal middle cerebral artery.

COURSE AND PROGNOSIS

Although the clinical prognosis after extracranial carotid or vertebral dissection depends on the severity of the initial neurologic injury, it is generally quite good (Tables 23.2 to 23.4).[19] Complete or excellent recovery occurs in 75% to

Table 23.4 Survey of Literature on Outcome of Management in 100 Patients

Presenting Features*	Patients' Outcomes		
	Normal	**Minor Deficit[†] or Death**	**Major Deficit**
Major stroke (18 cases)			
No Rx or APT	0/13	1/13	12/13
Anticoagulant	1/4	2/4	1/4
Surgery	0	1/1	0
Single TIA or minor stroke (45 cases)			
No Rx or APT	15/17	2/17	0
Anticoagulant	14/16	1/16	1/16
Surgery	6/12	5/12	1/12
Multiple TIA (15 cases)			
No Rx or APT	6/6	0	0
Anticoagulant	5/5	0	0
Surgery	3/4	1/4	0
Other (pain, tinnitus) (22 cases)			
No Rx or APT	18/20	1/20	1/20
Anticoagulant	2/2	0	0
Surgery	0	0	0
Total (in %)	70%	14%	16%

*Major complaint on presentation to physician, not necessarily the initial symptom.
[†]Nondisabling deficit; residual Horner's syndrome considered normal.
APT, antiplatelet therapy; Rx, medical therapy; TIA, transient ischemic attack.
Data from 100 cases from English language literature since 1975 on extracranial carotid artery dissection. Data from Hart RG, Easton JD: Dissections of cervical and cerebral arteries. Neurol Clin 1:155, 1993, plus references 85, 259–262.

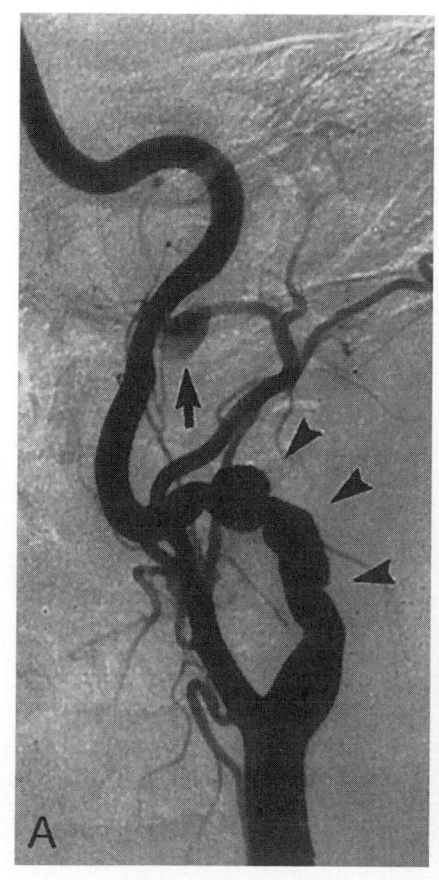
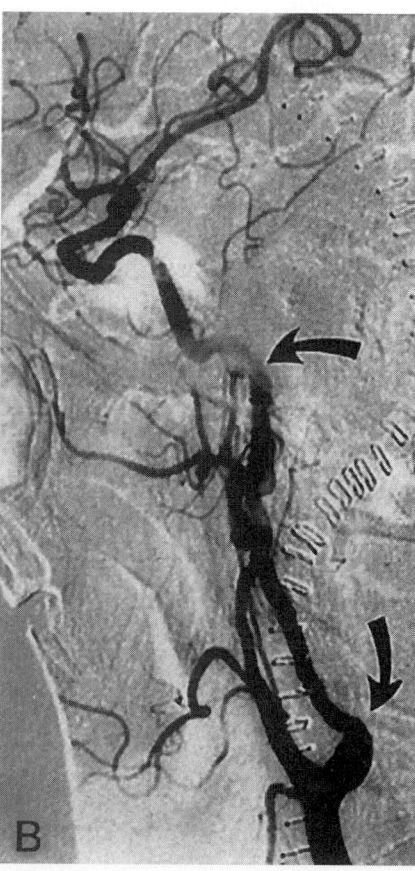

FIGURE 23–19 *A, A lateral left common carotid angiogram reveals a spontaneous dissecting aneurysm (arrow) of the internal carotid artery and evidence of fibromuscular dysplasia (arrowheads). B, A lateral left common carotid angiogram obtained after resection of the abnormal segment of artery and reconstruction with an interposition saphenous vein graft; arrows indicate the location of the anastomoses. (From Schievink WI: Spontaneous dissection of the carotid and vertebral arteries. N Engl J Med 344:898, 2001.)*

85% of patients.[26,105,106,244] Mortality is less than 5%,[116] and significant neurologic deficits persist in only 5% to 10% of patients.[26,105] Neurologic outcome is less favorable in patients with carotid artery occlusion,[132,245,246] traumatic dissections,[244] or intracranial dissection,[14,247] especially when it is associated with subarachnoid hemorrhage.[28,143,248] For example, 50% of survivors of intracranial carotid artery dissection have major residual deficits.[11,14,247] The prognosis of basilar artery dissection is particularly poor, with mortality exceeding 60%.[249] The risk of recurrent stroke more than 2 weeks after the diagnosis of dissection is exceedingly low (0.4% per year), being highest in the first year.[134] Persistent recurrent headaches or neck pain is not uncommon and tends to occur more commonly in patients with traumatic dissections.[26,244,250]

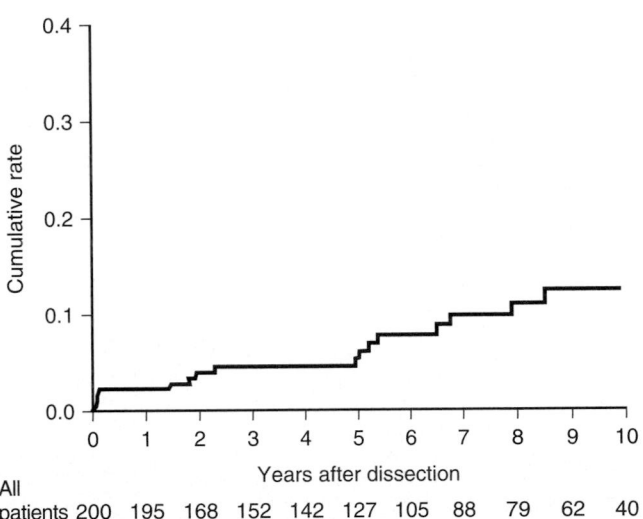

All patients   200   195   168   152   142   127   105   88   79   62   40

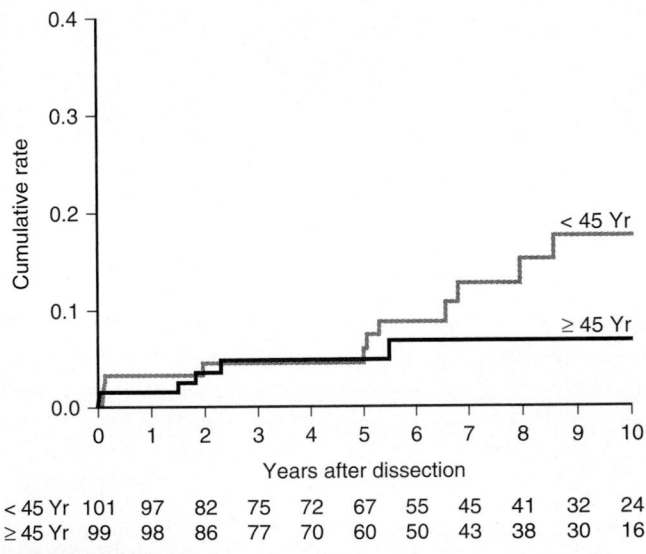

< 45 Yr	101	97	82	75	72	67	55	45	41	32	24
≥ 45 Yr	99	98	86	77	70	60	50	43	38	30	16

FIGURE 23–20 *Cumulative rate of recurrent arterial dissection in all patients* (upper panel) *and according to age* (lower panel). *The numbers shown below each panel are the numbers of patients at risk for recurrent dissection at each point. (From Schievink WI, Mokri B, O'Fallon M: Recurrent spontaneous cervical artery dissection. N Engl J Med 330:393, 1994.)*

Recurrent dissection in a previously involved artery is rare,[3–5,132,251] whereas the risk of recurrence in a previously uninvolved artery is low but not insignificant. Schievink and colleagues[3] reported a 2% recurrence risk in the first month with a 1% annual risk thereafter, and other series have reported similar figures, with equal rates for carotid and vertebral dissections.[4,5,19] In the Schievink series, risk declined with advancing age; the 10-year recurrence rate was 17% for patients younger than 45 years, and only 6% for patients older than 45 years (Fig. 23–20).[3] A family history of arterial dissection increased the risk of recurrence 6 times.[75] Presence of an underlying arteriopathy likewise raises the risk of recurrence.[4,5]

The angiographic prognosis of cervicocephalic dissection is favorable, although no correlation between angiographic and clinical prognosis has been found.[106,252] Angiographic stenoses improve or resolve in 80% to 90% of cases, with the rate of complete resolution averaging approximately 50% to 60% in published series.[26,105,106,175,177,191,244,252] Arterial occlusions recanalize in more than half of cases.[105,106,132,175,177,244] Complete resolution is seen in more than 20% of dissecting aneurysms,[105,174,177,191,244,253,254] and resolution or improvement in approximately 50%.[105,174,177,191,244,252,254] Angiographic improvement occurs within the first 2 to 3 months after the dissection and is rare after 6 months.[18,19,106,121,132,180,183,205] Persistent dissecting aneurysms do not rupture.[10,174,253]

References

1. Chan MT, Nadareishvili ZG, Norris JW: Diagnostic strategies in young patients with ischemic stroke in Canada. Can J Neurol Sci 27:120, 2000.
2. Giroud M, Fayolle H, Andre N, et al: Incidence of internal carotid artery dissection in the community of Dijon. J Neurol Neurosurgery Psychiatry 57:1443, 1994.
3. Schievink WI, Mokri B, O'Fallon M: Recurrent spontaneous cervical artery dissection. N Engl J Med 330:393, 1994.
4. Leys D, Moulin T, Stojkovic T, et al: Follow-up of patients with history of cervical artery dissection. Cerebrovasc Dis 4:43, 1995.
5. Bassetti C, Carruzzo A, Sturzenegger M, et al: Recurrence of cervical artery dissection: A prospective study of 81 patients. Stroke 27:1804, 1996.
6. Ducrocq X, Lacour JC, Debouverie M, et al: Accidents vasculaires cérébraux ischemiques du sujet jeune: Étude prospective de 296 patients ages 16 à 45 ans. Rev Neurol (Paris) 155:575, 1999.
7. Bogousslavsky J, Pierre P: Ischemic stroke in patients under age 45. Neurol Clin 10:113, 1992.
8. Gautier JC, Pradat-Diehl P, Loron P, et al: Accidents vasculaires cérébraux des sujets jeunes: Une étude de 133 patients age de 9 à 45 ans. Rev Neurol (Paris) 145:437, 1989.
9. Lisovoski F, Rousseaux P: Cerebral infarction in young people: A study of 148 patients with early cerebral angiography. J Neurol Neurosurgery Psychiatry 54:576, 1991.
10. Schievink WI, Mokri B, Jackers G: Spontaneous dissections of cervicocephalic arteries in childhood and adolescence. Neurology 44:1607, 1994.
11. Fullerton HJ, Johnston SC, Smith WS: Arterial dissection and stroke in children. Neurology 57:1155, 2001.
12. Leys D, Lucas C, Govert M, et al: Cervical artery dissections. Eur Neurol 37:3, 1997.
13. Hart RG, Easton JD: Dissections of cervical and cerebral arteries. Neurol Clin 1:155, 1983.
14. Bassetti C, Bogousslavsky J, Eskenasy-Cottier AC, et al: Spontaneous intracranial dissection in the anterior circulation. Cerebrovasc Dis 4:170, 1994.
15. Caplan LR, Zarins CK, Hemmat M: Spontaneous dissection of the extracranial vertebral arteries. Stroke 16:1030, 1996.

16. Hinse P, Thie A, Lachenmayer L: Dissection of the extracranial vertebral artery: Report of four cases and review of the literature. J Neurol Neurosurgery Psychiatry 54:853, 1991.

17. Bertram M, Ringleb P, Fieback J, et al: Das spectrum neurologischer symptome bei dissektionen hirnversorgender Arterien. Dtsch Med Wochensch 124:273, 1999.

18. Schievink WI: Spontaneous dissection of the carotid and vertebral arteries. N Engl J Med 344:898, 2001.

19. Saver JL, Easton JD: Dissections and trauma of cervicocerebral arteries. In Barnett HJM, Mohr JP, Stein BM, et al (eds): Stroke: Pathophysiology, Diagnosis and Management, 3rd ed. New York, Churchill Livingstone, 1998, p 769.

20. Caplan LR, Baquis GD, Pessin MS, et al: Dissection of the intracranial vertebral artery. Neurology 38:868, 1988.

21. Kawaguchi S, Sakaki T, Tsunoda S: Management of dissecting aneurysms of the posterior circulation. Acta Neurochir (Wien) 131:26, 1994.

22. Kitanaka C, Sasaki T, Eguchi T, et al: Intracranial vertebral artery dissections: Clinical, radiological features and surgical considerations. Neurosurgery 34:620, 1994.

23. Sasaki O, Ogawa H, Koike T, et al: A clinicopathologic study of dissecting aneurysms of the intracranial vertebral artery. J Neurosurg 75:874, 1991.

24. Bogousslavsky J: Dissections of the cerebral arteries clinical effects. Curr Opin Neurol Neurosurg 1:63, 1988.

25. Schievink WI: The treatment of spontaneous carotid and vertebral artery dissections. Curr Opin Cardiol 15:318, 2000.

26. Mokri B, Sundt TM, Houser OW, et al: Spontaneous dissection of the cervical internal carotid artery. Ann Neurol 19:126, 1986.

27. Berger M.S, Wilson CB: Intracranial dissecting aneurysms of the posterior circulation. Neurosurgery 61:882, 1984.

28. Friedman AH, Drake CG: Subarachnoid hemorrhage from intracranial dissecting aneurysm. J Neurosurg 60:325, 1984.

29. Halbach VV, Higashida R, Dowd CF, et al: Endovascular treatment of vertebral artery dissections and pseudoaneurysms. J Neurosurg 79:183, 1993.

30. Shimoji T, Bando K, Nakajima K, et al: Dissecting aneurysm of the vertebral artery: Report of seven cases and angiographic findings. J Neurosurg 61:1038, 1984.

31. Tsukahara T, Wada H, Satake K, et al: Proximal balloon occlusion for dissecting vertebral aneurysms accompanied by subarachnoid hemorrhage. Neurosurgery 36:914, 1995.

32. Beatty RA: Dissecting hematoma of the internal carotid artery following chiropractic manipulation. J Trauma 17:248, 1977.

33. Haldeman S, Kohlbeck F, McGregor M: Risk factors for vertebrobasilar artery dissection following cervical spine manipulation: A review of 60 cases. Neurology 46:A440, 1996.

34. Lee KP, Carlini WG, McCormick GF, et al: Neurologic complications following chiropractic manipulation: A survey of California neurologists. Neurology 45:1213, 1995.

35. Norris JW, Beletsky V, Nadareishvili ZG, et al: Sudden neck movement and cervical artery dissection. CMA J 163:38, 2000.

36. Haldeman S, Carey P, Murray T, et al: Arterial dissections following cervical manipulation: The chiropractic experience. CMA J 165:905, 2001.

37. Hufnagel A, Hammers A, Schonle PW, et al: Stroke following chiropractic manipulation of the cervical spine. J Neurol 246:683, 1999.

38. Mas JL, Henin O, Bousser MG, et al: Dissecting aneurysms of the vertebral artery and cervical manipulation: A case report with autopsy. Neurology (NY) 39:512, 1989.

39. Peters M, Bohl J, Thomke F, et al: Dissection of the internal carotid artery after chiropractic manipulation of the neck. Neurology 45:2284, 1995.

40. Rothwell DM, Bondy SJ, Williams JI: Chiropractic manipulation and stroke: A population-based case-control study. Stroke 32:1054, 2001.

41. Gould DB, Cunningham BS: Internal carotid artery dissection after remote surgery: Iatrogenic complications of anesthesia. Stroke 25:1276, 1994.

42. Schievink WI, Atkinson JLD, Bartleson JD, et al: Traumatic internal carotid dissections caused by blunt softball injuries. Am J Emerg Med 16:179, 1998.

43. Marks RL, Freed MM: Non-penetrating injuries of the neck in cerebrovascular accident. Arch Neurol 28:412, 1973.

44. Schneider RC, Gosch HH, Norell H, et al: Vascular insufficiency and differential distortion of the brain and spinal cord caused by cervical medullary football injuries. J Neurosurg 33:363, 1970.

45. Schneider RC: Serious and fatal neurosurgical football injuries. Clin Neurosurg 12:226, 1966.

46. Schneider RC, Gosch HH, Tareu JA, et al: Blood vessel trauma following head and neck injuries. Clin Neurosurg 19:312, 1972.

47. Ford FR: Syncope, vertigo, and disturbances of vision resulting from intermittent obstruction of the vertebral arteries due to deficit in the odontoid process and excessive mobility of the second cervical vertebrae. Johns Hopkins Med J 598:37, 1956.

48. Rogers L, Sweeney PJ: Stroke: A neurologic complication of wrestling. Am J Sports Med 7:352, 1979.

49. Vickers A, Zollman C: The manipulative therapies: Osteopathy and chiropractic. BMJ 319:1176, 1999.

50. Schievink WI, Mokri B, Piepgras DG, et al: Cervical artery dissections associated with chiropractic manipulation of the neck: The importance of pre-existing arterial disease and injury. J Neurol 243(Suppl 2):S92, 1996.

51. Fisher CM, Ojemann RG, Robertson GH: Spontaneous dissection of cervicocerebral arteries. Can J Neurol Sci 5:9, 1978.

52. Ringel SP, Harrison SH, Norenberg MD, et al: Fibromuscular dysplasia: Multiple "spontaneous" dissecting aneurysms of the major cervical arteries. Ann Neurol 1:301, 1977.

53. Schievink WI, Bjornsson J, Piepgras DG: Coexistence of fibromuscular dysplasia and cystic medial necrosis in a patient with Marfan's syndrome and bilateral carotid artery dissection. Stroke 25:2492, 1994.

54. Schievink WI, Michels VV, Piepgras DG: Neurovascular manifestations of heritable connective tissue disorders—a review. Stroke 25:889, 1994.

55. Schievink WI, Mokri B, Piepgras DG: Fibromuscular dysplasia of the internal carotid artery associated with alpha-1-antitrypsin deficiency. Neurosurgery 43:229, 1998.

56. Stanley JC, Fry WJ, Seeger JF, et al: Extracranial internal carotid and vertebral artery fibrodysplasia. Arch Surg 109:215, 1974.

57. Schievink WI, Wijdicks EFM, Michels VV, et al: Heritable connective tissue disorders in cervical artery dissections: A prospective study. Neurology 50:1166, 1998.

58. North KN, Whiteman DAH, Pepin MG, et al: Cerebrovascular complications in Ehlers-Danlos syndrome type IV. Ann Neurol 38:960, 1995.

59. Schievink WI, Limburg M, Dorthuys JE, et al: Cerebrovascular disease in Ehlers-Danlos syndrome type IV. Stroke 21:626, 1990.

60. Austin MG, Schaefer RF: Marfan's syndrome, with unusual blood vessel manifestations. Arch Pathol Lab Med 64:205, 1957.

61. Youl BD, Coutellier A, Dubois B, et al: Three cases of spontaneous extracranial vertebral artery dissection. Stroke 21:618, 1990.

62. Mokri B, Sundt TM Jr, Houser OW: Spontaneous internal carotid dissection, hemicrania, and Horner's syndrome. Arch Neurol 36:677, 1979.

63. Mayer SA, Rubin BS, Starman BJ, et al: Spontaneous multivessel cervical artery dissection in a patient with a substitution of alanine for glycine (G13A) in the alpha 1 (I) chain of type I collagen. Neurology 47:552, 1996.

64. Schievink WI, Prakash UBS, Piepgras DG. et al: Alpha 1-antitrypsin deficiency in intracranial aneurysms and cervical artery dissection. Lancet 343:452, 1994.

65. Brice JG, Crompton MR: Spontaneous dissecting aneurysms of the cervical internal carotid artery. BMJ 2:790, 1964.

66. Yuasa H, Tokito S, Izumi K, et al: Cerebrovascular moyamoya disease associated with an intracranial pseudoaneurysm. J Neurosurg 56:131, 1982.

67. Yamashita M, Tanaka K, Matsuo T, et al: Cerebral dissecting aneurysms in patients with moyamoya disease. J Neurosurg 58:120, 1983.

68. Adelman LS, Doe FD, Samat HB: Bilateral dissecting aneurysms of the internal carotid arteries. Acta Neuropathol 29:93, 1974.

69. Barbour PJ, Castaldo JE, Rae-Grant AD, et al: Internal carotid artery redundancy is signficantly associated with dissection. Stroke 25:1201, 1994.

70. Ben Hamouda-M'Rad I, Biousse V, Bousser MG, et al: Internal carotid artery redundancy is significantly associated with dissection. Stroke 26:1962, 1995.

71. Guillon B, Tzourio C, Biousse V, et al: Arterial wall properties in carotid artery dissection: An ultrasound study. Neurology 55:663, 2000.

72. Tzourio C, Cohen A, Lamisse N, et al: Aortic root dilatation in patients with spontaneous cervical artery dissection. Circulation 95:2351, 1997.

Specific Medical Diseases and Stroke

73. Schievink WI, Mokri B, Michels VV, et al: Familial association of intracranial aneurysms and cervical artery dissections. Stroke 22:1426, 1991.
74. Schievink WI, Mokri B, Piepgras DG: Angiographic frequency of saccular intracranial aneurysms in patients with spontaneous cervical artery dissection. J Neurosurg 76:62, 1992.
75. Schievink WI, Mokri B, Piepgras DG, et al: Recurrent spontaneous arterial dissections: Risk in familial versus nonfamilial disease. Stroke 27:622, 1996.
76. D'Anglejean-Chatillon J, Ribeiro V, Mas JL, et al: Migraine—a risk factor for dissection of cervical arteries. Headache 29:560, 1989.
77. Fisher CM: The headache and pain of spontaneous carotid dissection. Headache 22:60, 1982.
78. Grau AJ, Brandt T, Forsting M, et al: Infection-associated cervical artery dissection: Three cases. Stroke 28:453, 1997.
79. Grau AJ, Brandt T, Buggle F, et al: Association of cervical artery dissection with recent infection. Arch Neurol 56:851, 1999.
80. Constantinescu CS: Association of varicella-zoster virus with cervical artery dissection in 2 cases [letter]. Arch Neurol 57:427, 2000.
81. Wiebers DO, Mokri B: Internal carotid artery dissection after childbirth. Stroke 16:956, 1985.
82. Mas JL, Bousser MG, Corone P, et al: Dissecting aneurysm of the extracranial vertebral arteries and pregnancy. Rev Neurol (Paris) 143:761, 1987.
83. Gallai V, Caso V, Paciaroni M, et al: Mild hyperhomocyst(e)inemia: A possible risk factor for cervical artery dissection. Stroke 32:714, 2001.
84. Pezzini A, Del Zotto E, Archetti S, et al: Plasma homocysteine concentration, C677T *MTHFR* genotype, and 844ins68bp *CBS* genotype in young adults with spontaneous cervical artery dissection and atherothrombotic stroke. Stroke 33:664, 2002.
85. Mas JL, Goeau C, Bousser MG, et al: Spontaneous dissecting aneurysms of the internal carotid and vertebral arteries—two case reports. Stroke 16:125, 1985.
86. Mas JL, Bousser MG, Hasboun D, et al: Extracranial vertebral artery dissections: A review of 13 cases. Stroke 18:1037, 1987.
87. Schievink WI, Michels VV, Piepgras DG, et al: A familial syndrome of arterial dissections with lentiginosis. N Engl J Med 332:579, 1995.
88. Schievink WI, Mokri B: Familial aorto-cervicocephalic arterial dissections and congenitally bicuspid aortic valve. Stroke 26:1935, 1995.
89. Brandt T, Hausser I, Orberk E, et al: Ultrastructural connective tissue abnormalities in patients with spontaneous cervicocerebral artery dissections. Ann Neurol 44:281, 1998.
90. Brandt T, Orberk E, Weber R, et al: Pathogenesis of cervical artery dissections: Association with connective tissue abnormalities. Neurology 57:24, 2001.
91. Dunac A, Blecic S, Jeangette S, et al: Stroke due to artery dissection: Role of collagen disease. Cerebrovasc Dis 8(Suppl 4):18, 1998.
92. Brandt T, Grond-Ginsbach C: Spontaneous cervical artery dissection: From risk factors toward pathogenesis [editorial]. Stroke 33:657, 2002.
93. Grond-Ginsbach C, Weber R, Hausser I, et al: Familial connective tissue alterations in patients with spontaneous cervical artery dissections. Cerebrovasc Dis 10(Suppl 2):37, 2000.
94. Grond-Ginsbach C, Weber R, Haas J, et al: Mutations in the COL5A1 coding sequence are not common in patients with cervical artery dissections. Stroke 30:1887, 1999.
95. Kiuvaniemi H, Prockop DJ, Wu Y, et al: Exclusion of mutations in the gene for type III collagen (COL3A1) as a common cause of intracranial aneurysms or cervical artery dissections: Results from sequence analysis of the coding sequences of type III collagen from 55 unrelated patients. Neurology 43:2652, 1993.
96. van den Berg JS, Limburg M, Kappelle LJ, et al: The role of type III collagen in spontaneous cervical arterial dissections. Ann Neurol 43:494, 1998.
97. Grond-Ginsbach C, Thomas-Feles C, Weber R, et al: Mutations in the tropoelastine gene (ELN) were not found in patients with spontaneous cervical artery dissection. Stroke 31:1935, 2000.
98. Guillon B, Levy C, Bousser MG: Internal carotid artery dissection: An update. J Neurol Sci 153:146, 1998.
99. Pelkonen O, Tikkakoski T, Leinonen S, et al: Intracranial arterial dissection. Neuroradiology 40:442, 1998.
100. Frisoni GB, Anzola GP: Vertebrobasilar ischemia after neck motion. Stroke 22:1452, 1991.
101. Josien E: Extracranial vertebral artery dissection: Nine cases. J Neurol 239:327, 1992.
102. Bin Saeed A, Shuaib A, Al-Sulaiti G, et al: Vertebral artery dissection: Warning symptoms, clinical features and prognosis in 26 patients. Can J Neurol Sci 27:292, 2000.
103. Salari-Namin HR. Cohen SN: Management of Ischemic Stroke. New York, McGraw-Hill, 2000.
104. Manz HJ, Vester J, Laenstein B: Dissecting aneurysm of cerebral arteries in childhood and adolescence. Virchows Arch 384:325, 1979.
105. Mokri B, Houser OW, Sandock BA, et al: Spontaneous dissection of the vertebral arteries. Neurology 38:880, 1988.
106. Desfontaines P, Despland A: Dissection of the internal carotid artery: Aetiology, symptomatology, clinical and neurosonological follow-up and treatment in 60 consecutive cases. Acta Neurol Psych Belg 94:226, 1991.
107. Weiller C, Mullges W, Ringelstein EB, et al: Patterns of brain infarction in internal carotid artery dissections. Neurosurg Rev 14:111, 1991.
108. Steinke W, Schwartz A, Hennerici M: Topography of cerebral infarction associated with carotid artery dissection. J Neurol 243:323, 1996.
109. Lucas C, Moulin T, Deplanque D, et al: Stroke patterns of internal carotid artery dissection in 40 patients. Stroke 29:2646, 1998.
110. Baumgartner RW, Arnold M, Baumgartner I, et al: Carotid dissection with and without ischemic events: Local symptoms and cerebral artery findings. Neurology 57:827, 2001.
111. Srinivasan J, Newell DW, Sturzenegger M, et al: Transcranial Doppler in the evaluation of internal carotid artery dissection: Demonstration of a correlation between microemboli detected by transcranial doppler and stroke. Usefulness of this technique for the evaluation of anticoagulation efficacy. Stroke 27:1226, 1996.
112. Ast G, Woimant F, Georges B, et al: Spontaneous dissection of the internal carotid artery in 68 patients. Eur J Med 2:466, 1993.
113. Biousse V, D'Anglejean-Chatillon J, Touboul P-J, et al: Time course of symptoms in extracranial carotid artery dissections. Stroke 26:235, 1995.
114. Cox LK, Bertorini T, Laster RE: Headaches due to spontaneous internal carotid artery dissection. Headache 31:12, 1991.
115. Early TF, Gregory RT, Wheeler JR, et al: Spontaneous carotid dissection: Duplex scanning in diagnosis and management. J Vasc Surg 14:391, 1991.
116. Mokri B: Spontaneous dissections of internal carotid arteries. Neurologist 3:104, 1997.
117. Mullges W, Ringelstein EB, Leibold M: Non-invasive diagnosis of internal carotid artery dissections. J Neurol Neurosurg Psychiatry 55:98, 1992.
118. Ramadan NM, Tietjen GE, Levine SR, et al: Scintillating scotomata associated with internal carotid artery dissection. Neurology 41:1084, 1991.
119. Silbert PL, Mokri B, Schievink WI: Headache and neck pain in spontaneous internal carotid and vertebral artery dissections. Neurology 45:1517, 1995.
120. Sue DE, Brant-Zawadzki MN, Chance J: Dissection of cranial arteries in the neck: Correlation of MRI and arteoriography. Neuroradiology 34:273, 1992.
121. Sturzenegger M: Spontaneous internal carotid artery dissection: Early diagnosis and management in 44 patients. J Neurol 242:231, 1995.
122. Biousse V, D'Anglejean-Chatillon J, Touboul PJ, et al: Head pain in non-traumatic carotid artery dissections. Cephalgia 14:33, 1994.
123. Mokri B, Silbert PL, Schievink WI, et al: Cranial nerve palsy in spontaneous internal carotid and vertebral artery dissections. Neurology 46:356, 1996.
124. Francis KR, Williams DP, Troost BT: Facial numbness and dysesthesia: New features of carotid artery dissection. Arch Neurol 44:345, 1987.
125. Goodman JM, Zink WL, Cooper DF: Hemilingual paralysis caused by carotid artery dissection. Arch Neurol 40:653, 1983.
126. Guidetti D, Pisanello A, Giovanardi F, et al: Spontaneous carotid dissection presenting lower cranial nerve palsies. J Neurol Sci 184:203, 2001.
127. Panisset, M, Eidelman BH: Multiple cranial neuropathy as a feature of internal carotid artery dissection. Stroke 21:141, 1990.

128. Sturzenegger M, Huber P: Cranial nerve palsies in spontaneous carotid artery dissection. J Neurol Neurosurg Psychiatry 56:1191, 1993.

129. Waespe W, Niesper J, Imhof HG, et al: Lower cranial nerve palsies due to internal carotid dissection. Stroke 19:1561, 1988.

130. Gout O, Bonnaud I, Weill A, et al: Facial diplegia complicating a bilateral internal carotid artery dissection. Stroke 30:681, 1999.

131. Martin PJ, Humphrey PRD: Disabling stroke arising five months after internal carotid artery dissection. J Neurol Neurosurg Psychiatry 65:136, 1998.

132. Bogousslavsky J, Despland PA, Regli F: Spontaneous carotid dissection with acute stroke. Arch Neurol 44:137, 1987.

133. Rao TH, Schneider LB, Patel M, et al: Stroke 25:1271, 1994.

134. Saver JL, Easton JD: Dissections and trauma of cervicocerebral arteries. In Barnett HJM, Mohr JP, Stein BM, et al (eds): Stroke: Pathophysiology, Diagnosis and Management, 3rd ed. New York, Churchill Livingstone, 1998, p. 769.

135. Pozzati E, Galassi E, Godano U, et al: Regressing intracranial carotid occlusions in childhood. Pediatr Neurosurg 21:243, 1994.

136. Chang V, Rewcastle NB, Harwood-Nash DCF, et al: Bilateral dissecting aneurysms of the intracranial internal carotids in an 8-year-old boy. Neurology (NY) 25:573, 1975.

137. Nass R, Hays A, Chutorian A: Intracranial dissecting aneurysms in childhood. Stroke 13:204, 1982.

138. Adams HPJ, Aschenbrener CA, Kassell NF, et al: Intracranial hemorrhage produced by spontaneous dissecting intracranial aneurysm. Arch Neurol 39:773, 1982.

139. de Bray JM, Pennison-Besnier L, Dubas F, et al: Extracranial and intracranial vertebrobasilar dissections: Diagnosis and prognosis. J Neurol Neurosurg Psychiatry 63:46, 1977.

140. Provenzale JM, Morgenlander JC, Gress D: Spontaneous vertebral dissection: Clinical, conventional angiographic, CT, and MR findings. J Comput Assist Tomogr 20:185, 1996.

141. Takis C, Saver JL: Cerebrovascular Disease. Philadelphia, Lippincott-Raven, 1997, p 386.

142. Chiras J, Marciano S, Vega Molina J, et al: Spontaneous dissecting aneurysm of the extracranial vertebral artery (20 cases). Neuroradiology 27:327, 1985.

143. Caplan LR, Zarins CK, Hemmati M: Spontaneous dissection of the extracranial vertebral arteries. Stroke 16:1030, 1985.

144. de Bray JM, Pennison-Besnier I, Giroud M: Radiculopathie cervicale déficitaire au cours de trios cas de dissection de l'artère vertebrale. Rev Neurol (Paris) 154:762, 1998.

145. Crum B, Mokri B, Fulgham J: Spinal manifestations of vertebral artery dissection. Neurology 55:304, 2000.

146. Weidauer S, Claus D, Gartenschlager M: Spinal sulcal artery syndrome due to spontaneous bilateral vertebral artery dissection. J Neurol Neurosurg Psychiatry 67:550, 1999.

147. Goldsmith P, Rowe D, Jager R, et al: Focal vertebral artery dissection causing Brown-Sequard's syndrome. J Neurol Neurosurg Psychiatry 64:415, 1998.

148. Adams HPJ, Aschenbrener CA, Kassell NF, et al: Intracranial hemorrhage produced by spontaneous dissecting aneurysms of the internal carotid arteries. Acta Neuropathol 29:93, 1974.

149. Alexander CB, Burger PC, Goree JA: Dissecting aneurysms of the basilar artery in two patients. Stroke 10:294, 1979.

150. Farrell MA, Gilbert JJ, Kaufmann JC: Fatal intracranial arterial dissection: Clinical pathological correlation. J Neurol Neurosurg Psychiatry 48:111, 1985.

151. Arunodaya GR, Vani S, Shankar SK, et al: Fibromuscular dysplasia with dissection of basilar artery presenting as "locked-in-syndrome." Neurology 48:1605, 1997.

152. Berkovic SF, Spokes RL, Anderson RM, et al: Basilar artery dissection. J Neurol Neurosurg Psychiatry 46:126, 1983.

153. Brihaye J, Retif J, Jeanmart L: L'obstruction de l'artère basilaire chez le sujet jeune. Acta Neurochir 24:143, 1971.

154. Woimant F, Spelle L: Spontaneous basilar artery dissection: Contribution of magnetic resonance imaging to diagnosis. J Neurol Neurosurg Psychiatry 58:540, 1995.

155. Campiche PR, Anzil AP, Zander E: Aneurysme disséquant de tronc basilaire. Arch Suisse Neurol Neurochir Psychiatr 104:209, 1969.

156. Crosato F, Terzian H: Gli aneurismi dissecanti intracranici. Riv Pat Nerv Ment 82:450, 1961.

157. Escourolle R, Gautier JC, Rosa A, et al: Aneurysme disséquant vertébrobasilaire. Rev Neurol (Paris) 128:95, 1973.

158. Hayman JA, Anderson RM: Dissecting aneurysm of the basilar artery. Med J Aust 2:360, 1966.

159. Hosoda K, Fujita S, Kawaguchi T, et al: Spontaneous dissecting aneurysms of the basilar artery presenting with subarachnoid hemorrhage. J Neurosurg 75:628, 1991.

160. Hyland HH: Thrombosis of intracranial arteries. Arch Neurol Psychiatry 30:342, 1933.

161. Kulla L, Deymeer F, Smith TW, et al: Intracranial dissecting and saccular aneurysms in polycystic kidney disease. Arch Neurol 39:776, 1983.

162. Nozicka A: Zerebrovaskulare erkrankungen bei jungen leuten bedingt durch dissezierendes aneurysma der basalen hirnarterien. Hradec Kralove 25:225, 1972.

163. Pasquier B, Couderc P, Pasquier D, et al: Hemodissection parietale oblitérante ou anevrisme disséquant vertebro basilaire. Sem Hop Paris 52:2519, 1976.

164. Pasquier B, N'Golet A, Pasquier D, et al: Vertebro-basilar dissecting aneurysm. Sem Hop Paris 55:487, 1979.

165. Perier O, Cauchie G, Demanet JC: Hématome intramural par dissection parietale (aneurysme disséquant) du tronc basilaire. Acta Neurol Psych Belg 64:1064, 1964.

166. Perier O, Brihaye J, Dhaene R: Hemodissection parietale oblitérante (anevrisme disséquant) de l'artère basilaire. Acta Neurol Psych Belg 66:123, 1966.

167. Pozzati E, Andreoli A, Padovani R, et al: Dissecting aneurysms of the basilar artery. Neurosurgery 36:254, 1995.

168. Redondo-Marco JA, Walb D: Zur frage des aneurysma dissecans am intrakraniellen gefabsystem. Acta Neurochir 16:278, 1969.

169. Scholefield BG: A case of aneurysm of the basilar artery. Guys Hosp Rep 74:485, 1924.

170. Sekino H, Nakamura N, Katoh Y, et al: Dissecting aneurysms of the vertebro-basilar system: Clinical and angiographic observations. No Shinkei Geka 9:125, 1981.

171. Takita K, Shirato H, Akasaka T, et al: Dissecting aneurysm of the vertebro-basilar artery. No To Shinkei 31:1211, 1979.

172. Watson AJ: Dissecting aneurysm of arteries other than the aorta. J Pathol Bacteriol 72:439, 1956.

173. Wolman L: Cerebral dissecting aneurysms. Brain 82:276, 1958.

174. Djouhri H, Guillon B, Brunereau L, et al: MR angiography for the long-term follow-up of dissecting aneurysms of the extracranial internal carotid artery. AJR Am J Roentgenol 174:1137, 2000.

175. Kasner SE, Hankins LL, Bratina P, et al: Magnetic resonance angiography demonstrates vascular healing of carotid and vertebral artery dissections. Stroke 28:1993, 1997.

176. Kirsch EC, Kaim A, Engelter ST, et al: MR angriography in internal carotid artery dissection: Improvement of diagnosis by selective demonstration of the intramural hematoma. Neuroradiology 40:704, 1998.

177. Leclerc X, Lucas C, Godefroy O, et al: Preliminary experience using contrast-enhanced MRI angiography to assess vertebral artery structure for the follow-up of suspected dissection. Am J Neuroradiol 20:1482, 1999.

178. Provenzale JM: Dissection of the internal carotid and vertebral arteries: Imaging features. AJR Am J Roentgenol 165:1099, 1995.

179. Levy C, Laissy JP, Raveau V, et al: Carotid and vertebral artery dissections: Three dimensional time-of-flight MR angiography and MR imaging versus conventional angiography. Radiology 190:97, 1994.

180. Jacobs A, Lanfermann H, Neveling M, et al: MRI and MRA-guided therapy of carotid and vertebral artery dissection. J Neurol Sci 39:329, 1997.

181. Mascalchi M, Bianchi MC, Mangiafico S, et al: MRI and MRI angiography of vertebral artery dissection. Neuroradiology 39:329, 1997.

182. de Bray JM, Lhoste P, Dubas F, et al: Ultrasonic features of extracranial carotid dissections: 47 cases studied by angiography. J Ultrasound Med 13:659, 1994.

183. Sturzenegger M, Mattle HP, Rivoir A, et al: Ultrasound findings in carotid artery dissection: Analysis of 43 patients. Neurology 45:691, 1995.

184. Hoffman M, Sacco RL, Chan S, et al: Noninvasive detection of vertebral artery dissection. Stroke 24:815, 1993.

185. Sturzenegger M, Mattle HP, Rivoir A, et al: Ultrasound findings in spontaneous extracranial vertebral artery dissection. Stroke 24:1910, 1993.

186. Steinke W, Rautenberg W, Schwartz A, et al: Noninvasive monitoring of internal carotid artery dissection. Stroke 25:998, 1994.

187. Hennerici M, Steinke W, Rautenberg W: High-resistance Doppler flow pattern in extracranial carotid dissection. Arch Neurol 46:670, 1989.

188. Baumgartner RW, Baumgartner I, Mattle HP, et al: Transcranial color-coded duplex sonography in the evaluation of collateral flow through the circle of Willis. Am J Neuroradiol 18:127, 1997.

189. Leclerc X, Godefrey O, Pruvo JP, et al: Computed tomographic angiography for the evaluation of carotid artery stenosis. Stroke 26:1577, 1995.

190. Fredenberg P, Forbes K, Toye L, et al: Assessment of cervical vascular injury with CT angiography. BNI Q 17:44, 2001.

191. Houser OW, Mokri B, Sundt TM Jr, et al: Spontaneous cervical cephalic arterial dissection and its residuum: Angiographic spectrum. Am J Neuroradiol 5:27, 1984.

192. Lu C-J, Sun Y, Jeng J-S, et al: Imaging in the diagnosis and follow-up evaluation of vertebral artery dissection. J Ultrasound Med 19:263, 2000.

193. Rothrock JF, Lim V, Press G, et al: Serial magnetic resonance and carotid duplex examinations in the management of carotid dissection. Neurology (NY) 39:686, 1989.

194. Provenzale JM, Barboriak DP, Taveras JM: Exercise-related dissection of craniocervical arteries: CT, MR, and angiographic findings. J Comput Assist Tomogr 19:268, 1995.

195. Scazzeri F, Mascalchi M, Calabrese R, et al: Case report: MRI and MR angiography of basilar artery dissection in a child. Neuroradiology 39:654, 1997.

196. Stapf C, Elkind SV, Mohr JP: Carotid artery dissection. Annu Rev Med 51:329, 2001.

197. Silverboard G, Tart R: Cerebrovascular arterial dissection in children and young adults. Semin Pediatr Neurol 7:278, 2000.

198. Brugieres P, Castrec-Carpo A, Heran F, et al: Magnetic resonance imaging in the exploration of dissection of the internal carotid artery. J Neuroradiol 16:1, 1989.

199. Gelbert F, Assouline E, Hodes JE, et al: MRI in spontaneous dissection of vertebral and carotid arteries. Neuroradiology 33:111, 1991.

200. Hart RG: Vertebral artery dissection. Neurology (NY) 38:987, 1988.

201. Quint DJ, Spickler EM: Magnetic resonance imaging demonstration of vertebral artery dissection: Report of 2 cases. J Neurosurg 72:964, 1990.

202. Osborn AG, Anderson RE: Angiographic spectrum of cervical and intracranial fibromuscular dysplasia. Stroke 8:617, 1997.

203. Chiu N, DeLong GR, Heinz ER: Intracranial fibromuscular dysplasia in a 5-year-old child. Pediatr Neurol 14:262, 1996.

204. Mokri B, Houser OW, Stanson AW: Multivessel cervicocephalic and visceral arterial dissections: Pathogenic role of primary arterial disease in cervicocephalic arterial dissections. J Stroke Cerebrovasc Dis 1:117, 1991.

205. Treiman GS, Treima RL, Foran RF, et al: Spontaneous dissection of the internal carotid artery: A nineteen-year clinical experience. J Vasc Surg 24:597, 1996.

206. Schievink WI, Piepgras DG, McCaffrey TV, et al: Surgical treatment of extracranial internal carotid artery dissecting aneurysms. Neurosurgery 35:809, 1994.

207. Price RF, Sellar R, Leung C, et al: Traumatic vertebral arterial dissection and vertebrobasilar arterial thrombosis successfully treated with endovascular thrombolysis and stenting. Am J Neuroradiol 19:1677, 1998.

208. Derex L, Nighoghossian N, Turjman F, et al: Intravenous tPA in acute ischemic stroke related to internal carotid artery dissection. Neurology 54:2159, 2000.

209. Arnold M, Nedeltchev K, Sturzzenegger M, et al: Thrombolysis in patients with acute stroke caused by cervical artery dissection: Analysis of 9 patients and review of the literature. Arch Neurol 59:549, 2002.

210. Rudolf J, Neveling M, Grond M, et al: Stroke following internal carotid artery occlusion: A contraindication for intravenous thrombolysis. Eur J Neurol 6:51, 1999.

211. Sampognaro G, Turgut T, Connors JJ III, et al: Intra-arterial thrombolysis in a patient presenting with an ischemic stroke due to spontaneous internal carotid dissection. Cathet Cardiovasc Interv 48:312, 1999.

212. Ahmad HA, Gerraty RP, Davis SM, et al: Cervicocerebral artery dissections. J Accid Emerg Med 16:422, 1999.

213. Gomez CR, May AK, Terry JB, et al: Endovascular therapy of traumatic injuries of the extracranial cerebral arteries. Crit Care Clin 15:789, 1999.

214. Bejjani GK, Monsein LH, Laird JR, et al: Treatment of symptomatic cervical carotid dissections with endovascular stents. Neurosurgery 44:755, 1999.

215. Yadav JS, Roubin GS, Iyer S, et al: Elective stenting of the extracranial carotid arteries. Circulation 95:376, 1997.

216. Malek AM, Higashida RT, Phatouros CC, et al: Endovascular management of extracranial carotid artery dissection achieved using stent angioplasty. Am J Neuroradiol 21:1380, 2000.

217. Hemphill JC III, Gress DR, Halbach VV: Endovascular therapy of traumatic injuries of the intracranial cerebral arteries. Crit Care Clin 15:811, 1999.

218. Manninen HI, Koivisto T, Saari T, et al: Dissecting aneurysms of all four cervicocranial arteries in fibromuscular dysplasia: Treatment with self-expanding endovascular stents, coil, embolization, and surgical ligation. Am J Neuroradiol 18:1216, 1997.

219. Dorros G, Cohn JM, Palmer LE: Stent deployment resolves a petrous carotid artery angioplasty dissection. Am J Neuroradiol 19:392, 1998.

220. Horowitz MB, Miller G III, Meyer Y, et al: Use of intravascular stents in treatment of internal carotid and extracranial vertebral artery pseudoaneurysms. Am J Neuroradiol 17:693, 1996.

221. Perez-Cruet MJ, Patwardhan RV, Mawad ME, et al: Treatment of dissecting pseudoaneurysm of the cervical internal carotid artery using a wall stent and detachable coils: Case report. Neurosurgery 40:622, 1997.

222. Lenthall RK, White BD, McConachie NS: Endovascular management of complete vertebral artery dissection presenting with subarachnoid hemorrhage. Intervent Neuroradiol 5:161, 1999.

223. Siminonata F, Righi C, Scotti G: Post-traumatic dissecting aneurysm of extracranial internal carotid artery: Endovascular treatment with stenting. Neuroradiology 41:543, 1999.

224. Hurst RW, Haskal ZJ, Zager E, et al: Endovascular stent treatment of cervical internal carotid artery aneurysms with parent vessel preservation. Surg Neurol 40:313, 1998.

225. Singer RJ, Dake MD, Norbash A, et al: Covered stent placement for neurovascular disease. Am J Neuroradiol 18:507, 1996.

226. Hong MK, Satler LF, Gallino R, et al: Intravascular stenting as a definitive treatment of spontaneous carotid artery dissection. Am J Cardiol 79:538, 1997.

227. Matsuura JH, Rosenthall D, Jerius H, et al: Traumatic carotid artery dissection and pseudoaneurysm treated with endovascular coils and stent. J Endovasc Surg 4:339, 1997.

228. Mericle RA, Lanzino G, Wakhloo AK, et al: Stenting and secondary coiling of intracranial internal carotid artery aneursym: Technical case report. Neurosurgery 43:1229, 1998.

229. Klein GE, Szolar DH, Raith J, et al: Post-traumatic extracranial aneurysm of the internal carotid artery: Combined endovascular treatment with coils and stents. AJNR Am J Neuroradiol 18:1261, 1997.

230. Miyachi S, Ishiguchi T, Taniguchi K, et al: Endovascular stenting of a traumatic dissecting aneurysm of the extracranial internal carotid artery—a case report. Neurol Med Chir 37:270, 1997.

231. Yamashita M, Okamoto S, Kim C, et al: Emergent treatment of iatrogenic dissection of the internal carotid artery with the Palmaz-Shatz stent—case report. Neurol Med Chir 37:336, 1997.

232. DeOcampo J, Brillman,J, Levy DI: Stenting: A new approach to carotid dissection. J Neuroimag 7:187, 1997.

233. Scavee V, DeWispelaere JF, Mormont E, et al: Pseudoaneurysm of the internal carotid artery: Treatment with a covered stent. Cardiovasc Intervent Radiol 24:283, 2001.

234. Norris JW, Nadareishvili ZG, Rowe D, et al: Are the hazards of carotid stenting unacceptably high? Neurology 52(Suppl 2):A269, 1999.

235. Hobson RW II, Goldstein JE, Jamil Z, et al: Carotid restenosis: Operative and endovascular mangement. J Vasc Surg 29:228, 1999.

236. Vale FL, Fisher WS III, Jordan WD Jr, et al: Carotid endarterectomy performed after progressive carotid stenosis following angioplasty and stent placement: Case report. J Neurosurg 87:940, 1997.

237. Coumans JV, Watson VE, Picken CA, et al: Saphenous vein interposition graft for recurrent carotid stenosis after prior endarterectomy and stent placement: Case report. J Neurosurg 90:567, 1999.

238. Lyrer P, Engelter S: Antithrombotic drugs for carotid artery dissection (Cochrane Review). In: The Cochrane Library, Issue 2. Oxford: Update Software, 2003.

239. Painter TA, Hertzer NR, Beven EG, et al: Extracranial carotid aneurysms: Report of six cases and review of the literature. J Vasc Surg 2:312, 1985.

240. Sundt TM Jr, Pearson BW, Piepgras DG, et al: Surgical management of aneurysms of the distal extracranial internal carotid artery. J Neurosurg 64:169, 1986.

241. Coffin O, Maiza D, Galateau-Salle F, et al: Results of surgical management of internal carotid artery aneurysm by the cervical approach. Ann Vasc Surg 11:482, 1997.

242. Grubb RL, Derdeyn CP, Fritsch SM, et al: Importance of hemodynamic factors in the prognosis of symptomatic carotid occlusion. JAMA 280:1055, 1998.

243. Mokri B, Piepgras DG, Houser OW: Traumatic dissections of the extracranial internal carotid artery. J Neurosurg 68:189, 1988.

244. Mokri B: Traumatic and spontaneous extracranial internal carotid artery dissections. J Neurol 237:356, 1990.

245. Pozzati E, Giuliani G, Acciarri N, et al: Long-term follow-up of occlusive cervical carotid dissection. Stroke 21:528, 1990.

246. Milhaud K, de Freitas GR, van Melle G, et al: Occlusion due to carotid artery dissection. Arch Neurol 59:557, 2002.

247. de Bray JM, Pennison-Besnier L, Dubas F, et al: Extracranial and intracranial vertebrobasilar dissections: Diagnosis and prognosis. J Neurol Neurosurg Psychiatry 63:46, 1997.

248. Yamaura A, Ono J, Hirai S: Clinical picture of intracranial nontraumatic dissecting aneurysm. Neuropathology 1:85, 2000.

249. Saver JL, Easton JD, Hart RG: Dissections and trauma of cervicocerebral arteries. In Barnett HJM, Mohr JP, Stein BM, et al (eds): Stroke: Pathophysiology, Diagnosis and Management, 2nd ed. New York, Churchill Livingstone, 1992, p 67.

250. Arboix A, Massons J, Oliveres M, et al: Analisis de 1.000 pacientes consecutivos con enfermedad cerebrovascular aguda: Registro de patologia cerebrovascular de L'Alianza-Hospital Central de Barcelona. Med Clinic (Barc) 101:281, 1993.

251. Goldstein LB, Gray L, Hulette CM: Stroke due to recurrent ipsilateral carotid artery dissection in a young adult. Stroke 26:480, 1995.

252. Engelter ST, Lyrer PA, Kirsch EC, et al: Long-term follow-up after extracranial internal carotid artery dissection. Eur Neurol 44:199, 2000.

253. Guillon B, Brunereau L, Biousse V, et al: Long-term follow-up of aneurysms developed during extracranial internal carotid dissection. Neurology 53:117, 1999.

254. Touze E, Randoux B, Meary E, et al: Aneurysmal forms of cervical artery dissection: Associated factors and outcome. Stroke 32:418, 2001.

255. Benoit BG, Russell NA, Grimes JD, et al: Spontaneous dissection of carotid and vertebral arteries: Management considerations. Can J Neurol Sci 11:328, 1984.

256. Bogousslavsky J, Regli F, Despland A: Aneurysmes disséquants spontanes de l'artère carotide interne. Rev Neurol (Paris) 11:625, 1984.

257. Garcia-Merino JA, Gutierrez JA, Lopez-Lozano JJ: Double-lumen dissecting aneurysms of the internal carotid artery in fibromuscular dysplasia: A case report. Stroke 14:815, 1983.

258. Jackson MA, Hughes RC, Ward SC, et al: Headbanging and carotid dissection. BMJ 287:1262, 1983.

include fever, weight loss, fatigue, and malaise. Many patients have arthralgias, but frank arthritis is uncommon.[40] Dementia, confusion, and psychiatric symptoms, such as depression, have been reported.[33,41]

Polymyalgia Rheumatica

So named for its aching muscles and joints, polymyalgia rheumatica is a syndrome of limb girdle muscle pain and stiffness accompanied by systemic symptoms, including malaise, fever, weight loss, anorexia, and depression. Most patients with giant cell arteritis have symptoms of polymyalgia rheumatica for weeks to months before headache, jaw claudication, or visual loss develops.[42–46] Up to 44% of patients who present with polymyalgia rheumatica alone go on to have overt giant cell arteritis, and 23% have serious ophthalmologic or neurologic complications, such as visual loss, ophthalmoplegia, and stroke.[47] Patients with the clinical diagnosis of polymyalgia rheumatica frequently are found to have giant cell arteritis on temporal artery biopsy.[25,42] These findings support the notion that polymyalgia rheumatica and giant cell arteritis are not two distinct nosologic entities but, rather, different manifestations of a common disease.[45]

Ophthalmologic Complications

Visual loss is the most feared complication of giant cell arteritis. Anterior ischemic optic neuropathy, secondary to thrombosis of the posterior ciliary arteries, is the most common cause of visual loss.[25,48,49] Posterior ischemic optic neuropathy and central retinal artery occlusion also cause visual loss less commonly.[25,49–53] Homonymous hemianopia and cortical blindness may occur as a result of posterior circulation infarction (see later). Once established, the visual loss due to giant cell arteritis rarely improves, despite treatment with corticosteroids.[48,49]

Large series report visual loss in 40% to 50% of patients with giant cell arteritis.[40,45,49,54,55] Hollenhorst and associates[49] noted loss of vision within 2 to 3 months of onset of giant cell arteritis symptoms in one third of patients; all of the remaining patients destined to have this symptom suffered loss of vision within 10 months after the appearance of other symptoms.

Visual loss typically occurs suddenly, although 10% to 20% of patients with giant cell arteritis experience transient loss of vision (transient monocular blindness) before fixed visual deficits develop.[41,49,55] The loss is usually monocular, but bilateral involvement occurred in 33% of patients with visual loss reported by Jonasson and coworkers.[38] Visual loss in the second eye occurred simultaneously or within 24 hours after visual loss in the first eye in 36% of these patients, between the second and seventh days in 36%, and between 1 week and 1 month in the rest. Monocular or binocular positive visual phenomena ("scintillating scotoma") have been reported.[41]

Visual acuity is usually limited to hand motion or light perception, and most patients have reduced color perception. The disc is swollen and usually pale, flame hemorrhages may be seen, and disc atrophy subsequently develops. Afferent pupillary defects are common. Field defects are usually altitudinal and inferior, although inferior nasal defects, arcuate defects, and scotomas may be seen.[48,56]

Diplopia or *ophthalmoplegia*, usually transient, occurs in 10% to 15% of patients with giant cell arteritis.[45,49,54,57,58] Weakness of an extraocular muscle was demonstrable in only 10 of 22 patients who complained of double vision in one series.[49] Large clinical series have indicated that palsies of cranial nerves III and VI occur with roughly equal frequency in patients with giant cell arteritis.[54,55,58] Fisher[59] noted that ptosis was common. Ophthalmoplegia in giant cell arteritis is probably due to ischemic necrosis of extraocular muscles.[60] Giant cell arteritis may also cause "orbital infarction syndrome," in which orbital pain, blindness, ophthalmoplegia, and anterior and posterior segment ischemia occur as a result of global orbital ischemia.[61]

Stroke

Stroke is an uncommon but potentially lethal complication of giant cell arteritis. Although epidemiologic studies have not demonstrated an increased incidence of stroke among patients with giant cell arteritis,[25,37,38] studies from referral centers suggest that patients with giant cell arteritis may be at higher risk for stroke during the active phase of the disease.

Stroke due to giant cell arteritis may occur as the first indication of the disease. Usually, however, other symptoms, such as fever, weight loss, headache, and visual disturbance, precede giant cell arteritis–related stroke for periods of weeks to months. The erythrocyte sedimentation rate (ESR) is usually increased in patients with stroke due to giant cell arteritis, but temporal artery examination and biopsy results may be normal.[62] It is worrisome that several patients had strokes despite therapy with corticosteroids, sometimes within 2 weeks of initiation of treatment, and some have had stroke despite normalization of the erythrocyte sedimentation rate (ESR).[63]

Stroke in patients with giant cell arteritis may occur in the carotid or vertebrobasilar circulation. Compared with the foci usually affected by atherosclerosis, giant cell arteritis is more common in the brainstem and vertebral territories. Postmortem examinations in such patients most often document giant cell arteritis involving the extradural segments of the vessels only (Fig. 24–1),[62,64–68] although some have shown evidence of intradural involvement as well.[69–77] In some cases with intracranial vessel involvement, it may be difficult to distinguish giant cell arteritis from granulomatous angiitis of the central nervous system (CNS) (see later).[71,78–81] Clinical syndromes may include unilateral or bilateral occipital infarction, sometimes with top-of-the-basilar syndrome or cortical blindness from embolic occlusion of the distal basilar artery or posterior cerebral arteries. Others have had progressive and fatal infarction of the lower brainstem, sometimes heralded by initial development of a lateral medullary syndrome (Wallenberg's syndrome).[66]

Thrombotic occlusion due to arteritis in the internal carotid arteries, sometimes bilateral, has also been described in several autopsy-proven cases.[62,63,82] In each, the thrombus was found distal to the bifurcation. Sometimes the involved cavernous segments are completely occluded by thrombus, resulting in border zone "distal field" infarction.[63,67] Other patients have had artery-to-artery embolism with hemorrhagic infarction in the corresponding intracranial arterial territories.[82] Subclavian

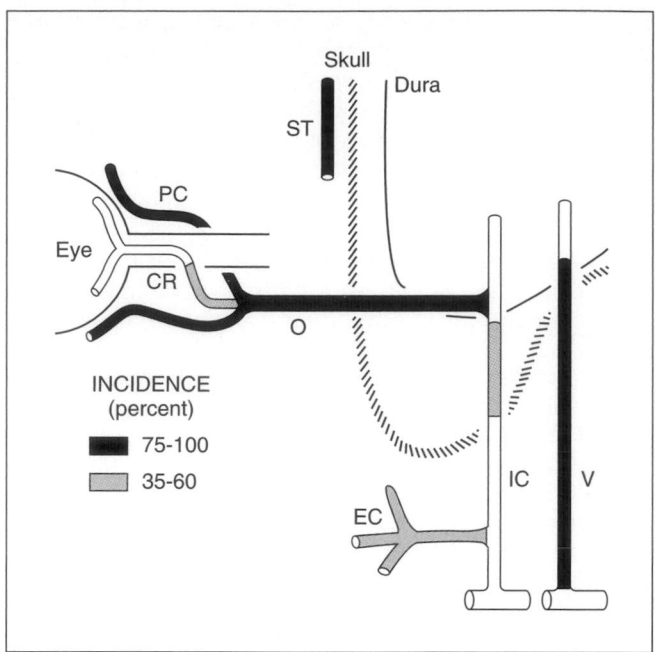

FIGURE 24–1 *Pattern of involvement of giant cell arteritis in head and neck arteries. Note the high incidence of involvement of vertebral artery (V), superior temporal artery (ST), ophthalmic artery (O), and posterior ciliary artery (PC). Intracranial arteries are rarely involved. CR, central retinal artery; EC, external carotid artery; IC, internal carotid artery. (From Wilkinson IMS, Russell RWR: Arteries of the head and neck in giant cell arteritis: A pathological study to show the pattern of arterial involvement. Arch Neurol 27:378, 1972.)*

steal,[83] aortic mural thrombus,[84] and myocardial infarction leading to cerebral embolism have also been reported.[85]

Diagnosis

The diagnosis of giant cell arteritis requires three of the following five criteria: age more than 50 years, new-onset localized headache, temporal artery tenderness or diminished pulse, ESR exceeding 50 mm/hr, and typical histologic findings on temporal artery biopsy.[86] Although the most common laboratory abnormality in patients with giant cell arteritis is a markedly increased ESR, a normal ESR value does not exclude the diagnosis.[87,88] In data from Olmsted County, Minnesota, the ESR in 9 of 167 patients (5.4%) who met criteria for diagnosis of giant cell arteritis was less than 40 mm/hr at the time of diagnosis. These patients had fewer systemic and visual symptoms, and none experienced blindness.[89] In another study, 10 of 248 patients (4%) had an ESR less than 50 mm/hr, but in none was it completely normal; the outcome was similar among those with and without ESR values less than 50 mm/hr.[90] Most patients have a mild to moderate normochromic or slightly hypochromic anemia. White blood cell counts are normal or moderately increased.[35,49] Mild abnormalities of liver enzymes have been reported.[91,92]

Temporal artery biopsy is the most specific diagnostic procedure. Biopsy is recommended for all patients in whom giant cell arteritis is suspected. Bilateral temporal artery biopsy is recommended for highest sensitivity. In a retrospective study of 190 patients clinically diagnosed with giant cell arteritis, biopsy findings were negative in 15.3%.[93] In one series of biopsy-proven cases, 86% were diagnosed through unilateral biopsy and the remaining 14% diagnosed only after biopsy of the other side.[94] A normal temporal artery biopsy does not exclude the diagnosis, however, because the disease may be segmental.[95] Other types of vasculitis may rarely cause inflammation of the temporal arteries and mimic the disease.[96,97] Complications of temporal artery biopsy are rare but include facial nerve injury, skin necrosis, eyebrow droop, and stroke.

Angiographic signs are uncommonly present, but the superficial temporal arteriogram may demonstrate areas of dilation and constriction along the length of the artery, and changes may also be seen in the internal carotid artery siphon segments. Angiographic abnormalities of intracranial arteries are rare and possibly represent cases of isolated granulomatous angiitis of the CNS.[78–80] Angiographic findings may be nonspecific, and arteriography offers no diagnostic advantage over the simple procedure of temporal artery biopsy. Color duplex ultrasonography has also been used in the diagnosis of giant cell arteritis. In one study, a typical dark halo was seen around the lumen of the superficial temporal artery in 73% of patients, an abnormality that disappeared with treatment.[98] Fludeoxyglucose positron emission tomography may also show abnormal tracer uptake in the aorta and its branches in patients with giant cell arteritis.[99] Brain magnetic resonance imaging (MRI) may rarely show multifocal dural enhancement and temporalis muscle enhancement.[100]

Treatment and Prognosis

Once the diagnosis of giant cell arteritis is suspected, the patient should be started on steroid therapy, and a temporal artery biopsy should be performed as soon as possible. Steroid therapy may be started before the biopsy is performed. An initial dosage of 40 to 60 mg/day of prednisone is recommended for the first month or until symptoms of the disease are controlled. Symptoms usually respond promptly to steroids, although visual loss and stroke may occur after the initiation of treatment. Steroids may be tapered while the symptoms and the ESR are monitored.

There is controversy about the duration of corticosteroid therapy. Rapid tapering of the dosage leads to relapse more often than slow tapering. Recurrence of symptoms or an increase in the ESR after initial control of the disease indicates relapse and should prompt resumption of higher doses of steroids. Relapse after withdrawal from steroids may not necessarily be accompanied by an increase in ESR, however.[101] In one series, the mean duration of steroid therapy was 5.8 years, 12.8 years being the maximum.[102] The relapse rate after withdrawal of treatment was 47%; relapse occurred in 46% of the patients within 1 month and in 96% within 1 year after cessation of treatment. The relapse rate after withdrawal of steroid therapy bore little relationship to the duration of treatment.[102] Alternate-day treatment regimens are thought to be less effective than daily administration of steroids.[103] Some investigators have advocated hospitalization and treatment with high-dose, pulsed intravenous administration of methylprednisolone for patients with acute visual loss.[104]

The role of steroid-sparing regimens in the treatment of giant cell arteritis is not clear, but a small (n = 42) single-center, randomized trial has shown that combination therapy with methotrexate reduces the cumulative dose of prednisone taken while also diminishing the likelihood of relapse from 84% to 45%.[105] Giant cell arteritis may cause death by stroke, myocardial infarction, or aortic rupture.[25,75,106] Epidemiologic studies and large clinical series, however, have not demonstrated shortened survival in patients with giant cell arteritis.[35,43]

ISOLATED ANGIITIS OF THE CENTRAL NERVOUS SYSTEM

Isolated angiitis of the CNS, or granulomatous angiitis of the CNS, is an inflammatory arterial disease restricted to the cerebral circulation. Unlike giant cell arteritis, isolated granulomatous angiitis of the CNS afflicts patients of any age, is characterized by neurologic disease out of proportion to systemic illness, preferentially involves smaller arteries and veins, and often responds poorly to steroids alone. The disease is rare, and much of the literature on the topic is based on case reports and small series, making definitive statements about prognosis and treatment difficult.

Pathology

As in giant cell arteritis, the pathologic process in isolated angiitis of the CNS is segmental. Any of the vessels of the brain and spinal cord may be involved, but most reports have noted a predilection for the small leptomeningeal vessels. The precapillary arterioles are most often affected. Some reports, however, have noted venular involvement.[107,108] Occasionally, the process may be quite focal, involving only one vessel or group of vessels. The inflammatory infiltrate is composed of lymphocytes, plasma cells, granulomas with multinucleated giant cells, and, occasionally, neutrophils and eosinophils.[109] These infiltrates may involve any portion of the vessel wall. Some investigators have noted more inflammation in the intima and adventitia than in the media.[107,110] Occasionally, thrombosis of larger intracranial arteries (internal carotid artery siphon, anterior cerebral, middle cerebral, posterior cerebral, and basilar arteries) is found.[111–113] Small aneurysms have also been reported.[114,115]

The etiology of granulomatous angiitis of the CNS is unknown. Because many cases appear to be related to specific underlying infections or other illnesses, it is likely that this condition encompasses a spectrum of different diseases characterized by a vascular inflammatory reaction to a foreign antigen rather than a single nosologic entity. A necrotizing angiitis of the CNS has been observed in brains of turkeys infected with *Mycoplasma gallisepticum*.[116,117] Other cases have been reported in association with Hodgkin's lymphoma, acquired immunodeficiency syndrome (AIDS),[118] primary intracerebral lymphoma, varicella encephalitis, leukemia, sarcoidosis, and cerebral amyloid angiopathy or as occurring after varicella zoster infection,[119] including herpes zoster ophthalmicus (Fig.

24–2).[120–126] In other cases in which no organisms were cultured, "virus-like" and "mycoplasma-like" particles were identified on electron microscopy in the brain.[111,127] Isolated angiitis of the nervous system has also been found in association with cerebral amyloid angiopathy, in which case the giant cells contain congophilic material immunoreactive for the Alzheimer A4 peptide, suggesting that the disease may be due to a foreign body reaction to A4 amyloid deposition in some patients.[128–131]

Clinical Features

The presentation of isolated CNS vasculitis is heterogeneous and requires a high index of clinical suspicion. Patients range in age widely, from 3 to 96 years. The duration of illness is variable. Death may occur within days after presentation in some patients, whereas others have an indolent course lasting years.[132–134] Headache, nausea, vomiting, dementia, amnesic states, disorientation, confusion, somnolence, encephalopathy, or coma occurs early in the course of the disease in many patients. Multifocal neurologic symptoms and signs may develop in a stepwise, progressive fashion, with episodes of quantitative and qualitative worsening, usually occurring after variable periods of stabilization (days, weeks, months, or sometimes years). Seizures are common. Ischemic or hemorrhagic stroke (or transient ischemic attack [TIA]) may occur.[113,115,135–137] Many patients demonstrate hemiplegia or extensor plantar responses, and some have spinal cord involvement (either alone or in association with brain involvement), including progressive or acute myelopathy with incontinence and paraplegia.[125,138,139] Papilledema is common.

Systemic symptoms, such as fever and weight loss, are uncommon, distinguishing this entity from most rheumatologic conditions that can cause stroke, such as giant cell arteritis or systemic lupus erythematosus. The ESR is usually not increased, and when abnormal, it is not as high as in giant cell arteritis. Blood cell counts, electrolyte levels, and results of serologic tests for collagen vascular disease are usually normal.

The most consistent cerebrospinal fluid (CSF) abnormality is an increase in protein (frequently >100 mg/dL), although CSF may occasionally be normal. Increased immunoglobulin values are occasionally reported. Varying numbers of red blood cells are frequently present. Opening pressure is increased in some but normal in others. Many patients have a moderate lymphocytic pleocytosis (usually <150 cells/μL). Isolated angiitis of the CNS may thus manifest as a chronic meningitis.[140,141]

Computed tomography (CT) scan findings may be heterogeneous, consisting of single or multiple infarcts, single or multiple hemorrhages, tumor with mass effect, tumor with hemorrhage, ring-enhancing lesions suggestive of abscess, and multiple areas of increased attenuation with surrounding decreased attenuation suggestive of multiple metastatic lesions. Brain MRI findings are equally heterogeneous and nonspecific; they include any combination of the following: multiple, bilateral white and gray matter infarcts, either sweeping and confluent or multiple and small white matter lesions with increased signal on T2-weighted images, diffuse nodular gadolinium enhancement, intraparenchymal hemorrhage, or gadolinium

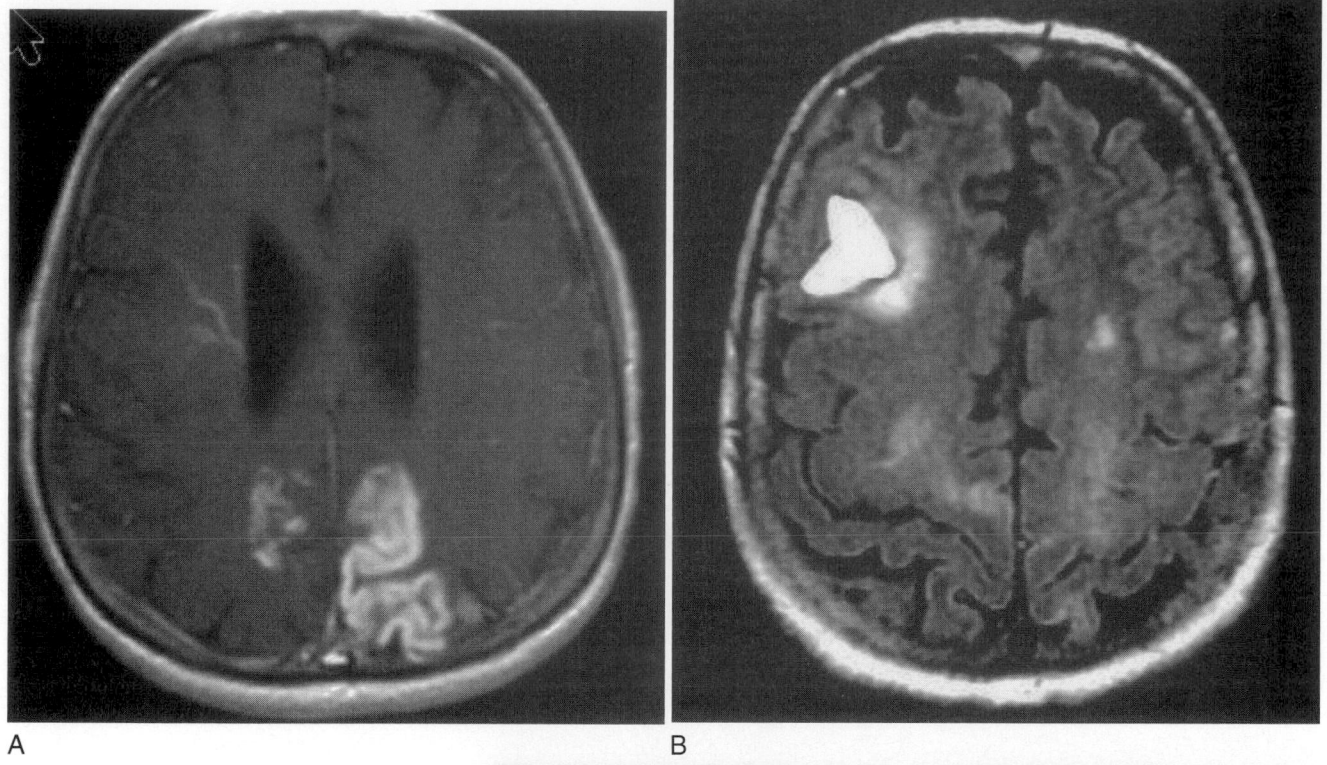

FIGURE 24–2 *Cerebral vasculopathy associated with varicella zoster infection. A, Contrast-enhanced MRI of the brain, demonstrating enhancement of infarctions in bilateral occipital lobes. B, Fluid-attenuated inversion recovery (FLAIR) MRI sequence showing increased signal in the right frontal lobe, a finding consistent with intracerebral hematoma. C, Cerebral angiogram. Note the beaded appearance of the middle cerebral and anterior cerebral artery branches (arrows), a finding consistent with vasculitis.*

enhancement of the meninges with little or no change in the brain parenchyma.[142–144] Some of these abnormalities may mimic multiple sclerosis, CNS lymphoma, or retinocochleocerebral vasculopathy (Fig. 24–3). Cerebral angiographic results are usually abnormal, with alternating segments of concentric arterial narrowing and dilatation.

However, cerebral angiographic findings may be normal at some time during the course of the disease.

Autopsy examination of visceral structures is usually normal but rarely may reveal small discrete foci of angiitis.[111,136,141,145–147] The most common neuropathologic finding is multiple small foci of infarction, followed by

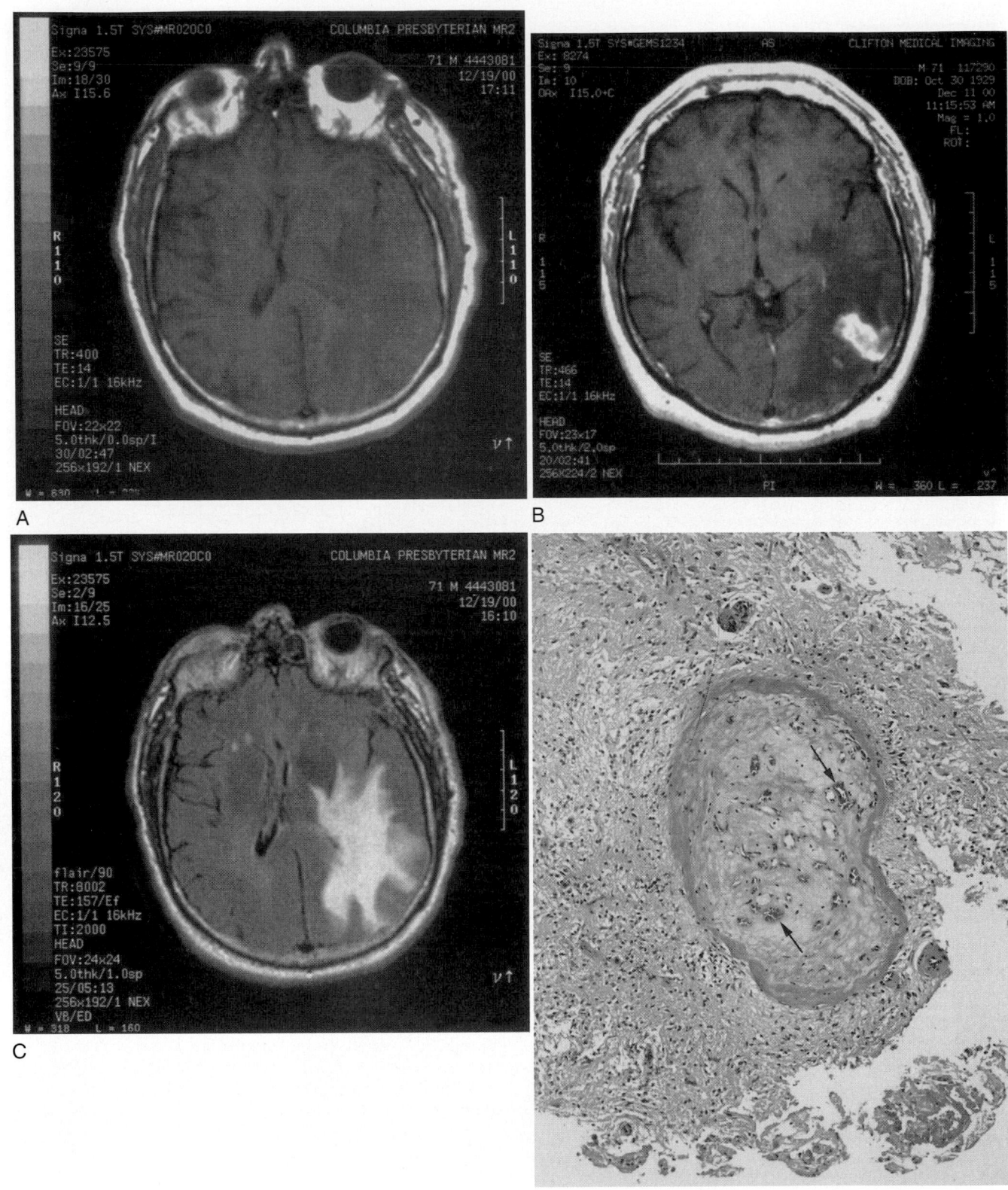

FIGURE 24–3 *Cerebral vasculitis presenting as a mass lesion. Precontrast (A) and postcontrast (B) T1-weighted MRI sequence showing the enhancement of a left temporoparietal mass lesion. C, T2-weighted MRI sequence showing extensive edema around the lesion. D, Pathologic specimen from brain biopsy demonstrates an intraparenchymal blood vessel with chronic occlusive changes, mural fibrosis, and recanalization by small, thin-walled vessels (arrows). The gray matter surrounding the blood vessel shows extensive gliosis and loss of neurons. Leukocytes, primarily lymphocytes, infiltrate the arterial adventitia and, to a lesser extent, the media, findings consistent with a chronic vasculitic process.*

multiple foci of hemorrhage ("brain purpura," "petechiae"). Large infarcts and, less often, large confluent intra-parenchymal hemorrhages may be present.[107,113,114,135–137] Occlusion of large or medium-sized vessels by thrombus is uncommon.[111,113,148] Subarachnoid blood and small aneurysms are rarely encountered.[115,135] Herniation (uncal or cerebellar) may occur secondary to massive edema or hemorrhage.

Diagnosis

None of the standard laboratory tests is diagnostic for granulomatous angiitis, and normal results of such tests do not exclude the diagnosis. Angiograms, in particular, may be normal; a pattern of alternating dilation and constriction ("beading") is a nonspecific sign that may be seen in various vasculitides (including those due to sarcoidosis, infection, and amphetamine-like drugs) and other noninflammatory conditions (such as intracranial atherosclerosis, especially in diabetic patients).[149–153] Laboratory tests may include blood cultures, CSF cultures, viral titers (including human immunodeficiency virus), serologic tests for syphilis, drug or toxicology screens, coagulation studies (prothrombin time, partial thromboplastin time, lupus anticoagulant), immunofixation electrophoresis, and tests for anticardiolipin antibodies, antinuclear antibodies, rheumatoid factor, complement, cryoglobulins, and antineutrophil cytoplasmic autoantibodies (ANCAs; also known as anticytoplasmic autoantibodies [ACPAs]) (to exclude alternative diagnoses such as polyarteritis nodosa and Wegener's granulomatosis).

Retrospective studies have indicated that brain biopsy is the best test for the diagnosis of primary CNS vasculitis[154,155] and is necessary to distinguish among tumor (especially lymphoma or intravascular malignant lymphomatosis), infection, and vasculitis (see Fig. 24–3). Because isolated granulomatous angiitis of the CNS has a predilection for leptomeningeal vessels, the procedure should include a leptomeningeal biopsy as well as a parenchymal biopsy. However, even these efforts are occasionally unrewarded; biopsy results have been negative in several subsequently autopsy-proven cases.[131,145,156–158]

Treatment

There is no standard treatment for isolated granulomatous angiitis of the CNS. Progression of the disease and death have frequently occurred despite treatment with high-dose steroids.[111,156] Remissions have been reported with the use of prednisone, in some cases combined with cyclophosphamide.[159,160] Methotrexate has also been used as a steroid-sparing agent with reported success in a child.[161] In one patient with Hodgkin's disease, stabilization of granulomatous angiitis of the CNS occurred after treatment of the lymphoma.[162]

HERPES ZOSTER OPHTHALMICUS AND DELAYED CONTRALATERAL HEMIPARESIS

Rarely, patients who have herpes zoster involving the first division of the trigeminal nerve (herpes zoster ophthalmi-cus) experience contralateral hemiparesis weeks to months later in relation to vasculitis affecting the cerebral vessels. The onset of hemiparesis may be acute and may be indistinguishable from stroke syndromes due to more conventional mechanisms, although some patients have more global mental status changes, suggesting an underlying meningoencephalitic process.[163,164] Occasionally, the hemiparesis may progress or may recur after a period of improvement. Central retinal artery occlusion,[165] optic neuritis,[166] and orbital pseudotumor syndrome[124] have also been reported with this syndrome.

Postmortem examinations have documented cerebral infarction in the ipsilateral carotid or middle cerebral artery territory secondary to a necrotizing (not granulomatous) arteritis with or without thrombosis,[163,164,167] although diffuse granulomatous angiitis of the CNS has been reported after herpes zoster ophthalmicus as well. One report documented an occlusive thrombotic vasculopathy without frank vasculitis.[168] One patient had cerebellar infarction ipsilateral to the involved trigeminal nerve, with a mild mononuclear infiltrate documented in the adventitia of the thrombosed superior cerebellar artery.[169] Swelling and lymphocytic infiltration of the ipsilateral trigeminal ganglion and nerve trunk have also been noted. Herpes-like virions have been identified in the smooth muscle of the middle cerebral artery.[167]

Cerebral angiography (including MR angiography) may be normal or may document segmental narrowing or occlusion in the ipsilateral supraclinoid internal carotid artery siphon segment, middle cerebral artery stem, anterior cerebral artery A_1 segment, and anterior cerebral artery A_2 segment beneath the genu of the corpus callosum (pericallosal). On rare occasions, the ipsilateral posterior cerebral artery P_1 segment and contralateral anterior cerebral artery A_1 segment have been involved.[170–172] Mycotic aneurysms and subarachnoid hemorrhage (SAH) have been reported.[173] One patient demonstrated aneurysmal dilatation of the intrapetrosal segment of the left internal carotid artery in association with ipsilateral Horner's syndrome, hearing loss, and ear pain.[174] CSF examination may disclose a mild to moderate pleocytosis and protein elevation.

The predilection for involvement of the ipsilateral intracerebral arteries at the base of the brain has led some researchers to suggest that the process may be due to spread of virus to the involved arteries via the intracranial branches of the ophthalmic division of the trigeminal nerve, but the exact pathogenesis remains unproven.[175,176] Therapy has included corticosteroids, acyclovir, and anticoagulants,[167,175] although recovery without treatment has been reported.

TAKAYASU'S ARTERITIS

Takayasu's arteritis (pulseless disease, idiopathic aortitis) is a large-vessel granulomatous arteritis that affects the aorta, its main branches, and, occasionally, the pulmonary artery. Although pathologic changes in the arteries are similar to those found in giant cell arteritis,[177] Takayasu's arteritis affects younger people, particularly women. Most cases have been reported from Asia, but the disease is found worldwide.[178] As in giant cell arteritis, constitutional symptoms (malaise, weight loss, fever) and increased ESR are

Specific Medical Diseases and Stroke

common in the acute phase of Takayasu's arteritis. Symptoms such as arm claudication and syncope occur more frequently than retinal or cerebral ischemia. Brachial pressures and pulses are commonly asymmetrical, and there may be asymmetry between pressures in the arms and legs.

Cerebrovascular complications occur in patients with more advanced disease, particularly those with retinopathy, hypertension secondary to renal artery stenosis, aortic regurgitation, or aortic aneurysms.[179] Cerebral infarction and retinal ischemia may occur subsequent to stenosis or occlusion of the extracranial carotid or vertebral arteries, but the intracranial arteries are rarely involved.[177] Subclavian steal also occurs, but this physiologic phenomenon is not always accompanied by symptoms of vertebrobasilar ischemia.[180] Intracerebral hemorrhage is usually related to hypertension.[181,182] In one case, SAH occurred; it was attributed to an aneurysm of the distal intracranial segment of one of the vertebral arteries.[183]

Treatment consists of corticosteroids, cytotoxic agents (cyclophosphamide), surgery, or a combination of these modalities. Regression of carotid stenosis has been reported after administration of corticosteroids.[179] Various surgical reconstructive and bypass procedures have been used,[184–186] with apparent success in some patients, although postoperative anastomotic stenoses may occur. Some investigators have advised delaying operation until after the inflammatory process can be controlled with corticosteroids,[178] but others have not found operating first to be problematic.[187] Some patients acquire unusual anastomotic vascular collateral patterns even without surgery, including collateral vessels from the right coronary artery to both vertebral arteries and the left internal carotid arteries.[188]

POLYARTERITIS NODOSA

Polyarteritis nodosa is a necrotizing angiitis of the medium-sized to small muscular arteries throughout the body. The peripheral nervous system is more commonly involved than the CNS, but in one series, 46% of patients had symptoms and signs referable to the CNS, and 13% had cerebral infarction or hemorrhage.[189] CNS complications tend to occur late in the course of the disease in the setting of renal failure, fever, and other systemic manifestations, and CNS involvement is not an independent predictor of death.[189,190] Diffuse or multifocal cerebral syndromes, such as headache, confusion, psychiatric syndromes, dementia, lymphocytic meningitis,[191] and generalized or focal seizures, are more common than stroke. Cerebral angiography in patients with CNS manifestations may demonstrate multiple saccular aneurysms similar to those visualized on visceral angiography.[192,193]

Necropsy has demonstrated necrotizing vasculitic changes in large cerebral arteries (internal carotid, middle cerebral, posterior cerebral),[194–197] small meningeal arteries,[195,196,198] or both. The size of the associated cerebral infarctions in these cases paralleled the size of the artery involved. SAH has been reported,[199] and in one instance, necropsy demonstrated massive SAH in the region of the anterior cerebral and anterior communicating arteries, with dissection into the frontal lobe and rupture into the ventricular system.[200] Necropsy-proven cases of cerebral infarction associated with necrotizing arteritis of the cerebral arteries have been reported in the setting of polyarteritis nodosa related to hepatitis B antigenemia.[201] The spinal cord may also be involved.[202,203]

Diagnostic studies in patients suspected of having polyarteritis nodosa should include serologic tests for hepatitis B and C and ANCA and may include visceral or cerebral angiography or biopsy of an organ system suspected of involvement. Treatment consists of corticosteroids and cyclophosphamide.[204,205] Infantile polyarteritis nodosa, a disease thought to be distinct from the adult form and possibly related to Kawasaki's disease, may cause stroke (infarction, aneurysmal SAH) in children.[206]

SYSTEMIC LUPUS ERYTHEMATOSUS

Reports on the neurologic manifestations of systemic lupus erythematosus (SLE) have long emphasized the high frequency of CNS complications, including stroke. Presence of neuropsychiatric disease is considered one of the 13 cardinal manifestations of SLE recognized in the American College of Rheumatology (ACR) criteria for the disease.[207] Of note, however, is that the two manifestations of neuropsychiatric disease considered are seizures and psychosis; cerebrovascular disease is not included. Pathologic series have documented various cerebrovascular lesions, but findings in the brain and cerebral vessels at autopsy infrequently correlate with clinical syndromes before death.[208] Several clinical and pathologic reports have called attention to potential embolic and prothrombotic mechanisms of stroke in SLE that were heretofore unrecognized or underemphasized.[208–213] These findings may have important therapeutic implications for some patients with SLE and stroke.

The percentage of patients with SLE in whom stroke develops is difficult to estimate from clinical series, which often originate from referral centers. In a prospective series of 150 patients, 4 patients had fatal stroke.[214] In another series, 5 of 140 patients with SLE had "typical cerebrovascular accidents."[215] Stroke occurred one third as often as seizures and one fifth as often as psychiatric illness, perhaps justifying the ACR criteria. Other reports have documented clinical syndromes of cerebrovascular disease in 5.6% to 15%,[210,213] and about 6% of patients with SLE die of stroke.[216] According to two series, stroke may be more likely to occur during the first 5 years after diagnosis of SLE.[210,213] Renal involvement, hypertension, and high titers of anti-DNA antibodies occur significantly more commonly in patients with SLE and stroke than in those with SLE but without stroke.[213] There appears to be no further increase in risk of stroke among patients with end-stage renal disease (ESRD) due to lupus compared with those with ESRD from other causes.[217] Patients with SLE and cardiac valvular disease seem to have a high risk of stroke (87%).[210] Few data exist on recurrence rates in patients with stroke in the setting of SLE, but in one series, it was alarmingly high—64%.[210]

Mechanisms of Cerebrovascular Disease in Patients with Systemic Lupus Erythematosus

Vasculitis

Although vasculitis is frequently mentioned as an important cause of stroke in patients with SLE, documented vasculitic changes in the vessels on postmortem examination are actually quite rare.[208,210,218,219] Johnson and Richardson[218] documented a high frequency of destructive and proliferative lesions in arterioles and capillaries associated with microinfarction and hemorrhage, but vasculitis was found in only 3 of their 24 cases and was thought to be either focal or reactive. In other series, vasculitis was found in only 7% of 57 cases,[219] in 1 of 10 brains,[220] and at autopsy in none of 50 patients with SLE.[208]

Cerebral Infarction

In the necropsy series reported by Johnson and Richardson,[218] widespread microinfarction in the cortex and brainstem occurred in the vast majority of patients (20 of 24 cases; 83%). This finding was thought to correlate with the predominant clinical features—seizures, "disturbances of mental function," and cranial nerve abnormalities. In contrast, macroscopically apparent areas of cerebral infarction occurred in only 4 cases (17%). The mechanisms of infarction in the few cases of macroscopic infarction in this series were not apparent. In another necropsy series, large infarcts (greater than 1 cm) were found in only 12%, usually in the distribution of the middle cerebral artery.[219] Angiographic studies have documented occlusions of large intracranial vessels (internal carotid artery, middle cerebral artery, anterior cerebral artery).[215,221,222] In other patients, tapering occlusions of the middle cerebral artery or internal carotid artery have been found.[222]

In their early communication describing an "atypical verrucous endocarditis" in patients with SLE (Fig. 24–4),

Libman and Sacks[223] suspected cerebral embolism in one of their patients. It has since become increasingly recognized that cardiogenic brain embolism (with or without associated nonbacterial thrombotic endocarditis) is an important mechanism of stroke in patients with SLE. Devinsky and coworkers[208] documented embolic brain infarcts in 10 (20%) of 50 patients with SLE, the cardiac sources being Libman-Sacks endocarditis in 5 patients, chronic valvulitis in 2 patients, and mural thrombus in 2 patients. Some patients with verrucous endocarditis also have antiphospholipid antibodies.[224–226] One study has also found that microembolic signals detected on transcranial Doppler ultrasonography testing, possibly indicating embolic material en route to the brain, were more common in patients with SLE who had neuropsychiatric symptoms than in those who had no CNS symptoms, raising the possibility that microemboli may play an even broader role in SLE than previously suspected.[227] Documentation of cardiac sources of emboli in patients with SLE and stroke might prompt treatment with anticoagulants.

Thrombotic thrombocytopenic purpura (thrombocytopenia, microangiopathic hemolytic anemia, fever, renal failure, CNS signs) is another important but underdiagnosed mechanism of stroke in the terminal stages of SLE. Thrombotic thrombocytopenic purpura was documented in 7 of the 50 patients (14%) in the necropsy series reported by Devinsky and coworkers.[208] This group found that 14 (28%) of their patients may have had thrombotic thrombocytopenic purpura during the terminal stages of

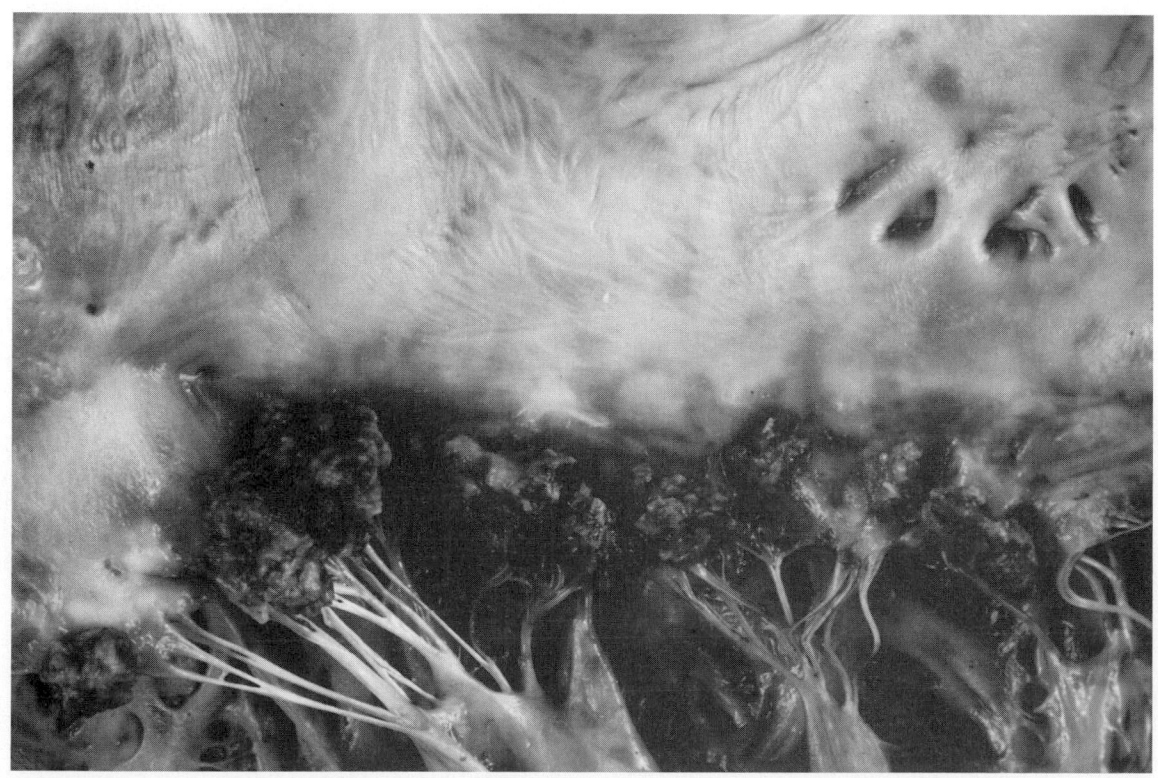

FIGURE 24–4 *Libman-Sacks endocarditis involving the mitral valve in a patient with systemic lupus erythematosus. (Courtesy of William D. Edwards, MD, Department of Laboratory Medicine and Pathology, Mayo Clinic, Rochester, MN.)*

the disease, but this diagnosis was made antemortem in only 1 patient.

Antiphospholipid antibodies, including anticardiolipin antibodies and the lupus anticoagulant, are a class of autoantibodies that bind to negatively charged phospholipid molecules.[228] Bowie and colleagues[229] noted the association of thrombotic events with the presence of the "circulating anticoagulant" in patients with lupus 30 years ago, but only in the last decade has attention been called to the association of antiphospholipid antibodies with cerebrovascular disease, systemic thrombotic events, spontaneous abortion, and thrombocytopenia.[230–239] These phenomena may be associated with antiphospholipid antibodies either in the setting of SLE or as a "primary" antiphospholipid syndrome.[240] In one series,[213] the lupus anticoagulant was detected in 38% and anticardiolipin antibody in 43% of patients with SLE and stroke who were investigated for these abnormalities. Documentation of a procoagulant state due to antiphospholipid antibodies in a patient with SLE and stroke may have important treatment implications, anticoagulants having been recommended by some investigators on the basis of anecdotal experience[241–243] or retrospective data[244] but not the results of controlled clinical trials. Vasculitis has only rarely been documented in patients with antiphospholipid antibodies.[230,239,245,246]

Additional possible causes of infarction in patients with SLE are hypertension and hyperlipidemia, both of which are overrepresented among such patients.[247] Confluent increased T2 signal abnormalities in white matter on brain MRI in some patients with SLE and dementing illness may represent perivascular demyelination rather than infarction.

Hemorrhage

Hemorrhage as a cause of stroke in patients with SLE is well documented clinically but appears to occur less often than infarction. In the series reported by Johnson and Richardson,[218] three patients died from intracerebral lobar hemorrhage. Intracerebral hemorrhage may be associated with hypertension and thrombocytopenia.[210,213] SAH is frequently found at autopsy, often in association with intraparenchymal hemorrhage.[219] Some patients with SLE do have clinical syndromes of SAH. In some instances, the SAH has been secondary to rupture of a berry aneurysm,[214,248] a possible chance association. On rare occasions, SAH has occurred secondary to rupture of a fusiform aneurysm, and associated transmural angiitis has been documented at necropsy.[249] Subdural hematoma has also been reported, but the mechanisms involved are uncertain.[208,250]

Cerebral Venous Thrombosis

Cerebral venous thrombosis is an uncommon but well-documented cerebrovascular complication in SLE.[251–254] The mechanism of venous thrombosis may be multifactorial, lupus anticoagulant and anticardiolipin antibody having been detected in some but not all affected patients.[252,254] Clinical syndromes have included focal cerebral signs, such as alternating hemiparesis, hemiplegia, and aphasia, but clinicians should be particularly alert to the fact that some patients have presented with headache, papilledema, and no focal neurologic signs ("pseudotumor

cerebri"). Cerebral angiography, MRI, or MR angiography may be necessary to confirm this diagnosis.

WEGENER'S GRANULOMATOSIS

Wegener's granulomatosis is a necrotizing granulomatous vasculitis involving the respiratory tract and other organ systems in association with glomerulonephritis.[255] Nervous system complications include peripheral neuropathy and mononeuritis multiplex, CNS infection, local invasion by destructive granulomatous lesions causing cranial nerve palsies,[407] and, rarely, CNS vasculitis.[256–260] Necrotizing granulomatous meningitis with leptomeningeal vasculitis may produce predominantly meningeal and encephalopathic syndromes or multiple cranial neuropathies, sometimes with prominent meningeal enhancement and confluent increased T2 signal abnormalities in white matter on brain MRI.[261–264]

Pathologically proven cerebrovascular complications include infarction, hemorrhage (including SAH), and cerebral venous thrombosis.[256,259,260,265–269] These complications typically occur in the setting of well-established extracranial disease, although stroke may rarely be the presenting manifestation of the disease.[270] In one autopsied case,[256] interhemispheric SAH and cerebral infarction in the distribution of the anterior cerebral artery occurred subsequent to panarteritic involvement of this artery. In another, the patient died of caudate hemorrhage with intraventricular rupture; at postmortem examination, the hemorrhage appeared to originate from vessels affected by necrotizing vasculitis.[271] Autopsy in a patient with bifrontal infarction showed thrombosis and fibrinoid necrosis of medium-sized to large branches of the anterior cerebral artery.[259] Necrotizing vasculitis and granulomatous lesions were present in the small arteries and veins in the frontal areas of the base of the brain, where a suppurative meningitis was also noted. Necrotizing cerebral thrombophlebitis accounted for cortical vein thrombosis in another reported case.[260] Cavernous sinus invasion may occur, and internal carotid artery occlusion has been documented in one case with such invasion.[272]

The presence of ANCAs facilitates the diagnosis of Wegener's granulomatosis.[273] These antibodies have high specificity and sensitivity, and increases in their titer may indicate a relapse.[274,275] CNS complications may have become less common with the advent of protocols combining cyclophosphamide and corticosteroids, which appear to be more effective than corticosteroids alone.[255,276]

Occasional reports of amaurosis fugax, ischemic optic neuropathy,[277] SAH,[278] and strokelike syndromes[279] have been reported in patients with various forms of necrotizing "allergic" angiitis (Churg-Strauss syndrome). In one patient, SAH was caused by vasculitis involving the choroid plexus, which was documented at autopsy.[276]

LYMPHOMATOID GRANULOMATOSIS

Lymphomatoid granulomatosis is an "angiocentric and angiodestructive lymphoreticular proliferative and granulomatous disease" that primarily involves the lungs and may involve the CNS in approximately 20% of cases.[280] The disease may mimic Wegener's granulomatosis,[281] and progression to lymphoma has sometimes occurred. Clinical manifestations of CNS involvement usually consist of subacute, progressive syndromes of focal brain parenchymal or cranial nerve involvement that mimic neoplasm, encephalitis, or multiple sclerosis, but rarely cerebrovascular disease.[282–289] Primary CNS involvement has been reported.[290]

SCLERODERMA

Only rarely does scleroderma (progressive systemic sclerosis) cause CNS manifestations directly.[291,292] Convulsions, stroke, and pathologic findings of arterial changes in the brains of patients with scleroderma may be the result of hypertension due to renal disease. Rarely, calcifications of cerebral vessels can be seen. Six percent of patients with scleroderma in one series[291] had cerebrovascular disease, but the mechanisms involved were obscure. Arteritis has only rarely been reported, and its relationship to the scleroderma may be coincidental in those cases.[293–295]

RHEUMATOID ARTHRITIS

CNS manifestations of rheumatoid arthritis are rare and tend to occur in the setting of long-established disease, with either clinical signs (fever, weight loss, active arthritis) or laboratory evidence (increase in rheumatoid factor titer or ESR) of disease activity. Rheumatoid meningitis ("pachymeningitis") has been reported as an asymptomatic finding at autopsy and may cause CNS symptoms and signs, including headache, visual loss, seizures, altered mental status, aphasia, memory loss, hemiparesis, and spinal cord compression.[296–303] Findings at autopsy include thickening and distension of the meninges with a proteinaceous fluid.[303] The dura and leptomeninges demonstrate foci of inflammatory mononuclear cells and multinucleated giant cells. Rheumatoid nodules similar to those found elsewhere in the body have been described in the meninges and the choroid plexus.[298,300,301]

CNS vasculitis, either isolated[304–307] or in association with systemic rheumatoid vasculitis,[308–311] has been documented on rare occasions. Some of the patients in these cases also had pachymeningitis. Usually, the small vessels of the leptomeninges are affected by fibrinoid necrosis, perivascular nodule formation (similar to that seen in polyarteritis nodosa), and "onion skin" proliferation. Small infarcts are the usual associated parenchymal findings, although hematoma formation has been seen along with necrotizing vasculitis involving the small and medium-sized arteries in at least one case,[307] and "patchy" subdural and subarachnoid hemorrhages were found in another instance, presumably related to vasculitis involving small vessels in the subarachnoid space.[431] Usually, affected patients have had encephalopathic syndromes, including seizures and altered mental status,[30,298,347,370,382] although the patient reported by Watson and colleagues[307] presented with acute signs and symptoms of stroke involving both the left frontal lobe and left pons, which were documented at autopsy to be secondary to hematomas.

One of the most feared neurologic complications of rheumatoid arthritis is compressive myelopathy secondary to C1-C2 vertebral subluxation. A well-documented complication of C1-C2 subluxation is massive vertebrobasilar territory infarction due to vertebral artery thrombosis. In two autopsy studies, patients presented with occipital headache and episodic vertigo that occurred with neck flexion or rotation or with syncope. Vertebral artery thrombosis was thought to have resulted from pinching of the vertebral artery between the odontoid and rim of the foramen magnum[312] or stretching of the vertebral arteries between the transverse foramina of the C1 and C2 vertebrae.[313] Precipitation of vertebrobasilar ischemic symptoms has been associated with neck flexion, extension, and rotation in patients with C1-C2 subluxation.[314,315] In some, angiography has documented narrowing or occlusion of the vertebral arteries with these maneuvers.[314,315] Formation of vertebral artery pseudoaneurysms has also been reported.[316]

One unusual case of brain embolism from an ulcerated and necrotic rheumatoid nodule of the aortic valve has been reported in a patient who tested seronegative for rheumatoid arthritis.[317] Instances of cerebral and ocular ischemia in the setting of rheumatoid arthritis have been associated with thrombocytosis[318,319] and hyperviscosity syndromes secondary to polyclonal gammopathy.[320]

SJÖGREN'S SYNDROME

Sjögren's syndrome (xerostomia and keratoconjunctivitis sicca) may be diagnosed in conjunction with other collagen vascular diseases that result in CNS complications. Anti-Ro (Sjögren's syndrome antigen A [SS-A]) antibodies are often present in patients with Sjögren's syndrome.[321] Primary Sjögren's syndrome is diagnosed when the disease is present in the absence of another collagen vascular disease. The frequency of CNS manifestations of primary Sjögren's syndrome is controversial because of the differences in populations studied and the difficulties of establishing the diagnosis and excluding other diseases.[322–331] Multiple sclerosis–like,[332] strokelike,[324,333,334] and dementing[335] syndromes have been reported, along with various CT and MRI findings.[336] In one series, 7 of 87 patients (8%) with primary Sjögren's syndrome had CNS involvement, but most cases were not due to focal disease.[337] In another series, subcortical hyperintensities on MRI were seen in 51.3% of patients with the disease, compared with only 36.6% of age- and sex-matched controls ($P < .001$).[338] Histopathologic documentation of the mechanisms involved is usually not available. In one case from Japan, a moyamoya-like progressive occlusion of bilateral carotid and vertebral arteries was present in a young woman for whom a parotid gland biopsy demonstrated Sjögren's syndrome.[334] Postmortem brain examination of three patients with primary Sjögren's syndrome demonstrated "diffuse polymorphous meningitis" in all three patients that was associated with microhemorrhages in two.[339] Necrotizing arteritis and spinal SAH have been reported in one patient with Sjögren's syndrome and cryoglobulinemia.[340] In another patient with the syndrome, positive antinuclear antibody results, aseptic meningitis, and SAH, vasculitis was seen in the basilar artery along with vesicoenteric leptomeningeal infiltrates.[341] Perivascular lymphocytic inflammation in leptomeningeal and parenchymal vessels was found in one patient with dementia, Sjögren's syndrome, and elevation in rheumatoid factor.[342]

SNEDDON'S SYNDROME

Livedo reticularis is a cutaneous condition characterized by a fixed, deep bluish red, reticulated pattern due to impaired superficial venous drainage of the skin (Fig. 24–5).[343] This cutaneous sign is found in several diseases, including polyarteritis nodosa, SLE, rheumatoid arthritis, dermatomyositis, and cryoglobulinemia.[343] Cerebrovascular disease in association with livedo reticularis is known as Sneddon's syndrome.[344,345] The original descriptions (including that of Champion and Rook, who described the syndrome 5 years before Sneddon) also included hypertension as part of a triad,[344,345] although not all patients have hypertension.[346] Approximately 40% of patients have antiphospholipid antibodies;[346–352] anti–endothelial cell antibodies may also be seen.[353] Patients with Sneddon's

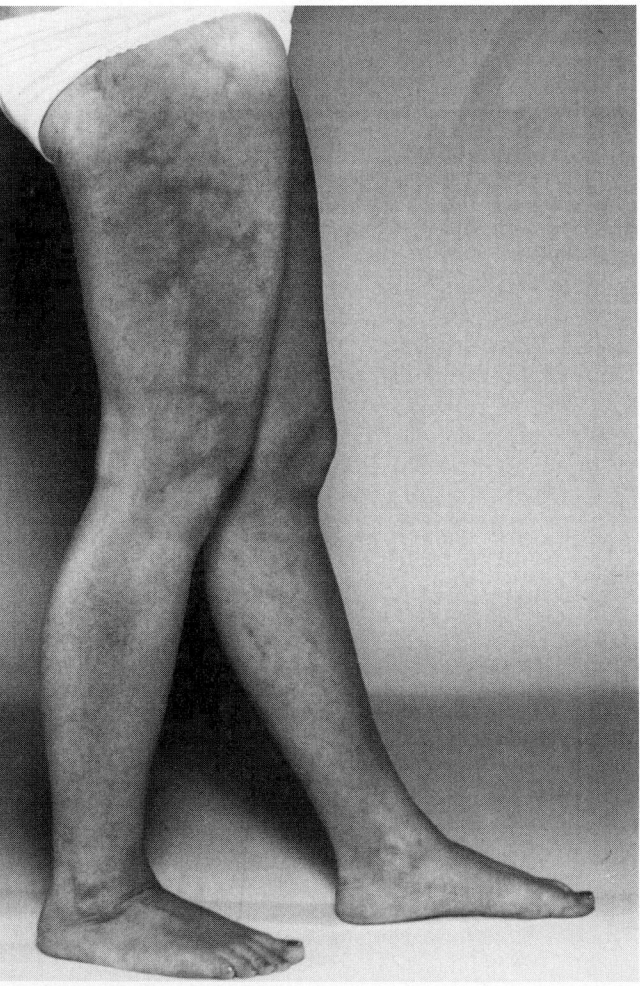

FIGURE 24–5 *Livedo reticularis in a patient with Sneddon's syndrome. (Courtesy of Department of Dermatology, Mayo Clinic.)*

syndrome may have a more progressive course than those with primary antiphospholipid antibody syndrome.[354] There is no consistent relationship between the presence of antiphospholipid antibodies and outcome.[346] Hypercoagulability is thought to play a role in many cases. Familial cases have also been reported.[355–358]

Livedo reticularis usually precedes neurologic involvement in patients with Sneddon's syndrome, but many present with stroke.[351] The most common cerebrovascular manifestation in this syndrome is recurrent cerebral infarction.[351,359–363] Transient ischemic attack, seizures, and dementia have been reported.[359,360] Dementia can be due to multiple small infarcts without overt acute clinical strokes,[364] but some patients appear to have dementia in the absence of infarction.[365] Various clinical stroke syndromes have been documented, frequently with prominent cortical signs. The mechanism of infarction in affected patients is for the most part unknown.

Brain CT and MRI frequently document infarction involving the cortex or white matter (Fig. 24–6).[356,358–361,366] Angiograms are either normal or demonstrate narrowing or occlusion of medium-sized arteries and their branches, sometimes with moyamoya-type collateral networks.[345,356,358–360,362,367,368] Asherson and colleagues[348] found cardiac valvular lesions in more than a third of patients with livedo reticularis associated with positive anticardiolipin antibodies. Similar skin lesions and stroke have also been reported as due to atrial myxoma, suggesting that echocardiography to exclude cardiac lesions should be performed in patients with suspected Sneddon's syndrome.[369] Skin biopsies have usually demonstrated an occlusive, noninflammatory vasculopathy involving medium-sized arteries along with focal and segmental intimal hyperplasia due to fibroelastic proliferation or subendothelial cell proliferation.[357,359] Some investigators have found inflammatory changes of the endothelium.[366,370] One patient had nonvasculitic granulomatous changes in the leptomeninges.[367] Instances of brain hemorrhage in Sneddon's syndrome have also been reported.[371,372] Various treatments used for this disease have included antiplatelet agents, warfarin, and plasmapheresis.[352,373]

MALIGNANT ATROPHIC PAPULOSIS

Malignant atrophic papulosis (Degos' disease, Köhlmeier-Degos disease) is a progressive vasculopathy that affects the skin, cerebral circulation, and other organ systems.[374] The characteristic skin lesion consists of an umbilicated, raised papule with a white center (Fig. 24–7). The appearance of cutaneous lesions usually precedes neurologic manifestations, sometimes by years.[375,376] In some patients, however, neurologic manifestations may precede or accompany the development of cutaneous lesions.[377,378] Bowel perforations may occur.[379,380]

Neurologic complications are varied. In some patients, the initial neurologic manifestations have been symptoms and signs of transient ischemic attack[376] or stroke.[381] Others have had progressive focal or multifocal deficits with stepwise quantitative and qualitative worsening.[377,382–384] Still others have shown evidence of spinal cord involvement.[375–377,385] Angiographic findings have included multiple branch occlusions and alternating segmental

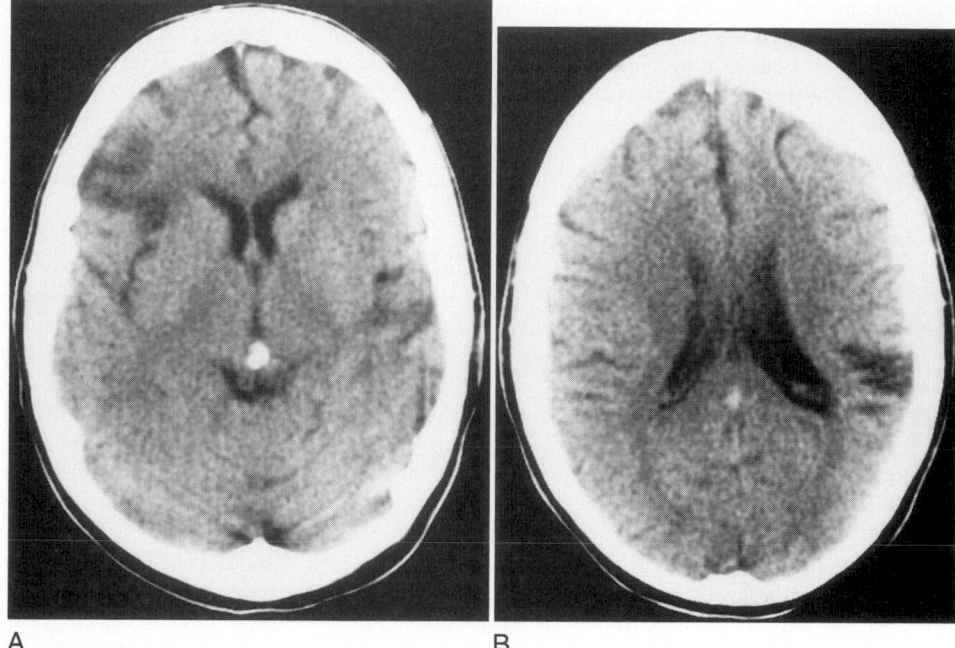

FIGURE 24–6 *CT scan demonstrates infarction in a patient with Sneddon's syndrome. A, Right frontal cortex. B, Left parietal cortex. (Courtesy of Dr. H. S. Luthra, Dr. A. J. D. Dale, Dr. J. Huston, and the Department of Diagnostic Radiology, Mayo Clinic, Rochester, MN.)*

A   B

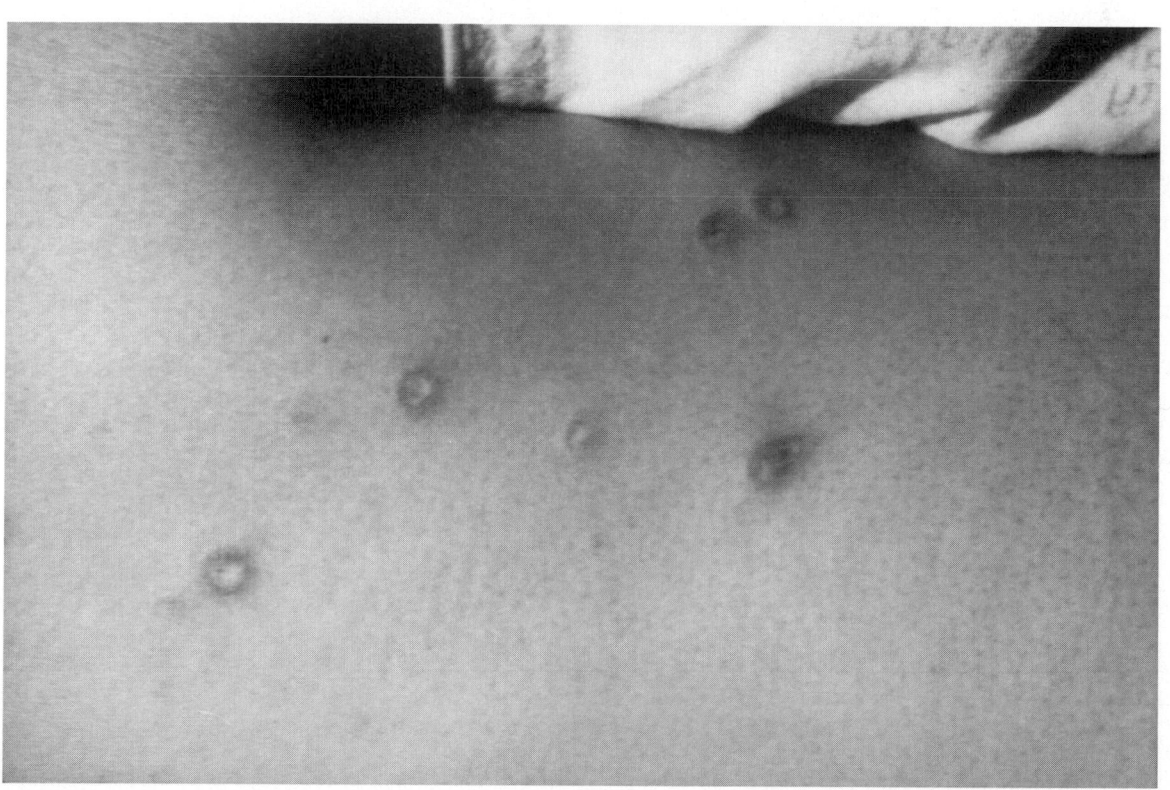

FIGURE 24–7 *Skin lesions of malignant atrophic papulosis (Degos' disease). (Courtesy of Department of Dermatology, Mayo Clinic, Rochester, MN.)*

Specific Medical Diseases and Stroke

constriction and dilatation. CT scans have demonstrated multifocal areas of infarction, hemorrhage, hemorrhagic infarction, and even subdural hemorrhage.[382,386]

Pathologic examination of brain vessels has documented a peculiar "fibrous intimal proliferation" or "deposition of fibrous material" between endothelium and internal elastic lamina, similar to vascular lesions in the skin.[375,377,381,385,386] This finding may be accompanied by thrombosis. Sparse lymphocytic vasculitis and perivascular lymphocytic infiltration were reported in one postmortem brain examination.[386] The small meningeal arteries are frequently involved, but medium-sized and even large arteries may also be affected. Multiple small infarcts, either hemorrhagic or bland, are often found.[377,383,385,386] These small infarcts may be confluent[387] and may involve the cortex[377] or cortex and deeper structures.[375] Less often, large infarction with shift and herniation is documented.[378,379] Venous thrombosis and hemorrhagic venous infarction have been reported.[386] Small parenchymal hemorrhages[375,381] and SAH[377] are occasionally documented.

The exact etiology of this proliferative and occlusive vasculopathy has not been established. Some investigators have reported increased platelet adhesiveness and aggregation,[388] but others have found no coagulation abnormalities.[389] The presence of anticardiolipin antibodies and lupus anticoagulant has been reported in at least one patient with Degos' disease.[390] Various therapies have been used, usually ineffectively, such as antiplatelet agents, anticoagulants, corticosteroids, and plasmapheresis.[377,385,391]

BEHÇET'S DISEASE

Behçet's disease is an inflammatory condition of unknown etiology characterized by the triad oral aphthous ulcers, genital ulcers, and uveitis. Other manifestations are arthritis, cutaneous vasculitis, thrombophlebitis, colitis, and CNS disease.[392,393] CNS complications usually occur in patients who have established cutaneous or ocular disease, but there are well-documented instances of neurologic presentation,[394–397] and some may have ocular and neurologic manifestations without oral or genital lesions.[398] Neurologic manifestations are varied, and few clinical features point to the underlying diagnosis in the absence of the cutaneous or ocular manifestations. Many patients present with a syndrome of aseptic meningitis or meningoencephalitis with fever and headache, with or without associated focal neurologic signs.[392,399] Many reports have emphasized a fluctuating course with exacerbations and remissions that are atypical for cerebrovascular disease.[392,400–403] Corticospinal tract signs, frequently bilateral, are common. Symptoms and signs of brainstem involvement and pseudobulbar palsy are frequently reported.[392,397,401,402,404,405] Less often, neurologic presentations are sudden in onset and suggest stroke.[394,395,400] Some patients have presented with symptoms and signs of increased intracranial pressure, occasionally with minimal or no focal findings, due to angiographically documented cerebral venous sinus thrombosis.[399,406–413] Retinal ischemia and vasculitis have also been reported.[395,399,414,415]

CSF examination frequently demonstrates a moderate pleocytosis, predominantly lymphocytic, as well as increased protein, usually less than 100 mg/dL. Anticardiolipin

antibodies have been reported in patients with Behçet's disease.[416] Brain imaging with CT and more recently MRI has demonstrated lesions that, in some respects, are atypical for more routine mechanisms of vascular disease.[414,417–422] CT scans show focal and circumscribed regions of decreased density that may be enhanced after administration of contrast medium.[418,421,422] Findings on MRI usually consist of increased signal intensity on T2-weighted images.[414,420,421] These lesions are usually found in the deep structures, including the brainstem, deep nuclei, and hypothalamus, and also in the hemispheric white matter, and they may be enhanced.[414,417,418,420,421] Unlike vascular lesions, these findings tend to resolve over time after treatment and frequently do not conform to a single arterial territory. These features, as well as leptomeningeal enhancement in some cases,[423] might be more suggestive of an inflammatory process as opposed to vascular occlusion. Cerebral hemorrhage has been reported, but the mechanisms involved are unclear.[424,425] Cerebral angiograms have usually been normal,[392] but occasional patients with a "vasculitic appearance" have been reported.[426] There is also a report of a large aneurysmal abnormality of the cervical segment of the internal carotid artery.[427]

The leptomeninges are frequently thickened and opacified.[401,402,404] Small regions of softening are most often found in the brainstem and basal ganglia, less often in the deep white matter, and least often in the cortex. Gliosis has been prominent in some reports.[397,402,404,428] Many patients have had varying degrees of lymphocytic perivascular infiltration, usually mild to moderate[397,401,404,428,429] and sometimes perivenular.[430] Small areas of perivascular necrosis and scarring are found, particularly in the brainstem, diencephalon, internal capsule, and basal ganglia. Most reports have emphasized the paucity of arterial lesions and thromboses. Small hemorrhages are also uncommonly documented.[400,405,425] Some reports have emphasized demyelination, both perivenular and diffuse.[397,401,428–430] On rare occasions, large areas of infarction, in either the cortex or the basal ganglia, with endarteritis and post-thrombotic recanalization have been reported.[404] Granulomatous or necrotizing angiitis does not appear to be a commonly documented mechanism of CNS involvement in Behçet's disease.

Various therapies have been used for Behçet's disease, including corticosteroids, anticoagulants (for venous thrombosis), cyclophosphamide, azathioprine, and chlorambucil.[393,412]

CRYOGLOBULINEMIA

There are rare reports of CNS complications in patients with mixed cryoglobulinemia.[431–434] CNS manifestations have included diffuse encephalopathic syndromes with focal signs, seizures, myelopathy, and, occasionally, ischemic stroke.[431–434] Two patients with cerebral ischemia due to an occlusive intracranial vasculopathy in the setting of hepatitis C virus infection, cryoglobulinemia, and hypocomplementemia have been reported.[432] Angiographic findings have included narrowing of the vertebral artery, occlusion of the posterior inferior cerebellar artery, occlusion of the left middle cerebral artery, and progressive stenosis of the distal internal carotid, anterior cerebral, and middle cerebral arteries with development of a moyamoya pattern of collateral vessels.[431,432] The exact underlying pathophysiologic mechanisms of vascular occlusions in these patients are unknown, and vasculitis has been documented only rarely.[435,436]

RETINOCOCHLEOCEREBRAL VASCULOPATHY (SUSAC'S SYNDROME)

Retinocochleocerebral vasculopathy is an unusual syndrome of small-vessel occlusions in the retina, cochlea, and brain.[437–450] Only about 60 cases have been reported. Approximately 85% of cases occur in women, and the mean age at presentation is 30 years.[451] Extracerebral clinical manifestations include multiple episodes of visual loss related to retinal arteriolar occlusions, sensorineural hearing loss in about two thirds of cases, and tinnitus.[451] Funduscopic examination demonstrates occlusion of multiple retinal arterioles with peculiar "long columns of white material" oscillating with the pulse. Neurologic manifestations, which occur in 44% of patients, consist of encephalopathy with prominent disturbances in cognition, memory, and behavior, dysarthria, pseudobulbar affect, ataxia, vertigo, hemiparesis, and hemisensory loss.[437,438,440,444–446,449,451]

CSF examinations may demonstrate a mild pleocytosis (predominantly lymphocytic) and increased protein concentration. Cerebral angiographic findings are usually normal. CT findings are also usually normal, but MRI findings are almost always abnormal, consisting of increased signal abnormalities on T2-weighted images in the white matter or white matter and deep gray matter (Fig. 24–8).[437,444,445] Brain biopsy has shown gliosis, microinfarcts, small-vessel sclerosis, and "healed arteritis." Results of tests for anticardiolipin antibody, lupus anticoagulant, protein C deficiency, protein S deficiency, and antithrombin III deficiency have been negative.[454] No definite underlying connective tissue disease has been identified in these patients. Other patients have been reported with partial syndromes of characteristic retinal arteriolar occlusions and cerebral manifestations without cochlear or vestibular symptoms.[446] The etiology remains obscure. Some cases have appeared to respond to steroids and immunosuppressants,[445,450] and others have progressed despite these treatments.[437,446] One patient's vision improved markedly after treatment with hyperbaric oxygen therapy.[452] The documentation of microangiopathic involvement of muscle in some patients[446] suggests that retinocochleocerebral vasculopathy may actually be a systemic disease with limited clinical expression.

Because Susac's syndrome affects young women and causes white matter abnormalities on MRI, the differential diagnosis includes multiple sclerosis. Unlike that of multiple sclerosis, however, the course of Susac's syndrome tends to be monophasic over 1 to 2 years, although late recurrences have been reported.[453,454] Several arteritides can also be associated with retinal vasculitis, including polyarteritis nodosa, SLE, Wegener's granulomatosis, and Behçet's disease, but the systemic manifestations of these diseases should distinguish them from retinocochleocerebral vasculopathy. Retinocochleocerebral vasculopathy should also be distinguishable from Cogan's syndrome,[455] which may produce visual loss due to interstitial keratitis as well as vestibulocochlear symptoms but rarely CNS involvement.[456] Anterior chamber inflammation, which is characteristic of Cogan's syndrome, is not seen in retinocochleocerebral vasculopathy. Acute posterior placoid pigment epitheliopathy is a retinal disease characterized by cream-colored posterior pole lesions[457–461] that may also occasionally be associated with cerebral vasculitis. The posterior pole lesions characteristic of this disorder are not seen in patients with retinocochleocerebral vasculopathy. Eales' disease produces visual loss in young men as a result of retinal vasculitis or periphlebitis and retinal hemorrhage and may also be associated with stroke.[462,463] Retinocochleocerebral vasculopathy is not typically associated with retinal venulitis or hemorrhage, however.

THE ROLE OF INFLAMMATION IN ATHEROSCLEROSIS AND STROKE

The role of inflammation in "garden variety" atherosclerosis and stroke has been receiving greater attention. According to the prevailing theory of atherosclerosis, developed by Sir Russell Ross[464] and others, atherosclerosis is predominantly an inflammatory condition produced by a "response to injury" (Fig. 24–9). Any of a number of toxic stimuli can lead to endothelial injury, which results in a cascade of events. First, there is adhesion of monocytes and lymphocytes to the endothelial surface, migration of those cells beneath the endothelial surface, and subsequent subendothelial localization. Then these inflammatory cells take up lipids, foam cells form, these and other macrophages are activated, and cytokines and growth factors are released. These events lead to smooth muscle cell proliferation and fibrous plaque formation, and the atherosclerotic process is under way. The range of proven and postulated causes of this endothelial injury is diverse and growing. Oxidized low-density lipoprotein is a well-recognized cause of endothelial injury, but other toxins, including homocysteine, toxic constituents of cigarette smoke, high shear force as is present in hypertension, and infections, have also been implicated.

Epidemiologic studies among patients with SLE and rheumatoid arthritis have demonstrated that the increased inflammation present in these conditions may contribute to atherosclerosis. For example, after data have been adjusted for age, sex, and conventional atherosclerotic risk factors, patients with rheumatoid arthritis are three times as likely to experience cardiovascular events, including stroke, as individuals without rheumatoid arthritis.[465] Although it is possible that medications used to treat rheumatoid arthritis or inactivity related to the disease is responsible for this increase in risk, there is also growing evidence that inflammatory mechanisms and cytokines involved in the pathogenesis of rheumatoid arthritis contribute to accelerated atherosclerosis. For example, a unique subset of T cells originally described in patients with rheumatoid arthritis, CD4+CD28−, is found in approx-

Specific Medical Diseases and Stroke

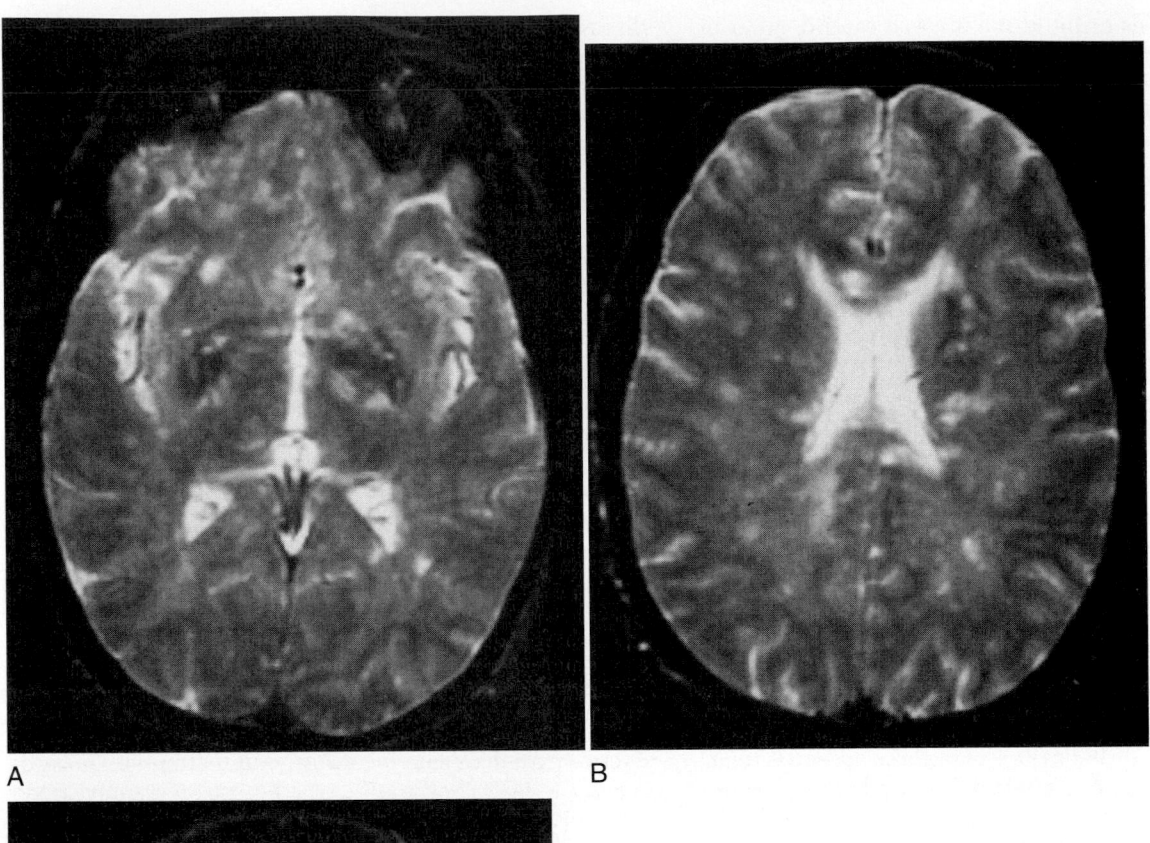

A

B

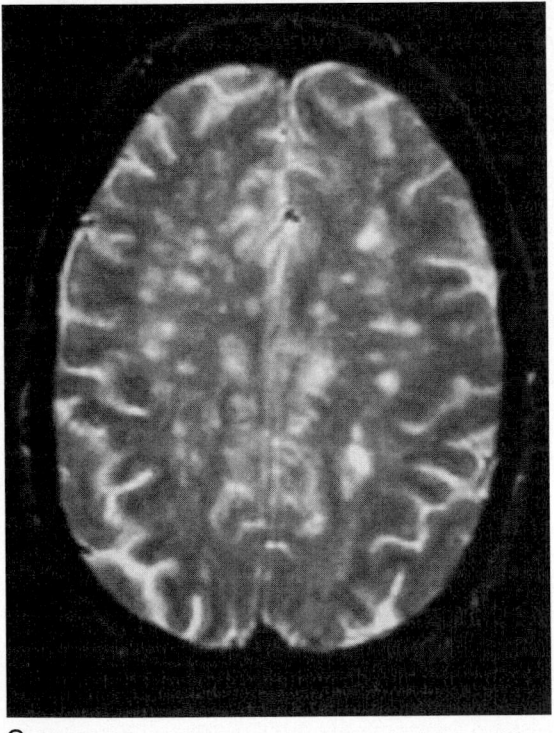

C

FIGURE 24–8　*T2-weighted MRI of the brain in a 40-year-old woman with retinocochleocerebral vasculopathy demonstrates small areas of increased signal intensity in the thalami (A), corpus callosum (B), and subcortical white matter (C). (Courtesy of Department of Radiology, Mayo Clinic, Rochester, MN.)*

imately 65% of patients with unstable angina but not in patients with stable angina or in normal controls.[466] In patients with rheumatoid arthritis, these cells are predominantly present in those with extra-articular manifestations of the disease. They are different from other helper T cells in several ways, including their ability to express high levels of interferon-γ, which stimulate monocyte activation and

could lead to increased levels of matrix metalloproteinases capable of proteolysis of plaque components, raising the likelihood of plaque rupture. Patients with rheumatoid arthritis also have elevated serum levels of C-reactive protein (CRP), interleukin-1 (IL-1), and tumor necrosis factor-α (TNF-α), all of which have been implicated in atherosclerosis. Patients with SLE also have accelerated

The response-to-injury hypothesis of atherosclerosis

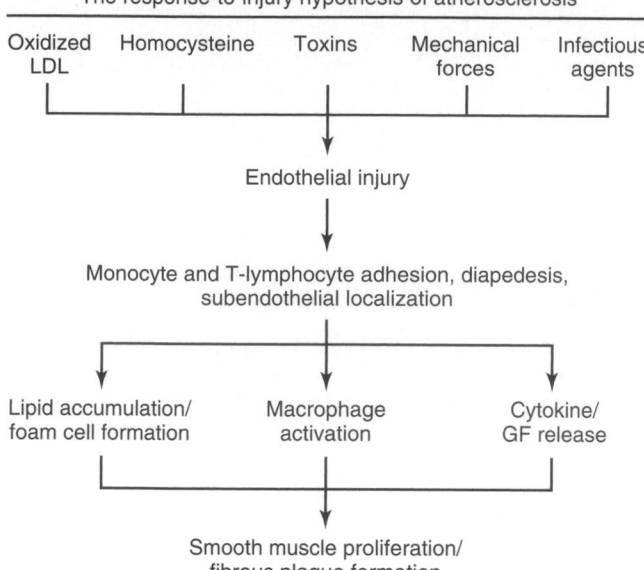

FIGURE 24–9 *The response-to-injury hypothesis of atherosclerosis. GF, growth factor; LDL, low-density lipoprotein. (Adapted from Ross R: Atherosclerosis—an inflammatory disease. N Engl J Med 340:115, 1999.)*

atherosclerosis and, like patients with rheumatoid arthritis, have a higher risk of cardiac events and stroke that is not fully explained by the presence of conventional risk factors.[467]

The role of inflammation in the atherosclerotic process can be divided into the following three phases: early development of atherosclerosis, progression of the atherosclerotic plaque, and acute plaque rupture. Monocyte-derived macrophages, and also T lymphocytes, have been found in human fatty streaks, the earliest stage of the disease process,[468–471] suggesting that immune processes may play an initiating or early role in the development of the lesion. Cytokines, including several interleukins, interferons, TNF, and several growth factors and colony-stimulating factors, have also been found within atheromatous lesions at all stages by means of various techniques.[472–476] Although the initial goal of the immune response, such as monocyte accumulation of oxidized low-density lipoprotein, is to contain the toxic exposure and prevent injury to the endothelium, activation of macrophages may propagate the inflammation through release of cytokines and growth factors.[477–479] Of note, granulocytes are not found within atherosclerotic lesions,[480] a situation similar to most (cirrhosis, glomerulosclerosis, pancreatitis) but not all (rheumatoid arthritis, pulmonary fibrosis) other chronic inflammatory conditions.

As this process continues, there is an increase of inflammatory cells in the atheroma, which are recruited from the blood as well as multiplication within the lesion itself.[481–484] Endothelium-derived leukointegrins cause adherence of monocytes and T cells, particularly at branch points of arteries, where turbulence is prominent.[485–487] Changes in shear stress at these sites lead to upregulation of the genes responsible for the production of these molecules.[488–491]

Animal studies confirm this data. Elevated levels of TNF-α and IL-1β increase monocyte recruitment into developing atherosclerotic lesions in mice.[492] Moreover, in knockout mice deficient in these adhesion molecules, atherosclerotic lesions are smaller despite lipid loading.[493] Blockage of certain immunomodulatory molecules, such as CD40 ligand, which is expressed by macrophages, T cells, endothelium, and smooth cells in atherosclerotic plaques, can reduce lesion formation.[494–497] Although this finding suggests that interference with inflammatory mechanisms could prevent the buildup of atherosclerotic lesions, the clinical implications remain uncertain in human beings. Metalloproteinase and metalloproteinase-like proteins in atherosclerotic plaques may also cleave adhesion molecules from leukocytes, allowing them to be measured in the serum as a marker of subclinical or clinical atherosclerotic disease.[498,499]

Plaque rupture, the acute precipitant of approximately 50% of clinical events related to large-vessel atherosclerosis, also involves inflammatory mechanisms. Rupture occurs at sites of the fibrous plaque where macrophages enter[500] and may be encouraged by destruction of the fibrous cap through upregulation and production of proteolytic enzymes, including metalloproteinases and collagenases derived from macrophages stimulated by activated T cells.[501] The profile of inflammatory cytokines in more advanced lesions, such as those taken from endarterectomy specimens, is predominantly a proinflammatory T-cell response.[502] Certain plaque inflammatory profiles may correlate with acute plaque instability as well. Plaques from patients with unstable angina show greater expression of P-selectin[503] and other cytokines, and the systemic cytokine profiles also differ in people with stable and unstable angina.[504] These data correlate with the clinical scenario in cerebrovascular disease; also, higher levels of macrophages and T cells[505] and intercellular adhesion molecule-1 and TNF-α[506,507] were found in endarterectomy specimens from patients with symptomatic carotid stenosis than in those with asymptomatic carotid stenosis. Other investigators have questioned the significance of these findings, however, because there can be great heterogeneity of inflammatory profiles within plaques.[508] Although the precise mechanisms by which these cytokines cause atherosclerosis remain unclear, there is little disagreement that inflammation plays an important role.

Of perhaps more direct interest to the clinician, epidemiologic studies have also generally shown that serologic evidence of inflammation is associated with atherosclerosis, coronary artery disease, and stroke. Leukocyte count is independently associated with carotid plaque thickness cross-sectionally[509] and progression of carotid intima-media thickness over time[510] as well as with risk of atherosclerotic heart disease[511–516] and stroke,[517,518] even after adjustment for smoking. Circulating levels of several cytokines have been associated with subclinical atherosclerosis, incident cardiovascular events, and prognosis after first myocardial infarction. As noted previously, proteolytic enzymes may cleave adhesion molecules from leukocytes or cytokines may diffuse from plaques into the blood stream, raising circulating levels of these markers. In a cross-sectional analysis, a CRP level higher than 0.55 mg/dL was significantly associated with a self-reported previous history of stroke.[519]

Specific Medical Diseases and Stroke

Prospective studies have also supported the role of inflammation in stroke. In a study among very elderly subjects (>85 years) in Europe, CRP was associated with a higher risk of fatal stroke but also with a risk of death from all causes.[520] CRP levels measured before the onset of clinical disease have been shown to be an independent predictor of first ischemic stroke (relative risk 1.9 for those in the quartile with highest CRP level [CRP > 2.1] versus those in the lowest quartile) in the Physicians' Health Study.[521] In the Framingham Study, during more than 10 years of follow-up, men in the highest CRP level quartile had twice the risk of stroke of those in the lowest, and women had three times the risk.[522] A few studies have looked at CRP and other markers as risk markers after stroke.[523-525] Beamer and associates[524] found that elevated levels of IL-6 and IL-1 receptor antagonist were associated with larger infarcts (>3 cm) and with nonlacunar infarct subtypes. A Scottish study found that in 228 patients with ischemic stroke, high CRP levels (>10.1 mg/L, the geometric mean) predicted mortality after stroke (hazard ratio, 1.23; 95% confidence level, 1.13–1.35).[523] In another study of 128 first-stroke patients, elevated CRP was independently predictive of death or a new vascular event, with subjects in the highest CRP level tertile having a 55% crude risk of an event after only 1 year.[525]

Elevations of inflammatory markers may also be important predictors of benefit from protective therapies, such as aspirin, because the benefit from aspirin was seen primarily in those in the highest CRP quartile in the Physicians' Health Study.[521] A novel approach to increased chronic inflammation may be the use of the cholesterol-lowering statin agents, or 3-hydroxy-3-methylglutaryl coenzyme A (hMG-CoA) reductase inhibitors. In clinical trials, patients with myocardial infarction who were randomly assigned to receive pravastatin had a significant decrease in levels of CRP, whereas those receiving placebo had elevations of CRP. These changes did not correlate with changes in lipid levels either, suggesting a potentially direct effect on the inflammatory parameters.[526] Future epidemiologic investigations and ongoing clinical trials should provide more robust information on the role of inflammatory mechanisms and anti-inflammatory therapies in risk for and prevention of stroke.

Specific Medical Diseases and Stroke

References

1. Machado EBV, Michet CJ, Ballard DJ, et al: Trends in incidence and clinical presentation of temporal arteritis in Olmsted County, Minnesota, 1950–1985. Arthritis Rheum 31:745, 1988.
2. Smith CA, Fidler WJ, Pinals RS: The epidemiology of giant cell arteritis: Report of a ten year study in Shelby County, Tennessee. Arthritis Rheum 26:1214, 1983.
3. Love DC, Rapkin J, Lesser GR, et al: Temporal arteritis in blacks. Ann Intern Med 105:387, 1986.
4. Lie JT: Aortic and extracranial large vessel giant cell arteritis: A review of 72 cases with histopathologic documentation. Semin Arthritis Rheum 24:422, 1995.
5. Machado EBV, Michet CJ, Ballard DJ, et al: Trends in incidence and clinical presentation of temporal arteritis in Olmsted County, Minnesota, 1950–1985. Arthritis Rheum 31:745, 1988.
6. Ostberg G: Morphological changes in the large arteries in polymyalgia arteritica. Acta Med Scand 533(Suppl):135, 1972.
7. Klein RG, Hunder GG, Stanson AW, Sheps SG: Large artery involvement in giant cell (temporal) arteritis. Ann Intern Med 83:806, 1975.
8. Cupps TR, Fauci AS: Giant cell arteritides: The vasculitides. Major Probl Intern Med 21:99, 1981.
9. Hunder GG, Hazleman BL: Giant cell arteritis and polymyalgia rheumatica. In Kelly WN, Harris ED Jr, Ruddy S, Sledge CB (eds): Textbook of Rheumatology. Philadelphia, WB Saunders, 1981.
10. Robbins SL, Cotran RS: Blood vessels. In Pathological Basis of Disease, 2nd ed. Philadelphia, WB Saunders, 1979, p 614.
11. Chakravarty K, Pountain G, Merry P, et al: A longitudinal study of anticardiolipin antibody in polymyalgia rheumatica and giant cell arteritis. J Rheumatol 22:1694, 1995.
12. Park JR, Jones JG, Harkniss GD, Hazleman BL: Circulating immune complexes in polymyalgia rheumatica and giant cell arteritis. Ann Rheum Dis 40:360, 1981.
13. Papaioannou CC, Gupta RC, Hunder GG, McDuffie FC: Circulating immune complexes in giant cell arteritis and polymyalgia rheumatica. Arthritis Rheum 23:1021, 1980.
14. Bonnetblanc JM, Adenis JP, Queroi M, Rammaert B: Immunofluorescence in temporal arteritis. N Engl J Med 298:458, 1978.
15. Chess J, Albert DM, Bhan AK, et al: Serologic and immunopathologic findings in temporal arteritis. Am J Ophthalmol 96:283, 1983.
16. Liang GC, Simkin PA, Mammik M: Immunoglobulins in temporal arteritis. Ann Intern Med 81:19, 1974.
17. Calamia KT, Moore SB, Elveback LR, Hunder GG: HLA-DR locus antigens in polymyalgia rheumatica and giant cell arteritis. J Rheumatol 8:993, 1981.
18. Asherson RA, Chan JKH, Harris EN, et al: Anticardiolipid antibody, recurrent thrombosis, and warfarin withdrawal. Ann Rheum Dis 44:823, 1985.
19. Fauchald P, Rygvold O, Oystese B: Temporal arteritis and polymyalgia rheumatica: Clinical and biopsy findings. Ann Intern Med 77:845, 1972.
20. Gonzalez-Gay MA: Genetic epidemiology: Giant cell arteritis and polymyalgia rheumatica. Arthritis Res 3:154, 2001.
21. Hunder GG, Taswell HF, Pineda AA, Elveback LR: HLA antigens in patients with giant cell arteritis and polymyalgia rheumatica. J Rheumatol 4:321, 1977.
22. Mattey DL, Hajeer AH, Dababneh A, et al: Association of giant cell arteritis and polymyalgia rheumatica with different tumor necrosis factor microsatellite polymorphisms. Arthritis Rheum 43:1749, 2000.
23. Salvarani C, Casali B, Boiardi L, et al: Intercellular adhesion molecule 1 gene polymorphisms in polymyalgia rheumatica/giant cell arteritis: Association with disease risk and severity. J Rheumatol 27:1215, 2000.
24. Machado EBV, Michet CJ, Ballard DJ, et al: Trends in incidence and clinical presentation of temporal arteritis in Olmsted County, Minnesota, 1950–1985. Arthritis Rheum 31:745, 1988.
25. Bengtsson BA, Malmvall BE: The epidemiology of giant cell arteritis including temporal arteritis and polymyalgia rheumatica. Arthritis Rheum 24:899, 1981.
26. Boesen P, Sorensen SF: Giant cell arteritis, temporal arteritis, and polymyalgia rheumatica in a Danish county: A prospective investigation, 1982–1985. Arthritis Rheum 30:294, 1987.
27. Galetta SL, Raps EC, Wulc AE, et al: Conjugal temporal arteritis. Neurology (NY) 40:1839, 1990.
28. Tanenbaum M, Tenzel J: Familial temporal arteritis. J Clin Neuro-Ophthalmol 5:244, 1985.
29. Rimenti G, Blasi F, Cosentini R, et al: Temporal arteritis associated with *Chlamydia pneumoniae* DNA detected in an artery specimen. J Rheumatol 27:2718, 2000.
30. Wagner AD, Gerard HC, Fresemann T, et al: Detection of *Chlamydia pneumoniae* in giant cell vasculitis and correlation with the topographic arrangement of tissue-infiltrating dendritic cells. Arthritis Rheum 43:1543, 2000.
31. Bonnet F, Morlat P, Delavaux I, et al: A possible association between *Chlamydiae psittaci* infection and temporal arteritis. Joint Bone Spine 67:550, 2000.
32. Duhaut P, Bosshard S, Dumontet C: Giant cell arteritis and polymyalgia rheumatica: Role of viral infections. Clin Exp Rheumatol 18(Suppl 20):S22, 2000.
33. Goodman BW: Temporal arteritis. Am J Med 67:839, 1979.
34. Hamilton CR, Shelley WM, Tumulty PA: Giant cell arteritis: Including temporal arteritis and polymyalgia rheumatica. Medicine (Baltimore) 50:1, 1971.
35. Hauser WA, Ferguson RH, Holley KE, Kurland LT: Temporal arteritis in Rochester, Minnesota, 1951 to 1967. Mayo Clin Proc 46:597, 1971.

36. Healey LA, Wilske KR: Manifestations of giant cell arteritis. Med Clin North Am 61:261, 1977.

37. Huston KA, Hunder GG: Giant cell (cranial) arteritis: A clinical review. Am Heart J 100:99, 1980.

38. Jonasson F, Cullen JF, Elton RA: Temporal arteritis: A 14-year epidemiological, clinical and prognostic study. Scott Med J 24:111, 1979.

39. Horton BT: Complications of temporal arteritis. BMJ 1:105, 1966.

40. Hamilton CR, Shelley WM, Tumulty PA: Giant cell arteritis: Including temporal arteritis and polymyalgia rheumatica. Medicine (Balt) 50:1, 1971.

41. Caselli RJ, Hunder GG, Whisnant JP: Neurologic disease in biopsy-proven giant cell (temporal) arteritis. Neurology (NY) 38:352, 1988.

42. Alestig K, Barr J: Giant-cell arteritis: A biopsy study of polymyalgia rheumatica, including one case of Takayasu's disease. Lancet 1:1228, 1963.

43. Bengtsson BA, Malmvall BE: Prognosis of giant cell arteritis including temporal arteritis and polymyalgia rheumatica. Acta Med Scand 209:337, 1981.

44. Fauchald P, Rygvold O, Oystese B: Temporal arteritis and polymyalgia rheumatica: Clinical and biopsy finding. Ann Intern Med 77:845, 1972.

45. Huston KA, Hunder GG, Lie JT, et al: Temporal arteritis: A 25-year epidemiologic, clinical and pathologic study. Ann Intern Med 88:162, 1978.

46. Ostberg G: On arteritis with special reference to polymyalgia arteritica. Acta Pathol Microbiol Scand 237(Suppl A):1, 1973.

47. Jones JG, Hazleman BL: Prognosis and management of polymyalgia rheumatica. Ann Rheum Dis 40:1, 1981.

48. Hayreh SS: Anterior ischemic optic neuropathy. Arch Neurol 38:675, 1981.

49. Hollenhorst RW, Brown JR, Wagener HP, Shick RM: Neurologic aspects of temporal arteritis. Neurology (NY) 10:490, 1960.

50. Boghen DR, Glaser JS: Ischaemic optic neuropathy. Brain 98:689, 1975.

51. Cardell BS, Hanley T: A fatal case of giant-cell or temporal arteritis. J Pathol 63:587, 1951.

52. Cohen DN, Damaske MM: Temporal arteritis: A spectrum of ophthalmic complications. Ann Ophthalmol 7:1045, 1975.

53. Crompton MR: The visual changes in temporal (giant cell) arteritis. Brain 82:377, 1959.

54. Graham E: Survival in temporal arteritis. Trans Ophthalmol Soc U K 100:108, 1980.

55. Russell RWR: Giant-cell arteritis: A review of 35.cases. Q J Med 28:471, 1959.

56. Miller NR: Anterior ischemic optic neuropathy: Diagnosis and management. Bull N Y Acad Med 56:643, 1980.

57. Dimant J, Grob D, Brunner NG: Ophthalmoplegia, ptosis, and myosis in temporal arteritis. Neurology (NY) 39:1054, 1980.

58. Meadows SP: Temporal or giant cell arteritis. Proc R Soc Med 59:329, 1966.

59. Fisher CM: Ocular palsy in temporal arteritis. Minn Med 42:1258, 1959.

60. Barricks ME, Traviesa DM, Glaser JS, Levy IS: Ophthalmoplegia in cranial arteritis. Brain 100:209, 1977.

61. Borruat FX, Bogousslavsky J, Uffer S, et al: Orbital infarction syndrome. Ophthalmology 100:562, 1993.

62. Howard GF, Ho SU, Kim KS, Wallach J: Bilateral carotid occlusion resulting from giant cell arteritis. Ann Neurol 15:204, 1984.

63. Wilkinson IMS, Russell RWR: Arteries of the head and neck in giant cell arteritis: A pathological study to show the pattern of arterial involvement. Arch Neurol 27:378, 1972.

64. Bogousslavsky J, Deruaz JP, Regli F: Bilateral obstruction of internal carotid artery from giant-cell arteritis and massive infarction limited to the vertebrobasilar area. Eur Neurol 24:57, 1985.

65. Whimster WF: Two neurological cases: Demonstration at the Royal College of Physicians of London. Br Med J 1:727, 1979.

66. Collado A, Santamaria J, Ribalta T, et al: Giant-cell arteritis presenting with ipsilateral hemiplegia and lateral medullary syndrome. Eur Neurol 29:266, 1989.

67. Gilmour JR: Giant-cell chronic arteritis. J Pathol 53:263, 1941.

68. Heptinstall RH, Porter KA, Barkley H: Giant cell (temporal) arteritis. J Pathol 67:507, 1954.

69. Gibb WRG, Urry PA, Lees AJ: Giant cell arteritis with spinal cord infarction and basilar artery thrombosis. J Neurol Neurosurg Psychiatry 48:945, 1985.

70. Greenfield JG: Giant cell arteritis. Proc R Soc Med 44:855, 1951.

71. Jellinger K: Giant cell granulomatous angiitis of the central nervous system. J Neurol 215:175, 1977.

72. Kjeldsen MH, Reske-Nielsen E: Pathological changes of the central nervous system in giant cell arteritis. Acta Ophthalmol Scand 46:49, 1968.

73. Missen GA: Involvement of the vertebrocarotid arterial system in giant cell arteritis. J Pathol 1972;106:2.

74. Morrison AN, Abitol M: Granulomatous arteritis with myocardial infarction. Ann Intern Med 42:691, 1955.

75. Säve-Söderbergh J, Malmvall BO, et al: Giant cell arteritis as a cause of death: Report of nine cases. JAMA 255:493, 1986.

76. Thystrup J, Knudsen GM, Mogensen AM, Fledelius HC: Atypical visual loss in giant cell arteritis. Acta Ophthalmol (Copenh) 72:759, 1994.

77. Verker R: Psychiatric aspects of temporal arteritis. J Mental Sci 98:280, 1952.

78. Enzmann D, Scott WR: Intracranial involvement of giant-cell arteritis. Neurology (NY) 27:794, 1977.

79. Hinck VC, Carter CC, Rippey GG: Giant cell (cranial) arteritis: A case with angiographic abnormalities. AJR Am J Roentgenol 92:769, 1964.

80. Hirsch M, Mayersdorf A, Lehman E: Cranial giant cell arteritis. Br J Radiol 47:503, 1974.

81. McCormick HM, Neuberger KT: Giant cell arteritis involving small meningeal and intracerebral vessels. J Neuropathol Exp Neurol 17:471, 1958.

82. Butt Z, Cullen JF, Mutlukan E: Pattern of arterial involvement of the head, neck, and eyes in giant cell arteritis: Three case reports. Br J Ophthalmol 75:368, 1991.

83. Pollack M, Blennerhasset JB, Clarke AM: Giant cell arteritis and the subclavian steal syndrome. Neurology (NY) 23:653, 1973.

84. Ostberg G: Temporal arteritis in a large necropsy series. Ann Rheum Dis 30:224, 1971.

85. Spencer WH, Hoyt WF: A fatal case of giant cell arteritis (temporal or cranial arteritis) with ocular involvement. Arch Ophthalmol 64:862, 1962.

86. Hunder GG, Bloch DA, Michel BA, et al: The American College of Rheumatology 1990 criteria for the classification of giant cell arteritis. Arthritis Rheum 33:1122, 1990.

87. Kausu T, Corbett JJ, Savino P, Schatz NJ: Giant cell arteritis with normal sedimentation rate. Arch Neurol 34:624, 1977.

88. Wong RL, Korn JH: Temporal arteritis without an elevated erythrocyte sedimentation rate: Case report and review of the literature. Am J Med 80:959, 1986.

89. Salvarani C, Hunder GG: Giant cell arteritis with low erythrocyte sedimentation rate: Frequency of occurrence in a population-based study. Arthritis Rheum 45:140, 2001.

90. Martinez-Taboada VM, Blanco R, Armona J, et al: Giant cell arteritis with an erythrocyte sedimentation rate lower than 50. Clin Rheumatol 19:73, 2000.

91. Hall GH, Hargreaves T: Giant cell arteritis and raised serum alkaline phosphate levels [letter]. Lancet 2:48, 1972.

92. Dickson ER, Maldonado JE, Sheps SG, Cain JA: Systemic giant-cell arteritis with polymyalgia rheumatica: Reversible abnormalities of liver function. JAMA 224:1496, 1973.

93. Gonzalez-Gay MA, Garcia-Porrua C, Llorca J, et al: Biopsy-negative giant cell arteritis: Clinical spectrum and predictive factors for positive temporal artery biopsy. Semin Arthritis Rheum 30:249, 2001.

94. Hall S, Hunder GG: Is temporal artery biopsy prudent? Mayo Clin Proc 59:793, 1984.

95. Klein RG, Campbell RJ, Hunder GG, Carney JA: Skip lesions in temporal arteritis. Mayo Clin Proc 51:504, 1976.

96. Hammoudeh M, Khan M: Cranial arteritis as the initial manifestation of malignant histiocytosis. J Rheumatol 9:443, 1982.

97. Morgan GJ Jr, Harris ED Jr: Non-giant cell temporal arteritis. Arthritis Rheum 21:362, 1978.

98. Schmidt WA, Kraft HE, Vorpahl K, et al: Color duplex ultrasonography in the diagnosis of temporal arteritis. N Engl J Med 337:1336, 1997.

99. Turlakow A, Yeung HW, Pui J, et al: Fludeoxyglucose positron emission tomography in the diagnosis of giant cell arteritis. Arch Intern Med 161:1003, 2001.

100. Joelsen E, Ruthrauff B, Ali F, et al: Multifocal dural enhancement associated with temporal arteritis. Arch Neurol 57:119, 2000.

Specific Medical Diseases and Stroke

101. Von Knorring J: Treatment and prognosis in polymyalgia rheumatica and temporal arteritis: A ten-year survey of 53 patients. Acta Med Scand 205:429, 1975.

102. Andersson R, Malmvall BE, Bengtsson BA: Long-term corticosteroid treatment in giant cell arteritis. Acta Med Scand 220:465, 1986.

103. Hunder GG, Sheps SG, Allen GL, Joyce JW: Daily and alternate-day corticosteroid regimens in treatment of giant cell arteritis: Comparison in a prospective study. Ann Intern Med 82:613, 1975.

104. Rosenfeld SI, Kosmorsky GS, Klingele TG, et al: Treatment of temporal arteritis with ocular involvement. Am J Med 80:143, 1986.

105. Jover JA, Hernandez-Garcia C, Morado IC, et al: Combined treatment of giant-cell arteritis with methotrexate and prednisone: A randomized, double-blind, placebo-controlled trial. Ann Intern Med 134:106, 2001.

106. Lie JT: Aortic and extracranial large vessel giant cell arteritis: A review of 72 cases with histopathologic documentation. Semin Arthritis Rheum 24:422, 1995.

107. Budzilovich GN, Feigin I, Siegel H: Granulomatous angiitis of the nervous system. Arch Pathol Lab Med 76:250, 1963.

108. Kolodny EK, Rebeiz JJ, Caviness VS, Richardson EP: Granulomatous angiitis of the central nervous system. Arch Neurol 19:510, 1968.

109. Cupps TR, Moore PM, Fauci AS: Isolated angiitis of the central nervous system. Am J Med 74:97, 1983.

110. Cravioto H, Feigin I: Non-infectious granulomatous angiitis with a predilection for the nervous system. Neurology (NY) 9:599, 1959.

111. Arthur G, Margolis G: Mycoplasma-like structures in granulomatous angiitis of the central nervous system: Case reports with light and electron microscope studies. Arch Pathol Lab Med 101:382, 1977.

112. Marsden HB: Basilar artery thrombosis and giant cell arteritis [abstract]. Arch Dis Child 49:75, 1974.

113. Nagaratnam N, James WE: Isolated angiitis of the brain in a young female on the contraceptive pill. Postgrad Med J 63:1085, 1987.

114. Sandhu R, Alexander S, Hornabrook RW, Stehbens WE: Granulomatous angiitis of the CNS. Arch Neurol 36:433, 1979.

115. Shuangshoti S: Localized granulomatous (giant cell) angiitis of brain with eosinophil infiltration and saccular aneurysm. J Med Assoc Thai 62:281, 1979.

116. Thomas L, David S, McClusky RT: Studies of PPLO infection. I: The production of cerebral polyarteritis by *Mycoplasma gallisepticum* in turkeys, the neurotoxic property of the mycoplasma. J Exp Med 123:897, 1966.

117. Clyde WA, Thomas L: Pathogenesis studies in experimental mycoplasma disease: *M. gallisepticum* infections of turkeys. Ann N Y Acad Sci 225:413, 1973.

118. Nogueras C, Sala M, Sasal M, et al: Recurrent stroke as a manifestation of primary angiitis of the central nervous system in a patient infected with human immunodeficiency virus. Arch Neurol 59:468, 2002.

119. Hayman M, Hendson G, Poskitt KJ, Connolly MB: Postvaricella angiopathy: Report of a case with pathologic correlation. Pediatr Neurol 24:387, 2001.

120. Blue MC, Rosenblum WI: Granulomatous angiitis of the brain with herpes zoster and varicella encephalitis. Arch Pathol Lab Med 107:126, 1983.

121. Borenstein D, Costa M, Jannotta F, Rizzoli H: Localized isolated angiitis of the central nervous system associated with primary intracerebral lymphoma. Cancer 62:375, 1988.

122. Gilbert GJ: Herpes zoster ophthalmicus and delayed contralateral hemiparesis: Relationship of the syndrome to central nervous system granulomatous angiitis. JAMA 229:302, 1974.

123. Ojeda VJ, Peters DM, Spagnolo DV: Giant cell granulomatous angiitis of the central nervous system in a patient with leukemia and cutaneous herpes zoster. Am J Clin Pathol 81:529, 1984.

124. Lexa FJ, Galetta SL, Yousem DM, et al: Herpes zoster ophthalmicus with orbital pseudotumor syndrome complicated by optic nerve infarction and cerebral granulomatous angiitis: MR-pathologic correlation. AJNR Am J Neuroradiol 14:185, 1993.

125. Inwards DJ, Piepgras DG, Lie JT, et al: Granulomatous angiitis of the spinal cord associated with Hodgkin's disease. Cancer 68:1318, 1991.

126. Yankner BA, Skolnik PR, Shoukimas GM, et al: Cerebral granulomatous angiitis associated with isolation of human T-lymphotropic virus type III from the central nervous system. Ann Neurol 20:362, 1986.

127. Reyes MG, Fresco R, Chokroverty S, Salud EQ: Virus-like particles in granulomatous angiitis of the central nervous system. Neurology (NY) 26:797, 1976.

128. Fountain NB, Eberhard DA: Primary angiitis of the central nervous system associated with cerebral amyloid angiopathy: Report of two cases and review of the literature. Neurology 46:190, 1996.

129. Gray F, Vinters HV, Le Noan H, et al: Cerebral amyloid angiopathy and granulomatous angiitis: Immunohistochemical study using antibodies to the Alzheimer A4 peptide. Hum Pathol 21:1290, 1990.

130. Probst A, Ulrich J: Amyloid angiopathy combined with granulomatous angiitis of the central nervous system: Report on two patients. Clin Neuropathol 4:250, 1985.

131. Ginsberg L, Geddes J, Valentine A: Amyloid angiopathy and granulomatous angiitis of the central nervous system: A case responding to corticosteroid treatment. J Neurol 235:438, 1988.

132. Beresford HR, Hyman RA, Shorer L: Self-limited granulomatous angiitis of the cerebellum. Ann Neurol 5:490, 1979.

133. Berger JR, Romano J, Menkin M, Norenberg M: Benign focal cerebral vasculitis: Case report. Neurology 45:1731, 1995.

134. Johnson MD, Maciunas R, Creasy J, Collins RD: Indolent granulomatous angiitis: Case report. J Neurosurg 81:472, 1994.

135. Biller J, Loftus CM, Moore SA, et al: Isolated central nervous system angiitis first presenting as spontaneous intracranial hemorrhage. Neurosurgery 20:310, 1987.

136. Burger PC, Burch JG, Vogel FS: Granulomatous angiitis: An unusual etiology of stroke. Stroke 8:29, 1977.

137. Koo EH, Massey EW: Granulomatous angiitis of the central nervous system: Protean manifestations and response to treatment. J Neurol Neurosurg Psychiatry 51:1126, 1988.

138. Caccamo DV, Garcia JH, Ho KL: Isolated granulomatous angiitis of the spinal cord. Ann Neurol 32:580, 1992.

139. Giovanini MA, Eskin TA, Mukherji SK, Mickle JP: Granulomatous angiitis of the spinal cord: A case report. Neurosurgery 34:540, 1994.

140. Anderson NE, Willoughby EW, Synek BJL: Leptomeningeal and brain biopsy in chronic meningitis. Aust N Z J Med 25:703, 1995.

141. Reik L, Grunnett ML, Spencer RP, Donalson JO: Granulomatous angiitis presenting as chronic meningitis and ventriculitis. Neurology (NY) 33:1609, 1983.

142. Ehsan T, Hasan S, Powers JM, Heiserman JE: Serial magnetic resonance imaging in isolated angiitis of the central nervous system. Neurology 45:1462, 1995.

143. Greenan TJ, Grossman RI, Goldberg HI: Cerebral vasculitis: MR imaging and angiographic correlation. Radiology 182:65, 1992.

144. Negishi C, Sze G: Vasculitis presenting as primary leptomeningeal enhancement with minimal parenchymal findings. AJNR Am J Neuroradiol 14:26, 1993.

145. Castleman B, McNeely BU: Case records of the Massachusetts General Hospital: Case 14-1967. N Engl J Med 276:741, 1967.

146. Castleman B, McNeely BU: Case records of the Massachusetts General Hospital: Case 26-1967. N Engl J Med 276:1432, 1967.

147. Frayne JH, Gilligan BS, Essex WB: Granulomatous angiitis of the central nervous system. Med J Aust 145:410, 1986.

148. Marsden HB: Basilar artery thrombosis and giant cell arteritis [abstract]. Arch Dis Child 49:75, 1974.

149. Ferris H: Cerebral arteritis: Classification. Radiology 109:327, 1973.

150. Giang DW: Central nervous system vasculitis secondary to infections, toxins, and neoplasms. Semin Neurol 14:313, 1994.

151. Hurst RW, Grossman RI: Neuroradiology of central nervous system vasculitis. Semin Neurol 14:320, 1994.

152. Leeds NE, Goldberg HI: Angiographic manifestations in cerebral inflammatory disease. Radiology 98:595, 1971.

153. Rumbaugh CL, Bergeron RT, Fang HC, McCormick R: Cerebral angiographic changes in the drug abuse patient. Radiology 101:335, 1971.

154. Alrawi A, Trobe JD, Blaivas M, Musch DC: Brain biopsy in primary angiitis of the central nervous system. Neurology 53:858, 1999.

155. Chu CT, Gray L, Goldstein LB, Hulette CM: Diagnosis of intracranial vasculitis: A multi-disciplinary approach. J Neuropathol Exp Neurol 58:30, 1998.

156. Harrison PE: Granulomatous angiitis of the central nervous system. J Neurol Sci 29:335, 1976.

157. Hughes JT, Brownell B: Granulomatous giant-celled angiitis of the central nervous system. Neurology (NY) 16:293, 1966.

158. Younger DS, Hays AP, Brust JCM, Rowland LP: Granulomatous angiitis of the brain: An inflammatory reaction of diverse etiology. Arch Neurol 45:514, 1988.

159. Moore PM: Diagnosis and management of isolated angiitis of the central nervous system. Neurology (NY) 39:167, 1989.

160. Cupps TR, Moore PM, Fauci AS: Isolated angiitis of the central nervous system. Am J Med 74:97, 1983.

161. Ebinger F, Mannhardt-Laakmann W, Zepp F: Cerebral vasculitis stabilised by methotrexate. Eur J Pediatr 159:712, 2000.

162. Greco FA, Kolins J, Rajjoub RK, Brereton HD: Hodgkin's disease and granulomatous angiitis of the central nervous system. Cancer 38:2027, 1976.

163. Gasperetti C, Son SK: Contralateral hemiparesis following herpes zoster ophthalmicus. J Neurol Neurosurg Psychiatry 48:338, 1985.

164. Hilt DC, Buchholz D, Krumholz A, et al: Herpes zoster ophthalmicus and delayed contralateral hemiparesis caused by cerebral angiitis: Diagnosis and management approaches. Ann Neurol 14:543, 1983.

165. Wilson CA, Wander AH, Choromokos EA: Central retinal artery obstruction in herpes zoster ophthalmicus and cerebral vasculopathy. Ann Ophthalmol 22:347, 1990.

166. Deane JS, Bibby K: Bilateral optic neuritis following herpes zoster ophthalmicus [letter]. Arch Ophthalmol 113:972, 1995.

167. Doyle PW, Gibson G, Dolman CL: Herpes zoster ophthalmicus with contralateral hemiplegia: Identification of cause. Ann Neurol 14:84, 1983.

168. Eidelberg D, Sotrel A, Horoupian DS, et al: Thrombotic cerebral vasculopathy associated with herpes zoster. Ann Neurol 19:7, 1986.

169. Filloux F, Townsend J: Herpes zoster ophthalmicus with ipsilateral cerebellar infarction. Neurology (NY) 35:1531, 1985.

170. Bourdette DN, Rosenberg NL, Yatsu FM: Herpes zoster ophthalmicus and delayed ipsilateral cerebral infarction. Neurology (NY) 33:1428, 1983.

171. Herkes GK, Storey CE, Joffe R, Mackenzie RA: Herpes zoster arteritis: Clinical and angiographic features. Clin Exp Neurol 64:169, 1987.

172. Sarazin L, Duong H, Bourgouin PM, et al: Herpes zoster vasculitis: Demonstration by MR angiography. J Comput Assist Tomogr 19:624, 1995.

173. O'Donohue JM, Enzmann DR: Mycotic aneurysm in angiitis associated with herpes zoster ophthalmicus. AJNR Am J Neuroradiol 8:615, 1987.

174. Görsoy G, Aktin E, Bahar S, et al: Post-herpetic aneurysm in the intrapetrosal portion of the internal carotid artery. Neuroradiology 19:279, 1980.

175. Mackenzie RA, Ryan P, Karnes WE, Okazaki H: Herpes zoster arteritis: Pathological findings. Clin Exp Neurol 23:219, 1987.

176. Martin JR, Mitchell WJ, Henken DB: Neurotropic herpesviruses, neural mechanisms and arteritis. Brain Pathol 1:6, 1990.

177. Nasu T: Takayasu's truncoarteritis in Japan: A statistical observation of 76 autopsy cases. Pathol Microbiol 43:140, 1975.

178. Hall S, Barr W, Lie JT, et al: Takayasu arteritis: A study of 32 North American patients. Medicine (Balt) 64:89, 1985.

179. Ishikawa K, Yonekawa Y: Regression of carotid stenoses after corticosteroid therapy in occlusive thromboaortopathy (Takayasu's disease). Stroke 18:677, 1987.

180. Yoneda S, Nukada T, Kunihiko T, et al: Subclavian steal in Takayasu's arteritis: A hemodynamic study by means of ultrasonic Doppler flowmetry. Stroke 8:264, 1977.

181. Vinijchaikul K: Primary arteritis of the aorta and its main branches (Takayasu's arteriopathy): A clinicopathologic autopsy study of eight cases. Am J Med 43:15, 1967.

182. Ishikawa K: Natural history and classification of occlusive thromboaortopathy (Takayasu's disease). Circulation 57:27, 1978.

183. Masuzawa T, Shimabukuro H, Furuse M, et al: Pulseless disease associated with a ruptured intracranial vertebral aneurysm. Neurol Med Chir 24:490, 1984.

184. Friedrich H, Laas J, Walterbusch G, Rickels E: Extra-intracranial bypass procedure with saphenous vein grafts. Thorac Cardiovasc Surg 34:57, 1986.

185. Giordano JM, Leavitt RY, Hoffman G, Fauci AS: Experience with surgical treatment of Takayasu's disease. Surgery 109:252, 1991.

186. Robbs JV, Human RR, Rajaruthnam P: Operative treatment of non-specific aortoarteritis (Takayasu's arteritis). J Vasc Surg 3:605, 1986.

187. Shelhamer JH, Volkman DJ, Parrillo JE, et al: Takayasu's arteritis and its therapy. Ann Intern Med 103:121, 1985.

188. Masugata H, Yasuno M, Nishino M, et al: Takayasu's arteritis with collateral circulation from the right coronary artery to intracranial vessels—a case report. Angiology 43:448, 1992.

189. Ford RG, Siekert RG: Central nervous system manifestations of periarteritis nodosa. Neurology (NY) 15:114, 1965.

190. Guillevin L, Lhote F, Gayraud M, et al: Prognostic factors in polyarteritis nodosa and Churg-Strauss syndrome: A prospective study in 342 patients. Medicine (Balt) 75:17, 1996.

191. Harle JR, Disdier P, Ali Cherif A, et al: Démence curable et panartérite noueuse. Rev Neurol (Paris) 147:148, 1991.

192. Beattie DK, Hellier WP, Powell MP: Stroke-induced cardiovascular changes: A rare cause of death from polyarteritis nodosa. Br J Neurosurg 9:223, 1995.

193. Travers RL, Allison DJ, Brettle RP, Hughes GRV: Polyarteritis nodosa: A clinical and angiographic analysis of 17 cases. Semin Arthritis Rheum 8:184, 1979.

194. Castaigne P, Cambier J, Escourolle R, Brunet P: Les manifestations nerveuses centrales de la périartérite noueuse: à propos d'une observation anatomo-clinique. Ann Med Interne 121:375, 1970.

195. Kernohan JW, Woltman HW: Periarteritis nodosa: A clinicopathologic study with special reference to the nervous system. Arch Neurol Neurosurg Psychiatry 39:655, 1938.

196. Parker HL, Kernohan JW: The central nervous system in periarteritis nodosa. Trans Am Neurol Assoc 72:54, 1947.

197. Parker HL, Kernohan JW: The central nervous system in periarteritis nodosa. Mayo Clin Proc 24:43, 1949.

198. Malamud N, Foster DB: Periarteritis nodosa: A clinicopathologic report, with special reference to the central nervous system. Arch Neurol Psychiatry 47:828, 1942.

199. Beattie DK, Hellier WP, Powell MP: Stroke-induced cardiovascular changes: A rare cause of death from polyarteritis nodosa. Br J Neurosurg 9:223, 1995.

200. Gherardi GJ, Lee HU: Localized dissecting hemorrhage and arteritis: Renal and cerebral manifestations. JAMA 199:187, 1967.

201. Sergent JS, Lockshin MD, Christian CL, Gocke DJ: Vasculitis with hepatitis B antigenemia: Long-term observations in nine patients. Medicine (Balt) 55:1, 1976.

202. Ojeda VJ: Polyarteritis nodosa affecting the spinal cord arteries. Aust N Z J Med 13:287, 1983.

203. Haft H, Finneson BE, Cramer H, Fiol R: Periarteritis nodosa as a source of subarachnoid hemorrhage and spinal cord compression. J Neurosurg 14:608, 1957.

204. Fauci AS, Katz P, Haynes BF, Wolff SM: Cyclophosphamide therapy of severe systemic necrotizing vasculitis. N Engl J Med 301:235, 1979.

205. Leib ES, Restivo C, Paulus HE: Immunosuppressive and corticosteroid therapy of polyarteritis nodosa. Am J Med 67:941, 1979.

206. Engel DG, Gospe SM Jr, Tracy KA, et al: Fatal infantile polyarteritis nodosa with predominant central nervous system involvement. Stroke 26:699, 1995.

207. Tan EM, Cohen AS, Fries JF, et al: The 1982 revised criteria for the classification of systemic lupus erythematosus. Arthritis Rheum 25:1271, 1982.

208. Devinsky O, Petito CK, Alonso DR: Clinical and neuropathological findings in systemic lupus erythematosus: The role of vasculitis, heart emboli, and thrombotic thrombocytopenic purpura. Ann Neurol 23:380, 1988.

209. Fox IS, Spence AM, Wheelis RF, Healey LA: Cerebral embolism in Libman-Sacks endocarditis. Neurology (NY) 30:487, 1980.

210. Futrell N, Millikan C: Frequency, etiology, and prevention of stroke in patients with systemic lupus erythematosus. Stroke 20:583, 1989.

211. Gorelick PB, Rusinowitz MS, Tiku M, et al: Embolic stroke complicating systemic lupus erythematosus. Arch Neurol 42:813, 1985.

212. Harris EN, Gharavi AE, Asherson RA, et al: Cerebral infarction in systemic lupus: Association with anticardiolipin antibodies. Clin Exp Rheumatol 2:47, 1984.

213. Kitagawa Y, Gotoh F, Koto A, Okayasu H: Stroke in systemic lupus erythematosus. Stroke 21:1533, 1990.

214. Estes D, Christian CL: The natural history of systemic lupus erythematosus by prospective analysis. Medicine (Balt) 50:85, 1971.

215. Feinglass EJ, Arnett FC, Dorsch CA, et al: Neuropsychiatric manifestations of systemic lupus erythematosus: Diagnosis, clinical spectrum, and relationship to other features of the disease. Medicine (Balt) 55:323, 1976.

Specific Medical Diseases and Stroke

216. Ward MM, Pyun E, Studenski S: Causes of death in systemic lupus erythematosus: Long-term follow-up of an inception cohort. Arthritis Rheum 38:1492, 1995.

217. Ward MM: Cardiovascular and cerebrovascular morbidity and mortality among women with end-stage renal disease attributable to lupus nephritis. Am J Kidney Dis 36:516, 2000.

218. Johnson RT, Richardson EP: The neurological manifestations of systemic lupus erythematosus: A clinical-pathological study of 24 cases and review of the literature. Medicine (Balt) 47:337, 1968.

219. Ellis SG, Verity MA: Central nervous system involvement in systemic lupus erythematosus: A review of neuropathologic findings in 57 cases, 1955–1977. Semin Arthritis Rheum 4:253, 1979.

220. Hanly JG, Walsh NM, Sangalang V: Brain pathology in systemic lupus erythematosus. J Rheumatol 19:732, 1992.

221. Silverstein A: Cerebrovascular accidents as the initial major manifestation of lupus erythematosus. N Y State J Med 5:2942, 1963.

222. Trevor RP, Sondheimer FK, Fessel WJ, Wolpert SM: Angiographic demonstration of major cerebral vessel occlusion in systemic lupus erythematosus. Neuroradiology 4:202, 1972.

223. Libman E, Sacks B: A hitherto undescribed form of valvular and mural endocarditis. Arch Intern Med 33:701, 1924.

224. D'Alton JG, Preston DN, Bormanis J, et al: Multiple transient ischemic attacks, lupus anticoagulant and verrucous endocarditis. Stroke 16:512, 1985.

225. Murphy JJ, Leach IH: Findings at necropsy in the heart of a patient with anticardiolipin syndrome. Br Heart J 62:61, 1989.

226. Young SM, Fisher M, Sigsbee A, Errichetti A: Cardiogenic brain embolism and lupus anticoagulant. Ann Neurol 26:390, 1989.

227. Kumral E, Evyapan D, Keser G, et al: Detection of microembolic signals in patients with neuropsychiatric lupus erythematosus. Eur Neurol 47:131, 2002.

228. Gharavi AE, Harris EN, Asherson RA, Hughes GRV: Anticardiolipin antibodies: Isotype distribution and phospholipid specificity. Ann Rheum Dis 46:1, 1987.

229. Bowie EJW, Thompson JH Jr, Pascuzzi CA, Owen CA Jr: Thrombosis in systemic lupus erythematosus despite circulating anticoagulants. J Lab Clin Med 62:416, 1963.

230. Clinical and laboratory findings in patients with antiphospholipid antibodies and cerebral ischemia. The Antiphospholipid Antibodies in Stroke Study Group. Stroke 21:1268, 1990.

231. Asherson RA, Mercey D, Phillips G, et al: Recurrent stroke and multi-infarct dementia in systemic lupus erythematosus: Association with antiphospholipid antibodies. Ann Rheum Dis 46:605, 1987.

232. Briley DP, Coull BM, Goodnight SH Jr: Neurological disease associated with antiphospholipid antibodies. Ann Neurol 25:221, 1989.

233. Coull BM, Bourdette DN, Goodnight SH Jr, et al: Multiple cerebral infarctions and dementia associated with anticardiolipin antibodies. Stroke 18:1107, 1987.

234. Coull BM, Goodnight SH: Antiphospholipid antibodies, prethrombotic states, and stroke. Stroke 21:1370, 1990.

235. Digre KB, Durcan FJ, Branch DW, et al: Amaurosis fugax associated with antiphospholipid antibodies. Ann Neurol 25:228, 1989.

236. Gastineau DA, Kazmier FJ, Nichols WL, Bowie EJW: Lupus anticoagulant: An analysis of the clinical and laboratory features of 219 cases. Am J Hematol 19:265, 1985.

237. Harris EN, Gharavi AE, Asherson RA, et al: Cerebral infarction in systemic lupus: Association with anticardiolipin antibodies. Clin Exp Rheumatol 2:47, 1984.

238. Hughes GRV, Asherson RA, Khamashta MA: The antiphospholipid syndrome—from theory to discovery. Postgrad Med J 65:691, 1989.

239. Levine SR, Deegan MJ, Futrell N, Welch KMA: Cerebrovascular and neurologic disease associated with antiphospholipid antibodies: 48 cases. Neurology (NY) 40:1181, 1990.

240. Asherson RA, Khamashta MA, Ordi-Ros J, et al: The "primary" antiphospholipid syndrome: Major clinical and serological features. Medicine (Balt) 68:366, 1989.

241. Asherson RA, Chan JKH, Harris EN, et al: Anticardiolipin antibody, recurrent thrombosis, and warfarin withdrawal. Ann Rheum Dis 44:823, 1985.

242. Briley DP, Coull BM, Goodnight SH Jr: Neurological disease associated with antiphospholipid antibodies. Ann Neurol 25:221, 1989.

243. Brey RL, Levine SR: Treatment of neurologic complications of antiphospholipid antibody syndrome. Lupus 5:473, 1996.

244. Khamashta MA, Cuadrado MJ, Mujic F, et al: The management of thrombosis in the antiphospholipid-antibody syndrome. N Engl J Med 332:993, 1995.

245. Lie JT, Kobayashi S, Tokano Y, Hashimoto H: Systemic and cerebral vasculitis coexisting with disseminated coagulopathy in systemic lupus erythematosus associated with antiphospholipid syndrome. J Rheumatol 22:2173, 1995.

246. Toussirot E, Figarella-Branger D, Disdier P, et al: Association of cerebral vasculitis with a lupus anticoagulant: A case with brain pathology. Clin Rheumatol 13:624, 1994.

247. Wierzbicki AS: Lipids, cardiovascular disease and atherosclerosis in systemic lupus erythematosus. Lupus 9:194, 2000.

248. Hashimoto N, Handa H, Taki W: Ruptured cerebral aneurysms in patients with systemic lupus erythematosus. Surg Neurol 26:512, 1986.

249. Kelley RE, Stokes N, Reyes P, Harik SI: Cerebral transmural angiitis and ruptured aneurysm: A complication of systemic lupus erythematosus. Arch Neurol 37:526, 1980.

250. Feit H, Frenkel EP, Dunn BR, et al: Acute subdural hematomas with lupus anticoagulant (procoagulant inhibitor). Neurology (NY) 34:519, 1984.

251. Enevoldson TP, Russell RW: Cerebral venous thrombosis: New causes for an old syndrome? Q J Med 77:1255, 1990.

252. Levine SR, Kieran S, Puzio K, et al: Cerebral venous thrombosis with lupus anticoagulants: Report of two cases. Stroke 18:801, 1987.

253. Shiozawa Z, Yoshida M, Kobayashi K, et al: Superior sagittal sinus thrombosis and systemic lupus erythematosus. Ann Neurol 20:272, 1986.

254. Vidailhet M, Piett JC, Wechsler B, et al: Cerebral venous thrombosis in systemic lupus erythematosus. Stroke 21:1226, 1990.

255. Fauci AS, Haynes BF, Katz P, Wolff SM: Wegener's granulomatosis: Prospective clinical and therapeutic experience with 85 patients for 21 years. Ann Intern Med 98:76, 1983.

256. Drachman DA: Neurological complications of Wegener's granulomatosis. Arch Neurol 8:145, 1963.

257. Anderson JM, Jamieson DG, Jefferson JM: Non-healing granuloma and the nervous system. Q J Med 41:309, 1975.

258. Scully RE, Mark EJ, McNeely WF, McNeely BU: Case records of the Massachusetts General Hospital: Case 12-1988. N Engl J Med 318:760, 1988.

259. Satoh J, Miyasaka N, Yamada T, et al: Extensive cerebral infarction due to involvement of both anterior cerebral arteries by Wegener's granulomatosis. Ann Rheum Dis 47:606, 1988.

260. Mickle JP, McLennan JE, Chi JG, Lidden CW: Cortical vein thrombosis in Wegener's granulomatosis: Case report. J Neurosurg 46:248, 1977.

261. Newman NJ, Slamovits TL, Friedland S, Wilson WB: Neuro-ophthalmic manifestations of meningocerebral inflammation from the limited form of Wegener's granulomatosis. Am J Ophthalmol 120:613, 1995.

262. Nishino H, Rubino FA, Parisi JE: The spectrum of neurologic involvement in Wegener's granulomatosis. Neurology 43:1334, 1993.

263. Tishler S, Williamson T, Mirra SS, et al: Wegener granulomatosis with meningeal involvement. AJNR Am J Neuroradiol 14:1248, 1993.

264. Weinberger LM, Cohen ML, Remler BF, et al: Intracranial Wegener's granulomatosis. Neurology 43:1831, 1993.

265. Enevoldson TP, Russell RW: Cerebral venous thrombosis: New causes for an old syndrome? Q J Med 77:1255, 1990.

266. Fred HL, Lynch EC, Greenberg SD, Gonzalez-Angulo A: A patient with Wegener's granulomatosis exhibiting unusual clinical and morphologic features. Am J Med 37:311, 1964.

267. Lucas FV, Benjamin SP, Steinberg MC: Cerebral vasculitis in Wegener's granulomatosis. Cleve Clin J Med 43:275, 1976.

268. MacFadyen DJ: Wegener's granulomatosis with discrete lung lesions and peripheral neuritis. Can Med Assoc J 83:760, 1960.

269. Tuhy JE, Maurice GL, Niles NR: Wegener's granulomatosis. Am J Med 25:638, 1958.

270. Nishino H, Rubino FA, DeRemee RA, et al: Neurological involvement in Wegener's granulomatosis: An analysis of 324 consecutive patients at the Mayo Clinic. Ann Neurol 33:4, 1993.

271. Lucas FV, Benjamin SP, Steinberg MC: Cerebral vasculitis in Wegener's granulomatosis. Cleve Clin J Med 43:275, 1976.

272. Goldberg AL, Tievsky AL, Jamshidi S: Wegener granulomatosis invading the cavernous sinus: A CT demonstration. J Comput Assist Tomogr 7:701, 1983.

273. Specks U, Wheatley CL, McDonald TJ, et al: Anticytoplasmic autoantibodies in the diagnosis and follow-up of Wegener's granulomatosis. Mayo Clin Proc 64:28, 1989.

274. Cohen Tervaert JW, van der Woude FJ, Fauci AS, et al: Association between active Wegener's granulomatosis and anticytoplasmic antibodies. Arch Intern Med 149:2461, 1989.

275. Nölle B, Specks U, Lüdemann J, et al: Anticytoplasmic autoantibodies: Their immunodiagnostic value in Wegener granulomatosis. Ann Intern Med 111:28, 1989.

276. Chang Y, Kargas SA, Goates JJ, Horoupian DS: Intraventricular and subarachnoid hemorrhage resulting from necrotizing vasculitis of the choroid plexus in a patient with Churg-Strauss syndrome. Clin Neuropathol 12:84, 1993.

277. Weinstein JM, Chui H, Lane S, et al: Churg-Strauss syndrome (allergic granulomatous angiitis): Neuro-ophthalmologic manifestations. Arch Ophthalmol 101:1217, 1983.

278. Lewis IC, Philpott MG: Neurological complications in the Schönlein-Henoch syndrome. Arch Dis Child 31:369, 1956.

279. Winkelmann RK, Ditto WB: Cutaneous and visceral syndromes of necrotizing or "allergic" angiitis: A study of 38 cases. Medicine (Balt) 43:59, 1964.

280. Liebow AA, Carrington CRB, Friedman PJ: Lymphomatoid granulomatosis. Hum Pathol 3:457, 1972.

281. Liebow AA: Pulmonary angiitis and granulomatosis. Am Rev Respir Dis 108:1, 1973.

282. Amin SN, Gibbons CM, Lovell CR, et al: A case of lymphomatoid granulomatosis with a protracted course and prominent CNS involvement. Br J Rheumatol 28:77, 1989.

283. Hogan PJ, Greenberg MK, McCarty GE: Neurologic complications of lymphomatoid granulomatosis. Neurology (NY) 31:619, 1981.

284. Hood J, Wilson ER Jr, Alexander CB, et al: Lymphomatoid granulomatosis manifested as a mass in the cerebellopontine angle. Arch Neurol 39:319, 1982.

285. Ironside JW, Martin JF, Richmond J, Timperley WR: Lymphomatoid granulomatosis with cerebral involvement. Neuropathol Appl Neurobiol 10:397, 1984.

286. Kapila A, Gupta KL, Garcia JH: CT and MR of lymphomatoid granulomatosis of the CNS: Report of four cases and review of the literature. AJNR Am J Neuroradiol 9:1139, 1988.

287. Kerr RSC, Hughes JT, Blamires T, Teddy PJ: Lymphomatoid granulomatosis apparently confined to one temporal lobe: Case report. J Neurosurg 67:612, 1987.

288. Patton WF, Lynch JP III: Lymphomatoid granulomatosis: Clinicopathologic study of four cases and literature review. Medicine (Balt) 61:1, 1982.

289. Whelan HT, Moore P: Central nervous system lymphomatoid granulomatosis. Pediatr Neurosci 13:113, 1987.

290. Schmidt BJ, Meagher-Villemure K, Del Carpio J: Lymphomatoid granulomatosis with isolated involvement of the brain. Ann Neurol 15:478, 1984.

291. Averbuch-Heller L, Steiner I, Abramsky O: Neurologic manifestations of progressive systemic sclerosis. Arch Neurol 49:1292, 1992.

292. Gordon RM, Silverstein A: Neurologic manifestations in progressive systemic sclerosis. Arch Neurol 22:126, 1970.

293. Estey E, Lieberman A, Pinto R, et al: Cerebral arteritis in scleroderma. Stroke 10:595, 1979.

294. Whittaker R, Barnett A, Ryan P: Antiphospholipid syndrome in scleroderma. J Rheumatol 20:1598, 1993.

295. Lee JE, Haynes JM: Carotid arteritis and cerebral infarction due to scleroderma. Neurology (NY) 17:18, 1967.

296. Bathon JM, Moreland LW, DiBartolomeo AG: Inflammatory central nervous system involvement in rheumatoid arthritis. Semin Arthritis Rheum 18:258, 1989.

297. Gutman L, Hable K: Rheumatoid pachymeningitis. Neurology (NY) 13:901, 1963.

298. Jackson CG, Chess RL, Ward JR: A case of rheumatoid nodule formation within the central nervous system and review of the literature. J Rheumatol 11:237, 1984.

299. Karam NE, Roger L, Hankins LL, Reveille JD: Rheumatoid nodulosis of the meninges. J Rheumatol 21:1960, 1994.

300. Kim RC: Rheumatoid disease with encephalopathy. Ann Neurol 7:861, 1980.

301. Kim RC, Collins GH, Parisi JE: Rheumatoid nodule formation within the choroid plexus: Report of a second case. Arch Pathol Lab Med 106:83, 1982.

302. Markenson JA, McDougal JS, Tsairis P, et al: Rheumatoid meningitis: A localized immune process. Ann Intern Med 90:786, 1979.

303. Spurlock RG, Richman AV: Rheumatoid meningitis: A case report and review of the literature. Arch Pathol Lab Med 107:129, 1983.

304. Mandybur TI: Cerebral amyloid angiopathy: Possible relationship to rheumatoid vasculitis. Neurology (NY) 29:1336, 1979.

305. Ouyang R, Mitchell DM, Rozdilsky B: Central nervous system involvement in rheumatoid disease: Report of a case. Neurology (NY) 17:1099, 1967.

306. Steiner JW, Gelbloom AJ: Intracranial manifestations in two cases of systemic rheumatoid disease. Arthritis Rheum 2:537, 1959.

307. Watson P, Fekete J, Deck J: Central nervous system vasculitis in rheumatoid arthritis. Can J Neurol Sci 4:269, 1977.

308. Johnson RL, Smyth CJ, Holt GW, et al: Steroid therapy and vascular lesions in rheumatoid arthritis. Arthritis Rheum 2:224, 1959.

309. Ramos M, Mandybur TI: Cerebral vasculitis in rheumatoid arthritis. Arch Neurol 32:271, 1975.

310. Rodman GP: Clinical pathological conference. J Rheumatol 11:855, 1984.

311. Singleton JD, West SG, Reddy VV, Rak KM: Cerebral vasculitis complicating rheumatoid arthritis. South Med J 88:470, 1995.

312. Jones MW, Kaufmann JCE: Vertebrobasilar artery insufficiency in rheumatoid atlantoaxial subluxation. J Neurol Neurosurg Psychiatry 39:122, 1976.

313. Webb FWS, Hickman JA, Brew DSJ: Death from vertebral artery thrombosis in rheumatoid arthritis. Br Med J 2:537, 1968.

314. Howell SJL, Molyneux AJ: Vertebrobasilar insufficiency in rheumatoid atlanto-axial subluxation: A case report with angiographic demonstration of left vertebral artery occlusion. J Neurol 235:189, 1988.

315. Robinson BP, Seeger JF, Zak SM: Rheumatoid arthritis and positional vertebrobasilar insufficiency: A case report. J Neurosurg 65:111, 1986.

316. Fedele FA, Ho G Jr, Dorman BA: Pseudoaneurysm of the vertebral artery: A complication of rheumatoid cervical spine disease. Arthritis Rheum 29:136, 1986.

317. Chatzis A, Giannopoulos N, Baharakakis S, et al: Unusual cause of a stroke in a patient with seronegative rheumatoid arthritis. Cardiovasc Surg 7:659, 1999.

318. Ehrenfeld M, Penchas S, Eliakim M: Thrombocytosis in rheumatoid arthritis: Recurrent arterial thromboembolism and death. Ann Rheum Dis 36:579, 1977.

319. Pines A, Kaplinsky N, Olchovsky D, et al: Recurrent transient ischemic attacks associated with thrombocytosis in rheumatoid arthritis. Clin Rheumatol 1:291, 1982.

320. Sarnat RL, Jampol LM: Hyperviscosity retinopathy secondary to polyclonal gammopathy in a patient with rheumatoid arthritis. Ophthalmology 93:124, 1986.

321. Harley JB, Alexander EL, Bias WB, et al: Anti-Ro (SS-A) and anti-La (SS-B) in patients with Sjögren's syndrome. Arthritis Rheum 29:196, 1986.

322. Alexander E, McFarland H: Sjögren's syndrome mimicking multiple sclerosis [letter]. Ann Neurol 17:586, 1990.

323. Alexander EL: Neurologic disease in Sjögren's syndrome: Mononuclear inflammatory vasculopathy affecting central/peripheral nervous system and muscle. A clinical review and update of immunopathogenesis. Rheum Dis Clin North Am 19:869, 1993.

324. Alexander GE, Provost TT, Stevens MB, Alexander EL: Sjögren syndrome: Central nervous system manifestations. Neurology (NY) 31:1391, 1981.

325. Binder A, Snaith ML, Isenberg D: Sjögren's syndrome: A study of its neurological complications. Br J Rheumatol 27:275, 1988.

326. Alexander EL, Ranzenbach MR, Kumar AJ, et al: Anti-Ro (SS-A) autoantibodies in central nervous system disease associated with Sjögren's syndrome (CNS-SS): Clinical, neuroimaging, and angiographic correlates. Neurology 44:899, 1994.

327. Miró J, Peña-Sagredo JL, Berciano J, et al: Prevalence of primary Sjögren's syndrome in patients with multiple sclerosis. Ann Neurol 27:582, 1990.

328. Moore PM, Lisak RP: Multiple sclerosis and Sjögren's syndrome: A problem in diagnosis or in definition of two disorders of unknown etiology? Ann Neurol 27:585, 1990.

329. Moutsopoulos HM, Sarmas JH, Talal N: Is central nervous system involvement a systemic manifestation of primary Sjögren's syndrome? Rheum Dis Clin North Am 19:909, 1993.

330. Noseworthy JH, Bass BH, Vandervoort MK, et al: The prevalence of primary Sjögren's syndrome in a multiple sclerosis population. Ann Neurol 25:95, 1989.

331. Noseworthy JH, Bass BH, Vandervoort MK, et al: Reply [letter]. Ann Neurol 27:587, 1990.

Specific Medical Diseases and Stroke

332. Alexander EL, Malinow K, Lejewski JE, et al: Primary Sjögren's syndrome with central nervous system disease mimicking multiple sclerosis. Ann Intern Med 104:323, 1986.

333. Gottfried JA, Finkel TH, Hunter JV, et al: Central nervous system Sjögren's syndrome in a child: Case report and review of the literature. J Child Neurol 16:683, 2001.

334. Nagahiro S, Mantani A, Yamada K, Ushio Y: Multiple cerebral arterial occlusions in a young patient with Sjögren's syndrome: Case report. Neurosurgery 38:592, 1996.

335. Caselli RJ, Scheithauer BW, Bowles CA, et al: The treatable dementia of Sjögren's syndrome. Ann Neurol 30:98, 1991.

336. Alexander EL, Beall SS, Gordon B, et al: Magnetic resonance imaging of cerebral lesions in patients with the Sjögren syndrome. Ann Intern Med 108:815, 1988.

337. Govoni M, Padovan M, Rizzo N, Trotta F: CNS involvement in primary Sjögren's syndrome: Prevalence, clinical aspects, diagnostic assessment and therapeutic approach. CNS Drugs 15:597, 2001.

338. Escudero D, Latorre P, Codina M, et al: Central nervous system disease in Sjögren's syndrome. Ann Intern Med 146:239, 1995.

339. de la Monte SM, Hutchins GM, Gupta PK: Polymorphous meningitis with atypical mononuclear cells in Sjögren's syndrome. Ann Neurol 14:455, 1983.

340. Alexander EL, Craft C, Dorsh C, et al: Necrotizing arteritis and spinal subarachnoid hemorrhage in Sjögren syndrome. Ann Neurol 11:632, 1982.

341. Giordano MJ, Commins D, Silbergeld DL: Sjögren's cerebritis complicated by subarachnoid hemorrhage and bilateral superior cerebellar artery occlusion: Case report. Surg Neurol 43:48, 1995.

342. Caselli RJ, Scheithauer BW, Bowles CA, et al: The treatable dementia of Sjögren's syndrome. Ann Neurol 30:98, 1991.

343. Quimby SR, Perry HO: Livedo reticularis and cerebrovascular accidents. J Am Acad Dermatol 3:377, 1980.

344. Champion RH, Rook A: Livedo reticularis. Proc R Soc Med 53:961, 1960.

345. Sneddon IB: Cerebro-vascular lesions and livedo reticularis. Br J Dermatol 77:180, 1965.

346. Tourbah A, Piette JC, Iba-Zizen MT, et al: The natural course of cerebral lesions in Sneddon syndrome. Arch Neurol 54:53, 1997.

347. Frances C, Papo T, Wechsler B, et al: Sneddon syndrome with or without antiphospholipid antibodies: A comparative study in 46 patients. Medicine 78:209, 1999.

348. Asherson RA, Mayou SC, Merry P, et al: The spectrum of livedo reticularis and anticardiolipid antibodies. Br J Dermatol 120:215, 1989.

349. Grattan CEH, Burton JL, Boon AP: Sneddon's syndrome (livedo reticularis and cerebral thrombosis) with livedo vasculitis and anticardiolipin antibodies. Br J Dermatol 120:441, 1989.

350. Jonas J, Kölble K, Völcker HE, Kalden JR: Central retinal artery occlusion in Sneddon's disease associated with antiphospholipid antibodies. Am J Ophthalmol 102:37, 1986.

351. Kalashnikova LA, Nasonov EL, Kushekbaeva AE, Gracheva LA: Anticardiolipin antibodies in Sneddon's syndrome. Neurology (NY) 40:464, 1990.

352. Levine SR, Langer SL, Albers JW, Welch KMA: Sneddon's syndrome: An antiphospholipid antibody syndrome? Neurology 38:798, 1988.

353. Francés C, Le Tonquéze M, Salohzin KV, et al: Prevalence of anti-endothelial cell antibodies in patients with Sneddon's syndrome. J Am Acad Dermatol 33:64, 1995.

354. Fetoni V, Grisoli M, Salmaggi A, et al: Clinical and neuroradiological aspects of Sneddon's syndrome and primary antiphospholipid antibody syndrome: A follow-up study. Neurol Sci 21:157, 2000.

355. Rehany U, Kassif Y, Rumelt S: Sneddon's syndrome: Neuroophthalmologic manifestations in a possible autosomal recessive pattern. Neurology 51:1185, 1998.

356. Geschwind DH, FitzPatrick M, Mischel PS, Cummings JL: Sneddon's syndrome is a thrombotic vasculopathy: Neuropathologic and neuroradiologic evidence. Neurology 45:557, 1995.

357. Lossos A, Ben-Hur T, Ben-Nariah Z, et al: Familial Sneddon's syndrome. J Neurol 242:164, 1995.

358. Pettee AD, Wasserman BA, Adams NL, et al: Familial Sneddon's syndrome: Clinical, hematologic, and radiographic findings in two brothers. Neurology 44:399, 1994.

359. Rebollo M, Val JF, Garijo F, et al: Livedo reticularis and cerebrovascular lesions (Sneddon's syndrome): Clinical, radiological and pathological features in eight cases. Brain 106:965, 1983.

360. Rumpl E, Neuhofer J, Pallua A: Cerebrovascular lesions and livedo reticularis (Sneddon's syndrome): A progressive cerebrovascular disorder? J Neurol 231:324, 1985.

361. Schulze-Lohff E, Krapf F, Bleil L, et al: IgM-containing immune complexes and antiphospholipid antibodies in patients with Sneddon's syndrome. Rheumatol Int 9:43, 1989.

362. Stephens WP, Ferguson IT: Livedo reticularis and cerebro-vascular disease. Postgrad Med J 58:770, 1982.

363. Thomas DJ, Kirby JDT, Britton KE, Galton DJ: Livedo reticularis and neurological lesions. Br J Dermatol 106:711, 1982.

364. Wright RA, Kokmen E: Gradually progressive dementia without discrete cerebrovascular events in a patient with Sneddon's syndrome. Mayo Clin Proc 74:57, 1999.

365. Adair JC, Digre KB, Swanda RM, et al: Sneddon's syndrome: A cause of cognitive decline in young adults. Neuropsychiatry Neuropsychol Behav Neurol 14:197, 2001.

366. Stockhammer G, Felber SR, Zelger B, et al: Sneddon's syndrome: Diagnosis by skin biopsy and MRI in 17 patients. Stroke 24:685, 1993.

367. Boortz-Marx RL, Clark HB, Taylor S, et al: Sneddon's syndrome with granulomatous leptomeningeal infiltration. Stroke 26:492, 1995.

368. Pellat J, Perret J, Pasquier B, et al: Etude anatomoclinique et angiographique d'une observation de thromboangiose disséminée a manifestations cérébrales prédominantes. Rev Neurol (Paris) 132:517, 1976.

369. Weisshaar E, Claus G, Friedl A, Gollnick H: Atrial myxoma syndrome mimicking Ehrmann-Sneddon syndrome. Dermatology 195:404, 1997.

370. Stockhammer GJ, Felber SR, Aichner FT, et al: Sneddon's syndrome and antiphospholipid antibodies: Clarification of a controversy by skin biopsy [letter]? Stroke 23:1182, 1992.

371. Dupont S, Fénelon G, Saiag P, Sirmai J: Warfarin in Sneddon's syndrome [letter]. Neurology 46:1781, 1996.

372. Uitdehaag BM, Scheltens P, Bertelsmann FW, Bruyn RP: Intracerebral haemorrhage in Sneddon's syndrome [letter]. J Neurol Sci 11:227, 1992.

373. Schulze-Lohff E, Krapf F, Bleil L, et al: IgM-containing immune complexes and antiphospholipid antibodies in patients with Sneddon's syndrome. Rheumatol Int 9:43, 1989.

374. Degos R, Delort J, Tricot R: Dermatite papulosquameuse atrophiante. Bull Soc Franc Dermat Syph 49:148, 1942.

375. Horner FA, Myers GJ, Stumpf DA, et al: Malignant atrophic papulosis (Kohlmeier-Degos disease) in childhood. Neurology (NY) 26:317, 1976.

376. Winkelmann RK, Howard FM Jr, Perry HO, Miller RH: Malignant papulosis of skin and cerebrum: A syndrome of vascular thrombosis. Arch Dermatol 87:94, 1963.

377. McFarland HR, Wood WG, Drowns BV, Meneses ACO: Papulosis atrophicans maligna (Köhlmeier-Degos disease): A disseminated occlusive vasculopathy. Ann Neurol 3:388, 1978.

378. Scully RE, Galdabini JJ, McNeely BU: Case records of the Massachusetts General Hospital: Case 43-1976. N Engl J Med 295:944, 1976.

379. Barlow RJ, Heyl T, Simson IW, Schulz EJ: Malignant atrophic papulosis (Degos' disease): Diffuse involvement of brain and bowel in an African patient. Br J Dermatol 118:117, 1988.

380. Strole WE Jr, Clark WH Jr, Isselbacher KJ: Progressive arterial occlusive disease (Köhlmeier-Degos): A frequently fatal cutaneosystemic disorder. N Engl J Med 276:195, 1967.

381. Dastur DK, Singhal BS, Shroff HJ: CNS involvement in malignant atrophic papulosis (Köhlmeier-Degos disease): Vasculopathy and coagulopathy. J Neurol Neurosurg Psychiatry 44:156, 1981.

382. Petit WA, Soso MJ, Higman H: Degos disease: Neurologic complications and cerebral angiography. Neurology (NY) 32:1305, 1982.

383. Culicchia CF, Gol A, Erickson EE: Diffuse central nervous system involvement in papulosis atrophicans maligna. Neurology (NY) 12:503, 1962.

384. Wolf SM, Schotland DL, Phillips LL: Involvement of nervous system in Behçet's syndrome. Arch Neurol 12:315, 1965.

385. Label LS, Tandan R, Albers JW: Myelomalacia and hypoglycorrhachia in malignant atrophic papulosis. Neurology (NY) 33:936, 1983.

386. Burrow JN, Blumbergs PC, Iyer PV, Hallpike JF: Köhlmeier-Degos disease: A multisystem vasculopathy with progressive cerebral infarction. Aust N Z J Med 21:49, 1991.

387. Warot P, Caron JC, Lehembre P, Houcke M: Maladie de Degos à forme cérébrale. Rev Neurol (Paris) 133:353, 1977.

388. Drucker CR: Malignant atrophic papulosis: Response to antiplatelet therapy. Dermatologica 180:90, 1990.

389. Magrinat G, Kerwin KS, Gabriel DA: The clinical manifestations of Degos' syndrome. Arch Pathol Lab Med 113:354, 1989.

390. Englert HJ, Hawkes CH, Boey ML, et al: Degos' disease: Association with anticardiolipin antibodies and the lupus anticoagulant. BMJ 289:576, 1984.

391. Shimazu S, Imai H, Kokubu S, et al: Long-term survival in malignant atrophic papulosis: A case report and review of the Japanese literature. Nippon Geka Gakkai Zasshi 89:1748, 1988.

392. O'Duffy JD, Goldstein NP: Neurologic involvement in seven patients with Behçet's disease. Am J Med 61:170, 1976.

393. O'Duffy JD, Robertson DM, Goldstein NP: Chlorambucil in the treatment of uveitis and meningoencephalitis of Behçet's disease. Am J Med 76:75, 1984.

394. Dobkin BH: Computerized tomographic findings in neuro-Behçet's disease. Arch Neurol 37:58, 1980.

395. Iraguli VJ, Maravi E: Behçet syndrome presenting as cerebrovascular disease. J Neurol Neurosurg Psychiatry 49:838, 1986.

396. Kozin F, Haughton V, Bernhard GC: Neuro-Behçet disease: Two cases and neuroradiologic findings. Neurology (NY) 27:1148, 1977.

397. Strouth JC, Dyken M: Encephalopathy of Behçet's disease: Report of a case. Neurology (NY) 14:794, 1964.

398. Lueck CJ, Pires M, McCartney AC, Graham EM: Ocular and neurological Behçet's disease without orogenital ulceration? J Neurol Neurosurg Psychiatry 56:505, 1993.

399. Rougemont D, Bousser MG, Wechsler B, et al: Manifestations neurologiques de la maladie de Behçet: Vingt-quatre observations. Rev Neurol (Paris) 138:493, 1982.

400. Kawakita H, Nishimura M, Satoh Y, Shibata N: Neurological aspects of Behçet's disease: A case report and clinico-pathological review of the literature in Japan. J Neurol Sci 5:417, 1967.

401. Lu AT, Barasch S: Neurological involvement in Behçet's syndrome: A case report with neuropathological data and a summary of the reported autopsied cases. Bull Los Angeles Neurol Soc 28:85, 1963.

402. Rubinstein LJ, Urich H: Meningo-encephalitis of Behçet's disease: Case report with pathological findings. Brain 86:151, 1963.

403. Wolf SM, Schotland DL, Phillips LL: Involvement of nervous system in Behçet's syndrome. Arch Neurol 12:315, 1965.

404. McMenemey WH, Lawrence BJ: Encephalomyelopathy in Behçet's disease: Report of necropsy findings in two cases. Lancet 2:353, 1957.

405. Scott D: Mucocutaneous-ocular syndrome (Behçet's syndrome) with meningoencephalitis: Report of a case with autopsy. Acta Med Scand 161:397, 1958.

406. Bank I, Weart C: Dural sinus thrombosis in Behçet's disease. Arthritis Rheum 27:816, 1984.

407. Cobby M, Hall CL, Higgs CMB: Behçet's syndrome presenting as intracranial hypertension in a Caucasian. J R Soc Med 81:478, 1988.

408. Harper CM Jr, O'Neill BP, O'Duffy JD, Forbes GS: Intracranial hypertension in Behçet's disease: Demonstration of sinus occlusion with use of digital subtraction angiography. Mayo Clin Proc 60:419, 1985.

409. Imaizumi M, Nukada T, Yoneda S, Abe H: Behçet's disease with sinus thrombosis and arteriovenous malformation in brain. J Neurol 222:215, 1980.

410. Pamir MN, Kansu T, Erbengi A, Zileli T: Papilledema in Behçet's syndrome. Arch Neurol 38:643, 1981.

411. Stern JM, Kesler SM: Raised intracranial pressure in a 16-year-old boy: Report of a case of Behçet's disease. S Afr Med J 75:243, 1989.

412. Wechsler B, Vidailhet M, Piette JC, et al: Cerebral venous thrombosis in Behçet's disease: Clinical study and long-term follow-up of 25 cases. Neurology 42:614, 1992.

413. Wilkins MR, Gove RI, Roberts SD, Kendall MJ: Behçet's disease presenting as benign intracranial hypertension. Postgrad Med J 62:39, 1986.

414. Al Kawi MZ, Bohlega S, Banna M: MRI findings in neuro-Behçet's disease. Neurology 41:405, 1991.

415. Besana C, Comi G, Del Maschio A, et al: Electrophysiological and MRI evaluation of neurological involvement in Behçet's disease. J Neurol Neurosurg Psychiatry 52:749, 1989.

416. Hull RG, Harris N, Gharavi AE, et al: Anticardiolipin antibodies: Occurrence in Behçet's syndrome. Ann Rheum Dis 43:746, 1984.

417. Banna M, el-Ramahl K: Neurologic involvement in Behçet disease: Imaging findings in 16 patients. AJNR Am J Neuroradiol 12:791, 1991.

418. Herskovitz S, Lipton RB, Lantos G: Neuro-Behçet's disease: CT and clinical correlates. Neurology (NY) 38:1714, 1988.

419. Kazui S, Naritomi H, Imakita S, et al: Sequential gadolinium-DTPA enhanced MRI studies in neuro-Behçet's disease. Neuroradiology 33:136, 1991.

420. Morrissey SP, Miller DH, Hermaszewski R, et al: Magnetic resonance imaging of the central nervous system in Behçet's disease. Eur Neurol 33:287, 1993.

421. Patel DV, Neuman JM, Hier DB: Reversibility of CT and MR findings in neuro-Behçet disease. J Comput Assist Tomogr 13:669, 1989.

422. Willeit J, Schmutzhard E, Aichner F, et al: CT and MR imaging in neuro-Behçet disease. J Comput Assist Tomogr 10:313, 1986.

423. Devlin T, Gray L, Allen NB, et al: Neuro-Behçet's disease: Factors hampering proper diagnosis. Neurology 45:1754, 1995.

424. Altinörs N, Senveli E, Arda N, et al: Intracerebral hemorrhage and hematoma in Behçet's disease: Case report. Neurosurgery 21:582, 1987.

425. Nagata K: Recurrent intracranial haemorrhage in Behçet disease. J Neurol Neurosurg Psychiatry 48:190, 1985.

426. Zelenski JD, Capraro JA, Holden D, Calabrese LH: Central nervous system vasculitis in Behçet's syndrome: Angiographic improvement after therapy with cytotoxic agents. Arthritis Rheum 32:217, 1989.

427. Dhobb M, Ammar F, Bensaid Y, et al: Arterial manifestations in Behçet's disease: Four new cases. Ann Vasc Surg 1:249, 1986.

428. Yamamori C, Ishino H, Inagaki T, et al: Neuro-Behçet disease with demyelination and gliosis of the frontal white matter. Clin Neuropathol 13:208, 1994.

429. Shimizu T, Ehrlich GE, Inaba G, Hayashi K: Behçet's disease (Behçet syndrome). Semin Arthritis Rheum 8:223, 1979.

430. Nishimura M, Satoh K, Suga M, Oda M: Cerebral angio- and neuro-Behçet's syndrome: Neuroradiological and pathological study of one case. J Neurol Sci 106:19, 1991.

431. Abramsky O, Slavin S: Neurologic manifestations in patients with mixed cryoglobulinemia. Neurology (NY) 24:245, 1974.

432. Petty GW, Duffy J, Huston J III: Cerebral ischemia in patients with hepatitis C virus infection and mixed cryoglobulinemia. Mayo Clin Proc 71:671, 1996.

433. Reik L Jr, Korn JH: Cryoglobulinemia with encephalopathy: Successful treatment by plasma exchange. Ann Neurol 10:488, 1981.

434. Ristow SC, Griner PF, Abraham GN, Shoulson I: Reversal of systemic manifestations of cryoglobulinemia: Treatment with melphalan and prednisone. Arch Intern Med 136:467, 1976.

435. Gorevic PD, Kassab HJ, Levo Y, et al: Mixed cryoglobulinemia: Clinical aspects and long-term follow-up of 40 patients. Am J Med 69:287, 1980.

436. Serena M, Biscaro R, Moretto G, Recchia E: Peripheral and central nervous system involvement in essential mixed cryoglobulinemia: A case report. Clin Neuropathol 10:177, 1991.

437. Bogousslavsky J, Gaio JM, Caplan LR, et al: Encephalopathy, deafness and blindness in young women: A distinct retinocochleocerebral arteriolopathy? J Neurol Neurosurg Psychiatry 52:43, 1989.

438. Coppeto JR, Currie JN, Monteiro MLR, Lessell S: A syndrome of arterial-occlusive retinopathy and encephalopathy. Am J Ophthalmol 98:189, 1984.

439. Gordon DL, Hayreh SS, Adams HP Jr: Microangiopathy of the brain, retina, and ear: Improvement without immunosuppressive therapy. Stroke 22:933, 1991.

440. Heiskala H, Somer H, Kovanen J, et al: Microangiopathy with encephalopathy, hearing loss and retinal arteriolar occlusions: Two new cases. J Neurol Sci 86:239, 1988.

441. Kaminska EA, Sadler M, Sangalang V, et al: Microangiopathic syndrome of encephalopathy, retinal vessel occlusion and hearing loss [abstract]. Can J Neurol Sci 2:241, 1990.

442. MacFadyen DJ, Schneider RJ, Chisholm IA: A syndrome of brain, inner ear and retinal microangiopathy. Can J Neurol Sci 14:315, 1987.

443. Manor RS, Ouaknine L, Ouaknine G: Susac-Red-M syndrome [abstract]. Presented as part of the proceedings of the Meeting of the International Neuro-Ophthalmological Society. Freiburg, Germany, June 1994.

444. Mass M, Bourdette D, Bernstein W, Hammerstad J: Retinopathy, encephalopathy, deafness associated microangiopathy (the RED M

Specific Medical Diseases and Stroke

syndrome): Three new cases [abstract]. Neurology (NY) 38(Suppl 1):215, 1988.

445. Monteiro MLR, Swanson RA, Coppeto JR, et al: A microangiopathic syndrome of encephalopathy, hearing loss, and retinal arteriolar occlusions. Neurology (NY) 35:1113, 1985.

446. Petty GW, Engel AG: Microangiopathic involvement of muscle in patients with retinocochleocerebral vasculopathy [abstract]. Neurology 45(Suppl 4):A312, 1995.

447. Pfaffenbach DD, Hollenhorst RS: Microangiopathy of the retinal arterioles. JAMA 225:480, 1973.

448. Schwitter J, Agosti R, Ott P, et al: Small infarctions of cochlear, retinal, and encephalic tissue in young women. Stroke 23:903, 1992.

449. Susac JO: Susac's syndrome: The triad of microangiopathy of the brain and retina with hearing loss in young women. Neurology 44:591, 1994.

450. Susac JO, Hardman JM, Selhorst JB: Microangiopathy of the brain and retina. Neurology (NY) 29:313, 1979.

451. O'Halloran HS, Pearson PA, Lee WB, et al: Microangiopathy of the brain, retina, and cochlea (Susac syndrome): A report of five cases and a review of the literature. Ophthalmology 105:1038, 1998.

452. Li HK, Dejean BJ, Tang RA: Reversal of visual loss with hyperbaric oxygen treatment in a patient with Susac syndrome. Ophthalmology 103:2091, 1996.

453. Papo T, Biousse V, Lehoang P, et al: Susac syndrome. Medicine 77:3, 1998.

454. Petty GW, Matteson EL, Younge BR, et al: Recurrence of Susac syndrome (retinocochleocerebral vasculopathy) after remission of 18.years. Mayo Clin Proc 76:958, 2001.

455. Cogan DG: Syndrome of nonsyphilitic interstitial keratitis and vestibuloauditory symptoms. Arch Ophthalmol 33:144, 1945.

456. Vollertsen RS, McDonald TJ, Younge BR, et al: Cogan's syndrome: 18 cases and a review of the literature. Mayo Clin Proc 61:344, 1986.

457. Sigelman J, Behrens M, Hilal S: Acute posterior multifocal placoid pigment epitheliopathy associated with cerebral vasculitis and homonymous hemianopia. Am J Ophthalmol 88:919, 1979.

458. Smith CH, Savino PJ, Beck RW, et al: Acute posterior multifocal placoid pigment epitheliopathy and cerebral vasculitis. Arch Neurol 40:48, 1983.

459. Stoll G, Reiners K, Schwartz A, et al: Acute posterior multifocal placoid pigment epitheliopathy with cerebral involvement. J Neurol Neurosurg Psychiatry 54:77, 1991.

460. Weinstein JM, Bresnick GH, Bell CL, et al: Acute posterior multifocal placoid pigment epitheliopathy associated with cerebral vasculitis. J Clin Neuro-Ophthalmol 8:195, 1988.

461. Wilson CA, Choromokos EA, Sheppard R: Acute posterior multifocal placoid pigment epitheliopathy and cerebral vasculitis. Arch Ophthalmol 106:796, 1988.

462. Gordon MF, Coyle PK, Golub B: Eales' disease presenting as stroke in the young adult. Ann Neurol 24:264, 1988.

463. Sawhney IM, Chopra JS, Bansal SK, Gupta AK: Eales' disease with myelopathy. Clin Neurol Neurosurg 88:213, 1986.

464. Ross R: Atherosclerosis—an inflammatory disease. N Engl J Med 340:115, 1999.

465. del Rincon ID, Williams K, Stern MP, et al: High incidence of cardiovascular events in a rheumatoid arthritis cohort not explained by traditional cardiac risk factors. Arthritis Rheum 44:2737, 2001.

466. Liuzzo G, Kopecky SL, Frye RL, et al: Perturbation of the T cell repertoire in patients with unstable angina. Circulation 100:2135, 1999.

467. Esdaile JM, Abrahamowicz M, Grodzicky T, et al: Traditional Framingham risk factors fail to fully account for accelerated atherosclerosis in systemic lupus atherosclerosis. Arthritis Rheum 44:2331, 2001.

468. Munro JM, van der Walt JD, Munro CS, et al: An immunohistochemical analysis of human aortic fatty streaks. Hum Pathol 18:375, 1987.

469. Napoli C, D'Armiento FP, Mancini FP, et al: Fatty streak formation occurs in human fetal aortas and is greatly enhanced by maternal hypercholesterolemia: Intimal accumulation of low density lipoprotein and its oxidation precede monocyte recruitment into early atherosclerotic lesions. J Clin Invest 100:2680, 1997.

470. Stary HC, Chandler AB, Glagov S, et al: A definition of initial, fatty streak, and intermediate lesions of atherosclerosis: A report from the Committee on Vascular Lesions of the Council on Arteriosclerosis, American Heart Association. Circulation 89:2462, 1994.

471. Simionescu N, Vasile E, Lupu F, et al: Prelesional events in atherogenesis: Accumulation of extracellular cholesterol-rich liposomes in the arterial intima and cardiac valves of the hyperlipidemic rabbit. Am J Pathol 123:109, 1986.

472. Mazzone A, De Servi S, Ricevuti G, et al: Increased expression of neutrophil and monocyte adhesion molecules in unstable coronary artery disease. Circulation 88:358, 1993.

473. Galea J, Armstrong J, Gadsdon P, et al: Interleukin-1β in coronary arteries of patients with ischemic heart disease. Arterioscler Thromb Vasc Biol 16:1000, 1992.

474. Barath P, Fishbein MC, Cao J, et al: Detection and localization of tumor necrosis factor in human atheroma. Am J Cardiol 65:297, 1990.

475. van der Wal AC, Das PK, Bentz van de Berg D, et al: Atherosclerotic lesions in humans: In situ immunophenotypic analysis suggesting an immune-mediated response. Lab Invest 61:166, 1989.

476. Nilsson J: Cytokines and smooth muscle cells in atherosclerosis. Cardiovasc Res 27:1184, 1993.

477. Quinn MT, Parthasarathy S, Fong LG, Steinberg D: Oxidatively modified low density lipoproteins: A potential role in recruitment and retention of monocyte/macrophages during atherogenesis. Proc Natl Acad Sci U S A 84:2995, 1987.

478. Rajavashisth TB, Andalibi A, Territo MC, et al: Induction of endothelial cell expression of granulocyte and macrophage colony-stimulating factors by modified low-density lipoproteins. Nature 344:254, 1990.

479. Leonard EJ, Yoshimura T: Human monocyte chemoattractant protein-1 (MCP-1). Immunol Today 11:97, 1990.

480. Stary HC: The histological classification of atherosclerotic lesions in human coronary arteries. In Fuster V, Ross R, Topol EJ (eds): Atherosclerosis and Coronary Artery Disease, vol 1. Philadelphia, Lippincott-Raven, 1996, p 463.

481. Jonasson L, Holm J, Skalli O, et al: Regional accumulations of T cells, macrophages, and smooth muscle cells in the human atherosclerotic plaque. Arteriosclerosis 6:131, 1986.

482. Gown AM, Tsukada T, Ross R: Human atherosclerosis II: Immunocytochemical analysis of the cellular composition of human atherosclerotic lesions. Am J Pathol 125:191, 1986.

483. Libby P, Ross R: Cytokines and growth regulatory molecules. In Fuster V, Ross R, Topol EJ (eds): Atherosclerosis and Coronary Artery Disease, vol 1. Philadelphia, Lippincott-Raven, 1996, p 585.

484. Raines EW, Rosenfeld ME, Ross R: The role of macrophages. In Fuster V, Ross R, Topol EJ (eds): Atherosclerosis and Coronary Artery Disease, vol 1. Philadelphia, Lippincott-Raven, 1996, p 539.

485. Chappell DC, Varner SE, Nerem RM, et al: Oscillatory shear stress stimulates adhesion molecule expression in cultured human endothelium. Circ Res 82:532, 1998.

486. Iiyama K, Hajra L, Iiyama M, et al: Patterns of vascular cell adhesion molecule-1 and intercellular adhesion molecule-1 expression in rabbit and mouse atherosclerotic lesions and at sites predisposed to lesion formation. Circ Res 85:199, 1999.

487. Tsuboi H, Ando J, Korenaga R, et al: Flow stimulates ICAM-1 expression time and shear stress dependently in cultured human endothelial cells. Biochem Biophys Res Commun 206:988, 1995.

488. Nagel T, Resnick N, Atkinson WJ, et al: Shear stress selectively upregulates intercellular adhesion molecule-1 expression in cultured human vascular endothelial cells. J Clin Invest 94:885, 1994.

489. Resnick N, Collins T, Atkinson W, et al: Platelet-derived growth factor B chain promoter contains a cis-acting fluid shear-stress–responsive element. Proc Natl Acad Sci U S A 90:4591, 1993.

490. Lin MC, Almus-Jacobs F, Chen HH, et al: Shear stress induction of the tissue factor gene. J Clin Invest 99:737, 1997.

491. Mondy JS, Lindner V, Miyashiro JK, et al: Platelet-derived growth factor ligand and receptor expression in response to altered blood flow in vivo. Circ Res 81:320, 1997.

492. Kim CJ, Khoo JC, Gillotte-Taylor K, et al: Polymerase chain reaction-based method for quantifying recruitment of monocytes to mouse atherosclerotic lesions in vivo: Enhancement by tumor necrosis factor alpha and interleukin-1beta. Arterioscler Thromb Vasc Biol 20:1976, 2000.

493. Hynes RO, Wagner DD: Genetic manipulation of vascular adhesion molecules in mice. J Clin Invest 98:2193, 1996.

494. Hollenbaugh D, Mischel-Petty N, Edwards CP, et al: Expression of functional CD40 by vascular endothelial cells. J Exp Med 182:33, 1995.

495. Mach F, Schonbeck U, Bonnefoy J-Y, et al: Activation of monocyte/macrophage functions related to acute atheroma complication by ligation of CD40: Induction of collagenase, stromelysin, and tissue factor. Circulation 96:396, 1997.

496. Schonbeck U, Mach F, Bonnefoy J-Y, et al: Ligation of CD40 activates interleukin 1(beta)-converting enzyme (capsase-1) activity in vascular smooth muscle and endothelial cells and promotes elaboration of active interleukin 1(beta). J Biol Chem 272:19569, 1997.

497. Mach F, Schonbeck U, Sukhova GK, et al: Reduction of atherosclerosis in mice by inhibition of CD40 signalling. Nature 394:200, 1998.

498. De Caterina R, Basta G, Lazzerini G, et al: Soluble vascular cell adhesion molecule-1 as a biohumoral correlate of atherosclerosis. Arterioscler Thromb Vasc Biol 17:2646, 1997.

499. Hwang S-J, Ballantyne CM, Sharrett AR, et al: Circulating adhesion molecules VCAM-1, ICAM-1, and E-selectin in carotid atherosclerosis and incident coronary heart disease cases: The Atherosclerosis Risk in Communities (ARIC) study. Circulation 96:4219, 1997.

500. Lee RT, Libby P: The unstable atheroma. Arterioscler Thromb Vasc Biol 17:1859, 1997.

501. Schonbeck U, Mach F, Sukhova GK, et al: Regulation of matrix metalloproteinase expression in human vascular smooth muscle cells by T lymphocytes: A role for CD40 signaling in plaque rupture? Circ Res 81:448, 1997.

502. Frostegard J, Ulfgren AK, Nyberg P, et al: Cytokine expression in advanced human atherosclerotic plaques: Dominance of pro-inflammatory (Th1) and macrophage-stimulating cytokines. Atherosclerosis 145:33, 1999.

503. Tenaglia AN, Buda AJ, Wilkins RG, et al: Levels of expression of P-selectin, E-selectin, and intercellular adhesion molecule-1 in coronary atherectomy specimens from patients with stable and unstable angina pectoris. Am J Cardiol 79:742, 1997.

504. Simon AD, Yazdani S, Wang W, et al: Inflammatory cytokine profiles in stable versus unstable angina. J Thromb Thrombol 9:217, 2000.

505. Jander S, Sitzer M, Schumann R, et al: Inflammation in high-grade carotid stenosis: A possible role for macrophages and T cells in plaque destabilization. Stroke 29:1625, 1998.

506. DeGraba TJ, Siren AL, Penix L, et al: Increased endothelial expression of intercellular adhesion molecule-1 in symptomatic versus asymptomatic human carotid atherosclerotic plaque. Stroke 29:1405, 1998.

507. DeGraba TJ: Expression of inflammatory mediators and adhesion molecules in human atherosclerotic plaque. Neurology 49(Suppl 4):S15, 1997.

508. Falkenberg M, Bjornheden T, Oden A, Risberg B: Heterogeneous distribution of macrophages, tumour necrosis factor alpha, tissue factor and fibrinolytic regulators in atherosclerotic vessels. Eur J Vasc Endovasc Surg 16:276, 1998.

509. Elkind MS, Cheng J, Boden-Albala B, et al: Elevated white blood cell count and carotid plaque thickness: The Northern Manhattan Stroke Study. Stroke 32:842, 2001.

510. Salonen R, Salonen JT: Progression of carotid atherosclerosis and its determinants: A population-based ultrasonography study. Atherosclerosis 81:33, 1990.

511. Friedman GD, Klatsky AL, Siegelaub AB: The leukocyte count as a predictor of myocardial infarction. N Engl J Med 290:1275, 1974.

512. Zalokar JB, Richard JL, Claude JR: Leukocyte count, smoking, and myocardial infarction. N Engl J Med 304:465, 1981.

513. Prentice RL, Szatrowski TP, Fujikura T, et al: Leukocyte counts and coronary heart disease in a Japanese cohort. Am J Epidemiol 116:496, 1982.

514. Grimm RH, Neaton JD, Ludwig W: Prognostic importance of the white blood cell count for coronary, cancer, and all-cause mortality. JAMA 254:1932, 1985.

515. Yarnell JWG, Baker IA, Sweetnam PM, et al: Fibrinogen, viscosity, and white blood cell count are major risk factors for ischemic heart disease. Circulation 83:836, 1991.

516. Kannel WB, Anderson K, Wilson PW: White blood cell count and cardiovascular disease: Insights from the Framingham Study. JAMA 267:1253, 1992.

517. Grau AJ, Buggle F, Becher H, et al: The association of leukocyte count, fibrinogen and C-reactive protein with vascular risk factors and ischemic vascular diseases. Thromb Res 82:245, 1996.

518. Prentice RL, Szatrowski TP, Kato H, Mason MW: Leukocyte counts and cerebrovascular disease. J Chronic Dis 35:703, 1982.

519. Ford ES, Giles WH: Serum C-reactive protein and self-reported stroke: Findings from the Third National Health and Nutrition Examination Survey. Arterioscler Thromb Vasc Biol 20:1052, 2000.

520. Gussekloo J, Schaap MC, Frolich M, et al: C-reactive protein is a strong but nonspecific risk factor of fatal stroke in elderly persons. Arterioscler Thromb Vasc Biol 20:1047, 2000.

521. Ridker PM, Cushman M, Stampfer MJ, et al: Inflammation, aspirin, and the risk of cardiovascular disease in apparently healthy men. N Engl J Med 336:973, 1997.

522. Rost NS, Wolf PA, Kase CS, et al: Plasma concentration of C-reactive protein and risk of ischemic stroke and transient ischemic attack. Stroke 32:2575, 2001.

523. Muir KW, Weir CJ, Alwan W, et al: C-reactive protein and outcome after ischemic stroke. Stroke 30:981, 1999.

524. Beamer NB, Coull BM, Clark WM, et al: Interleukin-6 and interleukin-1 receptor antagonist in acute stroke. Ann Neurol 37:800, 1995.

525. Di Napoli M, Papa F, Bocola V: Prognostic influence of increased C-reactive protein and fibrinogen levels in ischemic stroke. Stroke 32:133, 2001.

526. Ridker PM, Rifai N, Pfeffer MA, et al: Long-term effects of pravastatin on plasma concentration of C-reactive protein: The Cholesterol and Recurrent Events (CARE) Investigators. Circulation 100:230, 1999.

Specific Medical Diseases and Stroke

Chapter Twenty-Five

Moyamoya Disease

Junichi Masuda, Jun Ogata, and Takenori Yamaguchi

Moyamoya disease is an unusual form of chronic cerebrovascular occlusive disease that is characterized by angiographic findings of bilateral stenosis or occlusion at the terminal portion of the internal carotid artery together with the abnormal vascular network at the base of the brain (Fig. 25–1).[1–6] The first report of a patient with this disease was published in 1957 by Takeuchi and Shimizu[7] with the diagnosis "bilateral hypoplasia of the internal carotid arteries." This patient was a 29-year-old man who had been suffering from visual disturbance and hemiconvulsive seizures since the age of 10 years, and Takeuchi and Shimizu[7] considered this arterial occlusion to be congenital hypoplasia different from the atherosclerotic lesion on the basis of the histologic examination of a branch of the external carotid artery. Since then, similar cases have been reported, mainly among the Japanese, and a variety of names have been applied to this condition—"cerebral juxta-basal telangiectasia" by Sano,[8] "cerebral arterial rete" by Handa and colleagues,[9] "rete mirabile" by Weidner and associates,[10] and "cerebral basal rete mirabile" by Nishimoto and Takeuchi.[11] The terms "spontaneous occlusion of the circle of Willis," used by Kudo,[12] and "moyamoya disease" are now commonly used in the literature. The term *moyamoya disease* was proposed by Suzuki and Takaku,[13] taken from the characteristic angiographic findings of an abnormal vascular network at the base of the brain; the Japanese word *moyamoya*, meaning "vague or hazy puff of smoke," describes its appearance.

Extensive investigations of patients with this characteristic angiographic finding have been conducted mainly by Japanese neurosurgeons over the past 40 years. As a result, the clinical entity of this disease and its concept have now been established. It is well known, for example, that progression of stenosis or occlusion of the intracranial major arteries, including the distal ends of the internal carotid arteries, is the primary lesion of this disease and that the abnormal vascular network (moyamoya vessels) at the base of the brain is their collateral supply, developed secondary to brain ischemia, although this finding on angiography characterizes the clinical category (see Fig. 25–1).[2,4–6,14]

The guideline for the diagnosis of moyamoya disease was established and has been revised by the Research Committee on Spontaneous Occlusion of the Circle of Willis, organized by the Ministry of Health and Welfare, Japan (MHWJ), and the latest version (1996) was published not only in Japanese but also in English.[2,15] These publications help establish this disease as a clinical entity, and it is now known that moyamoya disease is widely distributed all over the world.[6,16,17] The epidemiology of moyamoya disease is discussed later.

The clinical features and radiologic findings have been sufficiently described in the previous edition of this textbook[6] and others,[4,14] so we shall use the present chapter to summarize the pathology and recent progress on the etiology and pathogenesis of moyamoya disease. The latest revision of the guideline for diagnosis in relation to magnetic resonance imaging (MRI) and angiography (MRA) is also addressed.

GUIDELINE FOR DIAGNOSIS

The guideline for the diagnosis of moyamoya disease has been developed by the MHWJ's Research Committee on Spontaneous Occlusion of the Circle of Willis (Tables 25.1 and 25.2).[2] It has been used not only for patient diagnosis but also for follow-up and further investigation into the etiology and pathogenesis of this unique and mysterious disorder.

Prior to 1995, the guideline stated that cerebral angiography is indispensable for the diagnosis in all but the autopsied cases.[6] Because the quality of the images of MRI and MRA has improved, the Research Committee conducted comparative studies to examine whether the MRI and MRA could be substituted for conventional cerebral angiography.[6,18–20] They concluded in 1995 that the diagnosis of moyamoya disease can be made without conventional cerebral angiography if MRI and MRA clearly demonstrate all the findings that indicate moyamoya disease. The diagnostic criteria applied to the MRI and MRA were added as a supplemented reference in the revision (see Table 25.2).[2] The substitution of noninvasive imaging methods for invasive is helpful for patients, especially children.

This revision also contains the addition of autoimmune disorders to the list of disorders that should be excluded in any patient being evaluated for moyamoya disease, to avoid confusing this disease with other disorders in which vascular lesions resembling those of moyamoya disease can form.

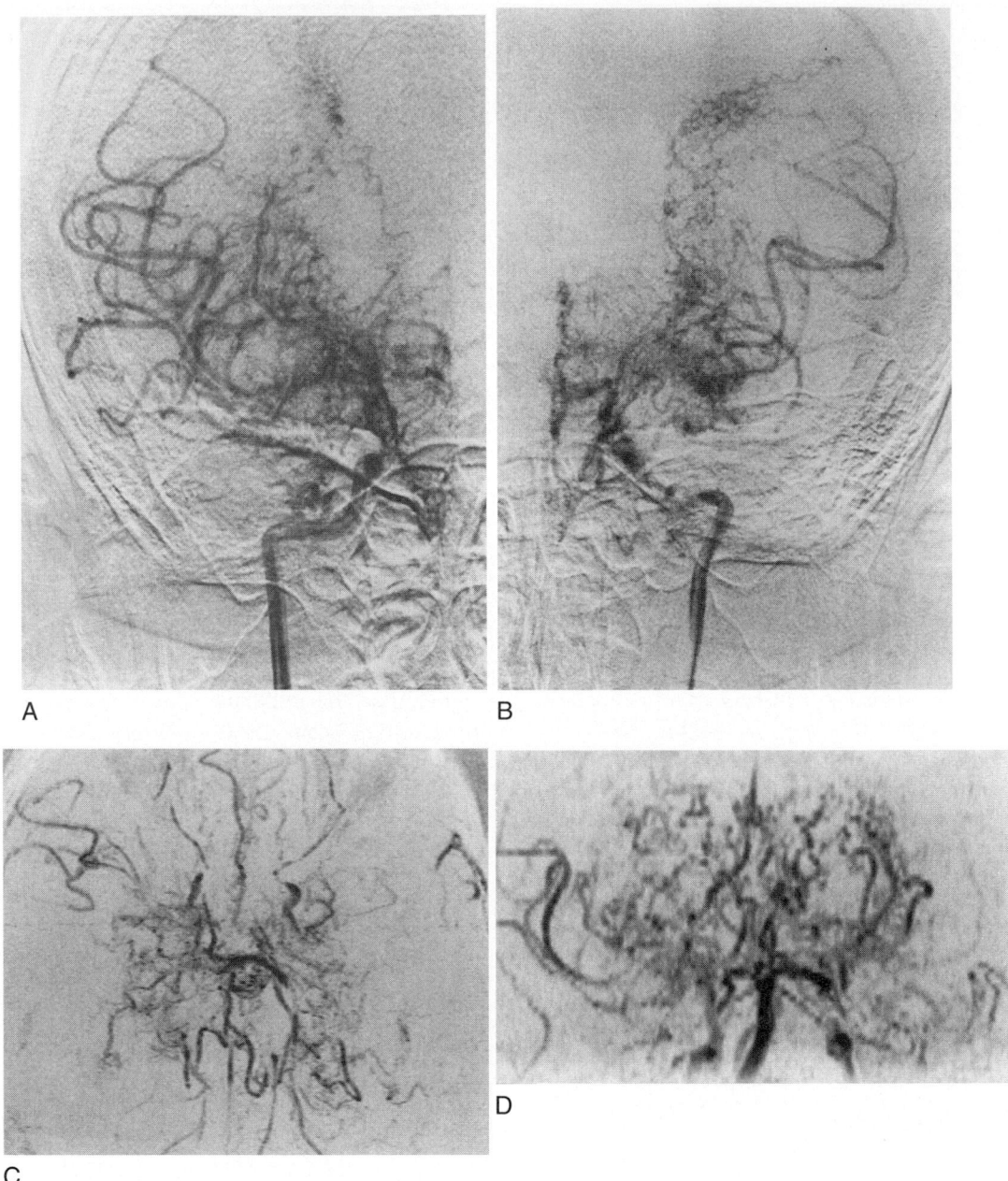

FIGURE 25–1 *Conventional cerebral angiography and magnetic resonance angiography in a 10-year-old boy with moyamoya disease. Anteroposterior views of conventional angiography show (A) severe stenosis of the right MCA and (B) nearly complete occlusion of the left MCA. Well-developed basal moyamoya vessels are also seen. Magnetic resonance angiography of this patient shows findings similar to those observed by conventional angiography. C, Basal view. D, Anteroposterior view. (From Houkin K, Aoki T, Takahashi A, et al: Diagnosis of moyamoya disease with magnetic resonance angiography. Stroke 25:2159, 1994.)*

EPIDEMIOLOGY

The incidence and prevalence of moyamoya disease in the Japanese have been surveyed by collaborative studies conducted by the research committees on the epidemiology of intractable diseases and on the spontaneous occlusion of the circle of Willis organized by the MHWJ in 1984, 1989, and 1994, and reported by Wakai and colleagues.[21] The estimated number of patients treated in Japan in 1994 was 3900 (95% confidence interval [CI], 3500 to 4400). The corresponding value surveyed in 1989 was 3300, but

small hospitals (<200 beds) had not been included, so the 1994 figure was recalculated to exclude small hospitals and re-estimated as 3200. Therefore, the prevalence is considered unchanged from 1989 to 1994, and the annual prevalence and incidence are calculated to be 3.16 and 0.35 per 100,000 population, respectively. Female preponderance has been reported[6] and was also confirmed in the patient survey of 1994 with a female-to-male ratio of 1.8 : 1.[21] The largest peak in age distribution was observed in patients 10 to 14 years old, and a smaller peak in patients in their 40s. The age at onset was younger than 10 in 47.8% of the

Table 25.1   Diagnostic Guidelines for Spontaneous Occlusion of the Circle of Willis (Moyamoya Disease)

(A) Cerebral angiography is indispensable for the diagnosis, and should present at least the following findings:
1. Stenosis or occlusion at the terminal portion of the internal carotid artery and/or at the proximal portion of the anterior and/or middle cerebral arteries.
2. Abnormal vascular networks seen in the vicinity of the occlusive or stenotic lesions in the arterial phase.
3. These findings should present bilaterally.

(B) When magnetic resonance imaging (MRI) and magnetic resonance angiography (MRA) clearly demonstrate all the findings described below, conventional cerebral angiography is not mandatory:
1. Stenosis or occlusion at the terminal portion of the internal carotid artery and at the proximal portion the anterior and middle cerebral arteries on MRA.
2. An abnormal vascular network in the basal ganglia on MRA. Note: an abnormal vascular network can be diagnosed when more than two apparent flow voids are seen in one side of the basal ganglia on MRI.
3. 1) and 2) are seen bilaterally. (Refer to Image Diagnostic Guidelines by MRI and MRA [Table 25.2].)

(C) Because the etiology of this disease is unknown, cerebrovascular disease with the following basic diseases or conditions should thus be eliminated:
1. Arteriosclerosis
2. Autoimmune disease
3. Meningitis
4. Brain neoplasm
5. Down syndrome
6. Recklinghausen's disease
7. Head trauma
8. Irradiation to the head
9. Others

(D) Instructive pathological findings:
1. Intimal thickening and the resulting stenosis or occlusion of the lumen are observed in and around the terminal portion of the internal carotid artery, usually on both sides. Lipid deposit is occasionally seen in thickened intima.
2. Arteries constituting the circle of Willis such as the anterior and middle cerebral and posterior communicating arteries often show stenosis of varying degrees or occlusion associated with fibrocellular thickening of the intima, a waving of the internal elastic lamina, and an attenuation of the media.
3. Numerous small vascular channels (perforators and anastomotic branches) are observed around the circle of Willis.
4. Reticular conglomerates of small vessels are often seen in the pia mater.

Diagnosis: In reference to A–D mentioned above, the diagnostic criteria are classified as follows: Autopsy cases not undergoing cerebral angiography should be investigated separately while referring to D.
1. Definite case: One which fulfills either A or B, and C. In children, however, a case which fulfills A-1 and A-2 (or B-1 and B-2) on one side and with remarkable stenosis at the terminal portion of the internal carotid artery on the opposite side is also included.
2. A probable case: One which fulfills A-1 and A-2 (or B-1 and B-2) and C (unilateral involvement).

From Fukui M: Guidelines for the diagnosis and treatment of spontaneous occlusion of the circle of Willis ("moyamoya" disease). Research Committee on Spontaneous Occlusion of the Circle of Willis (Moyamoya Disease) of the Ministry of Health and Welfare, Japan. Clin Neurol Neurosurg 99(Suppl 2):S238, 1997.

Table 25.2   Image Diagnostic Guidelines for Moyamoya Disease by MRI and MRA

(A) When magnetic resonance imaging (MRI) and magnetic resonance angiography (MRA) clearly demonstrate all the findings described below, conventional cerebral angiography is not mandatory:
1. Stenosis or occlusion at the terminal portion of the intracranial internal carotid artery and at the proximal portion of the anterior and middle cerebral arteries.
2. An abnormal vascular network in the basal ganglia.
3. 1) and 2) are seen bilaterally.

(B) Imaging methods and judgment.
1. More than a 1.0 tesla magnetic field strength is recommended.
2. There are no restrictions regarding MRA imaging methods.
3. The imaging paremeters, such as the magnetic field strength, the imaging methods and the use of contrast medium should be clearly documented.

4. An abnormal vascular network can be diagnosed when more than two apparent flow voids are seen on one side of the basal ganglia on MRI.
5. Either an over or under estimation of the lesion could be made according to the imaging conditions. To avoid a false-positive diagnosis, only definite cases should thus be diagnosed on the MRI and MRA findings.

(C) Because similar vascular lesions secondary to other disorders are sometimes indistinguishable from this disease in adults, a diagnosis based on MRI and MRA without conventional angiography is thus only recommended in pediatric cases.

From Fukui M: Guidelines for the diagnosis and treatment of spontaneous occlusion of the circle of Willis ("moyamoya" disease). Research Committee on Spontaneous Occlusion of the Circle of Willis (Moyamoya Disease) of the Ministry of Health and Welfare, Japan. Clin Neurol Neurosurg 99(Suppl 2):S238, 1997.

Specific Medical Diseases and Stroke

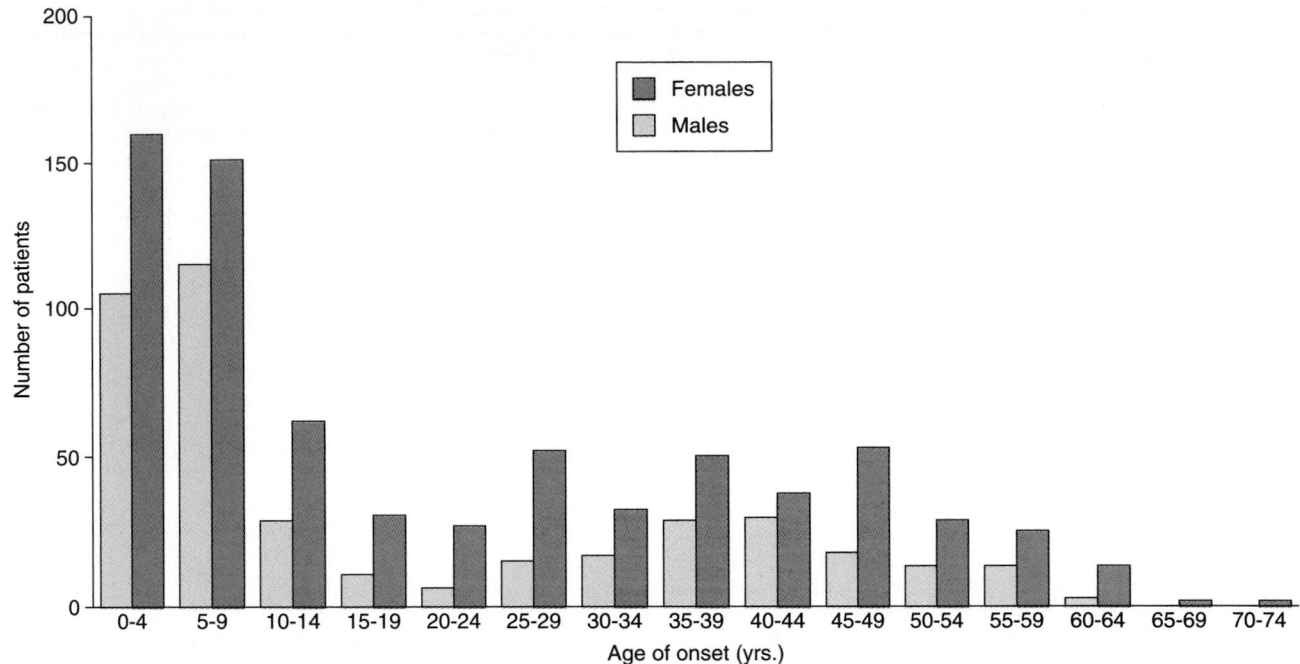

FIGURE 25–2   *Distribution of age-at-onset and sex of the patients with moyamoya disease. (From Wakai K, Tamakoshi A, Ikezaki K, et al: Epidemiological features of moyamoya disease in Japan: Findings from a nationwide survey. Clin Neurol Neurosurg 99[Suppl 2]:S1, 1997.)*

patients (childhood moyamoya), although the disease had developed in some patients between the ages of 25 and 49 years (adult-type moyamoya) (Fig. 25–2).

Evidence of the familial occurrence of this disease has been accumulating in the medical literature.[4,6,22–24] According to the previously mentioned nationwide survey, family histories of moyamoya disease were found to be present in 10% of patients, and 13 pairs of monovular twins were registered as having the disease.[21] The contribution of hereditary factors to the occurrence of moyamoya disease is discussed later, in the section on etiology and pathogenesis.

Although regional predilection has never been reported within Japan, there are remarkable regional differences in the frequencies of reported moyamoya patients in the world.[6,16,17] After the report by Taveras in 1969,[25] reports of moyamoya disease have been growing among non-Japanese people, including white and black people, although white patients are rare.[17,26] None of the races has as high an incidence as the Japanese, but relatively large numbers of patients have been found in Korea[27,28] and China.[29,30]

Korean neurosurgeons performed the first nationwide cooperative survey of moyamoya disease in their country in 1988, and 289 patients were registered.[27] The reported clinical features of these patients, however, were different from those of Japanese patients. Therefore, it is important to examine whether this heterogeneity suggests racial and regional differences or whether it is related to any differences between the criteria used for diagnosis of moyamoya disease in the two countries. In 1995, the Japanese neurosurgeons Ikezaki and Fukui and their associates organized a collaborative study with Korean neurosurgeon Han and colleagues, analyzing the patients registered in Korea on the basis of questionnaires about the angiographic findings.[15,28,31] Because the guideline established by the MHWJ Research Committee was not strictly applied to the diag-

nosis of moyamoya disease in Korea, Ikezakai and Fukui re-evaluated the registration records and divided the 451 registered Korean cases into definite (296), probable (103), and unlikely (52) cases. Analysis of the definite cases showed that the clinical features of the Korean patients were quite similar to those of the Japanese patients.[15,31] The pattern of distribution for the age at onset showed the same two peaks (<10 years and 25 to 49 years) the same as that of the Japanese, although the adult population was 20% larger in the Korean sample than in the Japanese. There was a slight female predominance (ratio 1.3 : 1), and the incidence of hemorrhage was higher in females than in males. The incidence of brain infarction and hemorrhage was significantly higher, whereas the rates of transient ischemic attacks and seizures were lower in Korean than in Japanese subjects. The incidence of infarction in children and that of hemorrhage in both children and adults were also statistically higher in Koreans.

From these results, the higher incidence of hemorrhage and adult-type moyamoya patients are suggested to be the features of moyamoya disease in Korean patients, but the diagnostic criteria and the interpretation of the angiography by neuroradiologists should be standardized in the two countries, and atherosclerotic cerebrovascular stenosis and occlusion should be excluded more carefully in the Korean patients before final conclusions are drawn. Such studies should be undertaken not only in Japan and Korea, but also in Western and other Asian countries for clarification of the racial significance and genetic background of this disease.

PATHOLOGY

Pathologic observations of approximately 100 autopsy cases of moyamoya disease revealed various forms of cerebrovascular lesions in the brain, and their macroscopic and microscopic findings have been accumulated and described in the literature.[9,32–39] The lesion observed most commonly at autopsy is intracranial hemorrhage, which is a major cause of death for patients with moyamoya disease.[38] Massive parenchymatous hemorrhage (intracerebral hemorrhage) occurs frequently in the basal ganglia, thalamus, hypothalamus, cerebral peduncle, and midbrain, and often extends and ruptures to the intraventricular spaces.[38] Subarachnoid hemorrhage (SAH) also occurs, but primary SAH caused by rupture of aneurysms seems to be not so frequent as described previously, and many cases appear to be secondary extensions of parenchymatous hemorrhage.[6] In addition, old brain infarction and focal cortical atrophy of the brain are not uncommon findings and are often found in multiple.[38,39] Furthermore, the infarcts are mostly small and localized in the basal ganglia, internal capsule, thalamus, and subcortex. The large and arterial territorial infarcts[40] are rare in moyamoya disease, although occlusion of the intracranial major arteries is present. This finding may suggest the function of moyamoya vessels as a collateral pathway after arterial occlusion. The frequency and distribution of intracranial hemorrhage and infarction found at autopsy may not represent those of patients with moyamoya disease, and the pathologic specimens obtained from the circle of Willis and moyamoya vessels are biased by the unavoidable clinical modifications related to their deaths. Nevertheless, the histologic and immunohistochemical analyses of the postmortem materials have provided a significant amount of valuable information relating to the etiology and pathogenesis of the lesion formation of this disease, and their findings are summarized herein.

The Circle of Willis and the Major Branches

In the guideline for the diagnosis of moyamoya disease, the pathologic findings in the intracranial arteries from autopsied patients are included as an aid for diagnosis at autopsy of the disease in patients who did not undergo angiography during life (see Table 25.1).[2,3] The histologic appearance of the circle of Willis and the major branches of the

patients with moyamoya disease are characteristic, but not peculiar to this disease.[34,35,39] Therefore, it is not always possible to diagnose moyamoya disease solely on the basis of pathologic findings.

On macroscopic observation, the circle of Willis and the major branches are tapered and narrowed entirely or partially with overgrown and dilated arteries branching from the circle of Willis (Fig. 25–3). The degree of tapering of arteries as well as the network formation of dilated arteries (moyamoya vessels) and their distributions vary from case to case. The distal ends of the internal carotid arteries are affected by severe narrowing or occlusion.

In conventional staining of specimens obtained from the circle of Willis or its major branches with lesion involvement, the arterial lumen is severely narrowed or occluded by fibrocellular intimal thickening (Fig. 25–4A and

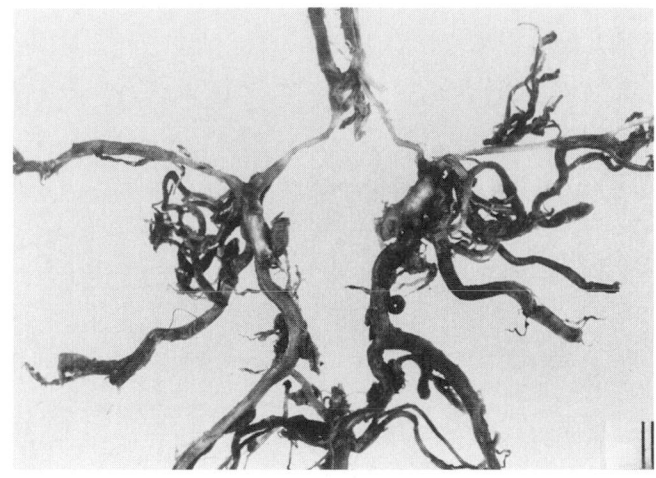

FIGURE 25–3 *Macroscopic appearance of the circle of Willis of a 66-year-old woman with moyamoya disease at autopsy. Tapering of anterior and middle cerebral arteries can be seen bilaterally with network formation of dilated arteries (basal moyamoya vessels).*

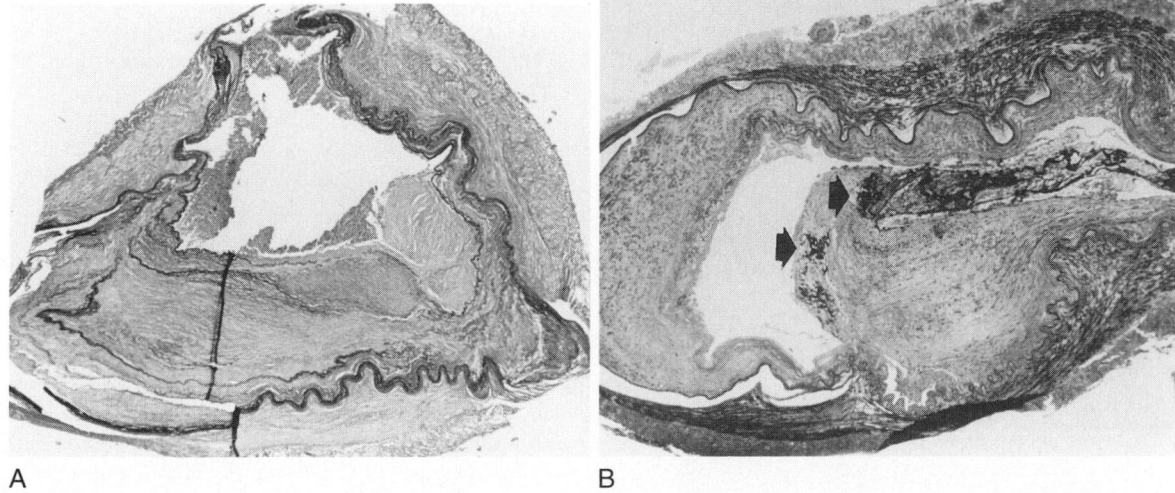

A   B

FIGURE 25–4 *Microscopic appearance of the circle of Willis of patients with moyamoya disease at autopsy. A, Intracranial portion of right internal carotid artery of a 60-year-old woman. (Elastica van Gieson stain.) B, Main trunk of the right middle cerebral artery of a 36-year-old man. Arrows indicate mural fibrin thrombi with its organization. (Mallory's phosphotungstic acid-hematoxylin [PTAH] stain.)*

Fig. 25–5A).[34,35,37,39] The thickened intima appears to be in a laminated structure with duplication or triplication of internal elastic lamina and a wavy appearance. These features closely resemble the structure noted focally at arterial branching portions in normal controls, the so-called intimal cushion. The outer diameter of the affected artery usually becomes smaller, and the underlying media are markedly attenuated. These histologic features are common to lesions at any site, although the extent of intimal thickenings and the distribution in the circle of Willis are variable in different patients.

Immunohistochemical staining of this lesion demonstrated that the thickened intima is composed mainly of smooth muscle cells (SMCs) (see Fig. 25–5B) that are phenotypically modulated from the contractile type to the synthetic.[37] With this immunohistochemical study, some of the SMCs in the intima were stained positively with the antibody for proliferating cell nuclear antigen (see Fig. 25–5C) and thereby were revealed to be proliferating. This evidence strongly suggests that SMC proliferation and phenotypic modulation contribute to the formation of fibrocellular intimal thickening in the circle of Willis in

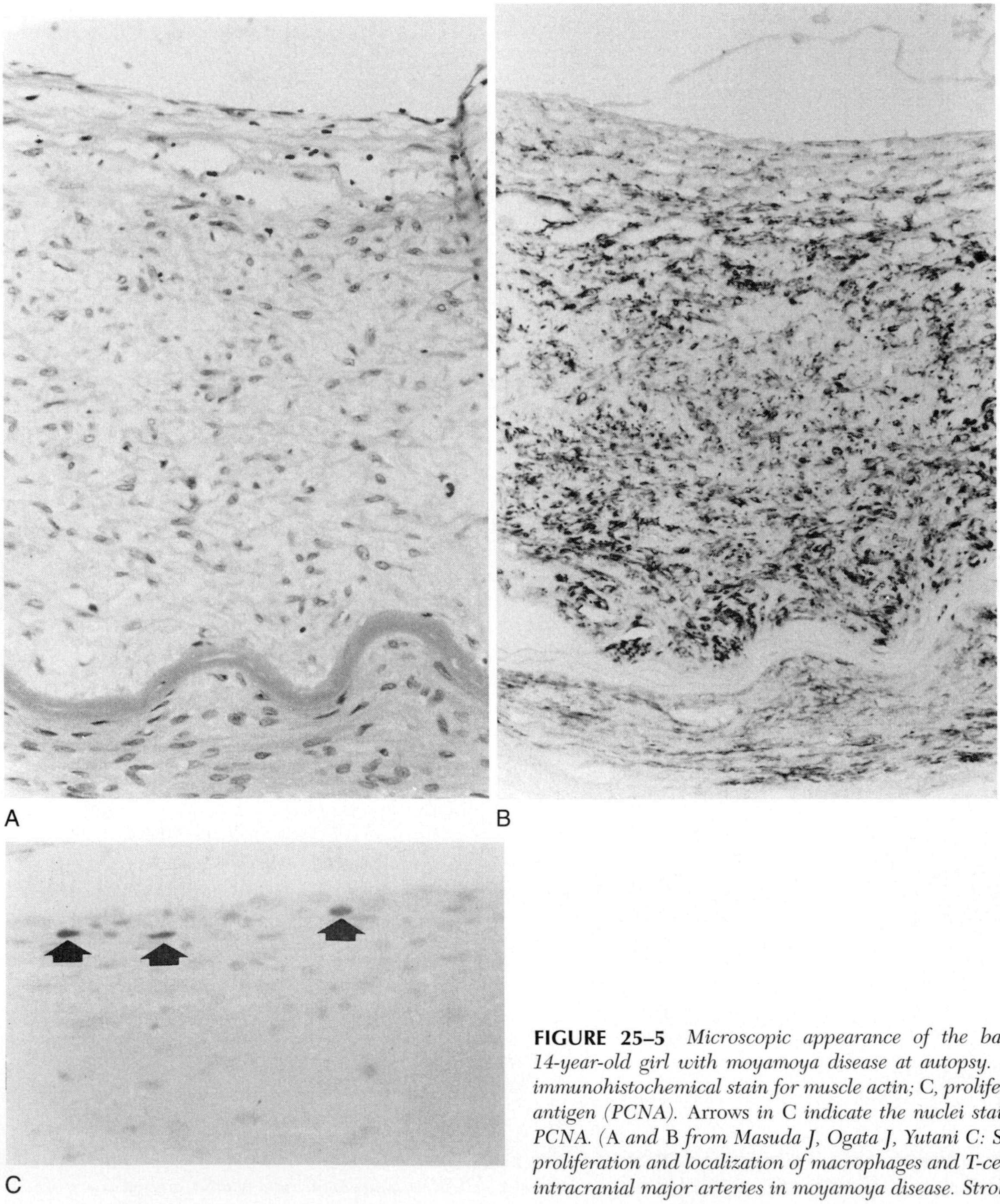

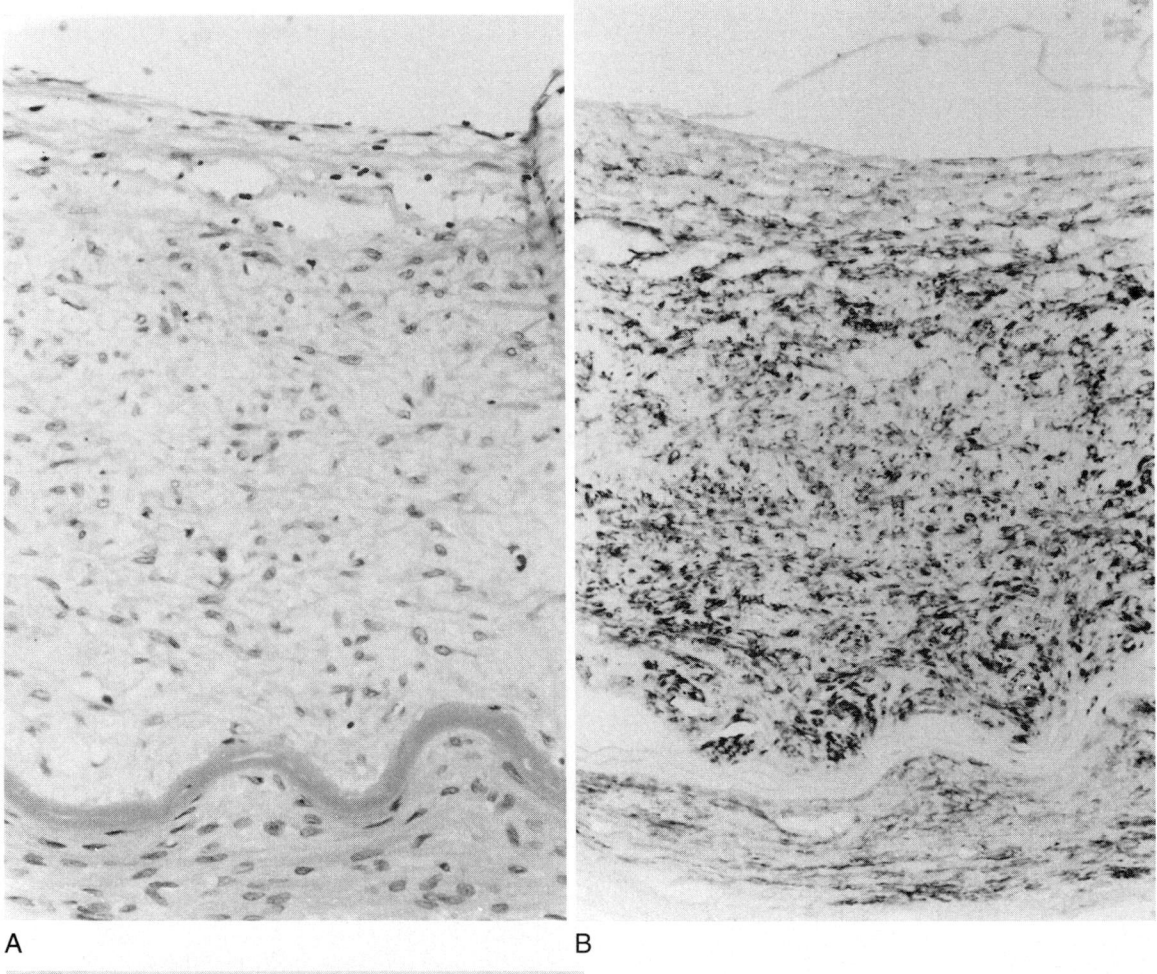

A

B

C

FIGURE 25–5 *Microscopic appearance of the basilar artery of a 14-year-old girl with moyamoya disease at autopsy.* A, *H&E stain;* B, *immunohistochemical stain for muscle actin;* C, *proliferating cell nuclear antigen (PCNA). Arrows in C indicate the nuclei stained positively for PCNA. (A and B from Masuda J, Ogata J, Yutani C: Smooth muscle cell proliferation and localization of macrophages and T-cells in the occlusive intracranial major arteries in moyamoya disease. Stroke 24:1960, 1993.)*

patients with moyamoya disease. Lipid deposition and lipid-containing macrophages (foam cells) have been found in some autopsy cases but are now considered features of atherosclerosis.[3]

Mural thrombi are often found in the stenotic lesions of the circle of Willis and the major branches (see Fig. 25–4B), but their frequency varies among the reports.[34,35,37,41] Judging from their histologic features, the organization of such thrombi appears to contribute to the pathogenesis of fibrocellular intimal thickening, which is discussed in the section on etiology and pathogenesis.

Aneurysm formation, a relatively common finding in the circle of Willis in patients with moyamoya disease, and its pathology are summarized later.

Perforating Arteries (Moyamoya Vessels)

The vascular network at the base of the brain consists of dilated, medium-sized or small muscular arteries branching off the circle of Willis, anterior choroidal arteries, intracranial portions of internal carotid arteries, and posterior cerebral arteries. These arteries form complex channels that usually connect to the distal portion of the anterior and middle cerebral arteries. Numerous small dilated and tortuous vessels originating from these channels enter into the base of the brain, corresponding to lenticulostriate and thalamoperforate arteries.

In microscopic observations, these perforating arteries in the brain parenchyma show various histologic changes. According to the morphometric analysis performed by Yamashita and colleagues,[39] the perforating arteries within the basal ganglia, thalamus, and internal capsule in patients with moyamoya disease can be divided into the following two groups, (1) a dilated artery with a relatively thin wall and (2) a thick-walled artery showing luminal stenosis. Dilatation of the arteries is more prominent in young patients than in adults. The majority of dilated arteries show fibrosis and marked attenuation of the media with occasional segmentation of the elastic lamina. With hemo-

dynamic stress or aging, the dilated arteries with attenuated walls may predispose to focal protrusion (microaneurysm formation) of the arterial wall, and its rupture is considered one of the mechanisms leading to the parenchymatous hemorrhage in patients with moyamoya disease (Fig. 25–6). The involvement by fibrinoid necrosis of the perforating arteries in the process of aneurysm formation has been shown in hypertensive parenchymatous hemorrhage but has never been confirmed pathologically in patients with moyamoya disease.

In contrast, the stenotic vessels are less common in young patients.[39] These vessels show concentric thickening of the intima with duplication of the elastic lamina and fibrosis of the tunica media (see Fig. 25–6). Partial dilatation with discontinuity of the elastic lamina and the occluding thrombus formation with its organization and recanalization are occasionally found. The presence of these histologic changes in the perforating arteries indicates that the arterial obstructive changes in patients with moyamoya disease are not limited to the circle of Willis and their major branches.

Leptomeningeal Vessels

The leptomeningeal anastomoses among the three main cerebral arteries and transdural anastomoses from the external carotid arteries are commonly observed as an abnormal vascular network on cerebral angiograms in patients with moyamoya disease (so-called vault moyamoya).[4,14,42] Kono and associates[43] performed a histopathologic and morphometric study of the leptomeningeal vessels in autopsied brains with moyamoya disease and compared them with vessels from age-matched controls. These researchers clarified that such anastomoses are not newly formed vessels but merely dilated preexisting ones in both arteries and veins. Attenuation or disruption of the internal elastic lamina is remarkable in patients with a short history of moyamoya disease, and fibrous intimal thickening is more prominent in patients with a longer history of the

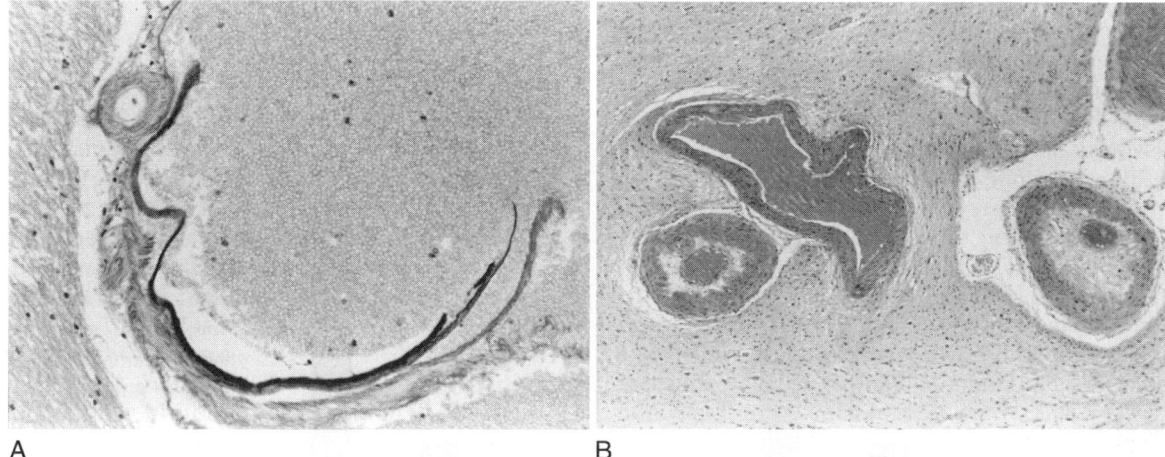

A   B

FIGURE 25–6 *Microscopic appearance of the perforating arteries of patients with moyamoya disease at autopsy. A, The artery in the right caudate nucleus of a 60-year-old woman with parenchymatous hemorrhage shows marked dilatation with rupture. (Elastica van Gieson stain.) B, Some of the arteries in the left thalamus of a 39-year-old woman show luminal stenosis due to fibrous and edematous intimal thickening. (Hematoxylin and eosin stain.)*

contribute to pathogenesis of the fibrocellular intimal thickening through its organization, and this hypothesis explains the lamellated structure of the thickened intima of the lesions. If endothelial injury really occurs as the initiation of the lesion formation, it is feasible to speculate that smooth muscle cell migration and proliferation in the intima are induced after the injury. There has been substantial evidence that endothelial injury provokes phenotypic modulation and proliferation of smooth muscle cells and leads to neointima formation, not only in experimental animals[75-78] but also in patients with angioplasty restenosis.[78,79] In moyamoya disease, however, it is unclear to what extent this process is responsible for the lesion formation. Furthermore, microthrombus is a nonspecific finding and reveals none of any specific etiologic factors in the endothelial injury.

None of the factors leading to endothelial injury has been identified in moyamoya disease. Ikeda and associates[80] detected loss of the endothelium covering the thickened intima in patients with moyamoya through the use of functional markers (thrombomodulin and von Willebrand factor). In relation to the hypotheses for the mechanisms of arterial injury, prothrombotic abnormalities, including inherited protein S deficiency and antiphospholipid antibodies, have been reported in some patients with moyamoya disease,[81,82] and chronic arteritis due to immunologic reactions may be implicated.[23,83] With cell type–specific immunohistochemistry, we previously demonstrated the presence of macrophages and T cells in the lesions, especially in the superficial layer of the thickened intima.[37] Such inflammatory cell infiltration observed in patients might, however, be a local reaction to microthrombi or a reflection of systemic inflammation or atherosclerotic changes unrelated to moyamoya disease. Therefore, it is not always easy to separate the histopathologic features of moyamoya disease from those of other pathologic changes, including atherosclerosis and various forms of arteritis.

In addition to the possible migration and proliferation of smooth muscle cells suggested in the genesis of intimal thickening and moyamoya vessel formation, many researchers have focused their attention on the growth factors and cytokines and their receptors, such as basic fibroblast growth factor (b-FGF),[84,85] platelet-derived growth factor (PDGF),[86] transforming growth factor-β (TGF-β),[87] interleukin-1 (IL-1), and prostaglandin E$_2$.[88] Immunohistochemical staining[84,85] and measurements of these proteins in the cerebrospinal fluid[89,90] have been attempted in patients with moyamoya disease. These approaches may help introduce methods of molecular biology and vascular biology that are now in rapid development in relation to the problem of angioplasty restenosis[77,79] and atherogenesis.[78] Genetic analysis and this work on candidate cytokines and their genes relevant to moyamoya disease may help identify the cause of the disorder.

CLINICAL SYMPTOMS AND SIGNS

Clinical symptoms and signs are manifested as a result of the cerebrovascular events that occur in relation to pathologic changes in cerebral arteries in patients with moyamoya disease. Initial symptoms occur abruptly as attacks of cerebrovascular events including TIA, brain infarction, intracranial hemorrhage, and, occasionally, epileptic seizures. Some patients have shown no overt symptoms, and their disease was diagnosed from the angiography performed because of the familial occurrence of the disease.[18]

The MHWJ's Research Committee has defined four clinical types of moyamoya disease, according to the initial symptoms and their frequencies in the registered patients accumulated until 1995,[91] as follows:

- Ischemic (63.4%)
- Hemorrhagic (21.6%)
- Epileptic (7.6%)
- Other (7.5%)

The ischemic type dominates in childhood moyamoya, representing 69% of cases in patients younger than 10 years; TIA occurs in 40% and infarction in 29% of patients manifesting a variety of symptoms, including motor paresis, disturbances of consciousness, speech disturbances, and sensory disturbances.[92] The course is sometimes repetitive and progressive and may result in cortical blindness, motor aphasia, or even a vegetative state within several years after onset. The ischemic symptoms, that is, transient weakness and paresis, are provoked by some conditions of hyperventilation, such as blowing to play wind instruments, blowing to cool something hot, and crying. They are considered to be induced by decreased cerebral blood flow (CBF) due to diminished PaCO$_2$. Ischemic deterioration is often precipitated by infection of the upper respiratory tract. Mental retardation and a low IQ during the long follow-up are other important problems for the children; this issue is further discussed in the section on disease progression and prognosis.

The hemorrhagic type is prevalent in adult patients, occurring in 66% of cases of the disease in adults, with a predominance of the hemorrhagic type in females.[92] Headache, disturbances of consciousness, and motor paresis are frequently encountered in the hemorrhagic type. Events triggering the bleeding are not identified, but hypertension and aging may be suggested as factors. Bleeding occurs often in multiple and repetitive intervals from several days to 10 years, and massive bleeding often leads to death.

Epilepsy was observed in about 5% of all patients, more than 80% of whom were children younger than 10 years.[92]

LABORATORY FINDINGS

Many groups have attempted to establish a diagnostic laboratory test for moyamoya disease, but none of the tests has proved successful. Some reports, however, showed fragments of data that provided valuable information concerning the etiology and pathogenesis of this disease. Infection by anaerobic bacteria such as *Propionibacterium acnes*,[71] cytomegalovirus, and Epstein-Barr virus,[70] for example, have been examined, with screening for specific antibodies and amplification of viral DNAs with polymerase chain reaction, and the reported data suggest positive correlation with moyamoya disease.

Prothrombotic abnormalities have been reported not only in patients with moyamoya disease but also in children with cerebrovascular diseases. Deficiency of protein S and protein C have been reported in some patients with moyamoya disease.[81-83] Anticardiolipin antibody, an autoantibody against phosphatidyl-glycerol, itself a component of cell membrane phospholipid, showed higher percentages in patients with moyamoya disease than in controls. These data suggest a possible connection between autoimmune mechanisms and moyamoya disease, because this antibody has been suggested to play an important role in arterial thrombi formation in brain infarction.[83,93]

RADIOLOGIC FINDINGS

Angiography

The fundamental angiographic finding in moyamoya disease is bilateral stenosis or occlusion at the intracranial portion of the internal carotid arteries together with a retiform arteriolar network (moyamoya vessels) at the base of the brain (see Figs. 25–1A and 25–1B). The stenotic or occlusive changes often extend along the arteries of the circle of Willis and their main branches. The vertebrobasilar system, however, has rarely been reported to be involved in this disease.[6,13,14] Formation of leptomeningeal collateral vessels, especially from the branches of the posterior cerebral artery, is frequently noted. Also usually present are transdural anastomoses via the ophthalmic artery, external carotid artery, and vertebral artery.

Suzuki and associates[13,14] divided the progression of moyamoya disease into the following six stages on the basis of angiographic findings as follows: (1) narrowing of the carotid forks, (2) initial appearance of moyamoya vessels, (3) intensification of moyamoya vessels, (4) minimization of moyamoya vessels, (5) reduction of moyamoya vessels, and (6) disappearance of moyamoya vessels with collateral circulation only from the external carotid arteries. Kitamura and associates[4] confirmed these chronologic changes of angiographic findings in their follow-up patients; i.e., as the narrowing of the main arteries advances, the moyamoya vessels increase in number, and they are later reduced when transdural anastomoses develop as disease progresses.

As noted previously, aneurysm formation is commonly seen in patients with moyamoya disease.

Computed Tomography

The features of moyamoya disease on computed tomography (CT) scans vary according to the clinical type. The most striking finding on conventional CT scans is high-density areas (HDAs) in the basal ganglia and thalamus, ventricular system, and subarachnoid spaces of the patients with the hemorrhagic type.[17,94] The HDAs resemble the topography of the hematoma in the internal type of hypertensive intracerebral hemorrhage.

In the ischemic type, CT scans reveal low-density areas (LDAs), which are relatively small and are usually confined to the cerebral cortex and subcortex, along with dilatation of cortical sulci and ventricles. Lacunar infarctions located in the basal ganglia and thalamus are sometimes seen in adults but are rare in children with the disease. Up to 40% of patients with the ischemic type, however, have no abnormalities on a conventional CT scan. Use of a contrast agent often visualizes tortuous and curvilinear vessels in the basal ganglia, which represent moyamoya vessels. The most proximal segments of the anterior and middle cerebral arteries are often poorly opacified.

Magnetic Resonance Imaging and Angiography

Because MRI and MRA are noninvasive techniques that can visualize various pathologic changes of the brain and the arterial tree, they have a big advantage over conventional angiography. MRI can demonstrate small subcortical lesions undetectable on CT. Brain infarctions in patients with moyamoya disease are usually small and located in the subcortex and are often multiple and bilateral. Brain atrophy and slight ventricular dilatation are also seen.[18-20,95] Stenotic or occlusive lesions at the distal ends of the internal carotid arteries can be demonstrated by MRA in most patients with this disease (see Figs. 25–1C and 25–1D). Apparent moyamoya vessels can be visualized as fine unusual vessels on MRA (see Figs. 25–1C and 25–1D) and also as a signal void on the MRI (Fig. 25–8), particularly in children. Small moyamoya vessels, however, are poorly visualized on both MRI and MRA, particularly in adults.

As described in the guideline for diagnosis of moyamoya disease, the MHWJ's Research Committee has concluded that this disease can be diagnosed without conventional angiography if MRI and MRA visualize the previously described findings bilaterally. To meet this agreement, the guideline was revised in 1995, and the diagnostic criteria on MRI and MRA were supplemented as shown in Table 25–2.[2] MRI and MRA have also shown to be useful imaging tools for postoperative assessment and longitudinal follow-up of patients with moyamoya disease.[19,96,97]

Electroencephalogram

Abnormal electroencephalogram (EEG) findings are found more frequently in patients with childhood onset of the disease than in adults. Such findings are related to permanent or transient ischemic changes due to a $PaCO_2$ variation that is not specific for moyamoya disease.[4,6,14] Yoshii and Kudo summarized the EEG findings as follows: (1) diffuse and bilateral abnormal low-voltage or slow waves and spike waves, (2) "buildup" with the appearance of delta waves during hyperventilation, and (3) no effect on photic stimulation.[99]

Other Clinical Examinations

Because the symptoms of the ischemic type and epileptic type of moyamoya disease are caused by impairment of CBF due to arterial stenosis or occlusion, regional CBF and metabolic distribution have been measured by xenon inhalation and visualized with CT methods, including stable xenon–enhanced computed tomography, dynamic computed tomography, positron emission computed tomography (PET), and single-photon emission computed

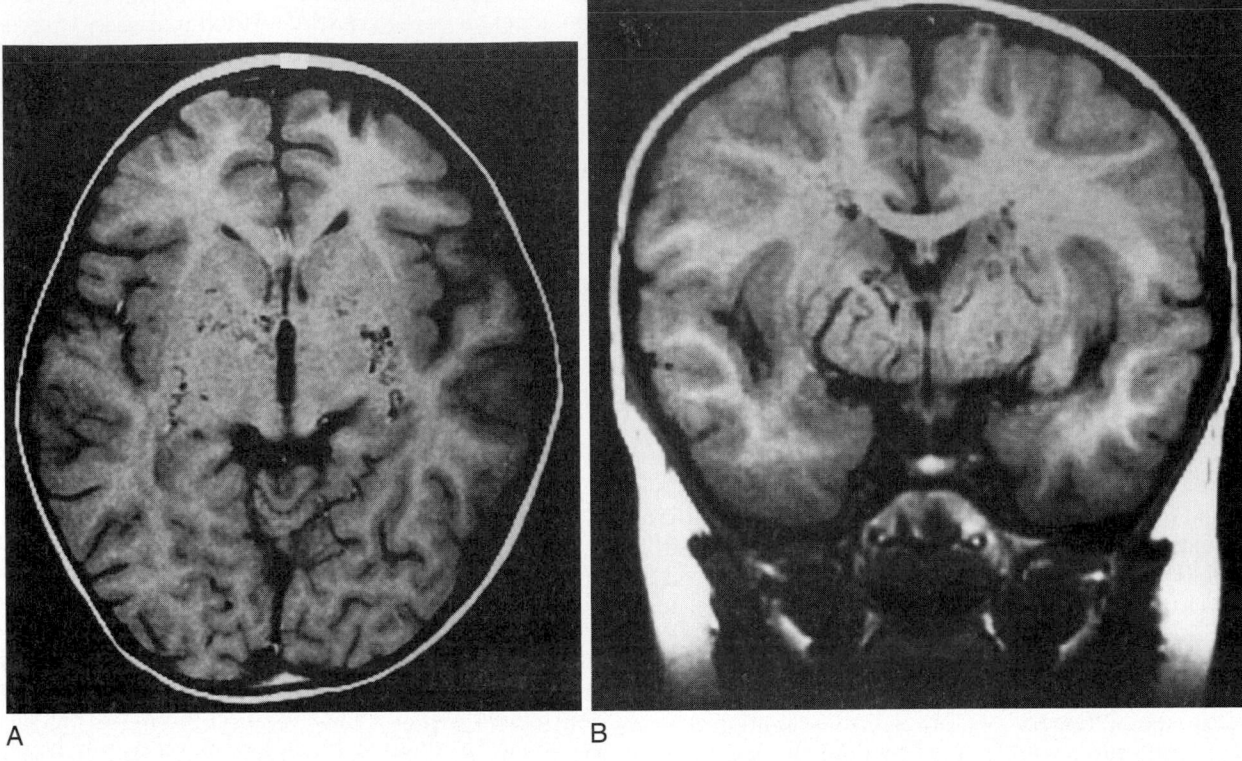

A   B

FIGURE 25–8   *Typical magnetic resonance images of moyamoya vessels. A, Axial image reveals multiple signal voids in the basal ganglia. B, Coronal image reveals well-developed basal moyamoya vessels in the bilateral basal ganglia. (From Houkin K, Aoki T, Takahashi A, et al: Diagnosis of moyamoya disease with magnetic resonance angiography. Stroke 25:2159, 1994.)*

tomography (SPECT). Measurements of these physiologic and morphologic parameters have been useful for the follow-up of patients as well as evaluation of medical and surgical treatment and determination of prognosis.[100–106]

DISEASE PROGRESSION AND PROGNOSIS

As regards disease progression and the prognosis of patients with moyamoya disease, there are remarkable differences between children and adults. In children, angiographic changes progress with time and sometimes rapidly,[107,108] and the formation of abnormal vascular networks at the base of the brain progresses from unilateral to bilateral during follow-up.[22,108,109] However, the prognosis for activities of daily life (ADLs) and life expectancy in children with moyamoya disease is generally fair, because irreversible ischemic and hemorrhagic complications are rarely encountered. More than 80% of such patients are in good health or in a state of independence, irrespective of treatment received. Nevertheless, many children are reported to be not well accommodated in social or school life because of poor intellectual ability, psychological impairment, and personality changes.[110–114] In general, the earlier the onset of the disease and the longer the period of suffering, the lower the mental function and quality of intelligence.

In adults, however, progression of angiographic changes is uncommon. Prognosis for ADLs and life expectancy,

however, is poor because multiple and repetitive intracranial hemorrhages occur in many patients.

TREATMENT

The majority of patients with moyamoya (77%) have been treated surgically by any of the revascularization operations, whereas patients with mild or transient symptoms tend to be observed and given conservative treatment.[91] The surgical treatment is more effective than conservative treatment for the improvement in CBF, according to the physiologic parameters revealed by regional CBF measurement and PET studies, and is generally believed to have an advantage for a better prognosis.[1,100,115]

Medical Treatment

Vasodilators, antiplatelet agents, antifibrinolytic agents, and fibrinolytic agents are used in patients with moyamoya disease. Other medications, including anticonvulsants and steroids, are used in patients with the epileptic type and in patients with increased cranial pressure, respectively.[92,94]

Steroids are considered to be effective in certain cases, especially (1) in patients with involuntary movements and (2) during the active phase of recurrent ischemic or hemorrhagic attacks. This effect is presumed to be related to influences of steroids on edema, regional CBF, and vasculitis.

Antiplatelet agents, acetylsalicylic acid, and ticlopidine chloride may also be prescribed to prevent recurrence of ischemic attacks and thrombosis of the circle of Willis and the main branches, which is thought to play an important role in the progression of moyamoya disease. Other drugs, such as vasodilators, antifibrinolytics, and fibrinolytics, are occasionally used for similar purposes. The efficacy of these drugs in patients with moyamoya disease, however, has never been tested thoroughly in clinical trials.

Surgical Treatment

Surgical revascularizations are classified into the following three categories of surgical procedures: direct bypass surgery, indirect bypass surgery, and a combination of the two (Fig. 25–9).[1,116] Surgical revascularization has been performed to give additional collateral flow to the ischemic brain and thereby to improve regional CBF and prevent or minimize irreversible brain damage during the follow-up. Also, collateral flow through the bypass is expected to have some effects in reducing hemodynamic stress on the moyamoya vessels and eventually to prevent the occurrence of hemorrhagic events. The evacuation of hematoma and ventricular drainage are performed in the acute stage of the hemorrhagic complication of moyamoya disease.

Superficial temporal artery–middle cerebral artery (STA-MCA) bypass is a direct revascularization surgery that was pioneered by Yasargil[117] and then applied to moyamoya disease by Karasawa and Kikuchi[118] and Reichman and colleagues[119] independently. It is now generally accepted that this direct revascularization surgery seems to achieve a remarkable improvement in CBF and a better prognosis than conservative treatment.[100,120] This technique, however, requires skill in microvascular surgery, and it is not always possible to find a cortical branch suitable for anastomosis. Furthermore, careful intraoperative monitoring of blood pressure and $PaCO_2$ is necessary; otherwise, there is a risk of perioperative ischemic complications.[101]

Indirect revascularizations are surgical procedures that aim to introduce external carotid flow into the internal carotid system via newly developed vascularization through the sutured tissues. Encephaloduroarteriosynan-giosis (EDAS)[121] and encephalomyosynangiosis (EMS)[122] are the two representative procedures most commonly used in patients with moyamoya disease. Other operative methods, such as encephaloarteriosynangiosis (EAS), dur-apexy, and omentum transplantation,[123] also belong to this category. These operations can be performed in patients who do not have a cortical branch suitable for anastomoses, although revascularization is not always sufficient to give a collateral flow sufficient to prevent ischemic symptoms. Therefore, the neurosurgeon often performs a *combination* of direct and indirect revascularization to obtain a better collateral flow.[120,124]

These surgical revascularizations are frequently performed in patients with the ischemic type of moyamoya disease (see Fig. 25–9), and the effect of surgery on improvement in regional CBF has been proved.[100,101,115,120,125] According to the follow-up study of registered patients who received surgery, surgical revascularization seems to be effective for the prevention of ischemic events and for improvement in ADLs and intellectual activity, as long as the surgical procedure is chosen properly and performed successfully.[91,96,114,124] There is controversy as to whether the introduction of collateral flow by revascularization raises the risk of hemorrhagic events[1,126,127]; therefore, bypass surgery is not commonly performed in patients with the hemorrhagic type (see Fig. 25–9).[91,128] Rebleeding ratio has been reported to be lower in patients receiving bypass procedures, but the difference was not significant.[129,130] During the follow-up study after surgery, however, moyamoya vessels actually diminished and often disappeared.[129] To evaluate the effect of bypass surgery in preventing recurrent bleeding, a prospective and randomized multi-center study, the Japan Adult Moyamoya (JAM) Trial, was initiated in January 2001.[131]

The long-term effects of the revascularization surgery on the prognosis, including prevention of relapse of the hemorrhagic events and the improvement in ADLs and intelligence, have never been evaluated accurately, and the natural course of patients with moyamoya disease remains to be clarified.

Specific Medical Diseases and Stroke

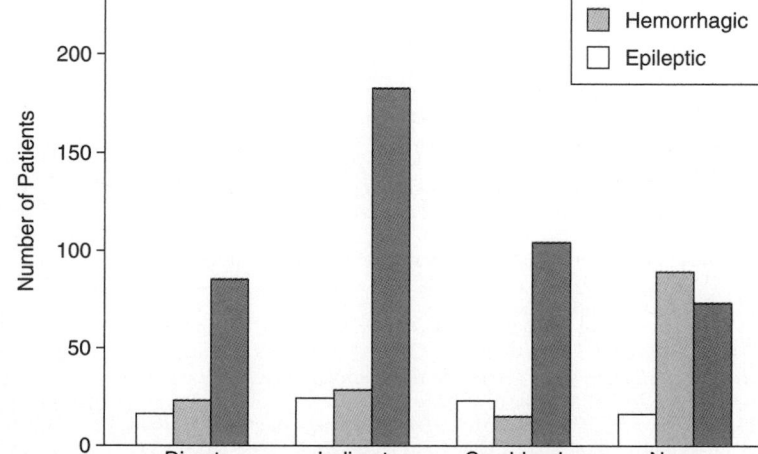

FIGURE 25–9 *Selection of surgical revascularization procedures for the patients with moyamoya disease according to the types of initial attacks. (Data from Fukui M, Kawano T: Follow-up study of registered cases in 1995. In Fukui M [ed]: Annual Report [1995] by the Research Committee on Spontaneous Occlusion of the Circle of Willis [Moyamoya Disease]. Ministry of Health and Welfare, Tokyo, Japan, 1996, p 12.)*

CONCLUSION AND FUTURE DIRECTIONS

As a result of the extensive investigation since the first report of this disease in 1957, moyamoya disease is now recognized as a true disease entity all over the world. Angiographic findings and pathophysiologic features of the disorder are well characterized, and the guidelines for diagnosis are also established, including the use of MRI and MRA.[2] Data concerning the epidemiology of the disease as well as the long-term effects of medical and surgical treatment on prognosis have been accumulating, and thus, need to be analyzed carefully and accurately.

As regards the etiology and pathogenesis of this disease, great advances have been achieved, and such data are expected to provide important clues to solve the genesis of this mysterious disorder. Newer techniques, including molecular genetics, cell biology, and experimental pathology, should be applied vigorously. The establishment of an experimental animal model of this disease will be extremely valuable.

References

1. Fukui M: Current state of study on moyamoya disease in Japan. Surg Neurol 47:138, 1997.
2. Fukui M: Guidelines for the diagnosis and treatment of spontaneous occlusion of the circle of Willis ("moyamoya" disease). Research Committee on Spontaneous Occlusion of the Circle of Willis (Moyamoya Disease) of the Ministry of Health and Welfare, Japan. Clin Neurol Neurosurg 99(Suppl 2):S238, 1997.
3. Fukui M, Kono S, Sueishi K, et al: Moyamoya disease. Neuropathology 20(Suppl):S61, 2000.
4. Kitamura K, Fukui M, Oka K, et al: Moyamoya disease. In Toole JF (ed): Handbook of Clinical Neurology, Volume 11: Vascular Diseases, Part III. Amsterdam, Elsevier, 1989, p 293.
5. Masuda J, Ogata J, Yamaguchi T: Moyamoya disease. In Barnett HJM, Mohr JP, Stein BM, Yatsu FM (eds): Stroke: Pathophysiology, Diagnosis, and Management, 3rd ed. New York, Churchill Livingstone, 1998, p 815.
6. Yonekawa Y, Goto Y, Ogata N: Moyamoya disease: Diagnosis, treatment, and recent achievement. In Barnett HJM, Mohr JP, Stein BM, Yatsu FM (eds): Stroke: Pathophysiology, Diagnosis, and Management, 2nd ed. New York, Churchill Livingstone, 1992, p 721.
7. Takeuchi K, Shimizu K: Hypoplasia of the bilateral internal carotid arteries. No To Shinkei 9:37, 1957.
8. Sano K: Cerebral juxta-basal telangiectasia. No To Shinkei 17:748, 1965.
9. Handa H, Tani K, Kajikawa H, et al: Clinicopathological study on an adult case with cerebral arterial rete. No To Shinkei 21:181, 1969.
10. Weidner W, Hanafee W, Markham C: Intracranial collateral circulation via leptomeningeal and rete mirabile anastomosis. Neurology 15:39, 1965.
11. Nishimoto A, Takeuchi S: Abnormal cerebrovascular network related to the internal carotid arteries. J Neurosurg 29:255, 1968.
12. Kudo T: Spontaneous occlusion of the circle of Willis: A disease apparently confined to Japanese. Neurology 18:485, 1968.
13. Suzuki J, Takaku A: Cerebrovascular "moyamoya disease": A disease showing abnormal net-like vessels in base of brain. Arch Neurol 20:288, 1969.
14. Suzuki J, Kodama N: Moyamoya disease: A review. Stroke 14:104, 1983.
15. Ikezaki K, Han DH, Kawano T, et al: A clinical comparison of definite moyamoya disease between South Korea and Japan. Stroke 28:2513, 1997.
16. Goto Y, Yonekawa Y: Worldwide distribution of moyamoya disease. Neurol Med Chir (Tokyo) 32:883, 1992.
17. Yonekawa Y, Ogata N, Kaku Y, et al: Moyamoya disease in Europe, past and present status. Clin Neurol Neurosurg 99(Suppl 2):S58, 1997.
18. Fukui M, Mizoguchi M, Matsushima T, et al: MR angiography in the families of moyamoya patients. In Fukui M (ed): Annual Report (1994) by Research Committee of Spontaneous Occlusion of the Circle of Willis (Moyamoya Disease). Ministry of Health and Welfare, Tokyo, Japan 1995, p 102.
19. Hasuo K, Mihara F, Matsushima T: MRI and MR angiography in moyamoya disease. J Magn Reson Imaging 8:762, 1998.
20. Houkin K, Aoki T, Takahashi A, et al: Diagnosis of moyamoya disease with magnetic resonance angiography. Stroke 25:2159, 1994.
21. Wakai K, Tamakoshi A, Ikezaki K, et al: Epidemiological features of moyamoya disease in Japan: Findings from a nationwide survey. Clin Neurol Neurosurg 99(Suppl 2):S1, 1997.
22. Kitahara T, Ariga N, Yamamura A, et al: Familial occurrence of moyamoya disease: Report of three Japanese families. J Neurol Neurosurg Psychiatry 42:208, 1979.
23. Kitahara T, Okumura K, Semba T, et al: Genetic and immunologic analysis of moyamoya disease. J Neurol Neurosurg Psychiatry 45:1048, 1982.
24. Yamada H, Nakamura S, Kageyama N: Moyamoya disease in monovular twins: Case report. J Neurosurg 53:109, 1980.
25. Taveras JM: Multiple progressive intracranial arterial occlusion: A syndrome of children and young adults. AJR 106:235, 1969.
26. Chiu D, Sheden P, Bratina P, et al: Clinical features of moyamoya disease in the United States. Stroke 29:1347, 1998.
27. Choi KS: Moyamoya disease in Korea—a cooperative study. In Suzuki J (ed): Advances in Surgery for Cerebral Stroke. Tokyo, Springer-Verlag, 1988, p 107.
28. Han DH, Kwon OK, Byun BJ, et al: A co-operative study: Clinical characteristics of 334 Korean patients with moyamoya disease treated at neurosurgical institutes (1976–1994). The Korean Society for Cerebrovascular Disease. Acta Neurochir (Wien) 142:1263, 2000.
29. Hung CC, Tu YK, Su CF, et al: Epidemiological study of moyamoya disease in Taiwan. Clin Neurol Neurosurg 99(Suppl 2):S23, 1997.
30. Matsushima Y, Qian L, Aoyagi M: Comparison of moyamoya disease in Japan and moyamoya disease (or syndrome) in the People's Republic of China. Clin Neurol Neurosurg 99(Suppl 2):S19, 1997.
31. Ikezaki K, Han DH, Kawano T, et al: Epidemiological survey of moyamoya disease in Korea. Clin Neurol Neurosurg 99(Suppl 2):S6, 1997.
32. Hanakita J, Kondo A, Ishikawa J, et al: An autopsy case of moyamoya disease. Neurol Surg 10:531, 1982.
33. Hirayama A, Kowada M, Fukasawa H, et al: Cerebrovascular moyamoya disease: A case report and review of 12 autopsy cases in Japan. No To Shinkei 26:1215, 1974.
34. Hosoda Y, Ikeda E, Hirose S: Histopathological studies on spontaneous occlusion of the circle of Willis (cerebrovascular moyamoya disease). Clin Neurol Neurosurg 99(Suppl 2):S203, 1997.
35. Hosoda Y: Pathology of so-called "spontaneous occlusion of the circle of Willis." Pathol Annu 19:221, 1984.
36. Maki Y, Nakata Y: Autopsy of a case with an anomalous hemangioma of the internal carotid artery at the skull base. No To Shinkei 17:764, 1965.
37. Masuda J, Ogata J, Yutani C: Smooth muscle cell proliferation and localization of macrophages and T-cell in the occlusive intracranial major arteries in moyamoya disease. Stroke 24:1960, 1993.
38. Oka K, Yamashita M, Sadoshima S, et al: Cerebral hemorrhage in moyamoya disease at autopsy. Virchows Arch 392:247, 1981.
39. Yamashita M, Oka K, Tanaka K: Histopathology of the brain vascular network in moyamoya disease. Stroke 14:50, 1983.
40. Masuda J, Yutani C, Ogata J, et al: Atheromatous embolism in the brain: A clinicopathologic analysis of 15 autopsy cases. Neurology 44:1231, 1994.
41. Yamashita M, Oka K, Tanaka K: Cervico-cephalic arterial thrombi and thromboemboli in moyamoya disease: Possible correlation with progressive intimal thickening in the intracranial major arteries. Stroke 15:264, 1984.
42. Kodama N, Fujiwara S, Horie Y, et al: Transdural anastomosis in moyamoya disease: Vault moyamoya. No Shinkei Geka 8:729, 1980.
43. Kono S, Oka K, Sueishi K: Histopathologic and morphometric studies of leptomeningeal vessels in moyamoya disease. Stroke 21:1044, 1990.
44. Herreman F, Nathal E, Yasui N, et al: Intracranial aneurysm in moyamoya disease: Report of ten cases and review of the literature. Cerebrovasc Dis 4:329, 1994.

45. Kodama N, Suzuki J: Moyamoya disease associated with aneurysm. J Neurosurg 48:565, 1978.
46. Konishi Y, Kadowaki C, Hara M, et al: Aneurysms associated with moyamoya disease. Neurosurgery 16:484, 1985.
47. Nagamine Y, Takahashi S, Sonobe M: Multiple intracranial aneurysms associated with moyamoya disease: Case report. J Neurosurg 54:673, 1981.
48. Pilz P, Hartjes HJ: Fibromuscular dysplasia and multiple dissecting aneurysms of intracranial arteries. A further cause of moyamoya syndrome. Stroke 7:393, 1976.
49. Yamashita M, Tanaka K, Matsuo T, et al: Cerebral dissecting aneurysms in patients with moyamoya disease: Report of two cases. J Neurosurg 58:120, 1983.
50. Yuasa H, Tokito S, Izumi K, et al: Cerebrovascular moyamoya disease associated with an intracranial pseudoaneurysm: Case report. J Neurosurg 56:131, 1982.
51. Ogata J, Masuda J, Nishikawa M, et al: Sclerosed peripheral-artery aneurysm in moyamoya disease. Cerebrovasc Dis 6:248, 1996.
52. Ikeda E: Systemic vascular changes in spontaneous occlusion of the circle of Willis. Stroke 22:1358, 1991.
53. Yamashita M, Tanaka K, Kishikawa T, et al: Moyamoya disease associated with renovascular hypertension. Hum Pathol 15:191, 1984.
54. Godin M, Helias A, Tadie M, et al: Moyamoya syndrome and renal artery stenosis. Kidney Int 15:450, 1978.
55. Goldberg HJ: Moyamoya associated with peripheral vascular occlusive disease. Arch Dis Child 49:964, 1974.
56. Yamano T, Onouchi Z, Shimada M: Moyamoya disease and renal hypertension: A case probably caused by fibromuscular dysplasia. Brain Dev 6:184, 1974.
57. Aoyagi M, Ogami K, Matsushima Y, et al: Human leukocyte antigen in patients with moyamoya disease. Stroke 26:415, 1995.
58. Seeler RA, Royal JE, Powe L, et al: Moyamoya disease in children with sickle cell anemia and cerebrovascular occlusion. J Pediatr 93:808, 1978.
59. Erickson RP, Wooliscroft J, Allen RJ: Familial occurrence of intracranial arterial occlusive disease (moyamoya) in neurofibromatosis. Clin Genet 18:191, 1980.
60. Lamas E, Diez Lobato R, Cabello A, et al: Multiple intracranial arterial occlusions (moyamoya disease) in patients with neurofibromatosis: One case report with autopsy. Acta Neurochir (Wien) 45:133, 1978.
61. Mito T, Becker LE: Vascular dysplasia in Down syndrome: A possible relationship to moyamoya disease. Brain Dev 14:248, 1992.
62. Nagasaka T, Shiozawa Z, Kobayashi M, et al: Autopsy findings in Down's syndrome with cerebrovascular disorder. Clin Neuropathol 15:145, 1996.
63. Fukuyama Y, Kanai N, Osawa M: Clinical genetic analysis on moyamoya disease. In Yonekawa Y (ed): Annual Report (1991) by Research Committee on Spontaneous Occlusion of the Circle of Willis. Ministry of Health and Welfare, Tokyo, Japan, 1992, p 141.
64. Fukuyama Y, Sugahara N, Osawa M: A genetic study of idiopathic spontaneous multiple occlusion of the circle of Willis. In Yonekawa Y (ed): Annual Report (1990) by Research Committee on Spontaneous Occlusion of the Circle of Willis. Ministry of Health and Welfare, Tokyo, Japan, 1991, p 139.
65. Inoue TK, Ikezaki K, Sasazuki T, et al: DNA typing of HLA in the patients with moyamoya disease. Jpn J Hum Genet 42:507, 1997.
66. Inoue TK, Ikezaki K, Sasazuki T, et al: Linkage analysis of moyamoya disease on chromosome 6. J Child Neurol 15:179, 2000.
67. Ikeda H, Sasaki T, Yoshimoto T, et al: Mapping of a familial moyamoya disease gene to chromosome 3p24.2-p26. Am J Hum Genet 64:533, 1999.
68. Yamauchi T, Tada M, Houkin K, et al: Linkage of familial moyamoya disease (spontaneous occlusion of the circle of Willis) to chromosome 17q25. Stroke 31:930, 2000.
69. Kasai N, Fujiwara S, Kodama N, et al: The experimental study on causal genesis of moyamoya disease: Correlation with immunological reaction and sympathetic nerve influence for vascular changes. No Shinkei Geka 10:251, 1982.
70. Tanigawara T, Yamada H, Sasaki N, et al: Studies on cytomegalovirus and Epstein-Barr virus infection in moyamoya disease. Clin Neurol Neurosurg 99(Suppl 2):S225, 1997.
71. Yamada H, Deguchi K, Tanigawa T, et al: The relationship between moyamoya disease and bacterial infection. Clin Neurol Neurosurg 99(Suppl 2):S221, 1997.
72. Fernandes-Alvares E, Pineda M, Royo C, et al: Moyamoya disease caused by cranial trauma. Brain Dev 1:133, 1979.
73. Bitzer M, Topka H: Progressive cerebral occlusive disease after radiation therapy. Stroke 26:131, 1995.
74. Rajakulasingam K, Cerullo LJ, Raimondi AJ: Childhood moyamoya syndrome: Postradiation pathogenesis. Childs Brain 5:469, 1979.
75. Bai H-Z, Masuda J, Sawa Y, et al: Neointima formation after vascular stent implantation: Spatial and chronological distribution of smooth muscle cell proliferation and phenotypic modulation. Arterioscler Thromb 14:1846, 1994.
76. Masuda J, Tanaka K: A new model of cerebral arteriosclerosis induced by intimal injury using a silicone rubber cylinder in rabbits. Lab Invest 51:475, 1984.
77. Reidy MA, Fingerle J, Lindner V: Factors controlling the development of arterial lesions after injury. Circulation 86(Suppl III):1845, 1992.
78. Ross R: The pathogenesis of atherosclerosis: A perspective for the 1990s. Nature 362:801, 1993.
79. Casscells W: Migration of smooth muscle and endothelial cells: Critical events in restenosis. Circulation 86:723, 1992.
80. Ikeda E, Maruyama I, Hosoda Y: Expression of thrombomodulin in patients with spontaneous occlusion of the circle of Willis. Stroke 24:657, 1993.
81. Bonduel M, Hepner M, Sciuccati G, et al: Prothrombotic disorders in children with moyamoya syndrome. Stroke 32:1786, 2001.
82. Takanashi J, Sugita K, Miyazato S, et al: Antiphospholipid antibody syndrome in childhood strokes. Pediatr Neurol 13:323, 1995.
83. Hughes GRV: The antiphospholipid syndrome: Ten years on. Lancet 342:341, 1993.
84. Hoshimaru M, Takahashi JA, Kikuchi H, et al: Possible roles of basic fibroblast growth factor in the pathogenesis of moyamoya disease: An immunohistochemical study. J Neurosurg 75:267, 1991.
85. Suzui H, Hoshimaru M, Takahashi JA, et al: Immunohistochemical reactions for fibroblast growth factor receptor in arteries of patients with moyamoya disease. Neurosurgery 35:20, 1994.
86. Aoyagi M, Fukui N, Sakamoto H, et al: Altered cellular responses to serum mitogens, including platelet-derived growth factor, in cultured smooth muscle cells derived from arteries of patients with moyamoya disease. J Cell Physiol 147:191, 1991.
87. Hojo M, Hoshimaru M, Miyamoto S, et al: Role of transforming growth-β1 in the pathogenesis of moyamoya disease. J Neurosurg 89:623, 1998.
88. Yamamoto M, Aoyagi M, Fukai N, et al: Increase in prostaglandin E(2) production by interleukin-1β in arterial smooth muscle cells derived from patients with moyamoya disease. Circ Res 85:912, 1999.
89. Takahashi A, Sawamura Y, Houkin K, et al: The cerebrovascular fluid in patients in moyamoya disease contains a high level of basic fibroblast growth factor. Neurosci Lett 160:214, 1993.
90. Yoshimoto T, Houkin K, Takahashi A, et al: Angiogenic factors in moyamoya disease. Stroke 27:2160, 1996.
91. Fukui M, Kawano T: Follow-up study of registered cases in 1995. In Fukui M (ed): Annual Report (1995) by Research Committee on Spontaneous Occlusion of the Circle of Willis (Moyamoya Disease). Ministry of Health and Welfare, Tokyo, Japan, 1996, p 12.
92. Handa H, Yonekawa Y, Goto Y, et al: Analysis of the filing data bank of 1500 cases of spontaneous occlusion of the circle of Willis and follow-up study of 200 cases for more than 5 years. In Handa H (ed): Annual Report (1984) by Research Committee on Spontaneous Occlusion of the Circle of Willis. Ministry of Health and Welfare, Tokyo, Japan, 1985, p 14.
93. Levine SR, Welch KMA: Cerebrovascular ischemia associated with lupus anticoagulant. Stroke 18:257, 1987.
94. Yamaguchi T, Tashiro M, Hasegawa Y: Collective analysis of the patients with spontaneous occlusion of the circle of Willis in Japan, registered from 1977 to 1982. In Gotoh F (ed): Annual Report (1982) by Research Committee on Spontaneous Occlusion of the Circle of Willis (Moyamoya Disease). Ministry of Health and Welfare, Tokyo, Japan, 1983, p 15.
95. Yamada I, Suzuki S, Matsushima Y: Moyamoya disease: Comparison with MR angiography and MR imaging versus conventional angiography. Radiology 196:221, 1995.
96. Houkin K, Kuroda S, Nakayama N: Cerebral revascularization for moyamoya disease in children. Neurosurg Clin N Am 12:575, 2001.

Specific Medical Diseases and Stroke

97. Yamada I, Nakagawa T, Matsushima Y, et al: High-resolution turbo magnetic resonance angiography for diagnosis of moyamoya disease. Stroke 32:1825, 2001.

98. Kodama N, Aoki Y, Hiraga H, et al: Electroencephalographic findings in children with moyamoya disease. Arch Neurol 36:16, 1979.

99. Yoshii N, Kudo T: Electroencephalographical study on occlusion of the Willis arterial ring. Rinsho Shinkeigaku 8:301, 1968.

100. Ikezaki K, Matsushima T, Kuwabara Y, et al: Cerebral circulation and oxygen metabolism in childhood moyamoya disease: A perioperative positron emission tomography study. J Neurosurg 81:843, 1994.

101. Iwama T, Hashimoto N, Yonekawa Y: The relevance of hemodynamic factors to perioperative ischemic complications in childhood moyamoya disease. Neurosurgery 38:1120, 1996.

102. Kuwabara Y, Ichiya Y, Otsuka M, et al: Cerebral hemodynamic changes in the child and adult with moyamoya disease. Stroke 21:272, 1990.

103. Kuwabara Y, Ichiya Y, Sasaki M, et al: Cerebral hemodynamics and metabolism in moyamoya disease—a positron emission tomography study. Clin Neurol Neurosurg 99(Suppl 2):S74, 1997.

104. Nariai T, Suzuki R, Hirakawa K, et al: Vascular reserve in chronic cerebral ischemia measured with acetazolamide challenge test: Comparison with positron emission tomography. AJNR Am J Neuroradiol 16:563, 1995.

105. Obara K, Fukuuchi Y, Kobari M, et al: Cerebral hemodynamics in patients with moyamoya disease and in patients with atherosclerotic occlusion of the major cerebral arterial trunks. Clin Neurol Neurosurg 99(Suppl 2):S86, 1997.

106. Taki W, Yonekawa Y, Kobayashi A, et al: Cerebral circulation and metabolism in adult's moyamoya disease—PET study. Acta Neurochir (Wien) 100:150, 1989.

107. Ezura M, Yoshimoto T, Fujiwara S, et al: Clinical and angiographic follow-up of childhood-onset moyamoya disease. Childs Nerv Syst 11:591, 1995.

108. Hirotsune N, Meguro T, Kawada S, et al: Long-term follow-up study of patients with unilateral moyamoya disease. Clin Neurol Neurosurg 99(Suppl 2):S178, 1997.

109. Kawano T, Fukui M, Hashimoto N, et al: Follow-up study of patients with "unilateral" moyamoya disease. Neurol Med Chir (Tokyo) 34:744, 1994.

110. Fukuyama Y, Mitsuishi Y, Umezu R: Intellectual prognosis of children with TIA type of spontaneous occlusion of the circle of Willis: With special reference to Wechsler's intelligence test and Benton's visual attention test. In Handa H (ed): Annual Report (1986) of Research Committee on Spontaneous Occlusion of the Circle of Willis. Ministry of Health and Welfare, Tokyo, Japan, 1987, p 43.

111. Imaizumi C, Imaizumi T, Osawa M, et al: Serial intelligence test scores in pediatric moyamoya disease. Neuropediatrics 30:294, 1999.

112. Imaizumi T, Hayashi K, Saito K, et al: Long-term outcomes of pediatric moyamoya disease monitored to adulthood. Pediatr Neurol 18:321, 1998.

113. Kurokawa T, Tomita S, Ueda K, et al: Prognosis of occlusive disease of circle of Willis (moyamoya disease) in children. Pediatr Neurol 12:288, 1969.

114. Matsushima Y, Aoyagi M, Nariai T, et al: Long-term intelligence outcome of post-encephalo-duro-arterio-synangiosis in childhood

moyamoya patients. Clin Neurol Neurosurg 99(Suppl 2):S147, 1997.

115. Nakashima H, Meguro T, Kawada S, et al: Long-term results of surgically treated moyamoya disease. Clin Neurol Neurosurg 99(Suppl 2):S156, 1997.

116. Ueki K, Meyer JB: Moyamoya disease: The disorder and surgical treatment. Mayo Clin Proc 69:749, 1994.

117. Yasargil MG: Microsurgery Applied to Neurosurgery. Stuttgart, Thieme, 1969.

118. Karasawa J, Kikuchi H, Furuse S, et al: Treatment of moyamoya disease with STA-MCA anastomosis. J Neurosurg 49:679, 1978.

119. Reichmann O, Anderson RE, Roberts TC, et al: The treatment of intracranial occlusive cerebrovascular disease by STA-cortical MCA anastomosis. In Handa H (ed): Microneurosurgery. Tokyo, Igaku Shoin, 1975, p 31.

120. Matsushima T, Inoue T, Suzuki SO, et al: Surgical treatment of moyamoya disease in pediatric patients: Comparison between the results of indirect and direct revascularization procedures. Neurosurgery 31:401, 1992.

121. Matsushima Y, Inaba Y: Moyamoya disease in children and its surgical treatment: Introduction of a new surgical procedure and its follow-up angiograms. Childs Brain 11:155, 1984.

122. Karasawa J, Kikuchi H, Furuse S: A surgical treatment of moyamoya disease: Encephalomyosynangiosis. Neurol Med Chir (Tokyo) 17:29, 1977.

123. Karasawa J, Touhou H, Ohnishi H, et al: Cerebral revascularization using omental transplantation for childhood moyamoya disease. J Neurosurg 79:192, 1993.

124. Matsushima T, Inoue TK, Suzuki SO, et al: Surgical techniques and the results of a fronto-temporo-parietal combined indirect bypass procedure for children with moyamoya disease: A comparison with the results of encephalo-duro-arterio-synangiosis alone. Clin Neurol Neurosurg 99(Suppl 2):S123, 1997.

125. Shirane R, Yoshida Y, Takahashi T, et al: Assessment of encephalo-galeo-myo-synangiosis with dural pedicle insertion in childhood moyamoya disease: Characteristics of cerebral blood flow and oxygen metabolism. Clin Neurol Neurosurg 99(Suppl 2):S79, 1997.

126. Aoki N: Cerebrovascular bypass surgery for the treatment of moyamoya disease: Unsatisfactory outcome in the patients presenting with intracranial hemorrhage. Surg Neurol 40:372, 1993.

127. Srinivasan J, Britz GW, Newell DW: Cerebral revascularization for moyamoya disease in adults. Neurosurg Clin N Am 12:585, 2001.

128. Ikezaki K, Fukui M, Inamura T, et al: The current status of the treatment for hemorrhagic type moyamoya disease based on a 1995 nationwide survey in Japan. Clin Neurol Neurosurg 99(Suppl 2):S183, 1997.

129. Houkin K, Kamiyama H, Abe H, et al: Surgical therapy for adult moyamoya disease: Can surgical revascularization prevent the recurrence of intracerebral hemorrhage? Stroke 27:448, 1996.

130. Yoshida Y, Yoshimoto T, Shirane R, et al: Clinical course, surgical management, and long-term outcome of moyamoya patients with rebleeding after an episode of intracerebral hemorrhage: An extensive follow-up study. Stroke 30:2272, 1999.

131. Miyamoto S: Study on the management of moyamoya disease with hemorrhagic onset. In Yoshimoto T (ed): Annual Report (2000) by Research Committee on Spontaneous Occlusion of the Circle of Willis. Ministry of Health, Labor, and Welfare, Tokyo, Japan, 2001, p 61.

Chapter Twenty-Six

Cervicocephalic Fibromuscular Dysplasia

Bartlomiej Piechowski-Józwiak and Julien Bogousslavsky

Fibromuscular dysplasia (FMD) is a rare nonatheromatous chronic systemic arteriopathy. The disease commonly affects young and middle-aged women. The pathologic changes it causes include segmental thickening of the arterial wall caused by fibrosis alternating with atrophy. The disease process usually affects multiple vessels (usually two or three arterial territories in one patient) of the body, including major aortic branches and their subdivisions, the renal arteries being most commonly involved. The disease process can also affect the distal portion of extracranial carotid arteries and vertebral arteries at the level of first and second cervical vertebrae, intracranial arteries, and splanchnic and iliac arteries. Fibromuscular dysplasia of these vessels may be an incidental finding in otherwise asymptomatic patients.

FMD can be associated with arterial dissection, aneurysm or fistula formation, thromboembolic phenomena, and hemodynamic failure in the affected arterial territory. In some patients with stroke, FMD can be considered a presumed cause of ischemic brain damage.

Leadbetter and Burkland[1] published the first report of a patient with FMD in 1938 under the diagnosis hypertension and renal artery stenosis. The patient was a child. These investigators found conglomerates of smooth muscle cells narrowing the lumen of the renal arteries. Subsequent reports of renal artery stenoses caused by abnormal intraluminal collections of smooth muscle cells appeared,[2] leading to the establishment of FMD as one of the surgically curable causes of arterial hypertension.[3-7] It took several years to document the presence of angiographic changes typical for FMD in the celiac artery and extracranial portion of the internal carotid artery.[7] In 1965, the first histologically proven case of internal carotid artery FMD was reported.[8] The same year, Connett and Lansche[9] presented a radiologic and histologic correlation in a patient with FMD in the internal carotid artery. Many reports have appeared since then documenting involvement of other vessels in the disease process, including vertebral[10,11] and intracranial[12-16] arteries.

The relationship between FMD of the cephalic arterial system and the occurrence of focal neurologic symptoms related to cerebrovascular incidents is still debated. How often otherwise symptomless and "benign" FMD can lead to vascular brain damage is not known. More than 500 cases of cephalic FMD associated with either transient cerebral ischemia, completed stroke, vascular malformations, or cerebral aneurysms have been published to date. Some researchers advocate conservative treatment, and others prefer either surgical repair or nonsurgical, transluminal dilatation of the diseased vessel. Because the natural history, etiology, and clinical-pathologic relationships of the disease are not well known and there is no consensus on treatment, FMD remains a mysterious and perplexing entity.

EPIDEMIOLOGY

Fibromuscular dysplasia is an uncommon disease, and there are no data in the literature concerning its overall incidence in a general population. In one study involving 819 autopsies, FMD of the renal arteries was found in 1.1% of cases.[17] In another study, the frequency of FMD assessed with digital subtraction angiography in 159 normotensive potential kidney donors was determined to be 4.4%.[18] Histologically confirmed FMD of the internal carotid artery is extremely rare, being found in only 0.02% of 20,244 serial autopsies.[19] The frequency of cerebral FMD based on approximately 23,000 angiograms is higher, ranging from 0.25% to 3.2%.[20-24] A single angiographic study showed a 10% frequency of cerebral FMD among patients with stroke.[25] FMD is more common in females at a ratio of 2:1; it is also more common in white people.[19,23,26] Cerebral FMD may occur at any age, being reported in the early postnatal period,[27] childhood,[28-34] and early adolescence,[35] but it most commonly affects middle-aged individuals (30 to 50 years).

PATHOLOGY

FMD is a nonatherosclerotic, noninflammatory arteriopathy. All three layers of the arterial wall—adventitia, media, and intima—can be involved in the disease process, and three histologic types of renal FMD can be differentiated: adventitial, medial, and intimal.[36,37] The *adventitial* type is the rarest histologic type. It leads to the vascular lumen narrowing by hypertrophy of adventitial and periarterial fibrous tissue.

The *intimal* type is more common, found in approximately 5% of cases. It usually affects younger patients—men and women equally. This type is characterized by intimal fibroplasia that leads to destruction of the internal part of the arterial elastic layer and concentric narrowing of the vascular lumen. It is found in rare cases of weblike stenosis, most often involving the carotid artery (carotid web).[38,39]

The most common is the *medial* type. It occurs in up to 95% of cases of renal FMD and is much more common in women. The medial type is characterized by the proliferation of fibrous tissue and hyperplasia of the smooth muscle component of the vascular wall. It leads to formation of fibromuscular rings that narrow the arterial lumen. The rings can be solitary and may occupy variable lengths of the vessel. Another histologic finding typical for this type of FMD consists of medial thinning and destruction of either external or internal elastic laminae or both that may lead to mural aneurysm formation. The areas of arterial wall thickening can alternate with medial thinning, producing an irregular pattern that gives a characteristic "string-of-beads" appearance on angiography (Figs. 26–1 to 26–3). In the postlesional part of the affected vessel, various forms of arterial wall dilatation—most often aneurysmal dilatation of renal artery branches—can be found. This pattern of histologic abnormalities is also present in approximately 90% of cases of cervicocephalic FMD.

At the subcellular level, all of the pathologic changes in these three types of FMD seem to be identical, differing only in the severity and localization. The main pathophysiologic process underlying the changes is the fibroblast-like transformation of smooth muscle cells. The modified

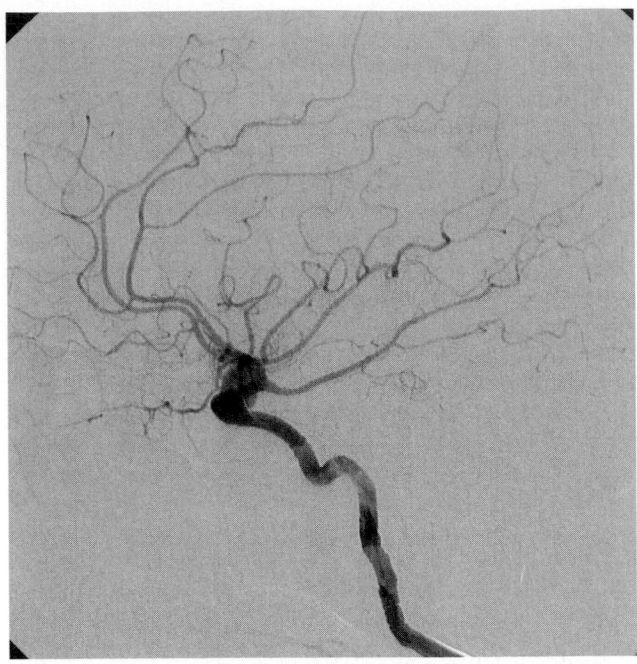

FIGURE 26–2   *Conventional lateral view angiogram of the left internal carotid artery, showing the "string-of-beads" appearance (base of picture, extracranial course) typical of fibromuscular hyperplasia and a large saccular aneurysm, partially hidden in the intracranial views of the circle of Willis.*

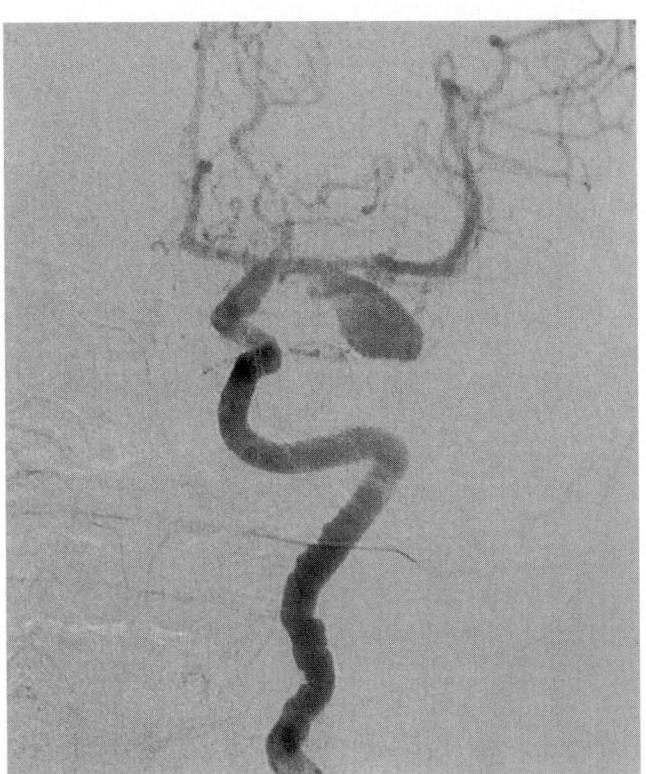

FIGURE 26–3   *Conventional anteroposterior view angiogram of the left internal carotid artery, showing the "string-of-beads" appearance (base of picture, extracranial course) typical of fibromuscular hyperplasia and a large saccular aneurysm, arising from the left side of the circle of Willis.*

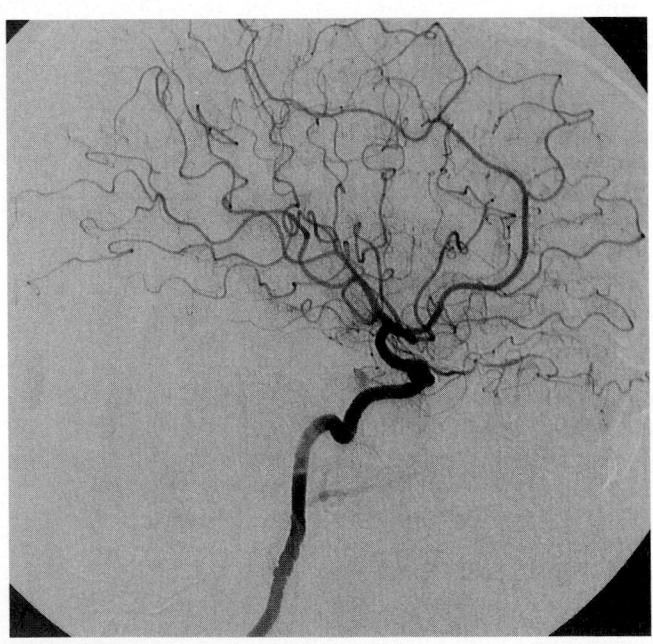

FIGURE 26–1   *Conventional lateral view angiogram of the right internal carotid artery, showing the "string-of-beads" appearance (base of picture, extracranial course) typical of fibromuscular hyperplasia.*

smooth muscle cells seem to be the source of abnormal connective tissue component synthesis. Along with the progression of the disease, the smooth muscle cells activate and increasingly synthesize collagen. Their cellular organelles—the nucleus, the granular endoplasmic reticulum—and the Golgi apparatus enlarge. When fibrous changes predominate, single fibroblasts can be found in the media. Concomitant with the continuous accumulation of collagen fibers, varying degrees of smooth muscle cell involution can be found. The other process that takes place is the diminution of the number of the elastic fibers in the media of the affected arteries that, especially in intimal FMD, destroys the inner elastic membrane of the arterial wall.[40]

In the cerebral form of FMD, extracranial arteries are more often affected than intracranial arteries. The disease typically affects multiple cerebral arteries, only rarely confined to one vessel. In the extracranial vessels, most of the lesions are located adjacent to the vertebral segments C1-C2, typically sparing the more proximal segments of these arteries. Thus, the proximal segment of the vertebral artery just after it branches from the subclavian artery and the proximal part of the internal carotid artery just above the carotid bifurcation are usually spared. The extracranial portion of the internal carotid artery is involved in 95% of all cases of cephalic FMD, and the disease affects both internal carotid arteries in 65% to more than 80%.[22,41,42] There are sporadic reports of the involvement of either the proximal internal carotid artery[38,43–45] or the distal intracranial portion of the internal carotid artery.[22,46,47] Involvement of the common carotid artery,[48–50] the carotid bifurcation,[51] and the external carotid artery[52] has also been reported. FMD affecting the vertebral artery is less often encountered than FMD of the carotid system. Rarely, a solitary cerebral vessel is affected.[28] Vertebral artery FMD is present in 10% to 43% of cases of cervicocephalic FMD[53] and can be either unilateral or bilateral.[54]

In addition to the involvement of intracranial portions of carotid arteries and vertebral arteries, the disease may affect other intracranial arteries. Isolated intracranial FMD is extremely rare. In most instances there is no histopathologic verification of the diagnosis, and intracranial vessels are usually affected concomitantly with extracranial vessels. The pathologic destruction of the vascular wall often starts at the extracranial or intracranial portion of the artery and further involves the branches of the circle of Willis in either a continuous or noncontinuous fashion.[34,55–57] The intracranial arteries in both the anterior and posterior circulation may be involved.[58] Most of the reported cases of intracranial vasculature involvement were diagnosed from the radiologic appearance rather than being microscopically proved; vessels affected included the middle,[59–61] anterior,[62] and posterior[23] cerebral arteries and the basilar artery.[16,63] Involvement of the long distal segments of the internal carotid arteries and the proximal branches of the circle of Willis may lead to the development of collateral circulation from the secondary anastomoses at the base of the brain or convexity, yielding a radiologic picture resembling that of moyamoya syndrome.[64,65]

The destruction of the different layers of the arterial wall in the course of FMD can lead to the following pathologic phenomena: internal carotid artery elongation and kinking, artery stenosis, dissection, and aneurysm and fistula formation.

In the extracranial cerebral vasculature, kinking and elongation have been described in the carotid system.[66] The arterial stenoses are most often located in the distal parts of the cervical arteries at the level of C1-C2 vertebrae. The internal carotid artery is affected just before it enters the skull. The stenoses are typically bilateral and may be very severe (>95%).[67,68] Unilateral or bilateral stenosis of the vertebral artery may accompany that of internal carotid artery(ies).[54] FMD of the extracranial portion of the internal carotid artery may be responsible for approximately 20% of spontaneous and also traumatic dissections, predominantly in young women.[69–72] Dissections of multiple cervical arteries in patients with FMD have been reported in the literature. The dissections are either spontaneous or post-traumatic, have involved either one or both internal carotid arteries and one or both vertebral arteries, and were in some cases complicated by aneurysm formation.[73–75] The arteriopathy due to FMD may also lead to dissection in other cerebral vessels—the middle cerebral,[76] anterior cerebral,[77] and superior cerebellar arteries.[78]

Weakening of the structure of the diseased arterial wall may cause dilatation of the vascular lumen and formation of an aneurysm (see Figs. 26–2 and 26–3, left internal carotid–middle cerebral junction). Saccular aneurysms of the extracranial vessels and saccular, berry, and fusiform aneurysms of the intracranial vessels are reported in patients with FMD. Aneurysms secondary to FMD are rare in the extracranial segments of the internal carotid artery; they preferentially occur at the level of second and third cervical vertebrae but may also involve the carotid artery at the level of skull base, causing paresis of lower cranial nerves and giving a clinical picture resembling the Collect-Sicard syndrome,[79] and in the cavernous portion of the artery.[80]

Different prevalence rates of internal carotid artery aneurysms due to FMD are reported by different investigators; the rates range from 3% to 50%, depending on the number of cases studied.[81–83] The major shortcomings of these studies are that they are retrospective and involve small numbers of patients. In the study that involved seven patients with internal carotid FMD, there was only one patient with a carotid aneurysm; in another paper assessing 30 cases of internal carotid FMD, there were no extracranial aneurysms.[24,84] The prevalence of cerebral aneurysms in patients with extracranial FMD is also debated in the literature. On the basis of one meta-analysis involving 615 cases of FMD affecting the internal carotid artery, vertebral artery, or both, the prevalence of incidental asymptomatic cerebral aneurysms was 7.3%, not significantly higher than in the general population (5.6%).[85]

Another phenomenon linked to FMD of cerebral vessels is spontaneous formation of arteriovenous fistulas. The fistulas may form between the intracranial segment of the internal carotid artery and the cavernous sinus[86–88] and between the vertebral artery and the paravertebral veins.[89–91] In two reported cases, there were coexisting carotid-cavernous and vertebral fistulas.[92]

ETIOLOGIC FACTORS

The smooth muscle cells seem to play a central role in the development of characteristic histopathologic changes. The transformation of smooth muscle cells into cells capable of producing extracellular matrix proteins—mainly collagen—appear to be crucial in pathogenesis of FMD. The issues that are not yet resolved are which mechanisms induce this kind of transformation and what the stimulus is for the smooth muscle cell to regain the properties of a myofibroblast that it abandoned during the cell maturation process. The role of genetic factors in FMD is accepted in the literature; an autosomal dominant trait with a variable penetrance was determined in familial cases of renal FMD.[93] In one study based on angiographic diagnosis of renal FMD, patients with renal FMD with a positive family history were typically found to have multifocal vascular lesions, more often bilateral than those with sporadic FMD.[94]

There are some episodic reports linking FMD with involvement of other systems into a genetically transmitted syndrome that may give further insight into the pathology of FMD. One such report describes a syndrome characterized by the simultaneous appearance of FMD in the renal, cerebral, splanchnic, and coronary arteries with congenital cardiac abnormalities, brachydactyly, syndactyly of the hands and feet, a mild form of osteogenesis imperfecta, and cognitive impairment. In this pedigree, four of nine siblings were affected. Each of the elements of this unique syndrome has its own way of transmission, a plausible explanation for this unique clustering of disorders being a parental gonadal mosaicism.[95] Some other reports investigated a possible association between FMD and skeletal deformities as well as connective tissue disorders such as Ehlers-Danlos syndrome and Marfan's syndrome, pointing to a mesenchymal disorder as a common denominator for these disorders.[96–98] One study further explored the hypothesis that the etiology of FMD is mesenchymally related. This study focused on linkage analysis of the elastin gene in 14 pedigrees of familial renal FMD that involved nine siblings, four trios, and one case of vertical transmission. The pedigree analysis showed an autosomal dominant mode of inheritance with an age- and sex-dependent incomplete penetrance. The role of the elastin gene in the pathogenesis of FMD was not demonstrated, however.[99]

An immune etiology of FMD has also been suggested. Several case reports show a coexistence of an autoimmune antiphospholipid syndrome and FMD confined to the cervical and intracranial vasculature.[100,101]

Another hypothesis for the pathogenesis of FMD concentrated on the role of the inhibitor of proteases, α_1-antitripsin. A higher prevalence of FMD in patients with α_1-antitripsin deficiency compared with patients without such a deficiency (33% vs. 0.3%) was demonstrated in a large autopsy study. Another interesting finding was that histopathologic changes in the arterial media were identical in patients with α_1-antitripsin deficiency and patients with FMD; these changes consisted of thickening of media and disorganization of muscular and connective tissue fibers.[102] α_1-Antitripsin is a major serum inhibitor of proteases (Pi) such as trypsin and elastases. In deficiency of α_1-antitripsin, an uninhibited action of proteases occurs, and in most cases, emphysema or liver cirrhosis develops. The gene for α_1-antitripsin is located on chromosome 14. There are more than 70 alleles, and their different combinations may give normal, reduced, or very low levels of α_1-antitripsin. The combination that gives the lowest levels is PiZZ. Several reports have shown a positive correlation between the different α_1-antitripsin deficiency phenotypes, such as PiMP,[76] PiMS,[103] PiMZ,[67] and PiSZ,[104] and the occurrence of cervicocephalic FMD.

Polymorphism of the renin-angiotensin system has also been implicated in the pathogenesis of multifocal renal FMD. Different phenotypes of angiotensin-converting enzyme (ACE) are characterized by different levels of circulating ACE. In one study using polymerase chain reaction (PCR), a positive correlation between the ACE I allele and occurrence of the multifocal renal form of FMD was demonstrated.[105] The ACE I phenotype is associated with lower levels of circulating ACE and lower tissue levels of angiotensin II, a strong modulator of smooth muscle cells growth and synthetic activity. Lower levels of angiotensin II in the ACE I phenotype could explain the improper remodeling of the medial arterial layer in the multifocal renal forms of FMD. Another interesting issue that points to the importance of the ACE phenotype in arterial disease is that the ACE D phenotype is linked with carotid intima-media complex thickening and coronary stent restenosis, both of which are typical of the atherosclerotic process and involve dysfunction of arterial intimal layer.

The theory of the etiopathologic role of vasospasm in FMD has also been discussed in the literature.[106] Some researchers have suggested that administration of ergot alkaloids might cause arterial vasospasm, which in turn may lead to the obstruction of the vas vasorum. These agents may also invoke an ischemic insult to the medial layer, giving a characteristic picture of the medial abnormalities seen in FMD. Segmental arterial mediolysis, a separate pathologic entity that is presumably caused by vasospasm, shares some pathologic features with FMD, in that smooth muscle cells of the medial layer are replaced by connective tissue. Segmental arterial mediolysis is confined to epicardial coronary arteries and the splanchnic arteries, however.[107] The role of ergot preparations in arterial wall dissection was also demonstrated in a few case reports. In one patient with chronic ergotism, spontaneous dissections of the cervicocephalic, renal, and hepatic arteries and of the descending aorta developed—the clinical picture and pattern of involvement and dissection of multiple vessels resembling that of multifocal FMD.[108] The separation of vasa vasorum from surrounding cellular elements in the medial arterial layer that was shown in some cases of FMD is further evidence of the importance of vessel wall ischemia in the disease process.[109] Results of experimental animal studies also confirm a plausible role for vascular wall ischemia in development of lesions similar to those of FMD.[110]

There is only one case-control study on FMD risk factors in a cohort of patients with angiographically proven renal FMD and kidney donors (n = 94).[111] Oral contraceptive preparations or markers of sex hormone dysfunction, mechanical stress to the renal artery wall, human lymphocytic antigen type, cigarette smoking, history of hypertension for more than 5 years, and family history of cardiovascular disease were assessed. A positive correlation between HLA-DRw6 and FMD, after adjustment for cigarette smoking (odds ratio [OR] 5.0; 95% confidence interval [CI], 1.3 to 19.6) was found. A positive (though not statistically significant) association was demonstrated between family history of cardiovascular disease and fibromuscular dysplasia (OR 1.7).

Many other elements may contribute to the development of FMD. The role of viral infections, as demonstrated in a domestic turkey model, has been reported.[112] Also, some researchers have pointed to the importance of the estrogens as stimulants of smooth muscle activity, considering the unquestionable preponderance of FMD in women and case reports documenting higher prevalence of the disease among women undergoing estrogen treatment.[113–116]

The etiology of FMD is probably multifactorial, and genetic predispositions can add to the external and internal factors in its development. These complicated associations are illustrated well in the case reports on the occurrence of FMD in patients with Turner's syndrome undergoing estrogen replacement therapy as well as in patients with Down's syndrome.[117,118]

DIAGNOSIS

The diagnostic technique that is considered a reference method for diagnosis of FMD is conventional catheter angiography (see Figs. 26–1 to 26–3).[119] Magnetic resonance angiography (MRA), both two-dimensional and three-dimensional time-of-flight and contrast-enhanced methods, is increasingly being used in the detection of arterial and venous disorders, including FMD, of the cervical and cerebral vasculatures.[120] An advantage of MRA over conventional angiography is that it allows for noninvasive and safe evaluation of patients with cerebrovascular diseases; in some instances, however, diagnosis may require verification with catheter angiography.[121,122]

Another method that is noninvasive and allows for visualization of the extracranial vessels in patients with FMD is duplex Doppler imaging with B-mode echotomography.[123,124] With this technique, it is also possible to visualize rare subtypes of FMD, such as intimal FMD.[125] With transcranial Doppler and transcranial color-coded Doppler ultrasonography, it is possible to assess the intracranial vasculature hemodynamically without visualization of the morphology of the large intracranial vessels.[126] Comparing the relative utility of conventional angiography, Doppler ultrasonography, and MRA for the diagnosis of diffuse disease of internal carotid arteries, especially in complicated cases, Wong and colleagues have concluded that catheter angiography is the reference method.[127]

There are three characteristic patterns of primary arterial lesions typical for FMD. The most common is the "string-of-beads" appearance, caused by alternation of areas of arterial wall thinning and dilatation with areas of vascular lumen constriction (see Figs. 26–1 to 26–3). In both the dilated and constricted segments, diameter of the artery is either wider or narrower than that of the healthy artery. These radiologic changes are most commonly encountered in the medial type of FMD, in which hyperplasia of the smooth muscle component of the vascular wall leads to formation of fibromuscular rings and medial thinning and destruction of elastic laminae weaken the walls of the arteries, causing their aneurysmal dilatation. Another and less common FMD pattern than that visualized on angiography is characterized by unifocal or multifocal tubular narrowing of the vascular lumen. This pattern has low diagnostic value for FMD histopathologic types because it may be associated with all three of them. The last and least common is the pattern that involves different, less common phenomena, such as diverticulum formation, aneurysmal dilatation of the arterial wall, and formation of an arterial web.

The other radiologic patterns are caused by complications related to primary FMD lesions. These are postlesional aneurysmal dilatations of the affected vessels or their branches, the string sign, and double flow or hematoma formation that are characteristic for arterial dissection. The angiographic signs of a functioning intracranial leptomeningeal and/or basal circulation fistula can also be seen; characteristically they resemble cigarette smoke, giving rise to a moyamoya-like appearance.[64,65] Also arteriovenous fistulas and pseudoaneurysms can be documented. Stenoses of either cervical or cephalic arteries are rarely found on angiographic evaluation of a patient with FMD.

Some of the following conditions manifesting similar angiographic phenomena of the cervical vasculature should be considered in the differential diagnosis of FMD. Stationary arterial waves may be caused by a distal obstacle to flow in the carotid artery, such as an occlusion of the vessel or flow stagnation due to intracranial hypertension.[128] Arterial segmental contractions may be caused by direct irritation of the arterial wall with the catheter. Differentiation of FMD from the arteritides of the major branches of aortic arch (such as Takayasu's arteritis) is based mainly on the involvement of more proximal arterial segments of the cervical vessels and the aortic arch in the arteritides. Cervical FMD is confined to the distal segments of the arteries in most cases at the level of C1 and C2. The same distinction can be made between FMD and cervical atherosclerotic lesions, which tend to involve proximal parts of the vertebral artery and internal carotid artery starting at the level of the carotid bifurcation. In the differential diagnosis of intracranial FMD, one should take into consideration atherosclerotic lesions, arteritides, and focal thromboembolic lesions.

CLINICAL SYMPTOMS

The relationship between FMD of the cephalic arterial system and the occurrence of focal neurologic symptoms related to ischemic brain damage is debated in the literature. How often otherwise symptomless and "benign" FMD can cause cerebrovascular disorders is not known. The clinical symptoms of nervous system dysfunction related to cervicocephalic FMD can be attributed either to focal cerebral ischemia and hemodynamic compromise of the cerebral circulation or to complications of FMD such as arterial dissection, mural aneurysm formation, and fistula formation.

The unambiguous correlation between FMD of the cervicocephalic arteries and the occurrence of ischemic stroke cannot be established in many patients, because the other concomitant disorders that are risk factors for ischemic stroke (cardiogenic source of emboli, atheromatous stenosis of internal carotid or vertebral artery, etc.) are more likely factors in ischemic stroke. Moreover, FMD of the cervicocephalic arteries is quite often an incidental finding in otherwise healthy individuals. The causal relationship between the stenosis of internal carotid arteries due to FDM and cerebral ischemia has seldom been shown in the literature.[129,130] The presence of a thrombus attached to the damaged arterial wall in a patient with the septal type of FMD and ischemic stroke has been reported, thus suggesting a thromboembolic mechanism of FMD-related ischemic stroke.[51,131] There is another report linking septal FMD with a thromboembolic etiology of ischemic stroke.[38] The other mechanism that may lead to ischemic brain damage in cervicocephalic FMD is cerebral hypoperfusion. The diseased arteries, in addition to having abnormal diameter and lumen constriction, may become elongated and kinked. The latter development predisposes to perfusion failure in distal arterial territory, which can be provoked, for example, by head turning. There are reports documenting circulatory insufficiency in the common carotid-internal carotid axis in patients with carotid FMD.[66,132]

Reports on stroke rates in patients with cervicocephalic FMD are conflicting. In a study by Corrin and associates,[23] during an average follow-up of 60 months in 79 patients (mean age 58 years) with proven carotid FMD, the rate of stroke was 3.8%, and the patients without stroke had no cerebrovascular episodes related to FMD. Other reports however, show higher rates of stroke in patients with carotid artery FMD. Wells and Smith,[133] for example, reported that in 16 female patients followed up for an average of 3.8 years, there were two ischemic strokes (12.5%). The highest rate of stroke in cervicocephalic FMD patients, 28.1%, was documented by So and colleagues.[51] The rate of transient ischemic attacks in patients with cervicocephalic FMD ranges from 7.6% to 67.5%.[23,134] The reasons for such discrepancies among these studies are that they (1) differ in methodology, study design (in most instances retrospective), and patient selection criteria, and (2) are usually based on a small sample sizes, and (3) vary in treatment regimens and demographic profile of studied groups. The selection bias probably is a reason for such divergent results.

Spontaneous arterial dissection (internal carotid and/or vertebral artery) is a rare condition but a well-recognized complication of FMD.[71] Internal carotid artery dissection may be complicated by arterial stenosis or occlusion that may lead to cerebral ischemia.[72] Typically, carotid dissection causes hemicrania, cervical pain, Horner's syndrome, and tinnitus. It may also lead to monocular ischemia and hemispheric symptoms. Sometimes the internal carotid dissection may be complicated by the formation of an aneurysm causing local mass effect and lower cranial nerves (IX to XII) palsy (Collet-Sicard syndrome).[135] Formation of a giant aneurysm on the intracranial portion of the internal carotid artery at the level of trigeminal ganglion may also lead to paratrigeminal oculosympathetic syndrome (Raeder's syndrome), which is characterized by trigeminal nerve involvement, neuralgic pain or sensory change, and ptosis or miosis or both but no anhidrosis. Some patients with intracranial carotid or vertebral FMD may also complain of persistent and pulsatile tinnitus.[136,137] A dissecting aneurysm of the intracranial portion of internal carotid and vertebral arteries may lead to subarachnoid hemorrhage.[74]

Another characteristic complication of FMD is spontaneous formation of arteriovenous fistulas. The fistulas usually couple the intracranial portion of the internal carotid artery with the cavernous sinus (carotid-cavernous fistula)[24,88,89] or the vertebral artery with paravertebral venous plexuses.[90–92] The clinical symptoms are related to entry of arterial blood at a high pressure straight into the venous system. The patient with a carotid-cavernous fistula may present with heart failure, pulsating exophthalmos, ophthalmoplegia, and headaches; and the patient with a vertebroparavertebral fistula may experience progressive cervical myelopathy and cervical bruit.

The association between extracranial FMD and the higher prevalence of cerebral aneurysms is debated in the literature. As already mentioned, one meta-analysis showed that the prevalence of incidental asymptomatic cerebral aneurysms was not significantly higher in patients with extracranial FMD than in the general population (7.3% vs. 5.6%).[86]

TREATMENT

The natural course of the cervicocephalic FMD has not been studied in a prospective manner. Most of the available information on the prevalence of FMD in otherwise healthy people and among patients with stroke as well as data concerning the progression of either treated or untreated disease originates usually from retrospective and small cohort studies. The important clinical questions are whether we should treat patients with FMD and, if we should, whether conservative or surgical treatment is superior. Unfortunately no randomized or controlled trials assessing these important issues have been performed. The only available data originate from several small cohort studies on progression of the arterial lesions and from follow-up studies after surgical or radiologic interventions or conservative treatment. In a cohort of 79 patients with cervical FMD monitored for an average of 60 months, there were only three ischemic strokes, which occurred in elderly patients 50 to 216 months after diagnosis and were not related to the FMD lesion.[23]

The natural history of FMD was also indirectly assessed in a study that involved 49 patients with angiographically proven internal carotid FMD.[138] Ischemic symptoms, either central or retinal, were present in 40.8% of the patients in this study, intracerebral hemorrhage in 6%, and nonlateralizing neurologic symptoms in 20%. There were four deaths; one patient had a massive ischemic stroke (as a complication of arteriography), and three patients had hemorrhagic strokes. More than 80% of cases were treated conservatively. In patients treated surgically, carotid endarterectomies and graduated internal dilatations were performed. In one case of occlusion that occurred after the dilatation procedure, an extracranial-to-intracranial bypass procedure was performed. There were no new neurologic complications after a mean 6.8 years of follow-up, irrespective of previous neurologic events and treatment. Three surgical procedures were repeated in these patients—one endarterectomy for asymptomatic carotid stenosis and two dilatation procedures in patients with general neurologic symptoms.[138] These results show that neither surgical nor conservative treatment influenced the rate of ischemic complications and that the course of the disease in untreated patients is rather benign.

Another study assessed the effectiveness of surgical interventions such as graduated internal dilatation and endarterectomy in 25 patients with internal carotid FMD. Transient ischemic attacks (including amaurosis fugax) were initially present in 68% of patients, and 92% of patients had severe internal carotid stenosis. There was one ischemic stroke in the perioperative period (5% morbidity). Of the 19 patients followed up for a mean 7.3 years, there were two recurrences of neurologic symptoms (10.5%).[131]

A direct comparison between the effectiveness of antiplatelet treatment and surgical dilatation procedures was conducted in a noncontrolled study[24] of 30 patients with carotid FMD who were retrospectively selected on the basis of the results of cerebral angiography. Sixty-three percent of patients presented with focal neurologic deficits. Antiplatelet treatment was started in 73% of patients, and the others underwent surgical dilatation procedures. There were no recurrences of neurologic symptoms in the surgically treated group. Recurrences were observed only in the conservatively treated group. The results of this study suggest that surgical dilatation procedures are superior for the prevention of recurrent cerebral ischemia in FMD.

The utility of surgical procedures in patients with multiple vessel involvement has also been assessed. Chiche and coworkers[54] reported on 70 patients with FMD of the carotid arteries, vertebral arteries, or both who underwent gradual intramural dilatation of the affected vessels. In 38.6% of cases, both carotid arteries and vertebral arteries were involved in the disease process. The positive history of antecedent ischemic stroke was established in 31.4% of cases, and 35.7% of the patients had a history of transient ischemic attack. Three strokes occurred in the perioperative period, one of which was fatal (4.2% morbidity and mortality rates). The patients were followed for a mean of 86.2 months. The actuarial survival rates at 5 and 10 years were 96.4% and 82.1%, respectively. The actuarial probabilities of stroke-free survival at 5 and 10 years were 94.2% and 88.6%, respectively.[54] In another study in which gradual intraluminal dilatation was performed in 79 cases of cervicocephalic FMD, the periprocedural morbidity (strokes and transient ischemic attacks) was 14%, and the stroke recurrence rate was 2.3%.[134]

Another method that can be used in the treatment of cervical FMD is stent grafting. There are some reports on the effectiveness and safety of angioplasty and stenting in patients with stenosis of one or both internal carotid arteries caused by dissection related to cervical FMD.[68,74,139] This technique is not free of complications, however, and strokes may occur during stent placement.[131] The precise data concerning the long-term effects of this treatment are lacking, and there have been no direct comparisons of stent implantation with surgical procedures in patients with cervical FMD. In the future, carotid stenting may become an interesting alternative to other surgical procedures used in internal carotid artery stenosis in patients with FMD.

Considering the lack of unambiguous data from large prospective studies as to the incidence of stroke and other outcomes as well as the effectiveness of different treatment strategies, no definitive recommendations on treatment in either asymptomatic or symptomatic patients with cervicocephalic FMD can be made. On the basis of available data, a conservative treatment is suggested.[140] Treatment is not recommended for patients who are asymptomatic, who have isolated bruit, or who have general nonfocal symptoms and in whom the lesions are discovered accidentally.

In patients with a history of focal neurologic deficits, the diagnosis and treatment should be focused on a plausible pathophysiologic mechanism presumed to be responsible for the symptoms. Other risk factors, such as atherosclerotic lesions, cardiogenic sources of emboli, and prothrombotic states, should be sought. When FMD is thought to be responsible for a thromboembolic phenomenon that caused focal neurologic symptoms, medical therapy is suggested (antiplatelets or anticoagulants). In case of hemodynamic compromise, direct surgical intervention or extracranial-to-intracranial bypass should be considered. In rare cases of septal FMD (e.g., carotid web), resection should be considered.

References

1. Leadbetter WF, Burkland CE: Hypertension in unilateral renal disease. J Urol 39:611, 1938.
2. Boyd CH, Lewis LG: Nephrectomy for arterial hypertension: Preliminary report. J Urol 39:627, 1938.
3. Wylie EJ, Wellington JS: Hypertension caused by fibromuscular hyperplasia of the renal arteries. Am J Surg 100:183, 1960.
4. Kincaid OW, Davis GD: Renal arteriography in hypertension. Proc Staff Meet Mayo Clin 36:689, 1961.
5. Perloff D, Sokolow M, Wylie EJ, et al: Hypertension secondary to renal artery occlusive disease. Circulation 24:1286, 1961.
6. Hunt JC, Harrison EG, Kincaid OW, et al: Idiopathic fibrous and fibromuscular stenoses of the renal arteries associated with hypertension. Proc Staff Meet Mayo Clin 37:181, 1962.
7. Palubinskas AJ, Perloff D, Wylie EJ, et al: Curable hypertension due to renal artery lesions. Radiol Clin 33:207, 1964.
8. Javid H: [Discussion]. Arch Surg 90:595, 1965.
9. Connett MC, Lansche JM: Fibromuscular hyperplasia of the internal carotid artery: Report of a case. Ann Surg 162:59, 1965.
10. Bergan JJ, McDonald JR: Recognition of cerebrovascular fibromuscular hyperplasia. Arch Surg 98:332, 1969.
11. Stanley JC, Gewertz BL, Bove EL, et al: Arterial fibrodysplasia: Histopathologic character and current etiologic concepts. Arch Surg 110:561, 1975.
12. Iosue A, Kier EL, Ostrow D: Fibromuscular dysplasia involving the intracranial vessels: Case report. J Neurosurg 37:749, 1972.
13. Frens DB, Petajan JH, Anderson R, Deblanc JH Jr: Fibromuscular dysplasia of the posterior cerebral artery: Report of a case and review of the literature. Stroke 5:161, 1974.
14. Rinaldi I, Harris WO Jr, Kopp JE, Legier J: Intracranial fibromuscular dysplasia: Report of two cases, one with autopsy verification. Stroke 7:511, 1976.
15. Garcia-Merino JA, Gutierrez JA, Lopez-Lozano JJ, et al: Double lumen dissecting aneurysms of the internal carotid artery in fibromuscular dysplasia: Case report. Stroke 14:815, 1983.
16. Hegedus K, Nemeth G: Fibromuscular dysplasia of the basilar artery: Case report with autopsy verification. Arch Neurol 41:440, 1984.

17. Heffelfinger MJ, Holley KE, Harrison EG, et al: Arterial fibromuscular dysplasia studied at autopsy. Am J Clin Pathol 54:274, 1970.

18. Andreoni KA, Weeks SM, Gerber DA, et al: Incidence of donor renal fibromuscular dysplasia: Does it justify routine angiography? Transplantation 73:1112, 2002.

19. Schievink WI, Bjornsson J: Fibromuscular dysplasia of the internal carotid artery: A clinicopathological study. Clin Neuropathol 15:2, 1996.

20. Harrington OB, Crosby VG, Nicholas L: Fibromuscular hyperplasia of the internal carotid artery. Ann Thorac Surg 9:516, 1970.

21. Momose KJ, New PF: Non-atheromatous stenosis and occlusion of the internal carotid artery and its main branches. Am J Roentgenol Radium Ther Nucl Med 118:550, 1973.

22. So EL, Toole JF, Dalal P, Moody DM: Cephalic fibromuscular dysplasia in 32 patients: Clinical findings and radiologic features. Arch Neurol 38:619, 1981.

23. Corrin LS, Sandok BA, Houser OW: Cerebral ischemic events in patients with carotid artery fibromuscular dysplasia. Arch Neurol 38:616, 1981.

24. Wesen CA, Elliott BM: Fibromuscular dysplasia of the carotid arteries. Am J Surg 151:448, 1986.

25. Chiras J, Bories J, Barth MO, et al: Cerebral angiography in ischemic strokes. Neuroradiology 27:521, 1985.

26. Mettinger KL: Fibromuscular dysplasia and the brain: Current concept of the disease. Stroke 13:53, 1982.

27. Kuchelmeister K, Schulz R, Bergmann M, et al: A probably familial saccular aneurysm of the anterior communicating artery in a neonate. Childs Nerv Syst 9:302, 1993.

28. Vles JS, Hendriks JJ, Lodder J, Janevski B: Multiple vertebro-basilar infarctions from fibromuscular dysplasia related dissecting aneurysm of the vertebral artery in a child. Neuropediatrics 21:104, 1990.

29. Nagaraja D, Verma A, Taly AB, et al: Cerebrovascular disease in children. Acta Neurol Scand 90:251, 1994.

30. Chiu NC, DeLong GR, Heinz ER: Intracranial fibromuscular dysplasia in a 5-year-old child. Pediatr Neurol 14:262, 1996.

31. Solder B, Streif W, Ellemunter H, et al: Fibromuscular dysplasia of the internal carotid artery in a child with alpha-1-antitrypsin deficiency. Dev Med Child Neurol 39:827, 1997.

32. Leventer RJ, Kornberg AJ, Coleman LT, et al: Stroke and fibromuscular dysplasia: Confirmation by renal magnetic resonance angiography. Pediatr Neurol 18:172, 1998.

33. Osseby G, Manceau E, Huet F, et al: 'Fou rire prodromique' as the heralding symptom of lenticular infarction, caused by dissection of the internal carotid artery in a 12-year-old boy. Eur J Paediatr Neurol 3:133, 1999.

34. DiFazio M, Hinds SR 2nd, Depper M, et al: Intracranial fibromuscular dysplasia in a six-year-old child: A rare cause of childhood stroke. J Child Neurol 15:559, 2000.

35. Puri V, Riggs G: Case report of fibromuscular dysplasia presenting as stroke in a 16-year-old boy. J Child Neurol 14:233, 1999.

36. Harrison EG Jr, McCormack LJ: Pathologic classification of renal arterial disease in renovascular hypertension. Mayo Clin Proc 46:161, 1971.

37. Stanley JC, Gewertz BL, Bove EL, et al: Arterial fibrodysplasia: Histopathologic character and current etiologic concepts. Arch Surg 110:561, 1975.

38. Morgenlander JC, Goldstein LB: Recurrent transient ischemic attacks and stroke in association with an internal carotid artery web. Stroke 22:94, 1991.

39. Watanabe S, Tanaka K, Nakayama T, et al: Fibromuscular dysplasia at the internal carotid origin: A case of carotid web. No Shinkei Geka 21:449, 1993.

40. Bragin MA, Cherkasov AP: Morphogenesis of fibromuscular dysplasia of the renal arteries (an ultrastructural study). Arkh Patol 41:46, 1979.

41. Luscher TF, Lie JT, Stanson AW, et al: Arterial fibromuscular dysplasia. Mayo Clin Proc 62:931, 1987.

42. Osborn AG, Anderson RE: Angiographic spectrum of cervical and intracranial fibromuscular dysplasia. Stroke 8:617, 1977.

43. Wirth FP, Miller WA, Russell AP: Atypical fibromuscular hyperplasia: Report of two cases. J Neurosurg 54:685, 1981.

44. Tan AK, Venketasubramanian N, Tan CB, et al: Ischaemic stroke from cerebral embolism in cephalic fibromuscular dysplasia. Ann Acad Med Singapore 24:891, 1995.

45. Kubis N, Von Langsdorff D, Petitjean C: Thrombotic carotid megabulb: Fibromuscular dysplasia, septae, and ischemic stroke. Neurology 52:883, 1999.

46. Zimmerman R, Leeds NE, Naidich TP: Carotid-cavernous fistula associated with intracranial fibromuscular dysplasia. Radiology 122:725, 1977.

47. Nakamura M, Rosahl SK, Vorkapic P: De novo formation of an aneurysm in a case of unusual intracranial fibromuscular dysplasia. Clin Neurol Neurosurg 102:259, 2000.

48. Goldstein M, Hanquinet P, Couvreur Y: A case of fibromuscular dysplasia in an unusual location. Acta Chir Belg 84:345, 1984.

48a. Wirth FP, Miller WA, Russell AP: Atypical fibrovascular hyperplasia: Report of the two cases. J Neurosurg 54:685, 1981.

49. Phadke RV, Taori KB, Divekar VK, et al: Fibromuscular dysplasia of common carotid artery: A case report. Australas Radiol 34:350, 1990.

50. Sandmann W, Schulte KM: Multivisceral fibromuscular dysplasia in childhood: Case report and review of the literature. Ann Vasc Surg 14:496, 2000.

51. So EL, Toole JF, Moody DM. et al: Cerebral embolism from septal fibromuscular dysplasia of the common carotid artery. Ann Neurol 6:75, 1979.

52. Cina C, Williamson C, Ameli FM: Fibromuscular dysplasia of the posterior auricular artery: An unusual aneurysmal lesion. J Cardiovasc Surg (Torino) 29:56, 1988.

53. Mettinger KL, Ericson K: Fibromuscular dysplasia and the brain: Observations on angiographic, clinical and genetic characteristics. Stroke 13:46, 1982.

54. Chiche L, Bahnini A, Koskas F, et al: Occlusive fibromuscular disease of arteries supplying the brain: Results of surgical treatment. Ann Vasc Surg 11:496, 1997.

55. Abdul-Rahman AM, Abu-Salih, Brun A, et al: Fibromuscular dysplasia of the cervico-cephalic arteries. Surg Neurol 9:217, 1978.

56. Bellot J, Gherardi R, Poirier J, et al: Fibromuscular dysplasia of cervico-cephalic arteries with multiple dissections and a carotid-cavernous fistula: A pathological study. Stroke 16:255, 1985.

57. Belen D, Bolay H, Firat M, et al: Unusual appearance of intracranial fibromuscular dysplasia: A case report. Angiology 47:627, 1996.

58. Slagsvold JE, Bergsholm P, Larsen JL: Fibromuscular dysplasia of intracranial arteries in a patient with multiple enchondromas (Ollier disease). Neurology 27:1168, 1977.

59. Mettinger KL, Ericson K: Fibromuscular dysplasia and the brain: Observations on angiographic, clinical and genetic characteristics. Stroke 13:46, 1982.

60. Feldmeyer JJ, Merendaz C, Regli F: Symptomatic stenoses of the middle cerebral artery. Rev Neurol 139:725, 1983.

61. Tripathi M, Santosh V, Nagaraj D, et al: Stroke in a young man with fibromuscular dysplasia of the cranial vessels with anticardiolipin antibodies: A case report. Neurol Sci 22:31, 2001.

62. Nomura S, Yamashita K, Kato S, et al: Childhood subarachnoid hemorrhage associated with fibromuscular dysplasia. Childs Nerv Syst 17:419, 2001.

63. Demirkaya S, Topcuoglu MA, Vural O: Fibromuscular dysplasia of the basilar artery: A case presenting with vertebrobasilar TIAs. Eur J Neurol 8:89, 2001.

64. Pilz P, Hartjes HJ: Fibromuscular dysplasia and multiple dissecting aneurysms of intracranial arteries: A further cause of moyamoya syndrome. Stroke 7:393, 1976.

65. Ashleigh RJ, Weller JM, Leggate JR: Fibromuscular hyperplasia of the internal carotid artery: A further cause of the 'moyamoya' collateral circulation. Br J Neurosurg 6:269, 1992.

66. Danza R, Baldizan J, Navarro T: Surgery of carotid kinking and fibromuscular dysplasia. J Cardiovasc Surg 24:628, 1983.

67. Schievink WI, Meyer FB, Parisi JE, et al: Fibromuscular dysplasia of the internal carotid artery associated with alpha1-antitrypsin deficiency. Neurosurgery 43:229, 1998.

68. Finsterer J, Strassegger J, Haymerle A, et al: Bilateral stenting of symptomatic and asymptomatic internal carotid artery stenosis due to fibromuscular dysplasia. J Neurol Neurosurg Psychiatry 69:683, 2000.

69. Brown OL, Armitage JL: Spontaneous dissecting aneurysms of the cervical internal carotid artery: Two case reports and a survey of the literature. Am J Roentgenol Radium Ther Nucl Med 118:648, 1973.

70. Ehrenfeld WK, Wylie EJ: Spontaneous dissection of the internal carotid artery. Arch Surg 111:1294, 1976.

71. Grotta JC. Ward RE, Flynn TC, Cullen ML: Spontaneous internal carotid artery dissection associated with fibromuscular dysplasia. J Cardiovasc Surg 23:512, 1982.

72. d'Anglejan Chatillon J, Ribeiro V, Mas JL, et al: Dissection of the extracranial internal carotid artery: 62 cases. Presse Med 19:661, 1990.

73. Lannuzel A, Moulin T, Amsallem D, et al: Vertebral-artery dissection following a judo session: A case report. Neuropediatrics 25:106, 1994.

74. Manninen HI, Koivisto T, Saari T, et al: Dissecting aneurysms of all four cervicocranial arteries in fibromuscular dysplasia: Treatment with self-expanding endovascular stents, coil embolization, and surgical ligation. Am J Neuroradiol 18:1216, 1997.

75. Eachempati SR, Sebastian MW, Reed RL 2nd: Posttraumatic bilateral carotid artery and right vertebral artery dissections in a patient with fibromuscular dysplasia: Case report and review of the literature. J Trauma 44:406, 1998.

76. Schievink WI, Puumala MR, Meyer FB, et al: Giant intracranial aneurysm and fibromuscular dysplasia in an adolescent with alpha 1-antitrypsin deficiency. J Neurosurg 85:503, 1996.

77. Hatayama K, Karasawa H, Naito H, et al: Anterior cerebral artery dissecting aneurysm associated with fibromuscular dysplasia (FMD): A case report. No Shinkei Geka 29:451, 2001.

78. Kalyan-Raman UP, Kowalski RV, Lee RH, et al: Dissecting aneurysm of superior cerebellar artery: Its association with fibromuscular dysplasia. Arch Neurol 40:120, 1983.

79. Bergentz SE, Ericsson BF, Linell F, et al: Carotid fibromuscular dysplasia and paresis of lower cranial nerves (Collect-Sicard syndrome): Case report. J Neurosurg 56:850, 1982.

80. Zimmerman R, Leeds NE, Naidich TP: Carotid-cavernous fistula associated with intracranial fibromuscular dysplasia. Radiology 122:725, 1977.

81. Miyauchi M, Shionoya S: Aneurysm of the extracranial internal carotid artery caused by fibromuscular dysplasia. Eur J Vasc Surg 5:587, 1991.

82. Faggioli GL, Freyrie A, Stella A, et al: Extracranial internal carotid artery aneurysms: Results of a surgical series with long-term follow-up. J Vasc Surg 23:587, 1996.

83. Rhee RY, Gloviczki P, Cherry KJ Jr, et al: Two unusual variants of internal carotid artery aneurysms due to fibromuscular dysplasia. Ann Vasc Surg 10:481, 1996.

84. Maiuri F, Gallicchio B, Gangemi M, et al: Fibromuscular dysplasia of the carotid arteries: Clinical and radiological considerations. Clin Neurol Neurosurg 90:57, 1988.

85. Cloft HJ, Kallmes DF, Kallmes MH, et al: Prevalence of cerebral aneurysms in patients with fibromuscular dysplasia: A reassessment. J Neurosurg 88:436, 1998.

86. Kaufman HH, Lind TA, Mullan S: Spontaneous carotid-cavernous fistula with fibromuscular dysplasia. Acta Neurochirurg 40:123, 1978.

87. Canova A, Esposito S, Patricolo A, et al: Spontaneous obliteration of a carotid-cavernous fistula associated with fibromuscular dysplasia of the internal carotid artery. J Neurosurg Sci 31:37, 1987

88. Hirai T, Korogi Y, Goto K, et al: Carotid-cavernous sinus fistula and aneurysmal rupture associated with fibromuscular dysplasia: A case report. Acta Radiol 37:49, 1996.

89. Reddy SV, Karnes WE, Earnest F 4th, et al: Spontaneous extracranial vertebral arteriovenous fistula with fibromuscular dysplasia: Case report. J Neurosurg 54:399, 1981.

90. Bahar S, Chiras J, Carpena JP, et al: Spontaneous vertebro-vertebral arterio-venous fistula associated with fibro-muscular dysplasia. Report of two cases. Neuroradiology 26:45, 1984.

91. Halbach VV, Higashida RT, Hieshima GB: Treatment of vertebral arteriovenous fistulas. AJR Am J Roentgenol 150:405, 1988.

92. Hieshima GB, Cahan LD, Mehringer CM, et al: Spontaneous arteriovenous fistulas of cerebral vessels in association with fibromuscular dysplasia. Neurosurgery 18:454, 1986.

93. Rushton AR: The genetics of fibromuscular dysplasia. Arch Intern Med 140:233, 1980.

94. Pannier-Moreau I, Grimbert P, Fiquet-Kempf B, et al: Possible familial origin of multifocal renal artery fibromuscular dysplasia. J Hypertens 15:1797, 1997.

95. Grange DK, Balfour IC, Chen SC, et al: Familial syndrome of progressive arterial occlusive disease consistent with fibromuscular dysplasia, hypertension, congenital cardiac defects, bone fragility, brachysyndactyly, and learning disabilities. Am J Med Genet 75:469, 1998.

96. Russo LS Jr: Fibromuscular hyperplasia of the extracranial arteries: Report of a case associated with intracranial aneurysm and skeletal deformities and a brief review of the literature. Mt Sinai J Med 40:60, 1973.

97. Sanchez Torres G, Contreras R: Fibromuscular dysplasia: A genetic entity related to Ehlers-Danlos syndrome. Arch Inst Cardiol Mex 44:571, 1974.

98. Schievink WI, Bjornsson J, Piepgras DG: Coexistence of fibromuscular dysplasia and cystic medial necrosis in a patient with Marfan's syndrome and bilateral carotid artery dissections. Stroke 25:2492, 1994.

99. Grimbert P, Fiquer-Kempf B, Coudol P, et al: Genetic study of renal artery fibromuscular dysplasia. Arch Mal Coeur Vaiss 91:1069, 1998.

100. Szpak GM, Kuczynska-Zardzewialy A, Popow J: Brain vascular changes in the case of primary antiphospholipid syndrome. Folia Neuropathol 34:92, 1996.

101. Tripathi M, Santosh V, Nagaraj D, et al: Stroke in a young man with fibromuscular dysplasia of the cranial vessels with anticardiolipin antibodies: A case report. Neurol Sci 22:31, 2001.

102. Schievink WI, Bjornsson J, Parisi JE, et al: Arterial fibromuscular dysplasia associated with severe alpha 1-antitrypsin deficiency. Mayo Clin Proc 69:1040, 1994.

103. Bofinger A, Hawley C, Fisher P, et al: Alpha-1-antitrypsin phenotypes in patients with renal arterial fibromuscular dysplasia. J Hum Hypertens 14:91, 2000.

104. Solder B, Streif W, Ellemunter H, et al: Fibromuscular dysplasia of the internal carotid artery in a child with alpha-1-antitrypsin deficiency. Dev Med Child Neurol 39:827, 1997.

105. Bofinger A, Hawley C, Fisher P, et al: Polymorphisms of the renin-angiotensin system in patients with multifocal renal arterial fibromuscular dysplasia. J Hum Hypertens 15:185, 2001.

106. Fievez ML: Fibromuscular dysplasia of arteries: A spastic phenomenon? Med Hypotheses 13:341, 1984.

107. Slavin RE, Saeki K, Bhagavan B, et al: Segmental arterial mediolysis: A precursor to fibromuscular dysplasia? Mod Pathol 8:287, 1995.

108. Garnier P, Michel D, Barral FG, et al: Roles of arterial dysplasia, chronic ergotism and other factors in a case of multiple spontaneous arterial dissections. Rev Med Interne 21:701, 2000.

109. Sottiurai VS, Fry WJ, Stanley JC: Ultrastructure of medial smooth muscle and myofibroblasts in human arterial dysplasia. Arch Surg 113:1280, 1978.

110. Nakata Y: An experimental study on the vascular lesions caused by obstruction of the vasa vasorum. Jpn Circ J 31:275, 1967

111. Sang CN, Whelton PK, Hamper UM, et al: Etiologic factors in renovascular fibromuscular dysplasia: A case-control study. Hypertension 14:472, 1989.

112. Julian LM: The occurrence of fibromuscular dysplasia in the arteries of domestic turkeys. Am J Pathol 101:415, 1980.

113. Ross R, Klebanoff SJ: Fine structural changes in uterine smooth muscle and fibroblasts in response to estrogen. J Cell Biol 32:155, 1967.

114. Ross R, Klebanoff SJ: The smooth muscle cell. I: In vivo synthesis of connective tissue proteins. J Cell Biol 50:159, 1971.

115. Bradley JR, Reynolds J, Williams PF, et al: Encephalopathy in renovascular hypertension associated with the use of oral contraceptives. Postgrad Med J 62:1031, 1986.

116. Mas JL, Bousser MG, Hasboun D, et al: Extracranial vertebral artery dissections: A review of 13 cases. Stroke 18:1037, 1987.

117. Fleisher GR, Buck BE, Cornfeld D: Primary intimal fibroplasia in a child with Down's syndrome. Am J Dis Child 132:700, 1978.

118. Lancman M, Mesropian H, Serra P, et al: Turner's syndrome, fibromuscular dysplasia, and stroke. Stroke 22:269, 1991.

119. Palmaz JC, Hunter G, Carson SN, et al: Postoperative carotid restenosis due to neointimal fibromuscular hyperplasia: Clinical, angiographic, and pathological findings. Radiology 148:699, 1983.

120. Heiserman JE, Drayer BP, Fram EK, et al: MR angiography of cervical fibromuscular dysplasia. Am J Neuroradiol 13:1454, 1992.

121. Phan T, Huston J, Matthew A, et al: Contrast-enhanced magnetic resonance angiography of the cervical vessels: Experience with 422 patients. Stroke 32:2282, 2001.

122. Johnston DC, Eastwood JD, Nguyen T, et al: Contrast-enhanced magnetic resonance angiography of carotid arteries: Utility in routine clinical practice. Stroke 33:2834, 2002.

123. Schlagenhauff RE, Khatri A: Fibromuscular dysplasia of internal carotid arteries: With Doppler ultrasonic studies. N Y State J Med 83:234, 1983.

124. Edell SL, Huang P: Sonographic demonstration of fibromuscular hyperplasia of the cervical internal carotid artery. Stroke 12:518, 1981.

125. Winter R, Ringleb P, Hacke W: Color-coded duplex ultrasound imaging of intimal fibromuscular dysplasia of the carotid artery. Nervenarzt 69:905, 1998.

126. Wong KS, Li H, Chan YL, et al: Use of transcranial Doppler ultrasound to predict outcome in patients with intracranial large-artery occlusive disease. Stroke 31:2641, 2000.

127. El-Saden SM, Grant EG, Hathout GM, et al: Imaging of the internal carotid artery: The dilemma of total versus near total occlusion. Radiology 221:301, 2001.

128. Kishore PRS, Lin JP, Kricheff H: Fibromuscular hyperplasia and stationary waves of the internal carotid artery. Acta Radiol 11:619, 1971.

129. Appleberg M: Graduated internal dilatation in the treatment of fibromuscular dysplasia of the internal carotid artery. S Afr Med J 51:244, 1977.

130. Starr DS, Lawrie GM, Morris GC: Fibromuscular disease of carotid arteries: Long term results of graduated internal dilatation. Stroke 12:196, 1981.

131. Balaji MR, DeWeese JA: Fibromuscular dysplasia of the internal carotid artery: Its occurrence with acute stroke and its surgical reversal. Arch Surg 115:984, 1980.

132. Rainer WG, Cramer GG, Newby JP, et al: Fibromuscular hyperplasia of the carotid artery causing positional cerebral ischemia. Ann Surg 167:444, 1968.

133. Wells RP, Smith RR: Fibromuscular dysplasia of the internal carotid artery: A long term follow-up. Neurosurgery 10:39, 1982.

134. Effeney DJ, Ehrenfeld WK, Stoney RJ: Why operate on carotid fibromuscular dysplasia? Arch Surg 115:1261, 1980.

135. Havelius U, Hindfelt B, Brismar J, et al: Carotid fibromuscular dysplasia and paresis of lower cranial nerves (Collect-Sicard syndrome): Case report. J Neurosurg 56:850, 1982.

136. Gruber B, Hemmati M: Fibromuscular dysplasia of the vertebral artery: An unusual cause of pulsatile tinnitus. Otolaryngol Head Neck Surg 105:113, 1991.

137. Dufour JJ, Lavigne F, Plante R, et al: Pulsatile tinnitus and fibromuscular dysplasia of the internal carotid. J Otolaryngol 14:293, 1985.

138. Stewart MT, Moritz MW, Smith RB, et al: The natural history of carotid fibromuscular dysplasia. J Vasc Surg 3:305, 1986.

139. DeOcampo J, Brillman J, Levy DI: Stenting: A new approach to carotid dissection. J Neuroimaging 7:187, 1997.

140. Sandok BA: Fibromuscular dysplasia of the cephalic arterial system. In Toole JF (ed): Handbook of Clinical Neurology, vol 11. Amsterdam, New York, Elsevier Science, 1989, p 283.

Specific Medical Diseases and Stroke

Chapter Twenty-Seven

Migraine and Stroke

H. C. Diener, K. M. A. Welch, and J. P. Mohr

Migraine is an episodic headache that is unilateral or bilateral in location, pulsating in quality, moderate to severe in intensity, and exacerbated by physical activity. Associated symptoms include nausea or vomiting, photophobia, and phonophobia. The prevalence of migraine is 12% to 18% in females and 6% to 8% in males.[1-4] The prevalence of migraine with aura (which includes familial hemiplegic migraine) is lower, around 4%.[5] Various forms of migraine are recognized; they are generally classified according to the transient, though sometimes persistent, neurologic deficits that may precede, accompany, or outlast the headache phase. The most accepted current classification was put forward in 1988 by the International Headache Society (IHS) (Table 27.1).[6] The new headache classification of the IHS is to be published in 2003.

A number of these clinical syndromes may mimic transient ischemic attack (TIA) or ischemic stroke, and a number may induce stroke or are associated with a greater risk of stroke. They include migraine with aura of different types, retinal or ocular migraine, ophthalmoplegic migraine, familial hemiplegic migraine, and basilar artery migraine. Each may be transient, prolonged, or persistent.[7] When the aura symptoms of a migraine attack persist for more than 24 hours, *migraine-induced stroke* is suspected. The clinical features of migraine that often mimic stroke are described later.

CLINICAL FEATURES

The most prevalent migraine syndromes are (1) typical headache without aura of neurologic deficit and (2) headache associated with aura of neurologic deficit.

Visual disturbances account for well over half the transient neurologic manifestations. Most commonly, these disturbances consist of "positive" phenomena, such as complex geometric patterns, including shapes like stars, spark photopsia, and, because of the wedge-shaped edges typical of French military forts built by Vauban, shapes that have been called Vauban fortification spectra. These positive phenomena may leave in their wake "negative" phenomena, such as increasing scotoma or slowly developing hemianopia. The symptoms are characteristically slow but steady in onset and slow in progression, although occasionally, the onset is more abrupt and may be confused with amaurosis fugax.[7] Visual symptoms sometimes progress to visual distortion or misperception, such as micropsia or dysmetropsia. The patterns of symptoms indicate the spread of neurologic dysfunction from the occipital cortex into the contiguous regions of the temporal or parietal lobes.[9-11] It is critical, differentiating migraine from stroke, to establish that the neurologic deficit in the aura of migraine actually crosses arterial territories, even if only to a slight extent.

The second most common symptoms are somatosensory, with a characteristic distribution to the hand and lower face (cheio-oral). Less frequently, the symptoms include aphasia, dysarthria, hemiparesis, and clumsiness of one limb. Characteristically, symptoms of the aura progress in a slow, marchlike progression.

CLASSIFICATION

The major problem that faces the diagnostician is a lack of consistency in the definition of migraine-related stroke in the studies conducted to date. Strict definition of terms is essential for future comprehensive epidemiologic or population-based studies. The following major questions arise:

- Does stroke occur in the course of the migraine attack, causing true migraine-induced cerebral infarction?
- Does migraine cause stroke because other risk factors for stroke are present to interact with the migraine-induced pathogenesis?
- Can stroke manifest as a migraine syndrome, that is, as symptomatic migraine?

Some developments in classification serve to clarify the association between migraine and stroke. The IHS classification has led to improved definitions of migraine and migraine-induced stroke in a more specific and comprehensive manner.[6] New techniques of brain imaging have provided insights into the relationship of the disorder through improved diagnosis.

Migrainous cerebral infarction is described in the IHS classification: (1) patient has previously fulfilled criteria for migraine with neurologic aura; (2) the present attack is typical of previous attacks, but neurologic deficits are not completely reversible within 7 days and/or neuroimaging demonstrates ischemic infarction in the relevant area; (3)

Table 27.1   Classification of Migraine Subtypes

International Headache Society Terminology (Previously Used Terms)	Main Features
Migraine without aura (common migraine)	Headache without focal neurologic symptoms
Migraine with aura	Headache with attacks of neurologic symptoms localizable to cerebral cortex or brainstem, developing gradually over 5–20 minutes and lasting <1 hour
Migraine with typical aura (ophthalmic, hemiparesthetic, hemiparetic, hemiplegic, or aphasic migraine, migraine accompaignée)	Aura consisting of homonymous visual disturbances, hemisensory symptoms, hemiparesis or dysphasia, or combinations thereof
Migraine with prolonged aura (complicated migraine, hemiplegic migraine)	Aura symptoms lasting >1 hour and ±7 days with normal brain imaging
Familial hemiplegic migraine	At least one first-degree relative has identical attacks
Basilar migraine (basilar migraine, Bickerstaff's migraine, syncopal migraine)	Aura symptoms originate from brainstem or both occipital lobes
Migraine aura without headache (migraine equivalents, acephelalgic migraine)	Aura unaccompanied by headache; when the onset is after 40 years, distinction from transient ischemic attacks may be difficult
Migraine with acute-onset aura	Aura developing fully in <5 minutes
Ophthalmoplegic migraine	Repeated attacks of headache associated with paresis of one or more ocular cranial nerves
Retinal migraine	Repeated attacks of monocular scotomata or blindness lasting <1 hour with headache
Childhood periodic syndromes that may be precursors to or associated with migraine	Poorly defined disorders of childhood, including benign paroxysmal vertigo and alternating hemiplegia
	Complications of migraine
	Headache lasting >72 hours with or without treatment and headache-free interval <4 hours
Status migrainosus	
Migrainous infarction (complicated migraine)	Aura symptoms not fully reversible lasting >7 days, and/or associated infarct on brain imaging

From the Headache Classification Committee of the International Headache Society: Classification and diagnostic criteria for headache disorders, cranial neuralgias and facial pain. Cephalalgia 8:1, 1988.

other causes of infarction have been ruled out by appropriate investigations. Table 27.1 presents an extended classification of stroke in association with migraine or migraine-related stroke. Included in this classification is migrainous infarction, for which the more precise term is *migraine-induced stroke*.

Migraine-Induced Stroke

The following criteria define *migraine-induced stroke*: (1) the neurologic deficit must exactly mimic the aura symptoms of previous attacks, (2) the stroke must occur during the course of a typical migraine attack, and (3) all other causes of stroke must have been excluded, although stroke risk factors may be present.

The major problem with this definition is that the IHS classification does not permit the diagnosis of migraine-induced stroke in patients who have migraine without aura (see definition). Perhaps, however, migraine without aura begins in "silent" brain areas and has the same pathogenesis as migraine with aura. This possibility is indicated by the blood flow measurements reported by Woods and colleagues,[11] who found a decrease in cerebral blood flow of 30% to 40% in the occipital lobe in a woman during an episode of migraine without aura. Migraine-induced stroke might occur in patients without other vascular risk factors.

Coexisting Stroke and Migraine

For the diagnosis of *coexisting stroke and migraine*, a clearly defined clinical stroke syndrome must occur remotely in time from a typical attack of migraine.

Stroke in the young is rare, and migraine is common. Clearly, the two conditions can coexist without migraine's being a contributory factor to stroke. When the two conditions coexist in the young, the true pathogenesis of stroke may be difficult to elucidate. A comorbidity of stroke risk in migraine sufferers seems apparent from the case-controlled series reviewed later in this chapter, in which none of the strokes was induced by the migraine attack. This finding increases the clinical significance of coincident stroke and should serve to raise clinical consciousness to the need for stroke risk factor awareness in all migraine sufferers.

Stroke with Clinical Features of Migraine

In *stroke with clinical features of migraine*, a structural lesion unrelated to migraine pathogenesis manifests clinical features typical of migraine.

In some cases, established structural lesions of the central nervous system (CNS) or cerebral vessels episodically cause symptoms typical of migraine with neurologic aura. Such cases should be termed *symptomatic migraine*.[12]

Cerebral arteriovenous malformations frequently masquerade as migraine with aura.[13] Migraine attacks associated with cerebral autosomal dominant arteriopathy with subcortical infarcts and leukoencephalopathy (CADASIL) may also be symptomatic of the membrane dysfunction associated with this disorder.[14,15] Subarachnoidal hemorrhage, venous-sinus thrombosis, and viral meningitis can mimic migraine attacks with or without aura in patients who have either migraine or a family history of migraine.

Stroke due to acute and progressing structural disease is accompanied by headache and a constellation of progressive neurologic signs and symptoms indistinguishable from those of migraine. This might best be termed a *migraine mimic*.

The diagnostic discrimination of a migraine mimic can be most difficult to define in patients with established migraine. Many of the cases described in the literature on the conceptual evolution of migraine-related stroke were likely migraine mimics, the diagnosis being hampered by limitations in investigative tools and uncertainty in the knowledge of migraine pathogenesis.

The issue of spontaneous carotid artery dissection is relevant, because patients with migraine are at increased risk for dissection. The occurrence of dissection as a typical migraine mimic has been reported.[16] Although the mechanism of pain production is not clearly understood, the occurrence of headache is an expected finding, present in 60% of patients,[17] and probably greater in vertebral artery dissection, along with a variable incidence of ischemic complications, a combination that may mimic migraine with aura.

Fisher[18] analyzed 21 selected cases of angiographically documented cervical carotid artery dissection, observing that almost all patients (19 of 21) had ipsilateral pain in one or more regions of the head, including forehead, orbit, temple, retro-orbit, side of head, and the frontal region. In addition, 12 patients had neck pain, usually in the upper neck and localized to a region including the mastoid, upper carotid, behind or below the angle of the jaw, and along the sternocleidomastoid muscle. The pain was usually severe, often sudden in onset, described equally as steady or throbbing, and occasionally accompanied by alterations in ipsilateral scalp sensation. The duration ranged from several hours to 2 years, with most cases lasting no longer than 3 to 4 weeks. About three fourths of Fisher's patients experienced ischemic complications, and in half, the headache preceded the ischemic event by a few hours to 4 days. Other common diagnostic findings were Horner's syndrome, subjective bruit, dysgeusia, and visual scintillations.

Uncertain Classification

Many migraine-related strokes cannot be categorized with certainty, because of complexity or multiple factors.

EPIDEMIOLOGY

Welch and Bousser[19] reviewed mostly uncontrolled hospital-based studies conducted before 1989 of patients younger than 50 years with a diagnosis of stroke. The review showed that between 1% and 17% of the strokes were attributed to migraine; in two thirds of these cases, the diagnosis of migraine was made in 1% to 8% of

patients; in one third of cases, the diagnosis was made in 11% to 17%.[20] A compilation of studies up to 1999 revealed a prevalence of 4% attributed to migraine in 448 total cases of stroke, 31% of which had an unknown cause. Stroke was more common in patients with migraine with aura than in those who had migraine without aura.[21,22] Most ischemic strokes occur in the territory of the posterior cerebral arteries.

Another controlled study of migraine with aura reported that 91% of patients who had strokes during an attack had no arterial lesions, as opposed to 9% of patients who had migraine with aura, who suffered stroke remote from a migraine attack, and 18% of patients with stroke who did not have a history of migraine.[23] A later study showed that elderly patients with migraine are not at increased risk for development of ischemic stroke.[24] In some instances, however, stroke risk factors increased stroke risk in migraine with aura.

The overall incidence of "migrainous infarction" has been estimated at 3.36 per 100,000 population per year (95% confidence interval (CI), 0.87 to 4.8); in the absence of other stroke risk factors, the incidence becomes 1.44 per 100,000 population per year (95% CI, 0.00 to 3.07).[25] This rate is similar to that reported later in subjects younger than 50 years,[26] in whom migrainous infarction accounted for 25% of cerebral infarcts. To place these data in context, the overall incidence of ischemic stroke in persons younger than 50 years ranges from 3 per 100,000 to 22.8 per 100,000.[27]

A large-scale prospective epidemiologic study of men and women in the United States showed that migraine as well as severe nonspecific headache was associated with a significantly higher risk of stroke.[28] The study involved more than 14,000 participants who were monitored for 10 years. At baseline, stroke rates in patients with migraine were 6.8% in men and 3.7% in women, compared with 4.5% and 2.6%, respectively, in patients without migraine. After the analysis was controlled for established stroke risk factors, the risk of stroke associated with migraine increased significantly. Migraine was associated with a risk ratio of 1.5.

A case-control study[29] found no overall association between migraine and ischemic stroke, but among women younger than 45 years, migraine and stroke were significantly associated; there was approximately a four-fold higher risk, which was even higher in women who smoked. When this study was extended to a larger population, the results were confirmed and strengthened.[29] The risk of stroke was three times that of controls for patients who had migraine without aura, and six times that of controls for patients who had migraine with aura. Further, young women with migraine who smoked increased their stroke risk to approximately 10 times that of controls, a value more than three times greater than the risk for young women without migraine who smoked.

In another case-control study of 308 patients with either TIAs or stroke, Carolei and associates[30] found that a history of migraine was more frequent in these patients than in controls (14.9% versus 9.1%). Migraine was the only significant risk factor (odds ratio [OR] 3.7) in women younger than 35 years. The risk figures appear startlingly high in both of these studies, but one must remember that the absolute risk of stroke for this patient population translates to around 19 per 100,000 per year, which is a low rate.

Chang and colleagues[31] reported the results of a later hospital-based case-control study involving five European centers, in which 291 women 20 to 40 years of age who had ischemic, hemorrhagic, or unclassified arterial stroke were compared with 736 age- and hospital-matched controls. Adjusted odds ratios associated with a personal history of migraine were 1.78 (95% CI, 1.14–2.77) for all strokes, 3.54 (95% CI, 1.30–9.61) for ischemic strokes, and 1.10 (95% CI, 0.63–1.94) for hemorrhagic strokes. Odds ratios for ischemic stroke were similar to those for migraine with aura (2.97; 95% CI, 1.26–11.5) and migraine without aura (2.97; 95% CI, 0.66–13.5). A family history of migraine irrespective of personal history was also associated with higher odds ratios, not only for ischemic stroke but also for hemorrhagic stroke. Use of oral contraceptives or a history of high blood pressure or smoking had greater than multiplicative effects on the odds ratios for ischemic stroke associated with migraine alone, although only the smoking effect was statistically significant. A change in the frequency or type of migraine associated with oral contraceptive use did not predict subsequent stroke. Between 20% and 40% of strokes may have been induced by a migraine attack. (This study should be interpreted with particular caution on the basis of the methods, working criteria for the classification, and questionnaire used. Concerns are related to (1) the higher numbers of patients who had migraine with aura compared with those who had migraine without aura and (2) the difficulty in diagnosing migraine by questionnaire in family members. Also, clinical experience would not support the high incidence of true migraine-induced stroke found in the study.)

The Physician's Health Study comprised 22,071 male physicians.[32,33] Physicians reporting migraine (n = 1479) had significantly higher risks of subsequent total stroke and ischemic stroke than those not reporting migraine. After adjustments were made for age, study medication (aspirin, beta carotene), and a number of cardiovascular risk factors, the relative risks were 1.84 (95% CI, 1.06–3.20) for total stroke and 2.00 for ischemic stroke (95% CI, 1.10–3.64). No associations were seen between ordinary nonmigraine headache and subsequent stroke.

Stroke Risk, Migraine, and Oral Contraceptive Use

Oral contraceptives are recognized to raise stroke risk in migraine sufferers and may cause coexisting stroke and migraine. In some instances, however, stroke occurs during the migraine attack, and the medication may have increased the risk of coagulopathy but may not have induced stroke in the absence of the migrainous process. The Cooperative Group for the Study of Stroke in Young Women used a case-control method to evaluate the risk of cerebrovascular disease in users of oral contraceptives.[34] The risk of cerebral thrombosis among women who used oral contraceptives was 9.5 times greater than that among those who did not. The role of migraine was assessed in both users and nonusers of contraceptives. Among migraineurs not exposed to birth control pills, the risk of stroke was equivocal, depending on the control group used

for comparison. The use of oral contraceptives in combination with migraine, however, increased the relative risk for thrombotic stroke from 2.0 to 5.9.

A study from Denmark found a multiplicative relationship between the risk of oral contraceptives and migraine.[35] A smaller French case-control study of women younger than 45 years found an increased ischemic stroke risk among women who had migraine without aura (OR 3.0; 95% CI, 1.5–5.8). The risk was even greater in women suffering from migraine with aura (OR 6.2; 95% CI, 2.1–18.0).[29] There was a dose-effect relationship between risk of stroke and the dose of estrogen: the odds ratio was 4.8 for pills containing 50 μg of estrogen, 2.7 for 30 to 40 μg, 1.7 for 20 μg, and 1 μg for progestogen. In none of these cases was the stroke induced by the migraine attack. Use of oral contraceptives in the absence of migraine resulted in an OR of 3.5. The combination of oral contraceptive use and migraine resulted in an OR of 13.9 (95% CI, 5.5–35.1).

Taking all these studies together, one can conclude that the absolute number of strokes in patients with migraine who are younger than 50 years is small (10–20 per 100,000).[36,37] Patients with migraine have an increased stroke risk, although the increase is small if one considers it in absolute numbers. The incidence of true migraine-induced strokes is low. Additional risk factors for stroke in patients with migraine are migraine with aura, use of oral contraceptives, and the presence of other vascular risk factors. Migraine leads to an increased risk only of ischemic stroke, not of cerebral hemorrhage.

NEUROIMAGING

In a radiologic series of selected patients who had migraine with or without focal neurologic deficits, the prevalence of computed tomography (CT) abnormalities ranged from 34% to 71%. Cala and Mastaglia[38] reported a large series, examining 94 patients with a history of "recurrent migrainous headaches," 6 of whom showed evidence of cerebral infarction. Of these 6 patients, 4 had fixed visual field defects with mesial occipital low densities. Cerebral edema, particularly in the periventricular white matter, was evident in another 6 patients. Of the 49 patients with migraine studied, 21 had evidence of low attenuation in the white matter, most extensive in the hemisphere on the side of the headache and contralateral to the sensory aura or signs.

Hungerford and associates[39] studied 53 patients who had "exceptionally severe" migraine or serious clinical complications, including hemiplegia. The abnormality most commonly encountered on CT scanning was cerebral atrophy, seen in 14 patients, 8 of whom showed focal changes. Well-defined hemispheric low-density lesions indicating infarction were seen in 6 patients. Of the 13 patients who had permanent neurologic deficits, 11 had CT abnormalities.

Rascol and colleagues[40] reported 10 patients with a mean age of 33 years and CT-confirmed cerebral infarction occurring in the course of a migrainous attack. These investigators required that the following three conditions be met before a diagnosis of complicated migraine or migrainous cerebral infarction was made: (1) there must be a previous history of migraine attacks conforming to the Ad Hoc Committee's definition; (2) there must be a close chronologic relationship between the migraine attack and the prolonged or persisting neurologic disorder; and (3) other vascular diseases or predisposing disorders must be excluded, such as vascular malformation, atherosclerotic risk factors (e.g., hypertension, diabetes, hyperlipidemia), atherosclerotic lesions on cerebral angiography, exposure to oral contraceptives, signs of ergotism, and infectious, inflammatory, hematologic, or immunologic diseases that might be associated with cerebral thrombosis. Of the 10 patients in this study, 6 had syndromes referable to the middle cerebral artery, and the other 4 had hemianopic defects due to posterior cerebral artery territory infarctions. Arteriography, performed in each patient at some point between 2 days and 6 months from stroke onset, gave an abnormal result in 9 patients, showing internal carotid artery occlusion in 1, middle or posterior cerebral artery stem occlusion in 4, and branch occlusions in the remaining 4.

Magnetic Resonance Imaging

The diagnosis of migraine-induced stroke has been greatly enhanced by the use of magnetic resonance imaging (MRI). From the research viewpoint, great interest was generated by observations on MRI of increased white matter lesions in approximately 30% of routinely studied patients with migraine compared with 0% of healthy controls.[41] Lesions were found in the centrum semiovale and frontal white matter, in some cases extending to deeper structures in the region of the basal ganglia. In some studies, such findings were more prevalent in patients with migraine subtypes associated with neurologic aura.[42] Not all case series found a greater incidence of such lesions in patients with migraine than in controls, however. DeBenedittis and colleagues[43] found a higher incidence of white matter lesions in patients with migraine and in patients with tension-type headache. The mechanisms of these changes remain to be determined. If relevant, they may represent small foci of ischemic infarction of obscure origin, or gliosis.

Positron Emission Tomography

Bousser and associates[44] provided confirmatory and novel evidence for an ischemic process using positron emission tomography (PET) in their study of a 45-year-old man with a long history of classic migraine. In this patient, the focal deficit, a pure right hemianopia, occurred upon awakening and was followed by severe generalized headache. The CT scan showed a contrast-enhancing low-density lesion in the left occipital lobe and an unenhanced lesion in the left temporal cortex, the latter suggesting a subclinical, old infarct. Cerebral angiography, performed 21 days after onset, was normal. Cerebral blood flow (CBF) and oxygen extraction, measured by the oxygen 15 inhalation technique, were both reduced in the left occipital cortex, findings typical of recent infarcts; in the temporal lobe, CBF was increased but oxygen extraction was normal. The finding of increased CBF was considered compatible with luxury perfusion, and normal oxygen extraction with reactive hyperemia. Unexplained supernormal oxygen extraction occurred in the asymptomatic right occipital lobe. Weiller and associates[45] found normal cortical blood flow during migraine attacks and after subcutaneous injection of 6 mg sumatriptan.

HEADACHE OF VASCULAR DISEASE

Not surprisingly, a major difficulty in differential diagnosis is that the symptom of head pain occurs in various forms of acute cerebrovascular disease, including ischemic stroke. The landmark experiments of Ray and Wolff[46] demonstrated that sensitivity to pressure, traction, and faradization occur in the intracranial internal carotid artery, the first 1 to 2 cm of the middle cerebral artery (MCA) stem, the first several centimeters of the anterior cerebral artery just beyond the A2 segment, and 1 to 2 cm of the vertebral, anterior, and posterior inferior cerebellar and pontine arteries. These sensitive structures, when electrically stimulated, provoke pain that is localized to specific areas of the scalp and face.

Fisher's clinicopathologic observations[18,47] extended these findings. A study of the headache syndromes due to ischemic cerebrovascular disease showed that most patients complained of the symptom at the onset of a persisting neurologic deficit, although in some cases, headache was premonitory or accompanied TIAs. The headache was usually not throbbing, was often localized, and was frequently lateralized ipsilateral to the presumed arterial occlusion; it was occasionally severe. Of special interest was the relatively high frequency of headache in posterior cerebral artery (PCA) territory infarctions compared with that seen in carotid or basilar disease. Headache was the exception in lacunar strokes with pure motor or pure sensory syndromes, and none occurred in any of the 58 patients with transient monocular blindness. Overall, the frequency of headache was 31% in carotid disease and 42% in vertebrobasilar disease. Mitsias and Ramadan[48] have extensively reviewed the literature on this topic up to 1997.

Drug-Induced Migraine-Related Stroke

Migraine-related stroke associated with ergot therapy is appropriately assigned to the category of drug-induced migraine-related stroke, because it is impossible to confidently exclude an interaction of the drug with the migrainous process to induce stroke. The mechanism of action of 5-hydroxytryptamine 1B/1D ($5HT_{1B/1D}$) agonists, such as ergotamine and the "triptans," may be neurogenic or vasoconstrictive; recorded cases have been associated with excessive dosage of these drugs, which presumably causes vasospasm.

Although rarely, ergot therapy even in therapeutic doses may produce focal and diffuse cerebral dysfunction. The peripheral vascular and central nervous system effects of ergot alkaloids in toxic doses, consisting of gangrene, seizures, encephalopathy, and coma, have long been recognized. The mechanism responsible for diffuse cerebral dysfunction is not settled and may be the result of either a direct central nervous system toxic effect or severe cerebral vasoconstriction, although in therapeutic doses, ergotamine usually has no effect on cerebral blood flow. Scattered reports have appeared that link ergotamine use to focal disturbances in the ophthalmic and cerebral circulations, which manifest as transient monocular blindness, bilateral papillitis, and sensorimotor deficits.[49–51] Since the introduction of the triptans, such as sumatriptan, there have also been scattered reports of strokelike events but, so far, none that has shown convincing evidence of primary involvement of the drug or can exclude the use of the drug in an event that mimics migraine. In most of the reported cases of stroke after injection of 6 mg sumatriptan, the time between the injection and the stroke ranged between 5 and 329 days.[52,53] Only one case of sinus thrombosis was reported with the use of sumatriptan.[54] Another case report described spinal cord infarction after use of zolmitriptan.[55]

Angiography

The precipitation of migraine-like signs and symptoms during cerebral angiography is not uncommon, and the disorder can potentially progress to stroke, although not all observers agree.[56] Angiography performed during migraine carries risk because of potential interaction with the migraine mechanism. Nevertheless, because arteriography can be complicated by stroke in all patients, the true pathogenesis of stroke cannot be attributed with certainty to migraine.

Hemorrhage

Cases of intracerebral hemorrhage due to migraine have been reported rarely and have been reviewed.[57] In our judgment, investigations have failed to establish true migraine-induced hemorrhage, most cases probably being symptomatic migraine or migraine mimics. From the viewpoint of pathogenesis, however, it is not unreasonable that ischemic softening of tissue during true migraine-induced cerebral infarction might become hemorrhagic, so dogmatism must be avoided. Experience with this entity in the context of the current IHS classification is awaited.

OTHER SETTINGS

Transient Focal Neurologic Events and Late-Onset Migraine Accompaniments

Headache is not an invariable occurrence in migraine. Adding to the potential for diagnostic confusion is the occurrence of migraine attacks consisting of visual disturbances or focal deficits not accompanied by typical headache, often termed "migraine sine hemicrania." Charcot identified an incomplete form of ophthalmic migraine as "migraines ophtalmiques frustes," consisting only of "les troubles oculaires."

More controversial has been the entity of migraine aura without headache, originally described by Whitty.[58] Fisher[7,59] emphasized that the migrainous syndrome, despite the absence of headache, could be diagnosed on the basis of characteristic clinical features. Since then, painless transient and persistent migraine accompaniments have become more widely recognized. The cause of late-onset migraine accompaniments has not been established. As the name of the syndrome suggests, the clinical features are essentially indistinguishable from those of migraine without headache. Brain imaging and cerebral arteriography do not reveal accountable structural lesions.

Retinal or Ocular Migraine

This group of disorders known as retinal or ocular migraine is designated as uncertain in classification because of limited clinical information. Most clinical case reports or series were described or published before the development of contemporary advanced neurologic investigation. Although transient homonymous scintillations or fortification scotoma are well-recognized cortical migrainous phenomena, monocular visual loss due to retinal involvement is less often a manifestation of migraine, although still a differential diagnostic point in the patient presenting with amaurosis fugax. Because both retinal and ciliary circulations may be affected, the term *ocular migraine* is preferred[60] and should be distinguished from the term *ophthalmic migraine*, which refers to any migrainous disturbance of vision whether ocular or cortical.

Migraine That Mimics Stroke

Hemiplegic Migraine

Living,[61] in 1893, first described transient hemiparesis associated with a migraine attack. Whitty[62] classified the disorder into hemiplegic migraine with a family history of migraine with or without aura and familial hemiplegic migraine (FHM) in which attacks occur with stereotypic features in family members, often with severe and long-lasting hemiparesis or other persistent aura symptoms and in an autosomal dominant inheritance pattern.

The IHS classifies hemiplegic migraine under "migraine with typical aura" (IHS 1.2.1) or "prolonged aura" (IHS 1.2.2.). FHM is classified as a subgroup of "migraine with aura" (IHS 1.2.3). The working definition includes the criteria for migraine with aura (1.2.1., 1.2.2.) with hemiplegic features that may be prolonged and at least one first-degree relative with identical attacks. As noted previously, the overall prevalence of migraine with aura is around 4%; this figure includes hemiplegic migraine.

Hemiplegic migraine attacks are characterized by hemiparesis or hemiplegia. The arm and leg are involved in the majority of attacks, often combined with face and hand paresis. Less often, isolated facial and arm paresis occurs. The progression of the motor deficit is slow with a spreading or marching quality. In most cases, symptoms are accompanied by homolateral sensory disturbance, particularly cheiro-oral in distribution, with a slowly spreading or marching quality. Infrequently, the hemiparesis may alternate from side to side, even during an attack.[63] Visual disturbance, which takes the form of hemianopic loss or typical visual aura, is common. Homolateral or contralateral localization of the visual disturbance is often obscure, however. When dysphasia occurs, it is more often expressive than receptive. The neurologic symptoms last 30 to 60 minutes and are followed by severe pulsating headache that is hemicranial or whole-head in distribution. Nausea, vomiting, photophobia, and phonophobia are associated features. In severe cases, the aura can persist throughout the headache phase.

Manifestations of severe hemiplegic migraine attacks are fever, drowsiness, confusion, and coma, all of which can be prolonged from days to weeks.[63] Severe hemiplegic migraine may lead rarely to persistent minor neurologic deficit, in which the cumulative effect of repeated attacks progresses to profound multifocal neurologic deficit, even dementia.

FHM is characterized by the neurologic deficit described previously that is identical in at least one other first-degree relative.[3] The disorder has an autosomal dominant inheritance pattern. Other neurologic deficits have been described in association with FHM. Most common is a syndrome of progressive cerebellar disturbance, dysarthria, nystagmus, and ataxia.[63] Retinitis pigmentosa, sensory neural deafness, tremor, dizziness, and oculomotor disturbances with nystagmus, ataxia, and coma have also been described.[64,65] These neurologic deficits are present between attacks and are not part of the aura. Hemiplegic migraine attacks also may be part of other familial disorders affecting other systems, such as MELAS (mitochondrial encephalomyopathy–lactic acidosis–and strokelike symptoms) and CADASIL. Attacks of hemiplegic migraine are less likely to be stereotyped in family members with these conditions, however, because the migraine attack is probably "symptomatic" of the underlying brain disorder.

A breakthrough in establishing the cause of FHM was achieved during the clinical investigation of the disease condition CADASIL.[66–68] This disorder is characterized by recurring small deep infarcts, dementia, and leukoencephalopathy. Some patients also experience recurrent attacks of severe migraine-like headache with aura symptoms that include transient headache and hemiparesis. Joutel and coworkers[69,70] identified the gene locus on chromosome 19. Ophoff and associates[71] and Joutel and colleagues[72] have isolated a gene, on chromosome 19p13.1, that encodes the alpha-1 subunit of a brain-specific, voltage-gated, P/Q-type neuronal calcium channel (CACNL1A4) from patients with FHM.

Several missense mutations were identified in the meantime.[73–75] The investigators also detected premature stop mutations predicted to disrupt the reading frame of CACNL1A4 in two unrelated patients with episodic ataxia type 2 (EA-2). Thus, FHM and EA-2 can be regarded as allelic channelopathies but of differing molecular mechanisms, the former involving a gain of function variant of the Ca^{2+} channel subunit and the latter a decrease in channel density. The results also indicate that different mutations in a single gene may cause phenotypic heterogeneity.[63,76]

Since this report, the same French group identified 10 different missense mutations in the Notch3 genes of 14 unrelated families with CADASIL. The Notch genes are intimately involved in intercellular signaling during development. Proteins belonging to the Notch family are transmembrane receptors. Nine of the ten mutations either added or mutated a cysteine residue in one of the epidermal growth factor (EGF)–like repeats; EGF-like motifs are to be found in the extracellular domain. It is likely that this mutation strongly affects protein conformation, although how this leads to CADASIL remains to be established. Possibly, however, membrane instability and abnormality of cell signaling could be the underlying basis of the migraine attacks in this disorder. The generalizability of the genetic findings in FHM, one of the rarest subtypes of migraine, to the more prevalent migraine subtypes remains to be established. It must be noted that cases of nonfamilial hemiplegic migraine studied by Ophoff and associates[71] failed to show mutations. Sometimes head trauma can lead to fatal brain edema in patients with FHM.[77]

Basilar Migraine

The concept of basilar artery migraine (IHS 1.2.4) was first proposed by Bickerstaff.[78,79] The diagnostic criteria include those for migraine with aura plus two or more aura symptoms of the following types:

- Visual symptoms in both the temporal and nasal fields of both eyes
- Dysarthria
- Vertigo
- Tinnitus
- Decreased hearing
- Double vision
- Ataxia
- Bilateral paresthesias
- Bilateral paresis
- Decreased level of consciousness

The absence of consistent evidence for basilar artery spasm during migraine attacks, and uncertainty about the origin of the mechanisms of the symptoms, prompted the IHS classification committee to remove the word "artery" from the terminology.

Reviewing a personal series of 300 cases, Bickerstaff[78] noticed 34 patients whose attacks were usually heralded by visual disturbances, either complete visual loss or positive phenomena such as teichopsia so dazzling as to obscure the entire field of vision. Other basilar symptoms followed, including dizziness or vertigo, gait ataxia, dysarthria, tinnitus, bilateral acral, perioral, and lingual numbness, and paresthesias. These symptoms persisted for 2 to 60 minutes and ended abruptly, although the visual loss generally recovered more gradually. After the premonitory phase subsided, a severe throbbing occipital headache supervened and was accompanied by vomiting. These patients recovered completely, and between such attacks, many had episodes of classic migraine. Typically affected were adolescent girls. Attacks were usually infrequent and strongly related to menstruation. In Bickerstaff's series, all but 2 patients were younger than 23 years, and 26 of 34 were girls. A clear-cut family history of migraine in close relatives was obtained in 82% of cases.

Lapkin and coworkers[80] encountered this entity in a younger population, reporting a group of 30 children with a mean age at onset of 7 years (range, 7 months to 14 years). The duration of episodes ranged from minutes to many hours; one patient was symptomatic for nearly 3 days. Unlike in the adolescent cases, the most common complaint for these patients was vertigo (73%), and visual disturbances occurred in 43% of cases. In more severely affected children, pyramidal tract dysfunction was observed as well as cranial nerve abnormalities, including internuclear ophthalmoplegia and facial nerve paresis. A family history of migraine was obtained for 86% of patients. During the follow-up period of 6 months to 3 years, none of the patients showed signs of progressive neurologic dysfunction, although 1 child was mentioned as having a permanent oculomotor nerve paralysis.

In the majority of cases of basilar migraine, the aura lasts between 5 and 60 minutes but can extend up to 3 days. Visual symptoms commonly occur first, predominantly in the temporal and nasal fields of vision. The visual disturbance may consist of blurred vision, teichopsia, scintillating scotoma, graying of vision, or total loss of vision. The features may start in one visual field and then spread to become bilateral. Bickerstaff[78] pointed out that when vision is not completely obscured, diplopia might occur, usually as a sixth nerve weakness. Some form of diplopia may occur in up to 16% of cases.[81] Vertigo and gait ataxia are the next most common symptoms, each occurring in 63% of patients in one series.[81] The ataxia can be independent of vertigo. Tinnitus may accompany vertigo. Dysarthria is as common as ataxia and vertigo. Tingling and numbness, in a typical cheiro-oral spreading pattern seen in migraine with aura, occurs in more than 60% of cases. This symptom is usually bilateral and symmetric but may alternate sides with a hemidistribution. Occasionally, dysesthesias extend to the trunk. Bilateral motor weakness occurs in more than 50% of cases.

The syndrome of basilar artery migraine (BAM) was later expanded to include alteration in consciousness. Bickerstaff[79] cited four cases in detail and recorded a total of 8 among 32 patients with previously diagnosed BAM. The onset of impaired consciousness occurred in the context of other basilar symptoms with a leisurely onset, not causing the patient to fall or incur self-injury, and was sometimes preceded by a dreamlike state. Ranging from drowsiness to stupor, the alteration in consciousness was akinetic and usually brief, lasting up to several minutes and not accompanied by rigidity, posturing, tongue biting, urinary incontinence, or changes in the respiratory pattern. As in the usual BAM, a throbbing headache occurred on recovery. Laboratory investigations were generally unrevealing, with normal results of cerebrospinal fluid analysis and electroencephalography (EEG).

Lee and Lance[82] encountered seven patients with a similar syndrome of altered consciousness, which they called *migraine stupor*. Unlike the brief episodes observed by Bickerstaff, the duration of stupor in Lee and Lance's patients ranged from 2 hours to 5 days. Four patients showed aggressive and hysteric behavior during the attacks of BAM, leading to initial psychiatric diagnoses. Although impairment of consciousness in some form is common, it progresses to stupor and prolonged coma. Other forms of altered consciousness are amnesia and syncope. Drop attacks are rare.

Headache occurs in almost all patients with BAM. It has an occipital location in the majority, has a throbbing, pounding quality, and is accompanied by severe nausea and vomiting. It is unusual for the headache to be unilateral or localized to the more anterior parts of the cranium. Photophobia and phonophobia occur in one third to one half of the patients. As with other forms of migraine, the symptoms may occur without headache, usually in no more than 4% of cases.[81] Seizures have been observed in association with basilar migraine. EEG changes in attacks of typical BAM but without seizures have also been described. In all, EEG abnormalities are detected in less than one fifth of patients with basilar migraine and are mostly independent of any clinical manifestation of the disorder.

Permanent brainstem deficits occurring as a result of BAM have been reported rarely. None of Bickerstaff's[79] patients had persisting neurologic disturbances; indeed, he stressed return to complete normality as a criterion for the diagnosis. Of the five cases of migraine-associated stroke uncovered in the literature, four have occurred in the vertebrobasilar territory, excluding the posterior cerebral artery. In Connor's[83] presentation of 18 cases of complicated migraine, three patients were considered to have lesions in the brainstem. In no instance did the transient episodes clearly resemble BAM as defined previously.

Cerebral infarction specifically affecting the brainstem circulation territory understandably has been offered as evidence for a primary vascular cause of basilar migraine. Skinhoj and Paulson,[84] in studies performed during the migraine aura, found angiographic results to be normal, despite a reduction in CBF, except for impaired filling in the top of the basilar artery. Cerebral angiography can itself precipitate migraine aura, however, although after a time lag of hours. Nevertheless, the combination of the clinical features plus the arteriographic studies previously mentioned emphasizes a primary vascular alternative for the cause of basilar migraine. Cerebrovascular disease is the most serious differential diagnosis of basilar migraine.

Ischemic stroke in the brainstem and posterior cortical regions, due to either cerebral embolism or thrombosis, manifests as a constellation of neurologic symptoms and signs of brainstem and posterior circulation defects that are accompanied in approximately a third of cases by headache. Basilar artery occlusive disease can, therefore, mimic basilar migraine. Another basilar migraine "mimic," and one for which patients with migraine are at increased risk, is vertebral artery dissection.

Transient ischemic attacks involving any part of the vertebrobasilar territory must also figure largely in the differential diagnosis, particularly if basilar migraine manifests for the first time in the later years of life. Certain familial disorders manifest as neurologic deficits in which attacks of hemiplegic or basilar migraine may be part of the symptom complex. This group includes CADASIL, MELAS, and variants of MELAS that are associated with seizures, particularly occipital in origin.

Mechanisms

From the preceding review, it should be apparent that migraine can mimic cerebrovascular disorders, especially ischemic stroke, and stroke can mimic migraine. This situation poses diagnostic problems for the clinician that in most cases are resolved. It is uncertain how much of the past literature on migraine-induced stroke described cerebrovascular disorders that were mistaken for migraine. This statement is meant not to criticize these earlier reports but to recognize that they were communicated at a time when diagnostic tools were less well developed and that concepts of migraine mechanisms have changed. It remains to be determined how a migraine attack can induce permanent neurologic deficit and brain damage. Perhaps even more intriguing is the question: What constitutes the comorbid increased risk for stroke between attacks? The latter is the more difficult to speculate on because, although comorbid factors may be present (such as increased platelet aggregation or mitral valve prolapse), many are uncertain risk factors for stroke. Indeed, when definite risk factors for stroke are present in a patient who has migraine, the stroke is attributed to this cause and not to migraine. On the basis of the epidemiologic data described, however, there must be stroke risk factors yet to be identified that are comorbid with migraine.

With regard to the mechanisms whereby stroke is induced during a migraine attack, available information provides some limited understanding. The current literature on CBF has been reviewed. To summarize, spreading cortical depression (SD) of Leao may induce short-lived increases in CBF followed by a more profound oligemia. Ischemic foci, however, may occasionally occur during attacks of migraine with aura. Possibly, SD is also associated with depolarization of intrinsic neurons that also supply intraparenchymal resistance microvessels, leading to constriction and a consequent flow reduction below the threshold for potassium ion (K^+) release from the neuron. Increased extracellular K^+ then might precipitate depolarization of contiguous cortical neurons.

Alternatively, the decreased extracellular space and brain swelling that accompany spreading cortical depression and possibly migraine could raise microvascular resistance by means of mechanical compression. Thus, low flow in major intracerebral vessels may be due to increased downstream resistance, not to major intracranial arterial vasospasm. Essentially, a low CBF and sluggish flow in large intracerebral vessels during the aura of migraine, when combined with factors predisposing to coagulopathy, could lead, although rarely, to intravascular thrombosis and, thus, migraine-induced cerebral infarction. Release of vasoactive peptides and endothelin, activation of cytokines, and upregulation of adhesion molecules during the neurogenically mediated inflammatory response that may be responsible for headache may also induce intravascular thrombosis. This possibility could explain why migraine-induced stroke usually respects intracranial arterial territories even though the aura involves more widespread brain regions. In addition, frequent aura, if due to spreading depression, could induce cytotoxic cell damage and gliosis based on glutamate release or excess intracellular calcium accumulation. This could explain persistent neurologic deficit without evidence of ischemic infarction due to selective neuronal necrosis. Increased extracellular K^+ that might precipitate rarely during episodes of migraine probably relates to variability in the coagulation status, extent of the neuronal and hemodynamic changes, and the interaction between/among these factors.

TREATMENT

Stroke Prevention in Patients with Migraine

Most patients with TIA or stroke receive antiplatelet treatment. Aspirin lowers stroke risk[85] and has a weak preventive action in migraine.[86,87] Clopidogrel, which is more effective than aspirin in the prevention of the combined endpoint of stroke, myocardial infarction, and vascular death,[88] can be given to patients with migraine. The combination of aspirin plus slow-release dipyridamole is more effective than aspirin in stroke prevention.[89] Dipyridamole may lead to headache in the first few days of intake. If the agent is tolerated for this period, however, the headache will improve. According to clinical experience, patients who used to suffer from migraine or patients from families with migraine have headache more often with dipyridamole than patients who have no history of migraine. Formal studies on how to treat the headache induced by dipyridamole are not available. Anticoagulation poses no problem for patients with migraine. In patients with significant carotid stenosis angiography, carotid endarterectomy or stenting with balloon dilation can induce migraine attacks in people who either had or still have migraine.

Patients with hypertension and migraine should be treated with β-blockers that have shown efficacy in migraine prophylaxis, such as propranolol, metoprolol, bisoprolol, and atenolol.[90] Whether angiotensin-converting enzyme (ACE) inhibitors, such as lisinopril, are effective in migraine prophylaxis is under debate.[91] Cholesterol-lowering drugs and antidiabetic treatment do not interfere with migraine or migraine treatment. Women who have migraine with aura, have other diseases, such as hypertension, diabetes, and obesity, and are smoking should receive treatment for these risk factors and should be advised about the risk of oral contraceptives.[92,93]

Migraine in Patients at Risk of Stroke or in Patients with Transient Ischemic Attack or Stroke

Treatment of migraine attacks with one of the triptans (almotriptan, eletriptan, frovatriptan, naratriptan, rizatriptan, sumatriptan, zolmitriptan) is contraindicated in patients with TIA or stroke and in patients with multiple vascular risk factors (Table 27.2). The reason is that triptans have a vasoconstrictive action[94-97] and might further reduce already decreased blood flow. Ergot alkaloids are also contraindicated, for the same reason.[97,98] Treatment of acute migraine attacks in patients at high risk of stroke is restricted to analgesic drugs. In some countries, aspirin is available as an intravenous injection for the treatment of acute migraine attack; 1000 mg aspirin given intravenously is inferior to 6 mg sumatriptan given subcutaneously in terms of efficacy but is better tolerated.[99]

Patients with frequent migraine attacks and vascular disease should receive migraine prophylaxis (Table 27.3). Drugs of first choice are β-blockers.[90] They are effective and also lower the increased blood pressure. Results of one study indicate that lowering the blood pressure might even prevent vascular events in patients with normal blood pressure.[100] Flunarizine is not available in all countries but can be given to most patients with vascular disease,[101] as can

Table 27.2   Treatment of Acute Migraine Attacks in Otherwise Healthy Patients with Transient Ischemic Attacks (TIAs), Stroke, or Risk of Stroke*

Drug	Dose (mg)	Patients without Vascular Risk	Patients with TIAs or Stroke
Aspirin	500–1000	+++	+++
Paracetamol, acetaminophen	500–1000	++	++
NSAIDs		+++	+++
Ergotamine, oral	1–2	++	Contraindicated
DHE, IV, SC	1–2	+++	Contraindicated
Sumatriptan	6 SC, 25, 50, 100 oral	+++	Contraindicated
Naratriptan	2.5	++	Contraindicated
Rizatriptan	10	+++	Contraindicated
Zolmitriptan	2.5, 5	+++	Contraindicated
Eletriptan	20, 40, 50, 80	+++	Contraindicated
Almotriptan	12.5	+++	Contraindicated
Frovatriptan	2.5	+	Contraindicated
Neuroleptics		+	+

*Plus signs indicate efficacy, from low (+) to high (+++) shown in clinical trials.
DHE, dihydroergotamine; IV, intravenous(ly); NSAIDs, nonsteroidal anti-inflammatory drugs; SC, subcutaneous(ly).

Table 27.3   Drugs for Migraine Prophylaxis in Otherwise Healthy Patients, Patients with Transient Ischemic Attacks (TIAs) or Stroke, and Patients at Risk of Stroke*

Drug	Dose (mg)	Patients without Vascular Risk	Patients with TIAs or Stroke
Metoprolol	50–200	+++	+++
Propranolol	40–160	+++	+++
Bisoprolol	5–10	++	++
Flunarizine	5–10	+++	+++
Valproic acid	500–600	+++	+++
Gabapentin	2400	++	++
Topiramate	50–200	+++	+++
Pizotifen	1.5	+	Contraindicated
Methysergide	4–8	++	Contraindicated
Magnesium	500	+	+
α-dihydrergocryptine	10	+	+
Aspirin	300	+	+

*Plus signs indicate efficacy, from low (+) to high (+ + +).

Specific Medical Diseases and Stroke

anticonvulsants.[102,103] Serotonin antagonists such as pizotifen and methysergide[104] are contraindicated in patients at risk of stroke. Aerobic exercise has migraine preventive action and lowers stroke risk.[105,106]

Patients who experienced cerebral hemorrhage or subarachnoidal hemorrhage should not use acetylsalicylic acid to treat migraine attacks and should not use nonsteroidal anti-inflammatory drugs for migraine prophylaxis. Triptans are contraindicated for treatment of headache after subarachnoidal hemorrhage. Valproic acid for migraine prophylaxis should be used only after the platelet count is under control. The treatment of the acute phase of cerebral hemorrhage and subarachnoidal hemorrhage is the same in patients with and without migraine.

ACKNOWLEDGMENTS

Petra Mummel assisted with literature research. The work of HCD is supported by a grant from the German Ministry of Science and Technology via the German Headache Consortium.

References

1. Lipton RB, Stewart WF: Epidemiology and comorbidity of migraine. In Goadsby PJ, Silberstein SD (eds): Headache. Boston, Butterworth-Heinemann, 1997, p 75.
2. Russel MB, Rasmussen BK, Thornvaldesen P, et al: Prevalence and sex ratio of the subtypes of migraine. Int J Epidemiol 24:612, 1995.
3. Stewart WF, Lipton RB, Celentano DD, et al: Prevalence of migraine headache in the United States—relation to age, race, income, and other sociodemographic factors. JAMA 267:64, 1992.
4. Stewart WF, Lipton RB, Celentano DD, et al: Prevalence of migraine headache in the United States: relation to age, income, race and other sociodemographic factors. JAMA 267:64, 1992.
5. Rasmussen BK, Olesen J: Migraine with aura and migraine without aura: An epidemiological study. Cephalalgia 12:221, 1992.
6. Headache Classification Committee of the International Headache Society: Classification and diagnostic criteria for headache disorders, cranial neuralgias and facial pain. Cephalalgia 8:1, 1988.

7. Fisher CM: Late-life migraine accompaniments as a cause of unexplained transient ischemic attacks. Can J Med Sci 7:9, 1980.
8. Queiroz AP, Rapaport AM, Weeks RE, et al: Characteristics of migraine visual aura. Headache 37:137, 1997.
9. Diener H: Positron emission tomography studies in headache. Headache 37:622, 1997.
10. Olesen J, Tfelt-Hansen P, Henriksen L, et al: Difference between cerebral blood flow reactions in classic and common migraine. In Rose FC (eds): Advances in Migraine Research and Therapy. New York, Raven Press, 1982, p 105.
11. Woods RP, Iacoboni M, Mazziotta JC: Bilateral spreading cerebral hypoperfusion during spontaneous migraine headache. N Engl J Med 331:1689, 1994.
12. Olesen J, Friberg L, Olsen TS, et al: Ischaemia-induced (symptomatic) migraine attacks may be more frequent than migraine-induced ischaemic insults. Brain 116:187, 1993.
13. Silvestrini M, Cupini LM, Calabresi P, et al: Migraine with aura-like syndrome due to arteriovenous malformation: The clinical value of transcranial Doppler in early diagnosis. Cephalalgia 12:115, 1992.
14. Chabriat H, Vahedi K, Iba-Zizen MT, et al: Clinical spectrum of CADASIL: A study of 7 families. Lancet 346:934, 1995.
15. Davous P: CADASIL: A review with proposed diagnostic criteria. Eur J Neurol 5:219, 1998.
16. Ramadan NM, Tietjen GE, Levine SR, et al: Scintillating scotoma associated with internal carotid artery dissection. Neurology 41:1084, 1991.
17. Sibert PL, Mokri B, Schievink WI: Headache and neck pain in spontaneous internal carotid and vertebral artery dissections. Neurology 45:1517, 1995.
18. Fisher CM: The headache and pain of spontaneous carotid dissection. Headache 22:60, 1982.
19. Welch KMA, Bousser M-G: Migraine and stroke. In Olesen J, Tfelt-Hansen P, Welch KMA (eds): The Headaches, 2nd ed. Philadelphia, Lippincott Williams & Wilkins, 2000, p 529.
20. Alvarez J, Matias Guiu J, Sumalla J, et al: Ischemic stroke in young adults. 1: Analysis of the etiological subgroups. Acta Neurol Scand 80:28, 1989.
21. Bogousslavsky J, Regli F: Ischemic stroke in adults younger than 30 years of age: Cause and prognosis. Arch Neurol 44:479, 1987.
22. Rothrock J, North J, Madden K, et al: Migraine and migrainous stroke: Risk factors and prognosis. Neurology 43:2473, 1993.
23. Bogousslavsky J, Regli F, Van Melle G, et al: Migraine stroke. Neurology 38:223, 1988.
24. Mosek A, Marom R, Korczyn AD, et al: A history of migraine is not a risk factor to develop an ischemic stroke in the elderly. Headache 41:399, 2001.
25. Henrich JB, Sandercock PAG, Warlow CP, et al: Stroke and migraine in the Oxfordshire Community Stroke Project. J Neurol 233:257, 1986.
26. Broderick JP, Swanson JW: Migraine-related strokes. Arch Neurol 44:868, 1987.
27. Bonita R: Epidemiology of stroke. Lancet 339:342, 1992.
28. Merikangas KR, Fenton BT, Cheng SH, et al: Association between migraine and stroke in a large-scale epidemiological study of the United States. Arch Neurol 54:362, 1997.
29. Tzourio C, Tehindrazanarivelo A, Iglesias S, et al: Case-control study of migraine and risk of ischemic stroke in young women. BMJ 310:830, 1995.
30. Carolei A, Marini C, DeMatteis G: History of migraine and risk of cerebral ischemia in young adults. The Italian National Research Council Study Group on Stroke in the Young. Lancet 347:1503, 1996.
31. Chang CL, Donaghy M, Poulter N, et al: Migraine and stroke in young women: Case-control study. BMJ 318:13, 1999.
32. Buring JE, Hebert P, Romero J, et al: Migraine and subsequent risk of stroke in the Physicians' Health Study. Arch Neurol 52:129, 1995.
33. Steering Committee of the Physicians' Health Study Research Group: Final report on the aspirin component of the ongoing Physicians' Health Study. N Engl J Med 321:129, 1989.
34. Collaborative Group for the Study of Stroke in Young Women: Oral contraception and stroke in young women: Associated risk factors. Collaborative Group for the Study of Stroke in Young Women. JAMA 231:718, 1975.
35. Lidegaard O: Oral contraceptives, pregnancy and the risk of cerebral thromboembolism: The influence of diabetes, hypertension,

migraine and previous thrombotic disease. Br J Obstet Gynaecol 102:153, 1995.
36. Kittner SJ: Stroke in young adults: Progress and opportunities. Neuroepidemiology 17:174, 1998.
37. Petitti DB, Sidney S, Quesenberry CP, et al: Incidence of stroke and myocardial infarction in women of reproductive state. Stroke 28:280, 1997.
38. Cala LA, Mastaglia FL: Computerized axial tomography findings in patients with migrainous headaches. BMJ 2:149, 1976.
39. Hungerford GD, Du Boulay GH, Zilkha KJ: Computerized axial tomography in patients with severe migraine: A preliminary report. J Neurol Neurosurg Psychiatry 39:990, 1976.
40. Rascol A, Cambier J, Guiraud B, et al: Accidents ischémiques cérébraux au cours de crises migraineuses: A propos des migraines compliquées. Rev Neurol (Paris) 135:867, 1979.
41. Igarashi H, Sakai F, Kan S, et al: Magnetic resonance imaging of the brain in patients with migraine. Cephalalgia 11:69, 1991.
42. Fazekas F, Koch M, Schmidt R, et al: The prevalence of cerebral damage varies with migraine type: A MRI study. Headache 32:287, 1992.
43. De Benedittis G, Lorenzetti A, Sina C, et al: Magnetic resonance imaging in migraine and tension type headache. Headache 35:264, 1995.
44. Bousser MG, Baron JC, Iba-Zizen MT, et al: Migrainous cerebral infarction: A tomographic study of cerebral blood flow and oxygen extraction fraction with the oxygen-15 inhalation technique. Stroke 11:145, 1980.
45. Weiller C, May A, Limmroth V, et al: Brain stem activation in spontaneous human migraine attacks. Nature Medicine 1:658, 1995.
46. Ray BS, Wolff HG: Experimental studies on headache: Pain- sensitive structures of the head and their significance in headache. Arch Surg 41:813, 1940.
47. Fisher CM: Headache in cerebrovascular disease. In Vinken PJ, Bruyn GW (eds): Handbook of Clinical Neurology, Vol. 5. Amsterdam, Elsevier, 1968, p 124.
48. Mitsias P, Ramadan NM: Headache in ischemic cerebrovascular disease. Part I: Clinical features. Cephalalgia 12:269, 1992.
49. Brohult J, Forsberg O, Hellstrom R: Multiple arterial thrombosis after oral contraceptives and ergotamine. Acta Med Scand 181:453, 1967.
50. Merhofff GC, Poter JM: Ergot intoxication: Historical review and description. Ann Surg 180:773, 1974.
51. Senter HJ, Liebermann AN: Cerebral manifestations of ergotism: Report of a case and review of the literature. Stroke 7:88, 1976.
52. O'Quinn S, Davis R, Guttermann D, et al: Prospective large-scale study of the tolerability of subcutaneous sumatriptan injection for the acute treatment of migraine. Cephalalgia 19:223, 1999.
53. Welch KMA, Mathew NT, Stone P, et al: Tolerability of sumatriptan: Clinical trials and post-marketing experience. Cephalalgia 20:687, 2000.
54. Cavazos JE, Carees JB, Chilukuri VR: Sumatriptan-induced stroke in sagittal sinus thrombosis. Lancet 343:1105, 1994.
55. Vijayan N, Peacock JH: Spinal cord infarction during use of zolmitriptan: A case report. Headache 40:57, 2000.
56. Shuaib A, Hachinski C: Migraine and the risks from angiography. 45:911, 1988.
57. Caplan L: Intracerebral hemorrhage revisited. Neurology 38:624, 1988.
58. Whitty CWM: Migraine without headache. Lancet 2:283, 1967.
59. Fisher CM: Migraine accompaniments versus arteriosclerotic ischemia. Trans Am Neurol Assoc 93:211, 1968.
60. Corbett JJ: Neuro-ophthalmic complications of migraine and cluster headaches. Neurol Clin 1:973, 1983.
61. Living E: On Megrim, Sick-Headache, and Some Allied Disorders: A Contribution to the Pathology of Nerve-Storms. London, J & A Churchill, 1893.
62. Whitty CWM: Familial hemiplegic migraine. J Neurol Neurosurg Psychiatry 16:172, 1953.
63. Ducros A, Denier C, Joutel A, et al: The clinical spectrum of familial hemiplegic migraine associated with mutations in a neuronal calcium channel. N Engl J Med 345:17, 2001.
64. Elliott MA, Peroutka SJ, Welch S, et al: Familial hemiplegic migraine, nystagmus, and cerebellar atrophy. Ann Neurol 39:100, 1996.
65. Vahedi K, Denier C, Ducros A, et al: CACNA1A gene de novo mutation causing hemiplegic migraine, coma and cerebellar atrophy. Neurology 55:1040, 2000.

Specific Medical Diseases and Stroke

66. Chabriat H, Tournier-Lasserve E, Vahedi K, et al: Autosomal dominant migraine with MRI white-matter abnormalities mapping to the CADASIL locus. Neurology 45:1086, 1995.

67. Chabriat H, Vahedi K, Iba-Zizen MT, et al: Clinical spectrum of CADASIL: A study of 7 families. Lancet 346:934, 1995.

68. Hutchinson M, Oriordan J, Javed M, et al: Familial hemiplegic migraine and autosomal dominant arteriopathy with leukoencephalopathy (CADASIL). Ann Neurol 38:817, 1995.

69. Joutel A, Corpechet C, Ducros A, et al: Notch3 mutations in CADASIL, a hereditary adult-onset condition causing stroke and dementia. Nature 383:707, 1996.

70. Joutel A, Corpechot C, Vayssière C, et al: Characterization of Notch3 mutations in CADASIL patients. Neurology 48:1729, 1997.

71. Ophoff RA, Terwindt GM, Vergouwe MN, et al: Familial hemiplegic migraine and episodic ataxia type-2 are caused by mutations in the Ca^{2+} channel gene CACNL1A4. Cell 87:543, 1996.

72. Joutel A, Bousser M, Biousese V, et al: A gene for familial hemiplegic migraine maps to chromosome 19. Nat Genet 5:40, 1993.

73. Carrera P, Piatti M, Stenirri S, et al: Genetic heterogeneity in Italian families with familial hemiplegic migraine. Neurology 53:26, 1999.

74. Terwindt GM, Ophoff RA, Haan J, et al: Familial hemiplegic migraine: A clinical comparison of families linked and unlinked to chromosome 19. Cephalalgia 16:153, 1996.

75. Terwindt GM, Ophoff RA, Haan J, et al: Variable clinical expression of mutations in the P/Q-type calcium channel gene in familial hemiplegic migraine. Neurology 50:1105, 1998.

76. Battistini S, Stenirri S, Piatti M, et al: A new CACNA1A gene mutation in acetazolamide-responsive familial hemiplegic migraine and ataxia. Neurology 53:38, 1999.

77. Kors EE, Terwindt GM, Vermeulen FLMG, et al: Delayed cerebral edema and fatal coma after minor head trauma: Role of CACNA1A calcium channel subunit gene and relationship with familial hemiplegic migraine. Ann Neurol 49:753, 2001.

78. Bickerstaff ER: Basilar artery migraine. Lancet i:15, 1961.

79. Bickerstaff ER: The basilar artery and migraine epilepsy syndrome. Proc R Soc Med 55:167, 1962.

80. Lapkin ML, French JH, Golden GS: The EEG in childhood basilar artery migraine. Neurology 27:580, 1977.

81. Sturzenegger MH, Meienberg O: Basilar artery migraine: A follow-up study of 82 cases. Headache 25:408, 1985.

82. Lee CH, Lance JW: Migraine stupor. Headache 17:32, 1977.

83. Connor RCR: Complicated migraine: A study of permanent neurological and visual defects caused by migraine. Lancet ii:1072, 1962.

84. Skinhoj E, Paulson OB: Regional cerebral blood flow in the internal carotid artery distribution during migraine. BMJ 3:569, 1969.

85. Antiplatelet Trialists Collaboration: Collaborative overview of randomised trials of antiplatelet therapy—I: Prevention of death, myocardial infarction, and stroke by prolonged antiplatelet therapy in various categories of patients. BMJ 308:81, 1994.

86. Bensenor IM, Cook NR, Lee I-M, et al: Low-dose aspirin for migraine prophylaxis in women. Cephalalgia 21:175, 2001.

87. Diener HC, Hartung E, Chrubasik J, et al: A comparative study of acetylsalicylic acid and metoprolol for the prophylactic treatment of migraine: A randomised, controlled, double-blind, parallel group phase III study. Cephalalgia 21:140, 2001.

88. CAPRIE Steering Committee: A randomised, blinded, trial of clopidogrel versus aspirin in patients at risk of ischaemic events (CAPRIE). Lancet 348:1329, 1996.

89. Diener HC, Cuhna L, Forbes C, et al: European Stroke Prevention Study 2: Dipyridamole and acetylsalicylic acid in the secondary prevention of stroke. J Neurol Sci 143:1, 1996.

90. Silberstein SD: Practice parameter: Evidence-based guidelines for migraine headache (an evidence-based review). Report of the Quality Standards Subcommittee of the American Academy of Neurology. Neurology 55:754, 2000.

91. Schrader H, Stovner LJ, Helde G, et al: Prophylactic treatment of migraine with angiotensin converting enzyme inhibitor (lisinopril): Randomised, placebo-controlled, crossover trial. BMJ 322:19, 2001.

92. Bousser M-G: Migraine, female hormones, and stroke. Cephalalgia 19:75, 1999.

93. MacGregor A: Gynaecological aspects of migraine. Rev Contemp Pharmacother 11:75, 2000.

94. Jansen I, Edvinson L, Mortensens A, et al: Sumatriptan is a potent vasoconstrictor in human dural arteries via a 5-HT1-like receptor. Cephalalgia 12:202, 1992.

95. Longmore J, Hargreaves RJ, Boulanger CM, et al: Comparison of the vasoconstrictor properties of the 5-HT1D-receptor agonists rizatriptan (MK-462) and sumatriptan in human isolated coronary artery: Outcome of two independent studies using different experimental protocols. Funct Neurol 12:3, 1997.

96. Longmore J, Hargreaves RJ, Boulanger CM, et al: Comparison of the vasoconstrictor properties of the 5-HT1D-receptor agonists rizatriptan (MK-462) and sumatriptan in human isolated coronary artery: Outcome of two independent studies using different experimental protocols. Funct Neurol 12:3, 1997.

97. Saxena PR, den Boer MO, Ferrari MD: The pharmacology of antimigrainous drugs. Clin Neuropharmacol 15:375A, 1992.

98. Saxena VK, De Deyn PP: Ergotamine: Its use in the treatment of migraine and its complications. Acta Neurol Napoli 14:140, 1992.

99. Diener HC: Efficacy and safety of intravenous acetylsalicylic acid lysinate compared to subcutaneous sumatriptan and parenteral placebo in the acute treatment of migraine: A double-blind, double-dummy, randomized, multicenter, parallel group study. The ASASUMAMIG Study Group. Cephalalgia 19:581, 1999.

100. Hansson L, Zanchetti A, Carruthers SG, et al: Effects of intensive blood-pressure lowering and low-dose aspirin in patients with hypertension: Principal results of the Hypertension Optimal Treatment (HOT) randomised trial. Lancet 351:1755, 1998.

101. Diener HC, Peters C, Rudizo M, et al: Ergotamine, flunarizine and sumatriptan do not change cerebral blood flow velocity in normal subjects and migraineurs. J Neurol 238:245, 1991.

102. Klapper J: Divalproex sodium in migraine prophylaxis: A dose-controlled study. Cephalalgia 17:103, 1997.

103. Mathew NT, Rapoport A, Saper J, et al: Efficacy of gabapentin in migraine prophylaxis. Headache 41:119, 2001.

104. Silberstein SD: Methysergide. Cephalalgia 18:421, 1998.

105. Sacco RL, Gan R, Boden-Albala B, et al: Leisure-time physical activity and ischemic stroke risk—The Northern Manhattan Stroke Study. Stroke 29:380, 1998.

106. Wannamethee G, Shaper AG: Physical activity and stroke in British middle aged men. BMJ 304:597, 1992.

Chapter Twenty-Eight

Hypertensive Encephalopathy

Catherine Lamy and Jean-Louis Mas

The term hypertensive encephalopathy was introduced by Oppenheimer and Fishberg[1] in 1928 to designate a constellation of neurologic symptoms that punctuate the course of severe hypertension. *Hypertensive encephalopathy* is currently defined as an acute syndrome characterized by elevated blood pressure associated with rapidly progressive signs and symptoms, including headache, seizures, altered mental status, visual disturbances, and other focal or diffuse neurologic signs. Its pathogenesis is still incompletely understood, although it seems to be related to breakthrough of autoregulation and endothelial dysfunction leading to cerebral edema. Recognition of this condition is important, because prompt control of blood pressure will usually cause reversal of the syndrome. If untreated, increasing intracranial pressure can be fatal.

PATHOGENESIS

The brain is protected from extremes of blood pressure by an autoregulation system that ensures constant perfusion over a wide range of systemic pressures (Fig. 28–1). In response to systemic hypotension, cerebral arterioles dilate to maintain adequate perfusion, whereas vessels constrict in response to high pressure. The basic mechanism of autoregulation of cerebral blood flow is still controversial.[2] The autoregulatory vessel caliber changes are most likely mediated by an interplay between myogenic and metabolic mechanisms.[3] The endothelium plays a central role in blood pressure homeostasis by secreting vasoactive substances such as nitric oxide and prostacyclin. In normotensive individuals, cerebral blood flow remains unchanged between mean blood pressures of 60 and 120 mm Hg.[4] At pressures above the upper limit of autoregulation, hypertensive encephalopathy may occur. Conversely, when cerebral perfusion pressure decreases below the lower limit of autoregulation, cerebral blood flow decreases, and cerebral ischemia occurs. There may be differences between individuals in the extent of hypertension that can give rise to autoregulatory dysfunction leading to encephalopathy as well as differences within a single person over time depending on comorbid factors. Longstanding hypertension causes a shift of the cerebral blood-flow curve to the right, presumably as a result of structural changes (vascular hypertrophy and inward remodeling)[5] and diminished responsiveness of resistance vessels.[6,7]

Therefore, sudden elevations to relatively higher blood pressure levels are required to produce hypertensive encephalopathy in a patient with chronic hypertension than in a normotensive person.[8] In children, the curve shifts to the left, leaving them more at risk for the development of hypertensive encephalopathy.[9,10]

Over the previous century, two theories were advanced to explain the pathogenesis of hypertensive encephalopathy. The conception that has historically been most widely advocated by clinicians postulated that the disorder results from spasm of the cerebral vasculature in response to acute hypertension (overregulation), leading to decreased cerebral blood flow and intra-arterial thrombosis. These developments, in turn, produce ischemia and cytotoxic edema in the border zones between arterial territories. The direct observation by Byrom[11] of alternating constriction and dilatation during episodes of acute rise in blood pressure in the hypertensive rat's pial vessels seemed to confirm this hypothesis.

Later investigations have implicated forced vasodilatation of cerebral vessels (autoregulation breakthrough), rather than vasoconstriction as the major component of hypertensive encephalopathy, that results in the extravasation of fluid into the interstitium, termed *vasogenic edema*. Patterns of cerebral blood flow with acute hypertension may be complex, with both low-flow and high-flow areas coexisting in adjacent cortical regions.[12] The concept of breakthrough of autoregulation has been initially characterized as a passive phenomenon, as the autoregulatory capacity of vessels is exceeded and the vessels dilate passively. Later evidence suggests that breakthrough of autoregulation may be an active process initiated by calcium-dependent potassium channels. This process generates reactive oxygen species and an active rise in permeability of the blood-brain barrier, as well as an increase in vesicular transport, rather than disruption of tight junctions.[5] Abnormalities in vasoactive factors released by the endothelium may contribute to the pathophysiology of hypertensive encephalopathy.[4] Ultimately, loss of endothelial fibrinolytic activity, activation of coagulation and platelets, and degranulation on damaged endothelium may promote further inflammation, thrombosis, and vasoconstriction.[4]

The preferential distribution of white matter lesions in posterior brain regions is recognized but not fully understood. One likely explanation involves the regional

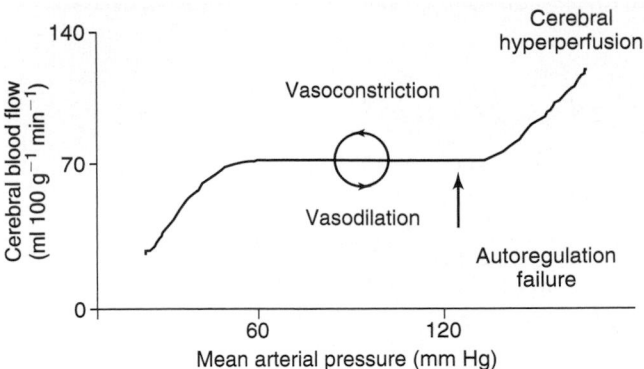

FIGURE 28–1 *Autoregulation of cerebral blood flow.*

heterogeneity of the sympathetic innervation.[13] The blood vessels of the pia are supplied by sympathetic nerves from the superior cervical sympathetic ganglion. Ultrastructural studies have shown that the density of sympathetic innervation is maximal in the internal carotid system, decreases posteriorly, and is lowest in the basilar artery and its branches. The penetrating vessels that supply deep gray and white matter receive scarce adrenergic innervation. Because of this anterior-to-posterior gradient of sympathetic innervation, a hyperperfusion state in perforating white matter arterioles might occur in hypertensive encephalopathy with a posterior-to-anterior gradient of edema.[14]

PATHOLOGIC FEATURES

The neuropathologic findings in hypertensive encephalopathy as shown in autopsy studies[15,16] consist of varying degrees of vascular alterations (fibrinoid necrosis of arterioles, thrombosis of arterioles and capillaries) and parenchymal lesions (microinfarcts, petechial hemorrhages, cerebral edema). Ring hemorrhages around a thrombosed precapillary compose the classic microscopic lesion. If hypertensive encephalopathy develops in a patient with long-standing hypertension, a variety of additional hypertensive cerebrovascular changes may be found, including medial atrophy, hyperplasia, hyalinization, and microaneurysms.

The lesions are most often multiple and bilateral, most prominent in the deep white matter and at the gray-white junction in the watershed and posterior areas; the brainstem is usually severely affected.[15] They may also be present in the basal ganglia, diencephalon, and cerebral cortex. Their extent and severity vary but are generally correlated with the severity of neurologic manifestations and blood pressure, especially during the terminal stage.[15] Brain swelling, occasionally sufficient to cause herniation of cerebellar tonsils through the foramen magnum, has been documented. The vascular changes are not confined to the brain but may also affect the eyes (retinal hemorrhages, papilledema), kidneys (fibrinoid arteriolar lesions of glomeruli), and other organs.[15] These findings, however, may not be representative of those in surviving patients,

instead representing the extreme of a spectrum of abnormalities.

CLINICAL FEATURES

The classic clinical manifestations of hypertensive encephalopathy include severe headache, nausea and vomiting, mental abnormalities including confusion and diminished spontaneity and speech, seizures, and visual disturbances.[8,15,17] Alterations in consciousness range in severity from mild somnolence to frank confusion, stupor, or coma in extreme cases. Lethargy and somnolence are often the first clinical signs. Temporary restlessness and agitation may alternate with lethargy. The mental functions are slowed; memory and the ability to concentrate are impaired, although severe amnesia is unusual. Abnormalities of visual perception are nearly always detectable. Patients often report blurred vision. Hemianopia, visual neglect, visual hallucinations,[18] and frank cortical blindness may occur. Papilledema may be present with flame-shaped retinal hemorrhages and exudates.[8] The tendon reflexes are often brisk, and some patients have weakness and incoordination. The onset is usually subacute but may be heralded by a seizure. Focal or generalized seizures may be the presenting manifestation.[19]

The electroencephalogram reflects an impaired level of consciousness through loss of normal alpha activity. Slow waves may be prominent in the occipital areas. Examination of the cerebrospinal fluid in patients with hypertensive encephalopathy has revealed elevated pressure,[17] mild pleocytosis, and elevated protein concentration.[8]

The differential diagnosis includes various neurologic conditions, such as stroke, venous thrombosis, encephalitis, and the reversible posterior leukoencephalopathy syndrome (see section on etiology), all of which can mimic hypertensive encephalopathy, and transient elevations of blood pressure may be the consequence of cerebral lesions. Therefore, patients with hypertension and altered neurologic status represent a difficult diagnostic problem, and hypertensive encephalopathy should remain a diagnosis of exclusion.

NEURORADIOLOGIC FEATURES

The most common abnormality found on neuroimaging is edema involving the white matter of the posterior portions of both cerebral hemispheres, especially the parieto-occipital regions. The calcarine and paramedian occipital lobe structures are usually spared, a finding that distinguishes hypertensive encephalopathy from bilateral infarction of the posterior cerebral artery territory.[20] Involvement of other posterior structures, such as the cerebellum and brainstem, are common. Predominance of posterior fossa lesions are infrequently reported.[21–23] In some rare cases, the posterior fossa lesions are severe enough to cause hydrocephalus.[22,24] Occasionally, the cortex, the basal ganglia, and the temporal and frontal regions are involved.[24–26] Although abnormalities tend to be symmetric, the involvement is often asymmetric. The abnormalities are often apparent on computed tomography (CT) scans[24] (Fig. 28–2), but they are best appreciated on magnetic resonance

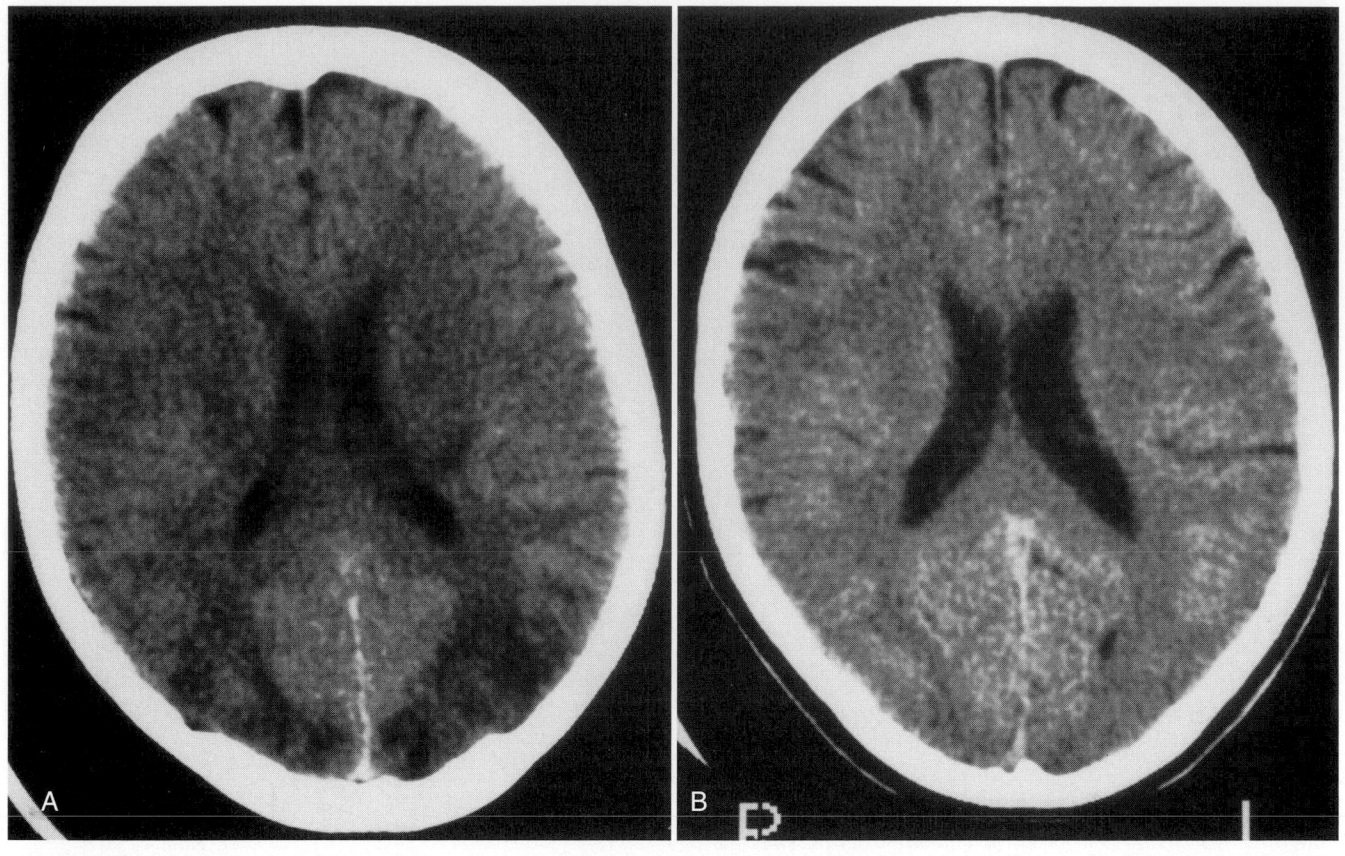

FIGURE 28–2 *Severe preeclampsia. Cortical blindness of sudden onset with complete clinical recovery after delivery. A, CT scan without contrast media, showing bilateral parieto-occipital hypodensities. B, Disappearance of the abnormalities on the follow-up CT scan.*

Specific Medical Diseases and Stroke

imaging (MRI) with T2 weighting or FLAIR (fluid-attenuated inversion recovery) sequences (Fig. 28–3).[26] Signal enhancement may be present, which can be explained by disruption of the blood-brain barrier.[26] In one patient, magnetic resonance spectroscopy showed a lower than normal ratio of N-acetyl-aspartate to creatinine in the occipital region, indicating neuronal dysfunction.[27] Gradient-echo imaging is the most sensitive technique for visualizing petechial hemorrhages.[24] Large parenchymal hemorrhages have been described in severe cases.[24,26,28]

Most patients studied by follow-up CT or MRI show improvement or resolution of white-matter abnormalities, suggesting transient edema rather than infarction. However, prospective differentiation between a reversible deficit and a permanent deficit is not possible with conventional MRI or CT. Diffusion-weighted imaging is a useful tool to distinguish between cytotoxic and vasogenic edema and therefore between permanent and potentially reversible lesions. Several studies using diffusion-weighted imaging and apparent coefficient diffusion maps in patients with hypertensive encephalopathy have shown increased diffusion consistent with vasogenic edema,[29–31] with a predominant watershed distribution.[32] The presence of both cytotoxic and vasogenic edema detected by diffusion-weighted imaging has also been reported in a woman with eclampsia; follow-up MRI showed that the regions of cytotoxic edema progressed to cerebral infarction.[33]

Both single-photon emission computed tomography (SPECT)[26] and perfusion imaging[10] have shown preserved or increased perfusion to edematous portions of the brain in patients with hypertensive encephalopathy. It is likely that these results depend on the time of imaging relative to the onset of therapy in patients with hypertensive encephalopathy. Current data tend to favor the theory that the condition begins with hyperperfusion, resulting in failure of autoregulation and breakthrough accumulation of vasogenic edema. In some severe cases, disturbed cerebral blood flow autoregulation may result in hypoperfusion and infarction, predominantly in the posterior border zones.

ETIOLOGY

Hypertensive encephalopathy occurs as a result of a sudden, sustained rise in blood pressure from any cause, sufficient to exceed the upper limit of cerebral blood flow autoregulation. Rapidly developing, fluctuating, or intermittent hypertension is associated with a particular risk for hypertensive encephalopathy. As would be predicted from the physiology of autoregulation (see earlier discussion), the extent of hypertension required to precipitate encephalopathy depends on the premorbid pressure.[7] Previously normotensive individuals can show signs of encephalopathy at blood pressures as low as 160 mm Hg

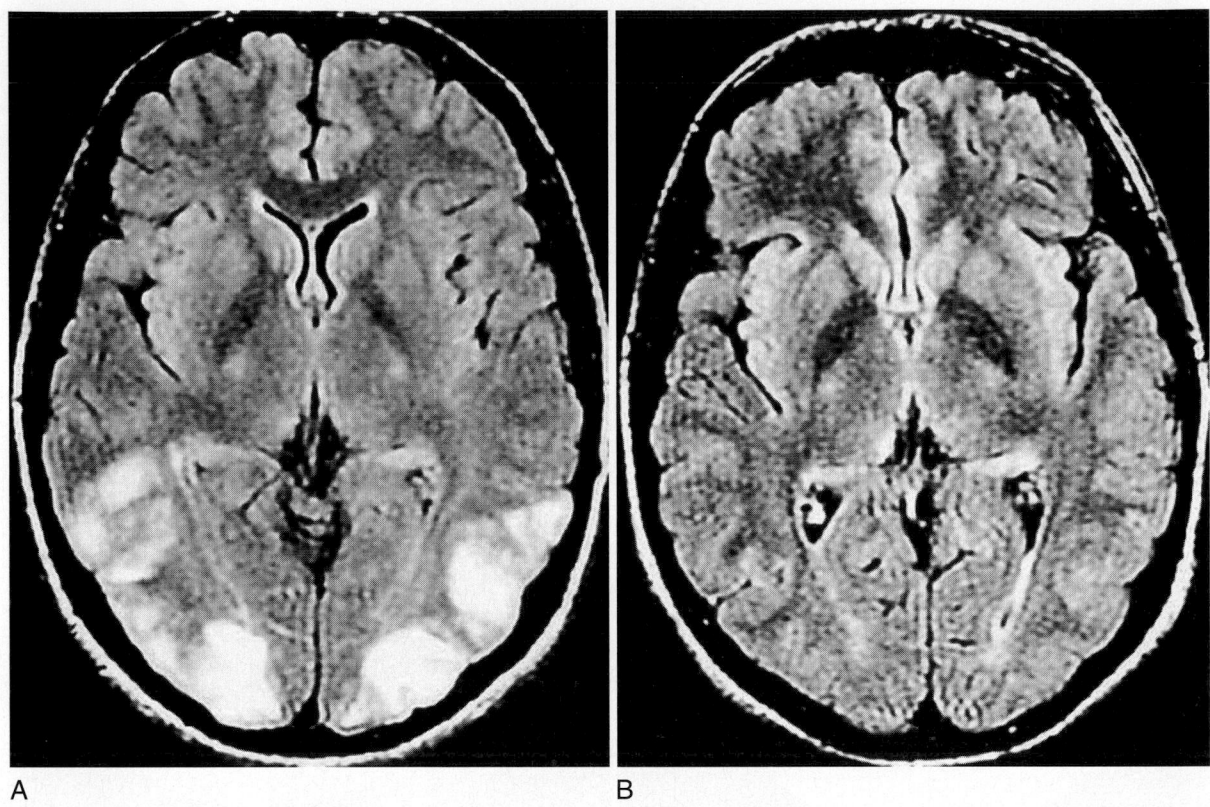

FIGURE 28–3 *Hypertensive encephalopathy in a 32-year-old man with thrombotic microangiopathy. A, MRI, axial FLAIR (fluid-attenuated inversion recovery) sequences. Bilateral high-signal areas in the occipital regions (normal diffusion-weighted images at similar level). B, Follow-up MRI 15 days later. Axial FLAIR sequences show complete regression of the lesions.*

systolic, 100 mm Hg diastolic (160/100 mm Hg).[4] The condition may occur at any age but is most common in the second to fourth decades of life.

Antihypertensive treatment has markedly reduced the incidence of hypertensive encephalopathy in individuals with known hypertension. However, abrupt elevations of blood pressure (characteristically, above 220/110 mm Hg) in patients with chronic hypertension who are receiving either no treatment or insufficient treatment or in patients whose treatment has been discontinued may cause hypertensive encephalopathy.[7] Acute or chronic renal diseases (glomerulonephritis,[24,34] nephrotic syndrome,[35] renal artery stenosis,[24] renal infarction,[36] renal failure[37]) are some of the most common causes of hypertensive encephalopathy. Whether the greater tendency toward development of hypertensive encephalopathy in patients with renal hypertension than in those with essential hypertension is related to increased circulating permeability factors or to endothelial damage remains to be determined.[38]

Eclampsia is usually considered a form of hypertensive encephalopathy, on the basis of similarities in clinical,[39] radiologic,[40,41] and pathologic features.[16,39] The fluid accumulation often observed during pregnancy may accentuate the tendency for brain edema to develop. The increase in peripheral resistance and blood pressure that characterizes preeclampsia may also be mediated, at least in part, by a substantial increase in sympathetic vasoconstrictor activity, as suggested by a study using intraneural recordings of sympathetic nerve activity in skeletal muscle nerve

fascicles of women with preeclampsia.[42] The precise mechanism underlying the increased sympathetic nerve activity remains to be determined, however. In eclampsia, a significant fall in cerebrovascular resistance and a loss of autoregulation resulting in cerebral overperfusion similar to that of hypertensive encephalopathy have been reported.[43] However, there is not always a good correlation between symptoms and signs of eclampsia and blood pressure levels.[44] Several findings suggest that vascular endothelial damage may play a role in eclampsia.[44,45] Endothelial damage is thought to be due to the secretion of trophoblastic cytotoxic factors originating from a poorly perfused fetal placental unit. Generalized endothelial dysfunction may lead to (1) increased sensitivity to normally circulating pressor agents and impaired synthesis of vasoactive compounds, which may result in vasospasm and reduced organ perfusion, (2) platelet activation with transitory platelet rich microvascular occlusion, (3) activation of the coagulation cascade, and (4) loss of fluid from the intravascular compartment.[46]

Other clinical situations associated with hypertensive encephalopathy are vasculitis (systemic lupus erythematosus,[47,48] polyarteritis nodosa[49]); endocrine disorders (pheochromocytoma,[23] primary aldosteronism[50]); porphyria[51]; thermal injury[52] and scorpion envenomation[53]; cocaine or amphetamine abuse[54]; and use of over-the-counter stimulants (phenylpropanolamine hydrochloride, ephedrine, pseudoephedrine, caffeine).[55] Hypertensive encephalopathy may also occur in previously normotensive patients after bilateral carotid endarterectomy in association with carotid baroreceptor failure syndrome.[56]

Hinchey and colleagues[20] reported on 15 patients with a reversible syndrome of headache, altered mental status, seizures, and visual loss, associated with posterior white matter changes on neuroimaging, that they termed reversible posterior leukoencephalopathy syndrome. Of the 15 patients, 7 were receiving immunosuppressive therapy (cyclosporine or tacrolimus) after transplantation or as treatment for aplastic anemia, 1 was receiving interferon-α for melanoma, 3 had eclampsia, and 4 had hypertensive encephalopathy. Most of these patients had an abrupt increase in blood pressure, but 3 of the 15 were normotensive.

This clinicoradiologic syndrome has been subsequently described in children[57] and has been recognized in a growing number of medical conditions, including disorders such as myeloproliferative disorders,[58] human immunodeficiency virus (HIV) infection,[59] thrombotic thrombocytopenic purpura,[60] and hemolytic-uremic syndrome[61]; treatment with erythropoeitin,[62] granulocyte-stimulating factor,[63] intravenous immune globulin,[64] interleukin,[65] cisplatin,[66] cytarabine,[67] and vincristine[68]; blood transfusion[69]; and exposure to contrast media.[70] Although most of the patients reported with these conditions had some degree of hypertension, blood pressure levels were usually lower than those typically encountered with pure hypertensive encephalopathy. In some patients, the lesions involved the gray matter and spread to the temporal and frontal regions, the brainstem and cerebellum, or both, and the reversibility of clinical and neuroradiologic abnormalities was not always complete.[27,57,71]

Failure of the autoregulatory capabilities of the cerebral vessels, itself resulting from various mechanisms such as hypertension and endothelial dysfunction, may represent a common pathophysiologic mechanism leading to this syndrome. Immunosuppressive drugs can damage the blood-brain barrier by various means—direct toxic effects on the vascular endothelium, vasoconstriction caused by release of endothelin, and increases in thromboxane and prostacyclin causing microthrombi.[20] The additional role of seizures has been suggested.[71] Seizures can result in elevations of blood pressure, regional hyperperfusion breakdown of the blood-brain barrier, and vasogenic edema.[72] Infectious or severe metabolic abnormalities (e.g., hyponatremia, hypomagnesemia, renal or hepatic dysfunction) may also be contributing factors.[73] Hypertension may therefore be the sole cause of the reversible posterior leukoencephalopathy syndrome or may act as a contributing factor.

TREATMENT

Hypertensive encephalopathy is one of the *hypertensive emergencies*, which are defined as situations requiring immediate blood pressure reduction (not necessarily to normal ranges) to prevent or limit target organ damage.[74] As there have been no large clinical trials, treatment of hypertensive encephalopathy is dictated by consensus.[4,74,75]

The aim should be to lower the mean arterial blood pressure by about 20% or the diastolic blood pressure to 100 mm Hg within the first hour.[4] If possible, the patient should be admitted to an intensive care unit, and the blood pressure lowered under constant monitoring. Intravenous administration of antihypertensive drugs is generally preferred. Excessive falls in pressure must be avoided, particularly in elderly patients and in patients with preexisting hypertension, because such drops may precipitate renal, cerebral, or coronary ischemia.[4,74] Although not based on evidence of efficacy, the use of anticonvulsants in patients with hypertensive encephalopathy who are having seizures is reasonable.[76]

Suitable agents in the management of hypertensive encephalopathy include sodium nitroprusside, labetalol, enalaprilat, and hydralazine.[4] Sodium nitroprusside, a short-acting arterial and venous dilator, should be given only by continuous intravenous infusion (0.25–10 μg/kg/min). It is commonly recommended as the first-line treatment for hypertensive emergencies, including hypertensive encephalopathy.[75] Although sodium nitroprusside has been reported to increase intracranial pressure, the contemporaneous fall in systemic vascular resistance seems to offset this effect. However, several of the following factors limit its use.[77] First, it is common for blood pressure to be unintentionally below a safe target level during treatment. Second, nitroprusside promotes baroreflex activation, causing tachycardia that can exacerbate acute coronary syndromes and heart failure. Another complication is cyanate or thiocyanate toxicity when the drug is given for a long period (days), especially in patients with hepatic or renal dysfunction. Finally, nitroprusside infusion requires intra-arterial monitoring of blood pressure, which may not otherwise be required.

Labetalol has both α-blocking and β-blocking activities.[78] The β-blocking effect of labetalol is about a fifth that of propranolol. It is administered as continuous infusion. Adverse effects include nausea, vomiting, and flushing. Bradycardia, heart block, bronchospasm, and heart failure can also complicate its use. Enalaprilat, an intravenously administered, rapidly acting angiotensin-converting enzyme inhibitor, can be used safely in hypertensive encephalopathy.[79] However, angiotensin-converting enzyme inhibitors should be used cautiously in patients who are hypovolemic or have underlying renal artery stenosis, because these agents can cause precipitous drops in blood pressure. Hydralazine, a direct-acting vasodilator, does not have adverse effects on renal function. Common side effects of this agent are reflex tachycardia, hypotension, and fluid retention. It may increase cardiac work and therefore must be given cautiously to patients with coronary artery disease. Other parenteral drugs used for hypertensive emergencies are nicardipine, a calcium channel antagonist, and fenoldopam, a selective post-synaptic dopamine$_1$ receptor agonist.[74] Reported side effects of fenoldopam include headache, flushing, and increased intraocular pressure. Clonidine should be avoided because it is a central nervous system depressant. Oral therapy should be instituted before parenteral agents are discontinued.

The management of hypertensive encephalopathy also includes early recognition and withdrawal of exacerbating factors such as immunosuppressive drugs.[4] Delivery is the ultimate cure for eclampsia. If convulsions have occurred, parenteral magnesium sulfate is the treatment of choice.[80] The role of prophylactic magnesium sulfate in preeclampsia is less clear. There is also long-standing experience with several suitable antihypertensive drugs. The parenteral

Specific Medical Diseases and Stroke

antihypertensive drugs most commonly used during pregnancy are hydralazine, labetalol, and nifedipine, but trials persistently show that hydralazine is inferior to the other two drugs.[51] Angiotensin-converting enzyme inhibitors and angiotensin receptor antagonists are contraindicated in pregnancy because of unacceptable fetal side effects.

References

1. Oppenheimer BS, Fishberg AM: Hypertensive encephalopathy. Arch Intern Med 41:264–278, 1928.
2. Strandgaard S, Paulson OB: Cerebral autoregulation. Stroke 15:413–416, 1984.
3. Paulson OB, Strandgaard S, Edvinsson L: Cerebral autoregulation. Cerebrovasc Brain Metab Rev 2:161–192, 1990.
4. Vaughan CJ, Delanty N: Hypertensive emergencies. Lancet 356:411–417, 2000.
5. Heistad DD: What's new in the cerebral microcirculation? Microcirculation 8:365–375, 2001.
6. Strangaard S, Paulson OB: Hypertensive disease and the cerebral circulation. In Laragh J, Brenner B (eds): Hypertension: Physiopathology, Diagnosis and Management. New York, Raven Press, 1990, pp 399–416.
7. Phillips SJ, Whisnant JP: Hypertension and the brain. National High Blood Pressure Education Program. Arch Intern Med 152:938–945, 1992.
8. Dinsdale HB: Hypertensive encephalopathy. Stroke 13:717–719, 1982.
9. Hulse JA, Taylor DSI, Dillon MJ: Blindness and paraplegia in severe childhood hypertension. Lancet 2(8142):553, 1979.
10. Jones BV, Egelhoff JC, Patterson RJ: Hypertensive encephalopathy in children. AJNR Am J Neuroradiol 18:101–106, 1997.
11. Byrom FB: The pathogenesis of hypertensive encephalopathy and its relation to the malignant phase of hypertension: Experimental evidence from the hypertensive rat. Lancet 2:201–211, 1954.
12. Dinsdale HB, Robertson DM, Haas RA: Cerebral blood flow in acute hypertension. Arch Neurol 31:80, 1974.
13. Sundt TJ: The cerebral autonomic nervous system: A proposed physiologic function and pathophysiologic response in subarachnoid hemorrhage and in focal cerebral ischemia. Mayo Clin Proc 48:127–137, 1973.
14. Beausang-Linder M, Bill A: Cerebral circulation in acute arterial hypertension: Protective effect of sympathetic nervous activity. Physiol Scand 111:193–199, 1981.
15. Chester EM, Agamanolis DP, Banker BQ, Victor M: Hypertensive encephalopathy: A clinicopathologic study of 20 cases. Neurology 28:928–939, 1978.
16. Richards A, Graham D, Bullock R: Clinicopathological study of neurological complications due to hypertensive disorders of pregnancy. J Neurol Neurosurg Psychiatry 51:416–421, 1988.
17. Healton EB, Brust JC, Feinfeld DA, Thomson GE: Hypertensive encephalopathy and the neurologic manifestations of malignant hypertension. Neurology 32:127–132, 1982.
18. Tallaksen CM, Kerty E, Bakke S: Visual hallucinations in a case of reversible hypertension-induced brain edema. Eur J Neurol 5:615–618, 1998.
19. Bakshi R, Bates V, Mechtler L, et al: Occipital seizures as the major clinical manifestation of reversible posterior leukoencephalopathy syndrome: Magnetic resonance imaging findings. Epilepsia 39:296–299, 1998.
20. Hinchey J, Chaves C, Appignani B, et al: A reversible posterior leukoencephalopathy syndrome. N Engl J Med 334:494–500, 1996.
21. Chang GY, Keane JR: Hypertensive brainstem encephalopathy: Three cases presenting with severe brainstem edema. Neurology 53:652–654, 1999.
22. Wang MC, Escott EJ, Breeze RE: Posterior fossa swelling and hydrocephalus resulting from hypertensive encephalopathy: Case report and review of the literature. Neurosurgery 44:1325–1327, 1999.
23. Sèze JD, Mastain B, Stojkovic T, et al: Unusual MR findings of the brainstem in arterial hypertension. AJNR Am J Neuroradiol 21:391–394, 2000.
24. Weingarten K, Barbut D, Filippi C, Zimmerman RD: Acute hypertensive encephalopathy: Findings on spin-echo and gradient-echo MR imaging. AJR 162:665–670, 1994.
25. Sanders TG, Clayman DA, Sanchez-Ramos L, et al: Brain in eclampsia: MR imaging with clinical correlations. Radiology 180:475–478, 1991.
26. Schwartz RB, Jones KM, Kalina P, et al: Hypertensive encephalopathy: Findings on CT, MR imaging, and SPECT imaging in 14 cases. AJR 159:379–383, 1992.
27. Pavlakis SG, Frank Y, Kalina P, et al: Occipital-parietal encephalopathy: A new name for an old syndrome. Pediatr Neurol 16:145–148, 1997.
28. Schwartz RB, Bravo SM, Klufas RA, et al: Cyclosporine neurotoxicity and its relationship to hypertensive encephalopathy: CT and MR findings in 16 cases. AJR 165:627–631, 1995.
29. Friese S, Fetter M, Küker W: Extensive brainstem edema in eclampsia: Diffusion-weighted MRI may indicate a favorable prognosis. J Neurol 247:465–466, 2000.
30. Schaefer PW, Buonanno FS, Gonzales RG, Schwamm LH: Diffusion-weighted imaging discriminates between cytotoxic and vasogenic edema in a patient with eclampsia. Stroke 28:1082–1085, 1997.
31. Schwartz RB, Mulkern RV, Gudbjartsson H, Jolesz F: Diffusion-weighted MR imaging in hypertensive encephalopathy: Clues to pathogenesis. AJNR Am J Neuroradiol 19:859–862, 1998.
32. Engelter ST, Provenzale JM, Petrella JR: Assessment of vasogenic edema in eclampsia using diffusion imaging. Neuroradiology 42:818–820, 2000.
33. Koch S, Rabinstein A, Falcone S, Forteza A: Diffusion-weighted imaging shows cytotoxic and vasogenic edema in eclampsia. AJNR Am J Neuroradiol 22:1068–1070, 2001.
34. Sheth RD, Riggs JE, Bodensteiner JB, et al: Parieto-occipital edema in hypertensive encephalopathy: A pathogenic mechanism. Eur Neurol 36:25–28, 1996.
35. Assadi FK, Lansky LL, John EG, et al: Acute hypertensive encephalopathy in minimal change nephrotic syndrome. Child Nephrol Urol 10:96–99, 1990.
36. Christophe JL, Plaen JFD, Goffette P, Lambert M: Severe hypertension and renal infarct: Physiopathology and treatment. Nephrologie 14:133–137, 1993.
37. Sharer K, Benninger C, Heimann A, Rascher W: Involvement of the central nervous system in renal hypertension. Eur J Pediatr 152:59–63, 1993.
38. Johansson BB: Hypertension and the blood-brain barrier. In Neewell E (ed): Implications of the Blood-Brain Barrier and its Manipulation, vol 2. New York, Plenum, 1989, pp 389–410.
39. Donaldson JO: Eclampsia. In Donaldson J (ed): Neurology of Pregnancy. London, WB Saunders, 1989, pp 269–310.
40. Digre KB, Varner MW, Osborn AG, Crawford S: Cranial magnetic resonance imaging in severe preeclampsia vs eclampsia. Arch Neurol 50:399–406, 1993.
41. Manfredi M, Beltramello A, Bongiovanni LG, et al: Eclamptic encephalopathy: Imaging and pathogenetic considerations. Acta Neurol Scand 96:277–282, 1997.
42. Schobel HP, Fischer T, Heuszer K, et al: Preeclampsia—a state of sympathetic overactivity. N Engl J Med 335:1480–1485, 1996.
43. Williams K, Wilson S: Persistence of cerebral hemodynamic changes in patients with eclampsia: A report of three cases. Am J Obstet Gynecol 181:1162–1165, 1999.
44. Schwartz RB, Feske SK, Polak JF, et al: Preeclampsia-eclampsia: Clinical and neuroradiographic correlates and insights into the pathogenesis of hypertensive encephalopathy. Radiology 217:371–376, 2000.
45. Mas JL, Lamy C: Severe preeclampsia/eclampsia: Hypertensive encephalopathy of pregnancy? Cerebrovasc Dis 8:53–58, 1998.
46. Roberts JM, Redman CWG: Pre-eclampsia: More than pregnancy-induced hypertension. Lancet 341:1447–1450, 1993.
47. Wong KL, Woo EK, Yu YL, Wong RW: Neurological manifestations of systemic lupus erythematosus. Q J Med 81:857–870, 1991.
48. Primavera A, Audenino D, Mavilio N, Cocito L: Reversible posterior leukoencephalopathy syndrome in systemic lupus and vasculitis. Ann Rheum Dis 60:534–537, 2001.
49. Vora J, Cooper J, Thomas JP: Polyarteritis nodosa presenting with hypertensive encephalopathy. Br J Clin Pract 46:144–145, 1992.
50. Kaplan NM: Primary aldosteronism with malignant hypertension. N Engl J Med 269:1282–1286, 1963.
51. Kupferschmidt H, Bont A, Schnorf H, et al: Transient cortical blindness and biocciptal brain lesions in two patients with acute intermittent porphyria. Ann Intern Med 123:598–600, 1995.
52. Popp MB, Friedberg DL, MacMillan BG: Clinical characteristics of hypertension in burned children. Ann Surg 191:473–478, 1980.

53. Sofer S, Gueron M: Vasodilatation and hypertensive encephalopathy following scorpion envenomation in children. Chest 97:118–120, 1990.

54. Grewal RP, Miller BL: Cocaine-induced hypertensive encephalopathy. Acta Neurol (Napoli) 13:279–281, 1991.

55. Lake CR, Gallant S, Masson E, Miller P: Adverse drugs effects attributed to phenylpropanolamine: A review of 142 case reports. Am J Med 89:195–208, 1990.

56. Ille O, Woimant F, Pruna A, et al: Hypertensive encephalopathy after bilateral endarterectomy. Stroke 26:488–491, 1995.

57. Pavlakis SG, Frank Y, Chusid R: Hypertensive encephalopathy, reversible occipitoparietal encephalopathy or reversible posterior leukoencephalopathy: Three names for an old syndrome. J Child Neurol 14:277–281, 1999.

58. Cooney M, Bradley W, Symko S, et al: Hypertensive encephalopathy: Complication in children treated for myeloproliferative disorders—report of three cases. Radiology 214:711–716, 2000.

59. Frank Y, Pavlakis S, Black K, Bakshi S: Reversible occipital-parietal encephalopathy syndrome in an HIV-infected child. Neurology 51:915–916, 1998.

60. Bakshi R, Shaikh Z, Bates V, Kinkel P: Thrombotic thrombocytopenic purpura: Brain CT and MRI findings in 12 patients. Neurology 52:1285–1288, 1999.

61. Taylor MB, Jackson A, Weller JM: Dynamic susceptibility contrast enhanced MRI in reversible posterior leukoencephalopathy syndrome associated with haemolytic uraemic syndrome. Br J Radiol 73:438–442, 2000.

62. Delanty N, Vaughan C, Frucht S, Stubgen P: Erythropoietin-associated hypertensive posterior leukoencephalopathy. Neurology 49:686–689, 1997.

63. Leniger T, Kastrup O, Diener HC: Reversible posterior leukoencephalopathy syndrome induced by granulocyte stimulating factor filgrastim. J Neurol Neurosurg Psychiatry 69:280–281, 2000.

64. Mathy I, Gille M, Raemdonck FV, et al: Neurological complications of intravenous immunoglobulin (IVIg) therapy: An illustrative case of acute encephalopathy following IVIg therapy and a review of the literature. Acta Neurol Belg 98:347–351, 1998.

65. Karp BI, Yang JC, Khorsand M, et al: Multiple cerebral lesions complicating therapy with interleukin-2. Neurology 47:417–424, 1996.

66. Ito Y, Arahata Y, Goto Y, et al: Cisplatin neurotoxicity presenting as reversible posterior leukoencephalopathy syndrome. AJNR Am J Neuroradiol 19:415–417, 1998.

67. Vaughn DJ, Jarvik JG, Hackney D, et al: High-dose cytarabine neurotoxicity: MR findings during the acute phase. AJNR Am J Neuroradiol 14:1014–1016, 1993.

68. Hurwitz RL, Mahoney DH, Armstrong DL, Browder TM: Reversible encephalopathy and seizures as a result of conventional vincristine administration. Med Pediatr Oncol 16:216–219, 1988.

69. Ito Y, Niwa H, Iida T, et al: Post-transfusion reversible posterior leukoencephalopathy syndrome with cerebral vasoconstriction. Neurology 49:1174–1175, 1997.

70. Sticherling C, Berkefeld J, Auch-Schwelk W, Landfermann H: Transient bilateral cortical blindness after coronary angiography. Lancet 351:570, 1998.

71. Dillon WP, Rowley H: The reversible posterior cerebral edema syndrome. AJNR Am J Neuroradiol 19:591, 1998.

72. Yaffe K, Ferriero D, Barkovitch AJ, Rowley H: Reversible MRI abnormalities following seizures. Neurology 45:104–108, 1995.

73. Ay H, Buonanno F, Schaefer P, et al: Posterior leukoencephalopathy without severe hypertension: Utility of diffusion-weighted MRI. Neurology 51:1369–1376, 1998.

74. Sixth report of the Joint National Committee on Prevention, Detection, Evaluation, and Treatment of High Blood Pressure. Arch Intern Med 157:2413–2446, 1997.

75. Calhoun DA, Oparil S: Treatment of hypertensive crisis. N Engl J Med 323:1177–1183, 1990.

76. Delanty N, Vaughan CJ, French JA: Medical causes of seizures. Lancet 352:383–390, 1998.

77. Blumenfeld JD, Laragh JH: Management of hypertensive crises: The scientific basis for treatment decisions. Am J Hypertens 14:1154–1167, 2001.

78. Wilson DJ, Wallin JD, Vlachakis ND: Intravenous labetalol in the treatment of severe hypertension and hypertensive emergencies. Am J Med 75 (Suppl):95–102, 1983.

79. Hirschl MM, Binder M, Bur A, et al: Clinical evaluation of different doses of intravenous enalaprilat in patients with hypertensive crisis. Arch Intern Med 155:2217–2223, 1995.

80. Duley L, Carroli G, Belizan J, et al: Which anticonvulsant for women with eclampsia? Lancet 345:1455–1463, 1995.

81. Walker JJ: Pre-eclampsia. Lancet 356:1260–1265, 2000.

Specific Medical Diseases and Stroke

Chapter Twenty-Nine

Vascular Cognitive Impairment and Dementia

Timo Erkinjuntti

Vascular dementias (VaDs) are the second most common cause of dementia.[1-5] Cerebrovascular disease (CVD) relates also to a high risk of cognitive impairment and dementia.[6,7] In addition, vascular factors such as coexisting stroke and white matter lesions (WMLs) relate to Alzheimer's disease (AD).[8] Thus, vascular causes are an important factor in cognitive impairment worldwide.[9]

The primary cause of clinical deficits in VaD is CVD with ischemic brain injury.[10] However, the multiplicity of vascular causes, associated risk factors, and clinical manifestations of dementia related to CVD make VaD a complex area of research.[10-12] Even though a number of sets of diagnostic criteria have been produced for epidemiologic studies of VaD, opinions are divided over the definition of VaD subtypes. How wide should the definition of VaD be, and which patients should be excluded from a diagnosis of VaD?

Further debate centers on difficulties in distinguishing dementia due to AD from that arising from CVD, because there are large overlaps in clinical signs and symptoms. Both result in cognitive, functional, and behavioral impairment. There are also similarities in the pathophysiologic mechanisms (e.g., WMLs, delayed neuronal death, apoptosis),[8,13,14] associated risk factors (e.g. age, education, arterial hypertension)[14,15] and neurochemical deficits (e.g., cholinergic dysfunction)[16,17] of these two causes of dementia.

Even more important, however, is the coexistence of AD and VaD in a large proportion of patients.[5,18,19] AD with CVD (sometimes referred to as *mixed dementia*) could manifest clinically either as AD with evidence of cerebrovascular lesions in brain imaging or with features of both AD and VaD.[20] On the basis of the findings from the Nun Study, it has been suggested that CVD may play an important role in determining the presence and severity of clinical symptoms of AD.[8] Either way, the prevalence of AD with CVD has previously been underestimated, and may exceed 30%.[18]

Aside from AD, the large number of different vascular etiologies and accessory risk factors in VaD introduce a high degree of heterogeneity in clinical subtypes of VaD. Varied progression paths are seen, so that abrupt onset and stepwise progression occur in some patients, but an insidious onset with a uniformly progressive course is observed in others.[21-23] This heterogeneity gives rise to difficulties in clinical and neuropathologic diagnosis as well as in the classification and monitoring of VaD. Neuroimaging findings of vascular lesions and the associated brain disease, combined with epidemiologic evidence from surveys of clinical deficits, are vital in establishing classifications of VaD subtypes. Findings from such studies have so far succeeded in identifying the most common types of cerebrovascular lesions associated with the onset of dementia. They include multiple corticosubcortical infarcts, strategically located single infarcts, and small vessel disease with lacunar infarcts and ischemic white matter disease. The clinical deficits commonly associated with these subtypes have also been elucidated.[23-25] VaD can now be seen as a group of syndromes rather than a single disease. Indeed, debate has now raised the possibility of using the "umbrella" term *vascular cognitive impairment* (VCI), which can apply in all patients with dementia associated with CVD and may or may not include AD with CVD.[5,20,25]

Critical elements of the concept and diagnosis of VaD include the identification of vascular changes and subsequent brain disease and a description of the characteristics of cognitive dementia syndrome (type, extent, and combination of impairments in different cognitive domains). Accessory clinical deficits, such as focal neurologic symptoms, also form an important part of the overall clinical picture in VaD. This chapter focuses on the pathology and clinical diagnosis of the most common VaD subtypes. It also addresses similarities and differences in AD in relation to differential diagnoses in VaD.

HISTORICAL BACKGROUND

As early as 1896, "arteriosclerotic dementia" (referring to VaD) was separated from "senile dementia" (referring to AD).[26] Alois Alzheimer, together with Otto Binswanger, recognized the heterogeneity of VaD by describing four clinicopathologic variants of VaD as well as vascular lesions in the Alzheimer brain. Nevertheless, until the 1960s and 1970s, cerebral atherosclerosis causing chronic strangulation of blood supply to the brain was thought to be the most common cause of dementia, and AD was regarded as a rare cause affecting only younger patients. Tomlinson and colleagues[27] redefined AD as the cause of dementia more common than arteriosclerosis. In 1979, Hachinski and associates[28] used the term *multi-infarct dementia* (MID) to describe the mechanism by which they considered VaD to be produced. As the pendulum swung in the direction of AD, vascular forms of dementia became relegated to a position of relative obscurity.[29]

Even though VaD was regarded as a dementia caused by small or large brain infarcts (MID) until the 1990s,[28,30] there is now a resurgence of interest in the whole spectrum of vascular causes of cognitive impairment and dementia.[31] The original findings of Alois Alzheimer have been "reinvented." New data have been collected that highlight complex interactions among vascular causes, changes in the brain, host factors, and cognition.[32–36] Recognition of the heterogeneity of VaDs has also fueled the discussion. Furthermore, the facts that vascular factors relate and coexist with AD have strengthened interest in the vascular burden of cognition.[14,18]

EPIDEMIOLOGY

Our understanding of the population distribution of VCI and its outcomes are subject to the variety of definitions used to identify it.[2,4] For example, if mixed AD-VaD is included in the definition, as argued elsewhere,[19] VCI may even be the most common cause of chronic progressive cognitive impairment in elderly people.

Prevalence

The prevalence of VCI has been estimated at 5% of people older than 65 years in the Canadian Study of Health and Aging (CSHA).[5] This figure included patients with VCI that did not meet the criteria for dementia. Such patients are a subset of the group said to have "Cognitive Impairment, No Dementia—CIND," which herein is called *vascular CIND*. The prevalence of vascular CIND in the CSHA was 2.4%, that of mixed AD-VaD 0.9%, and that of VaD 1.5%. By contrast, in the same study, the prevalence of AD without a vascular component was 5.1%, and at all ages up to 85 years, this disorder was less common than VCI. There was no clear sex differential in VCI or its subtypes.

As traditionally conceived, VaD is the second most common single cause of dementia, accounting for 10% to 50% of the cases, depending on the geographic location, patient population, and clinical methods used.[1,2,4] The prevalence of VaD has been reported as higher in China and Japan than in Europe and the United States.

The prevalence of VaD ranges from 1.2% to 4.2% in persons 65 years and older.[1] In a 1990s European collaborative study using population-based studies of persons 65 years and older, the age-standardized prevalence of dementia was 6.4% (all causes); that for AD was 4.4%, and that for VaD, 1.6%.[4] In this study, 15.8% of the patients had VaD and 53.7% had AD. The prevalence ranged from 0.0% to 0.8% in patients aged 65 to 69 years, and from 2% to 8.3% in patients 90 years and older in different studies. There was a difference in prevalence between men and women. In patients younger than 85 years, the prevalence

of VaD was higher in men compared than in women; thereafter, the prevalence was higher in women. The pooled prevalences for age groups were as follows:

65 to 69 years: 0.5% in men, 0.1% in women
70 to 74 years: 0.8% in men, 0.6% in women
75 to 79 years: 1.9% in men, 0.9% in women
80 to 84 years: 2.4% in men, 2.3% in women
85 to 89 years: 2.4% in men, 3.5% in women
90 years and older: 3.0 % in men, 5.8% in women

Incidence

The incidence of VaD has varied from 6 to 12 cases per year in 1000 persons aged 70 years and older.[1] The incidence of VaD rises with increasing age, without any substantial difference between men and women in a 2000 European collaborative study.[37] In that study, the pooled incidence rates of VaD per 1000 person-years were 0.7% in patients 65 to 69 years old; 1.2% in those 70 to 74 years old; 3.5% in those 75 to 79 years old; 5.9% in those 80 to 84 years old; 6.1% in those 85 to 89 years old; and 8.1% in those 90 years and older.[37]

Prognosis

In the CSHA, the mean duration of survival in VCI was 41 months.[5] The highest impact on mortality arose from VaD in women, for whom 5-year mortality rates were 60% in those aged 65 to 74 years old and 83% in those older than 85 years. Overall, the mortality rate ratio was highest for women with VaD aged 65 to 74 years, at 10.1 (95% confidence interval [CI], 5.27–19.4).[38] In general, survival for patients with VaD is around 5 years,[1] shorter than that for the general population or patients with AD.[39,40] Also, poststroke dementia is an independent predictor of mortality.[41] Detailed studies on the natural history of subcortical and cortical VaD are lacking, and little is known or can be predicted about the rate and pattern of cognitive decline and prognosis in VaD.[21]

STROKE AND DEMENTIA

Stroke and dementia show numerous points of interrelatedness. These intersections provide opportunities to advance our understanding of both syndromes.

Dementia after Stroke

Stroke raises the risk for dementia. The frequency of dementia in a Japanese community-based study was 27.2% in patients with history of stroke and 3.4% in controls.[42] In a New York study, the prevalence of dementia 3 months after an ischemic stroke in patients 60 years or older was 26.3%—a figure 9-fold higher than that in a stroke-free control group.[6] The risk was highest in patients 70 to 79 years of age, with an odds ratio (OR) of 31.2. In the Helsinki Stroke Aging Memory Study, the frequency of dementia, as defined by the DSM-III (American Psychiatric Association's *Diagnostic and Statistical Manual of Mental Disorders*, 3rd edition), 3 months after stroke was 25%; for patients aged 55 to 64 years, the frequency was

19%; for those 65 to 74 years, 24%; and for those 75 to 85 years, 32%.[43]

The frequencies of dementia reported after stroke in these studies are higher than those associated with any other known risk factor for dementia. In the New York study, stroke was the underlying cause of dementia in 56.1% of cases of dementia, whereas 36.4% of cases was presumably due to the cumulative effects of stroke and AD.[6] In the Helsinki study, the frequency of stroke-related dementia was 67.8 %.[43] Patients with stroke have also an increased risk of dementia; 1 year after stroke, the probability of new-onset dementia was 5.4% in patients older than 60 years, and 10.4% in patients older than 90 years.[36] Four years after a first lacunar infarct, 23.1% of patients demonstrate dementia—a rate 4 to 12 times that in controls.[44] Even after exclusion of patients who have dementia 3 months after an ischemic stroke, the relative risk of dementia within 4 years is 5.5.[7] In the community-based Rochester study, the standardized morbidity ratio for new-onset dementia was 8.6% for patients in the first year after stroke, and the rate of new-onset dementia doubled during the follow-up.[45] The incidence rate of AD after stroke is also doubled, suggesting that stroke may induce an earlier expression of AD.[45]

Stroke after Dementia

Interestingly, dementia also increases the risk of stroke. Two cohort studies have shown that prevalent dementia is associated with incident stroke, even after adjustment for other potential confounding variables.[46,47] An important interpretation of these data is that they may signal some forms of cognitive impairment as manifestations of cerebrovascular ischemia.

ETIOLOGY AND PATHOPHYSIOLOGY

VCI as a general entity includes many syndromes, which themselves reflect a variety of vascular mechanisms and changes in the brain with different causes and clinical manifestations. The pathophysiology of VaD incorporates interactions among vascular causes (CVD and vascular risk factors), changes in the brain (infarcts, WMLs, atrophy), host factors (age, education), and cognition.[32–36]

Causes of VaD consist of both CVDs and risk factors (Table 29–1). The main CVDs are large artery disease, cardiac embolic events, and small vessel and hemodynamic mechanisms.[48–52]

Risk factors in VaDs include risk factors for CVD, stroke, and WMLs, and also those for any cognitive decline and AD (see Table 29–1).[32]

Changes in the brain related to VaD include arterial territorial infarcts, distal field (watershed) infarcts, lacunar infarcts, ischemic WMLs, and incomplete ischemic injury.[35,36,48,49] In addition, both focal (around the ischemic lesion) and remote (disconnection, diaschisis) functional ischemic changes relate to VaD.[53]

Relationship between vascular factors and cognition is essential; thus, critical clinical issues include whether the identified vascular factors cause, compound, or only coexist with the VaD syndrome,[7,54] whether they contribute to the risk and clinical picture of AD,[8,33] and which type, extent,

Table 29.1   Causes of Vascular Dementia

Cerebrovascular disorders	Risk factors
Large artery disease	Arterial hypertension
Artery-to-artery embolism	Atrial fibrillation
Occlusion of an extracranial or	Cardiac abnormalities
intracranial artery	Myocardial infarction
Cardiac embolic events	Coronary heart disease
Small vessel disease	Diabetes
Lacunar infarcts	Generalized atherosclerosis
Ischemic white matter lesions	High cholesterol
Hemodynamic mechanisms	Smoking
Specific arteriopathies	Advamced age
Hemorrhages	Low education
Intracranial hemorrhage	
Subarachnoidal hemorrhage	
Hematologic factors	
Venous diseases	
Hereditary entities	

side, site, and tempo of vascular lesions in the brain relate to different types of VaD.[34–36,48]

CLINICAL CRITERIA

Since the 1970s, several clinical criteria for VaD have been used.[55–57] The criteria most widely used for VaD are as follows:

- American Psychiatric Association's *Diagnostic and Statistical Manual of Mental Disorders*, 4th ed (DSM-IV)[58]
- World Health Organization's International Classification of Diseases of the World, 10th revision (ICD-10), classification[59]
- State of California's Alzheimer's Disease Diagnostic and Treatment Centers (ADDTC) criteria[60]
- National Institute of Neurological Diseases and Stroke–Association Internationale pour la Recherche et l'Enseignement en Neurosciences (NINDS-AIREN) research criteria[61]

The two cardinal elements implemented in the clinical criteria for VaD are (1) the definition of the cognitive syndrome of dementia[62] and (2) the definition of the vascular cause of the dementia.[56,57,63] Variation in defining these two critical elements has meant that different definitions in use give different point prevalence estimates, identify different groups of subjects, and consequently also identify different types and distributions of brain lesions.[43,57,62,64,65] Further, this heterogeneity may have been a factor in the negative results reported for prior clinical trials on VaD.[66]

All the clinical criteria used are consensus criteria, which are neither derived from prospective community-based studies on vascular factors affecting the cognition nor based on detailed natural histories.[55,56,60,61,67] All the cited criteria are based mainly on the ischemic infarct concept and designed to have high specificity, although they have been poorly implemented and validated.[55,67]

The DSM-IV definition of VaD requires focal neurologic signs and symptoms or laboratory evidence of focal neurologic damage clinically judged to be related to the disturbance.[58] The course is specified by sudden cognitive and functional losses. The DSM-IV criteria do not detail brain imaging requirements. The DSM-IV definition for VaD is broad and lacks detailed clinical and radiologic guidelines.

The ICD-10 criteria require unequal distribution of cognitive deficits, focal signs as evidence of focal brain damage, and significant CVD judged to be etiologically related to the dementia.[59] The criteria do not detail brain imaging requirements. The shortcomings of these criteria include lack of detailed guidelines (e.g., unequal cognitive deficits and neuroimaging), lack of etiologic cues, and heterogeneity.[57,63]

The ADDTC criteria are used exclusively for ischemic vascular dementia (IVD).[60] They require either (1) evidence of two or more ischemic strokes in the history, neurologic signs, or neuroimaging studies (computed tomography [CT] or T1-weighted magnetic resonance imaging [MRI]) or (2) in the case of a single stroke, a clearly documented temporal relationship (not specified in detail), and, always, neuroradiologic evidence of at least one infarct outside the cerebellum. Ischemic WMLs on CT or MRI do not qualify as brain imaging evidence of probable IVD but may support a diagnosis of possible IVD. The criteria list features supporting the diagnosis, as well as a list of features casting doubt on a diagnosis of probable IVD.

The NINDS-AIREN research criteria for VaD include dementia syndrome, cerebrovascular disease, and a relationship between those.[61] CVD is defined as the presence of focal neurologic signs and detailed brain imaging evidence of ischemic changes in the brain. A relationship between dementia and cerebrovascular disorder is based either on the onset of dementia within 3 months after a recognized stroke or on abrupt deterioration in cognitive functions or fluctuating, stepwise progression of cognitive deficits. The criteria include a list of features consistent with the diagnosis as well as a list of features that make the diagnosis uncertain or unlikely. Also, different levels of certainty of the clinical diagnosis (probable, possible, definite) are included. The inter-rater reliability of the NINDS-AIREN criteria has been shown to be moderate to substantial (κ 0.46 to 0.72).[68]

Comparison of Clinical Criteria

The current criteria for VaD are not interchangeable; they identify different numbers and cluster of patients labeled as VaD. The DSM-IV criteria are less restrictive compared with the ICD-10, ADDTC, and the NINDS-AIREN criteria.[57,69] The ADDTC criteria seem to be more sensitive, and the NINDS-AIREN criteria more specific.[70]

Heterogeneity of patient populations derived through the use of current criteria has highlighted the need for an updated systematization. One suggestion has been that dividing VaD into subtypes would enable a more homogenous group of patients to be identified. A development in this area is the new research criteria for subcortical ischemic vascular disease and dementia (SIVD).[71]

MAIN SUBTYPES

The subtypes of VaD identified in current classifications are cortical VaD or MID, SIVD or small vessel dementia,

Table 29.2 Vascular Mechanisms and Changes in the Brain in Main Subtypes of Vascular Dementia

Vascular Mechanism	Changes in the Brain
Cortical vascular dementia or multi-infarct dementia	
Large vessel disease	Arterial territorial infarct
Cardiac embolic events	Distal field (watershed) infarct
Hypoperfusion	
Strategic infarct dementia	
Large vessel disease	Arterial territorial infarct
Cardiac embolic events	Distal field (watershed) infarct
Small vessel disease	Lacunar infarct
Hypoperfusion	Focal and diffuse white matter lesions
Subcortical vascular dementia or small vessel dementia	
Small vessel disease	Lacunar infarct
Hypoperfusion	Focal and diffuse white matter lesions
Incomplete ischemic injury	

and strategic infarct dementia.[49,51,61,72–75] Many researchers also include hypoperfusion dementia.[49,61,74,76] Further subtypes suggested are hemorrhagic dementia, hereditary vascular dementia, and AD with CVD (combined or mixed dementia).

Cortical VaD (MID) relates to large vessel disease, cardiac embolic events, and also hypoperfusion (Table 29–2). It shows predominantly cortical and cortico-subcortical arterial territorial and distal field (watershed) infarcts. Typical clinical features are lateralized sensori-motor changes and abrupt onset of cognitive impairment and aphasia.[73,77] In addition, some combination of different cortical neuropsychological syndromes has been suggested to be present in cortical VaD.[78]

In strategic infarct dementia, focal, often small, ischemic lesions involving specific sites critical for higher cortical functions have been classified separately. Of the cortical sites, the hippocampal formation, angular gyrus, and gyrus cinguli are examples. The subcortical sites include thalamus, fornix, basal forebrain, caudate, globus pallidus, and the genu or anterior limb of the internal capsule.[30,36,48] Depending on the strategic location in question, the time course and clinical features vary considerably.

SIVD with VaD incorporates two entities, "the lacunar state" and Binswanger's disease. It relates to small vessel disease and is characterized by lacunar infarcts, focal and diffuse ischemic WMLs, and incomplete ischemic injury.[73,78,79] The ischemic lesions in VaD affect especially the prefrontal subcortical circuit, and subcortical syndrome is the primary clinical manifestation.[71,80] Clinically, small vessel dementia is characterized by pure motor hemiparesis, bulbar signs and dysarthria, gait disorder, depression and emotional lability, and, especially, deficits in executive functioning.[78,79,81–83] The patient with subcortical VaD with multiple lacunes and extensive WMLs on neuroimaging often gives only a clinical history of prolonged transient ischemic attack (TIA) or multiple TIAs (which mostly are minor strokes) without residual symptoms and only mild focal findings (e.g. drift, reflex asymmetry, gait disturbance), further supporting the importance

Specific Medical Diseases and Stroke

of a requirement for neuroimaging in the criteria for this disorder.[71]

Clinical Features of the Main Subtypes

Early cognitive syndrome of SIVD is characterized by (1) dysexecutive syndrome, including slowed information processing, (2) memory deficit (may be mild), and (3) behavioral and psychological symptoms. The dysexecutive syndrome in SIVD consists of impairment in goal formulation, initiation, planning, organizing, sequencing, executing, set-sifting and set-maintenance as well as in abstracting.[74,78,84] The memory deficit in SIVD may be milder than that in AD, for example, and is specified by impaired recall, relative intact recognition, less severe forgetting, and better benefit from cues.[84] Behavioral and psychological symptoms in SIVD include, in particular, depression, personality change, emotional lability and incontinence, as well as inertia, emotional bluntness, and psychomotor retardation.[61,74,78]

Early cognitive syndrome of cortical VaD includes some memory impairment (by definition), which may be mild, mostly some heteromodal cortical symptoms, such as aphasia, apraxia, agnosia, and visuospatial or constructional difficulty. In addition, most patients have some degree of dysexecutive syndrome.

Clinical neurologic findings, especially early in the course of SIVD, comprise episodes of mild upper motor neuron signs (drift, reflex asymmetry, incoordination), gait disorder (apractic-atactic or small-stepped), imbalance and falls, urinary frequency and incontinence, dysarthria, and dysphagia as well as extrapyramidal signs (hypokinesia, rigidity).[61,73,79,81,82] However, these focal neurologic signs are often subtle.[85,86]

Patients with cortical VaD who have multiple cortico-subcortical infarcts often show visual field defect, lower facial weakness, lateralized sensorimotor changes, and gait impairment (hemiplegic, apractic-atactic).[73]

Onset and Course

In SIVD, the onset is variable. For example, in the study reported by Babikian and Ropper,[81] 60% of the patients had a slow, less abrupt onset, and only 30% an acute onset of cognitive symptoms. The course was gradual both without (40%) and with (40%) acute deficits, and acute stroke alone without progression was seen in 13%.[81]

Traditionally, cortical VaD (MID) has been characterized by a relative abrupt onset (days to weeks), a stepwise deterioration (some recovery after worsening), and a fluctuating course (e.g., difference between days) of cognitive functions.[60,61,79,85–87]

SUBCORTICAL ISCHEMIC VASCULAR DISEASE AND DEMENTIA

A more homogeneous subtype is SIVD.[88,89] In SIVD, small vessel disease is the chief vascular etiology, lacunar infarct and ischemic WMLs are the primary types of brain lesions, and lesions are primarily located in the subcortex, and subcortical syndrome is the primary clinical manifestation.[88]

Pathophysiology

The primary vascular mechanism in SIVD is small vessel disease.[90,91] The main risk factors for small vessel disease are age, arterial hypertension, diabetes, and genetic abnormality (e.g., cerebral amyloid angiopathy [CAA] and cerebral autosomal dominant arteriopathy with subcortical infarcts and leukoencephalopathy [CADASIL]). The main types of SIVD small vessel change are arteriolosclerosis (deep perforating arterioles, 40–200 μm, centrum semiovale and periventricular white matter, leading to WMLs), lipohyalinosis (small perforating arteries and arterioles, 40–200 μm, deep gray and white matter, leading to WMLs and lacunae), and intracerebral atherosclerosis (small perforating arteries, 200–850 μm, deep gray matter, leading to lacunae).[90,91] Functionally, small vessel disease causes obliteration and occlusion of the vessel, increased tortuosity and coiling, greater resistance, decreased autoregulation, endothelial changes, change in blood-brain barrier function, and perivascular changes.

Secondary SIVD risk factors are hemodynamic changes of systemic vascular, cardiac, and carotid origin. They include arterial hypotension, blood pressure fluctuations, cardiac failure, cardiac arrhythmia, and carotid stenosis. Small vessel disease may occur in two ways.[89] In the first, occlusion of a single arteriolar or arterial lumen leads to complete lacunar infarct; in the second, critical stenosis of multiple small vessels leads to hypoperfusion and incomplete infarcts. These complete infarcts give rise to acute and severe ischemia leading to cystic necrosis with loss of all tissue elements. Incomplete infarction causes more chronic, diffuse, and less severe ischemia leading to selective loss of tissue elements in order of their selective vulnerability—neuron, oligodendrocyte, myelinated axon, astrocyte, endothelial cell.[89] The neuropathologic picture of diffuse WMLs consists of araiosis, état criblé, demyelination, axonal loss, and changes in oligodendrocytes and glial cells as well as noncavitated and cavitated small infarcts.[90,92] Small vessel also involves atrophy, as severity of cognitive impairment in SIVD correlates with medial temporal lobe atrophy and WMLs correlate with both cortical atrophy and medial temporal lobe atrophy.[89,93] As previously state, SIVD incorporates two clinical entities, Binswanger's disease and "the lacunar state".[79,81,82]

Neuroimaging

The typical WMLs in SIVD consist of extending periventricular and deep WMLs affecting especially the genu or anterior limb of the internal capsule, anterior corona radiata, and anterior centrum semiovale. The lacunae are located mainly in the caudate, globus pallidus, thalamus, internal capsule, corona radiata, and frontal white matter. The brain imaging criteria in SIVD apply both to cases with predominantly WMLs (Binswanger type) and to cases with predominantly lacunar infarcts (lacunar state type).[88] Characteristics of two types or extremes of imaging changes include predominantly "white matter cases": extending periventricular and deep white matter lesions: extending caps (>10 mm as measured parallel to ventricle) or irregular halo (>10 mm broad, irregular margins and extending into deep white matter) *and* diffusely confluent hyperintensities (>25 mm, irregular shape) or extensive white matter change (diffuse hyperintensities without focal lesions), *and* lacunae in the deep gray matter. To include predominantly "lacunar cases": multiple (e.g., more than five) lacunae in the deep gray matter *and* at least moderate white matter lesions: extending caps or irregular halo or diffusely confluent hyperintensities or extensive white matter changes.[94]

Clinical Features

The ischemic lesions in SIVD affect especially the prefrontal subcortical circuit,[80] a feature that explains the main cognitive, behavioral, and clinical neurologic features.

The subcortical cognitive syndrome includes both the executive dysfunction and memory deficit. Executive dysfunction consists of impairment of goal formulation, initiation, planning, organizing, sequencing, executing, set-shifting and set-maintenance, and abstracting. Memory deficit, which can often be less severe, comprises impaired recall, relative intact recognition, less severe forgetting, and benefit from cues. Behavioral and psychological symptoms include depression, personality change, and psychomotor retardation.

Clinical Syndrome

The two traditional clinical syndromes related to SIVD are the "lacunar state" and Binswanger's disease.[79,81,82,89] Clinical features of the lacunar syndrome include hemiparesis (pure sensory and motor, and other lacunar syndromes), pseudobulbar palsy and affect, small-stepped gait, and urinary incontinence. Binswanger's disease consists of slowing of mental and motor processing, decreased initiative, depression, gait disturbance, and urinary incontinence. Early clinical features related to SIVD are episodes of mild upper motor signs (drift, reflex asymmetry, incoordination), gait disorder (small-step gait or marche à petits pas, magnetic, and apraxic-ataxic or Parkinsonian gait), imbalance, urinary frequency and incontinence, extrapyramidal signs (hypokinesia and rigidity), and depression and mood changes.

Onset and Cause

The onset is slow, less abrupt in 60% of cases, and gradual with or without acute deficits in 80% of cases.[81] This feature underlines the importance of neuroimaging criteria in the definitions of VaD.

Criteria

Clinical identification of patients with SIVD can be based on a modification of the NINDS-AIREN criteria for probable VaD.[88,95] The original NINDS-AIREN criteria for probable VaD also required a relationship between onset of dementia and CVD. In SIVD, the onset is often more insidious, and a strong relationship already exists among the cognitive syndrome, brain imaging features, and evidence of CVD. Accordingly, this requirement was omitted from the research criteria for SIVD. SIVD offers a solution to identify more homogenous and representative groups of patients and is expected to yield more predictable clinical

picture, natural history, outcomes, and treatment responses. Further empirical research is needed to define the syndrome and stages of SIVD, validate the brain imaging criteria for SIVD by clinical-pathologic correlation, as well as to elucidate the natural history and outcomes.

ALZHEIMER'S DISEASE AND CEREBROVASCULAR DISEASE

The presence of vascular risk factors per se does not offer diagnostic clues as to the etiology of dementia. Some studies have shown that many risk factors for vascular diseases, such as hypertension, diabetes, and high cholesterol, increase the risk of AD as well.[14] Moreover, comorbidity of AD and VaD is common, particularly in the very old.[8,18] There is substantial overlap of the patterns of cognitive impairment in vascular dementia and Alzheimer's disease, although some differences have been identified (Table 29–3). However, precise distinctions of cognitive impairment at specific levels of cognition in the two illnesses are still uncertain. The nature, extent, and progression of deterioration in functional abilities have been observed to differ in VaD and AD.[96] Analysis of data from the Canadian Study of Health and Aging showed that capabilities

Table 29.3 Differential Diagnosis Between Vascular Dementia and Alzheimer's Disease

Vascular Dementia	Alzheimer's Disease
Early cognitive syndrome Dysexecutive syndrome: impaired planning, sequencing, speed of processing	Impaired episodic memory: ineffective learning, increased forgetting, impaired recognition, poor response to cues, intrusion errors
Memory impairment (often mild): ineffective learning, less forgetting, preserved recognition, good response to cues, preservation	
Cortical symptom(s) (variable): aphasia, apraxia, agnosia, visuospatial and constructive difficulty	Anomia (mild) Visuospatial impairment (mild)

Early clinical features
  Mild upper motor neuron signs (motor deficit, decreased coordination, brisk tendon reflexes, Babinski's sign)
  Gait disorder, imbalance
  Urine frequency
  Dysarthria
  Mood changes, depression
	Absence of focal neurologic signs
	Dysthymia, mild depression

Onset Variable: relative abrupt, insidious	Insidious
Clinical course Variable: fluctuating, stepwise, progressive, stable	Progressive; may have plateaus

for motor functions, such as walking and getting into bed, were different in Alzheimer's disease and VaD, as opposed to nonmotor functions (e.g., handling of money, grooming, using the telephone, traveling, and taking medicine), for which no differences are seen.[97] Impairments in attention and visual perception are thought to be greater in early Alzheimer's disease than in VaD, which has been seen to produce differential effects on capabilities in complex activities (e.g., driving) in the two illnesses.[98]

Psychiatric comorbidity is a common feature of vascular dementia. The behavioral (neuropsychiatric) disorders often reported in patients with vascular disorders include depression, behavioral retardation, psychomotor slowing, anxiety, and apathy. Among these psychiatric comorbidities, most comparative studies have shown that depression occurs more frequently in vascular dementia than in AD.[96] The severity of behavioral symptoms generally increases with cognitive decline in both AD and vascular dementia. However, mood and personality changes can be more severe in vascular dementia,[99] and may occur earlier in the course of disease.[21]

The NINDS-AIREN criteria for the diagnosis of VaD have attempted to take some of the differences between AD and VaD into account. Probable VaD is characterized by NINDS-AIREN criteria as having an abrupt onset or a fluctuating and stepwise course with clinical signs of CVD and relevant CVD findings on brain imaging. In addition, it is specified that functional disability be distinguished as arising from cognitive deficit and not from physical disability related to brain disease. In contrast, AD is characterized in NINCDS Alzheimer's Disease and Related Disorders Association (ADRDA) criteria[100] as having insidious onset and a progressive course, without clinical signs of CVD or brain changes due to CVD on neuroimaging.

It is now becoming more clear that a continuum of disorders may exist whereby "pure" AD and VaD represent only the two extremes. Some studies have now suggested that mixed dementia, that is, AD with coexistent significant CVD, may be the most common cause of dementia in the very old.[5] Because these patients often show extensive WMLs and infarcts on brain imaging, the clinical diagnosis is difficult in the absence of defined biologic markers for AD. This fact may in the past have been a leading factor in the previous underestimation of this patient subgroup. Studies showing the frequency and possible causes of dementia after stroke have helped to define the link between dementia and CVD. Findings from studies in Japan and the United States and from the Helsinki Stroke Aging Memory Study have estimated the frequency of dementia after stroke at around 25%.[6,55,101] In the U.S. study, stroke was confirmed as the underlying cause of dementia in more than 50% of cases, and of these, approximately 36% were thought due to the cumulative effects of stroke and AD.[6]

The presence of CVD may play an important role in determining the presence and severity of the clinical symptoms of AD. The incidence rate of AD after stroke is doubled, suggesting that stroke may induce an earlier expression of AD.[45] Moreover, according to Henon and colleagues,[102] patients with stroke and mild AD experienced dementia syndrome during the first months after stroke, whereas pure vascular dementia may also develop at a later point after stroke. The Nun Study and other studies have shown that individuals meeting neuropathologic criteria for AD with additional evidence of CVD (e.g., lacunar infarcts) showed poorer cognitive performance and more prevalent dementia than those with AD and no evidence of brain infarcts.[8,103] These studies clearly demonstrate that many different disorders can contribute to the clinical symptoms of dementia in a single patient.

The identification of coexistent disorders in patients encountered in clinical practice is of great importance, particularly from a therapeutic aspect. In a study conducted by the Consortium for the Investigation of Vascular Impairment of Cognition (CIVIC), typical AD presentations with one or more features pointing to "vascular aspects" derived from the Hachinski Ischemia Scale score were used successfully in combination with neuroimaging of ischemic lesions to diagnose "mixed dementia."[5] Vascular risk factors and focal neurologic signs and symptoms were present more often in AD with CVD than in "pure" AD. Other visible clinical clues for a diagnosis of AD with CVD were gained from analyses of disease course characteristics and presentations of patchy cognitive deficits, early onset of seizures, or gait disorder.

The clinical recognition of patients with mixed dementia or AD with CVD is a problem. Such patients have a clinical history and signs of CVD, so they are clinically closer to VaD. A solution could be to find reliable biologic markers for clinical AD. Potential markers might be early and significant medial temporal lobe atrophy on MRI combined with bilateral parietal hypoperfusion on single photon emission computed tomography (SPECT) and changes in cerebrospinal fluid levels of beta-amyloid and tau-protein or the presence of apolipoprotein E_4 allele. In our search for therapeutic approaches, however, we may have to choose a new focus. Instead of being prisoners of old diagnostic dichotomies (pure AD vs. pure VaD), we should focus on etiopathogenic factors, measure both the vascular burden and the Alzheimer's burdens of the brain, and determine their consequences.

VASCULAR COGNITIVE IMPAIRMENT

Dementia criteria are typically modeled on AD criteria, whereby involvement of the medial temporal lobe results in dense episodic memory impairment. By contrast, patients with vascular lesions have no such predilection.[5,20] Furthermore, the emphasis on dementia may underestimate the vascular burden of cognition as well as distract focus from prevention and treatment. Accordingly, it has been suggested to abandon the "alzheimerized" dementia concept in the setting of CVD substituting a broader category of VCI.[5,20,25,104,105] In VCI, *vascular* refers to all causes of ischemic CVD, and cognitive impairment encompasses all levels of cognitive decline, from the earliest step to a more severe and broad, dementia-like cognitive syndrome.[25] VCI that does not meet the criteria for dementia has been labeled also as vascular cognitive impairment with no dementia or vascular CIND.[5,20] It is expected to apply to cases with cognitive impairment related to CVD (TIA, stroke), multiple cortico-subcortical infarcts, silent infarcts, strategic infarcts, small vessel disease with WMLs and lacunae, as well as AD disease with coexisting CVD lesions.

Still, the concept and definition of VCI or CIND are in evolution. The two main factors to be defined are the severity and the pattern of cognitive impairment. Especially, identification of a cognitive syndrome signaling a high risk for further cognitive decline, of vascular mild cognitive decline (VMCI), and of a group of patients similar to that for amnesic MCI as a risk state for AD,[106] is a challenge.

CLINICAL EXAMINATION

The clinical examination of a patient in whom vascular cognitive impairment is suspected has the following four objectives: (1) staging the severity of the disorder diagnosis of mild cognitive impairment or dementia, (2) identifying the vascular cause of the cognitive syndrome, (3) evaluating the specific cause of the CVD (e.g., causes and risk factors), and (4) examining secondary factors that may worsen the patient's cognitive function.

Examination of a patient with VaD should always include the assessment of the causes of and risk factors for CVD. Questions should be asked about the presence of smoking, cardiac diseases, hypertension, diabetes, and other possible risk factors for CVD. The basic evaluation of the cardiovascular system includes careful auscultation of heart and carotid vessels, measurement of heart rate and blood pressure, chest radiography, and electrocardiography. Further tests that may be needed in individual patients are the orthostatic test, 24-hour blood pressure monitoring, Holter monitoring, and two-dimensional echocardiography with additional radioisotope studies. Sonography of cervical vessels may also be useful in selected cases. In some cases, cerebral angiography, arterial biopsy, or even brain and leptomeningeal vessel biopsy may be needed, particularly in patients with suspected angiitis of brain vessels. Laboratory evaluation for risk factors in CVD includes measurements of blood glucose, cholesterol and lipid levels, and fibrinogen and blood coagulation tests in selected cases. Genetic tests, such as detection of Notch3 gene mutations if CADASIL is suspected, should be performed as indicated.

DIFFERENTIAL DIAGNOSIS

The differential diagnosis of VaD includes a number of other conditions in addition to VaD and AD (Table 29–4).

Alzheimer's Disease

AD has typical neuropathologic stages (transtentorial, limbic, and neocortical) corresponding to clinical stages (preclinical, early, and mild dementia).[107] Accordingly, AD is a typical stage concurrent disorder, progressing from mild cognitive impairment to early predementia AD and then to stages of AD dementia,[108] and is not a diagnosis of exclusion.

Taking the clinical series on differential diagnosis between AD and VaD into consideration, the main

Table 29.4 Differential Diagnosis of Vascular Dementia

Alzheimer's disease
Alzheimer's disease and cerebrovascular disease (mixed dementia)
Normal-pressure hydrocephalus
White matter lesions and dementia
Frontal lobe tumor
Intracranial mass
Lewy body dementia
Frontotemporal dementia
Parkinson's disease and dementia
Progressive supranuclear palsy
Multisystem atrophy

limitations have included (1) definition of the cognitive syndrome, the dementia syndrome, (2) definition of the cause of the dementia syndrome, and (3) heterogeneity of patient populations, especially that of VaDs.

The traditional concept of dementia has been based on the typical clinical features of AD.[100,109] The definition has been the prison of AD, because the focus has been early episodic memory impairment, a more or less global cognitive syndrome, with progressive course, and major restrictions of ADLs. These features are different from those of early VaD, and these criteria merely detect an end stage of VaD. One consequence has been that different definitions of dementia syndrome identify different groups of subjects in both epidemiologic studies[109] and clinical post-stroke series.[43]

The most widely used definition of the cause of the cognitive syndrome includes the NINDS-AIREN for probable VaD[61] and the NINCDS-ADRDA for probable AD.[100] These criteria define a stereotyped set of patient groups with either probable VaD characterized by abrupt onset or a fluctuating and stepwise course with clinical signs of CVD and relevant CVD on brain imaging. In contrast, AD is characterized by insidious onset and progressive course without clinical and brain imaging signs of CVD. Accordingly, in typical cases, the differentiation between probable VaD and AD using common clinical tools is direct.[54]

The Hachinski Ischemic Score has been widely used to differentiate patients with VaD and AD.[110] In most clinical series, the majority of the items differentiate VaD from probable AD—as a matter of fact, this is based on the clinical definitions used. However, in a large neuropathologically confirmed series reported by Moroney and associates,[111] the independent correlates of VaD were stepwise deterioration (odds ratio [OR] 6.1), fluctuating course (OR 7.6), history of hypertension (OR 4.3), history of stroke (OR 4.3), and history of focal neurologic symptoms (OR 4.4).

Alzheimer's Disease with Cerebrovascular Disease (Mixed Dementia)

The issue of mixed dementia is a challenge. Increasing evidence shows that different vascular factors are related to AD, and frequently, CVD coexists with AD.[14,18] This overlap is increasingly important in older populations. Clinical recognition of patients with mixed dementia or AD with CVD, however, is a problem. As detailed in the

Specific Medical Diseases and Stroke

neuropathologic series reported by Moroney and associates,[111] these patients have a clinical history and signs of CVD, being clinically closer to VaD. In fact, in this series, fluctuating course (OR 0.2) and history of strokes (OR 0.1) were the only items differentiating patients with AD from those with mixed dementia.

Problematic clinical examples include stroke unmasking AD in patients with post-stroke dementia, insidious onset, slow progressive course, or both in patients with VaD, and cases in which neuroimaging assessment of the role of less extensive WMLs or of distinct infarcts is difficult. This clinical challenge may be solved when a sensitive and specific antemortem marker for AD is available, and the distinction between AD and VaD could be supported by more detailed knowledge of which site, type, and extent of ischemic brain changes are critical for VaD and which extent and type of medial temporal lobe atrophy specify AD.

Normal-pressure hydrocephalus (NPH) is characterized by a slowly progressive apractic-atactic gait disorder, and urinary incontinence usually precedes cognitive impairment, psychomotor slowing, and abnormal executive function.[112] CT or MRI reveals large ventricles, a periventricular halo, and relatively narrow cortical sulci. Subcortical VaD and NPH may coexist. Cerebrospinal fluid analysis, monitoring of intraventricular pressure, and even installation of an intraventricular shunt are often needed for differential diagnosis.

White Matter Lesions and Dementia

Diffuse or patchy white matter lesions may also have a nonischemic etiology and be related to cognitive decline.[30,61] The causes include multiple sclerosis, encephalitis, neurosarcoidosis, leukodystrophies, brain irradiation, and nonischemic cerebral edema.

Frontal lobe tumors relate to disinhibition and behavioral changes, as in frontal lobe dementia, or slowing, indecision, and abnormal executive function, as in subcortical dementias. Symptoms and signs of increased intracranial pressure may arise. Occasionally, focal neurologic symptoms and signs are present. Brain imaging clarifies the diagnosis.

Intracranial Mass

Cognitive decline may relate to an intracranial mass lesion, such as tumor, metastasis, or cyst, as well as subdural hematoma. In some cases, focal neurologic symptoms and signs may be absent, and the course may be slowly progressive. Brain imaging clarifies the diagnosis.

Lewy Body Dementia

Lewy body dementia manifests as prominent attentional deficits, subcortical-frontal dysfunction, and visuospatial impairment with relative preservation of memory early in the course.[113] Fluctuating cognition with pronounced variations in attention and alertness is common, as are recurrent visual hallucinations, which are typically well formed and detailed. Patients show spontaneous motor features of parkinsonism, and experience repeated falls,

syncope, transient losses of consciousness, and neuroleptic sensitivity.

Frontotemporal Dementia

Frontotemporal dementia consists of progressive deterioration of personality and behavior, affective symptoms, speech disorders (reduced and stereotype speech, echolalia, late mutism), but relatively preserved spatial orientation and praxis. [114] Affected patients have early primitive reflexes and incontinence. They have frontal dysfunction on neuropsychological testing and frontal and anterior temporal atrophy on brain imaging; despite evident dementia, EEG in such patients is often normal.

Parkinson's Disease and Dementia

Extrapyramidal syndrome (tremor, hypokinesia, rigidity) usually precedes the cognitive impairment in Parkinson's disease with dementia. [115] Patients demonstrate subcortical dementia with apathy, poor concentration, and indecision. Parkinsonian features usually respond to dopaminergic drugs.

Progressive Supranuclear Palsy

Progressive supranuclear palsy is similar to Parkinson's disease and dementia, but parkinsonian features are not responsive to dopaminergic drugs.[116] Typical features are paralysis of upward gaze, downward gaze, or both, and truncal ataxia.

Multisystem Atrophy

Multisystem atrophy comprises slowly progressive dementia with any combination of pyramidal tract signs, extrapyramidal features, autonomic failure, and cerebellar ataxia.[117]

PREVENTION AND THERAPY

Primary prevention aims to reduce the incidence of disease by eliminating the causes or main risk factors.[118,119] Thus, in relation to vascular dementia, the targets of primary prevention are the risk factors for CVD and cognitive impairment but also putative protective factors.[32] Risk factors include arterial hypertension, atrial fibrillation, myocardial infarction, coronary heart disease, diabetes, generalized atherosclerosis, lipid abnormalities, and smoking. Putative protective factors are estrogen, anti-inflammatory agents, and antioxidants.[120] Knowledge of the effects of primary prevention of VaD is still scanty.[32,121] Some studies indicate that treatment of arterial hypertension could prevent cognitive decline.

Secondary prevention aims to keep a disease from progressing into a more serious outcome by means of early detection followed by treatment.[119] Preventive actions that should be taken in patients at risk for VCI and VaDs include (1) early diagnosis and treatment of acute stroke in order to limit the extent of ischemic brain changes and to promote recovery, (2) prevention of stroke recurrence according the type of stroke, and (3) intensification of the treatment of risk factors. Selection of treatment is guided by the cause of CVD, such as large artery disease (e.g., aspirin, dipyridamole, clopidogrel, carotid endarterectomy), cardiac embolic events (e.g., anticoagulation, aspirin), small vessel disease (e.g., antiplatelet therapy as in large vessel disease), and hemodynamic mechanisms (e.g., control of hypotension and cardiac arrhythmias).[50,67,72] Hypoxic ischemic events (cardiac arrhythmias, congestive heart failure, myocardial infarction, seizures, pneumonia) are an important risk factor for incident dementia in patients with stroke and should be taken into account in the secondary prevention of VaD.[122]

Detailed knowledge of the effects of secondary prevention of the vascular component of VaD is still scanty. In small series of patients with established VaD, control of high arterial blood pressure,[123] cessation of smoking,[123] and use of aspirin[124] have improved or stabilized cognition. It has been suggested that lowering of plasma viscosity could also have an effect in VaD.[125] Further, absence of progressive cognitive decline in patients receiving placebo in symptomatic treatment trials of VaD may also reflect an effect of intensified control of risk factors.[126]

Symptomatic Treatment or Tertiary Prevention

A number of drugs have been studied for symptomatic treatment of VaD, including cerebroactive and vasoactive drugs, nootropic agents, and some calcium antagonists, but these studies have largely shown negative results.[127] Such studies have mostly involved small numbers of patients, short treatment periods, and variations in diagnostic criteria and tools, have often included mixed populations, and have had variations in the application of clinical end points. Results of the use of nimodipine,[128] memantine,[129] and propentofylline[126] have raised expectations in the symptomatic treatment of VaD. It is possible that symptomatic treatment with acetylcholinesterase inhibitors[130] may prove effective also in the cognitive symptoms of VaD. Still, there currently is not a widely accepted standard symptomatic treatment for VaD.[3]

CONCLUSION

Vascular dementia is the second most common cause of dementia. VaD research, until recently overshadowed by research into Alzheimer's disease, is now developing rapidly, because it is an area that holds great promise for intervention. The following points summarize the present review on the subject:

- The pathophysiology of VaD incorporates interactions among vascular causes (CVD and vascular risk-factors), changes in the brain (infarcts, white matter lesions, atrophy), host factors (age, education), and cognition.
- Definitional heterogeneity—variations in defining the cognitive syndrome, in vascular causes, and in allowable brain changes—in current criteria have resulted in great variations in estimates of prevalence, identification of groups of subjects, and types and distribution of putative causal brain lesions.

- Should new criteria be developed? Ideally, in the construction of new criteria, the diagnostic elements should be tested with prospective studies with clinicopathologic correlation; we need to replace dogma with data. Meanwhile, focusing on more homogeneous subtypes of VaD and on imaging criteria could be a solution.
- In SIVD, small vessel disease is the chief vascular cause, lacunar infarct and ischemic white matter lesions are the primary types of brain lesions, lesions are primarily located in the subcortex, and subcortical syndrome is the primary clinical manifestation. The disorder incorporates two clinical entities, Binswanger's disease and "the lacunar state."
- Post-stroke dementia is common but is still often unrecognized. It has also been neglected in clinical trials of primary and secondary prevention of CVD.
- AD with VaD (mixed dementia) has been underestimated as a prevalent cause in the older population. In addition to simple coexistence, VaD and AD have closer interactions. Several vascular risk factors and vascular brain changes relate to clinical manifestation of AD, and they share also common pathogenetic mechanisms.
- Vascular cognitive impairment is a category aiming to replace the "alzheimerized" dementia concept in the setting of CVD, substituting a spectrum that includes subtle cognitive deficits of vascular origin, post-stroke dementia, and the complex group of the vascular dementias.
- There is no standard treatment for VaDs, and little is known as yet about primary prevention (brain at risk for CVD) and secondary prevention (CVD brain at risk for VCI or VaD). One focus in the future should be the assessment and treatment of the known distinct etiopathogenic factors, that is, the CVD and the AD burden of the brain.

References

1. Hebert R, Brayne C: Epidemiology of vascular dementia. Neuroepidemiology 14:240–257, 1995.
2. Rocca WA, Hofman A, Brayne C, et al: The prevalence of vascular dementia in Europe: Facts and fragments from 1980–1990 studies. EURODEM-Prevalence Research Group. Ann Neurol 30:817–824, 1991.
3. Doody RS, Stevens JC, Beck C, et al: Practice parameter: Management of dementia (an evidence-based review). Report of the Quality Standards Subcommittee of the American Academy of Neurology. Neurology 56:1154–1166, 2001.
4. Lobo A, Launer LJ, Fratiglioni L, et al: Prevalence of dementia and major subtypes in Europe: A collaborative study of population-based cohorts. Neurology 54(Suppl 5):S4–S9, 2000.
5. Rockwood K, Wenzel C, Hachinski V, et al: Prevalence and outcomes of vascular cognitive impairment. Neurology 54:447–451, 2000.
6. Tatemichi TK, Desmond DW, Mayeux R, et al: Dementia after stroke: Baseline frequency, risks, and clinical features in a hospitalized cohort. Neurology 42:1185–1193, 1992.
7. Tatemichi TK, Paik M, Bagiella E, et al: Risk of dementia after stroke in a hospitalized cohort: Results of a longitudinal study. Neurology 44:1885–1891, 1994.
8. Snowdon DA, Greiner LH, Mortimer JA, et al: Brain infarction and the clinical expression of Alzheimer disease. The Nun Study [see comments]. JAMA 277:813–817, 1997.
9. Hachinski V: Preventable senility: A call for action against the vascular dementias [see comments]. J Am Geriatr Soc 340:645–648, 1992.

10. Erkinjuntti T: Cerebrovascular dementia: A guide to diagnosis and treatment. CNS Drugs 1999.
11. Pohjasvaara T, Mäntylä R, Salonen O, et al: How complex interactions of ischemic brain infarcts, white matter lesions and atrophy relate to poststroke dementia. Arch Neurol 57:1295–1300, 2000.
12. Wallin A, Blennow K: Heterogeneity of vascular dementia: mechanisms and subgroups. J Geriatr Psychiatry Neurol 6:177–188, 1993.
13. Pantoni L, Garcia JH: Pathogenesis of leukoaraiosis: A review. Stroke 28:652–659, 1997.
14. Skoog I, Kalaria RN, Breteler MMB: Vascular factors and Alzheimer's disease. Alzheimer Dis Assoc Disord 13(Suppl 3):S106–S114, 1999.
15. Skoog I: Risk factors for vascular dementia: A review. Dementia 5:137–144, 1994.
16. Wallin A, Blennow K, Gottfries CG: Neurochemical abnormalities in vascular dementia. Dementia 1:120–130, 2002.
17. Togi H, Abe T, Kimura M, et al: Cerebrospinal fluid acetylcholine and choline in vascular dementia of Binswanger and multiple small infarct types as compared with Alzheimer-type dementia. J Neural Transm 103:1211–1220, 2002.
18. Kalaria RN, Ballard C: Overlap between pathology of Alzheimer disease and vascular dementia. Alzheimer Dis Assoc Disord 13(Suppl 3):S115–S123, 1999.
19. Rockwood K: Lessons from mixed dementia [editorial]. Int Psychogeriatr 9:245–249, 1997.
20. Rockwood K, Howard K, MacKnight C, Darvesh S: Spectrum of disease in vascular cognitive impairment. Neuroepidemiology 18:248–254, 1999.
21. Chui HC, Gonthier R: Natural history of vascular dementia. Alzheimer Dis Assoc Disord 13(Suppl 3):S124–130, 1999.
22. Desmond DW, Erkinjuntti T, Sano M, et al: The cognitive syndrome of vascular dementia: Implications for clinical trials. Alzheimer Dis Assoc Disord 13(Suppl 3):S21–S29, 1999.
23. Erkinjuntti T: Cerebrovascular dementia: Pathophysiology, diagnosis and treatment. CNS Drugs 12:35–48, 1999.
24. Hachinski VC, Lassen NA, Marshall J: Multi-infarct dementia: A cause of mental deterioration in the elderly. J Am Geriatr Soc 2:207–210, 1974.
25. Bowler JV, Steenhuis R, Hachinski V: Conceptual background to vascular cognitive impairment. Alzheimer Dis Assoc Disord 13(Suppl 3):S30–S37, 1999.
26. Berchtold NC, Cotman CW: Evolution in the conceptualization of dementia and Alzheimer's disease: Greco Roman period to the 1960s. Neurobiol Aging 19:173–189, 1998.
27. Tomlinson BE, Blessed G, Roth M: Observations on the brains of demented old people. J Neurol Sci 11:205–242, 1970.
28. Hachinski VC, Lassen NA, Marshall J: Multi-infarct dementia: A cause of mental deterioration in the elderly. Lancet 2(7874):207–210, 1974.
29. Brust JC: Vascular dementia is overdiagnosed. Arch Neurol 45:799–801, 1988.
30. Erkinjuntti T, Hachinski VC: Rethinking vascular dementia. Cerebrovasc Dis 3:3–23, 1993.
31. Hachinski VC: The decline and resurgence of vascular dementia. CMAJ 142:107–111, 1990.
32. Skoog I: Status of risk factors for vascular dementia. Neuroepidemiology 17:2–9, 1998.
33. Pasquier F, Leys D: Why are stroke patients prone to develop dementia? J Neurol 244:135–142, 1997.
34. Desmond DW: Vascular dementia: A construct in evolution. Cerebrovasc Brain Metab Rev 8:296–325, 1996.
35. Chui HC: Dementia: A review emphasizing clinicopathologic correlation and brain-behavior relationships. Arch Neurol 46:806–814, 1989.
36. Tatemichi TK: How acute brain failure becomes chronic: A view of the mechanisms and syndromes of dementia related to stroke. Neurology 40:1652–1659, 1990.
37. Fratiglioni L, Launer LJ, Andersen K, et al: Incidence of dementia and major subtypes in Europe: A collaborative study of population-based cohorts. Neurology 54(Suppl 5):S10–S15, 2000.
38. Ostbye T, Hill G, Steenhuis R: Mortality in elderly Canadians with and without dementia. Neurology 53:521–526, 2002.
39. Mölsä PK, Marttila RJ, Rinne UK: Long-term survival and predictors of mortality in Alzheimer's disease and multi-infarct dementia. Acta Neurol Scand 91:159–164, 1995.
40. Skoog I, Nilsson L, Palmertz B, et al: A population-based study of dementia in 85-year-olds. N Engl J Med 328:153–158, 1993.
41. Tatemichi TK, Paik M, Bagiella E, et al: Dementia after stroke is a predictor of long-term survival. Stroke 25:1915–1919, 1994.
42. Suzuki K, Kutsuzawa T, Nakajima K, Hatano S: Epidemiology of vascular dementia and stroke in Akita, Japan. In Hartmann A, Kuchinsky W, Hoyer S (eds): Cerebral Ischemia and Dementia. New York, Springer-Verlag, 1991, pp 16–24.
43. Pohjasvaara T, Erkinjuntti T, Vataja R, Kaste M: Dementia three months after stroke: Baseline frequency and effect of different definitions of dementia in the Helsinki Stroke Aging Memory Study (SAM) cohort. Stroke 28:785–792, 1997.
44. Loeb C, Gandolfo C, Croce R, Conti M: Dementia associated with lacunar infarction. Stroke 23:1225–1229, 1992.
45. Kokmen E, Whisnant JP, O'Fallon WN, et al: Dementia after ischemic stroke: A population-based study in Rochester, Minnesota (1960–1984). Neurology 46:154–159, 1996.
46. Ferrucci L, Guralnik JM, Salive ME, et al: Cognitive impairment and risk of stroke in the older population [see comments]. J Am Geriatr Soc 44:237–241, 1996.
47. Zhu L, Fratiglioni L, Guo Z, et al: Incidence of stroke in relation to cognitive function and dementia in the Kungsholmen Project. Neurology 54:2103–2107, 2002.
48. Erkinjuntti T: Clinicopathological study of vascular dementia. In Prohovnik I, Wade J, Knezevic S, et al (eds): Vascular Dementia: Current Concepts. Chichester, UK, John Wiley & Sons, 1996, pp 73–112.
49. Brun A: Pathology and pathophysiology of cerebrovascular dementia: Pure subgroups of obstructive and hypoperfusive etiology. Dementia 5:145–147, 1994.
50. Amar K, Wilcock G: Vascular dementia. BMJ 312:227–231, 1996.
51. Wallin A, Blennow K: The clinical diagnosis of vascular dementia. Dementia 5:181–184, 1994.
52. Pantoni L, Garcia JH: The significance of cerebral white matter abnormalities 100 years after Binswanger's report: A review. Stroke 26:1293–1301, 1995.
53. Mielke R, Herholz K, Grond M, et al: Severity of vascular dementia is related to volume of metabolically impaired tissue. Arch Neurol 49:909–913, 1992.
54. Erkinjuntti T, Haltia M, Palo J, et al: Accuracy of the clinical diagnosis of vascular dementia: A prospective clinical and post-mortem neuropathological study. J Neurol Neurosurg Psychiatry 51:1037–1044, 1988.
55. Rockwood K, Parhad I, Hachinski V, et al: Diagnosis of vascular dementia: Consortium of Canadian Centres for Clinical Cognitive Research consensus statement. Can J Neurol Sci 21:358–364, 1994.
56. Erkinjuntti T: Clinical criteria for vascular dementia: The NINDS-AIREN criteria. Dementia 5:189–192, 1994.
57. Wetterling T, Kanitz RD, Borgis KJ: Comparison of different diagnostic criteria for vascular dementia (ADDTC, DSM-IV, ICD-10, NINDS-AIREN). Stroke 27:30–36, 1996.
58. American Psychiatric Association: Diagnostic and Statistical Manual of Mental Disorders, 4th ed. Washington, DC, American Psychiatric Association, 1994.
59. World Health Organization: ICD-10 Classification of Mental and Behavioural Disorders: Diagnostic Criteria for Research. Geneva: WHO, 1993.
60. Chui HC, Victoroff JI, Margolin D, et al: Criteria for the diagnosis of ischemic vascular dementia proposed by the State of California Alzheimer's Disease Diagnostic and Treatment Centers [see comments]. Neurology 42:473–480, 1992.
61. Roman GC, Tatemichi TK, Erkinjuntti T, et al: Vascular dementia: Diagnostic criteria for research studies. Report of the NINDS-AIREN International Work Group. Neurology 43:250–260, 1993.
62. Erkinjuntti T, Ostbye T, Steenhuis R, Hachinski V: The effect of different diagnostic criteria on the prevalence of dementia. N Engl J Med 337:1667–1674, 1997.
63. Wetterling T, Kanitz RD, Borgis KJ: The ICD-10 criteria for vascular dementia. Dementia 5:185–188, 1994.
64. Skoog I, Nilsson L, Palmertz B, et al: A population-based study of dementia in 85-year-olds [see comments]. N Engl J Med 328:153–158, 1993.
65. Erkinjuntti T, Bowler JV, DeCarli C, et al: Imaging of static brain lesions in vascular dementia: Implications for clinical trials. Alzheimer Dis Assoc Disord 13(Suppl 3):S81–S90, 1999.

66. Inzitari D, Erkinjuntti T, Wallin A, et al: Subcortical vascular dementia as a specific target for clinical trials. Ann N Y Acad Sci 903:510–521, 2000.

67. Erkinjuntti T: Vascular dementia: Challenge of clinical diagnosis. Int Psychogeriatr 9(Suppl 1):51–58, 1997.

68. Lopez OL, Larumbe MR, Becker JT, et al: Reliability of NINDS-AIREN clinical criteria for the diagnosis of vascular dementia [see comments]. Neurology 44:1240–1245, 1994.

69. Verhey FR, Lodder J, Rozendaal N, Jolles J: Comparison of seven sets of criteria used for the diagnosis of vascular dementia. Neuro-epidemiology 15:166–172, 1996.

70. Gold G, Giannakopoulos P, Montes-Paixao JC, et al: Sensitivity and specificity of newly proposed clinical criteria for possible vascular dementia. Neurology 49:690–694, 1997.

71. Erkinjuntii T, Inzitari D, Pantoni L, et al: Research criteria for subcortical vascular dementia in clinical trials. J Neural Transm 59(Suppl 2):23–30, 2000.

72. Konno S, Meyer JS, Terayama Y, et al: Classification, diagnosis and treatment of vascular dementia. Drugs Aging 11:361–373, 1997.

73. Erkinjuntti T: Types of multi-infarct dementia. Acta Neurol Scand 75:391–399, 1987.

74. Cummings JL: Vascular subcortical dementias: Clinical aspects. Dementia 5:177–180, 1994.

75. Loeb C, Meyer JS: Vascular dementia: Still a debatable entity? J Neurol Sci 143:31–40, 1996.

76. Sulkava R, Erkinjuntti T: Vascular dementia due to cardiac arrhythmias and systemic hypotension. Acta Neurol Scand 76:123–128, 1987.

77. Erkinjuntti T, Haltia M, Palo J, et al: Accuracy of the clinical diagnosis of vascular dementia: A prospective clinical and post-mortem neuropathological study. J Neurol Neurosurg Psychiatry 51:1037–1044, 1988.

78. Mahler ME, Cummings JL: The behavioural neurology of multi-infarct dementia. Alzheimer Dis Assoc Disord 5:122–130, 1991.

79. Roman GC: Senile dementia of the Binswanger type: A vascular form of dementia in the elderly. JAMA 258:1782–1788, 1987.

80. Cummings JL: Fronto-subcortical circuits and human behavior. Arch Neurol 50:873–880, 1993.

81. Babikian V, Ropper AH: Binswanger's disease: A review. Stroke 18:2–12, 1987.

82. Ishii N, Nishihara Y, Imamura T: Why do frontal lobe symptoms predominate in vascular dementia with lacunes? Neurology 36:340–345, 1986.

83. Wallin A, Blennow K, Gottfries CG: Subcortical symptoms predominate in vascular dementia. Int J Geriatr Psychiatry 6:137–146, 1991.

84. Desmond DW, Erkinjuntti T, Sano M, et al: The cognitive syndrome of vascular dementia: Implications for clinical trials. Alzheimer Dis Assoc Disord 13(Suppl3):S21–S29, 1999.

85. Skoog I: Blood pressure and dementia. In Hansson L, Birkenhäger WH (eds): Handbook of Hypertension, Vol 18: Assessment of Hypertensive Organ Damage. Amsterdam, Elsevier Science, 1997, pp 303–331.

86. Fischer P, Gatterer G, Marterer A, et al: Course characteristics in the differentiation of dementia of the Alzheimer type and multi-infarct dementia. Acta Psychiatr Scand 81:551–553, 1990.

87. Erkinjuntti T: Differential diagnosis between Alzheimer's disease and vascular dementia: Evaluation of common clinical methods. Acta Neurol Scand 76:433–442, 1987.

88. Erkinjuntti T, Inzitari D, Pantoni L, et al: Research criteria for subcortical vascular dementia in clinical trials. J Neural Transm 59(Suppl 1):23–30, 2000.

89. Chui HC: Vascular dementia, a new beginning: Shifting focus from clinical phenotype to ischemic brain injury. Neuroloci Clin 18:951–977, 2001.

90. Erkinjuntti T, Pantoni L: Subcortical vascular dementia. In Gauthier S, Cummings JL (eds): Alzheimer's Disease and Related Disorders Annual. London, Martin Duniz, 2000, pp 101–133.

91. Pantoni L, Lammie A: Cerebral small vessel disease: Pathological and pathophysiological aspects in relation to vascular cognitive impairment. In Erkinjuntti T, Gauthier S (eds): Vascular Cognitive Impairment. London, Martin Duniz, 2001.

92. Erkinjuntti T, Benavente O, Eliasziw M, et al: Diffuse vacuolization (spongiosis) and arteriolosclerosis in the frontal white matter occurs in vascular dementia. Arch Neurol 53:325–332, 1996.

93. Fein G, DiSclafani V, Tanabe J, et al: Hippocampal and cortical atrophy predict dementia in subcortical ischemic vascular disease. Neurology 11:1626–1635, 2002.

94. Mantyla R, Erkinjuntti T, Salonen O, et al: Variable agreement between visual rating scales for white matter hyperintensities on MRI: Comparison of 13 rating scales in a poststroke cohort. Stroke 28:1614–1623, 1997.

95. Roman GC, Tatemichi TK, Erkinjuntti T, et al: Vascular dementia: Diagnostic criteria for research studies. Report of the NINDS-AIREN International Workshop [see comments]. Neurology 43:250–260, 1993.

96. Groves WC, Brandt J, Steinbeg M: VaD and Alzheimer's disease: Is there difference? A comparison of symptoms by disease duration. J Neuropsychiatr Clin Neurosci 12:305–315, 2000.

97. Gauthier S, Rockwood K, Gélinas I, et al: Outcome measures for the study of activities of daily living in vascular dementia. Alzheimer Dis Assoc Disord 13(Suppl 3):S143–S147, 1999.

98. Fitten LJ, Perryman KM, Wilkinson CJ, et al: Alzheimer and vascular dementias and driving: A prospective road and laboratory study [see comments]. JAMA 273:1360–1365, 1995.

99. Hargrave R, Geck LC, Reed B, Mungas D: Affective behavioural disturbances in Alzheimer's disease and ischemic vascular disease. J Neurol Neurosurg Psychiatry 68:41–46, 2000.

100. McKhann G, Drachman D, Folstein M, et al: Clinical diagnosis of Alzheimer's disease: Report of the NINCDS-ADRDA Work Group under the auspices of Department of Health and Human Services Task Force on Alzheimer's Disease. Neurology 34:939–944, 1984.

101. Pohjasvaara T, Erkinjuntti T, Vataja R, Kaste M: Dementia three months after stroke: Baseline frequency and effect of different definitions of dementia in the Helsinki Stroke Aging Memory Study (SAM) cohort. Stroke 28:785–792, 1997.

102. Henon H, Durie I, Guerouaou D, et al: Posttroke dementia: Incidence and relationship to prestroke cognitive decline. Neurology 57:1216–1222, 2001.

103. Heyman A, Fillenbaum GG, Welsh-Bohmer KA, et al: Cerebral infarcts in patients with autopsy-proven Alzheimer's disease. CERAD, part XVIII. Consortium to Establish a Registry for Alzheimer's Disease. Neurology 51:159–162, 1998.

104. Bowler JV, Hachinski V: Vascular cognitive impairment: A new approach to vascular dementia. Baillieres Clin Neurol 4:357–376, 1995.

105. Bowler JV, Hachinski V: Criteria for vascular dementia. Arch Neurol 57:170–171, 2000.

106. Petersen RC, Doody R, Kurz A, et al: Current concepts in mild cognitive impairment. Arch Neurol 58:1985–1992, 2002.

107. Braak H, Braak E: Neuropathological staging of Alzheimer-related changes. Acta Neuropathol (Berl) 82:239–259, 1991.

108. Petersen RC: Normal aging, mild cognitive impairment, and early Alzheimer's disease. Neurologist 1:326–344, 1995.

109. Erkinjuntti T, Ostbye T, Steenhuis R, Hachinski V: The effect of different diagnostic criteria on the prevalence of dementia. N Engl J Med 337:1667–1674, 1997.

110. Hachinski VC, Iliff LD, Zilhka E, et al: Cerebral blood flow in dementia. Arch Neurol 32:632–637, 1975.

111. Moroney JT, Bagiella E, Desmond DW, et al: Meta-analysis of the Hachinski Ischemic Score in pathologically verified dementias. Neurology 49:1096–1105, 1997.

112. Roman GC: White matter lesions and normal-pressure hydrocephalus: Binswanger disease or Hakim syndrome? AJNR Am J Neuroradiol 12:40–41, 1991.

113. McKeith IG, Galasko D, Kosaka K, et al: Consensus guidelines for the clinical and pathologic diagnosis of dementia with Lewy bodies (DLB): Report of the consortium on DLB International Workshop. Neurology 47:1113–1124, 1996.

114. Clinical and neuropathological criteria for frontotemporal dementia. The Lund and Manchester Groups. J Neurol Neurosurg Psychiatry 57:416–418, 1994.

115. Marder K, Tang MX, Cote L, et al: The frequency and associated risk factors for dementia in patients with Parkinson's disease. Arch Neurol 52:695–701, 1995.

116. Tolosa E, Valldeoriola F, Marti MJ: Clinical diagnosis and diagnostic criteria of progressive supranuclear palsy (Steele-Richardson-Olsewski syndrome). J Neural Transm Suppl 42:15–31, 1994.

Specific Medical Diseases and Stroke

117. Wenning GK, Be-Sholomon Y, Magalhaes M, et al: Clinicopathological study of 35 cases of multiple system atrophy. J Neurol Neurosurg Psychiatry 58:160–166, 1995.

118. Last JM (ed): A Dictionary of Epidemiology, 2nd ed. New York, Oxford University Press, 1988.

119. Skoog I: The possibility for secondary prevention of Alzheimer's disease. In Mayeux R, Christen Y (eds): The Epidemiology of Alzheimer's Disease: From Gene to Prevention. New York, Springer-Verlag, 1999.

120. Mortel KF, Meyer JS: Lack of postmenopausal estrogen replacement therapy and the risk of dementia. J Neuropsychiatry Clin Neurosci 7:334–337, 1995.

121. Skoog I: The relationship between blood pressure and dementia: A review. Biomed Pharmacother 51:367–375, 1997.

122. Moroney JT, Bagiella E, Desmond DW, et al: Risk factors for incident dementia after stroke: Role of hypoxic and ischemic disorders. Stroke 27:1283–1289, 1996.

123. Meyer JS, Judd BW, Tawaklna T, et al: Improved cognition after control of risk factors for multi-infarct dementia. JAMA 256:2203–2209, 1986.

124. Meyer JS, Rogers RL, McClintic K, et al: Randomized clinical trial of daily aspirin therapy in multi-infarct dementia: A pilot study. J Am Geriatr Soc 37:549–555, 1989.

125. Lechner H: Status of treatment of vascular dementia. Neuroepidemiology 17:10–13, 1998.

126. Rother M, Erkinjuntti T, Roessner M, et al: Propentofylline in the treatment of Alzheimer's disease and vascular dementia. Dementia Geriatr Cogn Disord 9(Suppl 1):36–43, 1998.

127. Knezevic S, Labs KH, Kittner B, et al: The treatment of vascular dementia: Problems and prospects. In Prohovnik I, Wade J, Knezevich J, et al (eds): Vascular Dementia: Current Concepts. Chichester, UK, John Wiley & Sons, 1996, pp 301–312.

128. Pantoni L, Carosi M, Amigoni S, et al: A preliminary open trial with nimodipine in patients with cognitive impairment and leukoaraiosis. Clin Neuropharmacol 19:497–506, 1996.

129. Görtelmeyer R, Erbler H: Memantine in treatment of mild to moderate dementia syndrome. Drug Res 42:904–912, 1992.

130. Erkinjuntti T, Kurz A, Gauthier S, et al: Galantamine is efficacious in probable vascular dementia and Alzheimer's disease combined with cerebrovascular disease. J Am Geriatr Soc 2001.

Chapter Thirty

Atherosclerotic Disease of the Proximal Aorta

Marco R. Di Tullio and Shunichi Homma

The role of atherosclerotic plaques in the aorta as a potential source of embolism has become increasingly evident. The proximal portion of the aorta, where the origin of blood vessels that supply the brain is located, has been shown to be the site of origin of cerebral embolism, providing an explanation for cerebral ischemic events otherwise considered of unknown etiology. In this chapter, we review the principal studies that have demonstrated the association of aortic plaques and ischemic stroke and discuss the related diagnostic and therapeutic issues.

FREQUENCY OF AORTIC PLAQUES IN THE GENERAL POPULATION

The atherosclerotic process in the aorta develops throughout life but becomes especially evident after the fourth decade of life; the prevalence and number of atherosclerotic lesions rise continuously thereafter. As discussed later, transesophageal echocardiography (TEE) is the most sensitive and widely used diagnostic technique to assess for aortic plaques. In the Stroke Prevention: Assessment of Risk in a Community (SPARC) study,[1] 588 volunteers older than 44 years underwent TEE. The prevalence of *simple plaques* (<4 mm in thickness, without ulceration or mobile debris) or *complex plaques* (≥4 mm thick or with complex features) was evaluated. Overall, aortic atherosclerosis of any degree and complex atherosclerosis in any segment of the aorta were present in 51.3% and 7.6% of subjects, respectively. Atherosclerosis of any degree was identified in the ascending aorta in 8.4%, in the aortic arch in 31.0%, and in the descending aorta in 44.9% of subjects; corresponding figures for complex atherosclerosis were 0.2%, 2.2%, and 6.0%, respectively. Atherosclerosis of any degree in any aortic segment was found to increase from approximately 17% in subjects 45 to 54 years old to more than 80% in subjects older than 75 years. Complex atherosclerosis was virtually absent in the younger subgroup but present in more than 20% of those older than 75 years. In a TEE study from Australia on healthy volunteers older than 59 years,[2] the prevalence of simple plaques in the aortic arch was 22%, and that of complicated plaques (≥5 mm in thickness or with irregular, ulcerated surface) was 4%.

AORTIC PLAQUES AND ISCHEMIC STROKE: PATHOLOGIC STUDIES

The first report of a strong association between aortic arch plaques and ischemic stroke came from a large autopsy case-control study conducted in France by Amarenco and colleagues.[3] These investigators found a much greater frequency of ulcerated aortic plaques in elderly patients who had died from a stroke than in patients who had died from other neurologic diseases (26% vs. 5%; age-adjusted OR [OR] 4.0; 95% CI, [CI,] 2.1 to 7.8). Importantly, the highest frequency of ulcerated plaques was observed in patients with unexplained (cryptogenic) stroke (61% vs 28%; adjusted OR 5.7; 95% CI, 2.4 to 13.6), thus providing a potential pathogenic mechanism for the stroke. In that study, the lack of association between ulcerated plaques and the presence of significant carotid artery stenosis and atrial fibrillation, two other important sources for brain embolism, suggested an independent role of aortic plaques in the risk of stroke. Among patients with ulcerated plaques, only 3% were younger than 60 years, indicating that ulcerated plaques could be a new potential stroke risk factor exclusively in elderly subjects.

In a later necropsy study on 120 unselected patients, Khatibzadeh and colleagues[4] found evidence of arterial embolization in 40 (33%). In that study, complicated aortic arch plaques were significantly associated with arterial embolism (OR 5.8; 95% CI, 1.1 to 31.7), independent of and with strength of association similar to that of severe ipsilateral carotid artery disease and atrial fibrillation.

IN VIVO STUDIES: TRANSESOPHAGEAL ECHOCARDIOGRAPHY

Transesophageal echocardiography is currently the most sensitive and most widely used technique for examining the proximal portion of the aorta. The technique has enabled the study of the association between aortic plaques and ischemic stroke in vivo. The proximity of the esophagus to the aorta and the absence of interposed structures allow the use of high-frequency ultrasound transducers, providing high-resolution images of the vessel. In the search for aortic plaques as the potential cause of ischemic stroke, the portion of aorta proximal to the takeoff of the left subclavian artery is the focus of the examination. Although the existence of retrograde diastolic flow has been demonstrated in the aorta,[5] its occurrence is probably an uncommon mechanism for embolization to the brain. Therefore, plaques that are located more distally in the aorta are unlikely causes of stroke.

The initial portion of the aorta can be accurately visualized by TEE from the aortic valve level to the initial curvature of the arch (Fig. 30–1). The middle and distal portions of the aortic arch are also visible in all patients (Fig. 30–2). A small portion of the vessel (proximal arch) cannot be visualized owing to the interposition of the trachea and is therefore a "blind spot" of the examination, although the introduction of multiplane transducers has allowed for a more complete visualization of the vessel in most patients. TEE allows an accurate assessment of the presence and thickness of plaques (Fig. 30–3) as well as the presence of ulcerations (Fig. 30–4) or superimposed thrombus (Figs. 30–5 through 30–7). TEE has been shown to be highly sensitive and specific in the detection of aortic

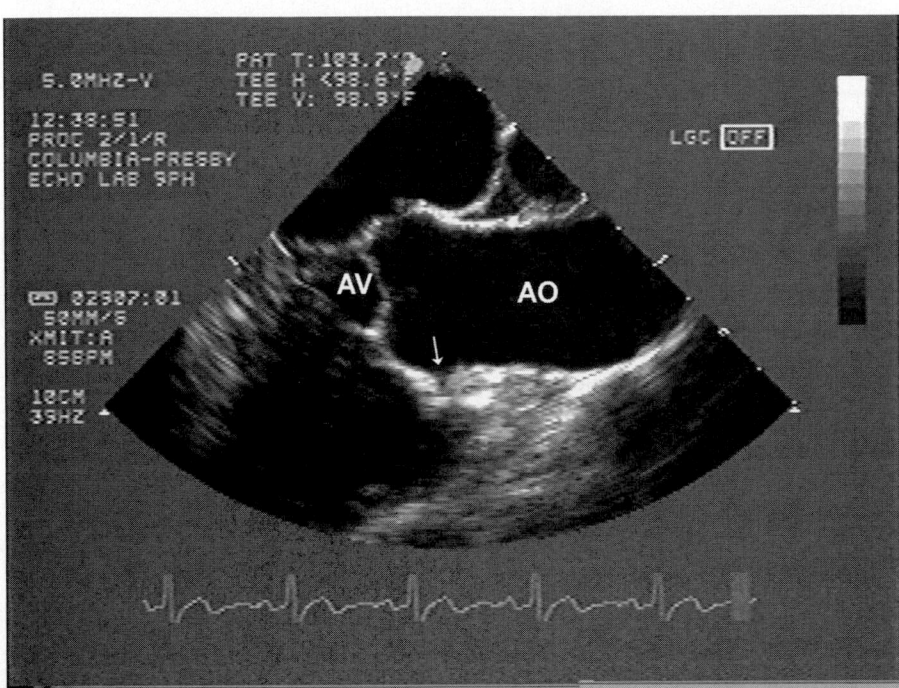

FIGURE 30–1 *Longitudinal view of the ascending aorta (AO) by transesophageal echocardiography (TEE). The entire ascending aorta is visualized, from the aortic valve (AV) to the initial curvature of the aortic arch. The takeoff of the right coronary artery is visible* (arrow).

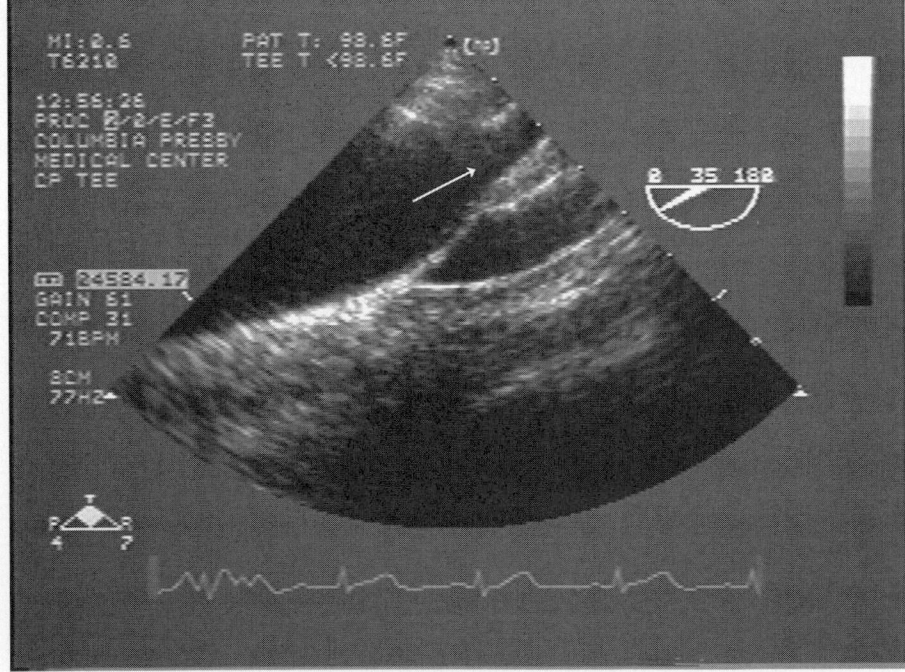

FIGURE 30–2 *Visualization by transesophageal echocardiography of the middle to distal portion of the aortic arch. The takeoff of the left subclavian artery is visible* (arrow).

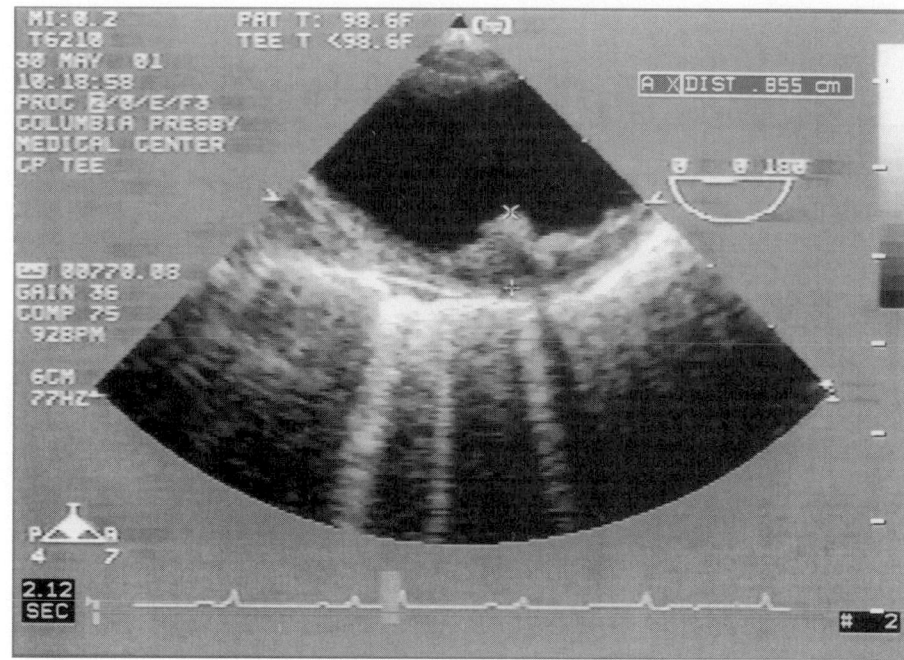

FIGURE 30–3 *Protruding atherosclerotic plaque in the distal aortic arch. Measurement of plaque thickness, perpendicular to the major axis of the aortic lumen, is shown. Plaque thickness (0.855 cm) is displayed in the upper right corner.*

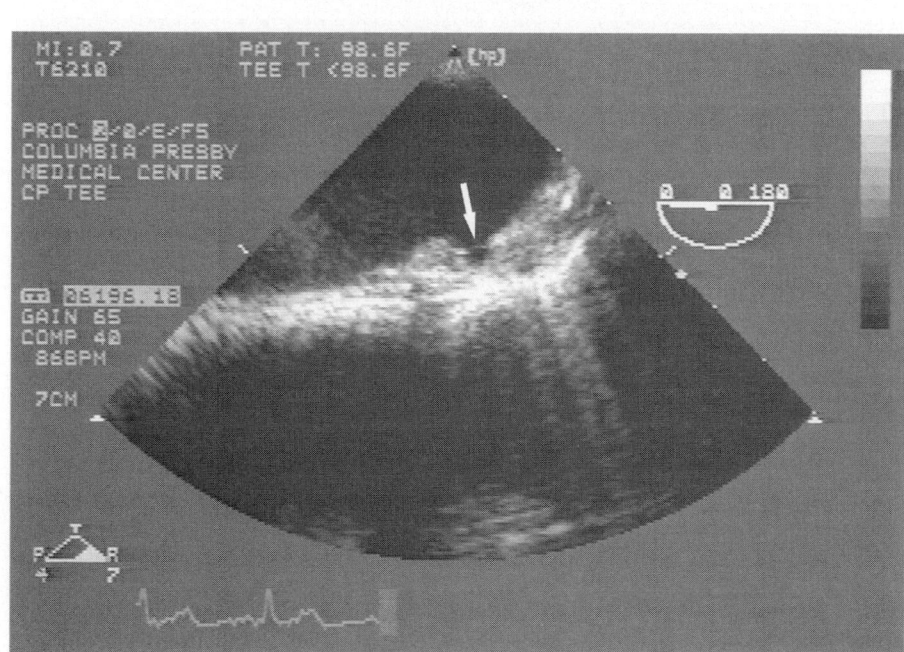

FIGURE 30–4 *Complex plaque in the distal aortic arch. A large ulceration (arrow) is visible.*

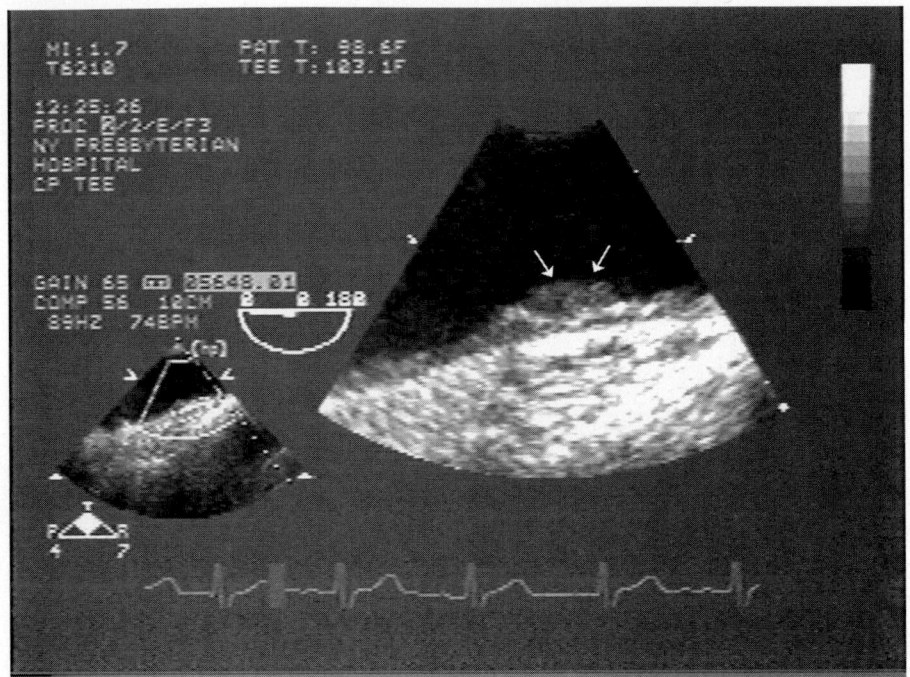

FIGURE 30–5 *Enlarged view of a plaque in the mid-portion of the aortic arch. Hypoechoic material suggestive of thrombus (arrows) appears superimposed on the brightly echogenic plaque.*

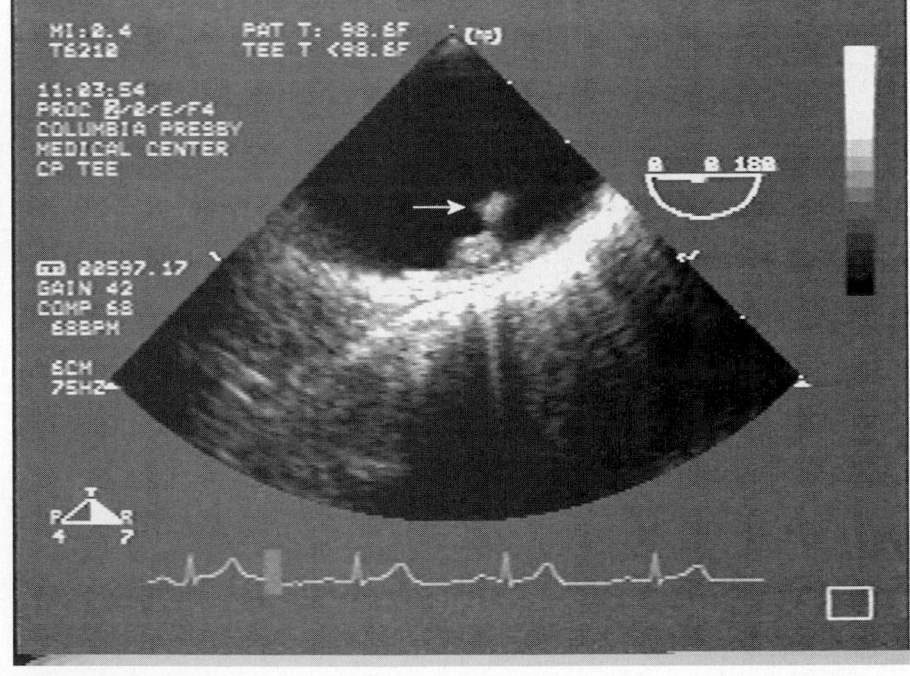

FIGURE 30–6 *Complex plaque in the mid-portion of the aortic arch. A large pedunculated portion is seen (arrow), which was highly mobile in real-time imaging.*

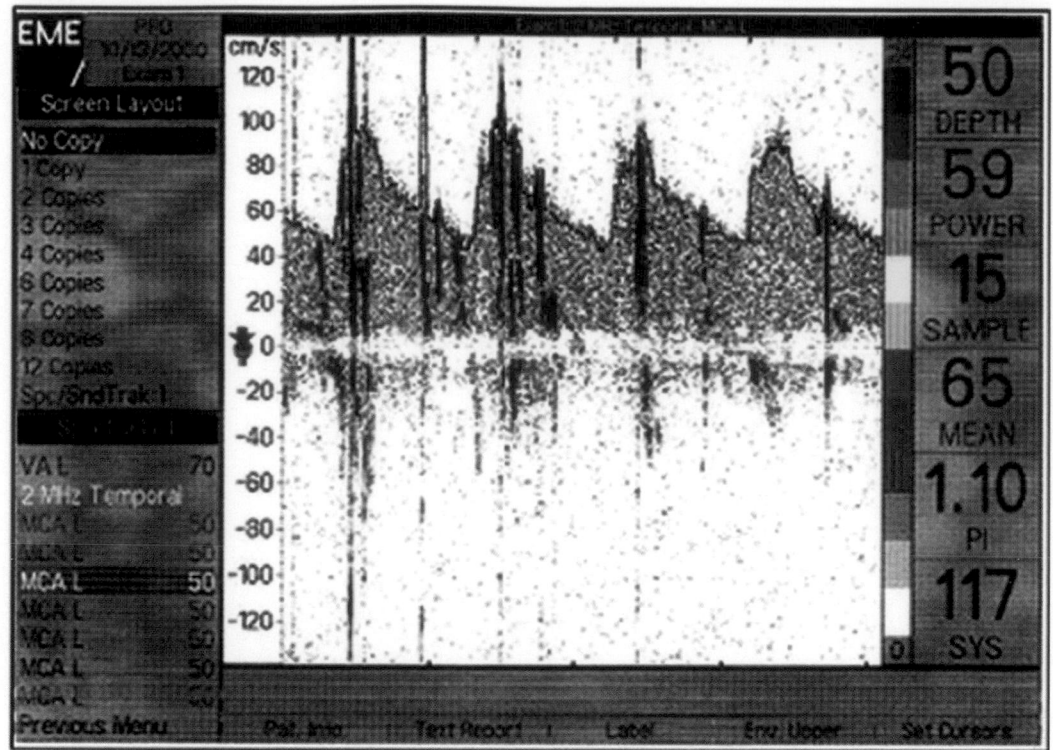

PLATE 30–1 *Transcranial Doppler ultrasonograph of the middle cerebral artery. High-intensity transient signals (HITSs) are visualized as vertical high-amplitude signals with narrow spectrum superimposed on the normal blood flow.*

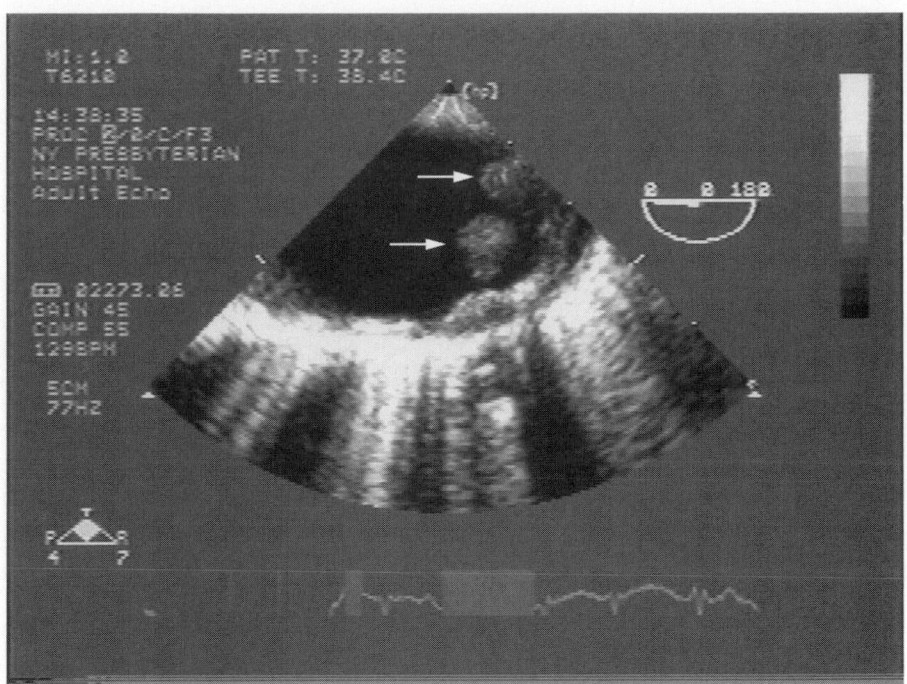

FIGURE 30–7 *Complex atherosclerotic plaque of the distal aortic arch. Two large thrombi* (arrows) *are visible.*

plaques.[6,7] Also, its diagnostic accuracy for presence of thrombus is high (sensitivity 91%, specificity 90%).[7] However, the sensitivity of TEE for detecting small ulcerations of the plaque surface, which may carry an additional risk for further embolic events,[2,8,9] has been described as less than optimal (approximately 75%).[6,7]

TEE is a safe, if semi-invasive, diagnostic test. Major complications are uncommon and mainly due to unsuspected preexisting esophageal disease. In a European series of more than 10,000 patients, one death was observed.[10] In an additional 2.7% of patients, the test could not be performed because of unsuccessful intubation (1.9%) or patient intolerance (0.8%). Similar results were obtained in a study from the Mayo Clinic of 15,381 consecutive patients, with 2 deaths (0.01%) and an overall incidence of complications of 1.7%.[11] In another series of 901 patients, intubation was unsuccessful in 1.2% of cases, and no deaths and a low incidence (0.6%) of major complications were observed.[12] Our experience in patients with stroke has shown no higher frequency of patient discomfort, unsuccessful intubation, or significant complications.[13] Moreover, the test can be safely performed even in patients of very advanced age.[14]

Case-Control Studies

In 1991, Tunick and associates[15] first reported on an increased frequency of aortic plaques 5 mm or larger in 122 patients referred for TEE with a history of arterial embolism compared with 122 age- and sex-matched patients with other cardiologic diagnoses (27% vs. 9%; OR 3.2; 95% CI, 1.6 to 6.5). This retrospective study, results of which were not adjusted for other potential embolic sources, was followed by other case-control studies that focused on the risk of ischemic stroke associated with TEE-detected aortic arch plaques. The principal studies in this category are summarized in Table 30.1. Amarenco and colleagues[16] studied 250 patients with acute ischemic stroke older than 60 years and 250 control subjects. These researchers found that arch plaques between 1 mm and

Table 30.1 Association Between Proximal Aortic Plaques and Ischemic Stroke: Transesophageal Echocardiographic Case-Control Studies

Study[*]	Cases/Controls (N)	Age (years)	Type of Atheroma	Controls (%)	Patients with Stroke (%)	Adjusted Odds Ratio (95% CI)[†]
Amarenco et al (1994)[16]	250/250	≥60	1–3.9 mm	22	46	4.4 (2.8–6.8)
			≥4 mm	2	14	9.1 (3.3–25.2)
Jones et al (1995)[2]	215/202	≥60	<5 mm, smooth	22	33	2.3 (1.2–4.2)
			≥5 mm, complex	4	22	7.1 (2.7–18.4)
Di Tullio et al (1996)[8]	106/114	≥40	≥5 mm	13	26	2.6 (1.1–5.9)
	30/36	<60		3	3	1.2 (0.7–20.2)
	76/78	≥60		18	36	2.4 (1.1–5.7)

[*]Superscript numbers indicate chapter references.
[†]Adjusted for conventional stroke risk factors (also see text); 95% CI = 95% confidence interval.

3.9 mm in thickness were associated with stroke after adjustment for conventional stroke risk factors (adjusted OR 4.4), but a sharp increase in risk was present for plaques 4 mm or larger (adjusted OR 9.1; 95% CI, 3.3 to 25.2). Also, only the stroke risk associated with plaques 4 mm or larger was independent of the presence of carotid stenosis and atrial fibrillation. The researchers speculated that the sharp increase in risk observed for larger plaques might depend on the more frequent presence on the plaques of superimposed thrombus, which would be included in the measurement of plaque thickness, as well as to a more frequent presence of mobile components, a circumstance also observed in other studies.[17] In this study, plaques 4 mm or thicker were also significantly more frequent in patients with cryptogenic stroke than in patients with stroke of determined origin (28.2% vs. 8.1%; OR 4.7; 95% CI, 2.2 to 10.1).[16]

Similar results, except for the association with cryptogenic stroke, were obtained in an Australian study by Jones and coworkers,[2] who studied 215 patients with stroke and 202 healthy volunteers older than 59 years (see Table 30.1). In that study, plaques 5 mm or more in thickness or with ulcerated or mobile components were associated with a much greater stroke risk (adjusted OR 7.1; 95% CI, 2.7 to 18.4) than smaller, smooth plaques (adjusted OR 2.3; 95% CI, 1.2 to 4.2). However, the frequency of large or complex plaques was similar in patients with cryptogenic stroke (20%) and in patients with stroke of determined origin (23%).

We also studied 106 patients with stroke older than 40 years and 114 age- and gender-matched controls[8]; we found an increased risk of stroke to be associated with aortic plaques 5 mm or more in thickness (adjusted OR 2.6; 95% CI, 1.1 to 5.9). The risk was entirely due to the subgroup of patients older than 59 years, whereas the prevalence of large plaques was very low (3%) both in patients with stroke and in controls 59 years or younger (see Table 30.1), emphasizing that large aortic plaques appear to represent a relevant clinical entity only in the elderly.

Using epiaortic ultrasonography instead of TEE, Davila-Roman and colleagues[18] studied the prevalence of aortic plaques in 1200 subjects older than 49 years who were undergoing cardiac surgery, 158 of whom had a previous embolic event. These investigators found plaques 3 mm or larger in 26.6% of patients with and 18.1% of patients without a previous cerebrovascular event. Aortic plaques, arterial hypertension, atrial fibrillation, and carotid artery stenosis were independently associated with neurologic events in that study.

In the SPARC study, the importance of the association between aortic atherosclerosis and cerebrovascular events has been questioned.[1] In 581 community-derived subjects who underwent TEE in that study, large (≥4 mm), ulcerated, or mobile plaques were associated with a history of coronary artery disease (OR 2.35; 95% CI, 1.1 to 5.0) but not with a history of ischemic stroke (OR 1.37; 95% CI, 0.44 to 4.3), leading the investigators to question the importance of aortic plaques as a risk factor for stroke in the community. However, the inclusion in that study of younger subjects (≥45 years) may have diluted the strength of the association observed between aortic plaques and stroke.

Prospective Studies

Other researchers have confirmed the role of aortic arch plaques as a risk factor for peripheral and cerebral embolization prospectively (Table 30.2), by monitoring patients who had a first stroke or other embolic event and comparing the embolic recurrence rate in patients with and without proximal aortic plaques. After a mean follow-up of 14 months, Tunick and colleagues[19] noted a significantly greater incidence of cerebral or peripheral embolic events in 42 patients with protruding aortic atheromas compared with control subjects matched for age, gender, and hypertension (33% vs. 7%; RR [RR] 4.3; 95% CI, 1.2 to 15.0). Similar results were reported by Mitusch and associates[20] in a group of 47 patients with large or mobile arch plaques and 136 patients with small or no atheroma. In that study, recurrence rate of embolic events was 13.7% per year in patients with plaques that were either at least 5 mm or mobile, and 4.1% per year in patients with plaques smaller than 5 mm (RR 4.3; 95% CI, 1.5 to 12.0). In a French multicenter study of 331 patients with stroke 60 years or older, arch plaques 4 mm or more in thickness were associated with an almost four-fold increase in the risk of recurrent stroke after adjustments were made for

Table 30.2 Recurrence Rate of Embolic Events and Stroke in Patients With and Without Proximal Aortic Plaques: Transesophageal Echocardiographic Prospective Studies

Study*	AP+/AP− (N)	Follow-up (months)	Type of Plaque	AP− (%)	AP+ (%)	Adjusted Relative Risk 95% CI†
Tunick et al (1994)[19]	42/42	14	≥4 mm	7	33	4.3 (1.2–15.0)
Mitusch et al (1997)[20]	47/136	16	≥5 mm/mobile vs. <5 mm	4.1/yr	13.7/yr	4.3 (1.5–12.0)
FAPS (1996)[21]‡	45/143	24–48	≥4 mm	2.8/yr	11.9/yr	3.8 (1.8–7.8)
				5.9/yr	26.0/yr	3.5 (2.1–5.9)

*Superscript numbers indicate chapter references.
AP+, Aortic plaque present; AP−, aortic plaque absent.
†Adjusted for conventional stroke risk factors (also see text).
‡Only study conducted on ischemic stroke patients. Data on first row refer to recurrence rate of stroke, data on the second row to recurrence rate of all embolic events.

the presence of carotid stenosis, atrial fibrillation, peripheral artery disease, and other conventional risk factors (see Table 30.2).[21] In the subgroup with large plaques, the recurrence rate was highest in patients whose index stroke was cryptogenic in nature (16.4 per 100 person-years). The incidence of all vascular events was also significantly greater in patients with large plaques (RR 3.5; see Table 30.2).[21]

PLAQUE MORPHOLOGY AND STROKE RISK

The role of aortic plaques as a risk factor for stroke in the elderly has been established mainly on the basis of the thickness of the plaque, with either 4 mm or 5 mm chosen as the threshold for increased risk. It is unclear, however, whether plaque thickness is directly related to the stroke mechanism or is rather a marker of diffuse atherosclerosis, which may in fact be responsible for the increased stroke risk. We have demonstrated that differences exist in the plaque-related stroke risk between genders.[22] In this study, aortic plaques 4 mm or larger were significantly more common in men than in women (31.5% vs. 20.3%; $P = .025$) and were associated with ischemic stroke in both men (adjusted OR 6.0; CI, 2.1 to 16.8) and women (adjusted OR 3.2; 95% CI, 1.2 to 8.8), after data were adjusted for other established stroke risk factors. Plaques 3 to 3.9 mm in thickness, however, were significantly associated with stroke in women (adjusted OR 4.8; 95% CI, 1.7 to 15.0) but not in men (adjusted OR 0.8; 95% CI, 0.2 to 3.0). This observation suggests that plaque thickness, instead of identifying the actual culprit lesion for the stroke, may be a marker of diffuse atherosclerosis, including intracranial atherosclerosis, or of other conditions that may differ between genders and are possibly related to the stroke mechanism.[21]

The complex morphology of a plaque appears to be more directly related to the stroke mechanism. As mentioned earlier, morphologic features of the plaque, such as ulceration and mobility, have been linked with an increased stroke risk,[1,4,6–9,17] especially in the case of cryptogenic stroke. Stone and colleagues[9] showed a significantly greater frequency of ulcerated plaques in 23 patients with cryptogenic

stroke than in 26 patients with stroke of determined origin (39% versus 8%; $P < .001$). In our experience in 152 elderly patients with stroke and 152 age-matched controls,[17] ulcerated or mobile plaques were found to be a much stronger risk factor for stroke than large but noncomplex plaques (Table 30.3). That study confirmed that plaques 4 mm or larger were indeed associated with an increased stroke risk (adjusted OR 4.3; 95% CI, 2.1 to 8.7); however, when these large plaques were divided on the basis of the presence or absence of ulceration (defined as a discrete indentation of at least 2 mm in width and depth) or mobile components, the stroke risk associated with those complex feature was exceedingly high (adjusted OR 17.1), whereas large but noncomplex plaques carried only a modest increase in risk (adjusted OR 2.4; see Table 30.3). This remained true even after patients with other conditions possibly related to stroke, such as atrial fibrillation, carotid stenosis of 60% or greater, and intracranial atherosclerosis, were excluded from the analysis.

Cohen and associates[23] studied the impact of plaque morphology (ulceration, hypoechoic components, or calcification) on the risk of recurrent vascular events in a prospective study in 334 patients with stroke older than 60 years who were monitored for 2 to 4 years. In patients with plaques 4 mm or larger, the presence of ulcerations or hypoechoic components was not found to increase the risk of vascular events. However, the absence of calcification was associated with the strongest increase in risk (adjusted RR 10.3; 95% CI, 4.2 to 25.2), whereas the presence of calcification decreased the risk of subsequent events (adjusted RR 1.2; 95% CI, 0.6 to 2.1), possibly signaling a more stable lesion. These observations suggest that although the thickness of a plaque represents the most readily available marker of the risk of embolization associated with an arch aortic plaque, the plaque's morphologic features strongly affect the embolic potential of the lesion, possibly opening the field to new therapeutic approaches in individual patients.

It should be remembered that any protruding, mobile component on a plaque identified by TEE represents thrombus superimposed on atherosclerotic material and usually occurs on ulcerated plaques. This observation has been confirmed by several studies that have correlated the TEE findings with data derived from the histopathologic

Specific Medical Diseases and Stroke

Table 30.3   Effect of Aortic Plaque Morphology on the Risk of Ischemic Stroke

	Patients with Stroke (N = 152)		Control Subjects (N = 152)		Unadjusted OR (95% CI)*	Adjusted OR (95% CI)*
	N	**(%)**	**N**	**(%)**		
No plaque	28	(18.4)	55	(36.2)	— —	— —
Small plaque (<4 mm)†	56	(36.8)	68	(44.7)	1.6 (0.9–2.9)	1.9 (1.0–3.6)
Large plaque (≥4 mm)	68	(44.8)	29	(19.1)	4.6 (2.5–8.6)	4.3 (2.1–8.7)
Noncomplex plaque	34	(22.4)	25	(16.5)	2.7 (1.3–5.3)	2.4 (1.1–5.1)
Complex plaque	34	(22.4)	4	(2.6)	16.7 (5.4–51.8)	17.1 (5.1–57.3)
Ulcerated	24	(15.8)	3	(2.0)	15.7 (4.4–56.7)	15.8 (4.1–61.4)
Mobile	10	(6.6)	1	(0.7)	19.6 (2.4–161.3)	21.3 (2.4–193.2)

CI, confidence interval; OR, odds ratio.
*Adjusted for age, gender, arterial hypertension, diabetes mellitus, and hypercholesterolemia.
†No complex forms were present among small plaques.

examination of the aorta.[4,24,25] Mobile components superimposed on an aortic plaque are infrequently seen in elderly patients with stroke, the rate ranging from 2.0% to 8.7% in different studies (Table 30.4).[2,6,9,16,17,26] However, when present, they represent a very strong risk factor for brain embolization. In our study,[17] mobile components superimposed on a plaque were present in 6.6% of elderly patients with stroke and were associated with a more than 20-fold increase in the risk of stroke, after adjustment for other conventional stroke risk factors (see Table 30.3). Occasionally, mobile thrombi without severe atherosclerotic changes can be seen in the aortic arch of patients younger than 60 years who present with an embolic event (23 cases out of 27,855 TEE examinations in a multicenter cardiology study).[27] These thrombi usually have an insertion site on small atherosclerotic plaques and appear to represent a rare variant of atherosclerotic disease associated with embolic events in younger patients.[27]

The potential for embolism to the brain of large plaques and, even more, of complex plaques, has been confirmed with transcranial Doppler ultrasonography. With this technique, it possible to monitor the blood flow into the middle cerebral arteries continuously. Monitoring can be done simultaneously on the arteries of both sides and can be maintained for prolonged periods. The passage of small particles in the area interrogated by the ultrasound beam produces a characteristic high-intensity transient signal, or HITS (Plate 30–1 following page 664); the identification of a HITS can be made more accurate through the application of appropriate filters. Using this technique over 30 minutes in 46 patients with acute ischemic stroke, Rundek and colleagues[28] showed the presence of HITSs in a much larger proportion of patients with stroke with plaques 4 mm or larger than of patients with small or no plaques, even in the absence of other TEE-detected possible embolic sources (70% vs. 18%; $P = .007$; Fig. 30–8). Moreover, all patients with large and complex plaques were found to have HITSs, compared with 39% of patients with large but noncomplex plaques ($P = .005$). Similar results for the association between plaques 4 mm or larger and HITSs were obtained in patients with cryptogenic stroke in a study by Castellanos associates,[29] in which data on plaque complexity were not reported.

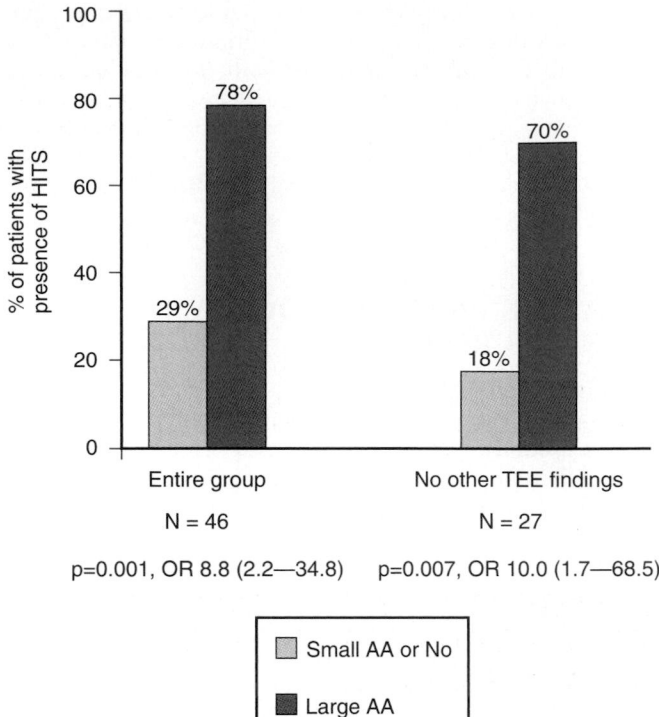

FIGURE 30–8   *Association between arch atheroma (AA) size and presence of high-intensity transient signals (HITSs). The significant association observed in the entire group was also observed after exclusion of 19 patients with atrial fibrillation (7 patients), patent foramen ovale (7), spontaneous echo contrast (9), and thrombus (2).*

In summary, aortic plaque thickness 4 mm or greater has been shown to be associated with increased stroke risk and remains a useful tool for risk stratification, although part of the risk may come from superimposed thrombus included in the measurement of plaque thickness. Plaque thickness is also a marker of diffuse atherosclerosis, which may play an important role in the stroke mechanism. The presence of complex morphologic features of a plaque, and especially mobile components, appears more directly related to stroke mechanism in individual patients.

NATURAL HISTORY OF AORTIC PLAQUES

The natural history of atherosclerotic plaques in the thoracic aorta has not been extensively studied. From the information available, however, it is appears that plaque size and morphology are important in determining the evolution of a plaque over time. Montgomery and coworkers[30] monitored 30 patients who had aortic atherosclerosis (12 with plaque <5 mm, 8 with plaques ≥5 mm, and 10 with plaques that had mobile components) on an initial TEE. A second TEE was performed at 12 months. Although no significant changes were seen in subjects with smaller plaques, 4 of 8 patients with plaques 5 mm or larger had a new mobile lesion. In patients who had a mobile lesion at the time of the initial study, such lesions had resolved in 70% of

Table 30.4   Prevalence of Mobile Thrombi Superimposed on Proximal Aortic Plaques in Patients with Ischemic Stroke

		Mobile Thrombi	
Study[a]	*Patients (N)*	**N**	**%**
Toyoda et al (1992)[6]	62	3	4.8
Nihoyannopoulos et al (1993)[26]	152	3	2.0
Jones et al (1995)[2]	202	11	5.4
Amarenco et al (1994)[16]			
Unselected	250	7	2.8
Cryptogenic	78	6	7.7
Stone et al (1995)[9]			
Unselected	49	2	4.1
Cryptogenic	23	2	8.7
Di Tullio et al (2000)[17]	152	10	6.6

[a]Superscript numbers indicate chapter references.

cases, but a new mobile lesion was observed in another 70%. Overall, although 20 of 30 patients (67%) had no change in the severity of atherosclerosis, there had been substantial changes in the plaque morphology. In another study of 78 patients with stroke or transient ischemic attack, progression of plaque over 9 months was observed in 37% of cases and was more common in the arch than in other aortic segments.[31] Using tr ansthoracic echocardiographic examination of the aortic arch from a suprasternal window, Geraci and Weinberger[32] studied plaque progression in 89 patients monitored for up to 18 months (mean 7.7 months). Although plaques smaller than 4 mm at baseline showed changes in thickness in only 23% of cases, plaques 4 mm or larger at baseline showed changes in thickness, either upward or downward, in 52% of cases. It therefore appears that large aortic plaques are extremely dynamic lesions whose appearance may change considerably over a relatively short time.

AORTIC PLAQUES IN PATIENTS OF DIFFERENT RACE-ETHNICITY WITH STROKE

Most studies on the association between atherosclerotic plaques in the proximal portion of the aorta and ischemic stroke have been conducted in white populations. Some information, however, is available about these associations in black and Hispanic persons that allows a comparison of plaque frequency, which is important in light of the different prevalence of risk factors for atherosclerosis in various race-ethnic groups. In a retrospective study of 1553 ischemic patients with stroke (889 white, 664 black), Gupta and associates[33] found a higher prevalence of aortic plaques in white than black subjects in the ascending aorta (14.7% vs. 11.1%; $P = .04$), aortic arch (67.7% versus 62.2%; $P = .03$) and descending aorta (58.4% versus 50.3%; $P = .002$). The *plaque burden*—sum of maximum plaque thickness at the three aortic locations—was also significantly higher in white subjects (4.97 mm vs. 4.28 mm; $P = .007$); in the aortic arch alone, the prevalences of plaques 4 mm or larger (25.9% vs. 18.7%; $P < .001$) and of complex plaques—defined as protruding, ulcerated, mobile or calcified regardless of plaque thickness— (26.3% vs. 19.0%; $P < .001$) were also significantly higher in white subjects. These findings were observed despite a higher prevalence of arterial hypertension and diabetes mellitus in the black subjects and cannot therefore be explained by differences in conventional stroke risk factor distribution.

In our case-control study in patients with ischemic stroke older than 59 years from the tri-ethnic community of Northern Manhattan,[17] non-complex plaques 4 mm or larger showed similar frequencies in white, black, and Hispanic subjects (24.1%, 20.0%, and 22.5%, respectively). However, complex plaques were twice as frequent in white (32.3%) than in black (15.6%) and Hispanic subjects (16.3%). Complex plaques were associated with a strong increase in stroke risk in all three race-ethnic subgroups. As in the Gupta study, the frequency of arterial hypertension and diabetes mellitus in our study was significantly lower in white subjects than in the other two race-ethnic subgroups, and that of hypercholesterolemia was significantly lower in

white than black subjects. The prevalence of plaques 4 mm or larger in the overall study population (44.8%) was much higher in our study than in a similar study from France (14.4%),[16] and also higher than the frequency of plaques 5 mm or larger and of complex plaques in a similar study from Australia (22%).[2] Therefore, even though the stroke risk associated with large or complex plaques appeared similar in the three studies, the attributable risk of stroke from proximal aortic plaques may be greater in the population of the United States, underscoring the need for effective preventive measures and risk factor reduction.

FACTORS ASSOCIATED WITH AORTIC PLAQUES IN PATIENTS WITH STROKE

Although differences in traditional risk factors for stroke and atherosclerosis alone do not seem to explain the race-ethnic differences in the frequency of aortic plaques, some of these risk factors are indeed associated with the presence of aortic plaques. Age is the strongest and universally accepted predictor of aortic atherosclerosis.[1–4,8,16–18,34,35] Cigarette smoking has consistently been shown to be associated with aortic atherosclerosis[2,16,18,34,35] and is the most important modifiable risk factor for the development of aortic plaques. Arterial hypertension has also been shown to be associated with proximal aortic atherosclerosis,[3,35] especially in the case of ulcerated lesions.[3] In the SPARC study, systolic and pulse pressure variables (office and ambulatory), but no diastolic variables were associated with atherosclerosis and complex atherosclerosis in the aorta after adjustments were made for age and smoking history.[35] The association between diabetes mellitus and aortic atherosclerosis has been supported in some studies[2] and negated in others,[34,35] at least after adjustment for other risk factors.[34] Hypercholesterolemia has been found to be associated with aortic atherosclerosis in some studies,[18,34,36] and treatment with 3-hydroxy-3-methylglutaryl coenzyme A (hMG-CoA) reductase inhibitors (statins) has been shown to induce regression of aortic atherosclerotic lesions in humans.[37–39]

Besides traditional risk factors, other variables have been identified that are associated with aortic atherosclerosis and are possibly cofactors in raising the embolic risk associated with aortic plaques. As mentioned earlier, the embolic potential of an aortic plaque is related at least in part to the presence of thrombus superimposed on the plaque. It is therefore conceivable that the coexistence of a hypercoagulable state in a patient with aortic arch plaque may increase the likelihood of superimposed thrombus formation and further enhance the embolic potential of the lesion. Procoagulant properties have been demonstrated in atherosclerotic aortas; increased tissue factor expression and activity has been observed in the atherosclerotic intima that may lead to thrombus formation as the result of its exposure to the flowing blood.[40] Among coagulation factors, an increased fibrinogen level has been shown to be a risk factor for cardiovascular disease and ischemic stroke[41,42] and to be associated with severity of carotid stenosis[43–45] as well as presence of abdominal aortic atheromas[43] and peripheral atherosclerotic disease.[46,47]

Specific Medical Diseases and Stroke

Atherogenic effects of fibrinogen have been described; they may result from its interactions with some lipoproteins. In fact, fibrinogen has been shown to modulate the atherogenic effects of lipoprotein(a)[48] (Lp[a]) and to increase the risk of severe carotid atherosclerosis and stroke in patients with low levels of high-density lipoprotein cholesterol.[49] The association between fibrinogen and carotid artery disease has been shown to be particularly strong in the elderly.[50] Moreover, interracial differences have been reported in the levels of fibrinogen, with black persons having higher levels than white persons[51] and both groups having higher levels than Asian persons.[52] Fibrinogen has also been shown to be independently associated with aortic atherosclerosis in a group of 148 patients who underwent TEE for evaluation of valvular heart disease.[34] In that study, there was a relationship between fibrinogen levels and severity of aortic atherosclerosis and of coronary artery disease.

Plasma homocysteine has also been found to be independently associated with aortic atherosclerosis diagnosed on TEE. In 82 patients with cardiac disease, Tribouilloy and colleagues[53] found, through a multivariate analysis including usual risk factors for atherosclerosis, that age, male gender, low-density lipoprotein (LDL) cholesterol, and homocysteine levels were the only factors independently associated with severity of aortic atherosclerosis. This finding suggests that homocysteine may be a marker of atherosclerotic lesions in large arterial vessels. Also, homocysteine was shown to be independently associated with progression of aortic arch atheromas over a period of 9 months in a group of 78 patients with stroke or TIA,[31] whereas no conventional risk factor for atherosclerosis was shown to have similar independent effect. Endothelial dysfunction causing plaque progression and a hypercoagulable state resulting in thrombus deposition were invoked as possible mechanisms for the finding.[31]

The embolic potential of an aortic atheroma is also related to its lipid content. Cholesterol crystal emboli have been documented on pathologic examination in peripheral arteries of patients in whom TEE demonstrated large atheromas.[54–56] In addition to the association of total and LDL cholesterol with aortic plaques mentioned earlier, Lp(a) has been shown to be an independent marker of aortic atherosclerosis.[57] Lp(a) is a complex between LDL and apoprotein(a) (Apo[a]). In spite of the close structural resemblance between LDL and Lp(a), these particles have very different metabolic properties. Serum Lp(a) levels are under strong genetic influence and are mainly determined by the synthetic rate of Apo(a), a protein with a striking similarity to plasminogen. This homology to plasminogen has prompted the speculation that Lp(a) may be an important risk factor for both atherosclerosis and thrombosis. It has been suggested that the atherogenic activity of Lp(a) might result from its inhibiting effect on plasminogen activation, with consequent decrease of plasmin formation, which in turn reduces the activation of transforming growth factor-beta, a potent inhibitor of smooth muscle cell proliferation.[58] In addition, Lp(a) has been detected in atherosclerotic plaques, where it combines with fibrin and attenuates the clearance of this protein, promoting atherogenesis and vascular dysfunction.[59]

In summary, some lipid and coagulation abnormalities are associated with proximal aortic atherosclerosis, an association that may be of importance in the progression of the atherosclerotic plaque, and are possibly implicated as cofactors in determining the plaque's embolic potential. The study and consequent better understanding of the relationships among lipid metabolism, coagulation, and proximal aortic atherosclerosis might provide indications for preventive and therapeutic measures in patients with proximal aortic plaques.

PROXIMAL AORTIC PLAQUES AND CAROTID ARTERY DISEASE

The relation between proximal aortic plaques and carotid artery disease, another important risk factor for ischemic stroke, has been investigated in several studies. In an autopsy study, Amarenco and coworkers[3] found ulcerated aortic plaques to be as common in patients with carotid stenosis of 75% or greater than in patients without it. In the same group's case-control TEE study, no correlation was observed between aortic plaques 4 mm or larger and carotid stenosis 70% or greater.[16] We observed that the frequency of carotid stenosis 60% or greater rose with increasing aortic plaque thickness[8]; however, the positive predictive value of carotid stenosis of 60% or greater for arch plaque 5 mm or larger was only 16%, suggesting that although a general correlation exists between aortic atherosclerosis and carotid atherosclerosis, one condition cannot be predicted on the basis of the other in individual patients. Jones and colleagues[2] obtained similar results, reporting a positive predictive value of carotid disease for aortic plaque of 57%. Kallikazaros and colleagues[60] found, in a group of 62 cardiac patients, that carotid plaque presence had good positive predictive value (83%) and acceptable sensitivity (75%) and specificity (74%) for aortic plaque presence, but lower negative predictive value (63%). In summary, a general correlation exists between carotid and aortic atherosclerosis, but one cannot be reliably predicted from the presence of the other, with the possible exception of patients with cardiac disease, in whom the relation appears to be closer.[60]

PROXIMAL AORTIC PLAQUES AND CORONARY ARTERY DISEASE

The relationship between aortic atherosclerosis and coronary artery disease has been extensively studied. In a TEE study on 61 patients who had previously undergone coronary angiography, Fazio and coworkers[61] found atherosclerotic plaques in the thoracic aorta in 37 of 41 patients (90%) with obstructive coronary disease (defined as 50% or greater stenosis in the left main coronary artery or 70% or greater stenosis in the left anterior descending, circumflex, or right coronary artery), but in only 2 of 20 patients (10%) with no or nonobstructive coronary disease. In that study, the demonstration of aortic plaque by TEE had 90% sensitivity and 90% specificity for obstructive coronary artery disease. In 153 consecutive patients undergoing coronary angiography and TEE, Khoury and colleagues[62] detected plaques in the aorta of 90 of 97 patients (93%) with coronary artery disease versus 12 of 55 patients (22%) with normal coronary arteries. The aortic arch had evidence of plaque in 80% of patients with coronary stenosis 50% or greater. In the SPARC study, aortic plaques were independently associated with history of myocardial infarction and coronary bypass surgery.[1] In the population-based Rotterdam Coronary Calcification Study, coronary calcification, assessed in 2013 subjects by electron beam computed tomography, showed a graded association with aortic calcification, considered a marker of atherosclerosis.[63] In that study, the association was stronger than that between coronary calcification and carotid disease.

Therefore, a strong association between aortic atherosclerosis and coronary artery disease has been widely documented. However, the strength of this association appears slightly lower in elderly patients. In the study reported by Khoury and colleagues,[62] the specificity of the presence of aortic plaques for the diagnosis of coronary artery disease was found to be lower in patients older than 63 years of age than in younger patients (64% vs. 90%). In another study in 84 patients with cardiac disease,[64] the presence of aortic plaques failed to predict significant coronary artery disease in patients older than 69 years but was a strong predictor in younger patients.

AORTIC PLAQUES AND ATHEROEMBOLISM

Besides being the site of origin of thromboembolism to the brain and the peripheral circulation, the atherosclerotic aorta can also give rise to atheroembolic phenomena, by which cholesterol crystal emboli are sent to various segments of the arterial circulation. Atheroembolism is generally characterized by small embolic particles that lodge in small arterioles (less than 200 μm in diameter)[65] and may occur spontaneously or after vascular surgery, arteriography, or anticoagulation.[66,67] The clinical consequences of atheroembolism vary according to the location of the target organ and the number and frequency of embolic episodes. Therefore, atheroembolism has a wide spectrum of clinical presentations, from clinically silent episodes recognized only during diagnostic procedures[68–70] to complex clinical pictures characterized by multiple organ involvement (brain, retina, kidneys, gastrointestinal tract, lower limbs).[71,72] The simultaneous or consecutive involvement of different body parts may, in fact, greatly facilitate a correct diagnosis in patients with subtle or subacute clinical presentation.

Older age is the strongest risk factor for atheroembolism from an aortic source. All 16 patients with atheroembolism reported by Gore and Collins[71] were older than 60 years. In their study, 12 of 13 autopsied patients had evidence of embolism to multiple sites. Older age and aortic atherosclerosis have major effects on the risk of atheroembolism after cardiac surgery, as discussed in the next section.

Proximal Aortic Plaques and Cardiac Surgery

Aortic atherosclerosis is widely recognized as a strong risk factor for atheroembolic events, and especially stroke, after cardiac surgery. As the mean age of the general population rises and indications for cardiac surgery in the elderly expand, an ever-increasing number of elderly subjects

undergo open-heart surgery, raising the number of subjects at high risk for atheroembolic events. Blauth and colleagues,[73] studying the autopsies of 221 subjects who had undergone cardiac surgery, identified embolic disease in 69 (31%), which was atheroembolic in nature in more two thirds of cases. The brain was the most common target organ (16%), followed by spleen (11%), kidney (10%), and pancreas (7%). Atheroembolism was multiple in 63% of subjects and was more common after coronary artery procedures than after valvular procedures (26% vs. 9%; $P = .008$). Atheroembolic events occurred in 37% of patients with severe atherosclerosis of the ascending aorta but only in 2% of patients without significant aortic disease ($P < .0001$), and 96% of patients who had evidence of atheroemboli had severe atherosclerosis of the ascending aorta. In that study, there was a strong relation between age, severe aortic atherosclerosis, and atheroembolism.

The consequences of atheroembolism during or after cardiac surgery may be devastating. One autopsy study found that in 6 of 29 patients (21%) with evidence of atheroemboli, death was directly attributed to the embolic event (intraoperative cardiac failure due to coronary embolization in 3, massive stroke in 2, and extensive gastrointestinal embolization in 1).[74] Proximal aortic atherosclerosis is also associated with the severity of postoperative neurologic complications. In a multicenter prospective study of 2108 patients from 24 U.S. institutions[75] on adverse cerebral outcomes after coronary bypass surgery, the most severe complications (focal injury, or stupor or coma at discharge) were predicted by proximal aortic atherosclerosis, history of neurologic disease, and older age.

In another study of 921 consecutive patients undergoing cardiac surgery, the incidence of postoperative stroke was 8.7% in patients with atherosclerotic disease of the ascending aorta and 1.8% in patients without it ($P < .0001$).[76] Logistic regression analysis indicated that aortic atherosclerosis was the strongest predictor of perioperative stroke. Aortic atherosclerosis was shown to be a predictor of both early (immediately after surgery) and delayed (after initial uneventful recovery) stroke in a third study of 2972 patients undergoing cardiac surgery.[77] In that study, 82% of early strokes and 71% of delayed strokes occurred in patients 65 years or older.

The increased risk of stroke during coronary artery bypass in patients with proximal aortic plaques has been related to the effects of cannulation of the aorta to establish extracorporeal circulation. Ura and colleagues[78] performed epiaortic echocardiography before cannulation and after decannulation in 472 patients undergoing cardiac surgery with extracorporeal circulation. In 16 patients (3.4%), these researchers found a new lesion in the intima of the ascending aorta after decannulation. In 10 of 16 patients (63%), the new lesions were severe, with mobile components or disruption of the intimal layer. Three patients in this group had a postoperative stroke. Thickness of the plaque near the site of aortic manipulation was associated with the development of a new lesion. The frequency of new lesion was 33.3% with plaque thickness 4 mm or more, 11.8% with plaque thickness 3 to 4 mm, and only 0.8% with plaque thickness less than 3 mm.

It has been suggested that the incidence of perioperative stroke and vascular events in patients with severe

Specific Medical Diseases and Stroke

proximal aortic atherosclerosis can be reduced by modifications of surgical approach. Trehan and colleagues,[79] who performed TEE in 3660 patients scheduled for coronary artery bypass surgery, found proximal aortic atheromas with mobile components in 104 (2.84%) of patients. In those patients, these investigators modified the surgical approach, the most common change being off-pump surgery (88 of 104 patients). The incidence of stroke and other vascular events at 1 week after all types of surgical procedures was 0.96% and 1.92%, respectively, and there were no embolic events in the 88 patients who had undergone surgery without the use of extracorporeal circulation. Therefore, preoperative TEE evaluation of the proximal aorta and evolution in surgical techniques may reduce the incidence of stroke associated with coronary artery bypass surgery.

Proximal Aortic Plaques and Cardiac Catheterization

The risk of embolism to the brain is high when severe proximal atherosclerosis is present in subjects undergoing catheter-based diagnostic or therapeutic procedures involving the aortic arch. Because a TEE examination of the aorta is not usually performed before intra-aortic procedures, the presence of aortic plaques is not known to the operator, a circumstance that raises the risk of embolic events after the procedure, especially in elderly patients. An awareness of the presence of aortic plaques, and the consequent modification of the catheterization technique, can be of great importance in reducing the risk of embolic sequelae. Karalis and associates[80] performed cardiac catheterization via the usual femoral approach in 59 patients with aortic atherosclerosis and in 71 control subjects. The incidence of embolic events was 17% in patients with aortic atherosclerosis and 3% in control subjects (P = .01). No embolic events occurred in 11 patients with aortic atherosclerosis in whom the femoral approach was replaced by a brachial approach. It is therefore evident that the identification of subjects at high risk for atheroembolism (elderly, history of prior embolic events or evidence of atherosclerosis in other body segments, or multiple risk factors for atherosclerosis) can be invaluable in identifying patients who should undergo TEE before intra-aortic procedures and could drastically reduce the incidence of embolic complications.

Obviously, the same considerations apply to therapeutic procedures involving the aorta. Keeley and Grines[81] evaluated the frequency of aortic debris retrieved during placement of guiding catheters in 1000 consecutive patients undergoing percutaneous revascularization procedures. In more than 50% of cases, guiding catheter placement was associated with scraping of debris from the aorta. These investigators emphasized that taking great care to allow debris to exit the back of the catheter was essential to preventing the injection of atheromatous debris into the blood stream. Karalis and colleagues[80] also compared the results of intra-aortic balloon pump placement in 10 patients with aortic atherosclerosis and 12 patients without it. An embolic event related to the procedure was observed in 5 patients (50%) in the former group, and in none in the latter (P = .02). These researchers concluded that when aortic debris is detected, and especially when mobile

components are identified, performing brachial rather than femoral catheterization and avoiding to placement of an intra-aortic balloon pump may reduce the risk of embolism.

TREATMENT OF PROXIMAL AORTIC PLAQUES

Although the role of proximal aortic plaques as a risk factor for cerebral and peripheral embolism has become increasingly evident in the past decade, no randomized clinical trials have so far been conducted to evaluate different treatment options for reducing the risk of a first or recurrent embolic event in patients with aortic plaques. Several preventive and therapeutic possibilities have been suggested, which we review in this section.

Systemic Anticoagulation

Because most embolic events associated with large or complex proximal aortic plaques are thought to be thromboembolic in origin, systemic anticoagulation has been suggested as an option to reduce their incidence in patients with such plaques. Dressler and colleagues[82] reported on the frequency of recurrent vascular events in 31 subjects presenting with a systemic embolic event and TEE demonstration of a mobile aortic plaque according to the use of warfarin. Patients were not randomly assigned for treatment with or without warfarin, and although 79% patients (11 of 14) with medium or large mobile components received warfarin, 47% (8 of 17) of those with small mobile components (diameter 1 mm or less) did not. Overall, 45% of patients not receiving warfarin had a vascular event over a mean follow-up period of approximately 10 months, compared with 5% of those receiving warfarin. Corresponding figures for stroke were 27% and 0, respectively. Annual incidence of stroke in the group not receiving warfarin was 32%. These researchers concluded that warfarin was protective against recurrent embolic events in patients with mobile plaques and that the dimension of the mobile component should not be used to assess the need for anticoagulation.

Prospective results from the Study on Prevention of Atrial Fibrillation (SPAF)[83] showed a significant reduction of embolic events in patients with protruding atheromas treated with adjusted-dose warfarin (international normalized ratio [INR] 2 to 3) compared with patients treated with low-intensity warfarin (INR 1.2 to 1.5) plus aspirin (325 mg/day). Overall, patients with complex aortic plaques had a four-fold higher stroke incidence than patients without plaques, and adjusted-dose warfarin reduced the risk by 75% (P = .005). Of course, all patients in that study had nonvalvular atrial fibrillation, a feature that precludes the direct extrapolation of its results to the general population.

Although the use of oral anticoagulation in patients with mobile plaques appears logical and is supported by the aforementioned studies, its use in patients with large but nonmobile lesions is more controversial. However, in 50 patients with atheromas that were 4 mm or larger but without mobile components who were monitored for 22 ±

10 months, Ferrari and coworkers[84] found a substantial incidence of stroke in patients treated with aspirin or ticlopidine (5/23, or 21.7%), compared with no stroke in 27 patients on warfarin (P = .01). Patients were not randomly assigned for treatment, but this study indicates that anticoagulation may be effective in patients who have large plaques even without mobile components.

The safety of systemic anticoagulation in patients with aortic plaques has traditionally been questioned,[85] because anticoagulation might induce bleeding within the plaque, with consequent ulceration and risk of embolization. Moreover, anticoagulation might remove the thrombin coating from ulcerated atheromas and therefore facilitate microembolization of cholesterol crystals.[86,87] Atheroembolism is a real clinical entity, and its sequelae[64–71] and association with anticoagulation[66,67] in patients with aortic atherosclerosis have been discussed earlier. However, the incidence of atherosclerosis after systemic anticoagulation appears to be rather low. In the SPAF, adjusted-dose treatment with warfarin (INR 2 to 3) was associated with an incidence of cholesterol embolization of 0.7% per year.[88]

Antiplatelet Medications

As mentioned earlier, antiplatelet therapy with aspirin or ticlopidine seems to be less protective against recurrent embolic events than warfarin therapy in patients with large or complex plaques.[82–84] However, the studies that have addressed this issue are few and without treatment randomization, except for the SPAF,[83] which was conducted in patients with atrial fibrillation. The combination of aspirin and clopidogrel is being tested against warfarin in patients with large plaques.[89] More data are therefore needed to assess the role of antiplatelet agents in the prevention of aortic plaque–related embolic events.

Thrombolysis

Thrombolysis has occasionally been used to treat large mobile plaques with seemingly very high embolic potential.[90] The high risk of major hemorrhagic complications, especially in elderly patients, and the questionable advantages of thrombolysis over anticoagulation make it an unlikely therapeutic choice in patients with mobile plaques and should be reserved for selected cases. Like systemic anticoagulation, thrombolysis has also been associated with atheroembolic complications in patients with aortic atherosclerosis,[91] although the incidence of this complication is probably rather low.[92]

Statins

The use of statins to prevent embolic events in patients with large or complex aortic plaques appears to have a powerful rationale, because these agents may induce plaque stabilization through the reduction of the lipid content, with consequent reduced frequency of ulceration and superimposed thrombus formation. As mentioned earlier, statins have been shown to induce plaque regression in humans.[37–39] To date, no randomized trial has assessed the efficacy of statins for this indication. The only available data come from Tunick and colleagues,[93] who

retrospectively identified 519 patients with severe thoracic aortic plaques and examined the incidence of embolic events according to treatment status (statins, warfarin, or antiplatelet medications). Patients were not randomly assigned for treatment, and those receiving each class of medication were matched with patients of similar age and embolic risk profile who were not receiving the medication. Over an average follow-up of 34 ± 26 months, embolic events occurred in 111 patients (21%). Multivariate analysis showed statin treatment to be independently protective against recurring events (P = .0001). In the matched analysis, the RR reduction was 59%. No protective effect was found for warfarin or antiplatelet medication. Given the limitations of the retrospective, nonrandomized design, this study represents preliminary evidence of the efficacy of statins in preventing embolic events in patients with severe aortic plaques that deserves confirmation in randomized, prospective studies.

Surgery

Aortic endarterectomy has been proposed as a preventive measure in patients with large mobile plaques in the proximal aorta at impending risk of embolism, especially when cardiac surgery is performed. However, the surgical procedure on the aorta carries in itself a high risk, especially for the potential to dislodge parts of the mobile component of the plaque and precipitate an embolic event. Stern and coworkers[94] performed intraoperative TEE in 3404 patients undergoing heart surgery, finding complex plaques (either ≥5mm or mobile) in 268 (8%). They performed arch endarterectomy in 43 patients in an attempt to prevent intraoperative stroke. The intraoperative stroke rate in the 268 patients was high (15.3%), as was mortality (14.9%). Multivariate analysis showed age and arch endarterectomy to be independently associated with intraoperative stroke. The OR for stroke of arch endarterectomy was 3.6 (P = .01). Therefore, the use of arch endarterectomy should be carefully considered only in carefully selected cases.

Rokkas and Kouchoukos[95] performed resection and graft replacement of a severely atherosclerotic segment of the ascending aorta in 81 patients (mean age 71 years) undergoing coronary bypass surgery. In that study, the 30-day mortality was 8.6% (7 patients). Perioperative strokes occurred in 4 patients (4.9%), and transient neurologic deficits in 2 (2.5%). During the follow-up, only one stroke occurred, 4 months after the procedure. However, 3-year survival was only 40%, with death being secondary mainly to complications of generalized atherosclerosis. In 17 patients who underwent graft replacement of the ascending aorta for severe atherosclerosis during elective coronary bypass grafting, King and colleagues[96] reported a hospital mortality of 23.5%, compared with only 2.3% in 89 patients who underwent replacement for ascending thoracic aortic aneurysm (P = .006). Cerebrovascular event rates were 17.6% and 3.4%, respectively (P = .05). Nonfatal postoperative complications were observed in 53% of the patients with atherosclerosis, compared with 20% of control subjects (P = .01).

From the cumulative evidence presented, one can conclude that surgical procedures on a severe atherosclerotic

Specific Medical Diseases and Stroke

proximal aorta are associated with substantial morbidity and mortality and should be reserved for carefully selected cases.

FUTURE DIRECTIONS

The most important advancements in the field of proximal aortic plaques and ischemic stroke will likely come from the results of randomized clinical trials to test preventive and therapeutic options in patients with proximal aortic atherosclerosis. As the general population ages, however, the number of subjects with atherosclerotic disease will increase, and the identification of subjects at high risk of embolic events to target for primary prevention measures will become more and more important. Better, easier, and noninvasive ways to identify high-risk aortic plaques will be needed. They may entail both a more accurate assessment of plaque morphology and attempts to identify plaques that are more likely to rupture and give origin to embolic events (vulnerable plaques).

Plaque Morphology: Newer Imaging Modalities

As mentioned earlier, the assessment of stroke risk in patients with proximal aortic plaques has been based on plaque thickness and morphology. The measure of plaque thickness, although very helpful for risk stratification, is a monodimensional measurement of a tridimensional lesion and may therefore not convey all the information on a plaque's embolic potential in an individual patient. Also, plaque thickness and morphology characteristics are usually evaluated with TEE, a semi-invasive technique that does not lend itself as a screening tool in asymptomatic elderly subjects. Transthoracic echocardiography performed from a suprasternal or supraclavicular approach would be much easier and more widely applicable,

provided that questions about its sensitivity in comparison with TEE, especially for identification of complex plaque morphology, can be addressed. Real-time three-dimensional echocardiographic equipment has become available that, with further technical refinements, might prove very useful in the noninvasive evaluation of the aortic arch. Figure 30–9 displays an example of an ulcerated plaque in the distal portion of the aortic arch, visualized by TEE (*A*), by commonly available transthoracic echocardiography (*B*), and by real-time three-dimensional echocardiography (*C*). The advantages of the three-dimensional technique over the traditional transthoracic image in displaying the actual extension of the plaque and the characteristics of its ulceration are apparent and allow a representation of the plaque characteristics that appears at least as good as that obtained by TEE. Further technical refinements, including transducers with smaller footprint to better fit into the suprasternal notch, and studies comparing the accuracy of the new technique with that of TEE are needed to evaluate the exact potential and applicability of this new technique.

Other noninvasive techniques have been shown to have excellent accuracy for the detection of proximal aortic plaques. Magnetic resonance imaging (MRI)[97] has been shown to correlate well with TEE for aortic plaque determination and to quantify accurately the fibrotic and lipidic components of the plaque in animal models.[98] Compared with TEE, dual-helical computed tomography has shown sensitivity of 87%, specificity of 82%, and overall accuracy of 84% for the detection of aortic plaques.[99]

Identification of the Vulnerable (High-Risk) Plaque

The noninvasive identification of the vulnerable plaque, or a plaque that is at higher risk of rupture and consequent superimposed thrombus formation because of its composition, would be of great importance in prevention of

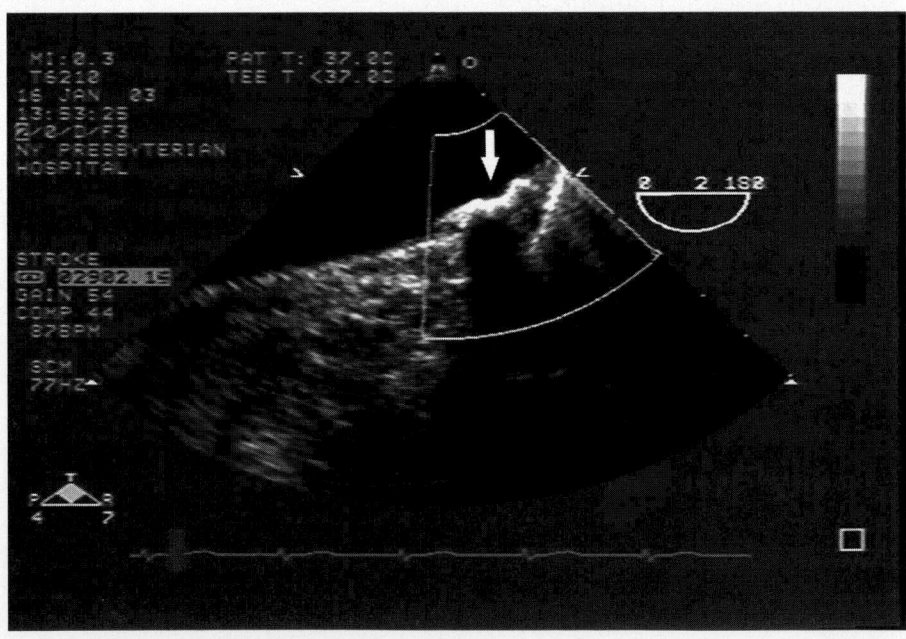

A

FIGURE 30–9 *A, Visualization by transesophageal echocardiography of a calcified plaque in the distal aortic arch. A large ulceration* (arrow) *is seen.*

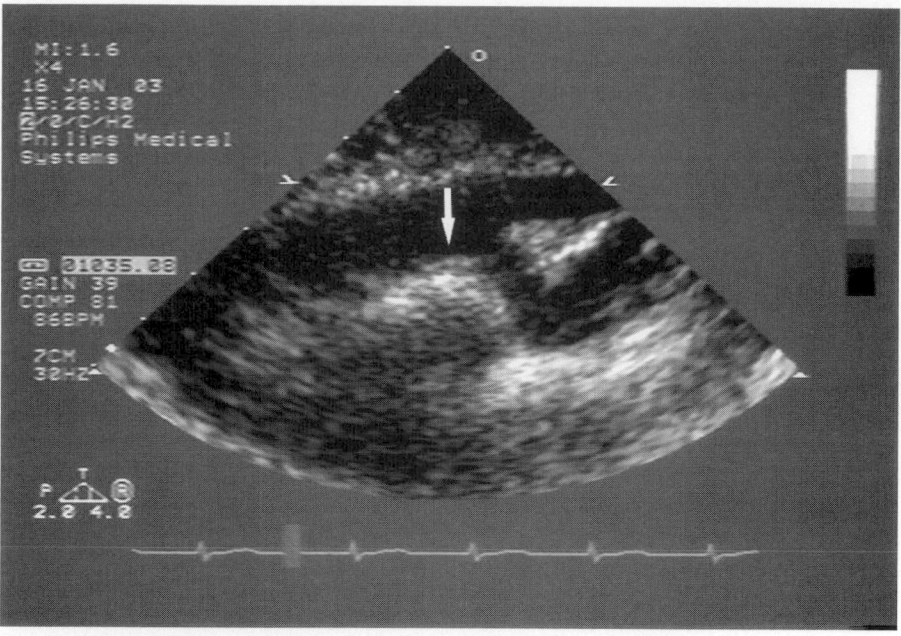

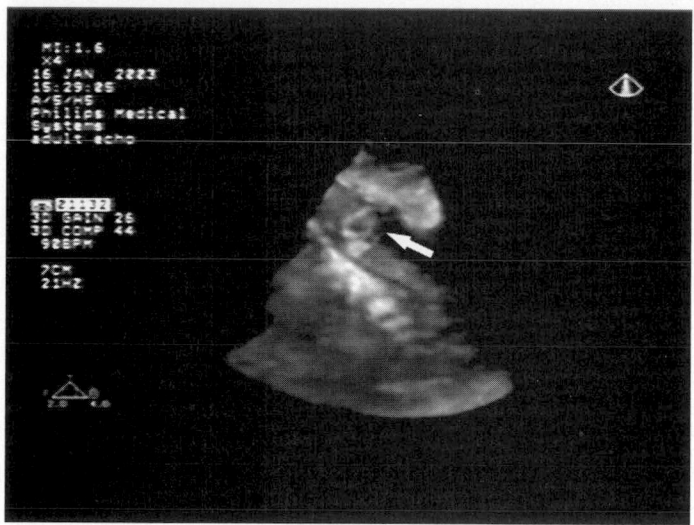

FIGURE 30–9, cont'd. B, *Same plaque visualized through the suprasternal transthoracic approach. No definite ulceration is visible.* C, *Transthoracic three-dimensional imaging of the same plaque. Rotation of transducer plane has allowed a better visualization of the plaque, and the entire area of ulceration (arrow) is now visible.*

embolic sequelae. As discussed, MRI has shown potential for identifying fibrotic and lipidic components of a plaque.[98] Contrast agents have now been introduced that may enhance this capability. Superparamagnetic iron oxide has been found to localize to aortic atherosclerotic plaques in animal models, allowing the detection of iron-laden macrophages in the aortic subendothelium[100] and therefore possibly providing a new noninvasive modality for imaging inflammatory aortic plaques. The accuracy of the method in detecting atherosclerotic lesions in mice has been described as good (between 85% and 88%) on comparison with histology[101] but limited by the elevated proportion of false-positive results (19%) and by a relatively low rate of interobserver agreement (67%).[101] Future optimization of the method should focus on improving the specificity of the test.

SUMMARY

Large and complex plaques in the proximal portion of the thoracic aorta have been established as a risk factor for ischemic stroke and other arterial embolic events in patients older than 60 years. The frequency of embolic events, both spontaneous and precipitated by diagnostic or therapeutic procedures on the aorta, has been defined. Progress has been made in aortic plaque imaging and in the understanding of morphologic characteristics that affect the plaque-related embolic risk. Further advancement is expected to come from improved techniques for the identification of high-risk plaques and from randomized treatment trials aimed at reducing the risk of embolic events associated with severe proximal aortic atherosclerosis.

References

1. Agmon Y, Khandheria BK, Meissner I, et al: Relation of coronary artery disease and cerebrovascular disease with atherosclerosis of the thoracic aorta in the general population. Am J Cardiol 89:262–267, 2002.

2. Jones EF, Kalman JM, Calafiore P, et al: Proximal aortic atheroma: An independent risk factor for cerebral ischemia. Stroke 26:218–224, 1995.

3. Amarenco P, Duyckaerts C, Tzourio C, et al: The frequency of ulcerated plaques in the aortic arch in patients with stroke. N Engl J Med 326:221–225, 1992.

4. Khatibzadeh M, Mitusch R, Stierle U, et al: Aortic atherosclerotic plaques as a source of systemic embolism. J Am Coll Cardiol 27:664–649, 1996.

5. Tenenbaum A, Motro M, Feinberg MS, et al: Retrograde flow in the thoracic aorta in patients with systemic emboli: A transesophageal echocardiographic evaluation of mobile plaque motion. Chest 118:1703–1708, 2000.

6. Toyoda K, Yasaka M, Nagata S, Yamaguchi T: Aortogenic embolic stroke: A transesophageal echocardiographic approach. Stroke 23:1056–1061, 1992.

7. Vaduganathan P, Ewton A, Nagueh SF, et al: Pathologic correlates of aortic plaques, thrombi and mobile "aortic debris" imaged in vivo with transesophageal echocardiography. J Am Coll Cardiol 30:357–363, 1997.

8. Di Tullio MR, Sacco RL, Gersony D, et al: Aortic atheromas and acute ischemic stroke: A transesophageal echocardiographic study in an ethnically mixed population. Neurology 46:1560–1566, 1996.

9. Stone DA, Hawke MW, LaMonte M, et al: Ulcerated atherosclerotic plaques in the thoracic aorta are associated with cryptogenic stroke: A multiplane transesophageal echocardiographic study. Am Heart J 130:105–108, 1995.

10. Daniel WG, Erbel R, Kasper W, et al: Safety of transesophageal echocardiography: A multicenter survey of 10,419 patients. Circulation, 83:817–821, 1991.

11. Oh JK, Seward JB, Tajik AJ: Transesophageal echocardiography. In The Echo Manual, 2nd ed. Philadelphia, Lippincott Williams & Wilkins, 1999.

12. Chee TS, Quek SS, Ding ZP, et al: Clinical utility, safety, acceptability and complications of transoesophageal echocardiography (TEE) in 901 patients. Singapore Med J 36:479–483, 1995.

13. Weslow RG, Di Tullio MR, Sacco RL, et al: Safety and tolerability of transesophageal echocardiography in stroke patients [abstract]. Cerebrovasc Dis 5:243, 1995.

14. Zabalgoitia M, Gandhi DK, Evans J, et al: Transesophageal echocardiography in the awake elderly patient: Its role in the clinical decision-making process. Am Heart J 20:1147–1153, 1990.

15. Tunick PA, Perez JL, Kronzon I: Protruding atheromas in the thoracic aorta and systemic embolization. Ann Intern Med 115:423–427, 1991.

16. Amarenco P, Cohen A, Tzourio C, et al: Atherosclerotic disease of the aortic arch and the risk of ischemic stroke. N Engl J Med 331:1474–1479, 1994.

17. Di Tullio MR, Sacco RL, Savoia MT, et al: Aortic atheroma morphology and the risk of ischemic stroke in a multiethnic population. Am Heart J 139:329–336, 2000.

18. Davila-Roman VG, Barzilai B, Wareing TH, et al: Atherosclerosis of the ascending aorta: Prevalence and role as independent predictor of cerebrovascular events in cardiac patients. Stroke 25:2010–2016, 1994.

19. Tunick PA, Rosenzweig BP, Katz ES, et al: High risk for vascular events in patients with protruding aortic atheromas: A prospective study. J Am Coll Cardiol 23:1085–1090, 1994.

20. Mitusch R, Doherty C, Wucherpfennig H, et al: Vascular events during follow-up in patients with aortic arch atherosclerosis. Stroke 28:36–39, 1997.

21. Atherosclerotic disease of the aortic arch as a risk factor for recurrent ischemic stroke. The French Study of Aortic Plaques in Stroke Group. N Engl J Med 334:1216–1221, 1996.

22. Di Tullio MR, Sacco RL, Savoia MT, et al: Gender differences in the risk of ischemic stroke associated with aortic atheromas. Stroke 31:2623–2637, 2000.

23. Cohen A, Tzourio C, Bertrand B, et al: Aortic plaque morphology and vascular events: A follow-up study in patients with ischemic stroke. Circulation 96:3838–3841, 1997.

24. Tunick PA, Culliford AT, Lamparello PJ, Kronzon I: Atheromatosis of the aortic arch as an occult source of multiple systemic emboli. Ann Intern Med 114:391–392, 1991.

25. Tunick PA, Lackner H, Katz ES, et al: Multiple emboli from a large aortic arch thrombus in a patient with thrombotic diathesis. Am Heart J 124:239–241, 1992.

26. Nihoyannopoulos P, Joshi J, Athanasopoulos G, Oakley CM: Detection of atherosclerotic lesions in the aorta by transesophageal echography. Am J Cardiol 71:1208–1212, 1993.

27. Laperche T, Laurian C, Roudat R, Steg PG: Mobile thromboses of the aortic arch without aortic debris: A transesophageal echocardiographic finding associated with unexplained arterial embolism. The Filiale Echocardiographie de la Societé Française de Cardiologie. Circulation 96:288–294, 1997.

28. Rundek T, Di Tullio MR, Sciacca RR, et al: Association between large aortic arch atheromas and high-intensity transient signals in elderly stroke patients. Stroke 30:2683–2686, 1999.

29. Castellanos M, Serena J, Segura T, et al: Atherosclerotic aortic arch plaques in cryptogenic stroke: A microembolic signal monitoring study. Eur Neurol 45:145–150, 2001.

30. Montgomery DH, Ververis JJ, McGorisk G, et al: Natural history of severe atheromatous disease of the thoracic aorta: A transesophageal echocardiographic study. J Am Coll Cardiol 27:95–101, 1996.

31. Sen S, Oppenheimer SM, Lima J, Cohen B: Risk factors for progression of aortic atheroma in stroke and transient ischemic attack patients. Stroke 33:930–935, 2002.

32. Geraci A, Weinberger J: Natural history of aortic arch atherosclerotic plaque. Neurology 54:749–751, 2000.

33. Gupta V, Nanda NC, Yesilbursa D, et al: Racial differences in thoracic aorta atherosclerosis among ischemic stroke patients. Stroke 34:408–412, 2003.

34. Triboulloy C, Peltier M, Colas L, et al: Fibrinogen is an independent marker for thoracic atherosclerosis. Am J Cardiol 81:321–326, 1998.

35. Agmon Y, Khandheria BK, Meissner I, et al: Independent association of high blood pressure and aortic atherosclerosis: A population based study. Circulation 102:2087–2093, 2000.

36. Di Tullio M, Savoia MT, Sacco RL, et al: Aortic arch atheromas and ischemic stroke in patients of different race-ethnicity [abstract]. Neurology 46:A441, 1996.

37. Pitsavos CE, Aggeli KI, Barbetseas JD, et al: Effects of pravastatin on thoracic aortic atherosclerosis in patients with heterozygous familial hypercholesterolemia. Am J Cardiol 82:1484–1488, 1998.

38. Corti R, Fayad ZA, Fuster V, et al: Effects of lipid-lowering by simvastatin on human atherosclerotic lesions: A longitudinal study by high-resolution, noninvasive magnetic resonance imaging. Circulation 104:249–252, 2000.

39. Corti R, Fuster V, Fayad ZA, et al: Lipid-lowering by simvastatin induces regression of human atherosclerotic lesions: Two-years' follow-up by high-resolution noninvasive magnetic resonance imaging. Circulation 106:2884–2887, 2002.

40. Sueishi K, Ichikawa K, Nakagawa K, et al: Procoagulant properties of atherosclerotic aortas. Ann N Y Acad Sci 748:185–192, 1995.

41. Qizilbash N: Fibrinogen and cerebrovascular disease. Eur Heart J 16(Suppl A):42–45, 1995.

42. Kannel WB, D'Agostino RB, Belanger AJ: Update of fibrinogen as a cardiovascular risk factor. Ann Epidemiol 2:457–466, 1992.

43. Levenson J, Giral P, Razavian M, et al: Fibrinogen and silent atherosclerosis in subjects with cardiovascular risk factors. Arterioscler Thromb Vasc Biol 15:1263–1268, 1995.

44. Heinrich J, Schulte H, Schonfeld R, et al: Association of variables of coagulation, fibrinolysis and acute-phase with atherosclerosis in coronary and peripheral arteries and those arteries supplying the brain. Thromb Haemost 73:374–379, 1995.

45. Agewall S, Wikstrand J, Suurkula M, et al: Carotid artery wall morphology, haemostatic factors and cardiovascular disease: An ultrasound study in men at high and low risk for atherosclerotic disease. Blood Coag Fibrinolys 5:895–904, 1994.

46. Smith FB, Lowe GD, Fowkes FG, et al: Smoking, haemostatic factors and lipid peroxides in a population case control study of peripheral arterial disease. Atherosclerosis 102:155–162, 1993.

47. Lassila R, Peltonen S, Lepantalo M, et al: Severity of peripheral atherosclerosis is associated with fibrinogen and degradation of cross-linked fibrin. Arterioscler Thromb 13:1738–1742, 1993.

Specific Medical Diseases and Stroke

48. Willeit J, Kiechl S, Santer P, et al: Lipoprotein(a) and asymptomatic carotid artery disease: Evidence of a prominent role in the evolution of advanced carotid plaques. The Bruneck Study. Stroke 26:1582–1587, 1995.

49. Szirmai IG, Kaimondi A, Magyar H, Juhasz C: Relation of laboratory and clinical variables to the grade of carotid atherosclerosis. Stroke 24:1811–1816, 1993.

50. Willeit J, Kiechl S: Prevalence and risk factors of asymptomatic extracranial carotid artery atherosclerosis: A population-based study. Arterioscler Thromb 13:661–668, 1993.

51. Folsom AR, Wu KK, Conlan MG, et al: Distribution of hemostatic variables in blacks and whites: Population reference values from the Atherosclerosis Risk in Communities (ARIC) Study. Ethn Dis 2:35–46, 1992.

52. Iso H, Folsom AR, Sato S, et al: Plasma fibrinogen and its correlates in Japanese and US population samples. Arterioscler Thromb 13:783–790, 1993.

53. Tribouilloy CM, Peltier M, Iannetta Peltier MC, et al: Plasma homocysteine and severity of thoracic aortic atherosclerosis. Chest 118:1685–1689, 2000.

54. Katz ES, Tunick PA, Kronzon I: The transesophageal echocardiographic demonstration of coronary flow augmentation and balloon function during intra-aortic balloon counterpulsation. Am J Cardiol 69:1635–1639, 1992.

55. Coy KM, Maurer G, Goodman D, Siegel RG: Transesophageal echocardiographic detection of aortic atheromatosis may provide clues to occult renal dysfunction in the elderly. Am Heart J 123:1684–1686, 1992.

56. Koppang JR, Nanda NC, Coghlan C, Sanyal R: Histologically confirmed cholesterol atheroemboli with identification of the source by transesophageal echocardiography. Echocardiography 9:379–383, 1992.

57. Peltier M, Iannetta Peltier MC, Sarano ME, et al: Elevated serum lipoprotein(a) is an independent marker of severity of thoracic atherosclerosis. Chest 121:1589–1594, 2002.

58. Bartens W, Wanner C: Lipoprotein(a): New insights into an atherogenic lipoprotein. Clin Invest 72:558–567, 1994.

59. Rabbani LE, Loscalzo J: Recent observations on the role of hemostatic determinants in the development of the atherothrombotic plaque. Atherosclerosis 105:1–7, 1994.

60. Kallikazaros IE, Tsioufis CP, Stefanidis CI, et al: Close relationship between carotid and ascending aortic atherosclerosis in cardiac patients. Circulation 102:III263–III268, 2000.

61. Fazio GP, Redberg RF, Winslow T, Schiller NB: Transesophageal echocardiographically detected atherosclerotic aortic plaque is a marker for coronary artery disease. J Am Coll Cardiol 21:144–150, 1993.

62. Khoury Z, Gottlieb S, Stern S, Keren A: Frequency and distribution of atherosclerotic plaques in the thoracic aorta as determined by transesophageal echocardiography in patients with coronary artery disease. Am J Cardiol 79:23–27, 1997.

63. Oei HH, Vliegenthart R, Hak AE, et al: The association between coronary calcification assessed by electron beam computed tomography and measures of extracoronary atherosclerosis: The Rotterdam Coronary Calcification Study. J Am Coll Cardiol 39:1745–1751, 2002.

64. Matsumura Y, Takata J, Yabe T, et al: Atherosclerotic aortic plaque detected by transesophageal echocardiography: Its significance and limitation as a marker for coronary artery disease in the elderly. Chest 112:81–86, 1997.

65. Soloway HB, Aronson SM: Atheromatous embolism to central nervous system. Arch Neurol 11:657–667, 1964.

66. Ben-Horin S, Bardan E, Barshack I, et al: Cholesterol crystal embolization to the digestive system: Characterization of a common, yet overlooked presentation of atheroembolism. Am J Gastroenterol 98:1471–1479, 2003.

67. Theriault J, Agharazzi M, Dumont M, et al: Atheroembolic renal failure requiring dialysis: Potential for renal recovery? A review of 43 cases. Nephron Clin Pract 94:c11–c18, 2003.

68. Bruno A, Russell PW, Jones WL, et al: Concomitants of asymptomatic retinal cholesterol emboli. Stroke 23:900–902, 1992.

69. Bruno A, Jones WL, Austin JK, et al: Vascular outcome in men with asymptomatic retinal cholesterol emboli: A cohort study. Ann Intern Med 122:249–253, 1995.

70. Mouradian M, Wijman CA, Tomasian D, et al: Echocardiographic findings of patients with retinal ischemia or embolism. J Neuroimaging 12:219–223, 2002.

71. Gore I, Collins DP: Spontaneous atheromatous embolization: Review of the literature and a report of 16 additional cases. Am J Clin Pathol 33:416–426, 1960.

72. Hauben M, Norwich J, Shapiro E, et al: Multiple cholesterol emboli syndrome: Six cases identified through spontaneous reporting system. Angiology 46:779–784, 1995.

73. Blauth CI, Cosgrove DM, Webb BW, et al: Atheroembolism from the ascending aorta: An emerging problem in cardiac surgery. J Thorac Cardiovasc Surg 103:1104–1111, 1992.

74. Doty JR, Wilentz RE, Salazar JD, et al: Atheroembolism in cardiac surgery. Ann Thorac Surg 75:1221–1226, 2003.

75. Roach GW, Kanchuger M, Mangano CM, et al: Adverse cerebral outcomes after coronary bypass surgery. Multicenter Study of Perioperative Ischemia Research Group and the Ischemia Research and Education Foundation Investigators. N Engl J Med 335:1857–1863, 1996.

76. van der Linden J, Hadjinikolau L, Bergman P, Lindblom D: Postoperative stroke in cardiac surgery is related to the location and extent of atherosclerotic disease in the ascending aorta. J Am Coll Cardiol 38:131–135, 2001.

77. Hogue CW Jr, Murphy SF, Schechtman KB, Davila-Roman VG: Risk factors for early or delayed stroke after cardiac surgery. Circulation 100:642–647, 1999.

78. Ura M, Sakata R, Nakayama Y, Goto T: Ultrasonographic demonstration of manipulation-related aortic injuries after cardiac surgery. J Am Coll Cardiol 35:1303–1310, 2000.

79. Trehan N, Mishra M, Kasliwal RR, Mishra A: Reduced neurological injury during CABG in patients with mobile aortic atheromas: A five year follow-up study. Ann Thorac Surg 70:1558–1564, 2000.

80. Karalis DG, Quinn V, Victor MF, et al: Risk of catheter-related emboli in patients with atherosclerotic debris in the thoracic aorta. Am Heart J 131:1149–1155, 1996.

81. Keeley EC, Grines CL: Scraping of aortic debris by coronary guiding catheters: A prospective evaluation of 1,000 cases. J Am Coll Cardiol 32:1861–1865, 1998.

82. Dressler FA, Craig WR, Castello R, Labovitz AJ: Mobile aortic atheroma and systemic emboli: Efficacy of anticoagulation and influence of plaque morphology on recurrent stroke. J Am Coll Cardiol 31:134–138, 1998.

83. Transesophageal echocardiographic correlates of thromboembolism in high-risk patients with nonvalvular atrial fibrillation. The Stroke Prevention in Atrial Fibrillation Investigators Committee on Echocardiography. Ann Intern Med 128:639–647, 1998.

84. Ferrari E, Vidal R, Chevallier T, Baudouy M: Atherosclerosis of the thoracic aorta and aortic debris as a marker of poor prognosis: Benefit of oral anticoagulants. J Am Coll Cardiol 33:1317–1322, 1999.

85. Moldveen-Geronimus M, Meriam JC Jr: Cholesterol embolization: From pathologic curiosity to clinical entity. Circulation 35:946–953, 1967.

86. Hollier LH, Kazmier FJ, Ochsner J, et al: "Shaggy" aorta syndrome with atheromatous embolization to visceral vessels. Ann Vasc Surg 5:439–444, 1991.

87. Hilton TC, Menke D, Blackshear JL: Variable effect of anticoagulation in the treatment of severe protruding atherosclerotic aortic debris. Am Heart J 127:1645–1647, 1994.

88. Blackshear JR, Zabalgoitia M, Pennock G, et al: Transesophageal echocardiography: Warfarin safety and efficacy in patients with thoracic aortic plaque and atrial fibrillation. SPAF TEE Investigators. Stroke Prevention in Atrial Fibrillation. Transesophageal echocardiography. Am J Cardiol 83:453–455, 1999.

89. Donnan GA, Davis SM, Jones EF, Amarenco P: Aortic source of brain embolism. Curr Treat Options Cardiovasc Med 5:211–219, 2003.

90. Hausmann D, Gulba D, Bargheer K, et al: Successful thrombolysis of an aortic arch thrombus patient after mesenteric embolism. N Engl J Med 327:500–501, 1992.

91. Geraets DR, Hoehns JD, Burke TG, Grover-McKay M: Thrombolytic-associated cholesterol emboli syndrome: Case report and literature review. Pharmacotherapy 15:441–450, 1995.

92. Aggarwal K, Tjahja IE: Atheroembolic disease following administration of tissue plasminogen activator (TPA). Clin Cardiol 19:906–908, 1996.

93. Tunick PA, Nayar AC, Goodkin GM, et al: Effect of treatment on the incidence of stroke and other emboli in 519 patients with severe aortic plaque. Am J Cardiol 90:1320–1325, 2002.

94. Stern A, Tunick PA, Culliford AT, et al: Protruding aortic arch atheromas: Risk of stroke during heart surgery with and without aortic arch endarterectomy. Am Heart J 138:746–752, 1999.

95. Rokkas CK, Kouchoukos NT: Surgical management of the severely atherosclerotic ascending aorta during cardiac operations. Semin Thorac Cardiovasc Surg 10:240–246, 1998.

96. King RC, Kanithanon RC, Shockey KS, et al: Replacing the atherosclerotic ascending aorta is a high-risk procedure. Ann Thorac Surg 66:396–401, 1998.

97. Fayad ZA, Nahar T, Fallon JT, et al: In vivo magnetic resonance evaluation of atherosclerotic plaques in human thoracic aorta: A comparison with transesophageal echocardiography. Circulation 101:2503–2509, 2000.

98. Helft G, Worthley SG, Fuster V, et al: Atherosclerotic aortic component quantification by noninvasive magnetic resonance imaging: An in vivo study in rabbits. J Am Coll Cardiol 15:1149–1154, 2001.

99. Tenenbaum A, Garniek A, Shemesh J, et al: Dual-helical CT for detecting aortic atheromas as a source of stroke: Comparison with transesophageal echocardiography. Radiology 208:153–158, 1998.

100. Litovsky S, Madjid M, Zarrabi A, et al: Superparamagnetic iron oxide-based method for quantifying recruitment of monocytes to mouse atherosclerotic lesions in vivo: Enhancement by tissue necrosis factor-alpha, interleukin-1beta, and interferon gamma. Circulation 107:1545–1549, 2003.

101. Schmitz SA, Taupitz M, Wagner S, et al: Iron-oxide-enhanced magnetic resonance imaging of atherosclerotic plaques: Postmortem analysis of accuracy, inter-observer agreement, and pitfalls. Invest Radiol 37:405–411, 2002.

Specific Medical Diseases and Stroke

Chapter Thirty-One

Binswanger's Disease and Vascular Dementia

Henning Mast and J. P. Mohr

With each succeeding edition of this book, the basis for acceptance of a disease process referred to as "Binswanger's disease" continues to change.[1] The first edition emphasized an historical review, but succeeding editions have witnessed a series of challenges to the notion of a Binswanger disease, per se, and an effort to determine whether there is an underlying disorder that justifies the continued use of the eponym. Some reviewers have argued that Binswanger's disease should not be considered a clinical entity and that vascular dementia should not bear Binswanger's name.[2–4] The majority of those interested in the pathology have followed Alzheimer's view that it is a form of atherosclerotic vascular disease.[5] Others have linked it to a form of lacunar disease,[2–4 6,7 8–10] and we have even suggested it may have been the first example of CADASIL and discussed issues of chronic ischemia.[10] For the majority of modern writers—too numerous to cite—Binswanger's disease has been accepted as an entity and has been used as the basis for study of some epidemiologic, clinical, radiographic, or laboratory aspects. Some researchers have even concluded it is a common entity,[8] one diagnosable from a triad of clinical, computed tomography (CT), and neuropathologic grounds.[9]

Binswanger's original report[11] did not include much morphologic detail and the cases he presented or reported having seen may well represent a different, even nonvascular, etiology—namely luetic encephalopathy. Much of the haggling over the issue of the pathologic basis for his conclusions can be set aside as tiresome arguments about the completeness of his original observations and their subsequent interpretations by Alzheimer,[5] who concluded that the disorder has a vascular basis. Although a lacunar hypothesis for Binswanger's disease is now popular, neither Binswanger nor Alzheimer made any reference to small, deep infarcts of the lacunar type. In addition to the progressive dementia, Binswanger's original cases featured an array of focal neurologic symptoms and signs, including hemiparesis, hemisensory loss, hemianopia, and aphasia as well as seizures (the latter three assigned to cortical rather than subcortical lesions in today's topologic thinking). The brain of Binswanger's original patient, as understood from reading of the original article, showed no lacunar lesions, but instead featured a white matter gliosis and atrophy mainly in the occipital and temporal lobes, a finding that may be more in line with the modern term *leukoaraiosis*.[12] Binswanger (and subsequently Alzheimer) proposed an underlying process of chronic cerebral ischemia (rather than infarction) induced by small vessel disease, but the closest modern reviewers might infer that the two original writers attributed the condition to a vascular disorder creating lacunar-type infarcts.

We propose that Binswanger's concept of chronic ischemia and dementia from arteriosclerotic small vessel disease may still prove valid and remains largely unexplored. Acceptance of the current view supports notions that infarction, not chronic ischemia, underlies the clinical syndromes, and that there may be a link with the condition currently known as CADASIL (cerebral autosomal dominant arteriopathy with subcortical infarcts and leukoencephalopathy; see Chapter 32), a condition unknown in Binswanger's time.

The review already undertaken in previous editions of this book was intended at least to put in one place as many of the published observations as we could find. Sadly, no distinctive picture has yet emerged as to lesion size, topography, severity, or underlying cause of Binswanger's disease.

BINSWANGER'S ORIGINAL CASE REPORT

In a now-famous lecture in 1894, before the Jahresversammlung des Vereins Deutscher Irrenaerzte in Dresden, Otto Binswanger set forth his concept of vascular dementia. Later published in three parts in the *Berliner Klinische Wochenschrift*,[11] his report delineated a heterogeneity of four dementia syndromes, starting with the then best-understood cause of dementia, syphilis (synonym: "progressive paralysis"). The other three syndromes were to have a major effect on the thinking about vascular disease and dementia in the century that followed.

Encephalitis subcorticalis chronica progressiva (ESCP) was the first of these subtypes, only later labeled "Binswanger's disease" and not always with the same elements as described by Binswanger. He started off by citing its rarity—he had seen only eight cases in the preceding

11 years—and summarized the macroscopic pathology with special emphasis on the severe white matter atrophy (WMA) which he found most pronounced in the occipital and temporal lobes. The atrophy was associated with ventricular enlargement, mainly of the inferior and posterior horns; "the main sites of the disease are the posterior brain segments." He found the cortex only slightly narrowed and noted it was otherwise not involved. The clinical picture featured gradual intellectual decline and focal signs such as aphasia, hemianopia, hemiparesis, and hemisensory loss. The severity of the focal syndromes could fluctuate at the onset of the disease process but reached a stable state toward the end. Seizures also occurred. Binswanger offered the opinion that ESCP usually started around the age of 50 years but one patient was 72 years old at onset. The course lasted for 10 or more years. Periods of clinical stability lasting several years were noted. Death was due to secondary causes (infection, cardiac failure) or "apoplectiform attacks."

Binswanger followed his general remarks with the only detailed clinicopathologic case report he was ever to publish. Using a purely macroscopic evaluation of the brain, he described the autopsy as revealing an asymmetric hemispheral WMA of the lower parietal as well as the upper and lateral temporal lobes. Measurements of both hemispheres after a coronal section through the posterior sylvian fissure showed a width of 8.7 cm for the right hemisphere, compared with 7.3 cm for the left hemisphere. The ventricles were enlarged, especially the lower horns. The frontal gray matter was described as only slightly narrowed. Contrary to his postulates as to the pathophysiology of ESCP from arteriosclerosis, his case showed no arteriosclerotic changes in the basal arteries. He did not describe the smaller vessels. Cavitary lesions were not mentioned (an important point differing from findings of subsequent writers; see later), and Binswanger explicitly stated that there were "nowhere signs of focal disease." The spinal cord showed diffuse pathologic changes throughout.

The clinical features of this case conformed fairly well to the syndrome he labeled ESCP. The patient had suffered for several years from "dizziness" (not further specified by Binswanger), visual decline of the right eye interpreted as "choroiditis disseminata," and "ptyalism." Beginning in his late forties, the patient suffered severe left-sided headache, paresthesias of the right arm and leg, fine motor disturbance of the right hand, and the complaint of "missing words," together with episodes of sudden loss of memory for remote events. More recent events were well remembered. Further symptoms were a depressed mood and, because the patient was fully aware of his state, a fear of becoming insane. No detailed neurologic examination is documented, but Binswanger stated that the strength of the right-sided extremities and results of sensory testing were normal. Calculation was impaired. (It remains unclear whether the initial history was taken by Binswanger himself or cited from notes of other physicians.) Because of a syphilitic infection the patient had acquired 26 years before, an "antiluetic" treatment was initiated and was believed to result in an incomplete remission of the syndrome.

The patient returned to his previous professional activity but never regained his previous level of intellectual performance. Instead, a gradual decline occurred, with increasing forgetfulness (especially for recent events) and paraphasic errors. Confusional states began about 5 years after the initial event and finally mandated hospital admission. The neurologic examination at that time showed a minimal right-sided central facial paresis and slight tongue deviation to the right. The pupils were normal in size and shape and reacted normally to light. Hearing was intact. No motor deficit was found in the arms, but the legs showed mild bilateral weakness that was more pronounced on the right. The patient could walk normally. Sensory testing showed normal pain perception. Other sensory qualities could not be evaluated reliably. The patient's speech, apparently fluent, was severely disturbed with a "completely meaningless stringing of words." The patient called a spoon a "school" (the corresponding German words *Loeffel* and *Schule* being phonetically farther apart than their English translation). The patient was unable to give the word for a watch (or clock); "that is ... I really don't know now—Erfurt—in Erfurt" (Erfurt is a German city). He called a hat "a hat," but then said of a ring, "That is also a hat." After being offered the correct term for spoon, the patient immediately agreed and mumbled repetitively "Loeffel." Repetition was intact. He followed simple commands (showing the tongue, lifting the right or left hand) correctly but made errors in more complex tasks (picking the wrong verbally named object; drawing a ring in the air when the investigator asked, "Show me *my* ring"). Reading and writing were also grossly impaired. The patient's behavior was "quite correct," and he struggled unsuccessfully to communicate his problems. In the following 4 years, nocturnal episodes of confusion and agitation became an increasing problem, and the neuropsychological deficits progressed. Stereotypical rubbing movements of the hands on the thighs and two generalized seizures were noted. The patient finally died in the course of an infection.

Binswanger then described two additional syndromes. Arteriosclerotic brain degeneration (ABD) was the second entity Binswanger advanced, which he considered separate from ESCP. The anatomical features were summarized as widespread large artery arteriosclerosis affecting the brain vessels as well as other organs with subsequent severe cardiac and renal changes. The weights of the brains in these cases were markedly reduced. He noted, "Generally, the vessel-holes are very enlarged. Already by macroscopic inspection, in the vicinity of the vessels in many areas of the cortex and the white matter the brain parenchyma is discolored light-gray to red-brown and slightly sunken in, especially in the area of the basal ganglia and internal capsule an état criblé is prominent." The white matter was discolored throughout, the cortex pale but only slightly narrowed, and the ventricles showed enlargement. "Miliary apoplexies" in the surrounding of arteriosclerotic vessels were pointed out. Microscopy revealed "simple atrophic or fatty degenerative" changes in small cortical and white matter arteries (and veins), in some "larger ones" with luminal narrowing (Binswanger described no specific microscopic findings for ESCP). In the area surrounding these vessels, neuronal and glia cell decline was found. The cortex showed a "degenerative-atrophic process" affecting cortical neurons. Myelinated cortical fibers were reduced in number.

The intellectual deficit in ABD was characterized by a more remittent course than in the cases of ESCP. Patients with ABD could show almost complete remission of memory deficits with more fluctuation than the patients with ESCP, whose deficits were either generally stable or relentlessly progressive. A variety of intermittent focal neurologic syndromes and episodes of loss of consciousness (seizures?) were also seen. Stable focal deficits, as in ESCP, were not listed. Binswanger further commented that "the close relationship" of ESCP and ABD allowed for intermediate forms that blurred the clinical discrimination.

Finally, in addition to these disseminated in situ arterial disorders, Binswanger noted "embolic and thrombotic" large artery occlusions leading to cerebral infarcts. This third form of vascular dementia he called "dementia post apoplexiam" with acute onset ("apoplectical insult") of intellectual and focal deficits with a stable nonremittant course, but no further anatomical details were given, and he cited no literature. Other nonvascular dementia forms, like "simple, pre-senile dementia" (the precursor of today's Alzheimer's disease) and alcoholic dementia were discussed by Binswanger, but are not dealt with further here. Although he promised future detailed descriptions, namely of ESCP, Binswanger did not write further on the topic.

PATHOLOGY

Several studies have attempted to define a neuropathologic basis for Binswanger's disease. In 1905, Bucholz[13] described five cases of Binswanger's ESCP, and in 1912, Ladame[14] reported one case. These writers concurred with the impression that the disease was a severe form of cerebral atherosclerosis. Few details were given. In 1920, Nissl[15] described the brain of a patient with a progressive mental deterioration punctuated by episodes of dysfunction attributable to numerous focal changes in the white matter, in the surface convolution as well as deep in the hemispheres, varying in size and associated with arteriosclerotic vessels of various calibers. He found vascular changes that consisted of severe and often extreme thickening of the vascular walls to such an extent that the distinction between the artery, vein, and capillary was not possible. The thickening was caused by concentric lamellae arranged in onionskin pattern. Nissl did not note a predilection of the lesions for the posterior half of the brain and described no focal lesions in the subcortical gray matter or in the brainstem. The work of Farnell and Globus[16] in 1932 echoed the previous descriptions, added no new data, and served mainly to continue earlier trends.

Davison,[17] in 1942, reported a very atypical case referred to as Binswanger's disease, which included swelling of the patchily involved white matter as well as some involvement of the overlying gray matter. Although atheromatous changes were seen in the small blood vessels of the white matter, it is unclear whether this case should be included among those classified as Binswanger's disease. Davison expressed uncertainty about whether Binswanger's disease existed as a pathologic entity. The 1947 case reported by Neuman[18] is usually listed in the Binswanger's disease literature but is also so atypical in course and pathologic

findings that it is more likely to be some type of other myelinoclastic disorder and is not further considered in our evaluation.

In 1965, Olszewski[19] published an important review of the tiny world literature on Binswanger's disease to that time and added two cases of his own. In this article, he published the translations of Binswanger's, Alzheimer's, and Nissl's descriptions of the disease. Olszewski took the position that the condition was an arteriosclerotic process preferentially affecting the vessels of the subcortical gray matter and the white matter and proposed the term "subcortical arteriosclerotic encephalopathy (Binswanger's type)". He attributed the demyelination to multiple areas of infarction with disruption of long tracts.

Jelgersma[20] described a case of Binswanger's subcortical arteriosclerotic encephalopathy (SAE) in 1964 that resembled previous cases clinically and pathologically. The vascular changes included relatively severe hyalinosis, hypertrophy of the media, atherosclerosis of the cerebral vessels, and état lacunaire of the basal nuclei; both the myelin sheaths and the axons had evidence of degeneration; the cortex and U fibers were normal. Although noting the vascular abnormalities, Jelgersma believed that the relative sparing of the cortex and U fibers argued against a vascular process. Few writers have followed this lead of a nonvascular cause of the disorder, but Jelgersma's work represents one definite etiologic path parallel with those for vascular disease.

In 1970, Biemond added two cases to the literature and concurred with most previous opinions that this was a vascular process.[21] He also noted patchy demyelination of the white matter. He appears to have been the first to suggest the possibility of diagnosing this condition antemortem on the basis of the typical clinical syndrome described by Binswanger. Burger and colleagues[22] described a patient in 1976 who appeared to have Binswanger's disease. They noted that his ventricles were large and that results of radioactive iodinated serum albumin (RISA) testing were abnormal, which suggested the diagnosis of normal-pressure hydrocephalus (NPH). The patient showed no response to shunting. He subsequently experienced a subdural hematoma, which required surgical drainage. In the last stages of disease, this patient had myoclonic jerks and demonstrated triphasic waves on electroencephalography (EEG). Electrolyte levels were reported to be normal. Results of neuropathologic examination were not consistent with Creutzfeldt-Jakob disease, but more consistent with Binswanger's disease. This case is somewhat atypical because of the presence of the myoclonic jerks and the triphasic waves.

White[23] subsequently reported another case with triphasic waves; this case also was atypical, in that the patient had a remarkably short course of 6 weeks. Autopsy revealed a large basilar territory infarct. The comments in White's discussion of neuropathologic findings include the finding of multiple lacunar infarctions in the subcortical white matter; no comments are made about the presence of other possible causes of triphasic waves. Brun and Englund[24] expressed a concern that the literature left unsettled whether Binswanger's disease could actually be said to exist.

In 1980, De Reuck and associates[6] reopened the issue of small, deep infarcts by equating those in the centrum semiovale with those known in deeper sites as lacunes. These investigators described four patients, three of whom had clinical histories very atypical for Binswanger's disease, having cystic or lytic lesions in the periventricular white matter (not noted by Binswanger in his original case material) surrounded by variable degrees of demyelination. They also had lacunes in the thalamus and basal ganglia (also lacking in Binswanger's original descriptions). Despite some of the atypical features, the neuropathologic changes were said to be the same as those seen in subacute arteriosclerotic encephalopathy. De Reuck and associates[6] expressed the opinion that these changes were the result of disease involving the lenticulostriate and medullary cerebral arteries. The sparing of the U fibers was ascribed to the direct derivation of their blood supply from the cortical vessels and not from the medullary, penetrating arteries. These investigators equated the lesions in the white matter with those of the lacunes seen in the basal ganglia. However, they did not believe that a primary arteriopathy such as that usually responsible for lacunes was the sole factor necessary for the development of Binswanger's disease. They expressed the view that the periventricular white matter is a watershed area, supplied by end arteries, the medullary arteries. They proposed that the combination of the severe penetrating vessel disease with hypoperfusion in the watershed area produces the pathologic picture of Binswanger's disease. This argument had been articulated years before by Lindenberg and Spatz,[24a] who said that demyelination in this area is the result of poor perfusion of these watershed areas during periods of hemodynamic crisis resulting in distal field infarction in the immediate periventricular area and less severe ischemic injury producing demyelination more proximally in the course of the medullary arteries.

Fisher[7] proposed a process of multiple lacunar infarcts as the morphologic basis underlying "subcortical arteriosclerotic encephalopathy (Binswanger's type)." This observation is at odds with his earlier work indicating only a low frequency of lacunar lesions in the centrum semiovale. Further, a central thesis for lacunes was that they occur mainly in the territories of very small vessels (e.g., thalamoperforators, lenticulostriates, paramedian branches of the basilar artery), which arise from very large ones, thus not being buffered from the effects of hypertension.

Furuta and coworkers[25] reported vascular changes seen in the medullary arteries (mainly those of the centrum semiovale) in 110 patients said to be nonneuropsychiatric patients, most of whom old but some in their 20s, and comparing the findings with those in 20 patients with subcortical arteriosclerotic encephalopathy (Binswanger's disease), and 20 with Alzheimer's disease. These researchers found on autopsy a prominent fibrohyaline thickening of the arterial walls, proportional in severity to the age in decades. The findings were the most prominent, in descending sequence, in the frontal, parietal, occipital, and temporal lobes, and were present in both the "nonneuropsychiatric" and demented groups. The intensity of the sclerotic changes correlated with the extent of ischemic white matter changes as well as with blood pressure. It may be important that the distribution of the vascular changes noted was in the opposite order to that stressed by Binswanger (parietal-occipital predominating), so it is not certain that these findings are the same as or different from those of Binswanger.

BINSWANGER'S DISEASE AND BRAIN IMAGING

Many studies of Binswanger's disease have focused mainly on CT or magnetic resonance imaging (MRI), with the autopsy and histopathologic details given less attention. Figure 31–1 is an example of the abnormalities found. Some of the earlier studies linked imaging with autopsy findings. Lotz and associates[26] performed a case-control study for the 82 patients in whom CT was performed prior to autopsy. Twenty had CT findings that these investigators took to represent changes consistent with SAE (as noted, often considered the same as Binswanger's disease). Microscopy was said to have confirmed the diagnosis in 18 patients. A point of special interest was the similar histologic vascular findings among 10 control patients showing normal cerebral white matter on CT, although the researchers considered the findings less severe than those for patients with SAE. Mathers and colleagues[27] reviewed their experience with 20 cases showing white matter changes on CT scan, which suggested a diagnosis of Binswanger's disease. They concluded that Binswanger's disease is probably due to chronic or acute-on-chronic white matter ischemia. They also noted the occurrence of lacunar infarctions in this group and differentiated Binswanger's disease clinically from multi-infarct dementia[12] on the basis of its time course.

Leifer and coworkers[28] reported their MRI and pathologic correlations in seven patients. Apart from the periventricular findings, the extensive subcortical changes on MRI were explained by multiple sclerosis in one case and by SAE (again equated with Binswanger's disease) in another, the latter showing widespread fiber loss and lacunar changes. Likewise, Revesz and associates[29] reported on four cases described as subcortical arteriosclerotic encephalopathy. They considered that a "firm" diagnosis was made clinically and pathologically, and a good correlation was observed between the extent and severity of the abnormal MRI signal and the pathologic changes. Microscopic signs of axonal and myelin loss with gliosis were found in the areas with signal abnormalities on MRI. The subcortical U fibers were spared. They attributed the abnormal MRI signal to increased tissue water attributable to gliosis and an expanded extracellular space. Subsequent studies have concentrated on leukoariosis,[30] even occult hydrocephalus[31] with little change in diagnostic criteria.

NONVASCULAR THESES

A few writers have been dissatisfied with the explanation that the demyelination occurs on a vascular basis and have proposed other causes. Feigen and Popoff[32] proposed that both vessel wall changes and the demyelination were the late effects of cerebral edema initiated by hypertensive disease. Although they commented that there was relatively little glial reaction in the areas of demyelination, they did not give any details about their cases, so it is difficult

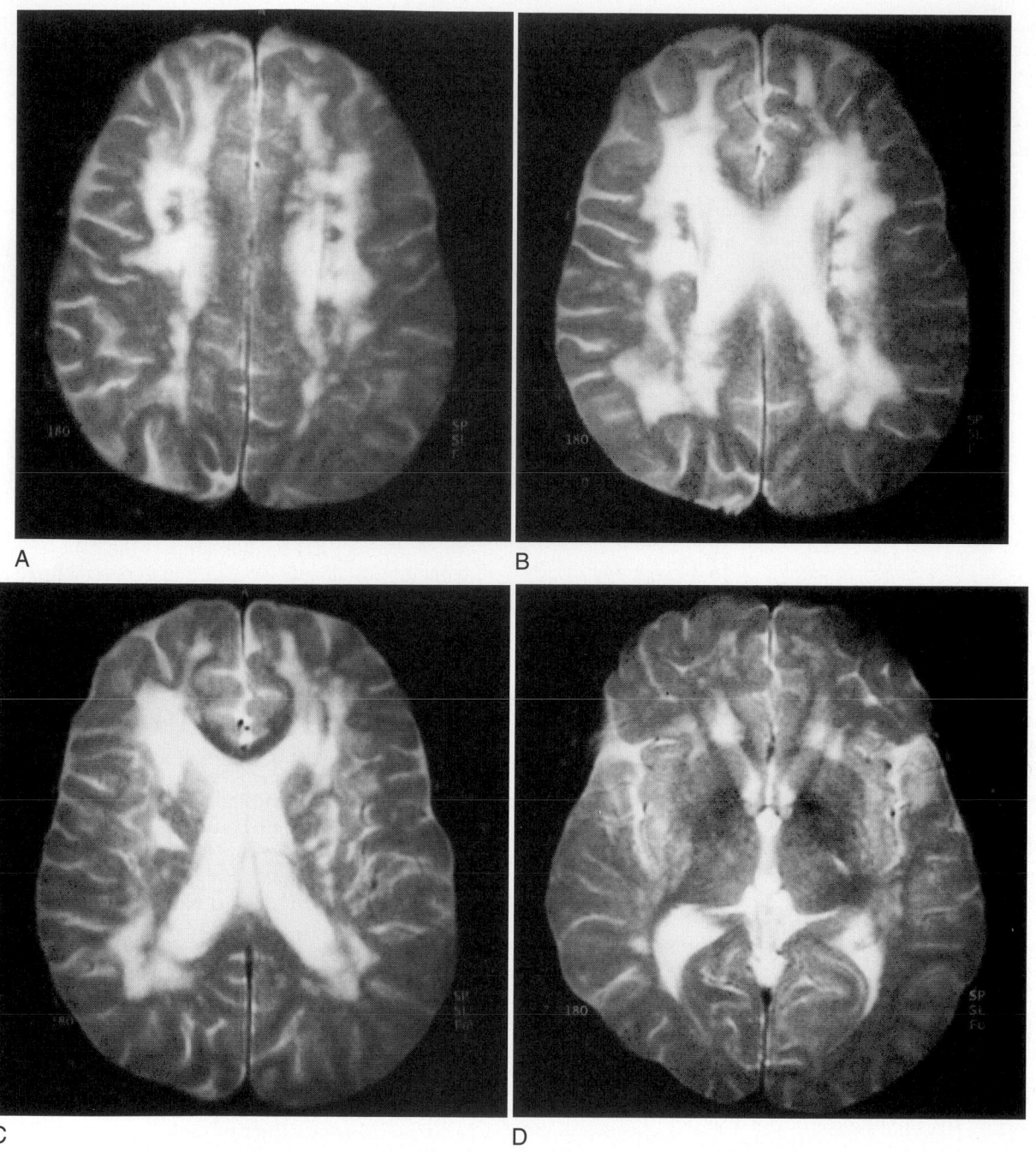

FIGURE 31–1 *A to D, T2-weighted MR images showing high signal changes in the centrum semiovale and corona radiata in a 35-year-old man with recurrent strokes and positive family history of early strokes. There is relative sparing of the basal ganglia and capsular structures.*

to interpret this remark. No data were offered to support this theory. Jellinger and Neumayer[33] thought there might have been an associated nutritional disturbance with organic damage of the blood vessels. Inzitari and colleagues[34] noted a difference between the histopathology of what they decided was leukoaraiosis and what they characterized as Binswanger's SAE. The findings in the first group did not seem to have a vascular basis, whereas those in the second group did. This study is a bit at odds with some of the other case series reported, adding to the

difficulties in settling the mechanisms of disease at work in this cohort.

Later studies have included two mechanisms of ischemic stroke that differ somewhat from older formulations, including demyelination and lacunar-type infarcts,[35] with rare reference to a role for astrocytes.[36] A possible mechanism of injury from vascular immunoreactivities has been put forward.[37,38] Even cerebrospinal fluid investigations have been pursued; Strittmatter and colleagues[39] attempted to distinguish Binswanger's from Alzheimer's disease but failed to find significant differences in the wide variety of items they measured.

ACCEPTABILITY OF BINSWANGER'S DISEASE AS AN ENTITY

A controversy about the mechanism and existence of Binswanger's disease dates back to the very beginning of the literature on the subject. Alzheimer's contribution relates to this dichotomy mainly through his separation of Binswanger's ESPC from cases that Alzheimer attributed to more visible arteriosclerosis. Many of Alzheimer's observations on "senile cortical atrophy" seem consistent with modern-day interpretations of distal field infarction from large carotid artery or middle cerebral artery stenosis or occlusion. His notion of small cortical wedge-shaped scars, which he attributed to arteriosclerosis of the small cortical vessels, resembles Pozzi's "granular cirrhosis of the brain"[40] and the old Winniwarter-Buerger concept of selective vulnerability to disease of vessels in the arterial borderzones.

Despite the ambiguities in the literature, the generally accepted altered definitions of Binswanger's disease are in line with the notions of ABD or the combined disease category offered by Binswanger and Alzheimer. If matters are to remain in this state, the Binswanger eponym is a misnomer and should be replaced by the names of other writers who contributed more to the knowledge of ABD (Klippel, Conso, Pactet, Marie, even Alzheimer).

Reports on cases of "true" ESCP are rare. For example, in only 1 of 84 autopsies of patients with dementia did Brun and Englund[24] find diffuse white matter atrophy with underlying fibrohyalinosis of the small penetrating arteries and arteriosclerosis of larger vessels. Lacunes, larger infarcts, or findings consistent with Alzheimer's disease were not seen in this case.

Later writers have tended more to "lump" rather than "split" the differing findings. In the 2nd edition of this book, Bogousslavsky[41] defined *Binswanger's disease* as diffuse white matter disease linked with "some infarcts, usually deep, but sometimes involving the cortex" with the internal capsule being "markedly spared."[41] Both Loeb[21] and Hachinski[2] are on record as doubting either the existence or the importance of the disorder.

CHRONIC ISCHEMIA

Apart from deciding whether there is a Binswanger's disease and how the white matter disease influences dementia, few writers have addressed or admitted the possibility of chronic ischemia, a concept that was central to the theses of Binswanger and Alzheimer. All through the work of these two investigators is a tacit assumption that diseased small vessels can cause a nutritional disorder, leading to atrophy, gliosis, and other injuries to the cerebrum, whether or not gross macroscopic or microscopic signs of infarction are found. This concept is at odds with much of the modern emphasis on energy failure thresholds, the two notions perhaps contrasting metaphorically as an incandescent light versus fluorescent light model of ischemia and infarction.

The importance of chronic ischemia may be supported by several studies, although these studies are not restricted to dementia cases. Using positron emission tomography (PET), Meguro and associates[42] found a reduction in cerebral blood flow in patients with diffuse white matter ischemic changes. The trend toward rising oxygen extraction fractions was consistent with chronic hypoperfusion. The finding of patchlike ischemic lesions in the periventricular regions and the centrum semiovale has led to the thesis of "incomplete ischemia" from hypoperfusion in the distal fields of the long, medullary branches.[6] Histopathologic investigations have shown hyalinization and concentric thickening of the media with proliferation and fibrosis of the intima[43] resulting in luminal narrowing especially involving the medullary arteries supplying the periventricular white matter.[25] In a combined MRI and histopathologic examination of arteriosclerotic vascular changes and white matter alterations, demyelination and astrogliosis correlated with white matter patches on MRI and was regularly associated with an increased ratio of wall thickness to the external diameter of arterioles.[44]

Angioarchitectural studies support the concept of zones of vulnerability in specific white matter regions related to the effects of aging and the pattern of collateral pathways.[45] Further pathologic studies have established that tortuosity, coiling, and spiraling of the perforating cortical arterioles occur commonly with aging, extending through the thickness of the cerebral cortex to the subcortical white matter.[46] The effect of increasing arterial tortuosity with age has been analyzed by computer modeling, an effort suggesting that resistance to flow is markedly elevated, thus raising the threshold of minimum pressure required for perfusion.[45] The long course of the medullary arteries already results in a large pressure drop, greater than that along short arteries that supply the cortex and corpus callosum. Thus, tortuosity and other arteriosclerotic changes further exacerbate this pressure drop, increasing the susceptibility of the centrum semiovale to chronic ischemic damage.

These findings suggest that there may be more to the concept of chronic ischemia than has been appreciated heretofore. In the end, Binswanger and Alzheimer might have made a greater contribution to pathophysiology through their notion of chronic ischemia than through any disease bearing either of their names.

SYNDROME EFFECTS OF PREDOMINANTLY CENTRUM SEMIOVALE INFARCTION

Apart from the disease underlying the centrum semiovale lesions, Binswanger's disease as a clinical entity prompts consideration of what is known of the effects of such lesions in the centrum semiovale on disturbances of higher cerebral function.[47] The problem bears on whether the lesions (whether from chronic ischemia or infarction) (1) serve mainly to reduce the number of fibers in a fashion that contributed to the volume effect suggested a generation ago by Lashley,[48] (2) produce specific syndromes supporting the older connectionist model of linkages between certain "centers," or (3) can be explained by yet other effects, such as injury to neurotransmitter pathways serving the likes of vasoreactivity.

It is a source of frustration that this field is plagued by problems segregating one from another of the many coexisting disease entities in the mainly elderly population affected by them. The common coexistence of focal ischemic lesions, leukoaraiosis, and histopathologic markers for Alzheimer's disease and Lewy body disease complicates the issue, and few attempts have been made to analyze the independent effects of diffuse and focal lesions in patients with dementia.

Differential effects of various diseases aside, the effect of focal ischemic lesions in the context of dementia remains largely unsettled. Lumping all disturbances in behavior under the unsatisfactory term "dementia," histopathologic investigations have suggested a rough relationship between sum-loss of brain tissue and dementia.[49] However, aggregate infarct volume studies based on brain imaging have failed to show a strong association.[47] Volume estimates in the latter studies included lacunes as well as large infarcts, so whatever role small, deep infarcts play could weigh toward or against a relationship between lesion volume and dementia in imaging studies.

Similar problems in correlating infarcts with dementia arise when the number of infarcts is taken into account. A clear correlation between multiple lacunar infarcts and dementia has not been established[50,51] and the concept of multi-infarct dementia (MID) is further obscured by its unclear definition. Some writers equate MID with multiple lacunes–état lacunaire, but others have used multifocal thrombotic or embolic infarcts as the characterizing elements or have proposed a combination of the two. In a controlled, prospective clinical and histopathologic study, leukoencephalopathy alone was not significantly associated with dementia; however, multiple lacunes and a sum-loss of more than 50 mL of brain tissue by small or larger infarcts was more common among the cases of dementia, suggesting that leukoaraiosis has a less prominent role than focal lesions in the etiology of dementia.[52] The finding of coexisting pathologic markers for nonvascular dementias (Alzheimer's disease, Lewy body disease) in many patients with vascular changes further complicates the issue, often making it impossible to assign the syndrome to one cause or the other.

The lack of better confirmation of the importance of vascular lesions in dementia might be the result, in part, of failure to take into account the *cerebral site* of lesions. Damage to the temporo-occipital or thalamic territory of the posterior cerebral artery, the basal ganglia bilaterally, the frontal brain in the anterior cerebral artery territory, and the caudate nucleus has been shown to induce dementia, but most of this evidence stems from acute stroke, in which such correlations are well-established. Binswanger and Alzheimer referred only in passing to acute dementia syndromes, and their work did not address specific brain areas carrying functions important for memory and cognition. The importance of these sites in progressive dementia has yet to be established, but an active literature is developing under the term *specific infarct dementia* (SID).[47] In passing, we note that any dementia attributed to deep lesions would run at odds with the cases described by Binswanger, in which no such findings were noted.

Work on CADASIL has reawakened interest in the variety of white matter syndromes and may serve to expand our understanding.[53,54] It may well be we can eventually understand whether the central white matter actually has tracts serving aspects of behavior that can be deranged in a focal manner, as is seen from lesions of the visual radiations, or whether volume effects are more important and less task specific. More work is in order.

References

1. Nichols F, Mohr JP: Binswanger's subacute arteriosclerotic encephalopathy. In Barnett HJM, Mohr JP, Stein BM, Yatsu FM (eds): Stroke: Pathophysiology, Diagnosis, and Management, vol 2. New York, Churchill Livingstone, 1986, pp 875–885.
2. Hachinski V: Binswanger's disease: Neither Binswanger's nor a disease. J Neurol Sci 103:1, 1991.
3. Pantoni L, Garcia JH: The significance of cerebral white matter abnormalities 100 years after Binswanger's report: A review. Stroke 26:1293, 1995.
4. Loeb C: Dementia due to lacunar infarctions: A misnomer or a clinical entity? Eur Neurol 35:187–192, 1995.
5. Alzheimer A: Neuere Arbeiten über die Dementia senilis und die auf atheromatöser Gefäßerkrankung basierenden Gehirnkrankheiten. Monatsschr Psychiatr Neurol 3:101, 1898.
6. De Reuck J, Crevits L, DeCoster W, et al: Pathogenesis of Binswanger's chronic subcortical encephalopathy: A clinical and radiological investigation. Neurology 30:920–928, 1980.
7. Fisher C. Binswanger's encephalopathy: a review. J Neurol 236:65–79, 1989.
8. Ramos-Estebanez C, Rebollo Alvarez-Amandi MR: [Binswanger disease: a common type of vascular dementia]. Rev Neurol 31:53–58, 2000.
9. Vega MG, Faccio EJ: [Binswanger's disease: evolution of thought and a proposed diagnostic triad]. Arq Neuropsiquiatr 53:518–525, 1995.
10. Mast H, Tatemichi TK, Mohr JP: Chronic brain ischemia: The contributions of Otto Binswanger and Alois Alzheimer to the mechanisms of vascular dementia. J Neurol Sci 132:4–10, 1995.
11. Binswanger O: Die Abgrenzung der allgemeinen progressiven Paralyse. Berl Klin Wochschr 31:1103-1105,1137–1139, 1180–1186, 1894.
12. Hachinski V, Lassen NA, Marshall J: Multi infarct dementia: A cause of mental deterioration in the elderly. Lancet 2:207–210, 1974.
13. Bucholz: Ueber die Geistesstoerungen bei Arteriosklerose und ihre Beziehungen zu den psychischen Erkrankungen des Seniums. Arch Psychiatr Nervenkr 39:499, 1905.
14. Ladame C: Encephalopathie sous-corticale chronique. Encephale 7:13, 1912.
15. Nissl: Zur Kasuistik der arteriosklerotischen Demenz (ein Fall von sogenannter "Encephalitis subcorticalis"). Ges Neuro 19:438, 1920.
16. Farnell F, Globus JH: Chronic progressive vascular subcortical encephalopathy. Arch Neurol Psychiatr 27:593, 1932.
17. Davison C: Progressive subcortical encephalopathy. J Neuropathol Exp Neurol 1:42, 1942.
18. Neumann M: Chronic progressive subcortical encephalopathy: Report of a case. J Gerontol 2:57, 1947.
19. Olszewski J: Subcortical arteriosclerotic encephalopathy: Review of the literature on the so-called Binswanger's disease and presentation of two cases. World Neurol 3:359, 1962.
20. Jelgersma H: A case of encephalopathia subcorticalis chronica (Binswanger's disease). Psychiatr Neurol Basel 147:81, 1964.
21. Loeb C: Binswanger's disease is not a single entity. Neurol Sci 21:343–348, 2000.
22. Burger PC, Burch JG, Kunze U: Subcortical arteriosclerotic encephalopathy (Binswanger's disease): A vascular etiology of dementia. Stroke 7:626–631, 1976.
23. White JC: Periodic EEG activity in subcortical arteriosclerotic encephalopathy (Binswanger's type). Arch Neurol 36:485–489, 1979.
24. Brun A, Englund E: A white matter disorder in dementia of the Alzheimer type: A pathoanatomical study. Ann Neurol 19:253–262, 1986.
24a. Lindenberg R, Spatz F: Über die thromboend-arteritis obliterans der Hernglässe. Virchows Arch Pathol Anat 305:531, 1940.

25. Furuta A, Ishii, N, Nishihara Y, Horie A: Medullary arteries in aging and dementia. Stroke 22:7–11, 1991.
26. Lotz PR, Ballinger WE Jr, Quisling RG: Subcortical arteriosclerotic encephalopathy: CT spectrum and pathologic correlation. AJR Am J Roentgenol 147:1209–1214, 1986.
27. Mathers SE, Chambers BR, Merory JR, Alexander I: Subcortical arteriosclerotic encephalopathy: Binswanger's disease. Clin Exp Neurol 23:67–70, 1987.
28. Leifer D, Buananno FS, Richardson EP Jr: Clinicopathologic correlations of cranial magnetic resonance imaging of periventricular white matter. Neurology 40:911–918, 1990.
29. Revesz T, Hawkins CP, du Boulay EP, et al: Pathological findings correlated with magnetic resonance imaging in subcortical arteriosclerotic encephalopathy (Binswanger's disease). J Neurol Neurosurg Psychiatry 52:1337–1344, 1989.
30. Ramos-Estebanez C, Hernandez Hernandez JL, Munoz Arrondo R, Alonso Valle H: [Binswanger's disease or multi-infarct dementia? Diagnostic keys in vascular dementia]. Rev Clin Esp 202:7–11, 2002.
31. Tullberg M, Hultin L, Ekholm S, et al: White matter changes in normal pressure hydrocephalus and Binswanger disease: Specificity, predictive value and correlations to axonal degeneration and demyelination. Acta Neurol Scand 105:417–426, 2002.
32. Feigen I, Popoff N: Neuropathological changes late in cerebral edema: The relationship to trauma, hypertensive disease, and Binswanger's encephalopathy. J Neuropathol Exp Neurol 22:500, 1963.
33. Jellinger K, Neumayer E: Progressive subcorticale vasculare Encephalopathie Binswanger. Eine Klinisch Neuropathologische Studie. Arch Psychiatr Nervenkr 205:523, 1964.
34. Inzitari D, Mascalchi M, Giordano GP, et al: Histopathological correlates of leukoaraiosis in patients with ischemic stroke. Eur Neurol 29:23–26, 1989.
35. Liu D, You G, Wei J, et al: [A clinico-pathological and etiological study of Binswanger's Disease]. Zhonghua Bing Li Xue Za Zhi 28:174–177, 1999.
36. Kibayashi K, Honjyo K, Higuchi A, Tsunenari S: Binswanger's disease: A rare cause of dementia in elderly persons. Nippon Hoigaku Zasshi 52:46–50, 1998.
37. Akiguchi I, Tomimoto H, Suenaga T, et al: Alterations in glia and axons in the brains of Binswanger's disease patients. Stroke 28:1423–1429, 1997.
38. Zhang WW, Olsson Y: The angiopathy of subcortical arteriosclerotic encephalopathy (Binswanger's disease): Immunohistochemical studies using markers for components of extracellular matrix, smooth muscle actin and endothelial cells. Acta Neuropathol (Berl) 93:219–224, 1997.
39. Strittmatter M, Hamann GF, Grauer MT, et al: Neurochemical differences in the CSF between Binswanger's and Alzheimer's disease. Dement Geriatr Cogn Disord 8:34–42, 1997.
40. Pozzi S: Sur un cas de cirrhose atrophique granuleuse disseminée des circonvolutions cerebrales. Encephale 3:155, 1883.
41. Bogousslavsky J: Binswanger's disease. In Barnett HJM, Mohr JP, Stein BM, Yatsu FM (eds): Stroke: Pathophysiology, Diagnosis, and Management, 2nd ed. New York, Churchill Livingstone 1992, pp 805–819.
42. Meguro K, Hatazawa, J, Yamaguchi T: Cerebral circulation and oxygen metabolism associated with subclinical periventricular hyperintensity as shown by magnetic resonance imaging. Ann Neurol 28:378–383, 1990.
43. Tomonaga M, Yamanouchi H, Tohgi H, Kameyama M: Clinicopathologic study of progressive subcortical vascular encephalopathy (Binswanger type) in the elderly. J Am Geriatr Soc 30:524–529, 1982.
44. van Swieten J, van den Hout JHW, van Ketel BA, et al: Periventricular lesions in the white matter on magnetic resonance imaging in the elderly: A morphometric correlation with arteriosclerosis and dilated perivascular spaces. Brain 114:761–771, 1991.
45. Moody DM, Bell MA, Challa VR: Features of the cerebral vascular pattern that predict vulnerability to perfusion or oxygenation deficiency: An anatomic study. AJNR Am J Neuroradiol 11:431–439, 1990.
46. Fang H: Observations on aging characteristics of cerebral blood vessels, macroscopic and microscopic features. In Terry RD, Gershon S (eds): Neurobiology of Aging. Philadelphia, Lippincott-Raven, 1976, pp 155–166.
47. Tatemichi TK: How acute brain failure becomes chronic: A view of the mechanisms of dementia related to stroke. Neurology 40:1652–1659, 1990.
48. Lashley K: Brain Mechanisms and Intelligence. Chicago, University of Chicago Press, 1929.
49. Brust J: Dementia and cerebrovascular disease. In Mayeux R, Rosen WG (eds): The Dementias. Philadelphia, Lippincott-Raven, 1983, pp 131–147.
50. Fields W: Multi-infarct dementia. Neurol Clin 74:405–413, 1986.
51. Meyer JS, McClintic KL, Rogers RL, et al: Aetiological considerations and risk factors for multi-infarct dementia. J Neurol Neurosurg Psychiatry 51:1489–497, 1988.
52. Crystal HA, Dickson DW, Sliwinski MJ, et al: Pathological markers associated with normal aging and dementia in the elderly. Ann Neurol 34:566-573, 1993.
53. Desmond DW, Moroney JT, Lynch T, et al: The natural history of CADASIL: A pooled analysis of previously published cases. Stroke 30:1230–1233, 1999.
54. Mohr JP: CADASIL and white matter syndromes. Ann Neurol 44:715–716, 1998.

Specific Medical Diseases and Stroke

Chapter Thirty-Two

CADASIL: Cerebral Autosomal Dominant Arteriopathy with Subcortical Infarcts and Leukoencephalopathy

H. Chabriat, A. Joutel, K. Vahedi, E. Tournier-Lasserve, and M. G. Bousser

CADASIL (cerebral autosomal dominant arteriopathy with subcortical infarcts and leukoencephalopathy)[1] is an inherited small artery disease of mid-adulthood that was identified during the past decade with the use of clinical, magnetic resonance imaging (MRI), pathologic, and genetic tools.[1] The disease is due to mutations of the *Notch3* gene on chromosome 19[2] that lead to an accumulation of the ectodomain of this receptor within the vascular wall. CADASIL is responsible for subcortical ischemic events and leads progressively to dementia with pseudobulbar palsy. The disease was first reported in European families. Today, CADASIL has been diagnosed in American, African, and Asiatic pedigrees and reported in all continents. The disease remains largely underdiagnosed.

HISTORY

In 1955, Van Bogaert[3] reported two sisters belonging to a family originating from Belgium who had a "subcortical encephalopathy of Binswanger's type of rapid course" with onset during mid-adulthood. Their clinical presentation included dementia, gait disturbances, pseudobulbar palsy, seizures, and focal neurologic deficits. Two other sisters had died at ages 36 and 43 years after a progressive dementia. The father had had a stroke at age 51 and died after a myocardial infarct. The pathologic examination revealed widespread areas of white matter rarefaction in the brain associated with multiple small infarcts mainly located in the white matter and basal ganglia.[3] These lesions were thought to be secondary to a familial arteriosclerosis of the brain similar to that reported by Mutrux[4] a few years earlier.

In 1977, Sourander and Walinder[5] coined the term "hereditary multi-infarct dementia" for a familial condition observed in a Swedish pedigree and characterized by dementia associated with pseudobulbar palsy occurring 10 to 15 years after recurrent stroke-like episodes.[6] Age of onset was between 29 and 38 years, and age at death varied from 30 to 53 years. These authors reported brain lesions identical to those observed by Van Bogaert in three cases also caused by a small vessel disease in the brain. The walls of the small arteries were thickened, causing a reduction in the lumen. Atherosclerosis of basal arteries was found only in one family member. In the pedigree, the condition followed an autosomal dominant pattern of transmission.

Up to 1993, several families having diseases close in presentation to the cases already described were reported, with various terms used for the diseases—hereditary multiinfarct dementia,[5] chronic familial vascular encephalopathy,[7] familiäre zerebrale arteriosklerose,[8] familiäre zerebrale Gefäberkrankung,[9] démence sous-corticale familiale avec leucoencéphalopathie artériopathique,[10] familial disorder with subcortical ischemic strokes, dementia and leukoencephalopathy,[11] and slowly progressive familial dementia with recurrent strokes and white matter hypodensities on CT scan.[12]

In 1976, we encountered a 50-year-old man with a clinical history of recurrent lacunar infarcts who presented with a large and widespread hypodensity of the white matter on CT scan. He had no vascular risk factor, in particular, no hypertension. Ten years later, his daughter came to see us for a long history of attacks of migraine with aura and transient ischemic attacks (TIAs) and for a recent minor stroke. Her computed tomography (CT) scan and MRI showed lesions in the white matter identical to those observed in her father. These two observations were the basis of the extensive clinical, MRI, and genetic studies of a whole family, which was a very large one, originating from the western part of France called Loire-Atlantique. The data were first described as "recurrent strokes in a family with diffuse white matter and muscular lipidosis—a new mitochondrial cytopathy,"[13] then as "autosomal dominant syndrome with stroke-like episodes and leukoencephalopathy,"[14] and later as "autosomal dominant leukoencephalopathy and subcortical ischemic strokes."[15] Because of the confusion raised by all these different names, we proposed in 1993 the acronym CADASIL to designate this disease and highlight its main characteristics.[1]

In 1993, we performed genetic analysis in our large family from Loire-Atlantique and demonstrated that the affected gene was located on chromosome 19 in a 12-centimorgan (cM) interval.[14] This finding was immediately confirmed in a second French affected pedigree.[1] The gene mapping was crucial to delineate the natural history of the disease. Since then, CADASIL has been recognized in several hundreds of families in all continents. In 1996, we demonstrated that various mutations of the Notch3 gene were responsible for the disease. This finding was a major step in the history of CADASIL, and genetic testing is currently used for its diagnosis. The gene identification is also crucial to understanding the pathophysiology of the disease necessary to open therapeutic avenues.

CLINICAL PRESENTATION

The earliest clinical manifestations of CADASIL are attacks of migraine with aura.[16] Despite their frequency in patients with the disease, which is four times that in the general population,[17,18] these manifestations are inconstant and are observed in as few as 20% to 30% of symptomatic subjects. They occur at a mean age of 28 ± 11 years.[19] The first attacks occasionally occur before the age of 20 years, before the appearance of MRI signal abnormalities.[20,21] Their frequency can vary greatly among the affected pedigrees.[22] The frequency of migraine attacks can also differ widely among affected subjects from one attack in life to several attacks per month.[23] As usually observed in migraine with aura, the most common neurologic symptoms associated with headache are visual, sensory, or both. However, the frequency of attacks with basilar, hemiplegic, or prolonged aura, according to International Headache Society (HIS) diagnostic criteria, is noticeably high.[16,17,21,23] A few patients have been reported with severe attacks, including unusual symptoms such as confusion, fever, meningitis, and coma,[23] which are only exceptionally reported in migraine with aura.[24,25]

Stroke is the most common clinical manifestation of the disease. Approximately two thirds of symptomatic subjects have had TIAs or a completed stroke.[19] These events occur at a mean age of 41 ± 9 years (extreme limits from 20 to 65 years).[17,19,26] Two thirds of them are classic lacunar syndromes, such as pure motor stroke, ataxic hemiparesis, pure sensory stroke, or sensory motor stroke. Other focal neurologic deficits of abrupt onset less frequently observed are dysarthria either isolated or associated with motor or sensory deficit, monoparesis, paresthesias in one limb, isolated ataxia, nonfluent aphasia, and hemianopia.[17] The onset of the neurologic deficit can be progressive over several hours. Some neurologic deficits occur suddenly and are associated with headache. When they are transient, they can mimic attacks of migraine with aura. Ischemic events usually occur in the absence of vascular risk factors. However, they are also observed in some patients with one or several vascular risk factors, most frequently in tobacco users and hypertensive subjects. The influence of such factors on the clinical or MRI phenotype remains unknown.[27]

About 20% of patients with CADASIL have a history of severe episodes of mood disturbances. Like that of migraine with aura, the frequency of such episodes varies widely among families.[23,28] Few patients have a severe depression of the melancholic type sometimes alternating with typical manic episodes.[21,23,26] The location of ischemic lesions in the basal ganglia or in the frontal white matter may play a key role in their occurrence.[29,30]

Dementia is the second most common clinical manifestation of CADASIL. It is reported in one third of symptomatic patients. The location of cerebral lesions explains the "subcortical" aspect of the cognitive deficit. The neuropsychological deficit is mainly responsible for attention deficit, apathy, and memory impairment.[10,17,31] Aphasia, apraxia, or agnosia is rare or is observed only at the end stage of the disease.[10,12] The cognitive deficit is often subtle, particularly at the onset of the disease, and can be detected only through the use of a battery of neuropsychological tests. Some tests can detect cognitive alterations even before the age of 35. In our experience, the Wisconsin card sorting test and the Trail Making test are the most sensitive examinations to detect a recent cognitive alteration.[32] The cognitive deficit can occur either suddenly or stepwise, but it can also occur progressively in the total absence of ischemic events, mimicking a degenerative dementia.[17,21]

The frequency and severity of the cognitive decline vary in different members of a given family. The variable location and the severity of cerebral tissue damage might play a key role. In a positron emission tomography (PET) study of two affected brothers, one demented and the other asymptomatic, we found a severe cortical metabolic depression in the demented subject, who had infarcts only within the basal ganglia and thalamus.[33] Furthermore, we observed that the severity of white matter microstructural damage is strongly related to the clinical status with CADASIL. This finding agrees with the correlations observed in patients between the clinical status and the load of T1 lesions within the white matter.[18] Therefore, the extent of tissue destruction or neuronal loss is crucial for the cognitive status of patients with CADASIL. When dementia is present—it occurs at a mean age of 60 years in patients with the syndrome—it is observed in the absence of any other clinical manifestations in only 10% of cases. Dementia is always associated with pyramidal signs, pseudobulbar palsy, gait difficulties, urinary incontinence, or a combination of such symptoms.[34] The cognitive and functional decline is usually progressive. The patient becomes bedridden and often dies as a result of pulmonary complications from swallowing difficulties. Baudrimont and colleagues[15] reported the death of one patient with CADASIL after the occurrence of a deep cerebral hematoma. Dementia is present in 90% of cases before death, which occurs at a mean age of 65 years (range, 30 to 77 years).

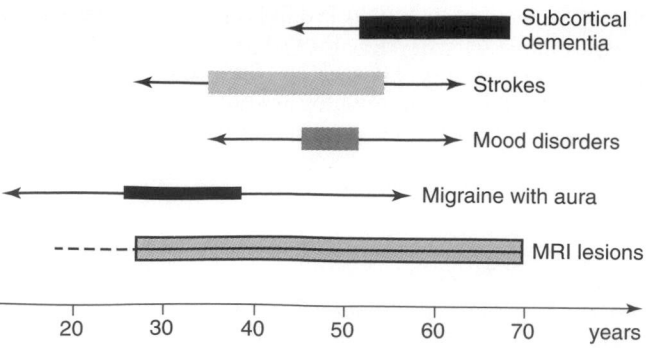

FIGURE 32–1 *A summary of the natural history of CADASIL (cerebral autosomal dominant arteriopathy with subcortical infarcts and leukoencephalopathy) summarized showing the different mean ages of occurrence of each symptom in the disease.*

Other neurologic manifestations have occasionally been reported in CADASIL. Focal or generalized seizures have been observed in 6% to 10% of cases.[17,26] Deafness of acute or rapid onset has been observed in several cases.[14] The lack of cranial nerve palsy, spinal cord disease, and symptoms of muscular origin is noteworthy in CADASIL. The cause of the radiculopathy reported in one patient by Ragno and associates[35] has not been determined.

Finally, the natural history of the disease is summarized in Figure 32–1. CADASIL starts between ages 20 and 30 years in one fifth of the patients as attacks of migraine with aura. Ischemic manifestations, observed in two thirds of patients, occur mainly during the fourth and fifth decades and are sometimes associated with severe mood disturbances. Dementia appears between ages 50 and 60 years and is found in nearly all cases before death, which occurs at a mean age of 65 years.

NEUROIMAGING

MRI is crucial for the diagnosis of CADASIL. The findings are always abnormal in symptomatic subjects.[1,17,36] In addition, the signal abnormalities can be detected during a presymptomatic period of variable duration. MRI signal abnormalities are observed in patients as young as 20 years. After age 35, all subjects having the affected gene have an abnormal MRI.[2,17] The frequency of asymptomatic subjects with abnormal MRI decreases progressively with aging among the gene carriers and becomes very low after 60 years.

T1-weighted images show punctiform or nodular hypointensity in the basal ganglia and white matter. T2-weighted images show hyperintensity in the same regions that are often associated with widespread areas of increased signal in the white matter.[36,37] The severity of the signal abnormalities is variable. These lesions dramatically increase with age in affected patients. In subjects younger than 40 years, the areas of hyperintensity on T2-weighted images are usually punctate or nodular with a symmetrical distribution, and they predominate in periventricular areas and in the centrum semiovale. Later in life, white matter lesions are diffuse and can involve the whole white

matter, including the U fibers under the cortex. Scores evaluating the severity of the lesions based on a semiquantitative rating scale significantly increase with age not only in the white matter but also in the basal ganglia and brainstem. The frontal and occipital periventricular lesions are constant when MRI is abnormal. The frequency of signal abnormalities in the external capsule (two thirds of cases) and in the anterior part of the temporal lobes (40% of cases) is noteworthy.[27,36,37] Brainstem lesions are observed mainly in the pons.[38] The medulla is usually spared. Cortical or cerebellar lesions are exceptional; they have been observed in only two patients older than 60 years. CT scanning can reveal the white matter and basal ganglia lesions but is much less sensitive than MRI.[39]

Findings of cerebral angiography performed in 14 patients belonging to seven affected families was normal except in one case with a detectable narrowing of small arteries.[17] Weller and associates[40] reported a worsening of the neurologic status in two patients with CADASIL in whom angiographic findings were normal with a possible vasospasm in one patient. One subject had a severe headache, vomiting, confusion, somnolence and a grand mal seizure that resolved within several hours. In a later report, other authors[18,41] later confirmed the high frequency of neurologic complications after angiography in patients with CADASIL. Results of ultrasound studies and echocardiography are usually normal. Cerebrospinal fluid examination results are also usually normal, but oligoclonal bands with pleocytosis have been reported.[39] An isolated increase in complement factor B has been reported in three patients with CADASIL.[42] Electromyographic parameters are essentially normal. A monoclonal immunoglobulin was detected in the serum of two cases in our first family but not in the other affected pedigrees.[14]

PATHOLOGY

Macroscopic examination of the brain shows a diffuse myelin pallor and rarefaction of the hemispheric white matter that spares the U fibers.[43,44] Lesions predominate in the periventricular areas and centrum semiovale. They are associated with lacunar infarcts located in the white matter and basal ganglia (lentiform nucleus, thalamus, caudate).[43,44] The most severe hemispheric lesions are the most profound.[10,15,44] In the brainstem, the lesions are more marked in the pons and are similar to the pontine rarefaction of myelin of ischemic origin described by Pullicino and associates.[45] Microscopic investigations show that the wall of cerebral and leptomeningeal arterioles is thickened with a significant reduction of the lumen.[15] Such abnormalities can also be detected by leptomeningeal biopsy.[46] Some inconstant features are similar to those reported in patients with hypertensive encephalopathy,[47]—duplication and splitting of internal elastic lamina, adventitial hyalinosis and fibrosis, and hypertrophy of the media. However, a distinctive feature is the presence of a granular material within the media and extending into the adventitia.[10,15,35,43–45,47–52] The positive response to periodic acid–Schiff (PAS) staining suggests the presence of glycoproteins; responses to staining for amyloid substance and elastin are negative.[15,44,53] Immunohistochemical analysis does not support the presence of immunoglobulins. By contrast, the endothelium of the vessels is usually spared.

Sometimes, the smooth muscle cells are not detectable and are replaced by collagen fibers.[47] On electron microscopy, the smooth muscle cells appear swollen and often degenerated, some of them with multiple nuclei. Gutierrez-Molina[43] described a granular, electron-dense, osmiophilic material within the media; according to Zhang and associates,[47] this material consists of granules of about 10 to 15 nm of diameter. It is localized close to the cell membrane of the smooth muscle cells, where it appears very dense. The smooth muscle cells are separated by large amounts of the unidentified material. In a single case, these vascular abnormalities were found in association with typical lesions of Alzheimer's disease.[54]

Ruchoux and colleagues[44,55] made the crucial observation that the vascular abnormalities seen in the brain were also detectable in other organs. The granular and osmiophilic material surrounding the smooth muscle cells in the brain is also present in the media of arteries located in the spleen, liver, kidneys, muscle, and skin and also in the walls of carotid and aortic arteries.[44,55] These vascular lesions can also be detected by nerve biopsy.[52] The presence of this material in the skin vessels now allows confirmation of the diagnosis of CADASIL in living patients through the use of punch skin biopsies,[56] although the sensitivity and specificity of this method have not yet been completely established.[44,51,55]

GENETICS

The study of the first and very large French family identified by our group allowed us to confirm the autosomal dominant pattern of transmission and to map the affected gene on chromosome 19 in 1993.[1] A crucial step for this mapping was the use of neuroimaging data for the genetic linkage analysis. Three years later, Joutel and associates identified 3 years later, different mutations of the *Notch3* gene as the cause of the disease.[2]

The clinical penetrance of the disease is related to age, approaching 100% at age 50 years. The penetrance based on MRI features reaches 100% at age 35 years. In the absence of a positive familial history, the diagnosis of CADASIL should not be ruled out because of possible de novo mutations of the *Notch3* gene.[57]

CADASIL is caused by stereotyped mutations of the *Notch3* gene. This gene is a 2321–amino acid protein, a transmembrane receptor with an extracellular domain containing 34 epidermal growth factor (EGF) repeats (including 6 cysteine residues) and 3 Lin repeats associated with an intracellular domain and a transmembrane domain. The stereotyped mis-sense mutations and deletions responsible for the disease are within EGF-like repeats and are located only in the extracellular domain of the Notch3 protein. In 70% of cases, the mutations are located within exons 3 and 4, which encode the first five EGF domains. All mutations in CADASIL lead to an uneven number of cysteine residues and presumably alter the function of the receptor.

The Notch3 protein is expressed exclusively in vascular smooth muscle cells.[58] The protein undergoes a proteolytic cleavage, leading to an extracellular and a transmembrane fragment. After cleavage, these two fragments form an heterodimer at the cell surface. The ectodomain of the Notch3 receptor accumulates within the vessel wall of affected subjects. This accumulation is found near but not within the characteristic granular osmiophilic material seen on electron microscopy. It is observed in all vascular smooth muscle cells and in pericytes within all organs (brain, heart, muscles, lungs, skin). An abnormal clearance of the Notch3 ectodomain from the smooth muscle cell surface is presumed to cause this accumulation.[58]

The identification of the CADASIL gene was a crucial step to develop a molecular diagnostic test that is now currently used for diagnosis of the disease. This genetic test is based on the sequencing of exons 3 and 4 to detect mutations that cause the loss or addition of a cysteine residue within EGF domains. The presence of such mutations enables one to ascertain the diagnosis because of the absence of similar mutations in control subjects. However, although the specificity of this test is actually excellent, its sensitivity remains insufficient (negative in 30% of cases).

For this reason, we evaluated another approach, based on the analysis of skin biopsies revealing an accumulation of Notch3 protein at the surface of skin vascular smooth muscle cells, to increase the sensitivity of diagnostic tests. We performed a comparative analysis of two groups of patients who are affected either by CADASIL or by a vascular leukoencephalopathy of another origin (negative screening of the totality of the Notch3 gene) using a specific monoclonal antibody directed against the extracellular domain of the receptor. This study showed the high sensitivity and specificity of immunostaining and its crucial diagnostic value when it was combined with the genetic test for the disease. The diagnosis of CADASIL can now be ruled out in a patient with absence of mutations in exons 3 and 4 when skin biopsy results are also negative, with an error risk lower than 5%. The complete sequencing of exons encoding EGF domains should now be requested only for a patient with a positive skin biopsy result and with a negative genetic test result.[59]

DIAGNOSIS

The diagnosis of CADASIL should be raised for any patient who has TIAs or strokes, severe mood disorders, or attacks of migraine with aura or dementia and in whom MRI shows widespread signal abnormalities in the subcortical white matter and basal ganglia. The association between such symptoms and these MRI findings should prompt a genealogic study of the family, including all first- and second-degree relatives. Clinical data, neuroimaging data, or both obtained from such relatives are crucial to confirm the hereditary origin of the disease. The diagnosis can be confirmed by genetic testing with or without skin biopsy, as previously described.

The clinical and MRI presentation of CADASIL is very close to that of Binswanger's disease (BD), but the two conditions differ on three points: Unlike CADASIL, BD (1) occurs most often in hypertensive patients, (2) is not associated with migraine with aura, and (3) is not recognized as an autosomal dominant condition.[60] It should be noted, however, that the familial character has not been systematically evaluated in most cases of BD and that, conversely, sporadic mutations of the *Notch3* gene are possible in the disease.[57] On MRI, the involvement of the external capsule and temporal lobes appears to be more common and more severe in CADASIL than in BD, a feature that may be useful for differential diagnosis.

Other causes of vascular leukoencephalopathies are easier to recognize. Amyloid angiopathies of hereditary origin can manifest as ischemic strokes and MRI white matter signal abnormalities but are essentially characterized by recurrent lobar cerebral hemorrhages and the presence of amyloid deposits within the walls of brain vessels.[61,62] Mitochondrial encephalomyopathy with lactis acidosis and stroke-like episodes (MELAS) often occurs in children or in early adult life. It is responsible for cortical and subcortical infarcts of asymmetrical distribution, sometimes outside a vascular territory, and is often associated with ragged-red muscle fibers. The disease is transmitted through a maternal inheritance.[63] The "familial young-onset arteriosclerotic leukoencephalopathy" reported in Japanese pedigrees is an autosomal recessive condition associated with alopecia and skeletal abnormalities, secondary to a thickening of the intima of small cerebral vessels.[64] The hereditary leukoencephalopathy reported by Lossos and coworkers,[65] a disorder with increased skin collagen content, leads to a progressive dementia and is associated with palmoplantar keratoderma.

CADASIL, particularly at onset, can be difficult to differentiate from multiple sclerosis. The autosomal dominant pattern of transmission of CADASIL, the absence of optic nerve or spinal cord involvement, and the symmetrical distribution of white matter signal abnormalities often associated with basal ganglia infarcts at MRI examination are the most helpful signs for recognizing the disease.[66] Also, adrenoleukodystrophy, an X-linked metabolic disorder with accumulation of very-long-chain fatty acids, can be observed in adults. Unlike CADASIL, however, adrenoleukodystrophy does not involve basal ganglia, and the cerebral disease is progressive and associated with spinal cord and peripheral nerve demyelination.

CONCLUSION

CADASIL is a systemic genetic disease of vascular smooth muscle cells. The developments in genetic and pathologic research suggest that the accumulation of the ectodomain of the Notch3 protein is associated with the severe ultrastructural alterations of the arteriolar wall observed in this disease. Other data suggest that the arteriolar wall changes may result in cerebral hypoperfusion, causing "chronic ischemia" and leading to the progressive accumulation of tissue lesions. These lesions predominate in the most vulnerable cerebral areas, possibly because of the distinctive angioarchitecture of the brain. Finally, both the variable severity of the tissue destruction within the white matter and basal ganglia and their different locations might be important sources of the variability of clinical severity among the members of a given family.

The research performed in CADASIL is crucial not only to determine the best target for future prevention of the disease. It is also important for a better understanding of the pathophysiology of small artery diseases. We believe that CADASIL should be considered a unique model for investigating the determinants of vascular dementia, the clinical correlates of ischemic white matter lesions, and the natural history of tissue damage associated with small artery diseases. Furthermore, the identification of the *Notch3* gene will be helpful in the dismantling of the group of cerebral vascular disorders associated with leukoaraïosis.

References

1. Tournier-Lasserve E, Joutel A, Melki J, et al: Cerebral autosomal dominant arteriopathy with subcortical infarcts and leukoencephalopathy maps to chromosome 19q12. Nat Genet 3:256–259, 1993.
2. Joutel A, Corpechot C, Ducros A, et al: Notch3 mutations in CADASIL, a hereditary adult-onset condition causing stroke and dementia. Nature 383(6602):707–710, 1996.
3. Van Bogaert L: Encephalopathie sous-corticale progressive (Binswanger) à évolution rapide chez deux soeurs. Med Hellen 24:961–972, 1955.
4. Mutrux S: Etude d'un cas familial de paralysie pseudo-bulbaire à forme ponto-cérebelleuse. Monatschr Psych U Neurol 122:349–355, 1951.
5. Sourander P, Walinder J: Hereditary multi-infarct dementia: Morphological and clinical studies of a new disease. Acta Neuropathol (Berl) 39:247–254, 1977.
6. Sonninen V, Savontaus ML: Hereditary multi-infarct dementia. Eur Neurol 27:209–215, 1987.
7. Stevens DL, Hewlett RH, Brownell B: Chronic familial vascular encephalopathy. Lancet 2:1364–1365, 1977.
8. Gerhard: Familiäre zerebrale Arteriosklerose. Zbl Allg Path Bd 124:163, 1980.
9. Colmant H: Familiäre zerebrale Gefäberkrankung. Zbl Allg Path Bd 124:163, 1980.
10. Davous P, Fallet-Bianco C: Démence sous-corticale familiale avec leucoencéphalopathie artériopathique: Observation clinico-pathologique. Rev Neurol (Paris) 5:376–384, 1991.
11. Mas JL, Dilouya A, De Recondo J: A familial disorder with subcortical ischemic strokes, dementia and leukoencephalopathy. Neurology 42:1015–1019, 1992.
12. Salvi F, Michelucci R, Plasmati R, et al: Slowly progressive familial dementia with recurrent strokes and white matter hypodensities on CT scan. Ital J Neurol Sci 13:135–140, 1992.
13. Bousser M, Tournier-Lasserve E, Aylward R, et al: Recurrent strokes in a family with diffuse white-matter abnormalities—a new mitochondrial cytopathy. J Neurol 235(suppl 1):S4–S5, 1988.
14. Tournier-Lasserve E, Iba-Zizen MT, Romero N, Bousser MG: Autosomal dominant syndrome with stroke-like episodes and leukoencephalopathy. Stroke 22:1297–1302, 1991.
15. Baudrimont M, Dubas F, Joutel A, et al: Autosomal dominant leukoencephalopathy and subcortical ischemic strokes: A clinico-pathological study. Stroke 24:122–125, 1993.
16. Classification and diagnostic criteria for headache disorders, cranial neuralgias and facial pain. Headache Classification Committee of the International Headache Society. Cephalalgia 7(suppl):8, 1988.
17. Chabriat H, Vahedi K, Iba-Zizen MT, et al: Clinical spectrum of CADASIL: A study of 7 families. Cerebral autosomal dominant arteriopathy with subcortical infarcts and leukoencephalopathy. Lancet 346(8980):934–939, 1995.
18. Dichgans M, Filipi M, Brüning R, et al: Quantitative MRI in CADASIL. Neurology 52:1361–1367, 1999.
19. Desmond DW, Moroney JT, Lynch T, et al: The natural history of CADASIL: A pooled analysis of previously published cases. Stroke 30:1230–1233, 1999.
20. Hutchinson M, O'Riordan J, Javed M, et al: Familial hemiplegic migraine and autosomal dominant arteriopathy with leukoencephalopathy (CADASIL). Ann Neurol 38(5):817–824, 1995.
21. Verin M, Rolland Y, Landgraf F, et al: New phenotype of the cerebral autosomal dominant arteriopathy mapped to chromosome 19: Migraine as the prominent clinical feature. J Neurol Neurosurg Psychiatry 59:579–585, 1995.

22. Vahedi K, Chabriat H, Ducros A, et al: Analysis of CADASIL clinical natural history in a series of 134 patients belonging to 17 families linked to chromosome 19. Neurology 46:A211, 1996.

23. Chabriat H, Tournier-Lasserve E, Vahedi K, et al: Autosomal dominant migraine with MRI white-matter abnormalities mapping to the CADASIL locus. Neurology 45:1086–1091, 1995.

24. Fitzimons RB, Wolfenden WH: Migraine coma: Meningitic migraine with cerebral oedema associated with a new form of autosomal dominant cerebellar ataxia. Brain 108:555–577, 1991.

25. Frequin STFM, Linssen WHJP, Pasman JW, et al: Recurrent prolonged coma due to basilar artery migraine: A case report. Headache 31:75–81, 1991.

26. Dichgans M, Mayer M, Uttner I, et al: The phenotypic spectrum of CADASIL: Clinical findings in 102 cases. Ann Neurol 44:731–739, 1998.

27. Chabriat H, Joutel A, Vahedi K, et al: CADASIL (cerebral autosomal dominant arteriopathy with subcortical infarcts and leukoencephalopathy). J Mal Vasc 21:277–282, 1996.

28. Chabriat H, Bousser MG, Pappata S: Cerebral autosomal dominant arteriopathy with subcortical infarcts and leukoencephalopathy: A positron emission tomography study in two affected family members. Stroke 26:1729–1730, 1995.

29. Aylward ED, Roberts-Willie JV, Barta PE, et al: Basal ganglia volume and white matter hyperintensities in patients with bipolar disorder. Am J Psychiatry 5:687–693, 1994.

30. Bhatia K, Marsden C: The behavioural and motor consequences of focal lesions of the basal ganglia in man. Brain 117:859–876, 1994.

31. Davous P, Bequet D: CADASIL: Un nouveau modèle de démence sous-corticale. Rev Neurol (Paris) 151:634–639, 1995.

32. Taillia H, Chabriat H, Kurtz A, et al: Cognitive alterations in non-demented CADASIL patients. Cerebrovasc Dis 8:97–101, 1998.

33. Chabriat H, Pappata S, Poupon C, et al: Clinical severity in CADASIL related to ultrastructural damage in white matter: In-vivo study with diffusion tensor MRI. Stroke 30:2637–2643, 1999.

34. Bousser M, Tournier Lasserve E: Summary of the First International Workshop on CADASIL. Stroke 25:704–707, 1994.

35. Ragno M, Tournier-Lasserve E, Fiori M, et al: An Italian kindred with cerebral autosomal dominant arteriopathy with subcortical infarcts and leukoencephalopathy (CADASIL). Ann Neurol 38:231–236, 1995.

36. Bousser MG, Tournier-Lasserve E: Summary of the proceedings of the First International Workshop on CADASIL. Paris, May 19–21, 1993. Stroke. 25:704–707, 1994.

37. Skehan SJ, Hutchinson M, MacErlaine DP: Cerebral autosomal dominant arteriopathy with subcortical infarcts and leukoencephalopathy: MR findings. Am J Neuroradiol 16:2115–2119, 1995.

38. Chabriat H, Mrissa R, Levy C, et al: Brain stem MRI signal abnormalities in CADASIL. Stroke 30:457–459, 1999.

39. Chabriat H, Joutel A, Vahedi K, et al: CADASIL: Cerebral autosomal dominant arteriopathy with subcortical infarcts and leukoencephalopathy. Rev Neurol (Paris) 153:376–385, 1997.

40. Weller M, Petersen D, Dichgans J, Klockgether Y: Cerebral angiography complications link CADASIL to familial hemiplegic migraine. Neurology 46:844, 1996.

41. Estes M, Chimowitz M, Awad I, et al: Sclerosing vasculopathy of the central nervous system in non-elderly demented patients. Arch Neurol 48:631–636, 1991.

42. Unlu M, de Lange RP, de Silva R, et al: Detection of complement factor B in the cerebrospinal fluid of patients with cerebral autosomal dominant arteriopathy with subcortical infarcts and leukoencephalopathy disease using two-dimensional gel electrophoresis and mass spectrometry. Neurosci Lett 282:149–152, 2000.

43. Gutierrez-Molina M, Caminero-Rodriguez A, Martinez Garcia C, et al: Small arterial granular degeneration in familial Binswanger's syndrome. Acta Neuropathol 87:98–105, 1994.

44. Ruchoux MM, Guerrouaou D, Vandenhaute B, et al: Systemic vascular smooth muscle cell impairment in cerebral autosomal dominant arteriopathy with subcortical infarcts and leukoencephalopathy. Acta Neuropathol 89:500–512, 1995.

45. Pullicino P, Ostow P, Miller L, et al: Pontine ischemic rarefaction. Ann Neurol 37:460–466, 1995.

46. Lammie GA, Rakshi J, Rossor MN, et al: Cerebral autosomal dominant arteriopathy with subcortical infarcts and leukoencephalopathy (CADASIL)—confirmation by cerebral biopsy in 2 cases. Clin Neuropathol 14:201–206, 1995.

47. Zhang W, Chun Ma K, Andersen O, et al: The microvascular changes in cases of hereditary multi-infarct disease of the brain. Acta Neuropathol 87:317–324, 1994.

48. Dichgans M, Petersen D: Angiographic complications in CADASIL [letter]. Lancet 349(9054):776–777, 1997.

49. Gray F, Robert F, Labrecque R, et al: Autosomal dominant arteriopathic leuko-encephalopathy and Alzheimer's disease. Neuropathol Appl Neurobiol 20:22–30, 1994.

50. Malandrini A, Carrera P, Ciacci G, et al: Unusual clinical features and early brain MRI lesions in a family with cerebral autosomal dominant arteriopathy. Neurology 48:1200–1203, 1997.

51. Sabbadini G, Francia A, Calandriello L, et al: Cerebral autosomal dominant arteriopathy with subcortical infarcts and leukoencephalopathy (CADASIL): Clinical, neuroimaging, pathological and genetic study of a large Italian family. Brain 118:207–215, 1995.

52. Schroder JM, Sellhaus B, Jorg J: Identification of the characteristic vascular changes in a sural nerve biopsy of a case with cerebral autosomal dominant arteriopathy with subcortical infarcts and leukoencephalopathy (CADASIL). Acta Neuropathol 89:116–121, 1995.

53. Ruchoux MM, Maurage CA: CADASIL: Cerebral autosomal dominant arteriopathy with subcortical infarcts and leukoencephalopathy. J Neuropathol Exp Neurol 56:947–964, 1997.

54. Gray F, Robert F, Labrecque R, et al: Autosomal dominant arteriopathic leuko-encephalopathy and Alzheimer's disease. Neuropath Appl Neurobiol 20:22–30, 1994.

55. Ruchoux MM, Chabriat H, Bousser MG, et al: Presence of ultrastructural arterial lesions in muscle and skin vessels of patients with CADASIL. Stroke 25:2291–2292, 1994.

56. Furby A, Vahedi K, Force M, et al: Differential diagnosis of a vascular leukoencephalopathy within a CADASIL family: Use of skin biopsy electron microscopy study and direct genotypic screening. J Neurol 245:734–740, 1998.

57. Joutel A, Dodick DD, Parisi JE, et al: De novo mutation in the Notch3 gene causing CADASIL. Ann Neurol 47:388–391, 2000.

58. Joutel A, Andreux F, Gaulis S, et al: The ectodomain of the Notch3 receptor accumulates within the cerebrovasculature of CADASIL patients [see comments]. J Clin Invest 105:597–605, 2000.

59. Joutel A, Favrole P, Labauge P, et al: Skin biopsy immunostaining with a Notch3 antibody for CADASIL diagnosis. Lancet 15(358):2049–2051, 2001.

60. Babikian V, Ropper A: Binswanger's disease: A review. Stroke:2–12, 1987.18

61. Greenberg S, Hyman B: Cerebral amyloid angiopathy and apolipoprotein E: Bad news for the good allele? Ann Neurol 41:701–702, 1997.

62. Greenberg S, Vonsattel J, Stakes J, et al: The clinical spectrum of cerebral amyloid angiopathy. Neurology 43:2073–2079, 1993.

63. Matthews PM, Tampieri D, Berkovic SF, et al: Magnetic resonance imaging shows specific abnormalities in the MELAS syndrome. Neurology 41:1043–1046, 1991.

64. Fukutake T, Hirayama K: Familial young-onset arteriosclerotic leukoencephalopathy with alopecia and lumbago without arterial hypertension. Eur Neurol 35:69–79, 1995.

65. Lossos A, Cooperman H, Soffer D, et al: Hereditary leukoencephalopathy and palmoplantar keratoderma: A new disorder with increased skin collagen content. Neurology 45:331–337, 1995.

66. Auer DP, Putz B, Gossl C, et al: Differential lesion patterns in CADASIL and sporadic subcortical arteriosclerotic encephalopathy: MR imaging study with statistical parametric group comparison. Radiology 218:443–451, 2001.

Chapter Thirty-Three

Cerebral Amyloid Angiopathy

Steven M. Greenberg

From a clinical perspective, cerebral amyloid angiopathy (CAA) can be defined as amyloid deposition in the cerebral vessels sufficient to cause symptomatic vascular dysfunction. The syndromes associated with CAA have become increasingly well recognized in clinical practice. The best characterized of these—vessel rupture and spontaneous intracerebral hemorrhage (ICH)—represent a notably severe and essentially untreatable form of stroke in the elderly. Data discussed here also point to the possibility that the β-amyloid peptide (Aβ) may alter normal vascular functioning and promote brain ischemia. Future investigations are thus likely to achieve further widening of the clinical spectrum of CAA.

In seeking to define diagnostic and treatment approaches to CAA, investigators have faced several obstacles. A leading obstacle is the inaccessibility of brain tissue during life, which generally forces clinicians to rely on indirect evidence for the diagnosis of CAA. Fortunately, much has been learned about the radiographic and genetic features of CAA, allowing a diagnosis of "probable CAA" in many clinical situations. Together with rapid progress in our understanding of the biology of Aβ, these emerging clinical insights into CAA form a promising foundation for identifying future treatments for this disorder.

EPIDEMIOLOGY AND RISK FACTORS

The difficulty of diagnosing CAA in living subjects makes precise figures on disease incidence or prevalence hard to ascertain. CAA *without* ICH is clearly a common phenomenon in the elderly brain. Analyses of brains from the Harvard Brain Tissue Resource Center (corrected for the overrepresentation of Alzheimer's disease among referred cases) indicate an estimated prevalence for moderate to severe CAA of 2.3% for patients age 65 to 74, 8.0% for those 75 to 84 years, and 12.1% for those 85 years or older.[1] When these figures are compared with the annual rate for *all* types of ICH, approximately 0.1% among North American and European elderly,[2-4] it is clear that only a minority of pathologically advanced CAA results in hemorrhagic stroke.

Despite the low frequency of hemorrhage, the hemorrhages produced by CAA account for a substantial pro-

portion of all spontaneous ICHs in elderly patients. Estimated rates of 11% to 15% emerged from autopsies of elderly patients with ICH (age ≥ 60 years) at the Japanese Yokufukai Geriatric Hospital between 1979 and 1990[5] and the Hawaiian Kuakini Hospital between 1965 and 1976.[6] Analysis of consecutively encountered clinical patients at the Massachusetts General Hospital (MGH) suggests an even greater proportion of hemorrhages, approximately 34%, attributable to CAA (Table 33.1). The apparently higher frequency of CAA in the MGH cohort might reflect either a lower incidence of hypertensive ICH in this Western population or secular improvements in blood pressure control as well as the methodologic differences between autopsy-based and clinic-based studies.

Examination of the clinical characteristics that predispose to CAA-related ICH (Table 33.2) suggests that its incidence is likely to rise with the aging of the population and is unlikely to be reduced through control of modifiable risk factors. *Advancing age* is the strongest clinical risk factor for CAA-related ICH, as predicted by the age dependence of the underlying disease.[1,7-9] All 26 patients identified with CAA-related ICH in three large autopsy series were older than 60 years, and 23 of 26 (88%) older than 70 years.[5,6,10] My colleagues and I at Massachusetts General Hospital found a similar pattern in consecutive patients analyzed for age at first CAA-related ICH, though with slightly younger age distribution as expected in a clinical series. Among 105 patients diagnosed with CAA between July 1994 and October 2001, first ICH occurred at a mean age of 76.1 ± 8.3 years (range 56 to 92 years). Ninety-seven percent of patients were older than 60 years at first hemorrhage, 75% older than 70 years, 39% older than 80 years, and 4% (4 of 105 patients) were in their 90s. There is no marked predilection for *gender* either in our clinical series (54% men, 46% women) or in pathologic cases (49% men, 51% women).[11]

Dementia has generally been considered a major risk factor for CAA-related ICH because of the close molecular relationship between CAA and Alzheimer's disease. Indeed, a pathologic study of 117 consecutive brains with Alzheimer's disease demonstrated advanced CAA to be common, with moderate to severe CAA disease in 25.6% of specimens and CAA-related hemorrhages in 5.1%.[12] Despite the frequent overlap of Alzheimer's disease with

Table 33.1 Estimated Prevalence of Cerebral Amyloid Arteriopathy (CAA)–Related Intracerebral Hemorrhage (ICH) in a Clinical Series of Elderly Patients

ICH Location (n = 355)	Percentage of Total[*]
Lobar	45.9 × 74%[†] = 34% of all primary ICHs in elderly due to CAA
Deep hemispheric	41.1
Brainstem	3.7
Cerebellum	8.5
Intraventricular	0.9

[*]Data from 355 consecutive patients age ≥55 presenting to Massachusetts General Hospital with spontaneous ICH.
[†]The estimated proportion of primary lobar ICH in the elderly caused by CAA, based on detection of advanced CAA in 29 of 39 consecutive pathology specimens of lobar ICH.[94]

Table 33.2 Risk Factors for Cerebral Amyloid Angiopathy (CAA)–Related Intracerebral Hemorrhage (ICH)[*]

Risk factors for CAA	Advanced age APOE ε2 or ε4 Alzheimer's disease
Risk factors for lobar ICH (not specifically linked to CAA)	Family history of ICH Frequent use of alcohol Previous ischemic stroke Low serum cholesterol

[*]See text for references.

CAA, approximately 60% to 80% of patients diagnosed with CAA-related ICH do *not* show clinical symptoms of dementia before their initial hemorrhagic stroke.[11,13,14] It is thus unclear from a clinical standpoint whether the presence or absence of dementia is useful to making the diagnosis of CAA. The association of CAA and Alzheimer's disease appears to be due in part to the shared genetic risk factor apolipoprotein E (APOE) ε4, although as discussed later, there are substantial differences between the roles of APOE in the two disorders.

Despite the clear importance of *hypertension* in promoting necrosis and rupture of the deep penetrating vessels,[15] there is little evidence for a similar role in CAA-related ICH. The estimated prevalence of hypertension in CAA is in the range of 32% (determined from 107 pathologic cases of CAA reviewed by Vinters[11]) to 52% (measured in our 105 consecutive clinical cases diagnosed as CAA), figures not much greater than the expected rate of hypertension for the general elderly population. Hypertension is significantly less common in lobar ICH than in ICH of the deep hemispheres, cerebellum, or pons in most[4,14,16,17] (though not all)[18,19] studies of the elderly. Further, a study of 71 consecutive survivors of an initial lobar ICH found that history of hypertension did not influence the rate of ICH recurrence, as discussed later.[20] These negative results are consistent with pathologic data showing no relationship between hypertension and the presence of CAA-related ICH.[21] Among other vascular factors, neither *diabetes mellitus* nor *coronary atherosclerosis* has demonstrated an elevated frequency in our CAA cohort.

Other clinical risk factors have been suggested for lobar ICH without specific evidence linking them to CAA. Midpoint analysis of the population-based Greater Cincinnati/Northern Kentucky study identified *family history of ICH, previous ischemic stroke,* and *frequent alcohol use* in addition to APOE genotype as predictors of lobar ICH in a multivariable model.[22] *Low serum cholesterol* has been found to be associated with ICH in several other population-based studies.[23–28] The few studies that have analyzed ICH according to location or presumed etiology have not indicated a specific relationship of cholesterol to CAA-related hemorrhages.[29,30]

PATHOPHYSIOLOGY AND EXPERIMENTAL SYSTEMS

CAA appears on pathologic analysis as a variable combination of vascular amyloid deposition and vessel wall breakdown (Fig. 33–1). Affected vessels are the capillaries, arterioles, and small- and medium-sized arteries primarily of the cerebral cortex, overlying leptomeninges, and cerebellum, with the white matter and deep gray structures largely spared. The distribution of CAA is typically patchy and segmental, such that heavily involved vessel segments may alternate with essentially amyloid-free regions (see Fig. 33–1C).[31] In its mildest detectable form, congophilic material accumulates at the border of the vessel's media and adventitia (see Fig. 33–1A). Amyloid-lined vacuoles often seen at this stage[31] may represent former sites of vascular smooth muscle cells that have died in apparent response to the surrounding amyloid. In moderately severe segments of CAA, vascular amyloid extends throughout the media to replace essentially the entire smooth muscle cell layer (see Fig. 33–1B).

The most advanced extent of CAA is marked not only by severe amyloid deposition but also by pathologic changes in

FIGURE 33–1 *Pathologic appearances of cerebral amyloid angiopathy (CAA). A, Vessel in longitudinal section. In mild stages of disease, amyloid appears at the outer edge of the vessel media, creating vesicle-like structures (arrows) at sites believed to be previously occupied by smooth muscle cells. B, Further amyloid deposition replaces the media and all smooth muscle cells. C, Specimen taken from a brain with the Iowa APP mutation. Amyloid deposits can cause marked thickening of vessel wall segments that alternate with skipped areas of normal caliber (arrows). Further vasculopathic changes in amyloid-laden vessels include concentric splitting of the vessel wall, creating a vessel-in-vessel appearance (D) and fibrinoid necrosis (E), signifying entry of plasma components into the wall. F, Some instances of advanced CAA are accompanied by visible inflammatory changes such as perivascular giant cell reaction (panel F). (A, D, and F stained by Luxol fast blue-hematoxylin-eosin; B and C by anti–β-amyloid immunostain with hematoxylin counterstain; and E with phosphotungstic acid–hematoxylin.)*

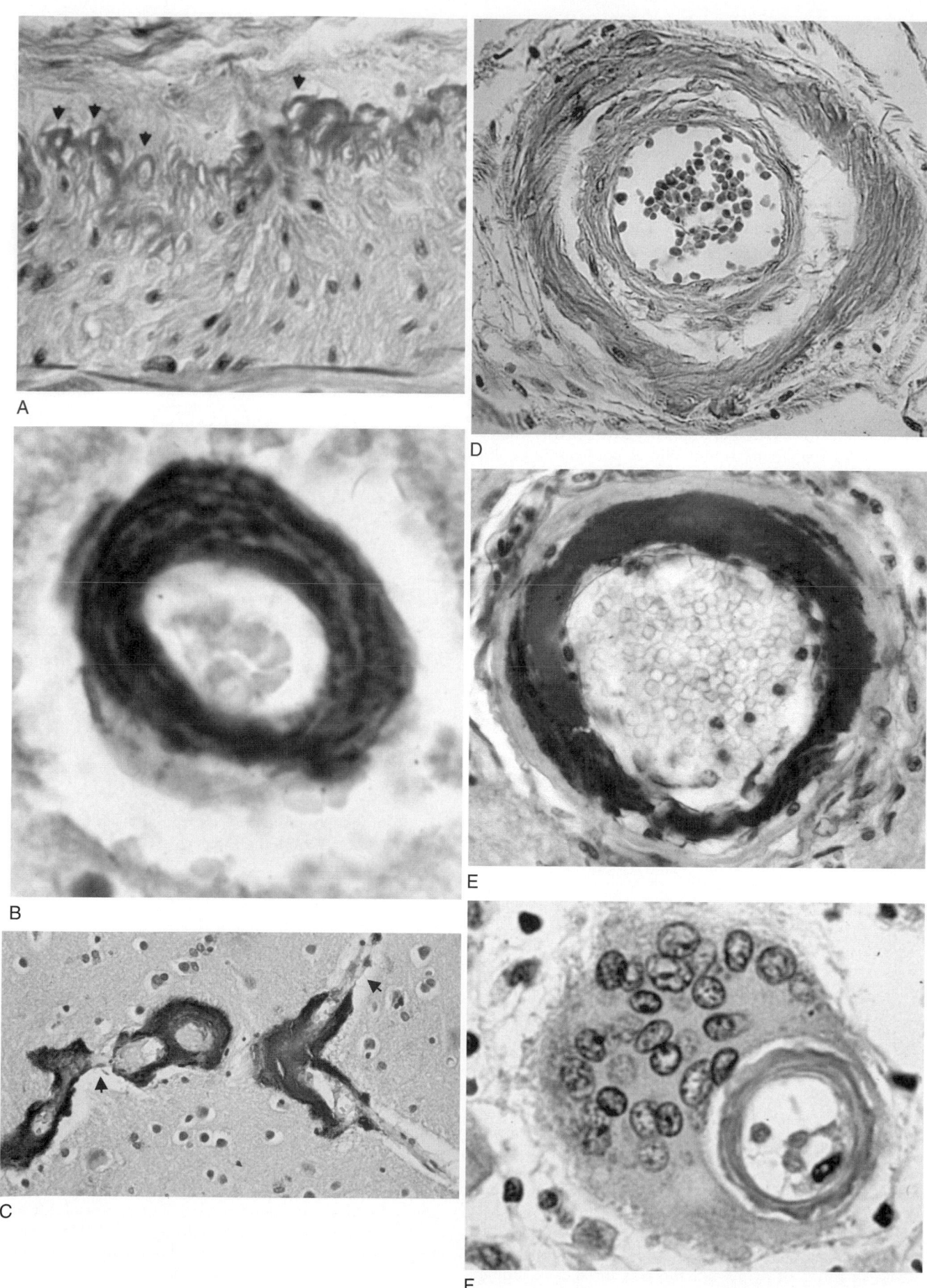

the amyloid-laden vessel wall. These vasculopathic changes can include microaneurysms, concentric splitting of the vessel wall (see Fig. 33–1D), chronic perivascular or transmural inflammation, and fibrinoid necrosis (see Fig. 33–1E).[13,31–35] CAA-related vasculopathic changes are often associated with paravascular red cells or hemosiderin deposits, suggesting ongoing leakage of blood. It is this combination of extensive amyloid deposition and breakdown of the amyloid-laden vessel walls that appears to act as the substrate for symptomatic hemorrhagic strokes.[13,31,36–38]

The principal constituent of both vascular amyloid in CAA and plaque amyloid in Alzheimer's disease is the β-amyloid peptide (Aβ). The Aβ peptides are 39– to 43–amino acid proteolytic fragments of the 695- to 770-residue β-amyloid precursor protein (APP). The subset of Aβ peptides with carboxyl termini extending to position 42 or 43 (denoted Aβ42) appears to be an important trigger to amyloid aggregation in both vessels and plaques.[39] In support of Aβ42 deposition as an early step in initiation of CAA is the observation that mildly affected vessels can stain positive for Aβ42 but stain negative for the more common Aβ fragments terminating at position 39 or 40 (Aβ40).[40,41] It is Aβ40, however, that appears to be the predominant species in more heavily involved vessel segments.[42–49] Quantitative analysis of brains with mild and severe CAA suggests a progressive addition of Aβ40 to previously seeded vessel segments.[49] A variety of other proteins or protein fragments can also be detected as components of vascular amyloid, though without a known pathogenic role in the breakdown of the vessel wall. These CAA-associated proteins include apolipoprotein E, cystatin C, alpha-synuclein, heparan sulfate proteoglycan, amyloid P component, and several complement proteins.[50–56]

The relationship of the pathology of CAA and APOE genotype provides an interesting window on the importance of both Aβ deposition and vessel breakdown to the pathogenesis of CAA-related ICH. The APOE ε2 and ε4 alleles, each a suggested risk factor for CAA-related ICH (see later), appear to act at these two distinct stages of CAA to promote hemorrhage. APOE ε4 associates in a dose-dependent manner with increased deposition of Aβ in vessels as it does in plaques[57–60]; APOE ε2 appears instead to promote the CAA-related vasculopathic changes such as concentric vessel splitting and fibrinoid necrosis.[38,61] The mechanism for this unexpected effect of APOE ε2 on vascular breakdown is unknown. The domain of the apolipoprotein E protein containing the ε2 determinant is present in both vessel and plaque amyloid deposits[56] but has not been linked to any specific pathogenic function.

One experimental approach to clarifying pathogenic mechanisms for CAA has been to study the effects of Aβ on vessel components in vitro. Aβ exerts toxic effects on a variety of vascular cells in culture, including cerebrovascular smooth muscle cells, endothelial cells, and pericytes.[62–65] Cell death is enhanced when the Aβ peptide used is either wild-type Aβ42 or mutant Aβ40 containing one of the amino acid substitutions associated with hereditary CAA,[66–68] suggesting that particular chemical properties of Aβ can specifically promote toxicity. Death of the cultured cerebrovascular smooth muscle cells appears to require a series of events on the cell surface, including

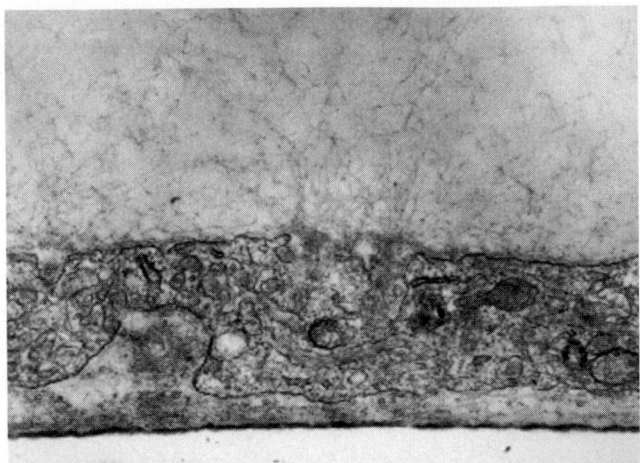

FIGURE 33–2 *Deposition of β-amyloid (Aβ) on cerebrovascular smooth muscle cell. This transmission electron micrograph shows a cultured human cerebrovascular smooth muscle cell treated with Dutch-type mutant Aβ40 for 6 days. Under these conditions, Aβ assembles into amyloid fibrils on the cell surface (seen at top). (Courtesy of William E. Van Nostrand.)*

assembly of Aβ into amyloid fibrils (Fig. 33–2) and accumulation of the secreted amino-terminal portion of APP.[69,70] Another in vitro property of Aβ is to stimulate tissue-type plasminogen activator (t-PA),[71,72] raising the intriguing possibility that CAA might promote ICH through direct effects on the coagulation-thrombolysis cascade as well as on the integrity of the vessel wall.

The pathogenesis of CAA has also been studied in transgenic mouse models (Fig. 33–3). Substantial CAA develops at advanced ages in lines of mice expressing high levels of mutant APP.[73–76] Affected vessels in these animals can demonstrate several pathologic features reminiscent of human CAA, including disruption or loss of the vascular smooth muscle, microaneurysms, and, in one mouse line, perivascular cerebral hemorrhages.[74,76,77] Because the expression of human APP in these animals is exclusively neuronal, the mice illustrate that Aβ produced by neurons is capable of remaining soluble in the extracellular space long enough to reach sites of deposition in the vessel; a similar pathway to the vessel walls has been proposed for human CAA.[78] Coexpression of APP and the cytokine transforming growth factor-β1 (TGF-1) leads to even more rapid and severe CAA.[79] The increase in CAA with TGF-β1 expression is associated with an unexpected decrease in plaque amyloid,[80] suggesting that inflammation might have opposing effects on the accumulation of Aβ in these two compartments.

One further insight to come from these transgenic studies is the possibility that Aβ may have specific effects on vessel physiology. In an investigation of living mice imaged by multiphoton microscopy, vessel segments that contained even mild Aβ deposits appeared significantly more dilated than segments of the same vessel without CAA.[75] Another set of studies using a different mouse line and measurement technique (laser Doppler flowmetry) found blunted cerebrovascular responses to both

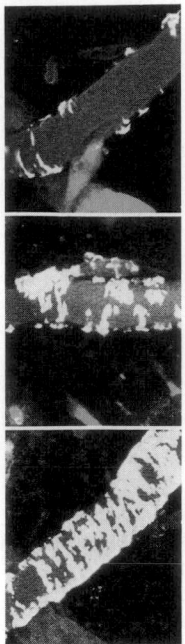

FIGURE 33–3 *Cerebral amyloid angiopathy in a transgenic mouse. Mice transgenic for mutant β-amyloid (Aβ) precursor protein driven by the platelet-derived growth factor promoter[164] demonstrate vessels with varying amounts of vascular Aβ deposition. Amyloid is visualized through topical application of thioflavine-S, and vessel lumens with intravenous Texas red–labeled dextran. In vivo imaging is performed by multiphoton fluorescent microscopy.[75] (Courtesy of Bradley T. Hyman.)*

Table 33.3 **Distribution of Cerebral Amyloid Angiopathy (CAA)–related Lobar Hemorrhages[°]**

Lobe	Number (n = 105)	Percentage of Total
Frontal	36	34
Parietal	28	27
Temporal	24	23
Occipital	17	16

[°]Data represent 105 hematomas from 100 consecutive patients diagnosed with CAA-related lobar intracerebral hemorrhage.

endothelium-dependent dilating agents and functional stimulation.[81,82] These hints of altered vascular physiology, raised as well by earlier studies of isolated vessel segments exposed to Aβ,[83] highlight the important possibility that even mild to moderate CAA might produce clinically significant dysfunction of blood flow.

CLINICAL PRESENTATION AND DIAGNOSIS

Spontaneous Intracerebral Hemorrhage

The best recognized clinical manifestation of CAA is spontaneous ICH. The hemorrhages largely follow the distribution of the vascular amyloid, appearing with highest frequency in the corticosubcortical or lobar regions and less commonly in cerebellum, and generally sparing the brainstem and deep hemispheric structures.[5,11] Lobar ICH in CAA is more likely to dissect into the subarachnoid space than into the lateral ventricles.[5,84–86] Despite extensive involvement of the leptomeningeal vessels, primary subarachnoid hemorrhage due to CAA is rare.[85,87]

CAA-related lobar ICH presents much like other types of lobar ICH,[88] with acute onset of neurologic symptoms and a variable combination of headache, seizures, and decreased consciousness according to hemorrhage size and location. Table 33.3 shows the various hematoma locations in 100 consecutive patients presenting at Massachusetts

General Hospital with lobar ICH that was diagnosed as CAA-related. Three of these patients presented with multiple hematomas (Fig. 33–4). The slight overrepresentation of frontal hemorrhages seen in Table 33.3 is almost identical to that noted in 107 autopsied brains reviewed by Vinters.[11] Whether this frontal predominance represents a true biological feature of CAA-related vessel rupture rather than an artifact of the methodology used for assigning hematoma location is unclear.

Many hemorrhagic lesions in CAA are small and clinically silent.[89] These small corticosubcortical lesions are well visualized by gradient-echo or T2°-weighted magnetic resonance imaging (MRI) techniques, which enhance the signal dropout associated with deposited hemosiderin.[90–93] By detecting even old hemorrhagic lesions, gradient-echo MRI provides a clinical method for demonstrating an individual's lifetime history of hemorrhage and thus for identifying the pattern of multiple lobar lesions characteristic of CAA (Fig. 33–5).

The Boston criteria for CAA codify the typical features of CAA-related ICH into the diagnostic categories "definite," "probable," and "possible" disease, as listed in Table 33.4.[14,94] Although diagnosis of definite CAA requires

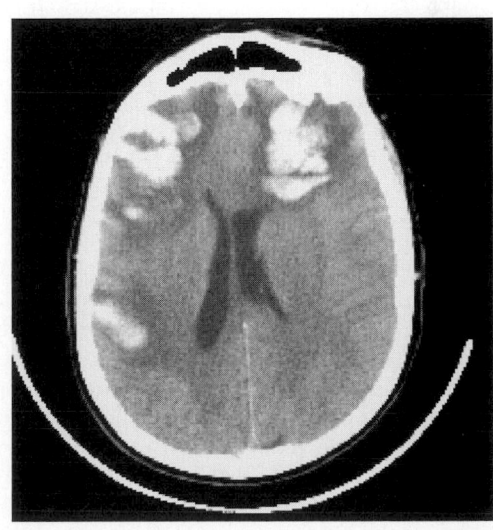

FIGURE 33–4 *Multiple concurrent cerebral amyloid angiopathy (CAA)–related hemorrhages. This computed tomography scan of a 66-year-old woman shows essentially simultaneous intracerebral hemorrhages in left frontal, right frontal, and right frontotemporal cortices. Subsequent cortical biopsy demonstrated severe CAA.*

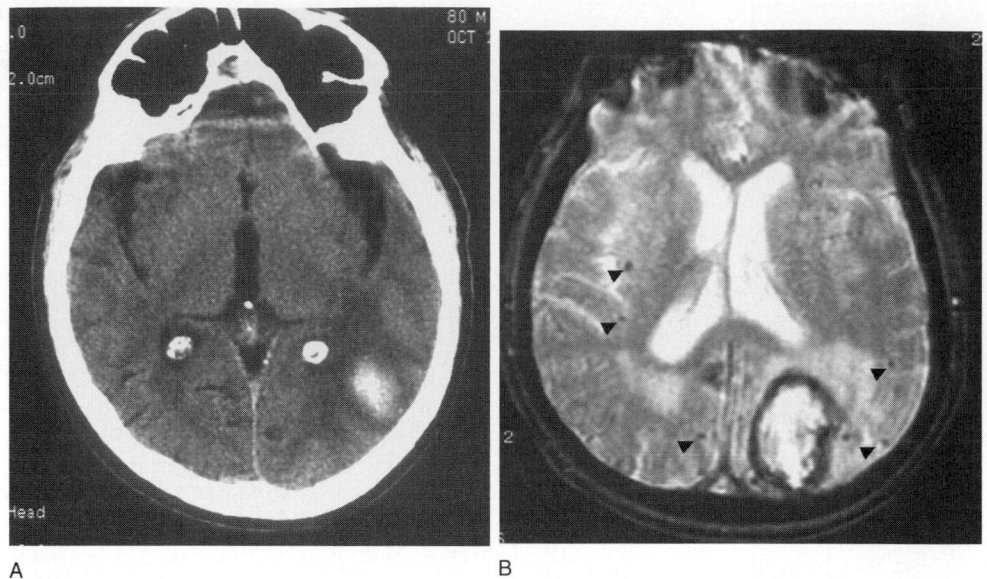

FIGURE 33–5 *Recurrent intracerebral hemorrhage (ICH). A, The computed tomography scan shows a left temporal ICH in an 80-year-old man with a history of previous cognitive decline. B, A gradient-echo magnetic resonance imaging sequence obtained 2 years later demonstrates recurrent ICH in the left parietal lobe as well as multiple punctate hypointense lesions (arrowheads) consistent with chronic asymptomatic hemorrhages. The presence of two or more strictly lobar hemorrhagic lesions is consistent with a diagnosis of probable cerebral amyloid angiopathy (see Table 33.4).*

Table 33.4   Boston Criteria for Diagnosis of Cerebral Amyloid Angiopathy–Related Intracerebral Hemorrhage

Definite CAA	Full postmortem examination of brain shows lobar ICH, severe CAA (see ref 31), and no other diagnostic lesion
Probable CAA with supporting pathologic evidence	Clinical data and pathologic tissue (evacuated hematoma or cortical biopsy specimen) showing some lobar CAA in pathologic specimen, and no other diagnostic lesion
Probable CAA	Clinical data and MRI or CT demonstration of two or more hemorrhagic lesions restricted to lobar regions (cerebellar hemorrhage allowed), patient age ≥ 55 yr, and no other cause of hemorrhage*
Possible CAA	Clinical data and MRI or CT demonstration of single lobar ICH, patient age ≥ 55 yr, and no other cause of hemorrhage*

*Other causes of ICH defined as excessive anticoagulation (INR > 3.0), antecedent head trauma or ischemic stroke, CNS tumor, vascular malformation or vasculitis, blood dyscrasia or coagulopathy. INR > 3.0 or other nonspecific laboratory abnormalities permitted for diagnosis of *possible* CAA.
CAA, cerebral amyloid angiopathy; CNS, central nervous system; CT, computed tomography; ICH, intracerebral hemorrhage; INR, International Normalized Ratio; MRI, magnetic resonance imaging.

demonstration of advanced disease through full postmortem examination, a clinical diagnosis of probable CAA can be reached during life through radiographic demonstration of at least two strictly lobar or corticosubcortical hemorrhagic lesions without other definite hemorrhagic process. In a small clinical-pathologic validation study, 13 of 13 subjects diagnosed clinically with probable CAA also had pathologic evidence of CAA,[94] suggesting that the criteria may be sufficiently specific to be useful in practice. In the same study, gradient-echo MRI detected the diagnostic pattern in 8 of 11 patients (73%) with pathologically documented CAA, providing an estimate for the sensitivity of the diagnosis. The Boston criteria propose a separate category of *probable CAA with supporting pathology* for patients with lobar ICH and an antemortem brain sample containing evidence of CAA (see Table 33.4). A validation

study for this diagnosis suggested that CAA of at least moderate severity in a random tissue sample was a reasonably specific marker for severe CAA in the brain as a whole.[1]

Iatrogenic Intracerebral Hemorrhage

Iatrogenic ICH occurring during anticoagulation or coronary thrombolysis is an especially important manifestation of CAA. Anticoagulation is hypothesized to promote ICH by allowing small leakages of blood to expand into large symptomatic hemorrhages[95] and might thus be particularly risky in the setting of advanced CAA. This possibility is supported by demonstration of advanced CAA in individual cases of ICH after either coronary thrombolysis[96–98] or anticoagulation.[99] The largest series of consecutive pathologic cases found CAA in 3 of 5 lobar ICHs after thrombolysis for acute myocardial infarction[100] and in 7 of 11 lobar ICHs occurring with warfarin therapy.[101] The association of CAA with anticoagulation-related ICH was further supported by a higher frequency of the APOE ε2 allele among patients with lobar ICH undergoing warfarin therapy compared with control patients without ICH who were also undergoing warfarin therapy.[101] The apparent link between CAA and iatrogenic ICH might partially explain the noted age dependence of these complications.[102-105] These observations raise the intriguing possibility that an individual's risk for CAA could ultimately be incorporated into the decision whether to treat with thrombolytic or anticoagulant agents.

Presentations Without Major Hemorrhage

Accumulating neuropathologic data suggest that advanced CAA may sufficiently affect blood flow to cause *ischemic infarction* as well as hemorrhagic infarction. Various types of ischemic lesions are reported in association with CAA, including punctate areas of gliosis in the cerebral cortex[89] and regions of myelin loss and focal gliosis in the white matter.[106] The white matter findings are ascribed to decreased perfusion via amyloid-laden overlying cortical vessels, because the white matter itself is largely spared from CAA. The relationship between CAA and ischemic damage was further strengthened by two neuropathologic studies of consecutive tissue samples. In a postmortem study of 145 brains of patients with Alzheimer's disease, severe CAA was associated with cortical infarctions with an odds ratio of 3.5.[107] A history of hypertension acted synergistically with CAA on risk of infarction in this study, suggesting the further possibility of an interaction between these two vascular processes. A second study looked at brain biopsy tissue and found CAA to be present in 14 of 108 (13%) samples from patients with cerebral or cerebellar infarction, compared with only 5 of 136 (3.7%) sample from patients of similar ages who underwent biopsy for other reasons.[108]

Despite the strength of this evidence (as well as the amyloid-related alterations in mouse blood flow noted previously), specific clinical syndromes resulting from CAA-related ischemia have remained difficult to define. A relatively rare presentation consisting of subacute cognitive decline, seizures, dramatic leukoencephalopathy, white matter edema, and mass effect[109,110] demonstrates the potential clinical impact of CAA-related ischemia. Another example of clinically significant ischemic damage is the leukoencephalopathy characteristic of several familial forms of CAA described later.[111,112] Given the clear role of vascular insufficiency and small strokes in exacerbating dementia,[113-115] it is reasonable to suspect that even smaller extents of CAA-related ischemia may cause substantial cognitive impairment.

One further group of patients with CAA and ischemic-type brain lesions are those with *vascular inflammation*. Although some increase in inflammatory cells may be a common feature of advanced CAA,[13,32] a minority of patients demonstrate more robust reactions ranging from perivascular giant cells (see Fig. 33–1F) to frank vasculitis.[116-119] These patients appear more likely to present with cognitive decline and focal or diffuse ischemic injury

rather than pure ICH. The reported response of at least some affected individuals to immunosuppressive treatment (particularly with cyclophosphamide)[117,120] suggests that CAA-related inflammation may be an important subtype to diagnose during life.

CAA can also manifest as *transient neurologic symptoms*,[109,121,122] another syndrome for which diagnosis during life is of particular practical importance. The neurologic symptoms can include focal weakness, numbness, paresthesias, or language abnormalities, often occurring in a recurrent and stereotyped pattern. Spells typically last for minutes and may spread smoothly from one contiguous body part to another during a single spell. Transient neurologic symptoms in CAA appear to be related to the hemorrhagic rather than the ischemic component of the disease, because gradient-echo MRI commonly demonstrates otherwise asymptomatic hemorrhage in the cortical region corresponding to the spell.[109] Spells often cease with anticonvulsant treatment. The major practical issue is to differentiate these episodes by clinical or radiographic means from true transient ischemic attacks, because administering anticoagulant agents to patients with advanced CAA may substantially raise the risk for future hemorrhagic stroke.

GENETICS

Familial Cerebral Amyloid Angiopathy

Several familial forms of CAA have been identified in which a protein entirely unrelated to Aβ accumulates in vessels, assumes amyloid conformation, and promotes vascular dysfunction. The clinical presentation of these familial CAAs differs from mutation to mutation, suggesting that each protein deposit provokes its own specific reaction. Substitution of glutamine for leucine at position 68 in the protease inhibitor cystatin C results in Icelandic CAA, which is characterized by very early deposition of a mutant protein fragment in vessel walls and symptomatic ICH by the third or fourth decade.[123,124] ICH is much less prominent in familial British dementia, a disorder caused by mutation in the BRI gene.[125] A single nucleotide substitution in the BRI stop codon causes cerebrovascular deposition of an abnormal carboxyl-terminus peptide fragment and a clinical syndrome of dementia and ataxia.[126] A third clinical presentation is associated with mutations in the transthyretin gene. When these mutations affect the central nervous system, they favor leptomeningeal and subependymal deposition, causing varying combinations of subarachnoid hemorrhage, seizures, hydrocephalus, cognitive changes, ataxia, and hearing loss.[127-131]

The other major forms of familial CAA are caused by mutations of the APP gene. Interestingly, the APP mutations associated with CAA cluster within the Aβ-coding region of APP (Fig. 33–6) rather than flanking the Aβ-coding segment like the Alzheimer's disease–associated mutations.[132] Dutch-type hereditary CAA caused by substitution of glutamate to glutamine at Aβ position 22[133,134] manifests as recurrent lobar ICH in the fifth or sixth decade and progresses to an early mortality.[135,136] A similar clinical picture is produced by the Italian substitution of lysine at this position.[67,137] Dementia and Alzheimer's

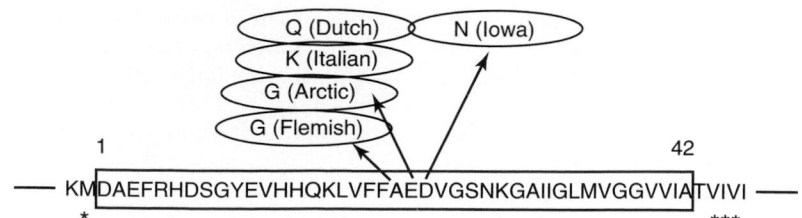

FIGURE 33–6   *Mutations of the APP (β-amyloid precursor protein) gene associated with familial cerebral amyloid angiopathy (CAA). The boxed segment of APP contains the region representing Aβ42 as well as the amino acid substitutions at positions 21 to 23 associated with familial CAA (see text for references). Asterisks indicate the positions of some of the mutations linked with early-onset Alzheimer's disease.*

disease–like neuritic pathology are more prominent features of two other CAA-associated mutations, the Flemish substitution of glycine at Aβ position 21[138,139] and the Iowa asparagine for aspartate substitution at residue 23.[112] Although differences have emerged among the various mutations in their effects on APP processing and Aβ bioactivity,[64,68] the precise mechanisms by which they predispose toward specific combinations of CAA and Alzheimer's disease pathology remain unclear.

Sporadic Cerebral Amyloid Angiopathy

The genes associated with familial CAA do not appear to play major roles as risk factors for sporadic CAA. Among 55 patients with sporadic CAA–related ICH examined for the cystatin C Icelandic mutation,[140–144] only one positive finding has been reported.[140] Similar searches for APP mutations at Aβ position 22 or 23 have yielded no instances in 111 reported patients with sporadic CAA.[112,140–143]

APOE has emerged as the strongest predictor of risk for sporadic CAA–related ICH. The APOE ε2 and ε4 alleles appear to promote CAA-related ICH at two distinct steps in the disease's pathogenesis, as previously described.[35,58–61,145] Each of these alleles was overrepresented more than twofold among 182 reviewed pathologic cases of CAA-related ICH.[146] The general importance of APOE to lobar ICH was further supported by the midpoint analysis of the Greater Cincinnati/Northern Kentucky cohort, in which presence of APOE ε2 or ε4 associated with an adjusted odds ratio for lobar ICH of 2.3.[22] The APOE alleles had an attributable risk for lobar ICH of 29% in this study, the largest proportion for any risk factor examined. APOE ε2 and ε4 appear to associate not only with greater risk for ICH occurrence but also with a younger age at first hemorrhage[61] and a shorter time until ICH recurrence (see later).[20]

CLINICAL COURSE AND TREATMENT

Initial Outcome and Risk of Recurrence

Despite improvements in the critical care of stroke, CAA-related lobar ICH remains a very serious clinical event. Among 103 consecutive patients with lobar ICH 55 years or older seen at Massachusetts General Hospital, in-hos-

pital mortality was 24%, and 6-month mortality 32%.[20] Factors contributing to poor outcome in these patients include advanced age[147] as well as a high prevalence of the APOE ε4 allele.[148,149]

Among the survivors of CAA-related ICH, the major neurologic risk is hemorrhage recurrence. A pooled analysis of patients monitored after lobar ICH reported a recurrence rate of 4.4% per year.[150] The value for cumulative ICH recurrence rate among the consecutive patients followed at Massachusetts General Hospital was approximately 10% per year,[20] perhaps reflecting a higher prevalence of CAA among the patients with lobar ICH in this population. Recurrent hemorrhages, like the initial hemorrhages, are typically lobar, though generally at a site distinct from that of the initial ICH (see Fig. 33–5).

The strongest risk factors for ICH recurrence are a history of previous recurrences and APOE genotype.[20] The risk ratio for ICH recurrence in the Massachusetts General Hospital series was 6.4 among patients with at least one hemorrhagic stroke before their index hemorrhage, suggesting that those with history of aggressive disease tend to remain on a high-risk course. Possession of either APOE ε2 or ε4 was associated with a risk ratio for recurrence of 3.8, the highest risk among the subgroup with the rare APOE ε2/ε4 genotype. These results suggest that risk for recurrence in CAA can be stratified according to a patient's baseline characteristics. In contrast, patient age, patient sex, and other vascular risk factors, such as hypertension and diabetes, had no apparent effect on risk of ICH recurrence.

Outcome is poor after a second ICH, as might be expected in an elderly population. For the 19 prospective recurrences among consecutive lobar hemorrhage patients at Massachusetts General Hospital, in-hospital mortality was 42%, and 6-month mortality 63%.[20] These observations underline the potential importance of secondary hemorrhage prevention as a treatment goal in CAA.

Approach to Treatment

No treatments for CAA have been established through clinical trial, leaving the clinician without clear guidelines for decision-making. This section describes our practice for managing patients with suspected CAA. The steps described are not offered as evidence-based treatment guidelines but rather as one potential approach based on the current understanding of the pathogenesis and course of CAA.

Acute Treatment of Intracerebral Hemorrhage

We use the general approach to acute medical and surgical management of ICH outlined by the American Heart Association Stroke Council[151] without any specific modification for CAA. Despite the differences in vascular pathology among ICH subtypes, the acute behavior of lobar hemorrhages due to CAA does not appear to differ from that of other types of ICH with regard to factors such as mass effect and hematoma expansion.[152] Patients with CAA who undergo hematoma resection show no excessive risk for acute rebleeding,[153–158] suggesting that the theoretical fragility of the amyloid-laden vessels need not deter surgical evacuation when indicated. Without fail, surgical specimens (including leptomeningeal tissue if available) should be examined through histochemical or immunochemical methods for the presence and severity of CAA.[1]

Diagnostic Testing

In the typical setting in which no neuropathologic tissue is available, we generally perform MRI with gradient-echo sequences when the patient is clinically stable. Although the absence of additional hemorrhagic lesions does not exclude CAA, their presence can support a diagnosis of probable CAA (see Table 33.4). MRI also helps exclude other potential causes of lobar ICH, such as underlying vascular malformation, tumor, and central nervous system vasculitis. We often perform MRI again 4 to 6 months after presentation to further rule out an underlying structural lesion if the diagnosis remains in doubt.

We pursue more aggressive diagnostic testing, such as cerebrospinal fluid examination, catheter angiography, and brain biopsy, only when a treatable entity is suggested by the clinical or radiographic presentation. The most relevant treatable entity is the CAA-related central nervous system vasculitis described previously. Although the clinical spectrum of this disorder remains to be fully established, its presence may be suggested by the finding of prominent white matter lesions or nonenhancing mass lesions on neuroimaging.[117–119]

Despite the association of APOE genotype with CAA, we do not routinely determine APOE genotype as part of the diagnostic evaluation. None of the APOE genotypes is either sensitive or specific for the diagnosis of CAA. APOE genotype could potentially prove useful in defining an individual's risk for ICH recurrence,[20] but whether this information is sufficient to alter clinical decisions remains unclear.

Outpatient Management

We generally advise patients to avoid anticoagulation therapy. This recommendation is based on the idea that the substantial risk of future hemorrhage[20] coupled with the very high morbidity and mortality associated with ICH during anticoagulation[95] outweigh virtually any projected benefit. Risk-benefit analyses of long-term anticoagulation therapy indeed indicate that even relatively small increments in the likelihood of hemorrhage can be sufficient to tip the balance against anticoagulation in most clinical situations.[159,160] The question of antiplatelet therapy appears less clear-cut, and we typically tailor our recommendation to the patient's cardiovascular risk profile. In the absence of a clear indication for antiplatelet agents, we recommend that they be avoided.

We also present a series of recommendations to patients regarding other medications and lifestyle issues. Although hypertension does not seem to affect the risk of CAA-related recurrence,[20] it is reasonable to keep the blood pressure under careful control. We also generally recommend against use of nonsteroidal anti-inflammatory agents because of their weak antiplatelet activity.[161] Acetaminophen and the nonacetylated salicylates, which appear to have the least effect on platelet activity,[162] may be useful alternatives. Limitation of alcohol consumption is recommended because of the possible role of alcohol use in predisposing to ICH. Finally, patients are advised that there is no known link between blood pressure fluctuations and rupture of amyloid-laden vessels and that they therefore need not avoid physical exertion, sexual activity, or emotional excitement.

The rapid gains in our understanding of the pathogenesis of CAA, occurring in tandem with advances in the field of Alzheimer's disease, offer the possibility that multiple therapeutic targets will emerge for future protective treatments. Treatment targets might include the processes of Aβ synthesis, deposition, toxicity, and clearance,[163] as well as other steps required for vessel breakdown. Therefore, several candidate drugs for prevention of recurrent ICH in CAA are likely to be developed, and prospects for developing effective therapies for this challenging disorder are good.

References

1. Greenberg SM, Vonsattel J-PG: Diagnosis of cerebral amyloid angiopathy: Sensitivity and specificity of cortical biopsy. Stroke 28:1418, 1997.
2. Brott T, Thalinger K, Hertzberg V: Hypertension as a risk factor for spontaneous intracerebral hemorrhage. Stroke 17:1078, 1986.
3. Broderick JP, Brott T, Tomsick T, et al: The risk of subarachnoid and intracerebral hemorrhages in blacks as compared with whites. N Engl J Med 326:733, 1992.
4. Schutz H, Bodeker RH, Damian M, et al: Age-related spontaneous intracerebral hematoma in a German community. Stroke 21:1412, 1990.
5. Itoh Y, Yamada M, Hayakawa M, et al: Cerebral amyloid angiopathy: A significant cause of cerebellar as well as lobar cerebral hemorrhage in the elderly. J Neurol Sci 116:135, 1993.
6. Lee SS, Stemmermann GN: Congophilic angiopathy and cerebral hemorrhage. Arch Pathol Lab Med 102:317, 1978.
7. Tomonaga M: Cerebral amyloid angiopathy in the elderly. J Am Geriatr Soc 29:151, 1981.
8. Vinters HV, Gilbert JJ: Cerebral amyloid angiopathy: Incidence and complications in the aging brain. II: The distribution of amyloid vascular changes. Stroke 14:924, 1983.
9. Masuda J, Tanaka K, Ueda K, et al: Autopsy study of incidence and distribution of cerebral amyloid angiopathy in Hisayama, Japan. Stroke 19:205, 1988.
10. Jellinger K: Cerebrovascular amyloidosis with cerebral hemorrhage. J Neurol 214:195, 1977.
11. Vinters HV: Cerebral amyloid angiopathy: A critical review. Stroke 18:311, 1987.
12. Ellis RJ, Olichney JM, Thal LJ, et al: Cerebral amyloid angiopathy in the brains of patients with Alzheimer's disease: The CERAD experience, Part XV. Neurology 46:1592, 1996.
13. Mandybur TI: Cerebral amyloid angiopathy: The vascular pathology and complications. J Neuropathol Exp Neurol 45:79, 1986.

14. Greenberg SM, Briggs ME, Hyman BT, et al: Apolipoprotein E e4 is associated with the presence and earlier onset of hemorrhage in cerebral amyloid angiopathy. Stroke 27:1333, 1996.

15. Fisher CM: Pathological observations in hypertensive cerebral hemorrhage. J Neuropathol Exp Neurol 30:536, 1971.

16. Bahemuka M: Primary intracerebral hemorrhage and heart weight: A clinicopathologic case-control review of 218 patients. Stroke 18:531, 1987.

17. Massaro AR, Sacco RL, Mohr JP, et al: Clinical discriminators of lobar and deep hemorrhages: The Stroke Data Bank. Neurology 41:1881, 1991.

18. Broderick J, Brott T, Tomsick T, et al: Lobar hemorrhage in the elderly: The undiminishing importance of hypertension. Stroke 24:49, 1993.

19. Thrift AG, McNeil JJ, Forbes A, et al: Three important subgroups of hypertensive persons at greater risk of intracerebral hemorrhage. Melbourne Risk Factor Study Group. Hypertension 31:1223, 1998.

20. O'Donnell HC, Rosand J, Knudsen KA, et al: Apolipoprotein E genotype and the risk of recurrent lobar intracerebral hemorrhage. N Engl J Med 342:240, 2000.

21. Ferreiro JA, Ansbacher LE, Vinters HV: Stroke related to cerebral amyloid angiopathy: The significance of systemic vascular disease. J Neurol 236:267, 1989.

22. Woo D, Sauerbeck LR, Kissela BM, et al: Genetic and environmental risk factors for intracerebral hemorrhage: Preliminary results of a population-based study. Stroke 33:1190, 2002.

23. Tanaka H, Ueda Y, Hayashi M, et al: Risk factors for cerebral hemorrhage and cerebral infarction in a Japanese rural community. Stroke 13:62, 1982.

24. Iso H, Jacobs DJ, Wentworth D, et al: Serum cholesterol levels and six-year mortality from stroke in 350,977 men screened for the multiple risk factor intervention trial [see comments]. N Engl J Med 320:904, 1989.

25. Yano K, Reed DM, MacLean CJ: Serum cholesterol and hemorrhagic stroke in the Honolulu Heart Program. Stroke 20:1460, 1989.

26. Gatchev O, Rastam L, Lindberg G, et al: Subarachnoid hemorrhage, cerebral hemorrhage, and serum cholesterol concentration in men and women. Ann Epidemiol 3:403, 1993.

27. Lindenstrom E, Boysen G, Nyboe J: Influence of total cholesterol, high density lipoprotein cholesterol, and triglycerides on risk of cerebrovascular disease: The Copenhagen City Heart Study [see comments]. BMJ 309:11, 1994; published erratum appears in BMJ 309:1619, 1994.

28. Iribarren C, Jacobs DR, Sadler M, et al: Low total serum cholesterol and intracerebral hemorrhagic stroke: Is the association confined to elderly men? Stroke 27:1993, 1996.

29. Giroud M, Creisson E, Fayolle H, et al: Risk factors for primary cerebral hemorrhage: A population-based study. The Stroke Registry of Dijon. Neuroepidemiology 14:20, 1995.

30. Segal AZ, Chiu RI, Eggleston-Sexton PM, et al: Low cholesterol as a risk factor for primary intracerebral hemorrhage: A case-control study. Neuroepidemiology 18:185, 1999.

31. Vonsattel JP, Myers RH, Hedley-Whyte ET, et al: Cerebral amyloid angiopathy without and with cerebral hemorrhages: A comparative histological study. Ann Neurol 30:637, 1991.

32. Yamada M, Itoh Y, Shintaku M, et al: Immune reactions associated with cerebral amyloid angiopathy. Stroke 27:1155, 1996.

33. Maat-Schieman ML, van Duinen SG, Rozemuller AJ, et al: Association of vascular amyloid beta and cells of the mononuclear phagocyte system in hereditary cerebral hemorrhage with amyloidosis (Dutch) and Alzheimer disease. J Neuropathol Exp Neurol 56:273, 1997.

34. Uchihara T, Akiyama H, Kondo H, et al: Activated microglial cells are colocalized with perivascular deposits of amyloid-beta protein in Alzheimer's disease brain. Stroke 28:1948, 1997.

35. Vinters HV, Natte R, Maat-Schieman ML, et al: Secondary microvascular degeneration in amyloid angiopathy of patients with hereditary cerebral hemorrhage with amyloidosis, Dutch type (HCHWA-D). Acta Neuropathol 95:235, 1998.

36. Maeda A, Yamada M, Itoh Y, et al: Computer-assisted three-dimensional image analysis of cerebral amyloid angiopathy. Stroke 24:1857, 1993.

37. Natte R, Vinters HV, Maat-Schieman ML, et al: Microvasculopathy is associated with the number of cerebrovascular lesions in hereditary cerebral hemorrhage with amyloidosis, Dutch type. Stroke 29:1588, 1998.

38. McCarron MO, Nicoll JA, Stewart J, et al: The apolipoprotein E epsilon2 allele and the pathological features in cerebral amyloid angiopathy-related hemorrhage. J Neuropathol Exp Neurol 58:711, 1999.

39. Jarrett JT, Berger EP, Lansbury PT: The carboxy terminus of the beta amyloid protein is critical for the seeding of amyloid formation: Implications for the pathogenesis of Alzheimer's disease. Biochemistry 32:4693, 1993.

40. Shinkai Y, Yoshimura M, Ito Y, et al: Amyloid β-proteins 1–40 and 1–42(43) in the soluble fraction of extra- and intracranial blood vessels. Ann Neurol 38:421, 1995.

41. Natte R, Yamaguchi H, Maat-Schieman ML, et al: Ultrastructural evidence of early non-fibrillar Abeta42 in the capillary basement membrane of patients with hereditary cerebral hemorrhage with amyloidosis, Dutch type. Acta Neuropathol (Berl) 98:577, 1999.

42. Iwatsubo T, Odaka A, Suzuki N, et al: Visualization of A beta 42(43) and A beta 40 in senile plaques with end-specific A beta monoclonals: Evidence that an initially deposited species is A beta 42(43). Neuron 13:45, 1994.

43. Mak K, Yang F, Vinters HV, et al: Polyclonals to beta-amyloid(1–42) identify most plaque and vascular deposits in Alzheimer cortex, but not striatum. Brain Res 667:138, 1994.

44. Gravina SA, Ho LB, Eckman CB, et al: Amyloid beta protein (a-beta) in Alzheimer's disease brain: Biochemical and immunocytochemical analysis with antibodies specific for forms ending at a-beta-40 or a-beta-42(43). J Biol Chem 270:7013, 1995.

45. Iwatsubo T, Mann DM, Odaka A, et al: Amyloid beta protein (A beta) deposition: A beta 42(43) precedes A beta 40 in Down syndrome. Ann Neurol 37:294, 1995.

46. Lemere CA, Blusztajn JK, Yamaguchi H, et al: Sequence of deposition of heterogeneous amyloid β-peptides and APO E in Down syndrome: Implications for initial events in amyloid plaque formation. Neurobiol Dis 3:16, 1996.

47. Castano EM, Prelli F, Soto C, et al: The length of amyloid-beta in hereditary cerebral hemorrhage with amyloidosis, Dutch type: Implications for the role of amyloid-beta 1–42 in Alzheimer's disease. J Biol Chem 271:32185, 1996.

48. Mann DM, Iwatsubo T, Ihara Y, et al: Predominant deposition of amyloid-beta 42(43) in plaques in cases of Alzheimer's disease and hereditary cerebral hemorrhage associated with mutations in the amyloid precursor protein gene. Am J Pathol 148:1257, 1996.

49. Alonzo NC, Hyman BT, Rebeck GW, et al: Progression of cerebral amyloid angiopathy: Accumulation of amyloid-β40 in already affected vessels. J Neuropathol Exp Neurol 57:353, 1998.

50. Snow AD, Mar H, Nochlin D, et al: Early accumulation of heparan sulfate in neurons and in the beta-amyloid protein-containing lesions of Alzheimer's disease and Down's syndrome. Am J Pathol 137:1253, 1990.

51. Vinters HV, Nishimura GS, Secor DL, et al: Immunoreactive A4 and gamma-trace peptide colocalization in amyloidotic arteriolar lesions in brains of patients with Alzheimer's disease. Am J Pathol 137:233, 1990.

52. Namba Y, Tomonaga M, Kawasaki H, et al: Apolipoprotein E immunoreactivity in cerebral amyloid deposits and neurofibrillary tangles in Alzheimer's disease and kuru plaque amyloid in Creutzfeldt-Jakob disease. Brain Res 541:163, 1991.

53. Kalaria RN, Kroon SN: Complement inhibitor C4-binding protein in amyloid deposits containing serum amyloid P in Alzheimer's disease. Biochem Biophys Res Commun 186:461, 1992.

54. Ueda K, Fukushima H, Masliah E, et al: Molecular cloning of cDNA encoding an unrecognized component of amyloid in Alzheimer disease. Proc Natl Acad Sci U S A 90:11282, 1993.

55. Verbeek MM, Eikelenboom P, de Waal RM: Differences between the pathogenesis of senile plaques and congophilic angiopathy in Alzheimer disease. J Neuropathol Exp Neurol 56:751, 1997.

56. Cho HS, Hyman BT, Greenberg SM, et al: Quantitation of apoE domains in Alzheimer disease brain suggests a role for apoE in Abeta aggregation. J Neuropathol Exp Neurol 60:342, 2001.

57. Schmechel DE, Saunders AM, Strittmatter WJ, et al: Increased amyloid beta-peptide deposition in cerebral cortex as a consequence of apolipoprotein E genotype in late-onset Alzheimer disease. Proc Natl Acad Sci U S A 90:9649, 1993.

58. Greenberg SM, Rebeck GW, Vonsattel JPV, et al: Apolipoprotein E e4 and cerebral hemorrhage associated with amyloid angiopathy. Ann Neurol 38:254, 1995.

59. Premkumar DR, Cohen DL, Hedera P, et al: Apolipoprotein E-epsilon4 alleles in cerebral amyloid angiopathy and cerebrovascular pathology associated with Alzheimer's disease. Am J Pathol 148:2083, 1996.

60. Olichney JM, Hansen LA, Galasko D, et al: The apolipoprotein E epsilon 4 allele is associated with increased neuritic plaques and cerebral amyloid angiopathy in Alzheimer's disease and Lewy body variant. Neurology 47:190, 1996.

61. Greenberg SM, Vonsattel JP, Segal AZ, et al: Association of apolipoprotein E epsilon2 and vasculopathy in cerebral amyloid angiopathy. Neurology 50:961, 1998.

62. Davis J, Van Nostrand WE: Enhanced pathologic properties of Dutch-type mutant amyloid beta-protein. Proc Natl Acad Sci U S A 93:2996, 1996.

63. Verbeek MM, de Waal RM, Schipper JJ, et al: Rapid degeneration of cultured human brain pericytes by amyloid beta protein. J Neurochem 68:1135, 1997.

64. Wang Z, Natte R, Berliner JA, et al: Toxicity of dutch (E22Q) and flemish (A21G) mutant amyloid beta proteins to human cerebral microvessel and aortic smooth muscle cells. Stroke 31:534, 2000.

65. Eisenhauer PB, Johnson RJ, Wells JM, et al: Toxicity of various amyloid beta peptide species in cultured human blood-brain barrier endothelial cells: Increased toxicity of Dutch-type mutant. J Neurosci Res 60:804, 2000.

66. Melchor JP, McVoy L, Van Nostrand WE: Charge alterations of E22 enhance the pathogenic properties of the amyloid beta-protein. J Neurochem 74:2209, 2000.

67. Miravalle L, Tokuda T, Chiarle R, et al: Substitutions at codon 22 of Alzheimer's abeta peptide induce diverse conformational changes and apoptotic effects in human cerebral endothelial cells. J Biol Chem 275:27110, 2000.

68. Van Nostrand WE, Melchor JP, Cho HS, et al: Pathogenic effects of D23N Iowa mutant amyloid beta-protein. J Biol Chem 276:32860, 2001.

69. Van Nostrand WE, Melchor JP, Ruffini L: Pathologic amyloid beta-protein cell surface fibril assembly on cultured human cerebrovascular smooth muscle cells. J Neurochem 70:216, 1998.

70. Melchor JP, Van Nostrand WE: Fibrillar amyloid beta-protein mediates the pathologic accumulation of its secreted precursor in human cerebrovascular smooth muscle cells. J Biol Chem 275:9782, 2000.

71. Kingston IB, Castro MJ, Anderson S: In vitro stimulation of tissue-type plasminogen activator by Alzheimer amyloid beta-peptide analogues. Nature Medicine 1:138, 1995.

72. Van Nostrand WE, Porter M: Plasmin cleavage of the amyloid beta-protein: Alteration of secondary structure and stimulation of tissue plasminogen activator activity. Biochemistry 38:11570, 1999.

73. Calhoun ME, Burgermeister P, Phinney AL, et al: Neuronal overexpression of mutant amyloid precursor protein results in prominent deposition of cerebrovascular amyloid. Proc Natl Acad Sci U S A 96:14088, 1999.

74. Van Dorpe J, Smeijers L, Dewachter I, et al: Prominent cerebral amyloid angiopathy in transgenic mice overexpressing the London mutant of human APP in neurons. Am J Pathol 157:1283, 2000.

75. Kimchi EY, Kajdasz S, Bacskai BJ, et al: Analysis of cerebral amyloid angiopathy in a transgenic mouse model of Alzheimer disease using in vivo multiphoton microscopy. J Neuropathol Exp Neurol 60:274, 2001.

76. Christie R, Yamada M, Moskowitz M, et al: Structural and functional disruption of vascular smooth muscle cells in a transgenic mouse model of amyloid angiopathy. Am J Pathol 158:1065, 2001.

77. Winkler DT, Bondolfi L, Herzig MC, et al: Spontaneous hemorrhagic stroke in a mouse model of cerebral amyloid angiopathy. J Neurosci 21:1619, 2001.

78. Weller RO, Massey A, Newman TA, et al: Cerebral amyloid angiopathy: Amyloid beta accumulates in putative interstitial fluid drainage pathways in Alzheimer's disease. Am J Pathol 153:725, 1998.

79. Wyss-Coray T, Masliah E, Mallory M, et al: Amyloidogenic role of cytokine TGF-ß1 in transgenic mice and in Alzheimer's disease. Nature 389:603, 1997.

80. Wyss-Coray T, Lin C, Yan F, et al: TGF-beta1 promotes microglial amyloid-beta clearance and reduces plaque burden in transgenic mice. Nature Med 7:612, 2001.

81. Iadecola C, Zhang F, Niwa K, et al: SOD1 rescues cerebral endothelial dysfunction in mice overexpressing amyloid precursor protein. Nat Neurosci 2:157, 1999.

82. Niwa K, Younkin L, Ebeling C, et al: Abeta 1-40-related reduction in functional hyperemia in mouse neocortex during somatosensory activation. Proc Natl Acad Sci U S A 97:9735, 2000.

83. Thomas T, Thomas G, McLendon C, et al: beta-amyloid-mediated vasoactivity and vascular endothelial damage. Nature 380:168, 1996.

84. Gilbert JJ, Vinters HV: Cerebral amyloid angiopathy: Incidence and complications in the aging brain. I: Cerebral hemorrhage. Stroke 14:915, 1983.

85. Yamada M, Itoh Y, Otomo E, et al: Subarachnoid haemorrhage in the elderly: A necropsy study of the association with cerebral amyloid angiopathy. J Neurol Neurosurg Psychiatry 56:543, 1993.

86. Miller JH, Wardlaw JM, Lammie GA: Intracerebral haemorrhage and cerebral amyloid angiopathy: CT features with pathological correlation. Clin Radiol 54:422, 1999.

87. Ohshima T, Endo T, Nukui H, et al: Cerebral amyloid angiopathy as a cause of subarachnoid hemorrhage. Stroke 21:480, 1990.

88. Kase CS: Lobar hemorrhage. In Kase CS, Caplan LR (eds): Intracerebral Hemorrhage. Boston, Butterworth-Heinemann, 1994, p 363.

89. Okazaki H, Reagan TJ, Campbell RJ: Clinicopathologic studies of primary cerebral amyloid angiopathy. Mayo Clin Proc 54:22, 1979.

90. Atlas SW, Mark AS, Grossman RI, et al: Intracranial hemorrhage: Gradient-echo MR imaging at 1.5 T. Comparison with spin-echo imaging and clinical applications. Radiology 168:803, 1988.

91. Greenberg SM, Finklestein SP, Schaefer PW: Petechial hemorrhages accompanying lobar hemorrhages: Detection by gradient-echo MRI. Neurology 46:1751, 1996.

92. Fazekas F, Kleinert R, Roob G, et al: Histopathologic analysis of foci of signal loss on gradient-echo T2*- weighted MR images in patients with spontaneous intracerebral hemorrhage: Evidence of microangiopathy-related microbleeds. AJNR Am J Neuroradiol 20:637, 1999.

93. Tsushima Y, Tamura T, Unno Y, et al: Multifocal low-signal brain lesions on T2*-weighted gradient-echo imaging. Neuroradiology 42:499, 2000.

94. Knudsen KA, Rosand J, Karluk D, et al: Clinical diagnosis of cerebral amyloid angiopathy: Validation of the Boston criteria. Neurology 56:537, 2001.

95. Hart RG, Boop BS, Anderson DC: Oral anticoagulants and intracranial hemorrhage: Facts and hypotheses. Stroke 26:1471, 1995.

96. Ramsay DA, Penswick JL, Robertson DM: Fatal streptokinase-induced intracerebral haemorrhage in cerebral amyloid angiopathy. Can J Neurol Sci 17:336, 1990.

97. Leblanc R, Haddad G, Robitaille Y: Cerebral hemorrhage from amyloid angiopathy and coronary thrombolysis. Neurosurgery 31:586, 1992.

98. Wijdicks EF, Jack CRJ: Intracerebral hemorrhage after fibrinolytic therapy for acute myocardial infarction. Stroke 24:554, 1993.

99. Melo TP, Bogousslavsky J, Regli F, et al: Fatal hemorrhage during anticoagulation of cardioembolic infarction: Role of cerebral amyloid angiopathy. Eur Neurol 33:9, 1993.

100. Sloan MA, Price TR, Petito CK, et al: Clinical features and pathogenesis of intracerebral hemorrhage after rt-PA and heparin therapy for acute myocardial infarction: The Thrombolysis in Myocardial Infarction (TIMI) II Pilot and Randomized Clinical Trial combined experience. Neurology 45:649, 1995.

101. Rosand J, Hylek EM, O'Donnell HC, et al: Warfarin-associated hemorrhage and cerebral amyloid angiopathy: A genetic and pathologic study. Neurology 55:947, 2000.

102. Anderson JL, Karagounis L, Allen A, et al: Older age and elevated blood pressure are risk factors for intracerebral hemorrhage after thrombolysis. Am J Cardiol 68:166, 1991.

103. De Jaegere PP, Arnold AA, Balk AH, et al: Intracranial hemorrhage in association with thrombolytic therapy: Incidence and clinical predictive factors. J Am Coll Cardiol 19:289, 1992.

104. Hylek EM, Singer DE: Risk factors for intracranial hemorrhage in outpatients taking warfarin. Ann Intern Med 120:897, 1994.

105. Bleeding during antithrombotic therapy in patients with atrial fibrillation. The Stroke Prevention in Atrial Fibrillation Investigators. Arch Intern Med 156:409, 1996.

106. Gray F, Dubas F, Roullet E, et al: Leukoencephalopathy in diffuse hemorrhagic cerebral amyloid angiopathy. Ann Neurol 18:54, 1985.

107. Olichney JM, Hansen LA, Hofstetter CR, et al: Cerebral infarction in Alzheimer's disease is associated with severe amyloid angiopathy and hypertension. Arch Neurol 52:702, 1995.

Specific Medical Diseases and Stroke

108. Cadavid D, Mena H, Koeller K, et al: Cerebral beta amyloid angiopathy is a risk factor for cerebral ischemic infarction: A case control study in human brain biopsies. J Neuropathol Exp Neurol 59:768, 2000.

109. Greenberg SM, Vonsattel JP, Stakes JW, et al: The clinical spectrum of cerebral amyloid angiopathy: Presentations without lobar hemorrhage. Neurology 43:2073, 1993.

110. Silbert PL, Bartleson JD, Miller GM, et al: Cortical petechial hemorrhage, leukoencephalopathy, and subacute dementia associated with seizures due to cerebral amyloid angiopathy. Mayo Clin Proc 70:477, 1995.

111. Bornebroek M, Haan J, van Buchem MA, et al: White matter lesions and cognitive deterioration in presymptomatic carriers of the amyloid precursor protein gene codon 693 mutation. Arch Neurol 53:43, 1996.

112. Grabowski TJ, Cho HS, Vonsattel JPG, et al: Novel amyloid precursor protein mutation in an Iowa family with dementia and severe cerebral amyloid angiopathy. Ann Neurol 49:697, 2001.

113. Snowdon DA, Greiner LH, Mortimer JA, et al: Brain infarction and the clinical expression of Alzheimer disease: The Nun Study. JAMA 277:813, 1997.

114. Esiri MM, Wilcock GK, Morris JH: Neuropathological assessment of the lesions of significance in vascular dementia. J Neurol Neurosurg Psychiatry 63:749, 1997.

115. Hofman A, Ott A, Breteler MM, et al: Atherosclerosis, apolipoprotein E, and prevalence of dementia and Alzheimer's disease in the Rotterdam Study. Lancet 349:151, 1997.

116. Gray F, Vinters HV, Le Noan H, et al: Cerebral amyloid angiopathy and granulomatous angiitis: Immunohistochemical study using antibodies to the Alzheimer A4 peptide. Hum Pathol 21:1290, 1990.

117. Mandybur TI, Balko G: Cerebral amyloid angiopathy with granulomatous angiitis ameliorated by steroid-cytoxan treatment. Clin Neuropharmacol 15:241, 1992.

118. Fountain NB, Eberhard DA: Primary angiitis of the central nervous system associated with cerebral amyloid angiopathy: Report of two cases and review of the literature. Neurology 46:190, 1996.

119. Case records of the Massachusetts General Hospital: Weekly clinicopathological exercises. Case 10-2000: A 63-year-old man with changes in behavior and ataxia [clinical conference]. N Engl J Med 342:957, 2000.

120. Fountain NB, Lopes MB: Control of primary angiitis of the CNS associated with cerebral amyloid angiopathy by cyclophosphamide alone. Neurology 52:660, 1999.

121. Smith DB, Hitchcock M, Philpott PJ: Cerebral amyloid angiopathy presenting as transient ischemic attacks: Case report. J Neurosurg 63:963, 1985.

122. Yong WH, Robert ME, Secor DL, et al: Cerebral hemorrhage with biopsy-proved amyloid angiopathy. Arch Neurol 49:51, 1992.

123. Palsdottir A, Abrahamson M, Thorsteinsson L, et al: Mutation in cystatin C gene causes hereditary brain haemorrhage. Lancet 2(8611):603, 1988.

124. Levy E, Lobez-Otin C, Ghiso J, et al: Stroke in Icelandic patients with hereditary amyloid angiopathy is related to a mutation in the cystatin C gene, an inhibitor of cysteine proteases. J Exp Med 169:1771, 1989.

125. Vidal R, Frangione B, Rostagno A, et al: A stop-codon mutation in the BRI gene associated with familial British dementia. Nature 399:776, 1999.

126. Mead S, James-Galton M, Revesz T, et al: Familial British dementia with amyloid angiopathy: Early clinical, neuropsychological and imaging findings. Brain 123:975, 2000.

127. Vidal R, Garzuly F, Budka H, et al: Meningocerebrovascular amyloidosis associated with a novel transthyretin mis-sense mutation at codon 18 (TTRD 18G). Am J Pathol 148:361, 1996.

128. Herrick MK, DeBruyne K, Horoupian DS, et al: Massive leptomeningeal amyloidosis associated with a Val30Met transthyretin gene. Neurology 47:988, 1996.

129. Petersen RB, Goren H, Cohen M, et al: Transthyretin amyloidosis: A new mutation associated with dementia. Ann Neurol 41:307, 1997.

130. Mascalchi M, Salvi F, Pirini MG, et al: Transthyretin amyloidosis and superficial siderosis of the CNS. Neurology 53:1498, 1999.

131. Brett M, Persey MR, Reilly MM, et al: Transthyretin Leu12Pro is associated with systemic, neuropathic and leptomeningeal amyloidosis. Brain 122:183, 1999.

132. Selkoe DJ: The origins of Alzheimer disease: A is for amyloid. JAMA 283:1615, 2000.

133. Levy E, Carman MD, Fernandez Madrid IJ, et al: Mutation of the Alzheimer's disease amyloid gene in hereditary cerebral hemorrhage, Dutch type. Science 248:1124, 1990.

134. Van Broeckhoven C, Haan J, Bakker E, et al: Amyloid beta protein precursor gene and hereditary cerebral hemorrhage with amyloidosis (Dutch). Science 248:1120, 1990.

135. Wattendorff AR, Frangione B, Luyendijk W, et al: Hereditary cerebral haemorrhage with amyloidosis, Dutch type (HCHWA-D): Clinicopathological studies. J Neurol Neurosurg Psychiatry 58:699, 1995.

136. Bornebroek M, Westendorp RG, Haan J, et al: Mortality from hereditary cerebral haemorrhage with amyloidosis–Dutch type: The impact of sex, parental transmission and year of birth. Brain 120:2243, 1997.

137. Tagliavini F, Rossi G, Padovani A, et al: A new βPP mutation related to hereditary cerebral haemorrhage. Alzheimer's Rep 2:S28, 1999.

138. Hendriks L, van Duijn CM, Cras P, et al: Presenile dementia and cerebral haemorrhage linked to a mutation at codon 692 of the beta-amyloid precursor protein gene. Nat Genet 1:218, 1992.

139. Cras P, van Harskamp F, Hendriks L, et al: Presenile Alzheimer dementia characterized by amyloid angiopathy and large amyloid core type senile plaques in the APP 692Ala–>Gly mutation. Acta Neuropathol (Berl) 96:253, 1998.

140. Graffagnino C, Herbstreith MH, Schmechel DE, et al: Cystatin C mutation in an elderly man with sporadic amyloid angiopathy and intracerebral hemorrhage. Stroke 26:2190, 1995.

141. Anders KH, Wang ZZ, Kornfeld M, et al: Giant cell arteritis in association with cerebral amyloid angiopathy: Immunohistochemical and molecular studies. Hum Pathol 28:1237, 1997.

142. Itoh Y, Yamada M: Cerebral amyloid angiopathy in the elderly: The clinicopathological features, pathogenesis, and risk factors. J Med Dental Sci 44:11, 1997.

143. Nagai A, Kobayashi S, Shimode K, et al: No mutations in cystatin C gene in cerebral amyloid angiopathy with cystatin C deposition. Mol Chem Neuropathol 33:63, 1998.

144. McCarron MO, Nicoll JA, Stewart J, et al: Absence of cystatin C mutation in sporadic cerebral amyloid angiopathy– related hemorrhage. Neurology 54:242, 2000.

145. Nicoll JA, Burnett C, Love S, et al: High frequency of apolipoprotein E epsilon 2 allele in hemorrhage due to cerebral amyloid angiopathy. Ann Neurol 41:716, 1997.

146. McCarron MO, Nicoll JAR: APOE genotype in relation to sporadic and Alzheimer-related CAA. In Verbeek MM, de Waal MW, Vinters HV (eds): Cerebral Amyloid Angiopathy in Alzheimer's Disease and Related Disorders. Dordrecht, Kluwer Academic Publishers, 2000, p 81.

147. Hemphill JC 3rd, Bonovich DC, Besmertis L, et al: The ICH score: A simple, reliable grading scale for intracerebral hemorrhage. Stroke 32:891, 2001.

148. Alberts MJ, Graffagnino C, McClenny C, et al: APOE genotype and survival from intracerebral haemorrhage. Lancet 346:575, 1995.

149. McCarron MO, Muir KW, Weir CJ, et al: The apolipoprotein E epsilon4 allele and outcome in cerebrovascular disease. Stroke 29:1882, 1998.

150. Bailey RD, Hart RG, Benavente O, et al: Recurrent brain hemorrhage is more frequent than ischemic stroke after intracranial hemorrhage. Neurology 56:773, 2001.

151. Broderick JP, Adams HP Jr, Barsan W, et al: Guidelines for the management of spontaneous intracerebral hemorrhage: A statement for healthcare professionals from a special writing group of the Stroke Council, American Heart Association. Stroke 30:905, 1999.

152. Brott T, Broderick J, Kothari R, et al: Early hemorrhage growth in patients with intracerebral hemorrhage. Stroke 28:1, 1997.

153. Greene GM, Godersky JC, Biller J, et al: Surgical experience with cerebral amyloid angiopathy. Stroke 21:1545, 1990.

154. Leblanc R, Preul M, Robitaille Y, et al: Surgical considerations in cerebral amyloid angiopathy. Neurosurgery 29:712, 1991.

155. Matkovic Z, Davis S, Gonzales M, et al: Surgical risk of hemorrhage in cerebral amyloid angiopathy. Stroke 22:456, 1991.

156. Kase CS: Cerebral amyloid angiopathy. In Kase CS, Caplan LR (eds): Intracerebral Hemorrhage. Boston, Butterworth-Heinemann, 1994, p 179.

157. Minakawa T, Takeuchi S, Sasaki O, et al: Surgical experience with massive lobar haemorrhage caused by cerebral amyloid angiopathy. Acta Neurochir 132:48, 1995.

158. Izumihara A, Ishihara T, Iwamoto N, et al: Postoperative outcome of 37 patients with lobar intracerebral hemorrhage related to cerebral amyloid angiopathy. Stroke 30:29, 1999.

159. Gustafsson C, Asplund K, Britton M, et al: Cost effectiveness of primary stroke prevention in atrial fibrillation: Swedish national perspective. BMJ 305:1457, 1992.

160. Eckman MH, Levine HJ, Salem DN, et al: Making decisions about antithrombotic therapy in heart disease: Decision analysis and cost-effectiveness issues. Chest 114:699S, 1998.

161. Schafer AI: Antiplatelet therapy. Am J Med 101:199, 1996.

162. Riendeau D, Charleson S, Cromlish W, et al: Comparison of the cyclooxygenase-1 inhibitory properties of nonsteroidal anti-inflammatory drugs (NSAIDs) and selective COX-2 inhibitors, using sensitive microsomal and platelet assays. Can J Physiol Pharmacol 75:1088, 1997.

163. Selkoe DJ: Translating cell biology into therapeutic advances in Alzheimer's disease. Nature 399:A23, 1999.

164. Games D, Adams D, Alessandrini R, et al: Alzheimer-type neuropathology in transgenic mice overexpressing v717f beta-amyloid precursor protein. Nature 373:523, 1995.

Specific Medical Diseases and Stroke

Chapter Thirty-Four

Coagulation Abnormalities in Stroke

Robin L. Brey and Bruce M. Coull

In normal circumstances, the coagulation system is balanced between maintaining the flow of blood in the vessels and stemming any leaks from disruptions in vessel integrity. However, many factors can upset that balance and result in thrombosis. Activation of blood coagulation with thrombosis is an obligatory event in almost all ischemic strokes. The formation of a thrombus most often ensues from the sudden and pathologic activation of the hemostasis that may be found with endothelial injury within an atherosclerotic precerebral artery or within the heart. Whereas many well-defined defects in hemostasis are associated with hemorrhagic stroke, most coagulation disorders that favor ischemic stroke remain less well characterized. A predisposition to thrombotic events is often called a "hypercoagulable state" by clinicians, but a better term when thrombosis is favored is *prothrombotic state*, which may involve activated blood coagulation, increased platelet reactivity, or impaired fibrinolysis.

PATHOGENESIS OF THROMBOSIS

Vascular Injury

As shown in Figure 34–1, prevention of intravascular thrombosis involves a dynamic interplay between the normal blood vessel and certain plasma proteins, platelets, fibrin formation, and fibrinolysis. Interactions among multiple plasma proteins, protein C, protein S, antithrombin III (ATIII), tissue factor pathway inhibitor, and normal vascular endothelial cells form an important barrier to thrombosis. A key protein, thrombomodulin, is expressed on the endothelial surface and promotes the activation of protein C. When protein C is combined with another natural anticoagulant, protein S, the resulting complex can rapidly inactivate activated factors V and VIII. Through the suppression of thrombin activation of thrombin-inducible fibrinolytic inhibitor, activated protein C may also have an indirect fibrinolytic effect.[1] Protein S is found in the plasma as both an active (free) and an inactive (C4b-binding protein–bound) form. A glycosaminoglycan, heparan, is also widely distributed on the normal endothelial surface. Heparan binds ATIII and enhances its anticoagulant function. Once bound to endothelial heparan, ATIII rapidly neutralizes the clotting enzyme thrombin as well as activated factor X and other prothrombotic serine proteases.[2–4]

Vascular endothelial cells also inhibit platelet adhesion and platelet aggregation. When the endothelium is activated by local injury, inflammation, or other thrombogenic stimuli, prostacyclin (PGI_2) is released. Prostacyclin causes vasodilatation and inhibits platelet plug formation. Blood vessels may also markedly enhance local fibrinolysis via the synthesis and release of tissue plasminogen activator (t-PA). Endothelium can synthesize and release nitric oxide, which is a potent platelet inhibitor.[5,6]

Although usually a barrier against thrombosis, the normal vascular endothelium may become a strong prothrombotic surface when injured.[5] Mediators of inflammation such as interleukin-1, tumor necrosis factor, and immune complexes may induce endothelial cells to express the prothrombotic tissue factor, expose binding sites for clotting factors, and downregulate thrombomodulin expression.[6] With severe injury, endothelial cells may be lost from the vascular surface altogether.[7,8] Brain vascular endothelium may not be as effective a barrier against thrombosis as vascular endothelium in other tissues. Results of some but not all studies suggest that the expression of thrombomodulin by brain vascular endothelium varies regionally within the brain and is limited in amount compared with systemic vessels.[9,10]

In established atherosclerosis, other prothrombotic factors also play a role. The atheromatous "gruel" that composes the inside of the plaque is rich in both tissue factor and lipids, which support coagulation reactions. For example, the rupture of an atherosclerotic plaque within a carotid or vertebral artery may expose the thrombogenic surface, promoting formation of mural thrombus. In addition, potent platelet-activating surfaces are exposed, leading to platelet deposition.

Factor V Leiden, Antithrombin III, Protein C, and Protein S Deficiencies and Prothrombin G20210a Polymorphism

Hereditary Deficiencies

There is little evidence that hereditary deficiencies of the main anticoagulant pathways of blood coagulation increase the risk of arterial thrombosis. However, studies show that

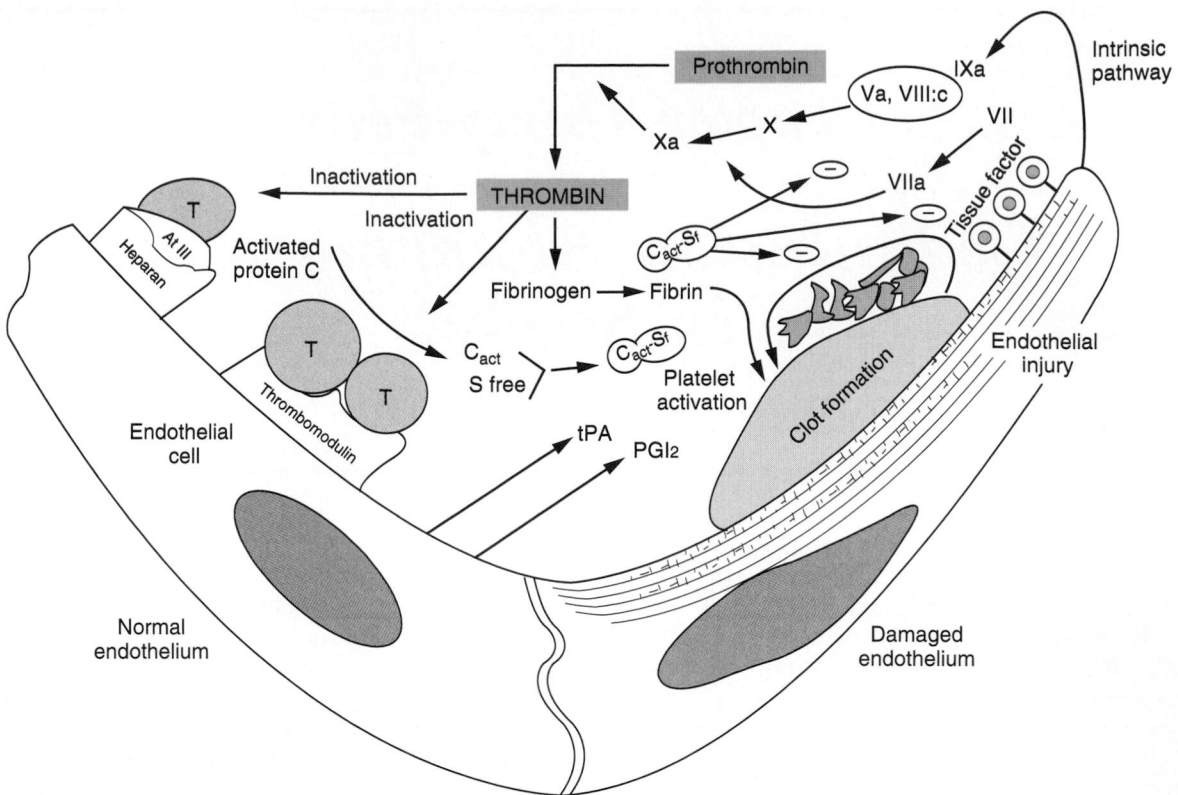

FIGURE 34–1 *When vascular endothelium is injured, clot formation is instigated by expression of tissue factor and activation of platelets and the coagulation pathways. The pivotal reaction is transformation of prothrombin to thrombin (T) with cleavage of fibrinogen to fibrin. The normal endothelium limits thrombosis by inactivating thrombin and by releasing prostacyclin (PGI$_2$), and tissue plasminogen activator (tPA). Activated protein C (C$_{act}$), when complexed with free protein S (S free), antagonizes platelet and factor X activation. See text for details.*

factor V Leiden,[11] activated protein C resistance,[12,13] and the prothrombin G20210A gene mutation[14] may contribute to stroke and myocardial infarction (MI) in selected groups of patients. By far the most common inherited defect leading to venous thrombosis is the clinical syndrome of hereditary resistance to activated protein C (APC) caused by the mutation in factor V (factor V Leiden), which renders activated factor V unable to be cleaved by APC. In white persons, factor V Leiden accounts for more than 95% of the total APC resistance. This defect is present in 5% to 7% of the normal population, 20% of patients experiencing a first episode of deep venous thrombosis, and 60% of patients with recurrent venous thromboses due to hypercoagulable states.

Although APC resistance due to factor V Leiden has a well-recognized association with cerebral venous thrombosis,[15,16] the relationship with arterial stroke is less clear. The Physician's Health Study showed that factor V Leiden does not increase the risk of stroke or MI.[17] In addition, a study of 489 patients with ischemic stroke and matched controls of all ages failed to find an association between APC resistance and acute ischemic stroke, supporting the findings of other, earlier prospective and case-control studies.[18] There was no difference in the prevalence of APC resistance between patients in younger and older age groups or within various stroke subtypes. In contrast,

another large study found factor V Leiden to be significantly more common in patients with large infarcts (13.6%; $P < .025$; confidence interval [CI], 1.16 to 4.34) than in the stroke-free control subjects (6.5%).[19] This study also found that the angiotensin-converting enzyme (ACE) D/D genotype was significantly more common in patients with small deep infarcts (40.3%; $P < .0005$; odds ratio [OR], 2.31; 95% CI, 1.49 to 3.57) than in the control group (22.6%). These two sets of results suggest that further study is warranted to explore more fully whether the Leiden mutation or ACE D/D genotype may predispose to underlying vascular pathophysiologic abnormality and stroke subtype.

Much less common are hereditary deficiencies or defects in protein C, protein S, and ATIII (approximately 1:1000 to 1:5000 persons). People who carry these defects have a higher incidence of thrombosis than people with factor V Leiden.[20] However, as with factor V Leiden, the majority of thrombotic episodes associated with the deficiencies are *venous*.[15] Protein C and protein S deficiencies, but not ATIII deficiency, can be associated with superficial thrombophlebitis.[21] The cerebral event most often associated with defects in these anticoagulant systems is also cerebral vein thrombosis, which may occur in 1% to 3% of affected patients, many of whom are young adults with these defects.[16,22-26] In the absence of an established explanation, patients with cerebral vein thrombosis should undergo testing for these coagulation abnormalities.

As for factor V Leiden, the association between inherited deficiencies in protein C, protein S, and ATIII and *arterial* thrombosis is less convincing. Activated protein C has been found to possess anti-inflammatory, antithrombotic, and neuroprotective effects in a murine model of focal ischemic stroke.[27] It would be logical to speculate that APC deficiency might contribute to increased stroke risk. In fact, the Atherosclerosis in Communities (ARIC) Study found no greater stroke risk associated with deficiencies in protein C (detected through measurement of protein C antigen) or ATIII activity.[28] Despite the negative results, the study found that higher stroke risk was associated with elevations of von Willebrand factor, factor VIIIc, and fibrinogen as well as high white blood cell count. D'Angelo and colleagues[29] reported that a reduced protein C level measured at the time of acute stroke was correlated with a poor outcome, but no differences in ATIII levels were found between survivors and nonsurvivors of stroke. When considering the results of this study, however, one must keep in mind that levels of these natural anticoagulants can be reduced in any acute inflammatory situation. For example, a case-control study found that low protein S levels were common in patients hospitalized for any reason,[30] making the role of this substance in stroke much more difficult to establish.

A single mutation in the 3′-untranslated region of the prothrombin gene resulting in a G-to-A (glycine-to-alanine) substitution has been associated with familial thrombophilia.[31] Prothrombin, or factor II, is the precursor of thrombin. A vitamin K–dependent zymogen, this protein is produced by the liver and has a central role in the conversion of fibrinogen to fibrin. Prothrombin has other functions in the body, such as limiting the hemostasis process. Thrombin also has regulatory functions that are important in the pathogenesis of atherosclerosis, such as initiating platelet aggregation and endothelial activation.

Factor II G20210A occurs in about 2.5% of the general population and in 6% of patients with a family history of venous thrombosis.[32] Like factor V Leiden mutation, this mutation is seen almost exclusively in white persons. Several studies have shown that in the presence of traditional vascular risk factors, the addition of factor II G20210A has a synergistic effect on the risk of MI, but results are conflicting (reviewed by Nguyen[31]). Few studies have investigated the role of factor II G20210A in stroke. A case-control study of consecutive patients with stroke or transient ischemic attack (TIA) found no difference in prevalence of the prothrombin mutation between the patients and controls.[33] Another study of 72 young patients with stroke and without traditional vascular risk factors found an increased prevalence in patients compared with controls (9.7% of patients had heterozygous mutation vs. 2.5% of controls; 2.8% of patients had homozygous mutation vs. 0% of controls).[14] The stroke risk associated with the heterozygous mutation was increased 3.8-fold, either mutation was increased 5.5-fold, and the homozygous mutation was increased 208-fold. Further studies are needed to clarify the role of this mutation in stroke and to determine whether the synergistic effect between the mutation and traditional vascular risk factors seen in MI is also seen in stroke.

Acquired Deficiencies

Acquired deficiencies of ATIII and proteins C and S have also been reported to produce a prothrombotic state related to brain infarction. Although extensive epidemiologic studies have not yet been performed, acquired anticoagulant protein deficiencies are usually associated with stroke in special clinical settings, many of which are listed in Table 34.1. Reductions of the anticoagulant proteins have been found in perioperative settings in women who are pregnant or taking oral contraceptives and in patients with malignancies, hepatic failure, or nephrotic syndrome. Acute fluctuations of anticoagulant protein levels can also follow plasmapheresis and hemodialysis. In a patient with any of the foregoing conditions who experiences TIA, stroke, or amaurosis fugax, careful evaluation may uncover one of these prothrombotic states.

Laboratory Investigation

Genetic tests are available for factor V Leiden and the prothrombin G20210A polymorphism.[34] For deficiencies of protein C, protein S, and antithrombin III, the underlying defect may be attributable to several different mutations, and DNA testing is not practical. In general, in situations for which genetic tests are unavailable (or their results would be negative in the case of acquired deficiencies), functional or activity-based assays should be used. Ten percent of defects are in the functional aspect of the molecule and would be missed with antigen assays.[34]

For protein C, functional assays are based on measurement of the anticoagulant activity of APS against the natural substrates, factors VIIIa and Va, or of the

Table 34.1 Acquired Deficiencies of Antithrombin III and Proteins C and S

Consumption coagulopathy
Disseminated intravascular coagulation (shock, sepsis)
Surgery
Preeclampsia
Liver dysfunction
Acute hepatic failure
Cirrhosis
Renal disease
Nephrotic syndrome
Hemolytic-uremic syndrome
Malignancies
Leukemia (acute promyelocytic leukemia)
Malnutrition or gastrointestinal loss
Vascular reconstruction (diabetes, age)
Protein-calorie deprivation
Inflammatory bowel disease
Drugs
Estrogens-progestins
Heparin
L-Asparaginase
Other
Vasculitis (? systemic lupus erythematosus)
Infection—neutropenia
Hemodialysis
Plasmapheresis

amidolytic activity against small synthetic substrates. The former should be the test of choice because it better mimics in vivo conditions.[34] These tests are commercially available but their results may be affected by conditions such as APC resistance and high concentrations of factor VIII and may be difficult to interpret.[35,36] These problems can be avoided through the use of amidolytic assays with snake venom as the activator. APC resistance can be assessed in plasma with activated partial thromboplastin time (aPTT)–based methods.[37] These are simple, inexpensive, and sensitive to the APC resistance syndrome as well as to factor V Leiden.[34]

For protein S, a functional assay should be theoretically superior to antigen measurement; however, available functional assays are based on the APC cofactor activity of protein S and are not very specific. The distribution of protein S in the plasma is 60% of the whole protein bound to C4b-binding protein, and 40% is free and active as APC cofactor.[38] The most common defect in protein S is a normal total protein S level but decreased levels of free protein S.[39] Thus, if one assays only the total protein S level, many cases of protein S defect will be missed. In a study of protein S deficiency established by genetic testing in a large kindred, levels of free protein S distinguished carriers from noncarriers much better than levels of the whole protein, suggesting that it may not be necessary to measure both free and total protein S.[40]

The measurement of antithrombin III antigen is not adequate to screen patients, because many patients with dysfunctional AT deficiency have normal antigen levels and they would not be diagnosed by ATIII antigen determination.[34] The two types of functional assays for ATIII deficiency are progressive inhibitory activity (performed without heparin) and heparin cofactor activity. Both may be performed with either thrombin or factor Xa as the target enzyme. The assay using heparin cofactor activity is able to detect all clinically relevant cases of ATIII deficiency. Factor Xa is probably a better target enzyme than thrombin because factor Xa is not affected by the presence of the other main plasma inhibitor of thrombin, heparin cofactor II.[41]

Activation of Hemostasis and Fibrin Formation

Simple assays are now available for measuring specific activation and breakdown products of coagulation.[42,43] When prothrombin is cleaved by factor Xa to form thrombin, the activation peptide ($F_{1.2}$) is cleaved off. The plasma levels of $F_{1.2}$ reflect ongoing activation of hemostasis. The conversion of fibrinogen to a cross-linked fibrin clot is a complex multistep process that is mediated by thrombin. In the first step, thrombin cleaves off fibrinopeptides A and B to form circulating fibrin monomers. The circulating fibrin monomer is then covalently cross-linked by thrombin-activated factor XIII. When the fibrin clot is lysed via fibrinolysis, specific breakdown products form; they include either nonspecific fibrin(ogen) degradation products or D dimer that is specific to fibrin degradation.[44–46]

During the acute phase of ischemic stroke, the intense activation of coagulation produces elevations of hemostatic markers, including prothrombin activation fragment $F_{1.2}$, fibrinopeptide A, and thrombin-antithrombin complex.[29,47–52] These elevations decline slowly but may persist for weeks to months.[47,50] Some studies have found persistent elevation of these markers in patients after stroke compared with controls.[52–54] One possible conclusion from these data is that there is an underlying prothrombotic state in patients with cerebrovascular disease. High levels of hemostatic markers have been found in patients with atrial fibrillation.[55–59] Levels of these markers are reduced by anticoagulation[60–63] and have been reported to decline after cardioversion.[64]

In the Edinburgh Artery Study, after adjustment for traditional vascular risk factors, several hemostatic factors were found to be associated with stroke and MI—plasma fibrinogen level, t-PA antigen, and fibrin–D dimer. This study also found that in older men and women, the presence of increased coagulation activity and disturbed fibrinolysis predicted future vascular events.[65] A later study confirmed these results and also found that levels of C-reactive protein, D dimer, and fibrinogen after an initial ischemic stroke were predictive of a new stroke.[66]

Fibrinogen itself is a strong independent risk factor for MI and stroke.[3,65,67–73] Fibrinogen levels increase after stroke,[74] and fibrinogen elevations are associated with an increased risk of further cardiovascular events in stroke survivors.[74,75] Patients with infection-associated stroke have higher levels of fibrinogen after stroke than those without a recent infection.[76] Possible mechanisms for the higher risk of stroke include activation of hemostasis, increased blood viscosity, a reflection of underlying inflammation, and decreased cerebral blood flow.[70,77] Fibrinogen also plays a critical role in platelet activation through binding to platelet glycoprotein IIb-IIIa membrane receptors,[78] which might be another mechanism favoring thrombosis.

Fibrinolysis

Homeostasis depends on the balance between clot formation and clot degradation, or *fibrinolysis*. Depression of fibrinolytic activity can tip the balance toward thrombosis. The fibrinolytic system is equilibrated between t-PA and its primary inhibitor, plasminogen activator inhibitor type 1 (PAI-1). Either reductions of t-PA or elevations of PAI-1 can inhibit fibrinolysis and predispose to thrombosis. Both of these mechanisms have been suggested as operating in venous thrombosis[79] but have not been comprehensively studied in stroke. Several rare inherited conditions are associated with depressed fibrinolysis, however, including plasminogen deficiency, qualitative plasminogen abnormalities, plasminogen activator deficiency, elevation of PAI-1, dysfibrinogenemia, and factor XII/prekallikrein deficiency.[80–86] These disorders usually manifest as venous thrombosis, but cases of arterial thrombosis including stroke have been described.

Fibrinolytic degradation products such as cross-linked D dimer are increased after stroke,[47,51,53,87,88] and their levels are correlated with infarct size, stroke severity, and subsequent mortality.[48] Peak levels of D dimer occur later than peak levels of fibrin markers, suggesting a relative excess of fibrin formation over fibrin(ogen)olysis in the acute phase of stroke. Functional assays have shown reduction in stimulatable fibrinolytic activity after stroke.[89,90]

Although elevations of both t-PA antigen and PAI-1 antigen have been observed after stroke,[52,91–93] the elevations of t-PA antigen do not necessarily indicate greater plasma fibrinolytic activity, because much of the t-PA antigen may be bound to PAI-1 antigen. Prospective population studies have demonstrated the seemingly paradoxical finding that elevations of t-PA antigen are associated with a greater risk of MI and stroke.[17,94,95] Elevations of t-PA antigen are also associated with the severity of carotid atherosclerosis.[96] Elevations of t-PA antigen do not necessarily denote increased fibrinolytic activity but instead may indicate an ongoing response to atherosclerosis and thrombosis and greater clot formation rather than a more effective fibrinolytic response. Furthermore, like the increase in prostacyclin seen in patients with atherosclerosis, t-PA antigen elevation may merely be a marker for ongoing endothelial damage.[97] These markers may eventually provide additional information for identifying patients at high risk of stroke.

At least one lipoprotein, lipoprotein (a)—or Lp(a)—can inhibit fibrinolysis in vitro and may have a similarly important effect in vivo.[98] Lp(a) has substantial homology to plasminogen, the precursor to plasmin.[99] Lp(a) also stimulates the release of PAI-1 from endothelial cells and effectively competes with plasminogen for binding either to fibrin or to the surface of vascular endothelial cells, inhibiting fibrinolysis.[100,101] Lp(a) levels have been found to be high in selected populations with cerebrovascular disease, and most, but not all, studies have shown Lp(a) elevation to be a potent risk factor for stroke, especially in young patients.[102–107] However, Lp(a) levels do not appear to be associated with stroke characteristics, recurrence, or prognosis.[100,101] Unfortunately, there is no established treatment for increased Lp(a) levels, and management consists of aggressively controlling other risk factors, especially lowering the low-density lipoprotein (LDL) cholesterol to less than 100 mg/dL.

Platelet Adhesion, Activation, and Aggregation

Platelet activation is related to cerebral ischemia, both as a potential cause of stroke and as a result of platelet exposure to the ischemic brain.[108] Atherothrombosis occurs when the vessel wall is damaged, for example, by rupture of an atherosclerotic plaque, exposing collagen fibers and subendothelial matrix proteins.[109] The first process in thrombosis is the adhesion of platelets to subendothelial matrix proteins, with activation of adhered platelets and stimulation of a large number of other platelets to form a platelet aggregate. Other coagulation proteins assemble on this aggregate and ultimately lead to thrombosis and possibly vessel occlusion.[110] Platelet activation, under certain conditions, can cause thrombus formation even in the absence of vessel wall injury; examples are thrombosis in disseminated coagulopathy and platelet activation as a stroke mechanism in some people with antiphospholipid antibodies.[108] Some conditions, such as cerebrovascular disease and MI, have been associated with a long-term increase in platelet activation, as evidenced by elevated serum levels of platelet release proteins[47,48,87,111–113] and by urinary metabolites of thromboxane.[114,115] There is some evidence that platelet activation occurs in ischemic brain tissue and continues for some time after the acute event.

Using a primate focal ischemia model, Del Zoppo and colleagues[116] have provided evidence that platelet activation occurs in the ischemic brain area. Whether the risk of stroke in people with persistent platelet activation is increased is not clear, however.

Patients with myeloproliferative disease (MPD), including polycythemia rubra vera (PV) and essential thrombocythemia (ET), have increases in platelet reactivity and platelet counts as well as large, dysfunctional platelets, which are strongly associated with stroke.[117–119] Thrombosis occurs more frequently in PV and ET than in acute myelocytic leukemia or chronic granulocytic leukemia and is a major cause of morbidity and mortality in patients with these myeloproliferative disorders. Up to 40% of patients with PV or ET experience a thrombotic episode, and the incidence of thrombosis could be as high as 75% per year. Arterial occlusions are more common than venous events,[119–124] and stroke is often the presenting feature of both PV and ET. At the time of diagnosis, 25% of patients with myeloproliferative syndromes manifest atherosclerosis, with 50% of patients having evidence of carotid intimal thickening. Increasing age, elevated hematocrit, and treatment with phlebotomy in PV all predispose to thromboembolism. Importantly, the magnitude of the elevation of the platelet count does not correlate with the risk of thrombosis. In one study, the average platelet count at the time of stroke was 600,000 cells/mm^3, but two thirds of patients had counts lower than 400,000 cells/mm^3. In the absence of MPD, secondary thrombocytosis is an occasional but much less common cause of stroke.[29,125]

Antiplatelet therapy, usually with aspirin, is recommended for treatment of patients with cerebral, coronary artery, or peripheral vascular thrombosis.[126] Aspirin irreversibly inhibits platelet cyclooxygenase through acetylation and attenuates thromboxane A$_2$, a potent stimulator of platelet activation.[108] Dipyridamole inhibits platelet activation through inhibition of platelet phosphodiesterase activity, ultimately blocking calcium-mediated platelet activation.[127] Ticlopidine and clopidogrel inhibit the excitatory receptor P2Y$_1$, thereby blocking adenosine diphosphate–induced platelet aggregation.[128] Platelet inhibitors also usually suppress the platelet hyper-reactivity associated with MPD and can prolong the usually shortened mean platelet survival time.[129] As well as its antithrombotic effects, aspirin may inhibit platelet secretion of vascular growth factors and inflammatory cytokines, thereby reducing chronic vascular damage.

In addition to pharmacologic antithrombotic measures, lowering of elevated platelet counts should be considered in patients with MPD and a history of thrombosis. Hydroxyurea (e.g., 1 g daily to start) has been shown in a randomized trial to prevent thrombotic complications in patients with essential thrombocytosis.[129,130] A platelet count of 250,000 to 450,000 cells/mm^3 is an appropriate target. The use of anagrelide to lower platelet counts should be considered for cases refractory to hydroxyurea or for patients unable to tolerate the drug.[129]

Heparin-Induced Thrombocytopenia

Heparin-induced thrombocytopenia (HIT) is an immune-mediated process in which antibodies against heparin are directed toward platelets, causing increased platelet activation.[131,132] Two classes of HIT have been described. Type I HIT is relatively common, occurring on the first day of heparin exposure. The platelet count may be as low as 50,000 cells/mm^3, but the syndrome resolves spontaneously without cessation of treatment. It is thought to arise directly from heparin-mediated platelet clumping.[131,132] Type II HIT occurs 6 to 10 days after heparin exposure and is associated with a significant reduction in platelet count and a high risk of thrombotic events, including stroke.[131-136] The incidence of HIT II is 1% to 5%. The risk is higher with higher doses of heparin but has been described after very low doses such as those used for intravenous line flushes.[137-140]

HIT II may provide some insight into immune mechanisms that promote thrombosis.[132,141] There is an interaction between heparin and platelet factor 4 (PF4), leading to platelet activation, endothelial damage, and thrombosis.[142] The HIT II antibodies are usually immunoglobulin (Ig) G antibodies that bind to a complex of heparin and platelet factor 4.[143] HIT II antibodies may also bind to heparan on the surface of endothelial cells and stimulate the production of tissue factor on the endothelial cell surface.[144] Heparin–platelet factor 4 complexes bind to FC gamma RII A receptors (CD 32) and induce platelet activation associated with more release of platelet factor 4, leading to a propagation of the HIT II process. An elevation of circulating adhesion molecules (selectins) has also been observed in HIT II.[145] Platelet-neutrophil complexes are mediated by P-selectin, which is also important in leukocyte adhesion. This finding supports a role for inflammation in the underlying pathophysiology of HIT II. Platelet activation leads to release of platelet microparticles, triggering an activation of the coagulation system.[145]

A 14-year retrospective review found that in patients diagnosed with isolated HIT II the 30-day risk of thrombosis was 53%.[139] Most thromboses were venous. Although platelet counts in HIT II may fall to as low as 20,000 cells/mm^3, hemorrhagic complications are uncommon. HIT II is often seen in postoperative settings, perhaps because of the combined influence of surgery-induced inflammation and heparin exposure. Atkinson and colleagues[134] have emphasized the relationship between HIT II and ischemic stroke after endarterectomy. Becker and Miller,[131] reviewing data on 29 patients with HIT II–related stroke from the literature, found that few patients had previous cerebrovascular disease and that most patients either died (25%) or were left disabled after their strokes. HIT II has also been associated with cerebral venous thrombosis.[146] Other risk factors for the development of HIT II are diabetes, neoplasm, heart failure, infection, antiphospholipid antibodies, and trauma.[142] The diagnosis of HIT II is based on a combination of clinical findings and demonstration of heparin-dependent antiplatelet antibodies.[139,147,148]

Prevention of HIT II is the best management strategy, and platelet counts should be closely monitored in patients undergoing heparin therapy. Once HIT II is recognized, heparin should be promptly discontinued; thrombosis risk is high in these patients, however, so some antithrombotic treatment must be given.[149] Because low-molecular-weight heparin will cross-react with antiheparin antibodies, this agent cannot be used for anticoagulation in patients with HIT II.[138] Currently, heparanoids and recombinant hirudins are appropriate treatments in patients with HIT II.[150-152] Thrombin inhibitors may have a role as well. Many patients need long-term anticoagulation with warfarin; however, this therapy cannot be initiated until platelet counts have normalized, because the acute drop in protein C in HIT II contraindicates early treatment with warfarin.[150,152]

Antiphospholipid Antibodies

Antiphospholipids (aPLs) are polyclonal, polyclass antibodies directed against certain phospholipids.[153-157] They are produced in a variety of clinical situations and are associated with a hypercoagulable state characterized primarily by thrombosis, thrombocytopenia, and fetal loss. It was noted in the 1950s that some patients with systemic lupus erythematosus (SLE) often had prolonged aPTTs and false-positive results on Venereal Disease Research Laboratory (VDRL) tests.[158] Despite the elevation of the aPTT, such patients did not experience hemorrhagic complications unless they also had hypoprothrombinemia or thrombocytopenia. Bowie and associates[159] first described the association of aPL and thrombosis in 1964. Feinstein and Rapaport,[160] in a 1972 review, called this phenomenon the "lupus anticoagulant." Harris and coworkers,[161] recognizing that cardiolipin is a major component of the VDRL test, developed and popularized the anticardiolipin (aCL) antibody test in 1983. Also in the 1980s, the fact that patients do not have to have SLE to have symptomatic disease from aPL became well recognized.

The lupus anticoagulant (LA) test is a functional measurement of aPL, whereas solid-phase immunoassays measure antibody concentration and binding avidity. Positive results of either test have been independently associated with thrombosis, and partial concordance is seen between the results of the two tests.[158] The preponderance of evidence, however, indicates that the LA test is more specific for patients at risk for thromboembolic events.[162] In contrast, the aCL antibody test is a more sensitive assay but is nonspecific, and positive results could also be found in various other patients, such as those who are healthy, those taking certain medications, and those with malignancies or infectious diseases.[163] Antibodies to antiphosphatidylserine, phosphatidylethanolamine, phosphatidylcholine, and phosphatidic acid have been less frequently studied, and their significance is still emerging.[164-166]

A major breakthrough in the field came in 1990, when three groups identified the need for a cooperative phospholipid-binding protein to detect most but not all aPL antibodies.[167-169] Shortly thereafter, coprecipitation and subsequent protein sequencing identified one serologic cofactor to be β_2 glycoprotein 1 (β_2GP1), or apolipoprotein H, a cationic plasma glycoprotein. Data strongly suggest that phospholipid membranes serve as a binding surface for the sequestration of the primary antigen, β_2GP1, in vivo.[170] One of the most promising aspects of the discovery of β_2GP1 as a target antigen for aPL is that β_2GP1, a minor natural anticoagulant, competes in vitro for available phospholipid surface area needed for assembly of the prothrombinase complex, thereby inhibiting prothrombinase activity. aPL may cross-link membrane-bound β_2GP1 and enhance β_2GP1's inhibitory abilities.[171] Commercial tests are available to detect antibodies to the aPL "cofactor," β_2GP1, directly. In some studies, the presence of β_2GP1 antibodies rivals the presence of LA in identifying patients with the highest risk for thrombosis.[172,173]

Diagnostic criteria for antiphospholipid-antibody syndrome (APS) include the presence of both thrombosis or recurrent, unexplained fetal loss and anticardiolipin antibodies (IgG or IgM isotype) of medium to high titers or lupus anticoagulants on at least two occasions at least 8 weeks apart.[174] Antibodies to other negatively charged phospholipids (phosphatidylserine, phosphatidylethanolamine) as well as to β_2GP1 are also associated with these and other clinical manifestations; however, with an evidence-based medicine approach, there are insufficient data for these antibodies to be included in a rigorous classification system. Other clinical manifestations that have been associated with aPL are livedo reticularis, optic changes, Addison's disease, and a variety of neurologic symptoms.[175] Once again, the strength of the association between these clinical manifestations and the presence of aPL was not strong enough for them to be included as diagnostic features.

Patients with APS but without SLE or other rheumatologic or autoimmune disorders have *primary APS* (PAPS). Patients with APS along with SLE or other collagen vascular diseases have *secondary APS*. Unlike those with secondary APS, patients with PAPS are more often male and typically have low or normal titers of antinuclear antibodies and no other criteria for SLE. In SLE and related rheumatic illnesses, aPLs impart an increased risk of thrombosis that is at least equal to and may be greater than that observed in PAPS.[162,176,177] The prevalence of aPLs in healthy adults rises with age and is estimated to be 2% to 12%, depending on the test used for detection.[178–180] Patients with aPL most often experience venous thrombosis, but an association with stroke and TIA is particularly well established in subjects with high levels of IgG aCL antibody or those with an LA.[181,182]

The largest study to evaluate the natural history and risk factors for recurrent thrombosis in patients with aPL comes from the Italian Registry.[183] In that study, 360 patients were studied prospectively for 4 years. Inclusion criteria were presence of aPL and availability of the subject for follow-up. aPL assays were performed clinically because of a thrombotic event, a disease known to be associated with APS, or a coagulation abnormality suggesting the presence of an LA. Thirty-four patients had thrombotic events over the 4-year period, including 10 strokes (1 fatal) and 6 TIAs. Treatment was at the discretion of the attending physician. Risk factors for thrombosis in this cohort included (1) aCL antibody titer higher than 40 GPL whits and prior thrombotic event and (2) aCL antibody titer higher than 40 GPL units and SLE. Other studies have also evaluated the association of APS with recurrent stroke.[60,183–188] Some[175,183,185–188] but not all[184] have suggested an association, with some studies finding the association to be true only in the presence of SLE.[189] Most of these studies are small to medium-sized case series, however, and their results thus cannot be considered

conclusive. It is crucial to know whether APS raises the risk for recurrent stroke.

Many case-control studies have shown an association between different types of aPL antibodies and both initial stroke[23,190–197] and MI,[198] but some have not.[199–201] The methodologic differences among studies, such as the type of aPL studied, sample size, and population studied, could explain discrepant results. It is interesting, however, that many of the larger studies find an association between aPL and incident stroke, whereas the association between aPL and recurrent stroke is weaker. The explanation is not clear but may be related to the higher importance of other stroke risk factors in the risk for recurrent stroke, which overshadow (or even negate) the recurrent stroke risk contributed by aPL.

Few prospective studies have examined the association between aPL and either an initial stroke or MI. These studies have been limited to performance of aCL antibody testing on only one occasion; therefore, patients included in the studies would not meet current criteria for APS.[182,202–204] Brey and colleagues[190] performed a prospective study of the association between aCL and stroke and MI over 20 years in men enrolled in the Honolulu Heart Program. Only presence of β_2GP1-dependent aCL of the IgG class was significantly associated with both incident ischemic stroke and MI. This association was attenuated in the last 5 years of follow-up. The risk factor–adjusted relative odds for men with presence versus absence of β_2GP1-dependent aCL of the IgG class were 2.2 (95% CI, 1.5 to 3.4) at 15 years and 1.5 (95% CI, 1.0 to 2.3) at 20 years. For MI, the adjusted relative odds were 1.8 (95% CI, 1.2 to 2.6) at 15 years and 1.5 (95% CI, 1.1 to 2.1) at 20 years. This is the first report of a prospective association between aCL and stroke. Two other studies did not show an association.[182,203]

Among the reports linking aCL to MI, results of two additional prospective studies suggest the possibility of a time-dependent association between aCL and MI in men.[203,204] In one study, the follow-up period was 5 years,[203] and in the other, a significant association was found only for the first 10 years of follow-up, even though there were more than twice as many MIs in the second 10 years of follow-up.[204] Such weakening of the association with time could be due to changes in risk factor status during follow-up, including aCL. It is unlikely that the observed associations between aCL and vascular disease are due to either chance or an artifact of study design. Prospective studies of MI[190,203,204] and stroke[190] preclude the possibility that the antibodies were a consequence of the vascular event but, as noted previously, do not exclude the possibilities that the antibodies are a consequence of preclinical disease and that other stroke risk factors must also be present for thrombosis to occur.

The clinical presentation of stroke and TIA associated with aPL has few distinguishing features. Both large and small cerebral arterial occlusions in the anterior and posterior circulations as well as venous occlusions are all reported to occur. Although deep lacunar infarctions and isolated white matter signal-enhancing lesions are detected on magnetic resonance imaging (MRI) and large brain infarctions occur, most strokes are relatively small and involve the cortex and subjacent white matter.[60] No single

Specific Medical Diseases and Stroke

mechanism for stroke associated with aPL has been established, but a few pathologic reports have demonstrated nonspecific microvascular platelet-fibrin plugs, suggesting possible thrombosis in situ. However, cardiac lesions, including mitral valve degeneration and nonbacterial thrombotic endocarditis, often accompany APS and could be responsible for these lesions as well.[205,206]

Sneddon's syndrome consists of stroke and livedo reticularis in the absence of systemic disease and is commonly associated with aPL.[207–209] Besides livedo reticularis, some patients with the syndrome have Raynaud's phenomenon and demonstrate acrocyanosis. Sneddon's syndrome is more common in women than in men and has been linked to tobacco use. Skin biopsy shows focal epidermal ulceration with chronic inflammatory infiltrates in the dermis, without evidence of vasculitis.[208] Vascular dementia, presumably from recurrent stroke, often ensues in patients with this syndrome. Although not all people with Sneddon's syndrome have aPLs, the finding of aPLs in such people probably augurs a worse prognosis.[210] Patients with Sneddon's syndrome are typically younger and have fewer stroke risk factors than typical patients with stroke, but patients with the syndrome report migraine-like headaches and have hypertension.

Progressive cognitive deterioration may occur with Sneddon's syndrome in the absence of a history of stroke-like episodes and despite antithrombotic therapy. This clinical course is reminiscent of the insights of both Sneddon[209] and Rebello and associates,[211] who emphasized that stroke with Sneddon's syndrome often leaves little neurologic deficit but the patients gradually became demented nonetheless. Unfortunately, except for the possible relationship to high aCL levels and presence of an LA, no specific findings identify those patients with the syndrome who are likely to experience recurrent ischemic events and progressive dementia. Many patients with Sneddon's syndrome eventually have complex partial seizures. Generalized seizures and status epilepticus are also the cardinal features of the syndrome of ischemic encephalopathy, which also includes altered mental status, diffuse systemic pulmonary and cardiac involvement, and dermatologic manifestations.[181,212]

Mechanisms underlying the aPL-associated vascular events, in the absence of SLE, are probably multifactorial and include case report and case series associations of strokes with valvular disease,[213,214] cerebral microemboli,[190,215,216] thrombosis and endothelial hyperplasia,[217–223] antibody to brain endothelium,[224,225] and adhesion molecule expression.[226] Some aPLs interfere with the vascular endothelial anticoagulant functions, whereas others directly activate endothelial thrombogenic mechanisms. Membranes of circulating white blood cells and platelets have also been implicated as a target for prothrombotic binding of aPLs. The thrombogenicity of aPLs may stem from their targeting of prothrombin on damaged membrane surfaces and their interference with the activated protein C pathway. aPLs can interfere with thrombomodulin-induced protein C activation and also with protein S cofactor function for protein C. The importance of platelet activation in the process is supported by analysis of brain tissue removed from patients with aPL-related stroke, in which small arteries and microvessels are occluded by platelet fibrin plugs. Single-photon emission computed tomography (SPECT)[227–230] and MRI spectroscopy[231] studies show diffuse damage that is compatible with many of these mechanisms. It is likely that the mechanism underlying the aPL-associated stroke in a given patient may affect treatment response. Animal models of stroke in APS exist[232,233] but are complex and therefore not yet suitable for evaluating therapy. There have been reports of strokes in animals immunized with β2GP1, but they seem to occur late in the disease and affect only a few animals.[234] Ziporen and coworkers[235] have suggested that microvascular thrombosis plays an important role in brain disease.

The thorough evaluation of patients in whom aPL is suspected often requires multiple testing procedures, because unfortunately, no one test can adequately screen a patient for aPL.[154,236] An effective initial screen is a sensitive aPTT test and the aCL assay. If results of these evaluations are negative but clinical suspicion remains high, further tests that should be performed are (1) kaolin clotting time, (2) dilute Russell viper venom time (dRVVT), and (3) lupus inhibitor screen (different aPTT reagents). One caveat about aPL testing is that levels of aPL may fall during thrombotic events, so tests may have to be repeated when the patient reaches a steady state. It cannot be stressed enough that all patients with suspected aPL-associated clinical manifestations should also be carefully evaluated for other potential causes.

Treatments such as platelet antiaggregant and anticoagulant therapy for secondary stroke prevention have been used in both APS and in cerebrovascular disease associated with aPL immunoreactivity. Khamashta and associates,[237] in a highly selected cohort studied retrospectively, found that high-dose anticoagulant therapy is associated with better outcomes. However, this potential benefit must be weighted against the considerably high hemorrhagic complication rate reported in that study. Further, the patients in the study did not undergo further aPL testing and would not fulfill current criteria for APS.

The largest study of recurrent stroke was performed by the prospective Antiphospholipid Antibody in Stroke Study group (APASS) trial. The APASS group completed the first prospective study of the role of aPL in recurrent ischemic stroke in collaboration with the Warfarin-Aspirin for Recurrent Stroke Study (WARSS) group.[238] This controlled and blinded study, initiated in 1993, compared the risk of recurrent stroke and other thromboembolic disease over a 2-year follow-up period in patients with ischemic stroke who were randomly assigned to receive either aspirin therapy, 325 mg per day, or warfarin therapy, at a dose to maintain the International Normalized Ratio (INR) between 1.4 and 2.8. The suggested target INR was 2.2. Exclusion criteria for WARSS included an indication for warfarin therapy (e.g., atrial fibrillation), a contraindication to warfarin therapy, and high-grade carotid stenosis, suggesting the need for carotid endarterectomy. The warfarin therapy group comprised 882 patients, and the aspirin therapy group, 890 patients. A single aPL determination was performed in each at study entry. In the warfarin group, 35.9% (23/64) of patients who tested positive for both aCL and LA had recurrent events, compared with 21.1% (27/128) of those who tested LAC-positive and aCL-negative; 26.6% (44/169) of those who tested

LAC-negative and aCL-positive; and 26.1% (136/521) who tested negative for both LAC and aCL. In the aspirin group, 26.8% (15/56) of patients who tested positive for both aCL and LAC had a recurrent event, compared with 18.2% (20/110) of those who tested LAC-positive and aCL-negative; 23.3% (45/193) of those who tested LAC-negative and aCL-positive; and 21.7% (115/531) of those who tested negative for both LAC and aCL. None of these differences were statistically significant. There were no differences in major bleeding complication rates between the treatment groups (presented at the American Stroke Association Meeting, San Antonio, Texas, USA, in review, 2002).

Thus, it appears that for patients who test positive for aPL in a single determination at the time of ischemic stroke (including those with low titers of aCL and/or IgA aCL) and who do not have either atrial fibrillation or high-grade carotid stenosis, aspirin therapy and warfarin therapy to achieve an INR of approximately 2.2 are equivalent in both efficacy and major bleeding complication rate. Both the INR value and the aspirin dose selected for this study were based on current treatment recommendations for secondary prevention of ischemic stroke in patients without aPL at the time the study was undertaken nearly 10 years ago. That is, the high INR–producing dose of warfarin that has been suggested (based on retrospective, limited data) as necessary for successful secondary prevention of aPL-associated thrombotic events was not used. Also, a lower dose of aspirin (60 to 81 mg) has theoretical advantages over the dose used in WARSS and currently is recommended over higher doses. It should be stressed that the analyses that are currently available from the WARSS or APASS data do not address the issue of whether meeting the proposed criteria for the diagnosis of definite APS is an important factor in stroke recurrence or therapeutic response. This is of clear importance, and these analyses will be available soon.

It remains possible, although unproven, that higher doses of warfarin can better prevent recurrence in aPL-associated ischemic stroke. Any benefit of higher doses of warfarin may be negated by a higher rate of major bleeding complications. To address this question, Ruiz Irastorza and colleagues[187] studied 66 patients with APS (58% of them with a previous stroke) undergoing high-intensity warfarin therapy and found a major bleeding rate of 6 cases per 100 patient-years; in no patient was the bleeding fatal, and only one patient had intracranial (subdural) hematoma. In all cases, bleeding was associated with a clear precipitating factor, including performance of a renal biopsy, internal hemorrhoids, or trauma. Interestingly, this group also found a high rate of thrombotic recurrences despite anticoagulant therapy, primarily in the same vascular territory as the original thrombotic episode (9.1 cases per 100 patient-years). In all but one case, patients were documented to have an INR lower than 3.0 at the time of recurrent thrombosis, suggesting that in patients with persistent medium-high titers of aCL, LA, or both, oral anticoagulation to a target INR of 2.5 (average INR in WARSS/APASS) may not be enough to prevent recurrent thrombotic events. Thus, whether warfarin therapy with this target INR can prevent recurrent stroke or other thrombotic episodes remains an open question. It is possible that subgroups of patients with different risks of recurrence will be identified in the coming years. With the current level of knowledge, however, patients with previous arterial thrombosis and persistent medium-high titers of aCL, LA, or both seem to be at the highest risk of recurrent events.

Although it is possible to suppress the LA with prednisone, this treatment, except as indicated for coexisting SLE or other connective tissue diseases, has not been effective in APS.[239] For a few patients who experience acute encephalopathy, seizures, or disseminated intravascular coagulation, plasmapheresis and immunosuppression therapy have been effective for short-term management.[178,240]

HOMOCYSTINURIA AND HOMOCYSTINEMIA

The 20-fold or higher increases in plasma homocysteine, homocystine, cysteine-homocysteine, and related mixed disulfides (together termed homocyst(e)ine [Hcy]) that typify homocystinuria produce premature atherosclerosis that is frequently complicated by early stroke or other large arterial occlusions.[241] Homocystinuria is a metabolic consequence of one of several inborn errors of metabolism that impair cystathionine β-synthase (CBS) and several other enzyme systems important for methionine metabolism (Fig. 34–2). These are autosomal recessive traits, and persons homozygous for CBS deficiency often have atherosclerosis and thromboembolic complications, including stroke, by age 30 years.[242] The classic phenotype of the child with homocystinuria consists of ocular, vascular, skeletal, and nervous system abnormalities. Affected individuals may have a marfanoid habitus, with arm spans greater than body height, setting-sun lenticular dislocations, and cognitive impairment. A malar flush and livedo reticularis are sometimes present, but the phenotypic expression varies considerably, and some individuals with homocystinuria exhibit none of these characteristics. About 0.3% to 1.5% of the general population may be heterozygous for CBS deficiency, with the estimated incidence of homocystinuria approximately 1 in 332,000 live births.[241] In obligate heterozygotes, CBS activity is reduced by 50%, but whether these individuals are at increased risk of stroke is not known.

In contrast to the striking plasma elevations found in homocystinuria, even modest elevations in plasma Hcy and related metabolites are now recognized as independent risk factors for ischemic stroke and related forms of atherosclerotic vascular disease.[202,240,243–247] Case-control studies suggest that as many as 30% of subjects with ischemic stroke have plasma levels of Hcy approximately 1.5 times higher than levels measured in healthy individuals of similar age and same sex.[248–250] Plasma Hcy is lower in premenopausal women than in men of similar age, but levels increase with age, and after menopause, gender differences disappear altogether. Clarke and associates[251] found plasma Hcy levels to be inversely related to red cell folate and serum vitamin B_2 levels. Other researchers have found a direct relationship between plasma Hcy levels and serum uric acid concentrations.[251] However, the association of

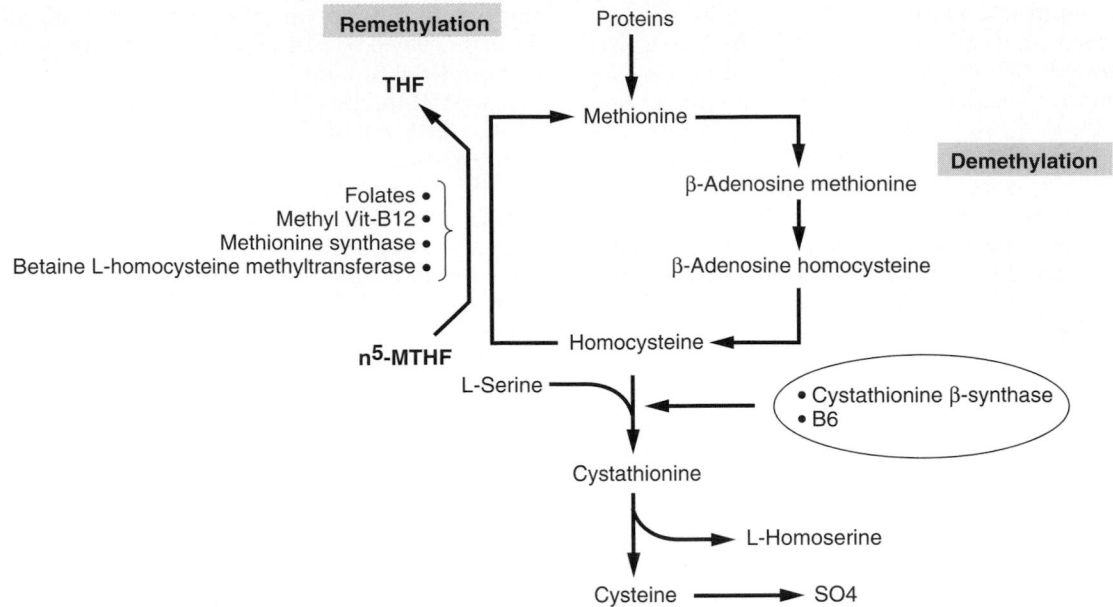

FIGURE 34–2 *Methionine metabolism and homocysteinemia. Plasma homocysteine levels may rise because of genetic or acquired metabolic deficiencies in pathways of methionine metabolism. The principal causes are dysfunction of the cystathionine β-synthase enzyme system for cysteine metabolism and dysfunction of remethylation tetrahydrofolate (THF) pathway, and may occur with folate or vitamin B$_{12}$ deficiencies. See text for details. B6, vitamin B$_6$; B12, vitamin B$_{12}$; n^5-MTHF, methyltetrahydrofolate.*

high plasma Hcy with other stroke risk factors, such as hypertension and diabetes mellitus, is weak, and the current consensus is that elevated plasma Hcy is an independent risk factor for stroke.[245,252] Malinow and colleagues[253] found that modest rises of Hcy (>10.5 μmol/L) in asymptomatic adults increased the odds of carotid intimal thickening more than threefold compared with subjects whose plasma Hcy levels were less than 5.88 μmol/L. For elderly subjects, plasma Hcy levels of 14 to 16 μmol/L signify a relative risk of stroke of approximately 2.8 compared with subjects with levels lower than 10 μmol/L. In the Rotterdam Study, the risk of stroke and MI rose in direct relationship with the total homocysteine level.[244] The Framingham Study also found nonfasting total Hcy levels to be an independent risk factor for incident stroke in the elderly.[254] On the basis of these findings, the attributable risk of stroke due to such modest increases in Hcy could be very significant because of the high prevalence of this mild Hcy elevation.

The range of normal for serum Hcy is controversial.[250,255,256] Folate deficiency raises Hcy levels. Before 1996, almost 90% of the population did not ingest the minimal 400 μg/day of folate needed to maximally decrease folate levels. Early that year, the U.S. Food and Drug Administration (FDA) published a regulation stating that by January 1998, all enriched-flour breads, rice, pasta, cornmeal, and other cereal grain products would be required to contain 140 μg of folic acid per 100 g of flour. The goal of this policy was to increase folic acid intake among women of childbearing potential and reduce the risk of neural tube defects in their children. Since that time, studies evaluating the effect of vitamin supplementation have shown only a modest further reduction in Hcy levels. Thus, the effect of what was once suspected to be a major health problem and

potential stroke risk factor may have been lessened by a change in public health policy.[205]

In addition to certain genetic predispositions, many individuals are at risk of hyperhomocysteinemia because of acquired defects in methionine metabolism. As shown in Figure 34–2, decreased CBS activity and reduced remethylation of Hcy may produce hyperhomocysteinemia via abnormalities in folate-, cobalamine-, or betaine-dependent metabolic pathways. Data from case-control studies of normal subjects as well as subjects with vascular disease indicate that an inverse relationship exists between plasma levels of folate and vitamin B$_{12}$ and plasma concentrations of Hcy.

A mutation in methylenetetrahydrofolate reductase (MTHFR) in the folate pathway has been correlated with an increase in plasma Hcy and may possibly be a risk factor for cardiovascular disease.[257] The common thermolabile MTHFR variant results from a C-to-T point mutation at nucleotide 677 (changing alanine to valine), which significantly reduces the enzyme's basal activity.[258] This mutation is prevalent in the population, with the frequency of heterozygotes being 40% to 50%, and of homozygotes, 5% to 15% in several populations. The presence of the mutation has been associated with elevated plasma Hcy and possibly an increase in rate of MI.[259,260] Studies on the T667C mutation as a risk factor for MIs and other vascular disease have given variable results. Kluijtmans and associates[260] reported an odds ratio of 3:1 for premature MI with the T667C mutation in a select group of patients. Gallagher and colleagues[259] also reported a higher risk in both heterozygotes and homozygotes for the T667C mutation. However, other studies have not shown an association between T667C and MI and other vascular diseases.[261] Data are currently lacking for support of this mutation as a risk factor for stroke.

Numerous studies indicate that homocysteinemia promotes the development of premature atherosclerosis, and the vascular pathology of large arteries from subjects with homocysteinemia demonstrates features typical of atherosclerosis, such as fibrous intimal plaques, medial fibrosis, and disruption of the internal elastic membranes.[262] Accumulation of lipids is less conspicuous in affected arteries, and despite the documentation of premature atherosclerosis, the vascular occlusive events appear to be disproportionate to the severity of arterial disease. Converging lines of evidence from experimental studies have demonstrated that Hcy damages vascular endothelial cells and interferes with the regulatory functions of endothelial cells in coagulation and nitric oxide generation.[263,264]

Probably all young persons with unexplained stroke and especially those with atherosclerosis should undergo plasma Hcy measurement.[246] A single plasma determination is probably an effective screen, but some researchers have advocated giving a methionine load beforehand, as doing so might increase the number of subjects testing positive by up to 30%. If an Hcy elevation is detected, first-degree relatives of the patient should also be tested. Because hyperhomocysteinemia is not limited to young people, elderly patients with stroke and TIA due to atherosclerosis should be considered for Hcy testing if an obvious cause for the atherosclerosis is lacking. As indicated in Figure 34–2, when an elevation of Hcy is detected, serum folate and vitamin B_{12} levels should also be measured. Establishing the presence of hyperhomocysteinemia has clinical utility, because even in the absence of low serum folate or B_{12} levels, plasma homocysteine may be lowered with dietary supplements of folic acid, biotin, and vitamins B_{12} and B_6.[246,253]

SICKLE CELL DISEASE

A critical single-point mutation that causes the substitution of valine for glutamic acid in the hemoglobin b chain underlies sickle cell anemia (SSA) and its consequent disease, sickle cell disease (SCD). Biochemically, because the solubility of deoxyhemoglobin S is lower than that of normal hemoglobin, HbS polymerization occurs when SSA erythrocytes are exposed to acidotic or hypoxic environments.[265,266] The extremely rigid, sickled erythrocyte produces a tremendous increase in blood viscosity that contributes to red blood cell sludging in the microcirculation during sickle crises. Even in the absence of crisis, SSA commonly causes a progressive systemic vasculopathy involving many organs, including the brain.[267] Fortunately, this untoward result happens in only about 30% of patients with SSA. Individuals with SCD experience vascular occlusive events, often recurrent, including catastrophic stroke as well as infarctions of the kidney, lung, bone, skin, and eye. Symptoms usually begin in early childhood, but occasionally, persons with SSA may live into early or middle adulthood before manifesting adverse effects.[242]

The prevalence of sickle trait (HbSA) in black Americans is estimated to be about 8.5%, with hemoglobin HbSS occurring in up to 0.16% and the variant HbSC in 0.21%. Roughly 10% of individuals with HbSS and 2% to 5% of those with HbSC experience symptomatic stroke.[268] The Cooperative Study of Sickle Cell Disease (CSSCD) has shown that 62 of 248 (25%) children with focal neurologic deficits have abnormalities on brain MRI compatible with ischemic injury.[269] These silent infarcts correlate with neuropsychological dysfunction and are also a strong independent risk factor for stroke in this population.[269,270] The CSSCD found the stroke rate to be 14-fold higher in patients with silent infarction on brain MRI than in those with normal brain MRI findings.[269] Other risk factors for stroke in patients with SCD are anemia, lack of thalassemia, recent or recurrent acute chest pain, elevated blood pressure, and high cerebral blood flow, as evidenced by transcranial Doppler (TCD) ultrasonography.[44,271,272] Unlike SCD, stroke with the sickle trait usually occurs in circumstances that cause severe hypoxia, heat stress, or dehydration.[273,274]

As SCD develops, there is a progressive segmental narrowing of the distal internal carotid artery and portions of the circle of Willis and proximal branches of the major intracranial arteries.[275] Pathologically, this large vessel arteriopathy demonstrates intimal proliferation and an increase in fibroblasts and smooth muscle cells within the arterial wall. The progressive nature of this occlusive arteriopathy is evidenced by the occasional development of the moyamoya phenomenon. In addition to disease in large arteries, sickled cell plugging of the microcirculation and cerebral veins is also well documented.[276] These alterations of arterial, capillary, and venous circulation raise the risk of both brain infarction and intracerebral hemorrhage (ICH). The incidence of brain infarction peaks at around age 10 years, and its rate outnumbers that of ICH, which occurs more often in older subjects, by a ratio of 3:1. Typically, infarctions include both deep and subcortical structures, but brainstem, spinal cord, and retinal infarctions as well as dural sinus thrombosis have all been reported. Pavlakis and colleagues[277] have emphasized the occurrence of watershed or borderzone infarctions particularly in territories of the middle cerebral artery. They speculate that a combination of occlusive arteriopathy and perfusion failure produces watershed strokes. ICH in SCD can result either from medial necrosis of cerebral arterioles with subsequent vascular rupture or from venous thrombosis. Increased cerebral blood flow, which is only partially explained by the underlying anemia, and increased cerebral blood volume may contribute to the predisposition to ICH.[278]

Although some asymptomatic persons with SSA may tolerate HbS of up to 50%, the mainstay of treatment for SCD is repeated exchange transfusion to maintain the concentration of HbSS at less than 30%. This treatment is highly effective for reducing the risk of stroke in SCD.[279] For children with previous stroke, the risk of stroke recurrence is exceedingly high if HbS levels are not suppressed. Powars and colleagues[280] reported a 67% recurrence in untreated persons, compared with a 10% incidence of recurrent stroke in patients who received repeated transfusions.

Transfusion therapy should be maintained over the long term, because one study showed that even after 10 years of treatment, the risk of stroke recurrence was 50% a year if transfusions were withheld.[270,271,281] The optimal duration of therapy remains controversial, however. A retrospective study of 137 pediatric patients who had received transfusion therapy for at least 5 years found that absence of an antecedent or concurrent medical event at the time of initial stroke was predictive of recurrent stroke.[282] Thirty-one patients (22%) had a second stroke (2.2/100 patient-years). Twenty-six patients had an antecedent or concurrent medical event at the time of initial stroke; none of these had a recurrent stroke 2 or more years after the initial stroke. The remaining 111 patients had an ongoing risk of recurrent stroke (1.9/100 patient-years) despite long-term transfusions ($P = .038$). These results suggest that in the 2-year period after an initial stroke, patients with SCD are particularly vulnerable to development of a second stroke, but that after 2 years, those with an antecedent or concurrent medical event at the time of initial stroke have a much lower recurrent stroke risk.

Bone marrow transplantation (BMT) is used to avoid the complications of repeated transfusions, but patients undergoing BMT are reported to experience stroke and other neurologic complications, especially during the phase of profound thrombocytopenia.[283] The timing of BMT is controversial. One would like to perform BMT before end-stage organ damage occurs yet limit BMT to patients destined to experience these complications. There is as yet no satisfactory answer to this dilemma.[284] The use of hydroxyurea has markedly decreased the incidence of sickle cell crisis in adults and children with severe disease.[285–287] However, it is too early to know whether the use of hydroxyurea will decrease the incidence of vascular complication.

SCREENING OF PATIENTS WITH STROKE FOR COAGULOPATHIES

There is no simple answer to the question of which patients with stroke should receive additional testing for coagulation abnormalities. Patients with stroke in whom the yield of screening is likely to be highest are those who are young, those who experience repeated unexplained strokes, and those with a prior history of thrombosis (particularly venous thrombosis). Patients with unexplained cerebral venous thrombosis (cortical vein or sagittal sinus thrombosis) should be investigated for hypercoagulable conditions, especially APC resistance. Patients with livedo reticularis and left heart valvular abnormalities and women with a history of spontaneous abortion should be screened for aPL antibodies. A hemoglobin electrophoresis should be considered in young black American patients. A suggested approach is summarized in Tables 34.2 and 34.3.

Table 34.2   Patients with Ischemic Stroke in Whom Additional Screening for Coagulopathies May Be Appropriate

Younger than 50 years with no obvious cause for stroke
Multiple unexplained strokes
Prior history of venous thrombosis
Family history of thrombosis
Abnormal findings of routine screening coagulation tests

Table 34.3   Laboratory Screening Tests for Coagulopathies in Selected Patients

Protein C, protein S, and antithrombin III measurements by functional assay
Free protein S antigen measurement
Anticardiolipin antibody assay by enzyme-linked immunosorbent assay (ELISA)
Functional assay for lupus anticoagulant
Hemoglobin electrophoresis (especially in black Americans)
Homocyst(e)ine measurement
Lipoprotein$_a$ measurement
Either factor V Leiden by polymerase chain reaction or functional assay for activated protein C resistance
Thrombin time for dysfibrinogenemia

References

1. Esmon CT: Molecular events that control the protein C anticoagulant pathway. Thromb Haemost 70:29, 1993.
2. Broze GJ Jr: Tissue factor pathway inhibitor and the revised theory of coagulation. Annu Rev Med 46:103, 1995.
3. Ernst E: Plasma fibrinogen: An independent cardiovascular risk factor. J Intern Med 227:365, 1990.
4. Esmon CT: Thrombomodulin as a model of molecular mechanisms that modulate protease specificity and function at the vessel surface. FASEB J 9:946, 1995.
5. Bombeli T, Mueller M, Haeberli A: Anticoagulant properties of the vascular endothelium. Thromb Haemost 77:408, 1997.
6. Wu KK, Thiagarajan P: Role of endothelium in thrombosis and hemostasis. Annu Rev Med 47:315, 1996.
7. Gimbrone MA Jr: Vascular endothelium: An integrator of pathophysiologic stimuli in atherosclerosis. Am J Cardiol 75:67B, 1995.
8. Schved JF, Gris JC, Ollivier V: Procoagulant activity of endotoxin or tumor necrosis factor activated monocytes is enhanced by IgG from patients with lupus anticoagulant. Am J Hematol 41:92, 1992.
9. Boffa MC: Thrombomodulin in human brain microvasculature [letter]. Lupus 4:165, 1995.
10. Tran ND, Wong VL, Schreiber SS, et al: Regulation of brain capillary endothelial thrombomodulin mRNA expression. Stroke 27:2304, 1996.
11. Rosendaal FR, Siscovick DS, Schwartz SM, et al: Factor V Leiden (resistance to activated protein C) increases the risk of myocardial infarction in young women. Blood 89:2817, 1997.
12. Press RD, Liu XY, Beamer N, Coull BM: Ischemic stroke in the elderly—role of the common factor V mutation causing resistance to activated protein C. Stroke 27:44, 1996.
13. Van der Bom JG, Bots ML, Haverkate F, et al: Reduced response to activated protein C is associated with increased risk for cerebrovascular disease. Ann Intern Med 125:265, 1996.
14. De Stefano V, Chiusolo P, Paciaroni K, et al: Prothrombin G20210A mutant genotype is a risk factor for cerebrovascular ischemic disease in young patients. Blood 91:3562, 1998.
15. Brey RL, Coull BM: Cerebral venous thrombosis: Role of activated protein C resistance and factor V gene mutation. Stroke 27:1719, 1996.
16. Dulli DA, Luzzio CC, Williams EC, Schutta HS: Cerebral venous thrombosis and activated protein C resistance. Stroke 27:1731, 1996.
17. Ridker PM, Vaughan DE, Stampfer MJ, et al: Endogenous tissue-type plasminogen activator and risk of myocardial infarction. Lancet 341:1165, 1993.
18. Zunker P, Hohenstein C, Plendl H-J, et al: Activated protein C resistance and acute ischemic stroke: Relation to stroke causation and age. J Neurol 248:701, 2001.
19. Szolnoki Z, Somogyvari F, Kondacs A, et al: Evaluation of the roles of the Leiden V mutation and ACE I/D polymorphism in subtypes of ischemic stroke. J Neurol 248:756, 2001.
20. Finazzi G, Barbui T: Different incidence of venous thrombosis in patients with inherited deficiencies of antithrombin III, protein C and protein S. Thromb Haemost 71:15, 1994.

21. Permpikul P, Rao LVM, Rapaport SI: Functional and binding studies of the roles of prothrombin and β-2-glycoprotein I in the expression of lupus anticoagulant activity. Blood 83:2878, 1994.
22. Bousser MG, Chiras J, Bories J, Castaigne P: Cerebral vein thrombosis: A review of 38 cases. Stroke 16:199, 1985.
23. Brey RL, Hart RG, Sherman DG, Tegeler CH: Antiphospholipid antibodies and cerebral ischemia in young people. Neurology (NY) 40:1190, 1990.
24. Enevoldson TP, Russel RWR: Cerebral vein thrombosis: New causes for an old syndrome? Q J Med 77:1255, 1990.
25. Hoffman CJ, Miller RH, Hultin MB: Correlation of factor VII activity and antigen with cholesterol and triglycerides in healthy young adults. Arterioscler Thromb 12:267, 1992.
26. Wintzen AR, Broekmans AW, Bertina RM, et al: Cerebral haemorrhagic infarction in young patients with hereditary protein C deficiency: Evidence for "spontaneous" cerebral venous thrombosis. BMJ 290:350, 1985.
27. Shibata M, Kumar SR, Amar A, et al: Anti-inflammatory, antithrombotic and neuroprotective effects of activated protein C in a murine model of focal ischemic stroke. Circulation 103:1799, 2001.
28. Folsom AR, Rosamond WD, Shahar E, et al: Prospective study of markers of hemostatic function with risk of ischemic stroke. Circulation 10:736, 1999.
29. D'Angelo A, Landi G, D'Angelo SV, et al: Protein C in acute stroke. Stroke 19:579, 1988.
30. Mayer SA, Sacco RL, Hurlet-Jensen A, et al: Free protein S deficiency in acute ischemic stroke: A case-control study. Stroke 24:224, 1993.
31. Nguyen A: Prothrombin G20210A polymorphism and thrombophilia. Mayo Clin Proc 75:595, 2000.
32. Poort SR, Rosendaal FR, Reitsma PH, Bertina RM: A common genetic variation in the 3'-untranslated region of the prothrombin gene is associated with elevated plasma prothrombin levels and an increase in venous thrombosis. Blood 88:3698, 1996.
33. Martinelli I, Franchi F, Akwan S, et al: The transition G to A at position 20210 in the 3'-untranslated region of the prothrombin gene is not associated with cerebral ischemia. Blood 90:3806, 1997.
34. Tripodi A, Mannucci PM: Laboratory investigation of thrombophilia. Clinical Chemistry 47:1597, 2001.
35. De Moerloose P, Reber G, Bouviar CA: Spuriously low levels of protein C with Protac activation clotting assay [letter]. Thromb Haemost 59:543, 1988.
36. Faioni EM, Franchi F, Asti D, Mannucci PM: Resistance to activated protein C mimicking dysfunctional protein C: Diagnostic approach. Blood Coagul Fibrinolysis 7:349, 1996.
37. Jorquera JI, Montoro JM, Fernandez MA, Aznar J: Modified test for activated protein C resistance [letter]. Lancet 344:1162, 1994.
38. Dahlback B: The protein C anticoagulant system: Inherited defects as basis for venous thrombosis. Thromb Res 77:1, 1995.
39. Comp PC, Doray D, Patton D, Esmon CT: An abnormal distribution of protein S occurs in functional protein S deficiency. Blood 67:504, 1986.
40. Simmonds RE, Ireland H, Lane DA, et al: Clarification of the risk for venous thrombosis associated with hereditary protein S deficiency by investigation of a large kindred with a characterized gene defect. Ann Intern Med 128:8, 1998.
41. Demers C, Henderson P, Blajchman MA, et al: An antithrombin III assay based on factor Xa inhibition provides a more reliable test to identify congenital antithrombin III deficiency than an assay based on thrombin inhibition. Thromb Haemost 69:231, 1993.
42. Leroy-Matheron C, Lamare M, Levent M, Gouault-Heilmann M: Markers of coagulation activation in inherited protein S deficiency. Thromb Res 67:607, 1992.
43. Schoene NW: Design criteria: Tests used to assess platelet function. Am J Clin Nutr 65(Suppl):1665S, 1997.
44. Alkjaersig N, Fletcher A: Catabolism and excretion of fibrinopeptide A. Blood 60:148, 1982.
45. Nossel H: Relative proteolysis of fibrin B chain by thrombin and plasmin as a determinant of thrombosis. Nature 291:165, 1981.
46. Owen J, Kvam D, Nossel H, et al: Thrombin and plasmin activity and platelet activation in the development of venous thrombosis. Blood 60:476, 1983.
47. Feinberg WM, Bruck DC, Ring ME, Corrigan JJ: Hemostatic markers in acute stroke. Stroke 20:592, 1989.
48. Feinberg WM, Erickson LP, Bruck D, Kittelson J: Hemostatic markers in acute ischemic stroke: Association with stroke type, severity, and outcome. Stroke 27:1296, 1996.
49. Jones SL, Close CF, Mattock MB, et al: Plasma lipid and coagulation factor concentrations in insulin dependent diabetics with microalbuminuria. BMJ 298:487, 1989.
50. Takano K, Yamaguchi T, Kato H, Omae T: Activation of coagulation in acute cardioembolic stroke. Stroke 22:12, 1991.
51. Takano K, Yamaguchi T, Uchida K: Markers of a hypercoagulable state following acute ischemic stroke. Stroke 23:194, 1992.
52. Tohgi H, Takahahi H, Chiba K, Tamura K: Coagulation-fibrinolysis system in poststroke patients receiving antiplatelet medication. Stroke 24:801, 1993.
53. Tohgi H, Kawashima M, Taa K, Suzuki H: Coagulation-fibrinolysis abnormalities in acute and chronic phases of cerebral thrombosis and embolism. Stroke 21:1663, 1990.
54. Yamazaki M, Uchiyama S, Maruyama S: Alterations of haemostatic markers in various subtypes and phases of stroke. Blood Coagul Fibrinolysis 4:707, 1993.
55. Asakura H, Hifumi S, Jokaji H, et al: Prothrombin fragment F 1+2 and thrombin-antithrombin complex are useful markers of the hypercoagulable state in atrial fibrillation. Blood Coagul Fibrinolysis 3:469, 1992.
56. Carter AM, Catto AJ, Grant PJ: Association of the alpha-fibrinogen Thr312Ala polymorphism with poststroke mortality in subjects with atrial fibrillation. Circulation 9:2423, 1999.
57. Feinberg WM, Bruck DC, Pearce LA: Intravascular coagulation in patients with atrial fibrillation [abstract]. Neurology (NY) 41:298, 1991.
58. Gustafsson C, Blomback M, Britton M, et al: Coagulation factors and the increased risk of stroke in nonvalvular atrial fibrillation. Stroke 21:47, 1990.
59. Kumagai K, Fukunami M, Ohmori M, et al: Increased intravascular clotting in patients with chronic atrial fibrillation. J Am Coll Cardiol 16:377, 1990.
60. Clinical and laboratory findings in patients with antiphospholipid antibodies and cerebral ischemia. Antiphospholipid Antibody in Stroke Study Group (APASS). Stroke 21:1268, 1990.
61. Feinberg WM, Cornell ES, Nightingale SD, et al: Relationship between prothrombin activation fragment F1.2 and international normalized ratio (INR) in patients with atrial fibrillation. Stroke 28:1101, 1997.
62. Kistler JP, Singer DE, Millenson MM, et al: Effect of low-intensity warfarin anticoagulation on level of activity of the hemostatic system in patients with atrial fibrillation. Stroke 24:1360, 1993.
63. Lip GYH, Lip PL, Zarafis J, et al: Fibrin D-dimer and β-thromboglobulin as markers of thrombogenesis and platelet activation in atrial fibrillation: Effects of introducing ultra-low-dose warfarin and aspirin. Circulation 94:425, 1996.
64. Lip GY: Fibrinogen and cardiovascular disorders. Q J Med 88:155, 1995.
65. Smith FB, Lee AJ, Fowkes FGR, et al: Hemostatic factors as predictors of ischemic heart disease and stroke in the Edinburgh artery study. Arterioscler Thromb Vasc Biol 17:3321, 1997.
66. Di Napoli M, Papa F, Villa Pini Stroke Data Bank Investigators: Inflammation, hemostatic markers, and antithrombotic agents in relation to long-term risk of new cardiovascular events in first-ever ischemic stroke patients. Stroke 33:1763, 2002.
67. Cook NS, Ubben D: Fibrinogen as a major risk factor in cardiovascular disease. Trends Pharmacol Sci 11:444, 1990.
68. Ernst E, Resch KL: Fibrinogen as a cardiovascular risk factor: A meta-analysis and review of the literature. Ann Intern Med 118:956, 1993.
69. Kannel WB, Wolf PA, Castelli WP, D'Agostino RB: Fibrinogen and risk of cardiovascular disease: The Framingham study. JAMA 258:1183, 1987.
70. Lowe GD, Lee AJ, Rumley A, et al: Blood viscosity and risk of cardiovascular events: The Edinburgh Artery Study. Br J Haematol 96:168, 1997.
71. Qizilbash N: Fibrinogen and cerebrovascular disease. Eur Heart J 16(Suppl A):42, 1995.
72. Wilhelmsen L, Svardsudd K, Korsan-Bengtsen K: Fibrinogen as a risk factor for stroke and myocardial infarction. N Engl J Med 311:50, 1984.
73. Yarnell JWG, Baker IA, Sweetnam PM, et al: Fibrinogen, viscosity, and white blood cell count are major risk factors for ischemic heart disease. Circulation 83:836, 1991.

Specific Medical Diseases and Stroke

74. Coull B, Beamer N, de Garmo P, et al: Chronic blood hyperviscosity in subjects with acute stroke, transient ischemic attack, and risk factors for stroke. Stroke 22:162, 1991.

75. Resch KL, Ernst E, Matrai A, Paulsen HF: Fibrinogen and viscosity as risk factors for subsequent cardiovascular events in stroke survivors. Ann Intern Med 117:371, 1992.

76. Ameriso SF, Wong VLY, Quismorio FP, Fisher M: Immunohematologic characteristics of infection-associated cerebral infarction. Stroke 22:1004, 1991.

77. Ernst E: Fibrinogen as a cardiovascular risk factor: Interrelationship with infections and inflammation. Eur Heart J 14(Suppl K):82, 1993.

78. Cahill M, Mistry R, Barnett DB: The human platelet fibrinogen receptor: Clinical and therapeutic significance. Br J Clin Pharmacol 33:3, 1992.

79. Juhan-Vague I, Valdier J, Alessi M, et al: Deficient t-PA release and elevated PA inhibitor levels in patients with spontaneous or recurrent deep venous thrombosis. Thromb Haemost 57:67, 1987.

80. Berdeaux D, Marlar R: Report of an American family with elevated PAI-1 as a cause of multiple thromboses responsive to prednisone [abstract]. Thromb Haemost 65:1044, 1991.

81. Dolan G, Greaves M, Cooper P, Preston FE: Thrombovascular disease and familial plasminogen deficiency: A report of three kindred. Br J Haematol 70:417, 1988.

82. Francis R: Clinical disorders of fibrinolysis: A critical review. Blut 59:1, 1989.

83. Furlan A, Lucas F, Craciun R, Wohl R: Stroke in a young adult with familial plasminogen disorder. Stroke 22:1598, 1991.

84. Hart RG, Kanter MC: Hematologic disorders and ischemic stroke: A selective review. Stroke 21:1111, 1990.

85. Jorgenson M, Bonnevie-Nielsen V: Increased concentration of the fast-acting plasminogen activator inhibitor in plasma associated with familial venous thrombosis. Br J Haematol 65:175, 1987.

86. Nagayama T, Shinohara Y, Nagayama M, et al: Congenitally abnormal plasminogen in juvenile ischemic cerebrovascular disease. Stroke 24:2104, 1993.

87. Feinberg WM, Bruck DC: Time course of platelet activation following acute ischemic stroke. J Stroke Cerebrovasc Dis 1:124, 1991.

88. Fisher M, Francis R: Altered coagulation in cerebral ischemia: Platelet, thrombin, and plasmin activity. Arch Neurol 47:1075, 1990.

89. Glueck C, Rorick M, Scherler M, et al: Hypofibrinolytic and atherogenic risk factors for stroke. J Lab Clin Med 125:319, 1995.

90. Kempter B, Peinemann A, Biniasch O, Haberl RL: Decreased fibrinolytic stimulation by short-term venous occlusion test in patients with cerebrovascular disease. Thromb Res 79:363, 1995.

91. Brockman MJ, Schwendemann G, Stief TW: Plasminogen activator inhibitor in acute stroke. Mol Chem Neuropathol 14:143, 1991.

92. Lindgren A, Lindoff C, Norrving B, et al: Tissue plasminogen activator and plasminogen activator inhibitor-1 in stroke patients. Stroke 27:1066, 1996.

93. Margaglione M, Di Minno G, Grandone E, et al: Abnormally high circulation levels of tissue plasminogen activator and plasminogen activator inhibitor-1 in patients with a history of ischemic stroke. Arterioscler Thromb Vasc Biol 14:1741, 1994.

94. de Bono D: Significance of raised plasma concentrations of tissue-type plasminogen activator and plasminogen activator inhibitor in patients at risk from ischaemic heart disease. Br Heart J 71:504, 1994.

95. Ridker PM: Plasma concentration of endogenous tissue plasminogen activator and the occurrence of future cardiovascular events. J Thromb Thrombolysis 1:35, 1994.

96. Salomaa V, Stinson V, Kark JD, et al: Association of fibrinolytic parameters with early atherosclerosis: The ARIC Study. Atherosclerosis Risk in Communities Study. Circulation 91:284, 1995.

97. Oates JA, FitzGerald GA, Branch RA, et al: Clinical implications of prostaglandin and thromboxane A2 formation. N Engl J Med 319:689, 1988.

98. Scott J: Lipoprotein (a): Thrombogenesis linked to atherosclerosis at last? Nature 341:22, 1989.

99. McLean JW, Tomlinson JE, Kuang WJ, et al: cDNA sequence of human apolipoprotein (a) is homologous to plasminogen. Nature 330:132, 1987.

100. Etingin OR, Hajjar DP, Hajjar KA, et al: Lipoprotein (a) regulates plasminogen activator inhibitor-1 expression in endothelial cells: A potential mechanism in thrombogenesis. J Biol Chem 266:2459, 1991.

101. Hajjar KA, Gavish D, Breslow JL, Nachman RL: Lipoprotein (a) modulation of endothelial cell surface fibrinolysis and its potential role in atherosclerosis. Nature 339:303, 1989.

102. Franceschini G, Cofrancesco E, Safa O, et al: Association of lipoprotein (a) with atherothrombotic events and fibrinolytic variables: A case-control study. Thromb Res 78:227, 1995.

103. Jürgens F, Költringer P: Lipoprotein (a) in ischemic cerebrovascular disease: A new approach to the assessment of stroke. Neurology (NY) 37:513, 1987.

104. Lassila R, Manninen V: Hypofibrinolysis and increased lipoprotein (a) coincide in stroke. J Lab Clin Med 125:301, 1995.

105. Schreiner PJ, Chambless LE, Brown SA, et al: Lipoprotein (a) as a correlate of stroke and transient ischemic attack prevalence in a biracial cohort: The ARIC study. Ann Epidemiol 4:351, 1994.

106. Shintani S, Kikuchi S, Hamaguchi H, Shiigai T: High serum lipoprotein (a) is an independent risk factor for cerebral infarction. Stroke 24:965, 1993.

107. Zenker G, Költringer P, Boné G, et al: Lipoprotein (a) as a strong indicator for cerebrovascular disease. Stroke 17:942, 1986.

108. Del Zoppo GL: The role of platelets in ischemic stroke. Neurology 51(Suppl 3):S9, 1998.

109. 1997 State of the Art: XVIth Congress of the International Society on Thrombosis and Haemostasis. Thromb Haemost 78:96, 1997.

110. Fitzgerald DJ: Vascular biology of thrombosis. Neurology 57(Suppl 2):S1, 2001.

111. Fisher M, Levine PH, Fullerton A, et al: Marker proteins of platelet activation in patients with cerebrovascular disease. Stroke 39:692, 1982.

112. Shah AB, Beamer N, Coull BM: Enhanced in vivo platelet activation in subtypes of ischemic stroke. Stroke 16:643, 1985.

113. Taomoto K, Asada M, Kanazaua Y, Matsumoto S: Usefulness of the measurement of plasma-thromboglobulin (beta-TG) in cerebrovascular disease. Stroke 14:518, 1983.

114. Koudstall P, Ciabattoni G, van Gijn J, et al: Increased thromboxane biosynthesis in patients with acute cerebral ischemia. Stroke 24:219, 1993.

115. Van Kooten F, Ciabattoni G, Patrono C, et al: Evidence for episodic platelet activation in acute ischemic stroke. Stroke 25:278, 1994.

116. Del Zoppo GL, Copeland BR, Harker LA, et al: Experimental acute thrombotic stroke in baboons. Stroke 17:1254, 1986.

117. Arboix A, Besses C, Acin P, et al: Ischemic stroke as first manifestation of essential thrombocythemia: Report of six cases. Stroke 26:1463, 1995.

118. Jabaily J, Iland HJ, Laszlo J, et al: Neurologic manifestations of essential thrombocythemia. Ann Intern Med 99:513, 1983.

119. Murphy S, Iland H, Rosenthal D, Laszlo J: Essential thrombocythemia: An interim report from the Polycythemia Vera Study Group. Semin Hematol 23:177, 1986.

120. Colombi M, Radaelli F, Zocchi L, Maiolo AT: Thrombotic and hemorrhagic complications in essential thrombocythemia: A retrospective study of 103 patients. Cancer 67:2926, 1991.

121. Johnson M, Gernsheimer T, Johansen K: Essential thrombocytosis: Underemphasized cause of large-vessel thrombosis. J Vasc Surg 22:443, 1995.

122. Murphy S, Peterson P, Iland H, Laszlo J: Experience of the Polycythemia Vera Study Group with essential thrombocythemia: A final report on diagnostic criteria, survival, and leukemic transition by treatment. Semin Hematol 34:29, 1997.

123. Riuniti O, Barbui T, Finazzi G, et al: Polycythemia vera: The natural history of 1213 patients followed for 20 years. Ann Intern Med 123:656, 1995.

124. Vadher BD, Machin SJ, Patterson KG, et al: Life-threatening thrombotic and haemorrhagic problems associated with silent myeloproliferative disorders. Br J Haematol 85:213, 1993.

125. Saxena VK, Brands C, Crols R, et al: Multiple cerebral infarctions in a young patient with secondary thrombocythemia. Acta Neurol 15:297, 1993.

126. Collaborative overview of randomized trials of antiplatelet therapy. I: Prevention of death, myocardial infarction, and stroke by prolonged antiplatelet therapy in various categories of patients. Antiplatelet Trialists' Collaboration. BMJ 308:81, 1994.

127. Hervey PS, Goa KL: Extended-release dipyridamole/aspirin. Drugs 58:469, 1999.

128. Quinn MJ, Fitzgerald DJ: Ticlopidine and clopidogrel. Circulation 100:1667, 1999.

129. Van Genderen PJJ, Mulder PGH, Waleboer M, et al: Prevention and treatment of thrombotic complications in essential thrombocythaemia: Efficacy and safety of aspirin. Br J Haematol 97:179, 1997.

130. Cortelazzo S, Finazzi G, Ruggeri M, et al: Hydroxyurea for patients with essential thrombocythemia and a high risk of thrombosis. N Engl J Med 332:1132, 1995.

131. Becker PS, Miller VT: Heparin-induced thrombocytopenia. Stroke 20:1449, 1989.

132. Kibbe MR, Rhee RY: Heparin-induced thrombocytopenia: Pathophysiology. Semin Vasc Surg 9:284, 1996.

133. Ansell J, Deykin D: Heparin-induced thrombocytopenia and recurrent thromboembolism. Am J Hematol 8:325, 1980.

134. Atkinson JL, Sundt TM Jr, Kazmier FJ, et al: Heparin-induced thrombocytopenia and thrombosis in ischemic stroke. Mayo Clin Proc 63:353, 1988.

135. Bell WR: Heparin-associated thrombocytopenia and thrombosis. J Lab Clin Med 111:600, 1988.

136. King DJ, Keltron JG: Heparin-associated thrombocytopenia. Ann Intern Med 100:535, 1984.

137. Fabris F, Ahmad S, Cella G, et al: Pathophysiology of heparin-induced thrombocytopenia: Clinical and diagnostic implications: A review. Arch Pathol Lab Med 124:1657, 2000.

138. Fabris F, Luzzatto G, Stefani PM, et al: Heparin-induced thrombocytopenia. Haematologica 85:72, 2000.

139. Warkentin TE, Kelton JG: Heparin and platelets. Hematol Oncol Clin North Am 4:243, 1990.

140. Warkentin TE, Levine MN, Hirsh J, et al: Heparin-induced thrombocytopenia in patients treated with low-molecular-weight heparin or unfractionated heparin. N Engl J Med 332:1330, 1995.

141. Aster R: Heparin-induced thrombocytopenia: Understanding improves but questions remain. J Lab Clin Med 127:418, 1996.

142. Goor Y, Goor O, Eldor A: Heparin-induced thrombocytopenia with thrombotic sequelae: A review. Autoimmun Rev 1:183, 2002.

143. Horsewood P, Warkentin TE, Hayward CP, Kelton JG: The epitope specificity of heparin-induced thrombocytopenia. Br J Haematol 95:161, 1996.

144. Cines DB, Tomasaki A, Tannenbaum S: Immune endothelial cell injury in heparin-associated thrombocytopenia. N Engl J Med 316:581, 1987.

145. Walenga JM, Jeske WP, Messmore HS: Mechanisms of venous and arterial thrombosis in heparin-induced thrombocytopenia. J Thromb Thrombolysis 10(Suppl):S13, 2000.

146. Kyritsis AP, Williams EC, Schutta HS: Cerebral venous thrombosis due to heparin-induced thrombocytopenia. Stroke 21:1503, 1990.

147. Spencer FA: Heparin-induced thrombocytopenia: Patient profiles and clinical manifestations. J Thromb Thrombolysis 10(Suppl):S21, 2000.

148. Warkentin TE: Heparin-induced thrombocytopenia: A clinicopathological syndrome. Thromb Haemost 82:439, 1999.

149. Wallis DE, Workman DL, Lewis BE, et al: Failure of heparin cessation as treatment for heparin-induced thrombocytopenia. Am J Med 106:629, 1999.

150. Greinacher A: Treatment of heparin-induced thrombocytopenia. Thromb Haemost 82:457, 1999.

151. Lewis BE, Walenga JM, Wallis DE: Anticoagulation with Novastan (argatroban) in patients with heparin-induced thrombocytopenia, and heparin-induced thrombocytopenia and thrombosis syndrome. Semin Thromb Hemost 23:197, 1997.

152. Lubenow N, Greinacher A: Management of patients with heparin-induced thrombocytopenia: Focus on recombinant hirudin. J Thromb Thrombolysis 10(Suppl):S47, 2000.

153. Emlen W: Antiphospholipid antibodies: New complexities and new assays. Arthritis Rheum 39:1441, 1996.

154. Goodnight SH: Antiphospholipid antibodies and thrombosis. Curr Opin Hematol 1:354, 1994.

155. Leéon-Velarde F, Ramos MA, Hernández JA: The role of menopause in the development of chronic mountain sickness. Am J Physiol 272:R90, 1997.

156. Mackworth-Young CG: The Michael Mason Prize Essay (1994): Antiphospholipid antibodies and disease. Br J Rheumatol 34:1009, 1995.

157. Shapiro SS: The lupus anticoagulant antiphospholipid syndrome. Annu Rev Med 47:533, 1996.

158. Arnout J, Vermylen J: Lupus anticoagulants: Mechanistic and diagnostic considerations. In Khamashta MA (ed): Hughes Syndrome: Antiphospholipid Syndrome. London, Springer-Verlag, 2000, p 225.

159. Bowie WEJ, Thompson JH, Pasacuzzi CA, Owen CA: Thrombosis in systemic lupus erythematosus despite circulating anticoagulants. J Clin Invest 62:416, 1963.

160. Feinstein DI, Rapaport SI: Acquired inhibitors of blood coagulation. Prog Hemost Thromb 1:75, 1972.

161. Harris EN, Boey ML, Mackworth-Young CG, et al: Anticardiolipin antibodies: Detection by radioimmunoassay and association with thrombosis in systemic lupus erythematosus. Lancet 2:1211, 1983.

162. Horbach DA, Oort EV, Donders RC, et al: Lupus anticoagulant is the strongest risk factor for both venous and arterial thrombosis in patients with systemic lupus erythematosus: Comparison between different assays for the detection of antiphospholipid antibodies. Thromb Haemost 76:916, 1996.

163. Campbell AL, Pierangeli SS, Wellhausen S, Harris EN: Comparison of the effects of anticardiolipin antibodies from patients with the antiphospholipid antibody syndrome and with syphilis on platelet activation and aggregation. Thromb Haemost 73:529, 1995.

164. Rauch J, Aminoff AS: Antiphospholipid antibodies against phospholipids other than cardiolipin: Potential roles for both phospholipid and protein. Lupus 5:498, 1996.

165. Rote NS, Dostal-Johnson D, Branch DW: Antiphospholipid antibodies and recurrent pregnancy loss: Correlation between the activated partial thromboplastin time and antibodies against phosphatidylserine and cardiolipin. Am J Obstet Gynecol 163:575, 1990.

166. Tuhrim S, Rand JH, Wu X, et al: Antiphosphatidylserine antibodies are independently associated with ischemic stroke. Neurology 53:1523, 1999.

167. Galli M, Comfurius P, Maassen C, et al: Anticardiolipin antibodies are directed not against cardiolipin but to a plasma cofactor. Lancet 335:1544, 1990.

168. Matsurra E, Igarashi Y, Fujimoto M, et al: Anticardiolipin cofactors and the differential diagnosis of autoimmune disease. Lancet 336:177, 1990.

169. McNeil HP, Simpson RJ, Chesterman CN, Krilis SA: Antiphospholipid antibodies are directed against a complex antigen that includes a lipid-binding inhibitor of coagulation β2 glycoprotein 1 (apolipoprotein H). Proc Natl Acad Sci U S A 87:4120, 1990.

170. Meroni PL, Del Papa N, Raschi E, et al: β2 glycoprotein 1 as a cofactor for antiphospholipid reactivity with endothelial cells. Lupus 5(Suppl):S44, 1998.

171. Roubey RAS, Eisenberg RA, Harper MF, Winfield JB: "Anticardiolipin" autoantibodies recognize β2 glycoprotein 1 in the absence of phospholipids: Importance of antigen density and bivalent binding. J Immunol 154:954, 1995.

172. Cabides J, Cabral A, Alarcon-Segovia D: Clinical manifestations of antiphospholipid antibody syndrome in systemic lupus erythematosus associated more strongly with anti-β2 glycoprotein 1 than antiphospholipid antibodies. J Rheumatol 22:1899, 1995.

173. Viard JP, Amoura Z, Bach JF: Association of anti-β2 glycoprotein 1 antibodies with lupus-type circulating anticoagulants and thrombosis in systemic lupus erythematosus. Am J Med 93:181, 1992.

174. Wilson WA, Gharavi AE, Koike T, et al: International Consensus Statement on Preliminary Classification Criteria for Definite Antiphospholipid Syndrome: Report of an International Workshop. Arthritis Rheum 2:1309, 1999.

175. Asherson RA, Khamashta MA, Gil A, et al: Cerebrovascular disease and antiphospholipid antibodies in systemic lupus erythematosus, lupus-like disease, and the primary antiphospholipid syndrome. Am J Med 86:391, 1989.

176. Goldstein R, Moulda JM, Smith CD, Sengar DP: MHC studies of the primary antiphospholipid antibody syndrome and of antiphospholipid antibodies in systemic lupus erythematosus. J Rheum 23:1173, 1996.

177. Toubi E, Khamashta MA, Panarra A, Hughes GR: Association of antiphospholipid antibodies with central nervous system disease in systemic lupus erythematosus. Am J Med 99:397, 1995.

178. Feldmann E, Levine SR: Cerebrovascular disease with antiphospholipid antibodies: Immune mechanisms, significance, and therapeutic options. Ann Neurol 37(Suppl 1):S114, 1995.

179. Fields RA, Toubbeh H, Searles RP, et al: The prevalence of anticardiolipin antibodies in a healthy elderly population and its association with antinuclear antibodies. J Rheumatol 16:623, 1989.

Specific Medical Diseases and Stroke

180. Shi W, Krilis SA, Chong BH, et al: Prevalence of lupus anticoagulant and anticardiolipin antibodies in a healthy population. Aust N Z J Med 20:231, 1990.

181. Briley DP, Coull BM, Goodnight SH Jr: Neurological disease associated with antiphospholipid antibodies. Ann Neurol 25:221, 1989.

182. Levine SR, Brey RL, Sawaya KL, et al: Recurrent stroke and thrombo-occlusive events in the antiphospholipid syndrome. Ann Neurol 38:119, 1995.

183. Finazzi G, Brancaccio V, Moia M, et al: Natural history and risk factors for thrombosis in 360 patients with antiphospholipid antibodies: A four-year prospective study from the Italian registry. Am J Med 100:530, 1996.

184. Anticardiolipin antibodies and the risk of recurrent thrombo-occlusive events and death. Antiphospholipid Antibody in Stroke Study (APASS) Group. Neurology 48:91, 1997.

185. Levine SR, Salowich-Palm L, Sawaya KL, et al: IgG anticardiolipin antibody titer > 40 GPL and the risk of subsequent thrombo-occlusive events and death: A prospective cohort study. Stroke 28:1660, 1997.

186. Rosove MH, Brewer PM: Antiphospholipid thrombosis: Clinical course after the first thrombotic event in 70 patients. Ann Intern Med 117:303, 1992.

187. Ruiz Irastorza G, Khamashta MA, Hunt BJ, et al: Bleeding and recurrent thrombosis in definite antiphospholipid syndrome: Analysis of a series of 66 patients treated with oral anticoagulation to a target international normalized ratio of 3.5. Arch Intern Med 162:1164, 2002.

188. Verro P, Levine SR, Tietjen GE: Cerebrovascular ischemic events with high positive anticardiolipin antibodies. Stroke 29:2245, 1998.

189. Love PE, Santoro SA: Antiphospholipid antibodies: Anticardiolipin and the lupus anticoagulant in systemic lupus erythematosus (SLE) and in non-SLE disorders. Ann Intern Med 112:682, 1990.

190. Brey RL, Abbott RD, Sharp DS, et al: Beta-2-glycoprotein 1-dependent (B2GP1-dep) anticardiolipin antibodies are an independent risk factor for ischemic stroke in the Honolulu Heart Cohort. Stroke 39:252, 1999.

191. Brey RL, Stallworth CL, McGlasson DL, et al: Antiphospholipid antibodies and stroke in young women. Stroke 33:2396, 2002.

192. Camerlingo M, Casto L, Censori B, et al: Anticardiolipin antibodies in acute nonhemorrhagic stroke seen within six hours after onset. Acta Neurol Scand 92:69, 1995.

193. Chakravarty KK, Byron MA, Webley M, et al: Antibodies to cardiolipin in stroke: Association with mortality and functional recovery in patients without systemic lupus erythematosus. Q J Med 79:397, 1991.

194. Kushner MJ: Prospective study of anticardiolipin antibodies in stroke. Stroke 21:295, 1990.

195. Nagaraja D, Christopher R, Manjari T: Anticardiolipin antibodies in ischemic stroke in the young: Indian experience. J Neurol Sci 150:137, 1997.

196. Nencini P, Baruffi MC, Abbate R, et al: Lupus anticoagulant and anticardiolipin antibodies in young adults with cerebral ischemia. Stroke 23:189, 1992.

197. Anticardiolipin antibodies are an independent risk factor for first ischemic stroke. The Antiphospholipid Antibodies and Stroke Study (APASS) Group. Neurology 43:2069, 1993.

198. Yilmaz E, Adalet K, Yilmaz G, et al: Importance of serum anticardiolipin antibody levels in coronary heart disease. Clin Cardiol 17:117, 1994.

199. Metz LM, Edworthy S, Mydlarski R, Fritzler MJ: The frequency of phospholipid antibodies in an unselected stroke population. Can J Neurol Sci 25:64, 1998.

200. Muir KW, Squire IB, Alwan W, Lees KR: Anticardiolipin antibodies in an unselected stroke population. Lancet 344:452, 1994.

201. Phadke KV, Phillips RA, Clarke DT, et al: Anticardiolipin antibodies in ischaemic heart disease: Marker or myth? Br Heart J 69:391, 1993.

202. Ridker PM, Manson JE, Buring JE, et al: Homocysteine and risk of cardiovascular disease among postmenopausal women. JAMA 281:1817, 1999.

203. Sletnes KE, Smith P, Abdolnoor M, et al: Antiphospholipid antibodies after myocardial infarction and their relation to mortality, reinfarction, and non-haemorrhagic stroke. Lancet 339:451, 1992.

204. Wu R, Nityanand S, Berglund L, et al: Antibodies against cardiolipin and oxidatively modified LDL in 50-year-old men predict myocardial infarction. Arterioscler Thromb Vasc Biol 17:3159, 1997.

205. Bouillanne O, Millaire A, De Groote P, et al: Prevalence and clinical significance of antiphospholipid antibodies in heart valve disease: A case-control study. Am Heart J 132:790, 1996.

206. Hojnik M, George J, Ziporen L, Shoenfeld Y: Heart valve involvement (Libman-Sacks endocarditis) in the antiphospholipid syndrome. Circulation 93:1579, 1996.

207. Coull BM, Bourdette DN, Goodnight SH, et al: Multiple cerebral infarctions and dementia associated with anti-cardiolipin antibodies. Stroke 18:1107, 1987.

208. Levine SR, Langer SL, Albers JW, Welch KMA: Sneddon's syndrome: An antiphospholipid antibody syndrome? Neurology (NY) 38:798, 1988.

209. Sneddon IB: Cerebrovascular lesions and livedo reticularis. Br J Dermatol 77:180, 1965.

210. Kalashnikova LA, Nasonov EL, Kushakhaeva AE, Grecheva LA: Anticardiolipin antibodies in Sneddon's syndrome. Neurology (NY) 40:464, 1990.

211. Rebello M, Val JF, Garijo F, et al: Livedo reticularis and cerebrovascular lesions (Sneddon's syndrome). Brain 106:965, 1983.

212. Asherson RA, Piette JC: The catastrophic antiphospholipid syndrome 1996: Acute multi-organ failure associated with antiphospholipid antibodies: A review of 31 patients. Lupus 5:414, 1996.

213. Barbut D, Borer JS, Wallerson D, et al: Anticardiolipin antibody and stroke: Possible relation of valvular heart disease and embolic events. Cardiology 79:99, 1991.

214. Kitagawa Y, Gotoh F, Koto A, Okayasu H: Stroke in systemic lupus erythematosus. Stroke 21:1533, 1990.

215. Rademacher J, Sohngen D, Specker C, et al: Cerebral microembolism: A disease marker for ischemic cerebrovascular events in the antiphospholipid syndrome of systemic lupus erythematosus? Acta Neurol Scand 99:356, 1999.

216. Specker C, Rademacher J, Sohngen D, et al: Cerebral microemboli in patients with antiphospholipid syndrome. Lupus 6:638, 1997.

217. Borowska-Lehman J, Bakowska A, Michowska M, et al: Antiphospholipid syndrome in systemic lupus erythematosus: Immunomorphological study of the central nervous system: Case report. Folia Neuropathol 33:231, 1995.

218. Ellison D, Gatter K, Heryet A, Esiri M: Intramural platelet deposition in cerebral vasculopathy of systemic lupus erythematosus. J Clin Pathol 46:37, 1993.

219. Hughson MD, McCarty GA, Sholer CM, Brumback RA: Thrombotic cerebral arteriopathy in patients with the antiphospholipid syndrome. Mod Pathol 6:644, 1993.

220. Jain R, Chartash E, Susin M, Furie R: Systemic lupus erythematosus complicated by thrombotic microangiopathy. Semin Arthritis Rheum 24:173, 1994.

221. Shoenfeld Y, Ziporen L: Lessons from experimental APS models. Lupus 7(Suppl 2):S158, 1998.

222. Westerman EM, Miles JM, Backonja M, Sundstrom WR: Neuropathologic findings in multi-infarct dementia associated with anti-cardiolipin antibody: Evidence for endothelial injury as the primary event. Arthritis Rheum 35:1038, 1992.

223. Ziporen L, Shoenfeld Y: Anti-phospholipid syndrome: From patient's bedside to experimental animal models and back to the patient's bedside. Hematol Cell Ther 40:175, 1998.

224. Hess DC, Sheppard JC, Adams RJ: Increased immunoglobulin binding to cerebral endothelium in patients with antiphospholipid antibodies. Stroke 24:994, 1993.

225. Lanir N, Zilberman M, Yron I, et al: Reactivity patterns of antiphospholipid antibodies and endothelial cells: Effect of antiendothelial antibodies on cell migration. J Lab Clin Med 131:548, 1998.

226. Kaplanski G, Cacoub P, Farnarier C, et al: Increased soluble vascular cell adhesion molecule 1 concentrations in patients with primary or systemic lupus erythematosus-related antiphospholipid syndrome: Correlations with the severity of thrombosis. Arthritis Rheum 43:55, 2000.

227. Hilker R, Thiel A, Geisen C, Rudolf J: Cerebral blood flow and glucose metabolism in multi-infarct dementia related to primary antiphospholipid antibody syndrome. Lupus 9:311, 2000.

228. Kao CH, Lan JL, Hsieh JF, et al: Evaluation of regional cerebral blood flow with 99m Tc-HMPAO in primary antiphospholipid antibody syndrome. J Nucl Med 40:1446, 1999.

229. Kato T, Nanbu I, Tohyama J, Ohba S: Evaluation of cerebral perfusion imaging with *N*-isopropyl-*p*-[123I]iodoamphetamine (IMP) in the cases of antiphospholipid syndrome. Kaku Igaku 32:31, 1995.

230. Maeshima E, Yamada Y, Yukawa S, Nomoto H: Higher cortical dysfunction, antiphospholipid antibodies and neuroradiological examinations in systemic lupus erythematosus. Intern Med 31:1169, 1992.

231. Sabet A, Sibbitt WL, Stidley CA, et al: Neurometabolite markers of cerebral injury in the antiphospholipid antibody syndrome of systemic lupus erythematosus. Stroke 29:2254, 1998.

232. Nowacki P, Ronin-Walknowska E, Ossowicka-Stepinska J: Central nervous system involvement in pregnant rabbits with experimental model of antiphospholipid syndrome. Folia Neuropathol 36:38, 1998.

233. Smith HR, Hansen CL, Rose R, Canoso RT: Autoimmune MRL-1 pr/1pr mice are an animal model for the secondary antiphospholipid syndrome. J Rheumatol 17:911, 1990.

234. Garcia CO, Kanbour-Shakir A, Tang H, et al: Induction of experimental antiphospholipid syndrome in PL/J mice following immunization with beta 2 GPI. Am J Reprod Immunol 37:118, 1997.

235. Ziporen L, Shoenfeld Y, Levy Y, Korczyn AD: Neurological dysfunction and hyperactive behavior associated with antiphospholipid antibodies: A mouse model. J Clin Invest 100:613, 1997.

236. Triplett DA: Antiphospholipid-protein antibodies: Laboratory detection and clinical relevance. Thromb Res 78:1, 1995.

237. Khamashta MA, Cuadrado MJ, Mujic F, et al: The management of thrombosis in the antiphospholipid-antibody syndrome. N Engl J Med 332:993, 1995.

238. The feasibility of a collaborative, double-blind study using anticoagulant: The Warfarin-Aspirin Recurrent Stroke Study (WARSS), the Antiphospholipid Antibody in Stroke Study (APASS), the Patent Foramen Ovale Study (PICSS) and the Hemostatic System Activation Study (HAS). WARSS, APASS, PICSS and HAS Study Groups. Cerebrovasc Dis 7:100, 1997.

239. Julkunen H, Hedman C, Kauppi M: Thrombolysis for acute ischemic stroke in the primary antiphospholipid syndrome. J Rheumatol 24:181, 1997.

240. Graham IM, Daly LE, Refsum HM, et al: Plasma homocysteine as a risk factor for vascular disease. JAMA 277:1775, 1997.

241. Mudd SH, Levy HL, Skouby F: Disorders of transsulfuration. In Scriver C, Beaudet AL, Sly WS, Valle D (eds): The Metabolic Basis of Inherited Disease, 6th ed, vol 1. New York, McGraw-Hill, 1989, p 693.

242. Moser FG, Miller ST, Bello JA: The spectrum of brain abnormalities in sickle-cell disease: A report from the Cooperative Study of Sickle Cell Disease. AJNR Am J Neuroradiol 17:965, 1996.

243. Bostom AG, Rosenberg IH, Silbershatz H, et al: Nonfasting plasma total homocysteine levels and stroke incidence in elderly persons: The Framingham Study. Ann Intern Med 131:352, 1999.

244. Bots ML, Launer LJ, Lindemans J, et al: Homocysteine and short-term risk of myocardial infarction and stroke in the elderly: the Rotterdam Study. Arch Intern Med 159:38, 1999.

245. Boushey CJ, Beresford SAA, Omenn GS, Motulsky AG: A quantitative assessment of plasma homocysteine as a risk factor for vascular disease—probable benefits of increasing folic acid intakes. JAMA 274:1049, 1995.

246. Fortin IJ, Genest J Jr: Measurement of homocyst(e)ine in the prediction of atherosclerosis. Clin Biochem 28:155, 1995.

247. Hogeveen M, Blom HJ, Van Amerongen M, et al: Hyperhomocysteinemia as a risk factor for ischemic and hemorrhagic stroke in newborn infants. J Pediatr 141:429, 2002.

248. Boers GHJ, Smals AGH, Trijbels FJM, et al: Heterozygosity for homocystinuria in premature peripheral and cerebral occlusive arterial disease. N Engl J Med 313:709, 1985.

249. Brattstrom LE, Israelsson B, Jeppson J-O, Hultberg BL: Folic acid: An innocuous means to reduce plasma homocysteine. Scand J Clin Lab Invest 48:215, 1988.

250. Coull BM, Malinow MR, Beamer N, et al: Elevated plasma homocyst(e)ine concentration as a possible independent risk factor for stroke. Stroke 21:572, 1990.

251. Clarke R, Daly L, Robinson K, et al: Hyperhomocysteinemia: An independent risk factor for vascular disease. N Engl J Med 324:1149, 1991.

252. Perry IJ, Refsum H, Morris RW, et al: Prospective study of serum total homocysteine concentration and risk of stroke in middle-aged British men. Lancet 346:1395, 1995.

253. Malinow MR, Nieto FJ, Szklo M, et al: Carotid artery intimal-medial wall thickening and plasma homocyst(e)ine in asymptomatic adults: The Atherosclerosis Risk in Communities Study. Circulation 87:1107, 1993.

254. Bostom AG, Selhub J, Jacques PF, Rosenberg IH: Power shortage: Clinical trials testing the "homocysteine hypothesis" against a background of folic acid-fortified cereal grain flour. Ann Intern Med 135:133, 2001.

255. Ubbink JB, Becker PJ, Vermaak WJH, Delport R: Results of B-vitamin supplementation study used in a prediction model to define a reference range for plasma homocysteine. Clin Chem 41:1033, 1995.

256. Verhoef P, Hennekens CH, Malinow MR, et al: A prospective study of plasma homocyst(e)ine and risk of ischemic stroke. Stroke 25:1924, 1994.

257. Kang SS, Passen EL, Ruggie N, et al: Thermolabile defect of methylenetetrahydrofolate reductase in coronary artery disease. Circulation 88:1463, 1993.

258. Frosst P, Blom HJ, Milos R, et al: A candidate genetic risk factor for vascular disease: A common mutation in methylenetetrahydrofolate reductase [letter]. Nature Genet 10:111, 1995.

259. Gallagher PM, Meleady R, Shields DC, et al: Homocysteine and risk of premature coronary heart disease: Evidence for a common gene mutation. Circulation 94:2154, 1996.

260. Kluijtmans LAJ, Van den Heuvel LPWJ, Boers GHJ, et al: Molecular genetic analysis of mild hyperhomocysteinemia: A common mutation in the methylenetetrahydrofolate reductase gene is a genetic risk factor for cardiovascular disease. Am J Hum Genet 58:35, 1996.

261. DeLoughery TG, Evans A, Sadeghi A, et al: Common mutation in methylenetetrahydrofolate reductase—correlation with homocysteine metabolism and late-onset vascular disease. Circulation 94:3074, 1996.

262. McCully KS: Vascular pathology of homocysteinemia: Implications for the pathogenesis of atherosclerosis. Am J Pathol 56:111, 1969.

263. Harpel PC, Zhang X, Borth W: Homocysteine and hemostasis: Pathogenic mechanisms predisposing to thrombosis. J Nutr 126(Suppl 4):1290S, 1996.

264. Upchurch GR Jr, Welch GN, Loscalzo J: Homocysteine, EDRF, and endothelial function. J Nutr 126(Suppl 4):1290S, 1996.

265. Green MA, Noguchi CT, Marwah SS, et al: Polymerization of sickle cell hemoglobin at arterial oxygen saturation impairs erythrocyte deformability. J Clin Invest 81:1669, 1988.

266. Keidan AJ, Sowter MC, Johnson CS, et al: Effect of polymerization tendency on hematological, rheological and clinical parameters in sickle cell anemia. Br J Haematol 71:551, 1989.

267. Rothman SM, Fulling KH, Nelson JS: Sickle cell anemia and central nervous system infarction: A neuropathological study. Ann Neurol 20:684, 1986.

268. Ohene-Frempong K, Weiner SJ, Sleeper LA, et al: Cerebrovascular accidents in sickle cell disease: Rate and risk factors. Blood 91:288, 1998.

269. Miller ST, Macklin EA, Pegelow CH, et al: Silent infarction as a risk factor for overt stroke in children with sickle cell anemia: A report from the cooperative study of sickle cell disease. J Pediatr 139:385, 2001.

270. Wang W, Enos L, Gallagher D, et al: Neuropsychologic performance in school-aged children with sickle cell disease: A report from the Cooperative Study of Sickle Cell Disease. J Pediatr 139:391, 2001.

271. Adams RJ, Nichols FT, Figueroa R, et al: Transcranial Doppler correlation with cerebral angiography in sickle cell disease. Stroke 23:1073, 1992.

272. Verlhac S, Bernaudin F, Tortrat D, et al: Detection of cerebrovascular disease in patients with sickle cell disease using transcranial Doppler sonography: Correlation with MRI, MRA and conventional angiography. Pediatr Radiol 25(Suppl 1):S14, 1995.

273. Radhakrishnan K, Thacker AK, Maloo JC, El-Mangoush MA: Sickle cell trait and stroke in the young adult. Postgrad Med J 66:1078, 1990.

274. Reyes MG: Subcortical cerebral infarctions in sickle cell trait. J Neurol Neurosurg Psychiatry 52:516, 1989.

275. Stockman JA, Nigro MA, Mishkin NM, et al: Occlusion of large cerebral vessels in sickle cell anemia. N Engl J Med 287:846, 1972.

276. Portnoy BA, Herion JC: Neurological manifestations in sickle cell disease. Ann Intern Med 76:643, 1972.

277. Pavlakis SG, Bello J, Prohovnik I, et al: Brain infarction in sickle cell anemia: Magnetic resonance imaging correlates. Ann Neurol 23:125, 1988.

Specific Medical Diseases and Stroke

278. Prohovnik I, Pavlakis SG, Piomelli S, et al: Cerebral hyperemia, stroke and transfusion in sickle cell disease. Neurology (NY) 39:334, 1989.

279. Pegelow CH, Adams RJ, McKie V, et al: Risk of recurrent stroke in patients with sickle cell disease treated with erythrocyte transfusions. J Pediatr 126:896, 1995.

280. Powars D, Wilson B, Imbus C, et al: The natural history of stroke in sickle cell disease. Am J Med 65:461, 1978.

281. Davies SC, Olatunji PO: Blood transfusion in sickle cell disease. Vox Sang 68:145, 1995.

282. Scothorn D, Price C, Schwartz D, et al: Risk of recurrent stroke in children with sickle cell disease receiving blood transfusion therapy for at least five years after initial stroke. J Pediatr 140:348, 2002.

283. Walters MC, Patience M, Leisenring W, et al: Bone marrow transplantation for sickle cell disease. N Engl J Med 335:369, 1996.

284. Platt OS, Guinan EC: Bone marrow transplantation in sickle cell anemia—the dilemma of choice. N Engl J Med 335:426, 1996.

285. Charache S, Terrin ML, Moore RD, et al: Effect of hydroxyurea on the frequency of painful crises in sickle cell anemia. Multicenter Study of Hydroxyurea in Sickle Cell Anemia Investigators. N Engl J Med 332:1317, 1995.

286. Claster S, Vichinsky E: First report of reversal of organ dysfunction in sickle cell anemia by the use of hydroxyurea: Splenic regeneration. Blood 88:1951, 1996.

287. Ferster A, Vermylen C, Cornu G, et al: Hydroxyurea for treatment of severe sickle cell anemia: A pediatric clinical trial. Blood 88:1960, 1996.

Chapter Thirty-Five

Stroke and Substance Abuse

John C. M. Brust

Drug dependence is "a state of psychic or physical dependence, or both, on a drug, arising in a person following administration of that drug on a periodic or continuous basis."[1] Drug abuse, on the other hand, implies a social judgment, whether or not the substance is taken continuously, periodically, or infrequently, and whether or not it is legally available. When alcohol and tobacco are included, millions of Americans are substance abusers, and many of them are at increased risk of stroke, either occlusive or hemorrhagic.[2–4] Mechanisms vary, including a higher incidence of atherosclerotic infarction in alcohol drinkers, cerebral complications of endocarditis common in parenteral drug abusers, and vasculitides affecting users of particular substances.[5,6]

OPIATES

It is estimated that heroin has been used at least once by more than 2 million Americans and that nearly 1 million are psychically or physically dependent.[7,8] The most common causes of death among heroin abusers are violence, overdose, acute adverse reactions, and acquired immunodeficiency syndrome (AIDS).[9] Stroke is another medical complication. Heroin is usually taken parenterally (and by addicts, more than once a day), and so infectious endocarditis is common,[10–15] especially with *Staphylococcus aureus* and *Candida*.[16] It affects the mitral, aortic, and tricuspid valves with equal frequency[17] and often causes cerebral emboli.

Stroke associated with endocarditis can be occlusive or hemorrhagic. Infarction follows embolic vessel occlusion or, less often, bacterial or fungal meningitis. Cerebral or subarachnoid hemorrhage usually occurs after rupture of a septic (mycotic) aneurysm.[18–20] Unlike saccular (berry) aneurysms, septic aneurysms are more likely to manifest with subtle or insidiously progressive neurologic or systemic symptoms (e.g., headache, fever, syncope, hemiparesis, aphasia) than with a sudden onset suggesting subarachnoid hemorrhage; also, cerebrospinal fluid (CSF) white cell pleocytosis may occur in asymptomatic patients with endocarditis days before a mycotic aneurysm ruptures.[21] The infrequency with which mycotic aneurysms spontaneously disappear during antimicrobial therapy, the high mortality associated with their rupture, and the relative ease (compared with berry aneurysms) of their

surgical removal support the view that cerebral angiography should be performed in patients with endocarditis who have either unexplained neurologic symptoms or abnormal CSF findings, and that, once found, most mycotic aneurysms should be promptly excised.[21,22] Mycotic aneurysms in heroin users have also occurred on the carotid and subclavian arteries.[23,23a]

Heroin users may also have hemorrhagic stroke secondary to hepatitis, liver failure, and deranged clotting, or to heroin nephropathy with uremia or malignant hypertension. Nine heroin addicts were reported from Harlem Hospital Center with stroke unassociated with endocarditis.[24] In three, ranging in age from 41 to 45 years, the relation of stroke to heroin was uncertain: one patient, while using heroin, had an intracerebral hemorrhage in the presence of probable heroin nephropathy and malignant hypertension; another, who was normotensive, had a basal ganglia hemorrhage 3 days after beginning methadone detoxification; the third, who was mildly hypertensive, had a probable capsular infarct 6 weeks after starting methadone maintenance. In the other six patients, ages 25 to 38 years, heroin appeared to be more directly causal. Four of the patients, all of whom were normotensive, had probable cerebral infarcts in association with loss of consciousness after intravenous injection of heroin. Cerebral angiography was normal in one of the patients but in another showed stenosis of the internal carotid artery at the siphon and of the proximal anterior cerebral artery, plus occlusion of the middle cerebral artery; the changes suggested primary vessel disease more than emboli. Cerebral infarctions occurred in the two remaining patients who were using heroin at the time, although the strokes were not related to overdose and did not follow recent injections. In one of these patients, who was normotensive, cerebral angiography suggested widespread small vessel arteritis. None of these patients was using oral contraceptives or had other illnesses that would predispose to stroke. Consistent with hypersensitivity, one patient had 10% eosinophilia, serum hypergammaglobulinemia, and a positive direct Coombs test result, and another had an erythrocyte sedimentation rate (ESR) of 94 mm/h and two positive latex fixation test results. Except for cocaine in one patient (whose stroke followed an acute reaction to heroin), these nine patients were using no other drugs.

Other reports of stroke in heroin abusers include that of a 19-year-old man who had taken heroin intravenously weekly for a year and had used lysergic acid diethylamide (LSD) intermittently; he experienced sudden global aphasia, and cerebral angiography suggested diffuse angiitis.[25] A 21-year-old woman demonstrated hemiparesis 2 weeks after starting daily heroin use and 6 hours after an intravenous injection.[26] Symptoms began with vomiting, headache, sweating, and shortness of breath, suggesting anaphylaxis, and cerebral angiography showed narrowing and irregularity of the distal internal carotid artery, suggesting arteritis. Eosinophilia and the fact that her husband had shared her heroin were consistent with hypersensitivity to heroin or to an adulterant. A normotensive 20-year-old man who had used heroin occasionally for 2 years took his first intravenous injection in 8 months and experienced sudden left homonymous hemianopia and incoordination; cerebral angiography showed "beading" of the right posterior cerebral artery.[27] Acute severe cerebellar ataxia followed intra-arterial injection of heroin in another patient.[28] Other heroin-associated infarcts resulted in aphasia and cortical blindness.[29,30] Ischemic stroke has also occurred after heroin sniffing[31]; in one such case, involving a 34-year-old man, cerebral angiography was normal.[32] A young German man had an intracerebral hemorrhage within minutes of intravenous injection of heroin.[33] Rupture of a cerebellar vascular malformation was reported in a woman who had sniffed heroin for many years.[34]

Heroin could cause stroke by a number of possible mechanisms.[24,35] Following heroin overdose, hypoventilation and hypotension can produce permanent brain damage with bilateral cerebral leukoencephalopathy.[36] Hemiplegia has appeared on awakening from naloxone-responsive coma[24,37]; overdose has also caused spastic quadriparesis, dementia, deafness, seizures, dystonia, and ballism.[38,39] Delayed postanoxic encephalopathy also occurs.[40–42] Bilateral globus pallidus infarction is commonly observed at autopsy in heroin users,[43–46] and hemichorea was present in a patient with heroin stroke.[24] In some cases an awkward position of the neck during overdose coma might have kinked the carotid artery and further decreased cerebral perfusion.[37] In no stroke patient, however, has hypotension been documented, nor has any had bibracheal palsy or other signs suggestive of border-zone ("watershed") infarction.[47,48]

Direct toxic injury from either heroin or an adulterant is another possibility. Heroin is often mixed with quinine and lactose or mannitol, as well, on occasion, as talc, starch, curry powder, abrasive cleanser, caffeine, or even strychnine.[35] Quinine caused amblyopia in a heroin addict[49] and may contribute to acute adverse reactions with pulmonary edema or sudden death after parenteral injection.[50,51] There is no evidence linking quinine to stroke, however.

Embolization of foreign material to the brain has not been observed in parenteral heroin users (even though the jugular vein is commonly used, with occasional accidental arterial injection) but has been documented at autopsy in abusers of other agents, including opiates.[52–54] Probably because of restricted heroin supply, pentazocine (Talwin) and tripelennamine (Pyribenzamine) ("Ts and Blues") were widely abused in Chicago and other Midwestern cities during the 1970s.[55,56] Oral tablets were crushed, suspended in water, passed through cotton or a cigarette filter, and injected intravenously, and cerebral infarcts and hemorrhages occurred in users.[57] Common at autopsy was pulmonary arteriolar occlusion by microcrystalline cellulose[58] or particulate magnesium silicate (talc),[59] which had been used to bind pentazocine and tripelennamine. Such microemboli also reached the brain, especially when multiple lung emboli produced pulmonary hypertension and opened "functional pulmonary arteriovenous shunts."[35] "Beaded arteries" were seen at cerebral angiography in "Ts and Blues" stroke patients, consistent with vasculitis, in turn secondary to "a granulomatous or immune process provoked by the injection of foreign material."[35]

Talc microemboli were also found at autopsy in the liver, spleen, and central nervous system of a parenteral paregoric abuser.[60] A young man who several times a day injected pulverized unfiltered meperidine tablets intravenously had occasional seizures after injection and then experienced difficulty with concentration, impaired memory, and visual blurring; fundal hemorrhages and areas of arterial occlusion were seen, and his symptoms improved with abstinence.[61]

Posterior cerebral artery occlusion followed intravenous injection of a melted hydromorphone (Dilaudid) suppository, the authors speculated that the mechanism was paradoxical fat embolism of the product's cocoa butter content.[62]

Some heroin strokes follow the first injection in weeks or months, and laboratory findings further suggest an immunologic cause. Heroin nephropathy may be immunologically mediated[63–66]; the C3 component of complement is reduced in patients with heroin pulmonary edema; and heroin addicts frequently have hypergammaglobulinemia[14, 67] (including elevated immunoglobulin IgM independent of IgG and IgA levels[68–71]), circulating immune complexes,[71] antibodies to smooth muscle and lymphocyte membranes,[69] false-positive serology,[67,72] and lymph node hypertrophy.[35] Opium, morphine, codeine, and meperidine, moreover, have caused urticaria, angioneurotic edema, and anaphylaxis.[73] Whether the offending antigen is the opiate or a contaminant is unclear, but morphine binding by gamma globulin is reported in addicts[74,75] and experimental animals.[76,77]

Relevant to heroin stroke and its possible mechanisms is heroin myelopathy. Acute paraparesis, sensory loss, and urinary retention have been reported in at least 16 heroin users, occurring shortly after injection and frequently following a period of abstinence.[15,78–83] In some, symptoms were present when they awakened from coma. Proprioception and vibratory sense were often preserved relative to loss of spinothalamic sensory modalities, suggesting infarction in the territory of the anterior spinal artery,[84–87] and in a patient with bilateral pallidal infarction, there was also magnetic resonance imaging (MRI) evidence of spinal cord border zone infarction.[44] Several hours after snorting heroin, a man awoke with flaccid paralysis of the legs and urinary retention; MRI showed midthoracic transverse myelitis.[88] Autopsy in another patient showed necrosis "confined almost entirely" to the upper thoracic spinal cord gray matter and in yet another demonstrated additional involvement of the anterior aspect of the posterior columns and a pyramidal tract in the lower thoracic cord.[79] If these lesions were cord infarcts, their possible causes, as with cerebral stroke in heroin users, include "watershed" infarction during a period of coma, hypoventilation, and hypotension[86] as well as hypersensitivity reaction. Consistent with the latter, one young man, remaining conscious, had several episodes of numbness and weakness of both legs for a few minutes after injection.[80]

Eleven days after injection an adolescent demonstrated a rash on the chest and feet and then, 6 days later, became paraplegic after a second injection.[82] Cord biopsy in another patient, moreover, showed vasculitis affecting mainly small arteries and arterioles, with "double refractile fragments" in inflamed tissue, including vessel walls.[89] (Such foreign particles are also seen in the skin of heroin addicts.[90]) A patient at Harlem Hospital had heroin injected into a vessel over his midthoracic spine and within 30 minutes experienced paraparesis and then urinary retention and sensory loss below that level. Myelography was normal. Whether the vessel injected was arterial or venous, the common intercostal origins of the posterior cutaneous and spinal arteries or veins would have allowed injected material direct access to the spinal cord[91,92]; that occurrence would not, however, distinguish whether the damage was direct toxicity, hypersensitivity, or embolism of foreign material.

A man using intravenous heroin for the first time in 2 years became comatose and apneic; after he received an opiate antagonist, quadriplegia, anarthria, dysphagia, and sensory loss consistent with a ventral pontine lesion developed over several hours.[93] Recovery was partial, and whether or not the lesion was vascular was not determined.

A heroin addict with unexplained clotting abnormalities was found to have high circulating levels of heparin, presumably added to her drug mixture[94]; if heparin becomes a common adulterant, addicts are obviously at increased risk for hemorrhagic stroke.

AMPHETAMINE AND RELATED AGENTS

Although their manufacture was greatly reduced after the 1972 Controlled Substances Act, amphetamine and similar stimulants are still produced in huge quantities.[95] There are two patterns of abuse. Housewives, truck drivers, or students may take it orally, often with sedatives or alcohol. Addicts more often take it intravenously, sometimes in doses of up to 300 mg every few hours over days. Strokes common to any parenteral drug abuse are therefore encountered. There are also strokes that may be unique to these agents.

Acutely amphetamine can cause excitement, hypertension, and a rectal temperature exceeding 109°F, followed by coma, vascular collapse, and death[96–101]; at autopsy, diffuse cerebral edema and petechiae are seen, without large infarcts or hematomas.[96,98,101–103] In dogs[104] or rabbits[105] given lethal doses of amphetamine, there was severe hyperpyrexia. At autopsy there was subendocardial and epicardial hemorrhage, myocardial fiber necrosis, and, in the brain, neuronal degeneration in the cerebral cortex and cerebellum.[104–106] Curare prevented the fever and the fatal course, suggesting that the hyperpyrexia was secondary to muscle hyperactivity and that death was secondary to heat stroke. Fever may have also contributed to similar brain

pathologic findings in cats receiving long-term methamphetamine over 2 weeks, although in that study, neuronal catecholamine depletion was suspected as the primary cause.[68,107]

Significant brain hemorrhage was not present in these experimental animals but has been found, along with focal neurologic signs, in animal and human cases of heat stroke,[108–111] often with severe clotting abnormalities, including decreased prothrombin activity, thrombocytopenia, hypofibrinogenemia, and fibrinolysis.[112] Hyperpyrexia and disturbed clotting have not been reported, however, with intracranial hemorrhage after amphetamine use. More than 30 patients have been reported, ages 16 to 60 years.[113–138] Eighteen had taken the drug orally, nine intravenously, two orally and intravenously, one nasally and intravenously, five by inhalation, and two by an uncertain route. Most were chronic users, but in five patients, stroke followed a first exposure. The dose was usually unknown but in one case was as low as 80 mg. Except for one instance each of diethylpropion and pseudoephedrine, all the reported patients took amphetamine or methamphetamine; seven also took methylphenidate, LSD, dimethoxymethylamphetamine ("STP"), cocaine, heroin, or barbiturates. Severe headache usually occurred within minutes of drug use. Blood pressure was elevated in 15 of the 26 patients in whom it was recorded, with diastolic pressures as high as 120 mm Hg in 5. Eight patients died, usually soon after admission. Computed tomography (CT), performed on 14 patients, variably showed intracerebral hemorrhage (frequently lobar), subarachnoid hemorrhage, or no abnormality. In 12 patients, angiography revealed irregular narrowing ("beading") of distal cerebral arteries, suggesting vasculitis; three of these patients had taken the drug only orally. Such vessel changes were present at autopsy in three patients (including one whose angiogram showed only an avascular mass). In another patient, a cerebral vascular malformation was seen on both angiography and CT.

Thus, some of these amphetamine-induced intracranial hemorrhages seem to have been secondary to acute hypertension, some to cerebral vasculitis, and some to a combination of the two, but in others neither feature was apparent. Although acute hypertension secondary to amphetamine could be causal, it might have been a transient result of the stroke in some patients.[139] Conversely, in other patients, fleeting blood pressure elevations could have been missed.

Amphetamine-induced cerebral vasculitis, which has caused occlusive as well as hemorrhagic strokes, appears to be of more than one type. Necrotizing angiitis, sometimes affecting the nervous system, occurred in 14 Los Angeles abusers of multiple drugs, including amphetamine, methedrine, barbiturates, chlordiazepoxide, diazepam, marijuana, hydroxyzine, LSD, heroin, meperidine, mescaline, oxycodone, oxymorphone, dimethoxymethylamphetamine, and strychnine.[140] All but two patients used intravenous methamphetamine, and one used it exclusively. Five patients were asymptomatic; in the others, symptoms included fever, weight loss, malaise, weakness, skin rash, pneumonitis, pulmonary edema, hematuria, proteinuria, renal failure, abdominal pain, pancreatitis, gastrointestinal hemorrhage, arthralgia, myalgia, peripheral neuropathy, anemia, leukocytosis, and hemolysis. One patient had renal failure, severe hypertension, papilledema, retinal detachment, "progressive encephalopathy," and, at autopsy, vasculitis affecting pontine arterioles. Another, who had demonstrated "mental obtundation" and hypertension at autopsy showed "recent and resolving cerebral and pontine infarction," "marked cerebellar hemorrhage," and vasculitis in the cerebrum, cerebellum, and brainstem. Vessel lesions consisted initially of fibrinoid necrosis of the media and intima, with infiltration by neutrophils, eosinophils, lymphocytes, and histiocytes; later, there was destruction of muscular and elastic components, replacement by collagen, and often "a nodular (nodose) bulge with nearly aneurysmal dilatation." The authors considered these lesions, which affected only muscular arteries and arterioles, typical for polyarteritis nodosa and distinguished them from hypersensitivity angiitis, which involves small arteries, capillaries, and venules.[140] They further noted that more than one drug or adulterant could have caused these lesions, and that, in contrast to polyarteritis nodosa,[141,142] the lesions observed in these patients were not associated with the presence of hepatitis antigen.[143]

Such brain lesions have been found pathologically in other polydrug (including amphetamine) abusers.[124, 144] In some, however, cerebral arteritis has been presumed on the basis of cerebral angiography,[113,114,118,128,138,145,146] and sometimes the relation to amphetamine abuse has been tenuous. In a report of three young men who experienced ischemic strokes in association with intranasal methamphetamine, cerebral angiography revealed supraclinoid beading of the internal carotid artery in one, occlusion of the internal carotid artery near its origin in another, and supraclinoid occlusion of the internal carotid artery in the third.[147] In another report, thalamic infarction followed intranasal methamphetamine use, but angiography was not performed.[148]

A radiographic study of 19 young drug abusers, most taking intravenous methamphetamine and hospitalized for coma or stroke, revealed widespread segmental constrictions of large and medium-sized cerebral arteries and stenosis or occlusion of many penetrating arterioles, consistent with either multiple emboli or vasculitis and thrombosis.[145] The same researchers then gave rhesus monkeys intravenous methamphetamine, 1.5 mg/kg (considered the lower limit of dosage for most abusers), and performed serial cerebral angiograms for 2 weeks.[149] Several animals studied 10 minutes after receiving the drugs showed irregularly decreased caliber of small cerebral vessels, with a return to normal at 24 hours. In others, these changes occurred in both small and large vessels and persisted for the 2-week period; in one animal, the changes actually worsened with time. Clinically, the animals had hypertension and behavioral change. Postmortem examination at 2 weeks revealed subarachnoid hemorrhage in some animals, with numerous brain petechial hemorrhages, infarcts, edema, microaneurysms, and perivascular white blood cell cuffing. In a later study, monkeys received intravenous methamphetamine three times weekly.[150] After either a month or a year, serial angiograms showed occlusions and slow blood flow in small cerebral arteries, and autopsy revealed attenuated and fragmented brain arterioles and capillaries, microaneurysms, dilated venules,

petechiae, neuronal loss, and gliosis. Talc crystals were present in capillaries (the drug was given as crushed methamphetamine hydrochloride [Desoxyn] tablets); but arguing against the notion that such particles play a critical role in the vasculitis was the finding that in the animals receiving crushed placebo tablets containing all the ingredients of Desoxyn except methamphetamine, vasculitis was minimal or absent.

In rats receiving 2 weeks of intravenous methamphetamine, electron microscopy showed that brain capillaries had abnormal "budding" from the luminal walls of endothelial cells and vesicles within the endothelial cell cytoplasm.[150] These changes affected vessels smaller than 100 μm and would therefore be missed on angiography. (The vulnerability of small vessels might be related to their separate innervation; large cerebral vessels are innervated by the peripheral sympathetic nervous system, but nerve terminals on smaller arteries appear to be from central noradrenergic neurons.[151])

Of three monkeys receiving intravenous methylphenidate (Ritalin) for a month, all had "a moderate degree of vascular change" on angiography, but only one had "some chromatolysis histologically."[152] Rats receiving methylphenidate, however, had the same severe degree of histologic brain damage as those receiving methamphetamine.

These lesions are different from those of polyarteritis nodosa, in which elastic arteries, capillaries, and veins are spared. Whether the lesions in methamphetamine users are the result of direct toxicity or of hypersensitivity is unclear, nor can the possibility be excluded that the early angiographic findings are secondary to subarachnoid hemorrhage (although beading of distal pial arteries in subarachnoid hemorrhage is rare).[114] In an adolescent amphetamine abuser with mononeuritis multiplex, sural nerve biopsy showed apparent hypersensitivity angiitis of medium and small muscular arteries, arterioles, venules, and veins, with fibrinoid necrosis and infiltration by polymorphonuclear leukocytes, lymphocytes, eosinophils, and plasma cells.[153] The central nervous system was clinically unaffected, however.

Phenylpropanolamine (PPA), a drug similar to but less potent than amphetamine, was marketed, sometimes with ephedrine or caffeine, in over-the-counter decongestants (e.g., Contac) and diet pills (e.g., Dex-a-diet, Dexatrim, Anorexin, Maxi-slim), as well as in drugs made deliberately to resemble amphetamine ("look-alike pills").[154,155] During the 1980s and 1990s, an estimated 5 billion doses of PPA were used in the United States annually.[156] Acute hypertension, severe headache, psychiatric symptoms, seizures, and hemorrhagic stroke occurred in users.[150,155,157-166] A case reported as "cerebral arteritis" in a PPA user was based simply on angiographic "beading."[167] PPA with caffeine, from a commercial diet preparation, produced subarachnoid hemorrhage in rats receiving it intraperitoneally at three to six times the recommended dose.[162]

In 2000, a case-control study involving 43 U.S. hospitals found that appetite suppressants containing PPA increase the risk of subarachnoid or intracerebral hemorrhage in women (odds ratio [OR], 16.58). No men in that study used PPA-containing diet pills, but a trend toward higher hemorrhagic stroke risk was observed in men and women using PPA-containing cough and cold remedies. The greater risk associated with diet pills was attributed to higher daily doses.[168] That year, the U.S. Food and Drug Administration (FDA) ordered products containing PPA to be withdrawn from the market.[169]

Ephedrine and pseudoephedrine are present in over-the-counter decongestants and bronchodilators. Complications of these agents include headache, tachyarrhythmia, hypertensive emergency, and hemorrhagic and occlusive stroke.[170–175] A young man who had previously used "speed" and LSD had a subarachnoid hemorrhage within an hour of ingesting pills that turned out to be ephedrine.[176] Cerebral angiography was initially normal, but angiography performed a week later showed beading and branch occlusions suggesting arteritis; a biopsy from grossly normal skin showed periluminal deposits of IgM and the C3 component of complement in dermal vessels, consistent with circulating immune complexes.

Dietary supplements containing ephedra alkaloids (ma huang) are popular in the United States for energy enhancement and weight reduction. An estimated 12 million people used these supplements in 1999. Cardiotoxicity (including sudden death) and ischemic and hemorrhagic strokes have been reported in users.[177–180] A review of 140 adverse events associated with ephedra use and reported to the FDA revealed stroke in 10 people and seizures in 7.[181] These products, bearing names such as "Shape-up Plus" and "Ultimate Orange," often contain caffeine, which, as an adenosine receptor antagonist, probably aggravates ephedra's vasoconstrictor and pressor actions.

Ischemic stroke was reported in two users of the anorexiant phentermine; one patient also used phendimetrazine.[182] Intracerebral hemorrhage occurred in a middle-aged woman taking fenfluramine and phentermine.[183] A cohort study of subjects taking appetite suppressants found that dexfenfluramine, fenfluramine, and phentermine increased the risk of stroke (OR, 2.4), but the confidence intervals were wide.[184] In 1998, all of these agents were withdrawn from the U.S. market because of reported cardiac valvular abnormalities associated with their use.[185]

Ischemic stroke occurred in a young man after intranasal use of amphetamine combined with caffeine.[186] Ischemic stroke has followed recreational use of 3,4-methylene-dioxymethamphetamine ("ecstasy").[187,188]

A young woman who injected crushed methylphenidate tablets into her jugular veins experienced immediate right hemiplegia after a left injection and, 2 months later, left hemiplegia after a right injection; presumably the injections were inadvertently made into the carotid artery, but the exact mechanism of stroke was not determined.[189] Intraretinal talc microemboli have been seen in the fundi of intravenous methylphenidate abusers.[52,190] In some there were retinal vascular and choroidal abnormalities, neovascularization, and vitreous hemorrhage,[190] and in one abuser, who had not had a clinical stroke, talc and cornstarch emboli were also present in arterioles, capillaries, and veins of the brain and lung.[52] Infarction of the medial medulla in a young woman occurred a few minutes after intravenous injection of methylphenidate; at autopsy there was systemic granulomatosis due to talc and talc deposits in small vessels around the medullary infarct.[53]

Mycotic subclavian and carotid aneurysms have been reported after inadvertant intra-arterial injection of phentermine.[191]

Death has followed parenteral[191a] or oral[192] abuse of propylhexedrine from nasal decongestant inhalers; stroke has not yet been reported in such patients, and the cause of death has been uncertain.

COCAINE

Use of cocaine became widespread in the United States in the 1980s. It was estimated in 1982, that 28% of people ages 18 to 25 years had used cocaine hydrochloride, usually intranasally but often parenterally (including cocaine-heroin mixtures, so-called "speedballs").[6] In 1985, the appearance of commercially prepared alkaloidal cocaine ("crack") led to acceleration of the epidemic. During 1998, nearly 2 million Americans were regular cocaine users.[193] Smokable "crack" produces a psychological "high" even more intense than that following intravenous injection of cocaine hydrochloride and is taken in larger and more frequent doses. Increasing morbidity and mortality, including stroke, have resulted.[194,195]

Parenteral cocaine users are at risk for stroke related to infection, including endocarditis, AIDS, and hepatitis. They also experience strokes caused directly by the drug itself, whether taken intranasally, intravenously, or intramuscularly or smoked as "crack."[196] The first report of a cocaine-related stroke appeared in 1977; a middle-aged, mildly hypertensive man injected cocaine intramuscularly after drinking a bottle of wine and an hour later abruptly experienced aphasia and right hemiparesis; CSF findings were normal, and cerebral angiography was refused.[197] The same year, fatal rupture of a cerebral saccular aneurysm occurred in a young man sniffing cocaine.[198] Further cases were not reported until the mid-1980s, but by the mid-1990s, more than 400 cases of cocaine-related stroke had been described, about half occlusive and half hemorrhagic.[53,152,199–271]

Ischemic strokes have included transient ischemic attacks and infarctions of cerebrum, thalamus, brainstem, spinal cord, retina, and peripheral oculomotor nerve.[211,232,272–280] Infarction has occurred in newborns whose mothers used cocaine shortly before delivery[204] and in pregnant women.[196,211,232,272] In some cases, cerebral infarction was attributed to vasculitis on the basis of angiographic findings[227]; such changes, however, may represent vasospasm after undiagnosed subarachnoid hemorrhage.[281] Autopsies usually show histologically normal cerebral vessels,[196,235,246] although in five cases, mild cerebral vasculitis was observed at biopsy or autopsy.[202,215,232,244] In these cases, cerebral angiography was normal. Conversely, in a man with multiple cerebral infarcts diagnosed both clinically and on MRI, angiography showed "multifocal areas of segmental stenosis and dilatation," yet brain biopsy revealed no evidence of vasculitis.[240] A young crack smoker had middle cerebral artery branch occlusion, cardiomyopathy, and a left atrial thrombus.[251] A 20-year-old with no other risk factors had superior cerebellar artery occlusion 6 months after the last use of cocaine, raising the possibility of delayed effects.[184]

In a 27-year-old occasional cocaine sniffer with "heaviness and paresthesias" in the legs and occasional "forgetfulness," MRI revealed multiple periventricular white matter lesions.[269] A young man who had used cocaine "regularly" for 10 years demonstrated progressively impaired cognition; CT revealed patchy areas consistent with infarction, and cerebral angiography showed marked stenosis of the internal carotid and middle cerebral arteries with moyamoya-like collateral vessels.[280] A young woman who had been using "crack" for 12 years experienced mental deterioration progressing to mutism over several weeks; CT showed diffuse cerebral atrophy, but single-photon emission computed tomography (SPECT) showed more focal reductions in perfusion.[282]

Intracerebral or subarachnoid hemorrhage has occurred during or within hours of cocaine use or has shown a less clear temporal relationship.[246,283–285] In some instances there has been other substance use, especially ethanol. Parenchymal hemorrhages have been located in the cerebrum, brainstem, and cerebellum.[246,271,275,276,279,286,287] Also described are superior saggital sinus thrombosis with hemorrhagic venous infarction, mycotic aneurysm rupture, dural arteriovenous fistula, spontaneous spinal epidural hematoma, and bleeding into embolic infarction or glioma.[270,275,288,289] Nearly half the patients with cocaine-associated intracranial hemorrhage who underwent angiography had saccular aneurysms or vascular malformations. Of 150 consecutive patients with subarachnoid hemorrhage, 17 had used cocaine within 72 hours, and mortality and morbidity were worse among the cocaine users, perhaps because of drug-aggravated vasospasm.[261] In another study, 27 of 440 patients with ruptured aneurysm had used cocaine within 72 hours, and although vasospasm was more likely among the cocaine users, there was no difference in clinical outcome.[290] Cerebral hemorrhages have occurred in newborns and postpartum women.[196,223,241] Autopsies on patients with cocaine-induced intracranial hemorrhage have revealed histologically normal cerebral vessels.[217,283]

A case-control study from Atlanta failed to find any association between crack use and stroke; this unexpected finding was probably related to lack of information regarding acute crack use in more than half of the subjects and controls.[291] In another case-control study from California, cocaine use was a strong risk factor for stroke (OR, 13.9).[292]

The mechanisms of cocaine-related stroke are diverse. Striking, if one considers that cocaine and amphetamine have similar actions and effects, is the high frequency of underlying aneurysm or vascular malformation in hemorrhagic strokes in cocaine users compared with amphetamine users, and, conversely, the frequency of vasculitis in amphetamine users compared with cocaine users.[293] Cocaine hydrochloride is more often associated with hemorrhagic than occlusive stroke, whereas hemorrhagic and occlusive strokes occur with roughly equal frequency in "crack" users, but the rising prevalence of stroke since the appearance of "crack" is probably attributable to wider use and higher dosage rather than to a peculiarity of "crack" itself.[294]

Coronary artery vasoconstriction has been documented during cardiac catheterization, and cocaine-induced myocardial infarction, cardiac arrhythmia, and cardiomyopathy carry a risk for embolic stroke.[295–301] More significant, however, is cocaine's effects on systemic and cerebral circulation. By blocking re-uptake of norepinephrine from sympathetic nerve endings (and probably also by affecting calcium flux and serotonin re-uptake), cocaine is a vasoconstrictor.[302–305] Acute hypertension can result, leading to intracranial hemorrhage, especially in subjects with underlying aneurysms or vascular malformations.[246] Cerebral vasoconstriction probably causes occlusive stroke, and it is possibly significant that cocaine metabolites, which in some long-term users are detectable in urine for weeks, also cause cerebral vasospasm.[306,307] In healthy young cocaine users, intravenous cocaine caused dose-related cerebral vasoconstriction (as detected by magnetic resonance angiography),[308] and Doppler ultrasonography revealed increased cerebrovascular resistance that persisted for at least one month during abstinence.[309]

The situation is complex, however, because cerebral and peripheral vessels frequently respond differently to similar stimuli. Whereas intraluminal cocaine constricted cat and rat pial vessels in vitro, topical cocaine dilated pial vessels in living cats,[302,306,310] and intravenous cocaine produced both vasoconstriction and vasodilatation of cerebral vessels in rabbits.[311,312] In swine, cocaine given intravenously caused carotid artery constriction, but there was no response in vitro, suggesting that at least in that species the vasoconstriction effect was indirect, through "release of humoral and/or neural vasoactive substances."[313] Other animal studies show either a central or a peripheral mechanism of action for cocaine-induced vasocontriction.[314,315]

In vitro studies with platelets are conflicting. Cocaine reportedly enhanced the response of platelets to arachidonic acid, thereby promoting aggregation.[316] It also, however, directly inhibited fibrinogen binding to activated platelets and caused dissociation of preformed platelet aggregates.[317] In rabbits, repeated cocaine injections caused arteriosclerotic aortopathy.[318] In a cocaine user with symptoms of coronary artery disease, protein C and antithrombin III levels were depleted but returned to normal, with clearing of symptoms, when use of the drug was discontinued.[298] In long-term cocaine users, immediate administration of cocaine caused erythrocytosis and increased levels of von Willebrand factor.[319]

Ethanol reportedly enhances cocaine toxicity; in the presence of ethanol, cocaine is metabolized to cocaethylene, which, perhaps even more powerfully than cocaine itself, binds to the synaptic dopamine transporter and blocks reuptake.[320] Cocaine and ethanol synergistically depress myocardial contraction.[321] The relevance of these observations to stroke in users of both cocaine and ethanol is uncertain.

It is controversial whether cocaine (or other psychostimulants) causes lasting mental abnormalities and, if so, whether they are a consequence of cerebrovascular disease. Human studies using controls suggest that long-term cocaine use produces subtle cognitive impairment.[322–325] Studies with positron emission tomography (PET) and SPECT in long-term cocaine users found irregularly decreased blood flow in the cerebral cortex; in some of these subjects, CT or MRI findings were normal, and in some (but not all), PET and SPECT abnormalities were associated with deficits on psychometric testing.[326–329] MRI studies in asymptomatic long-term cocaine users found abnormal cerebral white matter signals considered consistent with "subclinical vascular events."[330]

It is also controversial how cocaine affects the fetus. Perinatal and neonatal strokes—both occlusive and hemorrhagic—may be underrecognized in newborns exposed to cocaine in utero.[262,331] Cerebral blood flow studies during the first few days of life in cocaine-exposed neonates are consistent with persisting vasoconstriction.[332] Some investigators speculate that cocaine-induced vasospasm during the first trimester is responsible for CNS malformations (including encephalocele, holoprosencephaly, and hypoplastic cerebellum).[222] Others have doubted such causality.[333]

PHENCYCLIDINE

Phencyclidine (PCP, "angel dust") became a widely abused U.S. street drug in the 1970s; it can be smoked, eaten, or injected and is often misrepresented as marijuana or mescaline. A dose of 1 to 5 mg produces euphoria, emotional lability, and a feeling of diffuse numbness; 5 to 15 mg causes confusion, excitation, decreased sensory perception, and body distortion; higher doses cause psychosis, myoclonus, nystagmus, seizures, coma, and sometimes fatal respiratory and circulatory collapse.[334–337] Hypertension can occur both early and late during intoxication[336,338,339] and may be related to enhancement of the action of catecholamines and serotonin.[340] However, contractile responses to PCP of isolated basilar and middle cerebral arteries were not prevented or reversed by methysergide, phentolamine, atropine, diphenhydramine, or indomethacin, raising the possibility of PCP receptors on cerebral blood vessels.[341]

A 13-year-old boy became comatose after taking PCP; admission blood pressure was normal, and he became more alert. Three days later, however, his condition deteriorated with a blood pressure of 220/130 mm Hg. Autopsy revealed an intracerebral hemorrhage.[339] The urine of a 6-year-old boy who became unresponsive with seizures and right hemiparesis was found to contain PCP; CT demonstrated left parieto-occipital lucency and vessel enhancement, suggesting a vascular malformation. He recovered, and cerebral angiography was not performed.[338] A young man collapsed after smoking PCP; blood pressure was 180/100 mm Hg, and autopsy showed subarachnoid hemorrhage without parenchymal hematoma.[342] A 17-year-old boy with PCP in his blood died after perforation of the ventral surface of the basilar artery.[343] Hypertensive encephalopathy followed PCP ingestion in a young woman with systemic lupus erythematosus and a history of migraine.[344]

LYSERGIC ACID DIETHYLAMIDE

In high doses, LSD causes severe hypertension, obtundation, and convulsions.[345,346] In vitro spasm of cerebral vessel strips immersed in LSD-containing solution was prevented or reversed by methysergide.[341] After ingesting four LSD capsules, a 14-year-old boy experienced seizures and, 4 days later, left hemiplegia; carotid angiography showed progressive narrowing of the internal carotid artery from its origin to the siphon, with occlusion at its bifurcation.[347] A young woman demonstrated sudden left hemiplegia a day after oral ingestion of LSD; angiography showed marked constriction of the internal carotid artery at the siphon; 9 days later, the vessel was occluded at that level.[348] A 19-year-old with acute aphasia and cerebral angiographic findings consistent with arteritis had used both LSD and heroin, but the time relationship of either drug to the stroke was not stated in the report.[25] Another patient with angiographic evidence of vasculitis had used both LSD and "diet pills."[145]

MARIJUANA

Because marijuana is the most widely used illicit drug in the United States, it is hardly surprising that occlusive stroke affects marijuana users; causality is another matter. In fact, the diagnosis of stroke in some reports is dubious. Two young men had only conjugate deviation of the eyes for days or weeks after marijuana use,[349,350] and another young man awoke with dysarthria and hemiparesis the morning after smoking marijuana.[351] In none of these patients was imaging performed. Two young men, both hypertensive cigarette smokers, experienced hemiparesis during marijuana smoking, and CT showed cerebral infarction.[352] Another young smoker of tobacco and marijuana had three possible transient ischemic attacks and then hemiparesis and aphasia; CT showed a striatocapsular infarct.[353] Proposed mechanisms for alleged marijuana-induced stroke include systemic hypotension and cerebral vasospasm, but neither has been documented in clinical reports. In rats, delta-9-tetrahydrocannabinol (the psychoactive ingredient of marijuana) has vasoconstrictor action on systemic vessels.[354] In humans, marijuana has unpredictable effects on cerebral blood flow, either increasing or decreasing it.[355]

BARBITURATES

Usually abused orally, barbiturates and other sedatives and tranquilizers can cause cerebral infarction in association with overdose and diffusely decreased brain perfusion, but neither occlusive nor hemorrhagic stroke has otherwise been reported. A 20-year-old man taking a combination of secobarbital and strychnine ("M and Ms") orally became comatose with right hemiplegia, and cerebral angiography showed widespread segmental vascular irregularity consistent with arteritis; he had been taking other drugs as well for at least 10 years.[146] Cerebral vasculitis was also found in four other barbiturate abusers; two also abused chlorpromazine, one took other unidentified drugs, and the fourth apparently used only barbiturates, but whether orally or parenterally was not revealed.[145]

In monkeys receiving dissolved secobarbital (Seconal) capsules, 1.5 mg/kg intravenously three times a week for one year, cerebral angiography showed narrowing of small arteries. Histologic examination found scattered talc crystals in brain capillaries, without cellular reaction; one animal had a frontal lobe microinfarct.[146]

INHALANTS

Inhalation of vapors to achieve euphoric intoxication is common in the United States, especially among children. Substances include aerosols, enamels, paint thinners, lighter fluid, cleaning fluid, glues, cements, gasoline, and anesthetics. Death results from violence, accidents, suffocation, aspiration, or cardiac arrhythmia. A 12-year-old glue sniffer developed hemiplegia, and cerebral angiography showed occlusion of the middle cerebral artery; a proposed mechanism was vasospasm caused by trichloroethylene sensitization of vessel receptors to circulating catecholamines.[356] Radioisotope brain scanning in a boy with status epilepticus after toluene sniffing showed several wedge-shaped areas of increased uptake in both cerebral hemispheres, consistent with infarcts.[357]

ALCOHOL

Coronary artery disease and myocardial infarction are less prevalent in people who drink moderate amounts of alcohol than in those who do not.[358] The increased risk of coronary artery disease in heavy drinkers becomes an indirect risk for cardioembolic stroke secondary to cardiac wall hypokinesia or arrhythmia. Alcohol intoxication and withdrawal are also directly associated with cardiac arrhythmia ("holiday heart"),[359,360] and thromboembolism is a prominent feature of alcoholic cardiomyopathy.[52,201]

A large body of literature has addressed whether short-term or long-term alcohol use is a risk factor for stroke independent of its cardiac effects or other risk factors.[361–365] Retrospective studies, most notably from Finland, have found an association between recent heavy alcohol use and both occlusive and hemorrhagic strokes.[366–369] The Finnish studies, however, used population prevalence data as controls, and other similarly designed analyses have either not found such an association,[370] or, as in the National Institute of Neurological and Communicative Disorders and Stroke (NINCDS) Data Bank, have found an association only with intracerebral hemorrhage.[371] A study from Chicago found that the association between alcohol intoxication and stroke disappeared when data were corrected for cigarette smoking.[372,373] The same Finnish investigators, reporting that among young adults more strokes occurred during weekends and holidays than expected, observed a stronger association in young women than in young men, suggesting factors other than simply ethanol.

Numerous case-control and cohort studies have addressed the relationship of stroke to chronic alcohol use.[156,374–394] Contradictory findings are not surprising, for studies have differed in end points chosen (e.g., total stroke, occlusive stroke, hemorrhagic stroke, or stroke mortality), amount and duration of alcohol consumption, correction for other risk factors (especially hypertension and smoking), ethnicity and socioeconomics of populations being studied, and selection of controls. Drinkers tend to be overrepresented among hospitalized controls, leading to the impression that alcohol is protective against stroke; they tend to be underrepresented among community controls identified by a questionnaire, leading to the impression that alcohol is a risk factor for stroke.[395]

Among cohort studies, the Yugoslavia Cardiovascular Disease Study found increased stroke mortality among drinkers, and, although the association was especially strong for people with hypertension, it persisted with adjustment for blood pressure.[396,397] A reduced risk was found for modest drinkers. In the Honolulu Heart Study, heavy drinkers had a higher risk of hemorrhagic stroke independent of other risk factors, including hypertension and smoking.[398–401] There was no comparable risk for occlusive stroke. The Framingham Study described lower than expected stroke incidence among "moderate" drinkers and higher rates in both heavy drinkers and nondrinkers.[402]

In the Nurses' Health Study, independent of smoking and hypertension, there was an inverse association between modest alcohol intake (fewer than two drinks daily) and occlusive stroke, with a positive association at higher intake; subarachnoid hemorrhage was associated with both low and high alcohol intakes.[403] In the Lausanne Stroke Registry, severity of internal carotid artery stenosis inversely correlated with "light-to-moderate" alcohol intake; there were too few patients to assess heavy intake.[404] The Japanese Hisayama Study initially reported positive correlations[405]; later, the study found no independent association between alcohol and occlusive or hemorrhagic stroke after adjustments were made for other variables[406]; still later, study researchers found that heavy drinking conferred higher risk for cerebral hemorrhage in persons with hypertension, whereas light alcohol consumption reduced the risk of cerebral infarction.[407] A study of Japanese physicians found a positive association between stroke mortality and alcohol intake.[408,409] Three other Japanese studies found either independent associations between alcohol and hemorrhagic but not occlusive stroke,[410] no association between alcohol and occlusive stroke,[411] and a "J-shaped relationship" between alcohol intake and occlusive stroke—drinkers of less than 42 g/day ethanol had a lower risk, and heavy drinkers a higher risk, than "never drinkers."[412]

A review of 62 epidemiologic studies that examined the relation between stroke and "moderate" alcohol consumption (less than two drinks or less than 1 oz. of absolute ethanol) concluded that ethnicity played a role in the disparate results.[413] Among white people, moderate doses of alcohol seemed to protect against ischemic stroke, whereas higher doses increased risk. (This pattern is similar to that for alcohol and coronary artery disease.) Among the Japanese, little association seemed to exist between alcohol and ischemic stroke. In both populations, all doses of alcohol seemed to increase the risk of both intracerebral and subarachnoid hemorrhages. Some studies have suggested that the risk of hemorrhagic stroke declines with abstinence, but the evidence is insufficient to draw an association between stroke and recent intoxication per se.

An Australian case-control study found that low doses of ethanol (less than 20 g/day) were protective against "all strokes, all ischemic strokes, and primary intracerebral hemorrhage."[414] A British case-control study found that the protective effect of "light or moderate" drinking compared with nondrinking disappeared when data were corrected for exercise and obesity.[415] In an Italian case-control study, the role of alcohol as a risk factor for stroke "was practically lost" after correction for previous strokes, hypertension, diabetes, obesity, and hyperlipidemia.[374,416] A study from Denmark found that moderate wine drinking reduced the likelihood of stroke, moderate drinking of "spirits" increased the likelihood, and moderate drinking of beer had no effect in either direction.[417] Another Danish study found a decreased risk of stroke (ischemic, hemorrhagic, or not specified) in wine drinkers but not in beer or liquor drinkers.[418]

A Finnish study found that recent heavy drinking increased the risk of embolic stroke in patients with a source of thrombus in the heart or large cerebral vessels.[419] Another Finnish study found a higher risk for hemorrhagic stroke in binge-drinking young adults.[420]

In the Northern Manhattan Stroke Study, "moderate" ethanol intake (two drinks daily) protected against ischemic stroke, and the protection held for higher levels of consumption, up to five drinks daily. Seven drinks, however, increased the risk. There was no difference in benefit or risk between young and older subjects, between men and women, among white, black, and Hispanic people, or among drinkers of wine, beer, and liquor.[421]

In the U.S. Physicians' Health Study, the risk of ischemic stroke was significantly lower in subjects who had more than one drink weekly than in those who drank less. There was no difference in risk reduction between those who had one drink weekly and those who had one or more drinks daily.[422]

In the Framingham Study, when results were stratified according to age, ethanol intake reduced the risk of ischemic stroke only in subjects ages 60 to 69 years, and when results were stratified according to type of beverage, only wine was protective.[423] Remote but not current drinking of 12 or more grams of ethanol daily increased the risk of ischemic stroke in men but not women; these subjects were older and more often used tobacco, however.[424]

Studies with duplex ultrasonography and angiography have shown that heavy ethanol consumption raises the risk of carotid artery atherosclerosis, whereas low ethanol intake has a beneficial effect.[425] Similarly, a study using CT found that one to five drinks daily reduced the risk of leukoaraiosis in patients with stroke, whereas heavier alcohol consumption increased the risk.[426] The Japanese Hisayama study found alcohol to be an independent risk factor for "vascular dementia."[427] The U.S. Cardiovascular Health Study, in which adults 65 years of age and without a history of stroke underwent MRI of the brain, found a U-shaped relationship between alcohol consumption and white matter abnormalities, with one to seven drinks per week being most protective. Protection against frank infarction continued above 15 drinks per week.[428] Other studies describe a similar relationship between moderate ethanol consumption and improved cognitive performance; the degree to which such benefit is related to alcohol's effects on cerebral circulation is uncertain.[429–434] In the Rotterdam Study, alcohol was especially effective in reducing the risk for "vascular dementia."[435]

As with coronary artery disease, several mechanisms might explain the association between alcohol and stroke.[436] Alcohol acutely and chronically raises blood pressure,[396,398, 437–447] perhaps related to increased adrenergic activity and to increased blood levels of cortisol, renin, aldosterone, and vasopressin.[448] Corticotropin-releasing hormone is sympatho-excitatory when administered centrally; in normal subjects, dexamethasone blocked the increased sympathetic discharge and the increased blood pressure induced by intravenous ethanol.[449] The decline in systolic blood pressure seen during the first week after a stroke is greater in heavy drinkers than in light drinkers or abstainers,[450] and with abstinence, blood pressure may become normal.[451]

Perhaps related to its protective effects, alcohol lowers blood levels of low-density lipoproteins (LDLs) and elevates levels of high-density lipoproteins (HDLs).[452–455] One study found that alcohol seemed preferentially to protect large vessels from atherosclerosis, perhaps accounting for ethnic differences in patterns of protection or risk.[456] The relationship is uncertain, however, because alcohol may not raise blood levels of the more protective HDL-2 subfraction.[457,458] In the Northern Manhattan Stroke Study, the protective effect of moderate alcohol consumption on stroke risk was independent of the HDL cholesterol level.[421] In the Framingham Study, among men with the apolipoprotein E2 allele, LDL cholesterol was lower in drinkers than in nondrinkers; among those with the E4 allele, LDL cholesterol was higher in drinkers.[459]

Alcohol acutely decreases fibrinolytic activity, increases factor VIII level, increases platelet reactivity to adenosine diphosphate (ADP), and shortens bleeding time.[460–465] In one study, moderate ethanol consumption was associated with elevated endogenous tissue plasminogen activator.[466] Ethanol reportedly reduces plasma fibrinogen levels,[467] increases levels of prostacyclin,[468,469] decreases platelet function,[432, 470–474] and stimulates release of endothelin from endothelial cells.[475] In chronic alcoholics, diminished levels of clotting factors, excessive fibrinolysis, and platelet abnormalities appear to be secondary to liver disease.[448,476] During or after ethanol withdrawal, "rebound thrombocytosis" and platelet hyperaggregability have been observed.[477,478] In rats this rebound followed withdrawal in animals receiving ethanol or white wine but not in those receiving red wine.[479] In another report, however, alcoholic humans undergoing withdrawal had decreased platelet response to activators.[480] Withdrawal in humans was also associated with increased fibrinolytic activity as a result of decreased levels of tissue-type plasminogen activator inhibitor.[481]

Nondrinkers and heavy drinkers have higher blood levels of C-reactive protein than moderate drinkers, an observation relevant to the probable role of inflammation in atherosclerosis.[482]

Acute alcohol intoxication has been accompanied by cerebral vasodilatation[483] and blood-brain barrier leakage of albumin,[484] perhaps contributing to the severity of traumatic intracerebral hemorrhage during drinking.[45,484a] Increased cerebral blood flow has also been observed during alcohol withdrawal.[486] Chronic drinking is associated with diminished cerebral blood flow, mainly from reduced cerebral metabolism.[485] Alcohol-related hemoconcentration may also contribute to reduced cerebral blood flow.[448]

In vitro studies involving a variety of mammals have shown ethanol to be a potent vasoconstrictor of basilar and middle cerebral artery segments,[487] and in living rats, ethanol caused vasoconstriction of cerebral arterioles[488] and blocked the vasodilatation produced by acetylcholine, histamine, and ADP but not the vasodilatation produced by nitroglycerin or the vasoconstriction produced by a thromboxane analogue.[489] In cultured canine vascular smooth muscle cells, ethanol exposure caused depletion of intracellular magnesium ion.[490] Such an effect could lead to calcium ion overload, causing both hypertension and cerebral vasoconstriction, and, indeed, pretreatment of animals with magnesium ion prevents ethanol-induced strokes.[491–493]

Hyperhomocysteinemia is a risk factor for both myocardial ischemia and ischemic stroke, and alcoholics often have elevated blood homocysteine levels secondary to deficiency of folate, pyridoxine, or cobalamin.[494]

Studies suggesting a special protective benefit of wine—especially red wine—have led to speculation that the responsible constituents might be free radical scavengers in the form of polyphenols and flavonoids, which, by reducing oxidative damage to LDLs, might reduce altherogenesis.[495–498] Ethanol itself, however, is pro-oxidant.[498a]

Some investigators believe that snoring and sleep apnea are risk factors for stroke. To the extent that ethanol contributes to these conditions, it would increase that risk.[34]

TOBACCO

Epidemiologic studies show smoking to be a major risk factor for coronary artery and peripheral vascular diseases.[499–503] Although a few reports have found no such relationship or have demonstrated only insignificant trends toward higher risk of stroke among smokers,[504–507] most case-control and cohort studies have shown that smoking does raise the risk for both occlusive stroke and hemorrhagic stroke.[18,373,385, 509–532] In women smokers, the risk of occlusive and hemorrhagic stroke is greater in those taking oral contraceptives.[533–537] In a prospective cohort study of middle-aged women, smoking increased stroke risk in a dose-dependent fashion; for those smoking 25 or more cigarettes daily, the relative risk (RR) for all stroke was 3.7, and for subarachnoid hemorrhage 9.8, independent of other risk factors including oral contraceptives, hypertension, and alcohol.[538] In another report, smoking in hypertensive men and women carried a 15-fold risk for subarachnoid hemorrhage and was a greater risk than hypertension itself.[509] In another study, the treatment of hypertension reduced stroke incidence in nonsmokers but not in smokers.[539] Tobacco smoking, hypertension, and high blood cholesterol appear to interact synergistically as stroke risk factors.[540] Patients with ischemic stroke who smoke tend to be younger than those who do not.[541]

In the Honolulu Heart Program, stroke risk was independent of coronary artery disease.[542] The Framingham Study found smoking to be a risk factor for subarachnoid hemorrhage and, independent of age and hypertension, for both occlusive stroke and hemorrhagic stroke; this risk was dose-dependent and disappeared when smoking ceased.[543,544] Other researchers have confirmed reduction of stroke risk with cessation of smoking,[520,527,545] but a small long-term excess risk persists.[546] Smoking is a risk factor for central retinal artery occlusion as well as for aortic plaque formation.[547,548]

Among smokers, the risk of stroke mortality is reduced in those who smoke cigarettes with lower tar yield.[549] On the other hand, stroke was reported following application of a nicotine patch.[584] Stroke risk is raised by passive as well as active smoking.[546,550]

A study from the United Kingdom estimated that an intensive smoking reduction program (as had been adopted but then abandoned in California) would prevent 455 strokes during the year 2000 and 11,304 strokes by 2010.[551] A European study, noting a fall in stroke prevalence in Western Europe but a rise in Eastern Europe, attributed the difference to the higher prevalence of tobacco use in Eastern Europe.[552] A study from China estimated that (1) in 1990, 600,000 Chinese deaths (500,000 in men) were attributable to tobacco, (2) by 2000, this figure would rise to 800,000, and (3) of all Chinese males currently younger than 30 years of age, one third would die prematurely as a consequence of smoking and that 5% to 8% of their deaths would be caused by stroke.[553]

Several possible mechanisms could underlie tobacco's risk for stroke.[554] Smoking aggravates atherosclerosis. In a study of identical twins who were discordant for smoking, carotid plaques were significantly more prominent in the smokers, and in other reports, smoking correlated in dose-related fashion with severity of extracranial carotid atherosclerosis.[404,555–557] In the Atherosclerosis Risk in Communities (ARIC) Study, current cigarette smoking was associated with a 50% increase in the progression over 3 years of carotid artery atherosclerosis compared with that in never-smokers; past smoking was associated with a 25% increase, and passive exposure to environmental smoke with a 20% increase.[558] Smoking one cigarette causes transient increases in arterial wall stiffness that increase the likelihood of plaque formation.[559] The reduction in stroke risk with cessation of smoking argues against the possibility that such large vessel atherosclerosis is paramount, however.[544,560,561]

Carbon monoxide in cigarette smoke reduces blood's oxygen-carrying capacity, and nicotine constricts coronary arteries.[562,563] Coronary artery constriction and the greater myocardial oxygen demand induced by cocaine are exacerbated by concomitant tobacco smoking.[297] In animals, nicotine damages endothelium, and increased numbers of circulating endothelial cells are found in smokers.[564,565] A German study found that neonates and children during the first month of life who were exposed to environmental tobacco smoke already demonstrated endothelial cell damage.[566] In mice chronically exposed to nicotine, aortic walls exhibited subendothelial edema and swelling of endothelial cells and mitochondria.[565] Bovine endothelial cells exposed to nicotine demonstrated giant cell formation and cellular vacuolization.[567]

Smoking acutely raises blood pressure, systole more than diastole.[568,569] Whether smoking is a risk factor for chronic hypertension is less clear,[570] although it does accelerate the progression of chronic hypertension to malignant hypertension.[571,572] Smokers become tachycardic, and atrial fibrillation has been observed after chewing nicotine gum.[562] Demonstrating the complexity of interactions is a study in dogs in which ethanol followed by nicotine synergistically increased heart rate and blood pressure, yet these excitatory effects of nicotine were attenuated when ethanol was administered after nicotine.[573]

Smoking activates the coagulant pathway, increases platelet reactivity, and inhibits prostacyclin formation.[560,574-576,576a,576b] It raises blood fibrinogen levels, a linkage noted in several stroke studies, and polycythemia secondary to smoking increases blood viscosity.[577] In cultures of human brain endothelial cells, nicotine increased production of plasminogen activator inhibitor-1 (PAI-1).[577a] In rats, nicotine-induced depletion of tissue plasminogen activator was associated with enhanced focal ischemic brain injury.[577b] Increased plasma levels of PAI-1 are found in smokers.[578,579] The increased risk of subarachnoid hemorrhage in smokers has been blamed on greater elastolytic activity in the serum.[580]

The relative contributions of nicotine, tars, and the gaseous constituents of cigarette smoke to cardiovascular disease are uncertain.[581] Transdermal or oral nicotine produces plasma levels of platelet activation products (platelet factor 4 and β-thromboglobulin) and von Willebrand factor that are intermediate between those of smokers and non-smokers.[582,583] Although stroke was reported after application of a nicotine patch,[584] a meta-analysis of 35 clinical trials involving the transdermal nicotine patch found no excess incidence of myocardial infarction or stroke.[585]

Effects of tobacco smoke and nicotine on cerebral blood flow are complex, for nicotine has both direct and indirect effects on cerebral vessels themselves as well as on neuronal nicotinic receptors. In volunteers, several puffs on a lighted cigarette during a 5-minute period increased middle cerebral artery (MCA) flow velocity in all subjects; onset and offset were detected within a few seconds of starting and stopping smoking. The effect was independent of CO_2 autoregulation, and in fact, smoking suppressed CO_2-induced vasodilatation by 56% in men (but by only 5% in women).[586] In tobacco smokers who were abstinent overnight, nicotine nasal spray increased regional cerebral blood flow (rCBF) in the thalamus, pons, visual cortex, and cerebellum; it was noted that the increases did not necessarily correlate with the density of neuronal acetylcholine receptors in the different affected regions.[586a]

In rats, 2 minutes of exposure to tobacco smoke caused an increase in cerebral blood flow and an attenuation in CO_2-induced vasodilatation that lasted for an hour.[587] Cerebral vasodilatation induced by parenteral nicotine in rats was attenuated by destroying the nucleus basalis of Meynert and was abolished by the blocking nicotinic (but not muscarinic) receptors in brain parenchyma.[588] In rats, inhalation of tobacco smoke caused brief constriction of pial arterioles followed by dilatation; nicotine infusion caused only vasodilatation. The vasodilatation was considered the result of sympathetic activation; the vasoconstriction was considered partially the result of thromboxane A_2 induced by other constituents in cigarette smoke.[589] In lenticulostriate arterioles of rats with long-term exposure to nicotine, calcium channels were upregulated and calcium-activated potassium channels were downregulated; the effect was considered the result of decreased bioavailability of endogenous nitric oxide.[590] Nicotine-induced vasodilatation of porcine basilar arteries denuded of endothelium was abolished by the nitric oxide synthase inhibitor *N*-nitro-L-arginine; nicotine was considered to act on nicotinic receptors on presynaptic adrenergic nerve terminals, releasing norepinephrine, which in turn releases nitric oxide from neighboring nitric-oxidergic nerves.[591] In rats, a vasodilator area in the medulla is excited by hypoxia as well as by microinjections of nicotine.[592]

Progressive multifocal symptoms were observed in four young women who smoked and used oral contraceptives. Cerebral angiography demonstrated moyamoya vessels, and abnormal studies included elevated ESR, presence of antinuclear antibodies, and elevated CSF IgG. Disease progression ceased with discontinuation of oral contraceptives and reduction in smoking.[593] In another series of 39 patients with moyamoya disease, use of tobacco and oral contraceptives was also overrepresented.[594]

An elderly man had syncopal spells whenever he stood up after smoking a cigarette; the spells ceased when he stopped smoking. SPECT showed decreased cerebral perfusion "in the posterior circulation structures" after this patient smoked a cigarette or chewed nicotine gum.[595]

References

1. Eddy NB, Halbach H, Isbell H, Seevers MH: Drug dependence: Its significance and characteristics. Bull World Health Org 32:721, 1965.
2. Brust JCM: Neurological Aspects of Substance Abuse, 2nd ed. Newton, MA, Butterworth-Heinemann, 2003.
3. Kokkinos J, Levine SR: Stroke. Neurol Clin 11:577, 1993.
4. Patel AN: Self-inflicted strokes. Ann Intern Med 76:823, 1972.
5. Brust JCM: Stroke and drugs. In Toole JF (ed): of Handbook of Clinical Neurology, Rev Series II: Vascular Diseases, Part III, Vol 55. Amsterdam, Elsevier, 1989, p 517.
6. Brust JCM: Drug dependence. In Joynt RJ, Griggs R (eds): Clinical Neurology. New York, Harper & Row, 2002.
7. Halloway M: Treatment for addiction. Sci Am 265:94, 1991.
8. Kandel DB: Epidemiological trends and implications for understanding the nature of addiction. In O'Brien CP, Jaffe JH (eds): Addictive States. Res Publ Assoc Res Nerv Ment Dis 70:23, 1992.
9. Helpern M, Rho Y-M: Deaths from narcotism in New York City. NY State J Med 66:2391, 1966.
10. Banks T, Fletcher R, Ali N: Infective endocarditis in heroin addicts. Am J Med 55:444, 1973.
11. Cherubin CE: The medical sequelae of narcotic addiction. Ann Intern Med 67:23, 1967.
12. Louria DB, Hensle T, Rose J: The major medical complications of heroin addiction. Ann Intern Med 67:1, 1967.
13. Pearson J, Richter RW: Neuropathological effects of opiate addiction. In Richter RW (ed): Medical Aspects of Drug Abuse. Hagerstown, MD, Harper & Row, 1975, p 308.
14. Pearson J, Richter RW: Addiction to opiates: Neurologic aspects. In Vinken PJ, Bruyn GW (eds): Handbook of Clinical Neurology, Vol 37: Intoxications of the Nervous System. Amsterdam, North-Holland, 1979, p 365.
15. Richter RW, Pearson J, Bruun B, et al: Neurological complications of addiction to heroin. Bull N Y Acad Med 49:3, 1973.
16. Tuazon CU, Sheagren JN: Staphylococcal endocarditis in parenteral drug abusers: Source of the organism. Ann Intern Med 82:788, 1975.
17. Hubbell G, Cheitlin MD, Rapaport E: Presentation, management, and follow-up evaluation of ineffective endocarditis in drug addicts. Am Heart J 102:85, 1981.
18. Amine AB: Neurosurgical complications of heroin addiction: Brain abscess and mycotic aneurysm. Surg Neurol 7:385, 1977.
19. Gilroy J, Andaya L, Thomas VJ: Intracranial mycotic aneurysms and subacute bacterial endocarditis in heroin addiction. Neurology (NY) 23:1193, 1973.
20. Jara FM, Lewis JF, Magilligan DJ: Operative experience with infective endocarditis and intracerebral mycotic aneurysm. J Thorac Cardiovasc Surg 80:28, 1980.
21. Brust JCM, Dickinson PCT, Hughes JEO, Holtzman RNN: The diagnosis and treatment of cerebral mycotic aneurysms. Ann Neurol 27:238, 1990.

22. Frazee JG, Cahan LD, Winter J: Bacterial intracranial aneurysms. J Neurosurg 53:633, 1980.
23. Ledgerwood AM, Lucas CE: Mycotic aneurysm of the carotid artery. Arch Surg 109:496, 1974.
23a. Ho K, Rassekh Z: Mycotic aneurysm of the right subclavian artery: A complication of heroin addiction. Chest 74:116, 1978.
24. Brust JCM, Richter RW: Stroke associated with addiction to heroin. J Neurol Neurosurg Psychiatry 39:194, 1976.
25. Lignelli GJ, Buchheit WA: Angiitis in drug abusers. N Engl J Med 284:112, 1971.
26. Woods BT, Strewler GJ: Hemiparesis occurring six hours after intravenous heroin injection. Neurology (NY) 22:863, 1972.
27. King J, Richards M, Tress B: Cerebral arteritis associated with heroin abuse. Med J Aust 2:444, 1978.
28. Celius EG: Neurologic complications in heroin abuse: Illustrated by two unusual cases. Tidsskr Nor Laegeforen 117:356, 1997.
29. Kortikale Blindheit nach Heroin intoxication. Nukleomedizin 2:N16, 2000.
30. Munoz Casares FC, Serrano Castro P, Linan Lopez M, et al: Sudden aphasia in a young woman. Rev Clin Espanola 199:325, 1999.
31. Bartolomei F, Nicoli F, Swiader L, Gastaut JL: Accident vasculaire cérébral ischémique après prise nasale d'héroine: Une nouvelle observation. Presse Med 21:983, 1992.
32. Herskowitz A, Gross E: Cerebral infarction associated with heroin sniffing. South Med J 66:778, 1973.
33. Knoblauch AL, Buchholz M, Koller MG, Kistler H: Hemiplegie nach Injektion von Heroin. Schweiz Med Wochenschr 113:402, 1983.
34. Palomaki H, Partinen M, Erkinjuntti T, Kaste M: Snoring, sleep apnea syndrome, and stroke. Neurology 42(Suppl 6):75, 1992.
35. Caplan LR, Hier DB, Banks G: Stroke and drug abuse. Stroke 13:869, 1982.
36. Ginsberg MD, Hedley-Whyte ET, Richardson EP: Hypoxic-ischemic leukoencephalopathy in man. Arch Neurol 33:5, 1976.
37. Jensen R, Olsen TS, Winther BB: Severe non-occlusive ischemic stroke in young heroin addicts. Acta Neurol Scand 81:354, 1990.
38. Shoser BG, Groden C: Subacute onset of oculogyric crisis and generalized dystonia following intranasal administration of heroin. Addiction 94:431, 1999.
39. Vila N, Chamorro A: Ballistic movements due to ischemic infarcts after intravenous heroin overdose: Report of two cases. Clin Neurol Neurosurg 99:259, 1997.
40. Courville CN: The process of demyelination in the central nervous system. IV: Demyelination as a delayed residual of carbon monoxide asphyxia. J Nerv Ment Dis 125:534, 1957.
41. Plum F, Posner JB, Hain RF: Delayed neurologic deterioration after anoxia. Arch Intern Med 110:18, 1962.
42. Protass LM: Delayed postanoxic encephalopathy after heroin use. Ann Intern Med 74:738, 1971.
43. Anderson SN, Skullerud K: Hypoxic/ischemic brain damage, especially pallidal lesions, in heroin addicts. Forensic Sci Int 102:51, 1999.
44. Niehaus L, Roricht S, Meyer BU, Sander B: Nuclear magnetic resonance tomography detection of heroin-associated CNS lesions. Aktuelle Radiol 7:309, 1997.
45. Simonsen J: Traumatic subarachnoid hemorrhage in alcohol intoxication. J Forensic Sci 8:97, 1963.
46. Sturner WQ, Stressman G, Helpern M: Bilateral symmetrical encephalomalacia in the globus pallidus in drug addicts. Paper read at the meeting of the American Academy of Forensic Sciences, Chicago, February, 1968.
47. Adams JH, Brierley JB, Connor RCR, Treip CS: The effects of systemic hypotension upon the human brain: Clinical and neuropathological observations in 11 cases. Brain 89:235, 1966.
48. Brierley JB: The neuropathology of brain hypoxia. In Critchley M, O'Leary JL, Jennett B (eds): Scientific Foundations of Neurology. London, Heinemann, 1972, p 243.
49. Brust JCM, Richter RW: Quinine amblyopia related to heroin addiction. Ann Intern Med 74:84, 1971.
50. Baden MM: Pathology of the addictive states. In Richter RW (ed): Medical Aspects of Drug Abuse. Hagerstown, MD, Harper & Row, 1975, p 189.
51. Levine LH, Hirsch CS, White LW: Quinine cardiotoxicity: A mechanism for sudden death in narcotic addicts. J Forensic Sci 18:167, 1973.
52. Atlee W: Talc and cornstarch emboli in eyes of drug abusers. JAMA 219:49, 1972.
53. Mizutami T, Lewis R, Gonatas N: Medial medullary syndrome in a drug abuser. Arch Neurol 37:425, 1980.
54. Sapira JD: The narcotic addict as a medical patient. Am J Med 45:555, 1968.
55. Lahmeyer HW, Steingold RG: Pentazocine and tripelennamine: A drug abuse epidemic? Int J Addict 15:1219, 1980.
56. Wadley C, Stillie GD: Pentazocine (Talwin) and tripelennamine (pyribenzamine): A new drug abuse combination or just a revival? Int J Addict 15:1285, 1980.
57. Caplan LR, Thomas C, Banks G: Central nervous system complications of addiction to "T's and Blues." Neurology (NY) 32:623, 1982.
58. Houck RJ, Bailey G, Daroca P, et al: Pentazocine abuse. Chest 77:227, 1980.
59. Szwed JJ: Pulmonary angiothrombosis caused by "blue velvet" addiction. Ann Intern Med 73:771, 1970.
60. Butz WC: Disseminated magnesium and silicate associated with paregoric addiction. J Forensic Sci 15:581, 1970.
61. Lee J, Sapira JD: Retinal and cerebral microembolization of talc in a drug abuser. Am J Med Sci 265:75, 1973.
62. Biter S, Gomez CR: Stroke following injection of a melted suppository. Stroke 24:741, 1993.
63. Cunningham EE, Brentjens JR, Zielezny MA, et al: Heroin nephropathy: A clinicopathologic and epidemiologic study. Am J Med 68:47, 1980.
64. Friedman EA, Sreepada Rao TK, Nicastri AD: Heroin-associated nephropathy. Nephron 13:421, 1974.
65. Grishman E, Churg J, Porush JG: Glomerular morphology in nephrotic heroin addicts. Lab Invest 35:415, 1976.
66. Kilcoyne MM, Daly JJ, Gocke DJ, et al: Nephrotic syndrome in heroin addicts. Lancet 1(7740):17, 1972.
67. Becker C: Medical complications of drug abuse. Adv Intern Med 24:183, 1979.
68. Cushman P, Grieco MH: Hyperimmunoglobulinemia associated with narcotic addiction: Effects of methadone maintenance treatment. Am J Med 54:320, 1973.
69. Husby G, Pierce PE, Williams RL: Smooth muscle antibody in heroin addicts. Ann Intern Med 83:801, 1975.
70. Nickerson DS, Williams RL, Boxmeyer M, et al: Increased opsonic capacity of serum in chronic heroin addiction. Ann Intern Med 72:671, 1970.
71. Ortona L, Laghi V, Cauda R: Immune function in heroin addicts. N Engl J Med 300:45, 1979.
72. Boak RA, Carpenter CM, Miller JN: Biologic false-positive reactions for syphilis among narcotic addicts: A report on the incidence of BFP reactions as measured by the TPI test. JAMA 175:326, 1961.
73. Schoenfeld MR: Acute allergic reactions to morphine, codeine, meperidine hydrochloride, and opium alkaloids. N Y State J Med 60:2591, 1960.
74. Richter RW, Pearson J: Heroin addiction-related neurological disorders. In Richter RW (ed): Medical Aspects of Drug Abuse. Hagerstown, MD, Harper & Row, 1975, p 320.
75. Ryan JJ, Parker CW, Williams RL: Gamma-globulin binding of morphine in heroin addicts. J Lab Clin Med 80:155, 1972.
76. Ringle DA, Herndon BL: In vitro morphine binding by sera from morphine-treated rabbits. J Immunol 109:174, 1972.
77. Van Vanukis H, Wasserman E, Levine L: Specificities of antibodies to morphine. J Pharmacol Exp Ther 180:514, 1972.
78. Lee MC, Randa DC, Gold LH: Transverse myelopathy following the use of heroin. Minn Med 59:82, 1976.
79. Pearson J, Richter RW, Baden MM, et al: Transverse myelopathy as an illustration of the neurologic and neuropathologic features of heroin addiction. Hum Pathol 3:109, 1972.
80. Richter RW, Rosenberg RN: Transverse myelitis associated with heroin addiction. JAMA 206:1255, 1968.
81. Rodriguez E, Smokvina M, Sokolow J, Grynbaum BB: Encephalopathy and paraplegia occurring with use of heroin. N Y State J Med 71:2879, 1971.
82. Schein PS, Yessayun L, Mayman CI: Acute transverse myelitis associated with intravenous opium. Neurology (NY) 21:101, 1971.
83. Thompson WR, Waldman MB: Cervical myelopathy following heroin administration. J Med Soc NJ 67:223, 1970.
84. DiChiro G, Fried LC: Blood flow currents in spinal arteries. Neurology (NY) 21:1088, 1971.

85. Garland H, Greenburg J, Harriman DGF: Infarction of the spinal cord. Brain 89:645, 1966.

86. Henson RA, Parsons M: Ischemic lesions of the spinal cord: An illustrated review. Q J Med 36:205, 1967.

87. Turnbull IM: Microvasculature of the human spinal cord. J Neurosurg 35:141, 1971.

88. McCreary M, Emerman C, Hanna J, Simon J: Acute myelopathy following intranasal insufflation of heroin: A case report. Neurology 55:316, 2000.

89. Judice DJ, LeBlanc HJ, McGarry PA: Spinal cord vasculitis presenting as spinal cord tumor in a heroin addict. J Neurosurg 48:131, 1978.

90. Hirsch CS: Dermatopathology of narcotic addiction. Hum Pathol 3:37, 1972.

91. Anson BJ: Morris's Human Anatomy. New York, McGraw-Hill, 1966, p 728.

92. Pick TP, Howden R: Gray's Anatomy. Philadelphia, Running Press, 1974, p 548.

93. Hall JH, Karp HR: Acute progressive ventral pontine disease in heroin abuse. Neurology (NY) 23:6, 1973.

94. Maqbool Z, Billett HH: Unwitting heparin abuse in a drug addict. Ann Intern Med 96:790, 1982.

95. Treffert DA, Joranson D: Restricting amphetamines. JAMA 245:1336, 1981.

96. Bernheim J, Cox JN: Heat stroke and amphetamine intoxication in a sportsman. Schweiz Med Wochenschr 90:322, 1960.

97. Greenwood R, Peachey RS: Acute amphetamine poisoning: An account of three cases. Br Med J 1:742, 1957.

98. Jordan SC, Hampson F: Amphetamine poisoning associated with hyperpyrexia. Br Med J 2:844, 1960.

99. Lewis E: Hyperpyrexia with antidepressant drugs. Br Med J 2:1671, 1965.

100. Pretorius HPJ: Dexedrine intoxication of children: Two cases, one fatal. S Afr Med J 27:945, 1953.

101. Zalis EG, Parmley LF: Fatal amphetamine poisoning. Arch Intern Med 112:822, 1963.

102. Bonhoff C, Lewrenz H: Über Werkamine. Berlin, Springer-Verlag, 1954, p 144.

103. Harvey JK, Todd CW, Howard JW: Fatality associated with Benzedrine ingestion: A case report. Del Med 21:111, 1949.

104. Zalis EG, Lundberg GD, Knutson RA: The pathophysiology of acute amphetamine poisoning with pathologic correlation. J Pharmacol Exp Ther 158:115, 1967.

105. Kasirsky G, Zaidi IH, Tansy MF: LD50 and pathologic effects of acute and chronic administration of methamphetamine HCl in rabbits. Res Commun Chem Pathol Pharmacol 3:215, 1972.

106. Zalis EG, Kaplan G, Lundberg GD, Knutson RA: Acute lethality of the amphetamines in dogs and its antagonism with curare. Proc Soc Exp Biol Med 18:557, 1965.

107. Escalante OD, Ellinwood EH: Central nervous system cytopathological changes in cats with chronic methedrine intoxication. Brain Res 21:151, 1970.

108. Clowes GHA, O'Donnell TF: Heat stroke. N Engl J Med 291:564, 1974.

109. Ferris EB, Blankenhorn MA, Robinson HW, et al: Heat stroke: Clinical and chemical observations on 44 cases. J Clin Invest 17:249, 1938.

110. Freeman W, Dumoff S: Cerebellar syndrome following heat stroke. Arch Neurol Psychiatry 51:67, 1944.

111. Kumar P, Rathore CK, Nagar AM, et al: Hyperpyrexia with special reference to heat stroke: An analysis of 108 cases. J Indian Med Assoc 43:213, 1964.

112. Shibolet S, Coll R, Gilat T, Sohar E: Heatstroke: Its clinical picture and mechanism in 36 cases. Q J Med 36:525, 1967.

113. Cahill DW, Knipp H, Mosser J: Intracranial hemorrhage with amphetamine abuse. Neurology (NY) 31:1058, 1981.

114. Chynn KY: Acute subarachnoid hemorrhage. JAMA 233:55, 1973.

115. Coroner's Report: Amphetamine overdose kills boy. Pharm J 198:172, 1967.

116. Delaney P, Estes M: Intracranial hemorrhage with amphetamine abuse. Neurology (NY) 30:1125, 1980.

117. D'Souza T, Shraberg D: Intracranial hemorrhage associated with amphetamine use. Neurology (NY) 31:922, 1981.

118. Edwards K: Hemorrhagic complications of cerebral arteritis. Arch Neurol 34:549, 1977.

119. Gericke OL: Suicide by ingestion of amphetamine sulfate. JAMA 128:1098, 1945.

120. Goodman SJ, Becker DP: Intracranial hemorrhage associated with amphetamine abuse. JAMA 212:480, 1970.

121. Hall CD, Blanton DE, Scatliff JH, Morris CE: Speed kills: Fatality from the self administration of methamphetamine intravenously. South Med J 66:650, 1973.

122. Harrington H, Heller HA, Dawson D, et al: Intracerebral hemorrhage and oral amphetamine. Arch Neurol 40:503, 1983.

123. Kane FJ, Keeler MH, Reifler CB: Neurological crisis following methamphetamine. JAMA 210:556, 1969.

124. Kessler JT, Jortner BS, Adapon BD: Cerebral vasculitis in a drug abuser. J Clin Psychiatry 39:559, 1978.

125. Lloyd JTA, Walker DRH: Death after combined dexamphetamine and phenylzine. Br Med J 2:168, 1965.

126. LoVerme S: Complications of amphetamine abuse. In Culebras A (ed): Clini-Pearls Vol 2, No 8. Syracuse, NY, Creative Medical Publications, 1979, p 5.

127. Lukes SA: Intracerebral hemorrhage from an arteriovenous malformation after amphetamine injection. Arch Neurol 40:60, 1983.

128. Margolis MT, Newton TH: Methamphetamine ("speed") arteritis. Neuroradiology 2:179, 1971..

129. Matick H, Anderson D, Brumlik J: Cerebral vasculitis associated with oral amphetamine overdose. Arch Neurol 40:253, 1983

130. Olsen ER: Intracranial hemorrhage and amphetamine usage. Angiology 28:464, 1977.

131. Poteliakhoff A, Roughton BC: Two cases of amphetamine poisoning. Br Med J 1:26, 1956.

132. Shukla D: Intracranial hemorrhage associated with amphetamine use. Neurology (NY) 32:917, 1982.

133. Tibbetts JC, Hinck VC: Conservative management of a hematoma in the fourth ventricle. Surg Neurol 1:253, 1973.

134. Weiss SR, Raskind R, Morganstern NL, et al: Intracerebral and subarachnoid hemorrhage following use of methamphetamine ("speed"). Int Surg 53:123, 1970.

135. Yarnell PR: "Speed" headache and hematoma. Headache 17:69, 1977.

136. Yatsu FM, Wesson DR, Smith DE: Amphetamine abuse. In Richter RW (ed): Medical Aspects of Drug Abuse. Hagerstown, MD, Harper & Row, 1975, p 50.

137. Yen DJ, Wong SJ, Ju TH, et al: Stroke associated with methamphetamine inhalation. Eur Neurol 34:16, 1994.

138. Yu YJ, Cooper DR, Wellenstein DE, Block B: Cerebral angiitis and intracerebral hemorrhage associated with methamphetamine abuse: Case report. J Neurosurg 58:109, 1983.

139. Delaney P: Intracranial hemorrhage associated with amphetamine use. Neurology (NY) 31:923, 1981.

140. Citron BP, Halpern M, McCarron M, et al: Necrotizing angiitis associated with drug abuse. N Engl J Med 283:1003, 1970.

141. Gocke DJ, Christian CL: Angiitis in drug abusers. N Engl J Med 284:112, 1971.

142. Gocke DJ, Hsu K, Morgan C, et al: Association between polyarteritis and Australia antigen. Lancet 2(7684):1149, 1970.

143. Citron BP, Peters RL: Angiitis in drug abusers. N Engl J Med 284:112, 1971.

144. Bostwick DG: Amphetamine induced cerebral vasculitis. Hum Pathol 12:1031, 1981.

145. Rumbaugh CL, Bergeron RT, Fang HCH, McCormick R: Cerebral angiographic changes in the drug abuse patient. Radiology 101:335, 1971.

146. Rumbaugh CL, Fang HCH: The effects of drug abuse on the brain. Med Times 108:37S, 1980.

147. Rothrock JF, Rubenstein R, Lyden PD: Ischemic stroke associated with methamphetamine inhalation. Neurology (NY) 38:589, 1988.

148. Sachdeva K, Woodward KG: Caudal thalamic infarction following intranasal methamphetamine use. Neurology 39:305, 1989.

149. Rumbaugh CL, Bergeron T, Scanlon RL, et al: Cerebral vascular changes secondary to amphetamine abuse in the experimental animal. Radiology 101:345, 1971.

150. Rumbaugh CL, Fang HCH, Higgins RE, et al: Cerebral microvascular injury in experimental drug abuse. Invest Radiol 11:282, 1976.

151. Hartman BK, Zide D, Udenfriend A: The use of dopamine beta-hydroxylase as a marker for the central noradrenergic nervous system in rat brain. Proc Natl Acad Sci U S A 69:2722, 1972.

152. Mittleman RE, Wetli CV: Cocaine and sudden "natural" death. J Forensic Sci 32:11, 1987.

Specific Medical Diseases and Stroke

153. Stafford CR, Bogdanoff BM, Green L, Spector HB: Mononeuropathy multiplex as a complication of amphetamine angiitis. Neurology (NY) 25:570, 1975.

154. Blum A: Phenylpropanolamine: An over-the-counter amphetamine? JAMA 245:1346, 1981.

155. Mueller SM: Neurologic complications of phenylpropanolamine use. Neurology (NY) 33:650, 1983.

156. Lasagna L: Phenylpropanolamine: A Review. New York, Wiley, 1988.

157. Bernstein E, Diskant B: Phenylpropanolamine: A potentially hazardous drug. Ann Emerg Med 11:315, 1982.

158. Forman HP, Levin S, Stewart B, et al: Cerebral vasculitis and hemorrhage in an adolescent taking diet pills containing phenylpropanolamine: Case report and review of the literature. Pediatrics 83:737, 1989.

159. Kane FJ, Greene BQ: Psychotic episodes associated with the use of common proprietary decongestants. Am J Psychiatry 123:484, 1966.

160. King J: Hypertension and cerebral hemorrhage after trimolets ingestion. Med J Aust 2:258, 1979.

161. Lovejoy FH: Stroke and phenylpropanolamine. Pediatr Alert 12:45, 1981.

162. Mueller SM, Ertel PJ: Subarachnoid hemorrhage associated with over-the-counter diet medications. Stroke 14:16, 1983.

163. Mueller SM, Solow EB: Seizures associated with a new combination "pick-me-up" pill. Ann Neurol 11:322, 1982.

164. Ostern S, Dodson WH: Hypertension following Ornade ingestion. JAMA 194:472, 1965.

165. Schaffer CB, Pauli MW: Psychotic reaction caused by proprietary oral diet agents. Am J Psychiatry 137:1256, 1980.

166. Wharton BK: Nasal decongestants and paranoid psychosis. Br J Psychiatry 117:429, 1970.

167. Ryu SJ, Lin SK: Cerebral arteritis associated with oral use of phenylpropanolamine: Report of a case. J Formos Med Assoc 94:53, 1995.

168. Kernan WN, Viscdi CM, Brass LM, et al: Phenylpropanolamine and the risk of hemorrhagic stroke. N Engl J Med 343:1826, 2000.

169. Fleming GA: The FDA, regulation, and the risk of stroke. N Engl J Med 343:1886, 2000.

170. Bruno A, Nolte KB, Chapin J: Stroke associated with ephedrine use. Neurology 43:1313, 1993.

171. Garcia-Albea E: Subarachnoid hemorrhage and nasal vasoconstrictor abuse. J Neurol Neurosurg Psychiatry 46:875, 1983.

172. Loizou LA, Hamilton JG, Tsementzis SA: Intracranial hemorrhage in association with pseudoephedrine overdose. J Neurol Neurosurg Psychiatry 45:471, 1982.

173. Mariani PJ: Pseudoephedrine-induced hypertensive emergency: Treatment with labetalol. Am J Emerg Med 4:141, 1986.

174. Pentel P: Toxicity of over-the-counter stimulants. JAMA 252:1898, 1984.

175. Stoessl AJ, Young G, Feasby TE: Intracerebral hemorrhage and angiographic beading following ingestion of catecholaminergics. Stroke 16:734, 1985.

176. Wooten MR, Khangure MS, Murphy MJ: Intracerebral hemorrhage and vasculitis related to ephedrine abuse. Ann Neurol 13:337, 1983.

177. Adverse events associated with ephedrine-containing products–Texas, December 1993–September 1995. JAMA 276:1711, 1996.

178. Josefson D: Herbal stimulant causes U.S. deaths. BMJ 312:1378, 1996.

179. Theoharides TC: Sudden death of a healthy college student related to ephedrine toxicity from a ma huang–containing drink. J Clin Psychopharmacol 17:437, 1997.

180. Vahedi K, Domingo V, Amarenco R, Bousser MG: Ischemic stroke in a sportsman who consumed MaHuang extract and creatine monohydrate for body building. J Neurol Neurosurg Psychiatry 68:112, 2000.

181. Haller CA, Benowitz NL: Adverse cardiovascular and central nervous system events associated with dietary supplements containing Ephedra alkaloids. N Engl J Med 343:1833, 2000.

182. Kokkinos J, Levine SR: Possible association of ischemic stroke with phentermine. Stroke 24:310, 1993.

183. Wen PY, Feske SK, Teoh SK, Steig PE: Cerebral hemorrhage in a patient taking fenfluramine and phentermine for obesity. Neurology 49:632, 1997.

184. Deringer PM, Hamilton LL, Whelan MA: A stroke associated with cocaine use. Arch Neurol 47:502, 1990.

185. Gardin JM, Schumacher D, Constaine G, et al: Valvular abnormalities and cardiovascular status following exposure to dexfenfluramine or phentermine/fenfluramine. JAMA 283:1703, 2000.

186. Lambrecht GL, Malbrain ML, Chew SL, et al: Intranasal caffeine and amphetamine causing stroke. Acta Neurol Belg 93:146, 1993.

187. Manchanda S, Connolly MJ: Cerebral infarction in association with Ecstasy abuse. Postgrad Med J 69:874, 1993.

188. Reneman L, Habraken JB, Majoie CB, et al: MDMA ("Ecstasy") and its association with cerebrovascular accidents: Preliminary findings. Am J Neuroradiol 21:1001, 2000.

189. Chillar RK, Jackson AL: Reversible hemiplegia after presumed intracarotid injection of Ritalin. N Engl J Med 304:1305, 1981.

190. Tse DT, Ober RR: Talc retinopathy. Am J Ophthalmol 90:624, 1980.

191. Hamer R, Phelp D: Inadvertent intra-arterial injection of phentermine: A complication of drug abuse. Ann Emerg Med 10:148, 1981.

191a. Anderson RJ, Garza H, Garriott JC, Dimaio V: Intravenous propylhexedrine (Benzedrex) abuse and sudden death. Am J Med 67:15, 1979.

192. Riddick L, Reisch R: Oral overdose of propylhexedrine. J Forensic Sci 26:834, 1981.

193. Califano JA: Substance abuse and addiction—the need to know. Am J Public Health 88:9, 1998.

194. Kaku DA, Lowenstein DH: Emergence of recreational drug abuse as a major risk factor for stroke in young adults. Ann Intern Med 113:821, 1990.

195. Wetli C, Wright RK: Death caused by recreational cocaine use. JAMA 241:2519, 1979.

196. Levine SR, Brust JCM, Futrell N, et al: Cerebrovascular complications of the use of the "crack" form of alkaloidal cocaine. N Engl J Med 323:699, 1990.

197. Brust JCM, Richter RW: Stroke associated with cocaine abuse? N Y State J Med 77:1473, 1977.

198. Lundberg GD, Garriott JC, Reynolds PC, et al: Cocaine-related death. J Forensic Sci 22:402, 1977.

199. Altes-Capella J, Cabezudo-Artero JM, Forteza-Rei J: Complications of cocaine abuse. Ann Intern Med 107:940, 1987.

200. Baquero M, Alfaro A: Progressive bleeding in spontaneous thalamic hemorrhage. Neurologia 9:364, 1994.

201. Caplan LR, Hier DB, DeCruz I: Cerebral embolism in the Michael Reese Stroke Registry. Stroke 14:530, 1983.

202. Case records of the Massachusetts General Hospital. Weekly clinicopathological exercises. Case 27-1993: A 32-year-old man with the sudden onset of a right-sided headache and left hemiplegia and hemianesthesia. N Engl J Med 329:117, 1993.

203. Chadan N, Thierry A, Sautreaux JL, et al: Rupture aneurysmale et toxicomanie á la cocaine. Neurochirurgie 37:403, 1990.

204. Chasnoff IJ, Bussey ME, Savich R, Stack CM: Perinatal cerebral infarction and maternal cocaine use. J Pediatr 108:456, 1986.

205. Cregler LL, Mark H: Medical complications of cocaine abuse. N Engl J Med 315:1495, 1986.

206. Cregler LL, Mark H: Relation of stroke to cocaine abuse. NY State J Med 87:128, 1987.

207. Daras M, Tuchman AJ, Koppel BS, et al: Neurovascular complications of cocaine. Acta Neurol Scand 90:124, 1994.

208. Daras M, Tuchman AJ, Marks S: Central nervous system infarction related to cocaine abuse. Stroke 22:1320, 1991.

209. DeBroucker T, Verstichel P, Cambier J, De-Truchis P: Accidents neurologiqes après prise de cocaine. Presse Med 18:541, 1989.

210. Derby LE, Myers MW, Jick H: Use of dexfenfluramine, fenfluramine and phentermine and the risk of stroke. Br J Clin Pharmacol 47:565, 1999.

211. Devenyi P, Schneiderman JF, Devenyi RG, Lawby L: Cocaine-induced central retinal artery occlusion. CMAJ 138:129, 1988.

212. Devore RA, Tucker HM: Dysphagia and dysarthria as a result of cocaine abuse. Otolaryngol Head Neck Surg 98:174, 1988.

213. Dominguez R, Vila-Coro AA, Slopis JM, Bohan TP: Brain and ocular abnormalities in infants with in utero exposure to cocaine and other street drugs. Am J Dis Child 145:688, 1991.

214. Engstrand BC, Daras M, Tuchman AJ, et al: Cocaine-related ischemic stroke. Neurology (NY) 39(Suppl 1):186, 1989.

215. Fredericks RK, Lefkowitz DS, Challa VER, Troost BT: Cerebral vasculitis associated with cocaine abuse. Stroke 22:1437, 1991.

216. Golbe LI, Merkin MD: Cerebral infarction in a user of free-base cocaine ("crack"). Neurology (NY) 36:1602, 1986.

217. Green RS, Kelly KM, Gabrielson T, et al: Multiple intracerebral hemorrhages after smoking "crack" cocaine. Stroke 21:957, 1990.

218. Guidotti M, Zanasi S: Cocaine use and cerebrovascular disease: Two cases of ischemic stroke in young adults. Ital J Neurol Sci 11:153, 1990.

219. Hall JAS: Cocaine-induced stroke: First Jamaican case. J Neurol Sci 98:347, 1990.

220. Hamer JJ, Kamphuis DJ, Rico RE: Cerebral hemorrhages and infarcts following use of cocaine. Ned Tijdschr Geneeskd 135:333, 1991.

221. Harruff RC, Phillips AM, Fernandez GS: Cocaine-related deaths in Memphis and Shelby County: Ten-year history, 1980–1989. J Tenn Med Assoc 84:66, 1991.

222. Heier LA, Carpanzano CR, Mast J, et al: Maternal cocaine abuse: The spectrum of radiologic abnormalities in the neonatal CNS. AJR 157:1105, 1991.

223. Henderson CE, Torbey M: Rupture of intracranial aneurysm associated with cocaine use during pregnancy. Am J Perinatol 5:142, 1988.

224. Hoyme HE, Jones KL, Dixon SD, et al: Prenatal cocaine exposure and fetal vascular disruption. Pediatrics 85:743, 1990.

225. Jacobs IG, Roszler MH, Kelly JK, et al: Cocaine abuse: Neurovascular complications. Radiology 170:223, 1989.

226. Kaku DA, Lowenstein DH: Recreational drug use: A growing risk factor for stroke in young people. Neurology (NY) 39(Suppl 1):16, 1989.

227. Kaye BR, Fainstat M: Cerebral vasculitis associated with cocaine abuse. JAMA 258:2104, 1987.

228. Klonoff DC, Andrews BT, Obana WG: Stroke associated with cocaine use. Arch Neurol 46:989, 1989.

229. Konzen JP, Levine SR, Charbel FT, Garcia JH: The mechanisms of alkaloidal cocaine-related stroke. Neurology 42(Suppl 3):249, 1992.

230. Koppel BS, Kaunitz AM, Daras M, et al: Cocaine-associated stroke during pregnancy. Ann Neurol 32:239, 1992.

231. Kramer LD, Locke GE, Ogunyemi A, Nelson L: Neonatal cocaine-related seizures. J Child Neurol 5:60, 1990.

232. Krendel DA, Ditter SM, Frankel MR, Ross WK: Biopsy-proven cerebral vasculitis associated with cocaine abuse. Neurology (NY) 40:1092, 1990.

233. Lehman LB: Intracerebral hemorrhage after intranasal cocaine use. Hosp Physician 7:69, 1987.

234. Levine SR, Washington JM, Jefferson MF, et al: "Crack" cocaine-associated stroke. Neurology (NY) 37:1849, 1987.

235. Levine SR, Welch KM: Cocaine and stroke. Stroke 19:779, 1988.

236. Libman RB, Masters SR, de Paola A, Mohr JP: Transient monocular blindness associated with cocaine abuse. Neurology 43:228, 1993.

237. Lichtenfield PJ, Rubin DB, Feldman RS: Subarachnoid hemorrhage precipitated by cocaine snorting. Arch Neurol 41:223, 1984.

238. Lowenstein DH, Massa SM, Rowbotham MC, et al: Acute neurologic and psychiatric complications associated with cocaine abuse. Am J Med 83:841, 1987.

239. Mangiardi JR, Daras M, Geller ME, et al: Cocaine-related intracranial hemorrhage: Report of nine cases and reviews. Acta Neurol Scand 77:177, 1988.

240. Martin K, Rogers T, Kavanaugh A: Central nervous system angiopathy associated with cocaine abuse. J Rheumatol 22:780, 1995.

241. Mercado A, Johnson G, Calver D, Sokol RJ: Cocaine, pregnancy, and postpartum intracerebral hemorrhage. Obstet Gynecol 73:467, 1989.

242. Meza I, Estrad CA, Montalvo JA, et al: Cerebral infarction associated with cocaine use. Henry Ford Hosp Med J 37:50, 1989.

243. Moore PM, Peterson PL: Nonhemorrhagic cerebrovascular complications of cocaine abuse. Neurology (NY) 39(Suppl 1):302, 1989.

244. Morrow PL, McQuillen JB: Cerebral vasculitis associated with cocaine abuse. J Forensic Sci 38:732, 1993.

245. Nalls G, Disher A, Darabagi J, et al: Subcortical cerebral hemorrhages associated with cocaine abuse: CT and MR findings. J Comput Assist Tomogr 13:1, 1989.

246. Nolte KB, Brass LM, Fletterick CF: Intracranial hemorrhage associated with cocaine abuse: A prospective autopsy study. Neurology 46:1291, 1996.

247. Nolte KB, Gelman BB: Intracerebral hemorrhage associated with cocaine abuse. Arch Pathol Lab Med 113:812, 1989.

248. Nwosu CM, Nwabueze AC, Ikeh VO: Stroke at the prime of life: A study of Nigerian Africans between the ages of 16 and 45 years. East Afr Med J 69:384, 1992.

249. Peterson PL, Moore PM: Hemorrhagic cerebrovascular complications of crack cocaine abuse. Neurology (NY) 39(Suppl 1):302, 1989.

250. Peterson PL, Roszler M, Jacobs I, Wilner HI: Neurovascular complications of cocaine abuse. J Neuropsychiatry Clin Neurosci 3:143–149, 1991.

251. Petty GW, Brust JCM, Tatemichi TK, Barr ML: Embolic stroke after smoking "crack" cocaine. Stroke 21:1632, 1990.

252. Qureshi AI, Safdar K, Patel M, et al: Stroke in young black patients: Risk factors, subtypes, and prognosis. Stroke 26:1995, 1995.

253. Ramadan J, Levine SR, Welch KMA: Pontine hemorrhage following "crack" cocaine use. Neurology 41:946, 1991.

254. Reeves RR, McWilliams ME, Fitzgerald MJ: Cocaine-induced ischemic cerebral infarction mistaken for a psychiatric syndrome. South Med J 88:352, 1995.

255. Rogers JN, Henry TE, Jones AM, et al: Cocaine-related deaths in Pima Country, Arizona, 1982–1984. J Forensic Sci 31:1404, 1986.

256. Rowbotham MC: Neurologic aspects of cocaine abuse. West J Med 149:442, 1988.

257. Rowley HA, Lowenstein DH, Rowbotham MC, Simon RP: Thalamomesencephalic strokes after cocaine abuse. Neurology (NY) 39:428, 1989.

258. Sauer CM: Recurrent embolic stroke and cocaine-related cardiomyopathy. Stroke 22:1203, 1991.

259. Schwartz ICA, Cohen JA: Subarachnoid hemorrhage precipitated by cocaine snorting. Arch Neurol 41:705, 1984.

260. Seaman ME: Acute cocaine abuse associated with cerebral infarction. Ann Emerg Med 19:34, 1990.

261. Simpson RK, Fischer DK, Narayan RK, et al: Intravenous cocaine abuse and subarachnoid hemorrhage: Effect on outcome. Br J Neurosurg 4:27, 1990.

262. Singer LT, Yamashita TS, Hawkins S, et al: Increased incidence of intraventricular hemorrhage and developmental delay in cocaine-exposed, very low birth weight infants. J Pediatr 124:765, 1994.

263. Sloan MA, Kittner SJ, Rigamonti D, Price TR: Occurrence of stroke associated with use/abuse of drugs. Neurology 41:1358, 1991.

264. Sloan MA, Mattioni TA: Concurrent myocardial and cerebral infarctions after intranasal cocaine use. Stroke 23:427, 1992.

265. Spires MC, Gordon EF, Choudhuri M, et al: Intracranial hemorrhage in a neonate following prenatal cocaine exposure. Pediatr Neurol 5:324, 1989.

266. Tardiff K, Gross E, Wu J, et al: Analysis of cocaine-positive fatalities. J Forensic Sci 34:53, 1989.

267. Toler KA, Anderson B: Stroke in an intravenous drug user secondary to the lupus anticoagulant. Stroke 19:274, 1988.

268. Vivancos F, Diez-Tejedor E, Martinez N, et al: Stroke due to abuse of cocaine. J Neurol 24(Suppl 1):S39, 1994.

269. Weingarten KO: Cerebral vasculitis associated with cocaine abuse or subarachnoid hemorrhage? JAMA 259:1658, 1988.

270. Wojak JC, Flamm ES: Intracranial hemorrhage and cocaine use. Stroke 18:712, 1987.

271. Fessler RD, Esshaki CM, Stankewitz RC, et al: The neurovascular complications of cocaine. Surg Neurol 47:339, 1997.

272. Mody CK, Miller BL, McIntyre HB, et al: Neurologic complications of cocaine abuse. Neurology (NY) 38:1189, 1988.

273. DiLazzaro V, Restuccia D, Oliviero A, et al: Ischemic myelopathy associated with cocaine: Clinical, neurophysiological, and neuroradiological features. J Neurol Neurosurg Psychiatry 63:531, 1997.

274. Migita DS, Devereaux MW, Tomsak RL: Cocaine and pupillary-sparing oculomotor paresis. Neurology 49:1466, 1997.

275. Brown E, Prajer J, Lee HY, Ramsey RG: CNS complications of cocaine abuse: Prevalence, pathophysiology, and neuroradiology. AJR 159:137, 1992.

276. Mena I, Giombetti RJ, Miller BL, et al: Cerebral blood flow changes with acute cocaine intoxications: Clinical correlations with SPECT, CT, and MRI. NIDA Res Monogr 138:161, 1994.

277. Sawaya GR, Kaminski MJ: Spinal cord infarction after cocaine use. South Med J 83:601, 1990.

278. Strupp M, Hamann GF, Brandt T: Combined amphetamine and cocaine abuse caused mesencephalic ischemia in a 16-year boy -due to vasospasm? Eur Neurol 43:181, 2000.

279. Tolat D, O'Dell WO, Golamco-Estrella SP, Avella H: Cocaine-associated stroke: Three cases and rehabilitation considerations. Brain Inj 14:383, 2000.

280. Storen EC, Wijdicks EFM, Crum BA, Schultz G: Moyamoya-like vasculopathy from cocaine dependency. AJNR Am J Neuroradiol 21:1008, 2000.

Specific Medical Diseases and Stroke

281. Levine SR, Brust JCM, Welch KMA: Cerebral vasculitis associated with cocaine abuse or subarachnoid hemorrhage. JAMA 259:1648, 1988.

282. LaMonica G, Donatelli A, Katz JL: A case of mutism subsequent to cocaine abuse. J Subst Abuse Treat 17:109, 1999.

283. Aggarwal SK, Williams V, Levine SR, et al: Cocaine-associated intracranial hemorrhage: Absence of vasculitis in 14 cases. Neurology 46:1741, 1996.

284. Davis GG, Swalwell CI: The incidence of acute cocaine or methamphetamine intoxication in deaths due to ruptured cerebral (berry) aneurysms. J Forensic Sci 41:626, 1996.

285. Kibayashi K, Mastri AR, Hirsch CS: Cocaine-induced intracerebral hemorrhage: Analysis of predisposing factors and mechanisms causing hemorrhagic strokes. Hum Pathol 26:659, 1996.

286. Egido-Herrero JA, Gonzalez JL: Pontine hemorrhage after abuse of cocaine. Revista Neurol 25:137, 1997.

287. Oyesiku NM, Colohan AR, Barrow DL, Reisner A: Cocaine-induced aneurysmal rupture: An emergent factor in the natural history of intracranial aneurysms. Neurosurgery 32:518, 1993.

288. Samkoff LM, Daras M, Kleiman A, Koppell BS: Spontaneous spinal epidural hematoma: Another neurologic complication of cocaine? Arch Neurol 53:819, 1996.

289. Keller TM, Chappell ET: Spontaneous acute epidural hematoma precipitated by cocaine abuse: Case report. Surg Neurol 47:12, 1997.

290. Conway JE, Tamargo RJ: Cocaine use is an independent risk factor for cerebral vasospasm after aneurysmal subarachnoid hemorrhage. Stroke 32:2338, 2001.

291. Qureshi AI, Akbar MS, Czander E, et al: Crack cocaine use and stroke in young patients. Neurology 48:341, 1997.

292. Petitti DB, Sidney S, Quesenberry C, Bernstein A: Stroke and cocaine or amphetamine use. Epidemiology 9:596, 1998.

293. Brust JCM: Vasculitis owing to substance abuse. Neurol Clin 15:945, 1997.

294. Levine SR, Brust JCM, Futrell N, et al: A comparative study of the cerebrovascular complications of cocaine: Alkaloidal vs. hydrochloride. Neurology 41:1173, 1991.

295. Chokshi SK, Miller G, Rongione A, Isner JM: Cocaine and cardiovascular disease: The leading edge. Cardiology 3:1, 1989.

296. Lange RA, Cigarroa RG, Yancy CW, et al: Cocaine-induced coronary artery vasoconstriction. N Engl J Med 321:1557, 1989.

297. Moliterno DJ, Willard JE, Lange RA, et al: Coronary vasoconstriction induced by cocaine, cigarette smoking, or both. N Engl J Med 330:454, 1994.

298. Chokshi SK, Moore R, Pandian NG, Isner JM: Reversible cardiomyopathy associated with cocaine intoxication. Ann Intern Med 111:1039, 1989.

299. Smith HWB, Liberman HH, Brody SL, et al: Acute myocardial infarction temporally related to cocaine use: Clinical, angiographic, and pathophysiologic observations. Ann Intern Med 107:13, 1987.

300. Karch SB, Billingham ME: The pathology and etiology of cocaine-induced heart disease. Arch Pathol Lab Med 112:225, 1988.

301. Weiner RS, Lockhart JT, Schwartz RG: Dilated cardiomyopathy and cocaine abuse: Report of two cases. Am J Med 81:699, 1986.

302. Huang QF, Gebrewold A, Altura BT, Altura BM: Cocaine-induced cerebral vascular damage can be ameliorated by Mg^{2+} in rat brain. Neurosci Lett 109:113, 1990.

303. Isner JM, Chokshi SK: Cocaine and vasospasm. N Engl J Med 321:1604, 1989.

304. Konzen JP, Levine SR, Garcia JH: Vasospasm and thrombus formation as possible mechanisms of stroke related to alkaloidal cocaine. Stroke 26:1114, 1995.

305. Zhang X, Schrott LM, Sparber SB: Evidence for a serotonin-mediated effect of cocaine causing vasoconstriction and herniated umbilici in chicken embryos. Pharmacol Biochem Behav 59:585, 1998.

306. Powers RH, Madden JA: Vasoconstrictive effects of cocaine, metabolites and structural analogs on cat cerebral arteries. FASEB J 4:A1095, 1990.

307. Weiss RD, Gawin FH: Protracted elimination of cocaine metabolites in long-term, high-dose cocaine abusers. Am J Med 85:879, 1988.

308. Kaufman MJ, Levin JM, Ross MH, et al: Cocaine-induced cerebral vasoconstriction detected in humans with magnetic resonance angiography. JAMA 279:376, 1998.

309. Herning RI, King DE, Better WE, Cadet JL: Neurovascular deficits in cocaine abusers. Neuropsychopharmacology 21:110, 1999.

310. Dohi S, Jones D, Hudak ML, Traystman RJ: Effects of cocaine on pial arterioles in cats. Stroke 21:1710, 1990.

311. Diaz-Tejedor E, Tejada J, Munoz J: Cerebral arterial changes following cocaine IV administration: An angiographic study in rabbits. J Neurol 239(Suppl 2):S38, 1992.

312. Wang A-M, Suojanen JN, Colucci VM: Cocaine- and methamphetamine-induced acute cerebral vasospasm: An angiographic study in rabbits. Am J Neuroradiol 11: 1141, 1990.

313. Nunez BD, Miao L, Ross JN, et al: Effects of cocaine on carotid vascular reactivity in swine after balloon vascular injury. Stroke 25:631, 1994.

314. Mo W, Arruda JA, Dunea G, Singh AK: Cocaine-induced hypertension: Role of the peripheral nervous system. Pharmacol Res 40:139, 1999.

315. Vongpatanasin W, Monsour Y, Chavoshon B, et al: Cocaine stimulates the human cardiovascular system via a central mechanism of action. Circulation 100:497, 1999.

316. Togna G, Tempesta E, Togna AR, et al: Platelet responsiveness and biosynthesis of thromboxane and prostacyclin in response to in vitro cocaine treatment. Haemostasis 15:100, 1985.

317. Jennings LK, White MM, Sauer CM, et al: Cocaine-induced platelet defects. Stroke 24:1352, 1993.

318. Langner RO, Bement CL, Perry LE: Arteriosclerotic toxicity of cocaine. NIDA Res Monogr 88:325, 1988.

319. Siegel AJ, Sholar MB, Mendelson JH, et al: Cocaine-induced erythrocytosis and increase in von Willebrand factor: Evidence for drug-related blood doping and prothrombotic effects. Arch Intern Med 159:1925, 1999.

320. Randell T: Cocaine, alcohol mix in body to form even longer lasting, more lethal drug. JAMA 267:1043, 1992.

321. Wilson LD, Henning RJ, Suttheimer C, et al: Cocaethylene causes dose-dependent reductions in cardiac function in anesthetized dogs. J Cardiovasc Pharmacol 26:965, 1995.

322. O'Malley S, Adamse M, Heaton RK, Gawin FH: Neuropsychological impairment in chronic cocaine abusers. Am J Drug Alcohol Abuse 18:131, 1992.

323. Weinrieb RM, O'Brien CP: Persistent cognitive deficits attributed to substance abuse. Neurol Clin 11:663, 1993.

324. Bolla KI, Rothman R, Cadet JL: Dose-related neurobehavioral effects of chronic cocaine use. J Neuropsychiatry Clin Neurosci 11:361, 1999.

325. Smelson DA, Roy A, Santana S, Engelhart C: Neuropsychological deficits in withdrawn cocaine-dependent males. Am J Drug Alcohol Abuse 25:377, 1999.

326. Holman BL, Carvalho PA, Mendelson J, et al: Brain perfusion is abnormal in cocaine-dependent polydrug users: A study using technetium-99m-HMPAO and ASPECT. J Nucl Med 32:1206, 1991,

327. Strickland TL, Stein R: Cocaine-induced cerebrovascular impairment: Challenges to neuropsychological assessment. Neuropsychol Rev 5:69, 1995.

328. Tumeh SS, Nagel JS, English RJ, et al: Cerebral abnormalities in cocaine abusers: Demonstration by SPECT perfusion brain scintigraphy. Radiology 176:821, 1990.

329. Volkow ND, Fowler JS, Wolf AP, Gillespi A: Metabolic studies of drugs of abuse. In Harris L (ed): Problems of Drug Dependence, 1990. (NIDA Research Monograph 105.) Washington DC, US Department of Health and Human Services, 1991, p 47.

330. Bartzokis G, Beckson M, Hance DB, et al: Magnetic resonance imaging evidence of "silent" cerebrovascular toxicity in cocaine dependence. Biol Psychiatry 45:1203, 1999.

331. Dixon SD, Bejar R: Echoencephalographic findings in neonates associated with maternal cocaine and methamphetamine use: Incidence and clinical correlates. J Pediatr 115:770, 1989,

332. King TA, Perlman JM, Laptook AR, et al: Neurologic manifestations of in utero cocaine exposure in near-term and term infants. Pediatrics 96:259, 1995.

333. Volpe BJ: Effect of cocaine use on the fetus. N Engl J Med 327:399, 1992.

334. Burns RS, Lerner SE: Causes of phencyclidine-related deaths. Clin Toxicol 12:463, 1978.

335. Kessler GF, Demers LM, Brennan RW: Phencyclidine and fatal status epilepticus. N Engl J Med 291:979, 1974.

336. McCarron MM, Schultze BW, Thompson GA, et al: Acute phencyclidine intoxication: Incidence of clinical findings in 1000 cases. Ann Emerg Med 10:237, 1981.

337. Noguchi TT, Nakamura GR: Phencyclidine-related deaths in Los Angeles County, 1976. J Forensic Sci 23:503, 1978.

338. Crosley CJ, Binet EF: Cerebrovascular complications in phencyclidine intoxication. J Pediatr 94:316, 1979.

339. Eastman JW, Cohen SN: Hypertensive crisis and death associated with phencyclidine poisoning. JAMA 231:1270, 1975.

340. Illett KF, Jarrott B, O'Donnell SR, et al: Mechanism of cardiovascular actions of 1-(1-phenylcyclohexyl) piperidine hydrochloride (phencyclidine). Br J Pharmacol Chemother 28:73, 1966.

341. Altura B, Altura BM: Phencyclidine, lysergic acid diethylamide, and mescaline: Cerebral artery spasms and hallucinogenic activity. Science 212:1051, 1981.

342. Besson HA: Intracranial hemorrhage associated with phencyclidine abuse. JAMA 248:585, 1982.

343. Boyko OB, Burger PC, Heinz ER: Pathological and radiological correlation of subarachnoid hemorrhage in phencyclidine abuse: Case report. J Neurosurg 67:446, 1987.

344. Burns RS, Lerner SE: The effects of phencyclidine in man: A review. In Domino EF (ed): PCP (Phencyclidine): Historical and Current Perspectives. Ann Arbor, MI, NPP Books, 1981, p 449.

345. Bourne PG: Acute Drug Abuse Emergencies. San Diego, CA, Academic Press, 1976.

346. Stimmel B: Cardiovascular Effects of Mood-Altering Drugs. New York, Raven Press, 1979.

347. Sobel J, Espinas OE, Friedman SA: Carotid artery obstruction following LSD capsule ingestion. Arch Intern Med 127:290, 1971.

348. Lieberman AN, Bloom W, Kishore PS, Lin JP: Carotid artery occlusion following ingestion of LSD. Stroke 5:213, 1974.

349. Barrett CP, Braithwaite RA, Teale JD: Unusual case of tetrahydrocannabinol intoxication confirmed by radioimmunoassay. Br Med J 2:166, 1977.

350. Mohan H, Sood GC: Conjugate deviation of the eyes after cannabis intoxication. Br J Ophthalmol 48:160, 1964.

351. Cooles P: Stroke after heavy cannabis smoking. Postgrad Med J 63:511, 1987.

352. Zachariah SB: Stroke after heavy marijuana smoking. Stroke 22:406, 1991.

353. Barnes D, Palace J, O'Brien MD: Stroke following marijuana smoking. Stroke 9:1381, 1992.

354. Adams MD, Earnhardt JT, Dewcy WL, Harris LS: Vasoconstrictor actions of delta-8- and delta-9-tetrahydrocannabinol in the rat. J Pharmacol Exp Ther 196:649, 1976.

355. Mathew RJ, Wilson WH: Substance abuse and cerebral blood flow. Am J Psychiatry 148:292, 1991.

356. Parker MJ, Tarlow MJ, Milne-Anderson J: Glue sniffing and cerebral infarction. Arch Dis Child 59:675, 1984.

357. Lamont CM, Adams FG: Glue-sniffing as a cause of a positive radioisotope brain scan. Eur J Nucl Med 7:387, 1982.

358. Ahlawat SK, Siwach SB: Alcohol and coronary artery disease. Int J Cardiol 44:157, 1994.

359. Luck JC: Arrhythmias and social drinking. Ann Intern Med 93:253, 1983.

360. Thornton JR: Atrial fibrillation in healthy non-alcoholic people after an alcoholic binge. Lancet 2;1013, 1984.

361. Katsuki S, Omae T: Stroke prone profiles in the Japanese. In Engel A, Larsson T (eds): First Thule International Symposium on Stroke, 1966. Stockholm, Nordiska Bokhandein, 1967, p 215.

362. Klassen AC, Loewenson RB, Resch JA: Cerebral atherosclerosis in selected chronic disease states. Atherosclerosis 18:321, 1973.

363. Lee K: Alcoholism and cerebral thrombosis in the young. Acta Neurol Scand 59:270, 1979.

364. Okada H, Horibe H, Ohno Y, et al: A prospective study of cerebrovascular disease in Japanese rural communities, Akabane and Asahi. I: Evaluation of risk factors in the occurrence of cerebral hemorrhage and thrombosis. Stroke 7:599, 1976.

365. Ramanova MV, Romanov NS: Cerebral circulation disturbance in patients with chronic alcoholism. Sov Med 7:148, 1978.

366. Hillbom M, Kaste M: Does ethanol intoxication promote brain infarction in young adults? Lancet 2:1181, 1978.

367. Hillbom M, Kaste M: Ethanol intoxication: A risk factor for ischemic brain infarction in adolescents and young adults. Stroke 12:422, 1981.

368. Hillbom M, Kaste M: Alcohol intoxication: A risk factor for primary subarachnoid hemorrhage. Neurology (NY) 32:706, 1982.

369. Hillbom M, Kaste M: Ethanol intoxication: A risk factor for ischemic brain infarction. Stroke 14:694, 1983.

370. Hilton-Jones O, Warlow CP: The cause of stroke in the young. J Neurol 232:137, 1985.

371. Moorthy G, Price TR, Tuhrim S, et al: Relationship between recent alcohol intake and stroke type? The NINCDS Stroke Data Bank. Stroke 17:141, 1986.

372. Gorelick PB, Rodin MB, Langenberg P, et al: Is acute alcohol ingestion a risk factor for ischemic stroke? Results of a controlled study in middle-aged and elderly stroke patients at three urban medical centers. Stroke 18:359, 1987.

373. Gorelick PB, Rodin MB, Langenberg P, et al: Weekly alcohol consumption, cigarette smoking, and the risk of ischemic stroke: Results of a case-control study at three urban medical centers in Chicago, Illinois. Neurology (NY) 39:339, 1989.

374. Beghi E, Bogliun G, Cosso P, et al: Stroke and alcohol intake in a hospital population: A case-control study. Stroke 26:1691, 1995.

375. Boysen G, Nyboe J, Appleyard M, et al: Stroke incidence and risk factors for stroke in Copenhagen, Denmark. Stroke 19:1345, 1988.

376. Cullen K, Stenhouse NS, Wearne KL: Alcohol and mortality in the Busselton study. Int J Epidemiol 11:67, 1982.

377. Fuchs CS, Stampfer MJ, Colditz GA, et al: Alcohol consumption and mortality among women. N Engl J Med 332:1245, 1995.

378. Goldberg RJ, Burchfiel CM, Benfante R, et al: Lifestyle and biologic factors associated with atherosclerotic disease in middle-aged men: 20-year findings from the Honolulu Heart Program. Arch Intern Med 155:686, 1995.

379. Gordon T, Doyle JT: Drinking and mortality: The Albany Study. Am J Epidemiol 125:263, 1987.

380. Hansagi H, Romelsjo A, Gerhardsson de Verdier M, et al: Alcohol consumption and stroke mortality: 20 year follow-up of 15,077 men and women. Stroke 26:1768, 1995.

381. Herman B, Schmintz PIM, Leyten ACM, et al: Multivariate logistic analysis of risk factors for stroke in Tilburg, the Netherlands. Am J Epidemiol 118:514, 1983.

382. Khaw AL, Barrett-Connor E: Dietary potassium and stroke-associated mortality: A 12-year prospective study. N Engl J Med 316:235, 1987.

383. Kiechl S, Willeit J, Egger G, et al: Alcohol consumption and carotid atherosclerosis: Evidence of dose-dependent atherogenic and antiatherogenic effects. Results from the Bruneck Study. Stroke 25:1593, 1994.

384. Klatsky AL, Friedman GD, Siegelaub AB: Alcohol and mortality: A ten-year Kaiser-Permanente experience. Ann Intern Med 95:139, 1981.

385. Lee TK, Huang ZS, Ng SK, et al: Impact of alcohol consumption and cigarette smoking on stroke among the elderly in Taiwan. Stroke 26:790, 1995.

386. Oleckno WA: The risk of stroke in young adults: An analysis of the contribution of cigarette smoking and alcohol consumption. Public Health 102:45, 1988.

387. Paganini-Hill A, Ross RK, Henderson BE: Post-menopausal oestrogen treatment and stroke: A prospective study. Br Med J 297:519, 1988.

388. Palomaki H, Kaste M: Regular light-to-moderate intake of alcohol and the risk of ischemic stroke: Is there a beneficial effect? Stroke 24:1828, 1993.

389. Peacock PB, Riley CP, Lampton TD, et al: The Birmingham stroke, epidemiology, and rehabilitation study. In Stewart G (ed): Trends in Epidemiology: Applications to Health Service Research and Training. Springfield, IL, Charles C Thomas, 1972, p 231.

390. Rodgers H, Aitken PD, French JM, et al: Alcohol and stroke: A case-control study of drinking habits past and present. Stroke 24:1473, 1993.

391. Sasaki S, Zhang XH, Kesteloot H: Dietary sodium, potassium, saturated fat, alcohol, and stroke mortality. Stroke 26:783, 1995.

392. Semenciw RM, Morrison MI, Mao Y, et al: Major risk factors for cardiovascular disease mortality in adults: Results from the Nutrition Canada Survey Study. Int J Epidemiol 17:317, 1988.

393. Stemmermann GN, Hayashi T, Resch JA, et al: Risk factors related to ischemic and hemorrhagic cerebrovascular disease at autopsy: The Honolulu Heart Study. Stroke 15:23, 1984.

394. Taylor JR, Combs-Orme T: Alcohol and strokes in young adults. Am J Psychiatry 142:116, 1985

395. Ben-Shlomo Y, Markowe H, Shipley M, Marmot MG: Stroke risk from alcohol consumption using different control groups. Stroke 23:1093, 1992.

Specific Medical Diseases and Stroke

396. Kozararevic D, McGee D, Vojvodic N, et al: Frequency of alcohol consumption and morbidity and mortality: The Yugoslavia Cardiovascular Disease Study. Lancet 1(8169):613, 1980.

397. Kozarevic DJ, Vodvodic N, Gordon T, et al: Drinking habits and death: The Yugoslavia Cardiovascular Disease Study. Int J Epidemiol 12:145, 1983.

398. Blackwelder WC, Yano K, Rhoads GC, et al: Alcohol and mortality: The Honolulu Heart Study. Am J Med 68:164, 1980.

399. Donahue RP, Abbott RD, Reed DM, Yano K: Alcohol and hemorrhagic stroke: The Honolulu Heart Study. JAMA 255:2311, 1986.

400. Kagan A, Popper JS, Rhoads GG, Yano K: Dietary and other risk factors for stroke in Hawaiian Japanese men. Stroke 16:390, 1985.

401. Takeya Y, Popper JS, Shimizu Y, et al: Epidemiologic studies of coronary heart disease and stroke in Japanese men living in Japan, Hawaii, and California: Incidence of stroke in Japan and Hawaii. Stroke 15:15, 1984.

402. Wolf PA, D'Agostino RB, Odell P, et al: Alcohol consumption as a risk factor for stroke: The Framingham Study. Ann Neurol 24:177, 1988.

403. Stamfer MJ, Coditz GA, Willett WC, et al: A prospective study of moderate alcohol consumption and the risk of coronary disease and stroke in women. N Engl J Med 319:267, 1988.

404. Bogousslavsky J, Van Melle G, Despland PA, Regli F: Alcohol consumption and carotid atherosclerosis in the Lausanne Stroke Registry. Stroke 21:715, 1990.

405. Katsuki S: Hisayama study. Jpn J Med 10:167, 1971.

406. Ueda K, Hasuo Y, Kiyohara Y, et al: Hisayama: Incidence, changing pattern during long-term follow up, and related factors. Stroke 19:48, 1988.

407. Kiyohara Y, Kato I, Iwamoto H, et al: The impact of alcohol and hypertension on stroke incidence in a general Japanese population. The Hiseyama Study. Stroke 26:368, 1995.

408. Kono S, Ikeda M, Ogata M, et al: The relationship between alcohol and mortality among Japanese physicians. Int J Epidemiol 12:437, 1983.

409. Kono S, Ikeda M, Tokudome S, et al: Alcohol and mortality: A cohort study of male Japanese physicians. Int J Epidemiol 15:527, 1986.

410. Tanaka H, Ueda Y, Hayashi M, et al: Risk factors for cerebral hemorrhage and cerebral infarction in a Japanese rural community. Stroke 13:62, 1982.

411. Tanaka H, Hayaski M, Date C, et al: Epidemiologic studies of stroke in Shibata, a Japanese provincial city: Preliminary report on risk factors for cerebral infarction. Stroke 16:773, 1985.

412. Iso H, Kitamara A, Shimamoto T, et al: Alcohol intake and the risk of cardiovascular disease in middle-aged Japanese men. Stroke 26:767, 1995.

413. Camargo CA: Moderate alcohol consumption and stroke: The epidemiologic evidence. Stroke 20:1611, 1989.

414. Jamrozik K, Broadhurst RJ, Anderson CS, Stewart-Wynne EG: The role of lifestyle factors in the etiology of stroke: A population-based case-control study in Perth, Western Australia. Stroke 25:51, 1994.

415. Shinton R, Sagar G, Beevers G: The relation of alcohol consumption to cardiovascular risk factors and stroke: The West Birmingham Stroke Project. J Neurol Neurosurg Psychiatry 56:458, 1993.

416. Beghi E, Bogliun G, Cosso P, et al: Cerebrovascular disorders and alcohol intake: Preliminary results of a case-control study. Ital J Neurol Sci 13:209, 1992.

417. Gronback M, Deis A, Sorensen TI, et al: Mortality associated with moderate intakes of wine, beer, or spirits. BMJ 10:1165, 1995.

418. Truelson T, Gronbaek M, Schnohr P, Boysen G: Intake of beer, wine, and spirits and risk of stroke: The Copenhagen City Heart Study. Stroke 29:2467, 1998.

419. Hillbom M, Numminen H, Juvela S: Recent heavy drinking of alcohol and embolic stroke. Stroke 30:2307, 1999.

420. Juvela S, Hillbom M, Palomäki H: Risk factors for spontaneous intracerebral hemorrhage. Stroke 26:1558, 1995.

421. Sacco RL, Elkind M, Baden-Albala B, et al: The protective effect of moderate alcohol consumption on ischemic stroke. JAMA 281:53, 1999.

422. Berger K, Ajani UA, Case CS, et al: Light-to-moderate alcohol and the risk of stroke among U.S. male physicians. N Engl J Med 341:1557, 1999.

423. Djoussé L, Ellison RC, Beiser A, et al: Alcohol consumption and risk of ischemic stroke: The Framingham Study. Stroke 33:907, 2002.

424. Dulli DA: Alcohol, ischemic stroke, and lessons from a negative study. Stroke 33:890, 2002.

425. Palomaki H, Kaste M, Raininko R, et al: Risk factors for cervical atherosclerosis in patients with transient ischemic attack or minor ischemic stroke. Stroke 24:970, 1993.

426. Jorgensen HS, Nakagama H, Raaschou HO, Olsen TS: Leukoaraiosis in stroke patients: The Copenhagen Stroke Study. Stroke 26:588, 1995.

427. Yoshitake T, Kiyohara Y, Kato I, et al: Incidence and risk factors of vascular dementia and Alzheimer's disease in a defined elderly Japanese population: The Hisayama Study. Neurology 45:1161, 1995.

428. Mukamal KJ, Longstreth WT, Mittleman MA, et al: Alcohol consumption and subclinical findings on magnetic resonance imaging of the brain in older adults: The Cardiovascular Health Study. Stroke 32: 939, 2001.

429. Elias PK, Elias MF, D'Agostino RB, et al: Alcohol consumption and cognitive performance. Am J Epidemiol 150:580, 1999.

430. DeCarli C, Miller BL, Swan GE, et al: Cerebrovascular and brain morphologic correlates of mild cognitive impairment in the National Heart, Lung, and Blood Institute Twin Study. Arch Neurol 58: 43, 2001.

431. Herbert LE, Scherr PA, Beckett LA, et al: Relation of smoking and low-to-moderate alcohol consumption to change in cognitive function: A longitudinal study in a defined community of older persons. Am J Epidemiol 137:881, 1993.

432. Hendrie HC, Gao S, Hall KS, et al: The relationship between alcohol consumption, cognitive performance, and daily functioning in an urban sample of older black Americans. J Am Geriatr Soc 44: 1158, 1996.

433. Dufovil C, Ducimetierre P, Alperovitch A: Sex differences in the association between alcohol consumption and cognitive performance: EVA Study Group. Am J Epidemiol 146:405, 1997.

434. Lemeshow S, Letenneur L, Dartigues JF, et al: Illustration of analysis taking into account complex survey considerations: The association between wine consumption and dementia in the PAQUID Study. Am J Epidemiol 148;298, 1998.

435. Ruitenberg A, van Swieten JC, Witteman JCM, et al: Alcohol consumption and the risk of dementia: The Rotterdam Study. Lancet 359:281, 2002.

436. Hillbom M, Numminen H: Alcohol and stroke: Pathophysiologic mechanisms. Neuroepidemiology 17:281, 1998.

437. Beilin LJ: Alcohol and hypertension. Clin Exp Pharmacol Physiol 22:185, 1995.

438. Brackett, DJ, Gauvin DV, Lerner MR, et al: Dose- and time-dependent cardiovascular responses induced by ethanol. J Pharmacol Exp Ther 268:78, 1994.

439. Janssens E, Mounier-Vehier F, Hamon M, Leys D: Small subcortical infarcts and primary subcortical hemorrhages may have different risk factors. J Neurol 242:425, 1995.

440. Lip GY, Beevers DG: Alcohol, hypertension, coronary disease, and stroke. Clin Exp Pharmacol Physiol 22:189, 1995.

441. MacMahon S: Alcohol consumption and hypertension. Hypertension 9:111, 1987.

442. MacMahon SW, Norton RN: Alcohol and hypertension: Implications for prevention and treatment. Ann Intern Med 105:124, 1986.

443. Russell M, Cooper ML, Frone M, et al: Drinking patterns and blood pressure. Am J Epidemiol 128:917, 1988.

444. Tell GS, Rutan GH, Kronmal RA, et al: Correlates of blood pressure in community-dwelling older adults: The Cardiovascular Health Study. Hypertension 23:59, 1994.

445. Fuchs FD, Chambless LE, Whelton PK, et al: Alcohol consumption and the incidence of hypertension: The Atherosclerosis Risk in Communities Study. Hypertension 37:1242, 2001.

446. Cushman WC: Alcohol consumption and hypertension. J Clin Hypertension 3:166, 2001.

447. Okubo Y, Miyamoto T, Suwazano Y, et al: Alcohol consumption and blood pressure in Japanese men. Alcohol 23:149, 2001.

448. Gorelick PB: Alcohol and stroke. Stroke 18:268, 1987.

449. Randin D, Vollenweider P, Tappy L, et al: Suppression of alcohol-induced hypertension by dexamethasone. N Engl J Med 332:1733, 1995.

450. Harper G, Castleden CM, Potter JF: Factors affecting changes in blood pressure after acute stroke. Stroke 25:1726, 1994.

451. Longstreth WT, Koepsell TD, Yerby MS, van Belle G: Risk factors for subarachnoid hemorrhage. Stroke 16:377, 1985.

452. Baranoa E, Lieber CS: Alcohol and lipids. Rec Dev Alcohol 14:97, 1998.
453. Camargo CA, Williams PT, Vranizan KM, et al: The effect of moderate alcohol intake on serum apolipoproteins A-I and A-II: A controlled study. JAMA 253:2854, 1985.
454. Haskell WJ, Camargo C, Williams PT, et al: The effect of cessation and resumption of moderate alcohol intake on serum high-density lipoprotein subfractions: A controlled study. N Engl J Med 310:805, 1984.
455. Van Tol A, Hendriks HD: Moderate alcohol consumption: Effects on lipids and cardiovascular disease risk. Curr Op Lipid 12:19, 2001.
456. Reed DM, Resch JA, Hayashi T, et al: A prospective study of cerebral artery atherosclerosis. Stroke 19:820, 1988.
457. Avogaro P, Cazzolato G, Belussi F, Bittolo Bon G: Altered apoprotein composition of HDL-2 and HDL-3 in chronic alcoholics. Artery 10:317, 1982.
458. Gorelick PB: The status of alcohol as a risk factor for stroke. Stroke 20:1607, 1989.
459. Corella D, Tucker K, Lahoz C, et al: Alcohol drinking determines the effect of the APOE locus on LDL-cholesterol concentrations in men: The Framingham Offspring Study. Am J Clin Nutr 73:736, 2001.
460. Hillbom M, Kangasaho M, Kaste M, et al: Acute ethanol ingestion increases platelet reactivity: Is there a relationship to stroke? Stroke 16:19, 1985.
461. Hillbom M, Kaste M, Rasi V: Can ethanol intoxication affect hemocoagulation to increase the risk of brain infarction in young adults? Neurology (NY) 33:381, 1983.
462. Lang WE: Ethyl alcohol enhances plasminogen activator secretion by endothelial cells. JAMA 250:772, 1983.
463. Lee K, Nielsen JD, Zeeberg I, Gormsen J: Platelet aggregation and fibrinolytic activity in young alcoholics. Acta Neurol Scand 62:287, 1980.
464. Meade TW, Chakrabarti R, Haines AP, et al: Characteristics affecting fibrinolytic activity and plasma fibrinogen concentrations. Br Med J 1:153, 1979.
465. Numminen A, Syrjälä M, Benthin G, et al: The effect of acute ingestion of a large dose of alcohol on the hemostatic system and its circadian variation. Stroke 31:1269, 2000.
466. Ricker PM, Vaughn DE, Stampfer MJ, et al: Association of moderate alcohol consumption and plasma concentration of endogenous tissue-type plasminogen activator. JAMA 272:929, 1994.
467. DiMinno G, Mancini M: Drugs affecting plasma fibrinogen levels. Cardiovasc Drugs Ther 6:25, 1992.
468. Jakubowski JA, Vaillancourt R, Deykin D: Interaction of ethanol, prostacyclin, and aspirin in determining human platelet reactivity in vitro. Arteriosclerosis 8:436, 1988.
469. Landolfi R, Steiner M: Ethanol raises prostacyclin in vivo and in vitro. Blood 64:679, 1984.
470. Fenn CG, Littleton JM: Inhibition of platelet aggregation by ethanol: The role of plasma and platelet membrane lipids. Br J Pharmacol 73:305P, 1981.
471. Kangasaho M, Hillbom M, Kaste M, Vapaatalo H: Effects of ethanol intoxication and hangover on plasma levels of thromboxane B$_2$ and 6-keto-prostaglandin F$_{1\alpha}$ and on thromboxane B$_2$ formation by platelets in man. Thromb Haemost 48:232, 1982.
472. Quintana RP, Lasslo A, Dugdale ML, et al: Effects of ethanol and of other factors on ADP-induced aggregation of human blood platelets in vitro. Thromb Res 20:405, 1980.
473. Torres Duarte AP, Gong QS, Young J, et al: Inhibition of platelet aggregation in whole blood by alcohol. Thromb Res 78:107, 1995.
474. LaCoste L, Hung J, Lam JY: Acute and delayed antithrombotic effects of alcohol in humans. Am J Cardiol 87:82, 2001.
475. Tsaji S, Kawano S, Michida T, et al: Ethanol stimulates immunoreactive endothelin-1 and -2 release from cultured human umbilical vein endothelial cells. Alcohol Clin Exp Res 16:347, 1992.
476. Fujii Y, Takeuchi S, Tanaka R, et al: Liver dysfunction in spontaneous intracerebral hemorrhage. Neurosurgery 35:592, 1994.
477. Haselager EM, Vreeken J: Rebound thrombocytosis after alcohol abuse: A possible factor in the pathogenesis of thromboembolic disease. Lancet 1(8015):774, 1977.
478. Hutton RA, Fink FR, Wilson DT, Marjot DH: Platelet hyperaggregability during alcohol withdrawal. Clin Lab Haematol 3:223, 1981.
479. Ruf JC, Berger JL, Renaud S: Platelet rebound effect of alcohol withdrawal and wine drinking in rats: Relation to tannins and lipid peroxidation. Arterioscler Thromb Vasc Biol 15:140, 1995.
480. Neiman J, Rand ML, Jakowec DM, Packham MA: Platelet responses to platelet-activating factor are inhibited in alcoholics undergoing alcohol withdrawal. Thromb Res 56:399, 1989.
481. Delahousse B, Maillot F, Gabriel I, et al: Increased plasma fibrinolysis and tissue-type plasminogen activator/tissue-type plasminogen activator inhibitor ratios after ethanol withdrawal in chronic alcoholics. Blood Coag Fibrinolysis 12:59, 2001.
482. Imhof A, Froehlich M, Brenner H, et al: Effect of ethanol consumption on systemic markers of inflammation. Lancet 357:763, 2001.
483. McQueen JD, Sklar FK, Posey JB: Autoregulation of cerebral blood flow during alcohol infusion. J Stud Alcohol 39:1477, 1978.
484. Persson LI, Rosengren LE, Johansson BB, Hansson HA: Blood brain barrier dysfunction to peroxidase after air embolism, aggravated by acute ethanol intoxication. J Neurol Sci 42:65, 1979.
484a. Flamm ES, Demopoulos HB, Seligman ML, et al: Ethanol potentiation of central nervous system trauma. J Neurosurg 46:328, 1977.
485. Berglund M: Cerebral blood flow in chronic alcoholics. Alcoholism Clin Exp Res 5:295, 1981.
486. Hemmingsen R, Barry DL, Hertz MM, Klinken L: Cerebral blood flow and oxygen consumption during ethanol withdrawal in the rat. Brain Res 173:259, 1979.
487. Zhang A, Altura BT, Altura BM: Ethanol-induced contraction of cerebral arteries in diverse mammals and its mechanism of action. Eur J Pharmacol 248:229, 1993.
488. Gordon EL, Nguyen TS, Ngai AC, Winn HR: Differential effects of alcohols on intracerebral arterioles: Ethanol alone causes vasoconstriction. J Cerebral Blood Flow Metab 15:532, 1995.
489. Mayhan WG: Responses of cerebral arterioles during chronic ethanol exposure. Am J Physiol 262:H787, 1992.
490. Altura BM, Zhang A, Cheng TP, Altura BT: Ethanol promotes rapid depletion of intracellular free Mg in cerebral vascular smooth muscle cells: Possible relation to alcohol-induced behavioral and stroke-like effects. Alcohol 10:563, 1993.
491. Altura BM, Altura BT: Association of alcohol in brain injury, headaches, and stroke with brain tissue and serum levels of ionized magnesium: A review of recent findings and mechanisms of action. Alcohol 19:119, 1999.
492. Altura BM, Altura BT: Role of magnesium and calcium in alcohol-induced hypertension and strokes as probed by in vivo television microscopy, digital image microscopy, optical spectroscopy, 31P-NMR spectroscopy and a unique magnesium ion-selective electrode. Alcoholism Clin Exp Res 18:1057, 1994.
493. Altura BM, Gebrewold A, Altura BT, Gupta RK: Role of brain [Mg2+] in alcohol-induced hemorrhagic stroke in a rat model: A 31P-NMR in vivo study. Alcohol 12:131, 1995.
494. Cravo ML, Camilo ME: Hyperhomocysteinemia in chronic alcoholism: Relations to folic acid and vitamins B6 and B12 status. Nutrition 16:296, 2000.
495. Bell JR, Donovan JL, Wong R, et al: (+)-Catechin in human plasma after a single serving of reconstituted red wine. Am J Clin Nutr 71:103, 2000.
496. German JB, Walzam RK: The health benefits of wine. Annu Rev Nutr 20:561, 2000.
497. Malarcher AM, Giles WH, Croft JB, et al: Alcohol intake, type of beverage, and the risk of cerebral infarction in young women. Stroke 32:77, 2001.
498. Wollin SD, Jones PJ: Alcohol, red wine, and cardiovascular disease. J Nutrition 131:1401, 2001.
498a. Puddey IB, Croft KD: Alcohol, stroke, and coronary heart disease: Are there anti-oxidants and pro-oxidants in alcoholic beverages that might influence the development of atherosclerotic cardiovascular disease? Neuroepidemiology 18:292, 1999.
499. Aronow WS, Kaplan NM: Smoking. In Kaplan NM, Stamler J (eds): Prevention of Coronary Heart Disease. Philadelphia, WB Saunders, 1983, p 50.
500. Doll R, Hill AB: Mortality of British doctors in relation to smoking: Observations on coronary thrombosis. Natl Cancer Inst Monogr 19:205, 1966.
501. Kannel WB, D'Agostino RB, Belanger AL: Fibrinogen, cigarette smoking, and risk of cardiovascular disease: Insights from the Framingham Study. Am Heart J 113:1006, 1987.
502. Palmer JR, Rosenberg, Shapiro S: "Low yield" cigarettes and the risk of nonfatal myocardial infarction in women. N Engl J Med 320:1569, 1989.

Specific Medical Diseases and Stroke

503. Kroger K, Buss C, Govern M, et al: Risk factors in young patients with peripheral atherosclerosis. Int Angiol 19:206, 2000.

504. Davanipour Z, Sobel E, Alter M, et al: Stroke/transient ischemic attack in the Lehigh Valley: Evaluation of smoking as a risk factor. Ann Neurol 24:130, 1988.

505. Herman B, Leyten ACM, van Luuk JH, et al: An evaluation of risk factors for stroke in a Dutch community. Stroke 13:334, 1982.

506. Kannel WB, Dawber TR, Cohen ME, et al: Vascular disease of the brain—epidemiologic aspects. The Framingham Study. Am J Public Health 55:1355, 1965.

507. Nilsson S, Cartensen JM, Perhagen G: Mortality among male and female smokers: A 33 year follow up. J Epidemiol Commun Health 55: 825, 2001.

508. Bloch C, Richard JL: Risk factors for atherosclerotic diseases in the Prospective Parisian Study. I: Comparison with foreign studies. Rev Epidemiol Sante Publique 33:108, 1985.

509. Bonita R: Cigarette smoking, hypertension, and the risk of subarachnoid hemorrhage: A population-based case-control study. Stroke 17:831, 1986.

510. Bonita R, Scragg R, Stewart A, et al: Cigarette smoking and risk of premature stroke in men and women. Br Med J 293:6, 1986.

511. Candelise L, Bianchi F, Galligoni F, et al: Italian multicenter study on cerebral ischemic attacks. III: Influence of age and risk factors on cerebral atherosclerosis. Stroke 15:379, 1984.

512. U.S. Department of Health and Human Services: The Health Consequences of Smoking: Nicotine Addiction: A Report of the Surgeon General. (DHHS Publ No [CDC] 88-8406.) Washington, DC, US Government Printing Office, 1988.

513. Doll R, Gray R, Hafner B, et al: Mortality in relation to smoking: Twenty-two years' observations on female British doctors. Br Med J 1:967, 1980.

514. Hammond EC: Smoking in relation to mortality and morbidity: Finding in the first 34 months of follow-up in a prospective study started in 1959. JNCI 32:1161, 1964.

515. Hammond EC: Smoking in relation to death rates of one million men and women. Natl Cancer Inst Monogr 19:127, 1966.

516. Harmsen P, Rosengren A, Tsipogianni A, Wilhelmsen L: Risk factors for stroke in middle-aged men in Göteborg, Sweden. Stroke 21:223, 1990.

517. Herrschaft H: Prophylaxe zerbraler Durchblutungsstörungen. Fortschr Neurol Psychiatry 53:337, 1985.

518. Juvela S, Hillbom M, Numminen H, Koskinen P: Cigarette smoking and alcohol consumption as risk factors for aneurysmal subarachnoid hemorrhage. Stroke 24:639, 1993.

519. Kahn HA: The Dorn study of smoking and mortality among US veterans: Report on $8^{1}/_{2}$ years of observations. Natl Cancer Inst Monogr 19:1, 1966.

520. Koch A, Reuther R, Boos R, et al: Risikofactoren bei cerebralen Durchblutungsstörungen. Verh Dtsch Ges Inn Med 83:1773, 1977.

521. Kurtzke JF: Epidemiology of Cerebrovascular Disease. New York, Springer-Verlag, 1969.

522. Lakier JB: Smoking and cardiovascular disease. Am J Med 93:8S, 1992.

523. Love BB, Biller J, Jones MP, et al: Cigarette smoking: A risk factor for cerebral infarction in young adults. Arch Neurol 47:693, 1990.

524. Molgaard CA, Bartok A, Peddercord KM, et al: The association between cerebrovascular disease and smoking: A case-control study. Neuroepidemiology 5:88, 1986.

525. Paffenbarger RS Jr, Wing AL: Chronic disease in former college students. XI: Early precursors of nonfatal stroke. Am J Epidemiol 94:524, 1971.

526. Paffenbarger RS Jr, Wing A: Characteristics in youth predisposing to fatal stroke in later years. Lancet 1(7493):753, 1967.

527. Rogot E: Smoking and General Mortality Among US Veterans, 1954–1969. Bethesda MD, National Heart and Lung Institute, 1974.

528. Salonen JT, Puska P, Tuomilehto J, et al: Relation of blood pressure, serum lipids, and smoking to the risk of cerebral stroke: A longitudinal study in eastern Finland. Stroke 13:327, 1982.

529. Shinton R, Beevers G: Meta-analysis of relation between cigarette smoking and stroke. Br Med J 298:789, 1989.

530. Tuomilehto J, Bonita R, Stewart A, et al: Hypertension, cigarette smoking, and the decline in stroke incidence in eastern Finland. Stroke 22:7, 1991.

531. Benson RT, Sacco RL: Stroke prevention: Hypertension, diabetes, tobacco, and lipids. Neurol Clin 18:309, 2000.

532. Kissela BM, Saverbeck L, Woo D, et al: Subarachnoid hemorrhage: A preventable disease with a heritable component. Stroke 33:1321, 2002.

533. Collaborative Group for the Study of Stroke in Young Women: Oral contraception and increased risk of cerebral ischemia or thrombosis. N Engl J Med 288:871, 1973.

534. Frederiksen H, Ravenholt RT: Thromboembolism, oral contraceptives, and cigarettes. Public Health Rep 85:197, 1970.

535. Goldbaum GM, Kendrick JS, Hogelin GC, Gentry EM: The relative impact of smoking and oral contraceptive use on women in the United States. JAMA 258:1339, 1987.

536. Petitti DB, Wingerd J: Use of oral contraceptives, cigarette smoking, and risk of subarachnoid hemorrhage. Lancet 2(8083):234, 1978.

537. Royal College of General Practitioners: Oral Contraceptives and Health. London, Pitman, 1974.

538. Colditz GA, Bonita R, Stampfer MJ, et al: Cigarette smoking and risk of stroke in middle-aged women. N Engl J Med 318:937, 1988.

539. Medical Research Council Working Party: MRC Trial of treatment of mild hypertension: Principal results. Br Med J 291:97, 1985.

540. Pandey MR: Tobacco smoking and hypertension. J Indian Med Assoc 97: 367, 1999.

541. Christensen HK, Guasorra AD, Boysen G: Ischemic stroke occurs among younger smokers. Ugeskr Laeger 163:7057, 2001.

542. Abbott RD, Reed DM, Yano K: Risk of stroke in male cigarette smokers. N Engl J Med 315:717, 1986.

543. Sacco RL, Wolf PA, Bharucha NE, et al: Subarachnoid and intracerebral hemorrhage: Natural history, prognosis, and precursive factors in the Framingham Study. Neurology (NY) 34:847, 1984.

544. Wolf PA, D'Agostino RB, Kannel WB, et al: Cigarette smoking as a risk factor for stroke: The Framingham Study. JAMA 259:1025, 1988.

545. Wannamethee SG, Shaper AG, Whincup PH, Walker M: Smoking cessation and the risk of stroke in middle-aged men. JAMA 274:155, 1995.

546. Taylor BV, Oudit GY, Kalman PG, Liu P: Clinical and pathophysiological effects of active and passive smoking on the cardiovascular system. Can J Cardiol 14:1129, 1998.

547. Blackshear JL, Pearce LA, Hart RG, et al: Aortic plaque in atrial fibrillation: Prevalence, predictors, and thromboembolic implications. Stroke 30:834, 1999.

548. Framme C, Spiegel D, Roider J, et al: Central retinal artery occlusion: Importance of selective intra-arterial fibrinolysis. Ophthalmologe 98:725, 2001.

549. Tang JL, Morris JK, Wald NJ, et al: Mortality in relation to tar yield of cigarettes: A prospective study of four cohorts. BMJ 311:1530, 1995.

550. Bonita R, Duncan J, Truelsen T, et al: Passive smoking as well as active smoking increases the risk of acute stroke. Tob Control 8:156, 1999.

551. Naidoo B, Stevens W, McPherson K: Modelling the short term consequences of smoking cessation in England on the hospitalization rates for acute myocardial infarction and stroke. Tob Control 9:397, 2000.

552. La Vecchia C, Levi F, Lucchini F, Negri E: Trends in mortality from major diseases in Europe, 1980–1993. Eur J Epidemiol 14:1, 1998.

553. Liu BQ, Peto R, Chen ZM, et al: Emerging tobacco hazards in China. 1: Retrospective proportional mortality study of one million deaths. BMJ 317:1411, 1998.

554. Hawkins BT, Brown RC, Davis TP: Smoking and ischemic stroke: A role for nicotine? Trends Pharmacol Sci 23: 8, 2002.

555. Haapanen A, Koskenvuo M, Kaprio J, et al: Carotid arteriosclerosis in identical twins discordant for cigarette smoking. Circulation 80:10, 1989.

556. Whisnant JP, Homer D, Ingall TJ, et al: Duration of cigarette smoking is the strongest predictor of severe extracranial carotid atherosclerosis. Stroke 21:707, 1990.

557. Mast H, Thompson JLP, Lin I-F, et al: Cigarette smoking as a determinant of high-grade carotid artery stenosis in Hispanic, black and white patients with stroke or transient ischemic attack. Stroke 29:908, 1998.

558. Howard G, Wagenknecht LE, Burke GL, et al: Cigarette smoking and progression of atherosclerosis: The Atherosclerosis Risk in Communities (ARIC) Study. JAMA 279:119, 1998.

559. Kool MJ, Hoeks AP, Struijker Boudier HA, et al: Short and long-term effects of smoking on arterial wall properties in habitual smokers. J Am Coll Cardiol 22:1881, 1993.

560. Murchison LE, Fyfe T: Effects of cigarette smoking on serum lipids, blood glucose, and platelet adhesiveness. Lancet 2(7456):182, 1966.

561. Rogers RL, Meyer JS, Shaw TG, et al: Cigarette smoking decreases cerebral blood flow suggesting increased risk for stroke. JAMA 250:2796, 1983.

562. Benowitz NL: Pharmacologic aspects of cigarette smoking and nicotine addiction. N Engl J Med 319:1318, 1988.

563. Maouad J, Fernandez F, Barrillon A, et al: Diffuse or segmental narrowing (spasm) of coronary arteries during smoking demonstrated on angiography. Am J Cardiol 53:354, 1984.

564. Davis JW, Shelton L, Eigenberg DA, et al: Effects of tobacco and non-tobacco cigarette smoking on endothelium and platelets. Clin Pharmacol Ther 37:529, 1985.

565. Zimmerman M, McGreachie J: The effect of nicotine on aortic endothelium: A quantitative ultrastructural study. Atherosclerosis 63:33, 1987.

566. Haustein KO: Health consequences of passive smoking. Wien Med Wochenschr 150:233, 2000.

567. Talloss JH, Booyse FM: Effects of various agents and physical damage on giant cell formation in bovine aortic endothelial cell cultures. Microvasc Res 16:51, 1978.

568. Kubota K, Yamaguchi T, Abe Y: Effects of smoking on regional cerebral blood flow in neurologically normal subjects. Stroke 14:720, 1983.

569. Longstreth WT, Swanson PD: Oral contraceptives and stroke. Stroke 15:747, 1984.

570. Pardell H, Amario P, Hernandez R: Pathogenesis and epidemiology of arterial hypertension. Drugs 56(Suppl 2):1, 1998.

571. Green MS, Jucha E, Luz Y: Blood pressure in smokers and non-smokers: Epidemiologic findings. Am Heart J 111:932, 1986.

572. Isles C, Brown JJ, Cumming AM, et al: Excess smoking in malignant phase hypertension. Br Med J 1:579, 1979.

573. Mehta MC, Jain AC, Billie M: Combined effects of alcohol and nicotine on cardiovascular performance in a canine model. J Cardiovasc Pharmacol 31:930, 1998.

574. Belch JJ, McArdle BM, Burns P, et al: The effects of acute smoking on platelet behavior, fibrinolysis, and haemorheology in habitual smokers. Thromb Haemost 51:6, 1984.

575. Nadler JL, Velasso JS, Horton R: Cigarette smoking inhibits prostacyclin formation. Lancet 1(8336):1248, 1983.

576. Seiss W, Lorenz R, Roth P, Weber PC: Plasma catecholamines, platelet aggregation and associated thromboxane formation after physical exercise, smoking, or norepinephrine infusion. Circulation 66:44, 1982.j

576a. Miller GJ, Bauer KA, Cooper JA, Rosenberg RD: Activation of the coagulant pathway in cigarette smokers. Thromb Haemost 79:549, 1998.

576b. Nair S, Kulkarni S, Camoens NM, et al: Changes in platelet glycoprotein receptors after smoking—a flow cytometric study. Platelets 12:20, 2001.

577. Schwarcz TH, Hogan LA, Endean ED, et al: Thromboembolic complications of polycythemia: Polycythemia vera versus smokers' polycythemia. J Vasc Surg 17: 518, 1993,

577a. Zidovetski R, Chen P, Fisher M, Hofman FM: Nicotine increases plasminogen activator inhibitor-1 production by human brain endothelial cells via protein kinase C-associated pathway. Stroke 30:651, 1999.

577b. Wang L, Kittaka M, Sun N, et al: Chronic nicotine treatment enhances focal ischemic brain injury and depletes free pool of brain microvascular tissue plasminogen activator in rats. J Cereb Blood Flow Metab 17:136, 1997.

578. Margaglione M, Capucci G, d'Addedda M, et al: PAI-1 plasma levels in the general population without evidence of atherosclerosis: Relation to environmental and genetic determinants, Arterioscler Thromb Vasc Biol 18:562, 1998.

579. Simpson AJ, Gray RS, Moore NR, Booth NA: The effects of chronic smoking on the fibrinolytic potential of plasma and platelets. Br J Haematol 97:208, 1997.

580. Fogelholm R: Cigarette smoking and subarachnoid hemorrhage: A population-based case-control study. J Neurol Neurosurg Psychiatry 50:78, 1987,

581. Benowitz NL: The role of nicotine in smoking-related cardiovascular disease. Prev Med 26:412, 1997.

582. Benowitz NL, Fitzgerald GA, Wilson M, Zhang Q: Nicotine effects on eicosanoid formation and hemostatic function: Comparison of transdermal nicotine and cigarette smoking. J Am Coll Cardiol 22:1159, 1993.

583. Blann AD, Steele C, McCollum CN: The influence of smoking and of oral and transdermal nicotine on blood pressure, and haematology and coagulation indices. Thromb Haemost 78:1093, 1997.

584. Pierce JR: Stroke following application of a nicotine patch. Ann Pharmacol 28:402, 1994.

585. Greenland S, Satterfield MH, Lanes SF: A meta-analysis to assess the incidence of adverse effects associated with the transdermal nicotine patch. Drug Safety 18:297, 1998.

586. Boyajian RA, Otis SM: Acute effects of smoking on human cerebral blood flow: A transcranial Doppler ultrasonography study. J Neuroimag 10:204, 200.

586a. Domino EF, Minoshima S, Guthrie S, et al: Nicotine effects on regional cerebral blood flow in awake, resting tobacco users. Synapse 38:313, 2000.

587. Koskinen LO, Collin O, Bergh A: Cigarette smoke and hypoxia induce acute changes in testicular and cerebral microcirculation. Upsala J Med Sci 105:215, 2000.

588. Uchida S, Kagitani F, Nakayama H, Sato A: Effect of stimulation of nicotinic cholinergic receptors on cortical cerebral blood flow and changes in the effect during aging and in anesthetized rats. Neurosci Lett 228:203, 1997.

589. Iida M, Iida H, Dohi S, et al: Mechanisms underlying cerebrovascular effects of cigarette smoking in rats in vivo. Stroke 29:1656, 1998.

590. Gerzanich V, Zhang F, West GA, Simard JM: Chronic nicotine alters NO signaling of Ca (2+) channels in cerebral arterioles. Circ Res 88:359, 2001.

591. Zhang W, Edvinsson L, Lee TJ: Mechanism of nicotine-induced relaxation in the porcine basilar artery. J Pharmacol Exp Ther 284:790, 1998.

592. Golanov EV, Ruggiero DA, Reis DJ: A brainstem area mediating cerebrovascular and EEG responses to hypoxic excitation of rostral ventrolateral medulla in rat. J Physiol 529:413, 2000.

593. Levine SR, Fagan SC, Floberg J, et al: Moya-moya, oral contraceptives, and cigarette use. Ann Neurol 24:155, 1988,

594. Peerless SJ: Risk factors of moyamoya disease in Canada and the USA. Clin Neurol Neurosurg 99(Suppl 2):S45, 1997.

595. Fukada H, Kitani M, Omodani H: 99mTc-HMPAO brain SPECT imaging in a case of repeated syncopal episodes associated with smoking. Stroke 28:1461, 1997.

Specific Medical Diseases and Stroke

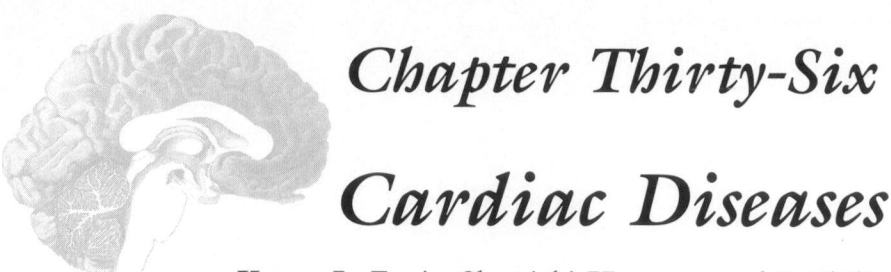

Chapter Thirty-Six

Cardiac Diseases

Karen L. Furie, Shunichi Homma, and J. Philip Kistler

EPIDEMIOLOGY

Embolism is the major mechanism of stroke in the United States, accounting for 60% of all ischemic strokes.[1] Up to 25% of these embolic strokes have a readily identifiable cause, atrial fibrillation (AF).[1] AF affects 9% of men aged 65 years and older.[2-4] In addition, approximately 25% to 30% of strokes in the young (younger than 45 years) can be attributed to cardiac embolism.[5,6] Table 36.1 estimates the prevalence of various cardiac conditions in embolic ischemia and infarction.[7] The economic toll of embolic strokes in the United States amounts to 18 billion dollars annually in both direct and indirect health care costs.[8,9]

In comparison with other subtypes of stroke, the prognosis after a cardioembolic stroke is poor.[10] There is a 6.5% risk of recurrence within 7 days, and the in-hospital mortality rate is 27.3%.[10] The 5-year mortality rate for cardioembolic stroke has been reported as high as 80%.[11]

Clinical Features of Cardioembolic Transient Ischemic Attack or Stroke

Cardioembolism as a proven cause of stroke has been a subject of long-standing argument. It can be inferred as the diagnosis and distinguished from other stroke subtypes on the basis of (1) the absence of a large artery stenosis or occlusion in the vessel supplying the ischemic territory, (2) a clinical syndrome or radiographic appearance inconsistent with a small vessel (lacunar) stroke, (3) absence of unusual precipitants of stroke (i.e., vasculitis), and (4) the absence of an atheroma of the aortic arch larger than 4 mm. Up to 18% of patients with presumed lacunar syndromes concomitantly have high-risk factors for cardioembolism.[12,13]

Clinical features of cardioembolic stroke are summarized in Table 36.2. Repetitive stereotyped transient ischemic attacks (TIAs), associated most commonly with low flow due to large vessel atherosclerotic disease, are unusual in embolic stroke, the onset of which is usually sudden. Less than a third of patients experience transient ischemic symptoms before the stroke.[14-17] The size of the emboli partially determines which vessels are affected. Small emboli can cause symptoms of retinal ischemia.[18-22] In a balloon catheter model of embolism, the majority of emboli were found to occlude the middle cerebral artery or one of its branches; next most common vessels were the

basilar artery and its branches and the anterior cerebral artery.[23] The size and composition of the embolus vary according to the underlying cardiac disorder (Table 36.3). Valvular lesions may result in the embolization of calcified particles.

Atrial myxomas can cause tumor emboli. In nonbacterial thrombotic endocarditis (NBTE), platelets are the main component, whereas emboli from left ventricular aneurysms contain mainly fibrinous material.[24]

The sudden onset of symptoms, observed in 25% to 82% of possible cardioembolic strokes, has low specificity, insomuch as onset is sudden in 66% of strokes due to other mechanisms.[14,15] Sudden onset and loss of consciousness are also insensitive for determining that symptoms are due to embolism.[14,10,25] In 1967, Fisher and Pearlman[26] described "non-sudden" cerebral embolism with stuttering progression, which they attributed to vacillating flow around an embolus lodged in the intracranial circulation. Seizures related to acute stroke are more common in patients with cardiac embolism.[27] There may be fluctuations in symptoms as the embolus lyses and fragments move downstream.[28] In addition, early clinical improvement or recovery may be due to the recruitment of collateral sources of blood flow.

Patients at high risk for cardioembolism are more likely to have large infarcts (half a lobe or larger) that involve both deep and superficial structures and are visible on initial head computed tomography (CT) (Fig. 36–1).[17,25,29,30] A pattern of multiple infarctions involving the anterior and posterior circulations is distinctive for embolism.[17,31,32] Cerebral or cerebellar surface branch occlusion by an embolus may lead to focal infarctions causing specific syndromes of focal motor deficits, isolated aphasia, or hemianopia.[17,33,34] Posterior cerebral artery territory infarcts, in particular, are often due to cardiac embolism.[35,36] Embolic strokes are believed to be more prone to hemorrhagic conversion, a complication detected on follow-up computed tomography in approximately 20% of cardioembolic strokes.[37] Hemorrhagic conversion occurs when there is spontaneous lysis of the thrombus with reperfusion of ischemic tissue (Fig. 36–2).

Between 30% and 60% of patients with ischemic stroke have a possible source of cardiac embolism.[24,38] It is important to recognize, however, that the detection of a potential cardiac source of embolism depends, to a large extent, on the thoroughness of the evaluation. For example, one

Table 36.1   Cardiac Conditions Associated with Cerebral Emboli

Source	Percentage of all Cardiogenic Emboli
Nonvalvular atrial fibrillation	45
Acute myocardial infarction	15
Ventricular aneurysm	10
Rheumatic heart disease	10
Prosthetic cardiac valve	10
Other	10

Table 36.2   Clinical Characteristics of Cardioembolic Stroke

Clinical features	Neurologic history and examination
	Sudden onset
	Isolated focal deficit
	Seizure at onset
	Loss of consciousness at onset
	Peak of deficit at onset
	Involvement of more than one vascular territory
	Evidence of systemic embolization
Neuroimaging findings	Multiple infarcts in more than one vascular territory
	Deep and superficial infarctions
	Hemorrhagic conversion
	Absence of large artery stenosis or occlusion in parent vessels
	Rapid recanalization of intracranial vessels on transcranial Doppler ultrasonography

Table 36.3   Characteristics of Emboli by Source

Source	Type	Size
Atrial fibrillation	Fibrin	Large
Left ventricular thrombus	Fibrin	Large
Myxoma	Myxomatous	Small or large
Infective endocarditis	Septic debris	Small or large
Degenerative valvular disease	Calcium	Small

study demonstrated that 15% of potential embolic sources were detected only after cardiac monitoring and two-dimensional (2D) transthoracic echocardiography.[39] In addition, ascribing a stroke to a definite cause can be difficult because of a coexistent mechanism involving a potential cardiac source of embolus (e.g., large vessel atherosclerosis in approximately 30% of cases).[17,24,40–43]

DIAGNOSTIC STUDIES

A thorough cardiac assessment of patients with stroke is necessary to accurately diagnose the mechanism of cerebral ischemia and to help establish prognosis. A standard 12-lead electrocardiogram (EKG) can identify patients who are in sustained AF and can detect acute myocardial ischemia; however, a 24- to 48-hour portable cardiac

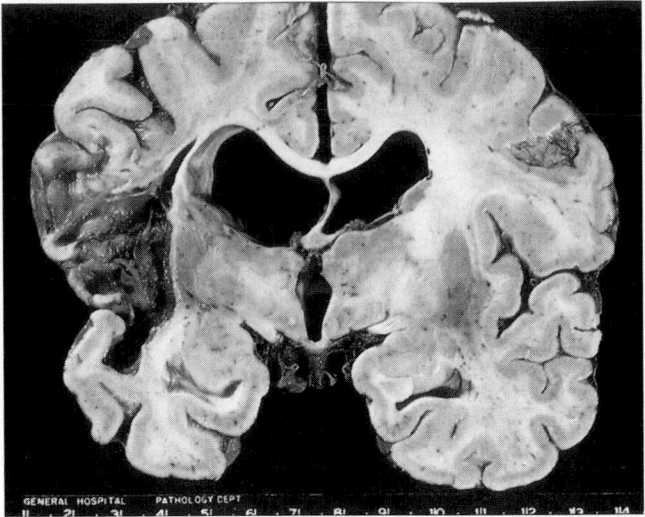

FIGURE 36–1   *Middle cerebral artery (MCA) territory infarction. A complete MCA territory infarction due to stem occlusion is common in embolic stroke. (From Rosenberg R [ed]: Atlas of Clinical Neurology. Philadelphia, Current Medicine, 1998.)*

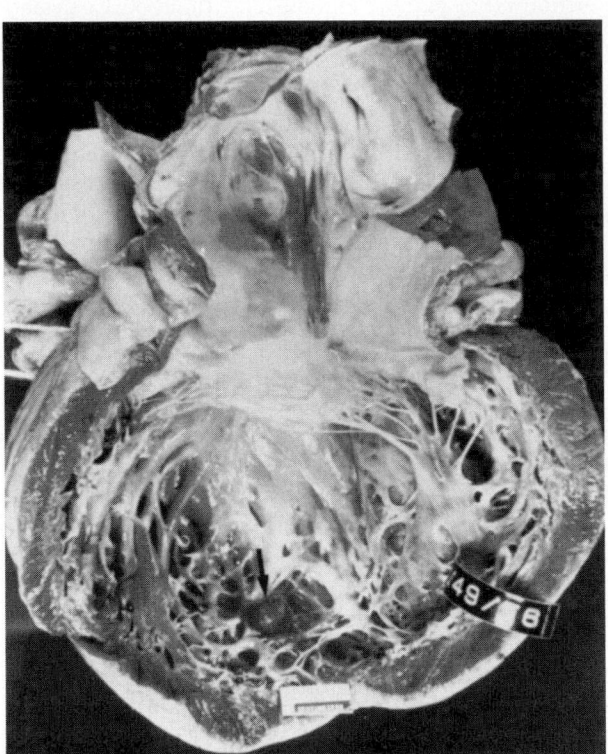

FIGURE 36–2   *Hypothetical mechanism of hemorrhagic transformation after embolic stroke caused by distal migration of embolus fragments with reperfusion of infarcted tissue. (From Barnett HJM: Heart in ischemic stroke—a changing emphasis. Neurol Clin 1:291, 1983.)*

monitor is essential to detect paroxysmal AF and the result is not always positive despite numerous such studies in the same patient.[39] A clinical history of angina pectoris or an abnormal EKG (anterior wall myocardial infarction [MI], left ventricular hypertrophy, and inverted T waves) have associated hazard ratios of 1.6 to 3.2 for nonfatal MI or cardiac death in patients with TIA or minor stroke.[44]

Transthoracic echocardiography (TTE) is an initial part of the embolic evaluation. M-mode and two-dimensional echocardiography can define the cardiac chambers, valves, and left ventricular function. The use of agitated saline allows for detection of an intracardiac shunt. TTE may be insensitive for masses and thrombi in the left atrium and upon the mitral valve, requiring further studies (see later).[45,46]

Transesophageal echocardiography (TEE) is more sensitive in detecting abnormalities in the left atrium and appendage, atrial septum, mitral valve, and aortic arch.[47–49] The cost effectiveness of performing TEE in all patients with stroke remains controversial.[50,51] This evaluation is recommended for patients with a suspected embolic stroke in whom cardiac monitoring and TTE findings are unremarkable and in young patients with stroke.

Embolus detection by *transcranial Doppler* (TCD) ultrasonography can be used to identify microemboli present in a variety of potential cardiac sources (AF, infectious endocarditis, cardiomyopathy, aortic stenosis, mitral stenosis, and patent foramen ovale).[52] The frequency of high-intensity transient signals (HITS) did not appear to vary according to echocardiographic diagnosis in one study, but another demonstrated a higher rate (33%) of microembolization in patients with high-risk sources of embolism (e.g., prosthetic valves) than in patients with other, lower-risk cardiac conditions (e.g., AF [15%]).[52,53]

APPROACH TO MANAGEMENT

Once the clinical presentation, radiographic appearance, and vascular and cardiac evaluations suggest or confirm cardioembolism, the focus shifts to management, mainly the question whether to use anticoagulant or antiplatelet therapy. Table 36.4 summarizes potential cardiac conditions according to the strength of indication for anticoagulation. Although the early period after stroke appears to be the highest risk period for recurrent embolization, it is also the period of greater risk of hemorrhagic conversion. One study examining the utility of immediate anticoagulation for a stroke due to any presumed mechanism, but occurring in a patient with AF did not demonstrate a benefit of anticoagulation in the first 2 weeks.[54] Still, in patients at higher risk for embolism, such as those with mechanical prosthetic valves or left ventricular thrombus, immediate anticoagulation should be considered.[55]

For long-term prevention of stroke, AF is the only condition for which warfarin has been shown to be superior to aspirin.[55] Still, anticoagulation is often used in situations with the potential for recurrent embolization. In the Warfarin Aspirin Recurrent Stroke Study (WARSS), warfarin was weakly (absolute risk reduction 9%) superior to aspirin therapy in patients in whom an embolic stroke was suspect but there was no evidence of a definite cardiac source; this difference was not statistically significant, however.[56] Currently, there are no data specifically comparing aspirin with other antiplatelet agents for the prevention of cardioembolic stroke.

Table 36.4 Classification of Cardioembolic Cerebral Ischemic Events

I. Definite cardioembolism
  A. Antithrombotic therapy considered the standard of practice
    1. Left ventricular thrombus
    2. Left atrial thrombus
    3. Recent transmural anterior myocardial infarction
    4. Rheumatic valvular disease
    5. Mechanical prosthetic valve
    6. Atrial fibrillation
  B. Antithrombotic therapy may be of value
    1. Nonbacterial thrombotic endocarditis
  C. Antithrombotic therapy contraindicated
    1. Bacterial endocarditis
    2. Atrial myxoma

II. Possible cardioembolism
  1. Mitral annular calcification
  2. Mitral valve prolapse
  2. Cardiomyopathy
  3. Patent foramen ovale
  4. Atrial flutter
  5. Sick sinus syndrome
  6. Valve strands
  7. Left atrial spontaneous echo contrast seen on transesophageal echocardiogram

SPECIFIC CARDIAC CONDITIONS CAUSING CEREBRAL EMBOLISM

The numerous structural and functional cardiac conditions associated with transient cerebral symptoms and infarction are described here in greater detail (see Table 36.1). Although cardiac testing can reveal a potential source, the neurologist must determine whether the symptoms, physical findings, and results of neuroimaging support the causal relationship. This determination includes analyzing whether the caliber of occluded vessel correlates with the expected embolus size.

Structural Cardiac Defects

Cardiomyopathy

The reported annual stroke rates, 1.3% to 3.5%, that were derived from cardiac trials likely underestimate the actual risk of stroke.[7,57–61] The risk of stroke is inversely related to the ejection fraction (EF), with as much as a 58% increase in thromboembolic events for every 10% decrease in EF, but not to the functional classification (New York Heart Association Functional Class).[60,62] There is a fourfold risk of stroke in patients who are 50 to 59 years old and have congestive heart failure.[4,63] The rate of stroke in patients with nonischemic dilated cardiomyopathy is approximately 1.5% to 3.5%.[58,64] In patients with cardiomyopathy, AF is often a complicating factor that further raises the risk of stroke. In the Survival and Ventricular Enlargement (SAVE) study, patients with EF values of 29% to 35% (mean 32%) had a stroke rate of 0.8% per year; the rate in patients with EF values of 28% or less (mean 23%) was 2.5% per year.[60]

Specific Medical Diseases and Stroke

Compared with placebo, warfarin has been shown to significantly reduce the risk of stroke by 40% to 55% in patients with ischemic and nonischemic cardiomyopathy.[65,66] However, the Sixties Plus study failed to show a significant risk reduction in stroke using an international normalized ratio (INR) value as high as 2.7 to 4.5.[67] A study comparing the efficacy of warfarin and aspirin for the prevention of stroke in patients with low EF is currently under way.[59]

Acute Myocardial Infarction

Within 2 to 4 weeks of an acute MI, 2.5% of patients suffer a stroke.[68,69] Stroke is more common with anterior wall MI (4% to 12% of cases) than with inferior wall infarction (1%) and usually occurs within the first 2 weeks.[68,69] Left ventricular thrombus develops in approximately 40% of patients with an anterior wall MI and can be detected with TTE. The thrombus usually develops in the first 2 weeks, coinciding with the period of highest risk of embolic stroke.[68–70] However, there have been reports of development of left ventricular thrombus as a late complication of anterior wall MI, and patients with low EF due to MI have a cumulative stroke risk of 8.1% after 5 years.[60,71] Despite the absence of clinical trial data, clinicians commonly choose to administer immediate anticoagulation, maintained for at least 3 to 6 months, when left ventricular thrombus is detected. The thrombus may resolve with anticoagulant therapy or may persist for several months. Intravenous tissue-type plasminogen activator (t-PA) has been used safely in patients with acute ischemic stroke and left ventricular thrombus.[72] After myocardial infarction, warfarin—alone for INR 2.1 or in combination with aspirin (75 mg daily)—resulted in fewer reinfarctions, thromboembolic events, or deaths compared with aspirin (160 mg daily) alone. However, the warfarin-treated patients had a fourfold higher risk of major hemorrhage.[72a]

Patent Foramen Ovale

Paradoxical embolism, or crossing of a venous thrombus into the arterial system, can occur in a patient with a patent foramen ovale (PFO) (Fig. 36–3).[73] The resultant right-to-left shunt may appear only in the setting of elevated right heart pressures, as occurs with a Valsalva's maneuver or with pulmonary hypertension (Fig. 36–4). PFOs are common in the general population, so care should be taken to establish a causal relationship of PFO with cerebral ischemic symptoms before PFO-specific treatment is initiated for secondary prevention of stroke.[73,74]

Strokes in association with PFO occur commonly in the pial convexity branches, as expected, but also in the basilar artery distribution.[75,76] Thrombus is believed to emanate from either a leg or pelvic vein. The latter should not be overlooked in the search for venous thrombus in the patient with a PFO and cerebral ischemic symptoms. In addition, there is conjecture that microthrombi can form within the PFO itself, particularly when there is a coexistent atrial septal aneurysm.[77]

In a study reported by Mas and colleagues,[78] the risk of recurrent stroke after 4 years of follow-up was 2.3% in patients with patent foramen ovale alone (95% confidence interval [CI], 0.3% to 4.3%), 15.2% among patients with both patent foramen ovale and atrial septal aneurysm (95% CI, 1.8% to 28.6%), and 4.2% in patients with neither (95% CI, 1.8% to 6.6%). These investigators found no recurrent strokes in patients with atrial septal aneurysms alone.

Larger defects (>2 mm) with greater shunting, as measured by the number of microbubbles crossing into the left atrium, have been associated with cryptogenic embolism.[75,79] The mean diameter of a PFO affects the risk of embolism, one study showing significantly larger diameters in patients with stroke or TIA than in control subjects. In that study, a PFO greater than 4 mm in diameter was associated with a higher risk of TIAs (odds ratio [OR], 3.4; 95% CI, 1.0 to 11; $P = .04$), ischemic strokes (OR, 12; 95% CI, 3.3 to 44; $P = .0001$), and multiple strokes (OR, 27; 95% CI, 4.7 to 160; $P = .0002$).[80] In the PFO in the Cryptogenic Stroke Study, there was no difference in rates of recurrent stroke or death in those with PFO (14.8%) or without (15.4%) in the entire population or the subset with a

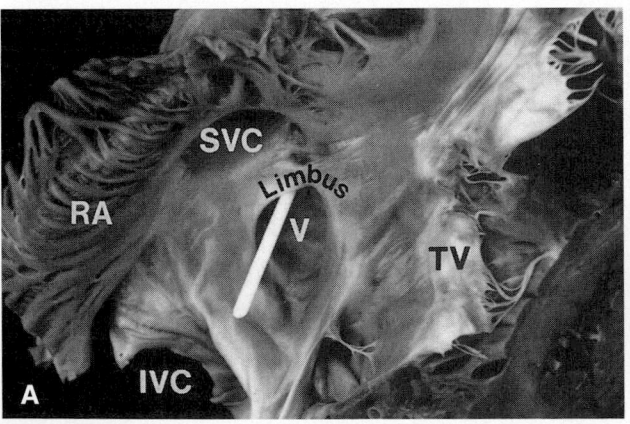
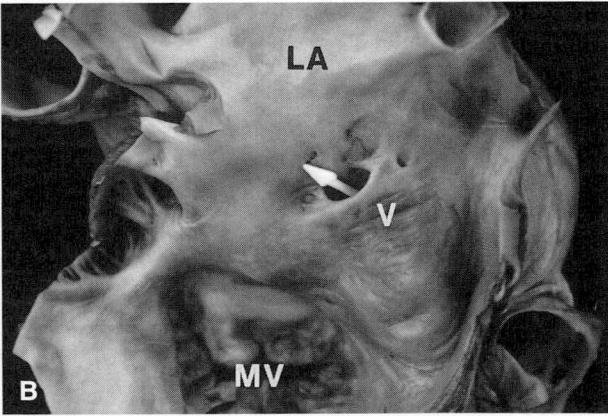

FIGURE 36–3 *Patent foramen ovale, shown in autopsy specimen. A, Right atrial (RA) view shows a probe in the foramen ovale, between limbus and valve (V) of fossa ovalis. B, Left atrial (LA) view shows the probe exiting through the ostium secundum, the prominent fenestration in the valve. Normally, when left atrial pressure exceeds right atrial pressure, the valve of the fossa ovalis is impressed against the limbus and closes the foramen ovale. IVC, inferior vena cava; MV, mitral valve; SVC, superior vena cava; TV, triscuspid valve. (From Hagen PT, Scholz DG, Edwards WD: Incidence and size of patent foramen ovale during the first 10 decades of life: An autopsy study of 965 normal hearts. Mayo Clin Proc 59:17, 1984.)*

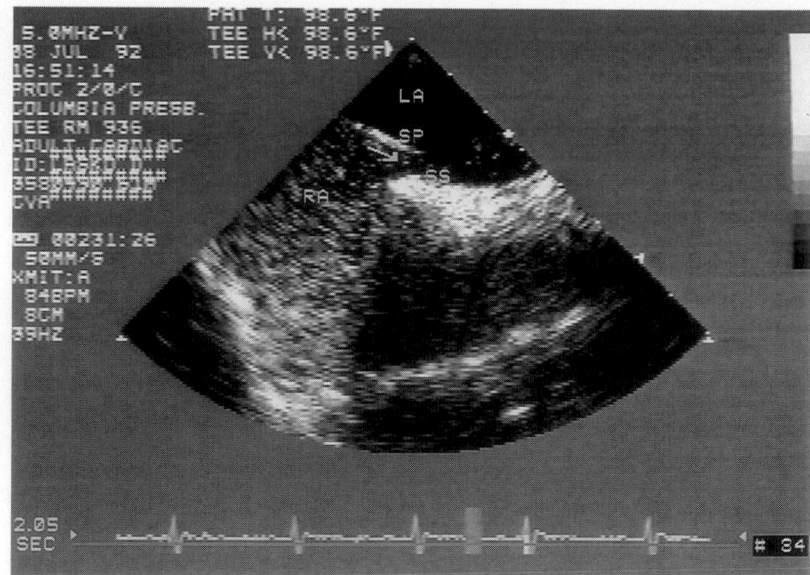

FIGURE 36–4 *Vertical transesophageal echocardiographic view of fossa ovalis area demonstrating the passage of microbubbles through the patent foramen ovale (arrow) from right atrium (RA) into left atrium (LA). Separation of septum primum (SP) from septum secundum (SS) is clearly visualized. (From Homma S, DiTullio MR, Sacco RL: Patent foramen ovale and ischemic stroke. In Barnett HJM, et al [eds]: Stroke: Pathophysiology, Diagnosis, and Management, 3rd ed. New York, Churchill Livingstone, 1998.)*

cryptogenic mechanism (14.3% versus 12.7%). Neither PFO size nor the association of an atrial septal aneurysm increased the risk of stroke or death. These patients were randomized as part of the Warfarin Aspirin Recurrent Stroke Study (WARSS) to receive either aspirin (325 mg daily) or warfarin (INR 1.4 to 2.8) for 2 years. Treatment did not affect time to primary endpoints in patients with PFO.[80a]

TEE is more sensitive than TTE with contrast agent in detecting a PFO.[81] However, TTE is risk free, and positive findings may eliminate the need for additional invasive testing.[82] Two-dimensional TEE measurement of PFO size may be more accurate than the traditionally used contrast technique.[83] Patients with cerebral ischemic symptoms and a PFO should undergo noninvasive studies of the legs to rule out deep venous thrombosis, and a pelvic vein magnetic resonance venogram (MRV) should be considered.[82]

It remains unclear whether warfarin is superior to aspirin for stroke prevention after an initial cerebral ischemic event. Current clinical trial data argue against anticoagulation for asymptomatic individuals with PFO. Transcatheter closure of patent foramen ovale is available; however, according to one series, there remains a risk of persistent shunting after such treatment in up to 20% of patients. After transcatheter closure, the annual risk of stroke or TIA has been reported to remain 3.2% per year.[84] This persistent risk may be explained in part by alternative mechanisms of stroke. Additional studies are needed to identify patients most likely to benefit from transcatheter closure of PFO and to improve performance of the devices used for the procedure.

Left Atrial Myxoma
An embolic event occurs in up to 3% to 50% of patients with atrial myxoma. Multiple events have been reported, some separated in time by months to years. The friability of the tumor lends itself to embolism of tumor fragments (Fig. 36–5).[85,86] Myxomas can be detected on TTE or TEE. The treatment is surgical resection.

Spontaneous Echo Contrast
Spontaneous echo contrast (SEC), a marker of disordered flow and hemostatic activation in the left atrium, is often seen on TEE in patients with AF.[50,87,88] SEC is associated with a higher risk of thromboembolism in mitral valve disorders.[89,90] Numerous studies have established an association between SEC and intracardiac thrombus formation, but SEC has not been shown to be an independent risk factor for embolic stroke.[89–92]

Mitral Valve Strands
Lambl's excrescences, or mitral valve strands, are filamentous processes on the ventricular surface of the aortic valve or the atrial surface of the mitral valve; they are detectable on TEE. Histologically, the strands are composed of endothelialized connective tissue. One study found that mitral valve strands were more common in patients with a history of recent cerebral ischemic events (6.3%) than in control subjects who had experienced neither (0.3%). In young patients in whom cardioembolic stroke was suspected, 16% had mitral valve strands, often without another identifiable cardiac source.[93] Other retrospective studies have shown that mitral valve strands are found more commonly in younger patients and in patients with a recent embolic event (10.6% to 53%) than in patients referred because of TEE for other reasons (2.3% to 15%).[94–96]

Dysrhythmias

Atrial Fibrillation
Thrombi in atrial fibrillation (AF) arise from the left atrium and atrial appendage. The combination of rheumatic heart disease and AF carries a stroke risk 17 times that in normal controls (who have neither AF nor RHD).[3] Of all the definite or possible mechanisms of cardioembolic stroke, AF has been the most extensively studied.[97–103] It is the most common cause of embolic stroke, accounting for 25% to 30% of all embolic strokes.[7] AF is the only cardioembolic

Specific Medical Diseases and Stroke

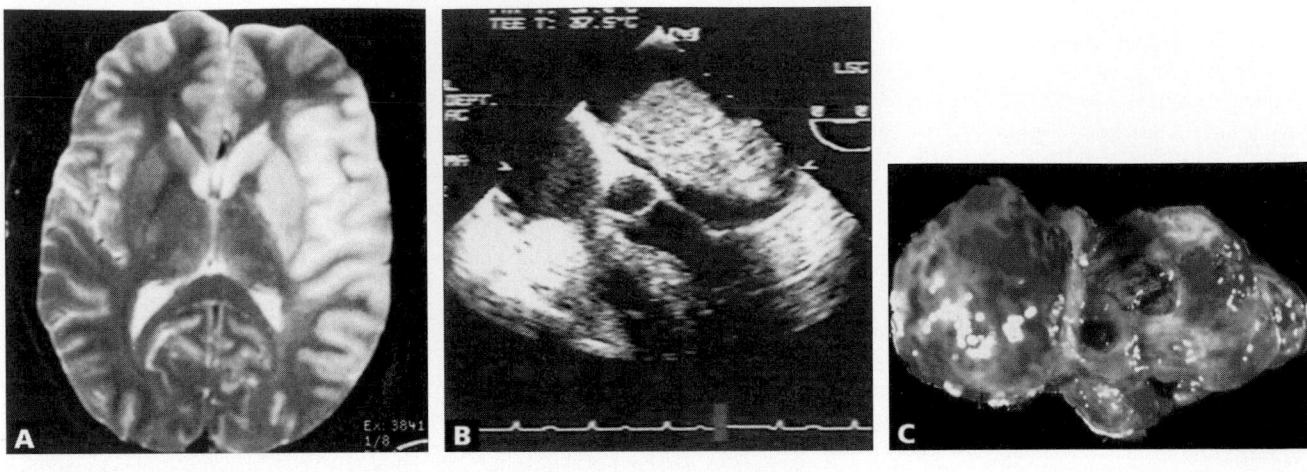

FIGURE 36–5   A, *T2-weighted MR image of the brain in a patient with left middle cerebral artery territory infarction due to atrial myxoma embolization. B, Echocardiogram showing a large atrial myxoma above the mitral valve during systole. C, Pathologic specimen showing a gelatinous atrial myxoma with numerous cysts. (From Rosenberg R [ed]: Atlas of Clinical Neurology. Philadelphia, Current Medicine, 1998.)*

source of stroke that has been subjected to randomized clinical trials evaluating the efficacy of antithrombotic and antiplatelet therapies for stroke prevention.[97–103] The rate of AF-related stroke rises with age.[3,4] Younger patients with AF who are free of cardiac disease, diabetes, and hypertension have an extremely low rate of stroke (1.3% per 15 years).[97,104] Beginning at age 65 years, however, the annual risk of stroke is 3% to 5% per year; the risk increases to 10% per year or greater by age 80 years, with women predominating.[4] The age-related risk is independent of other major risk factors (diabetes, hypertension, previous stroke, and congestive heart failure).[97]

The five aforementioned randomized primary and secondary prevention trials have demonstrated the efficacy and safety of warfarin in preventing AF-related stroke.[97–103] Pooled data from theses trials demonstrated a 68% reduction in ischemic stroke (95% CI, 50% to 79%) and an intracerebral hemorrhage rate of less than 1% per year. The data for aspirin suggested that it had a lesser effect, with a 36% risk reduction (95% CI, 4% to 57%). In addition, there is a small but definite risk of hemorrhage, particularly intracerebral hemorrhage, which is more common in elderly patients (>75 years).[97] Independent risk factors associated with an increased risk of stroke include age more than 65 years, previous history of stroke or TIA, hypertension, and diabetes mellitus. Impaired left ventricular function was identified as an additional risk factor in the Stroke Prevention in Atrial Fibrillation (SPAF) population. Despite these findings, only 30% to 60% of patients with AF receive appropriate anticoagulation therapy.[105]

TTE findings can also be factored into risk stratification. Moderate to severe impairment of left ventricular function is associated with a 2.5-fold greater risk of stroke. A left atrial anteroposterior diameter greater than 2.5 cm/m^2 was also found to be a predictor of cerebral embolism. In the SPAF study, 26% of patients had no clinical risk factor and normal echocardiographic (TTE) findings. These patients had a low risk of stroke(<1% per year). Approximately one third of patients considered at low risk according to

clinical criteria are reclassified as having a high risk on the basis of echocardiographic findings.[106–109]

TEE has greater sensitivity for detecting abnormalities in left atrium. SEC, reduced left atrial appendage emptying, and left atrial thrombus are markers of higher stroke risk. In addition, TEE is better able to visualize aortic plaque.[110,111] In patients with high-risk clinical factors, the presence of any left atrial abnormality or an aortic arch atheroma larger than 4 mm on TEE was found to raise the risk of stroke by as much as 20% per year.[112]

The use of anticoagulation for acute cardioembolic stroke due to AF is controversial. There is risk of hemorrhagic conversion of the acute infarction (1.7% to 4.4%), particularly with larger strokes.[113–116] Conversely, the risk of recurrent embolism ranges from 0.1% to 1.3% in the first 2 weeks.[54,117] A study of immediate therapy in patients with AF and ischemic stroke appeared to show no benefit of anticoagulation compared with antiplatelet therapy; however, a significant proportion of the strokes in this study were characterized as lacunar, suggesting that the mechanism of stroke may not have been cardioembolic.[54]

Sick Sinus Syndrome

Sick sinus syndrome (SSS), also referred to as tachycardia-bradycardia syndrome, is more common in older patients and is often attributed to ischemia, degeneration, or neuromuscular disease. Patients may experience atrial flutter and AF as part of this syndrome.[118] SSS has been associated with a higher risk of stroke; systemic embolism occurs in 16% of patients with SSS compared with 1.9% of patients with complete heart block.[119,120] The treatment of choice is surgical insertion of an atrial on-demand pacemaker.[121] Antithrombotic therapy has not been directly compared with antiplatelet therapy in this population, although clearly, in patients with paroxysmal AF, warfarin is recommended.

Atrial Flutter

In a study examining a large Medicare database, the stroke risk in patients with atrial flutter (relative risk [RR] 1.41) was determined to be higher than in a control group but lower than in patients with AF (RR 1.64). Patients with atrial flutter who subsequently had an episode of AF had a higher risk of stroke (RR 1.56) than patients with atrial flutter who never had a subsequent episode of AF (RR = 1.11).[122] Left atrial appendage velocities are similar in patients with AF and patients with atrial fibrillation-flutter (an intermediate form with elements of both AF and atrial flutter); thus, the risk of left atrial thrombus formation should be comparable in the two conditions.[123]

Largely because of the risk of intermittent AF in patients with atrial flutter, it is appropriate to consider anticoagulation in patients who present with atrial flutter and coexistent cardiac disease that predisposes to left atrial thrombus.[117]

Valvular Disease

Mitral Annular Calcification

Mitral annular calcification (MAC) has been associated with a higher risk of ischemic stroke.[124-126] This disorder is associated with aging, ischemic heart disease, and cardiac arrhythmias. Because patients with MAC are also at risk of stroke by other mechanisms, it is unclear whether there is a causal relationship (i.e., that thrombus calcific debris embolizes from the degenerated valve) or merely that mitral annulus calcification is a marker of systemic atherosclerosis and intrinsic cardiac dysfunction.

Prosthetic Valves

The rate of embolism in patients with mechanical prosthetic valves who are receiving anticoagulation approximates that of patients with bioprosthetic valves who are not, approximately 3% to 4% annually for mitral valves and 1.3% to 3.2% for aortic valves.[127-129] It is recommended that patients with bioprosthetic valves undergo anticoagulation either for the first 3 months or on a long-term basis if there is evidence of AF, left atrial thrombus, or previous emboli.[130] Adding aspirin to warfarin therapy in patients with mechanical valves and high-risk bioprosthetic valves is superior to warfarin alone in reducing rates of vascular mortality and systemic embolism (1.9% per year versus 8.5% per year, respectively) without a significant increase in major bleeding complications.[132]

Mitral Stenosis

Mitral stenosis, often related to rheumatic heart disease, is associated with left atrial thrombus in 15% to 17% of cases in autopsy series (Fig. 36–6).[133,134] The annual rate of stroke is approximately 2% in patients with mitral stenosis, and recurrent embolism is common. Warfarin should be considered when there is a strong suspicion of coexistent AF.[135]

Infective Endocarditis

Stroke occurs in 15% to 20% of infective endocarditis, usually within the first 48 hours (Fig. 36–7). Appropriate antibiotic therapy dramatically reduces the risk of stroke, and late embolism occurs in less than 5% of cases.[136,137] An elevated erythrocyte sedimentation rate in the setting of cerebral ischemic symptoms and fever or a new heart murmur should trigger a diagnostic evaluation including blood cultures, a transthoracic echocardiogram, and, if a high level of suspicion remains, TEE. Neurologic compli-

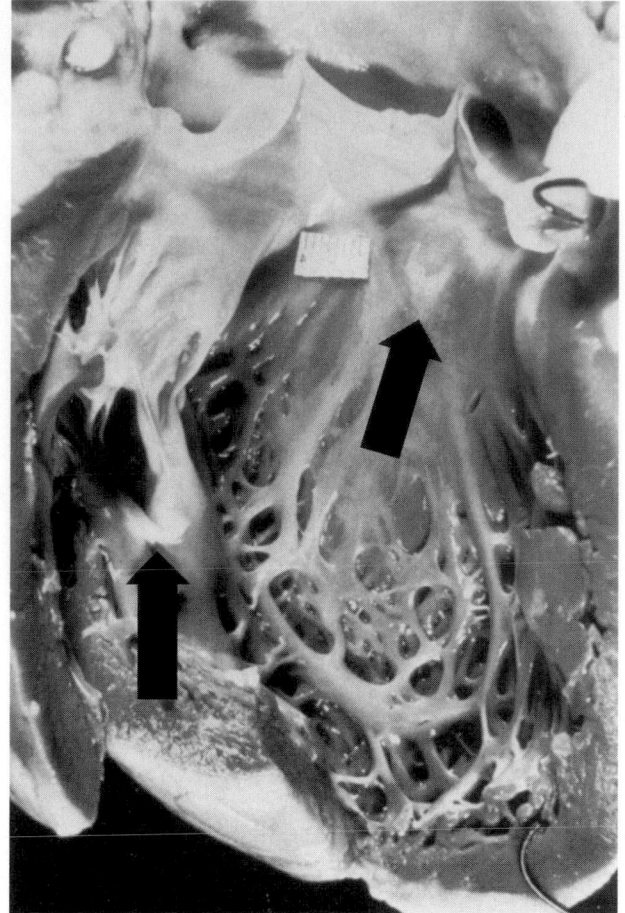

FIGURE 36–6 *Pathologic specimen showing mitral stenosis resulting from rheumatic heart disease with "jet lesions" (arrows) on the wall of the left ventricle. (From Hinchey JA, Furlan AJ, Barnett HJM: Cardiogenic brain embolism: Incidence, varieties, and treatment. In Barnett HJM [eds]: Stroke: Pathophysiology, Diagnosis, and Management, 3rd ed. New York, Churchill Livingstone, 1998.)*

cations of infective endocarditis, ischemic and hemorrhagic infarctions, toxic encephalopathy, arteritis, meningitis, and subarachnoid hemorrhage contribute to the high mortality rate (15% to 20%) associated with this condition despite antibiotic therapy.[138] Infective endocarditis can be complicated by mycotic aneurysms, which can rupture, causing subarachnoid hemorrhage. Mycotic aneurysms can be differentiated from berry aneurysms on the basis of their location distal to the first bifurcation of the intracranial vessels. When subarachnoid hemorrhage occurs in this setting, it is more superficial and is not generally complicated by vasospasm.

The most common organisms causing native valve endocarditis are streptococci, staphylococci, and enterococci. More rarely, other species of bacteria, fungi, spirochetes, and rickettsiae can infect valves.[139] Echocardiography has not been shown to be useful in predicting risk of embolism, and early antibiotic therapy remains the mainstay of treatment.[137,140] The risk of subarachnoid hemorrhage is considered by many to represent a contraindication to the use of

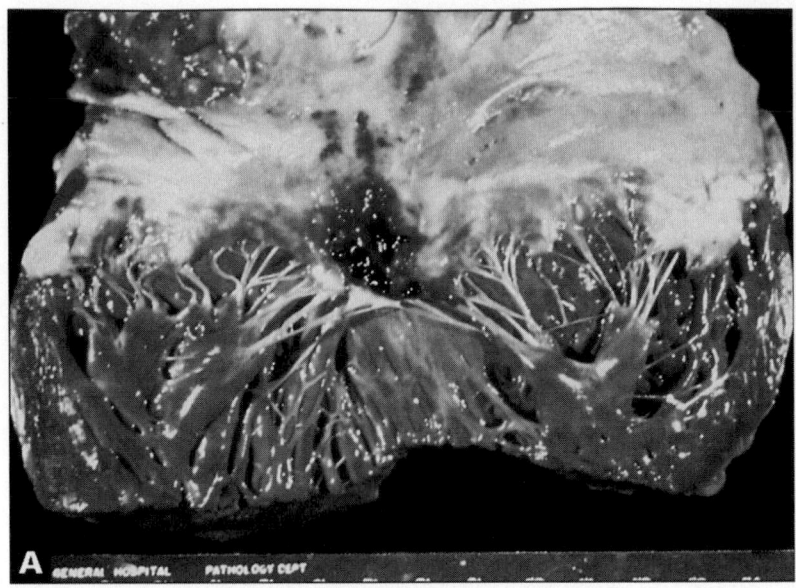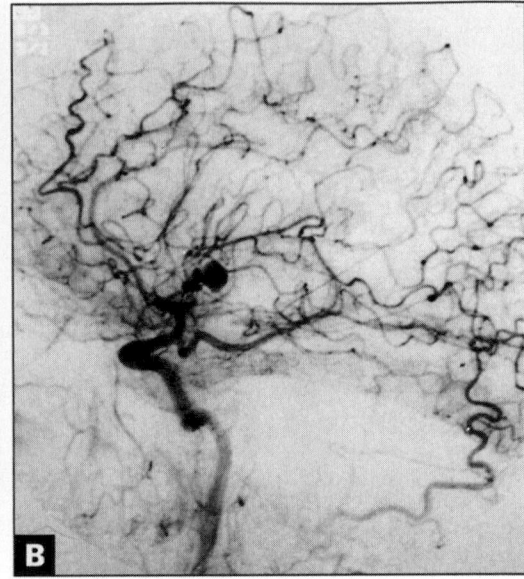

FIGURE 36–7 A, *Pathologic specimen showing a large hemorrhagic vegetation.* B, *Left common carotid angiogram showing an aneurysm of a proximal branch of the left middle cerebral artery. (From Rosenberg R [ed]: Atlas of Clinical Neurology. Philadelphia, Current Medicine, 1998.)*

anticoagulation in infectious endocarditis. Noninvasive arteriography with magnetic resonance or computed tomography angiography has largely replaced conventional transfemoral angiography in screening for mycotic aneurysms.[141]

Nonbacterial Thrombotic Endocarditis

Also known as marantic endocarditis, NBTE is associated with malignancy, often in combination with Trousseau's syndrome (Fig. 36–8).[142] The clinical manifestation may be one of focal deficits referable to one or more vascular territories, or a nonfocal encephalopathy.[143] NBTE should be suspected in all cases of stroke in patients with an underlying malignancy and is best diagnosed using echocardiography, either TEE or TTE.[144] Some clinicians recommend anticoagulation to prevent recurrent embolism, especially in a patient with a coexistent hypercoagulable state; however, efficacy of anticoagulation in this setting has not been proved.

Libman-Sacks endocarditis represents an atypical form of NBTE associated with systemic lupus erythematosus.[145,146] It is often associated with an antiphospholipid-mediated systemic hypercoagulable state. There are no proven treatment strategies for Libman-Sacks endocarditis and the antiphospholipid antibody syndrome.[145] Although anticoagulation is often used, particularly in patients with transient ischemic symptoms or stroke, the target INR range is debated.

Other Valvular Disorders

Mitral regurgitation is associated with a higher risk of stroke, largely because of coexistent AF in the majority of cases.[147,148] *Aortic stenosis* can also cause stroke, mainly through embolization of calcific material.[149] One case-control study demonstrated that *mitral valve prolapse* is considerably less common among young patients with stroke or transient ischemic symptoms than previously reported, yielding a crude OR of 0.70 in patients with mitral valve prolapse relative to controls (95% CI, 0.15 to 2.80; $P = 0.80$); after adjustment for age and sex, the OR was 0.59 (95% CI, 0.12 to 2.50; $P = 0.62$).[150] *Mitral valve papillary fibroelastoma* is a rare tumor detectable on echocardiography that can result in stroke and requires surgical resection.[151–153]

Cardiac Procedures

Coronary Artery Bypass Surgery–Related Embolism

Approximately 2% to 3% of patients undergoing coronary artery bypass grafting or valve replacement experience a perioperative stroke.[154,155] The mechanism of stroke may be cardioembolic, low-flow (distal field or watershed hypotensive ischemia), or artery-to-artery emboli from the aortic arch.[156] Most delayed strokes are due to postoperative AF, particularly in the setting of low EF.[154,157] Clinical factors such as age more than 75 years, recent MI or unstable angina, history of previous stroke, carotid artery disease, hypertension, diabetes, previous coronary artery surgery, postoperative AF, low EF, and history of pulmonary or renal insufficiency are associated with higher risk of stroke.[154,158,159] Diffusion-weighted magnetic resonance imaging is more sensitive than computed tomography for visualizing these acute infarcts, which are often multiple and may manifest as encephalopathy.[160] There appears to be a posterior circulation predominance to the pattern of infarction after coronary artery bypass grafting.[161]

Cardiac Catheterization

Cardiac catheterization can result in ischemic stroke, usually embolic. The embolus may occur artery-to-artery from the disruption of atherosclerotic plaque in the aorta

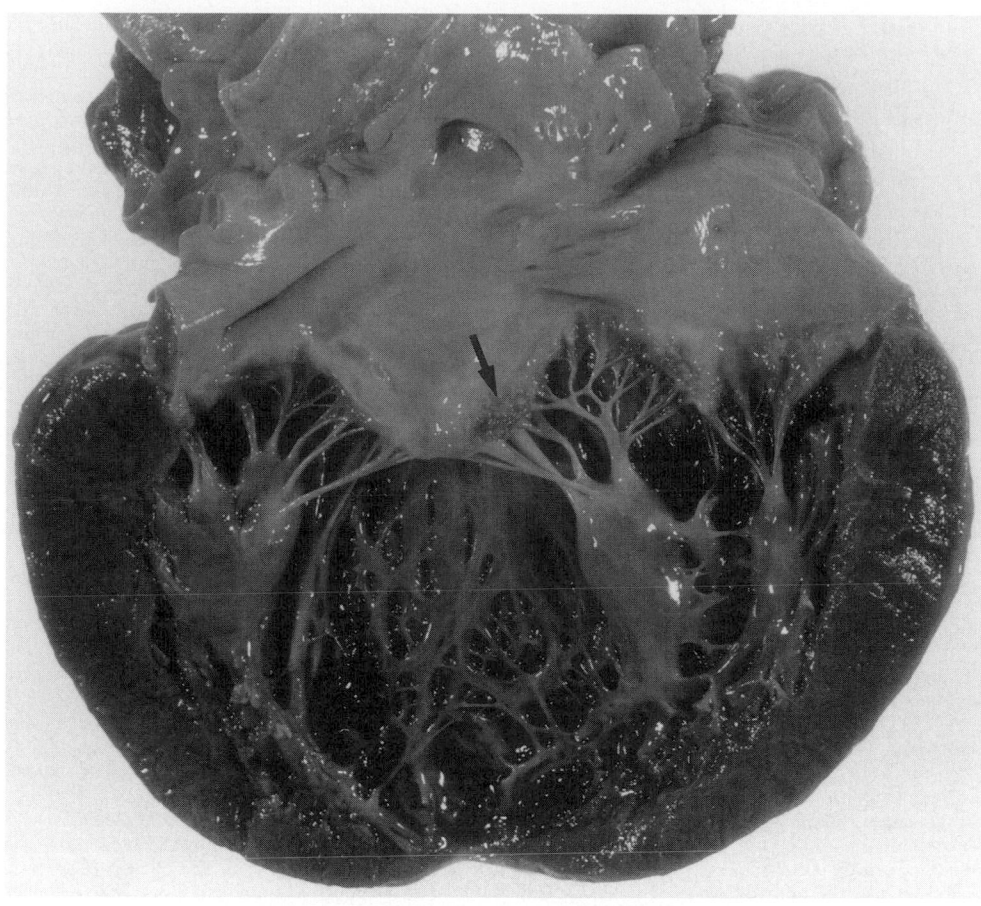

FIGURE 36–8 *Mitral valve vegetations of nonbacterial thrombotic endocarditis* (arrow). (*From Rogers LR, Cho ES, Kempin S, Posner JB: Cerebral infarction from nonbacterial thrombotic endocarditis: Clinical and pathological study including the effects of anticoagulation. Am J Med 83:746, 1987.*)

or may be secondary to cardiac injury during the procedure. The risk of stroke has been found to be significantly associated with the severity of coronary artery disease (OR 1.96) and the duration of fluoroscopy (OR 1.65). Diffusion-weighted magnetic resonance imaging was shown to be sensitive for detecting multiple silent infarcts and small vessel infarcts.[162] Hypertension, age more than 60 years, peripheral vascular disease, emergency performance of the procedure, and angioplasty raise the risk of catheterization-related thromboembolic complications.[163]

Cardiac Embolism and the Hemostatic System

AF, a model for embolic stroke, has been linked to alterations in the hemostatic system.[164–169] Local hemostatic factors in the endocardium are likely responsible for the development of left atrial thrombus.[170] As in other vascular beds, the regulation of this signaling is under genetic control, although a variety of external stimuli modulate the expression. In patients with AF, the level of prothrombin fragment F_{1+2}, a byproduct of the conversion of prothrombin to thrombin and thus a measure of thrombin generation, increases with age parallel with the rate of stroke.[171] The overwhelming majority of patients experience a dramatic reduction in stroke risk with warfarin, which correlates well with a reduction in the level of activity of the hemostatic system. In addition, aspirin has little effect on F_{1+2}, corresponding to its relative lack of efficacy in stroke prevention in patients with AF.

Other studies have confirmed that prothrombotic factor levels are increased in AF (factor VIII, fibrinogen, thrombin-antithrombin complex), as are those involved in fibrinolysis (tissue plasminogen activator, D dimer).[164–169] Von Willebrand factor levels are a marker of endothelial damage associated with AF as well.[168,169] Platelet activation has been shown to play a role in AF. Elevations in levels of platelet factor 4, β-thromboglobulin and P-selectin have been demonstrated in patients with AF.[164,168] This increased hemostatic activity is not unique to AF and suggests a common mechanism of stroke among other cardiac conditions associated with risk of embolism—left ventricular aneurysm,[172] mitral stenosis,[173] and heart failure.[174]

Therefore, it appears that aberrant flow in the heart secondary to structural disease may result in endothelial disruption, triggering local thrombus formation. The stability of the thrombus is mediated by the integrity of fibrin crosslinking. The genetic control regulating the interaction between the endothelium and the coagulation system may, in part, explain why some high-risk patients remain free of embolic events. These genetic influences may also be at play in cases of high-risk patients who experience emboli while undergoing therapeutic anticoagulation. The interaction between the endocardial surface and the coagulation system requires additional study.

References

1. Sacco RL, et al: Infarcts of undetermined cause: The NINCDS Stroke Data Bank. Ann Neurol 25:382–390, 1989.
2. Kannel WB, et al: Prevalence, incidence, prognosis, and predisposing conditions for atrial fibrillation: Population-based estimates. Am J Cardiol 82:2N–9N, 1998.
3. Wolf PA, et al: Epidemiologic assessment of chronic atrial fibrillation and risk of stroke: The Framingham study. Neurology 28:973–977, 1978.
4. Wolf PA, Abbott RD, Kannel WB: Atrial fibrillation: A major contributor to stroke in the elderly. The Framingham Study. Arch Intern Med 147:1561–1564, 1987.
5. Kittner SJ, et al: Cerebral infarction in young adults: The Baltimore-Washington Cooperative Young Stroke Study. Neurology 50:890–894, 1998.
6. Adams HP Jr, et al: Nonhemorrhagic cerebral infarction in young adults. Arch Neurol 4:793–796, 1986.
7. Cardiogenic brain embolism. Cerebral Embolism Task Force. Arch Neurol 43:71–84, 1986.
8. American Heart Association: Heart and Stroke Facts: Statistical Supplement. Dallas, American Heart Association, 1999.
9. Diringer MN, et al: Predictors of acute hospital costs for treatment of ischemic stroke in an academic center. Stroke 30:724–728, 1999.
10. Arboix A, et al: Cardioembolic infarction in the Sagrat Cor-Alianza Hospital of Barcelona Stroke Registry. Acta Neurol Scand 96:407–412, 1997.
11. Petty GW, et al: Ischemic stroke subtypes: A population-based study of functional outcome, survival, and recurrence. Stroke 31:1062–1068, 2000.
12. Horowitz DR, et al: Mechanisms in lacunar infarction. Stroke 23:325–327, 1992.
13. Staaf G, et al: Sensorimotor stroke: Clinical features, MRI findings, and cardiac and vascular concomitants in 32 patients. Acta Neurol Scand 97:93–98, 1998.
14. Ramirez-Lassepas M, et al: Can embolic stroke be diagnosed on the basis of neurologic clinical criteria? Arch Neurol 44:87–89, 1987.
15. Caplan LR, Hier DB, D'Cruz I: Cerebral embolism in the Michael Reese Stroke Registry. Stroke 14:530–536, 1983.
16. Foulkes MA, et al: The Stroke Data Bank: Design, methods, and baseline characteristics. Stroke 19:547–554, 1988.
17. Bogousslavsky J, et al: Cardiac sources of embolism and cerebral infarction—clinical consequences and vascular concomitants: The Lausanne Stroke Registry. Neurology 41:855–859, 1991.
18. Appen RE, Wray SH, Cogan DG: Central retinal artery occlusion. Am J Ophthalmol 79:374–381, 1975.
19. Babikian VL, et al: Cerebral microembolism and early recurrent cerebral or retinal ischemic events. Stroke 28:1314–1318, 1997.
20. Hankey GJ, Slattery JM, Warlow CP: Prognosis and prognostic factors of retinal infarction: A prospective cohort study. BMJ 302:499–504, 1991.
21. Babikian VL, et al: Clinical correlates of high-intensity transient signals detected on transcranial Doppler sonography in patients with cerebrovascular disease. Stroke 25:1570–1573, 1994.
22. Murkin JM: Etiology and incidence of brain dysfunction after cardiac surgery. J Cardiothorac Vasc Anesth 13(Suppl 1):12–77; discussion 36–37, 1999.
23. Gacs G, Merei FT, Bodosi M: Balloon catheter as a model of cerebral emboli in humans. Stroke 13:39–42, 1982.
24. Cardiogenic brain embolism. The second report of the Cerebral Embolism Task Force. Arch Neurol 46:727–743, 1989.
25. Timsit SG, et al: Brain infarction severity differs according to cardiac or arterial embolic source. Neurology 43:728–733, 1993.
26. Fisher CM, Pearlman A: The nonsudden onset of cerebral embolism. Neurology 17:1025–1032, 1967.
27. Kraus JA, Berlit P: Cerebral embolism and epileptic seizures: The role of the embolic source. Acta Neurol Scand 97:154–159, 1998.
28. Minematsu K, Yamaguchi T, Omae T: 'Spectacular shrinking deficit': Rapid recovery from a major hemispheric syndrome by migration of an embolus. Neurology 42:157–162, 1992.
29. Kittner SJ, et al: Features on initial computed tomography scan of infarcts with a cardiac source of embolism in the NINDS Stroke Data Bank. Stroke 23:1748–1751, 1992.
30. Ringelstein EB, et al: Computed tomographic patterns of proven embolic brain infarctions. Ann Neurol 26:759–765, 1989.
31. Bogousslavsky J, Bernasconi A, Kumral E: Acute multiple infarction involving the anterior circulation. Arch Neurol 53:50–57, 1996.
32. Bogousslavsky J, et al: Pathogenesis of anterior circulation stroke in patients with nonvalvular atrial fibrillation: The Lausanne Stroke Registry. Neurology 40:1046–1050, 1990.
33. Horowitz DR, Tuhrim S: Stroke mechanisms and clinical presentation in large subcortical infarctions. Neurology 49:1538–1541, 1997.
34. Bogousslavsky J, Van Melle G, Regli F: Middle cerebral artery pial territory infarcts: A study of the Lausanne Stroke Registry. Ann Neurol 25:555–560, 1989.
35. Yamamoto Y, et al: Posterior cerebral artery territory infarcts in the New England Medical Center Posterior Circulation Registry. Arch Neurol 56:824–832, 1999.
36. Pessin MS, et al: Clinical features and mechanism of occipital infarction. Ann Neurol 21:290–299, 1987.
37. Hart RG, Easton JD: Hemorrhagic infarcts. Stroke 17:586–589, 1986.
38. Mast H, et al: Cardiac sources of embolism in patients with pial artery infarcts and lacunar lesions. Stroke 25:776–781, 1994.
39. Rem JA, et al: Value of cardiac monitoring and echocardiography in TIA and stroke patients. Stroke 16:950–956, 1985.
40. Bogousslavsky J, et al: Cardiac and arterial lesions in carotid transient ischemic attacks. Arch Neurol 43:223–228, 1986.
41. Moncayo J, et al: Coexisting causes of ischemic stroke. Arch Neurol 57:1139–1144, 2000.
42. Hornig CR, et al: Specific cardiological evaluation after focal cerebral ischemia. Acta Neurol Scand 93:297–302, 1996.
43. Bogousslavsky J, et al: The etiology of posterior circulation infarcts: A prospective study using magnetic resonance imaging and magnetic resonance angiography. Neurology 43:1528–1533, 1993.
44. Pop GA, et al: Predictive value of clinical history and electrocardiogram in patients with transient ischemic attack or minor ischemic stroke for subsequent cardiac and cerebral ischemic events. The Dutch TIA Trial Study Group. Arch Neurol 51:333–341, 1994.
45. Popp RL: Echocardiography (2). N Engl J Med 323:165–172, 1990.
46. Popp RL: Echocardiography (1). N Engl J Med 323:101–109, 1990.
47. Pop G, et al: Transesophageal echocardiography in the detection of intracardiac embolic sources in patients with transient ischemic attacks. Stroke 21:560–565, 1990.
48. Hata JS, et al: Impact of transesophageal echocardiography on the anticoagulation management of patients admitted with focal cerebral ischemia. Am J Cardiol 72:707–710, 1993.
49. Pearson AC, et al: Superiority of transesophageal echocardiography in detecting cardiac source of embolism in patients with cerebral ischemia of uncertain etiology. J Am Coll Cardiol 17:66–72, 1991.
50. Warner MF, Momah KI: Routine transesophageal echocardiography for cerebral ischemia: Is it really necessary? Arch Intern Med 156:1719–1723, 1996.
51. McNamara RL, et al: Echocardiographic identification of cardiovascular sources of emboli to guide clinical management of stroke: A cost-effectiveness analysis. Ann Intern Med 127:775–787, 1997.
52. Sliwka U, et al: Occurrence of transcranial Doppler high-intensity transient signals in patients with potential cardiac sources of embolism: A prospective study. Stroke 26:2067–2070, 1995.
53. Tong DC, Bolger A, Albers GW: Incidence of transcranial Doppler-detected cerebral microemboli in patients referred for echocardiography. Stroke 25:2138–2141, 1994.
54. Berge E, et al: Low molecular-weight heparin versus aspirin in patients with acute ischaemic stroke and atrial fibrillation: A double-blind randomised study. HAEST Study Group. Heparin in Acute Embolic Stroke Trial. Lancet 355:1205–1210, 2000.
55. del Zoppo GJ: Antithrombotic treatments in acute ischemic stroke. Curr Opin Hematol 7:309–315, 2000.
56. Mohr JP, et al: A comparison of warfarin and aspirin for the prevention of recurrent ischemic stroke. N Engl J Med 345:1444–1451, 2001.
57. Katz SD, et al: Low incidence of stroke in ambulatory patients with heart failure: A prospective study. Am Heart J 126:141–146, 1993.

58. Fuster V, et al: The natural history of idiopathic dilated cardiomyopathy. Am J Cardiol 47:525–531, 1981.

59. Pullicino PM, Halperin JL, Thompson JL: Stroke in patients with heart failure and reduced left ventricular ejection fraction. Neurology 54:288–294, 2000.

60. Loh E, et al: Ventricular dysfunction and the risk of stroke after myocardial infarction. N Engl J Med 336:251–257, 1997.

61. Cleland JG: Anticoagulant and antiplatelet therapy in heart failure. Curr Opin Cardiol 12:276–287, 1997.

62. Dries DL, et al: Ejection fraction and risk of thromboembolic events in patients with systolic dysfunction and sinus rhythm: Evidence for gender differences in the studies of left ventricular dysfunction trials. J Am Coll Cardiol 29:1074–1080, 1997.

63. Kannel WB, Wolf PA, Verter J: Manifestations of coronary disease predisposing to stroke. The Framingham study. JAMA 250:2942–2946, 1983.

64. Segal JP, et al: Idiopathic cardiomyopathy: Clinical features, prognosis and therapy. Curr Probl Cardiol 3:1–48, 1978.

65. Effect of long-term oral anticoagulant treatment on mortality and cardiovascular morbidity after myocardial infarction. Anticoagulants in the Secondary Prevention of Events in Coronary Thrombosis (ASPECT) Research Group. Lancet 343:499–503, 1994.

66. Smith P, Arnesen H, Holme I: The effect of warfarin on mortality and reinfarction after myocardial infarction. N Engl J Med 323:147–152, 1990.

67. A double-blind trial to assess long-term oral anticoagulant therapy in elderly patients after myocardial infarction. Report of the Sixty Plus Reinfarction Study Research Group. Lancet 2:989–994, 1980.

68. Komrad MS, et al: Myocardial infarction and stroke. Neurology 34:1403–1409, 1984.

69. Puletti M, et al: Incidence of systemic thromboembolic lesions in acute myocardial infarction. Clin Cardiol 9:331–333, 1986.

70. Asinger RW, et al: Incidence of left-ventricular thrombosis after acute transmural myocardial infarction: Serial evaluation by two-dimensional echocardiography. N Engl J Med 305:297–302, 1981.

71. Stratton JR, Resnick AD: Increased embolic risk in patients with left ventricular thrombi. Circulation 75:1004–1011, 1987.

72. Derex L, et al: Thrombolytic therapy in acute ischemic stroke patients with cardiac thrombus. Neurology 57:2122–2125, 2001.

72a. Hurlen M, Abdelnoor M, Smith P, et al: Warfarin, aspirin, or both after myocardial infarction. N Engl J Med 347:969–974, 2002.

73. Sacco RL, Homma S, Di Tullio MR: Patent foramen ovale: A new risk factor for ischemic stroke. Heart Dis Stroke 2:235–241, 1993.

74. Di Tullio M, et al: Patent foramen ovale as a risk factor for cryptogenic stroke. Ann Intern Med 117:461–465, 1992.

75. Steiner MM, et al: Patent foramen ovale size and embolic brain imaging findings among patients with ischemic stroke. Stroke 29:944–948, 1998.

76. Barinagarrementeria F, Amaya LE, Cantu C: Causes and mechanisms of cerebellar infarction in young patients. Stroke 28:2400–2404, 1997.

77. Hanna JP, et al: Patent foramen ovale and brain infarct: Echocardiographic predictors, recurrence, and prevention. Stroke 25:782–786, 1994.

78. Mas JL, et al: Recurrent cerebrovascular events associated with patent foramen ovale, atrial septal aneurysm, or both. N Engl J Med 345:1740–1746, 2001.

79. Homma S, et al: Characteristics of patent foramen ovale associated with cryptogenic stroke: A biplane transesophageal echocardiographic study. Stroke 25:582–586, 1994.

80. Schuchlenz HW, et al: The association between the diameter of a patent foramen ovale and the risk of embolic cerebrovascular events. Am J Med 109:456–462, 2000.

80a. Homma S, Sacco RL, Di Tullio MR, et al: Effect of medical treatment in stroke patients with patent foramen ovale: Patent foramen ovale in Cryptogenic Stroke Study. Circulation 105:2625–2631, 2002.

81. Hausmann D, et al: Diagnosis of patent foramen ovale by transesophageal echocardiography and association with cerebral and peripheral embolic events. Am J Cardiol 70:668–672, 1992.

82. Lethen H, et al: Frequency of deep vein thrombosis in patients with patent foramen ovale and ischemic stroke or transient ischemic attack. Am J Cardiol 80:1066–1069, 1997.

83. Schuchlenz HW, et al: Transesophageal echocardiography for quantifying size of patent foramen ovale in patients with cryptogenic cerebrovascular events. Stroke 33:293–296, 2002.

84. Hung J, et al: Closure of patent foramen ovale for paradoxical emboli: Intermediate-term risk of recurrent neurological events following transcatheter device placement. J Am Coll Cardiol 35:1311–1316, 2000.

85. Sandok BA, von Estorff I, Giuliani ER: CNS embolism due to atrial myxoma: Clinical features and diagnosis. Arch Neurol 37:485–488, 1980.

86. Roeltgen DP, Weimer GR, Patterson LF: Delayed neurologic complications of left atrial myxoma. Neurology 31:8–13, 1981.

87. Zotz RJ, et al: Spontaneous echo contrast caused by platelet and leukocyte aggregates? Stroke 32:1127–1133, 2001.

88. Peverill RE, et al: Haematologic determinants of left atrial spontaneous echo contrast in mitral stenosis. Int J Cardiol 81:235–242, 2001.

89. Castello R, Pearson AC, Labovitz AJ: Prevalence and clinical implications of atrial spontaneous contrast in patients undergoing transesophageal echocardiography. Am J Cardiol 65:1149–1153, 1990.

90. Daniel WG, et al: Left atrial spontaneous echo contrast in mitral valve disease: An indicator for an increased thromboembolic risk. J Am Coll Cardiol 11:1204–1211, 1988.

91. Castello R, et al: Spontaneous echocardiographic contrast in the descending aorta. Am Heart J 120:915–919, 1990.

92. Comess KA, et al: Transesophageal echocardiography and carotid ultrasound in patients with cerebral ischemia: Prevalence of findings and recurrent stroke risk. J Am Coll Cardiol 23:1598–1603, 1994.

93. Tice FD, et al: Mitral valve strands in patients with focal cerebral ischemia. Stroke 27:1183–1186, 1996.

94. Freedberg RS, et al: Valve strands are strongly associated with systemic embolization: A transesophageal echocardiographic study. J Am Coll Cardiol 26:1709–1712, 1995.

95. Orsinelli DA, Pearson AC: Detection of prosthetic valve strands by transesophageal echocardiography: Clinical significance in patients with suspected cardiac source of embolism. J Am Coll Cardiol 26:1713–1718, 1995.

96. Roberts JK, et al: Valvular strands and cerebral ischemia: Effect of demographics and strand characteristics. Stroke 28:2185–2188, 1997.

97. Risk factors for stroke and efficacy of antithrombotic therapy in atrial fibrillation: Analysis of pooled data from five randomized controlled trials. Arch Intern Med 154:1449–1457, 1994.

98. Warfarin versus aspirin for prevention of thromboembolism in atrial fibrillation: Stroke Prevention in Atrial Fibrillation II Study. Lancet 343:687–691, 1994.

99. Adjusted-dose warfarin versus low-intensity, fixed-dose warfarin plus aspirin for high-risk patients with atrial fibrillation: Stroke Prevention in Atrial Fibrillation III randomised clinical trial. Lancet 348:633–638, 1996.

100. Patients with nonvalvular atrial fibrillation at low risk of stroke during treatment with aspirin: Stroke Prevention in Atrial Fibrillation III Study. The SPAF III Writing Committee for the Stroke Prevention in Atrial Fibrillation Investigators. JAMA 279:1273–1277, 1998.

101. The effect of low-dose warfarin on the risk of stroke in patients with nonrheumatic atrial fibrillation. The Boston Area Anticoagulation Trial for Atrial Fibrillation Investigators. N Engl J Med 323:1505–1511, 1990.

102. Stroke Prevention in Atrial Fibrillation Study: Final results. Circulation 84:527–539, 1991.

103. Secondary prevention in non-rheumatic atrial fibrillation after transient ischaemic attack or minor stroke. EAFT (European Atrial Fibrillation Trial) Study Group. Lancet 342:1255–1262, 1993.

104. Nabavi DG, et al: Absence of circulating microemboli in patients with lone atrial fibrillation. Neurol Res 21:566–568, 1999.

105. Albers GW, et al: Clinical characteristics and management of acute stroke in patients with atrial fibrillation admitted to US university hospitals. Neurology 48:1598–1604, 1997.

106. Asinger RW: Role of transthoracic echocardiography in atrial fibrillation. Echocardiography 17:357–364, 2000.

107. Egeblad H, et al: Role of echocardiography in systemic arterial embolism: A review with recommendations. Scand Cardiovasc J 32:323–342, 1998.

108. Predictors of thromboembolism in atrial fibrillation. II: Echocardiographic features of patients at risk. The Stroke Prevention in Atrial Fibrillation Investigators. Ann Intern Med 116:6–12, 1992.

Specific Medical Diseases and Stroke

109. Echocardiographic predictors of stroke in patients with atrial fibrillation: A prospective study of 1066 patients from 3 clinical trials. Arch Intern Med 158:1316–1320, 1998.

110. Abe Y, et al: Prediction of embolism in atrial fibrillation: Classification of left atrial thrombi by transesophageal echocardiography. Jpn Circ J 64:411–415, 2000.

111. Fagan SM, Chan KL: Transesophageal echocardiography risk factors for stroke in nonvalvular atrial fibrillation. Echocardiography 17:365–372, 2000.

112. Transesophageal echocardiographic correlates of thromboembolism in high-risk patients with nonvalvular atrial fibrillation. The Stroke Prevention in Atrial Fibrillation Investigators Committee on Echocardiography. Ann Intern Med 128:639–647, 1998.

113. Babikian VL, et al: Intracerebral hemorrhage in stroke patients anticoagulated with heparin. Stroke 20:1500–1503, 1989.

114. Rothrock JF, et al: Acute anticoagulation following cardioembolic stroke. Stroke 20:730–734, 1989.

115. Bogousslavsky J, Regli F: Anticoagulant-induced intracerebral bleeding in brain ischemia: Evaluation in 200 patients with TIAs, emboli from the heart, and progressing stroke. Acta Neurol Scand 71:464–471, 1985.

116. Lodder J, van der Lugt PJ: Evaluation of the risk of immediate anticoagulant treatment in patients with embolic stroke of cardiac origin. Stroke 14:42–46, 1983.

117. Stoddard MF: Risk of thromboembolism in acute atrial fibrillation or atrial flutter. Echocardiography 17:393–405, 2000.

118. Rubenstein JJ, et al: Clinical spectrum of the sick sinus syndrome. Circulation 46:5–13, 1972.

119. Fairfax AJ, Lambert CD, Leatham A: Systemic embolism in chronic sinoatrial disorder. N Engl J Med 295:190–192, 1976.

120. Fairfax AJ, Lambert CD: Neurological aspects of sinoatrial heart block. J Neurol Neurosurg Psychiatry 39:576–580, 1976.

121. Santini M, et al: Relation of prognosis in sick sinus syndrome to age, conduction defects and modes of permanent cardiac pacing. Am J Cardiol 65:729–735, 1990.

122. Biblo LA, et al: Risk of stroke in patients with atrial flutter. Am J Cardiol 87:346–349, 2001.

123. Santiago D, et al: Left atrial appendage function and thrombus formation in atrial fibrillation-flutter: A transesophageal echocardiographic study. J Am Coll Cardiol 24:159–164, 1994.

124. Nair CK, et al: Long-term follow-up of patients with echocardiographically detected mitral annular calcium and comparison with age- and sex-matched control subjects. Am J Cardiol 63:465–470, 1989.

125. Nishide M, et al: Cardiac abnormalities in ischemic cerebrovascular disease studied by two-dimensional echocardiography. Stroke 14:541–545, 1983.

126. de Bono DP, Warlow CP: Mitral-annulus calcification and cerebral or retinal ischaemia. Lancet 2:383–385, 1979.

127. Chesebro JH, Adams PC, Fuster V: Antithrombotic therapy in patients with valvular heart disease and prosthetic heart valves. J Am Coll Cardiol 8(Suppl B):41B–56B, 1986.

128. Kuntze CE, et al: Rates of thromboembolism with three different mechanical heart valve prostheses: randomised study. Lancet 1:514–517, 1989.

129. Kuntze CE, Blackstone EH, Ebels T: Thromboembolism and mechanical heart valves: A randomized study revisited. Ann Thorac Surg 66:101–117, 1998.

130. Olesen KH, et al: Long-term follow-up in 185 patients after mitral valve replacement with the Lillehei-Kaster prosthesis: Overall results and prosthesis-related complications. Eur Heart J 8:680–688, 1987.

131. Reference deleted.

132. Turpie AG, et al: A comparison of aspirin with placebo in patients treated with warfarin after heart-valve replacement. N Engl J Med 329:524–529, 1993.

133. Coulshed N, et al: Systemic embolism in mitral valve disease. Br Heart J 32:26–34, 1970.

134. Szekely P: Systemic embolism and anticoagulant prophylaxis in rheumatic heart disease. BMJ 1:1209–1212, 1964.

135. Szekely P: Rheumatic heart disease in three decades (1942–1971). Singapore Med J 14:417–419, 1973.

136. Salgado AV, et al: Neurologic complications of endocarditis: A 12-year experience. Neurology 39:173–178, 1989.

137. Hart RG, et al: Stroke in infective endocarditis. Stroke 21:695–700, 1990.

138. Pruitt AA, et al: Neurologic complications of bacterial endocarditis. Medicine (Baltimore) 57:329–343, 1978.

139. Karchmer AW: Infective endocarditis. In Braunwald E, Fauci AS, Kasper DL, et al (eds): Harrison's Principles of Internal Medicine, 15th ed. New York, McGraw-Hill, 2001.

140. Buda AJ, et al: Prognostic significance of vegetations detected by two-dimensional echocardiography in infective endocarditis. Am Heart J 112:1291–1296, 1986.

141. Salgado AV, Furlan AJ, Keys TF: Mycotic aneurysm, subarachnoid hemorrhage, and indications for cerebral angiography in infective endocarditis. Stroke 18:1057–1060, 1987.

142. Lopez JA, et al: Nonbacterial thrombotic endocarditis: A review. Am Heart J 113:773–784, 1987.

143. Rogers LR, et al: Cerebral infarction from non-bacterial thrombotic endocarditis: Clinical and pathological study including the effects of anticoagulation. Am J Med 83:746–756, 1987.

144. Lopez JA, Fishbein MC, Siegel RJ: Echocardiographic features of nonbacterial thrombotic endocarditis. Am J Cardiol 59:478–5=480, 1987.

145. Futrell N, Millikan C: Frequency, etiology, and prevention of stroke in patients with systemic lupus erythematosus. Stroke 20:583–591, 1989.

146. Gorelick PB, et al: Embolic stroke complicating systemic lupus erythematosus. Arch Neurol 42:813–815, 1985.

147. Pomerance A: Cardiac pathology and systolic murmurs in the elderly. Br Heart J 30:687–689, 1968.

148. Pomerance A: Cardiac pathology in the aged. Geriatrics 23:101–114, 1968.

149. Kapila A, Hart R: Calcific cerebral emboli and aortic stenosis: Detection of computed tomography. Stroke 17:619–621, 1986.

150. Gilon D, et al: Lack of evidence of an association between mitral-valve prolapse and stroke in young patients. N Engl J Med, 341:8–13, 1999.

151. Cesena FH, et al: Papillary fibroelastoma of the mitral valve 12 years after mitral valve commissurotomy. South Med J 92:1023–1028, 1999.

152. Muir KW, et al: Visualization of cardiac emboli from mitral valve papillary fibroelastoma. Stroke 27:1133–1134, 1996.

153. Kasarskis EJ, O'Connor W, Earle G: Embolic stroke from cardiac papillary fibroelastomas. Stroke 19:1171–1173, 1988.

154. Roach GW, et al: Adverse cerebral outcomes after coronary bypass surgery. Multicenter Study of Perioperative Ischemia Research Group and the Ischemia Research and Education Foundation Investigators. N Engl J Med 335:1857–1863, 1996.

155. Barbut D, Caplan LR: Brain complications of cardiac surgery. Curr Probl Cardiol 22:449–480, 1997.

156. Salazar JD, et al: Stroke after cardiac surgery: Short- and long-term outcomes. Ann Thorac Surg 72:1195–1201; discussion 1201–1202, 2001.

157. Hogue CW Jr, et al: Risk factors for early or delayed stroke after cardiac surgery. Circulation 100:642–647, 1999.

158. Newman MF, et al: Multicenter preoperative stroke risk index for patients undergoing coronary artery bypass graft surgery. Multicenter Study of Perioperative Ischemia (McSPI) Research Group. Circulation 94(Suppl):II74–II80, 1996.

159. Stamou SC, Corso PJ: Coronary revascularization without cardiopulmonary bypass in high-risk patients: A route to the future. Ann Thorac Surg 71:1056–1061, 2001.

160. Wityk RJ, et al: Diffusion- and perfusion-weighted brain magnetic resonance imaging in patients with neurologic complications after cardiac surgery. Arch Neurol 58:571–576, 2001.

161. Barbut D, et al: Posterior distribution of infarcts in strokes related to cardiac operations. Ann Thorac Surg 65:1656–1659, 1998.

162. Segal AZ, et al: Stroke as a complication of cardiac catheterization: Risk factors and clinical features. Neurology 56:975–977, 2001.

163. Jackson JL, Meyer GS, Pettit T: Complications from cardiac catheterization: Analysis of a military database. Mil Med 165:298–301, 2000.

164. Lip GY, et al: Fibrin D-dimer and beta-thromboglobulin as markers of thrombogenesis and platelet activation in atrial fibrillation: Effects of introducing ultra-low-dose warfarin and aspirin. Circulation 94:425–431, 1996.

165. Lip GY, et al: Fibrinogen and fibrin D-dimer levels in paroxysmal atrial fibrillation: Evidence for intermediate elevated levels of intravascular thrombogenesis. Am Heart J 131:724–730, 1996.

166. Lip GY, et al: Plasma fibrinogen and fibrin D-dimer in patients with atrial fibrillation: Effects of cardioversion to sinus rhythm. Int J Cardiol 51:245–251, 1995.

167. Lip GY, et al: Increased markers of thrombogenesis in chronic atrial fibrillation: Effects of warfarin treatment. Br Heart J 73:527–533, 1995.

168. Gustafsson C, et al: Coagulation factors and the increased risk of stroke in nonvalvular atrial fibrillation. Stroke 21:47–51, 1990.

169. Mitusch R, et al: Detection of a hypercoagulable state in nonvalvular atrial fibrillation and the effect of anticoagulant therapy. Thromb Haemost 75:219–223, 1996.

170. Rosenberg RD, Aird WC: Vascular-bed–specific hemostasis and hypercoagulable states. N Engl J Med 340:1555–1564, 1999.

171. Kistler JP, et al: Effect of low-intensity warfarin anticoagulation on level of activity of the hemostatic system in patients with atrial fibrillation. BAATAF Investigators. Stroke 24:1360–1365, 1993.

172. Lip GY, et al: Effects of warfarin therapy on plasma fibrinogen, von Willebrand factor, and fibrin D-dimer in left ventricular dysfunction secondary to coronary artery disease with and without aneurysms. Am J Cardiol 76:453–458, 1995.

173. Yamamoto K, et al: Coagulation activity is increased in the left atrium of patients with mitral stenosis. J Am Coll Cardiol 25:107–112, 1995.

174. Jafri SM, et al: Platelet function, thrombin and fibrinolytic activity in patients with heart failure. Eur Heart J 14:205–212, 1993.

Specific Medical Diseases and Stroke

Section V

Pathophysiology

Dennis Choi

The chapters in this thoroughly revised section present a current understanding of the pathogenesis of stroke. The field is in rapid evolution, but the authors, all distinguished authorities with active research programs, have skillfully summarized key principles while remaining in contact with the underlying data and providing more access to the experimental literature than typically found in major textbooks.

Since stroke begins as a disturbance in the brain's vasculature, the first four of the nine chapters in this section appropriately focus on blood vessels, atherosclerosis, and blood flow. The first chapter sets the stage by identifying mechanisms responsible for regulating cerebral arterial caliber under physiologic conditions, and then discussing how pathologic conditions relevant to stroke, such as chronic hypertension, atherosclerosis, inflammation, platelet activation, or hemorrhage alter these mechanisms. In keeping with the 4th Edition's emphasis on treatments, the chapter also describes how gene transfer to cerebral vessels may provide a means for the therapeutic modification of vascular regulation or proliferation. The next two chapters add substantial additional depth and breadth to the vascular story, describing the response of the microvasculature to ischemic insults as well as the biology of thrombus formation (and lysis). These events initiate and shape the evolution of ischemic infarction. The fourth chapter examines in detail the physiology of cerebral blood flow, including its relationship to oxygen consumption, and alterations associated with ischemic stroke or hemorrhage.

The next five chapters focus on the parenchymal consequences of ischemia, collectively providing modern insight into the classic question, "why is the brain so vulnerable to ischemia," and setting the stage for devising countermeasures. The first of the five chapters bridges back to standing concepts of ischemic brain damage, from the classic standpoint of histopathology. Of note, the author of this histopathology chapter challenges the emerging view—elegantly discussed in subsequent chapters—that apoptosis contributes substantially to ischemic cell death, an important reminder that the mechanisms underlying ischemic cell death have not yet been clarified to the point that all experts agree. The next four chapters delve into these mechanisms in considerable detail, each with a distinct center, but by necessity achieving overlapping coverage of interlocking pathways and interdependent consequences. As a group, they discuss experimental models of focal and global ischemia, excitotoxicity, apoptosis, inflammation, and the intracellular signaling cascades that position cells for death or survival. A major theme of these chapters is the substantial overlap in pathways that promote these opposing cell fates, beginning with the well known observation that sublethal ischemia can evoke tolerance to subsequent ischemic insults.

Chapter Thirty-Seven

Vascular Biology and Atherosclerosis of Cerebral Arteries

Christopher G. Sobey, Frank M. Faraci, and Donald D. Heistad

Cerebral perfusion is compromised by several pathophysiologic conditions that affect cerebrovascular reactivity and thrombosis and that are associated with an increased risk of stroke. Disease states may produce cerebral vascular abnormalities by a variety of mechanisms, including endothelial dysfunction, impaired relaxation of vascular muscle, and augmented vasoconstriction. Significant progress has been made in the understanding of mechanisms that normally regulate cerebral blood flow and of abnormalities of cerebral vascular function in pathophysiologic states.

This chapter summarizes the current understanding of some important mechanisms of cerebral vascular function and dysfunction. New developments in techniques and the potential therapeutic application of gene transfer to cerebral vessels are also briefly described. We do not, however, address some aspects of vascular biology, including vascular proliferation, remodeling, and formation of collateral vessels.

PHYSIOLOGIC DILATOR MECHANISMS IN CEREBRAL VESSELS

Nitric Oxide and Cyclic Guanosine Monophosphate–Mediated Mechanisms

Endothelium modulates vascular tone by producing and releasing potent vasoactive substances.[1–3] One of these important substances is endothelium-derived nitric oxide (NO), which diffuses to vascular muscle and produces relaxation through activation of the soluble form of guanylate cyclase, resulting in an increased intracellular concentration of cyclic guanosine monophosphate (cGMP) and relaxation. The NO–guanylate cyclase mechanism represents a major mechanism of cerebral vasodilatation.

NO is a potent dilator of cerebral vessels and may be produced by one of three isoforms of NO synthase (NOS) (neuronal/type I or nNOS, immunologic/type II or iNOS, and endothelial/type III or eNOS), each of which uses L-arginine as a substrate.[2,3] In blood vessels, NO is generated under basal conditions in the endothelium, by eNOS. Soluble guanylate cyclase, which is cytosolic, can also be activated by pharmacologic agents, including nitroglycerin and sodium nitroprusside.[3,4] Activity of NOS can be further stimulated by increases in intracellular calcium that occur in response to many receptor-mediated agonists, such as acetylcholine, or in response to rises in shear stress that are associated with increases in velocity of blood flow.[1,2]

Under normal conditions, NO is released both intraluminally and abluminally by endothelium. Endothelial release of both NO and prostacyclin, a product of arachidonic acid metabolism, into the vascular lumen contributes to the antithrombogenic properties of endothelium, because both of these substances inhibit aggregation of platelets and adherence of leukocytes to endothelium.

Particulate guanylate cyclase, the second form of guanylate cyclase in vascular muscle, can be activated by members of the natriuretic peptide family—atrial natriuretic peptide, brain natriuretic peptide, and C-type natriuretic peptide.[4] Administration of exogenous atrial and brain natriuretic peptides produces relaxation of cerebral blood vessels, but it is not clear whether endogenously produced natriuretic peptides contribute to regulation of cerebral vascular tone.

Although the endothelial and neuronal isoforms of NOS are constitutively expressed in blood vessels, the inducible or "immunologic" isoform is probably not expressed under normal conditions, but its expression may be induced in endothelium, vascular muscle, and other cell types in brain.[1,2] This inducible isoform of NOS can produce large amounts of NO during pathophysiologic conditions, such as ischemia–reperfusion, subarachnoid hemorrhage (SAH), and meningitis.

Cyclic Adenosine Monophosphate–Mediated Mechanisms

Activation of adenylate cyclase and production of cyclic adenosine monophosphate (cAMP) in vascular muscle mediate relaxation of blood vessels in response to a variety of endogenous substances[5]—representing a second major mechanism of vasodilatation in cerebral vessels. Stimuli that activate adenylate cyclase include prostanoids (prostacyclin and prostaglandin E_2), adenosine, calcitonin gene–related peptide (CGRP), vasoactive intestinal peptide, β-adrenergic agonists, pituitary adenylate cyclase activating peptide (PACAP), and adrenomedullin. A newer concept is that increases in intracellular cAMP in vascular muscle produce vasodilatation only in part by a direct effect and, in part, by activation of potassium ion (K^+) channels (see later).

K^+ Channels

A third vasodilator mechanism that has received considerable attention in the last decade involves activation of K^+ channels. Increases in activity of K^+ channels result in membrane hyperpolarization of vascular muscle.[2,6,7] At least four types of K^+ channels are present in cerebral blood vessels: ATP-sensitive K^+ (K_{ATP}) channels, large-conductance calcium-activated K^+ (BK_{Ca}) channels, voltage-dependent K^+ (K_V) channels, and inwardly rectifying K^+ (K_{IR}) channels.

K_{ATP} Channels

Activity of K_{ATP} channels is inhibited by intracellular ATP or an increased ratio of ATP to adenosine diphosphate (ADP). The intracellular concentration of ATP is normally sufficient to prevent opening of K_{ATP} channels, and in cerebral vascular muscle, these channels appear to be closed under normal conditions.[8] Because intracellular ATP levels are tightly regulated, it is likely that K_{ATP} channels are only rarely activated by reductions in ATP. Reductions in levels of intracellular pO_2 and pH also open these channels and produce vasorelaxation. Thus, activity of K_{ATP} channels appears to reflect, at least in part, the metabolic state of cells.[7]

Several endogenous substances produce hyperpolarization and relaxation of cerebral vascular muscle that is mediated, either fully or partly, by activation of K_{ATP} channels. These substances include CGRP,[9] norepinephrine,[10] and increased intracellular concentration of cAMP.[10] The concept that K_{ATP} channels may be activated by higher concentrations of cAMP is supported by evidence that dilatation of the basilar artery in response to forskolin, a direct activator of adenylate cyclase, can be attenuated with glibenclamide, a selective inhibitor of K_{ATP} channels.[9,10] In contrast, vasodilators that increase cGMP in cerebral vessels are usually not inhibited by glibenclamide in most studies.[8,11–13]

Systemic hypoxia is a potent cerebral dilator, and relaxation of cerebral vessels during hypoxia appears to involve activation of K^+ channels.[2,14] Relaxation during hypoxia of both large cerebral arteries in vitro and cerebral arterioles in vivo is inhibited by glibenclamide, suggesting that the response to hypoxia is mediated by activation of K_{ATP} channels.[8]

BK_{Ca} Channels

Activity of BK_{Ca} channels increases in response to elevations in intracellular calcium. BK_{Ca} channels in blood vessels appear to act as a negative feedback mechanism during increases in intracellular concentrations of calcium, so that these channels open more frequently during increases in blood pressure and with membrane depolarization. Tone of cerebral vessels, particularly during elevations of arterial pressure, may potentially be influenced by activity of BK_{Ca} channels (see later discussion of hypertension).[14] In contrast to K_{ATP} channels, BK_{Ca} channels may be active in large cerebral arteries under basal conditions, and selective inhibition of this channel (e.g., with tetraethylammonium or iberiotoxin) leads to constriction of cerebral arteries.[15–18]

BK_{Ca} channels are responsive to other stimuli in addition to the intracellular concentration of calcium. Activation of BK_{Ca} channels appears to contribute to relaxation of cerebral arterioles in response to activation of adenylate cyclase and accumulation of cAMP.[19,20] Because a variety of endogenous vasoactive stimuli raise the concentration of cAMP in vascular muscle, activation of BK_{Ca} channels by cAMP may play a major role in regulation of cerebral vascular tone. There is similar evidence that increases in cGMP, or of NO independent of cGMP,[21] can increase activity of BK_{Ca} channels in cerebral vessels.[18,19]

K_V Channels

Voltage-dependent K^+ (K_V) channels are activated in response to membrane depolarization, but this process occurs independently of the intracellular calcium concentration. These K^+ channels are also activated by elevations in arterial blood pressure and may thus modulate pressure-induced increases in cerebral artery tone.[22] Activation of K_V channels may also contribute directly to mechanisms that produce cerebral vasorelaxation in response to NO and endothelium-derived hyperpolarizing factor (EDHF).[23–25]

K_{IR} Channels

The name "inwardly rectifying K^+ channels" is based on the channels' properties that enable conduction of K^+ current into cells much more readily than outward K^+ current.[7,26,27] At physiologic membrane potential, however, a small rise above the normal extracellular K^+ (≈ 3 mM in cerebrospinal fluid) leads to an increase in the resting outward K^+ current through K_{IR} channels. Hence, a modest increase in extracellular K^+ (e.g., by <10 mmol/L), as may occur during neuronal or muscle activation,[28–30] can paradoxically lead to substantial vascular hyperpolarization and vasorelaxation because of K^+ efflux through K_{IR} channels.[31–36]

Reactive Oxygen Species

The cerebral circulation is unusual in terms of its acute vascular response to reactive oxygen species. In contrast to many extracranial vessels, in which oxygen radicals typically increase vascular tone,[37] cerebral arterioles relax in response to reactive oxygen species in vivo.[38–43] Stimuli such as bradykinin and arachidonic acid, which produce endogenous generation of reactive oxygen species, cause dilatation of cerebral arterioles that can be completely inhibited by indomethacin (implicating cyclooxygenase as the source of reactive oxygen species) or scavengers of reactive oxygen species.[40,41,44–48] Dilatation of cerebral arterioles in response to reactive oxygen species appears to be mediated by activation of BK_{Ca} channels[40,41] or K_{ATP} channels.[43] In large cerebral arteries, responses seem to be more complex, because reactive oxygen species can produce either relaxation[49,50] or contraction.[51-53] Some evidence suggests that low concentrations of reactive oxygen species produce relaxation of cerebral arteries but that high concentrations produce contraction.[54]

PATHOPHYSIOLOGIC ALTERATIONS IN CEREBRAL VESSEL FUNCTION

Platelets and Leukocytes

Activated platelets release potent vasoactive substances, including ADP (an endothelium-dependent vasodilator), serotonin (either a vasoconstrictor or an endothelium-dependent vasodilator, depending on vascular bed and vessel size) and thromboxane A_2 (a vasoconstrictor). In normal vessels, the vasomotor response to platelet products therefore may potentially be dilatation, constriction, or little net effect, depending on the relative influence of individual mediators. Under pathophysiologic conditions in which endothelial function is impaired, release of NO in response to ADP is reduced, and a greater portion of the net vasomotor response to platelet products is shifted to vasoconstrictor influences.

Polymorphonuclear leukocytes and monocytes also produce a variety of vasoactive agents, but the identity and conditions for release of many of these mediators are still poorly understood. In general, it is uncertain whether vasoconstrictor or vasodilator responses prevail in response to leukocytes.[55] Endothelium appears to mediate dilator responses, or to attenuate constrictor responses, to leukocytes (as well as platelets) in some vascular preparations. In contrast to platelets, however, leukocytes produce endothelium-dependent constriction of normal arteries.[55,56] The mechanism of this latter effect appears to be through inactivation or inhibition of NO that is released under basal conditions. The effect of endothelial dysfunction on vascular responses to leukocytes is therefore difficult to predict; evaluation of vasoactive influences of leukocytes on cerebral vessels under specific pathophysiologic conditions is an important issue.

Atherosclerosis

Endothelium-Dependent Relaxation in Atherosclerosis

Both basal and agonist-induced release or activity of NO is impaired in extracranial blood vessels by atherosclerosis.[2,57-61] Superoxide dismutase improves endothelium-dependent relaxation in atherosclerotic arteries,[60] suggesting that the mechanism of impairment involves excess generation of superoxide and inactivation of NO. In advanced atherosclerotic lesions, however, impairment of relaxation may also be related to reduced production of NO.

An important concept that has emerged in the past few years is that NADPH (reduced form of nicotinamide adenine dinucleotide phosphate) oxidase may be an important source of superoxide in vessels. Superoxide has many important vascular effects, including inactivation of NO. The phagocyte-like NADPH oxidase may play an important role in vascular consequences of atherosclerosis and

hypertension,[62] and a recent study suggests that an NADPH oxidase is present in cerebral vessels.[54] The role of NADPH in cerebral vascular disease is of great interest.

The effect of atherosclerosis on endothelium-dependent relaxation of cerebral vessels is less clear. Atherosclerosis seems to develop in intracranial vessels much more slowly than in extracranial vessels.[63] Relaxation of cerebral vessels to endothelium-dependent stimuli can be normal in the same atherosclerotic animals that exhibit marked impairment of endothelium-dependent relaxation in the aorta.[63-65] In contrast, some studies suggest that atherosclerosis or hypercholesterolemia produces cerebral endothelial dysfunction. For example, hypercholesterolemia is associated with impaired endothelium-dependent relaxation of the basilar artery,[66] and the influence of basal NO on vascular tone is reduced in cerebral arteries from atherosclerotic monkeys.[67] Administration of L-arginine, the substrate for NO synthesis, restores dilator responses of the basilar artery to acetylcholine to normal.[66] This finding is surprising, because it seems unlikely that L-arginine deficiency contributes to impairment of endothelial function in atherosclerosis. Evidence now suggests that the actions of endogenous inhibitors of NO synthesis, which compete with L-arginine for binding to NOS, may contribute to this phenomenon.[68]

Some studies now indicate that endothelial dysfunction is predictive of cardiovascular events.[69,70] It will be of great interest to determine whether endothelial dysfunction is predictive of stroke.

Cerebral Vascular Responses to Platelet and Leukocyte Products in Atherosclerosis

In the carotid and other large arteries supplying the brain, constrictor responses to serotonin and thromboxane A_2 are enhanced in the presence of atherosclerosis.[61,71-74] Collagen, which activates platelets, increases carotid blood flow normally but produces reductions in blood flow in the presence of atherosclerosis.[61] The normal increase in carotid blood flow produced by collagen is probably due largely to endothelium-dependent vasodilatation mediated by release of NO from small cerebral arteries in response to ADP,[75,76] a major product of platelet activation. Because NO normally inhibits constrictor responses of large cerebral arteries to serotonin, impairment of release or activity of NO may contribute to augmented vasoconstrictor responses during atherosclerosis.[77,78] Endothelial dysfunction alone, however, does not appear to be sufficient to account for all of the increases in constrictor responsiveness of large cerebral arteries to serotonin.[73,74]

Analogous results have been obtained concerning effects of leukocytes on cerebral arteries during atherosclerosis.[55] Leukocytes in vitro induce greater contraction of atherosclerotic arteries than of normal vessels.[55] Intravascular activation of leukocytes leads to prolonged contraction of cerebral arteries of the atherosclerotic monkey, whereas in normal animals, the constrictor effects of activated leukocytes are trivial.[71] Leukocytes from hypercholesterolemic rabbits release greater amounts of at least one unidentified contracting factor that inhibits NO-dependent vascular relaxation.[79]

Most transient ischemic attacks (TIAs) are thought to be produced by platelet adhesion, aggregation, and

Pathophysiology

embolization from plaques in large extracranial arteries.[80] Release of serotonin during aggregation of platelets, coupled with augmented constrictor responses to serotonin in atherosclerotic arteries, may produce pronounced vasoconstriction and perhaps contribute to cerebral ischemia.[74]

Importantly, vasoactive effects of platelets and leukocytes are likely to be closely interdependent. When leukocytes and platelets are activated together, there appears to be enhanced release of vasoactive products, and activation of leukocytes inhibits vasodilatation in response to platelets.[81] Furthermore, there is synergism in the action of platelet- and leukocyte-derived vasoconstrictors on vascular tone.[55] Abnormal cerebral vascular responses to activated platelets, and possibly leukocytes, may thus contribute to the pathophysiology of TIAs and cerebral ischemia in the presence of atherosclerosis.[73]

Effects of Therapy to Lower Plasma Cholesterol

Hypercholesterolemia is a major risk factor for coronary vascular events, but plasma cholesterol has been thought to have only a small effect on susceptibility to cerebrovascular events. Reduction in dietary cholesterol produces regression of atherosclerosis and restores endothelium-dependent relaxation of extracranial arteries toward normal in experimental animals.[58,59,61] Susceptibility to vasoconstriction in response to activation of platelets and leukocytes is reduced or abolished by regression of atherosclerosis.[82]

Augmented constrictor responses of large cerebral arteries to serotonin are also restored largely to normal during regression of atherosclerosis.[61,73] Significant functional improvement appears to precede structural regression and occurs within only a few months of dietary treatment of hypercholesterolemia in cerebral and noncerebral arteries of atherosclerotic monkeys.[61,83] Thus, the benefits of cholesterol-lowering therapy may occur relatively rapidly. Hypercholesterolemia alters platelets as well as blood vessels, and part of the rapid improvement in vascular responses during treatment of hypercholesterolemia may be related to normalization of platelet function.[84]

Of considerable interest is the finding that in patients with coronary heart disease who received a cholesterol-lowering agent for approximately 5 years, reduction of cholesterol reduced cerebrovascular events by one third.[85] The finding has been confirmed in other large trials using HMG (3-hydroxy-3-methylglutaryl)–coenzyme A reductase inhibitors. Pharmacologic lowering of plasma cholesterol using HMG–coenzyme A reductase inhibitors (i.e., statins) appears to provide additional benefits for vascular function, including increased expression of endothelial NOS and decreased activity of the proconstrictor enzyme Rho-kinase.[86,87] The response to statins is described as a "pleiotropic" effect, with some effects also occurring in normocholesterolemic animals and not due to reduction in plasma cholesterol (Fig. 37–1).[88] Upregulation of endothelial NOS by statins enhances cerebral blood flow and reduces stroke damage after cerebral ischemia.[86,87,89] Thus, statins improve vascular function, both by cholesterol lowering with regression of atherosclerosis and by a pleiotropic effect that is not related to reduction of cholesterol, and reduce cerebrovascular events.

Chronic Hypertension

Chronic hypertension is a major risk factor for numerous cardiovascular disorders and, for reasons that are not clear, is even more strongly associated with stroke than with myocardial infarction.[90] Hypertension may have profound deleterious effects on cerebral vascular function, the underlying mechanisms of which are still not well understood.

Endothelial Function in Chronic Hypertension

Endothelium-dependent relaxation is impaired in the cerebral circulation during chronic hypertension (Fig. 37–2). Dilatation of cerebral arterioles and the basilar artery in response to endothelium-dependent agonists such as acetylcholine and ADP is impaired in the chronically hypertensive rat.[2] Cerebral vasodilatation in response to endothelium-independent agonists (which act directly on vascular muscle) such as NO, nitroglycerin, and adenosine is not impaired during chronic hypertension, suggesting that endothelial function is impaired but vascular muscle relaxation is preserved.[2] Thus, the cAMP and cGMP mechanisms appear to be relatively normal during chronic hypertension.

Mechanisms that account for impaired endothelium-dependent relaxation during chronic hypertension appear to be different in cerebral arterioles and in the basilar artery. In cerebral arterioles, this impairment may be related to release of an endothelium-derived contracting factor (EDCF) that counteracts the normal dilator effects of NO (see Fig. 37–2).[91] This EDCF appears to be a prostanoid (and not, for example, endothelin), because indomethacin restores responses to endothelium-dependent agonists to or towards normal.[91] Impaired endothelium-dependent relaxation of the basilar artery, unlike that of the cerebral arterioles, does not appear to be due to production of an EDCF and is restored by L-arginine in stroke-prone, spontaneously hypertensive (SHRSP) rats.[92,93] The abnormality of endothelial function in the basilar artery during chronic hypertension may therefore be related to a reduction in production or activity of NO.

Altered responses of cerebral arterioles to endothelium-dependent agonists (acetylcholine and serotonin) in chronic hypertension may impair cerebral vasodilatation in response to vasoactive substances released by platelets. It is possible that, when platelets aggregate at plaques in the carotid arteries and release serotonin, impairment of endothelium-dependent responses during chronic hypertension may predispose to cerebral ischemia and stroke. Evidence consistent with that possibility is that serotonin produces greater constriction of large cerebral arteries in SHRSP rats than in Wistar Kyoto (WKY) rats.[94]

K⁺ Channels

Chronic hypertension has been the most extensively studied cardiovascular disease state in relation to changes to K^+ channel expression and function in cerebral arteries. There is evidence for abnormal function of several K^+ channel types in blood vessels during hypertension; this evidence has been reviewed.[2,6,94]

K_{ATP} Channels

Dilator responses of cerebral arteries of chronically hypertensive rats are impaired in response to activation of K_{ATP} channels (see Fig. 37–2).[96] Because K_{ATP} channels are

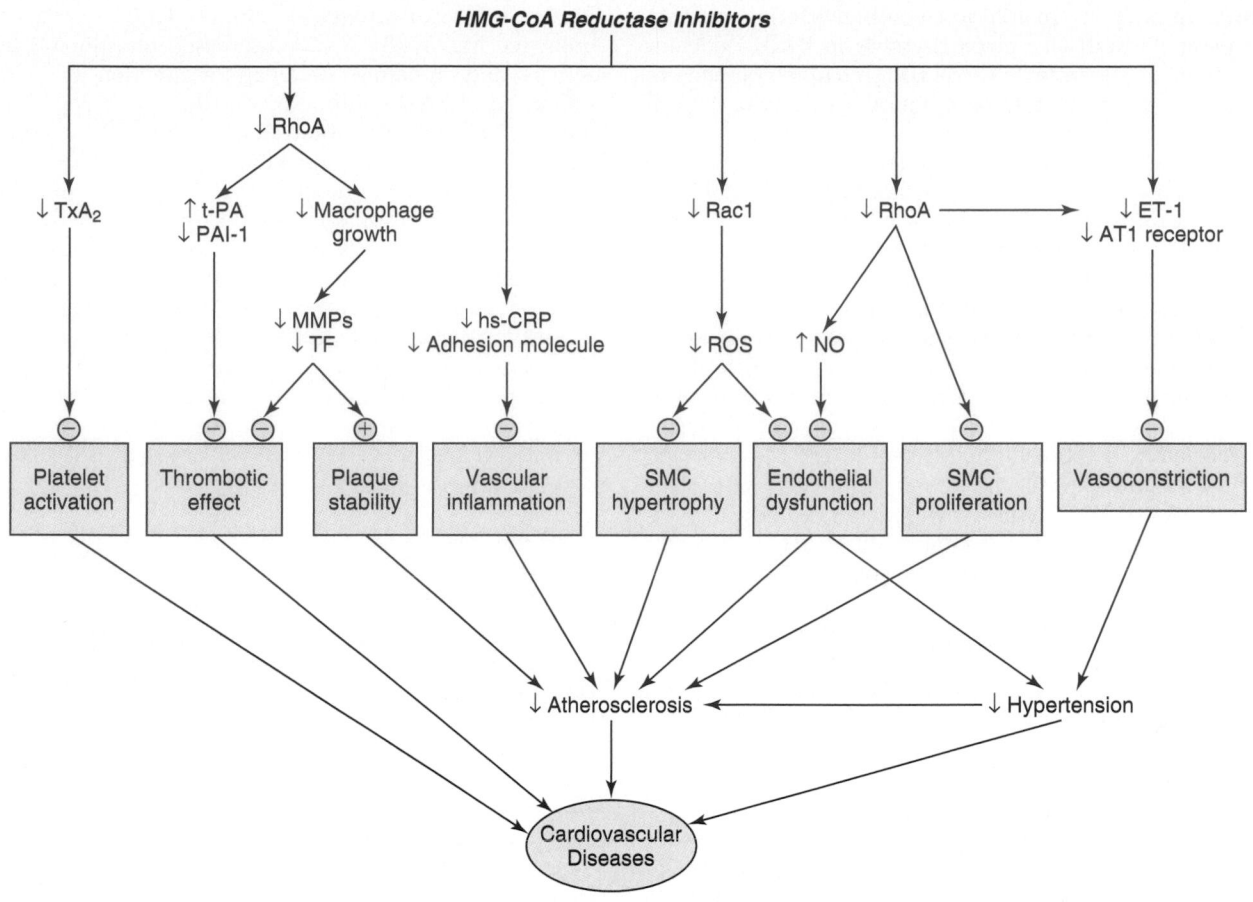

FIGURE 37–1 *HMG-CoA reductase inhibitors (statins) have multiple effects on blood vessels. Many of the effects are not produced by reduction of plasma cholesterol. AT1 receptor, angiotensin type 1 receptor; ET-1, endothelin-1; hs-CRP, C-reactive protein; MMPs, matrix metalloproteinases; NO, nitric oxide; PAI-1, plasminogen activator inhibitor-1; ROS, reactive oxygen species; SMC, smooth muscle cell; TF, tissue factor; t-PA, tissue-type plasminogen activator; TxA$_2$, thromboxane A$_2$. Adapted from Reference 87, with permission.*

FIGURE 37–2 *Some abnormalities in cerebral vessels during chronic hypertension. Decreased production or activity of nitric oxide (NO) may occur during chronic hypertension. Activity of ATP-sensitive potassium channels (K$_{ATP}$) may also be reduced during hypertension. Production of endothelium-derived contracting factors (EDCFs) may occur and counteract normal vasodilator mechanisms. Activity of large conductance calcium-activated K$^+$ channels appears to be increased during chronic hypertension, perhaps in response to increased levels of intracellular calcium.*

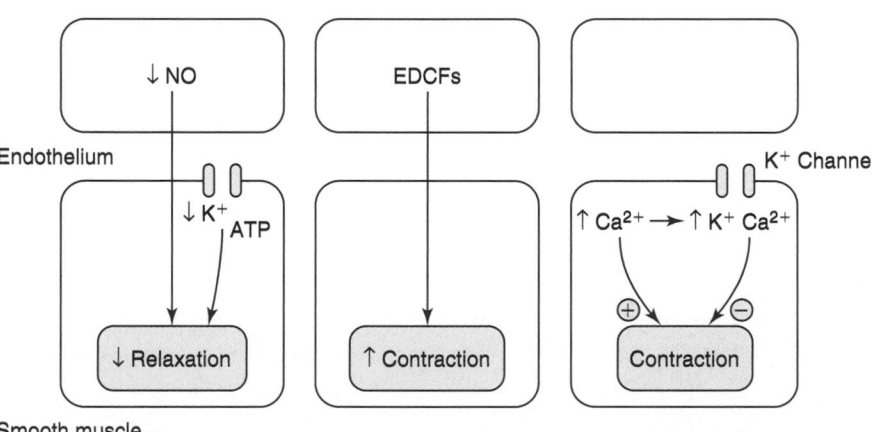

important mediators of vasodilator responses to hypoxia and hypotension, one might speculate that cerebral dilator responses to hypoxia and hypotension are impaired in chronic hypertension.[9,13]

BK$_{Ca}$ Channels
Specific inhibitors of BK$_{Ca}$ channels produce greater contraction of cerebral vessels in hypertensive than normotensive animals. Thus, basal activity of BK$_{Ca}$ channels appears to be increased in cerebral arteries during chronic hypertension.[17] Deficiency in expression of the BK$_{Ca}$ channel may itself result in cerebral artery dysfunction and systemic hypertension. Targeted deletion of the β1 subunit of the BK$_{Ca}$ channel, which renders the channel largely nonfunctional under physiologic conditions, produces hypertension (approx. 15 to 20 mm Hg higher than

Pathophysiology

normal) in mice.[97,98] In addition, cerebral arteries constrict to a greater extent at a given pressure in BKβ1-deficient mice than in controls.[97] Thus, BK_{Ca} channels appear to normally function to reduce cerebral artery tone as well as systemic blood pressure.

Consistent with such a function, studies have also demonstrated that in other experimental models of hypertension, expression and activity of the BK_{Ca} channel are increased in several vessels, including the carotid artery[15,99,100] and intracranial vessels.[17,101] Because of its role to limit vasoconstriction, BK_{Ca} channel function may be increased in vascular muscle as a protective negative feedback mechanism against increases in blood pressure. Such a mechanism would act to limit pressure-induced vasoconstriction and to preserve local blood flow. Potential clinical relevance of these findings may include the targeting of BK_{Ca} channels with therapeutic approaches to treat hypertension, and also investigation into whether mutations in genes encoding components of BK_{Ca} channels contribute to some types of human hypertension.

Subarachnoid Hemorrhage

Function of Endothelium and Soluble Guanylate Cyclase

Subarachnoid hemorrhage (SAH) produces several abnormalities of vascular function (Fig. 37–3). After SAH, cerebral vascular muscle is partially depolarized.[102] Depolarization of vascular muscle contributes to cerebral vasospasm, which often occurs after SAH.[103] Several mechanisms, including endothelial function, may contribute to vasospasm. Endothelium-dependent relaxation is impaired in large cerebral arteries in experimental models of SAH.[104] Similar impairment has been observed in the basilar artery from humans after SAH.[105]

Several mechanisms have been proposed to account for the impairment of endothelium-dependent relaxation after SAH.[103] Both the amount and activity of endothelial NOS protein are relatively unchanged in large cerebral arteries after SAH.[106,108] These findings are consistent with previous reports that release of NO is normal after SAH.[108–110]

Some findings suggest that impaired endothelium-dependent relaxation after SAH is due to reduction of protein levels, of activity of soluble guanylate cyclase, or both (see Fig. 37–3).[106,109,111] Increased phosphodiesterase activity and impaired K_V channel function in cerebral arteries after SAH could also contribute to this phenomenon.[112,113] In contrast, other studies report that vasorelaxation in response to nitrovasodilators is unaltered.[114,115]

The presence of hemoglobin in the cerebrospinal fluid may contribute to vasospasm after SAH by inactivation of NO. Hemoglobin avidly binds NO and thus may prevent diffusion of NO from endothelium to smooth muscle. In addition, hemoglobin may destroy NO through generation of superoxide.[103] Inactivation of NO by excessive generation of reactive oxygen species has also been suggested as a potentially important mechanism in cerebral vasospasm.[116,117] Thus, several mechanisms may contribute to impairment of endothelium-dependent relaxation of cerebral arteries after SAH.

Endothelin

Endothelin is a vasoconstrictor peptide that is produced by endothelial cells, and is thus an EDCF. It is not clear whether endothelin plays a role in physiologic regulation of the cerebral circulation.[2] Because endothelin-mediated constriction is long-lasting, it seems unlikely that endothelin contributes to the fine, short-term regulation of cerebral blood flow. Topical application of endothelin receptor antagonists does not alter diameter of cerebral vessels in vivo, suggesting that endothelin does not contribute to basal cerebrovascular tone.[118,119]

Several findings indicate that endothelin may contribute to cerebral vasospasm after SAH (see Fig. 37–3).[104] Hemoglobin and thrombin, which are present in cerebrospinal fluid after SAH, can enhance endothelin gene expression and endothelin release (see Fig. 37–3).[120–122] Concentrations of endothelin in the basilar artery and in cerebrospinal fluid are increased after SAH.[123–127] Intracisternal administration of endothelin-A (ET_A) receptor antagonists reduces vasospasm after SAH.[118,123,128–130] In contrast, other studies report no correlation between cerebrospinal fluid endothelin levels and cerebral vasospasm[131] and failure of ET_A receptor antagonists to reverse cerebral vasospasm.[132] However, most evidence is consistent with the concept that endothelin and activation of ET_A receptors contribute

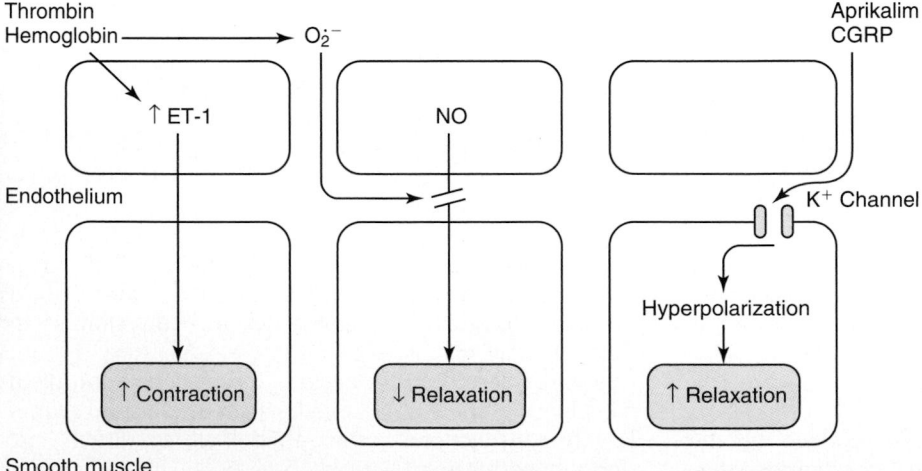

FIGURE 37–3 *Some abnormalities in cerebral vessels following subarachnoid hemorrhage. Thrombin and hemoglobin cause increased gene expression for endothelin-1 (ET-1), a potent vasoconstrictor. Superoxide anion ($O_2^{\cdot-}$) may be formed from hemoglobin, inactivate nitric oxide (NO), and thus impair relaxation. Vasodilatation in response to activation of ATP-sensitive K^+ channels (K_{ATP}) appears to be augmented following subarachnoid hemorrhage. This latter mechanism, in contrast to the first two, has implications for treatment of vasospasm following subarachnoid hemorrhage. CGRP, calcitonin gene-related peptide.*

to the onset or maintenance of cerebral vasospasm after SAH.

K⁺ Channel Function after Subarachnoid Hemorrhage

Another mechanism that may contribute to vasospasm after SAH may involve changes in activity of K⁺ channels in cerebral vessels. Partial depolarization of cerebral vascular muscle after SAH appears to be due to diminished membrane conductance to K⁺.[102,112] Depolarization and vasospasm can be inhibited by nicorandil,[15] a vasodilator that activates both K⁺ channels and soluble guanylate cyclase.[102] These findings suggest that activators of K⁺ channels in vascular muscle may have beneficial effects during vasospasm after SAH (see Fig. 37–3).

Consistent with these findings are reports that dilatation of the basilar artery in response to openers of K$_{ATP}$ channels is enhanced after SAH (see Fig. 37–3).[133,134] Interestingly, K$_{ATP}$ channel–mediated dilatation of large cerebral vessels may be especially enhanced after SAH during chronic hypertension.[133] Thus, augmented responses to activation of K⁺ channels despite the presence of hypertension are unusual and potentially therapeutically useful.

Hyperhomocysteinemia

Moderate elevation of plasma homocysteine appears to be an independent risk factor for stroke, and is associated with peripheral vascular disease and myocardial infarction.[135] Like hypercholesterolemia, hyperhomocysteinemia is caused by both genetic and dietary factors, and it may possibly contribute to vascular disease in a large number of patients.[136] Moderate elevations of plasma homocysteine can be decreased by dietary supplementation with folic acid, a finding suggesting that hyperhomocysteinemia may be a treatable risk factor for stroke and other vascular diseases.

Hyperhomocysteinemia produces vascular dysfunction, in both the carotid artery and the cerebral circulation. For example, acute elevation in homocysteine in the presence of copper (Cu^{2+}) inhibits NO-mediated cerebrovascular responses.[137] More modest, but chronic hyperhomocysteinemia produces endothelial dysfunction.[138–142] Both plasma levels of homocysteine and the extent of endothelial dysfunction are strongly influenced by dietary content of folate.[139] It is not entirely clear, however, to what extent vascular dysfunction is due to elevated homocysteine, folate deficiency, or other mechanisms. Importantly, a 2001 study suggests that endothelial dysfunction occurs in mice deficient in cystathionine β-synthase even in the absence of folate deficiency and is associated with increased S-adenosylmethionine levels.[142] These results suggest that altered S-adenosylmethionine–dependent methylation may contribute to the vascular pathophysiology of hyperhomocysteinemia.[142] In addition, studies with pharmacologic scavengers and genetically altered mice suggest that vascular dysfunction during hyperhomocysteinemia is at least partly mediated by oxidative stress.[141,143]

Diabetes Mellitus

Endothelial dysfunction also occurs in cerebral vessels during diabetes mellitus.[144–147] Mechanisms that account for impairment appear to be similar in diabetes to those observed during chronic hypertension. Altered responses of cerebral arterioles to endothelium-dependent agonists are probably due to production of an EDCF that activates a prostaglandin H₂–thromboxane A₂ receptor[146] with activation of protein kinase C.[147] In the basilar artery, impaired responses to endothelium-dependent stimuli are not due to production of a cyclooxygenase-derived EDCF.[145]

As in chronic hypertension, the activity of K$_{ATP}$ channels appears to be altered in diabetes. Dilatation of the basilar artery in response to aprikalim, an activator of K$_{ATP}$ channels, is reduced in diabetic rats, suggesting that function of K$_{ATP}$ channels may be abnormal in diabetes mellitus.[148]

Other findings indicate that hyperglycemia per se may produce impairment of endothelium-dependent dilatation of cerebral arterioles. This impairment of endothelium-dependent vasodilatation during acute elevations of glucose appears to involve activation of protein kinase C.[149]

GENE TRANSFER TO CEREBRAL BLOOD VESSELS

Gene transfer is a useful tool for study of vascular biology, and despite great obstacles, the application of such therapy to cerebrovascular disease has considerable potential.[150,151] The goal is to introduce complementary DNA (cDNA) into a cerebral artery or perivascular tissue and to stimulate production of a protein that favorably modulates vascular growth or function. Theoretically, this could be accomplished with the use of naked DNA, but the approach provides very inefficient gene transfer. Thus, more efficient vectors have been developed, including viral vectors (adenovirus, retrovirus, adeno-associated virus, and herpesvirus), complexes of DNA–cationic lipids, and viral conjugate vectors (liposomes with a viral coat).[150] Each of these vectors has specific advantages (related to efficiency, safety, trophism, and ease of preparation), and each has important limitations.[151] An "optimal" vector is not yet clearly identified.

Gene transfer can potentially be "targeted" to vascular tissues, such as adventitia or endothelium, or to specific receptors on endothelium.[152] Transgene expression may be driven by tissue-specific promoters, and regulated expression will be valuable. In addition, gene transfer can be used to express antisense oligonucleotides that inhibit expression of selected genes. For example, an antisense construct for astrocyte glial fibrillary acidic protein has been used to inhibit gliosis in astrocytes.[153]

It is now possible to accomplish gene transfer to cerebral vessels. Several studies demonstrate expression of functional proteins after gene transfer to carotid arteries and cerebral blood vessels.[154–160] Reporter genes, such as β-galactosidase, were used in some studies to demonstrate the feasibility of gene transfer.[154,161] In later studies proteins that modify vascular function, such as eNOS, have also been expressed in blood vessels through the use of gene transfer.[162–166]

Early approaches to producing gene transfer to blood vessels in vivo involved intraluminal methods that required stopping blood flow to allow uptake of vectors.[155] To avoid ischemia reperfusion after interruption of blood flow,

Pathophysiology

alternative methods have been developed to produce expression of transgene products in blood vessels. Promising methods are intracerebroventricular and intracisternal (cisterna magna) injection of viral vectors into cerebrospinal fluid.[161,167–169]

Gene transfer by intravenous injection of vectors results in high levels of transgene expression in liver and lung, but not in efficient expression in vessels. Protection against stroke has been reported, however, after gene transfer accomplished by intravenous gene transfer of atrial natriuretic peptide or kallikrein.[170,171] The mechanism of neural protection is not clear and may have resulted from reduction in blood pressure or response to circulating transgene products rather than from local effects of gene transfer to cerebral vessels. The studies nevertheless suggest that intravenous administration of vectors expressing some genes has potential for treatment or prevention of stroke.

One strategy for treatment of stroke assumes that progressive tissue injury, primarily in ischemic penumbral regions, may be inhibited. Thus, gene transfer may be useful in providing continuous local production of a therapeutic gene product to the penumbral region for several days after ischemia (Fig. 37–4).

Preliminary studies have been performed to evaluate the therapeutic potential of gene transfer to reduce ischemic brain injury. Adenovirus-mediated gene transfer of the *lacZ* gene, by direct injection into brain, produces high levels of expression of β-galactosidase in brain.[172] Thus, gene transfer can be accomplished in the brain after ischemia. This study is important in addressing the possibility that cerebral ischemia might impair synthesis of proteins after gene transfer.

Other studies report that intracerebroventricular injection of adenoviral vectors over-expressed an interleukin-1 receptor antagonist before ischemia and significantly reduced infarct size.[173] Neuroprotection against ischemic infarction has been reported after gene transfer of glial cell line–derived neurotropic factor[174] and atrial natriuretic peptide.[170] Many gene products have potential for therapeutic roles in protection against ischemic brain damage.

Another approach is to perform gene transfer to cells ex vivo and to surgically implant the transfected cells into blood vessels. In one study, tissue-type plasminogen activator protein (tPA)[175] was measurable in carotid arteries after implantation of cells exposed to adenoviral-mediated gene transfer ex vivo. Because tPA is used to treat ischemic stroke, the potential for gene therapy to express this substance is provocative.

Several studies suggest a future for gene therapy after SAH. Gene transfer to cerebral vessels can be accomplished after SAH,[176] suggesting that formation of a thrombus does not preclude intervention. Gene transfer of calcitonin gene–related peptide (CGRP), an extremely potent dilator of cerebral vessels, reduces vasospasm after SAH in rabbits.[177,178] Other laboratories have reported that gene transfer of eNOS attenuates vasospasm and improves vasodilator responses after SAH.[179,180] Thus, several interventions based on gene therapy may have therapeutic potential after embolic stroke and SAH.

Gene transfer might also be used to stimulate growth of collateral vessels in the presence of ischemia. This approach appears feasible in the peripheral circulation. Gene therapy might be used to treat brain tumors through inhibition of vascular proliferation, which thus would produce ischemia in the tumor.

Gene therapy might be useful for treatment of extracranial vascular disease, such as in the carotid or vertebral artery. Gene transfer approaches have been used to interrupt the cell cycle and thereby inhibit proliferation of vascular muscle. A goal of gene therapy might be to transfect an intracranial or extracranial artery after angioplasty with a gene that inhibits proliferation or remodeling. The problems related to inflammation and transient expression of transgenes provide major obstacles for the use of gene therapy at present.

SUMMARY

Abnormalities of cerebrovascular function occur in many disease states. Although the mechanisms are complex and

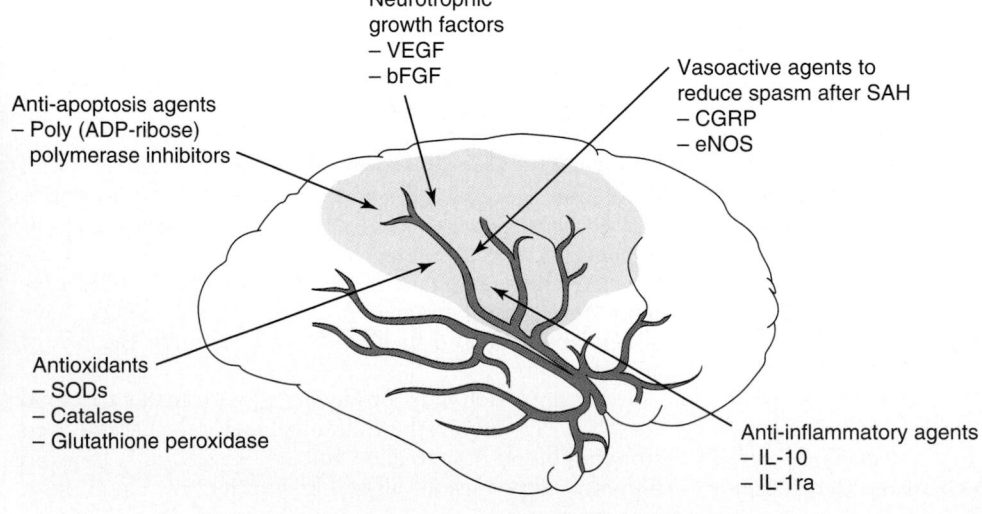

FIGURE 37–4 *Many gene products have potential for gene therapy in stroke by limiting the size of infarction or by reducing vasospasm. Some examples are bFGF, basic fibroblast growth factor; CGRP, calcitonin gene–related peptide; eNOS, endothelial NO-synthase; IL-10, interleukin-10; IL-1ra, interleukin-1 receptor antagonist; SODs, superoxide dismutases; VEGF, vascular endothelial growth factor; SAH, subarachnoid hemorrhage. (Adapted from Gunnett CA, Heistad DD: The future of gene therapy for stroke. Curr Hypertens Reports 3:36, 2001.)*

Neurotrophic growth factors
– VEGF
– bFGF

Vasoactive agents to reduce spasm after SAH
– CGRP
– eNOS

Anti-apoptosis agents
– Poly (ADP-ribose) polymerase inhibitors

Antioxidants
– SODs
– Catalase
– Glutathione peroxidase

Anti-inflammatory agents
– IL-10
– IL-1ra

Pathophysiology

multifactorial, a greater understanding of several mechanisms of cerebral vessel dysfunction has now been achieved. Many abnormalities of vasomotor function compromise regulation of cerebral blood flow and thus increase the risk of stroke. Therapy for cerebral vascular dysfunction focuses primarily on treatment of risk factors and, in addition, may involve pharmacologic or dietary interventions and potentially utilize gene therapy.

Acknowledgments

Original studies cited in this review were supported by NIH grants NS 24621, HL 38901, HL 14388, HL 16066, HL 62984, and AG 10269; by Research Funds from the Veterans Administration; and by a Project grant from the National Health and Medical Research Council of Australia (960672).

References

1. Faraci FM, Brian JE: Nitric oxide and the cerebral circulation. Stroke 25:692, 1994.
2. Faraci FM, Heistad DD: Regulation of the cerebral circulation: Role of endothelium and potassium channels. Physiol Rev 78:53, 1998.
3. Moncada S, Palmer RMJ, Higgs EA: Nitric oxide: Physiology, pathophysiology, and pharmacology. Pharmacol Rev 43:109, 1991.
4. Wong SK, Garbers DL: Receptor guanylyl cyclases. J Clin Invest 90:299, 1992.
5. Lincoln TM, Cornwell TL: Towards an understanding of the mechanism of action of cyclic AMP and cyclic GMP in smooth muscle relaxation. Blood Vessels 28:129, 1991.
6. Faraci FM, Sobey CG: Role of potassium channels in regulation of cerebral vascular tone. J Cereb Blood Flow Metab 18:1047, 1998.
7. Nelson MT, Quayle JM: Physiological roles and properties of potassium channels in arterial smooth muscle. Am J Physiol 268:C799, 1995.
8. Kitazono T, Faraci FM, Taguchi H, Heistad DD: Role of potassium channels in cerebral blood vessels. Stroke 26:1713, 1995.
9. Kitazono T, Heistad DD, Faraci FM: Role of ATP-sensitive K$^+$ channels in CGRP-induced dilatation of basilar artery in vivo. Am J Physiol 265:H581, 1993.
10. Kitazono T, Faraci FM, Heistad DD: Effect of norepinephrine on rat basilar artery in vivo. Am J Physiol 264:H178, 1993.
11. Faraci FM, Heistad DD: Role of ATP-sensitive potassium channels in the basilar artery. Am J Physiol 264:H8, 1993.
12. Onoue H, Katusic ZS: Role of potassium channels in relaxations of canine middle cerebral arteries induced by nitric oxide donors. Stroke 28:1264, 1997.
13. Taguchi H, Heistad DD, Kitazono T, Faraci FM: ATP-sensitive K$^+$ channels mediate dilatation of cerebral arterioles during hypoxia. Circ Res 74:1005, 1994.
14. Nelson MT, Cheng H, Rubart M, et al: Relaxation of arterial smooth muscle by calcium sparks. Science 270:633, 1995.
15. Asano M, Masuzawa-Ito K, Matsuda T: Charybdotoxin-sensitive K$^+$ channels regulate the myogenic tone in the resting state of arteries from spontaneously hypertensive rats. Br J Pharmacol 108:214, 1993.
16. Brayden JE, Nelson MT: Regulation of arterial tone by activation of calcium-dependent potassium channels. Science 256:532, 1992.
17. Paterno R, Heistad DD, Faraci FM: Functional activity of Ca^{2+}-dependent K$^+$ channels is increased in basilar artery during chronic hypertension. Am J Physiol 272:H1287, 1997.
18. Sobey CG, Faraci FM: Effect of nitric oxide and potassium channel agonists and inhibitors on basilar artery diameter. Am J Physiol 272:H256, 1997.
19. Paterno R, Faraci FM, Heistad DD: Role of Ca^{2+}-dependent K$^+$ channels in cerebral vasodilatation induced by increases in cyclic GMP and cyclic AMP in the rat. Stroke 27:1603, 1996.
20. Taguchi H, Heistad DD, Kitazono T, et al: Dilatation of cerebral arterioles in response to activation of adenylate cyclase is dependent on activation of Ca^{2+}-dependent K$^+$ channels. Circ Res 76:1057, 1995.
21. Onoue H, Katusic ZS: The effect of 1H-[1,2,4]oxadiazolo[4,3-a]quinoxalin-1-one (ODQ) and charybdotoxin (CTX) on relaxations of isolated cerebral arteries to nitric oxide. Brain Res 785:107, 1998.
22. Knot HJ, Nelson MT: Regulation of membrane potential and diameter by voltage-dependent K$^+$ channels in rabbit myogenic cerebral arteries. Am J Physiol 269:H348, 1995.
23. Dong H, Waldron GJ, Cole WC, et al: Roles of calcium-activated and voltage-gated delayed rectifier potassium channels in endothelium-dependent vasorelaxation of the rabbit middle cerebral artery. Br J Pharmacol 123:821, 1998.
24. Petersson J, Zygmunt PM, Hogestatt ED: Characterization of the potassium channels involved in EDHF-mediated relaxation in cerebral arteries. Br J Pharmacol 120:1344, 1997.
25. Sobey CG, Faraci FM: Inhibitory effect of 4-aminopyridine on responses of the basilar artery to nitric oxide. Br J Pharmacol 126:1437, 1999.
26. Nichols CG, Lopatin AN: Inward rectifier potassium channels. Ann Rev Physiol 59:171, 1997.
27. Quayle JM, Nelson MT, Standen NB: ATP-sensitive and inwardly rectifying potassium channels in smooth muscle. Physiol Rev 77:1165, 1997.
28. Caesar K, Akgoren N, Mathiesen C, et al: Modification of activity-dependent increases in cerebellar blood flow by extracellular potassium in anaesthetized rats. J Physiol (Lond) 520:281, 1999.
29. Iadecola C: Regulation of the cerebral microcirculation during neural activity: Is nitric oxide the missing link? Trends Neurosci 16:206, 1993.
30. Paulson OB, Newman EA: Does the release of potassium from astrocyte endfeet regulate cerebral blood flow? Science 237:896, 1987.
31. Chrissobolis S, Ziogas J, Chu Y, et al: Role of inwardly rectifying K$^+$ channels in K$^+$-induced cerebral vasodilatation in vivo. Am J Physiol 279:H2704, 2000.
32. Edwards FR, Hirst GDS, Silverberg GD: Inward rectification in rat cerebral arterioles: Involvement of potassium ions in autoregulation. J Physiol (Lond) 404:455, 1988.
33. Johnson TD, Marrelli SP, Steenberg ML, et al: Inward rectifier potassium channels in the rat middle cerebral artery. Am J Physiol 274:R541, 1998.
34. Knot HJ, Zimmerman PA, Nelson MT: Extracellular K$^+$-induced hyperpolarizations and dilatations of rat coronary and cerebral arteries involve inward rectifier K$^+$ channels. J Physiol (Lond) 492:419, 1996.
35. Quayle JM, McCarron JG, Brayden JE, et al: Inward rectifier K$^+$ currents in smooth muscle cells from rat resistance-sized cerebral arteries. Am J Physiol 265:C1363, 1993.
36. Zaritsky JJ, Eckman DM, Wellman GC, et al: Targeted disruption of Kir2.1 and Kir2.2 genes reveals the essential role of the inwardly rectifying K$^+$ current in K$^+$-mediated vasodilation. Circ Res 87:160, 2000.
37. Cosentino F, Sill JC, Katusic ZS: Role of superoxide anions in the mediation of endothelium-dependent contractions. Hypertension 23:229, 1994.
38. Leffler CW, Busija DW, Armstead WM, et al: H$_2$O$_2$ effects on cerebral prostanoids and pial arteriolar diameter in piglets. Am J Physiol 258:H1382, 1990.
39. Rosenblum WI: Effects of free radical generation on mouse pial arterioles: Probable role of hydroxyl radicals. Am J Physiol 245:H139, 1983.
40. Sobey CG, Heistad DD, Faraci FM: Mechanisms of bradykinin-induced cerebral vasodilatation in rats: Evidence that reactive oxygen species activate K$^+$ channels. Stroke 28:2290, 1997.
41. Sobey CG, Heistad DD, Faraci FM: Potassium channels mediate dilatation of cerebral arterioles in response to arachidonate. Am J Physiol 275:H1606, 1998.
42. Wei EP, Christman CW, Kontos HA, et al: Effects of oxygen radicals on cerebral arterioles. Am J Physiol 248:H157, 1985.
43. Wei EP, Kontos HA, Beckman JS: Mechanisms of cerebral vasodilation by superoxide, hydrogen peroxide, and peroxynitrite. Am J Physiol 271:H1262, 1996.
44. Busija DW, Heistad DD: Effects of indomethacin on cerebral blood flow during hypercapnia in cats. Am J Physiol 244:H519, 1983.
45. Ellis EF, Police RJ, Yancey L, et al: Dilation of cerebral arterioles by cytochrome P-450 metabolites of arachidonic acid. Am J Physiol 259:H1171, 1990.

Pathophysiology

46. Kontos HA, Wei EP, Povlishock JT, et al: Oxygen radicals mediate the cerebral arteriolar dilation from arachidonate and bradykinin in cats. Circ Res 55:295, 1984.

47. Leffler CW, Busija DW: Arachidonate metabolism on the cerebral surface of newborn pigs. Prostaglandins 30:811, 1985.

48. Wei EP, Ellis EF, Kontos HA: Role of prostaglandins in pial arteriolar response to CO_2 and hypoxia. Am J Physiol 238:H226, 1980.

49. Didion SP, Faraci FM: Effects of NADH on cerebral blood vessels [abstract]. FASEB J 15:A126, 2001.

50. Iida Y, Katusic ZS: Mechanisms of cerebral arterial relaxations to hydrogen peroxide. Stroke 31:2224, 2000.

51. Bryan RMJ, Steenberg ML, Marelli SP: The role of endothelium in shear stress-induced constrictions in the rat middle cerebral artery. Stroke 32:1394, 2001.

52. Katusic ZS, Schugel J, Cosentino F, et al: Endothelium-dependent contractions to oxygen-derived free radicals in the canine basilar artery. Am J Physiol 264:H859, 1993.

53. Madden JA, Christman NJT: Integrin signaling, free radicals, and tyrosine kinase mediate flow constriction in isolated cerebral arteries. Am J Physiol 277:H2264, 1999.

54. Didion SP, Faraci FM: Effects of NADH and NADPH on superoxide levels and cerebral vascular tone. Am J Physiol 282:H688, 2002.

55. Akopov S, Sercombe R, Seylaz J: Cerebrovascular reactivity: Role of endothelium/platelet/leukocyte interactions. Cerebrovasc Brain Metab Rev 8:11, 1996.

56. Sobey CG, Woodman OL: Myocardial ischaemia: What happens to the coronary arteries? Trends Pharmacol Sci 14:448, 1993.

57. Chester AH, O'Neil GS, Moncada S, et al: Low basal and stimulated release of nitric oxide in atherosclerotic epicardial coronary arteries. Lancet 336:897, 1990.

58. Faraci FM, Orgren K, Heistad DD: Impaired relaxation of the carotid artery during activation of ATP-sensitive potassium channels in atherosclerotic monkeys. Stroke 25:178, 1994.

59. Harrison DG, Armstrong ML, Freiman PC, et al: Restoration of endothelium-dependent relaxation by dietary treatment of atherosclerosis. J Clin Invest 80:1808, 1987.

60. Mugge A, Elwell JH, Peterson TE, et al: Chronic treatment with polyethylene-glycolated superoxide dismutase partially restores endothelium-dependent vascular relaxations in cholesterol-fed rabbits. Circ Res 69:1293, 1991.

61. Sobey CG, Faraci FM, Piegors DJ, et al: Effect of short-term regression of atherosclerosis on reactivity of carotid and retinal arteries. Stroke 27:927, 1996.

62. Griendling KK, Sorescu D, Ushio-Fukai M: NAD(P)H oxidase: Role in cardiovascular biology and disease. Circ Res 86:494, 2000.

63. Kanamaru K, Waga S, Tochio H, et al: The effect of atherosclerosis on endothelium-dependent relaxation in the aorta and intracranial arteries of rabbits. J Neurosurg 70:793, 1989.

64. Kitagawa S, Yamaguchi Y, Sameshima E: Differences in endothelium-dependent relaxation in various arteries from Watanabe heritable hyperlipidaemic rabbits with increasing age. Clin Exp Pharmacol Physiol 21:963, 1994.

65. Simonsen U, Ehrnrooth E, Gerdes LU, et al: Functional properties in vitro of systemic small arteries from rabbits fed a cholesterol-rich diet for 12 weeks. Clin Sci (Colch) 80:119, 1991.

66. Rossitch EJ, Alexander EI, Black PM, et al: L-Arginine normalizes endothelial function in cerebral vessels from hypercholesterolemic rabbits. J Clin Invest 87:1295, 1991.

67. Didion SP, Heistad DD, Faraci FM: Mechanisms that produce nitric oxide–mediated relaxation of cerebral arteries during atherosclerosis. Stroke 32:761, 2001.

68. Tsikas D, Boger RH, Sandmann J, et al: Endogenous nitric oxide synthase inhibitors are responsible for the L-arginine paradox. FEBS Lett 478:1, 2000.

69. Al Suwaidi J, Hamasaki S, Higano ST, et al: Long-term follow-up of patients with mild coronary artery disease and endothelial dysfunction. Circulation 101:948, 2000.

70. Schachinger V, Britten MB, Zeiher AM: Prognostic impact of coronary vasodilator dysfunction on adverse long-term outcome of coronary heart disease. Circulation 101:1899, 2000.

71. Faraci FM, Lopez JAG, Breese K, et al: Effect of atherosclerosis on cerebral vascular responses to activation of leukocytes and platelets in monkeys. Stroke 22:790, 1991.

72. Faraci FM, Williams JK, Breese KR, et al: Atherosclerosis potentiates constrictor responses of cerebral and ocular blood vessels to thromboxane in monkeys. Stroke 20:242, 1989.

73. Heistad DD, Breese KR, Armstrong ML: Cerebral vasoconstrictor responses to serotonin after dietary treatment of atherosclerosis: Implications for transient ischemic attacks. Stroke 18:1068, 1987.

74. Tamaki K, Armstrong M, Heistad D: Effects of atherosclerosis on cerebral vessels: Hemodynamic and morphometric studies. Stroke 17:1209, 1986.

75. Hardebo JE, Kahrstrom J, Owman C: P1- and P2-purine receptors in brain circulation. Eur J Pharmacol 144:343, 1987.

76. Vanhoutte PM, Houston DS: Platelets, endothelium, and vasospasm. Circulation 72:728, 1985.

77. Brian JE Jr, Kennedy RH: Modulation of cerebral arterial tone by endothelium-derived relaxing factor. Am J Physiol 264:H1245, 1993.

78. Faraci FM, Heistad DD: Endothelium-derived relaxing factor inhibits constrictor responses of large cerebral arteries to serotonin. J Cereb Blood Flow Metab 12:500, 1992.

79. Hart JL, Sobey CG, Woodman OL: Cholesterol feeding enhances vasoconstrictor effects of products from rabbit polymorphonuclear leukocytes. Am J Physiol 269:H1, 1995.

80. Barnett HJ: Progress towards stroke prevention: Robert Wartenberg lecture. Neurology 30:1212, 1980.

81. Kaul S, Waack BJ, Padgett RC, et al: Interaction of human platelets and leukocytes in modulation of vascular tone. Am J Physiol 266:H1706, 1994.

82. Padgett RC, Heistad DD, Mugge A, et al: Vascular responses to activated leukocytes after regression of atherosclerosis. Circ Res 70:423, 1992.

83. Benzuly KH, Padgett RC, Kaul S, et al: Functional improvement precedes structural regression of atherosclerosis. Circulation 89:1810, 1994.

84. Kaul S, Waack BJ, Padgett RC, et al: Altered vascular responses to platelets from hypercholesterolemic humans. Circ Res 72:737, 1993.

85. Randomised trial of cholesterol lowering in 4444 patients with coronary heart disease: The Scandinavian Simvastatin Survival Study (4S). Lancet 344:1383, 1994.

86. Laufs U, Endres M, Stagliano N, et al: Neuroprotection mediated by changes in the endothelial actin cytoskeleton. J Clin Invest 106:15, 2000.

87. Laufs U, Gertz K, Huang P, et al: Atorvastatin upregulates type III nitric oxide synthase in thrombocytes, decreases platelet activation, and protects from cerebral ischemia in normocholesterolemic mice. Stroke 31:2442, 2000.

88. Takemoto M, Liao JK: Pleiotropic effects of 3-hydroxy-3-methylglutaryl coenzyme A reductase inhibitors. Arterioscler Thromb Vasc Biol 21:1712, 2001.

89. Amin-Hanjani S, Stagliano NE, Yamada M, et al: Mevastatin, an HMG-CoA reductase inhibitor, reduces stroke damage and upregulates endothelial nitric oxide synthase in mice. Stroke 32:980, 2001.

90. Warlow CP: Epidemiology of stroke. Lancet 352(suppl III):1, 1998.

91. Mayhan WG: Role of prostaglandin H2-thromboxane A2 in responses of cerebral arterioles during chronic hypertension. Am J Physiol 262:H539, 1992.

92. Kitazono T, Faraci FM, Heistad DD: L-Arginine restores dilator responses of the basilar artery to acetylcholine during chronic hypertension. Hypertension 27:893, 1996.

93. Mayhan WG: Impairment of endothelium-dependent dilatation of basilar artery during chronic hypertension. Am J Physiol 259:H1455, 1990.

94. Mayhan WG: Responses of the basilar artery to products released by platelets during chronic hypertension. Brain Res 545:97, 1991.

95. Sobey CG: Potassium channel function in vascular disease. Arterioscler Thromb Vasc Biol 21:28, 2001.

96. Kitazono T, Heistad DD, Faraci FM: ATP-sensitive potassium channels in the basilar artery during chronic hypertension. Hypertension 22:677, 1993.

97. Brenner R, Perez GJ, Bonev AD, et al: Vasoregulation by the b1 subunit of the calcium-activated potassium channel. Nature 407:870, 2000.

98. Pluger S, Faulhaber J, Furstenau M, et al: Mice with disrupted BK channel b1 subunit gene feature abnormal $Ca(2+)$ Spark/STOC coupling and elevated blood pressure. Circ Res 87:e53, 2000.

99. Asano M, Masuzawa-Ito K, Matsuda T, et al: Functional role of Ca^{2+}-activated K^+ channels in resting state of carotid arteries from SHR. Am J Physiol 265:H843, 1993.

100. Kolias TJ, Chai S, Webb RC: Potassium channel antagonists and vascular reactivity in stroke-prone spontaneously hypertensive rats. Am J Hypertens 6:528, 1993.

101. Liu Y, Hudetz AG, Knaus H-G, et al: Increased expression of Ca^{2+}-sensitive K^+ channels in the cerebral microcirculation of genetically hypertensive rats: Evidence for their protection against cerebral vasospasm. Circ Res 82:729, 1998.

102. Harder DR, Dernbach P, Waters A: Possible cellular mechanism for cerebral vasospasm after subarachnoid hemorrhage in the dog. J Clin Invest 80:875, 1987.

103. Cook DA: Mechanisms of cerebral vasospasm in subarachnoid haemorrhage. Pharmacol Ther 66:259, 1995.

104. Sobey CG, Faraci FM: Subarachnoid haemorrhage: What happens to the cerebral arteries? Clin Exp Pharmacol Physiol 25:867, 1998.

105. Hatake K, Wakabayashi I, Kakishita E, et al: Impairment of endothelium-dependent relaxation in human basilar artery after subarachnoid hemorrhage. Stroke 23:1111, 1992.

106. Kasuya H, Weir BKA, Nakane M, et al: Nitric oxide synthase and guanylate cyclase levels in canine basilar artery after subarachnoid hemorrhage. J Neurosurg 82:250, 1995.

107. Naveri L, Stromberg C, Saavedra JM: Angiotensin IV reverses the acute cerebral blood flow reduction after experimental subarachnoid hemorrhage in the rat. J Cereb Blood Flow Metab 14:1096, 1994.

108. Kim P, Lorenz RR, Sundt TMJ, et al: Release of endothelium-derived relaxing factor after subarachnoid hemorrhage. J Neurosurg 70:108, 1989.

109. Kim P, Schini VB, Sundt TM, et al: Reduced production of cGMP underlies the loss of endothelium-dependent relaxations in the canine basilar artery after subarachnoid hemorrhage. Circ Res 70:248, 1992.

110. Kim P, Sundt TM, Vanhoutte PM: Alterations in endothelium-dependent responsiveness of the canine basilar artery after subarachnoid hemorrhage. J Neurosurg 69:239, 1988.

111. Chen AF, O'Brien T, Tsutsui M, et al: Expression and function of recombinant endothelial nitric oxide synthase gene in canine basilar artery. Circ Res 80:327, 1997.

112. Quan L, Sobey CG: Selective effects of subarachnoid hemorrhage on cerebral vascular responses to 4-aminopyridine in rats. Stroke 31:2460, 2000.

113. Sobey CG, Quan L: Impaired cerebral vasodilator responses to nitric oxide and PDE V inhibition after subarachnoid hemorrhage. Am J Physiol 277:H1718, 1999.

114. Kanamaru K, Weir BKA, Findlay JM, et al: Pharmacological studies on relaxation of spastic primate cerebral arteries in subarachnoid hemorrhage. J Neurosurg 71:909, 1989.

115. Katusic ZS, Milde JH, Cosentino F, et al: Subarachnoid hemorrhage and endothelial L-arginine pathway in small brain stem arteries in dogs. Stroke 24:392, 1993.

116. Kamii H, Kato I, Kinouchi H, et al: Amelioration of vasospasm after subarachnoid hemorrhage in transgenic mice overexpressing CuZn-superoxide dismutase. Stroke 30:867, 1997.

117. Shishido T, Suzuki R, Qian L, et al: The role of superoxide anions in the pathogenesis of cerebral vasospasm. Stroke 25:864, 1994.

118. Foley PL, Caner HH, Kassell NF, et al: Reversal of subarachnoid hemorrhage–induced vasoconstriction with an endothelin receptor antagonist. Neurosurgery 34:108, 1994.

119. Kitazono T, Heistad DD, Faraci FM: Enhanced responses of the basilar artery to activation of endothelin-B receptors in stroke-prone spontaneously hypertensive rats. Hypertension 25:490, 1995.

120. Cocks TM, Malta E, King SJ, et al: Oxyhaemoglobin increases the production of endothelin-1 (ET-1) by endothelial cells in culture. Eur J Pharmacol 196:177, 1991.

121. Kasuya H, Weir BKA, White DM, et al: Mechanism of oxyhemoglobin-induced release of endothelin-1 from cultured vascular endothelial cells and smooth muscle cells. J Neurosurg 79:892, 1993.

122. Ohlstein EH, Storer BL: Oxyhemoglobin stimulation of endothelin production in cultured endothelial cells. J Neurosurg 77:274, 1992.

123. Hirose H, Ide K, Sasaki T, et al: The role of endothelin and nitric oxide in modulation of normal and spastic cerebral vascular tone in the dog. Eur J Pharmacol 277:77, 1995.

124. Kraus GE, Bucholz RD, Yoon KW, et al: Cerebrospinal fluid endothelin-1 and endothelin-3 levels in normal and neurosurgical patients: A clinical study and literature review. Surg Neurol 35:20, 1991.

125. Masaoka H, Suzuki R, Hirata Y, et al: Raised plasma endothelin in aneurysmal subarachnoid haemorrhage. Lancet ii(8676):1402, 1989.

126. Suzuki H, Sato S, Suzuki Y, et al: Increased endothelin concentration in CSF from patients with subarachnoid hemorrhage. Acta Neurol Scand 81:553, 1990.

127. Yamaura I, Tani E, Maeda Y, et al: Endothelin-1 of canine basilar artery in vasospasm. J Neurosurg 76:99, 1992.

128. Clozel M, Watanabe H: BQ-123, a peptidic endothelin ET_A receptor antagonist, prevents the early cerebral vasospasm following subarachnoid hemorrhage after intracisternal but not intravenous injection. Life Sci 52:825, 1993.

129. Zuccarello M, Romano A, Passalacqua M, et al: Endothelin-1–induced endothelin-1 release causes cerebral vasospasm in-vivo. J Pharm Pharmacol 47:702, 1995.

130. Zuccarello MA, Lewis AI, Rapoport RM: Endothelin ETA and ETB receptors in subarachnoid hemorrhage–induced cerebral vasospasm. Eur J Pharmacol 259:R1, 1994.

131. Cosentino F, McMahon EG, Carter JS, et al: Effect of endothelin$_A$-receptor antagonist BQ-123 and phosphoramidon on cerebral vasospasm. J Cardiovasc Pharmacol 22:S332, 1993.

132. Gaetani P, Rodriguez y Baena G, Grignani G, et al: Endothelin and aneurysmal subarachnoid haemorrhage: A study of subarachnoid cisternal cerebrospinal fluid. J Neurol Neurosurg Psychiatry 57:66, 1994.

133. Sobey CG, Heistad DD, Faraci FM: Effect of subarachnoid hemorrhage on cerebral vasodilatation in response to activation of ATP-sensitive K^+ channels in chronically hypertensive rats. Stroke 28:392, 1997.

134. Sobey CG, Heistad DD, Faraci FM: Effect of subarachnoid hemorrhage on dilatation of basilar artery in vivo. Am J Physiol 271:H126, 1996.

135. Boushey CJ, Beresford SA, Omenn GS, et al: A quantitative assessment of plasma homocysteine as a risk factor for vascular disease: Probable benefits of increasing folic acid intakes. JAMA 274:1049, 1995.

136. Stampfer MJ, Malinow MR: Can lowering homocysteine levels reduce cardiovascular risk? N Engl J Med 332:328, 1995.

137. Zhang F, Slungaard A, Vercellotti GM, et al: Superoxide-dependent cerebrovascular effects of homocysteine. Am J Physiol 274:R1704, 1998.

138. Lentz SR, Sobey CG, Piegors DJ, et al: Vascular dysfunction in monkeys with diet-induced hyperhomocyst(e)inemia. J Clin Invest 98:24, 1996.

139. Lentz SR, Erger RA, Dayal S, et al: Folate dependence of hyperhomocysteinemia and vascular dysfunction in cystathionine beta-synthase–deficient mice. Am J Physiol 279:H970, 2000.

140. Symons JD, Mullick AE, Ensunsa JL, et al: Hyperhomocysteinemia evoked by folate depletion: Effects on coronary and carotid arterial function. Arterioscler Thromb Vasc Biol 22:772, 2002.

141. Eberhardt RT, Forgione MA, Cap A, et al: Endothelial dysfunction in a murine model of mild hyperhomocyst(e)inemia. J Clin Invest 106:483, 2000.

142. Dayal S, Bottiglieri T, Arning E, et al: Endothelial dysfunction and elevation of S-adenosylhomocysteine in cystathionine beta-synthase–deficient mice. Circ Res 88:1203, 2001.

143. Weiss N, Zhang YY, Heydrick S, et al: Overexpression of cellular glutathione peroxidase rescues homocyst(e)ine-induced endothelial dysfunction. Proc Natl Acad Sci U S A 98:12503, 2001.

144. Mayhan WG: Impairment of endothelium-dependent dilatation of cerebral arterioles during diabetes mellitus. Am J Physiol 256:H621, 1989.

145. Mayhan WG: Impairment of endothelium-dependent dilatation of the basilar artery during diabetes mellitus. Brain Res 580:297, 1992.

146. Mayhan WG, Simmons LK, Sharpe GM: Mechanism of impaired responses of cerebral arterioles during diabetes mellitus. Am J Physiol 260:H319, 1991.

147. Pelligrino DA, Koenig HM, Wang Q, et al: Protein kinase C suppresses receptor-mediated pial arteriolar relaxation in the diabetic rat. Neuroreport 5:417, 1994.

148. Mayhan WG: Effect of diabetes mellitus on response of the basilar artery to activation of ATP-sensitive potassium channels. Brain Res 636:35, 1994.

149. Mayhan WG, Patel KP: Acute effects of glucose on reactivity of cerebral microcirculation: Role of activation of protein kinase C. Am J Physiol 269:H1297, 1995.

150. Heistad DD, Faraci FM: Gene therapy for cerebral vascular disease. Stroke 27:1688, 1996.

Pathophysiology

151. Gunnett CA, Heistad DD: The future of gene therapy for stroke. Curr Hypertens Reports 3:36, 2001.

152. Chu Y, Heistad DD, Cybulsky MI, et al: Vascular cell adhesion molecule-1 augments adenovirus-mediated gene transfer. Arterioscler Thromb Vasc Biol 21:238, 2001.

153. Ghirnikar RS, Yu AC, Eng LF: Astrogliosis in culture. III: Effect of recombinant retrovirus expressing antisense glial fibrillary acidic protein RNA. J Neurosci Res 38:376, 1994.

154. Lund DD, Faraci FM, Ooboshi H, et al: Adenovirus-mediated gene transfer is augmented in basilar and carotid arteries of heritable hyperlipidemic rabbits. Stroke 30:120, 1999.

155. Kullo IJ, Mozes G, Schwartz RS, et al: Enhanced endothelium-dependent relaxations after gene transfer of recombinant endothelial nitric oxide synthase to rabbit carotid arteries. Hypertension 30:314, 1997.

156. Zoldhelyi P, McNatt J, Shelat HS, et al: Thromboresistance of balloon-injured porcine carotid arteries after local gene transfer of human tissue factor pathway inhibitor. Circulation 101:289, 2000.

157. Nishida T, Ueno H, Atsuchi N, et al: Adenovirus-mediated local expression of human tissue factor pathway inhibitor eliminates shear stress–induced recurrent thrombosis in the injured carotid artery of the rabbit. Circ Res 84:1446, 1999.

158. Mozes G, Mohacsi T, Gloviczki P, et al: Adenovirus-mediated gene transfer of macrophage colony stimulating factor to the arterial wall in vivo. Arterioscler Thromb Vasc Biol 18:1157, 1998.

159. Channon KM, Qian H, Neplioueva V, et al: In vivo gene transfer of nitric oxide synthase enhances vasomotor function in carotid arteries from normal and cholesterol-fed rabbits. Circulation 98:1905, 1998.

160. Ueno H, Yamamoto H, Ito S, et al: Adenovirus-mediated transfer of a dominant-negative H-ras suppresses neointimal formation in balloon-injured arteries in vivo. Arterioscler Thromb Vasc Biol 17:898, 1997.

161. Christenson SD, Lake KD, Ooboshi H, et al: Adenovirus-mediated gene transfer in vivo to cerebral blood vessels and perivascular tissue in mice. Stroke 29:1411, 1998.

162. Tsutsui M, Onoue H, Iida Y, et al: Effects of recombinant eNOS gene expression on reactivity of small cerebral arteries. Am J Physiol 278:H420, 2000.

163. Sato J, Mohacsi T, Noel A, et al: In vivo gene transfer of endothelial nitric oxide synthase to carotid arteries from hypercholesterolemic rabbits enhances endothelium-dependent relaxations. Stroke 31:968, 2000.

164. Lund DD, Faraci FM, Miller FJ Jr, et al: Gene transfer of endothelial nitric oxide synthase improves relaxation of carotid arteries from diabetic rabbits. Circulation 101:1027, 2000.

165. Kibbe M, Billiar T, Tzeng E: Nitric oxide synthase gene transfer to the vessel wall. Curr Opin Nephrol Hypertens 8:75, 1999.

166. Chen AF, O'Brien T, Tsutsui M, et al: Expression and function of recombinant endothelial nitric oxide synthase gene in canine basilar artery. Circ Res 80:327, 1997.

167. Toyoda K, Faraci FM, Russo AF, et al: Gene transfer of calcitonin gene–related peptide to cerebral arteries. Am J Physiol 278:H586, 2000.

168. Ooboshi H, Welsh MJ, Rios CD, et al: Adenovirus-mediated gene transfer in vivo to cerebral blood vessels and perivascular tissue. Circ Res 77:7, 1995.

169. Driesse MJ, Kros JM, Avezaat CJ, et al: Distribution of recombinant adenovirus in the cerebrospinal fluid of nonhuman primates. Hum Gene Ther 10:2347, 1999.

170. Lin KF, Chao J, Chao L: Atrial natriuretic peptide gene delivery reduces stroke-induced mortality rate in Dahl salt-sensitive rats. Hypertension 33:219, 1999.

171. Zhang JJ, Chao L, Chao J: Adenovirus-mediated kallikrein gene delivery reduces aortic thickening and stroke-induced death rate in Dahl salt-sensitive rats. Stroke 30:1925, 1999.

172. Abe K, Setoguchi Y, Hayashi T, et al: In vivo adenovirus-mediated gene transfer and the expression in ischemic and reperfused rat brain. Brain Res 763:191, 1997.

173. Betz AL, Yang GY, Davidson BL: Attenuation of stroke size in rats using an adenoviral vector to induce overexpression of interleukin-1 receptor antagonist in brain. J Cereb Blood Flow Metab 15:547, 1995.

174. Kitagawa H, Sasaki C, Sakai K, et al: Adenovirus-mediated gene transfer of glial cell line–derived neurotrophic factor prevents ischemic brain injury after transient middle cerebral artery occlusion in rats. J Cereb Blood Flow Metab 19:1336, 1999.

175. Kimura H, Sakata Y, Hamada H, et al: In vivo retention of endothelial cells adenovirally transduced with tissue-type plasminogen activator and seeded onto expanded polytetrafluoroethylene. J Vasc Surg 32:353, 2000.

176. Muhonen MG, Ooboshi H, Welsh MJ, et al: Gene transfer to cerebral blood vessels after subarachnoid hemorrhage. Stroke 28:822, 1997.

177. Toyoda K, Faraci FM, Watanabe Y, et al: Gene transfer of CGRP prevents vasoconstriction after subarachnoid hemorrhage. Circ Res 87:818, 2000.

178. Morishita R: Adventure of gene therapy into the brain: A new era for cardiovascular gene therapy. Circ Res 87:719, 2000.

179. Stoodley M, Weihl CC, Zhang ZD, et al: Effect of adenovirus-mediated nitric oxide synthase gene transfer on vasospasm after experimental subarachnoid hemorrhage. Neurosurgery 46:1193, 2000.

180. Onoue H, Tsutsui M, Smith L, et al: Expression and function of recombinant endothelial nitric oxide synthase gene in canine basilar artery after experimental subarachnoid hemorrhage. Stroke 29:1959, 1998.

Chapter Thirty-Eight

The Cerebral Microvasculature and Responses to Ischemia

G. F. Hamann and Gregory J. del Zoppo

ANATOMY OF THE CEREBRAL VASCULATURE

Regulation of vascular tone and circulatory hemostasis are important components of cerebral vascular physiology that are disrupted by ischemia. The cerebral vasculature has unique features for protection of the neuronal cells and preservation of their function through shifting of blood flow to regions of activation on demand and maintenance of an intravascular antithrombotic milieu.

The overall vascular strategy for protection of cortical and deep brain structures consists of the interconnection of territories of brain-supplying arteries via collateral anastomoses of the cerebral hemispheres and the circle of Willis. Pial and cortical penetrating arteries consist of (1) an endothelial cell layer, the basal lamina derived from the extracellular matrix (ECM), (2) layers of smooth muscle cells encased in ECM (myointima), and (3) an adventitia derived from the leptomeninges.[1] In the cortex, an extension of the subarachnoid space forms the Virchow-Robins space, which surrounds cortical penetrating arterioles until it disappears into the *glia limitans*, the abluminal boundary formed by the astrocyte end-feet. With further arborization of the microvasculature, the glia limitans at the capillary level fuses with the thin basal lamina. Cerebral capillaries are unique in that the endothelium and astrocyte end-feet are in close apposition, the adventitia being absent. Astrocytes serve both microvessels and neurons in this setting. The postcapillary venule network bears close ultrastructural resemblance to the capillaries, except for the presence of a limited myointimal layer. Another unique feature of the cerebral capillary is the permeability barrier, which prevents contact of the neuropil with the plasma column.

During normal blood flow, not all capillaries are perfused.[2] Observations also suggest the presence of a cerebrovascular reserve that can be recruited on short notice but does not involve neovascularization.[2,3] In contrast, direct measurements indicate that all capillaries of the pial and cortical circulation have plasma flow and that there is no capillary recruitment during forebrain ischemia.[4,5] Hence, the existence of a nascent microvascular bed that can be recruited in the early moments of focal ischemia remains uncertain.

THE BLOOD-BRAIN BARRIER AND MATRIX INTEGRITY

The permeability barrier characteristics of the cerebral microvasculature are represented by (1) inter–endothelial cell tight junctions (the blood-brain barrier) and (2) an intact subtending basal lamina. Both the permeability barrier and the basal lamina derive from the concerted interaction of the endothelial cells and astrocytes.[6–11] Cerebral microvessel endothelial cells display regional functional specialization along the microvascular axis.[12–16] In vitro co-culture studies suggest that this specialization depends on the interaction of its cellular components.[17–19] The proximity of the cellular components of intact cerebral capillaries implies ready communication between endothelial cells and astrocytes, and between astrocytes and neurons.[1,20] Flow alterations can be initiated by neuron stimulation or metabolic demand during arousal.[1]

The blood-brain barrier, the primary permeability barrier, is formed by endothelial cell tight junctions and limited endothelial cell pinocytosis and relies on the interactions of endothelial cells and astrocytes, as demonstrated by elegant xenograft experiments.[21] The primary barrier may involve adhesion of endothelial cells and astrocytes to the intervening matrix (basal lamina).[22–24] Astrocytes promote many microvessel blood-brain barrier properties, including endothelial cell tight junctions, Evan's blue exclusion from the neuropil and generation of the protein HT7-neurothelin.[23,25,26] It has been postulated that soluble factors generated by astrocytes maintain the endothelial characteristics of the blood-brain barrier, including the tight junctions, transendothelial resistance, and glucose–amino acid transport polarity.[19,21,27]

The secondary barrier involves integrin receptor cell–associated matrix adhesion and protects the brain parenchyma from hemorrhage.[22,28–32] The basal lamina separates the specialized endothelium from the astrocytes

Pathophysiology

and from their connections to neurons. The cerebral vascular basal lamina contains laminins, collagen type IV, fibronectin, and other components, including heparan sulfate proteoglycans (HSPGs), heparan sulfates, entactin, and nidogen.[7,11] Developmental interrelationships between the endothelium and astrocytes highlight the close functional association of endothelial cells and astrocytes in cerebral capillaries.[33]

Adhesion of both endothelial cells and astrocytes to the subtending basal lamina requires the interaction of cellular integrin receptors to their matrix ligands.[28,29] Haring and associates[29] described expression patterns of integrin subunits in normal central nervous system (CNS) microvessel subclasses.[29] Integrin $\alpha_1\beta_1$ on endothelial cells appears on all cerebral microvessels, including cerebral capillaries.[29,31,34–37] Integrins $\alpha_3\beta_1$ and $\alpha_6\beta_1$ are also expressed by cerebral endothelial cells. Integrin $\alpha_6\beta_4$ is expressed on astrocyte end-feet around select microvessels, whereas integrin $\alpha_1\beta_1$ is found on their fibers.[30,31] These relationships are perturbed by the loss of integrin-matrix attachments after middle cerebral artery occlusion (MCAO). Little is known, however, about the signaling functions of the integrins expressed in cerebral microvessels.

CEREBRAL MICROVESSEL RESPONSES TO FOCAL ISCHEMIA

During focal cerebral ischemia, a series of metabolic and morphologic alterations occur in the ischemic microvasculature.[38,39] They include loss of the endothelial cell permeability barrier, degradation or alteration of the vascular basal lamina, and extravasation of blood elements (Fig. 38–1). At least five responses of microvessels can be seen after cerebral ischemia; they are (1) loss of the barrier endothelial cell permeability with subsequent edema development, (2) loss of basal lamina and extracellular matrix, with subsequent hemorrhagic transformation, (3) alterations in microvessel cell-matrix adhesion, (4) loss of microvessel patency, and (5) expression of endothelial cell leukocyte adhesion receptors.

The capillary permeability barrier function is lost as early as 30 minutes after focal cerebral ischemia. This loss is associated with ultrastructural changes within the microvasculature such as swelling of endothelium and astrocytes, with cytoplasmic reorganization.[40–42] Garcia and colleagues[43] have also demonstrated that capillaries can expand and rupture. One consequence of the loss of

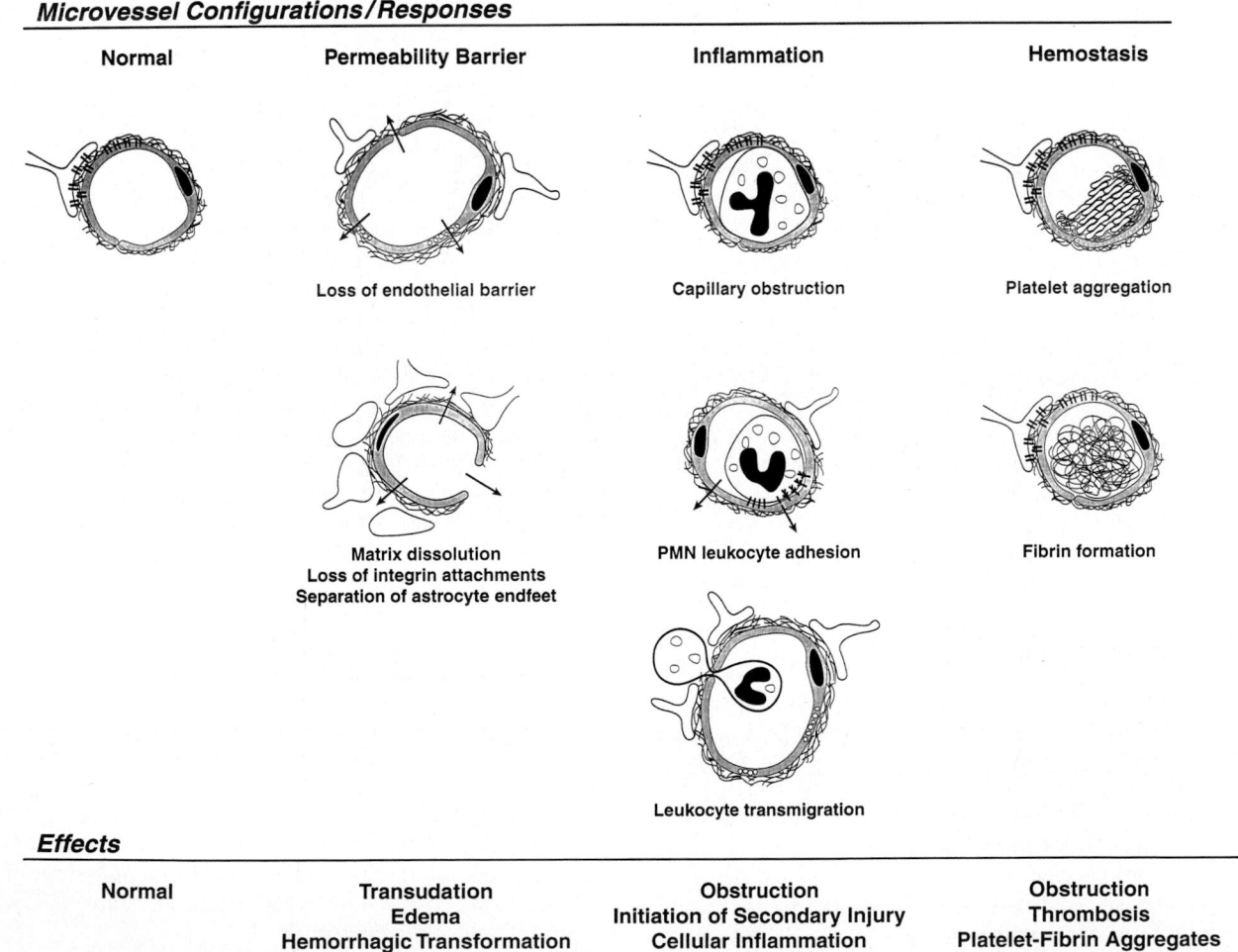

Microvessel Configurations/Responses

Normal **Permeability Barrier** **Inflammation** **Hemostasis**

Loss of endothelial barrier Capillary obstruction Platelet aggregation

Matrix dissolution
Loss of integrin attachments
Separation of astrocyte endfeet PMN leukocyte adhesion Fibrin formation

Leukocyte transmigration

Effects

Normal	Transudation	Obstruction	Obstruction
	Edema	Initiation of Secondary Injury	Thrombosis
	Hemorrhagic Transformation	Cellular Inflammation	Platelet-Fibrin Aggregates
		Transmigration	Vascular Permeability

FIGURE 38–1 *Early responses of cerebral microvessels in the target territory to focal ischemia. Not indicated are the appearance of activation antigens, and the signal proteins and receptors associated with neogenesis (see text).*

Pathophysiology

endothelial barrier function is the accumulation of transudate (edema) in the intercellular space of the neuropil, with the passage of albumin, immunoglobulins, and fibrinogen.[50] In both clinical and experimental settings, edema within the region of injury follows leakage of the vascular permeability barrier shortly after the onset of focal ischemia.[24,44-47] Loss of selective K^+ channels is associated with the swelling of astrocyte end-feet.[48-51] Swelling of the cellular compartments contributes to the "no-reflow" phenomenon.[52] There is evidence that loss of the blood-brain barrier and the microvascular ECM result from the actions of bradykinin,[53,54] vascular endothelial growth factor (VEGF),[55,56] thrombin,[44,54] active matrix metalloproteinases (MMPs),[57] proteases released by activated leukocytes,[58-61] and other protease activities.[62] Blockade of bradykinin receptors has been associated with reduced injury and edema formation.[63] Thrombin can increase edema formation through direct action on the cerebral microvascular endothelium.[54,64,65] VEGF disrupts the interendothelial cell tight junctions, which involve the gap junction complex containing connexin 43.[66]

The second functional microvascular barrier is the basal lamina, which prevents leakage of blood elements into the surrounding brain tissue. A gradual local decrease in the expression of the major vascular matrix components laminin-1 and laminin-5, collagen IV, and fibronectin (of cellular origin) is initiated by MCAO.[28,67] Hamann and associates[67] found a significant association between regional loss of microvascular matrix and the extravascular accumulation of hemoglobin (hemorrhagic transformation) within the regions of ischemic injury. The loss of microvascular ECM is also associated with the loss of endothelial cell reactivity during focal ischemia. Endothelial cell P-selectin and E-selectin and expression of β_1-integrin within the ischemic territory occur only on those microvessels with an intact basal lamina.[31,68]

Separate studies suggest that β_1 integrins, through their participation in cell matrix adherence, may play a role in preventing transudation and edema formation in conjunction with other contributors to the intact blood-brain barrier and might be disturbed during ischemia by action of cytokines locally generated by microglia and astrocytes.[69-71] How the loss of vascular integrins and of their matrix ligands in cerebral vessels are interconnected is unclear.

Focal Cerebral Ischemia and Proteolysis of the Microvascular Matrix

Alterations in the expression of the microvascular ECM can be explained by local proteolysis or conformational changes. Attention has focused on the expression and activity of MMPs and plasminogen activators (PAs) after experimental MCAO.[57,62,72-74] Loss of the basal lamina matrix in the primate ischemic striatum follows rapid increase in the regional expression of pro-matrix metalloproteinase-2 (pro-MMP-2), urokinase-type plasminogen activator (u-PA), and plasminogen activator inhibitor 1 (PAI-1).[57,62,72,74] Pro-MMP-2 is generated rapidly by the microvasculature, and by nonvascular cells during ischemia.[57,62,75-80] In the primate, increased pro-MMP-9 expression within the ischemic tissue is associated with hemorrhagic transfor-

mation.[57] Rosenberg and associates[80-82] have described a temporal correlation between pro-MMP-9 "activity" and edema formation in rat strains after MCAO. In contrast, in the nonhuman primate, early extravasation of plasma constituents coincides with expression of pro-MMP-2, u-PA, and PAI-1, but not of pro-MMP-9, by the cerebral microvasculature in the ischemic core.[57,62] Although it has been hypothesized that members of the PA and MMP families can contribute to matrix degradation, proof of pro-MMP activation is not available, and the manner of protease compartmentalization is not yet defined. Rosenberg and associates[72,80] have shown that MMP-2 antigen rests in select astrocytes around microvessels in the ischemic rat brain.

Significant alterations in the plasminogen activator axis have also been defined.[62] In rodent species, alterations in u-PA, PAI-1, and t-PA have been reported.[72,73] In the primate striatum, the very rapid increase in u-PA and PAI-1, and the early regional increase in t-PA·PAI-1 complex with a transient decrease in free t-PA, are consistent findings matching the rapid changes in other gene products in the microvasculature.[55,62] Secretion of u-PA has been attributed to stimulated endothelial cells, astrocytes, neurons, and microglia in vivo or in vitro,[83-88] and PAI-1 can be generated by endothelial cells, astrocytes, and neurons.[83-87,89-91] The differential upregulation of u-PA and PAI-1 in the ischemic parenchyma can be explained by stimulation by tumor necrosis factor-α (TNF-α), tumor growth factor-β (TGF-β), or interleukin-1β (1L-1β), none of which promotes endothelial cell t-PA synthesis or secretion.[84,87,92] The increase in PAI-1 in both plasma and tissue after ischemia is consistent with an endothelial cell source.[62]

Together, these observations suggest that proteases that could contribute to vascular and parenchymal matrix degradation are generated shortly after MCAO in the striatum and that microvascular cells are a likely local source of pro-MMP-2, u-PA, and PAI-1. Because protease generation may contribute to loss of cerebral microvessel integrity, strategies designed to protect basal lamina structures may be of benefit. Currently, there is interest in the possibility that inhibitors of matrix-degrading Zn^{+2} metalloproteases may provide a reduction in consequences of ischemic injury to the microvascular cells, including total hemorrhage.[93] However, this assertion has received only limited testing. Unresolved issues include the possible intersection of members of several protease families, the relative specificities of protease family inhibitors, and the impact of active proteases on hemostasis and intravascular cell interactions.

Focal Cerebral Ischemia and Microvessel Cell Adhesion

Cell adhesion receptors link the abluminal side of the endothelium and astrocyte end-feet with the basal lamina. Immunoreactivity of endothelial cell and astrocyte integrin $\alpha_1\beta_1$ and astrocyte integrin $\alpha_6\beta_4$ rapidly decreases after MCAO in the regions of neuron injury. Within the ischemic core, microvessel-related integrin $\alpha_1\beta_1$ expression has been found to decrease to 20% of baseline, also implying continued endothelial cell synthesis of integrin $\alpha_1\beta_1$ antigen on select microvessels.[31] The rapid fall and plateau of integrin expression could reflect injury to both endothelial cells and astrocytes initiated by ischemia, alterations of the matrix by processes involving microvessel endothelium or astrocytes with secondary changes in integrin expression, or both. Downregulation of β_1 integrin subunit expression in microvessels is in part due to shutdown of its transcription.[31] In the ischemic core, these changes are reflected topographically as multiple subregions of increased microvessel-associated integrin β_1 messenger RNA (mRNA) surrounding islands devoid of vascular integrin β_1 mRNA.[31] The β_1 subunit transcripts appear prominently over noncapillary microvessels. Importantly, the dynamic nature of microvessel integrin β_1 responses confirms the presence of viable microvascular endothelial cells within the ischemic core.

These changes suggest that despite widespread loss of integrin immunoreactivity, injury is not yet complete by 2 hours, in contrast to the commonly held view that striatal injury after MCAO is rapidly complete and irreversible. Furthermore, the spatial distribution of altered microvessel integrin expression is not homogeneous.[30,31,55] The early changes in microvessel expression of integrin β_1 and integrin $\alpha_6\beta_4$ appear heterogeneously interspersed among microvessels displaying apparently normal expression of these integrins.[30,31] Those observations as well as separate observations (see below) of microvessel integrin $\alpha_v\beta_3$ expression indicate that the early tissue injury within the ischemic core, where neuron injury is observed, is not homogeneous. Therefore, microvessels with apparently normal features may persist long after ischemia has been initiated, even in the most vulnerable territory.

THE FOCAL NO-REFLOW PHENOMENON AND SECONDARY INJURY

Experimental occlusion of a proximal cerebral artery significantly reduces the patency of the distal microvascular bed, initiating the focal no-reflow phenomenon.[94–96] This finding accords with regions of territorial vascular compromise after transient MCAO as demonstrated by carbon tracer techniques.[94–97] Although attributed to extrinsic compression from edema, endothelial cell swelling, and endothelial microvillus formation,[98] intravascular obstruction also occurs with the local activation of platelets, leukocytes, and coagulation (fibrin).[94] A differential effect on flow or patency appears between cortical regions and the basal ganglia, subject to ischemia.[99] Garcia and coworkers[100] emphasize that swelling of astrocytes after ischemia may contribute to secondary neuronal death, although the time delays suggest that the relation must be complex. Others have theorized that reactive astrocytes might contribute to impairment of microvessel perfusion in rodents, but technical issues have not been resolved.[101,102] It has been proposed that expansion of the regions of no-reflow by secondary injury recruits the peripheral zones into the ischemic core.[31]

Initiation of Cellular Inflammation

After ischemia, the microvasculature is a staging platform for the secondary injury processes associated with cellular inflammation. The interface between the vascular wall and the plasma compartment is significantly and swiftly altered by ischemia, which promotes microvascular obstruction by leukocyte (and platelet) activation and adhesion. Endothelial cell leukocyte adhesion receptors respond to focal ischemia in a rapid and orderly way. Transmigration of polymorphonuclear (PMN) leukocytes from microvessels in the ischemic core occurs as early as 1 hour after MCAO.[55] The appearance of P-selectin, intercellular adhesion molecule 1 (ICAM-1), and E-selectin on microvessel endothelium, together with their counter-receptors (e.g., P-selectin ligand glycoprotein-1 [PSGL-1], the β_2-integrin CD18) on PMN leukocytes, accompanies the initial movement of inflammatory cells into the ischemic region.[68,103,104] Observations in rodent models of focal cerebral ischemia have confirmed the appearance of leukocyte adhesion receptors on microvessels, but the details vary.[105,106]

The pro-inflammatory cytokines TNF-α and IL-1β are expressed in ischemic brain and influence microvascular responses to focal ischemia.[107–109] The leukocyte adhesion receptors P-selectin, ICAM-1, and E-selectin are stimulated by either TNF-α or IL-1β.[110,111] In rodent models, evidence of IL-1 and TNF-α transcription is seen by 6 hours after MCAO.[109] The actions of these cytokines can be pleiotropic, contributing to leukocyte adherence and transmigration, secondary injury, and protective processes.[107–109] For instance, although TNF binding protein (TNF-bp) or neutralizing antibodies to TNF-α can reduce injury in rodent models of focal ischemia,[112,113] TNF-α has been shown to contribute to ischemic tolerance in similar rodent models.[114,115] Whether the microvascular responses to these cytokines contribute to both their beneficial and injurious properties in the CNS is unclear at this time.

PMN leukocyte adhesion requires the interaction of leukocyte β_2-integrins (CD18) with the endothelial cell receptor ICAM-1 in the CNS as elsewhere.[103,104] Platelet-leukocyte interactions are mediated by platelet P-selectin—PMN leukocyte PSGL-1 binding, whereas platelet-fibrin binding requires the integrin $\alpha_{IIb}\beta_3$ on activated platelets.[116,117] The activation of PMN leukocytes may contribute to the focal no-reflow phenomenon.[94] Activated platelets begin to accumulate within the microvasculature of the ischemic territory within hours of MCAO.[103] Interference with either interaction by specific interventions against the β_2-integrin CD18 or integrin $\alpha_{IIb}\beta_3$ before reperfusion significantly increases residual microvessel patency (decreases focal no-reflow).[104,118] Separate work with knockout preparations and specific inhibitors has demonstrated that inhibition of the platelet-fibrin interactions can reduce microvessel obstruction and decrease tissue injury.[119,120] Monocytoid cells and lymphocytes also adhere and transmigrate,[121–123] processes that also require receptor activation. These interactions contribute to (1) loss of microvessel patency[94] and (2) proteolysis of the basal lamina matrix proteins.[98]

Fibrin Formation and Deposition

Activated platelets and fibrin(ogen) contribute to microvascular obstructions in both capillary and noncapillary sectors of the ischemic bed.[44,94,103,124] Fibrin is deposited in a growing proportion of microvessels with time after MCAO.[44,125] The accumulation of fibrin in the vascular lumen implies the intravascular generation of thrombin.[44] Tissue factor (TF), which is present preferentially in perivascular gray matter,[124] catalyzes fibrin formation when plasma fibrinogen is expressed to the TF that resides around noncapillary microvessels.[124,126,127] Blockade of the TF–factor VIIa complex significantly reduces fibrin deposition within the microvessel lumen and modestly increases microvessel patency.[44] Luminal fibrin implies locally increased permeability of the ischemic microvasculature.[44,128–130] Heparin has also been shown to improve outcome after experimental stroke; the underlying mechanisms may vary and may include increased intravascular patency.[131,132]

ANGIOGENESIS

The formation of new microvessels from existing vessels (*angiogenesis*) is a hallmark tissue response to injury.[133–136] The general observation is that immediately after MCAO, the cerebral microvasculature provides a scaffold for receptors and their ligands known to promote angiogenesis in other biological systems. New conduits are not formed immediately after MCAO,[2,4,5] but new capillaries begin to appear within the ischemic bed by 7 days after MCAO.[137,138]

It has been proposed that angiogenesis results from local hypoxia, leading to inhibition of degradation of hypoxia-inducible factor-1 (HIF-1) and its sustained expression, thereby stimulating expression of VEGF and integrin $\alpha_v\beta_3$.[139] VEGF promotes microvessel proliferation, which requires the expression of the two endothelial cell receptors flt-1 and flk/KDR.[140–142] Their interaction results in endothelial cell expression of integrin $\alpha_v\beta_3$. Integrin $\alpha_v\beta_3$ is necessary for angiogenesis, neovascularization in organ development, and tissue remodeling.[143,144] Endothelial cell migration and proliferation are stimulated by VEGF via the receptor flk-1,[140] but only smooth muscle cell (SMC) migration responds to VEGF.[145,146] After MCAO, all of these elements are set in motion.

Activation of cerebral microvessel cells in precapillary arterioles occurs within 1 to 2 hours of MCAO within the ischemic territory of the primate basal ganglia.[55] Okada and colleagues[147] first demonstrated the differential upregulation of angiogenesis-related elements, including integrin $\alpha_v\beta_3$ but not integrin $\alpha_v\beta_5$, on microvessels within the ischemic territory immediately after MCAO.[147] Integrin $\alpha_v\beta_3$ expression on cerebral microvessels has been found to be significantly and continuously associated with the intravascular deposition of fibrin.[147] Abumiya and co-workers[55] demonstrated highly significant co-expression of VEGF, proliferating cell nuclear antigen (PCNA), and integrin $\alpha_v\beta_3$ in microvessels consistent with pre-capillary arterioles immediately after MCAO. Other nonvascular sources of VEGF transcripts are leukocytes and microglia.[55] Kovacs and associates[148] and Hayashi and colleagues[149] described the appearance of VEGF on endothelial cells, neurons, and glial cells after MCAO in rodent models.

Another group of investigators demonstrated that hypoxia-induced VEGF expression precedes neovascularization in the borderzone of the ischemic neocortex in the rodent.[150] VEGF expression has also been found to increase in both microvessels and neurons by 24 hours, most prominently in the peri-infarct regions. Under those conditions, flt-1 increased in endothelial cells, neurons, and glial cells, and flk/KDR appeared in glial cells and endothelial cells.[151] Those findings indicate that the specific receptors for VEGF are expressed in concert with the ligand VEGF. A similar relationship of microvessel VEGF and integrin α_v to HIF-1α transcription has also been noted (T. Abumiya and G. J. del Zoppo, unpublished observations, 1999).

Other receptors associated with vasculogenesis appear in response to focal ischemia. Both angiopoietin-1 (ang-1) and ang-2 appear in endothelial cell vascular elements in the ischemic territory with some delay after MCAO in the rodent.[152,153] Similarly, the tyrosine kinase receptors tie-1 and tie-2 are expressed in the ischemic cortex, with tie-2 appearing on capillary-like structures in the outer cortical layers, and tie-1 detected in layers II through IV.[154] Although angiogenesis-neovascularization appears to be stimulated by hypoxia, proof of the entire process and how it affects microvessel integrity, neovascularization, and outcome after focal cerebral ischemia is still lacking.

AMYLOID DEPOSITION AND LIPOHYALINOSIS

Infiltration of cerebral microvessels can result from local insults, with resultant impairment of structural and functional integrity. Remodeling of vascular wall components may be a consequence.[155]

Amyloid precursor protein (APP) can accumulate within the cerebral vessel wall. APP mRNA has been detected in vascular endothelial cells, smooth muscle cells, and adventitial cells, and in cerebral vessels also in pericytes and perivascular cells.[156] Focal ischemia alters APP deposition in cerebral vessels. Cells that survive a focal ischemic insult or global cerebral hypoperfusion display an increased accumulation of APP.[157–159] The regional distribution of APP accumulation and its correlation with the level of cerebral blood flow reduction during cerebral ischemia have suggested the hypothesis that APP can contribute to selective neuronal vulnerability to ischemia.[160,161] APP has been shown to accumulate in the temporal neocortex, which is known to be sensitive to ischemia. However, APP has also been known to accumulate in the more resistant white matter tracts.[162,163] The ages of rodents undergoing reversible focal cerebral ischemia influence the accumulation of APP, particularly in microglial cells. Accumulation in astrocytes is greater in older rodents.[164] The vesicular deposition of APP during ischemia is characterized by an increase in its Kunitz protease inhibitor–bearing isoform (KPI-APP) but a decrease in APP.[6,89] The shift between the different RNA isoforms might explain neurodegenerative processes resulting from cerebral ischemia.[165]

Work in transgenic models has demonstrated that mice overexpressing APP have profound impairment in the endothelium-dependent cerebrovascular responses. These changes can be reproduced by infusion of APPβ-derived peptides Aβ 1-40, but not Aβ 1-42 in normal mice.[166] Therefore, the isoform Aβ 1-40 may contribute to functional impairment of cerebral vessels. Those animals overexpressing APP are also prone to development of severe ischemic lesions.[167] Reduced endothelium-dependent relaxation is thought to be an explanation for the greater

Pathophysiology

susceptibility of this murine line to ischemia. Mice over-expressing APP are more likely to have spontaneous hemorrhagic stroke, mimicking the findings in human cerebral amyloid angiopathy.[168] Clinical risk factors for the development of bleeding complications include advanced age, signs of severe microangiopathy (lacunar strokes, confluent white matter lesions), severe hypertension, diabetes mellitus, and vasculitides. Deposition of amyloid in the vessel wall (amyloid angiopathy) also leads to loss of vascular wall integrity, leakage, and later hemorrhagic changes.[169]

Lipohyalinosis or fibrinoid microangiopathy associated with hypertension has been classified in the following three states of severity: (1) sclerotic and hyalinotic thickening of the vessel wall which primarily affects arterioles 100 to 200 μm diameter, (2) disorganization of the vessel wall and disruption of the internal elastic lamina with occasional foam cell infiltration, and (3) fibrinoid degeneration of the vessel wall with thrombosis.[170] Most experimental models of focal cerebral ischemia do not mimic these age-dependent vascular disturbances, a lack that may also explain the rare occurrence of large hemorrhages in focal ischemia models compared with the frequency in humans. However, prolonged periods of ischemia or extended reperfusion can contribute to microvessel damage.

SUMMARY

Cerebral microvessels not only serve as conduits of blood but also respond dynamically to focal ischemia, initiating mechanisms important for cellular inflammation, secondary injury events, and potentially for vascular and tissue remodeling. The microvasculature is both a target and a platform for the interrelated processes ischemia, thrombosis, and inflammation.[98] All three processes stimulate protease secretion and activity. Consequences of their actions appear to be (1) loss of the primary blood-brain barrier, (2) alterations and degradation of the microvascular matrix (basal lamina), the second barrier, (3) microvascular hemorrhage, (4) edema formation, and (5) secondary alterations in the neuropil. Immediately after thrombotic occlusion of the arterial supply, integrins important for matrix adhesion of endothelial cells and astrocyte end-feet are lost, leukocyte adhesion receptors on endothelial cells of select vessels appear, leukocytes adhere and emigrate, and fibrin deposits and activated platelets accumulate within select microvessels. Activation of precapillary arterioles is accompanied by the expression of VEGF and integrin $\alpha_v\beta_3$, which are involved in angiogenesis. In the early moments after MCAO, these microvessel-dependent events occur together in a heterogeneous fashion adjacent to apparently normal microvessels throughout the ischemic region.

References

1. Peters A, Palay BL, Webster HD: The Fine Structure of the Nervous System: Neurons and Their Supporting Cells, 3rd ed. New York, Oxford University Press, 1991, pp 352–353.
2. Keyeux A, Ochrymowicz-Bemelmans D, Charlier AA: Induced response to hypercapnia in the two-compartment total cerebral blood volume: Influence on brain vascular reserve and flow efficiency. J Cereb Blood Flow Metab 15:1121–1131, 1995.
3. Weeks JB, Todd MM, Warner DS, Katz J: The influence of halothane, isoflurane, and pentobarbital on cerebral plasma volume in hypocapnic and normocapnic rats. Anesthesiology 73:461–466, 1990.
4. Pinard E, Engrand N, Seylaz J: Dynamic cerebral microcirculatory changes in transient forebrain ischemia in rats: Involvement of type I nitric oxide synthase. J Cereb Blood Flow Metab 20:1648–1658, 2000.
5. Seylaz J, Charbonne R, Nari K, et al: Dynamic in vivo measurement of erythrocyte velocity and flow in capillaries and of microvessel diameter in the rat brain by confocal laser microscopy. J Cereb Blood Flow Metab 19:863–870, 1999.
6. Janzer RC, Raff MC: Astrocytes induce blood-brain barrier properties in endothelial cells [letter]. Nature 325:353–355, 1987.
7. Bernstein JJ, Getz R, Jefferson M, Kelemen M: Astrocytes secrete basal lamina after hemisection of rat spinal cord. Brain Res 327:135–141, 1985.
8. Nagano N, Aoyagi M, Hirakawa K: Extracellular matrix modulates the proliferation of rat astrocytes in serum-free culture. GLIA 8:71–76, 1993.
9. Tagami M, Yamagata K, Fujino H, et al: Morphological differentiation of endothelial cells co-cultured with astrocytes on type-I or type-IV collagen. Cell Tissue Res 268:225–232, 1992.
10. Webersinke G, Bauer H, Amberger A, et al: Comparison of gene expression of extracellular matrix molecules in brain microvascular endothelial cells and astrocytes. Biochem Biophys Res Commun 189:877–884, 1992.
11. Kusaka H, Hirano A, Bornstein MB, Raine CS: Basal lamina formation by astrocytes in organotypic cultures of mouse spinal cord tissue. J Neuropathol Exp Neurol 44:295–303, 1985.
12. Spatz M, Bacic F, McCarron RM, et al: Human cerebromicrovascular endothelium: Studies in vitro. J Cereb Blood Flow Metab 9(Suppl):S393, 1989.
13. Spatz M, Micic D, Mrsulja BB, Klatzo I: Cerebral microvessels as mediators of cerebral transport. Adv Neurol 20:189–196, 1978.
14. Micic D, Swink M, Micic J, et al: The ischemic and postischemic effect on the uptake of neutral amino acids in isolated cerebral capillaries. Experientia 15:625–626, 1993.
15. McCarron RM, Merkel N, Bembry J, Spatz M: Cerebrovascular endothelium in vitro: Studies related to blood-brain barrier function. Proceedings of the eleventh International Congress of Neuropathy June (Suppl 4):785–787, 1991.
16. Honkanen RA, McBath H, Kushmerick C, et al: Barbiturates inhibit hexose transport in cultured mammalian cells and human erythrocytes and interact directly with purified GLUT-1. Biochemistry 34:535–544, 1995.
17. Tran ND, Schreiber SS, Fisher M: Astrocyte regulation of endothelial tissue plasminogen activator in a blood-brain barrier model. J Cereb Blood Flow Metab 18:1316–1324, 1998.
18. Wang L, Tran ND, Kittaka M, et al: Thrombomodulin expression in bovine brain capillaries: Anticoagulant function of the blood-brain barrier, regional differences, and regulatory mechanisms. Arterioscler Thromb Vasc Biol 17:3139–3146, 1997.
19. Minakawa T, Bready J, Berliner J, et al: In vitro interaction of astrocytes and pericytes with capillary-like structures of brain microvessel endothelium. Lab Invest 65:32–40, 1991.
20. Zonta M, Angulo M, Gobbo S, et al: Neuron-to-astrocyte signalling is central to the dynamic control of brain microcirculation. Nat Neurosci 6:43–50, 2003.
21. Hurwitz AA, Berman JW, Rashbaum WK, Lyman WD: Human fetal astrocytes induce the expression of blood-brain barrier specific proteins by autologous endothelial cells. Brain Res 625:238–243, 1993.
22. Risau W, Wolburg H: Development of the blood-brain barrier. Trends Neurosci 13:174–178, 1990.
23. Risau W, Hallmann R, Albrecht U, Henke-Fahle S: Brain astrocytes induce the expression of an early cell surface marker for blood-brain barrier specific endothelium. EMBO J 5:3179–3183, 1986.
24. Risau W, Esser S, Engelhardt B: Differentiation of blood-brain barrier endothelial cells. Pathol Biol 46:171–175, 1998.
25. Schlosshauer B, Herzog KH: Neurothelin: An inducible cell surface glycoprotein of blood-brain barrier specific endothelial cells and distinct neurons. J Cell Biol 110:1261–1274, 1990.
26. Lobrinus JA, Juillerat-Jeanneret L, Darekar P, et al: Induction of the blood-brain barrier specific HT7 and neurothelin epitopes in endothelial cells of the chick chorioallantoic vessels by a soluble factor derived from astrocytes. Brain Res Dev Brain Res 70:207–211, 1992.

27. Estrada C, Bready JV, Berliner JA, et al: Astrocyte growth stimulation by a soluble factor produced by cerebral endothelial cells in vitro. J Neuropathol Exp Neurol 49:539–549, 1990.

28. Hamann GF, Okada Y, Fitridge R, del Zoppo GJ: Microvascular basal lamina antigens disappear during cerebral ischemia and reperfusion. Stroke 26:2120–2126, 1995.

29. Haring H-P, Akamine P, Habermann R, et al: Distribution of the integrin-like immunoreactivity on primate brain microvasculature. J Neuropathol Exp Neurol 55:236–245, 1996.

30. Wagner S, Tagaya M, Koziol JA, et al: Rapid disruption of an astrocyte interaction with the extracellular matrix mediated by integrin $\alpha_6\beta_4$ during focal cerebral ischemia/reperfusion. Stroke 28:858–865, 1997.

31. Tagaya M, Haring H-P, Stuiver I, et al: Rapid loss of microvascular integrin expression during focal brain ischemia reflects neuron injury. J Cereb Blood Flow Metab 21:835–846, 2001.

32. Hamann GF, Liebetrau M, Martens H, et al: Microvascular basal lamina injury after experimental focal cerebral ischemia and reperfusion in the rat. J Cereb Blood Flow Metab 22:526–533, 2002.

33. Kozlova M, Kentroti S, Vernadakis A: Influence of culture substrata on the differentiation of advanced passage glial cells in cultures from aged mouse cerebral hemispheres. Int J Dev Neurosci 11:513–519, 1993.

34. Kramer RH, Cheng Y-F, Clyman R: Human microvascular endothelial cells use β_1 and β_3 integrin receptor complexes to attach to laminin. J Cell Biol 111:1233–1243, 1990.

35. Paulus W, Baur I, Schuppan D, Roggendorf W: Characterization of integrin receptors in normal and neoplastic human brain. Am J Pathol 143:154–163, 1993.

36. Gehlsen KR, Klier FG, Dickerson K, et al: Localization of the binding site for a cell adhesion receptor in laminin. J Biol Chem 264:19034–19038, 1989.

37. Korhonen M, Ylanne J, Laitinen L, Virtanen I: The alpha 1 and alpha 6 subunits of integrins are characteristically expressed in distinct segments of developing and adult human nephron. J Cell Biol 111:1245–1254, 1990.

38. Dietrich W: Neurobiology of stroke. Int Rev Neurobiol 42:55–101, 1998.

39. Dirnagl U, Iadecola C, Moskowitz M: Pathobiology of ischaemic stroke: An integrated view. Trends Neurosci 22:391–397, 1999.

40. Naganuma Y: Changes of the cerebral microvascular structure and endothelium during the course of permanent ischemia. Keio J Med 39:26–31, 1990.

41. Dietrich WD, Busto R, Ginsberg MD: Cerebral endothelial microvilli: Formation following global forebrain ischemia. J Neuropathol Exp Neurol 43:72–83, 1984.

42. Okumura Y, Sakaki T, Hiramatsu K, et al: Microvascular changes associated with postischaemic hypoperfusion in rats. Acta Neurochir (Wien) 139:670–676, 1997.

43. Garcia JH, Lowry SL, Briggs L, et al: Brain capillaries expand and rupture in areas of ischemia and reperfusion. In Reivich M, Hurtig HI (eds): Cerebrovascular Diseases. Raven Press, New York, 1983, pp 169–182.

44. Okada Y, Copeland BR, Fitridge R, et al: Fibrin contributes to microvascular obstructions and parenchymal changes during early focal cerebral ischemia and reperfusion. Stroke 25:1847–1854, 1994.

45. Olesen S-P: Rapid increase in blood-brain barrier permeability during severe hypoxia and metabolic inhibition. Brain Res 368:24–29, 1986.

46. Gotoh O, Asano T, Koide T, Takakura K: Ischemic brain edema following occlusion of the middle cerebral artery in the rat. I: The time courses of the brain water, sodium and potassium content and blood-brain barrier permeability to ^{125}I-albumin. Stroke 16:101–109, 1985.

47. Dietrich WD, Alonso O, Busto R: Moderate hyperglycemia worsens acute blood-brain barrier injury after forebrain ischemia in rats. Stroke 24:111–116, 1993.

48. Petito CK, Babiak T: Early proliferative changes in astrocytes in postischemic noninfarcted rat brain. Ann Neurol 11:510–518, 1982.

49. Maxwell K, Berliner JA, Cancilla PA: Stimulation of glucose analogue uptake by cerebral microvessel endothelial cells by a product released by astrocytes. J Neuropathol Exp Neurol 48:69–80, 1989.

50. Chan PH, Chu L: Mechanisms underlying glutamate-induced swelling of astrocytes in primary culture. Acta Neurochir Suppl 51:7–10, 1990.

51. Bender AS, Norenberg MD: Calcium dependence of hypoosmotically induced potassium release in cultured astrocytes. J Neurosci 14:4237–4243, 1994.

52. Ames A, Wright LW, Kowada M, et al: Cerebral ischemia. II: The no-reflow phenomenon. Am J Pathol 52:437–453, 1968.

53. Kamiya T, Katayama Y, Kashiwagi F, Terashi A: The role of bradykinin in mediating ischemic brain edema in rats. Stroke 24:571–575, 1993.

54. Aschner JL, Lum H, Fletcher PW, Malik AB: Bradykinin- and thrombin-induced increases in endothelial permeability occur independently of phospholipase C but require protein kinase C activation. J Cell Physiol 173:387–396, 1997.

55. Abumiya T, Lucero J, Heo JH, et al: Activated microvessels express vascular endothelial growth factor and integrin $\alpha_v\beta_3$ during focal cerebral ischemia. J Cereb Blood Flow Metab 19:1038–1050, 1999.

56. Zhang ZG, Zhang L, Jiang Q, et al: VEGF enhances angiogenesis and promotes blood-brain barrier leakage in the ischemic brain. J Clin Invest 106:829–838, 2000.

57. Heo JH, Lucero J, Abumiya T, et al: Matrix metalloproteinases increase very early during experimental focal cerebral ischemia. J Cereb Blood Flow Metab 19:624–633, 1999.

58. Garcia JH, Liu KF, Yoshida Y, et al: Influx of leukocytes and platelets in an evolving brain infarct (Wistar rat). Am J Pathol 144:188–199, 1994.

59. Armao D, Kornfeld M, Estrada EY, et al: Neutral proteases and disruption of the blood-brain barrier in rat. Brain Res 767:259–264, 1997.

60. Opdenakker G, Van den Steen PE, Dubois B, et al: Gelatinase B functions as regulator and effector in leukocyte biology. J Leuk Biol 69:851–859, 2001.

61. Hasty KA, Pourmotabbed TF, Goldberg GI, et al: Human neutrophil collagenase: A distinct gene product with homology to other matrix metalloproteinases. J Biol Chem 265:11421–11424, 1990.

62. Hosomi N, Lucero J, Heo JH, et al: Rapid differential endogenous plasminogen activator expression after acute middle cerebral artery occlusion. Stroke 32:1341–1348, 2001.

63. Relton JK, Beckey VE, Hanson WL, Whalley ET: CP-0597, a selective bradykinin β_2 receptor antagonist, inhibits brain injury in a rat model of reversible middle cerebral artery occlusion. Stroke 28:1430–1436, 1997.

64. Lee KR, Kawai N, Kim S, et al: Mechanisms of edema formation after intracerebral hemorrhage: Effects of thrombin on cerebral blood flow, blood-brain barrier permeability, and cell survival in a rat model. J Neurosurg 86:272–278, 1997.

65. Kubo Y, Suzuki M, Kudo A, et al: Thrombin inhibitor ameliorates secondary damage in rat brain injury: Suppression of inflammatory cells and vimentin-positive astrocytes. J Neurotrauma 2:163–172, 2000.

66. Suarez S, Ballmer-Hofer K: VEGF transiently disrupts gap junctional communication in endothelial cells. J Cell Sci 114:1229–1235, 2001.

67. Hamann GF, Okada Y, del Zoppo GJ: Hemorrhagic transformation and microvascular integrity during focal cerebral ischemia/reperfusion. J Cereb Blood Flow Metab 16:1373–1378, 1996.

68. Haring H-P, Berg EL, Tsurushita N, et al: E-selectin appears in nonischemic tissue during experimental focal cerebral ischemia. Stroke 27:1386–1392, 1996.

69. Liu T, McDonnell PC, Young PR, et al: Interleukin-1β mRNA expression in ischemic rat cortex. Stroke 24:1746–1751, 1993.

70. Buttini M, Appel K, Sauter A, et al: Expression of tumor necrosis factor alpha after focal cerebral ischaemia in the rat. Neuroscience 71:1–16, 1996.

71. Loddick SA, Rothwell NJ: Neuroprotective effects of human recombinant interleukin-1 receptor antagonist in focal cerebral ischaemia in the rat. J Cereb Blood Flow Metab 16:932–940, 1996.

72. Rosenberg GA, Navratil M, Barone F, Feuerstein G: Proteolytic cascade enzymes increase in focal cerebral ischemia in rat. J Cereb Blood Flow Metab 16:360–366, 1996.

73. Ahn MY, Zhang ZG, Tsang W, Chopp M: Endogenous plasminogen activator expression after embolic focal cerebral ischemia in mice. Brain Res 837:169–176, 1999.

74. Rosenberg GA: Matrix metalloproteinases in neuroinflammation. GLIA 39:279–291, 2002.

75. Norton WT, Cammer W, Bloom BR, Gordon S: Neutral proteinases secreted by macrophages degrade basic protein: A possible mecha-

Pathophysiology

nism of inflammatory demyelination. Adv Exp Med Biol 100:365–381, 1978.

76. Mackay AR, Corbitt RH, Hartzler JL, Thorgeirsson UP: Basement membrane type IV collagen degradation: Evidence for the involvement of a proteolytic cascade independent of metalloproteinases. Cancer Res 50:5997–6001, 1990.

77. McGuire PG, Seeds NW: The interaction of plasminogen activator with a reconstituted basement membrane matrix and extracellular macromolecules produced by cultured epithelial cells. J Cell Biochem 40:215–227, 1989.

78. Saksela O, Rifkin DB: Cell-associated plasminogen activation: Regulation and physiological functions. Annu Rev Cell Dev Biol 4:93–126, 1988.

79. Vassalli JD, Sappino AP, Belin D: The plasminogen activator/plasmin system. J Clin Invest 88:1067–1072, 1991.

80. Rosenberg GA, Cunningham LA, Wallace J, et al: Immunohistochemistry of matrix metalloproteinases in reperfusion injury to rat brain: Activation of MMP-9 linked to stromelysin-1 and microglia in cell cultures. Brain Res 893:104–112, 2001.

81. Rosenberg GA, Dencoff JE, McGuire PG, et al: Injury-induced 92-kilodalton gelatinase and urokinase expression in rat brain. Lab Invest 71:417–422, 1994.

82. Rosenberg GA, Navratil M: Metalloproteinase inhibition blocks edema in intracerebral hemorrhage in the rat. Neurology 48:921–926, 1997.

83. Nakajima K, Tsuzaki N, Shimojo M, et al: Microglia isolated from rat brain secrete a urokinase-type plasminogen activator. Brain Res 577:285–292, 1992.

84. van Hinsbergh VW, van den Berg EA, Fiers W, Dooijewaard G: Tumor necrosis factor induces the production of urokinase-type plasminogen activator by human endothelial cells. Blood 75:1991–1998, 1990.

85. Masos T, Miskin R: Localization of urokinase-type plasminogen activator mRNA in the adult mouse brain. Brain Res Mol Brain Res 35:139–148, 1996.

86. Tranque P, Naftolin F, Robbins R: Differential regulation of astrocyte plasminogen activators by insulin-like growth factor-I and epidermal growth factor. Endocrinology 134:2606–2613, 1994.

87. Schleef RR, Bevilacqua MP, Sawdey M, et al: Cytokine activation of vascular endothelium: Effects on tissue-type plasminogen activator and type 1 plasminogen activator inhibitor. J Biol Chem 263:5797–5803, 1988.

88. Vivien D, Buisson A: Serine protease inhibitors: Novel therapeutic targets for stroke? J Cereb Blood Flow Metab 20:755–764, 2000.

89. Vincent VA, Lowik CW, Verheijen JH, et al: Role of astrocyte-derived tissue-type plasminogen activator in the regulation of endotoxin-stimulated nitric oxide production by microglial cells. GLIA 22:130–137, 1998.

90. Patterson PH: On the role of proteases, their inhibitors and the extracellular matrix in promoting neurite outgrowth. J Physiol (Paris) 80:207–211, 1985.

91. Levin EG, del Zoppo GJ: Localization of tissue plasminogen activator in the endothelium of a limited number of vessels. Am J Pathol 144:855–861, 1994.

92. Docagne F, Nicole O, Marti H, et al: Transforming growth factor-b1 as a regulator of the serpins/t-PA axis in cerebral ischemia. FASEB J 13:1315–1324, 1999.

93. Rosenberg GA, Kornfeld M, Estrada E, et al: TIMP-2 reduces proteolytic opening of blood-brain barrier by type IV collagenase. Brain Res 576:203–207, 1992.

94. del Zoppo GJ, Schmid-Schönbein GW, Mori E, et al: Polymorphonuclear leukocytes occlude capillaries following middle cerebral artery occlusion and reperfusion in baboons. Stroke 22:1276–1284, 1991.

95. Little JR, Kerr FWL, Sundt TM, Jr: Microcirculatory obstruction in focal cerebral ischemia: Relationship to neuronal alterations. Mayo Clin Proc 50:264–270, 1975.

96. Little JR, Kerr FWL, Sundt TM Jr: Microcirculatory obstruction in focal cerebral ischemia: An electron microscopic investigation in monkeys. Stroke 7:25–30, 1976.

97. Sundt TM Jr, Grant WC, Garcia JH: Restoration of middle cerebral artery flow in experimental infarction. J Neurosurg 31:311–322, 1969.

98. del Zoppo GJ: Microvascular changes during cerebral ischaemia and reperfusion. Cerebrovasc Brain Metab Rev 6:47–96, 1994.

99. Wang CX, Todd KG, Yang Y, et al: Patency of cerebral microvessels after focal embolic stroke in the rat. J Cereb Blood Flow Metab 21:413–421, 2001.

100. Garcia JH, Liu KF, Yoshida Y, et al: Brain microvessels: Factors altering their patency after the occlusion of a middle cerebral artery (Wistar rat). Am J Pathol 145:728–740, 1994.

101. Zhang Z, Bower L, Zhang R, et al: Three-dimensional measurement of cerebral microvascular plasma perfusion, glial fibrillary acidic protein and microtubule associated protein-2 immunoreactivity after embolic stroke in rats: A double fluorescent labeled laser-scanning confocal microscopic study. Brain Res 844:55–66, 1999.

102. Zhang Z, Davies K, Prostak J, et al: Quantitation of microvascular plasma perfusion and neuronal microtubule-associated protein in ischemic mouse brain by laser-scanning confocal microscopy. J Cereb Blood Flow Metab 19:68–78, 1999.

103. Okada Y, Copeland BR, Mori E, et al: P-selectin and intercellular adhesion molecule-1 expression after focal brain ischemia and reperfusion. Stroke 25:202–211, 1994.

104. Mori E, Chambers JD, Copeland BR, et al: Inhibition of polymorphonuclear leukocyte adherence suppresses no-reflow after focal cerebral ischemia. Stroke 23:712–718, 1992.

105. Zhang RL, Chopp M, Li Y, et al: Anti-ICAM-1 antibody reduces ischemic cell damage after transient middle cerebral artery occlusion in the rat. Neurology 44:1747–1751, 1994.

106. Zhang R, Chopp M, Zhang Z, et al: The expression of P- and E-selectins in three models of middle cerebral artery occlusion. Brain Res 785:207–214, 1998.

107. Sirén AL, Heldman E, Doron D, et al: Release of proinflammatory and prothrombotic mediators in the brain and peripheral circulation in spontaneously hypertensive and normotensive Wistar-Kyoto rats. Stroke 23:1643–1651, 1992.

108. Wang X, Barone FC, Aiyar NV, Feuerstein GZ: Increased interleukin-1 receptor and receptor antagonist gene expression after focal stroke. Stroke 28:155–161, 1997.

109. Wang X, Yue T-L, Barone FC, et al: Concomitant cortical expression of TNF-α and IL-1β mRNA following transient focal ischemia. Mol Chem Neuropathol 23:103–114, 1994.

110. Wang X, Siren A-L, Liu Y, et al: Upregulation of intercellular adhesion molecule 1 (ICAM-1) on brain microvascular endothelial cells in rat ischemic cortex. Mol Brain Res 26:61–68, 1994.

111. Wang X, Yue T-L, Barone FC, Feuerstein GZ: Demonstration of increased endothelial-leukocyte adhesion molecule-1 mRNA expression in rat ischemic cortex. Stroke 26:1665–1669, 1995.

112. Dawson DA, Martin D, Hallenbeck JM: Inhibition of tumor necrosis factor-alpha reduces focal cerebral ischemic injury in the spontaneously hypertensive rat. Neurosci Lett 218:41–44, 1996.

113. Nawashiro H, Martin D, Hallenbeck JM: Neuroprotective effects of TNF-binding protein in focal cerebral ischemia. Brain Res 778:265–271, 1997.

114. Nawashiro H, Tasaki K, Ruetzler CA, Hallenbeck JM: TNF-alpha pretreatment induces protective effects against focal cerebral ischemia in mice. J Cereb Blood Flow Metab 17:483–490, 1997.

115. Tasaki K, Ruetzler C, Ohtsuki T, et al: Lipopolysaccharide pretreatment induces resistance against subsequent focal cerebral ischemic damage in spontaneously hypertensive rats. Brain Res 748:267–270, 1997.

116. Shattil SJ: Function and regulation of the beta 3 integrins in hemostasis and vascular biology. Thromb Haemost 74:149–155, 1995.

117. Shattil SJ: Signaling through platelet integrin αIIbβ3: Inside-out, outside-in, and sideways. Thromb Haemost 82:318–325, 1999.

118. Abumiya T, Fitridge R, Mazur C, et al: Integrin αIIbβ3 inhibitor preserves microvascular patency in experimental acute focal cerebral ischemia. Stroke 31:1402–1410, 2000.

119. Walder CE, Green SP, Darbonne WC, et al: Ischemic stroke injury is reduced in mice lacking a functional NADPH oxidate. Stroke 28:2252–2258, 1997.

120. Choudri TF, Hoh BL, Zerwes HG, et al: Reduced microvascular thrombosis and improved outcome in acute murine stroke by inhibiting GP IIb/IIIa receptor-mediated platelet aggregation. J Clin Invest 102:1301–1310, 1998.

121. Becker K, Kindrick D, Relton J, et al: Antibody to the α4 integrin decreases infarct size in transient focal cerebral ischemia in rats. Stroke 32:206–211, 2001.

122. McCarron RM, Racke M, Spatz M, McFarlin DE: Cerebral vascular endothelial cells are effective targets for in vitro lysis by encephalitogenic T lymphocytes. J Immunol 147:503–508, 1991.

Pathophysiology

123. de Jong AL, Green DM, Trial JA, Birdsall HH: Focal effects of mononuclear leukocyte transendothelial migration: TNF-alpha production by migrating monocytes promotes subsequent migration of lymphocytes. J Leukoc Biol 60:129–136, 1996.

124. del Zoppo GJ, Yu J-Q, Copeland BR, et al: Tissue factor location in non-human primate cerebral tissue. Thromb Haemost 68:642–647, 1992.

125. Thomas WS, Mori E, Copeland BR, et al: Tissue factor contributes to microvascular defects following cerebral ischemia. Stroke 24:847–853, 1993.

126. Mackman N, Morrissey JA, Fowler B, Edgington TS: Complete sequence of the human tissue factor gene: A highly regulated cellular receptor that initiates the coagulation protease cascade. Biochemistry 28:1755–1762, 1989.

127. Ruf W, Rehemtulla A, Morrissey JH, Edgington TS: Phospholipid independent and dependent interactions required for tissue factor receptor and cofactor function. J Biol Chem 266:2158–2166, 1990.

128. Mabuchi T, Kitagawa K, Ohtsuki T, et al: Contribution of microglia/macrophages to expansion of infarction and response of oligodendrocytes after focal cerebral ischemia in rats. Stroke 31:1735–1743, 2000.

129. Kitagawa K, Matsumoto M, Ohtsuki T, et al: The characteristics of blood-brain barrier in three different conditions—infarction, selective neuronal death and selective loss of presynaptic terminals—following cerebral ischemia. Acta Neuropathol 84:378–386, 1992.

130. Nordborg C, Sokrab TE, Johansson BB: The relationship between plasma protein extravasation and remote tissue changes after experimental brain infarction. Acta Neuropathol 82:118–126, 1991.

131. Li P, He Q, Siddiqui M, Shuaib A: Posttreatment with low molecular weight heparin reduces brain edema and infarct volume in rats subjected to thrombotic middle cerebral artery occlusion. Brain Res 801:220–223, 1998.

132. Quartermain D, Li Y, Jonas S: Enoxaparin: A low molecular weight heparin decreases infarct size and improves sensorimotor function in a rat model of focal cerebral ischemia. Neurosci Lett 288:155–158, 2000.

133. Hynes RO: A reevaluation of integrins as regulators of angiogenesis. Nat Med 8:918–921, 2002.

134. Carmeliet P: Mechanisms of angiogenesis and arteriogenesis. Nat Med 6:389–395, 2000.

135. Dvorak HF, Brown LF, Detmar M, Dvorak AM: Vascular permeability factor/vascular endothelial growth factor, microvascular hyperpermeability, and angiogenesis. Am J Pathol 146:1029–1039, 1995.

136. Papetti M, Herman IM: Mechanisms of normal and tumor derived angiogenesis. Am J Physiol 282:C947–C970, 2002.

137. Tsutsumi K, Shibata S, Inoue M, Mori K: Experimental cerebral infarction in the dog: Ultrastructural study of microvessels in subacute cerebral infarction. Neurol Med Chir (Tokyo) 27:73–77, 1986.

138. Tsutsumi K: Experimental cerebral infarction in the dog: Scanning electron microscopy with vascular endocasts of the microvessels in the ischemic brain. Neurol Med Chir (Tokyo) 26:595–600, 1986.

139. Namiki A, Brogi E, Kearney M, et al: Hypoxia induces vascular endothelial growth factor in cultured human endothelial cells. J Biol Chem 270:31189–31195, 1995.

140. Nicosia RF, Lin YJ, Hazelton D, Qian X: Endogenous regulation of angiogenesis in the rat aorta model: Role of vascular endothelial growth factor. Am J Pathol 151:1379–1386, 1997.

141. Straume O, Akslen LA: Expression of vascular endothelial growth factor, its receptors (FLT-1, KDR) and TSP-1 related to microvessel density and patient outcome in vertical growth phase melanomas. Am J Pathol 159:223–235, 2001.

142. Chan AS, Leung SY, Wong MP, et al: Expression of vascular endothelial growth factor and its receptors in the anaplastic progression of astrocytoma, oligodendroglioma, and ependymoma. Am J Surg Pathol 22:816–826, 1998.

143. Brooks PC, Montgomery AM, Rosenfeld M, et al: Integrin $\alpha_V\beta_3$ antagonists promote tumor regression by promoting apoptosis of angiogenic blood vessels. Cell 79:1157–1164, 1994.

144. Varner JA, Brooks PC, Cheresh DA: The integrin $\alpha_V\beta_3$: Angiogenesis and apoptosis. Cell Adhes Commun 3:367–374, 1995.

145. Wang Z, Castresana MR, Newman WH: Reactive oxygen and NF-kappaB in VEGF-induced migration of human vascular smooth muscle cells. Biochem Biophys Res Commun 285:669–674, 2001.

146. Grosskreutz CL, Anand-Apte B, Duplaa C, et al: Vascular endothelial growth factor-induced migration of vascular smooth muscle cells in vitro. Microvasc Res 58:128–136, 1999.

147. Okada Y, Copeland BR, Hamann GF, et al: Integrin $\alpha_V\beta_3$ is expressed in selected microvessels following focal cerebral ischemia. Am J Pathol 149:37–44, 1996.

148. Kovacs Z, Ikezaki K, Samoto K, et al: VEGF and flt: Expression time kinetics in rat brain infarct. Stroke 27:1865–1872, 1996.

149. Hayashi T, Abe K, Suzuki H, Itoyama Y: Rapid induction of vascular endothelial growth factor gene expression after transient middle cerebral artery occlusion in rats. Stroke 28:2039–2044, 1997.

150. Marti HJ, Bernaudin M, Bellail A, et al: Hypoxia-induced vascular endothelial growth factor expression precedes neovascularization after cerebral ischemia. Am J Pathol 156:965–976, 2000.

151. Lennmyr F, Ata KA, Funa K, et al: Expression of vascular endothelial growth factor (VEGF) and its receptors (Flt-1 and Flk-1) following permanent and transient occlusion of the middle cerebral artery in the rat. J Neuropathol Exp Neurol 57:874–882, 1998.

152. Beck H, Acker T, Wiessner C, et al: Expression of angiopoietin-1, angiopoietin-2, and tie receptors after middle cerebral artery occlusion in the rat. Am J Pathol 157:1473–1483, 2000.

153. Lin TN, Wang CK, Cheung WM, Hsu CY: Induction of angiopoietin and Tie receptor mRNA expression after cerebral ischemia-reperfusion. J Cereb Blood Flow Metab 20:387–395, 2000.

154. Lin TN, Nian GM, Chen SF, et al: Induction of Tie-1 and Tie-2 receptor protein expression after cerebral ischemia-reperfusion. J Cereb Blood Flow Metab 21:690–701, 2001.

155. Gibbons GH, Dzau VJ: The emerging concept of vascular remodeling. N Engl J Med 330:1431–1438, 1994.

156. Natte R, de Boer W, Maat-Schieman M, et al: Amyloid beta precursor protein-mRNA is expressed throughout cerebral vessel walls. Brain Res 828:179–183, 1999.

157. Stephenson D, Rash K, Clemens J: Amyloid precursor protein accumulates in regions of neurodegeneration following focal cerebral ischemia in the rat. Brain Res 593:128–135, 1992.

158. Kalaria R, Bhatti S, Lust W, Perry G: The amyloid precursor protein in ischemic brain injury and chronic hypoperfusion. Ann N Y Acad Sci 695:190–193, 1993.

159. Kalaria R, Bhatti S, Palatinsky E, et al: Accumulation of the beta amyloid precursor protein at sites of ischemic injury in rat brain. Neuroreport 4:211–214, 1993.

160. Lin B, Schmidt-Kastner R, Busto R, Ginsberg M: Progressive parenchymal deposition of beta-amyloid precursor protein in rat brain following global cerebral ischemia. Acta Neuropathol (Berl) 97:359–368, 1999.

161. Shi J, Panickar K, Yang S, et al: Estrogen attenuates over-expression of beta-amyloid precursor protein messenger RNA in an animal model of focal ischemia. Brain Res 810:87–92, 1998.

162. Dietrich W, Kraydieh S, Prado R, Stagliano N: White matter alterations following thromboembolic stroke: A beta-amyloid precursor protein immunocytochemical study in rats. Acta Neuropathol (Berl) 95:524–531, 1998.

163. Yam P, Takasago T, Dewar D, et al: Amyloid precursor protein accumulates in white matter at the margin of a focal ischaemic lesion. Brain Res 760:150–157, 1997.

164. Popa-Wagner A, Schroder E, Schmoll H, et al: Upregulation of MAP1B and MAP2 in the rat brain after middle cerebral artery occlusion: Effect of age. J Cereb Blood Flow Metab 19:425–434, 1999.

165. Kim H, Lee S, Kim S, et al: Post-ischemic changes in the expression of Alzheimer's APP isoforms in rat cerebral cortex. Neuroreport 16:533–537, 1998.

166. Niwa K, Carlson G, Iadecola C: Exogenous A beta 1-40 reproduces cerebrovascular alterations resulting from amyloid precursor protein overexpression in mice. J Cereb Blood Flow Metab 20:1659–1668, 2000.

167. Zhang F, Eckman C, Younkin S, et al: Increased susceptibility to ischemic brain damage in transgenic mice overexpressing the amyloid precursor protein. J Neurosci 17:7655–7661, 1997.

168. Winkler D, Bondolfi L, Herzig M, et al: Spontaneous hemorrhagic stroke in a mouse model of cerebral amyloid angiopathy. J Neurosci 21:1619–1627, 2001.

169. Vinters HV, Wang ZZ, Secor DL: Brain parenchymal and microvascular amyloid in Alzheimer's disease. Brain Pathol 6:179–195, 1996.

170. Brun A, Fredriksson K, Gustafson L: Pure subcortical atherosclerotic encephalopathy (Binswanger disease): A clinicopathological study. Cerebrovasc Dis 2:87–92, 1992.

Pathophysiology

Chapter Thirty-Nine

Mechanisms of Thrombosis and Thrombolysis

Gregory J. del Zoppo and Mary Kalafut

The processes of thrombosis—thrombus growth, dissolution, and migration—are inextricably connected. Thrombus formation involves activation of platelets, activation of the coagulation system, and the processes of fibrin dissolution. The central feature of each of these contributions is the action of thrombin to generate the fibrin network from circulating fibrinogen. Excess vascular fibrin formation or excess fibrin degradation can contribute to thrombus growth or hemorrhage, respectively. Plasminogen activators have been exploited to dissolve significant (symptomatic) thrombi; however, all substances that promote plasmin formation retain the potential to increase the risk of hemorrhage.

The use of plasminogen activators (PAs), when applied in the acute setting, has been associated with detectable clinical improvement in selected patients with symptoms of focal cerebral ischemia.[1–8] Thrombolysis has thus attained a limited place in the acute treatment of ischemic stroke. Currently, recombinant tissue-type plasminogen activator (rt-PA) is licensed in the United States and several other countries for the treatment of ischemic stroke within 3 hours of onset.[6]

The development of agents that promote fibrin degradation in the clinical setting stems from observations in the 19th century of the spontaneous liquefaction of clotted blood and the dissolution of fibrin thrombi.[9] A growing understanding of plasma proteolytic digestion of fibrin paralleled enquiry into the mechanisms of streptococcal fibrinolysis.[10,11] Streptokinase was first employed to dissolve closed space (intrapleural) fibrin clots,[12] but purified preparations were required for lysis of intravascular thrombi.[13] Development of PAs for therapeutic lysis of vascular thrombi has progressed in concert with insights into the mechanisms of thrombus formation and degradation.

THROMBUS FORMATION

The platelet-fibrin composition of a specific thrombus depends on the local development of fibrin, platelet activation, and regional blood flow or shear stress. Pharmacologic inhibition of the platelet activation and coagulation processes can alter thrombus composition and volume. At arterial flow rates thrombi are predominantly platelet rich,

whereas at lower shear rates characteristic of venous flow, activation of coagulation seems to predominate. It has been suggested that the efficacy of pharmacologic thrombus lysis depends on (1) the relative fibrin content and (2) the extent of fibrin cross-linking, which may reflect thrombus age.[14,15]

Thrombin (factor IIa) is the central player in clot formation (Fig. 39–1). Thrombin cleaves fibrinogen to generate fibrin, which forms the scaffolding for the growing thrombus.[16] Inter-fibrin strand cross-linking requires factor XIII, a transglutaminase bound to fibrinogen that is itself activated by thrombin and stabilizes the fibrin network (Fig. 39–2).[17–19] Thrombin-mediated fibrin polymerization leads to the generation of fibrin I and fibrin II monomers and to the release of fibrinopeptide A (FPA) and fibrinopeptide B (FPB).

Platelet activation is required for thrombus formation under arterial flow conditions and accompanies thrombin-mediated fibrin formation. Platelet membrane receptors and phospholipids form a workbench for the generation of thrombin through both the intrinsic and extrinsic coagulation pathways.[20] Platelets promote activation of the early stages of intrinsic coagulation by a process that involves the factor XI receptor and high-molecular-weight kininogen (HMWK)(see Fig. 39–1).[21] Also, factors V and VIII interact with specific platelet membrane phospholipids (receptors) to facilitate the activation of factor X to Xa and the conversion of prothrombin to thrombin on the platelet surface (the "tenase" complex).[22] Platelet-bound thrombin-modified factor V (factor Va) serves as a high-affinity platelet receptor for factor Xa.[23] These mechanisms accelerate the rate of thrombin generation, further catalyzing fibrin network formation.

This process also leads to the conversion of plasminogen to plasmin and the activation of *endogenous* fibrinolysis. Thrombin provides one direct connection between thrombus formation and plasmin generation through localized generation of PAs from endothelial cells. Active thrombin has been shown in vitro and in vivo to markedly stimulate release of tissue-type plasminogen activator (t-PA) from endothelial stores.[24–26] In one experiment, infusion of factor Xa and phospholipid into nonhuman primates resulted in a pronounced increase in circulating t-PA activity, suggesting that significant vascular stores of this PA may be released by

Pathophysiology

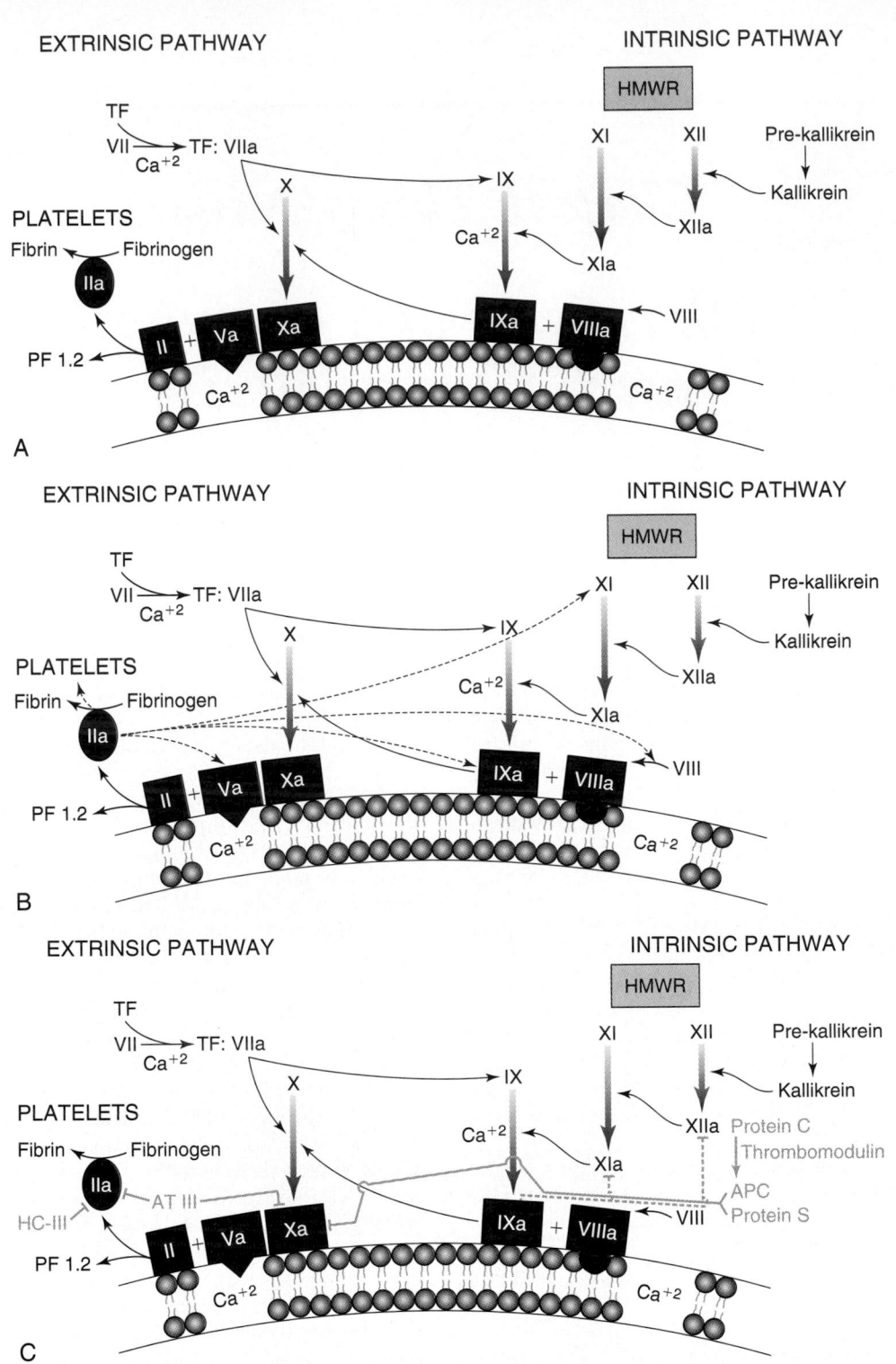

FIGURE 39–1 *Intrinsic and extrinsic coagulation pathways (see text). Phospholipid-containing membranes (e.g., platelets) provide the scaffold for acceleration of coagulation pathway activation. Both intrinsic and extrinsic pathways lead to prothrombin (factor II) activation, with fibrin generation from circulating fibrinogen. The extrinsic pathway initiates coagulation through the interaction of factor VII with tissue factor (TF) in the vascular adventitia, brain perivascular parenchyma, and activated monocytes. The TF:VIIa complex catalyzes activation of factor X and acceleration of thrombin generation. The extrinsic system involves activation of components within the vascular lumen. Initiation of coagulation through this pathway involves pre-kallikrein, kallikrein, high-molecular-weight kininogen (HMWK), and factors XI and XII. A, Thrombin generation. The intrinsic system activates factor X through the "tenase" complex (factors VIIIa and IXa, and Ca^{2+} on phospholipid). Both intrinsic and extrinsic pathways activate prothrombin through the common "prothrombinase" complex (factors Xa and Va, and Ca^{2+}). The platelet surface has receptors for factors Va and VIIIa. Cleavage of prothrombin generates the prothrombin fragment 1.2 (PF 1.2) and thrombin (factor IIa). B, Thrombin has multiple stimulatory positive feedback effects. It catalyzes activation of factors XI and VIII as well as the activities of the tenase and prothrombinase complexes. Thrombin also stimulates activation of platelets and granule secretion via specific thrombin receptors on their surface. C, Coagulation activation is regulated by interleaving inhibitor pathways. The effects of factors Va, Xa, and VIIIa are modulated by the protein C pathway. Activated protein C (APC), generated by the action of the endothelial cell receptor thrombomodulin on protein C, with its cofactor protein S, inhibit the action of factor V. AT-III, antithrombin-III; HC-III, heparin cofactor-III.*

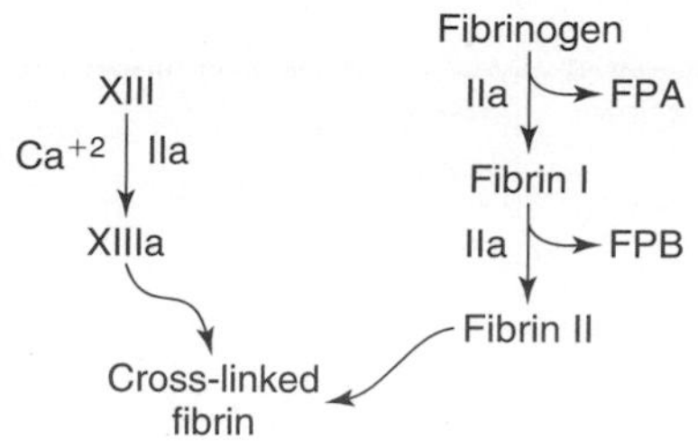

FIGURE 39-2 *Generation of cross-linked fibrin. Fibrinogen is cleaved successively to form fibrin I and fibrin II by thrombin (factor IIa) with the release of fibrinopeptides A and B (FPA and FPB). Thrombin activates factor XIII to the active transglutaminase, which promotes cross-linking of fibrin and stabilization of the growing thrombus.*

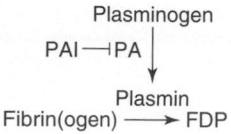

FIGURE 39-3 *Plasminogen activation and fibrin(ogen)olysis. Degradation of fibrinogen and fibrin is catalyzed by plasmin. Plasminogen activators (PAs), including tissue-type PA (t-PA), urokinase-type PA (u-PA), and novel constructs, cleave plasminogen to the active plasmin. Characteristic products of fibrin and fibrinogen degradation (FDP) are generated (see text). PAI, plasminogen activator inhibitor.*

active components of coagulation.[27] Other vascular and cellular stimuli may also augment PA release (see later), thereby pushing the balance toward thrombolysis.

Development of arterial or venous thrombi requires abrogation of the constitutive antithrombotic characteristics of endothelial cells.[28] In addition to both endothelial cell–derived antithrombotic properties and circulating anticoagulants (i.e., activated protein C, protein S), thrombus growth is limited by the *endogenous* thrombolytic system. Thrombus organization results from the preferential conversion of plasminogen to plasmin on the thrombus surface. There, fibrin binds t-PA in proximity to its substrate plasminogen, thereby accelerating local plasmin formation. In concert with local shear stress, these processes may also promote embolization into the downstream cerebral vasculature.[29] However, little is known about the endogenous generation and secretion of PAs within the cerebral vessels.[30] *Exogenous* application of pharmacologic doses of PAs accelerates conversion of thrombus-bound plasminogen to plasmin and can prevent thrombus formation, as discussed later.

FIBRINOLYSIS

Plasmin formation is central to lysis of vascular thrombi. The endogenous fibrinolytic system comprises plasmino-

gen, PAs, and their inhibitors. Plasmin mediates degradation of fibrin (and fibrinogen). Plasminogen, its activators, and their inhibitors contribute to the balance between vascular hemorrhage and thrombosis (Fig. 39–3; Tables 39.1 and 39.2).

Plasmin formation occurs (1) in the plasma, where it can cleave circulating fibrinogen and fibrin into soluble products,[31] and (2) on reactive surfaces (e.g., thrombi or cells). The fibrin network provides the scaffold for plasminogen activation, whereas various cells, including polymorphonuclear (PMN) leukocytes, platelets, and endothelial cells, express receptors for plasminogen binding.[32] Specific cellular receptors concentrate plasminogen and specific activators (e.g., urokinase-type plasminogen activators [u-PA]), thereby enhancing local plasmin production. Similar receptors on tumor cells (e.g., the urokinase plasminogen activator receptor [u-PAR], which concentrates u-PA) are also involved with the dissolution of basement membranes and the metastatic process. Plasmin can also cleave various basal lamina and extracellular matrix (ECM) ligands (e.g., laminins, collagen IV, fibronectin) in the central nervous system.

Plasminogen

The naturally circulating PAs, single-chain t-PA and single-chain u-PA (scu-PA or Pro-UK), catalyze plasmin formation.[33–36] Plasmin derives from the zymogen plasminogen, a single-chain 92-kDa glycosylated serine protease.[37,38]

Table 39.1 Plasminogen Activators (PAs)

Plasminogen Activators	Molecular Weight (kDa)	Chains	Plasma Concentration (mg/dL)	Plasma Concentration Half-Life ($t_{1/2}$)	Substrates
Endogenous					
Plasminogen	92	2	20	2.2 days	(Fibrin)
Tissue-type PA (t-PA)	68 (59)	1 → 2	5×10^{-4}	5–8 min	Fibrin/plasminogen
Single-chain urokinase-type PA (scu-PA)	54 (46)	1 → 2	$2–20 \times 10^{-4}$	8 min	Fibrin/plasmin(ogen)
Urokinase-type PA (u-PA)	54 (46)	2	8×10^{-4}	9–12 min	Plasminogen
Exogenous					
Streptokinase	47	1	0	41 and 30 min	Plasminogen, fibrin(ogen)
Anisoylated plasminogen-streptokinase activator complex (APSAC)	131	Complex	0	70–90 min	Fibrin(ogen)
Staphylokinase	16.5		0		Plasminogen

Table 39.2   Plasminogen Activator Inhibitors

Inhibitor	Molecular Weight (kDa)	Chains	Plasma Concentration (mg dL^{-1})	Plasma Concentration Half-Life $t_{1/2}$	Inhibitor Substrates
Plasmin inhibitors					
a$_2$-Antiplasmin	65	1	7	3.3 min	Plasmin
a$_2$-Macroglobulin	740	4	250		Plasmin (excess)
Plasminogen activator inhibitors					
PAI-1	48–52	1	5×10^{-2}	7 min	t-PA, u-PA
PAI-2	47, 70	1	$<5 \times 10^{-4}$	24 hr	t-PA, u-PA
PAI-3	50				u-PA, t-PA

PAI, plasminogen activator inhibitor; $t_{1/2}$, half-life; t-PA, tissue-type plasminogen activator; u-PA, urokinase-type plasminogen activator.

Structurally, plasminogen contains five kringles and a protease domain, two of which (K1 and K5) mediate the binding of plasminogen to fibrin through characteristic lysine-binding sites (Fig. 39–4).[37,39,40] Glu-plasminogen has an NH$_2$-terminal glutamic acid, and lys-plasminogen, which lacks an 8-kDa peptide, has an NH$_2$-terminal lysine. Plasmin cleavage of the NH$_2$-terminal fragment of glu-plasminogen generates lys-plasminogen.[41,42] Glu-plasminogen has a plasma clearance half-life ($t_{1/2}$) of about 2.2 days, whereas that of lys-plasminogen is 0.8 days.[13] Both t-PA and u-PA catalyze the conversion of glu-plasminogen to lys-plasmin through either of two intermediates, glu-plasmin or lys-plasminogen.[43] The lysine-binding sites of plasminogen mediate the binding of plasminogen to α$_2$-antiplasmin, thrombospondin, components of the vascular extracellular matrix, and histidine-rich glycoprotein (HRG).[38] α$_2$-Antiplasmin prevents binding of plasminogen to fibrin by this mechanism.[43] Partial degradation of the fibrin network enhances the binding of glu-plasminogen to fibrin, promoting further local fibrinolysis.

Plasminogen Activation

Plasminogen activation is tied to activation of the coagulation system and may involve secretion of physiologic PAs ("extrinsic activation"). It has been suggested that kallikrein, factor XIa, and factor XIIa, in the presence of HMWK, may directly activate plasminogen.[44,45] Several lines of evidence suggest that scu-PA activates plasminogen under physiologic conditions.[46–48] Tissue-type PA, which is secreted from the endothelium and other cellular sources, appears to be the primary PA in the vasculature.[13] Thrombin, generated by either intrinsic or extrinsic coagulation, stimulates secretion of t-PA from endothelial stores.[24,49,50]

Several serine proteases can convert plasminogen to plasmin by cleaving the arg^{560}-val^{561} bond.[38,51,52] Serine proteases have common structural features, including an NH$_2$-terminal "A" chain with substrate-binding affinity, a COOH-terminal "B" chain with the active site, and intrachain disulfide bridges. Plasminogen-cleaving serine proteases include the coagulation proteins factor IX, factor X, and prothrombin (factor II), protein C, chymotrypsin and trypsin, various leukocyte elastases, the plasminogen activators u-PA and t-PA, and plasmin itself.[38] Activation of plasminogen by t-PA is accelerated in a ternary complex with fibrin.[53–55] In the circulation, plasmin binds rapidly to the inhibitor α$_2$-antiplasmin and is thereby inactivated. Activation of thrombus-bound plasminogen also protects plasmin from the inhibitors α$_2$-antiplasmin and α$_2$-macroglobulin.[38] Here, the lysine-binding sites and the catalytic site of plasmin are occupied by fibrin, thereby blocking its interaction with α$_2$-antiplasmin.[53,54] Furthermore, fibrin and fibrin-bound plasminogen render t-PA relatively inaccessible to inhibition by other circulating plasma inhibitors.[56]

Thrombus Dissolution

Fibrinolysis occurs predominantly within the thrombus and at its surface but may be augmented by contributions from local blood flow.[57–60] During thrombus consolidation, plasminogen bound to fibrin and to platelets allows local release of plasmin.[61] In the *circulation*, plasmin cleaves the fibrinogen Aα chain appendage, generating fragment X (DED), Aα fragments, and Bβ 1-42. Further cleavage of fragment X leads to the generation of fragments DE, D, and E. Separately, degradation of the fibrin network generates YY/DXD, YD/DY, and the unique DD/E (fragment X = DED and fragment Y = DE).[31,57,62] Cross-linkage of DD with fragment E is vulnerable to further cleavage, producing D-dimer fragments. The measurement of D-dimer levels has clinical utility, in that the absence of circulating D dimer correlates with the absence of massive thrombosis.[63] Ordinarily, in the setting of focal cerebral ischemia, the thrombus load is small and the meaning of D-dimer elevations uncertain. The generation of the degradation products has the following two consequences: (1) incorporation of some of these products into the forming thrombus destabilizes the fibrin network and (2) reduced circulating fibrinogen and the generation of breakdown products of fibrin(ogen) limits the protection from hemorrhage.

PLASMINOGEN ACTIVATORS

All fibrinolytic agents are obligate plasminogen activators (see Table 39.1). Tissue-type PA, scu-PA, and u-PA are *endogenous* plasminogen activators involved in physiologic fibrinolysis. Recombinant t-PA, scu-PA, and u-PA, as well as streptokinase (SK), acylated plasminogen streptokinase activator complex (APSAC), staphylokinase, PAs of vampire bat origin, and other newer novel agents in clinical

Pathophysiology

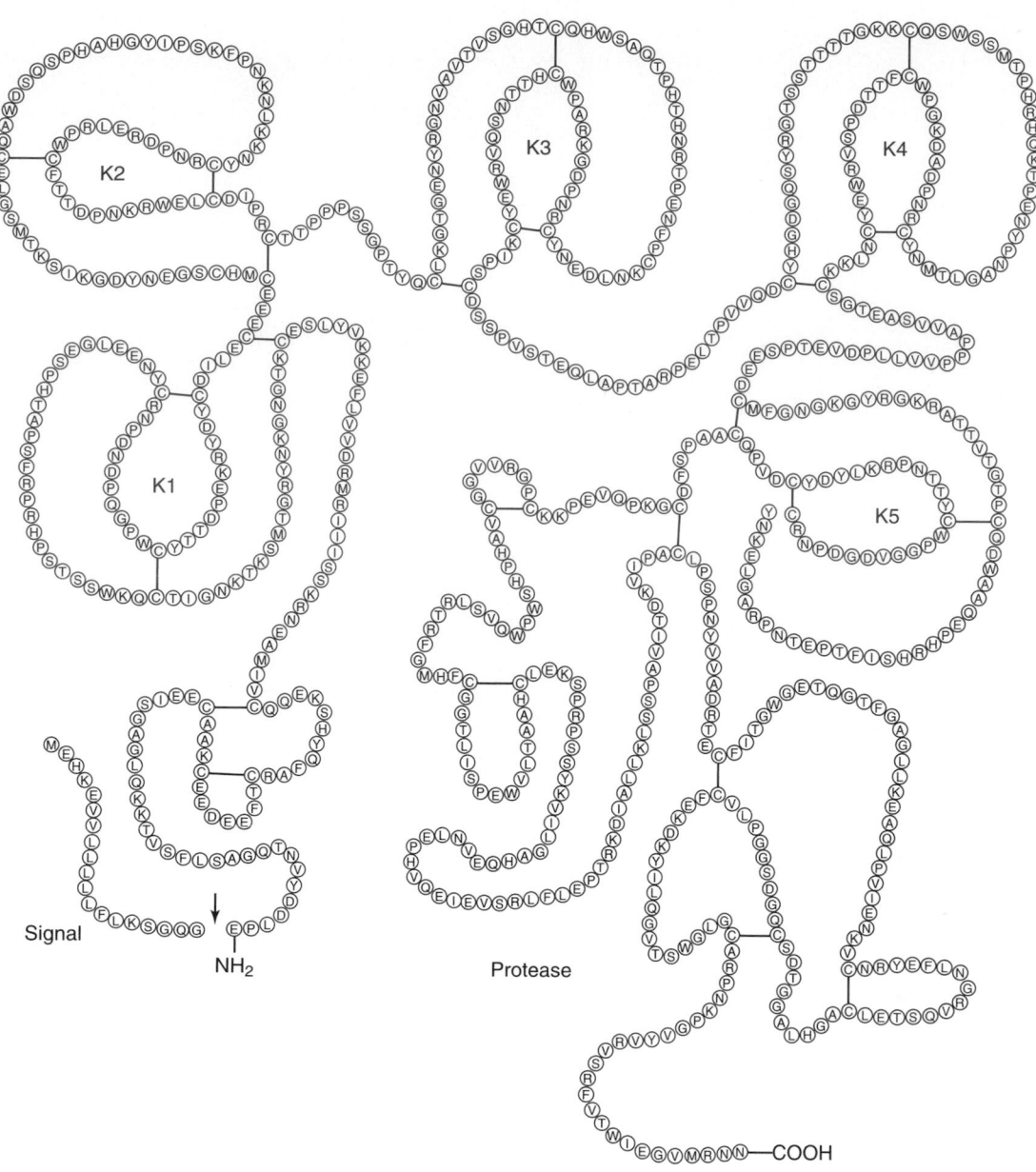

FIGURE 39–4 *The secondary structure of plasminogen.*

use, are *exogenous* plasminogen activators.[58–60] t-PA, scu-PA, and a number of novel agents have relative fibrin and thrombus specificity.[36,63]

Endogenous Plasminogen Activators

Tissue-Type Plasminogen Activator

Tissue-type PA is a 70-kDa, single-chain glycosylated serine protease that has four distinct domains—a finger (F-) domain, an epidermal growth factor (EGF) domain (residues 50–87), two kringle regions (K1 and K2), and a serine protease domain (Fig. 39–5).[51,64,65] The COOH-terminal serine protease domain contains the active site for plasminogen cleavage, and the finger and K_2 domains are responsible for fibrin affinity.[36,65,66] The two kringle domains are homologous to the kringle regions of plasminogen.

The single-chain form is converted to the two-chain form by plasmin cleavage of the arg^{275}-isoleu^{276} bond. Both single-chain and two-chain species are enzymatically active and have relatively fibrin-selective properties. Infusion studies in humans indicate that both single-chain and two-chain t-PA have circulating plasma $t_{1/2}$ values of 3 to 8 minutes,[36] although the biologic $t_{1/2}$ values are longer. Tissue-type PA is considered to be fibrin-dependent because of its favorable binding constant for fibrin-bound plasminogen and its activation of plasminogen in association with fibrin.[36,64] Significant inactivation of circulating factors V and VIII does not occur with infused rt-PA, and an anticoagulant state is generally not produced.[36] However, if sufficiently high dose rates are employed, clinically measurable fibrinogenolysis and plasminogen consumption can be produced.

Secretion of t-PA from cultured endothelial cells is stimulated by thrombin,[49,50,67] activated protein C (APC),[68]

Pathophysiology

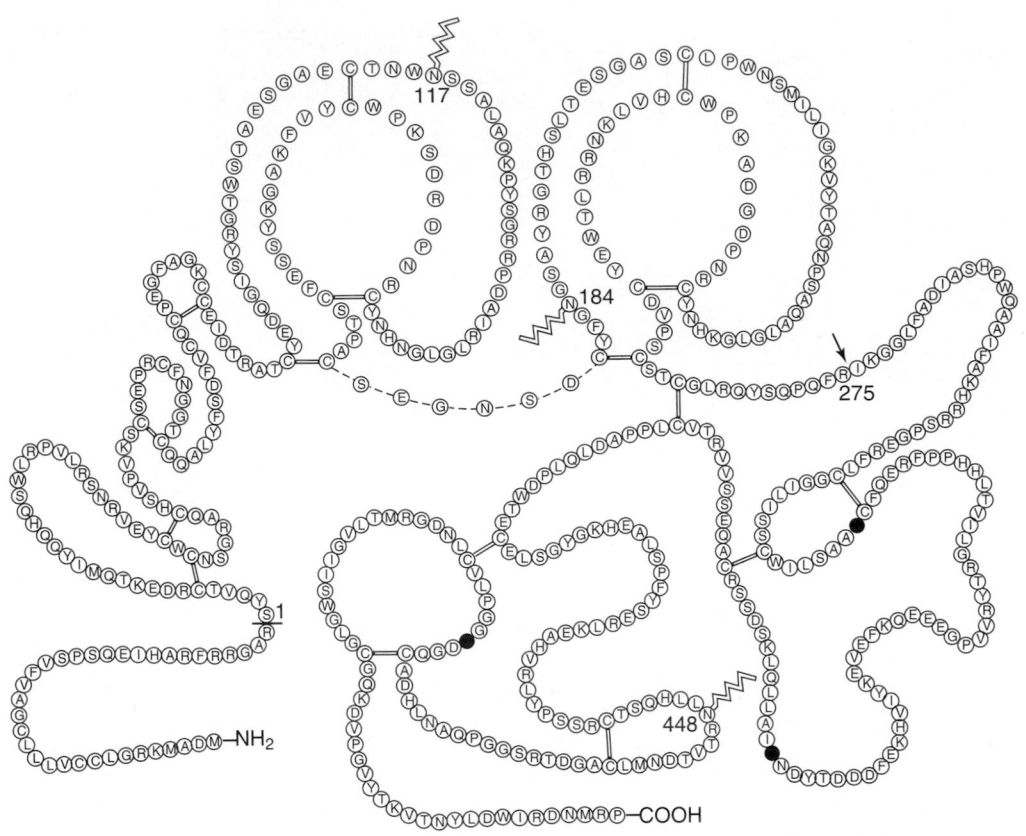

FIGURE 39–5   *The secondary structure of tissue-type plasminogen activator (t-PA). Conversion of single-chain t-PA to two-chain t-PA by plasmin occurs at the arg^{275}-isoleu^{276} bond (arrow).*

histamine,[49] phorbol myristate esterase, and other mediators.[69–73] However, the location of the in vivo storage pools of t-PA remains unclear. Physical exercise and certain vasoactive substances produce measurable increases in circulating t-PA levels, and 1-deamino(8-D-arginine) vasopressin (DDAVP) may produce a threefold to fourfold increase in t-PA antigen levels within 60 minutes of parenteral infusion in some patients.[74–76] Both t-PA and u-PA have been reported to be secreted by endothelial cells, neurons, astrocytes, and microglia in vivo or in vitro.[30,77–84] The reasons for this broad cell expression are not known, however.

Urokinase-Type Plasminogen Activator

Single-chain urokinase-type PA is a 54-kDa glycoprotein synthesized by endothelial and renal cells as well as by certain malignant cells (Fig. 39–6).[32] This single-chain proenzyme of u-PA is unusual in that it has fibrin-selective plasmin-generating activity[85,86] and also has been synthesized by recombinant techniques.[36,87]

The relationship of scu-PA to u-PA is complex: Cleavage or removal of lys^{158} from scu-PA by plasmin produces 54-kDa, two-chain u-PA. This PA consists of an A-chain (157 residues) and a glycosylated B-chain (253 residues), which are linked by the disulfide bridge at cys^{148} and cys^{279}. Further cleavages at lys^{135} and arg^{156} produce low-molecular-weight (31-kDa) u-PA.[65] Both high- and low-molecular-weight species are enzymatically active.

The 54-kDa urokinase (u-PA) activates plasminogen by first-order kinetics.[58,88] The two forms of u-PA exhibit measurable fibrinolytic and fibrinogenolytic activities in vitro and in vivo, and have plasma $t_{1/2}$ values of 9 to 12 minutes.[89,90] When infused as an *exogenous* therapeutic agent, u-PA leads to plasminogen consumption and inactivation of factors II (prothrombin), V, and VIII. The latter changes constitute the systemic lytic state.

It has been postulated that t-PA is primarily involved in the maintenance of hemostasis through the dissolution of fibrin, whereas u-PA is involved in generating pericellular proteolytic activity in relation to cells expressing the u-PA receptor, needed for degradation of extracellular matrix. The roles of these two PAs in central nervous system function are not yet fully known.

Exogenous Plasminogen Activators

Streptokinase

Streptokinase (SK) is a 47-kDa, single-chain polypeptide derived from group C β-hemolytic streptococci.[91] The active [SK-plasminogen] complex converts circulating plasminogen directly to plasmin and undergoes further activation to form [SK-plasmin]. The [SK-plasminogen], [SK-plasmin], and plasmin species circulate together.[92] The [SK-plasmin] complex not bound by the inhibitor α_2-antiplasmin and free circulating plasmin degrade both fibrinogen and fibrin and inactivate prothrombin, factor V, and factor VIII.[61] The kinetics of SK elimination are complex. Antistreptococcal antibodies formed from antecedent infections neutralize infused SK and arise

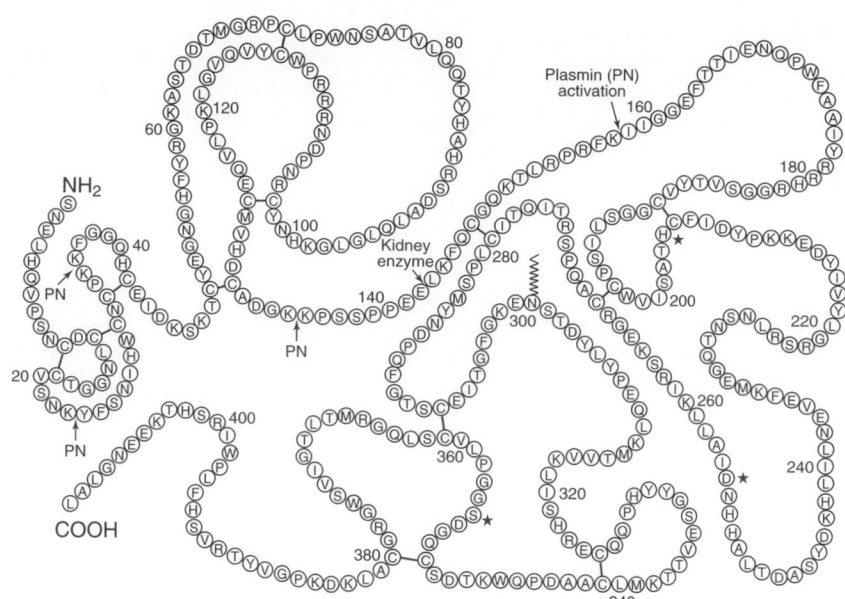

FIGURE 39–6 *The secondary structure of single-chain urokinase-type plasminogen activator (scu-PA; 54 kDa). Activation by plasmin takes place at the 158–159 bond (arrow). The zigzag line represents the glycosylation site.*

maximally by 4 to 7 days after initiation of an SK infusion. Therefore, the doses of SK required to achieve steady-state plasminogen activation must be individualized. Plasminogen depletion through conversion to plasmin and by as yet poorly understood clearance mechanisms for the [SK-plasminogen] complex can lead to hypoplasminogenemia. Generation of plasmin is limited at both low and high SK infusion dose rates because of inadequate plasminogen conversion and depletion of plasminogen, respectively.

APSAC (e.g., Anistreplase) is an artificial activator construct consisting of plasminogen and SK bound noncovalently. Fibrin selectivity relies on the fibrin-attachment properties of the plasminogen kringles.[36] The activity of APSAC depends on the deacylation rate of the acyl-plasminogen component. Hydrolytic activation of the acyl-protected active site of plasminogen allows plasmin formation by SK within the complex in the presence of fibrin. From those observations and on the basis of the terminal $t_{1/2}$ of SK and the $t_{1/2}$ for APSAC deacylation, APSAC has a longer circulation time than streptokinase.[93,94] APSAC has not found a place in the treatment of vascular thrombosis, however.

Staphylokinase
Staphylokinase (STK) is a 16.5-kDa polypeptide derived from certain strains of *Staphylococcus aureus*.[95–97] It combines stoichiometrically (1:1) with plasminogen to form an irreversible complex that activates free plasminogen. The binding of staphylokinase to plasmin has been worked out in detail.[95,97,98] Recombinant staphylokinase has been prepared from the known gene nucleotide sequence and has been tested in the setting of acute myocardial infarction, but it has not been used in ischemic stroke.

Plasminogen Activators Derived from *Desmodus rotundus*
Recombinant PAs identical to those derived from the saliva of *Desmodus* species are fibrin-dependent. The α form of *Desmodus* salivary PA (DSPA-α; desmoteplase) and vampire bat salivary plasminogen activator (bat-PA) are

more fibrin-dependent than t-PA and may be superior to t-PA in terms of sustained recanalization without fibrinogenolysis.[99–103] The plasma $t_{1/2}$ of DSPA is significantly longer than that of rt-PA.[99] Limited safety studies of desmoteplase in acute ischemic stroke have been performed.

Novel Plasminogen Activators
Efforts to alter the stability and thrombus selectivity of endogenous PAs have led to a lengthening list of possible pharmacologic agents. Point and deletion mutations in t-PA and u-PA have provided molecules with unique specificities.[104,105] For instance, t-PA sequences lacking the K1 and K2 domains possess fibrin specificity, normal specific activity, but reduced inhibition by PA inhibitor-1 (PAI-1).[66] In theory, the increased fibrin selectivity might provide greater thrombolytic effect; however, in studies of the use of this agent in coronary artery thromboses, significant advantages were not evident.

For the clinical target of myocardial ischemia, several t-PA mutants with prolonged $t_{1/2}$ and delayed clearance have been devised that may have benefit when infused as a single bolus.[106–108] Reteplase, a nonglycosylated PA consisting of the K2 and protease domains of t-PA, has a 4.5- to 12.3-fold longer $t_{1/2}$ owing in part to lower affinity for the hepatic cell t-PA receptor.[108,109] It also possesses lower fibrin selectivity. Tenectaplase (TNK-t-PA) differs from t-PA at three mutation sites (T103N, N117Q, and KHRR[296–299]AAAA), which alter two glycosylation sites and increase fibrin selectivity. The changes also result in decreased clearance and prolonged $t_{1/2}$.[110,111] Another t-PA mutant with greater $t_{1/2}$, lanoteplase (n-PA), derives from deletion of the fibronectin finger and epidermal growth factor domains and mutation of asn[117] to gln[117].[106,107] In addition to enhanced fibrin selectivity, TNK has relative resistance to inhibition by PAI-1.[112] A t-PA–like construct with moderate fibrin selectivity is monteplase (E6010).[113] This molecule differs from t-PA in the location and organization of disulfide bridges and the complexity of glycosylation. In contrast, the fibrin selectivity and specific activity of pamiteplase (YM866) are nearly identical to those of t-PA, but pamiteplase has a longer $t_{1/2}$.[114,115] These mutants have been developed for bolus infusion application in the setting of myocardial infarction (MI). Application of TNK to clinical ischemic stroke has not yet been formally tested, although experimental studies have been performed. What advantage delayed clearance or prolonged $t_{1/2}$ may have in acute application in ischemic stroke remains unclear.[116] Dose-adjustment studies in patients with stroke have not been reported. One unproven concern with long $t_{1/2}$ molecules is that they may augment the intercerebral hemorrhage risk in the setting of ischemic stroke.

A similar situation obtains for other novel PA constructs. These have included single-site mutants and variants of rt-PA and recombinant scu-PA; t-PA/scu-PA and t-PA/u-PA chimerae, u-PA/antifibrin monoclonal antibodies, u-PA/antiplatelet monoclonal antibodies, bifunctional antibody conjugates, and scu-PA deletion mutants.[117–121]

REGULATION OF ENDOGENOUS FIBRINOLYSIS

Endogenous fibrinolysis is modulated by several families of inhibitors of plasmin and of PAIs. In the circulation, α_2-antiplasmin is the primary inhibitor of fibrinolysis, which inhibits plasmin directly. Excess plasmin is inactivated by α_2-macroglobulin. The potential risk of vascular thrombosis then depends on the balance between plasminogen activation and plasmin activity and their respective inhibitors in the circulation. Thrombospondin interferes with fibrin-associated plasminogen activation by t-PA.[122] Inhibitors of the contact activation system and complement (C1 inhibitor) have an indirect effect on fibrinolysis. Histidine-rich glycoprotein (HRG) is a competitive inhibitor of plasminogen. Generally, though, these physiologic modulators of plasmin activity are overwhelmed by pharmacologic concentrations of PAs.

For streptokinase, APSAC, and staphylokinase, circulating neutralizing antibodies appear, which directly inhibit their activation of plasminogen.

α_2-Antiplasmin and α_2-Macroglobulin

Circulating plasmin generated in the plasma during fibrinolysis is bound by α_2-antiplasmin. The two forms of α_2-antiplasmin are (1) the native form, which binds plasminogen, and (2) a second form that cannot bind plasminogen.[123] Ordinarily, α_2-antiplasmin is found in either plasminogen-bound or free circulating forms.[124] Fibrin-bound plasmin is protected because of its interaction with fibrin and because α_2-antiplasmin is already occupied. Excess free plasmin is bound by α_2-macroglobulin. α_2-Macroglobulin is a relatively nonspecific inhibitor of fibrinolysis that inactivates plasmin, kallikrein, t-PA, and u-PA.[125]

Inhibitors of Plasminogen Activators and Fibrinolysis

Direct PAIs also reduce the activity of t-PA, scu-PA, and u-PA (see Table 39.2). PAI-1 specifically inhibits both plasma t-PA and u-PA. PAI-1 is derived from both endothelial cell and platelet compartments.[126–128] Several lines of evidence indicate that the K_2 domain of t-PA is responsible for the interaction between t-PA and PAI-1 and that this interaction is altered by the presence of fibrin.[129] PAI-1 is also an acute-phase reactant,[130] and deep venous thrombosis, septicemia, and type II diabetes mellitus are associated with elevated plasma PAI-1 levels. PAI-2 is derived from placental tissue, granulocytes, monocytes/macrophages, and histiocytes.[131,132] The kinetics of PA inhibition by PAI-2 differs from those for PAI-1. PAI-2, which is found in a 70-kDa form and a 47-kDa low-molecular-weight form, has a lower inhibition constant (Ki) for u-PA and two-chain t-PA. This inhibitor probably plays little role in the physiologic antagonism of t-PA, and is most important in the uteroplacental circulation.[133] PAI-3 is a serine protease inhibitor of u-PA, t-PA, and activated protein C (APC) found in plasma and urine.[134,135]

Thrombin-activable fibrinolysis inhibitor (TAFI) is an endogenous inhibitor of glu-plasminogen and, therefore, fibrinolysis.[136] TAFI is a precursor of plasma carboxypeptidase B and, when activated by thrombin in the plasma, produces an antifibrinolytic effect.

CONSEQUENCES OF THERAPEUTIC PLASMINOGEN ACTIVATION

Plasminogen activators given at pharmacologic doses significantly alter hemostasis. Urokinase-type PA, SK, and occasionally t-PA produce systemically detectable fibrinogen degradation, measured by a fall in fibrinogen concentration, and a reduction in circulating plasminogen and α_2-antiplasmin (through binding of the plasmin generated). Both u-PA and SK inactivate factors V and VIII, also contributing to the "systemic lytic state" or "anticoagulant state."[137] Fragments of fibrin(ogen) interfere with fibrin multimerization and contribute to thrombus destabilization, whereas the circulating fragments, hypofibrinogenemia, and factor depletion produce a transient anticoagulant state that limits thrombus formation and extension. The clinical consequences of u-PA or SK infusion include a progressive decrease or depletion of circulating plasminogen and fibrinogen, prolongation of the aPTT due to significant fibrinogen reduction, and inactivation of factors V and VIII.

Platelet function can also be affected. Clinical studies of rt-PA have demonstrated prolongation of standardized template bleeding times.[138] In experimental systems, infusion of rt-PA produces greater hemorrhage.[139,140] Furthermore, t-PA is known to cause disaggregation of human platelets through selective proteolysis of intraplatelet fibrin, which is inhibitable by α_2-antiplasmin.[141] Lys-plasminogen and glu-plasminogen can potentiate the platelet disaggregatory effect of rt-PA.[142] It is likely that the risk of intracerebral hemorrhage that attends PA infusion involves disruption of sustained platelet aggregation and lysis of fibrin formed at the site of vascular injury.

LIMITATIONS TO THE CLINICAL USE OF FIBRINOLYTIC AGENTS

The clinical setting in which PAs are used is an important and relevant variable for both the efficacy and the reduction of hemorrhage risk. Intracerebral hemorrhage is a known risk of the clinical use of PAs. The use of fibrinolytic agents in pharmacologic doses in the acute setting of ischemic stroke must conform to the original report,[6] as confirmed subsequently.[143] An abbreviated summary of strict contraindications to the use of fibrinolytic agents is as follows: (1) a history of previous intracranial hemorrhage, (2) septic embolism, (3) malignant hypertension or sustained diastolic or systolic blood pressure in excess of 180/110, (4) conditions consistent with ongoing parenchymal hemorrhage (e.g., gastrointestinal source), (5) pregnancy or parturition, (6) a history of recent trauma or surgery, and (7) known acquired (e.g., from anticoagulant use) and inherited hemorrhagic diatheses. These contraindications apply to the use of rt-PA in selected patients with ischemic stroke less than 3 hours after symptom onset[6] as well as other approved clinical indications for the use of rt-PA, u-PA, or SK.

PLASMINOGEN ACTIVATORS IN CEREBRAL TISSUE

Although current clinical interests focus on the use of PAs as therapeutic agents for vascular reperfusion, cerebral tissue also generates and uses PAs. PA activity has been associated with brain tissue development, vascular remodeling, cell migration, neuron viability, tumor development, and vascular invasion in the central nervous system. In normal cerebral tissue, t-PA antigen is associated with microvessels similar in size to those of the vasa vasorum of the aorta.[30] Expression of PA activity has been reported in nonischemic tissues of mice, spontaneously hypertensive and Wistar-Kyoto rats, and primates.[144,145] Tissue-type PA and u-PA are secreted by endothelial cells, neurons, astrocytes, and microglia in vivo or in vitro.[77-84] Urokinase-type PA mRNA is expressed in neurons and oligodendrocytes during process outgrowth in the rodent brain.[146] Although t-PA is expressed by neurons in many brain regions, extracellular proteolysis seems confined to specific, discrete brain regions.[147] Studies suggesting that t-PA mediates hippocampal neurodegeneration during excitotoxicity or following focal cerebral ischemia[148] have opened a discussion about whether PAs play roles in cellular viability outside the fibrinolytic system. Conflicting evidence of greater injury by t-PA in the hippocampus has been balanced against credible reports of no effect or infarct volume reduction in rodent models of focal cerebral ischemia (see later).[148,149]

PLASMINOGEN ACTIVATORS IN EXPERIMENTAL CEREBRAL ISCHEMIA

A limited number of experimental studies have tested the ability of PAs to increase arterial recanalization. Improved clinical (behavioral and/or neurologic) outcomes have been attributed to rodent models of focal cerebral ischemia treated with PAs (mostly rt-PA) very soon after thromboembolism.[150-153] Early infusion of rt-PA in a rabbit multiple-thromboembolism model demonstrated significant improvement in clinical outcome in comparison with untreated controls.[150] The use of rt-PA with putative inhibitors of polymorphonuclear leukocyte adhesion support this notion, although differences among rt-PA cohorts were observed in various experimental sets.[154,155] In an rt-PA dose-rate study in a nonembolic nonhuman primate model of stroke, no significant difference in clinical outcome was observed, according to a motor-weighted semiquantitated neurologic outcome score, in comparison with controls.[156,157] However, another study demonstrated a significant reduction in infarction volume after reperfusion of the middle cerebral artery territory in a single model.[158]

Focal cerebral ischemia rapidly initiates greater expression of u-PA and PAI-1 within striatal tissue of the primate.[159,160] Tissue-type PA decreases transiently as it binds PAI-1, but otherwise does not change. Urokinase-type PA is an indirect activator of pro-MMP-2, which is also generated early following middle cerebral artery occlusion.[160] The appearance of these proteases coincides with degradation of the extracellular matrix of the ischemic microvascular bed.[161,162] It has been postulated that loss of basal lamina integrity contributes to hemorrhagic transformation of the evolving infarction.[161,163] Whether exogenous PAs contribute to the loss in microvessel integrity is under study.

PLASMINOGEN ACTIVATORS AND RECANALIZATION IN ISCHEMIC STROKE

Experimental and clinical studies indicate that timely restoration of blood flow to the ischemic cerebral parenchyma is required for improved clinical outcome. Angiographic studies have provided valuable information about the anatomy of the vasculature, the magnitude of thrombus burden, and the success of recanalization with PAs. A series of angiographic studies have demonstrated occlusion of the symptomatic arterial territory within hours of symptom onset.[3,164-168] Further studies have documented that u-PA and rt-PA can contribute to arterial reperfusion as anticipated by their known activities (Table 39.3).

The frequency of arterial recanalization appears to be greater when the PA is administered by the intra-arterial route than by intravenous delivery (see Table 39.3). This observation is consistent with the notion that enhanced efficacy may be due to the higher local concentration of the PA at the thrombus surface.

Only a handful of studies have prospectively compared recanalization rates in PA-treated patients with a control group.[4,164,169,170] In those studies, recanalization was significantly greater in patients receiving the PA for angiographically proven occlusion of the middle cerebral artery. In a phase II study of recombinant scu-PA (pro-UK), the recanalization frequency was significantly improved by the co-administration of a heparin dose.[164] Many, but not all, subjects in those studies in whom early recanalization was documented experienced clinical improvement. Lack of clinical improvement despite recanalization may be influenced by poor collateralization or increased time to reperfusion, although this issue is unproven.

Table 39.3 Plasminogen Activators in Acute Ischemic Stroke: Carotid Territory

Study	Year	Agent	Patients (n)	Δ (T-0)[a] (hours)	Recanalization (%)	Total Hemorrhage (%)	Symptomatic Hemorrhage (%)
Intra-arterial Delivery							
del Zoppo et al[1]	1988	SK/u-PA	20	<24	90.0	20.0	0.0
Mori et al[2]	1988	u-PA	22	<7	45.5	18.2	9.1
Matsumoto et al[172]	1991	u-PA	39	<24	59.0	33.3	—
PROACT[164]	1997	scu-PA/h	26	<6	57.7	42.3	15.4
		C/h	14	<6	14.3	7.1	7.1
Gönner et al[173]	1998	u-PA	33	<6	58.0	21.2	6.1
PROACT II[169]	1999	scu-PA/h	121	<6	65.7	35.2	10.2
		-/h (IV)	59	<6	18.0	13.0	1.8
Intravenous Delivery							
Yamaguchi[174]	1991	rt-PA	58	<6	43.1	20.7	—
von Kummer and Hacke[175]	1991	rt-PA	32	<6	53.1	37.5	9.4
del Zoppo et al[3]	1992	rt-PA	93 (104)[b]	<8	34.4	30.8	9.6
Mori et al[4]	1992	rt-PA	19	<6	47.4	52.6	—
		C	12		16.7	41.7	—
Yamaguchi et al[5]	1993	rt-PA	47 (51)	<6	21.3	47.1	7.8
		C	46 (47)		4.4	46.8	10.6

[a]time from symptom onset to treatment
[b]intention to treat
C, control or placebo; h, heparin; rt-PA, recombinant tissue-type plasminogen activator; IV, intravenous; scu-PA, single-chain urokinase-type plasminogen activator; SK, streptokinase; u-PA, urokinase-type plasminogen activator.

PLASMINOGEN ACTIVATORS AND CEREBRAL HEMORRHAGE

Administration of PAs in the acute period can be complicated by the development of symptomatic parenchymal hemorrhage. A number of randomized studies have documented the greater risk of symptomatic hemorrhage associated with intravenous thrombolysis.[6-8,171] Rates of symptomatic hemorrhage for hemispheric stroke in the cerebral artery territory range from 3.3% to 9.6% in this setting.[3,7,8,143,164] In addition, the development of symptomatic hemorrhage in rt-PA–treated patients contributed to mortality in properly controlled trials, including the National Institute of Neurological Disorders and Stroke (NINDS) study.[6-8] Clinical features that have been associated with higher risk of hemorrhage include advancing age and signs of early infarction on initial cranial computed tomography. Early signs of infarct may reflect otherwise undetectable injury to the matrix of the microvascular bed.[6-8]

Despite the higher risk of hemorrhage associated with rt-PA, a robust clinical benefit has been demonstrated with proper use of this agent.[6] The results of two randomized trials of intra-arterial recombinant scu-PA are consistent with an effect of anticoagulation (heparin) to increase the risk of symptomatic cerebral hemorrhage.[164,169] Heparin dosage was lowered in the early stages of the phase II trial, before a significant excess of symptomatic hemorrhages would have been observed. A significant increase in recanalization rate also occurred in patients receiving the higher heparin dose. Nonetheless, there is no evidence that the increase in hemorrhage associated with the use of PAs was related to greater recanalization. Early infusion of a PA in selected patients is associated, however, with a decrease in hemorrhage risk.[3]

The experimental and clinical experience supports the view that careful intervention with PAs immediately after the onset of symptoms of focal ischemia can result in significant functional recovery, despite a possible increase in hemorrhagic transformation. This body of clinical evidence is consistent with the known pharmacologic properties of plasminogen activators.

References

1. del Zoppo GJ, Ferbert A, Otis S, et al: Local intra-arterial fibrinolytic therapy in acute carotid territory stroke: A pilot study. Stroke 19:307–313, 1988.
2. Mori E, Tabuchi M, Yoshida T, Yamadori A: Intracarotid urokinase with thromboembolic occlusion of the middle cerebral artery. Stroke 19:802–812, 1988.
3. del Zoppo GJ, Poeck K, Pessin MS, et al: Recombinant tissue plasminogen activator in acute thrombotic and embolic stroke. Ann Neurol 32:78–86, 1992.
4. Mori E, Yoneda Y, Tabuchi M, et al: Intravenous recombinant tissue plasminogen activator in acute carotid artery territory stroke. Neurology 42:976–982, 1992.
5. Yamaguchi T, Hayakawa T, Kikuchi H: Intravenous tissue plasminogen activator ameliorates the outcome of hyperacute embolic stroke. Cerebrovasc Dis 3:269–272, 1993.
6. Tissue plasminogen activator for acute ischemic stroke. The National Institutes of Neurological Disorders and Stroke rt-PA Stroke Study Group. N Engl J Med 333:1581–1587, 1995.
7. Hacke W, Kaste M, Fieschi C, et al: Intravenous thrombolysis with recombinant tissue plasminogen activator for acute hemispheric stroke: The European Cooperative Acute Stroke Study (ECASS). The ECASS Study Group. JAMA 274:1017–1025, 1995.
8. Hacke W, Kaste M, Fieschi C, et al: Randomised double-blind placebo-controlled trial of thrombolytic therapy with intravenous alteplase in acute ischaemic stroke (ECASS II). The Second European-Australasian Acute Stroke Study Investigators. Lancet 352:1245–1251, 1998.
9. Sherry S: The history and development of thrombolytic therapy. In Comerota AJ (ed): Thrombolytic Therapy for Peripheral Vascular Disease. Philadelphia, JB Lippincott, 1995, pp 67–86.

10. Christensen LR, MacLeod CM: A proteolytic enzyme of serum: Characterization, activation, and reaction with inhibitors. J Gen Physiol 28:559–583, 1945.
11. Kaplan MH: Nature and role of the lytic factor in hemolytic streptococcal fibrinolysis. Proc Soc Exp Biol Med 57:40–43, 1944.
12. Tillett WS, Sherry S: The effect in patients of streptokinase fibrinolysis (streptokinase) and streptococcal deoxyribonuclease on fibrinous, purulent and sanguineous pleural exudations. J Clin Invest 28:173–190, 1949.
13. Johnson AJ, Tillett WS: Lysis in rabbits of intravascular blood clots by the streptococcal fibrinolytic system (streptokinase). J Exp Med 95:449–464, 1952.
14. Schwartz ML, Pizzo SV, Hill RL, McKee PA: Human factor XIII from plasma and platelets: Molecular weight, subunit structures, proteolytic activation and cross-linking of fibrinogen and fibrin. J Biol Chem 248:1395–1407, 1973.
15. Gaffney PJ, Whittaker AN: Fibrin cross-links and lysis rates. Thromb Res 14:85–94, 1979.
16. Hermans J, McDonagh J: Fibrin: Structure and interactions. Semin Thromb Hemost 8:11–24, 1982.
17. Davie EW, Fujikawa K, Kisiel W: The coagulation cascade: Initiation, maintenance, and regulation. Biochemistry 30:10363–10370, 1991.
18. Nossel HL: Relative proteolysis of fibrin B-beta chain by thrombin and plasmin as a determinant of thrombosis. Nature 291:754–762, 1981.
19. Alkjaersig N, Fletcher AP: Catabolism and excretion of fibrinopeptide A. Blood 60:148–156, 1982.
20. Majerus PW, Miletich JP, Kane WP, et al: The formation of thrombin on the platelet surface. In Mann KG, Taylor FB (eds): The Regulation of Coagulation. New York, Elsevier/North Holland, 1980, p 215.
21. Kaplan AP: Initiation of the intrinsic coagulation and fibrinolytic pathways of man: The role of surfaces, Hageman factor, prekallikrein, high molecular weight kininogen, and factor XI. Prog Hemost Thromb 4:127–175, 1978.
22. Nesheim ME, Hibbard LS, Tracy PB, et al: Participation of factor Va in prothrombinase. In Mann KG, Taylor FB (eds): The Regulation of Coagulation. New York, Elsevier/North Holland, 1980, pp 145–159.
23. Miletich JP, Jackson CM, Majerus PW: Properties of the factor Xa binding site on human platelets. J Biol Chem 253:6908–6916, 1978.
24. Levin EG, Marzec U, Anderson J, Harker LA: Thrombin stimulates tissue plasminogen activator release from cultured human endothelial cells. J Clin Invest 74:1988–1995, 1984.
25. Van Hinsbergh VWM: Regulation of the synthesis and secretion of plasminogen activators by endothelial cells. Haemostasis 18:307–327, 1988.
26. Liesi P, Kirkwood T, Vaheri A: Fibronectin is expressed by astrocytes cultured from embryonic and early postnatal rat brain. Exp Cell Res 163:175–185, 1986.
27. Giles AR, Nosheim ME, Herring SW, et al: The fibrinolytic potential of the normal primate following the generation of thrombin in vivo. Thromb Haemost 63:476–481, 1990.
28. Nawroth PP, Stern DM: Endothelial cells as active participants in procoagulant reactions. In Gimbrone MA (ed): Vascular Endothelium in Hemostasis and Thrombosis. Edinburgh, Churchill Livingstone, 1986, pp 14–39.
29. Collen D, de Maeyer L: Molecular biology of human plasminogen. I: Physicochemical properties and microheterogeneity. Thromb Diath Haemorrhag 34:396–402, 1975.
30. Levin EG, del Zoppo GJ: Localization of tissue plasminogen activator in the endothelium of a limited number of vessels. Am J Pathol 144:855–861, 1994.
31. Gaffney PJ, Lane DA, Kakkar VV, Brahser M: Characterization of a soluble D-dimer-E complex in cross-linked fibrin digests. Thromb Res 7:89–99, 1975.
32. Plow EF, Felez J, Miles LA: Cellular regulation of fibrinolysis. Thromb Haemost 66:132–136, 1991.
33. Bachmann F, Kruithof IEKO: Tissue plasminogen activator: Chemical and physiological aspects. Semin Thromb Hemost 10:6–17, 1984.
34. Aoki N, Harpel PC: Inhibitors of the fibrinolytic enzyme system. Semin Thromb Hemost 10:24–41, 1984.
35. Collen D, Lijnen HR: New approaches to thrombolytic therapy. Arteriosclerosis 4:579–585, 1984.
36. Verstraete M, Collen D: Thrombolytic therapy in the eighties. Blood 67:1529–1541, 1986.
37. Forsgren M, Raden B, Israelsson M, et al: Molecular cloning and characterization of a full-length cDNA clone for human plasminogen. FEBS Lett 213:254–260, 1987.
38. Bachmann F: Molecular aspects of plasminogen, plasminogen activators and plasmin. In Bloom AL, Forbes CD, Thomas DP, Tuddenham EGD (eds): Haemostasis and Thrombosis. Edinburgh, Churchill Livingstone, 1994, pp 575–613.
39. Peterson LC, Serenson E: Effect of plasminogen and tissue-type plasminogen activator on fibrin gel structure. Fibrinolysis 5:51–59, 1990.
40. Tran-Thong C, Kruithof EKO, Atkinson J, Bachmann F: High-affinity binding sites for human glu-plasminogen unveiled by limited plasmic degradation of human fibrin. Eur J Biochem 160:559–604, 1986.
41. Wallen P, Wiman B: Characterization of human plasminogen. II: Separation and partial characterization of different molecular forms of human plasminogen. Biochim Biophys Acta 257:122–134, 1973.
42. Holvoet P, Lijnen HR, Collen D: A monoclonal antibody specific for lys-plasminogen: Application to the study of the activation pathways of plasminogen in vivo. J Biol Chem 260:12106–12111, 1985.
43. Thorsen S, Mullertz S, Svenson E, Kok P: Sequence of formation of molecular forms of plasminogen and plasminogen-inhibitor complexes in plasma activated by urokinase or tissue-type plasminogen activator. Biochem J 223:179–187, 1984.
44. Miles LA, Greengard JS, Griffin JH: A comparison of the abilities of plasma kallikrein, beta-factor XIIa, factor XIa and urokinase to activate plasminogen. Thromb Res 29:407–417, 1983.
45. Kluft C, Dooijewaard G, Emeis JJ: Role of the contact system in fibrinolysis. Semin Thromb Hemost 13:50–68, 1987.
46. Wun TC, Ossowski L, Reich E: A proenzyme of human urokinase. J Biol Chem 257:7262–2768, 1982.
47. Wun TC, Schleuning E, Reich E: Isolation and characterization of urokinase from human plasma. J Biol Chem 257:3276–3287, 1982.
48. Ichinose A, Fujikawa K, Suyama T: The activation of pro-urokinase by plasma kallikrein and its inactivation by thrombin. J Biol Chem 261:3486–3489, 1986.
49. Hanss M, Collen D: Secretion of tissue-type plasminogen activator and plasminogen activator inhibitor by cultured human endothelial cells: Modulation by thrombin endotoxin and histamine. J Lab Clin Med 109:97–104, 1987.
50. Levin EG, Stern DM, Nawrath PP, et al: Specificity of the thrombin-induced release of tissue plasminogen activator from cultured human endothelial cells. Thromb Haemost 56:115–119, 1986.
51. Robbins KC, Summaria L, Hsieh B, Shah RJ: The peptide chains of human plasmin. J Biochem 242:2333–2342, 1967.
52. Robbins KC: The plasminogen-plasmin system. In Comerota AJ (ed): Thrombolytic Therapy for Peripheral Vascular Disease. Philadelphia, JB Lippincott, 1995, pp 41–65.
53. Wiman B, Collen D: Molecular mechanism of physiological fibrinolysis. Nature 272:549–550, 1979.
54. Collen D: On the regulation and control of fibrinolysis. Thromb Haemost 43:77–89, 1980.
55. Hoylaerts M, Rijken DC, Lijnen HR, Collen D: Kinetics of the activation of plasminogen by human tissue plasminogen activator: Role of fibrin. J Biol Chem 257:2912–2919, 1982.
56. Wun T-C, Capugno A: Initiation and regulation of fibrinolysis in human plasma at the plasminogen activator level. Blood 69:1354–1362, 1987.
57. Bloom AL, Thomas DP: Haemostasis and Thrombosis. Edinburgh, Churchill-Livingstone, 1987.
58. Kakkar VV, Scully MF: Thrombolytic therapy. Br Med Bull 34:191–199, 1978.
59. Sharma GVRK, Cella G, Parish AF, Sasahara AA: Drug therapy: Thrombolytic therapy. N Engl J Med 306:1268–1276, 1982.
60. Verstraete M: Biochemical and clinical aspects of thrombolysis. Semin Hematol 15:35–54, 1978.
61. Castellino FJ: Biochemistry of human plasminogen. Semin Thromb Hemost 10:18–23, 1984.
62. Yasaka M, Yamaguchi T, Miyashita T, Tsuchiya T: Regression of intracardiac thrombus after embolic stroke. Stroke 21:1540–1544, 1990.
63. Bounameaux H, de Moerloose P, Perrier A, Reber G: Plasma measurement of D-dimer as diagnostic aid in suspected venous thromboembolism: An overview. Thromb Haemost 71:1–6, 1994.

Pathophysiology

64. Pennica D, Holmes WE, Kohr WJ, et al: Cloning and expression of human tissue-type plasminogen activator cDNA in *E. coli*. Nature 301:214–221, 1983.

65. Rijken DC: Structure/function relationships of t-PA. In Kluft C (ed): Tissue Type Plasminogen Activator (t-PA): Physiological and Clinical Aspects, Vol 1. Boca Raton, FL, CRC Press, 1988, pp 101–122.

66. Ehrlich HJ, Bang NW, Little SP, et al: Biological properties of a kringleless tissue plasminogen activator (t-PA) mutant. Fibrinolysis 1:75–81, 1987.

67. Gelehrter TD, Sznycer-Laszuk R: Thrombin induction of plasminogen activator-inhibitor in cultured human endothelial cells. J Clin Invest 77:165–169, 1986.

68. Sakata Y, Curriden S, Lawrence D, et al: Activated protein C stimulates the fibrinolytic activity of cultured endothelial cells and decreases antiactivator activity. Proc Natl Acad Sci U S A 82:1121–1125, 1985.

69. Moscatelli D: Urokinase-type and tissue-type plasminogen activators have different distributions in cultured bovine capillary endothelial cells. J Cell Biochem 30:19–29, 1986.

70. Bulens F, Nelles L, Van den Panhuyzen N, Collen D: Stimulation by retinoids of tissue-type plasminogen activator secretion in cultured human endothelial cells: Relations of structure to effect. J Cardiovasc Pharmacol 19:508–514, 1992.

71. Thompson EA, Nelles L, Collen D: Effect of retinoic acid on the synthesis of tissue-type plasminogen activator and plasminogen activator inhibitor-I in human endothelial cells. Eur J Biochem 201:627–632, 1991.

72. Saksela O, Moscatelli D, Rifkin DB: The opposing effects of basic fibroblast growth factor and transforming growth factor beta on the regulation of plasminogen activator activity in capillary endothelial cells. J Cell Biol 105:957–963, 1987.

73. Levin EG, Marotti KR, Santell L: Protein kinase C and the stimulation of tissue plasminogen activator release from human endothelial cells: Dependence on the elevation of messenger RNA. J Biol Chem 264:16030–16036, 1989.

74. Smith D, Gilbert M, Owen WG: Tissue plasminogen activator release in vivo in response to vasoactive agents. Blood 66:835–839, 1985.

75. Brommer EJP: Clinical relevance of t-PA levels of fibrinolytic assays. In Kluft C (ed): Tissue-Type Plasminogen Activator (t-PA): Physiological and Clinical Aspects, Vol 1, Part 2. Boca Raton, FL, CRC Press, 1988, p 89.

76. Agnelli G: The pharmacological basis of thrombolytic therapy. In Agnelli G (ed): Thrombolysis Yearbook 1995. Amsterdam, Excerpta Medica, 1995, pp 31–61.

77. Krystosek A, Seeds NW: Normal and malignant cells, including neurons, deposit plasminogen activator on growth substrata. Exp Cell Res 166:31–46, 1986.

78. Pittman RN: Release of plasminogen activator and a calcium-dependent metalloprotease from cultured sympathetic and sensory neurons. Dev Biol 110:91–101, 1985.

79. Vincent VA, Lowik CW, Verheijen JH, et al: Role of astrocyte-derived tissue-type plasminogen activator in the regulation of endotoxin-stimulated nitric oxide production by microglial cells. Glia 22:130–137, 1998.

80. Toshniwal PK, Firestone SL, Barlow GH, Tiku ML: Characterization of astrocyte plasminogen activator. J Neurol Sci 80:277–287, 1987.

81. Tsirka SE, Rogove AD, Bugge TH, et al: An extracellular proteolytic cascade promotes neuronal degeneration in the mouse hippocampus. J Neurosci 17:543–552, 1997.

82. Masos T, Miskin R: Localization of urokinase-type plasminogen activator mRNA in the adult mouse brain. Brain Res Mol Brain Res 35:139–148, 1996.

83. Tranque P, Naftolin F, Robbins R: Differential regulation of astrocyte plasminogen activators by insulin-like growth factor-I and epidermal growth factor. Endocrinology 134:2606–2613, 1994.

84. Nakajima K, Tsuzaki N, Shimojo M, et al: Microglia isolated from rat brain secrete a urokinase-type plasminogen activator. Brain Res 577:285–292, 1992.

85. Lijnen HR, Zamarron C, Blaber M, et al: Activation of plasminogen by pro-urokinase. I: Mechanism. J Biol Chem 261:1253–1258, 1986.

86. Peterson LC, Lund LR, Nielsen LS, et al: One-chain urokinase-type plasminogen activator from human sarcoma cells is a proenzyme with little or no intrinsic activity. J Biol Chem 263:11189–11195, 1988.

87. Gunzler WA, Steffens GJ, Otting F, et al: Structural relationship between human high and low molecular mass urokinase. Hoppe Seylers Z Physiol Chem 563:133–141, 1982.

88. White FW, Barlow GH, Mozen MM: The isolation and characterization of plasminogen activators (urokinase) from human urine. Biochemistry 5:2160–2169, 1966.

89. Fletcher AP, Alkjaersig N, Sherry S, et al: The development of urokinase as a thrombolytic agent: Maintenance of a sustained thrombolytic state in man by its intravenous infusion. J Lab Clin Med 65:713–731, 1965.

90. Stump DC, Mann KH: Mechanisms of thrombus formation and lysis. Ann Emerg Med 17:1138–1147, 1988.

91. Davies MC, Englert ME, De Rezo EC: Interaction of streptokinase and human plasminogen observed in the ultracentrifuge under a variety of experimental conditions. J Biol Chem 239:2651–2656, 1964.

92. Reddy KN, Marcus B: Mechanisms of activation of human plasminogen by streptokinase. J Biol Chem 246:1683–1691, 1972.

93. Standing R, Fears R, Ferres H: The protective effect of acylation on the stability of APSAC (Eminase) in human plasma. Fibrinolysis 2:157, 1988.

94. Ferres H: Preclinical pharmacological evaluation of Eminase (APSAC). Drugs 33(Suppl 3):33–50, 1987.

95. Lijnen HR, de Cock F, Matsuo O, Collen D: Comparative fibrinolytic and fibrinogenolytic properties of staphylokinase and streptokinase in plasma of different species in vitro. Fibrinolysis 6:33–37, 1992.

96. Collen D: Staphylokinase: A potent, uniquely fibrin-selective thrombolytic agent. Nat Med 4:279–282, 1998.

97. Jespers L, Vanwetswinkel S, Lijnen HR, et al: Structural and functional basis of plasminogen activation by staphylokinase. Thromb Haemost 81:479–484, 1999.

98. Lijnen HR, Van Hoef B, Matsuo O, Collen D: On the molecular interactions between plasminogen-staphylokinase, α_2-antiplasmin and fibrin. Biochim Biophys Acta 1118:144–148, 1992.

99. Witt W, Maass B, Baldus B, et al: Coronary thrombosis with *Desmodus* salivary plasminogen activator in dogs: Fast and persistent recanalization by intravenous bolus administration. Circulation 90:421–426, 1994.

100. Hare TR, Gardell SJ: Vampire bat salivary plasminogen activator promotes robust lysis of plasma clots in a plasma milieu without causing fluid phase plasminogen activation. Thromb Haemost 68:165–169, 1992.

101. Bergum PW, Gardell SJ: Vampire bat salivary plasminogen activator exhibits a strict and fastidious requirement for polymeric fibrin as its cofactor, unlike human tissue-type plasminogen activator: A kinetic analysis. J Biol Chem 267:17726–17731, 1992.

102. Mellot MJ, Stabilito II, Holahan MA, et al: Vampire bat salivary plasminogen activator promotes rapid and sustained reperfusion without concomitant systemic plasminogen activation in a canine model of arterial thrombosis. Arterioscler Thromb 12:212–221, 1992.

103. Witt W, Baldus B, Bringmann P, et al: Thrombolytic properties of *Desmodus rotundus* (vampire bat) salivary plasminogen activator in experimental pulmonary embolism in rats. Blood 79:1213–1217, 1992.

104. Lijnen HR, Collen D: Development of new fibrinolytic agents. In Bloom AL, Forbes CD, Thomas DP, Tuddenham EGD (eds): Haemostasis and Thrombosis. Edinburgh, Churchill Livingstone, 1994, pp 625–637.

105. Van de Werf F: New thrombolytic strategies. Aust N Z J Med 23:763–765, 1993.

106. Smalling RW: Pharmacological and clinical impact of the unique molecular structure of a new plasminogen activator. Eur Heart J 18(Suppl F):F11–F16, 1997.

107. Benedict CR, Refino CJ, Keyt BA, et al: New variant of human tissue plasminogen activator (TPA) with enhanced efficacy and lower incidence of bleeding compared with recombinant human TPA. Circulation 92:3032–3040, 1995.

108. Kohnert U, Horsch B, Fischer S: A variant of tissue plasminogen activator (t-PA) comprised of the kringle 2 and the protease domain shows a significant difference in the in vitro rate of plasmin formation as compared to the recombinant human t-PA from transformed Chinese hamster ovary cells. Fibrinolysis 7:365–372, 1993.

109. Fischer S, Kohnert U: Major mechanistic differences explain the higher clot lysis potency of reteplase over alteplase: Lack of fibrin

Pathophysiology

binding is an advantage for bolus application of fibrin-specific thrombolytics. Fibrinolysis Proteolysis 11:129–135, 1997.

110. Refino C, Paoni N, Keyt B, et al: A variant of t-PA T103N, KHRR 296–299 AAAA, that, by bolus, has increased potency and decreased systemic activation of plasminogen. Thromb Haemost 70:313–319, 1993.

111. Paoni N, Keyt B, Refino C, et al: A slow clearing, fibrin-specific, PAI-1 resistant variant of t-PA T103N, KHRR 296–299 AAAA. Thromb Haemost 70:307–312, 1993.

112. Keyt B, Paoni N, Refino C, et al: A faster-acting and more potent form of tissue plasminogen activator. Proc Natl Acad Sci U S A 91:3670–3674, 1994.

113. Kawai C, Suzuki S: Monteplase: Pharmacological and clinical experience. In Sasahara A (ed): New Therapeutic Agents in Thrombosis and Thrombolysis. New York, Marcel Dekker, 2002, pp 525–540.

114. Katoh M, Suzuki Y, Miyamoto I, et al: Biochemical and pharmacokinetic properties of YM866, a novel fibrinolytic agent. Thromb Haemost 65:1193, 1991.

115. Katoh M, Shimizu Y, Kawauchi Y, et al: Comparison of clearance rate of various tissue plasminogen activator (t-PA) analogues. Thromb Haemost 62:542, 1989.

116. Modi NB, Eppler S, Breed J, et al: Pharmacokinetics of a slower clearing tissue plasminogen activator variant, TNK-tPA, in patients with acute myocardial infarction. Thromb Haemost 79:134–139, 1998.

117. Runge MS, Bode C, Matsueda GR, Haber E: Antibody-enhanced thrombolysis: Targeting of tissue plasminogen activator in vivo. Proc Natl Acad Sci U S A 84:7659–7662, 1987.

118. Kasper W, Meinertz T, Hohnloser S, et al: Coronary thrombolysis in man with prourokinase: Improved efficacy with low dose urokinase. Klin Wochenschr 66:109–114, 1988.

119. Pierard L, Jacobs P, Gheysen D, et al: Mutant and chimeric recombinant plasminogen activators. J Biol Chem 262:11771–11778, 1987.

120. Bode C, Meinhardt G, Runge MS, et al: Platelet-targeted fibrinolysis enhances clot lysis and inhibits platelet aggregation. Circulation 84:805–813, 1991.

121. Jones RD, Donaldson IM, Parkin PJ: Impairment and recovery of ipsilateral sensory-motor function following unilateral cerebral infarction. Brain 112:113–132, 1989.

122. Bachmann F: Fibrinolysis. In Verstraete M, Vermylen J, Lijnen HR, Arnout J (eds): Thrombosis and Haemostasis. Leuven, ISTH/University of Leuven Press, 1987, pp 227–265.

123. Kluft C, Los N: Demonstration of two forms of α_2-antiplasmin in plasma by modified crossed immunoelectrophoresis. Thromb Res 21:65–71, 1981.

124. Winman B, Nilsson T, Cedergren B: Studies on a form of α_2-antiplasmin in plasma which does not interact with the lysine-binding sites in plasminogen. Thromb Res 28:193–200, 1982.

125. Aoki N, Harpel P: Inhibitors of the fibrinolytic enzyme system. Semin Hemostat Thromb 10:24–39, 1984.

126. Philips M, Juul AG, Thorsen S: Human endothelial cells produce a plasminogen activator inhibitor and a tissue-type plasminogen activator-inhibitor complex. Biochim Biophys Acta 802:99–110, 1984.

127. Loskutoff DJ, van Mourik JA, Erickson LA, Lawrence DA: Detection of an unusually stable fibrinolytic inhibitor produced by bovine endothelial cells. Proc Natl Acad Sci U S A 80:2956–2960, 1983.

128. Thorsen S, Philips M, Selmer J, et al: Kinetics of inhibition of tissue-type and urokinase-type plasminogen activator by plasminogen-activator inhibitor type 1 and type 2. Eur J Biochem 175:33–39, 1988.

129. Wilhelm OG, Jaskunas SR, Vlahos CJ, Bang NU: Functional properties of the recombinant kringle-2 domain of tissue plasminogen activator produced in Escherichia coli. J Biol Chem 265:14606–14611, 1990.

130. Juhan-Vague I, Moerman B, de Cock F, et al: Plasma levels of a specific inhibitor of tissue-type plasminogen activator (and urokinase) in normal and pathological conditions. Thromb Res 33:523–530, 1984.

131. Schleuning W-D, Medcalf RL, Hession C, et al: Plasminogen activator inhibitor 2: Regulation of gene transcription during phorbol ester-mediated differentiation of U-937 human histiocytic lymphoma cells. Mol Cell Biol 7:4564–4567, 1987.

132. Kruithof EKO, Tran-Thang C, Gudinchet A, et al: Fibrinolysis in pregnancy: A study of plasminogen activator inhibitors. Blood 69:460–466, 1987.

133. Bonnar J, Daly L, Sheppard BL: Changes in the fibrinolytic system during pregnancy. Semin Thromb Hemost 16:221–229, 1990.

134. Stump D, Thienpoint M, Collén D: Purification and characterization of a novel inhibitor of urokinase from human urine: Quantitation and preliminary characterization in plasma. J Biol Chem 261:12759–12766, 1986.

135. Heeb MJ, Espana F, Geiger M, et al: Immunological identity of heparin-dependent plasma and urinary protein C inhibitor and plasminogen activator inhibitor-3. J Biol Chem 262:15813–15816, 1987.

136. Bajzar L, Manuel R, Neshaim M: Purification and characterization of TAFI, a thrombin-activatable fibrinolysis inhibitor. J Biol Chem 270:14477–14484, 1995.

137. Marder VJ, Sherry S: Thrombolytic therapy: Current status (Parts 1 and 2). N Engl J Med 388:1512–1520; 1585–1595, 1988.

138. Gimple LW, Gold HK, Leinbach RC, et al: Correlation between template bleeding times and spontaneous bleeding during treatment of acute myocardial infarction with recombinant tissue plasminogen activator. Circulation 80:581–588, 1989.

139. Agnelli G, Buchanan MR, Fernandez F, et al: A comparison of the thrombolytic and hemorrhagic effects of tissue-type plasminogen activator and streptokinase in rabbits. Circulation 72:178–182, 1985.

140. Marder VJ, Shortell CK, Fitzpatrick PG, et al: An animal model of fibrinolytic bleeding based on the rebleed phenomenon: Application to a study of vulnerability of hemostatic plugs of different age. Thromb Res 67:31–40, 1992.

141. Loscalzo J, Vaughan DB: Tissue plasminogen activator promotes platelet disaggregation in plasma. J Clin Invest 79:1749–1755, 1987.

142. Chen LY, Muhta JL: Lys- and glu-plasminogen potentiate the inhibitory effect of recombinant tissue plasminogen activator on human platelet aggregation. Thromb Res 74:555–563, 1994.

143. Albers GW, Bates VE, Clark WM, et al: Intravenous tissue-type plasminogen activator for treatment of acute stroke: The Standard Treatment with Alteplase to Reverse Stroke (STARS) study. JAMA 283:1145–1150, 2000.

144. Danglet G, Vinson D, Chapeville F: Qualitative and quantitative distribution of plasminogen activators in organs from healthy adult mice. FEBS Lett 194:96–100, 1986.

145. Matsuo O, Okada K, Fukao H, et al: Cerebral plasminogen activator activity in spontaneously hypertensive stroke-prone rats. Stroke 23:995–999, 1992.

146. Dent MA, Sumi Y, Morris RJ, Seeley PJ: Urokinase-type plasminogen activator expression by neurons and oligodendrocytes during process outgrowth in developing rat brain. Eur J Neurosci 5:633–647, 1993.

147. Sappino A-P, Madani R, Huarte J, et al: Extracellular proteolysis in the adult murine brain. J Clin Invest 92:679–685, 1993.

148. Wang YF, Tsirka SE, Strickland S, et al: Tissue plasminogen activator (tPA) increases neuronal damage after focal cerebral ischemia in wild-type and tPA-deficient mice. Nat Med 4:228–231, 1998.

149. del Zoppo GJ: t-PA: A neuron buster, too [editorial]? Nat Med 4:148–150, 1998.

150. Zivin JA, Fisher M, DeGirolami U, et al: Tissue plasminogen activator reduced neurological damage after cerebral embolism. Science 230:1289–1292, 1985.

151. Zivin J, Fisher M, DeGirolami U, et al: Tissue plasminogen activator reduces neurological damage after cerebral embolism. Science 230:1289–1292, 1985.

152. Overgaard K, Sereghy T, Boysen G, et al: Reduction of infarct volume by thrombolysis with rt-PA in an embolic rat stroke model. Scand J Clin Lab Invest 53:383–393, 1993.

153. Hamann GF, del Zoppo GJ: Leukocyte involvement in vasomotor reactivity of the cerebral vasculature. Stroke 25:2117–2119, 1994.

154. Kunkel EJ, Jung U, Bullard DC, et al: Absence of trauma-induced leukocyte rolling in mice deficient in both P-selectin and intercellular adhesion molecule 1. J Exp Med 183:57–65, 1996.

155. Bowes MP, Rothlein R, Fagan SC, Zivin JA: Monoclonal antibodies preventing leukocyte activation reduce experimental neurologic injury and enhance efficacy of thrombolytic therapy. Neurology 45:815–819, 1995.

156. Spetzler RF, Selman WR, Weinstein P, et al: Chronic reversible cerebral ischemia: Evaluation of a new baboon model. J Neurosurg 7:257–261, 1980.

157. del Zoppo GJ, Copeland BR, Anderchek K, et al: Hemorrhagic transformation following tissue plasminogen activator in experimental cerebral infarction. Stroke 21:596–601, 1990.

158. Young AR, Touzani O, Derlon J-M, et al: Early reperfusion in the anesthetized baboon reduces brain damage following middle cere-

Pathophysiology

bral artery occlusion: A quantitative analysis of infarction volume. Stroke 28:632–638, 1997.

159. Heo JH, Lucero J, Abumiya T, et al: Matrix metalloproteinases increase very early during experimental focal cerebral ischemia. J Cereb Blood Flow Metab 19:624–633, 1999.

160. Hosomi N, Lucero J, Heo JH, et al: Rapid differential endogenous plasminogen activator expression after acute middle cerebral artery occlusion. Stroke 32:1341–1348, 2001.

161. Hamann GF, Okada Y, Fitridge R, del Zoppo GJ: Microvascular basal lamina antigens disappear during cerebral ischemia and reperfusion. Stroke 26:2120–2126, 1995.

162. Wagner S, Tagaya M, Koziol JA, et al: Rapid disruption of an astrocyte interaction with the extracellular matrix mediated by integrin $\alpha_6\beta_4$ during focal cerebral ischemia/reperfusion. Stroke 28:858–865, 1997.

163. Hamann GF, Okada Y, del Zoppo GJ: Hemorrhagic transformation and microvascular integrity during focal cerebral ischemia/reperfusion. J Cereb Blood Flow Metab 16:1373–1378, 1996.

164. del Zoppo GJ, Higashida RT, Furlan AJ, et al: PROACT: A phase II randomized trial of recombinant pro-urokinase by direct arterial delivery in acute middle cerebral artery stroke. The PROACT Investigators. Prolyse in Acute Cerebral Thromboembolism. Stroke 29:4–11, 1998.

165. Fieschi C, Argentino C, Lenzi GL, et al: Clinical and instrumental evaluation of patients with ischemic stroke within the first six hours. J Neurol Sci 91:311–321, 1989.

166. Solis OJ, Roberson GR, Taveras JM, et al: Cerebral angiography in acute cerebral infarction. Revist Interam Radiol 2:19–25, 1977.

167. Fieschi C, Bozzao L: Transient embolic occlusion of the middle cerebral and internal carotid arteries in cerebral apoplexy. J Neurol Neurosurg Psychiatry 32:236–240, 1969.

168. Irino T, Taneda M, Minami T: Angiographic manifestations in post-recanalized cerebral infarction. Neurology 27:471–475, 1977.

169. Furlan A, Higashida R, Wechsler L, et al: Intra-arterial prourokinase for acute ischemic stroke: The PROACT II Study: A randomized controlled trial. The PROACT Investigators. Prolyse in Acute Cerebral Thromboembolism. JAMA 282:2003–2011, 1999.

170. Yamaguchi T: Intravenous tissue plasminogen activator in acute thromboembolic stroke: A placebo-controlled, double-blind trial. In del Zoppo GJ, Mori E, Hacke W (eds): Thrombolytic Therapy in Acute Ischemic Stroke II. Heidelberg, Springer-Verlag, 1993, pp 59–65.

171. Clark WM, Wissman SAGW, Jhamandas JH, et al: Recombinant tissue-type plasminogen activator (alteplase) for ischemic stroke 3 to 5 hours after symptom onset. The ATLANTIS Study: A randomized controlled trial. Alteplase Thrombolysis for Acute Noninterventional Therapy in Ischemic Stroke. JAMA 282:2019–2026, 1999.

172. Matsumoto K, Satoh K: Topical intraarterial urokinase infusion for acute stroke. In Hacke W, del Zoppo GJ, Hirschberg M (eds): Thrombolytic Therapy in Acute Ischemic Stroke. Heidelberg, Springer-Verlag, 1991, pp 207–212.

173. Gonner F, Remonda L, Mattle H, et al: Local intra-arterial thrombolysis in acute ischemic stroke. Stroke 29:1894–1900, 1998.

174. Yamaguchi T: Intravenous rt-PA in acute embolic stroke. In Hacke W, del Zoppo GJ, Hirschberg M (eds): Thrombolytic Therapy in Acute Ischemic Stroke. Heidelberg, Springer-Verlag, 1991, pp 168–174.

175. von Kummer R, Hacke W: Safety and efficacy of intravenous tissue plasminogen activator and heparin in acute middle cerebral artery. Stroke 23:646–652, 1992.

Chapter Forty

Cerebral Blood Flow and Metabolism in Human Cerebrovascular Disease

Allyson R. Zazulia, Joanne Markham, and William J. Powers

ENERGY METABOLISM AND NORMAL CEREBRAL HEMODYNAMICS

Although brain cells do not perform mechanical work or external secretory activity, their metabolic energy requirements are substantial, accounting for about 20% of the total body basal oxygen consumption. Energy in the brain is used for maintenance of the membrane potential and ionic transport, maintenance of cell structure, biosynthesis and transport of neurotransmitters, and biosynthesis and transport of cellular elements. The brain performs work at the expense of adenosine triphosphate (ATP) energy, which it obtains by degrading exogenous compounds with a high energy content (primarily glucose) to simpler compounds with less energy content (CO_2 and H_2O). Because storage of substrates for energy metabolism in the brain is minimal, the brain is highly dependent on a continuous supply of oxygen and glucose from the blood for its functional and structural integrity and is exquisitely sensitive to even brief disturbances in this supply. Thus, in cardiac arrest, for example, complete interruption of the cerebral circulation results in loss of consciousness within 10 seconds.[1]

Methods of Measurement

Cerebral Blood Flow

Cerebral blood flow (CBF) is measured as volume of blood delivered to a defined mass of tissue per unit time, usually $mL/100\,g^{-1}/min^{-1}$. Quantitative CBF measurement methods employ an indicator that is introduced into the blood as a tracer for flow to the brain. Such indicators commonly are externally administered compounds that can be detected by radiation detection or other imaging devices. However, with some magnetic resonance or near infrared methods, an endogenous substance such as water or oxyhemoglobin may be used. The use of tracers to measure CBF requires a mathematical model that relates the measurement of the tracer to CBF. Although an increasing number of mathematical techniques are used to measure CBF, most are based on one of three fundamental tracer kinetic principles: the Fick principle, the central volume principle, and the compartmental principle.

Fick Principle

The Fick principle states that the change in the quantity of substrate in an organ $q(t)$ is equal to the arterial flow F times the arterial concentration $C_A(t)$ minus the venous flow times the venous concentration $C_V(t)$.[2,3] Because arterial flow equals venous flow, the equation can be written as follows:

1.
$$\frac{dq(t)}{dt} = F[C_A(t) - C_V(t)].$$

One can obtain $q(T)$, the total amount of tracer taken up by the brain at time T, by integrating Equation 1. When $q(0) = 0$, the following equation applies:

2.
$$F = \frac{q(T)}{\int_0^T (C_A(t) - C_V(t))dt}.$$

With this equation, the following three quantities must be known so as to compute flow: $q(T)$, $C_A(t)$, and $C_V(t)$.

The Fick principle was the basis for the first technique used to measure quantitative CBF in human subjects developed by Kety and Schmidt.[2] The Kety-Schmidt technique uses an inert inhaled gas (originally nitrous oxide in low concentration) as the tracer. Arterial and jugular venous concentrations are measured directly during the period of inhalation to determine the integral of the arterial-venous difference. Because Kety and Schmidt[2] could not directly measure $q(T)$ in the living human brain, they used a clever alternative approach to determine its value. First, they determined the value for the ratio of brain-to-blood nitrous oxide concentrations at equilibrium (the partition coefficient) in vitro. Then they multiplied the partition coefficient by the equilibrium blood concentration to determine $q(T)$ per unit brain volume.

The original Kety-Schmidt method permits only whole brain measurements in $mL/100 g^{-1}/min^{-1}$. Different adaptations of the Fick principle can be used to derive regional CBF measurements. Microsphere methods use tracers that are physically or metabolically trapped in the tissue, so that $C_V(t)$ is 0. The arterial concentration integral is measured directly. Regional tracer quantity $q(T)$ is measured directly by organ dissection[4] or by external radiation detection systems like single-photon emission computed tomography (SPECT).[5]

Autoradiographic techniques employ radioactive inert tracers that freely diffuse out of the blood into the brain.[6] Assuming instantaneous equilibration of the tracer in venous space with tissue tracer, the venous concentration can be expressed in terms of the tissue concentration $C_T(t)$ or amount through the following equation:

3.
$$C_V(t) = C_T(t)/\lambda = q(t)/(V_T\lambda)$$

where λ is the partition coefficient and V_T is the tissue volume. As with the microsphere method, the arterial time-radioactivity curve is measured directly, and the regional tracer quantity is measured by organ dissection or by external radiation detection systems like positron emission tomography (PET) or SPECT.

Central Volume Principle

The central volume principle is based on the concept of transit time. If a bolus of a tracer is introduced into arterial blood flowing through tissue, the tracer particles flow through and then out the venous drainage on the other side.[7] Because all particles do not take the same path, they need different times to transit the tissue. The mean transit time $\bar{t}$ for the particles is determined by the volume in which the tracer is distributed V_d and the flow F through the tissue, as follows:

4.
$$\bar{t} = \frac{V_d}{F}.$$

The mean transit time can be determined by measuring the total amount of tracer injected q_0 and the residue amount that remains in the tissue as a function of time $q(t)$, as follows:

5.
$$\bar{t} = \frac{\int_0^\infty q(t)dt}{q_0}.$$

With radioactive tracers, the residue function in the brain can be measured with external radiation detection devices. The integral of the residue function over time is equal to the numerator in equation 5. If the volume of the tracer injection is small enough and the injection is fast enough, all the tracer going to the tissue region under study is measured by the external detector during the initial portion of the residue curve. Thus, the initial height is equal to q_0. External radiation detection devices do not measure all the radioactivity emitted; some is absorbed by the tissue, and some exits the brain at angles not covered by the detector crystals. However, the efficiency of

detection e is the same for any amount of tracer in the tissue. Both the initial height and the remainder of the residue curve are measured at the same efficiency so $\bar{t}$ can be measured accurately. This is the strategy used to measure CBF by intracarotid bolus injection of freely diffusible tracers such as radioactive xenon.[8] In this case, the following equation applies:

6.
$$\bar{t} = \frac{e\int_0^\infty q(t)dt}{eq_0} = \frac{Area}{Height} = \frac{V_d}{CBF}.$$

The area and initial height of the residue curve are determined experimentally. If the volume of distribution of the tracer in the brain is known from previous in vitro experiments, CBF can be determined.

The central volume principle is valid for both diffusible and nondiffusible (intravascular) tracers. For intravascular tracers, V_d is the intravascular space or cerebral blood volume (CBV). Thus, the mean vascular transit time $\bar{t}_v$ is described by the following equation:

7.
$$\bar{t}_v = \frac{CBV}{CBF}.$$

Calculation of the mean transit time from the following equation is practical only for very limited conditions:

8.
$$\bar{t} = \frac{Area}{Height}.$$

The equation is accurate for a true bolus without recirculation of tracer and thus is most appropriate for tracers that wash out rapidly, such as intravascular tracers. Estimation of the height requires that all tracer be present in the region of interest at one time, and the area must be calculated over a relatively long period, a difficult requirement because of recirculation. Various techniques have been proposed for correcting the residue curve for the effects of recirculation, but none has been successful for all situations.[9]

The central volume principle is also valid for non–bolus-dispersed injections. However, q_0 cannot be measured from the initial height of the residue curve, because not all the tracer is within the field of view of the detector at once. Determining the total quantity of tracer delivered to the tissue region under these circumstances is difficult and limits the use of the central volume principle. Because the mean transit time cannot be determined from residue curves alone without accurate measurement of q_0, methods for deriving $\bar{t}_v$ based solely on the residue curve of intravenous injection do not yield accurate values.

It is important not to confuse residue detection with outflow detection in indicator dilution methods. The indicator dilution method is based on the measurement of the concentration of tracer in the venous outflow over time.[10] Equations for computation of mean transit time from outflow and from residue curves differ. Unfortunately, residue data are sometimes used in place of venous outflow data in these calculations. This can lead to erroneous calculation of $\bar{t}$, CBV, and CBF.[11,12]

Compartmental Models

Methods based on compartmental models differ from those based on the Fick and central volume principles because the methods make certain assumptions about the behavior of the tracer in the tissue. Compartmental models consist of a finite number of homogenous, well-mixed pools or compartments that interact through the exchange of material.[8,13] A fundamental assumption of compartmental models of tracer kinetics is that the concentration of the tracer is instantaneously the same everywhere once it is introduced into the compartment. The quantity of tracer at time t after introduction, $q(t)$, depends on the initial amount of tracer q_0, the volume of distribution of the tracer within the compartment V_d, and the flow F through the compartment, as shown in the following equation:

9.
$$q(t) = q_0 \exp(-\kappa t)$$

where $\kappa = F/V_d$. One-compartment models are reasonable approximations of the behavior of freely diffusible tracers in the brain and thus can be used for calculations of CBF from a residue curve if V_d is known.[8] The behavior of intravascular tracers in the brain does not conform to compartmental principles. Thus, compartmental models cannot be used to derive CBF or CBV from intravascular agents.[11]

Doppler devices measure the velocity of red blood cells moving toward them. The relationship of Doppler velocity to CBF can be given as shown in the following equation:

10.
$$\text{CBF} = \frac{V_m A \cos\theta}{M}$$

where θ is the angle between the Doppler device and the vessel, V_m is the mean velocity throughout the cardiac cycle of all red blood cells at a point in the vessel with cross-sectional area A, and M is the mass of brain perfused by the vessel. θ is difficult to measure accurately. Most Doppler devices do not measure V_m, only the velocity of the fastest flowing red blood cells. A is also difficult to measure accurately and varies as vessels dilate and constrict under the influence of changes in perfusion pressure and other stimuli. M may change as collateral channels develop. All of these factors mean that the measurement of red blood cell velocity with Doppler devices is only indirectly related to CBF.[14]

Cerebral Metabolism

The Fick principle can be used together with measurements of CBF to calculate substrate metabolism as follows:

11.
$$\text{CMR} = \text{CBF}(C_A - C_V)$$

where CMR (cerebral metabolic rate) is the steady-state rate of substrate utilization by the brain, CBF is the rate of cerebral blood flow in volume of blood per unit time, and $C_A - C_V$ is the steady-state difference between concentrations of the substance in arterial blood and cerebral venous blood. Because the Kety-Schmidt CBF technique requires measurement of arterial and jugular venous tracer concentrations to determine CBF, it is straightforward to measure substrate concentrations and determine CMR as well. Regional CBF techniques can also be combined with arterial-jugular venous difference measurements to try to measure regional metabolism, but the measurements are subject to error because the arterial-jugular venous differences may not be the same everywhere in the brain under pathologic conditions.[15]

The primary technique for measuring regional metabolism is PET. PET employs radiotracers and complicated mathematical models to measure both the cerebral metabolic rate of oxygen ($CMRO_2$) and the cerebral metabolic rate of glucose (CMRglc).[16,17]

Normal Values of CBF and CMR

On the basis of the Kety-Schmidt technique, healthy young adults have an average whole-brain CBF of approximately $46\,\text{mL}/100\,\text{g}^{-1}/\text{min}^{-1}$, a $CMRO_2$ of $3.0\,\text{mL}/100\,\text{g}^{-1}/\text{min}^{-1}$ ($134\,\mu\text{mol}/100\,\text{g}^{-1}/\text{min}^{-1}$), and a CMRglc of $25\,\mu\text{mol}/100\,\text{g}^{-1}/\text{min}^{-1}$.[18–21] The $CMRO_2$/CMRglc molar ratio is 5.4, rather than 6.0 as expected for complete oxidation, because of the production of a small amount of lactate by glycolysis.[18,20] CBF is approximately four times higher in gray matter ($80\,\text{mL}/100\,\text{g}^{-1}/\text{min}^{-1}$) than in white matter ($20\,\text{mL}/100\,\text{g}^{-1}/\text{min}^{-1}$).[22] Under normal resting physiologic conditions, regional blood flow is closely matched to the resting metabolic rate of the tissue.[23–25] Thus, the fraction of available oxygen extracted by the brain (oxygen extraction fraction, OEF) and glucose (glucose extraction fraction, GEF) is uniform. Approximately one third of the oxygen and one tenth of the glucose delivered to the brain by the blood is metabolized.[23,24,26–28]

The effects of aging on CBF and oxygen consumption have been well studied. Because brain maturation is incomplete at birth, it is not surprising that changes in flow and metabolism occur throughout infancy and childhood. Animal perinatal models demonstrate that CBF is quite low at 2 hours after birth and falls further by 24 hours.[29] In the third week of life, CBF increases 200% to 350%,[30] reaching adult levels by day 35.[31] Such data are scarce in the human preterm or term infant, because serial quantitative studies of cerebral hemodynamics in these patients are not so readily obtainable. Within the first 48 hours of life in the preterm neonate, mean global CBF is low, ranging from 6 to $35\,\text{mL}/100\,\text{g}^{-1}/\text{min}^{-1}$,[32–35] and remains low over the subsequent month.[36] In preterm infants with subsequently normal development at 6 months of age, CBF may be less than $10\,\text{mL}/100\,\text{g}^{-1}/\text{min}^{-1}$.[36] Global CBF in term infants ranges from 6 to $69\,\text{mL}/100\,\text{g}^{-1}/\text{min}^{-1}$.[36–38] Mean neonatal CBF in infants with abnormal childhood neurologic outcome is significantly higher than in those with normal childhood neurologic outcome (35.64 ± 11.80 versus $18.26 \pm 8.62\,\text{mL}/100\,\text{g}^{-1}/\text{min}^{-1}$), suggesting that CBF in normal term infants is substantially below that in adults.[39]

Data on global $CMRO_2$ in the normal newborn are even more limited. In one small study, $CMRO_2$ averaged 0 to $0.5\,\text{mL}/100\,\text{g}^{-1}/\text{min}^{-1}$ in preterm infants and 0 to $1.3\,\text{mL}/100\,\text{g}^{-1}/\text{min}^{-1}$ in term infants.[32] In two of the preterm infants with virtual absence of $CMRO_2$ ($0.06\,\text{mL}/100\,\text{g}^{-1}/\text{min}^{-1}$), minimal or no evidence of parenchymal brain injury was detected in the newborn period. Two term infants with no

Pathophysiology

neurologic disease had mean hemispheric $CMRO_2$ values of 0.4 and 0.7 mL/$100g^{-1}$/min^{-1} and were normal at 6 and 7 months, respectively. This finding indicates that energy requirements in fetal and newborn brains are minimal or can be met by nonoxidative metabolism. Mean CMRglc in the newborn has been reported to be 4 to 19 μmol/$100g^{-1}$/min^{-1}.[40–42]

Beyond the neonatal period, global CBF,[43–46] $CMRO_2$,[43] and CMRglc[47,48] progressively increase, reaching a maximum at 3 to 10 years. There is some disagreement about the magnitude of the peaks, with reports of CBF ranging from 60 to 120 mL/$100g^{-1}$/min^{-1}, of $CMRO_2$ ranging from 4.3 to 6.2 mL/$100g^{-1}$/min^{-1}, and of CMRglc ranging from 49 to 65 μmol/$100g^{-1}$/min^{-1}. By late adolescence, cerebral flow and oxygen and glucose metabolism decrease to adult levels.[44,45,48] Most studies report that CBF declines further from the third decade onward, albeit much more slowly than the decrease seen in adolescence.[15,49–51] This later decrease is probably region specific, affecting predominantly frontal, limbic, association, and insular cortices.[49,52] Further analysis of the decline in CBF indicates that the change occurs in gray matter only; blood flow in white matter remains relatively stable after age 1 to 2 years.[26,46,50,53]

The change in metabolic rate for oxygen and glucose with age is less clear. Several studies show a decrease[49,50,54–56] and others show no change.[57–59] In one study, the apparent decrease in CMRglc with age was less after brain atrophy and brain volume[60] were accounted for; this was not the case for $CMRO_2$.[55]

Control of Cerebral Blood Flow

Cerebral perfusion pressure (CPP) is equal to the difference between the arterial pressure driving blood into the brain and the venous back-pressure. Venous back-pressure is negligible unless intracranial pressure (ICP) is elevated or venous outflow is obstructed. Thus, under most circumstances, CPP is equal to the mean arterial pressure (MAP). CBF is regulated by CPP and the cerebrovascular resistance (CVR), as follows:

$$12. \qquad CBF = \frac{CPP}{CVR}.$$

Under conditions of constant CPP, any local or regional changes in CBF must occur as a result of changes in CVR. CVR is determined by blood viscosity, vessel length, and vessel radius. The cerebrovascular bed is not a static system. Rather, resistance vessels (primarily arterioles) dilate and constrict in response to a variety of stimuli.

Response of Cerebral Blood Flow to Changes in pCO_2

The sensitivity of the cerebral circulation to changes in arterial CO_2 tension has been well established. This relationship, in which a decrease in arterial pCO_2 to approximately 25 mm Hg via hyperventilation leads to a decrease in CBF of 30% to 35% and an increase in arterial pCO_2 to more than 50 mm Hg via CO_2 inhalation leads to an increase in CBF of about 75%, was initially described by Kety and Schmidt[61,62] and has been confirmed repeatedly.[63–65] The mechanism for the change in CBF is a change in CVR produced by vasodilation with increased pCO_2 and vasoconstriction with decreased pCO_2.[62] When the perturbation in arterial pCO_2 is maintained for a prolonged time, CBF gradually returns toward normal values.[65] With passive hyperventilation, CBF decreases, but there is no reduction in $CMRO_2$ or high-energy phosphate levels[66,67] despite the appearance of disturbances in consciousness[61]; however, with active hyperventilation, a slight increase in $CMRO_2$ has been reported.[61,62]

Response of Cerebral Blood Flow to Changes in pCO_2, CaO_2, Hemoglobin Content, and Blood Viscosity

The extent to which the partial pressure of oxygen in the blood (pO_2), arterial oxygen content (CaO_2), and blood viscosity influence cerebral oxygen delivery is disputed. The effect of pO_2 on the cerebral circulation has primarily been investigated through reduction in the inspired concentration of oxygen. In both humans and experimental animals, CBF does not increase until arterial pO_2 is reduced below about 30 to 50 mm Hg,[68,69] indicating that variations in pO_2 are unlikely to constitute an important mechanism for regulating CBF at physiologic levels of pO_2.

CaO_2 depends on the concentration of hemoglobin in the blood and the extent to which it is saturated with oxygen. Because of the sigmoid shape of the oxygen dissociation curve, a significant reduction in hemoglobin saturation and, hence, CaO_2 does not occur until arterial pO_2 falls to about 50 to 60 mm Hg.[68,70] The similarity between this number and the threshold for hypoxia-induced reduction in CBF suggests that it is primarily CaO_2 and not pO_2 that determines CBF. Reductions in CaO_2 due to hypoxemia or anemia cause vasodilation and compensatory increases in CBF.[18,62,68,71] Likewise, an excess of oxygen in arterial blood, as in polycythemia, is associated with a decrease in CBF.[72] In neither of these cases does cerebral metabolism change.[68,72] With chronic changes in CaO_2, there is a significant inverse relationship between CaO_2 and CBF throughout the range of oxygen content levels.[71] Sudden changes in CaO_2 due to reduction in hemoglobin or pO_2 produce a smaller increase in CBF than do long-term changes.[73,74]

Hematocrit is an important determinant of viscosity, and thus, viscosity often varies with CaO_2. Although an inverse relationship between viscosity and CBF has also been reported,[71,75] it is unlikely that viscosity is an independent determinant of CBF in most circumstances. In subjects with anemia and paraproteinemia in whom reduced CaO_2 is dissociated from changes in viscosity, no correlation is observed between viscosity and CBF, but there is a highly significant inverse relationship between CaO_2 and CBF.[76] In hematologically normal subjects, reduction of viscosity by plasma exchange without a concomitant change in hemoglobin concentration or CaO_2 does not increase CBF.[77] Finally, reducing CaO_2 via carbon monoxide inhalation without changing arterial pO_2 or viscosity has been shown to increase CBF.[78] Experimental data indicate that viscosity may have a more prominent effect on cerebral perfusion in the setting of preexisting vasodilation. In rats with increased CBF due to hemodilution, hypercapnia, and hypoxia, doubling the plasma viscosity reduced CBF by as much as half.[79,80] Similarly, in a middle cerebral artery (MCA) occlusion model in rats, CBF was lower in ischemic animals with decreased CaO_2 and greater in ischemic animals with decreased viscosity due to hemodilution but no change in CaO_2.[81]

Response of Cerebral Blood Flow to Changes in Blood Glucose Concentration

In contrast to the relationship of CBF with oxygen supply and demand, the balance between glucose supply and demand has little effect on CBF. In insulin clamp or bolus infusion experiments, decreasing the blood glucose concentration to 2.3 to 3 mmol/L in normal subjects resulted in no change in CBF.[82–85] However, more severe reductions in blood glucose, down to 1.1 to 2.2 mmol/L, produced a modest but significant increase in CBF.[86–90] This finding probably does not represent a compensatory mechanism to maintain glucose delivery to the brain. A blood glucose level of 2 mmol/L is well below the level at which brain dysfunction and counterregulatory hormone response occur.[83]

Furthermore, rises in CBF do not increase blood-brain glucose transport.[91,92] Glucose transport across the blood-brain barrier takes place by a stereospecific, saturable, carrier-mediated transport system. The amount of glucose transported from the blood into the brain depends on two factors, the capillary concentration and the transport capacity of the blood-brain barrier. As plasma glucose declines, forward transport diminishes. In order to maintain metabolism, a greater fraction of the transported glucose is metabolized. The net extraction rises from its normal value of 5% to 10%, but the rise is limited by the concomitant fall in forward transport. Even with profound acute hypoglycemia, net glucose extraction does not exceed 15%. Because the capillary glucose concentration is approximately halfway between arterial and venous concentrations, even doubling CBF and thus halving the extraction fraction would increase capillary concentration by less than 5%.

Transport can increase appreciably if either the number or affinity of the transporters rises. An enlargement in capillary surface area would effectively increase the number of transporters. Such capillary recruitment, although an intriguing possibility, has not been demonstrated.[93] Because vascular responses to other stimuli are preserved, this increase in CBF is not simply due to a general loss of vascular tone.[94,95]

Cerebral Blood Flow During Functional Activity

During functional activation of brain, regional CBF and CMRglc increase in the area of greater neuronal activity.[96] It was long assumed that similar rises in regional $CMRO_2$ would accompany increases in CBF during functional activation. However, two PET studies in humans revealed that large, stimulus-induced increases in CBF (30% and 50%) were accompanied by only small increases in $CMRO_2$ (5%).[97,98] It has been suggested that this apparent uncoupling of $CMRO_2$ and CBF occurs because disproportionately large increases in CBF are necessary to sustain even small increases in $CMRO_2$ during activation.[99] A later study has shown, however, that the magnitude of the regional CBF response to functional activation is not affected by either hypoglycemia or hypoxemia, indicating that the increase in blood flow associated with physiologic brain activation is not regulated by a mechanism that matches local cerebral glucose or oxygen supply to local demand.[74,100]

The sensor for the CBF increase with activity is not known. Ido and colleagues[101] offered the novel hypothesis that the accumulation of electrons in cytosolic free nicotinamide adenine dinucleotide (NAD) activates redox (oxidation-reduction) signaling pathways to augment blood flow. Because the ratio of cytosolic NADH (reduced form of NAD) and NAD+ (oxidized form of NAD) (NADH/NAD+) and the ratio of intracellular and extracellular lactate to pyruvate (L/P) are in near-equilibrium, the NADH/NAD+ ratio can be altered through a change in the L/P ratio. These researchers reported that elevated plasma L/P in normal rats augments blood flow increases in activated somatosensory (barrel) cortex. Increased flows were largely prevented by injection of pyruvate (to lower L/P). These findings suggest that the rise in CBF with functional activation serves to remove excess lactate generated by nonoxidative glycolysis, thus maintaining the redox state of the tissue.

Response of Cerebral Blood Flow to Changes in Cerebral Perfusion Pressure

Changes in CPP over a wide range from 70 to 150 mm Hg have little effect on CBF. Known as *autoregulation*, this compensatory mechanism is mediated by changes in CVR. When CPP decreases, vasodilation of the small arteries or arterioles reduces CVR.[102,103] This mechanism is effective at maintaining CBF in normal human subjects until MAP falls below the lower autoregulatory limit.[104,105]

Chronic hypertension shifts both the lower and upper limits of autoregulation to higher levels. In chronically hypertensive subjects, the lower autoregulatory limit is 100 to 120 mm Hg MAP.[104,106] This limit is variably and unpredictably affected by chronic antihypertensive drug treatment. Thus, acute reductions in MAP or CPP that would be safe in normotensive subjects may precipitate cerebral ischemia in patients with chronic hypertension.

Within the limits of autoregulation, a 10% decrease in MAP produces only a slight (2%–7%) decrease in regional CBF.[107,108] Reductions of CPP below the autoregulatory limit produce a much steeper fall in CBF. At this point, when the hemodynamic reserve has been exhausted, a second mechanism is invoked in an attempt to maintain $CMRO_2$—augmentation of oxygen extraction from the blood. Under normal circumstances, only 30% to 40% of oxygen delivered to the brain is used for energy production.[27,109] The unextracted fraction constitutes a reserve that can be used to maintain metabolism once the maximal vasodilatory capacity of the cerebral circulation has been exceeded. A progressive increase in the amount of oxygen extracted from the blood by the brain is manifested as an increase in the arterial-venous oxygen difference ($avDO_2$), resulting in a decrease in venous blood oxygen content and

Pathophysiology

an increase in OEF (Fig. 40–1). Once this mechanism becomes maximal and the increased OEF is no longer adequate to supply the energy needs of the brain, further reductions in CPP disrupt normal cellular metabolism and produce clinical evidence of brain dysfunction. This state may be reversible if circulation is rapidly restored. Persistent or further declines in CPP can lead to permanent tissue damage.[110]

Although reductions in CPP produce visible dilation of pial vessels, data regarding the response of CBV to reduced CPP are conflicting (see Fig. 40–1).[102,111–113] With experimental reductions in CPP, it is often possible to measure an increase in CBV that is presumed to be due to autoregulatory vasodilation.[114–116] CBV is composed of arterial, capillary, and venous segments. Veins account for some 80% to 85% of CBV, arteries for 10% to 15%, and capillaries for less than 5%.[117,118] Of these, arteries are the most responsive to autoregulatory changes in CPP. Veins respond less, and capillaries even less.[119,120] This increase in CBV to reduced CPP is not always evident, however,[121,122] and a decrease in CBV in response to severe reductions in CPP has even been observed.[123] Failure to demonstrate increased CBV in the setting of reduced CPP has been ascribed to a number of possible mechanisms in various situations, including differential vasodilatory capacity of different vascular beds, passive collapse of vessels due to low intraluminal pressures, small vessel

vasospasm, and resetting of vascular tone in response to a compensatory downregulation of $CMRO_2$.[124] The CBF/CBV ratio (or its reciprocal, the mean vascular transit time, MVTT) has been proposed to be a more sensitive indicator of reduced CPP than CBV alone.[121,125] Although it may be more sensitive, CBF/CBV is not reliable, because it may decrease in low-flow conditions with normal perfusion pressure, such as hypocapnia.[126,127]

When the cerebral blood vessels are already dilated, they are less responsive to further vasodilation induced by reduced CPP. Therefore, the autoregulatory response is attenuated or lost in the setting of preexisting hypercapnia, anemia, or hypoxemia.[128,129] The normal autoregulatory vascular responses may also be impaired or lost when the brain is damaged by ischemia or trauma. In such cases, CBF may fall when CPP is reduced even within the normal autoregulatory range.[130,131]

HEMODYNAMIC EFFECTS OF ARTERIAL OCCLUSIVE DISEASE

The importance of hemodynamic mechanisms in the pathogenesis of ischemic stroke remains unsettled.[132] Although it is clear that stenosis of a single artery produces no hemodynamic effect until a critical reduction of 60% to 70% in vessel lumen occurs, distal perfusion pressure with more severe stenosis is variable and may even remain normal with stenosis greater than 90%.[133] The reason is that hemodynamic effect depends not only on the degree of stenosis but also on the adequacy of the collateral circulation.

The importance of collateral circulation pathways in the prediction of ischemic events among patients with carotid occlusive disease is debated. The patency of primary collateral pathways (anterior and posterior communicating and ophthalmic arteries) has been shown to be associated with a lower incidence of ipsilateral stroke[134,135] and the presence of leptomeningeal collateral vessels with a higher incidence of ipsilateral stroke[136] in some studies. However, pattern of arteriographic collateral circulation to the MCA distal to an occluded carotid artery could not be used to identify patients with hemodynamic failure[122,135,137] or to predict stroke recurrence[122,137] in others. Vascular imaging techniques such as angiography and Doppler ultrasonography can detect the presence of these collateral vessels but not necessarily the adequacy of the blood supply they provide.[137] Likewise, measurement of CBF alone is inadequate to assess the cerebral hemodynamic effects of arterial occlusive disease states, for two reasons. First, normal values may be found when perfusion pressure is reduced but flow is maintained by autoregulatory vasodilation of distal resistance vessels. Second, CBF may be low when perfusion pressure is normal, such as when the metabolic demands of the tissue are reduced, as in the destruction of normal afferent or efferent fibers by a remote lesion (see later discussion of the remote metabolic effects of ischemia).

Identification of the hemodynamic effects of arterial stenosis or occlusion on the downstream perfusion pressure is of potential value in determining prognosis and in choosing or monitoring therapy for patients with

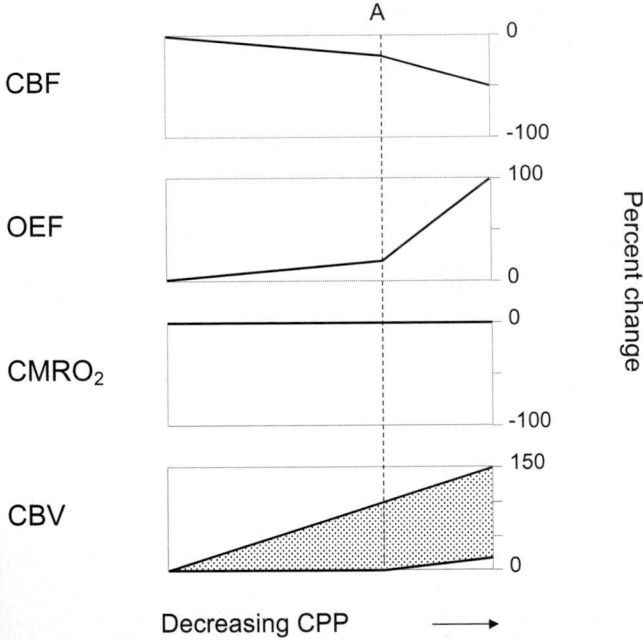

FIGURE 40–1 *Compensatory responses to reduced cerebral perfusion pressure (CPP). As CPP falls, cerebral blood flow (CBF) is initially maintained (with only slight reduction) by arteriolar dilation. When vasodilatory capacity has been exceeded, cerebral autoregulation fails, and CBF begins to decrease rapidly (A). A progressive increase in oxygen extraction (OEF) preserves cerebral oxygen metabolism ($CMRO_2$). The response of cerebral blood volume (CBV) to reduction in CPP is variable, ranging from a steady rise (of as much as 150%) to only a modest increase beginning at the point of autoregulatory failure.*

cerebrovascular disease. Because direct measurement of intravascular perfusion pressure is impractical, assessment of local cerebral hemodynamics depends on indirect evidence based on compensatory responses to reductions in CPP. Such responses have been determined by observation during global reductions in CPP due to systemic hypotension and increased ICP, as previously described; similar responses are assumed to occur with local reductions in CPP due to focal arterial stenosis.

Three-Stage Classification System of Cerebral Hemodynamics

On the basis of the known physiologic responses of CBF, CBV, and OEF to reductions in global CPP, a three-stage sequential classification system for local hemodynamic status using noninvasive measurements has been proposed.[138] Stage 0 consists of normal CPP with closely matched flow and metabolism such that OEF is normal. CBV and MVTT are not elevated, and the CBF response to vasodilatory stimuli is normal. Stage I is manifested by autoregulatory vasodilation of arterioles to maintain a constant CBF. Consequently, CBV and the MVTT are increased, and the CBF response to vasodilatory stimuli is diminished, but OEF remains normal. In Stage II or hemodynamic failure, autoregulatory capacity is exceeded, and there is an increase in OEF as CBF declines with respect to $CMRO_2$. This stage, which Baron and colleagues[139,140] have called "misery perfusion," is sometimes divided into two phases, that in which $CMRO_2$ is maintained (oligemia) and that in which $CMRO_2$ is reduced (ischemia).

Three clinical strategies are commonly used to determine hemodynamic status. The first relies on measurement of CBF at baseline and after application of a vasodilatory stimulus, such as CO_2 inhalation, breath-holding, acetazolamide administration, or physiologic activity (e.g., hand movement). Impairment of the normal increase in CBF or Doppler blood flow velocity in response to vasodilatory stimuli is assumed to reflect existing autoregulatory vasodilation due to reduced CPP. Responses to vasodilatory stimuli have been categorized into three grades of hemodynamic impairment as follows: (1) reduced augmentation (relative to contralateral hemisphere or normal controls), (2) absence of augmentation (same value as baseline), and (3) paradoxical reduction in regional blood flow compared with baseline measurement. This last category, also known as the "steal" phenomenon, can be identified only with quantitative CBF techniques.[141]

The second clinical strategy to determine hemodynamic status entails the quantitative measurement of regional CBV either alone or in combination with measurement of CBF at rest to detect the presence of autoregulatory vasodilation. Increases in CBV or the CBV/CBF ratio relative to the range observed in normal control subjects is assumed to indicate hemodynamic compromise, but the sensitivity and specificity of these measurements in detecting reduced CPP is unknown.

The third strategy, which involves direct measurement of regional OEF as an indicator of local autoregulatory failure, is currently possible only with PET. Magnetic resonance imaging (MRI) measurements using pulse

sequences sensitive to deoxyhemoglobin, which is increased in regions with increased oxygen extraction, are being developed to provide similar information.[142,143]

Correlation Among Methods

Although the three-stage classification scheme has been conceptually useful, it is too simplistic. First, as discussed previously, increases in CBV and MVTT are not reliable indices of reduced CPP. Second, CBF responses to different vasodilatory agents may vary within the same patient.[144-146] A normal vasodilatory response may occur in the setting of increased CBV.[147,148] Finally, according to the three-stage classification, all patients with increased OEF should have increased CBV and poor response to vasoactive stimuli; however, this increase in CBV is not always evident.[124] Normal or reduced CBV in the presence of increased OEF carries a lower risk of stroke[149] and may indicate preserved or regained vasodilatory capacity, but the mechanism remains obscure. The correlation between vasoreactivity and OEF is inconsistent.[148,150,151]

Taken together, these data indicate that evidence of hemodynamic impairment by one method of hemodynamic assessment does not predict an abnormal result by another. Different techniques rely on different physiologic mechanisms from which the presence of reduced perfusion pressure is inferred. Consequently, empirical proof linking each of these different measurements of hemodynamic compromise as risk factors to stroke risk is required.

Correlation with Stroke Risk and Effects of Cerebrovascular Surgery

Because carotid endarterectomy has been proven to reduce stroke risk in symptomatic high-grade extracranial carotid stenosis regardless of mechanism,[152] the discussion of the treatment implications of hemodynamic impairment in patients with such stenosis is of little clinical value. The benefit of carotid endarterectomy in asymptomatic stenosis is less convincing, with discordant results among the published randomized controlled trials.[153-156] Patients with asymptomatic carotid occlusion and impaired cerebral hemodynamics as measured by reduced vasodilatory response to inspired carbon dioxide may represent a subpopulation at greater risk for subsequent stroke.[157] Impaired vasoreactivity to either inspired carbon dioxide or breath-holding may also be a risk factor for subsequent stroke in patients with asymptomatic carotid stenosis.[157,158] No surgical treatment has proved to benefit patients with symptomatic carotid artery occlusion, who have a 2% to 7% annual risk of subsequent ipsilateral ischemic stroke.[159,160]

Several studies have explored the prognostic value of measurements of cerebral hemodynamics on stroke risk in symptomatic carotid occlusion. Despite earlier data suggesting a lack of predictive value of the CBV/CBF ratio,[161] two later studies have independently demonstrated that hemodynamic failure, defined as increased OEF distal to a symptomatic occluded carotid artery, is an independent predictor of subsequent ipsilateral ischemic stroke.[122,162,163] Data on vasomotor reactivity to acetazolamide or hypercapnia in predicting stroke have been inconsistent.[136,164-167]

Pathophysiology

Extracranial-intracranial (EC-IC) bypass surgery, in which an anastomosis is created between the superficial temporal and middle cerebral arteries, was developed in order to bypass a severe stenosis or occlusion of the internal carotid artery or proximal MCA that is not amenable to conventional endarterectomy and thereby to improve cerebral perfusion. After revascularization, improvement of the ipsilateral OEF to contralateral OEF ratio, in concert with postoperative improvement in CBF, can be demonstrated in most patients who had focally increased OEF before surgery (Plate 40–1 following page 808).[140,168] Similarly, impaired vasomotor reactivity has been shown to be reversible with revascularization.[169–171] Patients who have regions of increased MVTT without increased OEF preoperatively show a postoperative reduction in CBV with little change in CBF or CMRO$_2$,[172] implying that surgery has improved CPP and reduced the amount of vasodilation necessary to maintain normal CBF.

Although a large prospective randomized trial demonstrated no value for EC-IC bypass surgery in preventing subsequent stroke in patients with symptomatic extracranial or intracranial atherosclerotic disease of the internal carotid artery,[173] the trial's failure to demonstrate efficacy has been attributed to the inclusion of many patients with normal cerebral hemodynamics, a population that has a low risk of stroke.[174,175] Since the time of the trial, attempts have been made to identify the subgroup of patients with hemodynamic impairment who are most likely to benefit from revascularization. Determination of hemodynamic status is critical in selecting the subgroup of high-risk patients for a clinical trial to assess the efficacy of surgical revascularization in reducing stroke risk.

ACUTE ISCHEMIC STROKE

Evolution of Infarction

The evolution of changes in flow and metabolism after acute ischemic stroke has been established primarily through study of patients at different times after symptom onset. These data suffer from a lack of premorbid evaluation and are limited to capturing only discrete pictures of cerebral physiology during a highly dynamic process. Experimental studies in larger mammals have provided further information on the evolution of infarction, especially at very early times.

Sequential examinations before and after MCA occlusion in the baboon[176] and cat[177] demonstrate a prominent reduction in CBF and a concomitant increase in OEF in the MCA territory within 1 hour after occlusion. CMRO$_2$ is reduced somewhat but falls further over the subsequent 2 to 3 hours. Reflecting the declining CMRO$_2$, the initially markedly increased OEF decreases progressively, indicating the development of central necrosis. By 24 hours, CBF in the center of the MCA territory reaches its nadir, at less than 20% of baseline values, and CMRO$_2$ reaches 25% of baseline values. Also at this point, increased OEF is seen to develop outside the area of primary perfusion disturbance, in the tissue adjacent to the infarct core.[177] The volume of severely hypometabolic tissue remains stable between 1 and 7 hours after occlusion but enlarges by 24 hours and increases even more an average of 17 days after occlusion.[178]

Human data obtained at 2 to 24 hours after ictus show an area of reduced CBF, reduced CMRO$_2$, and high OEF within the core of the infarct (Plate 40–2 and Fig. 40–2).[179,180] Over the subsequent days, CBF in the infarct core usually increases. Spontaneous reperfusion occurs in about three quarters of patients. It may take place within a few hours of infarction[181] but peaks at day 14.[182] This rise in CBF occurs without a concomitant rise in CMRO$_2$; rather, CMRO$_2$ generally falls further. Consequently, a decrease in regional OEF below normal values mirrors the rise in CBF. This state, termed *luxury perfusion*,[183] indicates that the normal coupling of CBF to oxygen metabolism is deranged. Luxury perfusion may be absolute (Plate 40–3 bottom), with CBF values greater than normal. Alternatively, luxury perfusion may be relative (Plate 40–3 top), with low or normal CBF that is still in excess of that required to produce a normal OEF for the reduced CMRO$_2$.[184] Luxury perfusion is evident by 48 hours in one third of patients[185,186] and peaks at 1 to 2 weeks.[184] After this subacute period, CBF progressively declines and OEF normalizes such that the chronic stable infarct demonstrates flow and metabolism that are close to zero with OEF at or below baseline values (Plate 40–4).[187]

In the rim of tissue surrounding the infarct core, areas demonstrating reduced CBF and increased OEF with variable CMRO$_2$ can often be identified within hours after ictus and may persist for up to 17 hours.[188,189] In most cases, tissue regions demonstrating increased OEF go on to suffer progressive metabolic impairment despite stable

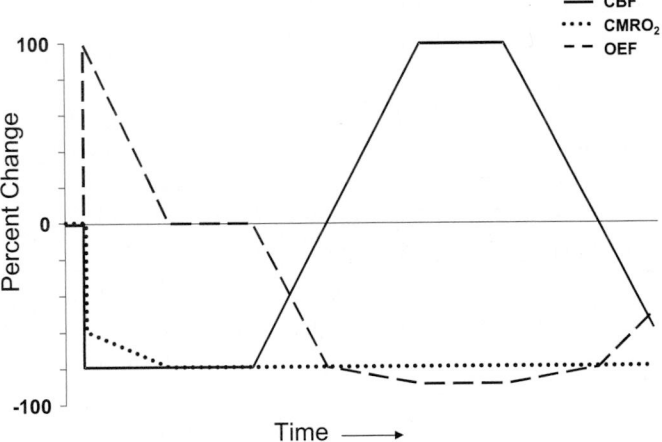

FIGURE 40–2 *Pathophysiologic changes in cerebral infarction. At the onset of ischemia, the initial drop in regional cerebral blood flow (CBF) is mirrored by a rise in regional oxygen extraction fraction (OEF). Because the increase in OEF is no longer able to maintain the energy needs of the brain, regional cerebral oxygen metabolism (CMRO$_2$) falls to the level of oxygen delivery. With time, CMRO$_2$ drops further, even though there is no further decrease in CBF, resulting in a decrease in OEF. Reperfusion via recanalization of the occluded artery or recruitment of collateral pathways results in an increase in CBF ("luxury perfusion") and a concomitant drop in OEF below baseline with no change in CMRO$_2$. With evolution to the stage of chronic infarction, CBF progressively declines, and OEF increases but often remains below baseline values.*

CBF, with a further reduction in $CMRO_2$ and a drop in OEF.

Determining the relationship between the metabolism of oxygen and that of glucose in acute ischemic stroke has been difficult because fluorodeoxyglucose ^{18}F (^{18}FDG), the PET tracer used for this purpose, can produce artifactually high values for CMRglc under ischemic conditions.[190,191] Studies with ^{18}FDG have shown evidence for uncoupling of oxidative and glucose metabolisms,[24,28,180,185] with better preservation of CMRglc such that the $CMRO_2$/CMRglc ratio is one third that for normal brain.[28] This finding of relatively increased glycolysis in the presence of adequate oxygen delivery has been attributed to glycolytic activity in neutrophils and macrophages.[28] An alternative explanation for the increased glucose consumption is spreading depression,[192] which is a reversible, slow (≈ 3 mm/min) wave of depolarization accompanied by a marked change in interstitial ion concentrations that occurs spontaneously during ischemia in association with the sustained increase of extracellular potassium and glutamate.[193] The frequency and severity of this excitation-induced spreading depression correlate with the ultimate extent of structural injury in experimental models.[194]

During the acute period after ischemic stroke, cerebrovascular control is deranged. The normal CO_2 vasodilatory response may disappear, and autoregulation can be impaired. Abnormalities of CO_2 response and autoregulation can occur together or can be dissociated. Reductions in CPP even within the normal range can produce reductions in CBF. Abnormalities of autoregulation occur in patients with and without persistent vessel occlusion. Other abnormalities, such as intracerebral steal (decreased CBF in ischemic area produced by vasodilation elsewhere), inverse steal (increased CBF in ischemic area due to vasoconstriction elsewhere), and false autoregulation (decreased CBF in ischemic area produced by increased CPP) also occur. These abnormalities in cerebrovascular control may persist for several weeks, even longer in cases of persistent occlusion.[195,196]

Predicting Tissue Viability

The ability to distinguish viable from irreversibly damaged tissue early in the course of ischemic stroke would have obvious value in assessing the efficacy of potential new treatments. Because tissue regions that demonstrate increased OEF are areas with reduced blood supply relative to oxygen demand but still with metabolically active cells, OEF has received much attention as the factor capable of predicting tissue viability. Such areas of increased OEF have been interpreted to represent the *ischemic penumbra*, defined as the tissue surrounding the dense core of irreversibly damaged cells that has preserved ionic homeostasis and reduced neuronal electrical activity but that may be salvageable with reperfusion.[197] Furthermore, the decline in OEF is often interpreted to signal the transition from reversible ischemia to irreversible infarction.[180,198] There is evidence that reperfusion occurring within 1 hour improves $CMRO_2$ in areas of increased OEF,[180] but reperfusion occurring at 6 hours does not improve $CMRO_2$, despite similar elevations in OEF prior to reperfusion.[199]

Other attempts to predict tissue viability involve determination of thresholds for CBF and $CMRO_2$ below which spontaneous tissue survivability is unlikely. All such attempts to determine thresholds suffer from a variety of technical problems, including small numbers of subjects, poor spatial resolution, lack of co-registration to CT, and poor counting statistics.[27,179,200] These limitations aside, thresholds for infarction have been reported as 0.87 to 1.7 mL/100 g^{-1}/min^{-1} for $CMRO_2$ and 8.4–19 mL/100 g^{-1}/min^{-1} for CBF.[27,179,200,201] The values at the lower end of the ranges were derived from single voxel measurements of both gray and white matter, whereas those at the higher end were determined from larger regions primarily in gray matter.

Perfusion deficits on acute perfusion-weighted MRI (PWI) have been reported to correlate with, but to regularly overestimate, final infarct size measured by T2-weighted MRI.[202–207] Threshold values ranging from 0.48 to 0.59 for mean relative CBF ratio on acute imaging have been reported to best discriminate areas of infarction and noninfarction on delayed imaging.[203,208] Given quantitative CBF thresholds, it is not surprising that the entire perfusion deficit does not go on to infarction and that a perfusion threshold is more predictive of final tissue status. In several of these studies, however,[202] assessment of final infarct volume occurred at a mean of 7 days after stroke onset.[203,204,206–208] Such assessments may be inaccurate, because lesion volume decreases between 7 days and 1 month after stroke in most patients.[209]

Predicting Clinical Outcome

The absolute values of $CMRO_2$ and CBF associated with poor tissue outcome do not necessarily correlate with poor clinical outcome because other factors, such as lesion location, patient characteristics, and brain plasticity, must be taken into consideration. Nevertheless, blood flow and metabolic patterns have been related to clinical outcome, with larger size and greater severity of the initial metabolic and blood flow disturbances being predictive of poor functional outcome independent of initial neurologic status.[186,210,211] Exceptions to this generalization consist of critically placed lacunar infarctions,[210] highlighting the importance of lesion location. Thresholds for predicting poor clinical outcome in patients with ischemic stroke have been reported to be 1.25 mL/100 g^{-1}/min^{-1} for $CMRO_2$ and 20 mL/100 g^{-1}/min^{-1} for CBF in the ischemic core.[184] In *non-infarcted penumbral tissue* (defined as tissue with increased OEF that escaped infarction), the volume of tissue with increased OEF has also been shown to correlate with 2-month neurologic recovery.[188] Finally, presence of a large volume of hypoperfused tissue on PWI performed in the acute period has been demonstrated to correlate with poor neurologic state during that period as well as with poor functional outcome in most,[205,206,209] but not all,[212] studies.

Thresholds for Ischemia in the Newborn Brain

Although it is generally accepted that the newborn brain is more resistant to ischemic injury than the adult brain, there have been no direct measurements of the tolerance

Pathophysiology

of the newborn human brain to reductions in either blood flow or substrate supply. As noted earlier, CBF as low as $5\,mL/100\,g^{-1}/min^{-1}$ has been observed in newborns with normal neurodevelopmental outcome[36,39] and EEG activity,[35] and virtual absence of $CMRO_2$ has been observed in newborns without evidence of parenchymal brain injury.[32] In one study of infants with hypoxic ischemic encephalopathy (HIE) after perinatal asphyxia, global CMRglc was inversely correlated with the severity of HIE, and infants who demonstrated cerebral palsy had a mean CMRglc of $18.1\,\mu mol/100\,g^{-1}/min^{-1}$, compared with $41.5\,\mu mol/100\,g^{-1}/min^{-1}$ in infants who demonstrated no neurologic sequelae at 2 years.[213]

REMOTE METABOLIC EFFECTS OF ISCHEMIA

A common finding from the earliest metabolic studies of stroke is the presence of areas of reduced blood flow and metabolism in structurally normal tissue distant from the site of infarction. Remote hypometabolism has been demonstrated for both oxygen consumption[184,214–216] and glucose utilization.[217,218] Metabolic values at these distant sites always remain higher than those within the ischemic core,[217] and flow is reduced to a slightly greater extent than metabolism, resulting in a slight increase in OEF.[219] Distinguished from misery perfusion, this situation has been interpreted to represent primary metabolic depression with secondary reduction in perfusion.

The remote hypometabolism is typically ascribed to a decrease in neuronal activity caused by interruption of afferent or efferent fiber pathways by the ischemic lesion, a phenomenon often termed *diaschisis*.[214] This term is not strictly accurate, though, because the word diaschisis refers to an acute and reversible functional depression at sites distant from but connected with the site of injury,[220] whereas the remote effects of ischemia are often stable for months[215,221] and may be permanent. Trans-synaptic neuronal degeneration has been proposed as an alternative explanation for the remote hypometabolism[216] and is supported by the fact that contralateral $CMRO_2$ often declines between early and later studies[222]; but this mechanism is unlikely to account for all cases because hypometabolism can be seen within hours of stroke.[223] In all probability, demonstrations of remote hypometabolism encompass a variety of reversible and irreversible processes.

Contralateral Cerebellar Hypometabolism

The best described remote metabolic effect of ischemia is contralateral cerebellar hypometabolism ("crossed cerebellar diaschisis"), which occurs in about 50% of patients with hemispheric lesions (Plate 40–5).[216,223] Several factors have been reported to influence its occurrence, although data are not consistent among the studies. Such hypometabolism may be more profound with deep MCA infarcts,[216] infarcts involving the frontal[215] or parietal lobes,[184] and those encompassing more than one lobe.[216,218,224] Although Lenzi and associates[184] found that "crossed cerebellar diaschisis was not evident in cases in which the dimensions of the infarct were small," Martin

and Raichle[215] reported no relationship between this finding and infarct size. Cerebellar hypometabolism has been shown to correlate with the presence,[187] but probably not the severity, of hemiparesis.[215] It also occurs in some patients who have no motor deficit.[216,218] Although contralateral cerebellar $CMRO_2$ and CMRglc values are reduced to the same degree immediately after stroke,[24] the reduction in CMRglc is greater than that in $CMRO_2$ over the long term in stroke (4 to 46 months), indicating an uncoupling of oxygen consumption and glucose utilization.[225]

Contralateral Cerebral Hypometabolism

Reduction in blood flow and metabolism in the hemisphere contralateral to cerebral infarction has also been described for both the homologous cortical area and the whole hemisphere.[184,226,227] Wise and associates[228] found that although patients with recent infarction had lower contralateral $CMRO_2$ values than normal control subjects, this difference vanished when the comparison group consisted of subjects who had extracranial cerebrovascular disease but did not have previous cerebral infarction. Nonhuman primate models of cerebral ischemia have not revealed evidence for contralateral hemispheric hypometabolism either in the acute period[176] or at delayed measurement (>2 weeks).[199]

Ipsilateral Cerebral Hypometabolism

Ipsilateral cerebral hypometabolism has been observed in the cortex overlying subcortical stroke and in the basal ganglia, thalamus, and distant sites in the cortex after cortical stroke,[217,226,229,230] probably occurring in a delayed fashion (>18 hours after clinical onset).[231] Because of the dense thalamocortical projections and interconnections between the thalamus and the brainstem, basal ganglia, and cerebellum, it is not surprising that this "intrahemispheric remote hypometabolism" is most commonly described with thalamic lesions.[198,217,232]

Clinical Relevance

The clinical correlate of the remote changes described in this section is unclear. Single case reports have suggested an association with focal neurologic deficits, including ataxia,[233,234] aphasia,[235,236] neglect,[237] and hemianopia,[226] but larger series of infarcts at various locations have revealed no such relationships.[216,238] In one study, stepwise regression analysis revealed that language performance depended mainly on parietotemporal metabolism irrespective of infarct location.[239] Impaired consciousness after stroke has been attributed to remote hypometabolism,[184,240] as has disordered higher cortical function.[210] Inconsistency of results may be at least partially explained by a failure to account for such confounding factors as patient age and lesion size as well as a failure to match control subjects for cerebrovascular risk factors in some of the studies.

Similarly, the predictive value of remote metabolic effects seen immediately after stroke is uncertain. Widespread metabolic disruption was a poor indicator of neurologic outcome (disability at 2 weeks to 3 months) in one

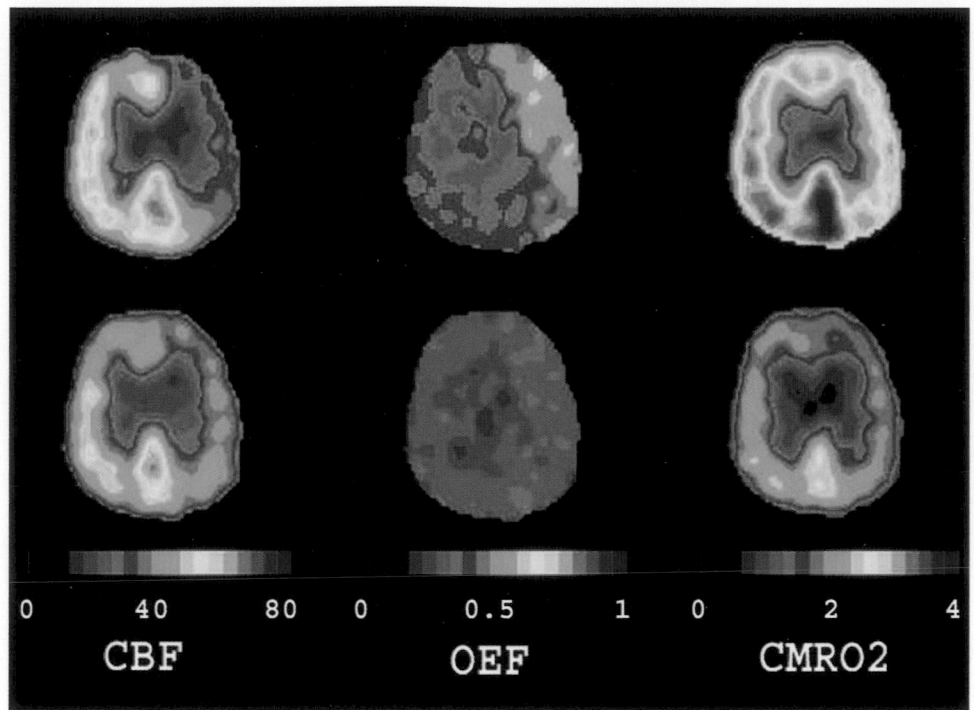

PLATE 40–1 *Normalization of oxygen extraction fraction (OEF) after extracranial-intracranial (EC-IC) bypass surgery in a 69-year-old man with symptomatic occlusion of the right carotid artery. The baseline positron emission tomography (PET) images (top row) demonstrate reduced cerebral blood flow (CBF) and increased OEF in the right hemisphere. A PET study performed 35 days after EC-IC bypass (bottom row) shows that ipsilateral CBF has improved and OEF has normalized. In all images, the right side of the brain is on the reader's right. CMRO₂, cerebral metabolic rate of oxygen.*

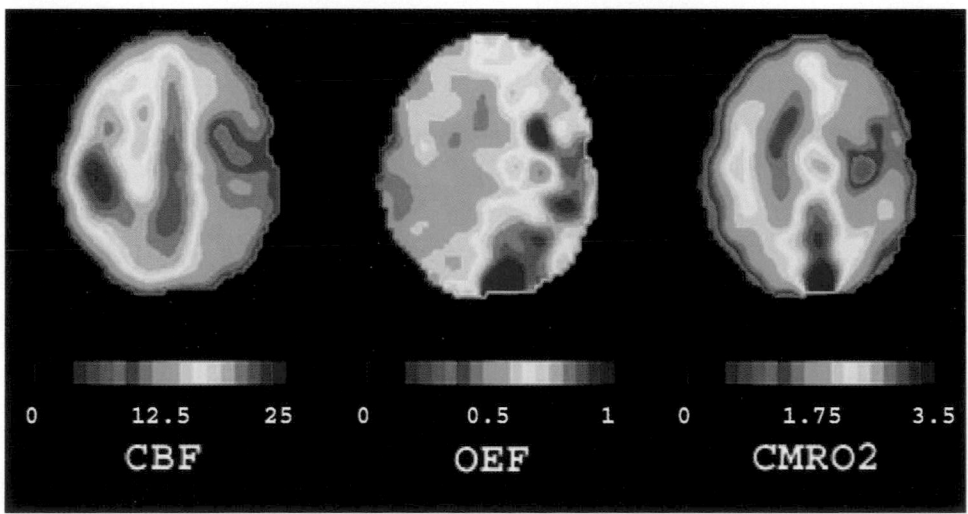

PLATE 40–2 *Positron emission tomography (PET) study in a 54-year-old woman who experienced left hemiparesis due to vasospasm 9 days after subarachnoid hemorrhage. Right hemispheric cerebral blood flow (CBF) and cerebral metabolic rate of oxygen (CMRO₂) are reduced, and oxygen extraction fraction (OEF) is increased, indicative of ischemia. In all images, the right side of the brain is on the reader's right.*

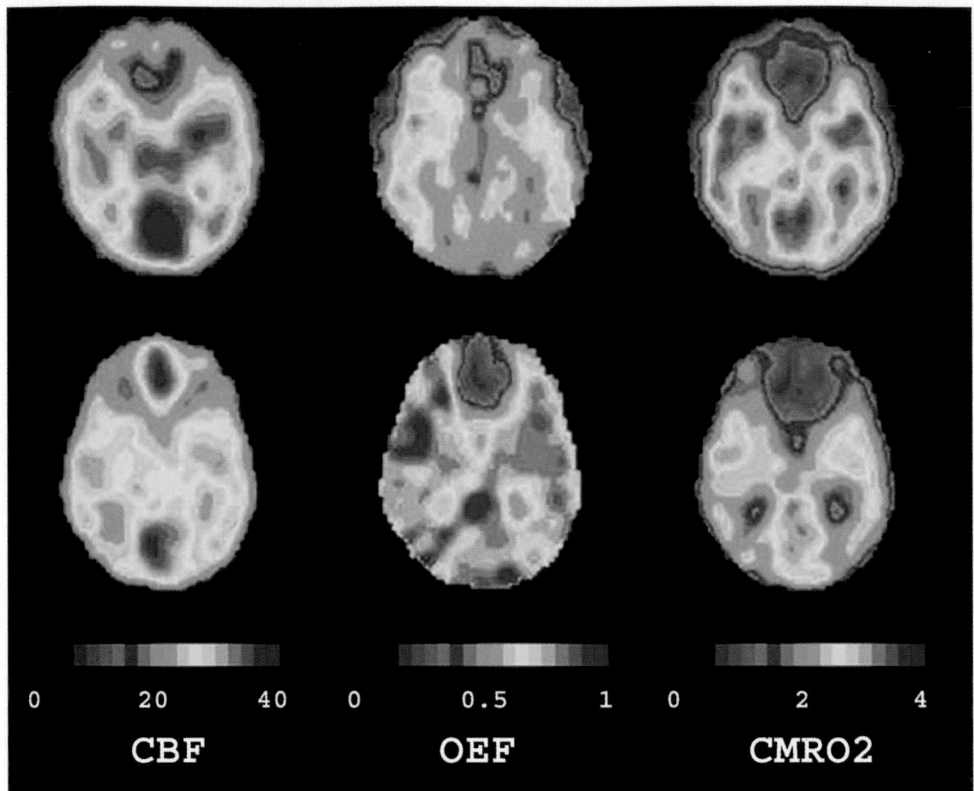

PLATE 40–3 *Sequential positron emission tomography (PET) studies in a 22-year-old woman with bifrontal infarcts associated with subarachnoid hemorrhage–induced vasospasm demonstrating luxury perfusion. The first study (top row), performed on day 6 after hemorrhage, reveals relative luxury perfusion: Cerebral blood flow (CBF) is reduced but is still in excess of oxygen requirements, as indicated by cerebral oxygen metabolism (CMRO₂), such that the oxygen extraction fraction (OEF) is diminished. The second study (bottom row), performed on day 20, shows increased CBF with reduced CMRO₂ and OEF, consistent with absolute luxury perfusion. In all images, the right side of the brain is on the reader's right.*

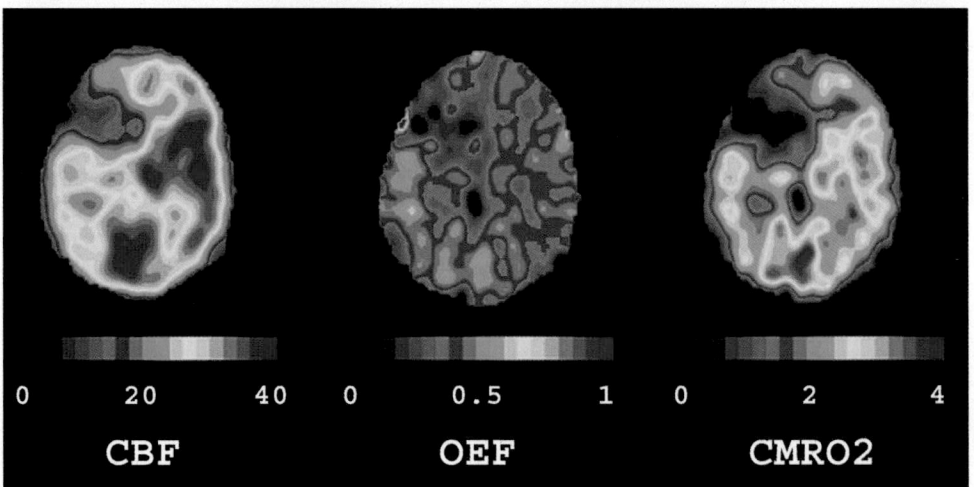

PLATE 40–4 *Positron emission tomography (PET) study performed 5 months after a left frontal infarct. Cerebral blood flow (CBF) and cerebral rate of oxygen (CMRO₂) are severely reduced, and the oxygen extraction fraction (OEF) is below normal. In all images, the right side of the brain is on the reader's right.*

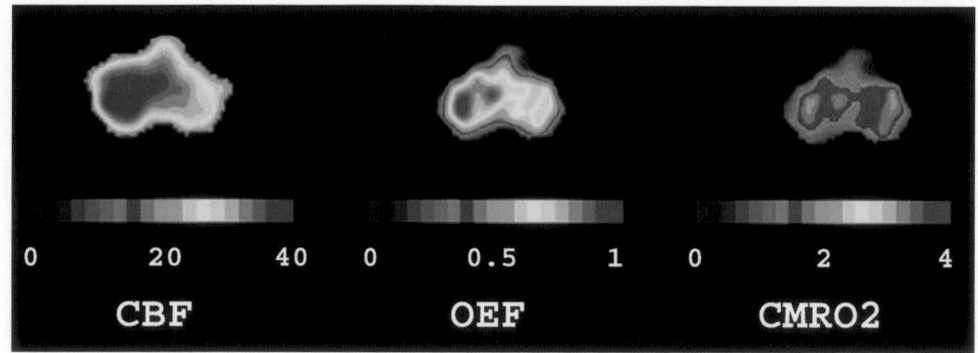

PLATE 40–5 *Positron emission tomography (PET) study performed 5 months after a left frontal infarct. Slices through the posterior fossa demonstrate crossed cerebellar hypometabolism with secondary hypoperfusion. In all images, the right side of the brain is on the reader's right. CBF, cerebral blood flow; OEF, oxygen extraction fraction; CMRO₂, cerebral oxygen metabolism.*

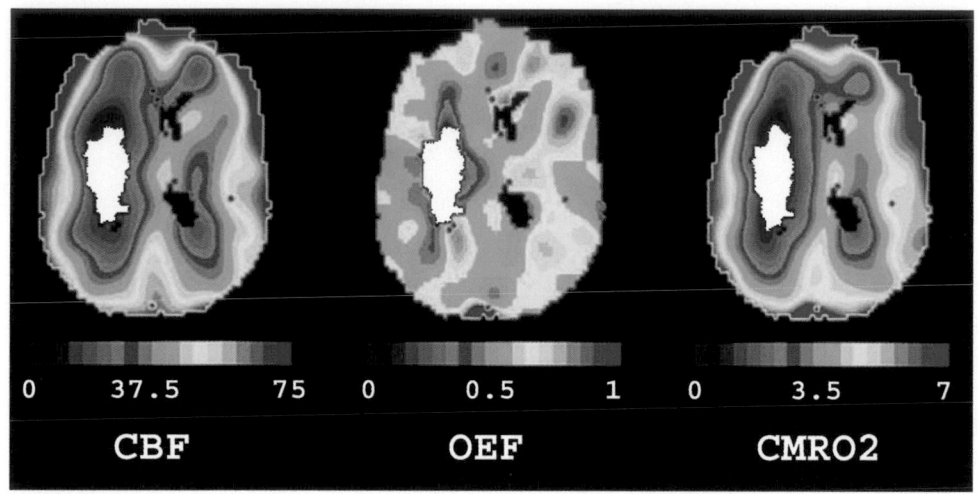

PLATE 40–6 *Partial volume–corrected positron emission tomography (PET) images of a 44-year-old hypertensive man with a left putaminal hemorrhage studied 21 hours after onset. Cerebral blood flow (CBF), cerebral oxygen metabolism (CMRO₂), and oxygen extraction fraction (OEF) around the clot are all reduced in comparison with the right hemisphere, suggestive of primary metabolic depression. In all images, the right side of the brain is on the reader's right, and the hemorrhage is depicted in white.*

study, regardless of CT findings.[210] In another, metabolism in structurally normal ipsilateral mesial-prefrontal tissue at 5 to 18 hours after MCA stroke was predictive of neurologic status at 3 weeks.[231] Furthermore, glucose metabolism in the left hemisphere 2 to 3 weeks after left MCA stroke has been found to predict both short-term (4 months) and long-term (2 years) recovery from aphasia.[241,242] Contralateral hemispheric or cerebellar $CMRO_2$ measured within 30 hours of MCA stroke has not, however, been found to correlate with either acute neurologic deficit or recovery at 15 to 60 days.[222,223]

INTRACEREBRAL HEMORRHAGE

Investigations of CBF and metabolic rate in intracerebral hemorrhage (ICH) have been less extensive than those in ischemic stroke. Bilateral hemispheric blood flow reduction has been reported in subacute hypertensive hemorrhage accompanied by bihemispheric increase in OEF in patients with very large clots (>40 mL), but not in those with smaller clots.[243] Insight into the cause for this increase in hemispheric OEF has now been gained. In a study of 19 hypertensive patients with acute ICH, OEF in the hemisphere ipsilateral to the hematoma was elevated in comparison with OEF in normal control subjects but not in comparison with that in hypertensive control subjects.[244] Thus, the higher hemispheric OEF in ICH may reflect the effects of chronic hypertension rather than increased ICP or other effects of the hematoma. Remote depression of CMRglc in morphologically intact brain structures in ICH has been compared with that in ischemic stroke. Studies have found that remote hypometabolism depends on size and location but not on the type of underlying lesion.[245,246] Comparison of those patients studied within 3 weeks of ICH with those studied more than 3 weeks after ICH showed that CMRglc in remote regions increased significantly with time.[246]

Blood flow investigations in ICH have now focused on the zone of tissue immediately surrounding the clot. Reduced CBF, determined on autoradiography or SPECT, has been demonstrated in this area in experimental models of ICH[247,248] and in patients with ICH,[249] although not always.[250,251] This reduction in CBF is often attributed to cerebral ischemia due to mechanical compression of the microvasculature surrounding the clot.[247,252] As in ischemic stroke, PET and SPECT studies of ICH suffer from the effect of partial volume averaging, which may cause regions of normal flow to appear reduced, depending on image resolution and the proximity to nonperfused tissue.[253,254] Unlike for ischemic stroke, there is a validated method permitting the correction for partial volume effects in ICH.[255] This method shows that a zone of hypoperfusion is still evident surrounding acute ICH.[255,256]

To determine whether this reduction in peri-clot flow indicates ischemia, evidence for increased OEF in peri-clot tissue has been sought. In 19 patients studied 5 to 22 hours after symptom onset, Zazulia and colleagues[256] found that peri-clot $CMRO_2$ was reduced to a greater degree than CBF, resulting in a decrease in OEF, rather than the increase that occurs in ischemia. This pattern was suggestive of a primary metabolic depression (Plate 40–6). These

data cannot exclude the possibility that regional ischemia occurs earlier than 5 hours. This possibility is doubtful, however, given that (1) in acute cerebral infarction, areas of increased OEF are demonstrable in the majority of patients studied within 24 hours,[198,257] and (2) in most patients with acute ischemic stroke who do not have increased OEF, CBF is elevated, suggesting reperfusion.[188,258]

Seeking to guide clinical decisions regarding the controversial issue of blood pressure management in patients with acute ICH,[259–261] several studies of CBF autoregulation in patients with recent ICH have been carried out.[262,263] Taken together, these studies demonstrate that regional autoregulation and global autoregulation are preserved after ICH down to a lower MAP limit, which averages 110 mm Hg or about 20% of the admission MAP but shows substantial individual variation. Reductions of MAP in excess of 20% or to less than 84 mm Hg may reduce CBF. None of these studies provided data on ICP, and with the exception of one in which hematoma size was not specified, all were carried out on patients with small to moderate-size hematomas. If ICP is elevated because of large hematomas or hydrocephalus, the lower limit of autoregulation may be shifted to a higher value. Calcium channel blockers and β-blockers have equivalent minimal effects on CBF within the autoregulatory range of MAP; ganglionic blockers may have a more profound effect on CBF. Although these data do not address the issue of whether early pharmacologic reduction in blood pressure is beneficial, they do challenge the assumption that such reductions are harmful, and they may provide useful guidelines when blood pressure treatment is deemed to be necessary in the patient with acute ICH.

Some workers have suggested that blood flow measurements might be used to identify candidates for surgical intervention in ICH. In one small SPECT study, perfusion in the ipsilateral hemisphere relative to the contralateral hemisphere improved by 3.87% after hematoma evacuation, whereas it decreased by 3.61% with conservative treatment. The importance of this finding is unclear, however, because a correlation between increased CBF and outcome after ICH has not been shown.[264]

Cerebral Blood Flow in Arteriovenous Malformations

Cerebral arteriovenous malformations (AVMs) are high-flow vascular structures lacking capillaries between arteries and veins, and as such, may induce marked hemodynamic disturbances in the surrounding tissue. Many[265–268] but not all[269] physiologic studies have demonstrated regions of decreased blood flow in the tissue adjacent to the AVM or even far removed in the ipsilateral or contralateral hemisphere. It has been postulated that decreased perfusion around the AVM may be responsible for ischemic symptoms through an intracerebral steal syndrome, in which blood flow is disproportionately shunted through the low-resistance AVM and away from other areas of the brain. This concept is controversial, because there is no uniform clinical definition of *steal*. Stable, nonprogressive focal neurologic deficits or seizures are sometimes included along with transient or progressive deficits. Furthermore, there is no clear relationship between regional CBF patterns and

Pathophysiology

symptoms.[270] Data linking the resolution of so-called steal-induced neurologic deficits after AVM obliteration to post-treatment resolution of hypoperfusion and return of normal vasoreactivity are rare.[271]

Similarly, it has been postulated that the occasionally encountered post-treatment complications of edema and hemorrhage are due to a sudden redistribution of previously shunted blood after removal of an AVM. This redistribution is termed *normal perfusion pressure break-through*[272] under the assumptions that (1) perfusion pressure is reduced below the lower limit of autoregulation by arterial hypotension and venous hypertension in neighboring vascular territories, (2) blood vessels in these territories are maximally dilated such that any decrease in perfusion pressure results in ischemia, (3) chronic hypoperfusion results in vasomotor paralysis and impaired autoregulatory capacity, and (4) reversal of arterial hypotension after treatment is not matched by a corresponding increase in CVR, leading to hyperemia and sometimes swelling and hemorrhage.[273–276]

Data counter to this theory have emerged, however, with several studies suggesting that autoregulation is intact in tissue adjacent to the AVM both before and after surgery[277,278] and that AVM removal may be associated with a decrease in regional CBF.[270] In addition, because feeding artery pressures are below the standard lower limit of autoregulation in the majority of patients with AVMs,[271] it would be expected that normalization of these pressures after AVM obliteration would result in a large number of "breakthrough" complications. Such complications are uncommon, however.[279–281] Finally, although there are some reports of impaired vascular reserve in tissue adjacent to and distant from the AVM,[282,283] others indicate that regional vasoreactivity may be preserved.[267,271] In fact, patients who experience hyperemic complications have been shown to exhibit *enhanced* vasoreactivity to acetazolamide.[267,281,283] Discrepant results may be partially explained by differing proportions of patients with prior AVM-associated hemorrhage, prior radiosurgery, and seizures, each of which features may be associated with altered perfusion and impaired vasoreactivity.[283–286] The preceding arguments notwithstanding, severely reduced regional perfusion and exhausted vasodilatory reserve occur at least in some patients with AVMs,[271,282] but it is not clear that the abnormal hemodynamic pattern is reversed after AVM obliteration.[283]

SUBARACHNOID HEMORRHAGE

When studied 1 to 4 days after aneurysmal subarachnoid hemorrhage (SAH), patients who have not undergone surgery and who do not have evidence for vasospasm, hydrocephalus, or ICH show significantly reduced $CMRO_2$, CBF, and CBV with normal OEF.[287,288] This pattern indicates that the reduction in metabolism at this stage is primary and that the reduction in CBF occurs secondary to reduced metabolic demands.

Vasospasm, defined as segmental or diffuse narrowing of the arteries at the base of the brain, can be detected angiographically in up to 70% of patients beginning 4 to 12 days after SAH and is a leading cause of delayed morbidity and

mortality after SAH.[289,290] This time course of angiographic vasospasm is paralleled by a progressive fall in CBF over the first 2 weeks and abnormally low CBF for at least 3 weeks after SAH as measured with daily xenon 133 inhalation.[291] Reduced CBF as measured by SPECT,[292,293] PET,[294] or xenon 133 clearance[295,296] correlates well with angiographically measured vessel diameter in SAH when the blood flow study and angiography are performed serially, preferably within 1 hour. However, in the case of focal angiographic vasospasm, the CBF reduction is global rather than restricted to the distribution of the spastic artery, arguing against vasospasm as the actual cause for the reduction in flow.[295]

The extent of CBF abnormality correlates well with the clinical severity of neurologic deficits after SAH, although there is a wide range of flows within each grade.[297–301] Patients with more severe neurologic deficits after SAH (Hunt and Hess clinical grades III and IV) have a more marked reduction in regional CBF than do patients with a more favorable clinical grade (Hunt and Hess grades I and II). Using regional CBF less than 20% of mean CBF as an indication of ischemia, Ishii[297] observed foci of ischemia in 39% of measurements in patients with grade I or II neurologic deficits, 64% of measurements in patients with grade III deficits, and 95% of measurements in patients with grade IV deficits. Presence of ischemic foci is also correlated with outcome, being seen in only one quarter of patients who ultimately recover but in two thirds of patients who die.[302] Similarly, there is a correlation between regional CBF and outcome; patients with a mean CBF of 41 to $42\,mL/100\,g^{-1}/min^{-1}$ have an excellent outcome, and those with a mean CBF of 25 to $33\,mL/100\,g^{-1}/min^{-1}$ have a poor outcome.[297,302]

Flow velocity as measured by transcranial Doppler (TCD) ultrasonography in the MCA progressively increases after SAH, from normal values of 30 cm/sec to 80 cm/sec,[303] peaking at 7 to 10 days and normalizing over the following 2 weeks.[304] In patients with lateralized aneurysms, the increase is higher on the side of the ruptured aneurysm.[305] TCD flow velocities in excess of 200 cm/sec are assumed to indicate a reduction in angiographic caliber of more than 50%.[304] Correlation between TCD flow velocity and angiographic vessel caliber is good when the velocity is either low (<120 cm/sec) or very high (≥200 cm/sec), but intermediate velocities, which are seen in more than half of patients with SAH, do not reliably predict severity of angiographic vasospasm.[306]

The use of TCD measurements of flow velocity to infer cross-sectional area of an artery assumes that flow is constant, an assumption that may be invalid if the tissue is infarcted or if different collateral channels are utilized. Many variables other than the diameter of the vessel may affect measured velocity, however, such as the overall resistance to flow of all downstream vessels,[307] ICP,[308] and hemodilution.[309] In addition, with severe vasospasm, flow may be reduced, resulting in a decrease in velocity with further reduction in vessel diameter.[310]

It is important to remember that TCD ultrasonography measures the velocity of red blood cells, which is not equivalent to CBF. CBF depends not only on the measured velocity (which depends on the insonation angle) but also on the cross-sectional area of the artery and the volume of tissue perfused. Thus, there is a poor correlation between TCD flow velocity and CBF.[311–313]

Measurement of velocity in the anterior and posterior cerebral arteries is limited, because these vessels have less favorable angles of insonation and more collateral flow than the MCA. Additionally, the sensitivity of detecting vasospasm in the anterior cerebral artery is poor because of the possibility of increased flow across the anterior communicating artery.[304]

The effects of SAH on cerebral blood flow and metabolism have not been completely defined. Depression of CBF and $CMRO_2$ has been reported by several investigators,[294,314–317] but OEF has been variably described as normal[294,315,317] or elevated.[316,318] Consequently, the reduced metabolism is interpreted to reflect primary metabolic depression or ischemia, respectively. Complicating the interpretation of these data are the effects of various confounding factors, such as associated ICH, hydrocephalus, sedative drugs, vasospasm, brain injury due to surgical retraction, and postoperative hemodilution. In patients with vasospasm who do not experience subsequent infarction,[287] CBF is decreased, $CMRO_2$ is normal, and OEF is increased, conditions that are consistent with ischemia.[287] With resolution of vasospasm, CBF increases.[316] Two groups of investigators have demonstrated reductions in CBF and $CMRO_2$ with no change in OEF in patients with SAH,[301,317] but because cerebral infarction or moderate to severe disability was reported in approximately two thirds of the patients in these two studies, the failure to find elevated OEF may be due to the inclusion of patients with subacute cerebral infarction in whom OEF had returned to normal (see preceding discussion of acute ischemic stroke.)

Studies of CBV in patients with SAH likewise have yielded conflicting results. Grubb and coworkers[294] reported a statistically significant higher CBV in patients with Hunt and Hess clinical grade III or IV with angiographic vasospasm than in normal volunteers. OEF values were not reported, but examination of the CBF and $CMRO_2$ data indicates that OEF was probably not higher in the patients with vasospasm than in those without it. In a PET study of SAH, Hino and associates[317] reported a significant increase in CBV in regions of symptomatic angiographic vasospasm. They did not, however, observe an elevation in regional OEF. In another PET study, regional CBF was lower than normal in patients with SAH with and without vasospasm as well as in patients with ipsilateral carotid occlusion ($P < .0001$).[288] Regional OEF was higher both during vasospasm and distal to carotid occlusion than in SAH without vasospasm or in normal volunteers ($P < .0001$). Regional CBV was lower than normal in regions with and without spasm, whereas it was increased ipsilateral to carotid occlusion ($P < .0001$). These findings, of reduced parenchymal CBV during vasospasm under conditions of tissue ischemia similar to those that produce increased CBV in patients with carotid occlusion, were interpreted as evidence that parenchymal vessels distal to arteries with angiographic spasm after SAH do not demonstrate normal autoregulatory vasodilation. The reason for the discrepancies among these studies in the measurement of CBV during vasospasm is not clear but it may reflect the variability of CBV changes during reduced CPP noted earlier.

In the absence of ICH, hydrocephalus, infarction, and vasospasm, autoregulation is probably preserved after SAH.[297,298,319] In the majority of patients with angiographic vasospasm of large arteries after aneurysmal SAH, the response of autoregulation to both reductions[297,298,319,320] and rises[321,322] in systemic arterial pressure is defective. Autoregulation is impaired even in patients with slight vasospasm (25% to 50% reduction of arterial caliber.)[319]

Because ischemia due to vasospasm may lead to infarction if blood flow is not restored to adequate levels, one of the primary goals of SAH management is to prevent or treat vasospasm. The calcium channel blocker nimodipine has been shown to reduce the incidence of cerebral ischemic deficits and to improve overall outcome after SAH,[323,324] but its effect on angiographic vasospasm is inconclusive.[325–328] Reports of the effect of nimodipine on CBF have been mixed.[329–331] Nimodipine had no effect on CO_2 reactivity in one small study of patients with SAH and Hunt and Hess clinical grade I or II[332] but improved CO_2 reactivity in another study of patients with SAH and Hunt and Hess grade III or IV.[331] Encouraging clinical results have also been achieved with hypertensive and/or hypervolemic hemodilution ("triple H") therapy,[333,334] but again, reports of the effects on CBF have been mixed.[321,335–338] Once the treatment for vasospasm that effects the greatest improvement in CBF can be determined, the next step will be to demonstrate that raising the CBF actually translates into an increase in oxygen metabolism in the areas of the brain that are deficient and that clinical improvement results. Obviously, if the tissue is permanently damaged, improved perfusion will have no clinical benefit.

Surgical retraction may have profound effects on cerebral metabolism. A small PET study before and after right frontotemporal craniotomies performed for clipping of ruptured anterior circulation aneurysms showed a 45% reduction in regional $CMRO_2$ and a 32% reduction in regional OEF without significant change in CBF in the region of retraction, but no change in the other hemisphere.[339] These changes indicate a primary reduction in metabolism and uncoupling of flow and metabolism (luxury perfusion). They are not suggestive of vasospasm, which produces diffuse changes respecting large vascular territories; these changes were focal in the area of retractor blade placement. Other studies have shown a reduction in CBF in the area of retraction.[340,341] In one of these, xenon 133 SPECT CBF measurements were made in patients with frontal lesions including infarction an average of 82 days after surgery.[340] As previously described, the long-term changes observed after cerebral ischemia include matched reductions in CBF and $CMRO_2$ and normal to slightly reduced OEF (see Plate 40–4). In two others,[341,342] CBF was measured with technetium 99m HM-PAO (hexamethyl-propyleneamineoxime), which requires intact metabolism for radiotracer uptake. Thus, when metabolism is reduced, this technique may yield artificially low CBF values.[343]

CONCLUSIONS

Measurements of CBF and CMR in ischemia and hemorrhage have provided valuable insight into the pathophysiology of stroke. Much has been learned about the compensatory responses of the brain to reductions in perfusion pressure and in the evolution of changes in blood flow and metabolism that occur when these mechanisms fail. Knowledge of these changes can help guide therapy when multiple factors, such as ischemia, hypoxemia, hypocarbia, or hypotension may be affecting cerebral blood flow. An understanding of the hemodynamic effects of arterial stenosis or occlusion on the downstream perfusion pressure has been instrumental in the design of new trials for treatment.[344] In acute ischemic stroke, measurements of CBF and metabolism have been used to define the ischemic penumbra and to predict both tissue and clinical outcomes, although the clinical utility of these markers of ischemia in distinguishing viable from irreversibly damaged tissue in the acute period remains to be proven.

Blood flow and metabolic studies in ICH have documented the integrity of autoregulation and suggested that hematomas exert a primary depression of metabolism rather than inducing ischemia in the surrounding tissue. This issue has important implications for future consideration of therapeutic interventions in this disease. Studies in SAH have differentiated the primary effects of the hemorrhage on cerebral hemodynamics and metabolism from those of vasospasm and surgical retraction. In addition, vasospasm-induced ischemia has been demonstrated to be reversible.

In summary, defining the pathophysiologic changes in CBF and metabolism in human cerebrovascular disease has provided and will continue to provide the basic foundation for development and testing of new treatment strategies.

Acknowledgments

This work was supported by grants from the National Institutes of Health (NS35966, 1K23NSO44885, and NS42167), and the Lillian Strauss Institute of Barnes-Jewish Hospital.

References

1. Rossen R, Kabat H, Anderson JP: Acute arrest of cerebral circulation in man. Arch Neurol Psychiatry 50:510–528, 1943.
2. Kety SS, Schmidt CF: The determination of cerebral blood flow in man by the use of nitrous oxide in low concentrations. J Clin Invest 143:53–66, 1945.
3. Kety SS, Schmidt CF: The nitrous oxide method for the quantitative determination of cerebral blood flow in man: Theory, procedure, and normal values. J Clin Invest 27:476–483, 1948.
4. Marcus ML, Heistad DD, Ehrhardt JC, Abboud FM: Total and regional cerebral blood flow measurement with 7–10-, 15-, 25-, and 50-mum microspheres. J Appl Physiol 40:501–507, 1976.
5. Kuhl DE, Barrio JR, Huang SC, et al: Quantifying local cerebral blood flow by N-isopropyl-p-[123I]iodoamphetamine (IMP) tomography. J Nucl Med 23:196–203, 1982.
6. Kety SS: Blood-tissue exchange methods: Theory of blood-tissue exchange and its application to measurement of blood flow. Methods Med Res 8:223–236, 1960.
7. Zierler KL: Equations for measuring blood flow by external monitoring of radioisotopes. Circ Res 16:309–321, 1965.
8. Hoedt-Rasmussen K, Sveinsdottir E, Lassen NA: Regional cerebral blood flow in man determined by intra-arterial injection of radioactive inert gas. Circ Res 18:237–247, 1966.
9. Larson KB, Snyder DL: Measurement of relative blood flow, transit-time distributions and transport-model parameters by residue

10. Zierler KL: Theoretical basis of indicator-dilution methods for measuring flow and volume. Circ Res 10:393–407, 1962.
11. Axel L: Cerebral blood flow determination by rapid-sequence computed tomography: Theoretical analysis. Radiology 137:679–686, 1980.
12. Weisskoff RM, Chesler D, Boxerman JL, Rosen BR: Pitfalls in MR measurement of tissue blood flow with intravascular tracers: Which mean transit time? Magn Reson Med 29:553–558, 1993.
13. Larson KB, Markham J, Raichle ME: Tracer-kinetic models for measuring cerebral blood flow using externally detected radiotracers. J Cereb Blood Flow Metab 7:443–463, 1987.
14. Powers WJ: Hemodynamics and metabolism in ischemic cerebrovascular disease. Neurol Clin 10:31–48, 1992.
15. Kety SS: Human cerebral blood flow and oxygen consumption as related to aging. J Chron Dis 3:478–486, 1956.
16. Baron JC, Frackowiak RS, Herholz K, et al: Use of PET methods for measurement of cerebral energy metabolism and hemodynamics in cerebrovascular disease. J Cereb Blood Flow Metab 9:723–742, 1989.
17. Powers WJ, Raichle ME: Positron emission tomography and its application to the study of cerebrovascular disease in man. Stroke 16:361–376, 1985.
18. Cohen PJ, Alexander SC, Smith TC, et al: Effects of hypoxia and normocarbia on cerebral blood flow and metabolism in conscious man. J Appl Physiol 23:183–189, 1967.
19. Madsen PL, Holm S, Herning M, Lassen NA: Average blood flow and oxygen uptake in the human brain during resting wakefulness: A critical appraisal of the Kety-Schmidt technique. J Cereb Blood Flow Metab 13:646–655, 1993.
20. Gottstein U, Bernsmeier A, Sedlmeyer I: Der kohlenhydratstoffwechsel des menschlichen gehirns. Klin Wochenschr 41:943–948, 1963.
21. Scheinberg P, Stead EA: The cerebral blood flow in male subjects as measured by the nitrous oxide technique: Normal values for blood flow, oxygen utilization, glucose utilization and peripheral resistance, with observations on the effect of tilting and anxiety. J Clin Invest 28:1163–1171, 1949.
22. McHenry LC Jr, Merory J, Bass E, et al: Xenon-133 inhalation method for regional cerebral blood flow measurements: Normal values and test-retest results. Stroke 9:396–399, 1978.
23. Lebrun-Grandie P, Baron JC, Soussaline F, et al: Coupling between regional blood flow and oxygen utilization in the normal human brain: A study with positron tomography and oxygen 15. Arch Neurol 40:230–236, 1983.
24. Baron JC, Rougemont D, Soussaline F, et al: Local interrelationships of cerebral oxygen consumption and glucose utilization in normal subjects and in ischemic stroke patients: A positron tomography study. J Cereb Blood Flow Metab 4:140–149, 1984.
25. Sette G, Baron JC, Mazoyer B, et al: Local brain haemodynamics and oxygen metabolism in cerebrovascular disease: Positron emission tomography. Brain 112:931–951, 1989.
26. Frackowiak RS, Lenzi GL, Jones T, Heather JD: Quantitative measurement of regional cerebral blood flow and oxygen metabolism in man using 15O and positron emission tomography: Theory, procedure, and normal values. J Comput Assist Tomogr 4:727–736, 1980.
27. Powers WJ, Grubb RL Jr, Darriet D, Raichle ME: Cerebral blood flow and cerebral metabolic rate of oxygen requirements for cerebral function and viability in humans. J Cereb Blood Flow Metab 5:600–608, 1985.
28. Wise RJ, Rhodes CG, Gibbs JM, et al: Disturbance of oxidative metabolism of glucose in recent human cerebral infarcts. Ann Neurol 14:627–637, 1983.
29. Richardson BS, Carmichael L, Homan J, et al: Regional blood flow change in the lamb during the perinatal period. Am J Obstet Gynecol 160:919–925, 1989.
30. Tuor UI: Local cerebral blood flow in the newborn rabbit: An autoradiographic study of changes during development. Pediatr Res 29:517–523, 1991.
31. Nehlig A, Pereira d, V, Boyet S: Postnatal changes in local cerebral blood flow measured by the quantitative autoradiographic [14C]iodoantipyrine technique in freely moving rats. J Cereb Blood Flow Metab 9:579–588, 1989.
32. Altman DI, Perlman JM, Volpe JJ, Powers WJ: Cerebral oxygen metabolism in newborns. Pediatrics 92:99–104, 1993.

detection when radiotracer recirculates. J Theor Biol 37:503–529, 1972.

33. Meek JH, Tyszczuk L, Elwell CE, Wyatt JS: Cerebral blood flow increases over the first three days of life in extremely preterm neonates. Arch Dis Child Fetal Neonatal Ed 78:F33–F37, 1998.

34. Pellicer A, Valverde E, Gaya F, et al: Postnatal adaptation of brain circulation in preterm infants. Pediatr Neurol 24:103–109, 2001.

35. Greisen G, Pryds O: Low CBF, discontinuous EEG activity, and periventricular brain injury in ill, preterm neonates. Brain Dev 11:164–168, 1989.

36. Altman DI, Powers WJ, Perlman JM, et al: Cerebral blood flow requirement for brain viability in newborn infants is lower than in adults. Ann Neurol 24:218–226, 1988.

37. Settergren G, Lindblad BS, Persson B: Cerebral blood flow and exchange of oxygen, glucose, ketone bodies, lactate, pyruvate and amino acids in infants. Acta Paediatr Scand 65:343–353, 1976.

38. Cross KW, Dear PR, Hathorn MK, et al: An estimation of intracranial blood flow in the new-born infant. J Physiol 289:329–345, 1979.

39. Rosenbaum JL, Almli CR, Yundt KD, et al: Higher neonatal cerebral blood flow correlates with worse childhood neurologic outcome. Neurology 49:1035–1041, 1997.

40. Powers WJ, Rosenbaum JL, Dence CS, et al: Cerebral glucose transport and metabolism in preterm human infants. J Cereb Blood Flow Metab 18:632–638, 1998.

41. Kinnala A, Suhonen-Polvi H, Aarimaa T, et al: Cerebral metabolic rate for glucose during the first six months of life: An FDG positron emission tomography study. Arch Dis Child Fetal Neonatal Ed 74:F153–F157, 1996.

42. Suhonen-Polvi H, Ruotsalainen U, Kinnala A, et al: FDG-PET in early infancy: Simplified quantification methods to measure cerebral glucose utilization. J Nucl Med 36:1249–1254, 1995.

43. Kennedy C, Sokoloff L: An adaptation of the nitrous oxide method to the study of the cerebral circulation in children: Normal values for cerebral blood flow and cerebral metabolic rate in childhood. J Clin Invest 36:1130–1137, 1957.

44. Chiron C, Raynaud C, Maziere B, et al: Changes in regional cerebral blood flow during brain maturation in children and adolescents. J Nucl Med 33:696–703, 1992.

45. Ogawa A, Nakamura K, Sugita Y, et al: Regional cerebral blood flow in children: Normal values and regional distribution of cerebral blood flow in childhood. J Cereb Blood Flow Metab 5(Suppl 1):S97–S98, 1985.

46. Ogawa A, Sakurai Y, Kayama T, Yoshimoto T: Regional cerebral blood flow with age: Changes in rCBF in childhood. Neurol Res 11:173–176, 1989.

47. Chugani HT, Phelps ME: Maturational changes in cerebral function in infants determined by 18FDG positron emission tomography. Science 231:840–843, 1986.

48. Chugani HT, Phelps ME, Mazziotta JC: Positron emission tomography study of human brain functional development. Ann Neurol 22:487–497, 1987.

49. Leenders KL, Perani D, Lammertsma AA, et al: Cerebral blood flow, blood volume and oxygen utilization. Normal values and effect of age. Brain 113(Pt 1):27–47, 1990.

50. Pantano P, Baron JC, Lebrun-Grandie P, et al: Regional cerebral blood flow and oxygen consumption in human aging. Stroke 15:635–641, 1984.

51. Dastur DK: Cerebral blood flow and metabolism in normal human aging, pathological aging, and senile dementia. J Cereb Blood Flow Metab 5:1–9, 1985.

52. Martin AJ, Friston KJ, Colebatch JG, Frackowiak RS: Decreases in regional cerebral blood flow with normal aging. J Cereb Blood Flow Metab 11:684–689, 1991.

53. Davis SM, Ackerman RH, Correia JA, et al: Cerebral blood flow and cerebrovascular CO2 reactivity in stroke-age normal controls. Neurology 33:391–399, 1983.

54. Kuhl DE, Metter EJ, Riege WH, Hawkins RA: The effect of normal aging on patterns of local cerebral glucose utilization. Ann Neurol 15(Suppl):S133–S137, 1984.

55. Marchal G, Rioux P, Petit-Taboue MC, et al: Regional cerebral oxygen consumption, blood flow, and blood volume in healthy human aging. Arch Neurol 49:1013–1020, 1992.

56. Yamaguchi T, Kanno I, Uemura K, et al: Reduction in regional cerebral metabolic rate of oxygen during human aging. Stroke 17:1220–1228, 1986.

57. de Leon MJ, George AE, Ferris SH, et al: Positron emission tomography and computed tomography assessments of the aging human brain. J Comput Assist Tomogr 8:88–94, 1984.

58. Duara R, Margolin RA, Robertson-Tchabo EA, et al: Cerebral glucose utilization, as measured with positron emission tomography in 21 resting healthy men between the ages of 21 and 83 years. Brain 106:761–775, 1983.

59. Duara R, Grady C, Haxby J, et al: Human brain glucose utilization and cognitive function in relation to age. Ann Neurol 16:703–713, 1984.

60. Yoshii F, Barker WW, Chang JY, et al: Sensitivity of cerebral glucose metabolism to age, gender, brain volume, brain atrophy, and cerebrovascular risk factors. J Cereb Blood Flow Metab 8:654–661, 1988.

61. Kety SS, Schmidt CF: The effects of active and passive hyperventilation on cerebral blood flow, cerebral oxygen consumption, cardiac output, and blood pressure of normal young men. J Clin Invest 25:107–119, 1946.

62. Kety SS, Schmidt CF: The effects of altered arterial tensions of carbon dioxide and oxygen on cerebral blood flow and cerebral oxygen consumption of normal young men. J Clin Invest 27:484–492, 1948.

63. Wollman H, Smith TC, Stephen GW, et al: Effects of extremes of respiratory and metabolic alkalosis on cerebral blood flow in man. J Appl Physiol 24:60–65, 1968.

64. Fencl V, Vale JR, Broch JA: Respiration and cerebral blood flow in metabolic acidosis and alkalosis in humans. J Appl Physiol 27:67–76, 1969.

65. Raichle ME, Posner JB, Plum F: Cerebral blood flow during and after hyperventilation. Arch Neurol 23:394–403, 1970.

66. Alexander SC, Smith TC, Strobel G, et al: Cerebral carbohydrate metabolism of man during respiratory and metabolic alkalosis. J Appl Physiol 24:66–72, 1968.

67. van Rijen PC, Luyten PR, van der Sprenkel JW, et al: 1H and 31P NMR measurement of cerebral lactate, high-energy phosphate levels, and pH in humans during voluntary hyperventilation: Associated EEG, capnographic, and Doppler findings. Magn Reson Med 10:182–193, 1989.

68. Shimojyo S, Scheinberg P, Kogure K, Reinmuth OM: The effects of graded hypoxia upon transient cerebral blood flow and oxygen consumption. Neurology 18:127–133, 1968.

69. Buck A, Schirlo C, Jasinsky V, et al: Changes of cerebral blood flow during short-term exposure to normobaric hypoxia. J Cereb Blood Flow Metab 18:906–910, 1998.

70. Lassen NA: Cerebral blood flow and oxygen consumption in man. Physiol Rev 39:183–238, 1959.

71. Brown MM, Wade JP, Marshall J: Fundamental importance of arterial oxygen content in the regulation of cerebral blood flow in man. Brain 108:81–93, 1985.

72. Lambertsen CJ, Kough RH, Cooper DY, et al: Oxygen toxicity: Effects in man of oxygen inhalation at 1 and 3.5 atmospheres upon blood gas transport, cerebral circulation and cerebral metabolism. J Appl Physiol 5:471–486, 1953.

73. Todd MM, Wu B, Maktabi M, et al: Cerebral blood flow and oxygen delivery during hypoxemia and hemodilution: Role of arterial oxygen content. Am J Physiol 267:H2025-H2031, 1994.

74. Mintun MA, Lundstrom BN, Snyder AZ, et al: Blood flow and oxygen delivery to human brain during functional activity: Theoretical modeling and experimental data. Proc Natl Acad Sci U S A 98:6859–6864, 2001.

75. Thomas DJ, Marshall J, Russell RW, et al: Effect of haematocrit on cerebral blood-flow in man. Lancet 2(8045):941–943, 1977.

76. Brown MM, Marshall J: Regulation of cerebral blood flow in response to changes in blood viscosity. Lancet 1(8429):604–609, 1985.

77. Brown MM, Marshall J: Effect of plasma exchange on blood viscosity and cerebral blood flow. BMJ 284:1733–1736, 1982.

78. Paulson OB, Parving HH, Olesen J, Skinhoj E: Influence of carbon monoxide and of hemodilution on cerebral blood flow and blood gases in man. J Appl Physiol 35:111–116, 1973.

79. Tomiyama Y, Brian JE Jr, Todd MM: Plasma viscosity and cerebral blood flow. Am J Physiol 279:H1949–H1954, 2000.

80. Rebel A, Lenz C, Krieter H, et al: Oxygen delivery at high blood viscosity and decreased arterial oxygen content to brains of conscious rats. Am J Physiol 280:H2591–H2597, 2001.

81. Cole DJ, Drummond JC, Patel PM, Marcantonio S: Effects of viscosity and oxygen content on cerebral blood flow in ischemic and normal rat brain. J Neurol Sci 124:15–20, 1994.

82. Powers WJ, Boyle PJ, Hirsch IB, Cryer PE: Unaltered cerebral blood flow during hypoglycemic activation of the sympathochromaffin system in humans. Am J Physiol 265:R883–R887, 1993.

Pathophysiology

83. Boyle PJ, Nagy RJ, O'Connor AM, et al: Adaptation in brain glucose uptake following recurrent hypoglycemia. Proc Natl Acad Sci U S A 91:9352–9356, 1994.

84. Gottstein U, Held K: The effect of insulin on brain metabolism in metabolically healthy and diabetic patients. Klin Wochenschr 45:18–23, 1967.

85. Boyle PJ, Kempers SF, O'Connor AM, Nagy RJ: Brain glucose uptake and unawareness of hypoglycemia in patients with insulin-dependent diabetes mellitus. N Engl J Med 333:1726–1731, 1995.

86. Tallroth G, Ryding E, Agardh CD: Regional cerebral blood flow in normal man during insulin-induced hypoglycemia and in the recovery period following glucose infusion. Metabolism 41:717–721, 1992.

87. Tallroth G, Ryding E, Agardh CD: The influence of hypoglycaemia on regional cerebral blood flow and cerebral volume in type 1 (insulin-dependent) diabetes mellitus. Diabetologia 36:530–535, 1993.

88. Neil HA, Gale EA, Hamilton SJ, et al: Cerebral blood flow increases during insulin-induced hypoglycaemia in type 1 (insulin-dependent) diabetic patients and control subjects. Diabetologia 30:305–309, 1987.

89. Kerr D, Stanley JC, Barron M, et al: Symmetry of cerebral blood flow and cognitive responses to hypoglycaemia in humans. Diabetologia 36:73–78, 1993.

90. Eckert B, Ryding E, Agardh CD: Sustained elevation of cerebral blood flow after hypoglycaemia in normal man. Diabetes Res Clin Pract 40:91–100, 1998.

91. Chen JL, Wei L, Acuff V, et al: Slightly altered permeability-surface area products imply some cerebral capillary recruitment during hypercapnia. Microvasc Res 48:190–211, 1994.

92. Chen JL, Wei L, Bereczki D, et al: Nicotine raises the influx of permeable solutes across the rat blood-brain barrier with little or no capillary recruitment. J Cereb Blood Flow Metab 15:687–698, 1995.

93. Kuschinsky W, Paulson OB: Capillary circulation in the brain. Cerebrovasc Brain Metab Rev 4:261–286, 1992.

94. Derrer SA, Sieber FE, Saudek CD, et al: Cerebrovascular and metabolic responses to hypoxia during hypoglycemia in dogs. Am J Physiol 258:H400–H407, 1990.

95. Sieber FE, Koehler RC, Derrer SA, et al: Hypoglycemia and cerebral autoregulation in anesthetized dogs. Am J Physiol 258:H1714–H1721, 1990.

96. Sokoloff L: Relationships among local functional activity, energy metabolism, and blood flow in the central nervous system. Fed Proc 40:2311–2316, 1981.

97. Fox PT, Raichle ME: Focal physiological uncoupling of cerebral blood flow and oxidative metabolism during somatosensory stimulation in human subjects. Proc Natl Acad Sci U S A 83:1140–1144, 1986.

98. Fox PT, Raichle ME, Mintun MA, Dence C: Nonoxidative glucose consumption during focal physiologic neural activity. Science 241:462–464, 1988.

99. Buxton RB, Frank LR: A model for the coupling between cerebral blood flow and oxygen metabolism during neural stimulation. J Cereb Blood Flow Metab 17:64–72, 1997.

100. Powers WJ, Hirsch IB, Cryer PE: Effect of stepped hypoglycemia on regional cerebral blood flow response to physiological brain activation. Am J Physiol 270:H554–H559, 1996.

101. Ido Y, Chang K, Woolsey TA, Williamson JR: NADH: Sensor of blood flow need in brain, muscle, and other tissues. FASEB J 15:1419–1421, 2001.

102. MacKenzie ET, Farrar JK, Fitch W, et al: Effects of hemorrhagic hypotension on the cerebral circulation. I: Cerebral blood flow and pial arteriolar caliber. Stroke 10:711–718, 1979.

103. Symon L, Pasztor E, Dorsch NW, Branston NM: Physiological responses of local areas of the cerebral circulation in experimental primates determined by the method of hydrogen clearance. Stroke 4:632–642, 1973.

104. Strandgaard S: Autoregulation of cerebral blood flow in hypertensive patients: The modifying influence of prolonged antihypertensive treatment on the tolerance to acute, drug-induced hypotension. Circulation 53:720–727, 1976.

105. Schmidt JF, Waldemar G, Vorstrup S, et al: Computerized analysis of cerebral blood flow autoregulation in humans: Validation of a method for pharmacologic studies. J Cardiovasc Pharmacol 15:983–988, 1990.

106. Strandgaard S, Olesen J, Skinhoj E, Lassen NA: Autoregulation of brain circulation in severe arterial hypertension. Br Med J 1:507–510, 1973.

107. Dirnagl U, Pulsinelli W: Autoregulation of cerebral blood flow in experimental focal brain ischemia. J Cereb Blood Flow Metab 10:327–336, 1990.

108. Heistad DD, Kontos HE: Cerebral circulation. In Shepherd JT, Aboud FM (eds): Handbook of Physiology, Section 2, Vol 3, Pt 1. Bethesda, American Physiological Society, 1983, pp 137–182.

109. Mies G, Paschen W, Hossmann KA: Cerebral blood flow, glucose utilization, regional glucose, and ATP content during the maturation period of delayed ischemic injury in gerbil brain. J Cereb Blood Flow Metab 10:638–645, 1990.

110. Sutton LN, McLaughlin AC, Dante S, et al: Cerebral venous oxygen content as a measure of brain energy metabolism with increased intracranial pressure and hyperventilation. J Neurosurg 73:927–932, 1990.

111. Fog M: Cerebral circulation: The reaction of pial arteries to a fall in blood pressure. Arch Neurol Psychiatry 37:351–364, 1937.

112. Wolfe HG, Forbes HS: The cerebral circulation. V: Observations of the pial circulation during changes in intracranial pressure. Arch Neurol Psychiatry 20:1035–1047, 1928.

113. Kato Y, Mokry M, Pucher R, Auer LM: Cerebrovascular response to changes of cerebral venous pressure and cerebrospinal fluid pressure. Acta Neurochir (Wien) 109:52–56, 1991.

114. Grubb RL Jr, Phelps ME, Raichle ME, Ter Pogossian MM: The effects of arterial blood pressure on the regional cerebral blood volume by X-ray fluorescence. Stroke 4:390–399, 1973.

115. Grubb RL Jr, Raichle ME, Phelps ME, Ratcheson RA: Effects of increased intracranial pressure on cerebral blood volume, blood flow, and oxygen utilization in monkeys. J Neurosurg 43:385–398, 1975.

116. Ferrari M, Wilson DA, Hanley DF, Traystman RJ: Effects of graded hypotension on cerebral blood flow, blood volume, and mean transit time in dogs. Am J Physiol 262:H1908–H1914, 1992.

117. Wiedeman MP: Dimensions of blood vessels from distributing artery to collecting vein. Circ Res 12:375–378, 1963.

118. Hilal SK: Cerebral hemodynamics assessed by angiography. In Newton TH, Potts DG (eds): Radiology of the Skull and Brain: Angiography. Volume 2, book 1. CV Mosby Company, St. Louis, 1974.

119. Auer LM, Ishiyama N, Pucher R: Cerebrovascular response to intracranial hypertension. Acta Neurochir (Wien) 84:124–128, 1987.

120. Kato Y, Auer LM: Cerebrovascular response to elevation of ventricular pressure. Acta Neurochir (Wien) 98:184–188, 1989.

121. Schumann P, Touzani O, Young AR, et al: Evaluation of the ratio of cerebral blood flow to cerebral blood volume as an index of local cerebral perfusion pressure. Brain 121:1369–1379, 1998.

122. Grubb RL Jr, Derdeyn CP, Fritsch SM, et al: Importance of hemodynamic factors in the prognosis of symptomatic carotid occlusion. JAMA 280:1055–1060, 1998.

123. Zaharchuk G, Mandeville JB, Bogdanov AA Jr, et al: Cerebrovascular dynamics of autoregulation and hypoperfusion: An MRI study of CBF and changes in total and microvascular cerebral blood volume during hemorrhagic hypotension. Stroke 30:2197–2204, 1999.

124. Derdeyn CP, Videen TO, Yundt KD, et al: Variability of cerebral blood volume and oxygen extraction: Stages of cerebral haemodynamic impairment revisited. Brain 125:595–607, 2002.

125. Gibbs JM, Wise RJ, Leenders KL, Jones T: Evaluation of cerebral perfusion reserve in patients with carotid-artery occlusion. Lancet 1:310–314, 1984.

126. Powers WJ: Is the ratio of cerebral blood volume to cerebral blood flow a reliable indicator of cerebral perfusion pressure? J Cereb Blood Flow Metab 13(Suppl 1):S325, 1993.

127. Grubb RL Jr, Raichle ME, Eichling JO, Ter Pogossian MM: The effects of changes in PaCO2 on cerebral blood volume, blood flow, and vascular mean transit time. Stroke 5:630–639, 1974.

128. Maruyama M, Shimoji K, Ichikawa T, et al: The effects of extreme hemodilutions on the autoregulation of cerebral blood flow, electroencephalogram and cerebral metabolic rate of oxygen in the dog. Stroke 16:675–679, 1985.

129. Haggendal E, Johansson B: Effect of arterial carbon dioxide tension and oxygen saturation on cerebral blood flow autoregulation in dogs. Acta Physiol Scand 66:27–53, 1965.

130. Meyer JS, Shimazu K, Fukuuchi Y, et al: Impaired neurogenic cerebrovascular control and dysautoregulation after stroke. Stroke 4:169–186, 1973.

131. Bouma GJ, Muizelaar JP: Cerebral blood flow, cerebral blood volume, and cerebrovascular reactivity after severe head injury. J Neurotrauma 9(Suppl 1):S333–S348, 1992.

132. Barnett HJ: Hemodynamic cerebral ischemia: An appeal for systematic data gathering prior to a new EC/IC trial. Stroke 28:1857–1860, 1997.

133. Sillesen H, Schroeder T, Steenberg HJ, Hansen HJ: Doppler examination of the periorbital arteries adds valuable hemodynamic information in carotid artery disease. Ultrasound Med Biol 13:177–181, 1987.

134. Henderson RD, Eliasziw M, Fox AJ, et al: Angiographically defined collateral circulation and risk of stroke in patients with severe carotid artery stenosis. North American Symptomatic Carotid Endarterectomy Trial (NASCET) Group. Stroke 31:128–132, 2000.

135. Vernieri F, Pasqualetti P, Matteis M, et al: Effect of collateral blood flow and cerebral vasomotor reactivity on the outcome of carotid artery occlusion. Stroke 32:1552–1558, 2001.

136. Klijn CJ, Kappelle LJ, van Huffelen AC, et al: Recurrent ischemia in symptomatic carotid occlusion: Prognostic value of hemodynamic factors. Neurology 55:1806–1812, 2000.

137. Derdeyn CP, Shaibani A, Moran CJ, et al: Lack of correlation between pattern of collateralization and misery perfusion in patients with carotid occlusion. Stroke 30:1025–1032, 1999.

138. Powers WJ: Cerebral hemodynamics in ischemic cerebrovascular disease. Ann Neurol 29:231–240, 1991.

139. Baron JC, Bousser MG, Comar D, Kellershohn C: Human hemispheric infarction studied by positron emission tomography and the 15O continuous inhalation technique. In Caille JM, Salamon G (eds): Computerized Tomography: INSERM Symposium, Bordeaux, September 20–22, 1979. New York, Springer-Verlag, 1980, pp 231–237.

140. Baron JC, Bousser MG, Rey A, et al: Reversal of focal "misery-perfusion syndrome" by extra-intracranial arterial bypass in hemodynamic cerebral ischemia: A case study with 15O positron emission tomography. Stroke 12:454–459, 1981.

141. Lassen NA, Palvolgyi R: Cerebral steal during hypercapnia and the inverse reaction during hypocapnia observed with the 133xenon technique in man. Scand J Clin Lab Invest 22(Suppl 102):13D, 1968.

142. Oja JM, Gillen JS, Kauppinen RA, et al: Determination of oxygen extraction ratios by magnetic resonance imaging. J Cereb Blood Flow Metab 19:1289–1295, 1999.

143. An H, Lin W, Celik A, Lee YM: Quantitative measurements of cerebral metabolic rate of oxygen utilization using MRI: A volunteer study. NMR Biomed 14:441–447, 2001.

144. Kazumata K, Tanaka N, Ishikawa T, et al: Dissociation of vasoreactivity to acetazolamide and hypercapnia: Comparative study in patients with chronic occlusive major cerebral artery disease. Stroke 27:2052–2058, 1996.

145. Inao S, Tadokoro M, Nishino M, et al: Neural activation of the brain with hemodynamic insufficiency. J Cereb Blood Flow Metab 18:960–967, 1998.

146. Pindzola RR, Balzer JR, Nemoto EM, et al: Cerebrovascular reserve in patients with carotid occlusive disease assessed by stable xenon-enhanced CT cerebral blood flow and transcranial Doppler. Stroke 32:1811–1817, 2001.

147. Hirano T, Minematsu K, Hasegawa Y, et al: Acetazolamide reactivity on 123I-IMP single photon emission computed tomography in patients with major cerebral artery occlusive disease: Correlation with positron emission tomography parameters. J Cereb Blood Flow Metab 14:763–770, 1994.

148. Nariai T, Suzuki R, Hirakawa K, et al: Vascular reserve in chronic cerebral ischemia measured by the acetazolamide challenge test: Comparison with positron emission tomography. AJNR Am J Neuroradiol 16:563–570, 1995.

149. Derdeyn CP, Yundt KD, Carpenter DA, et al: Time-related changes in cerebral blood volume in patients with increased oxygen extraction. Stroke 31:329, 2000.

150. Herold S, Brown MM, Frackowiak RS, et al: Assessment of cerebral haemodynamic reserve: Correlation between PET parameters and CO2 reactivity measured by the intravenous 133 xenon injection technique. J Neurol Neurosurg Psychiatry 51:1045–1050, 1988.

151. Powers WJ, Raichle ME, Grubb RL Jr: Positron emission tomography to assess cerebral perfusion. Lancet 1(8420):102–103, 1985.

152. Beneficial effect of carotid endarterectomy in symptomatic patients with high-grade carotid stenosis. North American Symptomatic Carotid Endarterectomy Trial Collaborators. N Engl J Med 325:445–453, 1991.

153. Carotid surgery versus medical therapy in asymptomatic carotid stenosis. The CASANOVA Study Group. Stroke 22:1229–1235, 1991.

154. Results of a randomized controlled trial of carotid endarterectomy for asymptomatic carotid stenosis. Mayo Asymptomatic Carotid Endarterectomy Study Group. Mayo Clin Proc 67:513–518, 1992.

155. Hobson RW, Weiss DG, Fields WS, et al: Efficacy of carotid endarterectomy for asymptomatic carotid stenosis. The Veterans Affairs Cooperative Study Group. N Engl J Med 328:221–227, 1993.

156. Endarterectomy for asymptomatic carotid artery stenosis. Executive Committee for the Asymptomatic Carotid Atherosclerosis Study. JAMA 273:1421–1428, 1995.

157. Markus H, Cullinane M: Severely impaired cerebrovascular reactivity predicts stroke and TIA risk in patients with carotid artery stenosis and occlusion. Brain 124:457–467, 2001.

158. Silvestrini M, Vernieri F, Pasqualetti P, et al: Impaired cerebral vasoreactivity and risk of stroke in patients with asymptomatic carotid artery stenosis. JAMA 283:2122–2127, 2000.

159. Hankey GJ, Warlow CP: Prognosis of symptomatic carotid artery occlusion. Cerebrovasc Dis 1:245–256, 1991.

160. Klijn CJ, Kappelle LJ, Tulleken CA, van Gijn J: Symptomatic carotid artery occlusion: A reappraisal of hemodynamic factors. Stroke 28:2084–2093, 1997.

161. Powers WJ, Tempel LW, Grubb RL Jr: Influence of cerebral hemodynamics on stroke risk: One-year follow-up of 30 medically treated patients. Ann Neurol 25:325–330, 1989.

162. Yamauchi H, Fukuyama H, Nagahama Y, et al: Evidence of misery perfusion and risk for recurrent stroke in major cerebral arterial occlusive diseases from PET. J Neurol Neurosurg Psychiatry 61:18–25, 1996.

163. Yamauchi H, Fukuyama H, Nagahama Y, et al: Significance of increased oxygen extraction fraction in five-year prognosis of major cerebral arterial occlusive diseases. J Nucl Med 40:1992–1998, 1999.

164. Webster MW, Makaroun MS, Steed DL, et al: Compromised cerebral blood flow reactivity is a predictor of stroke in patients with symptomatic carotid artery occlusive disease. J Vasc Surg 21:338–344, 1995.

165. Yokota C, Hasegawa Y, Minematsu K, Yamaguchi T: Effect of acetazolamide reactivity on long-term outcome in patients with major cerebral artery occlusive diseases. Stroke 29:640–644, 1998.

166. Vernieri F, Pasqualetti P, Passarelli F, et al: Outcome of carotid artery occlusion is predicted by cerebrovascular reactivity. Stroke 30:593–598, 1999.

167. Yonas H, Smith HA, Durham SR, et al: Increased stroke risk predicted by compromised cerebral blood flow reactivity. J Neurosurg 79:483–489, 1993.

168. Powers WJ, Martin WR, Herscovitch P, et al: Extracranial-intracranial bypass surgery: Hemodynamic and metabolic effects. Neurology 34:1168–1174, 1984.

169. Samson Y, Baron JC, Bousser MG, et al: Effects of extra-intracranial arterial bypass on cerebral blood flow and oxygen metabolism in humans. Stroke 16:609–616, 1985.

170. Laurent JP, Lawner PM, O'Connor M: Reversal of intracerebral steal by STA-MCA anastomosis. J Neurosurg 57:629–632, 1982.

171. Schmiedek P, Piepgras A, Leinsinger G, et al: Improvement of cerebrovascular reserve capacity by EC-IC arterial bypass surgery in patients with ICA occlusion and hemodynamic cerebral ischemia. J Neurosurg 81:236–244, 1994.

172. Gibbs JM, Wise RJ, Thomas DJ, et al: Cerebral haemodynamic changes after extracranial-intracranial bypass surgery. J Neurol Neurosurg Psychiatry 50:140–150, 1987.

173. Failure of extracranial-intracranial arterial bypass to reduce the risk of ischemic stroke. Results of an international randomized trial. EC/IC Bypass Study Group. N Engl J Med 313:1191–1200, 1985.

174. Ausman JI, Diaz FG: Critique of the Extracranial-Intracranial Bypass Study. Surg Neurol 26:218–221, 1986.

175. Day AL, Rhoton AL Jr, Little JR: The Extracranial-Intracranial Bypass Study. Surg Neurol 26:222–226, 1986.

176. Pappata S, Fiorelli M, Rommel T, et al: PET study of changes in local brain hemodynamics and oxygen metabolism after unilateral

Pathophysiology

middle cerebral artery occlusion in baboons. J Cereb Blood Flow Metab 13:416–424, 1993.

177. Heiss WD, Graf R, Wienhard K, et al: Dynamic penumbra demonstrated by sequential multitracer PET after middle cerebral artery occlusion in cats. J Cereb Blood Flow Metab 14:892–902, 1994.

178. Touzani O, Young AR, Derlon JM, et al: Sequential studies of severely hypometabolic tissue volumes after permanent middle cerebral artery occlusion: A positron emission tomographic investigation in anesthetized baboons. Stroke 26:2112–2119, 1995.

179. Ackerman RH, Lev MH, Mackay BC, et al: PET studies in acute stroke: Findings and relevance to therapy. J Cereb Blood Flow Metab 9(Suppl 1):S359, 1989.

180. Heiss WD, Huber M, Fink GR, et al: Progressive derangement of periinfarct viable tissue in ischemic stroke. J Cereb Blood Flow Metab 12:193–203, 1992.

181. Molina CA, Montaner J, Abilleira S, et al: Timing of spontaneous recanalization and risk of hemorrhagic transformation in acute cardioembolic stroke. Stroke 32:1079–1084, 2001.

182. Jorgensen HS, Sperling B, Nakayama H, et al: Spontaneous reperfusion of cerebral infarcts in patients with acute stroke: Incidence, time course, and clinical outcome in the Copenhagen Stroke Study. Arch Neurol 51:865–873, 1994.

183. Lassen NA: The luxury-perfusion syndrome and its possible relation to acute metabolic acidosis localised within the brain. Lancet 2(7473):1113–1115, 1966.

184. Lenzi GL, Frackowiak RS, Jones T: Cerebral oxygen metabolism and blood flow in human cerebral ischemic infarction. J Cereb Blood Flow Metab 2:321–335, 1982.

185. Hakim AM, Pokrupa RP, Villanueva J, et al: The effect of spontaneous reperfusion on metabolic function in early human cerebral infarcts. Ann Neurol 21:279–289, 1987.

186. Marchal G, Serrati C, Rioux P, et al: PET imaging of cerebral perfusion and oxygen consumption in acute ischaemic stroke: Relation to outcome. Lancet 341:925–927, 1993.

187. Baron JC, Bousser MG, Comar D, et al: Noninvasive tomographic study of cerebral blood flow and oxygen metabolism in vivo: Potentials, limitations, and clinical applications in cerebral ischemic disorders. Eur Neurol 20:273–284, 1981.

188. Furlan M, Marchal G, Viader F, et al: Spontaneous neurological recovery after stroke and the fate of the ischemic penumbra. Ann Neurol 40:216–226, 1996.

189. Marchal G, Beaudouin V, Rioux P, et al: Prolonged persistence of substantial volumes of potentially viable brain tissue after stroke: A correlative PET-CT study with voxel-based data analysis. Stroke 27:599–606, 1996.

190. Hawkins RA, Phelps ME, Huang SC, Kuhl DE: Effect of ischemia on quantification of local cerebral glucose metabolic rate in man. J Cereb Blood Flow Metab 1:37–51, 1981.

191. Gjedde A, Wienhard K, Heiss WD, et al: Comparative regional analysis of 2-fluorodeoxyglucose and methylglucose uptake in brain of four stroke patients: With special reference to the regional estimation of the lumped constant. J Cereb Blood Flow Metab 5:163–178, 1985.

192. Nedergaard M: Spreading depression as a contributor to ischemic brain damage. Adv Neurol 71:75–83, 1996.

193. Nedergaard M, Astrup J: Infarct rim: Effect of hyperglycemia on direct current potential and [14C]2-deoxyglucose phosphorylation. J Cereb Blood Flow Metab 6:607–615, 1986.

194. Hossmann KA: Viability thresholds and the penumbra of focal ischemia. Ann Neurol 36:557–565, 1994.

195. Fieschi C, Lenzi GL: Cerebral blood flow and metabolism in stroke patients. In Russell RWR (ed): Vascular Disease of the Central Nervous System, 2nd ed. New York, Churchill Livingstone, 1983, pp 101–127.

196. Meyer JS, Shimazu K, Fukuuchi Y, et al: Impaired neurogenic cerebrovascular control and dysautoregulation after stroke. Stroke 4:169–186, 1973.

197. Astrup J, Siesjo BK, Symon L: Thresholds in cerebral ischemia— the ischemic penumbra. Stroke 12:723–725, 1981.

198. Wise RJ, Bernardi S, Frackowiak RS, et al: Serial observations on the pathophysiology of acute stroke: The transition from ischaemia to infarction as reflected in regional oxygen extraction. Brain 106:197–222, 1983.

199. Young AR, Sette G, Touzani O, et al: Relationships between high oxygen extraction fraction in the acute stage and final infarction in reversible middle cerebral artery occlusion: An investigation in anesthetized baboons with positron emission tomography. J Cereb Blood Flow Metab 16:1176–1188, 1996.

200. Baron JC, Rougemont D, Bousser MG, et al: Local CBF, oxygen extraction fraction (OEF), and CMRO2: Prognostic value in recent supratentorial infarction in humans. J Cereb Blood Flow Metab 3(Suppl 1):S1–S2, 1983.

201. Marchal G, Benali K, Iglesias S, et al: Voxel-based mapping of irreversible ischaemic damage with PET in acute stroke. Brain 122:2387–2400, 1999.

202. Neumann-Haefelin T, Moseley ME, Albers GW: New magnetic resonance imaging methods for cerebrovascular disease: Emerging clinical applications. Ann Neurol 47:559–570, 2000.

203. Rohl L, Ostergaard L, Simonsen CZ, et al: Viability thresholds of ischemic penumbra of hyperacute stroke defined by perfusion-weighted MRI and apparent diffusion coefficient. Stroke 32:1140–1146, 2001.

204. Karonen JO, Vanninen RL, Liu Y, et al: Combined diffusion and perfusion MRI with correlation to single-photon emission CT in acute ischemic stroke: Ischemic penumbra predicts infarct growth. Stroke 30:1583–1590, 1999.

205. Barber PA, Darby DG, Desmond PM, et al: Prediction of stroke outcome with echoplanar perfusion- and diffusion- weighted MRI. Neurology 51:418–426, 1998.

206. Tong DC, Yenari MA, Albers GW, et al: Correlation of perfusion- and diffusion-weighted MRI with NIHSS score in acute (< 6.5 hour) ischemic stroke. Neurology 50:864–870, 1998.

207. Karonen JO, Liu Y, Vanninen RL, et al: Combined perfusion- and diffusion-weighted MR imaging in acute ischemic stroke during the 1st week: A longitudinal study. Radiology 217:886–894, 2000.

208. Liu Y, Karonen JO, Vanninen RL, et al: Cerebral hemodynamics in human acute ischemic stroke: A study with diffusion- and perfusion-weighted magnetic resonance imaging and SPECT. J Cereb Blood Flow Metab 20:910–920, 2000.

209. Beaulieu C, de Crespigny A, Tong DC, et al: Longitudinal magnetic resonance imaging study of perfusion and diffusion in stroke: Evolution of lesion volume and correlation with clinical outcome. Ann Neurol 46:568–578, 1999.

210. Kushner M, Reivich M, Fieschi C, et al: Metabolic and clinical correlates of acute ischemic infarction. Neurology 37:1103–1110, 1987.

211. Marchal G, Rioux P, Serrati C, et al: Value of acute-stage positron emission tomography in predicting neurological outcome after ischemic stroke: Further assessment. Stroke 26:524–525, 1995.

212. Schellinger PD, Fiebach JB, Jansen O, et al: Stroke magnetic resonance imaging within 6 hours after onset of hyperacute cerebral ischemia. Ann Neurol 49:460–469, 2001.

213. Thorngren-Jerneck K, Ohlsson T, Sandell A, et al: Cerebral glucose metabolism measured by positron emission tomography in term newborn infants with hypoxic ischemic encephalopathy. Pediatr Res 49:495–501, 2001.

214. Baron JC, Bousser MG, Comar D, Castaigne P: "Crossed cerebellar diaschisis" in human supratentorial brain infarction. Trans Am Neurol Assoc 105:459–461, 1980.

215. Martin WR, Raichle ME: Cerebellar blood flow and metabolism in cerebral hemisphere infarction. Ann Neurol 14:168–176, 1983.

216. Pantano P, Baron JC, Samson Y, et al: Crossed cerebellar diaschisis: Further studies. Brain 109:677–694, 1986.

217. Kuhl DE, Phelps ME, Kowell AP, et al: Effects of stroke on local cerebral metabolism and perfusion: Mapping by emission computed tomography of 18FDG and 13NH3. Ann Neurol 8:47–60, 1980.

218. Kushner M, Alavi A, Reivich M, et al: Contralateral cerebellar hypometabolism following cerebral insult: A positron emission tomographic study. Ann Neurol 15:425–434, 1984.

219. Yamauchi H, Fukuyama H, Kimura J: Hemodynamic and metabolic changes in crossed cerebellar hypoperfusion. Stroke 23:855–860, 1992.

220. Von Monakow C: Diaschisis. In Pribram KA (ed): Brain and Behavior I: Mood, States and Mind. Penguin Books, Baltimore, 1969, pp 27–36.

221. Lenzi GL, Frackowiak RS, Jones T, et al: CMRO2 and CBF by the oxygen-15 inhalation technique: Results in normal volunteers and cerebrovascular patients. Eur Neurol 20:285–290, 1981.

222. Iglesias S, Marchal G, Rioux P, et al: Do changes in oxygen metabolism in the unaffected cerebral hemisphere underlie early neurological recovery after stroke? A positron emission tomography study. Stroke 27:1192–1199, 1996.

223. Serrati C, Marchal G, Rioux P, et al: Contralateral cerebellar hypometabolism: A predictor for stroke outcome? J Neurol Neurosurg Psychiatry 57:174–179, 1994.

224. Kim SE, Choi CW, Yoon BW, et al: Crossed-cerebellar diaschisis in cerebral infarction: Technetium-99m-HMPAO SPECT and MRI. J Nucl Med 38:14–19, 1997.

225. Yamauchi H, Fukuyama H, Nagahama Y, et al: Uncoupling of oxygen and glucose metabolism in persistent crossed cerebellar diaschisis. Stroke 30:1424–1428, 1999.

226. Celesia GG, Polcyn RE, Holden JE, et al: Determination of regional cerebral blood flow in patients with cerebral infarction: Use of fluoromethane labeled with fluorine 18 and positron emission tomography. Arch Neurol 41:262–267, 1984.

227. Dobkin JA, Levine RL, Lagreze HL, et al: Evidence for transhemispheric diaschisis in unilateral stroke. Arch Neurol 46:1333–1336, 1989.

228. Wise R, Gibbs J, Frackowiak R, et al: No evidence for transhemispheric diaschisis after human cerebral infarction. Stroke 17:853–861, 1986.

229. Baron JC, Lebrun-Grandie P, Collard P, et al: Noninvasive measurement of blood flow, oxygen consumption, and glucose utilization in the same brain regions in man by positron emission tomography: Concise communication. J Nucl Med 23:391–399, 1982.

230. Heiss WD, Pawlik G, Wagner R, et al: Functional hypometabolism of noninfarcted brain regions in ischemic stroke. J Cereb Blood Flow Metab 3(Suppl 1):S582–S583, 1983.

231. Iglesias S, Marchal G, Viader F, Baron JC: Delayed intrahemispheric remote hypometabolism: Correlations with early recovery after stroke. Cerebrovasc Dis 10:391–402, 2000.

232. Szelies B, Herholz K, Pawlik G, et al: Widespread functional effects of discrete thalamic infarction. Arch Neurol 48:178–182, 1991.

233. Sakai F, Aoki S, Kan S, et al: Ataxic hemiparesis with reductions of ipsilateral cerebellar blood flow. Stroke 17:1016–1018, 1986.

234. Giroud M, Creisson E, Fayolle H, et al: Homolateral ataxia and crural paresis: A crossed cerebral-cerebellar diaschisis. J Neurol Neurosurg Psychiatry 57:221–222, 1994.

235. Metter EJ, Kempler D, Jackson C, et al: Cerebral glucose metabolism in Wernicke's, Broca's, and conduction aphasia. Arch Neurol 46:27–34, 1989.

236. Karbe H, Herholz K, Szelies B, et al: Regional metabolic correlates of Token test results in cortical and subcortical left hemispheric infarction. Neurology 39:1083–1088, 1989.

237. Perani D, Vallar G, Cappa S, et al: Aphasia and neglect after subcortical stroke: A clinical/cerebral perfusion correlation study. Brain 110:1211–1229, 1987.

238. Feeney DM, Baron JC: Diaschisis. Stroke 17:817–830, 1986.

239. Karbe H, Szelies B, Herholz K, Heiss WD: Impairment of language is related to left parieto-temporal glucose metabolism in aphasic stroke patients. J Neurol 237:19–23, 1990.

240. Pappata S, Mazoyer B, Tran DS, et al: Effects of capsular or thalamic stroke on metabolism in the cortex and cerebellum: A positron tomography study. Stroke 21:519–524, 1990.

241. Heiss WD, Kessler J, Karbe H, et al: Cerebral glucose metabolism as a predictor of recovery from aphasia in ischemic stroke. Arch Neurol 50:958–964, 1993.

242. Karbe H, Kessler J, Herholz K, et al: Long-term prognosis of poststroke aphasia studied with positron emission tomography. Arch Neurol 52:186–190, 1995.

243. Uemura K, Shishido F, Higano S, et al: Positron emission tomography in patients with a primary intracerebral hematoma. Acta Radiol Suppl 369:426–428, 1986.

244. Zazulia AR, Diringer MN, Videen TO, et al: Effects of acute ICH on hemispheric blood flow and metabolism. Stroke 32:338, 2001.

245. Heiss WD, Beil C, Pawlik G, et al: Non-traumatic intracerebral hematoma versus ischemic stroke: Regional pattern of glucose metabolism. J Cereb Blood Flow Metab 5(Suppl 1):S5–S6, 1985.

246. Dal-Bianco P: Positron emission tomography of 2(18F)-fluorodeoxyglucose in cerebral vascular disease: Clinicometabolic correlations in patients with nontraumatic spontaneous intracerebral hematoma and ischemic infarction. In Meyer JS, Lechner H, Reivich M, Ott EO (eds): Cerebral Vascular Disease 6: Proceedings of the World Federation of Neurology 13th International Salzburg Conference, September 25–27, 1986. Amsterdam, Excerpta Medica, 1987, pp 257–262.

247. Mendelow AD, Bullock R, Teasdale GM, et al: Intracranial haemorrhage induced at arterial pressure in the rat. Part 2: Short term changes in local cerebral blood flow measured by autoradiography. Neurol Res 6:189–193, 1984.

248. Nath FP, Jenkins A, Mendelow AD, et al: Early hemodynamic changes in experimental intracerebral hemorrhage. J Neurosurg 65:697–703, 1986.

249. Sills C, Villar-Cordova C, Pasteur W, et al: Demonstration of hypoperfusion surrounding intracerebral hematoma in humans. J Stroke Cerebrovasc Dis 6:17–24, 1996.

250. Qureshi AI, Wilson DA, Hanley DF, Traystman RJ: No evidence for an ischemic penumbra in massive experimental intracerebral hemorrhage. Neurology 52:266–272, 1999.

251. Mayer SA, Lignelli A, Fink ME, et al: Perilesional blood flow and edema formation in acute intracerebral hemorrhage: A SPECT study. Stroke 29:1791–1798, 1998.

252. Nath FP, Kelly PT, Jenkins A, et al: Effects of experimental intracerebral hemorrhage on blood flow, capillary permeability, and histochemistry. J Neurosurg 66:555–562, 1987.

253. Hoffman EJ, Huang SC, Phelps ME: Quantitation in positron emission computed tomography. 1: Effect of object size. J Comput Assist Tomogr 3:299–308, 1979.

254. Mazziotta JC, Phelps ME, Plummer D, Kuhl DE: Quantitation in positron emission computed tomography. 5: Physical-anatomical effects. J Comput Assist Tomogr 5:734–743, 1981.

255. Videen TO, Dunford-Shore JE, Diringer MN, Powers WJ: Correction for partial volume effects in regional blood flow measurements adjacent to hematomas in humans with intracerebral hemorrhage: Implementation and validation. J Comput Assist Tomogr 23:248–256, 1999.

256. Zazulia AR, Diringer MN, Videen TO, et al: Hypoperfusion without ischemia surrounding acute intracerebral hemorrhage. J Cereb Blood Flow Metab 21:804–810, 2001.

257. Baron JC: Pathophysiology of acute cerebral ischemia: PET studies in humans. Cerebrovasc Dis 1(Suppl 1):22–31, 1991.

258. Marchal G, Furlan M, Beaudouin V, et al: Early spontaneous hyperperfusion after stroke: A marker of favourable tissue outcome? Brain 119:409–419, 1996.

259. Wallace JD, Levy LL: Blood pressure after stroke. JAMA 246:2177–2180, 1981.

260. Powers WJ: Acute hypertension after stroke: The scientific basis for treatment decisions. Neurology 43:461–467, 1993.

261. Dandapani BK, Suzuki S, Kelley RE, et al: Relation between blood pressure and outcome in intracerebral hemorrhage. Stroke 26:21–24, 1995.

262. Kaneko T, Sawada T, Niimi T, et al: Lower limit of blood pressure in treatment of acute hypertensive intracerebral hemorrhage. J Cereb Blood Flow Metab 3:S51–S52, 1983.

263. Powers WJ, Zazulia AR, Videen TO, et al: Autoregulation of cerebral blood flow surrounding acute intracerebral hemorrhage. Neurology 57:18–24, 2001.

264. Siddique MS, Fernandes HM, Arene NU, et al: Changes in cerebral blood flow as measured by HMPAO SPECT in patients following spontaneous intracerebral haemorrhage. Acta Neurochir Suppl 76:517–520, 2000.

265. Batjer HH, Devous MD Sr, Seibert GB, et al: Intracranial arteriovenous malformation: Contralateral steal phenomena. Neurol Med Chir (Tokyo) 29:401–406, 1989.

266. Marks MP, O'Donahue J, Fabricant JI, et al: Cerebral blood flow evaluation of arteriovenous malformations with stable xenon CT. Am J Neuroradiol 9:1169–1175, 1988.

267. Batjer HH, Devous MD Sr: The use of acetazolamide-enhanced regional cerebral blood flow measurement to predict risk to arteriovenous malformation patients. Neurosurgery 31:213–217, 1992.

268. Homan RW, Devous MD Sr, Stokely EM, Bonte FJ: Quantification of intracerebral steal in patients with arteriovenous malformation. Arch Neurol 43:779–785, 1986.

269. Tyler JL, Leblanc R, Meyer E, et al: Hemodynamic and metabolic effects of cerebral arteriovenous malformations studied by positron emission tomography. Stroke 20:890–898, 1989.

270. Van Roost D, Schramm J, Solymosi L, Hartmann A: Presence and removal of arteriovenous malformation: Impact of regional cerebral blood flow, as assessed by xenon/CT. Acta Neurol Scand Suppl 166:136–138, 1996.

271. Hacein-Bey L, Nour R, Pile-Spellman J, et al: Adaptive changes of autoregulation in chronic cerebral hypotension with arteriovenous malformations: An acetazolamide-enhanced single-photon emission CT study. Am J Neuroradiol 16:1865–1874, 1995.

Pathophysiology

272. Spetzler RF, Wilson CB, Weinstein P, et al: Normal perfusion pressure breakthrough theory. Clin Neurosurg 25:651–672, 1978.

273. Nornes H, Grip A: Hemodynamic aspects of cerebral arteriovenous malformations. J Neurosurg 53:456–464, 1980.

274. Takeuchi S, Kikuchi H, Karasawa J, et al: Cerebral hemodynamics in arteriovenous malformations: Evaluation by single-photon emission CT. Am J Neuroradiol 8:193–197, 1987.

275. Barnett GH, Little JR, Ebrahim ZY, et al: Cerebral circulation during arteriovenous malformation operation. Neurosurgery 20:836–842, 1987.

276. Spetzler RF, Martin NA, Carter LP, et al: Surgical management of large AVM's by staged embolization and operative excision. J Neurosurg 67:17–28, 1987.

277. Young WL, Pile-Spellman J, Prohovnik I, et al: Evidence for adaptive autoregulatory displacement in hypotensive cortical territories adjacent to arteriovenous malformations. Columbia University AVM Study Project. Neurosurgery 34:601–610, 1994.

278. Young WL, Kader A, Prohovnik I, et al: Pressure autoregulation is intact after arteriovenous malformation resection. Neurosurgery 32:491–496, 1993.

279. Morgan MK, Johnston IH, Hallinan JM, Weber NC: Complications of surgery for arteriovenous malformations of the brain. J Neurosurg 78:176–182, 1993.

280. Heros RC, Korosue K, Diebold PM: Surgical excision of cerebral arteriovenous malformations: Late results. Neurosurgery 26:570–577, 1990.

281. Young WL, Kader A, Ornstein E, et al: Cerebral hyperemia after arteriovenous malformation resection is related to "breakthrough" complications but not to feeding artery pressure. The Columbia University Arteriovenous Malformation Study Project. Neurosurgery 38:1085–1093, 1996.

282. Tarr RW, Johnson DW, Rutigliano M, et al: Use of acetazolamide-challenge xenon CT in the assessment of cerebral blood flow dynamics in patients with arteriovenous malformations. Am J Neuroradiol 11:441–448, 1990.

283. Van Roost D, Schramm J: What factors are related to impairment of cerebrovascular reserve before and after arteriovenous malformation resection? A cerebral blood flow study using xenon-enhanced computed tomography. Neurosurgery 48:709–716, 2001.

284. Diehl RR, Henkes H, Nahser HC, et al: Blood flow velocity and vasomotor reactivity in patients with arteriovenous malformations: A transcranial Doppler study. Stroke 25:1574–1580, 1994.

285. Hasegawa S, Hamada J, Morioka M, et al: Radiation-induced cerebrovasculopathy of the distal middle cerebral artery and distal posterior cerebral artery—case report. Neurol Med Chir (Tokyo) 40:220–223, 2000.

286. Katayama S, Momose T, Sano I, et al: Temporal lobe CO2 vasoreactivity in patients with complex partial seizures. Jpn J Psychiatry Neurol 46:379–385, 1992.

287. Carpenter DA, Grubb RL Jr, Tempel LW, Powers WJ: Cerebral oxygen metabolism after aneurysmal subarachnoid hemorrhage. J Cereb Blood Flow Metab 11:837–844, 1991.

288. Yundt KD, Grubb RL Jr, Diringer MN, Powers WJ: Autoregulatory vasodilation of parenchymal vessels is impaired during cerebral vasospasm. J Cereb Blood Flow Metab 18:419–424, 1998.

289. Kassell NF, Sasaki T, Colohan AR, Nazar G: Cerebral vasospasm following aneurysmal subarachnoid hemorrhage. Stroke 16:562–572, 1985.

290. Heros RC, Zervas NT, Varsos V: Cerebral vasospasm after subarachnoid hemorrhage: An update. Ann Neurol 14:599–608, 1983.

291. Meyer CH, Lowe D, Meyer M, et al: Progressive change in cerebral blood flow during the first three weeks after subarachnoid hemorrhage. Neurosurgery 12:58–76, 1983.

292. Naderi S, Ozguven MA, Bayhan H, et al: Evaluation of cerebral vasospasm in patients with subarachnoid hemorrhage using single photon emission computed tomography. Neurosurg Rev 17:261–265, 1994.

293. Ohkuma H, Manabe H, Tanaka M, Suzuki S: Impact of cerebral microcirculatory changes on cerebral blood flow during cerebral vasospasm after aneurysmal subarachnoid hemorrhage. Stroke 31:1621–1627, 2000.

294. Grubb RL Jr, Raichle ME, Eichling JO, Gado MH: Effects of subarachnoid hemorrhage on cerebral blood volume, blood flow, and oxygen utilization in humans. J Neurosurg 46:446–453, 1977.

295. Jakobsen M, Overgaard J, Marcussen E, Enevoldsen EM: Relation between angiographic cerebral vasospasm and regional CBF in patients with SAH. Acta Neurol Scand 82:109–115, 1990.

296. James IM: Changes in cerebral blood flow and in systemic arterial pressure following spontaneous subarachnoid haemorrhage. Clin Sci 35:11–22, 1968.

297. Ishii R: Regional cerebral blood flow in patients with ruptured intracranial aneurysms. J Neurosurg 50:587–594, 1979.

298. Heilbrun MP, Olesen J, Lassen NA: Regional cerebral blood flow studies in subarachnoid hemorrhage. J Neurosurg 37:36–44, 1972.

299. Gelmers HJ, Beks JW, Journee HL: Regional cerebral blood flow in patients with subarachnoid haemorrhage. Acta Neurochir (Wien) 47:245–251, 1979.

300. Rosenstein J, Wang AD, Symon L, Suzuki M: Relationship between hemispheric cerebral blood flow, central conduction time, and clinical grade in aneurysmal subarachnoid hemorrhage. J Neurosurg 62:25–30, 1985.

301. Voldby B, Enevoldsen EM, Jensen FT: Regional CBF, intraventricular pressure, and cerebral metabolism in patients with ruptured intracranial aneurysms. J Neurosurg 62:48–58, 1985.

302. Geraud G, Tremoulet M, Guell A, Bes A: The prognostic value of noninvasive CBF measurement in subarachnoid hemorrhage. Stroke 15:301–305, 1984.

303. Aaslid R, Markwalder TM, Nornes H: Noninvasive transcranial Doppler ultrasound recording of flow velocity in basal cerebral arteries. J Neurosurg 57:769–774, 1982.

304. Macdonald RL, Weir BK: Radiology. In Macdonald RL, Weir BK (eds): Cerebral Vasospasm. San Diego, Academic Press, 2001, pp 176–220.

305. Hutchison K, Weir B: Transcranial Doppler studies in aneurysm patients. Can J Neurol Sci 16:411–416, 1989.

306. Vora YY, Suarez-Almazor M, Steinke DE, et al: Role of transcranial Doppler monitoring in the diagnosis of cerebral vasospasm after subarachnoid hemorrhage. Neurosurgery 44:1237–1247, 1999.

307. Giller CA, Hodges K, Batjer HH: Transcranial Doppler pulsatility in vasodilation and stenosis. J Neurosurg 72:901–906, 1990.

308. Klingelhofer J, Dander D, Holzgraefe M, et al: Cerebral vasospasm evaluated by transcranial Doppler ultrasonography at different intracranial pressures. J Neurosurg 75:752–758, 1991.

309. Brass LM, Pavlakis SG, DeVivo D, et al: Transcranial Doppler measurements of the middle cerebral artery: Effect of hematocrit. Stroke 19:1466–1469, 1988.

310. Newell DW, Winn HR: Transcranial Doppler in cerebral vasospasm. Neurosurg Clin North Am 1:319–328, 1990.

311. Romner B, Brandt L, Berntman L, et al: Simultaneous transcranial Doppler sonography and cerebral blood flow measurements of cerebrovascular CO2-reactivity in patients with aneurysmal subarachnoid haemorrhage. Br J Neurosurg 5:31–37, 1991.

312. Mizuno M, Nakajima S, Sampei T, et al: Serial transcranial Doppler flow velocity and cerebral blood flow measurements for evaluation of cerebral vasospasm after subarachnoid hemorrhage. Neurol Med Chir (Tokyo) 34:164–171, 1994.

313. Clyde BL, Resnick DK, Yonas H, et al: The relationship of blood velocity as measured by transcranial Doppler ultrasonography to cerebral blood flow as determined by stable xenon computed tomographic studies after aneurysmal subarachnoid hemorrhage. Neurosurgery 38:896–904, 1996.

314. Jakobsen M, Enevoldsen E, Bjerre P: Cerebral blood flow and metabolism following subarachnoid haemorrhage: Cerebral oxygen uptake and global blood flow during the acute period in patients with SAH. Acta Neurol Scand 82:174–182, 1990.

315. Hayashi T, Suzuki A, Hatazawa J, et al: Cerebral circulation and metabolism in the acute stage of subarachnoid hemorrhage. J Neurosurg 93:1014–1018, 2000.

316. Powers WJ, Grubb RL Jr, Baker RP, et al: Regional cerebral blood flow and metabolism in reversible ischemia due to vasospasm: Determination by positron emission tomography. J Neurosurg 62:539–546, 1985.

317. Hino A, Mizukawa N, Tenjin H, et al: Postoperative hemodynamic and metabolic changes in patients with subarachnoid hemorrhage. Stroke 20:1504–1510, 1989.

318. Kawamura S, Sayama I, Yasui N, Uemura K: Sequential changes in cerebral blood flow and metabolism in patients with subarachnoid haemorrhage. Acta Neurochir (Wien) 114:12–15, 1992.

Pathophysiology

319. Voldby B, Enevoldsen EM, Jensen FT: Cerebrovascular reactivity in patients with ruptured intracranial aneurysms. J Neurosurg 62:59–67, 1985.

320. Nornes H, Knutzen HB, Wikeby P: Cerebral arterial blood flow and aneurysm surgery. Part 2: Induced hypotension and autoregulatory capacity. J Neurosurg 47:819–827, 1977.

321. Darby JM, Yonas H, Marks EC, et al: Acute cerebral blood flow response to dopamine-induced hypertension after subarachnoid hemorrhage. J Neurosurg 80:857–864, 1994.

322. Touho H, Ueda H: Disturbance of autoregulation in patients with ruptured intracranial aneurysms: Mechanism of cortical and motor dysfunction. Surg Neurol 42:57–64, 1994.

323. Allen GS, Ahn HS, Preziosi TJ, et al: Cerebral arterial spasm—a controlled trial of nimodipine in patients with subarachnoid hemorrhage. N Engl J Med 308:619–624, 1983.

324. Pickard JD, Murray GD, Illingworth R, et al: Effect of oral nimodipine on cerebral infarction and outcome after subarachnoid haemorrhage: British aneurysm nimodipine trial. BMJ 298:636–642, 1989.

325. Neil-Dwyer G, Mee E, Dorrance D, Lowe D: Early intervention with nimodipine in subarachnoid haemorrhage. Eur Heart J 8(Suppl K):41–47, 1987.

326. Petruk KC, West M, Mohr G, et al: Nimodipine treatment in poor-grade aneurysm patients: Results of a multicenter double-blind placebo-controlled trial. J Neurosurg 68:505–517, 1988.

327. Philippon J, Grob R, Dagreou F, et al: Prevention of vasospasm in subarachnoid haemorrhage: A controlled study with nimodipine. Acta Neurochir (Wien) 82:110–114, 1986.

328. Feigin VL, Rinkel GJ, Algra A, et al: Calcium antagonists in patients with aneurysmal subarachnoid hemorrhage: A systematic review. Neurology 50:876–883, 1998.

329. Gaab MR, Haubitz I, Brawanski A, et al: Acute effects of nimodipine on the cerebral blood flow and intracranial pressure. Neurochirurgia (Stuttg) 28(Suppl 1):93–99, 1985.

330. Schmidt JF, Waldemar G, Paulson OB: The acute effect of nimodipine on cerebral blood flow, its CO2 reactivity, and cerebral oxygen metabolism in human volunteers. Acta Neurochir (Wien) 111:49–53, 1991.

331. Rasmussen G, Bergholdt B, Dalh B, et al: Effect of nimodipine on cerebral blood flow and cerebrovascular reactivity after subarachnoid haemorrhage. Acta Neurol Scand 99:182–186, 1999.

332. Seiler RW, Nirkko AC: Effect of nimodipine on cerebrovascular response to CO2 in asymptomatic individuals and patients with sub-arachnoid hemorrhage: A transcranial Doppler ultrasound study. Neurosurgery 27:247–251, 1990.

333. Kassell NF, Peerless SJ, Durward QJ, et al: Treatment of ischemic deficits from vasospasm with intravascular volume expansion and induced arterial hypertension. Neurosurgery 11:337–343, 1982.

334. Awad IA, Carter LP, Spetzler RF, et al: Clinical vasospasm after sub-arachnoid hemorrhage: Response to hypervolemic hemodilution and arterial hypertension. Stroke 18:365–372, 1987.

335. Yamakami I, Isobe K, Yamaura A: Effects of intravascular volume expansion on cerebral blood flow in patients with ruptured cerebral aneurysms. Neurosurgery 21:303–309, 1987.

336. Lennihan L, Mayer SA, Fink ME, et al: Effect of hypervolemic therapy on cerebral blood flow after subarachnoid hemorrhage: A randomized controlled trial. Stroke 31:383–391, 2000.

337. Egge A, Waterloo K, Sjoholm H, et al: Prophylactic hyperdynamic postoperative fluid therapy after aneurysmal subarachnoid hemorrhage: A clinical, prospective, randomized, controlled study. Neurosurgery 49:593–605, 2001.

338. Muizelaar JP, Becker DP: Induced hypertension for the treatment of cerebral ischemia after subarachnoid hemorrhage: Direct effect on cerebral blood flow. Surg Neurol 25:317–325, 1986.

339. Yundt KD, Grubb RL Jr, Diringer MN, Powers WJ: Cerebral hemodynamic and metabolic changes caused by brain retraction after aneurysmal subarachnoid hemorrhage. Neurosurgery 40:442–450, 1997.

340. Rousseaux M, Huglo D, Steinling M: Cerebral blood flow in frontal lesions of aneurysms of the anterior communicating artery. Stroke 25:135–140, 1994.

341. Tranquart F, Ades PE, Groussin P, et al: Postoperative assessment of cerebral blood flow in subarachnoid haemorrhage by means of 99mTc-HMPAO tomography. Eur J Nucl Med 20:53–58, 1993.

342. Rosen JM, Butala AV, Oropello JM, et al: Postoperative changes on brain SPECT imaging after aneurysmal subarachnoid hemorrhage: A potential pitfall in the evaluation of vasospasm. Clin Nucl Med 19:595–597, 1994.

343. Ahn CS, Tow DE, Yu CC, Greene RW: Effect of metabolic alterations on the accumulation of technetium-99m–labeled d,l-HMPAO in slices of rat cerebral cortex. J Cereb Blood Flow Metab 14:324–331, 1994.

344. Adams HP Jr, Powers WJ, Grubb RL Jr, et al: Preview of a new trial of extracranial-to-intracranial arterial anastomosis: The carotid occlusion surgery study. Neurosurg Clin North Am 12:613–624, 2001.

Pathophysiology

Chapter Forty-One

Histopathology of Cerebral Ischemia

Roland N. Auer

THE BIOLOGICAL LEVELS OF ORGANIZATION AND STROKE

The biologic levels of organization (Table 41.1) range from molecules, to subcellular organelles, cells, tissues, organs, and organisms, to terromes. Although organ dysfunction (brain dysfunction) and deficits at the organism level are what primarily concern us as end results, such disease inevitably comes about from events gone awry at lower levels of biologic organization. Pathology addresses damage mainly at the cellular and tissue levels. Diffuse cellular or subcellular (synaptic or chemical) lesions usually lead to behavioral deficits. Because of the extreme inhomogeneity of the brain compared with other organs, focal lesions in brain, even minor ones in some critical locations, can also lead to either behavioral or homeostatic brain dysfunction. The pathology of brain ischemia thus lies squarely between the molecular and the clinical levels.

We note here that not all events at lower biologic levels give rise to effects at higher levels. Thus, not all molecular events cause cellular dysfunction, and not all cellular or tissue lesions cause dysfunction of the organism. Stated differently, chemical changes can be silent at the cell or tissue level, and cytologic or histologic lesions can go undetected in the whole organism.

In this regard, it is important to remember that brain ischemia is not primarily a molecular dysfunction of the brain but, like brain trauma, is initiated by physical factors, in this case cessation of blood flow. Molecular events follow profound alterations in blood flow and cerebral metabolism, but the primary, initiating pathophysiologic event is at the tissue (not cellular, molecular, or whole organism) level. However, after being initiated by cessation of a fluid tissue (blood) flowing through a more formed tissue (brain), numerous potentially damaging molecular cascades are immediately set in motion. Which of these molecular events filters through to higher levels of biologic organization, to damage cells and tissues, is not always known. I focus in this chapter on events that occur at the cell and tissue levels and that are known to cause irreparable brain damage, teasing out only a few molecular mechanisms for which there is good evidence in the pathogenesis of ischemic brain damage.

One distinction deserves emphasis at the beginning: Behavioral tests in animals and clinical neurologic examination (or neuropsychologic testing) in humans all test the synapses of the brain. Classic neuropathology, in contrast, examines mainly the cell bodies of the brain, that is, the neuronal parenchyma in aggregate. This conceptual distinction is important. For example, ischemic brain damage may kill a few neurons in some places in the brain without causing a clinical neurologic deficit. This does not imply that neuronal death is not something to be avoided. It is insignificant or inconsequential by virtue of its location, not by the nature of the process.

Death of cells and tissues in the brain is always a serious event. Because the exact clinical consequences depend on the extent and precise location of the lesion, matters of pure chance (e.g., which arterial ramification receives an embolus) determine final end results, adding an unpredictable, stochastic element to ischemic brain damage. Clinical effects of lesions of roughly equal size are highly dependent on location within the brain. Thus, silent frontal lobe infarcts in humans[1] are not to be regarded as inconsequential, because had they occurred in slightly more posterior locations, merely by chance, they would have the potential to produce major and catastrophic clinical deficits. In this way, the highly inhomogeneous brain gives rise to considerable clinical variability in both the severity and the nature of the deficit for lesions of identical size.

One implication of the preceding discussion is that focusing on lesion size rather than direct clinical benefit requires fewer subjects to ascertain differences.[2] This issue underscores the value of the tissue burden of disease (e.g., infarct size measured pathologically or neuroradiologically). These considerations have implications for clinical trials.

SELECTIVE NEURONAL NECROSIS VERSUS INFARCTION

This discussion focuses on two grades of ischemic brain lesions, selective neuronal necrosis and infarction. Both kill neurons, the former exclusively so. The distinction rests on the physiologic severity of the lesion, in whatever brain

821

Table 41.1   Biological Levels of Organization and Stroke

Level	Tools Used
Terrome	—
Biome	—
Ecosystem	—
Community	Clinical
Organism	Clinical
Organ System	—
Organ	Gross observation, imaging
Tissue	Histopathology, imaging
Cell	Histopathology
Organelle [synapse]	Histopathology, E.M. [Clinical]
Supramolecular aggregate	—
Molecule	Drugs
Atom	—

location. Selective *neuronal necrosis* specifically denotes death of only neurons, sparing glia (Fig. 41–1A). *Infarction* refers to death of neurons *and* glia and is a much more serious tissue lesion (see Fig. 41–1B). The reason is that axonal sprouting, and any form of tissue regeneration, is precluded because all of the tissue dies. Infarction ultimately leaves a fluid-filled cyst, formed as a result of tissue breakdown and removal by macrophages. This cyst comes to contain only brain interstitial fluid, in direct exchange with cerebrospinal fluid (CSF).

It is important to remember that both grades of lesion severity can occur in the brainstem, cerebellum, or fore-brain. Thus, both selective neuronal necrosis and infarction can occur anywhere in the brain.

SELECTIVE VULNERABILITY

The concept of two degrees of severity of damage (selective neuronal necrosis and infarction) must be distinguished from the concept of selective vulnerability within the brain. The latter refers to the fact that the entire brain can be subjected to some primary insult, but only portions of the brain show damage. This is the rule rather than the exception in neuropathology. It applies fully to brain damage in ischemia. Elucidation of the basis of selective vulnerability gives clues to the mechanism of tissue damage in ischemia. Likewise, elucidation of the mechanism of selective neuronal necrosis or infarction also yields information useful to understanding and ultimately prevention of these two levels of tissue damage.

SELECTIVE NEURONAL NECROSIS

The concept of incomplete infarction has little support on close brain examination: it seems that either the entire local array of cells in the brain die en masse or only the neurons die, leaving the glia and neuropil intact. The neuropil is visible in histologic section as the finely reticulated or bubbly tissue that appears between cell bodies in central nervous tissue. Neuropil cannot be resolved at the light-microscopic level. Electron microscopy, however, reveals

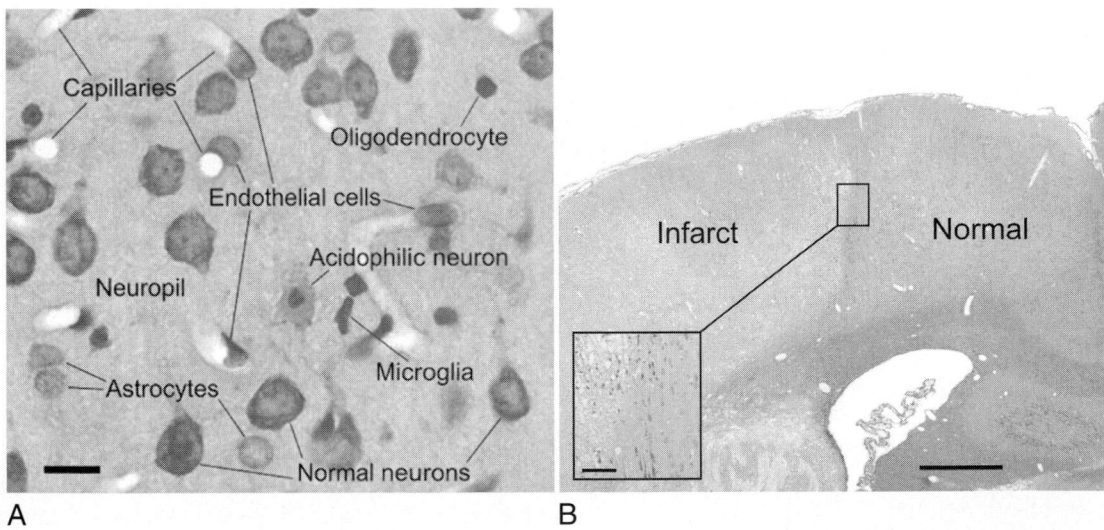

FIGURE 41–1   *A, Normal central nervous system histologic appearance and a single necrotic (acidophilic) neuron, showing selective neuronal necrosis. This tissue lesion spares glia as well as neuropil. The square nucleus above the rod-shaped microglia is also probably a microglial cell, from its nuclear shape as well as its position between the vessel and the dead neuron, suggesting recent emigration from the vessel. Axons, dendrites, and glial processes constitute the unresolvable (on light microscopy), finely reticulated neuropil. Astrocytes show characteristically pale nuclei compared with oligodendroglia and microglia. Cortex, global ischemia, 1 week survival, rat. (Hematoxylin and eosin; bar = 20 μm.) B, One of the most remarkable features of infarction, rarely receiving emphasis, is its characteristically geographic, sharply demarcated border, seen here running vertically through the neocortex in the center of the picture. Early, patchy cysts are seen (inset) as infarcted tissue is resorbed. Although a few dark neurons (inset, bottom) are seen at the infarct rim, there is rapid transition to normal neuropil, and normal neurons (inset, right). Note that inflammation is not yet seen. Focal ischemia, 24 hours survival, rat. (Hematoxylin and eosin; bars = 2 mm and 400 μm [inset].)*

Pathophysiology

the neuropil consists of axons, dendrites, and glial processes (Fig. 41–2).

Neuronal Acidophilia

At the cellular level, the pathology of cerebral ischemia has often focused on an ill-defined "ischemic cell change," really, in essence, neuronal death. But the hallmark of neuronal death at the light-microscopic level is an increased affinity for acid dyes. The reason for this neuronal acidophilia (see Fig. 41–1A) is uncertain. Because hematoxylin and eosin stain is the stain routinely used in pathology, acidophilia is often commonly referred to as "eosinophilia." The reason nuclei are blue and cytoplasm is pink in conventionally stained sections is that hematoxylin is a base and eosin is an acid. Because each component of the acid-base pair stains its opposite element in the tissue (i.e., acids stain basic tissue components, and bases stain acidic tissue components), death of neurons must be critically accompanied by some increase in chemically basic moieties of the molecular components of tissue. The nature of these basic tissue components that are revealed by acidic stains in neuronal death is uncertain but may involve binding of acid dyes to ε-amino groups of basic lysine residues in degenerating proteins.[3] Proteins constitute the bulk of stainable material in routine tissue sections and are, in fact, normally eosinophilic to some degree, because of the basic amino acid groups (ε-amino of lysine, guanidino of arginine, imidazole of histidine) in the residues of the polypeptide chain. This is the reason that neuropil, and the cytoplasm of neuronal cell bodies between the RNA, stain pink.

Alterations in protein are also suggested to explain acidophilia because of the electron-microscopic features of acidophilic neurons; mitochondrial flocculent densities (Fig. 41–3A) represent denatured protein.[4–6]

Conversely, nucleic acids stain blue owing to their affinity for basic dyes, such as hematoxylin. The nucleic acid–containing parts of a cell—nucleoli, nucleus, and cytoplasmic Nissl substance (composed of RNA)—all stain blue because of the affinity of nucleic acids for basic dyes in routine staining. For these reasons, we see nuclei as blue and cytoplasm as pink in normal histopathologic sections. In ischemic neuronal death, or indeed in any form of neuronal death, the acidophilia is not merely due to unmasking of basophilia by loss of nucleic acid staining.[3]

Neuronal acidophilia is not specific to neuronal death due to ischemia but merely indicates that the neuron has irreversibly succumbed from any cause. The etiology of cell death is clearly not revealed by the preceding description of acidophilic neurons, which have an identical acidophilic appearance whether cell death is caused by ischemia, hypoglycemia, epilepsy, or even neuronal infection by a virus. I thus decry the use of the term *ischemic cell change* for acidophilic neuronal death, because this is simply the nonspecific appearance of an irreversibly damaged or dead neuron, and the cell may not even have been exposed to ischemia.

Neurons Undergo a "Dendritic Death"

Electron microscopy gives some clue as to the nature of acidophilic neuronal death (see Fig. 41–2). Importantly, the neuropil surrounding neurons destined to die shows

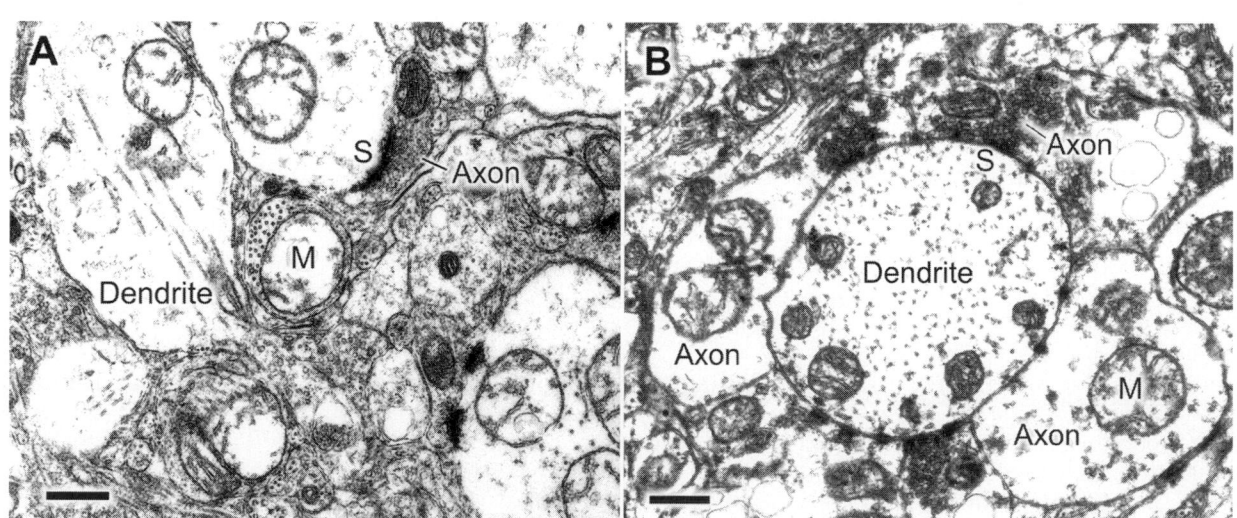

FIGURE 41–2 *Contrasting features of excitotoxic and hypermetabolic pathology. A, Excitotoxicity shows dendritic swelling, sparing axons. Dendritic microtubules are hollow and serve to definitively identify the cell process around the central mitochondrion as a dendrite. (Hypoglycemia, hippocampus; bar = 1 μm.) (From Auer RN, Kalimo H, Olsson Y, Weiloch T: The dentate gyrus in hypoglycemia: Pathology implicating excitotoxin-mediated neuronal necrosis. Acta Neuropathol [Berlin] 67:279–288, 1985; ©Springer-Verlag.) B, Hypermetabolism shows axonal swelling, sparing the central dendrite, which has axonal terminals surrounding it. Both the swollen axons and dendrites include swollen mitochondria (M). Synapses (S) are the darkest membranes in each picture, because of embedded proteins in the membrane, and can be seen to contain synaptic vesicles. (Epilepsy, substantia nigra, pars reticulata; bar = 1 μm.) (From Auer RN, Ingvar M, Nevander G, et al: Early axonal lesion and preserved microvasculature in epilepsy-induced hypermetabolic necrosis of the substantia nigra. Acta Neuropathol [Berlin] 71:207–215, 1985; ©Springer-Verlag.)*

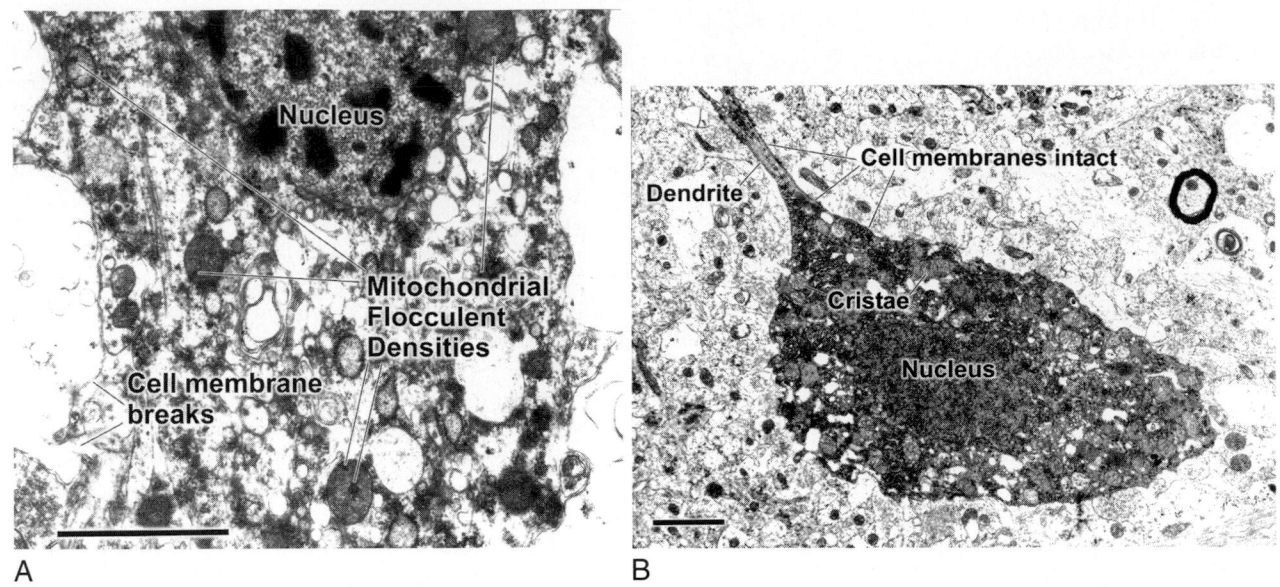

FIGURE 41–3 *Contrasting features of necrotic and apoptotic morphology. A, Necrosis shows mitochondrial flocculent densities, representing denatured cytochrome proteins. The nucleus shows coarse, stippled chromatin. The cytoplasm shows few recognizable organelles, consisting mainly of amorphous debris and membranous whorls. (Bar = 5 μm.) B, Three weeks after a hypoglycemic injury. The neuron shown here, one of only two such neurons found in my entire experience, was located in the hippocampus. Mitochondrial cristae are still visible, and there is early blebbing of the cytoplasm, with intact membranes. The nucleus is homogeneous, as would be expected in apoptosis, and contrasting with necrosis. There is generalized condensation of both nucleus and cytoplasm that gives rise to increased electron density, a feature compatible with apoptosis. The rarity of this deserves emphasis. (Bar = 5 μm.) (From Auer RN, Kalimo H, Olsson Y, Siesjö B: The temporal evolution of hypoglycemic brain damage. II: Light- and electron-microscopic findings in the hippocampal gyrus and subiculum of the rat. Acta Neuropathol [Berlin] 67:25–36, 1985; ©Springer-Verlag.)*

remarkably inhomogeneous damage to axons, dendrites, and glial processes. In the process of selective neuronal necrosis, dendrites swell selectively if attached to neurons destined to die, but intervening axons and glial processes are spared ultrastructurally (see Fig. 41–2A). This axon-sparing, dendritic lesion is the hallmark of the tissue action of endogenous excitatory amino acids or their chemical congeners. The selective dendritic swelling is due to the overwhelmingly dendritic location of excitatory amino acid receptors within the neuropil. Because excitatory amino acid receptors predominate on dendrites, ion and water fluxes are initiated there, and dendritic swelling results.

These axon-sparing, dendritic lesions are generally hard to find, because an appropriate part of the neuropil surrounding the neurons must be examined (i.e., a part of the neuropil containing dendrites that are activated by ischemia-released glutamate). Nevertheless, several independent laboratories have described axon-sparing dendritic lesions in ischemic neuronal death.[7,8] Although the excitatory amino acid released in ischemia is glutamate, identical lesions are seen in hypoglycemia,[9] in which aspartate[10] is released in greater quantities than glutamate. In epilepsy[11,12] and monosodium glutamate (MSG) neurotoxicity,[13] the neuropil has the same appearance through a similar mechanism.

It seems that the stage of selective dendritic swelling and calcium entry is reversible,[14] and may presage a more serious lesion, selective dendritic membrane breaks (see Figs. 41–2 and 41–4). This is evidenced by the entry of horseradish peroxidase (HRP) into the terminal dendrites

in swollen ischemic neuronal cell processes.[15] HRP has a molecular weight of approximately 40,000 to 60,000 daltons, and its entry into neurons indicates holes of considerable size in the cell membrane. Neuronal death can thus be envisaged as a series of membrane breaches beginning in dendrites, with initial swelling developing into cell membrane breaks (see Figs. 41–3 and 41–4). Provided that these breaches are limited to the distal dendritic tree and are not large and confluent, the neuron can survive their presence.[15] However, extension of cell membrane breaks into large portions of the neuronal perikaryon constitutes a subcellular lesion that is clearly irreversible.

At the time large and confluent perikaryal membrane breaches occur, mitochondrial flocculent densities appear (see Fig. 41–3A). These have been shown to represent trypsin-digestible proteins derived from the electron transport proteins of the mitochondrial matrix.[4–6] Mitochondrial flocculent densities and cell membrane breaks (in the neuronal perikaryon) constitute the electron-microscopic counterpart of the acidophilic neuron seen at the light microscopic level.

PAN-NECROSIS OR INFARCTION

Although selective neuronal necrosis seems related to the selective neuronal actions of glutamate or its congeners, pan-necrosis is a less discriminating cellular lesion that sweeps away neurons and glia alike. We can thus regard infarction, or pan-necrosis, as a tissue-level lesion rather

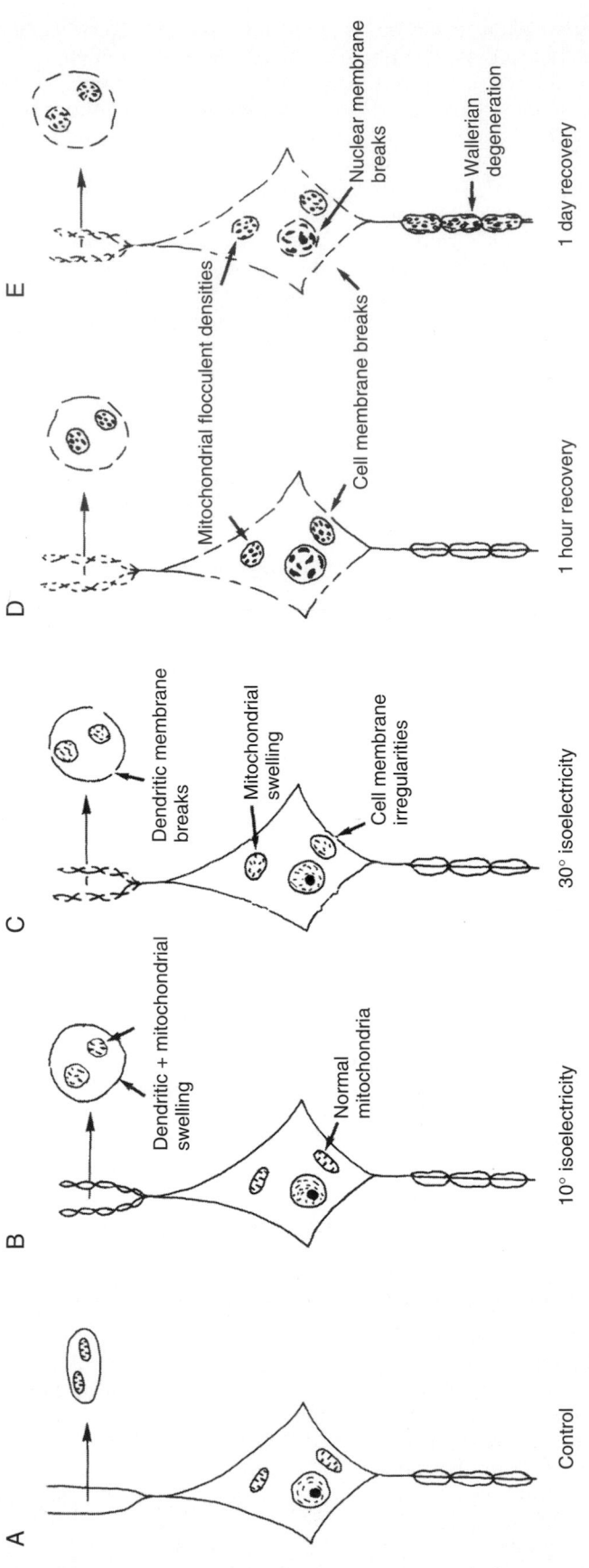

FIGURE 41–4 "*Dendritic death*" *of neurons, beginning as segmental dendritic swelling only and progressing to mitochondrial swelling in the perikaryon as well. Cell membrane breaks begin in dendrites and, once spread to the perikaryon, signify irreversible cellular injury and death. Wallerian degeneration of the axon and karyorrhexis/cytolysis follow over days to weeks. (Adapted from Auer RN, Kalimo H, Olsson Y, Weiloch T: The dentate gyrus in hypoglycemia: Pathology implicating excitotoxin-mediated neuronal necrosis. Acta Neuropathol [Berlin] 67:279–288, 1985; ©Springer-Verlag.)*

than a specific cellular lesion. The implication is that the cause of infarction is probably not related to the individually unique cytologic properties of the cells affected, because they are affected so indiscriminately. This lack of discrimination contrasts sharply with selective neuronal necrosis, in which cellular properties of neurons are critical in determining neuronal death. Indeed, infarction must be considered a consequence of primary interruption of blood flow to a brain region below critical cerebral blood flow thresholds. If this interruption is permanent, tissue events simply resemble autolysis. Permanent focal ischemia can thus be conceptually termed "autolytic infarction."

Hypermetabolism and Acidosis in Central Nervous System Tissue

There is, however, another mechanism for pan-necrosis, or cerebral infarction. Massive productions of hydrogen ions have been shown experimentally to indiscriminately kill all cell types in central nervous system (CNS) tissue.[16] The fact that H^+ ions, when injected into CNS tissue, can kill tissue components indiscriminately is only indirect evidence for acidosis-mediated tissue damage. However, there is more direct evidence from several CNS diseases that critical drops in pH cause pan-necrosis. These diseases are Wernicke's encephalopathy,[17] necrosis of the substantia nigra, pars reticulata in epilepsy,[18,19] and ischemia itself,[20,21] in which the necrotizing effect of enhanced tissue acidosis is best revealed by expansion of infarction at high glucose levels, which promote acidosis.[22,23] It is important to note that focal acidosis in brain can cause pan-necrosis[17,18,24] even with adequate local blood flow.[19,25] As in selective neuronal necrosis, pan-necrosis of identical appearance results from diverse initiating pathophysiologic states.

When experimental epilepsy is produced in rodents, high focal metabolic rates in the substantia nigra outstrip the capacity of the local blood supply to remove H^+ ions from the tissue. A marked increase in tissue lactate ensues, with an accompanying drop in pH.[19,26] Pan-necrosis occurs histologically, even though no hypoperfusion has taken place. The same process occurs in human encephalomyelopathies caused by mitochondrial abnormalities, in which acidotic brain infarcts occur in nonvascular distributions.[27,28]

In Wernicke's encephalopathy, there is a similar focal tissue acidosis due to thiamine deficiency.[17] The histologic appearance is noteworthy, consisting of selective necrosis of the neuropil, actually sparing cell bodies of all types. The sparing of neurons is especially remarkable. A similar histologic appearance is seen in Leigh's disease, another condition believed to be related to focal CNS acidosis.

In ischemia, pan-necrosis has salient histologic features identical to those seen in other acidosis-related causes of CNS necrosis. Specifically, the neuropil can be selectively affected, sparing neurons at infarct borders. This may account for the very narrow rim of penumbra seen in many studies (see Fig. 41–1B).[29] The production of acid equivalents by the neuropil is due to the location of glycolytic metabolism in the neuropil as opposed to the neuronal cell bodies. This metabolic correlate of micronecrosis and pan-necrosis in the neuropil derives from functional localization of glutamate-stimulated glycolysis[30,31] predominantly

to astrocytes and selective metabolism of lactate by neuronal processes in the neuropil.[32–34]

The consistent finding that infarcts have a sharp, well-demarcated border, without necessarily a rim of selective neuronal necrosis around an infarct (see Fig. 41–1B) implies that reduction of ischemic infarction may take place by shrinking of a relatively homogeneous area of tissue damage rather than through a decrease in grades of damage at the infarct border. This finding further supports the use of surrogate markers in clinical trials, because infarcts can be sharply demarcated and their volumes determined neuroradiologically. In spite of graded reductions of cerebral blood flow as one progresses outward from the core of an infarct, the resulting pathology has an "all or none" feature, suggesting a threshold effect. This pathology is consistent with acidosis below some critical threshold that gives rise to expanding pan-necrosis at the sharp rim of CNS infarction in ischemia,[22,23,35] as it does in the other CNS diseases already briefly reviewed.

Apoptosis in Ischemia

Since the description of apoptosis three decades ago,[36] an intense research effort has been made to demonstrate this phenomenon in adult nervous tissue subjected to ischemia. There are several reasons to believe that apoptosis is not a common occurrence in ischemia of the brain.

First, apoptosis is usually a counterforce to mitosis in biology. Thus, apoptosis balances mitosis in embryology, in tumors, and in normally proliferating epithelia of the body. Neurons lack mitosis, or a cell cycle. Indeed, it would be teleologically curious if apoptosis occurred in these important, post-mitotic cells.

Second, TUNEL labeling (terminal deoxyribonucleotidyl transferase [TDT]–mediated dUTP-digoxigenin nick end-labeling)[37] is often taken to support apoptosis, but results of TUNEL labeling are positive not only in apoptosis but in necrosis and autolysis as well,[38,39] likely representing nonspecific DNA degradation.

Third, electron-microscopic features of necrosis can be contrasted with those of apoptosis (Table 41.2) and are not seen in ischemia. Light microscopy is inadequate to resolve the features of the cell membrane and mitochondria. Thus, electron microscopy is required to determine the characteristic morphologic features of programmed cell death. Otherwise, karyorhectic and cytorhectic cell fragments may be mistaken for apoptotic bodies. In parts of the brain where there is a residuum of active neuronal regeneration, such as the dentate granule cell layer,[40] electron-

Table 41.2   Constrasting Features of Necrosis and Apoptosis

Feature	Necrosis	Apoptosis
Acidophilia	Early	Late
Cell volume change	Swelling	Shrinkage
Cell membrane breaks	Early	Late
Mitochondrial flocculent densities	Early	Late
Inflammation	Prominent (depending on severity of tissue injury)	Absent

microscopic evidence of apoptotic neuronal death (after adrenalectomy) has indeed been described.[41-43] Electron-microscopic studies specifically looking for features of apoptosis in ischemia, under conditions theoretically favoring apoptosis, have not found them.[44-46]

Fourth, inflammation is absent in apoptosis yet forms a prominent component of ischemic histopathology. Attempts to dampen inflammation and ameliorate ischemic damage have met with generally positive results[47-51] and also some negative results.[52,53] But whether or not it plays a role in cell death, the vigorous inflammatory response of ischemia argues against apoptosis.

Fifth, apoptosis in ischemic stroke would require the simultaneous cell suicide of neurons and all types of glia. The signaling necessary to accomplish this geographic coordination of cell suicide seems far from clear. Furthermore, the sharp line of demarcation of infarcts across the neuropil (see Fig. 41–1B) would require apoptosis of processes of cells and is a feature also incompatible with apoptosis. Sloviter[54] has proposed a conceptual framework for apoptosis.

Epilogue

The histopathology of cerebral ischemia derives its importance from being the mediator of clinical neurologic deficits resulting from ischemia. Global ischemia clinically occurs in the setting of cardiac arrest, and can be modeled by two-vessel occlusion,[55] four-vessel occlusion,[56] cardiac arrest, and aortic occlusion in animals. Focal cerebral ischemia is likewise easily modeled by either clip occlusion[57] or intraluminal occlusion models using an intraluminal suture[58] advanced into the middle cerebral artery in experimental animals. This suture mimics thromboembolic stroke as opposed to cardiac arrest.

In both cardiac arrest encephalopathy and focal ischemic infarction, it is necrosis of cells and tissue that causes clinical neurologic deficits. In global cerebral ischemia, selective neuronal necrosis occurs in the selectively vulnerable CA1 pyramidal neurons of the hippocampus, the clinical counterpart of which is persistent amnesia after cardiac arrest.[59,60] Focal cerebral ischemia gives rise to a very rich spectrum of potential neurologic disabilities dependent on the location of the infarct in the telencephalon or brain-stem-cerebellum. There is no precedent for acquired ischemic neurologic deficit without tissue necrosis of some kind. Thus, it is incumbent upon the clinician treating stroke to understand the causes of selective neuronal necrosis and infarction when attempting to mitigate these two tissue lesions wherever they may occur in the brain.

References

1. Norris JW, Zhu CZ: Silent stroke and carotid stenosis. Stroke 23:483–485, 1992.
2. de Courten-Myers GM, Kleinholz M, Wagner KR, Myers RE: Stroke assessment: Morphometric infarct size versus neurologic deficit. J Neurosci Meth 83:151–157, 1998.
3. Kiernan JA, Macpherson CM, Price A, Sun T: A histochemical examination of the staining of kainate-induced neuronal degeneration by anionic dyes. Biotech Histochem 73:244–254, 1998.
4. Trump BF, Goldblatt PJ, Stowell RE: Studies on necrosis of mouse liver in vitro: Ultrastructural alterations in the mitochondria of hepatic parenchymal cells. Lab Invest 14:343–371, 1965.
5. Trump BF, Strum JM, Bulger RE: Studies on the pathogenesis of ischaemic cell injury. I: Relation between ion and water shifts and cell ultrastructure in rat kidney slices during swelling at 0–4° C. Virch Arch B Cell Pathol 16:1–34, 1974.
6. Trump BF, McDowell EM, Arstila AU: Cellular reaction to injury. In Hill RB, LaVia MF (eds): Principles of Pathobiology, 3rd ed. New York, Oxford University Press, 1980, pp 20–111.
7. Johansen FF, Jørgensen MB, von Lubitz DKJE, Diemer NH: Selective dendrite damage in hippocampal CA1 stratum radiatum with unchanged axon ultrastructure and glutamate uptake after transient cerebral ischemia in the rat. Brain Res 291:373–377, 1984.
8. Yamamoto K, Hayakawa T, Mogami H, et al: Ultrastructural investigation of the CA1 region of the hippocampus after transient cerebral ischemia in gerbils. Acta Neuropathol (Berlin) 80:487–492, 1990.
9. Auer RN, Kalimo H, Olsson Y, Wieloch T: The dentate gyrus in hypoglycemia: Pathology implicating excitotoxin-mediated neuronal necrosis. Acta Neuropathol (Berlin) 67:279–288, 1985.
10. Sandberg M, Butcher SP, Hagberg H: Extracellular overflow of neuroactive amino acids during severe insulin-induced hypoglycemia: In vivo dialysis of the rat hippocampus. J Neurochem 47:178–184, 1986.
11. Ingvar M, Morgan PF, Auer RN: The nature and timing of excitotoxic neuronal necrosis in the cerebral cortex, hippocampus and thalamus due to flurothyl-induced status epilepticus. Acta Neuropathol (Berl) 75:362–369, 1988.
12. Griffiths T, Evans MC, Meldrum BS: Intracellular calcium accumulation in rat hippocampus during seizures induced by bicuculline or L-allylglycine. Neuroscience 10:385–395, 1983.
13. Olney JW, Sharpe LG, Feigin R: Glutamate-induced brain damage in infant primates. J Neuropathol Exp Neurol 31:464–488, 1972.
14. Griffiths T, Evans MC, Meldrum BS: Status epilepticus: The reversibility of calcium loading and acute neuronal pathological changes in the rat hippocampus. Neuroscience 12:557–567, 1984.
15. Diemer NH, von Lubitz DJKE: Cerebral ischaemia in the rat: Increased permeability of post-synaptic membranes to horseradish peroxidase in the early post-ischaemic period. Neuropathol Appl Neurobiol 9:403–414, 1983.
16. Kraig RP, Pulsinelli WA, Plum F: Carbonic acid buffer changes during complete brain ischemia. Am J Physiol 250:R348–R357, 1986.
17. Hakim AM: The induction and reversibility of cerebral acidosis in thiamine deficiency. Ann Neurol 16:673–679, 1984.
18. Ingvar M, Folbergrová J, Siesjö BK: Metabolic alterations underlying the development of hypermetabolic necrosis in the substantia nigra in status epilepticus. J Cereb Blood Flow Metab 7:103–108, 1987.
19. Ingvar M: Cerebral blood flow and metabolic rate during seizures. Ann N Y Acad Sci 462:194–206, 1986.
20. Hakim AM, Arrieta M: Cerebral acidosis in focal ischemia. I: A method for the simultaneous measurement of local cerebral pH with cerebral glucose utilization or cerebral blood flow in the rat. J Cereb Blood Flow Metab 6:677–675, 1986.
21. Hakim AM: Cerebral acidosis in focal ischemia. II: Nimodipine and verapamil normalize cerebral pH following middle cerebral artery occlusion in the rat. J Cereb Blood Flow Metab 6:676–683, 1986.
22. Nedergaard M: Transient focal ischemia in hyperglycemic rats is associated with increased cerebral infarction. Brain Res 408:79–85, 1987.
23. Nedergaard M, Diemer NH: Focal ischemia of the rat brain, with special reference to the influence of plasma glucose concentration. Acta Neuropathol (Berl) 73:131–137, 1987.
24. Auer RN, Ingvar M, Nevander G, et al: Early axonal lesion and preserved microvasculature in epilepsy-induced hypermetabolic necrosis of the substantia nigra. Acta Neuropathol (Berl) 71:207–215, 1986.
25. Hakim AM: Effect of thiamine deficiency and its reversal on cerebral blood flow in the rat: Observations on the phenomena of hyperperfusion, "no reflow," and delayed hypoperfusion. J Cereb Blood Flow Metab 6:79–85, 1986.
26. Folbergrová J, Ingvar M, Nevander G, Siesjö BK: Cerebral metabolic changes during and following flurothyl-induced seizures in ventilated rats. J Neurochem 44:1419–1426, 1985.
27. Kuriyama M, Umezaki H, Fukuda Y, et al: Mitochondrial encephalomyelopathy with lactate-pyruvate elevation and brain infarctions. Neurology 34:72–77, 1984.
28. Bogousslavsky J, Perentes E, Deruaz JP, Regli F: Mitochondrial myopathy and cardiomyopathy with neurodegenerative features and multiple brain infarcts. J Neurol Sci 55:351–357, 1982.

Pathophysiology

29. Nedergaard M, Gjedde A, Diemer NH: Focal ischemia of the rat brain: Autoradiographic determination of cerebral glucose utilization, glucose content, and blood flow. J Cereb Blood Flow Metab 6:414–424, 1986.

30. Pellerin L, Magistretti PJ: Glutamate uptake into astrocytes stimulates aerobic glycolysis: A mechanism coupling neuronal activity to glucose utilization. Proc Natl Acad Sci U S A 91:10625–10629, 1994.

31. Schurr A, Miller JJ, Payne RS, Rigor BM: An increase in lactate output by brain tissue serves to meet the energy needs of glutamate-activated neurons. J Neurosci 19:34–39, 1999.

32. Dringen R, Gebhardt R, Hamprecht B: Glycogen in astrocytes: Possible function as lactate supply for neighboring cells. Brain Res 623:208–214, 1993.

33. Sokoloff L, Takahashi S, Gotoh J, et al: Contribution of astroglia to functionally activated energy metabolism. Dev Neurosci 18:344–352, 1996.

34. Sokoloff L: Energetics of functional activation in neural tissues. Neurochem Res 24:321–329, 1999.

35. Anderson RE, Tan WK, Martin HS, Meyer FB: Effects of glucose and PaO$_2$ modulation on cortical intracellular acidosis, NADH redox state, and infarction in the ischemic penumbra. Stroke 30:160–170, 1999.

36. Kerr JFR: Shrinkage necrosis: A distinct mode of cellular death. J Pathol 105:13–20, 1971.

37. Charriaut-Marlangue C, Ben-Ari Y: A cautionary note on the use of the TUNEL stain to determine apoptosis. Neuroreport 7:61–64, 1995.

38. Grasl-Kraupp B, Ruttkay-Nedecky B, Koudelka H, et al: In situ detection of fragmented DNA (TUNEL assay) fails to discriminate among apoptosis, necrosis, and autolytic cell death: A cautionary note. Hepatology 21:1465–1468, 1995.

39. de Torres C, Munell F, Ferrer I, et al: Identification of necrotic cell death by the TUNEL assay in the hypoxic-ischemic neonatal rat brain. Neurosci Lett 230:1–4, 1997.

40. Palmer TD, Willhoite AR, Gage FH: Vascular niche for adult hippocampal neurogenesis. J Comp Neurol 425:479–494, 2000.

41. Sloviter RS, Valiquette G, Abrams GM, et al: Selective loss of hippocampal granule cells in the mature rat brain after adrenalectomy. Science 243:535–538, 1989.

42. Sloviter RS, Sollas AL, Dean E, Neubort S: Adrenalectomy-induced granule cell degeneration in the rat hippocampal dentate gyrus: Characterization of an in vivo model of controlled neuronal death. J Comp Neurol 330:324–336, 1993.

43. Sloviter RS, Dean E, Neubort S: Electron microscopic analysis of adrenalectomy-induced hippocampal granule cell degeneration in the rat: Apoptosis in the adult central nervous system. J Comp Neurol 330:337–351, 1993.

44. Deshpande J, Bergstedt K, Lindén T, et al: Ultrastructural changes in the hippocampal CA1 region following transient cerebral ischemia: Evidence against programmed cell death. Exp Brain Res 88:91–105, 1992.

45. Fukuda T, Wang H, Nakanishi H, et al: Novel non-apoptotic morphological changes in neurons of the mouse hippocampus following transient hypoxic-ischemia. Neurosci Res 33:49–55, 1999.

46. Colbourne F, Sutherland GR, Auer RN: Electron microscopic evidence against apoptosis as the mechanism of neuronal death in global ischemia. J Neurosci 19:4200–4210, 1999.

47. Bednar MM, Raymond S, McAuliffe T, et al: The role of neutrophils and platelets in a rabbit model of thromboembolic stroke. Stroke 22:44–50, 1991.

48. Bowes MP, Zivin JA, Rothlein R: Monoclonal antibody to the ICAM-1 adhesion site reduces neurological damage in a rabbit cerebral embolism stroke model. Exp Neurol 119:215–219, 1993.

49. Chen H, Chopp M, Bodzin G: Neutropenia reduces the volume of cerebral infarct after transient middle cerebral artery occlusion in the rat. Neurosci Res Comm 11:93–99, 1992.

50. Chopp M, Zhang RL, Chen H, et al: Postischemic administration of an anti-MAC-1 antibody reduces ischemic cell damage after transient middle cerebral artery occlusion in rats. Stroke 25:869–876, 1994.

51. Matsuo Y, Onodera H, Shiga Y, et al: Correlation between myeloperoxidase-quantified neutrophil accumulation and ischemic brain injury in the rat: Effects of neutrophil depletion. Stroke 25:1469–1475, 1994.

52. Schürer L, Grøgaard B, Gerdin B, et al: Leucocyte depletion does not affect post-ischaemic nerve cell damage in the rat. Acta Neurochir (Wien) 111:54–60, 1991.

53. Takeshima R, Kirsch JR, Koehler RC, et al: Monoclonal leukocyte antibody does not decrease the injury of transient focal cerebral ischemia in cats. Stroke 23:247–252, 1992.

54. Sloviter RS: Apoptosis: A guide for the perplexed. Trends Pharmacol Sci 23:19–24, 2002.

55. Smith M-L, Auer RN, Siesjö BK: The density and distribution of ischemic brain injury in the rat after 2–10 minutes of forebrain ischemia. Acta Neuropathol (Berl) 64:319–332, 1984.

56. Pulsinelli WA, Brierley JB: A new model of bilateral hemispheric ischemia in the unanesthetized rat. Stroke 10:267–272, 1979.

57. Tamura A, Graham DI, McCulloch J, Teasdale GM: Focal cerebral ischemia in the rat. 1: Description of technique and early neuropathological consequences following middle cerebral artery occlusion. J Cereb Blood Flow Metab 1:53–60, 1981.

58. Longa EZ, Weinstein PR, Carlson S, Cummins R: Reversible middle cerebral artery occlusion without craniectomy in rats. Stroke 20:84–91, 1989.

59. Longstreth WT Jr, Inui TS, Cobb LA, Copass MK: Neurologic recovery after out-of-hospital cardiac arrest. Ann Intern Med 98:588–592, 1983.

60. Longstreth WT Jr, Inui TS: High blood glucose level on hospital admission and poor neurological recovery after cardiac arrest. Ann Neurol 15:59–63, 1984.

Chapter Forty-Two

Molecular and Cellular Mechanisms of Ischemia-Induced Neuronal Death

R. Suzanne Zukin, Teresa Jover, Hidenori Yokota, Agata Calderone,
Monica Simionescu, and C. Geoff Lau

Ischemia is the condition or state in which a tissue such as brain is subjected to hypoxia or low oxygen because of an obstruction of the arterial blood supply or inadequate blood flow.[1] Brain ischemia can be broadly divided into two main classifications, global ischemia and focal ischemia. *Global ischemia* is the condition or state in which blood flow to the entire brain is transiently blocked, resulting in delayed, selective neuronal death. *Focal ischemia*, or cerebral infarction, is the condition or state in which a specific area of brain tissue undergoes injury as a consequence of a temporary or permanent obstruction of local blood supply. Focal ischemia results in death of both neurons and non-neuronal cells in contiguous areas of brain, usually representing a single vascular territory. In this chapter, we present the current understanding of the molecular and cellular mechanisms of neuronal death associated with brain ischemia. Table 42.1 defines the abbreviations used in the text.

GLOBAL ISCHEMIA

Global or brainwide ischemia arises most commonly in humans as a consequence of cardiac arrest, open-heart surgery, profuse bleeding, near-drowning, or carbon monoxide poisoning. Global ischemia associated with cardiac arrest affects 150,000 Americans each year and, in most cases, results in delayed onset of neurologic deficit.[1a–4] The most common neurologic deficits are cognitive impairments, of which memory loss is most notable. Although all forebrain areas experience oxygen and glucose deprivation (OGD) during the brief ischemic insult, only select neuronal populations degenerate and die in humans[1a–4] and in animals subjected experimentally to global ischemia.[5] Pyramidal neurons in the cornu ammonis 1 region of the hippocampus (CA1) are particularly vulnerable. Other neurons that may be damaged are hilar neurons of the dentate gyrus (DG), medium aspiny neurons of the striatum, pyramidal neurons in neocortical layers II, V, and VI, and Purkinje neurons of the cerebellum.[6,7] The molecular mechanisms underlying the cell-specific pattern of global ischemia–induced neuronal death are not well understood.

Histologic evidence of degeneration, or demonstration of the characteristics of apoptosis, is not observed until 2 to 3 days after ischemia in rats and 3 to 4 days in gerbils. At 1 week after induction of transient global ischemia, virtually complete ablation of the CA1 pyramidal cell layer can be observed. During the ischemic episode, cells exhibit a transient, early rise in intracellular calcium ion (Ca^{2+}), depolarize, and become inexcitable; ambient glutamate rises four-fold to $\approx 2\,\mu M$. After reperfusion, cells appear morphologically normal, exhibit normal intracellular Ca^{2+}, and regain the ability to generate action potentials for 24 to 72 hours after the insult. Ultimately, there is a late rise in intracellular Ca^{2+} and zinc ion (Zn^{2+}), and death of CA1 pyramidal neurons ensues. Although the molecular mechanisms underlying ischemia-induced death are not yet completely understood, the substantial delay between insult and onset of death suggests that transcriptional changes play a critical role. Candidate transcription factors that are thought to direct programs of gene expression changes after global ischemia include the cyclic adenosine monophosphate (cAMP) response element–binding protein (CREB), the Forkhead family of transcription factors, and the restrictive element (RE)1 gene–silencing transcription factor, also known as REST/neuron-restrictive silencer factor (NRSF).

FOCAL ISCHEMIA

Focal or localized ischemia arises in humans most commonly as a result of stroke, cerebral hemorrhage, or traumatic brain injury. Most strokes are caused by clots that either form at the site of occlusion in a cerebral artery or travel there from the heart (classic stroke), and the remainder are caused by a bursting of a weakened blood vessel in the brain and bleeding into the surrounding tissue (cerebral hemorrhage or traumatic brain injury). Stroke is the third leading cause of death in the United States and the primary cause of disabilities in adults. Of the approximately 600,000 new victims each year, nearly 30% die and 20% to 30% become severely and permanently disabled. Others

Table 42.1   Abbreviations Used in Chapter 42

AIF	Apoptosis-inducing factor	IRS-1	Insulin receptor substrate-1
Akt	Serine-threonine kinase, a proto-oncogenic ser-thr kinase; also known as protein kinase B	LTD	Long-term depression
		LTP	Long-term potentiation
AMP	Adenosine monophosphate	MAPK	Mitogen-activated protein kinase
AMPARs	α-Amino-3-hydroxy-5-methyl-4-isoxazole-propionic acid (AMPA) receptors	MCAO	Middle cerebral artery occlusion
		mGluR	Metabotropic GluR
Apaf-1	Apoptotic protease–activating factor 1	MKP-1	MAPK phosphatase-1
ATP	Adenosine triphosphate	MnSOD	Manganese superoxide dismutase
BAD	A proapoptotic member of the bcl-2 family of proteins	$NAD^{\dagger}$	β-Nicotinamide adenine dinucleotide, oxidized form
BCCO	Bilateral occlusion of the carotid arteries	NADPH	Nicotinamide adenine dinucleotide phosphate, reduced form
BDNF	Brain-derived neurotrophic factor		
BIR	Baculoviral IAP repeat	Naspm	Naphthyl acetyl spermine
CA1	Cornu ammonis 1 region of the hippocampus	NF-κB	Nuclear factor kappa B
CaMKIV	Ca^{2+}-calmodulin–dependent kinase IV	NGF	Nerve growth factor
CBP	CREB-binding protein	NMDARs	N-methyl-D-aspartate (NMDA) receptors
CREB	Cyclic AMP response element–binding protein	nNOS	Neural NOS
CREM	Cyclic AMP–response modulatory protein	NO	Nitric oxide
CSD	Cortical spreading depression	NOS	NO synthase
DG	Dentate gyrus area of the hippocampus	$\cdot O^{2+}$	Superoxide anion
DIABLO	Direct IAP–binding protein with low pI	NSRF	Neuron-restrictive silencer factor; also known as REST
DISC	Death-inducing signaling complex		
EDTA	Ethylenediaminetetraacetic acid	OGD	Oxygen and glucose deprivation
EEG	Electroencephalogram	$ONOO^-$	Peroxynitrite
ELK	Nuclear transcription factor	PARP-1	Poly (ADP-ribose) polymerase-1
EPSC	Excitatory postsynaptic current	PCD	Programmed cell death
ERα	Estrogen receptor-α	PCR	Polymerase chain reaction
ERE	Estrogen response element	PI3K	Phosphatidylinositol 3-kinase
ERK	Extracellular signal–regulated kinase	PKA	Protein kinase A
FADD	Fas-associated death domain	PP1	Protein phosphatase 1
GABA	Gamma-aminobutyric acid	PSD-95	Postsynaptic density protein of 95 kDa
GluR	Glutamate receptor	PV	Parvalbumin
GSK-3β	Glycogen synthase kinase-3β	REST	Repressor element gene silencing transcription factor; also known as NRSF
HDAC	Histone deacetylase		
HIF-1	Hypoxia-inducible factor-1	ROS	Reactive oxygen species
HSE	Heat shock element	Rsk	Ribosomal S6 kinase
HSP	Heat shock protein	RT-PCR	Reverse transcription-PCR
IAP	Inhibitor of apoptosis protein	SmaC	Second mitochondria–derived activator of caspases
ICAM-1	Intercellular adhesion molecule-1		
IEG	Immediate early gene	TNF	Tumor necrosis factor
IGF	Insulin-like growth factor	TRAIL	TNF-related apoptosis–inducing ligand
IGF-IR	IGF-I receptor	VDAC	Voltage-dependent anion channel
IκB	Inhibitor of NF-κB	VO	Vessel occlusion
IL-1β	Interleukin-1β	ZnT-3	Zn^{2+} transporter-3

suffer paralysis, reduced coordination, and neurologic deficits including impaired cognition, visual disturbance, and loss of sensation. People older than 65 years experience almost three fourths of all strokes. "Brain attack" can be studied through the implementation of focal ischemia on animal models.

Tissues at risk of harm from occlusion of a cerebral artery are the *core* or center of the stroke, which contains cells that are highly dependent on the blocked artery and receive essentially no blood, and the *penumbra* or surrounding region, which contains cells that receive some blood from other arteries (Plate 42–1C following page 840). Cells in the core die from several overwhelming causes and probably cannot be salvaged by any treatment short of immediate removal of the clot. Although the infarct starts in the core, at its maximum it encompasses both core and penumbra, generally after 6 to 24 hours of permanent ischemia.[8] The duration of the ischemic episode determines the extent or grade of damage, assessed 1 to 2 days after reperfusion.[9] At 10 to 20 minutes after induction of focal ischemia, only a few scattered dead neurons are observed in the core. At 1 hour, infarct is observed in the core, and the infarct size is maximal. The mechanisms underlying death of cells in the core are complicated but most certainly include glutamate receptor–mediated necrotic cell death (see later). Brain edema (as studied with magnetic resonance imaging [MRI] and computed tomography [CT]) serves as one of the earliest markers for the ensuing pathophysiology and is a key determinant of whether a patient survives beyond the first few hours after stroke.

EXPERIMENTAL MODELS OF GLOBAL AND FOCAL ISCHEMIA

A number of experimental models are currently used to study brain ischemia. The three main paradigms involving intact animals (in vivo ischemia) are global ischemia, focal ischemia, and hypoxia-ischemia, a condition that shares properties with both focal and global ischemia. In vivo models of global ischemia enable neuronal death to mature in an intact animal in which neural circuitry is preserved. Therefore, these models have greater physiologic validity and clinical relevance to global ischemia associated with cardiac arrest in humans than in vitro models.

In vitro models are also used to examine molecular and biophysical mechanisms of neuronal death. These models are particularly useful for suppression or overexpression of genes of interest. In vitro models involving organotypically cultured brain slices are particularly useful in that they afford preservation of neural circuitry.

In Vivo Models

Global Ischemia

Global ischemic insults consist of brief but nearly complete cessation of cerebral blood flow produced by permanent occlusion of the vertebral arteries and transient occlusion of the common carotid arteries (rats) or by transient occlusion of the common carotid arteries (gerbils and mice), followed by reperfusion.[10,11] The most commonly used models of global ischemia are (1) the four-vessel occlusion (4-VO) model in rats[12]; (2) the two-vessel occlusion (2-VO; also known as temporary bilateral common carotid occlusion, or BCCO) in gerbils[7,13] or (less commonly) mice[13,14]; and (3) two-vessel occlusion in combination with hypotension in rats.[10] Global ischemia can also be induced in large mammals such as monkeys[15] and goats.[16] Global ischemic insults are typically short (on the order of 5 to 20 minutes). During the ischemic episode, blood flow to the entire brain is reduced (to < 1%) essentially immediately and remains blocked until reperfusion. Adenosine triphosphate (ATP) is depleted in cells throughout the brain essentially immediately but recovers to near physiologic levels by the time of reperfusion.[17]

The 4-VO model in rats and the 2-VO model in gerbils differ from more severe models involving hypotension, in that neuronal death is extremely delayed and highly specific. Although all forebrain areas experience OGD during a brief ischemic insult, neuronal death elicited by a brief episode (10 minutes for 4-VO in rats; 5 minutes for 2-VO in gerbils) is largely restricted to pyramidal neurons of the hippocampal CA1 and hilar neurons (Plate 42–1B).[18] Inhibitory interneurons of the CA1 and most neurons in the nearby CA2 or transition zone, CA3, and DG survive. With the exception of a few scattered hilar neurons or pyramidal neurons in the cortex, no other neurons exhibit cell death. Although these models afford virtual ablation of the hippocampal CA1 by 7 days, the onset of histologically detectable neuronal death is not manifested until more than 48 hours in rats,[10,19] or more than 72 hours in gerbils,[7,20,21] after insult. Longer insults induce more widespread damage to areas such as medium aspiny striatal neurons, pyramidal neurons in neocortical layers II, V, and VI, and cerebellar Purkinje neurons.[6,7]

Advantages of the in vivo models of global ischemia are as follows:

1. They have clinical relevance to global ischemia associated with cardiac arrest in humans.

2. Neural circuitry is preserved.
3. The substantial delay between insult and neuronal death enables detailed molecular studies.
4. The specificity of cell death allows comparison of molecular changes in CA1 with those in CA3.
5. The cranium is completely blocked (rather than reduced by hypotension); thus, monitoring of blood flow is not necessary.
6. Animals exhibit no obvious behavioral manifestations, and the mortality rate is low.

The rare animals that do exhibit obvious behavioral manifestations (abnormal vocalization when handled, generalized convulsions, loss of greater than 20% of body weight by 3 to 7 days, hypoactivity) are excluded from the study.

Four-Vessel Occlusion Model in Rats

The 4-VO model is a well-established model of neuronal insult in which neuronal death is largely restricted to pyramidal neurons of the hippocampal CA1 and does not manifest until 3 to 4 days after insult.[12] A specific advantage of the rat model is that many available complementary DNA (cDNA) and RNA probes are directed to rat RNA, and many antibodies exhibit high specificity for rat tissue and may not recognize epitopes in other species. Age-matched male Sprague Dawley or Wistar rats, weighing 100 to 125 g are fasted overnight; the next day, animals are anesthetized with halothane. The vertebral arteries are exposed through a small incision in the neck and subjected to permanent electrocauterization. The common carotid arteries are exposed and isolated with a 3-0 silk thread, and the wound is sutured. Twenty-four hours later, the wound is reopened, and the common carotid arteries are subjected to temporary occlusion with surgical clasps (4 minutes for sublethal ischemia and 10 minutes for global ischemia), and anesthesia is discontinued (Plate 42–1A).[12,22] At the time of occlusion of the carotid arteries, blood flow is typically reduced to less than 3% of normal in the hippocampus, striatum, and neocortex.[23] The electroencephalogram (EEG) generally becomes isoelectric[24] and spontaneous cortical activity is abolished within 1 minute.[25] For sham operation, animals are subjected to the same anesthesia and surgical exposure procedures, except that the carotid arteries are not occluded. Although anesthesia is typically administered until occlusion of the carotid arteries, it is not essential to the surgical procedure.

Two-Vessel Occlusion with Hypotension in Rats

An alternative model of global ischemia in rats involves ligation of the common carotid (but not vertebral) arteries, together with systemic hypotension (50 mm Hg). Under these conditions, blood flow falls to 1% in the hippocampus, striatum, and neocortex,[26,27] and the EEG becomes isoelectric within 15 to 25 seconds.[28] Animals are subjected to anesthesia for the entire duration of the ischemic episode. Models of global ischemia involving systemic hypoxia and/or hypotension are more severe than the 4-VO model. These models cause a more rapid onset of generalized neuronal death, particularly in the cortex, striatum, and hippocampus, major behavioral manifestations, and a considerable death rate.

Pathophysiology

Two-Vessel Occlusion in Gerbils

Gerbils are advantageous for studies of global ischemia in that they lack posterior communicating arteries, structures that in humans and rats are necessary to complete the circle of Willis and permit collateral blood flow. Thus, global ischemia can be induced in gerbils by the relatively simple 2-VO model. In gerbils, 2-VO (5 minutes) elicits highly selective, extremely delayed neuronal death, with a pattern of cell specificity virtually identical to that in rats; neuronal death is not manifested until more than 72 hours after onset.[10,21] The 2-VO model is the model of global ischemia most commonly used for testing neuroprotective agents. Within 20 seconds of 2-VO, blood flow falls to 1% in neocortex and to 4% in hippocampus,[29] and the EEG becomes isoelectric.[30] Anesthesia is administered until occlusion of the carotid arteries.

Two-Vessel Occlusion in Mice

Mice offer advantages in that some strains (C57/BL6 and related strains) exhibit global ischemia in response to the relatively simple 2-VO model, enabling comparisons between animals with null mutations in a gene of interest and their wild-type littermates. However, strain differences in vulnerability to ischemic damage can complicate results.[31] In mice, 2-VO (20 minutes) elicits somewhat selective, delayed cell death. At 72 hours after ischemia, the majority of animals exhibit no detectable cell loss in the hippocampus; in one study, about 17% of animals exhibited minor cell loss and another 17% showed moderate cell loss in the CA1.[14] At 7 days after ischemia, nearly all animals exhibited marked loss in the pyramidal cell layer of CA1. In the majority of animals, CA3 exhibited at most slight cell loss, and the DG exhibited no cell loss at 7 days.

Focal Ischemia

Focal ischemia is the animal model that most nearly approximates stroke or cerebral infarction in humans.[32-34] Focal ischemia is produced experimentally by occlusion of the middle cerebral artery. Arterial occlusion can be permanent (arterial blockade maintained throughout the experiment) or temporary (occlusion for up to 3 hours, followed by reperfusion) and either proximal or distal (see later). These procedures induce a necrotic core of cells that are irreversibly damaged and a penumbra of cells that can be revived (see Plate 42–1C).[35] Focal ischemia is typically performed in rodents such as rats or mice. For rats, a preferred strain is the spontaneously hypertensive rat, which exhibits reduced collateral circulation during the ischemic episode.[36-38]

Proximal Occlusion

In the case of proximal occlusion, the middle cerebral artery (MCA) is subjected to occlusion close to its branching from the internal carotid, before the origin of the lenticulostriate arteries.[11,36] Proximal MCA occlusion (MCAO) is most commonly induced by ligation of the common carotid and external carotid arteries, followed by insertion of a suture into the internal carotid artery at the bifurcation of the common carotid and external carotid arteries. The suture is advanced intraluminally beyond the origin of the posterior communicating artery and past the origin of the MCA (see Plate 42–1A).[10,11,33] After MCAO, blood flow is nonuniformly reduced throughout the affected region. The center of the stroke, or core, is defined as the region in which blood flow is reduced to less than 15%; it encompasses the lateral portion of the caudate putamen and the parietal cortex. The penumbra, defined as the region in which blood flow is reduced to less than 40%, encompasses the remainder of the neocortex, the entorhinal cortex, and the medial caudate-putamen.

Distal Occlusion

In distal MCAO, blood flow to the basal ganglia is not interrupted; thus, damage is restricted to the neocortex. This type of occlusion can be induced surgically by means of a clip[37] or by inducing thrombotic clots[38,39] in combination with transient unilateral occlusion of the common carotid arteries.[28,40,41] The reduction of blood flow achieved in the core and penumbra with distal MCAO is similar to that achieved in the proximal model.

Hypoxia-Ischemia

The hypoxia-ischemia model involves transient unilateral occlusion of the common carotid artery in combination with systemic hypoxia, such that oxygen flow to the brain is reduced to 3% in adult rats or to 8% in neonates.[42-44] After 15 to 30 minutes of hypoxia, delayed neuronal death occurs in the hippocampal CA1 and CA3, striatum, and layer V of the neocortex in adults.[45] Young rats show delayed development of infarct, which can be induced by subjecting them to low levels of oxygen (8% of normal) for 60 minutes.[46]

In Vitro Models

Oxygen and glucose deprivation (OGD) of cell cultures or brain slices provides an in vitro model of global ischemia (Plate 42–2).[47-49] In vitro models require longer periods of OGD to induce cell death, and ATP levels do not fall as much as in in vivo models. The absence of blood vessels and blood flow simplifies interpretation of the results but renders the model less relevant than a model using an intact animal. Advantages of the in vitro OGD model are as follows:

1. Manipulations of the microenvironment can be more precise.
2. The model is amenable to patch clamp recording and detailed electrophysiologic analyses.
3. Prolonged survival of cultures permits molecular and genetic manipulations as, for example, ease of antisense suppression of a protein of interest by administration of antisense oligonucleotides.
4. It allows optical monitoring of changes in the same slice over days.
5. It enables internal control of a number of slices that can be obtained from the same animal.

Oxygen-Glucose Deprivation of Dissociated Neurons in Culture

In vitro OGD is performed in primary cultures of neurons or glia from the neocortex, hippocampus, cerebellum, and hypothalamus of embryonic or early postnatal rats or mice. Mixed neocortical specimens containing both neurons and glia are typically cultured from embryonic day 15 (E15) rats.[50] At 14 days in vitro (DIV), the culture medium is exchanged with deoxygenated, glucose-free salt solution to induce OGD. Cultures are deprived of oxygen and glucose for 90 to 100 minutes and then transferred to an oxygenated serum-free medium containing glucose and propidium iodide. Cell death is assayed at 24 and 48 hours.

Oxygen-Glucose Deprivation in Cultured Hippocampal Slices

Ischemic damage is also studied in organotypic hippocampal slice cultures from perinatal rats. Typically, hippocampal slices are obtained from rat pups (postnatal day 8, or P8) and maintained in vitro for 14 to 21 days.[51] Briefly, hippocampi are removed from rat brains, and transverse slices are cut with a tissue chopper in a sterile environment. Isolated slices are placed in ice-cold Hanks balanced salt solution supplemented with glucose and Fungizone and then transferred to humidified semiporous membranes. Slices are maintained in culture medium at 37°C and 95% air/5% CO_2. At 14 to 21 DIV, hippocampal slices are subjected to OGD by exposure to a serum-free medium devoid of glucose and saturated with 95% N_2/5% CO_2 for 30 to 60 minutes, then transferred to an oxygenated serum-free medium containing glucose and propidium iodide. Cell death is assayed at 48 and 72 hours. A 30-minute insult elicits selective death of CA1 neurons by 48 hours (see Plate 42–2). Neuronal death is typically assessed from permeability to dyes such as trypan blue and propidium iodide.[52] In vitro ischemia impairs synaptic transmission, protein synthesis, ATP production, and neuron morphology.

MODALITIES OF ISCHEMIC CELL DEATH

Cell death occurs by necrosis or apoptosis.[53,54] These two mechanisms have distinct histologic and biochemical signatures. In necrosis, the stimulus of death (e.g., ischemia) is itself often the direct cause of the demise of the cell. In apoptosis, however, the stimulus of death activates a cascade of events that orchestrate the destruction of the cell. Unlike necrosis, which is a pathologic process, apoptosis is part of normal development; however, aberrant apoptosis occurs in response to injurious stimuli.

Global ischemia induces neuronal death with hallmarks of both necrosis and apoptosis.[55] Ultrastructural studies indicate that global ischemia induces many of the morphologic features of necrotic cell death in CA1 neurons (see later) but do not detect critical hallmarks of apoptosis such as apoptotic bodies.[56] Thus, apoptosis as defined by stereotypic morphologic changes, especially evident in the nucleus where the chromatin condenses to compact an apparently simple geometric figure, does not occur. These and other studies cast doubt as to whether global ischemia elicits any of the morphologic features of apoptosis. Strong evidence in support of apoptosis, defined as activation of specific intracellular signaling cascades that result in cellular suicide,[53,57] comes from molecular studies that show mitochondrial release of cytochrome c and activation of the caspases, in particular caspase-3 (see later).

Focal ischemia also induces neuronal death with hallmarks of both necrosis and apoptosis.[11] Focal ischemia elicits early cell shrinkage and swelling of mitochondria,

followed by cell dispersal, shrinkage of the nucleus, the formation of cytoplasmic projections, and, ultimately, a shrunken, pyknotic nucleus without surrounding cytoplasm (the last remnant of the dead neuron). The early mitochondrial swelling and loss of integrity of the plasma membrane, with preservation of the nuclear membrane, are hallmarks of necrotic cell death. Evidence in support of apoptotic death in the penumbra has surfaced, including DNA fragmentation, activation of death receptors, mitochondrial release of cytochrome c, and activation of the caspase death cascade (see later).

Necrotic Cell Death

Necrosis is the death of a circumscribed area of tissue as a result of a wide variety of injuries. At the light-microscopic level, the morphologic hallmarks of necrotic cell death are early mitochondrial swelling and loss of integrity of the plasma membrane, with preservation of the nuclear membrane. At the ultrastructural level, the hallmarks of necrotic cell death are proliferation of endoplasmic reticulum, disaggregation of polyribosomes, selective swelling of dendrites, and dilation of organelles and intranuclear vacuoles. The necrotic tissue morphology is to a large extent due to postmortem events occurring after cell lysis. Necrotic cell death can be divided into two main states, edematous death, characterized by edema or organelle swelling, and ischemic death. The edematous state is characterized by swollen cytoplasm, the absence of dynamic plasma membrane blebbing of a dying cell (zeiosis), absence of microtubules, and presence of the endoplasmic reticulum, Golgi apparatus, and polysomes as incomplete structures. Although the nucleus appears nearly normal, irregular clumping of chromatin is seen.[58,59] These characteristics are observed for CA1 neurons undergoing delayed death in the rat and gerbil models of global ischemia.[60,61] By contrast, the ischemic state is characterized by darkening and shrinkage of the nucleus and cytoplasm[62–64]; the plasma and nuclear membranes become highly irregular, and the cell assumes a triangular shape. Cells undergoing ischemic cell change are acidophilic. In models of global ischemia, CA1 neurons exhibit edematous changes in the end stages of degeneration. In focal ischemia, cortical neurons in the core and penumbra exhibit morphologic changes before their demise.

Apoptotic Cell Death

Apoptosis, or programmed cell death (PCD), is the evolutionarily conserved process by which cells die as a result of an internally programmed series of events mediated by a dedicated set of gene products. Apoptotic cell death is essential during development (embryogenesis) and tissue homeostasis; when dysregulated, apoptotic cell death can result in cancer, abnormal neuronal death, or autoimmunity. A variety of injurious stimuli, including focal ischemia and global ischemia, can induce apoptosis if the insult is mild but will induce necrosis with a stronger insult. Apoptotic neurons exhibit characteristic morphologic features that differentiate them from necrotic neurons—cytoplasmic shrinkage, chromatin condensation, zeiosis (dynamic membrane blebbing), and apoptotic bodies. Unlike

Pathophysiology

necrotic cells, in which plasma membrane is damaged early, apoptotic cells exhibit intact plasma membranes until the last stages of death, at which time the membranes become permeable to normally retained solutes. A number of specific apoptotic death cascades involving downstream signaling molecules have now been identified. Molecular hallmarks of apoptosis include phosphatidylserine exposure (translocation from the inner leaflet to the outer surface of the plasma membrane), activation of the cell surface receptors such as Fas/CD95, a member of the tumor necrosis factor (TNF) family of death receptors,[65] mitochondrial release of cytochrome c,[66] activation of the caspases, notably caspase-3,[67] and DNA fragmentation.[68–70]

The Caspase Death Cascade

Caspases are a family of structurally related cysteine proteases that cleave target proteins just after an aspartate residue.[53] Because caspases are constitutively expressed as biologically inactive precursors or procaspases in most cells and can cleave their own procaspases, the caspase cascade is self-amplifying.

It had been thought that a key event (and "point of no return") in the execution of apoptosis was activation of the essential "terminator" protein, caspase-3. However, two recent studies provide compelling evidence that neurons can survive in the face of caspase-3 activation.[70a–b] In global ischemia, caspase-3 upregulation and activation occur 2 to 3 days before the onset of histologically detectable neuronal death.[71] The importance of early caspase-3 activation to global ischemia–induced neuronal death is underscored by the finding that Z-DEVD-FMK, a selective caspase-3 inhibitor, is neuroprotective if administered at the time of ischemia but not at 24 hours or later.[72] Thus, neurons become "committed" to die early in the postischemic period. Caspase-3 promotes cell death through proteolytic cleavage of downstream target proteins such as poly (ADP-ribose)polymerase (PARP), nuclear lamins, DNA-dependent protein kinase, and the inhibitory subunit of DNA fragmentation factor.[73,74] DNA fragmentation results in cell disintegration followed by engulfment by surrounding cells. The caspase cascade can be activated by either of two reversible and interacting pathways, an extrinsic or death receptor–dependent route (Plate 42–3) and an intrinsic (death receptor–independent) or mitochondrial route (Plate 42–4).

In the extrinsic or death receptor–dependent pathway, apoptotic stimuli trigger activation of death ligand–death receptor systems such as the FasL/Fas (also known as the Apo-1 or CD95) system.[75] Fas is a death domain-containing receptor and member of the TNF superfamily of cytokine receptors. Forkhead1 (FOXO-3A1 or FOXO-3A), a member of the Forkhead family of transcription factors, induces expression of target genes, such as the cytokine FasL (Fas ligand), that are implicated in the extrinsic receptor pathway of caspase activation.[76] FasL initiates apoptosis by binding to its cognate receptor Fas, triggering formation of a death-inducing signaling complex (DISC) within seconds of receptor engagement. Fas acts via its death domain to recruit the adaptor protein FADD (Fas-associated death domain). FADD, in turn, acts via its death domain to recruit procaspase-8 into the DISC. The signaling complex catalyzes the proteolytic cleavage and

transactivation of procaspase-8 to generate the "instigator" caspase, caspase-8. Once activated, caspase-8 is released from the DISC into the cytoplasm as a heterotetramer composed of two small subunits and two large subunits. Activated or processed caspase-8 can directly activate other members of the caspase family, paving the way for the execution phase of apoptosis. Caspase-8 additionally acts to induce the translocation of Bcl-2 family member BID to the mitochondria. When the abundance of BAX, BIM, BAD and BID exceeds that of anti-apoptotic Bcl-2 family members, cytochrome c is released from the mitochondria (see Plate 42–3).

In the death receptor–independent or mitochondrial route, apoptotic and necrotic death stimuli trigger the mitochondrial release of cytochrome c into the cytoplasm, an event that is blocked by Bcl-2 and its anti-apoptotic family members.[77] Once in the cytoplasm, cytochrome c assembles with the apoptotic protease activating factor 1 (Apaf-1), procaspase-9 and deoxy ATP to form a protein-signaling complex termed the *apoptosome*. Formation of the apoptosome promotes transactivation of procaspase-9 by Apaf-1. Activated caspase-9, in turn, cleaves procaspase-3 to generate the downstream "terminator" protein caspase-3. Thus, the apoptosome enables cytochrome c to jump-start the caspase self-amplifying cascade of proteolysis independently of ligand-activated death receptors (see Plate 42–4).

Both focal ischemia and global ischemia trigger the caspase death cascade in neurons destined to die. Global ischemia induces activation of death receptors, such as Fas[78] and p75[NTR, 79–81], and terminators, such as caspase-9 and caspase-3,[72,80,82] and the onset of DNA fragmentation, a marker for apoptotic cell death.[79,80,83] The observation that global ischemia triggers early release of cytochrome c from the mitochondria,[84] activation of caspase-9[82,84] and caspase-3,[71,80] and relatively late activation of Fas/FasL[78] provides strong support for activation of the caspases via an intrinsic pathway. In the case of focal ischemia, delayed neuronal death with many of the hallmarks of apoptosis are observed in the penumbra, including evidence of DNA fragmentation,[68–70] activation of the FasL/Fas receptor,[65] release of cytochrome c from the mitochondria,[66] and activation of caspase-3.[67]

Inhibitors of Apoptosis

The inhibitor of apoptosis proteins (IAPs) are a family of structurally related proteins that confer protection from death-inducing stimuli by potently binding and inhibiting activated caspases. IAPs, originally identified in the genome of baculovirus on the basis of their ability to suppress apoptosis in infected host cells, suppress apoptosis in mammalian cells by halting the caspase death cascade.[85–87] To date, eight human IAPs have been identified, including XIAP, c-IAP, c-IAP2, and survivin, and all exhibit anti-apoptotic activity in cell culture. The best-characterized IAP family member is the X-chromosome–linked protein XIAP. XIAP is an extremely potent suppressor of apoptosis, an effect mediated at least in part by its ability to bind and suppress active caspases. XIAP binds caspases -3, -7, and -9 reversibly and with high affinity, thereby masking the caspase active site. The main functional unit in the IAPs is the BIR (or baculoviral IAP repeat) domain, which contains about 80 amino acids folded around a zinc atom.

Most IAPs have multiple BIR domains that mediate specialized functions. For example, the linker region between BIR1 and BIR2 binds caspase-3 and caspase-7, BIR2 selectively targets caspase-7, and BIR3 targets caspase-9.

Under physiologic conditions, IAPs are present in mammalian cells, where they act as buffers or dampeners that suppress spurious spontaneous caspase activation. The actions of IAPs on neuronal survival are, however, not limited to caspase inhibition. Compelling data support additional roles for IAPs in protein degradation, cell cycle regulation and caspase-independent signaling cascades.[86] Emerging data indicate that the presence of a zinc-binding motif or RING domain at the distal end of the carboxy-termini in a subset of IAPs confers protein degradation activity.[88] These IAPs catalyze degradation of select target proteins via ubiquitylation. In this process, IAPs catalyze the sequential covalent addition of ubiquitin (a 76–amino acid protein) onto select lysine residues within target proteins. The modified residues can form multimeric poly-ubiquitin chains, which tag the protein and mark it for destruction.[88]

Injurious stimuli such as global ischemia elevate the expression of IAP proteins, which bind and reversibly inhibit the caspases. At the same time, injurious stimuli that are sufficiently potent promote the mitochondrial release of Smac (second mitochondria–derived activator of caspases)/DIABLO (direct IAP-binding protein with low pI) and cytochrome c. Whereas cytochrome c directly activates Apaf-1 and caspase-9 and forms the apoptosome, Smac/DIABLO binds to IAP family members and neutralizes their anti-apoptotic activity. Smac forms an elongated arch-shaped dimer more than 130 Å in length. The Smac dimer forms a stable complex with the BIR2 and BIR3 domains of XIAP. Structural studies involving nuclear magnetic resonance (NMR) and X-ray analyses reveal that the Smac *N*-terminal tripeptide (Ala-Val-Pro-Ile) recognizes a surface groove composed of highly conserved residues on the BIR3 domain.[89] The balance between the IAPs and Smac/DIABLO establishes a threshold for "lethal" caspase-3 activity. Only under conditions in which Smac/DIABLO is released from the mitochondria is activated caspase-3 liberated from IAPs and free to execute apoptotic cell death.

An alternative pathway to inhibit activated caspase-3 is via the anti-apoptotic protein Bcl-2.[90] Evidence indicates that the mammalian cell-death inhibitors Bcl-2 and Bcl-x$_L$, by analogy to the *Caenorhabditis elegans* cell-death inhibitor CED-9, might function as a pseudosubstrate inhibitor of activated caspase-3.[91] Studies of programmed cell death in *C. elegans* indicate that the CED-9 protein prevents apoptosis by direct inhibition of CED-3. CED-9 can be cleaved by CED-3 at two sites near its amino-terminus, at least one of which is important for complete protection by CED-9 against cell death. Ischemic preconditioning induces expression of Bcl-2 in CA1 neurons.[92] There is as yet no hard evidence, however, that mammalian Bcl-2 functions as an active site-directed inhibitor of caspase-3.

Poly(ADP-ribose)polymerase-1 and Apoptosis-Inducing Factor

Poly(ADP-ribose)polymerase-1 (PARP-1) is an abundant nuclear enzyme involved in DNA damage surveillance and DNA repair and is a critical downstream target of caspase-3. Under physiologic conditions, PARP-1 is critical for maintaining genomic integrity and may play a role in DNA replication and regulation of gene expression.[93] PARP acts via an amino-terminal DNA-binding motif to recognize nicks and breaks in the double-stranded nucleic acid. Upon binding to DNA strand breaks, PARP catalyzes the polyribosylation of β-nicotinamide adenine dinucleotide (NAD$^+$), generating branched polymers of ADP-ribose that it transfers to a subset of nuclear proteins, including histones, topoisomerases I and II, DNA polymerases, and PARP itself.[94–96] The obligatory triggers of PARP-1 activation are nicks and breaks in double-stranded DNA. Once activated, PARP-1 transfers between 50 and 200 molecules of ADP-ribose to target proteins, which may activate or inhibit their function. In the case of histones, poly(ADP-ribosyl)ation promotes chromatin relaxation.

Neuronal insults and other types of environmental stress effect the production of free radicals and oxidants. These agents induce DNA damage, which frequently triggers cell death by apoptosis. Apoptosis culminates in activation of caspase-3, which catalyzes the cleavage and activation of downstream targets including PARP-1. A major trigger for DNA damage in cerebral ischemia is peroxynitrite (ONOO$^-$), a cytotoxic oxidant formed by reaction between nitric oxide and superoxide (see Plate 42–4). Excessive activation of PARP-1 depletes the entire cell of its substrate NAD$^+$ (Plate 42–5B). NAD$^+$ depletion in mitochondria causes pronounced slowing of glycolysis, electron transport, and ATP formation, leading to energy failure and neuronal death. Observations that PARP-1 inhibition or gene inactivation may prevent the neuronal death associated with cerebral ischemia,[97,98] myocardial infarction,[99] inflammatory injury, reactive oxygen species–induced injury,[96] and glutamate excitotoxicity[100,101] have triggered an explosion of interest in the process of poly(ADP-ribosyl)ation.

Our understanding of the underpinnings of PARP-1-induced cell death was significantly advanced by the discovery that massive PARP-1 activation triggers apoptotic cell death mediated by apoptosis-inducing factor (AIF) (see Plate 42–5A).[102,103] AIF is a powerful cytotoxin that under normal conditions is confined to the mitochondrion together with cytochrome c and other pro-apoptotic molecules. Massive activation of PARP-1 promotes production of poly(ADP-ribose) and depletion of NAD$^+$, which appear to signal the release of AIF from the mitochondria.[103] Once released, AIF rapidly translocates to the cytoplasm and nucleus. Nuclear AIF promotes chromatin condensation, chromatin fragmentation, and, ultimately, apoptotic cell death via a caspase-independent pathway. Cytosolic AIF acts on the mitochondria to collapse the mitochondrial membrane potential and initiate the release cytochrome c, which activates caspase-3. However, caspase activation is apparently not required for PARP-1–initiated cell death, because caspase inhibitors do not afford protection.[103] Thus, PARP-1 activation is required for AIF translocation during cell death and AIF is essential for PARP-1–mediated cell death. Moreover, AIF-mediated cell death is caspase-independent.

Important unanswered questions are: Does NAD$^+$ depletion play a role in AIF release? Is the first step in

Pathophysiology

bidirectional signaling between the nucleus and mitochondria mediated by poly(ADP-ribosyl)ated molecules? and How does block of AIF afford protection in the presence of caspase-3 activation?

TRIGGERS OF ISCHEMIC CELL DEATH

Glutamate Excitotoxicity

Excitotoxicity refers to the ability of glutamate (and other excitatory amino acids) to destroy neurons by excessive activation of excitatory amino acid receptors.[104] Knowledge that glutamate is potentially toxic dates to observations by Lucas and Newhouse[105] nearly a half century ago that glutamate administered to animals in vivo caused death of retinal neurons. The concept of excitotoxic death was significantly advanced by Olney and Ho,[106] who used ultrastructural analysis to analyze the cytopathology of neurons exposed to glutamate. These studies revealed a characteristic pattern of glutamate-induced neuronal death in which postsynaptic structures such as dendrites and somata were destroyed but axons, presynaptic terminals, and nonneural cells survived. Other excitatory amino acids and glutamate analogues induced neuronal death with a rank order of potency similar to that for their ability to elicit excitatory transmission. With the advent of selective excitatory amino acid receptor antagonists in the 1980s and their application to studies of glutamate actions, excitatory amino acids were accepted as the major excitatory transmitters of the central nervous system (CNS) and, in high concentrations, as excitotoxins, capable of excessive activation of excitatory amino acid receptors and excitotoxic cell death.

The concept that glutamate plays a critical role in the pathogenesis of global and focal ischemia originated with observations that raising extracellular magnesium markedly reduced the vulnerability of cultured hippocampal neurons to anoxia[107,108] and that glutamate antagonists reduced neuronal injury in both in vitro and in vivo models of ischemia.[109,110] Over the past 15 to 20 years, accumulating evidence has mounted that glutamate antagonists afford neuroprotection in global and focal ischemia. It is now widely accepted that excitotoxicity plays a critical role in the neuronal death associated with these and many other neuronal insults and disorders.[104]

During the ischemic episode, anoxic depolarization triggers the massive release of synaptic glutamate.[111] Synaptically released glutamate activates the ionotropic glutamate receptors, α-amino-3-hydroxy-5-methyl-4-isoxazole-propionic acid receptors (AMPARs) and kainate receptors, which mediate the influx of Na^+ and thus further depolarize the postsynaptic membrane, and N-methyl-D-aspartate receptors (NMDARs) and GluR2-lacking AMPARs, which directly flux Ca^{2+} and Na^+ into postsynaptic cells.[112,113] Glutamate also activates group I metabotropic glutamate receptors (mGluRs). Group I mGluRs, consisting of mGluR1 and mGluR5, act via phospholipase C and inositol 1,4,5-triphosphate (InsP$_3$) to trigger release of Ca^{2+} from intracellular stores.[114] The massive rise in cytosolic Ca^{2+} causes cells to further depolarize and become inexcitable. Anoxic depolarization also drives the reverse operation of gluta-

mate transporters in astrocytes, contributing to the rise in extracellular glutamate. Glutamate toxicity induces reverse operation of the Na^+-Ca^{2+} exchanger in neurons and astrocytes, exacerbating the buildup of Ca^{2+}.[104,115] During global ischemia, extracellular glutamate rises from about $0.6\,\mu M$ to between 1 and $2\,\mu M$.[116] During focal ischemia, glutamate rises to between 16 and $30\,\mu M$ in the core.[117,118] A major consequence of the rise in extracellular glutamate is activation not only of synaptic but also of extrasynaptic ionotropic glutamate receptors (AMPARs, NMDARs, and kainate receptors), with consequent influx of toxic Ca^{2+} and shutoff of the CREB-initiated program of cell survival (see later).

NMDA Receptors

For nearly two decades, intense interest focused on NMDARs as the candidate mediator of Ca^{2+} entry into neurons destined to die.[119] NMDARs mediate the influx of toxic Ca^{2+} in a number of neurologic disorders, insults, and neurodegenerative diseases. Although it is well established that NMDARs are a critical player in focal ischemia–induced neuronal death, AMPARs appear to mediate the cell death associated with global ischemia. Although not completely understood, the following two factors are thought to reduce the contribution of NMDARs in postischemic neurons: (1) the rise in extracellular acidity, which inhibits NMDAR functional activity, and (2) the rise in extracellular Zn^{2+}, which potentiates currents mediated by AMPARs and inhibits those mediated by NMDARs.

Injurious stimuli, including hypoxia and transient ischemia, cause excessive activation of NMDARs, excessive Ca^{2+} influx, and excitotoxic cell death. Activation of NMDARs leads to neuronal death via nitric oxide (NO) signaling. NO is implicated as an important downstream mediator of NMDAR-induced excitotoxicity in postischemic neurons. At excitatory synapses, neuronal NO synthase (nNOS) is physically anchored to the NMDAR through the scaffolding protein postsynaptic density protein of 95kDa (PSD-95). NMDARs provide a direct route for entry of Ca^{2+} into the cell; once in the cell, Ca^{2+} binds calmodulin and rapidly activates nNOS. Upon stimulation, nNOS converts arginine to NO and citrulline. Overproduction of NO from excessive or inappropriate stimulation of nNOS is thought to mediate a major component of excitotoxic damage and focal ischemic cell death.

Under conditions of excessive glutamate release, activation of NMDARs further contributes to neuronal death via shutoff of the CREB-initiated program of gene expression. Under physiologic conditions, restricted Ca^{2+} influx via synaptic NMDARs activates CREB. CREB activates prosurvival target genes such as the neurotrophin brain-derived neurotrophic factor (BDNF). Ca^{2+} influx via synaptic NMDARs activates Ca^{2+}-calmodulin-dependent kinase IV (CaMKIV) and downstream kinases, which act in a coordinated manner to induce robust, sustained phosphorylation of Ser133 and activation of CREB.[120,121] In addition, CaMKIV phosphorylates and activates the co-adaptor protein CREB-binding protein (CBP) at Ser301. Upon activation, CREB recruits phosphorylated CBP to the promoter region of target genes, and the coactivator complex induces gene transcription.

Findings reported by Hardingham and colleagues[120] reveal that the location of Ca^{2+} entry into cells critically influences the fate of neurons. Whereas Ca^{2+} influx via synaptic NMDARs induces activation of CREB, Ca^{2+} influx via extrasynaptic NMDARs elicits dephosphorylation and inactivation of CREB.[122–124] Interestingly, contemporaneous activation of synaptic and extrasynaptic NMDARs by bath-applied NMDA also shuts off CREB, suggesting that extrasynaptic NMDARs act via a dominant, cell-death signal to override the CREB-promoting effects of synaptic NMDARs, L-type calcium channels and protein kinase A (PKA), or both.[122] Ca^{2+} influx via extrasynaptic NMDARs (and CREB shutdown) causes breakdown of the mitochondrial membrane potential, ATP depletion, and necrotic cell death. Thus, the cellular penalty of excess Ca^{2+} entry through extrasynaptic NMDARs is not only dysfunction of CREB signaling but also neuronal death.

The link between extrasynaptic NMDARs and mitochondrial dysfunction and neuronal death is particularly relevant to the pathophysiology of ischemia. Injurious stimuli such as focal ischemia and global ischemia cause excessive glutamate release and spillover; high extracellular glutamate stimulates extrasynaptic NMDARs, leading ultimately to cell injury or death. This model would explain severe, necrotic cell death in the ischemic core. Neurons experiencing shorter, less severe hypoxic-ischemic episodes or neurons in the penumbra may suffer only a transient and incomplete depolarization of the mitochondria. Their health could be compromised because of stimulation of extrasynaptic NMDARs. This model is consistent with findings of CREB shutoff and apoptosis in cells in the penumbra. Stroke-surviving neurons have sustained concentrations of CREB and elevated concentrations of BDNF.

An additional link between NMDARs and mitochondrial dysfunction has emerged. Mounting evidence suggests that efflux of K^+ leads to reduced intracellular K^+ concentrations and may be a critical driver of apoptosis.[55] NMDARs are an important route of K^+ efflux in cells undergoing apoptosis. Whereas NMDAR-mediated necrosis primarily involves influx of Na^+ and Ca^{2+}, NMDAR-mediated apoptosis primarily involves efflux of K^+.[125] Under normal conditions, excessive activation of NMDARs in cultured cortical neurons triggers necrotic cell death, characterized by prominent, acute swelling of cell bodies, little or no DNA laddering, and insensitivity to protein synthesis inhibitors. In contrast, under conditions of reduced extracellular Na^+ and Ca^{2+}, activation of NMDARs in the same cells induces apoptotic cell death, characterized by cell shrinkage, nuclear condensation, internucleosomal fragmentation, and sensitivity to protein synthesis inhibitors. The last is particularly relevant in the presence of low extracellular Na^+ and Ca^{2+}, as is observed after brain ischemia in vivo.[55]

Calcium-Permeable AMPA Receptors

AMPARs mediate fast synaptic transmission at excitatory synapses and play important roles in synaptic remodeling, activity-dependent synaptic plasticity, and excitotoxic cell death. The GluR2 subunit governs the biophysical properties of AMPARs, including Ca^{2+} permeability,[126,127] voltage-dependent block by intracellular polyamines, single channel conductance, and activity-dependent AMPAR recycling and targeting to the synapse.[128] Thus, an acute change in the level of GluR2 expression would be expected to have profound effects on synaptic activity and neuronal survival. The relative expression of GluR2 in neurons is not static but is regulated in a cell-specific manner during development and is remodeled by activity, anti-psychotics, drugs of abuse and corticosteroids, and after seizures[129,130] or ischemic insult.[131]

Considerable evidence implicates GluR2-lacking AMPARs in the neuronal death associated with global ischemia.[131] AMPAR antagonists, but not NMDAR antagonists, protect against global ischemia–induced cell death, even when administered hours after the ischemic insult.[132–134] GluR2-lacking AMPARs are an important route of Ca^{2+} and Zn^{2+} entry into insulted neurons.[135] In adult brain, principal neurons of the hippocampus express high levels of GluR2 and exhibit relatively low Ca^{2+} influx via AMPARs. Injurious stimuli such as global ischemia, severe limbic seizures, and spinal cord injury trigger suppression of GluR2 messenger RNA (mRNA) and protein expression in vulnerable CA1 neurons in a subunit-specific and cell-specific manner before onset of cell death (Plate 42–6). In hippocampal slices, CA1 neurons with robust action potentials exhibit greatly enhanced AMPA-elicited Ca^{2+} rises before onset of cell death.[136] Excitatory postsynaptic currents (EPSCs) at Schaffer collateral–CA1 synapses exhibit an enhanced Ca^{2+}-dependent component that may be mediated by GluR2-lacking AMPARs and marked inward rectification at late times after ischemia.[134a] These findings suggest an important role for GluR2-lacking AMPARs in ischemia-induced neuronal death. Consistent with this concept, acute gene suppression of GluR2 by in vivo administration of antisense oligonucleotides, even in the absence of an ischemic insult, causes selective death of pyramidal neurons.[137] A number of these events are replicated in in vitro models of hypoxia-ischemia. In hippocampal neurons, OGD triggers downregulation of GluR2 mRNA expression and a rise in intracellular Ca^{2+} that is blocked by 1-naphthyl acetyl spermine (Naspm, a channel blocker selective for GluR2-lacking AMPARs).[138]

Kainate Receptors

Although little attention has focused on the role of kainate-type glutamate receptors in global ischemia–induced neuronal death, one study provides convincing evidence that these receptors are also critical players. The kainate-selective drug decahydroisoquinoline LY377770 (a novel, soluble, systemically active Glu5 antagonist) affords robust protection against global ischemia–induced and focal ischemia–induced cell death, even when administered after occlusion.[139] A mechanism by which LY377770 may contribute to neuronal survival is by preventing glutamate release in focal ischemia. These findings suggest that kainate receptors play a central role in ischemic brain damage. Because NMDAR antagonists have a number of side effects, including psychotomimetic effects in humans, increased glucose utilization, and morphologic changes in the rat cingulate cortex, non-NMDAR antagonists may be better candidates for clinical use.

Pathophysiology

Calcium

The universal second messenger Ca^{2+} is a neuronal signaling molecule and critical player in ischemia-induced neuronal death. During the ischemic episode, CA1 pyramidal cells depolarize. Depolarization activates voltage-sensitive Ca^{2+} channels, which flux Ca^{2+} into the interior of cells, and triggers a massive release of synaptic glutamate. Synaptically released glutamate activates AMPARs and kainate receptors, which further depolarize the postsynaptic membrane, and NMDARs and GluR2-lacking AMPARs, which directly flux Ca^{2+} (as well as Na^+) into postsynaptic cells.[112,113] Glutamate also activates group I mGluRs. As already mentioned, group I mGluRs (mGluR1 and mGluR5) act via phospholipase C and $InsP_3$ to trigger release of Ca^{2+} from intracellular stores.[114] The massive rise in cytosolic Ca^{2+} causes cells to further depolarize and become inexcitable. Glutamate toxicity induces reverse operation of the Na^+-Ca^{2+} exchanger, exacerbating the buildup of Ca^{2+}.[104,115] At the same time, energy-dependent processes, such as presynaptic uptake of excitatory amino acids, are impeded, further contributing to the rise of glutamate in the extracellular space. Extracellular Ca^{2+} is depleted to less than 90% of its physiologic concentration. After reperfusion, Ca^{2+} homeostasis is restored; cells appear morphologically normal, exhibit normal intracellular Ca^{2+}, and regain the ability to generate action potentials for 24 to 72 hours after the insult. Ultimately, ambient glutamate elicits a late rise in intracellular Ca^{2+} and Zn^{2+} and death of CA1 neurons ensues, exhibiting hallmarks of apoptosis and necrosis.

Neuronal homeostasis requires that the intracellular concentration of Ca^{2+} be maintained in the range of 50 to 300 nM (or about four times lower than that of extracellular Ca^{2+}).[111] The massive rise in intracellular Ca^{2+} during the ischemic episode initiates a series of cytoplasmic and nuclear events that impairs cellular activity and damages tissue profoundly. High cytosolic Ca^{2+} activates Ca^{2+}-ATPase, which depletes the energy stores of the cell, and uncouples mitochondrial oxidative phosphorylation, which causes acute swelling of dendrites and cell bodies and subsequent cell death. Additionally, high Ca^{2+} activates Ca^{2+}-sensitive transcription factors, phospholipases, endonucleases, and proteases.[111] Proteases destroy cytoskeletal proteins such as actin and spectrin[140] as well as extracellular matrix proteins such as laminin.[141] High cytosolic Ca^{2+} also causes a derangement in signaling. A notable example is excessive activation of nitric oxide synthase, which promotes generation of free radicals. Free radicals destroy cell membranes by inhibition of critical membrane proteins, initiation of lipid peroxidation (see later),[115,142–145] damage of DNA, and induction of apoptosis.[115,146]

More severe insults elicit massive elevations in cytosolic Ca^{2+} and necrotic cell death,[115] and milder insults elicit less dramatic elevations in Ca^{2+} and may trigger apoptosis.[125] The "calcium set-point hypothesis" posits that whereas substantial elevations in cytosolic Ca^{2+} inhibit apoptosis,[147] lowering of cytosolic Ca^{2+} as, for example, by block or inactivation of voltage-sensitive Ca^{2+} channels, can induce apoptosis in otherwise healthy cells. Modest elevations in Ca^{2+} during the reperfusion period are implicated in the execution of apoptosis; possible targets of a late rise in Ca^{2+} include the cysteine proteases, such as caspase-3,[148] and endonucleases such as NUC18.[149]

Zinc

The transition metal Zn^{2+}, like Ca^{2+}, is a neuronal signaling molecule and critical player in ischemic cell death.[150] Zn^{2+} is present in cells throughout the body and serves as a tightly bound, functionally important component of many metalloenzymes and transcription factors. Free, chelatable Zn^{2+} is present at high concentrations in the presynaptic terminals of a subset of glutamatergic neurons and is particularly abundant in presynaptic vesicles. Zn^{2+} is colocalized with glutamate in a subset of vesicles in the presynaptic terminals of excitatory synapses of the neocortex layers I through III and V, hippocampus, subiculum, amygdala, thalamus, and striatum. Zn^{2+} is particularly abundant in vesicles at mossy fiber synapses of the hilar and CA3 region of the hippocampus (Plate 42–7A). Zn^{2+} is loaded into synaptic vesicles via a high-affinity transporter, Zn^{2+} transporter-3 (ZnT-3), which is highly expressed in hippocampus and cortex.[151] Zn^{2+} is released from nerve terminals in response to synaptic activity[152] or by exposure to high K^+ or kainate.[153–155] Upon release from presynaptic terminals, Zn^{2+} modulates the functional activity of excitatory and inhibitory amino acid receptors, including NMDARs, AMPARs and gamma-aminobutyric acid A ($GABA_A$) receptors. Whereas Zn^{2+} blocks currents mediated by NMDARs and $GABA_A$ receptors, it potentiates currents mediated by AMPARs.[150]

The notion that Zn^{2+}, like glutamate, might be neurotoxic emerged from findings that perforant path stimulation releases Zn^{2+} and that Zn^{2+} damages postsynaptic target hilar interneurons and CA3 pyramidal cells both in vivo[156,157] and in vitro.[158] Exposure of cortical neurons in culture to 300 µM Zn^{2+} for 15 minutes or to 1 mM Zn^{2+} for 5 minutes kills virtually all neurons. Moreover, vulnerability to Zn^{2+} is substantially enhanced by concurrent membrane depolarization. Studies also show that Zn^{2+} is a critical mediator of neuronal death associated with global ischemic insults[159] and prolonged seizures.[160] At late times after global ischemia (48 to 72 hours) or after status epilepticus (16 to 24 hours), Zn^{2+} accumulates in degenerating hilar and selectively vulnerable hippocampal neurons (see Plate 42–7). Studies with Zn^{2+} indicator dyes show that toxic levels of Zn^{2+} may reach as high as 0.5 µM. Channels that mediate this Zn^{2+} influx into CA1 neurons include voltage-sensitive Ca^{2+} channels, the Na^+-Zn^{2+} antiporter (exchanger), NMDARs, and GluR2-lacking AMPARs.[150] Administration of the membrane-impermeant Zn^{2+} chelator ethylenediaminetetraacetic acid (EDTA) substantially reduces the rise in intracellular Zn^{2+} in CA1 and hilar neurons and affords robust neuroprotection.[159] These observations implicate Zn^{2+} as a critical mediator of the neuronal death associated with global ischemia. Unresolved issues are (1) the pattern of global ischemia–induced neuronal death does not parallel the distribution of synaptic Zn^{2+} and (2) Zn^{2+} translocation precedes neuronal death in rodents (and probably humans) by 48 to 72 hours.

Mechanisms by which Zn^{2+} induces neurotoxicity include production of free radicals, disruption of mito-

Pathophysiology

chondrial function, including disruption of glycolysis and energy production and inhibition of respiration, and potentiation of AMPAR-mediated currents.[135] The ability of Zn^{2+} to shift excitotoxic injury from NMDAR-mediated injury and toward AMPAR-mediated injury is illustrated by preferential death of neurons with high NADPH (nicotinamide adenine dinucleotide phosphate, reduced form) diaphorase. These neurons exhibit resistance to NMDA toxicity and high susceptibility to AMPA toxicity,[161] consistent with the presence of GluR2-lacking AMPARs.[162] Ultimately, Zn^{2+} induces apoptotic cell death, necrotic cell death, or both, depending on the intensity of exposure. Zn^{2+} may also play a role in the cell death associated with focal ischemia.

MECHANISMS OF ISCHEMIC CELL DEATH

Metabolic Stress

A hallmark of cells undergoing ischemia is energy depletion with altered energy dynamics. Neurons and glia have relatively high consumptions of oxygen and glucose and depend almost exclusively on oxidative phosphorylation for energy production. During the ischemic episode, impairment of cerebral blood flow restricts the delivery of substrates, particularly oxygen and glucose, and impairs the energetics required to maintain ionic gradients.[49] Anoxic depolarization triggers the release of synaptic glutamate, which acts via ionotropic and metabotropic receptors to induce a massive rise in cytosolic Ca^{2+} (see previous discussion) and a resultant loss of extracellular Ca^{2+}.[163] At the same time, energy-dependent processes, such as presynaptic uptake of excitatory amino acids, are impeded, further contributing to the rise of glutamate in the extracellular space. Glutamate toxicity induces reverse operation of the Na^+-Ca^{2+} exchanger, exacerbating the buildup of Ca^{2+}.[104,115] Na^+ and Ca^{2+} influx drives a massive efflux of K^+, which flows out of neurons via NMDARs, leading to a rise in extracellular K^+.[164,165]

In global ischemia, ATP is depleted in cells throughout the brain essentially immediately but recovers to near physiologic levels by the time of reperfusion.[17,69] Low ATP levels encourage cells to die by necrosis by inducing depolarization of neurons, leading to synaptic release of glutamate from neurons and reverse operation of glutamate transporters in astrocytes, swelling of cells (edema), and rupture of the plasma membrane.[166] Because ATP is required for formation of the apoptosome that activates the caspase death cascade, ATP depletion prevents caspase activation and shifts the balance of death cascades in favor of necrosis. Nevertheless, insults such as global ischemia ultimately induce apoptosis. Apoptosis culminates in activation of caspase-3, which catalyzes the cleavage and activation of downstream targets, including PARP-1. Excessive PARP-1 activation depletes the entire cell of its substrate NAD^+. NAD^+ depletion in mitochondria causes pronounced slowing of glycolysis, electron transport, and ATP formation, resulting in further energy failure and cell demise.

Focal ischemia elicits different patterns of metabolic changes in the core and penumbra. Within 1 to 3 minutes, cells in the core exhibit a dramatic decline in ATP[94,95] as well as anoxic depolarization, which triggers release of synaptic glutamate. Na^+ enters neurons via NMDARs, AMPARs, and other channels permeable to monovalent ions. K^+ flows out of cells via NMDARs. Water follows passively, driven by the influx of Na^+ and Cl^-, which greatly exceeds the efflux of K^+. At the same time, as cells lose energy, energy-requiring pumps that normally force ions into and out of the cell in an attempt to maintain a concentration gradient either fail or operate in reverse. These factors induce a rise in extracellular $K^{+164,165}$ and a reduction in extracellular Ca^{2+}.[163,167] By 2 hours after temporary focal ischemia, extracellular K^+ is restored to a physiologic concentration.[164] The ensuing edema negatively affects perfusion of cells in the penumbra and affects more remote regions via long-range changes, including intracranial pressure, vascular compression, and herniation.

In contrast, cells in the penumbra experience a decline in energy[94] but do not exhibit anoxic depolarization or a rise in extracellular K^+.[94,95] In these cells, low ATP promotes necrosis by inducing failure or reverse operation of ion pumps, swelling of cells, and rupture of the plasma membrane.[166] ATP depletion inhibits formation of the apoptosome and tends to oppose caspase activation and the onset of apoptotic cell death. Nevertheless, apoptosis ensues in the penumbra. As in global ischemia, activated caspase-3 activates PARP-1, leading to NAD^+ depletion and further energy failure.

Mitochondrial Demise

Mitochondria house not only proteins involved in oxidative phosphorylation, but also pro-apoptotic proteins, including cytochrome c. Under physiologic conditions, cytochrome c is localized to the outer compartment of the mitochondria, where it serves as an electron carrier and participates in oxidative phosphorylation. Apoptotic (and necrotic) stimuli such as global ischemia disrupt the integrity of the outer mitochondrial membrane and cause the release of cytochrome c (see Plate 42–4). Upon release into the cytoplasm, cytochrome c forms the apoptosome (in a deoxy-ATP–mediated reaction), the signaling complex required for activation of caspase-9. Although the precise mechanisms by which the integrity of mitochondrial membrane breaks down are unknown, Bcl-2 family members are known to play a critical role.[75,168] For example, addition of pro-apoptotic Bcl-2 family members to purified mitochondria is sufficient to induce release of cytochrome c, and overexpression of anti-apoptotic Bcl-2 family members is sufficient to prevent it.

Many of the Bcl-2 family members are anchored in the outer membranes of mitochondria but oriented toward the cytosol. BAD, a pro-apoptotic member of this family, can heterodimerize with anti-apoptotic family members Bcl-2 and Bcl-x_L to initiate apoptosis. Injurious stimuli such as global ischemia induce sustained high cytoplasmic Ca^{2+}, which triggers activation of the serine-threonine phosphatase calcineurin.[169] Upon activation, calcineurin dephosphorylates BAD, promoting its release from cytosolic retention factor 14-3-3 and its translocation to the mitochondria, where it heterodimerizes with Bcl-x_L and initiates apoptosis.[169] Both apoptotic and necrotic stimuli are thought to converge upon Ca^{2+}-dependent destabilization of the mitochondrial membrane.[168] In contrast, growth factors and other pro-survival agents promote phosphorylation of BAD, impairing its binding to Bcl-x_L and abrogating its pro-apoptotic effect in cells. Ca^{2+}-dependent activation of calcineurin and dephosphorylation of BAD are thought to be critical to the change in mitochondrial membrane permeability and demise of mitochondria.[169]

How do Bcl-2 family members cause disruption of the outer mitochondrial membrane? One hypothesis is that Bcl-x_L, which is structurally similar to the pore-forming subunit of diphtheria toxin, might act by inserting into the outer mitochondrial membrane, where Bcl-2 family members could form channels or even large holes.[168] It is known that Bcl-2 family members insert into synthetic lipid bilayers, oligomerize, and form channels with discrete conductances. It is not clear, however, whether the holes are sufficiently large as to allow large proteins such as cytochrome c to pass through. In a second model, Bcl-2 family members would recruit other outer mitochondrial membrane proteins, such as voltage-dependent anion channel (VDAC), into forming a large pore channel. Such recruitment would likely involve a substantial conformational change in VDAC, which normally is permeable to much smaller molecules.

Nitric Oxide

The reactive gas NO is a diffusible signaling molecule present throughout cells of the body. In neurons, NO acts as an "aberrant transmitter," in that it is a small signaling molecule released by one cell that acts on another cell but is not released from vesicles and does not act via a classic membrane receptor.[170,171] NO is synthesized by nitric oxide synthetase nNOS, an enzyme that converts arginine to NO and citrulline. At excitatory synapses, nNOS is physically anchored to NMDARs in the postsynaptic membrane via PSD-95 (also known as synapse-associated protein-90, SAP-90). Activation of NMDARs triggers a rise in postsynaptic Ca^{2+}; intracellular Ca^{2+} binds calmodulin and rapidly activates nNOS, which synthesizes NO.[171,172] Thus, NO is an important downstream mediator of NMDARs and is critical to many forms of neuronal signaling and synaptic plasticity. Neuronal NOS is expressed in a small population of neurons throughout the CNS, with high densities in the accessory olfactory bulb and granule cells of the cerebellum.

NO is also implicated as an important downstream mediator of NMDA-induced excitotoxicity (see previous discussion). Injurious stimuli such as global and focal ischemia cause excessive stimulation of NMDARs and production of NO.[173] Some studies implicate the free radical form of NO and the superoxide anion ($\cdot O^{2-}$) in the oxidative damage of cellular DNA, lipid peroxidation (see later), and excitotoxic cell death.[174] NO reacts with the superoxide anion to form peroxynitrite, a cytotoxic oxidant that induces DNA damage (see Plate 42–4). DNA damage is a trigger of apoptotic cell death. Apoptosis culminates in activation of caspase-3, which catalyzes the cleavage and activation of downstream targets, including PARP-1. In addition to DNA damage, peroxynitrite contributes to cellular damage by several other mechanisms. It can nitrosylate cysteine residues in target proteins such as the NMDAR

and impair NMDAR-mediated synaptic transmission. Peroxynitrite oxidizes and destroys other critical neuronal proteins, such as mitochondrial cytochrome c oxidase complex,[175] and reacts with unsaturated fatty acids in membranes to initiate lipid peroxidation (see later).

NO contributes to cell damage via several additional mechanisms. It interferes with superoxide dismutase, thereby reducing its antioxidant action, and complexes with non-heme iron present in the form of iron-sulfur clusters within enzymes critical to DNA replication and mitochondrial energy production. NO is thought to damage DNA by diffusing from the mitochondria and cytoplasm to the nucleus, where it is cleaved to form hydroxyl radicals or singlet oxygen. Important evidence that NO is a critical mediator of neuronal death comes from studies that show that mice that either have a knockout of nNOS or have been treated with 7-nitroindazole, an inhibitor of nNOS, are protected against neuronal death in experimental models of stroke.[176]

Free Radicals and Lipid Peroxidation

Neuronal insults and other types of environmental stress induce the formation of free radicals such as the superoxide anion, hydroxyl radical, singlet oxygen, radical nitric oxide, and oxidants such as peroxynitrite. These agents, collectively termed *reactive oxygen species* (ROS), are implicated as critical mediators of neuronal injury.[174,177,178] NMDAR-mediated Ca^{2+} influx promotes production of free radicals by stimulation of NO, which reacts with superoxide free radical ($\cdot O^{2-}$) to form peroxynitrite (see earlier discussion). NMDAR-mediated influx of Ca^{2+} also activates phospholipase A_2. Phospholipase A_2 liberates arachidonic acid, an unsaturated fatty acid, and promotes production of free radicals via activation of the lipoxygenase and cyclooxygenase pathways.[179] Cyclooxygenase catalyzes the addition of two molecules of O_2 to arachidonic acid to produce prostaglandin PGG_2, which is rapidly peroxidized to PGH_2 with concomitant release of superoxide anion.[180] Metabolism of free arachidonic acid is thought to be a major source of superoxide anion. Zn^{2+} influx via GluR2-lacking AMPARs also promotes production of free radicals, such as mitochondrial superoxide, in injured neurons.[181]

Short exposure (10 to 90 minutes) to free radicals damages protein, lipids, and nucleic acids. In neurons, free radicals inactivate and damage critical membrane proteins such as Na^+ and Ca^{2+} pumps, creatine kinase and mitochondrial dehydrogenases, and promote oxidation of the Na^+-K^+-ATPase exchanger, rendering it susceptible to calpain-mediated proteolysis.[182] Free radicals damage proteins by oxidation of side chains and modification of disulfide bonds. Free radicals also inactivate and damage nucleic acids. Free radicals effect oxidative damage by causing single- and double-stranded breaks in DNA, chemically modifying nucleic acid bases, breaking the glycosylic bond between ribose and individual bases and crosslinking of protein to DNA strands.[174] If not repaired, such oxidative lesions disrupt nucleic acid elongation, alter the coding of DNA, or both, thus impairing DNA replication and transcription and contributing to the demise of cells.[183]

Free radicals also oxidize and damage unsaturated fatty acids. *Lipid peroxidation*, the oxidative deterioration of

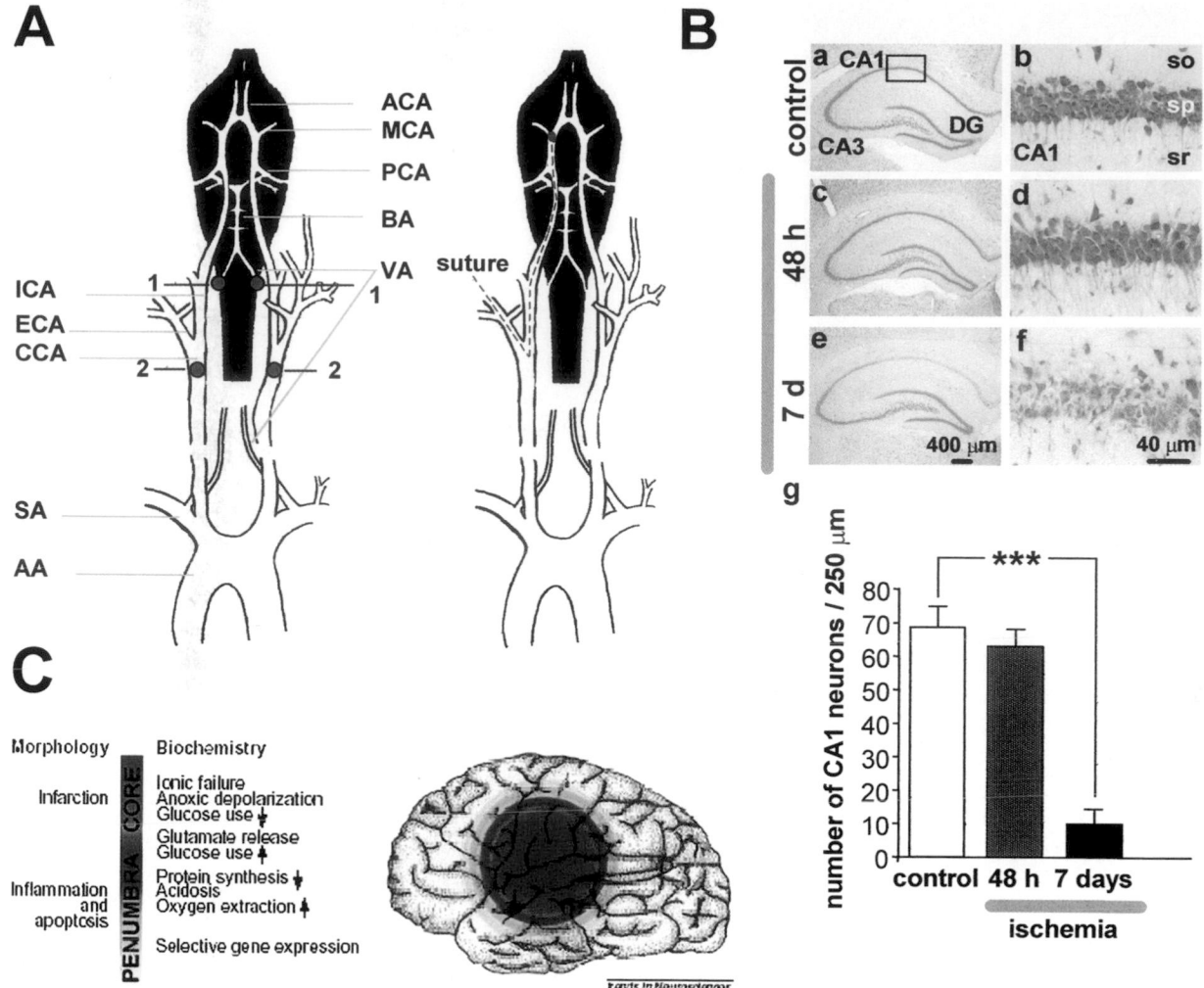

PLATE 42–1 *Global and focal ischemia elicits different spatiotemporal patterns of cell death. A, Diagram of the cerebrovascular anatomy of the rat, illustrating the permanent electrocauterization of the vertebral arteries (1) and the position of the surgical clips in the common carotid arteries (2) in a four-vessel occlusion (4-VO) model (left) and the intraluminal suture during occlusion in the temporary focal ischemia model (right). AA, arch of the aorta; ACA, anterior cerebral artery; BA, basilar artery; CCA, common carotid artery; ECA, external carotid artery; ICA, internal carotid artery; MCA, middle cerebral artery; PCA, posterior cerebral artery; SA, subclavian artery; VA, vertebral artery. B, Toluidine blue staining of coronal brain sections at the level of the dorsal hippocampus from control (a and b) and experimental male rats subjected to global ischemia at 48 hours (c and d) and 7 days (e and f) after ischemia. At 48 hours after global ischemia, there was no histologically detectable neuronal death in any hippocampal subfield. At 7 days after ischemia, the pyramidal cell layer of CA1 exhibited dramatic loss of neurons, whereas CA3 (region 3) and dentate gyrus showed no damage. so, stratum oriens; sp, stratum pyramidale; sr, stratum radiatum. (Scale bars: lower magnification, 400 μm; higher magnification, 40 μm.) View g shows quantitation of cell counts from brain sections illustrated in a through f. To assess hippocampal injury, the number of surviving neurons per 250-μm length in the pyramidal cell layer of the medial CA1 (cornu ammonis 1 region of the hippocampus) was counted under a light microscope at 40× magnification in sections. Neuronal counts from a minimum of four microscopic sections per animal were analyzed; comparisons among group means were made using the Student t-test (P < .001). C, The core and penumbra of ischemia are induced by focal blockade of cerebral arteries. A brain region of low perfusion in which cells have lost their membrane potential terminally (core) is surrounded by an area in which intermediate perfusion prevails (penumbra) and cells depolarize intermittently (peri-infarct depolarization". From the onset of the focal perfusion deficit, the core and penumbra are dynamic in space and time. Perfusion thresholds exist below which certain biochemical functions are impeded (color-coded scale). (A adapted from Longa EZ, Weinstein PR, Carlson S,, et al: Reversible middle cerebral artery occlusion without craniectomy in rats. Stroke 20:84–91, 1989; C from Dirnagl U, Iadecola C, Moskowitz MA: Pathobiology of ischaemic stroke: An integrated view. Trends Neurosci 22:391–397, 1999.)*

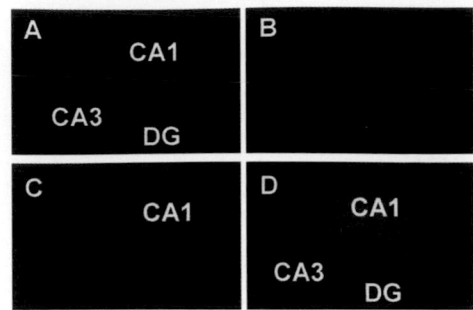

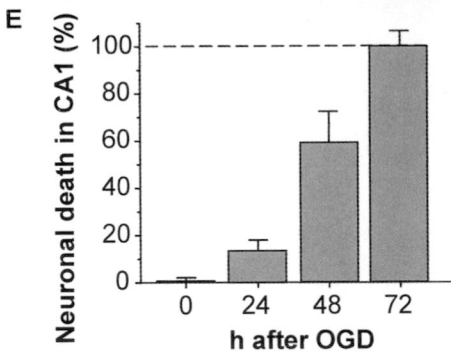

PLATE 42–2 *Oxygen-glucose deprivation (OGD) is a well-established in vitro model of global ischemia. Organotypically cultured hippocampal slices are maintained for 14 to 21 days in vitro (DIV) and subjected to OGD by exposure to serum-free medium devoid of glucose and saturated with 95% N₂/5% CO₂ for 30 to 60 minutes. Slices are then transferred to oxygenated, serum-free medium containing glucose and propidium iodide. OGD (20- to 30-minute insult) elicits delayed, selective neuronal death, primarily of CA1 (cornu ammonis 1 region of the hippocampus) neurons, as occurs after transient global ischemia in the intact animal. Cell death is assessed by propidium iodide uptake due to breakdown of the integrity of the plasma membrane as cells enter the initial stages of cell death. A, A control slice shows no uptake of propidium iodide. B to D, Time course of neuronal death in the CA1 subfield at 24 hours (B), 48 hours (C), and 72 hours (D) after OGD. DG, dentate gyrus. E, Quantitation of data like those shown in B to D. (K.M. Noh, unpublished observations, 2003).*

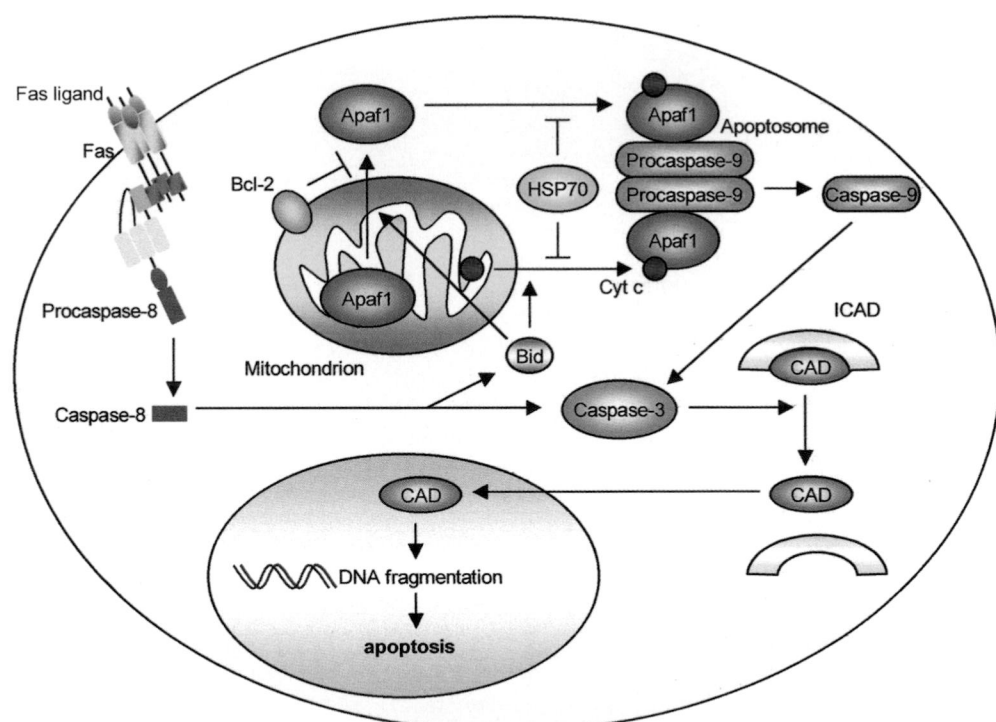

PLATE 42–3 *Signaling from the death receptor triggers the extrinsic pathway of apoptosis. Upon binding of Fas ligand, Fas is activated and recruits procaspase-8. The procaspase-8 transactivates, and the mature caspase cleaves and activates procaspase-3, leading to apoptosis. Signaling from the Fas receptor to mitochondria involves cleavage of the BH3-only protein BID by caspase-8. BID subsequently induces release of cytochrome c (cyt c) as well as downstream apoptotic events. Formation of the apoptosome leads to the activation of caspase-9 and subsequently caspase-3. Caspase-3, the "terminator" protein, exerts its apoptotic effects by several means, including the activation of caspase-activated DNase (CAD), which leads to the cleavage of genomic DNA and apoptosis. Heat shock protein 70 (HSP70) inhibits the oligomerization of apoptotic protease-activating factor-1 (Apaf1) and the release of cytochrome c from the mitochondria, thus inhibiting apoptosis. ICAD, inhibitor of CAD. Arrows indicate the activation of the targets, whereas lines with blunt ends indicate their inactivation. (Adapted from Zimmermann KC, Bonzon C, Green DR: The machinery of programmed cell death. Pharmacol Ther 92:57–70, 2001.)*

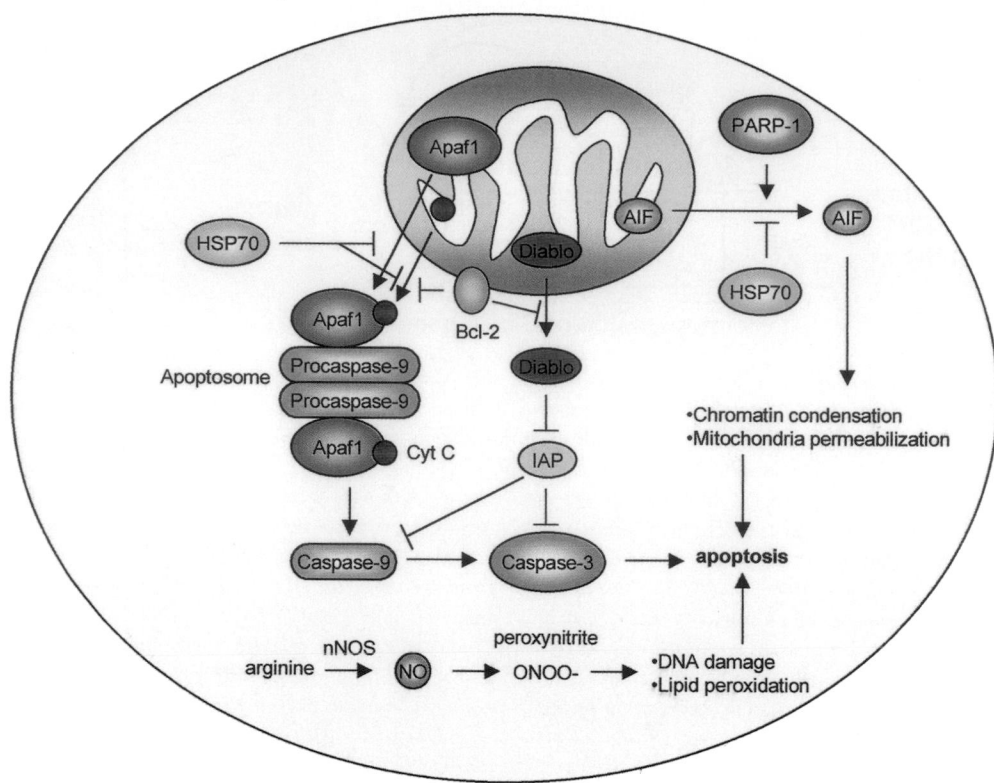

PLATE 42–4 *Mitochondrial demise induces apoptosis via the intrinsic pathway. Cellular stress induces pro-apoptotic Bcl-2 family members to translocate from the cytosol to the mitochondria, where they induce the release of cytochrome c. Cytochrome c (Cyt C) catalyzes the oligomerization of Apaf-1 (Apaf1), which recruits and promotes the activation of procaspase-9. This substance, in turn, activates procaspase-3, leading to apoptosis. Also illustrated is another mitochondrial activator of caspases, Smac/DIABLO (second mitochondria–derived activator of caspases/direct IAP [inhibitor of apoptosis protein] binding protein with low isoelectric point) (Diablo). Cytochrome c and Smac/DIABLO are released in a coordinated fashion from the mitochondria upon an apoptotic stimuli. While cytochrome c activates Apaf-1, Smac/DIABLO relieves the inhibition on caspases by binding to inhibitor of apoptosis proteins (IAPs). By this means, Smac/DIABLO disrupts the association of IAPs with processed caspase-9, allowing caspase-9 to activate caspase-3, leading to apoptosis. Heat shock protein 70 (HSP70) inhibits apoptosis via several pathways, (1) by preventing the release of cytochrome c and oligomerization of Apaf-1, thus inhibiting the formation of the apoptosome, and (2) by inhibiting the release of apoptosis-inducing factor (AIF). nNOS, neuronal nitric oxide synthase; ONOO⁻, peroxynitrite; PARP-1, Poly(ADP-ribose)polymerase-1. (Adapted from Zimmermann KC, Bonzon C, Green DR: The machinery of programmed cell death. Pharmacol Ther 92:57–70, 2001.)*

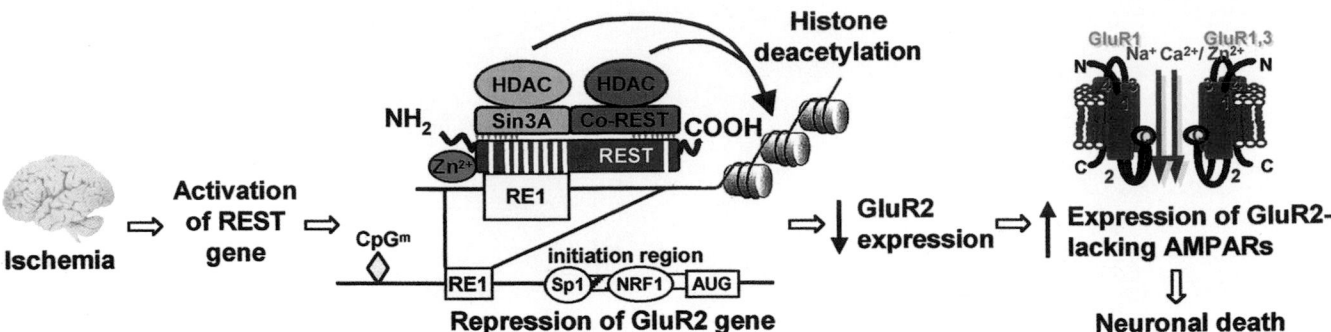

PLATE 42-5 *The poly(ADP-ribose)polymerase-1 (PARP-1) is an key player in ischemic neuronal death. A, Insults to cells such as ischemia and stress can activate PARP-1, resulting in the release of apoptosis-inducing factor (AIF) from the mitochondria. AIF can induce chromatin condensation and mitochondrial permeabilization independent of cytochrome c, thus triggering apoptotic cell death. PARP-1 can activate NF-κB, a transcription factor that has a crucial role in the regulation of genes involved in inflammatory responses. PARP-1 also transactivates p53, a transcription factor critical in the execution of apoptosis. B, A model of PARP overactivation-mediated cytotoxicity. Reactive oxygen species (ROS) such as nitric oxide (NO), superoxide anion (·O²⁻) and peroxynitrite (ONOO−) are generated during inflammation or ischemia-reperfusion. These ROS damage cellular molecules like proteins, lipids, and DNA. DNA damage activates PARP-1, synthesizing poly(ADP-ribose)polymer from its substrate β-nicotinamide adenine dinucleotide (NAD⁺). Limited amounts of DNA damage can be repaired by cellular DNA repair enzymes, and PARP-1, in this case, acts as a sensor for DNA damage, modulating the repair process. In apoptotic cell death, activated caspases cleave PARP-1 protein to inhibit a futile DNA repair process and preserve cellular adenosine triphosphate (ATP), which is essential for the apoptotic process. Extensive DNA damage can lead to overactivation of PARP. With excessive activation of PARP, NAD⁺ is depleted, and in efforts to resynthesize NAD⁺, ATP is also depleted. Hence, necrotic cell death involves energy loss. Depletion of ATP can transform an ongoing apoptotic process into necrosis with intracellular ATP levels regulating the mode of cell death. (A adapted from Chiarugi A: Poly(ADP-ribose) polymerase: Killer or conspirator? The 'suicide hypothesis' revisited. Trends Pharmacol Sci 23:122–129, 2002; B from Ha HC, Snyder SH: Poly(ADP-ribose) polymerase-1 in the nervous system. Neurobiol Dis 7:225–239, 2000.)*

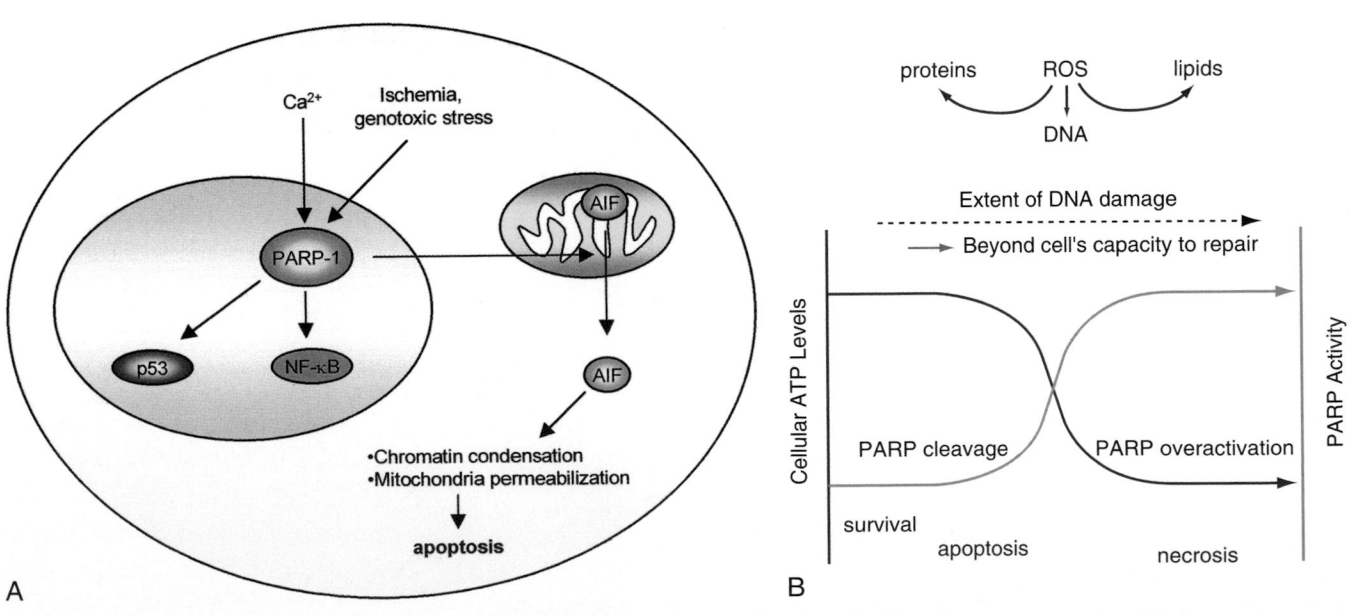

see legend on opposite page.

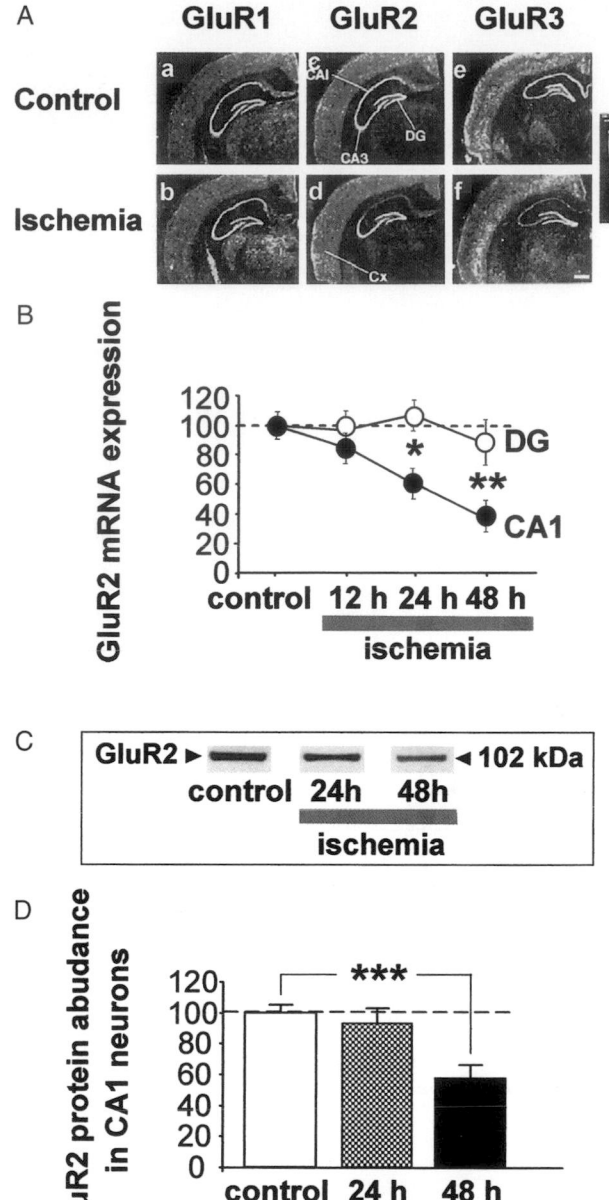

A GluR1 GluR2 GluR3

Control

Ischemia

B

C GluR2 ► control 24h 48h ◄ 102 kDa
ischemia

D

PLATE 42–7 *Zinc is translocated from the mossy fibers to the CA1 (cornu ammonis 1 region of the hippocampus) pyramidal neuron cell body after global ischemia, as revealed by TSQ staining. A, Fluorescent photomicrograph of a normal rat hippocampus after staining with TSQ, showing dense fluorescence in the hilus (H) and the stratum lucidum (SL) of CA3. In addition, TSQ staining is seen in the stratum radiatum (SR) and the stratum oriens (SO) of CA1. No Zn^{2+} fluorescence is seen in the stratum pyramidale (SP) or alveus (alv.) of CA1 (dark bands). DG, dentate gyrus. (Scale bar, 800 mm.) B, Twenty-four hours after a 10-minute forebrain ischemia, TSQ fluorescence is reduced in presynaptic terminals and is newly apparent in the cell bodies of some hilar neurons. (Scale bar, 200 mm.) C, The same hippocampal section as in B, with subsequent acid fuchsin staining. All the TSQ-fluorescent neurons in C exhibited ischemic acidophilic changes (pink cytoplasm, arrows). (Scale bar, 200 mm.) D, Seventy-two hours after a 10-minute period of ischemia, dense TSQ staining appeared in degenerating CA1 pyramidal neurons. (Scale bar, 100 mm.) E, The same section as in D, with acid fuchsin staining. All the CA1 neurons with Zn^{2+} fluorescence showed acidophilic changes. (Scale bar, 100 mm.) (From Koh JY, Suh SW, Gwag BJ, et al: The role of zinc in selective neuronal death after transient global cerebral ischemia. Science 272:1013–1016, 1996.)*

PLATE 42–6 *Global ischemia induces GluR2 messenger RNA (mRNA) and protein downregulation in the hippocampus. A, Global ischemia downregulates the mRNA expression of GluR2, as demonstrated by in situ hybridization. Pseudocolor display of densities of autoradiograms of GluR1, GluR2, and GluR3 mRNA localization in coronal sections of control and post-ischemic rat brains at the level of the hippocampus: a, GluR1 expression in control (sham-operated) brain; b, GluR1 expression in ischemic rats 24 hours after 10 minutes of global ischemia; c, GluR2 expression in control; d, GluR2 expression 24 hours after ischemia, showing dramatic and selective reduction in CA1 (cornu ammonis 1 region of the hippocampus) labeling; e, GluR3 expression in control brain; f, GluR3 expression 24 hours after ischemia, showing that reduction in CA1 is not as marked as in d and extends through CA3. Cx, neocortex; DG, dentate gyrus. (Scale bar, 1 mm.) B, The downregulation of GluR2 mRNA is apparent at 24 hours after ischemia. C and D, Ischemia reduces the protein expression of GluR2 in the CA1 area, as shown by Western blot analysis. (A from Pellegrini-Giampietro DE, Zukin RS, Bennett MV,, et al: Switch in glutamate receptor subunit gene expression in CA1 subfield of hippocampus following global ischemia in rats. Proc Natl Acad Sci U S A 89:10499–10503, 1992; B through D from Calderone A, Jover T, Noh KM, et al: Ischemic insults derepress the gene silencer REST in neurons destined to die. J Neurosci 23:2112–2121, 2003.)*

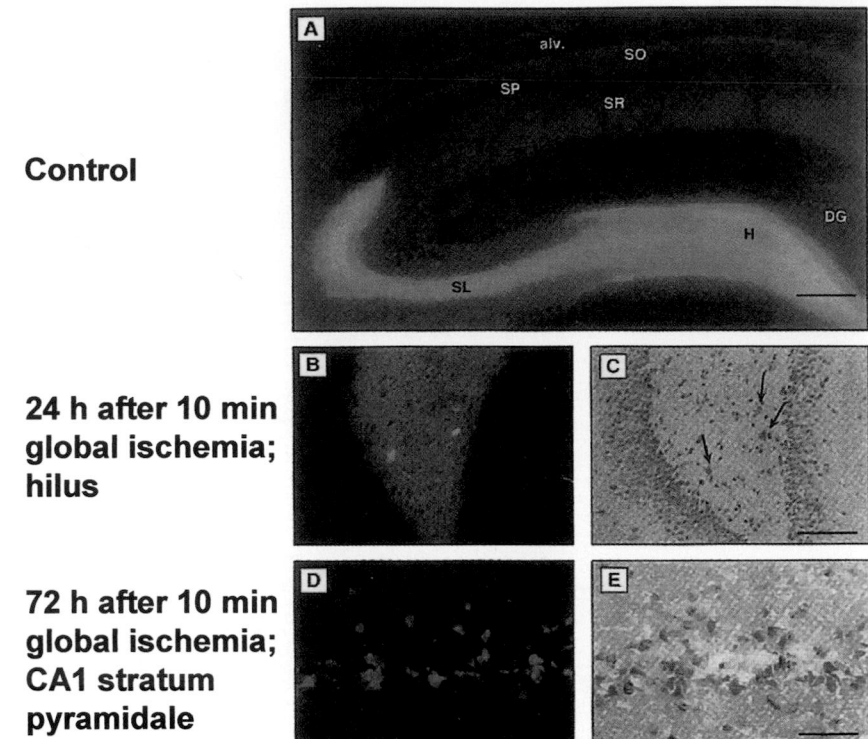

Control

24 h after 10 min global ischemia; hilus

72 h after 10 min global ischemia; CA1 stratum pyramidale

PLATE 42–8 *FOXO-3A/FKHRL1 is a member of the Forkhead family of transcription factors, which is implicated in death pathways in* Caenorhabditis elegans. *Within the nucleus, FOXO-3A triggers apoptosis by transactivation of target genes such as Fas ligand (FasL) and TRAIL. FasL, in turn, activates the cell surface death receptor Fas, which initiates the caspase death cascade via the extrinsic pathway of apoptotic cell death. In the presence of survival factors, the serine/threonine kinase Akt (PKB) phosphorylates FOXO-3A, leading to its association with 14-3-3 proteins and cytoplasmic retention and sequestration away from nuclear target genes. Ischemia promotes dephosphorylation (activation) of FOXO-3A in CA1, evident at 12 and 24 hours. Estrogen induces phosphorylation (inactivation) of FOXO-3A in control CA1 and attenuates ischemia-induced dephosphorylation of FOXO-3A. BDNF, brain-derived neurotrophic factor; DBD, DNA-binding domain of the FOXO-3A; IGF-1, insulin-like growth factor-1; NGF, nerve growth factor; NLS, nuclear localization signal; P, phosphate group; P13K, phosphotidylinositol 3-kinase; RTK, receptor tyrosine kinase. (Adapted from Burgering BM, Kops GJ: Cell cycle and death control: Long live Forkheads.* Trends Biochem Sci *27:352–360, 2002.) (Jover, et al., unpublished observations, 2003.)*

PLATE 42–10 *Neurotrophins promote cell survival by antagonizing apoptotic proteins. In the presence of survival factors, the PI3K-Akt/SGK pathway is activated. The serine/threonine kinase Akt and serum glucocorticoid inducible kinase (SGK) prevent the execution of apoptosis at several levels, in both transcription-dependent and transcription-independent manners. Akt and SGK phosphorylate and inhibit the transcription factor FOXO (or FKHRL1), and Akt indirectly inhibits p53 (a transcription factor critical in the execution of apoptosis), thereby preventing the expression of their target death genes. Akt also indirectly activates nuclear factor-kappa B (NF-κB), leading to the expression of survival genes, such as A1, Bcl-xL, and IAP. In addition, Akt acts at a step before cytochrome c release, preventing the association of the pro-apoptotic family member BAD with Bcl-xL, which allows Bcl-xL to promote cell survival. Furthermore, Akt may act at a step subsequent to cytochrome c release, possibly by phosphorylating caspase-9 (casp-9), apoptotic protease-activated factor (APAF-1), or the IAPs. BDNF, brain-derived neurotrophic factor; IGF-1, insulin-like growth factor-1; NGF, nerve growth factor; PDK1, phosphoinositide-dependent kinase-1; P13K, Phosphotidylinositol 3-kinase. Reproduced, with permission, from Brunet A, Datta SR, Greenberg ME: Transcription-dependent and -independent control of neuronal survival by the PI3K-Akt signaling pathway.* Curr Opin Neurobiol *11:297–305, 2001.)*

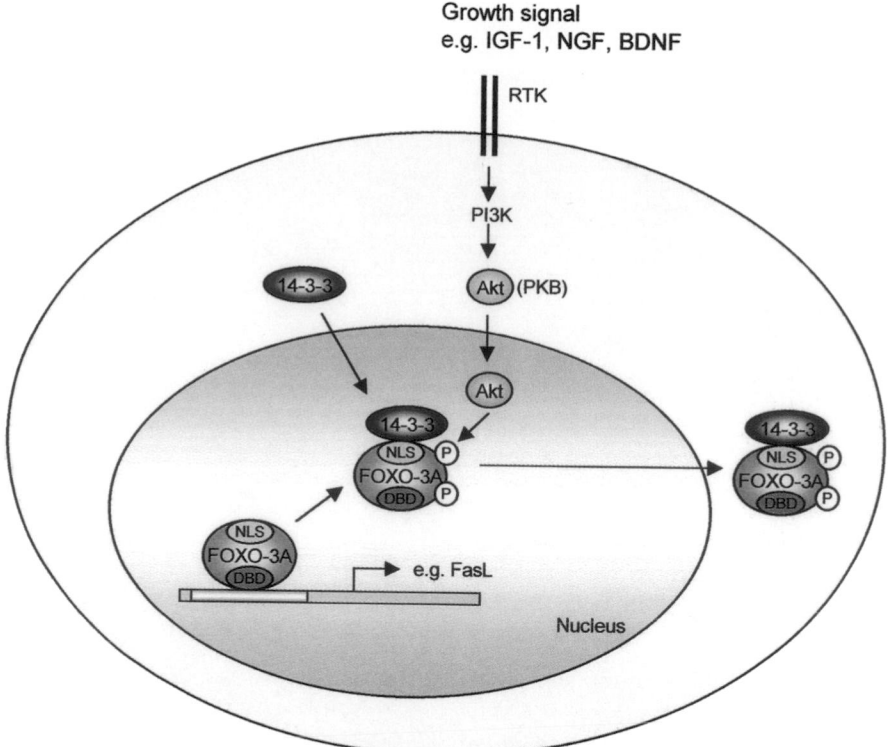

PLATE 42–9 *The neuronal repressor element-1 silencing transcription factor (REST) is critical to GluR2 downregulation and ischemia-induced neuronal death. Global ischemia induces REST, a member of the Gli-Krüppel family of zinc-finger transcriptional repressors containing nine noncanonical zinc finger motifs, through which it binds the cis-acting neuronal repressor element (RE1). REST associates with the co-repressors Sin3A and Co-REST, which in turn recruit histone deacetylases (HDAC) to the promoters of target genes, including the GluR2 gene subunit of the AMPA (α-amino-3-hydroxy-5-methyl-4-isoxazole-propionic acid) receptor (AMPAR). Deacetylation of histone proteins and tightening of the core chromatin complex restricts access of the transcription machinery required for gene activation. Decreased expression of GluR2 protein increases the Ca^{2+} permeability of AMPA-type glutamate receptors, exacerbating excitotoxicity and increasing the extent of neuronal death. AUG, start codon of GluR2; NRF1, nuclear respiratory factor-1; Sp1, regulatory transcription factor.*

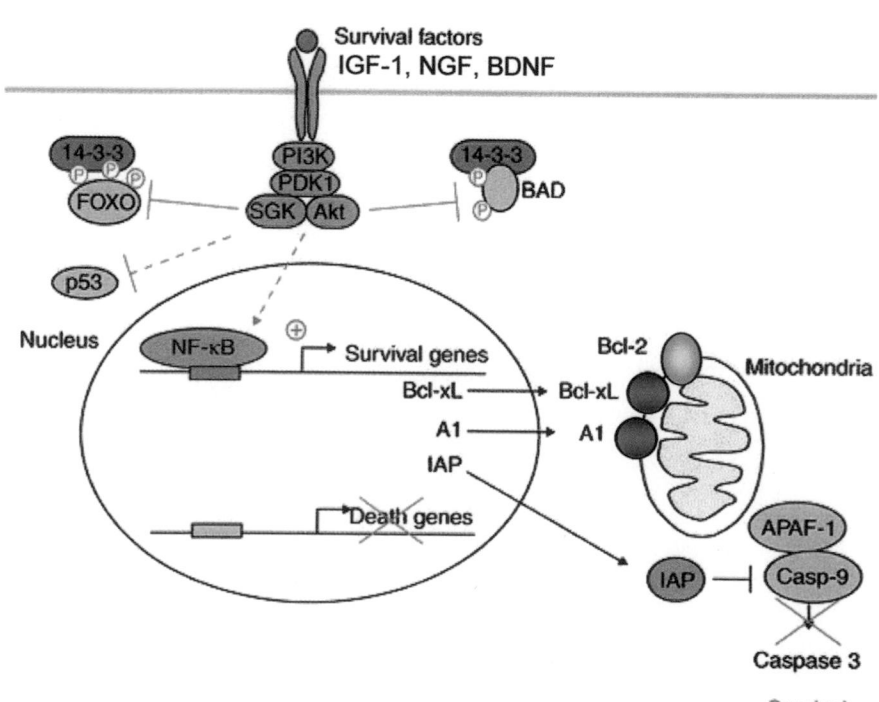

see legend on opposite page.

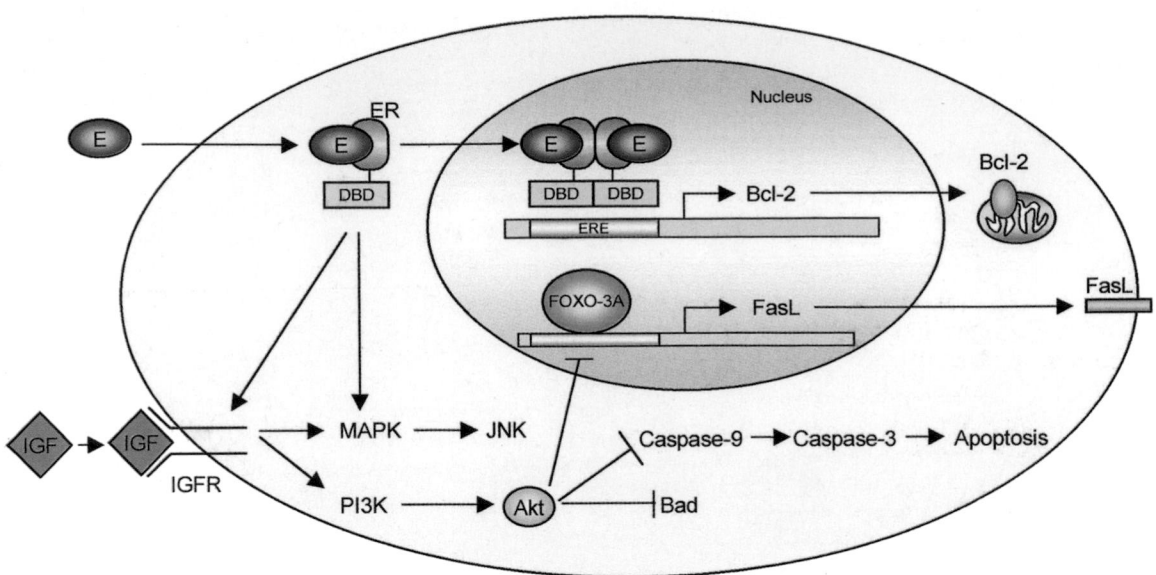

PLATE 42–11 *Estrogen acts via the PI3K (phosphotidylinositol 3-kinase) and/or MAPK (mitogen-activated protein kinase) signaling pathways to afford neuroprotection. Estrogen (E) exerts neuroprotection via genomic and nongenomic actions. In the classical, genomic model, Estrogen binds to estrogen receptor (ER) α and/or ERβ, and the activated receptor transactivates target genes, which contain the estrogen response element (ERE). Bcl-2 is a pro-apoptotic protein, and the bcl-2 gene is a critical estrogen target. Estrogen also acts in the cytosol to activate PI3K and/or MAPK signaling via nongenomic mechanisms. Cross-talk between estrogen and the insulin-like growth factor (IGF) signaling can occur nongenomically. Activation of ERα leads to formation of a supramolecular complex composed of the IGF receptor (IGFR), ERα, and PI3K, thereby activating PI3K. Activation of PI3K stimulates phosphorylation and activation of the serine/threonine kinase Akt (PKB). Akt, in turn, phosphorylates and inactivates the pro-apoptotic proteins FOXO-3A, Bad, and caspase-9 and thereby halts apoptosis. DBD, DNA-binding domain of the ER; JNK, c-jun N-terminal kinase.*

membrane unsaturated fatty acids, is caused by reaction of free radicals with unsaturated bonds in the side chains of polyunsaturated fatty acids.[184,185] These reactions spark a chain reaction leading to formation of peroxides, hydroperoxides, and aldehydes. Although superoxide anion is not itself a potent oxidizer, it promotes oxidation of ferric ion and release of ferrous iron from ferritin.[186] In the presence of transition metals such as copper and ferrous iron, these chain reactions can expand geometrically. Glial cells in the brain have abundant stores of oxidized iron,[187] mostly in the form of ferritin and transferrin.[117] Ultrastructural studies show that excessive generation of oxygen radicals, followed by lipid peroxidation, accelerates the structural damage of neurons.[188] Lipid peroxidation compromises the integrity of the neuronal plasma membrane by altering membrane permeability and fluidity and allowing ions such as Ca^{2+} to leak into the cell. Disruption of the membrane compromises the function of receptors, channels, transporters, and ion exchangers, adding further to the demise of injured cells. Specific populations of neurons are thought to be especially vulnerable to free radical–induced damage during reperfusion, either because they are deficient in glutathione peroxidase or because they are surrounded by iron-laden supporting cells that release iron during and after ischemia.

Transcription Factors

Injurious stimuli such as ischemia trigger a number of transcriptional pathways. Candidate transcription factors that are thought to direct programs of gene expression changes after global ischemia include (1) CREB and nuclear factor kappa B (NF-κB), which direct pro-survival programs, and (2) the Forkhead family of transcription factors and REST/NRSF, which direct pro-death pathways in adult neurons.

CREB is a stimulus-induced transcription factor that activates transcription of pro-survival (and pro-adaptive) target genes in response to a wide array of external stimuli, including NMDAR-mediated Ca^{2+} influx at synaptic sites.[121] Immediate early genes (IEGs), such as c-fos,[189] Bcl-2, IAPs, nNOS,[190] and BDNF,[191] are important to neuronal survival and are gene targets of CREB.[121] Upon activation, CREB plays an important role in promoting neuronal survival and adaptation in response to environmental cues. Consistent with this notion, targeted deletion of the genes encoding CREB and the cAMP-response element modulator (CREM) in neurons of the developing CNS elicits apoptosis. Postnatal ablation of CREB and CREM results in progressive neuronal degeneration in the adult brain.[121]

A member of the leucine-zipper superfamily of transcription factors, CREB is activated in response to external stimuli that activate intracellular signaling cascades, culminating in phosphorylation of CREB. Upon phosphorylation, CREB forms a functionally active dimer that binds the *cis*-acting CRE within the promoters of target genes.[121] As already mentioned, Hardingham and colleagues[120] have found that the location of Ca^{2+} signaling in neurons critically controls CREB activity. Ca^{2+} influx via synaptic NMDARs promotes the activation of Ca2+-calmodulin–dependent kinase IV (CaMKIV) and the Ras/mitogen–activated protein kinase (MAPK) pathway, which phosphorylates and activates the MAPK-activated kinases, the pp90 ribosomal S6 kinase (Rsk) family members. Rsks regulate gene expression by phosphorylating transcription factors such as CREB. These kinases act in a coordinated manner to induce robust, sustained phosphorylation of Ser133 and activation of CREB.[120,121] Whereas CaMKIV mediates the early phase of Ser133 phosphorylation, the MAPK pathway mediates prolonged Ser133 phosphorylation.[192] In addition, CaMKIV phosphorylates and activates the coadaptor protein CBP at Ser301. Upon activation, CREB recruits phosphorylated CBP to the promoters of CREB target genes, and the coactivator complex induces gene transcription. Considerable evidence indicates that phosphorylation of Ser142 and Ser143 also contributes to CREB activation, but inhibits the interaction of CREB with CBP.[192]

Although influx of Ca^{2+} via synaptic NMDARs induces activation of CREB and neuronal survival, influx of Ca^{2+} via extrasynaptic NMDARs elicits CREB shutoff.[122–124] At extrasynaptic sites, Ca^{2+} influx via NMDARs activates protein phosphatase 1 (PP1) and PP2A, which dephosphorylate and inactivate CREB. Interestingly, contemporaneous activation of synaptic and extrasynaptic NMDARs by bath-applied NMDA also shuts off CREB, suggesting that extrasynaptic NMDARs act via a dominant cell-death signal. Ca^{2+} influx via extrasynaptic NMDARs (and CREB shutdown) causes mitochondrial dysfunction, ATP depletion, and neuronal death.

NF-κB is expressed in nearly all mammalian cells. Under physiologic (resting) conditions, NF-κB exists as an inactive form composed of the transcription factor dimer and IκB (inhibitor of NF-κB) protein, which maintains NF-κB in an inactive form.[193] NF-κB is activated in response to a diverse range of external stimuli, including the cytokine TNF-α, neurotrophic factors such as nerve growth factor (NGF), neurotransmitters, cell adhesion molecules, and various types of stress. These stimuli activate NF-κB by phosphorylation and proteosomal degradation of IκB, releasing the active, dimeric NF-κB. Upon activation, NF-κB translocates to the nucleus, where it binds to upstream regulatory elements in κB-responsive genes. These include the Ca^{2+}-binding protein calbindin, cytokines such as TNF-α and interleukin-2β (IL-β2) the antioxidant enzyme manganese superoxide dismutase (MnSOD), the anti-apoptotic proteins Bcl-x$_L$ and Bcl-2, the IAPs, and BDNF.[193] Upon activation, NF-κB plays an important role in regulating cell survival and synaptic plasticity in neurons. Focal ischemia activates NF-κB and relocalizes it to the nucleus of ischemic neurons, where it binds target genes.[194] Targeted deletion of NF-κB significantly reduces ischemic damage, suggesting a cell death–promoting role of NF-κB in focal ischemia.[194]

As already mentioned, Forkhead1 (FOXO-3A or FKHRL-1), a member of the Forkhead family of transcription factors (FOXO-3A, FOXO-1, and AFX), induces expression of pro-apoptotic target genes.[76,195]). Under physiologic conditions, FOXO-3A resides in the cytosol away from target genes and is thus inactive. The neurotrophins (NGF, BDNF) and insulin-like growth factor-1 (IGF-I) act via the phosphatidylinositol 3-kinase (PI3K)/protein kinase B (Akt) pathway to promote FOXO-3A

Pathophysiology

phosphorylation.[196]). PI3K promotes neuronal survival by phosphorylation and activation of the serine-threonine kinase Akt. Akt promotes cell survival by phosphorylation and inactivation of target genes implicated in apoptotic cell death.[196] FOXO-3A is a critical target of Akt phosphorylation and inactivation.[197] Phosphorylation of FOXO-3A promotes its binding to the retention factor 14-3-3, which retains FOXO-3A in the cytoplasm, away from target genes such as FasL (Plate 42–8).[196]

Injurious stimuli trigger FOXO-3A dephosphorylation and nuclear translocation. Putative targets of FOXO-3A are the death cytokines FasL, TNF-α, and TRAIL (TNF-related apoptosis–inducing ligand) and their cognate death receptors, which are members of the TNF family of death receptors.[198] The death cytokines act via the extrinsic or death receptor–mediated pathway to initiate the caspase death cascade. Global ischemia triggers expression of FasL, which is implicated in the extrinsic or death-receptor pathway of caspase activation.[198] FasL, by binding to its cognate death receptor Fas, recruits caspase-8, which initiates the caspase death cascade.

The gene silencing transcription factor REST/NRSF is widely expressed during embryogenesis and plays a strategic role in terminal neuronal differentiation.[199,200] In neural progenitor cells and nonneural cells, REST actively represses a large array of neural-specific genes important to synaptic plasticity and synaptic remodeling, including synaptic vesicle proteins, structural proteins, voltage-sensitive ion channels, and neurotransmitter receptors.[201,202] Examples are synapsin I, superior cervical ganglion (SCG)—the protein also known as "SCG10", nicotinic acetyl choline receptor, muscarinic acetylcholine m4 receptor, μ-opioid receptor, the neuronal nicotinic acetylcholine receptor subunit β2, and the AMPAR subunit GluR2. As neural progenitors differentiate and migrate out of the ventricular zone, REST downregulation is essential for induction and maintenance of the neural phenotype. Perturbation of REST expression during embryogenesis causes cellular apoptosis, aberrant differentiation and patterning, and embryonic lethality.[203]

REST is a member of the Gli-Krüppel family of zinc-finger transcriptional repressors; it contains nine non-canonical zinc-finger motifs through which it binds the *cis*-acting RE1 (neuronal repressor element) within the promoter region of target genes.[201] REST associates with the co-repressors Sin3A and coREST, which in turn recruit histone deacetylase (HDAC) to the promoters of target genes.[204] The co-repressor complex silences gene transcription by deacetylation of core histone proteins and tightening of the core chromatin complex, thus restricting access of the transcription machinery required for gene activation.[201] Chromatin remodeling is a universal mechanism of transcriptional repression and is implicated in other histone-modulated processes, including DNA replication, recombination, and repair.

Dysregulation of REST and its target genes is implicated in the pathogenesis of Down's syndrome,[205] Alzheimer's disease,[206] a subset of medulloblastoma cells,[207] and global ischemia.[208] Global ischemia triggers a pronounced upregulation of REST mRNA and protein in selectively vulnerable CA1 neurons (Plate 42–9). Consistent with induction of REST, core histone proteins over the GluR2 promoter exhibit pronounced deacetylation, indicative of reduced

GluR2 promoter activity, and GluR2 mRNA and protein expression are suppressed in CA1 neurons. Because the GluR2 subunit governs AMPAR Ca^{2+} permeability and AMPARs are implicated in the excitotoxic death associated with global ischemia, these changes are expected to affect neuronal survival. Consistent with this concept, acute knockdown (suppression) of the REST gene by administration of antisense oligonucleotides directed to the REST mRNA administration rescues neurons from ischemic death. These findings suggest a causal relation between REST induction and neuronal death and implicate REST-dependent gene silencing and chromatin remodeling in transcriptional repression of GluR2 in neurons subjected to insult.

Inflammation

Considerable evidence indicates that inflammation exacerbates ischemic injury.[209,210] Ischemia-hypoxia triggers activation of transcription factors such as NF-κB, hypoxia-inducible factor-1 (HIF-1), interferon regulatory factor-1, and signal transducers and activators of transcription (STATs) STAT3. These, in turn, orchestrate expression of an array of proinflammatory target genes, such as platelet-activating factor and the cytokines TNF-α and IL-1β.[211] Cytokines are critical mediators of inflammation and are expressed within the first 2 hours after onset of ischemia. The first inflammatory response is the unleashing of resident immune cells such as microglia. Microglia become activated and exhibit characteristic ameboid morphology, owing to retraction of their processes by 24 hours.

Subsequently, invasion and infiltration of nonresident cells occur. Ischemia-hypoxia triggers expression of adhesion molecules such as intercellular adhesion molecule 1 (ICAM-1), P-selectins, and E-selectins, by endothelial cells on their luminal surfaces. The adhesion molecules interact with cognate receptors on neutrophils, guiding their migration across the vascular wall and inside the brain parenchyma to the site of injury. Neutrophils are present in high numbers in ischemic brain by 24 to 48 hours. Infiltration of lymphocytes, macrophages, and monocytes follows next. Lymphocytes release inflammatory cytokines such as TNF-α, which triggers production of chemokines such as IL-8 and monocyte chemoattractant protein-1[212] and thereby initiates the inflammatory reaction. Chemokines are a family of small, soluble adhesion molecules that rapidly recruit leukocytes (blood-borne inflammatory cells) from the circulation across the endothelial barrier to the site of injury by promoting their adhesion and chemotaxis. Macrophages appear in large quantity between 1 and 5 days after MCAO; by 5 to 7 days, they become the predominant cell type in the injured region, where they phagocytose dead cells. The triggering of inflammatory cascades and release of cytokines is thought to cause astrocyte death and exacerbate neuronal death.

Critical evidence that inflammatory responses are involved in the pathogenesis of ischemia-induced neuronal death comes from studies that show that ischemic injury is attenuated by preischemic induction of systemic neutropenia, pharmacologic block of adhesion molecules or their receptors, deletion of the ICAM-1 gene, anti-inflammatory steroids or antibody block of inflammatory mediators such as IL-1β or the transcription factor interferon regulatory factor-1.[210] Mounting evidence indicates that, in addition to its role as perpetrator of neuronal death, NO is a catalyst for microglial activation (see earlier discussion).

MECHANISMS OF NEUROPROTECTION

Immediate Early Genes

IEGs are early response genes that are coordinately activated (dynamically regulated) in response to neuronal activity and neuronal insults. Whereas some IEGs function as a network of constitutively expressed (and coordinately regulated) proteins that are upregulated in response to activity or insult, other IEGs are activated only in response to external stresses (stimuli). As such, IEGs are markers of neural activity. A striking feature of the IEG response is the broad functional repertoire of the molecules. These include growth factors, transcription factors, enzymes that synthesize neurotransmitters, synaptic vesicle proteins, and ion channel and structural proteins (scaffolding, adaptor, and cytoskeletal proteins). Examples are the proinflammation gene cyclooxygenase-2 (Cox-2), an enzyme implicated in synthesis of prostaglandins; neuronal activity-regulated pentraxin (Narp), implicated in the aggregation of AMPARs at excitatory synapses; activity-regulated cytoskeleton-associated protein (Arc), a component of the synaptic junctional complex; Homer, an adaptor protein that binds mGluRs via their carboxy-terminal tails and localizes them to excitatory synapses; and c-fos. A transcription factor, c-fos forms a heterodimer with a member of the Jun family of transcription factors and binds to the activator protein-1 (AP-1) promoter element to regulate gene expression. More than half of IEGs are transcription factors that act collectively to orchestrate expression of delayed response genes involved in neuronal plasticity.

Neuronal insults such as ischemia trigger activation of CREB, which in turn drives transcription of IEGs. Within minutes of ischemia, IEGs such as c-fos, c-jun, and zif268 are expressed in the entire hemisphere ipsilateral to the occluded MCA.[209] Focal ischemia also induces expression of nerve growth factors I-A, IB, and I-C, NF-κB, Nurr-1-activating transcription factor, and erg-2 and erg-3 within minutes of the ischemic episode.[213] Eng 1 is a member of the ether-a-gogo-related genes (ERG) family which encodes K⁺ channel subunits. During the inflammation response, cytokines induce expression of proinflammatory genes such as cox-2. Global ischemia induces expression of a number of stress genes, including the IEGs c-fos, c-jun, junB, knox, and zif268, within the first 30 minutes. In rats and gerbils, global ischemia induces IEG expression throughout the hippocampus, including vulnerable CA1 neurons.[214,215] Thus, whether or not IEGs play a protective role in ischemia is unclear.[213]

Heat Shock Protein and Stress Genes

Heat shock proteins (HSPs) are a highly conserved family of molecular chaperone proteins that play a role in the aggregation, assembly, transport, and folding of proteins. Under physiologic conditions, HSPs are critical to cell growth and maintenance and are thought to play a role in neuronal signaling, differentiation, and migration.

Harmful stresses such as ischemia trigger expression (or upregulation) of HSPs, which act collectively to sustain survival by limiting cellular damage and accelerate recovery by rescuing denatured proteins from degradation (the "stress response.")[216] Upon activation, HSPs act to prevent aggregation of denatured proteins and aid in their refolding to the correct tertiary structure.

HSPs are typically classified according to their molecular weight. Examples are HSP10, HSP27, HSP32, HSP47, HSP60, HSP70/72, HSP90, HSP100/105, and ubiquitin. Some heat shock proteins, such as HSP60 and HSP90, are constitutively expressed and associated with specific intracellular organelles. HSP70 and Hsc70 are cytosolic. HSP75 is associated with mitochondria, and the glucose-regulated protein (GRP78) gene with the endoplasmic reticulum. Others, such as HSP27 and HSP70, are rapidly induced in response to cellular stresses (see later).

HSPs are endowed with a modular structure that facilitates their regulatory actions on protein translocation, import, and folding.[216] HSPs act via a carboxy-terminal peptide-binding domain to bind stretches of hydrophobic residues exposed in unfolded proteins. The energy for these interactions is provided by an amino-terminal ATPase domain, which binds and hydrolyzes ATP. HSPs are a target of the serine-threonine kinase Akt, which phosphorylates and activates them by promoting trimerization. Trimeric HSPs binds to heat-shock elements (HSEs) within the promoter regions of target genes and stimulate transcription of pro-survival genes.

Injurious stimuli such as hyperthermia, oxidative stress, radiation, and ischemia can engage either or both of two fundamental responses, apoptosis and the HSP stress response, which functions to sustain survival by limiting cellular damage and accelerating recovery. Research indicates that a fine balance between these two opposing pathways may determine cellular susceptibility to damaging stresses.[217] Ischemia-hypoxia triggers pronounced upregulation of HSPs such as HSP70.[217,218–221] Focal ischemia induces a dramatic upregulation of HSP70 protein expression in cells of the ischemic penumbra but not in the core.[222,223] The induction of HSPs in the penumbra is correlated with tolerance to subsequent ischemic insults. Global ischemia triggers a massive upregulation of HSP70 mRNA and protein expression, although the cellular specificity of expression and its relation to neuronal vulnerability are unclear.[213] Thus, whether or not HSP70 is a major determinant of neuronal death associated with global ischemia remains unsettled.[213]

Evidence shows that HSP27, HSP70, and HSP90 exert their cytoprotective effects by halting the self-amplifying caspase death cascade and preventing apoptosis.[217] Heat shock proteins 70, 90, and 27 each possess the ability to prevent caspase-3 processing and activation. HSP70 and HSP90 interact with Apaf-1 to prevent the recruitment of caspase-9 to the apoptosome by directly associating with Apaf-1 and preventing its oligomerization (see Plate 42–4). HSP27 binds and sequesters cytosolic cytochrome c away from its target, Apaf-1.[224–226] Consistent with its presumptive role in neuroprotection, overexpression of HSP70 provides efficient protection against cell death triggered by harmful stresses. Transgenic mice that overexpress HSP70 exhibit significantly reduced infarct volumes compared with wild-type mice in models of focal ischemia,[227] and

Pathophysiology

HSP70.1 knockout mice exhibit significantly greater infarct volumes than wild-type mice.[228] HSP72 overexpression is neuroprotective, even when implemented after the onset of global ischemia.[229]

Spreading Depression

Cortical spreading depression (CSD) is a wave of sustained depolarization (neuronal inactivation) moving through intact brain tissue and associated with brain ischemia, migraine aura, and seizures.[230] Spreading depression elicits a temporary, but major, redistribution of ions between intracellular and extracellular compartments without causing irreversible damage. The ion redistribution becomes clinically significant under conditions of impaired brain metabolism, such as global or focal ischemia. Injurious stimuli such as hypoxia trigger spreading depression. As cells lose energy, energy-requiring pumps that normally force ions into and out of the cell in an attempt to maintain a concentration gradient either fail or operate in reverse. As previously described, these factors induce a rapid efflux of K^+, which flows out of neurons via NMDARs and a rise in extracellular K^+. The rapid rise in extracellular K^+ elicits neuronal excitation, followed by excessive depolarization and a period of electrical silence during which the potential at the brain surface becomes negative. Ca^{2+} ions flow in as the depolarization opens voltage-dependent Ca^{2+} channels and extracellular Ca^{2+} falls to abnormally low levels. Na^+ and Cl^- enter neurons. Water follows passively, driven by the influx of Na^+ and Cl^-, which greatly exceeds the efflux of K^+. The extracellular space is reduced, and edema ensues. Critical evidence that CSD is NMDAR dependent comes from studies that show that NMDAR antagonists block spreading depression completely in human neocortical tissue and delay the onset of spreading depression in rat hippocampus.[230]

Astrocytes are thought to play a critical role in the energy-dependent restitution of ion gradients that restores normal neuronal activity. Astrocytes actively take up glutamate during normal neuronal activity. They are coupled via gap junctions, which mediate spatial buffering of K^+. Cooperation between glia and neurons maintains normal extracellular ion and transmitter levels during neuronal activity. Under conditions of spreading depression, glutamate transporters operate in reverse and astrocytes release glutamate, prolonging the spreading depression. Ion fluxes are enhanced and highly synchronized. Astrocytic gap junctions are implicated in the synchronization of neuronal firing and propagation of spreading depression. Consistent with this notion, gap junction blockers prevent the formation and propagation of CSD, and astrocytes cultured from Cx43 knockout mice exhibit slow propagation of Ca^{2+} waves.[230] Curiously (and inexplicably), mice with a conditional Cx43 knockout in brain exhibit accelerated propagation of spreading depression.[231]

Growth Factors and Neurotrophins

Growth factor–induced signal transduction proceeds via a cascade of protein phosphorylation events that serve to relay environmental cues into cellular responses. These events ultimately culminate in activation of multiple nuclear transcription factors with a diverse range of target genes, many of which are involved in orchestrating cell survival and proliferation. Growth factors can initiate signaling via either the PI3K/Akt (protein kinase B) pathway, the Ras/MAPK signaling pathway, or both.[197]

The PI3K/Akt Pathway

Glutamate receptor activation can elicit the production and release of BDNF, which can signal through activation of the PI3K/Akt or Ras/MAPK pathway. The survival-promoting effects of neurotrophins (NGF, BDNF) and other growth factors (IGF-I) are executed, at least in part, through the PI3K/Akt pathway.[232-236] PI3K enzymes reside in the cytosol and catalyze the formation of the lipid 3′-phophorylated phosphoinositides, which regulate the localization and activity of a key component in neuronal survival, the serine-threonine kinase Akt. PI3K acts via 3′-phosphoinositol to phosphorylate and activate the serine-threonine kinase Akt (Plate 42–10). Upon activation, Akt is translocated to the nucleus, where it exerts its actions on gene expression. Akt promotes cell survival by suppressing genes implicated in apoptotic cell death.[196] In each case, Akt phosphorylates and thereby inactivates its target. Targets of Akt include the pro-apoptotic protein BAD (an inhibitor of Bcl-2), pro-caspase-9, which is processed to generate caspase-9 (an initiator of the caspase death cascade), and the transcription factor Forkhead-1 (FOXO-3A) (see Plate 42–8).[196,197]

Akt is uniquely endowed with a modular structure that enables it to translocate to the nucleus and phosphorylate target proteins in response to external stimuli. In addition to a centrally located kinase domain, Akt has an *N*-terminal pleckstrin homology domain, which mediates its interactions with proteins and phospholipids. Upon binding to lipids, Akt is translocated from the cytoplasm to the inner surface of the plasma membrane, which brings the kinase into close proximity with its activators. PI3K is also regulated by phospholipids. Thus, the lipid products generated by PI3K enzymes control the activity of Akt by regulating its location and activation. The ability of neurotrophins to promote neuronal survival requires functional PI3K/Akt signaling in the cell body and in distal axons that are in contact with the dendrites of target neurons. Critical evidence that Akt mediates neuronal survival comes from studies that show that Akt supports neuronal survival even in the absence of trophic factors and that a dominant mutation of Akt inhibits neuronal survival even in the presence of survival factors.[237]

Ras/MAPK Pathway

Neurotrophins and other growth factors also promote cell survival via the Ras/MAPK signaling pathway. The small guanosine triphosphate–binding protein Ras is a mitogen and key mediator of growth factor–dependent cell survival. Growth factors act via their cognate cell surface receptors to activate the MAPK signaling pathway, which entails a series of sequential phosphorylation events leading ultimately to phosphorylation of the MAPK-activated kinases known as Rsks.[238] The Rsks promote cell survival by a dual mechanism; they phosphorylate and inactivate the pro-apoptotic factor BAD and phosphorylate and potently activate the transcription factor CREB, which promotes transcription of pro-survival genes.[239] BDNF, a neurotrophin, acts via the Ras/MAPK pathway and extracellular signal–regulated kinases 1 and 2 to induce neuroprotection in an in vivo model of neonatal hypoxic-ischemic brain injury.[240]

In the CNS, the best-characterized targets of growth factor signaling are the extracellular signal–regulated kinases 1 and 2 (ERK1 and ERK2). ERK phosphorylates and activates nuclear transcription factors such as nuclear transcription factor ELK-1 and CREB. Other ERK targets are cytoskeletal proteins, cell adhesion molecules, ion channels, and transcription factors. CREB stimulates cell survival directly by activating transcription of bcl-2. In addition, CREB stimulates transcription of immediate early response genes, which in turn induce the delayed response genes that influence neuronal activity, including growth factors, enzymes that synthesize neurotransmitters, synaptic vesicle proteins, and ion channel and structural proteins. Thus, although there is a divergence in the survival signaling pathways downstream of neurotrophin receptors, both the PI3K and MAPK pathways converge on the same set of proteins, BAD and CREB, to inhibit apoptosis.

Interneurons

GABA-releasing inhibitory interneurons (or "local circuit" neurons) of the hippocampus and cortex are also thought to contribute to the selective spatial patterns of neuronal death in brain ischemia. Whereas pyramidal (or principal) neurons of the hippocampal CA1 die because of global ischemia, inhibitory interneurons of the CA1 (and other subfields) survive. Inhibitory interneurons are typically characterized by axons that make short-range projections and release GABA onto their targets.[241] Interneurons comprise a diverse array of anatomical and neurochemical subtypes. Interneurons have typically been characterized according to their neurochemical content (by calcium-binding proteins such as parvalbumin [PV], calbindin, and calretinin or by neuromodulator-transmitters such as somatostatin, neuropeptide Y, and nNOS). Many PV-positive interneurons are classified anatomically as basket cells or interneurons that send their axons to the cell body of the postsynaptic cell, surrounding it with a structure akin to a basket. Many somatostatin-positive interneurons are anatomically characterized as chandelier cells, a sub-class of inhibitory interneurons whose morphology resembles a chandelier, but there are many exceptions to the rule. Yet a third classification is by action potential firing patterns— for example, fast-spiking cells, low-threshold cells, and regular-spiking cells. Global ischemia kills pyramidal neurons of the hippocampal CA1, but interneurons in the CA1 survive. Studies have provided evidence for electrical coupling between like interneurons mediated via gap junctions.[242]

Gap junctions are conductive channels that connect the interiors of coupled cells.[242] Their large internal diameters (≈1.2 nm) allow the exchange of small ions and intracellular signaling molecules between neighboring cells. As a result, gap junctions synchronize activity of coupled cells and are thought to play an important role in intercellular signaling in brain development, morphogenesis, and pattern formation.[243–246] Gap junctions are composed of *connexins*, integral membrane proteins encoded by a gene family of at least 20 structurally related members in mammals. Although connexins share sequence similarity and a common membrane topology, they assemble to form channels that differ in gating and permeability properties and in temporal and spatial patterns of expression. Three gap junctional proteins, Cx32, Cx36, and Cx43, are expressed abundantly in mammalian brain but with differing cellular specificity. Whereas Cx43 is the most abundant connexin expressed by astrocytes, Cx32 is expressed predominantly in oligodendrocytes[247,248] and interneurons; Cx36 protein expression is neuron-specific.[249,250]

In CA1, PV-positive interneurons form a vast dendro-dendritic network extending many hundreds of microns and connected by anatomically identified electrical and mixed electrical-chemical synapses. This network of GABA-ergic interneurons is a candidate for the generator of synchronized oscillations in hippocampus. Electrophysiologic evidence indicates the presence of electrical coupling between GABA-ergic interneurons in the hippocampus and in visual cortex.[251,252] Reverse transcription–polymerase chain reaction (RT-PCR) studies indicate that electrical coupling between interneurons in these regions is likely to be mediated by Cx36 (and possibly Cx32), which exhibits high expression in bipolar interneurons in layers 2 and 3 of visual cortex, interneurons, and spiny stellate cells, and in layer 4 of barrel cortex and basket cells in DG.[252] Electrical coupling between interneurons is thought to mediate synchronous firing and thereby promote inhibitory transmission. These observations raise the possibility that Cx36 or Cx32 gap junction or both might play a role in the survival of hippocampal interneurons or the death of pyramidal neurons after ischemia.

A 2001 study[252a] indicates that global ischemia induces a selective upregulation of Cx36 (and Cx32) protein expression in PV-positive inhibitory interneurons in the vulnerable CA1 before the onset of neuronal death, consistent with a role in the survival of GABA-ergic interneurons.[253] Moreover, transgenic Cx32 null–mutant mice exhibit enhanced vulnerability to global ischemia–induced neuronal death. These findings provide a basis for understanding a role for neuronal gap junctions in defining cell-specific patterns of neuronal injury after global ischemia. Because global ischemia targets pyramidal neurons of the CA1 while sparing inhibitory interneurons, the findings just enumerated suggest the novel possibility that enhanced expression of Cx36 may play a critical role in the protection and survival of CA1 interneurons after global ischemia. One possibility is that coupling of inhibitory interneurons promotes their survival by mediating intercellular metabolic cooperation. Another possibility is that enhanced coupling of inhibitory interneurons represents a failed attempt of such interneurons to rescue CA1 neurons. The greater vulnerability of CA1 pyramidal cells in Cx32 knockout mice is consistent with observations that neocortical cells in these mice display enhanced intrinsic excitability and prolonged paroxysmal depolarizations, indicating dysfunction of inhibitory synaptic transmission.[253] Moreover, late-depolarizing glutamatergic excitatory postsynaptic potentials are enhanced, indicating reduced inhibitory input. Enhanced excitatory transmission and deficient inhibitory transmission would be

Pathophysiology

expected to increase pyramidal cell excitability and enhance vulnerability to excitotoxic cell death.

Astrocytes

Astrocytes are abundant glia (nonneural cells) present throughout the brain, where they are positioned in close association with neurons.[254,255] Astrocytes can enwrap synapses and play a critical role in transmitter uptake and release during normal neuronal activity. In the hippocampus, 57% of the synapses are associated with the process of an astrocyte. Astrocytes also have extensive contacts with endothelial cells from capillaries. Thus, astrocytes are well positioned to mediate signaling between neurons, between neurons and astrocytes, and between neurons and capillaries. Astrocytes respond to a variety of synaptically released transmitters, including glutamate, noradrenaline, histamine, acetylcholine, ATP and GABA. Application of any of these transmitters to astrocytes elicits sustained or oscillating elevations of intracellular Ca^{2+} concentration in the astrocytes. Ligands that evoke Ca^{2+} elevations in astrocytes can cause the release of glutamate from astrocytes in a Ca^{2+}-dependent manner. The three mechanisms that have been proposed to mediate the Ca^{2+}-dependent release of glutamate from astrocytes are reverse operation of glutamate transporters, an anion-channel dependent pathway induced by swelling, and Ca^{2+}-dependent exocytosis. Mounting evidence supports exocytosis as the key mechanism mediating glutamate release.

Astrocytes are thought to play a critical role in the neuronal death associated with focal ischemia.[254-256] Swelling of astrocytes contributes to infarct size in focal ischemia. Four to 6 hours after focal ischemia, astrocytes become hypertrophic and displace a greater volume. Both anti-excitotoxic and anti-apoptotic interventions reduce infarct volume, not just neuronal cell death, in animal models of focal ischemia. Astrocyte death may occur as a secondary consequence of neuronal death, possibly as a result of release of cytokines and the triggering of inflammatory cascades. In animal models of global ischemia, astrocytes survive and play an important role in reactive gliosis after neuronal loss.

Evidence supports a role for interastrocytic gap junctions in the spread of secondary injury associated with focal ischemia.[257-259] Astrocytic gap junctions remain functional in postischemic brain, and gap junction blockers limit the secondary expansion of infarcts after focal ischemia. In cultures, dying glia propagate cell death to healthy bystanders in proportion to their expression of gap junctions and functional coupling. Presumably, the "metabolic cooperation" mediated by gap junctions between healthy and dying cells provides too great a metabolic stress for the healthy cells. These findings suggest that astrocytic gap junctions might propagate and amplify neuronal death after global ischemia as well, and cooperativity in death of CA1 neurons after global ischemia has been proposed. Coupling of astrocytes can also attenuate neuronal death in some paradigms and appears to play a neuroprotective role in helping neurons to maintain Ca^{2+} homeostasis in the presence of oxidative stress. Administration of uncouplers of gap junctions, such as 18α-glycyrrhetinic acid (AGA), to slice cultures exacerbates neuronal death induced by oxidative stress.

A number of mechanisms have been proposed to explain the neuroprotective role of coupling between astrocytes; they include (1) enhanced synthesis and release of protective signaling molecules from astrocytes, (2) reduced synthesis and release of neurotoxic substances, (3) enhanced removal of glutamate from the intercellular space, and (4) spatial buffering of K^+. Astrocytes synthesize and release neurotrophic factors and cytokines, such as nerve growth factor, TNF-α, and basic fibroblast growth factor,[260] and are rich in the antioxidant enzyme catalase, which may increase survival after global ischemia.

NEUROPROTECTIVE STRATEGIES

Ischemic Tolerance

Ischemic tolerance is a well-known phenomenon in which brief ischemic insults (ischemic preconditioning) confer robust neuroprotection to hippocampal CA1 neurons against a subsequent severe ischemic challenge.[240,261-266] Ischemic tolerance can also be induced in vivo by spreading depression, hypoxia, and activation of A1 adenosine and inhibitors of oxidative phosphorylation and in vitro by exposure to excitotoxins. Although the molecular mechanisms underlying ischemic tolerance are not yet fully delineated, the considerable delay from the preconditioning stimulus until onset of ischemic tolerance is consistent with a role for transcriptional changes in adaptation. Ischemic preconditioning enhances expression of the anti-apoptotic factor Bcl-2, which can act upstream of caspase-3 to prevent initiation of the caspases and downstream to directly bind activated caspase-3 to halt the self-amplifying caspase death cascade.[90]

Ischemic tolerance is thought to require activation of NMDA-type ionotropic glutamate receptors and enhanced Ca^{2+} as well as opening of ATP-sensitive K^+ channels via activation of adenosine A_1 receptors. Ischemic preconditioning is known to activate c-fos and c-jun and a number of survival factors, HSP70, superoxide dismutase, NO, BDNF, and the anti-apoptotic factors Bcl-2 and Bcl-x_L.

Spreading depression can induce ischemic tolerance. CSD preconditioning induces expression of pro-survival genes such as nNOS, Ca^{2+}-independent protein kinase C, c-fos, junB, c-jun, and MAP kinase phosphatase-1 (MKP-1), and reduces infarct volume in animal models of focal ischemia.[267] The rise in intracellular Ca^{2+} associated with CSD activates nNOS, which promotes NO formation.[268] The rise in extracellular glutamate associated with spreading depression promotes phosphorylation and activation of ERK1 and ERK2.[267] Upon activation, ERK phosphorylates the synaptic vesicle protein synapsin I, which promotes transmitter release and a rise in extracellular glutamate.

Neuroprotection by Estrogen in Experimental Models of Stroke

Estradiol, the primary estrogen produced and secreted by the ovaries, has widespread actions on the brain.[269,270] Estradiol increases spine density, synapse number, and NMDA receptor NR1 subunit expression and potentiates kainate-elicited currents in CA1 pyramidal neurons. Moreover, estrogen affords neuroprotection in several experimental models of stroke.[269,271] Acute exogenous estrogen at physiologic levels protects against focal ischemia–induced cortical injury in estrogen-deprived female and male rats and mice.[271-277] To afford protection, estradiol must be present at physiologic concentrations at least 48 hours before focal ischemia. Clues as to the molecular mechanisms by which estrogen affords protection come from studies showing that estrogen acts via estrogen receptor-α (ERα) to afford neuroprotection in the focal ischemia model[278] and induces upregulation of ERα and the anti-apoptotic factor Bcl-2 neurons (Plate 42–11).[279]

Estrogen also provides neuroprotection in animal models of global ischemia. Acute estrogen at supraphysiologic concentrations protects against global ischemia–induced hippocampal injury[280,281] and improves behavioral outcome after ischemia in male gerbils with ischemia.[282] Moreover, long-term administration of estrogen at more physiologic concentrations typically used in hormone replacement therapy (HRT) gives robust protection.[80] In addition to direct actions on hippocampal neurons, estrogen may affect hippocampal neurons indirectly via ERs on basal forebrain cholinergic neurons, which innervate the CA1 or via a receptor-independent anti-oxidative mechanism to inhibit oxygen radical–induced lipid peroxidation. The importance of postmenopausal estrogen replacement therapy for protection against the neuronal death associated with cardiac arrest or stroke, however, remains controversial.

The classic mode of estrogen action on neurons involves binding to the intracellular estrogen receptors ERα and ERβ, which function as ligand-activated transcription factors.[269,271] Estrogen binding to ERα or ERβ induces a conformational change leading to release of HSPs and formation of a dimer with high affinity for specific DNA sequences known as estrogen response elements (EREs), which are located at the promoter region of target genes. EREs occur in a diverse set of genes involved in cell survival and cell proliferation. EREs include the growth factors NGF, BDNF, and IGF-I receptor (IGF-IR) and the anti-apoptotic factors Bcl-2 and Bcl-x_L. The estrogen receptor can also interact with transcription factors such as c-jun and c-fos, with transcriptional enhancers and repressors, and with other DNA elements, such as AP1 sites.[283,284] AP1 is a dimeric transcription factor complex AP1, whose key components are the proteins Fos and Jun.

In addition to its genomic actions, estrogen signals rapidly via the PI3K/Akt signaling pathway, the Ras/MAPK signaling pathway, or both.[285] PI3K phosphorylates and activates Akt, which promotes cell survival by suppression of pro-apoptotic target genes. These genes include the pro-apoptotic proteins BAD and pro-caspase-9 and FOXO-3A. FOXO-3A induces apoptosis by transactivation of the Fas ligand, which acts via the Fas receptor to initiate the caspase cascade. Akt phosphorylates FOXO-3A, eliciting its relocalization from the nucleus to the cytoplasm, away from target genes. Estrogen acts via the PI3K/Akt signaling pathway (see earlier discussion) to afford protection of cortical neurons in culture against glutamate toxicity. Findings also indicate that estrogen blocks apoptotic signaling cascades in a gerbil model of global ischemia.[80] An intriguing possibility is that estrogen acts via Akt to halt the caspase death cascade at the point of Forkhead activation.

Estrogen also signals rapidly via Ras/MAPK and the downstream kinases ERK1 and ERK2. MAPK signaling promotes cell survival via phosphorylation and inactivation of BAD and via phosphorylation and activation of CREB, which promotes transcription of pro-survival target genes. Estrogen rapidly phosphorylates ERK1 and ERK2, which phosphorylate and inactivate the downstream kinase glycogen synthase kinase-3β (GSK-3β). Estrogen is a powerful inducer of MAPK in various models, including neocortical explants, primary cortical neurons, and neuroblastoma cells.[269] Estrogen acts via the Ras/MAPK pathway and ERK1 and ERK2 to promote neuronal survival of cortical neurons against glutamate toxicity.[286,287]

Considerable evidence implicates crosstalk between ERα and IGF-I signaling in the actions of estrogen on neurons.[269,271] ERα and ERβ are colocalized with IGF-IRs in neurons and astrocytes throughout the brain. Estrogen and IGF-I each engage the PI3K/Akt and MAPK signaling cascades. Estrogen neuroprotection in vivo and in vitro requires growth factor signaling. Research has shed light on the molecular mechanisms underlying this unique codependence. Upon activation, ERα interacts with IGF-IR to form a supramolecular complex that includes ERα, IGF-IR, the p85 subunit of PI3K, and IRS-1.[288] Formation of such a supramolecular complex is likely to prove critical to the protective actions of estrogen against ischemic death.

Neuroprotection by Zinc Chelation

Considerable evidence indicates that a rise in intracellular Zn^{2+} to toxic levels in CA1 neurons contributes to global ischemia–induced neuronal death. Zn^{2+} chelation affords robust protection against global ischemia-induced neuronal death.[289] Koh and colleagues[159] were the first to demonstrate that Zn^{2+} translocation from presynaptic terminals to postsynaptic target neurons occurs relatively early after neuronal insult and is not restricted to CA3 and hilar neurons (see Plate 42–7). Moreover, exposure of cortical neurons to Zn^{2+} elicited a rise in intracellular Zn^{2+}, as assessed by the selective fluorescent indicator dye TSQ. To examine whether the rise in Zn^{2+} was causally related to neuronal death, Koh and colleagues injected the cell membrane impermeant chelator calcium disodium ethylenediaminetetraacetate (CaEDTA) into the lateral ventricles 30 minutes before global ischemia markedly reduced the rise in Zn^{2+} in CA1 (and hilar) neurons and abolished neuronal death. Although CaEDTA is not specific for Zn^{2+}, it has a higher affinity for Zn^{2+} than for Ca^{2+} or Mg^{2+}. Thus, CaEDTA can bind Zn^{2+} without significantly altering intracellular Ca^{2+} or Mg^{2+}. Moreover, CaEDTA blocks Zn^{2+} neurotoxicity in vitro but not the neurotoxicity of Cu^{2+} or Fe^{2+}. These findings suggest strongly that Zn^{2+} is a critical mediator of ischemia-induced cell death.

These observations raise the possibility of novel targets for neuroprotection. A major problem inherent with membrane-impermeant Zn^{2+} chelators is achieving adequate access of membrane-impermeable zinc chelators to the CNS. Alternative strategies include block of channels that mediate entry of Zn^{2+} into neurons; block or attenuation of release of synaptic Zn^{2+}; upregulation of transporters responsible for Zn^{2+} extrusion, sequestration, or both; upregulation of metallotransporters; and counteraction of downstream disturbances involved in neuronal death (e.g., block of mitochondrial respiration). Promising leads along these lines include dietary manipulation of synaptic zinc stores, intake of pyruvate to compensate for Zn^{2+}-induced blockade of glycolysis, and pharmacologic block of Zn^{2+}-induced apoptosis.[289]

Hypothermia

Hypothermic therapy (lowering of the body temperature during or after ischemic insult) affords robust neuroprotection against global ischemia induced neuronal death.[290] Prolonged, postischemic hypothermia provides robust and sustained neuronal survival and greatly reduces ischemia-induced cognitive deficits in rats and gerbils.[56,290,291] Brief forebrain ischemia kills more than 98% of CA1 pyramidal neurons. Prolonged, delayed hypothermia (induced 1 hour after ischemia and maintained for 48 hours) persistently (for as many as 60 days) preserves the ultrastructure of and protects more than 90% of CA1 neurons from ischemia-induced death. Hypothermia can be initiated as late as 12 hours after ischemia, although the neuroprotective effect is significantly less than when hypothermia is initiated 1 hour after ischemia. These findings support the potential clinical usefulness of postischemic hypothermia as a mode of intervention after global ischemia associated with cardiac arrest or cardiac surgery in humans.

Hypothermia decreases cerebral blood flow, intracranial pressure, and brain metabolism. It also reduces cerebral metabolic rate, which results in decreased consumption of glucose and oxygen. The reduction in energy demand slows the rate of high-energy phosphate (ATP) depletion and lactate accumulation and thereby lessens oxidative stress. Curiously, although hypothermia protects against global ischemia–induced neuronal death, it exacerbates neuronal injury associated with focal ischemia.

There are a number of mechanisms by which hypothermia protects against hypoxia. Only a few, however, are understood. During ischemia, there is a rise in extracellular K^+, in part due to efflux of K^+ from vulnerable neurons via NMDARs and in part due to breakdown and reverse operation of ion pumps such as the Na^+-K^+-ATPase.[292] Hypothermia reduces synaptic activity (the rate of neuronal firing) and, in effect, relieves the cell of its excessive extracellular K^+.[292] Findings also indicate that hypothermia promotes survival of neurons by accelerating recovery of ATP and other important sources of cellular energy in the mitochondria to physiologic levels.[293] Future studies will more completely elucidate the molecular mechanisms by which hypothermia affords protection.

References

1. On-line Medical Dictionary. Dept. of Medical Oncology, University of Newcastle. http://cancerweb.ncl.ac.uk/cgi-bin/omd?ischemia© 1997–2003.
1a. Petito CK, Feldmann E, Pulsinelli WA, et al: Delayed hippocampal damage in humans following cardiorespiratory arrest. Neurology 37:1281–1286, 1987.
2. Brillman J: Central nervous system complications in coronary artery bypass graft surgery. Neurol Clin 11:475–495, 1993.
3. Roach GW, Kanchuger M, Mangano CM, et al: Adverse cerebral outcomes after coronary bypass surgery: Multicenter Study of Perioperative Ischemia Research Group and the Ischemia Research and Education Foundation Investigators. N Engl J Med 335:1857–1863, 1996.
4. Swain JA, Anderson RV, Siegman MG: Low-flow cardiopulmonary bypass and cerebral protection: A summary of investigations. Ann Thorac Surg 56:1490–1492, 1993.
5. Schmidt-Kastner R, Freund TF: Selective vulnerability of the hippocampus in brain ischemia. Neuroscience 40:599–636, 1991.
6. Crain BJ, Westerkam WD, Harrison AH, et al: Selective neuronal death after transient forebrain ischemia in the Mongolian gerbil: A silver impregnation study. Neuroscience 27:387–402, 1988.
7. Kirino T: Delayed neuronal death in the gerbil hippocampus following ischemia. Brain Res 239:57–69, 1982.
8. Garcia JH, Yoshida Y, Chen H, et al: Progression from ischemic injury to infarct following middle cerebral artery occlusion in the rat. Am J Pathol 142:623–635, 1993.
9. Memezawa H, Smith ML, Siesjö BK: Penumbral tissues salvaged by reperfusion following middle cerebral artery occlusion in rats. Stroke 23:552–559, 1992.
10. Small DL, Buchan AM: Animal models. Br Med Bull 56:307–317, 2000.
11. Ginsberg MD, Busto R: Rodent models of cerebral ischemia. Stroke 20:1627–1642, 1989.
12. Pulsinelli WA, Brierley JB: A new model of bilateral hemispheric ischemia in the unanesthetized rat. Stroke 10:267–272, 1979.
13. Kitagawa K, Matsumoto M, Yang G, et al: Cerebral ischemia after bilateral carotid artery occlusion and intraluminal suture occlusion in mice: Evaluation of the patency of the posterior communicating artery. J Cereb Blood Flow Metab 18:570–579, 1998.
14. Oguro K, Jover T, Tanaka H, et al: Global ischemia-induced increases in the gap junctional proteins connexin 32 (Cx32) and Cx36 in hippocampus and enhanced vulnerability of Cx32 knockout mice. J Neurosci 21:7534–7542, 2001.
15. Nemoto EM: Monkey model of complete global ischemia. Stroke 24:328–329, 1993.
16. Torregrosa G, Barbera MD, Centeno JM, et al: Characterization of the cortical laser-Doppler flow and hippocampal degenerative patterns after global cerebral ischaemia in the goat. Pflugers Arch 435:662–669, 1998.
17. Pulsinelli WA, Duffy TE: Regional energy balance in rat brain after transient forebrain ischemia. J Neurochem 40:1500–1503, 1983.
18. Schmidt-Kastner R, Freund TF: Selective vulnerability of the hippocampus in brain ischemia. Neuroscience 40:599–636, 1991.
19. Pulsinelli WA, Brierley JB, Plum F: Temporal profile of neuronal damage in a model of transient forebrain ischemia. Ann Neurol 11:491–498, 1982.
20. Kirino T, Sano K: Fine structural nature of delayed neuronal death following ischemia in the gerbil hippocampus. Acta Neuropathol (Berl) 62:209–218, 1984.
21. Kirino T, Tamura A, Sano K: Selective vulnerability of the hippocampus to ischemia: Reversible and irreversible types of ischemic cell damage. Prog Brain Res 63:39–58, 1985.
22. Kinouchi H, Sharp FR, Koistinaho J, et al: Induction of heat shock hsp70 mRNA and HSP70 kDa protein in neurons in the 'penumbra' following focal cerebral ischemia in the rat. Brain Res 619:334–338, 1993.
23. Pulsinelli WA, Levy DE, Duffy TE: Regional cerebral blood flow and glucose metabolism following transient forebrain ischemia. Ann Neurol 11:499–502, 1982.
24. Raffin CN, Harrison M, Sick TJ, et al: EEG suppression and anoxic depolarization: influences on cerebral oxygenation during ischemia. J Cereb Blood Flow Metab 11:407–415, 1991.
25. Xu ZC, Pulsinelli WA: Responses of CA1 pyramidal neurons in rat hippocampus to transient forebrain ischemia: An in vivo intracellular recording study. Neurosci Lett 171:187–191, 1994.
26. Smith ML, Auer RN, Siesjö BK: The density and distribution of ischemic brain injury in the rat following 2–10 min of forebrain ischemia. Acta Neuropathol (Berl) 64:319–332, 1984.
27. Smith ML, Bendek G, Dahlgren N, et al: Models for studying long-term recovery following forebrain ischemia in the rat. 2: A 2-vessel occlusion model. Acta Neurol Scand 69:385–401, 1984.
28. Lipton P: Ischemic cell death in brain neurons. Physiol Rev 79:1431–1568, 1999.
29. Kato H, Araki T, Kogure K, et al: Sequential cerebral blood flow changes in short-term cerebral ischemia in gerbils. Stroke 21:1346–1349, 1990.
30. Suzuki R, Yamaguchi T, Li CL, et al: The effects of 5-minute ischemia in Mongolian gerbils. II: Changes of spontaneous neuronal

activity in cerebral cortex and CA1 sector of hippocampus. Acta Neuropathol (Berl) 60:217–222, 1983.

31. Schauwecker PE, Steward O: Genetic determinants of susceptibility to excitotoxic cell death: Implications for gene targeting approaches. Proc Natl Acad Sci U S A 94:4103–4108, 1997.

32. DeGirolami U, Crowell RM, Marcoux FW: Selective necrosis and total necrosis in focal cerebral ischemia: Neuropathologic observations on experimental middle cerebral artery occlusion in the macaque monkey. J Neuropathol Exp Neurol 43:57–71, 1984.

33. Longa EZ, Weinstein PR, Carlson S, et al: Reversible middle cerebral artery occlusion without craniectomy in rats. Stroke 20:84–91, 1989.

34. Nagasawa H, Kogure K: Correlation between cerebral blood flow and histologic changes in a new rat model of middle cerebral artery occlusion. Stroke 20:1037–1043, 1989.

35. Zhang RL, Chopp M, Chen H, et al: Temporal profile of ischemic tissue damage, neutrophil response, and vascular plugging following permanent and transient (2H) middle cerebral artery occlusion in the rat. J Neurol Sci 125:3–10, 1994.

36. McAuley MA: Rodent models of focal ischemia. Cerebrovasc Brain Metab Rev 7:153–180, 1995.

37. Buchan AM, Xue D, Slivka A: A new model of temporary focal neocortical ischemia in the rat. Stroke 23:273–279, 1992.

38. Kilic E, Hermann DM, Hossmann KA: A reproducible model of thromboembolic stroke in mice. Neuroreport 9:2967–2970, 1998.

39. Markgraf CG, Kraydieh S, Prado R, et al: Comparative histopathologic consequences of photothrombotic occlusion of the distal middle cerebral artery in Sprague-Dawley and Wistar rats. Stroke 24:286–292, 1993.

40. Brint S, Jacewicz M, Kiessling M, et al: Focal brain ischemia in the rat: Methods for reproducible neocortical infarction using tandem occlusion of the distal middle cerebral and ipsilateral common carotid arteries. J Cereb Blood Flow Metab 8:474–485, 1988.

41. Chen ST, Hsu CY, Hogan EL, et al: A model of focal ischemic stroke in the rat: Reproducible extensive cortical infarction. Stroke 17:738–743, 1986.

42. Petito CK: Early and late mechanisms of increased vascular permeability following experimental cerebral infarction. J Neuropathol Exp Neurol 38:222–234, 1979.

43. Rice JE, Vannucci RC, Brierley JB: The influence of immaturity on hypoxic-ischemic brain damage in the rat. Ann Neurol 9:131–141, 1981.

44. Roohey T, Raju TN, Moustogiannis AN: Animal models for the study of perinatal hypoxic-ischemic encephalopathy: A critical analysis. Early Hum Dev 47:115–146, 1997.

45. Salford LG, Plum F, Brierley JB: Graded hypoxia-oligemia in rat brain. II: Neuropathological alterations and their implications. Arch Neurol 29:234–238, 1973.

46. Williams GD, Towfighi J, Smith MB: Cerebral energy metabolism during hypoxia-ischemia correlates with brain damage: A 31P NMR study in unanesthetized immature rats. Neurosci Lett 170:31–34, 1994.

47. Dawson VL, Kizushi VM, Huang PL, et al: Resistance to neurotoxicity in cortical cultures from neuronal nitric oxide synthase-deficient mice. J Neurosci 16:2479–2487, 1996.

48. Goldberg MP, Choi DW: Combined oxygen and glucose deprivation in cortical cell culture: Calcium-dependent and calcium-independent mechanisms of neuronal injury. J Neurosci 13:3510–3524, 1993.

49. Martin RL, Lloyd HG, Cowan AI: The early events of oxygen and glucose deprivation: Setting the scene for neuronal death? Trends Neurosci 17:251–257, 1994.

50. Gottron FJ, Ying HS, Choi DW: Caspase inhibition selectively reduces the apoptotic component of oxygen-glucose deprivation-induced cortical neuronal cell death. Mol Cell Neurosci 9:159–169, 1997.

51. Pellegrini-Giampietro DE, Peruginelli F, Meli E, et al: Protection with metabotropic glutamate 1 receptor antagonists in models of ischemic neuronal death: Time-course and mechanisms. Neuropharmacology 38:1607–1619, 1999.

52. Strasser U, Fischer G: Protection from neuronal damage induced by combined oxygen and glucose deprivation in organotypic hippocampal cultures by glutamate receptor antagonists. Brain Res 687:167–174, 1995.

53. Friedlander RM: Apoptosis and caspases in neurodegenerative diseases. N Engl J Med 348:1365–1375, 2003.

54. Leist M, Jaattela M: Four deaths and a funeral: From caspases to alternative mechanisms. Nat Rev Mol Cell Biol 2:589–598, 2001.

55. Choi DW: Ischemia-induced neuronal apoptosis. Curr Opin Neurobiol 6:667–672, 1996.

56. Colbourne F, Sutherland GR, Auer RN: Electron microscopic evidence against apoptosis as the mechanism of neuronal death in global ischemia. J Neurosci 19:4200–4210, 1999.

57. Banasiak KJ, Xia Y, Haddad GG: Mechanisms underlying hypoxia-induced neuronal apoptosis. Prog Neurobiol 62:215–249, 2000.

58. Kalimo H, Garcia JH, Kamijyo Y, et al: The ultrastructure of "brain death." II: Electron microscopy of feline cortex after complete ischemia. Virchows Arch B Cell Pathol 25:207–220, 1977.

59. Kalimo H, Olsson Y, Paljarvi L, et al: Structural changes in brain tissue under hypoxic-ischemic conditions. J Cereb Blood Flow Metab 2(Suppl 1):S19–S22, 1982.

60. Kirino T, Sano K: Selective vulnerability in the gerbil hippocampus following transient ischemia. Acta Neuropathol (Berl) 62:201–208, 1984.

61. Petito CK, Pulsinelli WA: Sequential development of reversible and irreversible neuronal damage following cerebral ischemia. J Neuropathol Exp Neurol 43:141–153, 1984.

62. Brown AW, Brierley JB: Anoxic-ischaemic cell change in rat brain light microscopic and fine-structural observations. J Neurol Sci 16:59–84, 1972.

63. Brown AW: Structural abnormalities in neurones. J Clin Pathol Suppl (R Coll Pathol) 11:155–169, 1977.

64. Inamura K, Olsson Y, Siesjö BK: Substantia nigra damage induced by ischemia in hyperglycemic rats: A light and electron microscopic study. Acta Neuropathol (Berl) 75:131–139, 1987.

65. Martin-Villalba A, Herr I, Jeremias I, et al: CD95 ligand (Fas L/APO-IL) and tumor necrosis factor-related apoptosis-inducing ligand mediate ischemia-induced apoptosis in neurons. J Neurosci 19:3809–3817, 1999.

66. Fujimura M, Morita-Fujimura Y, Murakami K, et al: Cytosolic redistribution of cytochrome c after transient focal cerebral ischemia in rats. J Cereb Blood Flow Metab 18:1239–1247, 1998.

67. Namura S, Zhu J, Fink K, et al: Activation and cleavage of caspase-3 in apoptosis induced by experimental cerebral ischemia. J Neurosci 18:3659–3668, 1998.

68. Benveniste H, Drejer J, Schousboe A, et al: Elevation of the extracellular concentrations of glutamate and aspartate in rat hippocampus during transient cerebral ischemia monitored by intracerebral microdialysis. J Neurochem 43:1369–1374, 1984.

69. Cardell M, Koide T, Wieloch T: Pyruvate dehydrogenase activity in the rat cerebral cortex following cerebral ischemia. J Cereb Blood Flow Metab 9:350–357, 1989.

70. Tominaga T, Kure S, Narisawa K, et al: Endonuclease activation following focal ischemic injury in the rat brain. Brain Res 608:21–26, 1993.

70a. McLaughlin B, Hartnett KA, Erhardt JA, et al: Caspase-3 activation is essential for neuroprotection in preconditioning. Proc Natl Acad Sci USA 100(2):715–720, 2003.

70b. Garnier P, Ying W, Swanson RA: Ischemic preconditioning by caspase cleavage of poly(ADP-ribose) polymerase-1. J Neurosci 23(22):7967–7973, 2003.

71. Chen J, Nagayama T, Jin K, et al: Induction of caspase-3-like protease may mediate delayed neuronal death in the hippocampus after transient cerebral ischemia. J Neurosci 18:4914–4928, 1998.

72. Chen J, Nagayama T, Jin K, et al: Induction of caspase-3-like protease may mediate delayed neuronal death in the hippocampus after transient cerebral ischemia. J Neurosci 18:4914–4928, 1998.

73. Nicholson DW, Thornberry NA: Caspases: Killer proteases. Trends Biochem Sci 22:299–306, 1997.

74. Cohen GM: Caspases: The executioners of apoptosis. Biochem J 326:1–16, 1997.

75. Kroemer G, Reed JC: Mitochondrial control of cell death. Nat Med 6:513–519, 2000.

76. Burgering BM, Kops GJ: Cell cycle and death control: Long live Forkheads. Trends Biochem Sci 27:352–360, 2002.

77. Cryns V, Yuan J: Proteases to die for. Genes Dev 12:1551–1570, 1998.

78. Jin K, Graham SH, Nagayama T, et al: Altered expression of the neuropeptide-processing enzyme carboxypeptidase E in the rat brain after global ischemia. J Cereb Blood Flow Metab 21:1422–1429, 2001.

79. Bagum MA, Miyamoto O, Toyoshima T, et al: The contribution of low affinity NGF receptor (p75NGFR) to delayed neuronal death

Pathophysiology

after ischemia in the gerbil hippocampus. Acta Med Okayama 55:19–24, 2001.

80. Jover T, Tanaka H, Calderone A, et al: Estrogen protects against global ischemia-induced neuronal death and prevents activation of apoptotic signaling cascades in the hippocampal CA1. J Neurosci 22:2115–2124, 2002.

81. Lee TH, Abe K, Kogure K, et al: Expressions of nerve growth factor and p75 low affinity receptor after transient forebrain ischemia in gerbil hippocampal CA1 neurons. J Neurosci Res 41:684–695, 1995.

82. Krajewski S, Krajewska M, Ellerby LM, et al: Release of caspase-9 from mitochondria during neuronal apoptosis and cerebral ischemia. Proc Natl Acad Sci U S A 96:5752–5757, 1999.

83. MacManus JP, Buchan AM, Hill IE, et al: Global ischemia can cause DNA fragmentation indicative of apoptosis in rat brain. Neurosci Lett 164:89–92, 1993.

84. Ouyang YB, Tan Y, Comb M, et al: Survival- and death-promoting events after transient cerebral ischemia: Phosphorylation of Akt, release of cytochrome C and activation of caspase-like proteases. J Cereb Blood Flow Metab 19:1126–1135, 1999.

85. Deveraux QL, Reed JC: IAP family proteins—suppressors of apoptosis. Genes Dev 13:239–252, 1999.

86. Salvesen GS, Duckett CS: IAP proteins: Blocking the road to death's door. Nat Rev Mol Cell Biol 3:401–410, 2002.

87. Salvesen GS, Duckett CS: IAP proteins: Blocking the road to death's door. Nat Rev Mol Cell Biol 3:401–410, 2002.

88. Weissman AM: Themes and variations on ubiquitylation. Nat Rev Mol Cell Biol 2:169–178, 2001.

89. Shi Y: A structural view of mitochondria-mediated apoptosis. Nat Struct Biol 8:394–401, 2001.

90. Hengartner MO: The biochemistry of apoptosis. Nature 407:770–776, 2000.

91. Xue D, Horvitz HR: *Caenorhabditis elegans* CED-9 protein is a bifunctional cell-death inhibitor. Nature 390:305–308, 1997.

92. Shimazaki K, Ishida A, Kawai N: Increase in bcl-2 oncoprotein and the tolerance to ischemia-induced neuronal death in the gerbil hippocampus. Neuroscience Research 20:95–99, 1994.

93. D'Amours D, Desnoyers S, D'Silva I, et al: Poly(ADP-ribosyl)ation reactions in the regulation of nuclear functions. Biochem J 342:249–268, 1999.

94. Folbergrova J, Memezawa H, Smith ML, et al: Focal and perifocal changes in tissue energy state during middle cerebral artery occlusion in normo- and hyperglycemic rats. J Cereb Blood Flow Metab 12:25–33, 1992.

95. Folbergrova J, Zhao Q, Katsura K, et al: N-tert-butyl-alpha-phenylnitrone improves recovery of brain energy state in rats following transient focal ischemia. Proc Natl Acad Sci U S A 92:5057–5061, 1995.

96. Szabo C, Dawson VL: Role of poly(ADP-ribose) synthetase in inflammation and ischaemia-reperfusion. Trends Pharmacol Sci 19:287–298, 1998.

97. Eliasson MJ, Sampei K, Mandir AS, et al: Poly(ADP-ribose) polymerase gene disruption renders mice resistant to cerebral ischemia. Nat Med 3:1089–1095, 1997.

98. Endres M, Wang ZQ, Namura S, et al: Ischemic brain injury is mediated by the activation of poly(ADP-ribose)polymerase. J Cereb Blood Flow Metab 17:1143–1151, 1997.

99. Pieper AA, Walles T, Wei G, et al: Myocardial postischemic injury is reduced by polyADPribose polymerase-1 gene disruption. Mol Med 6:271–282, 2000.

100. Mandir AS, Poitras MF, Berliner AR, et al: NMDA but not non-NMDA excitotoxicity is mediated by poly(ADP-ribose) polymerase. J Neurosci 20:8005–8011, 2000.

101. Zhang J, Dawson VL, Dawson TM, et al: Nitric oxide activation of poly(ADP-ribose) synthetase in neurotoxicity. Science 263:687–689, 1994.

102. Chiarugi A, Moskowitz MA: Cell biology: PARP-1: A perpetrator of apoptotic cell death? Science 297:200–201, 2002.

103. Yu SW, Wang H, Poitras MF, et al: Mediation of poly(ADP-ribose) polymerase-1-dependent cell death by apoptosis-inducing factor. Science 297:259–263, 2002.

104. Choi DW: Calcium-mediated neurotoxicity: Relationship to specific channel types and role in ischemic damage. Trends Neurosci 11:465–469, 1988.

105. Lucas DR, Newhouse JP: The toxic effect of sodium L-glutamate on the inner layers of the retina. Arch Ophthalmol 58:193–201, 1957.

106. Olney JW, Ho OL: Brain damage in infant mice following oral intake of glutamate, aspartate or cysteine. Nature 227:609–611, 1970.

107. Kass IS, Lipton P: Mechanisms involved in irreversible anoxic damage to the in vitro rat hippocampal slice. J Physiol 332:459–472, 1982.

108. Rothman SM: Synaptic activity mediates death of hypoxic neurons. Science 220:536–537, 1983.

109. Rothman SM: The neurotoxicity of excitatory amino acids is produced by passive chloride influx. J Neurosci 5:1483–1489, 1985.

110. Simon RP, Swan JH, Griffiths T, et al: Blockade of N-methyl-D-aspartate receptors may protect against ischemic damage in the brain. Science 226:850–852, 1984.

111. Choi DW: Calcium-mediated neurotoxicity: Relationship to specific channel types and role in ischemic damage. Trends Neurosci 11:465–469, 1988.

112. Tsubokawa H, Oguro K, Masuzawa T, et al: Ca(2+)-dependent non-NMDA receptor-mediated synaptic currents in ischemic CA1 hippocampal neurons. J Neurophysiol 71:1190–1196, 1994.

113. Tsubokawa H, Oguro K, Robinson HP, et al: Intracellular inositol 1,3,4,5-tetrakisphosphate enhances the calcium current in hippocampal CA1 neurones of the gerbil after ischaemia. J Physiol (Lond) 497:67–78, 1996.

114. Oguro K, Nakamura M, Masuzawa T: Histochemical study of Ca(2+)-ATPase activity in ischemic CA1 pyramidal neurons in the gerbil hippocampus. Acta Neuropathol (Berl) 90:448–453, 1995.

115. Choi DW: Calcium: Still center-stage in hypoxic-ischemic neuronal death. Trends Neurosci 18:58–60, 1995.

116. Meldrum B, Garthwaite J: Excitatory amino acid neurotoxicity and neurodegenerative disease. Trends Pharmacol Sci 11:379–387, 1990.

117. Baker AJ, Zornow MH, Scheller MS, et al: Changes in extracellular concentrations of glutamate, aspartate, glycine, dopamine, serotonin, and dopamine metabolites after transient global ischemia in the rabbit brain. J Neurochem 57:1370–1379, 1991.

118. Mitani A, Kataoka K: Critical levels of extracellular glutamate mediating gerbil hippocampal delayed neuronal death during hypothermia: Brain microdialysis study. Neuroscience 42:661–670, 1991.

119. Lee JM, Zipfel GJ, Choi DW: The changing landscape of ischaemic brain injury mechanisms. Nature 399:A7–A14, 1999.

120. Hardingham GE, Fukunaga Y, Bading H: Extrasynaptic NMDARs oppose synaptic NMDARs by triggering CREB shut-off and cell death pathways. Nat Neurosci 5:405–414, 2002.

121. Lonze BE, Riccio A, Cohen S, et al: Apoptosis, axonal growth defects, and degeneration of peripheral neurons in mice lacking CREB. Neuron 34:371–385, 2002.

122. Hardingham GE, Bading H: The yin and yang of NMDA receptor signalling. Trends Neurosci 26:81–89, 2003.

123. Lonze BE, Ginty DD: Function and regulation of CREB family transcription factors in the nervous system. Neuron 35:605–623, 2002.

124. Riccio A, Ginty DD: What a privilege to reside at the synapse: NMDA receptor signaling to CREB. Nat Neurosci 5:389–390, 2002.

125. Yu SP, Canzoniero LM, Choi DW: Ion homeostasis and apoptosis. Curr Opin Cell Biol 13:405–411, 2001.

126. Hollmann M, Hartley M, Heinemann S: Ca2+ permeability of KA-AMPA–gated glutamate receptor channels depends on subunit composition. Science 252:851–853, 1991.

127. Verdoorn TA, Burnashev N, Monyer H, et al: Structural determinants of ion flow through recombinant glutamate receptor channels. Science 252:1715–1718, 1991.

128. Borges K, Dingledine R: AMPA receptors: Molecular and functional diversity. Prog Brain Res 116:153–170, 1998.

129. Friedman LK, Pellegrini-Giampietro DE, Sperber EF, et al: Kainate-induced status epilepticus alters glutamate and GABAA receptor gene expression in adult rat hippocampus: An in situ hybridization study. J Neurosci 14:2697–2707, 1994.

130. Prince HK, Conn PJ, Blackstone CD, et al: Down-regulation of AMPA receptor subunit GluR2 in amygdaloid kindling. J Neurochem 64:462–465, 1995.

131. Tanaka H, Grooms SY, Bennett MV, et al: The AMPAR subunit GluR2: Still front and center-stage. Brain Res 886:190–207, 2000.

132. Pulsinelli W, Sarokin A, Buchan A: Antagonism of the NMDA and non-NMDA receptors in global versus focal brain ischemia. Prog Brain Res 96:125–135, 1993.

133. Sheardown MJ: The pharmacology of AMPA receptors and their antagonists. Stroke 24:I146–I147, 1993.

134. Nurse S, Corbett D: Neuroprotection after several days of mild, drug-induced hypothermia. J Cereb Blood Flow Metab 16:474–480, 1996.

134a. Noh K, Yokota H, Castillo PE, et al: GluR2-lacking, calcium-permeable AMPA receptors in ischemia-induced delayed neuronal death in hippocampal CA1. Society for Neuroscience Abstract, 2002, Program No. 539.4.

135. Weiss JH, Sensi SL: Ca2+-Zn2+ permeable AMPA or kainate receptors: Possible key factors in selective neurodegeneration. Trends Neurosci 23:365–371, 2000.

136. Gorter JA, Petrozzino JJ, Aronica EM, et al: Global ischemia induces downregulation of Glur2 mRNA and increases AMPA receptor-mediated Ca2+ influx in hippocampal CA1 neurons of gerbil. J Neurosci 17:6179–6188, 1997.

137. Oguro K, Oguro N, Kojima T, et al: Knockdown of AMPA receptor GluR2 expression causes delayed neurodegeneration and increases damage by sublethal ischemia in hippocampal CA1 and CA3 neurons. J Neurosci 19:9218–9227, 1999.

138. Ying HS, Weishaupt JH, Grabb M, et al: Sublethal oxygen-glucose deprivation alters hippocampal neuronal AMPA receptor expression and vulnerability to kainate-induced death. J Neurosci 17:9536–9544, 1997.

139. O'Neill MJ, Bogaert L, Hicks CA, et al: LY377770, a novel iGlu5 kainate receptor antagonist with neuroprotective effects in global and focal cerebral ischaemia. Neuropharmacology 39:1575–1588, 2000.

140. Furukawa K, Fu W, Li Y, et al: The actin-severing protein gelsolin modulates calcium channel and NMDA receptor activities and vulnerability to excitotoxicity in hippocampal neurons. J Neurosci 17:8178–8186, 1997.

141. Chen ZL, Strickland S: Neuronal death in the hippocampus is promoted by plasmin-catalyzed degradation of laminin. Cell 91:917–925, 1997.

142. Choi DW: Cerebral hypoxia: Some new approaches and unanswered questions. J Neurosci 10:2493–2501, 1990.

143. Rothman SM, Olney JW: Glutamate and the pathophysiology of hypoxic-ischemic brain damage. Ann Neurol 19:105–111, 1986.

144. Siesjö BK, Bengtsson F: Calcium fluxes, calcium antagonists, and calcium-related pathology in brain ischemia, hypoglycemia, and spreading depression: A unifying hypothesis. J Cereb Blood Flow Metab 9:127–140, 1989.

145. Tsubokawa H, Oguro K, Robinson HP, et al: Abnormal Ca2+ homeostasis before cell death revealed by whole cell recording of ischemic CA1 hippocampal neurons. Neuroscience 49:807–817, 1992.

146. Takei N, Endo Y: Ca2+ ionophore-induced apoptosis on cultured embryonic rat cortical neurons. Brain Res 652:65–70, 1994.

147. Johnson EM Jr, Koike T, Franklin J: A "calcium set-point hypothesis" of neuronal dependence on neurotrophic factor. Exp Neurol 115:163–166, 1992.

148. Juin P, Pelletier M, Oliver L, et al: Induction of a caspase-3-like activity by calcium in normal cytosolic extracts triggers nuclear apoptosis in a cell-free system. J Biol Chem 273:17559–17564, 1998.

149. Gaido ML, Cidlowski JA: Identification, purification, and characterization of a calcium-dependent endonuclease (NUC18) from apoptotic rat thymocytes. NUC18 is not histone H2B. J Biol Chem 266:18580–18585, 1991.

150. Choi DW, Koh JY: Zinc and brain injury. Annu Rev Neurosci 21:347–375, 1998.

151. Palmiter RD, Cole TB, Quaife CJ, et al: ZnT-3, a putative transporter of zinc into synaptic vesicles. Proc Natl Acad Sci U S A 93:14934–14939, 1996.

152. Assaf SY, Chung SH: Release of endogenous Zn2+ from brain tissue during activity. Nature 308:734–736, 1984.

153. Howell GA, Welch MG, Frederickson CJ: Stimulation-induced uptake and release of zinc in hippocampal slices. Nature 308:736–738, 1984.

154. Li Y, Hough CJ, Frederickson CJ, et al: Induction of mossy fiber → Ca3 long-term potentiation requires translocation of synaptically released Zn2+. J Neurosci 21:8015–8025, 2001.

155. Aniksztejn L, Charton G, Ben Ari Y: Selective release of endogenous zinc from the hippocampal mossy fibers in situ. Brain Res 404:58–64, 1987.

156. Sloviter RS: A selective loss of hippocampal mossy fiber Timm stain accompanies granule cell seizure activity induced by perforant path stimulation. Brain Res 330:150–153, 1985.

157. Yanamoto H, Nagata I, Sakata M, et al: Infarct tolerance induced by intra-cerebral infusion of recombinant brain-derived neurotrophic factor. Brain Res 859:240–248, 2000.

158. Weiss JH, Hartley DM, Koh JY, et al: AMPA receptor activation potentiates zinc neurotoxicity. Neuron 10:43–49, 1993.

159. Koh JY, Suh SW, Gwag BJ, et al: The role of zinc in selective neuronal death after transient global cerebral ischemia. Science 272:1013–1016, 1996.

160. Grooms SY, Opitz T, Bennett MV, et al: Status epilepticus decreases glutamate receptor 2 mRNA and protein expression in hippocampal pyramidal cells before neuronal death. Proc Natl Acad Sci U S A 97:3631–3636, 2000.

161. Koh JY, Choi DW: Zinc alters excitatory amino acid neurotoxicity on cortical neurons. J Neurosci 8:2164–2171, 1988.

162. Weiss JH, Turetsky D, Wilke G, et al: AMPA/kainate receptor-mediated damage to NADPH-diaphorase-containing neurons is Ca2+ dependent. Neurosci Lett 167:93–96, 1994.

163. Harris RJ, Symon L, Branston NM, et al: Changes in extracellular calcium activity in cerebral ischaemia. J Cereb Blood Flow Metab 1:203–209, 1981.

164. Gido G, Kristian T, Siesjö BK: Extracellular potassium in a neocortical core area after transient focal ischemia. Stroke 28:206–210, 1997.

165. Nedergaard M, Hansen AJ: Characterization of cortical depolarizations evoked in focal cerebral ischemia. J Cereb Blood Flow Metab 13:568–574, 1993.

166. Nicotera P, Leist M, Fava E, et al: Energy requirement for caspase activation and neuronal cell death. Brain Pathol 10:276–282, 2000.

167. Harris RJ, Symon L: Extracellular pH, potassium, and calcium activities in progressive ischaemia of rat cortex. J Cereb Blood Flow Metab 4:178–186, 1984.

168. Hengartner MO: The biochemistry of apoptosis. Nature 407:770–776, 2000.

169. Wang HG, Pathan N, Ethell IM, et al: Ca2+-induced apoptosis through calcineurin dephosphorylation of BAD. Science 284:339–343, 1999.

170. Baranano DE, Ferris CD, Snyder SH: Atypical neural messengers. Trends Neurosci 24:99–106, 2001.

171. Bredt DS, Ferris CD, Snyder SH: Nitric oxide synthase regulatory sites. Phosphorylation by cyclic AMP-dependent protein kinase, protein kinase C, and calcium/calmodulin protein kinase: Identification of flavin and calmodulin binding sites. J Biol Chem 267:10976–10981, 1992.

172. Garthwaite J: Glutamate, nitric oxide and cell-cell signalling in the nervous system. Trends Neurosci 14:60–67, 1991.

173. Kumura E, Yoshimine T, Iwatsuki KI, et al: Generation of nitric oxide and superoxide during reperfusion after focal cerebral ischemia in rats. Am J Physiol 270:C748–C752, 1996.

174. Liu PK, Grossman RG, Hsu CY, et al: Ischemic injury and faulty gene transcripts in the brain. Trends Neurosci 24:581–588, 2001.

175. Bolanos JP, Heales SJ, Land JM, et al: Effect of peroxynitrite on the mitochondrial respiratory chain: Differential susceptibility of neurones and astrocytes in primary culture. J Neurochem 64:1965–1972, 1995.

176. Liu PK, Arora T: Transcripts of damaged genes in the brain during cerebral oxidative stress. J Neurosci Res 70:713–720, 2002.

177. Love S: Oxidative stress in brain ischemia. Brain Pathol 9:119–131, 1999.

178. Chan PH: Reactive oxygen radicals in signaling and damage in the ischemic brain. J Cereb Blood Flow Metab 21:2–14, 2001.

179. Aronowski J, Strong R, Grotta JC: Citicoline for treatment of experimental focal ischemia: histologic and behavioral outcome. Neurol Res 18:570–574, 1996.

180. Aguilar HI, Botla R, Arora AS, et al: Induction of the mitochondrial permeability transition by protease activity in rats: A mechanism of hepatocyte necrosis. Gastroenterology 110:558–566, 1996.

181. Sensi SL, Yin HZ, Carriedo SG, et al: Preferential Zn2+ influx through Ca2+-permeable AMPA/kainate channels triggers prolonged mitochondrial superoxide production. Proc Natl Acad Sci U S A 96:2414–2419, 1999.

182. Zolotarjova N, Ho C, Mellgren RL, et al: Different sensitivities of native and oxidized forms of Na+/K(+)-ATPase to intracellular proteinases. Biochim Biophys Acta 1192:125–131, 1994.

183. Liu PK: Ischemia-reperfusion-related repair deficit after oxidative stress: Implications of faulty transcripts in neuronal sensitivity after brain injury. J Biomed Sci 10:4–13, 2003.

Pathophysiology

184. Back T, Zhao W, Ginsberg MD: Three-dimensional image analysis of brain glucose metabolism-blood flow uncoupling and its electrophysiological correlates in the acute ischemic penumbra following middle cerebral artery occlusion. J Cereb Blood Flow Metab 15:566–577, 1995.

185. Back T, Ginsberg MD, Dietrich WD, et al: Induction of spreading depression in the ischemic hemisphere following experimental middle cerebral artery occlusion: Effect on infarct morphology. J Cereb Blood Flow Metab 16:202–213, 1996.

186. Baker CJ, Fiore AJ, Frazzini VI, et al: Intraischemic hypothermia decreases the release of glutamate in the cores of permanent focal cerebral infarcts. Neurosurgery 36:994–1001, 1995.

187. Baimbridge KG, Celio MR, Rogers JH: Calcium-binding proteins in the nervous system. Trends Neurosci 15:303–308, 1992.

188. Ashkenazi A, Dixit VM: Death receptors: Signaling and modulation. Science 281:1305–1308, 1998.

189. Sheng M, Greenberg ME: The regulation and function of c-fos and other immediate early genes in the nervous system. Neuron 4:477–485, 1990.

190. Sasaki M, Gonzalez-Zulueta M, Huang H, et al: Dynamic regulation of neuronal NO synthase transcription by calcium influx through a CREB family transcription factor-dependent mechanism. Proc Natl Acad Sci U S A 97:8617–8622, 2000.

191. Tao X, Finkbeiner S, Arnold DB, et al: Ca2+ influx regulates BDNF transcription by a CREB family transcription factor-dependent mechanism. Neuron 20:709–726, 1998.

192. Kornhauser JM, Cowan CW, Shaywitz AJ, et al: CREB transcriptional activity in neurons is regulated by multiple, calcium-specific phosphorylation events. Neuron 34:221–233, 2002.

193. Mattson MP, Camandola S: NF-kappaB in neuronal plasticity and neurodegenerative disorders. J Clin Invest 107:247–254, 2001.

194. Schneider A, Martin-Villalba A, Weih F, et al: NF-kappaB is activated and promotes cell death in focal cerebral ischemia. Nat Med 5:554–559, 1999.

195. Brunet A, Datta SR, Greenberg ME: Transcription-dependent and -independent control of neuronal survival by the PI3K-Akt signaling pathway. Curr Opin Neurobiol 11:297–305, 2001.

196. Datta SR, Brunet A, Greenberg ME: Cellular survival: A play in three Akts. Genes Dev 13:2905–2927, 1999.

197. Kaplan DR, Miller FD: Neurotrophin signal transduction in the nervous system. Curr Opin Neurobiol 10:381–391, 2000.

198. Brunet A, Datta SR, Greenberg ME: Transcription-dependent and -independent control of neuronal survival by the PI3K-Akt signaling pathway. Curr Opin Neurobiol 11:297–305, 2001.

199. Chong JA, Tapia-Ramirez J, Kim S, et al: REST: A mammalian silencer protein that restricts sodium channel gene expression to neurons. Cell 80:949–957, 1995.

200. Schoenherr CJ, Paquette AJ, Anderson DJ: Identification of potential target genes for the neuron-restrictive silencer factor. Proc Natl Acad Sci U S A 93:9881–9886, 1996.

201. Schoenherr CJ, Anderson DJ: Silencing is golden: Negative regulation in the control of neuronal gene transcription. Curr Opin Neurobiol 5:566–571, 1995.

202. Roopra A, Sharling L, Wood IC, et al: Transcriptional repression by neuron-restrictive silencer factor is mediated via the Sin3-histone deacetylase complex. Mol Cell Biol 20:2147–2157, 2000.

203. Chen ZF, Paquette AJ, Anderson DJ: NRSF/REST is required in vivo for repression of multiple neuronal target genes during embryogenesis [see comments]. Nat Genet 20:136–142, 1998.

204. Ballas N, Battaglioli E, Atouf F, et al: Regulation of neuronal traits by a novel transcriptional complex. Neuron 31:353–365, 2001.

205. Bahn S, Mimmack M, Ryan M, et al: Neuronal target genes of the neuron-restrictive silencer factor in neurospheres derived from fetuses with Down's syndrome: A gene expression study. Lancet 359:310–315, 2002.

206. Okazaki T, Wang H, Masliah E, et al: SCG10, a neuron-specific growth-associated protein in Alzheimer's disease. Neurobiol Aging 16:883–894, 1995.

207. Lawinger P, Venugopal R, Guo ZS, et al: The neuronal repressor REST/NRSF is an essential regulator in medulloblastoma cells. Nat Med 6:826–831, 2000.

208. Calderone A, Jover T, Noh KM, et al: Ischemic insults derepress the gene silencer REST in neurons destined to die. J Neurosci 23:2112–2121, 2003.

209. Iadecola C: Bright and dark sides of nitric oxide in ischemic brain injury. Trends Neurosci 20:132–139, 1997.

210. Dirnagl U, Iadecola C, Moskowitz MA: Pathobiology of ischaemic stroke: An integrated view. Trends Neurosci 22:391–397, 1999.

211. Ishibashi N, Prokopenko O, Reuhl KR, et al: Inflammatory response and glutathione peroxidase in a model of stroke. J Immunol 168:1926–1933, 2002.

212. Stevens SL, Bao J, Hollis J, et al: The use of flow cytometry to evaluate temporal changes in inflammatory cells following focal cerebral ischemia in mice. Brain Res 932:110–119, 2002.

213. Sharp FR, Massa SM, Swanson RA: Heat-shock protein protection. Trends Neurosci 22:97–99, 1999.

214. Kiessling M, Stumm G, Xie Y, et al: Differential transcription and translation of immediate early genes in the gerbil hippocampus after transient global ischemia. J Cereb Blood Flow Metab 13:914–924, 1993.

215. Dragunow M, Beilharz E, Sirimanne E, et al: Immediate-early gene protein expression in neurons undergoing delayed death, but not necrosis, following hypoxic-ischaemic injury to the young rat brain. Brain Res Mol Brain Res 25:19–33, 1994.

216. Parsell DA, Lindquist S: The function of heat-shock proteins in stress tolerance: Degradation and reactivation of damaged proteins. Annu Rev Genet 27:437–496, 1993.

217. Beere HM: Stressed to death: Regulation of apoptotic signaling pathways by the heat shock proteins. Sci STKE 93:RE1, 2001.

218. Papadopoulos M, Sun X, Cao J, et al: Over-expression of HSP-70 protects astrocytes from combined oxygen-glucose deprivation. Neuroreport 7:429–432, 1996.

219. Plumier J, Krueger A, Currie R, et al: Transgenic mice expressing the human inducible HSP70 have hippocampal neurons resistant to ischemic injury. Cell Stress Chaperones 2:162–167, 1997.

220. Wagstaff M, Collaco-Moraes Y, Smith J, et al: Protection of neuronal cells from apoptosis by HSP27 delivered with a herpes simplex virus-based vector. J Biol Chem 274:5069, 1999.

221. Yenari MA, Fink SL, Sun G, et al: Gene therapy with HSP72 is neuroprotective in rat models of stroke and epilepsy. Ann Neurol 44:584–591, 1998.

222. Kinouchi H, Sharp FR, Koistinaho J, et al: Induction of heat shock HSP70 mRNA and HSP70 kDa protein in neurons in the "penumbra" following focal cerebral ischemia in the rat. Brain Res 619:334–338, 1993.

223. Li Y, Chopp M, Zhang ZG, et al: Neuronal survival is associated with 72-kDa heat shock protein expression after transient middle cerebral artery occlusion in the rat. J Neurol Sci 120:187–194, 1993.

224. Bruey JM, Ducasse C, Bonniaud P, et al: Hsp27 negatively regulates cell death by interacting with cytochrome c. Nat Cell Biol 2:645–652, 2000.

225. Pandey P, Saleh A, Nakazawa A, et al: Negative regulation of cytochrome c-mediated oligomerization of Apaf-1 and activation of procaspase-9 by heat shock protein 90. EMBO J 19:4310–4322, 2000.

226. Saleh A, Srinivasula SM, Balkir L, et al: Negative regulation of the Apaf-1 apoptosome by HSP70. Nat Cell Biol 2:476–483, 2000.

227. Rajdev S, Hara K, Kokubo Y, et al: Mice overexpressing rat heat shock protein 70 are protected against cerebral infarction. Ann Neurol 47:782–791, 2000.

228. Lee S-H, Kim M, Yoon B-W, et al: Targeted HSP70.1 disruption increases infarction volume after focal cerebral ischemia in mice. Stroke 32:2905–2912, 2001.

229. Hoehn B, Ringer TM, Xu L, et al: Overexpression of HSP72 after induction of experimental stroke protects neurons from ischemic damage. J Cereb Blood Flow Metab 11:1303–1309, 2001.

230. James MF, Smith JM, Boniface SJ, et al: Cortical spreading depression and migraine: New insights from imaging? Trends Neurosci 24:266–271, 2001.

231. Theis M, Jauch R, Zhuo L, et al: Accelerated hippocampal spreading depression and enhanced locomotory activity in mice with astrocyte-directed inactivation of connexin43. J Neurosci 23:766–776, 2003.

232. Crowder RJ, Freeman RS: Phosphatidylinositol 3-kinase and Akt protein kinase are necessary and sufficient for the survival of nerve growth factor-dependent sympathetic neurons. J Neurosci 18:2933–2943, 1998.

233. Kuruvilla R, Ye H, Ginty DD: Spatially and functionally distinct roles of the PI3-K effector pathway during NGF signaling in sympathetic neurons. Neuron 27:499–512, 2000.

Pathophysiology

234. Philpott KL, McCarthy MJ, Klippel A, et al: Activated phosphatidylinositol 3-kinase and Akt kinase promote survival of superior cervical neurons. J Cell Biol 139:809–815, 1997.

235. Rosenmund C, Westbrook GL: Calcium-induced actin depolymerization reduces NMDA channel activity. Neuron 10:805–814, 1993.

236. Yao R, Cooper GM: Requirement for phosphatidylinositol-3 kinase in the prevention of apoptosis by nerve growth factor. Science 267:2003–2006, 1995.

237. Yuan J, Yankner BA: Apoptosis in the nervous system. Nature 407:802–809, 2000.

238. Pearson G, Robinson F, Beers GT, et al: Mitogen-activated protein (MAP) kinase pathways: Regulation and physiological functions. Endocr Rev 22:153–183, 2001.

239. Bonni A, Brunet A, West AE, et al: Cell survival promoted by the Ras-MAPK signaling pathway by transcription-dependent and—independent mechanisms. Science 286:1358–1362, 1999.

240. Nandagopal K, Dawson TM, Dawson VL: Critical role for nitric oxide signaling in cardiac and neuronal ischemic preconditioning and tolerance. J Pharmacol Exp Ther 297:474–478, 2001.

241. McBain CJ, Fisahn A: Interneurons unbound. Nat Rev Neurosci 2:11–23, 2001.

242. Galarreta M, Hestrin S: Electrical synapses between GABA-releasing interneurons. Nat Rev Neurosci 2:425–433, 2001.

243. Bennett MV, Barrio LC, Bargiello TA, et al: Gap junctions: New tools, new answers, new questions. Neuron 6:305–320, 1991.

244. Bruzzone R, White TW, Paul DL: Connections with connexins: The molecular basis of direct intercellular signaling. Eur J Biochem 238:1–27, 1996.

245. Dermietzel R, Spray DC: From neuro-glue ('Nervenkitt') to glia: A prologue. Glia 24:1–7, 1998.

246. Goodenough DA, Goliger JA, Paul DL: Connexins, connexons, and intercellular communication. Annu Rev Biochem 65:475–502: 475–502, 1996.

247. Kunzelmann P, Blumcke I, Traub O, et al: Coexpression of connexin45 and -32 in oligodendrocytes of rat brain. J Neurocytol 26:17–22, 1997.

248. Li J, Hertzberg EL, Nagy JI: Connexin32 in oligodendrocytes and association with myelinated fibers in mouse and rat brain. J Comp Neurol 379:571–591, 1997.

249. Rash JE, Staines WA, Yasumura T, et al: Immunogold evidence that neuronal gap junctions in adult rat brain and spinal cord contain connexin-36 but not connexin-32 or connexin-43. Proc Natl Acad Sci U S A 97:7573–7578, 2000.

250. Sohl G, Degen J, Teubner B, et al: The murine gap junction gene connexin36 is highly expressed in mouse retina and regulated during brain development. FEBS Lett 428:27–31, 1998.

251. Gibson JR, Beierlein M, Connors BW: Two networks of electrically coupled inhibitory neurons in neocortex. Nature 402:75–79, 1999.

252. Venance L, Rozov A, Blatow M, et al: Connexin expression in electrically coupled postnatal rat brain neurons. Proc Natl Acad Sci U S A 97:10260–10265, 2000.

252a. Oguro K, Jover T, Tanaka H: Global ischemia-induced increases in the gap junctional proteins connexin 3 (Cx32) and Cx36 in hippocampus and enhanced vulnerability of Cx32 knock out mice. J Neurosci 21(19):7534–7542, 2001.

253. Sutor B, Schmolke C, Teubner B, et al: TI-myelination defects and neuronal hyperexcitability in the neocortex of connexin 32-deficient mice. Cereb Cortex 10:684–697, 2000.

254. Haydon PG: Neuroglial networks: Neurons and glia talk to each other. Curr Biol 10:R712–R714, 2000.

255. Haydon PG: GLIA: Listening and talking to the synapse. Nat Rev Neurosci 2:185–193, 2001.

256. Lin B, Ginsberg MD, Busto R: Hyperglycemic exacerbation of neuronal damage following forebrain ischemia: Microglial, astrocytic and endothelial alterations. Acta Neuropathol (Berl) 96:610–620, 1998.

257. Rawanduzy A, Hansen A, Hansen TW, et al: Effective reduction of infarct volume by gap junction blockade in a rodent model of stroke. J Neurosurg 87:916–920, 1997.

258. Warner DS, Ludwig PS, Pearlstein R, et al: Halothane reduces focal ischemic injury in the rat when brain temperature is controlled. Anesthesiology 82:1237–1245, 1995.

259. Saito R, Graf R, Hubel K, et al: Reduction of infarct volume by halothane: Effect on cerebral blood flow or perifocal spreading depression-like depolarizations. J Cereb Blood Flow Metab 17:857–864, 1997.

260. Eckenstein FP: Fibroblast growth factors in the nervous system. J Neurobiol 25:1467–1480, 1994.

261. Kitagawa K, Matsumoto M, Kuwabara K, et al: 'Ischemic tolerance' phenomenon detected in various brain regions. Brain Res 561:203–211, 1991.

262. Liu Y, Kato H, Nakata N, et al: Protection of rat hippocampus against ischemic neuronal damage by pretreatment with sublethal ischemia. Brain Res 586:121–124, 1992.

263. Nishi S, Taki W, Uemura Y, et al: Ischemic tolerance due to the induction of HSP70 in a rat ischemic recirculation model. Brain Res 615:281–288, 1993.

264. Simon RP, Niiro M, Gwinn R: Prior ischemic stress protects against experimental stroke. Neurosci Lett 163:135–137, 1993.

265. Wu C, Zhan RZ, Qi S, et al: A forebrain ischemic preconditioning model established in C57Black/Crj6 mice. J Neurosci Methods 107:101–106, 2001.

266. Kirino T: Ischemic tolerance. J Cereb Blood Flow Metab 22:1283–1296, 2002.

267. Chow AK, Thompson CS, Hogan MJ, et al: Cortical spreading depression transiently activates MAP kinases. Brain Res Mol Brain Res 99:75–81, 2002.

268. Obrenovitch TP, Urenjak J, Wang M: Nitric oxide formation during cortical spreading depression is critical for rapid subsequent recovery of ionic homeostasis. J Cereb Blood Flow Metab 22:680–688, 2002.

269. Behl C: Oestrogen as a neuroprotective hormone. Nat Rev Neurosci 3:433–442, 2002.

270. McEwen B, Akama K, Alves S, et al: Tracking the estrogen receptor in neurons: Implications for estrogen-induced synapse formation. Proc Natl Acad Sci U S A 98:7093–7100, 2001.

271. Hurn PD, Macrae IM: Estrogen as a neuroprotectant in stroke. J Cereb Blood Flow Metab 20:631–652, 2000.

272. Culmsee C, Vedder H, Ravati A, et al: Neuroprotection by estrogens in a mouse model of focal cerebral ischemia and in cultured neurons: Evidence for a receptor-independent antioxidative mechanism. J Cereb Blood Flow Metab 19:1263–1269, 1999.

273. Dubal DB, Kashon ML, Pettigrew LC, et al: Estradiol protects against ischemic injury. J Cereb Blood Flow Metab 18:1253–1258, 1998.

274. Dubal DB, Zhu H, Yu J, et al: Estrogen receptor alpha, not beta, is a critical link in estradiol-mediated protection against brain injury. Proc Natl Acad Sci U S A 98:1952–1957, 2001.

275. Dubal DB, Wise PM: Neuroprotective effects of estradiol in middle-aged female rats. Endocrinology 142:43–48, 2001.

276. Rusa R, Alkayed NJ, Crain BJ, et al: 17beta-estradiol reduces stroke injury in estrogen-deficient female animals. Stroke 30:1665–1670, 1999.

277. Toung TJ, Traystman RJ, Hurn PD: Estrogen-mediated neuroprotection after experimental stroke in male rats. Stroke 29:1666–1670, 1998.

278. Dubal DB, Zhu H, Yu J, et al: Estrogen receptor alpha, not beta, is a critical link in estradiol-mediated protection against brain injury. Proc Natl Acad Sci U S A 98:1952–1957, 2001.

279. Dubal DB, Shughrue PJ, Wilson ME, et al: Estradiol modulates bcl-2 in cerebral ischemia: A potential role for estrogen receptors. J Neurosci 19:6385–6393, 1999.

280. Chen J, Adachi N, Liu K, et al: The effects of 17beta-estradiol on ischemia-induced neuronal damage in the gerbil hippocampus. Neuroscience 87:817–822, 1998.

281. Sudo S, Wen TC, Desaki J, et al: Beta-estradiol protects hippocampal CA1 neurons against transient forebrain ischemia in gerbil. Neurosci Res 29:345–354, 1997.

282. Kondo Y, Suzuki K, Sakuma Y: Estrogen alleviates cognitive dysfunction following transient brain ischemia in ovariectomized gerbils. Neurosci Lett 238:45–48, 1997.

283. McKenna NJ, O'Malley BW: Combinatorial control of gene expression by nuclear receptors and coregulators. Cell 108:465–474, 2002.

284. Nilsson S, Makela S, Treuter E, et al: Mechanisms of estrogen action. Physiol Rev 81:1535–1565, 2001.

285. Kelly MJ, Levin ER: Rapid actions of plasma membrane estrogen receptors. Trends Endocrinol Metab 12:152–156, 2001.

286. Harms C, Lautenschlager M, Bergk A, et al: Differential mechanisms of neuroprotection by 17beta-estradiol in apoptotic versus necrotic neurodegeneration. J Neurosci 21:2600–2609, 2001.

Pathophysiology

287. Honda K, Sawada H, Kihara T, et al: Phosphatidylinositol 3-kinase mediates neuroprotection by estrogen in cultured cortical neurons. J Neurosci Res 60:321–327, 2000.

288. Mendez P, Azcoitia I, Garcia-Segura LM: Estrogen receptor alpha forms estrogen-dependent multimolecular complexes with insulin-like growth factor receptor and phosphatidylinositol 3-kinase in the adult rat brain. Brain Res Mol Brain Res 112:170–176, 2003.

289. Canzoniero LM, Turetsky DM, Choi DW: Measurement of intra-cellular free zinc concentrations accompanying zinc-induced neuronal death. J Neurosci 19:RC31, 1999.

290. Colbourne F, Sutherland G, Corbett D: Postischemic hypothermia: A critical appraisal with implications for clinical treatment. Mol Neurobiol 14:171–201, 1997.

291. Colbourne F, Li H, Buchan AM: Indefatigable CA1 sector neuro-protection with mild hypothermia induced 6 hours after severe forebrain ischemia in rats. J Cereb Blood Flow Metab 19:742–749, 1999.

292. Sonn J, Granot E, Etziony R, et al: Effect of hypothermia on brain multi-parametric activities in normoxic and partially ischemic rats. Comp Biochem Physiol A Mol Integr Physiol 132:239–246, 2002.

293. Kimura T, Sako K, Tanaka K, et al: Effect of mild hypothermia on energy state recovery following transient forebrain ischemia in the gerbil. Exp Brain Res 145:83–90, 2002.

Pathophysiology

Chapter Forty-Three

Apoptosis in Cerebral Ischemia

Turgay Dalkara and Michael A. Moskowitz

PATHWAYS OF ISCHEMIC CELL DEATH

We have just begun to understand the basic pathways of ischemic neuronal death. Research over the past three decades has identified several mechanisms that can irreversibly damage brain tissue after ischemia, such as intracellular calcium overload, excitotoxicity, oxygen free radicals, excess generation of nitric oxide (NO), and peroxynitrite formation.[1,2] It is now generally accepted that although some cells readily die by swelling, osmotic disruption, and necrosis at the onset of focal ischemia, other cells die by apoptosis, and still others through a combination of apoptosis and necrosis.[3,4] The necrotic phenotype becomes more prevalent as the intensity and duration of ischemia increase (i.e., permanent focal ischemia and brief, transient focal ischemia form the two extremes of necrotic and apoptotic phenotypes, respectively).

Evidence now suggests, however, that apoptotic cell death and necrotic cell death are not entirely independent.[5-8] Early phases of cell death may involve a common pathway; when energy levels are severely compromised, cells dying by apoptosis may divert to dying instead by necrosis. Similarly, when cells dying by necrosis are incompletely treated, they may die by apoptosis. Growing evidence indicates that programmed cell death (PCD) has more than one apoptotic phenotype as well, interestingly, as a necrotic-like phenotype.[9] In these several types of cell death, the master control appears to be operating at the mitochondrial level.[10] Mitochondria can promote apoptotic and necrotic pathways, depending on the severity of insult.[11] After moderate but irreversible injury, mitochondria retain their membrane potential (at least partially) so they can continue synthesizing adenosine triphosphate (ATP), but they release cytochrome *c* and other pro-apoptotic factors to initiate apoptosis. Severe injury leads to loss of mitochondrial membrane potential, swelling and rupture of the inner and outer mitochondrial membranes, collapse of oxidative phosphorylation, and, hence, necrosis. Opening of the mitochondrial permeability transition pore triggers necrotic cell death through the loss of homeostasis and intramitochondrial milieu, although its role in inducing apoptosis by releasing mitochondrial macromolecules into cytoplasm is probably less important.[11-13] A considerable body of knowledge has now accumulated that establishes a role for oxidative stress, calcium overload, NO and peroxynitrite, cellular swelling, and inflammatory mediators in triggering apoptotic as well as necrotic pathways of cell death. In this chapter, we focus on the role of apoptotic mechanisms in ischemic cell demise within the brain.

MOLECULAR MECHANISMS OF APOPTOSIS

Apoptosis, a form of PCD, is biochemically and morphologically distinct from necrotic cell death.[14-16] Apoptosis requires expression of a set of genes and proteins and is characterized by internucleosomal cleavage of DNA, margination and condensation of chromatin in the nucleus, shrinkage of cytoplasm, and preservation of membrane integrity and mitochondrial ultrastructure. Eventually, the cell disintegrates with formation of apoptotic bodies, which are phagocytosed by neighboring cells, resident macrophages, and microglia without an overt inflammatory reaction. In contrast, necrotic cells die through swelling, rupture, loss of membrane integrity, and inflammation; DNA strands are randomly broken rather than precisely cleaved at internucleosomal linker points. The accidental form of necrotic death is considered to be most probably a passive process involving activation of only constitutively expressed enzymes with lytic activity, although damaged cells initially express some survival genes and proteins in an attempt to interrupt cell death.[9]

Apoptosis is the main form of cell death during development.[14,17] A great number of cells are eliminated during fetal life in this way. Involution of tissues like the thymus and pineal gland in adults also occurs via apoptosis, as does the death of rapidly dividing cell populations such as intestinal villi.[13,18] For proliferative tissues to maintain a constant size, older cells die by apoptosis. Similarly, cells die by apoptosis during regression of hyperplastic tissues, such as after liver hyperplasia induced by various chemicals. There is increasing evidence that apoptosis is implicated in neurodegenerative processes (e.g. Alzheimer's, Huntington's, and Parkinson's diseases; spinal muscular atrophy; amyotrophic lateral sclerosis),[19,20] although the role of apoptosis in these pathologic processes is still a matter of considerable controversy. One factor contributing to the controversy is that apoptotic cell demise is difficult to detect because it occurs rapidly over several hours. Given the longevity of neurons, cellular injury might build up over time to reach a threshold above which executioner programs are activated and promote the accelerated death of cells.[9]

Apoptosis may be triggered by developmental and environmental cues and is regulated by a complex balance between life- and death-promoting factors.[20] In the nematode *Caenorhabditis elegans*, the organism in which PCD has been extensively studied and which has become a prototype for understanding apoptosis in mammalians, apoptosis is regulated by a balance between the *ced-3* (cell death-3) and *ced-9* genes. The *ced-3* gene is indispensable for activating a cell death cascade, whereas the *ced-9* gene blocks PCD.[21,22] Another gene, *ced-4*, is also required for *ced-3* to execute cell death.

Caspases are a family of Ced-3 homologues in mammalian cells that dismantle a group of proteins essential for cell survival.[23] The mammalian counterpart of the anti-apoptotic *ced-9* gene is the *bcl-2* gene family, which has antiapoptotic as well as pro-apoptotic members. In mammalian cells, not only is each gene family diversified, but also several other pathways trigger cell death.[24] For example, death signals can be transduced from the extracellular medium into the cell via cell surface death receptors. Death-signaling cascades may also be initiated intracellularly from mitochondria, damaged DNA, or endoplasmic reticulum. In mammalian cells, mitochondria control apoptosis by sequestering apoptogenic proteins between the inner and outer mitochondrial membranes and then release them through pores or rupture of the outer mitochondrial membrane in the presence of apoptotic signaling.[10]

Mitochondrial Pathway

The interactions between the pro-apoptotic and anti-apoptotic Bcl-2 family proteins on the outer mitochondrial membrane are believed to play an important role in making the life-or-death "decision."[11,13] Normally, anti-apoptotic members such as Bcl-2 and Bcl-x_L are located on membranes of mitochondria, endoplasmic reticulum, and nucleus, and they protect mitochondria against several forms of injury, presumably by preventing release of apoptogenic mediators and, perhaps, opening of the permeability transition pore.[10,25]

Proapoptotic members such as Bax, Bad, and Bid are situated in the cytoplasm and are translocated to mitochondria on receiving death signals. Several mechanisms, such as dephosphorylation of Bad that is sequestered in the cytoplasm by the 14-3-3 protein and cleavage of Bid, may promote this translocation.[26,27] Activation of c-Jun N-terminal kinase (JNK) phosphorylates c-JUN, which in turn activates Bax via expression of DP5/Hrk, a Bcl-2 family protein.[20] Formation of homodimers and heterodimers among Bcl-2 family members on the outer mitochondrial membrane controls the release of proteins from the mitochondria, such as cytochrome *c*, apoptosis-inducing factor (AIF), endonuclease G (EndoG), and Smac/DIABLO.[10] Cytochrome *c*, deoxyadenosine triphosphate (dATP), and Apaf-1, the mammalian homologue of Ced-4,[28] form the apoptosome complex and catalyze conversion of pro-caspase-9 to its active form (Fig. 43–1).[10] Activated caspase-9 in turn cleaves and activates procaspase-3. Neurons can survive release of cytochrome *c* if apoptosis inhibitor proteins (IAP, NAIP, XIAP, survivin),[29] which suppress the caspase system, are not inactivated by the mitochondrial protein Smac/DIABLO.[10] AIF and EndoG migrate to the nucleus to degrade DNA.

How AIF initiates DNA fragmentation remains unclear.[10,30] AIF causes a lumpy and peripheral type of chromatin condensation and the formation of large DNA fragments that are independent of caspase activation; hence, AIF-induced PCD is called "caspase-independent apoptosis." Strong chromatin compaction characteristic of caspase activity is not seen after AIF-induced apoptosis.[10,31] Deficiency of AIF has profound effects during animal development; without this factor, the apoptosis necessary for the cavitation of embryoid bodies, which is essential for mouse morphogenesis, does not occur.[32] Unlike caspase homologues, AIF homologues are found in all metazoan kingdoms (animal, plant, and fungi), suggesting that AIF could be one of the phylogenetically oldest death effectors known.[31] Yu and colleagues[33] reported that activation of the DNA repair enzyme poly(ADP-ribose) polymerase-1 (PARP-1) after damage to DNA triggers release of AIF and, hence, promotes PCD through a caspase-independent pathway.

Death Receptor–Mediated Pathway

Cell surface receptors mediate apoptosis in a diverse set of disease states ranging from autoimmunity and acquired immunodeficiency syndrome (AIDS) to cancer.[9,34,35] These receptors, which belong to the tumor necrosis factor receptor (TNFR) superfamily, include TNFR-1, FAS (CD95/Apo-1), and p75^{NTR}. Death receptors share an evolutionarily conserved homologous amino acid sequence called the "death domain," through which they bind to death domain–containing adaptor molecules such as FADD (FAS-associating protein with death domain) and TRADD (TNFR-associating protein with death domain). Adaptor proteins also contain another sequence called the "death-effector domain," which binds to procaspase-8 by interacting with its death-effector domain.[36] On activation, FAS forms a death-inducing signaling complex (DISC) with FADD and procaspase-8 (see Fig. 43–1).[37,38] Binding of FAS ligand or TNF-α to their receptors leads to their oligomerization, which recruits and binds procaspase-8 and promotes its autoactivation. Active caspase-8 is released from the DISC complex and initiates downstream cleavage of caspase-3 by direct or mitochondrial-dependent mechanisms.[39] Bid, a cytosolic member of the Bcl-2 family of proapoptotic proteins, is cleaved by caspase-8 (see Fig. 43–1).[26,40] The truncated active form of Bid targets the outer mitochondrial membrane and induces release of cytochrome *c* by promoting pore formation via conformational changes in Bak and Bad within mitochondrial membranes.[41,42] In addition, activated caspase-3 may cleave procaspase-8, thereby amplifying the death process.[43]

Death receptors can also participate in necrosis.[9] That TNF-induced death can initiate either apoptosis or necrosis is well documented, and FAS receptor has also been shown to induce necrosis-like PCD.[9,44,45] To add to the

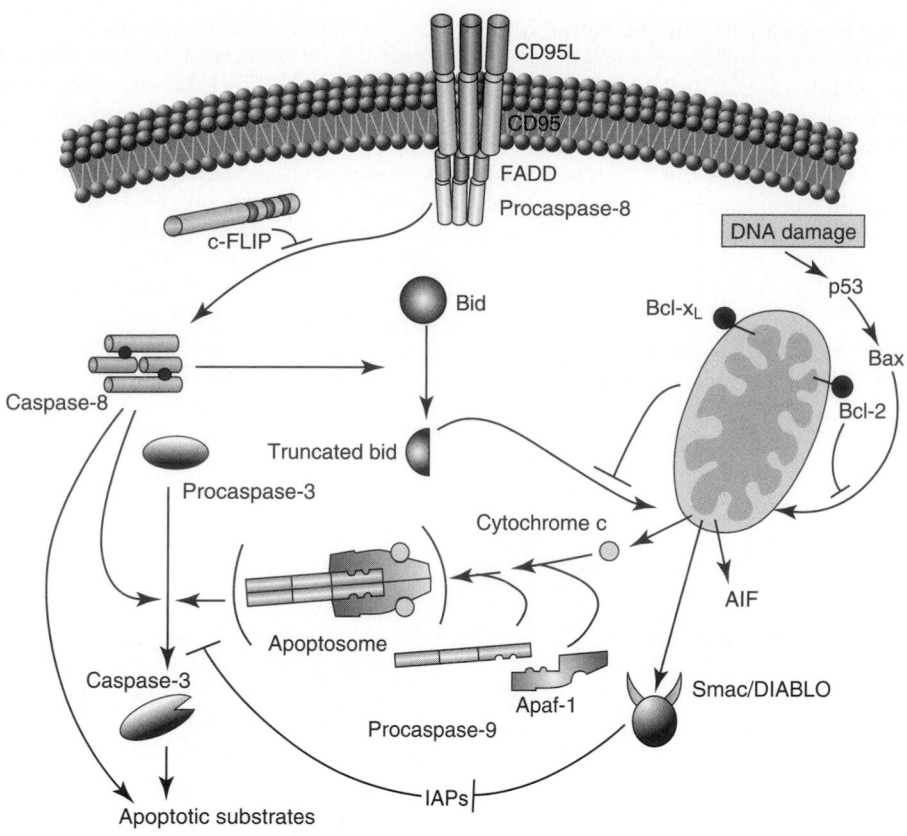

FIGURE 43–1 *The mitochondrial pathway* (right) *is initiated through the activation of proapoptotic members of the BCL-2 family, such as Bax, Bad, Bim, and Bid. On receiving proapoptotic signals, proapoptotic members are translocated to the mitochondria from cytosol, where they interact with antiapoptotic members like Bcl-2 and Bcl-x_L. This interaction leads to release of proteins such as cytochrome c, apoptosis-inhibiting factor (AIF), and Smac/DIABLO from the mitochondria. Cytochrome c associates with Apaf-1 and then procaspase-9 to form the apoptosome complex and activate caspase-9. Caspase-9, in turn, cleaves and activates procaspase-3. Caspase-3 activation and activity are antagonized by the inhibitors of apoptosis (IAPs), which themselves are inhibited by the Smac/DIABLO protein released from mitochondria. Active caspase-3 performs the ordered dismantling and removal of the cell.*

The death-receptor pathway is triggered by members of the death-receptor superfamily, such as CD95/FAS. Binding of CD95/FAS ligand induces receptor clustering and formation of a death-inducing signaling complex (DISC). This complex recruits multiple procaspase-8 molecules via the adaptor molecule FADD, resulting in caspase-8 activation. Caspase-8, in turn, cleaves and activates procaspase-3. Caspase-8 activation can be blocked by recruitment of the c-FLIP protein to the DISC.

Cross-talk between the death-receptor and mitochondrial pathways is provided by Bid, a proapoptotic Bcl-2 family member. Caspase-8-mediated cleavage of Bid results in its translocation to mitochondria and release of cytochrome c. (Redrawn from Hengartner MO: The biochemistry of apoptosis. Nature 407:770–776, 2000.)

complexity, FADD blocks TNFR-1–induced necrosis, probably by activating caspase-8.[45,46] So FADD might be a decision point between apoptotic and necrotic pathways triggered by TNF.[9] Similarly, the FAS inhibitor protein FLIP serves as a switch between cell proliferation and death signaling: When FLIP levels are low, caspase-8 is recruited to the DISC upon activation of FAS receptors.[35] In contrast, when FLIP levels are high, FLIP may outcompete procaspase-8 by preferentially binding to FADD and, hence, divert signals toward cell proliferation via the ERK and NF-κB pathways.

Nuclear Pathway

DNA damage, if irreparable, may activate the apoptotic suicide program, especially in cells with high replicative capacity. Kinases such as ATM, DNA-PKcs, and ATR

monitor and detect DNA damage.[47,48] On activation, ATM phosphorylates several cell cycle checkpoint proteins, including p53, to promote cell death.[49] In response to DNA damage, p53 stops the cell cycle in dividing cells. If the DNA damage is irreparable, p53 triggers apoptosis in part by promoting Bax expression. The short half-life of p53 is prolonged upon ATM-induced phosphorylation. Phosphorylated p53 cannot bind to Mdm2, a major inhibitor of p53 that binds to it and targets it for ubiquitin-mediated degradation.[50] Stabilized p53 upregulates expression of several modulators of the cell cycle (e.g., p21, GADD45, 14-3-3 proteins) as well as proapoptotic proteins such as Bax, Apaf-1, and death receptors, whereas it represses expression of the *bcl-2* gene.

DNA damage also leads to activation of the nuclear DNA repair enzyme PARP-1. PARP is a caspase substrate; however, studies on PARP knockout mice suggest that its cleavage is not essential for apoptosis.[51] Rapid activation of the enzyme in cells under stress depletes the cell of nicotinamide adenine dinucleotide (NAD) and ATP, which may result in cell death favoring a necrotic phenotype owing to collapse of energy metabolism.[52] Other evidence suggests, however, that PARP might also control the fate of cell death by regulating transcription factors such as NF-κB and p53 and by promoting release of mitochondrial AIF.[33,53,54]

Cell Survival Pathways

Cell death and cell survival pathways converge and interact at several points. For example, overexpression of

Bcl-2 not only inhibits apoptosis but also supports cell survival in response to a wide variety of insults as well as necrotic death.[55,56] Like all cells, neurons require trophic support for survival. Neuronal survival pathways are generally induced by the binding of neurotrophins (NTs) to tyrosine kinase receptors, which in turn activate phosphoinositide 3-kinase (PI3K) and the mitogen-activated protein kinase (MAPK) pathway (Fig. 43–2).[20,57] Activated PI3K phosphorylates Akt (protein kinase B), which suppresses expression of proapoptotic genes such as FAS ligand by activating forkhead transcription factors. Akt phosphorylates and inactivates the proapoptotic factors Bad and procaspase-9.[58,59] Phosphorylation of transcription factor

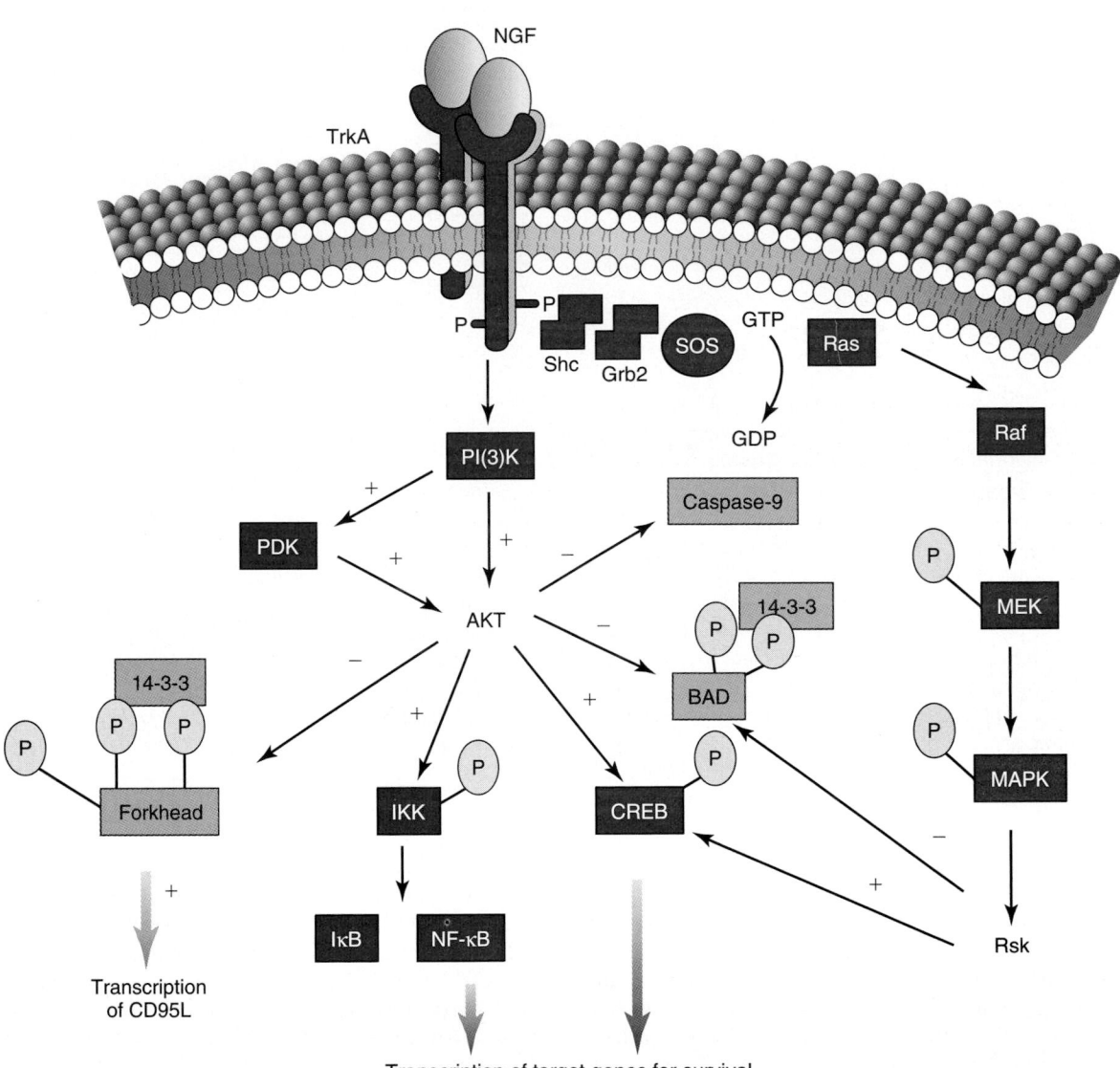

FIGURE 43–2 *Neuronal survival pathways are induced by the binding of nerve growth factor (NGF) to its receptor TrkA (tyrosine kinase A). NGF induces the autophosphorylation of TrkA, which activates phosphoinositide 3-kinase (PI(3)K) and the adaptor protein Shc. Activated PI(3)K phosphorylates Akt and phosphoinositide-dependent kinase (PDK), which in turn phosphorylates and activates Akt (protein kinase B). The phosphorylation of CREB and inhibitor kappa-B kinase (IKK) stimulates the transcription of prosurvival factors; whereas the phosphorylation of Bad, forkhead transcription factor, and caspase-9 inhibits the pro-apoptotic pathway. The interaction of Shc-Grb2 and SOS activates the mitogen-activated protein kinase (MAPK) pathway, resulting in the activation of Rsk. Proteins Bad and CREB are also the targets of Rsk that might act synergistically with Akt. (Redrawn from Yuan J, Yankner B: Apoptosis in the nervous system. Nature 407:802–809, 2000.)*

CREB and IκB kinase (IκB is the inhibitor of transcription factor NF-κB) stimulates the transcription of pro-survival factors such as Bcl-2. Triggering of the MAPK pathway by tyrosine kinase receptors leads to the activation of pp90 ribosomal S6 kinase pathway (Rsk), which phosphorylates Bad and CREB and, hence, acts synergistically with Akt. For example, basic fibroblast growth factor (bFGF) hinders the release of the pro-apoptotic Bcl-2 family member Bad that is sequestered by cytoplasmic 14-3-3 protein.[58] In addition, bFGF prevents translocation of Bad to mitochondria via the neurotrophin receptor–PI3K–Akt pathway and the MAPK pathway.[58] Basic FGF has also been shown to stimulate de novo synthesis of Bcl-x_L through activation of MAPK by phosphorylation of CREB.[60,61]

The PI3K-Akt pathway can also promote cell survival by decreasing transcription of FAS receptor and activating the transcription factor.[57] On stimulation, NF-κB dissociates from IκB and is translocated to the nucleus, where it activates anti-apoptotic or pro-apoptotic genes, depending on the circumstances in which it is activated.[62] However, NTs may protect cells against death via more than a single mechanism. For instance, bFGF may decrease N-methyl-D-aspartate (NMDA) receptor–mediated influx and excitotoxicity of Ca^{2+} and may upregulate the expression of free radical scavenging enzymes.[63,64] The stimulus for necrosis is thus diminished, as is the development of apoptosis for those cells less severely affected.

APOPTOSIS IN CEREBRAL ISCHEMIA

Linnik and associates[65] provided early pharmacologic evidence for involvement of PCD in cerebral ischemia based on the ability of the protein synthesis inhibitor cycloheximide to reduce brain injury. Cellular features of apoptosis have been documented after focal and global ischemia, including cytoplasmic shrinkage, chromatin condensation, nuclear segmentation, and apoptotic bodies,[66–69] although electron-microscopic studies indicate that ischemic neuronal death is characterized by a mixture of apoptotic and necrotic changes in ultrastructure.[70–72] Nevertheless, a substantial reduction in infarct volume after treatment by caspase inhibitors strongly suggests that the apoptotic cascade is activated in injured surviving cells.[74,99] Some biochemical markers conventionally thought to indicate necrosis (e.g., cathepsins, calpain) are also activated in ischemic cells, however, and inhibition of the markers confers resistance to ischemic injury, suggesting a complex interplay between apoptotic and necrotic death pathways in cerebral ischemia.[75,76]

DNA laddering, a biochemical hallmark of apoptotic cell death, was shown by gel electrophoresis along with terminal deoxynucleotidyl transferase–mediated deoxyuridine triphosphate (dUTP)–biotin nick-end labeling (TUNEL) staining.[65,68,77–82] Several markers of DNA damage–induced apoptosis (upregulation of p53, growth arrest and DNA damage protein 45 [GADD45], and MdM2) have also been detected in ischemic brains.[83] PARP is activated and NAD^+ levels become depleted in ischemic brain within minutes of reperfusion after occlusion of the middle cerebral artery (MCA). Inhibition of PARP activation or disruption of the *parp* gene confers protection after brain ischemia.[84,85] Ischemic neurons attempt to reenter the cell cycle after the loss of control over mitotic machinery in these terminally differentiated cells.[86] Upregulation of Bax, downregulation of Bcl-2/Bcl-x_L levels, and formation of Bax/Bcl-x_L dimers have also been demonstrated in early hours of ischemia, findings that may account for the activation of the mitochondrial pathway.[66,87–89] Events that occur downstream of the formation of Bax/Bcl-x_L dimers, such as release of cytochrome *c* from mitochondria and activation of caspase-9 and caspase-3, have been detected as well.[90–94]

CASPASE-MEDIATED CELL DEATH

With few exceptions, apoptosis in mammalian cells depends on the activation of caspases.[9,13,20,95] As alluded to previously, activation of caspases can be mediated through several pathways encompassing death receptors, mitochondria, DNA, or endoplasmic reticulum. In all apoptotic pathways, a group of caspases called "executioner caspases" appear to dismantle several cellular structures by their proteolytic activity once they are activated. Most of the 14 caspases discovered, except caspase-11 and caspase-12, are constitutively expressed as pro-enzymes (zymogens) in humans.[13,95] Caspases 1 through 3 and 7 through 9 have been detected in the brain. Caspase-1 (interleukin-converting enzyme [ICE]) family members—caspases 1, 4, and 5—are pro-inflammatory and pro-apoptotic. However, caspase-3 (CPP32) family members—caspases 2, 3, and 6 through 9—mediate apoptosis only. Caspases with death-effector domains (8 and 10) are activated after being recruited to death receptor complexes. Caspases with short prodomains (3, 6, and 7) are cleaved and activated by other caspases. Caspases with caspase-activating recruitment domains (CARDs), such as caspase-9, are probably activated after binding to a molecular complex such as apoptosome.

Caspase activity requires heterodimerization of the large and small cleavage products. Caspases have a catalytic site that contains a highly conserved sequence (QACXG) and cleave proteins at one or more sites but always after an aspartate residue.[95] They have a wide range of substrates, cleavage of which produces morphologic features characteristic of apoptosis. For example, caspase-mediated disintegration of the nuclear lamins may account for nuclear pyknosis and budding, whereas cleavage of cytoskeletal proteins like gelsolin, actin, and fodrin may cause cell shrinkage, and cleavage of the kinase PAK2 may mediate blebbing.[13] Caspase-3 cleaves the inhibitory subunit of the caspase-activated DNase (CAD) by translocating to the nucleus from cytoplasm.[96] CAD cleaves DNA at internucleosomal linker points, yielding multiple integers of 180 base-pair fragments that form the DNA ladder seen on DNA gel electrophoresis.

Caspase Activation During Focal and Global Ischemia

A considerable body of evidence suggests that caspase-1 and caspase-3 are processed after focal cerebral ischemia.[73,97–99] Hara and colleagues[73] found immunoreactive caspase-1 cleavage products (p20 and p10 bands) on

Pathophysiology

Western blot analyses in a 2-hour reversible filament occlusion model of focal ischemic injury. They also reported that interleukin-1β (IL-1β) levels peaked in brain 30 minutes to 1 hour after reperfusion and then decreased; this finding suggests that ICE (caspase-1) was transiently activated upon reperfusion. In line with these findings, mutant mice that are deficient in *ice* gene expression or that express a dominant negative ICE mutation are more resistant to ischemic.[73,100] However, IL-1β causes inflammation as well as apoptosis. Hence, it was difficult to establish whether ICE inhibition of inflammation or apoptosis or both were protective in these experiments.

The role of caspase-3 has been more convincingly characterized in focal ischemic brain damage. Asahi and coworkers[101] demonstrated upregulation of rat caspase-3 messenger RNA (mRNA) 1 hour after the induction of permanent ischemia. Namura and associates provided evidence for caspase-3 activation in the mouse brain subjected to 2-hour MCA occlusion.[91] They detected caspase-3 and its cleavage products (p20) in ischemic brain tissue soon after reperfusion. Caspase-like enzyme activity was also elevated for the first 3 hours of reperfusion. Cleavage of gelsolin, a substrate of caspase-like proteases, was detected by 6 hours of reperfusion, along with DNA laddering and positive response to TUNEL staining.[102] The p20 cleavage product (active caspase-3) was frequently visualized within TUNEL-positive cells, a finding that may account for CAD activation and DNA fragmentation. Cleavage of several other substrates of caspase activity (actin, PARP) have also been detected in brains after ischemia.[85,89,102] Hence, ischemia is accompanied by a time-dependent evolution of the mitochondrial apoptotic pathway, characterized by changes in Bcl-2 family proteins, cytochrome *c* release, caspase-like enzyme activation, and an associated increase in the cleaved active form (caspase-3 p20), which are followed several hours later by morphologic features of apoptosis and DNA fragmentation. The pace of caspase activation depends on the duration and severity of the insult. After brief periods of focal ischemia, caspase activation develops as late as 9 hours after reperfusion along with the appearance of caspase-3-p20 immunoreactive cleavage product.[103]

Detection of caspase-8 cleavage product in neurons suggests that death receptors are also activated upon ischemic injury.[93,104] In line with these findings, inhibition of TNF and FAS directly blocks stroke-related damage in addition to reducing secondary inflammatory injury.[105] Mice expressing dysfunctional FAS (CD95) ligand and TNF knockout mice demonstrate smaller infarcts after MCA occlusion.[106,107] Strikingly, hybrid mice lacking both cytokines showed a 93% reduction in infarct volume. A similar protection was observed in wild-type mice treated with antibodies that neutralize FAS ligand and TNF.[105] These remarkable findings underscore the role of death receptors in ischemic cell death.[108]

Death receptors may be activated by cytokines released from granulocytes infiltrating the infarct or by microglia that are activated within the first hours of ischemia.[109] The resistance of Bid knockout mice to ischemia suggests that there is cross-talk between the death receptor–induced and mitochondrial pathways during ischemic cell death.[110] Bid, after being cleaved by caspase-8, translocates to the

outer mitochondrial membrane and induces conformational changes in Bak and Bax; by so doing, it initiates cytochrome *c* release and caspase-3–mediated apoptosis.[26,40,111] Caspase-11 is upregulated and cleaved 12 hours after permanent ischemia.[112] A murine caspase not found in humans, caspase-11 appears uniquely able to bind and cleave caspase-1 as well as caspase-3, hence promoting both cytokine maturation and apoptosis.[94] Studies using a positional scanning combinatorial library method found that the optimal cleavage site of caspase-11 is (Ile/Leu/Val/Pro)EHD, similar to that of upstream caspases such as caspase-8 and caspase-9.[94] Caspase-11 knockout mice showed reduced caspase-3 cleavage within the ischemic cortex.[94] Contrary to activation of caspases 1, 3, 7, 8, and 9 with cerebral ischemia-reperfusion, caspase-2 protein levels remain unchanged after cerebral ischemia in the mouse. Also, mice deficient in caspase-2 are not protected from focal ischemic brain damage, despite the finding that caspase-2 mRNA is upregulated after 8 hours of transient focal and transient global ischemia.[101,113,114]

Similar changes have been reported in models of global ischemia. Caspase-3 is cleaved and activated, DNA laddering and positive response to TUNEL staining appear, and cells are protected by caspase inhibition.[74,115,116] Bhat and colleagues[117] found increases in caspase-1 mRNA and its corresponding protein within microglia of gerbil hippocampus several days after brief global ischemia. Other groups reported increased gene expression of caspases 2, 3, and 8 during the late stages of ischemia.[74,115,118–120] A change favoring Bax over Bcl-2 family proteins was convincingly documented in global ischemia.[66] Cytochrome *c* release was detected in hippocampal neurons after a global ischemic insult.[121–123] Caspase-9 activation and formation of apoptosome were also demonstrated.[92,124]

APOPTOSIS IN SPINAL CORD ISCHEMIA

Cell death due to spinal cord ischemia is also mediated in part by apoptotic mechanisms. Matsushita and coworkers[104] found that, as early as 90 minutes after transient ischemia, activated caspase-8 (p18) appeared within neurons in intermediate gray matter and in medial ventral horn. Cleaved caspase-8 appeared before the activation of caspase-3 and colocalized with FAS on motoneurons, possibly by formation of a DISC. The appearance of cytosolic cytochrome *c* and gelsolin cleavage along with numerous TUNEL-positive neurons containing cleaved forms of caspase-8 and caspase-3 were detected. These findings are consistent with the concept that transient spinal cord ischemia induces the formation of a DISC, which may participate in caspase-8 activation and sequential caspase-3 cleavage.

INHIBITION OF APOPTOTIC PATHWAYS REDUCES ISCHEMIC DAMAGE

Overexpression of anti-apoptotic proteins (e.g., Bcl-2) or knocking out of genes that encode pro-apoptotic proteins (e.g., Bid, Bax, p53, caspase-3, caspase-11) in transgenic animals confers resistance to ischemia,[20,94,125,126] emphasizing the role of apoptotic mechanisms in ischemic cell death. Similarly, pharmacologic inhibition of caspase activity leads to a reduction in cell death in focal as well global ischemia[74,99] and appears to be a promising therapeutic target. Loddick and associates[97] and Hara and colleagues[99] reported that z-VAD and z-DEVD, peptide inhibitors of caspases, protected brain from ischemic injury and improved neurologic deficits in rats and mice. Peptide inhibitors given intraventricularly afforded protection against loss of cells in the CA1 subfield of the hippocampus during global ischemia, and treated animals displayed a better performance on memory tests.[74,127]

Caspase inhibitors were effective if administered up to 1 hour after reperfusion following 2-hour MCA occlusion. After milder ischemia (30 minutes), z-DEVD-fmk protected the brain when injected up to 9 hours after restoration of blood flow.[103] The 9-hour treatment window corresponded to the onset of both DEVDase activation and caspase-3 cleavage, suggesting that activation of events downstream from caspase-3 may represent irreversible injury and that activation of execution caspases evolves slowly with delayed therapeutic opportunity in mild ischemia. In more severe ischemia (2 hours of occlusion), caspase inhibitors block cell death up to 2 hours after ischemia.[99,128] Although longer than for NMDA receptor antagonists, this time window is still shorter than desirable for clinical practice.

A synergy has been reported between an NMDA receptor antagonist and caspase inhibitors.[129] Not only did combination of subthreshold doses of the two agents protect against ischemia, but also the therapeutic window for caspase administration was extended. A similar synergy was also observed between a growth factor (bFGF) and caspase inhibitors.[130] The importance of interactions between survival factors and ischemic cell death is further exemplified by studies reporting that neurotrophin 4 (NT 4) and brain-derived neurotrophic factor (BDNF) exert a protective influence in cerebral ischemia, because mice lacking one allele of BDNF or both alleles of NT 4 are more vulnerable to ischemic injury.[131] Exogenous administration of NT 4 or BDNF, both of which bind to the TrkB (tyrosine kinase B) receptor, are also found to be protective in models of cerebral ischemia.[132–135]

APOPTOSIS IN HUMAN BRAIN

Most apoptosis-related proteins are expressed in the normal human brain (Table 43.1), suggesting a potential role for these proteins in disease. It should be noted, however, that cell death phenotypes may significantly vary according to the species, age, cell type, triggering factors, and coexisting conditions. Therefore, the biochemical characteristics of cell death in humans after ischemia, which may be different from that observed in experimental animals, need to be clarified. Love and colleagues[136] examined the brains of 35 patients who died of focal ischemic stroke. The group detected an early increase in pro-caspase-3 immunoreactivity followed by appearance of TUNEL-positive neurons especially at the edge of the

Table 43.1 Apoptosis-Related Proteins Detected in Normal Human Brain

Protein	Study(ies) Reporting Detection
Bcl-2 family	
Bcl-2	Marshall et al (1997),[144] Su et al (1997),[145] Vyas et al (1997),[146] Yachnis et al (1997),[147] Desjardins and Ledoux, (1998),[148] Kitamura et al (1998),[149] Clark et al (1999),[150] Henshall et al (2000),[151] Jarskog and Gilmore (2000)[152]
Bcl-x	Yachnis et al (1997),[147] Kitamura et al (1998)[149]
Mcl-1	Desjardins and Ledoux (1998)[148]
Bax	Su et al (1997),[145] Desjardins and Ledoux (1998),[148] Kitamura et al (1998),[149] Tatton (2000),[153] Engidawork et al (2001),[154] Hartmann et al (2001)[155]
Bad	Kitamura et al (1998)[149]
Bak	Kitamura et al (1998)[149]
Bim	Engidawork et al (2001)[154]
Caspases	
Caspase-1	Clark et al (1999),[150] Henshall et al (2000)[151]
Caspase-3	Engidawork et al (2001),[156] Clark et al (1999),[150] Hartmann et al (2000),[157] Henshall et al (2000)[151]
Caspase-8	Rohn et al (2001)[158]
Caspase-9	Engidawork et al (2001)[156]
Others	
Apaf-1	Engidawork et al (2001)[156]
Fas	Nishimura et al (1995),[159] de la Monte et al (1997),[160] Ferrer et al (2001)[161]
FLIP	Engidawork et al (2001),[156] Gulesserian et al (2001)[162]
DR-3,4,5	Newman et al (2000),[163] Dorr et al (2002)[143]
p53	de la Monte et al (1997)[160]
DFF45	Engidawork et al (2001),[156] Gulesserian et al (2001)[162]

infarct. Despite findings suggesting PCD activation in brain infarcts, the morphologic changes they observed were not those of classic apoptosis. These researchers also showed that the TUNEL labeling they observed was probably mediated by the release of endogenous endonucleases during protease or microwave pretreatment of the damaged tissue. Another study has also reported colocalization of TNF-α with TUNEL staining in neurons from autopsy specimens collected from patients with stroke.[137] DNA fragmentation was also detected by in situ nick-end labeling in cerebellar granular cells after global ischemia in two autopsy cases.[138]

Some of the biochemical steps of apoptosis may be activated in postmortem tissue.[136] Cell death may also be triggered in vulnerable neurons as a result of metabolic derangements during the premortem period.[139] Despite uncertainties in interpreting the data obtained from postmortem material, many studies performed on autopsy material have provided confirmation, such as colocalization of apoptotic changes with specific disease in contrast to generalized nonspecific activation of cell death in diverse cellular groups (Table 43.2). Studies performed on brain biopsy specimens, which lack some of the problems encountered with postmortem tissue, have more convincingly demonstrated apoptotic cell death in human neurodegenerative diseases.[140–143] These and other studies

Pathophysiology

Table 43.2 **Apoptotic Biochemical Alterations Detected in Human Brain**

Insultor Condition	Bcl-2 Family[*]	Caspase Activation[†]	DNA Fragmentation[‡]	Other[§]
Alzheimer's disease	O'Barr et al (1996)[164] Su et al (1997)[145]	Stadelmann et al (1999)[165] Rohn et al (2001)[158,168]	Su et al (1994)[166] Anderson et al (1996)[167]	Anderson et al (1996)[67] **(c-Jun)** de la Monte et al (1997)[160] **(p53 & Fas)**
			Su et al (1997)[145]	Yang et al (1998)[169] **(cleaved actin)** Rohn et al (2001)[158,168] **(cleaved fodrin)** Newman et al (2000)[163] **(death receptor-3)**
Parkinson's disease	Marshall et al (1997)[144] Tatton (2000)[153] Hartmann et al (2001)[155]	Hartmann et al (2000)[157] Tatton (2000)[153] Hartmann et al (2001)[155]	Mochizuki et al (1996)[170] Tatton (2000)[53]	—
Huntington's disease	—	—	Dragunow et al (1995)[171] Portera-Cailliau et al (1995)[172] Butterworth et al (1998)[173]	—
Acquired immunodeficiency syndrome	—	Garden et al (2002)[174]	Adle-Biassette et al (1995)[175] Shi et al (1996)[176]	—
Trauma (head injury)	Clark et al (1999)[150]	Clark et al (1999)[150]	Clark et al (1999)[150] Smith et al (2000)[178] Williams et al (2001)[179]	Qui et al (2002)[177] **(Fas and DISC)**

[*]Alterations detected in various members of the Bcl-2 family.
[†]Cleaved active forms of one or more caspases detected.
[‡]Usually detected with TUNEL method.
[§]Several other biochemical markers of apoptosis detected; specified in parentheses.

indicate that human brain cells have the potential to die by apoptotic mechanisms.

References

1. Dirnagl U, Iadecola C, Moskowitz MA: Pathobiology of ischaemic stroke: An integrated view. Trends Neurosci 22:391–397, 1999.
2. Lipton P: Ischemic cell death in brain neurons. Physiol Rev 79:1431–1568, 1999.
3. Schulz JB, Weller M, Moskowitz MA: Caspases as treatment targets in stroke and neurodegenerative diseases. Ann Neurol 45:421–429, 1999.
4. Graham SH, Chen J: Programmed cell death in cerebral ischemia. J Cereb Blood Flow Metab 21:99–109, 2001.
5. Hirsch T, Marchetti P, Susin SA, et al: The apoptosis-necrosis paradox: Apoptogenic proteases activated after mitochondrial permeability transition determine the mode of cell death. Oncogene 15:1573–1581, 1997.
6. Martin LJ, Al-Abdulla NA, Brambrink AM, et al: Neurodegeneration in excitotoxicity, global cerebral ischemia, and target deprivation: A perspective on the contributions of apoptosis and necrosis. Brain Res Bull 46:281–309, 1998.
7. Nicotera PLM, Manzo L: Neuronal death: A demise with different shapes. Trends Pharmacol Sci 20:46–51, 1999.
8. MacManus JP, Buchan AM: Apoptosis after experimental stroke: Fact or FAShion? J Neurotrauma 17:899–914, 2000.
9. Leist M, Jaattela M: Four deaths and a funeral: From caspases to alternative mechanisms. Nat Rev Mol Cell Biol 2:589–598, 2001.
10. Wang X: The expanding role of mitochondria in apoptosis. Genes Dev 15:2922–2933, 2001.
11. Kroemer G, Reed JC: Mitochondrial control of cell death. Nat Med 6:513–519, 2000.
12. Fiskum G: Mitochondrial participation in ischemic and traumatic neural cell death. J Neurotrauma 17:843–855, 2000.
13. Hengartner MO: The biochemistry of apoptosis. Nature 407:770–776, 2000.
14. Kerr JF, Wyllie AH, Currie A: Apoptosis: A basic biological phenomenon with wide-ranging implications in tissue kinetics. Br J Cancer 26:239–257, 1972.
15. Wyllie AH, Kerr JF, Currie AR: Cell death: The significance of apoptosis. Int Rev Cytol 68:251–306, 1980.
16. Majno G, Joris I: Apoptosis, oncosis, and necrosis: An overview of cell death. Am J Pathol 146:3–15, 1995.
17. Meier P, Finch A, Evan G: Apoptosis in development. Nature 407:796–801, 2000.
18. Renehan AG, Bach SP, Potten CS: The relevance of apoptosis for cellular homeostasis and tumorigenesis in the intestine. Can J Gastroenterol 15:166–76, 2001.
19. Mattson MP: Apoptosis in neurodegenerative disorders. Nat Rev Mol Cell Biol 1:120–129, 2000.
20. Yuan J, Yankner BA: Apoptosis in the nervous system. Nature 407:802–809, 2000.
21. Yuan JY, Horvitz HR: The *Caenorhabditis elegans* genes ced-3 and ced-4 act cell autonomously to cause programmed cell death. Dev Biol 138:33–41, 1990.
22. Metzstein MM, Stanfield GM, Horvitz HR: Genetics of programmed cell death in *C. elegans*: Past, present and future. Trends Genet 14:410–416, 1998.
23. Yuan J, Shaham S, Ledoux S, et al: The *C. elegans* cell death gene ced-3 encodes a protein similar to mammalian interleukin-1 beta-converting enzyme. Cell 75:641–652, 1993.
24. Joza N, Kroemer G, Penninger JM: Genetic analysis of the mammalian cell death machinery. Trends Genet 18:142–149, 2002.
25. Murphy AN, Fiskum G, Beal MF: Mitochondria in neurodegeneration: Bioenergetic function in cell life and death. J Cereb Blood Flow Metab 19:231–245, 1999.
26. Li H, Zhu H, Xu CJ, et al: Cleavage of BID by caspase 8 mediates the mitochondrial damage in the FAS pathway of apoptosis. Cell 94:491–501, 1998.
27. Wang HG, Pathan N, Ethell M, et al: Ca++ induced apoptosis through calcineurin dephosphorylation of BAD. Science 284:339–343, 1999.

28. Zou H, Henzel WJ, Liu X, et al: Apaf-1, a human protein homologous to *C. elegans* CED-4, participates in cytochrome c-dependent activation of caspase-3. Cell 90:405–13, 1997.

29. Stennicke HR, Ryan CA, Salvesen GS: Reprieval from execution: The molecular basis of caspase inhibition. Trends Biochem Sci 27:94–101, 2002.

30. Susin SA, Lorenzo HK, Zamzami N, et al: Molecular characterization of mitochondrial apoptosis-inducing factor. Nature 397:441–446, 1999.

31. Lorenzo HK, Susin SA, Penninger J, et al: Apoptosis inducing factor (AIF): A phylogenetically old, caspase-independent effector of cell death. Cell Death Differ 6:516–524, 1999.

32. Joza N, Susin SA, Daugas E, et al: Essential role of the mitochondrial apoptosis-inducing factor in programmed cell death. Nature 410:549–554, 2001.

33. Yu SW, Wang H, Poitras MF, et al: Mediation of poly(ADP-ribose) polymerase-1-dependent cell death by apoptosis-inducing factor. Science 297:259–263, 2002.

34. Eguchi K: Apoptosis in autoimmune diseases. Intern Med 40:275–284, 2001.

35. Budd RC: Death receptors couple to both cell proliferation and apoptosis. J Clin Invest 109:437–441, 2002.

36. Itoh N, Nagata S: A novel protein domain required for apoptosis: Mutational analysis of human FAS antigen. J Biol Chem 268:10932–10937, 1993.

37. Kischkel FC, Hellbardt S, Behrmann I, et al: Cytotoxicity-dependent APO-1 (FAS/CD95)-associated proteins form a death-inducing signaling complex (DISC) with the receptor. EMBO J 14:5579–5588, 1995.

38. Medema JP, Scaffidi C, Kischkel FC, et al: FLICE is activated by association with the CD95 death-inducing signaling complex (DISC). EMBO J 16:2794–2804, 1997.

39. Stennicke HR, Jurgensmeier JM, Shin H, et al: Pro-caspase-3 is a major physiologic target of caspase-8. J Biol Chem 273:27084–27090, 1998.

40. Luo X, Budihardjo I, Zou H, et al: Bid, a Bcl2 interacting protein, mediates cytochrome c release from mitochondria in response to activation of cell surface death receptors. Cell 94:481–490, 1998.

41. Korsmeyer SJ, Wei MC, Saito M, et al: Pro-apoptotic cascade activates BID, which oligomerizes BAK or BAX into pores that result in the release of cytochrome c. Cell Death Differ 7:1166–1173, 2000.

42. Wei MC, Zong WX, Cheng EH, et al: Proapoptotic BAX and BAK: A requisite gateway to mitochondrial dysfunction and death. Science 292:727–730, 2001.

43. Slee EA, Harte MT, Kluck RM, et al: Ordering the cytochrome c-initiated caspase cascade: Hierarchical activation of caspases-2, -3, -6, -7, -8, and -10 in a caspase-9-dependent manner. J Cell Biol 144:281–292, 1999.

44. Vercammen D, Brouckaert G, Denecker G, et al: Dual signaling of the FAS receptor: Initiation of both apoptotic and necrotic cell death pathways. J Exp Med 188:919–930, 1998.

45. Holler N, Zaru R, Micheau O, et al: FAS triggers an alternative, caspase-8-independent cell death pathway using the kinase RIP as effector molecule. Nat Immunol 1:489–495, 2000.

46. Khwaja A, Tatton L: Resistance to the cytotoxic effects of tumor necrosis factor alpha can be overcome by inhibition of a FADD/caspase-dependent signaling pathway. J Biol Chem 274:36817–36823, 1999.

47. Rich T, Allen RL, Wyllie AH: Defying death after DNA damage. Nature 407:777–783, 2000.

48. Zhou BB, Elledge SJ: The DNA damage response: Putting checkpoints in perspective. Nature 408:433–439, 2000.

49. Banin S, Mayal L, Shieh S, et al: Enhanced phosphorylation of p53 by ATM in response to DNA damage. Science 281:1674–1677, 1998.

50. Maya R, Balass M, Kim ST, et al: ATM-dependent phosphorylation of Mdm2 on serine 395: Role in p53 activation by DNA damage. Genes Dev 15:1067–1077, 2001.

51. Leist M, Single B, Kunstle G, et al: Apoptosis in the absence of poly-(ADP-ribose) polymerase. Biochem Biophys Res Commun 233:518–522, 1997.

52. Ha HC, Snyder SH: Poly(ADP-ribose) polymerase is a mediator of necrotic cell death by ATP depletion. Proc Natl Acad Sci U S A 96:13978–13982, 1999.

53. Chiarugi A: Poly(ADP-ribose) polymerase: Killer or conspirator? The 'suicide hypothesis' revisited. Trends Pharmacol Sci 23:122–129, 2002.

54. Chiarugi A, Moskowitz MA: Cell biology: PARP-1—a perpetrator of apoptotic cell death? Science 297:200–201, 2002.

55. Li H, Yuan J: Deciphering the pathways of life and death. Curr Opin Cell Biol 11:261–266, 1999.

56. Tamatani M, Che YH, Matsuzaki H, et al: Tumor necrosis factor induces Bcl-2 and Bcl-x expression through NFkappaB activation in primary hippocampal neurons. J Biol Chem 274:8531–8538, 1999.

57. Datta SR, Brunet A, Greenberg ME: Cellular survival: A play in three Akts. Genes Dev 13:2905–2927, 1999.

58. Datta SR, Dudek H, Tao X, et al: Akt phosphorylation of BAD couples survival signals to the cell-intrinsic death machinery. Cell 91:231–241, 1997.

59. Cardone MH, Roy N, Stennicke HR, et al: Regulation of cell death protease caspase-9 by phosphorylation. Science 282:1318–1321, 1998.

60. Bryckaert M, Guillonneau X, Hecquet C, et al: Both FGF1 and bcl-x synthesis are necessary for the reduction of apoptosis in retinal pigmented epithelial cells by FGF2: Role of the extracellular signal-regulated kinase 2. Oncogene 18:7584–7593, 1999.

61. Finkbeiner S: CREB couples neurotrophin signals to survival messages. Neuron 25:11–14, 2000.

62. Kaltschmidt B, Kaltschmidt C, Hofmann TG, et al: The pro- or anti-apoptotic function of NF-kappaB is determined by the nature of the apoptotic stimulus. Eur J Biochem 267:3828–3835, 2000.

63. Mattson MP, Scheff SW: Endogenous neuroprotection factors and traumatic brain injury: Mechanisms of action and implications for therapy. J Neurotrauma 11:3–33, 1994.

64. Mattson MP, Lovell MA, Furukawa K, et al: Neurotrophic factors attenuate glutamate-induced accumulation of peroxides, elevation of intracellular Ca^{2+} concentration, and neurotoxicity and increase antioxidant enzyme activities in hippocampal neurons. J Neurochem 65:1740–1751, 1995.

65. Linnik MD, Zobrist RH, Hatfield MD: Evidence supporting a role for programmed cell death in focal cerebral ischemia in rats. Stroke 24:2002–2008; 1993.

66. Krajewski S, Mai JK, Krajewska M, et al: Upregulation of bax protein levels in neurons following cerebral ischemia. J Neurosci 15:6364–6376, 1995.

67. Li Y, Chopp M, Jiang N, et al: Temporal profile of in situ DNA fragmentation after transient middle cerebral artery occlusion in the rat. J Cereb Blood Flow Metab 15:389–397, 1995.

68. Charriaut-Marlangue CMI, Represa A, Popovici T, et al: Apoptosis and necrosis after reversible focal cerebral ischemia: An in situ DNA fragmentation analysis. J Cereb Blood Flow Metab 16:186–195, 1996.

69. Chen J, Zhu RL, Nakayama M, et al: Expression of the apoptosis-effector gene, Bax, is up-regulated in vulnerable hippocampal CA1 neurons following global ischemia. J Neurochem 67:64–71, 1996.

70. Deshpande J, Bergstedt K, Linden T, et al: Ultrastructural changes in the hippocampal CA1 region following transient cerebral ischemia: Evidence against programmed cell death. Exp Brain Res 88:91–105, 1992.

71. van Lookeren Campagne M, Gill R: Ultrastructural morphological changes are not characteristic of apoptotic cell death following focal cerebral ischaemia in the rat. Neurosci Lett 213:111–114, 1996.

72. Colbourne F, Sutherland GR, Auer RN: Electron microscopic evidence against apoptosis as the mechanism of neuronal death in global ischemia. J Neurosci 19:4200–4210, 1999.

73. Hara H, Fink K, Endres M, et al: Attenuation of transient focal cerebral ischemic injury in transgenic mice expressing a mutant ICE inhibitory protein. J Cereb Blood Flow Metab 17:370–375, 1997.

74. Chen J, Nagayama T, Jin K, et al: Induction of caspase-3-like protease may mediate delayed neuronal death in the hippocampus after transient cerebral ischemia. J Neurosci 18:4914–4928, 1998.

75. Wang KK: Calpain and caspase: Can you tell the difference? Trends Neurosci 23:20–26, 2000.

76. Yamashima T: Implication of cysteine proteases calpain, cathepsin and caspase in ischemic neuronal death of primates. Prog Neurobiol 62:273–295, 2000.

77. Heron A, Pollard H, Dessi F, et al: Regional variability in DNA fragmentation after global ischemia evidenced by combined histological and gel electrophoresis observations in the rat brain. J Neurochem 61:1973–1976, 1993.

Pathophysiology

78. MacManus JP, Buchan AM, Hill IE, et al: Global ischemia can cause DNA fragmentation indicative of apoptosis in rat brain. Neurosci Lett 164:89–92, 1993.

79. Tominaga T, Kure S, Narisawa K, et al: Endonuclease activation following focal ischemic injury in the rat brain. Brain Res 608:21–26, 1993.

80. MacManus JP, Hill IE, Huang ZG, et al: DNA damage consistent with apoptosis in transient focal ischaemic neocortex. Neuroreport 5:493–496, 1994.

81. Charriaut-Marlangue C, Margaill I, Plotkine M, et al: Early endonuclease activation following reversible focal ischemia in the rat brain. J Cereb Blood Flow Metab 15:385–388, 1995.

82. Li Y, Chopp M, Jiang N, et al: Induction of DNA fragmentation after 10 to 120 minutes of focal cerebral ischemia in rats. Stroke 26:1252–1257; 1995.

83. Li Y, Chopp M, Powers C, et al: Apoptosis and protein expression after focal cerebral ischemia in rat. Brain Res 765:301–312, 1997.

84. Eliasson MJ, Sampei K, Mandir AS, et al: Poly(ADP-ribose) polymerase gene disruption renders mice resistant to cerebral ischemia. Nat Med 3:1089–1095, 1997.

85. Endres M, Wang ZQ, Namura S, et al: Ischemic brain injury is mediated by the activation of poly(ADP-ribose)polymerase. J Cereb Blood Flow Metab 17:1143–1151, 1997.

86. Katchanov J, Harms C, Gertz K, et al: Mild cerebral ischemia induces loss of cyclin-dependent kinase inhibitors and activation of cell cycle machinery before delayed neuronal cell death. J Neurosci 21:5045–5053, 2001.

87. Antonawich FJ, Krajewski S, Reed JC, et al: Bcl-x(l) Bax interaction after transient global ischemia. J Cereb Blood Flow Metab 18:882–886, 1998.

88. Isenmann S, Stoll G, Schroeter M, et al: Differential regulation of Bax, Bcl-2, and Bcl-X proteins in focal cortical ischemia in the rat. Brain Pathol 8:49–62; 1998.

89. Elibol B, Soylemezoglu F, Unal I, et al: Nitric oxide is involved in ischemia-induced apoptosis in brain: A study in neuronal nitric oxide synthase null mice. Neuroscience 105:79–86, 2001.

90. Fujimura M, Morita-Fujimura Y, Murakami K, et al: Cytosolic redistribution of cytochrome c after transient focal cerebral ischemia in rats. J Cereb Blood Flow Metab 18:1239–1247, 1998.

91. Namura S, Zhu J, Fink K, et al: Activation and cleavage of caspase-3 in apoptosis induced by experimental cerebral ischemia. J Neurosci 18:3659–3668, 1998.

92. Krajewski S, Krajewska M, Ellerby LM, et al: Release of caspase-9 from mitochondria during neuronal apoptosis and cerebral ischemia. Proc Natl Acad Sci U S A 96:5752–5757, 1999.

93. Velier JJ, Ellison JA, Kikly KK, et al: Caspase-8 and caspase-3 are expressed by different populations of cortical neurons undergoing delayed cell death after focal stroke in the rat. J Neurosci 19:5932–5941, 1999.

94. Kang SJ, Wang S, Hara H, et al: Dual role of caspase-11 in mediating activation of caspase-1 and caspase-3 under pathological conditions. J Cell Biol 149:613–622, 2000.

95. Thornberry NA, Lazebnik Y: Caspases: Enemies within. Science 281:1312–1316, 1998.

96. Zhang J, Xu M: Apoptotic DNA fragmentation and tissue homeostasis. Trends Cell Biol 12:84–89, 2002.

97. Loddick SA, MacKenzie A, Rothwell NJ: An ICE inhibitor, z-VAD-DCB attenuates ischaemic brain damage in the rat. Neuroreport 7:1465–1468, 1996.

98. Friedlander RM, Gagliardini V, Hara H, et al: Expression of a dominant negative mutant of interleukin-1 beta converting enzyme in transgenic mice prevents neuronal cell death induced by trophic factor withdrawal and ischemic brain injury. J Exp Med 185:933–940, 1997.

99. Hara H, Friedlander RM, Gagliardini V, et al: Inhibition of interleukin 1beta converting enzyme family proteases reduces ischemic and excitotoxic neuronal damage. Proc Natl Acad Sci U S A 94:2007–2012, 1997.

100. Schielke GP, Yang GY, Shivers BD, et al: Reduced ischemic brain injury in interleukin-1 beta converting enzyme-deficient mice. J Cereb Blood Flow Metab 18:180–185, 1998.

101. Asahi M, Hashimaru H, Uemura Y, et al: Expression of interleukin-1β converting enzyme gene family and Bcl-2 gene family in the rat brain following permanent occlusion of the middle cerebral artery. J Cereb Blood Flow Metab 17:11–18, 1997.

102. Endres M, Fink K, Zhu J, et al: Neuroprotective effects of gelsolin during murine stroke. J Clin Invest 103:347–354, 1999.

103. Fink K, Zhu J, Namura S, et al: Prolonged therapeutic window for ischemic brain damage caused by delayed caspase activation. J Cereb Blood Flow Metab 18:1071–1076, 1998.

104. Matsushita K, Wu Y, Qiu J, et al: FAS receptor and neuronal cell death after spinal cord ischemia. J Neurosci 20:6879–6887, 2000.

105. Martin-Villalba A, Hahne M, Kleber S, et al: Therapeutic neutralization of CD95-ligand and TNF attenuates brain damage in stroke. Cell Death Differ 8:679–686, 2001.

106. Martin-Villalba A, Herr I, Jeremias I, et al: CD95 ligand (FAS-L/APO-1L) and tumor necrosis factor-related apoptosis-inducing ligand mediate ischemia-induced apoptosis in neurons. J Neurosci 19:3809–3817, 1999.

107. Rosenbaum DM, Gupta G, D'Amore J, et al: FAS (CD95/APO-1) plays a role in the pathophysiology of focal cerebral ischemia. J Neurosci Res 61:686–692, 2000.

108. Mehmet H: Stroke treatment enters the FAS lane. Cell Death Differ 8:659–661, 2001.

109. Stoll G, Jander S, Schroeter M: Inflammation and glial responses in ischemic brain lesions. Prog Neurobiol 56:149–171, 1998.

110. Plesnila N, Zinkel S, Le DA, et al: BID mediates neuronal cell death after oxygen/glucose deprivation and focal cerebral ischemia. Proc Natl Acad Sci U S A 98:15318–15323, 2001.

111. Wei MC, Lindsten T, Mootha VK, et al: tBID, a membrane-targeted death ligand, oligomerizes BAK to release cytochrome c. Genes Dev 14:2060–2071, 2000.

112. Harrison DC, Davis RP, Bond BC, et al: Caspase mRNA expression in a rat model of focal cerebral ischemia. Brain Res Mol Brain Res 89:133–146, 2001.

113. Bergeron L, Perez GI, Macdonald G, et al: Defects in regulation of apoptosis in caspase-2-deficient mice. Genes Dev 12:1304–1314, 1998.

114. Kinoshita M, Tomimoto H, Kinoshita A, et al: Up-regulation of the Nedd2 gene encoding an ICE/Ced-3-like cysteine protease in the gerbil brain after transient global ischemia. J Cereb Blood Flow Metab 17:507–514, 1997.

115. Gillardon F, Bottiger B, Schmitz B, et al: Activation of CPP-32 protease in hippocampal neurons following ischemia and epilepsy. Brain Res Mol Brain Res 50:16–22, 1997.

116. Cheng Y, Deshmukh M, D'Costa A, et al: Caspase inhibitor affords neuroprotection with delayed administration in a rat model of neonatal hypoxic-ischemic brain injury. J Clin Invest 101:1992–1999, 1998.

117. Bhat RV, DiRocco R, Marcy VR, et al: Increased expression of IL-1beta converting enzyme in hippocampus after ischemia: Selective localization in microglia. J Neurosci 16:4146–4154, 1996.

118. Ni B, Wu X, Su Y, et al: Transient global forebrain ischemia induces a prolonged expression of the caspase-3 mRNA in rat hippocampal CA1 pyramidal neurons. J Cereb Blood Flow Metab 18:248–256, 1998.

119. Gillardon F, Kiprianova I, Sandkuhler J, et al: Inhibition of caspases prevents cell death of hippocampal CA1 neurons, but not impairment of hippocampal long-term potentiation following global ischemia. Neuroscience 93:1219–1222, 1999.

120. Ouyang YB, Tan Y, Comb M, et al: Survival- and death-promoting events after transient cerebral ischemia: Phosphorylation of Akt, release of cytochrome C and activation of caspase-like proteases. J Cereb Blood Flow Metab 19:1126–1135, 1999.

121. Antonawich FJ, Federoff HJ, Davis JN: BCL-2 transduction, using a herpes simplex virus amplicon, protects hippocampal neurons from transient global ischemia. Exp Neurol 156:130–137, 1999.

122. Nakatsuka H, Ohta S, Tanaka J, et al: Release of cytochrome c from mitochondria to cytosol in gerbil hippocampal CA1 neurons after transient forebrain ischemia. Brain Res 849:216–219, 1999.

123. Sugawara T, Fujimura M, Morita-Fujimura Y, et al: Mitochondrial release of cytochrome c corresponds to the selective vulnerability of hippocampal CA1 neurons in rats after transient global cerebral ischemia. J Neurosci 19:RC39, 1999.

124. Perez-Pinzon MA, Xu GP, Born J, et al: Cytochrome C is released from mitochondria into the cytosol after cerebral anoxia or ischemia. J Cereb Blood Flow Metab 19:39–43, 1999.

125. Chan PH: Reactive oxygen radicals in signaling and damage in the ischemic brain. J Cereb Blood Flow Metab 21:2–14, 2001.

126. Endres M, Hirt L, Moskowitz MA: Apoptosis and cerebral ischemia. In Rangnekar VM (ed): Apoptosis: Role in Disease, Pathogenesis and Prevention. Amsterdam, Elsevier Science, 2001, pp 137–167.

Pathophysiology

127. Himi T, Ishizaki Y, Murota S: A caspase inhibitor blocks ischaemia-induced delayed neuronal death in the gerbil. Eur J Neurosci 10:777–781, 1998.
128. Rothwell NJ, Loddick SA, Stroemer P: Interleukins and cerebral ischaemia. Int Rev Neurobiol 40:281–298, 1997.
129. Ma J, Endres M, Moskowitz MA: Synergistic effects of caspase inhibitors and MK-801 in brain injury after transient focal cerebral ischaemia in mice. Br J Pharmacol 124:756–762, 1998.
130. Ma J, Qiu J, Hirt L, et al: Synergistic protective effect of caspase inhibitors and bFGF against brain injury induced by transient focal ischaemia. Br J Pharmacol 133:345–350, 2001.
131. Endres M, Fan G, Hirt L, et al: Ischemic brain damage in mice after selectively modifying BDNF or NT4 gene expression. J Cereb Blood Flow Metab 20:139–144, 2000.
132. Beck T, Lindholm D, Castren E, et al: Brain-derived neurotrophic factor protects against ischemic cell damage in rat hippocampus. J Cereb Blood Flow Metab 14:689–692, 1994.
133. Tsukahara T, Yonekawa Y, Tanaka K, et al: The role of brain-derived neurotrophic factor in transient forebrain ischemia in the rat brain. Neurosurgery 34:323–331; 1994.
134. Chan KM, Lam DT, Pong K, et al: Neurotrophin-4/5 treatment reduces infarct size in rats with middle cerebral artery occlusion. Neurochem Res 21:763–767, 1996.
135. Schabitz WR, Schwab S, Spranger M, et al: Intraventricular brain-derived neurotrophic factor reduces infarct size after focal cerebral ischemia in rats. J Cereb Blood Flow Metab 17:500–506, 1997.
136. Love S, Barber R, Wilcock G K: Neuronal death in brain infarcts in man. Neuropathol Appl Neurobiol 26:55–66, 2000.
137. Sairanen T, Carpen O, Karjalainen-Lindsberg ML, et al: Evolution of cerebral tumor necrosis factor-alpha production during human ischemic stroke. Stroke 32:1750–1758, 2001.
138. Hara A, Yoshimi N, Hirose Y, et al: DNA fragmentation in granular cells of human cerebellum following global ischemia. Brain Res 697:247–250, 1995.
139. Kingsbury AE, Mardsen CD, Foster OJ: DNA fragmentation in human substantia nigra: Apoptosis or perimortem effect? Mov Disord 13:877–884, 1998.
140. Benjelloun N, Menard A, Charriaut-Marlangue C, et al: Case report: DNA fragmentation in glial cells in a cerebral biopsy from a multiple sclerosis patient. Cell Mol Biol (Noisy-le-grand) 44:579–583, 1998.
141. Anlar B, Soylemezoglu F, Elibol B, et al: Apoptosis in brain biopsies of subacute sclerosing panencephalitis patients. Neuropediatrics 30:239–242, 1999.
142. Ferrer I: Nuclear DNA fragmentation in Creutzfeldt-Jakob disease: Does a mere positive in situ nuclear end-labeling indicate apoptosis? Acta Neuropathol (Berl) 97:5–12, 1999.
143. Dorr J, Bechmann I, Waiczies S, et al: Lack of tumor necrosis factor–related apoptosis-inducing ligand but presence of its receptors in the human brain. J Neurosci 22:RC209, 2002.
144. Marshall KA, Daniel SE, Cairns N, et al: Upregulation of the anti-apoptotic protein Bcl-2 may be an early event in neurodegeneration: Studies on Parkinson's and incidental Lewy body disease. Biochem Biophys Res Commun 240:84–87, 1997.
145. Su JH, Deng G, Cotman CW: Bax protein expression is increased in Alzheimer's brain: Correlations with DNA damage, Bcl-2 expression, and brain pathology. J Neuropathol Exp Neurol 56:86–93, 1997.
146. Vyas S, Javoy-Agid F, Herrero MT, et al: Expression of Bcl-2 in adult human brain regions with special reference to neurodegenerative disorders. J Neurochem 69:223–231, 1997.
147. Yachnis AT, Powell SZ, Olmsted JJ, et al: Distinct neurodevelopmental patterns of bcl-2 and bcl-x expression are altered in glioneuronal hamartias of the human temporal lobe. J Neuropathol Exp Neurol 56:186–198, 1997.
148. Desjardins P, Ledoux S: Expression of ced-3 and ced-9 homologs in Alzheimer's disease cerebral cortex. Neurosci Lett 244:69–72, 1998.
149. Kitamura Y, Shimohama S, Kamoshima W, et al: Alteration of proteins regulating apoptosis, Bcl-2, Bcl-x, Bax, Bak, Bad, ICH-1 and CPP32, in Alzheimer's disease. Brain Res 780:260–269, 1998.
150. Clark RS, Kochanek PM, Chen M, et al: Increases in Bcl-2 and cleavage of caspase-1 and caspase-3 in human brain after head injury. FASEB J 13:813–821, 1999.
151. Henshall DC, Clark RS, Adelson PD, et al: Alterations in bcl-2 and caspase gene family protein expression in human temporal lobe epilepsy. Neurology 55:250–257, 2000.
152. Jarskog LF, Gilmore JH: Developmental expression of Bcl-2 protein in human cortex. Brain Res Dev Brain Res 119:225–230, 2000.
153. Tatton NA: Increased caspase 3 and Bax immunoreactivity accompany nuclear GAPDH translocation and neuronal apoptosis in Parkinson's disease. Exp Neurol 166:29–43, 2000.
154. Engidawork E, Gulesserian T, Seidl R, et al: Expression of apoptosis related proteins: RAIDD, ZIP kinase, Bim/BOD, p21, Bax, Bcl-2 and NF-kappaB in brains of patients with Down syndrome. J Neural Transm Suppl (61):181–192, 2001.
155. Hartmann A, Michel PP, Troadec JD, et al: Is Bax a mitochondrial mediator in apoptotic death of dopaminergic neurons in Parkinson's disease? J Neurochem 76:1785–1793, 2001.
156. Engidawork E, Gulesserian T, Yoo BC, et al: Alteration of caspases and apoptosis-related proteins in brains of patients with Alzheimer's disease. Biochem Biophys Res Commun 281:84–93, 2001.
157. Hartmann A, Hunot S, Michel PP, et al: Caspase-3: A vulnerability factor and final effector in apoptotic death of dopaminergic neurons in Parkinson's disease. Proc Natl Acad Sci U S A 97:2875–2880, 2000.
158. Rohn TT, Head E, Nesse WH, et al: Activation of caspase-8 in the Alzheimer's disease brain. Neurobiol Dis 8:1006–1016, 2001.
159. Nishimura T, Akiyama H, Yonehara S, et al: FAS antigen expression in brains of patients with Alzheimer-type dementia. Brain Res 695:137–145, 1995.
160. de la Monte SM, Sohn YK, Wands JR: Correlates of p53- and FAS (CD95)-mediated apoptosis in Alzheimer's disease. J Neurol Sci 152:73–83, 1997.
161. Ferrer I, Puig B, Krupinsk J, et al: FAS and FAS ligand expression in Alzheimer's disease. Acta Neuropathol (Berl) 102:121–31, 2001.
162. Gulesserian T, Engidawork E, Yoo BC, et al: Alteration of caspases and other apoptosis regulatory proteins in Down syndrome. J Neural Transm Suppl (61):163–179, 2001.
163. Newman SJ, Bond B, Crook B, et al: Neuron-specific localisation of the TR3 death receptor in Alzheimer's disease. Brain Res 857:131–140, 2000.
164. O'Barr S, Schultz J, Rogers J: Expression of the protooncogene bcl-2 in Alzheimer's disease brain. Neurobiol Aging 17:131–136, 1996.
165. Stadelmann C, Deckwerth TL, Srinivasan A, et al: Activation of caspase-3 in single neurons and autophagic granules of granulovacuolar degeneration in Alzheimer's disease: Evidence for apoptotic cell death. Am J Pathol 155:1459–1466, 1999.
166. Su JH, Anderson AJ, Cummings BJ, et al: Immunohistochemical evidence for apoptosis in Alzheimer's disease. Neuroreport 5:2529–2533, 1994.
167. Anderson AJ, Su JH, Cotman CW: DNA damage and apoptosis in Alzheimer's disease: Colocalization with c-Jun immunoreactivity, relationship to brain area, and effect of postmortem delay. J Neurosci 16:1710–1719, 1996.
168. Rohn TT, Head E, Su JH, et al: Correlation between caspase activation and neurofibrillary tangle formation in Alzheimer's disease. Am J Pathol 158:189–198, 2001.
169. Yang F, Sun X, Beech W, et al: Antibody to caspase-cleaved actin detects apoptosis in differentiated neuroblastoma and plaque-associated neurons and microglia in Alzheimer's disease. Am J Pathol 152:379–389, 1998.
170. Mochizuki H, Goto K, Mori H, et al: Histochemical detection of apoptosis in Parkinson's disease. J Neurol Sci 137:120–123, 1996.
171. Dragunow M, Faull RL, Lawlor P, et al: In situ evidence for DNA fragmentation in Huntington's disease striatum and Alzheimer's disease temporal lobes. Neuroreport 6:1053–1057, 1995.
172. Portera-Cailliau C, Hedreen JC, Price DL, et al: Evidence for apoptotic cell death in Huntington disease and excitotoxic animal models. J Neurosci 15:3775–3787, 1995.
173. Butterworth NJ, Williams L, Bullock JY, et al: Trinucleotide (CAG) repeat length is positively correlated with the degree of DNA fragmentation in Huntington's disease striatum. Neuroscience 87:49–53, 1998.
174. Garden GA, Budd SL, Tsai E, et al: Caspase cascades in human immunodeficiency virus-associated neurodegeneration. J Neurosci 22:4015–4024, 2002.
175. Adle-Biassette H, Levy Y, Colombel M, et al: Neuronal apoptosis in HIV infection in adults. Neuropathol Appl Neurobiol 21:218–227, 1995.

Pathophysiology

176. Shi B, De Girolami U, He J, et al: Apoptosis induced by HIV-1 infection of the central nervous system. J Clin Invest 98:1979–1990, 1996.

177. Qui J, Whalen MJ, Lowenstein P, et al: Upregulation of the FAS receptor death-inducing signaling complex after traumatic brain injury in mice and humans. J Neurosci 22:3504–3511, 2002.

178. Smith FM, Raghupathi R, MacKinnon MA, et al: TUNEL-positive staining of surface contusions after fatal head injury in man. Acta Neuropathol (Berl) 100:537–545, 2000.

179. Williams S, Raghupathi R, MacKinnon MA, et al: In situ DNA fragmentation occurs in white matter up to 12 months after head injury in man. Acta Neuropathol (Berl) 102:581–590, 2001.

Chapter Forty-Four

Molecular Pathophysiology of White Matter Anoxic-Ischemic Injury

Bruce R. Ransom, Aninda B. Acharya, and Mark P. Goldberg

Ischemia of the mammalian central nervous system (CNS), including the secondary vascular embarrassment that frequently accompanies traumatic brain and spinal cord insults,[1,2] damages both gray and white matter (Fig. 44–1). In fact, about 20% of ischemic strokes involve predominantly white matter, as a result of occlusion of small penetrating arteries that supply the deep areas of the cerebral hemispheres (see Chapter 11).[3] Clinically, damage to white matter can result in serious disability as seen in stroke, spinal cord and traumatic brain injury, and some forms of vascular dementia.[2,4] In spite of these facts, little attention had been paid to how white matter is injured by ischemia. Two reasons are foremost in explanation of this neglect; first, the brain of rodents, which is most often used to study stroke, has far less white matter than the human brain, and second, there is a tendency to think that protection of neuron cell bodies alone is sufficient to rescue stroke-imperiled brain tissue.

Great progress has been made in understanding the pathophysiology of ischemic white matter injury in the last decade. Models have been developed that allow white matter to be studied independently of gray matter. Basic knowledge about the ionic and molecular events initiated by ischemia in white matter is spawning testable hypotheses for protecting this unique part of the brain during stroke. Most importantly, there is a growing awareness about the importance of this topic to reach the goal of effective acute treatment for ischemic stroke. In this chapter, we review what is currently known about the cellular and molecular events triggered by ischemia in white matter and how these events lead to loss of function and irreversible injury.

WHITE MATTER ANATOMY AND PHYSIOLOGY

White matter of the mammalian CNS consists of the afferent and efferent axonal tracts that interconnect cortical and neuron cell body–containing nuclear areas of the brain and spinal cord. White matter contains no neuronal cell bodies or synapses. It consists of tightly packed glial cells and myelinated and unmyelinated axons; the presence of myelin lends a white appearance to this tissue. White matter regions vary widely with regard to the ratio of myelinated to unmyelinated axons; for example, all the axons of the optic nerve are myelinated, but only about 30% of those in the corpus callosum are myelinated.[5,6] The anatomy and physiology of myelinated axons are highly specialized and unique compared with those of unmyelinated axons.[7] It is not surprising, therefore, that regional differences have been noted in the pathophysiology of white matter injury.[8,9]

Most axons in cerebral white matter provide connections within cortical regions. They include short fiber bundles between adjacent cortical regions (U fibers) and longer axons projecting between contralateral hemispheres (callosal fibers) or distinct brain areas (association fibers). Output or input projections to basal ganglia, brainstem, or spinal cord are only a small proportion of total CNS score. Because most white matter axons connect cortical regions, the massive growth in cortical area from small lissencephalic animals to animals with larger, gyrencephalic brains is associated with a great expansion in white matter volume. White matter constitutes only a small fraction of forebrain volume in rodents (for mice, approximately 10% white matter; total forebrain volume $125\,mm^3$) but occupies a large proportion of the human brain (approximately 42%; total volume $1,000,000\,mm^3$) (Fig. 44–2).[10] This massive, four-fold expansion in the volume of brain occupied by white matter means that the human brain has far more white matter at risk during ischemia. It may also help explain why findings in animal models of stroke have not translated with fidelity to the clinical setting.

Although the role of glial cells in CNS function continues to evolve,[11] it is clear that astrocytes are crucial for ionic homeostasis of brain extracellular space (ECS) and glutamate uptake.[12] Only astrocytes contain glycogen, and they can provide neurons and axons with usable energy substrate in the form of lactate when glucose alone is restricted.[13] Because astrocytes are natural anaerobes and contain glycogen, they are the only cells in the brain that

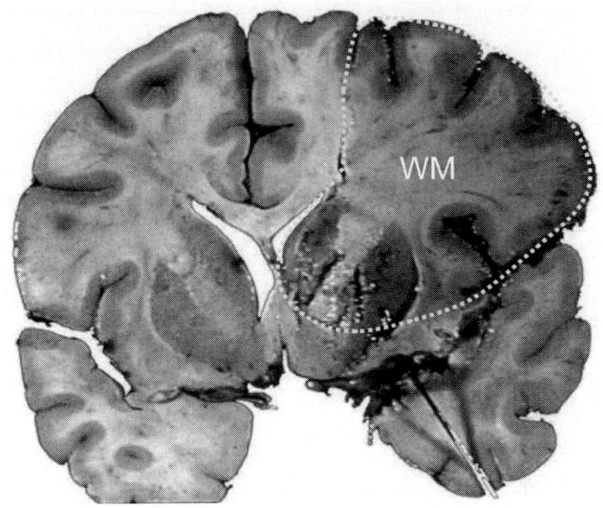

FIGURE 44–1 *Human stroke affects white matter and gray matter. Subacute infarct in vascular distribution of the middle cerebral artery demonstrates damage of a large volume of white matter (WM), including subcortical white matter, centrum semiovale, and internal capsule as well as gray matter structures such as neocortex and basal ganglia. (Image provided by Dr. Kevin A. Roth.)*

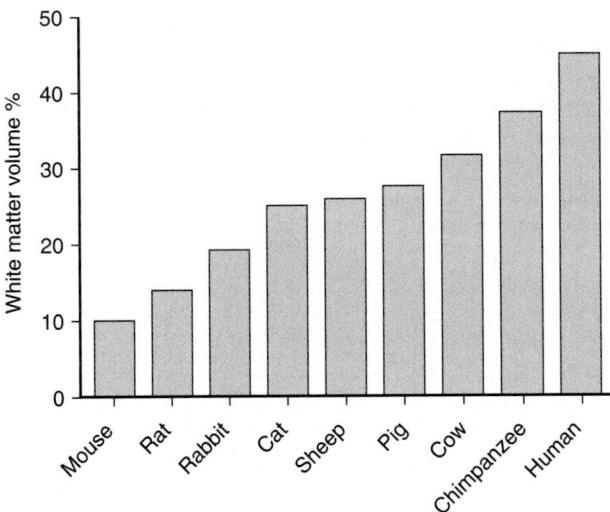

FIGURE 44–2 *The proportion of brain white matter greatly increases as brain size enlarges. Bars show the percentage of cerebral hemisphere volume composed of white matter in several mammals, ranging from mouse to human. (Data calculated from Zhang K, Sejnowski TJ: A universal scaling law between gray matter and white matter of cerebral cortex. Proc Natl Sci U S A 97:5621–5626, 2000.)*

are able to maintain enough adenosine triphosphate (ATP) to function during ischemia.[14,15] Oligodendrocytes provide myelin for CNS axons, and conduction fails in myelinated axons with injury to oligodendrocytes or their myelin. Ischemia will, of course, eventually affect all the elements in white matter, leading to axon-glial interactions that are important for understanding how injury occurs. These cellular interactions during ischemia have just begun to be explored in white matter. For example, microglial cells are thought to produce damaging free radical species during ischemia, and astrocytes are the key cell type capable of defending against free radical–mediated injury.[12] Little is known, however, about these topics as they pertain to ischemic injury in white matter.

It is essential to understand that an axon's energy metabolism is independent from that of its cell body of origin. Axons extend for great distances from their cell bodies and depend on local production of ATP to maintain ion gradients and sustain energy-consuming functions. This metabolic isolation also means that axons suffer energy deprivation in a manner that is independent of neuron cell bodies. The metabolic rate of white matter is about half that of gray matter on the basis of oxygen consumption.[16] Axons more than glial cells are calculated to contribute to this high metabolic rate.[17] The adult mammalian CNS is generally presumed to fail rapidly in the absence of oxygen. There are little actual data on this question because making an animal anoxic without compromising blood supply is challenging; Tekkök and associates,[18] however, have shown that a high percentage of myelinated axons in adult rodent optic nerve can function anaerobically. This finding implies that white matter could tolerate prolonged periods of pure anoxia without permanent injury.

Because white matter is less metabolically active than gray matter, it has a lower blood flow per volume of tissue. The blood flow in cerebral white matter averages 30 mL/100 mg/minute, compared with 50 mL/100 mg/minute in gray matter. White matter has a much less dense capillary network than gray matter. Much of the cerebral white matter is perfused by penetrating arterioles that originate from larger pial vessels. Deeper regions of the subcortical white matter are supplied by the striate arteries that arise from the circle of Willis. The most important of these are the medial striate arteries, which arise directly from the internal carotid artery and supply much of the internal capsule as it courses through the basal ganglia. As white matter tracts descend through the brainstem, they are perfused by penetrating arteries from the vertebral and basilar arteries or their circumferential branches.

Regions of white matter have distinct patterns of vascular supply (Fig. 44–3).[19] For example, in the centrum semiovale, the blood supply consists of long arterioles, which are characteristically terminal vessels with few anastomoses; occlusion of one of these vessels results in an area of ischemia that cannot be rescued by blood flow redistribution because there are no anastomotic connections with neighboring vessels. In contrast, the immediately subcortical association bundles (U fibers), corpus callosum, external capsule–claustrum, and extreme capsule are supplied by interdigitating arterioles derived from two or more pial vessels. Dual vascular supply may account for the relative resistance of these white matter areas to damage after anoxia or hypoperfusion.

MODEL SYSTEMS FOR STUDYING WHITE MATTER ISCHEMIA

Research in white matter ischemia requires experimental systems that appropriately model the cell biology and

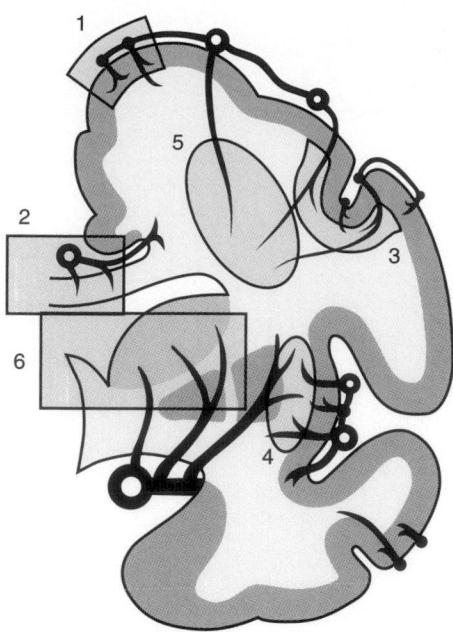

FIGURE 44–3 *Distinct patterns of vascular supply to the supratentorial brain. Regions: 1, cortex; 2, corpus callosum; 3, subcortical U fibers; 4, external capsule/claustrum/extreme capsule; 5, centrum semiovale; 6, basal ganglia and thalamus. Microradiography studies demonstrate much denser capillary beds in gray matter than in white matter structures. The regions of highest vulnerability to anoxic or hypoperfusion damage (cortex, centrum semiovale, basal ganglia, thalamus) are supplied by isolated penetrating arterioles with minimal overlap, whereas more resistant areas (U fibers, external capsule) have interdigitating vessels from two or more arterial supplies. (Redrawn from Moody DM, Bell MA, Challa VR: Features of the cerebral vascular pattern that predict vulnerability to perfusion or oxygenation deficiency: An anatomic study. AJNR Am J Neuroradiol 11:431–439, 1990.)*

physiology of myelinated axons and glia. Improved understanding of the pathways leading to white matter injury can lead to therapeutic approaches, to be tested in progressively more complex in vitro and in vivo systems and, ultimately, in clinical trials. However, it is important to understand the potential strengths and limitations of each model system and ensure that experiments appropriately examine specific facets of injury and recovery.

Cell Culture

Cell culture models provide the opportunity to examine individual cellular elements of white matter in isolation, separate from the effects of perfusion and vascular supply. Experiments in primary cultures allow assessment of enriched populations of brain cells to effects of energy deprivation, which is typically produced by transient removal of oxygen and glucose. Under these conditions, the relative vulnerabilities of cells, from greatest to least, are approximately as follows: neurons > oligodendrocytes = microglia > endothelial cells > astrocytes.[20–23] Within the oligodendrocyte lineage, immature oligodendrocytes are more vulnerable than mature cells to energy deprivation.[24] Reasons proposed for the high vulnerability of

oligodendrocytes to ischemic damage include their high metabolic demands, poor resistance to oxidative stress, and vulnerability to extracellular glutamate.[25]

Cell culture models provide excellent systems with which to study the molecular biology, pharmacology, and neurochemistry of ischemic injury, but important limitations must be considered. Most cultured cells are derived from brains of perinatal animals and so may reflect immature phenotypes not found in the adult brain. Relatively few studies of cultured central axons metabolically isolated from their neuronal cell bodies, as occurs in vivo, have been performed. More importantly, culture models generally exclude the important cell-cell interactions that characterize intact white matter. It is possible to address some of these concerns, because systems for isolating axons are well described[26] and oligodendrocytes selectively myelinate axons in co-culture.[27]

In Vitro Tissue Models

Many of the limitations of cell cultures are avoided by models that use acutely isolated, perfused preparations from intact white matter. Considerable progress in understanding white matter injury comes from studies of the isolated rodent optic nerve,[28–31] a CNS white matter tract consisting solely of myelinated axons. Similarly, later studies have examined preparations of other CNS white matter regions, such as preparations of isolated dorsal columns[32] and brain slices including corpus callosum.[8] Importantly, such preparations allow direct assessment of axon function (by measurement of compound action potential [CAP] propagation) as well as structure. Although these preparations are not suitable for studies of long-term outcomes after hypoxic or ischemic injury, the axons remain electrically functional for at least several hours in vitro, allowing assessment of short-term recovery.

In Vivo Models

Hundreds of studies of focal ischemia in rodent models have been conducted, but the extent of white matter injury has been examined in only a handful (see Pantoni and colleagues[33] and Dietrich and associates[34]).[35–37] This situation is in part due to the very small proportion of cerebral white matter in mice and rats (see Fig. 44–2); the most common outcome measure—infarct volume—is not significantly altered in such models whether white matter is or is not injured. Furthermore, a frequently used method of infarct volume assessment in rodent models involves staining with a vital dye, triphenyltetrazolium chloride, which provides little labeling of intact white matter.[38] Careful examination of white matter injury requires special histologic techniques to identify injury of axons, myelin, and glial cells.

EFFECTS OF ISCHEMIA ON WHITE MATTER

One can monitor white matter function by electrically evoking a CAP from constituent axons (Fig. 44–4A). Function (i.e., excitability) of CNS white matter fails rapidly during ischemia at 37° C.[8,39,40] In a completely myelinated white matter tract, the rat optic nerve, the CAP begins to

Pathophysiology

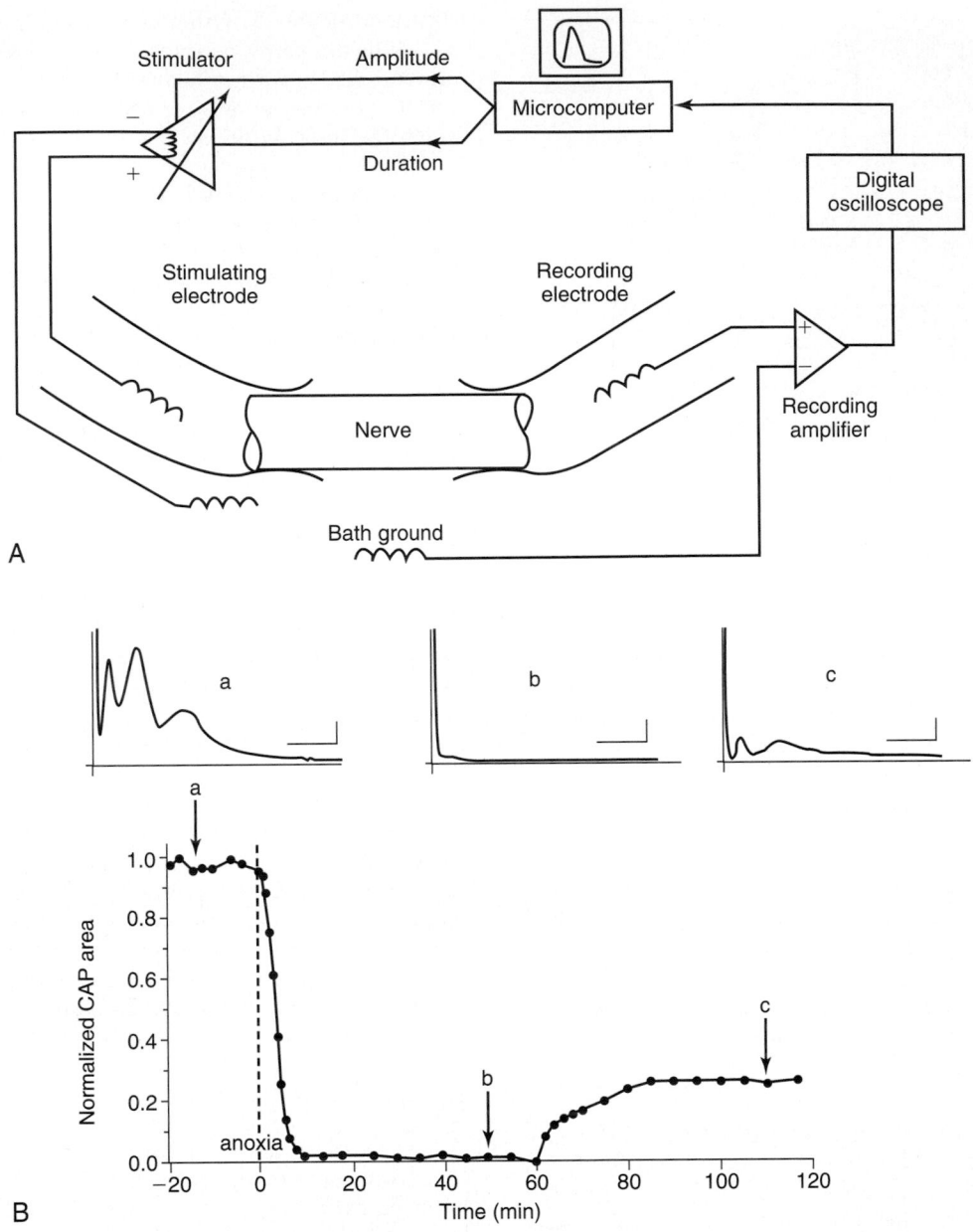

FIGURE 44–4 *Method of measuring rat optic nerve function before and after anoxia or ischemia. A, Diagram of recording arrangement. The rat optic nerve is stimulated with a supramaximal voltage pulse via one suction electrode. The compound action potential (CAP) is recorded from the other end of the nerve with a second suction electrode; signals are amplified, digitized, and transferred to a microcomputer for processing and storage. B, Effects of anoxia on white matter function. The function of the optic nerve was monitored as the area under the CAP (a to c); this is shown graphically as percentage of the control CAP integral. Anoxia was begun at time zero. CAP area rapidly declined, becoming virtually zero after 10 minutes of anoxia. A standard 60-minute period of anoxia or ischemia was used in most experiments. After O_2 was reintroduced, CAP area gradually recovered to a mean of about 30% of control in perfusate containing 2.0 mM $[Ca^{2+}]_o$. For quantification, postanoxic (or postischemic) CAP measurements were made 60 minutes after the end of the insult because recovery always reached a plateau by this time. Specimen records of the CAP under control (a), anoxic (b) and postanoxic (c) conditions are shown. Calibration marks are 1 ms and 1 mV. (Modified from Stys PK, et al: Role of extracellular calcium in anoxic injury of mammalian central white matter. Proc Natl Acad Sci U S A 87:4212–4218, 1990.)*

decline within 2 to 3 minutes of onset of ischemia or anoxia* and virtually disappears after 6 to 8 minutes (see Fig. 44–4B).[39] During reoxygenation after ischemia or anoxia, the CAP partially returns to a new stable level within 1 hour. The speed and magnitude of white matter recovery decrease as the duration of anoxia increases. Even after 60 minutes of ischemia, however, the mean recovery of function is about 30%.[39] This result is interpreted to mean that about 70% of the axons in the tract have been irreversibly injured. Indeed, electron-microscopic analysis

*For technical reasons, anoxia is essentially equivalent to ischemia in experiments on the rat optic nerve.[18] In this chapter, therefore, findings from anoxia experiments on rat optic nerve are considered relevant for ischemia

shows that a majority of axons subjected to 60 minutes of anoxia have severe structural changes.[41] Large axons are more severely affected than small ones. In vitro experiments imply that white matter recovers better from a given period of insult than gray matter.[39] The implication is that the therapeutic window for rescuing white matter from an ischemic insult is longer than that for gray matter.

There are regional differences in the pattern of white matter dysfunction due to ischemia. Ischemia causes a monophasic loss of function in both the optic nerve and the corpus callosum, but the pattern of CAP recovery is more complex in the corpus callosum (Fig. 44–5A). In the optic nerve, recovery of excitability is monophasic and stable after 30 to 60 minutes of restored glucose and oxygen. The corpus callosum, however, recovers excitability in a multiphasic fashion and shows a late progressive decline (see Fig. 44–5C). This difference remains unexplained.

Derangement of Transmembrane Ion Gradients

Rapid changes in brain extracellular ion concentrations occur with deprivation of oxygen, glucose, or both.[42] These changes reflect the metabolic state of local brain tissue[43]

and can have direct effects on neural behavior. Elevated extracellular potassium concentration ($[K^+]_o$) depolarizes neuronal membranes, reducing and then blocking action potentials, causes uncontrolled transmitter release,[44] induces cell swelling,[45] and may affect cerebral blood flow.[46] Elevated $[K^+]_o$ does not, in and of itself, reduce electrogenic glial uptake of the excitotoxin glutamate,[47] as was anticipated.[48] Extracellular acidosis can have direct toxic effects on both neuronal and glial membranes,[49,50] alters ion channel function,[51] and blocks currents generated by activation of n-methyl-D-aspartate (NMDA) receptors.[52] In the case of white matter, the extracellular ionic changes produced by anoxia predispose to other ionic events that are critical for injury (see later).

In white matter, anoxia or ischemia causes rapid changes in the extracellular concentrations of K^+ and H^+ that are qualitatively similar to those seen in gray matter, but smaller.[42,53,54] Within 3 or 4 minutes of the onset of anoxia, $[K^+]_o$ in the optic nerve begins to increase, reaching a final concentration of about 15 mM from a baseline of 3 mM. No spreading depression–like event occurs in white matter during anoxia, in contrast to most gray matter areas,[42,55] partially explaining why $[K^+]_o$ increases less in white matter than in gray matter.[54,56]

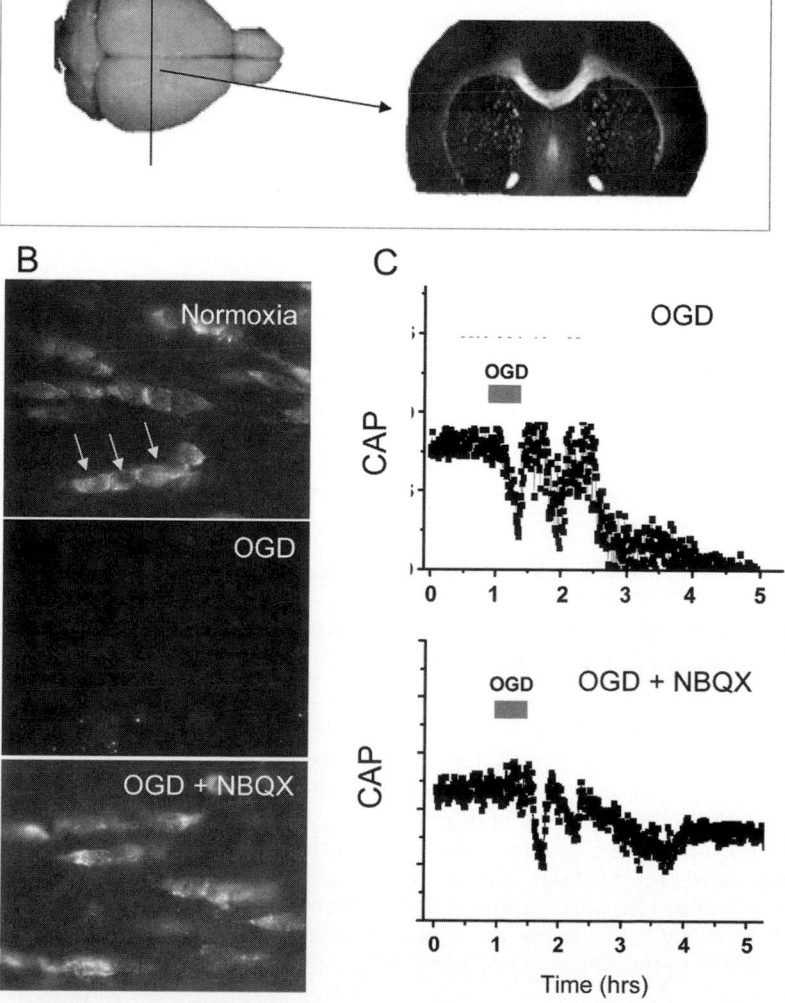

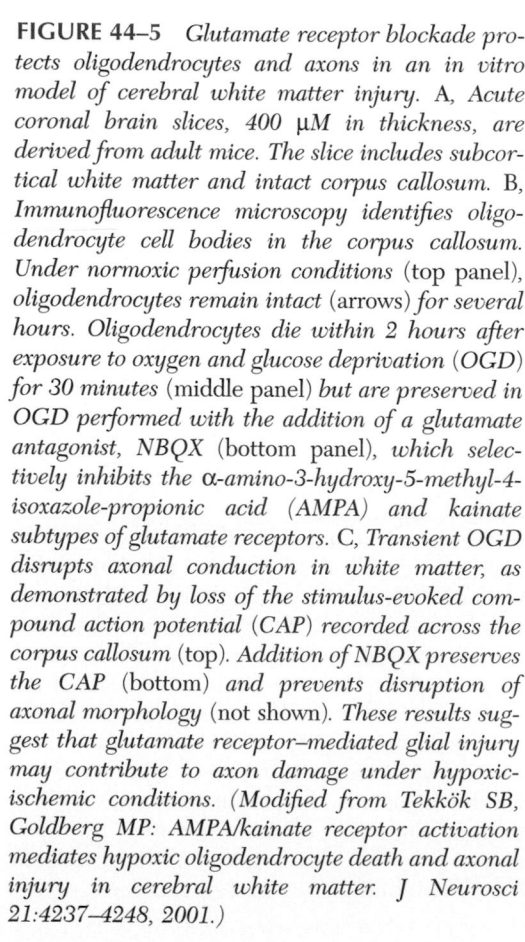

FIGURE 44–5 *Glutamate receptor blockade protects oligodendrocytes and axons in an in vitro model of cerebral white matter injury. A, Acute coronal brain slices, 400 μM in thickness, are derived from adult mice. The slice includes subcortical white matter and intact corpus callosum. B, Immunofluorescence microscopy identifies oligodendrocyte cell bodies in the corpus callosum. Under normoxic perfusion conditions (top panel), oligodendrocytes remain intact (arrows) for several hours. Oligodendrocytes die within 2 hours after exposure to oxygen and glucose deprivation (OGD) for 30 minutes (middle panel) but are preserved in OGD performed with the addition of a glutamate antagonist, NBQX (bottom panel), which selectively inhibits the α-amino-3-hydroxy-5-methyl-4-isoxazole-propionic acid (AMPA) and kainate subtypes of glutamate receptors. C, Transient OGD disrupts axonal conduction in white matter, as demonstrated by loss of the stimulus-evoked compound action potential (CAP) recorded across the corpus callosum (top). Addition of NBQX preserves the CAP (bottom) and prevents disruption of axonal morphology (not shown). These results suggest that glutamate receptor–mediated glial injury may contribute to axon damage under hypoxic-ischemic conditions. (Modified from Tekkök SB, Goldberg MP: AMPA/kainate receptor activation mediates hypoxic oligodendrocyte death and axonal injury in cerebral white matter. J Neurosci 21:4237–4248, 2001.)*

Pathophysiology

An acid shift in extracellular pH (pH_o) develops during anoxia with a maximum value of about 0.3 pH unit in standard physiologic solution.[54] After anoxia, pH_o returns slowly to its baseline level and exhibits a secondary acidification phase of unknown significance. The acid shifts in pH_o seen in white matter and gray matter during anoxia are probably the consequence of increased anaerobic metabolism leading to accumulation of extracellular lactic acid.[53,54,57] Lactic acid can exit cells by diffusion, in its undissociated form, or by a direct transport mechanism.[58] In vitro studies suggest that during anoxia, glial cells and neurons contain equivalent amounts of intracellular lactate but that glial cells transport more lactic acid to the ECS.[58] Astrocytes, but not neurons, contain glycogen, which is broken down and anaerobically metabolized to lactate during ischemia. Astrocytes may therefore have an important role in producing the acid shift in pH_o seen with anoxia or ischemia.[54]

Ischemia causes brain ATP to rapidly decline.[43,59] What is not well publicized is that ATP decline appears to be significantly slower in white matter than in gray matter.[60] The simple hypothesis for the slower loss of white matter ATP during ischemia is the lower metabolic rate of this tissue compared with gray matter. The implication is that white matter may retain sufficient ATP to prolong the time it can endure ischemia without sustaining irreversible injury. Reduction of ATP causes energy-dependent ion pumps to fail, including the Na^+-K^+ and Ca^{2+}-ATPases, and this failure would affect both axons and glial cells (see later). As a consequence, ions redistribute down their concentration gradients, leading to membrane depolarization that activates voltage-gated ion channels. Other K^+ channels may be activated and contribute to the increase in $[K^+]_o$, including Ca^{2+}-dependent K^+ channels, ATP-dependent K^+ channels, and Na^+-dependent K^+ channels.[42,61] Anoxia or ischemia causes the volume of the ECS of the rat optic nerve to decrease by as much as 20%,[62] probably because of glial swelling triggered by increases in $[K^+]_o$.[45]

In animal experiments, gray matter appears to suffer more damage when ischemia occurs in the presence of higher-than-usual glucose concentrations.[63,64] It is not known whether this observation is also true for white matter. During anoxia, however, white matter is functionally protected by elevated bath glucose,[54] even though it causes a greater acid shift, which is believed to worsen stroke outcome.[65] Curiously, in vitro studies, in contrast to in vivo studies, indicate that gray matter and white matter are both protected from anoxic injury by elevated glucose concentrations.[54,66]

Extracellular Ca^{2+} is Critical for Anoxic Injury in White Matter

The calcium hypothesis holds that unregulated increases in intracellular calcium concentration (Ca^{2+}) represent a "final common pathway" for cellular damage.[43,67] This hypothesis appears to be true whether the white matter damage is due to ischemia or anoxia.

Representative data indicating that extracellular Ca^{2+} is necessary for white matter injury are shown in Figure 44–6. Different concentrations of Ca^{2+} were applied to the in vitro rat optic nerve for a period extending from 10 minutes before the onset of anoxia to 10 minutes after the

end of anoxia (see Fig. 44–6B, inset). As the $[Ca^{2+}]$ of the test solution is decreased from 4 mM to zero, the extent of CAP recovery from anoxia gradually increases. Even a 50% reduction in $[Ca^{2+}]$, for instance, from 2 to 1 mM, results in significant enhancement of CAP recovery. The CAP area recovers to 100% of control with zero $[Ca^{2+}]$ perfusate (see Fig. 44–6), indicating that axons are strongly protected from anoxia-induced (i.e., 60-minute) injury. Injuries of other white matter preparations, of corpus callosum and spinal cord dorsal column, have similar dependencies on extracellular Ca^{2+}.[8,68]

These findings indicate that the presence of extracellular Ca^{2+} is critical for the development of irreversible anoxic injury in white matter and suggest that the severity of injury is related to the transmembrane Ca^{2+} gradient. Extracellular Ca^{2+}, therefore, probably acts as a source for inward flux of Ca^{2+} into a cytoplasmic compartment. This possibility is supported by the observation that extracellular calcium concentration (Ca^{2+}) falls during anoxia with a time course that fits well the development of irreversible injury.[69]

Because white matter axons become dysfunctional during anoxia, on the basis of the loss of the CAP, a damaging increase in intra-axonal $[Ca^{2+}]$ seems likely. Indeed, 60 minutes of anoxia causes striking pathologic alterations within axons.[41] Large vacuolar spaces appear between axons and their myelin sheaths, axoplasmic mitochondria are swollen and disrupted, and neurofilaments and microtubules disappear from the axoplasm (Fig. 44–7). Strengthening the argument that such changes are due to toxic increases in $[Ca^{2+}]_i$ is the observation that peripheral axons show similar ultrastructural abnormalities after a drug-induced increase in $[Ca^{2+}]_i$.[70] These changes are most prominent in large axons. Paranodal myelin retracts from the node in some fibers, a change that may adversely affect saltatory conduction (see Fig. 44–7B, arrow). Although some of the ultrastructural changes seen after 60 minutes of anoxia can partially recover after 60 minutes of reoxygenation, neurofilament and microtubule damage persists. There is a partial restitution in many fibers of the normal relation between axon membrane and paranodal myelin, which might represent the ultrastructural substrate for some of the postanoxic recovery that is measured as a partial return of the CAP (see Fig. 44–4B). We must emphasize, however, that the return of the CAP to a new steady level after anoxia is likely to be a multifactorial process and certainly involves the reestablishment of critical transmembrane ion gradients that are the basis of axonal excitability.[71]

If the nerve is exposed to anoxia in the absence of bath calcium, the ultrastructural abnormalities previously described are not seen.[72] The correlation, therefore, between changes in axonal structure and changes in axonal function (i.e., CAP area) is excellent; in the presence of normal extracellular Ca^{2+}, anoxia disrupts both axonal structure and function, whereas in the absence of extracellular Ca^{2+}, anoxia does not produce long-term disruption of either. The available evidence is indirect, but all of it points to the conclusion that during anoxia, Ca^{2+} rushes into axonal cytoplasm—probably at the nodes of Ranvier, where the axon membrane is most exposed—leading to the loss of normal architecture and excitability.

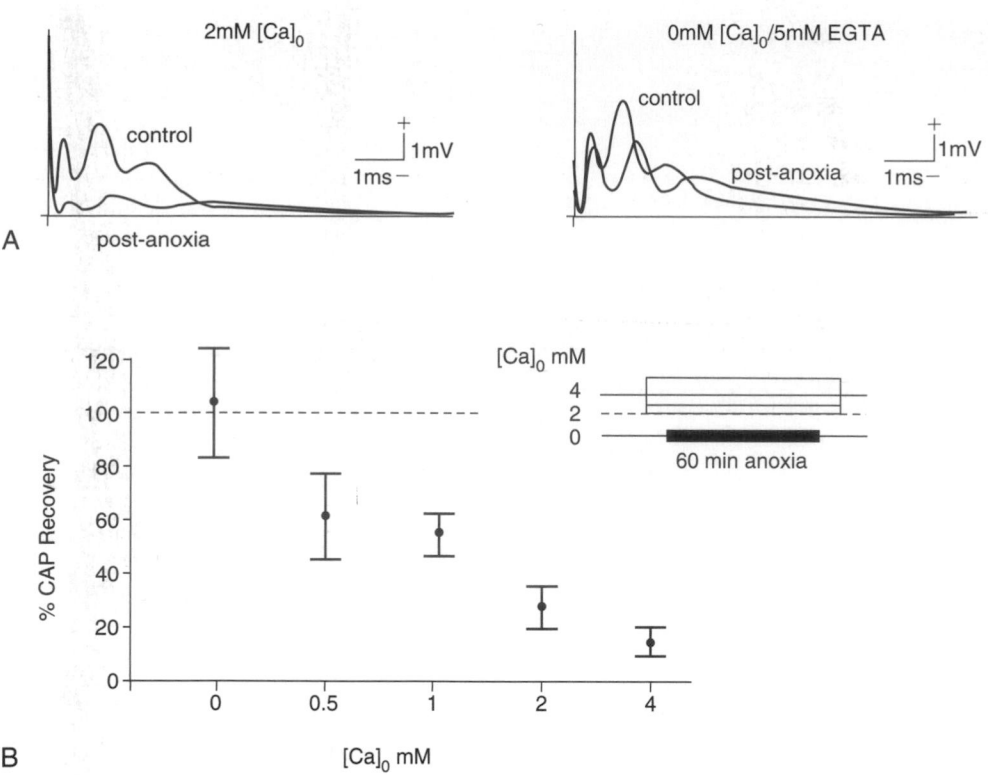

FIGURE 44–6 *Effect of perfusate extracellular calcium concentration ([Ca²⁺]) on recovery of compound action potential (CAP) from 60 minutes of anoxia. A, CAPs before ("control") and 60 minutes after anoxia in 2.0 mM [Ca²⁺] or zero [Ca²⁺]/5 mM EGTA are shown. CAP recovery from anoxia is enhanced in the zero Ca²⁺ solution. B, Graph showing average (± 1 S.D.) percentage CAP recovery after a 60-minute period of anoxia as a function of perfusate [Ca²⁺] during anoxia. Test solutions were begun 10 minutes before anoxia onset and continued until 10 min after the end of anoxia (see inset). The percentage recovery of the CAP gradually diminished as perfusate [Ca²⁺] increased from 0 to 4 mM. The mean recovery in 2.0 mM [Ca²⁺]ₒ was 28.5 ± 10.6%, whereas in zero [Ca²⁺]/5 mM EGTA, the area under the CAP recovered to 103 ± 23% of the control value. (Modified from Stys PK, et al: Role of extracellular calcium in anoxic injury of mammalian central white matter. Proc Natl Acad Sci U S A 87:4212–4218, 1990.)*

Ischemia also affects glial cells and myelin in white matter in a Ca²⁺-dependent manner.[8,68] In corpus callosum and dorsal column, oligodendrocytes and myelin are severely damaged according to histopathologic studies.[8,68] In general, the level of astrocyte injury seems minor for the durations of ischemia that have been evaluated. This finding probably reflects the ability of astrocytes to anaerobically manufacture ATP from their glycogen stores for tens of minutes during ischemia.[14] The ways in which these changes contribute to the pathophysiology of disrupted energy metabolism in white matter are still being worked out. Clearly, the disruption of myelin, and the cells that make it, would degrade signal transmission in white matter.

MECHANISMS OF WHITE MATTER INJURY

Ca²⁺ Entry into Axons During Ischemia or Anoxia

The central role of Ca²⁺ influx in mediating anoxic-ischemic damage in neuron cell bodies[73] and axons[69] is well established. In gray matter, where synapses abound, the predominant mechanism for Ca²⁺ entry into neurons is through NMDA-type glutamate receptors. White matter has no synapses and appears to be resistant to prolonged application of high concentrations of glutamate,[74] concentrations that would quickly kill neuron cell bodies. But the story of how white matter is disabled by ischemia has turned out to be more complicated and interesting than anticipated. Some early presumptions about white matter injury, most prominently that glutamate is not involved, have proved incorrect. There are still many unanswered questions about how white matter is injured, and the current model of ischemia-induced white matter injury will undoubtedly require major modifications. At present, there is good support for the hypothesis that ischemia injures both axons and glial cells in white matter and does so by very different mechanisms. Using this hypothesis as an organizing principle, we discuss axon and glial injuries separately.

The two ionic mechanisms that mediate pathologic entry of Ca²⁺ into axons during anoxia or ischemia are (1) reverse operation of the Na⁺-Ca²⁺ exchanger, a ubiquitous (with the exception of red blood cells) membrane protein that normally operates to extrude cytoplasmic Ca²⁺ in exchange for Na⁺ influx, and (2) voltage-gated Ca²⁺ channels.

Reversal of Na⁺-Ca²⁺ Exchange

The Na⁺-Ca²⁺ exchanger does not consume ATP and is driven primarily by the transmembrane Na⁺ gradient. The

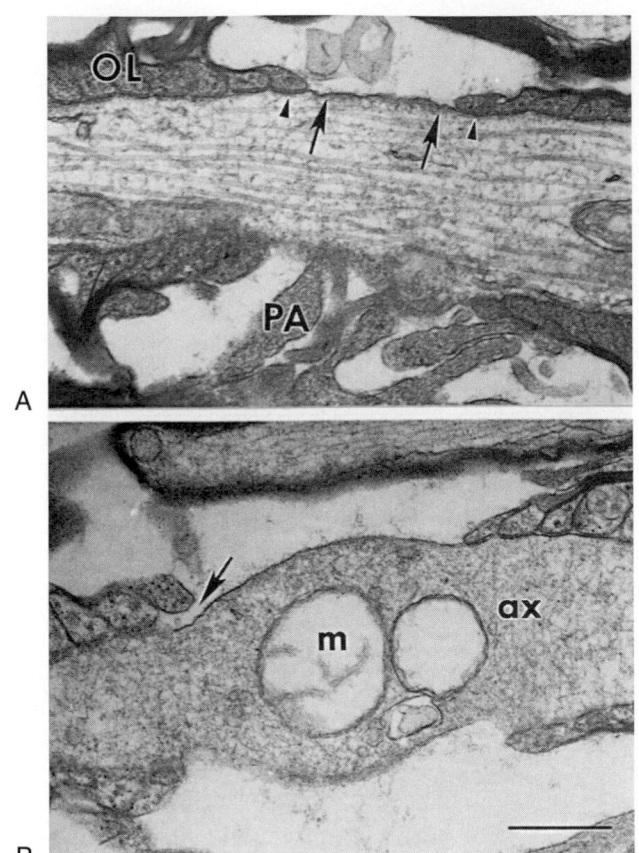

FIGURE 44–7 *Electron micrographs showing ultrastructural changes at nodes of Ranvier in the anoxic optic nerve. A, In the control optic nerve, note the close opposition of terminating oligodendroglial loops (OL) to the axon in the paranode (arrowheads), and the dense undercoating of the normal axon membrane (arrows). Perinodal astrocyte processes (PA) approach the node. The axoplasm contains a dense network of microtubules. B, In the anoxic optic nerve, there is occasional detachment of terminal myelin loops from the axon (arrow). Mitochondria are swollen with distorted cristae (m). There is destruction of microtubules within the axoplasm (ax). A and B, × 40,000; bar, 0.5 µm. (Modified from Waxman SG, et al: Ultrastructural concomitants of anoxic injury and early post-anoxic recovery in rat optic nerve. Brain Res 574:105–119, 1992.)*

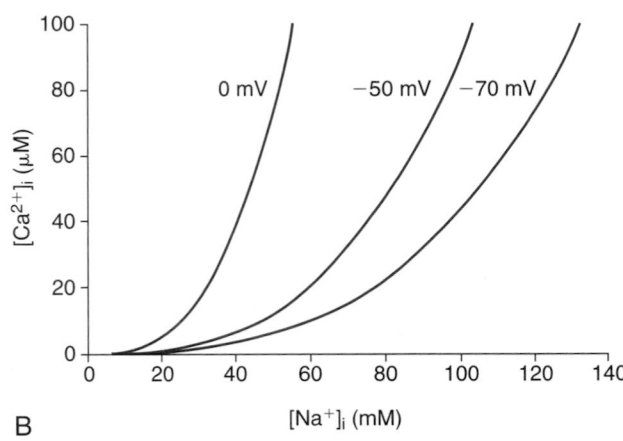

$$E_{NaCa} = \frac{n\,E_{Na} - 2\,E_{Ca}}{n-2} \qquad \text{eq.1}$$

$$[Ca]_i = [Ca]_0\ Exp\left[\frac{F\,Vm\,(n-2)}{RT}\right]\left[\frac{[Na]_i}{[Na]_0}\right]^n \qquad \text{eq.2}$$

A

B

FIGURE 44–8 *Effects of membrane potential and intracellular sodium ($[Na^+]_i$) on Na^+-Ca^{2+} exchange. A, Equations describing the behavior of the Na^+-Ca^{2+} exchanger.[3,64] E_{NaCa}, E_{Na}, and E_{Ca} are reversal potentials of the exchanger, Na^+ ions, and Ca^{2+} ions, respectively, and n represents the exchanger stoichiometry. The exchanger operates in the direction required to bring its reversal potential closer to membrane potential, V_m. At thermodynamic equilibrium, E_{NaCa} equals V_m. Substituting V_m into equation 1, expanding the expressions for E_{Na} and E_{Ca}, and rearranging, we obtain an expression (equation 2) for the intracellular calcium concertration ($[Ca^{2+}]_i$) that would be maintained by the Na^+-Ca^{2+} exchanger. B, Graphic representation of equation 2 at three values of membrane potential, assuming a stoichiometry of 3 Na^+:1 Ca^{2+}. With increasing $[Na^+]_i$ and/or membrane depolarization, both of which occur during anoxia, the Na^+-Ca^{2+} exchanger will tend to increase $[Ca^{2+}]_i$. (From Stys PK, Waxman SG, Ransom BR: Ionic mechanisms of anoxic injury in mammalian CNS white matter: Role of Na+ channels and Na[$^+$]-Ca^{2+} exchanger. J Neurosci 12:430–439, 1992.)*

exchanger can function equally well in forward and reverse directions and is a high-capacity, relatively low-affinity transporter of Ca^{2+}.[75] The typical stoichiometry of this process is that 3 Na^+ ions exchange for each Ca^{2+} ion; this exchange ratio causes the process to be electrogenic, and in fact, membrane current is generated by its operation.[76] For this reason, the exchanger is also influenced by membrane potential[77]; membrane depolarization favors reverse exchange (i.e., Na^+ efflux and Ca^{2+} influx). The manner in which $[Ca^{2+}]_i$ can be modulated by changes in the transmembrane Na^+ gradient, membrane potential, or both is illustrated in Figure 44–8.[9] It is important to note that relatively small changes in $[Na^+]_i$ (intracellular $[Na^+]$) or membrane potential can markedly alter $[Ca^{2+}]_i$. Specifically, increases in $[Na^+]_i$ and membrane depolarization lead to large increases in $[Ca^{2+}]_i$.

The hypothesized sequence of events leading to anoxic-ischemic injury of white matter axons is as follows. Anoxia-ischemia causes a rapid drop in ATP with an increase in $[K^+]_o$ (see earlier), resulting in axonal depolarization. Na^+ influx through voltage-dependent Na^+ channels would lead to an increase in $[Na^+]_i$ because the Na^+ pump function would be impaired.[78,79] Both membrane depolarization and the increase in $[Na^+]_i$ favor reverse operation of the Na^+-Ca^{2+} exchanger, which would continue until a higher, steady-state $[Ca^{2+}]_i$ is reached (see Fig. 44–8).

If reversal of Na^+-Ca^{2+} exchange mediates Ca^{2+} loading during anoxia in white matter, blocking the exchanger

Pathophysiology

during anoxia should improve outcome—and it does. Inhibitors of this transporter (e.g., bepridil or benzamil) markedly improve postanoxic recovery. The extent of postanoxic CAP recovery, seen after treatments that limit operation of the Na^+-Ca^{2+} exchanger, approaches the level of recovery seen when the nerve is bathed in zero-Ca^{2+} solution during anoxia. Additional proof that reverse operation of the Na^+-Ca^{2+} exchanger causes damaging Ca^{2+} influx into axons during anoxia is that the extent of $[Ca^{2+}]_o$ drop seen during anoxia is diminished by exchange inhibitors.[69]

It follows from the preceding sequence that increases in $[Na^+]_i$ strongly propel reverse Na^+-Ca^{2+} exchange. Axons accumulate net amounts of Na^+ during disruption of energy metabolism as a result of activation of voltage-dependent Na^+ channels (myelinated axons possess extremely high densities ($> 10^3/\mu m^2$) of nodal Na^+ channels).[7] Blocking Na^+ channels with tetrodotoxin (TTX) significantly improves CAP recovery after anoxia. Concentrations of TTX that do not significantly alter optic nerve excitability as measured by the CAP also protect against anoxic injury, but to a lesser extent than higher concentrations, which do block action potential electrogenesis.[80] TTX application during 60 minutes of anoxia yields at least 80% recovery of CAP area, compared with about 30% recovery under control conditions.

In the optic nerve, entry of Na^+ during anoxia continues throughout the entire period of exposure.[9] Conventional Na^+ channels quickly inactivate with depolarization and would not be available to mediate persistent Na^+ influx. Some Na^+ channels, however, inactivate slowly or not at all.[81] Non-inactivating Na^+ channels are present in optic nerve axons[80] and appear to account for the pathologic Na^+ influx that leads to axonal dysfunction in white matter.

Activation of Voltage-Gated Ca^{2+} Channels

Voltage-gated Ca^{2+} channels are known to participate in some models of anoxic injury.[82] Calcium channel blockers reduce the extent of this injury, presumably by preventing damaging influx of Ca^{2+} into neurons that are depolarized because of anoxia.[82,83] Initially, it appeared that organic and inorganic Ca^{2+} channel antagonists do not improve the outcome of white matter exposed to anoxia.[84] Subsequent studies, however, have clearly established that L-type Ca^{2+} channels are present on CNS myelinated axons[69] and mediate toxic Ca^{2+} influx during anoxia in CNS white matter.[69,85] Blockers of L-type Ca^{2+} channels applied during anoxia improve functional recovery. L-type Ca^{2+} channels are also present on white matter astrocytes.[69] Astrocytes, however, continue to produce ATP during brief periods of anoxia or ischemia (see earlier discussion) and would not depolarize to the extent necessary to activate high-threshold Ca^{2+} channels.

Reverse operation of the Na^+-Ca^{2+} exchanger and activation of Ca^{2+} channels may act in parallel to allow entry of Ca^{2+} into axons during anoxia. Alternatively, Ca^{2+} influx may be initiated through Ca^{2+} channels, leading to an increase in $[Ca^{2+}]_i$ that subsequently triggers reverse Na^+-Ca^{2+} exchange. For unclear reasons, higher-than-normal $[Ca^{2+}]_i$ is a necessary precondition for reversal of Na^+-Ca^{2+} exchange.[86] Axonal Ca^{2+} channels, therefore, might act to 'kick-start' the phase of Ca^{2+} accumulation mediated by the Na^+-Ca^{2+} exchanger.

A summary diagram of how ischemia leads to Ca^{2+} accumulation in white matter axons is shown in Figure 44–9. In the presence of oxygen and glucose, sufficient ATP is generated to operate the Na^+ pump. The Na^+ pump maintains a low $[Na^+]_i$ and prevents large increases in $[Na^+]_i$ with nerve action potentials.[79] It is also responsible for the axon's high negative resting membrane potential. These two conditions—normal transmembrane Na^+ gradient and negative membrane potential—dictate that the Na^+-Ca^{2+} exchanger operates in the "forward" mode, extruding Ca^{2+} (see Fig. 44–9A). In the absence of oxygen and glucose, ATP drops sharply in 2 to 3 minutes. The Na^+ pump, which consumes about half of all the energy used in neurons,[78] is no longer able to maintain transmembrane gradients of K^+ and Na^+. Increases in $[Na^+]_i$ secondary to influx through Na^+ channels can no longer be corrected.[79] Myelinated axons may be especially susceptible to this cascade of events, because their very high densities of Na^+ channels at nodes of Ranvier would predispose to large focal increases in $[Na^+]_i$. Increases in $[K^+]_o$ cause membrane depolarization and opening of non-inactivating, voltage-dependent Na^+ channels[28] that elevate $[Na^+]_i$. Ca^{2+} channels would be open persistently under these conditions, and the resulting Ca^{2+} influx would lead to elevation of $[Ca^{2+}]_i$. The progressive deterioration of membrane potential and transmembrane Na^+ gradient, along with an increase in $[Ca^{2+}]_i$, causes reverse operation of the Na^+-Ca^{2+} exchanger, leading to a rapid rise in $[Ca^{2+}]_i$[75] (see Fig. 44–8). This summary highlights the ionic disruptions that lead to increased $[Ca^{2+}]_i$ and ultimately to irreversible damage.[67] The "downstream" events promoted by increased $[Ca^{2+}]_i$ that are the ultimate cause of cell death[43,87,88] have yet to be defined in white matter. They are likely to include a set of biochemical reactions mediated by enzymes such as proteases and lipases as well as the generation of free radicals.[89]

Excitotoxic Pathways Injure Glia in White Matter

Release of endogenous glutamate and activation of neuronal glutamate receptors (*excitotoxicity*) is a major pathway leading to gray matter injury in ischemic stroke. Excitotoxicity might not be expected to contribute to white matter injury, because white matter lacks synapses and is devoid of the usual excitotoxic targets, neuronal cell bodies, and dendrites. This being said, compelling evidence supports a role for glutamate-mediated cell death in white matter injury associated with trauma and stroke, probably through activation of glutamate receptors on glial cells.

Like neurons, astrocytes and oligodendrocytes express functionally active α-amino-3-hydroxy-5-methyl-4-isoxazole-propionic acid (AMPA) and kainate (KA) glutamate receptor subunits.[90,91] The physiologic significance of these receptors remains to be established. In culture, oligodendrocyte lineage cells are highly vulnerable to glutamate excitotoxicity, and they can be rescued from hypoxic injury by glutamate receptor blockade.[21,24,92,93]

These in vitro studies raise the hypothesis that activation of AMPA/KA receptors contributes to hypoxic-ischemic death of oligodendrocytes in vivo and, in so doing, is a crucial step in white matter injury. However, cultured oligodendrocytes differ from their in vivo counterparts in

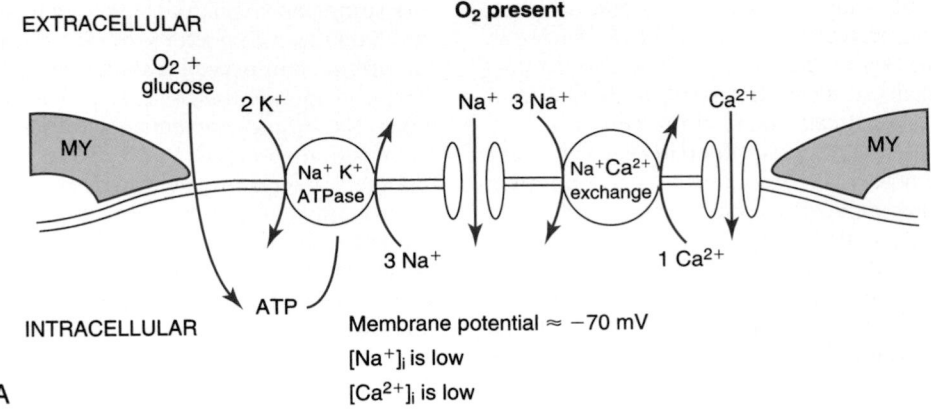

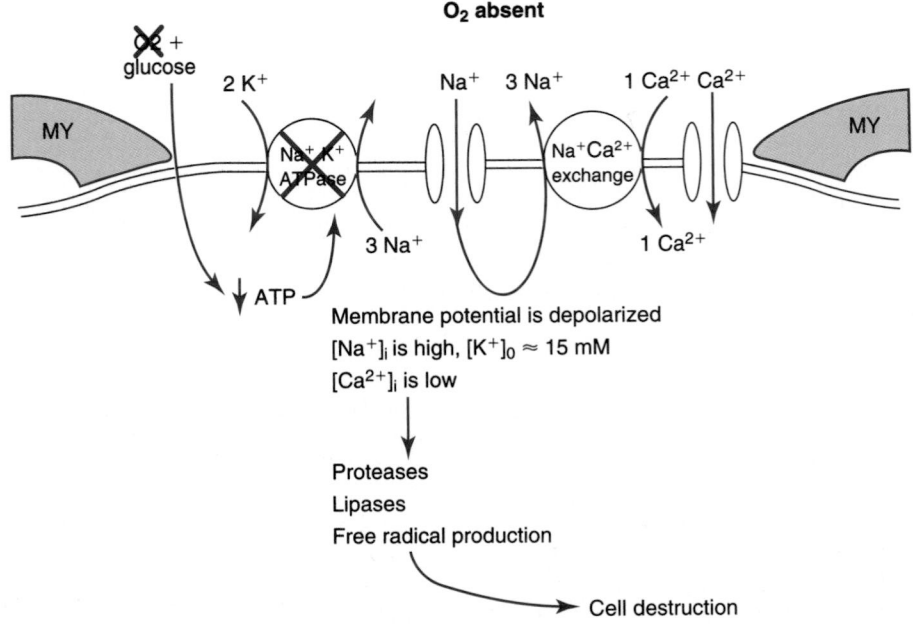

FIGURE 44–9   *Key ionic events that lead to intracellular Ca^{2+} accumulation during anoxia at nodes of Ranvier of central nervous system axons. A, Under normal conditions, sufficient oxygen and glucose are present to generate enough adenosine triphosphate (ATP) to operate the necessary ion pumps for maintaining excitability. If $[Na^+]_i$ increases because of action potentials, this increase is easily compensated by enhanced Na^+ pump activity. The steep Na^+ gradient produced by the Na^+ pump in conjunction with high negative membrane potential drives the high-capacity Na^+-Ca^{2+} exchanger in the forward direction, helping to maintain low $[Ca^{2+}]_i$. There is reason to believe that both the Na^+ pump and the Na^+-Ca^{2+} exchanger might be preferentially located at the nodes, because that is where activity-dependent ion fluxes occur in myelinated axons. Voltage-gated Ca^{2+} channels are also present but are not necessary for generation of action potentials. B, In the absence of oxygen, the generation of ATP is seriously reduced because it is now coming exclusively from glycolysis. The shortfall of ATP (the extent of which depends on glucose availability; see text) causes ion gradients to deteriorate, and the speed of deterioration is augmented by voltage-gated Na^+ channels, some of which are non-inactivating, increasing the workload on the Na^+ pump. As the transmembrane Na^+ gradient falls and the membrane depolarizes, the Na^+-Ca^{2+} exchanger is driven to work in reverse and begins loading the axon with Ca^{2+}. Ca^{2+} also enters the axon by way of voltage-gated Ca^{2+} channels. The ultimate destruction of cellular integrity is probably mediated by Ca^{2+}-activated destructive enzymes, such as proteases and lipases, and the generation of free radicals. (Modified from Ransom BR, Stys PK, Waxman SG: Anoxic injury of central myelinated axons: Ionic mechanisms and pharmacology. In Waxman SG [ed]: Molecular and Cellular Approaches to the Treatment of Brain Disease. New York, Raven Press, 1993, pp 121–151.)*

Pathophysiology

several important respects, including maturational state, receptor expression, and axonal-glial cellular interactions. Subsequent studies have confirmed a role for glutamate-mediated injury to oligodendrocytes in intact tissue preparations from mature white matter, including corpus callosum slices (see Fig. 44–5)[8] and spinal cord white matter.[32] Potential nonsynaptic sources for toxic glutamate release within ischemic white matter are axons,[32] astrocytes,[94,95] and oligodendrocytes.[24]

Blockade of AMPA/KA receptors has been found to reduce white matter injury in animal models of traumatic spinal cord injury,[96] spinal ischemia,[97] perinatal brain injury,[98] and focal cerebral ischemia.[99] In several experimental situations, AMPA/KA receptor blockade has been shown to protect axons as well as glial cells. Axons are not known to express functional glutamate receptors (but see

Brand-Schieber and Werner[100]), so the protective effects are likely to be mediated indirectly, through actions on associated glia.[8] These results support the hypothesis that glial cell injury mediated by glutamate, and axon injury mediated by ion channels or ion exchangers, are parallel pathways that interact, in currently unknown ways, to enhance white matter vulnerability to energy failure (Fig. 44–10). It is too early to conclude that this scheme applies to white matter everywhere in the brain. In fact, we predict that this will not be the case. It is logical to think that myelinated fibers would be more susceptible than unmyelinated fibers to failure and, perhaps injury, after oligodendrocyte and myelin damage, but this theory has not been critically tested. And what about the comparative time courses of these parallel pathways? In other words, does one proceed more quickly than the other? Answers to these questions

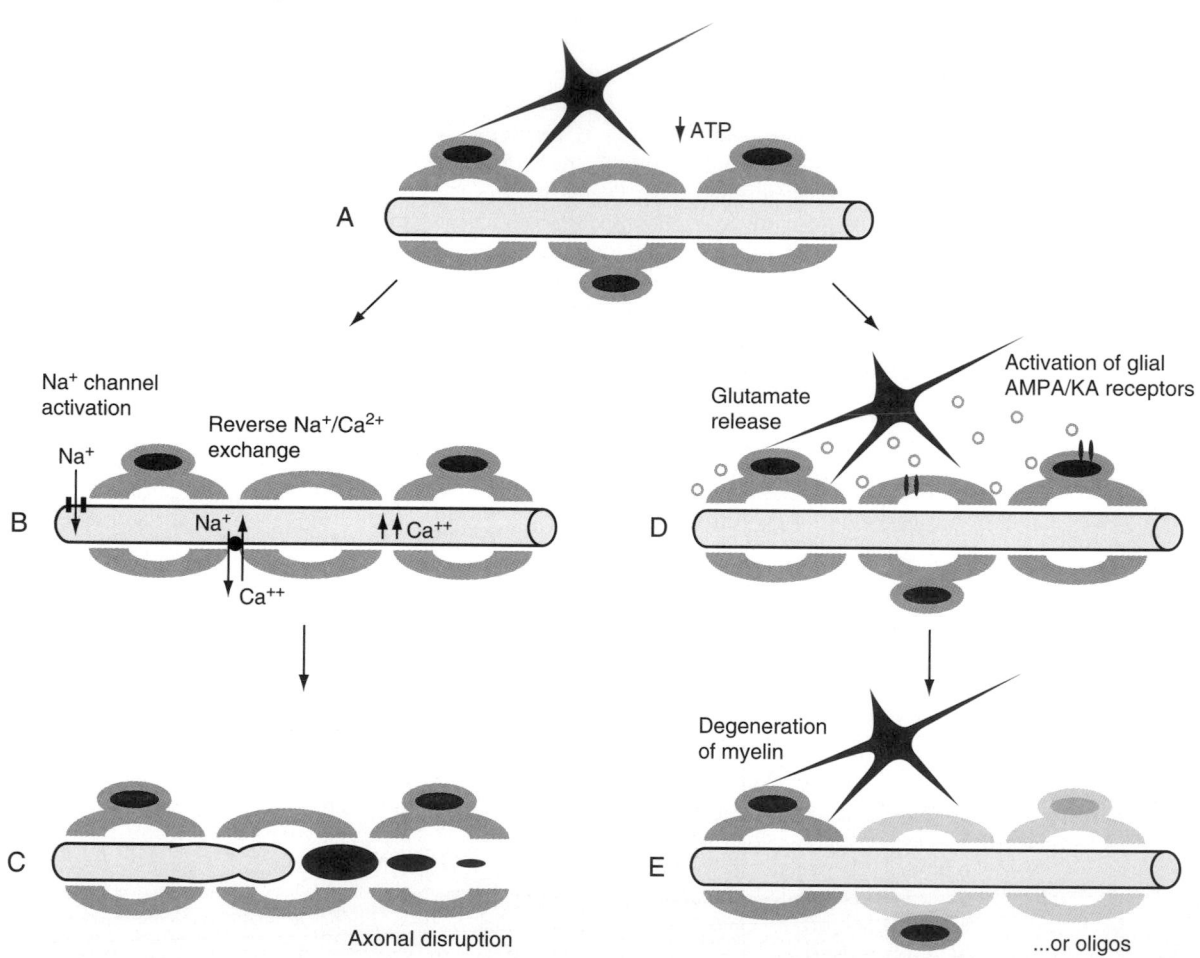

FIGURE 44–10 *Proposed axon and glial injury pathways in hypoxic-ischemic white matter injury. Schematic shows myelinated axon, oligodendrocytes (attached to myelin), and astrocytes (star-shaped). A, Hypoxia, ischemia, or glucose deprivation results in energy depletion and loss of adenosine triphosphate (ATP). B, Failure of Na/K-ATPase and depolarization leads to opening of noninactivating axon voltage-gated Na^+ channels. Ca^{2+} enters axons by reversal of Na-Ca exchange and activation of voltage-gated Ca^{2+} channels. Action potentials are halted reversibly by loss of ionic gradients. C, Excessive axoplasmic Ca^{2+} levels trigger destructive pathways, leading to degradation of axonal cytoskeleton and organelles, focal axonal swelling, and eventual interruption of axonal integrity. D, Another effect of energy deprivation is release of glutamate into extracellular space from axons, astrocytes, and/or oligodendrocytes. Glutamate activates ionotropic AMPA/KA (α-amino-3-hydroxy-5-methyl-4-isoxazole-propionic acid/kainate) receptors on glial cells. E, Sustained glutamate receptor activation triggers excitotoxic damage of oligodendrocyte processes (myelin) and death of oligodendrocytes. Myelin damage might result in conduction delay or block. (From Tekkök SB, Goldberg MP: AMPA/kainate receptor activation mediates hypoxic oligodendrocyte death and axonal injury in cerebral white matter. J Neurosci 21:4237–4248, 2001.)*

will be important to the development of therapeutic interventions.

AUTOPROTECTION IN WHITE MATTER

Nerve fiber tracts in the CNS do not contain synapses, but they do contain neurotransmitters and their cognate receptors. In addition to glutamate and glutamate receptors (see earlier discussion), white matter contains the neurotransmitters gamma-aminobutyric acid (GABA)[101] and adenosine[60] and their receptors.[102] Although the normal physiologic functions of GABA or adenosine in white matter are not known, both substances appear in extracellular fluid during ischemia.[60,103] Both GABA and adenosine, at very low concentrations, attenuate the severity of anoxia-induced white matter injury and therefore constitute a unique autoprotective system for this tissue.[104,105]

The effect of GABA on the extent of CAP recovery from a standard 60-minute period of anoxia is shown in Figure 44–11, from a study by Fern and colleagues.[105] Application of GABA (1 μM) to the optic nerve during anoxia significantly enhances improvement. These investigators found that the beneficial effect of GABA was mediated by GABA-B–type receptors; thus, GABA-induced protection was duplicated by the selective GABA-B agonist baclofen and blocked by the GABA-B antagonist phaclofen. High concentrations of GABA or baclofen did not afford protection, probably because of receptor desensitization.[104] These investigators also reported significantly worse outcome with use of the GABA-B receptor blocker phaclofen. This implied that GABA was being released from endogenous stores and was providing a protective action in the absence of bath application.[104]

GABA-B receptors are known to act through G-proteins, and G-protein antagonists blocked the protective effect of GABA against anoxic injury in the second study by Fern and colleagues.[104] The second messenger sequence of GABA's action was followed one step further and found to involve protein kinase C (PKC). Direct activation of PKC, in the absence of added GABA, mimicked the action of GABA, which is to say it was significantly protective.[104] Blockade of PKC prevented expression of GABA's protection action.

These findings suggest the following scheme: During ischemia-anoxia in white matter, GABA is released into the ECS, presumably from endogenous stores. The cellular origin of GABA under these conditions has not been determined, but glial cells contain GABA and have the capacity to release it if the ionic gradients that sustain uptake are degraded, as they would be during ischemia.[104] Once released, GABA acts at GABA-B receptors and through a G-protein/PKC pathway to partially protect the optic nerve from ischemia-induced injury. The protection is believed to be due to the phosphorylation by PKC of a critical protein within axons, but currently this target is not known. Phosphorylation and downregulation of the Na^+-Ca^{2+} exchanger would be one possibility. Curtailing the conductance of non-inactivating Na^+ channels or voltage-gated Ca^{2+} channels are other possibilities that could serve to lessen the impact of a period of ischemia.

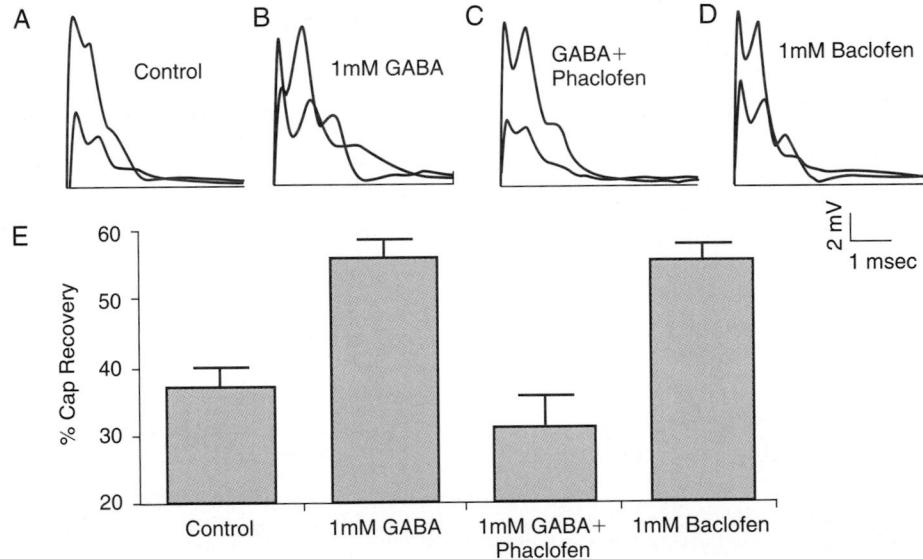

FIGURE 44–11   *The inhibitory neurotransmitter gamma-aminobutyric acid (GABA) acts at low concentrations to protect rat optic nerve axons from anoxia-induced damage. Superimposed preanoxic and postanoxic compound action potentials (CAPs) measured under control conditions and in the presence of various agents are shown along with a graphic summary of these results. The larger of each CAP pair is the preanoxic recording, and the smaller CAP is the postanoxic recovery. A, Under control conditions, the mean postanoxic CAP recovery is 36.5 ± 2.9%. B, GABA at 1 μM significantly increased recovery to a mean of 55.7 ± 2.5%. C, The selective GABA-B antagonist phaclofen (500 μM) blocked GABA's protective effect against anoxic injury. D, The selective GABA-B agonist baclofen (1 μM) protected against anoxic injury. E, Summarized results from numerous experiments like those shown in A through D. (Modified from Fern R, Waxman SG, Ransom BR: Endogenous GABA attenuates CNS white matter dysfunction after anoxia. J Neurosci 15:699–708, 1995.)*

Adenosine acts at specific receptors within white matter to reduce the extent of CAP loss associated with anoxic exposure and, in this way, closely mimics the behavior of GABA previously described.[104] In fact, GABA and adenosine act synergistically to protect white matter via the same G-protein/PKC pathway. Both are believed to be released at nanomolar concentrations during anoxia to recruit the "autoprotection" mechanism.[104] The extent to which this novel aspect of the pathophysiology of white matter damage can be pharmacologically manipulated remains to be investigated.

Strategies for Protecting White Matter from Anoxic-Ischemic Injury Are Diverse

The complexity of the injury process in white matter presents many potential strategies for therapeutic intervention. Experiments with isolated white matter have shown that inhibitors of voltage-gated Na^+ channels, voltage-gated Ca^{2+} channels, the Na^+-Ca^{2+} exchanger, and AMPA/KA receptors are all protective against anoxic-ishemic injury.[8,69,80,106] Potentiation of the GABA–adenosine autoprotective system is also protective in isolated white matter.[104,105] These pharmacologic manipulations act to block events that occur relatively early in the injury cascade. For example, the Na^+-Ca^{2+} exchanger inhibitor bepridil is protective because it prevents Ca^{2+} influx during anoxia, eliminating the downstream events that follow from high intracellular Ca^{2+}, such as the activation of destructive enzymes. In one sense this is advantageous, because interrupting the chain of events during the early stages represents the best opportunity for complete arrest of the injury process. The disadvantage of these drugs is that they must be present either before or immediately after the onset of an anoxic-ischemic event if they are to have a significantly protective effect. Therefore, identification of high-risk patients and long-term treatment with prophylactic concentrations of drugs may represent the most effective way of reducing the effect of white matter ischemic injuries such as lacunar infarcts. Such drugs would have to be very well tolerated and to have few side effects for their use in this preemptive way to be justified.

The utility of a therapeutic strategy will therefore be governed by both its efficacy and the extent to which it is tolerated by patients. Within these constraints, two types of intervention seem most promising. A number of drugs currently in clinical use for other conditions have been shown to protect white matter from anoxic-ischemic injury as a result of blocking Na^+ channels. They include antiarrhythmic drugs such as prajmaline and mexiletine[107,108] and the anti-epileptic drugs phenytoin and carbamazepine.[109] Some of these drugs have been shown to protect isolated white matter from injury at concentrations below those in current clinical use. For example, phenytoin improves recovery from a 60-minutes period of anoxia by about 80% at 1 μM, a concentration below that found in the cerebrospinal fluid of patients taking phenytoin to treat epilepsy.[109]

Drugs that interfere with GABA uptake and degradation represent a second way of interrupting the injury cascade with minimal side effects. These drugs, which include vigabatrin and gabapentin, have been developed to treat epilepsy and act by increasing the extracellular concentration of GABA.[110] Raising extracellular GABA is protective against anoxic injury in white matter,[104,105] suggesting a secondary use for these drugs in white matter ischemia. The relatively benign side effects of drugs such as gabapentin suggest that long-term treatment in patients at high risk of white matter injury may be possible.

Acknowledgments

Work in the authors' laboratories has been supported in part by grants from the National Institutes of Health (BRR, MPG), Eastern Paralyzed Veterans Association (BRR), American Heart Association (MPG), and the Juvenile Diabetes Research Foundation (MPG). An NINCDS (National Institute of Neurological and Communicative Disorders and Stroke) Training Grant supported ABA.

References

1. Young W: Blood flow, metabolic and neurophysiological mechanisms in spinal cord injury. In Becker D, Povlishock (eds): Central Nervous System Trauma Status Report. Bethesda, MD, National Institutes of Health/National Institute of Neurological and Communicative Disorders and Stroke, 1985, p 463.
2. Loizou LA, Kendall BE, Marshall J: Subcortical arteriosclerotic encephalopathy: A clinical and radiological investigation. J Neurol Neurosurg Psychiatry 44:294–304, 1981.
3. Fisher CM: Capsular infarcts: The underlying vascular lesions. Arch Neurol 36:65–73, 1979.
4. McQuinn BA, O'Leary DH: White matter lucencies on computed tomography, subacute arteriosclerotic encephalopathy (Binswanger's disease), and blood pressure. Stroke 18:900–905, 1987.
5. Foster RE, Connors BW, Waxman SG: Rat optic nerve: Electrophysiological, pharmacological and anatomical studies during development. Brain Res 255:371–386, 1982.
6. Sturrock RR: Myelination of the mouse corpus callosum. Neuropathol Appl Neurobiol 6:415–420, 1980.
7. Waxman SG, Ritchie JM: Organization of ion channels in the myelinated nerve fiber. Science 228(4707):1502–1507, 1985.
8. Tekkök SB, Goldberg MP: AMPA/Kainate receptor activation mediates hypoxic oligodendrocyte death and axonal injury in cerebral white matter. J Neurosci 21:4237–4248, 2001.
9. Stys PK, Waxman SG, Ransom BR: Ionic mechanisms of anoxic injury in mammalian CNS white matter: Role of Na^+ channels and $Na^{(+)}$-$Ca2^+$ exchanger. J Neurosci 12:430–439, 1992.
10. Zhang K, Sejnowski TJ: A universal scaling law between gray matter and white matter of cerebral cortex. Proc Natl Acad Sci U S A 97:5621–5626, 2000.
11. Ransom BR, Behar T, Nedergaard M: New roles for astrocytes (stars at last). Trends Neurosci 26:520–522, 2003.
12. Chen Y, Swanson RA: Astrocytes and brain injury. J Cereb Blood Flow Metab 23:137–149, 2003.
13. Wender R, et al: Astrocytic glycogen influences axon function and survival during glucose deprivation in central white matter. J Neurosci 20:6804–6810, 2000.
14. Rose CR, Waxman SG, Ransom BR: Effects of glucose deprivation, chemical hypoxia, and simulated ischemia on Na^+ homeostasis in rat spinal cord astrocytes. J Neurosci 18:3554–3562, 1998.
15. Ranson BR, Fern R: Anoxic-ischemic glial cell injury: Mechanisms and consequences. In Haddad GG (ed): Tissue Oxygen Deprivation. New York, Marcel Dekker, 1996, pp 617–652.
16. Nishizaki T, et al: Effects of temperature on the oxygen consumption in thin slices from different brain regions. Neurosci Lett 86:301–305, 1988.
17. Attwell D, Laughlin SB: An energy budget for signaling in the grey matter of the brain. J Cereb Blood Flow Metab 21:1133–1145, 2001.
18. Tekkök SB, Brown A, Ransom BR: Axon function persists during anoxia in mammalian white matter. J Cereb Blood Flow Metab 2003. In press
19. Moody DM, Bell MA, Challa VR: Features of the cerebral vascular pattern that predict vulnerability to perfusion or oxygenation defi-

ciency: An anatomic study. AJNR Am J Neuroradiol 11:431–439, 1990.

20. Lyons SA, Kettenmann H: Oligodendrocytes and microglia are selectively vulnerable to combined hypoxia and hypoglycemia injury in vitro. J Cereb Blood Flow Metab 18:521–530, 1998.

21. McDonald JW, et al: Oligodendrocytes from forebrain are highly vulnerable to AMPA/kainate receptor-mediated excitotoxicity. Nat Med 4:291–297, 1998.

22. Goldberg MP, Choi DW: Combined oxygen and glucose deprivation in cortical cell culture: Calcium-dependent and calcium-independent mechanisms of neuronal injury. J Neurosci 13:3510–3524, 1993.

23. Xu J, et al: Oxygen-glucose deprivation induces inducible nitric oxide synthase and nitrotyrosine expression in cerebral endothelial cells. Stroke 31:1744–1751, 2000.

24. Fern R, Moller T: Rapid ischemic cell death in immature oligodendrocytes: A fatal glutamate release feedback loop. J Neurosci 20:34–42, 2000.

25. Dewar D, Underhill SM, Goldberg MP: Oligodendrocytes and ischemic brain injury. J Cereb Blood Flow Metab 23:263–274, 2003.

26. Campenot RB: Local control of neurite development by nerve growth factor. Proc Natl Acad Sci U S A 74:4516–4519, 1977.

27. Lubetzki C, et al: Even in culture, oligodendrocytes myelinate solely axons. Proc Natl Acad Sci U S A 90:6820–6824, 1993.

28. Stys PK, et al: Role of extracellular calcium in anoxic injury of mammalian central white matter. Proc Natl Acad Sci U S A 87:4212–4216, 1990.

29. Ransom BR, Waxman SG, Stys PK: Anoxic injury of central myelinated axons: Ionic mechanisms and pharmacology. Res Publ Assoc Res Nerv Ment Dis 71:121–151, 1993.

30. Stys PK: Anoxic and ischemic injury of myelinated axons in CNS white matter: From mechanistic concepts to therapeutics. J Cereb Blood Flow Metab 18:2–25, 1998.

31. Garthwaite G, et al: Mechanisms of ischaemic damage to central white matter axons: A quantitative histological analysis using rat optic nerve. Neuroscience 94:1219–1230, 1999.

32. Li S, et al: Novel injury mechanism in anoxia and trauma of spinal cord white matter: Glutamate release via reverse Na(+)-dependent glutamate transport. J Neurosci 19:RC16, 1999.

33. Pantoni L, Garcia JH, Gutierrez JA: Cerebral white matter is highly vulnerable to ischemia. Stroke 27:1641–1647, 1996.

34. Dietrich WD, et al: White matter alterations after thromboembolic stroke: A beta-amyloid precursor protein immunocytochemical study in rats. Acta Neuropathol (Berl) 95:524–531, 1998.

35. Schabitz WR, Li F, Fisher M: The N-methyl-D-aspartate antagonist CNS 1102 protects cerebral gray and white matter from ischemic injury after temporary focal ischemia in rats. Stroke 31:1709–1714, 2000.

36. Yam PS, et al: NMDA receptor blockade fails to alter axonal injury in focal cerebral ischemia. J Cereb Blood Flow Metab 20:772–779, 2000.

37. Imai H, et al: Ebselen protects both gray and white matter in a rodent model of focal cerebral ischemia. Stroke, 32:2149–2154, 2001.

38. Goldlust EJ, et al: Automated measurement of infarct size with scanned images of triphenyltetrazolium chloride-stained rat brains. Stroke 27:1657–1662, 1996.

39. Fern R, et al: Axon conduction and survival in CNS white matter during energy deprivation: A developmental study. J Neurophysiol 79:95–105, 1998.

40. Stys PK, Ransom BR, Waxman SG: Compound action potential of nerve recorded by suction electrode: A theoretical and experimental analysis. Brain Res 546:18–32, 1991.

41. Waxman SG, et al: Ultrastructural concomitants of anoxic injury and early post-anoxic recovery in rat optic nerve. Brain Res 574:105–119, 1992.

42. Hansen AJ: Effect of anoxia on ion distribution in the brain. Physiol Rev 65:101–148, 1985.

43. Siesjö BK: Cell damage in the brain: A speculative synthesis. J Cereb Blood Flow Metab 1:155–185, 1981.

44. Benveniste H, et al: Elevation of the extracellular concentrations of glutamate and aspartate in rat hippocampus during transient cerebral ischemia monitored by intracerebral microdialysis. J Neurochem 43:1369–1374, 1984.

45. Kimelberg HK, Ransom BR: Physiological and pathological aspects of astrocytic swelling. In Federoff S, Vernadakis A (eds): Astrocytes. Orlando, FL, Academic Press, 1986, p 129.

46. Paulson OB, Newman EA: Does the release of potassium from astrocyte endfeet regulate cerebral blood flow? Science 237(4817):896–898, 1987.

47. Longuemare MC, et al: K(+)-induced reversal of astrocyte glutamate uptake is limited by compensatory changes in intracellular Na+. Neuroscience 93:285–292, 1999.

48. Schwartz EA, Tachibana M: Electrophysiology of glutamate and sodium co-transport in a glial cell of the salamander retina. J Physiol (Lond) 426:43–80, 1990.

49. Goldman SA, et al: The effects of extracellular acidosis on neurons and glia in vitro. J Cereb Blood Flow Metab 9:471–477, 1989.

50. Kraig RP, et al: Hydrogen ions kill brain at concentrations reached in ischemia. J Cereb Blood Flow Metab 7:379–386, 1987.

51. Tombaugh GC, Somjen GG: ph Modulation of voltage-gated ion channels. In Kaila K, Ransom BR (eds): ph and Brain Function. New York, Wiley-Liss, 1998, pp 395–416.

52. Traynelis SF: ph Modulation of ligand-gated ion channels. In Kaila K, Ransom BR (eds): pH and Brain Function. New York, Wiley-Liss, 1998, pp 417–446.

53. Kraig RP, Pulsinelli WA, Plum F: Hydrogen ion buffering during complete brain ischemia. Brain Res 342:281–290, 1985.

54. Ransom BR, et al: Anoxia-induced changes in extracellular K+ and pH in mammalian central white matter. J Cereb Blood Flow Metab 12:593–602, 1992.

55. Somjen GG, et al: Spreading depression-like depolarization and selective vulnerability of neurons: A brief review. Stroke 21(Suppl):III179–III183, 1990.

56. Kraig RP, Nicholson C: Extracellular ionic variations during spreading depression. Neuroscience 3:1045–1059, 1978.

57. Kraig RP, Ferreira-Filho CR, Nicholson C: Alkaline and acid transients in cerebellar microenvironment. J Neurophysiol 49:831–850, 1983.

58. Walz W, Mukerji S: Lactate release from cultured astrocytes and neurons: A comparison. GLIA 1:366–370, 1988.

59. Lowry OH, et al: Effect of ischemia on known substrates and cofactors of the glycolytic pathway in brain. J Biol Chem 239:18–30, 1964.

60. Dohmen C, et al: Adenosine in relation to calcium homeostasis: Comparison between gray and white matter ischemia. J Cereb Blood Flow Metab 21:503–510, 2001.

61. Haimann C, et al: Potassium current activated by intracellular sodium in quail trigeminal ganglion neurons. J Gen Physiol 95:961–979, 1990.

62. Ransom BR, Yamate CL, Connors BW: Activity-dependent shrinkage of extracellular space in rat optic nerve: A developmental study. J Neurosci 5:532–535, 1985.

63. Li PA, et al: Does long-term glucose infusion reduce brain damage after transient cerebral ischemia? Brain Res 912:203–205, 2001.

64. Plum F: What causes infarction in ischemic brain? The Robert Wartenberg Lecture. Neurology 33:222–233, 1983.

65. Siesjö BK, et al: Molecular mechanisms of acidosis-mediated damage. Acta Neurochir Suppl (Wien) 66:8–14, 1996.

66. Schurr A, et al: Increased glucose improves recovery of neuronal function after cerebral hypoxia in vitro. Brain Res 421:135–139, 1987.

67. Schanne FA, et al: Calcium dependence of toxic cell death: A final common pathway. Science 206(4419):700–702, 1979.

68. Li S, Stys PK: Mechanisms of ionotropic glutamate receptor-mediated excitotoxicity in isolated spinal cord white matter. J Neurosci 20:1190–1198, 2000.

69. Brown AM, et al: Axonal L-type Ca2+ channels and anoxic injury in rat CNS white matter. J Neurophysiol 85:900–911, 2001.

70. Schlaepfer WW: Structural alterations of peripheral nerve induced by the calcium ionophore A23187. Brain Res 136:1–9, 1977.

71. Hodgkin AL: The Conduction of the Nervous Impulse. London, Liverpool University Press, 1964.

72. Waxman SG, et al: Protection of the axonal cytoskeleton in anoxic optic nerve by decreased extracellular calcium. Brain Res 614:137–145, 1993.

73. Choi DW: Calcium-mediated neurotoxicity: Relationship to specific channel types and role in ischemic damage. Trends Neurosci 11:465–469, 1988.

74. Ransom BR, Waxman SG, Davis PK: Anoxic injury of CNS white matter: Protective effect of ketamine. Neurology 40:1399–1403, 1990.

75. Blaustein MP: Calcium transport and buffering in neurons. Trends Neurosci 11:438–443, 1988.

76. Lagnado L, Cervetto L, McNaughton PA: Ion transport by the Na-Ca exchange in isolated rod outer segray matterens. Proc Natl Acad Sci U S A 85:4548–4552, 1988.

77. Blaustein MP, Lederer WJ: Sodium/calcium exchange: Its physiological implications. Physiol Rev 79:763–854, 1999.

78. Ames AD, et al: Energy metabolism of rabbit retina as related to function: High cost of Na+ transport. J Neurosci 12:840–853, 1992.

79. Rose CR, Ransom BR: Regulation of intracellular sodium in cultured rat hippocampal neurones. J Physiol (Lond) 499(Pt:573–587, 1997.

80. Stys PK, et al: Noninactivating, tetrodotoxin-sensitive Na$^+$ conductance in rat optic nerve axons. Proc Natl Acad Sci U S A 90:6976–6980, 1993.

81. Taylor CP: Na$^+$ currents that fail to inactivate. Trends Neurosci 16:455–460, 1993.

82. Lipton SA: Calcium channel antagonists in the prevention of neurotoxicity. Adv Pharmacol 22:271–297, 1991.

83. Weiss JH, et al: The calcium channel blocker nifedipine attenuates slow excitatory amino acid neurotoxicity. Science 247:1474–1477, 1990.

84. Stys PK, Ransom BR, Waxman SG: Effects of polyvalent cations and dihydropyridine calcium channel blockers on recovery of CNS white matter from anoxia. Neurosci Lett 115:293–299, 1990.

85. Fern R, Ransom BR, Waxman SG: Voltage-gated calcium channels in CNS white matter: Role in anoxic injury. J Neurophysiol 74:369–377, 1995.

86. Dipolo R, Beauge L: Regulation of Na$^+$-Ca^{2+} exchange: An overview. Ann N Y Acad Sci 639:100–111, 1991.

87. Flamm ES, et al: Free radicals in cerebral ischemia. Stroke 9:445–447, 1978.

88. Nicotera P, et al: Ca^{2+}-activated mechanisms in cell killing. Drug Metab Rev 20:193–201, 1989.

89. Garthwaite G, et al: Soluble guanylyl cyclase activator YC-1 protects white matter axons from nitric oxide toxicity and metabolic stress, probably through Na($^+$) channel inhibition. Mol Pharmacol 61:97–104, 2002.

90. David JC, et al: AMPA receptor activation is rapidly toxic to cortical astrocytes when desensitization is blocked. J Neurosci 16:200–209, 1996.

91. Gallo V, Ghiani CA: Glutamate receptors in glia: New cells, new inputs and new functions. Trends Pharmacol Sci 21(7): p. 252–258, 2000.

92. Yoshioka A, et al: Alpha-amino-3-hydroxy-5-methyl-4-isoxazolepropionate (AMPA) receptors mediate excitotoxicity in the oligodendroglial lineage. J Neurochem 64:2442–2448, 1995.

93. Matute C, et al: Glutamate receptor-mediated toxicity in optic nerve oligodendrocytes. Proc Natl Acad Sci U S A 94:8830–8835, 1997.

94. Anderson CM, Swanson RA: Astrocyte glutamate transport: Review of properties, regulation, and physiological functions. GLIA 32:1–14, 2000.

95. Ye ZC, et al: Functional hemichannels in astrocytes: A novel mechanism of glutamate release. J Neurosci 23:3588–3596, 2003.

96. Wrathall JR, Choiniere D, Teng YD: Dose-dependent reduction of tissue loss and functional impairment after spinal cord trauma with the AMPA/kainate antagonist NBQX. J Neurosci 14:6598–6607, 1994.

97. Kanellopoulos GK, et al: White matter injury in spinal cord ischemia: Protection by AMPA/kainate glutamate receptor antagonism. Stroke 31:1945–1952, 2000.

98. Follett PL, et al: NBQX attenuates excitotoxic injury in developing white matter. J Neurosci 20:9235–9241, 2000.

99. McCracken E, et al: Grey matter and white matter ischemic damage is reduced by the competitive AMPA receptor antagonist, SPD 502. J Cereb Blood Flow Metab 22:1090–1097, 2002.

100. Brand-Schieber E, Werner P: AMPA/kainate receptors in mouse spinal cord cell-specific display of receptor subunits by oligodendrocytes and astrocytes and at the nodes of Ranvier. GLIA 42:12–24, 2003.

101. Van der Heyden JA, et al: GABA content of discrete brain nuclei and spinal cord of the rat. J Neurochem 33:857–861, 1979.

102. Bowery NG, Hudson AL, Price GW: GABAA and GABAB receptor site distribution in the rat central nervous system. Neuroscience 20:365–383, 1987.

103. Shimada N, et al: Ischemia-induced accumulation of extracellular amino acids in cerebral cortex, white matter, and cerebrospinal fluid. J Neurochem 60:66–71, 1993.

104. Fern R, Waxman SG, Ransom BR: Modulation of anoxic injury in CNS white matter by adenosine and interaction between adenosine and GABA. J Neurophysiol 72:2609–2616, 1994.

105. Fern R, Waxman SG, Ransom BR: Endogenous GABA attenuates CNS white matter dysfunction after anoxia. J Neurosci 15:699–708, 1995.

106. Ransom BR, Philbin DM Jr: Anoxia-induced extracellular ionic changes in CNS white matter: The role of glial cells. Can J Physiol Pharmacol 70(Suppl):S181-S189, 1992.

107. Stys PK, Lesiuk H: Correlation between electrophysiological effects of mexiletine and ischemic protection in central nervous system white matter. Neuroscience 71:27–36, 1996.

108. Stys PK: Protective effects of antiarrhythmic agents against anoxic injury in CNS white matter. J Cereb Blood Flow Metab 15:425–432, 1995.

109. Fern R, et al: Pharmacological protection of CNS white matter during anoxia: Actions of phenytoin, carbamazepine and diazepam. J Pharmacol Exp Ther 266:1549–1555, 1993.

110. Sayin U, Timmerman W, Westerink BH: The significance of extracellular GABA in the substantia nigra of the rat during seizures and anticonvulsant treatments. Brain Res 669:67–72, 1995.

111. Ransom BR, Stys PK, Waxman SG: Anoxic injury of central myelinated axons: Ionic mechanisms and pharmacology. In Waxman SG (ed): Molecular and Cellular Approaches to the Treatment of Brain Disease. New York, Raven Press, 1993, pp 121–151.

Pathophysiology

Chapter Forty-Five

Cerebral Ischemia and Inflammation

Costantino Iadecola, Sunghee Cho, Giora Z. Feuerstein, and John Hallenbeck

Ischemic stroke triggers an inflammatory reaction in the affected area, which progresses for days to weeks after the onset of symptoms. There is evidence that selected aspects of such inflammatory processes contribute to the progression of ischemic brain injury, leading to worsening of the tissue damage and exacerbation of neurologic deficits. Therefore, interventions aimed at suppressing postischemic inflammation offer attractive therapeutic strategies for human stroke, with a potentially wide therapeutic window. A large body of work has addressed the inflammatory process in the postischemic brain.[1-5] In this chapter, we review the basic cellular and molecular features of postischemic inflammation, focusing on recent advances and insights on the potential mechanisms by which such inflammation influences stroke outcome. We then analyze the potential therapeutic implications of modulators of specific inflammatory targets from the perspective of near-future translational approaches.

CEREBRAL ISCHEMIA, CYTOKINES, AND INFLAMMATION

Cerebral ischemia is associated with infiltration of inflammatory cells into ischemic territory. Histopathologic studies, investigations using biochemical markers of leukocytes, and human studies using radioactive indium–labeled circulating leukocytes have demonstrated that early accumulation of blood-borne inflammatory cells in the ischemic brain persists for hours and even days after the initial insult.[1] The infiltration of hematogenous cells into the ischemic territory is the hallmark of the inflammatory reaction, which parallels activation of brain microglia and astrocytes (Fig. 45–1).[6] Cytokines are important molecular signals in the inflammatory response to cerebral ischemia. In experimental models of stroke, ischemia induces expression of pro-inflammatory cytokines, such as tumor necrosis factor-α (TNF-α) , and interleukins (ILs) IL-6 and IL-1β, in the ischemic brain.[1] Increased production of cytokines has also been reported in patients with ischemic stroke.[7,8] Pro-inflammatory cytokines upregulate the expression of adhesion molecules, such as intercellular adhesion molecule-1 (ICAM-1), selectins (especially E-selectin and P-selectin), and integrins, on endothelial cells, leukocytes, and platelets.[1] Adhesion receptors mediate the interaction between endothelial cells and leukocytes that results in an initial "rolling" of leukocytes, which in turn leads to adhesion to the endothelium of venules, followed by leukocyte transmigration into the brain parenchyma.[2,9] Chemokines, the expression of which is upregulated in the ischemic territory, are believed to promote the infiltration of inflammatory cells toward the injured areas.[10]

Several lines of evidence suggest that postischemic inflammation has deleterious effects on the outcome of experimental cerebral ischemia (see Tables 45.1 through 45.4). First, interventions aimed at reducing the number of circulating neutrophils ameliorate ischemic damage in most studies, as indicated by reduction in infarct volume and improvement in functional outcome (Table 45.1).[11-13] Second, antibodies blocking the action of adhesion molecules reduce the influx of neutrophils and lessen tissue damage (Table 45.2).[14-19] Third, genetically engineered mice lacking adhesion molecules, such as ICAM-1 and P-selectin, are less susceptible to ischemic damage (see Table 45.2).[20-22] Furthermore, compounds that block the interaction of E-selectin with Sleu^x—the counterpart adhesion molecule on leukocytes that binds to E-selectin—reduce ischemic brain damage.[17] Fourth, interventions that inactivate cytokines or block cytokine receptors lessen ischemic damage (Table 45.3).[23-30]

MECHANISMS BY WHICH INFLAMMATION CONTRIBUTES TO ISCHEMIC BRAIN INJURY

The mechanisms by which postischemic inflammation contributes to cerebral ischemic damage are not well understood. Although infiltrating neutrophils and activated microglia may produce tissue damage by generating reactive oxygen species,[1] microvascular occlusion produced by intravascular neutrophils may also contribute by aggravating the ischemic insult.[3,5,9,31] However, a cause-and-effect

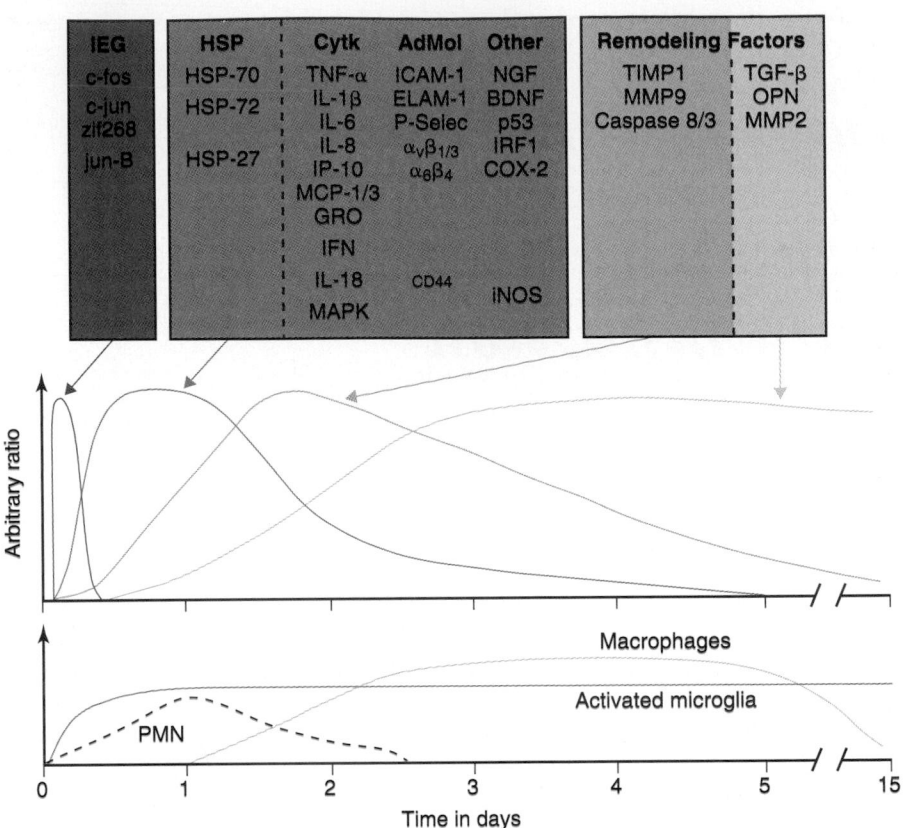

FIGURE 45–1   *Time course of the cellular and molecular events underlying postischemic inflammation.*

Table 45.1   **Effects of Leukocyte Depletion on the Outcome of Experimental Focal Cerebral Ischemia**

Intervention	Outcome	Selected Chapter Reference
Mechlorethamine and vinblastine	Improved histologic or functional outcome in models of focal ischemia	11
Antineutrophilic antibodies	Reduction in infarct size or edema in a rat model of focal cerebral ischemia	12
Neutrophil inhibitory factor	Reduction in infarct size in rats with transient middle cerebral artery occlusion	13
Leukocyte depletion	No effect on brain injury	140

Table 45.2   **Role of Adhesion Molecules in the Mechanisms of Experimental Focal Cerebral Ischemia**

Intervention	Outcome	Selected Chapter Reference
Anti–ICAM-1 antibodies	Reduction in infarct size in rats with transient MCAO	14
ICAM-1–null mice	Reduction in infarct size in transient and permanent MCAO	22
Anti-CD18 monoclonal antibodies	Increased reflow in microvessels of different sizes in primates	15
Anti-CD11b monoclonal antibody	Reduction in infarct size in rats with transient MCAO	16
Mac-1 (CD11b/CD18)–null mice	Reduction in infarct size in rats with transient MCAO	21
CY-1503, analog of sialyl-Lewis (x)	Reduction in infarct size in rats with transient MCAO	17
Synthetic oligopeptide corresponding to the lectin domain of selectins	Reduction in infarct size in rats with transient MCAO	18
P-selectin–null mice	Reduction in infarct size in rats with transient MCAO	20
Anti–P-selectin monoclonal antibody	Reduction in infarct size in rats with transient or permanent MCAO	19

ICAM-1, intercellular adhesion molecule-1; Mac-1, macrophage-1 antigen complex; MCAO, middle cerebral artery occlusion.

Table 45.3 Evidence that Cytokines Play a Role in the Mechanisms of Experimental Focal Cerebral Ischemia

Intervention	Outcome	Selected Chapter Reference(s)
TNF-α–soluble receptor type 1	Reduction in infarct size in rats and mice with permanent MCAO	23, 27
Anti–TNF-α monoclonal antibody	Reduction in infarct size in rats and mice with MCAO	24, 41
IL-1β administration	Increase in infarct size in rats with transient MCAO	25
IL-1 receptor antagonist	Reduction in infarct size in rats and mice with MCAO	26
IL-1 converting enzyme–null mice	Reduction in ICAM positive vessels in mice with permanent MCAO	28
IL-6 administration	Reduction in infarct size in rats with permanent MCAO	27
Anti–IL-8 monoclonal antibody	Reduction in infarct size in rabbits with transient ischemia	29
Anti-CINC antibody	Reduction in infarct size in rats with transient MCAO	30, 47
		61, 63
IL-IRI–null mice	Suppression of inflammation	47
	Reduced microglia activation	
	Reduced IL-1, IL-6, ICAM-1, Cox-2 expression	

CINC, cytokine-induced neutrophil chemoattractant; ICAM-1, intercellular adhesion molecule-1; IL, interleukin; MCAO, middle cerebral artery occlusion; TNF-α, tumor necrosis factor-α.

relationship between the extent of neutrophil trafficking and the severity of ischemic damage has not been firmly established.[3,5] Although intravascular adhesion of neutrophils is a relatively early postischemic event, parenchymal accumulation is generally observed late, when most of the ischemic damage may have already occurred.[5] In addition, no consistent relationship has been found between level of leukocyte infiltration and extent of ischemic damage.[32] These observations raise questions about the role of neutrophils in the mechanisms of ischemic brain injury and suggest that our understanding of the mechanisms and the pathophysiologic implications of postischemic leukocyte trafficking is rather limited.

New data have provided insight into additional mechanisms that may also play a role. In experimental models of stroke, TNF-α and IL-1β have been linked to the associated brain injury.[33–40] Intracerebral injection of TNF-α exacerbates ischemic injury, whereas anti–TNF-α monoclonal antibody or soluble TNF-receptor (TNF-binding protein) treatment reverses the effect.[41] Furthermore, the administration of IL-1 receptor antagonist (IL-1ra), a naturally occurring IL-1 inhibitor, or overexpression of IL-1ra in genetically engineered animals diminishes ischemic injury.[42–46] In addition, studies using IL-1 receptor I (IL-1RI) knockout mice suggest an involvement of this receptor in IL-1–mediated injury in brain trauma, possibly via microglia-macrophage activation as well as expression of cyclooxygenase-2 (COX-2), IL-1, and IL-6.[47]

However, there are instances in which cytokines ameliorate neuronal injury. For example, TNF-α can induce protection from subsequent ischemic injury (see later discussion of ischemic preconditioning) and TNF-α receptor knockout mice have greater sensitivity to brain injury.[48,49] In the case of TNF-α preconditioning, TNF-α is presumed to act as a noxious stimulus that activates feedback control mechanisms and confers tolerance to subsequent ischemia by generating cell survival agonists and cell death inhibitors. The response of TNF-α receptor knockout mice is more difficult to explain in light of the TNF-α inhibition studies just cited. One possible interpretation is that TNFRI/TNFRII-null mice are exposed to long-term deprivation because of TNF-α homeostatic effects and may

have developed compensatory mechanisms that render them different from wild-type mice that experience a sudden block of TNF-α activity. Such discrepancy may also be due to the specific TNF-α receptor involved in the process. For example, some studies indicate that different receptor subtypes (e.g., TNFRI and TNFRII) exert opposite roles in TNF-α–induced neuronal injury and survival.[50,51]

Another member of the TNF receptor superfamily, Fas, has been implicated in ischemic brain damage. In a seminal article, Martin-Villalba and associates[52] have reported that infarct volumes in both FasL (Fas ligand) and TNF-α knockout were 54% and 67% smaller, respectively, than those in controls. Hybrid mice lacking both cytokines showed a 93% reduction in infarct volume, and a combination of antibodies that neutralized FasL and TNF-α decreased infarct volume by 70%. Ligation of Fas by trimerized FasL leads to recruitment of adaptor proteins that form the death-inducing signaling complex (DISC) and, eventually, apoptosis. TNFRI recruits the TNF receptor–associated death domain protein (TRADD), which can interact with both Fas-associated death domain protein (FADD) and TNF receptor–associated factor 2 (TRAF2), that can activate nuclear factor-κB (NF-κB). Accordingly, these receptors can activate both pro-inflammatory and apoptotic pathways, a feature that may account for the potency of their dual blockade in ischemia.

NITRIC OXIDE AND INDUCIBLE NITRIC OXIDE SYNTHASE

A growing body of evidence suggests that inducible nitric oxide synthase (iNOS) is a critical effector of the damage produced by postischemic inflammation. Nitric oxide (NO), a free radical, acts as a signaling molecule in normal synaptic transmission as well as a neurotoxin in pathologic conditions. The following three isoforms of NOS have been identified: neuronal (NOS1), inducible (iNOS, NOS2), and endothelial NOS (NOS3). Both NOS1 and NOS3 are expressed constitutively, whereas NOS2 is induced in immune cells and neurons largely by stimuli

Pathophysiology

Therapy

evidence-based recommendations from the extensive clinical trial literature.

The section concludes with an enlightening review of all aspects of conducting clinical research studies in stroke prevention and treatment. This includes what constitutes phase 1, 2, and 3 studies, outcome measures, statistical power, inclusion criteria and quality assurance. Principles of data analysis are covered, and the chapter finishes by discussing the roles of the FDA, Institutional Research Boards, and informed consent.

Chapter Forty-Seven

Prehospital and Emergency Department Care of the Patient with Acute Stroke

Arthur M. Pancioli and Joseph P. Broderick

The Emergency Medical Services (EMS) community and emergency department (ED) team play important roles in the evaluation and management of patients with acute stroke. Because of the time-sensitive nature of acute stroke treatment, speed and accuracy of evaluation are critical for optimizing patient outcomes. Acute interventions aimed at reducing the morbidity and mortality from stroke can be initiated in both the prehospital arena and the ED. This chapter addresses the roles that prehospital care providers and ED teams play in the evaluation and management of patients with acute stroke.

THE COURSE OF EVENTS FOR THE ACUTE STROKE VICTIM

Speed and efficiency of initial management, diagnosis, and communication are significant components of the contribution to acute stroke care provided by prehospital and ED teams. An analysis of the course of events that transpire between the onset of a patient's symptoms and the delivery of definitive therapies is warranted. The major components in the evaluation and treatment process of patients with acute stroke can be divided into prehospital and ED phases, as follows.

Prehospital Components
1. Recognition of stroke symptoms by the patient or family members.
2. First contact with medical care (for example, phoning 911 in the United States).
3. Dispatch of appropriate level of prehospital care providers.
4. Prehospital evaluation, management, and transport.
5. Prehospital identification of stroke.
6. Prehospital notification of pending ED arrival.

Emergency Department
1. ED triage.
2. ED evaluation and management.

3. Divergence of pathway according to whether stroke is ischemic or hemorrhagic.
4. Disposition of patient from the ED.

The single largest component of the delay between symptom onset and definitive therapy exists between symptom onset and arrival at the ED. In one large multicenter study, which was designed to investigate patient delays in seeking care after stroke, the median prehospital delay was 2.6 hours with an interquartile range of 1.2 to 6.3 hours. The mean prehospital delay was 5.4 hours.[1] Thus, it is clear that to improve the number of patients eligible for acute therapies, the prehospital times must be decreased.

RECOGNITION OF STROKE SYMPTOMS BY THE PATIENT OR FAMILY MEMBERS

Possibly the largest component in the prehospital delay is failure of the patient or family members to recognize stroke symptoms and act accordingly. Factors that have been shown to be associated with delay in arrival at the ED are as follows[2-9]:

- The patient (or family member) initially phones the primary care physician instead of the local emergency service phone number.
- The patient lives alone.
- Stroke begins while the patient is asleep.
- Symptoms appear while the patient is at home versus at work.
- The stroke is mild rather than severe.

In addition, stroke often damages the areas of the brain that control either the patient's perception of a problem or the patient's ability to communicate. However, the major reasons for time-to-treatment delay appear to be the lack of recognition of stroke signs and symptoms and the lack of a proper response. In a 1996 Gallup Poll commissioned by the National Stroke Association, only 58% of U.S. residents older than 50 years recognized weakness of an arm or leg as a symptom of stroke, and only 32% recognized difficulties with speaking as a warning sign of stroke.[10] In another survey conducted in Greater Cincinnati, Ohio, only 37% of patients with stroke, their family members, or both knew at the onset of the patient's stroke that the symptoms were due to a stroke.[11] Of the 163 patients, 62 (38%) did not know a single warning symptom of stroke, and another 45 (28%) could identify only one symptom.

The lack of knowledge of the warning signs of and risk factors in stroke was quantified in a large telephone survey in the Greater Cincinnati, Ohio, area in 1995.[12] That survey assessed the level of stroke knowledge within a population whose demographics match those of patients with acute stroke. Using open-ended questions, the researchers in this study found that only 57% of the respondents were able to name even one warning sign of stroke. Similarly, only 68% could name even one risk factor for stroke. Persons older than 75 years were significantly less likely to be able to name one stroke warning sign or one risk factor than younger persons. Another survey was performed in 2000 within the same community and with the identical methodology in order both to reassess the level of stroke knowledge and to look for incremental change in the overall level of stroke knowledge in the public.[13] The researchers found an increase in the public knowledge of stroke warning signs, in that 70% of respondents in the 2000 survey were able to name at least one stroke warning sign. Although this survey population had a slightly higher number of respondents who described themselves as having at least "some college," which may account for the increase in knowledge of stroke warning signs, there was no change in the percentage of respondents who could name one risk factor.

Unfortunately, therefore, a significant portion of the general public still has minimal knowledge and understanding of stroke warning signs and risk factors. Inadequate public awareness of the importance of stroke symptoms may lead to significant delay in presentation of stroke victims for treatment. Such a relationship was noted in a multicenter study in Sweden. In the prospective study of factors influencing the time from onset of stroke or transient ischemic attack (TIA) to hospital arrival, both a lack of awareness of the need to seek medical attention and the failure to use direct ambulance transport were found to increase the prehospital delay.[14]

A study determining access to acute stroke care examined additional factors, including gender, ethnicity and access to care.[15] In that study, there was no relationship of ethnicity and time to arrival at the ED, with the median time to arrival being 222 minutes for African Americans, 230 minutes for non-Hispanic white Americans, and 280 minutes for Hispanic Americans. There was a trend toward longer prehospital time for women, and the time from ED arrival to evaluation by the ED physician was 49% longer for women (confidence interval [CI] 2.8%–116%). Having a primary care physician actually increased the delay to hospital arrival by 63% (CI 10%–141%) in the univariate analysis. This study also noted that use of an ambulance reduced the time to ED arrival by 55% (CI 34%–70%) in comparison with other methods of transport.

FIRST CONTACT WITH MEDICAL CARE

The EMS system is the point of first medical contact for 35% to 70% of people suffering acute stroke.[2,9,16,17] Although the symptomatology and presentation of many acute strokes are dramatic enough to lead patients or bystanders toward prompt action, less dramatic presentations often lead to significant delay. In a 1996 poll conducted by the Gallup organization for the National Stroke Association, individuals were asked what they would do if they believed that someone around them were having a stroke.[10] Ninety percent of respondents stated that they would immediately seek medical care. Forty-three percent of the total said that they would call 911. Twenty-six percent of respondents stated that they would call their family physician, and 11% stated they would go straight to a hospital ED.

Unfortunately, any action other than the immediate activation of the EMS system via 911 will lead to significant delays in treatment. In a study published in 1993, patients with stroke who arrived at the ED via the use of the EMS–911 system arrived with a median time from symptom onset to ED arrival of 84 minutes. For individuals who chose to first call the primary care physician, the median time from symptom onset to ED arrival was 270 minutes. Individuals who traveled to the ED using their own mode of transportation arrived within a median time of 210 minutes.[2] In a study performed in 1996–1997, use of the EMS system shortened time to arrival as well as time to treatment in patients with acute stroke. Patients arriving by ambulance were more likely to arrive earlier (odds ratio [OR] for arrival within 3 hours = 3.7) than individuals arriving via other modes of transport and were more likely to be seen by a physician within 15 minutes of arrival (OR = 2.3).[18] Thus, it is clear that the use of the EMS system is one critical link in reducing delay to ED arrival for patients with acute stroke.

DISPATCH OF APPROPRIATE LEVEL OF PREHOSPITAL PROVIDERS

Once the EMS–911 system is activated, EMS dispatchers gather initial information and dispatch prehospital care providers. Thus, the first triage by any form of medical provider occurs upon receipt of the 911 call. Yet, in one study, dispatchers without specific training in stroke can identify only 52% of verified cases of stroke.[19] Ambulance units were dispatched to the scene for preliminary diagnosis other than stroke in 48% of cases.[19]

In a retrospective review of San Francisco dispatcher performance for acute stroke or TIA calls, dispatchers were able to identify cases as "cerebrovascular accidents" only 31% of the time.[20] In the majority of cases in this study (59%), ambulances were dispatched at lower priority than they would have been for an identified stroke. Surprisingly, 51% of callers to 911 used the word *stroke* to describe their emergency, but only 48% of the patients for whom *stroke* was used in the 911 call were categorized by dispatchers as having cerebrovascular accidents.[20]

This decision about the level of prehospital provider to dispatch to a possible stroke victim is relatively important.

One study indicated that Advanced Life Support (ALS) transport might be better suited to the evaluation and transport of potential stroke victims. In that study, up to 29% of patients with acute ischemic stroke required pre-hospital interventions for treatable medical conditions, including compromised airway and cardiac instability. The patients transported by basic life-support units arrived at the hospital earlier (40 ± 1 minutes) than those transported by ALS units staffed by paramedics (45 ± 1 minutes; $P = .004$). However, patients transported by ALS units were seen by a physician sooner after arrival at the ED (10 ± 2 minutes) than those who arrived via basic life-support units (20 ± 4 minutes; $P = .02$). Thus, although the transport times were similar, the level of care for patients transported by ALS teams was higher. In that community, stroke is treated as a level I emergency equivalent to trauma and myocardial infarction. Not all local EMS networks treat stroke as a level I emergency.[21]

According to a presentation to the National Symposium on Rapid Identification and Treatment of Acute Stroke, sponsored in 1996 by the National Institute of Neurological Disorders and Stroke (NINDS),[22] dispatchers are charged with the responsibility of providing the 911 caller with "pre-arrival instructions" before prehospital care providers arrive on the scene. Initial steps, including gathering medication lists and determining time of symptom onset, can be performed by the dispatchers while the pre-hospital care providers are on their way.

PREHOSPITAL EVALUATION AND MANAGEMENT

Upon identification of a potential stroke victim, prehospital care providers must begin stabilization of the patient and measures aimed toward diagnosis (Table 47.1). An assessment of the patient's airway, breathing, and circulation (ABCs) with measurement of vital signs and pulse oximetry must be performed, and abnormalities addressed. The initial assessment should proceed with application of a cardiac monitor, measurement of the patient's serum glucose level, initiation of intravenous (IV) access, and application of supplemental oxygen. Notably, these measures should be performed during transport of the patient

Table 47.1 Guidelines for Prehospital Management of Stroke

Do . . .	*Do Not . . .*
• Determine time of onset	• Give large amounts of IV fluids
• Assess with Prehospital Stroke Scale	• Give dextrose without evidence of hypoglycemia
• Give supplemental oxygen	• Reduce blood pressure with vasoactive agents
• Attach cardiac monitor	• Delay transport
• Establish IV access	
• Measure blood glucose level	
• Perform ABCs (ensure airway, breathing, and circulation)	
• Treat hypotension	
• Give nothing by mouth (NPO)	
• Alert emergency department	
• Ensure rapid transport	

and, unless resuscitative measures are required, should not delay transport.[23]

One critical component of the prehospital care provider's assessment is to attempt to establish the exact time of onset of the patient's symptoms and to elicit the history of relevant events surrounding the episode, such as trauma, seizure activity, or migraine headache. Prehospital care providers have shown great creativity in eliciting key elements of the patient's history to help establish time of onset.

In addition to stabilization and establishing time of onset, prehospital care providers should pay specific attention to the management of blood pressure, fluid status, and glucose level. Interventions to lower blood pressure should not be attempted in the prehospital setting. The differentiation between acute hemorrhagic and acute ischemic stroke requires neurologic imaging and determines the aggressiveness of blood pressure management once the patient is in the ED.[24] Thus, elevations of blood pressure should not be treated prior to the patient's arrival in the ED.[25]

The prehospital administration of IV fluids to the patient with stroke should also be approached with caution. Dextrose containing fluids, such as 5% dextrose in water, should be administered only to patients with documented hypoglycemia. For resuscitation needs, isotonic crystalloid is the fluid of choice and should be given as needed to appropriately treat the patient with stroke and associated shock.[26]

Hypoglycemia is a potential stroke mimic that must be ruled out or treated. Ideally, hypoglycemia can be diagnosed in the prehospital setting by paramedics and other ALS providers. If hypoglycemia is documented and symptoms of stroke are present, administration of dextrose 50% in water is appropriate. The severity of the patient's symptoms, the time of glucose administration, and subsequent changes in the patient's clinical status must be documented by the EMS provider. Administration of glucose to a patient with suspected stroke but without documented hypoglycemia should be avoided, because elevations of serum glucose have been associated with worse outcomes after ischemic stroke.[27–29]

PREHOSPITAL IDENTIFICATION OF STROKE

Ideally, prehospital providers should be well versed in acute stroke recognition and can quickly initiate protocols for acute stroke.[30] Two tools, the Los Angeles Prehospital Stroke Scale (LAPSS) and the Cincinnati Prehospital Stroke Scale (CPSS), have emerged for use by prehospital care providers to allow for early stroke recognition and communication with hospital-based teams.

The LAPSS was created to be a stroke recognition tool specifically for prehospital care personnel (Fig. 47–1).[31] It is a one-page instrument that takes less than 3 minutes to perform. The LAPSS consists of four history items, three physical examination items, and a serum glucose test. In a prospective validation study of the LAPSS, paramedics identified acute stroke victims with a sensitivity of 91% and a specificity of 97%.[32]

Los Angeles Prehospital Stroke Screen (LAPSS)

1. Patient Name: _____   _____
                                    Last   First

2. Information History from:
   [ ] Patient
   [ ] Family Member _____   _____
   [ ] Other   Name   Phone

3. Last known time patient was at baseline or deficit free and awake: Military Time: _____
                                                                          Date: _____

SCREENING CRITERIA: Yes   Unknown   No
4. Age > 45   [ ]   [ ]   [ ]
5. History of seizures or epilepsy **absent**   [ ]   [ ]   [ ]
6. Symptom duration **less than** 24 hours   [ ]   [ ]   [ ]
7. At baseline, patient is **not** wheelchair bound or bedridden [ ]   [ ]   [ ]

                                                           Yes   No
8. Blood glucose between 60 and 400:   [ ]   [ ]

9. Exam: **LOOK FOR OBVIOUS ASYMMETRY**
                            Normal   Right   Left
   Facial Smile/Grimace: _   _ Droop   _ Droop

   Grip: _   _ Weak Grip   _ Weak Grip
                                      _ No Grip   _ No Grip

   Arm Strength   _   _ Drifts Down _ Drifts Down
                                      _ Falls Rapidly _ Falls Rapidly

                                                           Yes   No
Based on exam, patient has **only unilateral** (and not bilateral) weakness: [ ]   [ ]

10. **Items 4,5,6,7,8,9 all YES's (or unknown)   LAPSS screening**   Yes   No
    criteria met: [ ]   [ ]

11. If LAPSS criteria for stroke met, call receiving hospital with a "code stroke", if not, then return to the Appropriate Treatment Protocol. (Note: the patient may still be experiencing a stroke even if LAPSS criteria are not met).

FIGURE 47–1 *The Los Angeles Prehospital Stroke Screen. (From Kidwell CS, Saver JL, Schubert GB, et al: Design and retrospective analysis of the Los Angeles Prehospital Stroke Screen (LAPSS). Prehosp Emerg Care 2:267–273, 1998.)*

The CPSS is a three-item neurologic examination that was developed to assist prehospital care providers in identifying patients with stroke who may be candidates for thrombolysis (Table 47.2). The CPSS was derived via the selection of the three most sensitive and specific components of the National Institute for Health Stroke Scale (NIHSS)[33]—facial palsy, arm weakness, and speech abnormality. When performed by a trained physician, this scale has been shown to be effective in identifying such patients. The CPSS can be taught in approximately 10 minutes and performed in less than 1 minute.

The CPSS has also been shown to identify potential stroke victims accurately when performed by prehospital care providers.[34] Correlation for the total score (number of abnormal items) between prehospital care providers and physicians was excellent. The CPSS is valid in identifying

Table 47.2   The Cincinnati Prehospital Stroke Scale*

Facial Droop:	Have patient smile or show teeth
• Normal	Both sides move equally
• Abnormal	One side does not move as well
Arm Drift:	Patient closes eyes and holds both arms out
• Normal	Both sides move equally
• Abnormal	One side does not move as well
Speech:	Have patient say "you can't teach an old dog new tricks".
• Normal	Patient uses correct words without slurring
• Abnormal	Slurs words, uses inappropriate words, or is unable to speak

*Any one or more abnormal findings is suggestive of acute stroke.

patients with stroke (sensitivity, 66%; specificity, 87%), especially anterior circulation stroke (sensitivity, 88%). In the evaluation study, presence of a single abnormality on the CPSS identified all patients with anterior circulation stroke who would have been candidates for thrombolytic therapy. The addition of a test for ataxia to the CPSS would have identified 6 of the 10 patients with posterior circulation stroke who were not identified in this study. However, ataxia is one of the most poorly reproducible items on the NIHSS and is not included in the CPSS.

Both the LAPSS and the CPSS have been widely utilized in and are accepted tools for the EMS community. The LAPSS has greater overall sensitivity but requires slightly more time to perform. The CPSS is rapidly taught and performed but has a lower sensitivity for posterior circulation stroke.

PREHOSPITAL NOTIFICATION OF PENDING EMERGENCY DEPARTMENT ARRIVAL

So as to help diminish the time from symptom onset to definitive therapy for a patient with stroke, prehospital care providers can significantly facilitate rapid delivery of therapy via an advance notification call to the patient's destination hospital. Armed with tools such as the LAPSS or CPSS, prehospital care providers can, with very good accuracy, make a presumptive diagnosis of acute stroke and set an ED or "stroke team" into motion via advance notification.

Similar advance notification for acute myocardial infarction (AMI) has been demonstrated to dramatically diminish time from hospital arrival to definitive intervention. To improve results for patients with AMI, prehospital care providers were educated in the proper lead placement for generation of a true 12-lead electrocardiogram (ECG). Prehospital 12-lead ECG machines register and print a patient's 12-lead ECG and simultaneously send it by facsimile to the base hospital of choice. Time studies using the prehospital 12-lead ECG have shown that time from the arrival in the ED of a patient with AMI to balloon inflation for percutaneous angioplasty or administration of fibrinolytic therapy can be cut dramatically. The use of prehospital ECGs has been demonstrated to be feasible and accurate as well as to diminish time to definitive therapy for patients with AMI.[35-38]

Although no such controlled studies have been performed for either the LAPSS or the CPSS, the time from symptom onset to ED arrival is invariably the largest segment of the continuum from symptom onset to definitive therapy in the patient with acute stroke. Thus, measures that lead to an earlier activation of preparations for ED arrival of patients with acute stroke may ultimately translate into improved outcomes.

Organizations designed to improve stroke care have formally recognized the importance of EMS in systems such as "stroke centers." In a recommendation for the establishment of primary stroke centers, Alberts and colleagues[39] state, "It is vital that the EMS system be integrated with the stroke center. The stroke center should be able to communicate effectively with EMS personnel in the out-of-hospital setting during transportation of a patient experiencing an acute stroke. The ED should be able to efficiently receive and triage patients with stroke arriving via EMS. The stroke center staff should support and participate in educational activities involving EMS personnel." The community of prehospital care providers and the physician leaders in this field are committed to continuous improvement in stroke care and explicitly endorse ongoing efforts to include EMS in the continuum of acute stroke care.[40]

EMERGENCY DEPARTMENT TIME DELAYS

Delays in the ED are another barrier to the optimal triage and treatment of patients with acute stroke. Table 47.3 lists the recommendations of the NINDS-sponsored National Symposium on Rapid Identification and Treatment of Acute Stroke for time intervals from symptom onset to ED arrival for a patient with suspected stroke.[41]

This conference also provided a recommended algorithm for triage and the evaluation of patients with stroke in the ED. Triage of patients, which is based on stroke severity, available resources, and time from symptom onset, is one way to focus resources appropriately. For example, the patient with a mild or moderate stroke and stable neurologic deficit who presents more than 6 hours after symptom onset should be evaluated promptly, but it is more urgent to treat a patient who is a potential candidate for a thrombolytic agent within a very small time window (e.g., 3 hours).

Opportunities for physicians to intervene exist only for a limited time whether a patient is suffering an ischemic or a hemorrhagic stroke. Delays in patient arrival and delivery of care can significantly affect a patient's potential for a good outcome. Each element in the course of events for the patient with acute stroke previously present is discussed here.

Until the patient is stabilized and imaging is performed, the care of a patient with acute stroke should be kept on a course aimed at early intervention. Directing acute stroke care toward a rapid, aggressive path of intervention requires a "paradigm shift" from the approach used less than a decade ago. This shift is similar to the changes in practice mentality for AMI that occurred first upon the

Table 47.3 Guidelines for Rapid Evaluation of the Patient with Acute Stroke

Period Measured	Optional Time (min.)
From ED arrival to emergency physician evaluation	10
From ED arrival to CT scan	25
From ED arrival to CT scan interpretation	50
From ED arrival to initiation of therapy (80% compliance)*	60

*Target should be compliance with these guidelines in at least 80% of cases.
CT, computed tomography, ED, emergency department.

availability of thrombolytic agents and again with the advent of percutaneous intervention. A comparison of therapy for acute ischemic stroke with that of AMI is illustrative of the impediments to this "paradigm shift."

Despite reports that almost half the patients with ischemic stroke arrive at an ED within 3 hours of symptom onset, only 3.6% of more than 17,000 patients with potential stroke documented in the two NINDS studies were eligible for treatment (alteplase or placebo) within this time.[42] In contrast, approximately 33% of eligible patients with AMI, according to the National Registry for Myocardial Infarction II, are currently treated with a thrombolytic agent (26%) or alternative reperfusion methods (7%), such as invasive cardiac catheterization or angioplasty.[43]

Potential explanations for these differences in treatment for patients with stroke and those with AMI are shown in Table 47.4. Currently, the major difference is the perception among physicians and hospitals that myocardial infarction is a medical emergency but stroke is not. For example, in the NINDS study, the most ambitious stroke study performed thus far in terms of an early time-to-treatment criterion, the goal for time from patient arrival at the ED to treatment was 55 minutes.[42] In contrast, current guidelines for myocardial infarction recommend 30 minutes from arrival to treatment.[44]

To optimize the chance of successful treatment, management protocols for patients with stroke similar to those for patients with AMI or trauma must be designed. In patients with acute stroke, the average time in eight hospitals in Houston, Texas, from arrival in the ED to evaluation by a physician was 28 minutes; for patients brought to Greater Cincinnati hospitals, the elapsed time was 10 minutes for those who arrived by ALS units, and 20 minutes for patients brought by basic life-support units.[17,21] Times from patient arrival in an ED to performance of a computed tomography (CT) scan were 100 minutes in Houston and either 47 minutes (ALS unit transport) or 69 minutes (basic life-support unit transport) in Greater Cincinnati. In Houston, the availability of a designated "stroke team" shortened the time from arrival to examination by a physician by 13 minutes and to CT by 63 minutes. The results of these studies illustrate areas where delays currently occur in the evaluation of patients with stroke in the ED and the important effect that "stroke teams" can have in improving early evaluation and treatment.

EMERGENCY DEPARTMENT TRIAGE

Triage is derived from the French term *trier*, which means to sort or prioritize. This seemingly simple act of setting the patient's priority level via triage is one of the most important aspects of the ED management of an acute stroke. Like the decision a patient or family member makes about whether to call 911, the triage nurse's assignment of a patient with stroke to the critical care arena within an ED rather than to a "noncritical" bed entirely changes the dynamic of the patient's evaluation and treatment. Hospital-based systems seeking to improve the speed and efficiency of evaluation for patients with stroke must involve the ED nursing staff in the effort and must provide education to enable ED triage nurses to assign patients with acute stroke to receive the highest priority of care. It is also useful to give the ED nursing staff clear, concise guidelines for the triage of such patients. Similarly, having a well-understood and easily activated "acute stroke care pathway" with ED orders and a template for documentation can dramatically improve the management of acute stroke.[45,46]

EMERGENCY DEPARTMENT EVALUATION AND MANAGEMENT

The patient with a possible acute stroke must immediately be stabilized. The airway, breathing, and circulation (ABCs) assessment is primary. Simultaneously, the diagnostic evaluation must be initiated.

Airway

Airway compromise and the need for intubation may have multiple causes. They include diminished level of consciousness and inability to protect the airway, impairment of oropharyngeal mobility and sensation, and loss of protective reflexes due to ischemic or compressive brainstem dysfunction. Intubation and mechanical ventilation are the primary mechanism for airway protection in the ED setting.

The decision to intubate a patient is based on answering the following three fundamental clinical questions:

1. Is there a failure of airway maintenance or protection?
2. Is there a failure of ventilation or oxygenation?
3. What is the anticipated clinical course?

A common clinical error in airway assessment and management occurs when a patient is found to be "breathing

Table 47.4 Comparison of the Logistics of Treatment of Patients with Stroke and Patients with Acute Myocardial Infarction

Patients with Stroke	Patients with AMI
Current Treatment window of 3 hours (for alteplase)	Treatment window of at least 6 hours
Impairment of communication and perception is common	No impairment of communication and perception
Multiple presenting symptoms possible	A few presenting symptoms
Pain not a prominent factor of ischemic stroke	Pain and shortness of breath are often prominent
Poor public knowledge of stroke symptoms	Excellent public awareness of warning signs of AMI
Inconsistent designation of stroke as highest level of emergency by EMS	AMI designated highest level of emergency by EMS
Recommended time from ED arrival to treatment of 60 minutes (new goal, rarely reached at present)	Recommended time from ED arrival to treatment of 30 minutes (frequently attained)

AMI, acute myocardial infarction; ED; emergency department; EMS; emergency medical system.

on his or her own." Although they may be breathing, patients with stroke may be at serious risk for aspiration, at which point airway protection should be considered. If a patient cannot adequately maintain oxygen saturation despite supplemental oxygen or cannot properly eliminate carbon dioxide, mechanical ventilation is required. Finally, patients whose status can be expected to deteriorate or who require prolonged procedures such as angiography should be considered for early intubation under controlled circumstances.[47]

Prior to sedation and intubation, the emergency physician should take a few moments to perform as complete a neurologic examination as is safe for the patient. Once sedation and intubation are achieved, a significant component of the diagnostic and prognostic data is compromised because baseline neurologic data can no longer be obtained. It is therefore critical to record baseline neurologic status prior to these interventions.

If a patient requires intubation, rapid sequence intubation should be performed (Table 47.5). This process begins with careful preparation of all necessary equipment and medication so as to provide as controlled an environment as possible. During intubation, careful consideration must be given to avoiding raising the intracranial pressure (ICP).

The patient should be thoroughly preoxygenated and then should receive a sedative–induction agent. Etomidate and thiopental are commonly used as induction agents for rapid sequence intubation. Etomidate, an ultra–short-acting nonbarbiturate hypnotic, is a superb induction agent; it is given in a dose of 0.3 mg/kg IV. Etomidate causes very little alteration in hemodynamics and therefore has gained considerable favor in the induction of critically ill patients. Thiopental is a short-acting barbiturate that has been used for many years as an induction agent. It should be used only in hypertensive patients, if at all, because of its propensity to reduce systolic blood pressure, an effect that may be detrimental to the patient with acute stroke.

Additional premedication should include IV lidocaine (1.5 mg/kg), which is given for its ability to blunt the hemodynamic response and possibly blunt the rise in ICP that is associated with laryngoscopy. Blunting the hemodynamic response is necessary because of the rich sensory innervation of the supraglottic larynx. The use of the laryngoscope results in significant sympathetic activity and a marked catecholamine discharge. If autoregulation is

impaired, the hemodynamic response may result in an increase in ICP. Ideally, the lidocaine would be given at least 3 minutes prior to intubation. In addition, opiates can be used to decrease the sympathetic response. Fentanyl, given in a dose of 3 μg/kg, can be used as an adjunct to block the potential hemodynamic response and the potential rise in ICP due to laryngoscopy.[48]

A defasciculating dose of a nondepolarizing neuromuscular blocking agent should also be part of the premedication before laryngoscopy; an example is pancuronium or vecuronium, 0.01 mg/kg IV. Such an agent is given to blunt the rise in ICP that can occur in relation to the fasciculations that result from the use of a depolarizing neuromuscular blocking agent. Ideally, this dose is given 3 minutes before the use of a depolarizing neuromuscular blocking agent. Neuromuscular blockade should be achieved with a short-acting agent, such as succinyl choline, in a dose of 1.5 to 2.0 mg/kg IV. Prolonged paralysis is undesirable because of the loss of clinical signs and symptoms. Sedation must be maintained after intubation, however, to avoid agitation and elevation of ICP.

The ED team must be constantly aware that any patient with altered level of consciousness may have suffered trauma. A careful examination for evidence of injury is required. Cervical spine immobilization is required for all traumatized patients with altered level of consciousness.

Breathing

Once the airway has been addressed, the patient's respiratory status must be assessed. Patients may also have significant comorbidity, such as congestive heart failure, chronic obstructive pulmonary disease (COPD), or cancer. Oxygen delivery and oxygenation should be optimized. Patients commonly receive supplemental oxygen therapy, although there is no literature currently supporting the routine use of supplemental oxygen in patients with stroke but without hypoxia.[49] Because up to a third of patients with stroke experience pneumonia within 1 month of the stroke, aspiration pneumonia prevention must begin in the ED. Elevation of the head to 30 degrees, careful pulmonary toilet, and strict avoidance of any oral intake until a formal swallowing evaluation has been performed are imperative.

Circulation

Once a patient has been determined to be capable of protecting the airway or the airway has been secured and adequate ventilation and oxygenation have been established, attention is turned to the cardiovascular status. This assessment should address hypertension, hypotension, and ECG abnormalities.

Hypertension
Hypertension is extremely common in patients with acute stroke and should be treated cautiously, if at all.[25,50–52] The management of hypertension depends on the cause of the stroke. Hypertension in patients with presumed aneurysmal subarachnoid hemorrhage (SAH) or other vascular anomalies, in which the hypertension may actually be detrimental, should be treated more aggressively. Patients

Table 47.5 Rapid-Sequence Intubation

Preparation
Preoxygenation
Pretreatment:
   Lidocaine 1.5 mg/kg IV
   Vecuronium 0.01 mg/kg IV
   Fentanyl 3 μg/kg (over 1 minute)
Paralysis with induction:
   Etomidate 0.3 μg/kg IV
   Succinylcholine 1.5 mg/kg IV
Placement—confirm tube placement
Post-intubation management

Adapted from Walls R (ed): Manual of Emergency Airway Management. Philadelphia, Lippincott Williams & Wilkins, 2000.

with acute ischemic stroke, unless dramatically hypertensive, should be treated conservatively. If it is deemed critical to alter a patient's blood pressure, the following principles should guide the choice of agents and approach to the ED management of hypertension. First, short-acting, titratable agents should be used; examples are sodium nitroprusside, labetalol, nicardipine, and esmolol. Second, physicians should start with very low doses and titrate the dosage according to desired parameters. Third, physicians should avoid agents that may be harmful; diuretics should be avoided except in the setting of acute and compromising heart failure. Oral medications and unpredictable medications, such as sublingual nifedipine, should be avoided. Also, using more than one medication with different mechanisms of action in the acute setting may be particularly dangerous. The combination of two antihypertensive agents may have a summary effect significantly greater than the presumed individual effects of the two medications at their standard dosing. Finally, the goal should be a relatively slow and modest reduction in blood pressure to avoid a significant diminution in perfusion.

The lack of prospective controlled trials to support a specific target range for the safe treatment of blood pressure in acute stroke leaves the physician wanting.[50] Commonly used guidelines advocate using titratable short-acting vasoactive medications such as sodium nitroprusside when systolic pressure exceeds 230 mm Hg or diastolic blood pressure exceeds 140 mm/mc (the so-called hypertensive emergency). Systolic blood pressure lower than 230 or diastolic blood pressure lower than 140 can be treated with either careful observation or medications such as intravenous labetalol with careful dosage titration. The American Heart Association Guidelines recommend that the blood pressure not exceed 185 mm Hg systolic or 110 mm/mc diastolic at the time of initiation of intravenous thrombolytics.[53] The use of aggressive agents such as nitroprusside to lower the blood pressure into the "treatable range" is not advisable. Simple bedside maneuvers such as elevation of the head of the bed may help control hypertension by improving cerebral venous drainage.

Hypotension

Hypotension can decrease cerebral perfusion pressure and subsequently lead to a significant extension of an area of cerebral infarction. During an acute stroke, perfusion of ischemic areas is directly related to the mean arterial pressure. Hypotension should be evaluated and aggressively treated. As an initial intervention, putting the patient's head down flat can increase blood pressure and cerebral perfusion, and can sometimes result in clinical improvement. In addition, hypotension can be treated with intravenous fluids, inotropic agents, or vasopressors as necessary to maintain perfusion and prevent extension of an infarction. Physicians must search for a cause for a patient's relative hypotension. The emergency physician must be constantly vigilant for other diseases, such as AMI, gastrointestinal bleeding, occult trauma, aortic dissection, and sepsis.

Electrocardiographic Abnormalities

An evaluation of the patient's cardiac rhythm and an ECG are imperative. Cardiac rhythm can be significantly affected by acute stroke or may be the underlying cause of a patient's acute stroke. Cardiac rhythm disturbances such as atrial fibrillation are a significant risk factor for ischemic stroke. Similarly, acute or subacute myocardial infarction can precipitate either cardiovascular compromise leading to cerebral hyperperfusion or thrombus presenting as cerebrovascular embolism. Finally, acute dissection of the thoracic aorta may involve the carotid or vertebral arteries. Patients who have hemodynamic compromise or chest pain at the time of presentation with acute stroke should be evaluated for potential AMI or thoracic aortic dissection. In addition, patients who are mute or have significant difficulty communicating should be even more aggressively screened for these possibilities. Baseline ECG and chest radiograph should be considered. Conversely, cardiac rhythm and function can be affected by acute stroke. Hemispheric ischemic strokes that involve the insula and both SAH and intracerebral hemorrhage (ICH) can affect cardiac rhythm. ECG changes such as T wave inversion occur in 50% to 75% of patients with acute stroke.[54]

Other Issues

Management issues that must be addressed in the ED in addition to stabilization of the airway, breathing, and circulation are management of hyperglycemia, hyperpyrexia, seizures, and emesis.

Hyperglycemia

Patients with hyperglycemia at the time of the acute stroke have worse outcomes.[28] In the NINDS rt-PA Stroke Trial, a higher admission blood glucose level was associated with lower odds of desirable clinical outcome and a greater likelihood of a symptomatic ICH, regardless of recombinant tissue plasminogen activator (rt-PA) treatment.[27] Elevated glucose in patients with stroke may be partly due to a stress response. An alternative, speculative hypothesis is that elevated glucose may worsen brain injury, in part through the anaerobic metabolism of glucose in ischemic tissues with production of lactic acid. If this hypothesis is true, residual blood flow to the ischemic area would appear to be necessary for glucose-mediated injury. Glucose levels are not related to outcomes after lacunar infarcts.[29] For this reason, intravenous fluids should not include glucose, and patients with hyperglycemia should be treated with insulin to achieve euglycemia.

Hyperpyrexia

Temperature control is also important. Elevations in brain temperature have been shown to worsen cerebral ischemia and are associated with increases in stroke severity, infarct size, and mortality as well as worse outcome.[55,56] In a study of 390 patients with acute ischemic stroke, each temperature increase of 1°C raised the risk of poor outcome by a factor of 2.2.[57] Elevations in temperature have the greatest effect in the first 24 hours after stroke. Hyperthermia is easy to underestimate because brain temperature is higher than core body temperature and varies within regions of the brain.[58] Trials of hypothermia in patients who have experienced cardiac arrest have had encouraging results[59,60]; results of studies of the use of induced hypothermia in acute ischemic stroke have also been encouraging but are not definitive.[50] At this time, fever of any degree, even mild hyperthermia, should be treated with antipyretics (acetaminophen), and its cause should be investigated.

Seizures

Seizures can be a serious complication of acute stroke. They occur in approximately 5% of patients with acute ischemic stroke and may be related to involvement of the cerebral cortex or to very large strokes. The incidence of seizures in patients with ICH is approximately 25%. Seizures occur most commonly in patients with lobar hemorrhages or hemorrhages that extend into the cortex.[61] Seizures or seizure-like episodes occur in approximately 25% of patients with acute SAH.

Acute seizures are managed with benzodiazepines; if unsuccessful, these agents should be followed with barbiturates. Patients with acute stroke and seizure should receive a loading dose of phosphenytoin or phenytoin as soon as possible after the initiation of seizure activity. The principal advantage of phosphenytoin is that, unlike phenytoin, it can be dissolved in water. Phosphenytoin does not cause tissue necrosis if the patient suffers extravasation from an IV site and can be given intramuscularly. Both phenytoin and phosphenytoin can cause hypotension. The only significant detraction from the use of phosphenytoin is that it is significantly more expensive than phenytoin. Depakote, a commonly used anticonvulsant, should be avoided in the setting of ICH, because this agent has an antiplatelet effect, which may be deleterious in hemorrhagic stroke. In the setting of acute ischemic stroke, phenytoin should be administered after a seizure, but no evidence exists to support its prophylactic use.[50,62]

Emesis

Emesis is relatively common in acute hemorrhagic stroke, and because it may increase ICP, may be deleterious. Thus, throughout the ED phase of the patient's care, emesis should be avoided or controlled. Phenothiazine antiemetics such as promethazine (Phenergan) are usually adequate but do carry the theoretical burden of decreasing a patient's seizure threshold and causing sedation. The newer antiemetic agents known as the 5-hydroxytryptamine receptor antagonists (also known as the serotonin antagonists) are superior inhibitors of nausea and vomiting and neither decrease the seizure threshold nor cause sedation. The prototype agent in this class is ondansetron. The use of serotonin antagonists should be considered early in acute stroke if emesis occurs and are especially important for hemorrhagic stroke.

Diagnostic Studies

Basic diagnostic studies should be included in the initial evaluation of patients with acute stroke. The American Heart Association recommends an ECG, chest radiograph, complete blood count, platelet count, and measurements of partial thromboplastin time, prothrombin time, serum electrolyte levels, and serum glucose level.[50] Other laboratory studies (such as cardiac enzymes) should be ordered as indicated.

DIVERGENCE OF PATHWAYS BASED ON ISCHEMIC VERSUS HEMORRHAGIC STROKE

Once the initial stabilization and evaluation of a patient with stroke have been accomplished, laboratory and imaging data will lead to a divergence of potential pathways for treatment. First, the clinician is charged with ruling out stroke mimics while proceeding on the course toward rapid institution of stroke management. Second, although there is significant overlap in presentation, the management of acute ischemic stroke differs considerably from that of acute ICH and SAH.

Stroke Mimics

A number of stroke mimics may be encountered in an ED. The most common are hypoglycemia, seizure with a postictal paralysis, migraine headaches, mass lesion in the brain, systemic infection, trauma, positional vertigo, and metabolic derangements.[63] Because rapid stroke evaluation is labor intensive and costly and because the definitive therapies may carry significant risk, stroke mimics must be ruled out as early as possible in the ED.

Ischemic Stroke

Management

Currently, the optimal therapy for an appropriately selected patient with acute ischemic stroke is the initiation of thrombolysis. The ED's role in the treatment of ischemic stroke with thrombolytics is highly system dependent. The patient with undifferentiated stroke must be kept on the "fast track" toward therapy until either (1) the patient is either deemed an appropriate candidate and therapy is offered or (2) the patient is clearly excluded from thrombolytic intervention owing to a well-defined exclusion criterion.

A number of procedures can ensure that appropriate candidates are considered for therapy in the ED. First, the consistent and reinforced use of the NIHSS confirms and quantifies the extent of the stroke, facilitates discussions about risks and benefits, improves communication among colleagues, and allows for accurate reassessment of progress. Second, a stroke team whose role and availability are clearly defined has been shown to be one of the essential elements in optimizing rapid stroke treatment. Ideally, ED faculty would be members of this team.[39] Third, an agreed-upon clinical pathway should be developed and implemented by the institution along with emergency physicians and nurses, the stroke team, laboratory services, radiology services, and hospital administration; this pathway should be initiated in the ED.

The ED team can also provide a significant service to the patient with acute stroke by considering the possibility of and ruling out concomitant cardiovascular diseases such as AMI and dissection of a thoracic aortic aneurysm. Both of these entities can precipitate an acute ischemic stroke presentation, and both involve medical-surgical management issues that must be addressed. Thus, a chest radiograph and ECG are reasonable screening tools for these entities. Further diagnostic modalities, such as a CT scan of the chest with an intravenous contrast agent, may be required if a thoracic aortic dissection is suspected on either clinical or radiologic grounds.

Each hospital should develop a treatment plan for patients with acute stroke that reflects its abilities and limitations.[39] Hospitals without brain imaging facilities should never treat patients with a thrombolytic agent. Hospitals with easy access to brain imaging facilities, radiologic expertise, and an experienced physician should be able to treat appropriately identified patients with intravenous alteplase. However, in a hospital without an active intensive care unit or neurosurgical expertise, it is probably best that patients treated with alteplase be transferred immediately after treatment has begun to a hospital with these capabilities.

Teleradiography will likely play an increasingly important role in the treatment of patients with stroke in rural hospitals. In the future, treatment with neuroprotective agents that are safe and do not require a CT scan prior to administration could theoretically be given at any hospital, and possibly could be administered by paramedics before the patient arrives at the hospital. However, the realization of this possibility depends on results of ongoing and future randomized trials.

Prevention of Complications

The ED team may initiate the preventive measures so critical in the care of patients with acute stroke. Ideally, the measures would be initiated via the predefined stroke treatment pathway. They include keeping the patient on NPO status, initiating a consultation for a formal swallowing study, and beginning prophylaxis against deep venous thrombosis in patients not receiving thrombolytics. Because urosepsis is a significant risk, use of Foley catheters should be avoided whenever possible.[64] Finally, it cannot be overemphasized that the initiation of a stroke treatment pathway in the ED will help ensure complete and consistent care throughout a patient's hospitalization.

Special Consideration: Transient Ischemic Attacks

TIAs have been previously defined as "temporary focal brain or retinal deficits caused by vascular disease that clear completely in less than 24 hours."[64a] Neurovascular experts have now defined TIA as "a brief episode of neurologic dysfunction caused by focal brain ischemia, with clinical symptoms typically lasting less than 1 hour and without evidence of accompanying infarction on brain imaging."[64b] This newer definition should help clinicians avoid labeling mild strokes as TIAs.

TIAs are common and represent a significant warning of ischemic stroke.[65] On the basis of estimates of stroke incidence, approximately 300,000 TIAs occur each year in the United States.[66,67] In one study, 1 in 15 individuals older than 65 years reported a history of TIA.[68] Labeled by some clinicians as "unstable angina of the brain," this disease and its significance are becoming increasingly well understood.

Identification of TIAs in the ED is a complex and difficult task. TIAs often manifest as vague complaints that can be difficult to discern, especially in the patient without a classic medical history for the disease. Another problem is the fact that in the majority of cases of true TIA, the symptoms have abated by the time the patient is evaluated by an emergency physician. In addition, the differential diagnosis of TIAs is extensive; it includes syncope, seizure and/or Todd's paralysis, hypoglycemia, complicated migraines, multiple sclerosis, neuromuscular disorders, subarachnoid hemorrhage, Bell's palsy, neoplasm, hemorrhagic stroke, functional disorders, and vertigo. These factors combine to make the identification of TIAs difficult. It is important for the ED physician to realize that a TIA is the final common pathway of a number of disease processes and not necessarily an entity unto itself. For that reason, the history and physical examination are of paramount importance in diagnosis of the source of the TIA. Careful questioning of paramedics, family, friends, and other possible witnesses is usually required.

The role of the ED in the care of the patient with a suspected TIA has three primary components. The first is identification of the possibility of TIA and initiation of a rapid and aggressive evaluation to look for causes, a process aimed at reducing stroke risk. The second is prevention of ischemic stroke via the institution of antiplatelet or antithrombotic agents. Third is the disposition of the patient, with strong emphasis on admission to the hospital in order to facilitate monitoring and completion of the evaluation.

Hemorrhagic Stroke

Intracerebral Hemorrhage

ED management for patients with ICH consists of standard resuscitative techniques such as airway management and hemodynamic monitoring for stability. Blood pressure control is a primary directive of the emergency physician for patients with dramatic hypertension in the setting of ICH. This therapy should be thought of as an attempt to reduce the pressure driving the continuation of intracerebral bleeding.

The exact parameters for blood pressure control remain widely controversial, with some researchers advocating significant blood pressure drops, and other, more conservative workers advocating mean arterial pressure drops of 25%. Because nitroprusside, verapamil, and hydralazine are all cerebral vasodilators, these agents may be suboptimal in the setting of acute intracerebral pressure rises associated with intracerebral hematomas. Additional choices for blood pressure control in the setting of ICH appear to be labetalol, nicardipine, and an even more titratable agent, esmolol.

Intracerebral pressure management can be initiated in the ED. In the setting of an acute herniation syndrome, hyperventilation can be instituted. This measure acutely lowers cerebral blood flow and thereby decreases ICP. Hyperventilation should not be instituted for patients other than those with impending herniation syndrome, however, because of a theoretical concern that the perihematoma regions will suffer significant ischemia due to the decrease in intracerebral blood flow. Diuretics and mannitol can also be used but should be reserved for the patient with herniation syndrome or with a hematoma so large that herniation can be expected.

The ED team must remain vigilant for rapid changes in the neurologic status of patients with ICH. For many years, it was believed that ICH occurred over a brief time and that growth in hemorrhage volume was arrested very shortly after ictus. Brott and colleagues,[69] however, found that substantial growth in the volume of hematoma occurred in 26% of patients within the first hour after baseline CT. In addition, growth occurred in 12% of patients between 1 hour and 20 hours after baseline CT. Thus, 38% of patients had substantial growth (greater than one third of the volume) in the first 20 hours after baseline CT scanning. These results reveal a significant potential for a decline in a patient's neurologic status while the patient remains in the ED, and the treatment team must maintain a constant watch to be able to respond appropriately to such a change.

One role of the ED physician in consultation with neurologists and neurosurgeons is to provide prognostic information to families. The prognosis of ICH is quite poor, with a mortality of approximately 44%; half of the deaths occur in the first 48 hours.[70] There are, however, clinical indicators that can be used to aid in determining the prognosis of patients with ICH. The three most useful indicators appear to be (1) the volume of hemorrhage, (2) the level of consciousness upon arrival at the ED, and (3) the presence or absence of intraventricular extension.[71] On the basis of these three parameters, emergency physicians can assist in early decision-making both for family members and in concert with consultants.

Volume of ICH has been estimated by Lisk and associates[71] and Kothari and colleagues.[72] The formula for an ellipsoid is as follows:

$$4/3\pi\,(A/2)(B/2)(C/2)$$

where A, B, and C are the three dimensions of an ellipsoid that approximates the ICH.

This formula can be simplified by acknowledging that π is approximately 3 and then reducing the formula to $ABC/2$. For the bedside $ABC/2$ method, the CT slice with the largest area of hemorrhage is identified. The largest diameter (A) of the hemorrhage on this slice is measured. The largest diameter 90 degrees to A on the same slice is measured next (B). Finally, the number of slices upon which hemorrhage is seen multiplied by the slice thickness is calculated as the third dimension (C). If the hemorrhage area for a particular slice is greater than 75% of the area seen on the slice where the hemorrhage is largest, the slice is considered 1 hemorrhage slice for determining C. If the area is approximately 25% to 75% of the area, the slice is considered half a hemorrhage slice; and if the area is less than 25% of the largest hemorrhage, the slice is not considered a hemorrhage slice. The CT hemorrhage slice values are then added to determine the value for C. Multiplying A, B, and C together and dividing by 2 will give the approximate volume of the ICH. This method has been shown to be extremely accurate compared with computer modeling of the ICH volume.[72]

The next two components for prediction are the patient's Glasgow Coma Scale and the presence or absence of intraventricular extension of the hemorrhage. Using data from Broderick and colleagues,[70] the emergency physician can determine whether patients with ICH are at very high risk or relatively low risk for death, as follows:

The patient with an ICH volume > 60 cm³ and a Glasgow Coma Scale score < 8 has a 30-day predicted mortality of 91%.

The patient with an ICH volume < 30 cm³ and a Glasgow Coma Scale score > 9 has a predicted mortality of only 19%.

Although a 19% mortality is still high, it represents a particularly good prognosis for ICH.

Notably, morbidity remains quite high for ICH. In the study by Broderick and colleagues,[70] only 1 of 71 patients with an ICH volume greater than 30 cm³ could function independently at 30 days. As previously noted, intraventricular extension of the hemorrhage can also be used as a prognostic indicator; extension increases both morbidity and mortality from acute ICH.

Subarachnoid Hemorrhage

The most critical issue in the ED management of acute SAH is making the diagnosis. The diagnosis is not difficult in the setting of catastrophic SAH; nevertheless, hidden within the myriad patients with headache who present to an ED are those few individuals whose symptoms are limited to headache. Such patients have the best prognosis if the diagnosis is made but also the greatest likelihood that the diagnosis will be missed.

Patients with acute cephalgia account for approximately 1.2% of the more than 100 million ED encounters per year in the United States.[73] On the basis of this statistic, more than 1 million patients per year presenting to an ED are evaluated for acute headache. Buried within that group are approximately 30,000 patients with an aneurysmal SAH, of whom only 48% present with symptoms that would lead to their assignment to Hunt and Hess category 1 or 2.[74] Thus, patients with aneurysmal SAH who are assigned to Hunt and Hess category 1 or 2 at presentation represent approximately 1% of ED headache evaluations. It is exactly those patients in whom great vigilance is required to maximize their potential for a favorable outcome.

In the ED, the diagnosis is based on clinical suspicion followed by a non–contrast-enhanced head CT scanning; if CT does not yield a diagnosis, lumbar puncture is performed. There has been a debate in the emergency medicine literature regarding the need to perform lumbar puncture in all patients to rule out SAH if findings on head CT scanning performed with a third- or fourth-generation scanner are negative for SAH.[75-77] It is likely that latest-generation CT scanners are extremely sensitive for detection of SAH (reportedly 93.1% to 97.5% sensitive for scans obtained within 24 hours of ictus), they are unfortunately not 100% sensitive.[78,79] Thus, the standard evaluation for patients with sudden onset of severe (often termed "thunderclap") headache remains imaging, followed by lumbar puncture when imaging findings are normal.

Specific ED management of patients with nontraumatic SAH revolves around the basics of resuscitation and stabilization as well as management of the frequent complications of acute SAH. First, consultation with a neurosurgeon is required as soon as this diagnosis is made. Second, as with any potentially critically ill ED patient, the ED physician must begin with the ABCs of treatment. Patients with SAH frequently present with or progress to obtundation.

Therapy

Endotracheal intubation of obtunded patients protects them from aspiration caused by depressed airway protective reflexes and allows for hyperventilation if required.

Management of hypertension in the acute phase of SAH remains somewhat controversial. Recommendations have advocated blood pressure control for patients with significantly elevated blood pressure. Some experts have recommended antihypertensive agents for a systolic blood pressure (SBP) greater than 150 mm Hg.[80] Others have advocated keeping the mean arterial pressure (MBP) below 120 mm Hg; mean blood pressure is calculated from diastolic blood pressure and SBP as follows[81]:

$$MBP = \frac{(2 \times DBP) + SBP}{3}$$

When medications are required for blood pressure control, the clinician should use only agents that can be titrated rapidly. Patients receiving vasoactive agents require invasive arterial line monitoring, because labile blood pressure is common in high-grade SAH.

Cardiac Events, Electrocardiography, Dysrhythmias

Additional ED recommendations address adjunctive measures to prevent future complications. The ED team should monitor cardiac activity, oximetry, automated blood pressure measurements, and end-tidal carbon dioxide, and should avoid excessive or inadequate hyperventilation. The head of the patient's bed should be elevated to 30 degrees to facilitate intracranial venous drainage.

If the patient manifests evidence of herniation, a number of interventions should be started. The patient should receive osmotic agents, such as mannitol, and should be given a loop diuretic, such as furosemide, which will decrease ICP without increasing serum osmolality. Hyperventilation should be initiated or maintained.

DISPOSITION FROM THE EMERGENCY DEPARTMENT

Patients with hemorrhagic stroke or large ischemic stroke and all patients receiving rt-PA for an acute ischemic stroke should be admitted to a dedicated stroke care unit, if available, or the intensive care unit. Patients with smaller ischemic strokes who are deemed unlikely to be at risk for clinically significant cerebral edema would ideally be assigned to a monitored bed in a dedicated stroke unit. Because dedicated stroke units do not exist in many facilities, predesignated monitored beds should be assigned to where the acute stroke care pathway is well understood. Hospitals without the required capabilities should have a prearranged transfer agreement with a facility that can meet these requirements. It is rare for a patient with stroke to be discharged from the ED to other than an inpatient bed.

One area of considerable importance to the ED team is disposition of the patient with a suspected TIA. The disposition of the patient with a neurologic emergency such as TIA should be no different from that of any other patient with critical status and is in many ways analogous to that of the patient with unstable angina. Yet patients with neurologic emergencies commonly are not admitted and do not receive the urgent evaluation that data suggest they need to prevent recurrence or evolution of their medical problems. The disposition of an ED patient with a suspected TIA requires great care. TIAs represent a significant warning of potentially impending stroke.

When considering disposition of such a patient, the emergency physician must keep in mind the short-term prognosis after a suspected TIA. In an early incidence study from Rochester, Minnesota, investigators found a 10% incidence of ischemic stroke in the 3 months after a TIA.[82] In a study of 1707 patients evaluated for TIA in EDs, 10.5% experienced a stroke within 90 days of diagnosis, 2.6% were hospitalized for cardiac events, and 1.4% died of causes other than stroke.[82] This risk of stroke was more than 50 times that expected in a cohort of similar age.[65,66] Half of the strokes occurred within 2 days of the TIAs.[83]

One reason that the patient with a TIA might not receive an aggressive evaluation is the fact that symptoms commonly either have resolved by the time the patient is in the ED or resolve during the patient's ED stay. This fact, coupled with the difficulty of diagnosis of TIA by ED physicians, makes for a challenge. Given the known morbidity of TIA, few if any patients with TIA should be discharged from the ED. Emergency physicians would not hesitate to admit a patient with unstable angina, even if next-day follow-up and testing as an outpatient were available; yet, we do exactly that for the patients with similar disease in a different organ. Ideally, the emergency physician initiates the evaluation of a patient with TIA beyond a baseline CT when possible. The physician should also initiate or advance the patient's antiplatelet therapy. Then, the patient's care can be turned over to a primary care provider or neurologist for continuation of the observation and completion of the necessary evaluation.

The basis for admission is the rapid evaluation of these patients with TIA for the cause of disease. Given the known progression, it is not satisfactory to wait a week (for "rapid" outpatient evaluation) for diagnosis of the patient's carotid stenosis, atrial clot, or other disease. One possible solution for these patients is an observation unit with clinical protocols for diagnostic testing (carotid duplex ultrasonography, echocardiography, etc.) and rapid disposition with risk factor modification and follow-up. These protocols have yet to be implemented on a national scale but do hold promise for the treatment of TIA and other diseases.

It is critical that the emergency physician consider the literature that highlights the significant potential morbidity that TIA heralds. It is becoming clear that initial therapeutic intervention, thorough evaluation, initial testing, and admission with subsequent testing must be undertaken to prevent devastating harm to this group of patients. This change is truly a "paradigm shift" for many practitioners and consultants.

CONCLUSION

The care of a patient with an acute stroke should exist as a continuum from access to prehospital care through definitive therapies. Prehospital care providers are critical players in the pursuit of optimal care for acute stroke. As the point of first medical contact for many stroke victims, they serve as the first opportunity for identification of stroke and for the initiation of the cascade of events that must occur in order to optimize a patient's chance for recovery. The prehospital arena has been shown to be a part of a patient's care in which the greatest delays between symptom onset and definitive therapy occur. It is within this arena that symptom recognition and a decision to act based on symptom recognition make the difference between potential eligibility for acute therapy and automatic exclusion based on time. The fact that "all care begins prehospital" for the patient with acute stroke must not be lost on researchers and treating physicians. Improvements in public education, prehospital care provider education, protocol development, triage and communication, and destination selection can mean the difference between the implementation of advance therapies and a lost opportunity.

The ED is the next critical point in the care of a patient with stroke. In the ED, stabilization and a carefully coordinated evaluation, in concert with appropriate subspecialists, optimizes the patient's chance to receive the most appropriate definitive therapy in the shortest time. This process involves significant preplanning with the establishment of clear delineation of responsibilities and a well-designed "stroke care pathway." Thus, a major focus in the initial management of acute ischemic stroke revolves around well-orchestrated coordination of patient care to ensure that physician evaluation and diagnostic testing are performed very quickly. During this "golden hour of stroke," however, there remain multiple patient care issues for the clinician.[84]

Such system building, with the emphasis on prehospital and ED teams, represents a new paradigm in acute stroke care and will serve to create opportunities for patients to receive optimal therapies in an efficient manner.

References

1. Morris D, Rosamond WD, Madden K, et al: Prehospital and emergency department delays after acute stroke. The Genentech Stroke Presentation Survey. Stroke 31:2585–2590, 2000.
2. Barsan W, Brott T, Broderick J, et al: Time of hospital presentation in patients with acute ischemic stroke. Arch Intern Med 153:2558–2561, 1993.
3. Kay R, Woo J, Poon W: Hospital arrival time after onset of stroke. J Neurol Neurosurg Psychiatry 55:973–974, 1992.
4. Anderson N, Broad J, Bonita R: Delays in hospital admission and investigation in acute stroke. BMJ 311:162, 1995.
5. Fogelholm R, Murros K, Rissanen A, et al: Factors delaying hospital admission after acute stroke. Stroke 27:398–400, 1996.
6. Harper G, Haigh R, Potter J, et al: Factors delaying hospital admission after acute stroke in Leicestershire. Stroke 23:835–838, 1992.
7. Ferro J, Melo T, Oliveria V, et al: An analysis of the admission delay of acute strokes. Cerebrovasc Dis 4:71–75, 1994.
8. Jorgensen H, Nakauama H, Reith J, et al: Factors delaying hospital admission in acute stroke. Neurology 47:383–387, 1996.
9. Derex L, Adeleine P, Nighoghossian N: Factors influencing early admission in a French stroke unit. Stroke 33:153–159, 2002.
10. Gallup Poll, Sponsored by the National Stroke Association. USA. 1996.
11. Kothari R, Sauerbeck L, Jauch E, et al: Patients' awareness of stroke signs, symptoms, and risk factors. Stroke 28:1871–1875, 1997.
12. Pancioli A, Broderick J, Kothari R, et al: Public perception of stroke warning signs and potential risk factors. JAMA 279:1288–1292, 1998.
13. Schneider A, Pancioli A, Khoury J, et al: Trends in community knowledge of the warning signs and risk factors for stroke. JAMA 289:343–346, 2003.
14. Webster P, Radberg J, Lundgren B: Factors associated with delayed admission to hospital and in-hospital delays in acute stroke and TIA: A prospective, multicenter study. Stroke 30:40–48, 1999.
15. Menon SC, Pandey DK, Morgenstern LB: Critical factors determining access to acute stroke. Neurology 51:427–432, 1998.
16. Zweifler R, Drinkard R, Cunningham S, et al: Implementation of a stroke code system in Mobile, Alabama: Diagnostic and therapeutic yield. Stroke 28:981–983, 1997.
17. Bratina P, Greenberg L, Pasteur W, et al: Current emergency department management of stroke in Houston, TX. Stroke 26:409–414, 1995.
18. Lacy C, Suh D-C, Bueno M, et al: Delay in presentation and evaluation for acute stroke. Stroke Time Registry for Outcomes Knowledge and Epidemiology (STROKE). Stroke 32:63–69, 2001.
19. Kothari R, Barsan WG, Brott T, et al: Frequency and accuracy of prehospital diagnosis of acute stroke. Stroke 26:937–941, 1995.
20. Porteous G, Corry M, Smith W: Emergency medical services dispatcher identification of stroke and transient ischemic attack. Prehosp Emerg Care 3:211–216, 1999.
21. Kothari R, Barsan WG, Brott T, et al: The potential of pre-hospital care providers to impart early treatment in acute stroke: A pilot study. Stroke 26:937–941, 1995.
22. Sayre MR, Swor R, Honeycutt L: Prehospital identification and treatment. In Marler J, Winters-Jones P, Emr M (eds): Proceedings of a National Symposium on Rapid Identification and Treatment of Acute Stroke. Bethesda, MD, The National Institute of Neurological Disorders and Stroke, 1997, pp 35–45.
23. Pepe P, Zachariah BS, Sayre M, et al: Ensuring the chain of recovery for stroke in your community. Chain of Recovery Writing Group. Acad Emerg Med 5:352–358, 1998.
24. Alberts M: Stroke teams and intervention times. J Emerg Med Serv 22:25–30, 1997.
25. Broderick J, Brott T, Barsan WG, et al: Blood pressure during the first minutes of focal cerebral ischemia. Ann Emerg Med 22:96–101, 1993.
26. Kothari R: The biology of stroke and management of the stroke patient. J Emerg Med Serv 22:9–14, 1997.
27. Bruno A, Levine SR, Frankel M, et al: Relation between admission glucose level and outcome in the NINDS rt-PA Stroke Trial. Stroke 59:669–674, 2002.
28. Wass C, Lanier W: Glucose modulation of ischemic brain injury: Review and clinical recommendations. Mayo Clin Proc 71:801–812, 1996.
29. Bruno A, Biller J, Adams HP Jr, et al: Acute blood glucose level and outcome from ischemic stroke. Neurology 52:280–284, 1999.
30. Zachariah B, Van Cott C, Dunford J: Dispatch life support and the acute stroke patient: Making the right call. In Marler J, Winters-Jones P, Emr M (eds): Proceedings of a National Symposium on Rapid Identification and Treatment of Acute Stroke. Bethesda, MD, The National Institute of Neurological Disorders and Stroke, 1997, pp 29–33.
31. Kidwell CS, Saver JL, Schubert GB, et al: Design and retrospective analysis of the Los Angeles Prehospital Stroke Screen (LAPSS). Prehosp Emerg Care 2:267–273, 1998.
32. Kidwell CS, Starkman S, Eckstein M, et al: Identifying stroke in the fields. Prospective validation of the Los Angeles Prehospital Stroke Screen (LAPSS). Stroke 31:71–76, 2000.
33. Kothari R, Hall K, Brott T, et al: Early stroke recognition: Developing an out-of-hospital NIH Stroke Scale. Acad Emerg Med 4:986–990, 1997.
34. Kothari R, Pancioli A, Liu T, et al: Cincinnati Prehospital Stroke Scale: Reproducibility and validity. Ann Emerg Med 33:373–378, 1999.
35. Aufderheide T, Hendley GE, Thakur RK, et al: The diagnostic impact of prehospital 12-lead electrocardiography. Ann Emerg Med 19:1280–1287, 1990.
36. Aufderheide T, Hendley GE, Woo J, et al: A prospective evaluation of prehospital 12-lead ECG application in chest pain patients. J Electrocardiol 24:8–13, 1992.
37. Foster D, Dufendach JH, Barkdoll CM, et al: Prehospital recognition of AMI using independent nurse/paramedic 12-lead ECG evaluation: Impact on in-hospital times to thrombolysis in a rural community hospital. Am J Emerg Med 12:25–31, 1994.

38. Racht E: Prehospital 12-lead ECG: An evolving standard of care in EMS systems. Emerg Med Serv 30:105–107, 2001.

39. Alberts MJ, Hademenos G, Latchaw RE, et al: Recommendations for the establishment of primary stroke centers. JAMA 283:3102–3109, 2000.

40. Sahni R: Acute stroke: Implications for prehospital care. National Association of EMS Physicians Standards and Clinical Practice Committee. Prehosp Emerg Care 4:270–272, 2000.

41. Bock B: Response system for patients presenting with acute ischemic stroke. In Marler J, Winters-Jones P, Emr M (eds): Proceedings of a National Symposium on Rapid Identification and Treatment of Acute Stroke. Bethesda, MD, The National Institute of Neurological Disorders and Stroke, 1997, pp 55–57.

42. Anonymous: Tissue plasminogen activator for acute ischemia stroke. The National Institute of Neurological Disorders and Stroke rt-PA Stroke Study Group. N Engl J Med 333:1581–1587, 1995.

43. National Registry of Myocardial Infarction II (NRMI II). Quarterly Data Report, 1996: Ohio Data (September). San Francisco, Genentech, 1996.

44. Emergency department: Rapid identification and treatment of patients with acute myocardial infarction. National Heart Attack Alert Program Coordinating Committee, 60 Minutes To Treatment Working Group. Ann Emerg Med 23:311–329, 1994.

45. Baraff L, Lee TJ, Kader S, et al: Effect of a practice guideline on the process of emergency department care of falls in elder patients. Acad Emerg Med 6:1216–1223, 1999.

46. Bonnono C, Criddle LM, Lutsep H, et al: Emergi-paths and stroke teams: An emergency department approach to acute ischemic stroke. J Neurosci Nurs 32:298–305, 2000.

47. Walls R: The decision to intubate. In Walls R (ed): Manual of Emergency Airway Management. Philadephia, Lippincott Williams & Wilkins, 2000, pp 3–7.

48. Walls R, Murphy M: Increased intracranial pressure. In Walls R (ed): Manual of Emergency Airway Management. Philadephia, Lippincott Williams & Wilkins, 2000, pp 159–163.

49. Pancioli AM, Bullard MJ, Grulee ME, et al: Supplemental oxygen use in ischemic stroke patients: Does utilization correspond to need for oxygen therapy? Arch Intern Med 162:49–52, 2002.

50. Adams H, Brott T, Crowell R, et al: Guidelines for management of patients with acute ischemic stroke: A statement for healthcare professionals from a special writing group of the Stroke Council, American Heart Association. Stroke 25:1902–1914, 1994.

51. Lisk D, Grotta JC, Lamki LM, et al: Should hypertension be treated after acute stroke? A randomized controlled trial using single photon emission computed tomography. Arch Neurol 50:855–862, 1993.

52. Powers W: Acute hypertension after stroke: The scientific basis for treatment decisions. Neurology 43:461–467, 1993.

53. Adams H, Brott T, Furlan T, et al: Guidelines for thrombolytic therapy for acute stroke: A supplement to the Guidelines for the Management Of Patients With Acute Ischemic Stroke (AHA Medical/Scientific Statement). Circulation 94:1167–1174, 1996.

54. Dimant J, Grob D: Electrocardiographic changes and myocardial damage in patients with acute cerebrovascular accidents. Stroke 8:448–455, 1977.

55. Azzimondi G, Bassein L, Nonino F, et al: Fever in acute stroke worsens prognosis. A prospective study. Stroke 26:2040–2043, 1995.

56. Hajat C, Hajat S, Sharma P: Effects of post-stroke pyrexia on stroke outcome: A meta-analysis of studies in patients. Stroke 31:410–414, 2000.

57. Reith J, Jorgensen H, Pedersen PM, et al: Body temperature in acute stroke: Relation to stroke severity, infarct size, mortality, and outcome. Lancet 347:422–425, 1996.

58. Schwab S, Spranger M, Aschoff A, et al: Brain temperature monitoring and modulation in patients with severe MCA infarction. Neurology 48:762–767, 1997.

59. Bernard S, Gray TW, Buist MD, et al: Treatment of comatose survivors of out-of-hospital cardiac arrest with induced hypothermia. N Engl J Med 346:557–563, 2002.

60. Mild therapeutic hypothermia to improve the neurologic outcome after cardiac arrest. The Hypothermia After Cardiac Arrest Study Group. N Engl J Med 346:549–556, 2002.

61. Shah M, Biller J: Medical and surgical management of intracerebral hemorrhage. Semin Neurol 18:513–519, 1998.

62. McDowell F, Brott T, Goldstein M, et al: Stroke: The first hours, emergency evaluation, and treatment. National Stroke Association Consensus Statement. Stroke Clinical Update (Special Edition). Englewood, CO, National Stroke Association, 1997, pp 1–14.

63. Libman R, Wirkowski E, Alvir J, et al: Conditions that mimic stroke in the emergency department: Implications for acute stroke trials. Arch Neurol 52:1119–1122, 1995.

64. Roth EJ, Lovell L, Harvey RL, et al: Incidence of and risk factors for medical complications during stroke rehabilitation. Stroke 32:523–529, 2001.

64a. The Study Group on TIA Criteria and Detection: XI. Transient focal cerebral ischemia: Epidemiologic and clinical aspects. Stroke 5:277–284, 1974.

64b. Albers GW, Caplan LR, Easter JD, et al: Transient ischemic attack—proposal for a new definition. N Engl J Med 347:1713–1716, 2002.

65. Brown RJ, Petty GW, O'Fallon WM, et al: Incidence of transient ischemic attack in Rochester, Minnesota, 1985–1989. Stroke 29:2109–2113, 1998.

66. Broderick J, Brott T, Kothari R, et al: The Greater Cincinnati/Northern Kentucky Stroke Study: Preliminary first-ever total incidence rates of stroke among blacks. Stroke 29:415–421, 1998.

67. Williams G, Jiang JG, Matchar DB, et al: Incidence and occurrence of total (first-ever and recurrent) stroke. Stroke 30:2523–2528, 1999.

68. National Stroke Association: TIA/Mini Strokes: Public Knowledge and Experience—Roper Starch Worldwide Survey. Roper Starch Worldwide. Englewood, CO, National Stroke Association, 2000, p 55.

69. Brott T, Broderick J, Kothari R, et al: Early hemorrhage growth in patients with intracerebral hemorrhage. Stroke 28:1–5, 1997.

70. Broderick J, Brott T, Duldner J, et al: Volume of intracerebral hemorrhage: A powerful and easy-to-use predictor of 30-day mortality. Stroke 24:987–993, 1993.

71. Lisk D, Pasteur W, Rhoades H, et al: Early presentation of hemispheric intracerebral hemorrhage: Prediction of outcome and guidelines for treatment allocation. Neurology 44:133–139, 1994.

72. Kothari R, Brott T, Broderick J, et al: The ABCs of measuring intracerebral hemorrhage volume. Stroke 27:1304–1305, 1996.

73. Morgenstern L, Huber JC, Luna-Gonzales H, et al: Headache in the emergency department. Headache 41:537–541, 2001.

74. Whisnant JP, Sacco SE, O'Fallon WF, et al: Referral bias in aneurysmal subarachnoid hemorrhage. J Neurosurg 78:726–732, 1993.

75. Sidman R, Connolly E, Lemke T: Subarachnoid hemorrhage diagnosis: Lumbar puncture is still needed when the computed tomography scan is normal. Acad Emerg Med 3:827–831, 1996.

76. Edlow JA, Wyer PC: How good is a negative cranial computed tomographic scan result in excluding subarachnoid hemorrhage? Ann Emerg Med 36:507–517, 2000.

77. Prosser RL Jr, Edlow JA, Wyer PC: Feedback: Computed tomography for subarachnoid hemorrhage. Ann Emerg Med 37:679–680, 2001.

78. Sames TA, Storrow AB, Finkelstein JA, et al: Sensitivity of new-generation computed tomography in subarachnoid hemorrhage. Acad Emerg Med 3:16–20, 1996.

79. Morgenstern LB, Luna-Gonzales H, Huber JC, et al: Worst headache and subarachnoid hemorrhage: Prospective, modern computed tomography and spinal fluid analysis. Ann Emerg Med 32:297–304, 1998.

80. Bernardini GL, DeShaies RM: Critical care of intracerebral and subarachnoid hemorrhage. Curr Neurol Neurosci Rep 1:568–576, 2001.

81. Biller J, Godersky JC, Adams HP Jr: Management of aneurysmal subarachnoid hemorrhage. Stroke 19:1300, 1988.

82. Whisnant J, Matsumoto N, Elveback L: Transient cerebral ischemic attacks in a community—Rochester, Minnesota, 1955 through 1969. Mayo Clin Proc 48:194–198, 1973.

83. Johnston S, Gress DR, Browner WS, et al: Short-term prognosis after emergency-department diagnosis of transient ischemic attack. JAMA 284:2901–2906, 2000.

84. Thurman J, Jauch EC: Emergency department management of acute ischemic stroke. Emerg Med Clin North Am 20:609–630, 2002.

Therapy

Chapter Forty-Eight

Intravenous Thrombolysis

Lama Al-Khoury and Patrick D. Lyden

Thrombolysis offers the simplest and most direct treatment for thrombotic disorders, including most ischemic strokes. Plasminogen activators produce clinical improvement in patients with coronary artery thrombosis, peripheral vascular disease, venous thrombosis, pulmonary embolism, and acute ischemic stroke. According to the pivotal National Institutes of Neurological Disorders and Stroke (NINDS) study, intravenous (IV) tissue plasminogen activator (t-PA) improved the clinical outcome of all types of ischemic stroke (large artery, embolic, and small vessel or lacunar strokes) if treatment began within 3 hours of onset of symptoms.[1] Consequently, the U.S. Food and Drug Administration (FDA) approved recombinant t-PA (rt-PA) for the treatment of acute ischemic strokes within 3 hours of onset, excluding all patients with intracranial hemorrhage (ICH).

To date, other IV agents have proved useful also, but none is yet approved by the FDA for treatment of ischemic stroke. In this chapter we review the historical background of thrombolytic therapy in preclinical and clinical trials, summarize the different agents in previous as well as current use, and discuss the management protocol for thrombolytic treatment in patients with stroke.

THROMBOSIS AND THROMBOLYSIS

Thrombosis involves the processes of endothelial injury, platelet adherence and aggregation, and thrombin generation. Thrombin plays a major role in clot formation; it is responsible for cleaving fibrinogen to fibrin, which forms the clot matrix. Thrombin also activates factor XIII, which accomplishes interfibrin cross-linking.[2] Figure 48–1 illustrates the coagulation cascade.[3] In a process involving platelet membrane receptors and phospholipids, thrombin is generated locally by the extrinsic and intrinsic pathways. Factors V and XIII interact with specific platelet membrane phospholipids to facilitate activation of factor X to factor Xa, and the conversion of prothrombin to thrombin on the platelet surface. Platelet-bound thrombin-modified factor V (factor Va) serves as a high-affinity platelet receptor for factor Xa, which accelerates the rate of thrombin generation. The relative platelet-fibrin composition of a specific thrombus depends on regional blood flow or shear stress. At arterial flow rates, thrombi are predominantly platelet rich, whereas at lower venous flow rates, activation

of coagulation predominates. The efficacy of thrombolysis perhaps depends on the relative fibrin content and fibrin cross-linking, the latter possibly determined by the age of the thrombus. Theoretically, therefore, plasminogen activators may act less well on fibrin-poor clots, but such distinctions have not been observed clinically.

In addition to both endothelial cell–derived antithrombotic characteristics and circulating anticoagulants (activated protein C and protein S), thrombus growth is limited by the endogenous thrombolytic system, in which plasmin plays a central role. One effect of endogenous thrombolysis is continuous remodeling of the thrombus. This effect results from the preferential conversion of plasminogen to plasmin on the thrombus surface, where fibrin binds t-PA in proximity to its substrate plasminogen, accelerating plasmin formation. Plasminogen activation may also occur on cells that express plasminogen receptors and produce plasminogen activators, such as endothelial and polymorphonuclear cells. If sufficient quantities of plasminogen activators are produced or administered, plasminogen can be activated in plasma, where it cleaves circulating fibrinogen and fibrin to produce fibrin split products.

The naturally circulating plasminogen activators, t-PA and single chain urokinase-type PA (scu-PA) catalyze plasmin formation from plasminogen. In the circulation, plasmin rapidly binds to its inhibitor, α_2-antiplasmin, and is inactivated. Endogenous fibrinolysis is modulated by several inhibitors of plasmin and plasminogen activators. The half-life of plasmin in the circulation is estimated to be approximately 0.1 sec. α_2-Antiplasmin is the primary inhibitor of fibrinolysis through plasmin inhibition by binding to excessive plasmin. Thrombospondin interferes with the t-PA–mediated, fibrin-associated activation of plasminogen. Contact activation inhibitors and C1 inhibitor have indirect effects on thrombolysis.

A competitive inhibitor of plasminogen is histidine-rich glycoprotein (HRG). In addition to inhibitors of plasmin, there are specific plasminogen activator inhibitors that decrease the activity of t-PA, scu-PA, and urokinase (UK) plasminogen activator (u-PA). Both plasma t-PA and u-PA are inhibited by plasminogen activator inhibitor-1 (PAI-1), which is derived from platelets and endothelial cells. The potential risk for thrombosis reflects the relative concentrations of circulating PAI-1 and the endogenous plasminogen activators t-PA and u-PA. Other plasminogen activator inhibitors are derived from different tissues as

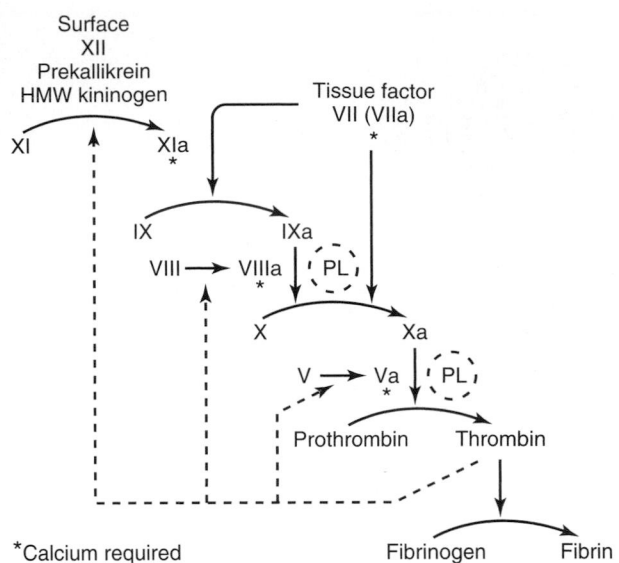

FIGURE 48–1 *Coagulation cascade. The different factors of the coagulation system are portrayed. The cascade culminates in the conversion of prothrombin to thrombin. The dashed lines show the autocatalytic action of thrombin. PL = phospholipids.[3] (From Douglas S: Coagulation history. Br J Haematol 107:22–32, 1999.)*

well. Within the thrombus, however, plasmin is protected from this inhibitor and the t-PA is also relatively protected from circulating plasma inhibitors. This is why plasmin and t-PA can achieve their fibrinolytic effect better within the clot than in serum, and also why clot lysis can be achieved with a relatively low risk of bleeding when these agents are used. Plasminogen activation is enhanced further by the complex formed by t-PA, fibrin, and plasminogen. The complex increases the clot-selective fibrinolytic activity of t-PA. Fibrinolysis occurs predominantly within the thrombus and at its surface. Lysis of thrombus is augmented by contributions from local blood flow.[2] During thrombus consolidation, plasminogen bound to fibrin and to platelets allows local release of plasmin. Within the circulation, plasmin cleaves the fibrinogen to different fragments, which incorporate into the fibrin and cause destabilization of its network, therefore allowing further degradation.[2]

All thrombolytic agents in current use are obligate plasminogen activators that act on fibrin and thrombin. Current thrombolytic agents are either endogenous plasminogen activators, which are involved in physiologic fibrinolysis, or exogenous plasminogen activators, which are not.[2]

Endogenous Plasminogen Activators

Tissue-Type Plasminogen Activator

Tissue-type plasminogen activator is a single-chain, 70-kilodalton (kDa), glycosylated serine protease. It has four domains: finger or F domain, growth factor or E domain, two kringle regions (K1 and K2), and a serine protease domain. The COOH-terminal serine protease domain has the active site for the cleavage of plasminogen. The two kringle domains of t-PA (Fig. 48–2) are similar to

the kringle domains on plasminogen. The finger domain residues and the K2 domain residues are responsible for fibrin affinity. The single t-PA chain is converted to the double-chain t-PA form by plasmin cleavage of the arginine (position 275)–isoleucine (position 276) bond. Both the single- and double-chain forms are enzymatically active and have fibrin-selective properties. The plasma half-life of the single- and double-chain forms is 3 to 8 minutes. Tissue-type PA is secreted by endothelial cells, neurons, astrocytes, and microglia. It is cleared by the liver. It is considered to be fibrin dependent because of favorable activation of plasminogen in association with fibrin. Exercise and certain vasoactive substances, such as desmopressin, raise t-PA levels. Heparin and heparan sulfate increase t-PA activity.[2] Recombinant DNA techniques are used to produce rt-PA for commercial use in both single-chain (alteplase) and double-chain (dulteplase) forms. Figure 48–2 illustrates the amino acid sequence of t-PA.[4]

Urokinase

Urokinase plasminogen activator and its precursor scu-PA, or pro-UK, are glycoproteins. Urokinase is synthesized by endothelial, renal, and malignant cells. The single-chain pro-UK possesses fibrin-selective plasmin-generating activity. Pro-UK has been synthesized by recombinant techniques to be used as an exogenous agent. Removal of the amino acid lysine at position 158 from scu-PA by plasmin produces the high-molecular-weight (HMW) double-chain u-PA (54 kDa) linked by the disulfide bridge, with further cleavage producing the low-molecular-weight (LMW) u-PA (31 kDa). Both LMW and HMW forms are enzymatically active. HMW u-PA activates plasminogen to plasmin directly. The half-life of the two forms is 9 to 12 minutes.[2] Pro-UK has been studied in patients with stroke but has not been approved for clinical use.

Exogenous Plasminogen Activators

Exogenous plasminogen activators are all the plasminogen activators that are produced or extracted from nonhuman sources, those produced by recombinant techniques such as rt-PA, and those produced through different mutations in the original physiologic plasminogen activator molecules, for example, TNK (see explanation in discussion of novel plasminogen activators).

Streptokinase

Streptokinase (SK) is a single-chain polypeptide derived from group C β-hemolytic streptococci. Streptokinase combines with plasminogen and the complex activates circulating plasminogen to plasmin, and in itself undergoes conversion to streptokinase-plasmin. This complex is not inhibited by α_2-antiplasmin, but streptokinase activity can be eliminated by the presence of streptokinase-neutralizing antibodies produced after previous infection with streptococci. The kinetics of streptokinase elimination are complex, consisting of an initial half-life of 4 minutes and a second half-life of 30 minutes.[2]

Anisoylated Plasminogen-Streptokinase Activator Complex

Anisoylated plasminogen-streptokinase activator complex (APSAC) consists of plasminogen and streptokinase bound

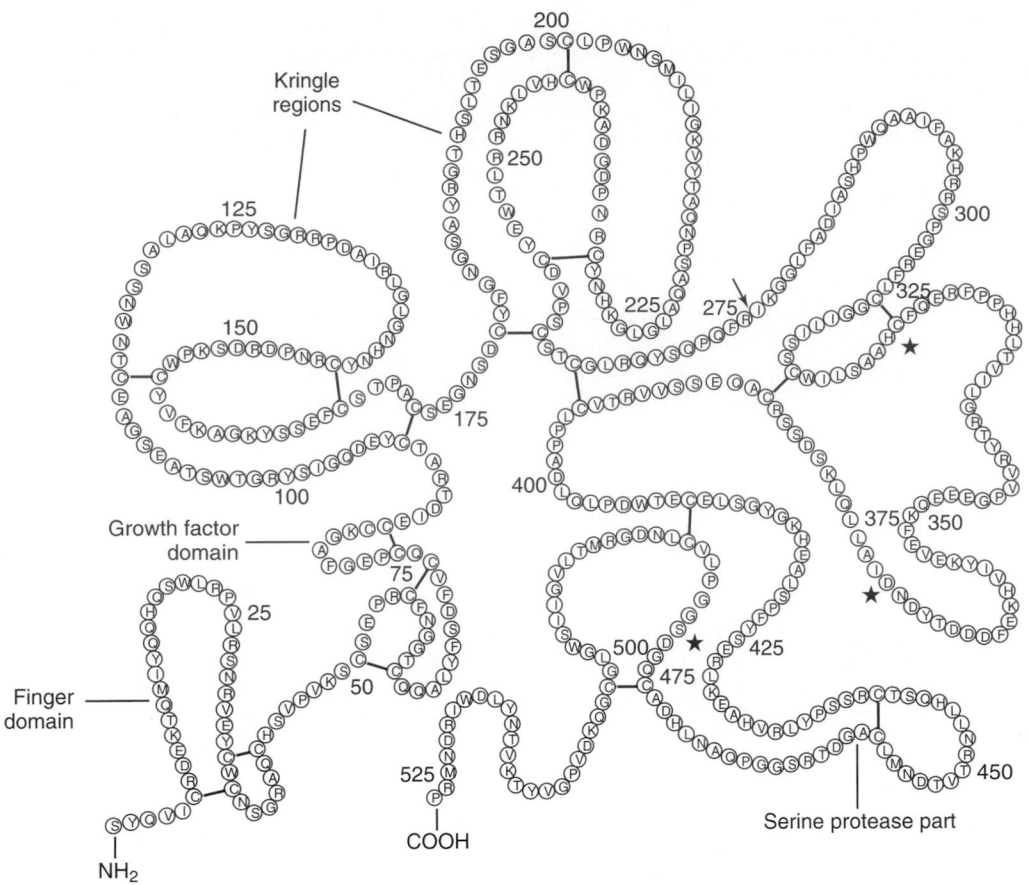

FIGURE 48–2　*Schematic representation of the amino acid sequence of t-PA. The amino acids are represented by their letter symbols. Black bars indicate the disulfide bonds. The active site residues histidine-322, asparagine-371, and serine-478 are indicated with an asterisk. The arrow indicates the plasmin cleavage site for conversion of single-chain to double chain t-PA.[4] (From Collen D: Fibrin-selective thrombolytic therapy for acute myocardial infarction. Circulation 93:857–865, 1996.)*

noncovalently. Its fibrin selectivity originates from its plasminogen-mediated fibrin-binding properties. In the presence of fibrin, streptokinase allows formation of plasmin within the complex, after activation of the acyl-protected active site of plasminogen.[2]

The half-life of APSAC is 70 minutes, which is longer than that of t-PA. APSAC has been studied in patients with cardiac disease. In a double-blind study published in December 1994, 382 patients with acute myocardial infarction (MI) were randomly assigned to receive APSAC, or t-PA, or a combination of both. The patency of the infarct-related artery at 1 hour and at 90 minutes and complete reperfusion rates were highest in the t-PA group. The rate of "unsatisfactory outcome," a composite of clinical endpoints assessed through hospital discharge, was lowest for the t-PA group although the difference was not statistically significant. The mortality rate at 6 weeks was lowest in the t-PA group (2.2% with t-PA, 8.8% with APSAC, and 7.2% with the combination treatment; P value for t-PA versus APSAC was .02, and that for t-PA versus combination therapy was .06).[5]

Both APSAC and streptokinase can be used in the thrombolytic treatment of acute MI. However, their longer half-lives, the production of anti-streptokinase antibodies to the two agents, and the higher frequency of the side effects hypotension and allergic reactions compared with t-PA give t-PA the priority as a thrombolytic agent. All three agents have been approved for use in treatment of acute MI.[6] APSAC has not yet been studied in patients with stroke.

Plasminogen Activators Derived from Saliva of *Desmodus rotundus*

The recombinant plasminogen activators that are identical to the ones derived from the saliva of the vampire bat (*Desmodus rotundus*) include an alpha form that is more fibrin dependent than t-PA. Its half-life is also longer than that of t-PA. Experimental studies have shown that the recombinant alpha-1 form and the bat plasminogen activator may be superior to t-PA in sustaining better recanalization with less fibrinogenolysis.[2]

Staphylokinase

Staphylokinase (STK) is a polypeptide derived from *Staphylococcus aureus*. It combines with plasminogen irreversibly and activates free plasminogen. The complex plasmin-staphylokinase has relative fibrin specificity, because in the absence of fibrin this complex is inhibited by α_2-antiplasmin. Recombinant STK has been used in experimental models of acute MI[2] but not of stroke.

Novel Plasminogen Activators

Different mutant forms of t-PA and u-PA have been developed through alteration of the original amino acid sequences by point mutations and deletions. These changes alter the specificity and stability of the molecules.

A good example is TNK-t-PA (tenecteplase), a mutant form of t-PA with delayed clearance and with a longer half-life than t-PA. In patients with MI, tenecteplase has a half-life of 17 ± 7 minutes, as compared with 3.5 ± 1.4 minutes for alteplase.[7] TNK has higher fibrin selectivity, has greater resistance to plasminogen-activator inhibitor with enhanced lytic activity on the thrombus, and induces earlier reperfusion than t-PA. The name TNK is derived from the fact that the molecule is produced through alter-ation of the amino acid sequence at the T, N, and K domains of t-PA, as portrayed in Figure 48–3, resulting in the improved characteristics already described.[8]

The ASSENT-1 study (Assessment of the Safety and Efficacy of New Thrombolytic Trial, study 1) evaluated the safety of TNK in 3325 patients with MI. The ICH rates were 0.7% with the 30-mg dose and 0.6% with the 40-mg dose of TNK, similar to rates for t-PA in previous MI trials. The rate of serious bleeding complications requiring trans-fusions was 1.4% for TNK compared with 7% for t-PA (statistically significant difference with the lesser bleeding rates in the TNK group).[9]

In ASSENT-2, 16,949 patients with acute MI were assigned to receive either a single-bolus dose of TNK or a

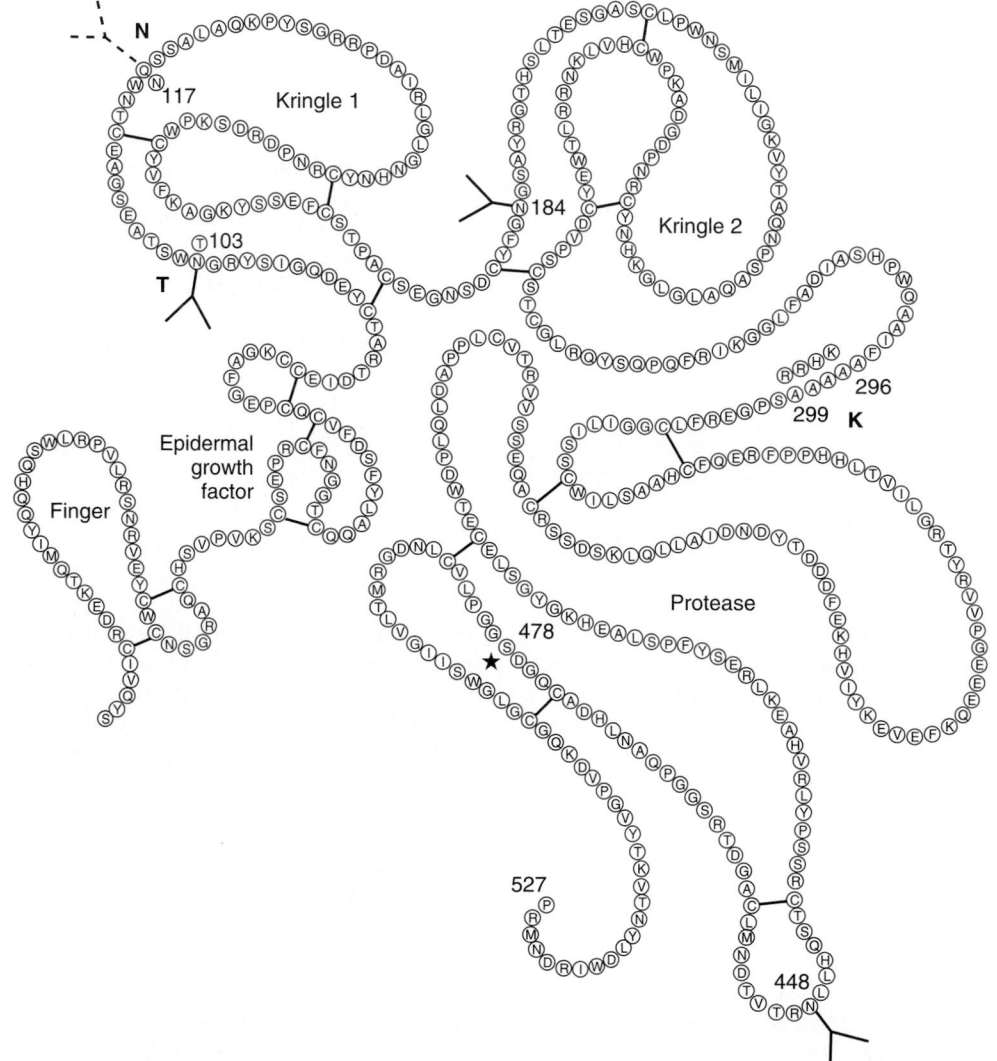

FIGURE 48–3 *The structure of the mutant form of t-PA called TNK-t-PA. This name is given to this compound because of substitu-tion at the T site (asparagine for threonine at position 103), N site (glutamine for asparagine at position 117), and K site (replacing one lysine, one histidine and 2 arginines with 4 alanines at positions 296 through 299) of the original t-PA molecule. The t-PA and TNK structures have the following domains: finger domain, epidermal growth factor domain, the two-kringle structures as well as the serine protease domain. Glycosylation sites are marked by a* Y. *(the star) marks the serine site where plasminogen activation occurs. There are short lines that show the bridging between the different loops of the molecule. The amino acid substitutions enhance the selectiv-ity and increase the half-life of the molecule as fully explained in the text.[8] (From Benedict CR, Refino CF, Keyt BA, et al: New variant of human tissue plasminogen activator [TPA] with enhanced efficacy and a lower incidence of bleeding compared with recombinant human TPA. Circulation 92:3032–3040, 1995.)*

30-minute infusion of t-PA. All patients received heparin and aspirin as well. The ICH rates were statistically similar in the two groups (0.93% in the TNK group, 0.94% in the t-PA group). However, there was a slightly but statistically significantly lower rate of major bleeding requiring transfusion with TNK (4.25% for the TNK group versus 5.49% for the t-PA group; P = .0003). The ASSENT-2 investigators concluded that TNK, which has higher fibrin specificity than t-PA and can be given as a single bolus, is associated with a lesser overall systemic bleeding rate but a similar ICH rate when given to patients with acute MI.[10]

Twenty-five patients were enrolled in each tier. Patients were followed up at 24 hours, at discharge, and at 3 months. Symptomatic intracranial hemorrhages within 36 hours from treatment did not occur in the first two tiers, but asymptomatic ICH occurred in 8% and 25% in the first two tiers, respectively. Clinical bleeding that did not require treatment occurred in 16% and 40%, respectively.[10a] Therefore, intravenous thrombolysis with TNK in acute stroke is feasible and safe. The data analysis of the higher doses is pending.

PRECLINICAL STUDIES OF THROMBOLYSIS FOR ACUTE STROKE

Considerable preclinical development showed that thrombolysis might be an effective stroke therapy. After recombinant technology was developed to produce large quantities of t-PA, animal studies could be conducted to show that t-PA, administered immediately after experimental embolic occlusion, caused reperfusion with significantly less neurologic damage. This development helped overcome the negative experience of early human use that accumulated before modern imaging techniques.

As early as 1963, Meyer and colleagues[11] studied embolic stroke models in cats and monkeys and administered IV or intra-arterial (IA) bovine or human plasmin; this treatment resulted in clot lysis without higher rates of hemorrhagic infarction.[11]

In 1983, del Zoppo and associates[12] demonstrated in baboons that after 3 hours of reversible balloon inflation compressing the middle cerebral artery (MCA), intracarotid administration of urokinase improved neurologic function and reduced infarct size without an increase in the rate of ICH detectable by computed tomography (CT). In 1985, Zivin and coworkers[13] documented that t-PA could substantially improve neurologic function after embolization with artificially made clots. These studies together suggested strongly that thrombolysis, by restoring blood flow soon after stroke onset, could prevent neurologic deficits.

Preclinical trials also yielded insights into the potential risks of thrombolysis. In 1986, del Zoppo and colleagues[14] studied t-PA–induced hemorrhagic transformation of ischemic baboon brains within 3.5 hours of MCA occlusion followed by 30 minutes of reperfusion. There was no significant difference in incidence or volume of infarct-related hemorrhage between any of the t-PA groups and the control group. In 1987, Slivka and Pulsinelli[15] investigated the hemorrhagic potential of both t-PA and streptokinase given 24 hours after experimental strokes in rabbits as well as that of streptokinase given 1 hour after experimental stroke. These investigators found that the thrombolytic agents increased the risk of ICH unless they were given early after the insult.[15] In 1989, Lyden and colleagues[16] found no difference in the frequency of hemorrhagic transformation in the ischemic brains of rabbits whether t-PA was administered 10 minutes, 8 hours, or even 24 hours after cerebral embolism. In 1991, Clark and associates[17] demonstrated that aspirin and t-PA act synergistically to cause intracranial bleeding in the rabbit embolism model.

To learn whether hemorrhagic risk was associated with thrombolytic agents in general or with a particular agent specifically, Lyden and coworkers[18] compared t-PA, streptokinase, and saline given after embolic stroke in rabbits. Streptokinase, but not t-PA, was associated with a significant increase in ICH rate and size. Table 48.1 demonstrates those results.[18] It should be noted that there was no clear dose-response effect for hemorrhages, and the doses used were comparable to the those used for cardiac disease

Table 48.1 Rates of Intracranial Hemorrhage and Thrombolysis in Rabbits with Embolic Strokes after Administration of Tissue-Type Plasminogen Activator (t-PA) as Compared with Streptokinase and Saline.*

Treatment	Dose	Time (min)	n	Hemorrhage		Thrombolysis	
				No.	%	No.	%
Saline	. . .	†	48	12	25	17	35
t-PA	3 mg/kg	90	16	5	31	9	56
t-PA	5 mg/kg	90	22	3	14	15	68
t-PA	10 mg/kg	90	11	4	36	10	91†
SK	30,000 units/kg	5	11	6	55	5	45
SK	30,000 units/kg	90	17	11	65‡	14	82†
SK	30,000 units/kg	300	12	10	83‡	10	83†

SK, streptokinase; Time, time after embolization that treatment was initiated; t-PA, tissue-type plasminogen activator.
*Results of t-PA treatment at 5 minutes and 4, 8, and 24 hours are contained in References 2 and 3.
†Saline-treated control rabbits were treated 5, 90, or 300 minutes after embolization.
‡p < 0.05 different from saline by x^2 test.
From Lyden PD, Madden KP, Clark WA, et al: Comparison of cerebral hemorrhage rates following tissue plasminogen activator or streptokinase treatment for embolic strokes in rabbits. Stroke 21: 981–983, 1990.

Therapy

in humans. Only the rabbits in which t-PA achieved thrombolysis had twice the frequency of ICH than those given placebo,[18] suggesting that reperfusion might be the basis for the higher rate of hemorrhagic transformation.

In summary, preclinical studies suggested that t-PA had reliably opened cerebral arteries in embolic experimental models. Considerable benefit was achieved if thrombolysis occurred early after occlusion onset. Hemorrhages occurred after thrombolysis and seemed to be related to the particular agent used, with streptokinase carrying a greater risk than t-PA.

CLINICAL STUDIES OF THROMBOLYSIS FOR ACUTE STROKE

The clinical development of thrombolysis for stroke proceeded logically from preclinical testing. Early experiments benefited from preclinical data and emphasized several factors: agent, dose, timing, and concomitant management. We review first-human-use studies that documented thrombolysis in humans after administration of thrombolytic agents.

Dose-ranging studies yielded important data about the dose of t-PA to use in pivotal trials; efficacy of the agents seemed to be counterbalanced by hemorrhages at higher doses. Large placebo-controlled trials confirmed the efficacy and hazards of these agents as well as observations from preclinical studies that streptokinase was more hazardous. Finally, after regulatory approval of t-PA for treatment of acute stroke, open-label studies confirmed the findings of the definitive trials and showed that IV thrombolysis is feasible and efficacious in a variety of settings. Data from experimental cerebral ischemia studies pointed to the need to treat acute stroke within a few hours, and this observation proved true in human trials as well.

Feasibility Studies

Results of early attempts to achieve thrombolysis for acute ischemic stroke were discouraging, especially in studies conducted without the benefit of brain CT to exclude hemorrhage; in these preliminary trials, patients were enrolled within significantly longer time windows than currently approved. In 1965, Meyer and coworkers[19] studied 73 patients with acute progressive strokes; the treatment group received streptokinase plus anticoagulation, and the control group received anticoagulation only. There was a higher incidence of death in the treatment group, and better clinical improvement in the control group.[19]

In 1976, Fletcher and associates[20] studied 31 patients with acute ischemic stroke who were treated with one of three different doses of IV urokinase; treatment was given within 36 hours of symptom onset. The study concluded that urokinase could be administered to patients in doses that achieve substantial thrombolysis without producing other than mild coagulation deficits; this study could not address the efficacy of the treatment, however, because the number of patients was too low. Mortality was 16%, and there was no placebo group for comparison. On the basis of these two studies, which were widely discussed, IV

thrombolysis for stroke was abandoned pending better agents and better selection procedures.

After the efficacy and safety of t-PA were proved in animal models, thrombolysis was pursued again in acute clinical stroke trials. In 1992, del Zoppo and associates[21] studied 139 patients with acute ischemic stroke who received different doses of IV t-PA within 8 hours of stroke onset. An angiogram confirmed occlusion of an extracranial or intracranial arterial cerebral blood supply in all patients. Exclusion criteria included a minor deficit, a transient ischemic attack (TIA), a clinically large stroke with a combination of hemiplegia, impaired consciousness, and forced gaze deviation, blood pressure higher than 200 mm Hg systolic, 120 mm Hg diastolic, and radiologic (CT) evidence of bleeding or radiologic evidence of significant mass effect or midline shift. Patients with early CT hypoattenuation changes were not excluded from the study. Primary endpoints were angiographic recanalization and ICH with neurologic deterioration. This landmark study reestablished the clinical promise of thrombolysis; 40% of all patients experienced recanalization of occluded arteries. Intriguingly, there was no relation between dose and recanalization, but patients with distal (i.e., smaller) clots showed higher recanalization rates. The frequency of all hemorrhages was 30.8%, although symptomatic hemorrhages occurred in 9.6% of all patients. Mortality during hospitalization was 12.5%. There was no increase in hemorrhage with the doses comparable to those used to achieve coronary reperfusion, though it could not be assumed that the safe and effective dose for acute coronary events would be the perfect dose for acute stroke treatment. Therefore, the effective and safe dose for stroke treatment was yet to be determined.

In 1992, the first in a series of government-sponsored trials appeared. In a dose-finding trial sponsored by the NINDS study, 74 patients with acute ischemic stroke received escalating doses of t-PA (0.35 to 1.08 mg/kg) within the time window of 90 minutes. Intracranial hematomas did not occur in any of the 58 patients who received doses of 0.85 mg/kg or less. Intracranial hematomas occurred with higher doses. Hemorrhages associated with neurologic deterioration (symptomatic hemorrhages) occurred in 3 of the 74 patients, although such hemorrhages did not occur at t-PA doses of less than 0.95 mg/kg. Major improvement, manifesting as a significant improvement in the National Institutes of Health Stroke Scale (NIHSS) score, occurred at 2 hours in 30% of the patients and at 24 hours in 46% of patients. Major neurologic improvement was not related to the dose of t-PA. The investigators concluded that the highest safe dose of t-PA was probably less than 0.95 mg/kg, but it is important to keep in mind that this conclusion was based on only three symptomatic hemorrhages occurring in a total experience of 74 patients. The distinct possibility remains that a higher dose could, in fact, prove to be safe and more efficacious.[22]

In 1992, Haley and associates[23] studied 20 patients with acute ischemic stroke in another dose-escalating trial in which t-PA treatment was given between 91 and 180 minutes after stroke onset. The risks of symptomatic ICH were 10% overall and 17% with the two higher dosage levels (the three doses used were 0.6 mg/kg, 0.85 mg/kg, and 0.95 mg/kg). Three patients (15%) improved by 4 points on the NIHSS at 24 hours.[23]

Mori and colleagues[24] conducted a trial in Japan in which either 6 million or 12 million units of IV t-PA or placebo was administered within 6 hours of stroke onset. Using angiograms before and after thrombolysis, these investigators confirmed that t-PA increased the rate of MCA recanalization. Of considerable importance is the fact that functional outcome measured by the Barthel Index (BI) was also significantly improved by thrombolysis. Like the del Zoppo trial, this trial established unequivocally that IV thrombolytics could open occluded cerebral vessels. Further, and perhaps even more important, the trial results suggested that angiographic confirmation of cerebral vessel occlusion might not be essential before IV thrombolysis.[24]

In 1993, in the "bridging trial," a forerunner of the definitive NINDS study, Haley and associates[25] studied 27 patients who received 0.85 mg/kg of IV t-PA or placebo within 3 hours of stroke onset. This was a randomized, double-blinded, placebo-controlled study. Despite the small sample size, there was suggestion of early neurologic improvement (at 24 hours) in the patients treated with t-PA. In the treatment arm in which therapy was given up to 90 minutes after stroke onset, 6 of the 10 patients who received t-PA improved by 4 or more points on the NIHSS, compared with 1 of the 10 patients given placebo. In the treatment arm in which therapy was given between 91 and 180 minutes after stroke onset, 2 patients in the t-PA group and 2 patients from the placebo subgroups improved by 4 or more points on the NIHSS at 24 hours.[25] The results of the bridging trial anticipated those of the larger NINDS study in a surprising number of respects. Nevertheless, large, rigorous, placebo-controlled, randomized trials were needed to confirm any beneficial effects afforded by IV thrombolytic agents.

Large, Randomized, Multicenter, Placebo-Controlled Trials

ECASS

Published in 1995, the European Cooperative Acute Stroke Study (ECASS) included 620 patients treated with 1.1 mg/kg of IV t-PA or placebo within 6 hours of stroke onset. The trial showed no significant efficacy in the intent-to-treat (ITT) primary analysis. Upon exclusion of patients with protocol violations (109 patients, 17.4%), a target population (TP) of 511 patients was selected for further analysis. Protocol violations consisted of inclusion of patients with large strokes (i.e., hypodensity of greater than one third of the MCA territory on CT), concurrent use of anticoagulants or volume expanders, detection of hemorrhage on baseline CT, uncontrolled hypertension, and lack of complete follow-up. The first hypothesis in this study was that there would be a 15-point difference in the BI between the two groups in the study, favoring the t-PA treatment group. The second hypothesis was that there would be a difference on the modified Rankin Scale (m-RS) score in favor of the t-PA group.

In the target population, there was a 1-point difference in the m-RS score between the two groups ($P = .035$) in favor of the t-PA group. There was no statistically significant difference in ICH rates between the groups but there was an increase in frequency of large parenchymal hem-

orrhages in the t-PA group and an increase in frequency of hemorrhagic infarcts in the placebo group. There was no statistically significant difference in mortality rates at 30 days.[26] Although ECASS failed to show a benefit (the hypothesis was not proved), subsequent analyses showed a significant treatment effect. In particular, on post hoc reanalysis of ECASS ITT using the NINDS global endpoint statistics, a statistically significant treatment effect was detected in the ITT group. This finding suggests that ECASS might have shown a beneficial effect of thrombolytic agents in stroke even though one cannot definitely reach that conclusion from a post hoc analysis.[27] Furthermore, when the patients treated within 3 hours were examined separately (38 given placebo, 49 given t-PA), a nonstatistically significant treatment effect (Fig. 48-4A) was demonstrated by the same statistical analysis methods used in the NINDS study (global odds ratio [OR] 2.3, $P = .07$).[28] The ECASS post hoc analyses suggested that an independent 3-hour trial might show a benefit for thrombolytic agents.

The NINDS Study

In December 1995, the NINDS study was published, a randomized, placebo-controlled, multicenter trial that showed the efficacy of t-PA in treating acute ischemic strokes within 3 hours of onset.[1] This NINDS study differed from ECASS in several respects besides the dose of t-PA and time to treatment. Most importantly, NINDS protocol required that the blood pressure had to be controlled to below 185 mm Hg systolic, 95 mm Hg diastolic. Table 48.2 summarizes the inclusion and exclusion criteria of the NINDS study.

The NINDS study had two parts with identical protocol but different endpoints. Part 1 tested whether t-PA showed clinical activity as indicated by a statistically significant difference on the primary endpoint, chosen arbitrarily to be either an improvement of 4 or more points on the NIHSS or complete resolution of the neurologic deficit within 24 hours. Part 2 used a global test statistic to assess clinical outcome after 3 months, based on scores on the BI, m-RS, Glasgow Outcome Scale (GOS), and NIHSS. Part 1 enrolled 291 patients (144 in the t-PA group, and 147 in the placebo group), and part 2, 333 patients (168 patients in the t-PA group and 165 patients in the placebo group). In part 1, on the primary endpoint, the number of patients improving by 4 or more points on the NIHSS at 24 hours was 67 (47%) in the t-PA group and 57 (39%) in the placebo group (not statistically significant, with a P value of .21).[1] Subsequent analysis showed that any other cutoff improvement in the 24-hour NIHSS, such as 5 or more points, would have yielded a statistically significant difference between the two groups (Fig. 48-5).[29]

In part 2 of the NINDS, benefit was observed on all four primary efficacy measures (NIHSS, BI, m-RS, GOS scores) at 3 months from onset of stroke. Figure 48-6 demonstrates the increase in proportion of patients with good clinical outcome in the t-PA group compared with the placebo group as measured by these scales. Patients treated with t-PA were 30% to 50% more likely to have minimal or no disability at 3 months, depending on the outcome measure. For example, the percentage of patients with an m-RS score of 1 or less at 3 months was 39% in

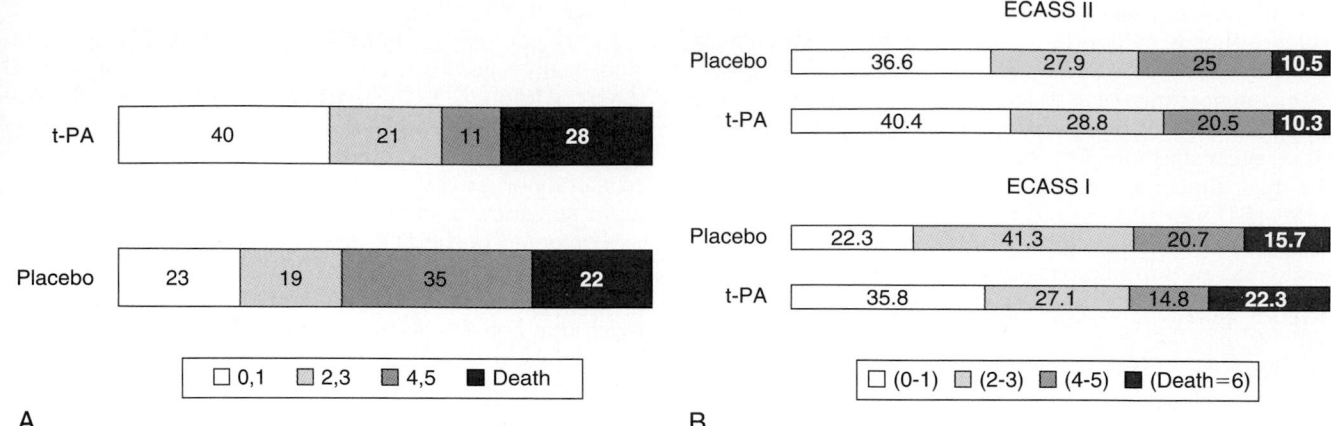

A

B

FIGURE 48–4 *A, Intention to treat subpopulation (N = 87, t-PA = 49, placebo = 38) in the ECASS-I patients who received treatment within 3 hours, using the same analysis method implemented previously in NINDS: global odds ratio is 2.3 (0.9, 5.3), P = 0.07.*[28] *The results are not statistically significant because of the small number of patients within 3 hours. B, Patient outcome by modified Rankin scale (m-RS) in ECASS-I and ECASS-II. Both ECASS-I and ECASS-II were positive for the endpoint of m-RS ≤ 2 (no disability to slight disability). Each bar shows the percent of patients with that grade. Grade 0: asymptomatic patients. Grade 1: no significant disability despite symptoms; patient is able to carry out all usual activities and duties. Grade 2: slight disability; the patient is unable to carry out all previous activities, but able to look after his or her affairs without assistance. Grade 3: moderate disability with the requirement of some help, but with preservation of the ability to walk without assistance. Grade 4: moderately severe disability with inability to walk without assistance and inability to attend to one's own bodily needs without assistance. Grade 5: severe disability; the patient is bedridden, incontinent, and requires constant nursing care and attention. Grade 6 is death.*

Table 48.2 Inclusion and Exclusion Criteria of the National Institute of Neurological Disorders and Stroke (NINDS) Study*

Inclusion Criteria of NINDS

Ischemic stroke of defined onset < 3 hours
Deficit measurable on NIHSS
Baseline CT of the brain without evidence of hemorrhage

Exclusion Criteria of NINDS

A prior stroke within the last 3 months prior to presentation (PTP)
Major surgery within the last 14 days PTP
Serious head trauma within the last 3 months PTP
History of intracranial hemorrhage (ICH)
Systolic blood pressure (bp) > 185 mm Hg or diastolic bp
 > 110 mm Hg or if aggressive treatment was required to
 lower the bp to below these limits
Rapidly improving or minor symptoms
Symptoms suggestive of subarachnoid hemorrhage (SAH)
Gastrointestinal bleeding or urinary tract hemorrhage within
 the 3 weeks PTP
Arterial puncture at a non-compressible site within the last
 7 days PTP
Seizure at the onset of symptoms
Anticoagulants or heparin within 48 hours before stroke onset
 or elevated PTT (partial thromboplastin time), or elevated
 PT (prothrombin time) > 15 sec
Platelet count < 100,000/mL
Blood glucose < 50 mg/dL or above 400 mg/dL

*Tissue Plasminogen Activator for Acute Ischemic Stroke
CT, computed tomography; NIHSS, National Institutes of Health Stroke Scale; NINDS, National Institute of Neurological Disorders and Stroke.
The National Institute of Neurological Disorders and Stroke rt-PA Stroke Study Group. N Engl J Med 333(24):1581–1587, 1995.

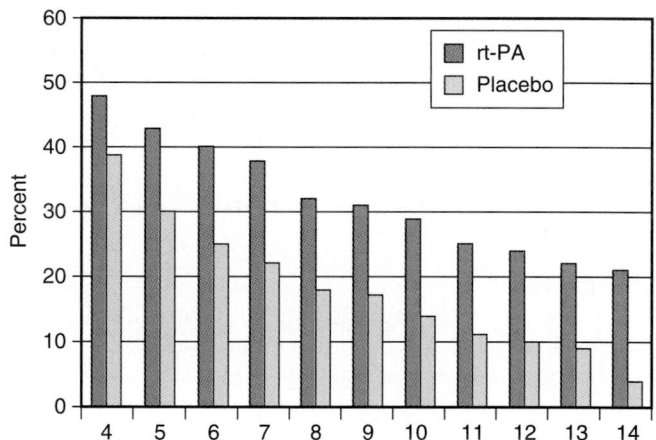

FIGURE 48–5 *The percentage of patients within each improvement category of NIHSS at 24 hours in Part 1 of NINDS. The improvement in NIHSS score at 24 hours was significantly better in the t-PA treated group as compared with placebo (p < 0.05) in each of the categories of improvement in the NIHSS score, except for a drop of NIHSS of ≥ 4 points (chosen as the primary end-point of Part I of NINDS). Therefore, had the primary endpoint been chosen to be a drop in NIHSS at 24 hours ≥ any number other than 4, Part 1 would have shown a statistically significant benefit of t-PA at 24 hours.*

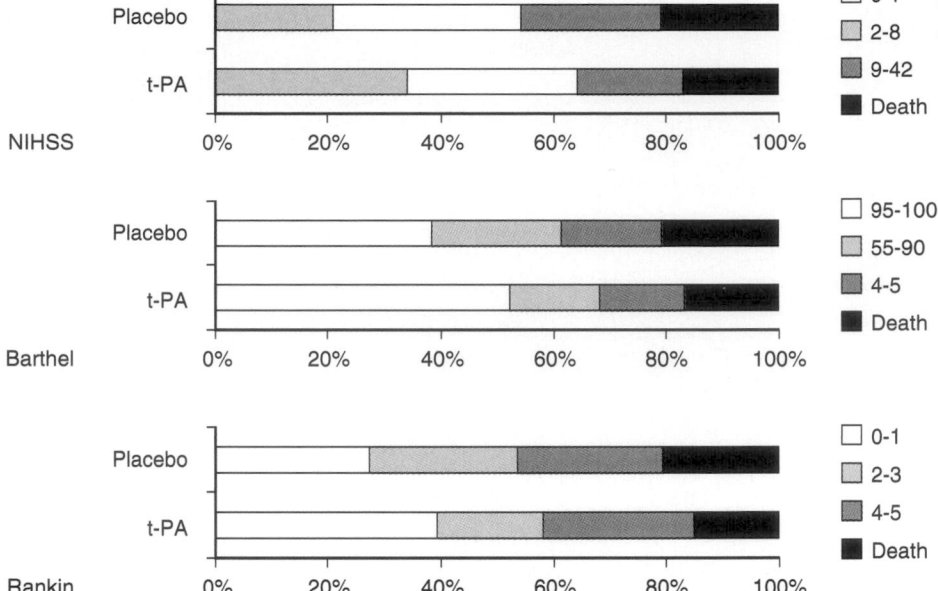

FIGURE 48–6 *Statistically significant improvement on all primary outcome measures at 3 months in NINDS, Part-2. NIHSS, Barthel Index, and m-RS at 3 months are depicted here and there is a statistically significant improvement in the t-PA treated patients as compared with placebo in each of these categories as well as in the Glasgow Outcome Scale (GOS) which is not shown here.*

the t-PA group versus 26% in the placebo group (statistically significant difference in favor of t-PA). Symptomatic ICH occurred in 6.4% of patients who received treatment, but only in 0.6% of patients who received placebo. Mortality at 3 months was not statistically different between the two groups, being 17% in the t-PA group and 21% in the placebo group.[1] Thus, despite an increased risk of hemorrhage, the mortality rate was not affected, and IV t-PA provided considerable benefit and improved outcome, as depicted in Figure 48–7. Furthermore, the NINDS data analysis showed that t-PA treatment resulted in a more favorable outcome regardless of the subtype of stroke (small-vessel, large-vessel, or cardioembolic stroke) diagnosed at baseline.[1]

Further subgroup analysis of the NINDS data showed that the only variables independently associated with an increased risk of symptomatic ICH in the t-PA–treated patients were the baseline severity of the stroke as measured by the NIHSS, brain edema defined by hypodensity on baseline CT, and mass effect on baseline CT (before treatment).[30]

Subsequent prespecified analyses of the NINDS database using the global statistical method showed sustained, statistically significant benefit at 6-month and 1-year follow-up points: The OR values for a favorable outcome in the t-PA group compared with the placebo group were 1.7 with a 95% confidence interval of 1.3 to 2.3 at 6 months, and the OR was 1.7 with a 95% confidence interval of 1.2 to 2.3 at 1 year. At 1 year, the range of absolute increase in the percentage of patients with a favorable outcome was 11% to 13%, and the range of relative increase in favorable outcome was 32% to 46% for the three outcome scales (m-RS, BI, GOS). Patients treated with t-PA were at least 30% more likely to be independent at 1 year than those given placebo. Importantly, favorable outcomes were not accompanied by an increase in severe disability or mortality. The proportion of patients surviving between 3 months and 12 months after stroke was consistently higher in the t-PA group than in the placebo group. However, there was no statistically significant difference in mortality at 6 months and 1 year. After adjustment for those variables, treatment with t-PA still offered better outcome.

As was the case for the 3-month follow-up data, there was no evidence of interaction between the subtype of stroke at baseline and treatment, meaning that all stroke subtypes (large-vessel, small-vessel, and embolic) benefitted from t-PA. Moreover, there was no significant difference in the incidence of recurrent stroke between the t-PA and placebo groups at 1 year.[31] Furthermore, another analysis of the NINDS data addressed finding the binary measures that predicted effectiveness of t-PA during the first 3 months. Measures using NIHSS and m-RS scores of 1 or less were the most sensitive discriminators of effectiveness of t-PA in the NINDS study. The best measure was NIHSS score of 2 or less at 24 hours. High-quality analysis of the volume of brain infarction as measured by CT was not as sensitive to detect a treatment effect as the clinical scale measures.[32]

ECASS II

ECASS II was a multicenter double-blind, randomized trial of 800 patients with acute stroke who received either 0.9 mg/kg t-PA (409 patients) or placebo (391 patients) within 6 hours of stroke onset. Exclusion criteria were similar to those for the NINDS, with the addition of evidence of early infarction changes on CT greater than one third of the MCA territory, coma or stupor, and hemiplegia with fixed eye deviation. Use of anticoagulants and antiplatelet agents was prohibited for the first 24 hours after random assignment of patients to treatment.

There were 72 protocol violations (17%), 34 in the t-PA group and 38 in the placebo group; the majority resulted from failure to abide by the CT criteria. There was no statistically significant difference in the proportion of favorable outcomes (m-RS score 0 to 1 at day 90) between the two groups, figures being 40.3% for the t-PA group and 36.6% for the placebo group ($P \geq .05$). However, a post hoc

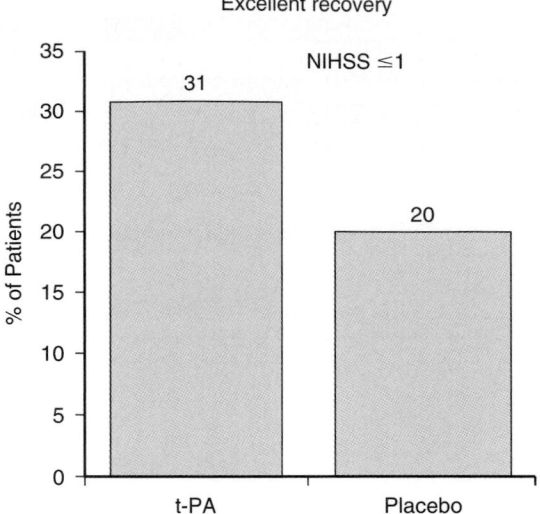

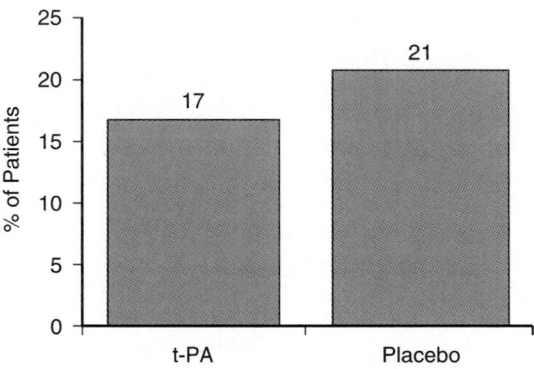

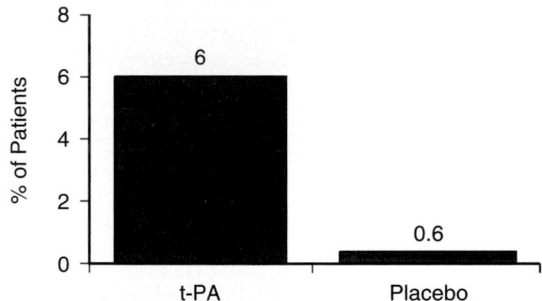

FIGURE 48–7 *Benefit and risk of t-PA in NINDS for acute stroke trial: benefit from t-PA is shown as a statistically significant higher percent of patients with NIHSS of 0–1 in the t-PA group as compared with placebo. Risk is depicted as a statistically significant increase in symptomatic intracranial hemorrhage at 36 hours that is attributable to t-PA treatment. Despite that risk, there is no significant difference in mortality between the t-PA and placebo groups at 3 months.*

analysis of the 90-day m-RS score, classifying each patient as either functionally independent (m-RS score ≤2) or dependent (m-RS score >2), found a statistically significant difference between the two groups in favor of t-PA (54.3% in the t-PA group versus 46.0% in the placebo group with an 8.3% absolute difference; $P = .024$). The incidence of symptomatic ICH was higher in the t-PA group (8.8%) than in the placebo group (3.4%).[33] Figure 48–4*B* shows the m-RS scores for the t-PA and placebo groups at 90 days in both ECASS-1 and ECASS-2.

Streptokinase Trials

Three clinical trials attempted to investigate the benefits and risks of streptokinase treatment in acute stroke. These trials were all terminated prematurely because of complications.

The Multicentre Acute Stroke Trial in Europe (MAST-E) was a double-blind, placebo-controlled, randomized study of streptokinase published in 1996.[34] Patients with acute MCA strokes presenting within 6 hours of onset received either 1.5 million units of IV streptokinase or placebo. There was no difference in the primary outcome measures (death and severe disability and m-RS score ≥ 3 at 6 months after treatment). In-hospital death and symptomatic ICH occurred more often in the streptokinase group. The use of anticoagulants or antiplatelet agents was allowed: 65% of patients given streptokinase and 75% of patients given placebo received heparin concomitantly with thrombolysis, and 20% of patients in each group also received aspirin. At 6 months, the mortality was slightly and nonsignificantly higher in the streptokinase group ($P = .06$). There was a trend toward less severe disability with streptokinase and significantly shorter rehabilitation or nursing home stay ($P = .003$). This study found no evident benefit from streptokinase treatment.[34]

The Multicentre Acute Stroke Trial in Italy (MAST-I), published in 1995, was a randomized, controlled trial that studied patients who received IV streptokinase, streptokinase plus aspirin, aspirin alone, or placebo within 6 hours of stroke onset. Anticoagulants were to be avoided in this trial, except for limited doses of subcutaneous heparin for prophylaxis of deep venous thrombosis. There was no proved benefit in any therapy group. Symptomatic hemorrhages were more common in the streptokinase groups than in the placebo and aspirin-only groups. Aspirin plus streptokinase therapy was associated with a statistically significant increase in early mortality compared with placebo.[35]

In the Australian Streptokinase (ASK) study,[36] 340 patients were randomly assigned to receive either placebo or streptokinase intravenously within 4 hours of stroke onset. The study had to be suspended because of poorer outcome in the streptokinase group. There was no relationship between the dose of streptokinase and the risk of hemorrhage. Hematoma rate was 9.6% in the streptokinase group and 0 in the placebo group for patients who received treatment within 3 hours of stroke onset. The streptokinase group had higher mortality, worse clinical outcome, and increased ICH rate. Hypotension was an adverse event that occurred in the streptokinase-treated patients. Subsequent analysis comparing the 70 patients treated within 3 hours and the 270 patients treated after 3 hours of stroke onset found that the earlier treatment was associated with better outcomes than was later treatment.[37]

A further multivariate meta-analysis of all patients from previous streptokinase studies (MAST-E, MAST-I, ASK, others) showed that concomitant use of aspirin increased the mortality in streptokinase-treated patients (17% without aspirin versus 91% with aspirin treatment, $P = .005$).[38]

The ATLANTIS Study

The Alteplase Thrombolysis for Acute Noninterventional Therapy in Ischemic Stroke (ATLANTIS) study, published in 1999, was a double-blind, randomized trial evaluating the efficacy and safety of treatment with 0.9 mg/kg of IV t-PA in patients with acute ischemic strokes within 6 hours of stroke onset (part A).[39] Later the treatment window was changed to 5 hours (part B),[40] because of concerns about safety in patients treated between 5 and 6 hours of onset. The trial ended prematurely in 1998 on the basis of analysis that the treatment was unlikely to be beneficial. In the final analysis of part B, the median time to treatment was 4.5 hours with the minority of patients receiving treatment within 3 hours. There was no difference in the primary end-point, that is, in the percentage of patients with NIHSS score of ≤1 at 90 days. The symptomatic ICH rate, however, was greater in the t-PA group.

Albers and coworkers[41] retrospectively evaluated data for the ATLANTIS patients who had received t-PA or placebo within the 3-hour time window. The primary end-point was the percentage of patients who had complete recovery with a NIHSS score of ≤1 at 90 days after treatment. Total number of patients was 61, with 38 in the placebo arm and 23 in the t-PA arm. The patients receiving t-PA were significantly more likely to have a favorable outcome, defined as a NIHSS score of ≤1 ($P = .01$); 60.9% of the t-PA group had an NIHSS score of ≤1 at 3 months versus only 26.3% in the placebo group, with an absolute difference of 34.6% (OR 4.4; $P < .01$). The symptomatic ICH rate was 13% in the t-PA group versus 0 in the placebo group (statistically significant difference, with $P = .05$). There was a trend toward higher mortality, in the t-PA group that did not reach statistical significance.[41]

COMMUNITY EXPERIENCE OF THROMBOLYSIS FOR ACUTE STROKE

On the basis of the results of the two NINDS studies and the post hoc analysis of the ECASS trials, the FDA approved t-PA as treatment for acute ischemic stroke in June 1996. Almost immediately, critics suggested that somehow the trials had been conducted only in specialized stroke centers and therefore the results could not be generalized to the larger stroke population. Despite the fact that the NINDS study included more patients randomly assigned for treatment at community medical centers than in academic centers, a need existed to demonstrate efficacy in community experience. Several such observational studies have now appeared, and the results nearly uniformly confirm those of the ECASS and NINDS studies. If the NINDS protocol is not followed, however, lower

response rates and higher hemorrhage rates can be observed. Table 48.3 summarizes the majority of the observational studies to date.

In 1998, Chiu and coworkers[42] published the first *Houston* community experience, which evaluated 30 patients with acute ischemic stroke who were treated with IV t-PA between December 1995 and December 1996 at a dose of 0.9 mg/kg. The rate of symptomatic ICH was 7%, and the rate of fatal ICH was 3%. On follow-up in December 1996, 37% of patients had recovered to fully independent function (BI 95 to 100), and 30% of patients had no disability (m-RS score 0 to 1). The 3-month mortality rate was 20% (compared with 17% in the corresponding NINDS group). Three patients were treated outside the 3-hour window. This study concluded that t-PA therapy is a feasible, safe, and effective treatment for acute ischemic stroke in one academic and three community medical centers. There was no difference in any outcome or safety measure between the two types of medical centers.[42]

In 1998, Grond and associates[43] published the *Cologne* community experience, in which 100 patients (22% of 453 patients with a presumed diagnosis of stroke) received t-PA; 26 were treated within 90 minutes of stroke onset. The average time from emergency department (ED) arrival to treatment (door-to-needle time) was 48 minutes, and the average arrival time from stroke onset was 78 minutes. At 3 months after t-PA therapy, 53% of patients had recovered with fully independent function (BI 95 to 100), 40% had no disability (m-RS score 0 to 1), and 42% had a NIHSS score of 0 to 1. Symptomatic ICH occurred in 5%, fatal ICH occurred in 1%, and total ICH, in 11%. The mortality rate was 12%. The investigators concluded that thrombolysis was effectively applied in acute stroke treatment with acceptable efforts and that the outcome and complication rates were comparable to those of the NINDS studies.

In 1999, the *Oregon* experience was published.[44] Thirty-three patients with acute ischemic stroke received t-PA within 3 hours of stroke onset. The exclusion criteria were the same as those for the NINDS study, with the addition of excluding patients with ischemic changes of more than one third of the MCA territory on CT. The mean baseline NIHSS score was 16.6, as compared with 14 in the NINDS study. The percentage of patients achieving full or almost full recovery at 3 months, as measured by m-RS score of 0 to 1, was 36.4%, compared with 39% in the NINDS study. Symptomatic ICH occurred in 9.1%, compared with 6.4% in the NINDS trial, and occurred in patients with severe strokes (NIHSS score ≥ 20). Mortality was 18.2% (6.1% secondary to ICH), versus 17% (3% secondary to ICH) in the NINDS study. The Oregon study results were compared with the NINDS study results, and t-PA was found to be a feasible and efficacious treatment.[44]

The initial *Cleveland* community experience with t-PA was published in 2000.[45] It showed more hemorrhages and fewer "responders" than the NINDS study. The objective was to estimate the rate of t-PA use in the community, the outcomes of t-PA treatment, and the incidence of ICH. The study was a chart review that enrolled patients from 29 hospitals in the metropolitan areas of Cleveland, Ohio. An attempt was made to collect all cases prospectively, but most of the cases were actually reviewed in retrospect. Of

Table 48.3 Summary of the Intravenous t-PA Studies in Stroke

Year	*Series*	*N(t-PA)*	*t-PA mg/kg*	*S. ICH*		*T. ICH*	*Outcome*
1992	NIH (<90 m)[23]	74	0.35–1.08	4%		—	46%[a]
1992	Haley et al (90–180 m)[24]	20	0.6–0.95	10%		—	15%[b]
1992	Mori et al, 6 h[25]	31(19)		PH	HI	T.ICH	mean HSS[c]
			20 MIU	*11%*	*56%*	*67%*	*–9(±18.6)*
			30 MIU	*10%*	*30%*	*40%*	*–20.3(±19.4)*
			Pl.	*8%*	*33%*	*42%*	*–29.7(±27.7)*
1993	Bridging Trial, 3 h[26]	27(14)	0.85	0% for t-PA < 90 min		—	57% t-PA 15% Pl.[d]
1995	ECASS, 6 h[27]	620(313)	1.1	—		t-PA43% Pl 37%	35.7% t-PA 29.3% Pl.[e]
1995	NINDS, 3 h[1]	624(312)	0.9	6.4% 0.6% Pl		—	39% t-PA 26% Pl.(ss)[f]
1997	ECASS-II 6 h[34]	800(409)	0.9	8.8% t-PA 3.4% Pl.		—	40.3% t-PA 36.6% Pl.[g]
1997	ECASS-II Post-hoc[34]	—	—	—		—	54.3% t-PA 46% Pl.(ss)[h]
1998	Houston, 3 h[43]	30	0.9	7%		10%	30%[i]
1998	Cologne, 3 h[44]	100	0.9	5%		11%	40%[j]
1998	Lyon, 7 h[54]	100	0.8			7%	45%[k]
1999	Oregon, 3 h[45]	33	0.9	9.1%			36.4%[l]
1999 (1991–1993)	ATLANTIS-A (6 h)[40]	142(71)	0.9	11% t-PA 0% Pl.		—	40% t-PA 21% Pl.[m]
1999 (1993–1998)	ATLANTIS-B (3–5 hr)[79]	547(272)	0.9	7% t-PA 1.1% Pl.		—	34% t-PA 32% Pl.[n]
2000	Cleveland, 3 h[46]	70	0.9	15.7%		—	Increased death[o]
2000	STARS, 3 h[48]	389	0.9	3.3%		11.5%	35%[p]
2000	Vancouver, 3 h[49]	46	0.9	2.2% (36 hr)		—	43%[q]
2001	Berlin, 3 h[51]	75	0.9	—		2.7%	40%[r]
2001	Calgary, 3 h[50]	84	0.9	7.1%		—	54%[s]
2001	Houston, 3 h[52]	269	0.9	5.6%[t]		—	—
2002	ATLANTIS < 3 hr patients[42]	61(23)	0.9	13% t-PA 0% Pl.		—	t-PA 60.9% Pl. 26.3%[u]
2002	CASES, 3 h[53,80]	1099	0.9	4.6%		—	46%[v]
In press	Lyon, 7 h[56]	200	0.8	5.5%			35%[w]

ATLANTIS, *alteplase thrombolysis for acute noninterventional therapy in ischemic stroke study*; ATLANTIS-A, *ATLANTIS Part A*; ATLANTIS-B, *ATLANTIS Part B*; CASES, Canadian Activase for Stroke Effectiveness Study; ECASS, European Cooperative Acute Stroke Study; h, hour; HI, *hemorrhagic infarct*; HSS, hemispheric stroke scale at day 30 (mean from baseline); m, minute; NIH, National Institutes of Health; N(t-PA), total number of patients (patients who received t-PA); *PH, parenchymal hematoma*; Pl., placebo; S. ICH, symptomatic intracerebral hemorrhage; STARS, *standard treatment with alteplase to reverse stroke*; TICH, total intracerebral hemorrhage; t-PA, tissue-type plasminogen activator. Superscript numbers indicate chapter references.

[a]NIHSS improvement ≥ 4 at 24 h.
[b]As in (a).
[c]Every 500,000 MIU of t-PA correspond to 1 mg. HT = hemorrhagic transformation. HSS = hemispheric stroke scale at day 30 (mean change from baseline). HSS ranges from 0 to 100.
[d]As in (a).
ICH was 0% for the group who received t-PA within 90 min from onset.
[e]Identical median mRS = 3 for t-PA and the placebo group.
35.7% of t-PA patients with mRS ≤ 2 versus 29.3% in the placebo group (intention to treat analysis).
[f]Percent of patients with mRS ≤ 1 at 3 months in the t-PA and placebo groups; ss = statistically significant difference (better in t-PA group).
[g]mRS ≤ 1 at 90 days. No statistically significant difference between t-PA and placebo.
[h]Statistically significant difference between t-PA and placebo groups for mRS ≤ 2.
[i]mRS ≤ 1 on follow-up in Dec 1996 of all 30 patients. Enrollment was between Dec 1995–Dec 1996.
[j]mRS ≤ 1 at 3 months.
[k]mRS ≤ 1 at day 90.
[l]mRS ≤ 1 at 3 months.
[m]NIHSS ≤ 1 at 90 days.
[n]NIHSS ≤ 1 at 90 days.
[o]Increased protocol violations and deaths. Only 1.8% were treated with t-PA.
[p]mRS ≤ 1 at 30 days.
[q]mRS ≤ 1 at 13 months.
[r]mRS ≤ 1 at 3 months.
[s]mRS ≤ 2 at 3 months.
[t]Mean baseline NIHSS 14.4(±6.1). At 24 hours mean NIHSS 10(±8). Mean discharge NIHSS 7(±7).
[u]NIHSS ≤ 1 at 90 days. Post-hoc analysis of the ATLANTIS patients who received t-PA within 3 hours from onset.
[v]Independent (mRS ≤ 2) at 90 days.
[w]mRS ≤ 1 at 3 months.

3948 patients with acute ischemic strokes presenting between 1997 and 1998, 17% were admitted within 3 hours of onset. Median NIHSS score was 12. Only 1.8% received t-PA treatment. Symptomatic hemorrhage occurred in 15.7% of the patients given t-PA, but 50% of the cases with t-PA treatment had protocol violations. Deviations from the protocol included use of antiplatelet agents or anticoagulants within 24 hours of treatment with t-PA, treatment beyond the 3-hour window, and deviation from the blood pressure guidelines. The in-hospital mortality rate and the length of hospital stay were significantly higher in the t-PA group.

The differences between the initial Cleveland community survey and all others probably are due in part to differences in methodology. In this trial, nurse abstractors attempted to find cases after the fact; a case ascertainment bias toward difficult cases with memorable adverse outcomes would be hard to avoid. In other series, cases of stroke were collected, prospectively, by the stroke team physicians.

The Cleveland group published a report of the Cleveland community experience with IV t-PA. This was a retrospective chart review of all patients with ischemic stroke who presented to the Cleveland Clinic Health System between June 2000 and June 2001. A stroke quality improvement (SQI) program had been implemented before that, starting in 1999. The SQI included very frequent review of acute stroke data, performance monitoring, implementation of stroke protocol in the emergency rooms, a 24-hour stroke beeper, and medical education about acute stroke management and IV t-PA use. The results showed that IV t-PA was given in 18.8% of patients who arrived within the 3-hour time window. Protocol deviations occurred in 19.1% of those patients who received t-PA; symptomatic ICH occurred in 6.4%, a rate that is comparable to that of the NINDS study. The authors concluded that IV t-PA could be given safely to appropriate patients with stroke at the community hospital level.[45a]

In summary, the higher rate of protocol violations in the initial Cleveland community experience had led to the higher frequency of adverse events. Moreover, after extensive education and retraining, the symptomatic ICH rate and protocol violations declined in Cleveland.

The results of the *STARS* (Standard Treatment with Alteplase to Reverse Stroke) study were published in March 2000; Albers and colleagues[46] looked at 389 consecutive patients with stroke enrolled between February 1997 and December 1998 from different academic and community hospitals in the United States. Those patients presented with acute ischemic stroke within 3 hours of onset. The median NIHSS score was 13. Protocol violations occurred in 127 patients (32.6%). The violations were anticoagulant use, treatment outside the recommended period, and nonadherence to blood pressure guidelines. Measure of recovery was m-RS score at 30 days after t-PA treatment; m-RS score was ≤1 in 35% of patients and ≤2 (independence) in 43% of patients. Symptomatic ICH occurred in 3.3% of patients, and asymptomatic ICH in 8.2%. This study showed favorable clinical outcome with t-PA treatment and a relatively low rate of symptomatic hemorrhage, comparable to that of the NINDS studies.[46]

In December 2000, the *Vancouver* study was published. Chapman and associates[47] studied 46 consecutive ischemic patients with stroke (combined retrospective and prospective study) who received t-PA within the 3-hour time window. The NINDS inclusion and exclusion criteria were applied. Symptomatic ICH at 36 hours occurred in 2.2% of patients. At 13-month follow-up, 22% of patients were dead (similar to NINDS results), and 43% of patients had a favorable outcome, consisting of m-RS score of 0 to 1, and 48% had a BI of 95 to 100.[47]

In April 2001, Barber and colleagues[48] published the *Calgary* experience, in which 2165 consecutive patients with acute stroke in Calgary, Canada, treated between October 1996 and December 1999 were studied. Of these patients, 1168 (53.9%) were diagnosed to have ischemic strokes. Hemorrhagic stroke was diagnosed in 31.8%, and transient ischemic attack (TIA) in 13.9%. Of the 1168 patients with ischemic stroke, 73.1% were excluded from the study because of delayed presentation. Causes for delay included uncertain time of onset (24.2%), waiting to see whether the deficit would improve (29%), transfer from another hospital (8.9%), and poor accessibility to the treating hospital—patient's home a long distance from the treating hospital or transfer of patients from an outlying hospital—(5.7%). Of the 1168 patients with ischemic stroke, 314 patients (27%) were admitted to the hospital within 3 hours of onset, and 84 of the 314 (26.7%) received IV t-PA. Exclusion from the study of the rest of the patients presenting within the 3-hour window was due to different reasons: 13.1% had mild strokes, 18.2% showed clinical improvement, 13.6% had other protocol exclusions, 8.9% experienced ED referral delay, and 8.3% had significant morbidity. At 3 months, 54% of the patients included in the study had an m-RS score ≤ 2 at 3 months. The symptomatic ICH rate was 7.1%. Only 4.7% of all patients presenting during the study period were treated with t-PA, the majority of t-PA treatment exclusions being related to delay in presentation. Of those patients whose strokes were considered too mild to be treated or who showed rapid improvement, 32% either remained dependent upon hospital discharge or died during hospital admission. This finding implied that a third of the patients who were excluded because of minimal deficits or dramatic improvement had bad outcome, raising the question whether such patients should also be treated.

In May 2001, the *Berlin* study was published.[49] Cases of acute ischemic stroke were collected over 2 years; only 75 of the patients, or 9.4%, received IV t-PA. Median baseline NIHSS score was 13 ± 6. Average time for initiation of thrombolysis was 144 minutes from onset; 17% of patients were treated after 3 hours from onset. Cerebral hemorrhages occurred in 2.7%. Outcome at 3 months was good (m-RS score 0 to 1) in 40%, moderate (m-RS score 2 to 3) in 32%, and poor (m-RS score 4 to 5) in 13%. Mortality rate was 15%. It was noticed in this study that over time, the median door-to-CT time and door-to-needle time shortened, and the number of patients treated per month increased from 2 to 4. The investigators, Koennecke and associates,[49] concluded that IV t-PA is safe and efficacious and that the performance of the stroke team and the number of patients enrolled can improve with time.

Therapy

In an article published in December 2001, Grotta and coworkers[50] described their own *Houston* community experience with t-PA treatment in patients with acute ischemic stroke between January 1996 and June 2000. The design was a prospective inception cohort registry of patients seen by the stroke team at the University of Texas–Houston Medical School and three community hospitals in addition to a retrospective medical record review of all patients treated with t-PA within the same 4-year period. A total of 269 patients were treated, representing 15% of all patients who presented with acute ischemic stroke during the study period. The mean door-to-needle time was 70 minutes, and 28% of patients were treated within 2 hours of onset. The symptomatic ICH rate was 4.5%. Protocol violations occurred in 13% of all treated patients, with an ICH rate of 15% in the patients with protocol violations. The mean NIHSS score was 14.4 ± 6.1 before treatment, 10 ± 8 at 24 hours, and 7 ± 7 upon discharge. In-hospital mortality rate was 15%. These investigators concluded that IV t-PA could be given in up to 15% of patients with acute ischemic stroke with a low risk for intracerebral bleeding; they also concluded that successful experience with such treatment depends on the experience and organization of the treating team and on following the treatment protocol.[50]

In May 2002, the final results of the Canadian Activase for Stroke Effectiveness Study (CASES) were published. A total of 1099 stroke patients who were treated with IV t-PA were enrolled between February 1999 and June 2001. The median baseline NIHSS was 15 (range 2 to 40). On follow-up evaluation at 90 days after the stroke, 30% of those patients had minimal or no residual neurologic deficit, and 46% were independent (m-RS 0 to 2). The ICH rate was 4.6%. Protocol violations occurred in 15%. Predictors of outcome were baseline NIHSS, baseline ASPECT score (evaluates the radiologic changes of stroke on brain CT), patient age, atrial fibrillation, and the patient's baseline serum sugar. Predictors of ICH were mean arterial blood pressure as well as baseline serum glucose. The CASES group concluded that IV Activase is safe and efficacious in Canada.[51]

The *Lyon* trial was a phase 2 trial of thrombolysis using a protocol that was very different from that of the NINDS study: The t-PA dose was 0.8 mg/kg, with 10% of the dose given as an IV bolus and the remaining 90% given as IV drip over 1 hour after that. The time window for t-PA administration was 7 hours after stroke, with the majority of patients receiving the t-PA within 3 to 6 hours. Heparin or LMW heparin was also given. The initial results of the first 100 patients were published in 1998[52]: At 90 days, 45% of the patients had good results (m-RS score 0 to 1), 18% had a moderate outcome (m-RS score 2 to 3), and 31% of patients had serious neurologic outcome (m-RS score 4 to 5). Of the 11 patients treated within 6 to 7 hours of stroke onset, 45% had good results. Death occurred in 6% of the patients, 2 of whom had intracerebral hematoma after having received intravenous heparin within the first 24 hours. The intracerebral hematoma rate was 7%. The results of the Lyon trial were updated in an abstract published in 2002.[53] The rate of good outcome (m-RS score ≤ 1) at 5 years was 37.4%. The mortality rate was 23.9%. Further later data analysis available to us, currently in press, evaluated a total of 200 patients in the Lyon trial.[54] The rate of good outcome (m-RS score 0 and 1) was 35% at 3 months. The rate of parenchymal anatomic hematoma within 7 days was 9%, and that of symptomatic hematomas, 5.5%. Mortality at 3 months occurred in 11.5%. Independent predictive factors of bad outcome appeared to be: structured hypodensity on day-1 CT, hyperdense MCS sign, internal carotid thrombosis, gray-white matter indistinction, no IV heparin within 24 hours or after 24 hours, use of low-molecular-weight heparin, and use of mannitol.

GUIDELINES FOR INTRAVENOUS THROMBOLYSIS IN ACUTE STROKE

Given the relationship between adverse events and protocol violations, it is important to understand the NINDS protocol for the use of t-PA in acute stroke. The study was originally intended to be a phase 2B confirmatory dose-finding and safety study, not a definitive phase 3 protocol, but because it proved efficacy, no further phase 3 trial was pursued. Therefore, the protocol contains some idiosyncrasies that were never intended to be included in the FDA package insert.

Treatment Protocol

Patients should present within the 3-hour window of stroke onset. Thrombolysis should not be implemented unless (1) the stroke diagnosis is established by a physician with expertise in stroke and (2) brain CT is assessed by a physician with expertise in reading this imaging study. A total dose of 0.9 mg/kg of recombinant t-PA is given, not to exceed a maximal dose of 90 mg. The first 10% of the dose is given as an IV bolus and the rest of the dose (90%) is given as an IV drip over the following hour. A list of inclusion and exclusion criteria is used to determine whether a patient should be given t-PA. These criteria were defined by the NINDS study (see Table 48–2) and were adopted nearly verbatim by the FDA even though they were not intended for clinical use.[55] At this time, it is important to follow these guidelines, but the physician's judgment is required in individual cases.

Patients are excluded for any of the exclusion criteria; we consider some of the more important criteria in the following discussion:

Use of Oral Anticoagulants, Prothrombin Time Longer than 15 Seconds, or International Normalized Ratio 1.7 or Greater. This criterion is obviously needed to exclude anticoagulated patients. In the original trial, any patient was excluded who had consumed any oral warfarin (Coumadin) in the previous day, no matter what the prothrombin time (PT) might be at the time of the stroke. The final package insert was written in such a way, however, as to allow thrombolysis even if the patient has taken warfarin recently; the criterion is only that the international normalized ratio (INR) be less than 1.7. The physician confronted with this situation must use judgment and must proceed thoughtfully, but generally, we recommend thrombolytic treatment if the INR is below the stated limit even if the patient has taken warfarin before the stroke occurred.

Use of Heparin in the Last 24 Hours with a Prolonged Partial Thromboplastin Time. This is an absolute contraindication, given the potential risk of hemorrhage. We are aware of anecdotal cases in which heparin was reversed with protamine and t-PA was given after the partial thromboplastin time (PTT) was recorded as normal. Because this approach has never been studied for safety, we cannot recommend it and do not use it routinely in our own practice. We are also aware of many cases in which reocclusion occurs after successful thrombolysis; preliminary data using serial transcranial ultrasonography has indicated that the reocclusion rate may be as high as 27%.[56] Certainly, after coronary thrombolysis, heparin is required to maintain vessel patency. We believe that further study on this point is warranted.

Platelet Count Less than 100,000 cells/mm³. The limit of 100,000 cells/mm³ for the platelet count is arbitrary and was chosen by the NINDS investigators on the basis of limited review of literature and consultation with hematologists. No one knows, however, how many functioning platelets are needed to protect a patient from hemorrhage during thrombolysis. The physician should exercise caution and judgment; in some situations, it may be wise to treat a patient with a platelet count below the limit.

Prior Stroke within the Last 3 Months. The time limit on prior stroke was set somewhat arbitrarily at 3 months, and no mention is made of severity. For example, does a minor motor lacune with signs lasting 3 days and resolving completely contraindicate thrombolytic therapy for 3 months? The physician must use considerable judgment in individual cases and consider the following questions:

How mild was the prior stroke?
Did it resolve completely, or partially?
How long ago was the prior stroke?
What is the potential for bleeding into the prior stroke if thrombolysis is used today?

There may be situations in which the benefit of treating the current stroke outweighs the risk due to recent, resolved minor stroke.

Head Trauma within the Last 3 Months. The considerations applying to this exclusion criterion are similar to those mentioned for prior stroke. The guidelines do not mention severity. The critical question is, how likely is the previous head trauma to predispose the patient to bleeding if thrombolysis is given now? The benefit of thrombolysis for the current event may outweigh the potential risks of bleeding after minor head trauma in the previous 3 months.

Major Surgery within the Last 14 Days. This contraindication is generally absolute, although we often consult with the surgeon who performed the surgery before making the decision. Often the devastation of the current stroke outweighs any harm that could be caused by rebleeding at the operative site. An individual exception to this exclusion rule could be considered in rare cases after careful consideration and discussion with the patient or family or both regarding the risks of hemorrhage.

Pretreatment Systolic Blood Pressure Greater than 185 mm Hg or Diastolic Blood Pressure Greater than 110 mm Hg. This exclusion criterion is absolute. If gentle antihypertensive therapy, such as 10 to 20 mg of IV labetalol, does not bring the blood pressure under the limits, no thrombolytic agents should be used. Hypertension at the time of thrombolysis has been shown to predict hemorrhagic transformation. On the other hand, the careful physician should be aware that most patients with stroke have an elevated blood pressure on arrival at the ED. The first blood pressure values obtained by paramedics or the triage nurse must not be used to exclude the patient from t-PA therapy. The patient should be allowed to acclimate to the ED for a few minutes; often, the blood pressure declines spontaneously. The patient who exhibits persistent hypertension despite the passage of time and gentle antihypertensive therapy should always be excluded from t-PA treatment.

Rapidly Improving Neurologic Signs. This exclusion criteria causes considerable discomfort for most physicians because stroke symptoms wax and wane over the first few hours. To qualify as rapidly improving, the symptoms must improve monotonically and dramatically. Patients whose deficits oscillate from severe to mild or who show only slight improvement should be treated. Generally, patients with TIA have complete resolution of symptoms within 1 or 2 hours. Patients who show only slight improvement over the first hour should be treated. The risk of ICH associated with thrombolytic treatment in a patient with TIA appears to be extremely low.[57]

Isolated Mild Neurologic Deficits. Patients with isolated mild neurologic deficits, such as isolated ataxia, isolated hemisensory loss, or isolated dysarthria, tend to recover completely with little residual effect. This criterion assumes a careful neurologic examination and a search for symptoms that could easily be overlooked, such as quadrantanopsia, hemispatial neglect, and mild expressive aphasia. The only patients who should be excluded from t-PA therapy are those with pure sensory or isolated ataxic symptoms. Also, individual judgment must be used; an isolated, mild expressive aphasia could end the career of a patient who speaks for a living. We routinely consider treating mild aphasia if the patient works in an occupation such as teaching, television broadcasting, or therapy. Likewise, an isolated hemianopsia could end some careers, such as truck or taxi driving, and treatment could be considered. Mild symptoms other than pure dysarthria or sensory deficit are associated with adverse outcomes. As mentioned earlier, of the patients studied by Barber and colleagues[48] whose deficits were considered mild or were rapidly improving, 32% were dependent at hospital discharge or died during hospital admission. Therefore, unless the symptoms are truly isolated to a purely sensory deficit or dysarthria, the patient should be treated.

Prior or Current Intracerebral Hemorrhage. This contraindication is absolute: If the patient has ever suffered an intracerebral hemorrhage, thrombolysis should not be used. Individual exceptions may be considered if the bleed was due to some nonrecurring condition, such as remote history of post-traumatic subdural hematoma that is proven to be resolved, but such circumstances must be exceedingly rare.

Blood Glucose Level Less than 50 mg/dL or Greater than 400 mg/dL. Hypoglycemia should be treated with glucose replacement; the deficit will most likely resolve, but if it does not, then thrombolysis could be considered. Hypoglycemia mimics stroke in 1.7% of cases.[58] On the other hand, incidental hypoglycemia could accompany a stroke and should not exclude the patient from therapy if the neurologic deficit persists despite blood glucose correction. Hyperglycemia is associated with increased hemorrhage risk and very low rates of successful outcome. Again, if insulin therapy brings the glucose value down to an acceptable level, it would theoretically be permissible to treat with t-PA. This approach has not been studied, however, and cannot be recommended in routine practice.

Seizure at the Onset of Stroke. The purpose of this exclusion is to ensure that patients with postictal paralysis are not mistaken as having stroke. In actual practice, some patients with stroke do suffer clonic jerks, which witnesses may report to paramedics or the physicians as seizures. Generally, postictal paralysis occurs in a patient with a known seizure disorder who has a typical tonic-clonic convulsion. Physicians must sort out from witnesses what actually occurred and whether the movements were tonic-clonic. There is probably little risk, however, in giving a thrombolytic to a patient with no stroke and postictal paralysis; one could argue for erring on the side of treatment, reasoning that failure to treat the patient with true ischemic stroke could result in much greater harm.

Gastrointestinal or Genitourinary Bleeding. Excluding patients with gastrointestinal (GI) or genitourinary (GU) bleeding from thrombolytic therapy is necessary because thrombolysis could activate bleeding from sources in the GI or GU tract. On the other hand, many patients consider blood loss inconsequential compared with the devastating effects of stroke. It is important to consider the nature of the bleeding, how recently it occurred, and how difficult it might be to control if it were to recur. Women with active menstruation and menometrorrhagia have been successfully and safely treated with t-PA for acute stroke, after consultation with the gynecologist, because an urgent uterine artery embolization or ligation could easily be performed to halt uncontrollable bleeding.[59] Giving such therapy to a patient with colonic polyposis or diverticulosis, however, could result in bleeding that would be far less easily controlled. Considerable physician judgment is required in this setting, and full discussion with the patient or family or both about the potential risks and benefits is essential.

Recent Myocardial Infarction. This is an absolute contraindication because of the possibility of pericardial rupture and tamponade. No specific time limit is specified, but "recent" is generally considered to be on the order of weeks. As with other exclusion criteria, one must consider the size of the myocardial infarct, the treatment given, and the current status of the patient in assessing the potential risk of cardiac rupture in a specific case.

Treatment Guidelines

Thrombolytic treatment should not be given unless ancillary care and the facility to handle bleeding complications are present, best provided in an intensive care unit setting. We are aware of many stroke units and "step-down" care units that are perfectly appropriate for monitoring patients

after thrombolysis. Vital signs and neurologic examinations (neuro-checks) are required to monitor the patient for blood loss (causing hypotension), hypertension above the post-treatment limits, neurologic deterioration (suggesting hemorrhage or reocclusion), and other complications of stroke.

Risks and benefits of thrombolytic treatment should be explained to the family, and consent should be obtained. Consent can be waived if the patient is not fit to give it and no family member is available. We recommend, however, that if any deviation from the protocol is contemplated, full consent from the family be obtained before it is initiated.

Early Computed Tomography Findings Are Not Contraindications to Treatment

In 1997, von Kummer and associates[60] analyzed the ECASS data and concluded that there could be an association between clinical severity of stroke and hemorrhagic infarction and that the risk of hemorrhagic infarction might be increased when early CT changes indicating hypoattenuation and mass effect are detected. It was clear that hemorrhage and death occurred more frequently in patients with early ischemic changes constituting more than one third of the MCA territory. They also concluded that rising age and treatment with t-PA were related to the risk of increased parenchymal hemorrhage. However, the analysis was post hoc and therefore should have served to generate hypotheses, not to guide patient care. Furthermore, the finding was not statistically significant, even in the first report. Unfortunately, the logical cautions expressed by these investigators in their report went unheeded, and the result has been widely applied as a common reason not to treat patients who would otherwise qualify.

In a retrospective analysis, the NINDS group looked at early ischemic changes (EICs) on baseline CT scans and tried to correlate them with outcome, CT lesion volume at 3 months, development of symptomatic ICH, and negative or positive interaction with t-PA treatment.[61] The EICs based on von Kummer's original report were (1) loss of distinction between gray matter and white matter, (2) hypodensity or hypoattenuation on baseline CT, or (3) compression of cerebrospinal fluid (CSF) spaces (sulcal effacement). The hyperdense MCA sign was not included. Overall, EICs were present in 35% of the patients given placebo and 28% of the patients given t-PA (similar in the two groups; $P = .09$). There was a strong association between stroke severity as measured by the NIHSS and the incidence of EICs; after correction for the NIHSS variable, however, there was no proven interaction between t-PA treatment and EIC. In other words, there was no higher risk associated with t-PA treatment when EICs were present on baseline CT. The patients given t-PA seemed to have a better outcome whether or not they had EICs. The findings are summarized in Figure 48–8. The investigators in this study concluded that the presence of EICs should not be critical in the decision for t-PA treatment if the patient otherwise meets eligibility criteria. They also commented that the analysis of the ECASS data and conclusions about EICs prohibiting treatment should have been established after correction for the variable of stroke severity. Gilligan and associates published similar results arising from the reanalysis of the Australian Streptokinase

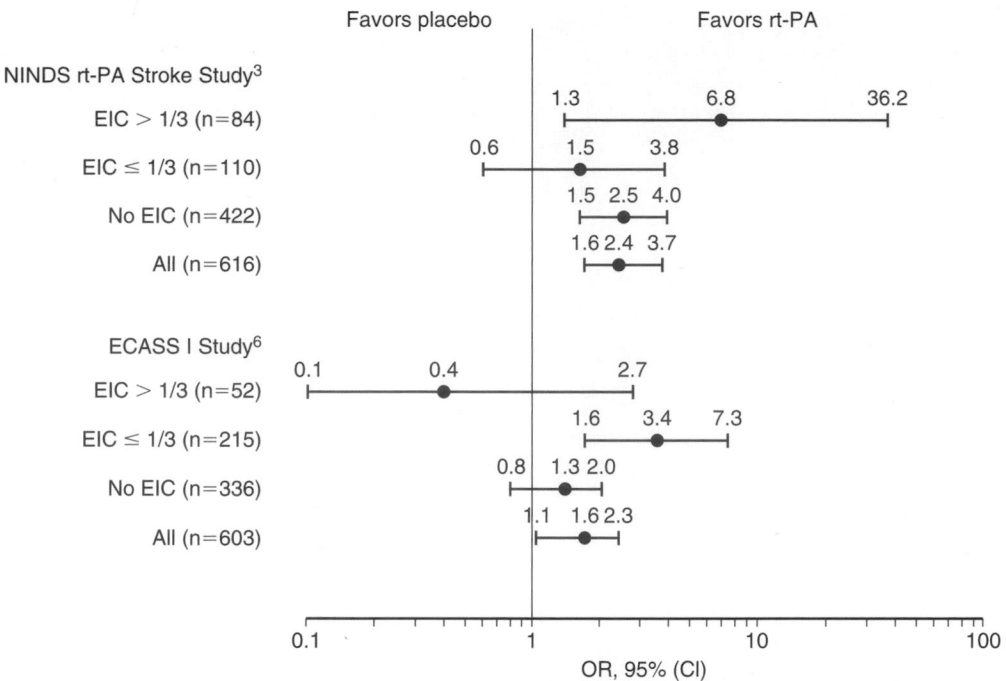

FIGURE 48–8 *Early ischemic changes (EIC) are not contraindications for t-PA treatment. The odds ratio from ECASS for patients with EIC of more than one third of the MCA vascular territory shows that there was no statistical difference in bad outcome between the t-PA and placebo groups in the presence of these early ischemic changes, but that there was benefit with t-PA treatment in the NINDS for acute stroke trial even in the presence of these early ischemic changes.[61] (From Patel S, Levine S, Tilley B, et al: Lack of clinical significance of early ischemic changes on computed tomography in acute stroke. JAMA 286:2830–2838, 2001.)*

trial in 2002.[62] The authors found that predictors of major hemorrhage were SK treatment and elevated systolic blood pressure prior to treatment (>165 mm Hg); however, EIC less than one third or more than one third of MCA territory was not associated with major hemorrhage.

In an attempt to reconcile the two positions and the contradiction between the analyses of the two studies (ECASS and NINDS), we may argue that the implication of more than one third of MCA territory-early CT changes might be different beyond 3 hours (ECASS) than they would be within 3 hours (NINDS). In the latter case, a substantial portion of the remaining two thirds of the MCA territory might be hypoperfused but still salvageable if lysis of the clot is successful, resulting in clinical benefit to offset the risk of bleeding. Beyond 3 hours, however, a smaller ischemic area might still be penumbral, with less of a hypothetical volumetric mismatch between the hypoperfused area and the irreversibly injured area.

It appears, therefore, that the CT findings should be used with caution in selecting patients for thrombolytic therapy. Certainly a hemorrhage contraindicates therapy. Areas of marked hypodensity, suggesting that the stroke is more than 3 hours old, should give the physician pause. Mild EIC such as sulcal effacement, loss of gray-white matter distinction, or loss of the so-called insular ribbon sign, no matter how large a portion of the MCA territory is involved, should not necessarily contraindicate therapy if the patient otherwise qualifies for treatment. Presence of the so-called hyperdense MCA sign, or hyperdense dot sign,[63] should not be regarded as a contraindication to therapy either, although the prospects for a good outcome are very low in this setting, regardless of the type of treat-

ment. Figure 48–9 demonstrates the CT of a 40-year-old man with the different CT signs mentioned and EICs at baseline and 24 hours after thrombolysis.

Considerable research is ongoing to find imaging parameters that may guide selection of treatment. It is probably true that strict adherence to the 3-hour time limit deprives many patients who could have remaining salvageable brain of useful treatment. Similarly, it is clear that many patients do not have salvageable brain even earlier than 3 hours after stroke onset. We need a truly reliable, rapid, and widely available imaging method that will indicate when brain becomes irretrievably damaged. Many techniques, such as diffusion and perfusion techniques of magnetic resonance imaging (MRI), have been proposed and are under intense evaluation. To date, however, no imaging modality has proved better for selection of patients for particular therapies than existing published clinical criteria.

Effect of Time to Thrombolytic Treatment

Thrombolytic therapy should be administered within 3 hours from time of onset, as discussed before, but a 2000 analysis of the NINDS study data showed that the benefit of treatment was higher when t-PA was given earlier in this time window. This analysis showed that patients treated within 90 minutes of stroke onset had greater odds of improvement at 24 hours and a higher favorable 3-month outcome than patients treated between 91 and 180 minutes after onset. The time of treatment within 3 hours had no effect on the ICH rate.[64] Therefore, the earliest possible treatment is recommended not for fear of ICH but of decreased benefit with later treatment. Figure

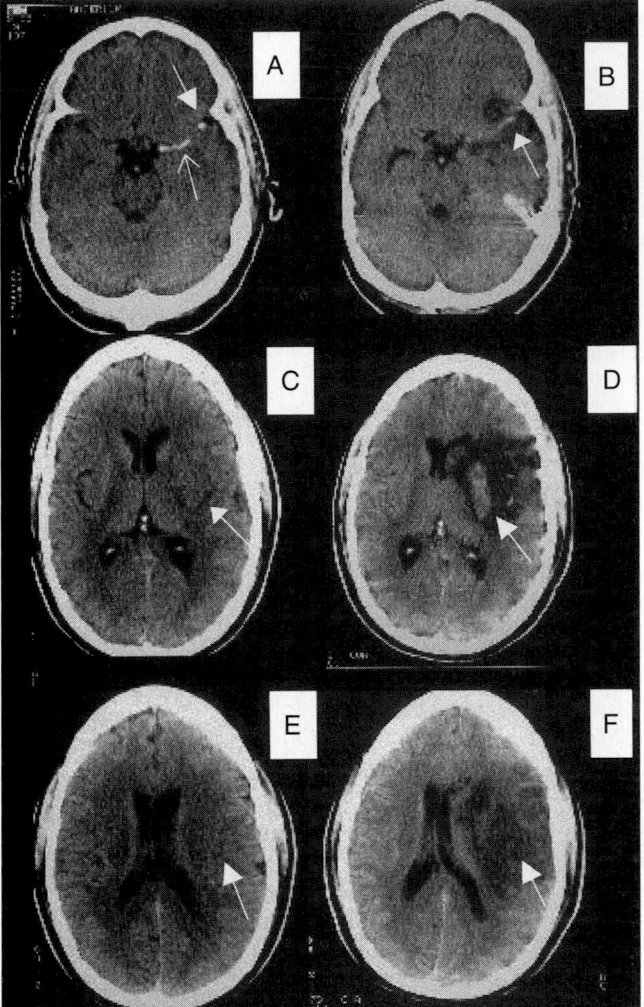

FIGURE 48–9 *Early ischemic changes (EIC) on CT are not contraindications for thrombolysis. This is the brain CT of a 40-year-old man with acute left hemispheric stroke on presentation (A, C, and E) and 48 hours post thrombolysis (B, D, and F). A, A linear hyperdense MCA sign (open head white arrow) and a hyperdense dot MCA sign (closed head white arrow), on presentation. B, The hyperdense MCA sign 48 hours later. C, Portrays loss of the left insular ribbon as one of the early ischemic changes. D, Portrays an island of relative hyperdensity within the stroke bed that might be either hemorrhagic transformation or an island of spared non-ischemic brain tissue within the ischemic bed at 24 hours post thrombolysis. E, Portrays ischemic related hypodense changes in the MCA territory on presentation. F, Portrays progression of the hypodense ischemic changes at 48 hours.*

48–10 shows that as the time to treatment approaches 3 hours, the odds ratio for a favorable outcome approaches 1 (the benefit of t-PA is greater than that of placebo if the odds ratio is greater than 1, as depicted in the graph).[64]

Generalized Efficacy of t-Pa for Acute Stroke

A post hoc analysis of the NINDS data was conducted to try to establish whether any factors might have had negative interactions with t-PA treatment or, in other words, to identify any pretreatment patient information that significantly affected the patient's response to t-PA treatment. The investigators included 27 baseline variables to check for possible interaction with t-PA treatment. These variables were age, race, sex, cigarette smoking, alcohol abuse, diabetes mellitus, hypertension, baseline NIHSS, percentage of correct t-PA dose received, history of atherosclerosis, history of atrial fibrillation, history of other cardiac disease, prior stroke, aspirin, baseline stroke subtype, early CT findings, presence or absence of thrombus, weight, percentage of correct dose, admission and baseline mean arterial blood pressure, admission and baseline systolic as well as admission and baseline diastolic blood pressure, centers of treatment, time from stroke onset to treatment, and admission temperature. This analysis also tested interactions among these factors and among confounding variables. Independent of t-PA therapy, outcome was related to age by deficit or age by NIHSS score, diabetes, age by blood pressure interaction, and early CT findings. These factors and their interactions altered the patient's long-term outcome but did not alter the likelihood of favorable response to t-PA treatment; the efficacy of t-PA as shown by the NINDS data were generalized to all subgroups. The investigators concluded that treatment for patients with acute stroke should be selected according to the NINDS guidelines and that further subselection is not supported.[65]

Recanalization and Arterial Reocclusion after t-Pa Treatment

Early studies by del Zoppo and colleagues[21] and Mori and associates,[24] as described earlier, showed that IV t-PA could recanalize the cerebral vessels on angiograms. Further data have been published to support their conclusions. In 2002, Alexandrov and coworkers[66] published the results of a series of 60 consecutively treated patients with occlusion of the M1 or M2 segment of the MCA who received t-PA (bolus followed by IV infusion) and were monitored by transcranial Doppler ultrasonography for 2 hours after t-PA treatment. Median pre-bolus NIHSS score was 16, and the median time to administration of the bolus was 120 minutes with 58% of patients receiving the t-PA within the first 2 hours. Recanalization was complete in 30% (18 patients), partial in 48% (29 patients), and null in 22% (13 patients). Early reocclusion occurred in 34% of patients given t-PA who experienced any initial recanalization, accounting for two thirds of deteriorations after improvement. Note that reocclusion occurred more often in patients with earlier and partial recanalization, with secondary neurologic deterioration and higher in-hospital mortality. Nevertheless, patients with reocclusion had better long-term outcomes than patients without any early recanalization.[66]

Management During and after Thrombolytic Treatment[55]

As mentioned before, the patient should be admitted to a skilled care unit, such as an intensive care unit or a stroke-care unit, that provides close observation, careful cardiovascular monitoring, and frequent neurologic evaluations. Blood pressure should be monitored and controlled care-

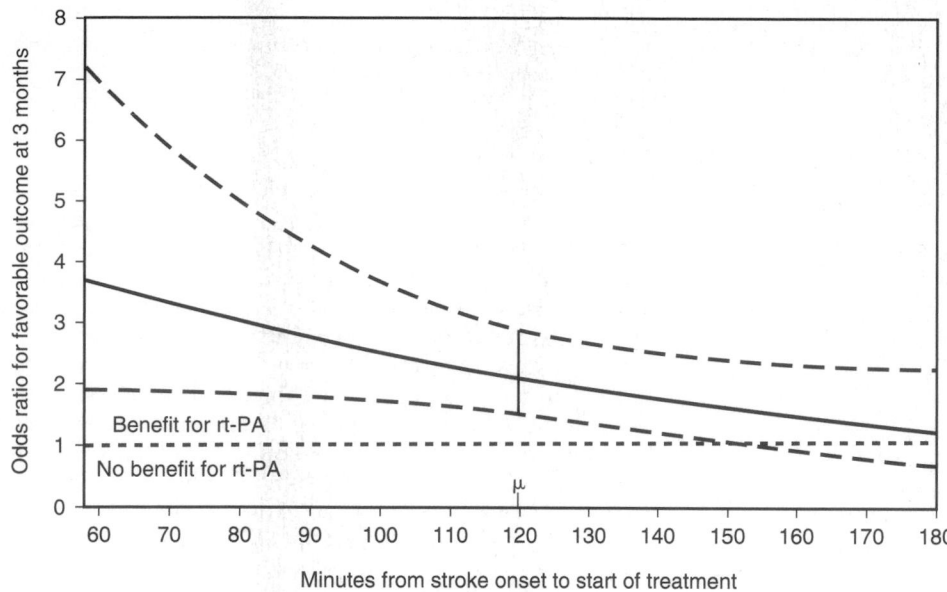

FIGURE 48–10 *Time to treatment effect: this figure shows that t-PA benefit disappears as the time from onset to t-PA treatment approaches 3 hours.*[61] *(From Marler J, Tilley B, Lu M, et al: Early stroke treatment associated with better outcome: The NINDS rt-PA Stroke Study. Neurology 55:1649–1655, 2000.)*

fully during the treatment and the following 24 hours. An excessively high blood pressure might predispose the patient to bleed intracranially, whereas low blood pressure might worsen cerebral ischemia. According to American Heart Association recommendations, blood pressure should be monitored every 15 minutes for 2 hours from the start of t-PA infusion, then every 30 minutes for 6 hours, then every 60 minutes over the rest of the 24 hours after initiation of t-PA treatment.[55]

The protocol for blood pressure treatment after thrombolysis is listed in Table 48.4. Recommended drugs listed in the table were selected because of their rapid onset of action and their predictable effects with low potential for overshoot.[67] Note that in the NINDS study, both of these medications were used, in addition to other medications such as IV nicardipine, hydralazine, sublingual nifedipine, and sustained-release or topical nitroglycerin.[68] Furthermore, although abrupt substantial declines in mean arterial pressure (MAP) have been shown to reduce cerebral flow, the threshold below which it is unsafe to lower MAP is unknown. The blood pressure eligibility criteria that were applied are similar to those used in the t-PA dose-finding trial. The blood pressure management algorithm was used because of the low incidence of symptomatic hemorrhage in the pilot study and recognition of the potential link between high blood pressure and ICH.[22,23]

Post hoc analyses of data from the NINDS study have shown that post-randomization but not pre-randomization blood pressure treatment was associated with a less favorable 3-month outcome in the t-PA group. However, because of the nonrandomized use of antihypertensive therapy, and the many post hoc comparisons leading to statistical errors, the significance of this observation was unclear, and the importance of controlling blood pressure after thrombolysis still holds because of the possible association of ICH with high blood pressure.[68]

Central lines and arterial puncture should be restricted in the first 24 hours after thrombolytic treatment. However, the physician should be aware that the serum

Table 48.4 Emergency Management of Arterial Hypertension for Patients Receiving Thrombolytic Treatment for Acute Ischemic Stroke: Method Used by the NINDS Study Group

Monitor arterial blood pressure during the first 24 hours after starting treatment.
- Every 15 minutes for 2 hours after starting the infusion, then
- Every 30 minutes for 6 hours, then
- Every 60 minutes until 24 hours after starting treatment.

If systolic blood pressure is 180–230 mm Hg or if diastolic blood pressure is 105–120 mm Hg for two or more readings 5–10 minutes apart:
- Give intravenous labetalol 10 mg over 1–2 minutes. The dose may be repeated or doubled every 10–20 minutes up to a total dose of 150 mg.
- Monitor blood pressure every 15 minutes during labetalol treatment and observe for development of hypotension.

If systolic blood pressure is >230 mm Hg or if diastolic blood pressure is in the range of 121–140 mm Hg for two or more readings 5–10 minutes apart:
- Give intravenous labetalol 10 mg over 1–2 minutes. The dose may be repeated or doubled every 10 minutes up to a total dose of 150 mg.
- Monitor blood pressure every 15 minutes during labetalol treatment and observe for development of hypotension.
- If no satisfactory response, infuse sodium nitroprusside (0.5–10 µg/kg per minute).°
- Continue monitoring blood pressure.

If diastolic blood pressure is >140 mm Hg for two or more readings 5–10 minutes apart:
- Infuse sodium nitroprusside (0.5–10 µg/kg per minute).°
- Monitor blood pressure every 15 minutes during infusion of sodium nitroprusside and observe for development of hypotension.

From Adams HP Jr, Brott TG, Furlan AJ, et al: Guidelines for Thrombolytic Therapy for Acute Stroke: A supplement to the guidelines for the management of patients with acute ischemic stroke. Circulation 94:1167–1174, 1996.

Therapy

half-life of t-PA is very short, and after 20 minutes, there is very little systemic thrombolytic activity. Therefore, if clinical circumstances require a central line or triple-lumen catheter for monitoring of cardiopulmonary pressures, such a line could be safely established an hour or more after thrombolysis was complete. Urinary tract instrumentation (placement of a Foley catheter) should be avoided during infusion of t-PA and at least 30 minutes after the infusion ends. Placement of a nasogastric tube should be avoided during the first 24 hours after initiation of treatment; as with central lines and arterial puncture, we routinely insert this catheter earlier if required by patient circumstances.[55]

For 36 hours after thrombolysis, hemorrhagic complications of t-PA are the major worry; these can be intracranial or extracranial hemorrhages. If bleeding is suspected, then a blood specimen is collected for measurement of hemoglobin level, hematocrit, partial thromboplastin time (PTT), prothrombin time (PT), international normalized ratio (INR), platelet count, and fibrinogen level. Blood should be typed and cross-matched when the need for transfusion arises. Arterial or venous sites should be compressed if they are the bleeding source.

If a major life-threatening bleed occurs, including ICH, gastrointestinal bleeding, and retroperitoneal bleed, thrombolytic treatment should be stopped if it is still going. Urgent CT of the brain should be obtained for suspected ICH.[55] Neurosurgical consultation for possible surgical intervention should also be obtained. Surgery should not be performed, however, unless the fibrinolytic state is corrected; such a correction usually requires both cryoprecipitate and fresh frozen plasma to overcome clotting factor deficiencies induced by the t-PA.

For major extracranial hemorrhages, the appropriate emergency imaging techniques should be performed, along with surgical consultations and interventions when appropriate. For 24 hours after IV t-PA treatment, patients should not receive aspirin, heparin, warfarin, or other antithrombotic or antiplatelet drugs.[55] As mentioned elsewhere, however, reocclusion may be a considerable problem after thrombolysis, and we are concerned that further studies of post-thrombolytic anticoagulation are lacking.

Predictors of Good Outcome with Thrombolytic Treatment

In a 2001 article, Demchuck and associates[69] analyzed data collected from 1205 patients treated in different centers in Germany, the United States, and Canada with IV t-PA as per NINDS protocol. Good outcome was defined as m-RS score 0 to 1, and poor outcome as m-RS score greater than 1. The independent predictors of good outcome in patients treated with IV t-PA, in relative order of decreasing magnitude, were milder baseline stroke severity, no history of diabetes mellitus, normal CT scan, normal pretreatment blood glucose, and normal pretreatment blood pressure. Confounding was observed among the variables: history of diabetes, CT scan appearance, baseline serum glucose level, and blood pressure (baseline mean arterial pressure), suggesting important relationships among these variables. Symptomatic ICH was associated with poor outcome. The

known risk factors for poor outcome in untreated patients, such as age and stroke mechanism, were not associated with outcome in this cohort study.

Risks of Thrombolysis

Plasminogen activators raise the risk of ICH by altering the framework of the platelet plug and by changing vascular permeability as well as the integrity of the vascular basal lamina at the site of injury; the latter two effects contribute to dissolution of the blood-brain barrier. Therefore, there is an increased risk of brain edema and ICH.[2] As mentioned before, subgroup analysis of the NINDS data showed that the only variables that were independently associated with increased risk of symptomatic ICH were baseline stroke severity as measured by NIHSS, the amount of edema defined by acute hypodensity, and mass effect on CT before treatment (baseline CT).[70] Table 48.3 summarizes the rates of ICH with t-PA in the various clinical studies.

Reperfusion injury is another hypothetical risk. It has been shown that reperfusion is associated with a secondary wave of glutamate and other neurotransmitter release, which result in calcium influx and excitotoxicity. Restoration of blood flow might allow synthesis of damaging proteins and other cytokines as well as supply oxygen to ischemic areas, providing a substrate for peroxidation of lipids and formation of free radicals. Moreover, thrombolysis might allow the clot to break and cause secondary embolization to a distal vascular distribution.[2]

Cost-Effectiveness of Thrombolysis

The cost-effectiveness of t-PA was demonstrated in 1998, in a study that used certain assumptions about stroke costs and outcomes based on data from the literature and from the NINDS study. Even though it shortened the stay at the hospital, t-PA therapy increased the hospital cost by $15,000 per patient for each additional patient who was discharged home rather than to a nursing home or inpatient rehabilitation center. On the other hand, t-PA reduced the costs of nursing home care and rehabilitation. The overall effect on both acute and long-term care costs (90% certainty) to the health care system is a net decrease of more than $4,000,000 for every 1000 patients treated.[71]

COMBINATION TREATMENT

Combining thrombolysis with other treatment regimens has not proved to be beneficial so far in clinical studies. Previous studies have combined anticoagulants with fibrinolysis. In the MAST-E study,[34] 65% of the patients who received streptokinase and 75% of the placebo group received heparin as well. There was no evidence of statistically significant benefit, and the study was terminated early because of increased ICH in the streptokinase group. It is recommended that no anticoagulants be given within 24 hours of t-PA treatment. Previous studies have shown that streptokinase with antiplatelet treatment (aspirin) is associated with a higher risk of ICH compared with streptokinase only or aspirin only (MAST-I).[35] Clinical studies have not tested t-PA in combination with aspirin. Experimental models, however, have shown that t-PA with heparin is safe and did not increase the rate of ICH.[17] A small group of patients (n = 30) received a combination of t-PA and heparin in a feasibility study described by von Kummer and associates[72]; these researchers concluded that when the combination treatment was given within 6 hours of stroke onset, the incidence of fatal ICH occurred in 9% of patients, whereas asymptomatic hemorrhagic infarction occurred in 28%. Reperfusion occurred in 34% of patients 90 minutes after initiation of thrombolysis and in 53% within 12 to 24 hours of thrombolysis initiation. Good clinical outcome correlated with reperfusion ($P < .05$). Future randomized controlled studies are needed to determine whether this or other anti-thrombotic strategies combined with IV t-PA are better than thrombolysis alone, weighing the benefit and risks involved.

Neuroprotective agents in combination with thrombolysis have been tested in experimental models and in clinical studies. Animal studies showed benefit in animals receiving neuroprotective agents within a short time window after the cerebrovascular occlusion. In 1991, Zivin and colleagues[73] used MK-801, a glutamate antagonist, followed by thrombolysis with t-PA and proved that such a combination was more effective than t-PA alone in reducing neurologic damage after stroke. MK-801 had no effect when used alone in the same stroke model. In 1999, Zhang and coworkers[74] showed that combining anti-CD18 antibodies, which prevent adhesion of white blood cells to the endothelium, with thrombolysis prolonged the effective time window of thrombolysis from 2 hours to 4 hours. Anti-CD18 antibodies alone had no effect. Neuroprotective agents can reduce the side effects of thrombolysis because they enhance the integrity of the vascular endothelium and protect the ischemic brain tissue from the hypothetical reperfusion injury discussed earlier. These results were not mirrored in clinical studies, most probably because these agents were given at a prolonged time from onset of stroke.

Several clinical studies combined thrombolysis with neuroprotective agents. However, the two latest studies have failed to show benefit. In October 2001, Grotta[75] published the results of a study in which patients received IV t-PA alone or t-PA plus the neuroprotective agent lubeluzole. This agent works via inhibition of the glutamate activated nitrous oxide (NO) pathway. Eighty-nine patients were randomly assigned for various treatments, but the study was terminated prematurely because another larger study using lubeluzole alone showed no benefit for such monotherapy. Note that lubeluzole was given before the end of the 1-hour t-PA drip (less than 4 hours from onset). There was no difference between the two treatment groups in the primary outcome measures: BI, mortality, ICH, and serious adverse events. This study showed that such a combination treatment is safe and feasible.

In October 2001, Lyden and coworkers[76] reported the results of a randomized study in which t-PA was given within 3 hours of stroke onset with or without clomethiazole administered within 12 hours of stroke onset. There was no significant difference between the two groups in the primary endpoints, serious adverse events and mortality at 3 months. This trial proved that such a combination was feasible and safe. There was no benefit in outcome as

measured by BI, m-RS, and NIHSS, with the combination treatment as compared to the t-PA group alone. However, there was benefit from the combination treatment in patients with total anterior circulation strokes (TACS), as well as decreased ICH on CT at 24 hours, even though the clomethiazole plus t-PA group had a higher frequency of edema and early ischemic changes on baseline CT. Future studies combining neuroprotective agents with thrombolysis should be pursued, keeping in mind that the neuroprotective agent should be administered earlier, and maybe earlier than the thrombolytic treatment, in light of animal models that show benefit only with very early administration of neuroprotective agents.

Hypothermia in combination with thrombolysis is under investigation. Future studies will evaluate whether hypothermia might prolong the time window of thrombolysis, so that benefit might be achieved from t-PA given in combination with induced hypothermia even later than 3 hours of stroke onset.

Intra-arterial thrombolysis in combination with IV thrombolysis is discussed in Chapter 49.

CONCLUSION

Thrombolysis using IV t-PA is safe and improves the outcome of patients with stroke despite a higher risk of ICH (but no increased mortality). The emphasis should be on (1) treating the patient as early as possible, but certainly within 3 hours of stroke onset; (2) excluding ICH on CT before treatment; and (3) controlling hypertension before and after treatment. A specialized unit setting is ideal for monitoring the patient. Treatment with anticoagulants and antiplatelet agents are forbidden within the first 24 hours after thrombolysis, according to the NINDS protocol. Newer-generation thrombolytic agents are currently under study for acute stroke treatment. Because they are more clot-selective, researchers hope to be able to increase the dose and rate of lysis with a lower risk for bleeding. It is hoped that future clinical studies using combination treatments of IV thrombolysis with intra-arterial lytics or mechanical clot disruption, anti-thrombotic therapy, or neuroprotective agents within a short time window might build on the positive results so far obtained with t-PA.

References

1. Tissue plasminogen activator for acute ischemic stroke: NINDS rt-PA Stroke Study Group. N Engl J Med 333:1581–1587, 1995.
2. Lyden PD: Thrombolytic Therapy for Stroke. Totowa, NJ, Humana Press, 2001.
3. Douglas S: Coagulation history. Br J Haematol 107:22–32, 1999.
4. Collen D: Fibrin-selective thrombolytic therapy for acute myocardial infarction. Circulation 93:857–865, 1996.
5. Cannon CP: Comparison of front-loaded recombinant tissue-type plasminogen activator, anistreplase and combination thrombolytic therapy for acute myocardial infarction: Results of the Thrombolysis in Myocardial Infarction (TIMI) 4 trial. J Am Coll Cardiol 24:1602–1610, 1994.
6. Cairns J, Fuster V, Gore J, Kennedy JW: Coronary thrombolysis. Cardiopulmon Crit Care J 108:401S–423S, 1995.
7. Verstraete M: Third generation thrombolytic drugs. Am J Med 109:52–58, 2000.
8. Benedict CR, Refino CJ, et al: New variant of human tissue plasminogen activator (tPA) with enhanced efficacy and a lower incidence

of bleeding compared with recombinant human tPA. Circulation 92:3032–3040, 1995.

9. Van de Werf F, Cannon C, Luyten A, et al: Safety assessment of single-bolus administration of TNK tissue-plasminogen activator in acute myocardial infarction: The ASSENT-1 trial. Am Heart J 137:786–791, 2000.

10. Van de Werf F, Barron HV, Armstrong P, et al: Incidence and predictors of bleeding events after fibrinolytic therapy with fibrin-specific agents. Eur Heart J 22:2253–2261, 2001.

10a. The TNK for Stroke Investigators: Pilot study in tenecteplase (TNK) in acute ischemic stroke: Preliminary report [Abstract]. Stroke 34:246, 2003.

11. Meyer JS, Gilroy J, Barnhart ME, et al: Therapeutic thrombolysis in cerebral thromboembolism. In Siekert W, Whisnant JGS (eds): Cerebral Vascular Diseases. Philadelphia, Grune & Stratton, 1963, pp 160–175.

12. del Zoppo G, Copeland BR, Waltz TA, et al: The beneficial effect of intracarotid urokinase on acute stroke in a baboon model. Stroke 17:638–643, 1986.

13. Zivin JA, Fisher M, DeGirolami U, et al: Tissue plasminogen activator reduces neurological damage after cerebral embolism. Science 230:1289–1292, 1985.

14. del Zoppo G, Copeland BR, Harker LA, et al: Experimental acute thrombotic stroke in baboons. Stroke 17:1254–1265, 1986.

15. Slivka A, Pulsinelli WA: Hemorrhagic complications of thrombolytic therapy in experimental stroke. Stroke 18:1148–1156, 1987.

16. Lyden PD, Zivin JA, Clark WA, et al: Tissue plasminogen activator mediated thrombolysis of cerebral emboli and its effect on hemorrhagic infarction in rabbits. Neurology 39:703–708, 1989.

17. Clark WM, Madden KP, Lyden PD, Zivin JA: Cerebral hemorrhagic risk of aspirin or heparin therapy with thrombolytic treatment in rabbits. Stroke 22:872–876, 1991.

18. Lyden PD, Madden KP, Clark WA, et al: Comparison of cerebral hemorrhage rates following tissue plasminogen activator or streptokinase treatment for embolic stroke in rabbits. Stroke 21:981–983, 1990.

19. Meyer JS, Gilroy J, Barnhart ME, Johnson JF: Therapeutic thrombolysis in cerebral thromboembolism: Randomized evaluation of intravenous streptokinase. In Millikan CH, Siekert RG, Whisnant JP (eds): Cerebral Vascular Diseases, Fourth Princeton Conference. New York, Grune & Stratton, 1965, pp 200–213.

20. Fletcher AP, Alkjaersig N, Lewis M, et al: A pilot study of urokinase therapy in cerebral infarction. Stroke 7:135–142, 1976.

21. del Zoppo G, Poeck K, Pessin MS, et al: Recombinant tissue plasminogen activator in acute thrombotic and embolic stroke. Ann Neurol 32:78–86, 1992.

22. Brott TG, Haley EC Jr, Levy DE, et al: Urgent therapy for stroke. Part I: Pilot study of tissue plasminogen activator administered within 90 minutes. Stroke 23:632–640, 1992.

23. Haley EC Jr, Levy DE, Brott TG, et al: Urgent therapy for stroke. Part II: Pilot study of tissue plasminogen activator administered 91–180 minutes from onset. Stroke 23:641–645, 1992.

24. Mori E, Yoneda Y, Tabuchi M, et al: Intravenous recombinant tissue plasminogen activator in acute carotid artery territory stroke. Neurology 42:976–982, 1992.

25. Haley EC, Brott TG, Sheppard GL, et al: Pilot randomized trial of tissue plasminogen activator in acute ischemic stroke. Stroke 24:1000–1004, 1993.

26. Hacke W, Kaste M, Fieschi C, et al: Intravenous thrombolysis with recombinant tissue plasminogen activator for acute hemispheric stroke: the European Cooperative Acute Stroke Study (ECASS). JAMA 274:1017–1025, 1995.

27. Hacke W, Bluhmki E, Steiner T, et al: Dichotomized efficacy end points and global end-point analysis applied to the ECASS intention-to-treat data set. Stroke 29:2073–2075, 1998.

28. Steiner T, Bluhmki E, Kaste M, et al: The ECASS 3-hour cohort. Cerebrovasc Dis 8:198–203, 1998.

29. Haley EC Jr, Lewandowski C, Tilley BC, et al: Myths regarding the NINDS rt-PA stroke trial: Setting the record straight. NINDS rt-PA Stroke Study Group. Ann Emerg Med 30:676–682, 1997.

30. Intracerebral hemorrhage after intravenous t-PA therapy for ischemic stroke. NINDS rt-PA Stroke Study Group. Stroke 28:2109–2118, 1997.

31. Kwiatkowski TG, Libman R, Frankel M, et al: Effects of tissue plasminogen activator for acute ischemic stroke at one year. N Engl J Med 340:1781–1787, 1999.

32. Broderick JP, Lu M, Kothari R, et al: Finding the most powerful measures of the effectiveness of tissue plasminogen activator in the NINDS tPA stroke trial. Stroke 31:2335–2341, 2000.

33. Hacke W, Kaste M, Fieschi C, et al: Randomised double-blind placebo-controlled trial of thrombolytic therapy with intravenous alteplase in acute ischaemic stroke (ECASS II). Lancet 352:1245–1251, 1998.

34. Multicenter Acute Stroke Trial—Europe Study Group (MAST-E): Thrombolytic therapy with streptokinase in acute ischemic stroke. N Engl J Med 335:145–150, 1996.

35. Randomised controlled trial of streptokinase, aspirin, and combination of both in treatment of acute ischaemic stroke. Multicentre Acute Stroke Trial-Italy (MAST-I) Group. Lancet 346:1509–1514, 1995.

36. Donnan GA, Davis SM, Chambers BR, et al: Streptokinase for acute ischemic stroke with relationship to time of administration: Australian Streptokinase (ASK) Trial Study Group. JAMA 276:961–966, 1996.

37. Donnan GA, Davis SM, Chambers BR, et al: ASK Trial: Unfavourable outcome if treated more than three hours after onset [abstract]. Cerebrovasc Dis 5:225–273, 1995.

38. Cornu C, Boutitie F, Candelise L, et al: Streptokinase in acute ischemic stroke: An individual patient data meta-analysis: The Thrombolysis in Acute Stroke Pooling Project. Stroke 31:1555–1560, 2000.

39. Clark WM, Albers GW, for the Atlantis Stroke Study Investigators: The ATLANTIS rt-PA (alteplase) acute stroke trial: Final results. 24th American Heart Association International Conference on Stroke and Cerebral Circulation; oral presentation [Abstract]. Stroke 30:234, 1999.

40. Clark W, Wissman S, Albers GW, et al: Recombinant tissue-type plasminogen activator (alteplase) for ischemic stroke 3 to 5 hours after symptom onset. JAMA 282:2019–2024, 1999.

41. Albers GW, Clark W, Madden K, Hamilton S: ATLANTIS Trial: Results for patients treated within 3 hours of stroke onset. Stroke 33:493–496, 2002.

42. Chiu D, Krieger D, Villar-Cordova C, et al: Intravenous tissue plasminogen activator for acute ischemic stroke feasibility, safety, and efficacy in the first year of clinical practice. Stroke 29:18–22, 1998.

43. Grond M, Stenzel C, Schmulling S, et al: Early intravenous thrombolysis for acute ischemic stroke in a community based approach. Stroke 29:1544–1549, 1998.

44. Egan R, Lutsep HL, Clark WM, et al: Open label tissue plasminogen activator for stroke: The Oregon experience. J Stroke Cerebrovasc Dis 8:287–290, 1999.

45. Katzan I, Furlan A, Lloyd L, et al: Use of tissue-type plasminogen activator for acute ischemic stroke: The Cleveland area experience. JAMA 283:1151–1158, 2000.

45a. Katzen IMM, Hammer MDM, Furlan AJM: Quality improvement and tissue-type plasminogen activator for acute stroke. A Cleveland update. Stroke 34:799–800, 2003.

46. Albers GW, Bates V, Clark W, et al: Intravenous tissue-type plasminogen activator for treatment of acute stroke: The Standard Treatment with Alteplase to Reverse Stroke (STARS) study. JAMA 283:1145–1150, 2000.

47. Chapman KM, Woolfenden AR, Graeb D, et al: Intravenous tissue plasminogen activator for acute ischemic stroke. Stroke 31:2920–2924, 2000.

48. Barber PA, Zhang J, Demchuk A, et al: Why are stroke patients excluded from TPA therapy? Neurology 56:1015–1020, 2001.

49. Koennecke HC, Nohr R, Leistner S, Marx P: Intravenous tPA for ischemic stroke team: Performance over time, safety and efficacy in a single center-2-year experience. Stroke 32:1074–1078, 2001.

50. Grotta J, Burgin WS, El-Mitwalli A, et al: Intravenous tissue-type plasminogen activator therapy for ischemic stroke. Arch Neurol 58:2009–2013, 2001.

51. Hill MD, Buchan AM: Canadian Activase for Stroke Effectiveness Study (CASES). Can J Neurol Sci 28:232–238, 2001.

52. Trouillas P, Nighoghossian N, Derex L, et al: Thrombolysis with intravenous rtPA in a series of 100 cases of acute carotid territory stroke. Determination of etiological, topographic, and radiological outcome factors. Stroke 29:2529–2540, 1998.

53. Trouillas P, Nighoghossian N, Derex L, Honnorat J: Prognosis at 5 years of acute cerebral infarcts of the carotid territory treated by intravenous rtPA: Data from the Lyon thrombolysis registry. Stroke 33:395, 2002.

54. Trouillas P, Nighoghossian N, Derex L, et al: Final results of the Lyon rtPA within 7 hours without radiological and clinical exclusions in carotid territory acute cerebral infarcts [Letter].

55. Adams HP Jr, Brott TG, Furlan AJ, et al: Guidelines for thrombolytic therapy for acute stroke: A supplement to the guidelines for the management of patients with acute ischemic stroke. Circulation 94:1167–1174, 1996.

56. Grotta J, Alexandrov AV: Early arterial re-occlusion in patients treated with 0.9 mg/kg IV TPA [abstract]. Stroke 33:354–354, 2002.

57. Lyden P, Lu M, Kwiatkowski TG, et al: Thrombolysis in patients with transient neurologic deficits. Neurology 57:2125–2128, 2001.

58. Hemmen TM, Meyer BC, Hayes KA, et al: Identification of "stroke mimics" among 411 code strokes at the UCSD Stroke Center from September 1998 to March 2001 [Abstract]. Stroke 33:385, 2002.

59. Wein TH, Hickenbottom SL, Morgenstern B, et al: Safety of tissue plasminogen activator for acute stroke in menstruating women. Stroke 33:2506–2508, 2002.

60. von Kummer R, Allen KL, Holle R, et al: Acute stroke: Usefulness of early CT findings before thrombolytic therapy. Radiology 205:327–333, 1997.

61. Patel S, Levine S, Tilley B, et al: Lack of clinical significance of early ischemic changes on computed tomography in acute stroke. JAMA 286:2830–2838, 2001.

62. Gilligan A, Markus R, Read S, et al: Baseline blood pressure but not early computed tomography changes predicts major hemorrhage after streptokinase in acute ischemic stroke. Stroke 33:2236–2242, 2002.

63. Barber P, Demchuk A, Hudon ME, et al: Hyperdense sylvian fissure MCA "dot" sign. Stroke 32:84–88, 2001.

64. Marler JR, Tilley BC, Lu M, et al: Early stroke treatment associated with better outcome: The NINDS rt-PA stroke study. Neurology 55:1649–1655, 2000.

65. Generalized efficacy of t-PA for acute stroke. NINDS rt-PA Stroke Study Group. Stroke 28:2119–2125, 1997.

66. Alexandrov AV, Grotta JC: Arterial reocclusion in stroke patients treated with intravenous tissue plasminogen activator. Neurology 59:862–867, 2002.

67. Brott TG, Reed RL: Antihypertensive therapy in stroke: Medical therapy of acute stroke. 117–141, 1989.

68. Brott T, Lu M, Kothari R, et al: Hypertension and its treatment in the NINDS rt-PA stroke trial. Stroke 29:1504–1509, 1998.

69. Demchuck AM, Tanne D, Hill MD, et al: Predictors of good outcome after intravenous tPA for acute ischemic stroke. Neurology 57:474–480, 2001.

70. The NINDS t-PA Stroke Study Group: Intracerebral hemorrhage after intravenous t-PA therapy for ischemic stroke. Stroke 28:2109–2118, 1997.

71. Fagen SC, Morgenstern LB, Petitta A, et al: Cost-effectiveness of tissue plasminogen activator for acute ischemic stroke. Neurology 50:883–890, 1998.

72. von Kummer R, Hacke W: Safety and efficacy of intravenous tissue plasminogen activator and heparin in acute middle cerebral artery stroke. Stroke 23:646–652, 1992.

73. Zivin J, Mazzarella V: Tissue plasminogen activator plus glutamate antagonist improves outcome after embolic stroke. Arch Neurol 48:1235–1238, 1991.

74. Zhang RL, Zhang ZG, Chopp M: Increased therapeutic efficacy with rt-PA and anti-CD18 antibody treatment of stroke in the rat. Neurology 52:273–279, 1999.

75. Grotta J: Combination therapy stroke trial. Cerebrovasc Dis 12:258–263, 2001.

76. Lyden P, Jacoby M, Schim J, et al: The Clomethiazole Acute Stroke Study in tissue-type plasminogen activator-treated stroke (CLASS-T): Final results. Neurology 57:1199–1205, 2001.

Chapter Forty-Nine

Intra-arterial Thrombolysis in Acute Ischemic Stroke

Anthony J. Furlan and Randall Higashida

INTRA-ARTERIAL THROMBOLYSIS

In the 1980s, several reports of intra-arterial thrombolysis (IAT) as therapy for acute ischemic stroke were published.[1-3] The thrombolytic agents used in these early series were urokinase (UK) and streptokinase (SK). More than a decade later, advances in technique and microcatheter technology now allow superselective catheterization of even distal branches of occluded intracranial vessels. Importantly, rapid technical advances have recently prompted the Accreditation Council for Graduate Medical Education[4] (ACGME) to standardize the training curricula in endovascular surgical neuroradiology (i.e., interventional neuroradiology) for neuroradiologists, neurosurgeons, and neurologists.

Studies of IAT for acute ischemic stroke were initially limited to uncontrolled protocols.[5,6] There was great variability in technique, and efficacy and complication rates varied among the reported series. As a result, in 1996, an American Heart Association (AHA) Special Writing Group published its recommendations for the use of thrombolytic agents in acute ischemic stroke. On the basis of the strength of the scientific evidence available at that time, the AHA group concluded that IAT "should be considered investigational and only used in the clinical trial setting," recommending "further testing of" IAT.[7]

Subsequently, the results of the first randomized multi-center controlled trials of IAT, the Prolyse in Acute Cerebral Thromboembolism trials, PROACT I[8] and PROACT II,[9] were reported in 1998 and 1999, respectively. PROACT II remains the only randomized, controlled, multicenter clinical trial to demonstrate the efficacy of IAT in patients with acute ischemic stroke of less than 6 hours' duration due to occlusion of the middle cerebral artery (MCA).

GENERAL TECHNIQUE OF INTRA-ARTERIAL THROMBOLYSIS

In patients with appropriate clinical and computed tomography (CT) criteria, a complete four-vessel cerebral angiogram should be performed from a transfemoral approach to evaluate the site of vessel occlusion, the extent of thrombus, the number of territories involved, and the collateral circulation. In this procedure, a diagnostic catheter is guided into the high cervical segment of the vascular territory to be treated, followed by the introduction of a 2.3-Fr coaxial microcatheter with a steerable microguidewire. Under direct fluoroscopic visualization, the microcatheter is gently navigated through the intracranial circulation until the tip is embedded within or through the central portion of the thrombus (Fig. 49–1).

Many variations in catheter design and delivery technique have been described.[10] Two types of microcatheters are being used most often for local cerebral thrombolysis, depending on the extent of clot formation. For the majority of intra-arterial procedures, a single–end-hole microcatheter is used, whereas for longer segments of clot formation, a microcatheter with multiple side-holes is used. Superselective angiography through the microcatheter is performed at regular intervals to assess for extent of clot lysis and to adjust the dosage and volume of the thrombolytic agent.

A superselective angiogram is performed, and if the clot is seen to be partially dissolved, the catheter is advanced into the remaining thrombus, where additional thrombolysis is performed. As the thrombus is dissolved, the catheter is advanced into more distal branches of the intracranial circulation, so that most the thrombolytic agent enters the occluded vessel and is not washed preferentially into adjacent open blood vessels. The goal is to achieve rapid recanalization with as little thrombolytic agent as possible to limit the extent of brain infarction and reduce the risk of hemorrhage. Common experience shows, however, that it can take up to 2 hours to achieve recanalization after the procedure begins, that thrombolytic agents alone (i.e., without mechanical manipulation) rarely achieve recanalization in less than 30 minutes, and that recanalization is often incomplete. Among other factors, clot composition plays a key role in the rapidity and extent of recanalization achieved with IAT.

Thrombolytic Agents

Recombinant prourokinase (r-proUK), the thrombolytic agent used in PROACT II (see later), is currently not approved by the U.S. Food and Drug Administration (FDA) and is not yet commercially available. Although some thrombolytic agents have theoretical advantages over others, there is no proof that one thrombolytic agent is superior to

Therapy

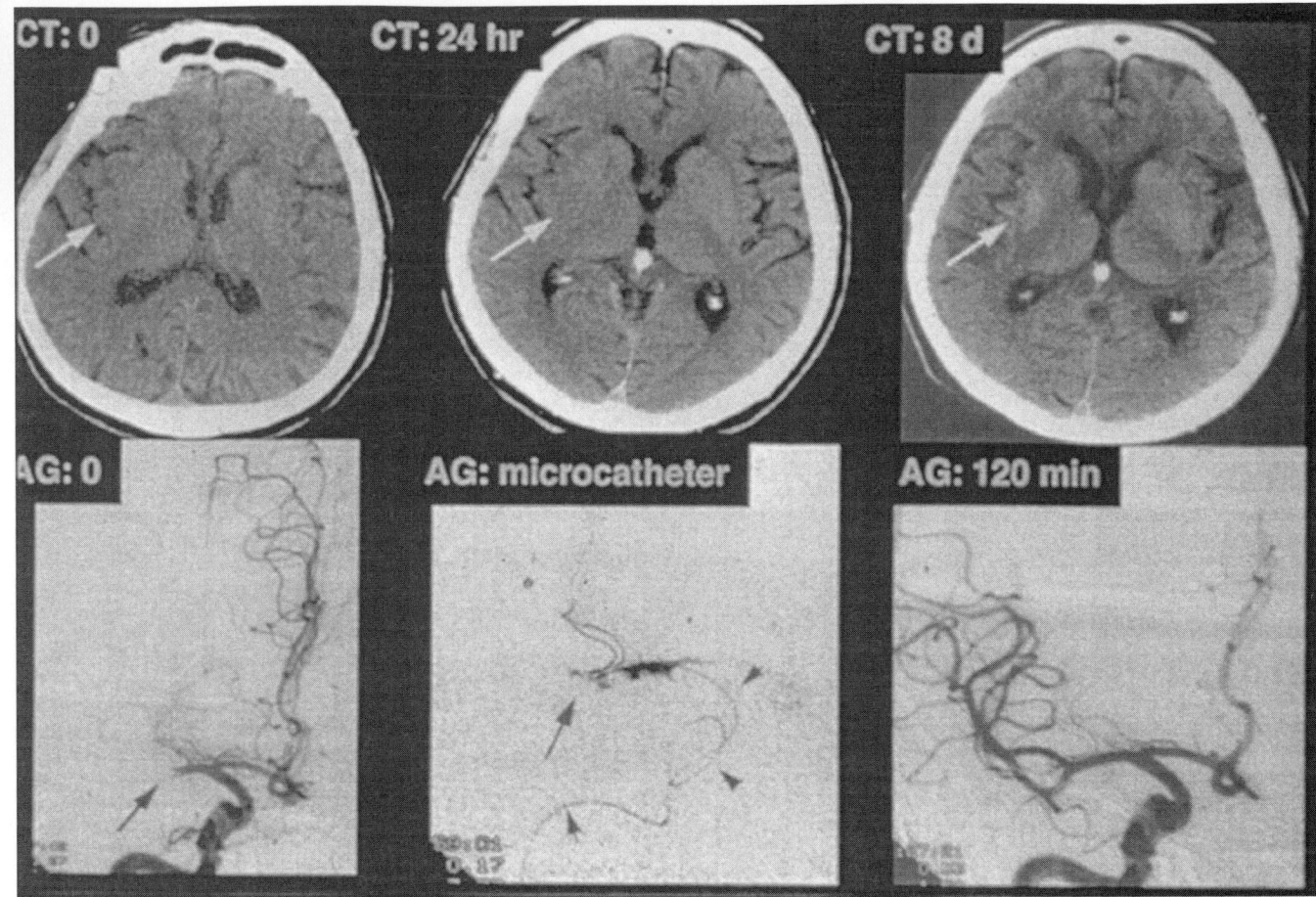

FIGURE 49–1 *Intra-arterial thrombolysis, with 9 mg r-proUK, 5.5 hours from stroke onset. A, Diagnostic angiogram (AG) shows complete TIMI 0 occlusion of the M1 MCA; minimal early infarct signs on baseline CT. B, Tip of the microcatheter embedded within proximal thrombus. Partial clot lysis after 1-hour infusion. C, Complete TIMI 3 recanalization at 2 hours. 24-hour CT shows minimal infarction. 8-day CT shows slight asymptomatic hemorrhagic conversion. (From Furlan A, Higashida R, Wechsler L, et al: Intra-arterial prourokinase for acute ischemic stroke: The PROACT II Study: A randomized controlled trial. JAMA 282:2003–2011, 1999.)*

another in terms of safety, recanalization rate, or clinical efficacy in acute ischemic stroke. Therefore it is not clear whether the results of PROACT II are applicable when agents other than r-proUK are used for IAT. Commercially available agents include urokinase (UK), tissue-type plasminogen activator (t-PA), reteplase (recombinant t-PA [rt-PA]), and tenectoplase (tNKase). These thrombolytic agents differ in stability, half-life, and fibrin selectivity. UK is not fibrin selective and therefore can cause systemic hypofibrinogemia. Both t-PA and r-proUK are fibrin selective and are active only at the site of thrombosis. However, r-proUK requires heparin for maximal thrombolytic effect. Newer agents, have long half-lives, allowing bolus administration, such as rt-PA, or are more fibrin selective, such as tNKase. However, the efficacy of second- and third-generation thrombolytic agents in acute ischemic stroke has not been demonstrated in a randomized controlled trial.[11]

Adjunctive Therapy

Intravenous (IV) heparin is given by most neuro-interventionists during IAT for stroke. Systemic anticoagulation with heparin reduces the risk of catheter-related embolism. Also, the thrombolytic effect of some agents,

such as r-proUK, is augmented by heparin. Another rationale for antithrombotic therapy is prevention of early reocclusion, which is probably more common with atherothrombosis than with cerebral embolism. These indications are counterbalanced by the higher risk of brain hemorrhage when heparin is combined with a thrombolytic agent.

The optimal dose of heparin during IAT for stroke has not been established. The PROACT I investigators reported a 27% rate of symptomatic brain hemorrhage when a conventional non–weight-adjusted heparin regimen (100 U/kg bolus followed by 1000 U/hr for 4 hours) was used with intra-arterial (IA) r-proUK.[8] Subsequently, a low-dose heparin regimen (2000 U bolus followed by 500 U/hr for 4 hours) was used with IA r-proUK, which reduced the rate of symptomatic brain hemorrhage to 7% in PROACT I and 10% in PROACT II. Unfortunately, the use of low-dose heparin therapy with IA r-proUK also cut the recanalization rate to half that for the original heparin regimen. Some neuro-interventionists now employ the PROACT low-dose heparin regimen during IAT. However, this dose of heparin does not prolong the activated partial thromboplastin time (APTT) or activated clotting time (ACT). Other neuro-interventionists employ weight-adjusted heparin dosage, keeping the ACT between 200 and 300 SEC.

The safety and efficacy of platelet glycoprotein (GP) IIb/IIIa inhibitor agents in patients with acute ischemic stroke undergoing IAT are unclear. Coronary doses of IV abciximab appear to be relatively safe in patients with acute ischemic stroke.[12] The risk of brain hemorrhage with the use of combined GP IIb/IIIa inhibitors and reduced-dose thrombolytic agents may be higher in patients older than 75 years.[13] The GP IIb/IIIa inhibitors abciximab and eptifibatide improve the efficacy of acute coronary interventions and have been used in patients undergoing cerebrovascular interventions.[14–16] The GP IIb/IIIa inhibitor dose can be adjusted to keep platelet inhibition between 50% and 80% during the intervention through monitoring of the platelet activation units (PAUs). However, GP IIb/IIIa inhibitors are not routinely employed during IAT for stroke. Adjunctive use of GP IIb/IIIa inhibition should be considered when the risk of acute reocclusion and endothelial injury is high as in angioplasty and stenting for basilar artery atherothrombosis. Concomitant use of clopidogrel and aspirin is usually avoided in acute stroke interventions because of the risk of brain hemorrhage.

THE PROLYSE IN ACUTE CEREBRAL THROMBOEMBOLISM TRIALS

Beginning in February 1994, patients were enrolled in the first placebo-controlled, double-blind multi-center trial of IAT in acute ischemic stroke, PROACT I.[8] The results were published in 1998. The thrombolytic agent used in PROACT I was recombinant prourokinase (r-proUK), which is not yet commercially available. This agent is a recombinant, single-chain zymogen of an endogenous fibrinolytic, either UK or urokinase-type plasminogen activator (u-PA).[17] Infusion of r-proUK does not lead to systemic dysfibrinogenemia with its associated higher risk of hemorrhagic side effects. Another clinically relevant characteristic of r-proUK is the facilitatory effect of co-administered heparin, which when given with r-proUK improves its fibrinolytic efficacy.

In PROACT I, the safety and recanalization efficacy of 6 mg r-proUK given IA was compared with IA administration of saline placebo in 40 patients with acute ischemic stroke of less than 6 hours' duration and due to MCA occlusion. Only patients in whom diagnostic cerebral angiography showed Thrombolysis in Acute Myocardial Infarction (TIMI) grade 0 or grade 1 occlusion of the M1 or M2 segment of the MCA were included. Another major inclusion criterion was a minimum National Institutes of Health Stroke Scale (NIHSS) score of 4 (except for isolated aphasia or hemianopsia) and a maximum score of 30. Major exclusion criteria were uncontrolled hypertension (blood pressure >180 mm Hg systolic/100 mm Hg diastolic), a history of hemorrhage, and recent surgery or trauma. CT evidence of early ischemic changes was not an exclusion criterion. Mechanical disruption of the clot was not permitted because the goal of the trial was to demonstrate the efficacy and safety of r-proUK. Patients also received IV heparin. The first 16 patients received the "high-dose" heparin regimen already mentioned. It consisted of a bolus of 100 IU/kg followed by a 1000 IU/hr infusion for 4 hours; anticoagulation was prohibited for the following 24 hours. On the basis of a recommendation from the external safety

committee, the heparin regimen was changed after the first 16 patients to a 2000-IU bolus followed by a 500 IU/hr infusion for 4 hours.

The recanalization rate was 57.7% in the r-proUK group and only 14.3% in the placebo group. In the "high-dose heparin" group receiving r-proUK, the recanalization rate was 81.8%, but the rate of symptomatic intracranial hemorrhage (ICH) was 27%. In contrast, the patients receiving r-proUK and "low-dose heparin" had a recanalization rate of 40%, but the ICH rate decreased to 6%. Overall, symptomatic ICH occurred in 15.4% of patients receiving treatment and in 14.3% of patients receiving placebo. Although PROACT I was not a clinical efficacy trial, there appeared to be a 10% to 12% higher rate of excellent outcomes in the IA r-proUK group than in the control group.

The follow-up clinical efficacy trial, PROACT II, was launched in February 1996, and the results were published in December 1999.[9] PROACT II was a randomized, controlled, multicenter trial but differed from PROACT I in that it employed open-label design with blinded follow-up. Patient selection was essentially the same as in PROACT I, with the major exception that patients with early signs of infarction in greater than one third of the MCA territory (the so-called ECASS [European Cooperative Acute Stroke Study] CT criterion)[18] on the initial CT scan were excluded. Additionally, a dose of 9 mg r-proUK was used instead of 6 mg, and "low-dose heparin" was given to both the treatment and control groups. A total of 180 patients were randomly assigned to receive either 9 mg of IA r-proUK plus low-dose IV heparin or low-dose IV heparin alone. Baseline stroke severity in the PROACT II patients was very high, with a median NIHSS score of 17. The median time from onset of symptoms to initiation of IAT was 5.3 hours.

The primary outcome measure was the proportion of patients who achieved a modified Rankin Scale score of 2 or less at 90 days, which signifies slight or no neurologic disability. For the group treated with r-proUK, there was a 15% absolute benefit ($P = .043$). The benefit was most noticeable in patients with a baseline NIHSS score between 11 and 20. On average, seven patients with MCA occlusion would require IAT for one of them to benefit. Recanalization rates were 66% at 2 hours for the treatment group and 18% for the placebo group (P < .001). Symptomatic brain hemorrhage occurred in 10% of the r-proUK group and 2% of the control group. Considering the later time to treatment and greater baseline stroke severity in PROACT II, the symptomatic brain hemorrhage rate compared favorably with that in the IV t-PA trials (6% in National Institutes of Neurological Disease and Stroke [NINDS],[17a] 9% in European Cooperative Acute Stroke Study [ECASS],[18] and 7% in Altephase Thrombolysis for Acute Noninterventional Therapy [ATLANTIS]).[18a] As in the NINDS trial, patients in PROACT II benefited overall from therapy despite the higher rate of brain hemorrhage, and there was no excess mortality (r-proUK, 24%; control, 27%).

DRAWBACKS OF INTRA-ARTERIAL THROMBOLYSIS

Access to facilities and a team of physicians (an interventionist and tertiary stroke team) capable of performing IAT is a limitation. Such expertise is not readily available in many developing countries or communities across the United States, usually being limited to large academic centers. Treatment delays are also inherent to IAT. In PROACT II, the median time from stroke onset to drug infusion was 5.3 hours, and the average time from the patient's arrival at the hospital to the initiation of IA r-proUK was 3 hours. IAT also involves costs and procedural risks not inherent to IV thrombolysis (IVT). However, serious procedural complications were uncommon in PROACT I and II; also, in experienced centers, cerebral angiography is associated with a morbidity of only 1.4% and rates of permanent complications and death of 0.1% and 0.02%, respectively.[19]

INTRA-ARTERIAL VERSUS INTRAVENOUS THROMBOLYSIS

IVT has the important advantages of time, ease of administration, and widespread availability. However, the difficulty in demonstrating a benefit when started more than 3 hours from stroke onset arises from a number of factors. The proportion of patients with major stroke who have salvageable brain decreases with time, whereas the brain hemorrhage rate with thrombolysis increases. A worse than expected outcome, owing to the inclusion of patients with early signs of infarction on CT, contributed to the negative results of ECASS I.[17] Conversely, a better than expected outcome made it difficult to demonstrate a benefit in ECASS II when such patients were excluded.[20] In the IVT trials, vascular imaging studies were not performed, so neither the sites of arterial occlusion nor the recanalization rates are known. Patients with ischemic stroke of less than 6 hours' duration have a wide variety of occlusion sites, and 20% have no visible occlusion, despite similar neurologic presentations.[21] Hence, the study populations in the IVT trials were relatively heterogeneous.

Although there have been no randomized studies comparing recanalization rates with outcomes of IVT and IAT, recanalization rates for cerebrovascular occlusions average 70% for IAT and 34% for IVT.[22] These differences in recanalization rates are most apparent with occlusions of large vessels such as the internal carotid artery (ICA), which is the vessel most resistant to thrombolysis, the carotid T segment, and the proximal (M1) segment of the MCA.

The greater recanalization efficacy for large vessel occlusions may help explain why the time window for successful IAT may be longer than that for IVT. On the basis of PROACT II, a 6-hour window appears to be a realistic goal for IA therapy in anterior circulation ischemia. For stroke in the vertebrobasilar circulation, there are some reports of successful therapy up to 48 hours after onset (see later).[23,24] The factors that determine individual susceptibility to ischemia are not completely understood, and there is clearly a great deal of variability in time from onset to irreversible damage among individuals. Even though a longer time window may be offered by IAT, it is critical to understand that urgency is paramount in ischemic stroke intervention and that the earlier recanalization is achieved with either IVT or IAT, the better the neurologic outcome.

IAT may be safer than IVT in patients with an excessive bleeding risk. Katzan and associates[25] reported the use of IAT in six patients with acute stroke after open heart surgery. Although this was only a small series, perioperative IAT appeared relatively safe, because only one minor bleeding complication occurred.

There are other special situations in which IAT can be employed. Weber and colleagues[26] and Padolecchia and associates[27] showed the safety and efficacy of superselective IAT in cases of central retinal artery occlusion. There were significant improvements in visual acuity with no hemorrhagic complications. In the series reported by Weber and colleagues,[26] 17.6% of patients recovered completely, a rate that is better than that in historical controls.

COMBINED INTRAVENOUS AND INTRA-ARTERIAL THROMBOLYSIS

It may be feasible to combine IVT and IAT to take advantage of the early infusion possible with IV administration and the greater recanalization efficacy of IA therapy. This approach was studied in the pilot Emergency Management of Stroke (EMS) Bridging Trial.[28] Patients with stroke of less than 3 hours' duration were given a loading dose (0.6 mg/kg) of IV t-PA or placebo followed by angiography and IAT if a vascular occlusion remained. In 70% of all patients, angiography showed clot after IV therapy. MCA recanalization improved in patients who then received IA t-PA, but the risk of life-threatening bleeding complications also rose. The results of the follow-up IV plus IA t-PA trial (Interventional Management of Stroke [IMS]) have been reported.[29] Among 62 patients with a baseline NIHSS score of 10 or more entered into IMS, 44 (71%) required both IV (0.6 mg/kg) and IA t-PA. The six symptomatic brain hemorrhages in the group receiving IV-IA combination therapy was 6.3%. A good outcome was achieved in 56% of patients younger than 80 years who received combination therapy, compared with 36% of patients with a baseline NIHSS score of 10 or higher who received IV t-PA alone in the NINDS t-PA Stroke Trial, and 40% in the PROACT II patients receiving IA r-proUK alone.

VERTEBROBASILAR INTRA-ARTERIAL THROMBOLYSIS

The natural history of basilar occlusion is extremely poor, with mortality rates ranging from 83% to 91%.[24,30] Because of this poor natural history, IAT has been preferred in patients with acute basilar artery occlusion. Approximately 278 cases have been reported, with an overall basilar recanalization rate of 60%. Basilar artery occlusions have a high incidence of residual stenosis, which often requires adjuvant therapies such as angioplasty and antithrombotic and antiplatelet treatments.

In a compilation of reported cases of vertebrobasilar thrombolysis, the mortality in patients in whom recanalization was not achieved was 90%, compared with 31% in patients in whom at least partial reperfusion was achieved.

Good outcomes are strongly associated with recanalization after thrombolytic therapy. The majority of patients with successful vertebrobasilar recanalization had mild or moderate disability, compared with less than 14% of patients whose vessels remained occluded.[31]

Success of recanalization depends on the location of the vertebrobasilar occlusion. Distal occlusions have higher recanalization rates than proximal occlusions. Emboli, which often lodge in the distal basilar artery, are easier to lyse than atherosclerosis-related thrombi, the usual cause of proximal basilar occlusions.[5,32] Short segment occlusions are easier to lyse than longer segment occlusions.[32] Patients who are younger have higher recanalization rates,[33,34] probably because they have a higher incidence of embolic occlusion.

The time window for thrombolysis may be longer in the posterior circulation. The presence of coma or tetraparesis for several hours portends poor prognosis despite recanalization. However, prolonged vertebrobasilar occlusion symptoms do not preclude survival and recovery. Many series have included patients not treated until 24,[3,35] 48,[32,36] or even 72 hours after symptom onset,[3,33] or patients with prolonged, stuttering courses.[37,38] An association between time to treatment and outcome has been suggested,[39] but other series do not support the finding.[32,40]

This great variability makes it difficult to predict the timing and outcome of thrombolysis in the vertebrobasilar circulation. Patients with vertebrobasilar artery occlusion often have chronic atherothrombotic disease, which allows collateral vessels to develop over time. As hypothesized by Cross and coworkers,[33] there may be two distinct populations of patients with vertebrobasilar occlusion. Paradoxically, patients with a progressive stuttering course may have better collateral circulation and better outcome after IAT despite later treatment than patients with sudden onset of a severe deficit but with poor collateral vessels who may actually be brought to treatment earlier.

Despite the apparently longer time window, the rate of hemorrhagic transformation after vertebrobasilar thrombolysis appears lower than in the anterior circulation. The average rate of symptomatic brain hemorrhage after vertebrobasilar IAT is 6.5%, compared with 8.3% for IAT in the anterior circulation. A lower rate of hemorrhagic transformation after vertebrobasilar thrombolysis may be due to higher ischemic tolerance in the posterior circulation, improved collateral circulation, or an increased density of white matter tracts.[41] There is no clear association between hemorrhage risk and time to treatment,[33] although 3 of the 18 symptomatic hemorrhages reported in the literature occurred when thrombolysis was initiated more than 48 hours after symptom onset.[3,40]

Some investigators believe that patients with CT evidence of brainstem infarction are not candidates for thrombolytic therapy,[3,32] but other researchers have found no correlation between this finding and neurologic outcome.[33,40] In two separate series, none of the patients who had CT evidence of ischemia had hemorrhage. However, because of the experience in the anterior circulation, caution should be used when one is considering vertebrobasilar thrombolysis in patients in whom CT reveals signs of early infarction.

RISK FACTORS FOR HEMORRHAGIC TRANSFORMATION

Several series have found no relationship between recanalization and hemorrhage risk.[42–44] However, these series do not address delayed recanalization or the status of recanalization at the time of brain hemorrhage.[45]

The amount of ischemic damage is a key factor in the development of hemorrhage after thrombolysis. Early extensive CT changes and severity of the initial neurologic deficit, both indicators of the extent of ischemic damage, are the best predictors of risk of hemorrhagic transformation (Fig. 49–2).[44,46] In ECASS I,[18] early CT changes in more than one third of the MCA territory correlated well with the frequency of hemorrhagic infarction. However, the so-called ECASS CT criterion is not present in all cases of hemorrhage, and there is considerable inter-reader variability in the interpretation of early CT changes. Furthermore, extensive early CT changes by themselves may be insufficient to exclude thrombolysis in specific patients.[47,48] An analysis of the PROACT II data indicates that patients with early (i.e., <6 hours) CT infarct volumes greater 100 mL do poorly.[49] However, estimated early CT changes (i.e., ECASS CT criterion) appear less predictive of outcome among homogeneous patients with MCA occlusion than in patients with mixed sites of arterial occlusion.[50] Furthermore, time may also be a key factor in interpreting early CT changes. In the NINDS trial, patients with early CT changes still benefited from t-PA administration, perhaps because of the earlier treatment time window.[44] Given the somewhat conflicting data, it would be prudent either (1) to avoid thrombolysis in patients with clear-cut and extensive early signs of infarction on CT and a NIHSS score higher than 20, especially those older than 75 years, or (2) to emphasize to the family of such a patient that the benefit-risk ratio is greatly reduced, even if treatment is begun within 3 hours of onset.

The amount of ischemic damage depends on the duration of occlusion and the amount of collateral blood flow. Both of these factors have been associated with increased risk of hemorrhage.[42,44,51] Ueda and coworkers[51] found that the amount of residual blood flow, as determined by single-photon emission CT (SPECT), was associated with hemorrhagic transformation, but they also used SPECT results to extend the thrombolytic time window beyond 6 hours in three patients. Improved perfusion after 3 hours of IV r-tPA has also been demonstrated with SPECT.[52]

Other factors that have been associated with hemorrhage after thrombolysis for both stroke and myocardial infarction (MI) are thrombolytic dose,[43,53] blood pressure,[54,55] advanced age, prior head injury,[44,56,57] and blood glucose level.[45] Age was the most important risk factor in one of the largest series of thrombolysis-related ICH. Because of the increased risk in elderly patients, an upper age limit was initially instituted for patients being considered for coronary thrombolysis. Older patients with MI were found to benefit from treatment, however, and the generally accepted age limit has been raised. A strong relationship between advanced age and hemorrhage was also demonstrated in the NINDS and ECASS trials. Although there is no strict age cutoff, physicians must take into account the greater risk of hemorrhage in patients 75 years and older when choosing to administer thrombolysis for stroke.

Intracerebral hemorrhage after thrombolysis for stroke can occur at sites distant from the ischemic region.[21] Cerebral amyloid angiopathy has been implicated as a causative

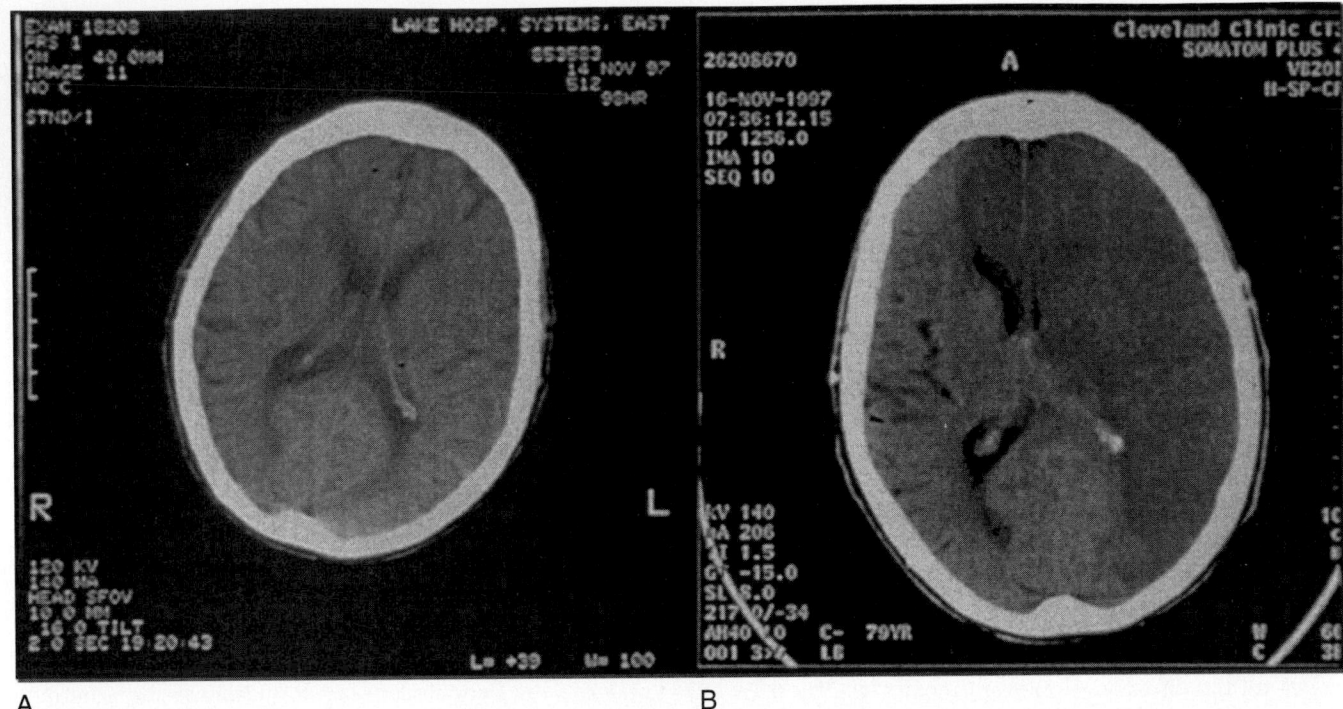

FIGURE 49–2 *Early infarct signs on CT scan. A 67-year-old man with acute right hemiplegia and aphasia. NIHSS 22. Internal carotid artery occlusion. A, Initial CT 4 hours after stroke onset shows sulcal effacement, loss of gray-white matter distinction, and loss of insular ribbon in more than one third of the left middle cerebral artery territory. (ECASS CT criteria.) B, Repeat CT at 25 hours shows massive left cerebral and right anterior cerebral artery infarcts.*

factor for brain hemorrhages after thrombolysis for MI.[58] Amyloid angiopathy is a well known cause of spontaneous hemorrhage in the elderly and is associated with dementia of the Alzheimer's type. Hence, thrombolytic therapy in elderly demented patients may carry a particularly high risk of brain hemorrhage. Hemorrhage into an arteriovenous malformation and unsuspected ischemic infarction have also been reported as causes of ICH after thrombolysis.[58]

OTHER FACTORS AFFECTING OUTCOMES WITH THROMBOLYSIS

Hacke[59] has described the ideal candidate for thrombolysis as follows: a young person with good collateral circulation who has an MCA occlusion distal to the lenticulostriates due to a fresh fibrin-rich thrombus that passed through a patent foramen ovale. The presence of collateral flow is one of the primary determinants of outcome.[60,61] Good leptomeningeal collaterals may limit the extent of ischemic damage and prolong the therapeutic window. Good collateral flow is also associated with higher rates of reperfusion, presumably because it allows a greater amount of thrombolytic agent to reach the clot.

Clot composition is a neglected factor in recanalization success rates.[62] Fresh thrombi, which are rich in fibrin and plasminogen, are easier to lyse than aged atherothrombi, which are more organized and have low fibrin and plasminogen contents and high amounts of platelets and cholesterol. Fresh cardiac emboli may therefore respond better to thrombolysis than atherothrombotic occlusion or calcific embolism.

Angiographic studies indicate that about 20% of patients presenting with a clinical picture consistent with acute ischemic stroke have no visible arterial occlusion.[21] There is controversy regarding the utility of thrombolysis in patients who have no large vessel occlusion.[63] The NINDS trial suggested a benefit of t-PA in patients with small vessel (i.e., lacunar) infarction, and it is possible that thrombolytic therapy may be effective in the recanalization of small vessels that are invisible on angiography. A meta-analysis of thrombolytic trials found no significant differences between studies that included patients with lacunar strokes and those that excluded such patients.[64]

NEW ENDOVASCULAR THERAPIES FOR ACUTE STROKE

The technique used in IAT, unlike IV administration, may be critical in achieving success and varies among interventionists. Direct intra-thrombus delivery of thrombolytic agent is preferred over regional infusion. However, the infusion process has been variable, ranging from continuous to pulsed infusion both with and without bolus administration. In some series, clot disruption by the microcatheter has been included in the protocol, theoretically to improve exposure of the thrombus to the thrombolytic agent and thereby speed clot lysis. Mechanical clot manipulation was prohibited in PROACT I and PROACT

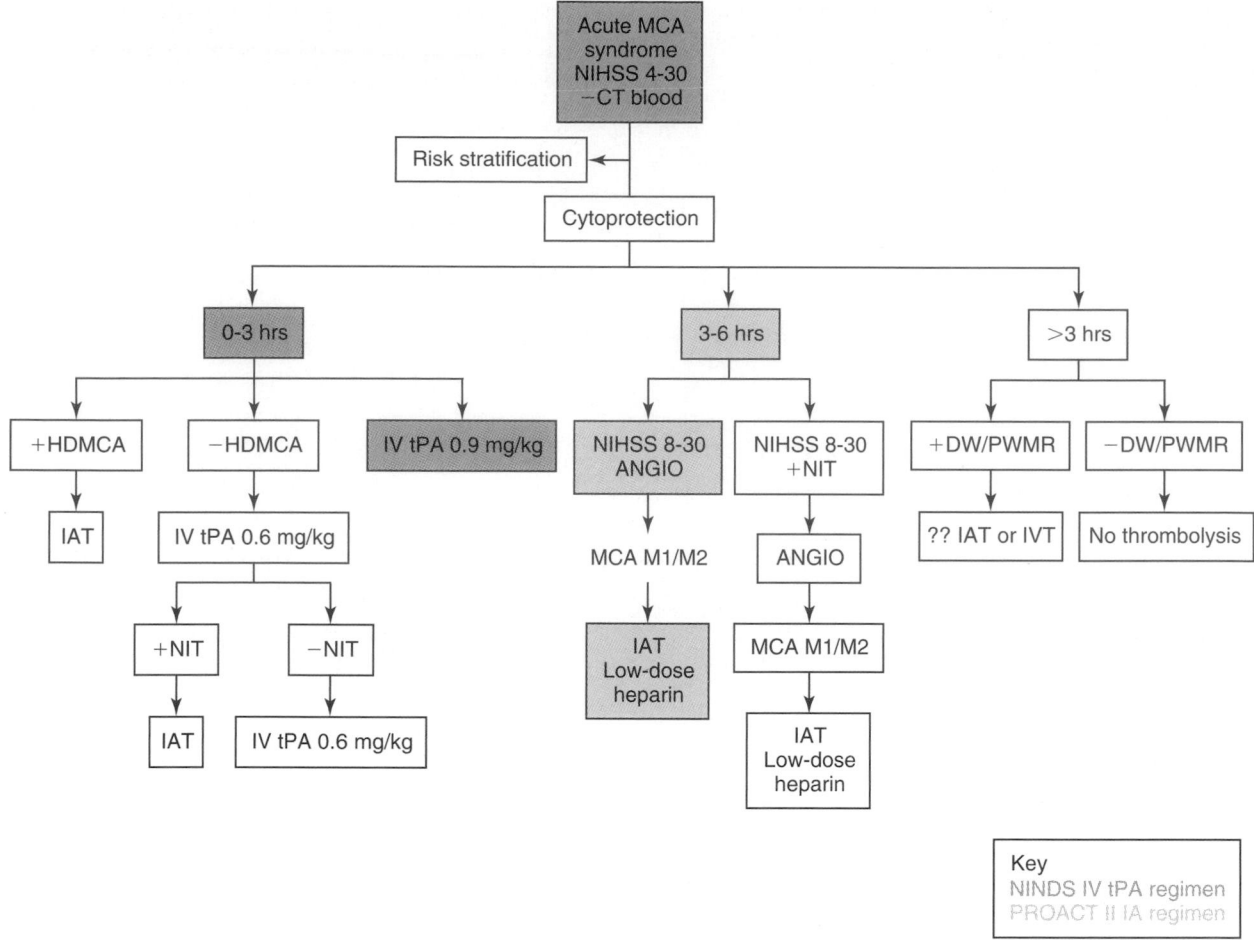

FIGURE 49–3 *Acute MCA syndrome potential treatment algorithm.* Plus sign *indicates positive result, and* minus sign *negative results, of the test.* CT, computed tomography (brain); DW/PWMR, diffusion/perfusion mismatch on MRI of the brain; ECASS, European Cooperative Acute Stroke Study; HDMCA, hyperdense middle cerebral artery; IAT, intra-arterial thrombolysis; IV, intravenous; IVT, intravenous thrombolysis; NIHSS, National Institutes of Health Stroke Scale; NIT, noninvasive tests; tPA, tissue-type plasminogen activator.

II. In some series, IAT was followed by percutaneous transluminal angioplasty (PTA) of the recanalized vessel.[65,66] To date, however, no prospective comparisons of any of these techniques have been conducted, so their relative merits remain unclear.

Several new interventional neuroradiologic techniques designed to improve the speed and completeness of recanalization in acute ischemic stroke have been described. These reports have all been individual case series from single institutions. The techniques include treatment of acute ischemic stroke by direct mechanical balloon angioplasty of the thrombus,[66–69] mechanical snaring of clot from the MCAs,[70] intravascular stenting of underlying occlusive atherosclerosis for restoring vessel patency,[71] use of suction thrombectomy devices for establishing reperfusion, laser-assisted thrombolysis of acute emboli to the brain, and power-assisted Doppler ultrasound thrombolysis.[72] As previously described, intravenous and intra-arterial GP IIb/IIIa inhibitors have also been used to enhance the effects of clot lysis during acute stroke.[12,15,16,73] These new technologies are in early feasibility and safety trials in both the United States and Europe and are still investigational. Phase 3 randomized controlled clinical trials must

be performed before specific recommendations as to the safety and efficacy of any of these methods can be made.

CURRENT STATUS OF INTRA-ARTERIAL THROMBOLYSIS

The fourth issue of the *Cochrane Database of Systematic Reviews* meta-analysis, which included data from PROACT I and PROACT II, concluded that overall, the risks of thrombolysis are offset by reductions in dependent survival, so that significantly more patients are alive and independent after treatment. Writers of this meta-analysis suggested, "The time window might extend to, or even beyond, six hours in selected patients."[74]

Diffusion-weighted and perfusion-weighted magnetic resonance imaging (MRI) studies have also provided pathophysiologic evidence linking MCA recanalization with smaller infarct volumes and improved clinical outcomes.[75–77] At least two ongoing trials of IVT (desmoteplase in acute stroke [DIAS], dose escalation of desmoteplase in acute stroke [DEDAS]) are exploring the feasibility of selecting patients for thrombolysis based on MRI diffusion/perfusion mismatch.

On the basis of this available evidence, the Second AHA International Evidence Evaluation Conference made a "major guideline change"[79]; IAT given within 3 to 6 hours after the onset of stroke symptoms is now a Class IIb recommendation (acceptable, clinically useful, alternative or optional treatment supported by good evidence). IAT has also been endorsed by other major medical societies.

Stroke specialists now routinely consider IAT in selected patients with acute ischemic stroke due to large cerebral vessel occlusions such as the MCA or basilar artery. Further evidence of the efficacy and safety of IAT is being collected through the Interventional Stroke Therapy Outcomes Registry (INSTOR).[80] As new options for acute stroke therapy emerge, an algorithmic approach to patient selection for IVT, IAT, cytoprotective, and combination therapies, analogous to that for acute coronary syndromes, may be required (Fig. 49–3).[81]

References

1. Nenci GG, Gresele P, Taramelli M, et al: Thrombolytic therapy for thromboembolism of vertebrobasilar artery. Angiology 34:561–571, 1983.
2. del Zoppo GJ, Ferbert A, Otis S, et al: Local intra-arterial fibrinolytic therapy in acute carotid territory stroke: A pilot study. Stroke 19:307–313, 1988.
3. Hacke W, Zeumer H, Ferbert A, et al: Intra-arterial thrombolytic therapy improves outcome in patients with acute vertebrobasilar occlusive disease. Stroke 19:1216–1222, 1988.
4. Accreditation Council for Graduate Medical Education. Program Requirements for Residence Education in Endovascular Surgical Neuroradiology. Available online at www.ACGME.org/RRC_progREQ/
5. Zeumer H, Freitag HJ, Zanella F, et al: Local intra-arterial fibrinolytic therapy in patients with stroke: Urokinase versus recombinant tissue plasminogen activator (rt-PA). Neuroradiology 35:159–162, 1993.
6. Nesbit GM, Clark WM, O'Neil OR, Barnwell SL: Intracranial intra-arterial thrombolysis facilitated by microcatheter navigation through an occluded cervical internal carotid artery. J Neurosurg 84:387–392, 1996.
7. Adams HP, Brott TC, Furlan AJ, et al: Guidelines for thrombolytic therapy for acute stroke: A supplement to the guidelines for the management of patients with acute ischemic stroke. A Statement for Healthcare Professionals from a Special Writing Group of the Stroke Council, American Heart Association. Stroke 27:1711–1718, 1996.
8. del Zoppo GJ, Higashida RT, Furlan AJ, et al: PROACT: A Phase II randomized trial of recombinant pro-urokinase by direct arterial delivery in acute middle cerebral artery stroke. Stroke 29:4–11, 1998.
9. Furlan A, Higashida R, Wechsler L, et al: Intra-arterial prourokinase for acute ischemic stroke—The PROACT II Study: A randomized controlled trial. JAMA 282:2003–2011, 1999.
10. Higashida RT, Halbach VV, Tsai FY, et al: Interventional neurovascular techniques in acute thrombolytic therapy for stroke. In T Yamagushi, E Mori, K Minematsu, GJ del Zoppo (eds): Thrombolytic Therapy in Acute Ischemic Stroke III. Tokyo, Springer-Verlag, 1995, pp 294–300.
11. Consensus Conference on Current Strategies for Intracerebral Fibrinolysis for Acute Stroke Therapy. Memphis, TN, Presented at Centocor, January 8–9, 2000.
12. Abciximab in acute ischemic stroke: A randomized, double-blind, placebo-controlled, dose-escalation study. The Abciximab in Ischemic Stroke Investigators. Stroke 31:601–609, 2000.
13. Reperfusion therapy for acute myocardial infarction with fibrinolytic therapy or combination reduced fibrinolytic therapy and platelet glycoprotein IIb/IIIa inhibition: The GUSTO V randomised trial. The GUSTO V Investigators. Lancet 357:1905–1914, 2001.
14. Wallace RC, Furlan AJ, Moliterno DJ, et al: Basilar artery rethrombosis: Successful treatment with platelet glycoprotein IIb/IIIa receptor inhibitor. Am J Neuroradiol 18:1257–1260, 1997.
15. Qureshi AI, Suri MF, Khan J, et al: Abciximab as an adjunct to high-risk carotid or vertebrobasilar angioplasty: Preliminary experience. Neurosurgery 46:1316–1324, 2000.
16. McDonald CT, O'Donnell J, Bemporad J, et al: The clinical utility of intravenous Integrilin combined with intra-arterial tissue plasminogen activator in acute ischemic stroke: The MGH experience [abstract]. Stroke 33:359, 2002.
17. Credo RB, Burke SE, Barker WM, et al: Recombinant glycosylated pro-urokinase: Biochemistry, pharmacology, and early clinical experience. In Sasahara AA, Loscalzo J (eds): New Therapeutic Agents in Thrombosis and Thrombolysis. New York, Marcel Dekker, 1997, pp 561–589.
17a. The National Institute of Neurological Disorders and Stroke t-PA Stroke Study Group: Tissue plasminogen activator for acute ischemic stroke. N Engl J Med 333:1581–1587, 1995.
18. Hacke W, Kaste M, Fieschi C, et al: Intravenous thrombolysis with recombinant tissue plasminogen activator for acute hemispheric stroke: The European Cooperative Acute Stroke Study (ECASS). JAMA 274:1017–1025, 1995.
18a. Clark WM, Wissman S, Albers GW, et al: Recombinant tissue plasminogen activator (Alteplase) for ischemic stroke 3 to 5 hours after symptom onset—the ATLANTIS Study: A randomized controlled trial. JAMA 282:2012–2026, 1999.
19. Waugh JR, Sacharis N: Arteriographic complications in the DSA era. Radiology 182:243, 1992.
20. Hacke W, Kaste M, Fieschi C, et al: Randomised double-blind placebo-controlled trial of thrombolytic therapy with intravenous alteplase in acute ischaemic stroke (ECASS II). Lancet, 352:1245–1251, 1998.
21. Wolpert SM, Bruckmann H, Greenlee R, et al: Neuroradiology evaluation of patients with acute stroke treated with recombinant tissue plasminogen activator. AJNR Am J Neuroradiol 14:3–13, 1993.
22. Pessin M, del Zoppo GJ, Furlan AJ: Thrombolytic treatment in acute stroke: Review and update of selective topics. In Moskowitz MA, Caplan LR (eds): Cerebrovascular Diseases: Nineteenth Princeton Stroke Conference. Boston, Butterworth-Heinemann, 1995, pp 409–418.
23. Hoffman AI, Lambiase RE, Haas RA, et al: Acute vertebrobasilar occlusion: Treatment with high-dose intraarterial urokinase. AJR Am J Roentgenol 172:709–712, 1999.
24. Hacke W, Zeumer H, Ferbert A, et al: Intra-arterial thrombolytic therapy improves outcome in patients with acute vertebrobasilar occlusive disease. Stroke 19:1216–1222, 1988.
25. Katzan IL, Masaryk TJ, Furlan AJ, et al: Intra-arterial thrombolysis for perioperative stroke after open heart surgery. Neurology 52:1081–1084, 1999.
26. Weber J, Remonda L, Mattle HP, et al: Selective intra-arterial fibrinolysis of acute central retinal artery occlusion. Stroke 29:2076–2079, 1998.
27. Padolecchia R, Puglioli M, Ragone MC, et al: Superselective intra-arterial fibrinolysis in central retinal artery occlusion. AJNR Am J Neuroradiol 20:565–567, 1999.
28. Lewandowski CA, Frankel M, Tomsick TA, et al: Combined intravenous and intra-arterial r-TPA versus intra-arterial therapy for acute ischemic stroke: Emergency Management of Stroke (EMS) Bridging Trial. Stroke 30:2598–2605, 1999.
29. Tomsick T, Broderick JP, Pancioli AP, et al: Combined IV-IA rtPA treatment in major acute ischemic stroke [abstract]. Stroke 33:359, 2002.
30. Brückmann H, Ferbert A, del Zoppo G, et al: Acute basilar thrombosis: Angiologic-clinical comparison and therapeutic implications. Acta Radiol 369(Suppl):38–42, 1987.
31. Katzan IL, Furlan AJ: Thrombolytic therapy. In Fisher M, Bogousslavsky J (eds): Current Review of Cerebrovascular Disease, 3rd ed. Boston, Butterworth Heinemann, 1999, pp 185–193.
32. Brandt T, von Kummer R, Muller-Kuppers M, et al: Thrombolytic therapy of acute basilar artery occlusion: Variables affecting recanalization and outcome. Stroke 27:875–881, 1996.
33. Cross DT, Moran CJ, Akins P, et al: Relationship between clot location and outcome after basilar artery thrombolysis. AJNR Am J Neuroradiol 18:1221–1228, 1997.
34. Huemer M, Niederwieser V, Ladurner G: Thrombolytic treatment for acute occlusion of the basilar artery. J Neurol Neurosurg Psychiatry 58:227–228, 1995.
35. Matsumoto K, Satoh K: Intraarterial therapy in acute ischemic stroke. In Yamaguchi T, Mori E, Minematsu K, et al (eds): Thrombolytic Therapy in Acute Ischemic Stroke III. Tokyo, Springer-Verlag, 1995, pp 279–287.
36. Clark W, Barnwell S, Nesbit G, et al: Efficacy of intra-arterial thrombolysis of basilar artery stroke [abstract]. J Stroke Cerebrovasc Dis 6:457, 1997.

Therapy

37. Wijdicks EF, Nichols DA, Thielen KR, et al: Intra-arterial thrombolysis in acute basilar artery thromboembolisms: The initial Mayo Clinic experience. Mayo Clin Proc 72:1005–1013, 1997.

38. Herderscheê D, Limburg M, Hijdra A, et al: Recombinant tissue plasminogen activator in two patients with basilar artery occlusion. J Neurol Neurosurg Psychiatry 54:71–73, 1991.

39. Zeumer H, Freitag HJ, Grzyska U, et al: Local Intraarterial Fibrinolysis in Acute Vertebrobasilar Occlusion. Neuroradiology, 31:336–340, 1989.

40. Becker KJ, Monsein LH, Ulatowski J, et al: Intraarterial thrombolysis in vertebrobasilar occlusion. AJNR Am J Neuroradiol 17:255–262, 1996.

41. Becker KJ, Purcell LL, Hacke W, et al: Vertebrobasilar thrombosis: Diagnosis, management, and the use of intra-arterial thrombolytics. Crit Care Med 24:1729–1742, 1996.

42. von Kummer R, Hacke W: Safety and efficacy of intravenous tissue plasminogen activator and heparin in acute middle cerebral artery stroke. Stroke 23:646–652, 1992.

43. Mori E, Yoneda Y, Tabuchi M, et al: Intravenous recombinant tissue plasminogen activator in acute carotid artery territory stroke. Neurology 42:976–982, 1992.

44. Levy DE, Brott TG, Haley EC, et al: Factors related to intracranial hematoma formation in patients receiving tissue-type plasminogen activator for acute ischemic stroke. Stroke 25:291–297, 1994.

45. Kase CS, Furlan AJ, Wechsler LR, et al: Hemorrhage after intra-arterial thrombolysis for ischemic stroke: The PROACT II Trial. Neurology 57:1603–1610, 2001.

46. Bozzao L, Angeloni U, Bastianello S, et al: Early angiographic and CT findings in patients with hemorrhagic infarction in the distribution of the middle cerebral artery. AJNR Am J Neuroradiol 12:1115–1121, 1991.

47. Grotta JC, Choi D, Patel SC, et al: Agreement and variability in the interpretation of early CT changes in stroke patients qualifying for intravenous tPA therapy. Stroke 30:1528–1533, 1999.

48. Patel SC, Levine SR, Tilley JC, et al: Lack of clinical significance of early ischemic changes on computed tomography in acute stroke. JAMA 286:2830–2838, 2001.

49. Roberts HC, Dillon WP, Furlan AJ, et al: Angiographic collaterals in acute stroke—relationship to clinical presentation and outcome: The PROACT II trial [abstract]. Stroke 32:336, 2001.

50. Kidwell CS, Saver JL, Duckwiler G, et al: Predictors of hemorrhagic transformation following intra-arterial thrombolysis [abstract]. Stroke 32:319, 2001.

51. Ueda T, Hatakeyama T, Kumon Y, et al: Evaluation of risk of hemorrhagic transformation in local intra-arterial thrombolysis in acute ischemic stroke by initial SPECT. Stroke 25:298–303, 1994.

52. Alexandrov AV, Bratina P, Grotta JC: tPA associated reperfusion after acute stroke demonstrated by HMPAO-SPECT [abstract]. Stroke 288, 1998.

53. Gore JM, Sloan M, Price TR, et al: Intracerebral hemorrhage, cerebral infarction, and subdural hematoma after acute myocardial infarction and thrombolytic therapy in the Thrombolysis in Myocardial Infarction Study: Thrombolysis in Myocardial Infarction, Phase II, Pilot and Clinical Trial. Circulation 83:448–459, 1991.

54. Selker HP, Beshansky JR, Schmid CH, et al: Presenting pulse pressure predicts thrombolytic therapy-related intracranial hemorrhage. Thrombolytic Predictive Instrument (TPI) Project Results. Circulation 90:1657–1661, 1994.

55. Simoons ML, Maggioni AP, Knatterud G, et al: Individual risk assessment for intracranial haemorrhage during thrombolytic therapy. Lancet 342:1523–1528, 1993.

56. Gebel JM, Sila CA, Sloan MA, et al: Thrombolysis-related intracranial hemorrhage: A radiographic analysis of 244 cases from the gusto-1 trial with clinical correlation. Stroke 29:563–569, 1998.

57. Larrue V, von Kummer R, del Zoppo G, et al: Hemorrhagic transformation in acute ischemic stroke, potential contributing factors in the European Cooperative Acute Stroke Study. Stroke 28:957–960, 1997.

58. Sloan MA, Price TR, Petito CK, et al: Clinical features and pathogenesis of intracerebral hemorrhage after rt-PA and heparin therapy for acute myocardial infarction: The Thrombolysis in Myocardial Infarction (TIMI) II pilot and randomized clinical trial combined experience. Neurology 45:649–658, 1995.

59. Hacke W: Thrombolysis: Stroke subtype and embolus type. In del Zoppo GJ, Mori E, Hacke W (eds): Thrombolytic Therapy in Acute Ischemic Stroke II. Berlin, Springer-Verlag, 1993, pp 153–159.

60. von Kummer R, Holle R, Rosin L, et al: Does arterial recanalization improve outcome in carotid territory stroke? Stroke 26:581–587, 1995.

61. Ringelstein EB, Biniek R, Weiler C, et al: Type and extent of hemispheric brain infarctions and clinical outcome in early and delayed middle cerebral artery recanalization. Neurology 42:289–298, 1991.

62. Chimowitz M, Pessin M, Furlan A, et al: The effect of source of cerebral embolus on susceptibility to thrombolysis [abstract]. Neurology 44(Suppl 2):A356, 1994.

63. Caplan LR, Mohr JP, Kistler JP, Koroshetz W: Thrombolysis–not a panacea for ischemic stroke. N Engl J Med 337:1309, 1997.

64. Wardlaw JM, Warlow CP, Counsell C: Systematic review of evidence on thrombolytic therapy for acute ischaemic stroke. Lancet 350:607–614, 1997.

65. Gönner F, Remonda L, Mattle H, et al: Local intra-arterial thrombolysis in acute ischemic stroke. Stroke 29:1894–1900, 1998.

66. Ueda T, Sakaki S, Nochide I, et al: Angioplasty after intra-arterial thrombolysis for acute occlusion of intracranial arteries. Stroke 29:2568–2574, 1998.

67. Mori T, Kazita K, Chokyu K, et al: Short-term arteriographic and clinical outcome after cerebral angioplasty and stenting for intracranial vertebrobasilar and carotid atherosclerotic occlusive disease. AJNR Am J Neuroradiol 21:249–254, 2000.

68. Nakayama T, Tanaka K, Kaneko M, et al: Thrombolysis and angioplasty for acute occlusion of intracranial vertebrobasilar arteries: Report of three cases. J Neurosurg 88:919–922, 1998.

69. Tsai FY, Berberaj B, Matovich V, et al: Percutaneous transluminal angioplasty adjunct to thrombolysis for acute middle cerebral artery rethrombosis. AJNR Am J Neuroradiol 15:1823–1829, 1994.

70. Chopko BW, Kerber C, Wong W, Georgy B: Transcatheter snare removal of acute middle cerebral artery thromboembolism: Technical case report. Neurosurgery 40:1529–1531, 2000.

71. Phatouros CC, Higashida RT, Malek AM, et al: Endovascular stenting of an acutely thrombosed basilar artery: Technical case report and review of the literature. Neurosurgery 44:667–673, 1999.

72. Alexandrov AV, Demchuk AM, Felberg RA, et al: High rate of complete recanalization and dramatic clinical recovery during tPA infusion when continuously monitored with 2-MHz transcranial Doppler monitoring. Stroke 31:610–614, 2000.

73. Lempert TE, Halbach VV, Malek AM, et al: Rescue treatment of acute parent vessel thrombosis with glycoprotein IIb/IIIa inhibitor during GDC coil embolization. Stroke 30:693–695, 1999.

74. Cochrane Database of Systematic Reviews, Issue 4, 1999.

75. Keir SL, Wardlaw JM: Systematic review of diffusion and perfusion imaging in acute ischemic stroke. Stroke 31:2723–2731, 2000.

76. Fisher M, Albers GW: Applications of diffusion-perfusion magnetic resonance imaging in acute ischemic stroke. Neurology 52:1750–1756, 1999.

77. Hacke W, Warach S: Diffusion-weighted MRI as an evolving standard of care in acute stroke. Neurology 54:1548–1549, 2000.

78. Guidelines 2000 for Cardiopulmonary Resuscitation and Emergency Cardiovascular Care. Part 7: The era of reperfusion. section 2: Acute stroke. The American Heart Association in collaboration with the International Liaison Committee on Resuscitation. Circulation 102(Suppl):I204-I216, 2000.

79. Emergency interventional stroke therapy: A statement from the American Society of Interventional and Therapeutic Neuroradiology and Society of Cardiovascular and Interventional Radiology. Am J Neuroradiol 22:54, 2001.

80. INSTOR: Interventional Stroke Therapy Outcomes Registry. Available online at www.strokeregistry.org/

81. Boden WE, McKay RG: Optimal treatment of acute coronary syndromes—an evolving strategy. N Engl J Med 344:1939-1942, 2001.

Therapy

Chapter Fifty

Antithrombotic Therapy for Acute Ischemic Stroke

Harold P. Adams, Jr., and Patricia H. Davis

Because most ischemic strokes are secondary to arterial thromboembolism, antithrombotic agents (anticoagulants and antiplatelet agents) are a leading component of medical treatment to prevent ischemic stroke. The utility of these medications in long-term management to prevent stroke or recurrent stroke has been established.[1] Oral anticoagulants are of proven efficacy in preventing cardioembolic stroke among patients with high-risk diseases of the heart, including atrial fibrillation. Antiplatelet agents are the mainstay of management for preventing stroke among patients with arterial diseases, including intracranial and extracranial atherosclerosis.[2] Because these medications are effective in long-term care and because most strokes are secondary to the formation of clots, there has been a strong interest in the emergency use of anticoagulant and antiplatelet medications in the setting of acute stroke.

Several antithrombotic agents have been prescribed (Table 50.1). In a survey of nonurban emergency departments in Texas, 9% of patients received heparin and 5% were given aspirin during acute treatment.[3] The rationale for using these medications comprise halting the propagation of an intra-arterial thrombosis, forestalling early recurrent embolization, and maintaining collateral flow to the ischemic focus. Finally, these agents might be used as adjuncts to thrombolytic agents. In addition, antithrombotic agents can help prevent deep vein thrombosis and pulmonary embolism—leading causes of morbidity or mortality among bedridden patients with stroke.

Despite the widespread use of antithrombotic agents, their administration in the emergency treatment of patients with recent ischemic stroke remains controversial. Experts have widely divergent opinions about the effectiveness and safety of these agents.[4-11] Surveys of physicians also produce a wide spectrum of opinions about the early administration of antithrombotic agents.[12,13] Physicians are unsure about which patients to treat and when to start antithrombotic therapy. They are uncertain about which medications to prescribe.

Despite the ambiguity of the data and lack of consensus in the medical community, physicians have been accused of medical malpractice when they have not administered antithrombotic agents, in particular heparin, within the first hours of stroke. In 1994, a panel of the Stroke Council of the American Heart Association (AHA) evaluated the information about the urgent use of antithrombotic agents in the setting of stroke.[14] The panel concluded that there was insufficient information to determine the efficacy (or lack thereof) of heparin or other short-acting antithrombotic agents to make a recommendation about their use. These conclusions held no matter the presumed vascular territory (carotid vs. vertebrobasilar circulation), the location of arterial disease (intracranial or extracranial), and the likely cause (including cardioembolism or arterial dissection). Fortunately, several clinical trials testing antithrombotic agents have been reported since 1994, and more definitive data are available to guide physicians' decisions about the use of these medications in the setting of acute ischemic stroke.

PHARMACOLOGY

Heparin, Low-Molecular-Weight Heparins, and Danaparoid

The glycosaminoglycans heparin, low-molecular-weight (LMW) heparin, and danaparoid have been used for more than 50 years, and they remain widely used medications for the treatment of patients with acute stroke. Heparin is a mixture of glycosaminoglycans that is obtained from porcine or bovine sources. Its molecular weight ranges from 5000 to 30,000 daltons (d). Heparin cannot be administered orally; it must be given either intravenously or subcutaneously. Because of the high risk of local bleeding, intramuscular injection of heparin is avoided. The agent has immediate antithrombotic effects when it is given intravenously in a bolus dose followed by a continuous intravenous infusion.[15-17] A lag of several hours in achieving antithrombotic responses can follow subcutaneous administration, and therapeutic levels cannot be reached within 24 hours.

Heparin binds to plasma proteins, platelet-derived proteins, and endothelial cells.[15] Differences in levels of these proteins might explain variations in clinical responses to heparin among patients. Heparin binds to and alters the conformation of antithrombin, which in turn increases the ability of antithrombin to inactivate thrombin, activated factor X (factor Xa), and activated factor IX (factor IXa). Heparin achieves these primary antithrombotic effects via

Table 50.1 Antithrombotic Agents That Could Be Used in the Management of Acute Ischemic Stroke

Anticoagulants	Heparin
	Low-molecular-weight heparins
	Danaparoid
	Direct thrombin inhibitors (argatroban, hirudin)
	Antithrombin
	Protein C
Antiplatelet agents	Aspirin
	Clopidogrel
	Glycoprotein IIb/IIIa receptor blockers

high-affinity pentasaccharides. Heparin does not directly affect either thrombin or factor Xa already incorporated in a formed thrombus, and, thus, it does not have thrombolytic effects.[18] The ratio of inhibition for activated thrombin and factor Xa is 1:1. Heparin prevents fibrin formation through its inhibition of thrombin-induced activation of platelets and factors V and VIII. Heparin also inactivates thrombin through heparin cofactor II, an action that occurs at high concentrations and that is independent from its effects on antithrombin. In addition, the higher molecular-weight components of heparin can alter endothelial modulation of clotting factors and interact with platelet factor IV.[18] Heparin's binding to von Willebrand factor also affects platelet function.[16,17]

Heparin binds to macrophages and endothelial cells. This binding, which is saturable, relates to the rapid clearance of heparin from the circulation, and this effect may explain variations in response among patients. In addition, an individual patient's response may change over time. Some of the differences in responses occur for no obvious reason. Heparin has a narrow therapeutic window; differences between safe but effective doses and dangerous levels are small.[18] There is a strong association between the risk of serious bleeding and increases in the dose of heparin. Some patients are relatively resistant to heparin (heparin resistance). This response can be secondary to a deficiency of antithrombin or to an elevation in heparin-binding proteins, fibrinogen, factor VIII, or platelet factor 4.[16]

The activated partial thromboplastin time (aPTT) is the most widely used test to monitor the biologic effects of heparin. This test measures responses to heparin's inhibition of thrombin, factor Xa, and factor IXa. The optimal level of anticoagulation is uncertain but is assumed to be approximately 1.5 times control values. The aPTT test has a number of serious limitations. Variability in reagents between institutions may lead to spurious aPTT results.[16] Patients with the lupus anticoagulant–antiphospholipid antibody syndrome often have falsely elevated aPTT values; in this situation, monitoring heparin therapy with this test can be problematic. Alternative ways to assess heparin's activity is to measure inhibition of factor Xa or to measure heparin levels via neutralization with protamine sulfate. However, the usual therapeutic level of heparin that achieves inhibition of factor Xa is 0.3 to 0.7 μ/mL.[15,16] The therapeutic heparin level obtained through protamine neutralization is estimated as 0.20 to 0.40 μ/mL.[16] These tests are not widely available and may be more difficult to perform than measurements of aPTT.

Most high-risk patients receive 5000 units of heparin twice a day for prevention of deep vein thrombosis. A different regimen is often given to patients with acute thromboembolic events. The usual dose is approximately 24,000 to 30,000 units of heparin daily to maintain a therapeutic antithrombotic effect. Traditionally, a bolus of heparin (usually 5000 units) is given to start treatment; thereafter heparin is given as a continuous intravenous infusion, usually in an hourly dose of 1000 units. Initially, the aPTT value is markedly prolonged, so follow-up assessments are usually delayed until 6 hours after the start of treatment. Depending on the results, the infusion is increased or decreased in increments of 100 U/hour, and the aPTT value is reassessed in 6 hours. This approach, although time-honored, has a number of limitations. It does not account for the marked variations in responses among patients. Some patients underwent excessive anticoagulation with an increased risk of bleeding, whereas others received insufficient anticoagulation with a resultant loss of efficacy. The patient's size is an important variable that affects responses to heparin. In response to this variable, weight-based nomograms have been developed to ease heparin administration (Table 50.2).[15,19,20]

Heparin has anti-inflammatory actions that may be different from the effects on coagulation.[10,11,21] In addition, heparin may have effects on major neurotransmitters in the brain.[22] The relationship between these effects and the potential utility of heparin for treatment of acute brain ischemia is not clear.

Because of the limitations of unfractionated (conventional) heparin, other parenterally administered, rapidly acting anticoagulant medications have been developed.[23] The leading alternatives are danaparoid and the LMW heparins. Potential advantages of these agents include a longer period of antithrombotic action and a more predictable dose–antithrombotic effect in comparison with unfractionated heparin. In addition, the medications have a weaker ability to inhibit thrombin and more selective antithrombotic effects on factor Xa. These agents of biologic origin have been largely created by the chemical or enzymatic depolarization of unfractionated heparin. The LMW heparins weigh approximately 1000 to 10,000 d. Danaparoid is a compound of similar molecular weight that differs slightly in that it consists primarily of heparan sulfate.[24] The reduction into lower-weight compounds leads to lessened binding to platelets, proteins, endothelial cells, and macrophages. These effects probably explain both the longer duration of effect of danaparoid and the LMW heparins as well as the more predictable responses to their use.[25]

The LMW heparins and danaparoid have a reduced effect on thrombin function than unfractionated heparin but the same inhibition of factor Xa. The ratio of inhibition for thrombin and factor Xa is estimated to be 1:2 to 1:4. Because these agents do not affect thrombin activity except in very high concentrations, assessment of the aPTT is unreliable. Rather, measuring inhibition of factor Xa tests the level of anticoagulation. The desired level is 0.3–0.7 U/mL. However, the reliability of laboratory measurements of anti–factor Xa activity is uncertain. Because these agents are excreted renally, the level of anticoagulation may rise in patients with renal failure.[17] An

Table 50.2 Weight-Based Nomogram for Intravenous Heparin Therapy Initial Dose: 80 U/kg Bolus Followed by Infusion at 18 U/kg/hr

aPTT Level	Modification(s)
<35 seconds (approximately <1.2 × control)	Administer another 80 U/kg bolus and increase infusion to 22 U/kg/h Increase hourly dose by 4 U/kg/h
35–45 seconds (approximately 1.2–2.5 × control)	Administer another 40 U/kg bolus and increase infusion to 20 U/kg/h Increase hourly dose by 2 U/kg/h
46–70 seconds (approximately 1.5–2.3 × control)	Continue infusion at 18 U/kg/h
71–90 seconds (approximately 2.3–3 × control)	Decrease infusion to 16 U/kg/h Decrease hourly dose by 2 U/kg/h
>91 seconds (approximately >3 × control)	Interrupt infusion for 1 h Restart infusion at 15 U/kg/h Decrease hourly dose by 3 U/kg/h

Check aPTT at 6 hours and adjust infusion in response to level of aPTT. Recheck aPTT at 6 hours after adjustment and modify regimen as shown.
aPTT, activated partial thromboplastin time.
Adapted from references 15, 19, and 20.

experimental study suggests that the LMW heparins might also have a neuroprotective effect.[26]

Although the LMW heparins and danaparoid can be given intravenously, most research has focused on the subcutaneously administered medications, particularly for prophylaxis against deep vein thrombosis. The usual regimen is an injection twice a day. Initial studies used a relatively uniform dose regardless of the patient's size. However, as with unfractionated heparin, there does appear to be a reason to use a weight-based nomogram in determining dosage for LMW heparins and danaparoid. The responses to the various LMW heparins are generally similar, but the specific pharmacologic effects can differ; thus, these agents should be evaluated individually. In particular, the ratio of antithrombin activity and anti–factor Xa activity can vary among the compounds. As a result, the data about the efficacy and safety of one LMW heparin might not be automatically applicable to another one.

Other Anticoagulants

Because of the lag between initiation of therapy with oral anticoagulants (vitamin K antagonists) and an antithrombotic effect, these agents have not been used in the setting of acute ischemic stroke. In addition, the transient prothrombotic effects of these medications—through initial inhibition of the actions of proteins C and S—limit their applicability.

Several other promising agents are being examined. Direct thrombin inhibitors can affect bound thrombin and produce a more reliable anticoagulant effect than unfractionated heparin. These agents also do not affect platelet function. Hirudin, originally derived from the leech, now is available through recombinant technology.[27,28] This agent is a potent and irreversible inhibitor of thrombin function. It has been used in the treatment of patients with unstable ischemic heart disease.[29] Argatroban is a selective inhibitor that competitively binds at the active site of thrombin. Argatroban has an immediate antithrombotic effect. It has a short half-life, approximately 50 minutes, so anticoagulation can be initiated and terminated more

rapidly with it than with unfractionated heparin or the LMW heparins.

Other natural, noncovalent and covalent thrombin inhibitors are also available.[27] In addition, direct or indirect inhibitors of activated factors VII, IX, and X are being examined.[27] None of these agents has been tested extensively. Activated protein C is produced by the complex of thrombin and thrombomodulin. It inactivates activated factors V and VIII. Several agents, including activated protein C concentrates, are being developed.[27,28] Thus, it is likely that several new anticoagulant agents might be available in the future.

Antiplatelet Agents

The pharmacology of aspirin has been examined extensively.[30–33] Aspirin irreversibly turns off the cyclooxygenase (COX) activity of prostaglandin (PG) H synthase 1 (COX-1) and 2 (COX-2) by the acetylation of a serine residue of the COX channel.[32] Aspirin's effects are approximately 170-fold more potent on platelet COX-1 than on monocyte COX-2.[33] The medication induces a permanent defect of thromboxane A_2–dependent platelet function that induces platelet aggregation and causes vasoconstriction. Aspirin also affects endothelial production of prostacyclin, an agent that inhibits platelet aggregation and induces vasodilation. The potentially prothrombotic effects of prostacyclin inhibition appear to be less clinically relevant, because the endothelium can regenerate new COX—unlike the anuclear platelet, in which COX inhibition is irreversible.[33]

Aspirin has antithrombotic effects in a broad range of doses. Because the effects on endothelial production of prostacyclin may be dose related, lower amounts of aspirin might be more effective than larger doses. Aspirin is readily absorbed, so peak plasma levels occur within 30 to 40 minutes, and inhibition of platelet aggregation is achieved within 1 hour.[32] Enteric coating delays absorption. A single dose of 100 mg of aspirin has an almost immediate effect on platelet aggregation.[34] These effects mean that aspirin might be useful in the setting of acute ischemic stroke. Lower doses of aspirin (<100 mg) might take longer than 24 hours to achieve maximal inhibition of COX.[33] Thus, the minimum initial dose appears to be at least 160 mg; this was the dose of aspirin used in the Chinese Acute Stroke Trial.[35] Additional antithrombotic actions of aspirin might be the result of its ability to facilitate inhibition of platelet activation by neutrophils, which is mediated by nitric oxide, and to enhance production of nitric oxide by the endothelium.[33,36] The utility of aspirin as a neuroprotective agent for use in acute stroke is not established, but there is evidence that strokes might be less severe among patients who have previously used aspirin.[37-39]

Dipyridamole blocks the actions of phosphodiesterase, an effect that in turn limits the re-uptake of adenosine in the platelets.[32] This agent also prolongs platelet survival[40] and produces vasodilation. The interval from initiation of treatment with dipyridamole to the achievement of antiplatelet effects is not established. Presumably, however, there is some lag; as a result, the medication will probably not be used to treat acute ischemic stroke.

Both ticlopidine and clopidogrel inhibit the platelet aggregation induced by adenosine diphosphate (ADP).[31] These medications affect the platelet receptor's interactions with fibrinogen.[19,41] The ability of clopidogrel to inhibit platelet aggregation occurs in a dose-dependent manner.[32,42] Inhibition of platelet function starts within 2 hours after ingestion of a loading dose. As a result, starting clopidogrel with a 300-mg dose might result in rapid achievement of inhibition of platelet aggregation. This attribute has led to the successful use of clopidogrel as treatment of patients with acute myocardial ischemia.[43]

The glycoprotein (integrin) IIB/IIIA receptor antagonists are potent blockers of platelet aggregation.[44-47] These agents do not block platelet adhesion, but they do have an effect on clot formation.[48,49] The new agents affect the binding of fibrinogen to the platelets.[47,49] Their pharmacologic effects vary.[46,50] Among these medications are monoclonal chimeric antibodies that block the receptor.[32] A bolus dose of abciximab can inhibit more than 80% of platelet receptors and maintain antiplatelet effects for several hours.[51] With blockade of more than 90% of platelet receptors, bleeding time is prolonged.[32] A bolus of dose of 0.25 mg/kg of abciximab can affect platelet function within 2 hours of administration.[32,51] Gradual recovery of platelet function occurs over the next 12 hours. An infusion of abciximab can maintain the effects during the subsequent hours. The antiaggregate effects of abciximab are increased by concomitant administration of aspirin.[52] Besides its antiplatelet effects, abciximab may inhibit thrombin formation.[32] The administration of abciximab in combination with other antithrombotics has been used successfully to treat patients with acute coronary artery syndromes.[50,53-57] In at least one trial, abciximab and stenting were superior to thrombolysis in promoting myocardial salvage among patients with acute coronary artery disease.[58]

Tirofiban is a nonpeptide derivative of tyrosine that selectively blocks the glycoprotein IIB/IIIA receptor.[32] The effects of tirofiban are rapid; marked inhibition of platelet aggregation and prolongation of the bleeding time occur within 5 minutes of the start of an intravenous infusion of the medication. These parameters begin to return to

normal within 1.5 hours after the infusion is stopped.[32] Tirofiban is being used to treat acute coronary artery diseases.[50,56] Eptifibatide is a heptapeptide with high affinity and specificity for the glycoprotein IIB/IIIA receptor[32] that also affects integrin-mediated binding of smooth muscle cells to thrombospondin and prothrombin.[59] After treatment of a bolus dose followed by an intravenous infusion of eptifibatide, platelet aggregation is markedly diminished within 1 hour.[32,60] This agent also has effects on thrombin generation and markedly prolongs the bleeding time. After treatment with eptifibatide is stopped, the bleeding time rapidly returns to normal. This agent is used to treat acute ischemic cardiac diseases.[50,56,61-63]

SAFETY OF THE TREATMENT OF ACUTE ISCHEMIC STROKE

Surveys of physicians emphasize their concerns about the safety of antithrombotic agents administered in the acute period of acute ischemic stroke.[12,13] Intracranial hemorrhage, including hemorrhagic transformation of the infarction, is the major complication of any therapy for acute ischemic stroke that exerts it primary effect on coagulation. The risks of major bleeding after treatment of stroke are highlighted by the trials of thrombolytic therapy, several of which were halted prematurely because of bleeding complications.[64-69] Fortunately, later trials of antithrombotic therapy have not been stopped prematurely for this reason.

Besides symptomatic hemorrhagic transformation of the infarction or other intracranial hemorrhage, bleeding complications can occur in other locations with antithrombotic therapy. In addition, some of the antithrombotic agents can be associated with nonhemorrhagic complications. In the past, solid information about the safety of some of these agents was limited. Fortunately, clinical trials have now provided safety data about their use.

Unfractionated Heparin

Although unfractionated heparin has been used extensively for treatment of patients with acute ischemic stroke, information about the associated risk of bleeding complications is limited. Studies performed in the 1960s give little information about bleeding risk.[70-75] Bleeding was not a major problem in the trial conducted by Duke and colleagues.[76] The Cerebral Embolism Study Group did not report bleeding complications related to heparin in a group of 45 patients with presumed embolic stroke.[77] In another report, the same group linked the risk of hemorrhagic complications to the severity of the stroke.[78,79] They also concluded that the use of a bolus dose to initiate heparin treatment might raise the risk of symptomatic intracranial hemorrhage.

Although asymptomatic hemorrhagic transformation is commonly observed after embolic stroke, Japanese investigators noted a higher risk of symptomatic hemorrhage in patients who were treated with heparin.[80] Slivka and Levy[81] reviewed the experience of heparin therapy in 69 patients with progressing stroke, noting that 2 patients had neurologic worsening secondary to intracerebral hemorrhage. In a meta-analysis of available data, Sandercock and associates[82] found that heparin is associated with a significant increase in the risk of hemorrhagic transformation. In 1994, the AHA Stroke Council panel concluded that the data about the safety of heparin in patients with acute stroke were insufficient.[14]

Later data on the safety of heparin are available (Table 50.3). Camerlingo and associates[83] administered heparin within 5 hours of onset of stroke to 45 patients, 2 of whom had symptomatic hemorrhages. A study performed in Spain involved administration of heparin to 83 patients within 72 hours after cardioembolic stroke.[84] Eight patients had symptomatic hemorrhages, which were fatal in 6. Two doses of subcutaneously administered heparin were tested in the International Stroke Trial.[85] Intracranial hemorrhage was diagnosed in 16 of 2429 (0.7%) patients given lower doses and in 43 of 2426 (1.8%) patients receiving higher doses of heparin. In a subgroup analysis of patients with atrial fibrillation, the risk of hemorrhage was listed as 1.3% and 2.8% for lower and higher doses of heparin, respectively.[86] Van den Berg and coworkers[87] reported major hemorrhagic complications in 0.8% of 664 patients who received heparin for treatment of acute cerebral ischemia. On the basis of the experience at the Mayo Clinic, Petty and colleagues[88] calculated that the risk of bleeding with

heparin was 0.3 per 100 person-days. The risk of bleeding with heparin is generally associated with the level of anticoagulation and the dose of medication.[89,90] In addition, the risk of bleeding complications of heparin is higher in women, in people older than 70 years, and in those with renal failure.[89,90]

Heparin has been given in conjunction with thrombolytic agents. Studies of intra-arterially administered prourokinase also included heparin as a concomitant therapy.[91-93] The risk of bleeding approached 10% and was increased with the larger of the two doses of heparin administered. On the other hand, two studies did not find higher risk of bleeding complications when heparin was given shortly after administration of recombinant tissue plasminogen activator (rt-PA).[94,95] Some of the experience accrued after approval of rt-PA by the U.S. Food and Drug Administration (FDA) demonstrated an unacceptably high risk of intracranial hemorrhage with the administration of this agent.[96] Part of the increase in risk in bleeding may be secondary to administration of heparin or other rapidly antithrombotic agents within 24 hours of treatment with rt-PA.

Nonneurologic bleeding can also complicate administration of heparin. In 1990, one study of heparin for

Table 50.3 Rates of Symptomatic Intracranial and Extracranial Hemorrhage with Antithrombotic Treatment of Acute Ischemic Stroke

Trial°	Agent	Intracranial Hemorrhage		Extracranial Hemorrhage	
		N	%	N	%
Unfractionated heparin					
Chamorro	Heparin	8/83	9.6	—	
Camerlingo	Heparin	2/45	4.4	0/45	0
IST	LD heparin	16/2429	0.7	10/2429	0.4
	HD heparin	43/2426	1.8	33/2426	1.4
LMW heparins or danaparoid					
FISS	LD nadroparin	0/100	0	4/100	4.0
	HD nadroparin	0/101	0	6/101	5.9
TOAST	Danaparoid	19/638	2.9	25/638	3.9
FISS-bis	LD nadroparin	10/271	3.7	—	
	HD nadroparin	15/245	6.1	—	
HAEST	Dalteparin	6/224	2.7	13/224	5.8
TOPAS	Certoparin	2/99	2.0	1/99	1.0
	Certoparin	1/102	0.9	0	0
	Certoparin	2/103	1.9	0	0
	Certoparin	4/100	4.0	5/100	5.0
TASIT	LD tinzaparin	3/507	0.6	2/507	0.4
	HD tinzaparin	7/486	1.4	4/486	0.8
Autiplatelet agents					
MAST	Aspirin	3/153	1.9	—	
IST	Aspirin	87/9720	0.9	109/9720	1.1
CAST	Aspirin	115/10335	1.1	86/10335	0.8
HAEST	Aspirin	4/225	1.8	4/225	1.8
TAIST	Aspirin	1/491	0.2	2/491	0.4
Abciximab	Abciximab	0/54	0	0/54	0

HD, high-dose; LD, low-dose; LMW, low-molecular-weight.
°Abciximab = Abciximab in Ischemic Stroke Study[121]; Camerlingo = Camerlingo et al[83]; CAST = Chinese Acute Stroke Trial[35]; Chamorro = Chamorro et al[84]; FISS = Fraxiparine Ischemic Stroke Study[114]; FISS-bis = Second Fraxiparine Ischemic Stroke Study[11]; HAEST = Heparin Aspirin Ischemic Stroke Trial[115]; IST = International Stroke Trial[85]; MAST = Multicenter Acute Stroke Trial–Italy[67]; TAIST = Tinzaparin in Acute Ischemic Stroke[112]; TOAST = Trial of Org 10172 in Acute Stroke Treatment[117]; TOPAS = Therapy of Patients with Acute Stroke.[116]

treatment of evolving stroke reported that 10 of 69 treated patients had bleeding complications; most did not involve intracranial hemorrhage (see Table 50.3).[81] In the International Stroke Trial, extracranial hemorrhage was diagnosed in 33 of 2426 (1.4%) patients given high-dose heparin and in 10 of 2429 patients (0.4%) receiving low-dose heparin (see Table 50.3).[85] The most common locations for serious bleeding are the gastrointestinal tract, urinary system, retroperitoneal space, and joints. These hemorrhages may lead to major morbidity or mortality. Minor hemorrhages, which might necessitate cessation of heparin therapy, include microscopic hematuria, epistaxis, bruising, and minor rectal bleeding.

Heparin should be discontinued if a patient experiences severe bleeding. Protamine sulfate can also be administered. The calculated dosage of protamine is based on the assumption that heparin has a half-life of 60 minutes and that the antidote can correspond to the amount of heparin given in the previous 90 minutes.[16] Approximately 1 mg of protamine sulfate negates the anticoagulant effects of approximately 100 units of heparin. Intravenous protamine sulfate should be administered slowly (at least over 10 minutes) because it can cause hypotension. Anaphylaxis can complicate administration of protamine sulfate.[16]

Osteoporosis can occur with prolonged use of heparin, but this potential complication should not be a major issue during short administration of the anticoagulant. A transient prothrombotic state might follow the sudden discontinuance of treatment with heparin. The frequency and importance of this phenomenon are not clear. However, Slivka and colleagues[97] reported recurrent ischemic events after cessation of heparin given as treatment for stroke.

Thrombocytopenia can complicate treatment with heparin. A modest decline in platelet count can occur in approximately 80% of patients who receive heparin for more than 3 days.[98] Ramirez-Lassepas and coworkers[99] reported a greater than 40% decline in platelet count in 21 of 137 patients with ischemic stroke who were treated with heparin. The decline in platelet count was asymptomatic in most cases. A more severe, autoimmune-mediated thrombocytopenia also can complicate use of heparin.[100–102] Because heparin is a foreign protein, abnormal immunoglobulin (Ig) G or IgM antibodies can be found in many patients exposed to heparin.[103] This finding usually develops between 5 and 15 days after the introduction of heparin.[98,104] However, the prior use of heparin may sensitize a patient, and a second exposure can induce a severe thrombocytopenia within hours. The autoimmune reaction can even complicate administration of a small dose of heparin.

The diagnosis of heparin-induced thrombocytopenia (HIT) is based on an unexplained drop in the platelet count of at least 50% or skin lesions at heparin injection sites and the presence of HIT antibodies. The white clot syndrome, leading to myocardial or cerebral ischemia, can result.[105] The neurologic complications can mimic those of thrombotic thrombocytopenia purpura.[105–107] Because of the considerable risk of thrombocytopenia, platelet counts should be performed every 2 to 3 days in patients receiving heparin. The medication should be stopped if a decline in platelet count is detected. Patients with heparin-associated thrombocytopenia and thrombosis could be treated with recombinant hirudin or argatroban until the platelet count recovers. These therapies should be considered even in patients without thrombosis because of the high risk of overt thrombosis in the week after heparin therapy is stopped.[16] Danaparoid, hirudin, or argatroban could be prescribed for a patient who needs anticoagulation but has a history of heparin-associated thrombocytopenia.[16,24,28,108,109]

Low-Molecular-Weight Heparins and Danaparoid

Bleeding is also the major potential complication of treatment with LMW heparins or danaparoid. Because of a more predictable dose-response relationship, the risk of bleeding might be less with these agents than with unfractionated heparin. Clinical studies in non-stroke settings have shown lower rates of bleeding with LMW heparins and danaparoid.[17,110] The long duration of their pharmacologic effects is a potential disadvantage if serious bleeding occurs. Clotting factors can be administered if a serious hemorrhage is diagnosed, but the effectiveness of this therapy is uncertain.

Several trials have tested the usefulness of a variety of LMW heparins in treatment of acute ischemic stroke (see Table 50.3).[111] All the trials tested subcutaneous administration of the agents, and two trials used a weight-based regimen for administration.[11,112] No major increase in risk of intracranial or extracranial hemorrhage was noted in the Hong Kong studies of nadroparin.[113,114] In a second trial of nadroparin, the risk of symptomatic intracranial hemorrhage was significantly higher.[11] Bleeding was diagnosed in 2.8% of 250 patients given placebo, in 3.7% of 271 patients administered a low dose of nadroparin, and in 6.1% of 245 patients give a higher dose of nadroparin.

In a study comparing aspirin and dalteparin in patients with stroke and atrial fibrillation, symptomatic bleeding was diagnosed in 2.7% of 224 patients given the LMW heparin and 1.8% of patients receiving aspirin.[115] Extracranial hemorrhage was also more common in patients receiving dalteparin. A German trial tested four different doses of certoparin.[116] The risk of symptomatic intracranial bleeding was greatest among the patients receiving the largest dose of the LMW heparin; this group also had a 5% rate of severe extracranial hemorrhage. In a trial testing two doses of tinzaparin in comparison with aspirin, the risk of symptomatic intracranial hemorrhage was 0.2% for aspirin, 0.6% for low-dose tinzaparin, and 1.4% for high-dose tinzaparin.[112] Serious extracranial hemorrhages were not a problem.

Another trial tested the utility of the intravenous administration of danaparoid.[117] The agent was given in a bolus dose followed by an intravenous infusion. The rate of the infusion was adjusted according to the levels of inhibition of factor Xa. Enrollment of patients with more than a moderately severe stroke (judged from the severity of neurologic impairments, as indicated by a score higher than 15 on the National Institutes of Health Stroke Scale [NIH Stroke Scale]) was stopped because of an unacceptably high rate of symptomatic hemorrhagic transformation in patients treated with danaparoid. Overall, the rate of symptomatic brain hemorrhage was 0.9% (6/628) for patients given placebo and 2.9% (19/638) for patients given danaparoid. Extracranial bleeding was also significantly higher with danaparoid (3.9%, vs. 1.1% for placebo). A meta-analysis that combined the results of most of the trials of LMW heparins and danaparoid supports the conclusion that these agents significantly raise the risks of both intracranial and extracranial hemorrhages.[111]

Although thrombocytopenia can complicate the administration of danaparoid and the LMW heparins, the risk appears lower than that for therapy with unfractionated heparin.[102,118] Because of the potential for cross-reactivity, patients who have experienced autoimmune heparin-associated thrombocytopenia should probably not receive the LMW heparins.

Other Antithrombotic Agents

The other rapidly acting antithrombotic agents have not been extensively tested in the setting of acute ischemic stroke. A study of antithrombin reported two hemorrhages among 20 patients who received the medication for treatment of cardioembolic stroke.[119] A study of argatroban was recently completed. Hirudin was tested in the treatment of patients with acute cardiovascular disease, but bleeding occurred with a relatively high frequency[28,29]; because of this high rate of bleeding, hirudin has not been used in treatment of patients with acute ischemic stroke.

Antiplatelet Agents

The long-term administration of aspirin is associated with an increased risk of hemorrhagic stroke.[120] Overall, the likelihood of serious intracranial bleeding is small. The safety of aspirin in the management of patients with acute ischemic stroke has been explored in several trials. Aspirin alone or in combination with streptokinase was tested in a clinical trial.[67] Bleeding was not increased among the patients given aspirin, but the combination of aspirin and streptokinase was associated with a very high rate of serious intracranial bleeding (see Table 50.3). In the Chinese Acute Stroke Trial, 115 bleeding events were reported in 10335 (1.1%) patients who received aspirin within 48 hours of onset of stroke.[35]

The International Stroke Trial examined the safety of aspirin given either alone or in combination with subcutaneously administered heparin.[85] Hemorrhages were reported in 87 of 9720 (0.9%) patients given aspirin. Among the 4858 patients who received only aspirin, the risk of hemorrhagic stroke was 0.5% (26 patients). LMW heparins were compared with aspirin in two trials; in both trials, the frequency of serious intracranial and extracranial bleeding was lower in those patients given aspirin.[112,115] Still, the evidence does show that aspirin is associated with a modest but significant increase (1.9 [standard error 1.0] per 1000 treated) in the risk of intracranial bleeding.[2] Serious extracranial bleeding also can complicate the use of antiplatelet agents.[2]

In another study, the chance of major bleeding complications was greater for patients receiving a combination of clopidogrel and aspirin for treatment of acute myocardial ischemia (3.7%) than in those receiving aspirin alone (2.7%), but the risks of life-threatening and intracranial hemorrhage were not higher.[43] This combination of

medications has not been tested in the setting of acute stroke. A pilot study of abciximab for treatment of acute ischemic stroke did not find symptomatic hemorrhagic transformation in patients receiving the antiplatelet agent, although the rate of asymptomatic hemorrhagic changes detected by CT was higher.[121] Further study of abciximab is under way, and more data about its safety are needed.

Additional experience about the safety of abciximab and other glycoprotein IIb/IIIa receptor blockers in treatment of patients with acute stroke is limited. Junghans and coworkers,[122] administering tirofiban to 17 patients with progressive stroke, noted no major increase in cerebral bleeding complications. Thrombocytopenia is a potential complication of the use of the new antiplatelet agents.[121] In some cases, the declines in platelet count have been profound. Monitoring for a drop in platelet count should therefore be a component of treatment with these new agents.

Conclusions

Clinical trials confirm that both anticoagulants and antiplatelet agents are associated with a modest but significant risk of serious bleeding complications. The odds for both intracranial and extracranial hemorrhage are greater with unfractionated heparin, the LMW heparins, and danaparoid than with aspirin. Information about the other anticoagulants and antiplatelet agents is too limited to make any firm conclusions about their safety.

Some other conclusions about the risk of hemorrhagic transformation of the infarction with anticoagulants can also be drawn from the results of several other studies. Although the risk of bleeding is relatively low with the anticoagulant medications, it is high enough to mandate that strong evidence for efficacy is needed to justify their use. The LMW heparins and danaparoid do not appear to be either more dangerous or safer than unfractionated heparin. The risk of serious bleeding complications increases with the dose of unfractionated heparin or LMW heparin. No data correlate the risk of bleeding with either subcutaneous or intravenous administration of heparin or the LMW compounds. The use of a bolus dose to start anticoagulation does not seem to be particularly dangerous. The likelihood of hemorrhage with heparin or LMW heparin is associated with the severity of neurologic impairments or the size of stroke on the initial brain imaging study. Anticoagulants probably cannot be given with a high level of safety to patients with findings of multilobar infarction. Patients with severe stroke (NIH Stroke Scale score >15) and those with a large area of hypodensity on CT probably should not be treated with either unfractionated heparin or any of the LMW compounds.

The initiation of treatment might be delayed for several days in patients with multilobar infarction; in this situation, an additional brain imaging study might be appropriate to screen for evidence of an asymptomatic hemorrhagic transformation of the ischemic lesion before antithrombotic agents are begun.

Physicians should also be alert to nonneurologic hemorrhagic complications. Patients with active bleeding or other illnesses that portend a high chance of serious bleeding (recent surgery or recent trauma) might be well served by not receiving anticoagulants. Agent-specific issues such as thrombocytopenia also should be kept in mind when administering antithrombotic agents to patients with acute ischemic stroke.

EFFICACY OF TREATMENT OF ACUTE ISCHEMIC STROKE

There has been considerable uncertainty about the efficacy of antithrombotic agents in improving outcomes after acute ischemic stroke. Unless there is strong evidence of efficacy, these medications, which can be associated with serious neurologic or medical complications, should not be administered. Although the medications are widely prescribed, strong clinical data on their efficacy are limited. Stroke treatment guidelines published in 1994 by the AHA Stroke Council panel concluded that there was no conclusive information about the efficacy or lack of efficacy of anticoagulants in the treatment of patients with acute ischemic stroke.[14] The panel could not find any compelling data for any subgroup of patients with stroke regardless of presumed vascular territory or presumed cause. A meta-analysis performed at approximately the same time demonstrated that heparin was effective in lowering the risk of deep vein thrombosis after stroke but that the

medication was not effective in improving outcomes.[82] Most physicians are not prescribing anticoagulants solely as a method to prevent deep vein thrombosis and pulmonary embolism. The goal has been to limit brain injury and improve neurologic outcome. In particular, these agents have been used to halt progressing stroke (*stroke-in-evolution*) or to prevent early recurrent thromboembolism. Some subgroups of patients, such as those with large artery atherosclerosis, cardioembolism, or arterial dissection, often have been preferentially treated with anticoagulants.

Unfractionated Heparin

Several studies of heparin were performed before the development of modern brain imaging methods (Tables 50.4 through 50.6).[70–75,123] In general, these studies' results suggested potential efficacy of emergency administration of heparin. Still, methodologic problems greatly weakened their data. Two studies included randomized assignment to treatment, but the numbers of patients were too few to produce any definitive results.[72,73] Three other studies used historical controls for comparisons.[70,74,75] In the 1980s, a randomized, placebo-controlled trial tested the potential utility of intravenously administered heparin.[76] Approximately 200 patients were enrolled, and most did not receive treatment until more than 24 hours after stroke. To

Table 50.4   Rates of Early Recurrent Stroke with Treatment of Acute Ischemic Stroke

Trial[°]	Agent	Treatment		Comparison Group		
		N	%	Type	N	%
Unfractionated heparin						
IST	LD heparin	78/2429	1.6	Control	214/4859	2.2
	HD heparin	86/2426	1.8			
IST—with atrial fibrillation						
	Heparin	44/1557	2.8	Control	79/1612	4.9
LMW heparins and danaparoid						
FISS	LD nadroparin	2/101	1.9	Placebo	5/105	4.7
	HD nadroparin	1/102	1			
TOAST	Danaparoid	7/638	1.1	Placebo	7/628	1.1
TOAST—cardioembolism						
	Danaparoid	0/143	0	Placebo	2/123	1.6
HAEST	Dalteparin	19/224	8.5	Aspirin	17/225	7.5
TOPAS	Certoparin	3/99	3.0			
	Certoparin	3/102	2.9			
	Certoparin	4/103	3.9			
	Certoparin	3/100	3.0			
TAIST	LD tinzaparin	24/507	4.7	Aspirin	15/491	3.1
	HD tinzaparin	16/486	3.3			
Antiplatelet agents						
MAST	Aspirin	1/153	0.6	Control	0/156	0
CAST	Aspirin	220/10335	2.1	Placebo	214/10320	2.5
IST	Aspirin	275/9719	2.8	Control	368/9714	3.8
HAEST	Aspirin	17/225	7.5	Dalteparin	19/224	8.5
TAIST	Aspirin	15/491	3.2	Tinzaparin	40/993	4.0
Abciximab	Abciximab	1/54	2.0	Placebo	1/20	5.0

HD, high-dose; LD, low-dose; LMW, low-molecular-weight.
[°]Abciximab = Abciximab in Ischemic Stroke Study[121]; CAST = Chinese Acute Stroke Trial[35]; FISS = Fraxiparine Ischemic Stroke Study[114]; HAEST = Heparin Aspirin Ischemic Stroke Trial[115]; IST = International Stroke Trial[85]; MAST = Multicenter Acute Stroke Trial–Italy[67]; TAIST = Tinzaparin in Acute Ischemic Stroke[112]; TOAST = Trial of Org 10172 in Acute Stroke Treatment[117]; TOPAS = Therapy of Patients with Acute Stroke.[116]

Table 50.5 Rates of Neurologic Worsening with Treatment of Acute Ischemic Stroke

| Trial* | Agent | Treatment Group | | Comparison Group | | |
		N	%	Type	N	%
LMW heparins and danaparoid						
TOAST	Danaparoid	63/635	10	Placebo	62/633	9.9
HAEST	Dalteparin	24/224	10.7	Aspirin	17/225	7.6
TAIST	LD tinzaparin	58/508	11.4	Aspirin	58/491	11.9
	HD tinzaparin	58/486	11.9			
Antiplatelet agents						
MAST	Aspirin	18/153	11.8	Control	21/156	13.4
CAST	Aspirin	545/10335	5.3	Placebo	614/10320	5.9
IST	Aspirin	567/4858	11.7	Control	604/4859	12.4
HAEST	Aspirin	17/225	7.6	Dalteparin	24/224	10.7
TAIST	Aspirin	58/491	11.9	Tinzaparin	116/993	11.7
Abciximab	Abciximab	6/54	11.0	Placebo	3/20	15.0

HD, high-dose; LD, low-dose; LMW, low-molecular-weight.

*Abciximab = Abciximab in Ischemic Stroke Study[121]; CAST = Chinese Acute Stroke Trial[35]; HAEST = Heparin Aspirin Ischemic Stroke Trial[115]; IST = International Stroke Trial[85]; MAST = Multicenter Acute Stroke Trial–Italy[67]; TAIST = Tinzaparin in Acute Ischemic Stroke[112]; TOAST = Trial of Org 10172 in Acute Stroke Treatment.[117]

Table 50.6 Rates of Favorable Outcomes with Antithrombotic Treatment of Acute Ischemic Stroke

| Trial* | Agent | Treatment | | Comparison group | | |
		N	%	Type	N	%
Unfractionated heparin						
IST	LD heparin	1776/4860	36.5	Control	3852/9718	36.9
	HD heparin	1802/4856	37.1			
LMW heparins and danaparoid						
FISS	LD nadroparin	48/101	47.5	Placebo	37/105	35.2
	HD nadroparin	57/102	55.8			
TOAST	Danaparoid	482/641	75.2	Placebo	467/634	73.6
FISS-bis	LD nadroparin	155/271	57.2	Placebo	142/250	56.8
	HD nadroparin	145/245	59.2			
HAEST	Dalteparin	76/224	33.9	Aspirin	79/225	35.1
TOPAS	Certoparin	37/96	38.5			
	Certoparin	38/97	39.2			
	Certoparin	36/98	36.7			
	Certoparin	42/96	43.7			
TAIST	LD tinzaparin	188/507	38.3	Aspirin	206/491	42.5
	HD tinzaparin	181/486	38.4			
Antiplatelet agents						
MAST	Aspirin	59/153	38.6	Control	50/156	32.1
CAST	Aspirin	7182/10335	69.5	Placebo	7054/10320	68.3
IST	Aspirin	1860/4858	38.3	Control	1795/4859	36.9
HAEST	Aspirin	79/225	35.1	Dalteparin	76/224	33.9
TAIST	Aspirin	206/491	42.5	Tinzaparin	369/993	38.3
Abciximab	Abciximab	24/54	44.0	Placebo	8/20	40.0

HD, high-dose; LD, low-dose; LMW, low-molecular-weight.

*Abciximab = Abciximab in Ischemic Stroke Study[121]; CAST = Chinese Acute Stroke Trial; FISS = Fraxiparine Ischemic Stroke Study[114]; FISS-bis = Second Fraxiparine Ischemic Stroke Study[11]; HAEST = Heparin Aspirin Ischemic Stroke Trial[115]; IST = International Stroke Trial[85]; MAST = Multicenter Acute Stroke Trial–Italy[67]; TAIST = Tinzaparin in Acute Ischemic Stroke[112]; TOAST = Trial of Org 10172 in Acute Stroke Treatment[117]; TOPAS = Therapy of Patients with Acute Stroke.[116]

be eligible for participation, the patients must have stable neurologic impairments. Not surprisingly, no net benefit of treatment was noted.

In a series of studies, the Cerebral Embolism Study Group[77–79] tested the potential utility of heparin. These studies showed a trend toward a lower rate of recurrent embolization. The investigators also estimated that the risk of recurrent embolization within the first week after stroke could be as high as 12%.[78] On the basis of a retrospective review of 44 patients with embolic stroke, Koller[124] estimated that heparin could halve the risk of early recurrent stroke. However, the meta-analysis performed by

Sandercock and associates[82] could not confirm the efficacy of heparin in improving outcomes after stroke or lowering the risk of recurrent embolism.

In a study that involved initiating treatment with heparin within 5 hours of stroke in 45 patients, improvement was noted in 23 patients.[83] In an uncontrolled study, Dahl and coworkers[125] administered heparin to 52 patients with progressing stroke, and neurologic worsening stopped in 38 patients; 11 patients experienced neurologic worsening despite heparin therapy. Haley and associates[126] found no benefit from heparin when it was administered to 36 patients with progressing stroke. Chamorro and colleagues[54] administered heparin to 231 patients with recent embolic stroke and noted recurrent events in 5 patients. In a historical control study, Roden-Jullig and Britton[127] compared outcomes among 314 patients not receiving heparin with those in 907 patients treated with the anticoagulant therapy. Progression of neurologic deficits was noted in 28% of patients who did not receive heparin and in 21% of those who did, and the investigators concluded that heparin did not improve outcomes. They judged that heparin was not effective in halting neurologic worsening. Another trial reported that recurrent strokes occurred in 2.4% of 664 patients who received heparin for treatment of acute ischemic stroke.[87]

In a very large study that enrolled approximately 20,000 participants, investigators of the International Stroke Trial tested two doses of subcutaneously administered heparin.[85] Within 48 hours of stroke, patients received either 5000 units (low-dose) or 12,500 units (high-dose) of heparin twice a day. Some patients also received aspirin (300 mg/day). The trial does have weaknesses in design. For a sizable number of patients enrolled in the trial, baseline brain imaging studies were not performed beforehand to exclude primary hemorrhage. Thus, some patients with de novo hemorrhage might have been treated. Both the treating physicians and the patients were aware of treatment allocation; this information might have biased the physicians' and patients' reporting of adverse experiences. No monitoring of the level of anticoagulation and no adjustment of doses of heparin were included. As a result, some patients might have received excessive doses of heparin that could raise the risk of major bleeding complications, whereas other patients might have received insufficient doses of heparin and, thus, the effectiveness of therapy might have been lost. The trial demonstrated a modest decline in the frequency of recurrent stroke within the first 14 days with the use of heparin. No reduction in mortality or improvement in the rate of favorable outcomes was seen. As a result, the trial found no net benefit from treatment with heparin. No net benefit from treatment with heparin was noted among the subgroup of patients who had atrial fibrillation.[86]

Low-Molecular-Weight Heparins and Danaparoid

Several trials have tested subcutaneously administered LMW heparins (see Tables 50.4 through 50.6). Two dosages of nadroparin (4100 anti–factor Xa units daily and 4100 anti–factor Xa units twice daily) were tested in a placebo-controlled trial performed by Kay and associates.[114]

Medications were started within 48 hours of stroke and continued for 10 days. No monitoring of anticoagulation or adjustment of doses was performed. Recurrent strokes occurred more frequently in the patients receiving placebo than in either group that received nadroparin. At an assessment performed at 6 months after stroke, excellent outcomes were significantly more common among the patients who received the larger dose of nadroparin than among those who received a placebo. However, no differences in favor of nadroparin were found at the end of treatment or at 3 months. The reason for differences in responses at 3 months and 6 months is not clear. A second trial of nadroparin tested two doses of the LMW heparin against placebo.[11] A weight-based treatment regimen was given, the lower dose was 85 anti–factor Xa units/day, and the larger dose was doubled. The medications were given within 24 hours of onset of stroke, but no monitoring or dose adjustments were included. No improvement in outcomes was noted.

A Norwegian trial tested dalteparin against aspirin in preventing recurrent stroke or improving outcomes in patients with stroke and atrial fibrillation.[115] The presence of the arrhythmia was used as a surrogate for the clinical diagnosis of cardioembolic stroke. Dalteparin was given subcutaneously for 10 days, and no monitoring of anticoagulation or adjustment in the dose of dalteparin was performed. Recurrent strokes occurred in 8.5% of 224 patients treated with dalteparin and 7.5% of 225 patients receiving aspirin. No differences between rates of favorable outcomes in the two treatment groups were seen. German investigators evaluated four doses of subcutaneously administered certoparin (3000 U/day, 3000 U/twice a day, 5000 U/twice a day, or 8000 U/twice a day) in a trial that enrolled approximately 400 patients.[116] Therapy was started within 12 hours of stroke. The levels of anticoagulation were not monitored, and adjustments were not made during the 12 to 16 days of treatment. No differences in the rates of recurrent strokes or favorable outcomes were seen among the groups. In a three-arm treatment trial that enrolled approximately 1500 patients, two different doses of tinzaparin (100 anti–factor Xa U/kg or 175 anti–factor Xa U/kg) were compared with aspirin (300 mg/day).[112] The doses of tinzaparin were not adjusted to the level of anticoagulation. Patients were treated within 48 hours of stroke. No reduction in mortality or improvement in the rate of favorable outcome was seen with either dose of tinzaparin. The presumed cause of stroke did not affect responses to treatment.

Intravenously administered danaparoid was compared with placebo in a randomized trial that enrolled approximately 1300 patients.[117] Patients were treated within 24 hours of stroke. Treatment with danaparoid was initiated with a bolus dose and continued with a continuous infusion for 7 days. Infusion rates were adjusted in response to levels of inhibition of factor Xa, but no weight-based dosage regimen was included. No differences were noted between the two treatment groups in the rates of neurologic worsening or recurrent ischemic stroke. The trial evaluated responses among subgroups of patients with different causes of stroke. Danaparoid did not lessen the risk of early recurrent stroke in the patients with cardioembolism. Although a trend in favor of treatment with danaparoid was noted during the 7 days of acute management, no sustained benefit from treatment was noted at 3 months. Patients with stroke secondary to large artery atherosclerosis seemed to benefit from treatment. This response was not replicated in the trial of tinzaparin described previously.[112] In a meta-analysis of the trials of LMW heparins and danaparoid, Bath and colleagues[111] could not establish efficacy of these agents in any group of patients with acute ischemic stroke.

Other Antithrombotic Agents

Little information is available about the efficacy of other antithrombotic agents. Yasaka and associates[119] administered antithrombin to 20 patients and noted no recurrent stroke events. Additional research is needed about the potential efficacy of these agents in the treatment of stroke.

Antiplatelet Agents

Aspirin has been examined in several clinical trials (see Tables 50.4 through 50.6). In one trial, the rate of favorable outcomes improved when aspirin was administered alone or in combination with streptokinase.[67] Recurrent stroke was observed in only 1 of 153 patients given aspirin alone. In the International Stroke Trial, aspirin 300 mg was given alone to 4858 patients and in conjunction with heparin to 4861 patients.[85] Recurrent stroke was diagnosed in 156 (3.2%) of the patients who received only aspirin and in 119 (2.4%) of the patients who received both aspirin and heparin. The reduction in recurrent events was statistically significant. The rates of recurrent stroke among patients treated with aspirin alone and with heparin, in comparison with the rate in those not receiving aspirin, are shown in Table 50.4. The rate of death or disability was modestly reduced in patients who were treated with either aspirin alone or the combination of heparin and aspirin. The significance of these results was borderline. In the randomized Chinese Acute Stroke Trial, which enrolled more than 20,000 patients, aspirin (160 mg/day) was compared with placebo.[35] Therapy was started within 48 hours of stroke and continued for 28 days. The long interval from onset of stroke to treatment and the long treatment period are sources of concern for this trial; in particular, the long treatment period during which the control group received placebo overlaps with the time that many physicians would consider that long-term stroke preventive medication should have been started. Aspirin reduced the risk of recurrent stroke (rate of stroke in aspirin group, 2.1% [220/10,335] and in placebo group, 2.5% [258/10,320]). The study showed a modest decline in mortality and disability with aspirin (30.5%, vs. 31.6% for placebo). The investigators in both the Chinese and international trials had prespecified a combined overview analysis. When the data from the two large trials were combined, aspirin was shown to have significant effects in preventing recurrent stroke (7 per 1000) with benefit in all subgroups of patients in improving outcomes after stroke.[35,128] In two trials of LMW heparins, aspirin was administered as the control therapy.[112,115] Outcomes were approximately the same in the aspirin and LMW heparin groups.

Small anecdotal studies have reported on the use of glycoprotein IIb/IIIa receptor blockers in a number of patients with ischemic cerebrovascular disease, including during angioplasty and stenting.[129,130] A pilot study of abciximab found that the agent might improve outcomes in patients treated within 24 hours after stroke.[121] The experience with tirofiban is also limited.[122] Additional research is needed to determine whether abciximab and other similarly acting antiplatelet agents are effective in treatment of stroke.

Conclusions

Prevention of Early Recurrent Stroke

The data from clinical trials provide conflicting evidence as to whether early administration of antithrombotic agents is effective in lowering the risk of recurrences during the first days after ischemic stroke. On the basis of information collected from several of the larger trials, the risk of early recurrent stroke is much lower than previously assumed.[35,85,117] A reasonable estimate is that approximately 2% of patients have a recurrent stroke within 1 week of the first event. By 2 weeks, the rate probably increases to between 3% and 4%. Although the risk of recurrent stroke is higher in patients with presumed cardioembolic stroke, the rates are approximately 2% to 8% in the first 7 to 14 days.[85,115,117] However, although the risk of early recurrent stroke is not high, the likelihood of a poorer neurologic outcome after a second event is considerable. Initiation of therapy to prevent this complication is important. Other critical issues are (1) when to start therapies to prevent recurrent stroke, (2) to maintain anticoagulation on a long-term basis, and (3) selection of the best agent for the individual patient.

Because the risk of recurrent embolism is relatively low, demonstration of the efficacy of anticoagulants in lessening the early risk of recurrent stroke will be difficult. Although some trials have not specifically evaluated the utility of anticoagulants in preventing recurrent stroke, others have not confirmed that unfractionated heparin, LMW heparins, or danaparoid is effective in lowering the risk. At present, early anticoagulation is not established as efficacious in preventing early recurrent stroke, including among patients with presumed cardioembolic stroke. No subgroup of patients with stroke who are judged as having a very high risk for recurrent stroke and who might benefit from emergency anticoagulation has been identified.

Results of the large trials of aspirin are somewhat conflicting. Although aspirin lowered the risk of early recurrent ischemic stroke, the benefit from aspirin was reduced when the aggregate of hemorrhagic or ischemic stroke was evaluated.[2,35,85,128] In two trials of LMW heparin, aspirin was administered as the control medication.[111,115] In the trial conducted by Berge and coworkers,[115] the rate of recurrent events in patients with atrial fibrillation and stroke who were treated with aspirin was slightly lower than that in those who were treated with dalteparin. Overall, the results suggest that aspirin started within 48 hours of stroke can produce a modest benefit in reducing the risk of early recurrent stroke.[128] Thus, starting aspirin within 48 hours of the event is a reasonable treatment option for most patients with ischemic stroke. The decision to start aspirin should be influenced by other therapies administered in the acute period. Aspirin should not be started in lieu of other effective treatments for acute stroke, such as rt-PA. Aspirin should not be started sooner than 24 hours after the administration of rt-PA.

Halting Neurologic Worsening (Stroke-in-Evolution)

Neurologic worsening is associated with a greater likelihood of poor neurologic outcome, so preventing this deterioration should be a primary focus of acute stroke care.[131] As a result, antithrombotic agents are often prescribed to patients who are judged to be at risk for neurologic deterioration. Although such worsening can occur in up to 40% of patients, exactly who will have deterioration cannot be predicted with certainty.[131,132] Some patients can be diagnosed through direct observation of stroke-in-evolution. Others can be judged as having a high risk for neurologic worsening on the basis of clinical findings. Neurologic decline seems to be more common with strokes in the vertebrobasilar circulation than in the carotid circulation.[133] Patients with multilobar or large brainstem strokes have a high risk for neurologic worsening. Unfortunately, these patients also have a high risk for hemorrhagic complications secondary to early administration of anticoagulants. In addition, neurologic worsening can be secondary to a number of medical or neurologic complications of stroke that might not be ameliorated by antithrombotic agents. Severe brain edema, acute hydrocephalus, seizures, electrolyte disturbances, and infections all are potential causes of neurologic decline.[134–137] None of these conditions is likely to be successfully treated with antithrombotic agents.

The clinical trials that have examined the impact of anticoagulants on halting neurologic worsening have reported negative results.[112,115,117] Overall, the risk of neurologic deterioration within the first 7 to 10 days after stroke was approximately 10% whether or not the patient received anticoagulation therapy. No superiority in reducing the likelihood of neurologic worsening was seen for anticoagulants in comparison with aspirin or placebo. These disappointing results are similar to those reported for uncontrolled trials in which anticoagulants were administered to patients with presumed stroke-in-evolution.[125–127] Overall, the data suggest that the effect of antithrombotic therapy in halting neurologic deterioration after stroke is likely to be small.

Improving Neurologic Outcomes

The data from the clinical trials of unfractionated heparin and LMW heparins or danaparoid are similar.[11,85,112,114,116,117] Overall, the trials do not demonstrate a net long-term benefit from initiation of anticoagulant therapy within the first 12 to 48 hours after stroke. There is no demonstrated decline in mortality or disability after stroke in patients receiving such therapy. Although there are real differences between the individual trials, probably reflecting the nature of the populations enrolled in the studies, all show a similar overall trend. The success with unfractionated heparin is not better or worse than that achieved with the LMW heparins. The likelihood of a therapeutic response does not seem to be influenced by the route of administration, the use of a bolus dose to start therapy, or the level of anticoagulation.

One trial noted a sustained favorable response to emergency anticoagulation in one subgroup of patients with acute stroke—those with symptomatic large artery atherosclerosis.[117] A subsequent trial was not able to confirm this finding.[112] Still, there is interest in the potential utility of anticoagulants for cases of symptomatic stenosis or occlusion of the internal carotid artery.[138] These cases might be recognized acutely through a combination of clinical findings, brain imaging, and noninvasive assessment of the carotid artery (carotid duplex ultrasonography, computed tomographic angiography, or magnetic resonance angiography). Additional testing of the role of anticoagulants in this group of patients is warranted.

Most of the information about the utility of aspirin comes from two large trials.[35,85] Although there are marked differences between the two studies in the rates of favorable outcomes, their aggregate data suggest that starting aspirin within 48 hours of stroke is associated with a modest improvement in the rate of favorable outcomes. The results are sufficiently positive that they can serve as a stimulus for future research on the usefulness of aspirin and other rapidly acting antiplatelet agents in the emergency treatment of stroke.

PREVENTION OF DEEP VEIN THROMBOSIS

Deep vein thrombosis and pulmonary embolism are potentially life-threatening complications of ischemic stroke.[134,139] The risk of these complications is greatest in bedridden patients with paralysis of the lower extremities. In this group of patients, the rate of deep vein thrombosis is estimated to be approximately 25% to 50%.[140,141] Pulmonary embolism accounts for approximately 5% to 25% of deaths after stroke.[141,142] Several measures, including early mobilization, can prevent deep vein thrombosis.[143]

Antithrombotic agents are the principal medical therapy for prevention or treatment of venous thromboembolism.[144–149] Kelly and associates[142] concluded that the short-term subcutaneous administration of low-dose unfractionated heparin did not have a sustained benefit in forestalling venous thromboembolic disease. However, other studies have concluded that there is a benefit from the early administration of these anticoagulants to patients with recent stroke.[82] Unfractionated heparin, the LMW heparins, and danaparoid are all effective and safe.[150–152] Some research has implied that the LMW compounds are superior to unfractionated heparin.[153,154] On the other hand, these medications are more expensive than conventional heparin.

The current evidence suggests that anticoagulants are effective in lowering the risk of deep vein thrombosis and, presumably, pulmonary embolism among high-risk bedridden patients with recent stroke. Guidelines for management recommend that an anticoagulant (usually subcutaneously administered heparin, LMW heparin, or danaparoid) be part of the ancillary care.[14,155] Anticoagulants might not be given to some patients at high risk of hemorrhagic transformation, such as those with a multilobar infarction. Aspirin also lowers the risk of deep vein thrombosis and pulmonary embolism.[156] Antiembolic stockings and external pneumatic calf compression devices can also reduce the risk of deep vein thrombosis and could be prescribed for a patient who cannot undergo anticoagulant therapy.[157] Intravenous infusions of heparin are usually prescribed to patients who experience pulmonary embolism.[158] Because of the gravity of the pulmonary complication, patients who are seriously ill from stroke are usually given such therapy; subsequently, they receive oral anticoagulants.

OTHER INDICATIONS

With initiation of therapy, warfarin affects levels of the antithrombotic factors proteins C and S before its effects on prothrombin activity are detected. Thus, a transient hypercoagulable state could occur during the first days after the start of warfarin therapy. This complication is most commonly detected among persons who have an inherited or acquired deficiency of protein C or protein S.[159,160] The purple toe syndrome is the leading clinical finding in this situation.[161] Neurologic worsening secondary to a transient warfarin-induced hypercoagulable state has not been described. Nevertheless, because of the concern about this risk, a brief course of intravenous anticoagulation with heparin can be used to protect the patient during the initiation of warfarin therapy.[162] The utility of this tactic is not known, however. An alternative approach is to start warfarin therapy with low doses of the medication so that inhibitions of both the prothrombotic and antithrombotic factors occur at approximately the same time.[163,164] Overall, this issue does not seem to be a primary indication for short-term intravenous anticoagulant therapy among patients with recent stroke.

Anticoagulation has been recommended for patients with stroke due to arterial dissection.[165] No randomized trials have compared anticoagulant treatment with antiplatelet therapy for extracranial carotid dissection, and a review of nonrandomized studies did not show any evidence of a significant difference. A randomized trial to answer this question would require at least 1000 patients in each treatment arm.[166]

CURRENT STATUS OF ANTITHROMBOTIC THERAPY

The latest clinical trials provide little support for the emergency administration of rapidly acting anticoagulant medications for treatment of patients with acute ischemic stroke.[7, 167,168] Anticoagulants are associated with a small but statistically significant risk of intracranial bleeding, including hemorrhagic transformation of the infarction. Still, the risk of bleeding is lower than that attributed to emergency administration of thrombolytic agents. Anticoagulant therapy is also accompanied by a risk of nonneurologic bleeding that can be potentially serious. Current data do not show that emergency anticoagulation has a therapeutic effect in preventing early recurrent stroke, halting neurologic worsening, or improving neurologic outcomes.

Although emergency anticoagulation is not established as efficacious, many physicians persist in prescribing anticoagulant therapy. Anticoagulants are often prescribed in the setting of neurologic worsening or a presumed high risk for recurrent stroke and for a patient who cannot be treated with other therapies, including rt-PA.[169] In this situation, the physician and patient should recognize that the value of emergency anticoagulation is not confirmed. If anticoagulants are prescribed, steps should be taken to assure the patient's safety. Anticoagulants should not be prescribed until the presence of a brain hemorrhage has been excluded on a CT scan. Anticoagulant therapy should be delayed for several days if the CT shows a multilobar infarction or if the patient has severe neurologic impairment. Anticoagulants should not be started within 24 hours of treatment with rt-PA; in this situation, a follow-up CT study should be performed to screen for asymptomatic hemorrhagic transformation of the stroke before anticoagulation is started. Monitoring of both the level of anticoagulation, to avoid overdose, and the platelet count should help reduce the risk of major complications. Determining the most likely cause of stroke and starting long-term stroke prophylactic therapies (either oral anticoagulants or antiplatelet agents) could limit the exposure to heparin.

The data suggest that aspirin provides a modest benefit in reducing recurrent events and improving outcomes among patients with recent stroke.[170] Its utility in the emergency management of stroke (within the first few hours) is not clear. Use of this agent should not be regarded as equal to thrombolytic therapy in improving outcomes after stroke. Still, starting treatment with aspirin within the first 48 hours after stroke seems prudent. Starting antiplatelet agents could eliminate the need for anticoagulants. There appear to be no particular limitations for starting aspirin with regard to severity of stroke as determined from clinical or CT criteria. Aspirin should not be given within the first 24 hours after treatment with rt-PA.

FUTURE OF ANTITHROMBOTIC THERAPY

Although the current data show that rapidly acting antithrombotic agents have a limited role in the immediate treatment of patients with acute ischemic stroke, research continues. Several clinical trials of anticoagulants are under way. Perhaps one or more of these trials will be able to establish the utility of anticoagulants. The rationale for the potential utility of these agents remains. There may be subgroups of patients, such as those with severe disease of the extracranial internal carotid artery, who benefit from treatment. Patients with acute occlusion of the internal carotid artery could have recurrent artery-to-artery embolism or hypoperfusion to the hemisphere that might be improved with anticoagulation. Some groups of patients with cardioembolic stroke, such as those with an intraventricular or intra-atrial thrombus, might be helped by anticoagulants.

Most of the later trials have enrolled patients whose strokes were relatively old (up to 48 hours); it is possible that emergency anticoagulation administered within a very short time is successful. The maximum interval from stroke until treatment is not known. However, Chamorro[10,11] is treating patients seen within 12 hours of onset of stroke, administering unfractionated heparin in a regimen similar to that used in the trial of danaparoid.[117] One of the reasons for testing heparin again is to search for any potential anti-inflammatory effect of the agent that might lessen the neurologic consequences of the infarction. Additional trials are testing promising antithrombotic agents, including argatroban and abciximab.

The primary role of antithrombotic agents in the future might be as part of a combination of interventions. Antiplatelet agents and anticoagulants already are given in combination or in conjunction with thrombolytic agents or angioplasty to patients with unstable coronary artery disease. A similar approach might be useful in patients with stroke. The medications could be given as an adjunct to mechanical or pharmacologic thrombolysis or neuroprotective therapies. The adjunctive use of these agents might maintain efficacy of thrombolytic agents while reducing the risk of major bleeding complications if the dose of the thrombolytic medication can be reduced. A few studies have used the combination of thrombolytic agents and anticoagulants or antiplatelet agents.[91,92,94,95] Although the preliminary data are promising, considerable additional research is needed. Several clinical trials testing thrombolytic therapy combined with either anticoagulants or antiplatelet agents will probably be performed in the future.

References

1. Albers GW, Amarenco P, Easton JD, et al: Antithrombotic and thrombolytic therapy for ischemic stroke. Chest 119:300S–320S, 2001.
2. Collaborative meta-analysis of randomised trials of antiplatelet therapy for prevention of death, myocardial infarction, and stroke in high risk patients. Antithrombotic Trialists' Collaboration. BMJ 324:71–86, 2002.
3. Burgin WS, Staub L, Chan W, et al: Acute stroke care in non-urban emergency departments. Neurology 57:2006–2012, 2001.
4. Phillips SJ: An alternative view of heparin anticoagulation in acute focal brain ischemia. Stroke 20:295–298, 1989.
5. Caplan LR: When should heparin be given to patients with atrial fibrillation-related embolic brain infarcts? Arch Neurol 56:1059–1060, 1999.
6. Chaves CJ, Caplan LR: Heparin and oral anticoagulants in the treatment of brain ischemia. J Neurol Sci 173:3–9, 2000.
7. Sandercock P: Intravenous unfractionated heparin in patients with acute ischemic stroke: A treatment to be used in the context of randomized trials only. Stroke 32:57, 2001.
8. Sandercock P: Is there still a role for intravenous heparin in acute stroke? No. Arch Neurol 56:1160–1161, 1999.
9. Chamorro A, Vila N, Ascaso C, Blanc R: Heparin in acute stroke with atrial fibrillation: Clinical relevance of very early treatment. Arch Neurol 56:1098–1102, 1999.
10. Chamorro A: Immediate anticoagulation in acute focal brain ischemia revisited: Gathering the evidence. Stroke 32:577–578, 2001.
11. Chamorro A: Heparin in acute ischemic stroke: The case for a new clinical trial. Cerebrovasc Dis 9(Suppl 3):16–23, 1999.
12. Marsh EE, Adams HP Jr, Biller J, et al: Use of antithrombotic drugs in the treatment of acute ischemic stroke: A survey of neurologists in practice in the United States. Neurology 39:1631–1634, 1989.
13. Anderson DC: How Twin Cities neurologists treat ischemic stroke: Policies and trends. Arch Neurol 50:1098–1103, 1993.
14. Adams HP Jr, Brott TG, Crowell RM, et al: Guidelines for the management of patients with acute ischemic stroke: A statement for healthcare professionals from a special writing group of the Stroke Council, American Heart Association. Circulation 90:1588–1601, 1994.
15. Hirsh J, Warkentin TE, Raschke R, et al: Heparin and low-molecular-weight heparin: Mechanisms of action, pharmacokinetics, dosing considerations, monitoring, efficacy, and safety. Chest 114:489S–510S, 1998.
16. Hirsh J, Anand SS, Halperin JL, Fuster V: Guide to anticoagulant therapy: Heparin. Circulation 103:2994–3018, 2001.
17. Hirsh J, Warkentin TE, Shaughnessy SG, et al: Heparin and low-molecular-weight heparin: Mechanisms of action, pharmacokinetics, dosing, monitoring, efficacy, and safety. Chest 119:64S–94S, 2001.
18. Fareed J, Callas D, Hoppensteadt DA, et al: Antithrombin agents as anticoagulants and antithrombotics: Implications in drug development. Med Clin N Am 82:569–586, 1998.
19. Becker RC, Ansell J: Antithrombotic therapy: An abbreviated reference for clinicians. Arch Intern Med 155:149–161, 1995.
20. Raschke RA, Reilly BM, Guidry JR, et al: The weight-based heparin dosing nomogram compared with a "standard care" nomogram: A randomized controlled trial. Ann Intern Med 119:874–881, 1993.
21. Lever R, Page C: Glycosaminoglycans, airways inflammation and bronchial hyperresponsiveness. Pulm Pharmacol Ther 14:249–254, 2001.
22. Kondashevskaya MV, Kudrin VS, Klodt PM, et al: New aspects of heparin effects. Bull Exp Biol Med 130:1134–1137, 2000.
23. Hirsh J, Weitz JI: New antithrombotic agents. Lancet 353:1431–1436, 1999.
24. Magnani HN: Heparin-induced thrombocytopenia (HIT): An overview of 230 patients treated with orgaran (Org 10172). Thromb Haemost 70:554–561, 1993.
25. Laposata M, Green D, Van Cott EM, et al: College of American Pathologists Conference XXXI on laboratory monitoring of anticoagulant therapy: The clinical use and laboratory monitoring of low-molecular-weight heparin, danaparoid, hirudin and related compounds, and argatroban. Arch Pathol Lab Med 122:799–807, 1998.
26. Mary V, Wahl F, Uzan A, Stutzmann JM: Enoxaparin in experimental stroke: Neuroprotection and therapeutic window of opportunity. Stroke 32:993–999, 2001.
27. Weitz JI, Hirsh J: New anticoagulant drugs. Chest 119:95S–107S, 2001.
28. Hirsh J: New anticoagulants. Am Heart J 142:S3–S8, 2001.
29. Topol EJ, Fuster V, Harrington RA, et al: Recombinant hirudin for unstable angina pectoris: A multicenter, randomized angiographic trial. Circulation 89:1557–1566, 1994.
30. Roth GJ, Calverley DC: Aspirin, platelets, and thrombosis: Theory and practice. Blood 83:885–898, 1994.
31. Harker LA: Therapeutic inhibition of platelet function in stroke. Cerebrovasc Dis 8(Suppl 5):8–18, 1998.
32. Patrono C, Coller B, Dalen JE, et al: Platelet-active drugs. Chest 119:39S–63S, 2001.
33. Awtry EH, Loscalzo J: Aspirin. Circulation 101:1206–1218, 2000.
34. Burch JW, Stanford N, Majerus PW: Inhibition of platelet prostaglandin synthetase by oral aspirin. J Clin Invest 61:314–319, 1978.
35. CAST: Randomised placebo-controlled trial of early aspirin use in 20,000 patients with acute ischaemic stroke. CAST (Chinese Acute Stroke Trial) Collaborative Group. Lancet 349:1641–1649, 1997.
36. Nagamatsu Y, Tsujioka Y, Hashimoto M, et al: The differential effects of aspirin on platelets, leucocytes and vascular endothelium in an in vivo model of thrombus formation. Clin Lab Haematol 21:33–40, 1999.
37. Grotta JC, Lemak NA, Gary H, et al: Does platelet antiaggregant therapy lessen the severity of stroke? Neurology 35:632–636, 1985.
38. Kalra L, Perez I, Smithard DG, Sulch D: Does prior use of aspirin affect outcome in ischemic stroke? Am J Med 108:205–209, 2000.
39. Wilterdink JL, Bendixen B, Adams HP Jr, et al: Effect of prior aspirin use on stroke severity in the Trial of Org 10172 in Acute Stroke Treatment (TOAST). Stroke 32:2836–2840, 2001.
40. Rivey MP, Alexander MR, Taylor JW: Dipyridamole: A critical evaluation. Drug Intell Clin Pharm 18:869–880, 1984.
41. Verstraete M, Zoldhelyi P: Novel antithrombotic drugs in development. Drugs 49:856–884, 1995.

42. Harker LA, Marzec UM, Kelly AB, et al: Clopidogrel inhibition of stent, graft, and vascular thrombogenesis with antithrombotic enhancement by aspirin in nonhuman primates. Circulation 98:2461–2469, 1998.

43. Yusuf S, Zhao F, Mehta SR, et al: Effects of clopidogrel in addition to aspirin in patients with acute coronary syndromes without ST-segment elevation. N Engl J Med 345:494–502, 2001.

44. Coller BS, Anderson K, Weisman HF: New antiplatelet agents: Platelet GPIIb/IIIa antagonists. Thromb Haemost 74:302–308, 1995.

45. Theroux P: Oral inhibitors of platelet membrane receptor glyco-protein IIb/IIIa in clinical cardiology: Issues and opportunities. Am Heart J 135:S107–S112, 1998.

46. Dickfeld T, Ruf A, Pogatsa-Murray G, et al: Differential antiplatelet effects of various glycoprotein IIb–IIIa antagonists. Thromb Res 101:53–64, 2001.

47. Proimos G: Platelet aggregation inhibition with glycoprotein IIb–IIIa inhibitors. J Thromb Thrombolysis 11:99–110, 2001.

48. Fintel DJ: From bench to bedside: GP IIb–IIIa inhibitors. Neurol-ogy 57:S12–S19, 2001.

49. Frelinger AL 3rd, Furman MI, Krueger LA, et al: Dissociation of glycoprotein IIb/IIIa antagonists from platelets does not result in fibrinogen binding or platelet aggregation. Circulation 104:1374–1379, 2001.

50. Bhatt DL, Topol EJ: Current role of platelet glycoprotein IIb/IIIa inhibitors in acute coronary syndromes. JAMA 284:1549–1558, 2000.

51. Tcheng JE, Ellis SG, George BS, et al: Pharmacodynamics of chimeric glycoprotein IIb/IIIa integrin antiplatelet antibody Fab 7E3 in high-risk coronary angioplasty. Circulation 90:1757–1764, 1994.

52. Schneider DJ, Baumann PQ, Holmes MB, et al: Time and dose dependent augmentation of inhibitory effects of abciximab by aspirin. Thromb Haemost 85:309–313, 2001.

53. Topol EJ, Califf RM, Weisman HF, et al: Randomised trial of coro-nary intervention with antibody against platelet IIb/IIIa integrin for reduction of clinical restenosis: results at six months. The EPIC Investigators. Lancet 343:881–886, 1994.

54. Topol EJ: Prevention of cardiovascular ischemic complications with new platelet glycoprotein IIb/IIIa inhibitors. Am Heart J 130:666–672, 1995.

55. Topol EJ, Mark DB, Lincoff AM, et al: Outcomes at 1 year and economic implications of platelet glycoprotein IIb/IIIa blockade in patients undergoing coronary stenting: Results from a multicentre randomised trial. Lancet 355:2019–2024, 2000.

56. Vernon SM: Glycoprotein IIb/IIIa antagonists and low-molecular-weight heparin in acute coronary syndromes. Cardiology Clinics 19:235–252, 2000.

57. Topol EJ, Moliterno DJ, Herrmann HC, et al: Comparison of two platelet glycoprotein IIb/IIIa inhibitors, tirofiban and abciximab, for the prevention of ischemic events with percutaneous coronary revascularization. N Engl J Med 344:1888–1894, 2001.

58. Schoning M, Klein R, Krageloh-Mann I, et al: Antiphospholipid antibodies in cerebrovascular ischemia and stroke in childhood. Neuropediatrics 25:8–14, 1994.

59. Lele M, Sajid M, Wajih N, Stouffer GA: Eptifibatide and 7E3, but not tirofiban, inhibit alpha(v)beta(3) integrin-mediated binding of smooth muscle cells to thrombospondin and prothrombin. Circula-tion 104:582–587, 2001.

60. Gilchrist IC, O'Shea JC, Kosoglou T, et al: Pharmacodynamics and pharmacokinetics of higher-dose, double-bolus eptifibatide in per-cutaneous coronary intervention. Circulation 104:406–411, 2001.

61. O'Shea JC, Hafley GE, Greenberg S, et al: Platelet glycoprotein IIb/IIIa integrin blockade with eptifibatide in coronary stent inter-vention: The ESPRIT trial: A randomized controlled trial. JAMA 285:2468–2473, 2001.

62. Marso SP, Bhatt DL, Roe MT, et al: Enhanced efficacy of eptifi-batide administration in patients with acute coronary syndrome requiring in-hospital coronary artery bypass grafting. PURSUIT Investigators. Circulation 102:2952–2958, 2000.

63. Lincoff AM, Harrington RA, Califf RM, et al: Management of patients with acute coronary syndromes in the United States by platelet glycoprotein IIb/IIIa inhibition: Insights from the platelet glycoprotein IIb/IIIa in unstable angina: Receptor suppression using Integrilin therapy (PURSUIT) trial. Circulation 102:1093–1100, 2000.

64. Donnan GA, Davis SM, Chambers BR, et al: Streptokinase for acute ischemic stroke with relationship to time of administration. Australian Streptokinase (ASK) Trial Study Group. JAMA 276:961–966, 1996.

65. Hommel M, Boissel JP, Cornu C, et al: Termination of trial of streptokinase in severe acute ischaemic stroke. MAST Study Group. Lancet 345:57, 1995.

66. Intracerebral hemorrhage after intravenous t-PA therapy for ischemic stroke. The NINDS t-PA Stroke Study Group. Stroke 28:2109–2118, 1997.

67. Randomised controlled trial of streptokinase, aspirin, and combina-tion of both in treatment of acute ischaemic stroke. Multicentre Acute Stroke Trial—Italy (MAST-I) Group. Lancet 346:1509–1514, 1995.

68. Thrombolytic therapy with streptokinase in acute ischemic stroke. Multicenter Acute Stroke Trial—Europe Study Group. N Engl J Med 335:145–150, 1996.

69. The National Institute of Neurological Disorders and Stroke rt-PA Stroke Study Group. Tissue plasminogen activator for acute ischemic stroke. N Engl J Med 333:1581–1587, 1995.

70. Millikan CH: Therapeutic agents—current status: Anticoagulant therapy in cerebrovascular disease. In Siekert RD, Whisnant JP (eds): Cerebral Vascular Disease, Fourth Conference. New York, Grune & Stratton, 1965, pp 181–184.

71. Millikan CH, McDowell FH: Treatment of progressing stroke. Stroke 12:397–409, 1981.

72. Carter AB: Anticoagulation treatment in progressing stroke. Br Med J 2:70–73, 1961.

73. Baker RN, Broward JA, Fong HC, et al: Anticoagulant therapy in cerebral infarction: Report on cooperative study. Neurology 12:823–835, 1962.

74. Fisher CM: Use of anticoagulants in cerebral thrombosis. Neurol-ogy 8:311–332, 1958.

75. Fisher CM: Anticoagulant therapy in cerebral thrombosis and cerebral embolism: A national cooperative study, interim report. Neurology 11:119–131, 1961.

76. Duke RJ, Bloch RF, Turpie AG, et al: Intravenous heparin for the prevention of stroke progression in acute partial stable stroke. Ann Intern Med 105:825–828, 1986.

77. Immediate anticoagulation and embolic stroke: A randomized trial. Cerebral Embolism Study Group. Stroke 14:668–676, 1983.

78. Immediate anticoagulation of embolic stroke: Brain hemorrhage and management options. Cerebral Embolism Study Group. Stroke 15:779–789, 1984.

79. Cardioembolic stroke, early anticoagulation, and brain hemorrhage. Cerebral Embolism Study Group. Arch Intern Med 147:636–640, 1987.

80. Okada Y, Yamaguchi T, Minematsu K, et al: Hemorrhagic transfor-mation in cerebral embolism. Stroke 20:598–603, 1989.

81. Slivka A, Levy D: Natural history of progressive ischemic stroke in a population treated with heparin. Stroke 21:1657–1662, 1990.

82. Sandercock PA, van den Belt AG, Lindley RI, Slattery J: Antithrom-botic therapy in acute ischaemic stroke: An overview of the com-pleted randomised trials. J Neurol Neurosurg Psychiatry 56:17–25, 1993.

83. Camerlingo M, Casto L, Censori B, et al: Immediate anticoagula-tion with heparin for first-ever ischemic strokes in the carotid artery territories observed within 5 hours of onset. Arch Neurol 51:462–467, 1994.

84. Chamorro A, Vila N, Saiz A, et al: Early anticoagulation after large cerebral embolic infarction: A safety study. Neurology 45:861–865, 1995.

85. The International Stroke Trial (IST): A randomised trial of aspirin, subcutaneous heparin, both, or neither among 19,435 patients with acute ischaemic stroke. International Stroke Trial Collaborative Group. Lancet 349:1581, 1997.

86. Saxena R, Lewis S, Berge E, et al: Risk of early death and recur-rent stroke and effect of heparin in 3169 patients with acute ischemic stroke and atrial fibrillation in the International Stroke Trial. Stroke 32:2333–2337, 2001.

87. van den Berg E, Lohmann N, Friedburg D, Rabe F: Report of general temporary anticoagulation in the treatment of acute cere-bral and retinal ischaemia. Vasa 26:222–227, 1997.

88. Petty GW, Brown RD Jr, Whisnant JP, et al: Frequency of major complications of aspirin, warfarin, and intravenous heparin for secondary stroke prevention. Ann Intern Med 130:14–22, 1999.

89. Levine M, Raskob GE, Landefeld CS, et al: Hemorrhagic complications of anticoagulant treatment. Chest 108(Suppl):276S–290S, 1995.

90. Levine MN, Raskob G, Landefeld S, Kearon C: Hemorrhagic complications of anticoagulant treatment. Chest 114(Suppl):511S–523S, 1998.

91. del Zoppo GJ, Higashida RT, Furlan AJ, et al: PROACT: A phase II randomized trial of recombinant pro-urokinase by direct arterial delivery in acute middle cerebral artery stroke. PROACT Investigators. Prolyse in Acute Cerebral Thromboembolism. Stroke 29:4–11, 1998.

92. Furlan AJ, Higashida R, Wechsler L, et al: Recombinant prourokinase (r-ProUK) in acute cerebral thromboembolism: Initial trial results. PROACT II Investigators. Stroke 30:234, 1999.

93. Furlan A, Higashida R, Wechsler L, et al: Intra-arterial prourokinase for acute ischemic stroke. The PROACT II Study: A randomized controlled trial. JAMA 282:2003–2011, 1999.

94. Grond M, Rudolf J, Neveling M, et al: Risk of immediate heparin after rt-PA therapy in acute ischemic stroke. Cerebrovasc Dis 7:318–323, 1997.

95. Trouillas P, Nighoghossian N, Derex L, et al: Thrombolysis with intravenous rtPA in a series of 100 cases of acute carotid territory stroke: Determination of etiological, topographic, and radiological outcome factors. Stroke 29:2529–2540, 1998.

96. Katzan IL, Furlan AJ, Lloyd LE, et al: Use of tissue-type plasminogen activator for acute ischemic stroke: The Cleveland area experience. JAMA 283:1151–1158, 2000.

97. Slivka A, Levy DE, Lapinski RH: Risk associated with heparin withdrawal in ischaemic cerebrovascular disease. J Neurol Neurosurg Psychiatry 52:1332–1336, 1989.

98. Horne MK, Alkins BR: Platelet binding of IgG from patients with heparin-induced thrombocytopenia. J Lab Clin Med 127:435–442, 1996.

99. Ramirez-Lassepas M, Cipolle RJ, Rodvold KA, et al: Heparin induced thrombocytopenia in patients with cerebrovascular ischemic disease. Neurology 34:736–740, 1986.

100. Atkinson JL, Sundt TMJ, Kazmier FJ, et al: Heparin-induced thrombocytopenia and thrombosis in ischemic stroke. Mayo Clin Proc 63:353–361, 1988.

101. Becker PS, Miller VT: Heparin-induced thrombocytopenia. Stroke 20:1449–1459, 1989.

102. Kappers-Klunne MC, Boon DM, Hop WC, et al: Heparin-induced thrombocytopenia and thrombosis: A prospective analysis of the incidence in patients with heart and cerebrovascular diseases. Br J Haematol 96:442–446, 1997.

103. Greinacher A, Potzsch B, Amiral J, et al: Heparin-associated thrombocytopenia: Isolation of the antibody and characterization of a multimolecular PF4-heparin complex as the major antigen. Thromb Haemost 71:247–251, 1994.

104. Gupta AK, Kovacs MJ, Sauder DN: Heparin-induced thrombocytopenia. Ann Pharmacother 32:55–59, 1998.

105. Boon DM, Michiels JJ, Tanghe HL, Kappers-Klunne MC: Heparin-induced thrombocytopenia with multiple cerebral infarctions simulating thrombotic thrombocytopenic purpura: A case report. Angiology 47:407–411, 1996.

106. Pohl C, Klockgether T, Greinacher A, et al: Neurological complications in heparin-induced thrombocytopenia. Lancet 353:1678–1679, 1999.

107. Pohl C, Harbrecht U, Greinacher A, et al: Neurologic complications in immune-mediated heparin-induced thrombocytopenia. Neurology 54:1240–1245, 2000.

108. Lewis BE, Walenga JM, Wallis DE: Anticoagulation with Novastan (argatroban) in patients with heparin-induced thrombocytopenia and heparin-induced thrombocytopenia and thrombosis syndrome. Semin Thromb Hemost 23:197–202, 1997.

109. Kanagasabay RR, Unsworth-White MJ, Robinson G, et al: Cardiopulmonary bypass with danaparoid sodium and ancrod in heparin-induced thrombocytopenia. Ann Thorac Surg 66:567–569, 1998.

110. Turpie AG, Gent M, Cote R, et al: A low-molecular-weight heparinoid compared with unfractionated heparin in the prevention of deep vein thrombosis in patients with acute ischemic stroke: A randomized, double-blind study. Ann Intern Med 117:353–357, 1992.

111. Bath PM, Iddenden R, Bath FJ: Low-molecular-weight heparins and heparinoids in acute ischemic stroke: A meta-analysis of randomized controlled trials. Stroke 31:1770–1778, 2000.

112. Bath PM, Lindenstrom E, Boysen G, et al: Tinzaparin in acute ischaemic stroke trial (TAIST): A randomised aspirin-controlled trial. Lancet 358:683–684, 2001.

113. Kay R, Wong KS, Woo J: Pilot study of low-molecular-weight heparin in the treatment of acute ischemic stroke. Stroke 25:684–685, 1994.

114. Kay R, Wong KS, Yu YL, et al: Low-molecular-weight heparin for the treatment of acute ischemic stroke. N Engl J Med 333:1588–1593, 1995.

115. Berge E, Abdelnoor M, Nakstad PH, et al: Low-molecular-weight heparin versus aspirin in patients with acute ischaemic stroke and atrial fibrillation: A double-blind randomised study. HAEST Study Group. Lancet 355:1205–1210, 2000.

116. Diener HC, Ringelstein EB, von Kummer R, et al: Treatment of acute ischemic stroke with the low-molecular-weight heparin certoparin. Stroke 32:22–29, 2001.

117. Low molecular weight heparinoid, ORG 10172 (danaparoid), and outcome after acute ischemic stroke: A randomized controlled trial. The Publications Committee for the Trial of ORG 10172 in Acute Stroke Treatment (TOAST) Investigators. JAMA 279:1265–1272, 1998.

118. Warkentin TE, Levine MN, Hirsh J, et al: Heparin-induced thrombocytopenia in patients treated with low-molecular-weight heparin or unfractionated heparin. N Engl J Med 332:1330–1335, 1995.

119. Yasaka M, Yamaguchi T, Moriyasu H, et al: Antithrombosis III and low-dose heparin in acute cardioembolic stroke. Cerebrovasc Dis 5:35–42, 1995.

120. He J, Whelton PK, Vu B: Aspirin and risk of hemorrhagic stroke. JAMA 280:1930–1935, 1998.

121. Abciximab in acute ischemic stroke: A randomized, double-blind, placebo-controlled, dose-escalation study. The Abciximab in Ischemic Stroke Investigators. Stroke 31:601–609, 2000.

122. Junghans U, Seitz RJ, Aulich A, et al: Bleeding risk of tirofiban, a nonpeptide GPIIb/IIIa platelet receptor antagonist in progressive stroke: An open pilot study. Cerebrovasc Dis 12:308–312, 2001.

123. Gentling E, Barnett HJM, Fields WS, et al: Cerebral ischemia: The role of thrombosis and antithrombotic therapy. Stroke 8:150–175, 1977.

124. Koller RL: Recurrent embolic cerebral infarction and anticoagulation. Neurology 32:283–285, 1982.

125. Dahl T, Sandset PM, Abildgaard U: Heparin treatment in 52 patients with progressive ischemic stroke. Cerebrovasc Dis 4:101–105, 1994.

126. Haley EC Jr, Kassell NF, Torner JC: Failure of heparin to prevent progression in progressing ischemic infarction. Stroke 19:10–14, 1988.

127. Roden-Jullig A, Britton M: Effectiveness of heparin treatment for progressing ischaemic stroke: Before and after study. J Intern Med 248:287–291, 2001.

128. Chen ZM, Sandercock P, Pan HC, et al: Indications for early aspirin use in acute ischemic stroke: A combined analysis of 40,000 randomized patients from the Chinese Acute Stroke Trial and the International Stroke Trial. On behalf of the CAST and IST collaborative groups. Stroke 31:1240–1249, 2000.

129. Qureshi AI, Suri FK, Khan J, et al: Abciximab as an adjunct to high-risk carotid or vertebrobasilar angioplasty: Preliminary experience. Neurosurgery 46:1316–1325, 2000.

130. Bednar MM, Gross CE: Antiplatelet therapy in acute cerebral ischemia. Stroke 30:887–893, 1999.

131. Roden-Jullig A: Progressing stroke: Epidemiology. Cerebrovasc Dis 7(Suppl 5):2–5, 1997.

132. Tai H, Uchiyama S, Ohara K, et al: Deteriorating ischemic stroke in 4 clinical categories classified by the Oxfordshire Community Stroke Project. Stroke 31:2049–2054, 2000.

133. Yamamoto H, Bogousslavsky J, Van Melle G: Different predictors of neurological worsening in different causes of stroke. Arch Neurol 55:481–486, 1998.

134. van der Worp HB, Kappelle LJ: Complications of acute ischaemic stroke. Cerebrovasc Dis 8:124–132, 1998.

135. Davalos A, Castillo J: Potential mechanisms of worsening. Cerebrovasc Dis 7(Suppl 5):19–24, 1997.

136. Davalos A, Cendra E, Teruel J, et al: Deteriorating ischemic stroke: Risk factors and prognosis. Neurology 40:1865–1869, 1990.

137. Castillo J: Deteriorating stroke: Diagnostic criteria, predictors, mechanisms and treatment. Cerebrovasc Dis 9(Suppl 3):1–8, 1999.

138. Adams HP Jr, Bendixen BH, Leira EC, et al: Antithrombotic treatment of ischemic stroke among patients with occlusion or severe stenosis of the internal carotid artery. Neurology 53:122–125, 1999.

139. Wijdicks EF, Scott JP: Pulmonary embolism associated with acute stroke. Mayo Clin Proc 72:297–300, 1997.

140. Warlow C, Ogston D, Douglas AS: Deep vein thrombosis in the legs after stroke. BMJ 1:1178–1188, 1976.

141. Oppenheimer S, Hachinski V: Complications of acute stroke. Lancet 339:721–724, 1992.

142. Kelly J, Rudd A, Lewis R, Hunt BJ: Venous thromboembolism after acute stroke. Stroke 32:262–267, 2001.

143. Langhorne P: Measures to improve recovery in the acute phase of stroke. Cerebrovasc Dis 9(Suppl 5):2–5, 1999.

144. Desmukh M, Bisignani M, Landau P, Orchard TJ: Deep vein thrombosis in rehabilitating stroke patients: Incidence, risk factors and prophylaxis. Am J Phys Med Rehabil 70:313–316, 1991.

145. McCarthy ST, Turner JJ, Robertson D, et al: Low-dose heparin as a prophylaxis against deep-vein thrombosis after acute stroke. Lancet 2:800–801, 1977.

146. McCarthy ST, Turner J: Low-dose subcutaneous heparin in the prevention of deep-vein thrombosis and pulmonary emboli following acute stroke. Age Ageing 15:84–88, 1986.

147. Sandset PM, Dahl T, Stiris M, et al: A double-blind and randomized placebo-controlled trial of low molecular weight heparin once daily to prevent deep-vein thrombosis in acute ischemic stroke. Semin Thromb Hemost 16(Suppl):25–33, 1990.

148. Turpie AG: Prophylaxis of venous thromboembolism in stroke patients. Semin Thromb Hemost 23:155–157, 1997.

149. Clagett GP, Anderson FA Jr, Geerts W, et al: Prevention of venous thromboembolism. Chest 114:531S–560S, 1998.

150. Turpie AG, Levine MN, Hirsh J, et al: Double-blind randomised trial of Org 10172 low-molecular-weight heparinoid in prevention of deep-vein thrombosis in thrombotic stroke. Lancet 1(8532):523–526, 1987.

151. Prandoni P, Lensing AW, Buller HR, et al: Comparison of subcutaneous low-molecular-weight heparin with intravenous standard heparin in proximal deep-vein thrombosis. Lancet 339:441–445, 1992.

152. Samama MM, Cohen AT, Darmon JY, et al: A comparison of enoxaparin with placebo for the prevention of venous thromboembolism in acutely ill medical patients. Prophylaxis in Medical Patients with Enoxaparin Study Group. N Engl J Med 793:800, 1999.

153. Gould MK, Dembitzer AD, Doyle RL, et al: Low-molecular-weight heparins compared with unfractionated heparin for treatment of acute deep venous thrombosis: A meta-analysis of randomized, controlled trials. Ann Intern Med 130:800–809, 1999.

154. Koopman MM, Buller HR: Low-molecular-weight heparins in the treatment of venous thromboembolism. Ann Intern Med 128:1037–1039, 1998.

155. Brott T, Bogousslavsky J: Treatment of acute ischemic stroke. N Engl J Med 343:710–722, 2000.

156. Prevention of pulmonary embolism and deep vein thrombosis with low dose aspirin: Pulmonary Embolism Prevention (PEP) trial. Pulmonary Embolism Prevention (PEP) Trial Collaborative Group. Lancet 355:1295–1302, 2000.

157. Kamran SI, Downey D, Ruff RL: Pneumatic sequential compression reduces the risk of deep vein thrombosis in stroke patients. Neurology 50:1683–1688, 1998.

158. Hyers TM, Agnelli G, Hull RD, et al: Antithrombotic therapy for venous thromboembolic disease. Chest 114:561S–578S, 1998.

159. Sallah S, Abdallah JM, Gagnon GA: Recurrent warfarin-induced skin necrosis in kindreds with protein S deficiency. Haemostasis 28:25–30, 1998.

160. Krahn MJ, Pettigrew NM, Cuddy TE: Unusual side effects due to warfarin. Can J Cardiol 14:90–93, 1998.

161. Hyman BT, Landas SK, Ashman RF, et al: Warfarin-related purple toes syndrome and cholesterol microembolization. Am J Med 82:1233–1237, 1987.

162. Litin SC, Gastineau DA: Current concepts in anticoagulant therapy. Mayo Clin Proc 70:266–272, 1995.

163. Harrison L, Johnston M, Massicotte MP, et al: Comparison of 5-mg and 10-mg loading doses in initiation of warfarin therapy. Ann Intern Med 126:133–136, 1997.

164. Crowther MA, Ginsberg JB, Kearon C, et al: A randomized trial comparing 5-mg and 10-mg warfarin loading doses. Arch Intern Med 159:46–48, 1999.

165. Schievink WI: Spontaneous dissection of the carotid and vertebral arteries. N Engl J Med 344:898–905, 2001.

166. Lyrer P, Engelter S: Antithrombotic drugs for carotid artery dissection. Cochrane Database Syst Rev CD000255, 2000.

167. Gubitz G, Counsell C, Sandercock P, Signorini D: Anticoagulants for acute ischaemic stroke. Cochrane Database Syst Rev CD000024, 2000.

168. Gubitz G, Sandercock P: Different doses of anticoagulant for acute ischaemic stroke. Cochrane Database Syst Rev Issue 1, 2001.

169. Grau AJ, Hacke W: Is there still a role for intravenous heparin in acute stroke? Yes. Arch Neurol 56:1159–1160, 1999.

170. Gubitz G, Sandercock P, Counsell C: Antiplatelet therapy for acute ischaemic stroke. Cochrane Database Syst Rev CD000029, 2001.

Chapter Fifty-One

General Stroke Management and Stroke Units

Markku Kaste and Risto O. Roine

Only thrombolytic therapy and stroke unit care have been shown to improve the outcome of stroke. Intravenous (IV) and intra-arterial delivery of thrombolysis were discussed in Chapters 48 and 49. This chapter characterizes stroke unit care, including all aspects of general stroke management that can optimally be delivered in stroke units. There is strong evidence that treatment of patients with ischemic stroke in stroke units significantly results in lower rates of death, dependency, and the need for institutional care than treatment on general medical wards (level I evidence). The acute stroke unit is a key element in the critical care pathway and the chain of recovery of a patient with stroke after emergency care in the emergency department.[1]

SHORT HISTORY OF STROKE UNITS

The first stroke units were established in North America in the 1960s. They were modeled after coronary care units but failed to have any effect on mortality or morbidity.[2–4] In the 1970s, rehabilitation stroke units were created, which involved multidisciplinary teams and staff education, but their effects were not evaluated critically.[5] Non–intensive care acute stroke units supplemented by early mobilization and rehabilitation were created in the 1970s and 1980s in North America,[6,7] the United Kingdom,[8] and Scandinavia.[9–11] At first they focused on diagnosis, prevention of complications, education of staff, and research but soon also included early rehabilitation, involvement of family, and multidisciplinary team work. Two studies verified that organized stroke care could improve the recovery of the patient with stroke.[8,11]

The findings of the two studies, demonstrating better functional outcome for patients treated in stroke units than for those treated on general medical wards, led to a number of randomized trials, the majority of which were carried out in the UK and Scandinavian countries.[10–24] Langhorne and coworkers,[25] the first to perform a meta-analysis on the results of these trials, showed that stroke unit care saves lives. The Stroke Unit Trialists' Collaboration then verified these results and demonstrated that organized care in stroke units also reduced the rate of both death or institutional care and death or dependency.[26]

STROKE UNIT DESIGN

The observed benefits are apparent for a wide variety of stroke services, including stroke centers, acute stroke units, combined acute and rehabilitation stroke units, rehabilitation stroke units admitting patients after a delay of 1 or 2 weeks, and mobile stroke teams.[27]

A *stroke center* consists of a comprehensive stroke service that offers the infrastructure to bring patients as quickly as possible to the stroke center. It provides immediate diagnosis and treatment as well as early rehabilitation, and refers patients to the appropriate further treatment, rehabilitation, and secondary prevention. A stroke center offers not only acute stroke unit services but also 24-hour availability of laboratory, neuroradiologic, and ultrasonographic diagnostic services as well as neurosurgical and cardiologic services (Table 51.1).[28] Stroke centers need a large catchment area, and most often, they are a part of a large teaching hospital located in a metropolitan area.

Stroke units provide a disease-specific service in a geographically defined area of a hospital ward and are exclusively dedicated to the management of patients with stroke. Such units can be organized in a variety of medical departments—neurology, internal medicine, geriatric medicine, and rehabilitation medicine. The most distinctive features are a coordinated multidisciplinary team, specialization (i.e. medical and nursing expertise in stroke and rehabilitation), educational programs for the staff, and involvement of caregivers. These basic principles of the Scandinavian model for a combined acute-rehabilitation stroke unit have been scientifically evaluated in Umeå, Sweden; Trondheim, Norway; and Helsinki, Finland.[11,19,22] Germany has established national guidelines for stroke units. According to the German guidelines, stroke units are divided into different levels according to equipment and staff, but they should all have computed tomography (CT) scanning and a diagnostic ultrasonography available 24 hours a day.[29,30]

Mixed assessment-rehabilitation units, which in essence are generic disability services, have an interest and expertise in the assessment and rehabilitation of disabling illnesses but do not exclusively manage patients with stroke. These units often combine acute admission with a period

Table 51.1   Requirements for Acute Stroke Units (modified from Kaste et al, 2000)

Minimum requirements for stroke centers	Written protocols for diagnostic and treatment guidelines and operational procedures for medical and nursing staff
	Availability of CT 24 hours a day
	Availability of blood tests 24 hours a day, including immediate availability of coagulation parameters
	Availability of neurosonographic investigations 24 hours a day (color-coded duplex ultrasonography of extracranial vessels and transcranial Doppler ultrasonography of intracranial vessels)
	Continuous or frequent monitoring of blood pressure, levels of blood gases and blood glucose, and body temperature
	Continuous ECG monitoring and availability of echocardiography within 24 hours
	Close cooperation of neurologists, internists, neuroradiologists, and neurosugeons in evaluation and treatment
	Trained nursing staff specialized in acute care of stroke
	Early rehabilitation, including physical therapy, speech therapy, neuropsychology, and occupational therapy
	Established network of rehabilitation facilities
Additional facilities recommended in acute stroke units	Diffusion and perfusion MRI and MRA
	CT angiography and perfusion CT
	Transesophageal echocardiography
	Cerebral angiography

CT, computed tomography; ECG, electrocardiogram; MRA, magnetic resonance angiography; MRI, magnetic resonance imaging. Modified from Kaste M, Skyhöj Olsen T, Bogousslavsky J, et al: Organization of stroke care: Education, stroke units, and rehabilitation. EUSI Executive Committee. Cerebrovas Dis 10 (Suppl 13): 1–11, 2000.

of rehabilitation, whereas delayed admission units admit patients after at least one week. The results of the Stroke Unit Trialists' Collaboration demonstrated that both types of units can positively influence outcome for patients with stroke.[31,32]

All the different models of stroke unit care incorporate specialist multidisciplinary team care coordinated through weekly meetings. The mixtures of staff available are similar in organized stroke unit settings and conventional care settings, consisting of medical nurses, physiotherapy staff, occupational therapists, speech therapists, and social workers.[33] The main difference is in the practice and organization of care. Stroke unit care most often includes a coordinated multidisciplinary team, staffing by people with an interest in stroke, staff education programs, routine provision of information to patients and caregivers, and involvement of caregivers as well as technical and human resources for delivering stroke unit care (Table 51.2). All members of the team must know the principles of good medical care and early rehabilitation and how to deliver it. The specialized rehabilitation personnel in conventional care settings usually work only during ordinary working hours, whereas at stroke units, the patients are treated 24 hours a day. Accordingly, all members of the staff in stroke units must be capable of participating in the rehabilitation.

EFFECTIVENESS OF STROKE UNIT CARE

Most randomized trials of stroke unit care have involved a relatively small number of patients and, accordingly, have not been able to verify differences in hard endpoints, such as case-fatality rates. A meta-analysis of those trials have verified, however, that patients receiving stroke unit care are more likely to survive, return home, and regain physical independence. Furthermore, secondary complications of stroke are less common in patients receiving stroke unit care.[31] Table 51.3 summarizes the results of the Stroke Unit Trialists' Collaboration.[31] In the United Kingdom, stroke unit care has been shown to be more effective than either stroke team or domiciliary management of stroke.[34]

WHO BENEFITS?

Subgroup analyses of randomized trials revealed that all patients, regardless of age, sex, and severity of stroke, benefit from stroke unit care (Table 51.4).[31] The only exceptions are patients admitted in coma, whose high case-fatality rate is not affected by stroke unit care. The numbers are relatively small but suggest that elderly patients and patients with severe stroke benefit most. Young patients and patients with mild strokes have better outcomes regardless of where they receive care.

Patients with mild strokes do not gain benefit from stroke unit care in terms of increased survival, but more survivors of mild stroke are independent in their daily lives. Approximately 25 mild strokes need to be treated in order for stroke unit care to result in more independent survivors (NNT [number of patients needed to be treated to make statistical difference] = 25). For patients with moderate stroke, the NNT is 17 for one more survivor and 33 for one more independent survivor. For patients with severe stroke, the NNT is 17 for one more survivor but 100 for one more independent survivor. Because of the small

Table 51.2 Characteristics of Stroke Unit Care and Conventional Care (Modified from Langhorne and Dennis, 1998)

Characteristic(s)	Stroke Unit Care	Conventional Care
Coordination of rehabilitation		
Multidisciplinary team and weekly meetings	All	Some
Caregivers routinely involved	Most	Some
Specialization of staff		
Physicians interested in stroke	Most	Some
Physicians interested in rehabilitation	Most	Some
Nurses interested in stroke	Most	Some
Nurses interested in rehabilitation	Most	Some
Education, training, and research		
Regular staff training	Most	Some
Routine information provision to Caregivers	Most	Some
Participation in stroke trials	Some	Some
Comprehensiveness of rehabilitation input		
All who need receive physical and occupational therapy	Most	Some
Earlier start of physical and occupational therapy	Most	Some
Protocol for medical investigations and treatment	Some	None
Intensity of input		
Enhanced nurse-to-patient ratio	Some	Some
More intensive physical and occupational therapy	Some	Some

Modified from Langhorne P, Dennis M: Stroke Units: An Evidence-Based Approach. London, BMJ Books, 1998.

Table 51.3 Stroke Unit Care versus Conventional Care: Outcome at the End of Follow-Up

Outcome	Stroke Unit (n/N)	Control (n/N)	Stroke Units Better°
Death	340/1626	417/1623	0.81 (0.68, 0.96)
Death or institutional care	640/1597	755/1600	0.75 (0.65, 0.87)
Death or dependency	843/1409	944/1421	0.71 (0.60, 0.84)

°Expressed as odds ratio (95% confidence interval fixed).
Modified from Langhorne P, Dennis M: Stroke Units: An Evidence-Based Approach. London, BMJ Books, 1998.

Table 51.4 Organized Stroke Unit Care versus Conventional Care: Death or Institutional Care at the End of Follow-up

			Stroke Units Better° (Risk of death or institutional care)	
	Stroke Unit (n/N)	Control (n/N)	OR	95 CI Fixed
Sex				
Female	172/418	193/384	0.77	(0.60, 0.98)
Male	120/366	158/364	0.66	(0.51, 0.85)
Age				
<75 years	241/839	273/796	0.77	(0.63, 0.94)
≥75 years	202/398	290/7422	0.69	(0.56, 0.85)
Severity				
Mild	36/287	47/273	0.95	(0.66, 1.36)
Moderate	279/649	317/627	0.70	(0.58, 0.84)
Severe	179/229	199/232	0.55	(0.38, 0.81)

°Expressed as odds ratio (95% confidence interval fixed).
Modified from Langhorne P, Dennis M: Stroke Units: An Evidence-Based Approach. London, BMJ Books, 1998.

numbers, all these figures are imprecise, and the 95% confidence interval (CI) includes the possibility of no benefit. However, the results suggest that there is no firm reason to exclude patients from stroke unit care on the basis of gender, age, or stroke severity.

Stroke unit care seems to be beneficial in all types of settings. In systematic review, the mean reduction in proportion of patients dead or institutionalized at late follow-up was 26% in geriatric medicine stroke units, 28% in general medicine stroke units, 28% in neurologic stroke units, and 33% in rehabilitation medicine stroke units.[33]

ARE THERE LONG-TERM BENEFITS OF STROKE UNIT CARE?

Both of the only trials of stroke unit care with a 5-year follow-up demonstrate that the odds ratio (OR) for adverse outcomes continue to favor stroke unit care.[35–37] The ORs are for death, 0.63 (0.45, 0.89); for death or institutional care, 0.62 (0.43, 0.89); and for death or dependency, 0.59 (0.38, 0.92). The first study extended the follow-up to 10 years after stroke and found a similar pattern of results. The ORs in this study are for death, 0.46 (0.23, 0.91); for death or institutional care, 0.40 (0.18, 0.86); and for death or dependency, 0.62 (0.26, 1.46).[38]

THE REBIRTH OF INTENSIVE CARE STROKE UNITS

With the advent of new invasive therapeutic modalities, such as hypothermia and hemicraniectomy in malignant middle cerebral artery infarction, the need for intensive stroke care has re-emerged.[39] Effectiveness of these therapies has not yet been documented in randomized trials, nor has the effectiveness of intensive care stroke units.

AVAILABILITY OF STROKE UNIT CARE

The Pan-European Consensus Meeting on Stroke Management, jointly organized by the World Health Organization (WHO) Regional Office for Europe and the European Stroke Council, recommended that stroke units should be established on a large scale throughout Europe, so that by the year 2005, all patients in Europe with acute stroke should have access to care in specialized stroke units or from stroke teams.[40] Development of such stroke units has begun, particularly in Germany and the Northern European countries. In Sweden, already about 70% of patients with stroke are treated in stroke units, according to the Swedish national quality assessment register for stroke care, Riks-stroke.[41] The Norwegian Board of Health has recommended that all hospitals treating patients with stroke should have stroke units. In Germany, patients with stroke are treated nationwide in stroke units, and according to the German Stroke Data Bank, the results are equally as good as those published by the Stroke Unit Trialists' Collaboration in 1997.[42]

GENERAL STROKE MANAGEMENT

A general recommendation of the European Stroke Initiative (EUSI) is that all patients with stroke should be treated in specialized stroke units.[28] The acute stroke unit is the third step in the critical pathway for stroke, after prehospital emergency care and care in the emergency department (see Chapter 47). Prevention of recurrent stroke and early rehabilitation are important aspects of stroke management in stroke units; these issues are thoroughly reviewed in Chapters 56 and 60. The main goals of stroke care at a stroke unit are shown in Table 51.5; the criteria for admission to an acute stroke unit are summarized in Table 51.6.

Vital Functions

The clinical condition of the patient with acute stroke should have been stabilized in the emergency department, before arrival at the acute stroke unit. For a patient in whom any of the ABCs of vital function (airway, breathing, and cardiovascular function) is compromised, intensive care facilities are used for as long as the clinical situation is unstable. The exceptions are patients in whom the prognosis is obviously poor, a fatal course is inevitable, or there are other reasons to withhold aggressive therapies. In other words, the patient should be stabilized in the emergency department before the next step of the critical pathway— to the acute stroke unit—is taken.

The decision where to treat the patient depends on local resources and the level of care and monitoring at the stroke unit; some stroke units do have intensive care facilities, such as continuous arterial blood pressure monitoring, central venous catheters, mechanical ventilators, and

Table 51.5 **Main Goals of Stroke Care in an Acute Stroke Unit**

Maintenance of vital functions
Recanalization of the occluded cerebral artery
Treatment of unstable cerebral ischemia and prevention of progressing stroke
Prevention and treatment of infarct edema
Prevention of acute medical complications
Prevention of recurrent stroke
Early rehabilitation

Table 51.6 **Criteria for Admission to an Acute Stroke Unit**

Acute large hemispheric stroke
Acute posterior stroke
Unstable cerebral ischemia with fluctuating or progressing symptoms
Thrombolytic and other therapies aiming at recanalization
Therapies targeted at improvement in cerebral perfusion pressure
Therapeutic trials in acute stroke
Unstable cardiovascular status
Compromised ventilatory function
Other imminent medical complications
Patient has a reasonable chance of independent recovery

continuous positive airway pressure (CPAP) ventilation. The vital functions of a patient with stroke are stable if (1) the patient has a secure airway and ventilatory function, (2) the blood pressure is not extremely high or low, (3) the cardiac rhythm is hemodynamically sufficient, and (4) unstable coronary ischemia is not present. Endotracheal intubation is indicated for patients with reduced consciousness, and controlled ventilation is needed for patients with spontaneous hypoventilating.

The patient with acute stroke, even the one with milder symptoms or with stable vital functions, must be recognized as an urgently ill medical patient.[43-45] Even transitory, rapidly resolving, or fluctuating symptoms may be associated with complete acute occlusion of the internal carotid artery (ICA) or even occlusion of the middle cerebral artery (MCA) trunk in patients with excellent collateral circulation. If the artery is not recanalized, the situation is likely to lead to embolic complications of the progressing thrombus and to worsening of the patient's clinical status. In some cases, hemodynamic ischemia may accentuate the symptoms, if the patient is dehydrated, hypotensive or is immediately mobilized without knowledge of the state of recanalization.

Recanalization

The first goal during the hyperacute stage at the scene and of the emergency medical services (EMS) personnel and again in the emergency department is to define whether the patient is a candidate for thrombolytic therapy . Intravenous and intra-arterial thrombolysis is extensively covered in other chapters and is not touched upon here (see Chapters 48 and 49).

Even if the patient is not a candidate for thrombolysis, the next step is to rapidly evaluate whether or not the occluded cerebral artery has already been recanalized.[46] Fortunately, several methods are readily available in most stroke centers. The intraluminal thrombus is often visible as a hyperdensity on the initial CT scan, showing as the characteristic dense media sign but also as the dense posterior, anterior, or basilar artery sign.[47] In borderline cases, the CT diagnosis can be difficult, and persistent arterial occlusion can be suspected only because of calcified atherosclerotic arteries. If the dense artery sign matches the perfusion defect in perfusion CT images, the artery has not recanalized.[48,49] CT angiography, if available, will answer this question. Magnetic resonance angiography (MRA) is also sensitive but is more time consuming and is not always readily available to diagnose lack of blood flow in the artery. The same holds true for single-photon emission computed tomography (SPECT) using fluorodeoxyglucose (FDG) or hexamethyl-propyleneamineoxime (HM-PAO) and for positron emission tomography (PET) using FDG.

The dynamic recanalization process calls for more feasible methods that can be repeated at the bedside or used in continuous monitoring mode. Transcranial Doppler (TCD) ultrasonography is a dynamic monitoring method available at the bedside; it is based on blood flow velocity measurement using Doppler ultrasonography (see Chapter 21). The demonstration of recanalization with TCD ultrasonography is very straightforward, and the method can be used to follow the recanalization process as

it is actually taking place.[50] Typical recanalization patterns of the MCA with repeated TCD ultrasonography measurements have been reported in patients.[51] A new Thrombolysis in Brain Ischemia (TIBI) classification, analogous to the angiographic Thrombolysis in Myocardial Ischemia (TIMI) classification to measure residual flow and recanalization of cardiac vessels, has been developed for noninvasive monitoring of intracranial vessel residual flow signals with TCD ultrasonography. TIBI classification as determined by emergency TCD ultrasonography correlated with initial stroke severity, clinical recovery, and mortality in patients with stroke who were treated with intravenous tissue-plasminogen activator (t-PA), and a flow-grade improvement has been found to correlate with clinical improvement.[51,52]

Unstable Cerebral Ischemia and Progressing Stroke

The unstable phase of cerebral ischemia generally extends up to the point that recanalization is complete and, in some cases, beyond, depending on the status of the cerebrovascular tree and the overall cardiopulmonary condition of the patient. The unstable phase is characterized both by persisting arterial occlusion and by fluctuating symptoms due to reduced perfusion or embolization of the thrombus that may or may not be accentuated if the blood pressure falls or as the patient is mobilized.[53]

"Progressing stroke" is an old concept, originated before the era of modern imaging technology. Development of the penumbral area into infarction has been demonstrated by several perfusion methods, including perfusion-weighted imaging (PWI), which is based on magnetic resonance imaging (MRI); deterioration of the clinical condition of the patient has many potential reasons, however, only a few of which are directly related to the thrombus itself.[54] Because of the heterogeneous nature of progressing stroke, it is not a feasible concept to use for research or clinical decision-making unless the diagnosis is based on recanalization, mismatched patterns on diffusion-weighted imaging (DWI) and PWI, or both. Treatment of progressing symptoms can be successful only if the pathophysiologic mechanism or multiple mechanisms behind the deterioration have been clarified. The main reasons for progressing stroke include most of the acute complications, which can be prevented in well-organized stroke unit care and, if they do occur, can be treated (Table 51.7).

Prevention and Treatment of Infarct Edema and Elevated Intracranial Pressure

Patients with large hemispheric strokes, defined as exceeding 50% of the MCA territory, are at risk for development of cerebral edema that could produce mass effect and may lead to herniation. The clinical picture is that of a progressive decline in level of consciousness, sighing, and vomiting, followed by decorticate or decerebrate posturing and pupillary dilation as the herniation proceeds. Intracranial pressure (ICP) is not usually elevated during the early phase of herniation, but there may be a gradient between the hemispheres that can be observed even noninvasively by TCD ultrasonography. Direct monitoring of

Table 51.7   **Reasons for Deterioration in Acute Ischemic Stroke**

Systemic causes	Dehydration
	Arterial hypotension
	Extreme degrees of arterial hypertension
	Increased body temperature, fever
	Hyperglycemia
	Hypoventilation, CO_2 retention
	Hypoxia
	Aspiration and pneumonia
	Sepsis, infection
	Pulmonary embolism
	Myocardial ischemia
	Cardiac arrhythmias
	Congestive heart failure
	Neurogenic pulmonary edema
	Hypoglycemia
	Epileptic seizure activity
	Hyponatremia and other disturbances of electrolyte balance
	Overhydration
	Thiamine deficiency
	Organic delirium
	Psychiatric factors
Causes related to arterial occlusion or cerebral infarct	Re-embolization
	Progressing thrombosis
	Reocclusion
	Infarct edema
	Increased intracranial pressure and reduced perfusion pressure
	Compartmental brain herniation
	Hemorrhagic transformation
	Decreasing collateral flow
	Reduced perfusion due to multiple stenosing arterial lesions
	Extension of the infarct core
	Extension of the penumbral area

ICP is generally not recommended but is being used in some intensive stroke care units.[55] Increased ICP is covered in more detail in Chapter 52. Close monitoring of neurologic status and serial CT scans are the diagnostic method of choice to guide interventions.

Ischemic brain edema occurs during the first 24 to 48 hours after ischemic infarcts. In younger patients, brain edema with elevated ICP may become a major complication, possibly leading to herniation and death.[56] Such patients usually show a rapid decline in consciousness and demonstrate the signs of herniation 2 to 4 days after onset of symptoms. Outcome is fatal in the majority of patients, the mortality being about 80% for standard treatment.[56–58]

According to historical studies, acute massive brain swelling with subsequent transtentorial herniation after MCA infarctions is found in 13% of autopsied patients with stroke, and raised ICP due to edema is common.[59,60] The time course of edema formation after stroke has been studied in patients already in their fifties.[61] Brain edema involving the gray and white matter surrounding the infarcted tissue could be seen within the 24 hours, reached its maximum on days 3 to 5, and then subsided completely within 2 weeks. In a paper exploring the effects of hemicraniectomy in the treatment of malignant MCA stroke, a

malignant MCA infarct has been defined as a space-occupying infarct of at least the total MCA territory, with signs of an increasing space-occupying effect on serial CT scans with a midline shift of more than 10 mm at the septum pellucidum level (see Chapters 52 and 75).[57,62] Such an infarct is almost always caused by an embolic occlusion of either the distal ICA or the proximal MCA trunk. Outcome is often fatal, and a mortality of up to 80% has been reported for standard care.[56,57]

Development of clinically significant edema in the infarct area, and especially the transformation into malignant MCA infarct, can often be predicted on clinical grounds as well as through the use of DWI or other perfusion methods, and several studies have addressed this question.[58,63–67] A lesion found on DWI that exceeds 145 cm³ has been demonstrated to be highly predictive of a malignant course with 100% sensitivity and 94% specificity, although with wide confidence intervals.[64]

Hemorrhagic transformation can be a factor in the unfavorable course of a large infarct. This phenomenon, however, is often asymptomatic. Because it has the potential to adversely affect the outcome, efforts to prevent hemorrhagic transformation seem justified.[68–71]

Basic management of elevated ICP after stroke usually consists of (1) placement of the patient in a semi-sitting position with elevation of the head and upper trunk to approximately 30 degrees, (2) avoidance of noxious stimuli, (3) pain relief, and (4) a low normal body temperature (36°C to 37°C). Because the head-up position may also lead to a decrease in mean arterial blood pressure (MAP), the head position should be individualized and adjusted to optimize cerebral perfusion pressure (MAP − ICP). Osmotherapy with 10% glycerol (250 mL of 10% glycerol over 60 minutes every 6 hours) or 15% mannitol (100 to 200 mL every 4 to 6 hours) is usually given intravenously at the first sign of space-occupying edema.[72] The effect of glycerol may last somewhat longer that that of mannitol and may be less commonly associated with a rebound increase in ICP. Hypertonic saline (up to 5% or more) has been used for the same purpose and has been reported to be more effective than mannitol.[73] Hypotonic and glucose-containing solutions are avoided, and a slightly negative fluid balance can be a target. One must keep in mind, however, that, especially in the early phase of an infarct, dehydration is known to be detrimental. Dexamethasone and other corticosteroids are useless and are relatively contraindicated.

A short-acting barbiturate such as thiopental given as a bolus results in rapid reduction in ICP but may be harmful if there is a significant drop in MAP and cerebral perfusion pressure (CPP). Propofol (10 mg/mL as a continuous infusion of 10 to 30 mL/hr) is commonly used for sedation of mechanically ventilated patients, but its effects on the ICP have not been well studied. In case of severe compromise of cerebral perfusion by rising ICP, the fastest way to restore intracranial circulation is volume loading with induction of hypertension by vasopressors. If the ICP is being directly measured, the CPP should be kept above 70 mm Hg. Alternatively, TCD ultrasonography monitoring may be used to ensure sufficient blood flow velocity and perfusion pressure, although absolute values are not available. During vasoactive treatment, continuous or intermittent monitoring of MCA blood flow by TCD ultra-sonography may also be used to exclude significant arterial spasm due to higher doses of vasopressors.

Only a few studies have addressed conservative treatment of infarct edema. Hypertonic saline with hydroxy-ethyl starch and glycerol have been reported to improve acute mortality in malignant MCA infarct.[73,74] A systematic review of the use of glycerol in ischemic stroke found a significant 35% OR reduction (95% CI 3% to 56%) in acute mortality, although only 601 patients were included in the meta-analysis. A single study of 173 patients that was both randomized and double-blinded showed a 60% reduction in acute mortality during the first week of intravenous glycerol therapy.[75] Thus, there is at least some evidence that glycerol may be helpful, but it has not been properly tested in the setting of malignant MCA infarct or in patients with infarct edema. Ten percent saline rapidly and effectively decreases ICP but may lead to cardiovascular compromise or osmotic injury, especially in the presence of hyponatremia, and so can hardly be recommended for general use.[73,74]

Hemicraniectomy is discussed in Chapters 52 and 75. It may have a role if all conservative means fail, but a proactive approach using all available conservative means to combat infarct edema and the rise in ICP may diminish the need for surgery. Most stroke neurologists believe that hemicraniectomy is very seldomly indicated.

Prevention of Acute Medical Complications

General Stroke Care

In addition to recanalization of the occluded vessel, there are other, almost as urgent goals in the acute management of stroke. Basically, the outcome of the patient depends heavily on the appearance of imminent medical complications involving different organ systems (cardiopulmonary system, gastrointestinal system, kidneys, skin, muscles, and peripheral and central nervous systems), fluid balance, coagulation, fibrinolysis, and nutritional and other disturbances of homeostasis (see Table 51.7). The subtype of stroke according to the TOAST (Trial of Org 10172 in Acute Stroke Treatment) classification is important, even for assessment of risk of recurrence and mortality, and affects secondary preventive strategies that should be initiated immediately.[76] Adequate treatment and preservation of vital functions constitute the basis of all therapeutic measures in acute stroke, not only in stroke units but also on normal wards. There is a consensus that management of general medical problems is the basis for stroke treatment.[45,77–80]

Fluid and Electrolyte Balance

Almost all patients with stroke are somewhat dehydrated on admission, a condition that has been found to correlate with less favorable outcome.[81] Several reasons may account for dehydration after acute stroke—swallowing, communication, and cognitive problems as well as immobility, infection, diuretic therapy, hyperthermia, and restlessness—and a preexisting dehydration for whatever cause may have had an acute prothrombotic effect that resulted in thromboembolic stroke. Especially patients who lay for hours or even days after stroke before being found and brought for treatment represent a subgroup of patients with stroke who are at very high risk for worsening and death. These patients commonly have multiple medical complications upon admission, such as severe dehydration, decubitus ulcer, aspiration pneumonia, urinary tract infection, rhabdomyolysis, renal insufficiency, and, possibly, imminent multiorgan failure. Although the issue has not been explicitly studied, it is commonly observed in a stroke unit that such patients have the worst overall prognosis.

In the prehospital care setting, one of the first things to be done for a patient with stroke is to establish an intravenous line with Ringer's irrigation or physiologic saline solution; rehydration will continue at the stroke unit. Intravenous fluid therapy is virtually always needed, and no patient with stroke should be deprived of it during the early phase. The fluid balance during the first 24 hours after stroke should be more or less positive, depending on the level of dehydration on admission, which can be assessed by measurement of hematocrit and osmolality. Because both volume depletion and volume overload should be avoided, the fluid balance of a patient with acute stroke must be closely monitored, especially during the unstable phase.

Sometimes more complex electrolyte disturbances ensue, in which low intake of salt or, very rarely, preexisting syndrome of inappropriate antidiuretic hormone (SIADH) may be a factor. It is our impression that the occurrence of SIADH is very exceptional after stroke and that hyponatremia and volume depletion are usually caused by the cerebral salt wasting (CSW) syndrome, which can be confused with SIADH. In these cases, the conventional recommendation to restrict fluids in order to correct hyponatremia carries a risk and may even prove fatal; instead, volume loading and sodium loading must be performed. As a rule, fluid restriction is virtually never indicated in acute stroke. In very severe stroke with compression or destruction of the hypothalamus, lack of antidiuretic hormone may lead to diabetes insipidus, which must be treated with vasopressin.

Cardiovascular Management

Cardiac arrhythmias and myocardial ischemia secondary to stroke are very common.

Significant alterations in the ST segments and the T waves on an electrocardiogram (ECG) may appear in the acute phase, representing true myocardial ischemia, sometimes in the absence of coronary disease.[82,83] Cardiac enzymes may be elevated in stroke, more commonly in severe stroke, including stroke due to intracerebral or subarachnoid hemorrhage.[84] The routine treatment for this phenomenon, which depends mainly on excess circulating catecholamines, is beta-blocker or alpha- and beta-blocker therapy. Beta-blockers are routinely administered to protect the myocardium, especially in more severe stroke. One must, however, abide by any preexisting and acute contraindications to this therapeutic modality, such as bronchoconstriction, congestive heart failure, severe bradycardia, and disturbances of atrioventricular or intraventricular conduction (i.e., prolonged PQ or QT interval).

An initial ECG should be performed in every patient with stroke. Continuous ECG monitoring is recommended at least in the patient with more severe stroke and, of course, for the patient with cardiac symptoms or hemodynamic instability, for as long as the patient stays in a bed with monitoring facilities and even in mild stroke for the first hours. Cardiac enzyme levels are routinely monitored for 24 hours and, in unstable patients, for several days. Etiologic studies, including echocardiography and invasive cardiologic evaluation, are an essential part of the diagnostic workup for many patients with stroke. Therefore, a cardiologist should be a frequent, almost daily, visitor in a large stroke unit.

Blood Pressure Management

A transient elevation of arterial blood pressure (BP) is the rule at the onset of stroke, occurring in 80% of patients with acute stroke.[85,86] This elevation has been viewed as a beneficial physiologic response to ischemia that does not need to be treated under most circumstances.[87] It has been attributed to a number of factors, such as catecholamine secretion in response to stress, neuroendocrine factors, alcohol, and topographic presentation of the infarct.[88–95] The BP usually declines during the first few days.[94–99] Although the general recommendation has been not to treat a moderate elevation in BP during the first few days, the issue is not entirely settled.[98] It is suggested that sudden lowering of the BP in the acute stage of occlusive stroke may either reduce the cerebral perfusion pressure in the ischemic portion of the brain or provoke an ischemic steal, especially with use of vasodilators such as calcium entry blockers.[45,97,100–103] Deficient autoregulation of cerebral blood flow (CBF) and watershed infarctions associated with critical internal carotid stenosis or occlusion may be accentuated after hypotensive therapy or acetazolamide administration, a possibility that should be kept in mind also for amaurosis fugax due to unilateral carotid stenosis.[96,101]

The natural course of BP in the acute phase of various subtypes of stroke is not very well known, but the elevation in BP is usually seen to decline spontaneously within a week after stroke without the use of intervening medications.[86] Chamorro and coworkers[98,104] conducted an observational study of 24-hour BP recordings in patients with strokes of various types and in hospital control subjects, immediately after presentation to the hospital and 7 days after admission. These researchers observed a lower incidence of brain edema in patients who received antihypertensive treatment during the acute phase of stroke than in those who did not, even when the mean arterial BP on admission was significantly higher in the former group. Complete recovery was more common in patients with edema who were treated with moderate blood pressure reduction.[104] It has been suggested that post-stroke hypertension could be deleterious, facilitating edema formation in the ischemic tissue. Pharmacologic elevation of BP as a therapeutic intervention has been studied, but the results are not conclusive.[105] This mode of therapy is used in intensive stroke units as a rescue therapy in acute situations when increasing ICP leads to rapid reduction of cerebral perfusion pressure. Invasive hemodynamic monitoring and intensive care facilities are needed for this therapy.

Increase in BP is a protective physiologic mechanism, and deficient autoregulation in the acute stage may lead to a severely reduced perfusion pressure in case of a sudden drop in BP. Some exceptions to this rule are acute congestive heart failure due to severe hypertension, hypertensive encephalopathy, subarachnoid hemorrhage, immediate or progressing hypertensive or anticoagulant-induced intracranial hemorrhage, hyperperfusion syndrome after carotid endarterectomy, myocardial ischemia, dissection of the thoracic or abdominal aorta, and the use of thrombolytic therapy.

Vasodilators typically cause a severe ischemic steal phenomenon and should be avoided except when strongly indicated as, for example, in myocardial ischemia. The drugs of choice for emergency intravenous antihypertensive treatment are (1) labetalol in boluses of 10 mg IV, which can be repeated as necessary, or as a continuous infusion at 30–60 mg/hr and (2) enalapril in repeated boluses of 1 mg every 15 to 30 minutes. Nicardipine can be used with a starting dose of 2 to 5 mg/hr as a continuous infusion (or nimodipine, 1 to 2 mg/hr); one must keep in mind, however, that calcium entry blockers can lead to steal of blood flow from ischemic to healthy regions of the brain and that the effect of a sharp drop in BP can be harmful. The use of peroral nifedipine is discouraged by most treatment guidelines, including those of the American Stroke Association. In resistant cases, sodium nitroprusside can be considered, although this agent carries the risk of severe compromise of cerebral perfusion with a sudden drop of blood pressure, reflex tachycardia, and myocardial ischemia. Either intravenous nimodipine or intravenous nitroglycerin effectively treats elevated BP when there is a special indication, such as subarachnoid hemorrhage or myocardial ischemia, for the use of either of these drugs.

According to the current recommendations of the American Heart Association (AHA) and the EUSI, BP values exceeding 220 mm Hg systolic, 130 mm Hg diastolic (220/130 mm Hg) should be treated actively even on admission.[45,106] The decision to treat also depends on the previous BP level as well as on the use of anticoagulants or thrombolytic therapy, during and after which BP readings of 180/100 mm Hg should not be exceeded. No recommendations currently exist on how to deal with BP in the setting of expansive infarct edema with or without increased ICP.

We use TCD ultrasonography to assess intracranial hemodynamics on an individual basis in order to optimize BP level according to the actual cardiopulmonary status of the patient. On the basis of current evidence, there is no need to revise existing recommendations. There may be a shift toward somewhat lower BP levels, but we believe that more aggressive lowering of BP necessitates monitoring of intracranial hemodynamics. The usual target systolic BP range in our stroke unit is 140 to 160 mm Hg, a value that has also been reported to be associated with the lowest mortality in the acute period (unpublished data from the Blood Pressure in Acute Stroke Collaboration [BASC], a prospective observational multicenter study that collects data on the use of antihypertensives and the BP in patients with acute stroke[107]).

Impressive progress has been made in the secondary prevention of stroke with antihypertensive treatment, although the topic is not within the scope of this chapter. Secondary prevention studies generally do not answer questions about how and when antihypertensive therapy should be used during the acute phase of stroke. However, a beneficial effect on long-term outcome has been convincingly demonstrated for diuretics, beta-blockers, and two angiotensin-converting enzyme (ACE) inhibitors, which makes them a logical choice also in acute care. ACE inhibitors carry less risk of accentuating cerebral ischemia and have been reported, thus protecting the brain from the ischemia associated with BP reduction.

There is some evidence for a deleterious effect of BP reduction on stroke. A word of caution about the use of dihydropyridine derivatives, such as nimodipine and nifedipine, to lower the BP is therefore appropriate. The Intravenous Nimodipine West European Stroke Trial (INWEST) found a correlation between nimodipine-induced reduction in BP and an unfavorable outcome of acute stroke.[108] Diastolic but not systolic BP reduction was associated with neurologic worsening after the intravenous administration of high-dose nimodipine for acute stroke.[100] It is unclear whether this negative effect was mediated through deficient autoregulation or reduced myocardial perfusion, which has a correlation to the diastolic BP. Nimodipine is highly effective in subarachnoid hemorrhage and is sometimes used for vasculitis, postpartum angiography, or cerebrovascular spasm of unknown cause, although there are no controlled studies to support this use. Oral nifedipine is contraindicated as emergency antihypertensive treatment in stroke according to most published guidelines, mainly because of the possibility of severe steal from ischemic regions and uncontrolled drop in BP.[45,106]

Respiratory Function and Prevention of Pulmonary Complications

In acute ischemic stroke, early changes in ventilatory drive and early respiratory disturbances due to reduced consciousness are rare. However, patients with complete MCA infarct, large supratentorial hemorrhage, or brainstem stroke may have early ventilatory problems. Patients with severe stroke are continuously monitored with pulse oxymetry, and supplemental oxygen should be used in the emergency and unstable phases, until stabilization of recanalization and later on, if needed, according to pulse oxymetry and arterial blood gas values or if signs of myocardial ischemia develop. Usually, 2 to 4 L/min administered via nasal tube are sufficient, but mask ventilation may be needed to deliver more oxygen. Temporary CPAP ventilation is sometimes necessary for refractory pulmonary edema.

The adequacy of ventilation must be ensured as part of any routine check of vital functions. Hypoxia must be excluded by oxygen saturation and with arterial blood gas measurement, if appropriate. Hypoventilation must be excluded especially in patients with even slightly decreased consciousness in case of aspiration pneumonia. The combination of hypoxia, hypoventilation, and low cerebral perfusion pressure is the worst case scenario.

If intubation is indicated, it should be preplanned and performed by an experienced anesthesiologist, because cerebral blood flow can be compromised during the procedure; such compromise may also provoke unwanted autonomic reflexes and blood pressure changes, thereby precipitating intracranial bleeding. The following findings are sufficient indications for intubation:

- Unconsciousness (Glasgow Coma Scale [GCS] score < 8)
- Inability to swallow or clear secretions from the mouth
- Absence of cough and gag reflexes
- Severe stridor

A patient with stroke should undergo intubation only if the possibility for independent recovery is present; that is, intubation should not be used only to prolong the terminal phase. Some patients clearly benefit from ventilator treatment, and independent recovery is possible.[109,110]

Chest radiographs show that most patients with acute stroke have at least slight pulmonary congestion or even pulmonary edema. The presence of either finding does not necessarily indicate volume overload or even congestive heart failure; the condition may be neurogenic and related to a burst of catecholamines. Neurogenic or catecholamine-induced edema often responds well to intravenous labetalol, especially in cases of extreme degrees of arterial hypertension. Slight pulmonary edema in a patient with acute stroke is generally not treated by fluid restriction or diuretics, unless the edema is severe or oxygenation is compromised.

One of the most important risks in the early phase after stroke is aspiration pneumonia. Bacterial pneumonia accounts for 15% to 25% of stroke-related deaths. The majority of the pneumonias are caused by aspiration.[111] Aspiration is commonly found in patients with reduced consciousness but also in patients with impaired gag reflexes or swallowing disturbances, which occur after conditions besides brainstem stroke. All patients who have severe stroke, who are initially unconscious or vomiting, or who lay for hours after stroke before being found and brought for treatment are assumed to have aspirated, implicating the need of antibiotics covering both the aerobic and anaerobic pathogens of aspiration pneumonia. It is not a good idea to wait for distinct signs of pneumonia, because the delay may worsen the outcome, and aspiration pneumonia is one of the most common medical complications of stroke.[112-115]

Nasogastric feeding may be helpful in the prevention of aspiration pneumonia, although it does not completely reduce the risk. Other reasons for pneumonia are poor cough (hypostatic pneumonia) and immobilization. Frequent changes of the patient's position in bed and pulmonary physical therapy may prevent this type of pneumonia.

Immobilization and Mobilization

Any patient with stroke should be mobilized as soon as considered safe. However, this is not an automatic routine, and the permission to mobilize the patient must be given by the treating physician. There are a number of situations in which mobilization is believed to carry a risk, although no evidence-based data derived from randomized clinical trials exist to support the belief.

Unstable cerebral ischemia, like unstable coronary ischemia, should be a contraindication for mobilization. Normally, the unstable phase ends as the vessel becomes recanalized, either spontaneously or as a result of thrombolytic therapy. Thrombolysis is followed by immobilization for 24 hours. Hemodynamic ischemia is typically enhanced by orthostatic hypotension. Volume depletion must, of course, be corrected before the patient is allowed to stand up. Intracerebral bleeding is progressive in a small number of patients, who should be immobilized for 24 hours or as long as progression is considered possible. Unstable cardiopulmonary status, coronary ischemia, and pulmonary embolism are typical contraindications to mobilization of a patient with stroke, but respiratory insufficiency is usually not because the ventilatory function commonly improves with sitting and upright positions.

Mobilization takes place in a controlled fashion, meaning that both vital functions and neurologic symptoms are monitored during the process, and possible sensorimotor or cognitive deficits are taken into account to protect the patient.

Urinary Tract Infection

Urinary tract infection is one of the most common medical complications of acute cerebral infarction. Urinary retention is common in the early phase after stroke. The majority of hospital-acquired urinary tract infections are associated with the use of indwelling catheters. A bladder catheter is usually needed, however, to ensure correct fluid balance and to follow diuresis hour by hour. Intermittent catheterization is not always feasible in the setting of severe stroke and incontinence, which may contribute to decubitus ulcer. Suprapubic catheters are considered to carry lower risk of infection. Acidification may reduce the risk of infection, whereas intermittent catheterization has not been shown to do so. Once urinary infection is seen, appropriate antibiotics should be started. However, prophylactic antibiotics are not recommended.

Pulmonary Embolism and Deep Venous Thrombosis

Pulmonary embolism is one of the most common causes of death in patients with ischemic cerebral infarction, even in patients who otherwise would have had an excellent recovery from the stroke.[112–115] The risk of deep venous thrombosis and pulmonary embolism can be reduced by early mobilization and by the use of subcutaneous heparin or low-molecular-weight heparin.[116] However, this effect seems to be counterbalanced by an increase in the rate of hemorrhagic complications.[117] Nevertheless, prophylaxis with subcutaneous low-dose heparin, 5000 IU every 12 hours, is recommended for bedridden patients with stroke until mobilization, as recommended by the EUSI.[106] Tachypnea, pain, and oxygen desaturation may be signs of pulmonary embolism or pneumonia. The lower extremities should be examined daily to detect signs of deep venous thrombosis, which can be excluded by venous ultrasonography. Physical therapy and the use of support stockings are suggested as an alternative to low-molecular-weight heparin.

Decubitus Ulcer

Frequent turning of immobilized patients is useful for prevention of decubitus ulcers. The skin of the incontinent patient must be kept dry. For patients at particularly high risk, an air- or fluid-filled oscillating mattress system should be used. If the decubitus ulcer does not respond to conservative treatment, antibiotic therapy for several days may be justified, before definitive surgical débridement.

Seizures

Partial (focal) or secondary generalized epileptic seizures may occur in the acute phase of ischemic stroke. Lorazepam (1 to 4 mg IV) or diazepam (5 to 10 mg IV) followed by intravenous fosphenytoin or carbamazepine is a common choice for the treatment of seizures. Monitoring with electroencephalography (EEG) is useful in some cases.

Delirium, Depression, and Psychiatric Problems

Acute organic delirium is common and must be recognized and treated promptly because of the high morbidity and mortality rates associated with it. Heavy use of alcohol, malnutrition, and infection are known predisposing factors, but delirium may develop in previously healthy patients as well. We use intravenous lorazepam in bolus doses of 1 to 2 mg or haloperidol in cases of severe restlessness, agitation, aggressiveness, and psychotic behavior. Parenteral thiamine substitution is started on admission for all patients at risk of delirium.

Treatment of depression is not within the scope of this discussion (see Chapter 56). Approximately one third of patients with stroke suffer from moderate to severe depression during the acute period after stroke. Citalopram lacks pharmacologic interactions and has been shown to be useful in the treatment of post-stroke depression.[118] The general attitude in the stroke unit is often the best way to combat depression,[119] but both antidepressive and anxiolytic medications must be used when indicated. A psychiatric consultation is rarely needed during the acute phase, except for an acute exacerbation of a preexisting psychiatric disorder.

Special Aspects

Body Temperature and Induced Hypothermia

Body temperature is commonly elevated to above 37.5°C in the early phase of stroke.[120–123] It may be a marker of stroke severity, may reflect infectious complications, or may be an independent prognostic factor adversely affecting morbidity and mortality. In experimental ischemia models, temperature is the main determinant of infarct size in both focal and global cerebral ischemia, and even postischemic hypothermia is neuroprotective.[124–127] There is now compelling evidence that even mild hyperthermia has a clear-cut, clinically significant deleterious effect in acute stroke and may lead to expanding infarct, edema, hemorrhage, and increased ICP.[121,123,124,128,129] A landmark work by Reith and coworkers[123] is the largest retrospective study showing that admission body temperature is highly correlated with initial stroke severity and infarct size as well as with poor outcome and mortality. These researchers found that the relative risk of poor outcome increased by a factor of 2.2 per each 1°C rise in body temperature. Furthermore, this relationship was independent of stroke severity, and the presence of infection was not independently predictive of poor outcome. The relationship between body temperature and outcome could be demonstrated even in mild stroke.[123]

The significance of elevated body temperature in stroke was probably first suggested in 1976 by Hindfelt[130] in a retrospective series of patients, although the beneficial effect of cool ambient temperature was anecdotally mentioned and even emphasized as a treatment modality in a Finnish home physician book more than 100 years ago.[131] Fever was confirmed as an independent predictor of unfavorable outcome in the 1990s.[121] As a result, interest in lowering body temperature of patients with acute stroke grew. Several pilot studies on hypothermia have been published, and some multicenter trials are to be launched shortly. Some studies favor either cooled air or blankets for external cooling or endovascular cooling catheters to decrease body temperature to between 32°C and 33°C for at least 24 hours or up to 3 days after the onset of stroke.[132] However, prolonged hypothermia may be deleterious, because the rate of infectious complications is believed to rise rapidly after the first day or so. In most hypothermia studies, relaxed general anesthesia was found to be necessary, except for one study favoring very mild hypothermia of 35°C to 36°C in conscious, lightly sedated patients who were given meperidine to control shivering.

Hypothermia is a promising approach to combat worsening edema and rising ICP.[129,133] This measure has been reported to markedly lower elevated ICP, although with a distinct rebound effect unless the hypothermia is tapered very slowly. So far, these approaches are not applicable for the majority of patients with stroke and might be reserved for patients with malignant MCA infarcts only until there is evidence from randomized, controlled trials that the therapy is safe and effective. However, if very mild hypothermia in awake patients, applicable in ordinary stroke units, proves safe and effective, it is likely to have a major impact on stroke care.[134] Even now, many stroke units combat fever aggressively, and routine administration of propacetamol or acetaminophen is common; for acetaminophen, a mean reduction of 0.4°C for 24 hours compared with placebo has been demonstrated.[135]

Mild hypothermia with brain temperatures between 33°C and 35°C was demonstrated to be safe and to reduce both mortality and ICP in a small number of patients with malignant MCA infarct.[136] Controlled randomized trials have demonstrated that therapeutic hypothermia is ineffective after head trauma but effective after cardiac arrest.[137–140] Even though the results of large-scale interventional studies in stroke are still awaited, the control of body temperature should be one of the top priorities in the acute care of stroke.

Blood Glucose and Hyperglycemia

More than 20% of patients with acute stroke are hyperglycemic on admission. Hyperglycemia has concomitant deleterious vascular and metabolic effects that increase infarct size and lead to hemorrhagic transformation in experimental reperfusion models.[141] There is less clinical information on this topic, but in general, published data seem to support an adverse impact of hyperglycemia on outcome of stroke. The mechanism of action of hyperglycemia is believed to be the endothelial expression of adhesion factors, promotion of vasospasm, production of reactive oxygen species, and upregulation of nuclear factor kappa-B (NF-κ_B) by oxidating products of glycosylation, leading to inflammation and metabolic tissue injury related to high lactate and low pH.[142]

Elevated blood glucose leads to a 12-fold increase in rate of hemorrhagic complications with intra-arterial thrombolysis, as reported by the second Prolyse in Acute Cerebral Thromboembolism trial (PROACT II) investigators.[143] There is some evidence that hyperglycemia may also enhance the hemorrhagic transformation in patients as it does in experimental reperfusion models.

Admission hyperglycemia is associated with increased infarct size.[144] The strong and consistent association between admission hyperglycemia and poor prognosis after stroke observed in nondiabetic patients suggests that glucose level is an important risk factor for morbidity and mortality after stroke.[145] After ischemic stroke, even a mildly elevated admission blood glucose level, of 110 to 126 mg/dL (6.1 to 7.0 mmol/L), was associated with an increased risk of 30-day mortality in nondiabetic patients only (relative risk = 3.28; 95% CI, 2.32 to 4.64). In nondiabetic patients, mild acute hyperglycemia seems to be associated with in-hospital mortality and a higher risk of poor functional recovery in stroke survivors.[145]

Elevated blood glucose is known to be a marker for poor outcome in ischemic stroke, subarachnoid hemorrhage, brain trauma, and global ischemia caused by cardiac arrest and to enhance edema in experimental ischemia models. No randomized studies have directly addressed the question whether the infarct edema can be controlled by insulin, although very strict blood glucose control (80 to 110 mg/dL [4.4 to 6.1 mmol/L]) has dramatically reduced the acute mortality of patients receiving general intensive care by 42% (95% CI 22% to 62%).[146]

What are the clinical implications of these data? Since the early 1990s, no glucose-containing solutions have been recommended to be given to patients with stroke, especially during the first few days and even longer if the situation remains unstable or there is threatening edema or hemorrhagic transformation. Blood glucose levels exceeding 144 mg/dL (8 mmol/L) are to be treated with small doses of rapidly acting subcutaneous insulin or, in resistant cases, intravenous insulin infusion.[106] In several stroke guidelines, including the recommendations of the EUSI, the cut-off value has been 180 mg/dL (10 mmol/L). There has been a shift toward lower values, but treatment levels lower than 144 mg/dL (8 mmol/L) may be possible only in the intensive care setting.[146] Nevertheless, control of blood glucose, especially during the early phase of stroke, should be another top priority probably equal in importance to the control of body temperature.

CONCLUSIONS

Stroke unit care is highly evidence-based medicine (especially in stroke units without intensive care facilities, mixed assessment/rehabilitation stroke units, or rehabilitation stroke units). Only one trial supports the effectiveness of a mobile stroke team[14]; accordingly, there is not enough data to reliably estimate the effectiveness of the mobile stroke team model. Such a team provides good service for delivering thrombolysis in a metropolitan area, but it does not have the advantages of ordinary stroke unit care in a geographically defined area provided by highly motivated multidisciplinary staff, the effectiveness of which has been verified.[32] Stroke unit care is cost-effective, saves lives, and reduces the likelihood of death or disability and the need for institutional care.[32,147–153] These benefits are not restricted to any special group of patients. All patients with stroke, regardless of age, sex, or severity of stroke, benefit from stroke unit care. The beneficial effect is long-standing for up to 5 to 10 years.[38]

The Pan-European Consensus Meeting on Stroke Management, organized by the WHO Regional Office for Europe together with the European Stroke Council, recommended in 1995 that all patients with acute stroke have easy access to stroke unit care by the year 2005.[40] The recommendations of the EUSI, on behalf of the European Stroke Council, the European Neurological Society, and the European Federation of Neurological Societies, state that acute stroke care should take place in stroke units.[78,154] Recommendations of the Advisory Working Group on Stroke Center Identification Options of the American Heart Association aim to improve the capacity of hospitals to provide organized care to patients with stroke.[155] Dedicated stroke unit care is already in large-scale practice in Germany and the Scandinavian countries, experience from which demonstrates that the results detected in the meta-analysis of Stroke Unit Trialists' Collaboration can be achieved on a population level.[41,42]

References

1. Critical pathways: A review. Committee on Acute Cardiac Care, Council on Clinical Cardiology, American Heart Association. Circulation 101:461–465, 2000.
2. Kennedy FB, Pozen TJ, Gableman EH, et al: Stroke intensive care—an appraisal. Am Heart J 80:188–196, 1970.
3. Drake WE, Hamilton MJ, Carlsson M, et al: Acute stroke management and patient outcome: The value of neurovascular care units (NCU). Stroke 4:933–945, 1973.
4. Pitner SE, Mance CJ: An evaluation of stroke intensive care: Results in a municipal hospital. Stroke 4:737–741, 1973.
5. Isaacs B: Five years' experience of a stroke unit. Health Bull 35:94–98, 1977.
6. McCann C, Cuthbertson RA: Comparison of two systems for stroke rehabilitation in a general hospital. J Am Geriatr Soc 24:211–216, 1976.
7. Feigenson JS, Gitlow HS, Greenberg SD: The disability oriented rehabilitation unit—a major factor influencing stroke outcome. Stroke 10:5–8, 1979.
8. Garraway WM, Akhtar AJ, Hockey L, Prescott RJ: Management of acute stroke in the elderly: Preliminary results of a controlled trial. BMJ 280:1040–1044, 1980.
9. Von Arbin M, Britton M, de Faire U, et al: A study of stroke patients treated in a non-intensive stroke unit or in general medical wards. Acta Med Scand 208:81–85, 1980.
10. Hamarin E: Early activation after stroke: Does it make a difference? Scand J Rehabil Med 14:101–109, 1982.
11. Strand T, Asplund K, Eriksson S, et al: A non-intensive stroke unit reduces functional disability and the need for long term hospitalization. Stroke 16:29–34, 1985.
12. Feldman DJ, Lee PR, Unterecker J, et al: A comparison of functionally orientated medical care and formal rehabilitation in the management of patients with hemiplegia due to cerebrovascular disease. J Chron Dis 15:297–310, 1962.
13. Gordon Ee, Kohn KH: Evaluation of rehabilitation methods in the hemiplegic patient. J Chron Dis 19:3–16, 1966.
14. Wood-Dauphinee S, Shapiro S, Bass E: A randomized trial of team care following stroke. Stroke 15:864–872, 1984.
15. Garraway WM, Alchtar AJ, Hockey L, Prescott RJ: Management of acute stroke in the elderly: Follow-up of a controlled trial. BMJ 281:827–829, 1980.
16. Fagerberg B, Blomstrand C: Do stroke units save lives? Lancet 342:992, 1993.
17. Hankey G, Deleo D, Stewart-Wynne EG: Acute hospital care for stroke patients: A randomized trial. Cerebrovasc Dis 5:228, 1995.
18. Ilmavirta M: Stroke Unit and Outcome of Brain Infarction [Dissertation]. Tampere, Finland, Acta Universitatis Tampereisis; series A, vol 410, 1994.
19. Indredavik B, Bakke F, Haheim LL, Holme I: Benefit of stroke unit: A randomised controlled trial. Stroke 22:1026–1031, 1991.
20. Juby LC, Lincoln NB, Berman P: The effect of a stroke rehabilitation unit on functional and psychological outcome: A randomised controlled trial. Cerebrovasc Dis 6:106–110, 1996.
21. Kalra L, Dale P, Crome P: Improving stroke rehabilitation: A controlled study. Stroke 24:1462–1467, 1993.
22. Kaste M, Palomäki H, Sarna S: Where and how should elderly stroke patients be treated? A randomized trial. Stroke 26:249–253, 1995.
23. Sivenius J, Pyörälä K, Heinonen OP, et al: The significance of intensity of rehabilitation after stroke: A controlled trial. Stroke 16:928–931, 1985.
24. Stevens RS, Ambler NR, Warren MD: A randomized controlled trial of a stroke rehabilitation ward. Age Ageing 13:65–75, 1984.
25. Langhorne P, Williams BO, Gilchrist W, Howie K: Do stroke units save lives? Lancet 342:395–398, 1993.
26. Collaborative systematic review of the randomised trials of organised in-patient (stroke unit) care after stroke. Stroke Unit Trialists' Collaboration. BMJ 314:1151–1159, 1997.
27. Langhorne P, Duncan P: Does the organisation of postacute stroke care really matter? Stroke 32:268–274, 2001.
28. Organization of stroke care: Education, stroke units and rehabilitation. European Stroke Initiative (EUSI). Cerebrovasc Dis 10(Suppl 3):1–11, 2000.
29. Diener HC: Future organisation of stroke service: A model for acute stroke management. In Wahlgren NG, Magnus von Arbin M (eds): Update on Stroke Therapy 1998–1999. Stockholm, 1999, pp 173–180.
30. Ringelstein EB, Berlit P, Busse O, et al: Konzepte der überregionalen und regionalen Schlaganfallversorgung in Deutschland. Akt Neurol 27:101–104, 2000.
31. Langhorne P, Dennis M: Stroke Units: An Evidence-Based Approach. London, BMJ Books, 1998.
32. Stroke Unit Trialists' Collaboration: Organised inpatient (stroke unit) care for stroke (Cochrane Review). In: The Cochrane Library, Issue 2. Oxford, Update Software, 2003.
33. Stroke Unit Trialists' Collaboration. How do stroke units improve patients' outcomes? A collaborative systematic review of the randomised trials. Stroke 28:2139–2144, 1997.
34. Kalra L, Evans A, Perez I, et al: Alternative strategies for stroke care: A prospective randomised controlled study of stroke unit, stroke team, and domiciliary management of stroke. Lancet 356:894–899, 2000.
35. Indredavik B, Slordahl SA, Bakke F, et al: Stroke unit treatment: Long-term effects. Stroke 28:1861–1866, 1997.
36. Indredavik B, Bakke F, Slordahl SA, et al: Stroke unit treatment improves long-term quality of life: A randomized controlled trial. Stroke 29:895–899, 1998.
37. Lincoln NB, Husbands S, Trescoli C, et al: Five year follow up of a randomised controlled trial of a stroke rehabilitation unit. BMJ 320:549, 2000.
38. Indredavik B, Bakke F, Slordahl SA, et al: Stroke unit treatment: 10-year follow-up. Stroke 30:1524–1527, 1999.
39. Hacke W, Schwab S, de Georgia M: Intensive care of acute stroke. Cerebrovasc Dis 4:385–392, 1994.
40. Aboderin I, Venables G: Stroke management in Europe. Pan-European Consensus Meeting on Stroke Management. J Intern Med 240:173–180, 1996.
41. Riks-Stroke—a Swedish national quality register for stroke care. Cerebrovasc Dis 15(Suppl 1):5–7, 2003.
42. Kostanalyse der Schlaganfall-Behandlung in Deutschland: Eine Auswertung der Schlaganfall-Datenbank der Stiftung Deutsche Schlaganfall-Hilfe. Ak Neurol 29:181–190, 2002.
43. Hacke W, Stingele R, Steiner T, et al: Critical care of acute ischemic stroke. Intensive Care Med 21:856–862, 1995.

44. Brott T, Fieschi C, Hacke W: General therapy of acute ischemic stroke. In Hacke W, Hanley DF, Einhäupl K, Bleck TP (eds): Neurocritical Care. Berlin, Springer Verlag, 1994, pp 553–577.

45. Adams HP, Brott T, Crowell RM, et al: Guidelines for the management of patients with acute ischemic stroke. Stroke 25:1901–1904, 1994.

46. Von Kummer R, Holle R, Rosin L, et al: Does arterial recanalization improve outcome in carotid territory stroke? Stroke 26:581–587, 1995.

47. Leys D, Pruvo JP, Godefroy O, et al: Prevalence and significance of hyperdense middle cerebral artery in acute stroke. Stroke 23:317–324, 1992.

48. Mayer TE, Hamann GF, Baranczyk J, et al: Dynamic CT perfusion imaging of acute stroke. Am J Neuroradiol 21:1441–1449, 2000.

49. Wolpert SM, Brückmann H, Greenlee R, et al: Neuroradiologic evaluation of patients with acute stroke treated with recombinant tissue plasminogen activator. The rt-PA Acute Stroke Study Group. AJNR Am J Neuroradiol 14:3–13, 1993.

50. Kaps M, Link A: Transcranial sonographic monitoring during thrombolytic therapy. AJNR Am J Neuroradiol 19:758–760, 1998.

51. Demchuk AM, Burgin WS, Christou I, et al: Thrombolysis in Brain Ischemia (TIBI) Transcranial Doppler flow grades predict clinical severity, early recovery, and mortality in patients treated with intravenous tissue plasminogen activator. Stroke 32:89–93, 2001.

52. Burgin SW, Malkoff M, Felberg RA, et al: Transcranial Doppler ultrasound criteria for recanalization after thrombolysis for middle cerebral artery stroke. Stroke 31: 1128–1132, 2000.

53. Alexandrov AV, Felberg RA, Demchuk AM, et al: Deterioration following spontaneous improvement: Sonographic findings in patients with acutely resolving symptoms of cerebral ischemia. Stroke 31:915–919, 2000.

54. Jansen O, Schellinger P, Fiebach J, et al: Early recanalisation in acute ischaemic stroke saves tissue at risk defined by MRI. Lancet 353:2036–2037, 1999.

55. Schwab S, Aschoff A, Spranger M, et al: The value of intracranial pressure monitoring in acute hemispheric stroke. Neurology 47: 393–398, 1996.

56. Hacke W, Schwab S, Horn M, et al: "Malignant" middle cerebral artery territory infarction: Clinical course and prognostic signs. Arch Neurol 53:309–315, 1996.

57. Rieke K, Schwab S, Krieger D, et al: Decompressive surgery in space occupying hemispheric infarction: Results of an open, prospective study. Crit Care Med 23:1576–1587, 1995.

58. Krieger DW, Demchuk AM, Kasner SE, et al: Early clinical and radiological predictors of fatal brain swelling in ischemic stroke. Stroke 30:287–292, 1999.

59. Ng LK, Nimmanniyta J: Massive cerebral infarction with severe brain swelling: a clinicopathological study. Stroke 1(3):158–163, 1970.

60. Christensen MS, Brodersen P, Olesen J, Powlson OB: Cerebral apoplexy (stroke) treated with or without prolonged artificial hyperventilation. 2. Cerebrospinal fluid acid-base balance and intracranial pressure. Stroke 4:620–631, 1973.

61. Shaw CM, Alvord EC, Berry GR: Swelling of the brain following ischemic infarction with arterial occlusion. Arch Neurol 1:161–177, 1959.

62. Schwab S, Steiner T, Aschoff A, et al: Early hemicraniectomy in patients with complete middle cerebral artery infarction. Stroke 29:1888–1893, 1998.

63. Steiger HJ: Outcome of acute supratentorial cerebral infarction in patients under 60: Development of a prognostic grading system. Acta Neurochir Wien 111:73–79, 1991.

64. Oppenheim C, Samai Y, Manai R, et al: Prediction of malignant middle cerebral artery infarction by diffusion-weighted imaging. Stroke 31:2175–2181, 2000.

65. Alexandrov AV, Black SE, Ehrlich LE, et al: Simple visual analysis of brain perfusion on HMPAO SPECT predicts early outcome in acute stroke. Stroke 27:1537–1542, 1996.

66. Berrouschot J, Barthel H, von Kummer R, et al: 99m technetium-ethyl-cysteinate-dimer single-photon emission CT can predict fatal ischemic brain edema. Stroke 29:2556–2562, 1998.

67. Andrefsky JA, Sila CA, Steiner CP, et al: Prediction of life-threatening brain swelling from large supratentorial hemispheric infarction comparing ellipsoid volume estimation (EVE) to computer assisted 3-D volumetric analysis (CAVA) within 48 hours of stroke onset. Neurology 52:101, 1999.

68. Berger C, Fiorelli M, Steiner T, et al: Hemorrhagic transformation of ischemic brain tissue asymptomatic or symptomatic? Stroke 32:1330–1335, 2001.

69. Molina CA, Montaner J, Abilleira S, et al: Timing of spontaneous recanalization and risk of hemorrhagic transformation in acute cardioembolic stroke. Stroke 32:1079–1084, 2001.

70. Morfis L, Schwartz RS, Poulos R, Howes LG: Blood pressure changes in acute cerebral infarction and hemorrhage. Stroke 28:1401–1405, 1997.

71. Broderick JP, Hagen T, Brott T, Tomsick T: Hyperglycemia and hemorrhagic transformation of cerebral infarcts. Stroke 26:484–487, 1995.

72. Righetti E, Celani MG, Cantisani T, et al: Glycerol for acute stroke (Cochrane Review). In The Cochrane Library, Issue 2. Oxford, Update Software, 2003.

73. Schwarz S, Schwab S, Bertram M, et al: Effects of hypertonic saline hydroxyethyl starch solution and mannitol in patients with increased intracranial pressure after stroke. Stroke 29:1550–1555, 1998.

74. Schwarz S, Georgiadis D, Aschoff A, Schwab S: Effects of hypertonic (10%) saline in patients with raised intracranial pressure after stroke. Stroke 33:136–140, 2002.

75. Bayer AJ, Pathy MS, Newcombe R: Double-blind randomised trial of intravenous glycerol in acute stroke. Lancet 1(8530):405–408, 1987.

76. Kolominsky-Rabas PL, Weber M, Gefeller O, et al: Epidemiology of ischemic stroke subtypes according to TOAST criteria: incidence, recurrence, and long-term survival in ischemic stroke subtypes: A population-based study. Stroke 32:2735–2740, 2001.

77. Recommendations on stroke prevention, diagnosis, and therapy. Report of the WHO Task Force on Stroke and Other Cerebrovascular Disorders. Stroke 20:1407–1431, 1989.

78. Hacke W, Kaste M, Olsen TS, et al: European Stroke Initiative recommendations for stroke management. Cerebrovasc Dis 10:335–351, 2000.

79. European strategies for early intervention in stroke. The European Ad Hoc Consensus Group. Cerebrovasc Dis 6:315–324, 1996.

80. Optimizing intensive care in stroke: A European perspective. A report of an Ad Hoc Consensus Group meeting. Cerebrovasc Dis 7:113–128, 1997.

81. Bhalla A, Sankaralingam S, Dundas R, et al: Influence of raised plasma osmolarity on clinical outcome after acute stroke. Stroke 31:2043–2048, 2000.

82. Norris JW, Hachinski VC, Myers MG, et al: Serum cardiac enzymes in stroke. Stroke 10:548–553, 1979.

83. Norris J: Effects of cerebrovascular lesions on the heart. Neurol Clin 1:87–101, 1983.

84. Kaste M, Somer H, Konttinen A: Heart type creatine kinase isoenzyme (CK MB) in acute cerebral disorders. Br Heart J 40:802–805, 1978.

85. Yatsu FM, Zivin J: Hypertension in acute ischemic strokes: Not to treat. Arch Neurol 42:999–1000, 1985.

86. Lavin P: Management of hypertension in patients with acute stroke. Arch Intern Med 146:66–68, 1986.

87. Waltz AG: Effect of blood pressure on blood flow in ischemic and in non-ischemic cerebral cortex. Neurology 18:613–621, 1968.

88. Ito A, Omae T, Katsuki S: Acute changes in blood pressure following vascular diseases in the brain stem. Stroke 4:80–84, 1973.

89. Carlberg B, Asplund K, Hägg E: High blood pressure in acute stroke: Is it white coat hypertension? J Intern Med 228:291–292, 1990.

90. Carlberg B, Asplund K, Hägg E: Course of blood pressure in different subsets of patients after acute stroke. Cerebrovasc Dis 1:281–287, 1991.

91. Carlberg B, Asplund K, Hägg E: Factors influencing admission blood pressure levels in patients with acute stroke. Stroke 22:527–530, 1991.

92. Olsson T, Marklund N, Gustafson Y, Nasman B: Abnormalities at different levels of the hypothalamic-pituitary-adrenocortical axis early after stroke. Stroke 23:1573–1576, 1992.

93. Myers MG, Norris JW, Hachinski VC, Sole MJ: Plasma norepinephrine in stroke. Stroke 12:200–203, 1981.

94. Jansen PAF, Schulte BPM, Poels EFJ, Gribnau FWJ: Course of blood pressure after cerebral infarction and transient ischemic attack. Clin Neurol Neurosurg 89:243–246, 1987.

95. Harper G, Castleden CM, Potter JF: Factors affecting changes in blood pressure after acute stroke. Stroke 25:1726–1729, 1994.

96. Wallace JD, Levy LL: Blood pressure after stroke. JAMA 246:2177–2180, 1981.
97. Britton M, Carlsson A, Faire UD: Blood pressure course in patients with acute stroke and matched controls. Stroke 17:861–864, 1986.
98. Chamorro A, Vila N, Ascaso C, et al: Blood pressure and functional recovery in acute ischemic stroke. Stroke 29:1850–1853, 1998.
99. Oppenheimer S, Hachinski V: Complications of acute stroke. Lancet 339:721–724, 1992.
100. Ahmed N, Näsman P, Wahlgren NG: Effect of intravenous nimodipine on blood pressure and outcome after acute stroke. Stroke 31:1250–1255, 2000.
101. Graham DI: Ischemic brain following emergency blood pressure lowering in hypertensive patients. Acta Med Scand 678(Suppl):61–69, 1982.
102. Power WJ: Acute hypertension after stroke: The scientific basis for treatment decisions. Neurology 43:461–467, 1993.
103. Jörgensen HS, Nakayama H, Raaschou HO, Olsen TS: Effect of blood pressure and diabetes on stroke in progression. Lancet 344:156–159, 1994.
104. Chamorro A: Blood pressure in acute ischemic stroke and functional recovery. In Wahlgren NG (ed): Update on Stroke Therapy 2001–2002. Stockholm, Repro Print AB, 2001, pp 193–203.
105. Rordorf G, Cramer SC, Efird JT, et al: Pharmacological elevation of blood pressure in acute stroke: Clinical effects and safety. Stroke 28:2133–2138, 1997.
106. Hacke W, Kaste M, Skyhöj Olsen T, et al: Acute treatment of ischemic stroke. European Stroke Initiative (EUSI). Cerebrovasc Dis 10(Suppl 3):22–33, 2000.
107. Bath FJ, Bath PMW: What is the correct management of blood pressure in patients with acute ischemic stroke? The Blood Pressure in Acute Stroke Collaboration. Cerebrovasc Dis 7:205–213, 1997.
108. Wahlgren NG, MacMahon DG, De Keyser J, et al: The Intravenous Nimodipine West European Trial (INWEST) of nimodipine in the treatment of acute ischemic stroke. Cerebrovasc Dis 4:204–210, 1994.
109. Grotta J, Pasteur W, Khwaja G, et al: Elective intubation for neurologic deterioration after stroke. Neurology 45:640–644, 1995.
110. Berrouschot J, Rössler A, Köster J, Schneider D: Mechanical ventilation in patients with hemispheric ischemic stroke. Crit Care Med 28:2956–2961, 2000.
111. Horner J, Massey E, Riski J, et al: Aspiration following stroke: Clinical correlates and outcome. Neurology 38:1359–1362, 1988.
112. Davenport RJ, Dennis MS, Wellwood I, Warlow CP: Complications after acute stroke. Stroke 27:415–420, 1996.
113. Langhorne P, Stott DJ, Robertson L, et al: Medical complications after stroke: A multicenter study. Stroke 31:1223–1229, 2000.
114. Roth EJ, Lovell L, Harvey RL, et al: Incidence of and risk factors for medical complications during stroke rehabilitation. Stroke 32:523–529, 2001.
115. Johnston KC, Li JY, Lyden PD, et al: Medical and neurological complications of ischemic stroke: Experience from the RANTTAS trial. RANTTAS Investigators. Stroke 29:447–453, 1998.
116. Kelly J, Rudd A, Lewis R, Hunt BJ: Venous thromboembolism after acute stroke. Stroke 32:262–267, 2001.
117. International Stroke Trial (IST): A randomised trial of aspirin, subcutaneous heparin, both, or neither among 19,435 patients with acute ischaemic stroke. International Stroke Trial Collaborative Group. Lancet 349:1569–1581, 1997.
118. Andersen G, Vestergaard K, Lauritzen L: Effective treatment of post-stroke depression with the selective serotonin reuptake inhibitor citalopram. Stroke 25:1099–1104, 1994.
119. Palomäki H, Kaste M, Berg A, et al: Prevention of post-stroke depression: One-year randomized placebo-controlled trial on mianserin with six months follow-up after therapy. J Neurol Neurosurg Psychiatry 66:490–494, 1999.
120. Christensen H, Boysen G, Christensen E: Body temperature in acute stroke. Cerebrovasc Dis 10(Suppl 2):101, 2000.
121. Castillo J, Martinez F, Leira R, et al: Mortality and morbidity of acute cerebral infarction related to temperature and basal analytic parameters. Cerebrovasc Dis 4:56–71, 1994.
122. Castillo J, Davalos T, Marrugat J, Noya M: Timing for fever-related brain damage in acute ischemic stroke. Stroke 29:2455–2460, 1998.
123. Reith J, Jörgensen HS, Pedersen PM, et al: Body temperature in acute stroke: Relation to stroke severity, infarct size, mortality, and outcome. Lancet 347:422–425, 1996.
124. Busto R, Globus MY, Dietrich WD, et al: Effects of mild hypothermia on ischemia-induced release of neurotransmitters and free fatty acids in rat brain. Stroke 20:904–910, 1989.
125. Yamamoto H, Hong SC, Soleau S, et al: Mild postischemic hypothermia limits cerebral injury following transient focal ischemia in rat neocortex. Brain Res 718:207–211, 1996.
126. Shimizu T, Naritomi H, Kakud W, et al: Mild hypothermia is effective for the treatment of acute embolic stroke if induced within 24 hours after onset but not in the later phase. J Cereb Blood Flow Metab 17:42, 1997.
127. Kawai N, Okauchi M, Morisaki K, Nagao S: Effects of delayed intraischemic and postischemic hypothermia on a focal model of transient cerebral ischemia in rats. Stroke 31:1982–1989, 2000.
128. Maher J, Hachinski V: Hypothermia as a potential treatment for cerebral ischemia. Cerebrovasc Brain Metab Rev 5:277–300, 1993.
129. Ginsberg MD, Busto R: Combating hyperthermia in acute stroke: A significant clinical concern. Stroke 29:529–534, 1998.
130. Hindfelt B: The prognostic significance of subfebrility and fever in ischaemic cerebral infarction. Acta Neurol Scand 53:72–79, 1976.
131. Wistrand AT: Kotilääkäri [English translation: Home Physician]. Helsinki, Sampo, 1901.
132. Georgiadis D, Schwarz S, Kollmar R, Schwab S: Endovascular cooling for moderate hypothermia in patients with acute stroke: First results of a novel approach. Stroke 32:2550–2553, 2001.
133. Ginsberg MD, Sternau LL, Globus MY, et al: Therapeutic modulation of brain temperature: Relevance to ischemic brain injury. Cerebrovasc Brain Metab Rev 4:189–225, 1992.
134. Kammersgaard LP, Rasmussen BH, Jorgensen HS, et al: Feasibility and safety of inducing modest hypothermia in awake patients with acute stroke through surface cooling: A case-control study. Stroke 31:2251–2256, 2000.
135. Kasner SE, Wein T, Piriyawat P, et al: Acetaminophen for altering body temperature in acute stroke: A randomized clinical trial. Stroke 33:130–135, 2002.
136. Schwab S, Schwarz S, Spranger M, et al: Moderate hypothermia in the treatment of patients with severe middle cerebral artery infarction. Stroke 29:2461–2466, 1998.
137. Marion DW, Penrod LE, Kelsey SF, et al: Treatment of traumatic brain injury with moderate hypothermia. N Engl J Med 336:540–546, 1997.
138. Clifton GL, Miller ER, Choi SC, et al: Lack of effect of induction of hypothermia after acute brain injury. N Engl J Med 344:556–563, 2001.
139. Zeiner A, Holzer M, Behringer W, et al: Mild resuscitative hypothermia to improve neurological outcome after cardiac arrest: A clinical feasibility trial. Hypothermia After Cardiac Arrest (HACA) Study Group. Stroke 31:86–94, 2000.
140. Mild therapeutic hypothermia after cardiac arrest. N Engl J Med 346:549–556, 2002.
141. Kawai N, Keep RF, Betz AL, Dietrich WD: Hyperglycemia and the vascular effects of cerebral ischemia. Stroke 28:149–154, 1997.
142. Kent TA, Soukup VM, Fabian RH: Heterogeneity affecting outcome from acute stroke therapy: Making reperfusion worse. Stroke 32:2318–2327, 2001.
143. Kase CS, Furlan AJ, Wechsler LR, et al: Symptomatic intracranial hemorrhage after intraarterial thrombolysis with recombinant prourokinase in acute ischemic stroke: The PROACT II Study. Neurology 54(Suppl 3):A260–A261, 2000.
144. Toni D, De Michele M, Fiorelli M, et al: Influence of hyperglycemia on infarct size and clinical outcome of acute ischemic stroke patients with intracranial arterial occlusion. J Neurol Sci 123:129–133, 1994.
145. Capes SE, Hunt D, Malmberg K, et al: Stress hyperglycemia and prognosis of stroke in nondiabetic and diabetic patients: A systematic overview. Stroke 32:2426–2432, 2001.
146. Van Den Berghe G, Wouters P, Weekers F, et al: Intensive insulin therapy in critically ill patients. N Engl J Med 345:1359–1367, 2001.
147. Gladman JRF: Stroke units: Are they cost effective? Br J Hosp Med 47:91–93, 1992.
148. Jörgensen HS, Nakayama H, Raaschou HO, et al: The effect of stroke units: Reductions in mortality, discharge rate to nursing home, length of hospital stay, and cost: A community-based study. Stroke 26:1178–1182, 1995.
149. Jörgensen HS, Nakayama H, Raaschou HO, Skyhöj Olsen T: Acute stroke care and rehabilitation: An analysis of direct cost and its clin-

ical and social determinants. The Copenhagen Stroke Study. Stroke 28:1138–1141, 1997.

150. Ronnig OM, Guldvog B: Stroke units versus general medical wards. I: Twelve and 18 month survival, a randomised controlled trial. Stroke 29:58–62, 1998.

151. Caro JJ, Huybrechts KF, Duchesne I: Management patterns and costs of acute ischemic stroke: An international study. Stroke Economic Analysis Group. Stroke 31:582–590, 2000.

152. Claesson L, Gosman-Hedström G, Johannesson M, et al: Resource utilization and costs of stroke unit care integrated in a care continuum: A 1-year controlled, prospective, randomized study in elderly patients. The Göteborg 701 Stroke Study. Stroke 31:2569–2577, 2000.

153. Fagerberg B, Claesson L, Gosman-Hedström G, Blomstrand C: Effect of acute stroke unit care integrated in a care continuum vs conventional treatment: A randomized 1-year study of elderly patients. The Göteborg 701 Stroke Study. Stroke. 31:2578–2584, 2000.

154. Brainin M: Neurological acute stroke care: The role of European neurology. European Federation of Neurological Societies Task Force. Eur J Neurol 4:435–441, 1997.

155. Adams R, Acker J, Alberts M, et al: Recommendations for improving the quality of care through stroke centers and systems: An examination of stroke center identification options from the Advisory Working Group on Stroke Center Identification Options of the American Stroke Association. Stroke 33:326, 2002.

Chapter Fifty-Two

Critical Care of the Patient with Acute Stroke

Dimitrios Georgiadis, Stefan Schwab, and Werner Hacke

GENERAL PRINCIPLES OF NEUROLOGIC CRITICAL CARE

Initial Assessment of Patients with Stroke

Initial clinical assessment of patients with severe stroke should concentrate on the following issues:

1. Vital functions (pulmonary function, heart rate, blood pressure)
2. Neurologic symptoms, severity of neurologic deficit based on validated stroke scales
3. Time of symptom onset, potential eligibility for specific treatment options
4. Blood sampling for electrolytes, full blood count, and coagulation studies

One should always bear in mind that most emergency measures depend on the cause of the stroke (ischemic versus hemorrhagic); even blood pressure management cannot be initiated before this determination. Thus, it is vital that appropriate neuroimaging studies not be unnecessarily delayed. Additionally, caution is warranted to avoid measures that have the potential to interfere with further treatment options (for example, insertion of a central venous line in a patient eligible for thrombolysis).

Ancillary Tests

A diagnostic tool for acute stroke should ideally enable differentiation between hemorrhage and ischemia and provide information on the exact anatomic localization and extent of the lesion as well as on the status of the basal cerebral arteries. The first two requirements are met by computed tomography (CT), which is currently used for the initial neuroradiologic evaluation of the vast majority of patients with acute stroke. Furthermore, the hyperdense middle cerebral artery (MCA) sign, brain swelling, and parenchymal hypodensity have been described as early CT signs of ischemic infarction.[1] Interobserver agreement in assessing early CT signs of cerebral infarction was reported as adequate[1-3]; specific training further improved diagnostic accuracy.[4] The extent of early parenchymal hypoattenuation has also been shown to predict outcome after thrombolytic therapy,[5] extent of irreversible brain damage,[6]

and cerebral infarct volume at 30 days.[7] Despite the high interobserver agreement in the diagnosis of early infarct signs on CT, their identification is not always straightforward, leading to incorrect estimates of the extent of hypoattenuation in approximately 9% and 5% of patients enrolled in European Cooperative Acute Stroke Study (ECASS) I[8] and ECASS II, respectively.[9]

Magnetic resonance imaging (MRI), however, appears to fulfill all the previous requirements; identification of intracerebral hemorrhage is feasible even within 2 hours of symptom onset through the use of susceptibility-weighted imaging.[10,11] Diagnosis of subarachnoid hemorrhage with fluid attenuation inversion recovery (FLAIR) MRI sequences is also possible.[12] Diffusion-weighted imaging (DWI) has been reported to be superior to CT for early identification of the extent and location of lesions in stroke patients[13,14]; although these results appear promising, large-scale studies are warranted to compare the diagnostic potential of the two techniques.

Perfusion-weighted imaging (PWI) provides an estimate of the extent of the hypoperfused—and thus dysfunctional—brain tissue. The combination of DWI and PWI not only has improved our understanding of the pathophysiology of stroke but also appears to provide clinically relevant information on the extent of potentially salvageable tissue: of the two observed mismatch patterns, one (DWI > PWI) has been shown to be associated with no further growth in infarct size, whereas the second (DWI < PWI) indicates the presence of hypoperfused areas without structural lesions.[15] Reports also suggest that the PWI/DWI mismatch can be used to predict patient outcome,[15,16] identify patients likely to benefit from thrombolysis[17,18] and assess the effectiveness of thrombolytic therapy.[19,20] Finally, MR angiography provides valuable information on the status of the intracranial vessels and visualizes relevant vessel occlusions.[21]

A combination of MR angiography and MRI incorporating susceptibility, T2, diffusion, and perfusion weighting provides all the information relevant in patients presenting with acute stroke and can potentially lengthen the time window for thrombolysis in selected patients. Still, this promising technique remains to be prospectively tested. Furthermore, the longer time required to perform this technique compared with CT (approximately 20 minutes) together with its limited availability, particularly on a 24-hour basis, restrict its applicability. The growing evidence for the clinical significance of MRI findings, particularly concerning DWI/PWI mismatch and the indication for thrombolysis, should lead to further integration of MRI into the treatment of patients with stroke patients.

Positron emission tomography (PET) can be used to distinguish hypoperfused but still salvageable tissue from tissue that has already been irreversibly damaged. Early PET studies were able to document the existence of the penumbra,[22,23] and further studies also provided ischemia and penumbra thresholds of cerebral blood flow (CBF)[24,25] in patients studied between 5 and 18 hours after stroke onset. Heiss and colleagues[26,27] have demonstrated that thrombolysis can salvage cerebral tissue with a CBF less than 12 mL/100 g/min if performed within 3 hours of stroke onset. Identification of the penumbra using PET could allow individual decision-making in acute stroke.

Single-photon emission computed tomography (SPECT) can also be used to assess brain perfusion. Initial reports suggested that differentiation between transient ischemic attacks and ischemic stroke within the first 6 hours of symptom onset using SPECT is feasible.[28] Furthermore, Berrouschot and associates[29] reported a high sensitivity and specificity for early (within 6 hours of stroke onset) SPECT findings in identifying patients in whom fatal ischemic brain edema developed; this finding could be of particular value in facilitating early patient selection for aggressive treatment.

Transcranial Doppler (TCD) ultrasonography offers a noninvasive, inexpensive method for evaluating the basal cerebral arteries. The suggestion that MCA insonation in patients with acute stroke could enhance the thrombolytic efficacy of recombinant tissue-plasminogen activator (rt-PA)[30] represents an intriguing novel application of MRI that merits further evaluation in controlled trials. Transcranial color-coded duplex ultrasonography has evolved as an attractive alternative to TCD ultrasonography for the acute evaluation of stroke patients. Further, for evaluation of the brain-supplying arteries, this technique can potentially differentiate between ischemic and hemorrhagic infarction[31] or identify hemorrhagic transformations.[32] Although CT remains the method of first choice for this purpose, transcranial color-coded duplex ultrasonography can be used for patients who are too unstable for transport or for follow-up studies. Finally, measurement of the dislocation of the midline allows an estimate of intracranial shift[33,34]; Gerriets and coworkers[35] demonstrate that midline shift in the first 12 hours after symptom onset can predict impending herniation and guide the decision for aggressive treatment.

Digital subtraction angiography (DSA) remains the standard for diagnosis of occlusion or severe stenosis of cerebral vessels. Despite the rapid improvements in MRA, DSA still has its applications in patients requiring endovascular therapy.[36–40]

It is of major importance that patients with severe stroke be accompanied by a physician during diagnostic procedures. Apart from frequently monitoring the neurologic state and vital signs, the physician must decide about the necessity for mild sedation if the patient is not cooperative enough for the procedure to be performed. In certain patients, intubation and mechanical ventilation may be required to allow acquisition of diagnostic studies of adequate quality. One should bear in mind, however, that the clinical evaluation of the patient is markedly limited after the use of these measures. It is thus of particular importance to weigh the potential relevance of the diagnostic information in the acute situation against the disadvantages caused by the later inability to monitor the patient's clinical course.

Pulmonary Function and Mechanical Ventilation

Maintenance of adequate oxygenation is essential in patients with acute stroke, because it potentially preserves metabolic turnover and reduces anaerobic processes, which could be deleterious for the ischemic penumbra. Avoidance of hypercapnia is of equal importance, as it potentially leads to vasodilation in the cerebral arterioles supplying healthy brain tissue, thereby reducing blood supply to the lesion site, where cerebral vessels are already maximally dilated under resting conditions. Transcutaneous evaluation of oxygen saturation constitutes the minimal requirement for monitoring of pulmonary function. Mechanical ventilation should be initiated when PO_2 values drop below 60 to 70 mm Hg, pCO_2 values exceed 50 to 60 mm Hg, or both. Other clinical signs of respiratory failure are tachypnea exceeding 35 breaths per minute, dyspnea with use of accessory muscles, and respiratory acidosis (Table 52.1).

Respiratory failure in patients with acute stroke is mostly associated with aspiration pneumonia, impaired central respiratory drive, or neurogenic pulmonary edema (NPE). During the course of the disease, however, respiratory function can be compromised by the development of various pathologic conditions, including atelectasis or pneumonia due to immobilization, decreased level of consciousness, epileptic seizures, and critical illness polyneuropathy. Additionally, patients with severe stroke undergo mechanical ventilation for performance of diagnostic or therapeutic interventions or airway protection when gag reflex is absent or reduced. The percentage of unselected patients with stroke who undergo mechanical ventilation has been reported as 10%.[41] Significant differences in rate of mechanical ventilation have been found to be related to the cause of stroke; Mayer and associates[41] reported that 5% of patients with ischemic stroke, 26% of patients with intracerebral hemorrhage (ICH), and 47% of patients with subarachnoid hemorrhage (SAH) underwent mechanical ventilation, whereas Gujjar and colleagues[42] found rates of 6% for ischemic stroke and 30% for ICH.

As the prognosis of patients with acute stroke undergoing mechanical ventilation is rather poor (mortality rates between 49% and 93%),[42–45] the identification of clinical predictors of adverse outcome is crucial. A Glasgow Coma Scale (GCS) score of less than 10 was found to predict mortality in most studies[41,44,46]; other factors were older age,[42,44] absence of brainstem reflexes,[42,46] intubation because of respiratory failure,[44] and bradycardia.[46] These data can obviously provide no guidelines for individual patients. Still, it is important to bear them in mind, particularly

Table 52.1   Indications for Mechanical Ventilation

PO_2 < 70 mm Hg despite O_2 administration via nasal probe or facial mask

PCO_2 > 60 mm Hg (except for patients with chronic obstructive airway disease and chronically elevated CO_2)

Vital capacity < 500–600 mL

Clinical signs of respiratory failure (tachypnea, use of accessory muscles)

Severe respiratory acidosis

Airway protection (gag and swallowing reflexes absent, level of consciousness decreased)

---

when one is discussing the issue of mechanical ventilation with a patient's family.

Orotracheal intubation is the approach of first choice because it enables the use of larger-diameter tubes, avoids the tube contamination that occurs during passage of oronasal tubes, and is associated with a lower prevalence of maxillary sinusitis.[47,48] Any drugs used before intubation should preferably be short-acting. We recommend sufentanil (70 μg), followed by etomidate (0.3–0.5 mg/kg) or propofol (1.5–3 mg/kg) in combination with a depolarizing neuromuscular blocking agent such as succinylcholine (1.2 mg/kg), given in rapid sequence, to avoid long-term influence on the hemodynamic situation. Continuous infusion of sedatives and analgesics is warranted for the duration of mechanical ventilation. Further details on sedation and analgesia are given in the next section of this chapter.

Ventilator settings should be adjusted to provide a PO_2 of 1.0 mm Hg and a pCO_2 between 38 and 42 mm Hg. Inspiration-to-expiration (I:E) ratio should initially be set at 1:2, and positive end-expiratory pressure (PEEP) at 4 mm Hg. Pressure- or volume-controlled ventilation modes can be applied. Inspiratory flow should be set at 30 L/min and tidal volume at 12 mL/kg. Higher PEEP levels are often necessary for adequate oxygenation of patients with pulmonary disorders, because PEEP improves oxygenation by preventing or reducing atelectasis, increasing functional residual capacity, and reducing pulmonary shunting. The assumption that use of higher PEEP levels causes an increase in intracranial pressure (ICP) could not be confirmed in a recent study.[49] Higher PEEP levels result in higher intrathoracic pressure and reduced venous return, and could affect cerebral perfusion pressure (CPP) by lowering mean arterial blood pressure (MAP). If one assumes a patent cerebral autoregulation, the MAP decrease would be compensated by a dilation of the cerebral arterioles, resulting in an increase in ICP. This effect, however, can be counteracted with a corresponding adjustment in the central venous pressure (CVP). Equally, it was shown that alterations of the I:E ratio from 1:2 to 1:1 do not influence ICP or CPP, and could therefore be readily applied in patients with acute stroke.[50]

Orotracheal or nasotracheal intubation is potentially associated with the risk of laryngeal or tracheal stenosis and phonation disability. Whited[51] described a 2% incidence of laryngeal stenosis in patients who had been intubated fewer than 6 days; the incidence rose to approximately 5% in patients intubated for 6 to 11 days. These findings were not confirmed in later studies. Colice and associates[52] described mucosal ulceration and varying severity of laryngeal edema in 94% of patients intubated longer than 4 days; these changes were mostly reversible, and duration of intubation did not influence the incidence of laryngeal lesions. Dunham and LaMonica[53] observed no differences in incidence of laryngeal complications whether patients underwent early or late tracheostomy.

In addition to reducing the risk of the complications just described, tracheostomy is associated with several advantages over orotracheal or nasotracheal intubation. They include patient comfort, a more secure airway, fewer complications due to unplanned extubation, easier reintubation, improved suctioning, and faster weaning from mechanical ventilation—all of which result in a shorter stay in the intensive care unit (ICU). It thus appears that patients who are not likely to be weaned from mechanical ventilation within 3 weeks would profit from early tracheostomy; identification of such patients is not always straightforward, however. Qureshi and associates[54] examined 69 mechanically ventilated patients with infratentorial lesions; unsuccessful weaning was found to be associated with a GCS lower than 7 as well as brainstem deficits. This study represents the only evaluation of predisposing factors for tracheostomy in patients with stroke.

Current guidelines suggest that tracheostomy is not indicated in patients requiring ventilatory support for less than 10 days but should be performed in patients who will require ventilatory support for more than 21 days. Still, tracheostomy should be performed earlier in patients who are likely to require ventilatory support for more than 21 days or who are without a functioning gag reflex and require tracheostomy for airway protection.

Sedation and Analgesia

Patients treated in the ICU are exposed to various stress factors, including anxiety, unfamiliar auditory and visual stimuli, awareness of severe illness, and sleep disturbances. Medical conditions such as pain, respiratory insufficiency, cardiovascular impairment, and sepsis constitute further stress factors; the same is true for several treatment options, particularly mechanical ventilation. Inadequate sedation and analgesia can cause postagression syndrome, which results in greater metabolic rate and oxygen consumption, potentially further endangering the ischemic penumbra. Furthermore, mechanical ventilation is greatly compromised, or even impossible, with inadequate sedation. Sedation is a major issue in intracranial hypertension, because coughing or straining raises ICP.

A variety of drugs are available for sedation of patients in ICU. Benzodiazepines, barbiturates, and neuroleptics constitute the most commonly administered drugs; for a list of drugs, dosages, and potential side effects, see Table 52.2. Midazolam and propofol are the drugs most commonly used for long-term sedation of patients in ICUs. Studies comparing their effects have reported a reliable, safe, and controllable sedation for both agents.[55–59] The main observed differences were (1) a higher incidence of arterial hypotension in patients receiving propofol[55,56,58] and (2) a faster recovery in patients treated with propofol,[55,56,58,59] also resulting in faster weaning.[57] The latter

Table 52.2   Sedatives Commonly Used in Patients Treated in Intensive Care Units

Drug	Doses	Characteristics
Midazolam	0.1–0.3 mg/kg/h	Antiepileptic properties Paradoxic reactions Contraindicated in myasthenia gravis Respiratory depression Liver dysfunction, agranulocytosis, hypotension Shorter half-life, higher effectiveness than diazepam
Propofol	5–10 mg (SD) 0.8–3 mg/kg/h	Short half-life, minimal accumulation Faster recovery Faster weaning Nutritional effect Antiepileptic properties Increases serum levels of triglycerides Hypotension, seizures, tachyphylaxia Contraindicated for children
Clonidine	0.3–1.2 mg/kg/h	Add on to reduce dose requirements of sedatives Withdrawal syndrome Initial hypertensive effect Reduces sympathetic tone Rebound phenomenon after discontinuation
Gamma-hydroxybutyric acid	50 mg/kg (SD) 10–20 mg/kg/h	Myoclonic seizures reported Hypernatremia Contraindicated in epilepsy, hypertension, renal failure, alcohol poisoning Less pronounced respiratory depression
Ketamine	1–2 mg/kg (SD) 0.5–4 mg/kg/h	Weak sedative potency Nightmares, hallucinations Sympathomimetic properties (inhibits re-uptake of catecholamines, bronchodilation) Analgesic potency Less pronounced respiratory depression Less pronounced depression of bowel motility
Haloperidol	5–15 mg IV (SD) 2.5–15 mg/h	Arterial hypotension Parkinsonoid syndrome [antidote: Biperiden] Arrhythmia, QT prolongation Antipsychotic properties Antiemetic properties Improvement of bowel motility
Thiopental	3–7 mg/kg (SD) 4–200 (to 900) mg/h	No ceiling effect Respiratory depression Liver dysfunction, agranulocytosis, hypotension Accumulation
Etomidate	0.15–0.3 mg/kg (repetitive injections up to 80 mg/day)	No hemodynamic effects Myoclonic seizures Dyskinesia Short sedation

IV, intravenous injection; SD, starting dose.

difference also outweighed the higher costs of propofol by reducing the duration of mechanical ventilation.[57] Use of midazolam infusion for treatment of refractory status epilepticus is well established; case reports suggest that propofol also possesses therapeutic potential for patients with this condition.[60] Additionally, initial comparisons have described no differences in antiepileptic properties between the two agents.[61]

Treatment of conditions with potential to aggravate the patient, particularly inadequate analgesia, is an important measure that may reduce the amount of sedation required. The same is true for nonmedical measures, such as communicating with and reassuring the patient and tempering psychological problems.

It must be stressed that sedation is never a substitute for adequate analgesia. Almost every patient in an ICU experiences pain at some point; the treatment of choice depends on the cause and severity of the pain. Non-opioids (paracetamol, salicylate, or nonsteroidal agents [indomethacin, ibuprofen, diclofenac]) may be adequate in some cases. Still, most patients require opioids for satisfactory pain control. The main advantage of opioids is their lack of cardiovascular side effects. These agents' respiratory depression and antitussive effects are of advantage in mechanically ventilated patients but limit their applicability in spontaneously breathing patients.

Two substances from this group are being routinely applied, fentanyl and sufentanil. Fentanyl possesses an approximately 100 to 150 times higher analgesic potency than morphine. The maximal effect is already reached 4 to 5 minutes after intravenous infusion. Fentanyl accumulates in fatty tissue. Its redistribution can cause significant rebound effects after its discontinuation, and even respiratory depression. Fentanyl is applied as a continuous intravenous infusion, at doses ranging between 0.05 and 0.3 mg/h, usually combined with midazolam or propofol.

Sufentanil is the most potent opioid, with an analgesic potency approximately 1000 higher than morphine's. It is reported to provide better patient comfort with less respiratory depression than fentanyl.[62] The effect of both substances on CBF remains uncertain.[63–65] Sufentanil has an additional sedative effect, which reduces the required dose of sedatives. It is applied as continuous intravenous infusion at rates of 0.5 to 0.75 μg/kg/hour. Because of the previously cited respiratory depression caused by opioids, tramadol, 50 to 100 mg given PO (orally), SC (subcutaneously), rectally, IM (intramuscularly), or IV (intravenously) or tilidine, 50 to 100 mg PO, should be applied in awake, spontaneously breathing patients.

Fluid Balance

Fluid and electrolyte disturbances are common findings in ICU patients. They may be due to (1) sympathetic responses to ischemic or hemorrhagic neuronal injury, (2) unbalanced fluid and electrolyte substitution (calculation of daily fluid requirement; see Table 52.3), (3) unbalanced nutritional regimen, or (4) administration of diuretics and other drugs (particularly osmotherapeutics). Sympathetic nervous system stimulation reduces renal blood flow, thus activating the renin-angiotensin system and increasing the secretion of aldosterone, an effect that in turn causes sodium retention and kaliuresis. Antidiuretic hormone (ADH) secretion may also be affected by central nervous system lesions, resulting in sodium and water retention and decreased urine output (syndrome of inappropriate antidiuretic hormone secretion [SIADH]) or in diabetes insipidus.

Fluid disturbances can be assessed by (1) clinical observation, (2) evaluation of fluid intake and output, (3) measurement of CVP via a central venous line or of pulmonary capillary wedge pressure via a pulmonary catheter, and (4) measurements of serum osmolarity, urine osmolarity, and serum sodium concentration. Sodium, the main electrolyte of the extracellular fluid, accounts for more than 90% of its osmolarity. There is a close relationship between

sodium and water shifts. Sodium concentrations and the hydration state of the patient provide the required information for diagnosis and the treatment of fluid imbalances. Isotonic volume depletion is the most common abnormality encountered. The treatment of choice is enteral or IV administration of isotonic fluids. Careful fluid balancing and monitoring of the CVP are warranted to allow determination of the amount of fluids needed. In patients with concomitant left ventricular failure, chest radiograph, echocardiography, or pulmonary wedge pressure should be used to avoid potentially deleterious fluid overload.

For hypernatremic or hyponatremic states, the therapeutic regimen depends on the hydration state of the patient. In the setting of a central diabetes insipidus, SC or IV administration of 2 to 5 units of aqueous vasopressin or 1 to 5 μg of its analog, desmopressin (DDAVP), effectively reduces water diuresis. Further details concerning fluid management are provided in textbooks of clinical medicine.

Nutrition

Nutrition in hospitalized patients with acute stroke is an often overlooked, though significant issue. Davalos and coworkers[66] reported protein-energy malnutrition in 16.3% of 104 patients admitted with acute stroke, and in 26.4% and 35% of the same population after the first and second weeks in hospital, respectively; additionally, malnutrition was identified as an independent predictor of poor outcome. Similar results were reported by Gariballa and associates[67]; they assessed 96 patients with acute stroke upon admission and after 2 weeks, and 51 of them again at 4 weeks. They found that nutritional status deteriorated significantly during the study period. Serum albumin concentrations showed a significant association with infective complications and were an independent predictor of death at 3 months. Davalos and coworkers[66] postulated a hypercatabolic state due to stress reaction or a neuroendocrine response to injury that modified the carbohydrate metabolism as possible explanation for the observed malnutrition. The demonstrated prognostic significance of malnutrition in patient outcome highlights the importance of an adequate caloric and protein supply in patients with acute stroke.

The resting energy expenditure is calculated by means of indirect calorimetry; although this technique constitutes the most reliable method, it is not readily available in neurological intensive care units (NICUs). Alternatively, the basal energy expenditure (BEE) is calculated on the basis of the Harris-Benedict equation. This value must consequently be multiplied by a factor determined by any concomitant diseases (Table 52.4). Fever further raises caloric requirements by 13% for every 1°C above 37°C. Caloric requirements are also increased by epileptic seizures, pain, and use of glucocorticoids and are decreased by hypothermia and barbiturate coma.

Essential amino acids, fatty acids, and vitamins are already included in standard parenteral and enteral feeding preparations. Protein requirements in critically ill patients are higher (1.2–1.5 g per kg body weight) than in nonstressed, healthy persons (0.8 g per kg body weight). Initial substitution with the preceding requirement should

Table 52.3 Assessment of Daily Fluid Requirement

Basal requirement	30 mL per kg body weight
+ Urinary output	Urine volume over last 24 hours
+ Stool water	Approximately 100 mL/day (more in diarrhea)
+ Insensible loss	Approximately 800 mL/day (spontaneously breathing patient)
	Approximately 400 mL/day (mechanically ventilated patient)
	Fever correction: add 500 mL per 1°C > 37°C

Table 52.4 Basal and Total Energy Expenditure

Harris-Benedict equation (W = weight in kg, H = height in cm,
  A = age in years):
  BEE (men) = 66.47 + 13.75 × W + 5.0 × H − 6.76 × A [kcal/d]
  BEE (women) = 655.1 + 9.56 × W + 1.85 × H − 4.68 × A [kcal/d]
Stress factors (Fs) (to be multiplied with BEE for estimated
  total calorie requirement):
  Critical care: F = 1.25
  Pneumonia: F = 1.5
  Large hemispheric infarction   F = 1.75
  Fever: F = 1.13 per 1°C > 37°C

BEE, Basal energy expenditure.

be adjusted to that calculated according to the urine urea nitrogen (N) test results, as follows:

$$\text{Amount of N output (gram)} = \text{Urea excreted (gram)} \times 0.45 \times 1.2$$

A 24-hour urine specimen should be collected at least once weekly for assessment of urea excretion. The value 0.45 in the preceding equation stands for the percentage of nitrogen in urea, and the 1.2 for nitrogen lost through skin and intestine. The supplied nitrogen is calculated as follows:

$$\text{N intake (gram)} = \text{Total Protein Intake}/6.25$$

In the acute phase of stroke, the stress reaction can be so prominent that a catabolic state cannot be prevented. Still, a slightly positive nitrogen balance should be achieved over the next few days.

Concepts now suggest that enteral rather than parenteral nutrition should be pursued in ICU patients. If possible, oral feeding should be allowed and carefully monitored to ensure adequate intake. If intake is consistently below 50% to 75% of the nutritional goals for 1 week, supplemental nutritional support should be initiated. Supplemental nutritional support is required in most patients treated in a neurocritical care unit because of depressed levels of consciousness, impaired swallowing function, or mechanical ventilation. For nutritional support, enteral nutrition with a nasogastric tube is the approach of first choice. The enteral route has several advantages, including simpler application, lower risk of infection, utilization of the normal physiologic functions of digestion and absorption, maintenance of the intestinal mucosa, and lower cost. Intestinal function and motility must be regularly monitored (bowel sounds, aspiration of gastric residuals) and, if necessary, supported by a stimulant such as metoclopramide or cisapride (although caution is warranted because of the risk of ventricular arrhythmias). If motility is still not restored, postpyloric feeding (endoscopically placed nasoduodenal or nasojejunal probe) or parenteral nutrition should be considered. Continuous pump-assisted infusion is better tolerated than bolus administration.

Patients who are bound to require long-term enteral nutritional support should be scheduled early for percutaneous endoscopic gastrostomy (PEG), which is better tolerated and causes fewer local complications. A common complication of enteral feeding is diarrhea, which occurs as a result of the hyperosmolar electrolyte solutions or of quick build-up of enteral feeding after an extended period of fasting or parenteral nutrition. Another potential complication is gastric retention, which enhances the risk of regurgitation and pulmonary aspiration.

Parenteral nutrition is indicated in cases of imminent intubation or operation, gastrointestinal leakage, ileus, pancreatitis, and other conditions in which a patient's gastrointestinal tract is unable to tolerate oral or enteral feeding for at least 5 to 7 days. A peripheral venous line is adequate for short-term parenteral nutrition, provided that the osmolarity of the infused solutions does not exceed approximately 1000 mOsm/kg. Long-term parenteral nutrition, meeting the patients' full calorie and protein requirements without giving an excess fluid volume, requires hyperosmolar formulas of up to 1800 mOsm/kg. These are very irritating to the venous endothelium and thus must be administered via central venous lines (see earlier discussion). Complications of parenteral feeding include the risks associated with the necessity of a central catheter as well as metabolic problems. Hyperglycemia, a common side effect, often requires continuous insulin infusion. Hypoglycemia after discontinuation of parenteral nutrition, on the other hand, can be prevented by a slow tapering of the formula. Liver function abnormalities, with mild to moderate elevations of serum liver enzyme activity and bilirubin, are also very common but usually benign and self-limiting.

Blood Pressure Control

A variety of drugs can be used for treatment of acute arterial hypertension. Modes of action and potential influence on ICP and CBF of the antihypertensive agents most commonly used in intensive care are described in this section. Dosages are listed in Table 52.5. Specific aspects of managing blood pressure according to cause of stroke and individual findings are covered later in the chapter.

Peripheral Vasodilators

Vasodilators cause relaxation of arterial and venous smooth muscle cells. This effect is accompanied by baroreceptor-

Table 52.5 Dosages of Commonly Used Antihypertensive Drugs

Drug	Dosage
Nitroprusside	IFR 0.5–2 µg/kg/min (up to 8 µg/kg/min for short periods possible)
Hydralazine	IV 10–20 mg; maximum IFR 30 mg/h
Labetalol	10–20 mg IV repeated q 10 min up to 80 mg IV. IFR 0.5–2.0 mg/min
Nicardipine	IFR 5–15 mg/h

IFR, infusion rate; IV; intravenous injection; OD, oral dose.

mediated tachycardia. These agents are also active in the cerebral vasculature, increasing CBF and ICP. In patients with acute stroke, cerebral vessels supplying the affected brain region are already maximally dilated. Thus, use of vasodilators can result in vasodilation of the vessels supplying unaffected brain regions, causing a redistribution of CBF (steal phenomenon) and potentially aggravating ischemic injury. Although this pathophysiologic concept has not been demonstrated in clinical studies, most institutions refrain from using vasodilators in patients with acute stroke.

The most commonly used vasodilators are nitroprusside, nitroglycerin, and dihydralazine. Nitroprusside and nitroglycerin, which have a fast onset and short duration of action, should be administered as continuous intravenous infusions. The main limitation of nitroprusside is the risk of cyanide intoxication, particularly in association with doses exceeding 18 μg/kg/hour or used longer than 48 to 72 hours. Nitroglycerin has been shown to dilate large cerebral arteries.[68] Rogers and colleagues[69] demonstrated significant ICP increases in association with the decrease in arterial blood pressure in a cat model. Cottrell and associates[70] reported similar findings in five anesthetized patients. Thus, the use of nitroglycerin is not indicated in patients with intracranial hypertension. Dihydralazine has a slower onset of action, although its effect after intravenous bolus administration lasts for approximately 4 hours. Like nitroprusside and nitroglycerin, dihydralazine is best administered as a continuous intravenous infusion. Studies on head-injured patients showed that dihydralazine administration is associated with increases in ICP.[71–73] To date, no clinical studies have examined the effect of dihydralazine in patients with acute stroke.

Adrenergic Agents

Urapidil is an alpha$_1$ receptor antagonist that has both a peripheral effect and a central effect. Owing to its central effect, administration of urapidil is not associated with tachycardia. Animal studies demonstrated that urapidil does not influence ICP when applied as a continuous intravenous infusion.[74,75] Results of bolus administration were not unanimous; one study described an ICP increase in cats with experimental cerebral cold lesions,[74] and the other described no ICP effects in dogs with intracranial hypertension.[75] Still, loss of cerebral autoregulation and significant decrease in cerebral perfusion pressure were reported.[76] A clinical study in eight patients undergoing craniotomy for intracerebral tumor showed that the decrease in systemic arterial blood pressure due to urapidil does not influence ICP.[77]

Clonidine stimulates alpha$_2$-adrenergic inhibitory neurons in the medulla, thus reducing sympathetic nervous system outflow. This reduction leads to decreases in arterial blood pressure, heart rate, and cardiac output. Clonidine also has sedative and analgesic properties.[78,79] It can be administered orally, subcutaneously, and as an intravenous infusion. Acute withdrawal results in rebound hypertension. The effects of clonidine on CBF remain unclear. Greene and coworkers[80] used clonidine in 13 patients with severe hypertension. Goal blood pressure was reached in 12 patients; a significant increase in CBF (>10%) occurred

in 5 patients, and a significant decrease in 4. The magnitude of CBF changes depended on the initial values, patients with initially low CBF experiencing an increase, and those with initially high CBF, a decrease. Asgeirsson and colleagues[81] found no effect of clonidine on CBF and ICP in six severely head-injured patients. Kanawati[82] and associates observed a significant reduction in CBF after administration of clonidine; because this effect could not be reproduced with use of a structural analogue of clonidine that does not cross the blood-brain barrier, these investigators suggested that the CBF response of clonidine is mediated by central mechanisms rather than by alterations in CPP. Favre and coworkers[83] observed significant changes in MAP and CPP in 12 patients who received clonidine during the preinduction period, while ICP remained unchanged. Ter Minassian and associates[84] also observed significant decreases in MAP and CPP after intravenous administration of clonidine; in contrast to the previous study, clonidine also resulted in a transient increase in ICP in 3 subjects. Thus, although thoroughly studied, the effects of clonidine on CBF remain unclear. The effect of clonidine on the cerebrovascular CO$_2$ response is also a matter of debate, with two studies reporting a reduced response[83,85] and another an increased response.[86]

Propranolol is a nonselective β-antagonist. Its administration results in decreases in blood pressure, heart rate, and cardiac output. No effect of propranolol on ICP was observed after oral administration in patients with intracerebral hemorrhage[87] or in patients with head injury.[71] Equally, no effect on CBF was noted in 31 hypertensive patients after long-term propranolol therapy.[88] No study has examined the effect of propranolol in patients with acute ischemic stroke. Because this agent can be administered either orally or by slow intravenous injection, it cannot be used for long-term control of hypertension in the ICU.

Labetalol is a mixed α- and β-antagonist. It can lower MAP by reducing systemic vascular resistance while preventing reflex tachycardia through the additional β-blockade. Labetalol can be administered as a continuous intravenous infusion, a feature that augments its applicability in ICU. This agent appears to have no effect on ICP in experimental studies using animal models[89,90] or in clinical studies in hypertensive patients.[91] Orlowski and associates[92] observed a slight but statistically significant ICP reduction in patients treated with nitroprusside alone compared with patients treated either with labetalol or with a combination of labetalol and nitroprusside. As with other agents in this category, studies examining the effectiveness of labetalol in patients with acute stroke are lacking.

Calcium Channel Blockers

Calcium channel blockers cause vasodilation (more pronounced in arteries than in veins) and decrease in heart rate, myocardial contractility, and conduction at the atrioventricular node. These effects can lead to myocardial depression, atrioventricular block, bradycardia, heart failure, and even cardiac arrest. Nifedipine and nicardipine are the most commonly used calcium channel blockers.

Nifedipine was shown to produce a discrete but statistically significant elevation in ICP when given intravenously to cats with normal baseline ICP; this increase, however, was larger in the presence of intracranial hypertension.[93] Similar results were reported by Anger and colleagues[94] in a further animal study; Wusten and associates[95] observed significant increase in ICP after administration of nifedipine but found that administration of urapidil did not influence ICP. Bertel and associates[96] compared oral nifedipine with placebo in 25 hypertensive patients who did not have intracranial disease. They observed significant reductions in MAP with nifedipine; furthermore, nifedipine administration resulted in CBF elevation in 4 of 5 patients in whom CBF was evaluated.[96] Still, Tateishi and coworkers[97] reported a significant ICP increase, ranging from 1 to 10 mm Hg, in 10 patients with head trauma or cerebrovascular disease.

Nicardipine is a potent vasodilator that also affects cerebral blood vessels. Its effect on CBF remains unclear. Sakabe and associates[98] observed significant postischemic rises in CBF in both nicardipine-treated and control animals; CBF significantly decreased in the control group but remained unchanged in the nicardipine-treated group. Kittawa and colleagues[99] observed no CBF changes with administration of nicardipine after an ischemic insult in rats; in contrast, in an animal model without intracranial disease, Tanaka and coworkers[100] saw CBF increases after administration of the agent. Interestingly, Sakabe and associates[98] observed no improvement in neurologic outcome in treated animals, but Kittawa and colleagues[99] reported significant decreases in neuron-specific enolase and in infarction and edema volume, which were associated with an improved neurologic outcome, with treatment. After topical application of nicardipine during extracranial-to-intracranial bypass procedures, Gaab and associates[101] observed a marked dilation in the small cortical arteries; a nicardipine infusion, however, was associated with an increase in cerebral PO$_2$. Akopov and colleagues[102] could demonstrate no consistent pattern in regional (r) global CBF changes in 75 hypertensive patients with symptoms of chronic ischemic cerebrovascular disorders.[102] Abe and coworkers,[103] however, reported a moderate increase in local CBF after administration of nicardipine.

Lisk and associates[104] examined the effect of nicardipine, captopril, or clonidine in hypertensive patients with acute ischemic stroke (treated within 72 hours of onset). Nicardipine administration resulted in the most marked drop in MAP. A total of four patients demonstrated an MAP decrease greater than 16%, which was associated with sustained or decreased CBF. Three of these four patients were treated with nicardipine. Administration of nicardipine also appears to increase ICP; Nishikawa and associates[105] observed significant rises in cerebrospinal fluid (CSF) pressure (approximately 5 mm Hg), which were associaated with significant decreases in MAP and CPP in 17 patients without intracranial disease. Interestingly, this effect was not influenced by the dose administered (0.1 to 0.3 mg/kg).

Angiotensin-Converting Enzyme Inhibitors

Various angiotensin-converting enzyme (ACE) inhibitors have been developed. Of those, enalapril is the only agent currently available for intravenous administration and therefore also the one relevant for use in neurocritical care units. Enalapril apparently has no effect on CBF in patients without intracranial disease[106,107] or in patients with a unilateral stenosis of the internal carotid artery greater than 70%.[108] Kobayashi and associates[109] observed a mean 8% CBF increase in patients with chronic cerebral infarction. These findings, together with its insignificant side effects, suggest that enalapril is an attractive alternative for treatment of arterial hypertension in patients with acute stroke.

Maintenance or Elevation of Arterial Blood Pressure

Patients with arterial hypotension should initially be assessed clinically, and underlying conditions (for example, arrhythmia or hypovolemia) treated accordingly, before catecholamines are administered. One should note that acute myocardial ischemia is a common cause of acute hypotension that should be excluded before other measures are initiated. Crystalloid or colloid fluids should be applied and fluid homeostasis maintained through precise evaluation of fluid intake and output. The target value of CVP lies between 8 and 12 cm H$_2$O. No studies have yet compared the efficacy or side effects of various catecholamines in patients with acute stroke, so no definitive recommendations are possible. Norepinephrine is our drug of choice, because its use is not associated with tachycardia or arrhythmia, as is the case with most catecholamines. Specific therapeutic concepts utilizing induced arterial hypertension are discussed later in the chapter.

Invasive Monitoring Procedures

Central Venous Line or Pulmonary Catheter

Venous access can be achieved by catheterizing a peripheral vein. Although several veins can be used, one must bear in mind that antecubital veins are not appropriate in awake and mobile patients because of discomfort and the risk of thrombosis; risk of thrombosis also prohibits the use of pedal veins, except for immobile bedridden patients. Central venous lines should be used (1) if no peripheral venous access can be obtained, (2) for administration of drugs that irritate peripheral veins or can cause tissue necrosis after extravasation, and (3) in unstable patients requiring several intravenous lines for drug administration.

The femoral, internal jugular, external jugular, and subclavian veins can be used for central venous access. Each approach has its own advantages and disadvantages. It is important to note that cannulation of the internal jugular vein should be avoided in patients with, or in danger of potential development of, intracranial hypertension, because of possible impairment of cerebral venous drainage. Puncture of the internal carotid artery is relatively common, but the incidence of pneumothorax is quite low. Cannulation of the subclavian vein bears an increased risk of pneumothorax; on the other hand, this vein does not collapse and can therefore be used in cases of shock or hypovolemia. Although cannulation of the femoral vein is relatively easy, this approach should be used only as a last resort, mainly because of the risk of infection. The position of all central venous lines, except for those inserted in the femoral artery, should be verified on a chest radiograph before they are used.

Pulmonary artery catheters provide important physiologic information for assessment of cardiac function, including intracardiac pressures, cardiac output, pulmonary arterial blood saturation, and right ventricular volume. Still, this information is usually not necessary for managing patients with acute stroke, with the exception of patients treated with moderate hypothermia or patients with complicated mechanical ventilation.

Invasive Monitoring of Arterial Blood Pressure

The main indications for peripheral arterial cannulation are continuous direct blood pressure measurement and access for blood sampling, particularly in patients whose peripheral veins are inadequate for repeated blood sampling. The radial artery is most commonly used. The pulse of the ulnar artery should be confirmed as palpable before cannulation of the radial artery is attempted. Alternatively, evaluation of the ulnar artery can be performed with Doppler ultrasonography.

Invasive Monitoring of Intracranial Pressure
Indications

ICP monitoring is essential in patients at risk for ICP increase during the course of their disease, particularly comatose or sedated patients, in whom clinical assessment is not feasible. ICP monitoring reduces the need for neuroradiologic examinations and allows evaluation of the effectiveness of diverse therapeutic approaches. ICP monitoring is routinely performed unilaterally; tissue shifts in the contralateral hemisphere are therefore detected with a certain temporal latency. The exact effects of this issue on the clinical relevance of ICP monitoring have not yet been systematically studied. Still, in our experience in patients undergoing bilateral ICP monitoring, the role of this latency is minor, because initial pressure gradients rapidly resolve. Furthermore, ICP transducers are mostly inserted in the affected hemisphere, so that ICP increases are readily recognized. Currently, monitoring can be performed with intraventricular, intraparenchymatous, or epidural catheters as well as subarachnoid bolts.

Intraventricular Catheters

Intraventricular catheters (IVCs) possess the highest accuracy. First introduced in 1953, they continue to constitute an attractive option for ICP monitoring, because they also allow CSF drainage. An IVC is mostly introduced through a skin incision and burr hole over the posterior frontal lobe of the nondominant hemisphere, and forwarded for 5 to 8 cm, until CSF is encountered. A three-way stopcock allows CSF drainage. The amount of CSF drained can be regulated by adjustment of the height of the reservoir. The external acoustic meatus usually serves as reference point for estimating reservoir height. Simultaneous performance of ICP monitoring and CSF drainage is a common mistake; the ICP measured under these conditions equals the atmospheric pressure. Thus, drainage must be temporarily interrupted to achieve an accurate measurement. The accuracy of the measured ICP can be compromised by accumulation of blood clots, debris, or air in the lumen of an IVC.

The major complication of IVCs is infection, the actual incidence of which varies widely among the different studies (0% to 21%).[110-113] The largest series was reported by Holloway and associates,[114] who undertook a retrospective analysis of 611 patients with closed head injuries and ventriculostomies; incidence rate of ventriculitis was 10.4%. Several factors in the risk of IVC-associated infection remain unclear, including (1) the potential influence of the duration of intraventricular catheterization and (2) the usefulness of prophylactic antibiotic treatment. In a prospective study of 172 consecutive neurosurgical patients, Mayhall and coworkers[110] identified ventricular catheterization for longer than 5 days as a risk factor for infection (ventriculitis or meningitis). Previous ventriculostomy, however, did not raise the risk of infection with subsequent procedures. These researchers thus concluded that an IVC should remain in place for up to 5 days, after which the catheter should be removed and re-inserted at a different site. These results were challenged by Holloway and associates,[114] who did not observe significant differences in infection rate between patients in whom catheters were replaced prior to 5 days and those whose catheters remained in place for longer periods; these results suggest that catheter exchange is not beneficial.

It must be noted that even the association between duration of IVC and infection is not unequivocally documented and remains a matter of debate. Prophylactic use of antibiotics was reported as beneficial by some investigators,[115] but not by others.[113,116] According to a 1999 survey, 72% of centers do use antibiotics (mainly cephalosporins and semisynthetic penicillins) in patients with IVCs.[117] This issue remains unclear and should be addressed in a randomized controlled trial.

Friedmann and Vries[118] reported that percutaneous tunneling of the IVC reduces the infection rate; they encountered no infections after 100 consecutive procedures in 66 patients, with a mean drainage duration of 6.2 days.[118] This finding was later confirmed by Khanna and associates,[119] who reported no infection during the first 16 days after IVC insertion in a series of 100 consecutive procedures; the overall infection incidence in their patients was quite low (4% for an average IVC duration of 18.3 days). Several studies have searched for factors associated with IVC infections—pneumonia,[112,114] sepsis,[112,114] intracerebral hemorrhage with intraventricular blood,[110,111,114] neurosurgical operation,[110,111,114] ICP higher than 20 mm Hg,[110] and depressed skull fracture.[114]

Parenchymal or subdural bleeding along the insertion site constitutes a further complication of IVC. Its incidence, however, is negligibly low.

Prior to removal of the IVC, it is vital to acquire some information about the CSF absorption. For this purpose, catheter drainage should be discontinued for 24 hours, and ICP values closely monitored. Provided that ICP values do not increase by more than 15 to 20 mm Hg during this period, removal of the catheter can be regarded as safe. The quantity of drained CSF is a further indicator for the patency of CSF absorption and the necessity of external drainage; CSF drainage less than 250 mL/day with the reservoir hanging 20 cm above the external acoustic meatus indicates an adequate CSF absorption.

Subarachnoid Catheter

Use of the subarachnoid catheter was introduced in 1973 by Vries and coworkers.[120] Its insertion involves perforating the dura with a thin needle, thus establishing the contact between catheter and subarachnoid space. The main advantages of this form of ICP monitoring lie in its minimal invasiveness and low infection risk; rates of less than 1% for ventriculitis and less than 2% local infections were reported in a series of 147 patients.[121] Aucoin and colleagues[113] reported an infection rate of 7.5% for the use of subarachnoid catheters, compared with 21% for IVCs. The occurrence of infection was always associated with flushing of the catheter.

Mendelow and associates[122] compared the ICP values acquired with a subarachnoid catheter with those acquired with an IVC in 10 patients with severe head injury. ICP values measured with the subarachnoid catheter corresponded to the ventricular fluid pressure in 48% of cases, were higher in 15%, and were lower in 27%. The observed tendency of the subarachnoid catheter to underestimate ICP was also reported by Dearden and coworkers.[123]

Epidural Catheters

Epidural ICP monitoring is the least invasive approach, in which bleeding complications or infections are extremely rare. Unfortunately, this method is also the most vulnerable to artifacts, and the results are therefore not reproducible. Kosteljanetz and associates[124] examined the efficacy of epidural catheters in 35 neurosurgical patients. Satisfactory catheter function was noted in approximately two thirds of cases. In 7 patients, ICP was simultaneously monitored with IVCs and epidural catheters; differences in measured ICP values of up to 25 mm Hg were noted. The researchers thus concluded that epidural catheters do not constitute an appropriate method for ICP monitoring.[124] Bruder and colleagues[125] reported similar findings; they observed no agreement between epidural and intraparenchymatous ICP values.

Intraparenchymal Microtransducers

Fiberoptic catheters can be used for parenchymal, subdural, or ventricular ICP monitoring but are mostly used as parenchymal monitoring devices. Their function is based on a device sensing changes in light reflection off a pressure-sensitive diaphragm. The first such device to be widely used was the Camino OLM ICP Monitor. ICP measurements with this catheter required a dedicated amplifier. The accuracy of the Camino transducer as compared with IVC catheters was found to be quite high; Gambardella and coworkers[126] reported a significant correlation between the ICP values acquired with the two catheters ($r = 0.946$) in 18 neurosurgical patients. Similar results were reported in two series, which evaluated 74 and 118 patients (104 parenchymal catheters), respectively.[127,128]

Munch and colleagues[128] reported a 0.7% incidence of infection associated with the use of Camino fiberoptic catheters in 118 patients (136 devices—104 parenchymal, 32 ventricular; average measuring time, 94 hours). Shapiro and coworkers[127] observed a single insertion site infection and two infected bone flaps in a series of 244 patients with intraparenchymal Camino catheters. Finally, Khan and associates[129] described a 0.6% incidence of infection in 52 patients with Camino catheters.

Although the risk of infection appears low, use of the Camino fiberoptic catheter is associated with some drawbacks. Reported incidence of fiberoptic breakage ranged from 5.1%[128] to 16%[127] in early studies; because current models are more flexible, this figure would be expected to be lower. The Camino catheter cannot be calibrated after insertion; the resultant significant ICP drift (inaccuracy of measurements over time) limits the accuracy of the recorded values. Crutchfield and associates[130] reported deviations of ±6 mm Hg after 5 days, and suggested that fiberoptic catheters should be replaced after this time. Bavetta and coworkers[131] described a wide range of bias (−12 to +14 mm Hg) already occurring in recordings obtained within the first 3 days of use, suggesting that zero drift is a significant problem reducing the reliability of fiberoptic catheters.[131]

The parenchymal transducers currently used are (1) fiberoptic (Camino OLM ICP Monitor), (2) piezoelectric (based on silicon chips, with pressure-sensitive resistors; Codmann MicroSensor ICP), and (3) pneumatic devices (based on a disposable air pouch plastic; Spiegelberg III). The Spiegelberg III transducer has the additional advantage that it performs an automatic in vivo calibration, further reducing the drift of measurements. Czosnyka and associates[132,133] obtained high-quality readings with both the Camino and Codmann microsensors and the Camino and Spiegelberg III microsensors during bench testing. Drift of all three sensors is currently estimated as ±2 mm Hg.

The Brain Trauma Foundation[134] has recommended the IVC as the device of choice for ICP monitoring, particularly in patients requiring CSF drainage. Parenchymal fiberoptic catheters should be used in patients in whom CSF drainage is not required or in patients with obstruction in the fluid couple. Because subarachnoid, subdural, and epidural devices do not yield accurate results, the Foundation concluded that their use cannot be recommended. One must bear in mind, however, that almost all studies of invasive ICP monitoring were conducted on neurosurgical patients. The extent of applicability of their results in patients with acute stroke is unclear.

Recanalizing Therapy

Publication of the National Institute of Neurological Disorders and Stroke (NINDS) trial in 1995 was the first report of an effective therapy for acute ischemic stroke,[135] leading to the U.S. Food and Drug Association (FDA) approval of intravenous rt-PA given within a 3-hour window. Two meta-analyses of thrombolytic studies also indicate a benefit for patients treated within a 6-hour window.[136,137] The results of a later controlled trial on intra-arterial thrombolytic therapy confirmed the efficacy and safety of intra-arterial treatment given within the first 6 hours.[138] Individual decision-making, based on clinical presentation and imaging findings, is warranted in the choice of thrombolytic drugs for a given patient as well as the appropriate mode of administration. The precise indications for thrombolytic therapy are discussed in Chapters 48 and 49.

Patients treated with intravenous thrombolytics do not necessarily require treatment in an intensive care setting. Nevertheless, careful monitoring is needed to detect potential neurologic deterioration. We routinely admit patients treated with intra-arterial thrombolysis to the neurocritical care unit for at least 24 hours. Close monitoring of vital functions, optimal blood pressure adjustment (depending on whether the occluded vessel has recanalized or not), and frequent neurologic evaluation are mandatory in these cases.

Treatment of Raised Intracranial Pressure

The main goal of ICP treatment is to minimize or, if possible, eliminate secondary ischemic insults and mechanical damage caused by shifts and local compression of brain tissue. The focus has hereby changed from the initially proposed regimen, which was purely ICP-oriented, to a regimen aiming at maintaining CPP. Sustained CPP drops can result in hypoperfusion of ischemic brain regions, because the supplying arterioles are maximally dilated and cerebral autoregulation is impaired (Figs. 52–1 and 52–2).

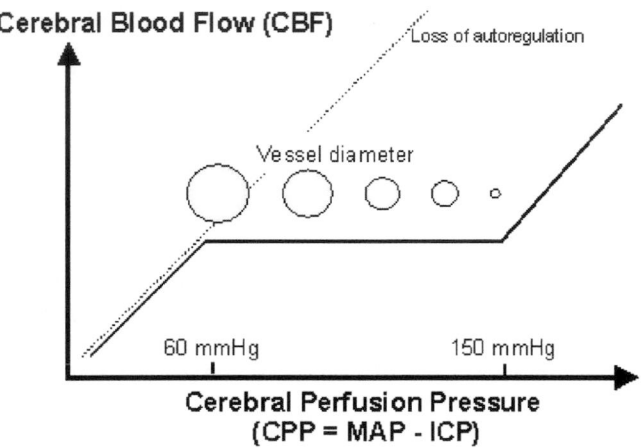

FIGURE 52–1 *Autoregulation of cerebral blood flow (CBF). The cerebral vascular bed is capable of maintaining a constant CBF from a mean arterial blood pressure of 60 to 150 mm Hg. This phenomenon of "autoregulation" is achieved either through a reduction (vasodilation) or an increase (vasoconstriction) of arterial resistances when the cerebral perfusion pressure (CPP) decreases or increases. If the autoregulation is impaired (dotted line), the CBF passively changes with the CPP.*

Basic Measures

Although the optimal blood pressure in patients with intracranial hypertension remains unknown, it is important to avoid sustained hypotensive episodes. Avoidance of hypovolemia is the simplest way to maintain blood pressure; in patients with a central line, CVP should be kept above 8 mm Hg. Crystalloid solutions, colloid solutions, and blood products can be used, in the order given. In patients with decreased peripheral resistance, vasopressors can be necessary; dopamine and epinephrine are the drugs of first choice. Dobutamine is the drug of choice when arterial hypotension is presumed to be caused by decreased cardiac output.

Keeping the patient's head elevated 15 to 30 degrees increases cerebral venous and CSF outflow, and could thus contribute to an ICP reduction. On the other hand, such a position compromises venous return to the heart, possibly decreasing arterial pressure. Ropper and colleagues[139] examined the influence of body position on ICP in 19 patients in ICU; ICP was lowest when the head was raised to 60 degrees in 10 patients and with the head horizontal in 2 patients; ICP remained unchanged in both positions in 5 patients. Rosner and Coley[140] examined the effect of various head positions (0 to 50 degrees, in steps of 10 degrees) on ICP and CPP. An average ICP decrease of 1 mm Hg was noted for each step but was associated with a reduction in CPP of 2 to 3 mm Hg; CPP was not beneficially affected by any degree of head elevation and was maximal in the horizontal position. Feldman and coworkers[141] observed no significant changes in CPP with elevation of the patient's head from horizontal to 30 degrees, and ICP was significantly reduced.[141] Similar results were reported by Meixensberger and associates,[142] who also found that tissue PO_2 remained unaffected by the body position. Moraine and colleagues,[143] however, observed no ICP changes when the patient's head was elevated from horizontal to 30 degrees; ICP values did drop, however, when the head was further elevated to 45 degrees. At the same time, CBF gradually decreased with head elevation from horizontal to 45 degrees, a change that these investigators attributed mainly to changes in arteriovenous pressure gradients.

It must be noted that all of the studies just summarized examined patients with severe head injury. In a study in 18

FIGURE 52–2 *Cerebral compliance. An increase of edematous brain tissue requires a compensatory decrease of the other two physiologic compartments contained in the skull, intravascular blood and cerebrospinal fluid (CSF). After the failure of these very limited compensatory mechanisms, the ICP rapidly rises, and even a small increase in the intracranial volume (Δ volumen) may substantially raise the ICP (Δ ICP). However, in this situation, even a small reduction in brain edema can dramatically lower the ICP.*

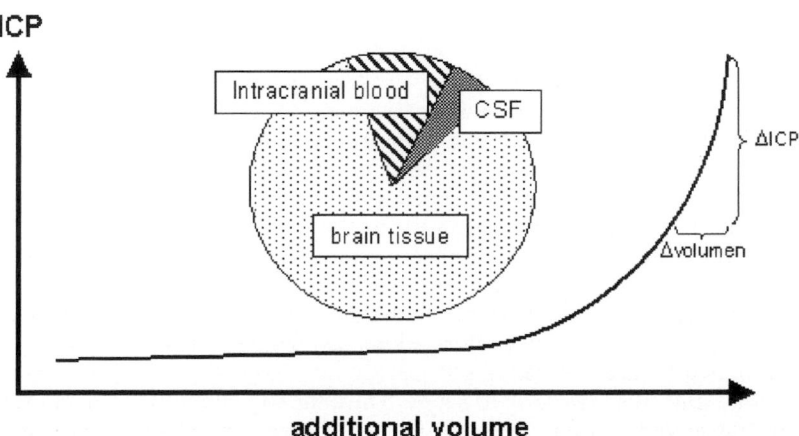

patients with acute stroke, we compared ICP, MAP, and CPP values when head position was changed from horizontal to 30 degrees of elevation. A mild but statistically significant reduction in ICP was evident; it was accompanied by a reduction in MAP of a much higher magnitude, so this maneuver mildly reduced ICP at the expense of a CPP reduction.[144] Like Ropper and colleagues,[139] we observed different behaviors of the monitored parameters among the patients studied. We thus suggest that optimal head positioning be decided on an individual basis, rather than routine positioning of all patients with 30-degree head elevation as is currently practiced in most ICUs.

Specific Treatment
Osmotherapy

Osmotherapeutic agents are hypertonic solutions of low molecular weight that increase serum osmolarity, thus creating an osmotic gradient between blood and brain tissue. An intact blood-brain barrier is essential for this osmotic gradient. Migration of osmotic substances through the damaged blood-brain barrier can reverse the osmotic gradient and aggravate brain edema (rebound effect). This result was demonstrated by Kaufmann and Cardoso,[145] in 23 cats with a cortical cold injury and vasogenic edema, and by Garcia-Sola and associates[146] in a goat model in which inflation of an epidural balloon was used to produce intracranial hypertension. Furthermore, volume reduction is more pronounced in the healthy hemisphere; this could potentially increase the pressure gradient between the two hemispheres and facilitate displacement and herniation of brain tissue. It must be noted, however, that such an increase in the pressure gradient constitutes a pathophysiologic model, which has not been substantiated in any animal or clinical studies. The increased intravascular volume also results in a hematocrit reduction, which improves the rheologic properties of blood.

Mannitol is the most commonly used osmotherapeutic agent. Its effectiveness was demonstrated in several studies examining patients with head injury.[147–152] Pollay and coworkers[153] also described a synergistic effect of mannitol and furosemide in reducing ICP, related to preferential excretion of water through the renal distal tubule, which sustains the osmotic gradient, and potentially also to reduced production of CSF.[153] Biestro and colleagues[154] compared the effectiveness of mannitol and glycerol for decreasing ICP, using a modified therapeutic intensity level to compare the two approaches. Although both agents were effective at reducing ICP, the duration of this effect was longer for glycerol, leading these investigators to suggest that glycerol should best be used as basic treatment and that a bolus of mannitol should be applied to counteract sudden increases in ICP. The relation of the occurrence of a rebound phenomenon to the osmotic agent used remains uncertain, because results of the few existing studies are conflicting.[146,155]

Bereczki and associates[156] evaluated the evidence for the effectiveness of mannitol in patients with acute ischemic stroke. They identified a total of four randomized studies, three of which were characterized as confounded. The fourth study demonstrated several methodologic drawbacks, significantly limiting its scope. Thus, the use of mannitol or glycerol in patients with acute ischemic stroke is based solely on the results of experimental studies or studies in patients with head trauma.

The effectiveness of hypertonic saline solutions in the treatment of intracranial hypertension after head trauma has been documented in several studies.[157–161] Gemma and colleagues[162] observed a comparable ICP decrease after the administration of 7.5% hypertonic saline or 20% mannitol in 50 patients during elective supratentorial procedures. In a similar study, Schwarz and associates[163] compared the effects of a combination of hypertonic saline–hydroxyethyl starch (HS-HES) and of mannitol; both substances were effective in reducing ICP. Qureshi and coworkers[164] reported a favorable trend toward ICP reduction after infusion of 3% saline/acetate in patients with head trauma (n = 8) or postoperative edema (n = 6), but not in patients with nontraumatic intracranial hemorrhage (n = 8) or ischemic stroke (n = 6). This result could not be reproduced, however, in a later study conducted in our department that examined the effect of hypertonic saline in 8 patients with stroke and increased ICP, in whom the standard mannitol treatment showed no effect; treatment with 75 mL of 10% saline over 15 minutes resulted in an ICP reduction in all cases.[165] Maximal ICP increase (mean, 9.9 mm Hg) was observed 20 minutes after the end of the infusion. No side effects were noted.[165] Thus, few studies have examined the effectiveness of hypertonic saline in patients with acute stroke, and their results, as described previously, were not unanimous.

Given the results already summarized, no evidence-based recommendation can be made on the use of osmotic agents in stroke. Regardless of the therapeutic regimen, it is vital to monitor serum electrolyte levels and osmolarity closely (at least twice daily) while osmotic agents are used. We initially use glycerol for control of intracranial hypertension. The potential for oral administration of glycerol gives it a significant advantage over mannitol. Side effects include hemolysis, hemoglobinuria, nausea, diarrhea, vomiting, and bleeding diathesis. If this treatment is ineffective, we add mannitol (100 mL of a 20% mannitol solution). This is given as bolus infusion (over 15 minutes), preferably through a central line. Because the half-life of mannitol is short (approximately 1 hour), several administrations (4 to 6 per day) are necessary. We aim for a target serum osmolarity of 320 mOsm/L, avoiding higher values in an effort to minimize the risk of acute tubular necrosis and because of the previously cited risk of rebound effect. We often combine mannitol with furosemide in an attempt to increase the osmotic gradient. Another osmotherapeutic agent would be one of the 40% sorbit solutions. Still, they have two major drawbacks: (1) they are metabolized through the liver, and thus cannot be used in patients with liver dysfunction, and (2) they are contraindicated in patients with fructose intolerance. For this reason, we refrain from their routine use. If mannitol therapy is not sufficient for ICP control, we use HS-HES, a hypertonic saline, or both.

Tromethamine

Tromethamine (Tham) has been shown to decrease ICP in animal models.[166] It acts by entering the CSF compartment, reducing cerebral acidosis, and causing vasoconstriction, thus reducing ICP. A prospective randomized clinical trial in 149 patients with severe head injury who received either Tham or placebo for 5 days demonstrated that the use of Tham was associated with (1) a significantly lower incidence of ICP values exceeding 20 mm Hg during the first two treatment days and (2) a significantly lower number of patients with barbiturate coma requiring treatment.[167] Nevertheless, no difference in outcome for the two groups was observed at 3, 6, or 12 months.

Tham should always be infused via a central line, because extravasation leads to severe tissue necrosis. Initially, the effectiveness of Tham should be assessed by infusing 1 mmol/kg in 100 mL of 5% glucose over 45 minutes. Continuous Tham infusion should be initiated only if the first application leads to an ICP reduction by approximately 10 to 15 mm Hg. The dose is adapted so as to achieve and then maintain blood pH between 7.5 and 7.55.

Hyperventilation

Hyperventilation results in reduction in arterial pressure of carbon dioxide ($PaCO_2$), which causes vasoconstriction, thus reducing CBF, cerebral blood volume, and, subsequently, ICP. This effect usually occurs within minutes of initiation of hyperventilation. It must be noted that metabolic autoregulation is not intact in ischemic brain regions, where brain arterioles are maximally dilated. Vasoconstriction is therefore limited to vessels supplying unaffected brain tissue, a feature that could theoretically lead to redistribution of CBF (reverse steal phenomenon). Michenfelder and Milde[1,68] examining the effect of hypocapnia in a primate model of acute ischemic stroke, found no differences in mortality or level of neurologic function, although they did note a tendency toward smaller infarct volumes. The applicability of hyperventilation is limited by the following major factors: (1) cerebral vasoconstriction can result in cerebral ischemia and (2) the induced elevation of CSF pH is compensated by the choroid plexus within hours, in contrast to the much slower compensation of blood pH, which can require several days. This latter finding implies that the effect of hyperventilation lasts for only a few hours, after which cerebral vessels regain their normal diameter. Termination of hyperventilation at this stage results in an increase of $PaCO_2$ in both blood and CSF, which in turn causes cerebral vasodilation, potentially leading to a rebound effect on ICP. In a randomized trial, Muizelaar and associates[169] examined the effects of hyperventilation alone, hyperventilation plus Tham, and normoventilation (control) in 113 patients with severe head injury, who were divided into two subgroups according to the initial motor score. These investigators observed a significantly worse outcome at 3 and 6 months after injury in patients with severe motor scores who were treated with hyperventilation alone. They also demonstrated that hyperventilation alone, in contrast to hyperventilation plus Tham, could not sustain CSF alkalinization.[169]

Hyperventilation is a treatment of choice for short interventions, to counteract sudden ICP elevations. Under these conditions, the risk of rebound is minimal. Hyperventilation is easily induced through an approximate 10% increase in tidal volume. Long-term hyperventilation under continuous Tham infusion could provide an attractive alternative for ICP control; still, its effectiveness in patients with acute stroke remains to be evaluated.

Barbiturates

The main effects of barbiturates are decreases in cerebral metabolism and CBF; the mechanism of these changes is unclear, although an enhancement of the binding of gamma-aminobutyric acid (GABA) to its receptor[170] and a direct effect on vascular tone have been postulated. The effect of barbiturates on ICP appears to be less uniform than that of other agents. ICP reductions were observed in 11 of 15 patients with nontraumatic lesions by Woodcock and associates[171]; in 14 of 21 patients with neurosurgical trauma by Lee and colleagues[172]; in 50 of 60 patients with acute ischemic stroke by Schwab and coworkers[173]; and in 57 of 67 patients with severe head injuries by Cormio and associates,[174] who found that ICP values were reduced but remained higher than 20 mm Hg in 27 of 67 patients. Schwartz and colleagues[175] found no differences in efficacy between barbiturate coma and mannitol in reducing ICP in 95 patients with head injury. Furthermore, only 5 of 60 (8%) patients treated with barbiturates survived in the study reported by Schwab and coworkers.[173] It must be noted, however, that barbiturates were mostly used as the last line of treatment, after failure of other treatment options; thus, outcome in some patients treated with barbiturates may already have been predetermined by the extent of brain lesions.

Because of several potential and partially severe side effects of barbiturate coma (marked arterial hypotension, myocardial damage, electrolyte disturbances, impairment of liver function, predisposition to infection), this treatment should only be used as a therapy of last choice, accompanied by invasive monitoring of arterial blood pressure and frequent evaluations of serum electrolyte and liver enzyme levels. Barbiturates should be infused over a separate venous line. Thiopental is the barbiturate used most in neurocritical care unit. It is advisable to apply a bolus injection of 100 mg of thiopental initially and to proceed with further applications only if a marked ICP reduction is observed. The barbiturate effect is monitored on the basis of the appearance of a burst-suppression pattern on electroencephalography (EEG). Serum levels of barbiturates are not reliable.

Glucocorticoids

Qizilbach and associates[176] have reviewed the use of corticosteroids for acute stroke. Seven trials involving 453 patients were chosen for analysis; the follow-up period varied between 1 and 12 months, and only one study utilized CT to exclude hemorrhagic stroke. The reviewers concluded that corticosteroid treatment did not influence mortality at 1 year or improve functional outcome in survivors. Reported adverse effects included gastrointestinal hemorrhage, infection, and hyperglycemia. A clinical study of corticosteroid therapy in 93 patients with supratentorial intracranial hemorrhage found no evidence of a beneficial effect, and the rates of complications already mentioned were significantly increased.[177] Obviously, the possibility that inclusion of patients with hemorrhagic infarcts may have influenced the results of early studies cannot be ruled out. Thus, it is possible that a subgroup of patients with ischemic stroke (particularly those with large infarcts and vasogenic edema) could potentially benefit from corticosteroid treatment. At the same time, the adverse effects observed in these early trials discourage the conduct of further research in this area.

Antiepileptics

Epileptic seizures occur in approximately 9% of patients with acute stroke.[178] MRI studies demonstrate that prolonged seizures are associated with formation of cerebral edema, which could potentially increase ICP.[179-182] The same is true for seizure-related cerebral vasodilation, and increases in oxygen and substrate demand can aggravate cerebral ischemia. Prophylactic application of antiepileptic drugs in patients with stroke remains a matter of debate. We administer antiepileptics only in patients who experience seizures.

Hemicraniectomy

First described by Cushing[183] in 1905, decompressive craniotomy has been established as an aggressive approach for treatment of intracranial hypertension in several experimental models of cerebral infarction.[184-186] The applicability of this approach in various stroke syndromes is discussed later in the chapter.

Hypothermia

Normal body temperature is 37°C, with a significant diurnal variation of ±0.6°C. Body core temperature can be measured at varying sites; the shell temperatures are measured either sublingually, axillary, or on the skin. Core temperatures reflect tympanic membrane, esophageal, rectal, bladder, and pulmonary artery temperature measurements. Hypothermia is defined as mild (>33°C), moderate (29–33°C), or deep (<29°C).

Physiology and Experimental Basis of Hypothermia. The systemic oxygen demand lessens when the core body temperature drops. Correspondingly, decreases in carbon dioxide production, plasma potassium levels, and carbohydrate metabolism are observed. Several studies have demonstrated a neuroprotective effect of moderate hypothermia in animal models of focal cerebral ischemia.[187-189] Potential underlying neuroprotective mechanisms include decrease in excitatory amino acid levels,[190-192] stabilization of the blood-brain barrier and cell membranes,[193-195] and a downregulation of cerebral metabolism.[196] Additionally, alteration of CBF during hypothermia may contribute to its neuroprotective effects.[196]

Nevertheless, patients with acute stroke are rarely treated with hypothermia within the first 12 hours after symptom onset, so neuroprotection is barely an issue in these cases. The rationale for hypothermia in patients with stroke is rather to attempt to reduce brain edema and thus control ICP. Although most of the studies cited did report a reduction of brain edema, none has yet specifically examined this issue. Additionally, animals were subjected to hypothermia before or shortly after cerebral ischemia, a practice that constitutes a major difference from the clinical use of the treatment.

Clinical Application. Deep hypothermia is routinely used during open heart surgery and also occasionally for cerebral protection during neurosurgical operations. Although initial clinical studies in patients with brain injury suggested a potential clinical benefit of moderate hypothermia,[197,198] these results could not be confirmed in a later multicenter trial.[199] Application of moderate hypothermia for ischemic stroke is detailed later in this chapter and in Chapter 53.

SPECIFIC TREATMENT OF VARIOUS STROKE SYNDROMES

Acute Large Middle Cerebral Artery Stroke

The clinical course of severe infarction of the MCA (malignant MCA syndrome) or of infarction of the MCA plus the anterior cerebral artery (ACA), the posterior cerebral artery (PCA), or both that is treated with medical therapy alone follows a predictable pattern in most patients.[200,201] Within the first few hours after onset of symptoms, patients with large supratentorial infarcts are typically fully awake, although some may show mild drowsiness. Bilateral motor signs, coma, posturing, and pupillary abnormalities are usually not observed in the very early phase of large supratentorial infarcts. Neurologic deterioration occurs during the first 24 hours in most patients with large supratentorial infarcts, corresponding to the development of brain edema. Such patients lose consciousness to varying degrees from drowsiness to coma. Pupillary enlargement and loss of pupillary reactivity—initially occurring only on the side of the infarction and later bilaterally—nausea, vomiting, posturing, and abnormal breathing patterns are signs of secondary brainstem dysfunction due to impending herniation. If ICP is being monitored, it is typically only moderately elevated (≈20 mm Hg), at the first onset of deterioration. ICP values subsequently rise over the next 24 to 48 hours. Elevated ICP is a reliable prognostic sign, and an ICP exceeding 30 mm Hg is usually associated with a fatal course.[202]

Most patients demonstrating neurologic deterioration within the first few hours after stroke onset eventually die. Various predictors for deterioration and poor clinical outcome have been identified. Regarding vascular disease, distal internal carotid artery (ICA) occlusion almost uniformly indicates fatal outcome. Proximal occlusion of the MCA stem is also an unfavorable radiologic finding, typically leading to a complete MCA infarction, including the basal ganglia, which are often spared in patients with a more distal MCA occlusion. It seems plausible that the extent of the infarcted area closely correlates with mortality. Complete MCA plus ACA infarcts and infarcts involving the complete hemisphere are usually lethal. Rapid onset of neurologic deterioration with loss of consciousness during the first 6 hours indicates an aggressive course of the disease and is associated with a high mortality.[200] The extent of brain edema depends largely on the size and location of the infarct but also shows substantial individual variability. As a general rule, young and middle-aged patients have less compensation capacity for space-occupying intracranial lesions than older patients with cerebral atrophy.

A large hemispheric infarct must be recognized in the emergency department as a life-threatening condition that requires prompt and massive intervention.[203] After stabilization of the airway, breathing, and circulation, the initial diagnostic evaluation and transfer of the patient to a neurocritical care unit should not be delayed. If indicated, early reperfusion therapies can be initiated in the emergency department. Venous access, continuous monitoring of blood pressure, electrocardiography (ECG), and pulse oxygenation are part of routine intensive care measures. Continuous ECG monitoring is especially important because neurogenic cardiac arrhythmias are commonly observed, particularly in patients with large infarcts of the right hemisphere. Although respiratory problems are uncommon upon presentation, their frequency sharply rises within the first 24 hours, reflecting increasing brain edema and brainstem dysfunction. Most patients with large infarcts require ventilatory support. To achieve sufficient cerebral oxygenation, oxygen should be insufflated via a face mask to achieve arterial PO_2 values greater than 90 mm Hg. Indications for intubation and mechanical ventilation were discussed earlier in the chapter.

Hemicraniectomy

Surgical decompression seems to be effective in lowering increased ICP, preventing transtentorial herniation, and reducing mortality in patients with malignant MCA infarction. Since 1988, eight studies involving a total of 133 treated patients with this disorder have been published

(see Table 52.6).[204–211] The overall mortality was 23.2%, and most patients demonstrated a Barthel index in excess of 60.

The surgical technique commonly used consists of removal of a bone flap with a diameter of 12 cm (including the frontal, parietal, temporal, and parts of the occipital squamae)(Figs. 52–3 and 52–4). The dura is initially fixed at the edge of the craniotomy, to prevent epidural bleeding, and subsequently opened. An adjusted, biconvex dural patch made of lyophilized cadaver dura or homologous temporal fascia is then placed into the incision. Although the size varies, dural patches 15 to 20 cm in length and 2.5 to 3.5 cm in width are generally used.

The ideal timing for decompressive surgery remains a matter of discussion; because the clinical course in patients with massive cerebral infarction (more than two thirds of the MCA territory) is highly predictable, it does not appear reasonable to wait for the appearance of clinical deterioration before performing surgery. One must also take into account that several hours may pass between the decision for surgery and its performance, and that the procedure itself requires approximately 3 hours. Thus, the patient may be unnecessarily exposed to the risk of mesencephalic ischemia, which greatly worsens clinical status and outcome. We advocate surgery within 24 hours of symptom

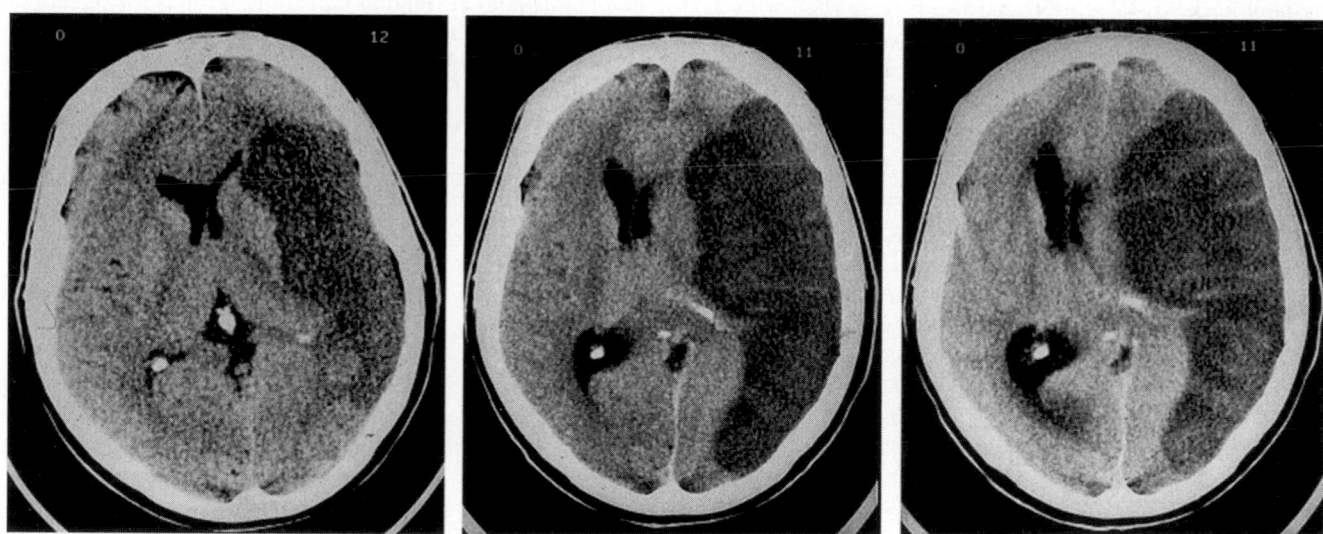

FIGURE 52–3 *Course of edema formation in complete infarction of the middle cerebral artery.*

Table 52.6 Clinical Studies on Hemicraniectomy in Patients with Acute Stroke

Study[a]	Year	No. of Patients	Age (yr)	Mortality (%)	Barthel Index (BI)
Kondziolka and Fazl[204]	1988	5	40	0	All BI > 60
Delashaw et al[205]	1990	9	57	11	BI > 60, n = 4
Jourdan et al[206]	1993	7	NA	28	All BI > 60
Kalia and Yonas[207]	1993	4	34	0	All BI > 60
Carter et al[208]	1997	14	49	21	BI > 60, n = 8
Schwab et al[209]	1998	63	50	27	Mean BI 65
Holtkamp et al[210]	2001	12	65	33	Mean BI 28, all < 60
Mori et al[211]	2001	19	63	16	28 ± 32
All		133		24	

[a]Superscript numbers indicate chapter references.

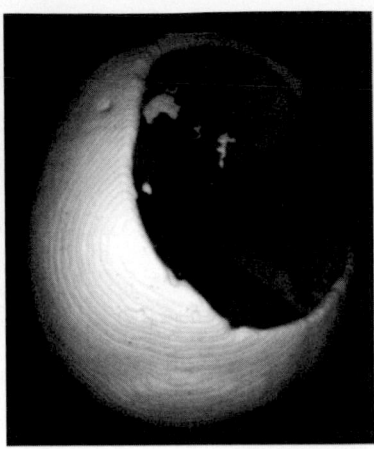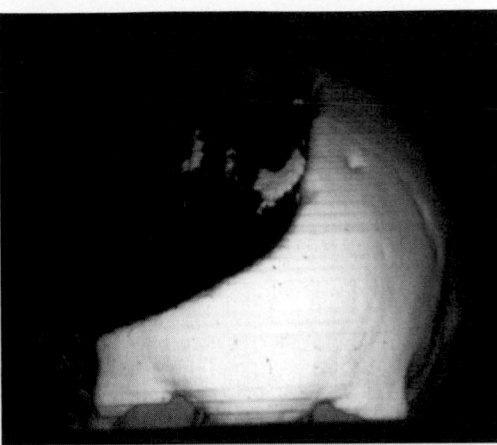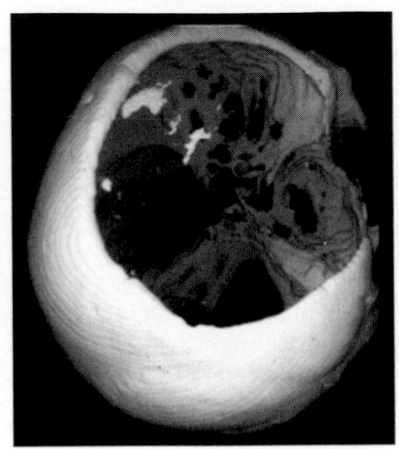

FIGURE 52–4   *Three-dimensional computed tomography reconstruction of decompressive surgery after space-occupying infarction of the middle cerebral artery. Note the extension of the bone flap.*

onset for any patient with (1) neuroradiologic signs of massive MCA infarction and (2) deterioration of clinical status since admission. We occasionally refrain from awaiting even this initial clinical deterioration in patients with complete MCA infarction. We also refrain from applying a rigid age limit for decompressive surgery, tending to rely on the health and social condition of each patient prior to the ischemic infarct. For patients with infarctions of the dominant hemisphere, we discuss prognosis—and particularly, probable residual deficit—with the family, in an attempt to assess the patient's viewpoint about disabled survival.

Moderate Hypothermia

The first clinical trial on the effect of moderate hypothermia (33°C) in patients with severe MCA infarction was reported by Schwab and colleagues[212] in 1998. Hypothermia was induced at a mean of 14 hours after symptom onset and maintained for 72 hours. Mortality was only 44%, and survivors had a favorable outcome, with a mean Barthel index of 70, even though all patients had met the criteria for diagnosis of a "malignant" MCA infarction. Although hypothermia significantly reduced ICP, a secondary rise in ICP, occasionally exceeding initial ICP levels and requiring additional treatment with osmotherapeutics, was observed upon rewarming. The rewarming period constitutes a critical phase, because metabolic needs potentially outstrip oxygen delivery. This ICP rebound after rewarming might be due to a hypermetabolic response after induced hypothermia, which has already been described after cardiopulmonary bypass surgery.

Schwab and colleagues[213] reported similar results in a multicenter observational study of 50 prospective patients with cerebral infarction involving at least the complete MCA territory who were treated with moderate hypothermia (33°C). Overall mortality was 38%; 8% of patients died during hypothermia, and 30% during rewarming owing to uncontrollable ICP increase. Neurologic outcomes were expressed as a score of 28 on the National Institute of Health Stroke Scale (NIHSS) was 28, and the modified Rankin Scale (mRS) 2.9, at 4 weeks and at 3 months after stroke, respectively. Krieger and associates[214] reported initial results in 10 patients with acute ischemic stroke

(NIHSS, 19.8 ± 3.3) who were treated with moderate hypothermia (32°C) after thrombolysis. Mortality was 33%, and the mean mRS at 3 months was 3.1 ± 2.3.

Side Effects

Hypothermia affects virtually every organ system. Ventricular ectopy and fibrillation limit the extent of hypothermia, but this effect is known to occur only at temperatures below 30°C. Pneumonia was the only severe side effect of moderate hypothermia in the first study reported by Schwab and colleagues.[212] The complications of moderate hypothermia most commonly described in the later multicenter trial were thrombocytopenia (70%), bradycardia (62%), and pneumonia (48%).[213] Four patients (8%) died during hypothermia, because of severe coagulopathy, cardiac failure, or uncontrollable intracranial hypertension. Complications in the 10 patients studied by Krieger and associates[214] were bradycardia ($n = 5$), ventricular ectopy ($n = 3$), hypotension ($n = 3$), melena ($n = 2$), fever after rewarming ($n = 3$), and infection ($n = 4$). Also, 4 patients with chronic atrial fibrillation experienced a rapid ventricular rate, and 3 patients had myocardial infarctions during hypothermia.[214]

Induction of Hypothermia

Initially, surface cooling with cooling blankets, alcohol applied to exposed skin, or application of ice bags to groin, axilla, and neck were used to induce hypothermia.[212–214] This approach, however, requires intensive effort from the medical and nursing staff for induction as well as for maintenance of the target temperature.

A novel technique using endovascular cooling has now been described.[215] It uses a central line with a single infusion lumen (ICY, Alsius Corporation, Irvine, CA, USA) and one further lumen that ends in three balloons, sized 8 mm, 5 mm, and 5 mm in diameter, located at the distal end of the catheter. The balloons are perfused with a sterile solution of normal saline via a closed-loop tubing system. The tubing is connected to a mobile temperature management device (CoolGard, Alsius Corporation, Irvine, CA, USA) placed at the patient's bedside. The device consists of a water bath with adjustable temperature; a pump circulates the saline solution through the water bath. The catheter is inserted into the femoral vein and advanced to the inferior vena cava. Initial results of this approach were promising, as target temperature was reached after 3 ± 1 hours (range, 2–4.5 hours) and deviations from the target temperature were minimal (>0.2°C or >0.3°C during 21% or 10% of the time, respectively).[215] The advantages of this approach over surface cooling remain to be evaluated in large-scale studies.

Comparison of Hemicraniectomy and Moderate Hypothermia

Hemicraniectomy and moderate hypothermia constitute promising treatment modalities for space-occupying cerebral infarction. To date, only one study has compared their effectiveness in controlling intracranial hypertension and reducing mortality.[216] In this study, a total of 36 patients with severe acute ischemic stroke were treated with hemicraniectomy (n = 17) or moderate hypothermia (n = 19). Allocation of a patient to undergo moderate hypothermia or to a hemicraniectomy group was decided according to the affected hemisphere, with hemicraniectomy being performed in patients with infarction of the nondominant hemisphere, and moderate hypothermia in those with infarctions of the dominant hemisphere. Age, sex, cranial computed tomography (CCT) findings, level of consciousness, and time to treatment were similar in the two groups. The significant differences initially noted in NIHSS score (20 [range, 18–22] for moderate hypothermia and 17 [range, 16–18] for hemicraniectomy) were not present when NIHSS score was corrected for aphasia (17 [range, 15–19] for moderate hypothermia and 17 [range, 16–18] for hemicraniectomy). Mortality was 12% for hemicraniectomy and 47% for moderate hypothermia; 1 patient treated with moderate hypothermia died on treatment complications (sepsis) and 3 on ICP crises that occurred during rewarming. Duration of mechanical ventilation and of neurocritical care unit stay did not significantly differ in the two groups, but duration of catecholamine use and maximal catecholamine dosage were significantly higher in the patients treated with moderate hypothermia. The researchers concluded that in patients with acute ischemic stroke, hemicraniectomy is associated with lower rates of both mortality and complications than moderate hypothermia.[216] These results remain to be confirmed in large-scale trials.

Blood Pressure Management

Blood pressure management is an intriguing issue in patients with acute stroke. Lisk and associates[217] demonstrated a significant relationship between reduction in arterial blood pressure and drop in CBF in 16 consecutive hypertensive patients with acute ischemic stroke (treated within 72 hours of onset).[217] According to American Heart Association (AHA) guidelines for acute stroke treatment, published in 2003, blood pressure should not be lowered in most patients; MAP values up to 130 mm Hg, or systolic blood pressure values up to 220 mm Hg, should be tolerated.[218] These guidelines are in accordance with the recommendations of the European Stroke Initiative published in 2000.[219]

Although the AHA guidelines have defined the values of spontaneous blood pressure that should be tolerated,

they provide no recommendations for normotensive or hypotensive patients with acute stroke. In a preliminary report, Rordorf and colleagues[220] observed an improvement of the NIHSS score in 7 of 13 patients with acute stroke during phenylephrine infusion and were able to establish a blood pressure threshold for this improvement in 6 patients. Schwarz and coworkers[221] examined the influence of sudden increases in MAP, which were induced by norepinephrine, during 47 monitoring sessions in 19 patients with severe ischemic stroke. These investigators noted a slight increase in ICP, accompanied by significant increases in CPP and in mean flow velocity of the MCA supplying the affected hemisphere. No hemorrhagic complications or other side effects were observed. This study suggests that induced hypertension could potentially improve the blood perfusion of the affected hemisphere. Confirmation of these intriguing results would have a major impact on blood pressure management in patients with acute stroke; evaluation through further studies is therefore warranted.

Acute Basilar Artery Occlusion

Occlusion of the basilar artery is associated with a grave prognosis; early studies reported a mortality rate in excess of 70%.[222–226] Hacke and associates[227] treated a series of 65 patients who had thrombotic vertebrobasilar occlusions with either local intra-arterial thrombolysis (n = 43) or conventional therapy (antiplatelet agents or anticoagulants; n = 22). A total of 48 patients (74%) died, 19 in the conventional treatment group and 29 in the group treated with local thrombolysis. Recanalization rate after thrombolysis was 44%, and recanalization was significantly associated with survival.

Brand and coworkers[228] retrospectively evaluated 51 consecutive patients treated with intra-arterial urokinase (n = 44) or intravenous or intra-arterial rt-PA (n = 7). Recanalization was achieved in 26 (51%) patients. Mortality was 46% in the patients in whom recanalization was achieved, and 92% in the patients in whom it was not. The cause of embolic stroke, length of basilar artery obstruction, and state of collateral circulation were identified as independent predictors of mortality. Functional outcome at 3 months was acceptable, with 10 survivors minimally, 5 moderately, and only 1 severely impaired.[228]

In contrast, Cross and associates[229] did not demonstrate a relationship between collateral circulation and mortality in 24 patients with symptomatic basilar thrombosis, although they did note a correlation between collateral circulation and neurologic outcome. A further study by the same group showed a significant relationship between clot location and survival; 5 of 7 patients with distal occlusion of the basilar artery were alive at 3 months, compared with only 2 of 13 patients with middle or proximal occlusion.[230] Interestingly, duration of symptoms before treatment, age, CT findings, and neurologic status at start of treatment were not found to predict outcome.

Levy and coworkers[231] performed a meta-analysis of six studies involving a total of 164 patients who were treated with urokinase or rt-PA. Complete recanalization was achieved in 91 patients (55%). Only 7% of patients with incomplete recanalization survived, compared with 57%

of those with complete recanalization. Additionally, survival was significantly higher in patients who were responsive at treatment (51%) than in those who were comatose (18%), and higher in patients with distal-third occlusions of the basilar artery (63%) than in those with occlusions of the vertebral artery or the proximal or middle third of the basilar artery (28%).

Few data comparing the efficacy of rt-PA and urokinase for intra-arterial fibrinolysis of basilar artery occlusion are available. Zeumer and colleagues[232] treated 28 patients who had vertebrobasilar clots with either 20 mg rt-PA or 750,000 units of urokinase; they observed no differences in recanalization and also no bleeding complications. Cross and associates,[233] however, reported spontaneous symptomatic hemorrhage in 3 of 4 patients treated with rt-PA (20 to 50 mg), compared with 3 of 20 patients treated with urokinase. Also, the extent of hemorrhage appeared to be greater in the rt-PA group. These investigators hypothesized that the difference could be due to the different dosages of rt-PA used, suggesting that 50 mg is too high. Intravenous heparin was administered to all patients in both studies, and there was no indication that this regimen significantly increased the rate of bleeding complications.

Implantation of flexible coronary stents for treatment of symptomatic basilar artery stenosis was recently published.[234] Phatouros and associates[235] implanted such a stent in a patient with acute thrombosis of the basilar artery after successful superselective intra-arterial thrombolysis of the vertebrobasilar clot and balloon angioplasty. This procedure could prove beneficial in preventing rethrombosis of the basilar artery after arterial thrombolysis, particularly in patients with underlying stenosis of this vessel. Junghans and coworkers[236] reported complete recanalization and good neurologic outcome in four patients with acute basilar artery thrombosis who were treated with a combination of intra-arterial rt-PA and a nonpeptide platelet glycoprotein IIb/IIIa inhibitor (tirofiban). Although this initial report could provide an attractive alternative for treatment of acute basilar artery occlusion, the efficacy of this approach remains to be confirmed in large-scale studies.

Patients with acute basilar artery occlusion should be treated in an ICU. In patients with impaired consciousness, immediate endotracheal intubation is mandatory. Our current treatment of choice consists of local thrombolysis with intra-arterial urokinase, 1.000.000 IU/hour under general anesthesia, followed by intravenous heparin. Another CT scan should be obtained after angiography to exclude intracerebral hemorrhage. Prognosis of patients who are already comatose upon admission and in whom somatosensory cortical-evoked potentials cannot be obtained is quite poor, barely justifying aggressive therapy.

Cerebellar Infarction

Cerebellar infarction constitutes 1.9 to 10.5% of cases in clinicopathologic series of patients with cerebral infarctions. Neurologic deterioration occurs as a result of a growing mass effect of the infarcted cerebellum in the posterior fossa. Therefore, patients with signs of increased pressure in the posterior fossa on CCT scan should be carefully monitored in a neurocritical care unit. One must always bear in mind that deterioration in such a patient can occur within minutes, although the clinical condition prior to this can appear stable or even to be improving. Additionally, deterioration can occur anytime within the first 2 weeks after onset of a cerebellar infarct and may be delayed compared with that in supratentorial stroke, indicating the need for prolonged monitoring in conservatively treated patients with cerebellar infarcts.

No controlled study has yet assessed the efficacy of decompressive surgery for cerebellar infarctions. Nevertheless, this is an important issue, because increasing mass effect of the infarcted cerebellum in the posterior fossa can lead to clinical deterioration and brainstem compression. Identifying patients with cerebellar infarctions who are bound to experience intracranial hypertension is not always straightforward; prognostic factors include underlying size of the infarction, hemorrhagic transformation, and poor collateral blood flow. One must keep in mind that neurologic deterioration can also be caused by occlusive hydrocephalus or progression of concurrent brainstem infarction. Close clinical monitoring and frequent CT scanning to estimate the severity of obstructive hydrocephalus are mandatory. In patients with fast decline of consciousness, decompressive surgery of the posterior fossa —with or without removal of infarcted cerebellar tissue—is significantly better than ventriculostomy.[237–239] Ventriculostomy alone may be a temporary measure, but great care must be taken in such a procedure because it may promote ascending herniation. We do not use this approach in patients with additional basilar artery thrombosis and large brainstem infarcts.

Because it is often difficult to clearly distinguish the mechanisms leading to further clinical deterioration, somatosensory evoked potentials (SSEPs) and brainstem auditory evoked potentials (BAEPs) provide further information for treatment decisions in those patients. Patients with normal BAEPs and SSEPs are usually treated with osmotherapeutics. Prolonged interpeak latencies in BAEPs and altered amplitudes in SSEPs indicate the need for decompressive surgery. Ventriculostomy is the treatment of choice in patients with CT findings indicating hydrocephalus alone.

Spontaneous Intracerebral Hemorrhage

Clinical Features

The clinical presentation of patients with ICH consists of general symptoms (mainly headache, vomiting and decreased level of consciousness) and focal deficits determined by the hematoma location and size. Focal symptoms in patients with ICH most commonly progress because of hematoma expansion; although symptom progression is usually of short duration (<30 minutes), late progression (up to 24 hours after onset) has also been reported.[240] Because ICH is the subject of a separate chapter (63), only issues related to ICU care are discussed here.

General Management

The current management of patients with ICH consists of stabilization of vital parameters, prevention of rebleeding, and surgical evacuation in certain subgroups. Patients with large, space-occupying ICH are at high risk for upper airway obstruction and aspiration because of weakness of upper airway muscles, impairment of airway and swallowing reflexes, and vomiting, thus requiring early endotracheal intubation. Constant monitoring of cardiac function and blood pressure and readiness for cardiopulmonary resuscitation are mandatory, because central vegetative disturbances such as bradycardia, tachycardia, hypotension, and hypertension are common in ICH.

Headache can be treated primarily with mild analgesics like paracetamol; aspirin and other agents that interfere with platelet function should be avoided. Opioids are often needed for proper pain control. Distressing anxiety can be alleviated with short-acting benzodiazepines (see earlier discussion). Stools should be kept soft with oral laxatives and an adequate fluid intake. Close monitoring and correction of glucose levels are important in patients with ICH. Body temperature must also be monitored closely, particularly because hyperthermia in such patients is due not only to infection but also to direct or indirect stimulation of the thermoregulatory center in the hypothalamus. Both blood glucose level and body temperature have been shown to affect long-term outcome after ICH.[241]

Like patients with ischemic stroke, patients with ICH can be mobilized early. Great care should be taken, however, with special monitoring of blood pressure to avoid abrupt and excessive elevations. Treatment of elevated ICP in patients with ICH does not differ from that used in patients with ischemic stroke (as discussed earlier).

Blood Pressure Management

Severe hypertension is commonly observed in patients with acute ICH. Although reduction of ICP may be sufficient to control arterial blood pressure, other pharmacologic treatment is often needed. Blood pressure lowering should not be too drastic; sudden or large drops in blood pressure could result in a decrease in CPP, which could enhance ischemic injury in patients with impaired cerebrovascular autoregulation. No specific guidelines for the treatment of hypertension in ICH have been developed from results of randomized, controlled studies, but there is agreement that diastolic blood pressure higher than 120 mm Hg and MAP higher than 125 to 135 mm Hg should be treated.[242,243] Pharmacologic agents that cause cerebral vasodilation, such as hydralazine, nitroglycerin, and nitroprusside, should be avoided because of the risk of further ICP increase. Appropriate agents are labetalol, captopril, clonidine, and urapidil (see earlier discussion).

Coagulation and Reversal of Anticoagulation

Early assessment and correction of the coagulation status of a patient with ICH are particularly important, because it may affect both the progression of cerebral bleeding and the incidence of early rebleeding. Patients with a prolonged activated partial thromboplastin time because of heparin therapy should be treated with protamine sulfate, 1 mg/100 IU of heparin. A prolonged prothrombin time due to phenprocoumon or warfarin therapy should be reversed with intravenous vitamin K, fresh frozen plasma, or both. If available, a prothrombin complex concentrate (prothrombin, proconvertin, Stuart-Prower factor, antihemophilic globulin B) should be administered, because such agents act more rapidly than vitamin K or fresh frozen

plasma[244]; however, use of such concentrates is associated with a potential risk of generalized thromboembolism.

A therapeutic dilemma arises in patients with warfarin-associated ICH and an underlying condition associated with a high risk of recurrent embolism. Wijdicks and colleagues[245] reviewed the medical records of 39 patients with prosthetic heart valves and ICH. A total of 13 patients (33%) died within 2 days of admission; the remaining 26 patients received fresh frozen plasma and vitamin K, and anticoagulation therapy was discontinued from 2 to 90 (median 8) days. No transient ischemic attacks (TIAs), ischemic strokes, systemic embolization, or valve thrombosis were observed in any patients.[245] A further study by the same group (Phan and coworkers[246]) reviewed records from 141 patients (group 1, 52 patients with prosthetic heart valves; group 2, 53 patients with atrial fibrillation and cardioembolic stroke; group 3, 36 patients with recurrent TIA or ischemic stroke). Overall mortality was 43%. Warfarin was discontinued for a median time of 10 days; only 3 patients had an ischemic stroke within 30 days of warfarin discontinuation, and the probability of an ischemic stroke at 30 days was 2.9% for group 1, 2.6% for group 2, and 4.8% for group 3. Re-initiation of warfarin therapy was not associated with recurrence of ICH during hospitalization.

These results were challenged by a smaller case series published by Bertram and associates,[247] who described 15 patients (10 with prosthetic heart valves; 5 with a high-risk cardioembolic source) presenting with ICH. The therapeutic regimen consisted of normalization of the INR (international normalized ratio) by administration of prothrombin complex, fresh frozen plasma, or vitamin K followed by administration of heparin (intravenous or subcutaneous). Three embolic complications were observed in patients with normalized INR values and insignificant elevation in partial thromboplastin time (PTT), and rebleeding occurred in 3 patients with INR values higher than 1.5 (2 of these patients were receiving full-dose heparin therapy). Interestingly, only 1 of the 15 patients died in the series reported by Bertram and associates,[247] for which the rate of cerebrovascular events was 40%; Phan and coworkers[246] reported 42% mortality as well as a 6% rate of cerebrovascular events in their 141 patients.

The number of patients per year who were receiving anticoagulation therapy and were admitted with ICH was 2.4 to 2.5 in the two studies, suggesting that the addressed issue is common in major referral centers. There appears to be agreement that warfarin treatment should be discontinued and the INR value normalized in patients with ICH. It also seems to be safe to resume oral anticoagulation within the first 7 to 14 days. The question whether to treat these patients with heparin in the interim phase cannot be answered, because the results of these two studies did not agree.

ICH is one of the most severe complications of thrombolytic therapy, occurring more commonly with streptokinase than with urokinase or rt-PA. According to AHA guidelines,[242] suspicion of hemorrhagic complications should lead to (1) discontinuation of ongoing infusion of a thrombolytic drug, (2) coagulation tests, (3) emergency CT scanning, (4) neurosurgical consultation (if necessary), and

(5) transfusion of 4 to 6 U of cryoprecipitate or fresh frozen plasma and 1 U of single-donor platelets. These guidelines are not evidence-based, however; we routinely use ε-aminocaproic acid (5 g over 15 to 30 min) and cryoprecipitate for ICH associated with thrombolytic therapy.

Hydrocephalus

Patients with ICH are at risk for hydrocephalus due to mass effects (blockade of the foramen of Monro, compression of the aqueduct or fourth ventricle, intraventricular blood). Phan and colleagues[248] demonstrated that the presence of obstructive hydrocephalus upon admission in a comatose patient with putaminal hemorrhage is a predictor of 30-day mortality. Decline in the level of consciousness is the major symptom of a developing hydrocephalus. External ventricular drainage is the treatment of choice; it should be considered early in any patient in whom the amount of intraventricular blood makes the development of a hydrocephalus likely.

Antiepileptic Therapy

During the first 3 days, epileptic seizures occur in 10% to 15% of patients with ICH in all locations and in 15% to 35% of patients with lobar hemorrhage[249]; seizures are less common in deep ICH (4% to 8%)[250] and very rare in thalamic ICH. Epileptic seizures should be treated initially with benzodiazepines, followed by phenytoin (18–20 mg/kg). If a second agent is needed, we usually add phenobarbital. If this combination is not sufficient for seizure control, thiopental can also be used; caution is needed with use of this agent, however, because of the potential for severe hypotensive episodes after its administration.

Surgery

The indication for surgery in supratentorial cerebral hematoma is still under dispute. Most of the information on this subject has been derived from clinical series with several methodologic flaws. There is no proof that evacuation of a hematoma by conventional surgery reduces residual deficits or speeds recovery. Randomized controlled surgical trials for spontaneous supratentorial ICH have been performed by six groups of investigators[251–256]; the essential data from their studies are summarized in Table 52.7. Current treatment strategies largely depend on (1) hemorrhage size and location and (2) clinical impairment and course.

Table 52.8 summarizes current recommendations regarding surgical or nonsurgical treatment in special subgroups of patients. New approaches, such as stereotactic or endoscopic aspiration of hematomas and thrombolytic therapy of intracerebral or intraventricular blood clots, offer promise[257–260]; except for stereotactically guided

---

Table 52.7   Summary of Surgical Trials for Spontaneous Intracranial Hemorrhage

Study*	Year	No. of Patients — Surgical Group	No. of Patients — Medical Group	Time Window (hrs)	Inclusion Criteria	Outcome — Surgical Group	Outcome — Medical Group
Juvela et al[252]	1989	26	26	<48	Unconscious; severe hemiparesis	M6: 46%	M6: 38%
Auer et al[253]	1989	50	50	<48	ICH > 10 mL	M6: 30%	M6: 70%
Batjer et al[254]	1990	8	13	<24	Putaminal location; ICH > 3 cm	M6: 50%	M6: 85%
Morgenstern et al[255]	1998	17	17	<12	ICH > 9 mL	M1: 6% / M6: 17%	M1: 24% / M6: 24%
Zuccarello et al[256]	1999	9	11	<27	ICH > 10 mL, GOS > 4	GOS > 3: 56%	GOS > 3: 36%

*Superscript numbers indicate chapter references.
GOS, percentage of patients with Glasgow Outcome Scale score; ICH, volume/size of hemorrhage; M1, mortality at 1 month; M6, mortality at 6 months.

Table 52.8   Recommendations for Surgical or Nonsurgical Treatment of Intracranial Hemorrhage

ICH	Clinical or CT features	Treatment
Putamen	Alert, small ICH (<30 mL)	Nonsurgical
	Comatose, large ICH (>60 mL)	Nonsurgical
	Drowsy, intermediate ICH (30–60 mL)	Consider evacuation
Caudate	Alert or drowsy, with intraventricular hemorrhage and hydrocephalus	Consider ventriculostomy
Thalamus	Drowsy or lethargic, with blood in the 3rd ventricle and hydrocephalus	Consider ventriculostomy
Lobar white matter	Drowsy or lethargic, with intermediate ICH (20–60 mL), progressive decline in level of consciousness	Consider evacuation
Pons, midbrain, medulla	—	Nonsurgical
Cerebellum	Noncomatose, with ICH > 3 cm in diameter, and/or hydrocephalus, and/or effacement of quadrigeminal cistern	Evacuation recommended, preceded by ventriculostomy if status is actively deteriorating

CT, computed tomography; ICH, intracranial hemorrhage.

endoscopic evacuation, however,[253] they have not yet been validated in randomized clinical trials. Very early surgical treatment for acute ICH is difficult to achieve but is feasible at specialized centers. The trend toward lower morbidity and mortality with surgical intervention in subgroups of patients with spontaneous supratentorial ICH warrants further investigation of very early clot removal in large randomized clinical trials.

Unlike with supratentorial hematomas, the indication for surgery in cerebellar hematomas is now undisputed, despite the complete lack of prospective trials. The prognosis rapidly worsens with a hematoma volume exceeding 20 mL (mean diameter of 3 cm). Surgery should be performed as soon as possible, because even patients with massive cerebellar hemorrhage can survive if they have been comatose for only a short time.[261] No recommendation can be made for surgical evacuation of brainstem hematomas, because the tissue destruction caused by the initial bleeding precludes any benefit. Anecdotal reports of successful surgical treatment of hematomas located in the vicinity of the fourth ventricle constitute neurosurgical rarities.

Intraventricular Hemorrhage

Primary intraventricular hemorrhages (IVHs) constitute a distinct entity, with symptoms similar to those of SAH (severe headache of acute onset, neck stiffness, depressed level of consciousness), although motor deficit is either absent or minimal. Secondary IVH occurs in up to 40% of all patients with ICH and in up to 20% of all patients with SAH. There is strong evidence that IVH contributes to mortality after cerebral hemorrhage. Routine clinical management consists of an external ventricular drainage, which lowers the ICP immediately, but the drainage has to be continued until the ventricular clot has dissolved, and CSF circulation normalized. The drainage prevents acute hydrocephalus but does not affect the clot resolution or the incidence of communicating hydrocephalus. Therefore, intraventricular thrombolysis was proposed as an effective measure to hasten the resolution of the intraventricular blood clot, reduce the duration of extraventricular drainage, decrease the severity and incidence of communicating hydrocephalus, and reduce IVH-associated mortality. Clinical experience with this approach has grown over the last 10 years, but data from randomized clinical trials are still lacking. We perform intraventricular lysis in patients with a large amount of intraventricular blood after ICH, giving 4 mg rt-PA every 12 hours over 2 days. Vascular malformations should be ruled out with either CT angiography (CTA) or conventional angiography before intraventricular lysis is initiated (Fig. 52–5).

Subarachnoid Hemorrhage

Systemic Causes

Several medical diseases can cause SAH. Association between sickle cell anemia and SAH has been reported; patients in such cases are mostly children. Angiography often shows occlusions of the distal branches of the intracranial vessel, and SAH is attributed to rupture of leptomeningeal collaterals. SAH can be seen in patients with a history of drug abuse. Amphetamines, cocaine, and other substances may cause changes to the arterial vessel wall, which then may lead to rupture and consequent SAH. Anticoagulant therapy may also cause SAH, which has a relatively poor outcome in the majority of patients.

Medical Therapy

SAH from the rupture of an intracranial aneurysm is often devastating and accounts for approximately one fourth of all cerebrovascular deaths. Despite great advances in the surgical, endovascular, and medical management of patients with aneurysmal SAH, the morbidity and mortality of this disease remain unacceptably high. Only about half of patients admitted to qualified neurosurgical centers with the diagnosis of aneurysmal SAH have a good clinical outcome.[262] Many patients die of the initial bleed or further complications associated with the disease. Of the survivors, about 50% are left disabled and dependent on the help of others.[263] Because the lesion is treatable and even curable at particular stages, management decisions are critical. Because loss of functional independence is a common consequence of aneurysmal bleeding despite surgical clipping or endovascular therapy of the aneurysm, the best medical management may complement efforts to improve outcome.

Outcome

Mortality and morbidity rates after SAH have improved but remain significant in spite of the development of better management and surgical techniques. The International Cooperative Study on the Timing of Aneurysm Surgery showed that less than 60% of all patients with aneurysmal SAH were able to return to their premorbid state.[264] However, case-fatality rates range from 32% to 76%, and of the patients who survive the bleed, almost one third remain dependent.[263] Persistent cognitive impairment is also a common sequela of SAH. There is a significant correlation between the affected arterial distribution and the neuropsychological deficit. For instance, damage to the anterior communicating artery commonly causes amnestic deficits or personality changes. The severity of the hemorrhage correlates well with cognitive impairment. Complications of SAH such as hydrocephalus, IVH, and parenchymatous hematoma also cause cognitive deficits and exacerbate the dysfunction due to SAH alone.[265]

Clinical Presentation and Prognosis

The clinical hallmark of SAH is the sudden onset of severe headache ("thunderclap"), which can be accompanied by a loss of consciousness. The patient often describes the headache as "the worst headache of my life." Patients usually also have neck stiffness, photophobia, and back pain as symptoms of meningeal irritation. Focal neurologic deficits, like cranial nerve deficits, hemiparesis, or aphasia, may occur as well. From 15% to 20% of all patients with SAH suffer a seizure as a result of a sudden rise in ICP or direct cortical irritation.[266]

Warning signs of impending SAH are present in more than 15% of all patients. These signs are usually attributed to either small leaks ("sentinel blood") or aneurysm expansion.[267] Warning signs occur in general within 1 to 3 months before the major hemorrhage.

Often, activities such as lifting heavy loads, sexual intercourse, and defecation can lead to a rise in blood pressure

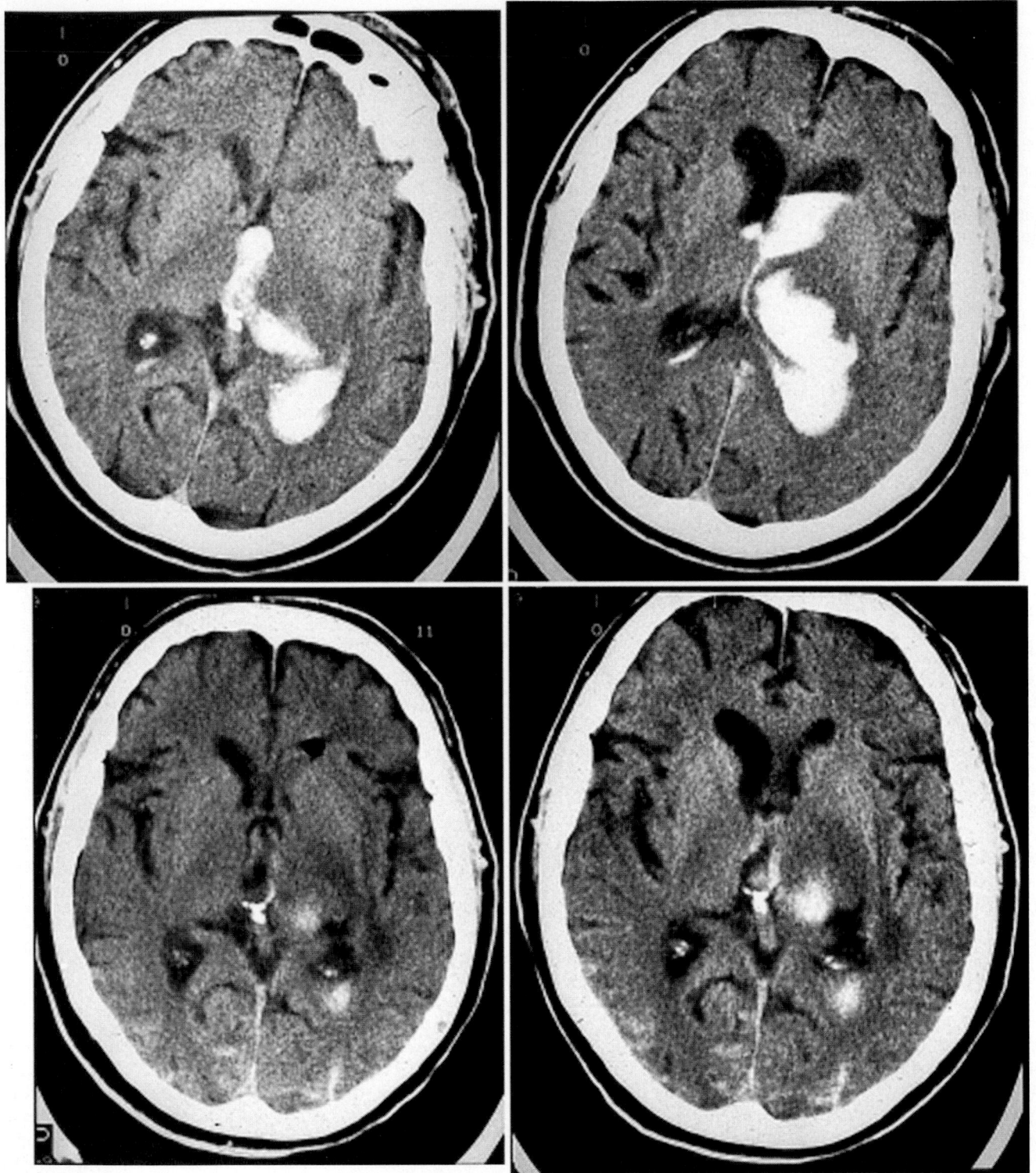

FIGURE 52–5   *Intraventricular thrombolysis after basal ganglia hemorrhage with intraventricular bleeding. Time course of therapy with recombinant tissue-plasminogen activator (rt-PA) for thrombolysis of intraventricular blood.* Top row, *before treatment;* bottom row, *after treatment.*

and thereby cause SAH. The clinical signs of SAH include headache, dizziness, and loss of consciousness. An elevation in ICP may lead to sixth nerve palsy. A complete or partial palsy of the third nerve can be seen in aneurysms of the internal carotid artery or at the origin of the poste-

rior communicating artery. However, the physical findings may be normal in some patients.

The clinical grading scale most widely used in SAH, developed by Hunt and Hess (Table 52.9),[268] is based on the presence or absence of neurologic deficits. Of all the

Table 52.9 Hunt and Hess Scale for Patients with Intracranial Aneurysms According to Surgical Risk

Grade	Criteria
I	Asymptomatic, mild headache and slight nuchal rigidity
II	Moderate to severe headache, nuchal rigidity, cranial nerve deficit
III	Drowsiness, confusion, lethargy
IV	Stupor, moderate or severe hemiparesis
V	Coma, decerebrate posturing

prognostic factors, initial neurologic condition, amount of subarachnoidal blood, and age are the most important. For clinical grading systems, the neurologic condition on admission is obviously the most important. Treatment protocols as well as prognostic estimation are based on this grading system.

Diagnostic Evaluation

Diagnostic evaluation of a patient with SAH is discussed in more detail in Chapter 14. In general, the diagnostic evaluation of a patient with suspected SAH consists of CT scan, lumbar puncture with CSF analysis, CTA, and cerebral angiography.

The first step in evaluation is non–contrast-enhanced CT scanning; this is the neuroradiologic investigation of choice to detect blood in the subarachnoid space. The pattern of blood distribution often gives clues to the location of the underlying aneurysm. Despite the presumed high sensitivity of this modality, initial CT findings can be normal in up to 5% of cases of SAH.[262,269,270] Improvements in MRI and magnetic resonance angiography (MRA) have increased their sensitivity considerably.[271,272] FLAIR sequences allow identification of extravasated blood, and MRA—like CTA—can visualize larger aneurysms noninvasively.

Lumbar puncture with CSF analysis is still an important step in the diagnosis of SAH. Every patient with a highly suggestive history of SAH and negative imaging results should undergo lumbar puncture. CSF is xanthochromic in a centrifuged specimen, provided that this is obtained at least 6 hours after the initial hemorrhage.

Cerebral angiography is still the standard for the detection of an aneurysm. Angiography is used to detect aneurysms and possible vasospasm. In general, a four-vessel angiography is essential to detect multiple aneurysms. If the initial angiogram could not demonstrate an aneurysm, the evaluation should be repeated within 2 weeks, when a possible thrombus or vasospasm has resolved. A second angiogram is probably not necessary for patients with a typical perimesencephalic hemorrhage.[273–275] In the future, a growing proportion of patients will probably undergo surgery for SAH after evaluation with CTA or MRA as the only imaging method, because these techniques continuously improve.

Cerebral Complications
Rebleeding
Medical management of patients with SAH should focus on (1) basic treatment and (2) prevention, close

monitoring, and treatment of complications of SAH, which are often fatal.

It is most important to avoid rerupture of the aneurysm. In the first few hours after the initial bleed, more than 10% of all patients demonstrate clinical deterioration, suggesting that rebleeding has occurred.[276,277] The mortality rate in SAH patients following rebleeding is approximately 50%.[278] To date, there is no method for identifying the patients with a higher risk for rebleeding. The probability of rebleeding is about 4% the first day after the bleed and about 1.5% per day thereafter.[279] Overall, the incidence of rebleeding is reportedly 20% in the first 2 weeks and 50% within the first 6 months after the initial bleed.[262,280] After this time, the risk gradually decreases to a level of 3% per year. Several predisposing factors for rebleeding have been identified.[279] They are female gender, early admission after SAH, poor neurologic grade, poor general medical condition, and with systolic blood pressure greater than 170 mm Hg.[279]

Clot formation and tissue damage stimulate fibrinolytic activity in the CSF, thus raising the risk of rebleeding; this observation constituted the rationale for the use of antifibrinolytic drugs. Aminocaproic acid and tranexamic acid were used. A randomized placebo-controlled trial, a non-randomized trial, and other reports assessing the efficacy of antifibrinolytic therapy showed a significantly lower incidence of rebleeding. However, mortality was not altered with this kind of therapy, which was associated with a higher incidence of ischemic stroke.[281–283] Important side effects of antifibrinolytic therapy were a greater tendency for bleeding after discontinuation of therapy, diuresis, diarrhea, abdominal discomfort, nausea, and dizziness.[284]

Other attempts to reduce the rebleeding rate, with fluid restriction, aggressive blood pressure reduction (induced hypotension), and prolonged bedrest, have not been shown to be effective.[285] Nevertheless, everything should be done to avoid stimulation of and agitation in patients with SAH. Patients should receive stool softeners, and nausea and vomiting should be treated vigorously. For pain control, analgesics such as meperidine, which does not interfere with patients' wakefulness, should be used.

Acute Hydrocephalus
Symptomatic obstructive hydrocephalus occlusus or malresorptivus occurs in 15% to 20% of patients with SAH.[286] A characteristic history consists of gradual obtundation after a lucid interval of a few hours. Insertion of an external ventricular catheter results in significant improvement within 1 or 2 days, even if it may carry a higher risk of rebleeding. The improvement can be explained by an abrupt decrease of ICP due to CSF drainage. Clinically, a slowly developing hydrocephalus can be assumed in a patient who demonstrates vertical gaze palsy, decline of cognitive functions, and progressive lethargy. Ventriculostomy is especially recommended in patients in Hunt and Hess grades IV or V.[287] A depression in level of consciousness indicates the need for CT scanning. If hydrocephalus is present, ventriculomegaly will be evident. It is best discerned through comparison of the current CT scan with earlier scans. In this situation, an external ventricular shunt is indicated. In patients with large amounts of intraventricular blood, intraventricular fibrinolysis therapy with low

doses of rt-PA (2 mg every 12 hours for 3 days) may improve clinical outcome, even though this observation needs confirmation in randomized clinical trials.[288] There is an association of shunt-dependent hydrocephalus and Hunt and Hess grade on admission, incidence of repeated SAH, anterior communicating artery (AcoA) aneurysm, and IVH.[289,290]

Infections are another serious concern after a drain has been in place for 5 days or more.[291,292] Most neurosurgeons try to remove or replace a ventricular drain by 7 days after insertion. Once a shunt is in place, it is monitored daily for amount of fluid drained and CSF cell count. After initial insertion, the shunt is set to drain at 5 to 10 cm H_2O. Over the next several days, the level of drainage is gradually increased as permitted by low CSF drainage amount and constant normal ventricular size as visualized on follow-up CT scans. Drainage of more than 250 mL of CSF per day indicates that there is still substantial obstruction of the CSF circulation and the patient is unlikely to tolerate elevation or even removal of the drainage level or even removal of the drain. The drain is clamped when ICP levels do not exceed 15 to 20 mm H_2O. If neurologic status and ventricular size remain stable, the extraventricular drain can be removed. If not, the drain should be changed 5 and 10 days after insertion or when there is evidence of ventriculitis. Ventriculitis should be suspected if CSF cell count increases over the days of drainage. In this case, local instillation of an antibiotic may be considered.

Vasospasm

Up to 25% of patients with a ruptured aneurysm experience delayed cerebral ischemia, mainly between day 5 and day 14 after the initial bleeding.[278,293] Ischemia is the prominent cause of death and disability after SAH. The total amount of subarachnoid blood is a strong risk factor, but its distribution does not predict the site of ischemia.[294] Thus, vasospasm occurs more commonly in patients with a poor Hunt and Hess grade SAH. The time course of vasospasm is consistent with an immune-mediated response, and later observations suggest that immunologic processes, including activation of the complement system, may be involved. Contraction of the arterial smooth muscle and morphologic changes in the vessel wall and along its endothelial surface occur in response to injury.[295] Studies examining the various components of blood for their potential to produce vasospasm have been reported.[293,295] Many of these components can cause vasospasm, although no single spasmogen has been identified. Other potential contributors to vasospasm are mechanical wall disruption, inflammation, and free radical formation. The clinical presentation of vasospasm is a gradual process, although it can also be abrupt on rare occasions or insidious with minor transient changes. Patients may complain of increased headache or may manifest meningism, seizures, decreased consciousness, or new focal neurologic deficits. A new deficit can range from a minor paresis to hemiplegia, aphasia, or behavioral change.[296]

The detection of vasospasm is possible with transcranial Doppler (TCD) ultrasonography, which demonstrates increased blood flow velocity due to arterial narrowing in the basal cerebral arteries. However, there is uncertainty about the diagnostic specificity of TCD ultrasonography.

Only flow velocities greater than 120 to 200 cm/sec are highly predictive for the diagnosis of vasospasm.[297] The sensitivity and specificity of TCD ultrasonography in diagnosing vasospasm in comparison with angiography were reported to be adequate in the MCA, but not in the ACA or PCA. Comparison of TCD ultrasonographic findings with rCBF measurements[298,299] indicates that the sensitivity and specificity of the modality may be inadequate to guide major medical decisions, although it may still be useful as a noninvasive screening tool. TCD ultrasonographic signs of vasospasm are listed in Table 52.10.

Triple-H Therapy

Treatment with hypervolemia, hemodilution, and induced hypertension therapy, also called triple-H therapy (see Table 52.11), aims to increase CBF and improve microcirculation by raising systolic blood pressure and cardiac output.[300] In the first larger patient series, reported by Kassell and associates,[301] the combination of induced hypertension and volume expansion reversed neurologic deficits in 43 of 58 patients. It is hypothesized that a defect in cerebral autoregulation renders the perfusion of the

Table 52.10   Findings of Transcranial Doppler Ultrasonography that Indicate Vasospasms

Intensity-weighted mean velocity	>3 kHz (120 cm/s) = borderline
	>4 kHz (160 cm/s) = significant
	>5 kHz (200 cm/s) = critical
Maximum systolic velocity	>4 kHz (160 cm/s) = relevant
	>7.5 kHz (300 cm/s) = critical
MCA/ICA index	>3.0
Velocity increase during the first 6 days	>50%/day or >1 kHz (40 cm/s)/day
Pulsatility of signals	Pulsatility index > 1.0
	Resistance index > 0.6

MCA/ICA index, mean flow velocity divided by ICA mean flow velocity.

Table 52.11   Definition of and Monitoring Requirements for Triple-H (Hypervolemia, Hemodilution, and Induced Hypertension) Therapy for Subarachnoid Hemorrhage

Monitoring requirements	High-volume colloidal infusion (hetastarch 500–1500 mL)
	Ringer's solution (5000–10,000 mL)
	Hemoglobin solution if necessary
	Sympathomimetics (norepinephrine, 0.2–1.2 mg/h, or dopamine, 10–30 mg/kg/min)
	Laboratory tests, including osmolarity of urine and serum
	Mean arterial blood pressure → systolic 160–180 mm Hg
	Central venous pressure → 10–12 mm Hg
	Fluid status and weight control → hematocrit 33%–38%
	Daily chest radiograph
	If available: wedge pressure (Swan-Ganz catheter) → <20 mm Hg
	Intracranial pressure and central perfusion pressure monitoring

brain passively dependent on systolic blood pressure. Triple-H therapy is indicated when severe vasospasm is found on TCD ultrasonography or a patient demonstrates progressive neurologic deterioration.

Hypervolemia is induced by infusion of isotonic saline or plasma expanders, aiming at a CVP of 10 to 14 mm Hg. If no clinical improvement is achieved, the additional use of vasopressors, such as dopamine, neosynephrine, or norepinephrine, should be considered for induced hypertension. Continuous infusion is titrated to achieve a mean increase in arterial blood pressure to 20 to 30 mm Hg above the baseline value, with systolic blood pressure values up to 180 mm Hg. Sometimes even systolic blood pressure as high as 240 mm Hg systolic is required to achieve adequate CPP. Although catecholamine-based vasopressor therapy is reported to occasionally reverse neurologic deficits, the cerebrovascular and metabolic effects of such agents in this situation are unclear. When catecholamines cross the blood-brain barrier, which is disrupted with vasospasm,[302] they have been reported to produce hypermetabolism and hyperemia in animals. Concomitant infusion of albumin and other fluids also leads to decreases in hematocrit value and blood viscosity. Animal studies have shown that the optimal hematocrit is 33%, because the oxygen–carrying capacity of the blood is not compromised.[303] This concept has been applied to clinical care in determining the endpoint for hemodilution therapy.[304]

Although the benefit of triple-H therapy has not yet been proven by randomized studies, the rate of permanent ischemic deficits seems to be lower than expected.[305] Triple-H therapy can be used either prophylactically or in the phase of reversible neurologic deficit with impending ischemia but without complete infarction.[296,306] Some evidence suggests that if infarction is present, triple-H therapy may cause further deterioration.[307] Also, pulmonary and cerebral edema, cardiac dysregulation due to volume overload, myocardial infarction, and the risk of rebleeding seem to be more common with this treatment. The overall incidence of systemic complications associated with triple-H therapy is 7% to 17% for pulmonary edema, 2% for myocardial infarction, 3% to 35% for dilutional hyponatremia, and 3% for coagulopathy.[308,309]

Calcium Antagonists

The use of calcium channel blockers is based on the assumption that they can reduce the frequency of vasospasm by inhibiting the calcium influx in the smooth muscle cells of the vasculature. Other factors may be preservation of oxidative metabolism, cell membrane stabilization, and microrheologic effects.[310] Nimodipine or nicardipine is the drug of choice. Nimodipine, which is more commonly used, significantly reduces delayed cerebral ischemia and improves outcome.[311,312] A systematic review of all randomized trials of calcium antagonist therapy in SAH showed a significant reduction in the frequency of poor outcome.[313] On the basis of these data, it is generally recommended that all patients with SAH receive nimodipine, 30 to 60 mg enterally every 4 to 6 hours or, in Europe, as an initial IV formula (1 mg/hr for 1 to 2 hours, followed by continuous infusion of 1 to 6 mg/hr); later, oral nimodipine (60 mg, 4–6 times per day) may be given for 2 to 3 weeks after SAH. Side effects include pulmonary right-to-left-shunt and hypotension, which affects the coronary blood flow and the digestive tract muscles.

Tirilazad, a potent in vitro inhibitor of free radical–mediated lipid peroxidation, has been studied in several trials.[314–316] The only beneficial effect on outcome was seen in a subgroup of men who were treated with a dosage of 6 mg/kg/day.[314] Another interesting therapeutic option is the use of antiplatelet agents such as aspirin, because several studies have demonstrated an activation of platelets within the first 3 days after SAH. Retrospective data suggest that patients who used salicylates before a hemorrhage had a significantly lower risk for delayed ischemia. Data from a pilot study suggest that this treatment is safe and feasible.[317]

Invasive approaches for the treatment of vasospasm include endovascular techniques such as balloon angioplasty, intra-arterial administration of papaverine, and a combination thereof.

Intra-arterial Papaverine

Papaverine is an alkaloid compound and a powerful vasodilator. It acts directly on the smooth muscle cells of the arterial wall by transendothelial absorption. Intra-arterial papaverine infusion is often associated with vasospasm in distal vessels.[318–320] Papaverine may be administered in patients with severe vasospasm who cannot be treated with angioplasty.[321] However, papaverine can transiently produce signs of neurologic deterioration during infusion, depending on the vascular territory infused, such as hemiparesis, seizures, pupillary changes, unconsciousness, increased ICP, and cardiovascular collapse.[319,322,323] Doses of approximately 300 mg may be intra-arterially infused for 20 minutes to 1 hour. On angiography notable changes in diameter are observed in 50% of patients, whereas clinical improvement is often less impressive (occurring in about one of four patients). The vasodilatory effect of papaverine is significantly reduced when vasospasm is present for several days and secondary histologic changes of the vessel have already occurred.[321,324]

Angioplasty and Stenting

When neurologic manifestations of delayed cerebral ischemia due to vasospasm cannot be reversed by medical therapy, balloon catheters may be used to dilate the narrowed arteries. Transluminal angioplasty has been shown to effectively reverse angiographic signs of vasospasm of proximal accessible vessels in 75% of cases refractory to conventional treatment with triple-H therapy.[325] The carotid artery, vertebral artery, proximal middle cerebral artery, and the entire basilar artery can be treated with transluminal angioplasty, whereas this technique does not seem safe to perform beyond the proximal portion of the anterior, middle, and posterior cerebral arteries.[326,327] Early results in patients with delayed ischemia who underwent angioplasty for vasospasm were very encouraging.[325–329] Delayed treatment as a salvage procedure seems to be less successful. Generally speaking, angioplasty is reserved for patients who have already undergone surgery or endovascular closure of the aneurysm. Obvious complications include rupture of an unclipped aneurysm, vessel rupture, arterial dissection, and vessel occlusion. Vessel stenting might be an option for the therapy of massive narrowing of the proximal portions of the three basal cerebral arteries.

Intracisternal Fibrinolysis

Intracisternal fibrinolysis aims to decrease the incidence of symptomatic vasospasm by injection of rt-PA in the basal cistern. Several studies showed that this therapy might decrease vasospasm but does not affect outcome after 3 months.[330–332] IVH occurs in up to 20% of patients with SAH. There is strong evidence that IVH contributes to mortality after cerebral hemorrhage or SAH.[333,334] Routine clinical management consists of an external ventricular drainage, which lowers the ICP immediately, but the drainage must be continued until the ventricular clot has dissolved and CSF circulation has normalized. Clotted blood often blocks the drain, necessitating its removal and insertion of a second catheter. Prolonged drainage, however, increases the risk of infection, with higher rates of ventriculitis after the first week of intraventricular catheter placement. The drainage itself prevents acute hydrocephalus but does not affect resolution of the clot or incidence of communicating hydrocephalus. Intraventricular thrombolysis was therefore proposed as an effective measure to hasten the resolution of the intraventricular blood clot, reduce the duration of extraventricular drainage, decrease the extent and incidence of communicating hydrocephalus, and thereby lower the death rate associated with IVH.

Clinical experience with this approach has grown over the last 10 years. However, a wide variety of dosages and substances (urokinase or rt-PA) have been used. To date, no randomized controlled trial results are available to show the beneficial effect of this therapy. To perform intraventricular thrombolysis in patients with a large amount of intraventricular blood after ICH, we use 4 mg rt-PA every 12 hours over 2 days. A multicenter trial is under way.[334] Before the initiation of thrombolysis, vascular malformations and aneurysms must be ruled out with either CTA or conventional angiography.

Extracranial Complications

A variety of extracranial complications arise as direct consequences of the SAH. They include abnormalities in cardiovascular, pulmonary, endocrine, and electrolyte homeostasis. Many of these abnormalities can be attributed to a post-SAH "hyperadrenergic state"—for example, myocardial infarction and cardiac dysrhythmia. Acute pulmonary edema can also result from massive sympathetic discharge. Other complications are gastrointestinal hemorrhage after stress ulcer after SAH.

Serum catecholamine levels rise dramatically after SAH; there seems to be a connection between the peak of vasospasm after SAH and symptom development corresponding to serum catecholamine levels.[335,336] Systemic hypertension can often be seen after SAH and is most likely related to elevations in catecholamine and renin levels secondary to the bleeding.[337] Other causes of hypertension are increased ICP, seizures, pain, agitation, and vasospasm. Severe arterial hypertension is associated with a higher rate of rebleeding, a higher incidence of vasospasm, and death.[338]

Cardiac arrhythmia and ECG changes are common problems in many patients after SAH. Arrhythmia can sometimes be severe and life-threatening, whereas ECG changes have a broad variety of patterns, some of which indicate myocardial ischemia. Morphologic changes of the ventricular wall consistent with myocardial ischemia have been observed after poor Hunt and Hess grade SAH. Neurogenic pulmonary edema is another rare complication of SAH.

Fluid and sodium imbalance represent a manifestation of hypothalamic dysfunction after SAH, which occurs in about one third of patients. Both hypovolemia and hyponatremia are common.[339,340] The clinical picture can be consistent with the syndrome of inappropriate antidiuretic hormone (SIADH) secretion.[341] In addition, the kidney may be unable to retain sodium,[342] an inability consistent with observed rises in atrial natriuretic factor, constituting the so-called "cerebral salt-wasting" syndrome.[343,344]

Fever is another common complication of SAH,[345] the etiology of which is unclear. Some reports indicate that fever is an indicator of developing vasospasm.[345] The presence of fever in patients with SAH may be even more deleterious, as fever is known to worsen the clinical course of cerebral ischemia.

Blood Pressure Management

SAH is accompanied by a hyperadrenergic state.[346] This is probably one contributing factor in the hypertension associated with SAH. A narrowed range of autoregulation of CBF after intracranial hemorrhage has been described. Such a narrower range makes perfusion of the brain dependent on arterial blood pressure. Therefore, it is advisable not to treat arterial hypertension after aneurysm rupture. Hypertension after SAH is regarded as a compensatory mechanism that should not be interfered with. This approach accords with the finding that the combined strategy of avoiding antihypertensive medication and increasing fluid intake lowers the risk of cerebral infarction.[273] Only extreme hypertensive blood pressure values (>200 mm Hg) should be treated with sympatholytic drugs such as beta blockers, clonidine, and ACE inhibitors. In addition, nimodipine or nicardipine may be advantageously used in this setting.

There is no consensus regarding the most appropriate vasopressor to use for therapy of hypotension. Theoretically, increasing cardiac output would improve CBF, supporting the use of dobutamine. However, the physiologic basis for this measure is not clear. An alternative approach is to use primarily vasoconstrictor drugs, such as phenylephrine and norepinephrine, in keeping with the idea that CBF in areas of vasospasm varies primarily as a function of perfusion pressure.

Management of Temperature

Fever occurs very commonly with SAH, particularly at about the time of worsening vasospasm or in patients with large amounts of intraventricular blood.[241] Body temperature in excess of 38.0° C should be aggressively treated with acetaminophen, paracetamol, or cooling blankets. When vasospasm is refractory to all therapy, hypothermia may be induced to about 33° C as a neuroprotective measure.[346] However, this approach has not yet undergone evaluation in this specific clinical setting.

Invasive Monitoring

Clear guidelines for instituting multimodal monitoring in patients with SAH have not yet been established. ICP monitoring may provide data for appropriate treatment of elevated ICP. However, ICP monitoring to evaluate CPP may not reflect the needs of the individual patient if it is the only method used. There is evidence that the continuous measurement of the partial oxygen pressure of brain tissue (pbrO$_2$) by microprobes within brain tissue of the frontal white matter may represent an important alternative in the monitoring of SAH patients, especially those who are at risk for vasospasm and delayed cerebral ischemia.[347,348] Several experimental studies have shown that the continuous measurement of the pbrO$_2$ in animals significantly reflects changes in blood oxygenation, ventilation, ICP, and CPP. Clinical experience with pbrO$_2$ monitoring has been gained mainly in patients with severe brain injury.[349]

New monitoring systems allow the insertion of several probes, such as those for ICP, temperature, and pbrO$_2$, either in the injured hemisphere or bilaterally within the white matter of the frontal lobe. A polarographic microprobe is used to register pbrO$_2$, and microprobes for continuous measurement of temperature. Data are processed in a computer to compensate for the temperature dependency of pbrO$_2$. Probes are inserted through one bolt and burr hole. The limitations of the cerebral oxygen probe are that although the measurements are accurate, they reflect only the tissue immediately surrounding the probe. Whether this technique is clinically useful to monitor for impending cerebral ischemia or vasospasm has yet to be established.

Endovascular Treatment of Aneurysms

Rapid technical advances in endovascular techniques over the past decade have opened new horizons for the treatment of intracranial aneurysms. Guglielmi and colleagues[350] introduced a coil design for embolization of aneurysms. Many observational studies have published data on complication rates, occlusion rate, and follow-up. Saccular aneurysms can be occluded angiographically by application of electrically detachable coils. Complications have occurred in 3.7% to 6.7% of patients, the most common being procedure-related ischemia.[351-353] The second important complication is perforation of the aneurysm, which occurs in 2% of all patients. Endovascular coiling was first applied in aneurysms for which surgical clipping is a high-risk procedure because of size or site, and patient's poor medical condition. Thus, most aneurysms treated with coils were located at the top of the basilar artery, internal carotid artery, and anterior communicating artery. Aneurysms at some sites are still the domain of surgical clipping, such as the MCA, especially at the MCA trifurcation, or the pericallosal arteries.

It remains to be established whether coiling will produce overall palliation in terms of prevention of SAH or limitation of mass effect. Reformation, expansion, and hemorrhage from coil-embolized aneurysms have been reported. Surgical treatment, however, is not definitive in some patients. The first study that compared endovascular coiling and surgical clipping for therapy of an aneurysm found no difference in outcome after 3 months.[354] However, endovascular treatment is a rapidly developing technology with data accumulating regarding efficacy, safety, and long-term results. This information will allow a better patient selection for the different therapeutic modalities (Figs. 52–6 through 52–8).

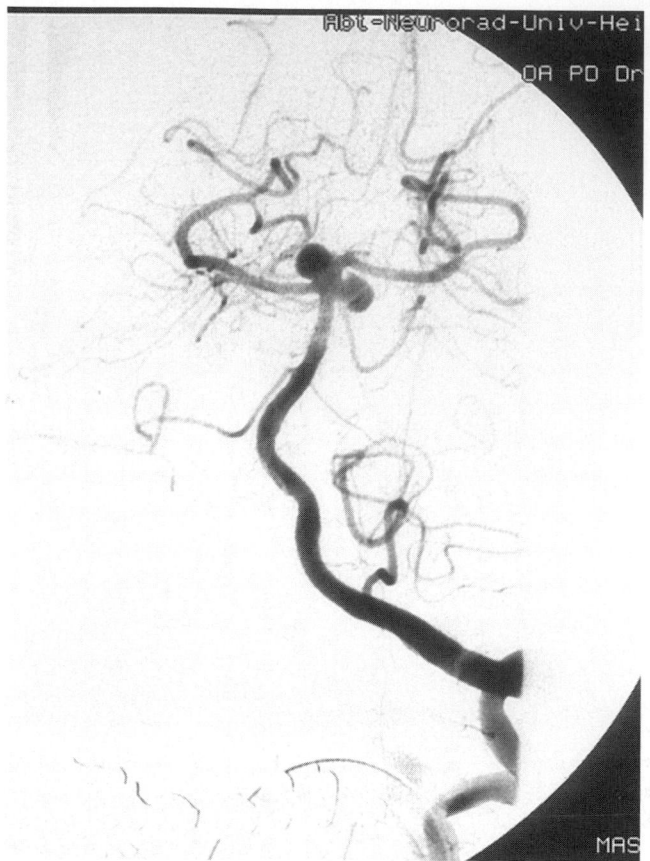

FIGURE 52–6 *Digital subtraction angiography (DSA) of a dumbbell-like aneurysm at the tip of the basilar artery.*

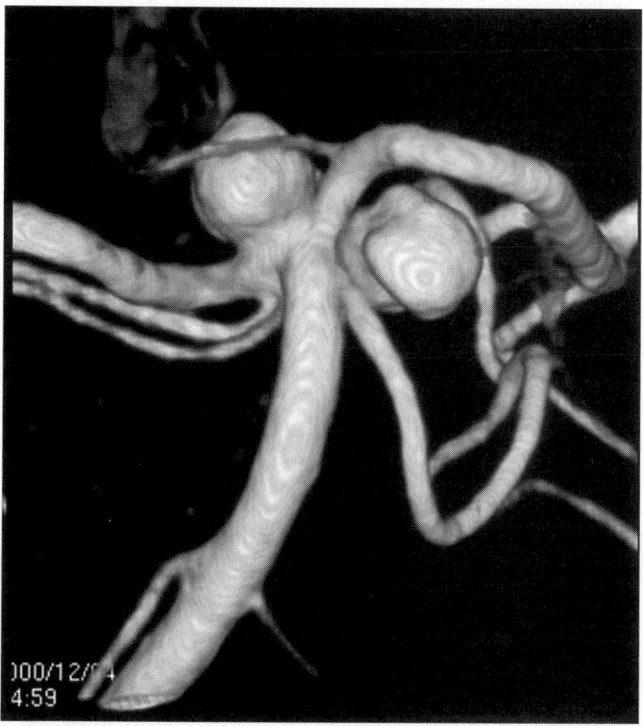

FIGURE 52–7 *Three-dimensional reconstruction of digital subtraction angiography (DSA) of a dumbbell-like aneurysm between the origin of the superior cerebellar arteries and posterior cerebral arteries.*

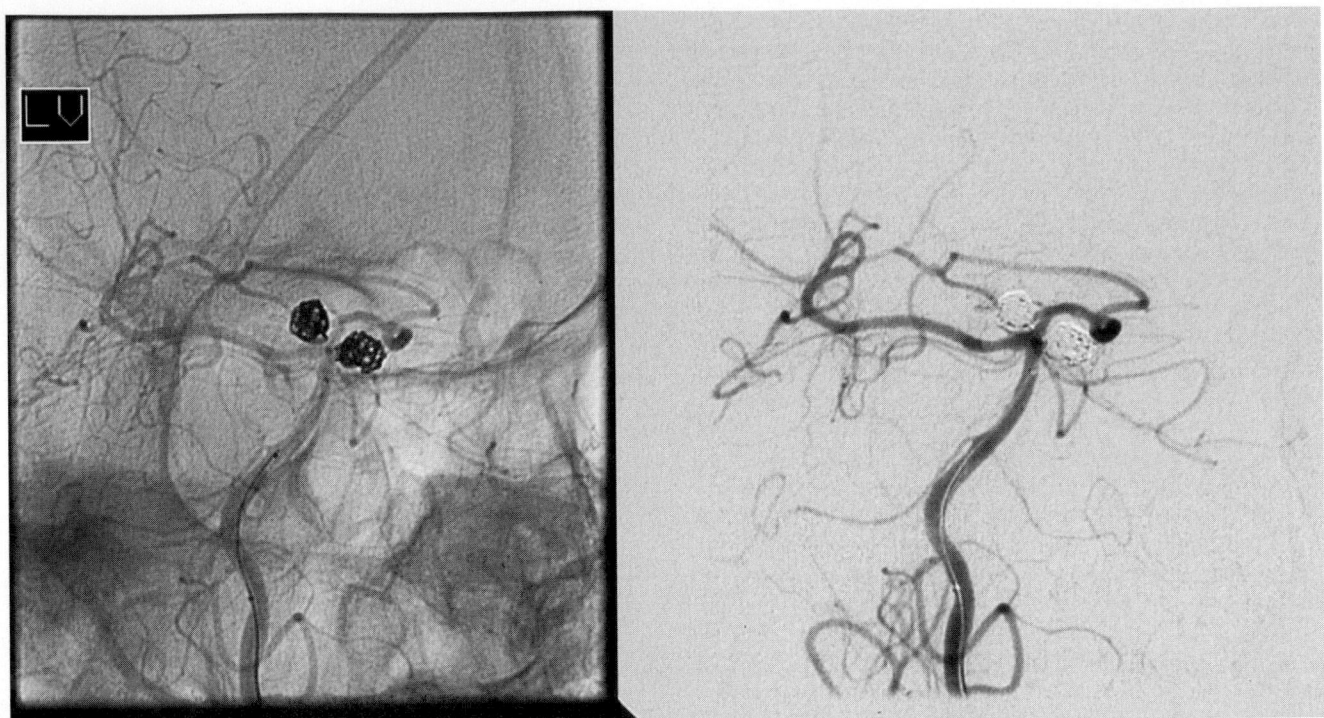

FIGURE 52–8   *Digital subtraction angiography after successful coiling of both compartments with guglielmi detachable coils (GDC). Unchanged compared with the preintervention angiography, complete perfusion of both superior cerebellar arteries and the left posterior cerebral artery (hypoplastic P1 segment on the right side).*

Surgical or Endovascular Treatment

Follow-up angiography has shown persistent occlusion in more than 90% of patients, and clinical results at up to 3 years were excellent.[355] Long-term follow-up studies must still be completed before this technique can be claimed as an alternative for surgical clipping of aneurysms. However, this approach may be particularly suitable for patients with a high associated medical comorbidity, high surgical risk, and a poor-grade SAH.

Intraparenchymatous bleeding with mass effect is an emergency indication for operative decompression to remove blood clots, stop the progression of bleeding, and reduce the risk of rebleeding by eliminating or clipping the vascular malformation. Early surgery to clip the aneurysm, once believed to be associated with a high perioperative complication rate, is now widely recommended for patients assigned Hunt and Hess grades I through IV. If an immediate intervention is not necessary, the patient is transferred to the ICU. The time for angiography depends on the intended operative treatment. For detailed information about surgical management of aneurysmal SAH, see Chapter 67.

Special Management Problems

Giant Aneurysms

There seems to be a correlation between size and incidence of complications during surgery for unruptured intracranial aneurysms. Aneurysms larger than 2.5 cm (giant aneurysm) in diameter have a 20% risk of significant surgical morbidity or poor outcome during surgical treatment. They constitute between 3% and 5% of all

aneurysms. Much of this morbidity can be attributed to giant basilar aneurysms, for which the rate of poor outcome was 50%. The recently introduced technique of deep hypothermic circulatory arrest may improve surgical results in patients with giant basilar aneurysms.

Different surgical strategies are a necessary component of therapy for giant aneurysms. Trapping and proximal ligation are usually the definitive treatment options, provided that the patient's collateral circulation can tolerate major vessel occlusion. Patients should undergo preoperative evaluation with temporary balloon occlusion to test their tolerance of trapping or proximal ligation. Major arterial branches leaving from the aneurysm dome can make proximal ligation the only therapeutic option. Different endovascular techniques may serve as adjuncts to surgical therapy and further improve treatment of giant aneurysms. In general, therapy of giant aneurysms should always arise from the combined therapeutic planning of neurosurgeons and neurointerventionists.

Mycotic Aneurysms

Mycotic aneurysms are generally found in the distal branches of the cerebral arteries and are usually caused by infectious endocarditis or aspergillosis. The most common organism causing mycotic aneurysms today is *Staphylococcus aureus*. Aneurysms caused by *Streptococcus*, *Salmonella*, *Klebsiella*, *Escherichia coli*, *Proteus*, and *Yersinia* have been reported as well. Pathogenic mechanisms include postoperative infection, septicemia, and, as already mentioned, endocarditis. Therapy consists of systemic application of antibiotics, which ensures aneurysm healing and disappearance over time. Surgery with wrapping of the aneurysm should be performed only if the aneurysm is observed to grow despite antibiotic therapy or in the case of recurrent hemorrhage.

Subarachnoid Hemorrhage in Vascular Malformations

Vascular malformations, including parenchymal arteriovenous malformations (AVMs), dural AVMs, venous angiomas, and cavernomas, can cause SAH. Parenchymal AVMs are often superficial and cause SAH, focal or generalized seizures, or both. Other symptoms are intracranial hemorrhage and a focal neurologic deficit referable to the mass effect. The incidence of intracranial aneurysms in AVMs is 10% to 20%. SAH is relatively rare in patients with AVMs. About 5% of all patients have subarachnoid blood after AVM rupture. SAH from AVM is much rarer than that from aneurysm and occurs in younger patients. The clinical presentation of SAH due to AVM differs little from that of aneurysmal SAH, except that the possibility of an associated intraparenchymal hemorrhage is much higher with an AVM. Surgery for AVMs is almost never performed in the acute stage, except in patients with life-threatening hematoma and severe mass effect. Diagnosis and preoperative evaluation of patients with SAH due to AVM consists of four-vessel selective angiography to visualize all possible feeding arteries and large draining veins.

Complete removal of the malformation is essential for rebleeding prophylaxis. However, some AVMs are too large or too deeply seated to be treated surgically. Probably the best management of such malformations consists of a combination of endovascular embolization and radiation therapy. For the first 2 years after irradiation, there is little difference in rate of recurrent hemorrhage between treated cases and the natural history of the disease. After this period of continued risk, irradiation causes obliteration of smaller lesions (<3.0 cm) by inducing histologic changes, considered radiation-induced necrosis of the vessel wall, thereby leading to a lower mortality.

Dural Arteriovenous Fistulas

Dural AVMs are arteriovenous shunts with dural arterial supply and venous drainage. Fistulas of the tentorium especially can cause a basal hemorrhage similar to SAH from aneurysm. Patients with direct cortical venous drainage, variceal venous dilatations, or both have a relatively higher risk for hemorrhage. Therapy consists of surgical resection or endovascular obliteration from either the arterial or the venous side.

Venous Angioma

Like cavernoma malformations, venous angiomas are benign in nature, causing SAH only in rare circumstances. For patients who have experienced a hemorrhage, surgery to remove the clot may be indicated.

Sinus Venous Thrombosis

Sinus venous thrombosis (SVT) is a rare disease; although not yet evaluated in epidemiologic studies, its incidence is approximately 0.5 cases per 100,000 people. On the other hand, SVT is the underlying cause for roughly 1% of strokes. The clinical presentation of SVT varies according to the localization of the thrombosis and the presence and extent of collateral pathways. The four most common clinical SVT syndromes are (1) focal motor or sensory deficits, headache, and epileptic seizures, (2) isolated intracranial hypertension with headache and papilledema, (3) sinus cavernosus syndrome with chemosis, ptosis, and painful ophthalmoplegia, and (4) subacute encephalopathy. Symptoms can occur simultaneously or in sequence.

Patients with SVT should always be admitted to the neurocritical care unit if they demonstrate (1) decreased level of consciousness, (2) increased ICP, (3) intracranial hemorrhage, and (4) focal or generalized epileptic seizures. Diagnostic evaluation consists of CCT, MRI, and MRA; the use of DSA is limited to selected cases.

Treatment

Anticoagulants

Intravenous anticoagulation is the first-line treatment for SVT. It must be noted that the efficacy of this treatment has been examined only in two studies. One of the studies, which reported a significant benefit of heparin,[356] was criticized because of the small number of recruited patients (n = 20) and several methodologic weaknesses. The other study, which used low-molecular-weight heparin (nadroparin), did not show any significant differences between the groups treated with nadroparin and placebo.[357] Analysis of the combined results of these studies, however, pointed to a "moderate, though clinically important benefit" for heparinization.[357] On the other hand, it appears quite clear that heparinization carries no significant risks for patients with SVT, even those with cerebral hemorrhage.

Several studies have described local use of thrombolytics in patients with SVT; an overview is presented in Table 52.12.[359–380] Although recanalization rate and speed appeared to be higher than for treatment with heparin alone, so did the incidence of hemorrhagic complications.

On the basis of the results of these studies, we suggest intravenous heparin as treatment of first choice in patients with SVT, even those with intracerebral hemorrhage or hemorrhagic transformation, followed by oral anticoagulation for 3 to 6 months. We aim for a partial prothrombin time (PTT) of 60 to 80 seconds. Local thrombolysis should be considered only in patients who demonstrate a clinical deterioration while on intravenous heparin therapy.

Anticonvulsants

Epileptic seizures are common in patients with SVT. Prophylactic antiepileptic treatment is used in some centers, under the assumption that occurrence of seizures could potentially cause or aggravate ischemic brain damage; other centers apply prophylactic treatment in specific cases, including women in the last trimester of pregnancy and puerperium and patients with abnormal EEG findings. No studies have examined this issue, and no recommendations can thus be provided. We do not apply antiepileptic treatment prophylactically but, rather, start it immediately after a seizure has occurred.

Intracranial Hypertension

Treatment of intracranial hypertension in patients with SVT remains an intriguing issue; various methods have

258. Matsumoto K, Hondo H: CT-guided stereotaxic evacuation of hypertensive intracerebral hematomas. J Neurosurg 61:440–448, 1984.

259. Niizuma H, Otzuki T, Juhkura H, et al: CT-guided stereotactic aspiration of intracerebral hematoma: Result of hematolysis method using urokinase. Appl Neurophysiol 48:427–430, 1985.

260. Schaller C, Rohde V, Meyer B, Hassler W: Stereotactic puncture and lysis of spontaneous intracerebral hemorrhage using recombinant tissue plasminogen activator. Neurosurgery 36:328–335, 1995.

261. Ott KH, Kase CS, Ojemann RG, Mohr JP: Cerebellar hemorrhage: Diagnosis and treatment: A review of 56 cases. Arch Neurol 31:160–167, 1974.

262. Kassell NF, Torner JC, Jane JA, et al: The International Cooperative Study on the Timing of Aneurysm Surgery. Part 2: Surgical results. J Neurosurg 73:37–47, 1990.

263. Hop JW, Rinkel GJ, Algra A, van Gijn J: Quality of life in patients and partners after aneurysmal subarachnoid hemorrhage. Stroke 29:798–804, 1998.

264. Kassell NF, Torner JC, Haley EC Jr, et al: The International Cooperative Study on the Timing of Aneurysm Surgery. Part 1: Overall management results. J Neurosurg 73:18–36, 1990.

265. Hutter BO, Kreitschmann-Andermahr I, Gilsbach JM: Cognitive deficits in the acute stage after subarachnoid hemorrhage. Neurosurgery 43:1054–1065, 1998.

266. Hart RG, Byer JA, Slaughter JR, et al: Occurrence and implications of seizures in subarachnoid hemorrhage due to ruptured intracranial aneurysms. Neurosurgery 8:417–421, 1981.

267. Bassi P, Bandera R, Loiero M, et al: Warning signs in subarachnoid hemorrhage: A cooperative study. Acta Neurol Scand 84:277–281, 1991.

268. Hunt WE, Hess RM: Surgical risk as related to time of intervention in the repair of intracranial aneurysms. J Neurosurg 28:14–20, 1968.

269. van der Wee N, Rinkel GJ, Hasan D, van Gijn J: Detection of subarachnoid haemorrhage on early CT: Is lumbar puncture still needed after a negative scan? J Neurol Neurosurg Psychiatry 58:357–359, 1995.

270. van Gijn J, van Dongen KJ: The time course of aneurysmal haemorrhage on computed tomograms. Neuroradiology 23:153–156, 1982.

271. Mitchell P, Wilkinson ID, Hoggard N, et al: Detection of subarachnoid haemorrhage with magnetic resonance imaging. J Neurol Neurosurg Psychiatry 70:205–211, 2001.

272. Noguchi K, Seto H, Kamisaki Y, et al: Comparison of fluid-attenuated inversion-recovery MR imaging with CT in a simulated model of acute subarachnoid hemorrhage. AJNR Am J Neuroradiol 21:923–927, 2000.

273. van Gijn J, Rinkel GJ: Subarachnoid haemorrhage: Diagnosis, causes and management. Brain 124:249–278, 2001.

274. Velthuis BK, Rinkel GJ, Ramos LM, et al: Perimesencephalic hemorrhage: Exclusion of vertebrobasilar aneurysms with CT angiography. Stroke 30:1103–1109, 1999.

275. Ruigrok YM, Rinkel GJ, Buskens E, et al: Perimesencephalic hemorrhage and CT angiography: A decision analysis. Stroke 31:2976–2983, 2000.

276. Kassell NF, Torner JC: Aneurysmal rebleeding: A preliminary report from the Cooperative Aneurysm Study. Neurosurgery 13:479–481, 1983.

277. Fujii Y, Takeuchi S, Sasaki O, et al: Ultra-early rebleeding in spontaneous subarachnoid hemorrhage. J Neurosurg 84:35–42, 1996.

278. Biller J, Godersky JC, Adams HP: Management of aneurysmal subarachnoid hemorrhage. Stroke 19:1300–1305, 1988.

279. Torner JC, Kassell NF, Wallace RB, Adams HP: Preoperative prognostic factors for rebleeding and survival in aneurysm patients receiving antifibrinolytic therapy: Report of the Cooperative Aneurysm Study. Neurosurgery 9:506–513, 1981.

280. Ojemann RG: Management of the unruptured intracranial aneurysm. N Engl J Med 304:725–726, 1981.

281. Vermeulen M, Lindsay KW, Murray GD, et al: Antifibrinolytic treatment in subarachnoid hemorrhage. N Engl J Med 311:432–437, 1984.

282. Kassell NF, Torner JC, Adams HP: Antifibrinolytic therapy in the acute period following aneurysmal subarachnoid hemorrhage: Preliminary observations from the Cooperative Aneurysm Study. J Neurosurg 61:225–230, 1984.

283. Roos Y: Antifibrinolytic treatment in subarachnoid hemorrhage: A randomized placebo-controlled trial. STAR Study Group. Neurology 54:77–82, 2000.

284. Glick R, Green D, Ts'ao C, et al: High dose epsilon-aminocaproic acid prolongs the bleeding time and increases rebleeding and intraoperative hemorrhage in patients with subarachnoid hemorrhage. Neurosurgery 9:398–401, 1981.

285. Solomon RA, Fink ME: Current strategies for the management of aneurysmal subarachnoid hemorrhage. Arch Neurol 44:769–774, 1987.

286. van Gijn J, Hijdra A, Wijdicks EF, et al: Acute hydrocephalus after aneurysmal subarachnoid hemorrhage. J Neurosurg 63:355–362, 1985.

287. Bailes JE, Spetzler RF, Hadley MN, Baldwin HZ: Management morbidity and mortality of poor-grade aneurysm patients. J Neurosurg 72:559–566, 1990.

288. Nieuwkamp DJ, de Gans K, Rinkel GJ, Algra A: Treatment and outcome of severe intraventricular extension in patients with subarachnoid or intracerebral hemorrhage: A systematic review of the literature. J Neurol 247:117–121, 2000.

289. Gruber A, Reinprecht A, Bavinzski G, et al: Chronic shunt-dependent hydrocephalus after early surgical and early endovascular treatment of ruptured intracranial aneurysms. Neurosurgery 44:503–509, 1999.

290. Kosteljanetz M: CSF dynamics in patients with subarachnoid and/or intraventricular hemorrhage. J Neurosurg 60:940–946, 1984.

291. Rebuck JA, Murry KR, Rhoney DH, et al: Infection related to intracranial pressure monitors in adults: Analysis of risk factors and antibiotic prophylaxis. J Neurol Neurosurg Psychiatry 69:381–384, 2000.

292. Paramore CG, Turner DA: Relative risks of ventriculostomy infection and morbidity. Acta Neurochir (Wien) 127:79–84, 1994.

293. Treggiari-Venzi MM, Suter PM, Romand JA: Review of medical prevention of vasospasm after aneurysmal subarachnoid hemorrhage: A problem of neurointensive care. Neurosurgery 48:249–261, 2001.

294. Shimoda M, Oda S, Tsugane R, Sato O: Prognostic factors in delayed ischaemic deficit with vasospasm in patients undergoing early aneurysm surgery. Br J Neurosurg 11:210–215, 1997.

295. Wilkins RH: Cerebral vasospasm. Crit Rev Neurobiol 6:51–77, 1990.

296. Heros RC, Zervas NT, Varsos V: Cerebral vasospasm after subarachnoid hemorrhage: An update. Ann Neurol 14:599–608, 1983.

297. Vora YY, Suarez-Almazor M, Steinke DE, et al: Role of transcranial Doppler monitoring in the diagnosis of cerebral vasospasm after subarachnoid hemorrhage. Neurosurgery 44:1237–1247, 1999.

298. Laumer R, Steinmeier R, Gonner F, et al: Cerebral hemodynamics in subarachnoid hemorrhage evaluated by transcranial Doppler sonography. Part 1: Reliability of flow velocities in clinical management. Neurosurgery 33:1–8, 1993.

299. Steinmeier R, Laumer R, Bondar I, et al: Cerebral hemodynamics in subarachnoid hemorrhage evaluated by transcranial Doppler sonography. Part 2: Pulsatility indices: Normal reference values and characteristics in subarachnoid hemorrhage. Neurosurgery 33:10–18, 1993.

300. Origitano TC, Wascher TM, Reichman OH, Anderson DE: Sustained increased cerebral blood flow with prophylactic hypertensive hypervolemic hemodilution ("triple-H" therapy) after subarachnoid hemorrhage. Neurosurgery 27:729–739, 1990.

301. Kassell NF, Peerless SJ, Durward QJ, et al: Treatment of ischemic deficits from vasospasm with intravascular volume expansion and induced arterial hypertension. Neurosurgery 11:337–343, 1982.

302. Germano A, d'Avella D, Imperatore C, et al: Time-course of blood-brain barrier permeability changes after experimental subarachnoid haemorrhage. Acta Neurochir (Wien) 142:575–580, 2000.

303. Wood JH, Kee DB: Hemorrheology of the cerebral circulation in stroke. Stroke 16:765–772, 1985.

304. Awad IA, Carter LP, Spetzler RF, et al: Clinical vasospasm after subarachnoid hemorrhage: Response to hypervolemic hemodilution and arterial hypertension. Stroke 18:365–372, 1987.

305. Wijdicks EFM: New management trends in aneurysmal subarachnoid hemorrhage. In Bogousslavsky J (ed): Acute Stroke Treatment. Martin Dunitz, 1997, pp 259–269.

306. Solomon RA, Fink ME, Lennihan L: Prophylactic volume expansion therapy for the prevention of delayed cerebral ischemia after early aneurysm surgery: Results of a preliminary trial. Arch Neurol 45:325–332, 1988.

307. Shimoda M, Oda S, Tsugane R, Sato O: Intracranial complications of hypervolemic therapy in patients with a delayed ischemic deficit attributed to vasospasm. J Neurosurg 78:423–429, 1993.

Therapy

308. Buckland MR, Batjer HH, Giesecke AH: Anesthesia for cerebral aneurysm surgery: Use of induced hypertension in patients with symptomatic vasospasm. Anesthesiology 69:116–119, 1988.

309. Hasan D, Wijdicks EF, Vermeulen M: Hyponatremia is associated with cerebral ischemia in patients with aneurysmal subarachnoid hemorrhage. Ann Neurol 27:106–108, 1990.

310. Siesjo BK: Cellular calcium metabolism, seizures, and ischemia. Mayo Clin Proc 61:299–302, 1986.

311. Hongo K, Kobayashi S: Calcium antagonists for the treatment of vasospasm following subarachnoid haemorrhage. Neurol Res 15:218–224, 1993.

312. Barker FG 2nd, Ogilvy CS: Efficacy of prophylactic nimodipine for delayed ischemic deficit after subarachnoid hemorrhage: A meta-analysis. J Neurosurg 84:405–414, 1996.

313. Feigin VL, Rinkel GJ, Algra A, et al: Calcium antagonists for aneurysmal subarachnoid haemorrhage. Cochrane Database Syst Rev CD000277, 2000.

314. Kassell NF, Haley EC Jr, Apperson-Hansen C, Alves WM: Randomized, double-blind, vehicle-controlled trial of tirilazad mesylate in patients with aneurysmal subarachnoid hemorrhage: A cooperative study in Europe, Australia, and New Zealand. J Neurosurg 84:221–228, 1996.

315. Haley EC Jr, Kassell NF, Apperson-Hansen C, et al: A randomized, double-blind, vehicle-controlled trial of tirilazad mesylate in patients with aneurysmal subarachnoid hemorrhage: A cooperative study in North America. J Neurosurg 86:467–474, 1997.

316. Lanzino G, Kassell NF, Dorsch NW, et al: Double-blind, randomized, vehicle-controlled study of high-dose tirilazad mesylate in women with aneurysmal subarachnoid hemorrhage. Part I: A cooperative study in Europe, Australia, New Zealand, and South Africa. J Neurosurg 90:1011–1017, 1999.

317. Hop JW, Rinkel GJ, Algra A, et al: Randomized pilot trial of postoperative aspirin in subarachnoid hemorrhage. Neurology 54:872–888, 2000.

318. Elliott JP, Newell DW, Lam DJ, et al: Comparison of balloon angioplasty and papaverine infusion for the treatment of vasospasm following aneurysmal subarachnoid hemorrhage. J Neurosurg 88:277–284, 1998.

319. Clouston JE, Numaguchi Y, Zoarski GH, et al: Intraarterial papaverine infusion for cerebral vasospasm after subarachnoid hemorrhage. AJNR Am J Neuroradiol 16:27–38, 1995.

320. Tsurushima H, Hyodo A, Yoshii Y: Papaverine and vasospasm. J Neurosurg 92:509–511, 2000.

321. Kaku Y, Yonekawa Y, Tsukahara T, Kazekawa K: Superselective intra-arterial infusion of papaverine for the treatment of cerebral vasospasm after subarachnoid hemorrhage. J Neurosurg 77:842–847, 1992.

322. Barr JD, Mathis JM, Horton JA. Transient severe brain stem depression during intraarterial papaverine infusion for cerebral vasospasm. AJNR Am J Neuroradiol 15:719–723, 1994.

323. Carhuapoma JR, Qureshi AI, Tamargo RJ, et al: Intra-arterial papaverine-induced seizures: Case report and review of the literature. Surg Neurol 56:159–163, 2001.

324. Kassell NF, Helm G, Simmons N, et al: Treatment of cerebral vasospasm with intra-arterial papaverine. J Neurosurg 77:848–852, 1992.

325. Newell DW, Eskridge J, Mayberg M, et al: Endovascular treatment of intracranial aneurysms and cerebral vasospasm. Clin Neurosurg 39:348–360, 1992.

326. Higashida RT, Halbach VV, Cahan LD, et al: Transluminal angioplasty for treatment of intracranial arterial vasospasm. J Neurosurg 71(Pt 1):648–653, 1989.

327. Eskridge JM, McAuliffe W, Song JK, et al: Balloon angioplasty for the treatment of vasospasm: Results of first 50 cases. Neurosurgery 42:510–516, 1998.

328. Bejjani GK, Bank WO, Olan WJ, Sekhar LN: The efficacy and safety of angioplasty for cerebral vasospasm after subarachnoid hemorrhage. Neurosurgery 42:979–986, 1998.

329. Polin RS, Coenen VA, Hansen CA, et al: Efficacy of transluminal angioplasty for the management of symptomatic cerebral vasospasm following aneurysmal subarachnoid hemorrhage. J Neurosurg 92:284–290, 2000.

330. Findlay JM, Weir BK, Kassell NF, et al: Intracisternal recombinant tissue plasminogen activator after aneurysmal subarachnoid hemorrhage. J Neurosurg 75:181–188, 1991.

331. Rohde V, Schaller C, Hassler WE: Intraventricular recombinant tissue plasminogen activator for lysis of intraventricular haemorrhage. J Neurol Neurosurg Psychiatry 58:447–451, 1995.

332. Nieuwkamp DJ, de Gans K, Rinkel GJ, Algra A: Treatment and outcome of severe intraventricular extension in patients with subarachnoid or intracerebral hemorrhage: A systematic review of the literature. J Neurol 247:117–121, 2000.

333. Mayfrank L, Hutter BO, Kohorst Y, et al: Influence of intraventricular hemorrhage on outcome after rupture of intracranial aneurysm. Neurosurg Rev 24:185–191, 2001.

334. Naff NJ, Carhuapoma JR, Williams MA, et al: Treatment of intraventricular hemorrhage with urokinase effects on 30-day survival. Stroke 31:841–847, 2000.

335. Minegishi A, Ishizaki T, Yoshida Y, et al: Plasma monoaminergic metabolites and catecholamines in subarachnoid hemorrhage: Clinical implications. Arch Neurol 44:423–428, 1987.

336. Staub F, Graf R, Gabel P, et al: Multiple interstitial substances measured by microdialysis in patients with subarachnoid hemorrhage. Neurosurgery 47:1106–1115, 2000.

337. Wijdicks EF, Vermeulen M, van Gijn J: Hyponatraemia and volume status in aneurysmal subarachnoid haemorrhage. Acta Neurochir Suppl (Wien) 47:111–113, 1990.

338. Disney L, Weir B, Grace M, Roberts P: Trends in blood pressure, osmolality and electrolytes after subarachnoid hemorrhage from aneurysms. Can J Neurol Sci 16:299–304, 1989.

339. Kurokawa Y, Uede T, Ishiguro M, et al: Pathogenesis of hyponatremia following subarachnoid hemorrhage due to ruptured cerebral aneurysm. Surg Neurol 46:500–507, 1996.

340. Diringer M, Ladenson PW, Stern BJ, et al: Plasma atrial natriuretic factor and subarachnoid hemorrhage. Stroke 19:1119–1124, 1988.

341. Nelson PB, Seif SM, Maroon JC, Robinson AG: Hyponatremia in intracranial disease: Perhaps not the syndrome of inappropriate secretion of antidiuretic hormone (SIADH). J Neurosurg 55:938–941, 1981.

342. Harrigan MR: Cerebral salt wasting syndrome: A review. Neurosurgery 38:152–160, 1996.

343. Oliveira-Filho J, Ezzeddine MA, Segal AZ, et al: Fever in subarachnoid hemorrhage: Relationship to vasospasm and outcome. Neurology 22;56:1299–1304, 2001.

344. Neil-Dwyer G, Walter P, Shaw HJ, et al: Plasma renin activity in patients after a subarachnoid hemorrhage—a possible predictor of outcome. Neurosurgery 7:578–582, 1980.

345. Hindman BJ, Todd MM, Gelb AW, et al: Mild hypothermia as a protective therapy during intracranial aneurysm surgery: A randomized prospective pilot trial. Neurosurgery 44:23–32, 1999.

346. Khaldi A, Zauner A, Reinert M, et al: Measurement of nitric oxide and brain tissue oxygen tension in patients after severe subarachnoid hemorrhage. Neurosurgery 49:33–38, 2001.

347. Charbel FT, Du X, Hoffman WE, Ausman JI: Brain tissue PO_2, PCO_2, and pH during cerebral vasospasm. Surg Neurol 54:432–437, 2000.

348. Kiening KL, Unterberg AW, Bardt TF, et al: Monitoring of cerebral oxygenation in patients with severe head injuries: Brain tissue PO_2 versus jugular vein oxygen saturation. J Neurosurg 85:751–757, 1996.

349. Guglielmi G, Vinuela F, Duckwiler G, et al: Endovascular treatment of posterior circulation aneurysms by electrothrombosis using electrically detachable coils. J Neurosurg 77:515–524, 1992.

350. Johnston SC, Wilson CB, Halbach VV, et al: Endovascular and surgical treatment of unruptured cerebral aneurysms: Comparison of risks. Ann Neurol 48:11–19, 2000.

351. Qureshi AI, Suri MF, Khan J, et al: Endovascular treatment of intracranial aneurysms by using Guglielmi detachable coils in awake patients: Safety and feasibility. J Neurosurg 94:880–885, 2001.

352. Cognard C, Weill A, Spelle L, et al: Long-term angiographic follow-up of 169 intracranial berry aneurysms occluded with detachable coils. Radiology 212:348–356, 1999.

353. Vanninen R, Koivisto T, Saari T, et al: Ruptured intracranial aneurysms: Acute endovascular treatment with electrolytically detachable coils—a prospective randomized study. Radiology 211:325–336, 1999.

354. Casasco AE, Aymard A, Gobin YP, et al: Selective endovascular treatment of 71 intracranial aneurysms with platinum coils. J Neurosurg 79:3–10, 1993.

355. Brilstra EH, Rinkel GJ, van der Graaf Y, et al: Treatment of intracranial aneurysms by embolization with coils: A systematic review. Stroke 30:470–476, 1999.

356. Einhäupl KM, Villringer A, Meister W, et al: Heparin treatment in sinus venous thrombosis. Lancet 338:597–600, 1991.

357. De Bruijn SFTM, Stam J: Randomized, placebo-controlled trial of anticoagulant treatment with low-molecular-weight heparin for cerebral sinus thrombosis. Stroke 30:484–488, 1999.

359. Scott JA, Pascuzzi RM, Hall PV, Becker GJ: Treatment of dural sinus thrombosis with local urokinase infusion: Case report. J Neurosurg 68:284–287, 1988.

360. Barnwell SL, Higashida RT, Halbach VV, et al: Direct endovascular thrombolytic therapy for dural sinus thrombosis. Neurosurgery 28:135–142, 1991.

361. Manthous CA, Chen H: Case report: Treatment of superior sagittal sinus thrombosis with urokinase. Conn Med 56:529–530, 1992.

362. Tsai FY, Higashida RT, Matovich V, Alfieri K: Acute thrombosis of the intracranial dural sinus: Direct thrombolytic treatment. AJNR Am J Neuroradiol 13:1137–1141, 1992.

363. Smith TP, Higashida RT, Barnwell SL, et al: Treatment of dural sinus thrombosis by urokinase infusion. AJNR Am J Neuroradiol 15:801–807, 1994.

364. Griesemer DA, Theodorou AA, Berg RA, Spera TD: Local fibrinolysis in cerebral venous thrombosis. Pediatr Neurol 10:78–80, 1994.

365. Horowitz M, Purdy P, Unwin H, et al: Treatment of dural sinus thrombosis using selective catheterization and urokinase. Ann Neurol 38:58–67, 1995.

366. Gurley MB, King TS, Tsai FY: Sigmoid sinus thrombosis associated with internal jugular venous occlusion: Direct thrombolytic treatment. J Endovasc Surg 3:306–314, 1996.

367. Spearman MP, Jungreis CA, Wehner JJ, et al: Endovascular thrombolysis in deep cerebral venous thrombosis. Am J Neuroradiol 18:502–506, 1997.

368. Gerszten PC, Welch WC, Spearman MP, et al: Isolated deep cerebral venous thrombosis treated by direct endovascular thrombolysis. Surg Neurol 48:261–266, 1997.

369. Smith AG, Cornblath WT, Deveikis JP: Local thrombolytic therapy in deep cerebral venous thrombosis. Neurology 48:1613–1619, 1997.

370. Holder CA, Bell DA, Lundell AL, et al: Isolated straight sinus and deep cerebral venous thrombosis: Successful treatment with local infusion of urokinase. Case report. J Neurosurg 86:704–707, 1997.

371. Rael JR, Orrison WW Jr, Baldwin N, Sell J: Direct thrombolysis of superior sagittal sinus thrombosis with coexisting intracranial hemorrhage. Am J Neuroradiol 18:1238–1242, 1997.

372. D'Alise MD, Fichtel F, Horrowitz M: Sagittal sinus thrombosis following minor head injury treated with continuous urokinase infusion. Surg Neurol 49:430–435, 1998.

373. Kuether TA, O'Neill O, Nesbit GM, Barnwell SL: Endovascular treatment of dural sinus thrombosis: Case report. Neurosurgery 42:1163–1166, 1998.

374. Kasner S, Gurian J, Grotta J: Urokinase treatment of sagittal sinus thrombosis with venous hemorrhagic infarction. J Stroke Cerebrovasc Dis 7:421–425, 1998.

375. Philips MF, Bagley LJ, Sinson GP, et al: Endovascular thrombolysis for symptomatic cerebral venous thrombosis. J Neurosurg 90:65–71, 1999.

376. Dowd CF, Malek AM, Phatouros CC, Hemphill JC 3rd: Application of a rheolytic thrombectomy device in the treatment of dural sinus thrombosis: A new technique. Am J Neuroradiol 20:568–570, 1999.

377. Gomez CR, Misra VK, Terry JB, et al: Emergency endovascular treatment of cerebral sinus thrombosis with a rheolytic catheter device. J Neuroimaging 10:177–180, 2000.

378. Novak Z, Coldwell DM, Brega KE: Selective infusion of urokinase and thrombectomy in the treatment of acute cerebral sinus thrombosis. Am J Neuroradiol 21:143–145, 2000.

379. Kim S, Suh J: Direct endovascular thrombolytic therapy for dural sinus thrombosis: Infusion of alteplase. Am J Neuroradiol 18:639–645, 1997.

380. Frey JL, Muro GJ, McDougall CG, et al: Cerebral sinus thrombosis: Combined intrathrombus rtPA and intravenous heparin. Stroke 30:489–494, 1999.

Chapter Fifty-Three

Pharmacologic Modification of Acute Cerebral Ischemia

Lise A. Labiche and James C. Grotta

BACKGROUND: PRECLINICAL AND CLINICAL CYTOPROTECTION

The Definition and Role of Cytoprotection

Pharmacologic therapy of acute ischemic stroke promises the opportunity to reduce brain injury and hence disability in a large proportion of patients with stroke. Treatments are needed that can be proven effective for important clinical outcomes in well-designed clinical trials. Optimally, these treatments should be low in morbidity, cost, and complexity so that they can be quickly and widely used in emergency settings of variable sophistication, as are common in the care of most patients with stroke worldwide.

Pharmacologic therapy of ischemic stroke can be split into broad groups on the basis of the sequence and location of physiologic events thought to occur upon occlusion of a cerebral artery, although as in most complex biologic systems, these events overlap both temporally and spatially. The first group of therapies targets the initial events occurring within the artery lumen, by reversing the arterial occlusion and restoring perfusion to damaged brain tissue. The prototypes of such therapy are thrombolytics, fibrinolytics, and anticoagulants. Reversing arterial occlusion has been the area of greatest clinical success to date in stroke treatment. Other therapies targeting later events will probably have much less impact on outcome than fast removal of the offending arterial occlusion, and it is even possible that further improvement in treatment cannot be achieved unless it is also accompanied by reperfusion of the damaged tissue. Much can be learned from the preclinical and clinical development of these "reperfusion" drugs, and the lessons will be brought into this chapter. However, such therapy is discussed in detail in Chapters 24, 25, and 26 and so is not specifically addressed further here.

The second broad category of pharmacotherapy for stroke targets the consequences of arterial occlusion on the blood vessel wall, neuron, glia, and neuronal environment. Although often labeled "neuroprotection," this approach to therapy actually has a wide variety of targets, many of which are non-neuronal, so a more appropriate term would be *cytoprotection*. Common to this approach is the effort to improve outcome by preventing progression to cellular death of tissue initially damaged by the ischemic event. Although unlikely to salvage irreversibly damaged cells, such therapies may "modify" the biologic perturbations induced at the cellular level in brain tissue whose fate still hangs in the balance. This type of pharmacotherapy is the subject of the present chapter.

A final category of stroke pharmacotherapy aims to augment recovery of brain function by targeting events during the restorative phase occurring after tissue damage is complete. This therapy is the subject of Chapter 32.

The concept of cytoprotection relies on the principle that delayed cellular injury occurs after ischemia. Neurons suffer irreversible damage after only a few minutes of complete cessation of blood flow. Such a condition might exist during cardiac arrest. In most instances of acute focal brain ischemia, however, if a state of zero blood flow occurs, it would only be in the core of the ischemic region. The larger surrounding penumbral area receives reduced blood flow, which causes loss of normal function that may lead to permanent cellular damage if uncorrected but allows for recovery if blood flow is restored by either clot lysis or collateral flow.

Because ischemia is clearly a process and not an instantaneous event, there is potential for modifying the process after the clinical ictus and altering the final outcome. It is equally apparent from experimental models that if cytoprotective treatments are to succeed, they must be instituted within a few minutes after the onset of ischemia. Previous clinical trials may have failed because such treatment was delayed and therefore unlikely to render a benefit.

The concept of cytoprotection is not new in the clinical domain. It has been known for years that hypothermia reduces ischemic neuronal injury. Accidental hypothermia can protect a drowning victim from otherwise fatal hypoxic-ischemic brain damage. Animal models of both global and focal ischemia confirm the beneficial effects of hypothermia. The benefit of hypothermia in treating global cerebral ischemic injury after cardiac arrest has also been dramatically demonstrated in humans. The importance of this result cannot be overemphasized because it is the first

Table 53.1 Past and Current Cytoprotective Clinical Trials

Drug	Phase	Latest Extent of Time Window (hr)	Adequate Power°	Adequate Dose	Dose-Limiting Adverse Effects	Homogeneous Patient Population	Linked to t-PA	Biologic Imaging Marker	Results
Calcium antagonists									
Nimodipine	3	6–48	+	?	Hypotension				Neutral
Nicardipine	2	12		?	Hypotension				Neutral
Glutamate antagonists									
Selfotel	3	6–12	+	No	Neuropsychological				Negative
Dextrorphan	2	48		Yes	Neuropsychological				Neutral
Aptiganel (Cerestat)	3	6–24	+	Yes	Hypertension				Negative
AR-R15696AR	2	12		Yes	Neuropsychological				Neutral
Magnesium	3†	2–12	+	Yes	No	+		+	?
AMPA antagonists									
YM872	2b	3–6	+	?	?	+	+	+	Neutral
ZK200775	2	24		?	Sedation			+	Negative
Indirect glutamate modulators									
Eliprodil	3	?	?	?	?	?	?	?	Negative
Gavestinel	3	6	+†	Yes	No	+			Neutral
Sipatrigine	2	12		?	Neuropsychological	+			Negative
Fosphenytoin	2/3	4	+	?	No				Neutral
BMS-204352	3	6	+	?	No	+		+	Neutral
Lifarizine	2	?		?	Hypotension				Neutral
Lubeluzole	3	4–8	+†	No	Cardiac	+	+		Neutral
Other neurotransmitter modulators									
Trazodone	2	?	?	?	?	?	?	?	Neutral
Repinotan	3†	6	+†	Yes	?	+			?
ONO-2506	2/3†	6	+	?	?	+			?
Opioid antagonists									
Naloxone	2	8–60		?	No				Neutral
Nalmefene	3	6	+†	?	No	+			Neutral
GABA agonists									
Clomethiazole	3	12	+†	Yes	Sedation	+			Neutral
Diazepam	3†	12	+	?	?				?
Free radical scavengers									
Tirilazad	3	6	+	?	No			+	Negative
Ebselen	3†	48	Yes	?	?	+			?
NXY-059	2b/3†	6	+†	?	?	+			?
Anti-inflammatory agents									
Enlimomab	3	6	+	Yes	Fever	+			Negative
LeukArrest	3	12	?	?	?				Neutral
FK-506	2†	12		?	?	+			?
Steroids	2	48		?	Infection				Negative
Membrane stabilizers, trophic factor									
GM$_1$	3	72	+	?	No				Neutral
Cerebrolysin	2	12–24		?	No				Positive trend
Citicoline	3	24	+†	?	No	+		+	Positive Post hoc
EPO	2a†								
bFGF	2/3	6	+	?	Hypotension	+			Negative
Hypothermia	2†	5–24		Yes	Pneumonia, arrhythmias, hypotension	+		+	?
Caffeinol	2†	4–6		Yes	No	+			?
Oxygen									
DCLHb	2	18		?	Hypertensive nephropathy				Negative
HBO	2/3†	24		?	?				Neutral

°Relevant only to phase 2b or 3 efficacy trial.
†Currently enrolling.
‡Not adequately powered for subgroup.
AMPA, α-amino-3-hydroxy-5-methyl-4-isoxazole proprionic acid; bFGF, basic fibroblast growth factor; DCLHb, diaspirin-cross-linked hemoglobin; EPO, erythropoietin; GABA, γ-aminobutyric acid; GM$_1$, genetic marker (monosialoganglioside); HBO, hyperbaric oxygen.

of nimodipine (30 mg PO every 6 hours) in the subgroup of patients who were treated earliest (within 12 hours).[63,67] Nimodipine appeared to prevent the early deterioration that occurred in many untreated patients with stroke. Theoretically, if "stroke progression" represents conversion of ischemic penumbra into infarction, it is logical to hypothesize that nimodipine protects the penumbra by maintaining calcium homeostasis. However, the latest and most extensive meta-analysis of 22 calcium antagonist trials, studying more than 6800 patients, did not demonstrate any beneficial effect of treatment, even in subgroups receiving early treatment (within 12 hours of stroke onset) (Fig. 53–1).[51] In addition, meta-analysis limited to the "good-quality" trials showed a statistically significant negative effect of calcium antagonists. A similar analysis of "poor-" and "moderate-quality" trials found that calcium antagonists exerted no effect on outcome. In fact, the results of this meta-analysis prompted the premature termination of the Very Early Nimodipine Use in Stroke (VENUS) trial, which was designed to determine the efficacy of nimodipine administered within 6 hours of stroke onset.[68] The interim analysis of 454 patients showed no effect of nimodipine; within the ischemic stroke subgroup, however, an increase in poor outcome at 3 months was found in the nimodipine-treated patients (relative risk [RR], 1.4; 95% confidence interval [CI], 1.0 to 2.1) (Table 53.2).

Another dihydropyridine calcium channel antagonist, *nicardipine*, has been tested in randomized placebo-controlled trials in aneurysmal subarachnoid hemorrhage.[69] IV nicardipine, given as an infusion of 0.15 mg/kg/hr for up to 14 days after hemorrhage, was shown to decrease the incidence of symptomatic and angiographic vasospasm. Nicardipine has also been tested in a pilot stroke study.[70] Hypotension was a common and dose-related side effect that could potentially negate the overall benefit of treatment.

In summary, given the weight of the evidence, calcium antagonists cannot be considered generally effective in improving the outcome of ischemic stroke and may even cause a worsened outcome. The lack of effect, or the presence of detrimental effect, may be due to the hypotension caused by blocking of the vascular smooth muscle cells. Blockade of L-type calcium channels in the setting of maximal vasodilation and impaired autoregulation within the ischemic region may cause a relative hypotension and a steal phenomenon with shunting of blood flow to nonischemic regions, thereby further decreasing perfusion to the penumbra.[71] Another plausible explanation for the failure of calcium antagonists is that neurotransmitter release is a proximal event in the excitotoxic cascade with immediate effects; therefore, any delay in administration of the drug precludes its theoretical efficacy in preventing cell necrosis. Delayed or prolonged use of L-type calcium antagonists may actually induce apoptotic cell death, because modest increases in calcium inhibit apoptosis.[72] This mechanism may overcome other protective actions of these agents. Ultra-early antagonism of other receptor subtypes, such as the N-type, may be more beneficial in penumbral preservation through inhibition of neurotransmitter release without undesired hypotension. Such agents have demonstrated cytoprotection in animal models, but they have not been extensively studied in humans owing to poor blood-brain barrier permeability of these

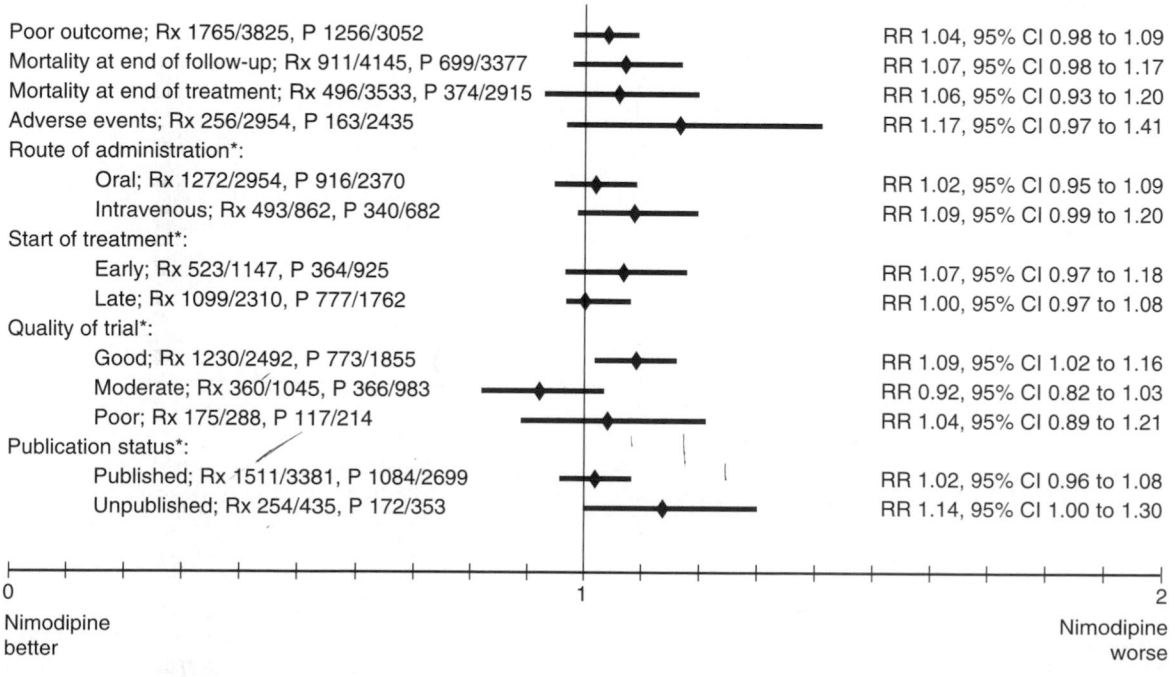

FIGURE 53–1 *Results from meta-analyses comparing nimodipine to placebo in acute ischemic stroke. 0, nimodipine better; 2, nimodipine worse; CI, confidence intervals; P, placebo group; RR, relative risk; Rx, treatment group; *, assessment of analyses indicated poor outcome. (Adapted from Horn J, Limburg M: Calcium antagonists for ischemic stroke: a systematic review. Stroke 32:570, 2001.)*

Table 53.2   Results from Very Early Nimodipine Use in Stroke (VENUS) Study Subgroup Analyses of Patients with Poor Outcome in Each Group*

	Nimodipine	Placebo	Relative Risk	95% Confidence Interval
Ischemic stroke	n = 133	n = 128		
Poor outcome at 3 mo	44 (34)	30 (24)	1.4	1.0–2.1
Hemorrhagic stroke	n = 20	n = 15		
Poor outcome at 3 mo	11 (58)	9 (60)	1.0	0.6–1.7
No computed tomography scan	n = 71	n = 79		
Poor outcome at 3 mo	16 (23)	21 (27)	0.8	0.5–1.5
Per protocol[†]	n = 179	n = 168		
Poor outcome at 3 mo	56 (31)	47 (28)	1.1	0.8–1.6

*Values given are number (%) of patients unless indicated otherwise.

[†]107 patients were excluded from this analysis because of the following exclusion criteria: 8, other diagnosis; 74, hemiparesis not severe enough; 8, age > 85 years; 10, swallowing disturbance; and 7, other exclusion criteria.

From Horn J, de Haan RJ, Vernenlen M, Linburg M: Very Early Nimodipine Use in Stroke (VENUS): A randomized, double-blind, placebo-controlled trial. Stroke 32: 461, 2001.

peptides.[73] We discuss methods to improve drug delivery at the end of the chapter.

Glutamate Antagonists

N-methyl-D-aspartate (NMDA) receptor antagonists were the first class of therapeutic agents for acute stroke to proceed from development in the laboratory to testing in humans that employed modern principles of clinical trial design, the most important being relatively early treatment. The potential utility of NMDA antagonists in stroke was first recognized when it was observed that a hypoxic or ischemic insult results in elevation of brain levels of the excitatory neurotransmitter glutamate. The excitotoxic theory of ischemic brain injury implicates glutamate as a pivotal mediator of cell death via ligand-gated receptors (NMDA and AMPA receptors), as reviewed previously. The NMDA receptor is a complex ligand-gated ion channel that requires activation by glutamate and glycine as well as concomitant membrane depolarization to overcome a voltage-dependent block by magnesium ions.

The complex structure of the NMDA receptor provides multiple sites for therapeutic inhibition. Competitive NMDA antagonists bind directly to the glutamate site of the NMDA receptor to inhibit the action of glutamate. Noncompetitive antagonists block the NMDA-associated ion channel in a use-dependent manner. Other sites on the NMDA receptor susceptible to antagonism are the glycine site and the polyamine site. Prototypes of these competitive and noncompetitive NMDA antagonists have been studied in phase 3 clinical trials for the treatment of stroke.

CGS19755 (*selfotel*) is a competitive NMDA receptor antagonist that limits neuronal damage in animal stroke models.[74-76] Selfotel was evaluated in a randomized, double-blind, placebo-controlled, ascending-dose, phase 2a study to determine its safety and tolerability and obtain pharmacokinetic and preliminary efficacy data.[77] Patients were treated within 12 hours of onset of ischemic hemispheric stroke. Adverse non-central nervous system (CNS) effects were uncommon and were not different in the selfotel and placebo groups. Adverse neuropsychiatric experiences were common, were dose-related, and lasted an

average of 24 hours; symptoms included hallucinations, agitation, confusion, dysarthria, ataxia, delirium, paranoia, and somnolence. There were no permanent sequelae. Two doses of 1 mg/kg were well tolerated. However, when the dose was increased to 2 mg/kg given either twice or even once, adverse experiences occurred in all patients. When the dose was decreased to 1.5 mg/kg, mild adverse experiences were noted in some patients but were easily managed with reassurance and low doses of lorazepam. For this reason, 1.5 mg/kg was deemed to be the maximal tolerated dose. There was no difference in mortality between the selfotel and placebo groups. The percent changes in both the NIHSS score and the BI score showed a trend toward greater improvement in treated patients. The improvement was comparable at all doses of selfotel.

On the basis of these data, phase 3 parallel studies of a single dose of 1.5 mg/kg of selfotel given within 6 hours of the onset of acute hemispheric stroke were begun in the United States and Europe; the studies were suspended after 31% of planned enrollment had been accomplished, however, because of an unfavorable efficacy-to-toxicity ratio.[78] Intention-to-treat analyses demonstrated that adverse events were more common and more often neurologic in the selfotel group (Table 53.3). In addition, the proportion of patients with neurologic progression or decreased arousal was higher in the selfotel group, as were both 8- and 30-day mortality rates. There was no difference between selfotel and placebo in the primary endpoint of functional independence even when stroke subtype subgroup analysis was performed (Table 53.4). Although there was no statistical difference in mortality during the entire study, post hoc analysis revealed a statistically significant increase in 8- and 30-day mortality rates in the selfotel group (Table 53.5). The computed probability of demonstrating efficacy if the trials were completed was very small, ranging from less than 1% to 32%.

We may conclude from these trials that selfotel is not efficacious as a cytoprotectant and may potentially exert a neurotoxic effect in patients with severe stroke. The selfotel trials exhibit an important principle of cytoprotectant failure—the narrow therapeutic index. Animal models determined that a plasma selfotel level of 40 μg/mL was

Table 53.3 Summary of the Most Frequently Occurring Adverse Experiences by Treatment Group*

Adverse Experience	Treatment Group		$P^†$
	Selfotel	**Placebo**	
Agitation	101 (36)	39 (1)	.001
Hallucination	59 (21)	13 (5)	.001
Fever	52 (19)	53 (19)	—
Hypertension	47 (17)	28 (10)	.015
Confusion	46 (16)	16 (6)	.001
Constipation	37 (13)	55 (19)	.052
Headache	35 (13)	55 (19)	—
Somnolence	30 (11)	29 (10)	—
Cerebrovascular disorder	29 (10)	13 (5)	.009
Urinary tract infection	29 (10)	36 (13)	—
Vomiting	19 (7)	30 (11)	—
Coma	15 (5.3)	7 (2.4)	.075
Stupor	12 (4.3)	0	.001

*Values given are number of patients (%) with adverse experiences.

†Adverse experiences were reported by ≥10% of patients treated with selfotel or placebo; by univariate analysis.
From Davis SM, Lees KR, Albers GW, et al: Selfotel in acute ischemic stroke: Possible neurotoxic effects of an NMDA agonist. ASSIST Investigators. Stroke 31: 347, 2000.

Table 53.4 Primary Outcome: Percentage of Patients With Total Barthel Index Score ≥60

Stroke Severity	Selfotel (%)	Placebo (%)	$P°$
3 months			
Mild/moderate	83	83	.981
Severe	48	43	.352
All patients	61	58	.490
3 months: Last observation carried forward			
Mild/moderate	79	78	.852
Severe	35	35	.981
All patients	50	50	.853

°By pooled protocols and intention-to-treat analysis.
From Davis SM, Lees KR, Albers GW, et al: Selfotel in acute ischemic stroke: Possible neurotoxic effects of an NMDA agonist. ASSIST Investigators. Stroke 31: 347, 2000.

cytoprotective. However, the highest tolerated level in human patients with stroke was only half of this target cytoprotective concentration ($21\,\mu g/mL$), and even these "subtherapeutic" levels produced marked neurologic and psychiatric effects.[79]

The noncompetitive NMDA antagonist *dextrorphan* was also evaluated in a pilot study.[80] Patients were enrolled in this study within 48 hours of the onset of hemispheric cerebral infarction. Initially, patients were treated with either dextrorphan or placebo, consisting of a 1-hour loading dose of 60 to 150 mg followed by a 23-hour ascending-dose maintenance infusion up to a maximal total dose of 3310 mg. Subsequently, additional patients were treated with dextrorphan in an open-label fashion; a 1-hour loading dose of 145 to 260 mg was followed by an 11-hour infusion of 30 to 70 mg/hour.

As with selfotel, adverse effects of dextrorphan occurred in a dose-dependent fashion. Some side effects were particularly prominent during the loading dose, including nystagmus, somnolence, nausea, and vomiting. Hypotension occurred at the highest loading doses (>200 mg/hr) but was not associated with neurologic deterioration. During the maintenance infusion, the most common side effects were agitation, confusion, hallucinations, and hypertension. There were no apparent differences in the outcome between patients receiving placebo and those receiving low-, medium-, or high-dose dextrorphan. Unlike with selfotel, the plasma concentrations of dextrorphan achieved were comparable to the cytoprotective level determined in cell culture and animal models. At present, no further clinical trials of dextrorphan are in progress.

A multicenter placebo-controlled, double-blind, randomized trial of the noncompetetive NMDA antagonist CNS1102 (aptiganel [Cerestat]) was then conducted to evaluate the safety and tolerability of escalating doses (3, 4.5, 6, and 7.5 mg) of aptiganel and to determine the pharmacokinetic properties of the drug.[82] Forty-six patients with ischemic carotid artery territory stroke (NIHSS score 4 to 20) were enrolled within 24 hours of symptom onset. In part A of the study, patients were randomly assigned in

Table 53.5 Relative Risk of Death for Stroke Patients Receiving Selfotel or Placebo, by Stroke Severity

Indication	Selfotel, % (n/N)	Placebo, % (n/N)	Relative Risk	Confidence Interval
All deaths				
All patients	22.1 (62/280)°	17.1 (49/286)	1.292	(0.923–1.809)
Patients with severe stroke	30.5 (57/187)	21.6 (40/185)	1.410	(0.994–1.999)
Patients with mild/moderate stroke	4.3 (4/92)	8.9 (9/101)	0.488	(0.156–1.531)
Deaths by day 8				
All patients	11.4 (32/280)°	5.9 (17/286)	1.923	(1.093–3.382)
Patients with severe stroke	16.6 (31/187)	9.2 (17/185)	1.804	(1.035–3.144)
Patients with mild/moderate stroke	0.6 (0/92)	0.0 (0/101)	—	—

°Includes one selfotel patient in selfotel group (Patient 402 in Protocol 10) who had no baseline stroke severity score and died on day 2.
Adapted from Davis SM, Lees KR, Albers GW, et al: Selfotel in acute ischemic stroke: Possible neurotoxic effects of an NMDA agonist. ASSIST Investigators. Stroke 31: 347, 2000.

a ratio of 3:1 to a single bolus of aptiganel or placebo. Doses up to 6 mg were well tolerated; however, 7.5 mg caused more frequent and more severe side effects (sedation, hallucination, confusion). In phase B, a constant, optimal bolus dose (6 mg as determined in part A) was followed by a 6- to 12-hour continuous infusion of 1 mg/hr. This dosing regimen was abandoned, however, because of hypertension and severe sedation that caused 5 of 6 patients to discontinue therapy. Thereafter, a lower-dose regimen was adopted (4.5-mg bolus followed by 0.75 mg/hr infusion). The lower-dose regimen successfully achieved the target cytoprotective plasma concentration, greater than 10 ng/mL, that had been identified in animal studies. This dose was associated with moderately increased systolic blood pressure (≈ 30 mm Hg), which responded to antihypertensive agents, and adverse neurologic experiences (mild sedation and confusion) that patients easily tolerated. However, no suggestion of treatment effect was found in this study.

On the basis of these results, a nested phase 2–phase 3 study was performed to compare low-dose (3-mg bolus then 0.5 mg/hr; total 9 mg) and high-dose (5-mg bolus then 0.75 mg/hr; total 14 mg) aptiganel regimens with placebo.[83] Patients with clinical diagnosis of ischemic stroke were randomly assigned to one of three treatment arms within 6 hours of symptom onset. There were no criteria for stroke severity or syndrome, and no stratified randomization procedure was used to enforce recruitment of patients within a 3-hour window. Phase 3 enrollment was terminated early, when analysis of the phase 2 data revealed an increase in mortality within the aptiganel cohort. Analysis of available phase 3 data (628 patients) showed no difference in 90-day outcome, as measured as by modified Rankin Scale (mRS), among the three groups. The difference in 90-day mortality was not significant, but mortality at 120 days was marginally increased in the high-dose group. Other secondary analyses showed a significant difference favoring placebo over high-dose aptiganel in multiple outcome measures, including 7-day NIHSS score, 30-day BI, and 30-day mRS. On the basis of this evidence, aptiganel is not efficacious when given within 6 hours of onset of stroke and may be harmful at higher doses.

Phase 2 studies have been conducted to study the safety and tolerability of a novel low-affinity, use-dependent NMDA antagonist, AR-R15696AR. The 2002 trial demonstrated that a dosing regimen capable of achieving cytoprotective concentrations produced a significant excess of side effects compared with placebo, including nausea, vomiting, fever, agitation, dizziness and hallucinations.[84] No positive treatment effect on BI or NIHSS score was observed at 1 month. As with other NMDA antagonists, the unfavorable efficacy-to-toxicity ratio has halted further investigation of this agent.[84]

Magnesium (Mg^{2+}) is theoretically an ideal neuroprotectant, because of its diverse mechanisms of action, low cost, ease of administration, wide therapeutic index, good blood-brain barrier permeability, and established safety profile. Mg^{2+} ions endogenously function as a physiologic voltage-dependent block of the NMDA receptor ion channel and inhibitor of ischemia-induced glutamate release.[85] In addition to these anti-excitotoxic actions, Mg^{2+} antagonizes voltage-gated calcium (Ca^{2+}) channels of all types,

promotes vasodilation, enhances mitochondrial buffering of calcium overload, prevents depletion of adenosine triphosphate (ATP), and inhibits the inflammatory response and calcium-mediated activation of intracellular enzymes.[85–87] Preclinical models show that magnesium sulfate ($MgSO_4$) consistently reduces infarct volume, a dose-response relationship being demonstrated within easily achieved serum levels (1.49 mmol/L).[88] Postischemic $MgSO_4$ treatment given 6 hours after embolization significantly reduces infarct volume by 48% compared with placebo.[88] This model refreshingly mimics the clinical reality, in which patients present for treatment hours after the onset of ischemia. However, as with previous agents, the benefit of Mg^{2+} has been shown only in some laboratories in some models.

The theoretical benefit of Mg^{2+} is augmented by the finding that up to 80% of patients with stroke have significantly decreased serum ionized Mg^{2+} levels and 15% show elevated ionized Ca^{2+}/Mg^{2+} ratio, a state promoting increased vascular tone.[89] Low cerebrospinal fluid Mg^{2+} levels have been associated with significantly larger cortical infarcts and greater likelihood of persistent neurologic deficit, whereas high cerebrospinal fluid Mg^{2+} levels are significantly correlated with neurologic improvement from baseline findings and smaller deficit at follow-up for patients with cortical or subcortical infarct.[90] These findings suggest that relative magnesium deficiency may play a role in the pathophysiology of ischemia and that magnesium treatment may have therapeutic utility.

Several pilot studies have already demonstrated the safety and tolerability of IV Mg^{2+} in patients with acute ischemic stroke.[86,91] Administration of $MgSO_4$ as a loading dose (8 to 16 mmol) followed by a 24-hour continuous infusion (65 mmol) has been studied in more than 3000 patients with stroke treated within 48 hours, in whom there were no significant adverse events. The majority of these studies have not revealed the significant hypotension or hyperglycemia that was experienced in some preclinical evaluations of $MgCl$.[92] The majority of reported adverse events were the expected complications of the initial stroke and did not differ from those reported in patients given placebo. A dose optimization study identified a dose (16 mmol bolus, 24-hour continuous infusion of 65 mmol) capable of achieving the minimum neuroprotective serum levels in all patients while producing no adverse events.[91] A systematic review of four phase 2 clinical trials disclosed a nonsignificant, 8% absolute reduction in the combined endpoint of death or functional dependence.[40]

One of the greatest impediments to translating experimental efficacy to a clinical reality is the delay in administration of potentially cytoprotective therapies. Ongoing trials of magnesium administration have been designed to specifically address this issue. The Field Administration of Stroke Therapy-Magnesium (FAST-MAG) pilot study was an open-label evaluation of the safety and feasibility of paramedic-initiated magnesium therapy to patients with stroke identified in the field by the Los Angeles Prehospital Stroke Screen (LAPSS).[43] The average time to treatment was only 29 minutes from symptom onset, the shortest onset-to-treatment interval reported to date. More than two thirds of patients had a good functional outcome.

A phase 3 multicenter, randomized, placebo-controlled trial is enrolling patients to evaluate the efficacy of field-administered, hyperacute Mg^{2+} therapy (given within 2 hours of stroke onset). Because patients are identified by the paramedics before neuroimaging, both ischemic and hemorrhagic strokes will be included. Analyses will be based on time-to-treatment stratification, and the primary endpoint is a global measure of functional outcome performed 90 days after treatment (BI, NIHSS, Stroke Impact Scale).[93]

Additionally, the IMAGES Study Group is conducting a large phase 3 trial of $MgSO_4$ administered within 12 hours of onset that is designed with sufficient statistical power to detect only a 5.5% absolute difference in death or dependence.[93a] Rigorous trial design has employed a randomization algorithm that maintains balanced group-allocation of patients based on prognostic variables, including age, laterality of stroke, time to randomization, and Oxfordshire Community Stroke Project classification, which differentiates clinical stroke presentation into prognostic categories on the basis of vascular territory. This study, which represents the single largest study of cytoprotective therapy to date, has enrolled more than 1800 patients, nearly half of whom have been treated within 6 hours of onset. An IMAGES substudy will employ MRI as a biologic surrogate for neuroprotective efficacy. The investigators hypothesize that magnesium will reduce infarct growth as measured by neuroimaging. Patients in this substudy will undergo baseline DWI and then T2-weighted imaging at 12 weeks. The change in lesion size in the magnesium- and placebo-treated patients will then be compared.

In summary, although preclinical studies of competitive and noncompetitive NMDA antagonists suggest that they can effectively protect penumbral regions, results of clinical studies have thus far been disappointing. Trial design, lacking forced time-to-treatment stratification and patient selection criteria for stroke homogeneity, may have contributed to these results. As with calcium antagonists, achieving neuroprotection by blocking glutamate-induced damage means interrupting events that are triggered almost immediately after the onset of ischemia, so that the time to treatment from onset must be brief. This small time window, seen in all animal studies, was ignored in all clinical trials of these drugs except for the FAST-MAG trial.

Even more important, the negative clinical results with NMDA antagonists may be attributed to the dose-limiting phencyclidine-like side effects, which prevent achievement of therapeutic drug levels in brain tissue. An understanding of the clinically apparent neurotoxicity of NMDA antagonists involves a condition described as "NMDA receptor hypofunction." NMDA antagonists have been shown to induce large vacuoles within the adult rodent brain that may signify irreversible damage.[94,95] Molecular experiments have demonstrated that an indirect complex network disturbance is responsible for the NMDA receptor hypofunction. Blockade of NMDA receptors on subcortical inhibitory neurons leads to disinhibition of glutamatergic and cholinergic cortical projections.[96] This disinhibited state, coupled with simultaneous stimulation of non-NMDA glutamate receptors, may lead to enhanced neurotoxicity. Concurrent administration of GABA-ergic or α-adrenergic agents appears to diminish the excitotoxic damage.[97] Finally, a model of immature rodents demonstrates that administration of NMDA antagonists during the period of synaptogenesis triggers diffuse apoptotic degeneration throughout the brain.[98]

These complex interactions indicate the potential problems with using drugs that target specific neurotransmitter function. Attempts have been made to develop strategies inhibiting glutamate-induced damage while avoiding the toxicity profile of direct NMDA receptor antagonism. Several agents with such properties have been tested in phase 2 and 3 trials, including polyamine site blockers, glycine antagonists, AMPA receptor antagonists, presynaptic glutamate release inhibitors, ion channel blockers, and GABA agonists. These agents are discussed individually in the following sections.

Agents Acting Indirectly on Glutamate

Eliprodil, an antagonist of the polyamine site of the NMDA receptor, has been evaluated in phase 2 and phase 3 trials involving patients with acute stroke. However, the data remain unpublished, and further investigation has stopped because of an unsatisfactory risk-to-benefit ratio.[99]

GV150526 (gavestinel) is a novel glycine site antagonist at the NMDA receptor complex. It exhibits neuroprotective effects in experimental stroke models at established plasma levels (10 to $30\,\mu g/mL$) with a paucity of toxicity and an extended time window (6 hours).[100] Gavestinel has no known antiplatelet or anticoagulant effects. Therefore, Bordi and colleagues[100] believe that this compound could be safely administered before performance and interpretation of neuroimaging in order to avoid treatment delays.

A phase 2 randomized, placebo-controlled, two-part ascending-dose trial evaluated the safety, tolerability, and pharmacokinetics of a gavestinel loading dose followed by continuous infusion given within 12 hours of stroke onset.[101] The first part involved administration of escalating loading doses (50, 100, 200, 400 or 800 mg) to determine the maximal tolerated dose of gavestinel. In the second part, the maximum tolerated loading dose from part one (800 mg) was followed by five maintenance infusions given every 12 hours (100, 200, or 400 mg bid). Sixty-six patients were enrolled (48 received active study drug). GV150526 produced no more hemodynamic or neuropsychiatric events than placebo. No consistently reported or dose-related side effects, serious adverse events, or deaths were attributed to administration of the drug. Mild anemia and asymptomatic, transient, dose-dependent elevations in liver function values were observed. Significantly higher serum glucose levels were found in patients receiving maintenance gavestinel, and the level of hyperglycemia was correlated with the volume of dextrose diluent used for infusion. All loading-dose regimens easily achieved plasma concentrations exceeding the predicted therapeutic levels from animal studies, and maintenance infusions of 200 or 400 mg bid sustained this neuroprotective level. These levels were well tolerated with no significant adverse events. The optimal dosage to be used for phase 3 efficacy studies was identified as an 800-mg loading dose followed by five 200-mg twice-daily infusions. Two additional phase 2 trials have corroborated the safety of this dosing regimen.[102,103]

Subsequently, two large phase 3 randomized, placebo-controlled, double-blind trials failed to demonstrate the efficacy of gavestinel despite statistical power adequate to detect even small differences. The GAIN Americas trial randomly assigned 1367 patients to treatment or placebo within 6 hours of stroke onset, and concomitant treatment with IV t-PA was allowed in eligible patients.[104] Treatment consisted of an 800-mg loading dose plus five maintenance doses (200 mg every 12 hours) of gavestinel or placebo. Patients were stratified at randomization by age (younger or older than 75 years) and initial stroke severity (NIHSS score 2 to 5, 6 to 13, or >13). Patients were well matched for baseline characteristics. Mean NIHSS score was 12, and median time to treatment was 5.2 hours. No statistically significant difference in mortality or 3-month outcome measures (BI, mRS, or NIHSS score) was found between the gavestinel and placebo groups (Fig. 53–2). Subgroup analysis revealed a significant treatment benefit in younger patients with mild stroke (<75 years, NIHSS 2 to 5) that persisted even after adjustment for age, baseline NIHSS score, use of t-PA, time from onset to treatment, and stroke subtype. However, no treatment effect was seen in either the t-PA–treated patients (n = 333) or the patients given gavestinel within 4 hours of onset (n = 244).

As previously described, the GAIN International trial recruited 1804 patients within 6 hours of stroke onset and used the same dosing regimen and stratified randomization schema as the GAIN Americas trial.[39] The primary efficacy measure, survival combined with 3-month BI, was analyzed only in the ischemic stroke population (721 patients given gavestinel, 734 placebo). Secondary endpoints were BI (at 7 days and 1 month), NIHSS score (at 7 days, 1 and 3 months), mRS (at 1 and 3 months), death within 3 months, and global statistical test of combined neurologic status (NIHSS 1 or less, BI score 95 or more,

mRS 1 or less) at 3 months. In comparison with placebo, gavestinel had no effect on primary or secondary outcome measures when baseline NIHSS score and age were included as covariates in proportional odds models. Minor adverse events (transient rises in liver function values and phlebitis) were seen more commonly in the gavestinel group, but no significant differences were found in rates of serious adverse events (Fig. 53–3).

The neutral results of the large gavestinel trials are disconcerting, for several reasons. First, the clinical testing closely mimicked the experimental models that had exhibited neuroprotection even after 6 hours of ischemia. Second, these trials incorporated an adequate number of patients to exclude a clinically significant benefit of gavestinel, a point that has been used to criticize previous trials. Second, these trials appropriately stratified patients according to baseline stroke severity and age, factors that may otherwise cause imbalances within treatment and placebo groups and thereby produce confounding results. Third, "supratherapeutic" levels of the neuroprotective agent were achieved with only minimal and tolerable side effects. Therefore, unlike with other modulators of glutamate activity, doses of gavestinel were not limited by intolerability of "therapeutic" doses.

The reason for the neutral results for gavestinel clinical trials remains to be identified. It is possible that the time window to effectively antagonize glutamate is simply less than 6 hours and that the neuroprotective benefit of infarct size reduction in animals does not translate into improved functional outcome measured in clinical trials. Just as likely, however, is that expectations for gavestinel were overinflated because only positive preclinical results were published (it is common for negative results in animal studies to go unreported). Mild beneficial effects were seen only in carefully standardized stroke models that do not reflect the heterogeneity of patients with stroke, in

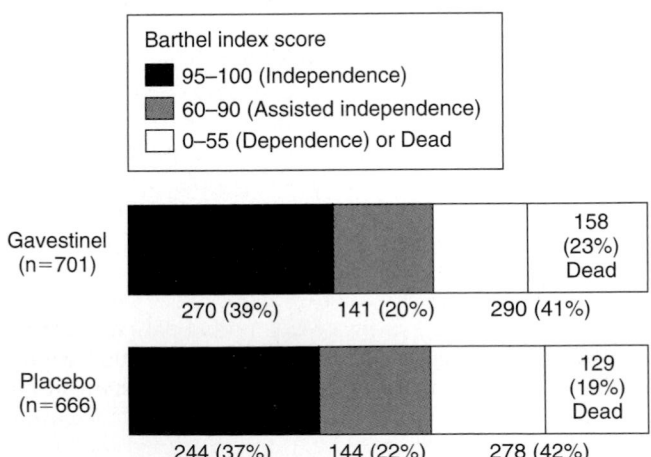

FIGURE 53–2 *Glycine antagonist in neuroprotection for patients with acute stroke—GAIN Americas. Primary outcome analysis, Barthel index score at 3 months. (Adapted from Sacco RL, DeRosa JT, Haley C, et al: Glycine antagonist in neuroprotection for patients with acute stroke: GAIN Americas: A randomized controlled trial. The GAIN Americas Investigators. JAMA 285:1719, 2001.)*

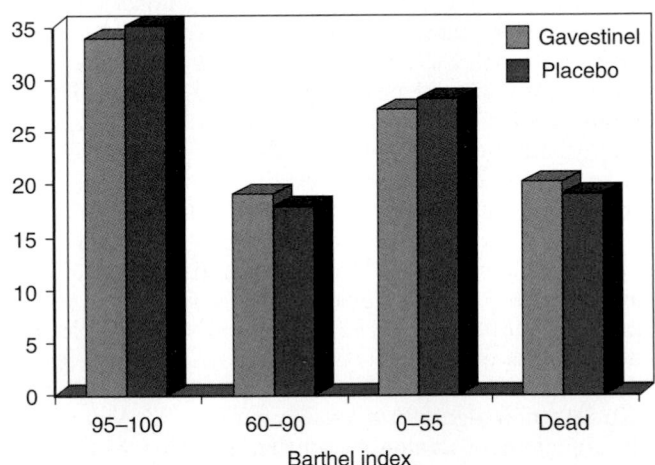

FIGURE 53–3 *Glycine antagonist in neuroprotection for patients with acute stroke—GAIN International. Primary outcome analysis, Barthel index score at 3 months. (Adapted from Lees KR, Asplund K, Carolei A, et al: Glycine antagonist [gavestinel] in neuroprotection [GAIN International] in patients with acute stroke: A randomized controlled trial. The GAIN International Investigators. Lancet 355:1949, 2000.)*

whom more robust efficacy would be needed to achieve clinical significance.

Blockade of glutamate-activated AMPA receptors represents another target of cytoprotection with several advantages over NMDA receptor antagonism. AMPA receptors are colocalized with NMDA receptors on cortical neurons but are also present on oligodendrocytes in the white matter.[105] These receptors are more permeable to sodium and mediate fast synaptic transmission and depolarization, thereby facilitating activation of NMDA receptors. Favorable attributes of AMPA antagonism include potential preservation of both cortical and subcortical regions as well as reduction of secondary activation of NMDA receptor and voltage-gated calcium channels. One promising AMPA antagonist, *YM872*, exhibits high-affinity competitive activity at the AMPA receptor as well as low affinity for the NMDA receptor, the glycine site on the NMDA receptor, and the kainate receptor. In animal models, this agent has demonstrated reduction of infarct volume comparable with that seen with NMDA receptor antagonists.[106] A phase 1 clinical trial showed that a 24-hour infusion of 1.25mg/kg/hour was tolerated in elderly volunteers, although central nervous system side effects limited the use of higher doses and longer infusion times.[107]

Enrollment has just been terminated prematurely in two concurrent YM872 clinical trials, the AMPA Receptor Antagonist Treatment in Ischemic Stroke (ARTIST) trials, on the basis of an interim futility analysis. These multicenter, randomized, double-blind, placebo-controlled trials were designed to "fill in the gaps" left by past neuroprotection trials—combination of reperfusion and neuroprotection strategies and use of a biologic marker of efficacy. The ARTIST+ trial compared the efficacy of YM872 plus t-PA with that of placebo plus t-PA. Preclinical data have demonstrated that co-administration of t-PA and YM872 within 2 hours of stroke imparts a higher level of cytoprotection than either agent alone.[108] Patients with acute hemispheric ischemic stroke and a moderate to severe deficit (NIHSS score 7 to 23, level of consciousness [LOC] score 0 to 1) treated with standard protocol t-PA were eligible. The planned enrollment was 600 patients, and more than 400 patients were enrolled. YM872 administration was started before the end of t-PA infusion and continued for 24 hours. Primary efficacy-outcome measures included neurologic function and disability scales.

The second trial, ARTIST MRI, evaluated the safety and potential efficacy of YM872 administered to patients with stroke within 6 hours of onset and used MRI as a surrogate marker of outcome. Baseline ischemic lesion volume on DWI was compared with final lesion volume on T2-weighted imaging with fluid-attenuated inversion recovery (FLAIR) to detect the effect of YM872 on lesion growth. The abandonment of these very well designed trials is disappointing. Further investigation of YM872 is not planned at this time.

Another approach to the biologic monitoring of neurotherapeutics is highlighted in a stroke trial investigating another AMPA antagonist, ZK200775.[109] This dose-finding trial utilized serum concentrations of S-100B and neuron-specific enolase as peripheral markers of glial and neuronal injury, respectively. The study found a significant worsening in the mean NIHSS score 48 hours after the start of treatment in the highest-dose group (525mg/48 hours). This neurologic deterioration was associated with a higher-than-expected elevation in serum S-100B in a multiple regression analysis controlling for stroke severity. There was no significant increase in neuron-specific enolase. Although these data suggest glial rather than neuronal damage, the oligodendrocytes are critical for neuronal homeostasis, and glial damage may contribute to neuronal dysfunction. These results provide corroborative evidence of the potential toxicity of glutamate antagonists suggested by the clinically apparent dose-related toxicity observed in previous trials. Such markers may be useful surrogate markers of cytoprotection and toxicity in future trials.

Inhibitors of glutamate release are a heterogeneous group of agents, including anticonvulsants and antidepressants. The proposed mechanism of action for these drugs is ion channel blockade.

The antiepileptic drug *lamotrigine* inhibits glutamate release and has shown beneficial effects in a rodent model of focal cerebral ischemia when administered immediately after ischemia.[110] However, a 2-hour delay of treatment produced no effect on infarct volume or neurologic outcome in two models.[110,111] To our knowledge, no clinical stroke trials of lamotrigine have been performed because the preclinical efficacy of immediate drug administration cannot be replicated in patients with stroke. Similarly, a derivative of lamotrigine, *sipatrigine (BW619C89)*, is a use-dependent sodium channel antagonist that inhibits presynaptic glutamate release. It has been shown to decrease glutamate release during ischemia[112]; like lamotrigine, however, sipatrigine reduced infarct volume only when administered at onset of ischemia.[113] This agent has been evaluated in phase 2 clinical trials in patients within 12 hours of stroke onset.[114] As with selfotel, continuous infusion of sipatrigine produced intolerable neuropsychiatric effects (sedation, agitation, confusion, hallucinations, and visual disturbances) while showing no trend to improve outcomes in a small cohort of 27 patients. A subsequent two-part trial evaluating the maximum tolerated dose and efficacy of sipatrigine was halted early by the trial sponsor, and further clinical development of the drug for stroke has ceased.[115]

Preclinical studies have shown that *phenytoin* can reduce neuronal injury, possibly by inhibiting spreading electrical depolarization in penumbral regions and thereby reducing postischemic glutamate release. Fosphenytoin, an aqueous-soluble rapidly injectable prodrug of phenytoin, is another sodium channel blocker. A multicenter combined phase 2–3 evaluation of IV fosphenytoin within 4 hours of acute stroke was terminated prematurely after interim analysis of 462 enrolled patients showed no difference between placebo and fosphenytoin in any of the functional or disability outcomes.[116]

A novel calcium-sensitive, maxi-K potassium channel opener, *BMS-204352 (MaxiPost)*, causes neuronal hyperpolarization, decreased calcium influx, and glutamate release.[117] Phase 1 and 2a studies revealed no safety concerns. However, a phase 3 trial, the Potassium-Channel Opening Stroke Trial (POST) of 1978 patients with moderate to severe cortical strokes (NIHSS score 6 to 20) treated within 6 hours of onset failed to show any significant beneficial effect compared with placebo, though these results have not yet been published. A substudy evaluated the change in lesion volume on MRI over a 12-week period as a biologic surrogate outcome marker.[118]

The pilot study of another ion channel blocker, *lifarizine*, also suggested reduced mortality and improved outcome, but because the drug causes hypotension, further clinical testing is not planned.[119]

Lubeluzole is a novel benzothiazole compound that has emerged as a neuroprotective agent in animal models of focal ischemia.[120–122] In some laboratories, lubeluzole has reduced infarct volume and improved neurologic outcome in animal models even when administered up to 6 hours after infarct induction.[120] Lubeluzole administered 1 hour after photochemically induced infarct attenuated the growth and density of ischemic damage in the periphery of infarct, the presumed penumbra, as measured by serial DWI with apparent diffusion coefficient (ADC) mapping.[122] There are several putative mechanisms by which lubeluzole protects the penumbral region in these models. First, lubeluzole normalizes neuronal activity in the peri-infarct region by inhibiting glutamate release possibly via blockade of non–L-type calcium channels.[123] Additionally, blockade of sodium channels and taurine release by lubeluzole suggests that it may reduce osmoregulatory stress in the peri-infarct zone.[124] Finally, lubeluzole downregulates the glutamate-induced NOS pathway and diminishes nitric oxide (NO)–related neurotoxicity.[125]

A phase 2 clinical trial of lubeluzole in acute ischemic stroke suggested that the agent lowers mortality and disability rates in some patients.[126] Two dosing regimens were compared with placebo. The low-dose treatment consisted of 7.5 mg of lubeluzole administered intravenously over 1 hour, followed by a continuous infusion of 10 mg/day for 5 days. The high-dose regimen was twice this dose (15 mg over 1 hour, then 20 mg/day for 5 days). Subjects clinically diagnosed with acute ischemic stroke in the MCA territory were treated within 6 hours of onset of symptoms. Prolongation of the QT interval on electrocardiography was observed at plasma drug concentrations of 100 ng/mL or greater in the phase 1 study but was not confirmed in this trial. The low-dose lubeluzole group experienced no excess of cardiac arrhythmias compared with the placebo group, although there was a higher incidence of ventricular fibrillation in the high-dose lubeluzole group. In patients with moderate to large strokes, mortality was 7% in the low-dose lubeluzole patients, and 20% in the placebo patients. Overall mortality was 6% for the low-dose regimen, 18% for placebo, and 35% for the high-dose regimen. The trial was terminated prematurely when a multivariate logistic regression analysis found this significant imbalance in the 28-day mortality favoring treatment with the low-dose regimen. The excess mortality in the high-dose group was partially due to imbalanced randomization of subjects, this group having more severe strokes. When multivariate regression analysis accounted for stroke severity, high-dose treatment had no effect on mortality. BI scores tended to be higher in the low-dose lubeluzole group, but no significant differences in efficacy measures were found among the groups.

On the basis of the results of this pilot study, subsequent phase 3 randomized, multicenter, double-blind, placebo-

controlled trials adopted the low-dose regimen to test the efficacy of lubeluzole in patients with acute ischemic stroke. However, it is essential to note that the low-dose regimen produced a mean plasma concentration (61 ± 22 ng/mL) that is below the minimal neuroprotective level established in animals (100 ng/mL).[127]

Three large-scale, multicenter, double-blind, placebo-controlled, randomized, phase 3 trials of low-dose lubeluzole in patients with stroke have produced conflicting results. The European and Australian trial, randomly assigning 725 patients to treatment within 6 hours of onset, demonstrated similar overall mortality, rates of adverse events, and clinical outcomes in all placebo- and lubeluzole-treated patients.[128] However, an unplanned post hoc analysis found that lubeluzole treatment decreased mortality among patients with mild to moderate stroke as measured by the Clinical Global Impression rating. The North American trial involved 721 patients treated within 6 hours of onset of moderate to severe hemispheric stroke (NIHSS score > 7).[129] The mean time to treatment was 4.7 hours. The extent of functional recovery (BI score) and disability (mRS) at 3 months significantly favored lubeluzole over placebo after the data were controlled for appropriate covariates. The odds of favorable outcome were 38% higher with lubeluzole according to the global test statistic. This study also found a nonsignificant improvement in mortality in the lubeluzole group and confirmed the safety of the low-dose regimen, reporting no significant differences in cardiac-related complications or adverse events.

The third trial evaluating the efficacy of low-dose lubeluzole randomly assigned to treatment a total of 1786 patients who were stratified according to time to treatment (0 to 6 hours and 6 to 8 hours).[130] During the trial, a target stroke population (core stroke group) was defined on the basis of results of a meta-analysis identifying patients who might benefit from treatment. The core stroke group consisted of patients with ischemic stroke, excluding patients 75 years or older with severe strokes, who were treated within 6 hours. Only the core stroke group was used in the primary efficacy analyses. Lubeluzole had no significant effect on mortality or 12-week functional status in the core stroke group. Similar neutral results were found in the nontarget population, including all patients treated within 6 to 8 hours of onset and patients 75 years or older with severe stroke. The most commonly reported adverse experiences were fever, constipation, and headache. Lubeluzole-treated patients experienced more cardiac events, including atrial fibrillation and QT interval prolongation, but this higher rate was not associated with increased mortality.

Finally, lubeluzole was the first potentially neuroprotective agent to be evaluated in a dedicated combination trial with t-PA. Patients who qualified for and received IV t-PA within 3 hours of symptom onset were randomly allocated 1:1 to receive either lubeluzole (7.5 mg IV over 1 hour, then a continuous 5-day infusion of 10 mg/day) or placebo.[42] The lubeluzole infusion was started before the end of the 1-hour t-PA infusion. Eighty-nine patients were enrolled before the trial was terminated early because of negative results of the previously described concurrent lubeluzole phase 3 trial.[130] In the enrolled patients (45% of the planned population), t-PA and the study drug were administered at a mean of 2.5 and 3.2 hours from symptom onset, respectively. There were no significant differences in rates of death (26%), intracerebral hemorrhage (10%), or serious adverse events (51%) or in functional outcomes (BI) between the lubeluzole and placebo groups. These results demonstrate the safety and feasibility of linking ultra-early neuroprotection with thrombolysis; however, the premature stoppage of enrollment led to a study with insufficient power to detect efficacy.

A systematic review of five randomized trials, involving a total of 3510 patients, found no evidence that lubeluzole given at any dose reduced the odds of death or dependency at the end of follow-up (odds ratio [OR], 1.03; 95% confidence interval, 0.91 to 1.19).[131] At any given dose, however, lubeluzole was associated with a significant excess of cardiac conduction disorders.

There are several reasons that the lubeluzole trials may have failed to show efficacy. As with many other agents, the time from stroke onset to drug administration is most likely too long to meaningfully inhibit glutamate release and action. Although an extended 6-hour time window for efficacious treatment has been reported, other animal models have failed to replicate the efficacy of lubeluzole initiated 30 minutes after ischemia. The discrepancy in results between the North American and European trials may be in part due to time to drug initiation. In the North American trial, the mean interval was 4.7 hours. Although a similar mean is not reported by the European trial, more than 80% of patients were treated after 4 hours, potentially leading to lessened efficacy. Also, dose-limiting side effects, primarily cardiac, led to a narrow therapeutic index with resultant serum drug levels below the minimum neuroprotective level reported in animal studies. A preliminary analysis of the pharmacokinetics-pharmacodynamics in the European trial found a trend toward improved functional outcome (mRS) in patients with a plasma drug concentration greater than 70 ng/mL. Variability in achieved plasma levels may have occurred to account for conflicting reports of efficacy. Although the combination trial of lubeluzole and t-PA required treatment within 4 hours, its early termination yielded a small sample size and a study with insufficient power to detect efficacy.

Other Neurotransmitter Modulators

Serotonin agonists may exert cytoprotection via several actions at presynaptic and postsynaptic 5-hydroxytrypta-mine-1A (5-HT$_{1A}$) receptors. Primarily, activation of this receptor causes neuronal membrane hyperpolarization by opening G protein–coupled potassium channels.[132] Activation of presynaptic serotonin receptors may lead to a reduction in glutamate release.[133] Lastly, these agents may inhibit apoptosis.[134]

One small trial of 49 patients with acute stroke failed to show greater efficacy of a serotonin reuptake inhibitor, *trazodone*, on mortality or neurologic deficit compared with placebo.[135] The neuroprotective efficacy, safety, and tolerability of another serotonergic agent are being studied in ongoing acute stroke trials. *Repinotan (BAY x 3702)* is a serotonin agonist of the 5-HT$_{1A}$ subtype that produces 55% reduction of infarct volume in experimental models of permanent focal ischemia.[136] A phase 2 trial of repinotan

identified 1.25 mg/day given for 3 days as a dose that is well tolerated by patients with stroke and may improve neurologic outcome at 3 months.[137] A double-blind, placebo-controlled phase 3 trial is currently randomly assigning patients with moderate to severe stroke (NIHSS scores 8 to 23) to receive either placebo or repinotan within 6 hours of symptom onset. Treatment with IV thrombolysis is allowed. The drug is administered at a rate of 1.25 mg/day for 72 hours, and doses are titrated to a targeted blood level of 5 to 20 μg/L. The primary outcome measure is the BI score at 3 months. Planned enrollment for this phase 3 trial is 600 patients.[138]

A safety and efficacy study of the novel neurotransmitter modulator *ONO-2506* is currently recruiting patients with stroke within 6 hours of onset of a radiographically confirmed cortical infarct. The proposed mechanism of action is modulation of glutamate transporter uptake capacity and expression of GABA receptors.[139]

The endogenous opioids act at the kappa (κ) opioid receptor as excitatory neurotransmitters and potentiators of ischemic injury. Opiate receptor antagonists have exhibited cytoprotective activity in preclinical focal and global models of ischemia.[140–142] Several small trials of *naloxone* have not conclusively shown efficacy in acute ischemic stroke.[143–147] The equivocal results are likely due to insufficient power of these small studies to detect small but significant treatment effects. Also, naloxone is relatively nonspecific for the kappa receptor. Attention has now shifted to *nalmefene*, an opiate antagonist that has relatively pure activity at the kappa receptor.

In a phase 2a trial, nalmefene (0.1 mg/kg) administered within 6 hours of stroke onset was found to be tolerable and possibly efficacious.[148] A subsequent phase 2b dose-comparison trial established that nalmefene doses up to 60 mg are safe in patients with stroke. Although no overall treatment effect was observed, a subgroup analysis suggested that nalmefene may confer a beneficial effect in young patients (<70 years old).[149]

On the basis of phase 2 data, a phase 3 trial was designed to study the safety and efficacy of 60 mg of nalmefene administered as a 10-mg bolus dose followed by continuous infusion of 50 mg over 24 hours.[150] A total of 368 patients were randomly assigned to undergo treatment within 6 hours of stroke onset. This sample size was constructed to detect a 15% improvement with treatment. Concomitant use of t-PA was allowed, but the patients who received t-PA were analyzed as a separate subgroup (n = 38) and were therefore excluded from the intention-to-treat analysis. The study found no significant treatment effect on 3-month outcome with any of the planned analyses, including secondary analyses in young patients and thrombolytic-treated patients. However, the small numbers of patients in both of these subgroups increases the likelihood that analysis would exclude a treatment effect that is actually present. Although the nalmefene-treated patients experienced more nausea, the study did not find a significant increase in incidence of neuropsychiatric effects.

There are several potential explanations for the negative results of the opioid antagonist trials. As with other upstream modulators of excitotoxicity, delayed treatment may not confer neuroprotection because the pivotal steps in the cascade have already occurred by the time of treatment. Also, the trial design did not enforce recruitment of adequate numbers of patients to the subgroups most likely to derive benefit (young patients, patients with moderate to severe deficits, patients eligible for thrombolytic treatment), resulting in insufficient power. Last, no pharmacokinetic studies were performed, so the adequacy of dosage is unknown.

Enhancement of GABA-induced inhibition may be a useful target of cytoprotection. *Clomethiazole* is a GABA agonist that theoretically prevents damage due to excessive excitatory neurotransmitters by enhancing inhibition at the $GABA_A$ receptor level.[151] Activation of the GABA receptor increases chloride conductance and membrane hyperpolarization, thereby depressing neuronal depolarization and excitability.[152] Clomethiazole has been shown to exhibit neuroprotection in several focal ischemia models.[153,154]

A dose-escalation trial demonstrated an acceptable safety profile in patients with acute stroke, with dose-related sedation observed.[155] In this study, 75 mg/kg of clomethiazole administered as a continuous infusion over 24 hours achieved plasma drug concentrations of 10 to 13 μmol/L, levels comparable to those producing experimental neuroprotection.[156] Therefore this dose was chosen for phase 3 trials.

The Clomethiazole Acute Stroke Study (CLASS) evaluated clomethiazole in a randomized, placebo-controlled fashion in patients with hemispheric ischemic stroke with a moderate to severe deficit who were treated within 12 hours of onset.[157] The study was powered to detect a 9% difference in the percentage of patients reaching relative functional independence with treatment. Efficacy analysis of 1353 patients revealed a nonsignificant 1.2% difference favoring clomethiazole in achievement of functional independence as assessed by BI. Sedation, the most common adverse event, led to withdrawal of treatment in 15.6% of patients. There was no difference in incidence of cardiopulmonary conditions or progressive stroke between the treatment and placebo groups. Onset-to-treatment interval had no effect on recovery between the groups after data were controlled for age and baseline stroke severity. Subgroup analyses found a significant beneficial effect of clomethiazole in two overlapping groups, patients with severe baseline neurologic deficit, and those classified as having a total anterior circulation stroke. An interaction between stroke syndrome classification and treatment was identified. In patients with total anterior circulation strokes, 40.8% of clomethiazole-treated patients reached relative functional independence compared with 29.8% of placebo-treated patients. This finding suggests that patients with the largest strokes may have a larger penumbra that may be salvaged by cytoprotective therapy.

Interestingly, CLASS did not require CT before patient enrollment. Ninety-five patients who were found on postrandomization CT to have intracerebral hemorrhage were enrolled in the study. A nonsignificant trend to favorable outcome was observed in the clomethiazole-treated patients in this group, with no increase in incidence of adverse events.[158]

The Clomethiazole Acute Stroke Study in Ischemic Stroke (CLASS-I) was designed to test the hypothesis generated by the previous CLASS trial, that clomethiazole is effective in patients with large ischemic anterior circulation strokes.[159] Patients with ischemic stroke who showed evidence of higher cortical dysfunction plus visual field and motor deficits were randomly assigned within 12 hours of onset to receive either placebo or clomethiazole (68 mg/kg over 24 hours, designed to achieve plasma concentration of 10 μmol/L). The mean NIHSS score was 16.9, and the mean time from onset to treatment was 7.7 hours. Plasma concentrations exceeded 5 μmol/L in 91% patients, and the population kinetic assay produced an average concentration of 11.9 μmol/L during the 24-hour infusion. There was no evidence of drug efficacy on any of the outcome variables, including NIHSS score, BI, mRS, and 30-day lesion volume.

The absence of treatment effect occurred despite adequate trial design based on sound preclinical data, appropriate patient selection, and adequate plasma drug concentrations. As with other trials, the lack of efficacy may be based on either the prolonged treatment time window (6 hours) or the inadequate prediction of human pharmacokinetics based on rodent data.

A large international trial is recruiting patients to study the effect of *diazepam*, a benzodiapine with established GABA-ergic activity, within 12 hours of stroke onset. There are no preliminary results thus far.[160]

In summary, a large number of drugs that target glutamate and other neurotransmitter functions have shown efficacy in preclinical studies but not in clinical trials. A major factor has been side effects that limit dose, but even in studies that have achieved therapeutic dose ranges and have been sufficiently powered, such as the GAIN and CLASS trials, results have been neutral or negative. Currently, the best remaining hope for this strategy is with ongoing trials of magnesium. However, taken in their entirety, the data suggest that monotherapy targeting a single neurotransmitter function may not offer sufficient neuroprotection to provide clinically meaningful benefit in stroke.

Free Radical Scavengers, Adhesion Molecule Blockers, Steroids, and Other Anti-Inflammatory Strategies

Other strategies of neuroprotection attack later stages of the ischemic cascade. NO synthesis is induced by stimulation of glutamate receptors, and NO in turn has a number of complex actions relevant to ischemia and cell injury. Endothelium-derived NO causes vasodilatation beneficial to ischemic brain, but neuronal NO generates oxygen free radicals that are toxic to cells. In animal models of stroke, NOS inhibitors have complex effects befitting the dual role of NO in cerebral ischemia. The usefulness of NO modulation in stroke will likely hinge on the ability to favorably manipulate the beneficial and deleterious effects of NO.

Reactive oxygen intermediates play a role in ischemic tissue damage and represent another target for cytoprotection. Free radical scavengers affect a late stage of the ischemic process. *Tirilazad mesylate* is a 21-aminosteroid free radical scavenger and potent membrane lipid peroxidation inhibitor that has shown neuroprotective promise in focal ischemia and subarachnoid hemorrhage models.[161,162] This agent protects the microvascular endothelium and maintains intact blood-brain barrier and cerebral autoregulatory mechanisms. Unfortunately, its penetration into the brain parenchyma is limited, possibly leading to unsatisfactory efficacy in stroke, as demonstrated by clinical trials to date.[163] However, a new group of antioxidants, pyrrolopyrimidines, with significantly improved blood-brain barrier penetrance, have demonstrated successful neuroprotection in focal ischemia with a postischemic treatment window of 4 hours.[163]

A sequential dose-escalation trial determined that tirilazad doses of up to 6 mg/kg/day for 3 days are safe and well tolerated when administered within 6 hours of acute stroke.[164] A phase 3 randomized trial of tirilazad therapy started within 6 hours of stroke onset was terminated prematurely after a preplanned interim analysis of 660 patients determined the futility of continued enrollment.[165] This study used an initial dose of 150 mg tirilazad IV over 10 to 30 minutes and maintenance doses of 1.5 mg/kg every 6 hours for 11 additional doses (total 6 mg/kg/day). No statistically significant difference was found in the proportion of patients demonstrating a favorable outcome because of tirilazad treatment administered at a median of 4.3 hours. The lack of drug efficacy in this trial was in part ascribed to inadequate dosing, especially in women, and a second tirilazad trial was designed using higher dosing regimens (10 mg/kg/day for 2 days in men; 15 mg/kg first day, then 12 mg/kg/day in women).[166] This trial was discontinued prematurely after safety concerns were raised in a concurrent European trial, despite trends toward reduced mortality and dependence in both men and women. A systematic review of six randomized, controlled trials involving more than 1700 patients included previously unpublished data from two large European trials with negative results.[167] This review found that tirilazad actually increases rates of death and disability by one fifth. Additionally, subgroup analyses demonstrated a significantly worse outcome in women and patients treated with lower doses of tirilazad as well as a trend for worse outcome in patients with mild to moderate stroke.

A substudy of the European trials determined that early tirilazad treatment (before 6 hours) had no significant effect on infarct volume in the whole population. Post hoc analysis did find that tirilazad significantly reduced infarct volume in men with cortical infarcts; however, this beneficial effect was no longer significant after data were adjusted for age and stroke severity.[168]

Whether tirilazad not only exhibits a lack of neuroprotection but may also induce worsening within specific populations of patients with stroke is still unclear. Potential reasons for these conclusions include controversial results of preclinical studies,[169] delay in drug administration (>75% of patients were treated >3 hours after stroke onset), thrombophlebitis causing a systemic inflammatory state, and inadequate blood-brain barrier permeability. Finally, it is possible that generation of free radicals plays a positive role in the recovery of patients with stroke.

Ebselen is another type (seleno-organic) of antioxidant that potentially inhibits lipid peroxidation through multiple mechanisms. These mechanisms include inhibition of lipoxygenase within the arachidonate cascade, blocked production of superoxide anions by activated leukocytes,[170] inhibition of inducible NOS,[171] and glutathione-like inhibition of membrane lipid peroxidation.[172] In animal ischemia models, pretreatment and concurrent treatment with ebselen have led to reduction in infarct size and a decrease in cerebral edema.[173]

A single randomized efficacy trial has shown that early treatment with ebselen improved outcome after acute ischemic stroke.[174] In this trial, ebselen was administered orally (150 mg bid) to patients within 48 hours of ischemic stroke onset (mean time to treatment 29.7 hours). There was no statistically significant difference in mortality. Intention-to-treat analysis demonstrated that ebselen therapy achieved a significantly better outcome at 1 month, but only a trend to improvement was observed at 3 months. Although the ebselen group contained slightly more patients with mild impairment than the placebo group, the difference was not significant, and the efficacy of ebselen was also demonstrated in patients with moderate to severe deficits. Ebselen treatment given within 24 hours significantly improved the likelihood of good recovery on the Glasgow Outcome Scale compared with placebo (42% versus 22%; $P = .038$), whereas treatment after 24 hours led to no significant differences between the groups. The ebselen-treated patients were marginally more likely to report adverse events, but the incidence was not significantly different from that in the placebo group. On the basis of the results of this adequately powered trial, ebselen is believed to be safe and possibly efficacious.

Currently, a multicenter phase 3 ebselen trial is recruiting patients. This trial will determine the efficacy of ebselen in patients with clinically and radiographically demonstrated cortical stroke when given within 24 hours of symptom onset. Planned enrollment is 390 patients, and primary outcome is the Glasgow Outcome Scale score at 3 months.

Free radicals are produced during ischemia and reperfusion and contribute to the neuronal injury after stroke. Several nitrone free radical–trapping agents (spin-trap agents) have demonstrated neuroprotection in rodent models of both transient and permanent focal ischemia.[175,176] *NXY-059* (disodium 4-[(*tert*-butylimino) methyl] benzene-1,3-disulfonate *N*-oxide) is a novel nitrone-based compound that has free radical–trapping properties. Despite its greater water solubility, NXY-059 has shown greater efficacy in reduction of infarct size and improvement in neurologic outcome than the free radical–trapping agent PBN (α-phenyl-*N*-tert-butyl nitrone) when given at equimolar doses.[177] The neuroprotective efficacy of NXY-059 is retained even when the agent is given up to 5 hours after onset of ischemia.[177] In a primate model of permanent focal ischemia, NXY-059 significantly decreased neurologic disability and reduced infarct volume in both cortical and subcortical regions.[178] Pharmacokinetic studies show that NXY-059 produces dose-dependent neuroprotection at unbound plasma concentrations of 30 to 80 μmol/L.[176]

A randomized, double-blind, placebo-controlled trial evaluated the tolerability and pharmacokinetics of two NXY-059 dosage regimens in patients with stroke.[180] Patients were randomly assigned to receive placebo, low-dose NXY-059 (250-mg loading dose, then 85 mg/hr), or high-dose NXY-059 (500-mg loading dose, then 170 mg/g) within 24 hours of stroke onset. Treatment was administered as a loading dose over 1 hour followed by a continuous infusion over 71 hours. The infusion rate was reduced by 50% in patients with impaired renal function (calculated creatinine clearance 50 to 59 mL/min). These dosage regimens were designed to reach a target plasma unbound drug concentration higher than 40 μmol/L, which has demonstrated neuroprotection in rodents. One hundred fifty patients were enrolled at a mean of 15 hours after symptom onset. Overall incidence of adverse events was no higher in the NXY-059 group than in the placebo group. However, more severe adverse events and deaths occurred in the low-dose group, in accordance with the higher number of primary intracerebral hemorrhages in this group. The common adverse events, hyperglycemia, headache, and fever, were not related to treatment. The mean unbound plasma concentrations were 25 and 45 μmol/L in the low-dose and high-dose groups, respectively.

As in the other phase 2 studies, these concentrations were well tolerated and below the target level. Therefore, study of higher NXY-059 doses was justified. A phase 2b/3 study is planned to determine the efficacy of a higher dosage regimen (2264-mg loading dose, then up to 947 mg/hr infusion over 71 hours). Planned enrollment is 1550 patients with acute stroke who will receive NXY-059 treatment within 6 hours of stroke onset; concurrent use of IV thrombolytics is to be allowed. Primary outcome measure will be the mRS.

Complex inflammatory processes mediate ischemic- and reperfusion-related brain injury, representing an ideal downstream target for cytoprotection. Modulation of cytokines, inflammatory-related enzymes (NOS), endothelial leukocyte interactions, leukocyte activation, and gene transcription factors has been investigated in experimental models and a few clinical trials.

Various models of focal ischemia have demonstrated greater expression of leukocyte-endothelial adhesion molecules,[181,182] and the absence of adhesion molecules in knockout mice significantly reduces infarct size.[183,184] Anti-adhesion molecule strategies have shown efficacy only in models of transient ischemia, supporting the belief that neuroprotection imparts significant benefit only if coupled with reperfusion.[185,186] Furthermore, animal studies have demonstrated that a combination of t-PA and anti-adhesion molecule therapy (antibodies to either intracellular adhesion molecule 1 [ICAM-1] or CD18) significantly reduces infarct volume and neurologic deficit score more than either agent alone even when administered up to 4 hours after induction of ischemia.[12,187]

Although there is contradictory evidence for upregulation of inflammatory adhesion molecules in patients with ischemic stroke, the majority of studies demonstrate elevations in circulating adhesion molecules (soluble [s] ICAM-1, soluble vascular cell adhesion molecule-1 [VCAM-1], sP-selectin, and sE-selectin).[188–190] Elevated ICAM-1 expression has been observed on microvessels within infarcts in patients surviving 15 hours to 6 days after stroke.[191]

Enlimomab is a murine monoclonal anti–ICAM-1 antibody that has undergone phase 3 testing in patients with stroke. A preliminary open-label pilot dose-ranging study identified a dose that was generally well tolerated and produced the target serum level thought to be

neuroprotective (>10 μg/mL).[192] A subsequent phase 3 trial compared the efficacy of this dosage regimen (160 mg on day 1 followed by a maintenance dose of 40 mg/day for 4 days) with that of placebo in 625 patients with ischemic stroke who received treatment within 6 hours of symptom onset.[193] Although patients with any stroke syndrome were enrolled, more than 85% of patients had MCA territory infarcts with a significant deficit (median NIHSS score 14). The target serum drug level was achieved in 96.6% of patients after the first dose, and adequate trough levels were maintained throughout the duration of treatment. Enlimomab treatment was associated with worse disability and greater mortality than placebo. This negative treatment effect was evident by day 5 of treatment and was confirmed with adjustments for age and stroke severity. The hazard of death averaged over the first 90 days was 43% higher in enlimomab-treated patients than placebo-treated patients. Adverse events reported more frequently by the active treatment group were fever, myocardial infarction, pulmonary edema, pneumonia, stroke progression, cardiac arrest, meningitis, cerebral edema, and intracerebral hemorrhage. Fever was reported twice as often in enlimomab-treated patients. However, the negative effect of treatment cannot be ascribed solely to the drug's propensity to cause fever, because stroke outcome was marginally better in febrile patients receiving enlimomab than in those receiving placebo, whereas afebrile patients receiving enlimomab had a worse outcome.

There are several possible explanations for the negative effect of enlimomab. First, enlimomab is a different type of antibody from that used in experimental models. Murine anti-ICAM antibody may have led to upregulation of endogenous adhesion molecules and precipitated a paradoxic inflammatory response. It has been shown that all enlimomab-treated patients develop anti-mouse antibodies.[192] An experimental model was subsequently designed to mimic the clinical trial that had negative results. Administration of this murine antibody to rats was shown to lead to production of host humoral response against the protein, consisting of the activation of compliment, neutrophils, and the microvascular system.[194] Second, no preclinical model delayed treatment for 6 hours or administered the drug for 5 consecutive days as in the clinical trial. Most important, animal studies showed no treatment benefit in permanent ischemia models. Only a minority of patients (4% to 24%) have spontaneous reperfusion, and hence most enrolled patients were not comparable to transient ischemia models, which were associated with treatment benefit. Therefore, the rational approach to future immunomodulatory therapies would be development of a humanized anti-adhesion molecule strategy with a revised (shorter) dosage regimen coupled with thrombolysis.

To this end, a humanized immunoglobulin (Ig) G1 antibody against human CD18 (*Hu23F2G* or rovelizumab [*LeukArrest*]) was developed to block leukocyte infiltration while avoiding the complications of enlimomab due to sensitization. Data from phase 1 and phase 2 studies revealed no safety concerns associated with LeukArrest. A phase 3 trial enrolled patients within 12 hours of stroke onset, allowed concomitant use of t-PA, and employed a reduced frequency of dosing schema compared with enlimomab:

The three groups received either a single dose at enrollment, the first dose at enrollment and a second dose 60 hours later, or placebo. The phase 3 trial of rovelizumab was terminated after interim futility analysis determined that treatment was unlikely to confer significant benefit if the trial were continued. To date, the data from this trial remain unpublished.[195]

Leukocyte activation is another event in the inflammatory process that may be interrupted. A recombinant protein inhibitor of CD11b/CD18 receptor (*UK-279,276*) blocks neutrophil activation and has shown neuroprotection in animal models of focal ischemia.[196] The unpublished preliminary results from a phase 2 trial of UK-279,276 in patients with acute stroke did not support further investigation of this drug in phase 3 studies.[197]

Promising new strategies are developing to target other "downstream" events of the ischemic-excitotoxic cascade—the calcium-dependent enzymatic reactions mediating necrotic and apoptotic cell death. Theoretically, because these processes occur "later" in the cascade, the therapeutic time window may be longer. Several important enzymes have been characterized as potential targets of neuroprotection. Calpain, a ubiquitous protease, mediates cell death via cleavage of structural and regulatory proteins. Caspase-3 is another protease that cleaves homeostatic proteins and may execute apoptosis.[198] Stress-activated mitogen–activated protein kinase is an enzyme that has been linked to inflammatory cytokine production and apoptosis.[199] Inhibition of these enzymes may be effective in preserving the structural integrity of neurons. Multiple experimental models have demonstrated the efficacy of calpain, caspase, and protein kinase inhibitors in reducing infarct volume when used up to 6 hours after onset of ischemia.[200–203] The inability of these large protein compounds to cross the blood-brain barrier, however, has thus far limited clinical development, although novel strategies are being developed to enhance delivery of neurotherapeutics to the brain.

Minocycline has demonstrated protective effects in hypoxic-ischemic, focal, and global ischemia models.[204,205] Minocycline, a semisynthetic second-generation drug of the tetracycline group, is a safe and readily available compound that exerts anti-inflammatory effects such as inhibition of microglial activation and production of other inflammation mediators. Furthermore, minocycline may inhibit the activity of matrix metalloproteinases (MMPs) and diminish permeability of the blood-brain barrier. An additional putative protective action of minocycline is inhibition of caspase, inducible NOS (iNOS), and p38 mitogen-activated protein kinase (MAPK).[206] The neuroprotective efficacy of minocycline has been demonstrated in animal models even when delayed up to 4 hours.[205] Minocycline appears to be an ideal neuroprotective candidate on the basis of its established safety profile, good central nervous system penetration, wide availability, and inexpensive cost and therefore deserves evaluation in clinical trials of acute ischemic stroke.

Tacrolimus (FK506) has been widely used for prevention of transplant organ rejection and is now being investigated as a potential neuroprotectant because of its immunosuppressive properties. Tacrolimus suppresses the calcium-dependent signal transduction pathway that promotes proliferation of helper T cells by inhibition of calcineurin.[207] Apoptotic cell death is also attenuated by tacrolimus.[208] Multiple animal models demonstrate the neuroprotective effects of this agent through both histologic and radiographic evidence of reduction in infarct volume.[209–213]

A new formulation of this agent, FK506 Lipid Complex-Gilead (FK506 LCG), has been developed for the acute stroke indication. Preliminary studies demonstrated a dose-dependent hypothermia and increase in blood pressure in animals and a transient increase in blood pressure and heart rate in humans. Overall, this compound was well tolerated, and a randomized, double-blind, placebo-controlled, dose-escalation study is planned to determine the safety, tolerability, and pharmacokinetics of FK506 LCG in patients with stroke. Criteria for enrollment include ischemic stroke detected and treated within 12 hours of onset, moderate to severe deficit (NIHSS score 6 to 25 for left and 4 to 25 for right hemispheric stroke), and clinical evidence of cortical involvement.

Corticosteroids theoretically may interrupt the inflammatory cascade that occurs during stroke. Experimental data suggest that corticosteroids activate endothelial NOS activity via a nontranscriptional pathway, thereby augmenting regional cerebral blood flow and reducing infarct volume.[214] Although corticosteroids substantially reduce stroke size in experimental models, trials using various routes of administration, dosage, and duration of treatment with *dexamethasone* have failed to demonstrate a beneficial effect of steroids.[215,216] Steroids do, however, raise rates of infection and hyperglycemic complications. A systematic review of published randomized trials comparing steroids with placebo in treatment given within 48 hours of onset concluded that there is insufficient evidence to justify corticosteroid use after ischemic stroke.[217] In this review, data from 453 patients within seven trials revealed that treatment did not reduce mortality or improve outcome. The substantial delay from stroke onset to drug administration is a possible culprit in the negative results. Additionally, the detrimental side effects of corticosteroids may be mediated by the transcriptional genomic activities of steroids, thereby limiting their clinical utility.[214] Therefore, novel compounds that selectively activate nontranscriptional glucocorticoid receptor activity may provide neuroprotection without the deleterious effects.[218] Such compounds are under development.

A growing interest in studying the pleiotropic effects of the 3-hydroxy-3-methylglutaryl coenzyme A (HMG CoA) reductase inhibitors ("*statins*") has uncovered a potential neuroprotective effect. A murine focal ischemia model demonstrated that long-term (14 to 28 days) or prophylactic treatment with mevastatin upregulates endothelial NOS, reduces infarct size, and improves neurologic deficit in a dose- and time-dependent manner independent of serum cholesterol levels.[219] Meta-analyses of clinical statin trials support a clinical benefit in humans through lowering of stroke risk by approximately 30%.[220] The possible mechanisms of neuroprotection include improved endothelial function, increased endothelial NOS activity, antioxidant effects, promotion of neovascularization, and anti-inflammatory properties. To our knowledge, there have been no preclinical or clinical trials to date that utilize statins in the acute setting.

Human serum albumin is a multifunctional protein with neuroprotective properties in experimental models of focal ischemia even when administered up to 4 hours after induction of reversible ischemia.[221] Several mechanisms have been speculated for its neuroprotective capacity, including inhibition of lipid peroxidation (antioxidant), maintenance of microvascular integrity, inhibition of endothelial cell apoptosis,[222] hemodilution, and mobilization of the free fatty acids required for restoration of damaged neurons.[223] Although non-albumin hemodilution trials have not demonstrated a benefit, these were designed to test efficacy of hemodilution, not of cytoprotection per se. A pilot study of albumin is under way.

Membrane "Stabilizers" and Trophic Factors

The monosialoganglioside *GM-1* is thought to limit excitotoxicity and facilitate nerve repair and regrowth. In a study of 792 patients with acute stroke, there was a nonsignificant trend toward greater recovery in patients treated for 3 weeks with GM-1 than in those given placebo.[224] Post hoc analysis showed a statistically significant difference in neurologic outcome favoring GM-1 in the subgroup of patients treated within 4 hours. There was no difference in mortality rates, and the drug had no significant side effects. To our knowledge, no further studies of gangliosides in acute stroke are planned.

Cerebrolysin is a compound consisting of free amino acids and biologically active small peptides that are products of the enzymatic breakdown of lipid free brain products. Experimental models have demonstrated neuroprotection although the mechanism of action is unclear.[225] Several small European trials have suggested that cerebrolysin administered as a continuous infusion (20 to 50 mL/day) for 20 days results in better motor function and global function than placebo.[226] Larger clinical trials would be required to confirm neuroprotection and determine the pharmacokinetics-pharmacodynamics of this peptide.

Energy failure and activation of phospholipases during ischemia lead to breakdown of cellular membranes and, ultimately, to neuronal death. *Cytidine-5′-diphosphocholine (citicoline)*, is the rate-limiting intermediate in the biosynthesis of phosphatidylcholine, is incorporated into the membrane of injured neurons and may prevent membrane breakdown into free radical–generating lipid byproducts. Citicoline has exhibited a neuroprotective effect in a variety of central nervous system injury models, including focal ischemia.[227] However, the neuroprotective capacity is modest and is lost if treatment is started beyond 3 hours after onset of injury.[228] Despite the extensive work performed with experimental models, the exact mechanism of action of citicoline remains elusive. However, it is believed to be due to increased phosphatidylcholine synthesis and inhibition of phospholipase A_2 within the injured brain. During ischemia, choline supply is limited, and membrane phospholipids are hydrolyzed to provide a source of choline for neurotransmitter synthesis. This autocannibalism ultimately leads to death of cholinergic neurons.[228] Additionally, there is evidence that citicoline reduces expression of procaspases and other proteins involved in apoptotic cell death after focal ischemia.[229]

Pharmacokinetic-pharmacodynamic studies show that orally administered citicoline is nearly completely absorbed, with blood levels peaking at 6 hours and brain uptake of citicoline metabolites as early as 30 minutes after dosing.[230] Although bioavailability is the same with oral and IV administration, brain uptake is approximately four times higher with the IV route (0.5% oral dose versus 2% IV dose). Encapsulation of citicoline within liposomes may increase brain availability to 23% of the administered dose.

A randomized dose-response trial in 259 patients found a significant difference in functional outcome (BI and mRS), neurologic function (NIHSS) and cognitive function (Mini-Mental State Examination) favoring oral citicoline.[231] Both 500 mg and 2000 mg citicoline had significant effects on favorable outcome at 3-month outcome (BI) after adjustment for initial stroke severity. There were no deaths and no dose-related serious adverse events, with the exception of mild dizziness experienced at 2000 mg/day. A subsequent phase 3 U.S. trial randomly assigned 394 patients with acute ischemic stroke to receive placebo or citicoline (500 mg PO daily) starting within 24 hours of stroke onset and continuing for 6 weeks. Patients with moderate to severe (NIHSS score > 4) strokes within the MCA territory were included.[232] An imbalance of stroke severity occurred, with significantly more patients with NIHSS scores less than 8 assigned to the placebo group. There was no statistical difference in planned secondary analyses, and the primary efficacy analysis was rendered unreliable because of the nonproportional distribution of patient Barthel Index scores. Post hoc analyses revealed that in the subgroup of patients with baseline NIHSS scores higher than 7, citicoline-treated patients were significantly more likely to achieve a full recovery (placebo 21%, citicoline 33%, $P = .05$). No difference between treatment arms was seen in patients with NIHSS scores of 7 or less.

Partly on the basis of this subgroup analysis, another large phase 3 trial was conducted to evaluate the efficacy of higher-dose citicoline (2000 mg/day) administered within 24 hours of onset to patients with baseline NIHSS scores higher than 7.[233] There was no difference between citicoline- and placebo-treated patients in the planned primary outcome, defined as improvement in NIHSS score of more than 7 points from baseline value. However, post hoc analyses found a significant positive effect of treatment on recovery and a global test of multiple outcomes. The neutral results of this trial are likely due to the chosen primary endpoint, which may not be reflective of recovery.

An important trial evaluating the effect of citicoline on MRI-demonstrated lesion volume showed the potential utility of neuroimaging as a surrogate marker of neuroprotective efficacy.[37] One hundred patients who had baseline NIHSS scores higher than 4 and who presented with an abnormality on DWI within 24 hours of stroke onset were randomly assigned to receive either placebo or citicoline, 500 mg/day for 6 weeks. Follow-up MRI was performed at 12 weeks. At 12 weeks, the ischemic lesion volume had expanded by 180% in the placebo group, compared with 34% in the citicoline group. Baseline predictors of change in lesion size included volume of perfusion deficit, baseline NIHSS score, initial DWI volume, arterial lesion on MRA, and elapsed time from onset (≤12 hrs versus >12 hrs). A significant association was found between reduction of lesion volume and improvement of NIHSS score by 7 points or more. This relationship between clinical outcome and lesion volume supports the use of DWI as a surrogate marker of neuroprotective efficacy.

Finally, IV citicoline at various doses (750 to 1000 mg/day) and treatment durations (10 to 30 days) has been evaluated in several non-U.S. trials, all of which showed significant improvements in recovery. A small pilot study comparing the efficacy of citicoline (1000 mg/day for 30 days) with that of placebo found that 71% of citicoline-treated patients improved from baseline compared with only 31% of placebo-treated patients.[234] The largest trial involved 272 patients randomly assigned to receive either citicoline (1000 mg/day for 14 days) or placebo. In this trial, a 26% relative difference on a global improvement rating scale favoring citicoline treatment over placebo was demonstrated.[235]

A meta-analysis of seven controlled clinical stroke trials showed that citicoline treatment was associated with significant reductions in rates of long-term death or disability.[236] A later pooled analysis of oral citicoline clinical trials in acute ischemic stroke sought to determine the effects of citicoline on neurologic recovery.[41] A systematic search identified all prospective, randomized, placebo-controlled, double-blind clinical trials of citicoline in patients with moderate to severe strokes (NIHSS score >8) and good prestroke functioning (mRS score <2). Individual patient data were extracted from four trials and pooled into a solitary database. Of 1652 total patients, 1372 fulfilled the inclusion criteria (583 placebo, 789 citicoline). Three-month recovery (composite NIHSS score <1, mRS score <1, BI value >95) was achieved in 25.2% citicoline-treated patients compared with 20.2% placebo-treated patients (Table 53.6). The largest difference in recovery was seen in patients treated with the highest dose (2000 mg) of citicoline. The promising results of these large-scale analyses will likely prompt further citicoline studies, because this meta-analysis of cytoprotective trials is the first to yield positive results.

Finally, the combination of citicoline and IV thrombolysis has been shown to significantly reduce infarct volume compared with either treatment alone in a rat embolic stroke model, although this treatment combination has not yet been tested in humans.[237] Given the positive results of the meta-analyses just described, clinical evaluation of the combination of citicoline and t-PA appears to be the logical next step.

Estrogen exerts a multifaceted modulation of neurons, and various injury models have demonstrated the neuroprotection imparted by this hormone.[238,239] Although the exact neuroprotective mechanism has not been determined, there are many candidate actions. They include induction of antiapoptotic Bcl-2 proteins,[240] complex interactions with neurotrophins, activation of the cyclic AMP (cAMP)-protein kinase A-cAMP response element binding protein (CREB) pathway (antiapoptotic), attenuation of glutamate receptor activation, and decrease in intracellular calcium.[241] Clinical and epidemiologic data indirectly support the neuroprotective role of estrogen in the finding that premenopausal women have fewer strokes and that tamoxifen (an estrogen receptor antagonist) increases stroke risk.[242,243] No acute neuroprotection trials have been conducted in human patients with stroke.

Erythropoietin (EPO) is a mediator of the physiologic response to hypoxia via activation of the erythropoietin receptor, a member of the cytokine receptor superfamily. Both astrocytes and neurons produce erythropoietin in response to hypoxia, and this glycoprotein has been demonstrated to cross the blood-brain barrier.[244] The overall result of erythropoietin receptor activation is cell proliferation, inhibition of apoptosis, and erythroblast differentiation.[245] Erythropoietin may also provide antioxidant activity and resistance to glutamate toxicity.[246,247]

Table 53.6   Meta-analyses of Citicoline Studies Intent-to-Treat Set: GEE-Estimated Probabilities of Global Recovery After 12 Weeks of Follow-Up

	Global Recovery at Week 12				
	Citicoline, %	**Placebo, %**	**OR**	**95% CI**	**P**
Citicoline vs placebo (4 trials, 1372 patients)°	25.2	20.2	1.33	1.10–1.62	.0034
Doses					
Citicoline 500 mg vs placebo					
Study 001a[231]	27.7	11.4	2.98	1.25–7.02	.0129
Study 007[232]	24.2	16.6	1.61	0.93–2.78	.0890
Study 010[37]	17.1	24.0	0.65	0.28–1.48	.3078
Overall	20.8	15.7	1.42	0.96–2.093	.0782
Citicoline 1000 mg vs placebo					
Study 001a[231]	9.1	10.7	0.84	0.35–2.15	.7096
Citicoline 2000 mg vs placebo					
Study 001a[231]	25.19	9.8	3.098	1.18–8.12	.0214
Study 018[233]	28.47	23.25	1.314	1.0–1.65	.0183
Overall	27.9	21.9	1.38	1.10–1.72	.0043

°Superscript numbers indicate chapter references.

CI, confidence interval; GEE, generalized estimating equation; OR, odds ratio.

From Davalos A, Castillo J, Alvarez-Sabin J, et al: Oral citicoline in acute ischemic stroke: An individual patient data pooling analysis of clinical trials. Stroke 33: 2850, 2002.

diagnosis with transcranial Doppler ultrasonography may be unreliable because of obliteration of the major intracranial cerebral vessels. When suspected, the diagnosis of vasospasm should be pursued with angiography and should be aggressively treated as already described; the utility of triple-H therapy or nimodipine in this setting is unknown, however.

For some patients, moyamoya disease is relatively benign, being limited to mild, transient symptoms, and conservative medical therapy may suffice.[131] However, in the majority of patients, these medical therapies offer very limited efficacy, and more aggressive surgical therapies should be considered.

Surgical revascularization procedures have two key goals, (1) improving regional cerebral blood flow to prevent ischemic complications, and (2) alleviating the pressure, flow, or both that exist in deep moyamoya collateral vessels, thus reducing the risk of hemorrhage. Direct bypass (such as anastomosis of the superficial temporal artery to the middle cerebral artery), indirect bypass (such as encephaloduroarteriosynangiosis and encephaloduroarteriomyosynangiosis), and a combination of the two procedures have all been described as effective treatments in a number of series and small uncontrolled studies.[132–140] However, their roles have never been studied in a randomized clinical trial. These surgical techniques and their proposed importance in moyamoya disease are described in detail elsewhere in this text.

Hyperhomocysteinemia and Homocystinuria

Elevated levels of the amino acid homocysteine appear to cause endothelial injury and proliferation of vascular smooth muscle cells, thereby leading to premature atherosclerosis.[141,142] In addition, homocysteine may interfere with endogenous anticoagulant mechanisms, resulting in a prothrombotic state.[143,144] Hyperhomocysteinemia appears to be independently associated with risk of ischemic stroke, although whether it is a cause or effect of vascular disease is debated.[141,142] Homocysteine levels can be reduced with folic acid (0.4 mg or more daily), pyridoxine (vitamin B_6, 25 to 50 mg daily), and cobalamin (vitamin B_{12}, 250 μg daily) supplementation, and controlled trials have shown some beneficial effects on surrogate indicators of vascular function.[145] However, these indicators may not directly correlate with clinical vascular events.[146] Two large randomized trials currently being conducted, the Vitamins to Prevent Stroke Study (VITATOPS) and the Vitamins in Stroke Prevention (VISP) study,[147] should determine whether multivitamin therapy reduces the rate of recurrent stroke and other major vascular events in patients with prior stroke or transient ischemic attack. Some investigators argue that until the results of these studies are available, widespread screening for, and treatment of, elevated homocysteine levels remains experimental and cannot be recommended.[142,147,148] On the other hand, vitamin therapy appears to be safe and inexpensive; thus, empiric treatment may offer a favorable benefit-to-risk profile until the results of the large trials are known.

Fabry's Disease

Fabry's disease is a rare X-linked inherited deficiency of the lysosomal enzyme α-galactosidase, which causes lipid deposition in the vascular endothelium and results in progressive vascular disease of the brain, heart, skin, and kidneys.[149] Angiokeratoma on the trunk is often the only early sign, but cerebral arteriopathy usually becomes clinically evident in young men with the disease by the fourth decade, and occasionally in older women.[150] The intracranial vertebrobasilar system is often dolichoectatic and may be the proximate source of ischemic stroke, although cardiogenic embolism and progressive small vessel occlusive disease with deep infarctions are also observed.[149,151,152]

Antiplatelet agents are believed to be useful in preventing ischemic events related to existing vascular disease, but the disease itself was untreatable and the prognosis was quite poor until recombinant α-galactosidase A became available. In a randomized controlled trial of 58 patients with Fabry's disease, α-galactosidase was given intravenously at a dose of 1 mg/kg every other week for 20 weeks.[153] New microvascular endothelial lipid deposits developed in only 31% of patients in the treated group after 20 weeks, compared with 100% of the patients in the placebo group ($P < .001$). In addition, after 6 months of open-label therapy, all patients in the former placebo group and 98% of the patients in the former recombinant α-galactosidase A group experienced clearance of microvascular endothelial deposits.

Because α-galactosidase A replacement therapy effectively clears endothelial deposits from affected organs in patients with Fabry's disease, it should arrest the disease process. This therapy should be instituted promptly after the diagnosis is established, and continued for 6 to 12 months. The safety and efficacy of longer-term therapy have not yet been evaluated, but some maintenance therapy is likely to be required. The major adverse effects of recombinant α-galactosidase A are fever and rigors, which may occur in 25% to 50% of treated patients; these effects may be minimized with slow infusion rates and premedication with acetaminophen and hydroxyzine.

Inflammatory Vasculopathies

Cerebrovascular disease may rarely occur as the result of derangement of cell-mediated and antibody-mediated immune responses. The vasculitides are a heterogeneous group of disorders in which inflammation of the blood vessels causes vascular narrowing, occlusion, or necrosis that may result in cerebral ischemia, infarction, or hemorrhage.[154] Vasculitis may be a primary process (isolated angiitis of the central nervous system) or may occur secondary to an identifiable systemic inflammatory disorder, infection, toxin, or neoplasm. Immunosuppression appears to be the key element of treatment (Table 54.4).

Isolated Angiitis of the Central Nervous System

Isolated angiitis of the central nervous system (IACNS) affects only the brain and spinal cord, having no systemic manifestations. Symptoms of IACNS include headache, seizure, stroke, and multifocal encephalopathy. In the early descriptions of IACNS, the prognosis was uniformly poor, but immunotherapy may alter the course of the disease. Clinical and angiographic improvement has been attributed to corticosteroids and cyclophosphamide, but because of the profound rarity of IACNS, randomized clinical trials have not been performed. In a review of the literature and description of eight additional cases, Calabrese

Table 54.4 Immunosuppressive Drugs Used in the Treatment of Inflammatory Vasculopathies

Drug	Indications	Dosing Regimens	Adverse Effects	Notes
Prednisone or methylprednisolone	IACNS GCA CVD-related ? Infection-related ? Toxin-related ? Neoplasm-related	*Induction:* 0.5–2 mg/kg/d orally *or* up to 1000 mg/d IV for acute or severe cases *Taper* as tolerated over 3–12 months *Maintenance:* 5–10 mg/d orally	Infections, cushingoid features, adrenal insufficiency, behavioral/mood changes, osteopenia, diabetes mellitus, many others	
Cyclophosphamide	IACNS CVD-related	*Induction:* 1–2 mg/kg/d orally *or* 750 mg/m² BSA IV monthly for acute, severe cases *Taper* as tolerated over 3–12 months *Maintenance:* Lowest dose without recurrent symptoms; consider switch to azathioprine	Bone marrow suppression, infections, malignancy, nausea/vomiting, alopecia, hemorrhagic cystitis, diarrhea, rash	
Azathioprine	IACNS GCA CVD-related	*Induction:* Not used as induction therapy *Maintenance:* Start 1 mg/kg/d orally; increase by 0.5 mg/kg/d every 4 weeks to maximum of 2.5 mg/kg/d	Bone marrow suppression, infections, hepatotoxicity, nausea/vomiting, diarrhea	Used as an alternative to cyclophosphamide
Methotrexate	GCA CVD-related	*Induction and maintenance:* 10 mg/d orally	Bone marrow suppression, hepatotoxicity, nephrotoxicity, nausea/vomiting, fatigue, fever/chills	Used in conjunction with corticosteroids

BSA, body surface area; CVD, collagen vascular disorder; GCA, giant cell (temporal) arteritis; IACNS, isolated angiitis of the central nervous system; IV, intravenous.

and Mallek[155] observed that nearly all untreated patients died or were persistently dependent, whereas 4 of 13 patients who were treated with steroids and 10 of 13 who were treated with both steroid and cyclophosphamide improved. In contrast, other researchers have found that corticosteroids alone offered at best a transient effect, and that combination therapy with cyclophosphamide was required for a clinical benefit.[156,157]

The appropriate dosages for both medications are unclear and vary among centers. For induction therapy, prednisone or prednisolone, 1 to 2 mg/kg/day, is recommended at the time of diagnosis, with tapering over 3 to 12 months to a minimal dose of 5 to 10 mg/day. Cyclophosphamide should be started at 1 to 2 mg/kg/day, but more aggressive treatment with intravenous cyclophosphamide may be useful for patients with more acute or severe symptoms, in the form of either 3 to 6 monthly pulses of 750 mg per m² of body surface area or 15 mg/kg.[154,158]

Patients may be monitored by means of serial neurologic examination, neuropsychiatric testing, cerebrospinal fluid examination, magnetic resonance imaging, or a combination of these methods, every 3 to 6 months. Serial angiography is seldom necessary. If remission or stabilization occurs, cyclophosphamide may be gradually tapered over several months and then replaced with the better-tolerated azathioprine, 2 mg/kg/day as maintenance therapy in some cases,[154] although the role of this agent is untested. These therapeutic regimens have been evaluated only for relatively brief terms (a few years), and their longer-term efficacy has not been described. Nevertheless, long-term therapy seems to be required for many patients, because relapses are common when immunotherapy is withdrawn. Medication doses should be titrated somewhat empirically according to each patient's clinical response. In patients undergoing cyclophosphamide or azathioprine therapy, careful monitoring of the leukocyte count for evidence of bone marrow suppression is required. In addition, oral fluid intake must be increased to minimize the risk of hemorrhagic cystitis. Antiemetics may be needed to manage nausea, particularly with intravenous pulse cyclophosphamide. Finally, patients must be monitored and treated for steroid-induced diabetes mellitus while taking steroids.

Other immunomodulatory approaches, including the use of other chemotherapeutic agents, plasma exchange, and intravenous immunoglobulin, have not been studied in IACNS beyond individual case reports. Similarly, the role of antithrombotic medication in this disease has not been evaluated.

Temporal (Giant Cell) Arteritis

Temporal (giant cell) arteritis is a systemic inflammatory vasculopathy that should be considered in any patient with stroke older than 50 years.[159] Treatment decisions must often be made before confirmation of the diagnosis. If the clinical features (described elsewhere) are present or the erythrocyte sedimentation rate (ESR) is elevated, a unilateral temporal artery biopsy should be performed. Corticosteroids, the mainstay of therapy, can be initiated before biopsy and will not affect the results if the procedure is performed within approximately 10 to 14 days.[159,160] For patients presenting with acute visual loss, immediate treatment with high-dose (up to 1000 mg daily) intravenous methylprednisolone for 3 to 5 days has been recommended on the basis of a favorable response in a single case report.[161] Other investigators have suggested that intravenous pulse steroid therapy offers no benefit over oral therapy but carries greater expense and risk.[162]

Chevalet and colleagues[163] performed a randomized clinical trial involving 164 patients with uncomplicated temporal arteritis. These researchers compared the following three dosage regimens: 240-mg intravenous pulse of methylprednisolone (IVMP) followed by 0.7 mg/kg/day of oral prednisone (group 1), 0.7 mg/kg/day of oral prednisone without an IV pulse (group 2), and 240 mg IVMP followed by 0.5 mg/kg/day of oral prednisone (group 3).[163] Steroid doses were then tapered starting 6 months after therapy. At 1 year, there were no significant differences among the three groups with regard to clinical symptoms, laboratory parameters, or steroid-related side effects. However, patients who did experience recurrent symptoms were regarded as corticosteroid-resistant and required higher cumulative doses of steroids during the follow-up period. The relative risks and benefits of this approach may differ in patients with acute ophthalmic or cerebrovascular symptoms. Chan and associates,[164] who performed a retrospective cohort study of 100 patients with acute visual loss due to giant cell arteritis, found a greater likelihood of improved vision in the group treated with intravenous steroids (40%) than in those receiving oral steroids (13%).[164] Thus, the role of intravenous steroids remains uncertain, and some investigators recommend using high-dose intravenous steroids only for those patients whose clinical condition progresses in spite of receiving oral steroid therapy.[165,166]

Maintenance therapy with daily oral prednisone, starting at 40 to 80 mg daily (0.5 to 1.0 mg/kg),[167] should then be initiated, with a gradual tapering of dosage. The goal of maintenance therapy is to prevent subsequent ischemic events, and the tapering should likely be adjusted to the patient's clinical response, ESR, and C-reactive protein value. There is great controversy about the duration of therapy and the rapidity of the taper. However, in a cohort study involving 90 patients, the timing of cessation of therapy had no effect on the risk of recurrent symptoms.[168] If symptoms recur or there is an increase in ESR or C-reactive protein value during dosage tapering, the prednisone dose should be increased by 20 to 40 mg/day for 2 to 3 weeks, after which the tapering can be resumed.

Experience with other immunosuppressive agents for temporal arteritis is limited. Methotrexate has been studied in a randomized clinical trial involving 42 patients with new-onset giant cell arteritis confirmed by biopsy.[169] All patients were initially treated with high-dose steroids, were started on steroid dosage tapering, and then were randomly assigned to receive either methotrexate or placebo for 2 years. Compared with steroids alone, the addition of methotrexate, 10 mg orally per day, reduced the risk of relapse from 84% to 45% ($P = 0.02$). Methotrexate was also steroid sparing, in that the cumulative dose of steroids was reduced in the methotrexate group, but the overall incidence of side effects was similar in the two groups. The role of methotrexate as immediate treatment is unclear.[162] Further research regarding methotrexate is needed, but it should be considered a possible alternative

or adjunctive to steroid therapy in any patient for whom steroid-related side effects are intolerable. Azathioprine was shown to reduce the required dose of corticosteroids in a randomized trial involving 31 patients,[170] but its efficacy is unproven, and further study is necessary. Cyclosporine offered no benefit over steroids alone in a small open trial.[171]

Cerebral Vasculitis Related to Collagen Vascular Disorders

Systemic vasculitides include polyarteritis nodosa (PAN), Sjögren's disease, Churg-Strauss angiitis, Wegener's granulomatosis, Henoch-Schönlein purpura, cryoglobulinemia, systemic lupus erythematosus, scleroderma, and rheumatoid arthritis, each of which is characterized by the pattern of involvement of other organ systems.[172–184] Neurologic involvement is variable in each of these disorders and is typically less prominent than the other features, but it may be the initial manifestation in some cases. Further, neurologic symptoms, when present, are rarely due to cerebral vasculitis or cerebritis but, rather, are more commonly related to cardiac emboli (such as nonbacterial thrombotic endocarditis), hypercoagulable states (such as antiphospholipid antibody syndrome), or atherosclerosis (due to renovascular hypertension or steroid-induced diabetes mellitus).[185,186] Treatment of the cerebral component is, in general, dictated by the treatment of the systemic disease and often includes corticosteroids and other immunosuppressant agents.[172] When the diagnosis of concomitant cerebral vasculitis exists and persists despite treatment of the systemic process, more aggressive treatment as for IACNS may be warranted; however, data to support this approach are lacking.

Cerebral Vasculitis Related to Infection

Among the secondary causes of vasculitis, infectious causes include meningovascular syphilis, tuberculous meningitis, other bacterial (*Streptococcus pneumoniae*, *Neisseria*) meningitis, fungal (*Aspergillus*, *Candida*, *Coccidioides*, *Cryptococcus*, *Histoplasma*, *Mucor*) meningoencephalitides, neurocysticercosis, varicella-zoster virus (VZV) encephalitis, and human immunodeficiency virus (HIV).[187–219] Specifically directed antimicrobial therapy is advisable for each of these disorders and may improve the vasculopathic angiographic features,[193] although this approach may not necessarily have any effect on the clinical course.[220] Immunosuppressive regimens are often used in patients with persisting vasculopathy[193,220]; the efficacy of this approach is unproven, however. The roles of antiplatelet agents, anticoagulation, and thrombolysis in infection-related vasculopathy are also uncertain, and caution with their use is advised because there may be a necrotizing component of the vasculitis as well as dysfunction of the blood-brain barrier, thereby increasing the risk of ICH.[221]

Cerebral Vasculitis Related to Toxins

Toxins implicated in cerebral vasculitis include cocaine, amphetamines, heroin, lysergic acid diethylamide (LSD), and inhaled volatile solvents (glue sniffing), although all of these agents may result in a process more like vasospasm after SAH than a true inflammatory vasculitis.[222–227] Other sympathomimetic agents, such as ephedrine and phenyl-propanolamine, may have similar effects.[228-230] In the setting of acute ischemic stroke associated with drug use (cocaine, in particular), there is evidence to suggest that a combination of vasospasm and superimposed thrombosis may occur.[231] In such cases, thrombolysis may be a reasonable therapeutic option in the first few hours, and antiplatelet therapy may be appropriate later.[232]

No specific therapy has been shown to improve the vasculopathy, but the offending agent should certainly be removed.[227] Patients should be closely monitored and treated for symptoms of drug withdrawal. Because many abusers of illicit drugs also abuse alcohol, the clinical approach should include a low threshold for initiating benzodiazepines for symptoms or signs of alcohol withdrawal.

Ideal therapy for ongoing vasculitis among users of methamphetamine has not been identified, in part because the pathogenesis of the vasculitis is unclear. Steroid therapy has been used in some patients on a short-term basis, but there is little evidence to suggest that it is beneficial.[227] Calcium channel blockers have been advocated for the treatment of cocaine users with vasospasm or vasculitis, but there are no formal data regarding their efficacy.

Long-term secondary stroke prevention strategies should include cessation of the identified abused drug. Antiplatelet therapy is probably indicated for patients with ischemic stroke, although data specifically applicable to stroke in the setting of drug abuse are limited.

Cerebral Vasculitis Related to Neoplasms

Arteriopathies may rarely complicate the course of systemic neoplasms. The small and medium-sized intracranial arteries may be affected by carcinomatous or lymphomatous meningitis as well as endovascular (angiotrophic large cell) lymphoma. The prognosis is quite poor in these cases. Steroids and palliative chemotherapy may offer some transient benefit for the inflammatory vasculopathy, although in some cases, this approach has led to acute worsening of symptoms.[233-235]

HEMATOLOGIC DISORDERS

Ischemic stroke may be associated with a number of hereditary and acquired prothrombotic states, including abnormalities of red blood cell or platelet function, coagulation factors, and endogenous fibrinolysis (see Table 54.2). These disorders are uncommon but are overrepresented among young stroke victims and should be considered when no alternative cause is identified.[1-4]

Prothrombotic Disorders

Disorders of the Coagulation System

The most common inherited disorder of coagulation, present in up to 8% of the normal population, is factor V Leiden mutation, which causes resistance to activated protein C.[236,237] However, the role of factor V Leiden mutation in stroke is uncertain. Stroke is also associated with inherited deficiencies of protein C, protein S, and antithrombin III, which are far less common; acquired deficiencies may occur, however, because these factors

may be depleted in nephrotic syndrome, hepatic disease, and pregnancy. Prothrombotic tendencies are also found in association with oral contraceptive use, systemic inflammatory disorders, and malignancies. Hyperhomocysteinemia may also predispose to thrombosis, as described previously.

In the setting of acute ischemic stroke, these underlying inherited or acquired disorders may not be recognized, and patients may be treated with standard thrombolytic or antithrombotic therapy.[238] Long-term anticoagulation is often recommended for secondary prevention among stroke survivors with a confirmed prothrombotic state, although this approach remains rather controversial.[239] Those rare patients with known protein C or protein S deficiencies should not be treated initially with warfarin unless heparin is given concurrently, because there is a small risk of inducing a transient hypercoagulable state with warfarin alone.[240]

Antiphospholipid Antibody Syndrome

Antiphospholipid antibodies (APLAs) may occur either with systemic disorders or in isolation. They appear to be an independent risk factor for both arterial and venous thromboembolism in some but not all studies, because their presence may be confounded by other disorders or medications.[241-251] The mechanism by which APLAs may lead to thrombosis is uncertain, but they appear to interfere with endogenous anticoagulants, protein C, and platelet homeostasis. Moreover, APLAs are relatively common, occurring in up to 10% of the normal population,[252,253] suggesting that not all patients with this laboratory abnormality require specific treatment. In most asymptomatic patients with APLAs, there is no well-defined role for primary prevention. However, asymptomatic patients with systemic lupus erythematosus and APLAs appear to be at very high risk for thromboembolic events[254] and should perhaps receive prophylactic treatment, although this issue has not been directly studied. Finally, a distinction should be made between the mere presence of APLAs and the APLA syndrome, which is characterized by the occurrence of multiple thromboembolic events.

In the acute setting, t-PA has been used for stroke due to APLA syndrome.[238] However, assessment of the eligibility of such patients for thrombolysis may be obscured if the partial thromboplastin time (PTT) is spuriously prolonged owing to the presence of APLAs. Prolonged PTT is an exclusion criterion for the use of intravenous t-PA, but only if the patient has received heparin or has a known predisposition to bleed (such as a factor deficiency).[255] This is not the case with APLAs, so patients with falsely prolonged PTT due to APLAs should still be considered candidates for thrombolysis. Anti–t-PA antibodies have been identified in patients with APLA syndrome[256]; these antibodies may theoretically attenuate the potential effect of thrombolysis, but this issue has not been evaluated.

Preventive strategies for patients who have experienced stroke or other thromboembolic events include antithrombotic and immunomodulatory therapies. The prospective Antiphospholipid Antibody Stroke Study (APASS) specifically addressed the role of APLAs in a large population of patients with non-cardioembolic, non–carotid-related stroke as part of the Warfarin versus Aspirin for Recurrent

Chapter Fifty-Five

Medical Therapy of Intracerebral and Intraventricular Hemorrhage

Lewis B. Morgenstern

Blood frightens people. Although acute hemorrhage is white rather than red on a CT scan, it usually prompts an emergency department physician to rapidly call a tertiary referral center to transfer the patient. The physician accepting the call at the referral center is frequently left wondering what the referral center can do for the patient that the local community hospital cannot. The good news is that although we still have no "magic bullet" to treat intracerebral and intraventricular hemorrhage, aggressive therapy is likely to reduce mortality and improve outcome. Surgery remains controversial, and many therapies can be provided at any hospital with a good intensive care unit and neurologic or neurosurgical expertise.

This chapter discusses medical therapy of spontaneous intracerebral hemorrhage (ICH) and intraventricular hemorrhage (IVH) in adults. Epidemiology, clinical presentation, imaging and surgical treatment are covered elsewhere in this book. Care for ICH or IVH begins in the community with prompt recognition, transport, and triage of the patient with acute stroke. In the emergency department, after a *stat* head computed tomography (CT) scan determines that a spontaneous cerebral hemorrhage has occurred and a search for the cause begins, therapy commences with blood pressure control and assessment of cerebral edema. A watchful eye for hydrocephalus and intensive care unit (ICU) complications are critical. Early feeding and rehabilitation are important.

This chapter begins with emergency department management of the patient with acute ICH or IVH, which is followed by a discussion of the utility of specialized wards for patients with ICH or IVH and the importance of aggressive medical therapies. Edema, hydrocephalus, and ventricular drainage procedures are then discussed; instillation of "lytics" is considered in this section. Next is a discussion of rebleeding and the steps to prevent this serious complication. Brief consideration is given to the circumstances special to warfarin-related cerebral hemorrhage. Finally, patient selection for surgical interventions and the predictors of outcome are dealt with. Primary IVH is rare.[1] One study found that primary IVH accounted for only 3% of all cases of IVH.[2] We therefore discuss ICH and IVH as one entity.

EMERGENCY DEPARTMENT MANAGEMENT

Table 55–1 reviews the steps in the care of patients with ICH or IVH. Initial concerns should focus on the "ABCs" of emergency therapy. The patient who has brainstem injury or in whom aspiration or trauma is associated with the cerebral bleed may have compromise of airway or breathing. These complications are treated with airway management (with adequate cervical spine protection for those in whom trauma is suspected) and intubation as discussed later. Patients who have been immobile for long periods before they are brought to the emergency department may have rhabdomyolysis and renal failure; these possibilities should be kept in mind.[3]

THE IMPORTANCE OF AGGRESSIVE MEDICAL THERAPIES

Stroke Units and Intensive Care Units

Patients with ICH or IVH should be cared for in specialized units where personnel are familiar with both intensive care procedures and neurologic injury. At the minimum, this statement implies training of nurses to perform neurologic examinations and to promptly recognize deterioration so that rescue therapies can be instituted to halt worsening. The evidence in support of providing care in specialized hospital areas comes from the data on stroke units[4-6] and specific studies on the role of stroke units in caring for patients with ICH. Ronning and colleagues[7] randomly assigned 121 patients with ICH to an acute stroke unit or a general medical ward. Thirty-day mortality rates

Therapy

Table 55.1   Emergency Department Considerations for Suspected Intracerebral Hemorrhage (ICH)

1. Secure airway, breathing, and circulation.
2. History of recent head trauma, hypertension, tumor arteriovenous malformation (AVM), aneurysm, clotting disorder, or chemotherapy?
3. Order *stat* head CT scan.
4. Collect and send specimens for complete blood count, prothrombin time, partial thromboplastin time, chemistry panel, and urine drug screen.
5. Insert intravenous and Foley bladder catheters.
6. If CT confirms ICH: reduce blood pressure slowly by no more than 15%–20% to mean arterial pressure of 100–110 mm Hg if possible.
7. Obtain neurologic and neurosurgical consultations.
8. Suspect aneurysm or AVM if CT shows subarachnoid hemorrhage, hemorrhage in an atypical location, or the patient is not known to have hypertension.
9. Watch patient closely for signs of deterioration; repeat CT if deterioration occurs.
10. Invoke intracranial pressure protocol if Glasgow Coma Scale score is less than 14.
11. Consider early surgery (see text).
12. Treat fever and hyperglycemia or hypoglycemia.

Table 55.2   Representative Standard Orders for Patients Admitted to an Intensive Care Unit or Stroke Unit with Cerebral Hemorrhage

Admit to Intensive Care Unit/Stroke Unit
Diagnosis: intracerebral hemorrhage
Condition: critical
Vital signs: q1h with neurologic checks and pulse oximetry
Activity: bedrest; have patient up with therapists after 24 hours if stable
Call physician if: temp >38.0°C (obtain chest x-ray, urinalysis and culture, blood culture × 2, and give acetaminophen, 1 g q6h, and cooling blanket to keep temp <38.0°C); mean arterial blood pressure >120 mm Hg; finger-stick glucose q6h, call if glucose >150 or <70 mg/dL for sliding scale; pulse <60, >120 bpm; respirations <8, >24 min; change in National Institutes of Health Stroke Scale score of ≥ 2 points
Diet: NPO until cleared by speech pathologist
Allergies: ?
Lab tests: electrolytes, blood chemistry
IV fluids: normal saline at 80 mL/hour
Pneumatic compression stockings; may switch to heparin, 5000 usc q12h after 48 hours
Ventillator settings as needed
Histamine₂ blocker

in the stroke unit patients were 39%, compared with 63% in the general medical ward group. No difference between the groups was found for the proportions of patients discharged home and patients requiring placement in long-term facilities.

The decision to assign patients to a neurologic ICU rather than a general ICU is also supported by a study that examined outcome in 1000 patients with ICH in 43 ICUs in the United States.[8] Those who were *not* in a neurologic ICU had a higher odds ratio (OR) for mortality, of 3.4 (95% confidence interval [CI], 1.7–7.6). Patients in the ICUs that had a full-time intensivist on staff had a lower mortality rate (OR 0.39; 95% CI, 0.2–0.7).

Fever

Stroke units not only provide rescue treatment for patients with worsening neurologic signs but also give prophylaxis against complications and avoid conditions that are toxic to damaged neurons. Representative standard orders are shown in Table 55–2. Fever is an independent predictor of poor outcome in ICH.[9] No studies have been performed to document that lowering body temperature improves outcome, but there is good evidence that patients with stroke do worse if they have fever.[10,11] In patients with elevated temperatures, an infectious source should be sought assiduously. Prompt use of acetaminophen, and mechanical cooling devices (blankets) is advocated.

Hyperglycemia

Elevated serum glucose concentration also appears to detrimentally affect injured neurons.[12] A high serum glucose level may also predispose to ICH after intravenous administration of recombinant tissue-type plasminogen activator (rt-PA) for acute ischemic stroke.[13] Ensuring

metabolic homeostasis by striving for normal glucose levels is also desirable.

Hypertension

Blood pressure management of the patient with acute ICH or IVH remains controversial, but a consensus is emerging. Although lowering the blood pressure in acute hemorrhage holds the theoretical promise of preventing rebleeding, many researchers have worried that perihematomal ischemia may be worsened. Evidence now suggests that this is a moot point. Experimental laboratory data in dogs first showed that lowering mean arterial pressure within normal limits of cerebral autoregulation did not detrimentally affect regional cerebral blood flow or intracranial pressure (ICP).[14] Positron emission tomography (PET) also fails to demonstrate tissue hypoxia surrounding cerebral hematomas in humans.[15] Powers and colleagues[16] performed a controlled trial of blood pressure reduction in acute patients with ICH and measured perihematomal and global cerebral blood flow; neither declined.

Some researchers suggest that the goal for mean arterial blood pressure should be gradually lowered to less than 130 mm Hg but that reductions of more than 20% should be avoided, and mean arterial blood pressures should not be reduced to less than 84 mm Hg.[3,17] Choice of agent may be important.[18] Intravenous labetalol[19] or nicardipine may provide smooth onset of action and allow physician control of blood pressure in patients without cardiac contraindications to these agents. Nitrates theoretically may worsen cerebral edema owing to their vasodilatory properties.

Mechanical Ventilation

The decision for mechanical ventilation of patients with ICH or IVH relies on a diverse group of indications. One study found that intubation is five times more common in patients with ICH than in those with ischemic stroke.[20] Hypoxia and hypercarbia can damage neurons, contributing to poor outcome. Pulmonary indications include hypoxia related to pneumonia and exacerbated preexisting pulmonary or cardiac conditions. Hypercarbia may be related to central or pulmonary causes. Airway protection in the obtunded patient is also important to avoid aspiration. Intubation is one way of protecting the airway, but an oropharyngeal or nasopharyngeal airway is less invasive. Such an airway is adequate for the patient who has good oxygenation and ventilation but impaired consciousness or brainstem dysfunction that prohibits keeping the airway clear.

Endotracheal intubation has some advantages over simply providing an airway. Intubation further protects against aspiration, allows suctioning of upper respiratory structures, and provides for the administration of some drugs. The stimulation provided during intubation may lead to abrupt elevations in ICP. These elevations may be avoided with a rapid induction procedure using a short-acting neuromuscular blocker, barbiturate, and lidocaine. Supplemental oxygen and the placement of nasogastric or orogastric tubes are important to prevent aspiration.[3]

Deep Venous Thrombosis

Prevention of deep venous thrombosis is critical. Admitted patients should be immediately fitted with pneumatic compression stockings. After a few days, this treatment can be replaced by subcutaneous heparin.

Steroids

Two randomized trials have examined the role of steroids in ICH.[21,22] Both failed to demonstrate a benefit for steroids in patients with ICH. In fact, in one study,[21] patients treated with steroids had more infectious complications than those who did not receive the agents.

Anticonvulsants

No studies have been performed to guide the use of prophylactic anticonvulsants in ICH, although some guidelines recommend their use for a month.[3] It may be prudent to reserve the use of anticonvulsants to patients who exhibit a first seizure, to avoid unnecessarily treating patients who will never have a seizure.

Other Therapies

Critically ill patients should be monitored for infection, and appropriate antibiotics should be instituted if necessary. Frequent change of positioning reduces pressure sores. Gastrointestinal hemorrhage is common in the high stress of an ICU stay. Use of prophylactic histamine$_2$ (H$_2$) blockers is suggested. Early rehabilitation is advisable but has not been well studied. Avoidance of sedation except in patients with documented increased ICP allows the patient to take a more active participation in rehabilitation and neurologic changes to be observed and managed.

PREVENTION OF REBLEEDING

Evidence now suggests that much of the morbidity and mortality in ICH stems from early rebleeding. The first report of the regrowth of cerebral hematomas came from Fujii and associates.[23] They observed that of their 419 patients with ICH who presented within 24 hours of symptom onset, hematoma growth was observed in 14% when imaging was repeated within 24 hours of admission. Patients who presented earliest with larger hemorrhages were likely to have regrowth. Liver disease, an irregularly shaped hematoma on CT, and coagulation abnormalities were also associated with hematoma expansion.

Kazui and associates[24] reported that 36% of 74 patients who underwent imaging within 3 hours had hematoma expansion on later imaging studies. Even after 6 hours, 17% had rebleeding, but none showed rebleeding after 24 hours. This group analyzed potential factors associated with risk of rebleeding.[25] They found that hematoma growth was independently associated with a history of ischemic stroke, liver disease, interaction of either elevated blood glucose (>141 mg/dL) or glycosylated hemoglobin concentration (>5.1%) with systolic blood pressure (>200 mm Hg).

In another study, Brott and colleagues[26] performed head CT scanning in patients with ICH upon emergency department presentation, 1 hour later, and 20 hours later. These researchers found that 26% of the 103 study subjects experienced rebleeding consisting of more than 33% of the initial hematoma volume within 1 hour of hospital arrival. The mean time from hospital arrival to initial CT scan was 89 minutes. This finding implies that a quarter of patients with ICH or IVH rebled within 2.5 hours of the initial bleeding. Brott and colleagues[26] reported that 12% of the remaining patients experienced rebleeding between the 1-hour and 20-hour CT scans.

It seems that hematoma growth happens early, in the majority of cases within the first minutes to hours of the initial bleed. Rebleeding after 6 hours is rare. Patients who have coagulation disorders or a hepatic predisposition for coagulation deficits are at risk. An initial large size and irregularity of the hematoma should raise concern about rebleeding. The roles of blood pressure and glucose are also potential factors.

One possible way to directly determine whether hemostasis has not yet occurred is through CT perfusion imaging. Becker and associates[27] found that extravasation of contrast material in patients with ICH suggested that the hemorrhage was still growing. Extravasation of contrast material can also be demonstrated on magnetic resonance imaging (MRI), with the same correlation with rebleeding.[28] This finding suggests that the group of patients with imaging evidence of continued bleeding are candidates for local or systemic therapies to promote clotting. However, clinical studies are required before such therapies can be advocated. We must also consider that the injection of large volumes of contrast material may exacerbate problems with hemostasis. The safety of contrast material administration in ICH has not been well studied.

The coagulation factors related to the occurrence and growth of hemorrhage remain unknown. Finding specific therapies to intervene in the acute period requires an understanding of the natural phenomena in patients with ICH. One study found that normal systemic hemostatic activation does not occur unless the cerebral hematoma extends into the ventricular system or subarachnoid space.[29] A trial is currently under way to investigate the effect of factor VIIa, which is used in bleeding disorders such as hemophilia, on the prevention of rebleeding in acute ICH. Future areas of research to limit clot enlargement might be preventing lysis of the hemostatic plug, enhancing the formation of the hemostatic plug, and more aggressive lowering of blood pressure during the first 24 hours.

MANAGEMENT OF CEREBRAL EDEMA AND HYDROCEPHALUS

Significant causes of mortality in ICH or IVH are cerebral edema and hydrocephalus. There are therapies for these conditions, and their results are mixed.

Cerebral Edema

Cerebral edema is a well-recognized complication of ICH. Whether the edema is due to an acute space-occupying lesion or the toxic effects of blood is unknown. An intriguing finding is that patients with thrombolysis-related ICH have far less cerebral edema than patients with spontaneous ICH.[30] This finding suggests that something in the clotting process may be directly responsible for the cerebral edema seen in patients with spontaneous ICH. Mass effect and midline shift maximize around 48 hours after symptom onset and, perhaps, during a second peak 2 to 3 weeks after hemorrhage.[31] Despite the success of antiedema therapies in controlling ICP in animal models,[32] the therapeutic value of these agents has not been borne out in human studies. Two randomized trials of therapy for cerebral edema in patients with ICH have been performed. The first utilized intravenous glycerol.[33] A total of 216 patients were randomly assigned to receive either glycerol or a placebo. There was no difference in 6-month mortality rates or functional outcomes between the two groups. A similar trial of hemodilution in ICH compared with the best medical therapy failed to demonstrate an advantage for hemodilution treatment.[34]

Hydrocephalus

Hydrocephalus is an independent predictor of poor outcome from ICH or IVH.[35,36] Hydrocephalus can occur because of obstruction of cerebrospinal fluid (CSF) flow in patients with ventricular clot or communicating hydrocephalus from a variety of causes. The treatment is placement of a ventriculostomy for external drainage of CSF and blood in the ventricular system. Most devices now allow simultaneous measurement of ICP. When the device is first placed, measurement of opening pressure is important. The drain is usually set at 15 cm above the ear to facilitate drainage. The risk of infection rises with time, so a ventricular fluid specimen is collected every other day for analysis to monitor cell count, differential cell counts, and glucose and protein levels as well as for bacterial culture.

The drain should remain in place until the pressure returns to normal (<20 cm H_2O).

Often, when ventricular blood is copious, hydrocephalus becomes chronic, and the patient is drain dependent. Conversion of the ventriculostomy to an internalized shunt must be timed properly. If the externalized shunt is internalized when too much blood still remains, there is the danger of blockage of the shunt by clotting. Waiting too long, however, raises the risk of ventriculitis. In general, when the CSF visually clears of blood and the CSF protein level has decreased towards the normal range, it is time to consider a shunt in a patient who cannot maintain a normal ICP after a trial of 7 to 10 days.

Observational studies suggest that external drainage is associated with a 25% reduction in risk of death and poor outcome compared with conservative treatment.[37] Although ventriculostomy is clearly indicated for patients with hydrocephalus, their outcome is extremely poor. Good outcome in patients with hydrocephalus perhaps occurs only in those with small hemorrhages.[38] Unfortunately, no trials have been conducted to guide our management of hydrocephalus.

An intriguing possibility is lysis of the clot in the ventricular system to improve hydrocephalus. A systemic review suggested a 92% reduction in risk of death and poor outcome compared with conservative treatment.[37] In one study, 10 patients with IVH received direct intraventricular injection of rt-PA and subsequent CSF drainage.[39] Forty percent of patients made a good recovery, and only 1 died. In another group of 20 patients treated with intraventricular urokinase, the mortality was 20%, compared with a predicted mortality of 68%.[40] This large reduction in mortality for a modest number of patients has prompted a larger trial of ventricular clot lysis that is currently under way.

Intracranial Pressure Considerations

Cerebral edema and hydrocephalus are two causes of increased ICP. ICP must be maintained below 20 cm H_2O. To accomplish this goal, evaluation of the underlying cause of the elevation in ICP should proceed. If it is not possible to remove the underlying cause (e.g., surgical removal of the hematoma), an algorithm for treatment of ICP should be followed (Fig. 55–1). It is important to remember that cerebral blood flow depends on adequate cerebral perfusion pressure. *Cerebral perfusion pressure* is the difference between mean arterial blood pressure and ICP. Cerebral perfusion pressure should be kept above 70 mm Hg.[41] If ICP is high, lowering the systemic blood pressure could be deleterious.

When ICP is increased, deterioration in consciousness follows quickly. Patients with elevated ICP should be intubated with ICP precautions as discussed previously. The goal for the pCO_2 is 35 to 40 torr. Hyperventilation to a pCO_2 of 30 to 35 torr decreases cerebral blood flow and reduces edema. The problem is that this effect is short-lived, so it should be reserved for the period immediately before a definitive therapy such as hematoma evacuation.[42,43] The rebound effect from reversal of hyperventilation may dramatically worsen cerebral edema and elevate

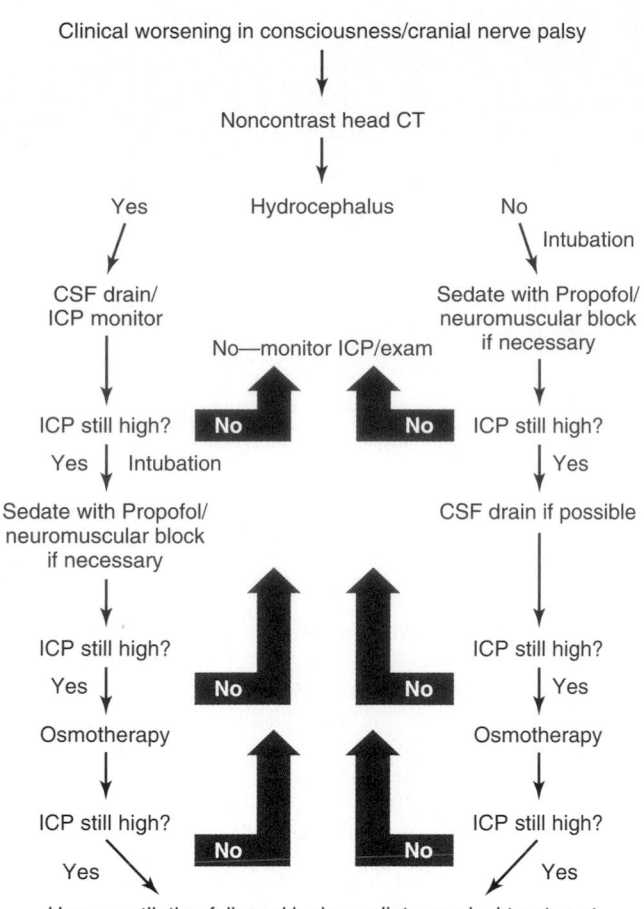

Clinical worsening in consciousness/cranial nerve palsy

Noncontrast head CT

Hydrocephalus

Yes → CSF drain/ICP monitor

No → Intubation → Sedate with Propofol/neuromuscular block if necessary

No—monitor ICP/exam

ICP still high? No
ICP still high? No

Yes | Intubation

Sedate with Propofol/neuromuscular block if necessary

CSF drain if possible

ICP still high? Yes
ICP still high? Yes

No | No

Osmotherapy
Osmotherapy

ICP still high?
ICP still high?

No | No

Yes
Yes

Hyperventilation followed by immediate surgical treatment

FIGURE 55–1 *Suggested algorithm for the management of intracranial pressure in intracerebral hemorrhage. ICP, intracranial pressure; CSF, cerebrospinal fluid.*

ICP.[3] Sedation is accomplished with a continuous drip of intravenous propofol, a short-acting agent that can be turned off for intermittent neurologic examinations. Neuromuscular paralysis may be added (vecuronium is a good choice) but should never be given without proper sedation.

When ICP corrections are needed, osmotherapy is often used. Mannitol is the best-known treatment. Therapy is commenced with an infusion of 1 g/kg, followed by 25 to 50 g every 6 hours to titrate the serum osmolality to 310 to 320 mOsm/kg. Mannitol tends to deplete the intravascular space and therefore to lower mean arterial pressure. An alternative osmotherapy combination is colloid plus furosemide. The choices of colloid are albumin, dextran, and hydroxyethyl starch. The colloid substances allow maintenance of the intravascular space. The risk is pulmonary edema. Careful monitoring of central venous pressures and a critical care specialist consultation are highly recommended. Like hyperventilation, the effect of osmotherapy is short-lived, and rebound elevations in cerebral edema and ICP are likely if the therapy is not tapered slowly.[3]

Mechanical devices to measure ICP are controversial.[44,45] Monitoring ICP is necessary when ventricular drainage is proceeding. In patients with a Glasgow Coma Scale (GCS) score of less than 9 it is also advisable.[3] Because ICH is an asymmetric disease, pressures in the skull may vary, unlike in a global condition such as hepatic failure. Patients may undergo various herniation syndromes while the ICP monitor continues to record a "normal" number. The clinical examination should always be the mainstay for detection of progression and institution of emergency imaging and therapy for patients with progressing cerebral edema and mass effect.

Two experimental therapies may hold promise in the future for the management of cerebral edema and increased ICP. Hypothermia dramatically lowers ICP in animal models. Studies are ongoing for the use of hypothermia in patients who have experienced cardiac arrest, ischemic stroke, and closed-head injury.[46] Its use in ICH seems a logical next step. One potential side effect of hypothermia is coagulopathy, so studies must be performed before this therapy can be advocated for ICH. The other therapy is hemicraniectomy and duraplasty. This treatment involves removing a large portion of the skull and making a broad incision in the dura to allow the brain to swell without added tissue pressure inside the enclosed skull cavity. Impressive results have been reported for small case series of patients with large hemispheric infarctions.[47] The application of hemicraniectomy in ICH has not been reported.

SPECIAL CONSIDERATIONS IN WARFARIN-RELATED INTRACRANIAL HEMORRHAGE

Outcome of warfarin-related ICH is related most to the size of the hemorrhage.[48] Ensuring that the bleeding has stopped is imperative. Emergency hematology consultation should be obtained. Vitamin K should be administered urgently, but it takes a while to work. Fresh-frozen plasma (FFP) has been the "gold standard" of treatment. In a series of 13 patients randomly assigned to receive either FFP or factor IX complex concentrate, coagulopathy reversed significantly faster in the group receiving factor IX than in the group receiving FFP. Neurologic outcomes were the same in the two groups, but the factor IX group had fewer complications.[49]

The issue of how to manage anticoagulation in high-risk patients (e.g., those with prosthetic heart valves or atrial fibrillation) who have an ICH requires further study. One study found that the risk of ischemic stroke within 30 days after cessation of warfarin was less than 5%, but that in the 35 subjects in whom warfarin was quickly restarted, the risk of recurrent ICH was zero during hospitalization.[50] Long-term studies are needed to assess the risks of this therapy.

SELECTION OF PATIENTS FOR SURGERY

Several small studies have investigated surgical treatment of ICH. This discussion concentrates on the overall benefits of surgery and which patients should have surgery. The best reported benefits for hematoma evacuation come from surgical removal of thrombolytic-related ICH. In an observational study, patients treated with surgery had a 65% 30-day survival, compared with a 35% survival for patients treated medically ($P < 0.001$).[51] For patients with spontaneous hemorrhage, it seems that operating long after symptom onset does not improve outcome. The goals of early surgery are to reduce mortality and to improve functional outcome.[52] One randomized study of 20 patients treated within 24 hours of symptom onset found a nonsignificant trend toward better outcome in those treated medically.[53]

In a randomized trial of 34 patients undergoing either medical treatment or surgery within 12 hours of symptom onset for spontaneous supratentorial ICH, Morgenstern and colleagues[54] reported mortality to be 24% in the medical group and 19% in the surgical group (the difference was not statistically significant).[54] Functional outcome was unchanged. When these researchers added another surgical arm to the study, involving operation within 4 hours of symptom onset, they found that early postoperative rebleeding was a problem.[55] Figure 55–2 shows examples of a successful clot evacuation and an evacuation complicated with postoperative hematoma reaccumulation. Clearly, residual hematoma volume is directly related to poor outcome,[54] suggesting that if early surgery could be performed with good hemostasis, the procedure might be of benefit. Achieving hemostasis is probably related in part to the compulsiveness of the surgeon in identifying bleeding of microvessels and to careful coagulation.[56,57]

Earlier attempts at synthesizing the evidence to determine the relative value of surgery in spontaneous supratentorial ICH usually concluded that the evidence was insufficient to allow any conclusions to be drawn.[58,59] The additional data just described, however, indicate that surgery may be beneficial. Systematic reviews now suggest a modest benefit for surgery in reducing death and dependency compared with best medical therapy (OR 0.63; 95% CI, 0.35–1.14).[60] A large, multicenter trial in Europe, the Surgical Trial in Intracerebral Hemorrhage, should provide added insights into the relative benefit of surgery in acute ICH.[61]

From the inclusion criteria of these studies, it appears that surgical benefit may be found for patients who (1) receive early treatment, (2) have moderate-size hematomas (20–80 mL in volume), (3) have GCS scores greater than 4, (4) are younger, (5) are not very ill with other malignant conditions, (6) do not have large amounts of intraventricular blood, and (7) are treated in centers with "compulsive" surgeons. Surgical technique requires further study. Stereotactic approaches allow less disruption of tissue than open craniotomy for deep hemorrhages, but they cannot remove enough hematoma volume in a timely manner. Stereotactic approaches coupled with local thrombolysis may be promising.

For patients with infratentorial hemorrhage the indications for surgery are different. Patients with cerebellar hemorrhage may experience brainstem compression syndromes quickly at any time within the first 3 weeks after the event. Suboccipital craniotomy with removal of the clot is life-saving, and patients recover well if the procedure is carried out at the earliest threat of brainstem compression, before frank herniation occurs.[62]

PREDICTORS OF OUTCOME

Although many researchers have offered complicated formulas, hematoma volume is the most important predictor of outcome from ICH.[63] Initial GCS score is also a potent predictor of outcome.[63,64] In patients with a hematoma volume exceeding 30 mL both morbidity and mortality rates are high. Some workers have tried to replicate the success of ischemic stroke rating scales, such as the National Institutes of Health Stroke Scale score, with an "ICH Score."[65] Predicting which patients will experience deterioration after initial presentation is difficult. Studies attempting to identify clinical predictors have been unsuccessful.[64,66]

Becker and colleagues[67] considered the role of withdrawal of care in patients with ICH. They found that the level of medical support was the biggest predictor of outcome, and that a "Do Not Resuscitate" status is likely to bias outcome data and lead to self-fulfilling prophecies.

New measures of quality of life after ICH are important barometers of recovery and should guide future clinical trial results.[68] Determining whether to use antiplatelet therapy in patients after initial ICH is an important concern. In one study, patients with ICH had a 2.4% yearly risk of recurrence and a 3.0% risk of subsequent ischemic stroke.[69] In a systemic review, the risk of recurrent ICH was 2.3% per year (95% CI, 1.9%–2.7%). For patients with lobar ICH, the risk was almost double—the rate of ischemic stroke was 1.1% per year (95% CI, 0.8%–1.7%).[70]

CONCLUSIONS

Although ICH is a devastating disease, aggressive medical therapy can make a large difference in outcome. Much of the therapy is "supportive," but it is also intensive and must be started urgently. A nihilistic approach to the care of patients with ICH is quickly dissipating. When care is limited, recovery is all but impossible. Future studies of surgery, neuroprotection, and strategies to prevent rebleeding will likely revolutionize ICH therapy.

In the interim, aggressive but reasonable treatment of the patient with ICH is warranted. Conservative control of blood pressure, treatment of fever, and glucose regulation are important. Patients with ICH or IVH should be cared for on specialized wards with well-trained personnel. When elevated ICP is suspected, head CT should be performed, and an ICP treatment algorithm invoked. Early feeding and rehabilitation are also important. Prevention of complications such as pneumonia, ventriculitis, and deep venous thrombosis are necessary. Compulsive attention to these intensive medical therapies are of great value for the patient with ICH, whose life and functional status are clearly related to the level of care provided by the physician in charge of the case.

Acknowledgment

The author wishes to thank Dr. Marc D. Malkoff for reviewing this chapter.

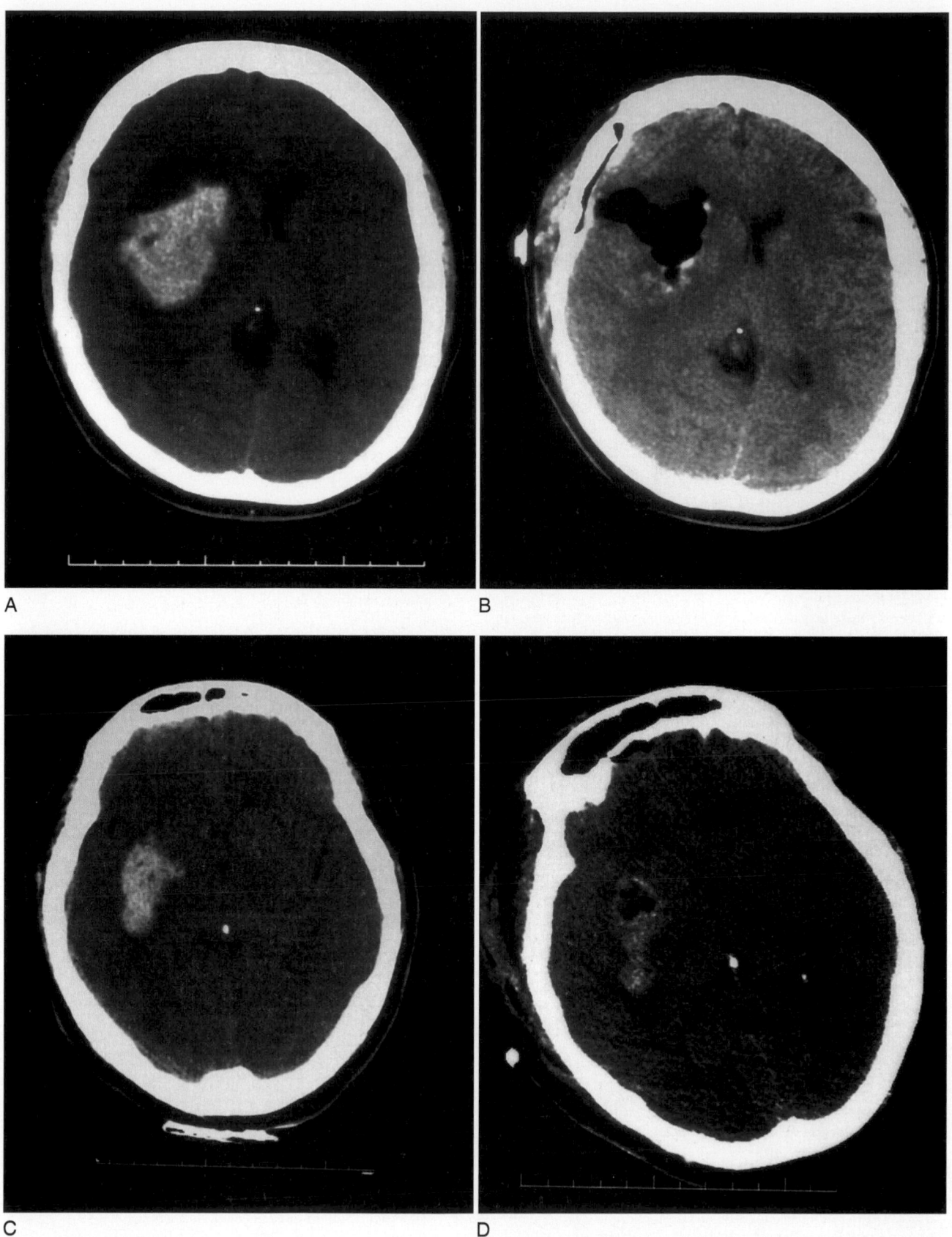

FIGURE 55–2 *Surgical clot removal by craniotomy for intracranial hemorrhage within 4 hours of symptom onset in two patients. Baseline head CT scan (A) and 24-hour postoperative CT scan (B) of a patient in whom clot evacuation was successful. Dark areas in the hematoma cavity represent gel foam and air, which subsequently reabsorbed. Baseline head CT scan (C) and 24-hour postoperative CT scan (D) of a patient in whom hematoma regrowth occurred after clot evacuation.*

References

1. Marti-Fabregas J, Piles S, Guardia E, et al: Spontaneous primary intraventricular hemorrhage: Clinical data, etiology and outcome. J Neurol 246:287–91, 1999.
2. Darby DG, Donnan GA, Saling MA, et al: Primary intraventricular hemorrhage: Clinical and neuropsychological findings in a prospective stroke series. Neurology 38:68–75, 1988.
3. Broderick JP, Adams HP, Barsan W, et al: Guidelines for the management of spontaneous intracerebral hemorrhage. Stroke 30:905–915, 1999.
4. Langhorne P, Dennis M (eds): Stroke Units: An Evidence Based Approach. London, BMJ Publishing Group, 1998.
5. Ronning OM, Guldvog B: Stroke units versus general medical wards. I: 12 and 18 month survival: a randomized controlled trial. Stroke 29:58–62, 1998.
6. Ronning OM, Guldvog B: Stroke units versus general medical wards. II: Neurological deficits and activities of daily living. Stroke 29:586–592, 1998.
7. Ronning, OM, Guldvog, B, Stavem K: The benefit of an acute stroke unit in patients with intracranial hemorrhage: A controlled trial. J Neurol Neurosurg Psychiatry 70:631–634, 2001.
8. Diringer MN, Edwards DF: Admission to a neurologic/neurosurgical intensive care unit is associated with reduced mortality rate after intracerebral hemorrhage. Crit Care Med 29:635–40, 2001.
9. Schwarz S, Hafner K, Aschoff A, et al: Incidence and prognostic significance of fever following intracerebral hemorrhage. Neurology 54:354–61, 2000.
10. Azzimondi G, Bassein L, Nonino F, et al: Fever in acute stroke worsens prognosis: A prospective study. Stroke 26:2040, 1995.
11. Reith J, Jorgensen HS, Pedersen PM, et al: Body temperature in acute stroke: Relation to stroke severity, infarct size, mortality, and outcome. Lancet 347:422, 1996.
12. Pulsinelli WA, Levy DE, Sigsbee B, et al: Increased damage after ischemic stroke in patients with hyperglycemia with or without established diabetes mellitus. Am J Med 74:540, 1983.
13. Demchuk AM, Morgenstern LB, Krieger DW, et al: Serum glucose level and diabetes predict tissue plasminogen activator-related intracerebral hemorrhage in acute ischemic stroke. Stroke 30:34–9, 1999.
14. Qureshi AI, Wilson DA, Hanley DF, et al: Pharmacologic reduction of mean arterial pressure does not adversely affect regional cerebral blood flow and intracranial pressure in experimental intracerebral hemorrhage. Crit Care Med 27:965–971, 1999.
15. Hirano T, Read SJ, Abbott DF, et al: No evidence of hypoxic tissue on 18F-fluoromisonidazole PET after intracerebral hemorrhage. Neurology 53:2179–2182, 1999.
16. Powers, WJ, Zazulia AR, Videen TO, et al: Autoregulation of cerebral blood flow surrounding acute (6 to 22 hours) intracerebral hemorrhage. Neurology 57:18–24, 2001.
17. Morgenstern LB, Yonas H: Lowering blood pressure in acute intracerebral hemorrhage. Neurology 57:5–6, 2001.
18. Kuronda K, Kuwata N, Sato N, et al: Changes in cerebral blood flow accompanied with reduction of blood pressure treatment in patients with hypertensive intracerebral hemorrhages. Neurological Research 19:169–173, 1997.
19. Patel RV, Kertland HR, Jahns BE, et al: Labetalol: Response and safety in critically ill hemorrhagic stroke patients. Ann Pharmacother 27:180–181, 1993.
20. Gujjar AR, Deibert E, Manno EM, et al: Mechanical ventilation for ischemic stroke and intracerebral hemorrhage: Indications, timing, and outcome. Neurology 51:447–451, 1998.
21. Poungvarin N, Bhoopat W, Viriyavejakul A, et al: Effects of dexamethasone in primary supratentorial intracerebral hemorrhage. N Engl J Med 316:1229–1233, 1987.
22. Tellez H, Bauer R: Dexamethasone as treatment in cerebrovascular disease. 1: A controlled study in intracerebral hemorrhage. Stroke 4:541–546, 1973.
23. Fujii Y, Tanaka R, Takeuchi S, et al: Hematoma enlargement in spontaneous intracerebral hemorrhage. J Neurosurg 80:51–57, 1994.
24. Kazui S, Naritomi H, Yamamoto H, et al: Enlargement of spontaneous intracerebral hemorrhage. Stroke 27:1783–1787, 1996.
25. Kazui S, Minematsu K, Yamamoto H, et al: Predisposing factors to enlargement of spontaneous intracerebral hematoma. Stroke 28:2370–2375, 1997.
26. Brott T, Broderick J, Kothari R, et al: Early hemorrhage growth in patients with intracerebral hemorrhage. Stroke 28:1–5, 1997.
27. Becker KJ, Baxter AB, Bybee HM, et al: Extravasation of radiographic contrast is an independent predictor of death in primary intracerebral hemorrhage. Stroke 30:2025–2032, 1999.
28. Murai Y, Ikeda Y, Teramoto A, et al: Magnetic resonance imaging: Documented extravasation as an indicator of acute hypertensive intracerebral hemorrhage. J. Neurosurg 88:650–655, 1998.
29. Fujii Y, Takeuchi S, Harada A, et al: Hemostatic activation in spontaneous intracerebral hemorrhage. Stroke 32:883–890, 2001.
30. Gebel J, Brott T, Sila C, et al: Deceased perihematomal edema in thrombolysis—related intracerebral hemorrhage compared with spontaneous intracerebral hemorrhage. Stroke 31:596–600, 2000.
31. Zazulia A, Diringer M, Derdeyn C, et al: Progression of mass effect after intracerebral hemorrhage. Stroke 30:1167–1173, 1999.
32. Qureshi AI, Wilson DA, Traystman RJ: Treatment of elevated intracranial pressure in experimental intracerebral hemorrhage: Comparison between mannitol and hypertonic saline. Neurosurgery 44:1055–1063, 1999.
33. Yu YL, Kumana CR, Lauder IJ, et al: Treatment of acute cerebral hemorrhage with intravenous glycerol: A double-blind, placebo-controlled, randomized trial. Stroke 23:967–971, 1992.
34. Italian Acute Stroke Study Group: Haemodilution in acute stroke: Results of the Italian haemodilution trial. Lancet 1(8581):318–321, 1988.
35. Phan TG, Vierkant RA, Wijdicks EF: Hydrocephalus is a determinant of early mortality in putaminal hemorrhage. Stroke 31:2157–62, 2000.
36. Diringer MN, Edwards DF, Zazulia AR: Hydrocephalus: A previously unrecognized predictor of poor outcome from supratentorial intracerebral hemorrhage. Stroke 29:1352–1357, 1998.
37. Nieuwkamp DJ, deGans K, Rinkel GJ, et al: Treatment and outcome of severe intraventricular extension in patients with subarachnoid or intracerebral hemorrhage: A systematic review of the literature. J Neurol 247:117–21, 2000.
38. Adams RE, Diringer MN: Response to external ventricular drainage in spontaneous intracerebral hemorrhage with hydrocephalus. Neurology 50:519–23, 1998.
39. Goh KY, Poon WS: Recombinant tissue plasminogen activator for the treatment of spontaneous adult intraventricular hemorrhage. Surg Neurol 50:526–31, 1998.
40. Naff NJ, Carhuapoma JR, Williams MA, et al: Treatment of intraventricular hemorrhage with urokinase. Stroke 31:841–847, 2000.
41. Diringer MN: Intracerebral hemorrhage: Pathophysiology and management. Crit Care Med 21:1591–1603, 1993.
42. Fortune JB, Feustel PJ, Graca L, et al: Effect of hyperventilation, mannitol, and ventriculostomy drainage on cerebral blood flow after head injury. J Trauma 39:1091–1097, 1995.
43. Van Santbrink H, Maas AJR, Avezaat CJJ: Continuous monitoring of partial pressure of brain tissue oxygen in patients with severe head injury. Neurosurgery 38:21–31, 1996.
44. Frank J: Large hemispheric infarction, deterioration, and intracranial pressure. Neurology 45:1286–1290, 1995.
45. Schwab S, Aschoff A, Spranger M, et al: The value of ICP monitoring in acute hemispheric stroke. Neurology 47:393–398, 1996.
46. Clifton GL, Miller ER, Choi SC, et al: Lack of effect of induction of hypothermia after acute brain injury. N Engl J Med 344:556–563, 2001.
47. Schwab S, Steiner T, Aschoff A, et al: Early hemicraniectomy in patients with complete middle cerebral artery infarction. Stroke 29:1888–1893, 1998.
48. Berwaerts J, Dijkhuizen RS, Robb OJ, et al: Prediction of functional outcome and in-hospital mortality after admission with oral anticoagulant-related intracerebral hemorrhage. Stroke 31:2558–62, 2000.
49. Boulis NM, Bobek MP, Schmaier A, et al: Use of factor IX complex in warfarin-related intracranial hemorrhage. Neurosurgery 45:1113–1119, 1999.
50. Phan TG, Koh M, Wijdicks EFM: Safety of discontinuation of anticoagulation in patients with intracranial hemorrhage at high thromboembolic risk. Arch Neurol 57:1710–1713, 2000.
51. Mahaffey KW, Granger CB, Sloan MA, et al: Neurosurgical evacuation of intracranial hemorrhage after thrombolytic therapy for acute myocardial infarction: Experience from the GUSTO-I Trial. Am Heart J 138:493–9, 1999.
52. Fujitsu K, Muramoto M, Ikeda Y, et al: Indications for surgical treatment of putaminal hemorrhage. J Neurosurg 73:518–525, 1990.

53. Zuccarello M, Brott T, Derex L, et al: Early surgical treatment for supratentorial intracerebral hemorrhage: A randomized feasibility study. Stroke 30:1833–1839, 1999.

54. Morgenstern LB, Frankowski RF, Shedden P, et al: Surgical treatment for intracerebral hemorrhage (STICH). Neurology 51:1359–1363, 1998.

55. Morgenstern LB, Demchuk AM, Kim DH, et al: Rebleeding leads to poor outcome in ultra-early craniotomy for intracerebral hemorrhage. Neurology 56:1294–1299, 2001.

56. Kaneko M, Tanaka K, Shimada T, et al: Long-term evaluation of ultra-early operation for hypertensive intracerebral hemorrhage in 100 cases. J Neurosurg 58: 838–842, 1983.

57. Kaneko M, Koba T, Yokoyama T: Early surgical treatment for hypertensive intracerebral hemorrhage. J Neurosurg 46:579–583, 1977.

58. Hankey GJ, Hon C: Surgery for primary intracerebral hemorrhage: Is it safe and effective? Stroke 28:2126–2132, 1997.

59. Prasad K, Browman G, Srivastava A, et al: Surgery in primary supratentorial intracerebral hematoma: A meta-analysis of randomized trials. Acta Neurol Scand 95:103–110, 1997.

60. Fernandes HM, Gregson B, Siddique S, et al: Surgery in intracerebral hemorrhage the uncertainty continues. Stroke 31:2511–2516, 2000.

61. Mendelow AD: Surgical Trial in Intracerebral Hemorrhage (STICH). Acta Neurochir 76:521–522, 2000.

62. Montes JM, Wong JH, Fayad PB, Awad IA: Stereotactic computed tomographic-guided aspiration and thrombolysis of intracerebral hematoma: Protocol and preliminary experience. Stroke 31:834–840, 2000.

63. Broderick JP, Brott TG, Duldner JE, et al: Volume of intracerebral hemorrhage: A powerful and easy-to-use predictor of 30-day mortality. Stroke 24:987–993, 1993.

64. Flemming, KD, Wijdicks EF, St. Louis EK, et al: Predicting deterioration in patients with lobar hemorrhages. J Neurol Neurosurg Psychiatry 66:600–605, 1999.

65. Hemphill JC, Bonovich DC, Besmertis L, et al: The ICH score: A simple, reliable grading scale for intracerebral hemorrhage. Stroke 32:891–897, 2001.

66. Mayer SA, Sacco RL, Shi T, et al: Neurologic deterioration in noncomatose patients with supratentorial intracerebral hemorrhage. Neurology 44:1379–1384, 1994.

67. Becker KJ, Cohen WA, Bybee HM, et al: Withdrawal of support in intracerebral hemorrhage may lead to self-fulfilling prophecies. Neurology 56:766–72, 2001.

68. Hanedani AG, Wells CK, Brass LM, et al: A quality-of-life instrument for young hemorrhagic stroke patients. Stroke 32:687–695, 2001.

69. Hill MD, Silver FL, Austin PC, et al: Rate of stroke recurrence in patients with primary intracerebral hemorrhage. Stroke 31:123–127, 2000.

70. Bailey RD, Hart RG, Benavente O, et al: Recurrent brain hemorrhage is more frequent that ischemic stroke after intracranial hemorrhage. Neurology 56:773–777, 2001.

Chapter Fifty-Six

Rehabilitation and Recovery of the Patient with Stroke

Bruce H. Dobkin

OVERVIEW OF NEUROLOGIC REHABILITATION

The rehabilitation of the patient with stroke aims to lessen physical and cognitive impairments, increase functional independence, lessen the burden of care provided by significant others, reintegrate the patient into the family and community, and restore the patient's health-related quality of life. Rehabilitation differs from usual neurologic care in that its long-term goal is to lessen disability and to give patients the opportunity to participate in their typical roles and activities. Despite this soft-sounding edge, neurologic rehabilitation draws heavily from the neuroscientific bases for learning and neural adaptability.

Physicians who consider the management of stroke a "done deal" beyond the first 3 hours or few days after a disabling brain injury are abandoning their obligation to provide best patient care. Along with offering interventions to prevent another stroke, stroke neurologists and other clinicians who treat acute stroke ought to be familiar with the short-term and long-term interventions that may prevent complications of immobility, reduce impairments and disabilities, and improve quality of life for their patients.

Specialized Assessment and Outcome Measures

To grasp the special concerns of neurorehabilitation services and outcomes, the clinician must be familiar with certain jargon.

Impairments such as hemiplegia and hemineglect are measured by the clinical and neurologic examination or by standard scales such as the National Institutes of Health Stroke Scale (NIHSS) and the Fugl-Meyer Assessment of Sensorimotor Recovery. The Fugl-Meyer Assessment measures both selective and synergistic movements.

Disabilities are the functional restrictions induced by impairments, such as the inability to walk without physical assistance. The Barthel Index (BI) (Table 56.1) and the Functional Independence Measure (FIM) (Table 56.2) are commonly used ordinal scales for the semiquantification of the level of independence in activities of daily living (ADLs).

On admission to inpatient rehabilitation, the majority of patients have a moderate level of disability, with a BI of 40 to 60 or a total FIM score of 40 to 80. These impairment and disability scales do not reflect fine motor function, the ease of completion, quality of execution, or time for completion of a task, or whether an affected upper extremity is used to carry it out. Patients who score 100 on the BI or more than 60 on the motor subscore of the FIM are continent and can feed, bathe, and dress themselves; get up out of bed and chairs; walk at least 150 feet, but usually a block or more; and ascend and descend stairs. A maximum score does not imply that such people can cook, keep house, live alone, and meet the public, but they usually get along without attendant care. A BI of less than 60 at hospital discharge predicts a level of dependence that makes discharge to home less likely. Since 2002, scores on the FIM serve as an economic modifying factor in the Medicare payment system for inpatient rehabilitation in the United States.

A general relationship exists between motor impairment and disability scores. The NIHSS performed 7 days after a stroke forecasts good recovery or severe disability at 3 months.[1] The NIHSS score also describes the severity of impairment observed during inpatient stroke rehabilitation.[2] The Orpington Prognostic Scale is a bit easier to use than the NIHSS and may be modestly better as a predictor of ADLs at 3 to 6 months after a mild to moderate stroke.[3]

Handicaps arise from impairments and disabilities but are driven by barriers in the environment. They include the disadvantages that limit or prevent the fulfillment of a usual role or activity. The scales of handicap describe how well subjects participate in home, work, and community activities, which are called *instrumental ADLs*. They can be measured, in part, by the Frenchay Activities Index.[4]

Health-related quality of life (QOL), which includes a patient's perception of his or her physical functioning as well as mental, psychosocial, and emotional state, has been measured most often with the Sickness Index Profile and the Medical Outcomes Study Short Form-36 (SF-36).[5] The SF-12 generates the physical and mental component summary scores of the SF-36 in some groups of patients after a stroke.[6] The Stroke-Specific QOL (SS-QOL) scale

Table 56.1   The Barthel Index

	Needs Help	Independent
1. Feeding (If subject's food must be cut up, score as "needs help").	5	10
2. Moving from wheelchair to bed and return (includes sitting up in bed).	5–10	15
3. Personal toilet (wash face, comb hair, shave, clean teeth).	0	5
4. Getting on and off toilet (handling clothes, wipe, flush).	5	10
5. Bathing self.	0	5
6. Walking on level surface (or, if unable to walk, propelling wheelchair).	10	15
	0°	5°
7. Ascend and descend stairs.	5	10
8. Dressing (include tying shoes, fastening fasteners).	5	10
9. Controlling bowels.	5	10
10. Controlling bladder.	5	10

°Score only if unable to walk.

Table 56.2   Functional Independence Measure (FIM) Items

Self-care	Eat
	Groom
	Bathe
	Dress upper body
	Dress lower body
	Toileting
Sphincter	Bladder management
	Bowel management
Mobility	Bed-to-chair and wheelchair-to-chair transfer
	Toilet transfer
	Tub and shower transfer
Locomotion	Walk or use wheelchair
	Climb stairs
Social cognition	Social interaction
	Problem solving
	Memory
	Communication
	Comprehension
	Expression

Score	Burden of Care
7	Complete independence (timely, safely)
6	Modified independence (device)
5	Supervision
4	Minimal assistance (subject does at least 75% of task)
3	Moderate assistance (subject does at last 50% of task)
2	Maximal assistance (subject does at least 25% of task)
1	Total assistance (subject does <25% of task)

contains 12 questions about problems walking and using a wheelchair and 9 about functional use of the affected upper extremity.[7] A 54-item QOL scale for young patients who suffer a hemorrhagic stroke (HSQuale) has seven domains, covering work and financial status, social and leisure activities, and relationships.[8] Caregiver strain may be another dimension of QOL for the patient and family.[9,10]

Some scales used in stroke studies, such as the Rankin Scale, mix the domains of impairment, disability, and handicap into five or fewer general outcomes. Such scales are better for large trials than for the assessment of individual patients. A newcomer, the Stroke Impact Scale (SIS)—available online at www2.kumc.edu/coa—is a self-report measure with 64 items that assess eight domains and covers strength, hand function, ADLs, instrumental ADLs,

mobility, communication, memory, emotion, thinking, and participation.[11] Its reliability, validity, and responsiveness between 1 and 6 months after stroke are good, and the tool may not have the floor and ceiling effects of the BI and the SF-36 (see later). A clinically meaningful change in the SIS score is about 10 to 15 points. A 16-item SIS is available.

Another instrument is the American Heart Association's Stroke Outcome Classification (AHA.SOC).[12] This scale rates impairments, basic self-care skills, and instrumental ADLs. The number of impairments and the severity of impairments are graded on a scale of 3 to 0 for motor, sensory, visual, affective, cognitive, and language deficits. Five levels, from independence to complete dependence, are graded for the combination of basic ADLs (feeding, swallowing, grooming, dressing, bathing, continence, toileting, and mobility) and instrumental ADLs (using the telephone, handling money, using transportation, maintaining a household or job, participating in leisure activities). Many other scales may be of use as assessment and outcome measures for neurorehabilitation interventions.[13]

Mechanisms for Gains

A decrease in impairments and disabilities over the first 3 to 6 months after a stroke is often called *spontaneous recovery*. Resolution of edema, heme, ion fluxes, cell and axon physiologic dysfunction, and diaschisis from transsynaptic and neurotransmitter dysfunction may lead to *restitutive* intrinsic biologic activity and gains over several weeks. Rehabilitation interventions may aim for *substitutive* extrinsic drives to manipulate biologic activity.[13] Although finger pinch or walking may improve with restitutive mechanisms, the multilevel effects of activity-dependent plasticity associated with practice and learning have become increasingly clear from molecular, electrophysiologic, and morphologic studies in recovering animals, and from serial functional neuroimaging studies in humans.[14,15] Patients make gains by experience-driven changes within partially spared pathways, within flexible neuronal assemblies that represent movements, sensation, and cognition, and within multiple representational maps in parallel, distributed networks.[13]

Rehabilitation approaches often emphasize *compensatory strategies* for impairments and disabilities. Patients are trained to make a greater effort to employ a defective skill, substitute a latent skill, learn a new way to accomplish a goal or alter the environment to make a task easier, or change their expectations about performing a particular task. Most compensatory approaches require learning, and gains may be reflected in experience-dependent plasticity.

The optimal duration and intensity of training are uncertain for human rehabilitation strategies. More intensive, task-oriented practice seems to enhance learning and performance.[16,17] Most patients, however, receive no more than a few months of formal inpatient and outpatient retraining. *Intensive rehabilitation* often amounts to less than 20 hours of engagement in physical, occupational, or speech therapy. Each therapist works at many tasks for 2 to 4 weeks of inpatient care and 2 to 4 months of outpatient care. This modest amount of practice may be far less than what is needed to, say, regain the ability to walk at a speed that permits community activities or to improve word-finding skills.[18–21]

Organization of Services

The focus of rehabilitation on enhancing gains across a wide range of impairments and disabilities requires an interdisciplinary group of participants, including physicians such as neurologists and physiatrists; nurses with special competence in rehabilitation teaching and care; physical, occupational, recreational, and speech-language therapists; social workers; neuropsychologists; orthotists; dietitians; and biomedical engineers.

Patients who are at a supervised or minimally assisted level of self-care are usually discharged from the acute hospital setting to the home. They may then receive outpatient therapy. By the end of the first 2 weeks after a stroke, from 12% to 20% of patients in the United States are referred for inpatient rehabilitation. These patients need ongoing supervision by physicians and nurses, have enough stamina to participate in rehabilitation therapies for at least 3 hours a day, and have adequate psychosocial supports, so the rehabilitation team can anticipate discharge to the home or to a board-and-care facility. Further criteria for inpatient rehabilitation are adequate motivation and cognition for learning. Patients who do not meet these criteria may receive therapies in a skilled nursing facility.

Although the issue is difficult to study formally, the literature suggests that the earlier the initiation of an inpatient rehabilitation program (within 20 days of onset of stroke, compared with 20 to 60 days in subjects with similar levels of disability), the better the outcomes.[22] Length of stay in inpatient rehabilitation is determined during weekly conferences in which the team reassesses the patient's progress toward reasonable functional goals. The discharge from inpatient or outpatient rehabilitation should be scheduled with adequate notice for the family to make preparations. Patients need appropriate durable medical equipment, such as a lightweight wheelchair, a cane, an ankle-foot orthosis, and a tub bench, along with follow-up medical and disability-oriented community care.

A number of studies have tried to establish the best locus and time for acute and subacute rehabilitation care. At least 20 trials have compared outcomes between patients managed on specialized stroke or rehabilitation units and those receiving standard medical ward care. In general, these subjects were not too low-level or high-level in function for inpatient rehabilitation as practiced in the United States today. The milieu of a dedicated stroke unit that provides rehabilitation or of a dedicated rehabilitation unit appears to improve outcomes. Although some of the benefit relates to acute care interventions,[23] some benefit derives from the focus on prevention of medical complications related to immobility, on retraining in functional activities,[24] on family training, on the intensity of retraining, on early recognition of mood disorders, and on outpatient follow-up.[25] One prospective study showed that patients admitted to a rehabilitation hospital were significantly more likely to return to the community and recover ADLs than patients sent to nursing facilities for therapy.[26] Case management may not add any benefit to a multidisciplinary approach.[27]

Inpatient rehabilitation is expensive and removes patients from their usual psychosocial and physical environment. Studies with good designs for trials of outpatient therapy suggest that the organization and intensity of services may be related to better outcomes. However, several nonrandomized European community studies of all stroke survivors found that patients who receive therapy either in the hospital or through an organized outpatient approach perform, overall, as well as those who receive little or no remedial treatment.[28] This result is likely to vary with the severity of stroke and the availability of medical and home supports. A short-term inpatient stay that enables patients to become independent enough to be treated at home, followed by outpatient therapy at home, in a clinic, or in a day program may best meet the functional, cognitive, and psychosocial needs of patients.

One large randomized trial compared patients who had rehabilitation at home after an average 12-day inpatient stay with patients who had an additional week of inpatient care followed by hospital-based outpatient treatment.[29] Subjects who lived alone were independent in transfers when they left the hospital or they were assisted by a caregiver. Similar outcomes at 12 months after stroke were achieved in both groups, but at lower cost because of less use of hospital beds by the early discharge group. An intention-to-treat randomized trial with 250 subjects showed that rehabilitation on an inpatient unit after a brief stay in an acute stroke unit or general medical ward produced better outcomes in moderate to severely disabled patients (BI <50) than rehabilitation treatment in the community.[30] No differences in QOL were found, and instrumental ADLs were not measured. Smaller trials confirm similar positive outcomes at 3 to 6 months for home versus various forms of outpatient care, with the home groups having fewer in-hospital days[31] and greater gains in instrumental ADLs.

Community mobility, cooking and cleaning skills, leisure activities, social isolation, and support for caregivers often continue to be problematic for 2-year survivors of a stroke.[32] The clinician should either ask about instrumental ADLs or use an assessment that has patients rate the difficulty they perceive in carrying out these tasks,[33] so that an appropriate rehabilitation prescription may be ordered. A pulse of therapy carried out beyond 6 months after stroke, especially if focused on training in specific skills such as walking and using the affected arm, often improves the ADLs that the patient practices.[18,34]

Overview of Practices

At the time of admission to inpatient rehabilitation, the following features are unfavorable prognosticators for functional gains and for a discharge back to the home: advanced age and neurologic impairments such as profound paresis, loss of proprioception, visuospatial hemineglect, gaze palsy, dementia, and bowel and bladder incontinence. Also, the higher the admission BI or FIM score, the higher the discharge score and the greater the likelihood that the patient resumes living at home.

An epidemiologic report from the Framingham Study is one of the very few studies to compare functional disabilities in survivors of stroke with a control group matched for age and sex.[35] About 80% of the subjects were older than 65 years. Of the 148 patients who had survived for 6 months after stroke, testing with the BI revealed that 20% were dependent in ambulation, one third were dependent in ADLs, and more than two thirds socialized much less than they had before the stroke. These disabilities were significantly greater than any in the stroke-free control subjects. The control subjects, however, had a high level of disability. About 28% did not socialize inside or outside the home, 20% were limited in household tasks, 9% were dependent in self-care activities, and 6% were dependent in mobility. Thus, premorbid functional disabilities may account for limitations in recovery when superimposed upon stroke-induced impairments.

Table 56.3 shows descriptor data and outcomes based on the FIM score for patients admitted for inpatient rehabilitation from more than 500 sites reporting to the Uniform Data Services for Medical Rehabilitation. Most patients had a moderate to maximally assisted level of function and improved to minimally assisted ADLs or better.

Table 56.3 First Admission for Stroke Rehabilitation: Typical Functional Independence Measure (FIM) Results, Patient Characteristics, and Discharge Reports by Uniform Data System for Medical Rehabilitation[189]

Average FIM Scores	At Admission	At Discharge
Self-care	3.5	5.2
Sphincter	3.7	5.4
Mobility	3.0	5.0
Locomotion	2.1	4.3
Communication	4.2	5.2
Social cognition	3.5	4.6
Total	62	86
Patient Characteristics		
Age (yrs)	70	
Onset (days)	12	
Stay (days)	20	
Discharge Destination (%)		
Community	76	76
Long-term care	15	14
Acute care	7	6

Adapted from Iwanenko W, Fielder R, Granger C, et al: The Uniform Data System for Medical Rehabilitation. Am J Phys Med Rehabil 80:56–61;2001.

Do neurorehabilitation practices lessen residual impairments and disabilities? One may better ask whether global neurorehabilitation services have benefits or whether specific interventions for clearly defined impairments and disabilities really work.[36] After reviewing 124 investigations drawn from a literature search of studies performed from 1960 through 1990, Ottenbacher and Janell[37] carried out a meta-analysis on 36 of them. These trials, which included hemiparetic patients with stroke who were given a rehabilitation service, compared at least two groups or conditions for change in a functional measure that could be quantified.[37] Outcomes included gait, hand function, ADLs, response times, and visuoperception. The average patient who received a program of focused stroke rehabilitation or a particular procedure performed better than about 65% of the patients in the comparison group. Larger treatment effect was associated with an earlier intervention and younger patients. The review could not, however, assess the intensity of the interventions or how well they were carried out, detect systematic biases, or account for missing data.

REHABILITATION-RELATED MEDICAL COMPLICATIONS

The time from onset of a stroke to transfer to inpatient rehabilitation has decreased by more than half over the past 20 years at centers in the United States. Physicians and nurses are increasingly responsible for managing new medications started during the acute hospitalization, which often means adjusting dosages of anticoagulant, antihypertensive, and diabetes medications, diagnosing a deep vein thrombosis or sleep apnea, and providing therapy to people who have had a myocardial infarction. Medical complications often interfere with a patient's ability to participate in therapy.[38–41] During inpatient rehabilitation, about one third of patients have a urinary tract infection, urinary retention, musculoskeletal pain, or depression. Up to 20% fall, experience a rash, or need continuous management of blood pressure, hydration, nutrition, or glucose levels. About 10% have a transient toxic-metabolic encephalopathy, pneumonia, cardiac arrhythmias, pressure sores, or thrombophlebitis. Up to 5% have a pulmonary embolus, seizures, gastrointestinal bleeding, heart failure, or other medical complications. Prophylactic measures for these potential problems, when feasible, are essential.

Bladder Dysfunction

Urinary incontinence occurs in up to 60% of patients in the first week after a stroke, but the rate tends to decline to less than 25% at hospital discharge without a specific medical treatment.[42] Urinary dribbling and involuntary bladder emptying, however, affect 30% of healthy, noninstitutionalized people older than 65 years. Across studies, about 18% of those who were incontinent at 6 weeks after stroke are still so at 1 year. Urinary tract infections develop in about 40% of patients during acute stroke and rehabilitation care.

In patients with retention of urine volumes greater than 250 mL, intermittent bladder catheterization with a clean

Table 56.4 Pharmacologic Manipulation of Bladder Dysfunction

Medication and Dosage	Indication	Mechanism of Action
Bethanechol, 25 mg bid to 50 mg qid	Facilitate emptying	Increase detrusor contraction
Prazosin, 1 mg bid to 2 mg tid	Decrease outlet obstruction	Alpha blockade of external sphincter to decrease tone
Tamsulosin, 0.4 mg qd	Prostatic hypertrophy	
Oxybutinin, 2.5 mg hs to 5 mg qid	Urge incontinence Frequency	Relax detrusor; increase internal sphincter tone
Tolterodine, 2 mg bid		
Imipramine, 25–50 mg hs	Urge incontinence Enuresis	Increase internal sphincter tone; decrease detrusor contractions

technique probably lessens the risk of an infection, although there is no evidence for this claim. Perineal cleanliness should lessen the risk of infection by fecal contamination. If urinary retention persists, an indwelling catheter is best for the short run. Most patients with incontinence after a hemispheric stroke either have a small bladder and are unable to suppress the micturition reflex or become aware of filling too late to void in a urinal, commode, or toilet. Scheduled voiding is one good approach. Urodynamic testing may point to an abnormality of urine filling and storage, bladder emptying, or a combination of both, making the choice of medication more rational (Table 56.4). Use of an anticholinergic agent, such as 5 mg of oxybutynin, before sleep may allow greater filling and less urgency or incontinence overnight. Persistent lack of bladder control is often secondary to an unstable detrusor muscle or to detrusor-sphincter dyssynergia.[43] Medications may reduce outlet obstruction in men, but prostatic surgery may be indicated once the patient is a stable outpatient.

Musculoskeletal and Central Pain

Pain is common after a stroke and can limit participation in therapy. Central pain may become a major source of disability, especially after a thalamoparietal stroke, but affects fewer than 5% of all patients with stroke. Some patients only need assurance that the pain or dysesthesia does not represent a serious complication or a warning signal of another stroke. Patients need to assist their physicians in setting goals about moderating the severity, frequency, duration, and time of day of the pain. Musculoskeletal pain is far more common.

Shoulder pain at the hemiparetic arm develops in 5% to 50% of patients.[44] Pain exacerbates hypertonicity and may trigger flexor and extensor spasms and dystonic postures. A painful shoulder may cause the hemiplegic arm to flex at the elbow and wrist. A placebo-controlled, randomized

trial of 37 patients with chronic hemiplegic shoulder pain found that three intra-articular injections of triamcinolone over 4 weeks did not produce a statistically significant reduction in pain.[45] The shoulder-hand syndrome with reflex sympathetic dystrophy or complex regional pain[46] has been described in up to 25% of patients in prospective studies.[47] This rate is much higher than expected from clinical experience and may reflect a lack of patient education as well as physician enthusiasm to always manage limb pain immediately with analgesia, anti-inflammatory medication, and range-of-motion exercises.

During rehabilitation and later, many patients suffer with cervical, lumbar, hip, knee, or ankle pain secondary to musculoligamentous injuries, overuse, overstretching, and poor resting postures. Thus, pain may arise from errors of omission and commission by patients, families, and hospital staff. Physical modalities, analgesics, anti-inflammatory agents, and local anesthetics or steroids may reduce most sources of musculoligamentous pain. Examples of prevention of further injury are using an orthotic to hold the wrist and fingers in extension, especially for the patient who has a hemineglect, and controlling hyperextension-induced pain at the knee with an ankle-foot orthosis.

Burning or nonburning spontaneous central pain arises most often from a lesion in the ventroposterolateral nucleus of the thalamus.[48] A variety of drugs may diminish dysesthetic or lancinating pain. In one randomized controlled trial, lamotrigine, 200 mg per day, had a significant, if moderate effect on reducing symptoms of pain.[49] Tricyclic antidepressants have also shown efficacy in randomized trials.[50] Many anecdotal reports find value in using one or a combination of drugs. The clinician must establish a global pain scale with a patient and initiate trials of medication with a gradual titration of the dosage. If a tricyclic antidepressant such as amitriptyline or desipramine fails to work at doses up to 100 mg, which may not be tolerated, a reasonable series of trials can progress as follows: gabapentin, lamotrigine, carbamazepine, baclofen, clonidine, and mexiletine. Trazodone before sleep or use of a serotonin-specific reuptake inhibitor (SSRI) antidepressant may augment the effectiveness of these drugs.

Depression

Depression is common in late life[51] and after a stroke. The community-based Framingham Study diagnosed depression in 47% of 6-month stroke survivors, with no difference being found in the incidence between subjects with left- and right-sided lesions.[52] Depression was simultaneously diagnosed in 25% of age- and sex-matched controls, however. Other studies suggest a predisposition to depression after left anterior and right posterior infarcts, primarily soon after a stroke.[53] In a population-based cohort of Swedish patients with stroke whose mean age was 73 years, the prevalence of major depression was 25% at hospital discharge, 30% at 3 months after stroke, 16% at 1 year, 19% at 2 years, and 29% at 3 years.[54] A left anterior infarct, dysphasia, and living alone may predict depression. By 3 months after stroke, greater dependence in ADLs and social isolation have been associated with depression. In another large study conducted in Finland, major depression affected 26%, and minor depression 14%, of 486 consecutive patients with stroke from 3 to 4 months after the infarction.[55] Premorbid depression was a strong risk factor for major depression after stroke.

Counseling during rehabilitation may lessen the risk for depression, especially when directed towards concerns that patients have about becoming a burden on others.

Clinical trials reveal the efficacy of treatment of depression with tricyclic or SSRI antidepressants. Methylphenidate can also alleviate the mood disorder and improve rehabilitation outcomes.[56–60] The specific medication used depends on the patient's medical risk factors (anticholinergic side effects might cause cardiac arrhythmias, drowsiness, confusion, or urinary retention), the presence of anxiety (some SSRI and tricyclic antidepressants appear to be more useful for this factor), insomnia (a tricyclic antidepressant may aid sleep), and speed of onset (methylphenidate can act within a few days). Small clinical trials reveal the efficacy of citapralam.[56] If depression and apathy limit a patient's participation during inpatient rehabilitation, I most often start with methylphenidate, 10 mg after breakfast, and build up to 20 mg at 8 AM and 2 PM. An SSRI antidepressant such as fluoxetine, 10 mg, or sertraline, 25 to 50 mg, is started several days later, then increased as needed.

Dysphagia

Swallowing disorders may cause malnutrition, dehydration, and aspiration pneumonia. The stroke and any associated toxic-metabolic encephalopathy may combine to cause lethargy, inattention, poor judgment, and impaired control or sensitivity of the tongue and cheek. These problems often impair the oral stage of swallowing. Patients cannot form a bolus, food is pocketed in the cheek, the swallowing reflex may be delayed, the bolus slides over the base of the tongue and collects in the valleculae and hypopharynx, and sometimes the pharyngeal constrictor muscle malfunctions. Patients may take too much food or liquid in a bolus, which then enters the airway before triggering a swallow reflex. Slow oral intake, a cough or wet voice after swallowing, and a rising blood urea nitrogen level point to the potential for the clinical complications of dysphagia.

A videofluoroscopic modified barium swallow (MBS) study provides the best information about the safety and efficacy of the stages of swallowing. An MBS performed with less than a teaspoonful of thin barium, the same of thickened barium, and a test of swallowing with a barium-coated piece of cookie help document problems at the oral, pharyngeal, and esophageal stages. The therapist can simultaneously assess the effect of changes in head and neck position on deglutition. During inpatient rehabilitation, an abnormal MBS result reveals the greater risk for pneumonia in aspirators compared to nonaspirators.[61] Nasogastric feeding tubes and gastrostomies do not appreciably lessen the risk of aspiration, probably because of gastric reflux, aspiration of oral secretions, and errors in tube placement.

Therapy by a speech or occupational therapist is indicated when delayed swallow, cough, residual barium in the vallecula, or aspiration are noted during the MBS study. Therapies include compensatory head repositioning such as flexing or turning to one side, tongue and sucking exercises, double swallowing, and supraglottic and dry coughing. Most patients fed with pureed foods and thickened liquids have adequate nutrition. Nasogastric feedings can supplement oral intake, especially if given after each meal so they do not blunt the patient's appetite. If dysphagia persists near the time of discharge from inpatient rehabilitation, a gastrostomy or gastrojejunostomy tube is a comfortable portal for nutrition. Because a gastrostomy tube must stay in place for at least 6 weeks after insertion, clinicians should be certain that this approach is warranted in the first week after a stroke. Recovery from dysphagia may be associated with a greater motor representation for the pharyngeal muscles in the uninjured hemisphere that evolves over time and with practice in swallowing.[62]

Skin Ulcers

Education in skin management during rehabilitation provides an important opportunity to prevent morbidity and mortality. Ischemia of the skin and underlying tissues occurs particularly in weight-bearing areas adjacent to bony prominences. Sores related to sitting are most commonly associated with the ischial tuberosities, where tissue pressure can exceed 300 mm Hg when the patient sits on an unpadded seat. A 2-inch-thick foam pad may decrease that local pressure to 150 mm Hg. Capillary and venule pressures are 11 to 33 mm Hg.

A four-stage classification for degrees of integument breakdown, prophylactic measures, and wound care is available from the Agency for Health Care Policy and Research.[63] No particular intervention for a pressure sore, other than antibiotics and débridement for stage 3 to 4 ulcers, appears to be better than another.[64]

Sexual Dysfunction

After stroke, sexual desire may persist, but many men and women who had been sexually active experience sexual dysfunction.[65] Premorbid problems from diabetes, medications, vascular disease, and psychogenic causes can be exacerbated by new neural dysfunction, decreased mobility, pain, and new medications. Counseling and education with patient and spouse help. Medication such as sildenafil and prostheses for men assist erectile dysfunction. Such medication may be contraindicated in patients with clinically significant coronary artery disease.

Sleep Disorders

During rehabilitation, insomnia, sleep apnea, and excessive daytime sleepiness can interfere with attention and perhaps with learning.[66] Medications, pain, anxiety, depression, and chronically poor sleep habits contribute to sleep deficits. Reversed sleep-wake cycles are common in patients with cognitive dysfunction in the first days of inpatient rehabilitation. Up to one third of patients receiving inpatient stroke rehabilitation may have a sleep disorder.

Central and obstructive types of sleep apnea have been associated with a higher risk for stroke. Pharyngeal muscle weakness and impairment of neural control of the nasopharyngeal and pharyngolaryngeal muscles due to a stroke contribute to the risk for new onset of obstructive apnea. Polysomnography is indicated when the rehabilitation team observes a hypersomnolent, confused, and snoring or apneic patient. The number of oxygen desaturation events and the oximetry measures during sleep-disordered breathing correlates with poorer functional recovery scores at 1 and 12 months after stroke.[67–69]

Insomnia during the first week or two of rehabilitation can be managed with short-acting hypnotic agents such as chloral hydrate, zolpidem, and zaleplon, nighttime non-narcotic analgesics, and careful positioning in bed. Nocturia more than two times that awakens the patient can be diminished by avoiding liquid intake after dinner and using medications that lessen activation of the bladder detrusor muscle. Melatonin may help correct a reversed day-night sleep cycle. A positive-pressure breathing apparatus will prevent the complications of sleep apnea.

Spasticity

A number of still ill-defined mechanisms after stroke alter membrane properties and morphologically and physiologically reorganize spinal circuits, leading to hypertonicity, clonus, spasms, and contractures.[70,71] Spasticity can lead to dystonic postures and, in some instances, limit function. However, the paresis, slowness, and fatigability that accompany an upper motor neuron (UMN) syndrome are usually more serious contributors to impairment and disability than hypertonicity. The difficulty in quantifying spasticity and measuring a functional consequence has made research and drug testing difficult. The Ashworth Scale is most often used, but the score it produces is little more than an extension of the clinical examination of resistance to passive movement. Also, the properties of joints, ligaments, tendons, and muscles change with paresis after a UMN injury and contribute to the alteration in resistance to joint stretch.[72]

The neurophysiologic schools of physical therapy hold that exercise may induce hypertonicity. Small trials of modest exercise therapy have not revealed any increase in tone, however.[73–75] Indeed, clonus and spasms often diminish with weight bearing on the leg or arm. Excessive resistance exercises, however, that only flex the arm, as in performing curls, or that only extend the leg may drive flexor or extensor postures, respectively, and produce a dystonic arm or leg. Nevertheless, experimental studies suggest that hemiparetic subjects can increase force output when pushing against higher loads, such as when pedaling to gain muscular force output, without inducing a decline in motor control.[73,76,77] Use of the large leg muscles by pedaling against resistance at less than 20 cycles per minute or by walking on a treadmill also improves cardiovascular fitness in patients who have at least fair motor control.[78,79]

Pathologically increased muscle tone in patients with hemiplegia can usually be managed by aiming to maintain the normal length of the muscle and soft tissue across a joint and by helping patients avoid abnormal flexor and extensor patterns at rest and during movement. Spasticity should be treated more aggressively when it interferes with nursing care and perineal hygiene or contributes to contractures and pressure sores.

No studies offer convincing evidence of functional benefits on movement from systemic antispasticity

Table 56.5 Dosages of Medications for Symptomatic Spasticity

First Line
  Dantrolene, 25 mg bid to 50 mg qid
  Baclofen, 5 mg bid to 40 mg qid
  Clonidine, 0.05 mg qd to 0.2 mg tid
  Tizanidine, 2 mg bid to 8 mg qid
  Clonazepam, 0.5 to 2 mg bid to tid
Useful Additions
  Gabapentin, 300 mg tid to 600 mg qid
  Phenytoin, serum concentration 10 to 20 mg%
  Cyproheptadine, 4 mg bid to 8 mg qid
  Levodopa/carbidopa, 25/100 mg bid to qid
Injectables
  Intramuscular botulinum toxin A or B
  Intramuscular phenol
Intrathecal baclofen, 50 μg trial dose
Intrathecal clonidine

medications after a stroke. Dantrolene, baclofen, a benzodiazepine such as clonazepam, and tizanidine[80,81] can reduce hypertonicity-related spasms and flexor postures of the upper limb or extensor postures of the lower extremity (Table 56.5). A clear effect should be evident, and after further physical therapy, attempts should be made to eliminate the drug.

As a last resort, chemical agents such as phenol have been injected into a nerve, motor point, or muscle to lessen inappropriate muscle co-contraction, spasms, and dystonic postures. Because motor point blocks can partially spare voluntary movement and reduce reciprocal inhibition when given to an antagonist muscle, they may improve some aspects of motor control. Intramuscular injections of ethanol or botulinum toxin reduce local features of spasticity for about 3 months, especially flexor postures of the arm and hand and equinovarus foot positioning.[82–86] These agents may improve the Ashworth Scale score, but they do not improve motor control or the torque around a joint. Such injections should be followed by physical therapy to try to maintain range of motion and improve selective motor control. For dystonic postures that do not respond to oral medications, intrathecal baclofen may be of value.[87]

Although surgery is rarely needed after a stroke, a variety of surgical procedures, including tendon lengthening, tenotomy, and tendon transfer, can correct deformities induced by spasticity and, sometimes, improve function. Tendon lengthening of the hamstrings, Achilles, and toe or finger and wrist flexors is an occasional consideration to improve range of motion. A gait analysis with electromyography (EMG) helps determine which procedure might aid mobility. Physical therapy must be administered after surgery.

COGNITIVE REHABILITATION

Cognitive impairments may accompany a cortical or subcortical stroke. Disabilities arise from aphasia and hemineglect as well as from faltering attention, visuoperception, memory, and executive functions. Lesions within the frontal-subcortical circuit that include the caudate, basal ganglia, or thalamus may lead to deafferentiation of the dorsolateral prefrontal cortex and impair working memory, judgment, problem-solving skills, and creative thought. Neuropsychological tests help define these problems. A modest number of randomized clinical trials have studied specific interventions for cognitive retraining.[88]

Memory Disorders

Patients are called upon to encode and retrieve new information during rehabilitation. Memory disturbances impede compensatory learning that underlies much of the rehabilitation process. The incidence and risk factors for memory loss and dementia caused by one or more strokes are increasingly being appreciated.[89–93] Up to 30% of all stroke survivors have a disturbance in memory. Community-based studies report dementia in 15% to 30% of patients after stroke within 3 months to 1 year and in 33% within 5 years.[89,94,95]

Cognitive remediation for memory disorders aims to train compensatory strategies such as rehearsal, visual imagery, semantic elaboration, and memory aids, including notebooks, calendars, and electronic devices. In normal subjects who are learning a new skill, constant feedback enhances immediate performance, but an intermittent schedule of reinforcement that allows errors and gradual processing of how to perform may improve long-term retention. The optimal way to enhance learning in a particular person with brain injury may depend on what type of memory, attention, or other cognitive processes have been affected. Amnestic subjects and at least some subjects with impaired episodic memory do worse with trial-and-error training; more frequent feedback and errorless learning may improve retention in these subjects.[96] In general, patients with stroke have good procedural or motor learning abilities.[97,98]

Visuospatial and Attentional Disorders

In one study, visual neglect was found in 38% of 150 consecutive patients with moderate disability after a new stroke, but severe neglect was rare beyond 6 months.[99] Patients with anosognosia, visual neglect, tactile extinction, motor impersistence, or auditory neglect at 10 days after stroke have the lowest BI at 1 year, even after the data are adjusted for initial ADL scores and for post-stroke rehabilitation.[100] Recovery is most rapid within the first 2 weeks, regardless of the side of the stroke, and visual neglect improves by 3 months in most patients. Many patients have more subtle impairments that are found by testing.

Treatments for left hemi-inattention aim to engage attention to the left, disengage attention to the right, shift spatial coordinates to the left, and increase arousal. Well-described behavioral interventions for visuospatial retraining have been employed to improve attention to the left.[101,102] The techniques include a stimulus such as a red ribbon on the left to anchor attention followed by a gradual withdrawal of left-sided spatial cues, work on sensory awareness to physical stimuli on the left, and tasks to aid spatial organization. Intensive practice involving a variety of pencil and paper and physical tasks for left-sided

Table 56.6   Interventions For Hemineglect*

Multisensory visual and sensory cues, then fading cues[101]
Verbal elaboration of visual analysis[97]
Visual imagery[190]
Environmental adaptations
Video feedback[191]
Monocular and binocular patches[192–195]
Prisms[194,196]
Left limb movement in left hemispace[99,107]
Head and trunk midline adjustments[106,197,198]
Left cerebral transcranial magnetic stimulation[199]
Vestibular stimulation[200,201]
Optokinetic stimulation[202]
Reduce hemianopic defects[203]
Computer-assisted training[204,205]

*Superscript numbers indicate references.

attention may help the subject with moderate to severe neglect.[103,104] Visual scanning training[105] and scanning combined with trunk rotation,[106] self-cuing by movement of the left arm,[99,107] or a warning tone to increase alertness to space have improved scores on tests of left hemispace awareness.[108] These interventions do not necessarily improve left hemiattention during ADLs. Table 56.6 lists some of the techniques that have been tried with some success, though usually not in a double-blinded randomized trial.

Pharmacotherapy

Medications that affect neurotransmitters and neuromodulators may have positive or negative effects on domains of cognition. Some may affect general processes like attention and memory. Others, such as stimulants of the noradrenergic projections from the locus ceruleus, may modulate the signal-to-noise ratio for attended stimuli. Other drugs may enable gains in some aspect of cognition when their use is combined with task-oriented practice. Investigators and clinicians have tested many drugs in small trials after stroke and traumatic brain injury. Hemineglect may improve with a dopamine agonist[109] but may make some patients, perhaps those with a striatal lesion, worse.[110] Cholinesterase inhibitors may improve memory in patients with vascular dementia.[110a]

Table 56.7 lists some of the adjunct pharmacologic interventions used in patients with stroke and traumatic brain injury that have been found useful in case reports and small series. The number in each column is the order in which I tend to put the drugs into an n-of-1 trial for patients. Therapy specific to targeted goals is provided during these trials. Potential classes of drugs that may contribute to recovery include neurotrophins and molecules associated with the cascades of proteins and genes required for short-term and long-term memory storage and maintenance.[111,112]

Speech and Language Therapies

The Copenhagen Stroke Study was a community-based population study that prospectively monitored about 1200 patients admitted for acute stroke, and nearly all of the 800

Table 56.7   Drugs That May Enhance Activity-Dependent Gains: A Clinical Algorithm for Use

| Drug | Targeted Impairment or Disability | | | | |
	Aphasia	Motor Function	Neglect	Memory	Depression
Amphetamine	3	6	4		
Methylphenidate	4	5	3	2	1
L-Dopa		4	2		
Dopamine agonists	5		1		
Anticholinesterases	2	1		1	
Tricyclics					3
Serotoninergics	6	2	5	3	2
Piracetam	1	3			

1, first choice; 2, second choice; 3, third choice; 4, fourth choice; 5, fifth choice; 6, sixth choice.

survivors. The investigators reported that 38% of 881 patients were aphasic on admission and 20% of the admissions were rated as severe on the Scandinavian Stroke Scale (SSS).[113] Nearly half of the patients with severe aphasia died early after stroke onset, and half of those with mild aphasia recovered by 1 week. Only 18% of community survivors were still aphasic at the time of acute and rehabilitation hospital discharges. Up to 28% received early speech therapy as needed. Patients were retested for 6 months. The investigators found that the best predictor of recovery is a lesser severity of aphasia close to the time of the stroke. Ninety-five percent of subjects with mild aphasia reached their best level of recovery by 2 weeks, those with a moderate aphasia by 6 weeks, and those with severe aphasia by 10 weeks. Only 8% of the severely aphasic patients fully recovered on the scoring system by 6 months. In this study, mild language deficits and changes undetected by the limited sensitivity of the SSS were not ascertained. Functional communication was not a measured outcome. This natural history data does not imply that aphasic patients cannot improve in aspects of comprehension and expression for months, even years after stroke onset.

Interventions

For the aphasic patient, speech therapists attempt to find ways to circumvent, deblock, or compensate for impairments in the comprehension and expression of language. Visual and verbal cuing techniques include picture matching and sentence completion tasks. Frequent repetition and positive reinforcement are used as the patient approaches the desired responses. A large variety of approaches for particular language and linguistic impairments have evolved. Melodic intonation therapy for nonfluent aphasics who have good comprehension, for example, may enhance expression.[114]

A meta-analysis performed on 55 interventional trials of speech-language therapy in aphasic patients after stroke offers insights into the effectiveness of language therapies.[115] Significant benefits were found in treated patients compared with untreated patients at all stages of recovery. The benefit appeared most evident in patients who started speech therapy soon after stroke. Total treatment amounts of more than 2 hours per week achieved greater gains than lesser amounts. Patients with severe aphasia showed greater improvement when treated by a speech-language pathologist than by family members or assistants. Only one

defined intervention, multimodal stimulation, was tested in enough cases to show its greater average effect. Any differential effects of treatment for differing types of aphasia could not be assessed by this analysis because too few studies have been published.[115]

The intensity and specificity of practice may be most important in testing a particular therapy. One well-designed study employed a picture card game in which a group of aphasic subjects were prompted to request and provide cards of depicted objects from their hands of cards. The results suggest that behaviorally relevant mass practice for at least 3 hours a day for 10 days that also constrained the use of nonverbal communication and reinforced appropriate responses within a group setting could improve comprehension and naming skills more effectively than less intensive and formalized therapy.[21] The cortical response to an intervention may be monitored during activation studies by means of functional neuroimaging.[116–118]

Computer software offers other forms of practice. An uncontrolled case series of patients with chronic aphasia showed that repetitive practice with a therapist and at home with a microcomputer-based symbolic language device led to improvements on several tests of language function.[119] A visual iconic computer-based interface also improved the ability of subjects with chronic aphasia to relearn the use of past-tense verbs and to comprehend passive-voice sentences, pointing to an approach to lessen agrammatism and syntactic deficits.[120]

Pharmacotherapy

Clinical trials in modest numbers of patients with amphetamine,[121] piracetam,[117,122] and cholinergic[123] and dopaminergic[124,125] agents have suggested efficacy of these agents for particular aphasic syndromes and language impairments. The neurotransmitter systems stimulated by such drugs may affect a variety of pathways for attention, memory, reward, and learning.[126–128] Clinicians can try any of these agents in an n-of-1 series of trials. A few standard tests that can detect changes in perseveration, word finding, simple sentence comprehension, and social communication may serve as measures of efficacy. I tend to start with an anticholinesterase agent in a dose typical for use in patients with Alzheimer's disease and to follow it with levodopa/carbidopa, 25 mg and 100 mg, twice during the day, and then with 10 mg of amphetamine every other day before speech therapy.

Therapeutic strategies are needed that combine analytic approaches from speech pathology, neurolinguistics, neuropsychology, neuroimaging, pharmacology, and computer sciences. Theory-based treatments will define the short-term and long-term benefits of a specific intervention for a particular aspect of language. Single-case studies and clinical trials must also address the optimal intensity, duration, and learning paradigm for a specific intervention.

MOBILITY TRAINING

Natural History

In the Copenhagen Stroke Study, 51% of patients were initially unable to walk, 12% walked with assistance, and 37% were independent.[129,130] At discharge after acute and rehabilitative care, 22% of survivors could not walk, 14% walked with assistance, and 64% walked independently. About 80% of those who were initially nonwalkers reached their best walking function within 6 weeks, and 95% within 11 weeks. Of patients who initially walked with physical assistance, 80% reached best function within 3 weeks, and 95% within 5 weeks. Independent walking was achieved by 34% of the survivors who had been dependent and by 60% of those who initially required assistance. Recovery of ambulation correlated directly with residual leg strength. Within the first week after onset, patients who improved leg strength by several points on the SSS within the first 2 to 3 weeks after stroke almost always became ambulatory.[131] In general, patients who can flex the hip and extend the hemiparetic knee against gravity after stroke will be able to ambulate without human assistance.

More detailed information about outcomes in relationship to impairment and disability was reported in a prospective study of 95 consecutive inpatients admitted to a rehabilitation center after a hemispheric stroke.[132] Patients were followed up until they reached a plateau of recovery. Life-table analyses of the probability of recovering BI functions were made; patients were divided into three groups according to impairment and examined at 2-week intervals. More than 90% of patients with a pure motor (M) deficit became independent in walking 150 feet by week 14, but only 35% of those with motor and proprioceptive (SM) loss did so by week 24, and 3% of those with motor, sensory and hemianopic deficits (SMH) did so by week 30. The probability of walking more than 150 feet with assistance increased to 80% by week 8 and to 100% by week 14 in those with M impairment. The probability of walking with physical help exceeded 90% in those with SM and SMH loss by 28 weeks after the stroke. Table 56.8 shows recovery data according to impairment group for another cohort of patients with stroke.

Interventions

Sensorimotor impairments and disabilities in mobility and other ADLs are managed by four general approaches:

- Exercise and selective muscle group strengthening
- Facilitation and neurophysiologic techniques drawn from various schools of facilitative therapy, including those of Bobath and Brunnstrom
- Compensatory training to adapt to disability
- Task-oriented retraining that emphasizes principles for learning and intensive practice

When compared with one another, no differences in outcomes have been found among the traditional schools of facilitative therapy. Strengthening exercises seem to be mildly more beneficial than facilitation alone.[133] Task-oriented activity with optimal schedules of practice and reinforcement looks promising as part of a physical and occupational therapy strategy.[16,19]

Range of motion in the paretic arm and leg is maintained with positioning, splints, and slow rhythmic rotation and stretch of all joints several times a day, along with weight bearing as soon as possible. Patient and family are taught to assist. Flexion at the hip, knee, and ankle are encouraged by mat exercises that include rolling onto the side and bringing the knee to the chest. Once the patient has adequate endurance and stability to stand in the parallel bars or at a hemibar with the therapist's help to control the paretic leg, gait training begins. The therapist concentrates on the most prominent deviations from normal during the gait cycle, such as circumduction of the hip, pelvic drop, hyperextension or flexor give-way of the knee, inadequate dorsiflexion of the ankle, and toe clawing. The physical therapist also encourages heel strike at initial stance, greater weight bearing on the paretic leg, push-off at the end of stance, at least 5 to 10 degrees of hip extension in late stance, and a longer step length.

The hemiparetic patient who cannot control ankle movement, whose foot tends to turn over during gait, or who lacks enough knee control to prevent the knee from snapping back is fitted with a polypropylene ankle-foot orthosis. As inpatient therapy for gait progresses away from the parallel bars to increasing distances walked with an assistive device such as a quadcane, then to stair climbing and outdoor ambulation on uneven surfaces, therapy continues in the outpatient setting, where mobility in the home and community is stressed.

Table 56.8   Recovery of Walking in Patients Grouped by Impairments at Onset of Stroke

Impairment Group	Onset (%)	1 Month (%)	3 Months (%)	6 Months (%)
Motor	18	50	75	85
Sensorimotor	10	48	72	72
Motor, hemianopia	7	28	68	75
Sensorimotor, hemianopia	3	16	33	38

Data from Kaplan-Meier graphs in reference 206.

Task-Oriented Approaches

Treadmill walking is a task-oriented approach for ambulation. Body weight–supported treadmill training (BWSTT), if carried out optimally, allows the spinal cord and supraspinal locomotor regions to experience sensory inputs akin to those of ordinary stepping, unlike the atypical inputs created by compensatory gait deviations and difficulty with loading a paretic limb during conventional locomotor training. The therapist employs different levels of weight support and treadmill speed and, most important, assists the step pattern with physical and verbal cues to optimize the temporal, kinematic, and kinetic parameters of the step cycle. The more normal input may improve the timing and increase the activation of residual descending locomotor outputs on spinal motor pools. Sensory inputs related to the level of loading of the stance leg and to extension of the hip before swing, as well as to treadmill speed, have been shown to modulate the EMG output during BWSTT, even when the legs are fully assisted during the step cycle.[134,135] This finding, which is similar to the results of studies of cats after experimental low thoracic spinal cord transection, points to the powerful modulation by sensory inputs of spinal locomotor neuronal pools and the ability of the spinal cord to learn from rhythmic inputs.[136]

In subjects with a chronic hemiparetic stroke who walk slowly, 12 sessions of BWSTT at 2 mph increases overground walking speed by 30% to 50%.[137] Two randomized trials of ambulatory patients with stroke show that progressive increase in the treadmill speed as physiologically tolerated enables patients to achieve overground walking speeds that are significantly higher than when they are trained at a modest increment of speed or treated with conventional overground training.[137,138] Higher walking speeds are associated with greater likelihood of community ambulation. This approach also leads to a reorganization of activity in the supplementary motor cortex and primary sensorimotor cortex, associated with increases in walking speed and in selective control of ankle dorsiflexion.[139,140] As with any task-oriented approach, the intensity and specificity of practice drive functional gains for the practiced motor skill.

Small studies[141] and a larger, randomized Canadian clinical trial[142] suggest that BWSTT increases the likelihood of achieving more independent ambulation and at greater speeds compared with both treadmill training without weight support and conventional locomotor therapy.[18] When BWSTT was carried out at slow treadmill speeds in a randomized trial of patients 3 weeks after stroke, the intervention improved outcomes equal to those of conventional gait training provided for a half-hour a day for a median of 10 weeks.[143] However, mean treadmill training speeds after 4 and 8 weeks of training in this Swedish trial were only 0.9 mph. Subjects walked overground at a mean of 0.7 mph 10 months after stroke. Thus, the training methodology used by the investigators did not take advantage of step training at the higher speeds made possible by BWSTT.

EMG, visual, and auditory biofeedback to increase muscle contractions or lessen co-contractions may improve the pattern of arm or leg movements and improve balance,[144] but no technique has come into common usage. Gains during biofeedback sessions may not generalize to movements during walking. Electrical stimulation of leg muscles is sometimes used, mostly to aid ankle dorsiflexion. This peroneal nerve stimulation may improve foot clearance and may modestly improve walking speed. Case reports suggest that some patients may benefit from electrical stimulation of the gluteal and quadriceps muscles for hip stability and knee extension, but this approach is limited to research laboratories.

Selective muscle strengthening,[20] treadmill walking to improve strength and endurance,[145] and rhythmic practice entrained by the temporal elements of music[146] may also improve walking speed and the symmetry of both stance and swing phases of gait.

UPPER EXTREMITY AND SELF-CARE SKILLS

The occupational therapist brings to the rehabilitation team expertise with assistive devices for ADLs and often works with the neuropsychologist in addressing visuospatial inattention, memory loss, apraxia, dysphagia, and difficulties in problem solving. Tables 56.1 and 56.2 provide an overview of the ADL tasks that the therapist addresses, especially during inpatient rehabilitation. Community and leisure activities are addressed during outpatient therapy. Outcomes for prospective studies of patients undergoing rehabilitation, as well as for the overall population of patients admitted for acute care after a first stroke, suggest that 60% to 70% of patients recover the ability to manage basic ADLs, although the majority do not return to their premorbid level of socialization.

Natural History

Using the BI and SSS, the Copenhagen Study graded recovery before and after acute and rehabilitative inpatient stays and at 6 months. Within the same facility, all patients who needed rehabilitation received services for an average stay of 35 days (S.D. 41). By then, 11% had severe impairment, 11% had moderate impairment, and 78% had mild or no deficits. At the same time, 20% had severe, 8% moderate, and 26% mild disability, and 46% had no disability. ADL scores plateaued by 9 weeks in patients with initially mild strokes, within 13 weeks in those with moderate strokes, within 17 weeks in those with severe strokes, and within 20 weeks in those with most severe stroke.[129] The study by Reding and Potes,[132] of patients admitted to one rehabilitation inpatient program, found that 65% of subjects achieved a BI of more than 95 by 15 weeks if they had only M deficits and by 26 weeks with SM loss, but only 10% of those with SMH deficits scored that high by 18 to 30 weeks. However, 100% of patients with M loss achieved a BI higher than 60 by 14 weeks, 75% of those with SM deficits, by 23 weeks, and 60% of those with SMH loss, by 29 weeks.

Functional recovery of the upper extremity was assessed in the Copenhagen Stroke Study using BI subscores for feeding and grooming for the affected arm.[147] Within 9 weeks, 95% of patients achieved their best function. With mild paresis, this was accomplished by 6 weeks after stroke onset. In those with severe paresis, best function was achieved by 11 weeks. The ability to shrug or abduct the affected shoulder within the first few weeks after stroke may predict outcomes better than synergistic hand function.[148] Patients who have no movement of the hand by several weeks after onset of the stroke most often do not recover independent feeding and dressing with that hand. Patients who have some voluntary finger and wrist extension within the first few weeks may show improvement in hand coordination for practiced tasks for 12 months or more.

Interventions

Occupational therapy to improve upper extremity function first puts an emphasis on visually and manually patterning the patient through parts of a task and then through the entire task with frequent positive feedback. Techniques that conserve energy and promote independence in dressing, grooming, bathing, and toileting involve relearning how to carry out the task with compensation when using the unaffected arm and adaptive strategies with the affected arm. The therapist also provides a wheelchair with proper seating, a clear plastic lap board or arm trough to rest the paretic limb where it can be seen by the patient, an arm sling if shoulder subluxation or pain arises, a compression glove to reduce hand edema if elevation and massage fail to do so, and static and dynamic splints to maintain wrist and finger position in extension. A visit to the home of a patient who is less than fully independent is the best way to establish the need for assistive devices, such as grab bars, rails, ramps, and environmental controls, as well as architectural changes such as widening a doorway to allow wheelchair access.

Acupuncture appeared to improve motor impairments or functional outcomes in several quasi-experimental and randomized clinical trials.[149] Two well-designed randomized trials that used a sham procedure did not find any improvement in performance of ADLs.[150,151]

Task-Oriented Approaches

Most therapists take a task-oriented approach to retraining ADLs supplemented by Bobath and other techniques. One trial randomly assigned 185 patients within 1 month of stroke either to up to 5 months of home-based therapy with an occupational therapist or to no therapy.[17] The number of visits ranged from 1 to 15, with a mean of only 6 visits per patient. None of the subjects had been admitted to a hospital for the stroke, and median BI values were 18 (about 90 on the American version of the test), so they were minimally disabled. Blinded assessment of outcomes revealed significant gains with the therapy. The group that received therapy improved in instrumental ADLs and handicap, and made modest gains in ADLs, and caregiver strain decreased in this group.

Failed early attempts to use the affected limb may suppress subsequent use. Forced use of the affected arm and gradual shaping of a variety of functional movements to overcome what is theorized as learned nonuse of the paretic limb may increase the incorporation of the affected arm into daily activities.[152] In one study, 9 patients with

chronic stroke who could extend the wrist and fingers at least 10 degrees spent about 7 hours a day for up to 2 weeks practicing a variety of guided upper extremity movements and wore a sling or glove that prevented use of the unaffected upper extremity for the rest of the day. Much of the improvement in daily use of the affected arm was evident within 1 to 2 days of restraint of the unaffected arm plus therapy; this finding suggests that a latent capability had succumbed to learned nonuse.[153,154] Constraint-induced movement therapy (CIMT) is associated with primary motor cortex reorganization in some but not all studies, suggesting that the approach can induce activity-dependent plasticity.[155]

A well-designed randomized trial of 66 subjects with chronic stroke compared CIMT with bimanual hand training based on the neurodevelopmental program developed by Patricia Davies.[156] After 2 weeks of training, the CIMT group scored modestly better in the functional use and amount of daily use of the affected arm. The difference in amount of use did not persist 1 year later. Subjects with sensory loss and hemi-inattention appeared to do better with CIMT, a finding that bears further study. A pilot study of 20 patients with acute stroke compared 2 hours of daily CIMT for 2 weeks with standard occupational therapy that did not emphasize use of the affected arm.[157] Functional outcomes appeared better for the CIMT group. A randomized trial of CIMT is in progress in the United States for subjects who, at 3 to 9 months after their stroke, can extend several fingers and the wrist at least 10 degrees.

CIMT is a form of intensive, task-oriented practice for patients who have at least modest motor control of the upper extremity. The intervention does not define any particular approach to motor learning. In any controlled trial, CIMT must be compared with an equally active program of upper extremity management. When brief, intensive therapy of various types has been provided to subjects with recent or chronic stroke, aspects of upper extremity function related to the practiced task have usually improved.[16,44,98,158-160] Practice also improves aspects of motor function in the ipsilesional upper extremity,[161] which is often a bit weaker or slow in its movements compared with the upper extremity in normal, healthy subjects.[162]

Robotic and other mechanical assistive training devices have also improved the performance for reaching, usually in the plane of practice or across the joints most used.[163-165] Trials that do not succeed in augmenting the amount of practice time generally produce negative results.[166] In a randomized trial that began about 3 weeks after onset of stroke in 56 subjects undergoing inpatient rehabilitation, robot-trained subjects used a low-inertia, back-drivable device for 25 hourly sessions and 1500 repetitions of assisted movement in the horizontal plane for the shoulder and elbow, whereas the control group used the device for the unaffected arm or for the affected arm without a robotic assist.[167] The robotically trained group, which had significantly less motor and cognitive impairment as indicated by FIM score at the start, had a modest but statistically significant increase in FIM motor score compared with the control group. The FIM tasks were not necessarily carried out by the affected arm, however.

Although available for nearly 20 years, EMG-triggered neuromuscular stimulation procedures that produce modest gains in wrist extensor strength have not come into general use. Two randomized trials provided from 15 to 24 sessions of electrical stimulation of the wrist and finger extensors in response to the feedback of the low-amplitude EMG signal elicited by attempted wrist extension during inpatient rehabilitation for stroke.[168,169] Functional wrist extension improved more in the group undergoing feedback therapy than in those receiving routine therapy, but the positive effects did not persist by 24 weeks after stimulation stopped. A randomized study of 11 subjects with chronic hemiparesis achieved significantly better hand extensor strength and, in a rare demonstration, improved the ability of subjects to pick up small objects.[170] Up to 25% of patients discontinue this form of functional electrical stimulation because the evoked response induces pain.

Five weeks of functional electrical stimulation may also reduce shoulder pain related to subluxation from paresis and may improve shoulder function,[171] perhaps by allowing pain-free practice. Orthotic devices placed across the wrist and designed to electrically stimulate a grasp or pincer movement have not yet been used widely.[172,173] Virtual reality systems that augment feedback about the position of the hand in space represent a potentially powerful form of practice, offering feedback information about knowledge of performance and of results using parameters such as velocity, trajectory, and accuracy of the reaching movement. The optimal style, daily intensity, and overall duration of training and the best outcome measures, in terms of sensitivity to change and relevance to useful movements, are a work in progress for all interventions.

Pharmacotherapy

When combined with physical therapies, several monaminergic agents have lessened motor impairments and improved ADLs. These attempts to develop a pharmacotherapy for neurorehabilitation are drawn from animal studies of enhanced learning and neuroplasticity,[174–176] although the leap from biologic responses in rats to those in humans after focal brain injury is a precarious one.[177] In small randomized trials, amphetamine,[178,179] methylphenidate,[180] levodopa,[181] and fluoxetine[182,183] have shown modest levels of success for improving strength or motor control, but the trials did not necessarily improve ADLs.

Amphetamine has received the most acclaim. Investigators have rejected at least 20 patients for every patient who met the criteria for these trials.[178,179] Best results were achieved when physical therapy relevant to the outcome measure was combined with the drug. Side effects of amphetamine, using 10 mg every other morning, have been minimal, and most studies have probably used exclusion criteria that were too strict. In another double-blind, placebo-controlled trial of D-amphetamine, however, no effect of drug was found in 9 patients who received 10 mg of drug every morning for 14 days and then 5 mg daily for 3 days during inpatient rehabilitation.[184] A later trial randomly assigned 39 geriatric patients with stroke to 10 therapy sessions combined with 10 mg of amphetamine or placebo during 5 weeks of rehabilitation.[185] No differences between the amphetamine group and the placebo group were found for motor function or ADLs.

A well-designed trial randomly assigned 53 patients admitted for inpatient rehabilitation to 100 mg of levodopa and carbidopa or to placebo.[181] Subjects received their assigned medication every morning before physiotherapy for 3 weeks and then continued therapy for another 3 weeks. Regardless of the initial level of motor dysfunction as indicated by the Rivermead Motor Assessment, subjects receiving levodopa improved a statistically significant 2 points on the 15-point subscale for the arm. Improvement persisted 3 weeks later. The relative improvement, however, does not necessarily correlate with a difference in strength, coordination, or functional use of the arm. Other quasi-experimental studies using, for example, the norepinephrine precursor L-threo-3,4-dihydroxyphenylserine,[186,187] reported gains. Drugs that enhance cerebral activation during a task carried out during functional magnetic resonance imaging[127,188] may help predict whether an agent is likely to be of benefit in promoting activity-dependent plasticity.

Should clinicians routinely try pharmacologic adjuncts to enhance motor gains? Such an approach may be worthwhile in patients with some sensorimotor function who are undergoing active rehabilitation and in whom motor control lags and limits gains in walking or use of the upper extremity. As shown in Table 56.7, it is best to start with drugs that tend to have the fewest side effects, such as the anticholinesterase inhibitors donepezil or galantamine at typical doses used in Alzheimer's disease, followed by a trial of an SSRI such as sertraline, 50 mg, or the dopaminergic agent levodopa and carbidopa, 25 mg and 100 mg.

CONCLUSIONS

The milieu and focus on functional gains provided by an inpatient rehabilitation team lead to better outcomes than those achieved by general medical care and less organized services.

Patients may improve by spontaneous processes at first, but important gains are likely related to intrinsic biologic mechanisms that are driven by external stimuli. Task-oriented practice may be a critical element for successful motor and cognitive retraining. Practice sessions must include learning paradigms and problem-solving techniques with optimal cues and reinforcers. Practice must be relevant to the subject, frequent, and of adequate duration. The goals of therapy include an increase in functional independence and renewed social reintegration into the family and community.

To improve motor performance, practice should engage the patient and aim to improve selective movements, motor control, skill, strength, endurance for an activity, and generalized fitness. This approach to training may lead to synaptic and morphologic changes associated with activity-dependent plasticity at the levels of the spinal cord, brainstem, and cerebral hemispheres.[13] Certain pharmacologic interventions may help drive experience-induced learning and neural adaptations for specific tasks, but clinical trials to date offer only modest support for this theory. The physician with expertise in neurorehabilitation should help therapists develop training paradigms drawn from an integration of basic neuroscience, cognitive neuroscience, clinical neuromedicine, clinical research study designs, and outcomes research.

Therapy

Therapy

References

1. Adams H, Davis P, Leira E, et al: Baseline NIH Stroke Scale score strongly predicts outcome after stroke. Neurology 53:126–131, 1999.
2. Heinemann A, Harvey R, McGuire J, et al: Measurement properties of the NIH Stroke Scale during acute rehabilitation. Stroke 28:1174–1180, 1997.
3. Lai S-M, Duncan P, Keighley J: Prediction of functional outcome after stroke: Comparison of the Orpington Prognostic Scale and the NIH Stroke Scale. Stroke 29:1838–1842, 1998.
4. Pedersen P, Jorgensen H, Nakayama H, et al: Comprehensive assessment of activities of daily living in stroke: The Copenhagen Stroke Study. Arch Phys Med Rehabil 78:161–165, 1997.
5. Golomb B, Vickrey B, Hays R: A review of health-related quality-of-life measures in stroke. Pharmacoeconomics 19:155–185, 2001.
6. Pickard A, Johnson J, Penn A, et al: Replicability of SF-36 summary scores by the SF-12 in stroke patients. Stroke 30:1213–1217, 1999.
7. Williams L, Weinberger M, Harris L, et al: Development of a stroke-specific quality of life scale. Stroke 30:1362–1369, 1999.
8. Hamedani A, Wells C, Brass L, et al: A quality-of-life instrument for young hemorrhagic stroke patients. Stroke 32:687–695, 2001.
9. Bugge C, Alexander H, Hagen S: Stroke patients informal caregivers: Patients, caregiver, and service factors that affect caregiver strain. Stroke 30:1517–1523, 1999.
10. Knapp P, Hewison J: Disagreement in patient and carer assessment of functional abilities after stroke. Stroke 30:934–938, 1999.
11. Duncan W, Wallace D, Lai M, et al: The Stroke Impact Scale Version 2.0. Stroke 30:2131–2140, 1999.
12. Kelly-Hayes M, Robertson J, Broderick J, et al: The American Heart Association Stroke Outcome Classification. Stroke 29:1274–1280, 1998.
13. Dobkin B: The Clinical Science of Neurologic Rehabilitation. New York, Oxford University Press, 2003.
14. Dobkin B: Activity-dependent learning contributes to motor recovery. Ann Neurol 44:158–160, 1998.
15. Dobkin B: Functional rewiring of brain and spinal cord after injury: The three R's of neural repair and neurological rehabilitation. Curr Opin Neurol 13:655–659, 2000.
16. Kwakkel G, Wagenaar R, Twisk J, et al: Intensity of leg and arm training after primary middle cerebral artery stroke: A randomised trial. Lancet 354:191–196, 1999.
17. Walker M, Gladman J, Lincoln N, et al: Occupational therapy for stroke patients not admitted to hospital: A randomised controlled trial. Lancet 354:278–280, 1999.
18. Dobkin B: Overview of treadmill locomotor training with partial body weight support: A neurophysiologically sound approach whose time has come for randomized clinical trials. Neurorehabil Neural Repair 13:157–165, 1999.
19. Kwakkel G, Wagenaar R, Koelman T, et al: Effects of intensity of rehabilitation after stroke: A research synthesis. Stroke 28:1550–1556, 1997.
20. Nugent J, Schurr K, Adams R: A dose-response relationship between amount of weight-bearing exercise and walking outcome following cerebrovascular accident. Arch Phys Med Rehabil 75:399–402, 1994.
21. Pulvermuller F, Neininger B, Elbert T, et al: Constraint-induced therapy of chronic aphasia after stroke. Stroke 32:1621–1626, 2001.
22. Paolucci S, Antonucci G, Grasso M, et al: Early versus delayed inpatient stroke rehabilitation: A matched comparison conducted in Italy. Arch Phys Med Rehabil 81:695–700, 2000.
23. How do stroke units improve patient outcomes? A collaborative systematic review of the randomized trials. Stroke Unit Trialists' Collaboration. Stroke 28:2139–2144, 1997.
24. Kalra L, Eade J: Role of stroke rehabilitation units in managing severe disability after stroke. Stroke 26:2031–2034, 1995.
25. Indredavik B, Fjaertoft H, Ekeberg G, et al: Benefit of an extended stroke unit service with early supported discharge. Stroke 31:2989–2994, 2000.
26. Kramer A, Steiner J, Schlenker R, et al: Outcomes and costs after hip fracture and stroke: A comparison of rehabilitation settings. JAMA 277:396–404, 1997.
27. Sulch D, Perez I, Melbourn A, et al: Randomized controlled trial of integrated (managed) care pathway for stroke rehabilitation. Stroke 31:1929–1934, 2000.
28. Wade D, Skilbeck C, Bainton D, et al: Controlled trial of a home-care service for acute stroke patients. Lancet XX:323–326, 1985.
29. Rudd A, Wolfe C, Tilling K, et al: The effectiveness of a package of community care on one year outcome of stroke patients. BMJ 315:1039–1044, 1997.
30. Ronning OM, Guldvog B: Outcome of subacute stroke rehabilitation: A randomized controlled trial. Stroke 29:779–784, 1998.
31. Holmqvist L, von Koch L, Kostulas V, et al: A randomized controlled trial of rehabilitation at home after stroke in southwest Stockholm. Stroke 29:591–597, 1998.
32. Nilsson A, Aniansson A, Grimby G: Rehabilitation needs and disability in community living stroke survivors two years after stroke. Top Stroke Rehabil 6:30–47, 2000.
33. Grimby G, Andren E, Daving Y, et al: Dependence and perceived difficulty in daily activities in community-living stroke survivors 2 years after stroke: A study of instrumental structures. Stroke 29:1843–1849, 1998.
34. Taub E, Uswatte G, Pidikiti R: Constraint-induced movement therapy: A new family of techniques with broad application to physical rehabilitation—a clinical review. Rehabil Res Develop 36:237–251, 1999.
35. Gresham GE, Phillips TF, Wolf PA: Epidemiologic profile of long-term stroke disability: The Framingham Study. Arch Phys Med Rehabil 60:487–491, 1979.
36. Dobkin B: Focused stroke rehabilitation programs do not improve outcome. Arch Neurol 46:701–703, 1989.
37. Ottenbacher K, Jannell S: The results of clinical trials in stroke rehabilitation research. Arch Neurol 50:37–44, 1993.
38. Dobkin B: Neuromedical complications in stroke patients transferred for rehabilitation before and after DRGs. J Neurol Rehabil 1:3–8, 1987.
39. Dromerick A, Reding M: Medical and neurological complications during inpatient stroke rehabilitation. Stroke 25:358–361, 1994.
40. Langhorne P, Stott D, Robertson L, et al: Medical complications after stroke: A multicenter study. Stroke 31:1223–1229, 2000.
41. Roth E, Lovell L, Harvey R, et al: Incidence of and risk factors for medical complications during stroke rehabilitation. Stroke 32:523–529, 2001.
42. Brittain K, Peet S, Castleden C: Stroke and incontinence. Stroke 29:524–528, 1998.
43. Gelber D, Jozefczyk P, Good D, et al: Urinary retention following acute stroke. J Neurol Rehabil 8:69–74, 1994.
44. Sunderland A, Tinson D, Bradley E, et al: Enhanced physical therapy improves recovery of function after stroke: A randomised controlled trial. J Neurol Neurosurg Psychiatry 55:530–535, 1992.
45. Snels I, Beckerman H, Twisk J, et al: Effect of triamcinolone acetonide injections on hemiplegic shoulder pain: A randomized clinical trial. Stroke 31:2396–2401, 2000.
46. Rowbotham MC: Complex regional pain syndrome type I (reflex sympathetic dystrophy). Neurology 51:4–5, 1998.
47. Werner R, Priebe M, Davidoff G: Reflex sympathetic dystrophy syndrome associated with hemiplegia. Neuro Rehabil 2:16–22, 1992.
48. Bowsher D, Leijon G, Thuomos K: Central poststroke pain: Correlation of MRI with clinical pain characteristics and sensory abnormalities. Neurology 51:1352–1358, 1998.
49. Vestergaard K, Andersen G, Gottrup H, et al: Lamotrigine for central poststroke pain. Neurology 56:184–190, 2001.
50. Leijon G, Boivie J: Central poststroke pain—a controlled trial of amitriptyline and carbamazepine. Pain 36:27–36, 1989.
51. Gallo J, Coyne J: The challenge of depression in late life. JAMA 284:1570–1572, 2000.
52. Wolf P, Bachman D, Kelly-Hayes M, et al: Stroke and depression in the community: The Framingham Study. Neurology 40(Suppl 1):416, 1990.
53. Robinson R, Kubos K, Starr L, et al: Mood disorders in stroke patients: Importance of location of lesion. Brain 187:81–93, 1984.
54. Astrom M, Adolfsson R, Asplund K: Major depression in stroke patients: A 3-year longitudinal study. Stroke 24:976–982, 1993.
55. Pohjasvaara T, Leppavuori A, Siira I, et al: Frequency and clinical determinants of poststroke depression. Stroke 29:2311–2317, 1998.
56. Andersen G, Vsetergaard K, Lauritzen L: Effective treatment of poststroke depression with the selective serotonin reuptake inhibitor citalopram. Stroke 25:1099–1104, 1994.
57. Lazarus L, Moberg P, Langsley P, et al: Methylphenidate and nortriptyline in the treatment of poststroke depression: A retrospective comparison. Arch Phys Med Rehabil 75:403–406, 1994.

58. Reding M, Orto L, Winter S, et al: Antidepressant therapy after stroke. Arch Neurol 43:763–765, 1986.

59. Whooley M, Simon G: Managing depression in medical outpatients. N Engl J Med 343:1942–1950, 2000.

60. Wiart L, Petit H, Joseph P, et al: Fluoxetine in early poststroke depression: A double-blind placebo-controlled study. Stroke 31:1829–1832, 2000.

61. DePippo K, Holas M, Reding M, et al: Dysphagia therapy following stroke: A controlled trial. Neurology 44:1655–1660, 1994.

62. Hamdy S, Aziz Q, Rothwell J, et al: Recovery of swallowing after dysphagic stroke relates to functional reorganization in the intact motor cortex. Gastroenterology 115:1104–1112, 1999.

63. Agency for Health Care Policy and Research: Pressure ulcers in adults: Prediction and prevention. In: U.S. Department of Health and Human Services, 1992.

64. Epstein F: Cutaneous wound healing. New Engl J Med 341:738–746, 1999.

65. Boldrini P, Basaglia N, Calanca M: Sexual changes in hemiparetic patients. Arch Phys Med Rehabil 72:202–207, 1991.

66. Maquet P, Laureys S, Peigneux P, et al: Experience-dependent changes in cerebral activation during human REM sleep. Nature Neurosci 3:831–836, 2000.

67. Bassetti C, Aldrich M, Quint D: Sleep-disordered breathing in patients with acute supra- and infratentorial strokes: A prospective study of 39 patients. Stroke 28:1765–1772, 1997.

68. Good D, Henkle J, Gelber D, et al: Sleep-disordered breathing and poor functional outcome after stroke. Stroke 27:252–259, 1996.

69. Mohsenin V, Valor R: Sleep apnea in patients with hemispheric stroke. Arch Phys Med Rehabil 76:71–76, 1995.

70. Dietz V: Supraspinal pathways and the development of muscle-tone dysregulation. Dev Med Child Neurol 41:708–715, 1999.

71. Hiersemenzel L-P, Curt A, Dietz V: From spinal shock to spasticity. Neurology 54:1574–1582, 2000.

72. Hufschmidt A, Mauritz K: Chronic transformation of muscle in spasticity: A peripheral contribution to increased tone. J Neurol Neurosurg Psychiatry 48:676–685, 1985.

73. Brown D, Kautz S: Increased workload enhances force output during pedaling exercise in persons with poststroke hemiplegia. Stroke 29:598–606, 1998.

74. Sharp S, Brouwer B: Isokinetic strength training of the hemiparetic knee: Effects on function and spasticity. Arch Phys Med Rehabil 78:1231–1236, 1997.

75. Smith G, Silver K, Goldberg A, et al: "Task-oriented" exercise improves hamstring strength and spastic reflexes in chronic stroke patients. Stroke 30:2112–2118, 1999.

76. Benecke R, Conrad B, Meinck H, et al: Electromyographic analysis of bicycling on an ergometer for evaluation of spasticity of lower limbs in man. In Desmedt J (ed): Motor Control Mechanisms in Health and disease. New York, Raven Press, 1983.

77. Brown D, Kautz S, Dairaghi C: Muscle activity adapts to anti-gravity posture during pedalling in persons with post-stroke hemiplegia. Brain 120:825–837, 1997.

78. Macko R, Smith G, Dobrovolny C, et al: Treadmill training improves fitness reserve in chronic stroke patients. Arch Phys Med Rehabil 82:879–884, 2001.

79. Potempa K, Lopez M, Braun L, et al: Physiological outcomes of aerobic exercise training in hemiparetic stroke. Stroke 26:101–105, 1995.

80. Bes A, Eysette M, Pierrot-Deseilligny E: A multi-centre, double-blind trial of tizanidine in spasticity associated with hemiplegia. Curr Med Res Opin 10:709–718, 1988.

81. Gelber D, Good D, Dromerick A, et al: Open-label dose-titration safety and efficacy study of tizanidine hydrochloride in the treatment of spasticity associated with chronic stroke. Stroke 32:1841–1846, 2001.

82. Bakheit A, Thilmann A, Ward A, et al: A randomized, double-blind, placebo-controlled, dose-ranging study to compare the efficacy and safety of three doses of botulinum toxin type A (Dysport) with placebo in upper limb spasticity after stroke. Stroke 31:2402–2406, 2000.

83. Hesse S, Krajnik J, Luecke D, et al: Ankle muscle activity before and after botulinum toxin therapy for lower limb extensor spasticity in chronic hemiparetic patients. Stroke 27:455–460, 1996.

84. Reiter F, Danni M, Lagalla G, et al: Low-dose botulinum toxin with ankle taping for the treatment of spastic equinovarus foot after stroke. Arch Phys Med Rehabil 79:532–535, 1998.

85. Brashear A, Gordon M, Elovic E, et al: Intramuscular injection of botulinum toxin for the treatment of wrist and finger spasticity after stroke. N Engl J Med 347:395–400, 2002.

86. Simpson D, Alexander D, O'Brien C, et al: Botulinum toxin type A in the treatment of upper extremity spasticity: A randomized, double-blind, placebo-controlled trial. Neurology 46:1306–1310, 1996.

87. Meythaler J, Guin-Renfroe S, Hadley M: Continuously infused intrathecal baclofen for spastic/dystonic hemiplegia. Am J Phys Med Rehabil 78:247–254, 1999.

88. Cicerone K, Dahlberg C, Kalmar K, et al: Evidence-based cognitive rehabilitation: Recommendations for clinical practice. Arch Phys Med Rehabil 81:1596–1615, 2000.

89. Desmond D, Moroney J, Paik M, et al: Frequency and clinical determinants of dementia after ischemic stroke. Neurology 54:1124–1131, 2000.

90. Gorelick P: Status of risk factors for dementia associated with stroke. Stroke 28:459–463, 1997.

91. Moroney J, Bagiella E, Desmond D, et al: Risk factors for incident dementia after stroke. Stroke 27:1283–1289, 1996.

92. Rockwood K, Wentzel C, Hachinski V, et al: Prevalence and outcomes of vascular cognitive impairment. Neurology 54:447–451, 2000.

93. Tatemichi T, Desmond D, Stern Y, et al: Cognitive impairment after stroke: Frequency, patterns, and relationship to functional abilities. J Neurol Neurosurg Psychiatry 57:202–207, 1994.

94. Henon H, Pasquier F, Durieu I, et al: Preexisting dementia in stroke patients. Stroke 28:2429–2436, 1997.

95. Pohjasvaara T, Erkinjuntti T, Vataja R, et al: Dementia three months after stroke: Baseline frequency and effect of different definitions of dementia in the Helsinki Stroke Aging Memory Study (SAM) Cohort. Stroke 28:785–792, 1997.

96. Wilson B, Baddeley A, Evans J, et al: Errorless learning in the rehabilitation of memory impaired people. Neuropsychol Rehabil 4:307–326, 1994.

97. Hanlon R: Motor learning following unilateral stroke. Arch Phys Med Rehabil 77:811–815, 1996.

98. Winstein C, Merians A, Sullivan K: Motor learning after unilateral brain damage. Neuropsychologia 37:975–987, 1999.

99. Kalra L, Perez I, Gupta S, et al: The influence of visual neglect on stroke rehabilitation. Stroke 28:1386–1391, 1997.

100. Marshall R, Sacco R, Lee S, et al: Hemineglect predicts functional outcome after stroke [abstract]. Ann Neurol 36:298, 1994.

101. Ben-Yishay Y, Diller L: Cognitive remediation in traumatic brain injury: Update and issues. Arch Phys Med Rehabil 74:204–213, 1993.

102. Gordon W, Diller L, Lieberman A, et al: Perceptual remediation in patients with right brain damage: A comprehensive program. Arch Phys Med Rehabil 66:353–359, 1985.

103. Pizzamiglio L, Antonucci G, Judica A, et al: Chronic rehabilitation of the hemineglect disorder in chronic patients with unilateral right brain damage. J Clin Exp Neuropsychol 14:901–923, 1992.

104. Pizzamiglio L, Perani D, Cappa S, et al: Recovery of neglect after right hemisphere damage. Arch Neurol 55:561–568, 1998.

105. Young G, Collins D, Hren M: Effect of pairing scanning training with block design training in the remediation of perceptual problems in left hemiplegics. J Clin Neuropsychol 5:201–212, 1983.

106. Wiart L, Bon Saint Come A, Debelleix X, et al: Unilateral neglect syndrome rehabilitation by trunk rotation and scanning training. Arch Phys Med Rehabil 78:424–429, 1997.

107. Robertson I, North N: Spatio-motor cueing in unilateral neglect: The role of hemispace, hand and motor activation. Neuropsychologia 30:553–563, 1992.

108. Robertson I, Mattingley J, Rorden C, et al: Phasic alerting of neglect patients overcomes their spatial deficit in visual awareness. Nature 395:169–172, 1998.

109. Fleet W, Valenstein E, Watson R, et al: Dopamine agonist therapy for neglect in humans. Neurology 37:1765–1770, 1987.

110. Grujic Z, Mapstone M, Gitelman D, et al: Dopamine agonists reorient visual exploration away from the neglected hemispace. Neurology 51:1395–1398, 1998.

110a. Erkinjuntti T, Kurz A, Gauthier S, et al: Efficacy of galantamine in probable vascular dementia and Alzheimer's disease combined with cerebrovascular disease: a randomised trial. Lancet 359:1283–1290, 2002.

111. Glazewski S, Giese K, Silva A, et al: The role of alpha-CaMKII autophosphorylation in neocortical experience-dependent plasticity. Nature Neurosci 3:911–917, 2000.

112. Kandel E: The molecular biology of memory storage: A dialogue between genes and synapses. Science 294:1030–1038, 2001.

113. Pedersen P, Jorgensen H, Nakayama H, et al: Aphasia in acute stroke: Incidence, determinants, and recovery. Ann Neurol 38:659–666, 1995.

114. Benson D, Dobkin B, Rothi L, et al: Assessment: Melodic intonation therapy. Neurology 44:566–568, 1994.

115. Robey R: A meta-analysis of clinical outcomes in the treatment of aphasia. J Speech Lang Hear Res 41:172–187, 1998.

116. Damasio H, Grabowski TJ, Tranel D, et al: Neural correlates of naming actions and of naming spatial relations. Neuroimage 13:1053–1064, 2001.

117. Kessler J, Thiel A, Karbe H, et al: Piracetam improves activated blood flow and facilitates rehabilitation of poststroke aphasic patients. Stroke 31:2112–2116, 2000.

118. Musso M, Weiller C, Kiebel S: Training-induced brain plasticity in aphasia. Brain 122:1781–1790, 1999.

119. Aftonomos L, Steele R, Wertz R: Promoting recovery in chronic aphasia with an interactive technology. Arch Phys Med Rehabil 78:841–846, 1997.

120. Weinrich M, Boser K, McCall D, et al: Training agrammatic subjects on passive sentences: Implications for syntactic deficit theories. Brain Lang 76:45–61, 2001.

121. Walker-Batson D, Curtis S, Natarajan R, et al: A double-blind placebo-controlled study of the use of amphetamine in the treatment of aphasia. Stroke 32:2093–2098, 2001.

122. Huber W, Willmes K, Poeck K, et al: Piracetam as an adjuvant to language therapy for aphasia: A randomized double-blind placebo-controlled pilot study. Arch Phys Med Rehabil 78:245–250, 1997.

123. Tanaka Y, Albert M, Yokoyama E, et al: Cholinergic therapy for anomia in fluent aphasia. Ann Neurol 50(Suppl 1):S61–S62, 2001.

124. Gold M, VanDam D, Silliman E: An open-label trial of bromocriptine in nonfluent aphasia: A qualitative analysis of word storage and retrieval. Brain Lang 74:141–156, 2000.

125. Dobkin B: Greater plasticity through chemicals and practice. Neurol Network Comment 2:171–174, 1998.

126. Fried I, Wilson C, Morrow J, et al: Increased dopamine release in the human amygdala during performance of cognitive tasks. Nature Neurosci 4:201–206, 2001.

127. Mattay V, Callicott J, Bertolino A, et al: Effects of dextroamphetamine on cognitive performance and cortical activation. Neuroimage 12:268–275, 2000.

128. Waelti P, Dickinson A, Schultz W: Dopamine responses comply with basic assumptions of formal learning theory. Nature 412:43–48, 2001.

129. Jorgensen H, Nakayama H, Raaschou H, et al: Outcome and time course of recovery in stroke. Part II: Time course. The Copenhagen Stroke Study. Arch Phys Med Rehabil 76:406–412, 1995.

130. Jorgensen H, Nakayama H, Raaschou H, et al: Outcome and time course of recovery in stroke. Part I: Outcome. The Copenhagen Stroke Study. Arch Phys Med Rehabil 76:399–405, 1995.

131. Wandel A, Jorgensen H, Nakayama H, et al: Prediction of walking function in stroke patients with initial lower extremity paralysis: the Copenhagen Stroke Study. Arch Phys Med Rehabil 81:736–738, 2000.

132. Reding M, Potes E: Rehabilitation outcome following initial unilateral hemispheric stroke: Life table analysis approach. Stroke 19:1354–1364, 1988.

133. Giuliani C: Strength training for patients with neurological disorders. Neurology Report 19:29–34, 1995.

134. Dobkin B, Harkema S, Requejo P, et al: Modulation of locomotor-like EMG activity in subjects with complete and incomplete chronic spinal cord injury. J Neurol Rehabil 9:183–190, 1995.

135. Harkema S, Hurley S, Patel U, et al: Human lumbosacral spinal cord interprets loading during stepping. J Neurophysiol 77:797–811, 1997.

136. Harkema S, Dobkin B, Edgerton V: Pattern generators in locomotion: Implications for recovery of walking after spinal cord injury. Top Spinal Cord Inj Rehabil 6:82–96, 2000.

137. Sullivan K, Knowlton B, Dobkin B: Step training with body weight support: Effect of treadmill speed and practice paradigms on poststroke locomotor recovery. Arch Phys Med Rehabil 83:683–691, 2002.

138. Pohl M, Mehrholz J, Ritschel C, et al: Speed-dependent treadmill training in ambulatory hemiparetic stroke patients. Stroke 33:553–558, 2002.

139. Dobkin B, Sullivan K: Sensorimotor cortex plasticity and locomotor and motor control gains induced by body weight–supported treadmill training after stroke. Neurorehabil Neural Repair 15:258–259, 2001.

140. Dobkin BH: Functional MRI: A potential physiologic indicator for stroke rehabilitation interventions. Stroke 34:23–28, 2003.

141. Hesse S, Bertelt C, Jahnke M, et al: Treadmill training with partial body weight support compared with physiotherapy in nonambulatory hemiparetic patients. Stroke 26:976–981, 1995.

142. Visintin M, Barbeau H, Korner-Bitensky N, et al: A new approach to retrain gait in stroke patients through body weight support and treadmill stimulation. Stroke 29:1122–1128, 1998.

143. Nilsson L, Carlsson J, Danielsson A, et al: Walking training of patients with hemiparesis at an early stage after stroke: A comparison of walking training on a treadmill with body weight support and walking training on the ground. Clin Rehabil 15:515–527, 2002.

144. Moreland J, Thomson M, Fuoco A: Electromyographic biofeedback to improve lower extremity function after stroke: A meta-analysis. Arch Phys Med Rehabil 79:134–140, 1998.

145. Macko R, DeSouza C, Tretter L, et al: Treadmill aerobic exercise training reduces the energy expenditure and cardiovascular demands of hemiparetic gait in chronic stroke patients. Stroke 28:326–330, 1997.

146. Thaut M, Kenyon G, Schauer M, et al: The connection between rhythmicity and brain function. IEEE Eng Med Biol March/April:101–108, 1999.

147. Nakayama H, Jorgensen H, Raaschou H, et al: Recovery of upper extremity function in stroke patients: The Copenhagen Stroke Study. Arch Phys Med Rehabil 75:394–398, 1994.

148. Katrak P, Bowring G, Conroy P, et al: Predicting upper limb recovery after stroke: The place of early shoulder and hand movement. Arch Phys Med Rehabil 79:758–761, 1998.

149. Johansson K, Lingren I, Widner H, et al: Can sensory stimulation improve the functional outcome in stroke patients? Neurology 43:2189–2192, 1993.

150. Gosman-Hedstrom G, Claesson L, Klingenstierna U, et al: Effects of acupuncture treatment on daily life activities and quality of life. Stroke 29:2100–2108, 1998.

151. Johannson B, Haker E, von Arbin M, et al: Acupuncture and transcutaneous nerve stimulation in stroke rehabilitation: A randomized, controlled trial. Stroke 32:707–713, 2001.

152. Taub E, Wolf S: Constraint induced movement techniques to facilitate upper extremity use in stroke patients. Top Stroke Rehabil 3:38–61, 1997.

153. Miltner W, Bauder H, Sommer M, et al: Effects of constraint-induced movement therapy on patients with chronic motor deficits after stroke. Stroke 30:586–592, 1999.

154. Taub E, Miller N, Novack T, et al: Technique to improve chronic motor deficit after stroke. Arch Phys Med Rehabil 74:347–354, 1993.

155. Liepert J, Bauder H, Miltner W, et al: Treatment-induced cortical reorganization after stroke in humans. Stroke 31:1210–1216, 2000.

156. van der Lee J, Wagenaar R, Lankhorst G, et al: Forced use of the upper extremity in chronic stroke patients: Results from a single-blind randomized clinical trial. Stroke 30:2369–2375, 1999.

157. Dromerick A, Edwards D, Hahn M: Does the application of constraint-induced movement therapy during acute rehabilitation reduce arm impairment after ischemic stroke? Stroke 31:2984–2988, 2000.

158. Butefisch C, Hummelsheim H, Denzler P, et al: Repetitive training of isolated movements improves the outcome of motor rehabilitation of the centrally paretic hand. J Neurol Sci 130:59–68, 1995.

159. Dean C, Shepherd R: Task-related training improves performance of seated reaching tasks after stroke. Stroke 28:722–728, 1997.

160. Feys H, De Weerdt W, Selz B, et al: Effect of a therapeutic intervention for the hemiplegic upper limb in the acute phase after stroke. Stroke 29:785–792, 1998.

161. Pohl P, Winstein C: Practice effects on the less-affected upper extremity after stroke. Arch Phys Med Rehabil 80:668–675, 1999.

162. Colebatch J, Gandevia S: The distribution of muscular weakness in upper motor neuron lesions affecting the arm. Brain 112:749–763, 1989.

163. Reinkensmeyer D, Kahn L, Averbuch M, et al: Understanding and treating arm movement impairment after chronic brain injury: Progress with the ARM guide. J Rehab Res Develop 37:653–662, 2000.

164. Volpe B, Krebs H, Hogan N, et al: Robot training enhanced motor outcome in patients with stroke maintained over 3 years. Neurology 53:1874–1876, 1999.

165. Whitall J, Waller S, Silver K, et al: Repetitive bilateral arm training with rhythmic auditory cueing improves motor function in chronic hemiparetic stroke. Stroke 31:2390–2395, 2000.

166. Lincoln N, Parry R, Vass C: Randomized, controlled trial to evaluate increased intensity of physiotherapy treatment of arm function after stroke. Stroke 30:573–579, 1999.

167. Volpe B, Krebs H, Hogan N, et al: A novel approach to stroke rehabilitation: Robot-aided sensorimotor stimulation. Neurology 54:1938–1944, 2000.

168. Chae J, Bethoux F, Bohinc T, et al: Neuromuscular stimulation for upper extremity motor and functional recovery in acute hemiplegia. Stroke 29:975–979, 1998.

169. Powell J, Pandyan A, Granat M: Electrical stimulation of wrist extensors in poststroke hemiplegia. Stroke 30:1384–1389, 1999.

170. Cauraugh J, Light K, Kim S, et al: Chronic motor dysfunction after stroke: Recovering wrist and finger extension by electromyography-triggered neuromuscular stimulation. Stroke 31:1360–1364, 2000.

171. Chantraine A, Baribeault A, Uebelhart D, et al: Shoulder pain and dysfunction in hemiplegia: Effects of functional electrical stimulation. Arch Phys Med Rehabil 80:328–331, 1999.

172. Jizerman M, Stoffers T, Groen I, et al: The NESS Handmaster orthosis: Restoration of hand function in C5 and stroke patients by means of electrical stimulation. J Rehabil Sci 9:86–90, 1996.

173. Popovic D, Stojanovic A, Pjanovic A: Clinical evaluation of the bionic glove. Arch Phys Med Rehabil 80:299–304, 1999.

174. Rossignol S, Chau C, Brustein E, et al: Pharmacological activation and modulation of the central pattern generator for locomotion in the cat. Ann N Y Acad Sci 860:346–359, 1998.

175. Stroemer R, Kent T, Hulsebosch C: Enhanced neocortical neural sprouting, synaptogenesis and behavioral recovery with *d*-amphetamine therapy after neocortical infarction in rats. Stroke 29:2381–2395, 1998.

176. Sutton R, Feeney D: Alpha-noradrenergic agonists and antagonists affect recovery and maintenance of beam walking ability after sensorimotor cortex ablation in the rat. Restor Neurol Neurosci 4:1–11, 1992.

177. Dobkin B: Experimental brain injury and repair. Curr Opin Neurol 10:493–497, 1997.

178. Crisostomo E, Duncan P, Propst M, et al: Evidence that amphetamine with physical therapy promotes recovery of motor function in stroke patients. Ann Neurol 23:94–97, 1988.

179. Walker-Batson D, Smith P, Curtis S, et al: Amphetamine paired with physical therapy accelerates motor recovery after stroke. Stroke 26:2254–2259, 1995.

180. Grade C, Redford B, Chrostowski J, et al: Methylphenidate in early poststroke recovery: A double-blind, placebo-controlled study. Arch Phys Med Rehabil 79:1047–1050, 1998.

181. Scheidtmann K, Fries W, Muller F, et al: Effect of levodopa in combination with physiotherapy on functional motor recovery after stroke: A prospective, randomised, double-blinded study. Lancet 358:787–790, 2001.

182. Dam M, Tonin P, De Boni A, et al: Effects of fluoxetine and maprotiline on functional recovery in poststroke hemiplegic patients undergoing rehabilitation therapy. Stroke 27:1211–1214, 1996.

183. Pariente J, Loubinoux I, Carel C, et al: Fluoxetine modulates motor performance and cerebral activation of patients recovering from stroke. Ann Neurol 50:718–729, 2001.

184. Reding M, Solomon B, Borucki S: Effect of dextroamphetamine on motor recovery after stroke. Neurology 45(Suppl 4):A222, 1995.

185. Sonde L, Nordstrom M, Nilsson C, et al: A double-blind placebo-controlled study of the effects of amphetamine and physiotherapy after stroke. Cerebrovasc Dis 12:253–257, 2001.

186. Miyai I, Saito T, Nozaki S, et al: A pilot study of the effect of L-threodops on rehabilitation outcome of stroke patients. Neurorehabil Neural Repair 14:141–147, 2000.

187. Nishino K, Sasaki T, Takahashi K, et al: The norepinephrine precursor L-threo-3-4-dihydroxyphenylserine facilitates motor recovery in chronic stroke patients. J Clin Neurosci 8:547–550, 2001.

188. Loubinoux I, Carel C, Alary F, et al: Within-session and between-session reproducibility of cerebral sensorimotor activation: A test-retest effect evidenced with functional MRI. J Cereb Blood Flow Metab 21:592–607, 2001.

189. Iwanenko W, Fiedler R, Granger C, et al: The Uniform Data System for Medical Rehabilitation. Am J Phys Med Rehabil 80:56–61, 2001.

190. Smania N, Bazoli F, Piva D, et al: Visuomotor imagery and rehabilitation of neglect. Arch Phys Med Rehabil 78:430–436, 1997.

191. Tham K, Tegner R: Video feedback in the rehabilitation of patients with unilateral neglect. Arch Phys Med Rehabil 78:410–413, 1997.

192. Beis J-M, Andre J-M, Baumgarten A, et al: Eye patching in unilateral spatial neglect: Efficacy of two methods. Arch Phys Med Rehabil 80:71–76, 1999.

193. Butter C, Kirsch N: Combined and separate effects of eye patching and visual stimulation on unilateral neglect following stroke. Arch Phys Med Rehabil 73:1133–1139, 1992.

194. Rossi P, Kheyfets S, Reding M: Fresnel prisms improve visual perception in stroke patients with homonymous hemianopia or unilateral visual neglect. Neurology 40:1597–1599, 1990.

195. Serfaty C, Soroker N, Glicksohn J, et al: Does monocular viewing improve target detection in hemispatial neglect? Restor Neurol Neurosci 9:7–13, 1995.

196. Rossetti Y, Rode G, Pisella L, et al: Prism adaptation to a rightward optical deviation rehabilitates left hemispatial neglect. Nature 395:166–169, 1998.

197. Mennemeier M, Chatterjee A, Heilman K: A comparison of the influences of body and environment centred reference frames on neglect. Brain 117:1013–1021, 1994.

198. Simon E, Hegarty A, Mehler M: Hemispatial and directional performance biases in motor neglect. Neurology 45:525–531, 1995.

199. Oliveri M, Rossini P, Traversa R, et al: Left frontal transcranial magnetic stimulation reduces contralesional extinction in patients with unilateral right brain damage. Brain 122:1731–1739, 1999.

200. Rode G, Charles N, Perenin M-T, et al: Partial remission of hemiplegia and somatoparaphrenia through vestibular stimulation in a case of unilateral neglect. Cortex 28:203–208, 1992.

201. Vallar G, Sterzi R, Bottini G, et al: Temporary remission of left hemianesthesia after vestibular stimulation: A sensory neglect phenomenon. Cortex 26:123–131, 1990.

202. Pizzamiglio L, Frasca R, Guariglia C, et al: Effects of optokinetic stimulation in patients with visual neglect. Cortex 26:535–540, 1990.

203. Kerkhoff G, MunBinger U, Meier E: Neurovisual rehabilitation in cerebral blindness. Arch Neurol 51:474–481, 1994.

204. Gray J, Robertson I, Pentland B, et al: Microcomputer-based attentional retraining after brain damage: A randomised group controlled trial. Neuropsychol Rehabil 2:97–115, 1992.

205. Robertson I, Gray J, Pentland B, et al: Microcomputer-based rehabilitation for unilateral left visual neglect: A randomized controlled trial. Arch Phys Med Rehabil 71:663–668, 1990.

206. Patel A, Duncan P, Lai S, et al: The relation between impairments and functional outcomes poststroke. Arch Phys Med Rehabil 81:1357–1363, 2000.

Chapter Fifty-Seven

Antiplatelet Therapy for Secondary Prevention of Stroke

Babette B. Weksler

Cerebral ischemia tends to recur after a primary episode of either transient ischemia attack (TIA) or stroke. Most commonly, cerebral ischemia is caused by thromboemboli that form on damaged vascular surfaces of extracranial or intracerebral arteries. Local activation of platelets on the walls of diseased arteries initiates thrombus formation under conditions of high flow typical of arteries, because activated platelets not only clump together but also directly catalyze thrombin generation. These thrombi are classically considered "white clots," that is, they are composed mainly of platelets plus some fibrin. These platelet-rich thrombi that form on atherosclerotic plaques may either occlude small arterioles directly or embolize into intracerebral endarteries, producing vascular occlusion that results in neurologic dysfunction.

Because platelet activation is causally linked to episodes of cerebral arterial ischemia, therapies that diminish or block the early steps in hemostasis that are platelet-dependent are used in patients with TIAs or stroke to prevent further episodes of cerebral ischemia. However, despite the use of a variety of antithrombotic therapies for secondary prevention of stroke, risk reduction has been disappointing, only about 15% to 20% in most large clinical trials.[1] Increasing the intensity of treatment, either antiplatelet therapy or anticoagulation (or both together), has the important adverse effect of increasing intracerebral and systemic hemorrhage and negates net therapeutic benefit. Thus, current antithrombotic therapies for secondary prevention of stroke are considerably less successful than the same therapies used for secondary prevention of acute cardiac ischemic events; the latter respond very well to antiplatelet therapy. The modest success of antiplatelet drugs in reducing the recurrence of ischemic stroke further incorporates the fact that bleeding is less common during antiplatelet therapy than during anticoagulant therapy.

In contrast to arterial thrombi, venous thrombi form under conditions involving vascular stasis, consist mainly of fibrin and erythrocytes, and are much less dependent on platelet activation. Venous thrombosis, including cerebral venous thrombosis, thus is better prevented by anticoagulation than by antiplatelet therapy.[2] This is also true for cardioembolic stroke associated with atrial fibrillation (AF). However, the distinctions between factors contributing to arterial versus venous thrombi are far from absolute. Both platelet-dependent phases and coagulation factor–dependent phases of hemostasis intermingle to a considerable extent, for example, because of the prominent role played by platelets in catalyzing thrombin generation.

Moreover, combining antiplatelet and anticoagulant agents in the search for more powerful effects during long-term, secondary prevention of cerebral ischemia has been notably unsuccessful, because when the drug combinations are used at doses that effectively block both platelet function and blood coagulation, an unacceptably high incidence of intracerebral and extracranial bleeding ensues.[3]

UNDERSTANDING PLATELET PHYSIOLOGY IN THE PLANNING OF ANTIPLATELET THERAPY

The evidence is clear that persons at increased risk of stroke have excessively active platelets, and that even normal platelet activation in the setting of arterial disease imparts thromboembolic risk. This provides the pathophysiologic basis for antiplatelet therapy in secondary reduction of stroke risk. To understand the rationale for using particular antiplatelet drugs, it is important first to consider how platelets regulate normal hemostasis. *Hemostasis* is defined as the appropriate physiologic response to vascular injury that provides prompt control of blood loss. In contrast, *thrombosis* is excessive or inappropriate blood clotting. Platelet hemostatic function needs then to be contrasted with platelet prothrombotic function, that is, how platelets promote inappropriate formation of blood clots in the setting of arterial vascular disease. Because platelets interact with the blood vessel wall in both hemostasis and thrombosis, the status of the arterial endothelial lining is an important determinant of platelet behavior. Normal vascular endothelium is nonthrombogenic and prevents platelet interactions with it, and with other platelets or leukocytes, by multiple mechanisms including secretion of prostaglandins and nitric oxide, surface expression of anticoagulant heparan sulfate and adenosine diphosphate (ADP)–metabolizing enzymes, and facilitation of smooth, nonturbulent blood flow.

Normal Functions of Platelets in Hemostasis

Normal platelets circulate for about 7 to 10 days after being released from megakaryocytes in the bone marrow, even though they lack nuclei and are almost incapable of protein synthesis. The youngest platelets are the most hemostatically active. The relatively long life of platelets in the blood has permitted effective, once-daily dosing with several antiplatelet drugs. Circulating platelets do not normally interact with one another with other blood cells, nor with the surface of the normal vascular endothelium. If a blood vessel is injured and endothelial continuity is broken, however, platelets undergo, within seconds, a rapid series of coordinated activation changes that quickly leads to a hemostatic platelet plug. This primary hemostatic plug prevents bleeding at the injury site without blocking blood flow through the vessel (Fig. 57–1).

These activation steps (shown in *italics*) start with *adhesion* of single platelets to the damaged vessel wall, in which the platelets change in shape from flat, unreactive discs to "spiny spheres" that spread out over the surface. Next is *aggregation*, in which additional platelets join into masses or clumps on top of the original spread layer of platelets,

blocking blood loss. During this process, the now activated platelets *release* vasoactive substances from storage granules, including adhesive glycoproteins, procoagulants, agonists for platelet activation, enzymes, and inflammatory mediators (Table 57.1). Moreover, once platelets are

Table 57.1   Platelet-Derived Vasoactive Mediators

Dense granule contents	Adenosine diphosphate, adenosine triphosphate, Ca^{++}, serotonin
Alpha granule contents	*Adhesive proteins*: fibronectin, fibrinogen, thrombospondin, vitronectin
	Coagulation factors: von Willebrand factor, factor V, factor X
	Growth factors: fibroblast growth factor, platelet-derived growth factor, transforming growth factor-β
	Membrane proteins: P-selectin, amyloid precursor protein
	Others: albumin, immunoglobulin G, antibacterial proteins, platelet inhibitor activator-1
Lysosomes	Acid hydrolases, neutral proteases, elastase, complement-activating enzymes, heparitinase
Peroxisomes	Catalase
Lipid mediators (not preformed)	Prostaglandin endoperoxides, thromboxane A_2 prostaglandin D_2, 12-hydroxyeicosatetraenoic acid isoprostanes

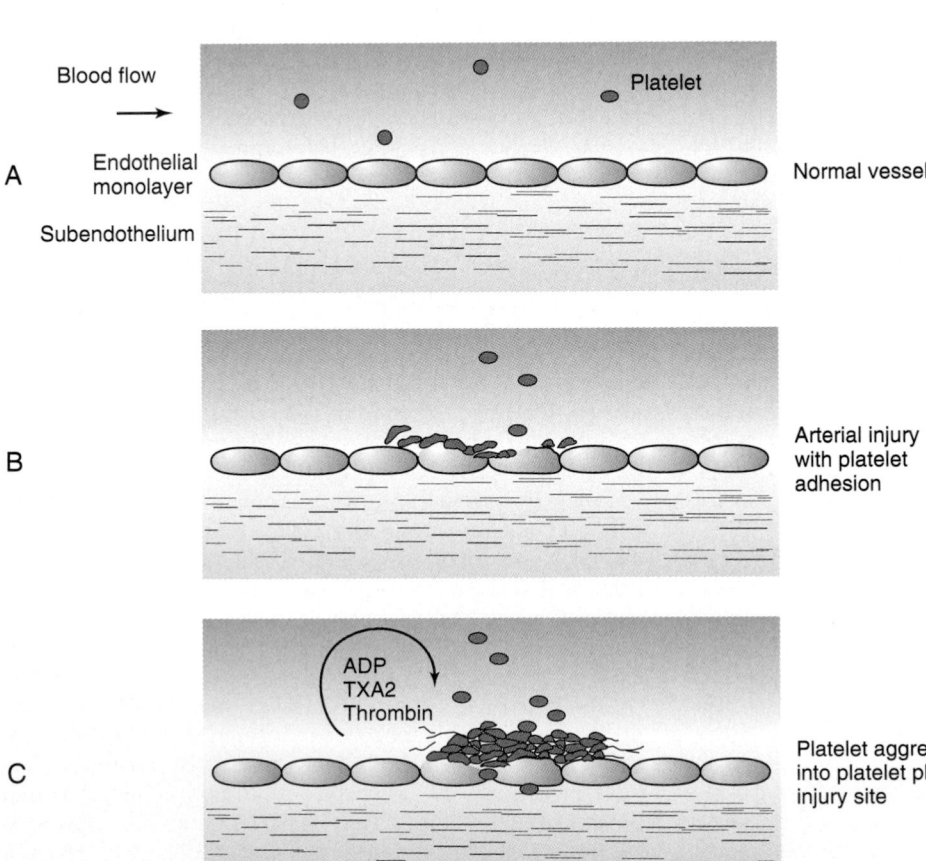

FIGURE 57–1 *Platelets and primary hemostatic plug formation. Sequence of events in primary hemostasis after arterial injury. A, Blood flow over normal arterial endothelium. No interaction of platelets with the vascular wall. B, Immediately after injury that disrupts the arterial endothelium, platelets adhere to the subendothelium exposed at the injury site, forming a platelet monolayer, change shape, spread out, and begin to release vasoactive substances. C, Within a few minutes, activated platelets aggregate on the first layer of spread platelets, clumping together, releasing vasoactive mediators such as adenosine diphosphate (ADP) and thromboxane A_2 (TXA2), and catalyze generation of thrombin, so that fibrin strands (designated by wavy lines) form and stabilize the platelet plug.*

activated, vasoactive lipids, such as thromboxane A$_2$ and leukotrienes, are rapidly synthesized and released. Many of these substances either recruit other platelets or produce vascular contraction, functions that help stop bleeding promptly at the injury site. Most importantly, the surface membranes of activated platelets *catalyze thrombin generation* with great efficiency, so that activated platelets serve to initiate, augment, and localize fibrin formation, further amplifying thrombotic potential as well as participating in *clot stabilization*.

Participants in the Initial Platelet Response to Vascular Injury

In both hemostasis and thrombosis, the major signal for platelet activation is a local injury to endothelium, which leads to exposure to the blood of prothrombotic components, usually localized in the subendothelial matrix. Whereas normal, intact endothelium displays numerous antithrombotic functions and repels platelets, subendothelium is rich in prothrombotic substances such as collagen and adhesive molecules, including von Willebrand factor (vWF), thrombospondin, and fibronectin. In addition, subtle endothelial dysfunction produced by turbulent blood flow, hyperlipidemia, inflammation, or atherosclerosis—without any physical discontinuity in the endothelial monolayer lining the blood vessels—can also activate platelets. Moreover, once activated, platelets themselves recruit additional platelets by releasing vasoactive mediators and catalyzing thrombin formation; in turn, thrombin is a potent platelet activator. Platelet activation is therefore an exponential and interactive, rather than linear, process.

Platelet Membrane Components Mediating Platelet Activation

Platelet activation involves changes in both the morphologic and biochemical state of the platelet membrane, including conformational changes in adhesion receptors, binding of adhesive proteins, mobilization of intracellular granule contents, interactions with the cytoskeleton, initiation of signaling, and platelet-platelet interaction. Glycoprotein (GP) platelet adhesion receptors mediate attachment of platelets to substrate proteins. Adhesion receptors that are important for normal hemostasis and so represent potential therapeutic targets for preventing thrombosis include the following: GPIa, a collagen receptor; GPIb, a receptor for vWF; the GPIIb/IIIa complex, a major receptor for fibrinogen, fibronectin, and vWF; GPIV, a thrombospondin receptor, required for irreversible platelet activation; glycoproteins V and IX; and $\alpha_v\beta_3$, a receptor for vitronectin, fibrinogen, and fibronectin. These receptors are all functional on resting platelets except for GPIIb/IIIa, which requires platelet activation in order to undergo the conformational change that permits this complex to bind fibrinogen.

Many of the adhesive glycoproteins that are ligands for these receptors share the peptide sequence RGD (R, arginine; G, glycine; D, aspartic acid), which is directly involved in cell-cell adhesion.

Platelet Adhesion

Adhesion of platelets to other platelets, to the subendothelium exposed by vascular injury, or to activated endothelium is the first major step in the platelet activation sequence. Platelet adhesion is mediated by a complex of GPIb-V-IX, which binds to matrix vWF at high shear rates and is also a binding site for thrombin, thus acting to amplify platelet responses to thrombin.[4,5] GPIb-V-IX is mainly involved in platelet activation resulting from abnormal shear stress, such as is found in arteries narrowed by atherosclerosis. Changes in conformation of the GPIbα component of the complex or of vWF can induce interaction between these two molecules. Binding of vWF to collagen induces small conformational changes in vWF that permit its binding to GPIb. Furthermore, binding of vWF to GPIb causes redistribution of the GPIb-V-IX glycoprotein complex within platelets, linking the complex to the cytoskeleton and activating phosphorylating enzymes that regulate actin polymerization and the activation of the GPIIb/IIIa complex. Therefore, inhibition of platelet adhesion should be antithrombotic. Peptides that block GPIb-V-IX function are under development as novel antiplatelet drugs. Activation of GPIb-V-IX in a thromboxane-independent manner accounts for part of the "resistance" to aspirin that is observed in connection with the presence of atherosclerotic risk factors. Absence or dysfunction of GPIb is characteristic of a rare platelet disorder involving soft tissue bleeding, the Bernard-Soulier syndrome. At low shear, the GPIIb/IIIa complex also participates in platelet adhesion to surfaces through binding of fibrinogen.

Platelet Aggregation

Aggregation is the step in the platelet activation process most relevant to the pathogenesis of occlusive vascular events in an oxygen-sensitive arterial bed. During aggregation, activated platelets clump together atop an initial, adherent layer of platelets deposited at a site of injury or diseased vascular wall. These white thrombi, composed mainly of platelets and fibrin, may be transient or may become stabilized by further fibrin deposition, forming the nidus of bulkier clots in which erythrocytes and leukocytes also become trapped. During normal hemostasis, such platelet plugs halt bleeding from injured microvessels without obstructing blood flow, but in diseased vessels (e.g., in atherosclerosis or vasculitis, or after irradiation), excessive platelet plug formation can occlude cerebral vasculature, producing TIA or stroke.

Platelet Membrane Receptors in Aggregation

The most important membrane receptor for aggregation is the integrin GPIIb/IIIa, a bimolecular membrane complex unique to platelets and megakaryocytes. Platelet aggregation by all known pathways depends on conformational changes in GPIIb/IIIa induced by platelet agonists.[6,7] Three main physiologic pathways independently triggered by different ligands can activate the GPIIb/IIIa complex; one pathway is activated by arachidonic acid leading to thromboxane A$_2$ (TXA$_2$) formation, the second by ADP, and the third by thrombin (Fig. 57–2).[8–10] All of these signaling pathways converge in a final common mechanism to produce a conformational change in GPIIb/IIIa that exposes a high-affinity fibrinogen binding site. The activated GPIIb/IIIa complex thus markedly increases fibrinogen binding, becomes associated with cytoskeletal

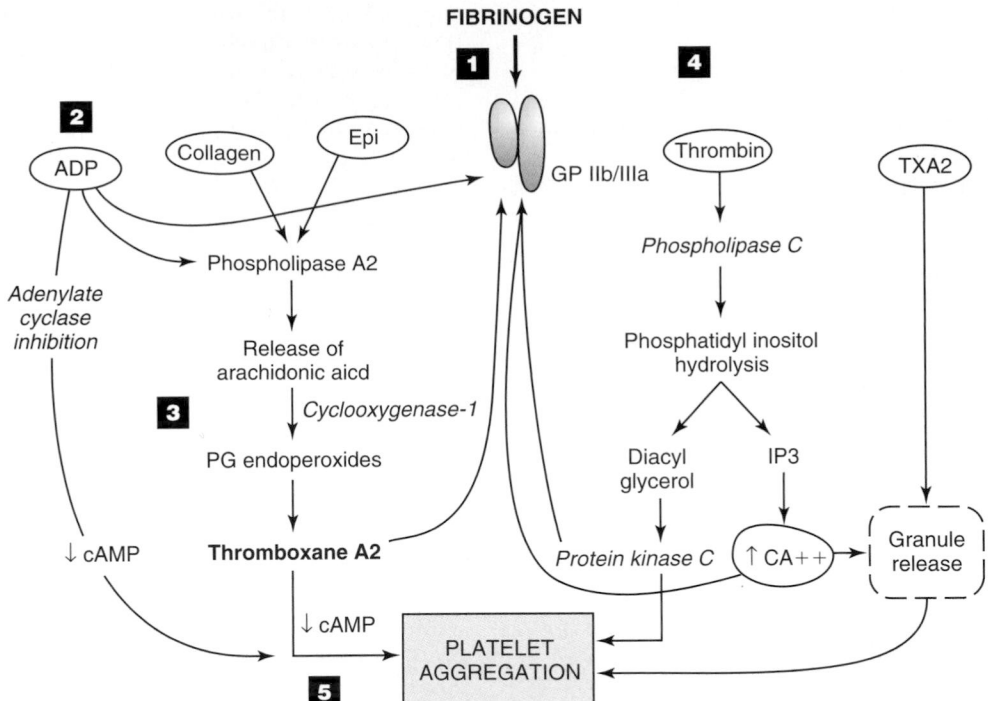

FIGURE 57–2 *Platelet activation pathways and their inhibition. Specific, seven-transmembrane–spanning, G-protein–linked receptors on the platelet surface (depicted as ellipses) are activated by binding of their specific ligands and initiate different pathways for platelet activation, which converge upon the conformational activation of the glycoprotein (GP) IIb/IIIa receptor complex to increase fibrinogen binding. These pathways lead to activation of the arachidonic acid pathway, hydrolysis of phosphatidyl inositol, increase in intraplatelet calcium ion (CA++) concentration, release of vasoactive substances from platelet granules, synthesis of vasoactive lipids, and platelet aggregation. Mechanisms of inhibition of specific activation mechanisms by antiplatelet drugs (numbers in boxes) are (1) blocking of GPIIb/IIIa function and therefore of fibrinogen binding and platelet aggregation; (2) blocking of the adenosine diphosphate (ADP) receptor; (3) inhibition of cyclooxygenase-interrupting arachidonic acid metabolism and prevention of the production of thromboxane A$_2$ (TXA2); (4) blocking of thrombin action and thrombin receptor activation; (5) maintenance of high intraplatelet cyclic adenosine monophosphate (cAMP), which prevents platelet aggregation. Not depicted is inhibition of thromboxane A$_2$ synthase or thromboxane A$_2$ receptor function, because drugs with these activities have not been clinically useful. Epi, epinephrine; IP3, inositol 1,4,5-triphosphate; PG, prostaglandin.*

proteins and signaling kinases (e.g., pp60[c-src]), forms receptor clusters, and becomes phosphorylated. All of these functions favor platelet-platelet interactions. Both outside-inside signaling (e.g., agonist-driven) and inside-outside signaling (i.e. kinase/phosphatase-driven) are involved in this activation process.

Because the final common pathway for platelet activation requires the GPIIb/IIIa complex, therapeutic blockade of the complex inhibits all further platelet activation. In contrast, drugs that inhibit only one of the three pathways, such as aspirin inhibition of the thromboxane pathway or clopidogrel inhibition of the ADP pathway, do not prevent GPIIb/IIIa activation. Drugs that directly block the functions of the GPIIb/IIIa complex thus have profound inhibitory effects on platelet function and are currently used to treat acute cardiac ischemia. Development of the monoclonal antibody abciximab (ReoPro), of peptides such as eptifibatide (Integrilin), and of peptidomimetics such as tirofiban (Aggrastat), which inhibit GPIIb/IIIa function when administered intravenously, has permitted highly successful antiplatelet therapy in acute cardiac interventions. Used over a short interval in combination with heparin and aspirin, these GPIIb/IIIa inhibitors prevent early thrombosis and deter vascular reocclusion after coronary angioplasty and stent placement. Unfortunately the use of oral GPIIb/IIIa inhibitors for long-term prevention of cardiac thrombosis has been unsuccessful to date in numerous clinical trials, in which administration of such agents has been accompanied by higher rates of thrombosis or bleeding. A single clinical trial testing the safety of abciximab in treatment of acute stroke has been published (see later). Indeed, the Blockage of the Glycoprotein IIb/IIIa Receptor to Avoid Vascular Occlusion (BRAVO) study of lotrafiban (an oral GPIIB/IIIa inhibitor) and heparin for prevention of cardiovascular and cerebrovascular events, initiated in 2000, had to be discontinued because of excess occurrences of thrombosis.[3]

Multiple Independent Pathways to Aggregation

Each of the three independent biochemical pathways of platelet aggregation provides a separate potential for therapeutic intervention. One major pathway involves metabolism of arachidonic acid, which is released from membrane phospholipids during platelet activation (see Fig. 57–2, center left). This pathway is sensitive to aspirin and other nonsteroidal anti-inflammatory drugs (NSAIDs). Receptor engagement by various platelet agonists activates phospholipase C to cleave membrane bound phosphatidyl inositol to IP_3 (inositol 1,4,5-triphosphate) and diacylglycerol. IP_3 in turn releases stored calcium ions, permitting activation of platelet phospholipase A_2, which releases esterified arachidonic acid from membrane phospholipids. The enzyme cyclooxygenase-1 in platelets rapidly converts the released arachidonic acid to prostaglandin endoperoxides that are isomerized to thromboxane A_2 (TXA_2), a potent platelet agonist and vasoconstrictor. The TXA_2 diffuses out of the platelets and binds to its specific seven-transmembrane receptor on the platelet surface, signaling further activation of phospholipase C. Concomitantly, the liberated diacylglycerol activates protein kinase C, which translocates to the platelet plasma membrane and triggers activation of GPIIb/IIIa, exposing its fibrinogen binding site and thereby permitting platelet aggregation and secretion of platelet granule contents (see Fig. 57–2, right side). Aspirin, which irreversibly binds to cyclooxygenase-1, blocks the formation of TXA_2 for the entire life span of circulating platelets, because platelets are incapable of synthesizing new cyclooxygenase protein.

Platelets that cannot produce TXA_2 can still be activated via the ADP-dependent and thrombin-dependent activation pathways. Platelet aggregation can be initiated via two interacting ADP receptors by ADP that is released by platelets or derived from extra-platelet sources such as red blood cells, even in the presence of aspirin.[9,10] Thrombin acts upon several specific protease-activated membrane receptors (PARs) that signal the activation of phospholipase C and irreversible platelet aggregation and the release reaction that is independent of arachidonic acid metabolism.[8] Similarly, platelet activation by the phosphorylcholine derivative platelet-activating factor (PAF), which is produced by leukocytes or by disturbed endothelial cells, is also aspirin-insensitive. The existence of these separate pathways for platelet aggregation may be regarded as representing fail-safe or redundant mechanisms to avoid hemorrhage.

Platelet Release Reaction

Release of vasoactive contents of platelet storage granules normally accompanies platelet activation, augments platelet aggregation, and accelerates localized clot formation, vasoconstriction, and the initiation of wound healing. Not only are preformed glycoprotein mediators, ADP, vasoactive amines, growth factors, calcium ions, and serotonin released into the blood or displayed on the surface membrane; short-lived lipid mediators are also synthesized and released during platelet activation. The extent of the release reaction can be modulated by antiplatelet drugs.

Several types of granules rich in substances that participate in blood coagulation, cell-cell interactions, and wound repair are present in platelets (see Table 57.1). The different granule types—dense granules, alpha granules, lysosomes, and peroxisomes—can be morphologically distinguished and are also functionally characterized by their contents and the ease of release of their contents. For example, weak platelet stimuli, such as ADP, adenosine triphosphate (ATP), serotonin, and calcium—all of which participate in potentiating irreversible platelet aggregation— release the contents of the dense granules. By contrast, strong stimuli are required for release of alpha granule contents; fibrinogen, fibronectin, vWF, platelet-derived growth factor (PDGF), epidermal growth factor (EGF), transforming growth factor-β (TGF-β), platelet factor-4 (PF-4) and β-thromboglobulin. Alpha granules also contain albumin, immunoglobulins, antibacterial proteins, and a complement inhibitor. The membrane of the alpha granules contains P-selectin and the amyloid precursor protein; upon platelet activation, P-selectin is transferred to the surface of the platelets, where it mediates cell-cell interactions with leukocytes and plays an important role in inflammatory reactions. Platelet lysosomes, the last granule type to be released, contain acid hydrolases, neutral proteases, elastase, enzymes that activate complement, and a heparitinase. Peroxisomes contain catalase.

In general, release of components of both dense bodies and alpha granules usually accompanies platelet aggregation but may also occur from platelets that are adherent to damaged endothelium or subendothelium, even without formation of platelet aggregates.

Platelet Synthesis of Vasoactive Lipid Mediators

In contrast to the release of preformed proteins or amines from platelet granules, vasoactive lipid mediators are not stored by platelets but instead are rapidly synthesized and released upon platelet activation. Most of these lipids are oxygenated metabolites of arachidonic acid, which is mobilized from membrane phospholipids when agonists interact with platelet membrane receptors. The released arachidonate is the substrate for several different metabolic pathways producing eicosanoids and hydroxylated fatty acids. TXA_2 is the major platelet product of arachidonic acid metabolism by the eicosanoid pathway, and its synthesis occurs very rapidly—within seconds—upon platelet activation. G-protein linked, seven-membrane-spanning receptors for TXA_2 are present on platelets, leukocytes, and vascular cells.[11] These receptors bind TXA_2 and also its endoperoxide precursors, which have similar vasoconstrictor properties. Signal transduction via TXA_2 receptors initiates platelet activation and causes vasoconstriction.

Platelets also synthesize hydroxylated fatty acids from arachidonate via a separate enzymatic pathway involving lipoxygenase. The major product of this pathway in platelets is 12-hydroxyeicosatetraenoic acid (12-HETE), an inflammatory mediator that is chemotactic for leukocytes, stimulates vascular smooth muscle proliferation, and can be converted to additional inflammatory mediators, di-HETEs, by leukocytes. In contrast to the rapid burst of TXA_2 synthesis by activated platelets, the production of 12-HETE occurs continuously over a long period. Nonenzymatic, vasoactive metabolites of arachidonate, isoprostanes are also formed by oxidation; they can inactivate vascular or platelet nitric oxide (NO).

Interactions among different cell types can produce additional arachidonic acid products via transcellular metabolism, yielding products that are not made by a single cell type alone. Thus, platelet-released arachidonic acid can be converted into other vasoactive products by

Acute Changes in Platelet Reactivity

Because inflammation by itself can produce increased platelet activation, better methods to distinguish between the inflammatory effects of a stroke and a preexisting state of chronic platelet activation are being actively sought. This distinction is very difficult. Increased levels of fibrinogen, factor VIII, vWF, and C-reactive protein as well as leukocyte counts accompany ischemic stroke.[23] Cytokines released during inflammation that have prothrombotic effects may engender platelet hyperreactivity, activation of prothrombotic properties of endothelium, and heightened platelet-leukocyte interactions. Even so, not all markers of inflammation correlate with risk of active coronary artery disease; for example, in one study, levels of soluble P-selectin (which can be released from platelets, endothelium, or leukocytes), intercellular adhesion molecule-1 (ICAM-1), vascular cell adhesion molecule-1 (VCAM-1), and E-selectin were found to be unrelated.[38]

Chronic Changes in Platelet Reactivity

The question whether greater platelet reactivity in patients with stroke merely reflects the body's inflammatory response to tissue damage is, however, clearly answered with a "no." Increases in platelet activation not only may follow an acute stroke for many months but also may be chronically present before an episode of cerebral ischemia. In adults, increased platelet aggregability after atherosclerotic stroke has been demonstrated to continue for at least 3 to 9 months after the acute event in 60% of patients; this time extends well beyond that required for resolution of the acute inflammatory changes typical of cerebral tissue damage.[23,36] Similar changes in platelet aggregability are not observed after stroke caused by cardiac emboli, even though brain tissue damage may be extensive. Chronic increase in platelet aggregation after acute cerebral ischemia correlates with poorer outcome. In some unusual circumstances, oxidative stress has been correlated with chronic platelet activation. In familial stroke, infants presenting with stroke can be shown to have a chronic platelet hyperreactivity that is not blocked by NO; such infants lack the plasma enzyme glutathione peroxidase and, therefore, have low blood antioxidant potential that counters the protective effect of NO on platelets.[39] In most cases of adult ischemic stroke, however, no such simple correlation between oxidative stress and platelet hyperreactivity can be made.

The pathologic consequences of greater platelet reactivity in the stroke-prone patient clearly show that more is not better. In normal arteries, hemostasis rapidly controls bleeding, and the damaged area is soon precisely repaired, whereas in a diseased arterial bed, even this normal hemostatic response may have the unwanted consequences of arterial thrombosis. This dysequilibrium between hemostasis and thrombosis appears to be particularly true in vessels vulnerable to even temporary occlusion, such as the endarteries of the brain. Furthermore, normal platelet contributions to wound repair can similarly be detrimental in stroke-prone patients, where platelet-derived mediators promote excessive vascular cell proliferation that accelerates intimal hyperplasia and vascular narrowing.[23,40]

CHOICE OF ANTIPLATELET DRUGS FOR SECONDARY PREVENTION OF STROKE

The sequential steps in platelet activation are sensitive to different pharmacologic interventions. Antiplatelet drugs that mainly affect platelet aggregation and mediator release tend to block platelet-initiated thrombosis without much depression of hemostasis and, therefore, involve a smaller chance of hemorrhagic complications; however, they have limited efficacy in preventing stroke. On the other hand, antiplatelet drugs that block platelet adhesion, the initial step in platelet activation at a vascular surface, or the GPIIb/IIIa complex and, thus, all aggregation pathways, are highly effective in preventing thrombosis but so far impose an unacceptable risk of bleeding, particularly in the brain. Only direct inhibitors of thrombin, factor Xa, or both block the capacity of platelets to catalyze thrombin generation. Such agents also pose a major bleeding risk with long-term use in secondary prevention of cerebral ischemia.

Antiplatelet drugs in current use for secondary prevention of stroke include aspirin, clopidogrel, ticlopidine, dipyridamole, and various combinations of these agents (Table 57.2). Intravenous GPIIb/IIIa inhibitors, widely used in secondary prevention of coronary artery thrombosis after acute cardiac interventions, have just begun to be used in cerebral ischemia. Although aspirin and dipyridamole have been used for several decades, controversies about dose and efficacy remain active. Moreover, antiplatelet therapy has not reduced the severity of a subsequent stroke in patients treated after an initial episode, although it did lengthen the stroke-free interval.[41] The current consensus is that the modest efficacy of available drugs may improve if various combinations are used but that an ideal, effective secondary prevention of stroke has not yet been achieved. For this reason, a discussion of new antiplatelet drugs now under development that affect ADP metabolism, GPIb, or NO is provided later in the chapter.

In clinical settings in which platelets are not major factors in the production of vaso-occlusive arterial emboli, anticoagulation is an effective form of secondary prevention of stroke. The foremost of settings is cardioembolic stroke associated with nonvalvular AF and valvular heart disease, the incidence of which is rising rapidly as the population ages.[2] Other important causes of stroke that are relatively independent of platelets are cholesterol emboli released from ulcerated atherosclerotic plaques, patent foramen ovale, fibrin-rich emboli from intracardiac mural thrombus, "bland" cardiac valve vegetations in inflammatory disease, thalassemia, and sickle cell disease[42–46]; these causes together represent about 15% of cerebral ischemic episodes. Even in some of these settings, antiplatelet agents may have a role in stroke prevention if anticoagulation alone does not suffice or if the patient also has atherosclerotic risk factors for stroke.

Aspirin

Mechanism of the Antiplatelet Effect of Aspirin

Aspirin has long been known to prolong bleeding time. That the lengthened bleeding time involves decreased

Table 57.2   Actions of Antiplatelet Drugs

Activity	Effect on Platelets	Drug
Inhibition of membrane GPIb receptor	Block GPI-V-IX function, prevent adhesion and aggregation	S-nitroso-AR545C°
Inhibition of membrane GPIIb/IIIa receptor	Prevent bending of fibrinogen	Abciximab
	Prevent platelet-platelet interaction	RGD peptide analogues Disintegrins
Inhibition of membrane ADP P2Y$_{12}$ receptor	Prevent binding of ADP	Ticlopidine, clopidogrel
	Prevent ADP-mediated aggregation	AR-C69931 MX[†]
	Decrease GPIIb/IIIa activation	
Inhibition of membrane ADP P2Y$_1$ receptor	Prevent binding of ADP	Adenosine 3′-phosphate,
	Prevent calcium mobilization	5′-phosphosulfate[†]
Catabolism of ADP	Prevent ADP-mediated aggregation	Soluble recombinant CD39°
	Foster disaggregation	
Inhibition of cyclooxygenase-1	Prevent TXA$_2$ generation	Aspirin (irreversible effect)
	Inhibit arachidonic acid–mediated platelet aggregation and secretion	NSAIDs (competitive effect)
Stimulate adenylate cyclase	Raise platelet cAMP, preventing aggregation and secretion	Epoprostenol, Iloprost Fish oils, ϖ-3 fatty acids°
Inhibition of phosphodiesterase	Maintain elevated cAMP once raised	Dipyridamole Methylxanthines°
Stimulate guanylate cyclase	Raise platelet cGMP, preventing aggregation and secretion	NO, NO-donors, e.g. S-nitroso-glutathione, nitroglycerin
Inhibit calcium flux	Prevent calcium mobilization	Ca^{++} channel blockers°
	Decrease aggregation and secretion	Local anesthetics° Beta-blockers°
Inhibit thrombin generation or action	Inhibit aggregation and secretion	Heparins, hirudin
	Inhibit procoagulant activity	Antithrombin peptides[†]

°Weak or adjunctive effect.
[†]Under development.
ADP, adenosine diphosphate; CA^{++}, calcium ion; cGMP, cyclic guanosine monophosphate; NO, nitric oxide; NSAID, nonsteroidal anti-inflammatory drug; TXA$_2$, thromboxane A$_2$.

platelet aggregation was first demonstrated in the 1960s. In 1971, aspirin was first shown to affect platelet function by irreversible acetylation and thus inactivation of the platelet enzyme cyclooxygenase-1 (prostaglandin endoperoxide synthase-1), thus preventing the addition of molecular oxygen to arachidonic acid to form prostaglandin endoperoxides G$_2$ and H$_2$ and blocking downstream formation of TXA$_2$ from endoperoxides.[47–49] Because platelets do not synthesize proteins, platelet functions that depend on TXA$_2$ activity are inhibited for the life span of the platelet. The separate peroxidase function of cyclooxygenase, not involved in eicosanoid synthesis, remains unaffected by aspirin. Very small doses of aspirin rapidly (within minutes) block platelet cyclooxygenase in vivo.[50] Certain peculiarities of platelet kinetics favor the profound and long-lasting effect of aspirin. Platelets circulate for 7 to 10 days, but once exposed to aspirin, they are permanently unable to produce TXA$_2$. Because only about 10% of circulating platelets are replaced each day by new platelets released from bone marrow megakaryocytes, a single daily dose of aspirin produces virtually complete inhibition of platelet cyclooxygenase. Therefore, high, persistent blood levels of aspirin are not required for the inhibitory effect on platelet function, even in patients with cerebral ischemia.[51]

In contrast to platelets, other cells in vascular endothelium, cells in kidney or lung epithelium, and monocytes are capable of rapid resynthesis of cyclooxygenase. The inhibitory effect of aspirin on eicosanoid synthesis in cells other than platelets is therefore much briefer. Moreover, these other tissues also synthesize cyclooxygenase-2, a related isoform inducible by inflammatory stimuli and cytokines. Platelets neither contain nor synthesize cyclooxygenase-2. Cyclooxygenase-2 is also inhibited by aspirin, but because of its rapid resynthesis in many cell types (monocytes, vascular endothelium, and smooth muscle), net eicosanoid production by these cells is less durably inhibited by aspirin.[52] In terms of the vascular bed, once-daily dosage with aspirin selectively inhibits platelet function usually without impairing production by the blood vessel wall of vasoprotective prostaglandins such as prostacyclin and prostaglandin (PG) E$_2$.

Pharmacokinetics

After oral administration, aspirin is rapidly absorbed from the stomach and upper small intestine, reaching a peak plasma level 30 minutes after a single dose. It is rapidly deacetylated in the liver to salicylate. Although salicylate has little or no antiplatelet efficacy, it does have independent anti-inflammatory effects through modulation of NFκB-regulated genes. By 3 hours after oral ingestion of aspirin, the plasma acetylsalicylate level is negligible. However, because aspirin exposure inactivates platelet cyclooxygenase within minutes, even a brief exposure of circulating platelets to aspirin produces full inactivation of cyclooxygenase and depresses platelet function. Intravenous aspirin works even faster.[53]

As little as 1 mg aspirin taken orally per hour, a dose completely deacetylated on first pass through the liver, fully inhibits platelet cyclooxygenase within about 12 hours, because platelets traveling through the portal circulation encounter sufficient newly absorbed aspirin to inhibit their cyclooxygenase.[50] In clinical studies, an initial dose of 162 mg fully blocks platelet cyclooxygenase in an adult, and 81 mg/day (one pediatric aspirin tablet) maintains full inhibition.[54] As little as 30 mg taken once daily for several days builds to the same net effect with a week, because the antiplatelet effects of aspirin are cumulative over time.[55] Effects of enteric-coated aspirin are similar to those of plain aspirin except for a slightly slower onset of action.[56]

Dose-Response Effects

Antiplatelet effects of aspirin usually maximize at 81 to 325 mg/day, and higher doses do not inhibit platelet function any further.[57] Only in persons with a very rapid rate of platelet turnover are higher or more frequent doses needed for full effect (see later). TXA_2 synthesis must be decreased by 95% for full inhibitory effects of aspirin on platelet function to be achieved.[50] Aspirin was approved by the U.S. Food and Drug Administration (FDA) in 1980 for the prevention of transient ischemic attacks and stroke, and in 1985 for the prevention of unstable angina and secondary prevention of MI; the recommended dosage is 50 to 325 mg/day.

At these doses, the bleeding time lengthens to about double the baseline time in at least 60% of individuals; larger doses of aspirin do not prolong bleeding time further. Indeed, very high doses may slightly shorten the bleeding time because of inhibition of vascular cyclooxygenase. Prolongation of bleeding time by aspirin correlates poorly with either gastric irritation or gastrointestinal bleeding. After aspirin is stopped, bleeding time returns to normal within 1 to 2 days regardless of the dose administered. Concomitant alcohol ingestion can further lengthen aspirin-induced prolongation of bleeding time and slows recovery; this factor may contribute to the incidence of gastrointestinal bleeding in aspirin users.

Once aspirin is stopped, platelet aggregation and TXA_2 formation return to normal levels within 7 to 10 days with linear kinetics after a 1- to 2-day lag that likely reflects the acetylation of megakaryocyte cyclooxygenase, resulting in release of aspirin-impaired platelets during the first 2 days. In patients at major risk of stroke, such as those with high-grade carotid stenosis, doses of aspirin up to 1300 mg/day have been tried, but the data obtained do not show greater clinical efficacy of doses higher than 325 mg (see later).[58–60]

NSAIDs inhibit platelet cyclooxygenase in a reversible, competitive manner, so their antiplatelet effects all depend on maintenance of a high blood level of drug. Therefore, their duration of antiplatelet activity is relatively brief. However, the co-administration of an NSAID, such as ibuprofen or naproxen, with low-dose aspirin can *decrease* the irreversible effects of aspirin on platelet cyclooxygenase by competition, and may impair the antiplatelet efficacy of aspirin.[61]

In contrast, the "coxib" cyclooxygenase-2 inhibitors do not block the ability of aspirin to acetylate platelet cyclooxygenase-1 and so do not diminish the antiplatelet effects of aspirin.[62] No definitive data are currently available on incidence of cardiovascular events and stroke, in particular, in patients taking both aspirin and cyclooxygenase-2 inhibitors, although patients taking only the latter have been reported in some studies to have a higher incidence of MI; more information is clearly needed.[63]

Range and Limits of Aspirin Effects on Platelet Function

The effects of aspirin on platelet activation all result from cyclooxygenase inhibition. They are blocking of TXA_2 production, complete inhibition of arachidonate-induced platelet aggregation, a decreased release reaction that is reflected in diminished and slowed platelet responses to collagen and epinephrine, and reduced platelet aggregation to low-dose ADP. In contrast, aspirin does not affect platelet adhesion, prolong the shortened platelet life span, decrease secretion of vascular growth factors from platelets, or block thrombin-induced platelet activation. Because TXA_2, the major eicosanoid produced by blood platelets, is a strong stimulus for platelet aggregation and release and a powerful vasoconstrictor, all of the aspirin-induced changes in platelet activation previously listed are related to blocking of the TXA_2 pathway of platelet activation.

Because thrombin affects platelets in a cyclooxygenase-independent manner, activation of platelets by thrombin is not inhibited by aspirin. Even so, use of aspirin (325 to 500 mg/day) has been reported to reduce platelet-dependent thrombin generation in vitro and in vivo.[64] The inhibitory effect of aspirin on thrombin generation is weaker in hypercholesterolemic patients, who are known to have a hypercoagulable state and who often show enhanced platelet TXA_2 generation.[65] It is postulated that the antithrombinogenic effect of aspirin may involve acetylation of platelet membrane proteins, but the mechanism is not yet clear. The clinical relevance of aspirin-induced impairment of thrombin generation remains to be assessed.

Aspirin has little or no effect upon the lipoxygenase pathway of arachidonic acid metabolism, and thus, 12-HETE production by platelets is not altered. Production of epoxyeicosatrienoic acids (EETs) and isoprostanes, which are formed nonenzymatically, is also unaltered by aspirin.

Aspirin Resistance

In patients with rapid platelet turnover, such as those with severe atherosclerosis, once-daily dosing with aspirin may not achieve complete inhibition of cyclooxygenase, and more frequent or larger doses may occasionally be needed. High levels of fibrinogen may also diminish the antiplatelet effects of aspirin,[27] as may high levels of circulating catecholamines. Such "aspirin resistance," however, is uncommon. Because the efficacy of aspirin is low in stroke prevention, the question has been raised whether some patients might be "nonresponders" to aspirin therapy. Unlike the case with acute cardiac ischemic syndromes, in which a low dose of aspirin is clearly as useful as higher doses, the controversy about the optimal dose for stroke-prone patients remains unresolved.[56,65,66] A proportion of patients receiving aspirin therapy after a first episode of cerebral ischemia experience recurrent stroke.[67] One large study classified the reason for admission in 5.7% of patients consecutively admitted for ischemic stroke as failure of aspirin therapy, because the patients were taking aspirin at the time they had a stroke. Pertinent characteristics of these cases included significant hyperlipidemia, ischemic heart disease, and lower dose of aspirin, suggesting that individuals with greater risk factors for occlusive vascular disease might benefit less from aspirin.[68]

In another study, to test whether "aspirin resistance" might develop over time, post-stroke patients prescribed aspirin were repeatedly tested at 6-month intervals for aspirin's effects on platelet aggregation.[69] At the outset, 75% of 306 patients had a maximal effect and 25% a partial effect of aspirin; but on repeated testing, only 33% continued to show good inhibition. Increasing the aspirin dose restored maximal inhibition in about two thirds of the others, but only temporarily. Neither compliance with dosing nor lipid status was directly assessed, except that patients were reminded to take aspirin on the day of testing. Overall, about 8% of patients showed aspirin resistance even at 1300 mg/day. Results of yet another study indicated that about 10% of outpatients who were prescribed aspirin or ticlopidine as antiplatelet therapy were noncompliant with medication and showed a decreased inhibition of platelet aggregation on repeat testing.[70,71] Another possible source of apparent platelet resistance to aspirin may stem from concomitant use of NSAIDs. Regular dosage of naproxen or ibuprofen may compete with aspirin for binding sites on platelet cyclooxygenase and so may diminish the irreversible antiplatelet effects of aspirin, leading to apparent resistance to the drug.[61]

Other Potential Hemostatic Effects of Aspirin

In addition to effects on platelet activation, aspirin has been reported to have effects on fibrinolysis that may add to its antithrombotic effect.[72,73] Long-term aspirin administration is associated with shortening of plasma clot lysis time, likely through acetylation of fibrinogen that impedes factor XIII–induced fibrin cross-linking and so permits fibrinolysis to occur more easily.[73] Conversely, large doses of aspirin may block release of tissue plasminogen activator from venous endothelium without impeding release of plasminogen activator inhibitor-1.[74] This effect would be predicted to inhibit fibrinolysis, but whether the net effects of aspirin on fibrinolysis are clinically important has not been clearly established. At very high concentrations, such as those used to treat rheumatic fever or rheumatoid arthritis, aspirin can induce hypoprothrombinemia and can inhibit synthesis of vitamin K–dependent clotting factors. These effects are more likely due to high levels of blood salicylate and can be reversed with vitamin K. At the usual antiplatelet doses of aspirin, no significant depression of vitamin K dependent clotting factors is seen.

Clinical Evaluation of Antithrombotic Effects of Aspirin in Stroke Prevention

Many controlled clinical trials of aspirin therapy for prevention of TIA, stroke, unstable angina, and MI have been conducted and repeatedly analyzed. These trials show an overall risk reduction of these clinical end points ranging from 13% to 25% for prevention of stroke,[75-77] to 20% to 25% for MI,[1] to 40% to 50% for progression of unstable angina to MI or sudden death.[1] In addition, aspirin treatment has lowered the incidence of pulmonary embolism after hip surgery as well as the rate of early coronary rethrombosis after bypass graft surgery or other cardiac interventions.[1] Major meta-analyses have confirmed the interpretations in single trials of the extent of risk reduction for many types of vascular end points, including stroke, and have shown that aspirin reduces risk similarly in both sexes, although there are many more clinical data about men.[78]

For secondary prevention of TIA and ischemic stroke, aspirin has been beneficial in the elderly as well as in younger patients[79]; however, for prevention of embolic stroke in subjects older than 75 years who have nonvalvular AF, aspirin is less effective than anticoagulation.[80-82] A similar extent of clinical benefit has been documented over a dose range between 160 and 1300 mg/day in numerous studies, but there have been very few direct comparisons of different aspirin doses. In the Dutch TIA Trial of secondary prevention of stroke that compared two low doses of aspirin, 30 mg/day and 283 mg/day, the two doses appeared to have similar efficacy.[55] Controversy remains over the optimum dose of aspirin to use in the prevention of cerebral ischemia in high-risk patients, and some neurologists maintain that 1300 mg/day (4 aspirin tablets) is needed, although no controlled clinical trials of stroke prevention have compared high and low doses except in patients undergoing carotid endarterectomy, a particularly high-risk group. The one study in such patients compared doses of aspirin from 81 to 1300 mg/day and found no significant differences in efficacy.[59]

There are few data supporting the use of low-dose aspirin in primary prevention of stroke. In the Physicians Health Study, in which 325 mg aspirin every other day was administered to more than 20,000 healthy men, there was a clear benefit in primary prevention of MI but not in prevention of stroke; indeed, a slight increase in hemorrhagic stroke was reported in that study that did not reach statistical significance.[83]

Aspirin Toxicity

Gastrointestinal irritation and bleeding, well-known side effects of aspirin, can cause major or fatal bleeding, partly through a direct irritant action and partly through blocking the production of protective prostaglandins in the gastric mucosa. Risk increases with dose and duration of use.[1,50] Reexamination of the occurrence of hemorrhagic stroke, the major central nervous system toxicity of aspirin as an antithrombotic agent, in a meta-analysis of more than 55,000 subjects enrolled in 16 clinical trials of secondary prevention of vascular events showed that aspirin use gave an absolute risk reduction per 10,000 persons of 137 MIs and 39 ischemic strokes, which was offset by an absolute risk increase of 12 hemorrhagic strokes.[78] These were all statistically significant effects (in each case, $P < .001$). The risk of hemorrhagic stroke did not depend on aspirin dose.[78] Thus, in this later, more focused analysis, as in the analysis by the Antiplatelet Trialists' Collaboration,[1] a real increase in hemorrhagic stroke was clearly observed in patients taking aspirin; this adverse effect was considerably less, however, than the decreases in both MI and ischemic stroke seen when patients with extensive vascular disease took aspirin prophylactically.

Carotid Endarterectomy

In patients with asymptomatic carotid artery stenosis of more than 50%, aspirin has been studied to ascertain whether it could prevent ischemic effects such as TIA, stroke, MI, unstable angina, and death. Among 372 patients who were given placebo or aspirin 325 mg/day and monitored for more than 2 years, the rate of ischemic events or death was 12.3% for the placebo group and 11.0% for the aspirin group (P = .61), suggesting no significant benefit of aspirin use.[84] In the North American Symptomatic Carotid Endarterectomy trial (NASCET, 1415 patients) of carotid endarterectomy for high-grade, symptomatic carotid stenosis, the incidence of perioperative stroke was lower in patients self-reporting aspirin intake of 650 to 1300 mg/day (1.8%) than in patients reporting intake of 0 to 325 mg/day (6.9%); this, however, was a retrospective analysis.[85] In the ASA and Carotid Endarterectomy (ACE) Trial (2804 patients), which compared doses of enteric-coated aspirin ranging from 81 mg to 1300 mg/day starting 2 days before and continuing to 90 days after carotid surgery, no correlation was observed between aspirin dosage and occurrence of stroke, MI, or death during the study period.[60] Patients taking low doses had an event rate of 4.7% at 30 days, and those taking high doses, 6.1%. Rates of hemorrhagic stroke rates ranged from 0.6% in the lowest-dose group to 1.1% in the highest-dose group.

Prevention of Early Stroke Recurrence

Aspirin given within 48 hours after an ischemic stroke has been documented to decrease stroke recurrence in two very large studies, the Chinese Acute Stroke Trial (CAST, 20,655 patients)[86] and the International Stroke Trial (IST, 19,435 patients).[87] In the CAST, patients were randomly assigned to receive either 160 mg/day aspirin or placebo starting within 48 hours of the stroke (in some, as early as 6 hours) and continuing for 4 weeks. Death or recurrent nonfatal stroke occurred in 5.3% of aspirin-treated patients and in 5.9% of patients receiving placebo, translating into a significant absolute risk reduction (0.68%; 2P = 0.03)—in other words, a decrease of 7 strokes per 1000 patients treated. The absolute risk reduction for ischemic stroke (0.47%; 2P = .01) was offset by a small excess of hemorrhagic strokes (0.21%; 2P > .1), 2 per 1000 patients treated.[86]

The IST examined the safety and efficacy of 300 mg/day aspirin, subcutaneous unfractionated heparin, or both drugs together in preventing recurrent stroke; treatment was started within 48 hours of the first ischemic event and continued for 14 days. Aspirin therapy in the IST led to an absolute reduction of 1.1% (2P < .001) for recurrent ischemic strokes without an increase in risk of hemorrhagic stroke, although the risk of other bleeding rose significantly. Heparin use significantly increased the risk of hemorrhagic stroke or fatal extracranial bleeding, and although it did reduce the risk of recurrent ischemic stroke, this benefit was negated by an equal increase in hemorrhagic stroke. Functional status at 6 months was not altered by early post-stroke use of aspirin in either CAST or IST.

A later analysis combined data from both CAST and IST to evaluate the effects of early aspirin use after ischemic stroke on the balance between reduced risk of recurrent ischemic stroke and risk of hemorrhagic stroke.[88] Among all treated subgroups examined, the absolute risk reduction of about 7 recurrent ischemic strokes per 1000 was similar (1.6% recurrent strokes with aspirin versus 2.3% without aspirin; 2P < .01), and the benefit from early aspirin treatment did not vary with respect to patient age or sex, level of consciousness, CT findings, blood pressure, stroke subtype, prognostic category, or concomitant heparin use. Neither AF nor treatment assignment without a prior CT scan (which occurred in 9000 patients, or 22%) altered the net benefit of aspirin treatment. The risk reduction for those taking aspirin was similar whether or not they also received heparin. Overall, there was an absolute decrease of 4 deaths per 1000 without further stroke, and the increase in hemorrhagic stroke averaged about 2 per 1000. In aspirin-treated patients, there was a 1.0% rate of hemorrhagic stroke or hemorrhagic transformation, whereas the placebo group had a rate of 0.8% (2P = .07). Extracranial bleeding that required transfusion was significantly more common in patients receiving aspirin, especially in those also receiving heparin (1.8% of those taking aspirin plus heparin versus 0.9% of those taking aspirin alone; excess bleeds occurred in 9 per 1000 treated; 2P = .0001). Most of the cases of hemorrhage were nonfatal. Indeed, among 800 patients inadvertently randomly assigned to receive aspirin after a hemorrhagic stroke, there was no evidence of net hazard, including further stroke and death. The conclusions of this meta-analysis of the CAST and IST data are that low-dose aspirin started early after an acute ischemic stroke produces a definite reduction of recurrent ischemic stroke that is of net benefit to a wide range of patients. Of particular interest is that the benefit was also observed in patients who started aspirin therapy without a prior CT scan, who might have been expected to have a higher incidence of intracranial bleeding. Patients of both sexes, older patients, patients with AF, and hypertensive patients all benefited. It was also concluded that the reduction of further stroke or death from early aspirin use within 1 month of the first event compared favorably with the monthly benefits previously reported for long-term antiplatelet therapy.

Comparison with Anticoagulation in Ischemic Stroke Prevention

The latest large-scale, randomized, double-blind study of prevention of early stroke recurrence, the Warfarin-Aspirin Recurrent Stroke Study (WARSS, 2206 patients), compared aspirin and warfarin treatment in patients who had suffered an ischemic, noncardiogenic stroke within 30 days and were monitored for 2 years.[89] In the WARSS, 92% of entering patients had Glasgow Outcome Scale scores of 4 or 5, indicating moderate disability; 40% were female; 59% were older than 60 years; and their ethnic diversity was broad, consisting of 57% white, 31% African-American, and 10% Hispanic subjects. Aspirin dosage was 325 mg/day, and warfarin was given to achieve an International Normalized Ratio (INR) range of 1.4 to 2.8. In both of the study arms, placebo tablets were used for the alternative therapy. Two-year end-point status was established for more than 98% of the patients.

The overall rate of the primary end point of death or recurrent ischemic stroke was 16.9% and did not significantly differ in the treatment groups (warfarin 17.8%, and aspirin 16.0%; $P = 0.25$). The rates of major hemorrhage were low, at 2.2 per 100 patient-years for warfarin and 1.49 per 100 patient-years for aspirin, with more minor hemorrhages in the warfarin group. Thus, no significant difference in prevention of recurrent stroke or death was observed between aspirin and anticoagulant treatment of adult patients with prior ischemic stroke.

These results contrasted markedly with those of studies comparing the effects of antiplatelet and anticoagulant therapies for prevention of cardioembolic stroke, in which anticoagulation was generally preferred. In fact, in the WARSS, warfarin was slightly less effective than aspirin, was more costly, and required closer monitoring. Aspirin was slightly but not significantly superior for large-vessel and lacunar strokes. The possibility that using higher warfarin dosages to achieve higher INR values was not addressed for safety reasons, because the Stroke Prevention in Reversible Ischemia Trial (SPIRIT), in which an INR of 3.0 to 4.5 was used, had to be stopped owing to high rates of major bleeding.[90]

Ticlopidine and Clopidogrel, Thienopyridine Inhibitors of ADP-Mediated Platelet Activation

Mechanism of Action

Thienopyridine drugs, specifically ticlopidine (Ticlid) and a closely related compound, clopidogrel (Plavix, Iscover), have been clinically tested as antiplatelet agents that are chemically and functionally unrelated to prior classes of antiplatelet drugs.[91,92] These drugs block the binding of ADP to one specific type of purinergic receptor on platelets ($P2Y_{12}$) and therefore inhibit ADP-mediated platelet activation and G_i protein association with platelet membranes.[10] Thienopyridines therefore prevent the activation of GPIIb/IIIa, the fibrinogen receptor, to its high-affinity form but do not inhibit ADP-induced calcium flux or changes in platelet shape. Ticlopidine and clopidogrel have similar antiplatelet effects but differ in potency and pharmacokinetics.[92]

Bleeding time is prolonged much more by thienopyridines than by aspirin, and the prolongation is dose-dependent.[92] When ticlopidine or clopidogrel is given together with aspirin, the effects on bleeding time are additive. The prolongation of bleeding time due to thienopyridines can be reversed by the administration of corticosteroids, although the antiplatelet effects are not reversed. In emergency situations—for example, when urgent surgery is required in a patient taking a thienopyridine—the prolongation of bleeding time can be reversed quickly by desmopressin or by a bolus dose of dexamethasone (20 mg). The newer agent, clopidogrel, is more potent, can be rapidly effective, and is safer than ticlopidine and so is rapidly taking the place of ticlopidine in clinical practice.

In addition to decreasing binding of ADP and fibrinogen to platelet membranes, thienopyridines decrease platelet adhesion to artificial surfaces, reduce platelet deposition on atheromatous plaque,[93] and restore abnormally short platelet survival toward normal. In contrast, they do not affect platelet arachidonic acid metabolism or decrease TXA_2 synthesis. Thienopyridines also reduce plasma fibrinogen levels and blood viscosity and enhance red cell deformability, suggesting possibly beneficial rheologic properties.[92] They can oppose the action of several vasoconstrictors, such as endothelin and TXA_2, presumably by acting on vascular purinergic receptors.[94] In many different experimental thrombosis systems, these drugs have been shown to reduce thrombosis and to improve outcome whether or not platelets are important in the pathogenesis of the thrombosis. There is no gender nor age difference in response to the drugs.

Pharmacokinetics and Dosing

Both drugs are administered orally, ticlopidine at 250 mg bid and clopidogrel at 75 mg/day. Although ticlopidine and clopidogrel block ADP-mediated platelet activation processes in vivo, they are prodrugs inactive in vitro, indicating that their antiplatelet activity depends on drug metabolites. Both of these prodrugs are activated by hepatic metabolism. Clopidogrel is converted to active metabolites on first pass through the liver and therefore develops antiplatelet efficacy within a few hours when a loading dose (300 mg) is used. In contrast, ticlopidine circulates as the parent drug and requires several days for effective formation of active metabolites and a week for development of maximal antiplatelet effects. Thus, ticlopidine does not have a rapid onset of antiplatelet action. The antiplatelet effects of both drugs last for up to a week after administration is stopped, because their effect on circulating platelets is not reversible and active metabolites are slowly cleared.

Clinical Studies of Thienopyridine Use for Stroke Prevention

Ticlopidine

Ticlopidine hydrochloride was shown to prevent recurrent cerebral ischemia in two large randomized clinical trials, the Ticlopidine-Aspirin Stroke Study (TASS, 3069 subjects)[95] and the Canadian-American Ticlopidine Study (CATS, 1072 subjects).[96] The dose used in both was 250 mg bid, and average follow-up time exceeded 3 years. In the TASS, ticlopidine appeared to be slightly more effective (20%) than 1300 mg/day aspirin in preventing TIA, stroke, or death after an initial TIA or reversible stroke.[95] Maximum benefit occurred during the first year of treatment, and the difference between groups remained, but diminished, over time. In the CATS, ticlopidine produced a 23% risk reduction for recurrent TIA or stroke compared with placebo by intention-to-treat analysis, and a 30% risk reduction by efficacy analysis.[96] Patients with reversible cerebral ischemia also benefited.[97] A subgroup analysis of TASS data indicated that nonwhite patients had a 48% reduction in risk of nonfatal stroke or death with ticlopidine and a 60% risk reduction in fatal or nonfatal stroke.[98] The drug also decreased MI and stroke in patients with peripheral vascular disease.[99,100] Subsequently, ticlopidine was widely adopted by cardiologists as a key antithrombotic agent in combination with aspirin for maintaining arterial patency in acute cardiac interventions such as coronary artery angioplasty and stenting.[92]

Adverse effects of ticlopidine, however, have discouraged its long-term use. In published studies of ticlopidine prophylaxis for cerebral ischemia, treatment was discontinued before the end of the study in almost 50% of treated subjects because of side effects, necessity for other treatment modalities, or cerebral ischemic events.[95,96] More importantly, serious safety concerns have limited the overall use of ticlopidine because of unpredictable early, severe neutropenia or thrombocytopenia in up to 2.4% of recipients as well as rarer cases of aplastic anemia, and a high incidence of potentially fatal thrombotic thrombocytopenic purpura (TTP), estimated as 1 in 1500 to 1 in 4000 persons exposed.[101] Although the bone marrow depression resulting in neutropenia and thrombocytopenia is generally seen within the first 6 weeks of the start of ticlopidine therapy (requiring close monitoring of blood counts in all patients) and is usually reversible when the drug is stopped, TTP can occur at any time during ticlopidine use and may be fatal. These multiple adverse effects have also contributed to the clinical replacement of ticlopidine by clopidogrel.

Clopidogrel

Clopidogrel was established as an antiplatelet agent that is slightly more effective than aspirin by the randomized, international Clopidogrel versus Aspirin in Patients at Risk of Ischaemic Events (CAPRIE) study[102] and was approved by the FDA in 1997. In this study, secondary prevention of stroke, MI, or vascular death was evaluated in 19,185 subjects, all of whom had a prior atherosclerotic vascular event and who were assigned to a single daily dose of either 75 mg clopidogrel or 325 mg aspirin. An 8.7% greater risk reduction in combined end point (P = .043) was observed for clopidogrel in comparison with aspirin. In patients randomly assigned for therapy in the CAPRIE study after prior stroke, the average event rates per year were similar in the two treatment groups, 7.15% for clopidogrel versus 7.71% for aspirin; most strokes occurred in this subgroup of enrollees.

Rash and diarrhea were the major adverse effects of clopidogrel use. There was significantly less gastrointestinal hemorrhage in patients treated with clopidogrel than in those receiving aspirin, although no difference in cerebral hemorrhage or hemorrhagic stroke was observed. The CAPRIE study showed that the safety profile of clopidogrel is distinctly better than that of ticlopidine; severe neutropenia or thrombocytopenia did not occur, and there appeared to be less rash and diarrhea than with ticlopidine. Clopidogrel has rapidly taken over ticlopidine's role in short-term antithrombotic therapy during and after acute cardiac interventions. However, whether clopidogrel is preferable to aspirin in long-term prophylaxis, especially considering the high cost of the new agent, remains a therapeutic question in patients who can tolerate either drug.[3, 103] An excess of cytopenias has not been observed during the broader use of clopidogrel, confirming the general safety of the drug observed in the CAPRIE study. However, in post-marketing experience, a small number of cases of TTP have been associated with the use of clopidogrel, although a causal relationship has not yet been clearly established.[104,105]

Inhibitors of Platelet Membrane GPIIb/IIIa Activation

Two major membrane receptor complexes are involved in signaling platelet activation, GPIb-V-IX and GPIIa/IIIb. As detailed earlier, the GPIb-V-IX complex, which is important in shear-stress–mediated platelet activation, mediates platelet adhesion via vWF, so there has been considerable concern that blocking adhesion would result in hemorrhage. GPIIa/IIIb, in contrast, mediates platelet aggregation induced by all physiologic agonists but is not involved in platelet adhesion. This finding has suggested that blocking GPIIa/IIIb function might have antithrombotic effects while sparing hemostasis.[106] The successful use of this concept in preventing thrombosis during and immediately after acute coronary artery interventions such as angioplasty and stenting implies that a short-term, profound decrease in platelet reactivity has a marked, acute antithrombotic effect.[107]

Critical sites on the GPIIb/IIIa complex can be blocked (1) by monoclonal antibodies to epitopes exposed in the activated GPIIb/IIIa complex or (2) by small molecular "disintegrins" based on peptides or peptidomimetics containing the RGD motif. The humanized monoclonal antibody abciximab (c7E3Fab, ReoPro), binds to and blocks GPIIb/IIIa function.[106] Abciximab has been widely successful in preventing acute cardiac ischemic events. In the Evaluation of c7E3Fab in the Prevention of Ischemic Complications trial (EPICS, >2000 patients), a 12-hour infusion of abciximab (in addition to aspirin and heparin) in patients undergoing coronary angioplasty or atherectomy reduced the incidence of MI and the need for emergency revascularization by 35%.[107] Restenosis was also decreased, but this effect remains controversial.[108]

Efficacy of abciximab requires greater than 80% blockade of GPIIb/IIIa receptors. Antithrombotic effects of abciximab extend beyond GPIIb/IIIa blockade to inhibition of thrombin formation triggered by tissue factor and inhibition of the vitronectin receptor.[109] In a platelet-dependent model system, abciximab not only inhibited thrombin generation by 50% but also inhibited the formation of thrombin-antithrombin complexes (TAT), generation of prothrombin F1+2, release of growth factors and PF4 from platelets, incorporation of thrombin into clots, and formation of procoagulant platelet microparticles.[109,110] These observations suggest that blockade of platelet integrins leads to a decrease in most of the indicators of hypercoagulability that have been described as markers of acute or chronic cerebral ischemia.

Comparison between abciximab and eptifibatide or tirofiban, small molecule competitive inhibitors of GPIIb/IIIa, indicates that abciximab has a much longer duration of action because of multiple cycles of binding to these receptors, but that small molecule GPIIb/IIIa inhibitors used intravenously also provide effective platelet inhibition during cardiac interventions.[110] The latter do not, however, bind the vitronectin receptor or Mac-1 on leukocytes, activities of abciximab that may broaden its effectiveness.

Major risks of abciximab therapy include enhanced bleeding risk and production of anti–mouse immunoglobulin (Ig) G antibodies, the latter preventing reuse of the drug. However, in the EPICS trial, no excess of strokes or cerebral hemorrhage was observed among abciximab-treated patients once heparin dosage had been lowered.[107]

Whether the antithrombotic effects observed in the heart are clinically transferable to the cerebral circulation without incurring excess bleeding remains a key question.

Because patients with Glanzmann's thrombasthenia, whose platelet GPIIb/IIIa function is genetically defective, experience mainly mucocutaneous bleeding and rarely central nervous system bleeding, it was hoped that GPIIb/IIIa antagonists could also be used in prevention. In experimental focal cerebral ischemia, an inhibitor of GPIIb/IIIa blocked platelet accumulation in and occlusion of target cerebral microvascular beds.[111]

Abciximab in Stroke Prevention

To date, a single, multicenter safety trial of abciximab in treatment of acute cerebral ischemia has been published.[112] Escalating doses of abciximab versus placebo were evaluated in a randomized, double-blind, placebo-controlled manner in 74 adults (54 receiving drug) presenting within 24 hours of ischemic stroke onset. All patients underwent a baseline head CT scan before random assignment to treatment arm, and all had a minimum National Institutes of Health Stroke Scale (NIHSS) score of 4. Neurologic status was assessed daily for 5 days or until discharge and again at 3 months, and another head CT scan was obtained by 36 hours after the study agent was stopped. Platelet counts were monitored because thrombocytopenia is a side effect of abciximab. Twelve patients died during the study, 2 within the first 2 days (9/54 patients given abciximab and 3/20 patients given placebo), but none died from intracranial hemorrhage (ICH). Asymptomatic parenchymal ICH was detected on post-therapy CT scans in 4 of 54 patients receiving abciximab and 1 of the 20 patients receiving placebo patients, and 6 more asymptomatic ICHs were detected in abciximab recipients on later brain imaging. Thus, 19% of patients receiving abciximab and 5% of patients receiving placebo had asymptomatic ICH during the 3-month study ($P = .07$). Additional antithrombotic drugs were used in 11 subjects with hemorrhagic transformation of ischemic infarcts—heparin in 3, aspirin in 1, and heparin plus aspirin in 6.

The rates of nonneurologic bleeding episodes were similar in the two groups. Moderate thrombocytopenia occurred in 7 of the 54 abciximab recipients without ICH. Overall neurologic improvement was similar in the two groups, but neurologic disability was minimal at 3 months in 35% of the abciximab group versus 20% of the placebo group. The study investigators concluded that abciximab could safely be used in treating early stroke and that a bolus dose plus 0.25 μg/kg/hr—the usual dose in cardiology settings—was feasible.[112]

An independent trial was planned to evaluate abciximab use within 6 hours of stroke onset using a bolus of 0.22 μg/kg followed by 9 μg/min infused for 12 hours and permitting concomitant use of oral antiplatelet agents. However, the second patient entered in the trial experienced massive hemorrhagic transformations of both new and old cerebral infarct sites within the first 24 hours of treatment and died. The study was subsequently halted. The investigators concluded that concomitant use of other antithrombotic medications during administration of abciximab should probably be avoided.[113]

Other GPIIb/IIIa Inhibitors

Other studies of intravenous GPIIb/IIIa inhibitors in cardiovascular settings using the synthetic disintegrin eptifibatide or a nonpeptide GPIIb/IIIa antagonist, lamifiban, had also showed decrease in acute ischemic end points.[110] Theoretical advantages of these and similar small molecule inhibitors—especially the newer oral preparations—were ease of administration, absence of antibody formation, and protracted use as preventive therapy.[114] However, all cardiologic trials using oral GPIIb/IIIa inhibitors have been prematurely halted and abandoned because of high bleeding rates plus an excess of ischemic events. As already mentioned, the later BRAVO trial of lotrifiban and heparin in secondary prevention of cardiac or cerebral ischemia also had to be discontinued because of similar adverse events.[3,115] Evidence now suggests that patients expressing the Pl^{A2} allele on GPIIIa have excessive platelet activation in the presence of fiban-type GPIIb/IIIa inhibitors, perhaps accounting for the excess of ischemia in these trials.[3] As a consequence of this negative clinical experience, no trials with GPIIb/IIIa inhibitors for secondary prevention of cerebral ischemia are currently envisaged. The oral inhibitors have not been beneficial, and it appears that intravenous abciximab regimens that are effective in the coronary circulation for secondary prevention of acute ischemic events cannot be safely used for secondary prevention of stroke.

COMBINATIONS OF ANTIPLATELET AGENTS

Aspirin and Thienopyridines

Because aspirin and the thienopyridines have quite different modes of action, there has been considerable interest in combining these drugs to improve antiplatelet activity. This goal has been achieved with use of aspirin and ticlopidine for acute cardiac interventions, without excessive hemorrhage during a relatively brief period of use (generally 2 to 4 weeks). Completed studies in which aspirin and clopidogrel have been combined are few and mainly concern acute cardiac procedures rather than stroke prevention.[116] The Clopidogrel Aspirin Stent International Cooperative Study (CLASSICS) compared safety (and, secondarily, efficacy) of clopidogrel plus aspirin with or without a loading dose with ticlopidine plus aspirin after successful coronary stenting in 1020 subjects who were randomly assigned to receive one of these drug regimens for 28 days.[117] The study demonstrated that use of clopidogrel plus aspirin use is associated with a significantly lower rate of noncardiac adverse events such as bleeding, cytopenias, early discontinuation of the study drug (4.6%) compared with use of ticlopidine plus aspirin (9.1%), yielding a relative risk ratio of 0.50 ($P = .005$; CI = 0.31–0.87). The rates of major adverse cardiac events, including death, MI, and the need for revascularization, ranged between 0.9% and 1.5% for all treatments (P not significant).

In a later, secondary prevention study, the Clopidogrel in Unstable Angina to Prevent Recurrent Events (CURE) trial, the long-term efficacy of clopidogrel plus aspirin was compared with that of aspirin alone in patients who had acute coronary syndromes without ST elevation.[118] In the CURE trial, 12,562 patients presenting within 24 hours of symptoms were assigned aspirin (75 to 325 mg) daily and either clopidogrel 300 mg immediately followed by

75 mg daily or placebo for up to 12 months. The primary outcome—cardiovascular death, MI, or stroke—was significantly less frequent in patients receiving both clopidogrel and aspirin (9.3%) than in patients receiving aspirin alone (11.4%), yielding a relative risk (RR) of 0.80 (confidence interval [CI] 0.72 to 0.90; P < .001) for clopidogrel compared with placebo. The incidences of refractory angina and need for revascularization were also less in the clopidogrel plus aspirin group; rates of major bleeding episode were increased but those of hemorrhagic stroke were not. Patients undergoing percutaneous coronary intervention followed by long-term therapy with clopidogrel plus aspirin had significantly lower rates of cardiovascular death, MI, or need for revascularization after 30 days and also after a mean of 8 months, suggesting long-term benefit from the drug combination. Cardiovascular death or MI with the combination decreased by 31% (P = .002), and no significant difference in major bleeding was observed between the two treatment groups. No specific information on the incidence of stroke was available in this study.[119]

Results with clopidogrel plus aspirin in 139 consecutive patients undergoing carotid artery stenting at a single center were compared with those in 23 similar patients who received ticlopidine plus aspirin.[120] The cumulative 30-day rate of death, stroke, TIA, or MI was 4.3% in patients receiving clopidogrel plus aspirin versus 13% in those receiving ticlopidine plus aspirin (P = .01). Although these data might suggest that the use of clopidogrel plus aspirin in patients with carotid stenting is associated with a low rate of ischemic events and that clopidogrel might be better than ticlopidine in this high-risk group, these are results of a small, unblinded study, so caution is important. Whether the results in cardiac studies like the CURE trial can be successfully extrapolated to stroke prevention is a key question currently being addressed in the Management of Atherosclerosis with Clopidogrel in High-Risk Patients (MATCH) study, a large randomized trial comparing clopidogrel plus aspirin with clopidogrel alone in high-risk patients enrolled after a TIA or stroke.[121] This study is empowered to assess both efficacy and safety of the drug combination in a population with cerebrovascular disease. The MATCH study is particularly important because the data from the CAPRIE study suggested that clopidogrel might be much more effective in secondary prevention of MI than in secondary prevention of stroke.

Aspirin and Dipyridamole

Dipyridamole, a pyrimidopyrimidine derivative, inhibits platelet phosphodiesterases that destroy cAMP, therefore permitting platelet cAMP levels to remain elevated once they have risen, leading to cAMP-mediated inhibition of platelet activation.[122] Dipyridamole also blocks adenosine uptake by platelets and vascular cells, decreases platelet adhesion to the vascular wall, prolongs abnormally shortened platelet survival, and is a vasodilator.[122] Long prescribed for its theoretical antiplatelet effects, dipyridamole alone was not effective in preventing stroke when tested in controlled clinical trials carried out mainly in the 1980s. No additional benefit from dipyridamole was observed either in the Accidents Ischémiques Cérébraux Liés a

L'Athérosclerose study (AICLA), which compared aspirin alone with aspirin plus dipyridamole (400 subjects),[76] or in the American-Canadian Cooperative Study Group trial (890 subjects).[77] Because dipyridamole is a short-acting drug, requiring four daily doses for effective blood levels, and frequently causes headache because of its vasodilatory action, compliance problems might have contributed to the apparent lack of efficacy observed.

The European Stroke Prevention Study (ESPS-1, 2500 subjects) showed that the combination of high-dose aspirin and dipyridamole was superior to placebo in preventing TIA and stroke over a 2-year period, reducing rates of stroke and death by 33.5%, but no aspirin-only group was compared.[123]

A fixed combination of low-dose aspirin and slow-release dipyridamole (Aggrenox, Asasantin Retard) was then studied for secondary prevention of stroke in the second European Stroke Prevention Study (ESPS-2).[124] In ESPS-2, 6602 subjects who had had prior TIA or ischemic stroke were randomly assigned to receive aspirin only, dipyridamole only, both aspirin and dipyridamole, or placebo; they were monitored for 2 years for primary end points of stroke, death, or stroke/death. The combination of aspirin 25 mg plus extended-release dipyridamole 200 mg twice daily was significantly better than either agent alone in preventing stroke and TIA, yielding a 37% relative risk reduction (P < .001) by efficacy analysis comparing it with placebo.[124] The drug combination did not appear to cause an excess of cerebral hemorrhage.[125] Smaller but significant risk reductions were also observed with dipyridamole only (16.3%) and aspirin only (18.1%). A fairly high percentage of patients taking the drug combination (29%) withdrew from treatment during the study. Headache, palpitations, and gastrointestinal symptoms are common side effects, as is bleeding; indeed, headache is a common reason given by patients for discontinuing treatment. Several cost-benefit analyses have subsequently suggested that this drug combination is cost effective in stroke prevention.[103]

To confirm whether dipyridamole plus aspirin is superior to aspirin alone or to anticoagulation for secondary prevention of stroke, the international European/Australian Stroke Prevention in Reversible Ischemia Trial (ESPRIT) was launched in 2000.[126] In ESPRIT, 4500 subjects with prior TIA or minor ischemic stoke are being randomly assigned to one of the following three regimens: 400 mg/day dipyridamole plus 30 to 325 mg/day aspirin, aspirin only, or oral anticoagulants adjusted to maintain an INR of 2.0 to 3.0. Mean follow-up is planned to take 3 years, and the planned primary outcome is the composite of vascular death, nonfatal stroke, nonfatal MI, or major bleeding.

Combinations of Antiplatelet Agents with Anticoagulants

Anticoagulation has traditionally been used to prevent cardioembolic stroke in patients with AF. Several Stroke Prevention in Atrial Fibrillation (SPAF) trials have compared both the efficacy and safety of aspirin and warfarin. Results of SPAF I suggested that warfarin was more effective, but the overall number of cerebral ischemic events was small, making interpretation difficult.[127,128] SPAF II examined age effects of these two regimens (warfarin to maintain INR at 2.0 to 4.5 or aspirin 325 mg/day) in patients younger than and older than 75 years in the prevention of ischemic stroke and systemic embolism.[82] The absolute rate of the primary events varied with age. In treated low-risk patients younger than 75, the primary event rate per year was 1.3% for those taking warfarin and 1.9% for those taking aspirin (RR 0.67, P = .24). In treated patients older than 75, the primary event rate was 3.6% per year with warfarin and 4.8% with aspirin (RR 0.73; P = .39). However, for the older group, despite greater effectiveness of anticoagulation in preventing thromboembolic stroke, the rate per year of all strokes (ischemic plus hemorrhagic) with residual deficit was 4.6% with warfarin and 4.3% with aspirin. Thus, although warfarin may be more effective than aspirin for preventing ischemic stroke in older patients with AF or in high-risk younger patients, the overall rate of stroke in warfarin-treated patients remains high, reflecting bleeding complications due to the intervention itself. These results in patients with AF are similar to those observed several decades ago in the Sixty Plus Reinfarction Study, in which elderly patients who received anticoagulation therapy after one MI were observed to have fewer ischemic strokes but more hemorrhagic strokes, so that no net benefit in stroke prevention resulted, whereas the incidence of recurrent MI was clearly decreased.[129]

Many clinical trials have assessed whether the combination of an antiplatelet agent with an anticoagulant improves secondary protection against stroke, but the results have been disappointing. Either no benefit has ensued, or the combination results in increased intracerebral bleeding, negating the benefit. Dose is an important consideration in these studies. For example, the Coumadin Aspirin Reinfarction Study (CARS, 2028 subjects) showed that fixed-dose warfarin (1 or 3 mg) plus aspirin (80 mg/day) after an MI was no better than aspirin alone for the prevention of recurrent MI, stroke, or cardiovascular death.[59] In particular, the incidence of ischemic stroke was lower in patients treated with 160 mg/day aspirin than in those treated with warfarin 1 mg/day plus aspirin 80 mg/day (0.6% versus 1.1%; P = .0534). The highest-risk group, patients with Q-wave MI and male patients, had greater benefit from aspirin alone. This clinical trial was prematurely discontinued for lack of efficacy.

In SPAF III (1085 subjects), patients with AF who had at least one thromboembolic risk factor had a worse outcome if they took a combination of fixed-dose warfarin plus aspirin than if they took adjusted-dose warfarin alone.[130] This trial was stopped because of the higher rate of strokes and systemic embolism in the combined-therapy group (7.9% per year) compared with the adjusted-dose warfarin group (1.9% per year), although the incidences of bleeding were similar in the two groups.

Risk stratification of patients with nonvalvular AF indicates that patients who can be prospectively identified as having a low risk of stroke, particularly disabling ischemic stroke, benefit from aspirin therapy and so may not require anticoagulation with its higher adverse event rates. Specifically, in patients with AF who have no history of hypertension and none of the following four thromboembolic risk factors, the ischemic stroke risk is no greater than that of the general population of similar age (namely ~1%/yr):

(1) recent congestive heart failure or left ventricular dysfunction, (2) prior thromboembolism, (3) systolic blood pressure higher than 160 mm Hg, and (4) female sex with age greater than 75 years. Although patients with nonvalvular AF are usually considered to be at increased risk for cardioembolic stroke—for which anticoagulation is clearly indicated—they may also be at risk for ischemic stroke. Further modulating factors for stroke risk in patients from the aspirin-only arm of SPAF trials I through III trials (2012 subjects) were consumption of 14 or more alcoholic drinks per week (decreased stroke risk), prior stroke or TIA (increased stroke risk), and estrogen hormone replacement therapy (increased stroke risk).[131]

The combination of anticoagulants with antiplatelet drugs has been beneficial in several clinical settings that do not directly involve the cerebral circulation, heart valve replacements, coronary stents thrombolysis, and angioplasty.[132] Benefit in terms of reduced mortality, especially from vascular causes, and decreased embolic rates, without severe increase in bleeding was achieved in the patients with prosthetic heart valves.[133] A comparison of the results of four separate trials of patients treated with aspirin (doses between 75 and 1000 mg/day combined with moderate anticoagulation to an INR of 1.5 to 4.5) indicated that the rate of bleeding complications correlated more with higher aspirin dose than with INR level, suggesting that aspirin dose should be kept low if the combination were to be used.[134] However, later studies have clearly shown that this combination cannot be used for stroke prevention without incurring unacceptable rates of intracerebral hemorrhage.

NEW ANTIPLATELET STRATEGIES

Exploiting natural antithrombotic defenses represents another strategy for stroke prevention therapy. Antiplatelet effects of vascular endothelium involve several separate mechanisms, as follows:

1. Heparin-like molecules, or natural anticoagulants.
2. Secretion of prostacyclin, which stimulates platelet adenylate cyclase, raises cAMP, and blocks platelet aggregation.
3. Release of NO, which stimulates platelet guanylate cyclase, raises cGMP, and blocks platelet aggregation.
4. Presence of an endothelial membrane enzyme, an ectonucleotidase/ADP hydrolase that metabolizes ATP and ADP released from platelets to AMP, which in turn is cleaved by 5-nucleotidase to adenosine, an inhibitor of platelet activation.

All the antiplatelet substances—prostacyclin, NO, and adenosine—are vasodilators. Each has been explored for possible antithrombotic efficacy, particularly for antiplatelet effects.

Direct Thrombin Inhibitors

Thrombin is the most potent physiologic platelet activator. Because thrombin bound to the surface of a clot is not readily inactivated by heparin, platelets localized in thrombi are particularly resistant to aspirin- or heparin-based antithrombotic therapies. Direct antithrombin agents may be a more effective therapy to halt thrombin-mediated, platelet-dependent occlusive events taking place on diseased arteries.[135,136] How to target platelet recruitment to ongoing arterial thrombi without impairing normal hemostasis is a difficult task, and bleeding, particularly hemorrhagic strokes, has halted some cardiologic clinical trials, such as the Global Utilization of Streptokinase and Tissue Plasminogen Activator for Occluded Arteries (GUSTO) and Thrombolysis in Myocardial Infarction (TIMI) 9 trials, which employed hirudin, a direct thrombin inhibitor.[3]

The major current approaches under study use several antithrombin peptides. Antithrombin peptides containing D-Phe-Pro-Arg (RGD-inhibitory) sequences interact with the catalytic site of thrombin to block thrombin-induced platelet aggregation and fibrinogen cleavage in vitro and in vivo. Bivalirudin, a bifunctional antithrombin peptide that combines part of the hirudin sequence with the active site inhibitory peptide, and oral antithrombins are also under development as new anticoagulants. Clinical trials of bivalirudin in angioplasty models and of argatroban—the latter now approved for treatment of heparin-induced thrombocytopenia—are in process. Development of inhibitors of extrinsic pathway or tissue factor–mediated thrombus formation may yield the antithrombotic specificity required, sparing hemostasis. An oral prodrug, ximelagatran, which liberates a direct antithrombin metabolite, melagatran, in vivo, has been shown to be as effective as warfarin in early clinical trials for prophylaxis of venous thrombosis.[137] Ximelagatran also is capable of blocking thrombin-mediated platelet activation.

Antiplatelet Effects of Polyunsaturated Fatty Acids and Prostacyclin

Interest in the antiplatelet and antithrombotic effects of dietary modification, other than that involving cholesterol, has focused on the effects of highly polyunsaturated ω-3 fatty acids present in oils of cold-water fish like salmon and mackerel. Administration of fish, fish oil, or the ω-3 fatty acids has been shown to decrease platelet aggregation, prolong bleeding time, and decrease TXA_2 production but to increase vascular prostacyclin levels.[138,139] In addition, ω-3 fatty acids have anti-inflammatory effects on neutrophil and monocyte functions. However, although diets including regular intake of fish have been associated with decreased coronary artery disease mortality, no association has been found between fish intake and stroke incidence in several epidemiologic studies.[140] A possible explanation for the difference between effects of ω-3 fatty acids in coronary disease and in cerebrovascular disease may reside in the antiarrhythmic effects of these fatty acids.[141,142]

The prostaglandins epoprostenol (prostacyclin, PGI_2) and PGE_1, produced by vascular endothelium, smooth muscle cells, and monocytes, are direct inhibitors of platelet aggregation. By stimulating adenylate cyclase, PGI_2 and PGE_2 increase platelet cAMP, activating cAMP-dependent protein kinases and enhancing uptake of Ca^{2+} into intracellular storage pools. The resulting lowered platelet Ca^{2+} levels oppose platelet activation. However, these prostaglandins do not offer useful stroke prevention therapy; oral preparations of PGI_2 are not available, and

intravenous PGI_2 causes hypotension at concentrations required to inhibit platelet aggregation and desensitizes or downregulates vascular PGI_2 receptors, enhancing platelet adhesion to endothelium. Parenteral PGI_2 or synthetic congeners such as iloprost can support hemodialysis in bleeding patients in whom heparin could not be used, can substitute for heparin during cardiac surgery, and can be used in long-term treatment of primary pulmonary hypertension. There is no effort to develop these drugs for stroke prevention. Antagonists of TXA_2 or of thromboxane synthase have not been clinically effective antithrombotic agents in early trials and currently are not being tested for stroke prevention.

Nitric Oxide Derivatives as Antiplatelet Agents

NO produced by normal endothelium via nitric oxide synthase (eNOS) has antiplatelet and vasodilator effects.[17] NO stimulates platelet guanylate cyclase and consequently elevates platelet cGMP, which blocks platelet activation. Platelets also contain NO synthase, and their own production of NO downregulates platelet activation and inhibits both cyclooxygenase and 12-lipoxygenase.[143] Considerable evidence supports a role for endogenous NO in platelet regulation. Platelet-derived NO inhibits platelet recruitment into arterial thrombi.[144] In animal models of pulmonary thromboembolism due to platelet aggregates, administration of arginine, a precursor of NO, decreases platelet accumulation in pulmonary vessels in response to aggregating stimuli, whereas the eNOS inhibitor L-NAME aggravates formation of platelet emboli and, in a different model, potentiates cerebral ischemia.[17,145] NO itself is very unstable in vivo, but stable S-nitrosothiol derivatives of NO inhibit both thrombin-induced and endoperoxide-induced activation of GPIIb/IIIa complexes on platelets and can induce platelet disaggregation by blocking activation and translocation of PI_3 kinase.[17] NO indirectly blocks platelet adhesion to collagen and interferes with interactions between GPIIb/IIIa and vWF but does not directly block GPIb/IX function. In vivo correlates of these effects include the observations that atherosclerotic human arteries show decreased NO production and impaired vasodilation, and that mice lacking NO synthase have short bleeding times and enhanced hemostatic reactions to injury.[146] Conversely, platelets from patients with acute coronary syndromes produce less NO than platelet from patients with stable angina, suggesting that the NO deficiency may contribute to acute, platelet-dependent thrombosis.[147]

Therefore, interest has developed in the use of NO donation as an antiplatelet strategy. Inhaled NO is already used in acute lung syndromes such as adult respiratory distress syndrome (ARDS) and in the acute chest syndrome of sickle cell anemia to improve vascular perfusion. Intravenous S-nitroso (SNO) glutathione given to patients undergoing carotid endarterectomy (together with heparin and aspirin) has produced a marked decrease in asymptomatic cerebral embolic signals compared with aspirin and heparin alone; these embolic signals are thought to represent platelet thrombi.[148] During coronary angioplasty, infusion of SNO-glutathione causes inhibition of platelet activation at concentrations of the drug that did not lower blood pressure. Statins upregulate NOS in platelets and protect mice from cerebral ischemia, activities that may explain some of the antithrombotic effects of statins that are independent of their cholesterol-lowering properties.[149] In a rat model of stroke, administering sildenafil within the first few days after middle cerebral artery occlusion decreased the extent of neurologic disability and stimulated neuronal proliferation.[150] Sildenafil is a vasodilatory drug that, by inhibiting a specific phosphodiesterase, acts to increase cGMP and NO.

One novel approach to future antiplatelet therapy involves an *S*-nitrosated derivative of a recombinant vWF fragment, termed AR545C.[151] The SNO-glutathione compound inhibits both platelet adhesion and aggregation in vitro and in vivo in animal models of thrombosis, without producing significant hypotension and shows synergic effects compared with either SNO-glutathione or heparin alone.[152] The vWF fragment portion of this compound blocks GPIb-mediated platelet adhesion, whereas the SNO group raises platelet cGMP, inhibiting aggregation. Combining these two actions in the same molecule has synergetic effects in blocking platelet activation. Whether this or similar NO-containing drugs can be utilized in secondary stroke prevention awaits further testing.

Soluble CD39 as an Antiplatelet Agent that Inhibits Released ADP

Among endothelial mechanisms that control platelet activation is the ecto-ADPase CD39, which breaks down ATP and ADP to AMP.[16,153] Not only does this enzymatic action remove key platelet agonists released by activated platelets, but also, the further conversion of AMP to adenosine by endothelial 5′-nucleotidase provides high local concentrations of adenosine, a platelet antagonist and vasodilator. The pathophysiologic relevance of this system to stroke is illustrated by a CD39-knockout strain of mice, which have a normal phenotype except that transient carotid artery injury results in larger ischemic strokes and lower post-ischemic cerebral perfusion in these animals than in CD39-normal mice.[154] Infusion of soluble CD39 into CD39-knockout animals prevents large strokes without causing bleeding, whereas aspirin fails to protect against stroke and increases bleeding in the brain.[154] Soluble, recombinant CD39 retaining the ADPase activity inhibits platelet activation in vitro and prevents platelet activation in vivo in mice.[151] In an arterial thrombosis model in pigs, soluble CD39 is antithrombotic, has a prolonged duration of action, yet does not induce bleeding.[16] This novel molecule, developed through extrapolation of a natural antiplatelet function of endothelium, has promising antithrombotic potential in stroke prevention.

Simultaneous Blockade of Platelet P2Y$_{12}$ and P2Y$_1$ ADP Receptors

Shear-stress–induced platelet aggregation in arteries, which is important in the genesis of arterial thrombosis, requires the participation of platelet ADP as well as binding of large vWF molecules to GPIbα and activation of GPIIb/IIIa.[155] ADP appears to stabilize platelet aggregates. Data now indicate that two different types of platelet ADP receptors, the P2Y$_{12}$ receptor, which is blocked by thienopyridines, and the P2Y$_1$ receptor, which is not blocked by thienopyridines but is blocked by certain ATP analogues, are both needed for shear-stress–induced platelet aggregation and platelet procoagulant activity.[156–158] P2Y$_1$ platelet ADP receptors are also important in mediating collagen-induced platelet activation. Combining inhibitors of both P2Y$_{12}$ and P2Y$_1$ types of ADP receptors markedly decreases mural thrombosis in arterial flow models using whole blood, whereas an inhibitor to either ADP receptor type alone fails to block thrombosis. Specific nucleotide analogue inhibitors of both the P2Y$_{12}$ and P2Y$_1$ receptors are under development. One of these, AR-C69931MX (2-trifluoropropylthio, nn-(2-[methylthio]ethyl-β,γ-dichloromethylene ATP), a specific inhibitor of the P2Y$_{12}$ ADP receptor, was more potent than GPIIb/IIIa inhibitors in abolishing thrombus-related cyclic flow variations in the Folts model.[159] In patients with unstable angina or non–Q-wave infarction, AR-C69931MX produced greater inhibition of ADP-induced platelet activation than did clopidogrel and had a rapid onset of action and short half-life.[160] These data suggest the potential for combined ADP receptor blockade in a future therapeutic approach to stroke prevention; as with other therapies useful in the cardiac setting, however, both the efficacy and safety of the approach must be established for the cerebral circulation.

References

1. Collaborative overview of randomised trials of antiplatelet therapy. I: Prevention of death, myocardial infarction and stroke by prolonged antiplatelet therapy in various categories of patients. Antiplatelet Trialists' Collaboration. Br Med J 308:8, 1994.
2. Warfarin versus aspirin for prevention of thromboembolism in atrial fibrillation: Stroke Prevention in Atrial Fibrillation II study. Stroke Prevention in Atrial Fibrillation Investigators. Lancet 343:687, 1994.
3. Bousser M-G: Antithrombotic strategy in stroke. Thromb Haemost 86:1, 2001.
4. Andrews RK, Shen Y, Gardiner EE, et al: The glycoprotein Ib-IX-V complex in platelet adhesion and signaling. Thromb Haemost 82:357, 1999.
5. Fitzgerald DJ: Vascular biology of thrombosis: The role of platelet-vessel wall adhesion. Neurology 57:S1, 2001.
6. Shattil SJ, Brass LP: Induction of the fibrinogen receptor on human platelets by intracellular mediators. J Biol Chem 262:992, 1987.
7. Plow EF, Cieniewski CS, Xiao Z, et al: $\alpha_{11b}\beta_3$ and its antagonism at the new millennium. Thromb Haemost 86:34, 2001.
8. Coughlin SR: Thrombin signalling and protease-activated receptors. Nature 407:258, 2000.
9. Gachet C: ADP receptors of platelets and their inhibition. Thromb Haemost 86:222, 2001.
10. Hollopeter G, Jntwen HM, Vincent D, et al: Identification of the platelet ADP receptor targeted by antithrombotic drugs. Nature 409:202,2001.
11. Shen RF, Tai HH: Thromboxanes: Synthase and receptors. J Biomed Sci 5:153, 1998.
12. Hajjar KA: Cellular receptors in the regulation of plasmin generation. Thromb Haemost 74:294, 1995.
13. Miles LA, Ginsberg MH, White JG, Plow EF: Plasminogen interacts with human platelets through two distinct mechanisms. J Clin Invest 77:2001, 1986.
14. Schafer AI, Adelman B: Plasmin inhibition of platelet function and of arachidonic acid metabolism. J Clin Invest 75:456, 1985.
15. Fitzgerald DJ, Wright F, FitzGerald GA: Increased thromboxane biosynthesis during coronary thrombolysis: Evidence that platelet activation and thromboxane A2 modulate the response to tissue-type plasminogen activator in vivo. Circ Res 65:83, 1989.

16. Marcus AJ, Broekman MJ, Drosopoulos JHF, et al: Thromboregulation by endothelial cells: Significance for occlusive vascular diseases. Arterioscler Thromb Vasc Biol 21:178, 2001.

17. Loscalzo J: Nitric oxide insufficiency, platelet activation, and arterial thrombosis. Circ Res 88:756, 2001.

18. Yao S-K, Ober JC, Krishnaswami A, et al: Endogenous nitric oxide protects against platelet aggregation and cyclic flow variations in stenosed and endothelium-injured arteries. Circulation 86:1302, 1992.

19. Zwaginga JJ, Sixma JJ, DeGroot PG: Activation of endothelial cells induces platelet thrombus formation on their matrix. Arteriosclerosis 10:49, 1990.

20. Feinberg WM, Erickson LP, Bruck D, Kittelson J: Hemostatic markers in acute ischemic stroke: Association with stroke type, severity and outcome. Stroke 27:1296, 1996.

21. Uchiyama S, Yamazaki M, Hara Y, et al: Alteration of platelet, coagulation and fibrinolysis markers in patients with acute ischemic stroke. Semin Thromb Haemost 23:535, 1997.

22. Zeller T, Tschoepe D, Kessler C: Circulating platelets show increased activation in patients with acute cerebral ischemia. Thromb Haemost 81:373, 1999.

23. Folsom AR, Rosamond WD, Shahar E, et al: Prospective study of markers of hemostatic function with risk of ischemic stroke. The Atherosclerosis Risk in Communities (ARIC) study investigators. Circulation 100:736, 1999.

24. Haddar HB, Cortes J, Salomaa V, et al: Correlation of specific platelet activation markers with carotid arterial wall thickness. Thromb Haemost 74:943, 1995.

25. Tofler GH, Brezinski D, Schafer AI, et al: Concurrent morning increase in platelet aggregability and the risk of myocardial infarction and sudden cardiac death. N Engl J Med 316:1514, 1987.

26. Marler JR, Price TR, Clark GL, et al: Morning increase in onset of ischemic stroke. Stroke 20:473, 1989.

27. Ernst E, Resch KL: Fibrinogen as a cardiovascular risk factor: A meta-analysis and review of the literature. Ann Intern Med 118:956, 1993.

28. Becher H, Grau A, Steindorf K, et al: Previous infection and other risk factors for acute cerebrovascular ischemia: Attributable risks and the characterisation of high risk groups. J Epidemiol Biostat 5:277, 2000.

29. Woodhouse PR, Khaw K, Plummer M, et al: Seasonal variations of plasma fibrinogen and factor VII activity in the elderly: Winter infections and death from cardiovascular disease. Lancet 343:435, 1994.

30. Grau AJ, Buggle F, Becher H, et al: Recent bacterial and viral infection is a risk for cerebrovascular ischemia. Neurology 50:196, 1998.

31. Kristensen SD, Roberts KM, Kishk YT, Martin JF: Accelerated atherogenesis occurs following platelet destruction and increases in megakaryocyte size and DNA content. Eur J Clin Invest 20:239, 1990.

32. O'Malley T, Langhorne P, Elton RA, Stewart MD: Platelet size in stroke patients. Stroke 26:995, 1995.

33. Cortelazzo S, Finazzi G, Ruggeri M, et al: Hydroxyurea for patients with essential thrombocythemia and a high risk of thrombosis. N Engl J Med 332:1132, 1995.

34. Koudstaal PJ, Ciabattoni G, van Gijn J, et al: Increased thromboxane synthesis in patients with acute cerebral ischemia. Stroke 24:219, 1993.

35. van Kooten F, Ciabattoni G, Patrono C, et al: Evidence for episodic platelet activation in acute ischemic stroke. Stroke 25:278, 1994.

36. van Kooten F, Ciabattoni G, Koudstall PJ, et al: Increased platelet activation in the chronic phase after cerebral ischemia and intracerebral hemorrhage. Stroke 30:546, 1999.

37. Michelson AD: Flow cytometry: A clinical test of platelet function. Blood 87:4925, 1996.

38. Malik I, Danesh J, Whincup P, et al: Soluble adhesion molecules and prediction of coronary heart disease: A prospective study and meta-analysis. Lancet 358:971, 2001.

39. Kenet G, Freedman J, Shenkman B, et al: Plasma glutathione peroxidase deficiency and platelet insensitivity to nitric oxide in children with familial stroke. Arterioscler Thromb Vasc Biol 19:2017, 1999.

40. Knapp HR, Reilly IA, Alessandrini P, FitzGerald GA: In vivo indexes of platelet function and vascular function in patients with atherosclerosis. N Engl J Med 314:937, 1986.

41. Sivenius J, Cunha L, Diener H-C, et al: Antiplatelet treatment does not reduce the severity of subsequent stroke. Neurology 53:825, 1999.

42. Amarenco P, Cohen A, Tzourio C, et al: Atherosclerotic disease of the aortic arch and the risk of ischemic stroke. N Engl J Med 331:1474, 1994.

43. Orgera M, O'Malley P, Taylor AJ: Secondary prevention of cerebral ischemia in patent foramen ovale: Systematic review and meta-analysis. South Med J 94:699, 2001.

44. Gunning AJ, Pickering GW, Robb-Smith AH, Russell RR: Mural thrombosis of the internal carotid artery and subsequent embolization. Quart J Med 33:155, 1964.

45. Eldor A, Rachmilewitz EA: The hypercoagulable state in thalassemia. Blood 99:36, 2002.

46. Barnett JHM, Eliasziw M, Meldrum HE: Drugs and surgery in the prevention of ischemic stroke. N Engl J Med 332:238, 1995.

47. Smith JB, Willis AL: Aspirin selectively inhibits prostaglandin production in human platelets. Nature 231:235, 1971.

48. Vane JR: Inhibition of prostaglandin synthesis as a mechanism of action for aspirin-like drugs. Nature 231:232, 1971.

49. Roth GJ, Stanford N, Majerus PW: Acetylation of prostaglandin synthetase by aspirin. Proc Natl Acad Sci U S A 72:3073, 1975.

50. Patrono C, Coller B, Dalen JE, et al: Platelet-active drugs: The relationships among dose, effectiveness and side effects. Chest 114:S470, 1998.

51. Weksler BB, Kent JL, Rudolph D, et al: Effects of low-dose aspirin on platelet function in patients with recent cerebral ischemia. Stroke 16:5, 1985.

52. Weksler BB, Tack-Goldman K, Subramanian VA, et al: Cumulative inhibitory effect of low dose aspirin on vascular prostacyclin and platelet thromboxane production in patients with atherosclerosis. Circulation 71:332, 1985.

53. Goertler M, Baemer M, Kross R, et al: Rapid decline of cerebral microemboli of arterial origin after intravenous acetylsalicylic acid. Stroke 30:66, 1999.

54. Kyrle PA, Eichler HG, Jager U, Lechner K: Inhibition of prostacyclin and thromboxane A_2 generation by low-dose aspirin at the site of plug formation in man in vivo. Circulation 75:1025, 1987.

55. A comparison of two doses of aspirin (30 mg vs 283 mg a day) in patients after a transient ischemic attack or minor ischemic stroke. The Dutch TIA Trial Study Group. N Engl J Med 325:1261, 1991.

56. Ali M, McDonald JWD, Thiessen JJ, Coates PE: Plasma acetylsalicylate and salicylate and platelet cyclooxygenase activity following plain and enteric-coated aspirin. Stroke 11:9, 1980.

57. Patrono C, Roth GJ: Aspirin in ischemic cerebrovascular disease: How strong is the case for a different dosing regimen? Stroke 27:756, 1996.

58. Tohgi H, Konno S, Tamura K, et al: Effect of low-to-high doses of aspirin on platelet aggregability and metabolites of thromboxane A2 and prostacyclin. Stroke 23:1400, 1993.

59. O'Connor CM, Gattis WA, Hellkamp AS, et al: Comparison of two aspirin doses on ischemic stroke in post-myocardial infarction patients in the warfarin (Coumadin) Aspirin Reinfarction Study (CARS). Am J Cardiol 88:541, 2001.

60. Taylor DW, Barnett JHM, Haynes RB, et al: Low-dose and high-dose acetylsalicylic acid for patients undergoing carotid endarterectomy: A randomized clinical trial. ASA and Carotid Endarterectomy (ACE) Trial Collaborators. Lancet 353:2179, 1999.

61. Catella-Lawson F, Reilly MP, Kapoor S, et al: Cyclooxygenase inhibitors and the antiplatelet effects of aspirin. N Engl J Med 345:1809, 2001.

62. Ouellet M, Riendeau D, Percival MD: A high level of cyclooxygenase-2 inhibitor selectivity is associated with a reduced interference of platelet cyclooxygenase-1 inactivation by aspirin. Proc Natl Acad Sci U S A 98:14583, 2001.

63. Cardiovascular safety of cox-2 inhibitors. Med Lett 43:99, 2001.

64. Szeczklik A, Krzanowski M, Gora P, Radwan J: Antiplatelet drugs and generation of thrombin in clotting blood. Blood 80:2006, 1992.

65. Szeczklik A, Musial J, Undas A, et al: Aspirin inhibits thrombogenesis in normocholesterolemic but not in hypercholesterolemic man. Thomb Haemost 69:798, 1993.

66. Hart RG, Harrison MJG: Aspirin wars: The optimal dose of aspirin to prevent stroke. Stroke 27:585, 1996.

67. Grotemeyer KH, Schorafinski HW, Husstedt IW: 2-year followup of aspirin responders and aspirin non-responders—a pilot study including 180 post-stroke patients. Thromb Res 71:397, 1993.

68. Bornstein NM, Karpov VG, Aronovich BD, et al: Failure of aspirin treatment after stroke. Stroke 25:275, 1994.

69. Helgason CM, Bolin KM, Hoff JA, et al: Development of aspirin resistance in persons with previous ischemic stroke. Stroke 25:2331, 1994.

70. Komiya T, Kudo M, Urabe T, Mizuno Y: Compliance with antiplatelet therapy in patients with ischemic cerebrovascular disease: Assessment by platelet aggregation testing. Stroke 25:2337, 1994.

71. Sappok T, Faulstich A, Stuckert E: Compliance with secondary prevention of ischemic stroke: A prospective evaluation. Stroke 32:1884, 2001.

72. Moroz L: Increased blood fibrinolytic activity after aspirin ingestion. N Engl J Med 296:525, 1977.

73. Bjornsson TD, Schneider DE, Berger H Jr: Aspirin acetylates fibrinogen and enhances fibrinolysis: Fibrinolytic effect is independent of changes in plasminogen activator levels. J Pharm Exp Ther 250:154, 1989.

74. Levin RI, Harpel PC, Harpel JG, Recht PA: Inhibition of tissue plasminogen activator activity by aspirin in vivo and its relationship to levels of tissue plasminogen activator antigen, plasminogen activator inhibitor and their complexes. Blood 74:1635, 1989.

75. A randomized trial of aspirin and sulfinpyrazone in threatened stroke. Canadian Cooperative Study Group. N Engl J Med 299:53, 1978.

76. Bousser MG, Eschwege E, Haguenau M, et al: "AICLA" controlled trial of aspirin and dipyridamole in the secondary prevention of atherothrombotic cerebral ischemia. Stroke 14:5, 1983.

77. Persantine Aspirin Trial in cerebral ischemia. Part II: Endpoint results. American-Canadian Co-operative Study Group. Stroke 16:418, 1985.

78. He J, Whelton PK, Vu B, et al: Aspirin and risk of hemorrhagic stroke: A meta-analysis of randomized controlled trials. JAMA 280:1930, 1998.

79. Sivenius J, Riekkinen PH, Laakso M, et al: European Stroke Prevention Study (ESPS): Antithrombotic therapy is also effective in the elderly. Acta Neurol Scand 87:111, 1993.

80. Report of the Stroke Prevention in Atrial Fibrillation study. N Engl J Med 322:863, 1990.

81. Patients with nonvalvular atrial fibrillation at low risk of stroke during treatment with aspirin. Stroke Prevention in Atrial Fibrillation III Study. The SPAF III Writing Committee for the Stroke Prevention in Atrial Fibrillation Investigators. JAMA 279:1273, 1998.

82. Warfarin versus aspirin for prevention of thromboembolism in atrial fibrillation: SPAF II. Stroke Prevention in Atrial Fibrillation Investigators. Lancet 343:687, 1994.

83. Final report on the aspirin component of the ongoing Physicians' Health Study. Steering Committee of the Physicians' Health Study Research Group. N Engl J Med 321:129, 1989.

84. Cote R, Battista RN, Abrahamowicz M, et al: Lack of effect of aspirin in asymptomatic patients with carotid bruits and substantial carotid narrowing. The Asymptomatic Cervical Bruit Study Group. Ann Intern Med 123:649, 1995.

85. Barnett HJM, Taylor DW, Eliasziw M, et al: Benefit of carotid endarterectomy in patients with symptomatic moderate or severe stenosis. North American Symptomatic Carotid Endarterectomy Trial Collaborators. N Engl J Med 339:1415, 1998.

86. CAST: A randomised placebo-controlled trial of early aspirin use in 20,000 patients with acute ischemic stroke. Chinese Acute Stroke Trial Collaborative Group. Lancet 349:1641, 1997.

87. The International Stroke Trial (IST): A randomized trial of aspirin, subcutaneous heparin, both or neither among 19,435 patients with acute ischemic stroke. International Stroke Trial Collaborative Group. Lancet 349:1569, 1997.

88. Chen Z-M, Sanderock P, Pan H-C, et al: Indications for early aspirin use in acute ischemic stroke: A combined analysis of 40,000 randomized patients from the Chinese Acute Stroke Trial and the International Stroke Trial. Stroke 31:1240, 2000.

89. Mohr JP, Thompson JL, Lazar RM, et al: A comparison of warfarin and aspirin for the prevention of recurrent ischemic stroke. N Engl J Med 345:1444, 2001.

90. Gorter JW: Major bleeding during anticoagulation after cerebral ischemia: Patterns and risk factors. Stroke Prevention in Reversible Ischemia Trial (SPIRIT). European Atrial Fibrillation Trial (EAFT) study groups. Neurology 54:1319, 1999.

91. Schror K: The basic pharmacology of ticlopidine and clopidogrel. Platelets 4:252, 1991.

92. Sharis PJ, Cannon CP, Loscalzo J: The antiplatelet effects of ticlopidine and clopidogrel. Ann Intern Med 129:394, 1998.

93. Isaka K, Kiurma K, Etani H, et al: Effect of aspirin and ticlopidine on platelet deposition in carotid atherosclerosis. Stroke 17: 1215-20, 1986.

94. Yang LJ, Hoppensteadt D, Fareed J: Modulation of vasoconstriction by clopidogrel and ticlopidine. Thromb Res 92:83, 1998.

95. Hass WK, Easton JD, Adams HP, et al: A randomized trial comparing ticlopidine hydrochloride with aspirin for the prevention of stroke in high-risk patients. Ticlopidine Aspirin Stroke Study Group. N Engl J Med 321:501, 1989.

96. Gent M, Easton JD, Hachinski VC, et al: The Canadian-American Ticlopidine Study (CATS) in thromboembolic stroke. Lancet 8649:1215, 1989.

97. Bellavance A: Efficacy of ticlopidine and aspirin for prevention of reversible cerebrovascular ischemic events: The Ticlopidine Aspirin Stroke Study. Stroke 24:1452, 1993.

98. Weisberg LA: The efficacy and safety of ticlopidine and aspirin in non-whites: Analysis of a patient subgroup from the Ticlopidine Aspirin Stroke Study. Neurology 43:27, 1993.

99. Janzon I, Bergquist D, Boberg J, et al: Prevention of myocardial infarction and stroke in patients with intermittent claudication: Effects of ticlopidine. Results from the STIMS, the Swedish Ticlopidine Multicentre Study. J Intern Med 227:301, 1990.

100. Balsano F, Rizzon P, Violi F, et al: Antiplatelet treatment with ticlopidine in unstable angina, a controlled multicenter trial. The Studio della Ticlopidina nell'Angina Instabile Group. Circulation 82:17, 1990.

101. Bennett CL, Davidson CJ, Raisch DV, et al: Thrombotic thrombocytopenic purpura associated with ticlopidine in the setting of coronary artery stents and stroke. Arch Intern Med 159:2524, 1999.

102. A randomized, blinded trial of clopidogrel versus aspirin in patients at risk of ischaemic events (CAPRIE). CAPRIE Steering Committee. Lancet 348:1329, 1996.

103. Hankey GJ, Sudlow CLM, Dunbabin DW: Thienopyridines or aspirin to prevent stroke and other serious vascular events in patients at high risk of vascular disease: A systematic review of the evidence from randomized trials. Stroke 31:1779, 2000.

104. Bennett CL, Connors JM, Carwile JM, et al: Thrombotic thrombocytopenic purpura associated with clopidogrel. N Engl J Med 342:1773, 2000.

105. Nara W, Ashley I, Rosner F: Thrombotic thrombocytopenic purpura associated with clopidogrel administration: Case report and brief review. 322:170, 2001.

106. Coller BS, Anderson K, Weisman HF: New antiplatelet agents: Platelet GPIIb/IIIa antagonists. Thromb Haemost 74:302, 1995.

107. Use of a monoclonal antibody directed against the platelet glycoprotein IIb/IIIa receptor in high-risk coronary angioplasty. The EPICS Investigation. N Engl J Med 330:956, 1994.

108. Topol EJ, Califf RM, WEisman HF, et al: Randomized trial of coronary intervention with antibody against platelet IIB/IIIa integrin for reduction of clinical restenosis: Results at six months. Lancet 343:881, 1994.

109. Reverter JC, Beguin S, Kessels H, et al: Inhibition of platelet-mediated, tissue factor-induced thrombin generation by the mouse/human chimeric 7E3 antibody: Potential implications for the effect of c7E3 Fab treatment on acute thrombosis and clinical restenosis. J Clin Invest 98:863, 1996.

110. Coller BS: Anti-GP IIb/IIIa drugs: Current strategies and future directions. Thromb Haemost 86:427, 2001.

111. Abumiya T, Fitridge R, Mazur C, et al: Integrin alpha IIb beta 3 inhibitor preserves microvascular patency in experimental acute focal cerebral ischemia. Stroke 31:1402, 2000.

112. Abciximab in acute ischemic stroke: A randomized, double-blind, placebo-controlled, dose-escalation study. The Abciximab in Ischemic Stroke Investigators. Stroke 31:601, 2000.

113. Cheung RTF, Ho DS: Fatal hemorrhagic transformation of acute cerebral infarction after the use of abciximab [letter]. Stroke 31: 2518, 2000.

114. Coutre S, Leung L: Novel antithrombotic therapeutics targeted against platelet glycoprotein IIb/IIIa. Ann Rev Med 46:257, 1995.

115. Topol EJ, Easton JD, Amarenco P, et al: Design of the blockade of the glycoprotein IIb/IIIa receptor to avoid vascular occlusion (BRAVO) trial. Am Heart J 139:927, 2000.

116. Cadroy Y, Bossavy JP, Thalamas C, et al: Early potent antithrombotic effect with combined aspirin and a loading dose of clopidogrel on experimental arterial thrombogenesis in humans. Circulation 101:2823, 2001.

117. Bertrand ME, Rupprecht H-J, Urban P, et al: Double-blind study of the safety of clopidogrel with and without a loading dose in combination with aspirin compared with ticlopidine in combination with aspirin after coronary stenting. The Clopidogrel Aspirin Stent International Study (CLASSICS). Circulation 102:624, 2000.

118. Yusuf S, Zhao F, Mehta SR, et al: Effects of clopidogrel in addition to aspirin in patients with acute coronary syndromes without ST-segment elevation. N Engl J Med 345:494, 2001.

119. Mehta SR, Yusuf S, Peters R, et al: Effects of pretreatment with clopidogrel and aspirin followed by long-term therapy in patients undergoing percutaneous coronary intervention: The PCI-CURE study. Lancet 358:527, 2001.

120. Bhatt DL, Kapadia SR, Bajzer CT, et al: Dual antiplatelet therapy with clopidogrel and aspirin after carotid artery stenting. J Invasive Cardiol 13:767, 2001.

121. Albers GW, Amarenco P: Combination therapy with clopidogrel and aspirin: Can the CURE results be extrapolated to cerebrovascular patients. Stroke 32:2948, 2001.

122. FitzGerald GA: Dipyridamole. N Engl J Med 316:1247, 1987.

123. The European Stroke Prevention study (ESPS). Principal endpoints. The ESPS Group. Lancet 8572:1351, 1987.

124. Diener HC, Cunha L, Forbes C, et al: European Stroke Prevention Study 2: Dipyridamole and acetylsalicylic acid in the secondary prevention of stroke. J Neurol Sci 143:1, 1996.

125. Diener HC, Lowenthal A: Reply to Dr. G. Hart and Dr. Benavente. J Neurol Sci 153:112, 1997.

126. DeSchryver EL: Design of ESPRIT, an international randomized trial for secondary prevention after non-disabling cerebral ischaemia of arterial origin. European/Australian Stroke Prevention in Reversible Ischaemia Trial (ESPRIT) group. Cerebrovasc Dis 10:147, 2000.

127. Muller TH: Inhibition of thrombus formation by low-dose acetylsalicylic acid, dipyridamole and their combination in a model of platelet-vessel wall interaction. Neurology 57:S8, 2001.

128. Preliminary report of the Stroke Prevention in Atrial Fibrillation study. N Engl J Med 322:863, 1990.

129. A double blind trial to assess long-term oral anticoagulant treatment in elderly patients after myocardial infarction. Report of the Sixty Plus Reinfarction Study Research Group. Lancet 8202:989, 1980.

130. Adjusted-dose warfarin versus low- intensity fixed-dose warfarin plus aspirin for high-risk patients with atrial fibrillation: Stroke Prevention in Atrial Fibrillation III randomised clinical trial. Lancet 348:633, 1996.

131. Hart RG, Pearce LA, McBride R, et al: Factors associated with ischemic stroke during aspirin therapy in atrial fibrillation. The Stroke Prevention in Atrial Fibrillation (SPAF) Investigators. Stroke 30:1223, 1999.

132. Cappelleri JC, Fiore LD, Brophy MT, et al: Efficacy and safety of combined anticoagulant and antiplatelet therapy versus anticoagulant monotherapy after mechanical heart-valve replacement: A meta-analysis. Am Heart J 130:547, 1995.

133. Turpie AG, Gent M, Laupacis A, et al: A comparison of aspirin with placebo in patients treated with warfarin after heart-valve replacement. N Engl J Med 329:524, 1993.

134. Fiore LD, Ezekowitz M, Brophy MT, et al: Department of Veterans Affairs Cooperative Studies Program clinical trial comparing combined warfarin and aspirin with aspirin alone in survivors of acute myocardial infarction: primary results of the CHAMP study. Circulation 105:557, 2002.

135. Goodnight S: Antiplatelet therapy with aspirin: from clinical trials to practice. Thromb Haemost 74:401, 1995.

136. Lefkowitz J, Topol EJ: Direct thrombin inhibitors in cardiovascular medicine. Circulation 90:1522, 1994.

137. Heit JA, Colwell CW, Francis CW, et al: Comparison of the oral direct thrombin inhibitor ximelegatran with enoxaparin as prophylaxis against venous thromboembolism after total knee replacement. Arch Int Med 161:2215, 2001.

138. DeCaterina R, Giannessi D, Mazzone A, et al: Vascular prostacyclin is increased in patients taking fish oil n-3 polyunsaturated fatty acids prior to coronary bypass surgery. Circulation 82:428, 1990.

139. Morris M, Manson J, Rosner B, et al: Fish consumption and cardiovascular disease in the Physicians Health Study: A prospective study. Am J Epidemiol 142:166, 1995.

140. Orencia AJ, Daviglus M, Dyer AR, et al: Fish consumption and stroke in men: 30-year findings of the Chicago Western Electric Study. Stroke 27:204, 1996.

141. Billman GF, Hallaq A, Leaf A: Prevention of ischemia-induced ventricular fibrillation by ω-3 fatty acids. Proc Natl Acad Sci U S A 91:4427, 1994.

142. Kang JX, Leaf A: Prevention of fatal cardiac arrhymias by polyunsaturated fatty acids. Am J Clin Nutr 71:202S, 2000.

143. Boulos C, Jiang H, Balazy M: Diffusion of peroxynitrite into the human platelet inhibits cyclooxygenase via nitration of tyrosine residues. J Pharmacol Exp Ther 293:222, 2000.

144. Freedman JE, Loscalzo J, Barnard MR, et al: Nitric oxide release from activated platelets inhibits platelet recruitment. J Clin Invest 100:350, 1997.

145. Stagliano NE, Zhao W, Prado R, et al: The effect of nitric oxide synthase inhibition on acute platelet accumulation and hemodynamic depression in a rat model of thromboembolic stroke. J Cereb Blood Flow Metab 17:1182, 1997.

146. Freedman JE, Sauter R, Battinelli EM, et al: Deficient platelet-derived nitric oxide and enhanced hemostasis in mice lacking the NOSIII gene. Circ Res 84:1416, 1999.

147. Freedman JE, Ting B, Hankin B, et al: Impaired platelet production of nitric oxide predicts presence of acute coronary syndromes. Circulation 98:1481, 1998.

148. Molloy J, Martin J, Baskerville P, et al: S-nitrosoglutathione reduces the rate of embolisation in humans. Circulation 98:830, 1998.

149. Laufs U, Gertz K, Huang P, et al: Atorvastatin upregulates type III nitric oxide synthase in thrombocytes, decreases platelet activation and protects from cerebral ischemia in normocholesterolemic mice. Stroke 31:2442, 2000.

150. Wang Y, Zhang RL, Zhang ZG, et al: Sildenafil citrate increases proliferation of progenitor cells in the subventricular zone and improves functional recovery after focal cerebral ischemia in the rat. Stroke 33:397, 2002.

151. Inbal A, Gurevitz O, Tamarin I, et al: Unique antiplatelet effects of a novel S-nitrosoderivative of a recombinant fragment of von Willebrand factor, AR545C: In vitro and ex vivo inhibition of platelet function. Blood 94:1693, 1999.

152. Gurevitz O, Eldar M, Skutelsky E, et al: S-nitrosoderivative of a recombinant fragment of von Willebrand factor (S-nitroso-AR545C) inhibits thrombus formatin in guinea pig carotid artery thrombosis model. Thromb Haemost 84:912, 2000.

153. Marcus AJ, Broekman M, Drosopoulos J, et al: The endothelial cell ecto-ADPase responsible for inhibition of platelet function is CD39. J Clin Invest 99:1351, 1997.

154. Pinsky DJ, Broekman MJ, Peschon JJ, et al: Elucidation of the thromboregulatory role of CE39/ectoapyrase in the ischemic brain. J Clin Invest 109:1031, 2002.

155. Moake JL, Turner NA, Stathopoulos NA, et al: Shear-induced platelet aggregation can be mediated by vWF released from platelets, as well as by endogenous large or unusually large vWF multimers, requires adenosine diphosphate and is resistant to aspirin. Blood 71:1366, 1988.

156. Foster CJ, Prosser DM, Agans JM, et al: Molecular identification and characterization of the platelet ADP receptor targeted by thienopyridine antithrombotic drugs. J Clin Invest 107:1591, 2001.

157. Jin J, Kunapuli SP: Coactivation of two different G protein-coupled receptors is essential for ADP-induced platelet aggregation. Proc Natl Acad Sci U S A 95:8070, 1998.

158. Turner NA, Moake JL, McIntire LV: Blockade of adenosine diphosphate receptors P2Y(12) and P2Y(1) is required to inhibit platelet aggregation in whole blood under flow. Blood 98:3340, 2001.

159. Huang J, Driscoll EM, Gonzales MI, et al: Prevention of arterial thrombosis by intravenously administered platelet P2T receptor antagonist AR-C69931MX in a canine model. J Pharmacol Exp Ther 295:492, 2000.

160. Storey F: The P2Y12 receptor as a therapeutic target in cardiovascular disease. Platelets 12:197, 2001.

Chapter Fifty-Eight

Long-Term Medical Management of Ischemic Stroke and Transient Ischemic Attack Due to Arterial Disease

Cathie Sudlow and Charles P. Warlow

In this chapter, we deal with the long-term management of patients with ischemic strokes and transient ischemic attacks (TIAs) due either to disease of the large and medium-sized extracranial and intracranial arteries supplying the brain, or to "small (intracranial) vessel disease." We focus on the secondary prevention of serious vascular events among such patients, drawing whenever possible on the guidance available from the results of relevant randomized trials and their systematic reviews.

Most large and medium-sized arterial disease is due to *atherothromboembolism*, a term encompassing the pathologic processes of atherosclerosis, thrombus formation in association with atheromatous plaques, and artery-to-artery thromboembolism. These processes probably account for about half of all ischemic strokes and TIAs, at least in white people.[1,2] In situ occlusion by atherosclerosis with complicating thrombus may occur, especially in the posterior circulation.[3,4] More commonly in the anterior circulation, artery-to-artery emboli from thrombus overlying atheroma in the extracranial arteries (particularly at the origin of the internal carotid artery) occlude large intracranial arteries more distally.[5–7]

About a quarter of ischemic cerebrovascular events are said to be "lacunar" and are caused by occlusion of one of the small, deep, perforating arteries—"small vessel disease."[1,2] When symptomatic, infarcts arising from such occlusions are generally associated with one of the lacunar syndromes (see Chapter 11).[8] The vascular pathology underlying small vessel occlusion is not well understood, mainly because of the paucity of informative autopsy studies (patients with lacunar infarction have a very low early case-fatality rate) and the difficulty in imaging the very small arteries involved. Much of what we do know comes from Miller Fisher's meticulous clinicopathologic studies of 68 lacunar infarcts in 18 postmortem brains.[9] These studies suggested that atheromatous plaques, with or without complicating thrombus, accounted for most *symptomatic* lacunar infarcts, arising from the occlusion of arteries about 200 to 800 μm in diameter. The vascular pathology underlying most *asymptomatic* lacunar infarcts, arising from the occlusion of arteries about 40 to 200 μm in diameter, appeared be "lipohyalinosis," a destructive small vessel lesion characterized in the acute phase by fibrinoid necrosis and in the healed phase by loss of normal wall architecture, collagenous sclerosis, and mural foam cells.[9,10] Thus, at least on the basis of the evidence available, it seems that most symptomatic cerebrovascular events due to arterial disease occur as a result of some combination of atheroma, thrombosis, and artery-to-artery embolism.

The management of ischemic strokes that are thought to be due to emboli from the heart or to arise from one of the much rarer nonatherothromboembolic causes of arterial occlusion is dealt with elsewhere (see Chapters 54 and 60).

AIMS OF LONG-TERM MANAGEMENT

Patients who have had an ischemic stroke or TIA are at high risk of a subsequent stroke. Community and hospital-based series, in which patients were generally assessed some days after the ischemic cerebrovascular event, found this risk to be about 10% in the first year and about 5% annually thereafter.[11] But for series in which some patients had experienced one or more TIAs a few days prior to an ischemic stroke, the very early prognosis may have been missed. Studies focusing on this early period have suggested a particularly high early stroke risk. 5% of patients with TIA presenting to an emergency department in the United States had a stroke within 2 days, and 10% within 90 days[12]; and, in a re-analysis of data from a community-based study of stroke incidence in the United Kingdom, the risk of stroke in the first 30 days after an ischemic stroke or TIA may have been as high as 12%.[13] In addition, a community-based study of first-ever ischemic stroke in the United States found that the risk of early recurrence was especially high among patients with severe extracranial arterial disease.[14] Because atherosclerosis is a systemic vascular disease, patients who have experienced an ischemic cerebrovascular event are also at risk of serious vascular events other than stroke. In particular, their annual risk of myocardial infarction (MI) is about 3%, and about half of such patients eventually die from ischemic heart disease.[11]

The aims of long-term management should therefore be to start proven secondary preventive treatments as early as possible, in an attempt to avoid the high early stroke recurrence risk as well as the longer-term risk of serious vascular events affecting cerebral and noncerebral parts of the arterial tree.

ORGANIZATION AND SERVICE PROVISION

These long-term management aims require a service that can respond quickly and so needs to include the following:

- Prompt clinical assessment of all patients with a suspected stroke or TIA by an experienced stroke specialist physician (a large proportion of suspected acute cerebrovascular events turn out to be something else[15])
- Rapid access to appropriate diagnostic investigations (including blood tests, cardiac investigations, brain imaging, and imaging of the extracranial arteries in the neck) and to reliable reporting of their results
- A streamlined system for referring appropriately selected patients for further specialist input when required (e.g., to a cardiologist for cardiac disorders or to a vascular surgeon if carotid endarterectomy is being considered)
- An effective and quick way of communicating investigation results and management advice to other specialists and family doctors when required
- An appropriate means of providing information to patients and their relatives or caregivers.

Depending on the local health care setting and the particular patient, these requirements may best be met by a "one-stop" specialist outpatient clinic or via the hospital emergency department. Either way, the very high early recurrence rate means that patients with nondisabling ischemic strokes or TIAs who do not require hospital admission should nonetheless be treated as having medical emergencies and should be assessed on the day—or at the very least within a few days—of the onset of the attack. Achieving this goal requires both very good health service organization and public education programs. For patients with disabling ischemic strokes who must be admitted to the hospital, appropriate acute management requires that admission and assessment be performed as soon as possible after onset (see Chapter 47), but longer-term secondary prevention strategies must not be forgotten and should also be considered at an early stage.

Of course, long-term secondary prevention needs not only to begin early but also to be maintained. How such maintenance is achieved depends very much on the local system of health care provision. Nevertheless, the essential components are ongoing clinical review and the education and support of the patients and their families and care givers.

ANTITHROMBOTIC TREATMENT

Atherothrombosis and thromboembolism cause most arterial occlusive disease, including the majority of ischemic cerebrovascular events and MIs. Therefore, drugs that inhibit thrombus formation by interfering with platelet function (antiplatelet drugs) or with the coagulation cascade (anticoagulants) may well have a role in the secondary prevention of serious vascular events after an ischemic stroke or TIA. Because antithrombotic drugs also increase the risk of both intracranial and extracranial hemorrhage, however, the balance of benefits and risks must be carefully considered.

Antiplatelet Treatment in General

The role of antiplatelet treatment among patients at high risk of serious vascular events, including those with a previous ischemic stroke or TIA, has been addressed in a large number of randomized trials conducted over the last several decades. Data from trials available by the end of 1997 were summarized in a large systematic review published in 2002 by the Antithrombotic Trialists'(ATT) Collaboration.[16]

Benefits

The ATT overview identified 195 randomized trials comparing an antiplatelet regimen (mostly aspirin alone) versus no antiplatelet treatment in about 135,000 individuals at high risk of vascular disease. In the 21 trials among about 20,000 patients with a prior ischemic stroke or TIA, antiplatelet treatment produced a relative reduction in the odds of the primary outcome of a serious vascular event (stroke, MI, or vascular death) of 22% (95% confidence interval [CI], 15% to 27%) (Fig. 58–1). For every 1000 such patients treated for about 3 years, this relative odds reduction corresponded to the prevention (or delay) of 36 serious vascular events (25 nonfatal strokes, 6 nonfatal MIs, and 7 vascular deaths), or about one such event per month. There was also a statistically significant reduction in all-cause mortality (Fig. 58–2). The relative reductions in serious vascular events were similar in a wide range of patients with conditions conferring a high risk of subsequent serious vascular events (although the relative reduction was somewhat smaller in the first few weeks after an acute ischemic stroke) (see Fig. 58–1).[16] Previous analyses found that the relative benefits of antiplatelet treatment among such high-risk patients were also similar irrespective of age, gender, blood pressure, and presence or absence of diabetes.[17]

Risks

The most serious risk of antiplatelet treatment is that of hemorrhage. Intracranial hemorrhages are frequently fatal

Stroke, MI, or Vascular Death

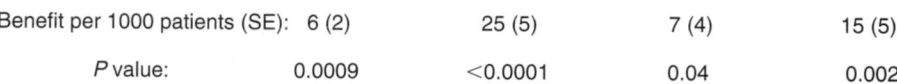

Category	Trials	Antiplatelet (%)	Control (%)	Odds Ratio (and CI)	% Odds Reduction (SE)
Prior MI	12	1345/9984 (13.5)	1708/10022 (17.0)		25% (4)
Acute MI	15	1007/9658 (10.4)	1370/9644 (14.2)		30% (4)
Prior stroke/TIA	21	2045/11493 (17.8)	2464/11527 (21.4)		22% (4)
Other high risk	140	1683/20359 (8.0)	2102/20543 (10.2)		26% (3)
All high risk excluding acute stroke	188	6035/51494 (11.7)	7644/51736 (14.8)		**25% (2)**
Acute stroke	7	1670/20418 (8.2)	1858/20403 (9.1)		11% (3)

Heterogeneity of odds reductions between four high risk categories excluding acute stroke:
$\chi^2_{3df} = 3.4$; $P = $ NS

0   0.5   1   1.5   2

Antiplatelet better   Antiplatelet worse

FIGURE 58–1 *Relative effects of antiplatelet treatment versus control on vascular events (stroke, myocardial infarction [MI] or vascular death). The typical odds ratio for each category is shown as red square (size of square proportional to statistical weight of category) together with its 99% confidence interval (CI) (horizontal line). The typical odds ratio for the subtotal is shown as a diamond, with 95% CI equal to the width of the diamond. NS, not significant; SE, standard error; TIA, transient ischemic attack. (Adapted from Collaborative meta-analysis of randomised trials of antiplatelet therapy for the prevention of death, MI, and stroke in high risk patients. Antithrombotic Trialists' Collaboration. BMJ 324:71–86, 2002.)*

Previous Stroke or Transient Ischemic Attack (Mean Treatment Duration 3 Years)

Benefit per 1000 patients (SE):	6 (2)	25 (5)	7 (4)	15 (5)
P value:	0.0009	<0.0001	0.04	0.002

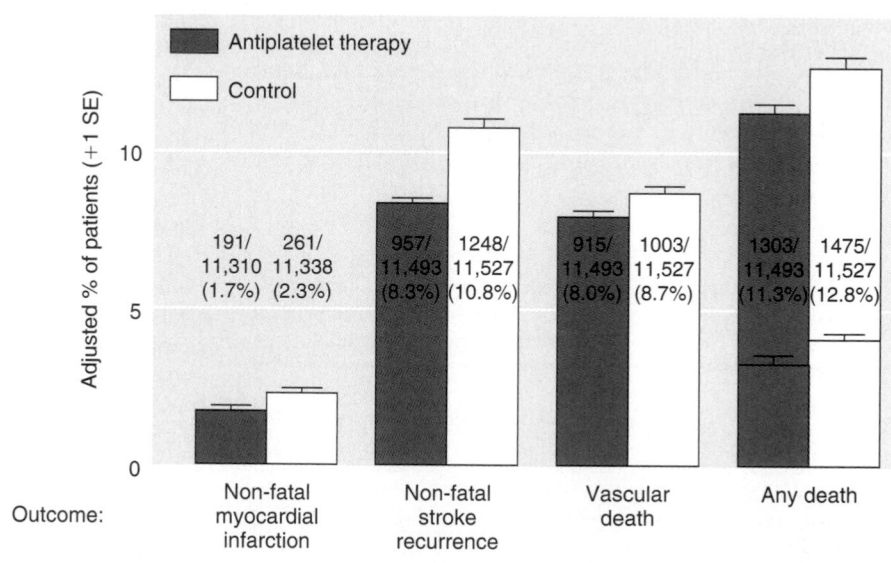

FIGURE 58–2 *Absolute effects of antiplatelet treatment on various outcomes in patients with previous ischemic stroke or transient ischemic attack. In the* Any death *column, nonvascular deaths are represented by lower horizontal lines (and the number may be calculated by subtracting the number of vascular deaths from the number of any deaths). SE, standard error. (From Collaborative meta-analysis of randomised trials of antiplatelet therapy for the prevention of death, MI, and stroke in high risk patients. Antithrombotic Trialists' Collaboration. BMJ 324:71–86, 2002.)*

or permanently disabling,[18] whereas most extracranial hemorrhages are gastrointestinal and far less likely to cause death or permanent disability.[19] In the trials recruiting patients with a prior ischemic stroke or TIA included in the ATT overview, about half of all intracranial hemorrhages and about 20% of major extracranial hemorrhages (generally defined as those that were fatal or required hospital admission or blood transfusion) recorded were fatal.[16] The overview found that antiplatelet treatment increased the relative odds of intracranial hemorrhage by about one

fifth and of major extracranial hemorrhage by about 60%, corresponding to an absolute excess of about one intracranial hemorrhage and about five major extracranial hemorrhages per 1000 patients who had a prior ischemic stroke or TIA and had been treated for about 3 years.[16]

Balance of Benefits and Risks

When considering the balance of benefits versus risks using the ATT data, one must note that all intracranial hemorrhages, as well as all fatal extracranial hemorrhages (defined as vascular deaths), were included in the serious vascular events (the primary outcome). Thus, to evaluate net benefit, only the excess nonfatal major extracranial hemorrhages must be weighed against the reduction in serious vascular events. It is clear that the benefits of antiplatelet treatment among patients with a previous ischemic stroke or TIA greatly outweigh the risks (Table 58.1). The generalizability of the results of randomized trials is sometimes questioned on the grounds that the patients included were likely to have a lower risk of treatment-related adverse effects than those commonly encountered in day-to-day clinical practice. However, even if the risks in a nontrial population of patients were twice as high as those seen in the randomized trials, there would still be a substantial net benefit (see Table 58.1).[16]

Aspirin

Overall Balance of Benefits and Risks

Aspirin therapy alone is by far the most widely tested antiplatelet regimen. Indeed, in the ATT overview, more than two thirds of all the high-risk patients—and almost half of all patients with a prior ischemic stroke or TIA—who were assigned to receive an antiplatelet regimen in trials of antiplatelet treatment versus control received aspirin alone. The relative effects of aspirin as well as the absolute balance of benefits and risks in the various categories of high-risk patients, including those with a prior ischemic stroke or TIA, were very similar to those found for antiplatelet treatment in general (see Table 58.1).[16]

Different Daily Doses of Aspirin
Benefits

Until recently, and perhaps even still today, there has been a wide variation in the dosage of aspirin used for long-term secondary prevention after an ischemic stroke or TIA, with daily doses ranging from 30 to 1500 mg.[20-22] The earliest

Table 58.1 Antiplatelet Treatment versus Control: Balance of Absolute Benefits and Risks in Patients with a Prior Ischemic Stroke or Transient Ischemic Attack*

	Vascular Events[†]	Intracranial Hemorrhage[‡]	Major Extracranial Hemorrhage[§]
Any antiplatelet regimen versus control	↓ 36 (5)	↑ 1 (1)	↑ 5 (2)
Aspirin alone versus control	↓ 28 (8)	↑ 3 (2)	↑ 5 (2)

*Number of patients out of 1000 treated with an antiplatelet regimen for 3 years who would avoid (↓) or suffer (↑) an event. Standard error (SE) given in parentheses.
[†]Stroke, myocardial infarction, or vascular death.
[‡]Fatal and nonfatal events accounted for within vascular events.
[§]Fatal events (~20% of total) accounted for within vascular events.
Data from collaborative meta-analysis of randomized trials of antiplatelet therapy for the prevention of death, myocardial infarction, and stroke in high risk patients. Antiplatelet Trialists' Collaboration. BMJ 324: 71–86, 2002.

trials used doses of more than 1000 mg daily.[16,23-25] Laboratory studies have shown, however, that because of the irreversible nature of aspirin's inhibition of platelet cyclooxygenase, daily doses as low as 30 to 50 mg daily have a cumulative inhibitory effect, resulting in virtually complete suppression of thromboxane A_2 biosynthesis after 7 to 10 days. Such doses could have a greater antithrombotic effect than higher doses, because lower doses may spare the production of prostacyclin (which inhibits platelet aggregation and induces vasodilation) from endothelial cells yet suppress thromboxane A_2 production by platelets; this hypothesis has never actually been shown to be of clinical relevance in vivo.[26,27] These theoretical arguments, along with the suggestion that the adverse effects of aspirin may be dose-related, led to the use of lower daily doses in later trials, although the effects of doses less than 75 mg daily have not been extensively studied.[16,28-30]

In assessing the evidence from randomized trials for the relative effects of different doses of aspirin, one must consider two types of comparison, direct and indirect. *Direct* head-to-head comparisons of different daily doses are the most reliable, but the numbers of patients (and, importantly, outcome events) involved in such comparisons has been limited. The ATT overview identified ten trials that directly compared different daily doses of aspirin in almost 7000 patients at high risk of serious vascular events (about two thirds of whom had a prior ischemic stroke or TIA). There were no statistically significant differences among the various doses in their effects on serious vascular events, but too few events were recorded to rule out small but clinically important differences.[16] The Aspirin in Carotid Endarterectomy (ACE) trial, the results of which were not available in time to be included in the ATT overview, directly compared lower with higher doses of aspirin (81 mg or 325 mg daily versus 625 mg or 1300 mg daily) among about 3000 patients undergoing carotid endarterectomy. The combined risk of stroke, MI, or death within 3 months of carotid endarterectomy was (just) significantly lower in the lower dose group (6.2% versus 8.4%, $2P = .03$).[31]

There were more data in the ATT overview for making *indirect* comparisons between different aspirin doses in trials of aspirin versus control (no aspirin), although such comparisons are intrinsically less reliable. (One can appreciate this concept by reflecting that it is less reliable to compare the French and English football teams from their respective performances against the German team than in a match in which they play each other). Among a total of almost 60,000 high-risk patients, the relative reduction in vascular events was 19% with 500 to 1500 mg daily, 26% with 160 to 325 mg daily, and 32% with 75 to 150 mg daily. However, daily doses of less than 75 mg seemed to produce a somewhat smaller relative reduction, 13% (Fig. 58–3).[16]

Risks

Neither the ATT overview nor other systematic reviews revealed any significant differences in the risks of intracranial or major extracranial hemorrhage with different daily aspirin doses.[16,32] Indirect comparisons in a systematic review of randomized trials of aspirin versus control found no clear variation in risk of gastrointestinal hemorrhage between different daily doses.[33] Direct randomized comparisons did, however, show a trend toward an excess of

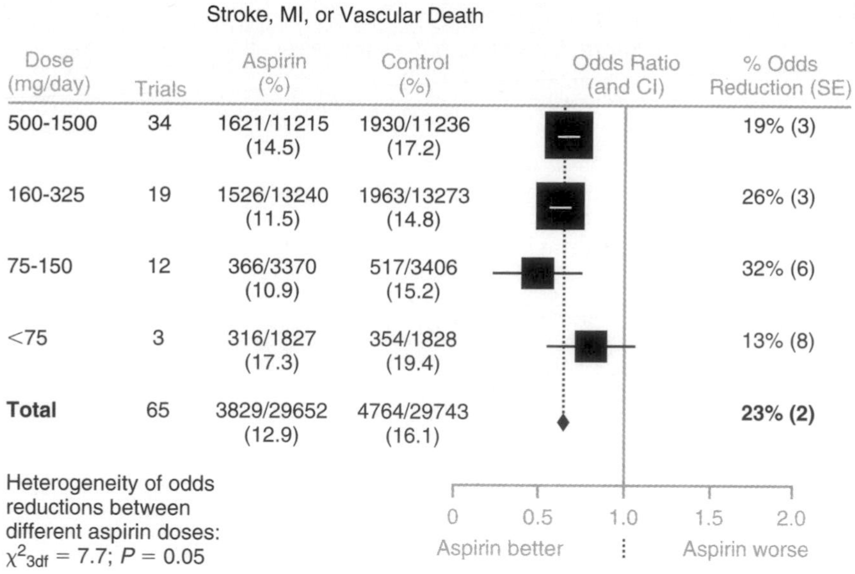

FIGURE 58–3 *Relative effects of different daily doses of aspirin on vascular events (stroke, myocardial infarction [MI], or vascular death) in high-risk patients (excluding those with acute stroke). The typical odds ratio for each category is shown as a red square (size of square proportional to statistical weight of category) together with its 99% confidence interval (CI) (horizontal line). The typical odds ratio for the total is shown as a diamond, with 95% CI equal to the width of the diamond. SE, standard error. (Adapted from Collaborative meta-analysis of randomised trials of antiplatelet therapy for the prevention of death, MI, and stroke in high risk patients. Antithrombotic Trialists' Collaboration. BMJ 324:71–86, 2002.)*

Stroke, MI, or Vascular Death

Dose (mg/day)	Trials	Aspirin (%)	Control (%)	Odds Ratio (and CI)	% Odds Reduction (SE)
500–1500	34	1621/11215 (14.5)	1930/11236 (17.2)		19% (3)
160–325	19	1526/13240 (11.5)	1963/13273 (14.8)		26% (3)
75–150	12	366/3370 (10.9)	517/3406 (15.2)		32% (6)
<75	3	316/1827 (17.3)	354/1828 (19.4)		13% (8)
Total	65	3829/29652 (12.9)	4764/29743 (16.1)		**23% (2)**

Heterogeneity of odds reductions between different aspirin doses: $\chi^2_{3df} = 7.7$; $P = 0.05$

0   0.5   1.0   1.5   2.0
Aspirin better : Aspirin worse

gastrointestinal hemorrhage and a definite excess of upper gastrointestinal symptoms for daily doses of 500 to 1500 mg compared with 75 to 325 mg (odds ratio [OR] 1.3; 95% CI 1.1 to 1.5).[31,34,35] In support of this finding, an overview of five observational studies assessing the gastrointestinal risks of different daily doses of aspirin suggested greater risks for daily doses higher than 300 mg daily.[36] There were no definite differences, however, between the medium and very low doses in one trial comparing daily doses of 283 mg and 30 mg.[30]

Finally, there is no clear evidence of a protective advantage of enteric-coated preparations or other formulations from randomized trials or observational studies.[33,36]

Balance of Benefits and Risks

The available evidence from randomized trials therefore suggests that daily doses of 75 to 150 mg are as effective as higher doses, but there is insufficient evidence to be certain that daily doses lower than 75 mg are as effective. Because data from both randomized trials and observational studies suggest that the adverse effects of aspirin are less frequent at lower doses, at least down as far as 75 to 300 mg daily, there is no clear evidence to support the use of higher doses in long-term secondary prevention. Also, although more expensive enteric-coated aspirin preparations are widely used, there is no clear evidence that they reduce symptomatic adverse effects.

Alternative Antiplatelet Regimens

Aspirin is cheap, widely available, relatively safe, and easy to use. But a range of other antiplatelet drugs acting through different pathways to inhibit platelet aggregation (see Chapter 57) may conceivably be more beneficial than aspirin, if used either instead of or in combination with aspirin. The combination approach, involving the inhibition of more than one platelet metabolic pathway, seems more likely to produce clinically meaningful differences as long as any excess risk of hemorrhage does not negate

any added benefit. Realistically, however, any differences in effects on clinically important outcomes between antiplatelet regimens are likely to be small (perhaps no more than about a 10% relative difference in serious vascular events), and their reliable detection would require randomization of very large numbers (tens of thousands) of patients.[37]

Indirect comparisons of different antiplatelet regimens in the ATT overview found no significant differences among a variety of different regimens, and most direct comparisons between aspirin alone and some alternative antiplatelet regimen involved far too few patients to be informative about clinically important outcomes.[16] However, several thousand or more high-risk patients were included in randomized comparisons between the thienopyridine antiplatelet drugs (ticlopidine and clopidogrel) and aspirin, and between the combination of aspirin plus dipyridamole and aspirin alone.[16] The evidence for the use of these potential alternatives to aspirin is therefore worth more detailed consideration.

The Thienopyridines (Ticlopidine and Clopidogrel)

More than 22,000 high-risk patients have been involved in randomized trials comparing one of the thienopyridine antiplatelet drugs with aspirin. Most of these patients were subjects of the Clopidogrel versus Aspirin to Prevent Ischemic Events (CAPRIE) trial, in which about 19,000 patients with a prior MI, ischemic stroke, or peripheral arterial disease were randomly allocated to received either 75 mg of clopidogrel or 300 mg of aspirin daily.[38] A systematic review of these trials found that the effects of ticlopidine and clopidogrel, in comparison with those of aspirin, were very similar. The thienopyridines produced a reduction in the relative odds of a serious vascular event of 9% (95% CI, 2% to 16%), corresponding to the prevention or delay of 11 (95% CI, 2 to 19) events per 1000 patients treated for 2 years (Fig. 58–4). The effect on vascular events among the subgroup of about 10,000 patients

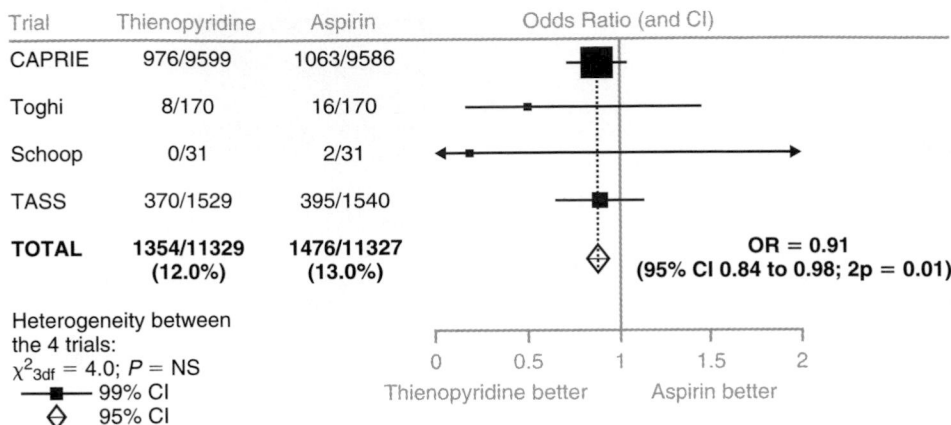

FIGURE 58–4 *Relative effects of the thienopyridines and aspirin on vascular events (stroke, myocardial infarction [MI], or vascular death) in high-risk patients. Odds ratio (OR) for each trial is shown as a red square (size of square proportional to statistical weight of trial) together with its 99% confidence interval (horizontal line). Typical odds ratio for the total shown is as a diamond, with the 95% confidence interval (CI) equal to the width of the diamond. CAPRIE, Clopidogrel versus Aspirin in Patients at high Risk of Ischemic Events; NS, not significant; TASS, Ticlopidine Aspirin Stroke Study. (Adapted from Hankey GJ, Sudlow CLM, Dunbabin DW: Thienopyridines or aspirin to prevent stroke and other serious vascular events in patients at high risk of vascular disease? A systematic review of the evidence from randomized trials. Stroke 31:1779–1784, 2000.)*

recruited on the basis of a history of ischemic stroke or TIA was similar to that seen overall (relative odds reduction 10%, with 95% CI 0 to 19%; absolute reduction 14 events per 1000 over 2 years, with 95% CI −1 to 29).[39,40] However, the wide 95% CIs for all of these results demonstrate substantial uncertainty about the size of any additional benefit of replacing aspirin with a thienopyridine in high-risk patients, especially for any particular subgroup of interest.

In terms of adverse effects, the review found no detectable difference between the thienopyridines and aspirin in either intracranial or major extracranial bleeding although it did find that the thienopyridines produced less gastrointestinal hemorrhage and other upper gastrointestinal symptoms than aspirin (Fig. 58–5). However, all of the trials reviewed used a daily aspirin dose of 325 mg or higher. Lower aspirin doses (down to 75 mg daily) might compare more favorably with a thienopyridine, because lower doses should produce similar benefits to higher doses of aspirin but less gastrointestinal toxicity (see earlier discussion on different daily doses of aspirin). Furthermore, compared with aspirin, clopidogrel produced about a one-third relative increase in—and ticlopidine more than doubled—the odds of both diarrhea and rash. Ticlopidine, but not clopidogrel, produced an excess of neutropenia compared with aspirin (see Fig. 58–5).[39,40] In addition, observational studies have demonstrated a higher risk of both thrombocytopenia and thrombotic thrombocytopenic purpura among patients receiving ticlopidine, but no definite excess of hematologic problems with clopidogrel.[41–44] Finally, randomized trials directly comparing ticlopidine with clopidogrel (both given along with aspirin) among patients undergoing coronary artery stent insertion have shown similar effectiveness but a favorable safety profile for clopidogrel.[45–47]

The results have recently become available from one further relevant, randomized trial, the African-American Antiplatelet Stroke Prevention Study (AAASPS). The

AAASPS compared ticlopidine 500 mg daily with aspirin 650 mg daily in 1800 African-American patients with a recent noncardioembolic ischemic stroke. It found no statistically significant difference between trilopidine and aspirin in the prevention of vascular events or of stroke alone, but confidence intervals for these estimates of effect were wide.[48] This trial will now need to be included in an updated meta-analysis of thienopyridines versus aspirin. However, its relatively small size makes it unlikely that this will lead to material alterations in the conclusions already made from previous reviews.[39,40]

Thus, the thienopyridines appear to be at least as effective as aspirin and *possibly* somewhat more so. Clopidogrel is preferred over ticlopidine on the grounds of safety and tolerability and seems to be as safe as aspirin. Because it is considerably more expensive than aspirin, however, clopidogrel is best used as an alternative antiplatelet treatment for patients who are genuinely unable to tolerate aspirin.

The potential of combining the antiplatelet effects of clopidogrel and aspirin seems a more promising option.[49] Two large randomized trials have assessed the effects of adding clopidogrel to aspirin for several months to a year in a total of about 15,000 high-risk patients with ischemic heart disease.[50,51] Both demonstrated clear benefits of the combination, and another large, ongoing randomized trial is currently comparing this combination with aspirin alone in patients with acute MI.[52] We do not yet know whether the benefits extend to patients with ischemic cerebrovascular disease, but a further large randomized trial addressing the effectiveness of clopidogrel plus aspirin compared with aspirin alone in 15,000 high-risk patients (including those with a prior ischemic stroke or TIA) is under way.[53] One other ongoing randomized trial, the Management of ATherothrombosis with Clopidogrel in High-risk patients with recent transient ischemic attack or ischemic stroke (MATCH) trial, is comparing clopidogrel plus aspirin with

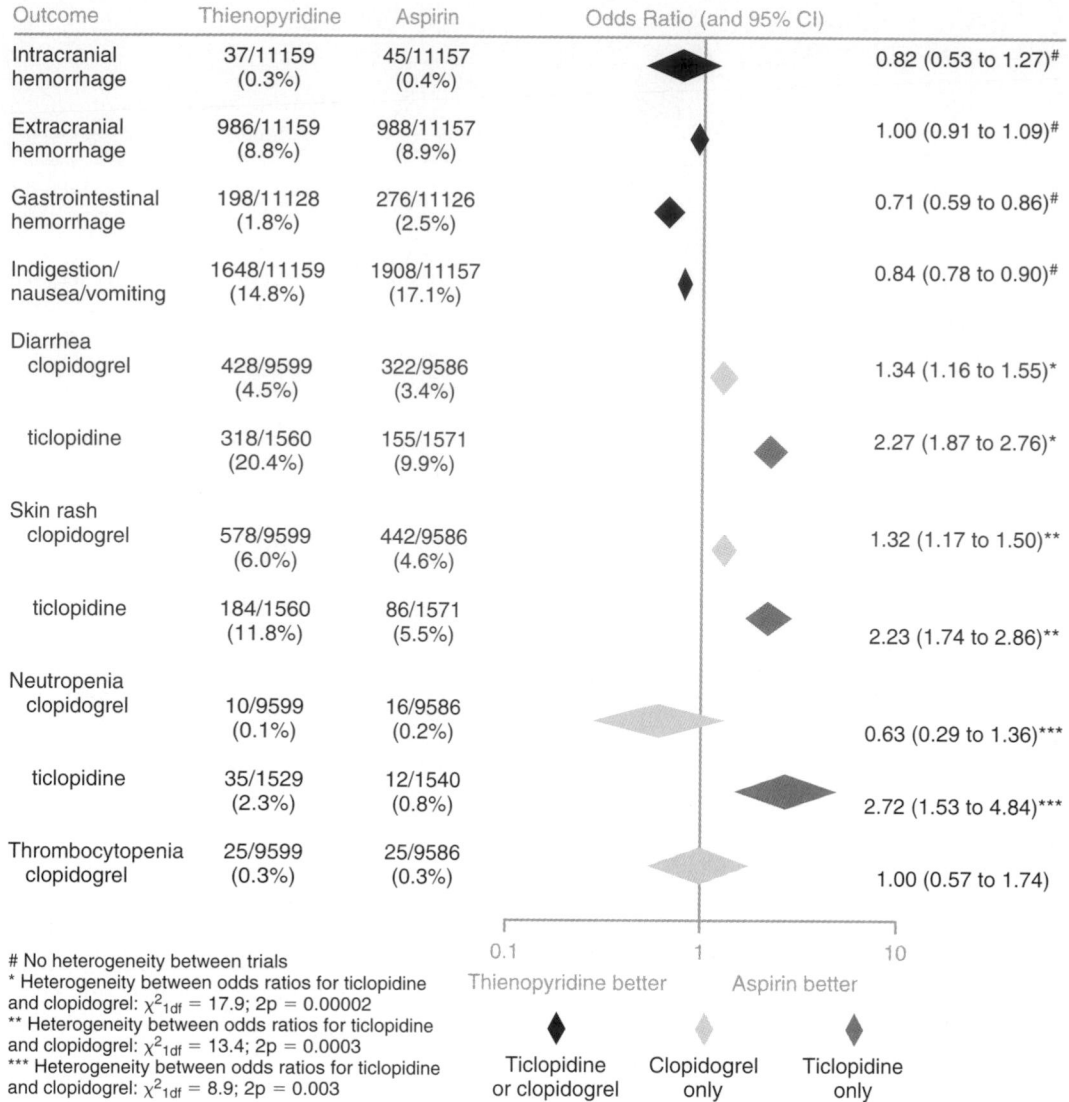

Outcome	Thienopyridine	Aspirin	Odds Ratio (and 95% CI)
Intracranial hemorrhage	37/11159 (0.3%)	45/11157 (0.4%)	0.82 (0.53 to 1.27)#
Extracranial hemorrhage	986/11159 (8.8%)	988/11157 (8.9%)	1.00 (0.91 to 1.09)#
Gastrointestinal hemorrhage	198/11128 (1.8%)	276/11126 (2.5%)	0.71 (0.59 to 0.86)#
Indigestion/ nausea/vomiting	1648/11159 (14.8%)	1908/11157 (17.1%)	0.84 (0.78 to 0.90)#
Diarrhea clopidogrel	428/9599 (4.5%)	322/9586 (3.4%)	1.34 (1.16 to 1.55)*
ticlopidine	318/1560 (20.4%)	155/1571 (9.9%)	2.27 (1.87 to 2.76)*
Skin rash clopidogrel	578/9599 (6.0%)	442/9586 (4.6%)	1.32 (1.17 to 1.50)**
ticlopidine	184/1560 (11.8%)	86/1571 (5.5%)	2.23 (1.74 to 2.86)**
Neutropenia clopidogrel	10/9599 (0.1%)	16/9586 (0.2%)	0.63 (0.29 to 1.36)***
ticlopidine	35/1529 (2.3%)	12/1540 (0.8%)	2.72 (1.53 to 4.84)***
Thrombocytopenia clopidogrel	25/9599 (0.3%)	25/9586 (0.3%)	1.00 (0.57 to 1.74)

No heterogeneity between trials
* Heterogeneity between odds ratios for ticlopidine and clopidogrel: $\chi^2_{1df} = 17.9$; $2p = 0.00002$
** Heterogeneity between odds ratios for ticlopidine and clopidogrel: $\chi^2_{1df} = 13.4$; $2p = 0.0003$
*** Heterogeneity between odds ratios for ticlopidine and clopidogrel: $\chi^2_{1df} = 8.9$; $2p = 0.003$

0.1   1   10
Thienopyridine better   Aspirin better

Ticlopidine or clopidogrel   Clopidogrel only   Ticlopidine only

FIGURE 58–5   *Relative effects of the thienopyridines and aspirin on adverse events in high-risk patients. The typical odds ratios are shown as diamonds, with 95% confidence intervals (CIs) equal to the width of the diamonds. (Adapted from Hankey GJ, Sudlow CLM, Dunbabin DW: Thienopyridines or aspirin to prevent stroke and other serious vascular events in patients at high risk of vascular disease? A systematic review of the evidence from randomized trials. Stroke 31:1779–1784, 2000.)*

clopidogrel alone in 7600 patients who have experienced a recent ischemic stroke or TIA considered to be of atherothrombotic origin and who have ischemic heart disease, diabetes, symptomatic peripheral arterial disease, or a combination of these disorders.[54] Because clopidogrel (and not aspirin) is the single antiplatelet drug comparator, however, this trial will not inform us about the effects of adding clopidogrel to the most widely tested and frequently used "gold standard" antiplatelet drug, aspirin.

Dipyridamole

Too few patients (about 3500) have been included in randomized head-to-head comparisons between dipyridamole and aspirin for any reliable conclusions to be drawn from the results, but more than 10,000 high-risk patients have been involved in 25 trials comparing the combination of aspirin plus dipyridamole with aspirin alone. Meta-analy-

sis of these latter studies found that the addition of dipyridamole was not associated with a significant reduction in the odds of a serious vascular event (Fig. 58–6).[16] When the component outcomes comprising serious vascular events were considered separately, adding dipyridamole to aspirin appeared to reduce the odds of nonfatal stroke (odds reduction 24%) but not of nonfatal MI or of vascular death (see Fig. 58–6).[16] The apparent reduction in nonfatal stroke was derived mainly from one large trial, the second European Stroke Prevention Study (ESPS-2), in which about 6000 patients with a prior ischemic stroke or TIA were randomly assigned to receive aspirin 50 mg daily, modified-release dipyridamole 400 mg daily, both, or neither for 2 years.[29] The result for nonfatal stroke in this trial was not supported by the findings in the other trials or by the overall findings for nonfatal MI or vascular death.[16] The potential explanations for the apparent reduction in stroke

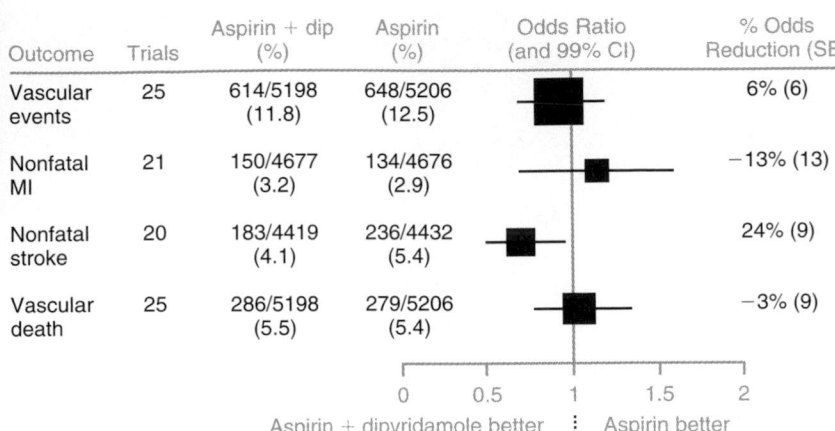

Outcome	Trials	Aspirin + dip (%)	Aspirin (%)	Odds Ratio (and 99% CI)	% Odds Reduction (SE)
Vascular events	25	614/5198 (11.8)	648/5206 (12.5)		6% (6)
Nonfatal MI	21	150/4677 (3.2)	134/4676 (2.9)		−13% (13)
Nonfatal stroke	20	183/4419 (4.1)	236/4432 (5.4)		24% (9)
Vascular death	25	286/5198 (5.5)	279/5206 (5.4)		−3% (9)

Aspirin + dipyridamole better ⋮ Aspirin better

FIGURE 58–6 *Relative effects of aspirin + dipyridamole and aspirin on various outcomes in high-risk patients. The typical odds ratio for each outcome is shown as a* red square *(size of square proportional to statistical weight) together with its 99% confidence interval (CI) (horizontal line). SE, standard error. (Data from Collaborative meta-analysis of randomised trials of antiplatelet therapy for the prevention of death, MI, and stroke in high risk patients. Antithrombotic Trialists' Collaboration. BMJ 324:71–86, 2002.)*

with the addition of dipyridamole to aspirin in the ESPS-2 are as follows:

- The reduction may be real and may relate to the particular dose and modified-release formulation of dipyridamole used. (The other trials generally used lower doses of non–modified-release dipyridamole.)
- It may be due to the use of a daily dose of aspirin (50 mg) that was too low to be maximally effective (see earlier discussion of the benefits of different doses of aspirin).
- It could be a finding related entirely to the play of chance.
- A blood pressure–lowering—rather than an antiplatelet—effect of dipyridamole (which is also a vasodilator) might explain why the risk of stroke, but not MI, was reduced.
- A combination of both antiplatelet and cardiotoxic effects of dipyridamole could even explain the observed pattern.

In summary, although the addition of modified-release dipyridamole to aspirin *may* have a role in the prevention of stroke, uncertainties remain. In addition, the ESPS-2 showed higher risks of both adverse effects (whether major, minor, or trivial) and of premature cessation of study treatment with the combination than with aspirin alone (16% versus 9%).[29] These uncertainties may be resolved when the results of the ongoing European and Australian Stroke Prevention in Reversible Ischaemia Trial (ESPRIT) become available. In this trial, 4500 patients with a prior TIA or minor ischemic stroke are being randomly assigned to receive aspirin alone, aspirin plus modified-release dipyridamole, or oral anticoagulation.[55]

Oral Anticoagulants

Although there is an established role for long-term oral anticoagulant therapy in appropriately selected patients with atrial fibrillation, both with and without a prior ischemic (generally presumed cardioembolic) stroke (see relevant Chapter 60), the situation for patients with a prior ischemic stroke or TIA of presumed arterial origin remains unclear.

Oral Anticoagulants versus No Oral Anticoagulants

A *Cochrane Database Systematic Review* found that only about 2500 patients with a previous ischemic stroke presumed to be of arterial origin had been included in eleven randomized trials comparing anticoagulation with a control group for long-term secondary prevention.[56] The trials reviewed were generally of limited methodologic quality, and most predated both the advent of computed tomography (CT) scanning to exclude hemorrhagic stroke and the use of the International Normalized Ratio (INR) for monitoring anticoagulant control. The review found no clear benefits of anticoagulants on the risks of stroke, death, or death and dependency, but did find definite increased risks of intracranial hemorrhage (absolute excess, 11 per 1000 patients treated per year) and of major extracranial hemorrhage (absolute excess, 25 per 1000 patients treated per year).[56] Thus, these results do not support the routine use of oral anticoagulants in patients with noncardioembolic ischemic stroke or TIA. Given the established benefits of antiplatelet treatment, the questions of clinical importance are (1) whether oral anticoagulants alone are superior to antiplatelet treatment alone and (2) whether anticoagulation adds worthwhile benefit to antiplatelet treatment without an unacceptable increase in the risk of hemorrhage.

Oral Anticoagulants versus Antiplatelet Treatment

A few randomized trials have compared oral anticoagulants with antiplatelet treatment in patients with prior presumed arterial ischemic stroke or TIA. The Stroke Prevention In Reversible Ischemia Trial (SPIRIT) compared high-intensity anticoagulation (INR, 3.0 to 4.5) with aspirin, 30 mg daily, among patients with a prior nondisabling ischemic stroke or TIA.[57] This trial was stopped early, after only 1316 of the intended sample of 3000 patients had been recruited, because of a more than twofold rise in the risk of the primary outcome cluster of vascular death, nonfatal stroke, nonfatal MI, or nonfatal major hemorrhage among patients allocated to anticoagulant therapy (81 of 651 patients allocated to receive anticoagulants versus 36 of 665 allocated to receive aspirin; hazard ratio [HR] 2.3; 95% CI, 1.6 to 3.5). Anticoagulants also approximately doubled the risks of vascular death and of all-cause mortality, but there was no detectable difference in major ischemic events (HR anticoagulants versus aspirin 1.03; 95% CI, 0.6 to 1.75). The excess risk in the anticoagulant group was mainly due to a substantial increase in risk of major hemorrhage (53 of 651 patients in the anticoagulant group versus 6 of 665 patients in the aspirin group; HR 9.3; 95% CI, 4.0 to 22), amounting to an excess of about 30 major extracranial hemorrhages and about 30 intracranial hemorrhages for every 1000 patients treated for a year with oral anticoagulants rather than aspirin.[57] The rate of major bleeding complications rose steeply with achieved INR. Higher age and the presence of leukoaraiosis on the baseline CT scan also appeared to be important risk factors for intracranial hemorrhage. The excess bleeding risk may have been overestimated for the following reasons: (1) the trial was stopped early (when, by chance, the results may have been more extreme than they would have been in the long run); (2) only the outcome assessment was "blinded"; the patients and treating physicians were not; and (3) the total number of major hemorrhages was small. However, these reasons seem unlikely to explain all of the substantial excess. The trialists concluded that, for patients with a prior ischemic stroke or TIA of presumed arterial origin, antiplatelet treatment remained the antithrombotic treatment of first choice; that high-intensity oral anticoagulation should be avoided because of the bleeding risks; and that the role of medium-intensity oral anticoagulation remained uncertain.[57,58]

Several randomized trials have also addressed the question whether oral anticoagulants at a lower intensity than assessed in SPIRIT have a beneficial advantage over aspirin without an excessive bleeding risk.[58-60] A *Cochrane Database Systematic Review* identified three small trials that compared medium-intensity anticoagulation (target INR 2.1 to 3.6) with antiplatelet treatment, but the total number of patients was only 493 and the results were inconclusive.[58] The much larger Warfarin-Aspirin Recurrent Stroke Study (WARSS) was a randomized, placebo-controlled trial of medium-intensity warfarin (target INR 1.4 to 2.8, mean achieved INR 2.1) versus aspirin (325 mg daily) in 2200 patients who had recent noncardioembolic ischemic stroke and were followed for 2 years.[60] The researchers found no definite difference between warfarin and aspirin for the primary outcome of recurrent ischemic stroke or death (OR for warfarin versus aspirin 1.13; 95% CI, 0.92 to 1.38), but the results were compatible with anything from a small advantage of warfarin to a more substantial advantage of aspirin. In addition, there was a trend toward an increase in major hemorrhage with warfarin (OR 1.28; 95% CI, 0.78 to 2.10) and a significant increase in minor hemorrhage (OR 1.51; 95% CI, 1.22 to 1.87).[60]

At present, therefore, there seems to be no clear role for oral anticoagulants in secondary prevention after a noncardioembolic ischemic cerebrovascular event. Several ongoing trials should provide data from a few thousand more patients in due course.[55,61,62] Perhaps the slightly higher INR range that these trials are assessing, 2.0 to 3.0, will provide the hoped-for net benefit over aspirin, but the size of any such benefit is likely to be small, and its reliable detection to require randomized trials involving many thousands of patients.

Implications for Clinical Practice

No antithrombotic (antiplatelet or anticoagulant) alternative to aspirin has been shown to be clearly superior in the long-term prevention of serious vascular events among patients with a prior presumed arterial ischemic stroke or TIA. We therefore continue to favor aspirin as first-line antiplatelet treatment for such patients. In the immediate aftermath of an ischemic cerebrovascular event, we advocate daily doses of 160 to 300 mg, because such doses have a rapid onset of action and were used in the relevant, large randomized trials of aspirin in acute ischemic stroke.[63] After the first few days and in the long term, however, a daily dose of 75 to 150 mg daily is sufficient. If patients are genuinely unable to tolerate aspirin, we substitute clopidogrel, 75 mg daily.

Breakthrough Events with Aspirin Therapy

There is no specific evidence from randomized trials to guide the management of patients who have ischemic cerebrovascular events even though they are taking aspirin and adhering to all other appropriate secondary preventive measures. Such cases are commonly referred to as "aspirin failures," implying that the aspirin is not working. Studies of platelet function have suggested that the effects of aspirin on platelet function vary between individuals; it may therefore be tempting to increase the dose of aspirin in those who seem to be "aspirin resistant."[64-66] There is no clear evidence, however, that doing so will affect clinically important outcomes, and there is secure evidence that increasing aspirin doses raises the risk of adverse effects (see earlier discussion on the risks of different aspirin doses). Furthermore, it is incorrect to assume that an ischemic event in a patient taking aspirin necessarily means that the aspirin is not working. After all, platelet function is not abolished altogether by aspirin (and we would not want it to be!), and platelets are not the only important factor in arterial occlusion. Breakthrough events in association with any secondary preventive treatment occur in the highest-risk patients, in whom the combination of several factors leads to an event despite the lowering of their risk. Without treatment, more—or perhaps more severe—events might have occurred.

We remain uncertain about the role of adding either clopidogrel or dipyridamole to aspirin and await with interest the results of the various planned or ongoing trials addressing this question, although it is unclear how much information they will provide on the specific issue of breakthrough events during aspirin therapy. However, the promising (albeit somewhat uncertain) results of the ESPS-2 trial have led us to add modified-release dipyridamole (400 mg daily) to aspirin (75 to 150 mg daily) in some patients who have experienced breakthrough events while taking aspirin, provided that the combination of the two antiplatelet drugs is well tolerated.

BLOOD PRESSURE REDUCTION

Blood Pressure Reduction Among People Without a History of Stroke or Transient Ischemic Attack

The positive and continuous relationship of both systolic and diastolic blood pressure (BP) with stroke risk and the similar but less steep relationship with ischemic heart disease are well established.[67-69] There is also clear evidence, from overviews of randomized trials, that lowering of BP reduces the risks of both stroke and ischemic heart disease among individuals without a history of vascular disease.[70-72] In keeping with the epidemiologic relationships, the evidence from randomized trials suggests that the relative benefits increase with larger reductions in BP, and there appears to be little, if any, difference in the relative benefits of different classes of antihypertensive drugs.[72-74]

Blood Pressure Reduction Among Patients with a Prior Stroke or Transient Ischemic Attack

Until very recently, many stroke specialists were cautious about extrapolating this evidence to patients who had already had a stroke or TIA. Some observational data, albeit in rather small numbers of patients, suggested that lower BP among such patients may produce an increased risk of further stroke, perhaps because of reduced cerebral perfusion (Fig. 58–7A).[75,76] But this relationship, which is J-shaped when plotted on a graph, may have arisen by chance or because severe strokes are associated both with a fall in BP and, independently, with a higher risk of

recurrence.[77] If the latter explanation were the case, then one might expect the relationship between BP and stroke risk among patients with minor cerebrovascular disease to be positive and continuous, similar to that seen among individuals with no history of vascular disease. Such a relationship is exactly what was found in an analysis of data from almost 2500 patients with a history of minor ischemic stroke or TIA in the United Kingdom Transient Ischaemic Attack (UK-TIA) aspirin trial (Fig. 58–7B).[76]

Really reliable evidence from randomized trials of the effects of BP lowering among patients with a history of stroke or TIA did not appear, however, until the beginning of the 21st century. Two small randomized trials published in the early 1970s examined the effects of diuretic-based antihypertensive treatment in a total of about 500 such patients with hypertension.[78,79] Two further randomized trials published in the 1990s assessed the effects of the beta-blocker atenolol in a total of about 2200 such patients with a range of BPs, mostly in the nonhypertensive range.[80,81] When the data were considered together in a meta-analysis, active treatment in these four studies produced an average BP reduction of 6 mm Hg systolic/3 mm Hg diastolic and a nonsignificant 19% reduction in the relative risk of stroke (Fig. 58–8).[82] A much larger randomized trial conducted among 5665 Chinese patients with a history of stroke or TIA found that, compared with

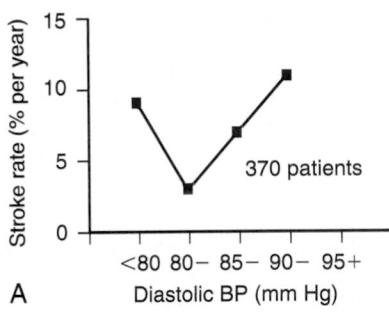

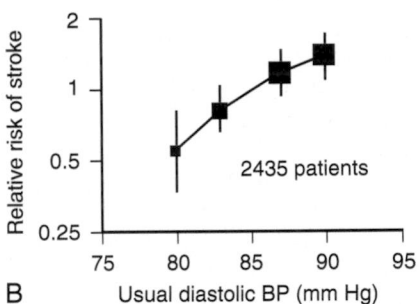

FIGURE 58–7   A, *J-shaped relationship between post-stroke diastolic blood pressure (BP) and stroke recurrence rate.* B, *Relative risk of stroke according to usual diastolic blood pressure in patients with minor ischemic stroke or transient ischemic attack.* Vertical lines represent 95% confidence intervals, and solid squares *are proportional to the number of strokes in each category.* (A *adapted from Irie K, Yamaguchi T, Minematsu K, Omae T: The J-curve phenomenon in stroke recurrence.* Stroke 24:1844–1849, 1993; B *adapted from Rodgers A, MacMahon S, Gamble G, et al: Blood pressure and risk of stroke in patients with cerebrovascular disease. The United Kingdom Transient Ischaemic Attack Collaborative Group.* BMJ 313:417, 1996.)

Trial	Subjects	OR (and CI)	% Odds Reduction (SE)
Carter	97		66% (27)
HSCSG	452		27% (20)
TEST	720		0% (19)
Dutch TIA	1473		16% (8)
Total	2472		19% (10) 2p = 0.07
Heterogeneity between the four trials: $\chi^2_{3df} = 5.5$; *P* = NS		Treatment better Treatment worse	

FIGURE 58–8   *Relative effects of blood pressure–lowering treatment and control (no blood pressure–lowering treatment) on stroke in patients with a history of stroke or transient ischemic attack (TIA). The odds ratio (OR) for each trial is shown as a red square (size of square proportional to statistical weight of trial) together with its 99% confidence interval (CI) (horizontal line). The typical odds ratio for the total is shown as a red diamond, with 95% CI equal to the width of the diamond. NS, not significant; SE, standard error. Chapter references for listed trials are: Carter,[78] HSCSG,[79] TEST,[81] and Dutch TIA.[80] (Adapted from Blood pressure lowering for the secondary prevention of stroke: Rationale and design for PROGRESS. PROGRESS Management Committee.* J Hypertens 14[Suppl 2]:S39–S46, 1996.)

placebo, about 2 years of therapy with the thiazide diuretic indapamide produced a 5 mm Hg/2 mm Hg reduction in BP and a 29% (95% CI, 12% to 42%) reduction in the relative risk of stroke. These very promising results have only ever been published, however, in a preliminary report.[83]

The results of two later large randomized trials have now clarified the issue. In the PROtection aGainst REcurrent Stroke Study (PROGRESS), about 6000 patients with a history of stroke or TIA were randomly assigned either active treatment with the angiotensin-converting-enzyme (ACE) inhibitor perindopril (4 mg daily), with the addition of the diuretic indapamide at the discretion of the treating physicians, or placebo. There were no BP entry criteria; baseline diastolic BPs ranged from 55 to 125 mm Hg, and systolic BPs from 100 to 240 mm Hg, with a mean of 147 mm Hg/86 mm Hg.[84] Only about half of the patients had hypertension (defined as a baseline BP higher than 160 mm Hg/90 mm Hg). During 4 years of follow-up, active treatment lowered BP by 9 mm Hg/4 mm Hg on average, and reduced the relative risks of the primary outcome of stroke by 28% (95% CI, 17% to 38%) (Fig. 58–9) and of all major vascular events (stroke, MI, or vascular death) by 26% (95% CI, 16% to 34%). These results correspond to avoidance of stroke in 11 patients and of a major vascular event in 14 patients out of every 1000 receiving active treatment for a year. The relative reductions in both ischemic and hemorrhagic strokes were similar, and the relative benefits of treatment were similar regardless of whether patients were hypertensive at baseline or not. In keeping with the relationship between BP and stroke risk in patients with a history of stroke or TIA, the greater BP-lowering effects of combination treatment with perindopril and indapamide were associated with larger reductions in stroke risk than treatment with perindopril alone.[85]

In the Heart Outcomes Prevention Evaluation (HOPE) study, about 9000 high-risk patients (age 55 years or older with a history of vascular disease or diabetes plus at least one other cardiovascular risk factor) were randomly assigned to receive the ACE inhibitor ramipril (10 mg daily) or placebo for a mean of 5 years. About 1000 patients had a history of stroke or TIA, more than half were normotensive, and the average baseline BP among all patients included was 139 mm Hg/70 mm Hg. Compared with placebo, ramipril lowered mean blood pressure by 3 mm Hg/2 mm Hg and reduced the relative risks of the combined primary outcome of stroke, MI, and cardiovascular death by 22% (95% CI, 14% to 30%), and of stroke alone by 32% (95% CI, 16% to 44%). There were also statistically significant reductions in the separate outcomes of MI, cardiovascular death, and all-cause mortality.[86] The relative effects of ramipril on the primary outcome and on stroke alone were similar in patients both with and without a history of cerebrovascular disease and regardless of baseline BP.[87] Because of the small mean reduction in BP, the HOPE investigators suggested that the benefits of ramipril could not be accounted for by BP lowering alone and that additional cardiovascular actions were likely to be important.[86,88] However, trial treatment in HOPE (but not in other large antihypertensive trials) was given at bedtime, with BP measurements taken during daytime study visits. A substudy of 24-hour BP recordings in 38 patients enrolled in HOPE demonstrated that ramipril lowered BP more at night than during the day and reduced the average 24-hour blood pressure by 10 mm Hg/4 mm Hg compared with placebo.[89] Thus, the timing of drug intake in relation to BP measurement in HOPE may have led to an underestimation of its effects on BP in comparison with the effects measured in other trials of antihypertensive agents. If this substudy result applies to the HOPE trial in general, very similar BP reductions in HOPE and in PROGRESS produced very similar relative reductions in the risk of stroke.

Implications for Clinical Practice

The implications of these two trials for clinical practice are that BP-lowering treatment should be considered routinely for patients with a history of stroke or TIA, whether or not they would classically be regarded as hypertensive. The benefits appear to be related to the extent of BP reduction rather than to any specific drug or drug class. However, because most of the available evidence in patients with stroke or TIA comes from PROGRESS, the combination of a thiazide diuretic and an ACE inhibitor seems an appropriate first choice. We tend to start with a thiazide, ensure that it is well tolerated, and then introduce an ACE inhibitor, keeping a check on blood urea, creatinine, and electrolyte levels.

It seems perfectly reasonable to use other classes of antihypertensive drugs if the patient experiences adverse effects with either thiazides or ACE inhibitors or if these agents are otherwise contraindicated. The results of PROGRESS and HOPE do not imply any particular target BP but rather suggest that, at least within the range of BPs tested, the lower the blood pressure, the lower the stroke risk. Therefore, the aim should probably be to gently lower the BP as far as possible as long as adverse effects of treatment do not occur. We do not tend to aim for lower than about 120/70 mm Hg, however, given that relatively small

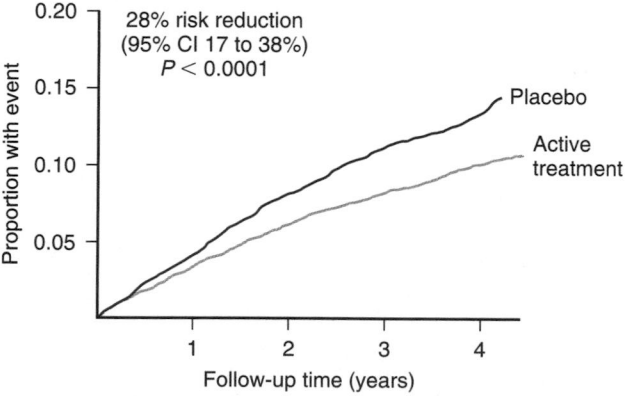

FIGURE 58–9 *Results of the PROtection aGainst REcurrent Stroke Study (PROGRESS) for the primary outcome of stroke. Cumulative incidence of stroke among active treatment and placebo groups. CI, confidence interval. (Adapted from Randomised trial of a perindopril-based blood-pressure–lowering regimen among 6105 individuals with previous stroke or transient ischemic attack. PROGRESS Collaborative Group. Lancet 358: 1033–1041, 2001.)*

numbers of patient with stroke or TIA achieved BPs of this level or below in the trials. And we continue to be particularly cautious with antihypertensive treatment in patients with known severe stenosis or occlusion of one or more extracranial neck arteries.

CHOLESTEROL REDUCTION

Relationship Between Cholesterol and Stroke

In contrast to the positive and continuous observed relationship between plasma cholesterol level and ischemic heart disease, prospective observational studies in individuals without a history of vascular disease found no overall association between plasma cholesterol level and stroke risk.[69,90] This situation may be the result of a balance between a suggested positive association with ischemic stroke and a negative association with hemorrhagic stroke.[69]

Randomized Trials of Cholesterol Lowering and Stroke

Before the 2000s, only a couple of very small trials in a total of about 600 patients had examined the role of cholesterol lowering specifically among patients with a prior ischemic stroke or TIA. The drug used (clofibrate in both cases) produced only a small drop in the mean plasma cholesterol level, and the results were inconclusive.[91,92] However, tens of thousands of patients who either had a history of ischemic heart disease or were considered to be at high risk of ischemic heart disease because of a raised plasma cholesterol or other risk factors had been entered into trials designed to assess the effects of cholesterol-lowering treatments on coronary events. Many of these trials also reported on stroke as an outcome. The trials that assessed the effects of a variety of nonstatin treatments (fibrates, resins, surgery, or dietary regimens) found that a relative reduction of about 10% in mean cholesterol over an average of 5 to 6 years had no significant effect on stroke but produced a reduction of about one quarter in coronary events.[93–96] By contrast, those trials that assessed the effects of a statin in comparison with placebo found a substantially larger relative reduction in mean cholesterol, 21% over an average of 4 years, which reduced the relative odds of stroke by 24% (and the relative odds of coronary events by a third) (Table 58.2).[94,97] The differences in effectiveness between nonstatin treatments and statins seem likely to be related to the extent of cholesterol lowering.[95]

Even though cholesterol lowering with a statin appeared to reduce the risk of stroke among patients with a history—or at high risk—of ischemic heart disease, direct evidence for the effects among patients with a prior ischemic stroke or TIA was lacking, and evidence for the effects of statins among elderly patients and patients with below-average cholesterol levels for Western populations was limited. Furthermore, concerns remained that, although the overall stroke risk appeared to be reduced, there was a possible increase in fatal stroke (see Table 58.2). Because hemorrhagic strokes are more likely than ischemic strokes to be fatal, this finding might imply a higher risk of hemorrhagic stroke from cholesterol lowering with a statin (as suggested by the observational studies described earlier). This issue could not be examined directly, however, because the trials so far available had not generally reported results for hemorrhagic strokes separately.[94,97]

Many of the uncertainties have now been resolved by the results of the Heart Protection Study (HPS).[98] This large randomized trial compared simvastatin 40 mg daily with placebo among about 20,000 patients 40 to 80 years

Table 58.2 Effects of Cholesterol Lowering with a Statin on Risk of Stroke: Results of a Systematic Review and Subsequent Randomized Trials

	No Participant	No. Strokes	Mean Pretreatment Cholesterol* (mmol/L)	Average Follow up Duration* (years)	Mean Reduction in Cholesterol* (%)	Summary Odds Ratio for Active Treatment versus Control[†]	
						Fatal or Nonfatal Stroke	**Fatal Stroke**
Overview of 15 trials before HPS[94,97]	38,000	827	6.3	4	21	0.76 (0.66–0.87)	0.99 (0.67–1.45)
HPS[98]	20,000	1029	5.9	5	20	0.75 (0.66–0.85)	0.81 (0.62–1.1)
PROSPER[99]	6000	266	5.7	3.2	20[‡]	1.02 (0.80–1.31)	1.66 (0.86–3.24)
ALLHAT[99a]	10,000	440	5.8	4.8	9.6	0.90 (0.75–1.09)	0.95 (0.65–1.38)
ASCOT-LLA[99b]	10,000	210	5.5	3.3	19	0.73 (0.55–0.96)	—
All trials	84,000	2772	6.0	4.2	19	0.80 (0.74–0.86)	0.93 (0.77–1.11)

ALLHAT, Antihypertensive and Lipid-Lowering treatment to prevent Heart Attack Trial; ASCOT-LLA, Anglo-Scandinavian Cardiovascular Outcomes Trial-Lipid Lowering Arm; CI, confidence interval; HPS, Heart Protection Study; OR, odds ratio; PROSPER, PROspective Study of Pravastatin in the Elderly at Risk.
*Weighted by trial size.
[†]95% confidence interval given in parentheses.
[‡]Estimated from reduction in low-density lipoprotein (LDL) cholesterol.

of age who had ischemic heart disease, other occlusive vascular disease, or diabetes, and whose nonfasting blood total cholesterol levels were more than 3.5 mmol/L. Among those recruited to the trial were 3000 patients with a history of ischemic stroke or TIA, more than 4000 patients with pretreatment cholesterol levels below 5.0 mmol/L, and almost 6000 more than 70 years of age. Treatment lowered mean total cholesterol by 20% over 5 years and reduced the relative odds of stroke by a quarter (see Table 58.2). A much larger number of strokes (>1000) occurred in this study than in any previous cholesterol-lowering trial, and the study investigators collected information on pathologic type of stroke. Simvastatin produced a definite and substantial reduction in risk of ischemic stroke, and the results provided some reassurance about the effects of statin drugs on hemorrhagic stroke, which affected similar numbers of patients in the treatment and placebo groups. In addition, simvastatin significantly reduced the rates of coronary events and vascular and total mortality. The composite outcome of major vascular events (major coronary events, strokes, and coronary or non-coronary revascularizations) was about a quarter lower in the treatment group (relative reduction in event rate, 24%; 95% CI, 19% to 28%). The relative reductions in major vascular events were similar in patients with different pretreatment concentrations of cholesterol and triglycerides, in all age groups, and regardless of prior history of ischemic stroke or TIA, ischemic heart disease, peripheral arterial disease, or diabetes. Not all of the patients in the treatment group actually took their statin throughout the trial, and some of the placebo group patients actually took non-study statin treatment. Allowing for the noncompliance, the results assess the effects of about two thirds of the simvastatin-assigned patients actually taking 40 mg simvastatin daily. Actual use of the regimen tested would probably reduce major vascular events by about one third, corresponding to the prevention of about 70 to 100 such events per 1000 people treated for 5 years among the many types of high-risk patients studied.[98]

The HPS was large enough to be able to provide substantially more data than had previously been available about the potential adverse effects of lowering cholesterol with a statin. The results were very reassuring. Active treatment was not associated with any excess of cancer, elevated liver or muscle enzymes, myopathy, neuropsychiatric disorder, or respiratory disease. The investigators plan to continue follow-up for several more years to detect any delayed effects on cancers or other major outcomes.[98]

Since the results of the HPS became available, further evidence supporting the benefits of lowering cholesterol with a statin has emerged from three large randomized trials, two of which included patients with a prior ischemic stroke or TIA.[99,99a,99b,99c] In the Pravastatin in the Elderly at Risk (PROSPER) trial, almost 6000 patients aged 70–82 years with a history of or risk factors for vascular disease, were randomly assigned to receive either pravastatin 40 mg daily or placebo and were followed up for about 3 years.[99] About 650 of the subjects had a history of ischemic stroke or TIA. Pravastatin reduced the incidence of the composite primary outcome of coronary death, non-fatal myocardial infarction, and fatal or non-fatal stroke by 15% (95% CI 3% to 26%), consistent with the results of the HPS and other

previous statin trials. Stroke risk appeared to be unaffected, but because only 266 strokes were recorded, statistical power to detect a reduction in stroke risk was limited, so the results may reflect the play of chance (see Table 58.2). Moreover, the observation of a borderline-significant relative reduction of one quarter in the risk for a TIA does suggest that treatment had an effect on ischemic cerebrovascular events. Although a slight excess of cancers with pravastatin treatment was observed in PROSPER, this was not confined to any particular site, suggesting that the excess may have been due to chance. And reassuringly, a meta-analysis of cancer incidence in all the major statin trials, including PROSPER, did not show any excess risk of cancer either with pravastatin, or with the statins in general.[99,103]

The lipid-lowering component of the Antihypertensive and Lipid-Lowering treatment to prevent Heart Attack Trial (ALLHAT) was a randomized, non-blinded comparison of the effects of pravastatin 40 mg daily versus usual care in about 10,000 participants aged over 55 years with moderately raised cholesterol, hypertension, and at least one additional risk factor for ischemic heart disease.[100] After a mean follow-up of about 5 years, there was a modest, non-significant reduction in the relative risk of stroke (see Table 58.2), with a similar, non-significant reduction in coronary events. These modest and non-significant reductions may be because a substantial proportion of those allocated usual care in this open trial were prescribed a statin, so there was only a 9.6% reduction in mean total cholesterol level in the pravastatin group relative to the usual care group.[100] The Anglo-Scandinavian Cardiovascular Outcomes Trial-Lipid Lowering Arm (ASCOT-LLA) assessed the effects of atorvastatin 10 mg daily versus placebo in about 10,000 patients with hypertension and at least three other cardiovascular risk factors.[101] About 1000 of these patients had a prior stroke or TIA. After about 3 years of follow-up, active treatment produced a 19% relative reduction in total cholesterol, and clear reductions in the risks both of stroke and of coronary events (see Table 58.2).[101]

Implications for Clinical Practice

There is good evidence to support the use of cholesterol-lowering therapy with a statin among a range of individuals at high risk of vascular events, including those with a history of ischemic stroke or TIA and the elderly. Among all the statin trials, the HPS involved the largest number of patients with a prior ischemic stroke or TIA, and so for such patients, we generally favor simvastatin 40 mg daily, the active treatment used in the HPS.[98] For patients who are already taking and tolerating simvastatin at a lower dose, we would generally recommend increasing to 40 mg daily. For patients who are already taking and tolerating a different statin drug, however, we would generally suggest that it should be continued in a daily dose equivalent to 40 mg of simvastatin, because the evidence from overviews of cholesterol-lowering trials suggest that it is probably the size of the cholesterol reduction with statin treatment, not the particular drug used, that is beneficial.[95,98,102]

Because the relative benefits of treatment are similar regardless of baseline cholesterol level (at least down as far as 3.5 mmol/L; lower levels are rarely encountered in Western populations), there does not seem to be any particular target cholesterol level to treat or to aim for. Rather, it makes sense to consider treatment routinely for all patients at high risk whose pretreatment cholesterol level is 3.5 mmol/L or higher, because it is those patients at highest absolute risk of recurrent ischemic stroke and other vascular events who have the most to gain. In addition, monitoring of the response of the cholesterol level to treatment is likely to be most useful for motivation, checking compliance, and picking up those few patients with persistently very high cholesterol levels (say, >7.5 mmol/L) who may benefit from referral to a specialist lipid clinic.

The reassuring absence of an association between statin treatment and liver or muscle problems in the HPS suggests to us that routine monitoring of blood levels of liver and muscle enzymes is not necessary. However, statin treatment should still be avoided in patients with active liver or muscle disease, and patients should be advised to report any unexplained muscle symptoms.

For physicians who remain uncertain, the Cholesterol Treatment Trialists' prospectively planned meta-analyses of the results of all large-scale randomized trials of cholesterol-lowering therapy should provide even more reliable assessments of the effects of statins on important vascular outcomes and adverse events in particular patient subgroups.[104] Further information will also become available from the ongoing Stroke Prevention by Aggressive Reduction in Cholesterol Levels (SPARCL) study, a randomized trial of atorvastatin versus placebo in 4200 patients with a prior stroke or TIA.[105]

MANAGEMENT OF DIABETES

Diabetes mellitus raises the risk of stroke, ischemic heart disease, and peripheral arterial disease. In addition, after a stroke or MI, patients with diabetes have a worse prognosis, with a higher risk of death and of recurrent vascular events.[106–108] The relative benefits of antiplatelet treatment, BP reduction, and cholesterol reduction with a statin are similar in the presence or absence of diabetes.[17,86,85,98] Diabetic patients who have experienced an ischemic stroke or TIA attributable to arterial disease should therefore receive all of these treatments unless there is some definite contraindication, particularly because their higher risk of a serious vascular event will lead to a greater absolute benefit.

Randomized trials among a few thousand individuals with type 1 and type 2 diabetes (mainly without a history of vascular disease) found that improved glycemic control reduced the risk of microvascular complications (such as nephropathy and retinopathy). There was no definite evidence of a reduced risk of stroke or of macrovascular complications in general, although there were favorable, nonstatistically significant trends. More intensive treatment increased the risk of hypoglycemic episodes and weight gain, but there were no clear adverse effects on neuropsychological outcomes or quality of life.[109,110] These results suggest that careful glycemic control is likely to improve long-term outcome. Of course, for a particular patient with diabetes and a history of stroke or TIA, a number of factors, such as age, stroke- and diabetes-related disability, and unawareness of hypoglycemia (which increases the risk of more intensive treatment),

help determine the most appropriate goals and strategies for glycemic control. It is usually appropriate to involve in such judgments a diabetologist or other physician with considerable experience in the management of diabetes.

VITAMIN SUPPLEMENTS

Folic Acid (and Vitamins B_{12} and B_6) to Reduce Plasma Homocysteine Levels

Observational studies have shown an association between rising plasma levels of the amino acid homocysteine and an increased risk of stroke and ischemic heart disease. However, the relative lack of prospective studies and the possibility of residual confounding by factors independently associated both with vascular disease and with plasma homocysteine make it difficult to be sure that homocysteine is truly an independent and causal risk factor.[111–113] If it is, then lowering homocysteine levels might lead to reductions in the risk of stroke and heart disease, particularly among patients at high risk. Folic acid–based vitamin supplementation appears to be a cheap and simple way to lower blood homocysteine concentrations. Homocysteine metabolism depends on an adequate supply of folic acid, vitamin B_{12}, and, under some conditions, vitamin B_6. Thus, plasma homocysteine levels are inversely related to dietary intake and plasma levels of folate, vitamin B_{12}, and, to a lesser extent, vitamin B_6.[112]

The results of a meta-analysis of randomized trials of homocysteine-lowering treatment with folic acid–based supplements suggested that a daily dose of at least 0.5 mg of folic acid with about 0.5 mg of vitamin B_{12} should reduce homocysteine levels by about a quarter to a third in typical Western populations.[114] However, we do not yet know whether this reduction will lower the risk of clinically important vascular outcomes. Several large randomized trials are currently assessing the effects on serious vascular events of lowering homocysteine with folic acid–based supplements in patients at high risk.[112] Two of these (the VITAmins TO Prevent Stroke [VITATOPS] and the Vitamin Intervention for Stroke Prevention [VISP] trials) will provide data on the effects of vitamin supplementation (with folic acid, B_{12}, and B_6) in comparison with placebo among a total of more than 10,000 patients with a previous stroke or TIA.[115,116] At present, however, there is no indication for routine folic acid–based supplementation among such patients.

Antioxidants

A number of observational studies, mainly among individuals without a history of vascular disease, have suggested that dietary or supplementary antioxidant vitamins (beta carotene, vitamin C, vitamin E) may protect against stroke and other vascular events. However, large randomized trials of antioxidant vitamin supplementation have consistently failed to show any evidence of benefit on vascular or other outcomes, either in previously healthy individuals or in patients at high risk for or with preexisting arterial disease.[117–122] It seems likely that the lower risks of vascular outcomes among individuals with higher intake of antioxidant vitamins found in observational studies are due to confounding by other differences in lifestyle associated with vitamin intake. The results of the HPS, which randomly assigned about 20,000 high-risk patients with preexisting arterial disease or diabetes to either antioxidant vitamin supplementation (with vitamin E, vitamin C, and beta carotene) or placebo (and, in a factorial design, to either simvastatin or placebo; see earlier discussion), did provide reassurance that these vitamins are safe in such patients.[122] However, the evidence from randomized trials does not support the routine use of antioxidant vitamins among patients at high risk of vascular disease, including those with a prior stroke or TIA.

HORMONE REPLACEMENT THERAPY

Use of hormone replacement therapy (HRT) has risen among postmenopausal women in Western countries over the past few decades. The main reasons for prescribing HRT are relief of menopausal symptoms and prevention or management of osteoporosis. In addition, evidence about the long-term effects on vascular disease and cancer has gradually accumulated, first from observational studies and later from randomized trials set up to study these outcomes, comparing estrogen alone or estrogen-progestagen combinations with placebo in postmenopausal women followed up for several years.[123,124]

Results are now available from one trial involving almost 700 women with a recent ischemic stroke or TIA, two trials studying a total of 3800 women with ischemic heart disease, one small trial in 140 women with previous venous thromboembolic disease, and one trial of about 16,600 healthy women.[123,125] For some outcomes, the combined results of these randomized trials broadly confirm those of observational studies—an increased risk of breast cancer and venous thromboembolism and a reduced risk of colorectal cancer and femoral neck fracture.[123] Although observational studies generally suggested that rates of ischemic heart disease were lower among HRT users, with rather less consistent results for stroke, the ever-present possibility of confounding (i.e., women taking HRT might be at lower risk of arterial disease for some other reason) made the results difficult to interpret. In contrast, the randomized trials showed no evidence of benefit of HRT on coronary events (possibly even a slightly increased risk) and about a one-third increase in the relative risk of stroke, although there was no reliable information about the effects on different pathologic types of stroke.[123]

The absolute balance of benefits and risks for these long-term outcomes in a particular woman depends on her baseline risk of development of each one of them (and so on her age, medical history, etc). For most healthy postmenopausal women, the overall long-term risks of HRT probably outweigh the benefits, but the average net absolute risk is very small.[123] For women who have had an ischemic stroke or TIA, the absolute excess risk of stroke is greater, thus weighing the balance further against HRT. Therefore, there is certainly no evidence to support a role for starting HRT for secondary prevention after a stroke or TIA. Also, the apparent higher risk of recurrent stroke, along with the other long-term risks, suggests to us that most women with a history of cerebrovascular disease should be advised to stop taking HRT if they are already taking it, unless there are compelling reasons (such as severe menopausal symptoms) to continue it.

MODIFYING RISK FACTORS WITH LIFESTYLE CHANGES

Stopping Smoking

The adverse health effects of smoking (which include ischemic cerebrovascular disease) are so clearly established that all people who use tobacco in any form (cigarettes, pipe, cigars, etc.) should be advised to stop.[126] Patients who have had any type of stroke are at high risk of serious vascular events, and observational studies suggest that their risk is likely to decline within several years of stopping smoking.[127] *Cochrane Database Systematic Reviews* of large numbers of randomized trials among several tens of thousands of participants in a variety of settings have found that a number of different interventions increase smoking quit rates by about 1.5 to 2.5 times compared with control. These interventions include various types of advice and counseling from health care professionals (physicians, nurses, trained counselors) to stop smoking, different forms of nicotine replacement therapy, and the antidepressants buproprion and nortriptyline.[128-134] Although advice and counseling are not associated with any harm, both nicotine replacement therapy and antidepressants can be associated with a number of adverse effects, although they are almost all minor and reversible.[134] In practice, the most appropriate strategy for helping individual patients give up smoking depends on their motivation and personal preference, their experience of any previous attempts to quit, and the local availability of the various helpful interventions.

Dietary Changes

Assessing the effects of various components of diet on the risk of stroke and vascular disease is very difficult because of problems in measuring or recording dietary intake accurately as well as the ever-present potential for confounding by other dietary or lifestyle factors in observational studies. Even in very large randomized trials, it may be difficult to achieve sufficient change with dietary advice to demonstrate any detectable effect on clinically important outcomes, even if very small benefits do occur. Randomized trials have often focused on the effects of dietary change on risk factors rather than on vascular outcomes. For example, systematic reviews of randomized trials have shown that advice to eat a diet low in saturated fat and cholesterol can achieve small relative reductions in blood cholesterol concentrations—3% to 5% in individuals living in the community, and perhaps a little more in those with a history of vascular disease.[121,134] However, no clear effect of cholesterol-lowering diet on vascular outcomes has been demonstrated. Similarly, randomized trials have shown that dietary advice to restrict salt intake, or to reduce weight in obese individuals, produces small reductions in blood pressure, but the effects on important clinical outcomes have not been studied.[121,134]

Therapy

Observational studies have also shown that a diet rich in fruit and vegetables is associated with a lower risk of stroke and of ischemic heart disease, but lack of evidence from randomized trials means that the size and nature of any real protective effect are uncertain.[119,135] There is some evidence from randomized trials among patients with ischemic heart disease that advice to eat more oily fish, fruit and vegetables, bread, pasta, olive oil, and rapeseed margarine (i.e., a Mediterranean diet) may reduce mortality, but there are no such trials among patients with cerebrovascular disease.[121]

In practice, although there is very limited randomized trial evidence to support dietary modifications, advising patients to modify their diet by reducing total fat and salt content, replacing saturated with unsaturated fats, and increasing the intake of fruit, vegetables, and oily fish may well be beneficial and seems highly unlikely to be harmful. However, the role of such advice in the overall management of an individual patient who has survived a stroke or TIA depends on such factors as age, cognitive function, lifestyle, motivation, and level of dependency. Such dietary modifications may be particularly difficult or inappropriate in particular patients and, when such is not the case, it is important to ensure that the modifications do not detract from secondary preventive interventions of clearly established effectiveness.

Exercise

Observational studies indicate that physical activity is associated with lower risks of stroke and ischemic heart disease.[136] There is some evidence from randomized trials that sedentary people can be encouraged to increase their physical activity; that aerobic exercise reduces blood pressure; and that cardiac rehabilitation, including exercise, reduces the risk of major cardiac events after an MI.[121,134,137] However, the effects of exercise programs after a stroke or TIA on further vascular events are unknown, and the levels of physical activity likely to produce a reduction in risk may not be achievable in many cases. It seems appropriate, however, to encourage such patients to return to normal physical activities as much as they can.

Alcohol

It seems unlikely that there will ever be any randomized trials of the effects of different levels of alcohol intake on stroke or other vascular outcomes, either in healthy individuals or in those with a history of disease. Data from observational studies suggest that the relationships between alcohol consumption and the risk of stroke, ischemic heart disease, and mortality, when plotted on graphs, are probably all U- or J-shaped, so that the lowest risk occurs in persons with a modest alcohol intake.[138-142] The mechanisms behind these observations are uncertain, but studies suggest that high levels of alcohol intake are associated with high blood pressure and that moderate alcohol intake has beneficial effects on serum lipid levels and hemostatic factors.[139,143]

The optimal level of consumption is difficult to gauge, both because self-reported alcohol intake is often inaccurate and because the balance between the benefits and risks of different levels of alcohol intake vary with age, gender,

medical history, and a variety of risk factors for vascular and other diseases. In middle and old age in Western populations, benefits probably outweigh harms with up to four drinks per day in men and somewhat less in women.[138] Thus, it makes sense to advise patients who have had a stroke or TIA to avoid heavy alcohol intake but to reassure those with a modest intake that they need not abstain altogether.

SELECTING PATIENTS FOR CAROTID ENDARTERECTOMY

Carotid endarterectomy is highly beneficial for selected patients with a recent nondisabling ischemic stroke or TIA affecting the territory of a carotid artery with stenosis. Pooled individual patient data meta-analyses are now available from more than 6000 patients followed up for an average of 6 years in the three randomized trials of carotid endarterectomy for recently symptomatic carotid stenosis (the European Carotid Surgery Trial [ECST], the North American Symptomatic Carotid Endarterectomy Trial [NASCET], each contributing about 3000 patients, and the much smaller Veterans Affairs Trial 309).[144] Comparable definitions of outcomes and consistent measurement of angiographic stenosis using the NASCET method (calculated by dividing the minimal residual luminal diameter at the point of most severe stenosis by the luminal diameter of the normal internal carotid artery beyond the stenosis) demonstrated very similar results for the two largest trials. The pooled analyses showed that, provided that the 30-day operative risk of stroke or death is no higher than the 7% recorded in the trials and patients are willing to take this initial risk, then the effectiveness of surgery is as follows:

- Highly effective for patients with more than 70% stenosis without near-occlusion; the combined outcome of any stroke or operative death at 5 years was avoided in 150 of 1000 operated patients at 5 years, and net benefits started to accrue within the first year (Fig. 58–10).
- Moderately effective for patients with 50% to 69% stenosis; 80 patients of 1000 operated patients avoided any stroke or operative death at 5 years, but patients were at higher risk during the first 2 years, and net benefits did not start to accrue until the third year (see Fig. 58–10).

Surgery tended to be harmful for patients with less than 30% stenosis and was of no net benefit for patients with 30% to 49% stenosis. Also, pooled estimates showed no significant net benefits for patients with near-occlusion (if the artery distal to the stenosis begins to collapse). This situation may be explained by the fact that their unoperated risk of stroke was lower than in patients with severe stenosis but no near-occlusion, probably because of good collateral circulation. Because the pooled data included only 262 such patients, however, the benefits and risks of surgery in this group could not be estimated reliably; the 95% confidence interval for the estimate of the overall effect on any stroke or operative death is consistent with either net benefit or net harm (see Fig. 58–10).[144]

Although the degree of stenosis is a major determinant of the effectiveness of surgery, the decision about whether or not to operate is finely balanced and also depends on

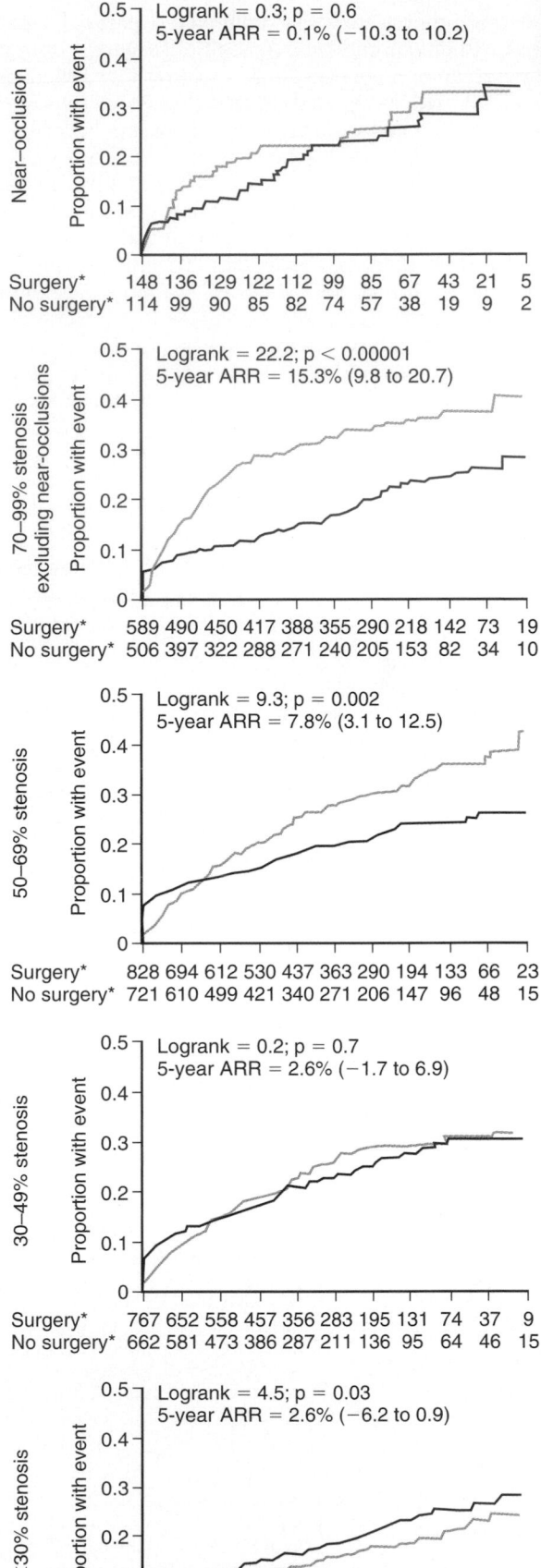

FIGURE 58–10 *Effects of surgery on any stroke or operative death according to degree of symptomatic carotid stenosis in an analysis of pooled data from the European Carotid Surgery Trial (ECST), the North American Symptomatic Carotid Endarterectomy Trial (NASCET), and Veterans Affairs Trial 309. °, Numbers at risk. Solid lines represent surgical treatment. ARR, absolute risk reduction. (From Rothwell PM, Eliasziw M, Gutnikov S, et al: Analysis of pooled data from the randomised controlled trials of carotid endarterectomy for symptomatic carotid stenosis. Lancet 361:107–116, 2003.)*

several other factors that influence a particular patient's risk without surgery or as a result of surgery. For example, operative risk appears to be greater in women and in patients with peripheral arterial disease or hypertension, whereas the risk without surgery is particularly high early after the most recent ischemic stroke or TIA (especially in those with severe stenosis) and is higher after cerebral than after ocular events.[145] Predicted life expectancy (and so age and gender) is also important in determining the tradeoff between earlier risks and later benefits, particularly in patients with moderate stenosis.[146] Interestingly, although the results of several studies suggest that ipsilateral internal carotid artery stenosis seems to be an innocent bystander in carotid territory lacunar infarction, the trials suggest that surgery benefits patients with lacunar as well as nonlacunar infarction in the territory of a stenosed internal carotid artery.[147,148] So, at present, there is no compelling evidence to support the notion that patients with infarcts resulting from small vessel occlusion do not benefit from endarterectomy.

Because inclusion of patients in the endarterectomy trials required prerandomization intra-arterial carotid angiography, care should be taken in applying these results to current clinical practice. Many centers no longer perform intra-arterial angiography routinely, because (1) it is not risk free, especially in older patients with symptomatic vascular disease, (2) it may delay surgery if there is any wait before the procedure, and (3) rapidly improving alternative noninvasive imaging techniques (carotid Doppler ultrasonography, magnetic resonance angiography, and CT angiography) for assessing stenosis are now available. These newer techniques must be properly validated, however, against the "gold standard," intra-arterial angiography.[149] With an experienced operator using

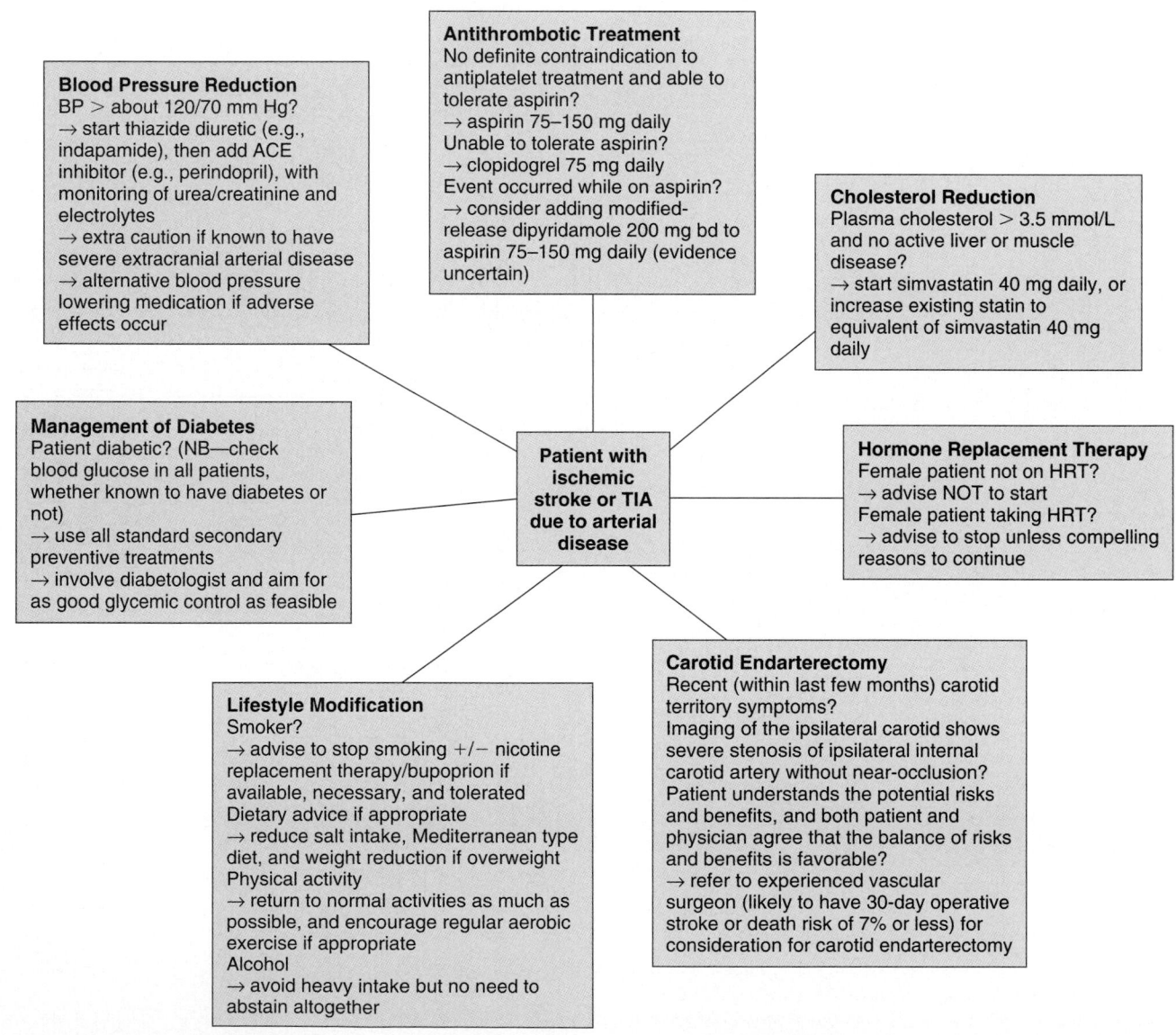

FIGURE 58–11 *Summary of long-term secondary preventive management for patients with ischemic stroke or transient ischemic attack (TIA) due to arterial disease. ACE, angiotensin-converting enzyme; BP, blood pressure; HRT, hormone replacement therapy; NB, nota bene.*

modern equipment, carotid Doppler ultrasonography is quick, practical, relatively inexpensive, and reliable.[150] Thus, a reasonable strategy is to obtain an ultrasonogram first and, if severe stenosis is suspected, arrange a further confirmatory noninvasive imaging test (magnetic resonance angiogram, CT angiogram, or another ultrasonogram) by an independent observer. If the two imaging findings disagree, adding a third noninvasive test would result in very few misclassified carotid stenoses, and this minor loss of accuracy may well more than offset the disadvantages of intra-arterial angiography.[151]

Angioplasty (with or without stenting) may turn out to be as effective and durable as (or more so than) endarterectomy for carotid stenosis or to have a role in the management of severe stenosis in the vertebrobasilar system, although these issues remain uncertain. The Carotid and Vertebral Transluminal Angioplasty Study (CAVATAS) is the only reasonably large randomized trial so far available comparing carotid angioplasty with endarterectomy for symptomatic patients. The study was too small (500 patients) for reliable conclusions to be drawn about the relative merits of the two approaches, although it identified no significant differences in major procedural risks or in overall early outcome. CAVATAS also randomly assigned 16 patients with vertebral artery stenosis to undergo either vertebral angioplasty or best medical treatment, but this comparison will have to be evaluated in many more patients before reliable estimates of the relative effectiveness of the two approaches can be made.[152] Further information on the relative effects of carotid artery angioplasty with stenting and carotid endarterectomy for symptomatic stenosis will be provided by two ongoing trials, the Carotid Revascularization Endarterectomy versus Stenting Trial (CREST) and the International Carotid Stenting Study (ICSS).[153,154] Until then, there is really no good evidence to support the routine use of angioplasty as an alternative to endarterectomy.

CLINICAL PRACTICE SUMMARY

Figure 58–11 summarizes the various recommendations for clinical practice that we make in this chapter.

References

1. Sandercock PAG, Warlow CP, Jones LN, Starkey IR: Predisposing factors for cerebral infarction: The Oxfordshire Community Stroke Project. BMJ 298:1460–1465, 1989.
2. Bamford J, Sandercock P, Dennis M, et al: Classification and natural history of clinically identifiable subtypes of cerebral infarction. Lancet 337:1521–1526, 1991.
3. Castaigne P, Lhermitte F, Gautier J, et al: Arterial occlusions in the vertebrobasilar system: A study of 44 patients with post-mortem data. Brain 93:231–258, 1973.
4. Caplan LR, Tettenborn B: Vertebrobasilar occlusive disease: Review of selected aspects. 2: Posterior circulation embolism. Cerebrovasc Dis 2:320–326, 1992.
5. Lhermitte F, Gautier JC, Derouesne C: Nature of occlusions of the middle cerebral artery. Neurology 20:82–88, 1970.
6. Bogousslavsky J, Hachinski VC, Boughner DR, et al: Cardiac and arterial lesions in carotid transient ischemic attacks. Arch Neurol 43:223–228, 1986.
7. Lammie GA, Sandercock PAG, Dennis MS: Recently occluded intracranial and extracranial carotid arteries: Relevance of the unstable atherosclerotic plaque. Stroke 30:1319–1325, 1999.
8. Bamford J: Lacunar syndromes: Are they still worth diagnosing? In Donnan G, Norrving B, Bamford J, Bogousslavsky J (eds): Subcortical Stroke, 2nd ed. Oxford, Oxford University Press, 2002, pp 161–174.
9. Fisher CM: Lacunar infarcts—a review. Cerebrovasc Dis 1:311–320, 1991.
10. Lammie GA: Pathology of lacunar infarction. In Donnan G, Norrving B, Bamford J, Bogousslavsky J (eds): Subcortical Stroke, 2nd ed. Oxford, Oxford University Press, 2002, pp 37–46.
11. Warlow CP, Dennis MS, van Gijn J, et al: Preventing recurrent stroke and other serious vascular events. In Stroke: A Practical Guide to Management. Oxford, Blackwell Science, 2001, pp 653–722.
12. Johnston SC, Gress DR, Browner WS, Sidney S: Short-term prognosis after emergency department diagnosis of TIA. JAMA 284:2901–2906, 2000.
13. Lovett JK, Dennis MS, Sandercock PAG, et al: High early risk of stroke after a first transient ischaemic attack [abstract]. J Neurol Neurosurg Psychiatry 74:402–403, 2003.
14. Petty GW, Brown RD, Whisnant JP, et al: Ischemic stroke subtypes: A population-based study of functional outcome, survival and recurrence. Stroke 31:1062–1068, 2000.
15. Warlow CP, Dennis MS, van Gijn J, et al: Is it a vascular event and where is the lesion? Identifying and interpreting the symptoms and signs of cerebrovascular disease. In Stroke: A Practical Guide to Management. Oxford, Blackwell Science, 2001, pp 28–105.
16. Collaborative meta-analysis of randomised trials of antiplatelet therapy for the prevention of death, MI, and stroke in high risk patients. Antithrombotic Trialists' Collaboration. BMJ 324:71–86, 2002.
17. Collaborative overview of randomised trials of antiplatelet therapy—I: Prevention of death, MI, and stroke by prolonged antiplatelet therapy in various categories of patients. Antiplatelet Trialists' Collaboration. BMJ 308:81–106, 1994.
18. Bamford J, Sandercock P, Dennis M, et al: A prospective study of acute cerebrovascular disease in the community: The Oxfordshire Community Stroke Project, 1981–1986: Incidence, case fatality rates and overall outcome at one year of cerebral infarction, primary intracerebral haemorrhage and subarachnoid haemorrhage. J Neurol Neurosurg Psychiatry 53:16–22, 1990.
19. Roderick PJ, Wilkes HC, Meade TW: The gastrointestinal toxicity of aspirin: An overview of randomised controlled trials. Br J Clin Pharmacol 35:219–26, 1993.
20. Dyken ML, Barnett HJM, Easton D, et al: Low-dose aspirin and stroke: "It ain't necessarily so." Stroke 23:1395–1399, 1992.
21. Barnett HJM, Kaste M, Meldrum H, Eliasziw M: Aspirin dose in stroke prevention: Beautiful hypotheses slain by ugly facts. Stroke 27:588–592, 1996.
22. Patrono C, Roth G: Aspirin in ischemic cerebrovascular disease: How strong is the case for a different dosing regimen? Stroke 27:756–760, 1996.
23. Fields WS, Lemak NA, Frankowski RF, Hardy RJ: Controlled trial of aspirin in cerebral ischemia. Stroke 8:301–314, 1977.
24. Fields WS, Lemak NA, Frankowski RF, Hardy RJ: Controlled trial of aspirin in cerebral ischemia. Part II: Surgical group. Stroke 9:309–318, 1978.
25. A randomized trial of aspirin and sulfinpyrazone in threatened stroke. Canadian Co-operative Study Group. N Engl J Med 299:53–59, 1978.
26. Patrono C: Aspirin as an antiplatelet drug. N Engl J Med 330:1287–1294, 1994.
27. Patrono C, Coller B, Dalen JE, et al: Platelet-active drugs: The relationship among dose, effectiveness, and side effects. Chest 114(Suppl):470S–88S, 1998.
28. Swedish aspirin low-dose trial (SALT) of 75mg aspirin as secondary prophylaxis after cerebrovascular ischaemic events. SALT Collaborative Group. Lancet 338:1345–1349, 1991.
29. Diener HC, Cunha L, Forbes C, et al: European stroke prevention study 2: Dipyridamole and acetylsalicylic acid in the secondary prevention of stroke. J Neurol Sci 143:1–13, 1996.
30. A comparison of two doses of aspirin (30mg vs 283mg a day) in patients after a transient ischemic attack or minor ischemic stroke. Dutch TIA Trial Study Group. N Engl J Med 325:1261–1266, 1991.
31. Taylor DW, Barnett HJM, Haynes RB, et al: Low-dose and high-dose acetylsalicylic acid for patients undergoing carotid endarterectomy: A randomised controlled trial. Lancet 353:2179–2184, 1999.

32. He J, Whelton PK, Vu B, Klag MJ: Aspirin and risk of hemorrhagic stroke: A meta-analysis of randomized controlled trials. JAMA 280:1930–1935, 1998.

33. Derry S, Loke YK: Risk of gastrointestinal haemorrhage with long term use of aspirin: A meta-analysis. BMJ 321:1183–1187, 2000.

34. The United Kingdom transient ischaemic attack (UK-TIA) aspirin trial: Final results. UK-TIA Study Group. J Neurol Neurosurg Psychiatry 54:1044–1054, 1991.

35. Sudlow C: Update on antiplatelet drugs. Proc R Coll Physicians Edinb 31(Suppl 8):6–10, 2001.

36. García Rodríguez LA, Hernández-Díaz S, de Abajo FJ: Association between aspirin and upper gastrointestinal complications: Systematic review of epidemiologic studies. Br J Clin Pharmacol 52:563–571, 2001.

37. Collins R, MacMahon S: Reliable assessment of the effects of treatment on mortality and major morbidity. I: Clinical trials. Lancet 357:373–380, 2001.

38. Gent M, Beaumont D, Blanchard J, et al: A randomised, blinded, trial of clopidogrel versus aspirin in patients at risk of ischaemic events (CAPRIE). Lancet 348:1329–1338, 1996.

39. Hankey GJ, Sudlow CLM, Dunbabin DW: Thienopyridines or aspirin to prevent stroke and other serious vascular events in patients at high risk of vascular disease? A systematic review of the evidence from randomized trials. Stroke 31:1779–1784, 2000.

40. Hankey GJ, Sudlow CLM, Dunbabin DW: Thienopyridine derivatives (ticlopidine, clopidogrel) versus aspirin in preventing stroke and other serious vascular events in high vascular risk patients. Cochrane Database Syst Rev CD001246, 2003.

41. Moloney BA: An analysis of the side effects of ticlopidine. In Hass WK, Easton JD (eds): Ticlopidine, Platelets and Vascular Disease. New York, Springer, 1993, pp 117–139.

42. Bennett CL, Davidson CJ, Raisch DW, et al: Thrombotic thrombocytopenic purpura associated with ticlopidine in the stenting of coronary artery stents and stroke prevention. Arch Intern Med 159:2524–2528, 1999.

43. Bennett CL, Connors JM, Carwile JM, et al: Thrombotic thrombocytopenic purpura associated with clopidogrel. N Engl J Med 342:1773–1777, 2000.

44. Hankey GJ: Clopidogrel and thrombotic thrombocytopenic purpura. Lancet 356:269–270, 2000.

45. Müller C, Büttner HJ, Petersen J, Roskamm H: A randomized comparison of clopidogrel and aspirin versus ticlopidine and aspirin after the placement of coronary-artery stents. Circulation 101:590–593, 2000.

46. Bertrand ME, Rupprecht H-J, Urban P, et al: Double-blind study of the safety of clopidogrel with and without a loading dose in combination with aspirin compared with ticlopidine in combination with aspirin after coronary stenting. The Clopidogrel Aspirin Stent International Cooperative Study (CLASSICS). Circulation 102:624–629, 2000.

47. Taniuchi M, Kurz H, Lasala JM. Randomized comparison of ticlopidine and clopidogrel after intracoronary stent implantation in a broad patient population. Circulation 104:539–543, 2001.

48. Gorelick PB, Richardson D, Kelly M, et al: Aspirin and ticlopidine for prevention of recurrent stroke in black patients: A randomized trial. The African-American Antiplatelet Stroke Prevention Study (AAASPS). JAMA 289:2947–2957, 2003.

49. Born GVR, Collins R: Aspirin versus clopidogrel: The wrong question? Lancet 349:806, 1997.

50. Effects of clopidogrel in addition to aspirin in patients with acute coronary syndromes without ST-segment elevation. The Clopidogrel in Unstable Angina to Prevent Recurrent Events (CURE) Trial Investigators. N Engl J Med 345:494–502, 2001.

51. Steinhubl SR, Berger PB, Mann JT, et al: Early and sustained dual oral antiplatelet therapy following percutaneous coronary intervention: A randomized controlled trial. The CREDO Investigators. JAMA 288:2411–2420, 2002.

52. Rationale, design and organisation of the Second Chinese Cardiac Study (CCS-2): A randomised trial of clopidogrel plus aspirin, and of metoprolol, among patients with suspected acute MI. Second Chinese Cardiac Study (CCS-2) Collaborative Group. J Cardiovasc Risk 7:435–441, 2000.

53. Clopidogrel for High Atherothrombotic Risk and Ischemic Stabilization, Management and Avoidance (CHARISMA). Information available online at: http://www.clinicaltrials.gov

54. Major ongoing stroke trials: Management of ATherothrombosis with Clopidogrel in High-risk patients with recent transient ischemic attack or ischemic stroke (MATCH). Stroke 33:1733, 2002.

55. Major ongoing stroke trials: Anticoagulants versus aspirin and the combination of aspirin and dipyridamole versus aspirin only in patients with transient ischemic attacks or nondisabling ischemic stroke: ESPRIT (European/Australian Stroke Prevention in Reversible Ischemia Trial). Stroke 33:1728, 2002.

56. Sandercock P, Mielke O, Lui M, Counsell C: Anticoagulants for preventing recurrence following presumed non-cardioembolic ischaemic stroke or transient ischaemic attack. Cochrane Syst Database Rev CD000248, 2003.

57. A randomized trial of anticoagulants versus aspirin after cerebral ischemia of presumed arterial origin. The Stroke Prevention in Reversible Ischemia Trial (SPIRIT) Study Group. Ann Neurol 42:857–865, 1997.

58. Algra A, De Schryver ELLM, van Gijn J, et al: Oral anticoagulants versus antiplatelet therapy for preventing further vascular events after transient ischaemic attack or minor stroke of presumed arterial origin. Cochrane Database Syst Rev CD001342, 2003.

59. Hankey GJ: Warfarin-Aspirin Recurrent Stroke Study (WARSS) trial: Is warfarin really a reasonable alternative to aspirin for preventing recurrent noncardioembolic ischemic stroke? Stroke 33:1723–1726, 2002.

60. Mohr JP, Thompson JLP, Lazar RM, et al: A comparison of warfarin and aspirin for the prevention of recurrent ischemic stroke. The Warfarin-Aspirin Recurrent Stroke Study Group. N Engl J Med 345:1444–1451, 2001.

61. Major ongoing stroke trials: Warfarin vs Aspirin for Symptomatic Intracranial Disease (WASID). Stroke 33:1737, 2002.

62. Internet Stroke Center Stroke Trials Directory. Available online at http://www.strokecenter.org/trials/

63. Chen ZM, Sandercock P, Pan HC, et al: Indications for early aspirin use in acute ischemic stroke: A combined analysis of 40,000 randomized patients from the Chinese Acute Stroke Trial and the International Stroke Trial. On behalf of the CAST and IST collaborative groups. Stroke 31:1240–1249, 2000.

64. Cambria-Kiely JA, Ghandi PJ: Possible mechanisms of aspirin resistance. J Thrombos Thrombolys 13:49–56, 2002.

65. Eikelboom JW, Hirsh J, Weitz JI, et al: Aspirin-resistant thromboxane biosynthesis and the risk of MI, stroke, or cardiovascular death in patients at high risk for cardiovascular events. Circulation 105:16650–1655, 2002.

66. Gum PA, Kottke-Marchant K, Poggio ED, et al: Profile and prevalence of aspirin resistance in patients with cardiovascular disease. Am J Cardiol 88:230–235, 2001.

67. MacMahon S, Peto R, Cutler J, et al: Blood pressure, stroke, and coronary heart disease. Part 1: Prolonged differences in blood pressure: Prospective observational studies corrected for the regression dilution bias. Lancet 335:765–774, 1990.

68. Age-specific relevance of usual blood pressure to vascular mortality: A meta-analysis of individual data for one million adults in 61 prospective studies. Prospective Studies Collaboration. Lancet 360:1903–1913, 2002.

69. Blood pressure, cholesterol and stroke in eastern Asia. Eastern Stroke and Coronary Heart Disease Collaborative Group. Lancet 352:1801–1807, 1998.

70. Collins R, MacMahon S: Blood pressure, antihypertensive drug treatment, and the risks of stroke and of coronary heart disease. Br Med Bull 50:272–298, 1994.

71. Psaty BM, Smith NL, Siscovick DS, et al: Health outcomes associated with antihypertensive therapies used as first-line agents: A systematic review and meta-analysis. JAMA 277:739–745, 1997.

72. Wright JM, Lee C-H, Chambers GK: Systematic review of antihypertensive therapies: Does the evidence exist in choosing a first-line drug? Can Med Assoc J 161:25–32, 1999.

73. Staessen JA, Wang J-G, Thijs L: Cardiovascular protection and blood pressure reduction: A meta-analysis. Lancet 358:1305–1315, 2001.

74. Effects of ACE inhibitors, calcium channel antagonists, and other blood-pressure–lowering drugs: Results of prospectively designed overviews of randomised trials. Blood Pressure Lowering Treatment Trialists' Collaboration. Lancet 356:1955–1964, 2000.

75. Irie K, Yamaguchi T, Minematsu K, Omae T: The J-curve phenomenon in stroke recurrence. Stroke 24:1844–1849, 1993.

76. Rodgers A, MacMahon S, Gamble G, et al: Blood pressure and risk of stroke in patients with cerebrovascular disease. The United Kingdom Transient Ischaemic Attack Collaborative Group. BMJ 313:417, 1996.

77. Carlsson A, Britton M: Blood pressure after stroke. Stroke 24:195–199, 1993.

78. Carter AB: Hypotensive therapy in stroke survivors. Lancet 7645:1485–1489, 1970.

79. Effect of antihypertensive treatment on stroke recurrence. Hypertension Stroke Cooperative Study Group. JAMA 229:409–418, 1974.

80. Trial of secondary prevention with atenolol after transient ischemic attack or non-disabling ischemic stroke. Dutch TIA Trial Study Group. Stroke 24:543–548, 1993.

81. Eriksson S, Olofsson BO, Wester PO: Atenolol in secondary prevention after stroke. The TEST study group. Cerebrovasc Dis 5:21–25, 1995.

82. Blood pressure lowering for the secondary prevention of stroke: Rationale and design for PROGRESS. PROGRESS Management Committee. J Hypertens 14(Suppl 2):S39–S46, 1996.

83. Post-stroke Antihypertensive Treatment Study: A preliminary result. PATS Collaborating Group. Chinese Med J 108:710–717, 1995.

84. PROGRESS—Perindopril Protection Against Recurrent Stroke Study: Characteristics of the study population at baseline. PROGRESS Management Committee. J Hypertens 17:1647–1655, 1999.

85. Randomised trial of a perindopril-based blood-pressure–owering regimen among 6105 individuals with previous stroke or transient ischaemic attack. PROGRESS Collaborative Group. Lancet 358:1033–1041, 2001.

86. Effects of an angiotensin-converting-enzyme inhibitor, ramipril, on cardiovascular events in high-risk patients. The Heart Outcomes Prevention Evaluation Study Investigators. N Engl J Med 342:145–153, 2000.

87. Bosch J, Yusuf S, Pogue J, et al: Use of ramipril in preventing stroke: Double blind randomised trial. The HOPE Investigators. BMJ 324:1–5, 2002.

88. Sleight P, Yusuf S, Pogue J, et al: Blood pressure reduction and cardiovascular risk in HOPE. The Heart Outcomes Prevention Evaluation (HOPE) Study Investigators. Lancet 358:2130–2131, 2001.

89. Svensson P, de Faire U, Sleight P, et al: Comparative effects of ramipril on ambulatory and office blood pressures: A HOPE substudy. Hypertension 38:e28–e32, 2001.

90. Cholesterol, diastolic blood pressure, and stroke: 13,000 strokes in 450,000 people in 45 prospective cohorts. Prospective Studies Collaboration. Lancet 346:1647–1653, 1995.

91. Acheson J, Hutchinson EC: Controlled trial of clofibrate in cerebral vascular disease. Atherosclerosis 15:177–183, 1972.

92. The treatment of cerebrovascular disease with clofibrate. Veterans Administration Cooperative Study Group. Stroke 4:684–693, 1973.

93. Hebert PR, Gaziano JM, Hennekens CH: An overview of trials of cholesterol lowering and risk of stroke. Arch Intern Med 155:50–55, 1995.

94. Sudlow C: Stroke prevention: Cholesterol reduction. Clin Evid 9:226–227, 2003.

95. Di Maschio R, Marchioli R, Tognoni G: Cholesterol reduction and stroke occurrence: An overview of randomized clinical trials. Cerebrovasc Dis 10:85–92, 2000.

96. Rubins HB, Robins SJ, Collins D, et al: Gemfibrozil for the secondary prevention of coronary heart disease in men with low levels of high-density lipoprotein cholesterol. N Engl J Med 341:410–418, 1999.

97. Hebert PR, Gaziano JM, Chan KS, Hennekens CH: Cholesterol lowering with statin drugs, risk of stroke, and total mortality: An overview of randomized trials. JAMA 278:313–321, 1997.

98. MRC/BHF Heart Protection Study of cholesterol lowering with simvastatin in 20 536 high-risk individuals: A randomised placebo-controlled trial. Heart Protection Study Collaborative Group. Lancet 360:7–22, 2002.

99. Shepherd J, Blauw GJ, Murphy MB, et al: Pravastatin in elderly individuals at risk of vascular disease (PROSPER): A randomised controlled trial. The PROSPER study group. Lancet 360:1623–1230, 2002.

100. The ALLHAT officers and coordinators for the ALLHAT collaborative research group: Major outcomes in moderately hypercholesterolemic, hyperten-sive patients randomized to pravastatin versus usual care. The Antihypertensive and Lipid-Lowering Treatment to Prevent Heart Attack Trial (ALLHAT-LLT). JAMA 288:2998–3007, 2002.

101. Sever PS, Dahlöf B, Poulter NR, et al: Prevention of coronary and stroke events with atorvastatin in hypertensive patients who have average or lower-than-average cholesterol concentrations, in the Anglo-Scandinavian Cardiac Outcome Trial–Lipid Lowering Arm (ASCOT-LLA): A multicentre randomized controlled trial. Lancet 361:1149–1158, 2003.

102. Armitage J: Cholesterol lowering for the prevention of stroke. Practical Neurology 3:224–233, 2003.

103. Collins R, Armitage J: High-risk elderly patients PROSPER from cholesterol-lowering therapy. Lancet 360:1618–1619, 2002.

104. Protocol for a prospective collaborative overview of all current and planned randomized trials of cholesterol treatment regimens. Cholesterol Treatment Trialists' (CTT) Collaboration. Am J Cardiol 75:1130–1134, 1995.

105. Major ongoing stroke trials: Stroke Prevention by Aggressive Reduction in Cholesterol Levels (SPARCL). Stroke 33:1736, 2002.

106. Laakso M, Lehto S: Epidemiology of macrovascular disease in diabetes. Diabetes Rev 5:294–315, 1997.

107. Kanters SDJM, Banga J-D, Stolk RP, Algra A: Incidence and determinants of mortality and cardiovascular events in diabetes mellitus: A meta-analysis. Vasc Med 4:67–75, 1000.

108. Beckman JA, Creager MA, Libby P: Diabetes and atherosclerosis: Epidemiology, pathophysiology, and management. JAMA 287:2570–2581, 2002.

109. Herman W: Glycaemic control in diabetes. Clin Evid (7):523–557, 2002.

110. Malcolm J, Meggison H, Sigal R: Cardiovascular disease in diabetes. Clin Evid (8):541–568, 2002.

111. Boushey CJ, Beresford SA, Omenn GS, Motulsky AG: A quantitative assessment of plasma homocysteine as a risk factor for vascular disease: Probable benefits of increasing folic acid intake. JAMA 274:1049–1057, 1995.

112. Eikelboom JW, Lonn E, Genest J, et al: Homocysteine and cardiovascular disease: A critical review of the epidemiologic evidence. Ann Intern Med 131:363–375, 1999.

113. Perry IJ: Homocysteine and risk of stroke. J Cardiovasc Risk 4:235–240, 1999.

114. Lowering blood homocysteine with folic acid based supplements: Meta-analysis of randomised trials. Homocysteine Lowering Trialists' Collaboration. BMJ 316:894–898, 1998.

115. Major ongoing stroke trials: Vitamin Intervention for Stroke Prevention (VISP). Stroke 33:1736, 2002.

116. The VITATOPS (Vitamins to Prevent Stroke) Trial: Rationale and design of an international, large, simple, randomised trial of homocysteine-lowering multivitamin therapy in patients with recent transient ischaemic attack or stroke. The VITATOPS Trial Study Group. Cerebrovasc Dis 13:120–126, 2002.

117. Lonn EM, Yusuf S: Is there a role for antioxidant vitamins in the prevention of cardiovascular diseases? An update on epidemiological and clinical trials data. Can J Cardiol 13:957–965, 1997.

118. Ness AR, Powles JW, Khaw KT: Vitamin C and cardiovascular disease: A systematic review. J Cardiovasc Risk 3:513–521, 1997.

119. Ness A, Powles J: The role of diet, fruit and vegetables and antioxidants in the aetiology of stroke. J Cardiovasc Risk 6:229–234, 1999.

120. Hooper L, Ness AR, Davey Smith G: Antioxidant strategy for cardiovascular diseases. Lancet 357:1705, 2001.

121. Sudlow C, Lonn E, Pignone M, et al: Secondary prevention of ischaemic cardiac events. Clin Evid 9:166–205, 2003.

122. MRC/BHF Heart Protection Study of antioxidant vitamin supplementation in 20,536 high-risk individuals: A randomised placebo-controlled trial. Heart Protection Study Collaborative Group. Lancet 360:23–33, 2002.

123. Beral V, Banks E, Reeves G: Evidence from randomised trials on the long-term effects of hormone replacement therapy. Lancet 360:942–944, 2002.

124. Rossouw JE: Hormones for coronary disease—full circle. Lancet 360:1996–1997, 2002.

125. Oestrogen therapy for prevention of reinfarction in postmenopausal women: A randomised placebo controlled trial. The ESPRIT team. Lancet 360:2001–2008, 2002.

126. Ezzati M, Lopez A, Rodgers A, et al: Selected major risk factors and global and regional burden of disease. The Comparative Risk Assessment Collaborative Group. Lancet 360:1347–1360, 2002.

127. Murphy M, Foster C, Sudlow C, et al: Primary prevention. Clin Evid 9:132–165, 2003.

128. Rice VH, Stead LF: Nursing interventions for smoking cessation. Cochrane Database Syst Rev CD001188, 2003.

129. Silagy C, Stead LF. Physician advice for smoking cessation. Cochrane Database Syst Rev CD000165, 2003.

130. Lancaster T, Stead LF: Individual behavioural counselling for smoking cessation. Cochrane Database Syst Rev CD001292, 2003.

131. Stead LF, Lancaster T: Group behaviour therapy programmes for smoking cessation. Cochrane Database Syst Rev CD001007, 2003.

132. Silagy C, Lancaster T, Stead L, et al: Nicotine replacement therapy for smoking cessation. Cochrane Database Syst Rev CD000146, 2003.

133. Hughes JR, Stead LF, Lancaster T: Antidepressants for smoking cessation. Cochrane Database Syst Rev CD000031, 2003.

134. Thorogood M, Hillsdon M, Summerbell C: Cardiovascular disorders: Changing behaviour. Clin Evid 9:72–94, 2003.

135. Murphy M, Foster C, Sudlow C, et al: Primary prevention. Clin Evid 9:132–165, 2003.

136. Murphy M, Foster C, Sudlow C, et al: Primary prevention. Clin Evid 9:132–165, 2003.

137. Murphy M, Foster C, Sudlow C, et al: Primary prevention. Clin Evid 9:132–165, 2003.

138. Doll R: One for the heart. BMJ 315:1664–1668, 1997.

139. Hillbom M, Juvela S, Numminen H: Alcohol intake and risk of stroke. J Cardiovasc Risk 6:223–228, 1999.

140. Berger K, Ajani UA, Kase CS, et al: Light-to-moderate alcohol consumption and the risk of stroke among US male physicians. N Engl J Med 341:1557–1564, 1999.

141. Hommel M, Jaillard A: Alcohol for stroke prevention? N Engl J Med 341:1605–1606, 1999.

142. Gaziano JM, Gaziano TA, Glynn RJ, et al: Light-to-moderate alcohol consumption and mortality in the Physicians' Health Study enrollment cohort. J Am Coll Cardiol 35:96–105, 2000.

143. Rimm EB, Williams P, Fosher K, et al: Moderate alcohol intake and lower risk of coronary heart disease: Meta-analysis of effects on lipids and haemostatic factors. BMJ 319:1523–1528, 1999.

144. Rothwell PM, Eliasziw M, Gutnikov S, et al: Analysis of pooled data from the randomised controlled trials of carotid endarterectomy for symptomatic carotid stenosis. Lancet 361:107–116, 2003.

145. Rothwell PM, Warlow CP: Prediction of benefit from carotid endarterectomy in individual patients: A risk-modelling study. The European Carotid Surgery Trialists' Collaborative Group. Lancet 353:2105–2110, 1999.

146. Randomised trial of endarterectomy for recently symptomatic carotid stenosis: Final results of the MRC European Carotid Surgery Trial (ECST). European Carotid Surgery Trialists' Collaborative Group. Lancet 351:1379–1387, 1998.

147. Mead GE, Lewis SC, Wardlaw JM, et al: Severe ipsilateral carotid stenosis and middle cerebral artery disease in lacunar ischaemic stroke: Innocent bystanders? J Neurol 249:266–271, 2002.

148. Inizitari D, Eliasziw M, Sharpe BL, et al: Risk factors and outcome of patients with carotid artery stenosis presenting with lacunar stroke. The North American Symptomatic Carotid Endarterectomy Trial Group. Neurology 54:660–666, 2000.

149. Rothwell PM, Pendlebury ST, Wardlaw JM, Warlow CP: A critical appraisal of the design and reporting of studies of imaging and measurement of carotid stenosis. Stroke 31:1444–1450, 2000.

150. Zweibel WJ: Duplex carotid sonography. In Zweibel WJ (ed): Introduction to Vascular Ultrasonography, 3rd ed. Philadelphia, WB Saunders, 1992.

151. Patel SG, Collie D, Wardlaw JM, et al: Outcome, observer reliability, and patient preferences if CTA, MRA, or Doppler ultrasound were used, individually or together, instead of digital subtraction angiography before carotid endarterectomy. J Neurol Neurosurg Psychiatry 73:21–28, 2002.

152. Endovascular versus surgical treatment in patients with carotid stenosis in the Carotid and Vertebral Transluminal Angioplasty Study (CAVATAS): A randomised trial. CAVATAS Investigators. Lancet 357:1729–1737, 2001.

153. Major ongoing stroke trials: Carotid Revascularization Endarterectomy versus Stenting Trial (CREST). Stroke 33:1730, 2002.

154. Major ongoing stroke trials: International Carotid Stenting Study (ICSS). Stroke 33:1732, 2002.

Chapter Fifty-Nine

Carotid Stenting

Gary S. Roubin, Sriram S. Iyer, Jiri J. Vitek, and Giora Weisz

Carotid artery stenting has evolved rapidly over the last decade and is currently being practiced in many medical centers. Since the pioneering work of Dotter[1] and Gruentzig[2] on percutaneous vascular intervention some 30 years ago, few procedures have met the vigorous scrutiny and criticism that has been encountered by carotid artery stenting. Given the potential for procedural neurologic complications and the existence of a well-validated surgical therapy, caution has always been warranted. But in the case of carotid artery stenting, opposition based on less valid motives[3] has caused delays in the federal approval of advanced devices and techniques, slowed progress in clinical trials, created confusion in reimbursement policy, and has resulted in inequitable access for patients who might benefit. Despite resistance, carotid artery stenting has become widely accepted as a viable alternative to carotid endarterectomy (CEA). In this chapter, we review the development of the technique, the clinical and technical management of patients who undergo carotid artery stenting, current results, and future directions.

HISTORICAL PERSPECTIVE

Pioneered in the early 1950s, CEA has been demonstrated in at least three prospective randomized trials to reduce the risk of stroke in patients with carotid stenoses.[4-6] These trials, not completed until the late 1980s and early 1990s, confirmed the large body of prospective observational data that suggested a benefit for surgery over medical therapy, depending on symptom status and severity of stenosis. Millions of patients were treated by competent surgeons before the availability of data from these randomized trials and likely benefited from the operation. The trial data confirmed the view that if periprocedural stroke and mortality risk was low, patients benefited. Rigorous prospective multicenter trials however, documented a significant perioperative risk not generally highlighted by the surgeons. In the North American Symptomatic Carotid Endarterectomy Trial (NASCET), perioperative cranial nerve damage (5.6%), medical complications (8.1%), myocardial infarction (1.2%), and congestive heart failure (1.2%) characterized the adverse events associated with an open surgical procedure that usually required general anesthesia.

The mission to develop safer, percutaneous solutions to arterial stenoses was pioneered by Dotter[1] and Gruentzig[2];

by 1980, interventional radiologists were cautiously treating the brachiocephalic and carotid arteries. Mathias and colleagues[7] first reported balloon angioplasty of the carotid bifurcation. In 1983, Vitek and associates[8] described angioplasty of the innominate artery with distal occlusion balloon protection of the common carotid artery (CCA). In 1986, Russian investigators Rabkin and coworkers[9] described the use of primitive nitinol stents in the carotid artery, and Theron and coworkers[10] began pivotal work with distal balloon protection during carotid bifurcation angioplasty.

As was the case with other arterial sites,[11] the evolution and availability of arterial stents transformed Gruentzig's less predictable balloon procedure, and by the early 1990s, prospective observational studies of carotid artery stenting had been initiated.[12,13] Careful patient selection and technique minimized neurologic complications, and from the outset, carotid artery stenting performed by experienced operators produced acceptable outcomes in terms of low rates of disabling periprocedural stroke and death (both less than 1%). Nondisabling neurologic events (7%) were evident, being more common in patients with advanced age and more complex and severe stenoses.[14]

All of the carotid artery stenting studies were initiated with prospective preprocedure and postprocedure (24-hour) evaluation of patients by a board-certified neurologist and completion of an objective National Institutes of Health Stroke Scale (NIHSS) data form. This level of rigorous adjudication had never been applied to CEA. The NASCET and Asymptomatic Carotid Atherosclerosis Study (ACAS) involved independent prospective neurologic evaluation of patients at 30 days after surgery. In addition, early studies were heavily biased towards patients at high risk of an adverse event because of their general medical status and risk profile for CEA. It became clear early in the development of carotid artery stenting that comparable patient selection and equivalent documentation of adverse events would be necessary to a fair comparison of the procedure with CEA.

The incidence of emboli-induced nondisabling neurologic events was not entirely unexpected, given the nature of the carotid lesion. This situation led to the development of embolic protection techniques and devices and expertise in patient selection to limit the occurrence of such events. In Europe, Henry and associates[15] perfected Theron's technique with a low-profile occlusion balloon system for embolic protection, and Iyer and colleagues independently developed distal embolic filter devices, a concept proposed earlier by Wholey.[15a] Parodi and coworkers[20] focused on proximal occlusion devices that facilitated embolic protection by temporarily reversing flow in the internal carotid artery (ICA).

Availability of embolic protection systems and randomized data from the Carotid and Vertebral Artery Transluminal Angioplasty Study (CAVATAS)[16] dramatically increased interest in carotid artery stenting. This study was completed without embolic protection, and "bail-out" stenting was used in only about 30% of patients. Although periprocedural neurological complications were higher than would be expected today with distal embolic protection, they were not different from those observed in the surgical cohort. This first "head-to-head" comparison of CEA and carotid artery stenting in comparable patients randomly assigned to treatment was encouraging and engendered interest in carotid artery stenting.

After the availability of embolic protection systems, many single-center studies and multicenter registries confirmed the ability of experienced operators to achieve good results from carotid artery stenting with a remarkably low risk of stroke and death.[15,17–24] The simplicity of this less invasive approach and the acceptable low morbidity have accelerated its acceptance in many medical centers.

INDICATIONS

In general, the indications for intervention with carotid artery stenting are similar to those for carotid surgery with respect to symptomatic status and severity of carotid artery stenosis. The American Heart Association/Society for Vascular Surgery (AHA/SVS) guidelines for CEA apply to stenting; accordingly, individual operator experience and documented 30-day outcomes must be known before an informed decision can be made about a treatment option.

This approach to patient management is based on documented prospective outcomes assessment from many experienced operators and centers that we discuss later in the chapter. It also assumes that the prospective multicenter randomized studies now in progress will continue to support at least equivalence if not superiority of carotid artery stenting in relation to CEA in terms of 30-day outcomes. If prospective independent neurologic audit at any center shows, for example, in a group of surgically eligible symptomatic or asymptomatic patients, that the 30-day death and disabling stroke rate is less than 1% and total 30-day neurologic event rate is less than 3%, stenting should be an attractive therapeutic option.

There are notable exceptions to these therapeutic principles. Some subsets of patients are being recognized as better candidates for stenting, and others as better candidates for CEA. It is now becoming important for the neurologic community to understand the relative indications and contraindications. Patients who have comorbid medical conditions that increase their risk from an open surgical approach or the use of general anesthesia are one important group who probably should be primary candidates for stenting. On the basis of the results of the Stenting & Angioplasty with Protection in Patients at High Risk for Endarterectomy (SAPPHIRE) study,[25] these conditions include advanced age, cardiac and pulmonary disease, and a variety of other medical disabilities (Table 59.1).

In addition, any condition that raises the risk of operative exposure also represents a probable indication for stenting. Such conditions are prior ipsilateral endarterectomy, prior neck dissection or irradiation, high lesions that need extensive cephalad dissection, and low lesions that require thoracic exposure. Patients with contralateral carotid artery occlusion also should be included in this group, given their inclusion in the SAPPHIRE study and the documented 14% rate of 30-day mortality and stroke in this subset of patients in NASCET. Even the most facile surgeon takes a few minutes to shunt lesions during CEA. For patients with "isolated hemispheres" (i.e., with limited collateral flow), neurologic consequences are not unexpected. The use of embolic protection filters during stenting facilitates constant perfusion of the brain. Balloon inflation used during stenting is necessary for only 10 seconds to 20 seconds. Another advantage of stenting is that the angiographic status (anatomy, collateral circulation, intact circle of Willis, intracranial lesions, and flow characteristics) is usually well defined during or before the stenting procedure. For experienced operators, the risk of angiography is minimal, and as stent use increases, so will the angiographic skills and experience in the interventional community.

Although not emphasized in carotid surgery trials, the incidences of cranial nerve damage, wound hematoma, and infection were significant and must be considered before a patient is referred for neck surgery. Additionally, complications from the general anesthesia that is still being utilized in 90% of CEA procedures performed in the United States must be carefully weighed. Although the risk of stroke or death favored stenting in all categories in the SAPPHIRE study, the number of events did not allow the difference to reach statistical significance.[25] Perioperative myocardial infarction, however, was twice as common for patients undergoing surgery as for those undergoing

Table 59.1 Conditions That Raise Surgical Risk for Carotid Endarterectomy

- Congestive heart failure (class III or IV) and/or severe left ventricular dysfunction with ejection fraction <30%
- Open heart surgery needed within 6 weeks
- Recent myocardial infarction (>24 hours and <4 weeks)
- Unstable angina (Canadian Cardiovascular Society class III or IV)
- Severe pulmonary disease
- Contralateral carotid occlusion
- Contralateral laryngeal nerve palsy
- Radiation therapy
- Previous ipsilateral carotid endarterectomy with recurrent stenosis
- Higher cervical internal carotid artery lesions or common carotid artery lesions below the clavicle
- Severe tandem lesions not easily accessible by surgery
- Patient age >80 years

stenting, and overall, complication rates significantly favored stenting.

Carotid artery stenting also has a number of notable relative contraindications (Table 59.2). The experience with stenting over the last decade has defined the circumstances that raise the risk of the procedure. First, patients who are intolerant of or allergic to a combination of antiplatelet agents may be more safely managed with endarterectomy. Experience has shown that a combination of aspirin and clopidogrel or aspirin and ticlopidine is mandatory adjunctive therapy to prevent platelet aggregation and embolization during and for at least 3 to 4 weeks after stenting. The details of how these agents should be administered are discussed later.

Similarly, if there is has a compelling reason for a patient to undergo a major surgical procedure within 3 weeks to 4 weeks that will require the cessation of antiplatelet therapy, endarterectomy may be a better option. The most common clinical situation in which this is encountered is the patient with critical carotid disease and critical coronary disease requiring coronary artery bypass grafting (CABG). Given the risks of endarterectomy in this setting or the risks of a combined procedure (CABG plus CEA), careful consideration is required. For the vast majority of patients, stenting followed by CABG in 3 to 4 weeks, after cessation of antiplatelet therapy, is the option of choice. Very few patients with coronary disease cannot be safely "settled down" for 3 to 4 weeks with aggressive antiplatelet therapy and anti-ischemic cardiac medical therapy.

In rare instances, (e.g., critical disease of the left main coronary artery in combination with critical bilateral carotid artery disease), patients must proceed to CABG soon after stenting. Carotid artery stenting may still be the initial procedure of choice. Stenting must be performed with optimal modulation of blood pressure and heart rate support and even the use of intra-aortic balloon pump support. Many cardiothoracic surgeons are able to operate successfully in a patient receiving aggressive antiplatelet therapy, but greater use of blood and blood products is usually required. It is of note that cessation of antiplatelet therapy soon after stenting and in combination with cardiac surgery has been associated with stent thrombosis.

Chronic renal failure is another relative contraindication to carotid artery stenting, although it has also been shown to raise the risk of endarterectomy. Experienced operators who are placing stents in patients with good anatomy can complete the procedure with 50 to 75 mL of contrast agent. If the patient is well hydrated and managed with mitigating adjunctive therapy, acceleration of renal failure is usually not a concern. If, however, the patient has complex vascular anatomy that may prolong the procedure and necessitate the use of large volumes of contrast agent, endarterectomy may be a safer option.

A third clinical contraindication is the presence of an extremely high-grade stenosis and a recent (<14 days) cerebral infarction. The more critical the stenosis, particularly in a hypertensive patient, the larger the volume of infarction, and the closer the time to the index event, the greater the risk of hemorrhagic conversion after the stenoses are relieved. Of course, the same risk applies to CEA. In addition, lesions that have recently embolized are typically more likely to shower debris from the unstable plaque and could potentially overwhelm embolic protection systems. Medical therapy for a period of 10 to 14 days allows the plaque and cerebral tissue to heal before intervention. The risk of cerebral hemorrhage has been mitigated by the use of minimal doses of antithrombin therapy during the procedure. Heparin, 4000 IU (activated clotting time [ACT], 200 to 300 sec), or a newer antithrombin agent, such as bivalirudin (Angiomax), may be used. Bivalirudin has been shown to be associated with lower rates of hemorrhagic complications in other types of interventions. Management of hypertension at the time the stenosis is opened is important in avoiding this devastating complication. It is noteworthy that for elective carotid artery stenting using the protocol described in this chapter, the risk of cerebral hemorrhage is less than 3 in 1000.

ANATOMIC CONTRAINDICATIONS TO STENTING

There are important relative anatomic contraindications that increase the risk of carotid artery stenting and make alternative therapies, medical or surgical, better options. The first is difficult vascular access. Stenting can be performed from a brachial approach but requires advanced skills.[26] The procedure is generally much more straightforward with femoral access; if the femoral approach is not possible because of severe occlusive vascular disease, other options should be explored. Similarly, severe diffuse disease, calcification, and tortuosity of the proximal great vessels and aortic arch make access to the carotid bifurcation difficult and dangerous (Fig. 59–1). Discrete lesions at the origins of the great vessels can be safely treated, usually in a separate index procedure before the bifurcation lesion is approached.

Severe tortuosity in the region of the carotid bifurcation is another anatomic finding that poses a high risk for stenting (Fig. 59–2). The placement of embolic protection

Table 59.2 Relative Contraindications to Stenting

Clinical contraindications	Allergy or intolerance to available combinations of antiplatelet therapy
	Absolute need for a major surgical procedure within 3 weeks
	Moderate or large ischemic or hemorrhagic stroke within 2 weeks
	Severe renal impairment and complex anatomy necessitating a >60 mL "contrast load"
Anatomic contraindications	Poor vascular access
	Diffuse and severe disease of the aortic arch vessels
	Tortuosity of the common carotid artery
	Tortuosity of the internal carotid artery
	Evidence of large volumes of mobile thrombus
	Severe concentric calcification in presence of severe tortuosity of vessels

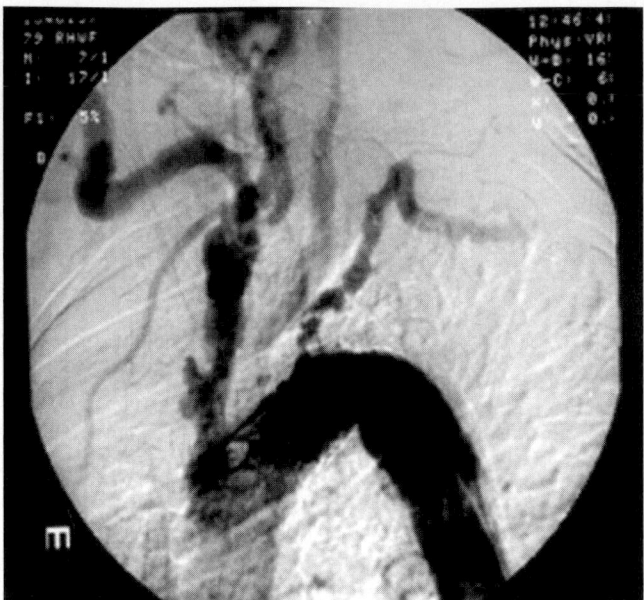

FIGURE 59–1 *Atheromatous aortic arch and proximal great vessel represents a contraindication for carotid artery stenting.*

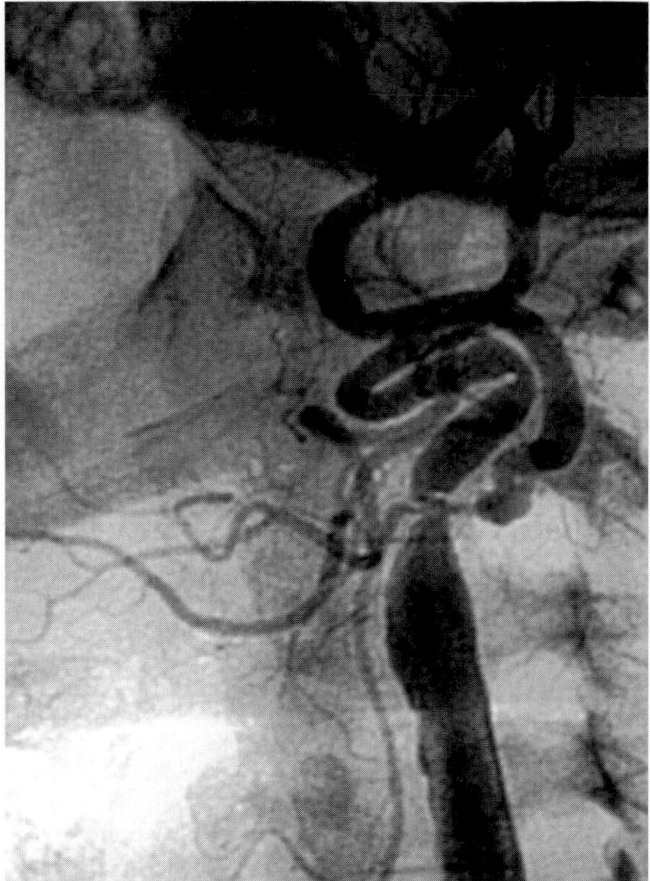

FIGURE 59–2 *This carotid artery with a significant lesion in the origin of the internal carotid artery manifests 5 adverse morphological features for carotid artery stenting: (1) Significant extension of the lesion into the common carotid artery, (2) 90 degree take-off of the ICA, (3) severe tortuosity of the ICA, (4) severe concentric calcification, and (5) luminal filling defect that may represent mobile thrombus. In combination, 2 or more of these morphological features may make the lesion unsuitable for stenting.*

systems, wire guides, and stents is much more complicated with such anatomy. The tortuosity may increase substantially after the placement of a carotid access sheath or guiding catheter (Fig. 59–3). Accordingly, the final decision to proceed with carotid artery stenting is always made after placement of the guiding sheath and final angiographic assessment of anatomy (Fig. 59–4).

Other relative anatomic contraindications are the presence of multiple, high-grade, complex lesions in a bifurcation with an acute takeoff of the ICA and severe tortuosity distal to the lesion. If the disease involves the CCA and the external carotid origin, the risks are enhanced (see Fig. 59–2). Severe calcifications further complicate the procedure. Individually, any of these features can be handled by experienced operators, but if all are present, the patient may be better treated with other therapies.

The ideal lesion for carotid artery stenting is a discrete subcritical stenosis in an up-going, straight segment of the ICA (Figs. 59–5 and 59–6). With the use of embolic protection, severe ulceration is not a contraindication, but the patient with a large mobile thrombus either should undergo surgery or should be given 3 weeks of combination antiplatelet therapy and warfarin or subcutaneous heparin before the stent procedure.

Fibromuscular dysplasia with severe stenosis, spontaneous dissection, high lesions, and diffuse disease are not contraindications to carotid artery stenting. "String sign" lesions can be treated if the distal vessel reconstitutes to a well-sized, normal appearing vessel well below the entry into the skull base and there is a clear segment in which to place an embolic protection device once the lesion is crossed. Intracranial stenoses are not a contraindication, nor is arteriovenous malformation or stable aneurysmal disease. In a patient with the last condition, close control of hypertension and modulation of anticoagulation are mandatory.

EVALUATION AND MANAGEMENT OF THE PATIENT UNDERGOING STENT PLACEMENT

Preprocedure Evaluation

The majority of patients are referred for carotid artery stenting after clinical evaluation and duplex ultrasonography have demonstrated the presence of a significant stenosis at the carotid bifurcation. Good-quality magnetic resonance angiography (MRA) studies are very helpful in evaluation the severity of the lesion and detecting the presence of other disease in the extracranial and intracranial vessels. After assessment of the relative benefits and risks of alternative strategies, the patient is scheduled for carotid angiography and stenting. Every patient is informed that if the angiographic severity of the lesions merits intervention and if the lesion is anatomically suitable, stenting will proceed in the same session. Angiography usually takes 15 to 20 minutes, and stenting 15 to 20 minutes longer.

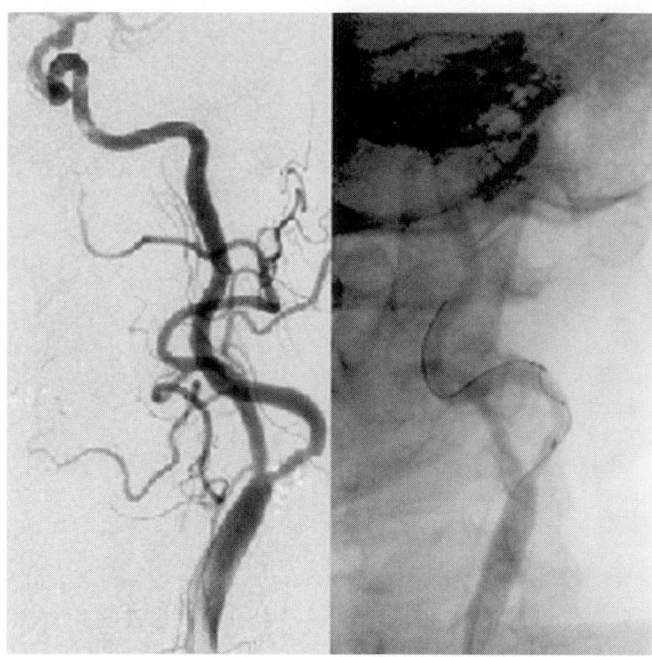

FIGURE 59–3 A, *Moderate tortuosity on initial diagnostic angiograms.* B, *After placement of the guiding sheath tortuosity is increased. In this patient with severe tortuosity of the internal carotid artery, the operator had difficulty in advancing the distal protection device.*

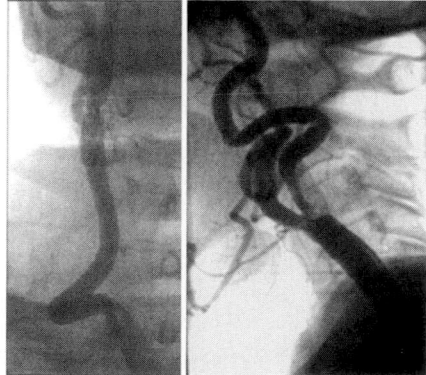

FIGURE 59–4 Left, *severe tortuosity of the proximal common carotid artery. After placement of the guiding sheath; right, tortuosity was transmitted distally, making the vessel unsuitable for stenting. In such a patient, the procedure should be terminated and patient referred for elective endarterectomy.*

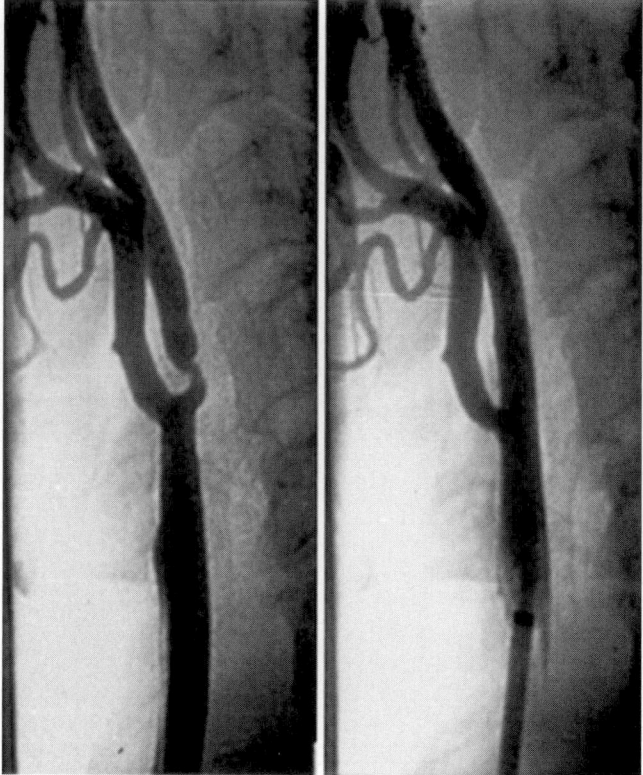

FIGURE 59–5 *An ideal lesion for carotid artery stenting. Left, an 80% post CEA restenosis. Note lack of tortuosity that may complicate the procedure; right, post stenting.*

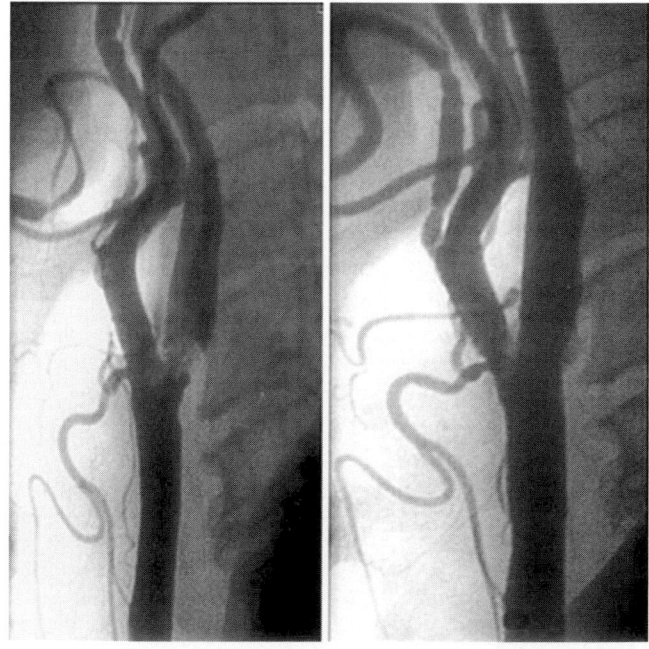

FIGURE 59–6 *Despite the presence of an ulcerated, critical lesion, the straight, up-going anatomy makes this an ideal lesion for stenting with embolic protection. Left, baseline; right, post stent.*

For experienced operators, the angiography required for carotid artery stenting is associated with minimal risk (1 in 1000) of a neurologic complication. Alternatively, it is notable that in a sizable percentage of patients referred to us with significant lesions as documented by duplex ultrasonography, MRA, or both, angiography shows insignificant stenosis according to NASCET criteria (Fig. 59–7).[27] The large majority of these patients are asymptomatic. They are discharged the same day with optimal medical therapy, and they are at no short- or intermediate-term risk of stroke. It is important to realize that if these patients had been referred to a vascular surgeon and had not under-

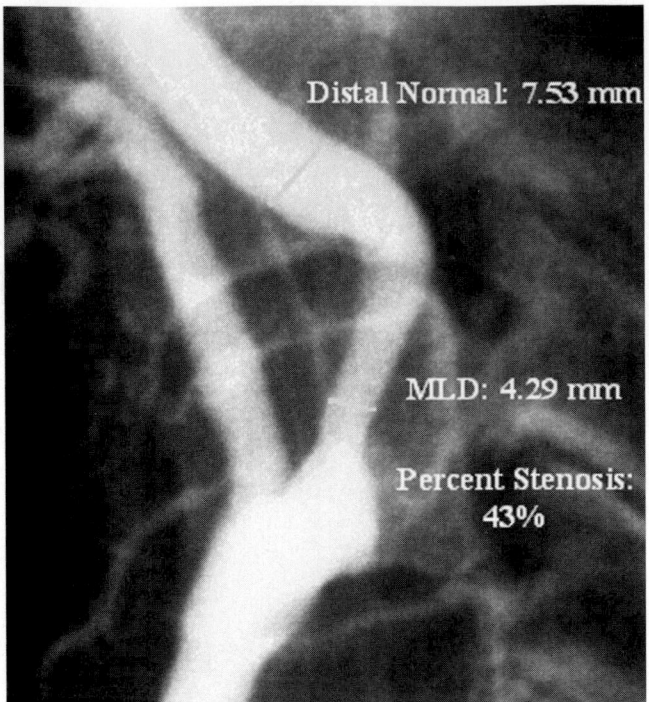

Distal Normal: 7.53 mm

MLD: 4.29 mm

Percent Stenosis: 43%

FIGURE 59–7 *Carotid angiography will reduce unnecessary CEA. This patient was referred for carotid artery stenting, based on a duplex study demonstrating a "critical" internal carotid stenosis: systolic velocity was 268mm/sec, diastolic 100mm/sec (ratio of 2.68), indicating ICA stenosis of 70–90%. Carotid angiography revealed 43% stenosis. No intervention was done, and the patient was discharged home on medical therapy, the same day. MLD, minimal lumen diameter, 4.29 mm.*

gone angiography, most would have been subjected an unnecessary operation with its attendant risks.

Of the patients with angiographically critical stenosis, approximately 5% have anatomy not suitable for stenting (usually vessel tortuosity). After angiography, such patients are discharged, to be scheduled for elective endarterectomy at an appropriate time.

General preprocedure clinical assessment includes evaluation of peripheral vascular and cardiovascular status. If evaluation of iliac and coronary anatomy is needed, it can be done at the time of carotid angiography, particularly if the interventionist is a cardiologist. Not infrequently, critical coronary stenosis is documented. When it is, a relative risk assessment is performed; coronary intervention can be prioritized as the index procedure, and the patient rescheduled for carotid intervention. Alternatively, the carotid stenosis is treated, and the patient rescheduled for subsequent coronary intervention. This type of coordinated cardiovascular assessment leads to efficient and better management of the patient's problems. Combined carotid and coronary interventions or carotid and iliac interventions can be done at the same sitting,[28,29] but for a variety of reasons, particularly procedure time and contrast agent load, they are best performed as separate procedures. Bilateral carotid stenoses can be treated in the same procedure,[30] but if both lesions are critical, there is a risk of inducing a hyperperfusion syndrome and prolonged

hypotension. Procedure time and contrast agent load are also relevant in this situation.

In patients with renal dysfunction, contrast agent load should be minimized and angiography focused on evaluation of ipsilateral extracranial and intracranial arteries. If embolic filter devices are to be used, evaluation of collateral supply is not mandatory. If distal- or proximal-occlusion embolic protection systems are to be used, assessment of the contralateral or posterior circulation and documentation of a functioning circle of Willis may be necessary. When necessary, experienced operators with access to good digital angiographic equipment can generally perform carotid artery stenting with minimal volumes of contrast agent. All patient with chronic renal impairment should be well hydrated and should be pretreated with (*N*-acetylcysteine [Mucomyst]).[31]

Preprocedure antiplatelet therapy is an important element of the intervention. Ideally, patients should receive a combination of aspirin, 325 mg, plus clopidogrel, 75 mg, daily for 5 to 7 days before the procedure. A loading dose can be used but must be given at least 6 hours before stenting. Studies have shown that 600-mg and 450-mg doses of clopidogrel are superior to 300 mg in producing effective platelet inhibition.[32] A study demonstrated in coronary intervention that clopidogrel significantly reduces ischemic events but only if given in sufficient doses before stenting.[33] The potential for platelet clumping on the large metallic stents placed in the carotid bifurcation is marked, and the use of antiplatelet therapy cannot be overemphasized. Patients who are taking warfarin should be told to stop doing so 5 days before intervention, instead given aspirin plus clopidogrel therapy for 5 days (Table 59.3).

Because stenting of the carotid bifurcation "pressurizes" the carotid baroreceptors and naturally induces hypotension, patients taking large doses of antihypertensive medication should not take the agent on the morning of the procedure. If necessary, blood pressure can be controlled during surgical preparation of the patient with intravenous nitroglycerin, but this agent should be stopped 10 minutes before stenting, after dilation of the stent, and again before post-stenting dilation of the stent.

Mild sedation may be offered to anxious patients before the procedure, but for the vast majority, gentle reassurance is all that is necessary and facilitates continuous, accurate neurologic monitoring before, during, and after the procedure. Conscious sedation is not necessary for carotid artery stenting.

Intraprocedural Care

The interventionist can accomplish intraprocedural monitoring by talking to the patient and having the patient

Table 59.3 Preprocedure Checklist for Carotid Endarterectomy

- Adequate dual-antiplatelet therapy (sufficient dose for sufficient time before procedure)
- Hold of all antihypertensive agents
- Good hydration
- Atropine, phenylephrine, nitroglycerin available for immediate use
- Activated clotting time (ACT) analysis available in laboratory

count and intermittently use a squeeze toy in the contralateral hand. Pulse oximetry, intra-arterial pressure monitoring, and heart rate monitors are essential. Careful control of hemodynamics is a critical element of the procedure. Atropine, 0.6 to 1 mg, should be administered to every patient at the start of the procedure. If the blood pressure remains elevated after the stenosis has been relieved, it should be rapidly lowered with the use of intravenous nitroglycerin, nitroprusside, or another appropriate, rapidly acting agent. If an occlusion balloon embolic protection system is being used, blood pressure should be lowered before the protection balloon is deflated.

Usually, substantial hypotension is noted after postplacement dilatation of the stent, particularly in elderly patients with highly calcified stenoses. This hypotension is invariably quite benign and does not require aggressive treatment. However, in patients with other critical disease in intracranial, extracranial, or coronary vessels, the hypotension must be treated. Phenylephrine (Neo-Synephrine), 100 mg as an intravenous bolus, hydration, and sometimes dopamine infusions are necessary.

The bradycardia, and rarely, asystole, observed with balloon inflation can be abolished or blunted with atropine. Severe bradycardia or asystole resolves immediately on balloon deflation. In elderly patients with preclinical conduction system disease, bradycardias may be seen for 3 to 5 days after the procedure. Intraprocedural temporary cardiac pacing is rarely, if ever, necessary. On rare occasions, carotid artery stenting precipitates the need for permanent cardiac pacing after the procedure.

Anticoagulation during stenting is critical, but only modest anticoagulation levels (ACT 200 to 300 sec) are necessary. ACTs must be monitored during the intervention. Heparin, usually 4000 IU, is used, depending on body weight. A new antithrombin agent, bivalirudin has a very short half-life and requires a bolus injection followed by an infusion, depending on the duration of the procedure. This extremely reliable antithrombin agent has the potential to limit cerebral and femoral access bleeding. In the usual procedure completed in 10 to 15 minutes, only the bolus injection is required. It should be administered just before placement of the guiding sheath or catheter. Intravenous glycoprotein (GP) IIb/IIIa receptor antagonists are not routinely used.

Current technique requires use of 6F femoral access sheaths that facilitate the use of femoral closure systems. The use of short-acting anticoagulants also facilitates the use of femoral closure devices before the patient leaves the intervention suite. Accordingly, patients can sit up and begin to move immediately. This approach allows full neurologic assessment, and the catecholamine release associated with activity naturally counters much of the bradycardia and hypotension associated with stent placement.

Postprocedure Care

Intensive care monitoring after the procedure is not necessary. The patient should be managed in a step-down, monitored bed with nursing staff familiar with post-intervention patients, groin observations, and care. If sheaths are not removed in the interventional suite

with femoral closure systems, they should be removed as soon as possible by experienced personnel once the ACT has fallen below 150 sec.

Patients do not require prolonged heparinization, and if the access site is stable, they do not need bed rest, sedation, or narcotics. All of these measures exacerbate hypotension and mitigate against rapid ambulation and recovery. Hypotension may continue for up to 3 days. Patients' families and nursing staff should be reassured. Patients, particularly the elderly, should be assisted with ambulation if there are additional postural effects. If necessary, standard pseudoephedrine tablets, every 6 hours, can be given to raise the blood pressure as a temporary intervention. All patients with hypotension should be well hydrated and should undergo routine hemoglobin and hematocrit checks as well as groin examination. It is important that other major causes of hypotension, such as retroperitoneal bleeding, not be overlooked. Patients for whom the procedure was uncomplicated and who have femoral anatomy suitable for a percutaneous closure device can be discharged on the same day as the procedure. Al-Mubarak and colleagues[34] reported the results in 100 consecutive patients who met these criteria and were able to be safely discharged without any untoward consequences.

Hospital Discharge and Follow-Up

At discharge, patients are started on a combination of clopidogrel, 75 mg, and aspirin, 325 mg, for 1 month. After this time, either aspirin or clopidogrel should be continued indefinitely, depending on other indications for antiplatelet therapy and individual patient tolerance. Aggressive antiplatelet regimens appear to be important in preventing stent thrombosis and should not be stopped for elective surgery for at least 3 to 4 weeks after stenting. If this drug combination cannot be tolerated, alternatives include aspirin plus ticlopidine, clopidogrel plus dipyridamole, and large doses of a combination of aspirin and dipyridamole (Aggrenox).

Depending on arterial puncture site considerations, patients may travel or return to work immediately. Some patients notice neck stiffness for a period of 2 weeks and may need mild analgesic support.

A baseline duplex ultrasonographic study should be performed within 1 month to serve as a reference for future follow-up evaluations. Not infrequently, despite the good results documented by angiography, blood flow velocities are elevated after stenting. Evidence to date suggests that this finding predicts neither excessive progression of neointimal proliferation nor an adverse clinical outcome. Such early measurements, however, do clarify later readings recorded at 6- and 12-month follow-up. Angiographic follow-up correlation studies have shown that although low velocity measurements denote favorable angiographic findings, moderately elevated velocities are not well correlated with significant restenoses.[35] In correlative studies, 80% of patients undergoing follow-up angiography because of high duplex ultrasonography blood velocity measurements had less than 50% stenosis. Only a small minority, 5%, had greater than 80% stenosis.[36] Efforts to redefine the optimal methodology (velocity plus B-mode analysis) to examine the carotid bifurcation are undergoing intensive investigation. The problem appears to be associated with a relatively long (3-cm) length of the stented vessel in which a moderate layer of intimal proliferation develops to cover the stent. Although this layer of tissue effectively sequesters the underlying atheromatous plaque and appears to bestow a favorable clinical outcome, it confounds the duplex ultrasonographic follow-up surveillance. Importantly, this neointimal layer is thickest at 4 to 6 months and does not appear to progress over time.

MRA is not useful for follow-up purposes because of the signal dropout associated with the metallic stent. Computed tomography (CT) angiography has shown some promise and may prove to be the follow-up modality of choice. Significant angiographic restenosis (>80%), an uncommon finding, is rarely associated with clinical symptoms. Restenosis is seen more commonly in patients in whom the original stenosis was associated with radiation-induced injury. Patients undergoing carotid artery stenting for recurrent stenosis after CEA also tend to have higher chances of recurrence after stenting. If restenosis occurs after stenting, it can be managed with a second balloon dilatation and, occasionally, additional stenting.

STENTING TECHNIQUE

The details of the stenting technique have been covered in many interventional texts.[37,38] In principle, the intervention should be as brief as possible and should be performed with minimum manipulation of the lesion and the vessel. If significant difficulty is encountered at any point during placement of the guiding sheath or with attempts to initially pass a guidewire or embolic protection device, the decision to proceed must be reassessed. Given the availability of an alternative surgical option for many patients, operators must be aware of their technical limitations and limitations caused by the patient's anatomy. The procedure can safely be terminated at any time before pre–stent placement dilatation of the lesion and the patient referred for elective surgery. In our experience, emergency surgical backup has never been required or utilized for carotid artery stenting. Surgery should be scheduled for a later date, when the heavy antiplatelet effects have subsided.

Transcranial Doppler ultrasonography has shown that few particles are generated during placement of the sheath or crossing of the lesion with an embolic protection system.[39–41] Transcranial Doppler ultrasonography studies performed before use of embolic protection showed that pre-placement dilatation of the lesion caused release of a modest number of particles, and stent deployment release of more particles. Release of the largest number of particles occurred during post-placement dilatation of the stent. These findings support the view that if an embolic protection system cannot be easily passed through the lesion in a safe and expeditious manner, the procedure should be abandoned. Operators should be reassured that this situation is encountered by the most experienced carotid interventionists. A proximal-occlusion, flow-reversal embolic protection systems can be used in such a case if the patient has (1) an intact circle of Willis

and, thus, good collateral supply and (2) suitable iliac and proximal carotid anatomy so as to facilitate placement of the higher-profile device.

Transcranial Doppler ultrasonography has also demonstrated the importance of minimum manipulation of the lesion with balloon dilatation and stent placement. Pre-placement dilatation of the lesion with a low-profile, 4.0 mm × 40 mm coronary balloon reduces movement of the balloon during inflation. Only a single, brief inflation is required. Pre-placement dilatation reduces risk of embolization during advancement of the higher-profile stent delivery system across the lesion. Using good land-marking or "road mapping," the interventionist positions the stent in one movement; it must be of sufficient length to cover the lesion from normal distal vessel to the CCA. There is no disadvantage to covering the external carotid artery origin or leaving excess stent in the CCA.

Post-placement dilation should be done with a single, well-positioned inflation with a conservatively sized balloon (5.0 or 5.5 mm × 20 mm). A second inflation in the same position has the effect of "shearing off" large amounts of plaque through the stent struts. Embolic protection systems are extremely effective in abolishing or markedly reducing the volume of particles reaching the brain, but all devices can be overwhelmed by sub-optimal techniques that release a large volume of debris. The variety of embolic protection systems and the data supporting their efficacy are discussed later.

The stenting technique begins with diagnostic carotid angiography, the extent of which can be tailored to the anatomic information gained from preceding noninvasive duplex ultrasonography and MRA studies. The assessment should be performed by experienced angiographers familiar with the use of low-profile, atraumatic, and safe neuroradiology diagnostic catheters and coated guidewires. The Vitek catheter (Cook, Inc.) with a 0.038-inch, angle-tipped Glide wire (Meditech, Inc.) is recommended. The minimum information required consists of the severity and anatomy of the bifurcation lesion to be treated, ipsilateral intracranial anatomy in anteroposterior cranial and lateral views, and an assessment of disease and or tortuosity involving the CCA. The last item is important in determining safety of access with a guiding sheath. If occlusion-type embolic protection systems are to be used, assessment of collateral supply from the contralateral vessel and posterior circulation is useful, and complete cerebral angiography is recommended.

The stenting procedure itself has the following four components:

1. The 6F guiding sheath is advanced over an atraumatic wire into the distal CCA. The tip of the wire should ideally be placed in the external carotid branch. Definitive angiograms are obtained to reassess the lesion anatomy and enhanced tortuosity that is commonly encountered. At this point, the procedure may be terminated if anatomy is unfavorable. The long sheath must be carefully flushed and anticoagulation given as soon as the sheath is in the circulation.
2. The lesion is crossed with an embolic protection device, which is deployed in a distal segment of the cervical ICA.

3. The lesion is dilated before stent placement with a single inflation, the stent is placed, and then the lesion is dilated with a conservatively sized balloon.
4. The embolic protection system is removed, and final extracranial and intracranial angiography is performed.

With the use of a contemporary, rapid-exchange filter, balloon, and stent system, the entire process can take as little as 10 to 15 minutes (Fig. 59–8).

EMBOLIC PROTECTION SYSTEMS

Embolic protection devices come in two types of design: filters and balloons (Fig. 59–9). The first type have umbrella- or windsock-like micropore filters that are compressed in low-profile sheaths and deployed distal to the lesion. With appropriate sizing and positioning, these devices provide good wall apposition and filtration efficiency. Numerous studies have documented the ability of these devices to capture plaque, thrombus, and even cholesterol crystals ranging in size from 1 to 5000 μm (average 290 μm) (Fig. 59–10).[15,17,18,20–23] After post-placement dilatation of the stent, such devices are collapsed

through a variety of innovative technological means and removed.

The advantages of the filter systems are that they provide continuous perfusion to the brain. The disadvantages are the somewhat higher profile than that of distal balloon occlusion systems, a difficulty in negotiating more angulated bifurcations and tortuous vessels, and the theoretical issue of missing very small particles. A number of embolic protection devices will be available in the near future, which will probably be approved by the U.S. Food and Drug Administration (FDA) for both CEA and carotid artery stenting in high-risk patients.

The second type of embolic protection, balloon occlusion devices, are available in two systems. The most commonly used system is a very-low-profile, soft latex balloon that occludes the distal ICA below the siphon. Blood containing any debris is aspirated after the stent has been dilated. The balloon is then deflated and removed. This device has a very low profile and is "trackable" (can be manipulated) through tortuous vessels. Theoretically, the aspiration removes all particles. The principal disadvantage of the balloon device is that 5% to 10% of patients do not tolerate vessel occlusion. To be certain that a patient can tolerate the device, one must obtain complete cerebral

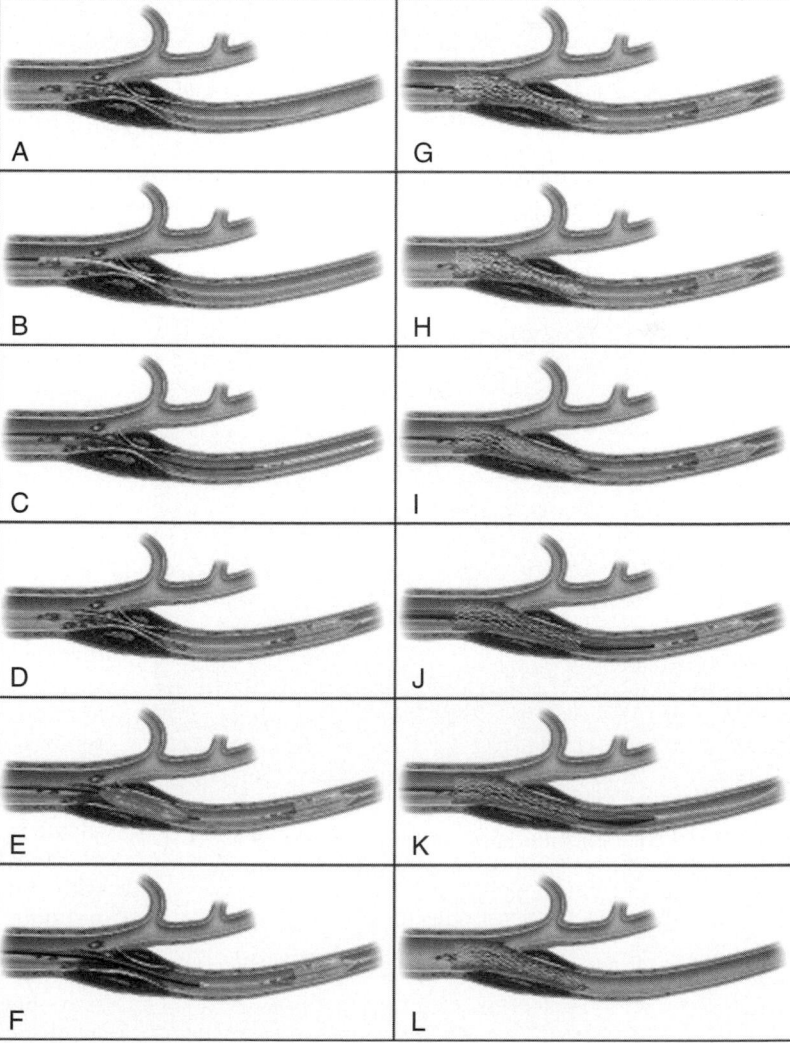

FIGURE 59–8 *Carotid artery stenting technique using a filter for distal protection. A, After placement of a guiding catheter in the common carotid artery, the lesion is crossed with a guidewire. B and C, Specially designed filter guidewire. The lesion is crossed with the distal protection filter delivery catheter, which can be easily advanced over the guidewire by means of a rapid-exchange system. D, Opening of the filter. E, Balloon (4-mm diameter) dilatation before stent placement. F, Positioning of the stent. G, Deployment of self-expanding stent. The self-expanding nature of the stent allows the cover to appose the vessel wall without inducing the trauma often associated with balloon dilation. H, The self-expanding stent is deployed, but the vessel sill is stenosed. I, Dilatation (5.0-mm to 5.5-mm diameter balloon) after stent placement allows further dilatation of the stenosed segment. J, Advancement of the retrieval catheter. K, Retrieval of the filter that contains the embolic debris into the retrieval catheter. L, The stent is fully deployed with good apposition to vessel wall.*

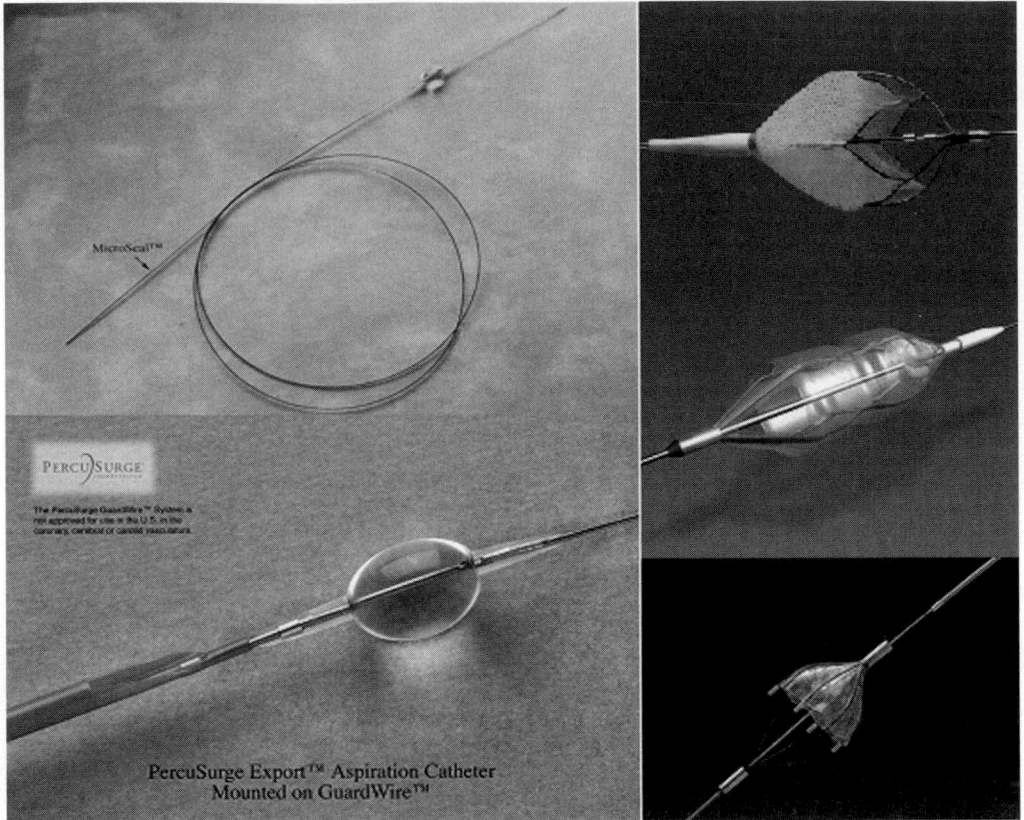

FIGURE 59–9   *Some of the distal protection devices available.* Left, upper and lower, *the GuardWire (Medtronic) balloon distal occlusion. Wire and balloon are placed distal to the lesion. Inflation of the balloon results in occlusion of the distal blood vessel. All the debris that is dislodged from the lesion is than aspirated by the Export aspiration catheter. With the filters, the embolic material is caught in the filter umbrella. Retrieval of the filter includes entrapment of the debris inside the filter using a special retrieval catheter.* Upper right, *the Accunet (Guidant) filter.* Middle right, *Neuroshield (Mednova) filter.* Lower right, *Angioguard (Cordis) filter.*

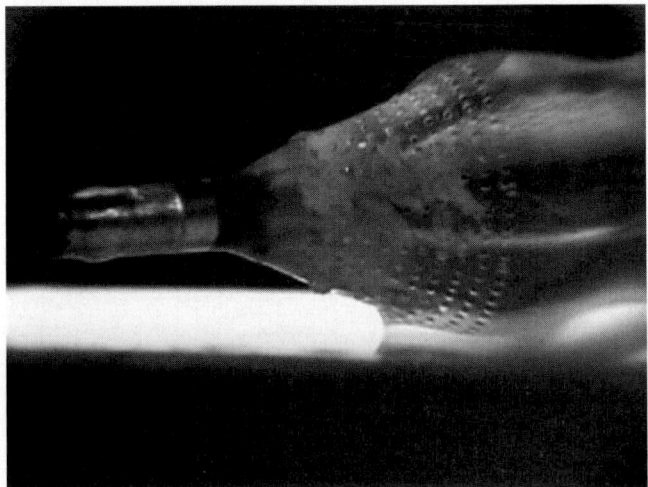

FIGURE 59–10   *Embolic material inside the Mednova Neuroshield filter after stenting of an 80% stenosis in the internal carotid artery of a 64-year-old woman.*

angiography. In addition, particles can be diverted up the external carotid artery and reach the cerebral tissue via ophthalmic or vertebral collateral vessels. Retinal infarction has also been noted. Rarely, significant dissection of the distal ICA has occurred.

An alternative, proximal occlusion system utilizes a more complicated device that features a cuff balloon surrounding the guiding sheath. The sheath thus occludes the distal CCA. A side port allows placement of a latex balloon that occludes the external carotid artery. In patients with a collateralization from the circle of Willis, flow in the ICA is reversed. Blood is shunted back through the guiding sheath and via a filter to a small catheter placed in the femoral vein. The theoretical advantage of this approach is removal of all particles, even those that may be produced when the lesion is crossed. The disadvantages include the large profile of the guiding catheter, necessitating an 11F sheath in the femoral artery, and the somewhat more complicated setup procedure. Again, 5% to 10% of patients with "isolated hemispheres" do not have the physiology to promote reversal of flow and do not tolerate the absence of cerebral perfusion.

From a practical perspective, all of the devices described have been studied in well-conducted prospective trials involving hundreds, even thousands of patients. When used by experienced operators in anatomically appropriate situations, all of the embolic protection devices have demonstrated excellent recovery of debris and superior procedural outcomes.

RESULTS

Interpreting Outcomes

Clinical decisions for patients with carotid bifurcation stenosis must be made with a clear understanding of the outcomes that may be expected for each of the three treatment modalities available—medication, stenting, and surgery.

Stenting outcomes must be interpreted first, in an environment of rapidly evolving technology and experience. Procedural outcomes documented several years ago[95–98,200] are not relevant in consideration of what might be expected with the use of distal embolic protection systems, enhanced access sheaths, lower-profile, more "trackable" stents and balloons, and adjunctive antiplatelet therapy. Collective and individual operator understanding of patient selection and technical issues has also improved dramatically over the last decade.

As with any interventional procedure, outcomes are predicated on operator expertise and experience. There is a steep learning curve for physicians beginning carotid artery stenting. The interventional and clinical skills required for optimal results are not found within the confines of any traditional medical discipline. Neuroradiologists generally lack experience in large vessel intervention, especially stenting, clinical management of patients, and the attending hemodynamic and cardiovascular issues. Cardiologists may have this expertise but lack specific neuroradiology and neuroscience backgrounds. Vascular surgeons and neurosurgeons generally do not have the required interventional skills. Interventional radiologists often have little experience in the carotid vessels and lack the clinical skills.

Through interdisciplinary collaboration and focused training, many physicians from diverse disciplines have gained the experience and skills needed to produce excellent outcomes of carotid artery stenting. Cardiologists, vascular surgeons, neurosurgeons, neuroradiologists, interventional radiologists, and neurologists are all performing carotid artery stenting. For optimal results, operators should have a minimal experience of 20 to 30 procedures and should maintain a case volume of 5 to 10 procedures per month. Results must be audited by independent neurologic oversight, and objective performance criteria—30-day stroke and death rates—must be rigorously monitored. Objective performance criteria (OPC) for carotid stent operators and endarterectomy operators must be defined and constantly monitored.

Choosing stenting therapy for an individual patient requires an understanding of outcomes expected from alternative approaches. It is important to appreciate how results of carotid artery stenting have been more rigorously scrutinized that those of surgical therapies. Current AHA/SVS guidelines for performance of endarterectomy in symptomatic and asymptomatic patients were based on the results of surgery in the NASCET and ACAS. Independent, prospective stroke scale assessment by a neurologist at 24 hours was not undertaken in any of the surgical trials. In contradistinction, all of the credible carotid stent studies have included this protocol-driven outcome assessment. The importance of this difference cannot be overemphasized. The vast majority of neurologic events seen after stenting are mild and resolve completely by 30 days, which was the independent neurologic assessment point for ACAS and NASCET.

An equally important issue has been the inclusion in early carotid artery stenting series of patients never subjected to rigorous prospective study by endarterectomy trials. The generally low-risk patients studied in the NASCET and ACAS have been studied in only the latest carotid stent series. Outcomes in these younger patients with fewer co-morbidities, presented in the next section, confirm the importance of patient population profiles in outcomes assessment. Ultimately, prospective randomized trials will "level the playing field" and provide comparable results. Some randomized trial data are already available and support the results of observational studies. Results of the Carotid Revascularization Endarterectomy vs Stent Trial (CREST) and second CAVATAS (CAVATAS II), however, are a number of years away. For the present, neurologists and others making decisions about carotid revascularization must depend on single-center and multi-center observational series results and individual operator experience.

CURRENT RESULTS

Procedural: 30-Day Outcomes

A large number of centers and operators throughout the world have now gained experience in many hundreds of carotid artery stenting procedures. Two groups have extensive experience with well over 1000 cases, and examination of their outcomes provides insight into the progress that has been made over the last 10 years, particularly the influence of embolic protection devices.

From September 1994 through March 2003, we completed more than 1397 carotid stent procedures in 1268 patients. Outcomes have been prospectively recorded on the basis of independent neurologic examination of patients within 24 hours of the stent procedure. The database has been maintained as the group moved from the University of Alabama at Birmingham to the Lenox Hill Heart and Vascular Institute (LHHVI) in New York. This large data set is constantly being updated and analyzed to evaluate the outcomes that can be expected when an experienced group of operators perform stenting on a well-selected subset of patients.

The data set has been used to examine the impact of the routine use of embolic protection devices and outcomes that may be expected in various populations of low- and high-risk patients. In this population of 1268 patients, the mean age was 71 ± 9 years; 205 (16%) of the patients were 80 years or older. Thirty-four percent were female, 56% had severe coronary artery disease, 16% had undergone prior CEA, and 45% had bilateral disease. Thirty-nine percent had prior symptoms of stroke, transient ischemic attack, or amaurosis fugax, and 61% had high-grade asymp-

Therapy

Table 59.4   Comparison of 30-Day Outcomes Before and After Availability of Embolic Protection

	Before Embolic Protection		After Embolic Protection	
	No.	%	No.	%
Procedures	809	—	588	—
Outcomes				
Minor stroke	33	4.1	7	1.2
Major stroke	8	1.6	2	0.3
Fatal stroke	4	0.5	2	0.3
Non–stroke-related death	5	0.6	3	0.5
Total fatal or nonfatal strokes	45	5.6	11	1.9
Total strokes & deaths	50	6.2	14	2.4

tomatic lesions. First, we examined outcomes in the 551 patients (588 separate vessel-hemispheric interventions) since the availability of embolic protection devices in comparison to our previous experience (Table 59.4). There was a significant reduction in the 30-day incidence of any stroke and death from 6.2% to 2.4%. The difference was seen for both the rate of major and fatal strokes (from 1.5% to 0.6%) and that of non-disabling stroke (from 4.1% to 1.2%) ($P < .05$).

Next, we examined the same outcomes in a provocative group of octogenarians and older patients treated during the same period. Previous analyses have demonstrated that for a variety of reasons related to extent of disease, severity of lesions, and diminished cerebral vascular reserve, this group has had a higher incidence of neurologic events.[14] The use of embolic protection devices in this population of patients showed dramatic benefit. Disabling and non-disabling stroke rates decreased dramatically from 15.4% to 2.3%. We also examined the 30-day outcomes in a group of "ACAS-like" patients, whose carotid stenosis was asymptomatic and who were considered at low risk for CEA (Table 59.5). In this group, the current stroke risk is 1.07%. Accordingly, when counseling such patients on the relative merits of stenting and endarterectomy, we are able to demonstrate a stroke risk of 1% for stenting without the operative risks of a surgical procedure. The total 30-day risk of stroke and mortality from any cause was 1.6%.

Table 59.5   Outcomes of Carotid Stenting in 187 Low-Risk "ACAS-Like"* Patients[†]

Outcome	Number	Percentage
Minor stroke	2	1.07
Major stroke	0	—
Fatal stroke	0	—
Myocardial infarction	0	—
Any death	1	0.53
Total strokes & deaths	3	1.6

*With asymptomatic carotid stenosis and considered at low risk for carotid endarterectomy, as patients in the Asymptomatic Carotid Atherosclerosis Study.
[†]At Lenox Hill Heart and Vascular Institute, 2001–2003.

In all of these analyses, we noted a slight rise in the incidence of retinal embolic events. These events were related to the dominant use of distal occlusion embolic protection devices during this time and potential for directing particles to the external carotid artery and, in some patients, the ophthalmic artery collateral vessels. These events have not been seen in our later experience with distal filter systems. Multivariate analysis demonstrated two positive predictors of a procedural stroke during stenting, (1) history of hypertension and (2) age greater than 80 years. A significant negative predictor was use of an embolic protection system.

These LHHVI results from a highly experienced group of operators are important, because they provide insight into what can be expected for many other operators who have received training and are rapidly gaining experience with the technique. Embolic protection devices, even in an early stage of development, improve outcomes. The results are most dramatic in patients at higher risk of events–those who are elderly, are recently symptomatic, or have very severe stenoses and long, bulky lesions. Stenting can have outcomes equivalent to those of historical surgical controls, and even to the best results reported for endarterectomy, without the risks of neck operation, general anesthesia, and the attending complications. In patients at higher risk with CEA, the stent procedure is clearly a safer option. In patients for whom CEA poses a low risk, the stent procedure appears to be as safe and is much more acceptable to the patient.

The second large single-center experience is also worth discussing in detail. Mathias and associates in Dortmund, Germany, were also early investigators of percutaneous carotid stenosis intervention and have accumulated an extensive and powerful data set for analysis. These results are entirely concordant with the LHHVI experience (see Table 59.4). From 1984 to 1998, they treated 1222 arteries (hemispheres) with carotid angioplasty and, more recently, stenting without embolic protection (K Mathias, Dortmund, Germany, personal communication, 2002). In this population, minor stroke was 2.1%, major stroke 1.1%, and death 0.5%, for a total 30-day death and stroke rate of 3.8%. Since 1998, this group has treated 577 more patients with the inclusion of embolic protection devices. The minor stroke rate was 0.9%, the major stroke rate 0.4%, and the 30-day mortality rate 0.2%; thus, the total 30-day stroke and death rate was 1.7%.

Overall, this group also observed a dramatic reduction in rate of stroke events associated with the introduction of embolic protection systems, from 3.3% to 1.3%. Of importance to patients and neurologists alike is that the incidence of major, disabling stroke has been 0.35% in this large series. This rate is similar to that observed in our series and suggests a reduction from the rate observed for endarterectomy surgery, after which stroke events are most frequently disabling. The Dortmund group reported a procedure-related stroke and death rates of 2.8% in symptomatic patients and 1.75% in asymptomatic patients.

Can these results from large centers with long experience be translated to the community? The outcome analyses from large multicenter and multinational studies strongly suggest that they are applicable. The German Quality Assurance Program (Prospective Registry) is one good example of what might be expected.[47] The program, under the auspices of the German Societies of Angiology and Radiology, compiled data and prospectively audited outcomes from 35 centers in Germany, Austria, and Switzerland. During the first 30 months, 2142 planned carotid interventions were registered. Of these, 57% were performed for symptomatic stenosis, and 43% for asymptomatic stenosis. In 98% of cases, stents were used. Embolic protection systems were introduced as they became available and monitored in the last half of the series; the devices were selectively used in 55% of interventions, and since that time, the overall stroke and death rate was 3.0%. Individual rates were 0.7% mortality rate, 1.4% major stroke rate, and 0.8% minor stroke rate. The investigators concluded that the outcomes represented a realistic view of carotid intervention in the community and suggested that this less traumatic approach is a realistic alternative to CEA.[47]

Wholey and associates[48] conducted a retrospective, multicenter, multinational registry of 24 centers throughout the world and have updated their results to include more than 10,000 cases. The multiple centers included both high-volume and low-volume operators. These researchers were able to examine procedural outcomes in both symptomatic and asymptomatic patients and also to study the beneficial influence of embolic protection devices (Table 59.6).

Al-Mubarak and colleagues[18] reported the combined outcomes of procedures from three experienced centers in the United States, United Kingdom, and Italy using the same embolic protection filter device. All data were collected prospectively according to regulations of the appropriate governmental agencies. The study was completed with the use of early versions of the device, which has subsequently been markedly improved. Of 162 patients studied, 48% were symptomatic. The overall 30-day stroke and death rate was 2%. There were no major strokes and two minor strokes, one death from cerebral hemorrhage, and one cardiac death, the cause of which was not related to the procedure.

Procedures with Embolic Protection in Single-Center Studies

A large body of evidence now confirms the premise that carotid artery stenting performed by experienced operators using contemporary equipment, including embolic

Table 59.6   Global Registry of Carotid Endarterectomy Procedures

	Number of Cases	Total 30-Day Stroke & Death Rate (%)
Without embolic protection		
Symptomatic	4223	6.97
Asymptomatic	2465	4.78
With embolic protection		
Symptomatic	1949	3.25
Asymptomatic	2056	2.54

From Wholey MH, Wholey M, Mathias K, et al. Global experience in cervical carotid artery stent placement. Catheter Cardiovasc Interv 50:160–167, 2000.

protection systems, can produce safety results comparable to, or even superior to, those of CEA. Henry and coworkers[15] were the first to report results from a large series using a commercially available balloon distal occlusion system (PercuSurge; Medtronic Inc., Minneapolis, MN). In a consecutive series of 150 patients, they observed rates of 1.3% for non-disabling strokes and 1.6% for disabling strokes as well as a single fatal stroke (0.75%) at 30 days. Parodi and associates[20] described results of a series of 46 consecutive procedures; they reported a 9.5% complication rate in the first 23 patients, in whom no embolic protection was used, and no complications in the subsequent 23 patients treated with the benefit of embolic protection. Reimers and colleagues[21] reported on 84 consecutive patients treated with three different embolic protection systems; non-disabling strokes occurred in 1.2% of patients, and disabling strokes in none. In 164 patients undergoing 194 stenting procedures (hemispheres treated), 92% of whom were symptomatic, Guimaraens and associates[24] observed a stroke rate of 1.3% and a 30-day mortality of 1.9%. These investigators concluded that stenting of with embolic protection produced salutary results and that its use should probably not be restricted to patients with symptomatic stenosis.

Early Randomized Trials

Early randomized trials of carotid artery stenting conducted before the introduction of embolic protection devices are also worthy of note.

The first CAVATAS[16] (CAVATAS I) was conducted between 1992 and 1997. It was included before suitable carotid stent devices were available, and the majority of the patients had balloon angioplasty alone. The ability of stents to overcome the problems of acute vessel recoil and lesion dissection may explain the overall incidence of angioplasty complications. The trial is noteworthy because of its extremely valuable late outcome results, which are discussed later.

Another early trial of note is commonly known as the "Wallstent Trial."[45] This study was an early industry-sponsored, randomized trial using the self-expanding Wallstent device. No embolic protection systems were available, and operators were required to perform only three "lead-in" procedures before beginning randomization of patients to treatment. Given the learning curve associated with stenting as well as other poorly managed protocol issues, the event rate in the group receiving stents was excessive. The company that acquired the Wallstent technology decided to abandon the trial and await availability of an embolic protection system before proceeding with another trial.

Naylor and associates[44] reported on a stopped "randomized trial" of 15 patients from Leicester, United Kingdom. Of the 8 patients who received stents, 6 experienced a neurologic event. Clearly, the stent operator lacked the knowledge and skill to perform carotid stenosis intervention, and this study was also underpowered. This study underscores the danger of relying on small single-center trials to assess safety and outcome of a new procedure or device.

In another larger single-center study, surgeons, collaborating with skilled interventional cardiologists and neurologists, were able to produce markedly different results.

Brooks and associates[49] conducted a single-center randomized study in 104 symptomatic patients and showed comparable and low (1%) rates of neurologic event in the stenting and CEA cohorts. In another randomized study of asymptomatic patients, the same investigators have convincingly demonstrated that both skilled carotid artery stenting and CEA can produce excellent outcomes in this low-risk cohort of patients.[50]

Special Patient Subsets

Shawl and coworkers[51] reported the immediate and medium-term outcomes in a consecutive series of 170 patients undergoing 192 interventions (arteries-hemispheres) from 1995 to 1998. No patient was treated with the benefit of an embolic protection device. The population included 61% symptomatic patients and was largely a subset for whom CEA would have posed high risk, with 76% having co-morbidities that would have excluded them from NASCET. The 30-day stroke rate was 2.9%, accounted for by one major and four minor strokes.

Gupta and colleagues[52] reported results of stenting in 100 elderly (>65 years) patients. Most (85%) were symptomatic, 24% were women, and 80% had concomitant coronary artery disease. As in the previous study, this series was completed without the use of embolic protection devices. One patient had a disabling stroke (1%), and 5 had non-disabling strokes (5%). All were resolved within 30 days. There were no deaths in the first 30 days.

New and coworkers[53] examined outcomes in a subset of patients with previous ipsilateral CEA and restenosis. A total of 358 arteries underwent stenting in 14 centers in the United States. The overall 30-day stroke and death rate was 3.7%. The minor stroke rate was 1.7%, the major disabling stroke rate 0.8%, and the fatal stroke rate 0.3%. The rate of non–stroke-related deaths within 30 days was 0.9%. Overall 3-year freedom from all fatal and non-fatal strokes was 96 ± 1% (± SEE [standard error of estimate]).

Randomized Trials in High-Risk Patients

The first prospective, randomized, multicenter trial using embolic protection devices has confirmed the utility of stenting compared with endarterectomy, particularly in patients believed to be at moderate to high risk from CEA.[25] The SAPPHIRE Study, as previously mentioned, randomly assigned 307 patients deemed to be at increased risk from CEA to undergo either CEA or carotid artery stenting. In the total cohort, approximately 30% were symptomatic and 70% were male. As defined, severe comorbidities were common; 80% of patients had coronary disease, approximately one third had undergone CABG and had myocardial infarction, and 20% had congestive heart failure, unstable angina, and prior CEA. This first credible "head-to-head" comparison using contemporary stenting techniques confirmed that for every adverse outcome measure, stenting was safer than endarterectomy: Death rates were 0.6% for stenting versus 2.0% for CEA; stroke rates, 3.8% vs. 5.3%, respectively; and rates of major ipsilateral stroke, 0 vs 1.3%, respectively (Table 59.7). The rate of myocardial infarction was 2.6% for stenting and 7.3% for CEA (*P* = .07), and the rate for combined predetermined endpoint of death/stroke/MI was 5.8% for stenting and 12.6% for CEA (*P* = .047). In addition, there was a 5.3% incidence of cranial nerve injury in the surgical group, and no such injuries in the stent group.

Late Outcomes

Late outcomes after carotid artery stenting have been consistently favorable and competitive with if not superior to those after CEA (M Wholey, Shadyside Hospital, Pittsburgh, PA: Personal communication, 2000; K Mathias, Dortmund, Germany: Personal communication, 2002).[16,24,51,54–58] Numerous studies have shown that neurologic events are rare once the patients leave the procedure room. The exception may be in patients inadequately pretreated with antiplatelet therapy. Rates of late ipsilateral strokes and stroke-related deaths have also been consistent with those seen after endarterectomy. Rates of restenosis by angiographic definition have also been very low (less than 5%), as have those for the need for second intervention on the stented artery (3% or less) (Figs. 59–12 through 59–14).

Roubin and colleagues[54] prospectively monitored the first 528 consecutive patients they treated with carotid artery stenting over 5 years. Clinical follow-up was 99.6% complete and ranged from 6 months to 5 years. First, there was a marked reduction in periprocedural events over the study period, from 7% rate of minor stroke in the first year

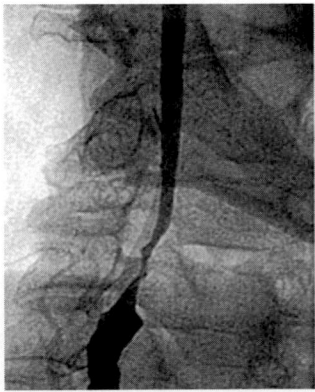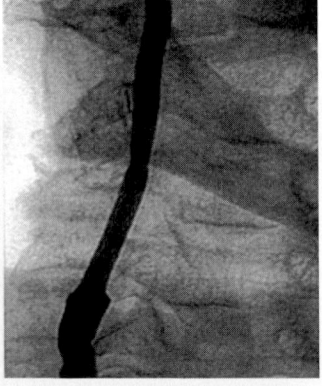

FIGURE 59–11   Left, *Restenosis after carotid endarterectomy.* Right, *Following stenting of the restenosis lesion.*

Table 59.7 Outcomes (%) of a Prospective, Randomized Trial of Stenting and Embolic Protection vs. Carotid Endarterectomy (CEA) in "High-Risk" Patients*

Outcome	Stenting + Embolic Protection	CEA
Death	0.6	2.0
Any stroke	3.8	5.3
Major ipsilateral stroke	0	1.3
Myocardial infarction (MI)	2.6	7.3
Any death/stroke/MI	5.8	12.6
Cranial nerve palsy	0	5.3

*Data from Yadav JTSI: Stenting and angioplasty with protection in patients at high risk for endarterectomy: The SAPPHIRE Study. Circulation 106:2, 2002.

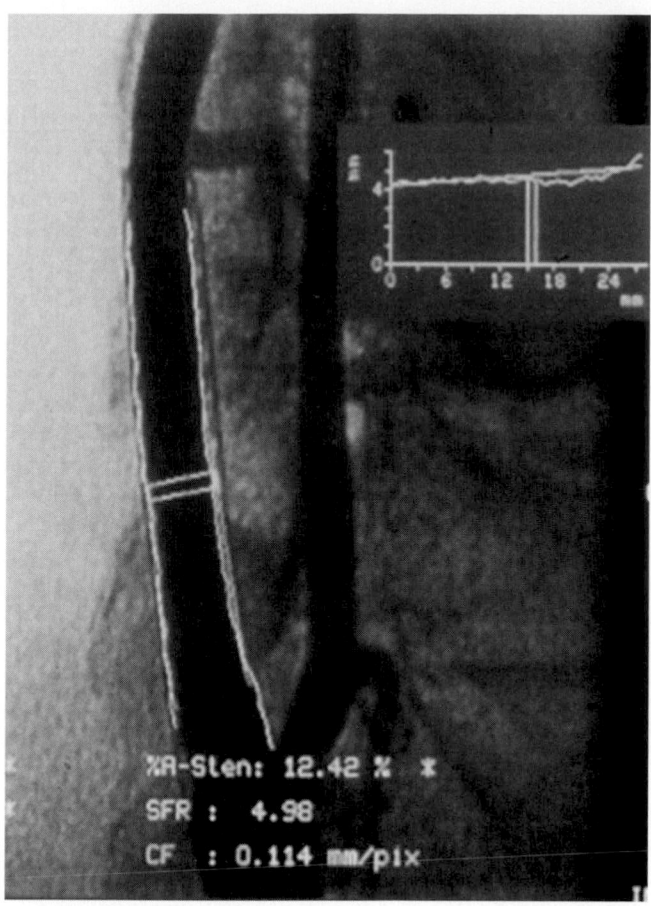

FIGURE 59–12 *Angiographic follow-up 9 months after stenting. There is minimal formation of neointima. This process is favorable and plays a role in stabilizing the atheromatous plaque.*

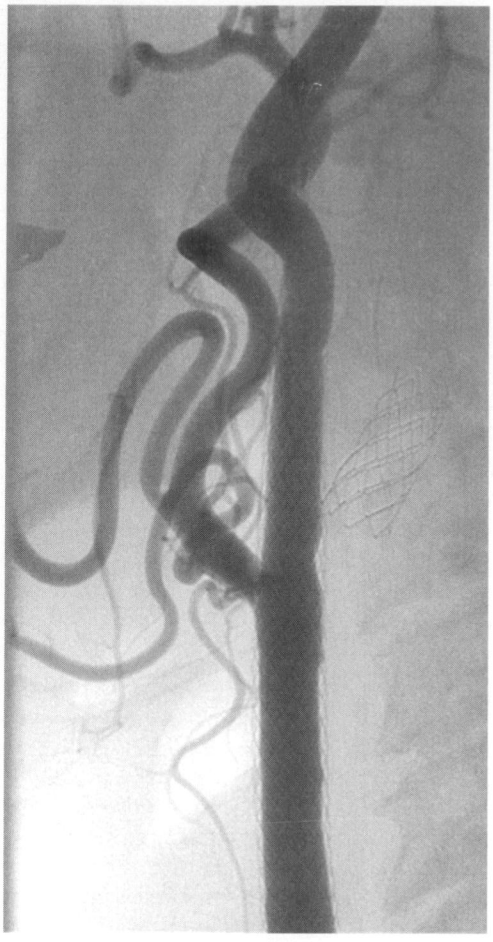

FIGURE 59–13 *Angiographic follow-up 6 years after stenting. There is minimal formation of neointima.*

to 3.1% in the last year (before availability of embolic protection devices). The rate of procedure-related disabling stroke averaged 1% over the study period. Given the dramatic decrease in 30-day event rate that has occurred over the last 9 years, particularly with the current routine use of embolic protection devices, it is relevant to examine the outcomes after 30 days. In this series, the rate of freedom from all fatal and nonfatal ipsilateral strokes was 99 ± 1% (±S.E.E) at 3 years (Fig. 59–15). Even including the 30-day events, the rate of freedom from all fatal and nonfatal ipsilateral strokes was 95 ± 2% at 3 years. Of importance, outcomes were equally favorable for symptomatic and asymptomatic patients and for men and women. Comparison with late outcomes from surgical series is difficult because the NASCET and ACAS studied a low-risk group and did not include patients older than 80 years. Despite this bias against the stent population, the late outcomes appear extremely favorable. Clinically relevant restenosis was uncommon.

Mathias and associates reported 6-month follow-up studies on 1487 treated carotid arteries (K Mathias, Dortmund, Germany, personal communication, 2002). Of the treated patients, 94% were available for follow-up. All-cause mortality was 1.8%. Five patients (0.4%) had suffered an ipsilateral stroke. The rate of restenosis (>50%) was 4.3%; 0.5% of patients with restenosis had complete

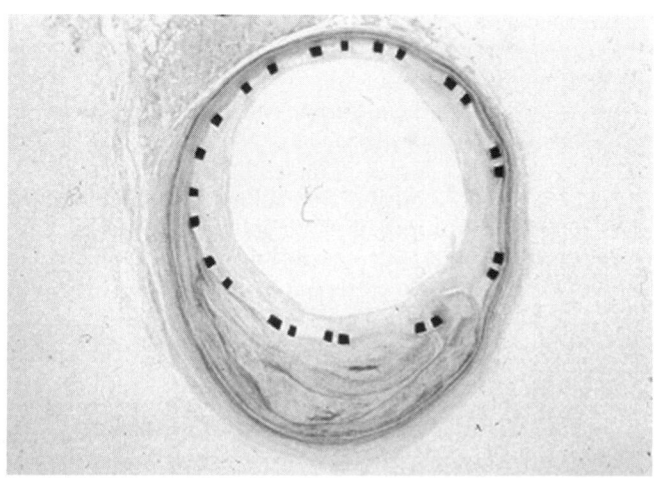

FIGURE 59–14 *Self-expanding nitinol stent showing excellent healing and sequestration of the cholesterol-laden plaque behind stent struts and neointimal tissue.*

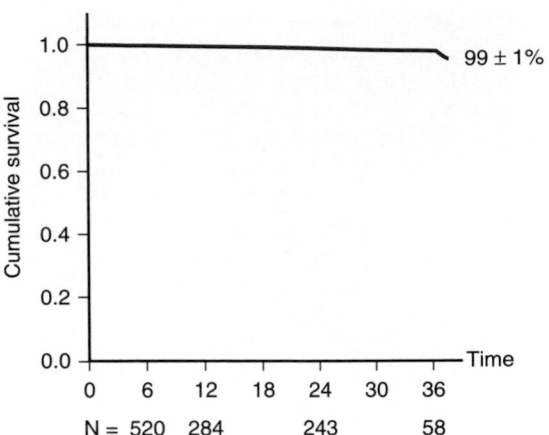

FIGURE 59–15 *Rate of survival free of ipsilateral stroke and fatal stroke after discharge from hospital. (From Roubin GS, New G, Iyer SS, et al: Immediate and late clinical outcomes of carotid artery stenting in patients with symptomatic and asymptomatic carotid artery stenosis: A 5-year prospective analysis. Circulation, 103:532–537, 2001.)*

occlusion. A second intervention was required in 1.4% of patients at 5-year follow-up, and the rate of patency, defined as less than 50% stenosis, was 89.2%. The ipsilateral stroke rate was 2.3%. Gray and coworkers,[55] who monitored 136 consecutive patients undergoing stent procedures, demonstrated rates of 3.1% for 6-month angiographic restenosis and 100% for 2 years of freedom from ipsilateral major stroke. Wholey and colleagues have followed their patients from large experience in Pittsburgh, PA (USA) (M Wholey, Shadyside Hospital, Pittsburgh, PA: Personal communication, 2000). Mean follow-up was 21 months (range 0 to 5.6 years) and was 94% complete. In 464 consecutive patients, the cumulative rate of freedom from stroke or neurologic death at 3 years was 96% for patients given self-expanding stents and 95% for those given balloon-expandable stents (early cases) (Fig. 59–16).

The most powerful evidence of the efficacy of carotid artery stenting in terms of late outcomes comes from CAVATAS I.[16] This prospective, multicenter, randomized trial compared carotid artery stenting with CEA. The carotid interventions were performed by operators in the learning phases of their experience and without the benefit

of embolic protection devices, contemporary appreciation for use of aggressive antiplatelet therapy, or state-of-the-art stents and ancillary equipment. Periprocedural stroke and death rates were identical, and so are the long-term outcomes. Rates of death and disabling stroke and ipsilateral stroke have been the same for both treatment groups (Fig. 59–17). In the CAVATAS follow-up, carotid duplex ultrasonography showed higher rates of blood flow velocities in the nonsurgical group. No angiographic correlations were performed, however, and the relevance of elevated blood flow velocity and its prognostic implications are in dispute.

A number of other studies with excellent follow-up have confirmed the low incidence of clinical events and stent restenosis.[24,51] Shawl and associates[51] monitored 170 consecutive patients who underwent stenting in 192 arteries (hemispheres); during a mean follow-up of 19 months, 3 patients (2%) had asymptomatic restenosis. The rate of freedom from any stroke was 95%. Bergeron[56] carefully monitored 148 patients who received stents from 1994. Over the next 5-years, freedom from stroke was 96% post procedure. The annual risk of stroke at 5 years was competitive with that reported for the NASCET and European Carotid Surgery Trial (ECST). The rate of in-stent restenosis (50%), as detected by duplex ultrasonography, contrast-enhanced CT, and contrast angiography, was 4%. This surgical group concluded that the "efficiency" of protection from stroke from stenting was comparable to that for endarterectomy.

FUTURE DIRECTIONS

Ongoing Clinical Trials

Interpreting clinical trial results requires an understanding of the research strategies undertaken in each study and the different populations of patients undergoing investigation. Attention in these trials is being directed toward the following three general groups of patients:

1. Symptomatic patients who are good candidates for CEA: Carotid Revascularization Endarterectomy versus Stent Trial (CREST) and CAVATAS II.
2. Asymptomatic patients who are good surgical candidates: CArotid Revascularization with Endarterectomy or Stenting Systems (CARESS).

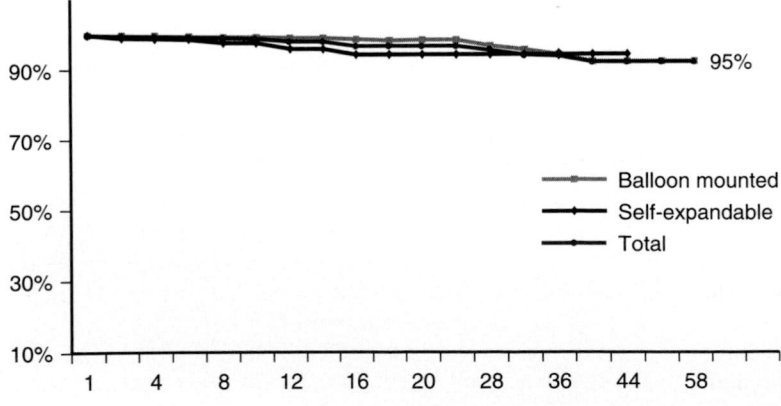

FIGURE 59–16 *Survival free of stroke and neurologic death in 464 patients with mean follow-up of 21 months. (Courtesy of M. Wholey, Shadyside Hospital, Pittsburgh, PA. Personal communication, 2002.)*

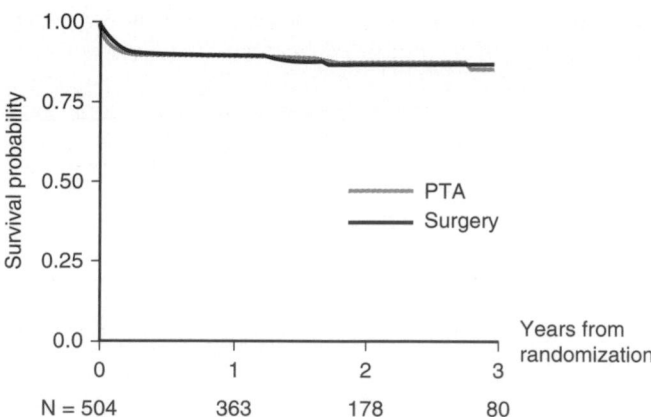

FIGURE 59–17 *Survival free of ipsilateral stroke. Late outcome from the CAVATAS. Follow-up is now extended up to 5 years, showing comparable clinical outcomes.(From Brown MM, Venables G, Clifton A, et al: Carotid endarterectomy vs carotid angioplasty. Lancet 349:880–881, 1997.)*

3. Symptomatic and asymptomatic patients who are either not technically suitable for operation or are deemed to be at increased risk from endarterectomy: FDA- and industry-sponsored studies, BEACH, MAVERICK, SAPPHIRE, SECURITY, and Acculink for Revascularization of Carotids in High Risk Patients (ARCHeR).

There will be some overlap among studies. For example, the CREST study is recruiting patients older than 80 years and patients with contralateral carotid occlusion. The definition of "high risk" for CEA varies from study to study. In some trials, merely age greater than 80 years is accepted as a high-risk designation, but in others, an additional comorbidity, such as poor left ventricular function, is needed for the classification.

CREST is a prospective multicenter study sponsored by the National Heart Lung and Blood Institute (NHLBI) and conducted primarily in North America.[59] The trial compares the two revascularization techniques in a cohort of symptomatic patients comparable to the group studied in the NASCET. CREST, however, will depart from the NASCET by also randomly assigning symptomatic patients older than 80 years to either treatment. The major endpoints in CREST will be the composite endpoints of death/stroke/myocardial infarction at 30 days and ipsilateral stroke at 5 years. Another departure from the NASCET is the requirement that all patients be examined by an independent neurologist 24 hours after stenting or CEA. In the trial, stent operators and CEA surgeons are rigorously credentialed to ensure optimal technical performance. To date, 50 study centers have been identified and are contributing lead-in cases for operator credentialing purposes.

Fifteen sites are actively assigning patients to the CREST protocol. The results in the "open label" lead-in patients receiving stents provide insight into the possible final outcome of this trial. The lead-in cohort (for credentialing purposes) represents the learning curve with neuroprotection devices for many of the operators. In addition, high-risk, noneligible, and asymptomatic patients with high-grade stenoses were included to expedite the recruitment process. All data were rigorously collected per protocol. The 30-day composite endpoint rate was 3.6% for asymptomatic patients and 6.6% for symptomatic patients. These very preliminary data demonstrate clinical equivalence with similar historical data for CEA and highlight the importance of completing this important study.

The CREST is an ambitious attempt to compare two quite different clinical strategies. The first is direct referral to endarterectomy on the basis of duplex ultrasonographic evidence of significant stenosis; neither MRA nor contrast angiography is mandated. The second strategy is referral for angiography and stenting usually in the same procedure. Stenting is not mandated, and if the angiographic anatomy is not suitable, the patient has the secondary option of elective endarterectomy. Analysis, however, will be based on intention-to-treat and will compare the benefits and risks of operating without the information provided by angiography with the "intention to stent" if anatomically suitable strategy. The CREST will allow secondary analysis examining the frequency of mismatch between duplex ultrasonographic and angiographic measurements (in the stent arm). Both sets of studies will be subjected to centralized analysis. They will also provide a contemporary look at the non-stroke morbidity associated with surgery and stenting outcomes in females and the elderly, who were not well represented in previous trials. Cost-benefit comparisons will also be performed.

CAVATAS II, sponsored by the British Heart Foundation, the National Health Service (NHS) Management Executive, and the Stroke Association, is a similar prospective randomized study in the United Kingdom and other European centers. To date, the trial has recruited more than 300 patients. Along with the North American study, this trial will provide successful level one evidence on the equivalence or otherwise of carotid artery stenting and endarterectomy.

The CARESS Study is a prospective multicenter trail examining outcomes in patients with asymptomatic stenosis and those not eligible for the CREST. This trial, conducted in the United States, will study a cohort of "real-world" patients representing the large majority of subjects currently being treated by endarterectomy. Conducted by the International Society of Endovascular Specialists (ISES), the study will compare two contemporaneously treated, nonrandomized cohorts of patients undergoing CEA and stenting at the same institution. Any baseline differences in demographics, clinical presentation, or comorbidities will be analyzed, and sophisticated statistical models will allow appropriate comparisons. The pilot phase of this study has been successfully completed, and a pivotal trial using multiple embolic protection devices and stents is planned.

Technical Developments

From a technical perspective, carotid artery stenting is in an extremely rapid phase of development. The CREST was initiated with a first-generation embolic protection device but will soon move on to the incorporation of second-, third-, and fourth-generation devices. The SAPPHIRE Study was completed with the use of a first-generation embolic protection device, and the outcomes in the stenting cohort in that trial are already being questioned, given the availability of new technology.

Iterative improvements include lower profile, better "trackability," improved particle capture efficiency, and ease of retrieval. Embolic protection devices and stents are evolving to rapid-exchange technology, which further expedites the procedure. The future will produce carotid artery stents with antiplatelet and antithrombin coatings as well as antiproliferative agents. These devices are already available for use in coronary arteries. Much work is still to be done to define the optimal adjunctive antiplatelet and anticoagulant therapy for carotid artery stenting.

Most importantly, experience and expertise with carotid intervention will grow, and as with all medical procedures, the technique will evolve to provide more effective and safer therapy.[60,61] As the medical management of carotid artery stenosis progresses, the need for reevaluation of stenting in comparison with medical therapy will arise.

The next major federally sponsored trial should probably compare carotid artery stenting with optimal contemporary medical management in asymptomatic patients with moderate (60% to 80% of diameter) carotid stenoses. Such a trial, however, must await a collective community experience with stenting in low-risk patients that demonstrates a periprocedural complication rate of 2% or less.

Given the progress with stenting that has been made to date, such a trial should be a reality within the next 5 years. In combination with aggressive community-based and individual approaches to primary prevention, there is a significant potential for this emerging technology to have a profound benefit on prevention of stroke. In the final analysis, the availability of a much less invasive, patient-friendly, outpatient procedure is likely to gain widespread acceptance.

References

1. Dotter C: Transluminal angioplasty: A long view. Radiology 135:561–564, 1980.
2. Gruentzig A: Percutane rekanalisation chronischer arterieller verschlusse mit einem neven dilatationskatheter. Tsch Med Wochenschr 99:2502, 1974.
3. Roubin G: Angioplasty and stenting should not be restricted to clinical trials. Stroke 33:2520–2522, 2002.
4. Beneficial effect of carotid endarterectomy in symptomatic patients with high-grade carotid stenosis. North American Symptomatic Carotid Endarterectomy Trial Collaborators. N Engl J Med 325:445–453, 1991.
5. Endarterectomy for asymptomatic carotid artery stenosis: Executive Committee for the Asymptomatic Carotid Atherosclerosis Study. JAMA 273:1421–1428, 1995.
6. Randomised trial of endarterectomy for recently symptomatic carotid stenosis: Final results of the MRC European Carotid Surgery Trial (ECST). Lancet 351:1379–1387, 1998.
7. Mathias K: Ein neuartiges Kathetersystem zur perkutanen transluminalen Angioplastie von Karotisstenosen. Fortschr Med 95:1007–1011, 1977.
8. Vitek JJ, Raymon BC, Oh SJ: Innominate artery angioplasty. Am J Neuroradiol 5:113–114, 1984.
9. Rabkin I, Germashev VG: [Five-year experience with roentgenologically controlled endovascular nitinol prothesis] [in Russian]. Kardiologiia 30:11–17, 1990.
10. Theron JG, Payelle GG, Coskun O, et al: Carotid artery stenosis: Treatment with protected balloon angioplasty and stent placement. Radiology 201:627–636, 1996.
11. Roubin GS, Black AJ, King SB III: Intracoronary stenting for acute closure following percutaneous transluminal coronary angioplasty (PTCA). Circulation 78:II407, 1988.
12. Yadav SS, Roubin GS, Iyer SS, et al: Application of lessons learned from cardiac interventional techniques to carotid angioplasty. J Am Coll Cardiol 25:380A, 1995.
13. Roubin GS, Yadav S, Iyer SS, Vitek J: Carotid stent-supported angioplasty: A neurovascular intervention to prevent stroke. Am J Cardiol 78:8–12,1996.
14. Mathur A, Roubin GS, Iyer SS, et al: Predictors of stroke complicating carotid artery stenting. Circulation 97:1239–1245, 1998.
15. Henry M, Amor M, Klonaris C, et al: Angioplasty and stenting of the extracranial carotid arteries. Tex Heart Inst J 27:150–158, 2000.
15a. Tan WA, Bates MC, Wholey MH: Cerebral protection systems for distal emboli during carotid artery interventions. J Interv Cardiol Review. Aug: 14;(4):465–474, 2001.
16. Brown MM, Venables G, Clifton A, et al: Carotid endarterectomy vs carotid angioplasty. Lancet 349:880–881, 1997.
17. Jaeger H, Mathias K, Drescher R, et al: Clinical results of cerebral protection with a filter device during stent implantation of the carotid artery. Cardiovasc Intervent Radiol 24:249–256, 2001.
18. Al-Mubarak N, Colombo A, Gaines PA, et al: Multicenter evaluation of carotid artery stenting with a filter protection system. J Am Coll Cardiol 39:841–846, 2002.
19. Iyer SS, Roubin GS, Vitek JJ, et al: Carotid artery stenting with neuroprotection. Circulation 39:30A, 2002.
20. Parodi JC, La Mura R, Ferreira LM, et al: Initial evaluation of carotid angioplasty and stenting with three different cerebral protection devices. J Vasc Surg 32:1127–1136, 2000.
21. Reimers B, Corvaja N, Moshiri S, et al: Cerebral protection with filter devices during carotid artery stenting. Circulation 104:12–15, 2001.
22. Tubler T, Schluter M, Dirsch O, et al: Balloon-protected carotid artery stenting: Relationship of periprocedural neurological complications with the size of particulate debris. Circulation 104:2791–2796, 2001.
23. Angelini A, Reimers B, Della Barbera M, et al: Cerebral protection during carotid artery stenting: Collection and histopathologic analysis of embolized debris. Stroke 33:456–461, 2002.
24. Guimaraens L, Sola MT, Matali A, et al: Carotid angioplasty with cerebral protection and stenting: Report of 164 patients (194 carotid percutaneous transluminal angioplasties). Cerebrovasc Dis 13:114–119, 2002.
25. Yadav J: Stenting and angioplasty with protection in patients at high risk for endarterectomy: The Sapphire Study. Circulation 106:2, 2002.
26. Al-Mubarak N, Vitek JJ, Iyer SS, et al: Carotid artery stenting with distal-balloon protection via the transbrachial approach. J Endovasc Ther 8:571–575, 2001.
27. New G, Roubin GS, Oetgen ME, et al: Validity of duplex ultrasound as a diagnostic modality for internal carotid artery disease. Catheter Cardiovasc Interv 52:9–15, 2001.
28. Mathur A, Roubin GS, Yadav JS, et al: Combined coronary and bilateral carotid artery stenting: A case report. Cathet Cardiovasc Diagn 40:202–206, 1997.
29. Shawl FA: Carotid artery stenting in patients with symptomatic coronary artery disease: A preferred approach. J Invasive Cardiol 10:432–442, 1998.
30. Al-Mubarak N, Roubin GS, Vitek JJ, Gomez CR: Simultaneous bilateral carotid artery stenting for restenosis after endarterectomy. Cathet Cardiovasc Diagn 45:11–15, 1998.
31. Baker C: Prevention of radiocontrast-induced nephropathy. Cathet Cardiovasc Interv 57:532–538, 2003.
32. Muller I, Seyfarth M, Rudiger S, Wolf B, et al: Effect of a high loading dose of clopidogrel on platelet function in patients undergoing coronary stent placement. Heart 85:92–93, 2001.
33. Steinhubl SR Bergeron PB, Mann JT 3rd, Fry ET, et al: Early and sustained dual oral antiplatelet therapy following percutaneous coronary intervention: A randomized controlled trial. JAMA 288:2411, 2002.
34. Al-Mubarak N, Roubin GS, Vitek JJ, et al: Procedural safety and short-term outcome of ambulatory carotid artery stenting. Stroke 32:2305–2309, 2001.
35. Robbin ML, Lockhart ME, Weber TM, et al: Carotid artery stents: Early and intermediate follow-up with Doppler US [see comments]. Radiology 205:749–756, 1997.
36. Roffi M, Mukherjee D, Chan A, Yadav J: Can ultrasound accurately predict restenosis after carotid artery stenting? Circulation 104:II-583, 2001.

37. Roubin GS, Vitek J, Iyer SS, New G: Carotid artery intervention. In Stack RS, Rubin GS, O'Neill WW (eds): Interventional Cardiovascular Medicine, 2nd ed. Philadelphia, Churchill Livingstone, 2002, p 959.

38. Henry M, Amos M, Theron J, Roubin G: Carotid Angioplasty and Stenting. Essey-les-Nancy, FR, Groupe Composer, 1998.

39. Al-Mubarak N, Roubin GS, et al: Effect of the distal-balloon protection system on microembolization during carotid artery stenting. Circulation 104:1999–2002, 2001.

40. Al-Mubarak N, Roubin G, Vitek J, Iyer S: Microembolization during carotid artery stenting with the distal-balloon antiemboli system. Interv Angiol 21:344–348, 2002.

41. Beebe HG, Archie JP, Baker WH, et al: Concern about safety of carotid angioplasty. Stroke 27:197–198, 1996.

42. Jordan WD Jr, Voellinger DC, Fisher WS, et al: A comparison of carotid angioplasty with stenting versus endarterectomy with regional anesthesia. J Vasc Surg 28:397–403, 1998.

43. Jordan WD Jr, Roye GD, Fisher WS 3rd, et al: A cost comparison of balloon angioplasty and stenting versus endarterectomy for the treatment of carotid artery stenosis. J Vasc Surg 27:16–24, 1998.

44. Naylor AR, Bolia A, Abbott RJ, et al: Randomized study of carotid angioplasty and stenting versus carotid endarterectomy: A stopped trial. J Vasc Surg 28:326–334, 1998.

45. Alberts M: Results of a multicenter prospective randomized trial of carotid artery stenting vs carotid endarterectomy. Stroke 32:325, 2001.

46. Golledge J, Mitchell A, Greenhalgh R, Davies A: Systematic comparison of the early outcome of angioplasty and endarterectomy for symptomatic carotid artery disease. Stroke 31:1439–1443, 2000.

47. Theiss W, Mathias K, et al: Pro-Cas: A Prospective Registry of Carotid Angioplasty and Stenting. Munich, German Societies of Angiology and Radiology, 2002, p 19.

48. Wholey MH, Wholey M, Mathias K, et al: Global experience in cervical carotid artery stent placement. Catheter Cardiovasc Interv 50:160–167, 2000.

49. Brooks W, McClure RR, Jones M, et al: Carotid angioplasty and stenting versus carotid endarterectomy: Randomized trial in a community hospital. J Am Coll Cardiol 38:1589–1595, 2001.

50. Brooks W, McClure RR, Jones M, et al: Carotid angioplasty and stenting versus carotid endarterectomy for treatment of asymptomatic carotid stenosis. Personal communication, 2003.

51. Shawl F, Kadro W, Domanski M, Lapetina F, et al: Safety and efficacy of elective carotid artery stenting in high-risk patients. J Am Coll Cardiol 35:1721–1728, 2000.

52. Gupta A, Bhatia A, Ahuja A, Shalev Y, et al: Carotid artery stenting in patients older than 65 years with inoperable carotid artery disease: A single-center experience. Cathet Cardiovasc Interv 50:1–8, 2000.

53. New G, Roubin GS, Iyer SS, et al: Safety, efficacy, and durability of carotid artery stenting for restenosis following carotid endarterectomy: A multicenter study. J Endovasc Ther 7:345–52, 2000.

54. Roubin GS, New G, Iyer SS, et al: Immediate and late clinical outcomes of carotid artery stenting in patients with symptomatic and asymptomatic carotid artery stenosis : A 5-year prospective analysis. Circulation 103:532–537, 2001.

55. Gray WA, White HJ Jr, Barrett DM, et al: Carotid artery stenting and endarterectomy: A clinical and cost comparison of revascularization strategies. Stroke 33:1063–1070, 2002.

56. Bergeron P, Bergeron A, Pietri P, Khanoyan P, et al: Long term results of carotid angioplasty and stenting. In Amos M, Bergeron P, Mathias K, Raithel D (ed): Carotid Artery Angioplasty and Stenting. Torino, Edizioni Minerva Medica, 2002.

57. Cremonesi A, Castriota F, Manetta R, et al: Endovascular treatment of carotid atherosclerotic disease: Early and late outcome in a non-selected population. Ital Heart J 1:801–809, 2000.

58. Dietz A, Burkefeld J, Theron J, et al: Endovascular treatment of symptomatic carotid stenosis using stent placement: Long term follow-up of patients with a balanced surgical risk/benefit ratio. Stroke 32:1855–1859, 2001.

59. Hobson RW II, Goldstein JE, Jamil Z, et al: Carotid restenosis: Operative and endovascular management. J Vasc Surg 29:228–238, 1999.

60. Heyer E, Sharma R, Rampersad A, et al: A controlled prospective study of neuropsychological dysfunction following carotid endarterectomy. Arch Neurol 59:217–221, 2002.

61. Crawley F, Stygall J, Lunn S, Harrison M, et al: Comparison of microembolism detected by transcranial doppler and neuropsychological sequelae of carotid surgery and percutaneous transluminal angioplasty. Stroke 31:1329–1334, 2000.

Chapter Sixty

Secondary Prevention of Cardioembolic Stroke

Oscar Benavente and David Sherman

Cardioembolic stroke is an important stroke subtype, accounting for approximately one fifth of all ischemic strokes.[1] Advances in imaging techniques have led to easier recognition of cardiac disorders potentially responsible for embolic stroke. Because the underlying cardiac condition is often evident before stroke occurs and antithrombotic therapies are notably effective, cardiogenic emboli to the brain are among the most preventable causes of stroke.

With a thorough cardiac evaluation, a potential source of cardiogenic emboli can be identified in at least 30% of all patients with ischemic stroke.[2,3] However, potential cardioembolic sources often coexist with other cardiovascular disease risk factors.[4-6] During the past two decades, new and better noninvasive cardiac imaging became available; therefore new potential cardioembolic sources have been recognized. This situation is reflected in the increased frequency of cardioembolic stroke over time. Aggregate data from stroke registries conducted between 1988 and 1994 show mean frequency of cardioembolic stroke to be 20% (range 17% to 28%).[4,7-11] Data from later stroke registries (1995 to 2001) showed a higher mean prevalence of cardioembolic stroke, 25% (range 16% to 38%).[12-18]

Cardioembolic stroke is caused by a variety of cardiac disorders, each with a unique natural history and a variable response to antithrombotic therapy (Fig. 60–1).

The embolic material originating from the heart and proximal aorta can be quite diverse. The thrombi may be composed of varying proportions of platelets and fibrin, cholesterol fragments, tumor particles, or bacterial clusters. The natural history and response to antithrombotic therapy of each of these conditions are unique, and consequently, each source of cardioembolic strokes should be considered separately. Thus cardioembolic stroke is not a single disease; it is a syndrome with diverse causes (see Figure 60–1).

The incidence of ischemic stroke associated with cardioembolic sources varies greatly. Cardioembolic sources of stroke can be divided according to their stroke risk potential as "major-risk sources," for which the risk for stroke is well established, or "minor-risk sources," for which the risk for stroke has been incompletely established (Table 60.1). The major-risk sources of cardioembolic carry a substantial annual risk of emboli and a high risk of recurrence, and usually, antithrombotic therapy is warranted for stroke prevention. Conversely, the so-called minor sources of emboli can cause stroke but have a low or uncertain risk of embolism and are more often coincidental than casual; therefore, antithrombotic therapy is usually reserved for selected cases.

The conditions leading to cardioembolic stroke are described in more detail in Chapters 30 and 36. In this chapter, we discuss conditions in reference to the indications for and choices of treatment for stroke prevention.

ATRIAL FIBRILLATION

Atrial fibrillation (AF) is the most common cardiac arrhythmia, affecting 0.7% of the general population of the United States (1.8 million people). Its prevalence increases with age, being present in about 5% of persons at age 65 years and in 10% at age 80 years. AF is equally distributed in men and women, and the mean age of individuals affected is about 75 years.[19]

Nonvalvular AF is responsible for about 16% (range 11% to 29%) of all ischemic strokes.[4,5,20-23] AF is present in more than one third of patients older than 70 years with ischemic stroke.[24] Nonvalvular AF is a recognized independent powerful risk factor for ischemic stroke.[25] The risk of ischemic stroke increases five-fold (from 1% to 5% per year) in elderly patients (mean age 70 years) with nonvalvular AF, and about 18-fold in patients with AF and rheumatic mitral stenosis.[25] AF accounts for about half of presumed cardioembolic strokes. Patients with AF are typically older and have large middle cerebral artery strokes associated with a high mortality rate during the first 30 days.[26,27]

Most embolic strokes in patients with AF are caused by the embolization of thrombi forming in the appendage of the left atrium. About 70% of ischemic strokes in patients with AF are embolic, but up to 30% are secondary to intrinsic cerebrovascular disease, atheromas of the proximal aorta, or other cardioembolic sources.[28-32] The formation of thrombi in the left atrium appendage in patients with AF is precipitated by the sluggish flow from ineffective atrial contraction. However, AF alone may not be enough to promote thrombi formation. Other factors may also contribute, because associated cardiovascular disease

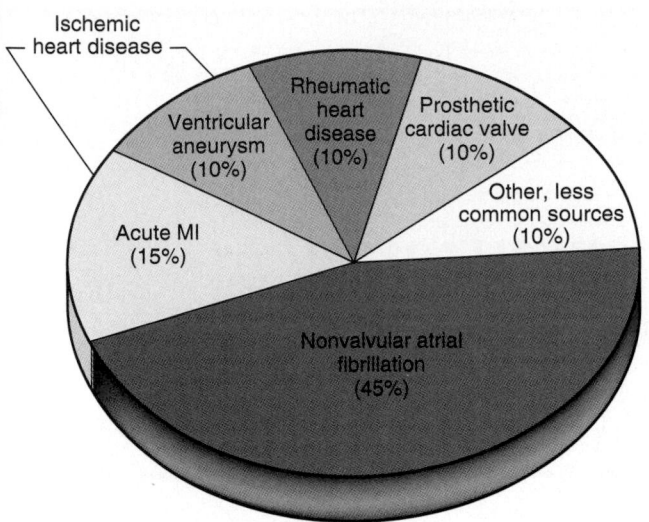

FIGURE 60–1 *Sources of cardioembolic stroke.*

Table 60.1 Cardioembolic Sources

Location	Major-Risk Sources	Minor-Risk Sources
Atrial	Atrial fibrillation	Patent foremen ovale
	Left atrial thrombus	Atrial septal aneurysm
	Left atrial myxoma	
	Sustained atrial flutter	
Valvular	Mitral stenosis	Mitral valve prolapse
	Prosthetic cardiac valves	Calcific aortic stenosis
	Infective endocarditis	Mitral annular calcification
	Marantic endocarditis	Fibroelastoma
		Giant Lambl's excrescences
Ventricular	Left ventricular thrombus (mobile or protruding)	Left ventricular regional wall abnormalities
	Recent anterior wall myocardial infarction	Congestive heart failure
	Nonischemic dilated cardiomyopathy	Akinetic ventricular wall segment

and age appear to influence the stroke risk in AF and, hence, also to influence the formation of atrial appendage thrombi. This variable risk is reflected by the wide range of stroke risk in patients with AF ("lone AF") compared with other "high-risk" groups. Temporal variation in factors that influence thrombus formation may explain the intermittency of embolism in different patients with AF and even within each patient. Embolic events are intermittent in AF, sometimes separated by years. A balance between the formation and inhibition of clot is likely present in the atrial appendage of such patients. This balance is influenced by atrial size, appendage flow velocities, and coagulation factors. Therefore, the type and intensity of antithrombotic therapy needed to inhibit appendage thrombi may differ among patients with AF and over time for the same patient.

The overall incidence of ischemic stroke among people with AF is about 5% per year. The rate of stroke varies

widely, however, ranging from 0.5% per year in young patients with "lone AF" to 12% per year in those with prior transient ischemia attack (TIA) or stroke. This variation depends on coexisting cardiovascular disorders.[28,32,33] Identification of subgroups of patients with AF with relatively high versus low absolute rates of stroke is important for selecting prophylactic antithrombotic therapy.[34–36] Prospective studies have shown that hypertension, prior TIA or stroke, and left ventricular systolic dysfunction are independently predictive of stroke in patients with AF.[37,38] Echocardiographic studies identified left ventricular systolic dysfunction to be strongly, consistently, and independently associated with subsequent stroke in patients with AF (Table 60.2).[34] Stratification schemes are particularly important for the identification of appropriate antithrombotic therapy.[39]

The short-term risk of stroke recurrence after an acute stroke in patients with AF has not been well characterized. However, data from three randomized clinical trials indicate that patients treated with aspirin at different doses administered at different times after stroke have a risk of recurrent stroke of 5% in 2 weeks, a value much lower than previously thought.[40–43]

Stroke Prevention in Atrial Fibrillation

The efficacy of antithrombotic therapies to prevent stroke in nonvalvular AF has been well established by randomized clinical trials.[44–46] An aggregate analysis showed that anticoagulation with warfarin reduces ischemic stroke by 60% compared with the rate in untreated patients, and an efficacy analysis indicated an even greater benefit. Warfarin was effective in preventing disabling stroke by 59% and non-disabling stroke by 61%. This analysis included one trial for secondary stroke prevention, the rest being trials for primary prevention. The rate of stroke among patients receiving placebo was about 5% per year in

Table 60.2 Predictors of Stroke in Patients with Atrial Fibrillation

Consistent independent predictors	Age (some studies at age 65 years, others at age >75 years)
	Hypertension
	Prior ischemic stroke or transient ischemic attack
	Left ventricular dysfunction
Possible independent predictors	Diabetes mellitus
	Systolic blood pressure >160 mm Hg
	Women older than 75 years
	Coronary artery disease/prior myocardial infarction
	Transesophageal echocardiography: appendage thrombi, spontaneous dense echocontrast
Not independently predictive	Left atrial diameter
	Paroxysmal atrial fibrillation

Adapted from Flaker GC, Fletcher KA, Rothbort RM, et al: Clinical and echocardiographic features of intermittent atrial fibrillation that predict recurrent atrial fibrillation. Stroke Prevention in Atrial fibrillation (SPAF) Investigators. Am J Cardiol 76: 355–358, 1995.

patients without prior stroke or (primary prevention) and 12% per year in patients with a prior stroke or TIA (secondary prevention). For patients being treated as primary prevention), warfarin showed a 59% reduction in events; the reduction with warfarin therapy was 68% for those with prior ischemic events. The absolute risk reduction for all stroke was 3% per year for primary prevention (numbered needed to treat [NNT] for 1 year to prevent one stroke = 37) and 8% per year for secondary prevention (NNT for 1 year = 12).[44] In addition, the increase in rate of major bleeding among elderly patients with AF undergoing anticoagulation in these trials was only 0.3% to 2.0% per year with a target internationalized ratio (INR) of 1.5 to 4.0. Participants in these trials were carefully selected to minimize bleeding risks and were monitored closely by means of clinical trial protocols.[44-47] The risk of major hemorrhage in elderly patients with AF who are taking oral anticoagulants seems to be related to the intensity of anticoagulation, patient age, and fluctuation in INR.[47] The optimal intensity of anticoagulation to prevent ischemic stroke and minimize the risk of bleeding probably varies according to individual stroke risk. Low-intensity anticoagulation (INR target range 2.0 to 3.0) is effective in primary stroke prevention for patients with AF. However, warfarin proved to be more effective in high-risk patients with prior TIAs or strokes when a higher INR target (2.5–4.2) was used.[32,48,49]

The efficacy of aspirin, with doses ranging from 50 mg to 1300 mg per day, for stroke prevention in patients with AF has been tested in six randomized clinical trials. Pooled analysis showed a risk reduction of 22% (confidence interval [CI] 2% to 38%), with an absolute risk reduction of 1.5% per year (NNT = 67) for primary prevention and 2.5% per year for secondary prevention compared with placebo. Aspirin tends to reduce the risk primarily of nondisabling stroke. The rate of intracerebral hemorrhage with aspirin therapy was 0.2% per year.[44] A meta-analysis

compared the efficacy of oral anticoagulants with that of aspirin in patients with AF. A pool analysis of individual patient data from six randomized clinical trials showed that patients assigned to receive oral anticoagulation were significantly less likely to experience stroke (2% vs. 5% per year; CI 0.43–0.71) but were more likely to experience major bleeding (2% vs. 1% per year; CI 1.21–2.41) than those taking aspirin. In short, treating 1000 patients with AF for 1 year with oral anticoagulants rather than aspirin would prevent 23 ischemic strokes but cause nine additional episodes of major bleeding.[50]

The higher benefit of warfarin for secondary stroke prevention can be explained by the fact that in patients who have experienced TIA or prior stroke, the underlying mechanism for stroke is more likely an embolus from a thrombus originating in the left atrium.[28,31,32] The effect of antithrombotic therapy varies according the mechanism of the ischemic stroke in patients with AF. Aspirin reduces the risks of noncardioembolic strokes more than cardioembolic strokes in patients with AF, whereas adjusted-dose warfarin is much more efficacious than aspirin for prevention of cardioembolic stroke.[29-31]

Unquestionably, warfarin is highly efficacious for preventing stroke in patients with AF and relatively safe for selected patients. Aspirin offers less benefit, possibly by decreasing noncardioembolic strokes in these patients. The choice of antithrombotic prophylaxis is based on the risk stratification (Table 60.3). Long-term anticoagulation cannot be recommended for all unselected patients with AF, because most of them would not experience strokes even if untreated. Patients with AF with a relatively low risk of subsequent stroke would not substantially benefit from the use of warfarin, because the absolute risk reduction would be small (≈1% per year). In these patients, anticoagulation may not be warranted. On the contrary, patients with AF who have a high risk for ischemic stroke (>7%) because of

Table 60.3   Risk Stratification Schemes for Stroke Prevention in Atrial Fibrillation

Stratification Scheme	Definition of Risk		
	High	**Moderate**	**Low**
Atrial Fibrillation Investigators (1994)°	Prior stroke/TIA Age >65 yr History of HTN Diabetes mellitus		Age <65 yr No high risk features
American College of Chest Physicians (2001)°	Prior stroke/TIA Age >75 yr History of HTN Left ventricular dysfunction More than one moderate factor	Age 65–75 yr Diabetes Thyrotoxicosis Coronary disease	Age <65 yr No risk factors
Stroke Prevention in Atrial Fibrillation (SPAF) (1995)†	Prior stroke/TIA Women >75 yr Systolic BP >160 mm Hg Left ventricular dysfunction	History of HTN No high-risk features	
SPAF Exploratory Analysis (1999)†	Prior stroke/TIA Women >75 yr Systolic BP >160 mm Hg HTN + age >75 yr	HTN + age >75 yr Diabetes No high-risk features	No risk factors

°Untreated patients.
†Aspirin-treated patients.
HTN, hypertension; TIA, transient ischemic attack.

a history of hypertension, prior TIA or stroke, or ventricular dysfunction would have a significantly lower stroke rate if they received anticoagulation.

High-risk patients who are good candidates for anticoagulation realize remarkable benefit from warfarin. For high-risk patients 75 years old or younger, a target INR of 2.5 (range 2.0 to 3.0) is effective and safe; for those older than 75 years, choosing a slightly lower target (INR 2.0), with the hope of minimizing bleeding complications, appears appropriate. For secondary prevention, a target closer to an INR of 3.0 may be optimal. Patients younger than 60 years with "lone" AF may not require long-term anticoagulation, and because their intrinsic risk for stroke is small, aspirin may be sufficient. Higher intensities of anticoagulation may be required to prevent ischemic stroke in patients with multiple risk factors.

Paroxysmal atrial fibrillation (PAF), with underlying causes similar to those in sustained or constant AF, constitutes between 25% and 60% of all cases of AF. A clinical concern is whether patients with PAF face the same risk of stroke as those with sustained AF.[51] Epidemiologic data have suggested that the risk of stroke for patients with PAF is intermediate between those of patients with constant AF and patients with sinus rhythm. However, when controlling for stroke risk factors, PAF involves a stroke risk similar to that of constant AF.[52,53] Because the awareness of AF among patients with PAF varies greatly, it is difficult to stratify the stroke risk on the basis of the duration of the reported AF episodes; hence every patient with PAF should be assumed to have frequent episodes of AF and should be treated accordingly. The risk-to-benefit ratio for antithrombotic therapy in patients with PAF has not been evaluated in clinical trials. Therefore, the recommendations are based on indirect data form AF trials, so the approach to patients with PAF should be the same as that to patients with sustained AF.[33,51]

New antithrombotic therapies are currently being tested in patients with AF; the preliminary results of the Stroke Prevention Using an Oral Thrombin Inhibitor in Atrial Fibrillation (SPORTIF III) trial were presented. More than 7000 patients with AF were randomly assigned, in an open-label study, to therapy with either adjusted-dose warfarin (INR 2 to 3) or fixed-dose ximelagatran (36 mg bid). In a non-inferiority analysis (intention-to-treat), patients allocated to ximelagatran therapy had fewer strokes and systemic emboli than those receiving warfarin (1.6% vs. 2.3% per year, respectively). The efficacy analysis showed a 44% relative risk reduction in event rate in patients assigned to ximelagatran (1.3% per year, vs. 2.2% per year for warfarin). The rate of intracranial and major bleeds was lower in patients receiving ximelagatran. However, these patients showed a significant increase in liver enzyme values.[54] Direct thrombin inhibitors such as ximelagatran appear to have several advantages over warfarin, (1) fixed dose, (2) no need for monitoring levels of anticoagulation and (3) almost no drug or food interactions. The safety profile and cost-effectiveness of ximelagatran will be most likely the determining factors in selection of this agent over warfarin for stroke prevention in patients with AF.

It has been theorized that the reversal of AF and maintenance of sinus rhythm might reduce the risk of stroke. The Atrial Fibrillation Follow-up Investigation of Rhythm

Management (AFFIRM) study compared the outcomes of patients with AF randomly assigned to treatment with either a rhythm-control strategy or a rate-control strategy.[55] One objective of this study was to describe any differences in stroke occurrence in the two groups. The AFFIRM study was designed to compare mortality rates of patients managed with rate control only and those managed with rhythm control utilizing cardioversion and pharmacologic efforts along with anticoagulation. All patients had AF and at least one additional feature that put them at high risk for stroke. The AFFIRM study enrolled 4060 patients with a mean age of 69 years. Clinical stroke risk factors included hypertension (71%), history of congestive heart failure (CHF) (23%), history of TIA or stroke (13%), and diabetes mellitus (20%). The rat-control and rhythm-control groups did not differ significantly in the primary endpoint, that is, mortality ($P = .078$). Two hundred eleven patients (8%) had at least one stroke event. Ischemic stroke occurred in 6%, primary intraparenchymal hemorrhage in 1.2%, and subdural or subarachnoid hemorrhage in 0.8% of patients.[56] The most common ischemic stroke mechanism was cardioembolic in 37 patients. Eighty-nine patients had an ischemic stroke of unknown mechanism. At 5 years, 94% of patients in both treatment arms remained free of ischemic stroke. Treatment assignment had no significant effect on the occurrence of ischemic stroke. Age, history of TIA or stroke, history of diabetes, AF during follow-up, and absence of warfarin use were positively associated with ischemic stroke. After adjustment of data for other factors, patients with AF at the time of follow-up had a 72% greater chance of having ischemic stroke than those without AF. Taking warfarin reduced the chance of having ischemic stroke by 68%. The AFFIRM study therefore showed that the presence of AF increased ischemic stroke risk and the use of warfarin reduced stroke risk regardless of assigned treatment strategy.

Systemic embolization is the most serious complication of cardioversion of AF. Most of the embolic phenomena occur during the first 72 hours after cardioversion, most likely as a result of emboli arising from the left atrium at the time of cardioversion.[57] Prospective studies have shown an incidence of systemic emboli of 5% in patients with cardioversion who were not receiving anticoagulants versus 0.8% in those who were receiving oral anticoagulants.[58] The current recommendations for patients with AF undergoing cardioversion include anticoagulant therapy (INR 2.5) for 3 weeks before and at least 4 weeks after the procedure. Alternatively, patients with AF should be started on anticoagulation, undergo transesophageal echocardiogram, and then have cardioversion without delay if no thrombus is seen. Oral anticoagulation should be continued until normal sinus rhythm has been maintained for at least 4 weeks.[33]

CARDIOMYOPATHIES

A cardiomyopathy is the second most common cause of cardiogenic stroke after AF, with a three-fold increase in relative risk.[59] Cardiac failure affects some 4.5 million Americans, and its prevalence is increasing substantially as the population ages.[60]

The ejection fraction (EF) is a reliable measurement of left ventricular function, with the normal value between 50% and 70%. A decline in EF produces an elevated left ventricular filling pressure and a drop in stroke volume with a consequent reduction of systemic blood flow. The reduced stroke volume creates relative stasis within the left ventricle that promotes thrombus formation and an increased risk of thromboembolic events. Cardiomyopathies can be dilated or hypertrophic. Dilated cardiomyopathy is present if the diastolic dimension of the left ventricle becomes enlarged and hypertrophic when wall thickness is increased.

The relative risk for stroke in patients with heart failure is about 4% at age 60 years and decreases to about 2% by age 80 to 89 years.[59,61] In patients with CHF who are treated with aspirin or warfarin, the aggregate stroke risk per year has been found to be between 1% and 4%.[62–66] The stroke rate was inversely proportional to the EF in two studies.[62,67] In the Survival And Ventricular Enlargement trial (SAVE), patients with EF of 32% had a stroke rate of 1% per year, with EF of 28% or less, the rate increased up to 2% per year. This translates in an 18% increment in the risk of stroke for every 5% decline in EF.[63] Factors that raise the risk of stroke in patients with ischemic cardiomyopathy are the presence of AF and left ventricular thrombus. Stasis of blood in a poorly functioning left ventricle is thought to predispose to formation of ventricular thrombus; patients with chronic heart failure may also have hemostatic abnormalities.[68]

Dilated Cardiomyopathy

Ventricular thrombus formation occurs in about 30% to 50% of patients with dilated cardiomyopathy.[69] Systemic embolism occurs in 10% to 20% of patients with dilated cardiomyopathy, representing an annual risk of systemic embolization of 3% to 4%.[70,71] The thrombi present in dilated cardiomyopathy are less well anchored than those in acute myocardial infarction (MI) and often embolize before they can be visualize by echocardiogram. Thrombi in the left ventricle are distributed throughout the diffusely hypokinetic ventricle and are not localized to any particular region, as they are with saccular dyskinetic areas in patients after MI. The underlying mechanism for thrombus formation in patients with dilated cardiomyopathy is probably complex and multifactorial, including mechanical factors such as low velocity in the left ventricle and activation of hemostatic factors.[72,73] The intracavitary flow velocity is chronically reduced in these patients; therefore the risk of thrombus formation is constant.

There is a lack of prospective studies assessing the use of anticoagulants in patients with cardiomyopathy. However, in view of the high risk of systemic embolization in such patients, long-term anticoagulation with a target INR of 2 to 3 is recommended in patients with global left ventricular hypokinesis and an ejection fraction of less than 35%, especially in elderly subjects, regardless of cause.[63,74]

MYOCARDIAL INFARCTION

The stroke rate in survivors of MI is about 1% to 2% per year. Because coronary artery atherosclerosis often coexists with atherosclerotic cerebrovascular disease, not all the strokes in these individuals are cardioembolic.[75,76] The risk of stroke is particularly high during the first 3 months after MI.[77,78]

The use of long-term anticoagulants after MI is associated with a 75% risk reduction in the incidence of stroke; however, this value represents an absolute risk reduction of only 1% per year. At the same time, anticoagulation (INR 2.5 to 4.5) has an associated 10-fold increased risk of intracerebral hemorrhage (ICH), or 0.4% per year. In addition, ICHs have a higher mortality and are more disabling than ischemic strokes.[79] In summary, we would need to treat 1000 unselected MI survivors to prevent approximately 10 strokes per year, and of those 1000 patients treated, 4 would suffer a disabling or fatal ICH; therefore, the net benefit is minimal. The risks and benefits of a lower-intensity anticoagulation (INR 1.6 to 2.5) have not been tested in this setting.[80] Aspirin reduces the incidence of stroke in patients with prior MI, with a relative risk reduction of 30% but a very small absolute risk reduction (<0.5%). Because of such small net benefit, oral anticoagulation cannot be routinely recommended to prevent stroke in unselected MI survivors.

There are, however, specific subsets of patients with prior MI at higher risk of ischemic stroke who benefit from anticoagulation. Patients suffering anterior wall MI have a higher risk for stroke than patients with MI in other locations.[76,78,81] The presence of left ventricular thrombi after MI is associated with a much higher incidence of embolic stroke (approximately 5% to 10% over the following 6 to 12 months).[1,82] Left ventricular mural thrombus occurs in 20% of all MIs and up to 40% of anterior infarctions involving the apex. Formation of mural thrombi is almost exclusively limited to mural infarctions.[83] More than 90% of mural thrombi involve the left ventricular apex, and in acute MI, the formation of mural thrombi is directly related to the location and size of infarction and to the presence of ventricular failure.[84] Stasis associated with dyskinesias of the ventricle is an essential factor for formation of thrombi. Endothelial injury in the area of the infarction also plays an important role in thrombus formation. Finally, a hypercoagulable state during the acute phase of MI contributes to the development of thrombus.[85,86]

The risk of thromboembolism is greatest in the first week after infarction. Approximately half to two thirds of thrombi are detected within 48 hours of symptom onset, and two thirds of systemic emboli occur in the first 4 weeks after infarction.[82,87] The presence of thrombus mobility, proximity to a hypokinetic segment, and protrusion appear to raise the risk of embolism.[88] Additional risk factors predisposing to thrombus formation are EF less than 35%, apical dyskinesia, and anterior infarction.[82] In about 35% of cases, the thrombus disappears without treatment; however, the use of warfarin for 6 months is associated with thrombus disappearance. Systemic embolization has been documented in 20% of patients with echocardiographically proven thrombi, compared with 2% without visualization of thrombi. In a study from the Mayo Clinic, the presence of thrombus correlated inversely with the duration of anticoagulation. Anticoagulation is associated with a low incidence of embolization because with anticoagulation, the thrombus organizes, becomes endothelialized, and attaches to the ventricular wall.[89–91]

In short, when ventricular thrombus is present, anticoagulants reduce the stroke risk by 60%. Therefore, anticoagulation therapy is indicated for 3 to 6 months after detection of ventricular thrombi. Chronic thrombi (>6 months old) have less emboligenic potential, so anticoagulation after this period would be reasonable only for a patient in whom a thrombus is mobile or protruding.[92,93]

The presence of AF in MI survivors markedly raises the risk for embolic stroke.[78,94,95] Therefore, anticoagulation is routinely recommended in this situation. The risk of stroke increases by 1% to 2% per year when CHF is present in MI survivors. Even though the incidence of stroke in patients with CHF is double that in patients without CHF, the risk is still relatively low, and anticoagulation may not be of substantial benefit.[64,96]

In summary, oral anticoagulation (INR 2.5 to 4.8) to prevent stroke does not substantially benefit unselected patients with acute MI. The value of lower-intensity anticoagulation (INR 1.6 to 2.5) and antiplatelet agent therapy for stroke prevention in this setting is still unproven. On the other hand, patients with prior MI and AF or acute left ventricular thrombi are at higher risk of embolic stroke; anticoagulation (INR 2.0 to 3.0) is routinely recommended for stroke prevention in these patients. On the basis of the available evidence, oral anticoagulation in the patient with left ventricular thrombus should be administered for at least 6 months; the patient should then be reassessed for the presence and characteristics of left ventricular thrombi by means of echocardiography.

VALVULAR HEART DISEASE

Before the use of surgical replacement of heart valves, valvular disease, especially rheumatic mitral valve disease, was associated with a very high risk of systemic emboli. Now almost all the patients with congenital or acquired valvular disease undergo surgical implantation of prosthetic heart valves. Hence, for most patients with valvular heart disease, the requirement for antithrombotic therapy depends on the thromboembolic risk associated with valve replacement. Data on antithrombotic therapy in patients with native valvular disease is limited, and all published recommendations are based on clinical experience.

Rheumatic Mitral Valve Disease

Of all native valvular diseases, rheumatic mitral valve disease carries the highest risk of systemic emboli. The incidence of systemic emboli ranges from 2% to 5% per year.[97,98] In short, it can be assumed that a patient with rheumatic mitral valve diseases has at least one chance in five of having a symptomatic systemic embolus during his or her life.[99] Mitral stenosis carries a higher risk of embolization than mitral regurgitation, and the presence of atrial fibrillation increases the risk of embolism by about seven-fold.[98,100] In addition, the risk of systemic emboli in patients with rheumatic heart disease increases with age and is higher in those with associated low ejection fraction.[97,101,102] After a first episode of embolization, recurrent emboli occur in 30% to 65% of patients; and more than half of recurrences are seen during the first year, most during the first 6 months.[99,103]

Although long-term anticoagulation was never examined in randomized trials in this population, observational studies have established the effectiveness of this intervention in reducing systemic emboli. Szekely[98] observed a significant reduction in the proportion of emboli in patients receiving anticoagulation in comparison with patients receiving no treatment (3% vs. 10% per year, respectively). The annual incidence of systemic emboli in 217 patients who were undergoing anticoagulation and had with mitral stenosis was reported to be as low as 0.8% per year.[104,105] In patients with mitral stenosis and ischemic stroke who were monitored for 20 years, there was significant reduction in death associated with cerebral emboli; 13 deaths occurred in the untreated patients, and 4 in the patients receiving anticoagulation.[106]

In view of these data, all patients with rheumatic mitral valve disease and AF should be treated with long-term anticoagulation if possible. Patients with rheumatic heart disease and prior ischemic stroke should also receive anticoagulation in view of the high recurrence rate.[99,103] The intensity of anticoagulation is recommended as a target INR of 2.5. If recurrent embolism occurs despite adequate anticoagulation, the target INR should be increased to 3.0 or aspirin, 81 mg per day, should be added. For patients intolerant of aspirin, the addition of clopidogrel could be an option, although there are no data to support this recommendation.[107]

PROSTHETIC CARDIAC VALVES

Despite advances in valve design and effective anticoagulant therapy, systemic embolism remains a serious threat in patients who have undergone heart valve replacement. The rate of embolism is high in patients with mechanical prosthetic cardiac valves, being 2% to 4% per year even in those with proper anticoagulation.[108-113] The risk of embolism is higher with tilting disk prosthetic valves in the mitral position than in the aortic position. Embolism occurs at estimated rates of 0.5% per year with prosthetic aortic valves, 1% per year with mitral valves, and 1.5% per year for both.[114] Embolism is more frequent with valves in the mitral position, with multiple valves, and with cage-ball valves. Atrial stasis, a risk factor for thrombogenicity, is influenced by valve type and position, coexistent AF, and ventricular pacemakers. AF and enlargement of the left atrium are more frequent in patients with mitral valve disease.[106,115]

Permanent anticoagulation is generally recommended to prevent embolic stroke and valve thrombosis with all mechanical prosthetic valves. In addition, anticoagulation is also recommended for bioprosthetic valves in the mitral position in the patient with AF, enlarged (>5.5 cm) left atrium, ventricular pacemakers, or evidence of atrial thrombi or prior thromboembolism.[109]

Long-term anticoagulation may not be required for bioprosthetic valves in the aortic position in patients with sinus rhythm because the stroke rate is relatively low. Warfarin (INR 2.0 to 3.0) is recommended for a period of 3 months after valve implantation, because the frequency of thromboembolism is increased (about 6%) in patients who do not receive anticoagulation.[107,109]

Thrombogenicity of specific valves varies, as do factors influencing thromboembolic risk; thus, multiple factors should be considered in the selection of prophylactic antithrombotic therapy. In the past, the intensity of anticoagulation for mechanical valves was a target INR between 3.0 and 4.5. Now it is believed that a lower intensity (INR 2.5 to 3.5) would be as effective; however, this issue remains controversial. Adding an antiplatelet agent such as aspirin or dipyridamole to warfarin further reduces embolism risk; however, this therapeutic strategy may raise the risk of bleeding (mostly minor bleeds when aspirin is added).[110]

The success of antithrombotic therapy in primary stroke prevention in patients with prosthetic valves is influenced by the type of prosthesis, factors associated with left atrial stasis, underlying cardiovascular disease, and tolerability of antithrombotic therapies. The optimal or appropriate intensity of anticoagulation and the decision to use additional antiplatelet agents in individual patients depends on the presence of some of the previously mentioned risk factors and the valve type.

The current recommendations are as follows: Oral anticoagulation with a target INR between 2 and 3 should be used in all patients with mechanical prosthetic valves (St. Jude Medical bileaflet valve or Medtronic ball tilting disk mechanical valve) in the aortic position and with sinus rhythm. For patients with tilting disk valves and bileaflet mechanical valves in the mitral position, the intensity of anticoagulation is a target INR of 2.5 to 3.5. The same intensity of anticoagulation is recommended for patients with AF who are given prosthetic valves in the aortic position. An alternative therapeutic option is to add aspirin, 81 to 100 mg per day, to warfarin (target INR 2.0 to 3.0) in patients at high risk of embolization (i.e., valves in mitral position, AF, tilting disk valves). For those with caged-ball or caged-disk valves or additional risk factors, a higher target INR (2.5 to 3.5) plus low-dose aspirin is recommended.[107,109]

In patients with full anticoagulation, the incidence of stroke is about 1% per year, and most of the emboli are minor, leaving mild residual deficits.[112,113,116] When stroke occurs in patients receiving anticoagulation, transesophageal echocardiography (TEE) should usually be performed to search for infective valve vegetations, thrombi, spontaneous echodensities, and atrial thrombi.[117] Anticoagulation may be increased if embolism from the left atrium is suspected, but adding an antiplatelet agent might be useful if the stroke is attributed to associated cerebrovascular disease or valve-related thrombi.[110]

In patients at high risk of thromboembolism, the interruption of anticoagulant therapy before invasive procedures often presents a challenge to clinicians. No randomized controlled trial has assessed this situation, but data from small nonrandomized studies favor the use of low-molecular-weight (LMW) heparin for safety and economic reasons.[118–120] It is recommended that warfarin therapy be stopped approximately 4 days before surgery, allowing the INR to return to a normal level. Full-dose LMW heparin is begun as the INR falls (about 2 days before surgery). The LMW heparin can be stopped about 12 hours before surgery and restarted between 8 and 12 hours after the procedure.[121,122]

PATENT FORAMEN OVALE

The high frequency of patent foramen ovale (PFO) is in part the result of advances that have been made in cardiac imaging techniques. PFO has been associated with stroke in several case-control studies, particularly in young individuals without an alternative recognized cause of stroke. PFO is a potential conduit for paradoxical embolism.[123–127] However, its relationship to stroke, its prognosis, and the therapeutic implications are not clearly established. Precordial contrast echocardiography detects some interatrial shunting in about 18% of normal controls,[123,128–131] especially during early systole or Valsalva maneuver–provoking activities such as coughing.[132,133] The fossa ovalis and the size of PFO can be directly visualized by TEE, considered the diagnostic "gold standard."[134–136] Transcranial Doppler (TCD) ultrasonography can detect injected microbubbles that bypass the pulmonary capillaries and enter the cerebral circulation, an observation that correlates well with the TEE evidence of PFO in the majority of patients.[137–140] The size of the PFO patency varies from 1 to 9 mm at autopsy.[141] The volume of shunting depends on the size of the PFO and the difference in atrial pressures. Contrast-enhanced TCD ultrasonographic assessment of the middle cerebral artery is highly specific compared with contrast TEE in detecting right-to-left shunt.[142]

Several studies have now shown that the prevalence of PFO in young adults with TIA or ischemic stroke is increased ($\approx$ 40%, range 32% to 48%),[123–127,143] especially among those with cryptogenic ischemic stroke, in whom its prevalence in some series exceeds 50%.[126,131,141] The wide range of PFO prevalence may reflect in part the interobserver variability in the diagnosis of septal abnormalities. Hence, the frequency of PFO is increased two to threefold among young adults with cerebral ischemia, and PFO is clearly associated with cryptogenic stroke in young adults, who are less likely to have traditional risk factors for stroke. The difference in risk factors suggests differing stroke mechanisms in patients with and without PFO.[124] In older patients with stroke, the prevalence of PFO is lower, probably because its importance as an independent risk factor is offset by the higher prevalence of other stroke mechanisms.[144–147] In a meta-analysis of case control studies comparing patients with stroke and control subjects, PFO was significantly associated with ischemic stroke only in patients younger than 55 years. The odds ratio of stroke was 3 (95% CI 2–4).[148]

Because PFO is also common in normal subjects, it is important to characterize the cases associated with stroke. Therefore, it is possible that patients with PFO plus atrial septal aneurysm (ASA) constitute a subgroup of patients at increased risk of stroke.[124] The mechanism of PFO-associated stroke is thought to be due to paradoxical embolism in many patients. Paradoxical embolism occurs when embolic material originating in the venous system or right heart chambers migrates into the systemic circulation through vascular shunts that bypass the pulmonary vasculature. However, this mechanism has been well documented in only a few cases, in which the embolus was seen in its passage through a PFO. A venous source of thromboembolism is rarely found in patients with stroke and PFO.[149,150] The failure to document a venous source does

Therapy

not rule out paradoxical emboli, because in many cases, deep venous thrombosis in the pelvis or legs is under-recognized. Another potential mechanisms for stroke is direct embolization from thrombi formed locally within the PFO or in an associated ASA.[151] It is also postulated that patients with PFO are more prone to develop supraventricular arrhythmias that may predispose to thrombus formation.[131] Emboli can arise from thrombi in the crural pelvic veins or in the right heart chamber; however, the source of embolism is often not found.

In short, paradoxical embolism may not be the most common underlying mechanism of stroke in patients with PFO. First, in patients with isolated PFO, the shunting during Valsalva maneuver involves only a small fraction of the cardiac output, and the chances that this level of shunting will result in recurrent emboli is remote.[152] Second, deep venous thrombosis is identified in only about 10% of PFO-associated strokes. Further, PFO is associated with mitral valve prolapse and ASA, both of which are independent potential cardioembolic sources of emboli. ASAs are present in about 25% of young patients with PFO-associated stroke,[124,153] and their presence alone has been associated with a higher risk of embolic stroke. It is possible that in as many as half of patients with PFO-associated stroke, PFO and stroke coexist by chance.

In addition to the unclear mechanism of stroke in patients with PFO, the risk of recurrent stroke remains unsettled owing to the lack of prospective data. Most studies are retrospective and without control subjects.[131,153–155] Two studies reported stroke recurrence between 1% and 2% in patients with PFO.[156,157] A prospective study of 581 patients with cryptogenic stroke treated with aspirin reported that at 4 years, the risk of recurrent stroke was 2% in those with PFO (n = 216), 15% in those with both PFO and ASA (n = 51), and 4% in those with neither. Only 10 patients in the study had ASA alone, and no recurrence was seen in this group. In this study, only the presence of both abnormalities was associated with a significant risk of stroke (relative risk [RR] 4; 95% CI 1–12). PFO alone, regardless its size, did not influence the risk of stroke.[158]

Results of the Patent Foramen Ovale in Cryptogenic Stroke Study (PICSS), a substudy of the Warfarin-Aspirin Recurrent Stroke Study (WARSS), were reported in 2002. The 630 patients first underwent TEE, which documented PFO in 34%, and then were randomly assigned to receive either warfarin (INR 2.0) or aspirin. The stroke rates were similar for the two interventions, and the presence of PFO did not alter the event rate when associated with all or cryptogenic strokes. There was no benefit in using warfarin in patients with large PFO or in those with PFO and ASA (12% of the total).[142]

In short, the role of PFO as a cause of stroke is still unsettled; therefore, the optimal treatment remains undetermined. On the basis of current evidence, every patient with stroke and PFO should receive antiplatelet therapy. In addition, if there is evidence of deep venous thrombosis, pulmonary embolism, or recurrent stroke, the use of long-term anticoagulation seems appropriate.

It is sensible to speculate that closure of PFO by surgical or device-mediated procedures would prevent stroke recurrence in patients with paradoxical emboli. Device closure seems to be effective, safe, and cost-effective.[159–164]

Its value is still unclear, however, given the uncertainties in pathogenesis, recurrence rate of stroke, and comparative efficacy against antithrombotic agents. Before this procedure is widely used for stroke prevention, it must be compared in randomized clinical trials with medical treatment. Currently, the Randomized Evaluation of recurrent Stroke comparing PFO closure to Established Current standard of care Treatment (RESPECT) trial (AGA Medical Corp) is recruiting patients with prior stroke or TIA and PFO without other known cause. A total of 500 patients will be assigned to either percutaneous closure of PFO using the Amplatzer PFO Occluder device or to best medical treatment (oral anticoagulants or antiplatelet agents), with follow-up for up to 5 years.[165] Until the results of clinical trials are available, patients with PFO should be treated with antithrombotic agents and encouraged to participate in randomized trials testing different interventions.

ANTICOAGULANT AGENTS

Heparin, Low-Molecular-Weight Heparin, and Heparinoids

Heparin is the most commonly used parenteral anticoagulant. Unfractionated heparin is derived from bovine lung or porcine gut tissue. A glycosaminoglycan of varying molecular weight, heparin binds to antithrombin III to inactivate factors IIa and Xa.[2] Its major anticoagulant effect comes from a unique pentasaccharide with high-affinity binding to antithrombin. Unfractionated heparin is quite heterogeneous, containing saccharides ranging in molecular weight from 5000 to 30,000 daltons. Only about one third of the unfractionated heparin molecules have anticoagulant activity. This heterogeneity is one of the reasons for the variability in the anticoagulant effect of heparin administration among individuals.

The most common side effect of heparin administration is bleeding. Other complications are thrombocytopenia, osteoporosis, skin necrosis, alopecia, hypersensitivity reactions and hypoaldosteronism. Thrombocytopenia is somewhat more common with heparin derived from bovine lung than from porcine gut. The thrombocytopenia is thought to occur because of the binding of immunoglobulin (Ig) G to heparin. Thrombocytopenia occurs in between 0.3% (in prophylactic use) and 2.4% (with higher therapeutic doses) of treated patients.

LMW heparin represents a fragment of a standard heparin with lower molecular weight, higher bioavailability, longer half-life, and more predictable anticoagulant effects. LMW heparin is said to have fewer bleeding complications and fewer interactions with platelets, but this issue remains somewhat controversial. Heparinoids are analogues of heparin that inhibit factor Xa, have a longer half-life than unfractionated heparin, and cause fewer bleeding complications. LMW heparin is as effective as, if not more effective than, unfractionated heparin, has the advantage of being given in fixed subcutaneous doses, and does not require monitoring or dose adjustment.[166]

Warfarin

Warfarin, an oral anticoagulant, is the most commonly used coumarin. Warfarin acts as a vitamin K antagonist, interfering with the production of vitamin K–dependent proteins, including the coagulation factors II, VII, IX, and X. The dose of warfarin ranges typically between 2 and 10 mg per day and must be individualized and adjusted to achieve the desired INR. Therapy is initiated with an estimated daily maintenance dose, such as 5 mg per day. Lower initial doses (3 to 4 mg/day) may be used in elderly and small individuals. The prothrombin time and INR are monitored frequently until values are in the target range and stable. Thereafter, stable patients are typically monitored at least monthly. The target INR for most indications is 2.5 (range 2.0 to 3.0). The target is increased to 3.0 (range 2.5 to 3.5) in patients with high-risk mechanical prosthetic cardiac valves and in patients with the antiphospholipid antibody syndrome.[167,168]

Warfarin therapy is contraindicated in patients at risk for major hemorrhage. Commonly acknowledged contraindications include active bleeding, recent surgery, pregnancy, esophageal varices, thrombocytopenia, concurrent use of thrombolytic agents, recent lumbar puncture, and congenital clotting defects. Patients at increased risk for falls or other trauma may not be candidates for long-term anticoagulation therapy. The importance of compliance dictates that unreliable or demented patients should receive warfarin therapy only if their therapy and INR monitoring can be adequately supervised.

Warfarin has the potential to interact with numerous agents (Table 60.4). Some potentiate and others inhibit the anticoagulant effects of warfarin. In addition, foods high in vitamin K can inhibit the effects of warfarin. Other substances, such as alcohol, may increase bleeding risk. The best course is to monitor the INR after any change in medications in a patient receiving warfarin and adjust the dose as needed. In addition, patient education about the potential effects of over-the counter-preparations and foods is an important element of warfarin management.

The main potential side effect of warfarin is bleeding. The only other serious side effect is skin necrosis. This uncommon complication, seen on the third to eighth day of therapy, is caused by thrombosis of venules and capillaries within the subcutaneous fat. A number of factors influence bleeding risk with warfarin therapy. The intensity of anticoagulation is directly related to bleeding risk, the rate of major bleeds increasing dramatically with INR levels exceeding 4.0. Patients older than 75 years have a higher risk of hemorrhage, particularly ICH. Patients with cerebrovascular disease are at greater risk for ICH than patients without a history of ischemic cerebrovascular disease. Other comorbid conditions that increase bleeding risk are hypertension, heart disease, renal insufficiency, and malignancy. Alcoholism and liver disease are also considered by many to raise the risk of bleeding associated with warfarin therapy.

Oral Anticoagulants Combined with Antiplatelet Agents

The risks and benefits of combination of an oral anticoagulant and an antiplatelet agent compared with an oral anticoagulant alone for secondary prevention of cardioembolic stroke has not been clearly established. Turpie and colleagues[110] studied young patients with prosthetic valves and showed a significant reduction of embolic events in those assigned to combination therapy and no significant increase in the incidence of ICH (7 patients vs. 3 patients, respectively).[110] However, in view of the occurrence of only a few events and the patients' ages, these results cannot be generalized to different group of patients (i.e., elderly with established cerebrovascular disease).

A meta-analysis of six randomized clinical trials that compared warfarin plus aspirin versus warfarin alone in different populations found that the addition of aspirin to warfarin significantly increased the risk of ICH (relative risk, 2.3; 95% CI 1.1–4.8). The increased risk of ICH was seen even in trials that used lower doses of aspirin.[169] It is possible that the risk-to-benefit ratio of combination therapy for elderly patients with prior ischemic strokes may be higher than that for young patients with prosthetic valvular disease. For those at high risk of suffering ICH during anticoagulation (i.e., older than 75 years, white matter abnormalities, prior stroke), the addition of aspirin could offset the benefit of reducing ischemic events. Therefore, we recommended that aspirin not be added routinely to oral anticoagulant therapy in elderly patients with established cerebrovascular disease until additional data define the risks and benefits.

INTRACEREBRAL HEMORRHAGE ASSOCIATED WITH ANTICOAGULATION

Intracerebral hemorrhage (ICH) is the most serious complication of anticoagulant therapy because of its high associated mortality. Anticoagulation with INR targets

Table 60.4 Drug Interactions with Warfarin: Effect of Drugs on International Normalized Ratio (INR)

Drug	Effect
Major Effects on INR	
Amiodarone	↑
Antithyroid drugs	↓
Barbiturates	↓
Co-trimoxazole	↑
Danazol	↑
Disulfiran	↑
Metronidazole	↑
Phenylbutazone	↑
Rifampin	↓
Sulfinpyrazone	↑
Thyroid hormones	↑
Moderate effects on INR	
Allopurinol	↑
Antidiabetics	↑
Carbamazepine	↓
Cephalosporins	↑
Cimetidine	↑
Fluconazole	↑
Griseofulvine	↑↓
Ketoconazole	↑
Miconazole	↑
Penicillins	↑↓
Phenytoin	↑↓
Vitamin C	↓
Vitamin E	↑
"Statins"	↑

between 2.5 and 4.5 increase the risk of ICH 7 to 10 times,[170-172] representing an absolute rate of 1% per year in stroke-prone patients.[47] The mortality in patients with ICH related to oral anticoagulants exceeds 50%. The cerebellum is frequently involved, and simultaneous ICHs at multiple sites can occur, particularly with excessive anticoagulation. One of the unique features of intracerebral hematomas related to anticoagulation is that they can continue to enlarge for 12 to 24 hours; therefore, anticoagulation should be reversed immediately, even in patients with minimal deficits and small hematomas. ICH-related anticoagulation is usually managed by the following approaches:

- Cessation of anticoagulation therapy.
- Administration of vitamin K; the INR is not affected for several hours, and the dose should not exceed 10 mg because higher doses lead to refractoriness to further anticoagulant therapy for days.
- Administration of plasma derivatives containing vitamin K–dependent clotting factors, such as fresh frozen plasma (FFP) and cryoprecipitates.

FFP reverses anticoagulation immediately, but it has the disadvantage of requiring a large infusion to correct the INR, which could be a problem in patients with poor cardiac function. Factor concentrates (factor II, VII, IX, and X) are an alternative for patients who cannot tolerate large volume of fluids but should not be used in patients with liver failure. The hemostatic agent recombinant activated factor VII (rFVIIa) has been used for the management of hemorrhages in the central nervous system associated with anticoagulation. The clinical experience indicates that rFVIIa may be safe and effective for rapid reversal of anticoagulation in patients with ICH.[173]

Well-established risk factors for ICH in patients who have been receiving anticoagulants include advanced age (particularly >75 years), hypertension, prior ischemic stroke,[174] and intensity of anticoagulation (perhaps also fluctuations in the level of anticoagulation).[37,172,175] The significance of high INR levels in influencing the development of ICH was demonstrated in an observational study and in the Stroke Prevention in Reversible Ischemia Trial (SPIRIT) study. In this trial, the absolute rate of ICH was 3% per year in patients receiving anticoagulation, particularly those with INR values exceeding 4.0.[176,177]

White matter abnormalities, identified by neuroimaging studies in patients with established cerebrovascular disease, were found to be an independent risk factor for ICH associated with anticoagulation.[176,178,179] Small hemosiderin deposits (indicative of asymptomatic "microbleeds") are frequently detected by gradient-echo magnetic resonance imaging (MRI) in patients with stroke, particularly those with small vessel disease (i.e., lacunar stroke, primary ICH, and white matter abnormalities).[180,181] It is likely that the presence of microbleeds predisposes to ICH in patients taking anticoagulants; so far, this predisposition has been reported only in patients receiving antiplatelet agents.[182] It is sensible to speculate that white matter abnormalities and microbleeds represent manifestations of a vasculopathy that predisposes to development of ICH in patients receiving anticoagulants.[183] Currently, the pres-

ence of white matter abnormalities or microbleeds does not preclude the use of anticoagulants; more data are needed to stratify risk of ICH on the basis of MRI findings.

ANTICOAGULATION IN ACUTE CARDIOEMBOLIC STROKE

Hemorrhagic transformation is defined as the presence of petechiae or confluent petechial hemorrhage confined to the ischemic zone. It is a relatively common consequence of developing cerebral infarction, being present in about 15% of all ischemic strokes and up to 30% of cardioembolic strokes.[184-186] The proposed mechanism for hemorrhagic transformation is the distal migration or lysis of an embolus resulting in reperfusion of the ischemic tissue which can become hemorrhagic depending on the extent of the ischemic vascular injury.

Detection of hemorrhagic transformation depends on the neuroimaging technique used. MRI with T2-weighted sequences as well as diffusion- and perfusion-weighted imaging have higher sensitivity than computed tomography (CT) for early detection of hemorrhagic transformation.[187,188] A prospective MRI study that imaged patients 3 weeks after cardioembolic stroke reported a 60% incidence of hemorrhagic transformation.[185] Autopsy series showed hemorrhagic transformation in even higher numbers (50% to 70%) of patients undergoing anticoagulation.[189] The great majority of hemorrhagic transformations are asymptomatic in patients not receiving anticoagulants.

The visualization of hemorrhagic transformation in a patient with ischemic stroke is important, in that it may provide guidance as to the possible underlying mechanism of stroke (i.e., cardioembolic) and may influence the selection of antithrombotic therapy. Because of the high incidence of secondary hemorrhagic transformation in patients with cardioembolic stroke, early anticoagulation is potentially risky. At present, it is impossible to formulate firm guidelines for anticoagulation in acute cardioembolic stroke because of a paucity of adequate data. The risk-benefit ratio of early anticoagulation is influenced by the specific cardioembolic source of the stroke as well as the size of the infarct.

In the past, the risk of early recurrent stroke or systemic embolism after a recent cardioembolic stroke in untreated patients was estimated to be around 10% during the first week[1] and to be especially high during the first 5 or 6 days after an acute cardioembolic stroke.[190,191] However these data were not supported by recent studies, in which the risk of recurrent stroke within the first 14 days of stroke in patients with AF was between 5% and 8% without anticoagulation.[43]

Pooled data from case series and one small controlled trial suggest that heparin reduces early stroke recurrence by about 70% in patients with cardioembolic stroke. However, the increased risk of symptomatic ICH in patients in whom anticoagulation is begun early offsets the benefit conveyed by the therapy.[192,193]

The relationship between anticoagulants and clinically significant delayed hemorrhage is controversial. The occurrence and timing of asymptomatic hemorrhagic transformation do not seem to be affected by anticoagulation[194]; however, the magnitude and likelihood of associated clinical deterioration are augmented.[194,195] The incidence of symptomatic hemorrhagic transformation in patients receiving early anticoagulation varies widely (from 1% to 25%).[196,197]

Patients with a large infarct, excessive anticoagulation, and detection of hemorrhagic infarction on initial CT scan are at higher risk for symptomatic hemorrhagic transformation. Small case series have advocated the use of anticoagulants even in patients with early CT visualization of hemorrhagic infarction.[198,199] It appears that hemorrhagic infarction may not be an absolute contraindication to anticoagulation, especially in individual patients who are at high risk of recurrent embolism. Given the lack of prospective studies and the relatively small number of patients in these case series, however, early anticoagulation in hemorrhagic infarction cannot be routinely recommended without assessment of the risk of recurrent stroke. Delaying the start of anticoagulation for 1 to 2 weeks after detection of hemorrhagic infarction may be prudent.

For patients at relatively low risk for early stroke recurrence, including those with nonvalvular AF or recent MI without associated ventricular thrombi, deferring anticoagulation for several weeks may reduce the risk of hemorrhagic deterioration, particularly for patients with moderate to large infarcts or uncontrolled hypertension. Initiation of anticoagulation with oral warfarin (without the use of heparin) is an alternative for these patients. Thus, the "typical" patient with ischemic stroke and AF is unlikely to benefit from initiation of anticoagulation within the first day or two, especially if the stroke is large. In the interest of management efficiency, some physicians initiate oral anticoagulation within the first day or two, assuming that therapeutic, and therefore dangerous, levels of anticoagulation will not be achieved for a few days, when the period of increased risk for symptomatic hemorrhage has past. Some patients with AF might benefit from early anticoagulation because their recurrent stroke risk is increased—for example, the patient with documented thrombi in the left atrium. The randomized clinical trials that included patients with AF have not studied this subgroup and other potentially important subgroups to establish with certainty whether atrial thrombi or other predictors might identify a subpopulation at sufficiently increased risk of early stroke recurrence to justify prompt initiation of anticoagulation.[43]

For patients at high risk for recurrent embolization (i.e., mechanical prosthetic valve, intracardiac thrombus, AF with valvular disease or CHF), early anticoagulation is recommended, particularly if there are no associated risk factors for brain hemorrhage. Intravenous boluses of heparin and excessive anticoagulation should be avoided.

The value of antiplatelet agents and low-dose subcutaneous heparin in this setting has not been systematically assessed. Both could be alternatives to intravenous heparin, particularly in patients at low risk of early recurrent stroke (e.g., nonvalvular AF).

Patients with prosthetic valves who in full anticoagulation at the time of stroke represent a management challenge. Reversing anticoagulation should be considered in patients with large infarcts or with infarcts already visible on early CT scan (<6 to 12 hours). Anticoagulation is not indicated for embolic stroke secondary to infective endocarditis of native valves.

RESUMPTION OF ANTICOAGULATION IN THE PRESENCE OF INTRACEREBRAL HEMORRHAGE

The risk of ICH in the general population ranges from 0.5% to 2% per year. In patients undergoing anticoagulation, the risk of hemorrhage is about 10 times higher.[47,200] However, the risk of cerebral emboli in patients with major cardioembolic sources (e.g., left ventricular thrombi, prosthetic valve disease) without protection offered by anticoagulation is high. Therefore, it is essential to estimate the risks and benefits of anticoagulation in this particular group of patients. So far, data are insufficient for firm recommendations to be made in these situations. Results of several small series and retrospective studies have suggested that, when absolutely necessary, resumption of oral anticoagulation after 1 or 2 weeks is associated with a low short-term risk of embolism and no major complications, worsening, or recurrence of ICH.[201-207]

The use of intravenous heparin or continuation of oral anticoagulant therapy in a patient who has ICH or a cerebral with hemorrhagic transformation and a high-risk embolic source is less clear and continues to be a challenge for physicians. Two small case series reported good outcome in patients with ICH and therapy with early intravenous heparin.[199,204] Despite these encouraging results, it is difficult to draw firm conclusions from these studies because of their small sample size and potentially biased selection.

In short, when to initiate anticoagulation and whether to continue anticoagulant therapy in patients with ICH remain controversial, and it is unlikely that these important issues will be settled by a large study. In view of the lack of evidence, we recommend that each case be assessed individually through balancing of the risks and benefits of the intervention. For instance, in patients who have hemorrhagic transformation or small intracerebral hematoma but are clinically stable and have a high risk of cardioembolic stroke, the use of antiplatelet agents during the first days and initiation of oral anticoagulation seems to be appropriate.

SUMMARY

Emboli arising from the heart account for at least 20% of ischemic strokes. Cardiac sources of emboli are being detected with increasing ease with modern echocardiography. The common clinical dilemma is whether the detection of one of the "minor" cardiac sources of emboli bears any responsibility for causing a stroke in a given patient. Long-term oral anticoagulation is highly effective in preventing recurrent stroke in patients with "major" cardiac abnormalities including AF, in patients who have received prosthetic cardiac valves, and in patients with intracardiac thrombi due to myocardial infarction or cardiomyopathy.

Therapy

References

1. Cardiogenic brain embolism: The second report of Cerebral Embolism Task Force. Arch Neurol 46:727–741, 1989.
2. Comess KA, DeRook FA, Beach KW, et al: Transesophageal echocardiography and carotid ultrasound in patients with cerebral ischemia: Prevalence of findings and recurrent stroke risk. J Am Coll Cardiol 23:1598–603, 1994.
3. Albers GW, Comess KA, DeRook FA, et al: Transesophageal echocardiographic findings in stroke subtypes. Stroke 25:23–28, 1994.
4. Bogousslavsky J, Cachin C, Regli F, et al: Cardiac sources of embolism and cerebral infarction—clinical consequences and vascular concomitants: The Lausanne Stroke Registry. Neurology 41:855–859, 1991.
5. Hornig CR, Brainin M, Mast H: Cardioembolic stroke: Results from three current stroke data banks. Neuroepidemiology 13:318–323, 1994.
6. Ramirez-Lassepas M, Cipolle RJ, Bjork RJ: Can embolic stroke be diagnosed on the basis of neurological clinical criteria? Arch Neurol 44:87–89, 1987.
7. Foulkes MA, Wolf PA, Price TR, et al: The Stroke Data Bank: Design, methods, and baseline characteristics. Stroke 19:547–554, 1988.
8. Lindgren A, Roijer A, Norrving B, et al: Carotid artery and heart disease in subtypes of cerebral infarction. Stroke 25:2356–2362, 1994.
9. Czlonkowska A, Ryglewicz D, Weissbein T, et al: A prospective community-based study of stroke in Warsaw, Poland. Stroke 25:547–551, 1994.
10. Moulin T, Tatu L, Crepin-Leblond T, et al: The Besançon Stroke Registry: An acute stroke registry of 2,500 consecutive patients. Eur Neurol 38:10–20, 1997.
11. Ward G, Jamrozik K, Stewart-Wynne E: Incidence and outcome of cerebrovascular disease in Perth, Western Australia. Stroke 19:1501–1506, 1988.
12. Vemmos KN, Takis CE, Georgilis K, et al: The Athens Stroke Registry: Results of a five-year hospital-based study. Cerebrovasc Dis 10:133–141, 2000.
13. Vemmos KN, Bots ML, Tsibouris PK, et al: Stroke incidence and case fatality in southern Greece: The Arcadia Stroke Registry. Stroke 30:363–370, 1999.
14. Lee BI, Nam HS, Heo JH, Kim DI: Yonsei Stroke Registry. Analysis of 1,000 patients with acute cerebral infarctions. Cerebrovasc Dis 12:145–151, 2001.
15. Arboix A, Vericat MC, Pujades R, et al: Cardioembolic infarction in the Sagrat Cor-Alianza Hospital of Barcelona Stroke Registry. Acta Neurol Scand 96:407–412, 1997.
16. Amarenco P, Cohen A, Hommel M, et al: Causes of cerebral infarcts in 250 consecutive elderly patients [abstract]. Stroke 26:162, 1995.
18. Grau AJ, Weimar C, Buggle F, et al: Risk factors, outcome, and treatment in subtypes of ischemic stroke: The German stroke data bank. Stroke 32:2559–2566, 2001.
19. Feinberg WM, Blackshear JL, Laupacis A, et al: Prevalence, age distribution, and gender of patients with atrial fibrillation. Arch Intern Med 155:469–473, 1995.
20. Broderick JP, Philips SJ, O'Fallon WM, et al: Relationship of cardiac disease to stroke occurrence, recurrence and mortality. Stroke 23:1250–1256, 1992.
21. Mohr JP, Caplan LR, Melski JW: The Harvard Cooperative Stroke Registry: A prospective registry. Neurology 28:754–762, 1978.
22. Sandercock P, Bamford J, Dennis M, et al: Atrial fibrillation and stroke: Prevalence in different types of stroke and influence on early and longterm prognosis. Oxfordshire Community Stroke Project. BMJ 305:1460–1465, 1992.
23. van Merwijk G, Lodder J, Bamford J, Kester ADM: How often is non-valvular atrial fibrillation the cause of brain infarction. J Neurol 237:205–207, 1990.
24. Asplund K, Carlberg B, Sundstrom G: Stroke in the elderly. Cerebrovasc Dis 2:152–157, 1992.
25. Wolf PA, Abbot RD, Kammel WB: Atrial fibrillation as an independent risk factor for stroke: The Framingham Study. Stroke 22:983–988, 1991.
26. Saxena R, Lewis S, Berge E, et al: Risk of early death and recurrent stroke and effect of heparin in 3169 patients with acute ischemic stroke and atrial fibrillation in the International Stroke Trial. Stroke 32:2333–2337, 2001.
27. Lamassa M, Di Carlo AA, Pracucci G, et al: Characteristics, outcome, and care of stroke associated with atrial fibrillation in Europe: Data from a multicenter multinational hospital-based registry (The European Community Stroke Project). Stroke 32:392–398, 2001.
28. Hart RG, Halperin JL: Atrial fibrillation and stroke: Concepts and controversies. Stroke 32:803–808, 2001.
29. Miller VT, Rothrock JF, Pearce LA, et al: Ischemic stroke in patients with atrial fibrillation: Effect of aspirin according to stroke mechanism. Stroke Prevention in Atrial Fibrillation Investigators. Neurology 43:32–36, 1993.
30. Miller VT, Pearce LA, Feinberg WM, et al: Differential effect of aspirin versus warfarin on clinical stroke types in patients with atrial fibrillation. Stroke Prevention in Atrial Fibrillation Investigators. Neurology 46:238–240, 1996.
31. Hart RG, Pearce LA, Miller VT, et al: Cardioembolic vs. noncardioembolic strokes in atrial fibrillation: Frequency and effect of antithrombotic agents in the stroke prevention in atrial fibrillation studies. Cerebrovasc Dis 10:39–43, 2000.
32. Hart RG, Halperin JL: Atrial fibrillation and thromboembolism: A decade of progress in stroke prevention. Ann Intern Med 131:688–695, 1999.
33. Albers GW, Dalen JE, Laupacis A, et al: Antithrombotic therapy in atrial fibrillation. Chest 119:194S–206S, 2001.
34. Flaker GC, Fletcher KA, Rothbart RM, et al: Clinical and echocardiographic features of intermittent atrial fibrillation that predict recurrent atrial fibrillation. Stroke Prevention in Atrial Fibrillation (SPAF) Investigators. Am J Cardiol 76:355–358, 1995.
35. Predictors of thromboembolism in atrial fibrillation. I: Clinical features of patients at risk. The Stroke Prevention in Atrial Fibrillation Investigators. Ann Intern Med 116:1–5, 1992.
36. Predictors of thromboembolism in atrial fibrillation. II: Echocardiographic features of patients at risk. The Stroke Prevention in Atrial Fibrillation Investigators. Ann Intern Med 116:6–12, 1992.
37. Stroke Prevention in Atrial Fibrillation Study: Final results. Circulation 84:527–539, 1991.
38. van Latum JC, Koudstaal PJ, Venables GS, et al: Predictors of major vascular events in patients with a transient ischemic attack or minor ischemic stroke and with nonrheumatic atrial fibrillation. European Atrial Fibrillation Trial (EAFT) Study Group. Stroke 26:801–806, 1995.
39. Pearce LA, Hart RG, Halperin JL: Assessment of three schemes for stratifying stroke risk in patients with nonvalvular atrial fibrillation. Am J Med 109:45–51, 2000.
40. Berge E, Abdelnoor M, Nakstad PH, Sandset PM: Low molecular-weight heparin versus aspirin in patients with acute ischaemic stroke and atrial fibrillation: A double-blind randomised study. HAEST Study Group. Heparin in Acute Embolic Stroke Trial. Lancet 355:1205–1210, 2000.
41. Randomised placebo-controlled trial of early aspirin use in 20,000 patients with acute ischaemic stroke. CAST (Chinese Acute Stroke Trial) Collaborative Group. Lancet 349:1641–1649, 1997.
42. A randomised trial of aspirin, subcutaneous heparin, both, or neither among 19,435 patients with acute ischaemic stroke. International Stroke Trial Collaborative Group. Lancet 349:1569–1581, 1997.
43. Hart RG, Palacio S, Pearce LA: Atrial fibrillation, stroke, and acute antithrombotic therapy: Analysis of randomized clinical trials. Stroke 33:2722–2727, 2002.
44. Hart RG, Benavente O, McBride R, Pearce LA: Antithrombotic therapy to prevent stroke in patients with atrial fibrillation: A meta-analysis. Ann Intern Med 131:492–501, 1999.
45. Benavente O, Hart R, Koudstaal P, et al: Oral anticoagulants for preventing stroke in patients with non-valvular atrial fibrillation and no previous history of stroke or transient ischemic attacks. Cochrane Database Syst Rev (2):CD001927, 2000.
46. Benavente O, Hart R, Koudstaal P, et al: Antiplatelet therapy for preventing stroke in patients with non-valvular atrial fibrillation and no previous history of stroke or transient ischemic attacks. Cochrane Database Syst Rev (2):CD001925, 2000.
47. Hart RG, Boop BS, Anderson DC: Oral anticoagulants and intracranial hemorrhage: Facts and hypotheses. Stroke 26:1471–1477, 1995.
48. Hart RG: Anticoagulation for nonrheumatic atrial fibrillation. N Engl J Med 336:441–442, 1997.

49. Hart RG: Intensity of anticoagulation to prevent stroke in patients with atrial fibrillation. Ann Intern Med 128:408, 1998.

50. van Walraven C, Hart RG, Singer DE, et al: Oral anticoagulants vs aspirin in nonvalvular atrial fibrillation: An individual patient meta-analysis. JAMA 288:2441–2448, 2002.

51. Lip GY, Hee FL: Paroxysmal atrial fibrillation. Q J Med 94:665–678, 2001.

52. Hart RG, Pearce LA, Rothbart RM, et al: Stroke with intermittent atrial fibrillation: Incidence and predictors during aspirin therapy. Stroke Prevention in Atrial Fibrillation Investigators. J Am Coll Cardiol 35:183–187, 2000.

53. Risk factors for stroke and efficacy of antithrombotic therapy in atrial fibrillation: Analysis of pooled data from five randomized controlled trials. Arch Intern Med 154:1449–1457, 1994.

54. Diener HC: Ximelagatran compared with Warfarin for prevention of stroke and systemic embolism in patients with atrial fibrillation. N Engl J Med 347:1825–1833, 2002.

55. Wyse DG, Waldo AL, DiMarco JP, et al: A comparison of rate control and rhythm control in patients with atrial fibrillation. N Engl J Med 347:1825–1833, 2002.

56. Sherman DG, Kim S, Boop BS, et al: The occurrence and characteristics of stroke events in the AFFIRM Study. Neurology 60(Suppl 1):A326, 2003.

57. Berger M, Schweitzer P: Timing of thromboembolic events after electrical cardioversion of atrial fibrillation or flutter: A retrospective analysis. Am J Cardiol 82:1545–1547, 1998.

58. Bjerkelund CJ, Orning OM: The efficacy of anticoagulant therapy in preventing embolism related to D.C. electrical conversion of atrial fibrillation. Am J Cardiol 23:208–216, 1969.

59. Kannel WB, Wolf PA, Verter J: Manifestations of coronary disease predisposing to stroke: The Framingham study. JAMA 250:2942–2946, 1983.

60. Pullicino PM, Halperin JL, Thompson JL: Stroke in patients with heart failure and reduced left ventricular ejection fraction. Neurology 54:288–294, 2000.

61. Wolf PA, Abbott RD, Kannel WB: Atrial fibrillation: A major contributor to stroke in the elderly: The Framingham Study. Arch Intern Med 147:1561–1564, 1987.

62. Dries DL, Rosenberg YD, Waclawiw MA, Domanski MJ: Ejection fraction and risk of thromboembolic events in patients with systolic dysfunction and sinus rhythm: Evidence for gender differences in the studies of left ventricular dysfunction trials. J Am Coll Cardiol 29:1074–1080, 1997.

63. Loh E, Sutton MS, Wun CC, et al: Ventricular dysfunction and the risk of stroke after myocardial infarction. N Engl J Med 336:251–257, 1997.

64. Katz SD, Marantz PR, Biasucci L, et al: Low incidence of stroke in ambulatory patients with heart failure: A prospective study. Am Heart J 126:141–146, 1993.

65. Cioffi G, Pozzoli M, Forni G, et al: Systemic thromboembolism in chronic heart failure: A prospective study in 406 patients. Eur Heart J 17:1381–1389, 1996.

66. Effects of enalapril on mortality in severe congestive heart failure: Results of the Cooperative North Scandinavian Enalapril Survival Study (CONSENSUS). The CONSENSUS Trial Study Group. N Engl J Med 316:1429–1435, 1987.

67. Loh E, Sutton MS, Wun CC, et al: Ventricular dysfunction and the risk of stroke after myocardial infarction. N Engl J Med 336:251–257, 1997.

68. Sbarouni E, Bradshaw A, Andreotti F, et al: Relationship between hemostatic abnormalities and neuroendocrine activity in heart failure. Am Heart J 127:607–612, 1994.

69. Fuster V, Gersh BJ, Giuliani ER, et al: The natural history of idiopathic dilated cardiomyopathy. Am J Cardiol 47:525–531, 1981.

70. Falk RH, Foster E, Coats MH: Ventricular thrombi and thromboembolism in dilated cardiomyopathy: A prospective follow-up study. Am Heart J 123:136–142, 1992.

71. Gottdiener JS, Gay JA, VanVoorhees L, et al: Frequency and embolic potential of left ventricular thrombus in dilated cardiomyopathy: Assessment by 2-dimensional echocardiography. Am J Cardiol 52:1281–1285, 1983.

72. Randomised trial of late thrombolysis in patients with suspected acute myocardial infarction. EMERAS (Estudio Multicentrico Estreptoquinasa Republicas de America del Sur) Collaborative Group. Lancet 342:767–772, 1993.

73. Maze SS, Kotler MN, Parry WR: Flow characteristics in the dilated left ventricle with thrombus: Qualitative and quantitative Doppler analysis. J Am Coll Cardiol 13:873–881, 1989.

74. Loh E, Sutton MS: Anticoagulation and left ventricular dysfunction: Friend or foe? Eur Heart J 18:1039–1041, 1997.

75. Stratton JR, Nemanich JW, Johannessen KA, Resnick AD: Fate of left ventricular thrombi in patients with remote myocardial infarction or idiopathic cardiomyopathy. Circulation 78:1388–1393, 1988.

76. Martin R, Bogousslavsky J: Mechanism of late stroke after myocardial infarct: The Lausanne Stroke Registry. J Neurol Neurosurg Psychiatry 56:760–764, 1993.

77. Dexter DD Jr, Whisnant JP, Connolly DC, O'Fallon WM: The association of stroke and coronary heart disease: A population study. Mayo Clin Proc 62:1077–1083, 1987.

78. Tanne D, Goldbourt U, Zion M, et al: Frequency and prognosis of stroke/TIA among 4808 survivors of acute myocardial infarction. The SPRINT Study Group. Stroke 24:1490–1495, 1993.

79. Bleeding during antithrombotic therapy in patients with atrial fibrillation. The Stroke Prevention in Atrial Fibrillation Investigators. Arch Intern Med 156:409–416, 1996.

80. Long-term anticoagulant therapy after myocardial infarction. United States Veterans Administration. JAMA 243:661–669, 1980.

81. Bodenheimer MM, Sauer D, Shareef B, et al: Relation between myocardial infarct location and stroke. J Am Coll Cardiol 24:61–66, 1994.

82. Keren A, Goldberg S, Gottlieb S, et al: Natural history of left ventricular thrombi: Their appearance and resolution in the posthospitalization period of acute myocardial infarction. J Am Coll Cardiol 15:790–800, 1990.

83. Friedman MJ, Carlson K, Marcus FI, Woolfenden JM: Clinical correlations in patients with acute myocardial infarction and left ventricular thrombus detected by two-dimensional echocardiography. Am J Med 72:894–898, 1982.

84. Delemarre BJ, Visser CA, Bot H, Dunning AJ: Prediction of apical thrombus formation in acute myocardial infarction based on left ventricular spatial flow pattern. J Am Coll Cardiol 15:355–360, 1990.

85. Merlini PA, Bauer KA, Oltrona L, et al: Persistent activation of coagulation mechanism in unstable angina and myocardial infarction. Circulation 90:61–68, 1994.

86. Johnson RC, Crissman RS, DiDio LJ: Endocardial alterations in myocardial infarction. Lab Invest 40:183–193, 1979.

87. Stratton JR, Resnick AD: Increased embolic risk in patients with left ventricular thrombi. Circulation 75:1004–1011, 1987.

88. Jugdutt BI, Sivaram CA: Prospective two-dimensional echocardiographic evaluation of left ventricular thrombus and embolism after acute myocardial infarction. J Am Coll Cardiol 13:554–564, 1989.

89. Reeder GS, Tajik AJ, Seward JB: Left ventricular aneurysm, thrombus, and embolism. Chest 79:369, 1981.

90. Reeder GS, Tajik AJ, Seward JB: Left ventricular mural thrombus: Two-dimensional echocardiographic diagnosis. Mayo Clin Proc 56:82–86, 1981.

91. Reeder GS, Lengyel M, Tajik AJ, et al: Mural thrombus in left ventricular aneurysm: Incidence, role of angiography, and relation between anticoagulation and embolization. Mayo Clin Proc 56:77–781, 1981.

92. Ohman EM, Harrington RA, Cannon CP, et al: Intravenous thrombolysis in acute myocardial infarction. Chest 119:253S–277S, 2001.

93. Cairns JA, Theroux P, Lewis HD Jr, et al: Antithrombotic agents in coronary artery disease. Chest 119:228S–252S, 2001.

94. Behar S, Tanne D, Zion M, et al: Incidence and prognostic significance of chronic atrial fibrillation among 5,839 consecutive patients with acute myocardial infarction. The SPRINT Study Group. Secondary Prevention Reinfarction Israeli Nifedipine Trial. Am J Cardiol 70:816–818, 1992.

95. Komrad MS, Coffey CE, Coffey KS, et al: Myocardial infarction and stroke. Neurology 34:1403–1409, 1984.

96. Dunkman WB, Johnson GR, Carson PE, et al: Incidence of thromboembolic events in congestive heart failure. The V-HeFT VA Cooperative Studies Group. Circulation 87:VI94–VI101, 1993.

97. Dervall PB, Olley PM, Smith DR: Incidence of stenosis embolism before and after mitral valvotomy. Thorax 23:530–540, 1968.

98. Szekely P: Systemic embolism and anticoagulants prophylaxis in rheumatic heart disease. BMJ 1:209–212, 1964.

99. Levine HJ: Which atrial fibrillation patients should be on chronic anticoagulation? J Cardiovasc Med 6:483–487, 1981.

100. Hinton RC, Kistler JP, Fallon JT, et al: Influence of etiology of atrial fibrillation on incidence of systemic embolism. Am J Cardiol 40:509–513, 1977.

101. Daley R, Mattingly TW, Holt C: Systemic arterial embolism in rheumatic heart disease. Am Heart J 42:566–581, 1951.

102. Cassella K, Abelmann WH, Ellis LB: Patients with mitral stenosis and systemic emboli. Arch Intern Med 114:773, 1964.

103. Carter AB: Prognosis of cerebral embolism. Lancet 2:514–519, 1965.

104. Fleming HA, Bailey SM: Mitral valve disease, systemic embolism and anticoagulants. Postgrad Med J 47:599–604, 1971.

105. Fleming HA: Anticoagulants in rheumatic heart-disease. Lancet 2:486, 1971.

106. Adams GF, Merrett JD, Hutchinson WM, Pollock AM: Cerebral embolism and mitral stenosis: Survival with and without anticoagulants. J Neurol Neurosurg Psychiatry 37:378–383, 1974.

107. Salem DN, Daudelin HD, Levine HJ, et al: Antithrombotic therapy in valvular heart disease. Chest 119:207S–219S, 2001.

108. Saour JN, Sieck JO, Mamo LA, Gallus AS: Trial of different intensities of anticoagulation in patients with prosthetic heart valves. N Engl J Med 322:428–432, 1990.

109. Stein PD, Alpert JS, Bussey HI, et al: Antithrombotic therapy in patients with mechanical and biological prosthetic heart valves. Chest 119:220S–227S, 2001.

110. Turpie AG, Gent M, Laupacis A, et al: A comparison of aspirin with placebo in patients treated with warfarin after heart-valve replacement. N Engl J Med 329:524–529, 1993.

111. Butchart EG, Lewis PA, Grunkemeier GL, et al: Low risk of thrombosis and serious embolic events despite low-intensity anticoagulation: Experience with 1,004 Medtronic Hall valves. Circulation 78:I66–I77, 1988.

112. Kuntze CE, Blackstone EH, Ebels T: Thromboembolism and mechanical heart valves: A randomized study revisited. Ann Thorac Surg 66:101–107, 1998.

113. Kuntze CE, Ebels T, Eijgelaar A, Homan van der Heide JN: Rates of thromboembolism with three different mechanical heart valve prostheses: Randomised study. Lancet 1:514–517, 1989.

114. Cannegieter SC, Rosendaal FR, Wintzen AR, et al: Optimal oral anticoagulant therapy in patients with mechanical heart valves. N Engl J Med 333:11–17, 1995.

115. Coulshed N, Epstein EJ, McKendrick CS, et al: Systemic embolism in mitral valve disease. Br Heart J 32:26–34, 1970.

116. Altman R, Rouvier J, Gurfinkel E, et al: Comparison of two levels of anticoagulant therapy in patients with substitute heart valves. J Thorac Cardiovasc Surg 101:427–431, 1991.

117. Scott PJ, Essop R, Wharton GA, Williams GJ: Left atrial clot in patients with mitral prostheses: Increased rate of detection after recent systemic embolism. Int J Cardiol 33:141–148, 1991.

118. Tinmouth A, Kovacs M, Cruickshank M: Outpatient peri-operative and peri-procedure treatment with dalteparin for chronically anticoagulated patients at high risk for thromboembolic complications. Thromb Haemost 82(Suppl):662, 1999.

119. Kearon C, Hirsh J: Management of anticoagulation before and after elective surgery. N Engl J Med 336:1506–1511, 1997.

120. Johnson J, Turpie AG: Temporary discontinuation of oral anticoagulants: Role of low molecular weight heparin. Thromb Haemost 82(Suppl):62–63, 1999.

121. Ansell J, Hirsh J, Dalen J, et al: Managing oral anticoagulant therapy. Chest 119:22S–38S, 2001.

122. Hirsh J, Dalen J, Anderson DR, et al: Oral anticoagulants: Mechanism of action, clinical effectiveness, and optimal therapeutic range. Chest 119:8S–21S, 2001.

123. Di Tullio M, Sacco RL, Gopal A, et al: Patent foramen ovale as a risk factor for cryptogenic stroke. Ann Intern Med 117:461–465, 1992.

124. Cabanes L, Mas JL, Cohen A, et al: Atrial septal aneurysm and patent foramen ovale as risk factors for cryptogenic stroke in patients less than 55 years of age: A study using transesophageal echocardiography. Stroke 24:1865–73, 1993.

125. Lechat P, Lascault G, Mas JL, et al: [Prevalence of patent foramen ovale in young patients with ischemic cerebral complications]. Arch Mal Coeur Vaiss 82:847–852, 1989.

126. Lechat P, Mas JL, Lascault G, et al: Prevalence of patent foramen ovale in patients with stroke. N Engl J Med 318:1148–1152, 1988.

127. Webster MW, Chancellor AM, Smith HJ, et al: Patent foramen ovale in young stroke patients. Lancet 2:11–12, 1988.

128. Louie EK, Konstadt SN, Rao TL, Scanlon PJ: Transesophageal echocardiographic diagnosis of right to left shunting across the foramen ovale in adults without prior stroke. J Am Coll Cardiol 21:1231–1237, 1993.

129. Langholz D, Louie EK, Konstadt SN, et al: Transesophageal echocardiographic demonstration of distinct mechanisms for right to left shunting across a patent foramen ovale in the absence of pulmonary hypertension. J Am Coll Cardiol 18:1112–1117, 1991.

130. Konstadt SN, Louie EK, Black S, R, et al: Intraoperative detection of patent foramen ovale by transesophageal echocardiography. Anesthesiology 74:212–216, 1991.

131. Hausmann D, Mugge A, Daniel WG: Identification of patent foramen ovale permitting paradoxic embolism. J Am Coll Cardiol 26:1030–1038, 1995.

132. Strunk BL, Cheitlin MD, Stulbarg MS, Schiller NB: Right-to-left interatrial shunting through a patent foramen ovale despite normal intracardiac pressures. Am J Cardiol 60:413–415, 1987.

133. Lynch JJ, Schuchard GH, Gross CM, Wann LS: Prevalence of right-to-left atrial shunting in a healthy population: Detection by Valsalva maneuver contrast echocardiography. Am J Cardiol 53:1478–1480, 1984.

134. Comess KA, DeRook FA, Beach KW, et al: Transesophageal echocardiography and carotid ultrasound in patients with cerebral ischemia: Prevalence of findings and recurrent stroke risk. J Am Coll Cardiol 23:1598–1603, 1994.

135. Albers GW, Comess KA, DeRook FA, et al: Transesophageal echocardiographic findings in stroke subtypes. Stroke 25:23–28, 1994.

136. DeRook FA, Comess KA, Albers GW, Popp RL: Transesophageal echocardiography in the evaluation of stroke. Ann Intern Med 117:922–932, 1992.

137. Jauss M, Kaps M, Keberle M, et al: A comparison of transesophageal echocardiography and transcranial Doppler sonography with contrast medium for detection of patent foramen ovale. Stroke 25:1265–1267, 1994.

138. Jauss M, Schleime C, Hugens-Penzel M, et al: Disclosure of paradoxical brain embolism in two stroke patients with ultrasound test for right-to-left shunt and diffusion-weighted MRI. Cerebrovasc Dis 14:267–269, 2002.

139. Karnik R, Stollberger C, Valentin A, et al: Detection of patent foramen ovale by transcranial contrast Doppler ultrasound. Am J Cardiol 69:560–562, 1992.

140. Klotzsch C, Janssen G, Berlit P: Transesophageal echocardiography and contrast-TCD in the detection of a patent foramen ovale: Experiences with 111 patients. Neurology 44:1603–1606, 1994.

141. Hagen PT, Scholz DG, Edwards WD: Incidence and size of patent foramen ovale during the first 10 decades of life: An autopsy study of 965 normal hearts. Mayo Clin Proc 59:17–20, 1984.

142. Homma S, Sacco RL, Di Tullio MR, et al: Effect of medical treatment in stroke patients with patent foramen ovale: Patent foramen ovale in Cryptogenic Stroke Study. Circulation 105:2625–2631, 2002.

143. Sacco RL, Homma S, Di Tullio MR: Patent foramen ovale: A new risk factor for ischemic stroke. Heart Dis Stroke 2:235–241, 1993.

144. Jones EF, Calafiore P, Donnan GA, Tonkin AM: Evidence that patent foramen ovale is not a risk factor for cerebral ischemia in the elderly. Am J Cardiol 74:596–599, 1994.

145. de Belder MA, Tourikis L, Leech G, Camm AJ: Risk of patent foramen ovale for thromboembolic events in all age groups. Am J Cardiol 69:1316–1320, 1992.

146. Stollberger C, Finsterer J, Slany J: Why is venous thrombosis only rarely detected in patients with suspected paradoxical embolism? Thromb Res 105:189–191, 2002.

147. Stollberger C, Slany J, Schuster I, et al: The prevalence of deep venous thrombosis in patients with suspected paradoxical embolism. Ann Intern Med 119:461–465, 1993.

148. Overell JR, Bone I, Lees KR: Interatrial septal abnormalities and stroke: A meta-analysis of case-control studies. Neurology 55:1172–1179, 2000.

149. Lamy C, Giannesini C, Zuber M, et al: Clinical and imaging findings in cryptogenic stroke patients with and without patent foramen ovale: The PFO-ASA Study. Atrial Septal Aneurysm. Stroke 33:706–711, 2002.

150. Ranoux D, Cohen A, Cabanes L, et al: Patent foramen ovale: Is stroke due to paradoxical embolism? Stroke 24:31–34, 1993.

151. Silver MD, Dorsey JS: Aneurysms of the septum primum in adults. Arch Pathol Lab Med 102:62–65, 1978.

152. Falk RH: PFO or UFO? The role of a patent foramen ovale in cryptogenic stroke. Am Heart J 121:1264–1266, 1991.
153. Hanna JP, Sun JP, Furlan AJ, et al: Patent foramen ovale and brain infarct: Echocardiographic predictors, recurrence, and prevention. Stroke 25:782–786, 1994.
154. Cujec B, Mainra R, Johnson DH: Prevention of recurrent cerebral ischemic events in patients with patent foramen ovale and cryptogenic strokes or transient ischemic attacks. Can J Cardiol 15:57–64, 1999.
155. De Castro S, Cartoni D, Fiorelli M, et al: Morphological and functional characteristics of patent foramen ovale and their embolic implications. Stroke 31:2407–2413, 2000.
156. Bogousslavsky J, Garazi S, Jeanrenaud X, et al: Stroke recurrence in patients with patent foramen ovale: The Lausanne Study. Lausanne Stroke with Paradoxal Embolism Study Group. Neurology 46:1301–1305, 1996.
157. Mas JL, Zuber M: Recurrent cerebrovascular events in patients with patent foramen ovale, atrial septal aneurysm, or both and cryptogenic stroke or transient ischemic attack. French Study Group on Patent Foramen Ovale and Atrial Septal Aneurysm. Am Heart J 130:1083–1088, 1995.
158. Mas JL, Arquizan C, Lamy C, et al: Recurrent cerebrovascular events associated with patent foramen ovale, atrial septal aneurysm, or both. N Engl J Med 345:1740–1746, 2001.
159. Baker SS, O'Laughlin MP, Jollis JG, et al: Cost implications of closure of atrial septal defect. Catheter Cardiovasc Interv 55:83–87, 2002.
160. Bruch L, Parsi A, Grad MO, et al: Transcatheter closure of interatrial communications for secondary prevention of paradoxical embolism: Single-center experience. Circulation 105:2845–2848, 2002.
161. Wahl A, Meier B, Haxel B, et al: Prognosis after percutaneous closure of patent foramen ovale for paradoxical embolism. Neurology 57:1330–1332, 2001.
162. Wahl A, Windecker S, Eberli FR, et al: Percutaneous closure of patent foramen ovale in symptomatic patients. J Interv Cardiol 14:203–209, 2001.
163. Zahn EM, Wilson N, Cutright W, Latson LA: Development and testing of the Helex septal occluder, a new expanded polytetrafluoroethylene atrial septal defect occlusion system. Circulation 104:711–716, 2001.
164. Latson LA, Zahn EM, Wilson N: Helex septal occluder for closure of atrial septal defects. Curr Interv Cardiol Rep 2:268–273, 2000.
165. www.amplatzer.com/respecttrial.
166. Hirsh J, Warkentin TE, Shaughnessy SG, et al: Heparin and low-molecular-weight heparin: Mechanisms of action, pharmacokinetics, dosing, monitoring, efficacy, and safety. Chest 119:64S–94S, 2001.
167. Ansell J, Hirsh J, Dalen J, et al: Managing oral anticoagulant therapy. Chest 119:22S–38S, 2001.
168. Hirsh J, Dalen J, Anderson DR, et al: Oral anticoagulants: Mechanism of action, clinical effectiveness, and optimal therapeutic range. Chest 119:8S–21S, 2001.
169. Hart R, Benavente O, Pearce LA: Increased risk of intracranial hemorrhage when aspirin is combined with warfarin: A meta-analysis and hypothesis. Cerebrovasc Dis 9:215–217, 1999.
170. Fogelholm R, Eskola K, Kiminkinen T, Kunnamo I: Anticoagulant treatment as a risk factor for primary intracerebral haemorrhage. J Neurol Neurosurg Psychiatry 55:1121–1124, 1992.
171. Franke CL, de Jonge J, van Swieten JC, et al: Intracerebral hematomas during anticoagulant treatment. Stroke 21:726–730, 1990.
172. Wintzen AR, de Jonge H, Loeliger EA, Bots GT: The risk of intracerebral hemorrhage during oral anticoagulant treatment: A population study. Ann Neurol 16:553–538, 1984.
173. Lin J, Hanigan WC, Tarantino M, Wang J: The use of recombinant activated factor VII to reverse warfarin-induced anticoagulation in patients with hemorrhages in the central nervous system: Preliminary findings. J Neurosurg 98:737–740, 2003.
174. Torn M, Algra A, Rosendaal FR: Oral anticoagulation for cerebral ischemia of arterial origin: high initial bleeding risk. Neurology 57:1993–1999, 2001.
175. Hylek EM, Singer DE: Risk factors for intracranial hemorrhage in outpatients taking warfarin. Ann Intern Med 120:897–902, 1994.
176. A randomized trial of anticoagulants versus aspirin after cerebral ischemia of presumed arterial origin. The Stroke Prevention in

177. Hylek EM, Skates SJ, Sheehan MA, Singer DE: An analysis of the lowest effective intensity of prophylactic anticoagulation for patients with nonrheumatic atrial fibrillation. N Engl J Med 335:540–546, 1996.
178. Smith EE, Rosand J, Knudsen KA, et al: Leukoaraiosis is associated with warfarin-related hemorrhage following ischemic stroke. Neurology 59:193–197, 2002.
179. Gorter JW: Major bleeding during anticoagulation after cerebral ischemia: Patterns and risk factors. Stroke Prevention in Reversible Ischemia Trial (SPIRIT). European Atrial Fibrillation Trial (EAFT) study groups. Neurology 53:1319–1327, 1999.
180. Kato H, Izumiyama M, Izumiyama K, et al: Silent cerebral microbleeds on T2°-weighted MRI: Correlation with stroke subtype, stroke recurrence, and leukoaraiosis. Stroke 33:1536–1540, 2002.
181. Kim DE, Bae HJ, Lee SH, et al: Gradient echo magnetic resonance imaging in the prediction of hemorrhagic vs ischemic stroke: A need for the consideration of the extent of leukoariosis. Arch Neurol 59:425–429, 2002.
182. Wong KS, Chan YL, Liu JY, et al: Asymptomatic microbleeds as a risk factor for aspirin-associated intracerebral hemorrhages. Neurology 60:511–513, 2003.
183. Hart RG: What causes intracerebral hemorrhage during warfarin therapy? Neurology 55:907–908, 2000.
184. Hart RG, Easton JD: Hemorrhagic infarcts. Stroke 17:586–589, 1986.
185. Hornig CR, Bauer T, Simon C, et al: Hemorrhagic transformation in cardioembolic cerebral infarction. Stroke 24:465–468, 1993.
186. Molina CA, Montaner J, Abilleira S, et al: Timing of spontaneous recanalization and risk of hemorrhagic transformation in acute cardioembolic stroke. Stroke 32:1079–1084, 2001.
187. Nighoghossian N, Hermier M, Berthezene Y, et al: Early diagnosis of hemorrhagic transformation: Diffusion/perfusion-weighted MRI versus CT scan. Cerebrovasc Dis 11:151–156, 2001.
188. Hermier M, Nighoghossian N, Derex L, et al: MRI of acute post-ischemic cerebral hemorrhage in stroke patients: Diagnosis with T2°-weighted gradient-echo sequences. Neuroradiology 43:809–815, 2001.
189. Okada Y, Yamaguchi T, Minematsu K, et al: Hemorrhagic transformation in cerebral embolism. Stroke 20:598–603, 1989.
190. Immediate anticoagulation of embolic stroke: Brain hemorrhage and management options. Cerebral Embolism Study Group. Stroke 15:779–789, 1984.
191. Yasaka M, Yamaguchi T, Oita J, et al: Clinical features of recurrent embolization in acute cardioembolic stroke. Stroke 24:1681–1685, 1993.
192. Sandercock P: Full heparin anticoagulation should not be used in acute ischemic stroke. Stroke 34:231–232, 2003.
193. Koller RL: Recurrent embolic cerebral infarction and anticoagulation. Neurology 32:283–285, 1982.
194. Cardioembolic stroke, early anticoagulation, and brain hemorrhage. Cerebral Embolism Study Group. Arch Intern Med 147:636-640, 1987.
195. Calandre L, Ortega JF, Bermejo F: Anticoagulation and hemorrhagic infarction in cerebral embolism secondary to rheumatic heart disease. Arch Neurol 41:1152–1154, 1984.
196. Shields RW Jr, Laureno R, Lachman T, Victor M: Anticoagulant-related hemorrhage in acute cerebral embolism. Stroke 15:426–437, 1984.
197. Chamorro A, Vila N, Saiz A, et al: Early anticoagulation after large cerebral embolic infarction: A safety study. Neurology 45:861–865, 1995.
198. Rothrock JF, Dittrich HC, McAllen S, et al: Acute anticoagulation following cardioembolic stroke. Stroke 20:730–734, 1989.
199. Pessin MS, Estol CJ, Lafranchise F, Caplan LR: Safety of anticoagulation after hemorrhagic infarction. Neurology 43:1298–1303, 1993.
200. Gebel JM, Broderick JP: Intracerebral hemorrhage. Neurol Clin 18:419–438, 2000.
201. Crawley F, Bevan D, Wren D: Management of intracranial bleeding associated with anticoagulation: Balancing the risk of further bleeding against thromboembolism from prosthetic heart valves. J Neurol Neurosurg Psychiatry 69:396–398, 2000.
202. Bertram M, Bonsanto M, Hacke W, Schwab S: Managing the therapeutic dilemma: Patients with spontaneous intracerebral hemor-

Reversible Ischemia Trial (SPIRIT) Study Group. Ann Neurol 42:857–865, 1997.

Samples sizes in most therapeutic trials are smaller than those needed for the prevention trials. The follow-up periods tend to be shorter, usually 3 months after stroke.

WHEN CAN A STROKE-RELATED TRIAL BE CONDUCTED?

Ethical conduct of a randomized clinical trial requires equipoise. A clinical trial can be conducted only at that point in time at which the treatment is acceptable to administer to humans but there is still uncertainty about treatment outcome. If the consensus of potential participants or clinicians is that a treatment or procedure is beneficial (or harmful), randomization becomes impractical and possibly unethical. In the EC/IC Bypass Study, some of the original participating centers' investigators decided that they could not ethically randomly assign potential participants away from surgery.[22] Enough centers continued to enroll participants in the trial for it to continue, and at the conclusion, surgery was not found to be better than best medical care.

Ethical considerations also prohibit conducting a clinical trial to evaluate risk factors. For example, the magnitude of the stroke-related risk of cigarette smoking cannot be evaluated in the context of a clinical trial with participants randomly assigned to smoking as an intervention. This prohibition does not preclude clinical trials comparing approaches to changing stroke-related risk factors. Clinical trials are generally not used to determine long-term adverse effects of a treatment, because such a purpose would require long-term maintenance of participants on ineffective treatment. In the latter situation, post-marketing surveillance of patients receiving the beneficial treatment is the usual approach.

DEVELOPMENT OF A DRUG OR BIOLOGICS: FROM LABORATORY TO MARKETING

An average time from development of a drug in the laboratory to marketing is approximately 7.5 years.[23] Initial drug development in the laboratory is referred to as the *nonclinical* or *preclinical phase*, encompassing pharmacology, toxicology, and formulation processes. The preclinical phase involves experimentation in different species of animals. When the new drug is ready to be tested in humans, an Investigational New Drug (IND) application is submitted, and once U.S. Food and Drug Administration (FDA) grants the drug developer permission to proceed, clinical testing begins.

Clinical testing, on average, takes about 75% of the drug development resources[24] and generally consists of three phases before marketing. Although the nomenclature and definition of the phases are, in general, not standardized, the three phases are Phase I (dose finding and safety), Phase II (determination of futility, feasibility, and safety), and Phase III (efficacy or effectiveness). In the development of therapies for stroke, these phases are often not distinct. Phases I and II or Phases II and III may be combined. After FDA approval for marketing, Phase IV (post-marketing surveillance) is often conducted, particularly if

such a phase is a condition of FDA approval. Phase IV is generally a large population study to assess long-term effects of the new treatment and monitor subsequent adverse reactions. Phase IV studies are also used for cost-effectiveness assessment and marketing purposes.

PHASE 1 TRIALS

Phase I trials establish a safe dose in humans with an acceptable level of toxicity, establish a route of administration, and determine the clinical pharmacology. Sample sizes usually range from 20 to 80 participants. In studies of cancer chemotherapy, the intent of a Phase I trial is to discover the maximum tolerated dose (MTD) on the basis of the premise that the maximum benefit (efficacy) would be observed with the highest tolerable dose. The occurrence of toxicity that is unacceptable is termed dose-limiting toxicity (DLT). Hence, the MTD is determined by the absence of DLT.[25] In stroke, there is no consensus regarding the need to escalate the dose to the MTD. The level of escalation chosen for a Phase I trial would be treatment specific.

Another ambiguity in Phase I studies for stroke is the definition of DLT. Oncology clinical trials use standard definitions for the varying levels of toxicity.[25] Stroke has no such guidelines. A Phase I study funded by NINDS aims to establish the MTD of human serum albumin as a neuroprotective agent for participants with recent ischemic stroke (http://crisp.cit.nih.gov/crisp; 5R01NS0406). A Safety Evaluation Committee, consisting of a team of neurologists and cardiologists, evaluates participants' records at each dose level according to prespecified guidelines to determine whether severe and serious adverse events occurred during the 72 hours after ictus. The existence of DLT is determined by a consensus after each member of the committee has reviewed the charts of all the participants at each dose level.

Design of Phase I Trials

Dixon and Mood[26] developed the up-and-down method for Phase I trials, the traditional and most often implemented design. A design proposed by Storer,[27] which is adapted from the Dixon and Mood design, utilizes a set of prespecified dose levels. The choice of the initial dose is based either on animal experiments for a drug that has never been used in humans or on previous studies in humans for an existing drug. The common approach starts from one tenth of the dose causing 10% mortality in the rodents (LD_{10}). The dose is increased by a smaller percentage each time, often using a modified Fibonacci scheme (Table 61.1). If a trial is stopped because of a DLT, the MTD is one dose level below the dose at which the DLT was noted.[25]

O'Quigley and associates[28-30] proposed the continual reassessment method (CRM) as an alternative design for a Phase I study. CRM uses information gathered in the trial from a previous increase in dose to estimate the probability of DLT at the next dose level. Simulation studies show that the MTD may be reached sooner with CRM than with the up-and-down method. However, Goodman and colleagues showed CRM has a tendency to use higher doses in a greater proportion of participants, increasing the chances of serious toxicity.[31] They proposed a modification

Table 61.1 Idealized Modified Fibonacci Search Scheme Approach to Dose Escalation in a Phase 1 Study

Drug Dose*	Percentage Increase Above Preceding Dose Level
n	—
2.0 n	100
3.3 n	67
5.0 n	50
7.0 n	40
9.0 n	33
12.0 n	33
16.0 n	33

*n, starting dose (mg/m^2).
Adapted from Von Hoff DD, Kohn J, Clark GM: Design and conduct of phase I trials. In Buyse M, Staquet MJ, Sylvester RJ (eds): Cancer Clinical Trials. New York, Oxford University Press, 1984.

yielding accurate estimation of MTD with fewer toxicities. Also, O'Quigley and Shen[30] proposed a modification of the CRM to efficiently emulate the up-and-down method, putting fewer participants at risk from higher doses.

PHASE II TRIALS

Phase II studies primarily rule out clearly ineffective treatments—that is, they assess futility. Phase II studies also assess side effects and toxicity, logistics of administration and cost, and provide information used to plan a scientifically sound Phase III study.[32] Traditional Phase II trials use data previously collected on historical controls and are considered single-arm studies. Placebo data from trial participants with recent ischemic stroke are available on the Web from the NINDS rt-PA study through the National Technological Service (http://www.ntis.gov/search/product.asp?ABBR=PB2003500017&starDB=GRAHIST) and can be obtained by request from numerous other clinical trials. Phase II studies do not seek to draw definitive conclusions about the treatment effectiveness, instead, they look for evidence to justify proceeding to a Phase III study.

A single-arm Phase II study is appropriate when the follow-up period to obtain the primary outcome can be short or when surrogate endpoints can be used to minimize follow-up time. In studies involving cancer, tumor size shrinkage 3 to 6 months after initiation of chemotherapy is used as an outcome of interest in most Phase II studies, whereas survival or disease-free survival is used as the primary outcome in the Phase III studies. In stroke prevention trials, a surrogate outcome such as reduction in some risk factor would be required because the primary outcome, new stroke or death, takes years to ascertain. Therapeutic Phase II stroke trials do not generally require a surrogate outcome, because the primary outcome is usually ascertained at 3 months.

Phase II studies have been underutilized in stroke. New therapies often are studied in Phase I trials and then studied in underpowered Phase III trials, sometimes called *Phase II studies*. Traditional Phase II trials have the advantage of requiring smaller sample sizes (generally four-fold smaller) than a controlled study with the same error and

effect size parameters. Therefore, implementation and completion of Phase II trials require less time and fewer resources. More new treatments may be explored at this stage of drug development. A single-arm Phase II design is especially attractive when availability of participants is limited in relation to the rate of development of new treatments.

Design of Phase II Trials

Sample size for Phase II trials can be computed through the use of standard methods for one-sided tests with modification to the type I and type II error. In Phase II trials, the null hypothesis is that the treatment equals some minimal acceptable success measure or maximum acceptable failure measure, a single number derived from historical data (proportion or mean). The alternative hypothesis is that the treatment is worse than the historical control rate.[33] Based on study results, if the null hypothesis is rejected by the trial investigator, the therapy will not be studied further. If the null hypothesis is not rejected, the therapy is carried forward into a Phase III trial. Thus, false-positive treatments are tested further in a Phase III study, in which the treatment effect is scrutinized with smaller error probabilities at the expense of a larger sample size. One-tailed alpha (chance of calling effective treatment ineffective) and beta (chance of missing an ineffective treatment) levels in the range of 0.10 to 0.15 are recommended.[32]

In December 1993, the Alteplase ThromboLysis for Acute Noninterventional Therapy in Ischemic Stroke (ATLANTIS) Part B Study[33] began to evaluate the efficacy of giving intravenous recombinant t-PA (rt-PA), or alteplase, for ischemic stroke 3 to 5 hours after symptom onset. The primary favorable outcome measure was a National Institutes of Health (NIH) Stroke Scale (NIHSS) score of 0 or 1 at 90 days after stroke. Thirty-two percent of participants receiving placebo and 34% of participants receiving alteplase had favorable outcome at 3 months (P = .65). The estimated sample size for the Phase III trial was 968, but only 613 participants were enrolled. The data and safety monitoring committee terminated participant enrollment in the trial for lack of efficacy.

We used the effect sizes from the original trial, with one-sided alpha = 0.10 and beta = 0.15, to estimate the required sample size for a Phase II trial of 169 participants. We estimated the sample size for this two-stage Phase II design, allowing one look at the data halfway through the study, through the use of EAST 2000 (Cytel Software Corporation) with an O'Brien-Fleming stopping boundary,[34] as described later (see "Interim Analysis"). Under this Phase II design, after enrollment of 85 consecutively treated participants, the study would continue if the number of positive outcomes (NIHSS score ≤1 at 90 days after stroke) was 29 or higher. In the Phase III trial, the observed number of successes in the first 85 consecutively treated patients was 27. If we used these Phase III data as if they were from a Phase II trial, the same conclusion would have been reached as was reached in the Phase III trial, but with 85 rather than 613 participants.[35] Broderick and colleagues[36] completed a Phase II trial of combined intravenous and intra-arterial t-PA using the design just described and determined continuing to Phase III was worthwhile.

PHASE III TRIALS

In Phase I trials, there is generally no control group, and in Phase II trials, the control group can be an historical cohort (i.e., Phase II can be a single-arm study). Generally, in a Phase III clinical trial, whether preventive or therapeutic, each participant is randomly assigned to an intervention or control (placebo, usual care, best medical treatment for the condition, etc.). Hence, a Phase III trial is generally a multiple-arm study. A well-designed, well-executed, randomized, concurrently controlled Phase III clinical trial is the ultimate proof (or lack thereof) of the strength of association between the treatment and a clinical effect. For stroke, the intervention could be a chemical or biologic agent, a device, surgery, dietary instructions, reading materials, or simply additional prevention or care directions given orally by a health professional.

The dose and dosing schedule adopted in Phase III are determined in Phase I studies, Phase II studies, or both. A variety of outcome measures are employed in randomized therapeutic clinical trials for stroke to assess clinical outcomes, usually at 90 days from the onset of stroke symptoms.

The remainder of this chapter focuses on methods for Phase III trials as well as ethical and regulatory considerations.

Outcome Measures

All clinical trials begin with a clear definition of the question to be studied and a definition of the expected outcomes. Most primary and secondary prevention trials use new stroke occurrence and stroke-related mortality or overall mortality. The outcome measure is generally not mortality alone, because most people who experience a stroke do not die in the first 3 months. For example, incidence data from two areas in the southeastern Stroke Belt of the United States yield case-fatality rates of 12.8% and 14.7%.[37]

Prevention trials generally must obtain sufficient information from multiple clinical sites to define new stroke occurrence and, where applicable, stroke-related mortality, at a cost low enough to allow the trial to be conducted. In planning a new trial, investigators can draw on the experience of other large prevention trials. Investigators in the ACAS, for example, devised a symptom-based questionnaire and algorithm for detecting TIAs and other neurologic illness[38] but recommended that positive results be confirmed by neurologic evaluation. The three SPAF trials questioned participants every 3 months.[39] Reported stroke events were verified and categorized into stroke subtypes by a blinded (see later) central events committee using a clinical classification scheme.[40] In the WARSS,[10] local centers reported possible outcomes to the data management center and submitted clinical summaries with supporting imaging studies. An independent neurologist who was blinded as to treatment assignments reviewed the images, and five neurologists also blinded to treatment assignments adjudicated the events to a majority verdict. The WEST[11] used the ACAS questionnaire already described, along with questions about the occurrence of specific events of interest. Investigators blinded as to treatment assignment reviewed medical records for patients reporting possible events.

Adjudication of events is usually accompanied through some local chart audits by an outside monitor to ensure that there is no under-reporting of events. This process of adjudication is costly and time consuming. Classifying deaths as stroke-related adds an additional level of complexity to the review of events.

Acute stroke treatment trials generally use some measure of post-stroke recovery as the outcome measure rather than mortality or new stroke. Participants who have died are given the worst score on an outcome measure or some weighted score.[41] In the NINDS rt-PA Study, in which participants were classified as having a favorable or unfavorable outcome on four outcome measures, participants who died were considered to have an unfavorable outcome.[16]

There is no single accepted outcome measure of recovery after stroke. Generally, acute stroke treatment trials use a combination of outcome measures, such as the modified Rankin Scale (mRS),[42] Barthel Index,[43] NIHSS,[44] and Glasgow Outcome Scale.[45] These measures are correlated with each other, but not perfectly (Table 61.2). For example, a participant could obtain a score high on the Barthel Index, which measures performance of activities of daily living, but have severe aphasia, as indicated by the NIHSS. Analytic techniques to address the statistical issues posed by these correlated outcome measures are discussed later.

If a trial is planned to use a new outcome measure or to use an existing outcome measure in a new population, the measure should be validated in patients similar to possible trial participants before it is used in the trial. Hanston[46] describes the considerations for and required approaches to validating new outcome measures for stroke trials.

Sample Size

Both Lachin[47] and Friedman and colleagues[1] offer general methods for calculating sample size for most trial outcomes. NQuery Advisor,[48] a user-friendly software

Table 61.2 Percentage Agreement and Correlations Among Outcome Measures Used in the National Institute of Neurological Disorders and Stroke Recombinant Tissue-Type Plasminogen Activator Stroke Trial*

Measures(s)	% Agreement	Phi Coefficient
Barthel & NIHSS	77	0.55
Barthel & Rankin	87	0.76
Barthel & Glasgow	89	0.78
NIHSS & Rankin	86	0.67
NIHSS & Glasgow	85	0.69
Rankin & Glasgow	94	0.88

*Measures are binary; correlation is measured by Phi coefficients.[71]

Barthel, Barthel Index; Glasgow, Glasgow Outcome Scale; NIHSS, National Institutes of Health Stroke Scale; Rankin, Rankin Scale.

Adapted from Tilley BC, Marler J, Geller N, et al: Using a global test for multiple outcomes in stroke trials with application to the NINDS t-PA Stroke Trial. Stroke 27:2136–2141, 1996.

package, and STPLAN, free shareware developed at M.D. Anderson in Houston,[49] implement approaches to calculation of sample size. Applying these general methods to clinical trials in stroke entails consideration of the distributions of stroke outcomes as well as of the usual parameters required to develop an estimate of sample size.

J-Shaped Distribution

In therapeutic stroke trials, many of the outcome measures take on a J- or U-shaped distribution. Figure 61–1 shows a typical example using the Barthel Index. This J- or U-shaped distribution does not lend itself to transformation into a distribution that is less skewed or more normally distributed. To analyze a J- or U-shaped distribution, some investigators have dichotomized the outcome into success or failure by choosing a value or cut point in the distribution. In Figure 61–1, a cut point at 95 could be chosen. Values at 95 and to the left could be considered successes, and values to the right of 95 could be considered failures.[16]

The choice of a cut point depends on the question of interest. The goal of the NINDS t-PA Stroke Study was to achieve recovery with minimal or no disability as defined by a set of four outcome measures. For the Barthel Index, a score of 95 or 100 (the Barthel Index was measured in 5-point increments between 0 and 100) was considered a favorable outcome. A participant with a score lower than 95 was considered to have an unfavorable outcome. In other studies in which more moderate success is expected, the cut point may be lower in the scale. If a decision is made to dichotomize the outcome, the cut point must be chosen before the start of the study and used in calculating the sample size.

Sample size estimates depend highly on the approach to analysis of the outcome measure when it has a J-shaped distribution. Data from the NINDS t-PA Stroke Study provide an example. Ranking the data using a Wilcoxon rank sum test to detect a difference in the Barthel Index between the t-PA group and the placebo group at the α = 0.05 level (two-tailed) of the magnitude observed in that trial with power of 90% would require 507 participants per group. If the Barthel Index is dichotomized (95 or 100 versus <95), the binomial test comparing proportions at the same alpha and power to detect the effect observed in the t-PA trial would require 335 participants per group.

One-Tailed or Two-Tailed Tests

The choice of a one-tailed or two-tailed test also affects sample size calculations. A one-tailed test requires a smaller sample size to achieve the same effect with the same power. Generally, to avoid the appearance that a one-tailed test was chosen only because statistical significance was not achieved with a two-tailed test, investigators avoid one-tailed tests. Also, it is usually important to understand whether the treatment group has an outcome better or worse than that of the control group. The EC/IC Bypass Study was an exception to this generality.[8] Investigators designed the study using a one-tailed test to compare surgery with best medical care. Because of the cost of surgery, if the trial indicated that surgery was no better than best medical care, surgery would not be recommended in the future. Investigators did not consider showing that surgery was worse than best medical care to be clinically meaningful.

Power and Alpha Level

In large multicenter Phase III stroke trials, power (1 chance of missing a true difference) is usually set high (90% or greater) to allow interpretation of a negative result or lack of a treatment effect. If the investigators are willing to accept a greater chance of missing a true difference, power can be as low as 80% (i.e., a 20% chance of missing the hypothesized treatment effect). The alpha level (chance of calling an ineffective treatment effective) is usually 0.05, but if multiple groups are being compared, the alpha level may be set to a smaller value. O'Brien[50] makes the argument that if the comparisons represent separate questions (i.e., assessment of the impact of the intervention on two or three different outcomes), they can be considered separate experiments with no need for adjustment of the alpha level. Where an overall hypothesis and a subgroup hypothesis are being tested (e.g., all stroke patients and patients with severe NIHSS at baseline), Moye[51] suggests spending some alpha on this overall comparison (0.04) and less on the subgroup (0.0). Where all possible pair-wise comparisons were to be made among a series of treatments, some adjustment of the alpha level for multiple comparisons would be required. Simes' correction,[52] a step-down approach, is less conservative than the Bonferroni approach, which uses alpha divided by the number of comparisons.[53] For example, if alpha = 0.05, and

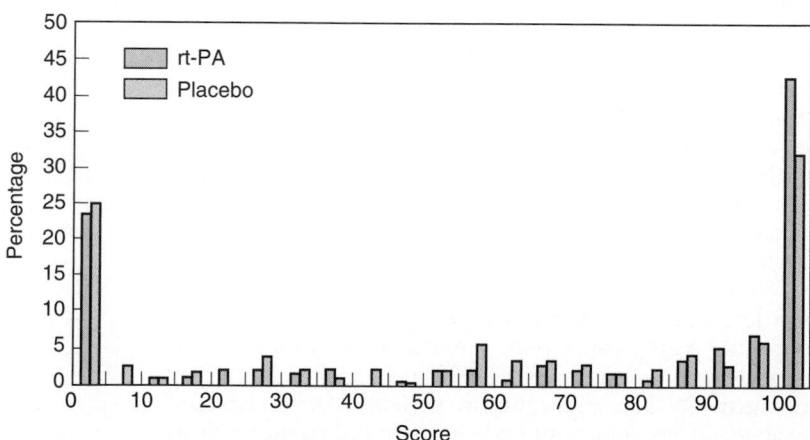

FIGURE 61–1 *Distribution of the Barthel Index. (Data from NINDS t-PA Stroke Study.[8,9])*

there are 5 comparisons, the critical level for testing is 0.01 (i.e., 0.05/5). If the analytical approach is analysis of variance, other methods for multiple comparisons are available in most standard statistical packages such as SAS or Stata.

Equivalence

Studies to demonstrate the equivalence of one therapy to another require special attention to sample size computations. These studies require specialized approaches to analysis[54] and high power. If the probability of missing a true difference is high, negative study results are difficult to interpret. The software package NQuery Advisor[48] has the ability to calculate sample size for equivalence studies.

Adjusting for Drop-Outs and Drop-Ins

Drop-outs (patients who are stopping the study therapy) and drop-ins (patients changing over to a study treatment different from their original assignment) must be considered in calculation of sample size. Inflating the sample size by the proportion expected to drop out or drop in may underestimate the size needed. Lachin[47] suggests inflating the calculated sample size by using the formula $1/(1-R)^2$, where R is the drop-out or drop-in rate. Because the inflation factor greatly enlarges the sample size, efforts should be made to keep these rates as low as possible (see later discussion of adherence).

Midcourse Modifications to Sample Size

Several papers have been written on approaches to modifying sample size when the control rate or the expected treatment difference varies from what is expected. This type of adjustment should be carefully considered, especially its impact on the credibility of the trial, before such a modification is made. Proschan and coworkers[55] review some of the newest approaches and suggest setting a minimal clinically meaningful effect prior to doing any adjustment of the sample size.

Inclusion and Exclusion Criteria for Phase III Trials

Inclusion and exclusion criteria define the trial population to be studied. Investigators may wish to give a treatment its "best chance to succeed" by excluding participants who do not "do well," such as those who are older or have high NIHSS scores, subtle computed tomography (CT) findings, or certain stroke subtypes. If one suspects that patients *with* a risk factor will have a *poorer* outcome with treatment than with placebo and patients *without* a risk factor would have a *better* outcome with treatment than with placebo, a *treatment–risk factor interaction* is implied. It would be difficult to justify randomly assigning treatment for those with the risk factor. If no interaction with treatment is expected—patients with the risk factor are expected to do worse than those without it, *regardless* of treatment assignment—there is no strong rationale to exclude these participants.

The more restrictive the criteria for entry into the trial, the less generalizable are the results. Trials that exclude potential participants with specific stroke subtypes or include participants only from large specialty clinics may not provide data applicable to patients seen in general practice of neurology, and if the treatment appears efficacious, a wider range of patients than that used in the trial

may receive the treatment. Additionally, because the treatment has not yet been proven to be efficacious (or the trial would not be conducted), there is some uncertainty about the usefulness of the eligibility criteria.

A better approach, unless there are well-documented treatment interactions, is to have broad eligibility criteria and include prespecified exploratory post hoc subgroup analyses (see later discussion of subgroups). Additionally, overly restrictive entry criteria may limit enrollment of older adults and minority populations who are more likely to have comorbidities and who are most in need of the new approaches to stroke prevention or therapy. Potential participants at higher risk of unfavorable outcomes are also potential "responders" to treatment.

Table 61.3 shows published data from the NINDS t-PA Stroke Study. The percentage of participants with a favorable outcome decreased with age and with increasing NIHSS score, but the t-PA–treated group always had a higher percentage of favorable outcomes, except for a few random fluctuations, than the placebo-treated group. In the oldest patients, with the highest NIHSS scores, there were no favorable outcomes in either treatment group, but 74% of the t-PA–treated patients and 86% of the placebo-treated patients experienced severe disability or death.

To demonstrate the impact of exclusion criteria, we computed the sample size required to detect the observed effect on the mRS using combined data from Parts 1 and 2 of the NINDS t-PA Stroke Study. In the combined trials,

Table 61.3   **Proportions of Favorable Outcomes at Three Months by Baseline and Age Subgroups***

Variable	% Patients with Favorable Outcome	
	t-PA	**Placebo**
Age ≤ 60 yr		
Baseline NIHSS Score		
0–9 (n = 46)	59	42
10–14 (n = 35)	38	18
5–20 (n = 49)	41	27
>20 (n = 26)	22	12
Age 61–68 yr		
NIHSS Score		
0–9 (n = 44)	60	37
10–14 (n = 28)	25	25
15–20 (n = 39)	0	25
>20 (n = 30)	7	0
Age 69–75 yr		
NIHSS Score		
0–9 (n = 41)	50	54
10–14 (n = 45)	39	27
15–20 (n = 40)	26	0
>20 (n = 35)	8	0
Age >75 yr		
NIHSS Score		
0–9 (n = 46)	67	36
10–14 (n = 28)	27	15
15–20 (n = 43)	23	6
>20 (n = 49)	0	0

NIHSS, National Institutes of Health Stroke Scale; t-PA, tissue-type plasminogen activator.

*Favorable outcome = NIHSS Score of 0 or 1 at 3 months. The categories for age and baseline NIHSS represent quartiles of the range of each variable. From NINDS t-PA Study Group.[58]

42.6% of the t-PA–treated group and 26.6% of placebo-treated group had favorable outcome (scores of 0 or 1) on the mRS.[16] Assuming α = 0.05, two-tailed test, and power = 90%, a sample size of 184 per group would be required to detect an effect of that size in a new study. If only those younger than 75 years or with an NIHSS score less than 20 were included, the power to detect a difference of the observed magnitude in the subgroup described (46.8% favorable outcomes for t-PA versus 28.2% for placebo) would increase to 95% for the sample size (184 per group). Although this step offers some gain in power, excluding either patients 75 years and older or patients with NIHSS scores of 20 and higher, both of whom may show some benefit from treatment, would leave the treatment untested in groups at high risk of unfavorable outcomes after stroke as well as in a growing population of older people. Patients with a mild stroke (NIHSS scores ≤ 5) are thought to potentially have little benefit from the treatment and so are sometimes excluded from trials on the grounds that inclusion of such patients dilutes the treatment effect. With the NINDS data again used as an example, if only those with an NIHSS score higher than 5 were included, the power to detect the observed effect in the subgroup described (37.0% favorable outcome for t-PA versus 23.7% for placebo) would decrease to 80% if the sample size of 184 per group were used. In both cases, generalizability is affected, and in the latter case, the sample size for the trial would have to be larger to achieve the required 90% power.

If potential participants in a specific subgroup are excluded, reports on the trial should clearly state that results do not apply to the group excluded. The North American Symptomatic Carotid Endarterectomy Trial (NASCET)[56] excluded patients who either had carotid artery stenosis of less than 30% severity or were asymptomatic. The NASCET studied participants as two groups—those with high-grade stenosis (70% to 99% narrowing) and those with moderate or severe stenosis (30% to 69%). When an article was published on the results of the trial in symptomatic participants with high-grade stenosis, the authors were careful to clarify that conclusions could be drawn only for that subgroup.[56]

To minimize problems with missing data (see discussions of adherence and on analyses of missing data), investigators may consider excluding potential participants with characteristics that might prevent the participants from completing the study or from being compliant with the study medication. For example, if a health status assessment at a weekly clinic visit is an essential component of the study, enrollment of patients who live out of town could easily lead to high rates of noncompliance. However, potential participants should not be unnecessarily excluded on the basis of preconceptions. For example, excluding all homeless persons from a trial as a matter of policy may not be necessary if study staff has a means of regular contact with some of the potential homeless participants.

Randomization

Randomization is the method of allocating participants to the different treatment arms of a randomized clinical trial. Simple randomization is similar to flipping an unbiased coin and using heads or tails to assign a participant to one of two treatment arms. Using alternating assignment of participants to treatment or control as they come in to a study is not a random assignment, because once the first participant is randomly assigned to treatment, the treatment assignments for subsequent participants are predetermined. If a participant's treatment assignment in the sequence of alternating assignments is revealed, all other participants' assignments can be ascertained. To ensure randomness, a random number generator, available in most statistical software packages, is generally used to conduct the randomization.

Stratification

Simple randomization may result in imbalances in the risk factors associated with outcome or in the number of participants in each treatment arm. In stroke treatment trials, as in all trials, investigators desire balance in factors associated with treatment outcome to ensure that one group does not inadvertently have an advantage over another. To obtain balance, one solution is to stratify participants before randomization into specific subgroups and then to randomly assign participants to treatment arms within each subgroup. Another goal of stratification is to improve the precision of the statistical analysis.

The EC/IC Bypass Study stratified participants on the basis of clinical center, type of underlying vascular lesion (two categories), presence or absence of a related neurologic deficit; participants with internal carotid occlusion were stratified according to presence or absence of related symptoms after angiographic demonstration of occlusion.[8,9] In WEST, a secondary prevention trial,[11] participants were stratified according to clinical center and a baseline risk group as previously defined by a validated clinical index.[57]

In therapeutic trials with smaller samples, a smaller number of strata must be used. For the NINDS t-PA Stroke Study, there was limited knowledge about the predictors of stroke outcome in patients treated soon after stroke (within 180 minutes of stroke onset), so a decision was made to stratify only according to clinical site and time from stroke outcome to treatment (0–90 minutes or 91–180 minutes).

There is a rapid increase in the number of subgroups as the number of variables used for stratification rises. For example, post hoc analyses of the NINDS t-PA Stroke Study data showed that in addition to treatment, the age × NIHSS score interaction (see later), a history of diabetes, the age × mean admission blood pressure interaction, time from stroke onset × treatment interaction, and the presence of early CT findings are all associated with 3-month stroke outcome.[58,59] In a trial that did not take all of these covariates into account, but stratified only on the basis of time from stroke onset (early, late), clinical center (8 locations), NIHSS score (3 levels), and age (3 levels), there would be 144 subgroups. In a study with 300 participants, this scheme could at best result in only about 1 participant per treatment arm if the participants were uniformly distributed across the strata, an unlikely scenario because some combinations are much less likely to occur. With a large number of subgroups, a small number of participants could be unequally assigned to treatment groups within strata, inducing an overall imbalance in the treatment arms. A complex randomization scheme also makes it more likely that clinics will make errors in the randomization.

Another concern is stratification on risk factors that *interact* with treatment. If a participant with the risk factor has an enhanced treatment effect, the risk factor might be considered a stratifying variable. If instead the risk factor interacts with treatment to produce an adverse effect, patients with the risk factor should not be enrolled in the trial (see earlier discussion of inclusion and exclusion criteria).

Most treatment trials and prevention trials have sufficient sample size to make stratification unnecessary except on the basis of one or two influential variables. There is little gain in statistical precision once the number of participants per group exceeds 50, with the greatest gains from stratification for trials with 20 or fewer participants per treatment arm.[3,60,61] Generally, the most important stratifying variable in multiple-site trials is the clinical site.

If the overall sample size is small and stratification by site may lead to imbalances in treatment groups, one solution is *minimization*, a statistical approach to balancing the treatment arms to the extent possible after each participant's entry criteria are ascertained.[62] When a study uses stratification, the stratifying variables should be included in the primary analysis (see later discussion of analysis).

Blocking

Simple randomization may yield unequal proportions of participants in the arms of a two-arm study. Blocking is the process of forcing the proportion in each of the two treatment arms to be fixed, usually at 0.5. Other options may include randomizing a higher proportion to treatment. Blocking also ensures balance in the treatment arms through time; that is, blocking provides balance on unknown temporal variables. A block size of 4 in a trial with equal randomization to the two treatment arms would imply that after every four participants are randomly assigned, there would be two participants in each treatment arm. Generally, the selected block size is large enough to make it difficult for an investigator to guess the next treatment assignment. Often the block size is randomly chosen from a range of block sizes (e.g., 4, 6, or 8) called permuted blocks, to make it more difficult to detect the end of a block. Block sizes are used within strata.

If a study such as a stroke prevention trial of treatment versus control continues for many years, blocking will protect against a simple randomization scheme such that a greater proportion of the participants are randomized to treatment early in the trial, and a greater proportion of controls are randomized later in the trial. In the NINDS t-PA Stroke Study, randomly chosen block sizes of 4, 6, and 8 were used, resulting in 144 rt-PA and 147 placebo participants in Part I and 168 rt-PA and 165 placebo participants in Part II. In the WEST,[11] block sizes of 4 were used. In trials for which a design paper describing trial methodology is published before the end of the trial, the block size usually is not discussed so that the blinding (see later) is protected.

Blinding

Blinding (sometimes referred to as *masking*) is an approach used to reduce bias in the assessment of the trial outcome measures. In a single-blind study, either the participant or the investigator is blinded to (prevented from learning) the treatment assignment of the participant. In double-blind study, neither the participant nor the investigator knows the treatment assignment. When the outcome is death, it is more difficult to introduce bias unless the outcome must be classified as stroke-related death. Bias in classifying a participant as having a new stroke (or stroke-related death) could inadvertently be introduced if the rater assessing outcomes knows the treatment assignment or if differing amounts of effort were put into finding information about the event, depending on treatment group. For many of the other outcome measures of post-stroke recovery, some inherent subjectivity is built into the scale assessment. Even if the rater does not introduce bias, there can be a perception of bias on the part of those who review the trial report if the study was not blinded.

A traditional approach to blinding is to formulate the intervention in such a way that neither physician nor participant can determine what treatment is being given to the participant. If this approach is not possible (e.g., surgery versus medical care), efforts must be made to collect outcome data in as unbiased a way as possible. Also as noted previously, block sizes used in randomization should not be revealed to investigators. If the block size is known and one or two patients in a block are unblinded (their treatment assignment is revealed to them) because of side effects or other reasons, there is a potential for the treatment assignment of others in the block to be ascertained.

In the WARSS,[10] periodic dose adjustments were needed for many participants receiving warfarin. The decision to change dose was made in the study's central laboratory and then was transmitted to the investigators. To maintain the blind, the coordinating center fabricated clinically plausible international normalized ratio values for participants in the aspirin-placebo treatment arm. A message to change the placebo dose for some patients was sent from the laboratory to the investigator. The frequency and amount of change for participants on placebo was determined through the use of a complex algorithm that mimicked the frequency and direction of changes in the warfarin-treated group.

In the NINDS t-PA Study, although the placebo formulation was identical in appearance and method of administration to rt-PA, possible bleeding at the site of rt-PA injection could potentially unblind an observer as to the participant's treatment group. To avoid ascertainment bias by a potentially unblinded rater, all follow-up data collected after randomization were assessed by a health professional who was not present at the time of randomization.[16]

For some interventions, such as surgery, participants generally cannot be blinded, and it is unlikely that the investigator can be blinded. Thus, efforts must be made to use as unbiased an approach as possible in collecting outcome data. In the EC/IC Bypass Study, which was a surgical trial, the primary outcome was fatal or nonfatal stroke.[8,9] A neurologist and a neurosurgeon independently adjudicated the cause of death and the occurrence and severity of stroke. Both adjudicators were blinded to treatment and to each other's judgments. Neither delivered medical care to any participants in the study. Disagreements were resolved by discussion and development of a consensus.

Recruitment

Proper planning help ensure recruitment on the timetable projected. This is particularly important for acute stroke therapy trials, in which participant eligibility must be quickly assessed and time from admission to treatment needs to be minimized. In the NINDS t-PA Stroke Study, methods of total quality improvement were used to flow-chart the process in each emergency department and to engage those involved in the process (CT technicians, laboratory technicians, nurses, pharmacists, neurologists, emergency department physicians and staff) in helping determine how to enroll patients more quickly.[63] Even in prevention trials, flow-charting the recruitment process may identify barriers before the start of the study. This process of flow-charting is ideally site specific, because the problems that affect recruitment are generally local ones.

Another important aspect of recruiting is engagement of the community. For acute stroke trials, cooperation of the community emergency medical services is essential in facilitating prompt arrival of prospective trial participants at participating emergency departments.[64] For both prevention and therapeutic studies, it is also important to inform the community at large. In acute stroke trials, the yield of participants from community presentations is low, but communication remains important to create a climate of trust. Also, community consent may be needed in order to meet institutional review board (IRB; see later) requirements for randomization in the emergency department (see later section on informed consent). Community presentations have the side benefit of improving awareness of stroke as well as of strategies for its prevention and treatment. For prevention trials, especially those conducted in groups of participant who are not acutely ill, the special efforts made to engage the community may have a greater effect on recruitment. In particular, some minority groups may be willing to participate in treatment trials, but often are less willing to participate in prevention trials unless a climate of trust has been developed in the community by the study investigators.

There is a growing literature on recruitment of minority participants, but little rigorous research has been conducted that tests recruitment methodologies. In a 2000 survey, Napoles-Springer and coworkers[65] identified factors associated with willingness to participate. These factors included altruism and tangible benefits to the participant, knowledge of both of which could be beneficial to the planning of a recruitment approach.

Adherence to Treatment and Trial Follow-up

Friedman and colleagues[1] have presented a detailed plan to maintain participant adherence that is generally applicable to stroke trials. They suggest that investigators can minimize or prevent potential adherence problems before a participant is enrolled in the trial by (1) keeping the study design and intervention simple, (2) selecting the appropriate participants, (3) maintaining close contact with participants after enrollment, (4) truly informing the patient, family, or both about the trial before randomization, and (5) when possible, conducting a "run-in" period that mimics the study before randomization to eliminate "noncompli-

ers" before they are entered into the trial. A run-in period may be feasible for long-term stroke prevention trials but would not be possible in therapeutic trials for acute stroke, in which treatment must be given as quickly as possible. A run-in period before randomization may also be limited by carryover drug effects that could influence the outcome in the group eventually assigned to receive placebo.

Chamberlaine (personal communication, 2003) suggests a counseling approach for patients who are not complying with medication regimens or with study visits (Table 61.4). Patients are rated on each activity required by the trial protocol (see Table 61.4). Not all trials will have all items listed in the example. The rating scores are listed in column 1 and the score for each activity is recorded at the bottom of the column representing that activity. The scores are summed to give a total adherence score. The intensity of the adherence intervention is given in column 6 and may vary by activity. Counseling is non-judgmental and is directed at ascertaining barriers to compliance and helping the participant find solutions. The total score is a measure of overall adherence and can be used in analysis or by those monitoring trial performance. This strategy has not yet been validated in stroke trials.

In both stroke prevention and therapeutic trials, all participants should be monitored to the end of a trial even if they no longer take study medications or participate in other aspects of the intervention. For an acute stroke trial with a one-time dose, the possibility of drop-out from therapy is minimal; however, completeness of follow-up remains an important issue. At a minimum, participants should be encouraged to return for the final visit, regardless of whether they are receiving the intervention, to avoid the problem of missing outcome data (see later discussion on missing data).

Measuring Adherence to Treatment

If treatment is, for example, an educational intervention to reduce stroke risk factors or an exercise rehabilitation program, a participant's adherence to the regimen can be estimated with process measures (e.g., number of sessions attended) or by changes in his or her knowledge, attitudes, and beliefs. If laboratory tests are applicable, reliable, and affordable, the most accurate assessment of medication compliance may be measurement of blood, saliva, or urine levels of the drug; if, however, a participant is generally noncompliant but takes medication more often close to the next clinic visit, such a measurement would not reflect the true level of adherence. Other standard adherence measures for medication trials are making pill counts of returned medication at each visit and counting the number of times the bottle was opened (collected through a miniaturized electronic device in the lid of the pill bottle). Both methods are only estimates, however, subject to under- and over-counting, and the electronic device is expensive to purchase.

Morisky and associates[66] suggest posing a set of questions as a better measure of compliance than a pill count (Table 61.5). The usefulness of these questions in stroke trials needs validation. Counts of missed visits, missed forms, and missed items on forms, and the adherence score from Table 61.4 may also be useful in monitoring adherence to treatment.

Table 61.4   Clinical Record: Adherence Measurements and Interventions*

Adherence Score	Pills Taken	Calendar Completed	Appointments Kept/Missed	Lab Studies Done	Prescribed Interventions
1	85–100%	Complete 75–100%	Kept as appointed	Done within 7 days	Research nurse: Thanks and congratulations on each task well done
2	75–84%	50–74%	Kept within 14 days	Done 8–14 days	Research nurse: Identify deficiency, briefly discuss, thanks for the specific tasks well done
3	65–74%	24–49%	Kept 15–30 days	Done 15–30 days	Research nurse: Identify deficiencies, nurse counseling, if repeated add physician counseling. Corrective action with telephone reminders.
4	<65%	<25%	Kept >30 days	Done >30 days	Research nurse + physician: Identify deficiencies, physician counseling. Corrective action with telephone reminders.
5	None	None	None	None	Research nurse or physician: Telephone inquiry and counseling
Score	P____	C____	A____	L____	

*Calculations:

$$\frac{(\text{Bottles} \times \text{number of pills per bottle}) - \text{Pills returned}}{\text{Days} \times \text{number of pills required per day}} = \underline{\quad}\%$$

$$\frac{\text{Calendar days w/notes}}{\text{Days since last visit}} = \underline{\quad}\%$$

Form adapted from Chamberlaine, personal communication, 2003.

Table 61.5   Self-Reported Medication Taking

1. Do you ever forget to take your medicine?
2. Are you careless at times about taking your medicine?
3. When you feel better, do you sometimes stop taking your medicine?
4. Sometimes if you feel worse when you take your medicine, do you stop taking it?

Adapted from Morisky DE, Green LW, Levine DM: Concurrent and predictive validity of a self-reported measure of medication adherence. Med Care 24:67–74, 1986.

Data Collection and Quality Assurance

General

Both Meinert and Tonascia[3] and Friedman and colleagues[1] provide detailed plans for study data collection and quality assurance applicable to stroke trials. Key approaches include study documentation, timely applications of range and consistency checks, and prompt communication of data errors to the study coordinators for resolution.

Protocol and Manual of Procedures

A trial has two key documents, the protocol and the manual of procedures. Both are essential to trial management.

The *protocol* is the blueprint for the trial. It is the document that is sent to the IRB and, when necessary, the FDA. Changes to the protocol generally require new IRB approval and often notification of the FDA. Because protocol changes reflect basic changes in study design, the implications of a change in terms of previously collected data should be seriously considered before the change is instituted. Such actions as expanding the entry or exclusion criteria, modifying the laboratory testing required, and modifying an outcome measure would require a protocol change.

Procedural changes, such as deciding to improve adherence by offering participants transportation to study visits, would be reflected in the *manual of procedures* documenting how a study is conducted and would not require a protocol change or new approvals. The manual of procedures contains study instruments (i.e., forms for data collection), detailed instructions for completing the study instruments, and other instructions for data collection, follow-up, laboratory procedures, and so on. (Note: Changes to study instruments administered to patients may require IRB approval.) The manual documents answers to questions raised by investigators conducting the trial in the field so that answer to the same question is consistent over time. The protocol and manual of procedures provide sufficient detail to allow someone who has not been participating in the trial to replicate it in another setting.

Training

An important aspect of quality assurance is training of the people collecting data for the trial. In therapeutic stroke trials, the NIHSS is particularly difficult to standardize. In the TOAST and the NINDS t-PA Stroke Study, video training programs were developed along with programs to test the people who would be administering the NIHSS.[67,68] To maintain consistency of measurement over time, investigators in the NINDS Study were re-certified through the use of additional testing tapes. The same approach could be used for other scales, such as the mRS and Barthel Index.

Data Analyses

Intent to Treat

The guiding principle in clinical trials is the use of intent-to-treat analysis.[69] In this approach to analysis, all participants are analyzed in the group to which they are randomized, and all participants who are randomized are included in the primary analysis, whether or not they withdraw or deviate from the protocol. In a surgical trial, under an intent-to-treat analysis, participants randomized to surgery, whether or not they received surgery, would be analyzed in the surgical group, and participants randomized to medical care whether or not they received medical care or surgery would be analyzed in the medical care group. In the EC/IC Bypass Study methodology paper, it appeared that the intent-to-treat principle would not be followed (see discussion of crossovers in the article),[8] but in the article presenting the trial results, the analytic approach was changed, and the intent-to-treat principle was followed.[9]

In stroke trials, several difficult issues arise. If it is necessary to randomly assign participants to treatment before an entry criterion is completely ascertained—for example, before magnetic resonance imaging can be performed—how are participants who do not meet the entry criteria counted in the analysis? Friedman and colleagues[1] suggest that no withdrawals be allowed and that analyses include all participants who were randomized. Gillings and Koch[69] describe other approaches. Subgroup analyses (see later) would be conducted as well. If results of subgroup analyses agree with the analyses of the full trial data set, the interpretation is clear. If results do not agree, caution is needed in presenting the results, and emphasis should generally be placed on the analysis of the full data set. The ECASS investigators presented a subgroup analysis of a target group of participants who were deemed to meet all the entry criteria on the basis of a postrandomization CT review; these results differed from those of the intent-to-treat analysis.[17] The intent-to-treat analysis, which included all participants randomized, was considered the primary analysis for the trial. When many ineligible participants are expected to be enrolled, the effect on the trial sample size should be considered in the trial design.

Gillings and Koch[69] describe several other complex situations relevant to stroke trials. In some trials, participants who do not receive the first dose are excluded. This number should be small, less than 5%, in a well-conducted trial. If the number is larger, there some sort of bias may be operating. If the number is small, the more conservative approach would be to include these participants in the analysis, but from the clinical perspective, doing so makes little sense. Either way, including or excluding this small number of participants should have little effect on the results, but if there are differences, the analysis of the complete study cohort should be considered the primary analysis.

In general, all participants, even those no longer receiving treatment, should be monitored to the end of the trial, and their final outcomes should be used as the primary trial outcomes. Methods for imputing data in order to include participants with missing follow-up and adherence to the intent-to-treat principle are described in a later section in the chapter.

The terms "completer" analysis, "on-treatment analysis," and "analyzable population" are generally used to describe a situation in which participants who stop treatment, did not adhere to protocol, or have incomplete follow-up are excluded. Biased analyses can be used as secondary measures of treatment efficacy, but these analyses are not replacements for primary analyses by intent to treat. "On-

treatment analysis" has also been used by some investigators at the FDA to describe the situation in which through some administrative error, a participant received a different drug from that planned. If there are a small number of such participants, and if the administrative error is not based on the background of these participants or their prognosis, Gillings and Koch[69] recommend that data from such participants be analyzed according to the treatment they received and would not consider doing so to result in a biased, on-treatment analysis.

General Approaches

Friedman and colleagues[1] summarize the analytic approaches used in clinical trials. These standard approaches, such as analyses of time to new stroke or death, are generally useful in prevention trials for which the outcome is usually binary (yes, no; each participant either survived stroke-free or had a new stroke or died).

Global Tests

Trials of acute therapy present a special problem. As noted previously, the outcome of therapeutic trials is often recovery from stroke, for which there is no one accepted measure. Thus, trials are usually designed with a set of correlated outcome measures. These measures can be analyzed separately, but interpretation of the set of outcomes with respect to an overall effect of treatment is difficult. Requiring all outcomes to be statistically significant may be asking too much. As noted in the discussion of sample size, testing of multiple individual outcomes may require some adjustment for multiple comparisons and larger sample sizes than needed for a single outcome tested at the 0.05 level. After adjustment for multiple comparisons, if one outcome is highly significant (treatment is beneficial) and the remaining outcomes strongly favor the control group, the treatment would be considered a success. Yet what is of interest is the overall effect of treatment considering all outcomes.

To aid in this interpretation of an overall effect, a global test for multiple outcomes was used in the NINDS rt-PA Stroke Study.[16,70] This global test was based on the categorization of the outcomes into minimal or no disability (yes, no). Data from the NINDS t-PA Stroke Trial show the observed correlations among the outcome measures used in that trial as measured by a phi coefficient because the outcomes are binary (see Table 61.2).[71] The global test for binary outcomes uses a logit model (a mathematical formulation used for binary outcomes and described in the appendix to the article by Tilley and colleagues[70]) and generalized estimating equations. This approach is used to take the correlations among outcomes into account in developing an odds ratio for favorable outcome—that is, minimal or no disability.[72,73] Generally, when the global test is reported, the odds ratios for the individual outcomes are also given to help interpretation of the global test (Table 61.6).

The global test differs from the multivariate t-test (Hotelling's T^2)[74] that tests association among outcomes but does not consider the direction of the association. A treatment that is significantly better on one outcome and significantly worse on another could have a statistically significant result when Hotelling's T^2 is used.

Global tests can also be conducted for continuous outcomes with the approaches of O'Brien[75] or Pocock and

Table 61.6　NINDS t-PA Stroke Trial, Part II Data*

Outcome	Proportion with Favorable Outcome		Odds Ratio[†]	95% Confidence Intervals	P Value
	t-PA (N = 168)	Placebo (N = 165)			
Barthel Index Value	50	38	1.63	1.06–2.49	0.026
Modified Rankin Scale Score	39	26	1.68	1.09–2.59	0.019
Glasgow Outcome Scale Score	44	32	1.64	1.06–2.53	0.025
NIH Stroke Scale Score	31	20	1.72	1.05–2.84	0.033
Global			1.73	1.16–2.60	0.008

*Intent-to-treat. Those with missing values scored as having unfavorable result for that outcome.

[†]Odds ratios, confidence intervals, and *P* values for single outcomes calculated using Mantel Haenszel approach and for global test using generalized estimating equations and Wald test statistic. Strata for all analyses included center and time from stroke onset to initiation of treatment (0–90, 91–180 minutes).

NIH, National Institutes of Health; NINDS, National Institute of Neurological Disorders and Stroke; t-PA, tissue-type plasminogen activator.

Adapted from: Tissue plasminogen activator for acute ischemic stroke. National Institute of Neurological Disorders and Stroke (NINDS) rt-PA Stroke Study Group. N Engl J Med 333:1581–1587, 1995.

associates.[76] O'Brien's test is based on a nonparametric approach that ranks patients across treatment and control groups on each outcome, sums the ranks across outcomes for each patient, and then uses a *t*-test or other statistical procedure to compare treatment and control groups. Additionally, both O'Brien[75] and Pocock and associates[76] present a weighted least-squares approach. Global tests can be constructed using any set of clinically meaningful outcomes. If the global test is the primary outcome, the variables included must be pre-specified prior to the start of the trial.

Clustering

Special analytic issues arise in the analyses of clustered data, i.e., data where there is some correlation or association among participants. An example is a clinical trial in which the unit of randomization is a physician's practice rather than a patient. This type of trial might be used in testing a new approach to stroke prevention in which the provider receives the intervention, such as feedback on progress in reducing stroke-related risk factors for the patients in his or her practice. In this sort of trial, providers are randomly assigned to receive the intervention or control condition. In the analysis of clustered data, assuming there is a positive correlation among patients in the provider's practice (patients in a practice are more like one another than like patients in other practices in terms of risk factor modification), the variance unadjusted for clustering is smaller than the variance adjusted for clustering. Thus, by ignoring the clustering, the investigator may falsely reject a null hypothesis and claim treatment benefit. Lafata and colleagues[77] discuss issues in the design and analysis of such trials of clustered data.

Missing Data

In spite of excellent study design, precise execution, and attention to adherence as already described, a certain amount of missing data is inevitable in all clinical trials. All courses of action should be taken to avoid missing data; however, when data are missing, a variety of statistical methods may be used either to perform analysis with some data to be omitted or to impute values for missing data before analysis.

There are two patterns of missing data in longitudinal clinical trials: intermittent (e.g., due to a single missed clinic visit) and monotone (e.g., due to participant withdrawal or loss to follow-up).

Little and Rubin[78] have classified missing data according to the following three mechanisms, which are explained with the assumption that the missing data of interest are outcome data:

- Missing completely at random (MCAR): Data that are missing because of an event, circumstances, or measure completely independent of the outcome of interest or other participant-specific measures collected in the study.
- Missing at random (MAR): Data that are missing because of an event, circumstances, or measure independent of the outcome of interest but related to another participant-specific measure.
- Missing not at random (MNAR or non-ignorable): The data are missing because of the unobserved outcome of interest.

For example, if a participant's 3-month NIHSS score is missing because (1) the investigational staff simply forgot to evaluate the participant on the NIHSS at 3 months or (2) the participant's car broke down on his way to the clinic for his 3-month visit, the missing information is MCAR. If, however, the 3-month NIHSS score is missing because the participant was feeling depressed and did not wish to make the clinic visit, it is MAR (depression is not measured by NIHSS score). If the 3-month NIHSS score is missing because the participant's neurologic condition (which is measured by the NIHSS score) had deteriorated to the extent that the participant was unable to travel to the clinic, the missing data are non-ignorable.

Statistically, MCAR and MAR data are not problematic, because standard statistical methods as well as various imputation methods can be applied with minimal or no bias. If all missing data are MCAR, they can be ignored, and analysis using only the observed data can be conducted without bias because the missing data in this case are considered a representative sample of the observed data. However, if more than a minimal amount of data is missing, this approach leads to reduction in statistical power. For statistical analysis with MAR data, a multiple imputation method is recommended before analysis, because the method designates some uncertainty for the imputed value, thereby allowing for more appropriate variance estimation.[78,79] Alternatively, when appropriate, repeated measures analysis can be conducted with MAR data without imputing, if all other assumptions are met.

Non-ignorable missing data are more problematic for analysis. Application of standard statistical methods may yield biased results. Model-based procedures, such as the pattern mixture model, in which non-ignorable missing data are modeled separately from observed data, are often adopted. These models are likelihood-based with sophisticated assumptions and mathematical complexity.[78]

Of particular concern for missing data in clinical trials is the biased use only of those participants for whom there is complete outcome data. Bias may arise because the participants who provided data may have a better response to treatment than those who did not, even those in the placebo group. Therefore, a subgroup of fully compliant participants ("completers") is not a random sample of the original sample. Patterns of missing data (i.e., rate, time to withdrawal, and reason for withdrawal) may differ among treatment groups, contributing bias to study results. Furthermore, the amount of missing data may differ between treatment groups. If a substantial proportion of data (e.g., >20%) is unobserved, especially in the primary outcome of interest, the integrity and quality of the entire study could be questioned, regardless of the approach taken to adjust for the missing data. Therefore, unless participants withdraw consent, regardless of compliance with the study protocol, the participants should be monitored to the end of the study period. All of their assessments should be performed and the results collected according to protocol.

In general, using the intent-to-treat principle of statistical analysis, data from all randomized participants must be included in the primary analysis. If there are missing data, various multiple imputation methods are available to substitute values for the missing data items,[78,79] many of which have good statistical properties. Computer software is available to implement these methods.[80]

In the WARSS, the primary outcome (recurrent ischemic stroke or death from any cause) for 2173 of the 2206 participants was assessed at the end of the trial.[10] For the remaining 33, an innovative approach to imputation was used. Those for whom outcome data were missing classified on the basis of their case records by a senior clinician who was blinded to treatment assignments. The clinician classified the participants into three categories for which the following decisions were made:

1. Endpoint eminent; an endpoint was assumed to have occurred at the time the participant was lost to follow-up (N = 1).
2. Data missing for reason unrelated to study (e.g., participant moved to Puerto Rico with daughter); participant was censored at the date of loss to follow-up (i.e., participant's outcome was considered unknown after the date specified and participant does not contribute information after that point in time) (N = 20).

3. Data missing for reason possibly related to study (e.g., TIAs occur, then participant lost to follow-up); use methods of multiple imputation to impute a value for time to outcome using baseline covariates (N = 12). Of the 12 participants for whom multiple imputation was used, a primary outcome was imputed for 2, and an event-free follow-up imputed for 10.[81]

NINDS t-PA Stroke Study participants who died before the 3-month follow-up visit were given the worst possible score on the four primary 3-month outcome measures. Surviving participants who missed the 3-month follow-up visit were given any outcome data available after 3 months. For participants for whom no data beyond the 3-month visit were available, data from the time point closest to 3 months but more than 7 days after randomization were used; otherwise, participants were given the worst possible score on the missing 3-month outcome measures (N = 1 in Part I of the study, and N= 4 in Part II).[58,64]

Interim Analysis

Almost all clinical trials are longitudinal in nature, and participants are enrolled sequentially. In the last three decades, interim analysis of clinical trial data has steadily gained popularity. Ethical, economic, and administrative reasons drive the analyses. By conducting interim analyses, investigators are better able to ensure participant safety. Stopping the study early because of overwhelming evidence of the efficacy of a drug means earlier access to an efficacious treatment for patients and earlier profit for the pharmaceutical industry. Stopping a study early because of negative results ensures that participants are not unnecessarily exposed to inferior or ineffective treatment and prevents wasting of resources. Evidence either for or against treatment effectiveness of a drug allows for informed management decisions about the allocation of limited research and development funds. Administratively, interim analyses of data help ensure that the study is being executed as planned and that only the appropriate participants are enrolled. Interim analyses may also uncover the presence of unanticipated problems, such as noncompliance, that can be remedied. Interim analysis allows the investigators and statisticians to evaluate assumptions made in the design of the trial, such as participant accrual rate and the parameters used for sample size estimation.

The concept of interim analysis arose in the late 1920s among practitioners of quality assurance for manufacturing production. In the 1940s, Wald[82] developed a fully sequential study design and analysis method—sequential probability ratio test (SPRT)—whereby data were analyzed after an outcome was obtained for each unit of observation. Armitage[83] pioneered the use of group sequential design in medical studies. A modification of the SPRT, group sequential design requires that interim analysis be conducted at prespecified times or after a prespecified amount of information (e.g., number of participants) has been gathered, rather than after pairs of participants (treatment and control) are entered.

All methods of interim analysis provide quantitative guidelines for early termination of the study and a penalty for early termination in the form of an adjusted critical value (type I error). Figure 61–2 gives examples of three

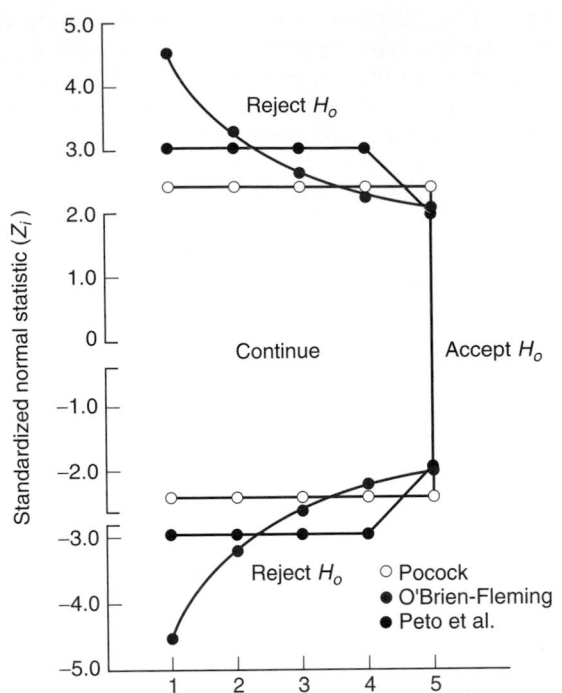

FIGURE 61–2 *Guidelines for stopping a clinical trial. (Adapted from Friedman LM, Furberg CD, DeMets DL: Fundamentals of Clinical Trials, 3rd ed. New York, Springer Verlag, 1998.)*

different guidelines for stopping a trial. Peto and colleagues[84] and O'Brien and Fleming[34] use more conservative guidelines early in the study, so that the final alpha level for testing is close to the planned overall alpha (0.05). Pocock[85] uses a less conservative guideline, but the final comparison for the trial would be made at an alpha level less than 0.05, potentially less acceptable to investigators.

Any interim analysis adds a level of complication to the planning and execution of the study. For example, the randomization scheme must ensure even distribution according to a prespecified ratio among the treatment groups at all times. Blocking, as described earlier in this chapter, would help accomplish this balance. There is also a data management burden. The statistician must be given data in a timely manner that is complete and correct to the cut-off date for the interim analysis. Care must be taken to ensure that no unblinding occurs as a result of interim analysis.

Investigators must weigh the value of interim analysis when participant follow-up is long compared with the participant accrual rate. For instance, many stroke therapeutic trials adopt the 90-day neurologic assessment as the primary outcome. If all needed participants are quickly entered into the trial by the time the first or the second interim analysis is conducted, further interim analyses may be unnecessary. An example is the Interventional Management of Stroke Study,[36] a Phase II trial with a planned sample size of 80 and a planned interim analysis. Accrual was expected to be slow, so interim analyses were planned to allow early stopping of a futile treatment. Surprisingly, the trial sites enrolled 10 patients per month and enrollment was completed in 8 months, making the planned interim analyses unnecessary.

There are two types of stopping guidelines, one based only on the current evidence at the time of interim analysis and the other based on prediction of the future outcome (referred to as stochastic curtailment procedure [SCP]). An example of the former, and the method most commonly adopted in clinical trials today, is the Lan-DeMets group sequential method[86] with the stopping boundaries as described above by O'Brien and Fleming.[34] The Lan-DeMets method differs from the original O'Brien and Fleming approach in that it allows more flexibility in the choice of time points when interim analyses are conducted but still uses the O'Brien and Fleming spending function method of using the alpha allocated for testing. Under Lan-DeMets guidelines, one must observe extreme differences in the treatment effect between the groups in order to reject the null hypothesis in the early stages of the study, because it spends the type I error (alpha) conservatively.

Stochastic curtailment originated in the quality control field for manufacturing, where an entire batch of products would be rejected if a certain number of defective items was found; if and when that number is reached, the rest of the batch is not inspected. Given current data, SCP measures the chance of statistical significance (i.e., rejection of the null). In clinical trials, SCP is used to determine whether proceeding further with the study would be unlikely to have a statistically significant result. These analyses are completed separately from analyses of efficacy. An SCP is usually implemented using the B-statistic as described in Ellenberg and colleagues.[87] The section on "stopping rules" in the design paper describing the VISP Trial is an example of a typical write-up for a study protocol.[13] Bayesian rules, derived from subjective prior information, have also been developed for stochastic curtailment and have been used more frequently in trials of cancer therapies than in trials of stroke prevention and therapy.[88]

Guidelines provided by the FDA and International Conference on Harmonization (ICH; see later) state require that (1) investigators assess the effects of any interim analysis performed, (2) any and all interim analyses, formal or informal, be described in full, even if they are performed by blinded investigators, and (3) the plan for interim analysis be provided in the study protocol.

Analysis of Covariance

Unless most participants in one treatment arm of a study have the risk factor and most participants in the other arm do not have the risk factor, it is possible to adjust statistically for imbalances between treatment groups by including the risk factor in a model testing for a treatment effect.[89] If the imbalance in the risk factor explains away the treatment benefit, the benefit has been artificially enhanced by the imbalance. If the treatment benefit remains or is enhanced after adjustment for the risk factor, the imbalance was not artificially inflating the treatment benefit. One danger in such post hoc analyses is that many variables may be tested in an attempt to bring out a positive treatment outcome, making the end result less credible. Investigators can avoid this "data dredging" by prespecifying the variables to be included as covariates.[90]

The odds ratio for a favorable outcome in the second NINDS rt-PA Stroke Study (Part II) was 1.7 (95% confidence interval [CI] 1.2–2.6). Post hoc analyses of covariance were conducted with adjustment for the three variables (age, weight, and aspirin use before stroke) that were imbalanced (P <.05) between the two treatment groups. These post hoc analyses suggested an even greater benefit of t-PA (odds ratio for a favorable outcome, 2.0 (95% CI, 1.3–3.1).[16]

Subgroup Analyses and Interactions

After the completion of a trial, multiple analyses are often performed to determine whether there are subgroups in which the treatment might have been beneficial or harmful. To avoid bias, subgroups should be "proper"— that is, defined by characteristics measured at baseline— before treatment.[91] For example, in the NINDS t-PA Stroke Study, each participant's stroke subtype was determined 7 to 10 days after stroke from CT scans taken 24 hours after thrombolytic treatment and clinical data collected at baseline.[92] The therapy could affect the 24-hour CT findings through both its clot-busting properties and its potential hemorrhagic side effects. The grouping of patients by this postrandomization classification of stroke subtype, rather than reflecting the effect of treatment, could reflect the characteristics of patients that led to a particular response or side effect.

In addition to choosing a proper subgroup, there are statistical issues in the analyses of subgroups. The more subgroups examined, the more likely the analyses will lead to an alpha error (i.e., detection of a difference by chance alone). If ten mutually exclusive subgroups are studied, there is a 20% chance that the treatment will be better than control in one group and the converse will be true in another group. To protect against bias and alpha errors, Yusuf and colleagues[91] recommend two approaches, one relating to specification of hypotheses and the other to statistical

methodology. First, predefined subgroups based on a clearly justified rationale and specified hypothesis can be identified in the protocol before the start of the trial. These a priori subgroups are less subject to bias than subgroups defined after study results are known (post hoc). Second, analyses can be adjusted for multiple comparisons, with the potential for greatly reduced power, depending on the number of subgroups. If there are a small number of predefined subgroups in the study protocol, there is less need to adjust for multiple comparisons in exploring these subgroup hypotheses. Additionally, to protect against bias and alpha error, testing for a treatment interaction before subgroup analyses are conducted provides a more stringent approach.

An interaction between treatment and the subgrouping variable is present if (1) the treatment is harmful in one subgroup but beneficial in another (see next paragraph) or (2) the magnitude of treatment benefit differs among subgroups (see Table 61.7 and later discussion). Generally, interactions are tested at the 0.1 rather than 0.05 alpha level in recognition that most studies are not designed with high power to test for treatment interactions.

Meade and Brennan[93] conducted subgroup analyses of patients in a thrombosis prevention trial with emphasis on detecting subgroups who might derive the most benefit in terms of stroke prevention. These investigators presented analyses with tests of interactions suggesting that participants who had baseline systolic blood pressures 145 mm Hg and higher and were receiving aspirin therapy were at a higher risk of stroke than those with similar blood pressure levels who were receiving placebo, whereas participants with lower blood pressures experienced a protective effect (P value for the interaction, 0.006).

Table 61.7 gives another example of a treatment interaction.[94] In this example, trial participants given t-PA who

Table 61.7   Three-Month Outcomes of t-PA Therapy by Apolipoprotein E2 and E4 Phenotype, Adjusted for Baseline Covariate*

Treatment Arm and Apolipoprotein Phenotype	No. of Patients	Odds Ratio	95% CI	P Values for Interaction
t-PA treatment group				
Apolipoprotein E2 phenotype				0.01
Apo E2-positive	27	6.4	2.4–12.1	
Apo E2-negative	190	2.0	1.2–2.6	
Apolipoprotein E4 phenotype				0.49
Apo E4-positive	53	2.0	1.2–3.9	
Apo E4-negative	164	2.6	1.4–3.2	
Placebo group				
Apolipoprotein E2 phenotype				0.01
Apo E2-positive	31	0.8	0.5–2.0	
Apo E2-negative[‡]	161	1.0	NA	
Apolipoprotein E4 phenotype				0.49
Apo E4-positive	58	1.1	0.6–2.1	
Apo E4-negative	134	1.0	NA	

*Adjusted for baseline covariates, age (categorized), rank of the actual weight, rank of total dose delivered, baseline pulse pressure, prior aspirin use, NIHSS score (5 groups), hypertension, race, cardiac history, age × NIHSS score, admission MBP, age × admission MBP, diabetes, and the variable early CTT.
[†]Global test for multiple outcomes.
[‡]Reference group for calculation of odds ratio.
CI, confidence interval; CTT, computed tomography; MBP, mean blood pressure; NIHSS, National Institutes of Health Stroke Scale; t-PA, tissue-type plasminogen activator.
Adapted from Broderick J, Lu M, Jackson C, et al: Apolipoprotein E phenotype and the efficacy of intravenous tissue plasminogen activator in acute ischemic stroke. Ann Neurol 49:736–744, 2001.

had the apolipoprotein (Apo) E2 factor had an odds of a favorable outcome, based on the global test and adjusted for covariates, of 6.4 compared with participants who were given placebo and did not have the Apo E2 factor. In contrast, those given t-PA who did not have the Apo E2 factor had an odds ratio of only 2.0 compared with the placebo group without the Apo E2 factor. This differential effect is reflected in the *P* value of 0.01 testing for the presence of the interaction. In contrast, for the Apo E4 factor, no interaction is detected. The beneficial effect of treatment with t-PA compared with placebo is clear but does not differ in patients with and without the Apo E4 factor. On the basis of the statistical analysis, the difference in magnitude of benefit is not sufficient to consider there to be an Apo E4 treatment interaction. A graphical approach to depicting interaction when the patient characteristic is continuous is given in Figure 61–3, in which a time from stroke onset to treatment interaction is demonstrated.

In summary, the pitfalls in reporting subgroup analyses in stroke trials can be avoided by (1) prespecifying subgroup hypotheses in the protocol, (2) testing for treatment by participant characteristic (subgroup) interactions, (3) clearly differentiating between the patient characteristics that lead to poorer outcome in both intervention and control groups and the characteristics that lead to differential treatment effect in the intervention group, and (4) carefully reporting post hoc subgroup analyses as generating hypotheses that need further confirmation in other studies.

Meta-analysis

Meta-analysis is the statistical synthesis of different research studies addressing a similar question. The goals of meta-analysis are to obtain more reliable estimates of treatment effects and to provide a convenient way to summarize information from multiple studies. Results of a meta-analysis are usually displayed as odds ratios and confidence limits for the individual studies along with pooled odds ratio and confidence limits for the studies combined. It is well known that meta-analysis can suffer from selection bias reflecting the researcher's choice of studies to include, ascertainment bias (not all relevant studies can be found), publication bias (only positive studies are in print), and from follow-up bias (some studies follow patients longer than others). Meta-analyses can also be affected by differences between study protocols, such as dosage or route of administration of treatment, inclusion-exclusion criteria, and definition of outcome measures.[95]

In therapeutic trials for stroke, selection bias, ascertainment bias, and publication bias are less of a problem than for trials in many other diseases. There is high interest among investigators in this field in both positive and negative studies as well as a close international community of investigators who perform stroke-related clinical trials research and are aware of one another's work. Follow-up differences are also less of an issue in clinical trials for stroke. Patients with stroke tend to stabilize by 3 months, leading to minimal differences between outcome data at 3 months and outcome data at 6 months. The major issue in meta-analysis of clinical trials for stroke is the potential for differences in outcome measures and treatment protocols.

In contrast to trials of treatments for myocardial infarction, for which the outcome is often death, the outcome of therapeutic trials in stroke is usually some measure of post-stroke disability. Unlike rheumatoid arthritis (RA), for which a core set of measures of outcome has been identified for use in all therapeutic trials,[96] there is no agreed-upon core set of stroke outcome measures to be used in the meta-analyses (see earlier discussion of outcome measures).

In trials of thrombolytic agents, the time from stroke onset has been shown to interact with treatment,[59] making it difficult to interpret comparisons of trials with differing times from stroke onset to treatment. Other protocol differences are variations in dose and in eligibility criteria, such as differences in exclusions based on early CT findings. Statistical approaches to meta-analysis such as stratified analyses lack power to detect strata × treatment interactions (see previous discussion of subgroup analyses and interactions) and generally cannot adjust away protocol differences, especially if an interaction is present. If interactions are present, separate analyses within strata must be conducted, or the positive effects of treatment in one stratum maybe obfuscated by the negative effects of treatment in another stratum, further reducing the power of the

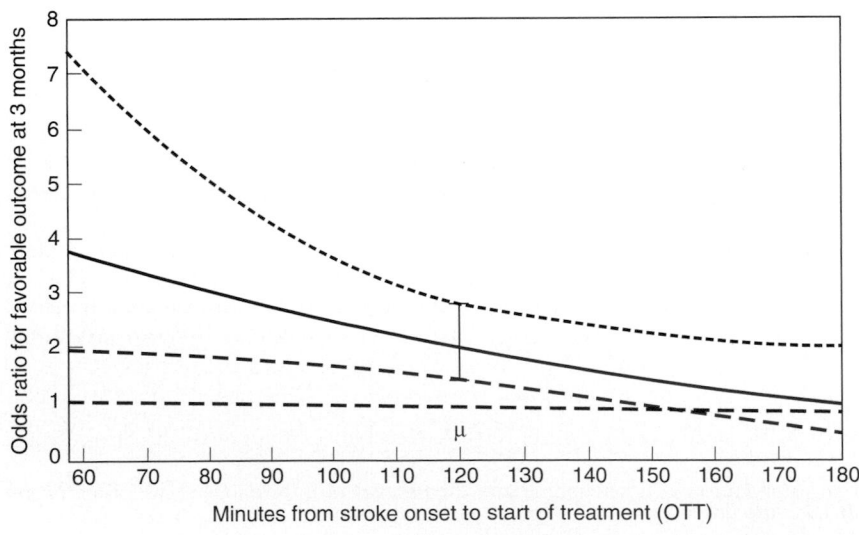

FIGURE 61–3 *Graph of model estimating odds ratio for favorable outcome at 3 months in patients treated with recombinant tissue-type plasminogen activator (rt-PA) and those given placebo by onset-to-treatment time (OTT) with 95% confidence intervals (CIs), after adjustment for the baseline National Institutes of Health (NIH) Stroke Scale score. Odds ratio > 1 indicates greater odds that rt-PA–treated patients will have a favorable outcome at the 3 months than the placebo-treated patients. Range of OTT was 58–180 minutes with a mean (μ) of 119.7 minutes. (Adapted from Marler JR, Tilley BC, Lu M, et al: Early stroke treatment associated with better outcome. NINDS rt-PA Stroke Study Group. Neurology 55:1649–1655, 2000.)*

comparisons. LeLorier and colleagues[97] suggest that summarizing all information from a set of trials into a single odds ratio can be an oversimplification of a complex issue.

Flather and associates[95] and LeLorier colleagues[97] contend that meta-analyses of large trials or individual analyses of large single trials are preferred because the estimates are more stable. In stroke prevention trials, the definition of "large" as used in cardiovascular trials may apply, because mortality or new stroke plus mortality is the usual outcome. In therapeutic trials with post-stroke disability at the outcome, "large" should be defined by the expected effect sizes and sample sizes required to obtain high power to detect such a difference between treatment and control. Generally, this sample size is much smaller than for cardiovascular trials.

Federal Regulations

This section of the chapter deals with regulations in the United States. Investigators conducting trials outside the United States must work with the regulating agencies within each country to determine what is required. (See also the section on international guidelines).

In the United States, the two main federal agencies responsible for regulations of stroke-related clinical trials are the U.S. Department of Health and Human Services (DHHS) and the FDA. The DHHS 45 *Code of Federal Regulations* (CFR) §46 applies to all clinical investigations, and FDA 21 CFR §50 and 56 apply to studies involving FDA-regulated products. Additional regulations and policies (such as those of the ICH's Good Clinical Practice, Department of Veterans Affairs, and the Joint Commission on Accreditation of Health Care Organization) may also apply, depending on the source of funding or the purpose of the investigation.

Federal regulations govern all clinical trials that are funded by federal money or are conducted in institutions that (1) receive federal money, (2) have federal project–wide assurances, or (3) conduct studies of investigational drugs with human participants. Any clinical trial of drugs, biologic products, or medical devices involving interstate shipping or marketing requires prior submission to and approval from the FDA (see Federal Food Drug And Cosmetic Act 5.05I1A and 21 CFR §50, 56, 312, and 314). "Interstate shipping" is broadly defined. If the container or label or gel that holds the medication or anything related to the product is shipped across state lines, interstate shipping is considered to be involved.

Studies of dietary supplements do not require FDA review if the supplements are not approved by the FDA as drugs. The FDA does not regulate surgery unless a device is used and does not regulate many behavioral and dietary interventions. If there is a question about the need for FDA review, investigators should contact the agency for clarification. Even if FDA approval is not required, DHSS regulations may still apply, as noted previously, if studies are funded through federal sources.

FDA-Regulated Research

The FDA, formed in 1931, is a subcabinet organization within the DHHS. Its website is *www.fda.gov*. As described in FDA's Mission Statement, formalized in the FDA Modernization Act of 1997, the agency's purpose is to ensure that "food is safe, wholesome, sanitary, and properly labeled; human and veterinary drugs are safe and effective; there is reasonable assurance of the safety and effectiveness of devices intended for human use; cosmetics are safe and properly labeled; and public health and safety are protected from electronic product radiation."[98] In 1938, a Federal Food, Drugs and Cosmetics Act was passed that requires the pharmaceutical companies to submit full reports of investigations on the safety of new drugs.

New drugs are the responsibility of the Center for Drug Evaluation and Research (CDER) or the Center for Biologics Evaluation and Research (CBER) at the FDA. Their purview includes IND submissions as well as submissions of New Drug Applications (NDAs), Biologics Licensing Applications (BLAs) and Abbreviated New Drug Applications (ANDAs) for studies of new drugs or biologics or new uses for an existing drug or biologic. Biologics include viruses, therapeutic serums, toxins, antitoxins, vaccines, blood and blood components, blood derivatives, and allergenic products. Recombinant t-PA, a genetically engineered pharmaceutical studied in several stroke trials, was considered a biologic and was submitted for approval through the CBER.

An IND must be submitted to the FDA before a new drug or biologic can be used in humans for the first time and must be filed when an already marketed drug is evaluated in humans for a new indication (21 CFR §312). The investigator-sponsor holds an IND for a drug while it is under investigation for a new indication. The FDA reviews the NDA; if the NDA is approved, the drug can be marketed for the new indication. Holding an IND means that the investigator-sponsor is permitted to ship drug from state to state and gather the data on the clinical safety and effectiveness needed for an NDA or BLA. The CDER or CBER reviews the IND to evaluate whether the risk of exposure to the drug or biologic is reasonable on the basis of previous animal and human (if available) testing, methods of manufacturing, and a well-developed clinical research plan that minimizes the risk to the participants.

After all the phases of clinical trials through phase 3 are completed, an NDA or BLA is submitted. An NDA or BLA is usually submitted with results from at least two adequate, well-controlled clinical studies conducted in humans to demonstrate substantial evidence of the effectiveness and safety of the drug. The FDA accepts a single trial on a case-by-case basis; acceptance of a single trial is more likely when there is no other treatment for the condition or disease. The FDA accept some trials of surrogate outcomes but usually requires post-marketing surveillance in these cases.

The Center for Devices and Radiological Health (CDRH) oversees clinical trials of devices (e.g., instruments such as micro-catheters, apparatus, implements, machine contrivances, implants, and in vitro reagents). CDRH requires an investigator to submit an Investigational Device Exemption (IDE) in order to perform clinical trials and either a Pre-market Approval of Medical Devices (PMA), or a Product Development Protocol (PDP), similar to the IND and NDA, respectively, for approval to market a device.

For each of the specific drug classes and subspecialties (e.g., neurologics, anti-inflammatory agents, vaccines), the FDA has established an independent external review group. The FDA Advisory Committee consists of clinical, pharmacologic, and statistical experts and at least one consumer advocate. These committee members are responsible for reviewing data from completed trials and recommending the product to the FDA as approvable to market, approvable to market with some conditions, or not approvable to market.

Participant Safeguards

Ethics and the Protection of Human Subjects

Ethical concerns about experimentation with human subjects as a result of Nazi atrocities,[99] the Public Health Services Syphilis Study,[100,101] and several other notorious studies led to the development of laws and guidelines. The Declaration of Helsinki is a code of research ethics created in 1964 by the World Medical Association.[102] It is a code of conduct adapted specifically for medical research, especially for studies of therapeutic intent. The ethical principles detailed in the Declaration of Helsinki guide the oversight responsibilities of the institutional review board (see later). The Belmont Report provided further clarification.[103] It addresses the principles of respect for persons (including the rules of obtaining informed consent and respect for privacy), beneficence (including the use of research designs to minimize harm and maximize benefits and competence of researchers), and justice (including equal opportunity for each subject to be selected into the study and avoidance of exploiting vulnerable populations, such as children and prisoners). The CFR ensures that these ethical principles and guidelines for the protection of human subjects are adhered to in all clinical investigations.

Institutional Review Board

An Institutional Review Board (IRB) is a group designated to review and monitor biomedical research involving human subjects. Clinical trials coming under 21 CFR §56.101 and clinical trials funded by government agencies, such as the National Institutes of Health (NIH), require approval from an IRB or an equivalent committee consisting of scientists and non-scientists. If an IRB does not exist at the institution in which the research involving human subject is conducted, oversight is conducted by an external established (independent or institutional) IRB. IRBs have the authority to approve, require modification of, or disapprove research as well as to observe and audit a study. The sponsor of a clinical trial is responsible for obtaining IRB approval for the study before recruitment of any participant into an FDA-regulated trial (21 CFR §812.40).

NIH policies on trials funded by NIH also require that participating investigators receive training on the ethical conduct of research in human subjects. A widely used course from the University of Miami is available online (*www.ci4.miami.edu*), although a person using this website for testing must be affiliated with an institution subscribing to the University of Miami's service.

Informed Consent

The federal regulations for the protection of human subjects in research require that such subjects give their informed consent to participate. The purpose of the informed consent is to protect participants, to ensure that potential participants clearly understand the risks and benefits associated with their participation in the study, and to provide them with all information they need to make a decision to participate or not. The required elements of informed consent are as follows:

1. Disclosure of research with an explanation of its purpose, duration, and procedures.
2. Description of risks or discomforts to the participant.
3. Description of benefits to the participant and others.
4. Disclosure of alternative treatments and/or procedures that may be advantageous to the participant.
5. Description of how confidentiality of records will be maintained.
6. Description of financial compensation, if any, for participation, and financial responsibilities.
7. Description of contact information—specific office, name(s), and telephone number(s)—for further information and questions.
8. A statement that participation is voluntary, that refusal to participate involves no penalty or loss of benefits, and that the participant may discontinue participation at any time.

An informed consent involves more than the signature of the potential participant on a written document. It is the investigator's responsibility to ensure that every participant understands the risks and benefit of participating in the study. Ensuring compliance with informed consent regulations is the responsibility of the Office of Human Research Protection in the DHSS (45 CFR §46), the FDA (21 CFR §50), and the IRB.

In clinical trials of stroke therapies, the informed consent process may be difficult because stroke may involve a emergency situation in which a participant's life is in peril. In 1996, criteria to waive the informed consent requirement (45 CFR §46.116; 21 CFR §50.23 and 50.24) were established for research in emergency settings. These criteria provide exception to the requirement of informed consent from each participant or legally authorized representative before experimental intervention in situations in which the participant cannot provide informed consent because of a life-threatening medical condition and absence of his or her legally authorized representative. The IRB may permit informed consent waiver upon review of the life-threatening situation, existence of clinical equipoise (i.e., the relative benefits and risks of the proposed intervention, as compared with standard therapy, are unknown), and the need for the collection of valid scientific evidence to determine safety and effectiveness of the intervention under study. The IRB must also consider the feasibility, or lack thereof, of obtaining informed consent from the participant or legally authorized representative as well as the prospect of direct benefit to the participant through participation in the trial (also see the discussion under Recruitment of Community Consent).

Furthermore, for a waiver to be obtained, additional protection of the rights and welfare of participants must be provided, including at least a consultation with the representatives of the communities in which the study is to be conducted and from which the potential participants will be recruited. The IRB is also responsible for approving recruiting materials used to provide the information about the clinical trial to the public. In addition, for studies with an informed consent waiver, an independent data monitoring committee must be established to oversee the clinical investigation. The NIH is now also requiring the establishment of independent data and safety monitoring committees for most of the trials that NIH funds. The role of this committee was described in the section on interim analysis.

In clinical trials in which the treatment must be administered in the shortest possible time after stroke and for which informed consent is still required, some IRBs are willing to use the process to waive consent. Other IRBs do not allow waiver of consent but in emergency situations do accept a family member's consent by telephone (if followed by written documentation) when the potential participant is unable to give or withhold consent. The issue of who can give consent in trials of urgent stroke therapy or whether consent can be waived as described above must be resolved on a case-by-case basis by each IRB.

Table 61.8 List of Responsibilities for Research Investigators

- Protect the rights and welfare of study participants.
- Understand the ethical standards and regulatory requirements of conducting research.
- Inform the research staff of the regulations.
- Ensure that all research activities have institutional review board (IRB) approval before human participants are involved.
- Ensure that research activities follow the approved protocol or investigational plan and applicable regulations.
- Ensure that drugs and devices are used in participating participants only under the investigator's supervision or under the supervision of a recognized co-investigator.
- Obtain informed consent of participants before they are involved in the research.
- Maintain written records of IRB reviews and decisions, and informed consent of the participants or their legally authorized representative.
- Maintain good records of the dispensation of the drug or device, and return unused materials at the end of the study.
- Obtain IRB approval for any proposed change to the research protocol.
- Notify the IRB of any physical or psychological adverse events, emergent or potential problems experienced by a participant because of his/her participation in the study, and any Investigational New Drug (IND) safety reports received.
- Obtain continuation approval from the IRB on the schedule specified at the time of the initial review.
- Make provisions for the safe retention of complete research records and all research materials.
- Ensure the confidentiality and security of all information obtained from and about the participants.
- Provide progress and safety reports, financial disclosure to the sponsor and regulatory agencies, as appropriate.
- In collaborative studies, verify that the IRB approval has been obtained from all participating institutions.
- Notify the IRB regarding the emergency use of an investigational drug or device within 5 working days of the administration of the drug or device.

From U.S. Food and Drug Administration (FDA) website, at www.fda.gov

International Guidelines for Conducting Clinical Trials

The International Conference on Harmonization, established in 1990, is a tripartite harmonization of technical requirements for the registration of pharmaceutical products in the United States, the European Union, and Japan. The ICH is the result of a need to standardize the regulatory requirements among the countries because of globalization of the pharmaceutical industry, arbitrary differences in regulations, and the need for a process to allow more timely access to new drugs for patients. The website for the ICH is *www.ifma.org/ich1.html/.*

The Good Clinical Practice (GCP) is a set of guidelines for design, conduct, analysis, quality control, and reporting of clinical studies to achieve and maintain high-quality clinical research in a responsible and ethical manner. It is a part of the ICH document (Section E6). Compliance with the GCP ensures that the rights and safety of trial participants are guaranteed and that the results produced by the clinical trials are credible. All clinical trial personnel (i.e., clinicians, research nurse, study coordinators, statisticians, data managers, project managers, quality assurance personnel) should follow the GCP. A copy of the GCP can be obtained from the website, at *http://www.fda.gov/oc/gcp/.*

Table 61.8 summarizes the responsibilities of research investigators. Possible consequences of ignoring the regulations are suspension of the research project, of the PI of the research project, or both; inability to publish study results; notification of noncompliance to the sponsors and the FDA; debarment by the FDA from using investigational products; inability to receive funding from federal grants; termination of employment; loss of licenses; and immediate closure of all research at the institution.

References

1. Friedman LM, Furberg CD, DeMets DL: Fundamentals of Clinical Trials, 3rd ed. New York, Springer Verlag, 1998.
2. Piantadosi S: Clinical Trials: A Methodologic Perspective. New York, John Wiley and Sons, 1997.
3. Meinert CL, Tonascia S: Clinical Trials Design, Conduct, and Analysis. New York, Oxford University Press, 1986.
4. Medical Research Council's General Practice Research Framework. Thrombosis Prevention Trial: Randomized low-dose aspirin in the primary prevention of ischaemic heart disease in men at increased risk. Lancet 351:233–241, 1998.
5. Gullov AL, Koefoed BG, Petersen P, et al: Fixed mini-dose warfarin and aspirin alone and in combination vs adjusted-dose warfarin for stroke prevention in atrial fibrillation. Arch Intern Med 158:1513–1521, 1998.
6. Asymptomatic Carotid Atherosclerosis Study Group. Study design for randomized prospective trial of carotid endarterectomy for asymptomatic atherosclerosis. Stroke 20:844–849, 1989.
7. Stroke Prevention in Atrial Fibrillation Investigators. Adjusted-dose warfarin versus low-intensity, fixed-dose warfarin plus aspirin for high-risk patients with atrial fibrillation: The Stroke Prevention in Atrial Fibrillation III randomised clinical trial. Lancet 348:633–638, 1996.
8. EC/IC Bypass Study Group. The International Cooperative Study of Extracranial/Intracranial Arterial Anastomosis (EC/IC Bypass Study): Methodology and entry characteristics. Stroke 16:397–406, 1985.
9. EC/IC Bypass Study Group. Failure of extracranial-intracranial arterial bypass to reduce risk of ischemic stroke. Results of an international randomized trial. N Engl J Med 313:1191–2000, 1985.
10. Mohr JP, Thompson JLP, Lazar RM, et al: A comparison of warfarin and aspirin for the prevention of recurrent ischemic stroke. N Engl J Med 345:1444–1451, 2001.

Therapy

11. Viscoli CM, Brass LM, Kernan WN, et al: A clinical trial of estrogen-replacement therapy after ischemic stroke. N Engl J Med 345:1243–1249, 2001.

12. VITATOPS Trial Study Group. The VITATOPS (Vitamins to Prevent Stroke) Trial: Rationale and design of an international, large, simple, randomised trial of homocysteine-lowering multivitamin therapy in patients with recent transient ischaemic attack or stroke. Cerebrovasc Dis 13:120–126, 2002.

13. Spence JD, Howard VJ, Chambless LE, et al: Vitamin Intervention for Stroke Prevention (VISP) Trial: Rationale and design. Neuroepidemiology 20:16–25, 2001.

14. Edvardsson N, Juul-Moller S, Omblus R, Pehrsson K: Effects of low-dose warfarin and aspirin versus no treatment on stroke in a medium-risk patient population with atrial fibrillation. J Intern Med 254:95–101, 2003.

15. Little KM, Alexander MJ: Medical versus surgical therapy for spontaneous intracranial hemorrhage. Neurosurg Clin North Am 13:339–347, 2002.

16. Tissue plasminogen activator for acute ischemic stroke. National Institute of Neurological Disorders and Stroke (NINDS) rt-PA Stroke Study Group. N Engl J Med 333:1581–1587, 1995.

17. Hacke W, Kaste M, Fieschi C, et al: Intravenous thrombolysis with recombinant tissue plasminogen activator for acute hemispheric stroke: The European Cooperative Acute Stroke Study (ECASS). ECASS Study Group. JAMA 274:1017–1025, 1995.

18. Hacke W, Kaste M, Fieschi C, et al: Randomised double-blind placebo-controlled trial of thrombolytic therapy with intravenous alteplase in acute ischaemic stroke (ECASS II). Second European-Australasian Acute Stroke Study Investigators. Lancet 352:1245–1251, 1998.

19. Adams HP Jr, Woolson RF, Clarke WR, et al: Design of the Trial of Org 10172 in Acute Stroke Treatment (TOAST). Control Clin Trials 18:358–377, 1997.

20. Nilsson L, Carlsson J, Danielsson A, et al: Walking training of patients with hemiparesis at an early stage after stroke: A comparison of walking training on a treadmill with body weight support and walking training on the ground. Clin Rehabil 15:515–527, 2001.

21. Scheidtmann K, Fries W, Muller F, Koenig E: Effect of levodopa in combination with physiotherapy on functional motor recovery after stroke: A prospective, randomised, double-blind study. Lancet 358(9284):787–790, 2001.

22. Goldring S, Zervas N, Langfiti T: The Extracranial-Intracranial Bypass Study: A report of the committee appointed by the American Association of Neurological Surgeons to examine the study. N Engl J Med 316:817–820, 1987.

23. Millard, SP: Applied Statistics in the Pharmaceutical Industry With Case Studies Using S-Plus. New York, Springer Verlag, 2000, p 7.

24. Chow SC, Liu JP: Design and Analysis of Clinical Trials: Concepts and Methodologies. New York, Wiley, 1998, p 7.

25. Von Hoff DD, Kuhn J, Clark GM: Design and conduct of phase I trials. In Buyse M, Staquet MJ, Sylvester RJ (eds): Cancer Clinical Trials. New York, Oxford University Press, 1984.

26. Dixon WJ, Mood AM: A method for obtaining and analyzing sensitivity data. J Am Stat Assoc 43:109–126, 1948.

27. Storer E: Design and analysis of phase I trials. Biometrics 45:925–937, 1989.

28. O'Quigley J, Pepe M, Fisher L: Continual reassessment method: A practical design for phase I clinical trials in cancer. Biometrics 46:33–48, 1990.

29. O'Quigley J, Chevret S: Methods for dose finding studies in cancer clinical trials: A review and results of Monte Carlo study. Stat Med 10:1647–1664, 1991.

30. O'Quigley J, Shen LZ: Continual reassessment method: A likelihood approach. Biometrics 52:673–684, 1996.

31. Goodman SN, Zahurak ML, Piantadosi S: Some practical improvements in continual reassessment method for phase I studies. Stat Med 14:1149–1161, 1995.

32. Herson J: Predictive probability early termination plans for phase II clinical trials. Biometrics 35:775–783, 1979.

33. Clark WM, Wissman S, Albers GW, et al: Recombinant tissue-type plasminogen activator (Alteplase) for ischemic stroke 3 to 5 hours after symptom onset. JAMA 282:2019–2026, 1999.

34. O'Brien PC, Fleming TR: A multiple testing procedure for clinical trials. Biometrics 35:549–556, 1979.

35. Palesch YY, Tilley BC, Broderick JP: Value of a single-arm phase II futility design for acute stroke therapy. Presented to the American Academy of Neurology, Honolulu, March 29–April 5, 2003.

36. IMS Study Investigators: Combined intravenous and intra-arterial recanalization for acute ischemic stroke: The Interventional Management of Stroke (IMS). Stroke, in press.

37. Lackland DT, Bachman DL, Carter TD, et al: The geographic variation in stroke incidence in two areas of the Southeastern Stroke Belt: The Anderson and Pee Dee Stroke Study. Stroke 29:2061–2068, 1998.

38. Karanjia PN, Nelson JJ, Lefkowitz DS, et al: Validation of the ACAS TIA/stroke algorithm. Neurology 48:346–351, 1997.

39. Hart RG, Pearce LA, McBride R, et al: Factors associated with ischemic stroke during aspirin therapy in atrial fibrillation: Analysis of 2012 participants in the SPAF I–III clinical trials. Stroke 30:1223–1229, 1999.

40. Miller VT, Rothrock JF, Pearce LA, et al: Ischemic stroke in patients with atrial fibrillation: Effect of aspirin according to stroke mechanism. Neurology 43:32–36, 1993.

41. Hallstrom AP, Litwin PE, Weaver WD: A method of assigning scores to components of a composite outcome: An example from the MITI trial. Control Clin Trials 13:148–155, 1992.

42. Rankin J: Cerebral vascular accidents in patient over the age of 60. II: Prognosis. Scott Med J 2:200–215, 1957.

43. Mahoney FI, Barthel DW: Functional evaluation: The Barthel Index. Md State Med J 14:61–65, 1965.

44. Brott T, Adams HP, Olinger CP: Measurements of acute cerebral infarction: A clinical examination scale. Stroke 20:864–870, 1989.

45. Jennet B, Bond M: Assessment of outcome after severe brain injury: A practical scale. Lancet 1:480–484, 1975.

46. Hantson L: Neurological scales in assessment of stroke. In Grotta J, Miller LP, Buchan AM (eds): Ischemic Stroke: Recent Advances in Understanding Stroke Therapy. Southborough, MA, International Business Communications, 1985, pp 42–54.

47. Lachin JM: Introduction to sample size determination and power analysis for clinical trials. Control Clin Trials 2:93–113, 1981.

48. Elashoff JD: NQuery Advisor® 4.0. Statistical Solutions Ltd, Boston, MA, info@statsolusa.com, 2000.

49. Brown BW, Brauner C, Chan A, et al: Calculations for sample sizes and related problems. University of Texas Cancer Center, 1996. Available online at http://odin.mdacc.tmc.edu/anonftp/

50. O'Brien P: The appropriateness of analysis of variance and multiple comparison procedures. Biometrics 39:787–794, 1983.

51. Moye LA: Alpha calculus in clinical trials: considerations and commentary for the new millennium. Comment in Stat Med 19:763–766, 2000.

52. Simes RJ: An improved Bonferroni procedure for multiple tests of significance. Biometrika 73:751–754, 1988.

53. Miller RG Jr: Simultaneous Inference. New York, McGraw-Hill, 1966.

54. Ebbutt AF, Frith L: Practical issues in equivalence studies. Stat Med 17:1691–1701, 1998.

55. Proschan MA, Liu Q, Hunsberger S: Practical midcourse sample size modification in clinical trials. Control Clin Trials 24:4–15, 2003.

56. North American Symptomatic Carotid Endarterectomy Trial Collaborators. Beneficial effect of carotid endarterectomy in symptomatic patients with high-grade carotid stenosis. N Engl J Med 325:445–453, 1991.

57. Kernan WN, Horwitz RI, Brass LM, et al: A prognostic system for transient ischemia or minor stroke. Ann Intern Med 114:552–557, 1991.

58. National Institute of Neurologic Disorders and Stroke (NINDS) rt-PA Stroke Study Group. Generalized efficacy of t-PA for acute stroke: subgroup analysis of the NINDS t-PA Stroke Trial. Stroke 28:2109–2118, 1997.

59. Marler JR, Tilley BC, Lu M, et al: Early stroke treatment associated with better outcome. Neurology 55:1649–1655, 2000.

60. Meier P: Stratification in the design of a clinical trial. Control Clin Trials 1:355–361, 1981.

61. Grizzle JE: A note on stratifying versus complete random assignment in clinical trials. Control Clin Trial 3:365–368, 1982.

62. Scott NW, McPherson GC, Ramsay CR, Campbell MK: The method of minimization for allocation to clinical trials: A review. Control Clin Trials 23:662–674, 2002.

63. Tilley BC, Lyden PD, Brott TG, et al: Total quality improvement methodology reduces delays between emergency department

admission and treatment of acute ischemic stroke. Arch Neurol 54:1466–1474, 1997.

64. National Institute of Neurologic Disorders and Stroke (NINDS) rt-PA Stroke Study Group. A systems approach to immediate evaluation and management of hyperacute stroke: Experience at eight centers and implications for community practice and patient care. Stroke 28:1530–1540, 1997.

65. Napoles-Springer AM, Grumbach K, Alexander M, et al: Clinical research with older African Americans and Latinos. Res Aging 22:668–691, 2000.

66. Morisky DE, Green LW, Levine DM: Concurrent and predictive validity of a self-reported measure of medication adherence. Med Care 24:67–74, 1986.

67. Lyden P, Brott T, Tilley BC, et al: Improved reliability of the NIH Stroke Scale using video training. NINDS t-PA Stroke Study Group. Stroke 25:2220–2226, 1994.

68. Adams RJ, Meador KS, Sethi KD, et al: Graded neurologic scale for use in acute hemispheric stroke treatment protocols. Stroke, 18:665–669, 1987.

69. Gillings D, Koch G: The application of the principle of intention-to-treat to the analysis of clinical trials. Drug Inf J 25:411–424, 1991.

70. Tilley BC, Marler J, Geller N, et al: Using a global test for multiple outcomes in stroke trials with application to the NINDS t-PA Stroke Trial. Stroke 27:2136–2141, 1996.

71. Cohen J, Cohen P: Bivariate correlation and regression. In Applied Multiple Regression/Correlation Analysis for the Behavioral Sciences, 2nd ed. Hillsdale, NJ, Lawrence Erlbaum Associates, 1983, p 39.

72. Lefkopoulou M, Moore D, Ryan L: The analysis of multiple correlated binary outcomes: Application to rodent teratology experiments. J Am Stat Assoc 84:810–815, 1989.

73. Lefkopoulou M, Ryan L: Global tests for multiple binary outcomes. Biometrics 49:975–988, 1993.

74. Hotellings H: The generalization of Student's ratio. Ann Math Stat 2:360–378, 1931.

75. O'Brien PC: Procedures for comparing samples with multiple endpoints. Biometrics 40:1079–1087, 1984.

76. Pocock SJ, Geller NL, Tsiatis AA: The analysis of multiple endpoints in clinical trials. Biometrics 43:487–498, 1987.

77. Lafata JE, Tilley BC, Nerenz D: Considerations in deciding when and how to evaluate provider group interventions. Health Services and Outcomes Research Methodology 1:49–62, 2000.

78. Little RJA, Rubin DB: Statistical Analysis with Missing Data. New York, Wiley, 1987, p 9.

79. Schafer JL: Multiple imputation: A primer. Stat Methods Med Res 8:3–15, 1999.

80. Schafer JL: Software for Multiple Imputation. University Park, PA, The Pennsylvania State University Department of Statistics, 1999. Available online at http://www.stat.psu.edu/~jls/misoftwa.html/

81. Thompson JLP, Levin B, Sciacca RR, et al: Statistical Considerations in the WARSS Collaboration. Presented to American Heart Association Stroke Meeting, San Antonio, February 7–9, 2002.

82. Wald A: Sequential Analysis. New York, John Wiley & Sons, 1947.

83. Armitage P: Sequential tests in prophylactic and therapeutic trials. Q J Med 23:255–274, 1954.

84. Peto R, Pike MC, Armitage P, et al: Design and analysis of randomized clinical trials requiring prolonged observation of each patient. I: Introduction and design. Br J Cancer 34:585–612, 1976.

85. Pocock SJ: Size of cancer clinical trials and stopping rules. Br J Cancer 38:757–766, 1978.

86. Lan KKG, DeMets DI, Halperin M: Stochastically curtailed tests in long-term clinical trials. Communications in Statistics: Sequential Analysis 1:207–219, 1982.

87. Ellenberg S, Fleming TR, DeMets DL: Data Monitoring Committees in Clinical Trials: A Practical Perspective. John Wiley and Sons, New Jersey, 2002, pp. 129–133.

88. Berry DA, Ho C-H: One-sided sequential stopping boundaries for clinical trials: A decision theoretic approach. Biometrics 44:219–227, 1988.

89. Egger MJ, Coleman ML, Ward JR, et al: Uses and abuses of analysis of covariance in clinical trials. Control Clin Trials 6:12–24, 1985.

90. Koch GG, Davis SM, Anderson RL: Methodological advances and plans for improving regulatory success for confirmatory studies. Stat Med 17:1675–1690, 1998.

91. Yusuf S, Wittes J, Probstfield J, Tyroler HA: Analysis and interpretation of treatment effects in subgroups of patients in randomized clinical trials. JAMA, 266:93–98, 1991.

92. National Institute of Neurological Disorders and Stroke (NINDS) rt-PA Stroke Study Group. Effect of intravenous recombinant tissue plasminogen activator on ischemic stroke lesion size measured by computed tomography. Stroke 31:2912–2919, 2000.

93. Meade T, Brennan PJ: Determination of who may derive most benefit from aspirin in primary prevention: Subgroup results from a randomised controlled trial. BMJ 321(7252):13–17, 2000.

94. Broderick J, Lu M, Jackson C, et al: Apolipoprotein E phenotype and the efficacy of intravenous tissue plasminogen activator in acute ischemic stroke. Ann Neurol 49:736–744, 2001.

95. Flather MD, Farkouh ME, Pogue JM, Yusuf S: Strengths and limitations of meta-analysis: Larger studies may be more reliable. Control Clin Trials 18:568–579; discussion 661–666, 1997.

96. Felson DT, Anderson JJ, Boers M, et al: The American College of Rheumatology preliminary core set of disease activity measures for rheumatoid arthritis clinical trials. Arthritis Rheum 36:729–740, 1993.

97. LeLorier J, Grégoire G, Benhaddad A, et al: Discrepancies between meta-analyses and subsequent large randomized, controlled trials. N Engl J Med 337:536–542, 1997.

98. U.S. Food and Drug Administration: Mission Statement formalized in the FDA Modernization Act of 1997). Available online at: www.fda.gov/opacom/morechoices/mission.html/

99. Annas GJ, Grodin MA: The Nazi Doctors and the Nuremberg Code: Human Experimentation. New York, Oxford University Press, 1992.

100. Brandt AM: Racism and research: The case of the Tuskegee Syphilis Study. Hastings Cent Rep 8:21–29, 1978.

101. U. S. Department of Health, Education, and Welfare: Final Report on the Tuskegee Syphilis Study Ad Hoc Advisory Panel. Washington, DC, Government Printing Office, 1973.

102. World Medical Association: Declaration of Helsinki: Recommendations Guiding Medical Doctors in Biomedical Research Involving Human Subjects (revised 1975, 1983, and 1989). Helsinki, World Medical Association, 1964.

103. National Commission for Protection of Human Subjects of Biomedical and Behavioral Research. The Belmont Report: Ethical principles and guidelines for the protection of human subjects of research. DHEW Publication Number (OS) 78-0012; Appendix I, DHEW Publication No. (OS) 78-0013; Appendix II, DHEW Publication No. (OS) 78-0014. Washington, DC, US Department of Health, Education and Welfare, 1978.

Therapy

Section VI

Therapy

B: Surgical Therapy

Bryce Weir

The majority of strokes of all types are not amenable to surgical treatment. Notwithstanding this fact a very significant constellation of pathological entities producing hemorrhage and/or ischemia have as their best treatment, sometimes their only treatment, operative management. In this section these entities and their therapies are presented.

While some procedures have stood the test of time, and their conduct is much as has been described in previous editions, others are new and could scarcely even have been imagined in the eighties when Barnett and his colleagues launched this book.

When I began my career, neurosurgeons carried out neuroradiological procedures such as ventriculography and angiography more commonly than our radiological confreres. No longer! As well, with the advent of coils and stents, we have had to make room for our neuroradiological (and cardiological and neurological) partners who are taking a much more active role in treating many conditions causing strokes. Territorial squabbling has been gratifyingly mute and privileges generally reflect training, knowledge and experience rather than specialty affiliation. Some vascular neurosurgeons have eagerly embraced the challenge of the catheter world and have worked shoulder to shoulder with neuroradiological colleagues in bringing about the stunning progress of the past decade. Teams of multiple specialists with different talents, working cooperatively in high volume institutions, probably offer the patient with an unusual vascular brain lesion the optimal chance of preservation of function and life.

Despite phenomenal technical advances, the surgical therapy of stroke continues to be based on a sparse outcomes database. Important studies are underway and year by year the uncertainty is lessened. In the following chapters the reader will be brought the latest available information regarding significant ongoing studies. Among the skills required by contemporary neurosurgeons is a level of sophistication in the assessment of medical evidence. Randomized trials, rigid protocols, blinded observers, and avoidance of statistical errors are now taken for granted in contemporary medical science. This does not mean that individual clinical experience and common sense are anachronisms. Some elaborate investigations in the field of stroke have in retrospect been found to be fatally flawed or to suffer from severe limitations. This is not to say that we should not strive to subject contentious clinical questions to such analyses. The inexorable march of science sometimes (and fortunately) throws into question even apparently established tenets. In our field of study, what is `true' at a few months follow-up may be `untrue' decades later; or what is applicable in one large population may not be so in another.

Because a lesion can be operated upon does not automatically mean it should be. The contributors to the "Surgical Therapy" section have delineated as clearly as possible the sometimes unclear boundaries of certainty in the decision to operate. Experienced and compassionate surgeons will weigh individual situations and attach the greatest importance in therapeutic recommendations to the factors arising from the individual patient and then to the pathology. Unruptured aneurysms which are too small, arteriovenous malformations and intracerebral hematomas which are too large, cavernous malformations too far

Therapy

from the brain stem surface; particularly in patients who are too old or too deteriorated to have a significant chance of meaningful recovery, should be spared the rigors of surgery. In this difficult decision making what is required is knowledge of the natural history of the disease, willingness to consult with and sometimes defer to colleagues, courage to operate in the face of daunting pathology, and humility in the face of certain defeat.

Two exemplary studies have recently been published.[1,2] The International Study of Unruptured Intracranial Aneurysms[1] presented the 5-year cumulative rupture rates for patients who did not have a previous subarachnoid hemorrhage, of whom 1692 did not have aneurysm repair, 1917 had open surgery, and 451 had endovascular procedures. For aneurysms on the internal carotid, anterior communicating or anterior cerebral, or middle cerebral artery the supture rates were 0%, 2.6%, 14.5%, and 40% for aneurysms less than 7 mm, 7–12 mm, 13–24 mm, and 25 mm or greater, respectively, compared with 2.5%, 14.5%, 18.4%, and 50% for the same size categories involving posterior circulation and posterior communicating artery aneurysms. Outcomes were influenced by age, aneurysm size, and location. Risks of either type of treatment of unruptured aneurysms may well exceed the risks of rupture. Unlike the initial report from this group, further analysis and longer follow-up do not support the view that size of less than 10 mm should automatically preclude treatment for an unruptured aneurysm in a patient with no previous history of subarachnoid hemorrhage. It also remains a possibility that even longer follow-up will be associated with higher rupture rates than those observed at 5 years.

The International Subarachnoid Aneurysm Trial[2] of neurosurgical clipping versus endovascular coiling showed patients who had definite subarachnoid hemorrhage within the previous 28 days, demonstration of the responsible aneurysm, a clinical state that justified treatment, and doubt as to which modality constituted the best treatment. Results at 1 year were presented on 793 patients allocated to neurosurgery and 801 receiving endovascular treatment. These groups emerged from 9,559 patients with subarachnoid hemorrhage who were assessed. Patients at follow-up who had significant restriction of lifestyle or poorer status comprised 25.4% of the endovascular treatment group and 36.4% of the surgical group. Will these results be reproducible in all aneurysms and at all treatment centers? Further studies are clearly indicated in which all ruptured aneurysms in the study are randomized and long-term follow-ups check the durability of each treatment modality. Obviously, however, endovascular therapy is a legitimate way of treating ruptured aneurysms in some circumstances; whether it is the best way to treat all aneurysms is not yet demonstrated.

The presentation of a segregated surgical section in this book should not be construed as support for a subspecialized approach to stroke. Stroke is a huge catchword, perhaps as scientific a term as dropsy was a couple of centuries or so ago. The sophisticated reader will derive some pleasure from comparing the different approaches from neurologists, radiologists and neurosurgeons. Despite the varied nuances there is broad consensus developing between the specialties, based on real data, as to how best to treat specific cerebral vascular diseases.

I hope that the enormous experience represented by the surgical contributors to this section will be of substantial assistance to the neurosurgeons "in the trenches" who ultimately bear the burden of the neurosurgical care of stroke.

References

1. Wiebers DO, Whisnant JP, Huston J 3rd. et al: Unruptured intracranial aneurysms: Natural history, clinical outcomes, and risks of surgical and endovascular treatment. Lancet 362:103–110, 2003.
2. International Subarachnoid Aneurysm Trial (ISAT) Collaborative Group: International Subarachnoid Aneurysm Trial (ISAT) of neurosurgical clipping versus endovascular coiling in 2143 patients with ruptured intracranial aneurysms: A randomized trial. Lancet 360: 1267–1274, 2002.

Chapter Sixty-Two

Familial Vascular Diseases of Neurosurgical Significance

Antti Ronkainen and Juha Hernesniemi

Inherited or familial vascular diseases are rare. The most significant familial neurovascular disease is the familial occurrence of intracranial aneurysms. The incidence of familial intracranial aneurysms (FIAs) is probably as high as 10% among aneurysmal SAH patients. The inheritance pattern for cases of FIA is still unknown. Familial cavernous malformations occur most often among Mexican American people; nearly half of the patients with these malformations are of Mexican American heritage. Familial occurrence of moyamoya disease has been reported mostly in the Japanese population. Only a very few familial arteriovenous malformations (AVMs) have been reported in the literature.

DEFINITION

A vascular disease is commonly regarded as familial or inherited when there are more affected members in a family than would be expected by chance. This usually means there are at least two affected persons among third-degree relatives—siblings, parents, grandparents, uncles, aunts, and first cousins. *Familial vascular diseases* is a better term than *inherited vascular diseases*, because the term familial does not require an exact knowledge of the inheritance patterns. *Familial* is therefore commonly used in clinical daily practice. Use of *inherited vascular disease* might exclude almost all clinically important vascular diseases because of the lack of information about the mode of inheritance. By using *familial*, we can include both vascular diseases that are suspected and those that are confirmed to be inherited.

FAMILIAL INTRACRANIAL ANEURYSMS

History and Epidemiology

The information about the clustering of aneurysms in some families is well known. O'Brien[1] published the first report in 1942, describing subarachnoid hemorrhage (SAH) in identical twins. A review of the English literature reveals that there are more than 100 papers on FIA or familial SAH.[1-35]

The incidence of FIA in patients with SAH has been studied in different populations. The first population-based study was carried out in North Sweden by Norrgård and colleagues,[11] who found the occurrence of FIA to be 7%. In two studies from the states of Washington and Minnesota in the United States, the occurrence rates for FIA were 11% and 20%, respectively.[24,27] In East Finland, the incidence of FIA was 10% among patients with aneurysmal SAH.[20] In comparing the outcomes of FIA cases and sporadic SAH cases, Bromberg and associates[36] found that FIA cases have a greater risk of poor outcome. On the other hand, Ronkainen and coworkers[37] did not find any differences in outcomes between patients with FIA and those with sporadic SAH.

In most of the reported FIA families, only two affected family members have documented SAH, so the familial aggregation of intracranial aneurysms might be fortuitous. There are no means to separate truly familial cases from sporadic cases in families with only two affected individuals. For the study by Schievink and colleagues[31] from the Mayo Clinic in Rochester, Minnesota, and a separate study by Ronkainen and coworkers[38] in Kuopio, Finland, the relative risk was calculated to be about 4 for those having two affected persons in the same family compared with the general population from the same catchment area. This result supports the hypothesis that in most familial aggregations of SAH, even in families with only two affected members, these cases are not caused by chance alone. A family history of SAH, without confirmation by medical documents, is an insufficiently accurate tool to prove or disprove the diagnosis of FIA.[39]

Gender and Age

A female preponderance seems to be a constant finding in FIA, as in sporadic SAH.[11,20,24,27,34,35,40] In the work by Norrgård and associates[11] from Sweden, 70% of patients were female. Schievink and colleagues[24] reported that 73% of their affected patients were female, and Bromberg and associates,[36] 55%. In both studies, the difference in gender was not significant compared with that for the sporadic cases. Two later studies have also confirmed the preponderance of females in patients with FIA.[34,35] Leblanc,[40] in a study of 14 FIA families, found a statistically significant difference in the gender distribution. He also noticed that the gender bias is age related. Of the patients 49 years or younger, 78% were female; in the group aged 50 to 70 years, 83% were female.

The other constant finding is that the mean age at the time of SAH is lower for FIA than for the sporadic type,[11,20,24,36,40] the difference ranging from 2 to 9 years.[11,24,40] Another interesting finding reported in two studies is that rupture occurs within the same decade twice as frequently among siblings as in randomly selected pairs of patients with sporadic SAH.[8,40,41]

Familial Aneurysms

In population-based studies of FIAs, the middle cerebral artery (MCA) and internal carotid artery (ICA) seem to be the most common locations.[8,11,24,34,41] The finding of a higher frequency of mirror intracranial aneurysms in patients FIA than in those with sporadic SAH has not been confirmed.[8,34,41] The proportion of cases with multiple intracranial aneurysms does not differ from that of sporadic aneurysms. The FIAs rupture at a smaller size, especially in women.[8,40,41] These differences have been small and were statistically insignificant. The problem of studying FIAs is the small number of aneurysms present in homogeneous study groups. Observations made from a large group of heterogeneous, small families from different populations do not give reliable results.

The prevalence of intracranial aneurysms in asymptomatic members of FIA families has been evaluated in only a few studies.[28,32,42] One of the first studies was carried out by Nakagawa and associates[32] in 179 volunteers with family history of intracranial aneurysm; 18% of the volunteers had incidental intracranial aneurysm. In another screening study from Finland, the prevalence of intracranial aneurysms among asymptomatic members of FIA families was 8.2% of 438.[28]

Inheritance Patterns

Inheritance patterns of FIA have not been found. There are reports of the occurrence of intracranial aneurysms in identical twins, which support the possible genetic background of FIA.[1,43,44] Autosomal dominant, autosomal recessive, and multifactorial inheritance patterns have all been reported in the literature.[22,29,45–47] The main problem in studying the inheritance patterns of FIA is that these lesions are acquired, and an unknown percentage of intracranial aneurysms remains asymptomatic. The lack of well-organized screening studies of asymptomatic FIA family members is unfortunate. Another problem is that in most of the reported families only two family members are affected, so the possibility of fortuitous aggregation of intracranial aneurysms is difficult to exclude.

Schievink and colleagues[22] performed a meta-analysis of the literature using a segregation analysis to interpret the inheritance pattern for FIA. Several inheritance patterns without a single mendelian model could explain the inheritance of intracranial aneurysm. These researchers concluded that there is a genetic heterogeneity for FIA instead of mendelian inheritance. Onda and associates[48] published the first genome-wide linkage study of intracranial aneurysms in 104 Japanese affected sib pairs; they documented positive evidence of linkage on chromosome 7q11. This is the first study in which intracranial aneurysms could be connected to a particular chromosome in a human genome. This preliminary study needs to be confirmed.

Intracranial Aneurysms and Genetically Related Diseases

Intracranial aneurysms have been associated with some rare heritable disorders, such as autosomal dominant polycystic kidney disease, fibromuscular dysplasia, Ehlers-Danlos syndrome type IV, Marfan's syndrome, pseudoxanthoma elasticum disease, neurofibromatosis type I, and various other groups of heritable diseases. Only autosomal dominant polycystic kidney disease has clinical importance.[22,49]

Autosomal Dominant Polycystic Kidney Disease

Polycystic kidney disease (PKD) is divided into two groups, autosomal dominant PKD (ADPKD) and autosomal recessive PKD. PKD is characterized by bilateral multiple renal cysts. Cysts may also be seen in many other parts of the body. Vascular complications are described in cases of ADPKD. ADPKD is the most common genetic disease, its prevalence being 1 in 400 to 1 in 1000 population. The mode of inheritance is an autosomal dominant pattern.[50–52] In about 80% of cases, the gene is localized on chromosome 16, with the second gene located on chromosome 4.[50,53] SAH is the most common extrarenal complication in patients with ADPKD.[54–56] There are some differences between patients with intracranial aneurysms who have ADPKD and those with intracranial aneurysms who do not have ADPKD; males predominate, and intracranial aneurysms rupture at an earlier age.[57,58] The prevalence of intracranial aneurysms among patients with ADPKD is 5% to 12% when studied with magnetic resonance angiography (MRA), three-dimensional (3D) computed tomography (CT), or angiography. In only 14% of such patients is the intracranial aneurysm larger than 6mm, and about half the patients have a positive family history for SAH.[57,59–64]

Fibromuscular Dysplasia

Fibromuscular dysplasia affects medium-sized arteries, causing irregular thickening of the vessel through proliferation of smooth muscle and fibrous tissue of the media, which narrows the lumen.[65] The most common clinical manifestation is renovascular hypertension caused by involvement of the renal arteries. Other symptoms are strokes, migraine, and impaired hearing. Fibromuscular dysplasia typically produces symptoms at a young age and may occur predominantly in females.[66,67] The prevalence of fibromuscular dysplasia is not known. It is believed that fibromuscular dysplasia is underdiagnosed in clinical practice, and only re-investigation of angiograms could give a correct estimation of the prevalence of fibromuscular dysplasia in a population. As many as 30% to 50% of patients with fibromuscular dysplasia may have the familial form of the disease. The inheritance pattern is believed to be autosomal dominant with variable penetrance. Cloft and associates[68] found the prevalence of aneurysms to be only about 7% instead of the previously accepted 25% to 50%.[66] They combined data from their own 117 patients with fibromuscular dysplasia and data from a meta-analysis of the literature to obtain this figure.

Ehlers-Danlos Syndrome

Ehlers-Danlos syndrome is a heterogeneous group of connective tissue disorders. Typical clinical manifestations are joint laxity, dystrophic scarring, bruising, and hyperextensibility of the skin. There are several subtypes of the syndrome, classified according to clinical manifestations and genetic criteria. Intracranial aneurysms are associated with Ehlers-Danlos syndrome type IV, which was first recognized in 1967.[51,69,70] Type IV is the most life-threatening form of the syndrome because of its vascular manifestations. Survival beyond 50 years is uncommon.[51] The prevalence of Ehlers-Danlos syndrome type IV is estimated to be 1/50,000 to 1/500,000 per year.

The clinical diagnosis of Ehlers-Danlos syndrome type IV is difficult, but vascular events, spontaneous rupture of the intestines at an early age, and uterine rupture during pregnancy can be the hallmarks. The molecular defect is an abnormality of type III collagen, which is the major component of the extracellular matrix of distensible tissues. The inheritance pattern is autosomal dominant. Ehlers-Danlos syndrome type IV is associated more with intracavernous intracranial aneurysms and carotid-cavernous fistula formation than with saccular intracranial aneurysms.[31]

Marfan's Syndrome

Clinical manifestations of Marfan's syndrome consist of a combination of skeletal, ocular, and cardiovascular abnormalities. Typical manifestations are tall stature, long and thin fingers, prognathism, kyphoscoliosis, pectus excavatum, and joint hypermobility.[51,71] Myopia and ectopia are common ocular manifestations. Insufficiency of the aortic and mitral valves and dissection of the aorta are the most common cardiovascular manifestations.[72] The usual cause of death in children is aortic or mitral insufficiency, and in adults, acute aortic dissection.[72] The prevalence of Marfan's syndrome is 1/10,000 to 1/20,000. The disease is inherited as an autosomal dominant trait, but in one third of cases, the cause is a new mutation.[71] In 10% to 20% of cases of Marfan's syndrome, an aortic dissection extending into the innominate and common carotid arteries may cause ischemic symptoms, and involvement of spinal arteries may result in paraparesis. The basic molecular defect of this syndrome is a deficiency in the protein fibrillin, one of the major components of elastin-associated microfibrils. The gene encoding for fibrillin has been localized to chromosome 15; also, several mutations of this gene have been characterized.[51] The association of intracranial aneurysms with Marfan's syndrome may be fortuitous.[73] There have only been a few case reports in which intracranial aneurysms and Marfan's syndrome were both present.

Pseudoxanthoma Elasticum

Pseudoxanthoma elasticum is a disorder affecting elastic fibers in the skin, ocular system, and cardiovascular system.[51] The cardiovascular changes are stenotic, but aneurysms may develop in medium-sized peripheral arteries. The prevalence of pseudoxanthoma elasticum is around 1 per 100,000 in the population. The pathogenesis of pseudoxanthoma elasticum is not known, but abnormalities of elastic fibers are suspected to be the cause of the clinical manifestations. The disease is genetically heterogeneous, having autosomal dominant and autosomal recessive types.[74] Cerebral infarction caused by stenotic or occlusive disease of the carotid or vertebral arteries is the most common neurovascular manifestation of pseudoxanthoma elasticum.[75] Intracranial aneurysms have been associated quite frequently with pseudoxanthoma elasticum. The location is often the cavernous sinus, leading to ocular motor nerve palsies without SAH.

Neurofibromatosis

Neurofibromatosis has been divided into two types. Neurofibromatosis 2 (NF2) is characterized by bilateral vestibular schwannomas and other tumors of the central or peripheral nervous system, with or without mild skin manifestation.[51] Neurofibromatosis 1 (NF1) is characterized by a wide variety of organ system involvement—café au lait spots and freckling of the skin, Lisch nodules in the eyes, central nervous system gliomas, meningiomas, scoliosis, pheochromocytomas, vascular stenosis and occlusion, and rupture of aneurysms or fistula formation in medium-sized or large arteries.[76]

Clinically, NF1 is more common than NF2. Renal artery stenosis is the most common vascular lesion associated with neurofibromatosis 1. The prevalence of neurofibromatosis is around 1/3000. The inheritance pattern is autosomal dominant, but in half of the cases, neurofibromatosis is caused by a new mutation. The incidence of saccular intracranial aneurysms with NF1 is unknown. There are reports of patients with fusiform aneurysms of the petrous and cavernous segments.

Osteogenesis Imperfecta

Bone fragility and blue sclera are the most typical clinical manifestations of osteogenesis imperfecta.[51] The more severe form of the disorders includes skeletal deformity and hearing loss. Neurovascular and cardiovascular manifestations are less evident in osteogenesis imperfecta than in Marfan's syndrome. The prevalence is estimated to be 1/10,000. Both dominant and recessive autosomal inheritance patterns have been described.

Miscellaneous Disorders

A great variety of diseases are associated with intracranial aneurysms. A few examples are α-glucosidase deficiency, α_1-antitrypsin deficiency, alkaptonuria, Anderson-Fabry disease, hereditary hemorrhagic telangiectasia, Noonan's syndrome, tuberous sclerosis, and Wermer's syndrome. Intracranial aneurysms are also associated with abdominal aortic aneurysms, sickle cell anemia, and Graves' disease.[22,51,77–79]

FAMILIAL CAVERNOUS MALFORMATIONS

Cavernous malformations are reported to account for about 1% of all intracranial vascular lesions and 15% of all cerebrovascular malformations. At the time of the diagnosis of cavernous malformation, one third of the patients have seizures, one third hemorrhage, and one third mass lesions.[80] The number of detected cavernous malformations is growing with the increasing use of magnetic resonance imaging (MRI). CT and angiography are unreliable methods for identification of cavernous malformations.

At least two members of the same family should have the characteristic appearance of cavernous malformations on MRI or MRA before the diagnosis of a familial cavernous malformation is made. The familial form is inherited as an autosomal dominant trait, and the lesions are multiple in the central nervous system. When MRI is used to identify phenotypes in asymptomatic family members, the penetrance approaches 100%.[81] Multiple lesions are seen in 10% to 15% of patients with sporadic cavernous malformation, and in 85% of patients with the familial form. A high frequency of the familial form of cavernous malformations is seen in Mexican Americans. Half of the patients with cavernous malformation may have a strong family history of the disorder. Dubovsky and colleagues[82] were able to connect familial cavernous malformation with chromosome 7. Later studies have shown a high genetic heterogeneity among familial cavernous malformations.[83–85]

Familial intracavernous malformations seem to be dynamic lesions that tend to change over time. In a follow-up study of patients with the disorder, more than one third showed alterations in lesion size and signal intensity.[86] Performance of MRI studies of symptomatic individuals at 12-month intervals is recommended as routine follow-up.

Operative treatment of patients with familial cavernous malformation who have multiple lesions is recommended if clinically significant hemorrhage, uncontrollable seizures, or progressive neurologic deterioration occurs.

FAMILIAL MOYAMOYA DISEASE

The etiology of the occlusion of the circle of Willis and adjacent vessels (moyamoya disease) is unknown. Moyamoya disease is most common among Japanese and Korean people.[87] In Japan, the annual incidence is 0.35 per 100,000 population.[87] The male-to-female ratio is estimated to be about 1:1.7. In the Japanese population, the familial occurrence is approximately 10%.[87–89] Moyamoya disease most often causes clinical symptoms related to cerebral ischemia and hemorrhage.[87] Diagnosis is made through angiography studies, MRI, or MRA.

Pathologic and epidemiologic studies of moyamoya disease suggest that a genetic factor is more important than acquired factors.[90] The pathogenesis of moyamoya disease is most likely polygenic. Moyamoya disease has been connected to chromosome 6, chromosome 17, and chromosome 3.[90–92] Reports of affected twin pairs support the possible genetic etiology of this disease.[88,93,94]

FAMILIAL ARTERIOVENOUS MALFORMATION

Only ten reports of familial occurrence of AVM were found in the literature as of 2003. Familial AVMs manifest at a somewhat younger age than do AVMs in general. In the familial AVMs, there is a female preponderance.[94,95] In reports of familial AVMs, 74% were supratentorial, 5% deep-seated, and 7% infratentorial. The number of reported familial AVM cases is so low that conclusions regarding the possibility that a genetic factor controls the occurrence of AVMs are not possible.

References

1. O'Brien JG: Subarachnoid hemorrhage in identical twins. BMJ 607–609, 1942.
2. Bannerman RM, Ingall GB, Graf CJ: The familial occurrence of intracranial aneurysms. Neurology 20l:283–292, 1970.
3. Chakravorty BG, Gleadhill CA: Familial incidence of cerebral aneurysms. BMJ: 1(5480):147–148, 1966.
4. Endtz IJ: Familial incidence of intracranial aneurysms. Acta Neurochir 19:297–305, 1968.
5. Fox JL: Familial intracranial aneurysms. J Neurosurg 57:416–417, 1982.
6. Jain KK: Familial intracranial aneurysms: Review of literature and presentation of six new cases. Acta Neurochir: Wien) 30:129–137, 1974.
7. Kak VKM, Gleadhill CA, Bailey IC: The familial incidence of intracranial aneurysms. J Neurol Neurosurg Psychiatry 33:29–33, 1970.
8. Lozano AM, Leblanc R: Familial intracranial aneurysms. J Neurosurg 66:522–528, 1987.
9. Mellergård P, Ljunggren B, Brandt L, et al: HLA-typing in a family with six intracranial aneurysms. Br J Neurosurg 3:479–486, 1989.
10. Morooka Y, Waga S: Familial intracranial aneurysms: Report of four families. Surg Neurol 19:260–262, 1983.
11. Norrgård TM, Ångquist KA, Fodstad H, et al: Intracranial aneurysms and heredity. Neurosurgery 20:236–239, 1987.
12. Shigemori M, Nakayama K, Oshima Y, et al: Familial intracranial aneurysms. Kurume Med J 32:209–213, 1985.
13. Stavenow L: Familial occurrence of intracranial aneurysms. Acta Med Scand 206:197–200, 1979.
14. Sakai N, Sakata K, Yamada H, et al: Familial occurrence of intracranial aneurysms. Surg Neurol 2:25–29, 1974.
15. Ikeda H, Sakugawa H, Ueda S, Morisada A: Familial cases of cerebral aneurysm. No To Shinkei 23:201–205, 1971.
16. Acosta-Rua G: Familial incidence of ruptured intracranial aneurysms. Arch Neurol 35:675–677, 1978.
17. ter Berg HWM, Dippel DWJ, Limburg M, et al: Familial intracranial aneurysms: A review. Stroke 23:1024–1030, 1992.
18. Alberts MJ: Genetic aspects of cerebrovascular disease. Stroke 25:25–30, 1990.
19. Hashimoto I: Familial intracranial aneurysms and cerebral vascular anomalies. J Neurosurg 46:419–427, 1977.
20. Ronkainen A, Hernesniemi J, Ryynänen M: Familial subarachnoid hemorrhage in East Finland 1977–1990. Neurosurgery 33:787–797, 1993.
21. Ronkainen A, Hernesniemi J, Ryynänen M, et al: Ten percent prevalence of asymptomatic familial intracranial aneurysms: Preliminary report on 110 magnetic resonance angiography studies in members of 21 Finnish familial intracranial aneurysm families. Neurosurgery 35:208–213, 1994.
22. Schievink WI, Schaid DJ, Rogers HM, et al: On the inheritance of intracranial aneurysms. Stroke 25:2028–2037, 1994.
23. Bailey IC: Familial subarachnoid hemorrhage. Ulster Med J 62:119–126, 1993.
24. Schievink WI, Schaid DJ, Michels VV, Piepgras DG: Familial aneurysmal subarachnoid hemorrhage: A community-based study. J Neurosurg 83:426–429, 1995.
25. Alberts MJ, Quinones A, Graffagnino C, et al: Risk of intracranial aneurysms in families with subarachnoid hemorrhage. Can J Neurol Sci 22:121–125, 1995.
26. Bromberg JEC, Rinkel GJE, Algra A, et al: Subarachnoid hemorrhage in first and second degree relatives of patients with subarachnoid hemorrhage. BMJ 311:288–289, 1995.
27. Wang PS, Longstreth WT, Koepsell TD: Subarachnoid hemorrhage and family history: A population-based case-control study. Arch Neurol 52:202–204, 1995.

28. Ronkainen A, Hernesniemi J, Puranen M, et al: Familial intracranial aneurysms. Lancet 349:380–384, 1997.

29. Bromberg JEC, Rinkel GJE, Algra A, et al: Familial subarachnoid hemorrhage: Distinctive features and patterns of inheritance. Ann Neurol 38:929–934, 1995.

30. Leblanc R, Melanson D, Tampieri D, Guttmann RD: Familial cerebral aneurysms: A study of 13 families. Neurosurgery 37:633–639, 1995.

31. Schievink WI: Genetics of intracranial aneurysms. Neurosurgery 40:651–663, 1997.

32. Nakagawa T, Hashi K, Kurokawa Y, Yamamura A: Family history of subarachnoid hemorrhage and the incidence of asymptomatic, unruptured cerebral aneurysms. J Neurosurg 91:391–395, 1999.

33. Gaist D, Vaeth M, Tsiropoulos I, et al: Risk of subarachnoid hemorrhage in first degree relatives of patients with subarachnoid hemorrhage: Follow up study based on national registries in Denmark. BMJ 320:141–145, 2000.

34. Kasuya H, Onda H, Takeshita M, et al: Clinical features of intracranial aneurysms in siblings. Neurosurgery 46:1301–1306, 2000.

35. Connolly ES Jr, Choudhri TF, Mack WJ, et al: Influence of smoking, hypertension, and sex on the phenotypic expression of familial intracranial aneurysms in siblings. Neurosurgery 48:64–69, 2001.

36. Bromberg JEC, Rinkel GJE, Algra A, et al: Outcome in familial subarachnoid hemorrhage. Stroke 26:961–963, 1995.

37. Ronkainen A, Niskanen M, Piironen R, Hernesniemi J: Familial subarachnoid hemorrhage: Outcome study. Stroke 30:1099–1102, 1999.

38. Ronkainen A, Miettinen H, Karkola K, et al: Risk of harboring an unruptured intracranial aneurysm. Stroke 29:359–362, 1998.

39. Bromberg JEC, Rinkel GJE, Algra A, et al: Validation of family history in subarachnoid hemorrhage. Stroke 27:630–632, 1996.

40. Leblanc R: Familial cerebral aneurysms: A bias for women. Stroke 27:1050–1054, 1996.

41. Ronkainen A, Hernesniemi J, Tromp G: Special features of familial intracranial aneurysms: Report of 215 familial aneurysms. Neurosurgery 37:43–47, 1995.

42. Risks and benefits of screening for intracranial aneurysms in first-degree relatives of patients with sporadic subarachnoid hemorrhage. The Magnetic Resonance Angiography in Relatives of Patients with Subarachnoid Hemorrhage Study Group. N Engl J Med 341:1344–1350, 1999.

43. Fairburn B: "Twin" intracranial aneurysms causing subarachnoid hemorrhage in identical twins. BMJ 1(5847):210–211, 1973.

44. Parekh HC, Gurusinghe NT, Sharma RR: Cerebral berry aneurysms in identical twins: A case report. Surg Neurol 38:277–279, 1992.

45. Fox JL, Ko JP: Familial intracranial aneurysms: Six cases among 13 siblings. J Neurosurg 52:501–503, 1980.

46. Shinton R, Palsingh J, Williams B: Cerebral hemorrhage and berry aneurysm: Evidence from a family for a pattern of autosomal dominant inheritance. J Neurol Neurosurg Psychiatry 54:838–840, 1991.

47. Evans TW, Venning MC, Strang FA, Donnai D: Dominant inheritance of intracranial berry aneurysm. BMJ 283:824–825, 1981.

48. Onda H, Kasuya H, Yoneyama T, et al: Genome-linkage and haplotype-association studies map intracranial aneurysm to chromosome 7q11. Am J Hum Gen 69:804–819, 2001.

49. Fox JL: Intracranial Aneurysms. New York, Springer-Verlag, 1983, pp 410–411 and pp 1433–1438.

50. Gabow PA: Autosomal dominant polycystic kidney disease: More than a renal disease. Am J Kidney Dis 16:403–413, 1990.

51. Schievink WI, Michels VM, Piepgras DG: Neurovascular manifestations of heritable connective tissue disorders: A review. Stroke 25:889–903, 1994.

52. Iglesias CG, Torres VE, Offord KP, et al: Epidemiology of adult polycystic kidney disease, Olmsted County, Minnesota, 1935–1980. Am J Kidney Dis 2:630–639, 1983.

53. van Dijk MA, Chang PC, Peters DJM, Breuning MH: Intracranial aneurysms in polycystic kidney disease linked to chromosome 4. J Am Soc Nephrol 6:1670–1673, 1995.

54. Ryu SJ: Intracranial hemorrhage in patients with polycystic kidney disease. Stroke 21:291–294, 1990.

55. Fehlings MG, Gentili F: The association between polycystic kidney disease and cerebral aneurysms. Can J Neurol Sci 18:505–509, 1991.

56. Chauveau D, Pirson Y, Verellen-Dumoulin C, et al: Intracranial aneurysms in autosomal dominant polycystic kidney disease. Kidney Int 45:1140–1146, 1994.

57. Schievink WI, Torres VE, Piepgras DG, Wiebers DO: Saccular intracranial aneurysms in autosomal dominant polycystic kidney disease. J Am Soc Nephrol 3:88–95, 1992.

58. Lozano AM, Leblanc R: Cerebral aneurysms and polycystic kidney disease: A critical review. Can J Neurol Sci 19:222–227, 1992.

59. Bigelow NH: The association of polycystic kidneys with intracranial aneurysms and other related disorders. Am J Med Sci 225:485–494, 1953.

60. Brown RAP: Polycystic disease of the kidneys and intracranial aneurysms: The etiology and interrelationship of these conditions: Review of recent literature and report of seven cases in which both conditions coexisted. Glasgow Med J 32:333–348, 1951.

61. Chapman AB, Rubinstein D, Hughes RY, et al: Intracranial aneurysms in autosomal dominant polycystic kidney disease. N Engl J Med 327:916–920, 1992.

62. Huston J III, Torres VE, Sulivan PP, et al: Value of magnetic resonance angiography for the detection of intracranial aneurysms in autosomal dominant polycystic kidney disease. J Am Soc Nephrol 3:1871–1877, 1993.

63. Ruggieri PM, Poulos N, Masaryk TJ, et al: Occult intracranial aneurysms in polycystic kidney disease: Screening with MR angiography. Radiology 191:33–39, 1994.

64. Pirson Y, Chauveau D: ADPKD-associated intracranial aneurysm: New insights and unanswered questions. Contrib Nephrol 115:53–58, 1995.

65. Bergan JJ, MacDonald JR: Recognition of cerebrovascular fibromuscular hyperplasia. Arch Surg 98:332–335, 1969.

66. Mettinger KL, Ericson K: Fibromuscular dysplasia and the brain: Observations on angiographic, clinical and genetic characteristics. Stroke 13:46–52, 1982.

67. Rushton AR: The genetics of fibromuscular dysplasia. Arch Intern Med 140:233–236, 1980.

68. Cloft HJ, Kallmes DF, Kallmes MH, et al: Prevalence of cerebral aneurysms in patients with fibromuscular dysplasia: A reassessment. J Neurosurg 88:436–440, 1998.

69. Rubinstein MK, Cohen NH: Ehlers-Danlos syndrome associated with multiple intracranial aneurysms. Neurology 14:125–132, 1964.

70. Majamaa K, Savolainen E-R, Myllylä VV: Synthesis of structurally unstable type III procollagen in patients with cerebral artery aneurysm. Biochim Biophys Acta 1138:191–196, 1992.

71. Finney HL, Roberts TS, Anderson RE: Giant intracranial aneurysm associated with Marfan's syndrome: Case report. J Neurosurg 45:342–347, 1976.

72. Marsalese DL, Moodie DS, Vacante M, et al: Marfan's syndrome: Natural history and long-term follow-up of cardiovascular involvement. J Am Coll Cardiol 14:422–428, 1989.

73. van den Berg Js, Limburg M, Hennekam RC: Is Marfan syndrome associated with symptomatic intracranial aneurysms? Stroke 27:10–12, 1996.

74. Pope FM: Historical evidence for the genetic heterogeneity of pseudoxanthoma elasticum. Br J Dermatol 92:493–509, 1975.

75. Iqbal A, Alter M, Lee SH: Pseudoxanthoma elasticum: A review of neurological complications. Ann Neurol 4:18–20, 1978.

76. Tomsick TA, Lukin RR, Chambers AA, Benton C: Neurofibromatosis and intracranial arterial occlusive disease. Neuroradiology 11:229–234, 1976.

77. Levey AS, Pauker SG, Kassirer JP: Occult intracranial aneurysms in polycystic kidney disease: When is cerebral angiography indicated? N Engl J Med 308:986–994, 1983.

78. Norrgård Ö, Ängqvist KA, Fodstad H, et al: Co-existence of abdominal aortic aneurysms and intracranial aneurysms. Acta Neurochir 87:34–39, 1987.

79. Oyesiku NM, Barrow DL, Eckman JR, et al: Intracranial aneurysms in sickle-cell anemia: Clinical features and pathogenesis. J Neurosurg 75:356–363, 1991.

80. Simard JM, Garcia-Bengochea F, Ballinger WE Jr, et al: Cavernous angioma: A review of 126 collected and 12 new clinical cases. Neurosurgery 18:162–172, 1986.

81. Rigamonti D, Hadley MN, Drayer BP, et al: Cerebral cavernous malformations: Incidence and familial occurrence. N Engl J Med 319:343–347, 1988.

82. Dubovsky J, Zabramski JM, Kurth J, et al: A gene responsible for cavernous malformations maps to chromosome 7q. Hum Mol Genet 4:453–458, 1995.

83. Labauge P, Laberge S, Brunereau L, et al: Hereditary cerebral cavernous angiomas: Clinical and genetic features in 57 French

families. Société Francaise de Neurochirurgie. Lancet 352:1892–1897, 1998.

84. Siegel AM, Andermann F, Badhwar A, et al: Anticipation in familial cavernous angioma: Ascertainment bias or genetic cause. Acta Neurol Scand 98:372–376, 1998.

85. Gil-Nagel A, Dubovsky J, Wilcox KJ, et al: Familial cerebral cavernous angioma: A gene localized to a 15-cM interval on chromosome 7q. Ann Neurol 39:807–810, 1996.

86. Zabramski JM, Wascher TM, Spetzler RF, et al: The natural history of familial cavernous malformations: Results of an ongoing study. J Neurosurg 80:422–432, 1994.

87. Fukui M, Kono S, Sueishi K, Ikezaki K: Moyamoya disease. Neuropathology 20(Suppl):S61–S64, 2000.

88. Kaneko Y, Imamoto N, Mannoji H, Fukui M: Familial occurrence of moyamoya disease in the mother and four daughters including identical twins. Neurol Med Chir 38:349–354, 1998.

89. Yamauchi T, Houkin K, Tada M, Abe H: Familial occurrence of moyamoya disease. Clin Neurol Neurosurg 99(Suppl 2):S162–S167, 1997.

90. Ikeda H, Sasaki T, Yoshimoto T, et al: Mapping of a familial moyamoya disease gene to chromosome 3p24.2-p26. Am J Hum Genet 64:533–537, 1999.

91. Yamauchi T, Tada M, Houkin K, et al: Linkage of familial moyamoya disease: Spontaneous occlusion of the circle of Willis to chromosome 17q25. Stroke 31:930–935, 2000.

92. Inoue TK, Ikezaki K, Sasazuki T, et al: Linkage analysis of moyamoya disease on chromosome 6. J Child Neurol 15:179–182, 2000.

93. Andreone V, Ciarmiello A, Fusco C, et al: Moyamoya disease in Italian monozygotic twins. Neurology 53:1332–1335, 1999.

94. Tanghetti B, Capra R, Giunta F, et al: Moyamoya syndrome in only one of two identical twins. J Neurosurg 59:1092–1094, 1983.

95. Yokoyama K, Asano Y, Murakawa T, et al: Familial occurrence of arteriovenous malformation of the brain. J Neurosurg 74:585–589, 1991.

96. Aberfeld DC, Rao KR: Familial arteriovenous malformation of the brain. Neurology 31:184–186, 1981.

Chapter Sixty-Three

Intracerebral Hemorrhage

Alexander David Mendelow

The burden of intracerebral hemorrhage (ICH) in the community is growing because of (1) the more common use of antiplatelet therapy for the primary and secondary prevention of atherosclerosis, (2) the increasing use of anticoagulation, particularly in the elderly population, and (3) the more frequent use of thrombolysis for both myocardial infarction and ischemic stroke. It has been estimated that between 1% and 2% of the population is now undergoing warfarin therapy,[1] and that the total number of intracerebral hemorrhages occurring throughout the world each year is 1,500,000.[2] Almost half of the affected patients die without recovering, and more than half of the survivors remain permanently disabled. The cost to healthcare systems and to communities is great and probably represents the greatest burden of stroke.

There are considerable controversies about the prevention of rebleeding as well as the medical management and surgical treatment of this condition. Surgical fashions vary in different countries of the world, with high rates of surgical evacuation for spontaneous intracerebral hemorrhage found in some centers in Lithuania and Sweden, and low rates in some centers in Hungary (Fig. 63–1).[3] The main controversy is about whether or not to evacuate supratentorial ICH and, although eight small randomized, controlled trials have been reported to date, the International Surgical Trial in Intracerebral Haemorrhage (ISTICH) had not completed follow-up at the time of writing (1033 patients from 27 countries randomly assigned to treatment worldwide). Other controversies relate to cerebellar hemorrhage, treatment of the underlying cause (arteriovenous malformation [AVM] or aneurysm), and initial medical treatment. The International Subarachnoid Hemorrhage Aneurysm Trial (ISAT) to determine the relative benefits of endovascular coiling and clipping should resolve some of the issues about treating the cause of ICH, and the 1-year follow up results have indicated a 7% absolute benefit from endovascular coiling compared with clipping,[69] but the ISAT trial did not set out to evaluate endovascular coiling in the context of ICH.

"Unruptured" aneurysms are now being diagnosed with increasing frequency, and there is great controversy about whether or not to intervene in such cases. One of the greatest tragedies in medicine is a fatal hemorrhage in a patient with a known unruptured aneurysm in whom the previous medical advice was "wait and see." All clinicians who deal with such patients must know the natural history of unruptured aneurysms and must keep up to date with new studies, such as the International Study of Unruptured Intracranial Aneurysms (ISUIA), as reports appear.[4,5] From these presentations, it has now become clear that the critical size is 6 mm; for aneurysms larger than this threshold, the risk of hemorrhage rises towards 1% per year.

EPIDEMIOLOGY AND ETIOLOGY

Incidence

The incidence of ICH varies as a percentage of all strokes, being highest in Asia and lowest in the United States. Estimates of the crude incidence of ICH per 100,000 per year vary from 6 in Kuwait to 411 in China.[2]

Varying Effect of Age

Life expectancy varies greatly among countries.[6] Countries with a longer life expectancy are more likely to have a greater percentage of ischemic strokes than intracerebral hemorrhage.

Changing Patterns

With the greater use of anticoagulants in elderly patients, particularly in the treatment of atrial fibrillation in patients with symptomatic cerebrovascular disease, intracerebral and subdural hemorrhages are occurring more frequently. Similarly, antiplatelet therapy is being used for both primary and secondary prevention of stroke and atherosclerosis; antiplatelet agents also raise the incidence of ICH. More frequent use of recombinant tissue-type plasminogen activator (rt-PA) in both myocardial infarction and stroke has also been shown to increase the incidence of ICH. The reduction in poor outcomes in patients with ischemic stroke receiving rt-PA is offset by a ten-fold increase in the number of patients with ICH.[7] The use of "recreational" drugs has resulted in a new epidemic of intracerebral hematomas in young patients and teenagers.[8] The surgical treatment of ICH has to be considered in the context of these pharmacologic environments, which influence bleeding, the rate of bleeding and, most important of all to the surgeon, the efficacy of hemostasis. This issue is particularly important because the rate of postoperative

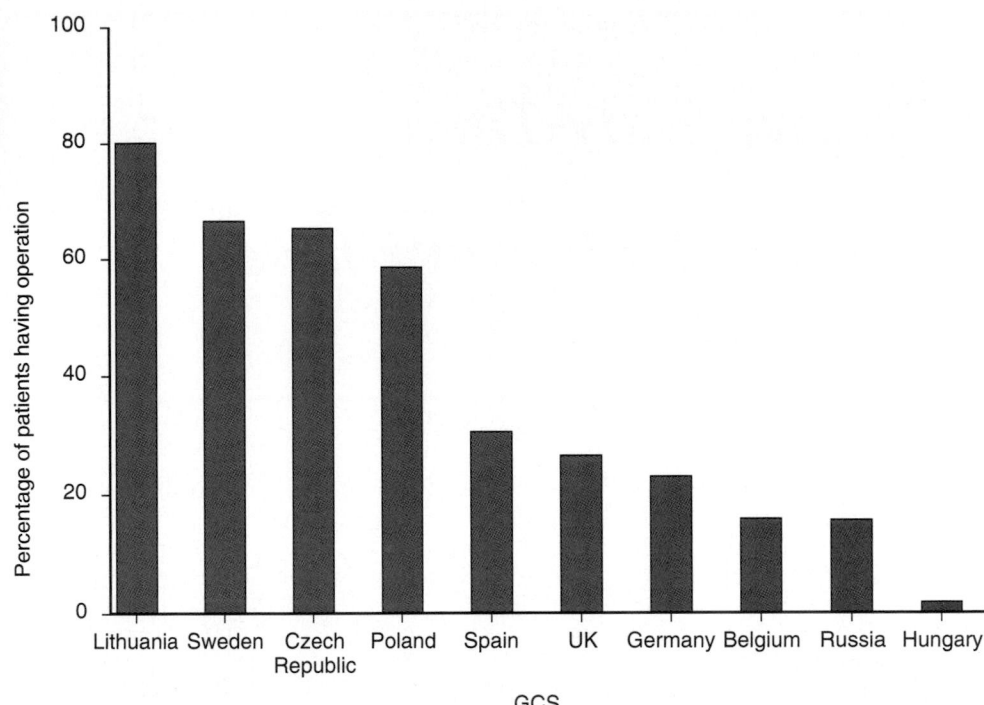

FIGURE 63–1 *Graph showing rates of operation in centers from different countries.*

hemorrhage after craniotomy for ICH is about 4% even without a bleeding disorder.[9]

Causes of Intracerebral Hemorrhage

The causes of ICH are listed in Table 63.1. The most common cause is thought to be chronic hypertension, but it is not acceptable to simply regard an acute elevation of blood pressure at the time of the ictus as the cause. Often an ICH induces an acute rise in blood pressure, as Cushing[10] so elegantly showed more than 100 years ago. Therefore, great care must be taken in defining the cause of the ICH, which modern imaging often shows to be a structural vascular lesion. The underlying cause of ICH is also critical to the choice of surgical treatment. For example, Heiskanen and colleagues[11] showed that surgical evacuation of ICH due to an aneurysm was much more effective than conservative treatment.

IMAGING IN THE DIAGNOSIS OF INTRACEREBRAL HEMORRHAGE

The difficulty of differentiating ischemic stroke from ICH is well known. Although the sudden onset of severe headache, coma, or epilepsy is more likely to be due to ICH, urgent imaging is essential to avoid the danger of using thrombolytic therapy for ischemic stroke in a patient with an ICH. Computed tomography is perfectly adequate for diagnosing ICH, although magnetic resonance imaging (MRI) is similarly diagnostic in the acute phase.

Computed Tomography

In the acute phase, spontaneous ICH is easy to recognize on CT scan as a high-density mass. Subsequently, the area

Table 63.1   Causes of Intracerebral Hemorrhage

Idiopathic
Hypertension
Amyloid angiopathy
Cerebral aneurysms
Cerebral arteriovenous malformations
Cerebral arteriovenous fistulae
Cavernous malformations
Brain tumors (primary and secondary)
Anticoagulants/antiplatelet agents/tissue-type plasminogen
   activator
Recreational drugs
Unrecognized trauma
Postoperatively (remote and cerebellar)
Post-infarction (hemorrhagic conversion)
Hereditary hemorrhagic telangiectasia
Blood dyscrasias (e.g., hemophilia, leukemia)

around the ICH develops low-density changes as a result of brain edema. The volume of the hematoma can be calculated with the use of the approximation of an ellipse, from the following equation described by Brott and Broderick:[12]

$$\frac{4}{3}\pi r^2 \approx \frac{A \times B \times C}{2}$$

where r is the radius, and *A*, *B*, and *C* are the diameters in three planes.

The volume of the hematoma determines the outcome, larger hematomas having a much poorer prognosis than smaller hematomas.[13] Now that CT scanning is performed more frequently in patients with stroke, a greater number of patients with ICH will be discovered. This trend should help to differentiate these two completely different disorders that have, in the past, often been lumped together as "stroke."

Sites of Hemorrhage

Lesions at certain sites are more likely to be associated with aneurysmal ICH—interhemispheric and sylvian (Figs. 63–2 and 63–3). The classic hypertensive ICH occurs in the basal ganglia, whereas lobar hematomas are more likely with amyloid angiopathy. The CT scan may also demonstrate evidence of underlying tumor or trauma. Adjacent or remote calcification may also give an indication that there is an underlying cerebral AVM or tumor. Contrast-enhanced CT scanning and CT angiography may display aneurysms or cerebral AVMs. Cerebellar hematomas can produce noncommunicating obstructive hydrocephalus, which may need urgent treatment in its own right.

Magnetic Resonance Imaging

MRI easily differentiates ischemic stroke from ICH. However, the MRI appearances will change as the time from ictus increases (Table 63.2). MRI with diffusion-weighted imaging (DWI) also displays the development of brain edema.

Angiography

Some surgeons prefer to obtain an angiogram routinely before undertaking surgery. This step is taken to prevent the unexpected discovery of an otherwise difficult-to-treat AVM. Similarly, for the patient in whom an aneurysm is suspected, most neurosurgeons would recommend angiography to display the aneurysm. CT angiography may be an acceptable alternative to intra-arterial angiography. Magnetic resonance angiography (MRA) is becoming more readily available as an urgent investigation in some centers, and the addition of gadolinium enhancement may be sufficient to exclude an underlying structural vascular lesion.

Blood Flow Mapping with SPECT and PET

Single-photon emission computer tomography (SPECT) using technetium hexamethyl-propyleneaminoeoxime (HM-PAO) has been shown to display a penumbra of functionally impaired but potentially recoverable tissue around an ICH. Through the use of the difference-based

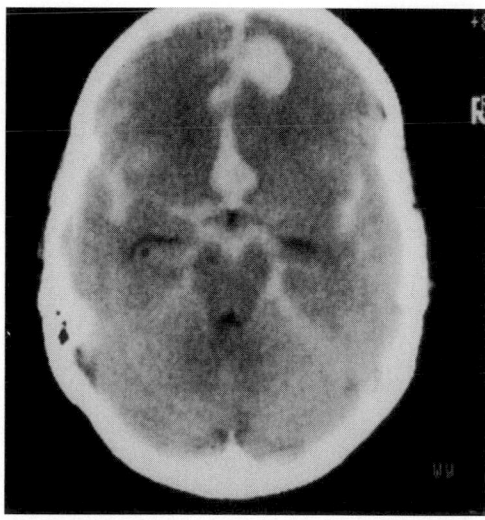

FIGURE 63–2 *Computed tomography scan showing interhemispheric hematoma from a ruptured anterior communicating artery aneurysm.*

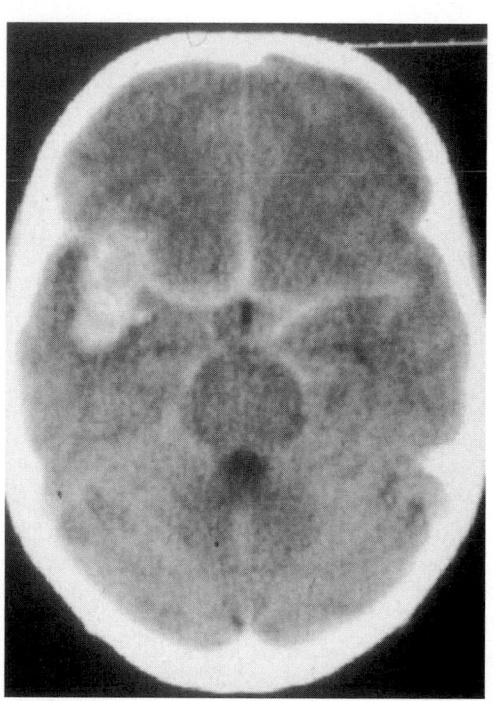

FIGURE 63–3 *Computed tomography scan showing intracerebral and subarachnoid hemorrhage from a ruptured middle cerebral artery aneurysm.*

Table 63.2   **Magnetic Resonance Imaging Characteristics of Hemorrhage**

Time from ictus	Clinical Phase	Appearance on T1-weighted Images	Appearance on T2-weighted Images	Hemoglobin State
Immediate	Hyperacute	Isointense	Bright	Intracellular oxyhemoglobin
6 hr	Acute	Isointense	Dark	Intracellular deoxyhemoglobin
6–48 hr	Early subacute	Bright	Dark	Extracellular deoxyhemoglobin
2 wk	Late subacute	Bright	Bright	Extracellular methemoglobin
>3 wk	Chronic	Dark	Dark	Hemosiderin

region-growing (DBRG) method, the penumbra has been objectively identified in patients with supratentorial ICH.[20] Similarly, positron emission tomography (PET) has been used to identify a penumbra around ICH,[15,16] although this issue remains controversial.[17-19] The importance of demonstrating a penumbra around an ICH is the recognition of the potential for reversal of the ischemic process by either pharmacologic or surgical means. It is the demonstration of the penumbra that makes the case for the intervention. In some patients, there may be no penumbra, whereas in others it is still present. An understanding of this issue is therefore essential to appreciating the possible role for surgery in a particular case; the next section contains a discussion of this matter.

PATHOPHYSIOLOGY OF THE PENUMBRA

Controversy exists as to whether or not there is a penumbra around an ICH.[15-20] The importance of the issue is that if such a penumbra exists, there is the potential for medical or surgical intervention to minimize the brain damage in the area surrounding the ICH. Histologic studies have established that there is ischemic neuronal damage in the tissue around the ICH. Later studies, using KU80 and fractin antibody stains, have shown that there is apoptosis in the tissue around an ICH (Fig. 63–4). This finding implies that some cells have undergone programmed cell death (apoptosis) and that these cells, having initially survived, may be potential targets for urgent therapeutic intervention.[2]

The first experimental evidence of a large penumbra around an ICH came from experiments in rats in which blood was introduced into the caudate nucleus under arterial pressure (Fig. 63–5).[21,22] Carbon 14–iodoantipyrene autoradiography demonstrated a large ischemic area (Fig. 63–6). Similarly, in a study using an inflatable and deflat-

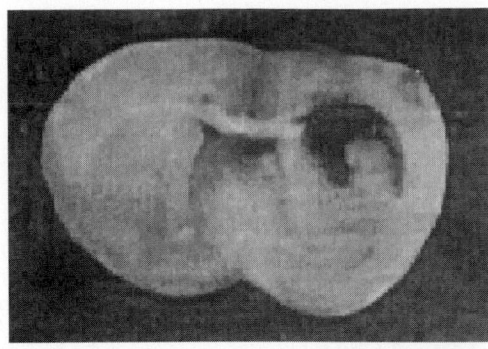

FIGURE 63–5   *Section of rat brain showing caudate intracerebral hemorrhage.*

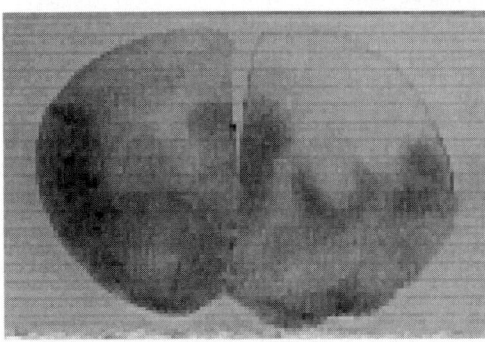

FIGURE 63–6   *Carbon 14 autoradiograph showing large perfusion defect around caudate intracerebral hemorrhage.*

able microballoon (50 µL), deflation of the microballoon 2 hours after inflation produced a much smaller infarct than when the balloon was left inflated for a full 2 hours.[22] These experimental studies provide a background for clinical studies, which have also revealed a penumbra in some patients with ICH (Plate 63–1 following page 1224). Reduced cerebral blood flow (CBF) has also been demonstrated around ICH in patients by means of dynamic CT perfusion techniques.[23] Other clinical studies using MRI and PET have similarly demonstrated a penumbra.[15,16,20]

By contrast, some clinical studies have not shown a penumbra.[17-19] It may well be that a penumbra is present in some patients with ICH but not in others. Therefore, the patient with a penumbra is likely to benefit from surgical decompression; if such patients could be identified, selective surgery could be applied. Kanno and Nonomura[24] have shown that the use of hyperbaric oxygen leads to an improvement in the clinical condition of (and thus demonstrates the existence of penumbra) in some patients. They have used this approach in the selection of patients for surgery. Similarly, microdialysis methods have demonstrated very high glutamate levels in the penumbra around ICH (confirming the preceding studies that suggest an ischemic process around the ICH). Microdialysis has also found elevated lactate pyruvate ratios in the penumbra.[13]

Measurements of intracranial pressure (ICP) and cerebral perfusion pressure (CPP) in ICH have shown that patients with high ICP and reduced CPP have poorer outcomes than those with normal values.[13] Reduction of blood

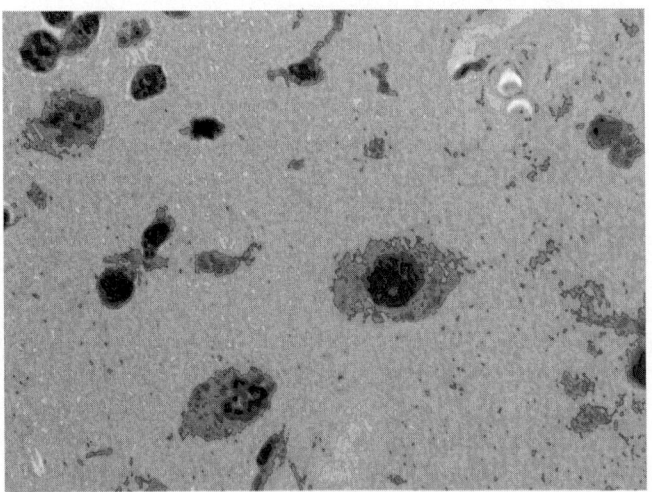

FIGURE 63–4   *Photomicrograph of brain around an intracerebral hemorrhage stained with KU80 antibody to show evidence of apoptosis. (This finding indicates programmed cell death and therefore supports the concept of a penumbra.)*

pressure and, therefore, CPP may be hazardous in patients with ICH. Heiss and coworkers[25] have clearly shown that a penumbra does exist in some patients. The challenge, therefore, is to define which patients have a penumbra and which do not. Also, with time, the penumbra changes and perihematoma edema progresses, adversely affecting outcome.[26,27] As discussed previously, if a penumbra can be identified, surgery is more likely to be beneficial if undertaken rapidly, before permanent secondary processes take place.

Underlying Pathology

In some patients with ICH, the underlying disease (e.g., tumor or cerebral AVM) causes the hemorrhage. Similarly, amyloid angiopathy is associated with amyloid deposits in the area around small cerebral vessels. It is thought that the weakening in the wall associated with this vasculo-pathic process results in the classic lobar parieto-occipital hematomas that occur in the elderly. Of the various tumors, metastatic melanomas are most likely to bleed. For this reason, every ICH should be investigated to exclude underlying disease.

MEDICAL MANAGEMENT AND TREATMENT

The following four aspects of ICH must be considered:

1. Early expansion of the hematoma with further bleeding into the cavity
2. Associated acute hypertension
3. Rebleeding from an underlying abnormality such as a cerebral AVM or aneurysm
4. Complications that develop around the hematoma itself

Expansion of the Hematoma

From the many studies that show that hematomas enlarge in the hours immediately after hemorrhage,[28] it is clear that prevention of expansion may have a role to play in treatment of ICH. However, no prospective, randomized controlled studies have yet been conducted to confirm this concept. Prevention of expansion through alteration of the clotting mechanisms seems an attractive approach; it may take two forms, treatment of underlying coagulation disorders (reversal of warfarin or cessation of heparin therapy) or actively giving treatment that would improve coagulation. This latter approach would include the use of fresh frozen plasma and vitamin K. Also, recombinant factor VIIa is being studied in phase 2 trials at present, and a phase 3 trial is planned. Recombinant factor VIIa has been shown to be effective in reducing extracranial hemorrhage in patients with hemophilia, but recommendations for its use in spontaneous ICH must await the results of the phase 3 studies.

Treatment of Acute Hypertension

The most controversial aspect of initial therapy for ICH is treatment of the acute reactive hypertension with which it is usually associated. The proponents of active treatment point out that control of the hypertension prevents further bleeding into the cavity. Also, autoregulation may be preserved in some patients.[17] Opponents of this approach are concerned about lowering the CPP and thereby aggravating the ischemic brain damage. No recommendations can be made at this stage, and treatment of reactive hypertension remains an option. Treatment of this acute reactive hypertension, however, must not be confused with the treatment of chronic hypertension, which has been shown to reduce the occurrence of ICH in the first place. In the presence of an unsecured aneurysm, the case for lowering blood pressure before definitive treatment is strongest.

Treatment of the Underlying Cause

Treatment of the underlying cause, such as a cerebral AVM or aneurysm, must also be considered. The calcium antagonist nimodipine has been claimed to reduce rebleeding from aneurysms in patients with subarachnoid hemorrhage,[29] but its role in spontaneous ICH has not been established in relation to rebleeding. Also, Heiskanen and coworkers[11] showed that when an ICH is due to an aneurysm, the aneurysm should be treated; the mortality in their patients receiving nonoperative treatment was 80%, whereas that in patients undergoing aneurysm clipping was 27%. Kerr and associates[31] have also suggested that securing the aneurysm with endovascular coiling may prevent rebleeding in patients with ICH. Once again, no prospective randomized controlled trial of endovascular coiling in patients with ICH and associated aneurysms has been undertaken. These investigators,[31] in an observational study, reported a favorable outcome (Glasgow Outcome Scale [GOS] score 1 or 2) in 48% of patients and a mortality of 21%, values that compare very favorably with results of most other surgical series. Ruptured aneurysms should be clipped at the time the associated clot is removed. Large AVMs are usually best treated in a delayed fashion after acute clot removal.

Treatment of the Complications of Intracerebral Hemorrhage

Because ischemic neuronal damage occurs in the brain surrounding an intracerebral hematoma, the use of neuroprotective agents that are effective in preventing ischemic neuronal damage is an attractive concept. Such agents include calcium antagonists and N-methyl-D- aspartate (NMDA) receptor antagonists. These agents prevent pathologic calcium influx through the cell membrane, and a small randomized controlled trial of nimodipine has shown promise.[30] Experimental evidence has suggested that NMDA receptor antagonists and the 21-amino steroid tirilazad reduce the ischemic neuronal damage associated with ICH.[32,33]

In patients with elevated ICP, the use of osmotic diuretics like mannitol may reduce ICP. Randomized controlled trials have shown that mannitol is useful in patients undergoing surgery for traumatic hematomas,[61,62] but the agent's effectiveness has not yet been shown in spontaneous ICH. Nevertheless, it would seem logical to use mannitol in patients with high ICP during the wait for surgery. Treatment with dexamethasone has not yet been shown to be effective in patients with ICH, although the appearance of a large area of low density around the hematoma on CT scan seems to justify setting up trials of dexamethasone in such patients.

Careful monitoring of patients with ICH is a logical approach, and a prospective randomized controlled trial of monitoring in patients with stroke has shown improved outcomes, particularly in the elderly.[34] The majority of these patients had ischemic stroke, but some patients with spontaneous ICH were included in the trial.[34] More invasive monitoring with arterial lines and ICP monitors would also seem sensible. In studies my colleagues and I have conducted at the University of Newcastle-Upon-Tyne, patients with high ICP and pressure CPP had worse outcomes than patients with normal values.[13]

A literature search for class I evidence from controlled trials of medical treatment has uncovered five small trials,[2] but none provides convincing evidence for any medical intervention.[35-39]

SURGICAL TREATMENT

One of the greatest controversies in neurosurgery is whether or not to operate on a patient with supratentorial ICH. Although it is clear that some patients need operation and that others do not, there is an area of uncertainty between these extremes. For example, a young patient with ICH in the nondominant hemisphere who is initially conscious and talking but who subsequently deteriorates with a lobar ICH would warrant surgical treatment. By contrast, an elderly dependent patient with a large ICH in the dominant hemisphere and extending into the thalamus who is in coma from the outset has such a poor prognosis that surgery would not be considered. Surgery would also not be considered for the patient with a very small volume ICH who has a minimal focal deficit with no disturbance of consciousness, particularly if the clot is deep-seated. It is, therefore, clear that some patients would not undergo surgery because they are too well and others would not undergo surgery because the prospects are hopeless. These two negative aspects in relation to surgery have resulted in confusion about the indications, particularly as there are some patients, as in the example already given, who would clearly benefit. It is the patients between these extremes for whom uncertainty about performing surgery exists.

Prospective Randomized Controlled Trials and Observational Studies

Class I Evidence

In the original review about surgical treatment for ICH reported by Prasad and Shrivastava,[40] four prospective randomized trials were cited. In a subsequent meta-analysis, Fernandes and colleagues[41] summarized seven prospective randomized controlled trials, results of which have shown that there is no certainty about treatment because most of the trials were too small to produce meaningful conclusions (Fig. 63–7). A further small trial of stereotactic aspiration has also failed to demonstrate improved outcome from thrombolytic assisted aspiration.[42] For this reason, the International Surgical Trial in Intracerebral Hemorrhage (ISTICH) was begun in 1995 and, at the time of writing, recruitment has stopped (1033 have been randomly assigned to the different treatment arms). It is likely that the final results of this trial will be known towards the end of 2003. A report of the pooled and blinded results describes the demographic and clinical data so far,[43] but analyses of the results from the two groups in the trial (early surgery versus initial conservative treatment) cannot be done until all the patients have been randomly assigned for treatment (February 2003) and all the 6-month follow-up data have been gathered (September 2003).

When supratentorial ICH is associated with a ruptured aneurysm, surgical treatment is undoubtedly better, yielding a much lower mortality (27%) than that for conservative treatment (80%).[11] The probability of sudden death from a ruptured intracranial aneurysm has been subject to a systematic review with meta-analysis by Huang and van Gelder.[44]

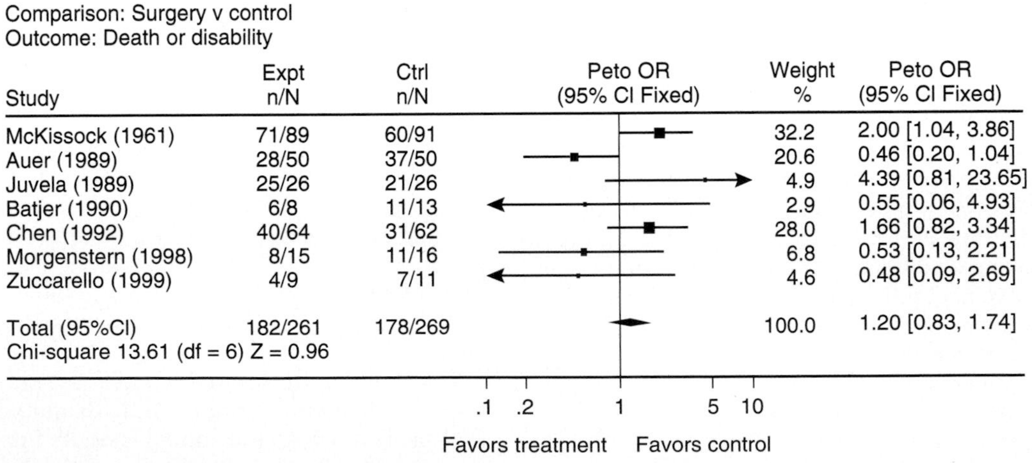

Comparison: Surgery v control
Outcome: Death or disability

Study	Expt n/N	Ctrl n/N	Peto OR (95% CI Fixed)	Weight %	Peto OR (95% CI Fixed)
McKissock (1961)	71/89	60/91		32.2	2.00 [1.04, 3.86]
Auer (1989)	28/50	37/50		20.6	0.46 [0.20, 1.04]
Juvela (1989)	25/26	21/26		4.9	4.39 [0.81, 23.65]
Batjer (1990)	6/8	11/13		2.9	0.55 [0.06, 4.93]
Chen (1992)	40/64	31/62		28.0	1.66 [0.82, 3.34]
Morgenstern (1998)	8/15	11/16		6.8	0.53 [0.13, 2.21]
Zuccarello (1999)	4/9	7/11		4.6	0.48 [0.09, 2.69]
Total (95%CI)	182/261	178/269		100.0	1.20 [0.83, 1.74]

Chi-square 13.61 (df = 6) Z = 0.96

.1　.2　　　1　　　5　10

Favors treatment　　Favors control

FIGURE 63–7　*Meta-analysis of randomized controlled trials of the effect of surgery after a supratentorial spontaneous intracerebral hemorrhage, with death and disability combined. (Modified from Fernandes HM, et al: Surgery in intracerebral hemorrhage: The uncertainty continues. Stroke 31:2511–2516, 2000.)*

With cerebellar ICH, no class I evidence exists of the efficacy of any treatment, but it is generally accepted that these patients may do well with surgical intervention. With cerebellar ICH, the treatment of hydrocephalus also must be considered, because hydrocephalus may lead to disturbance of consciousness. Correction of the hydrocephalus with external ventricular drainage may therefore dramatically improve the level of consciousness. Whether or not to remove the cerebellar ICH has been considered, and an algorithm has been offered for its management (Fig. 63–8).[45] In some patients with supratentorial ICH who may have suffered a head injury, it may be difficult to know whether or not the lesion is traumatic or spontaneous. No trials have been conducted to ascertain whether surgical treatment should be undertaken in patients with traumatic ICH. It is clear that patients with traumatic ICH (TICH) differ from patients with spontaneous ICH (SICH), and these differences have been characterized by Siddique and colleagues.[46] By and large, patients with traumatic ICH have better outcomes perhaps because as a group they are younger than patients with spontaneous ICH.

Class II and Class III Evidence

Many observational studies (yielding class II and class III evidence) have been performed to examine treatment of ICH. Retrospective studies that either compare results of surgery and nonoperative management or are "pure" surgical series without controls are numerous, and more than 60 such studies were reported by Fernandes.[13] In general, the reports of "new" surgical techniques are encouraging. Such techniques include the well-established and standard craniotomy,[47–50] stereotaxic aspiration,[51–53] and ultrasonic aspirations.[54] Fernandes[13] also summarized the class II evidence, which came from 32 papers comparing medical and surgical treatments prospectively but in a nonrandomized way. The results of these studies were mixed with some finding better results from surgery,[55] some finding no difference,[56] and others finding surgery worse.[57]

In the largest series to date, Kanaya and Kuroda[58] reported on more than 7000 patients in the Japanese ICH register; these investigators found that patients with deep coma and very large ICHs faired badly with surgical treatment. Craniotomy was better for hematomas of greater than 50 mL, whereas aspiration was better for smaller clots. Other studies have similarly concluded that surgical results in patients with large hematomas were poor, particularly because the patients were selected for surgery because of their comatose state and large hematomas. It is possible to draw completely the wrong conclusion from results of these observational studies, however, because they were nonrandomized studies in which the less severely affected patients underwent medical treatment.[47]

Craniotomy

The majority of neurosurgeons around the world still favor a craniotomy for the evacuation of a hematoma. Generally, surgeons are more inclined to operate if the ICH is in the nondominant hemisphere, if the patient deteriorates, and if the clot is lobar and near the surface.[59] If the clot is lobar and polar, especially in the nondominant hemisphere, surgery is easier and a larger internal decompression is possible at less risk to function.

Some surgeons prefer a large craniotomy because it leaves open the option of external decompression if there is a lot of brain swelling. Although this technique is gaining favor in traumatic ICH and with larger infarcts from ischemic stroke, it has not been formally evaluated in randomized controlled trials except in one small trial of decompressive craniectomy for traumatic brain swelling in children.[60] This trial was subjected to several interim analyses, so the improved result with decompression was not

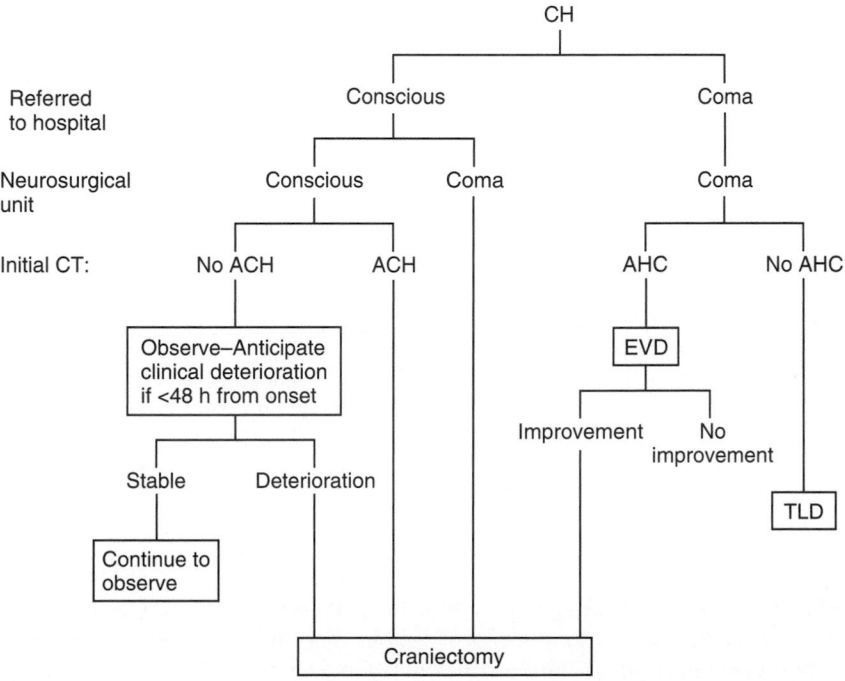

FIGURE 63–8 *Recommendations for neurosurgical management of cerebellar hematomas. ACH, acute hydrocephalus; CH, cerebellar hemorrhage; EVD, external ventricular drainage; TLD, treatment-limiting decision. (Redrawn from Mathew P, et al: Neurosurgical management of cerebellar hematoma and infarct. J Neurol Neurosurg Psychiatry 59:287–292, 1995.)*

quite significant, although as new trials are reported, the results of this small trial will be useful in a meta-analysis. There are no ongoing or planned trials of external decompression for spontaneous supratentorial ICH at present; the technique must therefore remain unproved in patients with ICH.

For the procedure, patients are usually positioned supine with the head rotated, but in elderly patients with osteoarthritic necks, the lateral position may be preferred, especially if the clot is occipital as often occurs with amyloid angiopathy in the elderly. A large bolus of IV mannitol is given preoperatively; Cruz and associates[61,62] have demonstrated in prospective randomized controlled trials that such a bolus is effective. A craniotomy is made over the hematoma, with avoidance of eloquent areas of the brain such as the motor strip and speech areas of the cortex.

If the dura is very tight even after administration of mannitol, repositioning, and correction of any other problem such as high CVP or hypercapnia, the clot should be gently aspirated with a Dandy-type cannula so that the dura can be opened without trauma to the cortex, which may otherwise herniate alarmingly through the durotomy. Removal of even a few milliliters of clot in this way may move the patient's condition down the pressure-volume curve. It is better to correct all of these problems quickly while aspirating to minimize the ischemia, which would otherwise persist in any penumbra surrounding the hematoma. The sooner reperfusion is restored, the smaller the ultimate ischemic damage is likely to be.

Once the dura is open, the clot may be visible or the flattened pale overlying gyri may be obvious. If not, image guidance or ultrasonography may prove helpful. A cortical window that avoids arteries and major venous structures is created, rather than a cortical incision. The window avoids or reduces the need for retraction; also, it is my belief that if access through noneloquent cortex has been planned, the ultimate damage will be less with a cortical window.

Once located, the clot is entered and easily removed with gentle suction and irrigation, with Hartman's solution rather than saline because it more closely resembles cerebrospinal fluid (CSF). Use of the operating microscope, which allows access to all parts of the hematoma through a relatively small cortical window, is highly recommended. Self-retaining retractors facilitate access to all parts of the cavity. Hemostasis is secured with bipolar diathermy. Hemostatic materials can be used but only after the surgeon has ensured that all arterial and venous bleeding points have been attended to.

Usually, the brain will have become slack, and the dura can be closed and the bone flap replaced. If the brain is very swollen, however, leaving the dura open with removal of the bone flap is an option. Alternatively, the bone flap can be left riding with dura open, and the noneloquent cortex covered with a hemostatic material. If the clot has ruptured into the ventricle, it is reasonable practice to leave an external ventricular drain in situ; the drain either can be used to drain CSF postoperatively at a relatively high pressure (e.g., 20 cm CSF) or can be connected to a pressure transducer and opened to drainage only if the ICP rises or the CPP drops below an acceptable threshold (e.g., below a CPP of 65 mm Hg in an adult or 55 mm Hg in a child).[63]

Postoperative neurologic monitoring must be continued until the patient shows signs of recovery of consciousness, because the postoperative rebleeding rate is high. In some units, postoperative CT scanning, ICP monitoring, or both are routine, but neither of these critical care measures has been formally evaluated in trials.

Other methods of surgical evacuation have been evaluated, including endoscopy, ultrasonic aspiration, and intracavity thrombolysis.

Endoscopic Removal of Hematoma

Auer and coworkers[64] showed, in a prospective randomized controlled trial conducted in one center and published in 1989, that endoscopic removal was superior to medical treatment. Other observational reports have also favored endoscopy, and with stereotactic guidance and real-time ultrasonographic imaging, very encouraging results have been obtained with smaller clots (<30 mL). In later studies, such techniques have been tried with greater success in larger hematomas (K. Kuroda, et al: personal communication, 2003). This technique is not generally applied at present. Nevertheless, variations on the theme of stereotactic aspiration abound.[65] In some reports the laser has been used as a hemostatic tool through the endoscope, again with encouraging results. All these technological advances have yet to be formally evaluated in prospective randomized controlled trials.

Ultrasonic Aspiration

Hondo and associates[54] have reported success with a stereotactic aspiration of supratentorial ICH using an ultrasonic aspirator. Studies of this procedure are observational, and the method has not yet been subjected to prospective randomized controlled trials.

Intracavity Thrombolysis

Blaauw and colleagues undertook a small prospective randomized controlled trial in patients with supratentorial ICH; these investigators introduced urokinase into the cavity of the ICH and, after a specified period, aspirated the contents. This small prospective randomized controlled trial was stopped early; preliminary results show no benefit in terms of mortality,[42,66] although there was a possible benefit in a small number of patients analyzed using multivariate analysis.[67] In some patients, in whom ICH has ruptured into the ventricle, external ventricular drainage (EVD) may be useful. Like the other methods described, this technique has never been subjected to prospective randomized controlled trials, but observational studies have highlighted the poor prognoses in these patients.[68]

PREVENTIVE TREATMENT OF THE UNDERLYING CAUSE

Aneurysmal Intracerebral Hemorrhage

Heiskanen and colleagues[11] showed in a prospective randomized controlled trial that the mortality was significantly lower for surgery than for medical treatment. For this

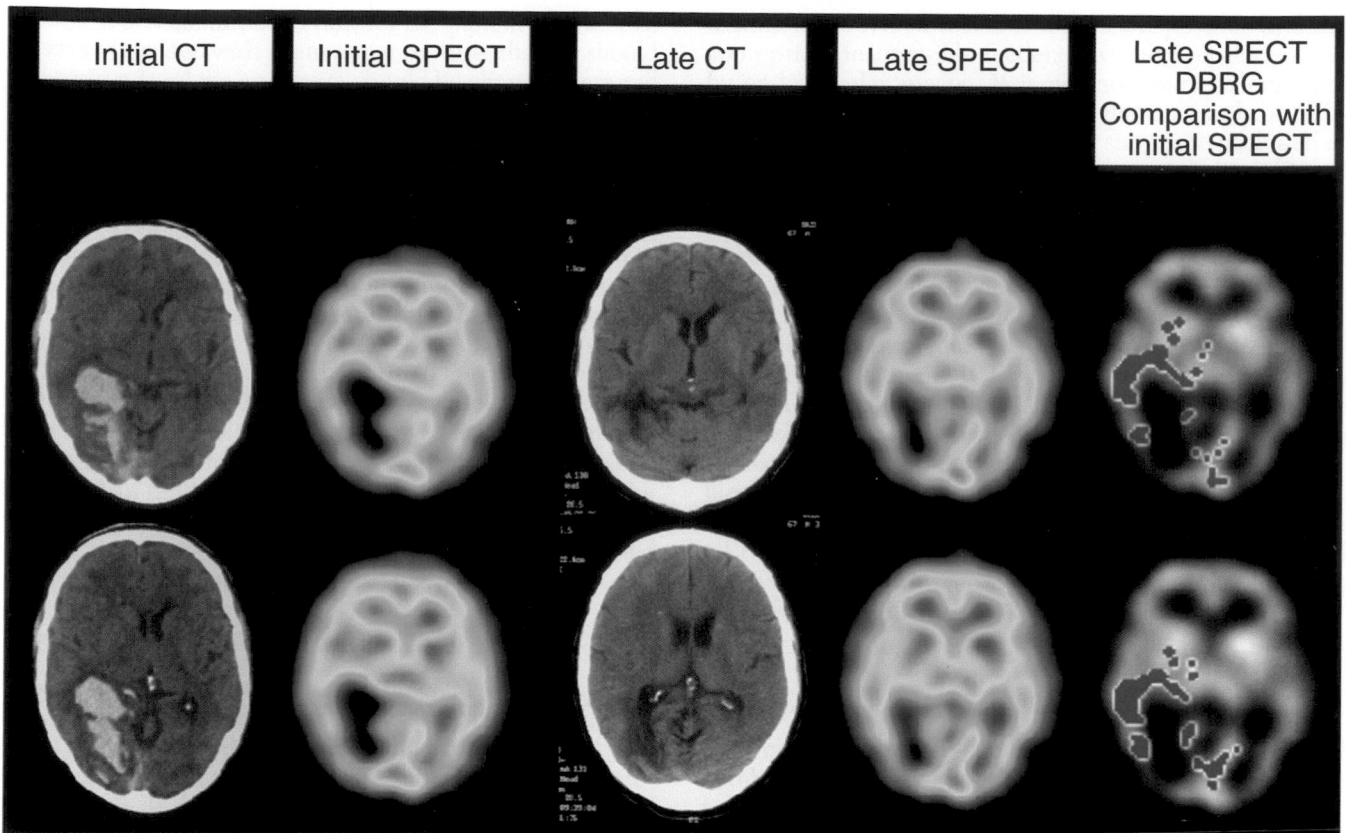

PLATE 63–1 *Hexamethyl-propyleneaminoeoxime (Hm-PAO) single-photon emission computed tomography (SPECT) scans with matching computed tomography scans at the time of the ictus (left) and months later (right). Scans were compared through the use of the difference-based region growing method of comparison to show the "penumbra" (red areas on the extreme right). (From Siddique MS, et al: Reversible ischemia around intracerebral hemorrhage: A single-photon emission computerized tomography study. J Neurosurg 96:736–741, 2002.)*

orrhages respond well to surgery, but the effect of hydro-cephalus must be considered separately. There are no randomized controlled trials on which to base management decisions. However, Mathew and coworkers[45] have proposed an algorithm for management that is sensible and easy to use (see Fig. 63–8). As with supratentorial ICH, underlying causes of cerebellar hemorrhage should be sought and treated.

With rapid treatment, the outcome of cerebellar hemorrhage with appropriate management of hydrocephalus may be surprisingly good.[45,70–78] Nevertheless, one should not underestimate the morbidity and mortality associated with posterior fossa surgery, which carries a high complication rate compared with ventricular drainage for hydrocephalus, which is relatively straightforward. The counter-argument is that very poor outcomes result from an overly conservative approach.[45,79] Indeed conservative management is condemned by some clinicians, but the reason may be that their patients had particularly severe clinical presentations with large hematomas diagnosed in the pre-CT era.[80,81]

PROGNOSIS AND FOLLOW-UP

In general, many studies using multivariate analyses of cases of cerebral ICH have shown that patients in deep coma, with advancing age, or with very large hematomas tend to do poorly. Kanaya and Kuroda[58] analyzed more than 7000 patients from Japan and classified them into five groups. They recommended that no surgery should be undertaken in patients in groups IVb and V (patients in coma or with herniation).

Our own studies at Newcastle-Upon-Tyne have confirmed that elderly patients in coma with large hematomas fair poorly. We treated 440 patients with spontaneous supratentorial ICH between May 1993 and August 1999. Of these, 56% were men, and only 24% had favorable scores on the Glasgow Outcome Scale. Multivariate analysis of patients in the prospectively collected database (including patients not in the International Surgical Trial of Intracerebral Hemorrhage) has confirmed these findings (Table 63.3).

Epilepsy

Patients with ICH may present with epilepsy for the first time, and epilepsy may be the cause of sudden unexplained death.[82] Faught and associates[83] reported that in patients with ICH, seizure incidence was more common with cortical lobar hemorrhage than with basal ganglia or subcortical hemorrhage and that no epilepsy was found if the bleed was thalamic.[83] Chronic epilepsy after ICH has been reported in 2.5% to 25% of patients,[84–86] partial seizures being the most common type.[87]

Risk of Rebleeding

Most hematomas enlarge in the first few hours whatever the cause of the initial bleed,[28] but delayed rebleeding or continued oozing is more likely to occur with a structural vascular cause such as an aneurysm or AVM or with an underlying tumor. Emergency angiography is, therefore, necessary if an aneurysm is suspected. After clot evacuation, delayed angiography should be considered to eliminate an AVM. This step must not be forgotten in a patient who makes a reasonable recovery, because the results of a second hemorrhage are often worse than those of the first.

Assessment of Dependence and Disability

Unfortunately, the quality of life in survivors of ICH is often poor. Most neurosurgeons prefer to use the GOS[88]; as assessed with this scale, good recovery occurs in only 5% of patients, with 10% moderately disabled (independent) and 40% remaining severely disabled (SD) (dependent).[46] Stroke physicians prefer to use the Rankin and Barthell Scales; once again, very few patients become independent when rated on these scales.

The GOS was originally developed by Jennett and Bond[88] for use in head injury studies. "Severe disability" was used for patients who were dependent on daily support because of mental disability, physical disability, or both. Patients with "moderate disability" could travel by public transport and could work in a sheltered environment, could shop independently, and were therefore independent as far as daily life was concerned. Moderately disabled patients could have residual disabilities such as hemiparesis, dysphasia, memory deficits, or personality changes, but this category did not include patients who were able only to care for themselves in their own homes; such patients were described instead as being severely disabled. "Good

Table 63.3   Logistic Regression Analysis of Independent Predictors of Outcome from 440 Newcastle Patients with Intracerebral Hemorrhage in the Prospectively Collected Database (Dec 1993–Aug 1999)

	P	Odds Ratio	95% Confidence Interval Lower	95% Confidence Interval Upper
Age	<0.0001	0.9493	0.9277	0.9715
Verbal Glasgow Coma Scale score	0.0013	1.4697	1.1630	1.8574
Location: basal ganglia or lobar	<0.0001	7.0618	3.3713	14.7922
Hematoma volume <20 mL compared with >40 mL	<0.0001	7.9539	3.3807	18.7132
Hematoma volume 20–40 mL compared with >40 mL	0.0035	3.6871	1.5344	8.8598
Basal cisterns (open)	0.0251	12.2821	1.3685	110.2258

From Siddique MS: Intracerebral Hemorrhage: The global magnitude of the problem and the scientific basis for intervention in the acute phase.

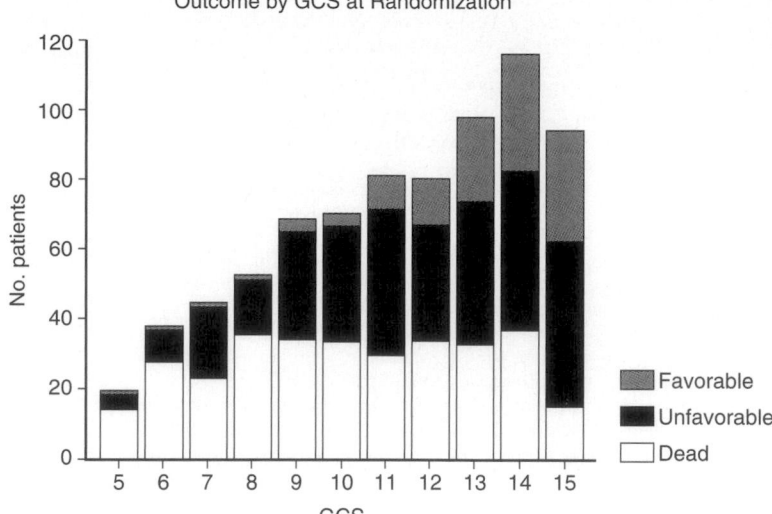

FIGURE 63–10 *Outcome plotted against Glasgow Coma Scale (GCS) score in relation to random assignment to treatment for patients in the Surgical Trial in Intracerebral Hemorrhage (STICH).*

recovery" implied a resumption of normal life, including the capacity to return to work, to leisure, and family relationships. When Jennett and Bond[88] used this classification in their study of more than 500 survivors of severe head injury, 7% were classified as vegetative, 29% as severely disabled, and 33% as moderately disabled, and 31% made a good recovery. To compare groups treated in different ways, the scale was dichotomized into unfavorable outcome (dead, vegetative, or severely disabled) and favorable outcome (moderate disability or good recovery).

With time, the GOS has been used more and more frequently to measure outcome in patients with conditions other than head injury, including stroke, aneurysmal subarachnoid hemorrhage, and spontaneous ICH. The use of this scale in such patient groups must take into account the differences in age, health, and social independence before the event and, hence, the potential for recovery. For many elderly patients, it is clear that independence *within* the home should be regarded as a favorable outcome, but this independence might not include the ability to use public transportation or to shop independently. Such an outcome would certainly be considered favorable for patients who initially present in coma. For patients with ICH, traditional classification to an outcome of severe disability would apply to three quarters of the group, but the category would vary widely from people who were able to look after themselves all day within their own homes to those who were bedridden and needed total care. The GOS should therefore be modified for use in patients with stroke and ICH to take into account these widely differing abilities.

The extended GOS (GOS-E) provides a finer classification of outcome because it subdivides each of the categories into an upper and lower level of disability.[89] It is clear that patients with ICH who are admitted to the hospital in coma very rarely achieve a good recovery or moderate disability whatever treatment they receive, whereas those with ICH and an admission Glasgow Coma Scale score of 14 or 15 may achieve these outcome levels (Fig. 63–10). Thus, a single dichotomous outcome division, uniform for the whole patient group, is less sensitive than measures that take into account the severity of the condi-

tion at the outset and the varying potential for improvement in individual patients. A sliding dichotomy has therefore been proposed,[14] with the breakpoints between moderate disability and severe disability for the groups with the best prognoses and between upper and lower severe disability for the groups with the worst prognoses. This clinical logic has been ignored in the analysis of most stroke trials, which have tended to lump all patients into just one category. Outcome analysis by statisticians should, therefore, recognize this stratification of initial severity, especially with hemorrhagic stroke, although ischemic strokes also differ in initial severity.

Rehabilitation

For all patients with stroke who survive, rehabilitation is critical and should begin early. The very poor outcomes with hemorrhagic stroke place a great burden on rehabilitation staff, who should recognize that extra time and effort are required for these patients with ICH and that unsatisfactory final results may be predestined. An integrated multidisciplinary approach is desirable, especially in patients with ICH.

References

1. Sudlow M, et al: Prevalence of atrial fibrillation and eligibility for anticoagulants in the community. Lancet 352:1167–1171, 1998.
2. Siddique MS: Intracerebral hemorrhage: The global magnitude of the problem and the scientific basis for intervention in the acute phase. In Department of Neurosurgery (MD Thesis). Newcastle-upon-Tyne, UK, University of Newcastle-upon-Tyne, 2003, pp 39–78.
3. Gregson BA, et al: Variation in rates of surgery in centres in different countries in the International STICH trial. Stroke. Submitted, 2003.
4. Wiebers DO: Assessing risks of treating patients with unruptured intracranial aneurysms: The International Study Of Unruptured Intracranial Aneurysms. Cerebrovasc Dis 13(Suppl 3):0427, 2002.
5. Brown RDJ: The natural history of unruptured intracranial aneurysms: Prospective data from the International Study Of Unruptured Intracranial Aneurysms. Cerebrovasc Dis 13(Suppl 3):0426, 2002.
6. Mathers C, et al: Healthy life expectancy in 191 countries, 1999. Lancet 357:1685–1691, 2001.

Therapy

7. Tissue plasminogen activator for acute ischemic stroke. The National Institute of Neurological Diseases and Stroke rt-PA Stroke Study Group. N Engl J Med 333:1581–1587, 1995.

8. Qureshi AI, et al: Crack cocaine use and stroke in young patients. Neurology 48:341–345, 1997.

9. Palmer J, Sparrow OC, Ianotti F: Postoperative hematoma: A 5-year survey and identification of avoidable risk factors. Neurosurgery 35:1064–1065, 1994.

10. Cushing H: Some experimental and clinical observations concerning states of increased intracranial tension. Am J Med Sci 124:375–400, 1902.

11. Heiskanen O, et al: Acute surgery for intracerebral hematomas caused by rupture of an intracranial arterial aneurysm: A prospective randomized study. Acta Neurochir (Wein), 90:81–83, 1988.

12. Broderick JP, et al: Volume of intracerebral hemorrhage: A powerful and easy-to-use predictor of 30-day mortality [see comments]. Stroke 24:987–993, 1993; comment in Stroke 24:1761, 1993.

13. Fernandes HM: Primary intracerebral hemorrhage: A study of its effects upon intracranial hemodynamics, current surgical practice and a trial of early surgery. In Department of Neurosurgery (MD Thesis). Newcastle-upon-Tyne, UK, University of Newcastle-upon-Tyne, 2002, p 280.

14. Murray G, et al: Design and Analysis of Phase III trials with ordered outcome scales: The concept of the sliding dichotomy. (In submission) 2002.

15. Heiss W-D, et al: Nontraumatic intracerebral hematoma versus ischemic stroke: Regional pattern of glucose metabolism. J Cereb Blood Flow Metab 5:S5–S6, 1985.

16. Uemura K, et al: Positron emission tomography in patients with a primary intracerebral hematoma. Acta Radiol Suppl 369:426–428, 1986.

17. Powers WJ, et al: Autoregulation of cerebral blood flow surrounding acute (6 to 22 hours) intracerebral hemorrhage. Neurology 57:18–24, 2001.

18. Videen TO, et al: Correction for partial volume effects in regional blood flow measurements adjacent to hematomas in humans with intracerebral hemorrhage: Implementation and validation. J Comput Assist Tomogr 23:248–256, 1999.

19. Zazulia AR, et al: Hypoperfusion without ischemia surrounding acute intracerebral hemorrhage. J Cereb Blood Flow Metab 21:804–810, 2001.

20. Siddique MS, et al: Reversible ischemia around intracerebral hemorrhage: A single-photon emission computerized tomography study. J Neurosurg 96:736–741, 2002.

21. Bullock R, et al: Intracranial hemorrhage induced at arterial pressure in the rat. Part 1: Description of technique, ICP changes and neurological findings. Neurol Res 6:184–188, 1984.

22. Mendelow AD, et al: Intracranial hemorrhage induced at arterial pressure in the rat. Part 2: Short term changes in local cerebral blood flow measured by autoradiography. Neurol Res 6:189–193, 1984.

23. Rosand J, et al: Dynamic single-section CT demonstrates reduced cerebral blood flow in acute intracerebral hemorrhage. Cerebrovasc Dis 14:214–220, 2002.

24. Kanno T, Nonomura K: Hyperbaric oxygen therapy to determine the surgical indication of moderate hypertensive intracerebral hemorrhage. Minim Invasive Neurosurg 39:56–59, 1996.

25. Heiss WD: Ischemic penumbra: Evidence from functional imaging in man. J Cereb Blood Flow Metab 20:1276–1293, 2000.

26. Gebel JM, et al: Relative edema volume is a predictor of outcome in patients with hyperacute spontaneous intracerebral hemorrhage. Stroke 33:2636–2641, 2002.

27. Gebel JM, et al: Natural history of perihematomal edema in patients with hyperacute spontaneous intracerebral hemorrhage. Stroke 33:2631–2635, 2002.

28. Brott TG, et al: Early hemorrhage growth in patients with intracerebral hemorrhage. Stroke 28:1–5, 1997.

29. Pickard JD, et al: The effect of oral nimodipine on cerebral infarction and outcome after subarachnoid hemorrhage. British Aneurysm Nimodipine Trial. Br Med J 298:636–642, 1989.

30. Chandra B: Small intracerebral bleedings: To treat or not to treat? Cerebrovasc Dis 13(Suppl 3):0188, 2002.

31. Kerr R, et al: Intracerebral hematoma due to aneurysmal rupture: Endovascular treatment followed by clot evacuation. In 12th World Congress of Neurosurgery. Sydney, World Federation of Neurosurgical Societies, 2001.

32. Stevenson J, Jenkins A, Mendelow A: Experimental intracerebral hemorrhage—U74006F (tirilazad mesylate) reduces ischemic neuronal damage. J Neurosurg 82:359, 1995.

33. Kane PJ, et al: Cerebral oedema following intracerebral hemorrhage: The effect of the NMDA receptor antagonists MK-801 and D-CPPene. Acta Neurochir Suppl 60:561–563, 1994.

34. Davis M, et al: Age and the risk of stroke progression in the acute stroke monitoring trial. Cerebrovasc Dis 13(Suppl 3):0424, 2002.

35. Meyer JS, Bauer RB: Medical treatment of spontaneous intracerebral hemorrhage by the use of hypotensive drugs. Neurology 12:36–47, 1962.

36. Yu YL, et al: Treatment of acute cerebral hemorrhage with intravenous glycerol: A double-blind, placebo-controlled, randomized trial. Stroke 23:967–971, 1992.

37. Hemodilution in acute stroke: Results of the Italian hemodilution trial. Italian Acute Stroke Study Group. Lancet 1(8581):318–321, 1988.

38. Tellez H, Bauer RB: Dexamethasone as treatment in cerebrovascular disease. 1: A controlled study in intracerebral hemorrhage. Stroke 4:541–546, 1973.

39. Poungvarin N, et al: Effects of dexamethasone in primary supratentorial intracerebral hemorrhage. N Engl J Med 316:1229–1233, 1987.

40. Prasad K, Shrivastava A: Surgery for primary supratentorial intracerebral hemorrhage. Cochrane Database Syst Rev CD00200, 2000.

41. Fernandes HM, et al: Surgery in intracerebral hemorrhage: The uncertainty continues. Stroke 31:2511–2516, 2000.

42. Teernstra OPM, et al: Stereotactic aspiration of intracerebral haematoma by means of a plasminogen activator. A multicentric randomized controlled trial (SKHPA). Stroke 34: 968–974, 2003.

43. Mendelow AD, et al: The International STICH trial: An update. In Brain Edema XII. Kurion A, et al (eds). Acta Neurochirurgica (In press) 2003.

44. Huang J, van Gelder JM: The probability of sudden death from rupture of intracranial aneurysms: A meta-analysis. Neurosurgery 51:1101–1107, 2002.

45. Mathew P, et al: Neurosurgical management of cerebellar hematoma and infarct. J Neurol Neurosurg Psychiatry 59:287–292, 1995.

46. Siddique MS, et al: Comparative study of traumatic and spontaneous intracerebral hemorrhage. J Neurosurg 96:86–89, 2002.

47. Chen X, Yang H, Cheng Z: The comparative study of the total medical and surgical treatment of hypertensive intracerebral hemorrhage. Acta Academia Medicinae Shanghai 19:234–240, 1992.

48. Chen B, Hou D: Surgical treatment of hypertensive intracerebral hemorrhage. Chin Med J 94:723–728, 1981.

49. McKissock W, Richardson A, Taylor J: Primary intracerebral hemorrhage: A controlled trial of surgical and conservative treatment in 180 unselected cases. Lancet 2:221–226, 1961.

50. Pia HW: The surgical treatment of intracerebral and intraventricular hematomas. Acta Neurochir 27:149, 1972.

51. Zunghui L, et al: Evacuation of hypertensive intracerebral hematoma by a stereotactic technique. Stereotact Funct Neurosurg 54:451–452, 1990.

52. Niizuma H, et al: Results of stereotactic aspiration in 175 cases of putaminal hemorrhage. Neurosurgery 24:814–819, 1989.

53. Mohadjer M: Computed tomographic-stereotactic evacuation and fibrinolysis of spontaneous intracerebral hematomas. In Lorenz R, Klinger M, Brock M (eds): Advances in Neurosurgery. Berlin, Springer-Verlag, 1993, pp 47–51.

54. Hondo H, et al: Computed tomography controlled aspiration surgery for hypertensive intracerebral hemorrhage: Experience of more than 400 cases. Stereotact Funct Neurosurg 54:432–437, 1990.

55. Kanaya H, et al: A neurological grading for patients with hypertensive intracerebral hemorrhage and a classification for hematoma location of computer tomography. Presented at 7th Conference of Surgical Treatment of Stroke, Japan, 1978, pp 265–270.

56. Kanno T, et al: Role of surgery in hypertensive intracerebral hematoma: A comparative study of 305 nonsurgical and 154 surgical cases. J Neurosurg 61:1091–1099, 1984.

57. Coraddu M, et al: Considerations about the surgical indication of the spontaneous cerebral hematomas. J Neurosurg Sci 34:35–39, 1990.

58. Kanaya H, Kuroda K: Intracerebral hematomas: Development in Neurosurgical Approaches to Hypertensive Intracerebral Hemorrhage in Japan. Kaufmann H. H. (Ed.) Intracerebral Hematomas. New York, Raven Press, 1992, pp 197–209.

59. Fernandes HM, Mendelow AD: Spontaneous intracerebral hemorrhage: A surgical dilemma. Br J Neurosurg 13:389–394, 1999.

60. Taylor A, Butt W, Rosenfeld J, et al: A randomized trial of very early decompressive craniectomy in children with traumatic brain injury and sustained intracranial hypertension. Childs Nerv Syst 17:154–162, 2001.

61. Cruz J, Minoja G, Okuchi K: Improving clinical outcomes from acute subdural hematomas with the emergency preoperative administration of high doses of mannitol: A randomized trial. Neurosurgery 49:864–871, 2001.

62. Cruz J, Minoja G, Okuchi K: Major clinical and physiological benefits of early high doses of mannitol for intraparenchymal temporal lobe hemorrhages with abnormal pupillary widening: A randomized trial. Neurosurgery 51:628–637, 2002.

63. Chambers IR, Treadwell L, Mendelow AD: The determination of threshold levels of cerebral perfusion pressure and intracranial pressure in severe head injury using receiver operator characteristic curves: An observational study on 291 patients. J Neurosurg 94:412–416, 2001.

64. Auer LM, et al: Endoscopic surgery versus medical treatment for spontaneous intracerebral hematoma: A randomized study. J Neurosurg 70:530–535, 1989.

65. Marquardt G, Wolff R, et al: Manual stereotactic aspiration of spontaneous deep-seated intracerebral hematomas in non-comatose patients. Br J Neurosurg 15:126–131, 2001.

66. Teernstra O, et al: Stereotactic Treatment of Intracerebral Hematoma by means of a Plasminogen Activator, a multicentre randomised controlled trial (SICHPA). In 4th World Stroke Conference. Melbourne, Australia: American Heart Association, 2000.

67. Teernstra OPM, et al: SICHPA: Stereotactic Treatment of Intracerebral Hematoma by Means of a Plasminogen Activator: A Multicentre Randomised Controlled Trial. In 12th World Congress of Neurosurgery. Sydney, World Federation of Neurosurgical Societies, 2001.

68. Arene NU, et al: Intraventricular hemorrhage from spontaneous intracerebral hemorrhage and aneurysmal rupture: In von Wild HRH (Ed.): Pathophysiological principles and controversies in neurointensive care. W. Zuckschwerdt Verlag (Munchen) 134–138, 1998.

69. Molyneux A, Kerr R, Stratton I, Sandercock P, et al: International Subarachnoid Aneurysm Trial (ISAT) of neurosurgical clipping versus endovascular coiling in 2143 patients with ruptured intracranial aneurysms: a randomised trial. International Subarachnoid Aneurysm Trial (ISAT) Collaborative Group. Lancet 360:1267–1274, 2002.

70. Auer LM, Auer T, Sayama I: Indications for surgical treatment of cerebellar hemorrhage and infarction. Acta Neurochir 79:74–79, 1986.

71. Donauer E, et al: Prognostic factors in the treatment of cerebellar hemorrhage. Acta Neurochir 131:59–66, 1994.

72. Dunne JW, Chakera T, Kermode S: Cerebellar hemorrhage: Diagnosis and treatment: A study of 75 consecutive cases. Q J Med 64:739–754, 1987.

73. Firsching R, Huber M, Frowein RA: Cerebellar hemorrhage: Management and prognosis. Neurosurg Rev 14:191–194, 1991.

74. Gerritsen van der Hoop R, Vermeulen N, van Gijn J: Cerebellar hemorrhage: Diagnosis and treatment. Surg Neurol 29:6–10, 1988.

75. Heros RC: Cerebellar hemorrhage and infarction. Stroke 29:6–10, 1982.

76. Koziarski A, Frankiewicz E: Medical and surgical treatment of intracerebellar hematomas. Acta Neurochir 110:24–28, 1991.

77. Lui T, et al: Surgical treatment of spontaneous cerebellar hemorrhage. Surg Neurol 23:555–558, 1985.

78. Waidhauser E, Hamburger C, Marguth F: Neurosurgical management of cerebellar hemorrhage. Neurosurg Rev 13:211–217, 1990.

79. Ott KH, et al: Cerebellar hemorrhage: Diagnosis and treatment. A review of 56 cases. Arch Neurol 31:160–167, 1974.

80. Brennan RW, Bergland RM: Acute cerebellar hemorrhage: Analysis of clinical findings and outcome in 12 cases. Neurology 27:527–532, 1977.

81. Fisher CM, et al: Acute hypertensive cerebellar hemorrhage: Diagnosis and surgical treatment. J Nerv Mental Dis 140:38–57, 1965.

82. Black M, Graham D: Sudden unexplained death in adults caused by intracranial pathology. J Clin Pathol 55:44–50, 2002.

83. Faught E, et al: Seizures after primary intracerebral hemorrhage. Neurology 39:1089–1093, 1989.

84. Lancman M, et al: Risk factors for developing seizures after a stroke. Epilepsia 34:141–143, 1993.

85. Sung C, Chu NS: Epileptic seizures in intracerebral hemorrhage. J Neurol Neurosurg Psychiatry 52:1273–1276, 1989.

86. Arboix X, et al: Predictive factors of early seizures after cerebrovascular disease. Stroke 28:1590–1594, 1997.

87. Cervoni L, et al: Epileptic seizures in intracerebral hemorrhage: A clinical and prognostic study of 55 cases. Neurosurg Rev 17:185–188, 1994.

88. Jennett B, Bond M: Assessment of outcome after severe brain damage. Lancet 1(7905):480–484, 1975.

89. Wilson JT, Pettigrew LE, Teasdale GM: Structured interviews for the Glasgow Outcome Scale and the extended Glasgow Outcome Scale: Guidelines for their use. J Neurotrauma 15:573–585, 1998.

Therapy

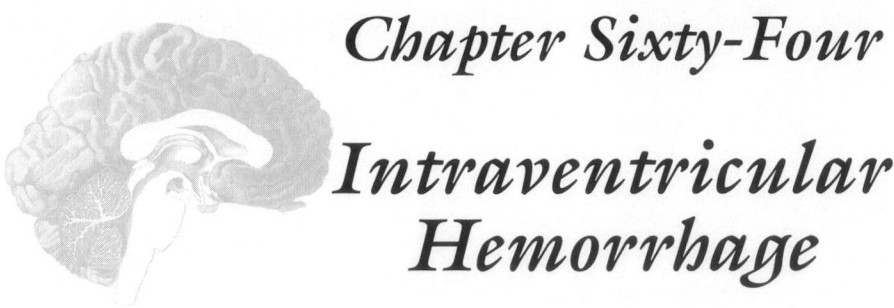

Chapter Sixty-Four

Intraventricular Hemorrhage

J. Max Findlay

Bleeding directly into the ventricles from a source or lesion that is in contact with or is part of a ventricular wall, such as a vascular malformation or neoplasm, is classified as *primary intraventricular hemorrhage* (IVH). This type of IVH without an associated parenchymal hematoma is rare, accounting for only about 3% of all spontaneous intracerebral hemorrhages (ICHs).[1] Much more commonly, IVH is secondary either to intracerebral bleeding that dissects through brain parenchyma to reach a ventricle or to bleeding into the subarachnoid space that spreads into the ventricles through the fourth ventricular foraminae. Primary or secondary IVHs can fill one or more ventricles and, when of sufficient volume and density, can result in formed ventricular blood clots, or *hematocephalus*. Blood that refluxes into the ventricles from the subarachnoid space often remains unclotted and settles in dependent parts of the ventricular system. Although the presence of IVH per se does not always correlate with neurologic condition or prognosis, IVH is an independent and important clinical problem when clots distend the ventricular system, compress adjacent brain, or obstruct cerebrospinal fluid (CSF) flow to cause hydrocephalus and elevated intracranial pressure (ICP).

As shown in Table 64.1, many causes of spontaneous ICH can result in IVH, but the most common are hypertensive ICH, saccular aneurysms, and arteriovenous malformations (AVMs).[2–8] IVH resulting from germinal matrix hemorrhage in the newborn and traumatic IVH are not reviewed in this chapter.

PRIMARY INTRAVENTRICULAR HEMORRHAGE

Spontaneous, primary IVH is most often due either to a vascular malformation that contacts the ependyma of one of the ventricular chambers (Fig. 64–1) or to an intraventricular or periventricular neoplasm.[7] There have been rare reports of primary IVH due to ruptured intraventricular aneurysms, which arise from distal lenticulostriate or choroidal arteries that reach the ventricular lining or choroid plexus.[9] Aneurysms have been reported on penetrating arteries enlarged by moyamoya disease.[10–12] In some cases, no cause of primary IVH can be established, and it

has been proposed that in these instances, bleeding may be from rupture of arterioles located in the immediate periventricular region that have been weakened by chronic hypertension. Primary IVH can be due to any type of bleeding disorder, including anticoagulation[8] and fibrinolytic treatment.[13,14] My colleagues and I have treated one patient with a large IVH due to hemorrhagic infarction of the choroid plexus (Fig. 64–2).

The most common brain neoplasm that bleeds spontaneously is malignant astrocytoma. Rarer tumors causing primary IVH are ependymoma,[15] subependymoma,[16] choroid plexus papilloma,[17] intraventricular meningioma,[18,19] pituitary tumors that erode through the floor of the third ventricle,[20] neurocytoma,[21] granular-cell tumor,[22] and metastasis.[23] It is likely that any cause of primary ICH can be responsible for direct bleeding in the ventricles.

HYPERTENSIVE BRAIN HEMORRHAGE AND INTRAVENTRICULAR HEMORRHAGE

Spontaneous hypertensive ICHs are associated with secondary IVH in one third to one half of patients.[24] The most significant risk factor for this arteriopathy, which most commonly affects the lenticulostriate and thalamoperforating arterioles, is chronic arterial hypertension; other risk factors are moderate to heavy alcohol intake and anticoagulant treatment.[25] IVH most often complicates thalamic, putaminal, or caudate bleeding that spreads into the lateral or third ventricles (Fig. 64–3). Not surprisingly, IVH in this setting has been associated with larger parenchymal hematomas, midline shift of brain structures, and worse clinical outcome.[26,27]

ANEURYSMAL INTRAVENTRICULAR HEMORRHAGE

Of patients who survive rupture of an intracranial aneurysm, IVH is seen in roughly 15% of the entire group, in 25% of those with severe subarachnoid hemorrhage (SAH), and in 40% of those who subsequently die from the

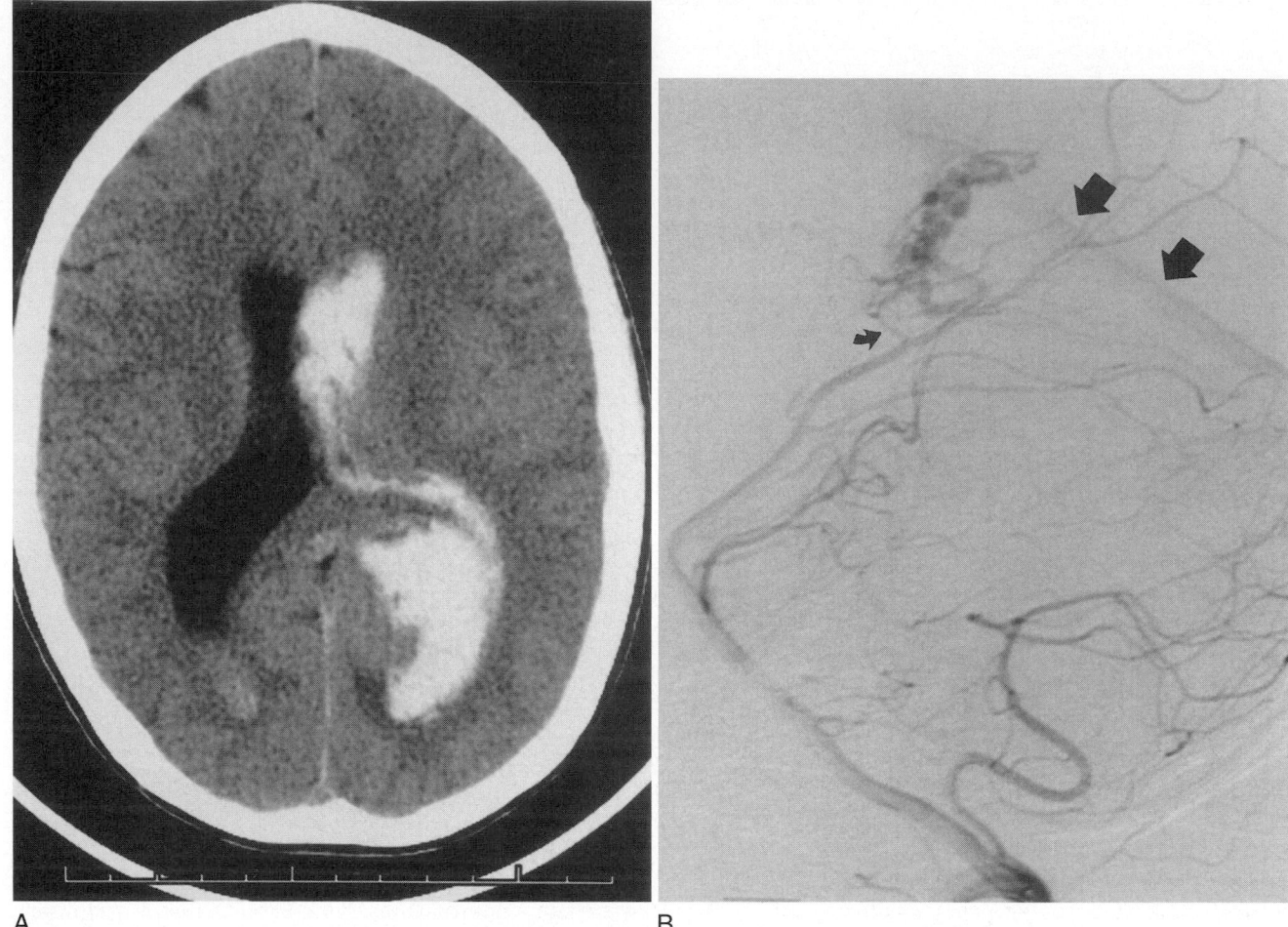

FIGURE 64–1   *A large left-sided lateral ventricular primary ventricular hemorrhage* (A), *arising from a ruptured trigonal arteriovenous malformation fed by the lateral posterior choroidal artery* (small arrow in B), *in an 11-year-old patient. Note the deep venous drainage via the vein of Galen and straight sinus* (large arrows).

Table 64.1   Causes of Intraventricular Hemorrhage

Primary intraventricular hemorrhage	Germinal matrix hemorrhage in the premature newborn
	Intraventricular or periventricular vascular malformation (i.e., arteriovenous malformation, cavernous malformation)
	Intraventricular or periventricular tumor (i.e., papilloma, meningioma, subependymoma, astrocytoma)
	Coagulation or platelet disorder
	Trauma
	Insertion or removal of ventricular catheter
	Intraventricular or periventricular arterial aneurysm (rare)
	Idiopathic
Secondary intraventricular hemorrhage	Hypertensive brain hemorrhage
	Aneurysm (i.e., saccular, mycotic)
	Vascular malformation
	Tumor (i.e., metastasis, malignant astrocytomas)
	Pituitary apoplexy
	Coagulation or platelet disorder
	Vasculitis and amyloid angiopathy
	Trauma
	Hemorrhagic cerebral infarction
	Illicit drug use (i.e., amphetamines)

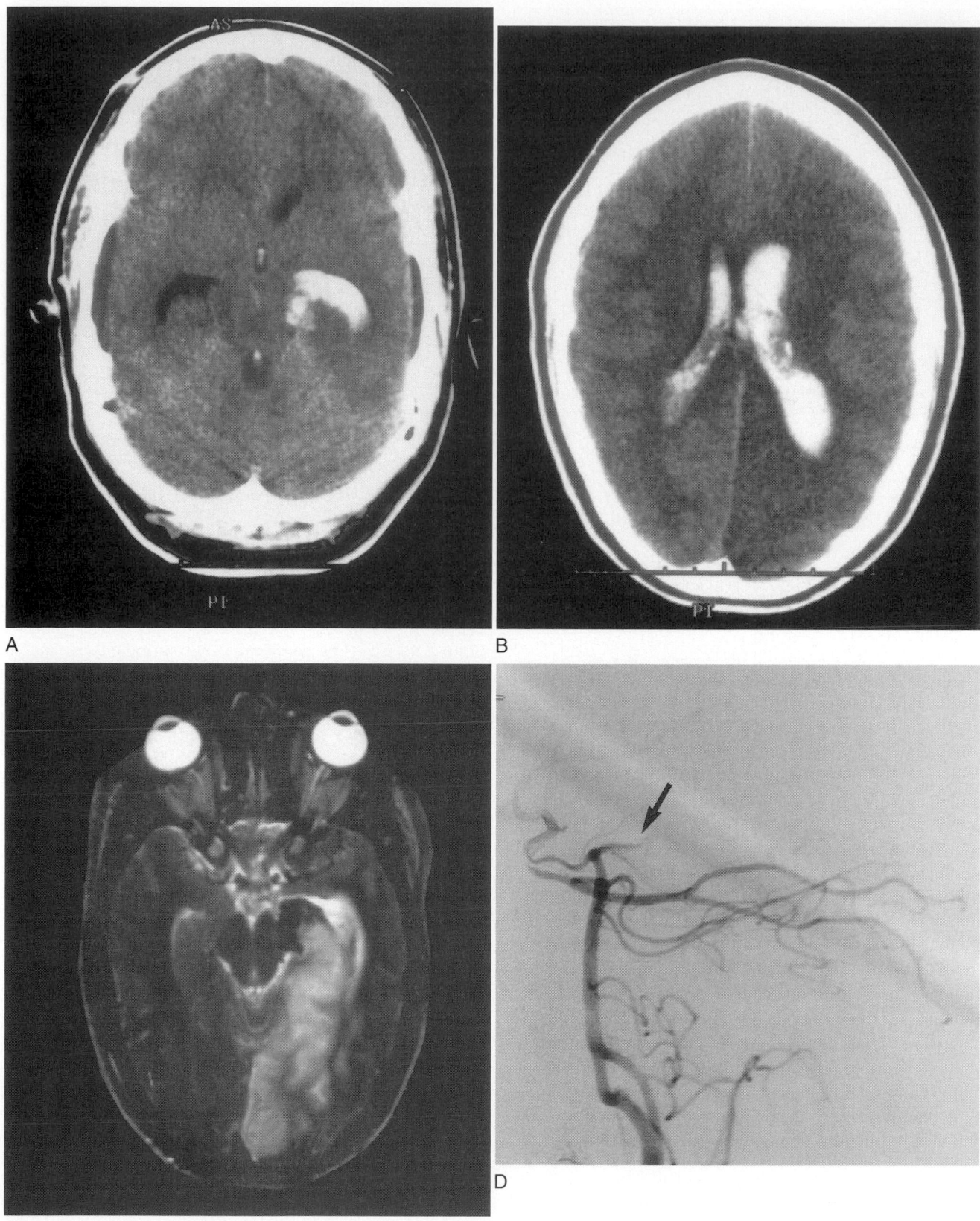

FIGURE 64–2   A and B, A previously healthy 20-year-old man presented with a sudden loss of consciousness due to a large primary intraventricular hemorrhage that appeared to arise in the left trigone. C, Repeat CT scanning and MRI revealed infarction in the distribution of the left posterior cerebral artery. D, Cerebral angiography showed occlusion of the proximal left posterior cerebral artery (arrow), the underlying cause of the infarctions of the left occipital cortex and choroid plexus, the latter of which became hemorrhagic. Despite a detailed cardiologic and vascular disease evaluation, the underlying cause of the vessel occlusion was not found.

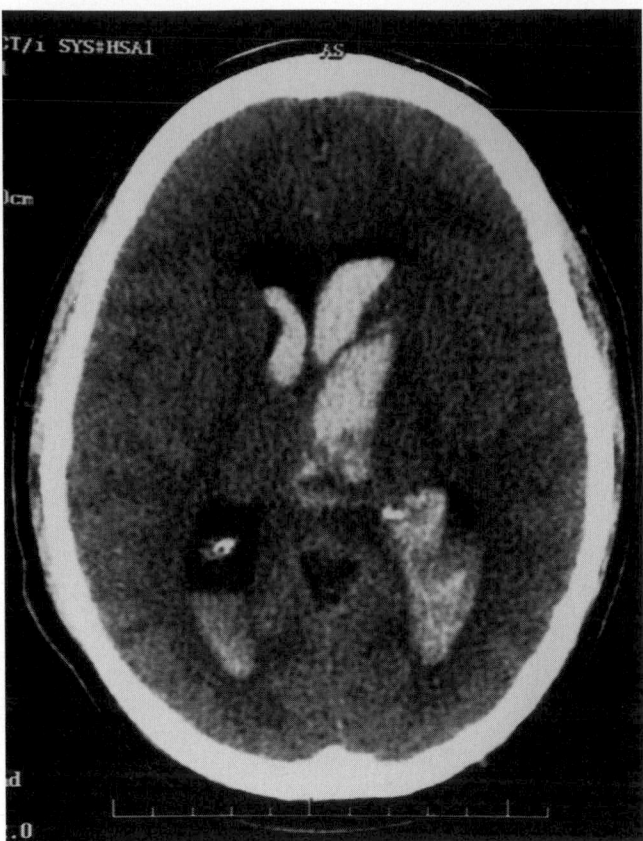

FIGURE 64–3 *A hypertensive left thalamic intracerebral hemorrhage with secondary extension into the third ventricle and both lateral ventricles.*

rupture.[28] Aneurysmal IVH is associated with an up to 50% chance of requiring a ventriculoperitoneal shunt (Fig. 64–4).[29,30] Aneurysm rupture can cause IVH through several different mechanisms.[31] Blood can reflux into the ventricular system from an aneurysm in any location, but disproportionate or isolated fourth ventricular hemorrhage in association with SAH is especially suggestive of a posterior circulation aneurysm situated closer to the fourth ventricular foraminae. Up to one half of posterior inferior cerebellar artery (PICA) aneurysm ruptures have an accompanying IVH.[32]

Sudden death from aneurysmal SAH is commonly associated with IVH, and in some patients, the mechanism may be acute fourth ventricular dilatation.[33,34]

Aneurysms also cause secondary IVH when forceful hemorrhage dissects through intervening brain parenchyma to reach the ventricular system. This occurrence is most commonly seen with anterior communicating aneurysms.[35] With a 25% incidence of associated IVH, this aneurysm is the most common type to cause IVH. Blood can break directly through the lamina terminalis into the third ventricle or can pass superiorly beneath the rostrum of the corpus callosum to leak into the septum pellucidum, distending it and then rupturing into the lateral ventricles. Frontal hemorrhages resulting from anterior communicating or middle cerebral artery aneurysms can spread into the anterior horn of the lateral ventricles.

Internal carotid artery aneurysm, at the origin of either the posterior communicating or the anterior choroidal arteries, can rupture into the temporal horn of the lateral ventricles. Basilar apex aneurysms can rupture directly through the hypothalamus to reach the third ventricle, usually with serious clinical consequences.

VASCULAR MALFORMATIONS AND INTRAVENTRICULAR HEMORRHAGE

Subependymal, choroid plexus, and cerebral AVMs that extend to the ventricular wall commonly rupture primarily into the ventricles, although cerebral AVMs more commonly bleed into both parenchyma and ventricle. Ventricular hemorrhage is particularly associated with deep venous drainage. In a prospective AVM database, 16% of first AVM hemorrhages were intraventricular, and 31% occurred in combined locations.[36] Periventricular cavernous malformations and dural arteriovenous fistulas with transcerebral venous drainage can also cause IVH.

NATURAL CLEARANCE OF INTRAVENTRICULAR HEMORRHAGE

Normally, the CSF contains little fibrinolytic activity, although fibrinolysis becomes detectable after bleeding into the CSF. As in plasma, the principal fibrinolytic enzyme in the CSF is plasmin, which is carried into the ventricles in its precursor form, plasminogen, as a normal constituent of blood. It is converted to its active form by tissue plasminogen activator (t-PA). Tissue plasminogen activator is released from the endothelium of small vessels in the meninges and ependyma, and leukocytes and platelets within the ventricular thrombi are additional sources of plasminogen activator enzymes. These various activators diffuse into clot, bind to fibrin, and activate plasminogen incorporated into the coagulum. The degree of fibrinolytic activity is meager relative to plasma, but appears proportional to the volume of blood clots, and is balanced by the presence of inhibitors also released by irritated leptomeninges.[37] Changes in CSF coagulation and fibrinolysis have been studied in the context of SAH but are probably similar to changes seen after IVH.[38]

The resolution of intraventricular blood clot appears to follow first-order kinetics, such that the daily percentage rate of clot breakdown and clot half-life is constant and the absolute amount of clot broken down per day rises with increasing IVH volume.[39] The clearance of erythrocytes from CSF is accomplished by several mechanisms. The first is hemolysis, which begins within hours and reaches a plateau 2 to 10 days after IVH, depending on the size of the hemorrhage. Another is phagocytosis by macrophages, which occurs both in the leptomeninges irritated by blood and in arachnoid granulations engorged with erythrocytes.

CLINICAL FEATURES

Spontaneous and primary IVH manifests as sudden headache, vomiting, and sometimes decreased consciousness.[5]

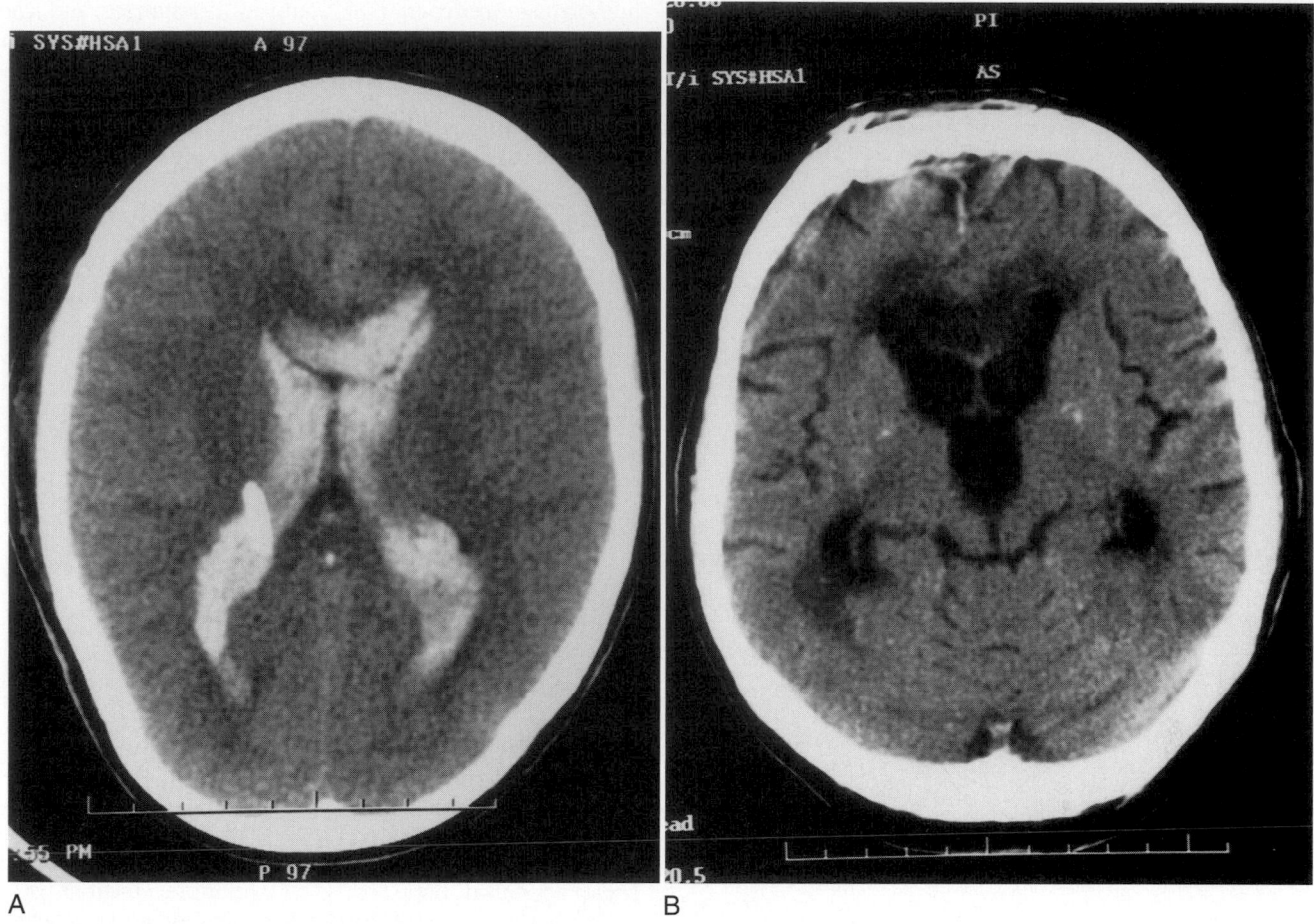

FIGURE 64–4 A, *A distal anterior cerebral artery aneurysm arising at the origin of the left pericallosal branch caused hemorrhage through the corpus callosum and secondary intraventricular bleeding.* B, *Three months later, the 64-year-old patient presented again with lethargy and obtundation because of delayed posthemorrhagic hydrocephalus.*

A generalized seizure may occur, but without any significant associated ICH, focal signs are generally absent. Symptoms from even a large primary IVH can sometimes be surprisingly minimal, provided that the ventricles have not become distended and the ICP remains normal. The total volume of CSF in adults is approximately 150 mL, and the normal ventricular volume is 20 to 30 mL. The possible connections among acute fourth ventricular distention after aneurysm rupture with brainstem compression, advanced neurologic deterioration, and early death have already been mentioned.

With secondary IVH, presenting symptoms are usually due to the associated ICH or SAH. The nature and magnitude of the symptoms and signs correspond to the location and size of the hemorrhage.

Symptomatic vasospasm of the anterior and middle cerebral arteries after an AVM-related IVH has been described,[40,41] but the complication is exceptional after hemorrhage restricted to the ventricles. Delayed-onset cerebral vasospasm after aneurysm rupture depends on thick blood clots deposited in the basal subarachnoid cisterns and left in prolonged contact with the adventitial surface of arteries. The presence of thick subarachnoid hematoma with blood clots also in both lateral ventricles

may predict an even higher risk of delayed cerebral ischemia after aneurysm rupture.[42]

Noncommunicating hydrocephalus can occur acutely after IVH if clots obstruct CSF drainage within the ventricular system, and communicating hydrocephalus may develop more gradually or even in a very delayed fashion because of obstruction and then scarring of the arachnoid granulations from blood elements carried to them by CSF flow. The risk of hydrocephalus correlates with the severity of the IVH and is greater if there is blood in the third or fourth ventricle or if there is associated SAH. In spontaneous supratentorial ICH, secondary IVH correlates with the presence of acute hydrocephalus and poor outcome.[43] Acute hydrocephalus is seen in roughly 15% of patients with ruptured aneurysms, and its presence is also significantly related to the computed tomography (CT) features of IVH.[44]

DIAGNOSIS

Intraventricular hemorrhage is usually diagnosed on CT scanning, and several different scoring systems have been devised to quantitate the extent of spontaneous adult IVH seen on CT scan (Table 64.2).[45] Although IVH numerical

Table 64.2   Grading System for Severity of Intraventricular Hemorrhage*

Score	Criterion II
1	Less than half of ventricle filled with blood
2	More than half of ventricle filled with blood
3	Ventricle filled and distended with blood

*Third ventricle, fourth ventricle, and each lateral ventricle are scored separately. All the scores are then summed (maximum total score = 12).

scores are useful in comparing volumes of IVH among patients, clinical condition and prognosis are more closely related to ventricular distention, associated parenchymal damage, and the underlying cause of bleeding.

If CT scanning shows IVH secondary to a deep (thalamic or ganglionic) parenchymal hemorrhage in an older patient, a small vessel cause can usually be assumed, and further investigation can be avoided. Similarly, if the primary hemorrhage is lobar and is strongly suspected to be secondary to a bleeding disorder, amyloid angiopathy, or conversion of a cardioembolic infarct, angiography is often unwarranted. If the underlying cause of IVH remains uncertain, angiography, magnetic resonance imaging (MRI), or both are indicated, especially if thrombolytic therapy (discussed in the next section) is being considered (Fig. 64–5). Further imaging is firmly recommended for any patient with primary IVH and no apparent cause, and for any patient younger than 45 years who has an IVH.[6, 45]

TREATMENT

Management is directed at any identified underlying cause of IVH (aneurysm repair, AVM or tumor excision, blood pressure control, correction of bleeding disorder, etc.) as well as external ventricular drainage to relieve any associated hydrocephalus and help manage raised ICP. Surgical evacuation through a frontal corticotomy of lateral ventricles packed with clot after aneurysm rupture was judged not to be useful,[46] but there has been one case report of an apparently successful fourth ventricle decompression.[47]

A common complication of ventriculostomy for IVH is catheter occlusion with blood clot, necessitating irrigation or replacement of the catheter. With obstruction of the foramen of Monro, bilateral ventricular drainage tubes are sometimes necessary. Infection becomes a risk among patients with IVH in whom prolonged drainage is required.[48] In addition, ventricular drainage alone has a limited ability to relieve cerebral compression due to intraventricular blood clots themselves.

Intraventricular fibrinolytic treatment using urokinase or recombinant tissue plasminogen activator (rt-PA) has been tested. Experiments in a dog model of IVH showed that repeated ventricular injections of urokinase without ventricular drainage could speed the clearance of ventricular clots and reduce hydrocephalus.[49,50] A single intraventricular injection of recombinant t-PA (rt-PA) in pigs with experimental IVH also accelerated clot clearance and restored normal ventricular size.[51] An injection of rt-PA in the cisterna magna of cats after experimental subarachnoid

hemorrhage reduced CSF outflow resistance, and the reestablishment of normal CSF absorption pathways reduced morphologic hydrocephalus.[52,53]

A number of reports have studied fibrinolytic treatment for IVH in humans. Injections or infusions of urokinase or rt-PA, administered through external ventricular drainage catheters, have been used to treat IVH from a variety of causes, including aneurysm and AVM rupture, chronic hypertension, ventricular catheter insertion, trauma, and germinal matrix hemorrhage in the newborn.[54-65] The total dose of fibrinolytic agent and number of days they have been given have varied, but collectively, these preliminary studies have suggested that fibrinolytic treatment accelerates the clearance of ventricular blood clots. Ventricles clear within several days, usually beginning in the third and fourth ventricles, accompanied by normalization of ventricular size. One series has indicated that treatment helps control elevated ICP.[66] A systematic review of studies reporting on either conservative, external drainage or external drainage plus fibrinolysis concluded that ventricular drainage combined with fibrinolytic therapy may improve outcome, although that impression was derived from indirect comparison between observational studies.[67] Another cohort study compared patients who received urokinase with those who were treated with ventriculostomy alone.[68] Nearly all patients had suffered hypertensive ICHs with secondary IVH, and treatment consisted of 10,000 U urokinase, given every 12 hours through a frontal ventricular catheter, combined with intervening ventricular drainage. Urokinase was stopped when the third ventricle appeared open on CT. Urokinase resulted in a significantly faster rate of ventricular clearance, a lower mortality rate, and a trend toward more favorable outcomes (67% rate of poor outcome in untreated patients compared with 32% in urokinase-treated patients).

Another multicenter trial indicated better 30-day survival for urokinase-treated patients with spontaneous IVH.[64] Most studies have indicated that the treatment is quite safe, but there has been one report describing two patients (out of a total of eight treated) who had intraventricular rebleeding from hypertensive thalamic hemorrhages after rt-PA treatment, although one of these patients received additional rt-PA to clear the increased IVH without further complications.[69]

Urokinase is no longer available for clinical use, so currently, intraventricular fibrinolysis is generally accomplished with rt-PA.[56,57,64] Intraventricular rt-PA can be considered for patients with large IVHs that expand and occlude the ventricular system but without large parenchymal hematomas or clinical conditions that would predict an unfavorable outcome. Although clinical judgment must be applied to each case, most physicians would not undertake fibrinolytic treatment in a patient in whom CT showed deep or dominant brain destruction, a patient with severely elevated ICP, or a patient with rapidly failing brainstem activity.

One protocol is to begin treatment after CT confirmation of results of uncomplicated surgery for aneurysm or AVM repair (if applicable) and satisfactory ventricular catheter placement. A 2- to 4-mg (1 mg/mL) dose of rt-PA is given slowly through the ventricular catheter with frequent checks of ICP to ensure that it does not reach

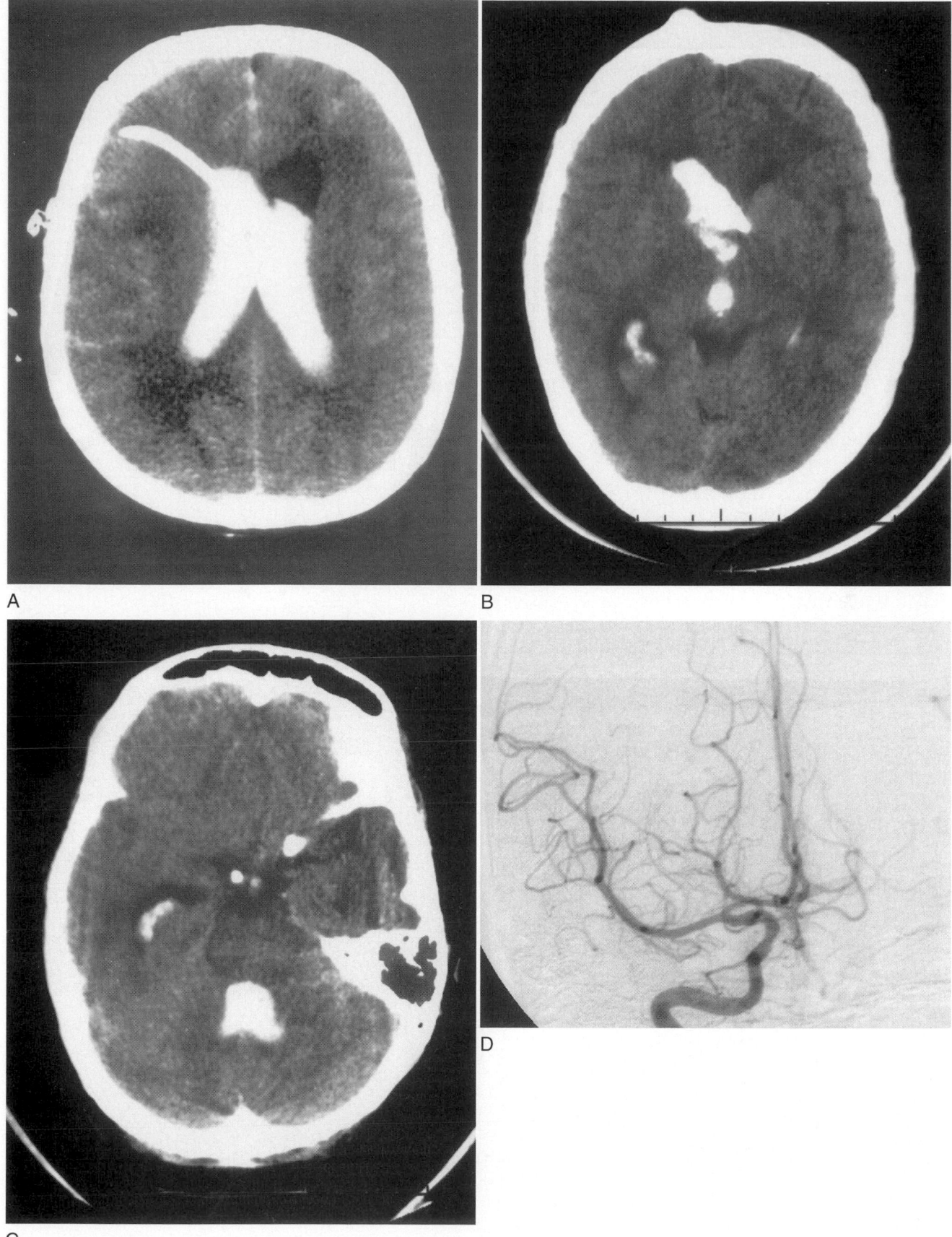

FIGURE 64–5   *A to C, At presentation, a previously healthy nonhypertensive 40-year-old Asian woman was unconscious with a pan-ventricular hemorrhage. Cerebral angiography, (D) and MRI (E) (on next page) did not reveal an underlying cause. The patient was treated with a total of 8 mg of recombinant tissue plasminogen activator (rt-PA) through a ventriculostomy over 2 days.*

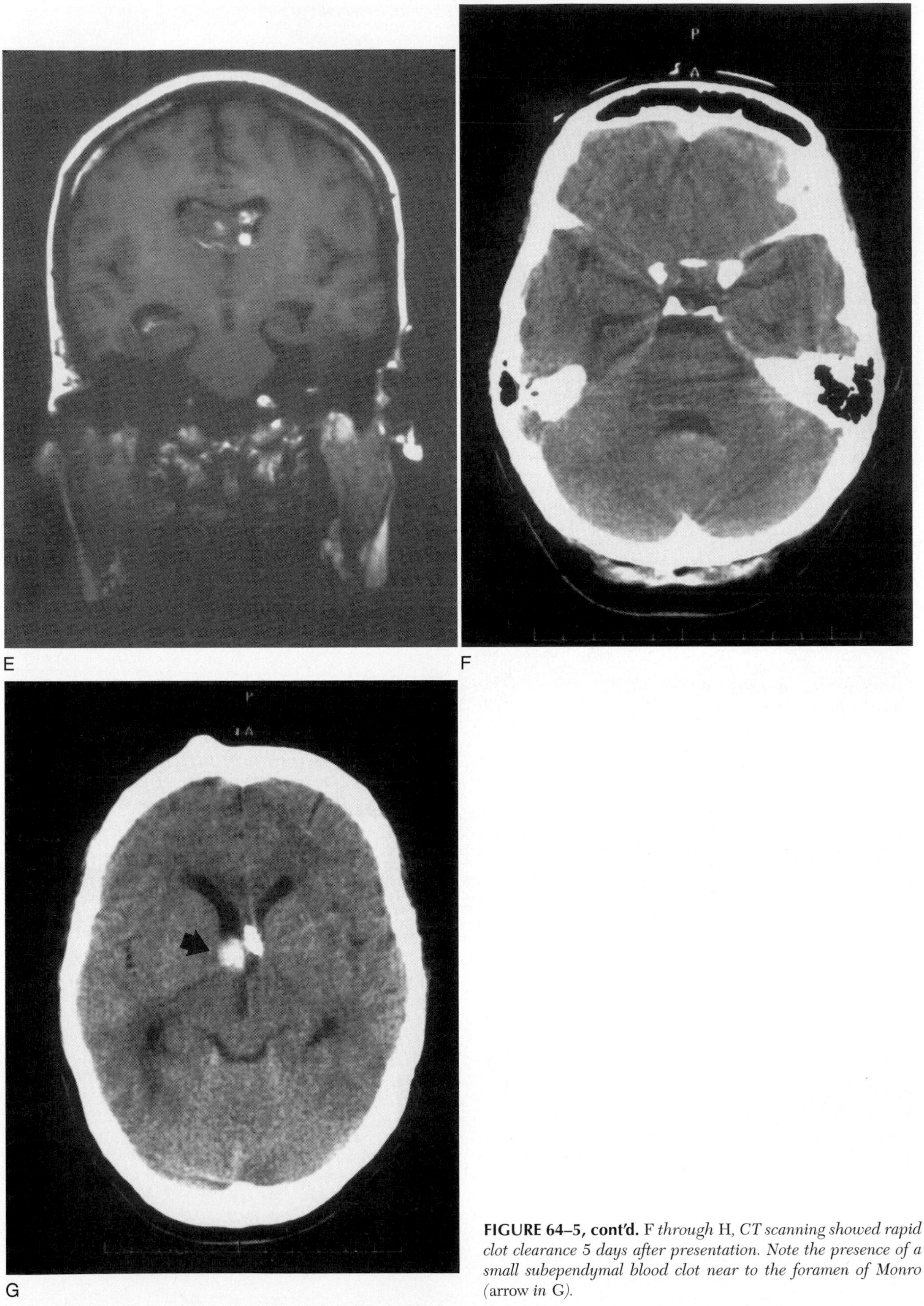

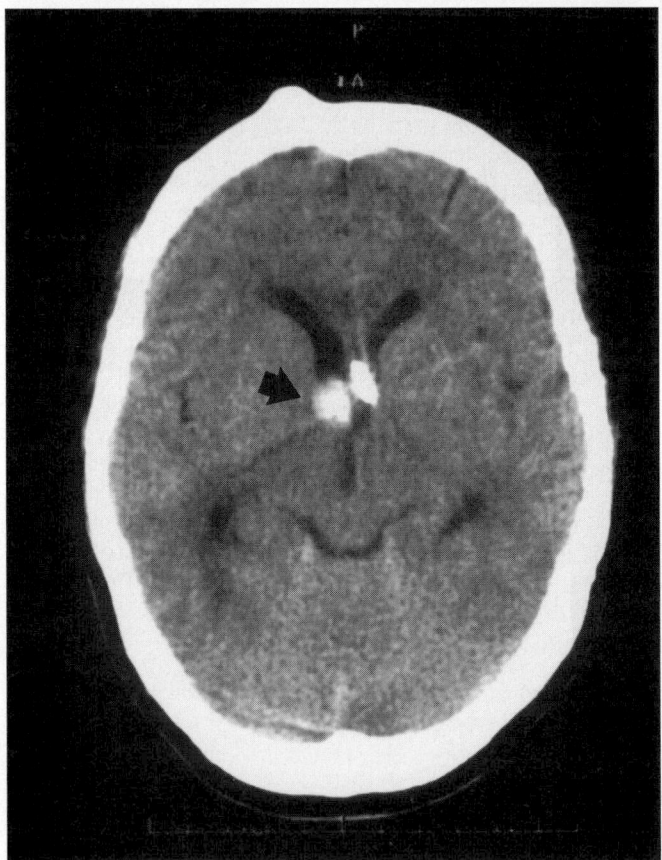

E

F

G

FIGURE 64–5, cont'd. *F through* H, *CT scanning showed rapid clot clearance 5 days after presentation. Note the presence of a small subependymal blood clot near to the foramen of Monro (arrow in* G).

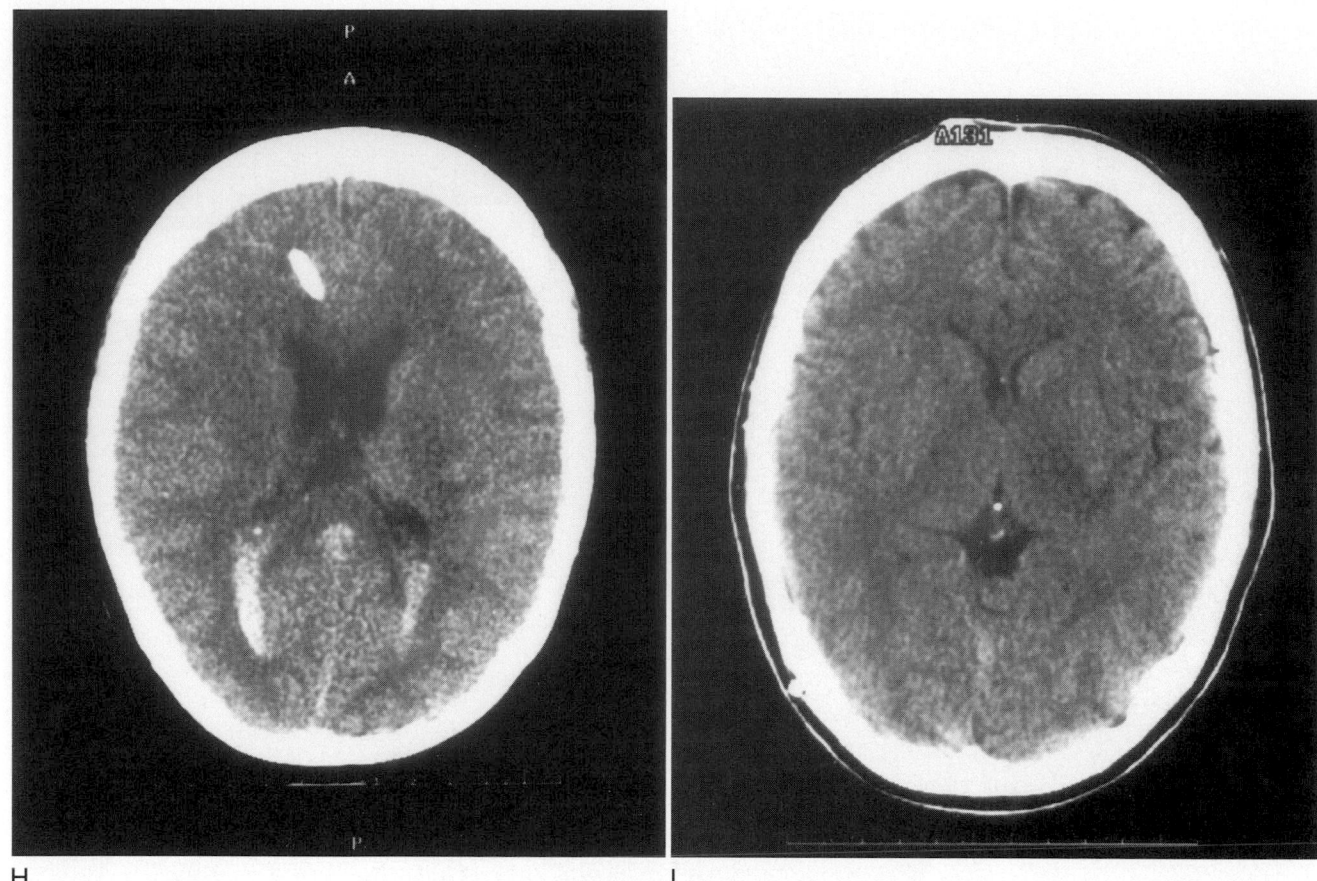

H　　　　　　　　　　　　　　　I

FIGURE 64–5, cont'd. *Several months later, both CT (I) and MRI findings were normal.*

dangerous levels, which would compromise cerebral perfusion pressure. If the patient tolerates only a portion of the 4-mg dose, the rest can be given several hours later. The ventricular drain is closed for 1 hour and is then opened to drain against a pressure gradient of 1 to 2 cm (above the level of the external auditory canal) for 1 hour. The drain is then opened and closed during alternating hours for the next 24 hours. CT scanning is performed daily for the first several days, and additional rt-PA can be given if necessary, with the goal being to open ventricular pathways (especially the foramen of Monro, the third and the fourth ventricles), restore normal ventricular size, treat intracranial hypertension, and maintain catheter patency (Fig. 64–6). Complete clearance of clot settled in dependent parts of the ventricular chambers is not necessary.

Tissue plasminogen activator is supplied as a 50-mg lyophilized powder cake that must be reconstituted with sterile water for use. In order to prevent waste of unused rt-PA and reduce cost, the hospital pharmacy can reconstitute the cake, divide the rt-PA solution into 10 mg (10-mL) aliquots, and store them in syringes in a freezer at −80°C. Under these conditions, the enzyme remains active for up to 12 months. Once a single syringe is thawed for use, the rt-PA solution within that syringe remains active for several weeks if stored in a refrigerator, and a single syringe usually provides sufficient rt-PA for a single patient with IVH.

As shown in Table 64.3, most patients that my colleagues and I have treated required one to two injections of rt-PA to establish patency of the ventricular system within 2 to 3 days. There have been two complications of intracerebral hemorrhage in our series; one patient had multifocal parenchymal hemorrhages and concomitant disseminated intravascular coagulation, and another patient experienced a frontal hemorrhage adjacent to the ventricular catheter. Neither patient required surgery for the ICH. Results of CSF culture have been positive in two patients during rt-PA treatment but while they were still undergoing ventricular drainage; neither patient experienced clinical ventriculitis. No patient has required ventricular drain replacement for obstruction once treatment has begun, but roughly one-third of the treated patients have gone on to require ventriculoperitoneal shunting in follow-up (longest follow-up, 8 years).

PROGNOSIS

The presence of IVH does not necessarily portend a poor prognosis in every patient, as was once thought. Even quite large primary IVHs can be associated with a good clinical condition and a good outcome.[70,71] However, secondary IVHs associated with large subarachnoid or intracerebral hemorrhage or anticoagulant treatment are associated with

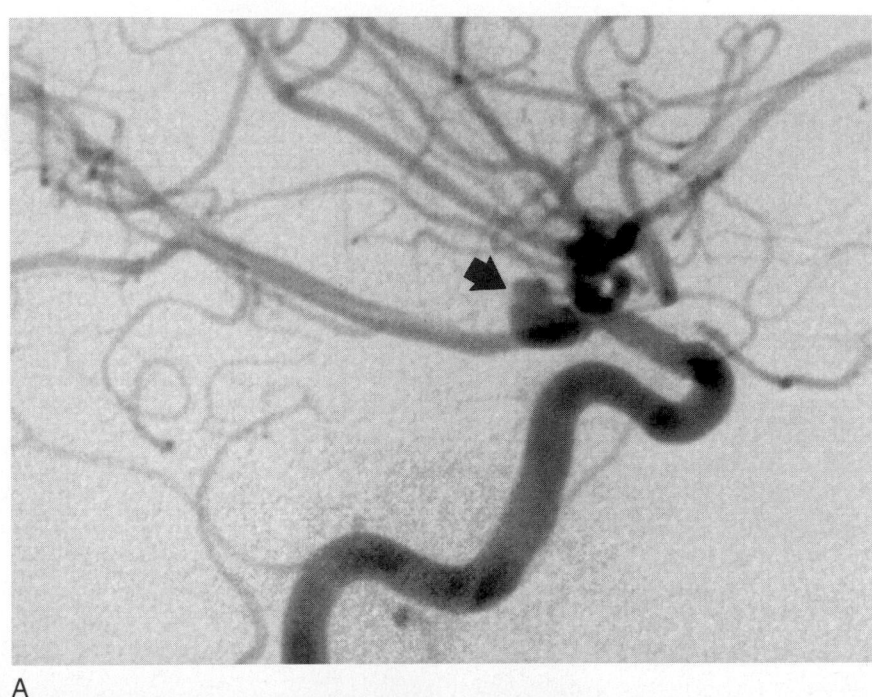

A

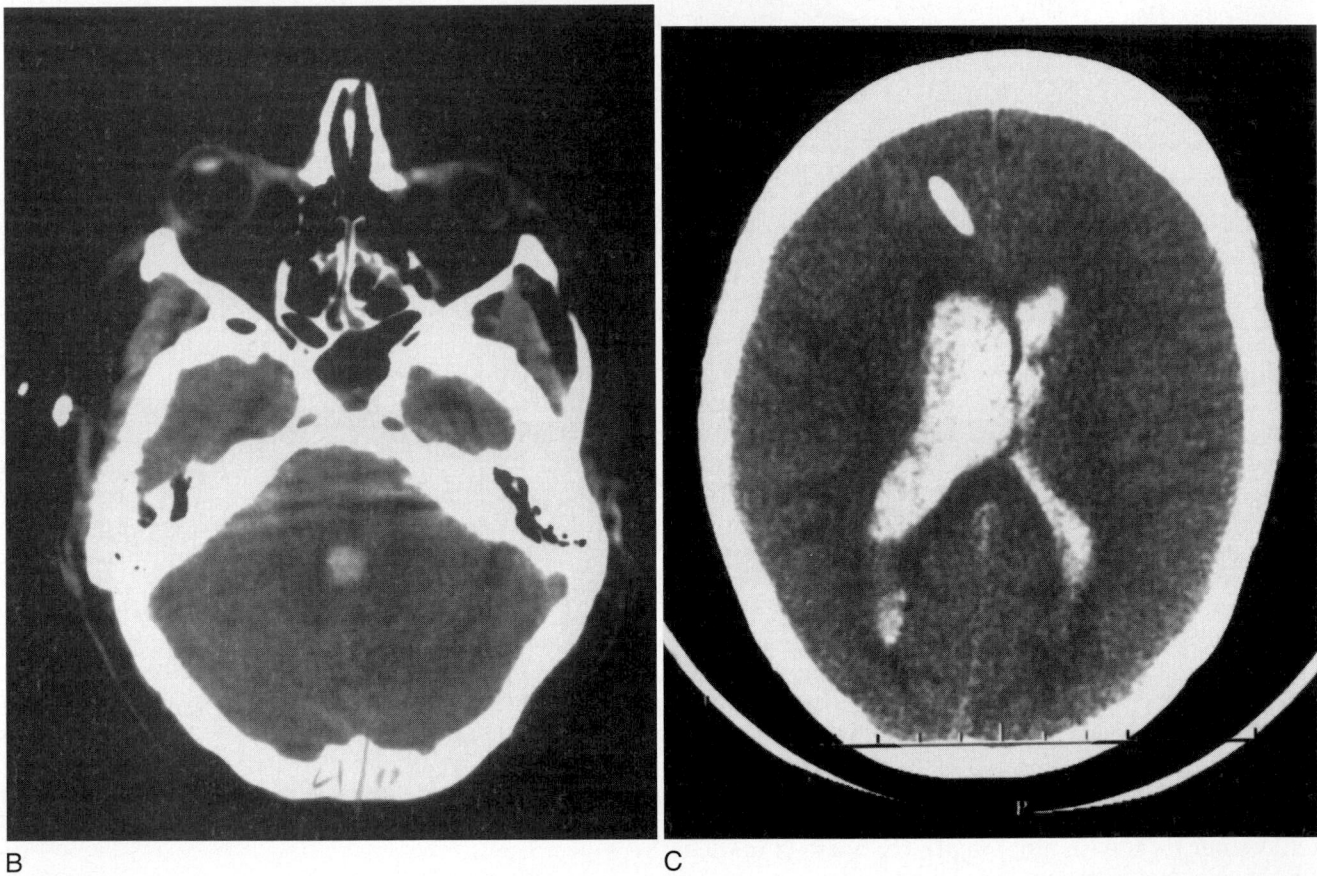

B   C

FIGURE 64–6   *A 44-year-old man experienced sudden loss of consciousness from the rupture of a right internal carotid–posterior communicating artery aneurysm (arrow in A), which resulted in a right temporal lobe and panventricular hemorrhage (B and C).*

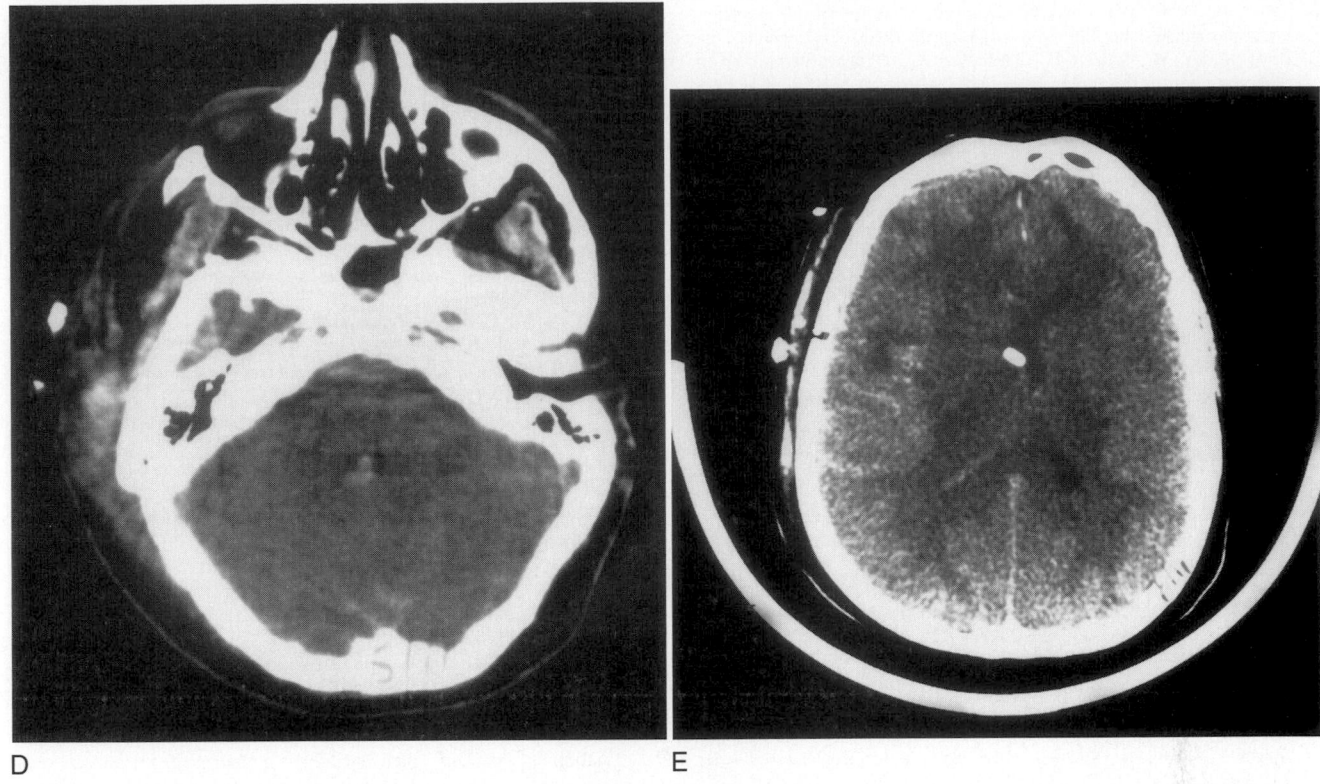

D E

FIGURE 64–6, cont'd. *After ventriculostomy and microsurgical clip repair of the aneurysm, 4 mg of intraventricular recombinant tissue plasminogen activator (rt-PA) resulted in fourth ventricular clot lysis (D), and a second injection of the same dose resulted in rapid clearance of the third and lateral ventricular hematomas by the third day after aneurysm rupture and surgical repair (E).*

Table 64.3 Treatment of 36 Patients with Intraventricular Hemorrhage (IVH) with Recombinant Tissue Plasminogen Activator (rt-PA)*

Etiology of IVH		
Aneurysm	22	(61%)
Arteriovenous malformation	4	(11%)
Hypertension	5	(14%)
Ventriculostomy	2	(6%)
Uncertain	3	(8%)
Number of rt-PA injections per patient		
1	18	(50%)
2	14	(39%)
3	4	(11%)
Total dose of rt-PA (mg) per patient		
2–4	18	(50%)
5–8	14	(39%)
9–12	3	(8%)
15	1	(3%)
Number of days from treatment onset to opening of ventricular system[†]		
1	5	(14%)
2	11	(31%)
3	15	(42%)
4	5	(14%)
Ventriculoperitoneal shunt required	12	(33%)
Treatment complication[‡]	2	(6%)
Outcome[§]		
Good	13	(36%)
Moderate disability	14	(39%)
Severe disability	6	(17%)
Death	3	(8%)

*Series of patients treated at the University of Alberta, 1990–2001.
[†]Opening defined as patency within all ventricles, IVH score <2 per ventricle.
[‡]See text for details.
[§]Glasgow Outcome Scale (see reference 75).

poorer neurologic condition on presentation and a worse outcome.[72–74] Massive IVH that produces fourth ventricular distention and periventricular cerebral compression is an especially ominous sign associated with early death.[32]

Patients with large IVHs who survive hemorrhage without vital brain destruction are potential candidates for fibrinolytic treatment. Intraventricular fibrinolysis helps maintain ventriculostomy patency, promotes rapid IVH clearance, and sometimes facilitates ICP management. Whether or not fibrinolysis reduces long-term shunt requirements is uncertain. These issues as well as the effect of intraventricular fibrinolysis on long-term patient outcome, may be clarified in a randomized controlled trial.[64]

References

1. Darby DG, Donnan GA, Saling MA, et al: Primary intraventricular hemorrhage: Clinical and neuropsychological findings in a prospective stroke series. Neurology 38:68–75, 1988.
2. Pia HW: The surgical treatment of intracerebral and intraventricular haematomas. Acta Neurochir 27:149–164, 1972.
3. Little JR, Blomquist GA Jr, Ethier R: Intraventricular hemorrhage in adults. Surg Neurol 8:143–149, 1977.
4. Donauer E, Reif J, Al-Khalaf E, et al: Intraventricular haemorrhage caused by aneurysms and angiomas. Acta Neurochir 122:23–31, 1993.
5. Angelopoulos M, Gupta SR, Azat KB: Primary intraventricular hemorrhage in adults: Clinical features, risk factors, and outcome. Surg Neurol 44:433–436, 1995.
6. Chang DS, Lin CL, Howng SL: Primary intraventricular hemorrhage in adult—an analysis of 24 cases. Kao Hsiung I Hsueh Ko Hsueh Tsa Chih 14:633–638, 1998.
7. Marti-Fabregas J, Piles S, Guardia E, Marti-Vilalta JL: Spontaneous primary intraventricular hemorrhage: Clinical data, etiology and outcome. J Neurol 246:287–291, 1999.

Therapy

8. Taheri SA, Wani MA, Lewko J: Uncommon causes of intraventricular hemorrhage. Clin Neurol Neurosurg 92–3:195–202, 1990.

9. Bergsneider M, Grazee JG, DeSalles AA: Thalamostriate artery aneurysm within the third ventricle. J Neurosurg 81:463–465, 1994.

10. Hamada J, Hashimoto N, Tsukahara T: Moyamoya disease with repeated intraventricular hemorrhage due to aneurysm rupture. J Neurosurg 80:328–331, 1994.

11. Newman P, Al-Menar A: Intraventricular hemorrhage in pregnancy due to Moyamoya disease. J Neurol Neurosurg Psychiatry 64:686, 1998.

12. Larrazabal R, Pelz D, Findlay JM: Endovascular treatment of a lenticulostriate artery aneurysm with N-butyl cyanoacrylate. Can J Neurol Sci 28:256–259, 2001.

13. Szabo K, Sommer A, Gass A, et al: Rapid resorption of intraventricular hemorrhage after thrombolytic therapy of ischemic stroke. Cerebrovasc Dis 12:144, 2001.

14. Gebel JL, Sila CA, Sloan MA, et al: Thrombolysis-related intracranial hemorrhage: A radiographic analysis of 244 cases from the GUSTO-1 trial with clinical correlation. Stroke 29:563–569, 1998.

15. Toffol GJ, Biller J, Adams HP Jr: Nontraumatic intracerebral hemorrhage in young adults. Arch Neurol 44:483–485, 1987.

16. Lindboe CF, Stolt-Nielsen A, Dale LG: Hemorrhage in a highly vascularized subependymoma of the septum pellucidum: Case report. Neurosurgery 31:741–745, 1992.

17. Matsushima M, Yamamoto T, Motomochi M, Ando K: Papilloma and venous angioma of the choroid plexus causing primary intraventricular hemorrhage. J Neurosurg 39:666–670, 1973.

18. Lang I, Jackson A, Strang FA: Intraventricular hemorrhage caused by intraventricular meningioma: CT appearance. AJNR Am J Neuroradiol 6:1378–1381, 1995.

19. Murai Y, Yoshida D, Ikeda Y, et al: Spontaneous intraventricular hemorrhage caused by lateral ventricular meningioma—case report. Neurol Med Chir (Tokyo) 36:586–589, 1996.

20. Challa VR, Richards F II, Davis CH Jr: Intraventricular hemorrhage from pituitary apoplexy. Surg Neurol 16:360–361, 1981.

21. Okamura A, Goto S, Sato K, Ushio Y: Central neurocytoma with hemorrhagic onset. Surg Neurol 43:252–255, 1995.

22. Graziani N, Dufour H, Figarella-Branger D, et al: Suprasellar granular-cell tumor, presenting with intraventricular haemorrhage. Br J Neurosurg 9:97–102, 1995.

23. Mandybur TI: Intracranial hemorrhage caused by metastatic tumors. Neurology 27:650–655, 1977.

24. Young WB, Lee KP, Pessin MS: Prognostic significance of ventricular blood in supratentorial hemorrhage: A volumetric study. Neurology 40:616–619, 1990.

25. Juevela S, Hillbom M, Palomäki: Risk factors for spontaneous intracerebral hemorrhage. Stroke 26:1558–1564, 1995.

26. Broderick JP, Brott TG, Duldner JE, et al: Volume of intracerebral hemorrhage: A powerful and easy-to-use predictor of 30-day mortality. Stroke 24:987–993, 1993.

27. Ruscalleda J, Peiró A: Prognostic factors in intraparenchymatous hematoma with ventricular hemorrhage. Neuroradiology 28:34–37, 1986.

28. Findlay JM: Intraventricular hemorrhage. Neurosurg Q 10:182–195, 2000.

29. Vale FL, Bradley EL, Fisher WS III: The relationship of subarachnoid hemorrhage and the need for postoperative shunting. J Neurosurg 86:462–466, 1997.

30. Graff-Radford NR, Torner J, Adams HP Jr, Kassell NF: Factors associated with hydrocephalus after subarachnoid hemorrhage. Arch Neurol 46:744–752, 1989.

31. Inagawa T, Hirano A: Ruptured intracranial aneurysms: An autopsy study of 133 patients. Surg Neurol 33:117–123, 1990.

32. Ruelle A, Cavazzani P, Andrioli G: Extracranial posterior inferior cerebellar artery aneurysm causing isolated intraventricular hemorrhage: A case report. Neurosurgery 23:774–777, 1988.

33. Schievink WI, Wijdicks EFM, Parisi JE, et al: Sudden death from aneurysmal subarachnoid hemorrhage. Neurology 45:871–874, 1995.

34. Shapiro SA, Campbell RL, Scully T: Hemorrhagic dilation of the fourth ventricle: An ominous predictor. J Neurosurg 80:805–809, 1994.

35. Mohr G, Ferguson G, Khan M, et al: Intraventricular hemorrhage from ruptured aneurysm: Retrospective analysis of 91 cases. J Neurosurg 58:482–487, 1983.

36. Hartmann A, Mast H, Mohr JP, et al: Morbidity of intracranial hemorrhage in patients with cerebral arteriovenous malformation. Stroke 29:931–934, 1998.

37. Findlay JM, Weir BKA, Kanamaru K, et al: Intrathecal fibrinolytic therapy after subarachnoid hemorrhage: Dosage study in a primate model and review of the literature. Can J Neurol Sci 16:28–40, 1989.

38. Ikeda K, Asakura H, Futami K, Yamashita J: Coagulative and fibrinolytic activation in cerebrospinal fluid and plasma after subarachnoid hemorrhage. Neurosurgery 41:344–350, 1997.

39. Naff NJ, Williams MA, Rigamonti D, et al: Blood clot resolution in human cerebrospinal fluid: Evidence of first-order kinetics. Neurosurgery 49:614–621, 2001.

40. Yanaka K, Hyodo A, Tsuchida Y, et al: Symptomatic cerebral vasospasm after intraventricular hemorrhage from ruptured arteriovenous malformation. Surg Neurol 38:63–67, 1992.

41. Maeda K, Kurita H, Nakamura T, et al: Occurrence of severe vasospasm following intraventricular hemorrhage from an arteriovenous malformation: Report of two cases. J Neurosurg 87:436–439, 1997.

42. Classen J, Bernardini GL, Kreiter K, et al: Effect of cisternal and ventricular blood on risk of delayed cerebral ischemia after subarachnoid hemorrhage: The Fisher Scale revisited. Stroke 32:2012–2020, 2001.

43. Diringer MN, Edwards DF, Zazulia AR: Hydrocephalus: A previously unrecognized predictor of poor outcome from supratentorial intracerebral hemorrhage. Stroke 29:1352–1357, 1998.

44. Mohr G, Ferguson G, Khan M, et al: Intraventricular hemorrhage from ruptured aneurysm: Retrospective analysis of 91 cases. J Neurosurg 58:482–487, 1983.

45. Graeb DA, Robertson WD, Lapointe JS, et al: Computed tomographic diagnosis of intraventricular hemorrhage. Radiology 143:91–96, 1982.

46. Shimoda M, Oda S, Shibata M, et al: Results of early surgical evacuation of packed intraventricular hemorrhage from aneurysm rupture in patients with poor-grade subarachnoid hemorrhage. J Neurosurg 91:408–414, 1999.

47. Lagares A, Putman CM, Ogilvy CS: Posterior fossa decompression and clot evacuation for fourth ventricle hemorrhage after aneurysmal rupture: Case report. Neurosurgery 49:208–211, 2001.

48. Mayhall CG, Archer NH, Lamb VA, et al: Ventriculostomy-related infections: A prospective epidemiologic study. N Engl J Med 310:553–559, 1984.

49. Pang D, Sclabassi RJ, Horton JA: Lysis of intraventricular blood clot with urokinase in a canine model: Part 1: Canine intraventricular blood cast model. Neurosurgery 19:540–546, 1986.

50. Pang D, Sclabassi RJ, Horton JA: Lysis of intraventricular blood clot with urokinase in a canine model: Part 2: In vivo safety study of intraventricular urokinase. Neurosurgery 19:547–552, 1986.

51. Mayfrank L, Kissler J, Raoofi R, et al: Ventricular dilatation in experimental intraventricular hemorrhage in pigs: Characterization of cerebrospinal fluid dynamics and the effects of fibrinolytic treatment. Stroke 28:141–148, 1997.

52. Brinker T, Seifert V, Stolke D: Effect of intrathecal fibrinolysis on cerebrospinal fluid absorption after experimental subarachnoid hemorrhage. J Neurosurg 74:789–793, 1991.

53. Brinker T, Seifert V, Dietz H: Subacute hydrocephalus after experimental subarachnoid hemorrhage: Its prevention by intrathecal fibrinolysis with recombinant tissue plasminogen activator. Neurosurgery 31:306–312, 1992.

54. Shen PH, Matsuoka Y, Kawajiri K, et al: Treatment of intraventricular hemorrhage using urokinase. Neurol Med Chir (Tokyo) 30:329–333, 1990.

55. Todo T, Usui M, Takakura K: Treatment of severe intraventricular hemorrhage by intraventricular infusion of urokinase. 74:81–86, 1991.

56. Findlay JM, Grace MGA, Weir BKA: Treatment of intraventricular hemorrhage with tissue plasminogen activator. Neurosurgery 32:941–947, 1993.

57. Findlay JM, Weir BKA, Stollery DE: Lysis of intraventricular hematoma with tissue plasminogen activator. J Neurosurg 74:803–807, 1991.

58. Mayfrank L, Lippitz B, Groth M, et al: Effect of recombinant tissue plasminogen activator on clot lysis and ventricular dilatation in the treatment of severe intraventricular hemorrhage. Acta Neurochir 122:32–38, 1993.

59. Rhode V, Schaller C, Hassler WE: Intraventricular recombinant tissue plasminogen activator for lysis of intraventricular haemorrhage. J Neurol Neurosurg Psychiatry 58:447–451, 1995.

60. Akdemir H, Selcuklu A, Pasaoglu A, et al: Treatment of severe intraventricular hemorrhage by intraventricular infusion of urokinase. Neurosurg Rev 18:95–100, 1995.
61. Rainov NG, Burkert WL: Urokinase infusion for severe intraventricular haemorrhage. Acta Neurochir 134:55–59, 1995.
62. Grabb PA: Traumatic intraventricular hemorrhage treated with intraventricular recombinant -tissue plasminogen activator: Technical case report. Neurosurgery 43:966–969, 1998.
63. Goh KY, Poon WS: Recombinant tissue plasminogen activator for the treatment of spontaneous adult intraventricular hemorrhage. Surg Neurol 50:526–531, 1998.
64. Naff NJ, Carhuapoma JR, Williams MA, et al: Treatment of intraventricular hemorrhage with urokinase: Effects on 30-day survival. Stroke 31:841–847, 2000.
65. Haines SJ, Lapointe M: Fibrinolytic agents in the management of post hemorrhagic hydrocephalus in preterm infants: The evidence. Childs Nerv Syst 15:226–234, 1999.
66. Findlay JM, Grace MG, Weir BKA: Lysis of intraventricular hematoma with tissue plasminogen activator. Neurosurgery 32:941–947, 1993.
67. Nieuwkamp DJ, de Gans K, Rinkel GJE, et al: Treatment and outcome of severe intraventricular extension in patients with subarachnoid hemorrhage: A systematic review of the literature. J Neurol 247:117–121, 2000.
68. Coplin WM, Vinas FC, Agris JM, et al: A cohort study of the safety and feasibility of intraventricular urokinase for nonaneurysmal spontaneous intraventricular hemorrhage. Stroke 29:1573–1579, 1998.
69. Schwarz S, Schwab S, Steiner H, Hacke W: Secondary hemorrhage after intraventricular fibrinolysis: A cautionary note: A report of two cases. Neurosurgery 42:659–663, 1998.
70. Verma A, Maheshwari MC, Bhargava S: Spontaneous intraventricular haemorrhage. J Neurol 234:233–236, 1987.
71. Roos YB, Hasan D, Vermeulen M: Outcome in patients with large intraventricular haemorrhages: A volumetric study. J Neurol Neurosurg Psychiatry 58:622–624, 1995.
72. De Weerd AW: The prognosis of intraventricular hemorrhage. J Neurol 222:45–51, 1979.
73. Juvela S: Risk factors for impaired outcome after spontaneous intracerebral hemorrhage. Arch Neurol 52:1193–2000, 1995.
74. Sjoblom L, Hårdemark HG, Lindgren A, et al: Management of prognostic features of intracerebral hemorrhage during anticoagulant therapy: A Swedish multicenter study. Stroke 32:2567–2574, 2001.
75. Jennett B, Bond M: Assessment of outcome after severe brain damage. A practical scale. Lancet 1:480–484, 1975.

Therapy

Chapter Sixty-Five

Carotid Endarterectomy

J. Max Findlay and B. Elaine Marchak

Since it was first conceived a little more than a half-century ago, the surgical correction of carotid artery stenosis to prevent stroke gradually grew to great popularity, was then seriously questioned with respect to its efficacy, resulting in a dramatic drop in its performance, and finally was scientifically validated in randomized clinical trials. Carotid endarterectomy (CEA) has now once again become the most commonly performed peripheral vascular operation in North America, although it now faces a new challenge, comparison with endovascular correction of carotid stenosis with angioplasty and stenting. In addition to its relative merit in different patient groups, the technique of CEA continues to be the subject of much study. Numerous variations in anesthesia, monitoring, and surgical technique have been described. In this chapter we review indications for CEA, outline perioperative care and surgical techniques, and discuss complications of CEA and their management.

HISTORICAL REVIEW

Between 1856 and 1914, Savory,[1] Gowers,[2] Chiari,[3] Guthrie and Mayou,[4] and Hunt[5] all described patients who experienced neurologic deficits and were subsequently found at autopsy to have occlusion of the cervical carotid arteries. Hunt in particular emphasized the relation between episodes of cerebral ischemia and partial carotid obstruction, which he described in analogy as "cerebral intermittent claudication."[5] The next major step in appreciating extracranial carotid disease was made possible with the introduction of carotid angiography and roentgenographic visualization of the carotid bifurcation by Moniz[6] in 1927.

It was not until 1951, however, that the neurologist C. Miller Fisher[7] fully elucidated the concept of carotid thrombosis and embolism from atherosclerotic plaques as a cause of stroke. In a detailed clinicopathologic and radiologic analysis of eight patients suffering transient ischemia and stroke from carotid bifurcation atheroma, Fisher also foreshadowed an era of carotid reconstruction, postulating that "it is even conceivable that some day that vascular surgery will find a way to by-pass the occluded portion of the artery during the period of ominous fleeting symptoms. Anastomosis of the external carotid artery, or one of its branches, with the internal carotid artery (ICA)

above the area of narrowing should be feasible."[7] Further reports from Fisher confirming the importance of extracranial carotid disease in stroke appeared in 1952 and 1954.[8,9]

In 1951, Carrea and associates[10] in Buenos Aires did what Fisher suggested, resecting the diseased segment of an ICA and connecting the external carotid to the distal normal ICA, although they did not report the experience until 1955. In 1953, Gurdjian and Webster[11] in Detroit described 30 patients with stroke resulting from cervical internal carotid thrombosis, 15 of whom underwent surgical exposure of the carotid bifurcation and excision of the thrombosed portion of the artery. They speculated that if seen early enough, patients might be treated with thrombectomy and reestablishment of flow in the carotid artery. In 1953, Hamelin and colleagues[12] at the Massachusetts General Hospital in Boston resected a severely stenotic segment of the left ICA from a 50-year-old woman, 5 weeks after she had suffered a left hemispheric stroke, and anastomosed the common carotid artery (CCA) with the distal ICA; this successful procedure was not reported until 1958. Strully and coworkers[13] reported a failed attempt at carotid thromboendarterectomy in 1953 but predicted that such an operation would be successful in patients in whom there was a patent distal vessel.

The same operation described by Hamelin and colleagues,[12] a left internal carotid arterectomy and end-to-end anastomosis of the common and internal carotid arteries, was performed by the vascular surgeons Eastcott and Rob, at St. Mary's Hospital in London in May, 1954; Pickering, the third author of the report on the procedure, was the attending neurologist.[14] According to the report, which was published in November 1954, the patient, a 66-year-old woman who presented with transient ischemic attacks, was neurologically well a month after surgery, aside from bouts of angina pectoris. This was the first report of successful carotid artery reconstruction to appear in the medical literature.

In 1955, Denman and colleagues[15] in Houston described the staged resection of internal carotid bifurcations and insertion of preserved arterial homografts to reconnect the common and distal internal carotid arteries in a patient, a remarkable surgical achievement at the time. Cooley and associates[16] performed and first reported on a true carotid endarterectomy in 1956. The patient was a 71-year-old man with a cervical bruit and stenosis that was removed through a transverse incision across the carotid bulb.

Although the surgeons used a needle-pointed polyvinyl shunt to provide cerebral circulation around the temporary carotid occlusion (making their report also the first to describe carotid shunting), the patient awoke with signs of having experienced a small stroke. Two years later, Crawford and coworkers[17] made reference to a successful carotid artery repair that they had performed in 1953 (prior to the endarterectomy described by Cooley and associates[16]); in a 1965 publication, the same group of surgeons stated that this repair had been a thromboendarterectomy, which they therefore believed was the world's first.[18]

The first reports of large series of patients undergoing CEA with good results set the stage for development and adoption of surgical management of extracranial carotid disease to prevent stroke.[19–21] A multicenter, cooperative, "joint" study examining the role of surgery for cerebrovascular insufficiency was established in 1959 by a group of physicians and surgeons led by William Fields.[22] The joint study registry eventually numbered almost 5000 patients, yielded 10 journal articles in total, and served to refine the investigation of carotid disease, identify reasonable candidates for CEA, and determine clear contraindications for the operation.[23] However, it did not prove the superiority of endarterectomy over medical management alone.

By 1980, CEA had become the most commonly performed peripheral arterial operation in the United States, reaching a peak of 107,000 operations in 1985.[24] A relatively straightforward surgical procedure for a common condition, it was practiced by vascular, general, neurologic, and cardiac surgeons. In the mid-1980s, however, concerns were raised about a possibly profligate use of the procedure. In 1976, the first of many trials demonstrating efficacy of platelet inhibition in reducing the risk of stroke appeared,[25] establishing a proved, alternative medical treatment for carotid atherosclerosis. There were disturbing reports of high complication rates associated with CEA in community and hospital surveys[26–30] as well as descriptions of the use of the procedure for what appeared to be inappropriate indications.[31] Finally, another "stroke operation," extracranial-to-intracranial bypass grafting, was found to have no benefit over medical therapy in a randomized trial for symptomatic intracranial occlusive disease.[32] Leaders in the stroke field began to seriously question the enthusiastic practice of CEA.[33,34] The result was a surprisingly prompt decline in the rate of CEA in the United States by the late 1980s.[35]

In response to uncertainty about the danger of CEA, multicenter, randomized controlled trials were launched by several groups that went on to validate the use of the procedure under certain circumstances.[36–42] Several of the key investigators in this scientific reevaluation of CEA have been Charles Warlow from the Western General Hospital in Edinburgh, and Henry Barnett of the University of Western Ontario and the John P. Roberts Research Institute in London, Ontario. In the years after the publication of the results of these trials, there has been a dramatic resurgence in the rates of CEA, which in some areas either matched or exceeded the rates seen in the early 1980s.[43–47] Along with this renewed interest in CEA, reassessments have been made of carotid artery investigation, risk

stratification for the natural history and surgical treatment of different stenosis subgroups, perioperative management and surgical techniques, and complications of CEA and their management—all topics to be discussed in this chapter. Also, CEA has begun to be compared in terms of efficacy, risk, and cost with the endovascular correction of carotid artery stenosis by means of balloon angioplasty with or without stenting.[48]

CAROTID ARTERY STENOSIS AND STROKE RISK

Randomized trials examining the role of CEA in different patient subgroups have provided information about the risk of carotid stenosis treated with medical therapy alone. Although not representing the untreated, "natural history" of such lesions, these patients undergoing solely medical therapy demonstrate the risks with which the risks and long-term outcome of CEA must be compared. At this point, we should note that unless otherwise stated, the percentage stenoses referred to throughout this chapter are those determined by what has become known as the "NASCET method,"[49] from the North American Symptomatic Carotid Endarterectomy Trial (NASCET). In this method, the narrowest diameter of the residual lumen (on the angiographic view showing the greatest stenosis) (N) is compared with the luminal diameter of the ICA well beyond the bulb, where the walls of the artery have become parallel (D); the percentage of stenosis is calculated as follows:

$$\% \, \text{Stenosis} = \frac{1 - N}{D} \times 100$$

In NASCET, 26% of 331 patients who presented with transient carotid ischemia or a nondisabling stroke and stenosis between 70% and 99% and were treated with medical therapy (primarily aspirin) had an ipsilateral stroke within 2 years; 32% suffered any type of stroke or died during the same period.[36] Among the 428 patients with 50% to 69% symptomatic stenosis, the 5-year risk for ipsilateral stroke was 22%, and for any stroke or death, 43%.[42] The risk of ipsilateral stroke is highest immediately after the initial ischemic event, and for patients with both moderate stenosis and severe stenosis (all those in the 50% to 99% stenosis range), the annual ipsilateral event rate drops to about 3% within 2 to 3 years. Another study found that 11% of 1707 patients diagnosed with a transient ischemic attack (TIA) in an emergency room returned to the emergency room with a stroke within 90 days, and half of these strokes occurred in the first 2 days.[50] Age more than 60 years, diabetes mellitus, duration of symptoms longer than 10 minutes, and hemispheric symptoms (weakness or speech impairment) were independently associated with ensuing stroke, and combining these factors identified subgroups with a short-term stroke risk as high as 34%.

Within these broad ranges of stenosis, additional risk factors for stroke have been identified for symptomatic patients. The severity of stenosis correlates with risk, the highest risk being for patients with 90% to 94% stenosis

(35% at 1 year), and lower for both less severe stenosis and "near-occlusions"; the 1-year stroke risks for 70% to 79% stenosis and for near-occlusions are both close to 11%.[36,51] Results of the post hoc subgroup analysis of the European Carotid Surgery Trial (ECST) were similar. Researchers in that study found that post-stenotic narrowing of the ICA (a "slim sign" due to reduced distal intra-arterial perfusion pressure) was associated with a lower risk of ipsilateral stroke with medical treatment, only 8% at 5 years.[52] The lower risk associated with near-occlusion may be due to the presence of superior collateral vessels in many of these cases. In NASCET, the presence of angiographic collateral vessels in 339 patients with severe stenosis (70% to 99%) who were treated medically more than halved the 2-year stroke risk, lowering it from 28% to 11%.[53]

Plaque ulceration has a significant bearing on prognosis for symptomatic stenosis. The 2-year risk of ipsilateral stroke in medically treated patients with ulcerated plaques in NASCET (230 of 659 patients) rose incrementally from 26% to as high as 73% as the severity of stenosis associated with the ulcer increased from 75% to 95%.[54] Again, ECST results were similar, with angiographic plaque surface irregularity an independent predictor of ipsilateral ischemic stroke with medical treatment for all levels of stenosis severity.[55]

Data from the medical arm of NASCET showed that the presence of an occluded carotid artery contralateral to a symptomatic stenosis more than doubles the risk of ipsilateral stroke over 2 years.[56] Also, intracranial atherosclerosis distal to carotid stenosis was also found to be an independent risk factor for stroke, raising the 3-year risk of a stenosis in the 85% to 99% range from 25% to 46%, for example.[57]

In symptomatic patients, certain presenting symptoms and patient-related variables correlate with stroke risk. In NASCET, patients presenting with hemispheric symptoms who underwent medical treatment (n = 417) were about twice as likely to suffer a stroke over 3 years than the group presenting with monocular blindness who received medical treatement (n = 198).[58] Results from NASCET also indicated that in symptomatic patients, stroke risk is higher for men than women (particularly in the group with 50% to 69% severity, in whom the 5-year ipsilateral stroke risk is 25% for men and 15% for women) and that the risk is higher for patients who present with stroke rather than TIA.[42]

In summary, the risk associated with a symptomatic carotid artery stenosis varies considerably, depending on the severity of stenosis, the presence of plaque irregularity or ulceration, the presence of distal disease, the quality of collateral flow to the hemisphere, the status of the contralateral carotid artery, and the symptoms at presentation (Table 65.1). A conservative estimate of the 2-year stroke risk associated with an irregular or ulcerated 75% to 80% stenosis that causes a hemispheric TIA is about 50%, and as the patient's age at presentation increases from 65 to 75 years, his or her lifetime risk falls from nearly 100% to 86%, assuming a 4% annual risk after the first 2 years.

In general, the risks for asymptomatic stenosis are less than half of those for an equivalent symptomatic stenosis. Unfortunately, only 20% of patients are warned of impending stroke by a TIA.[59]

Table 65.1   Risk Factors for Increased Stroke Risk: Symptomatic Stenosis Treated Medically*

Increasing degree of stenosis (until "near-occlusion," when the stroke risk falls somewhat)[36,51,52]
Absence of angiographic evidence of collateral vessels to affected hemisphere[53]
Plaque ulcerations or irregularity[54,55]
Contralateral carotid occlusion[56]
Presence of intracranial atherosclerosis ("tandem" disease)[57]
Presence of intraluminal thrombus[146]
Hemispheric symptoms more than amaurosis fugax[58]
Male gender[42]
Stroke more than transient ischemic attack presentation[42]

*Superscript numbers indicate chapter references.

INVESTIGATION OF CAROTID STENOSIS

Computed tomography (CT) or magnetic resonance imaging (MRI) of the brain is useful and is indicated for most patients with carotid symptoms being considered for CEA. A possible exception is the patient with classic amaurosis fugax and no hemispheric symptoms.[60] Brain imaging is particularly important in patients with persisting sensorimotor or speech deficits, in order to confirm infarction, rule out hemorrhage, and exclude an intracranial mass lesion, such as a subdural hematoma or tumor, that can rarely cause stroke-like symptoms.

Debate surrounds the need for catheter angiography in assessing patients for CEA. Although the technique is considered the "gold standard" for providing a precise measurement of carotid stenosis, one can argue that carotid ultrasonography indicating severe carotid stenosis is sufficient to make decisions regarding treatment in many patients, especially if it is combined with a confirmatory (and also noninvasive) investigation, such as magnetic resonance angiography (MRA) or CT angiography.[61-64] Ultrasonography alone has been found to have only moderate accuracy in most vascular laboratories, making it more valuable as a screening test than as a means of assigning stroke risk and determining treatment.[65,66] Similarly, CT angiography[67] and conventional MRA[68,69] have been found, by themselves, to be sometimes inaccurate compared with catheter angiography; overestimation of the extent of stenosis is the most common error. A critical appraisal of 40 different studies of imaging and measurement of carotid stenosis performed up to 1997 found that the majority had insufficient methods and standards to inform clinical practice.[70]

As suggested previously, some clinicians choose to combine two noninvasive tests and, if the results agree, to formulate a treatment plan without subjecting the patient to catheter angiography. Others believe that the less than 1% major complication risk of disabling stroke associated with catheter angiography[71] is tolerable, in view of the high degree of accuracy angiography provides for stenosis measurement and treatment selection based on randomized trial data.[66,72] Other distinct advantages of catheter angiography are optimal demonstration of plaque morphology such as ulceration and plaque length, detection of intraluminal thrombus, assessment of intracranial atherosclerosis, determination of the location of the carotid bifurcation in the neck, and information about collateral circulation to the distal ICA through the communicating arteries and circle of Willis. This information not only helps in the determination of stroke risk but also informs the surgeon of the relative risks and difficulties that might be encountered at surgery. It is hoped that a noninvasive or minimally invasive imaging technique, such as contrast-enhanced MRA,[73,74] will be developed to provide the same information and to supplant catheter angiography altogether.

INDICATIONS FOR CAROTID ENDARTERECTOMY

Symptomatic Stenosis

For patients with symptomatic high-grade stenosis, CEA was shown to have a beneficial effect in NASCET.[36] The first report from the trial, published in 1991, showed that for patients who had either TIAs or nondisabling stroke within 120 days before entry into the trial and a stenosis of between 70% and 99% of normal lumen diameter on cerebral angiography, CEA was clearly superior to drug therapy (primarily with antiplatelet agents) in preventing stroke, lowering the 2-year risk of ipsilateral stroke from 26% to 9% ($P < .001$). The risk of stroke in patients treated with drugs rose with a higher severity of carotid stenosis; correspondingly, the benefit from surgery was greater for patients with more severe stenosis. The rate of perioperative stroke and death was 5.8% (within 30 days of surgery) in the surgical group, which totaled 328 patients. NASCET had a number of inclusion and exclusion criteria for patient enrollment; we detail the more important ones. Patients were excluded from the study if they (1) had an intracranial lesion that was more severe than the surgically accessible lesion, (2) had a cerebral infarction that deprived them of all useful function in the affected territory, or (3) were 80 years or older. Patients were temporarily ineligible if they (1) had uncontrolled hypertension, diabetes mellitus, or unstable angina, (2) had had a myocardial infarction within the previous 6 months, or (3) had signs of progressive neurologic dysfunction.

The final results of NASCET, published in 1998, included the results for 2226 patients with symptomatic stenosis less than 70% as well as the 8-year CEA results for 659 patients with stenosis 70% or greater.[42] There was no benefit from surgery for stenosis less than 50%, which had a 5-year stroke risk of between 15% and 19% in both treatment groups. Among patients with moderate stenosis (between 50% and 69%; 858 patients), the 5-year stroke rate following treatment with CEA was 15.7%, compared with 22.2% for medical treatment, indicating a significant benefit from surgery (absolute risk reduction, 6.5% over 5 years; $P = .045$). The overall rate of perioperative stroke and death within 30 days in patients with moderate stenosis was 6.7%. Patients with severe stenosis had a durable benefit from surgery after 8 years of follow-up. If one combines the surgical results of both the moderate and severe stenosis groups, the combined stroke and death rate 90 days from surgery was 6.4%, and the rate for disabling stroke and death was 2.0%.

In NASCET, CEA was of much greater benefit for patients with severe stenosis, only six of whom needed to undergo CEA so that one ipsilateral stroke could be prevented in 2 years (the number needed to treat [NNT], which is the inverse of the absolute risk reduction value). For moderate stenosis (between 50% and 69%), 21 patients needed to undergo the procedure to prevent one stroke at 2 years (Table 65.2).[75] In this moderate stenosis group, surgical benefit appeared greatest in men, in patients with recent stroke as a qualifying event (vs. TIA), in patients with hemispheric rather than retinal symptoms (amaurosis fugax), and in patients taking 650 mg or more of aspirin per day.[42] NASCET data showed that the risk of stroke with medical therapy alone and the benefit from surgery both were greater for patients with higher grades of stenosis, except for stenosis between 95% and 99%, for which the risk declined slightly.[42,51] Contralateral carotid occlusion and plaque ulceration appear to raise the stroke

Table 65.2 Two-Year Risk of Ipsilateral Stroke and Number Needed to Treat by Carotid Endarterectomy: Symptomatic Patients

Stenosis*	No. of Patients	Risk at 2 yr (%) Medical	Risk at 2 yr (%) Surgical	Absolute Risk Reduction (%)	Relative Risk Reduction (%)	NNT	Perioperative Stroke and Death Rate (%)
70%–99%							
NASCET[37]	659	24.5	8.6	15.9	65	6	5.8
ECST[38]	501	19.9	7.0	12.9	65	8	5.6
50%–69%							
NASCET[43]	858	14.6	9.3	5.3	36	19	6.9
ECST[42]	684	9.7	11.1	−1.4	−14	—	9.8
<50%							
NASCET[43]	1368	11.7	10.2	1.5	13	67	6.5
ECST[42]	1822	4.3	9.5	5.2	−109	—	6.1

*Stenoses according to NASCET measurement method. Superscript numbers indicate chapter references.
ECST, European Carotid Surgery Trial; NASCET, North American Symptomatic Carotid Endarterectomy Trial; NNT, number of patients needed to treat by endarterectomy to prevent one additional ipsilateral stroke in 2 years after the procedure, compared with medical therapy alone; data not applicable.
Adapted from Barnett HJM, Meldrum HE, Eliasziw M, for the North American Symptomatic Carotid Endarterectomy Trial (NASCET) Collaborators: The appropriate use of carotid endarterectomy. CMAJ 166:1169–1179, 2002.

risk with medical therapy as well as the operative stroke risk, but patients still benefit from CEA.[54,56] The presence of intracranial (tandem) atherosclerotic lesions and absence of collateral pathways to the distal, symptomatic ICA predict a higher risk of stroke with medical therapy and indicate a greater benefit from CEA, despite a slightly higher operative risk.[53,57] Patients older than 75 years who have symptomatic carotid stenosis appear to benefit more from CEA over 2 years than younger patients; therefore, CEA is recommended for otherwise fit elderly patients.[76,77]

The results of ESCT, a parallel trial examining symptomatic patients in Europe, are strikingly similar to those of NASCET, especially when the stenosis measurements from ECST are converted to equivalent NASCET values.[37,41] ECST, which involved a total of 3024 patients, found clinical benefit of surgery compared with drug therapy for stenoses greater than 70%, a measurement equivalent to roughly 45% by NASCET methods. Patients in ESCT with less severe stenosis were harmed by CEA.

Carotid Endarterectomy and Coronary Bypass Surgery

There is a strong association between carotid atherosclerosis and coronary artery atherosclerosis,[78] although the evidence that the presence of isolated asymptomatic stenosis is an independent risk factor for ipsilateral stroke in patients undergoing coronary bypass surgery is limited.[79-82] More convincing are studies showing that symptomatic stenosis puts patients undergoing coronary bypass at increased risk of perioperative stroke.[79,83] Even more clearly established is the fact that symptomatic carotid stenosis 70% or greater is usually best treated with CEA for long-term stroke prevention, quite separate from the stroke risk associated with coronary bypass (see preceding section on symptomatic carotid stenosis).

Patients with coronary symptoms and disease that warrant aortocoronary bypass are not often symptomatic from carotid stenosis at the same time, but when the situation does arise, options include staged carotid and coronary procedures,[82,84] combined coronary bypass surgery and CEA,[85-87] and finally, endovascular treatment of either the carotid or coronary artery before surgical repair of the other artery.[88,89] The choice is usually determined by the preference and expertise of individual surgeons and institutions as well as the characteristics of the individual patients. Many commentators on this subject have concluded that only randomized controlled trials could establish credible recommendations for patients with concomitant coronary and carotid disease. The preference in our center when both operations are judged to be indicated is a combined procedure; CEA is performed in the usual fashion (described later), at the same time as saphenous vein harvesting but before cardiopulmonary bypass, and the neck incision is closed entirely before sternotomy is begun.

Summary

In the past two decades, large randomized trials have evaluated the benefit and risk of CEA for patients with symptomatic and asymptomatic stenosis of the ICA. Sufficient

Table 65.3 Guidelines for Performance of Carotid Endarterectomy (CEA)

CEA is appropriate for patients with	Symptomatic, 70% to 99% stenosis
Appropriateness of CEA is uncertain for patients with	Symptomatic, 50% to 69% stenosis Asymptomatic, 60% to 99% stenosis
CEA is inappropriate for patients with	Symptomatic, <50% stenosis Asymptomatic, <60% stenosis Unstable medical or neurologic status Recent large cerebral infarction Decreased level of consciousness Surgically inaccessible stenosis

time has passed since the publication of these studies to allow full analysis of their results and implications and for general recommendations to be made about the application of CEA on the basis of current knowledge (Table 65.3). A number of organizations and experts have published their analyses of the trials and made general recommendations for the use of CEA.[75,90-95]

CEA is highly appropriate for patients with symptomatic, severe stenosis (70% to 99% using the NASCET method) that is causing either TIAs or nondisabling stroke. The maximum allowable rate of all strokes or death in this group of patients is 6%. The appropriateness of CEA for patients with symptomatic stenosis in the 50% to 69% range, and those with asymptomatic stenosis, is uncertain in general; such patients may benefit, however, if they are selected carefully for CEA on the basis of additional features indicative of a higher stroke risk. These features are male gender, higher degrees of stenosis, plaque ulceration, contralateral carotid occlusion, a hemispheric as opposed to retinal TIA presentation, a stroke as opposed to TIA presentation, and a younger age at presentation; additional features have yet to be identified. Asymptomatic patients benefit less from CEA, and to achieve any benefit at all, surgery must be performed with particularly low stroke rates, in the range of 2% or 3% (no more than half the stroke rate for symptomatic patients). Patients for whom CEA would be inappropriate include those with less than 50% symptomatic stenosis or less than 60% asymptomatic stenosis and those with unstable medical or neurologic conditions, such as unstable angina, recent myocardial infarction, uncontrolled congestive heart failure, and progressing or major stroke. CEA for acute carotid occlusion is discussed later. "Chronic ocular ischemia" is an uncertain indication for this procedure.[96]

TIMING OF CAROTID ENDARTERECTOMY

After a minor and nondisabling cerebral infarct due to carotid stenosis, there is no need to wait weeks or months to perform surgery, as was once thought necessary.[97] Patients with smaller infarcts (usually <2 cm) and clinically more minor strokes marked by monoparesis or mild hemiparesis followed by improvement face no additional risk if they undergo surgery early; indeed, they are afforded

Table 65.7   Avoiding Complications During Carotid Endarterectomy

Complication	How to Avoid
Hypoglossal nerve injury	The nerve can be applied to an overlying facial vein (especially a higher one) and should be avoided each time a vein overlying the carotid bifurcation is divided. When the nerve must be moved for ICA exposure, cut the descendens hypoglossi and mobilize rather than retract. If inadvertently divided, the nerve should be reanastomosed with microsutures.
Vagus nerve injury	Leave the nerve adherent to the internal jugular vein and protect with overlying cottonoid strip.
Facial nerve (or branch) injury	Avoid dissection into the parotid gland and replace excessive manual retraction of the apex of the wound (with a right-angle retractor) with fish-hooks.
Accessory nerve injury	Avoid excessive posterior mobilization of the proximal sternomastoid muscle.
Intraoperative embolization	Avoid excessive mobilization of the carotid bifurcation from its bed during dissection, expel all air from the ICA by deoccluding the ECA prior to final arteriotomy closure, and declamp the ECA, CCA, and ICA *in that sequence* to send any debris from the CCA into the ECA.
Incomplete removal of plaque or rough distal end	Ensure ample distal ICA exposure and access before arteriotomy, and use magnification for plaque bed inspection.
Cross-clamp ischemia	Aim for 30 minutes or less. Consider shunting if EEG, SSEP, or TCD ultrasonography monitoring suggests distal ischemia, if there is scant reflux of blood down the ICA on temporary declamping, or in the setting of contralateral ICA occlusion or a hypoplastic anterior precommunicating artery.
Distal subintimal dissection	Use tack-down sutures on loose or prominent distal intimal shelves.
Stenosing arteriotomy closure	Prevent the arteriotomy from slipping into the crotch of the carotid bifurcation. Use magnification and patch liberally (narrow arteries, long or repeat endarterectomies, and problematic distal ends).
Neck hematoma	Maintain absolute hemostasis throughout (bi-and monopolar cautery dissection and/or hemostatic scalpel). Use suture ligatures rather than simple suture ties on facial veins. Pay special attention to patients on ticlopidine preoperatively.

CCA, common carotid artery; ECA, external carotid artery; EEG, electroencephalography; ICA, internal carotid artery; SSEP, somatosensory evoked potential; TCD, transcranial Doppler.

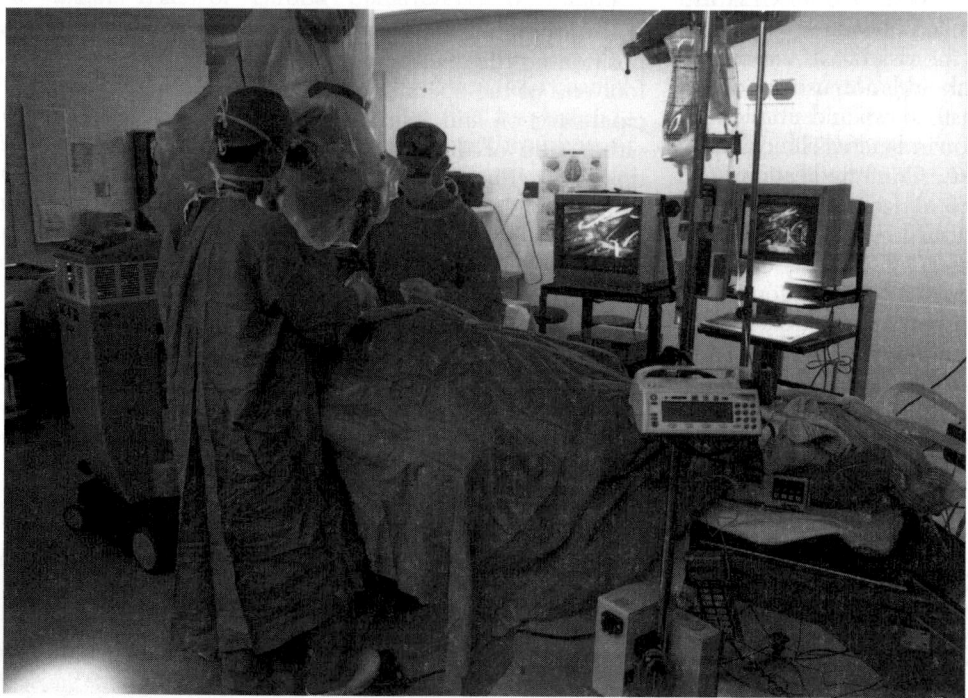

FIGURE 65–1 *After exposure of the carotid bifurcation, the operating microscope is positioned in line with the cephalad end of the operating table. A diploscope arrangement gives both surgeons comfortable and unrestricted access to the operative field.*

often requires division of the great auricular nerve or one of its branches, resulting in a variable amount of numbness of the submandibular region and tragus. Some surgeons avoid this division by making a transverse skin incision centered over the midsection of the SCM muscle, believing that it also offers a better cosmetic result. The limitation of a transverse incision is possible inadequate distal exposure of the ICA in some patients.

The plane beneath the investing fascia of the neck is opened under the SCM muscle, which is mobilized by means of a monopolar cautery needle or thermal scalpel. The underlying areolar tissue is exposed with blunt-toothed self-retaining retractors. Beneath this tissue lie the internal jugular vein and carotid sheath. Strict hemostasis with frequent use of bipolar cautery prevents blood staining and obscuration of the tissue planes and cranial nerves. Lymphatic tissue is mobilized on a broad pedicle in the direction of the internal jugular vein to expose the carotid arteries beneath.

The superior belly of the omohyoid muscle marks the inferior extent of the exposure, and the carotid sheath above it is opened to allow CCA exposure and control with an encircling polymeric silicone (Silastic) vessel loop. The common facial vein is usually encountered next in the proximal to distal exposure of the arteries, bridging over the bifurcation and draining into the internal jugular vein. This vein is skeletonized, clamped, ligated with clips or silk suture-ligatures, and divided. The jugular vein is then retracted posteriorly with the blunt-toothed self-retaining retractors.

Dissection continues distally, and a high exposure of the ICA is sought, often to the level of the posterior belly of the digastric muscle, another useful anatomic landmark. This high exposure sometimes requires additional maneuvers. The hypoglossal nerve is identified as it loops forward anteriorly, lateral to the carotid arteries. This nerve is often tethered in its position by two structures. The first is the descending hypoglossal nerve, which arises from the genu of the hypoglossal nerve and passes inferiorly to the ansa cervicalis, supplying the strap muscles. The second is an arterial branch to the SCM muscle, usually arising from the occipital artery, which passes posteriorly over the top of the hypoglossal nerve. Occasionally, the occipital artery itself can act as the arterial tether. The descending hypoglossal nerve and the SCM arterial branch can be divided without consequence to allow anterior and superior mobilization of a low-lying hypoglossal nerve, providing better exposure of the underlying distal carotid arteries.

Vessel loops are passed around the ICA and the external carotid artery (ECA), and the first arterial branch of the ECA (superior thyroidal artery) is occluded with an additional loop, which is fastened with a mosquito clamp to adjacent drapes to apply caudal traction to the bifurcation. The ICA is not manipulated or displaced too much from its bed, lest thrombus be dislodged into the cerebral circulation. The vagus and hypoglossal nerves are protected from injury, as is the accessory nerve if it is exposed.

Initial exposure should include at least 5 mm of ICA beyond where it is estimated the ICA plaque ends. Such an estimate is based on both the angiographic appearance of the plaque with respect to the bifurcation and the external appearance of the ICA. Atheroma within the ICA can cause a yellowish discoloration of the vessel wall as well as adventitial inflammation and adherence to the carotid sheath. Large fish-hooks applied to the skin edges at the upper end of the incision can improve an otherwise cramped distal exposure. We have not found it necessary to sublux the mandible for distal exposure of the ICA.[121]

Endarterectomy Technique

If used, the operating microscope is introduced at this point. The surgical instruments that we find useful for this part of the procedure are shown in Figure 65–2. After heparinization (heparin, 100 U per kg of body weight), an occlusive clamp such as a small DeBakey is used to occlude the CCA at a point where palpation rules out a hard, calcified plaque that might fracture with clamp application. Some surgeons prefer to occlude the ICA first, and large aneurysm clips are used to clamp both the ICA and ECA (Fig. 65–3). The ECA can also be occluded through tightening of the vessel loop encircling it. An arteriotomy is made with a No. 11 blade held cutting edge up, followed by Pott's scissors; it is important to stay in the middle of

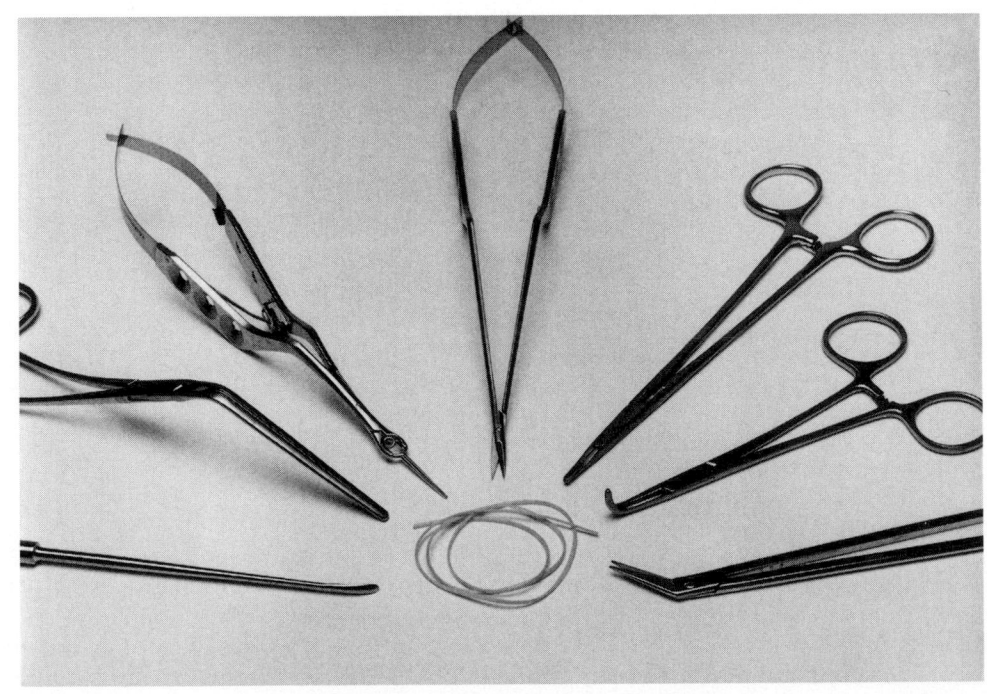

FIGURE 65–2 *Instruments useful in the microsurgical part of the procedure include, from left to right, a No. 4 Penfield elevator, a small DeBakey vascular clamp (for occlusion of the common carotid artery), a large aneurysm clip applier and clip (aneurysm clips are used for temporary occlusion of both the external and internal carotid arteries), microscissors, a Rider vascular needle driver, a small Lauer clamp, and Pott's scissors. Coiled in the center is an elastic vessel loop.*

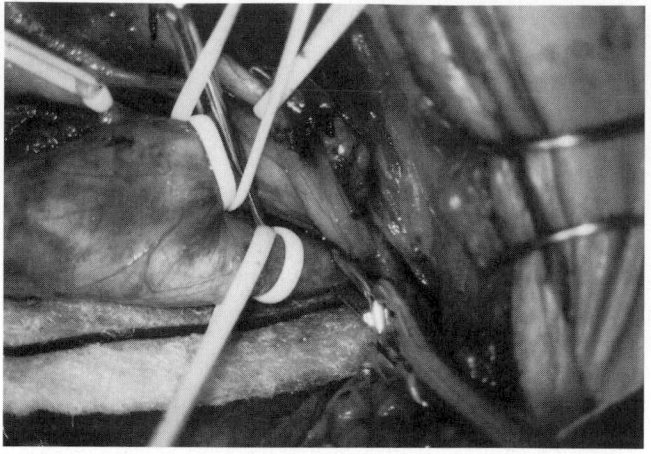

FIGURE 65–3 *A large aneurysm clip is placed on the left internal carotid artery distal to the encircling vessel loop.*

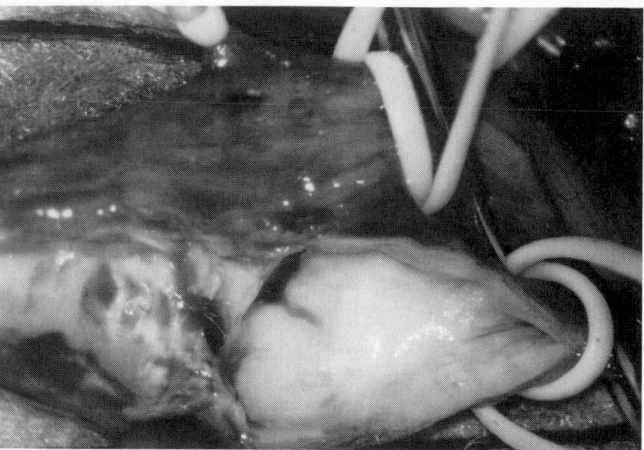

FIGURE 65–5 *The arteriotomy is continued several millimeters past the distal end of the internal carotid artery plaque.*

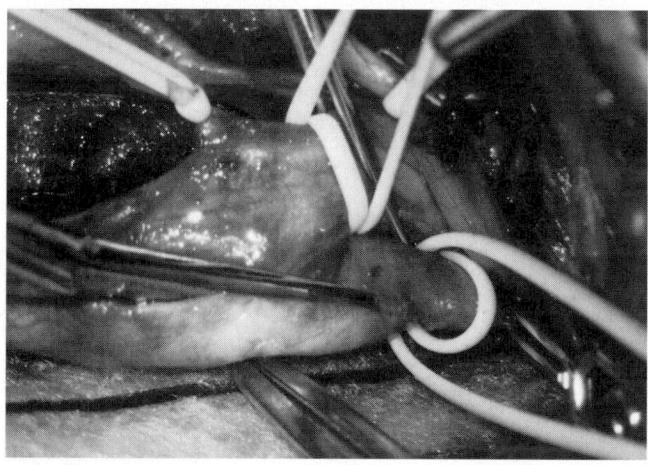

FIGURE 65–4 *The arteriotomy is continued with small Pott's scissors, cutting through both artery wall and atheroma. Care is taken to keep the cut in the middle of the lateral surface of the internal carotid artery and away from the bifurcation of the common carotid artery.*

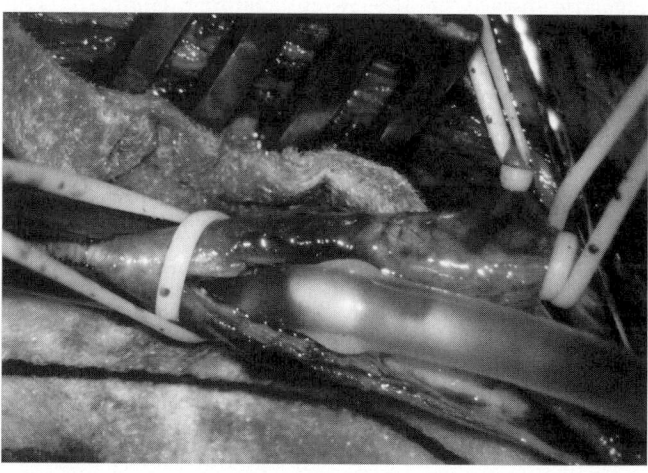

FIGURE 65–6 *The proximal end of a carotid bypass shunt is inserted into the common carotid artery and past the loosened vessel loop. It will be passed proximal to the released small DeBakey vascular clamp.*

the lateral exposure of the ICA and away from the apex of the carotid bifurcation (where scissors have a tendency to slip) (Fig. 65–4). The arteriotomy is continued several millimeters past the stenosis because a tapering tongue of atheroma extends more distally on the medial side of the artery (Fig. 65–5). Persistent bleeding from the arteriotomy despite adequate occlusion of the carotid arteries usually means that a low branch of the ECA, often the ascending pharyngeal artery with an origin medial to the bifurcation, requires identification and temporary occlusion with a small aneurysm clip.

If used, an arterial shunt is inserted at this stage of the operation. The proximal end is first quickly slid into the artery past the loosened CCA loop and the briefly released clamp, with suction in the wound (Fig. 65–6). The CCA encircling vessel loop is then tightened, and the ends of the loop are attached to nearby drapes with a mosquito clamp, securing the proximal limb of the shunt in place.

The clamp occluding flow through the shunt is then released briefly, expelling any air trapped in the tubing. Then the distal end of the shunt is inserted and secured in the ICA in the same manner (Fig. 65–7). High exposure of the ICA and magnification improve the accuracy and safety of shunt placement.

The surgeon can assess retrograde back-bleeding down the ICA before beginning plaque dissection by temporarily removing the ICA aneurysm clip. Vigorous bleeding provides additional assurance that good collateral blood flow is present in the distal ICA (in addition to evidence of good collateral vessels from angiography, the condition of the patient while under local anesthesia, and the results of intraoperative neurologic monitoring with the patient while under general anesthesia), whereas scant back-bleeding might prompt insertion of a shunt. Shunts are used routinely by some surgeons and selectively by others, according to different criteria to be discussed later.

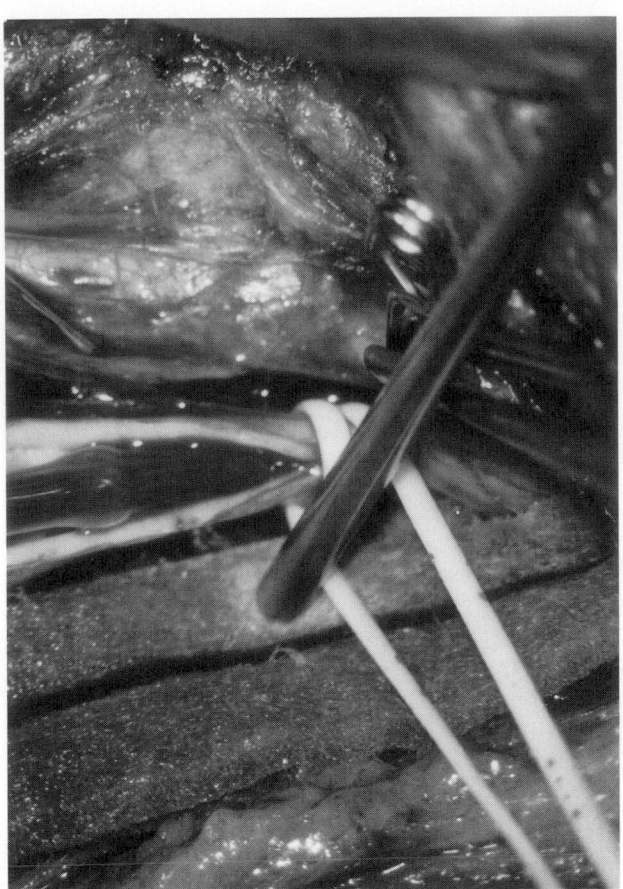

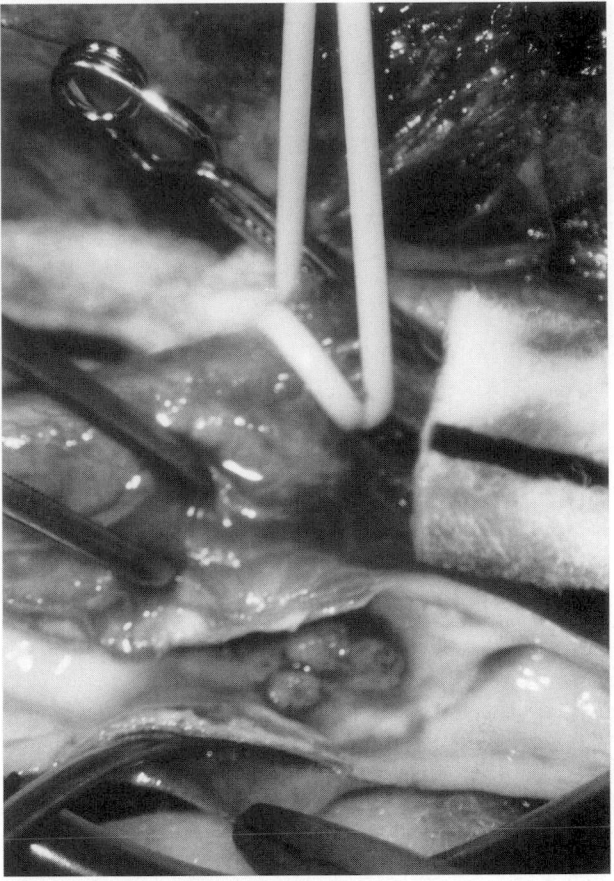

FIGURE 65–7 *The shunt tubing has been declamped briefly, expelling all air and debris from the tubing, and now is being introduced distally into the internal carotid artery.*

FIGURE 65–8 *The plane between the atheroma and outer arterial wall is established with a Penfield dissector at the point where the plaque is thickest, usually midway along its length.*

With a small Penfield elevator, atheroma is separated from the outer arterial wall along the edge of the arteriotomy (Fig. 65–8). The correct plane is first defined, where the plaque is thickest. Plaque can be detached from the distal end first, where in the best of circumstances, it feathers out to a tapered end on the medial side of the luminal wall. In this situation, the plaque often separates readily with no more than gentle, rolling traction applied to the plaque as it is held with vascular forceps and countertraction is applied to the arteriotomy edge (Figs. 65–9 through 65–11). If this part of the plaque does not come out smoothly, the artery should be opened more distally to improve the distal repair. Sometimes microscissors are used to begin the distal plaque excision, and if the plaque does not have a tapering end, microscissors can be used to cut a clean shallow step between the plaque bed and distal intima. Any significant distal intimal step or shelf not firmly adherent to the arterial wall should be tacked down with 7-0 monofilament sutures, with knots tied on the outside of the vessel wall (Figs. 65–12 and 65–13). Magnification improves the surgeon's appreciation of these distal intimal steps.

It can be hazardous to pull a plaque down and away from the ICA from above the level of the arteriotomy blindly, because a loose intimal attachment, vulnerable

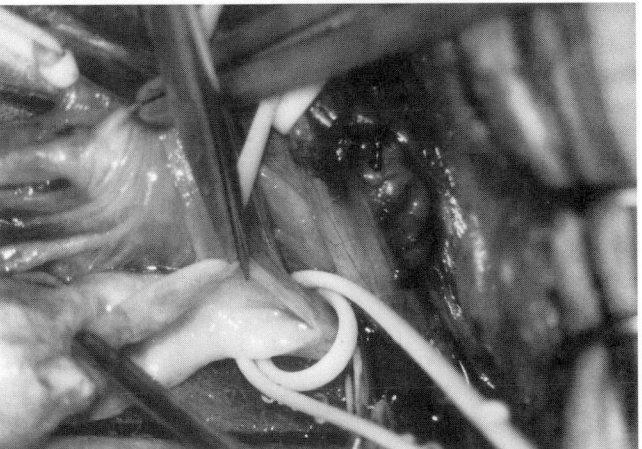

FIGURE 65–9 *The distal plaque excision is begun with microscissors; here, a film of intima that stretches from the plaque surface to the distal, normal part of the internal carotid artery is being cut.*

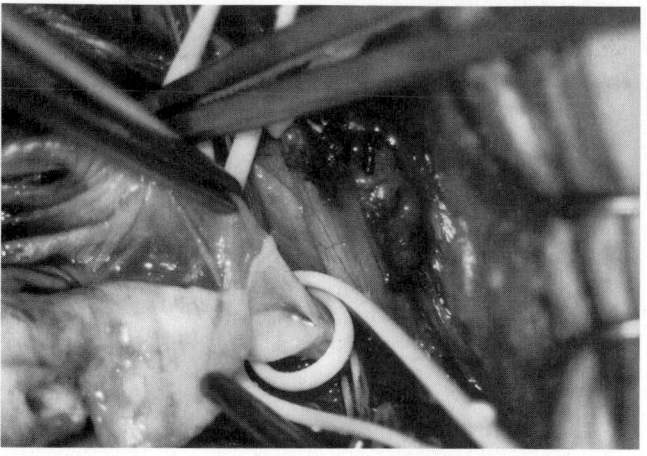

FIGURE 65–10 *The tapering end of the plaque is then pulled from the internal carotid artery with a rolling, downward traction applied against countertraction on the vessel wall.*

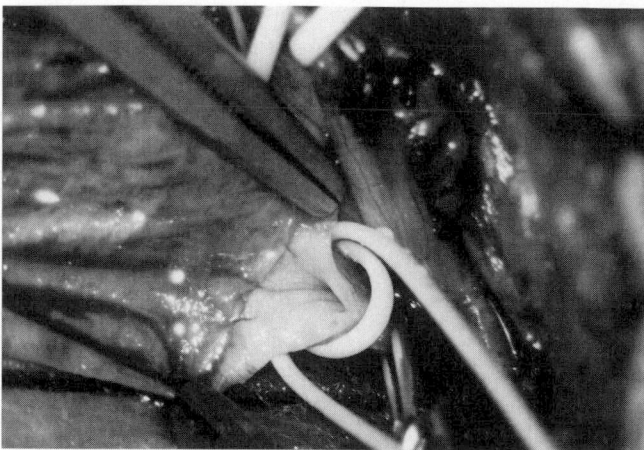

FIGURE 65–13 *A total of three tack-down sutures have been placed between the plaque bed and the distal intima, with the suture knots on the outside of the vessel.*

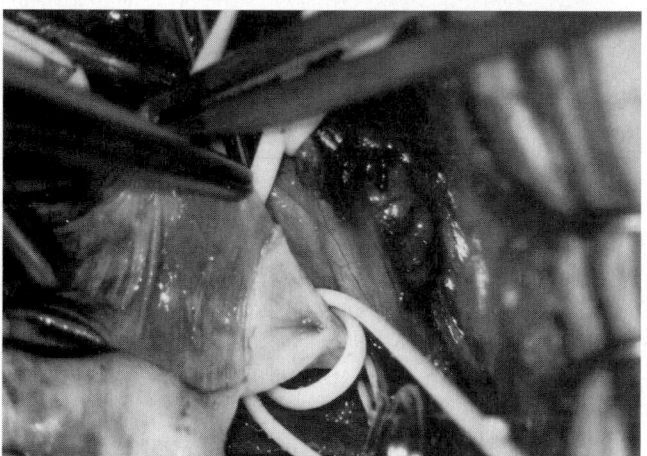

FIGURE 65–11 *Plaque removal is complete.*

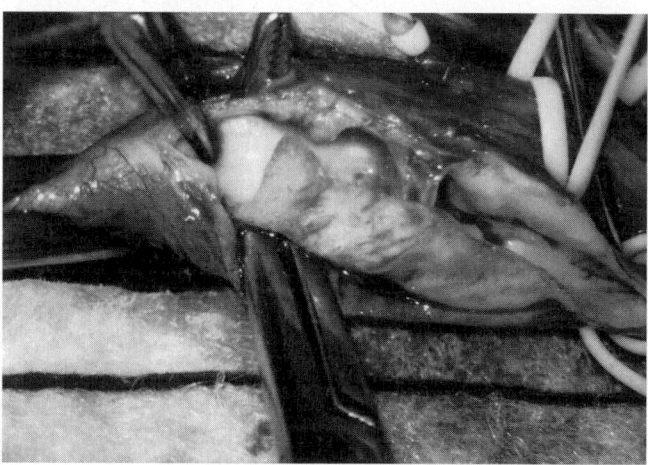

FIGURE 65–14 *The circumferential incision separating the plaque from the common carotid artery is complete in the same plane with the assistance of a small Mixter clamp inserted between the plaque and outer arterial wall.*

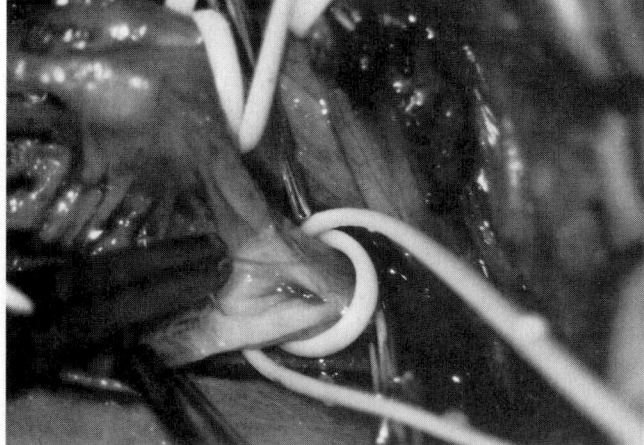

FIGURE 65–12 *Excision of this plaque has left a prominent distal shelf between the plaque bed and the intima of the distal internal carotid artery. A 7-0 polypropylene tack-down suture is being inserted.*

to subintimal dissection and carotid occlusion, cannot be fully appreciated or properly repaired in this location.

Atheroma thickens the CCA wall circumferentially, and a clean incision begun at the proximal end of the arteriotomy, well below the stenosis, is made with Pott's scissors. The correct dissection plane can be made with a small right-angled clamp, either a Mixter or Lauer, passed between the plaque and the outer vessel wall until its tips protrude at the opposite margin of the arteriotomy (Fig. 65–14). The goal is to create a clean step from the proximal atheromatous but nonstenotic CCA to the plaque bed. The difficulty with dissecting and cutting the plaque independently from both the arteriotomy margins is that the planes of dissection started from either edge of the arteriotomy may not meet.

The plaque, now freed at its distal and proximal ends, is everted out of the ECA orifice as far as possible. If the plaque does not detach cleanly, it can be cut flush from the outer artery wall with either Pott's scissors or microscissors (Fig. 65–15).

With intermittent heparinized saline irrigations, all loose plaque remnants are stripped from the plaque bed with fine vascular forceps (Fig. 65–16).

The artery is then closed primarily with a fine, non-stenosing 6-0 monofilament running suture, usually begun at the distal end with a double-armed technique and with the knot placed above the level of the arteriotomy (Figs. 65–17 and 65–18). If a patch is used, closure is also begun at the distal end with a double-armed technique (Fig. 65–19). If desired, an anchoring stitch can be placed at the heel of the patch as well (Figs. 65–20 and 65–21).

Just before the arteriotomy is closed and after the shunt has been removed, the clip on the ECA is removed or its

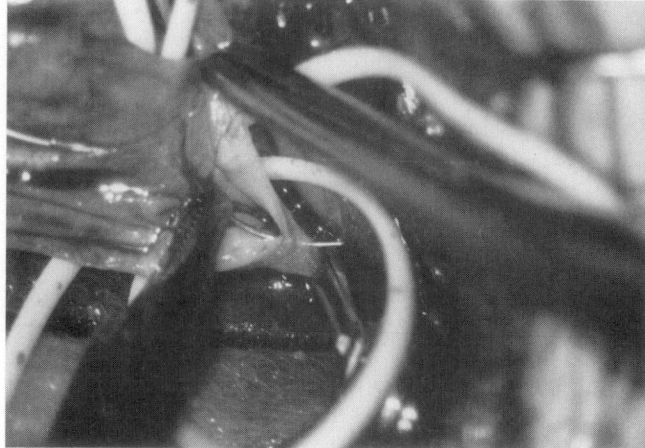

FIGURE 65–17 *The arteriotomy closure is begun with a double-armed 6-0 polypropylene suture.*

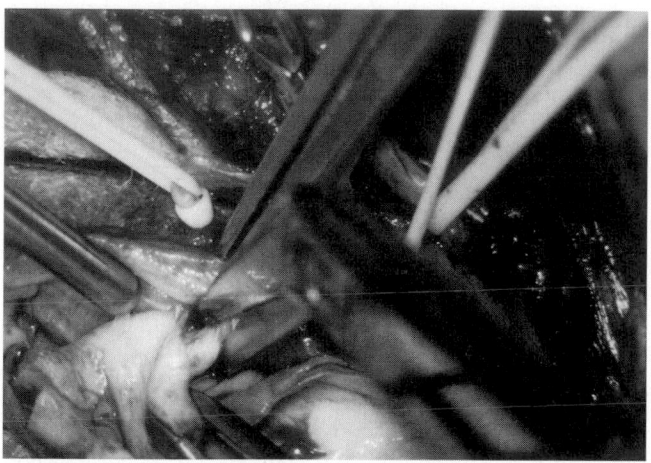

FIGURE 65–15 *Plaque extending into the origin of the external carotid artery is grasped circumferentially and everted from the artery for several millimeters, whereupon it is cut sharply at its distal extremity with inverted Pott's scissors.*

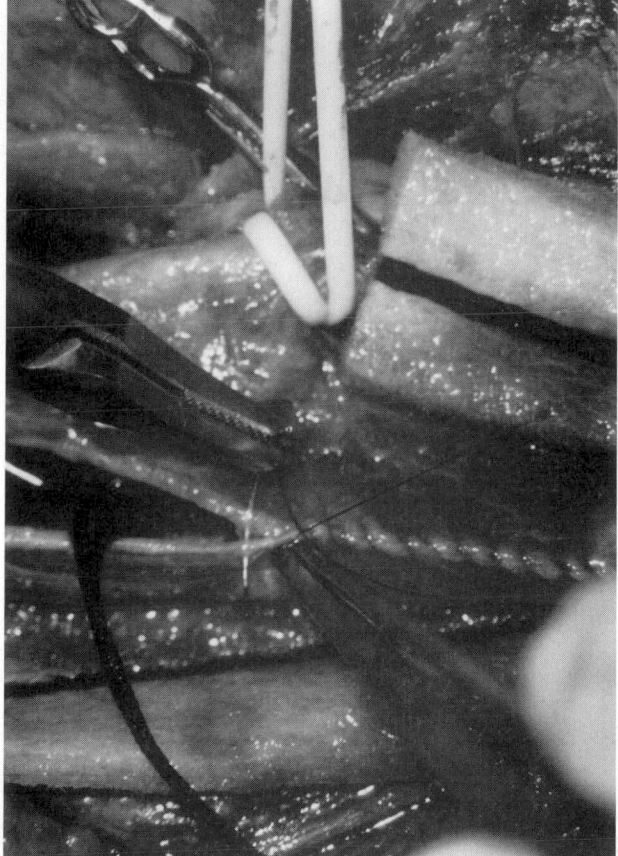

FIGURE 65–18 *Simple arteriotomy closure continues with fine bites, over an indwelling carotid bypass shunt.*

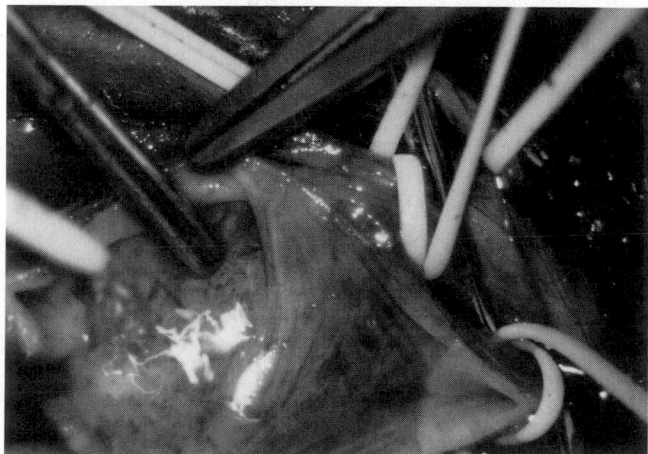

FIGURE 65–16 *Under a stream of heparinized saline irrigation, all loose atheroma tags and filaments are identified and stripped from the plaque bed.*

encircling loop is loosened briefly, and any air within the lumen is expelled. Irrigation is used to flush and fill the reconstituted arterial lumen.

The declamping sequence is specific and important. The aneurysm clip is removed, and the loop is loosened on the ECA. Occlusive fingertip pressure is applied to the ICA

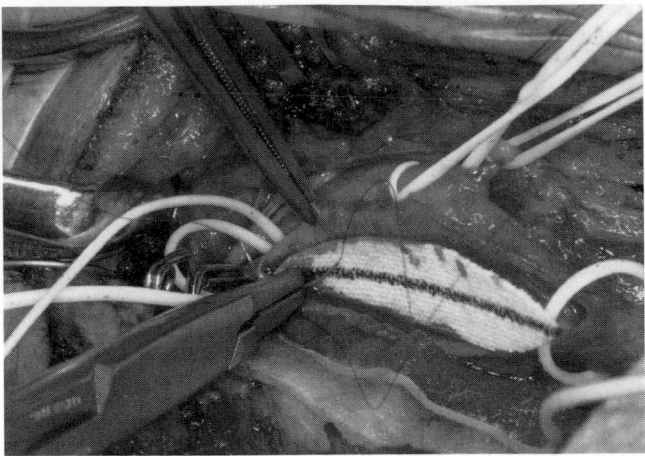

FIGURE 65–19   *Insertion of a fabric patch is begun at the distal end of the arteriotomy.*

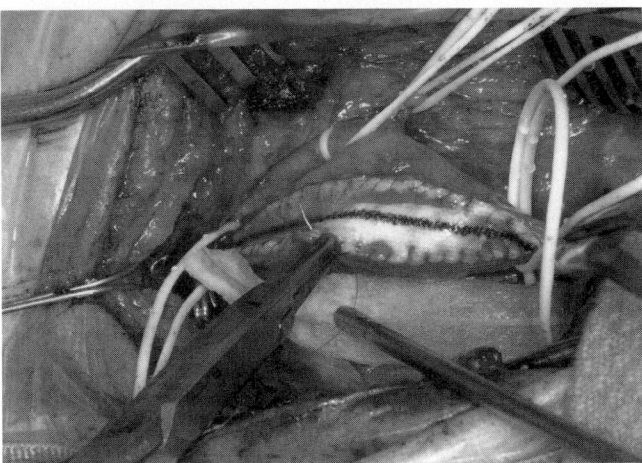

FIGURE 65–20   *Patch closure is near completion.*

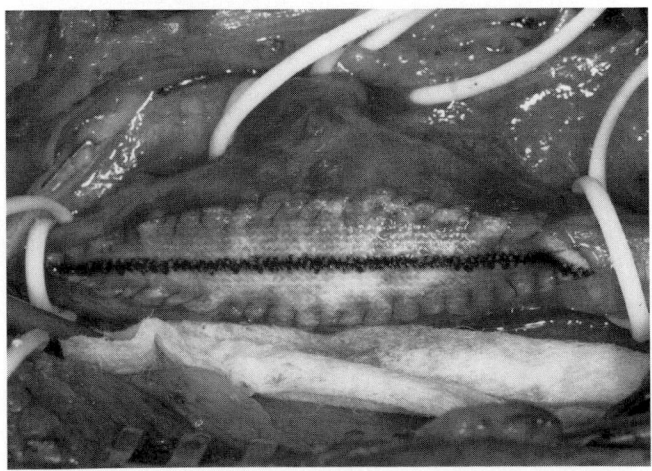

FIGURE 65–21   *Patch closure after declamping of external, common, and internal carotid arteries (in that order).*

proximal to its clip, and the CCA clamp is slowly removed, restoring blood flow to the ECA. Any missed debris or air is washed up the ECA rather than the ICA. Fingertip pressure, the loop, and the aneurysm clip are released from the ICA, and the suture line is inspected for leaks. A slow ooze will spontaneously stop, but more active bleeding requires an additional interrupted suture, with care being taken not to create an arterial stenosis.

Practice varies with respect to reversal of heparinization and the use of a drain in the wound; for example, we normally use neither procedure. Platysma and skin are closed in layers.

Eversion Endarterectomy

Eversion endarterectomy is a technique in which the ICA is transected at its origin from the CCA, the atheroma within is grasped, and the outer adventitial vessel wall layer is peeled and everted over the ICA plaque to its distal end. An intact tube of ICA atheroma is removed, and the ICA is reanastomosed to the carotid bulb with a running suture. This technique is inappropriate for patients with significant CCA atheroma and stenosis, and the use of a shunt is more difficult with this procedure than with conventional CEA, but proponents of eversion endarterectomy consider the procedure faster and the risk of recurrent stenosis less.[122–125] This procedure has been compared with standard CEA in a randomized trial in Europe, without any clear differences emerging either from that trial or from a systematic review of a number of studies.[126,127]

Patch Closure

The use of patch closure in CEA is debated. Possible benefits from the augmented lumen diameter resulting from a patching include a reduced acute thrombosis (and stroke) risk as well as a lower incidence of longer-term restenosis. Commonly used patch materials include autologous saphenous vein, various synthetic materials such as polytetrafluoroethylene (PTFE, Gore-Tex) and the polyester fabric Dacron, and bovine pericardium.[128] Vein grafts provide an endothelialized luminal surface and the suture lines are especially hemostatic; however, harvesting and a second wound are required, and there have been rare reports of postoperative rupture and aneurysm formation in association with vein patches.[129] Collagen-impregnated fabric grafts have been shown to be a satisfactory alternative.[130]

Some surgeons use a patch closure routinely, some never, and others in selected patients, such as those undergoing a second CEA procedure or those with either small ICAs or long plaques. In NASCET, a simple closure was used in 79% of 1415 patients, a fabric patch in 10%, and a vein patch in 10%.[104] Patch closure was performed more commonly by vascular surgeons than by neurosurgeons but did not correlate with perioperative stroke risk. Patch closure was used in 28% of 1729 operations in ECST; there was no association with its use and the risk of stroke or death.[131]

In a small study of 74 patients undergoing bilateral CEAs, in whom patch closure was performed on one side (either PTFE or saphenous vein) and primary closure on the other (staged operations in a random sequence), it was found that patching was associated with a lower operative stroke risk (4% for primary closure versus 0 for patching), a lower incidence of ultrasonographically detected restenosis (22% versus 1%, respectively) and a better cumulative patency rate; all of these differences were statistically significant.[132] These results concur with both the results of a previous randomized trial conducted by the same researchers in which the two techniques were compared in different patients,[133] and the results of a systematic analysis of the literature on the subject.[134] Two randomized trials compared synthetic with saphenous vein patches; the incidence of postoperative microemboli detected by transcranial Doppler ultrasonography was not significantly different in one trial,[135] and stroke and mortality rates did not differ for patch types in either.[135,136] In another randomized trial of bilateral procedures, eversion endarterectomy was found to be superior to patching with conventional techniques in terms of cumulative patency.[137]

On the basis of available evidence, there appears to be benefit to a liberal or even routine use of patching, but the choice of graft material is less important. A graft is certainly not essential in an elderly patient with an already large bifurcation and ICA. Our own practice is to insert a collagen-impregnated fabric graft patch in (1) any patient with a small-in-diameter ICA or an especially long plaque (usually subjective intraoperative determinations, but ICA diameters < 5 mm are considered small, and arteriotomies > 20 mm are considered long), (2) any patient in whom the endarterectomy has been technically difficult (such as an arteriotomy that has slipped into the "crotch" of the bifurcation), (3) any patient undergoing a repeat endarterectomy, and (4) any patient considered relatively "young" for CEA. This last indication has been arbitrarily set at an age of less than 65 years and accounts for the largest group of patients given patches in our own series. Given the number of variables involved, it is understandable that some surgeons have adopted a simple "patch all" policy. Immediately available synthetic grafts simplify the decision even further.

Bilateral Carotid Endarterectomy

Several groups have reported successful simultaneous bilateral CEAs.[138–140] The appropriate indication for this surgical undertaking remains unclear, however, because it is very uncommon for bilateral carotid stenoses to be symptomatic at the same time. The most important risks of simultaneous CEAs aside from stroke are bilateral neck edema or hematomas causing airway compromise and bilateral recurrent laryngeal nerve palsies predisposing to aspiration. For patients in whom bilateral CEAs are judged to be truly indicated, most carotid surgeons plan staged procedures, repairing the symptomatic side first.

Carotid Occlusion

A number of studies have proved the feasibility of reopening acutely occluded ICAs. Successful cases usually involve patients who present with a TIA or minor stroke (and therefore have collateral blood flow adequate to prevent a major hemispheric infarct with the loss of the ICA) who are found on angiography to have retrograde reflux filling from collateral sources to the level of the petrous or distal cervical ICA.[141–144] To be successful, de-occlusion must be undertaken early, preferably within several days. Whether or not the benefit of reopening a carotid artery outweighs the risk to a patient who has tolerated the loss of the artery is open to question. Advocates point to studies indicating a roughly 5% annual stroke risk distal to an occluded ICA.[145]

The specifics of carotid thrombectomy, as opposed to endarterectomy, require description, partly because an important indication is post-endarterectomy occlusion. After exposure of the carotid bifurcation, passage of vessel loops around the CCA, ECA, and ICA, and systemic heparinization, only the CCA and ECA are occluded. An arteriotomy is made (or reopened, for post-CEA thrombosis), exposing a column of thrombus distal to the stenosis or the plaque bed, as the case may be. In the best of circumstances, suction and mechanical traction on the thrombus retrieve the entire column of clot from the ICA, which is propelled and followed by retrograde bleeding. In most patients, however, a No. 2 Fogarty catheter must be passed up the ICA 10 to 12 cm (or until any resistance is felt, whereupon the catheter is withdrawn 1 cm), its balloon is inflated, and the catheter is withdrawn, retrieving thrombus and, one hopes, followed by back-bleeding. If after several attempts, little or no back-bleeding is established, the ICA should be ligated. If retrograde bleeding is established, a regular CEA should be carried out, and flow restored up the ICA. In these circumstances, an intraoperative completion angiogram is useful. A danger specific to this maneuver is the creation of a carotid-cavernous fistula, so care must be taken not to advance the catheter too far or against any resistance.

Intraluminal Thrombus

The presence of an intraluminal filling defect on angiography, suggestive of thrombus, is a significant risk factor for both medical and surgical treatment. In NASCET, 6% of patients with stenoses between 85% and 99% in severity had an associated intraluminal thrombus.[146] Endarterectomy is associated with the risk of dislodging thrombus into the cerebral circulation, so some authorities have recommended anticoagulation as treatment. In NASCET, however, the 30-day risk of stroke or death for medically treated patients with a clot was triple that for those without a clot. At 1 year, the risk of ipsilateral stroke was 16% among surgically treated patients, and 25.3% among those treated medically.[146] Therefore, despite the markedly increased risk associated with surgery, it is still safer than medical treatment.

In the presence of suspected intraluminal thrombus, care should be taken to manipulate the ICA as little as possible. Our own preference in patients whose distal ICA is not readily accessible is to avoid an ICA clip until after an arteriotomy is made and the stenosis and thrombus have been visualized. Other surgeons prefer to first place a clip on the distal ICA in every case.

For the rare patient with a long, pedunculated clot propagating well up the ICA and a very high risk of embolization during surgery, we have adopted another strategy. We perform a small frontotemporal craniotomy and microsurgical supraclinoid ICA exposure before cervical exposure. After CCA exposure and heparinization but before ICA dissection in the neck, we move the microscope back to the cranial exposure and place a temporary aneurysm clip across the supraclinoid ICA, temporarily occluding flow. The cervical ICA dissection, arteriotomy, and thromboendarterectomy are then performed, after which the intracranial clip is removed, permitting back-bleeding down the ICA. The addition of the craniotomy prolongs the procedure and adds risks of its own, and we consider this option only in patients in whom angiography also demonstrates the potential for collateral blood supply to the intracranial ICA (i.e., a patent anterior or posterior circle of Willis).

Intraoperative Vascular Imaging

Some surgeons consider intraoperative vascular imaging with either ultrasonography, angioscopy, or angiography useful for ruling out technical errors in the repair, such as an intimal flap, although the usefulness of imaging in reducing operative stroke risk has not been shown.[147–150]

ANESTHESIA AND MONITORING FOR CAROTID ENDARTERECTOMY

Patients presenting for CEA commonly provide a challenging array of problems for the anesthesiologist. The patients are often elderly with ischemic heart disease, peripheral vascular disease, and hypertension. Obesity, diabetes, and respiratory disease are also common. Such multiple comorbidities in association with a history of stroke or TIA put the patients at significant risk for perioperative neurologic and cardiopulmonary complications.

The traditional approach to the management of CEA has been with general anesthesia. In NASCET and ECST, the proportions of patients receiving general anesthesia were 93% and 97%, respectively.[104,151] Surveys in the United States and the United Kingdom indicate that general anesthesia remains the predominant anesthetic technique.[152,153] The goals in the management of patients undergoing general anesthesia for CEA are (1) to maintain cerebral perfusion pressure without unduly increasing myocardial oxygen demands and (2) to achieve rapid emergence of the patient from anesthesia and return to an alert state to allow prompt postoperative neurologic assessment. The relatively recent availability of ultra–short-acting narcotics, volatile anesthetics with low solubility, and muscle relaxants without hemodynamic effects makes these goals more easily attainable.

The advantages of general anesthesia are guaranteed patient immobility, optimum patient positioning, lack of pressure to complete a procedure in a patient who is restless or uncomfortable, and excellent control of oxygenation and ventilation. Most general anesthetics reduce the cerebral metabolic rate of oxygen ($CMRO_2$) and may improve cerebral tolerance to ischemia. The major disadvantage of general anesthesia is the loss of the ability to assess the adequacy of cerebral perfusion, particularly at the time of carotid clamping.

Monitoring

The availability of a monitor that accurately detects significant impairment of cerebral perfusion could direct therapeutic interventions such as deliberate hypertension, the use of potentially neuroprotective drugs, and shunting. Unfortunately a highly sensitive and specific monitor of cerebral perfusion for intraoperative use does not exist at this time. The monitoring modalities that have been studied in CEA are described here.

Stump Pressure

One of the earliest techniques used to estimate the adequacy of collateral flow after carotid clamping is stump pressure. European studies report the use of stump pressure in approximately 40% of patients,[151,153] whereas in North America, the modality is used in 10% to 15%.[104,152] The threshold stump pressure considered to be of significance varies widely among studies, ranging from less than 25 mm Hg to less than 50 mm Hg. The sensitivity and specificity of stump pressure for predicting new neurologic deficits vary with the threshold value chosen as abnormal, but the overall predictive value is low.[154]

Electroencephalography

Electroencephalography (EEG) is probably the most commonly used monitor for detection of alterations in cerebral perfusion during CEA. EEG primarily reflects changes in cortical activity and may not reflect ischemia in subcortical structures. Cortical activity is monitored only in the areas beneath the overlying scalp electrode; therefore, positioning of leads is very important. EEG changes, which begin to appear at cerebral blood flows lower than 20 mL per 100 g per min, commonly consist of a decrease in fast wave, an increase in slow wave activity, and loss of signal amplitude. In processed EEG, the analog raw EEG signal is digitized, and amplitude of the signal in each frequency spectrum is displayed on a time axis. This EEG form is somewhat easier for non-neurophysiologists to interpret.

Reduction of the spectral edge frequency by more than 50% and more than 30% loss of total power have been considered markers for cerebral ischemia. Interpretation of both raw and processed EEG is complicated by anesthetic agents,[155] changes in anesthetic depth, and preexisting cerebral infarction stroke. Early reports of a high degree of sensitivity for EEG in predicting immediate postoperative neurologic deficit[156] have not been widely duplicated.

Somatosensory Evoked Potentials

Somatosensory evoked potentials (SSEPs) have been used as indicators of cerebral ischemia during CEA, although far less commonly than EEG. In NASCET, 7% of patients were monitored with SSEPs.[104] Unlike EEG, SSEPs are sensitive to both cortical and subcortical ischemias. Cerebral compromise may be suggested by loss of amplitude or increase in latency of the SSEP signal. There is no uniform agreement as to the degree of amplitude loss that should be regarded as significant, but decreases ranging from 30%

to more than 50% have been used as markers for ischemia. Advantages of SSEP monitoring include less sensitivity to anesthetic effect than EEG and some utility in the patient with previous stroke.[157] Electrode placement is time consuming, and a dedicated technician is usually required. Reported sensitivities and specificities of SSEPs for predicting postoperative neurologic deficits are variable.

Transcranial Doppler Ultrasonography

Changes in MCA flow velocity as measured by transcranial Doppler (TCD) ultrasonography have been used as markers for cerebral ischemia during CEA. As with previously discussed monitoring modalities, it has been difficult to establish definitive thresholds in TCD ultrasonography that indicate cerebral ischemia. Reductions in MCA flow velocity ranging from more than 50%[157] to more than 90%[158] have been used, with variable sensitivities and specificities. At least 10% of patients have no acoustic window through the temporal bone, making the study impossible.

The major advantage of TCD ultrasonography is in the real-time detection of cerebral emboli, which are common during carotid dissection prior to cross-clamping, during shunt insertion, and during carotid artery closure. Detection of emboli allows alterations to be made in surgical technique.

Significant numbers of emboli on closure may represent luminal thrombi and impending occlusion; their appearance may warrant intraoperative and early postoperative studies and intervention.[159] TCD ultrasonography may also be useful in predicting postoperative hyperperfusion syndrome.[160]

Cerebral Oximetry

In cerebral oximetry measured by near-infrared spectroscopy (NIRS), an emitter-sensor is placed in direct contact with the scalp. Oxygen saturation of hemoglobin contained in arteries, veins, and capillaries at a calculated depth beneath the sensor is measured.

Although cerebral oximetry instrumentation has improved, inaccuracies related to differentiating blood from intracranial and extracranial sources do occur. Sensor location is important, because oxygen saturation is measured only in the area limited by sensor range and regional discrepancies in perfusion would not be detected. The requirement for direct scalp contact may necessitate removal of hair for appropriate placement of the emitter-sensor. Individual baseline variations in regional oxygen saturation are wide, making thresholds for identification of ischemia difficult to define.[161] Cerebral oximetry during CEA with use of regional anesthesia shows high negative predictive value but low positive predictive value with respect to intraoperative neurologic deficit.[162]

Jugular Venous Oxygen Saturation

Measurement of jugular venous oxygen saturation during CEA has been studied in a limited fashion. Its clinical utility in this setting is uncertain.

Summary

All of the cerebral monitoring modalities for CEA currently available have predictable limitations. Efforts at monitoring cerebral perfusion during CEA have been directed primarily at preventing hemodynamic strokes. The failure of available monitoring modalities to predict all and even immediately postoperative neurologic deficits may relate in part to the occurrence of focal embolic events. With most monitors, the criteria or thresholds for identifying ischemia have been difficult to define. Sensitivity and specificity vary widely among studies, depending on the thresholds chosen. No monitoring modality has emerged as clearly superior, and consequently, there is a wide variation in clinical practice.

A recent UK survey reported no cerebral monitoring by 37% of responding clinicians who used general anesthesia for CEA.[153] In contrast, multiple modalities are used routinely in some centers. At present there is no clear evidence that the use of any monitoring modality can alter the incidence of intraoperative hemodynamic stroke.

Regional Anesthesia

Interest in the use of regional anesthesia for CEA has been growing. The following approaches are possible: (1) deep cervical plexus block, (2) superficial cervical plexus block, (3) combined superficial and deep cervical plexus blocks, (4) local infiltration, and (5) cervical epidural anesthetic. A combination of deep and superficial cervical plexus block appears to be used most commonly. Deep cervical plexus block can be associated with a number of complications, including inadvertent injection of local anesthetic into the vertebral artery, subarachnoidally, or epidurally.

Phrenic nerve block with regional anesthesia is usual and may compromise respiratory function in patients with preexisting lung disease. Recurrent laryngeal nerve block can also occur. One study has reported that superficial block alone may be as effective as combined block, without the potential complications associated with deep block.[163]

In patients with high carotid bifurcations, or in whom carotid plaque extends very distally, mandibular retraction is required. This maneuver produces troublesome jaw pain, which may be reduced by additional placement of a mandibular nerve block.[164] The major advantage to regional anesthesia is the ability to continuously monitor neurologic function, obviating additional cerebral monitoring and allowing for highly selective shunt placement. The disadvantages are difficult airway access in emergency circumstances, frequent intraoperative hypertension, and the requirement for a cooperative patient.

Debate continues as to the influence of anesthetic technique upon postoperative morbidity and mortality. To date, the number of randomized controlled trials is insufficient to address this issue definitively. There is no clear evidence that postoperative stroke rates are influenced by anesthetic technique. Results of nonrandomized trials suggest that the incidences of stroke, death, and cardiopulmonary complications as well as the length of hospital stay may be less with regional anesthesia. However, these studies are potentially biased, and this issue can be settled only by a large prospective randomized trial.[165]

PERIOPERATIVE MANAGEMENT

Unless already admitted to hospital for investigation of TIAs or stroke, patients undergoing CEA on our service are admitted on the same day as the operation. Those with a history of significant medical problems, such as ischemic heart disease, undergo a preoperative medical or anesthetic consultation. All patients should receive antiplatelet agents before CEA, usually aspirin, at least 81 mg per day, to reduce the risk of postoperative stroke.[166] Intravenous heparin can be continued right until the time of surgery, although oral anticoagulation should be completely reversed; patients receiving clopidogrel preoperatively can undergo surgery, but they do require special attention with respect to wound hemostasis.

The "routine" postoperative care of patients who have undergone CEA has changed significantly with the realization that invasive postoperative monitoring in intensive care units followed by several days of hospitalization on a general ward is excessive and expensive.[167,168] On the other hand, patients who have undergone CEA have a high incidence of coexistent cardiac disease and hypertension; on the whole, they demonstrate a higher amount of hemodynamic instability postoperatively than most surgical patients. A safe compromise is a step-down or close-observation unit, where patients can receive close monitoring by a nurse assigned to just several patients overnight, with discharge after a total of 1 or 3 days in the hospital.

On our service, patients are monitored in a close-monitoring unit after surgery for at least 12 hours. If a patient demonstrates any hemodynamic instability in the first several postoperative hours, the indwelling arterial line inserted at surgery is left in until the next day. Continuous electrocardiographic monitoring is maintained in all patients, but they are otherwise allowed to sit, stand, and ambulate to the bathroom. Patients for whom there is no concern about neck swelling are allowed dinner on the day of surgery. Neurologic signs are assessed hourly for 10 hours, every 4 hours for the next 24 hours; then such assessments are discontinued. Antiplatelet agents and other regular medications are prescribed postoperatively. Patients are discharged home on the first or second postday of surgery, depending on their age, general condition, whether or not they live a distance from the hospital, and their wishes. Anxious patients are encouraged to stay 2 nights in the hospital.

The first 12 hours are the most critical in terms of postoperative complications, and during this time, both hypertension and hypotension are commonly encountered.[169] Systolic blood pressure lower than 100 mm Hg is treated with intravenous atropine if there is an associated bradycardia, or with intravenous fluid infusions if the heart rate exceeds 60 beats/min. Care is taken not to induce hypervolemia if the patient has a history of congestive heart failure. A vasopressor agent is rarely required. Significant hypertension (a value that is variable and is based on the patient's preoperative blood pressure record) usually responds to intravenous labetalol, although rarely, a nitroprusside infusion is required for adequate blood pressure control.

Many surgeons order postoperative carotid ultrasonography to document carotid patency, although the utility and cost-effectiveness of this practice, as well as yearly follow-up ultrasound examination thereafter to detect restenosis, have been questioned.[170]

NECK HEMATOMAS

Neck hematomas complicating CEA can be life-threatening. Of the 1415 surgical patients in NASCET, neck hematomas were recorded in 101 (7.1%), but only roughly half of the hematomas were significant—delaying discharge or requiring a return to the operating room—and there were two deaths due to airway obstruction.[104] An arteriotomy or carotid patch dehiscence (carotid "blow-out"), which can be rapidly fatal, is fortunately very rare. Patients should be checked and rechecked during the first few hours after CEA. The use of drains does not eliminate the risk.

Mild or moderate hematomas that do not cause pain or breathing difficulty may stabilize with sandbag pressure, but any hematoma that is causing any degree of stridor or respiratory distress is most safely treated by surgical evacuation of the clot. In more extreme circumstances, such as frank hypoxia with imminent respiratory arrest, intubation should be preformed by a skilled anesthetist in the operating room if at all possible. Intubation may be difficult, and urgent surgery must follow. If the hematoma causes enough airway distortion to prevent visualization of the vocal cords, the wound should be opened immediately to decompress the airway. Tracheostomy under these circumstances is a last resort, because the trachea is difficult to locate. It is sometimes hard to locate the precise source of bleeding in these patients. Intubation should continue at least overnight and until swelling begins to subside and an air leak is detected around the endotracheal tube when its cuff is deflated.

POSTOPERATIVE STROKE

Stroke complicating CEA has several possible causes, including thrombotic occlusion of the ICA, embolism from the endarterectomy site, cerebral ischemia during carotid cross-clamping for arterial repair, and intracranial hemorrhage. The majority of operative strokes occur during or within 12 hours of surgery, and ICA thrombosis or thromboembolism accounts for the majority.[171] Hemorrhage is a rare cause of postoperative stroke, often related to repair of a critical stenosis in the presence of a distal infarct in a hypertensive patient.[102] In NASCET's 1415 surgical patients (albeit carefully selected), there were only two postoperative intracerebral hemorrhages.[104]

In the setting of an acute postoperative stroke causing hemiparesis or hemiplegia, most authorities have recommended either urgent surgical reexploration or cerebral angiography with the goal of reopening occluded vessels and correcting flaws in the arterial repair. However, there is some question as to the efficacy of this approach in reversing stroke. The surgical results of NASCET include ten patients who underwent emergency reoperation for major hemispheric strokes, eight of whom had occluded arteries that were reopened, but none benefited.[104] Other investigators have reported more favorable results from an aggressive surgical approach to acute postoperative

Table 65.8 Management of Postendarterectomy Neurologic Deficits

Hemispheric deficits (hemiplegia, forced eye deviation)	Immediate carotid angiography or reexploration to detect and reverse acute carotid occlusion
Focal deficits	In setting of preexisting neurodeficit (prior stroke), temporize for 30 minutes, because postoperative exacerbation of deficit is common, and gradual movement will be noted
	If no preoperative deficit was present, postoperative deficit may indicate cerebral angiography and possibly intra-arterial thrombolysis of distal thromboemboli
	Perform CT scanning if angiographic findings are negative for thromboembolism (to rule out intracranial hemorrhage)

stroke.[172] A review of 700 consecutive CEA procedures examined in detail 13 patients who experienced major hemispheric deficits (hemiplegia with or without aphasia, forced eye deviation, and decreased consciousness) that prompted either immediate surgical reexploration or cerebral angiography with reoperation on the basis of angiogram results.[101] Approximately half of the patients had an underlying, correctable lesion (endarterectomy site occlusion or stenosis), and in these patients, stroke typically occurred after they awoke from surgery. Approximately half of these patients with occlusion or stenosis improved as a result of immediate reopening of occluded arteries, although new infarcts were seen in almost all patients on CT scanning.

The options for an aggressive approach to postoperative stroke are immediate carotid artery imaging with ultrasonography or contrast angiography, surgical reexploration of the operative site, and, perhaps, a combination of the two if intraoperative cerebral angiography is available. If available, prompt cerebral angiography best directs further management, which might include endovascular management with thrombolysis or stents.[173–176] CT of the brain is less profitable in the first several hours after CEA, given the rarity of acute intracerebral hemorrhage after this procedure. The course of action chosen, usually on the basis of the suspected cause of stroke, the timing of its onset, and the speed with which either angiography or surgery can be performed, is aimed at detecting and correcting carotid artery occlusion or significant residual stenosis (Table 65.8). As with all types of acute and potentially reversible ischemic stroke, speed is of the essence. On occasion, immediate operation can result in an important, early neurologic improvement.

CAROTID ENDARTERECTOMY VERSUS CAROTID ANGIOPLASTY AND STENTING

Used for several decades in the treatment of peripheral and coronary artery disease, percutaneous transluminal angioplasty is a technique in which an endovascular balloon catheter is used to mechanically dilate a stenosed artery, and a metallic stent can be deployed afterwards along the dilated segment to help maintain vascular patency. It was first reported in the carotid artery in the early 1980s for atherosclerosis and fibromuscular dysplasia,[177–181] and the first series of patients who underwent carotid angioplasty was described later in the same decade.[182,183] Since then, its use has grown remarkably, performed primarily by interventional cardiologists and radiologists and, to a lesser extent, by specially trained neurologists, neurosurgeons, and vascular surgeons. A multicenter registry has published information on more than 5000 patients who have been treated with carotid angioplasty world-wide.[184] Less invasive than open surgery, angioplasty with stenting avoids the potential wound complications associated with CEA, such as infection, cranial neuropathies, and neck hematomas.

Periprocedural stroke risk in some uncontrolled, single-institution case-series has been similar to or lower than the risk associated with CEA.[185–187] In angioplasty for severe carotid stenosis, however, a guidewire and catheter must be passed across the narrowing and the plaque must be distended, a maneuver that can be associated with cerebral embolism. A systematic comparison of 30-day outcome of CEA and angioplasty with or without stenting and for symptomatic carotid disease reported in single-center studies published between 1990 and 1999 (13 angioplasties and 20 CEAs) found a significantly higher risk of stroke or death with angioplasty.[188] Several randomized controlled trials comparing angioplasty with stenting and CEA have been reported to date. Two were stopped early because of significantly worse outcomes among patients randomly assigned to angioplasty and stenting.[189,190] A third, the Carotid and Vertebral Artery Transluminal Angioplasty Study (CAVATAS) randomly assigned 253 patients to undergo surgery and 251 to receive endovascular treatment in Europe. Although there were no significant differences in outcomes, the results were relatively poor, with a 10% stroke rate in both groups, and rates of 5.9% and 6.4% for disabling stroke and death in the surgery and endovascular treatment groups, respectively.[191]

The durability of carotid angioplasty and stenting has been a concern,[192] and the procedure does not appear to be consistently less costly than CEA.[193,194] Commentaries have concluded that current evidence does not support the incorporation of carotid angioplasty and stenting into routine clinical practice at present, although the situation may change in the future.[194–196] Special circumstances may warrant its current use, such as radiation-induced stenosis, high cervical and surgically inaccessible stenosis, and symptomatic stenosis in a patient with a significant medical contraindication to surgery, such as recent myocardial infarction. Carotid angioplasty with stenting is a promising technique, particularly with the development of devices that can protect the brain from microembolization of plaque during the procedure,[197–199] improved stent technology, and greater operator experience. It is hoped that another randomized, controlled trial currently under way, the Carotid Revascularization Endarterectomy versus Stent Trial (CREST), comparing CEA and carotid angioplasty with stenting in symptomatic patients who have at least 70% stenosis, will help clarify the role of this intervention in the management of carotid artery disease.[48]

PERFORMANCE OF CAROTID ENDARTERECTOMY: AUDITING AND OUTCOMES ANALYSIS

CEA is well suited for examination of its outcomes, complications, and appropriateness. Indications for CEA have become reasonably well defined, and the major events that can complicate CEA—stroke and death—are readily detected from reviews of hospital records and contact with patients for follow-up. In addition to studies that have documented a large resurgence in the use of CEA,[43–47,200] studies have characterized the increases in terms of patient demographics and geographic locations, indications for and appropriateness of surgery, complication rates, and outcomes as they relate to provider or surgeon volumes.

Higher CEA rates have also been noted in women and elderly patients,[45,47] and marked geographic variations between countries and between regions within countries have been recorded, probably reflecting regional clinical practice and supply of services.[43,201–204] Indications for surgery also vary among study populations, although many studies from North America have documented high rates of surgery for asymptomatic stenosis, ranging between 25% and nearly 60% in various parts of Canada or the United States.[205–210] These high rates for an uncertain indication have been a cause of some disquiet, as discussed previously in this chapter.

Despite concerns that the complication rates seen in the randomized trials might not be matched in regular practice, several population-based studies examining this issue have reported acceptable outcomes.[206–214] A number of studies have tried to correlate surgical results with surgical volumes, some showing higher complication rates in low-volume centers or among surgeons with extremely low annual volumes (less than 5 or 10 procedures per year),[208,214,215] but some having found no clear relation between the number of procedures performed and the outcome.[207,216–218] Other surgeon characteristics have been considered, including specialty (vascular surgery versus neurosurgery) and various surgical techniques, also with conflicting results.[104,219,220]

For the clinician faced with a patient possibly requiring CEA, more important than results from studies or other centers are local and individual surgeon results, information that is usually not readily available.[221] When local audits are conducted, the results are generally kept confidential. A regular auditing process providing direct feedback of surgical indications and operative results to operating surgeons, however, has been found to result in significant improvements in both indications for and results of CEA.[210]

References

1. Savory WS: Case of a young woman in whom the main arteries of both upper extremities and of the left side of the neck were throughout completely obliterated. Med-Chir Tr Lond 39:205–219, 1856.
2. Gowers WR: On a case of simultaneous embolism of central retinal and middle cerebral arteries. Lancet 2:794, 1976.
3. Chiari H: Uber das Verhalten des Teilungswinkels der Carotis communis bei der Endarteriitis chronica deformans. Verhandl D Deutsch Path Gesellsch 9:326, 1905.
4. Guthrie LG, Mayou S: Right hemiplegia and atrophy of left optic nerve. Proc R Soc Med 1:180, 1908.
5. Hunt JR: The role of the carotid arteries in the causation of vascular lesions of the brain, with remarks on certain special features of the symptomatology. Am J Med Sci 147:704–713, 1914.
6. Moniz E: Encephalographic artérielle son importance dans la localisation des tumeurs cérébrales. Rev Neurol (Par) 2:72–90, 1927.
7. Fisher M: Occlusion of the internal carotid artery. Arch Neurol Psych 65:346–377, 1951.
8. Fisher M: Transient monocular blindness associated with hemiplegia. Arch Ophthalmol 47:167–203, 1952.
9. Fisher M: Occlusion of the carotid arteries. Arch Neurol Psych 72:187–204, 1954.
10. Carrea R, Mollins M, Murphy G: Surgical treatment of spontaneous thrombosis of the internal carotid artery in the neck: Carotid-carotideal anastomosis—report of a case. Acta Neurol Latino Am 1:71, 1955.
11. Gurdjian ES, Webster JE: Stroke resulting from internal carotid artery thrombosis in the neck. JAMA 151:541–545, 1953.
12. Hamlin H, Sweet WH, Lougheed WM: Surgical reconstruction of occluded cervical carotid artery. J Neurosurg 15:427–437, 1958.
13. Strully KJ, Hurwitt ES, Blankenberg HW: Thrombo-endarterectomy for thrombosis of the internal carotid artery in the neck. J Neurosurg 10:474–482, 1953.
14. Eastcott HHG, Pickering GW, Rob CG: Reconstruction of internal carotid artery in a patient with intermittent attacks of hemiplegia. Lancet 267:994–996, 1954.
15. Denman FR, Ehni G, Duty WS: Insidious thrombotic occlusion of cervical carotid arteries, treated by arterial graft. Surgery 38:569–577, 1955.
16. Cooley DA, Al-Naaman YD, Carton CA: Surgical treatment of arteriosclerotic occlusion of common carotid artery. J Neurosurg 13:500–506, 1956.
17. Crawford ES, De Bakey ME, Fields WS: Roentgenographic diagnosis and surgical treatment of basilar artery insufficiency. JAMA 168:509–514, 1958.
18. DeBakey ME, Crawford ES, Cooley DA, et al: Cerebral arterial insufficiency: One to 11-year results following arterial reconstructive operation. Ann Surg 161:921–945, 1965.
19. Thompson JE, Austin DJ: Surgical treatment of arteriosclerotic occlusions of the carotid artery in the neck. Surgery 51:74–83, 1962.
20. Murphey F, Maccubbin DA: Carotid endarterectomy: A long-term follow up study. J Neurosurg 23:156–168, 1965.
21. Lougheed WM, Elgie RG, Barnett HJM: The results of surgical management of extracranial internal carotid artery occlusion and stenosis. CMAJ 95:1279–1293, 1966.
22. Fields WS, North RR, Hass WK, et al: Joint study of extracranial arterial occlusion as a cause of stroke: Organization of study and survey of patient population. JAMA 203:955–960, 1968.
23. Fields WS, Maslenikov V, Meyer JS, et al: Joint study of extracranial arterial occlusion. V: Progress report of prognosis following surgery or nonsurgical treatment for transient cerebral ischemic attacks and cervical carotid artery lesions. JAMA 211:1993–2003, 1970.
24. Dyken ML, Pokras R: The performance of endarterectomy for disease of the extracranial arteries of the head. Stroke 15:948–950, 1984.
25. A randomized trial of aspirin and sulfinpyrazone and threatened stroke. Canadian Cooperative Stroke Study Group. N Engl J Med 299:53–59, 1978.
26. Brott T, Thalinger K: The practice of carotid endarterectomy in a large metropolitan area. Stroke 15:950–955, 1984.
27. Slavish LG, Nicholas GG, Gee W: Review of a community hospital experience with carotid endarterectomy. Stroke 15:956–959, 1984.
28. Muuronen A: Outcome of surgical treatment of 110 patients with transient ischemic attacks. Stroke 15:959–964, 1984.
29. Fode NC, Sundt TM Jr, Robertson JT, et al: Multicenter retrospective review of results and complications of carotid endarterectomy in 1981. Stroke 17:370–376, 1986.
30. Merrick NJ, Brook RH, Fink A, et al: Use of carotid endarterectomy in five California Veterans Administration medical centers. JAMA 256:2531–2535, 1986.

31. Winslow CM, Solomon DH, Chassin MR, et al: The appropriateness of carotid endarterectomy. N Engl J Med 318:721–727, 1988.
32. Failure of extracranial-intracranial arterial bypass to reduce the risk of ischemic stroke: Results of an international randomized trial. The EC/IC Bypass Study Group. N Engl J Med 313:1191–1200, 1985.
33. Warlow C: Carotid endarterectomy:does it work? Stroke 15:1068–1076, 1984.
34. Barnett HJ, Plum F, Walton JN: Carotid endarterectomy: An expression of concern. Stroke 15:941–943, 1984.
35. Pokras R, Dyken ML: Dramatic changes in the performance of endarterectomy for diseases of the extracranial arteries of the head. Stroke 19:1289–1290, 1988.
36. Beneficial effect of carotid endarterectomy in symptomatic patients with high-grade carotid stenosis. North American Symptomatic Carotid Endarterectomy Trial Collaborators. N Engl J Med 325:445–453, 1991.
37. MRC European Carotid Surgery Trial: Interim results for symptomatic patients with severe (70–99%) or with mild (0–29%) carotid stenosis. European Carotid Surgery Trialists' Collaborative Group. Lancet 337:1235–1243, 1991.
38. Hobson RW, Weiss DG, Fields WS, et al: Efficacy of carotid endarterectomy for asymptomatic carotid stenosis. Veterans Affairs Cooperative Study Group. N Engl J Med 328:221–227, 1993.
39. Mayberg MR, Wilson SE, Yatsu F, et al: Carotid endarterectomy and prevention of cerebral ischemia in symptomatic carotid stenosis. Veterans Affairs Cooperative Studies Program 309 Trialist Group. JAMA 266:3289–3294, 1993.
40. Endarterectomy for asymptomatic carotid artery stenosis. Executive Committee for the Asymptomatic Carotid Atherosclerosis Study. JAMA 273:1421–1428, 1995.
41. Endarterectomy for moderate symptomatic carotid stenosis: Interim results from the MRC European Carotid Surgery Trial. Lancet 347:1591–1593, 1996.
42. Barnett HJM, Taylor DW, Eliaziw M, et al: Benefit of carotid endarterectomy in patients with symptomatic moderate or severe stenosis. North American Symptomatic Carotid Endarterectomy Trial Collaborators. N Engl J Med 339:1415–1425, 1998.
43. Tu JV, Hannan EL, Anderson GM, et al: The fall and rise of carotid endarterectomy in the United States and Canada. N Engl J Med 339:1441–1447, 1998.
44. Hsia DC, Moscoe LM, Krushat WM: Epidemiology of carotid endarterectomy among medicare beneficiaries: 1985–1996 update. Stroke 29:346–350, 1998.
45. Holloway RG Jr, Witter DM Jr, Mushlin AI, et al: Carotid endarterectomy trends in the patterns and outcomes of care at academic medical centers, 1990 through 1995. Arch Neurol 55:25–32, 1998.
46. Gross CP, Steiner CA, Bass EB, et al: Relation between prepublication release of clinical trial results and the practice of carotid endarterectomy. JAMA 284:2886–2893, 2000.
47. Morasch MD: Carotid endarterectomy: Characterization of recent increases in procedure rates. J Vasc Surg 31:901–909, 2000.
48. Hobson RW II: Carotid angioplasty-stent: Clinical experience and role of clinical trials. J Vasc Surg 33:S117–S123, 2001.
49. Fox AJ: How to measure carotid stenosis. Radiology 186:316–318, 1993.
50. Johnston SC, Gress DR, Browner WS, et al: Short-term prognosis after emergency department diagnosis of TIA. JAMA 284:2901–2906, 2000.
51. Morgenstern LB, Fox AJ, Sharpe BL, et al: The risks and benefits of carotid endarterectomy in patients with near occlusion of the carotid artery. Neurology 48:911–915, 1997.
52. Rothwell PM, Warlow CP: Low risk of ischemic stroke in patients with reduced internal carotid artery lumen diameter distal to severe symptomatic carotid stenosis: Cerebral protection due to low poststenotic flow? European Carotid Trialists' Collaborative Group. Stroke 31:622–630, 2000.
53. Henderson RD, Eliasziw M, Fox AJ, et al: Angiographically defined collateral circulation and risk of stroke in patients with severe carotid artery stenosis. Stroke 31:128–132, 2000.
54. Eliasziw M, Streifler JY, Fox AJ, et al: Significance of plaque ulceration in symptomatic patients with high-grade carotid stenosis. Stroke 25:304–308, 1994.
55. Rothwell PM, Gibson R, Warlow CP: Interrelation between plaque surface morphology and degree of stenosis on carotid angiograms and the risk of ischemic stroke in patients with symptomatic carotid

stenosis. European Carotid Trialists' Collaborative Group.Stroke 31:615–621, 2000.
56. Gasecki AP, Eliasziw M, Ferguson GG et al: Long-term prognosis and effect of endarterectomy in patients with symptomatic severe carotid stenosis and contralateral carotid stenosis or occlusion: Results from NASCET. J Neurosurg 83:778–782, 1995.
57. Kappelle LJ, Eliasziw M, Fox AJ, et al: Importance of intracranial atherosclerotic disease in patients with symptomatic stenosis of the internal carotid artery. Stroke 30:282–286, 1999.
58. Benavente O, Eliaszw M, Streifler JY, et al: Prognosis after transient monocular blindness associated with carotid artery stenosis. N Engl J Med 345:1084–1090, 2001.
59. Liapis CD, Kakisis JD, Kostakis AG: Carotid stenosis: Factors affecting symptomatology. Stroke 32:2782–2786, 2001.
60. Culebras A, Kase CS, Masdeu JC, et al: Practice guidelines for the use of imaging in transient ischemic attacks and acute stroke. A report of the Stroke Council, American Heart Association. Stroke 28:14801497, 1997.
61. Johnston DCC, Goldstein LB: Clinical carotid endarterectomy decision making: Noninvasive vascular imaging versus angiography. Neurology 56:1009–1015, 2001.
62. Larkin M: Should endarterectomy decisions be based on noninvasive imaging? Lancet 357:1343, 2001.
63. Collier, PE: Changing trends in the use of preoperative carotid arteriography: The community experience. J Cardiovasc Surg 6:485–489, 1998.
64. Guzman RP: Appropriate imaging before carotid endarterectomy. Can J Surg 41:218–223, 1998.
65. Eliasziw M, Rankin RN, Fox AJ, et al: Accuracy and prognostic consequences of ultrasonography in identifying severe carotid artery stenosis. North American Symptomatic Carotid Endarterectomy Trial (NASCET) Group. Stroke 26:1747–1752, 1995.
66. Qureshi AI, Suri FK, Ali Z, et al: Role of conventional angiography in evaluation of patients with carotid artery stenosis demonstrated by Doppler ultrasound in general practice. Stroke 32:2287–2291, 2001.
67. Anderson GB, Ashforth R, Steinke DE, et al: CT angiography for the detection of characterization of carotid bifurcation disease. Stroke 31:2168–2174, 2000.
68. Wardlaw JM, Lewis SC, Humphrey P, et al: How does the degree of carotid stenosis affect the accuracy and interobserver variability of magnetic resonance angiography? J Neurol Neurosurg Psychiatry 71:155–160, 2001.
69. Ozaki CK, Irwin PB, Flynn TC, et al: Surgical decision making for carotid endarterectomy and contemporary magnetic resonance angiography. Am J Surg 178:182–184, 1999.
70. Rothwell PM, Pendlebury ST, Wardlaw J, et al: Critical appraisal of the design and reporting of studies of imaging and measurement of carotid stenosis. Stroke 31:1444–1450, 2000.
71. Hankey GJ, Warlow CP, Molyneus AJ: Complications of cerebral angiography for patients with mild carotid territory ischaemia being considered for carotid endarterectomy. J Neurol Neurosurg Psychiatry 53:542–548, 1990.
72. Chaturvedi S, Policherla PN, Femino, L: Cerebral angiography practices at US teaching hospitals: Implications for carotid endarterectomy. Stroke 28:1895–1897, 1997.
73. Ruehm SG, Goyen M, Barkhausen J, et al: Rapid magnetic resonance angiography for detection of atherosclerosis. Lancet 357:1086–1091, 2001.
74. Phan T, Huston J, Bernstein MA, et al: Contrast-enhanced magnetic resonance angiography of the cervical vessels: Experience with 422 patients. Stroke 32:2282–2286, 2001.
75. Barnett HJM, Meldrum HE, Eliasziw M, et al: The appropriate use of carotid endarterectomy. CMAJ 166:1169–1179, 2002.
76. Alamowitch S, Eliasziw M, Algra A, et al: Risk, causes, and prevention of ischaemic stroke in elderly patients with symptomatic internal-carotid-artery stenosis. Lancet 357:1154–1160, 2001.
77. Rothwell PM: Carotid endarterectomy and prevention of stroke in the very elderly. Lancet 457:1142–1143, 2001.
78. Kallikazaros I, Costas T, Sideris S, et al: Carotid artery disease as a marker for the presence of severe coronary artery disease in patients evaluated for chest pain. Stroke 30:1002–1007, 1999.
79. Gerraty RP, Gates PC, Doyle JC: Carotid stenosis and perioperative stroke risk in symptomatic and asymptomatic patients undergoing vascular or coronary surgery. Stroke 24:1115–1118, 1993.

80. Ricotta JJ, Faggioli GL, Castilone A, et al: Risk factors for stroke after cardiac surgery: Buffalo Cardiac-Cerebral Study Group. J Vasc Surg 21:359–363, 1995.

81. Palerme LP, Hill AB, Obrand D, et al: Is Canadian cardiac surgeons' management of asymptomatic carotid artery stenosis at coronary artery bypass supported by the literature? A survey and a critical appraisal of the literature. Can J Surg 43:93–103, 2000.

82. Das SK, Brow TD, Pepper J: Continuing controversy in the management of concomitant coronary and carotid disease: An overview. Int J Cardiol 74:47–65, 2000.

83. Takach TJ, Reul GJ Jr, Cooley DA, et al: Is an intergrated approach warranted for concomitant carotid and coronary artery disease? Ann Thorac Surg 64:16–22, 1997.

84. Borger MA, Fremes SE, Weisel RD, et al: Coronary bypass and carotid endarterectomy: Does a combined approach increase risk? A metaanalysis. Ann Thorac Surg 68:14–20, 1999.

85. Darling RC III, Dylewski M, Chang BB, et al: Combined carotid endarterectomy and coronary artery bypass grafting does not increase the risk of perioperative stroke. Cardiovasc Surg 6:448–452, 1998.

86. Minami K, Fukahara K, Boethig D, et al: Long-term results of simultaneous carotid endarterectomy and myocardial revascularization with cardiopulmonary bypass used for both procedures. J Thorac Cardiovasc Surg 119:764–773, 2000.

87. Estes JM, Khabbaz KR, Barnatan M, et al: Outcome after combined carotid endarterectomy and coronary artery bypass is related to patient selection. J Vasc Surg 33:1179–1184, 2001.

88. Landesberg G, Wolf Y, Schechter D, et al: Preoperative thallium scanning, selective coronary revascularization, and long-term survival after carotid endarterectomy. Stroke 29:2541–2548, 1998.

89. Lopes DK, Mericle RA, Lanzino G, et al: Stent placement for the treatment of occlusive atherosclerotic carotid artery disease in patients with concomitant coronary artery disease. J Neurosurg 96:490–496, 2002.

90. Kistler JP, Furie KL: Carotid endarterectomy revisited. N Engl J Med 342:1693–1700, 2000.

91. Gorelick PB, Sacco RL, Smith DB, et al: Prevention of a first stroke: A review of guidelines and a multidisciplinary consensus statement from the National Stroke Association. JAMA 281:1112–1120, 1999.

92. Moore WS, Barnett HJM, Beebe HG, et al: Guidelines for carotid endarterectomy: A multidisciplinary consensus statement from the Ad Hoc Committee, American Heart Association. Stroke 26:188–201, 1995.

93. Findlay JM, Tucker WS, Ferguson GG, et al: Guidelines for the use of carotid endarterectomy: Current recommendations from the Canadian Neurosurgical Society. CMAJ 157:653–659, 1997.

94. Wolf PA, Clagett GP, Easton JD, et al: Preventing ischemic stroke in patients with prior stroke and transient ischemic attack: A statement from healthcare professionals from the Stroke Council of the American Heart Association. Stroke 30:1991–1994, 1999.

95. Albers GW, Hart RG, Lutsep HL, et al: Supplement to the guidelines for the management of transient ischemic attacks: A statement from the Ad Hoc Committee on Guidelines for the Management of Transient Ischemic Attacks, Stroke Council, American Heart Association. Stroke 30:2502–2511, 1999.

96. Kawaguchi S, Okuno S, Sakaki T, et al: Effect of carotid endarterectomy on chronic ocular ischemic syndrome due to internal carotid artery stenosis. Neurosurgery 48:328–332, 2001.

97. Little JR, Moufarrij NA, Furlan AJ: Early carotid endarterectomy after cerebral infarction. Neurosurgery 24:334–338, 1989.

98. Gasecki AP, Ferguson GC, Eliasziw M: Early endarterectomy for severe carotid artery stenosis after a nondisabling stroke: Results from the North American Symptomatic Carotid Endarterectomy Trial. J Vasc Surg 2:288, 1994.

99. Hoffman M, Robbs J: Carotid endarterectomy after recent cerebral infarction. Eur J Vasc Surg 18:6–10, 1999.

100. Blaser T, Hofmann K, Buerger T, et al: Risk of stroke, transient ischemic attack, and vessel occlusion before endarterectomy in patients with symptomatic severe carotid stenosis. Stroke 33:1057–1062, 2002.

101. Findlay JM, Marchak BE: Reoperation for acute hemispheric stroke after carotid endarterectomy: Is there any value? Neurosurgery 50:486–492, 2002.

102. Henderson RD, Phan TG, Piepgras, DG: Mechanisms of intracerebral hemorrhage after carotid endarterectomy. J Neurosurg 95:964–969, 2001.

103. Zannetti S, Parente B, De Rango P, et al: Role of surgical techniques and operative findings in cranial and cervical nerve injuries during carotid endarterectomy. Eur J Vasc Endovasc Surg 15:528–531, 1998.

104. Ferguson GG, Eliasziw M, Barr HW, et al: The North American Symptomatic Carotid Endarterectomy Trial: Surgical results in 1415 patients. Stroke 30:1751–1758, 1999.

105. Rothwell PM, Slattery J, Warlow CP: A systematic review of the risks of stroke and death due to endarterectomy for symptomatic carotid stenosis. Stroke 27:260–265, 1996.

106. Lanzino G, Couture D, Andreoli A, et al: Carotid endarterectomy: Can we select surgical candidates at high risk for stroke and low risk for perioperative complications? Neurosurgery 49:913–924, 2001.

107. Sundt TM Jr, Sandok BA, Wisnant JP: Carotid endarterectomy: Complications and preoperative assessment of risk. Mayo Clin Proc 50:301–306, 1975.

108. Sieber FE, Toung TJ, Diringer MN, et al: Preoperative risks predict neurological outcome of carotid endarterectomy related stroke. Neurosurgery 30:847–854, 1992.

109. McCrory DC, Goldstein LB, Samsa GP, et al: Predicting complications of carotid endarterectomy. Stroke 24:1285–1291, 1993.

110. Rothwell PM, Slattery J, Warlow CP: Clinical and angiographic predictors of stroke and death from carotid endarterectomy: Systematic review. BMJ 315:1571–1577, 1997.

111. Goldstein LB, Samsa GP, Matchar DB, et al: Multicenter review of preoperative risk factors for endarterectomy for asymptomatic carotid artery stenosis. Stroke 29:750–753, 1998.

112. Kucey DS, Bowyer B, Iron K, et al: Determinants of outcome after carotid endarterectomy. J Vasc Surg 28:1051–1058, 1998.

113. Bond R, Narayan SK, Rothwell PM, et al: Clinical and radiological risk factors for operative stroke death in the European Carotid Surgery Trial. Eur J Vasc Surg 23:108–116, 2001.

114. Rothwell PM, Slattery J, Warlow CP: A systematic comparison of the risks of stroke and death due to carotid endarterectomy for symptomatic and asymptomatic stenosis. Stroke 27:266–269, 1996.

115. Dardik A, Bowman HM, Gordon TA, et al: Impact of race on the outcome of carotid endarterectomy: A population-based analysis of 9,842 recent elective procedures. Ann Surg 232:704–709, 2000.

116. Meyer FB, Piepgras DG, Fode NC: Surgical treatment of recurrent carotid artery stenosis. J Neurosurg 80:781–787, 1994.

117. AbuRahma AF, Jennings TG, Wulu JT, et al: Redo carotid endarterectomy versus primary carotid endarterectomy. Stroke 32:2787–2792, 2001.

118. Hill BB, Olcott C IV, Dalman RL, et al: Reoperation for carotid stenosis is as safe as primary carotid endarterectomy. J Vasc Surg 30:26–35, 1999.

119. Johnson CA, Tollefson DFJ, Olsen SB, et al: The natural history of early recurrent carotid artery stenosis. Am J Surg 177:433–436, 1999.

120. Findlay JM, Lougheed W: Microsurgical endarterectomy. Tech Neurosurg 3:34–44, 1997.

121. Simonian GT, Pappas PJ, Padberg FT Jr, et al: Mandibular subluxation for distal internal carotid exposure: Technical considerations. J Vasc Surg 30:1116–1120, 1999.

122. Shah DM, Darling RC 3rd, Chang BB, et al: Carotid endarterectomy by eversion technique: Its safety and durability. Ann Surg 228:471–478, 1998.

123. Peiper C, Nowack J, Ktenidis K, et al: Eversion endarterectomy versus open thromboendarterectomy and patch plasty for the treatment of internal carotid artery stenosis. Eur J Vasc Endovasc Surg 20:317–318, 2000.

124. Green RM, Greenberg R, Illig K, et al: Eversion endarterectomy of the carotid artery: Technical considerations and recurrent stenoses. J Vasc Surg 32:1052–1061, 2000.

125. Katras T, Baltazar U, Rush DS, et al: Durability of eversion carotid endarterectomy: Comparison with primary closure and carotid patch angioplasty. J Vasc Surg 34:453–458, 2001.

126. Cao P, Giordano G, De Rango P, et al: Eversion versus conventional carotid endarterectomy: Late results of a prospective multicenter randomized trial. J Vasc Surg 31:19–30, 2000.

127. Cao PG, de Rango P, Zannetti S, et al: Eversion versus conventional carotid endarterectomy for preventing stroke. Cochrane Database Syst Rev CD001921, 2001.

128. Jackson MR, Clagett GP: Use of vein or synthetic patches in carotid endarterectomy. In Loftus CM, Kresowik TK (eds): Carotid Artery Surgery. New York, Thieme, 1999, pp 281–290.

129. Yamamoto Y, Piepgras DG, Marsh WR, et al: Complications resulting from saphenous vein patch graft after carotid endarterectomy. Neurosurgery 39:670–675, 1996.

130. Meyer FB, Windschitl WL: Repair of carotid endarterectomy with collagen-impregnated fabric graft. J Neurosurg 88:647–649, 1998.

131. Bond R, Narayan SK, Rothwell PM, et al: Clinical and radiographic risk factors for operative stroke and death in the European Carotid Surgery Trial. Eur J Vasc Endovasc Surg 23:108–116, 2002.

132. AbuRahma AF, Robinson PA, Saiedy S, et al: Prospective randomized trial of bilateral carotid endarterectomies: Primary closure versus patching. Stroke 30:1185–1189, 1999.

133. AbuRhama AF, Robinson PA, Saiedy S, et al: Prospective randomized trial of carotid endarterectomy with primary closure and patch angioplasty with saphenous vein, jugular vein, and polytetrafluoroethylene: Perioperative (30-day) results. J Vasc Surg 24:998–1007, 1996.

134. Counsell CE, Salinas R, Naylor R, et al: A systematic review of the ramdomised trials of carotid patch angioplasty in carotid endarterectomy. Eur J Vasc Endovasc Surg 13:345–354, 1997.

135. Hayes PD, Allroggen H, Steel S, et al: Randomized trial of vein versus Dacron patching during carotid endarterectomy: Influence of patch type on postoperative embolization. J Vasc Surg 33:994–1000, 2001.

136. O'Hara PJ, Hertzer NR, Mascha EJ, et al: A prospective, randomized study of saphenous vein patching versus synthetic patching during carotid endarterectomy. J Vasc Surg 35:324–332, 2002.

137. Ballotta E, Renon L, Da Giau G, et al: A prospective randomized study on bilateral carotid endarterectomy: Patching versus eversion. Ann Surg 232:119–125, 2000.

138. Dimakakos PB, Kotsis T, Tsiligiris B, et al: Comparative results of staged and simultaneous bilateral carotid endarterectomy: A clinical study and surgical treatment. Cardiovasc Surg 8:9–17, 2000.

139. Kumar SM, Wang JCC, Barry MC, et al: Carotid stump syndrome: Outcome from surgical management. Eur J Vasc Endovasc Surg 21:214–219, 2001.

140. Farsak B, Oc M, Boke E: Simultaneous bilateral carotid endarterectomy: Our first experience. Ann Thorac Cardiovasc Surg 7:292–296, 2001.

141. Hugenholtz H, Elgie RG: Carotid thromboendarterectomy: A reappraisal. J Neurosurg 53:776783, 1980.

142. Meyer FB, Sundt TM, Piepgras DG, et al: Emergency carotid endarterectomy for patients with acute carotid occlusion and profound neurological deficits. Ann Surg 203:82–89, 1986.

143. McCormick PW, Spetzler RF, Bailes JE, et al: Thromboendarterectomy of the symptomatic occluded internal carotid artery. J Neurosurg 76:752–758, 1992.

144. Kasper GC, Wladis AR, Lohr JM, et al: Carotid thromboendarterectomy for recent total occlusion of the internal carotid artery. J Vasc Surg 33:242–249, 2001.

145. Cote R, Barnett HJM, Taylor DW: Internal carotid occlusion: A prospective study. Stroke 14:898, 1983.

146. Villarreal J, Silva T, Eliasziw M, et al: Prognosis of patients with an intraluminal thrombus in the internal carotid artery. North American Symptomatic Carotid Endarterectomy Trial (NASCET) Group. Stroke 29:276, 1998.

147. Lennard N, Smith JL, Gaunt ME, et al: A policy of quality control assessment helps to reduce the risk of intraoperative stroke during carotid endarterectomy. Eur J Vasc Surg 17:234–240, 1999.

148. Zannetti S, Cao P, De Rango P, et al: Intraoperative assessment of technical perfection in carotid endarterectomy: A prospective analysis of 1305 completion procedures. Collaborators of the EVEREST study group. Eversion versus standard carotid endarterectomy. Eur J Vasc Surg 18:52–58, 1999.

149. Padayachee TS, McGuinness CL, Modareski KB, et al: Value of intraoperative duplex imaging during supervised carotid endarterectomy. Br J Surg 88:389–392, 2001.

150. Panneton JM, Berger MW, Lewis BD, et al: Intraoperative duplex ultrasound during carotid endarterectomy. Vasc Surg 35:1–9, 2001.

151. Bond R, Warlow CP, Naylor AR, Rothwell PM: Variation in surgical and anesthetic technique with operative risk in the European Carotid Surgery Trial: Implications for trials of ancillary techniques. Eur J Vasc Surg 23:117–126, 2002.

152. Cheng MA, Theard MA, Tempelhoff R: Anesthesia for carotid endarterectomy: A survey. J Neurosurg Anes 9:211–216, 1997.

153. Knighton JD, Stoneham MD: Carotid endarterectomy: A survey of anaesthetic practice. Anaesthesia 55:475–488, 2000.

154. Finocchi C, Gandolfo C, Tiziana C, et al: Role of transcranial Doppler and stump pressure during carotid endarterectomy. Stroke 28:2448–2452, 1997.

155. Wellman BJ, Loftus CM, Kresowick TF, et al: The differences in electroencephalographic changes in patients undergoing carotid endarterectomies while under local versus general anesthesia. Neurosurgery 43:769–773, 1998.

156. Sundt TM, Sharbrough FW, Piepgras DG, et al: Correlation of cerebral blood flow and electroencephalographic changes during carotid endarterectomy. Mayo Clin Proc 56:533–543, 1981.

157. Manninen PH, Tan TK, Sarjeant RM: Somatosensory evoked potential monitoring during carotid endarterectomy in patients with a stroke. Anesth Analg 93:39–44, 2001.

158. McCarthy RJ, McCabe AE, Walker R, et al: The value of transcranial Doppler in predicting cerebral ischemia during carotid endarterectomy. Eur J Vasc Endovasc Surg 21:408–412, 2001.

159. Ackerstaff RGA, Moons KGM, van de Vlasakker CJW, et al: Association of intraoperative transcranial Doppler variables with stroke from carotid endarterectomy. Stroke 31:1817–1823, 2000.

160. Dalman JE, Beenakkers ICM, Moll FL, et al: Transcranial Doppler monitoring during carotid endarterectomy helps to identify patients at risk of postoperative hyperperfusion. Eur J Vasc Endovasc Surg 18:222–227, 1999.

161. Beese U, Langer H, Lang W, et al: Comparison of near infrared spectroscopy and somatosensory evoked potentials for the detection of cerebral ischemia during carotid endarterectomy. Stroke 29:2032–2037, 1998.

162. Samra SK, Dy EA, Welch K, et al: Evaluation of a cerebral oximeter as a monitor of cerebral ischemia during carotid endarterectomy. Anesthesiology 93:964–970, 2000.

163. Pandit JJ, Bree S, Dillon P, et al: A comparison of superficial versus combined (superficial and deep) cervical plexus block for carotid endarterectomy: A prospective, randomized study. Anesth Analg 91:781–786, 2000.

164. Bourke DL, Thomas P: Mandibular nerve block in addition to cervical plexus block for carotid endarterectomy. Anesth Analg 87:1034–1036, 1998.

165. Tangkanakul C, Counsell C, Warlow C: Local versus general anesthesia for carotid endarterectomy (Cochrane Review). In: The Cochrane Library, Issue 2, 2002.

166. Taylor DW, Barnett HJ, Haynes RB, et al: Low-dose and high-dose acetylsalicylic acid for patients undergoing carotid endarterectomy: A randomised controlled trial: ASA and Carotid Endarterectomy (ACE) trial collaborators. Lancet 353:2179–2184, 1999.

167. Rigdon EE, Manajjem N, Rhodes RS: Criteria for selective utilization of the intensive care unit following carotid endarterectomy. Ann Vasc Surg 11:220–237, 1997.

168. Harbaugh KS, Harbaugh RE: Early discharge after carotid endarterectomy. Neurosurgery 37:219–225, 1995.

169. Wong JH, Findlay JM, Suarez-Almazor ME: Hemodynamic instability after carotid endarterectomy: Risk factors and associations with operative complications. Neurosurgery 41:35–41, 1997.

170. Post PN, Kievit J, van Baalen JM, et al: Routine duplex surveillance does not improve the outcome after carotid endarterectomy: A decision and cost utility analysis. Stroke 33:749–755, 2002.

171. Radak D, Popovic AD, Radicevic S, et al: Immediate reoperation for perioperative stroke after 2250 carotid endarterectomies: Differences between intraoperative and early post operative stroke. J Vasc Surg 30:245–251, 1999.

172. Rockman CB, Castillo J, Adelman MA, et al: Carotid endarterectomy in female patients: Are the concerns of the asymptomatic carotid atherosclerosis study valid? J Vasc Surg 33:236–240, 2001.

173. Barr JD, Horowitz MB, Mathis JM, et al: Intraoperative urokinase infusion for embolic stroke during carotid endarterectomy. Neurosurgery 36:606–611, 1995.

174. Winkelaar GB, Salvian AJ, Fry PD, et al: Intraoperative intraarterial urokinase in early postoperative stroke following carotid endarterectomy: A useful adjunct. Ann Vasc Surg 13:566–570, 1999.

175. Perler BA, Murphy K, Sternbach Y, et al: Immediate postoperative thrombolytic therapy: An aggressive strategy for neurologic salvage when cerebral thromboembolism complicates carotid endarterectomy. J Vasc Surg 31:1033–1037, 2000.

176. Anzuini A, Briguori C, Roubin GS, et al: Emergency stenting to treat neurological complications occurring after carotid endarterectomy. J Am Coll Cardiol 15:2074–2079, 2001.

Therapy

Therapy

177. Kerber CW, Hornwell LD, Loehden OL: Catheter dilatation of proximal carotid stenosis during distal bifurcation endarterectomy. AJNR Am J Neuroradiol 1:348–349, 1980.

178. Hasso AN, Bird CR, Zinke DE, et al: Fibromuscular dysplasia of the internal carotid artery: Percutaneous transluminal angioplasty. AJR 136:955–960, 1981.

179. Garrido E, Montoya J: Transluminal dilation of the internal carotid artery in fibromuscular dysplasia: A preliminary report. Surg Neurol 16:469–471, 1981.

180. Bockenheimer SA, Mathias K: Percutaneous transluminal angioplasty in arteriosclerotic internal carotid artery stenosis. AJNR Am J Neuroradiol 4:791–792, 1983.

181. Wiggl U, Gratzl O: Transluminal angioplasty of stenotic carotid arteries: Case reports and protocol. AJNR Am J Neuroradiol 4: 793–795, 1983.

182. Tsai FY, Matovich V, Hieshima G, et al: Percutaneous transluminal angioplasty of the carotid artery. AJNR Am J Neuroradiol 7:349–358, 1986.

183. Freitag G, Freitag J, Koch KE, et al: Percutaneous angioplasty for carotid artery stenosis. Neuroradiology 28:126–127, 1986.

184. Wholey MH, Wholey M, Mathias K, et al: Global experience in cervical carotid artery stent placement. Cathet Cardiovasc Interv 50:160–167, 2000.

185. Roubin GS, New G, Lyer SS, et al: Immediate and late clinical outcomes of carotid artery stenting in patients with symptomatic and asymptomatic carotid artery stenosis: A 5-year prospective analysis. Circulation 103:532–537, 2001.

186. Dietz A, Berkefeld J, Theron JG, et al: Endovascular treatment of symptomatic carotid stenosis using stent placement: Long-term follow-up of patients with a balanced surgical risk/benefit ratio. Stroke 32:1855–1859, 2001.

187. Gray WA, White HJ Jr, Barnett DM, et al: Carotid stenting and endarterectomy: A clinical and cost comparison of revascularization strategies. Stroke 33:1063–1070, 2002.

188. Golledge J, Mitchell A, Greenhalgh RM, et al: Systematic comparison of the early outcome of angioplasty and endarterectomy for symptomatic carotid artery disease. Stroke 31:1439–1443, 2000.

189. Naylor AR, Bolia A, Abbott RJ, et al: Randomized study of carotid angioplasty and stenting versus carotid endarterectomy: A stopped trial. J Vasc Surg 28:326–334, 1998.

190. Alberts MJ, for the publication committee of the WALLSTENT: Results of a multicenter prospective randomized trial of carotid artery stenting vs carotid endarterectomy. Stroke 32:325, 2001.

191. Endovascular versus surgical treatment in patients with carotid stenosis in the Carotid and Vertebral Artery Transluminal Angioplasty Study (CAVATAS): A randomised trial. Lancet 357:1729–1737, 2001.

192. Chakhtoura EY, Hobson RW, Oldstein J, et al: In-stent restenosis after carotid angioplasty-stenting: Incidence and management. J Vasc Surg 33:220–226, 2001.

193. Jordan WD, Roye GD, Fischer WS, et al: A cost comparison for balloon angioplasty and stenting versus endarterectomy for the treatment of carotid artery stenosis. J Vasc Surg 27:16–22, 1998.

194. Pelz DM, Lownie SP: Carotid angioplasty and stenting: Current status. CMAJ 162:1451–1454, 2000.

195. Spence D, Eliasziw M: Endarterectomy or angioplasty for treatment of carotid stenosis? Lancet 357:1722–1723, 2001.

196. Perler BA: Carotid endarterectomy: The "gold standard" in the endovascular era. J Am Coll Surg 194:S2–8, 2002.

197. Crawley F, Clifton A, Buckenham T, et al: Comparison of hemodynamic cerebral ischemia and mircoembolic signals detected during carotid endarterectomy and carotid angioplasty. Stroke 28:2460–2464, 1997.

198. Angelini A, Reimers B, Barbera MD, et al: Cerebral protection during carotid artery stenting: Collection and histopathologic analysis of embolized debris. Stroke 33:456–461, 2002.

199. Al-Mubarak N, Colombo A, Gaines PA, et al: Multicenter evaluation of carotid artery stenting with a filter protection system. J Am Coll Cardiol 39:841–846, 2002.

200. Huber TS, Wheelers KG, Cuddeback JK, et al: Effect of the Asymptomatic Carotid Atherosclerosis Study on carotid endarterectomy in Florida. Stroke 28:1099–1105, 1998.

201. Kresowick TF, Breztler D, Karp HR, et al: Multistate utilization, processes, and outcomes of carotid endarterectomy. J Vasc Surg 33:227–235, 2001.

202. Oliver SE, Thomson RG: Are variations in the use of carotid endarterectomy explained by population need? A study of health service utilisation in two English health regions. Eur J Vasc Endovasc Surg 17:501–506, 1999.

203. Feasby TE, Quan H, Ghali WA: Geographic variation in the rate of carotid endarterectomy in Canada. Stroke 32:2417–2422, 2001.

204. Ferris G, Roderick P, Smithies A, et al: An epidemiological needs assessment of carotid endarterectomy in an English health region. Is the need being met? BMJ 317:447–451, 1998.

205. Wong JH, Findlay JM, Suarez-Almazor ME: Regional performance of carotid endarterectomy: Appropriateness, outcomes, and risk factors for complications. Stroke 28:891–898, 1997.

206. Karp HR, Flanders WD, Shipp CC, et al: Carotid endarterectomy among medicare beneficiaries: A statewide evaluation of appropriateness and outcome. Stroke 29:46–52, 1998.

207. Mayo SW, Eldrup-Jorgensen J, Lucas FL, et al: Carotid endarterectomy after NASCET and ACAS: A statewide study. North American Symptomatic Carotid Endarterectomy Trial. Asymptomatic Carotid Artery Stenosis Study. J Vasc Surg 27:1017–1022, 1998.

208. Cebul RD, Snow RJ, Pine R, et al: Indications, outcomes, and provider volumes for carotid endarterectomy. JAMA 279:1282–1287, 1998.

209. Kresowick TF, Hemann RA, Grund SL, et al: Improving the outcomes of carotid endarterectomy: Results of a statewide quality improvement project. J Vasc Surg 31:918–926, 2000.

210. Findlay JM, Nykolyn L, Lubkey TB, et al: Auditing carotid endarterectomy: A regional experience. Can J Neuro Sci 29:326–332, 2002.

211. Johna S, Gaw F, Berten R, et al: Carotid endarterectomy for severe asymptomatic Carotid stenosis: A perioperative experience at a community hospital. Am Surg 66:1046–1048, 2000.

212. Wong JH, Lubkey TB, Suarez-Almazor ME, et al: Improving the appropriateness of carotid endarterectomy: Results of a prospective city-wide study. Stroke 30:12–15, 1999.

213. Hallett JW Jr: Managed care: Future good news or bad news for vascular surgeons. J Vasc Surg 28:365–369, 1998.

214. Perler BA, Dardik A, Burleyson GP, et al: Influence of age and hospital volume on the results of carotid endarterectomy: A statewide analysis of 9918 cases. J Vasc Surg 27:25–31, 1998.

215. Hannan EL, Popp AJ, Tranmer B, et al: Relationship between provider volume and mortality for carotid endarterectomies in New York state. Stroke 29:2292–2297, 1998.

216. Wennberg DE, Lucas FL, Birkmeyer JD, et al: Variation in carotid endarterectomy mortality in the Medicare population: Trial hospitals, volume, and patient characteristics. JAMA 279:1278–1281, 1998.

217. Peck C, Peck J, Peck A: Comparison of carotid endarterectomy at high- and low-volume hospitals. Am J Surg 181:450–453, 2001.

218. Shackley P, Slack R, Booth A, et al: Is there a positive volume-outcome relationship in peripheral vascular surgery? Results of a systematic review. Eur J Vasc Endovasc Surg 20:326–335, 2000.

219. O'Neill L, Lanska DJ, Hartz A: Surgeon characteristics associated with mortality and morbidity following carotid endarterectomy. Neurology 55:773–781, 2000.

220. Hannan EL, Popp AJ, Feustel P, et al: Association of surgical specialty and processes of care with patient outcomes for carotid endarterectomy. Stroke 32:2890–2897, 2001.

221. Goldstein LB, Moore WS, Robertson JT, et al: Complication rates for carotid endarterectomy: A call to action. Stroke 28:889–890, 1997.

Chapter Sixty-Six

Asymptomatic Carotid Occlusive Disease

Edwin J. Cunningham and Marc R. Mayberg

Of the approximately 700,000 new strokes per year occurring in the United States, 5% to 12% result from angiographically demonstrated carotid occlusive disease.[1–3] Of these carotid atheroembolic strokes, 75% to 80% occur without a warning stroke or transient oculocerebral ischemic symptoms.[1,2,4] Asymptomatic carotid stenosis is, therefore, a significant cause of stroke morbidity and mortality in America. Management of patients with asymptomatic carotid stenosis has been the subject of controversy for more than 20 years, and the publication of four randomized controlled trials comparing best medical therapy with endarterectomy has not resolved the issue in many clinicians' minds.

This chapter commences with a discussion of the stroke risk associated with asymptomatic carotid stenosis and a summary of the major studies comparing medical management with carotid endarterectomy (CEA). Then, the four common clinical scenarios related to the incidental finding of asymptomatic stenosis are discussed, followed by a summary of our recommendations for managing this important cause of stroke.

RISK OF STROKE ASSOCIATED WITH ASYMPTOMATIC CAROTID STENOSIS

Several retrospective and prospective studies have quantified the stroke risk associated with asymptomatic internal carotid artery (ICA) stenosis (Tables 66.1 and 66.2). The annual risk of stroke appears to be between 2% and 4% for stenoses greater than 60%, although individual studies cannot be directly compared. The majority of published studies include ischemic strokes in both carotid distributions in their risk assessment.[5–8] The inclusion of strokes in the contralateral carotid distribution falsely inflates the risk of stroke due to ipsilateral carotid stenosis. Moreover, many of the studies found that the stroke risk in patients with severe stenosis was evenly distributed between carotid distributions.[6,7,9] For example, Bock and associates[9] prospectively followed 242 patients with asymptomatic, unoperated carotid stenosis by means of duplex ultrasonography. At a mean follow-up of 27.4 months, patients with 80% to 99% stenosis had a 21% annual rate of risk of transient ischemic attack (TIA) and stroke, compared with

4.8% in patients with less than 80% stenosis ($P = .002$). However, only 5.1% of the events in patients with severe stenosis occurred in the carotid distribution affected by the stenosis (i.e., the majority occurred in the other carotid or vertebrobasilar distribution).

Other studies, however, have reported a strong correlation between asymptomatic stenosis and ipsilateral stroke.[5,8] Roederer and colleagues[8] prospectively followed a selected cohort of 167 patients with asymptomatic carotid bruits by means of annual ultrasound exams. The presence of or progression to greater than 80% stenosis was highly correlated with either the development of total carotid occlusion or new symptoms. Nine of ten neurologic events occurred in patients with greater than 80% stenosis (all ipsilateral to the lesion). Similarly, Chambers and Norris[5] found that 27 of 31 (87%) carotid ischemic events in previously asymptomatic patients occurred either in the carotid distribution ipsilateral to the stenosis in patients with unilateral disease or in either carotid distribution in patients with bilateral stenosis. Only four events (13%) occurred in a carotid distribution without proximal stenosis.

The natural history of the progression of stenosis in asymptomatic patients has also been described. Muluk and associates[10] prospectively studied 1004 asymptomatic patients with serial duplex ultrasonography over a mean follow-up period of 28 months (mean number of scans, 2.9/patient). The annual rate of stenosis progression for the group was 9.3%. Risk factors for progression of stenosis by multivariate analysis included baseline ipsilateral ICA stenosis greater than 50%, baseline ipsilateral external carotid artery (ECA) stenosis greater than 50%, baseline contralateral ICA stenosis greater than 50%, and systolic blood pressure higher than 160 mm Hg. Ipsilateral stroke or TIA occurred in 14% of the patients and was strongly correlated with progression of ICA stenosis.

The natural history data from these single-institution studies have been supplemented by data from multicenter randomized controlled trials.[11,12] In addition to the advantages of a rigorous trial design, these studies are more meaningful to current practitioners because all the patients received conventional medical therapy (aspirin plus aggressive modification of risk factors). Thus, the stroke risk in the medical arm of these studies serves as a

Therapy

Table 66.1 Summary of Natural History Studies and Clinical Trials Evaluating the Annual Risk of Stroke in Patients with Asymptomatic Carotid Stenosis

Study[*]	Design[†]	Year	Measurement Method	Stenosis (%)	No. Patients	Annual Stroke Risk (%)[‡]
Roederer et al[8]	Prospective	1984	Duplex US	<80	262	0
				>80	24	5.6
Chambers and Norris[5]	Prospective	1986	Doppler US	0–29	230	1.3
				30–74	157	1.9
				75–100	113	5.3
Hennerici et al[6]	Prospective	1987	Doppler US	50–80	199	2.0
				>80	36	8.3
Meissner et al[7]	Retrospective	1987	Ocular PPG	Normal	348	1.5
				Abnormal	292	3.4
Bock et al[9]	Prospective	1993	Duplex US	0–15	49	0
				16–49	99	1.8
				50–79	61	2.7
				80–99	13	8.8
				Occluded	20	6.5
Veterans Administration Cooperative Study[12]	RCT	1993	Angiogram	>50	233	2.3
Asymptomatic Carotid Atherosclerosis Study (ACAS)[11]	RCT	1995	Doppler US	60–99	834	2.2
European Carotid Surgery Trial (ECST)[13]	Retrospective	1995	Angiogram	0–29	1270	0.6
				30–69	843	0.7
				70–99	127	1.9
				Occlusion	55	1.2
North American Symptomatic Carotid Endarterectomy Trial (NASCET)[14]	Retrospective	2000	Angiogram	1–60	1604	1.6
				>60	216	3.2

PPG, pneumoplethysmography; RCT, randomized controlled trial (data are from medical arm); US, ultrasonography.
[*]Superscript numbers indicate chapter references.
[†]ECST and NASCET data on asymptomatic disease were derived from retrospective studies.
[‡]Annual stroke risks for VA Study, ACAS, ECST and NASCET are in the carotid distribution of the most severe asymptomatic stenosis. For all other studies, risk applies to bilateral carotid distributions.

Table 66.2 Natural History of Asymptomatic Carotid Stenosis*

- Annual risk of ipsilateral large artery stroke for asymptomatic carotid stenosis <60% is <1%.[4,9,13]
- Annual risk of ipsilateral large artery stroke for asymptomatic carotid stenosis of 60% to 99% is ≈2%.[11,12]
- Risk of stroke within 60% to 99% range appears to be directly proportional to the degree of stenosis.[4,9,10,13]
- 80% of patients who experience ipsilateral large artery stroke with a previously asymptomatic stenosis do so without antecedent TIA.[1,4]
- Annual risk of ultrasonographic progression of asymptomatic carotid stenosis is ≈10%.[10]
- Risk factors for large artery stroke in patients with >60% stenosis include silent cerebral infarction, diabetes, higher degree of stenosis, and progression of stenosis.[4]

*Superscript numbers indicate chapter references.

practical estimate for patients who may be managed with standard medical therapy.

In the Veterans Administration (VA) Cooperative Study it was found that for asymptomatic stenosis 50% or greater in severity, the annual risk of ipsilateral stroke in patients in the medical treatment arm was 2.2%. The risk for patients in the medical arm who had 60% or greater

stenosis was nearly identical, at 2.3% per year, in the Asymptomatic Carotid Atherosclerosis Study (ACAS). Neither study analyzed the cause of ischemic stroke in the study groups (e.g., cardioembolism vs. large artery) or demonstrated a relation between severity of stenosis and risk of stroke.

Though reviewed retrospectively and applicable only to patients with a concurrent history of contralateral symptomatic stenosis, data from the North American Symptomatic Carotid Endarterectomy Trial (NASCET) show similar results.[4] For this cohort of patients, the annual stroke risk in the distribution of an asymptomatic stenosis greater than 60% was 3.2%. Approximately 55% of these events were large artery strokes (i.e., due to carotid thromboembolism). Importantly, 80% of the infarctions were not preceded by TIA. This figure is nearly identical to the 78% value for stroke without warning reported by Foulkes and coworkers[1] from the Stroke Data Bank. Risk factors for large artery stroke were prior silent brain infarction, diabetes, and more severe stenosis. The annual risk of ipsilateral stroke for asymptomatic stenosis less than 60% was 1.6%. Approximately half of these strokes were cardioembolic or lacunar. Thus, the true risk of ipsilateral stroke due to carotid artery disease in asymptomatic stenosis measuring 60% or less is lower than 1% per year.

In summary, the presence of asymptomatic carotid stenosis is a significant risk factor for stroke in general, although the risk of ipsilateral stroke is only slightly increased. Patients with asymptomatic carotid stenosis should be thoroughly evaluated for stroke risks, and medical measures for stroke risk reduction (aspirin, serum lipid management, treatment of hypertension and diabetes, cessation of smoking) should be aggressively instituted.

RISK OF STROKE FOR ASYMPTOMATIC CAROTID OCCLUSION

The annual risk of ipsilateral stroke for a previously asymptomatic carotid occlusion, based on data from NASCET and the European Carotid Surgery Trial (ECST), is approximately 1% to 2%.[4,13] A more recent prospective study suggests a more benign prognosis for patients who have an occlusion at the time of their initial evaluation. Powers and Derdeyn[14] followed 30 previously asymptomatic patients with carotid occlusion. Over a mean follow-up period of 34 months, no strokes occurred in the ipsilateral carotid distribution in these patients. Similarly, Bornstein and coworkers[15] reported a 0 annual risk of stroke for 19 patients with asymptomatic occlusion who were followed for a mean duration of 48 months. For patients whose disease progressed from high-grade stenosis to occlusion during the study (N = 21), the annual stroke risk was 3.8% in the ipsilateral carotid distribution. On the basis of findings in these last two studies, there appear to be two categories of carotid occlusion—occlusion at the time of initial evaluation (negligible risk of large artery stroke ipsilateral to occlusion) and progression to occlusion during follow-up (3% to 4% annual risk of ipsilateral stroke). The higher risk in the latter group may reflect an initial 2- to 3-year period of near occlusion in which trace flow of blood through the lesion provides a small risk of embolic stroke.

The preceding data support the concept that stroke related to carotid stenosis is usually not hemodynamically mediated. The brain is highly adept at developing collateral circulation and generally tolerates high-grade carotid stenosis or occlusion. Carotid stenosis causes stroke because emboli tend to form at this site. When the carotid plaque is "active" because of ulceration or intraplaque thrombus, the risk of embolic stroke rises dramatically. In this setting, (symptomatic stenosis), higher severity of stenosis increases the propensity for embolus formation. In asymptomatic stenosis, however, the risk of de novo embolus formation is substantially less, even in the setting of hemodynamically significant stenosis.

EFFICACY OF THERAPY

Nonrandomized Studies

Most nonrandomized studies comparing medical therapy with endarterectomy were undertaken in the 1980s and focused on patients with severe stenosis. Moneta and associates[16] prospectively identified 129 asymptomatic carotid stenoses of 80% to 99% severity in 115 patients from a larger group of patients with vascular disease who underwent noninvasive testing. In this nonrandomized study, 56

endarterectomies were performed, and 73 lesions were followed nonsurgically. One perioperative stroke occurred in the surgical group, and nine ipsilateral strokes occurred without warning in the nonsurgical group. These results contradict the data of Chambers and Norris,[5] who reported that the majority of patients with high-grade asymptomatic stenoses suffered ischemic symptoms prior to infarction.

Freischlag and coworkers[17] also provide evidence to support a benefit for endarterectomy. In their retrospective review of 141 consecutive endarterectomies in patients with asymptomatic stenoses greater than 75%, there were no perioperative deaths. At a mean follow-up of 5 years, two patients had experienced strokes (neither in the distribution of the endarterectomy) and one had experienced TIA due to restenosis. These researchers contend that their results are significantly better than the natural history of the disease, given the 5% annual risk of stroke for stenoses greater than 75%.

Randomized Controlled Trials

The first published multicenter randomized controlled trial for CEA, the Carotid Artery Stenosis with Asymptomatic Narrowing Operation Versus Aspirin (CASANOVA) study, has been criticized for several methodologic flaws.[18] Asymptomatic patients were screened with Doppler ultrasonography and arteriography, and randomly assigned to a treatment arm of the study if severity of stenosis was between 50% and 90%. The investigators excluded patients with greater than 90% stenosis on the basis of the contention that these patients clearly benefited from endarterectomy. Both treatment groups received 330 mg aspirin and 75 mg dipyridamole three times daily. In the intention-to-treat analysis, there were no significant differences between the groups for the study endpoints, which were ischemic neurologic deficit exceeding 24 hours and death due to operation or stroke (Table 66.3). On the basis of these results, the CASANOVA investigators recommended medical therapy for stenoses less than 90%. However, 22% of patients randomly assigned to the surgical treatment arm did not undergo endarterectomy, and 42% of patients randomly assigned to medical therapy underwent endarterectomy during the course of follow-up. The high proportion of crossovers and the exclusion of patients with greater than 90% stenosis have undermined the validity of the conclusions; this study has not significantly influenced clinical decision-making.

The Mayo Asymptomatic Carotid Endarterectomy (MACE) study was designed to compare the efficacy of medical treatment using low-dose aspirin (80 mg/day) with CEA in patients with an asymptomatic carotid stenosis 50% or greater.[19] Patients randomly assigned to undergo surgery did not receive aspirin unless they had known cardiac disease. Primary endpoints were any TIA, stroke, and death. Secondary endpoints included myocardial infarction and coronary artery bypass for symptomatic coronary artery disease. The trial was terminated at a mean follow-up of 23.6 months, when interim analysis determined that eight of 36 surgical patients had suffered myocardial infarctions compared with none in the medical arm ($P = 0.037$). Four of the eight myocardial infarctions occurred before surgery, two on the day of surgery, one 7

Table 66.3 Summary of the Major Randomized Controlled Trials for Asymptomatic Carotid Stenosis (Best Medical + Endarterectomy vs. Best Medical)

Trial[*]	Year	Stenosis (%)	No. Patients	Medical Treatment	Mean Follow-Up (months)	Primary Endpoints	Results
Carotid Artery Stenosis with Asymptomatic Narrowing Operation vs. Aspirin (CASANOVA)[18]	1991	50–90	410	ASA 330 mg tid Dipyridamole 75 mg tid	42 m	Ischemic neurologic deficit >24 hours death	No surgical benefit
Mayo Asymptomatic Carotid Endarterectomy (MACE)[19]	1992	>50	71	ASA 80 mg qd in medical arm; ASA withheld in surgical arm unless patient had preexisting heart disease	24 m	TIA, stroke, death	Trial terminated because of high incidence of myocardial infarction in surgical arm
Veterans Affairs Cooperative Study[12]	1993	>50	444	ASA 650 mg bid	48 m	TIA, stroke, death	No surgical benefit for stroke or death Surgical benefit for TIA
Asymptomatic Carotid Atherosclerosis Study (ACAS)[11]	1995	60–90	1659	ASA 325 mg qd	32 m	Ipsilateral stroke, any stroke, death	Surgical benefit for all patients with >60% stenosis (relative risk reduction for surgical arm = 53%)

ASA, acetylsalicylic acid (aspirin); bid, twice daily; qd, once daily; tid, three times daily; TIA, transient ischemic attack.
[*]Superscript numbers indicate chapter references.

days after surgery, and one 5 months after surgery. There was no significant difference between the groups in the number of TIAs (three in the medical group, one in the surgical group) or strokes (zero medical, three surgical; $P = .086$). Although the early termination of the trial precluded an adequate comparison of primary endpoints between the treatment groups, the study was significant in that it highlighted the cardiac protection conferred by antiplatelet therapy for many patients who have significant underlying coronary artery disease. The investigators recommended continuous use of aspirin during the perioperative and postoperative periods.

The VA Study randomly assigned 444 men with asymptomatic lesions with more than 50% stenosis to either optimal medical therapy (including aspirin 1300 mg/day) plus endarterectomy (N = 211) or optimal medical therapy alone (N = 233).[12] Primary endpoints were TIA, transient monocular blindness, and nonfatal and fatal strokes ipsilateral to carotid stenosis. The incidence of these primary endpoints was significantly ($P < 0.001$) lower for endarterectomy than for medical therapy (8.0% vs. 20.6%; relative risk 0.38, 95% confidence interval [CI] 0.22 to 0.67). However, there were no differences between the groups in incidences of ipsilateral strokes, all strokes, or all strokes and deaths. The study has been criticized for its inclusion of TIAs and transient monocular blindness as primary endpoints, which accounted for the difference in outcome between the groups. It should be noted that both NASCET and ECST have demonstrated that TIAs are a strong risk factor for subsequent stroke. Some clinicians view the results of the VA Study as justification for endarterectomy for asymptomatic lesions, whereas others

maintain that the study demonstrated only a reduction in TIAs for patients who undergo surgery. Ultimately, because of either a small sample size or a true absence of a difference, the study failed to demonstrate that endarterectomy was more effective in preventing stroke than medical therapy alone.

Asymptomatic Carotid Atherosclerosis Study

The largest and latest randomized controlled trial of endarterectomy for asymptomatic carotid stenosis was the ACAS.[11] Despite a more rigorous design, which avoided methodologic flaws of previous trials, the results of ACAS and its interpretation have generated substantial controversy. Thirty-nine U.S. and Canadian centers recruited patients from vascular ultrasonography laboratories, practitioners who auscultated carotid bruits, and physicians who found carotid stenosis during preoperative evaluation or in the setting of contralateral symptomatic stenosis. All patients had 60% to 99% stenosis as defined by arteriography or Doppler ultrasonography. In patients randomly assigned to undergo surgery, arteriography was performed prior to surgery; this evaluation was not performed in medically treated patients. If the stenosis was less than 60% on the preoperative arteriogram, the patient did not undergo surgery but was kept in the surgical group for comparison.

Treatment in the ACAS was either best medical therapy plus endarterectomy (N = 825) or best medical therapy alone (N = 834). Best medical therapy consisted of aspirin 325 mg/day and modification of stroke risk factors. In patients who were to undergo surgery, CEA was performed within 2 weeks of assignment to this treatment. The primary endpoints were any stroke and death within

30 days of surgery (within 42 days of random assignment for the medical cohort) and ipsilateral stroke during the 5 years of follow-up. The trial reached a stopping boundary at a median follow-up of 2.7 years. At that time, follow-up was 5 years for 9% of the patients, 4 years for 26%, and more than 3 years for 44%. During the 6 years of the study, more than 42,000 patients were screened, and 1662 patients were randomly assigned to the study (4% of patients screened). Two thirds of the patients were men, and the mean age was 67 years.

For the surgery cohort, the risk of stroke or death during the perioperative period (including complications of angiography) was 2.3% (95% CI, 1.28% to 3.32%) compared with 0.4% for the medical cohort (95% CI, 0.0% to 0.8%). The 5-year Kaplan-Meier estimate of risk for ipsilateral stroke and any perioperative stroke or death were 5.1% for the surgical cohort and 11.0% for the medical cohort (*P* = .004), for an absolute risk reduction of 5.9% (Fig. 66–1). The relative reduction in risk for the surgical group was 53% (95% CI, 22% to 72%). In men, endarterectomy reduced the 5-year event rate by 66%, and in women by 17%, but the difference between genders was not significant (*P* = .10). There was no apparent relationship between severity of stenosis and stroke risk, although the study was not powered to address that question.

Interpreting Results

Many clinicians rejected the findings of ACAS for various reasons.[20–23] Some cited the lower than 3% surgical morbidity and mortality rate achieved in the trial as "not generalizable" to community surgeons. Others suggested that careful patient selection eliminated those with a high risk of surgical complications. Still others doubted the validity of results that did not show a graded benefit for increasing stenosis on subanalysis. Finally, the statistical analyses of the study were called into question.[23] The ACAS investigators addressed these criticisms and others in several publications.[24–26]

Do the results of ACAS indicate that all patients with greater than 60% carotid stenosis should undergo endarterectomy? A close analysis of the study and several subsequent publications supports a more cautious approach.[27] First, the very low surgical complication rate achieved by the ACAS surgeons (1.5% stroke and death rate) was the determining factor in demonstrating a benefit for the procedure. This rate is lower than that achieved in other contemporary trials. The VA Study found a 4.7% 30-day risk of permanent stroke and death (surgical plus arteriographic complications) for patients with asymptomatic stenosis.[12] In the ACAS, the risk of permanent stroke or death due to arteriography was 1.2%; thus, nearly half of the combined 2.7% risk of stroke and death was contributed by arteriography. Routine substitution of noninvasive imaging (e.g., magnetic resonance arteriography [MRA]) for arteriography will eliminate the arteriographic risk and thereby improve the risk reduction derived from endarterectomy. Until that goal is achieved, however, the risk of stroke or death from arteriography and surgery should be less than 3% if CEA is to show benefit over the best medical therapy. This 3% risk may be difficult for some centers to achieve if their volume of cases is low. Post hoc analysis of ACAS data found that diabetes,

contralateral siphon stenosis, and never consuming alcohol were associated with a higher risk of perioperative stroke.[28] If these risk factors are validated prospectively, their use should refine further patient selection for CEA.

Other factors to be considered are gender and race. Although the result is not statistically significant, CEA reduced the 5-year event rate in women by only 17% (vs. 55% in men [*P* = .10]). The loss of benefit was due primarily to higher procedural morbidity and mortality in women (3.6%, vs. 1.7% in men [*P* = .12]). The reasons for the pronounced trend toward greater procedural risk for women are unclear, but these findings from the study should be borne in mind when one is considering CEA for the individual patient. Also, nonwhite people represented only 5% of the patients studied in the ACAS; the results of the study therefore may not apply to African Americans, Hispanic people, and Asian Americans.

SCREENING FOR ASYMPTOMATIC CAROTID STENOSIS

Noninvasive screening of the general population with Doppler ultrasonography for carotid stenosis is neither cost-effective nor efficacious. In 1994, the Stroke Prevention Patient Outcome Research Team estimated the cost of noninvasive screening for 50% of the U.S. population older than 60 years at $7 billion.[29] Only 4% of patients screened for the ACAS met eligibility criteria and were enrolled in the trial. Additionally, asymptomatic stenosis in the medical treatment arm of ACAS was associated with a relatively low annual rate of ipsilateral stroke (approximately 2% per year) compared with that observed for symptomatic high-grade stenosis (>10% per year). If one applies these data, it would be necessary to perform 19 endarterectomies in asymptomatic patients with carotid stenosis to prevent one stroke for a cohort of patients surviving 5 years. Five to six procedures would be required to prevent one stroke in symptomatic patients who were followed for 2 years.[30]

PATTERNS OF PRESENTATION FOR ASYMPTOMATIC CAROTID STENOSIS

The incidental finding of an asymptomatic carotid lesion is usually made in one of the following four settings:

- Asymptomatic carotid bruit detected on routine examination
- Silent cerebral infarction demonstrated by CT or magnetic resonance imaging (MRI)
- Contralateral asymptomatic stenosis detected during evaluation of symptomatic carotid stenosis
- Carotid lesion discovered during preoperative evaluation for a major surgical procedure, usually cardiac or vascular

Asymptomatic Carotid Bruit

The incidence of asymptomatic carotid bruit in patients older than 45 years is 3% to 7%. Several population studies have addressed the natural history of bruits.[5,31,32] In the

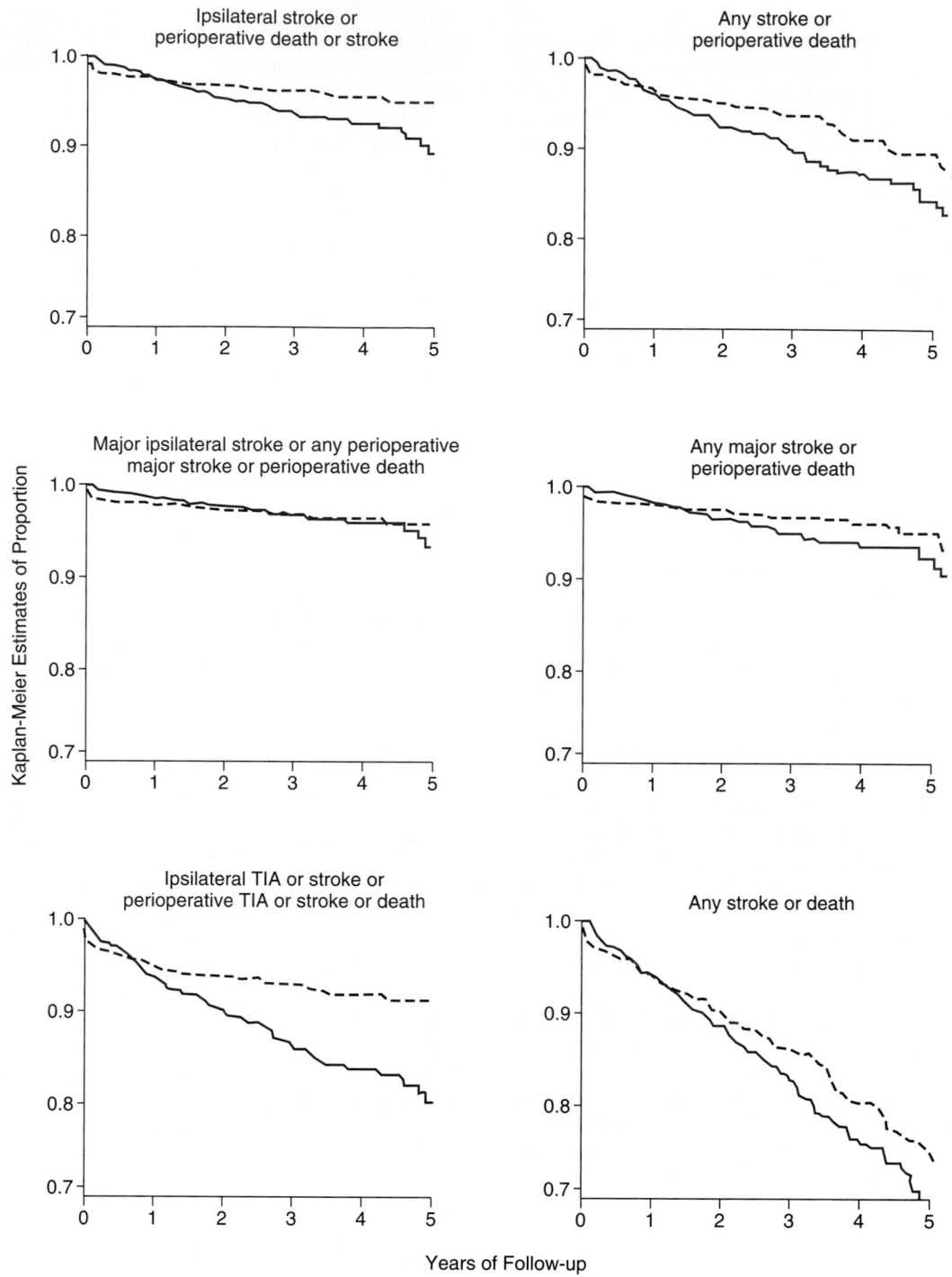

FIGURE 66–1 *Kaplan-Meier estimates from the Asymptomatic Carotid Artery Study. Proportion of patients without endpoint at a given time during follow-up, by treatment group, using the Kaplan-Meier estimation method.* Solid line *indicates medical patients;* broken line, *surgical patients. TIA, transient ischemic attack. (From Endarterectomy for asymptomatic carotid artery stenosis. Executive Committee for the Asymptomatic Carotid Atherosclerosis Study. JAMA 273:1421–1428, 1995.)*

Evans County, Georgia, study conducted by Heyman and colleagues,[31] 13.9% of patients with asymptomatic bruit suffered a stroke during the 6-year follow-up period, compared with only 3.4% of patients without bruit. Seven of the ten strokes in the bruit group, however, did not occur in the carotid distribution ipsilateral to the bruit. Heyman and colleagues[31] concluded that bruits identify patients at increased risk of stroke but are not associated with a higher stroke risk for the vascular distribution distal to the bruit.

In the Framingham Study, Wolf and associates[32] monitored 171 patients with asymptomatic bruits for 8 years. Twenty-one strokes (12.3%) occurred in the group; most of the events were not in the distribution of the bruit. The bruit group also had twice the risk of myocardial infarction and a higher mortality than an age-matched group without carotid bruit. Wolf and associates[32] concluded that bruits are a sign of systemic vasculopathy but do not pose a significantly increased risk of stroke in the distribution of the bruit. On the basis of their findings, the investigators of both of these population studies did not recommend prophylactic endarterectomy for asymptomatic carotid bruits.

Results of observational studies that include carotid ultrasonography in the evaluation of asymptomatic bruits have been conflicting. As described previously, Roederer and colleagues[8] prospectively studied 167 patients with asymptomatic carotid bruits by means of annual ultrasonography examinations. The presence of or progression to greater than 80% stenosis was highly correlated with either the development of total carotid occlusion or new symptoms. Nine of ten neurologic events (all ipsilateral to the bruit) occurred in patients with greater than 80% stenosis. These investigators recommended serial Doppler ultrasonography scanning of patients with asymptomatic bruits and endarterectomy for those with progression to greater than 80% stenosis.

Similarly, Hennerici and associates[6] followed 339 patients with asymptomatic carotid bruit by means of annual Doppler ultrasonography examinations. The group had a high annual mortality at 7%, but 80% of the deaths were due to cardiac disease. The risk of stroke without premonitory TIA was only 0.4% per year. Over a median follow-up period of 29 months, progression of stenosis was noted in 36% of patients. Among a number of clinical and ultrasonographic variables assessed, only progression of stenosis raised the risk of stroke. Because of the very low risk of stroke without premonitory TIA, Hennerici and associates[6] did not recommend prophylactic endarterectomy in patients with asymptomatic carotid bruit.

In a study with similar results, Chambers and Norris[5] monitored 500 patients with asymptomatic bruit for 4 years by means of Doppler ultrasonography. The overall risk of stroke was 1.7% at 1 year, but the rate was 5.5% for a subset of patients who had greater than 75% stenosis on the initial ultrasonography examination. Although the risk of cerebral infarction was significantly higher in patients with severe stenosis, most strokes in this cohort were preceded by TIA. On the basis of this finding, Chambers and Norris[5] did not recommend serial ultrasonography or prophylactic endarterectomy for asymptomatic bruits.

As discussed in the first section of the chapter, the results of the single-institution studies have been superseded by the publication of ACAS. Seventy-five percent of patients randomized in ACAS were enrolled following the discovery of an asymptomatic bruit.

Silent Cerebral Infarction

The prognostic significance of silent cerebral infarction in patients with asymptomatic stenosis remains poorly defined because of conflicting data from retrospective studies. The prevalence of silent infarction in patients with asymptomatic stenosis appears to be 15% to 20%, and many studies report the lesions as being small, centrally located, and evenly distributed between the ipsilateral and contralateral hemispheres.[33–35] Brott and colleagues,[35] in a review of the ACAS data, did not find severity of stenosis to be associated with an increased risk of silent infarction. Taken collectively, the findings of these retrospective studies imply that many silent infarcts in the setting of asymptomatic stenosis are not related to thromboembolism from carotid disease, but more likely reflect small vessel disease (i.e., lacunae). The results of other studies, however, contradict this conclusion.

Norris and Zhu[36] compared CT scans and carotid Doppler ultrasonography in 137 patients with asymptomatic stenosis and silent infarctions. Thirty percent of asymptomatic patients were found to have silent infarctions, 70% of which were ipsilateral to the stenosis. Univariate analysis showed the highest proportion of patients with silent infarcts to be the group with greater than 75% stenosis ($P < .001$). A multivariate analysis was not performed in the study. As previously mentioned, Inzitari and colleagues[4] found that silent cerebral infarction was an independent risk factor for large artery stroke in patients with carotid stenosis.

Although the data on the significance of silent cerebral infarction are conflicting, the results of the Inzitari study[4] are the most convincing, especially in light of the findings from ACAS demonstrating a benefit for endarterectomy in patients with greater than 60% stenosis. Patients who have asymptomatic severe stenosis and one or more ipsilateral silent infarcts may be at higher risk for thromboembolic stroke and should be considered for endarterectomy.

Contralateral Asymptomatic Stenosis

Sixty-three percent of patients enrolled in NASCET for a symptomatic lesion had contralateral asymptomatic stenoses ranging in severity from 0% to 99%.[4] Contralateral stenosis of 60% to 99% severity was found in 12% of this group (8% of all patients enrolled). Over 5 years of follow-up, the annual risk of ischemic stroke in the distribution of an asymptomatic stenosis of less than 60% was 1.6%, and approximately half of the strokes were cardioembolic or lacunar in etiology. The annual risk of stroke for patients with greater than 60% stenosis was 3.2%; the majority of strokes were attributed to large artery disease. Importantly, 80% of first strokes were not preceded by TIA. As stated previously, independent risk factors for large artery stroke in this study included higher severity of carotid artery stenosis, silent cerebral infarction, and a history of diabetes.

In ECST, the 3-year risk of stroke in the distribution of an asymptomatic contralateral stenosis ranging from 0% to 99% in severity was 2.1%.[13] The risk for patients with 80% to 89% stenosis was 9.8% (3.3% annual risk), and that for patients with 90% to 99% stenosis was 14.4% (4.8% annual risk). The numbers of patients in these two subgroups, however, were too low for the differences to reach statistical significance.

The data from NASCET and to a lesser extent, ECST suggest that patients with coexisting *severe* asymptomatic stenosis in the carotid artery contralateral to a symptomatic lesion are at an increased risk of stroke on the asymptomatic side (3% to 5% per year). Most of the strokes have a large artery cause and are not preceded by TIA. Both the overall results and the results of subgroup analyses from the ACAS demonstrate that these patients are best managed with endarterectomy.[11] Thirty percent (N = 504) of patients in the ACAS presented with a symptomatic lesion in one carotid artery and were enrolled in the study when a contralateral asymptomatic stenosis was discovered. For this subgroup, 5-year risks for stroke or death from the asymptomatic side were 12.6% in the medical cohort and 4.5% in the surgical cohort.

Asymptomatic Carotid Stenosis in the Preoperative Patient

The incidence of asymptomatic bruits in randomly evaluated preoperative patients is approximately 15%.[37–40] Most of the patients in the studies cited were undergoing evaluation before planned coronary artery or peripheral artery revascularization. The risk of perioperative stroke in this cohort was about 1%, but there was no correlation between the presence or location of carotid bruits and the risk of stroke. Other studies have also failed to demonstrate a correlation between the severity of stenosis as measured on preoperative ultrasonography and the risk of perioperative stroke.[41–44] Furlan and Craciun[45] reviewed a group of patients who were to undergo coronary bypass surgery and in whom angiography demonstrated asymptomatic stenosis greater than 50%. In the group, perioperative stroke risk was not increased for patients with less than 90% stenosis or total ICA occlusion. The number of patients with 90% to 99% stenosis was insufficient, however, to allow a statistical conclusion.

Gerraty and colleagues[43] prospectively studied patients who were to undergo planned vascular or coronary surgery. Preoperative carotid duplex ultrasonography was performed in all patients. Of 53 patients with asymptomatic stenoses greater than 50% (in 28 patients, stenosis was >80%), none had a perioperative stroke. Conversely, of the 10 patients with a history of cerebral ischemia and an ipsilateral carotid stenosis of greater than 50%, three suffered perioperative stroke. The numbers of patients in this prospective study were small, but the results were similar to those of earlier retrospective studies.

The results of all of these studies taken collectively do not support routine prophylactic endarterectomy in preoperative patients in whom either asymptomatic cervical bruit or asymptomatic carotid stenosis is detected on ultrasonography or angiography. From the available data, it appears that CEA may be safely deferred in patients with asymptomatic stenosis who are to undergo other major surgical procedures, although some surgeons have demonstrated low perioperative stroke and death rates when both procedures are performed in one stage.[46,47]

RECOMMENDATIONS FOR MANAGEMENT OF ASYMPTOMATIC CAROTID STENOSIS

Patients who present with an asymptomatic cervical bruit or silent cerebral infarction may be evaluated initially with noninvasive scanning (i.e., duplex ultrasonography). It is important to emphasize that the accuracy of duplex ultrasonography depends heavily on the training and experience of the individual technician.[48] One should refer patients only to a validated and standardized laboratory.[49,50] Patients with asymptomatic stenosis contralateral to a symptomatic lesion have likely already undergone a carotid ultrasonography, MRA, or digital subtraction angiography (DSA).

On the basis of the results of the ACAS, CEA should be considered as an option for all patients with ultrasonographic stenoses greater than 60% (assuming that further imaging studies verify >60% stenosis). As emphasized previously in the discussion of the ACAS, it is critical to have objective data from the local institution regarding the risk of stroke and death from angiography and CEA for asymptomatic patients being evaluated and treated there.

Selection of patients with asymptomatic stenoses greater than 60% who would most benefit from CEA remains difficult, because prospective risk analysis studies are lacking. Several of the published post hoc analyses have been described in this chapter,[4,28,51] but none of the reported risk factors has been validated in a prospective study. In spite of the inherent limitations of post hoc analyses, their findings provide helpful information to guide decision-making. As described, the study by Inzitari and colleagues[4] assessing risk factors for stroke with medical therapy suggests that patients with silent cerebral infarction, diabetes, and a greater severity of stenosis are at higher risk of stroke with medical therapy. It has not been demonstrated that the increased stroke risk for these patients is eliminated by CEA, but endarterectomy may be more efficacious in this setting. Post hoc analysis of ACAS data showed that diabetes, contralateral siphon stenosis, and never consuming alcohol were associated with a higher risk of perioperative stroke.[28] In a separate prospective multicenter study, risk factors for stroke or death after CEA included female gender, age greater than 75 years, history of congestive heart failure, and prophylactic endarterectomy.[51] The finding of increased operative risk for women was also seen in the ACAS. The data from these studies must be taken into consideration when one is counseling the individual patient.

After a thorough evaluation and discussion with the patient of his or her risk profile and the risks and benefits of each treatment option, a decision is made to proceed with CEA or medical therapy. If CEA is chosen, further imaging of the carotid lesion is necessary.[52,53] Although DSA provides the most accurate anatomical information at present, it contributed half of the morbidity associated with endarterectomy in the ACAS.[28] Many centers routinely use MRA in place of DSA.[54,55] If data from MRA and duplex ultrasonography are not concordant, DSA should be considered.

References

1. Foulkes MA, Wolf PA, Price TR, et al: The Stroke Data Bank: Design, methods, and baseline characteristics. Stroke 19:547–554, 1988.
2. Bogousslavsky J, Van Melle G, Regli F: The Lausanne Stroke Registry: Analysis of 1,000 consecutive patients with first stroke. Stroke 19:1083–1092, 1988.

3. Timsit SG, Sacco RL, Mohr JP, et al: Early clinical differentiation of cerebral infarction from severe atherosclerotic stenosis and cardioembolism. Stroke 23:486–491, 1992.
4. Inzitari D, Eliasziw M, Gates P, et al: The causes and risk of stroke in patients with asymptomatic internal- carotid-artery stenosis. North American Symptomatic Carotid Endarterectomy Trial Collaborators. N Engl J Med 342:1693–1700, 2000.
5. Chambers BR, Norris JW: Outcome in patients with asymptomatic neck bruits. N Engl J Med 315:860–865, 1986.
6. Hennerici M, Hulsbomer HB, Hefter H, et al: Natural history of asymptomatic extracranial arterial disease: Results of a long-term prospective study. Brain 110:777–791, 1987.
7. Meissner I, Wiebers DO, Whisnant JP, O'Fallon WM: The natural history of asymptomatic carotid artery occlusive lesions. JAMA 258:2704–2707, 1987.
8. Roederer GO, Langlois YE, Jager KA, et al: The natural history of carotid arterial disease in asymptomatic patients with cervical bruits. Stroke 15:605–613, 1984.
9. Bock RW, Gray-Weale AC, Mock PA, et al: The natural history of asymptomatic carotid artery disease. J Vasc Surg 17:160–171, 1993.
10. Muluk SC, Muluk VS, Sugimoto H, et al: Progression of asymptomatic carotid stenosis: A natural history study in 1004 patients. J Vasc Surg 29:208–216, 1999.
11. Endarterectomy for asymptomatic carotid artery stenosis. Executive Committee for the Asymptomatic Carotid Atherosclerosis Study. JAMA 273:1421–1428, 1995.
12. Hobson RW 2nd, Weiss DG, Fields WS, et al: Efficacy of carotid endarterectomy for asymptomatic carotid stenosis. The Veterans Affairs Cooperative Study Group. N Engl J Med 328:221–227, 1993.
13. Risk of stroke in the distribution of an asymptomatic carotid artery. The European Carotid Surgery Trialists Collaborative Group. Lancet 345:209–212, 1995.
14. Powers WJ, Derdeyn CP, Fritsch SM, et al: Benign prognosis of never-symptomatic carotid occlusion. Neurology 54:878–882, 2000.
15. Bornstein NM, Norris JW: Benign outcome of carotid occlusion. Neurology 39:6–8, 1989.
16. Moneta GL, Taylor DC, Nicholls SC, et al: Operative versus nonoperative management of asymptomatic high-grade internal carotid artery stenosis: Improved results with endarterectomy. Stroke 18:1005–1010, 1987.
17. Freischlag JA, Hanna D, Moore WS: Improved prognosis for asymptomatic carotid stenosis with prophylactic carotid endarterectomy. Stroke 23:479–482, 1992.
18. Carotid surgery versus medical therapy in asymptomatic carotid stenosis. The CASANOVA Study Group. Stroke 22:1229–1235, 1991.
19. Results of a randomized controlled trial of carotid endarterectomy for asymptomatic carotid stenosis. Mayo Asymptomatic Carotid Endarterectomy Study Group. Mayo Clin Proc 67:513–518, 1992.
20. Irvine CD, Baird RN, Lamont PM, Davies AH: Endarterectomy for asymptomatic carotid artery stenosis. BMJ 311:1113–1114, 1995.
21. Kase CS, Wolf PA: Endarterectomy for asymptomatic carotid artery stenosis. BMJ 312(7028):442–443, 1996.
22. Perry JR, Szalai JP, Norris JW: Consensus against both endarterectomy and routine screening for asymptomatic carotid artery stenosis. Canadian Stroke Consortium. Arch Neurol 54:25–28, 1997.
23. Barnett HJ, Eliasziw M, Meldrum HE, Taylor DW: Do the facts and figures warrant a 10-fold increase in the performance of carotid endarterectomy on asymptomatic patients? Neurology 46:603–608, 1996.
24. Castaldo JE, Nicholas GG: Endarterectomy on asymptomatic patients. Neurology 48:1742–1743, 1997.
25. Chambless LE, Hosking JD, Kronmal R, et al: Clearing up misunderstandings about clinical trial methodology: A reply to Barnett et al's commentary on the ACAS Trial. ACAS Executive Committee, ACAS Data and Safety Monitoring Committee. Neurology 48:1743–1748, 1997.
26. Toole JF: Quality-based medicine. Arch Neurol 54:23–24, 1997.
27. Mayberg MR, Winn HR: Endarterectomy for asymptomatic carotid artery stenosis: Resolving the controversy. JAMA 273:1459–1461, 1995.
28. Young B, Moore WS, Robertson JT, et al: An analysis of perioperative surgical mortality and morbidity in the asymptomatic carotid atherosclerosis study. ACAS Investigators. Asymptomatic Carotid Arteriosclerosis Study. Stroke 27:2216–2224, 1996.
29. Matchar DB: Carotid endarterectomy: Decision-making and cost analysis. Presented at the Congress of Neurological Surgeons Annual Meeting, October 3, 1994, Chicago.
30. Clinical alert: Benefit of carotid endarterectomy for patients with high-grade stenosis of the internal carotid artery. National Institute of Neurological Disorders and Stroke, Stroke and Trauma Division. North American Symptomatic Carotid Endarterectomy Trial (NASCET) investigators. Stroke 22:816–817, 1991.
31. Heyman A, Wilkinson WE, Heyden S, et al: Risk of stroke in asymptomatic persons with cervical arterial bruits: A population study in Evans County, Georgia. N Engl J Med 302:838–841, 1980.
32. Wolf PA, Kannel WB, Sorlie P, McNamara P: Asymptomatic carotid bruit and risk of stroke. The Framingham Study. JAMA 245:1442–1445, 1981.
33. Ricotta JJ, Ouriel K, Green RM, DeWeese JA: Use of computerized cerebral tomography in selection of patients for elective and urgent carotid endarterectomy. Ann Surg 202:783–787, 1985.
34. Berguer R, Sieggreen MY, Lazo A, Hodakowski GT: The silent brain infarct in carotid surgery. J Vasc Surg 3:442–447, 1986.
35. Brott T, Tomsick T, Feinberg W, et al: Baseline silent cerebral infarction in the Asymptomatic Carotid Atherosclerosis Study. Stroke 25:1122–1129, 1994.
36. Norris JW, Zhu CZ: Silent stroke and carotid stenosis. Stroke 23:483–485, 1992.
37. Evans WE, Cooperman M: The significance of asymptomatic unilateral carotid bruits in preoperative patients. Surgery 83:521–522, 1978.
38. Treiman RL, Foran RF, Cohen JL, et al: Carotid bruit: A follow-up report on its significance in patients undergoing an abdominal aortic operation. Arch Surg 114:1138–1140, 1979.
39. Treiman RL, Foran RF, Shore EH, Levin PM: Carotid bruit: Significance in patients undergoing an abdominal aortic operation. Arch Surg 106:803–805, 1973.
40. Carney WI Jr, Stewart WB, DePinto DJ, et al: Carotid bruit as a risk factor in aortoiliac reconstruction. Surgery 81:567–570, 1977.
41. Barnes RW, Liebman PR, Marszalek PB, et al: The natural history of asymptomatic carotid disease in patients undergoing cardiovascular surgery. Surgery 90(6):1075–1083, 1981.
42. Breslau PJ, Fell G, Ivey TD, et al: Carotid arterial disease in patients undergoing coronary artery bypass operations. J Thorac Cardiovasc Surg 82:765–767, 1981.
43. Gerraty RP, Gates PC, Doyle JC: Carotid stenosis and perioperative stroke risk in symptomatic and asymptomatic patients undergoing vascular or coronary surgery. Stroke 24:1115–1118, 1993.
44. Turnipseed WD, Berkoff HA, Belzer FO: Postoperative stroke in cardiac and peripheral vascular disease. Ann Surg 192:365–368, 1980.
45. Furlan AJ, Craciun AR: Risk of stroke during coronary artery bypass graft surgery in patients with internal carotid artery disease documented by angiography. Stroke 16:797–799, 1985.
46. Terramani TT, Rowe VL, Hood DB, et al: Combined carotid endarterectomy and coronary artery bypass grafting in asymptomatic carotid artery stenosis. Am Surg 64:993–997, 1998.
47. Darling RC 3rd, Dylewski M, Chang BB, et al: Combined carotid endarterectomy and coronary artery bypass grafting does not increase the risk of perioperative stroke. Cardiovasc Surg 6:448–452, 1998.
48. Curley PJ, Norrie L, Nicholson A, et al: Accuracy of carotid duplex is laboratory specific and must be determined by internal audit. Eur J Vasc Endovasc Surg 15:511–514, 1998.
49. Howard G, Chambless LE, Baker WH, et al: A multicenter validation study of Doppler ultrasound versus angiogram. J Stroke Cerebrovasc Dis 1:166–173, 1991.
50. Ranke C, Creutzig A, Becker H, Trappe HJ: Standardization of carotid ultrasound: A hemodynamic method to normalize for interindividual and interequipment variability. Stroke 30:402–406, 1999.
51. Goldstein LB, Samsa GP, Matchar DB, Oddone EZ: Multicenter review of preoperative risk factors for endarterectomy for asymptomatic carotid artery stenosis. Stroke 29:750–753, 1998.
52. Qureshi AI, Suri MF, Ali Z, et al: Role of conventional angiography in evaluation of patients with carotid artery stenosis demonstrated by Doppler ultrasound in general practice. Stroke 32:2287–2291, 2001.

Therapy

53. Johnson MB, Wilkinson ID, Wattam J, et al: Comparison of Doppler ultrasound, magnetic resonance angiographic techniques and catheter angiography in evaluation of carotid stenosis. Clin Radiol 55:912–920, 2000.

54. Back MR, Wilson JS, Rushing G, et al: Magnetic resonance angiography is an accurate imaging adjunct to duplex ultrasound scan in patient selection for carotid endarterectomy. J Vasc Surg 32:429–440, 2000.

55. Liberopoulos K, Kaponis A, Kokkinis K, et al: Comparative study of magnetic resonance angiography, digital subtraction angiography, duplex ultrasound examination with surgical and histological findings of atherosclerotic carotid bifurcation disease. Int Angiol 15:131–137, 1996.

Chapter Sixty-Seven

Intracranial Aneurysms

G. Edward Vates, Joseph M. Zabramski, Robert F. Spetzler, and
Michael T. Lawton

An *aneurysm* is an abnormal dilatation of an artery, and in the brain, most aneurysms are thin-walled sacs protruding from the arteries of the circle of Willis or its major branches. Usually these lesions are discovered after they rupture, producing subarachnoid hemorrhage (SAH). Less commonly, intracranial aneurysms manifest as the signs and symptoms of a mass lesion or are discovered incidentally when cerebral angiography, computed tomography (CT), or magnetic resonance imaging (MRI) is performed for other diagnostic purposes (Figs. 67–1 and 67–2).

The modern history of intracranial aneurysms began with Charles Symonds,[1] who suggested that SAH could be diagnosed during life and investigated the matter at the request of his mentor, Harvey Cushing.[2] Symonds coined the term subarachnoid hemorrhage, described the use of lumbar puncture for diagnosis of SAH, and brought the relationship between SAH and rupture of intracranial aneurysms to the attention of the medical community. With the introduction of cerebral angiography by Moniz[3] in 1927, ruptured aneurysms could be diagnosed and localized accurately. By 1933, Dott[4] reported the clinical and angiographic findings in eight patients and the operative treatment of two of them. Dandy[5] performed the first intracranial clipping of an aneurysm in 1937 and, with this bold approach, opened the doors to the surgical therapy of intracranial aneurysms.

In this chapter, we first review issues surrounding diagnosis and perioperative management of patients presenting with aneurysmal SAH. We then address the management of unruptured aneurysms, which has been the focus of considerable controversy over the past decade. Finally, we review the surgical approaches to aneurysms in different locations in the brain.

INCIDENCE OF ANEURYSMAL SUBARACHNOID HEMORRHAGE

Aneurysmal SAH is a major health care problem throughout the world. In the United States, the annual incidence rate is approximately 10 per 100,000 population. Incidence rates vary widely, with Finland and Japan reporting the highest values.[6–16] Women outnumber men by a ratio of 1.6:1 in most large series,[17–24] although in patients younger than 50 years, men predominate.[25] Jellinger[26] reviewed 12 postmortem studies, totaling 87,772 examinations, and noted aneurysms in approximately 2% of cases, but the frequency varies considerably from one report to another. Much of this variation results from disagreement about the size at which an arterial outpouching is considered an aneurysm. If microaneurysms (2 mm or smaller) are included as aneurysms, as many as 17% of routine autopsies reveal intracranial aneurysms.[27] However, if the cutoff is 4 mm, the apparent rate decreases to less than 2%. The problem is further complicated by evidence that aneurysm size may be significantly underestimated during routine autopsy examinations. In an elegant study, McCormick and Acosta-Rua[28] demonstrated that perfusing the intracranial vessels with saline under a pressure of 70 mm Hg caused aneurysm size to increase from 30% to 60%.

In the United States, the peak age for aneurysm rupture is between 40 and 60 years.[16,21,22,29–32] Intracranial aneurysms are rare in children and adolescents.[33–49] In postmortem studies, the prevalence of intracranial aneurysms increases with age and reaches a peak in the fifth or sixth decade of life.[16,28,50] The annual incidence rates for SAH parallel this change in prevalence, increasing from 3 per 100,000 population in the third decade to 30 per 100,000 in the sixth decade.[6–16] When intracranial hemorrhage does occur in children, an arteriovenous malformation (AVM) is usually the culprit; in persons older than 20 years, hemorrhage is more likely the result of a ruptured aneurysm (Fig. 67–3).

SAH during pregnancy is one of the leading causes of maternal deaths in North America.[51–63] The frequency is reported to vary between 1 and 5 per 10,000 pregnancies.[53,60] Arteriovenous malformations tend to rupture during early pregnancy or delivery, whereas aneurysms tend to rupture during the third trimester; aneurysms rupture rarely during labor,[51,53,60,64–67] although this is the period of maximum risk. The evaluation and treatment of SAH in a pregnant patient should be the same as in any other patient. The medical welfare of the mother should not be jeopardized by withholding essential procedures because of the fear of detrimental effects on the fetus.[62] Craniotomy and clipping of the aneurysm are the most appropriate forms of therapy,[52,53,56,62,64,68] although some reports suggest that endovascular treatment is an option.[58] Although prophylactic cesarean section has been recommended for the management of pregnant women with

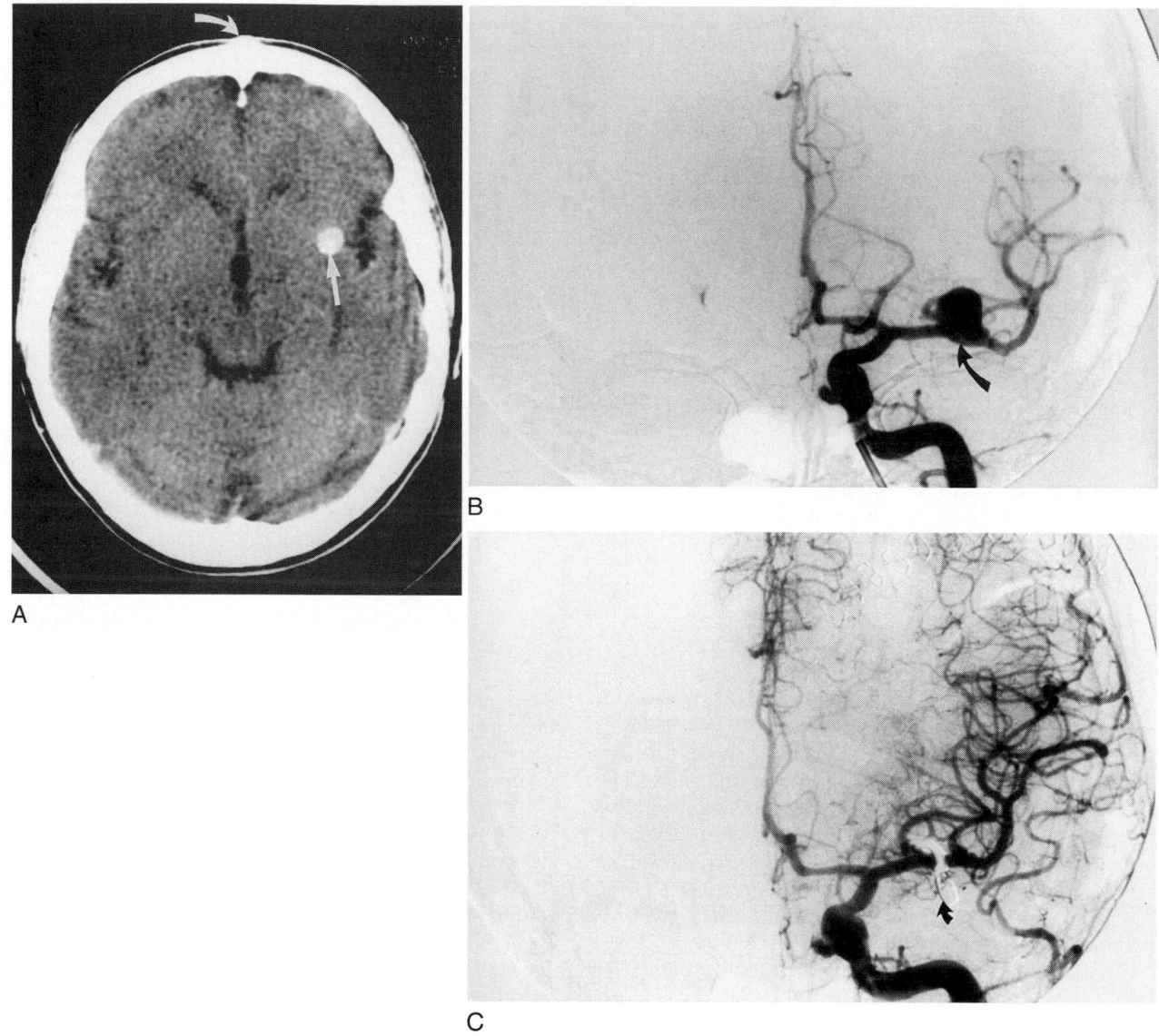

FIGURE 67–1   *A 64-year-old woman sought evaluation by a plastic surgeon for treatment of a bony prominence in the mid-forehead. A, As part of her evaluation, a basic head CT scan was obtained. CT findings included a focal area of increased density (straight arrow) in the left sylvian fissure compatible with a partially calcified middle cerebral artery aneurysm. There was no history consistent with previous subarachnoid hemorrhage. Note the small bony prominence (curved arrow) in the frontal region. B, Anteroposterior view of the left internal carotid artery angiogram reveals a large, irregularly shaped, left middle cerebral artery aneurysm (arrow). The patient underwent pterional craniotomy with clipping of the aneurysm (see Fig. 67–11). C, The postoperative angiogram demonstrates complete obliteration of the aneurysm with no compromise of the parent vessels. A slightly curved aneurysm clip (arrow) is faintly visible in this subtracted image.*

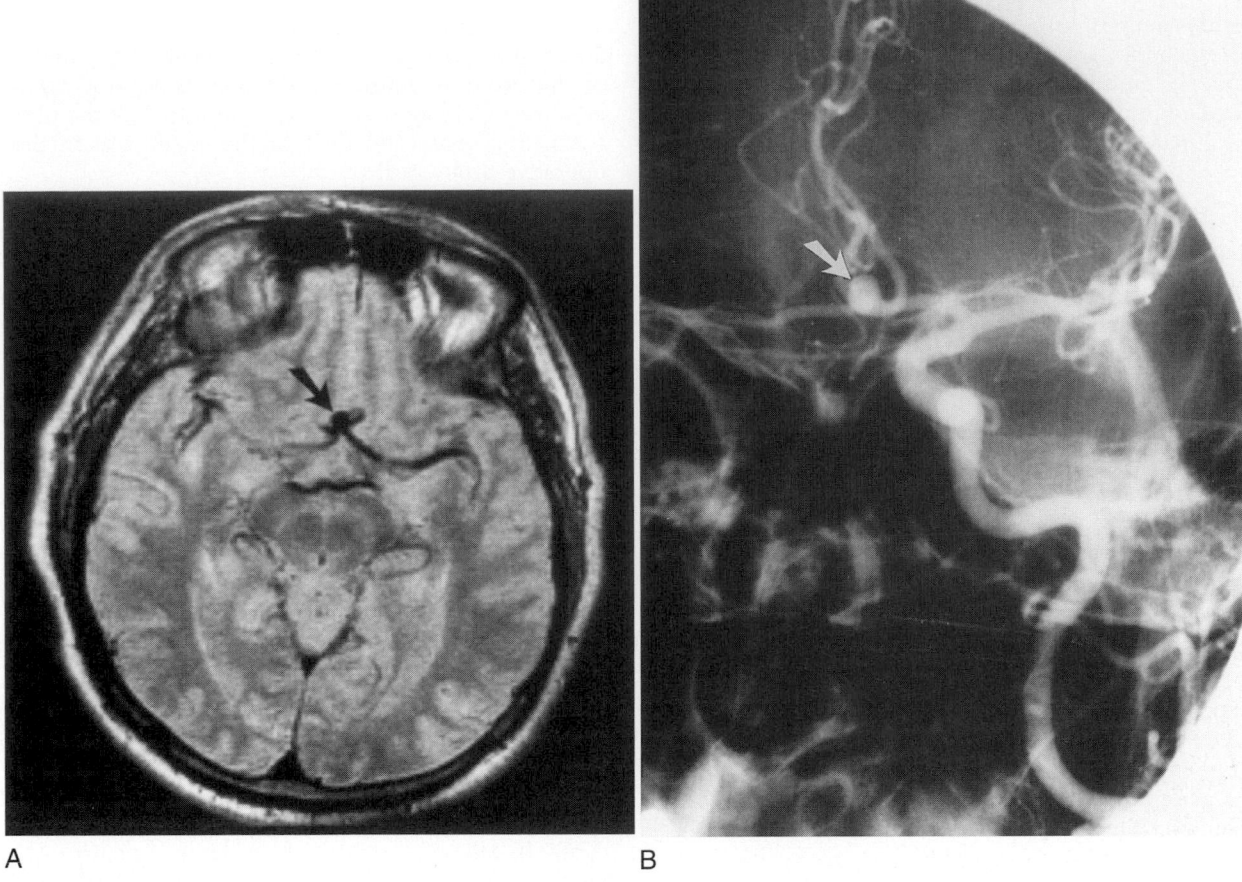

A   B

FIGURE 67–2 *A 34-year-old man had severe recurrent headaches after a motor vehicle accident. A, Transverse T1-weighted MR image taken through the base of the brain demonstrates a flow-related vascular defect consistent with an anterior communicating artery aneurysm (arrow). B, Oblique view of the left common carotid artery angiogram confirms the presence of a small (approximately 6-mm) anterior communicating artery aneurysm (arrow). The patient underwent elective clipping of the aneurysm without complication.*

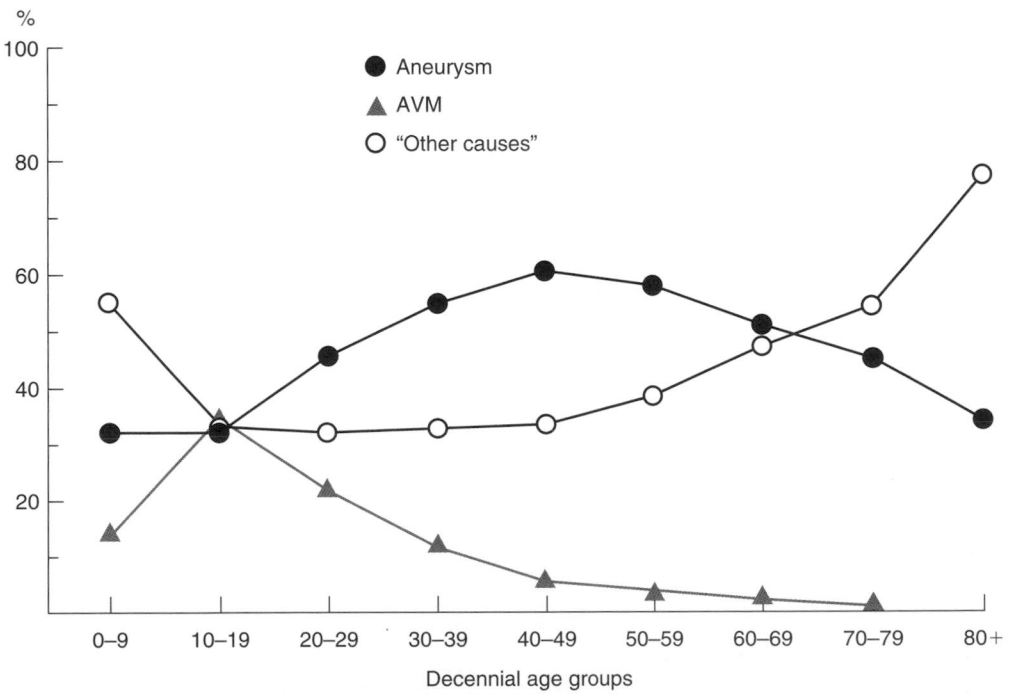

FIGURE 67–3 *Relative probability of major causes of subarachnoid hemorrhage in each decade of life. AVM, arteriovenous malformation. (From Locksley HB: Natural history of subarachnoid hemorrhage, intracranial aneurysms and arteriovenous malformations: Based on 6368 cases in the cooperative study. J Neurosurg 25:219, 1966.)*

untreated aneurysms, vaginal delivery with lumbar epidural anesthesia appears to be equally safe and effective and is therefore the method of choice.[62] Cesarean section is recommended if the mother is moribund and the child appears viable.[69]

DISTRIBUTION OF INTRACRANIAL ANEURYSMS

Aneurysms arise at a branch site on the parent artery, where it turns, and the aneurysm dome points in the direction of the maximal hemodynamic thrust in the pre-aneurysmal segment of the parent artery.[70–72]

The International Cooperative Study on the Timing of Aneurysm Surgery constitutes the most extensive series that has evaluated patients for the distribution of ruptured aneurysms.[21,32] This study was the collaborative effort of 213 neurosurgeons at 68 medical centers in 15 countries. Altogether 3521 patients with documented aneurysmal SAHs were enrolled. Unlike in earlier studies of this type, patients in this series underwent complete angiographic evaluation that included the posterior circulation.

The anterior communicating artery was the most common aneurysm site, accounting for 34% of cases, followed by the internal carotid artery (ICA) (30%) and the middle cerebral artery (22%; Table 67.1). Aneurysms of the ICA were most often found at the origin of the posterior communicating artery, followed by the carotid bifurcation and the origin of the ophthalmic artery. Basilar tip

Table 67.1   Distribution of Ruptured Aneurysms

Artery	No. of Cases	(%) Total
Internal carotid		
Cavernous	11	0.3
Ophthalmic	89	2.5
Posterior communicating	807	23.0
Carotid bifurcation	144	4.1
Anterior cerebral		
Proximal to anterior communicating	59	1.7
Anterior communicating	1184	34.0
Distal to anterior communicating	131	3.7
Middle cerebral		
Proximal (M_1) segment	101	2.9
At tri/bifurcation	662	19.0
Distal to tri/bifurcation	23	0.7
Posterior cerebral		
P_1	11	0.3
P_2 at posterior communicating	10	0.3
Distal posterior cerebral	10	0.3
Vertebral		
Posterior inferior cerebellar	88	2.5
Vertebral junction	18	0.5
Basilar		
Trunk	7	0.2
Superior cerebellar	16	0.4
Bifurcation (tip)	106	3.0
Other	44	1.2
Total	3521	

Data from Kassell NF, Torner JC, Haley EC Jr, et al. The International Cooperative Study on the Timing of Aneurysm Surgery. Part 1: Overall management results. J Neurosurg 80:788, 1994.

aneurysm was the most common posterior circulation aneurysm, followed by aneurysms of the vertebral origin of the posterior inferior cerebellar artery and the other basilar trunk branches. Overall, aneurysms of the posterior circulation composed 7.6% of the aneurysms in the Cooperative Study series.

Interestingly, a subsequent study to determine the risk of rupture in unruptured intracranial aneurysms (International Study of Unruptured Intracranial Aneurysms; ISUIA) found a different distribution of unruptured aneurysms among 2621 patients.[73] In this study, ICA aneurysms were the most common, followed by middle cerebral artery and anterior communicating artery aneurysms. Aneurysms of the posterior circulation composed 10% to 11% of aneurysms in the ISUIA. These differences likely reflect differences in the risk of aneurysms in different locations.

Multiple aneurysms are found in 20% to 30% of patients with aneurysmal SAH.[73–78] Risk factors associated with the formation of multiple aneurysms are hypertension, smoking, female sex, and age.[73,78–80] When more than one aneurysm is discovered at angiography, the lesion responsible for the hemorrhage must be correctly identified so that it can be treated first.[75,77,81–85] In a retrospective analysis of 205 aneurysms in 69 patients, Nehls and colleagues[75] found that irregularity of contour was the most reliable indicator for aneurysm ruptured, although size and location were also helpful. With aneurysms of similar size, the more irregular of the aneurysms was the site of rupture in 93.3% of cases. In only one instance did a larger but less irregular aneurysm rupture. When aneurysms had smooth walls, the largest and most proximal aneurysm was the most likely culprit. Finally, when all other factors were equal, the most common site of rupture was the posterior communicating artery, followed by the anterior communicating artery, the middle cerebral artery, and other ICA branch points.

Focal spasm in the area of an aneurysm is a rare but highly reliable angiographic sign for localizing the site of rupture. CT or MRI can also help identify the aneurysm responsible for hemorrhage.[86–88] Focal accumulations of subarachnoid blood (e.g., within the interhemispheric or sylvian fissures) are the most indicative signs (Fig. 67–4). Overall, the offending aneurysm can be identified correctly in more than 90% of cases.[89,90] When multiple aneurysms exist, surgery should focus on obliterating the ruptured aneurysm first. If other aneurysms can be treated simultaneously without adding to operative risk, they should also be approached.[77,81–85,91] This aggressive stance, however, may be inappropriate, in patients who have poor clinical grade or multiple posterior circulation aneurysms, patients who are elderly, and in operations of long duration or with complications. In such cases, surgical obliteration of the ruptured aneurysm, combined with either conservative or endovascular management of the unruptured aneurysms, may be preferred.[77,81,83,84,92] This issue is addressed further later.

NATURAL HISTORY OF RUPTURED ANEURYSMS: RATIONALE FOR WHOM AND WHEN TO TREAT

Numerous retrospective studies prove that the natural history of untreated aneurysmal SAH is grim. Attempts to

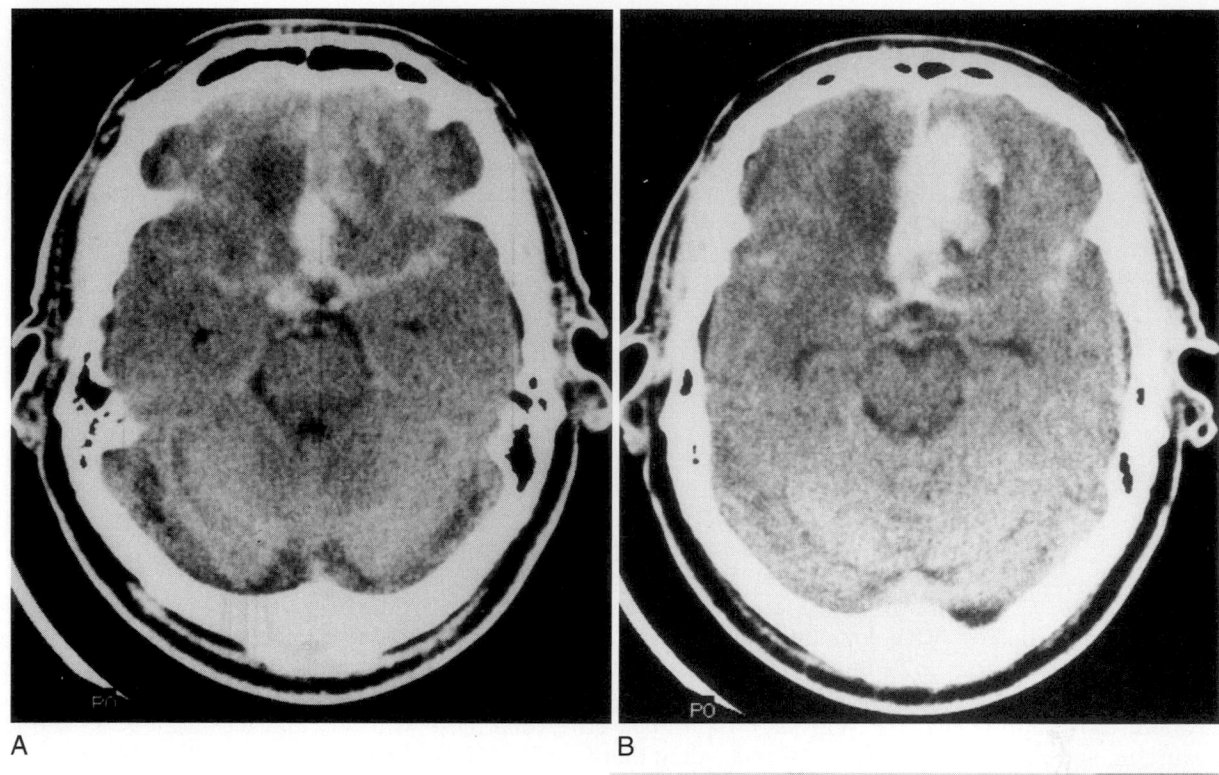

A B

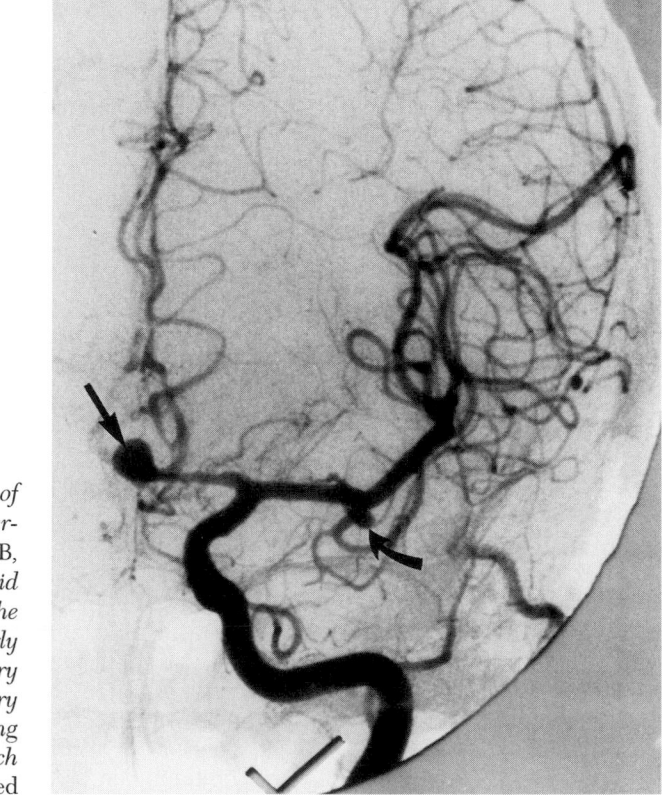

FIGURE 67–4 *A 56-year-old man presented with sudden onset of severe headache, nausea, and photophobia. On evaluation in the emergency room, the patient was mildly lethargic and confused. A and B, Basic head CT scans at two levels demonstrate a severe subarachnoid hemorrhage with a large collection of blood within and adjacent to the interhemispheric fissure. Hemorrhage in this distribution is nearly pathognomonic for rupture of an anterior communicating artery aneurysm. C, Anteroposterior view of the left internal carotid artery angiogram reveals an approximately 7-mm anterior communicating artery aneurysm (straight arrow) as well as the presence of a much smaller, incidental left middle cerebral artery aneurysm (curved arrow).*

C

assemble a representative series have been hampered by the problem of evaluating patients who receive no treatment because of selection criteria and by the lack of complete angiographic evaluation in many historical studies. Despite these difficulties, various researchers have collected valuable data that shed light on the factors affecting the prognosis of patients with ruptured aneurysms. The results of several population studies suggest that 25% to 35% of patients are found dead after the initial hemorrhage.[8,80,93-95] For patients who initially survive the acute hemorrhage, data from multiple cooperative studies suggest that the mortality rate for untreated patients during the first 2 weeks is 20% to 30%, with an additional morbidity rate of about 20%.[21,29,31]

Rebleeding is a major cause of death and disability in the untreated patient. The risk of rebleeding is approximately 20% during the first 2 weeks after hemorrhage, increasing to 33% at 1 month and 50% at 6 months.[21,29,96-102] The mortality rate associated with this second hemorrhage is at least 40% to 50%. The risk of rebleeding diminishes with time but never reaches zero. Annually, approximately 3% of long-term survivors can be expected to experience rebleeding.[95-97] Even considering the limitations of the accumulated data, the mortality rate is almost 50% during the first year after rupture of an aneurysm, and the continuing threat of rebleeding thereafter is 3% annually.

In addition to the risk of rebleeding, patients with aneurysmal SAH are at risk for electrolytic abnormalities, delayed ischemic neurologic deficits due to vasospasm, and hydrocephalus. Medical complications of SAH and vasospasm are discussed in detail elsewhere, but these sequelae are the major causes of nonoperative complications and death after aneurysm occlusion.[103] The exact incidence of vasospasm is unknown. As judged from angiography and transcranial Doppler (TCD) ultrasonography, however, vasospasm occurs in 50% to 70% of patients with aneurysmal SAH and is symptomatic in 40% to 60% of patients.[15,23,104-110] In most contemporary series, as many as 15% of patients suffer stroke or death from vasospasm despite maximal therapy.[17,32,106,107,111-113] Mortality from vasospasm alone is currently less than 5%. Various medical consequences of acute illness caused by SAH (e.g., electrolytic abnormalities, cardiovascular dysfunction, pneumonia, deep venous thrombosis, pulmonary edema, sepsis) occur in 25% to 50% of patients, even those in good clinical condition.[21,103,114-119]

Given that a quarter of patients die before receiving medical attention and that morbidity and mortality approach 30% to 50% for patients who survive and are taken to the hospital still die, it is important to identify which patients will benefit most from aggressive treatment. A clinical grading scale cannot encompass all of the different interrelated factors that can affect outcome after SAH, such as severity of the initial ictus, rebleeding, perioperative medical complications, and the timing and technical success of any attempt to obliterate the aneurysm. Nonetheless, a number of different grading schemes have been proposed to help predict prognosis for patients with SAH on the basis of clinical presentation or radiographic findings.[120-123] One of the most widely used grading systems is the Hunt and Hess classification (Table 67.2).[121] The scale heavily emphasizes level of consciousness, which is

Table 67.2　Hunt and Hess Clinical Grading Scale

Group	Condition
0	Unruptured aneurysm
1	Asymptomatic or minimal headache and slight nuchal rigidity
2	Moderate or severe headache and nuchal rigidity; no neurologic deficit other than cranial nerve palsy
3	Drowsiness, confusion, or mild focal deficit
4	Stupor, moderate to severe hemiparesis
5	Deep coma, decerebrate posturing, moribund appearance

the most important factor in predicting outcome.[21,123] The clinical grade of a patient should not be calculated until maximal cardiopulmonary resuscitation and control of elevated intracranial pressure (ICP) are achieved. Historically, however, the correlation between Hunt and Hess grade and outcome has been calculated without these provisions.

In consideration of outcome as it relates to clinical grade, patients are commonly divided into those with good clinical status (Hunt and Hess clinical grades 1, 2, and 3) and those with poor clinical status (Hunt and Hess grades 4 and 5).[124] Unfortunately, 20% to 40% of patients with aneurysmal SAH have poor clinical status, and the association between poor outcome and poor clinical grade after SAH is clear.[124-126] Despite the grim prognosis, however, some patients with poor clinical grade may benefit from aggressive treatment. This issue is intimately related to timing of surgery, because the decision whether and when to perform surgery after aneurysmal rupture strongly affects the ability to prevent or treat some of the deadly complications of SAH.[98]

The decision whether and when to operate can be distilled as the following dilemma: whether to operate immediately to avoid aneurysmal rerupture and place an injured brain at risk or to wait until either the effects of the initial hemorrhage subside or the patient's condition declares surgery a lost cause. During the last 20 years, there has been a shift in policy regarding the timing of surgery from that of delayed management to minimize the risks of surgical complications to one of early surgery to prevent rebleeding and improve overall outcome. This change reflects the evolution of neurosurgical techniques.

Before the development of microsurgical techniques and contemporary neuroanesthesia, the risks of early operative intervention for the clipping of ruptured aneurysms outweighed any potential benefit. In the late 1970s and early 1980s, a number of workers reported good outcomes in patients undergoing early surgery for ruptured aneurysms.[6,127-133] Simultaneously, the emphasis of outcome studies in aneurysmal SAH shifted from operative morbidity and mortality to overall management outcome.

To assess the risks and benefits of early versus delayed surgery, the International Study on the Timing of Aneurysm Surgery (ISTAS) was launched.[21,32,134] Between January 1981 and June 1983, 3521 patients who were hospitalized within 3 days of SAH were enrolled in the cooperative multi-institutional, intention-to-treat protocol. When a patient was admitted and enrolled, the surgeon was required to specify the time of surgery; the intervals that could be chosen were days 0 to 3, days 4 to 6, days 7 to 10, days 11 to 14, and days 15 to 32 after SAH; no surgery was also an option. Principal outcome measures were the patient's neurologic and disability status 6 months after SAH, rates of vasospasm and rebleeding, and medical and surgical complications during hospitalization.

The study concluded that patients who had surgery on days 7 to 10 after SAH had the least favorable outcomes and the highest mortality rate, but surgical morbidity and mortality rates for all other intervals were similar. In addition, the incidence of focal ischemic deficits due to vasospasm was higher for patients who underwent surgery later than day 7 after SAH. The overall comparison demonstrated that the mortality rate attributable to intervening events during the wait for delayed surgery (rerupture, ischemia due to vasospasm) almost equaled the postoperative mortality rate for early surgery. However, when results from North American participants were examined separately, the good recovery rate was significantly greater in the group that underwent surgery during the first 3 days after SAH. This finding reflected the more prevalent use of hypertensive-hypervolemic therapy in North American centers. As a consequence, early surgery is now the standard of care for most patients. This standard has been reinforced by studies demonstrating that, in patients with good clinical status (Hunt and Hess grades 1 to 3), the combination of early surgery, calcium antagonists, and hypervolemic-hypertensive therapy can reduce overall management mortality to 10% or less, with good outcomes in 75% or more of the patients who survive.[19,94,132,135–141]

We now recommend surgery for all patients with good clinical status (Hunt and Hess grades 1 to 3), regardless of the time of presentation, and we exert extra care to prevent hypovolemia and hypotension in patients who present later than 3 days after SAH. Although some surgeons delay surgery if a patient's initial angiogram shows evidence of vasospasm, we do not believe that angiographic evidence of vasospasm, except of an extreme degree in comatose

patients, should be considered a contraindication to surgery. Special care must be taken to limit the risks of further ischemic injury in these patients. Blood pressure (BP) should be maintained within 10 to 15 mm Hg of preoperative values during surgery. Once the aneurysm is controlled proximally, the surgeon can safely apply papaverine to the exposed vessels to relieve arterial spasm and improve blood flow while dissection and clipping proceed.

The decision when and whether to operate on patients with poor clinical status (Hunt and Hess grades 4 and 5) after aneurysmal hemorrhage is still controversial. Data suggest that 35% to 50% of such patients can have a reasonable neurologic outcome with aggressive therapy,[124–126,142,143] and clinical and radiographic findings are commonly inaccurate predictors of outcome.[109,124,126,143–147] In addition, most patients with poor clinical status who survive and have a good outcome are able to follow commands within 5 days of aneurysm rupture.[124–126,147] We have concluded that we cannot accurately predict the future for individual patients with poor clinical status. Although early surgery and aggressive treatment are costly and fruitless in more than half the patients, we must still treat all comers at the outset and let the course of the disease dictate who lives and who dies despite our best efforts. Worsening neurologic function, lack of improvement after surgery, persistently increased ICP, and evidence of certain types of structural brain injury on CT or MRI can be used to determine when to abandon hope.

We have developed a protocol for selecting operative candidates on the basis of CT data, ICP measurements, and angiographic findings (Fig. 67–5). Briefly, a ventriculostomy is placed in all patients presenting with SAH in grades 4 and 5, except those with radiographic evidence of irreversible brain destruction. For example, a large hematoma in the dominant basal ganglia would preclude active treatment. In addition, operative intervention is withheld for the following three reasons after ventriculostomy:

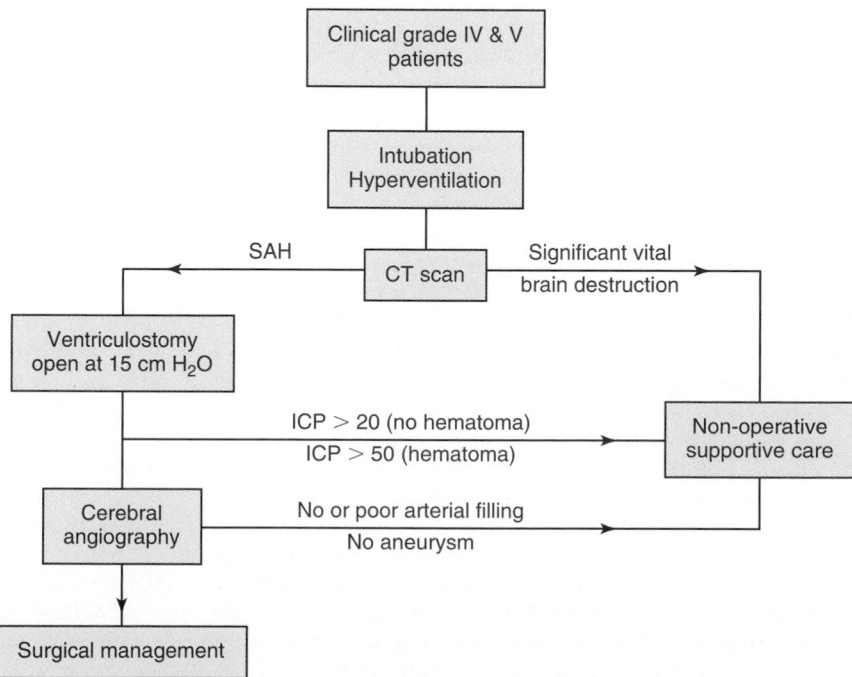

FIGURE 67–5 *Treatment algorithm for the management of patients with poor clinical status and aneurysmal subarachnoid hemorrhage. CT, computed tomography; ICP, intracranial pressure; SAH, subarachnoid hemorrhage. (Adapted from Bailes JE, Spetzler RF, Hadley MN, et al: Management morbidity and mortality of poor-grade aneurysm patients. J Neurosurg 72:559, 1990.)*

- If ICP cannot be controlled and kept below 20 mm Hg in a patient without hematoma.
- If ICP is greater than 50 mm Hg in a patient with a hematoma.
- If intracranial filling is poor or absent on angiography.

The remaining patients undergo early surgery for aneurysm clipping, irrespective of their neurologic status. Postoperatively, patients are treated with calcium antagonists and aggressive hypervolemic-hypertensive therapy.

MANAGEMENT OF INCIDENTAL ANEURYSMS

Because of the widespread use and increasing sensitivity of imaging technology, a growing number of patients are diagnosed with unruptured, asymptomatic intracranial aneurysms. How these patients should be counseled is a hotly debated issue,[80,145-163] with much of the controversy coming from the initial results of the International Study of Unruptured Intracranial Aneurysms (ISUIA.).[73] Patients with unruptured aneurysms have potentially devastating abnormalities in their brains, but selection of optimal treatment requires knowledge of the following issues:

1. How likely is an unruptured aneurysm to rupture?
2. What are the consequences of rupture?
3. What risks are posed by intervention?
4. What is the cost to the patient of watchful waiting?

The consequences of rupture are well described and grim; SAH is a horrible disease, as previously detailed. As for the other three questions, the answers are still uncertain.

The ISUIA was a combined retrospective and prospective study that enrolled 2621 patients in 53 centers worldwide.[73] In the retrospective arm, 1449 patients with 1937 aneurysms were identified from all centers (diagnosed between 1970 and 1991) through review of records and acquisition of hard copies of angiograms for evaluation. The study centered on quantifying the characteristics of the aneurysms in these patients (size and location) and on quantifying patient characteristics that could serve as predictors for subsequent hemorrhage (age, medical comorbidities, family history, social habits). Patients were divided into two groups, those without a history of SAH (727 patients; group 1) and those with a history of SAH from another aneurysm (722 patients; group 2). Follow-up information was obtained by means of an annual standardized questionnaire and a review of medical records. Detailed information was obtained on all endpoints (definite or questionable SAH or intracerebral hemorrhage and death). Estimates of the risk of hemorrhage were made with life-table methods, and data from patients were censored at last follow-up. Predictors of hemorrhage were ascertained by means of a proportional-hazards regression model. The mean follow-up was 8.3 years.

Among group 1 patients (without history of SAH), those with giant aneurysms at the basilar tip, vertebrobasilar or posterior cerebral artery, or posterior communicating artery sites had a 45% risk of hemorrhage over 7.5 years.[164] Large aneurysms (10 to 24 mm) and small aneurysms (<10 mm) in the same locations had 15% and 2% risks of hemorrhage, respectively, over 7.5 years. For patients with aneurysms in all other locations, the risk of hemorrhage over 7.5 years for giant, large, and small aneurysms were 8%, 3%, and 0, respectively. In other words, the annual rates of rupture for small, large, and giant aneurysms were 0.05%, 1%, and 6%, respectively, excluding intracavernous aneurysms.[73,165] Predictors of rupture identified from this arm of the study were increasing size and location (as described previously).

For group 2 patients (history of SAH from a different aneurysm), the annual rates of rupture for small and large aneurysms were almost the same (0.5% and 1%, respectively), and there were too few giant aneurysms in this group to permit a separate analysis (3 patients). The predictors of rupture for group 2 patients were location (basilar tip aneurysms stood alone as having significantly higher risk) and age, although the effect of age was much weaker than that of location.[73]

The goals of the prospective component of the ISUIA were to delineate the risks of morbidity and mortality associated with treatment of unruptured aneurysms and to determine whether these risks were higher for some patients than others. This arm enrolled 1172 patients between 1991 and 1995. As in the prospective arm, patients were divided into those without a history of SAH (961 patients; group 1) and those with a history of SAH from a different aneurysm (211 patients; group 2). Baseline assessments using the Rankin scale and Mini-Mental State Examination were compared with similar measures at follow-up (Rankin scale, Mini-Mental State Examination, or the Telephone Interview for Cognitive Status); follow-up intervals were 7 days after intervention, at discharge, at 30 days, and then annually. Factors that were analyzed included survival, morbidity (as defined by a Rankin score of 3 to 5, a Mini-Mental State Examination score <24, or a Telephone Interview for Cognitive Status score <27), and mortality at 30 days and 1 year. Survival estimates were calculated by life-table methods, and factors related to overall morbidity and mortality were determined with logistic regression.

In group 1, 798 patients (83%) underwent surgical obliteration of the aneurysm. The rest were treated with various endovascular procedures. The rate of procedure-related morbidity and mortality was 17.5% at 1 month and 15.7% at 1 year. In group 2, 198 patients (94%) had surgery and the rest were treated endovascularly. The overall morbidity and mortality rate was 13.6% at 1 month and 13.1% at 1 year. The only significant predictor of poor surgical outcome was increased age.[73] The study had insufficient power to allow assessment of other potential predictors, such as aneurysm location and size and the difference between surgery and endovascular treatments.

On the basis of these findings, a position paper regarding recommendations for treatment of unruptured aneurysm was published,[150] and is summarized here. The following patients should be considered for treatment, especially with aneurysms of the posterior circulation:

- Patients with additional unsecured aneurysms of all sizes who have previously undergone treatment of another ruptured aneurysm.

- Patients with symptomatic but unruptured aneurysms of any size and location (including cavernous carotid aneurysms).
- Patients with asymptomatic aneurysms >10 mm in diameter.

In contrast, patients with asymptomatic cavernous carotid aneurysms and asymptomatic aneurysms less than 10 mm in diameter should be observed, although youth, unusual aneurysm shape (daughter sac formation), and a family history of SAH would argue in favor of special consideration for treatment. Untreated aneurysms should be observed at regular intervals. If a specific symptom arises or if the aneurysmal size or configuration changes, treatment should be considered.

The findings of the ISUIA and the treatment recommendations based on these findings struck many neurosurgeons as premature and possibly flawed because of concerns about bias in the ISUIA data.° Two criticisms are common. First, the population studied by the ISUIA may not be representative of the population commonly seen by practicing neurosurgeons. Second, the comparison of natural history from a retrospective study of patients selected for nonoperative intervention with treatment outcomes from a prospective study of patients selected for surgical intervention is inherently incorrect. The retrospective group might represent only a small proportion of the total number of patients with unruptured aneurysms diagnosed between 1970 and 1991. Patients with the highest risk of rupture may have been excluded, thereby introducing data collection bias and artificially decreasing the annual hemorrhage rate for unruptured aneurysms. Also, the endpoints of the retrospective arm of the study (hemorrhage or death) were different from those of the prospective arm (death, surgical morbidity, or cognitive dysfunction), and a comparison of these endpoints is biased against patients undergoing surgery. No explanation was offered for the apparent discrepancy between the ISUIA finding that aneurysms less than 10 mm in diameter had a very low risk of rupture even though the overwhelming majority of ruptured aneurysms are less than 10 mm in diameter. No correlation was observed between treatment morbidity-mortality and aneurysm size, a finding that is counterintuitive to the experience of most practicing neurosurgeons. Finally, if most aneurysms are less than 10 mm in diameter and their annual risk of rupture is 0.05% as the ISUIA states, the incidence of SAH (approximately 30,000/year) would require that almost one of every six adults (>30 years old) who are at risk for aneurysm formation has an aneurysm, a rate that seems preposterously high.[161]

The ISUIA investigators have presented data to refute the issue of population bias. By the criteria of age, race, aneurysm size, and other characteristics, the ISUIA population seems almost identical to the population of patients in most published series.[153] The ISUIA investigators have also pointed out that the data presented in the first report are preliminary, especially in the comparison of natural history with surgical outcome, and that the study is continuing to enroll patients for a prospective natural history component (phase II).[162,174] As for correlations between aneurysm characteristics and the risk of surgery, these data are being compiled for both phases of the study and may yet provide a correlation between aneurysm size or location and the risk of surgical morbidity and mortality. As for the correlation between aneurysm size and the risk of rupture, recent data suggest that the risk of rupture increases gradually as aneurysm diameter increases. There is no sudden bump in risk as an aneurysm crosses the 10-mm threshold. This finding may lead to a revision of the ISUIA-recommended size threshold for strongly considering surgery from 10 mm or larger to 8 mm or larger. How these adjustments in the size-risk ratio affect the population-derived calculation offered by Winn and colleagues[161] is not yet known.

Problems with the ISUIA still remain. The life-table analyses published in the preliminary report show that only 242 of the 727 group 1 patients enrolled at the beginning of the study period remained in the study by the 7.5 year time-point. Why the data from the other 485 patients were censored was not specified.[73] That data from so many patients were censored makes the value of 8.3-year mean follow-up time dubious; the median follow-up as well as the specific follow-up intervals for group 1 and group 2 patients with small, large, and giant aneurysms would be more meaningful. That data from so many patients were censored raises other questions: Why were those data censored? How many patients died of causes seemingly unrelated to hemorrhage? How many were "lost to follow-up"? What effort was made to search for patients? What techniques were used to determine whether "lost" patients may have died suddenly out of the study's view? How was the validity of cause of death determined? The issues of the number of patients who died, the causes of death, and the sensitivity of the study's data-capturing mechanisms are critical for this study. Of the 727 group 1 patients in the retrospective arm of the study, 424 patients had aneurysms less than 10 mm in diameter (58.3%), but only one patient had a documented aneurysm rupture. However, if most of these patients were censored by the 7.5-year time point, and if a small number of those censored were "lost to follow-up" and may have had a hemorrhage, then the annual risk of hemorrhage calculated in the ISUIA may be spurious. When the number of events is so small and the number of patients censored is so high, an analysis of the censored patients is essential to interpreting the validity of the study's conclusions or, at the very least, for estimating confidence intervals for the calculated annual hemorrhage risk.

There is also no discussion of the discrepancy between the morbidity and mortality rates observed by ISUIA and the morbidity and mortality rates reported in many surgical series. The implication of the ISUIA is that the investigators provided a more reproducible and representative (i.e., "truer") measure of surgical outcome by using the Rankin score, Mini-Mental State Exam, and the Telephone Interview of Cognitive Status. This attitude is dismissive of the many experienced surgeons who have reported their results and suggests that surgeons are incapable of providing or unwilling to provide meaningful follow-up information about their patients, a conclusion we firmly dispute.

Since the ISUIA results were published, other natural history studies have appeared with results that are more congruent with the previously reported annual risk of

---

°80,148,151–153,155,158,159,161,163,166–173

rupture from unruptured aneurysms(1% to 5%). As with many single-institution studies, the number of patients in these studies is small, so interpretation of their results is difficult. Nonetheless, following so closely on the heels of the surprising ISUIA results, these studies emphasize that the risk of rupture from incidental aneurysms is still undefined to the degree that specific recommendations cannot be made for patients. The decision to treat an unruptured aneurysm can be made only by patients who are aware of (1) the treatment options available and their attendant risks, (2) the data available so far about the risk of rupture, and (3) the controversy about treatments.

PREOPERATIVE AND OPERATIVE MANAGEMENT

Our discussion of preoperative management is limited, as the topic is reviewed thoroughly elsewhere in this text. The present discussion focuses on the highlights of our management techniques as they relate to diagnosing SAH, particular management issues with specific types of aneurysms (e.g., mycotic aneurysms, giant aneurysms), and operative approaches and special techniques (e.g., bypass, hypothermic cardiac standstill).

Diagnosis

The most common complaint with aneurysmal SAH is a sudden severe headache.[175] If alert, the patient often describes the pain as "the worst headache of my life" or "like something exploded in my head." Nuchal pain and rigidity, nausea, vomiting, and altered mental status are also common. Twenty percent of patients suffer a sudden loss of consciousness, which may be accompanied by apnea and circulatory arrest. Patients with less severe symptoms may not recognize the severity of the episode or may be misdiagnosed if they do seek medical evaluation. Careful attention to the patient's history and the sudden, unheralded onset of the symptoms readily separates SAH from other causes of headache.

Focal neurologic findings can result from intraparenchymal hemorrhage, from SAH with clot formation causing mass effect, or from distal embolization from partially thrombosed aneurysms that may or may not have ruptured.[125,176–183] Although intraparenchymal bleeding is common with aneurysms of the anterior circulation, it is rarely seen with posterior circulation aneurysms, perhaps because of the tough pial envelope of the brainstem and the absence of aneurysm-enfolding brain, such as that around the interhemispheric and sylvian fissures.

Both anterior and posterior circulation aneurysms can cause cranial nerve deficits, with or without SAH. Often, these deficits arise when an aneurysm approaches giant dimensions (>2.5 cm); giant aneurysms are discussed later. However, nongiant aneurysms in both the anterior and posterior circulation can cause cranial nerve deficits. Anterior circulation aneurysm most commonly manifest as visual or oculomotor abnormalities, whereas a posterior circulation aneurysm can manifest as cranial nerve deficit that corresponds to the origin of the aneurysm. Aneurysms of the basilar apex, superior cerebellar artery, and upper basilar artery can cause oculomotor dysfunction. An ante-

rior inferior cerebellar artery aneurysm can cause hearing loss or facial palsy. Aneurysms of the vertebrobasilar junction or lower basilar trunk can cause swallowing or tongue dysfunction.

When SAH is suspected, evaluation should consist of the following steps: (1) clinical history, (2) general physical and neurologic examination, (3) routine laboratory evaluation (electrocardiography, electrolyte measurements, complete blood count, coagulation tests), (4) CT, (5) lumbar puncture (if CT results are negative), and (6) four-vessel cerebral angiography.

The initial evaluation of a patient with suspected SAH invariably includes CT, which usually clinches the diagnosis. In about 95% of patients with rupture of an intracranial aneurysm, the initial CT scan shows evidence of hemorrhage if the study is obtained within 24 hours of hemorrhage.[184] The number of scans positive for blood decreases progressively over the ensuing days to about 75% on day 3 after hemorrhage. The distribution of blood occasionally gives clues to the location of the aneurysm. Anterior communicating artery aneurysms often bleed into the interhemispheric fissure, septum pellucidum, and adjacent medial frontal lobe ("flame" hemorrhage). Middle cerebral artery aneurysms can manifest as a clot in the sylvian fissure and temporal lobe. Basilar tip aneurysms can cause a large amount of clot in the interpeduncular cistern. If the jet of rupture is directed through the floor of the third ventricle, intraventricular hemorrhage results. When posterior inferior communicating artery (PICA) aneurysms rupture, the resultant subarachnoid blood may be limited to the lower regions of the posterior fossa, but associated small amounts of blood in the third and fourth ventricles is common.

Although CT is the initial procedure of choice for the evaluation of patients with suspected SAH, negative CT scan results do not rule out SAH. When CT fails to demonstrate SAH in a patient with a history suggestive of an aneurysmal bleed, lumbar puncture is the next step. CT results can be negative if the patient has suffered a small (or sentinel) hemorrhage or if the patient presents more than 2 or 3 days after rupture. Soon after rupture of an aneurysm, cerebrospinal fluid (CSF) is reddish-orange, and it becomes more yellow as oxyhemoglobin is increasingly converted to bilirubin. Depending on the severity of the hemorrhage, blood may not be detected in a lumbar CSF sample until several hours after rupture of the aneurysm. Evidence of aneurysmal hemorrhage in the CSF persists for 1 to 2 weeks, depending on the severity of the bleed. The blood from a traumatic spinal tap tends to clear with successive collection tubes, but this observation is an unreliable sign that the patient does not have SAH. With very rare exceptions, the presence of xanthochromia in the spun supernatant of a fresh CSF specimen is diagnostic of SAH, regardless of the cell counts.

Patients with confirmed SAH should undergo cerebral angiography as soon as possible. High-quality four-vessel angiography in multiple projections remains the standard for diagnosis and surgical planning. Preoperative angiographic studies determine the following five key features: (1) the aneurysm's vessel of origin, (2) the aneurysm's size, shape, and relationship to parent and adjacent arteries, (3) the presence or absence and location of vasospasm, (4) the displacement of adjacent vessels suggesting mass effect from hematoma or partial thrombosis of an aneurysmal sac whose dimensions are much larger than that seen on angiography (angiography-CT mismatch), and (5) the presence of other aneurysms or other vascular abnormalities. Angiography should be performed by an experienced team using biplanar magnification views. Digital subtraction angiography (DSA) has replaced conventional film angiography at most institutions. DSA has several advantages, including increased sensitivity of contrast over standard film techniques and the enhancement of details that would otherwise be hidden by overlying bone. Suspicion about the location of the ruptured aneurysm can guide which of the major vessels is injected first; however, 20% to 30% of patients have multiple aneurysms, so a complete four-vessel study should be performed unless a patient's condition dictates otherwise.

CT angiography is gaining acceptance as an alternative to conventional arteriography for the diagnosis and localization of intracranial aneurysms.[185-198] Although it may not be as sensitive for small aneurysms and infundibula as conventional angiography, CT angiography has the advantage of providing reconstructed views that better display the three-dimensional relationships among the aneurysm and afferent and efferent vessels. CT angiography is also better at showing intraluminal thrombus and calcification. Finally, CT angiography may be useful in patients with poor clinical status and a large intracerebral hemorrhage. In these patients, clot removal must be performed as an emergency procedure, and there is no time to allow standard angiography. In most cases, CT angiography can provide sufficient information to allow safe clipping of the aneurysm. Data suggest that saving time in this manner can help save patients who are otherwise near death.[199]

In as many as 15% of cases, cerebral angiography does not demonstrate a source for SAH.[32,200,201] Aneurysms may be obscured on an angiogram because of vasospasm, hypoperfusion, poor imaging technique, or spontaneous thrombosis. Undetected aneurysms are found in many such patients on examinations performed 2 to 4 weeks after the first study.[202,203] The most commonly missed aneurysm is also the most commonly ruptured aneurysm (anterior communicating artery). Rarely, MR angiography (MRA) demonstrates an aneurysm not visualized by digital subtraction angiography. A high index of suspicion for aneurysm rupture is essential in patients with typical aneurysmal SAH patterns on CT (e.g., anterior interhemispheric blood, clot in the lateral sylvian fissure, or intraventricular hemorrhage) and negative results on initial studies. In these patients, we recommend obtaining a second angiogram 2 to 3 weeks after the first.

A subset of patients with SAH and normal angiograms, however, has a distinctive pattern of blood that has been called a variety of names (e.g., perimesencephalic SAH, benign nonaneurysmal SAH).[204] In these patients, SAH is limited to the perimesencephalic and prepontine cisterns and is not associated with blood in the ventricles or lateral sylvian fissure. Patients with this type of SAH tend to be younger, nonhypertensive, and male and to have good clinical status.[200,201,205-207] A second angiogram is nondiagnostic in 95% of such patients. They have a good prognosis with very little risk of rebleeding or vasospasm.[201,208,209]

General Care of Patients with Aneurysmal Subarachnoid Hemorrhage

The goals of perioperative care of patients with aneurysmal SAH are (1) to minimize the risk of recurrent hemorrhage before aneurysm obliteration and (2) to accelerate clinical recovery before and after surgery. Aggressive perioperative management can reduce the incidence and severity of vasospasm and effectively deal with the neurologic and medical complications associated with aneurysmal SAH. Patients with SAH are critically ill, and their management can be quite complex because the most important threat to a patient's well-being shifts with time after SAH. Before surgery, treatment is focused on cardiopulmonary stabilization, management of ICP, diagnosis, and prevention of re-rupture. After surgery, the focus shifts to recognizing and treating brain ischemia due to vasospasm, managing hydrocephalus, and dealing with the other medical problems commonly found in the seriously ill (fluid and electrolyte disturbances, thromboembolic complications, infections, gastrointestinal hemorrhage).

Cardiopulmonary Care

The initial assessment of patients in whom SAH is suspected or confirmed has similarities to that of patients with acute trauma: Airway, breathing, and circulation are prerequisites of life and must be addressed first. Patients with SAH can be obtunded or comatose on presentation, and the airway must be protected in patients with a Glasgow Coma Scale score of 8 or less. Intubation prevents hypoventilation, hypoxia, and hypercapnia, all of which can aggravate ischemia and swelling in the injured brain. It also reduces complications due to vomiting and aspiration in a patient unable to protect the airway. Intubating patients with a ruptured aneurysm is not trivial; endotracheal intubation can cause wide fluctuations in BP and should be attempted only by an anesthesiologist or intensivist who shares the neurosurgeon's concern about preserving brain perfusion without causing aneurysm re-rupture.[210,211]

Hemodynamic management is complex in patients with aneurysmal SAH. Patients should be admitted to an intensive care unit and should undergo cardiac monitoring and placement of an arterial line for BP monitoring. Hypertension in the immediate postrupture period may be due to increased ICP, pain, or anxiety. BP often returns to normal after the patient has been admitted to the hospital and these problems have been addressed by bed rest in a quiet room as well as by sedation and pain medication as needed. For sedation and control of pain, we prefer small intravenous doses of morphine sulfate (1 to 4 mg/hr) or fentanyl (25 to 100 μg/hr); both of these agents have a short half-life and their effects can be readily reversed if necessary to evaluate apparent changes in mental status. These issues must be addressed quickly because hypertension has been linked with the risk of re-rupture. Review of the Cooperative Aneurysm Study data shows that the risk of re-rupture was 9% in patients when systolic BP was maintained between 94 and 169 mm Hg but increased to 16% when systolic BP was allowed to range between 170 and 240 mm Hg.[212]

In general, we treat hypertension in patients before surgery only when systolic BP exceeds 150 mm Hg. We routinely prescribe nimodipine, which can lower systemic BP and also increase cerebral blood flow. Treatment with nimodipine (60 mg q4h, orally) for the first 21 days after hemorrhage significantly improves outcomes and decreases the incidence of delayed ischemic deficits in patients with ruptured aneurysms.[1,23,108–110,213] It is the only agent currently approved by the U.S. Food and Drug Administration (FDA) for the prevention and treatment of delayed cerebral ischemic injury. The exact mechanism of action of nimodipine is unknown. Initially, the agent was given to patients in an attempt to reduce the incidence of vasospasm by blocking smooth muscle contraction. However, subsequent study has shown that nimodipine has no effect on angiographic or clinical incidence of vasospasm. Instead, nimodipine appears to prevent the death of neurons at risk by preventing the influx of calcium from the extracellular space; alternatively, it may reduce the ease with which intracellular calcium is mobilized in marginally ischemic neurons. Occasionally, patients can be very sensitive to nimodipine, particularly elderly patients and patients who were taking antihypertensive medications before admission. Therefore, we begin nimodipine therapy with 30 mg (orally or by nasogastric tube) every 4 hours and increase this dose to 60 mg every 4 hours if the patient remains clinically stable. If, despite sedation and nimodipine, BP consistently remains higher than 150 mm Hg before surgical clipping of the ruptured aneurysm, small doses of labetalol can be given intravenously. Labetalol, however, should be used carefully, because patients with SAH and high ICP are prone to secondary cerebral insults, much like head-injured patients after trauma.[214]

After the aneurysm has been obliterated surgically, cardiovascular management must shift gears; rather than a struggle to keep systolic BP controlled to prevent aneurysm re-rupture, the goal becomes maintenance of adequate BP to guard against or treat vasospasm. This topic is reviewed more extensively elsewhere in this volume, but the mainstay of treatment is hypervolemia and hypertension.[215–219] Our general strategy is outlined in Table 67.3; we use crystalloid to maintain mild hypervolemia, with a target central venous pressure (CVP) between 8 and 10 mm Hg. For patients with cardiac dysfunction from either preexisting heart disease or SAH,

placement of a pulmonary artery catheter-monitor can help guide management. The goal is a pulmonary artery wedge pressure between 10 and 16 mm Hg. During the first 14 days after aneurysm rupture and after the aneurysm has been obliterated, hypertension is left untreated unless systolic BP exceeds 200 mm Hg.

If a patient is unable to maintain systolic BP above 120 mm Hg, we use an intravenous phenylephrine (Neo-Synephrine) infusion to keep the systolic BP between 120 and 160 mm Hg. Cardiac consultation and placement of a pulmonary artery catheter should be considered if hypotension fails to respond to fluids and low-dose phenylephrine (<100 μg/min). Anemia during this period of prolonged intensive care management is common and is treated with transfusion of paced red blood cells to maintain the hematocrit between 28% and 34%.

If a patient demonstrates clinical evidence of vasospasm or has transcranial Doppler or angiographic evidence of severe vasospasm, the intensity of hypervolemic-hypertensive therapy is increased (Table 67.4), including placement of a pulmonary artery catheter (if not already in use) and elevation of systolic blood pressure to a range of 160 to 200 mm Hg. If this strategy fails to ameliorate clinical deficits related to vasospasm, then more intensive treatment is indicated (endovascular angioplasty or administration of intra-arterial papaverine).

Intracranial Pressure

Increased ICP after SAH is usually caused by acute hydrocephalus, but it can also be caused by intracerebral hematoma or cerebral edema.[124,220–225] Although other factors may be of significance, continued obtundation after SAH is primarily related to elevated ICP. Without measuring ICP, one cannot manage it. When CT reveals evidence of hydrocephalus or intraventricular hemorrhage

---

Table 67.3   Prophylactic Hypervolemic Fluid Therapy

Low-risk vasospasm protocol (CT scan—Fisher grade 1 or 2)
  Normal saline—150 mL/hr
  Serum sodium level daily
    If serum sodium <135 mEq/L, switch to high-risk protocol
High-risk vasospasm protocol (CT scan—Fisher grade 3)
  Swan-Ganz catheter
    Continuous monitoring of PADP
    Cardiac output and parameters twice daily
  Normal saline 150 mL/hr
  Plasmanate (5% plasma protein fraction [human], Miles Inc.)
    100 mL/hr prn PADP or PCWP <10 mm Hg
  Serum sodium level twice daily
    If serum sodium <135 mEq/L, begin 3% saline solution at
    30–50 mL/hr; hold for PADP >16 mm Hg

CT, computed tomography; PADP, pulmonary artery diastolic pressure; PCWP, pulmonary capillary wedge pressure.

Table 67.4   Hypervolemic-Hypertensive Treatment Protocol for Clinically Symptomatic Vasospasm

Swan-Ganz catheter
  Constant monitoring of PADP
  Cardiac output and parameters at 8-hour intervals
Normal saline—150 mL/hr
Plasmanate (5% plasma protein fraction [human], Miles Inc.)
    100 mL/hr prn PADP or PCWP <12 mm Hg
    DDAVP injection (desmopressin acetate, Rhône-Poulenc
    Rorer Inc.), 1 mL IV at 12-hour intervals if urine output
    >200 mL/hr for two consecutive hours (hold if PADP
    >16 mm Hg or serum sodium <135)
Phenylephrine (Neo-Synephrine) infusion (50 mg in 250 mL
    normal saline)
  Titrate to maintain blood pressure between 180 and
    220 mm Hg systolic and reverse ischemic deficits (maintain
    systemic vascular resistance <1500 dyne/s/m²)
Dopamine infusion
  Titrate to maintain cardiac output ≥5 L/min (hold for heart
    rate >120 beats/min)
Serum sodium level twice daily
  If serum sodium level <135 mEq/L, begin 3% sodium
    chloride solution at 30 to 50 mL/hr (hold for PADP
    >16 mm Hg)

PADP, pulmonary artery diastolic pressure; PCWP, pulmonary capillary wedge pressure.

or when the level of consciousness is depressed (i.e., Hunt and Hess grades 3 to 5), an external ventriculostomy drain (EVD) should be placed. The drain not only provides a direct measurement of ICP but also provides a means of treatment should the ICP become elevated by draining CSF. Other familiar measures for controlling elevated ICP are raising the head of the bed to 25 to 30 degrees, maintaining cerebral perfusion pressure at 70 mm Hg, mannitol therapy, and, if needed in the acute period, hyperventilation to maintain pCO_2 at 30 to 35 mm Hg.

After the EVD is placed, the ventriculostomy is initially closed to drainage and monitored. If ICP rises above 20 cm H_2O, the drain is opened at a level 10 cm above the external auditory meatus. This level of drainage maximizes cerebral perfusion and often improves clinical status by 1 or 2 Hunt and Hess grades.[124,226,227] Patients who improve within 24 hours of EVD placement are more likely to experience a favorable outcome.[228] However, a good outcome does not always correlate with improvement after EVD placement, and presence or absence of improvement is not a reliable way of differentiating between patients with poor clinical status who would benefit from surgery and those who would not.[146,147,228–230] After surgery, the drain is opened to constant drainage at 10 to 15 cm H_2O, until CSF output drops to less than 60 to 80 mL/day or until the 14th day after hemorrhage; then the drain is elevated intermittently to wean the patient from the ventriculostomy.

Risk of infection from an external ventriculostomy can be minimized by combining meticulous sterile technique during placement of the catheter with the use of prophylactic antibiotics (we prefer intravenous ceftriaxone, 2 g given immediately before placement of the catheter) and routine tunneling of the ventriculostomy catheter a minimum of 4 cm subcutaneously from the insertion site. Finally, the catheter must be connected to a closed drainage system that does not need to be opened directly to air for zeroing or obtaining CSF samples (Becker External Drainage System, PS Medical, Goleta, CA 93117). CSF samples are obtained twice weekly on a routine basis for cell counts, Gram stain, and culture, and more frequently in patients with nonspecific signs of infection (fever, leukocytosis). We routinely leave EVD catheters in place for as long as 2 to 3 weeks and have had a 3% to 5% incidence of infection.[230a] This practice is supported by studies that have examined best practices for surveillance and management of ventriculostomy infections.[231–234]

Patients with acute hydrocephalus after SAH are certainly at risk of chronic hydrocephalus requiring permanent CSF diversion. The condition is not inevitable, however, and a substantial number of patients do not experience hydrocephalus until days or weeks after SAH. Consequently, CT should be performed in any patient with a history of SAH and declining neurologic function to rule out progressive ventriculomegaly. The decision to place a shunt should be guided by clinical parameters.

Fluid and Electrolyte Management

The most common electrolyte and intravascular fluid abnormalities in SAH are hypovolemia and hyponatremia. Hyponatremia occurs in 10% to 35% of patients after SAH and is most often associated with cerebral salt wasting caused by atrial natriuretic factor release.[114,235–241] Previ-ously, this hyponatremia was incorrectly attributed to the syndrome of inappropriate antidiuretic hormone (SIADH) secretion. It can exacerbate the hypovolemia found in about half of patients with SAH during the first 6 days after hemorrhage.[115] Together, these factors combine to cause volume contraction that can increase the risk of delayed vasospasm.[115,236,242–244] For this reason, hypervolemic therapy with normal saline, use of hypertonic saline to replace sodium lost by SAH-related natriuresis, and the occasional use of desmopressin to expand intravascular volume are essential features of our proactive regimen for treating SAH (see Table 67.4).

Antifibrinolytic Therapy

Aminocaproic acid (Amicar) and other antifibrinolytic agents that were once widely used to reduce the incidence of early rebleeding during the wait for surgery (usually 10 to 14 days) no longer constitute standard treatment. With modern microsurgical techniques, early clipping or coiling of aneurysms is performed without increased rates of operative morbidity and mortality. More important, however, is evidence from a number of studies showing that although antifibrinolytic therapy reduces the risk of early rebleeding by as much as 50%, its use is associated with an equally significant rise in the risk of strokes.[245–247] In addition, antifibrinolytic agents have been linked to a higher incidence of hydrocephalus.[220,246,248] Together, these findings suggest that antifibrinolytic treatment is contraindicated in most cases.

General Operative Considerations

Although we strongly recommend the early clipping of ruptured aneurysms, we believe that surgery in these difficult cases is best performed by a well-rested, experienced team. Surgery should be performed within 12 to 24 hours of admission. This short delay allows enough time for complete radiographic evaluation and medical stabilization. In our experience, many patients with poor clinical status show improvement during this period. The patient with an intracerebral or extra-axial hematoma who shows deterioration is an obvious exception and requires emergency surgical intervention.

The anesthesiologist should be experienced in the management of neurosurgical patients and familiar with the surgeon's preferences for intraoperative management (i.e., use of mannitol, barbiturates; see next section). He or she should assist with the operative positioning of the patient, including padding of all pressure points. In all but the most urgent cases, surface electrodes are placed for recording electroencephalographic (EEG) potentials and somatosensory evoked potentials (Fig. 67–6). Both adjuncts are necessary for monitoring burst suppression during barbiturate administration. In addition, we monitor motor-evoked potentials during surgery for basilar tip aneurysms and anterior choroidal aneurysms. This modality may be a more sensitive indicator of thalamoperforator occlusion during placement of clips.

Anesthesia for Aneurysm Surgery

Advances in neuroanesthesia have reduced the risks of early intracranial surgery in patients with ruptured

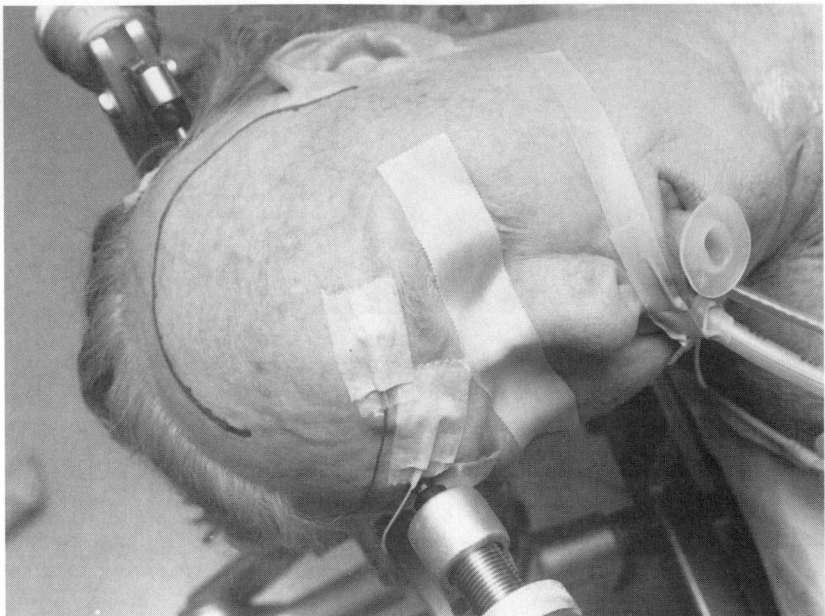

A

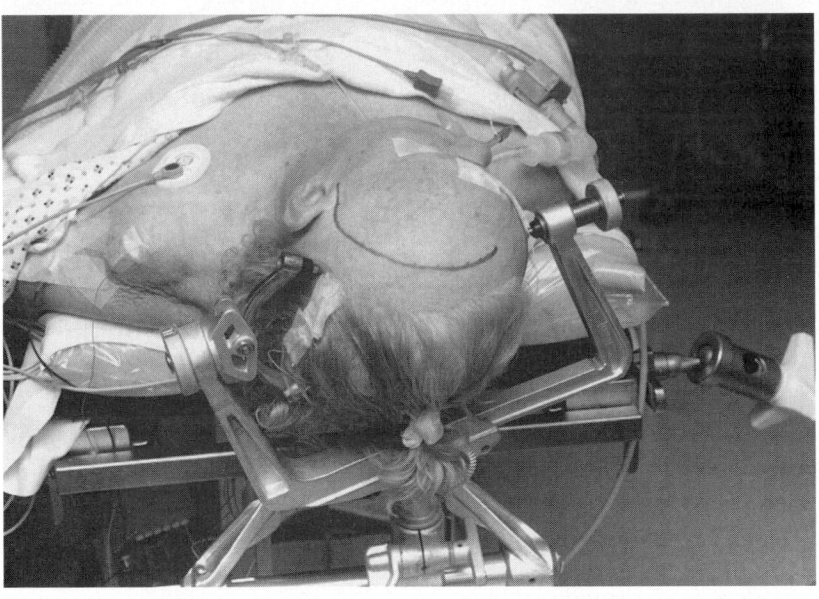

B

FIGURE 67–6 *A and B, Surface electrode placement for compressed spectral analysis monitoring of electroencephalogram activity and for median nerve somatosensory evoked potentials. The planned craniotomy incision has been outlined with a skin marker.*

aneurysms.[211] Modern anesthetic management begins before the patient is transferred to the surgical suite, with a complete review of the patient's history and current medical problems. In the alert patient, mild sedation can reduce stress and fluctuations in mean BP before the induction of anesthesia. Anesthesia is usually induced through a combination of agents, with the goal of avoiding significant swings in BP and heart rate. Hypotension in the clinically compromised patient could significantly reduce cerebral blood flow, and hypertension could raise the risk of recurrent aneurysmal hemorrhage.

A sedative such as midazolam combined with sodium thiopental and lidocaine is used for induction and is followed by complete neuromuscular blockade with vecuronium before intubation is attempted. The patient is ventilated to maintain end tidal pCO_2 between 35 and

40 mm Hg until brain retraction is begun; it is then lowered to 30 mm Hg. Anesthesia is maintained with a combination of inhalational agents, such as isoflurane and nitrous oxide, and small intravenous doses of sufentanil (or fentanyl in patients with cardiac instability) are used to keep BP and heart rate within 10% of preoperative values. Mannitol (25 to 50 g) is delivered intravenously if the brain is not already slack when the dura is opened. Ventricular drainage and barbiturate therapy are also valuable means of further reducing brain volume before retraction. These guidelines are consistent with anesthetic parameters described in the literature (see Dangor and Lam[211] for a review).

Previously, moderate systemic hypotension was routinely employed to reduce the risks of rupture during the dissection and clipping of aneurysms. This level of hypotension would normally result in little or no change in cerebral blood flow. In patients with aneurysmal SAH, however, particularly those with a depressed level of consciousness or vasospasm, impaired cerebral autoregulation can lead to significant, generalized cerebral ischemia.[249–254] Most surgeons have abandoned the use of systemic hypotension in favor of short periods of temporary vessel occlusion to reduce the risk of premature aneurysm rupture or to control hemorrhage after rupture.[255–258] In general, temporary occlusion of the major intracranial vessels is well tolerated for 10 to 20 minutes.[257–263] Moderate hypothermia (33°C to 34°C), common with general anesthesia, also increases the brain's tolerance of ischemia. We routinely combine this level of hypothermia with deep barbiturate anesthesia. Barbiturate administration is begun just before brain retraction; thiopental is administered as a loading dose of 5 to 10 mg per kg of body weight, followed by a continuous infusion titrated to produce 10 to 20 seconds of complete EEG burst suppression (Fig. 67–7). BP is maintained within 10% of preoperative values with small doses of phenylephrine if necessary. Clinical and laboratory evidence suggests that barbiturates reduce the risk of ischemic injury during temporary vessel occlusion.[259,264–270]

Direct Clipping of Aneurysms

The treatment of choice for most intracranial aneurysms is direct clipping of the aneurysm neck. Advances in microsurgical technique, skull base approaches to aneurysms previously considered unreachable, and the availability of a wide spectrum of aneurysm clips have increased the percentage of aneurysms suitable for direct neck obliteration. Aneurysms that are unsuitable for direct clipping can be approached in various ways, as discussed later.

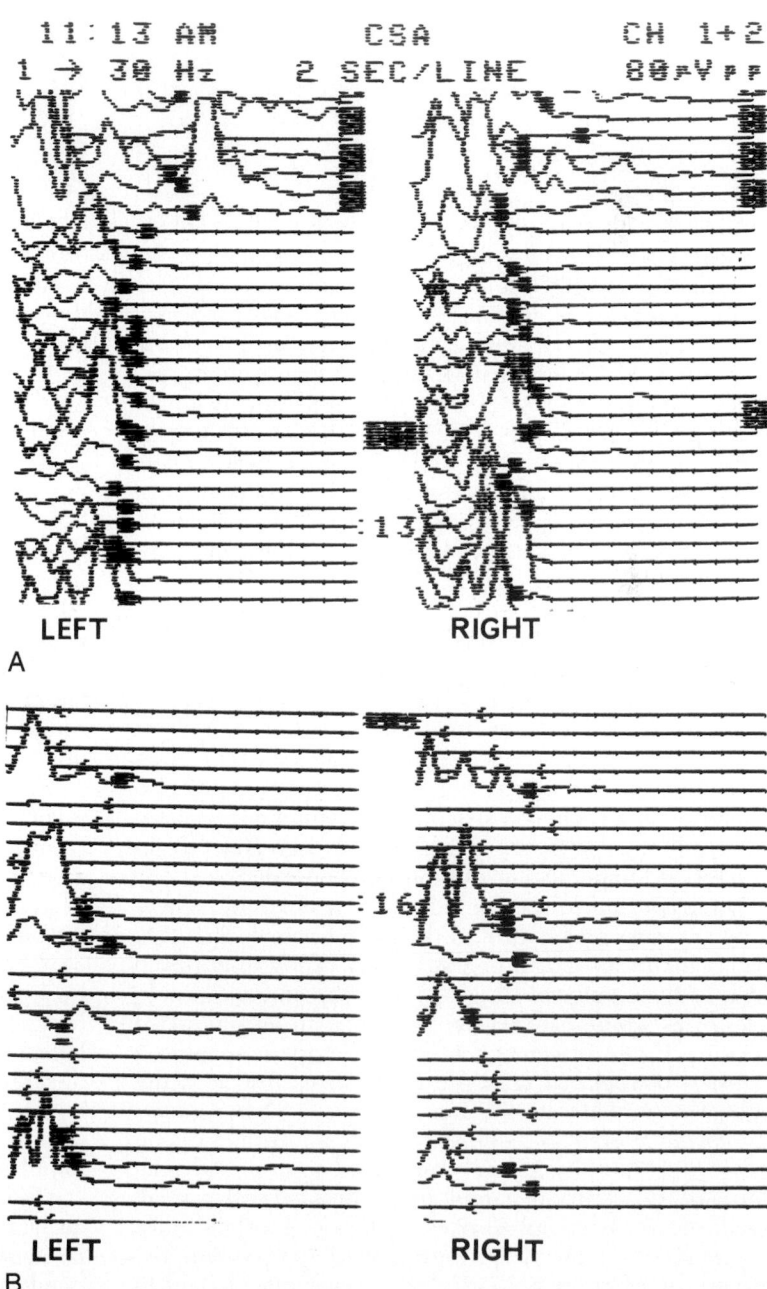

FIGURE 67–7 *Compressed spectral analysis (CSA) of electroencephalogram (EEG) activity during surgery for elective clipping of an incidental aneurysm. CSA before (A) and after (B) initiation of deep barbiturate coma with EEG burst suppression. Each line of the display represents a 2-second frequency spectrum analysis of EEG activity between 0 and 30 Hz. The flat lines represent periods of complete EEG burst suppression.*

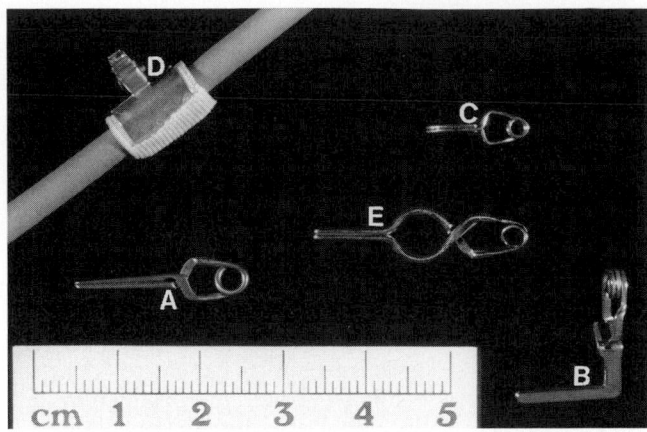

FIGURE 67–8 *Types of aneurysm clips available to the surgeon. A to C, Clips with parallel blades in various shapes and sizes that are placed directly across the aneurysm neck. D, Circumferential clips that enclose the parent vessel completely and obliterate the aneurysm neck between the ends of concave jaws. E, Clips that combine parallel jaws for obliterating the aneurysm neck with a proximal aperture through which an artery or nerve may pass.*

The three types of spring-loaded clips (Fig. 67–8) are (1) clips with parallel blades placed directly across the neck of the aneurysm, which come in all lengths, curves, and bayonet shapes, (2) circumferential clips, which enclose the parent vessel to obliterate the aneurysm neck between the ends of the concave jaws, and (3) fenestrated clips, which combine the parallel, long, thin jaws of the first type with a proximal round aperture through which an artery or nerve may pass. These clips, in combination with the new thin appliers, can accurately obliterate the aneurysm neck even in narrow, awkward locations. Special clips with lower closing pressures designed to prevent intimal injury are also available for temporary vessel occlusion.

Certain principles govern surgical management of acutely ruptured aneurysms. The operating room staff should be experienced in microsurgical techniques. Exposed surfaces of the brain should be covered and protected from dehydration and trauma (we prefer Telfa strips). CSF drainage and mannitol can facilitate brain retraction. The induction of barbiturate burst suppression when the dura is opened also encourages brain relaxation, raises tolerance to ischemia, and affords a greater margin of safety if temporary vessel occlusion is needed.

The approach to a ruptured aneurysm should include early exposure and control of the parent vessel. The neck of the aneurysm should be completely exposed. With the neck of the aneurysm dissected free, the surgeon should select the appropriate clip and apply it in an unhurried manner. If clip placement is unsatisfactory, it should be adjusted or replaced until the right clip is placed in the right way to obliterate the aneurysm neck while preserving flow in afferent and efferent vessels. After the surgeon is satisfied that the clip has been placed appropriately, the dome of the aneurysm can be decompressed with a small needle to verify complete neck occlusion. Last and most important, if the aneurysm ruptures before occlusion, the surgeon must resist the impulse to react quickly and to place the clip hurriedly. Instead, a suction tip can control the ruptured dome with gentle tamponade by means of a small cotton patty; then, controlled dissection can continue, or a temporary clip can be placed across the parent vessels, and dissection completed.

Broad-necked aneurysms often call for multiple clips. The wide variety of fenestrated Sugita clips (SIMS Surgical Inc., Keene, NH) and Sundt-Kees clips (Codman, Johnson & Johnson, Randolph, MA) are particularly well adapted for the occlusion of awkward aneurysm necks. Fenestrated, straight, or right-angle clips can be placed serially over the parent vessel to extend the length of neck occlusion (Fig. 67–9).

Specific Operative Techniques

Aneurysms of the Anterior Circulation

Anterior circulation aneurysms are those that arise from the ICA or its two terminal branches, the anterior cerebral and middle cerebral arteries. Most aneurysms of the anterior circulation are readily treated through a pterional craniotomy (Fig. 67–10). Minor modifications may be helpful for exposing specific lesions, but the general approach is the same for all. Because the pterional approach is most commonly used for aneurysm surgery, it is presented in detail. We are beginning to use the orbitozygomatic approach more regularly for anterior communicating artery aneurysms; this approach is more thoroughly discussed in approaches to posterior circulation aneurysms.

After the induction of general anesthesia, the patient's head is positioned using three-point skeletal fixation and rotated 30 to 60 degrees off midline toward the shoulder of the unaffected side. The degree of rotation depends on the specific lesion, being greatest for anterior communicating artery aneurysms and least for aneurysms involving the posterior communicating artery and the ICA bifurcation (further discussed later). The head is also extended 10 to 20 degrees so that the maxillary prominence is the highest point in the field. This position helps maximize gravitational retraction of the frontal lobe once the craniotomy is complete. Lumbar subarachnoid drainage is not routinely used because CSF in the basal cisterns can be drained readily before brain retraction is needed.

The skin is incised from the posterior margin of the zygomatic process, 1 cm in front of the tragus. The incision is carried forward and superiorly in a gently curving arc to a point just behind the hairline in the middle of the forehead (see Fig. 67–10). The bone flap need not extend to the midline, but the skin incision is extended to the midline or just beyond so that the scalp flap can be retracted inferiorly to drill the pterion thoroughly. The scalp and underlying muscle are elevated together, with a small fascial cuff left along the insertion of the temporalis muscle to be used during closure to firmly secure the temporalis muscle in its normal anatomic position. This maneuver reduces postoperative temporomandibular joint dysfunction and improves cosmetic appearance (see Fig. 67–10).

The soft tissues are retracted with low-profile fishhooks on elastic bands, and a free frontotemporal bone flap is fashioned with a high-speed drill through a single temporal burr hole near the root of the zygoma. The frontal

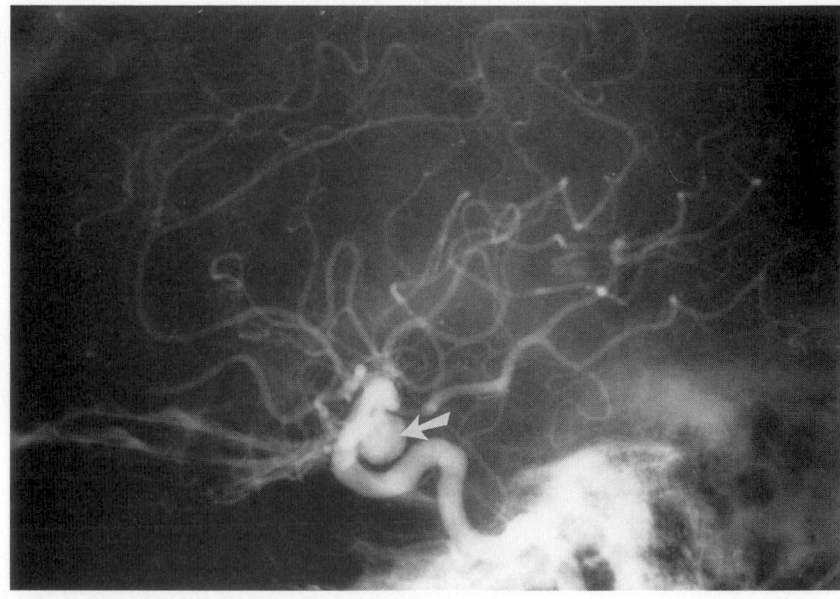

A

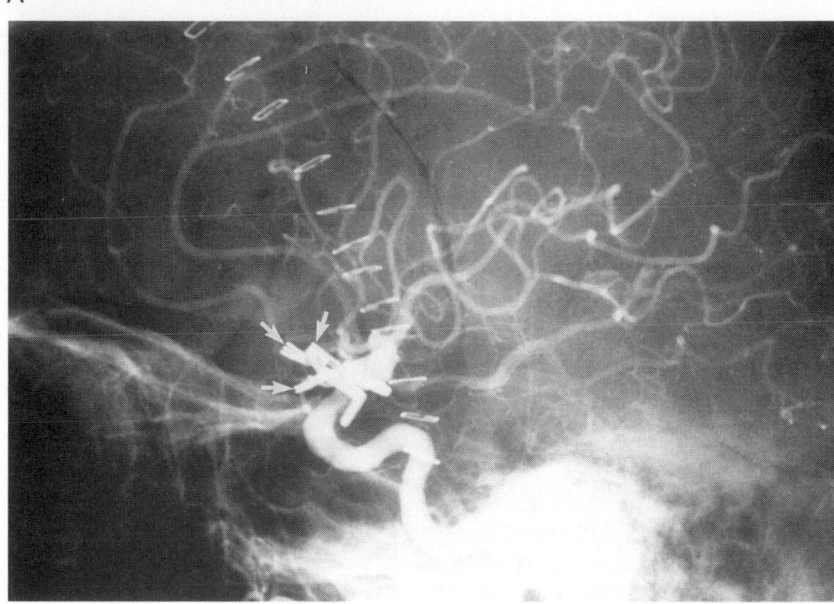

B

FIGURE 67–9 *A 53-year-old woman was referred for evaluation after experiencing transient ischemic attacks that affected her right arm. A, Lateral view of the left internal carotid artery angiogram demonstrates a large, wide-necked, left internal carotid artery aneurysm (arrow). Cardiac and extracranial vascular evaluations did not show other possible embolic sources. B, Lateral view of the postoperative left internal carotid artery angiogram shows good clipping of the aneurysm. Note that a combination of three clips (arrows) has been used to obliterate the aneurysm neck and reconstruct the parent vessel.*

cut extends medially to the foramen of the supraorbital nerve and inferiorly to the floor of anterior cranial fossa (Fig. 67–11). Because the craniotomy is centered on the pterion, this approach facilitates further resection of the pterion, exposes the sylvian fissure, and creates a corridor down to the ICA. The pterion is drilled extensively to remove the lesser wing of the sphenoid bone, the base of the anterior clinoid process, the bony ridges of the orbital roof, the inner table of the inferior frontal bone over the superior orbital rim, and the squamosal portion of the temporal bone inferiorly to the middle fossa floor. After drilling is complete, the dural fold of the superior orbital fissure is skeletonized. The extensive bone removal around the pterion creates a flat corridor with ample space under the frontal and temporal lobes in the sylvian fissure.

The dura is then incised to create a curvilinear flap based over the orbit (see Fig. 67–11). With the appropri-

ate extradural bone removal, the bony prominences at the base of the anterior clinoid process that normally obscure the optic nerve and carotid artery are gone, and these structures can be seen with minimal brain retraction. The dura is elevated and retracted with stay sutures over the muscle to sweep the dura and muscle out of the surgical corridor. The brain should be covered to prevent drying and trauma from retractors and instruments; as previously mentioned, we prefer Telfa strips, which can be readily cut to different sizes. The frontal lobe is gently elevated with a self-retaining retractor (see Fig. 67–11). If necessary, another small, thin retractor can be placed over the temporal lobe at its junction with the sylvian fissure.

If there is any resistance to retraction, brain relaxation can be increased with mannitol, barbiturates, and CSF drainage. In the patient without a ventricular catheter, incising the arachnoid around the optic nerve and ICA

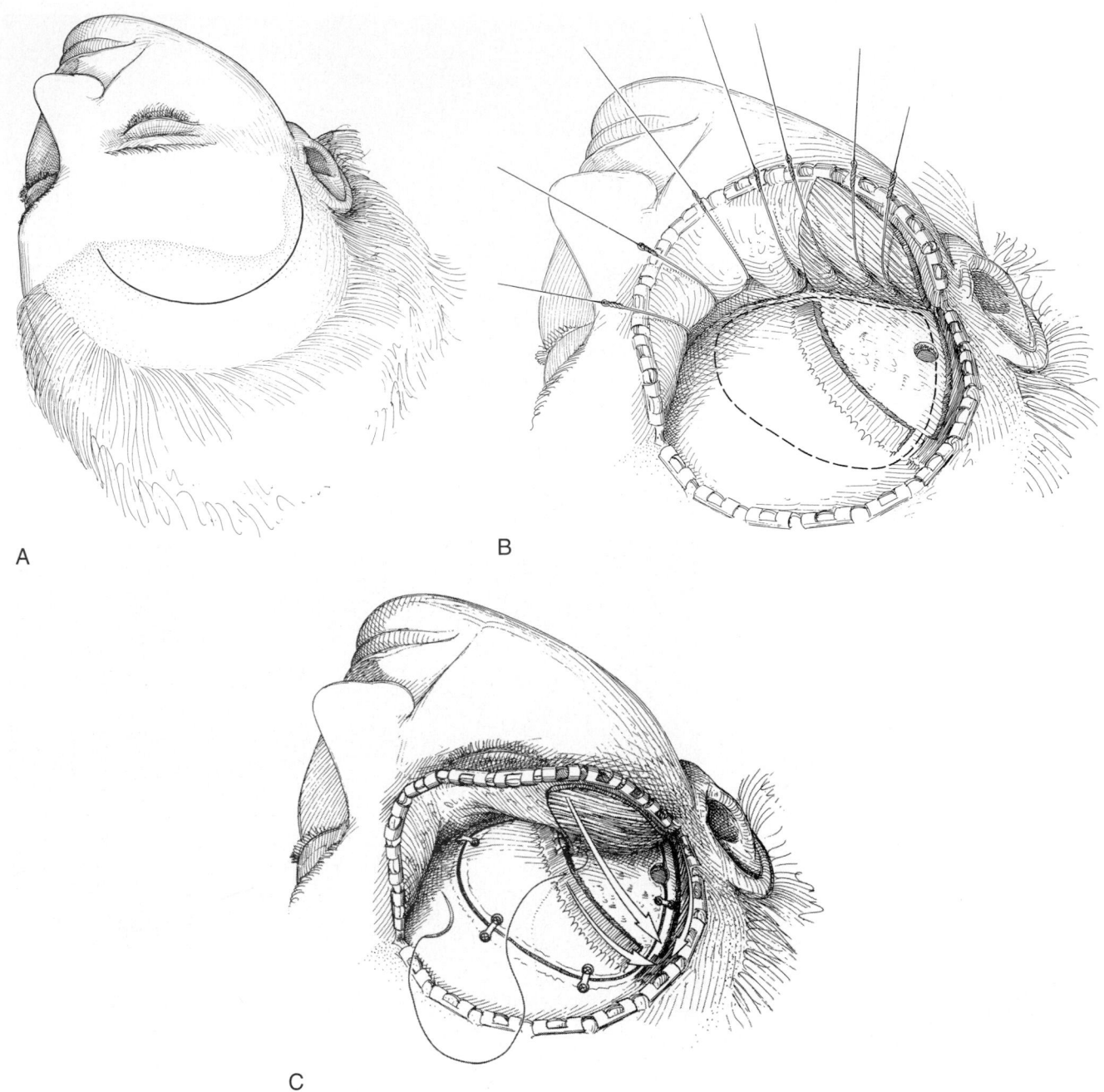

FIGURE 67–10 *Pterional approach to anterior circulation aneurysms (see text for details). A, Outline of scalp incision. B, The scalp flap and underlying temporalis muscle have been elevated together, with the exception of a small fascial cuff along the insertion of the temporalis muscle. Fishhooks have been used to retract the scalp and temporalis muscle flaps. Note the outline for the planned bone flap, which is brought to the midpupillary line and as close to the frontal fossa floor as possible. This type of bony dissection helps minimize the extent of brain retraction needed to visualize the basal cisterns. C, The intracranial portion of the procedure has been completed, and the bone flap has been replaced and fixed securely in position with miniplates and screws. The cut edges of the temporalis fascia are being approximated with a running suture. This closure helps ensure normal anatomic function of the temporalis muscle as well as improve the postoperative cosmetic appearance of the temporal fossa region. (Adapted from Spetzler RF, Lee KS: Reconstruction of the temporalis muscle for the pterional craniotomy: Technical note [see comments]. J Neurosurg 73:636, 1990.)*

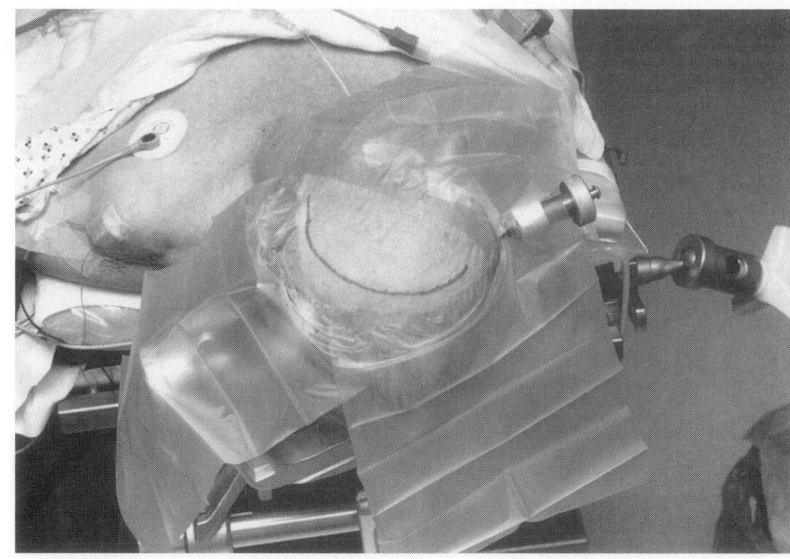

A

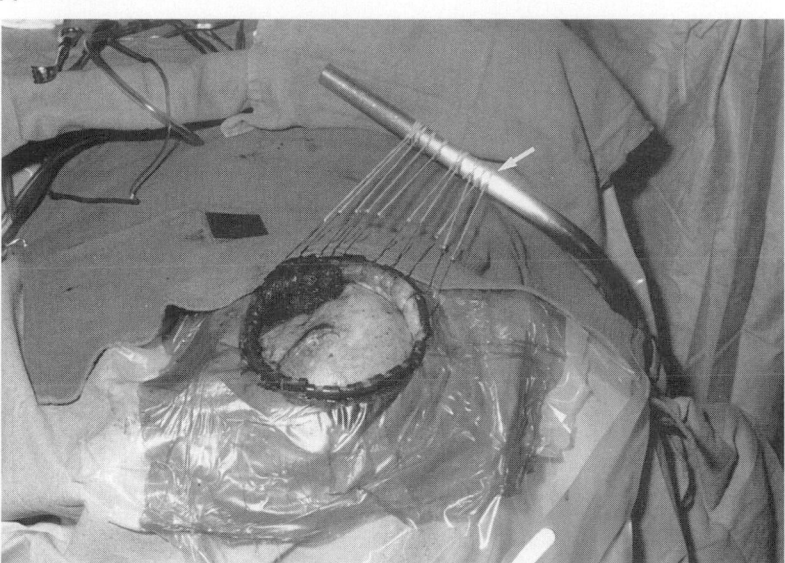

B

FIGURE 67–11 *Surgical treatment of the incidental left middle cerebral artery aneurysm in the 64-year-old woman presented in Figure 67-1. A, The patient has been positioned for a pterional craniotomy, and the incision outlined. Self-adhering sterile drapes help isolate the field and protect the electrodes used for intraoperative monitoring from moisture. B, The scalp flap has been elevated, and the skin and muscle are being retracted with fishhooks attached to rubber bands, which are, in turn, secured to a Leyla bar (arrow). C, The craniotomy bone flap has been turned and elevated, exposing the underlying dura. Dural tackup sutures have been placed at regular intervals around the margin of the bone flap to control bleeding. The lateral wall of the sphenoid wing has been removed with a high-speed drill to bring the bony dissection flush with the frontal fossa floor (arrows). The removal of bone minimizes the retraction needed to visualize the basal cisterns and aneurysm.*

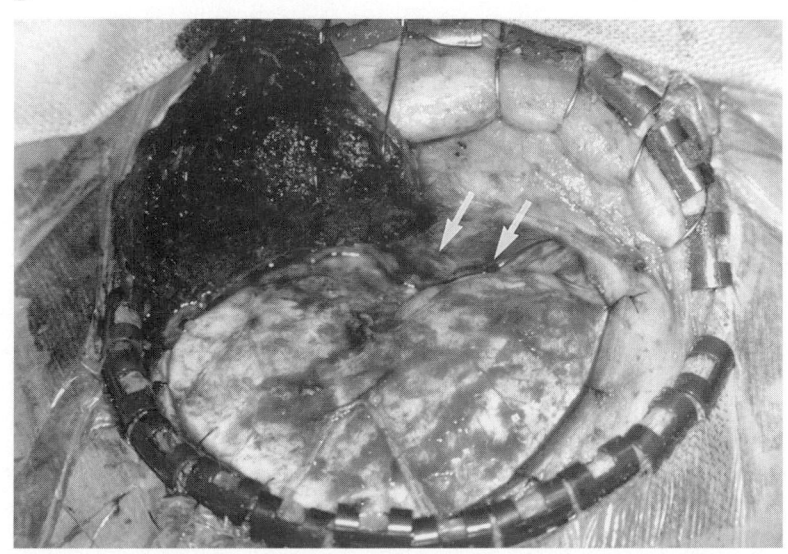

C

Continued

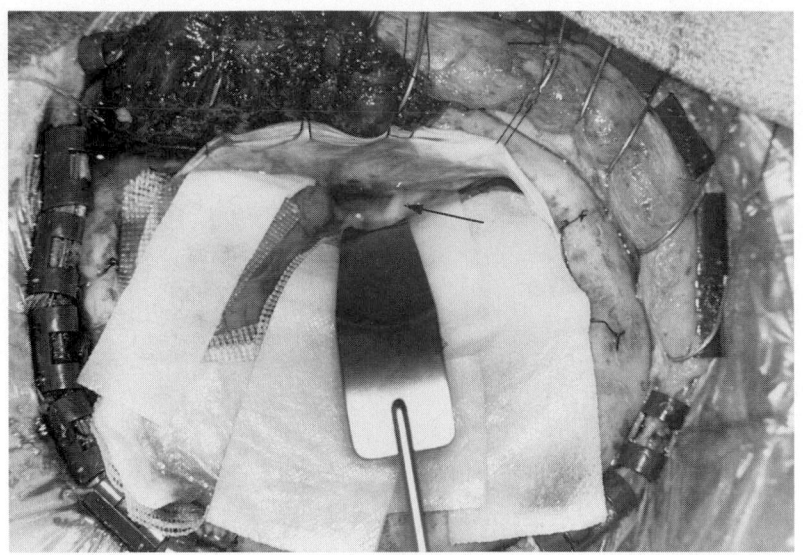

D

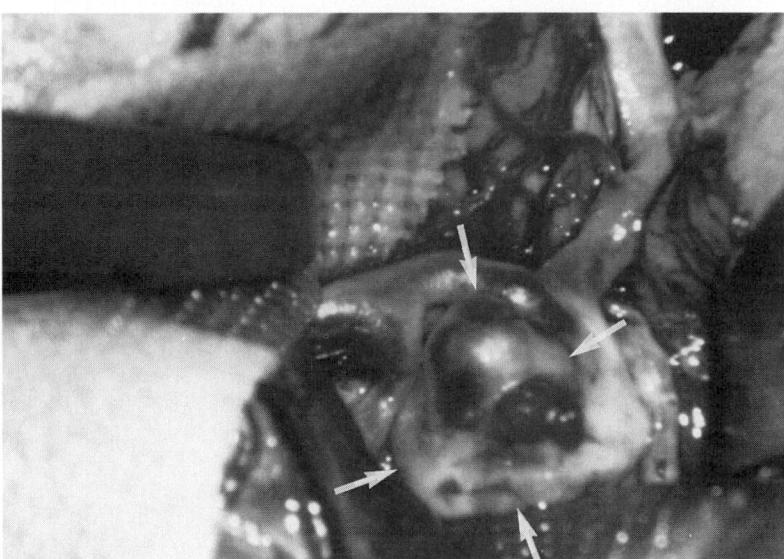

E

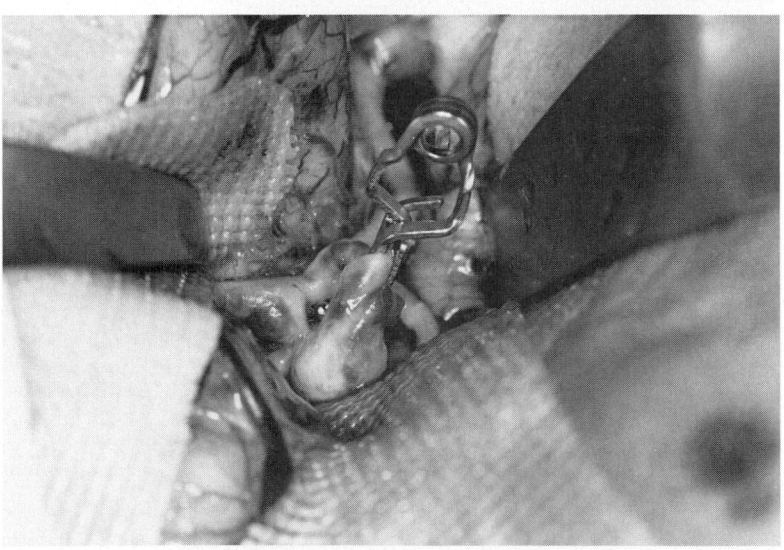

F

FIGURE 67–11, cont'd. D, *The dura has been opened and retracted with stay sutures. The brain surface is covered with Telfa strips to protect it from drying and trauma. The frontal lobe is being gently elevated to expose the basal cisterns. The pristine white silhouette of the optic nerve (arrow) is faintly visible through an intact vale of arachnoid at the tip of the retractor blade. E, The sylvian fissure has been widely opened, and the aneurysm at the middle cerebral artery bifurcation exposed (arrows). Note the marked irregularity of the aneurysm dome. At surgery, blood could be readily visualized swirling through the thinned outpouchings of the aneurysm surface. F, The aneurysm has been dissected free of the surrounding vessels, and its neck obliterated with a single clip. The dome of the aneurysm has been punctured and collapsed to ensure that it no longer fills.*

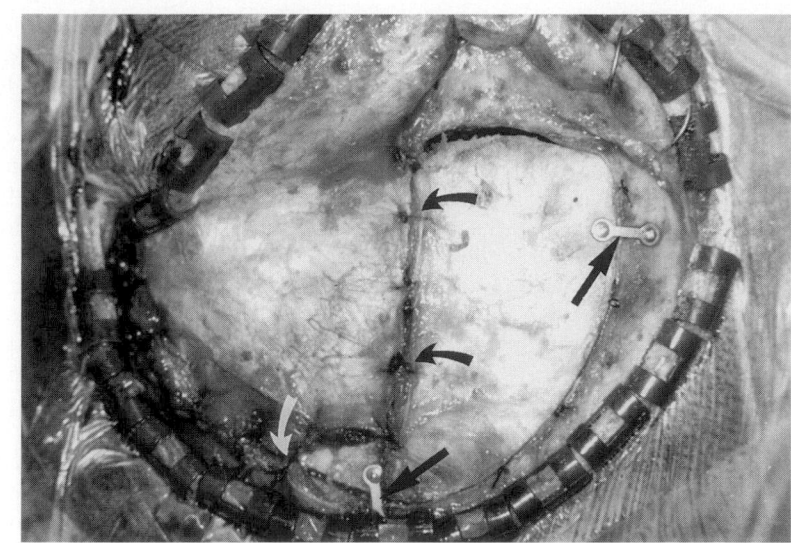

FIGURE 67–11, cont'd. G, *The craniotomy bone flap has been replaced and secured in position with miniplates and screws* (straight arrows). *The cut edges of the temporalis fascia have been reapproximated* (curved arrows), *and only the scalp closure remains to be completed.*

G

provides a pathway for ample CSF drainage. We prefer to perform this maneuver after the sylvian fissure has been split as needed, because the fissure is more easily dissected when it is filled with CSF. Depending on the aneurysm's location, the fissure is either split from lateral to medial or vice versa. The extent of fissure splitting is also dictated by the aneurysm's location. Nonetheless, the essential feature of successful anterior circulation aneurysm surgery is careful arachnoid dissection, especially in the region of the sylvian fissure (see Fig. 67–11). During lateral to medial dissection, the least traumatic strategy is to use either a No. 11 blade scalpel or fine microscissors to separate the superficial adhesions between the frontal and temporal lobes along the frontal lobe side of the sylvian veins. Once an M_2 branch of the middle cerebral artery is found, the surgeon can follow it down deeply into the fissure toward the insula by gently spreading the bipolar forceps and cutting tenacious arachnoid adhesions with microscissors. When a deeper cleft has been created by following an M2 branch to the bottom of the fissure, the fissure can be opened in an inside-out fashion, as one separates the sections of an orange. Depending on the needs of aneurysm exposure, the fissure dissection can proceed medially or laterally. One critical point is that the trans-sylvian veins should be spared as long as possible, especially those that drain into the sphenoparietal sinus. If these veins are sacrificed early in the sylvian fissure dissection, venous congestion makes the frontal and temporal surfaces friable and prone to hemorrhage, which is potentially devastating.

Carotid-ophthalmic aneurysms and aneurysms originating from the carotid artery as it winds around the anterior clinoid process have been classified many different ways (superior hypophyseal, dorsal variant). However, they are all near the carotid rings, the anterior clinoid process, and the optic strut, and this proximity makes their treatment challenging and their intracranial proximal control tricky.[271–277] Proximal control is best achieved at the cervical segment of the carotid artery. We routinely include the cervical carotid area in the sterile draping for paraclinoidal aneurysms and then proceed with a standard pterional

craniotomy and extradural resection of the sphenoid ridge. It is possible to remove the anterior clinoid process extradurally, but we prefer to remove it intradurally because the remnants of the anterior clinoid process left after the pterion is removed are best seen intradurally, especially in relation to the optic nerve and aneurysm fundus.

We start by opening the arachnoid over the optic nerve and carotid artery, a maneuver that allows the brain to relax by CSF removal. After the terrain around the anterior clinoid and the aneurysm has been surveyed, an incision is made along the medial sphenoid ridge to the tip of the anterior clinoid process. Another incision proceeds from this first incision medially toward the falciform ligament. Once these leaves of dura have been dissected free from the underlying bone, the anterior clinoid process and optic strut can be thinned with a high-speed drill, small rongeurs, and microdissectors. Bleeding from the cavernous sinus is easily controlled with hemostatic agents and pressure. Finally, the falciform ligament over the optic nerve is completely transected to prevent optic nerve compression and, if needed, to allow the optic nerve to be mobilized superiorly off the origin of the ophthalmic artery. Clipping then proceeds as dictated by the particular anatomy of the aneurysm. During closure, any communications with the sphenoid sinus must be occluded, usually with a combination of absorbable gelatin sponge (Gelfoam), a muscle plug, and fibrin glue to prevent CSF leakage.

The same surgical approach is used for aneurysms of the posterior communicating artery, anterior choroidal artery, and ICA bifurcation because of their anatomic proximity. The posterior communicating artery emerges from the posteromedial surface of the ICA as the carotid bends upward toward its bifurcation, and most aneurysms arising at the posterior communicating origin point posteriorly and inferiorly. Posterior communicating aneurysms, however, can be broken into the following two subcategories: (1) aneurysms that project medially to the tentorial incisura and cause oculomotor nerve compression where the nerve enters the dura at the tentorial edge and (2) aneurysms that project laterally above the tentorium and can manifest as temporal lobe hematomas after they rupture.[278] The origin of the anterior choroidal artery is only a few millimeters further along the ICA from the posterior communicating artery, so the hemodynamic factors that lead to aneurysms in the two regions are similar. However, the anterior choroidal artery arises on the lateral surface of the carotid and swings laterally and posteriorly, beside the optic tract, before entering the choroidal fissure. Aneurysms of the ICA bifurcation project in the direction of terminal carotid flow, toward the anterior perforated substance, and usually project anterosuperiorly or straight superiorly. The perforators at the apex of the ICA bifurcation are invariably swept posteriorly by the fundus of the aneurysm, and they may be tightly adherent to its wall.

A standard pterional craniotomy and removal of the sphenoid ridge with the head turned 30 degrees toward the shoulder of the unaffected side is adequate for aneurysms in these locations. Opening the sylvian fissure provides a view of the distal carotid artery and essential branches and perforators in this region. However, the dissection should proceed carefully as the temporal lobe is freed of adhesions. Laterally projecting posterior communicating aneurysms are often tightly adherent to the medial temporal lobe, and excessive movement of the temporal tip can avulse the aneurysm dome, with catastrophic results. In addition, with posterior communicating artery aneurysms manifesting as oculomotor palsy, a portion of the fundus often projects below the incisura and is adherent to the compressed oculomotor nerve. The aneurysm can rupture as the clip blades close around the aneurysm's neck, but bleeding will stop as the blades of the clip close tightly and the neck is obliterated.

Once the neck is closed, dissection should proceed to ensure that thalamoperforators and the anterior choroidal artery (which may have duplicate origins) are not occluded by the blades of the clip. Infarcts caused by occlusion of the anterior choroidal artery or perforators off the posterior communicating artery are poorly tolerated. In contrast, occlusion of the posterior communicating segment may be unavoidable. Such occlusion is usually well tolerated as long as there is collateral flow to the perforators exiting the communicating segment by way of the posterior circulation. However, the opposite is not true if the posterior communicating segment is a fetal variant.

Aneurysms of the anterior communicating artery and proximal anterior cerebral arteries are the most common intracranial aneurysms, are the aneurysms most commonly missed on angiography, and are some of the most surgically challenging in terms of anatomy. Most anterior communicating artery aneurysms are associated with a dominant A_1 segment. Consequently, they point toward the contralateral hemisphere as a continuation of the dominant A_1 direction of flow. There is wide variability in the anatomy of the anterior communicating artery region. For example, there may be two or more communicating arteries, each with multiple perforating branches, only one A_2 segment (azygos A_2), or three A_2 segments.

The following nine landmarks form the road map for safe surgery of an anterior communicating artery aneurysm: the proximal (A_1) and distal (A_2) branches of both anterior cerebral arteries, the anterior communicating artery, and the frontopolar branches and recurrent arteries of Heubner to both hemispheres. Failure to see

these vessels and protect them from occlusion can lead to serious neurologic morbidity. Anterior communicating artery aneurysms usually point either anteroinferiorly, below the A_2 vessels and toward the planum sphenoidale, or posterosuperiorly, between the A_2 vessels into the interhemispheric fissure.[279] Those that point inferiorly obscure the contralateral A_2 and are best approached on the side of the dominant A_1, even if the patient's functionally dominant hemisphere must be opened. In contrast, anterior communicating artery aneurysms that point superiorly are tucked away between the hemispheres and leave the view of both A_1 branches unobstructed. These aneurysms can be approached safely from whatever side is thought to put less functional brain at risk.

With the patient's head turned 60 degrees to the unaffected side, a standard pterional craniotomy with sphenoid ridge resection provides the lateral corridor needed to reach the ipsilateral and contralateral sides of the anterior communicating artery complex. Initial arachnoid dissection is directed to the optic nerve and ICA until the ipsilateral A_1 segment is identified. The A_1 segment is then followed to the anterior communicating artery complex. After all nine of the pertinent vessels are identified (both A_1 and A_2 segments, the anterior communicating artery, both recurrent arteries, and both frontopolar arteries) as well as the much smaller perforators that emerge from the A_1 segments and anterior communicating artery, clipping can proceed safely. Adhesions between the frontal lobe and the temporal lobe sometimes prevent adequate retraction. In this case, the sylvian fissure should be split adequately to untether the frontal pole. Great care should be exerted during elevation of the frontal lobe in patients with inferiorly projecting anterior communicating aneurysms. The aneurysm may be adherent to the visual apparatus and can be inadvertently avulsed by frontal lobe elevation. For superiorly projecting aneurysms, resection of a small portion of the gyrus rectus immediately adjacent to the anterior communicating complex can make visualization much easier. This maneuver preserves the recurrent arteries and small perforators exiting the A_1 and anterior communicating artery and brings the proximal A_2 segments into view. We have started to use the orbitozygomatic craniotomy approach for some anterior communicating artery aneurysms that point superiorly, because removal of the orbit provides a superior trajectory with less brain retraction.

Middle cerebral artery aneurysms most commonly occur where the artery bifurcates into superior and inferior trunks, immediately before the vessels make an elbow turn to run along the surface of the insula. Most middle cerebral artery aneurysms therefore project laterally and anteriorly between the two trunks into the sylvian fissure and toward the temporal pole. When they rupture, these aneurysms usually produce clot in the sylvian fissure or anterior temporal pole, with relatively less blood in the basal cisterns. These aneurysms are best approached through a standard pterional craniotomy with sphenoid ridge resection, with the patient's head turned 45 degrees. It is essential to open the sylvian fissure widely to see and protect the major trunks of the middle cerebral bifurcation adequately as well as any small perforators that may originate from the M_1 segment. The advantage of proceeding with dissection from the medial end of the fissure is early proximal control. The advantages of starting from the lateral end of the fissure are as follows: First, the fissure is easier to open because the basal cisterns have not been opened and the fissure remains filled with CSF. Second, less retraction is needed. Finally, the trans-sylvian veins draining into the sphenoparietal sinus are at less risk, minimizing the chance of sacrificing these veins and causing pial engorgement that makes subarachnoid dissection more difficult. Before the fissure is opened, it is important to note in which direction the aneurysm points (frontally or temporally) and to proceed along the M_2 trunk on the opposite side, so that the aneurysm fundus is not encountered unexpectedly.

Once the middle cerebral bifurcation is identified and the M_1 segment is in view, the fissure can be split more widely to adequately expose the aneurysm neck, the proximal M_2 trunks, and any perforators off of the M_1 segment. If the aneurysm ruptures during lateral sylvian dissection, the basal cisterns should be opened quickly, and a temporary clip applied to the ICA. Then the medial portion of the sylvian fissure can be opened. When the M_1 segment of the middle cerebral artery comes into view, the temporary clip can be repositioned, and dissection can proceed.

Pericallosal Aneurysms

Pericallosal aneurysms are relatively uncommon, composing about only 3% of aneurysms in most major series.[95,280–282] The distal segments of the anterior cerebral artery run immediately adjacent to each other, tightly apposed to the corpus callosum deep within the interhemispheric fissure. The distal anterior cerebral arteries branch along the genu of the corpus callosum into (1) the callosomarginal arteries that run in the cingulate sulcus and (2) the pericallosal arteries that are the terminal continuation of the distal anterior cerebral arteries running along the surface of the corpus callosum. Aneurysms of the distal anterior cerebral branches are best clipped through an intrahemispheric approach. A bifrontal scalp incision located behind the hairline permits the scalp flap to be reflected forward and inferiorly to expose the anterior third of the cranium.

The bone flap should be sufficiently anterior to allow proximal control of the parent vessel before the aneurysm is encountered, but the flap should also be long enough to allow a suitable trajectory between bridging veins. In right-handed patients, a right-sided approach is usually preferred by right-handed surgeons, but the final choice should be the side with more space between draining veins, because whether the approach is ipsilateral or contralateral to such medially located aneurysms is relatively unimportant. To minimize retraction of the frontal lobe, the bone flap should continue across the sagittal sinus. The dura is opened so that it remains hinged along the edge of the sinus and is retracted with stay sutures to maximize midline exposure with minimal frontal lobe retraction. The parent vessel is exposed proximally and followed until the aneurysm can be dissected and clipped.

Aneurysms of the Posterior Circulation
Basilar Bifurcation Aneurysms

The basilar apex is best targeted from an anterosuperior trajectory. The craniotomy-transcranial route is either subtemporal-incisural, pterional–trans-sylvian, or orbitozygomatic-pterional, a sequence that reflects both the genealogy of surgical approaches and an increasingly anterior trajectory. These cranial exposures can be combined to vary the direction of approach as needed, and the surgeon can expand the mesial part of the exposure by removing adjacent bony obstructions (e.g., the anterior and posterior clinoid processes, the dorsum sella–upper clivus, and medial petrous apex) or by working through the cavernous sinus or tentorium.

Subtemporal Approach. The subtemporal approach and the surgical treatment of basilar tip aneurysms in general were pioneered by Drake.[283–291] This approach uses a lateral trajectory and requires elevation of the temporal lobe. Dissection proceeds between the medial temporal lobe and the tentorial edge. In most cases, the subtemporal trajectory parallels the long axis of the aneurysm neck; this facilitates clip placement, because the posterior perforating arteries, whose preservation is perhaps the most crucial aspect of the procedure, can be visualized best. However, the lateral trajectory precludes exposure of the contralateral anatomy (posterior cerebral artery, superior cerebellar artery, and oculomotor nerve), places the ipsilateral oculomotor nerve in the center of the operative field, and requires potentially dangerous retraction of the temporal lobe and vein of Labbé.

Typically, the approach is from the patient's right unless there are mitigating factors, such as aneurysmal anatomy that favors a left-sided approach, a preexisting left oculomotor nerve palsy, right hemiparesis, coexisting vascular disease, or known right hemispheric dominance. The patient is placed in either the lateral decubitus or supine position. The head is rotated until the midline plane parallels the floor, and the head is angled 15 degrees downward to achieve a line of sight parallel to the floor of the middle fossa. A lumbar subarachnoid drain permits CSF drainage and brain relaxation to facilitate temporal lobe retraction during the approach to the tentorial incisura.

A linear incision that extends superiorly 7 cm from the zygomatic arch and 1 cm anterior to the tragus, or a horseshoe-shaped flap based over the ear, is used. Depending on the skin incision, the temporalis muscle is either divided and held apart, or flapped inferiorly. A 4 × 4–cm craniotomy is made in the temporal bone, and additional temporal squamosal bone is drilled inferiorly until the cranial exposure is flush with the floor of the middle fossa (Fig. 67–12). This bony removal is crucial because any lip of bone remaining above the middle fossa floor would block the surgical corridor and necessitate greater retraction of the temporal lobe.

Using the operating microscope, the surgeon positions a self-retaining retractor to elevate the temporal lobe and expose the tentorial incisura (see Fig. 67–12). The arachnoid over the interpeduncular and ambient cisterns is opened, and the oculomotor nerve is identified. The surgeon can enlarge the opening into the interpeduncular cistern by pulling the edge of the tentorium laterally with a tacking suture placed between the oculomotor nerve and the trochlear nerve. Additional inferior exposure in the posterior fossa can be gained through division of the tentorium behind the entry of the trochlear nerve. Manipulation of the oculomotor nerve is minimized, but it is often conveniently retracted superiorly because of its adhesions to the medial temporal lobe. The superior cerebellar and poste-

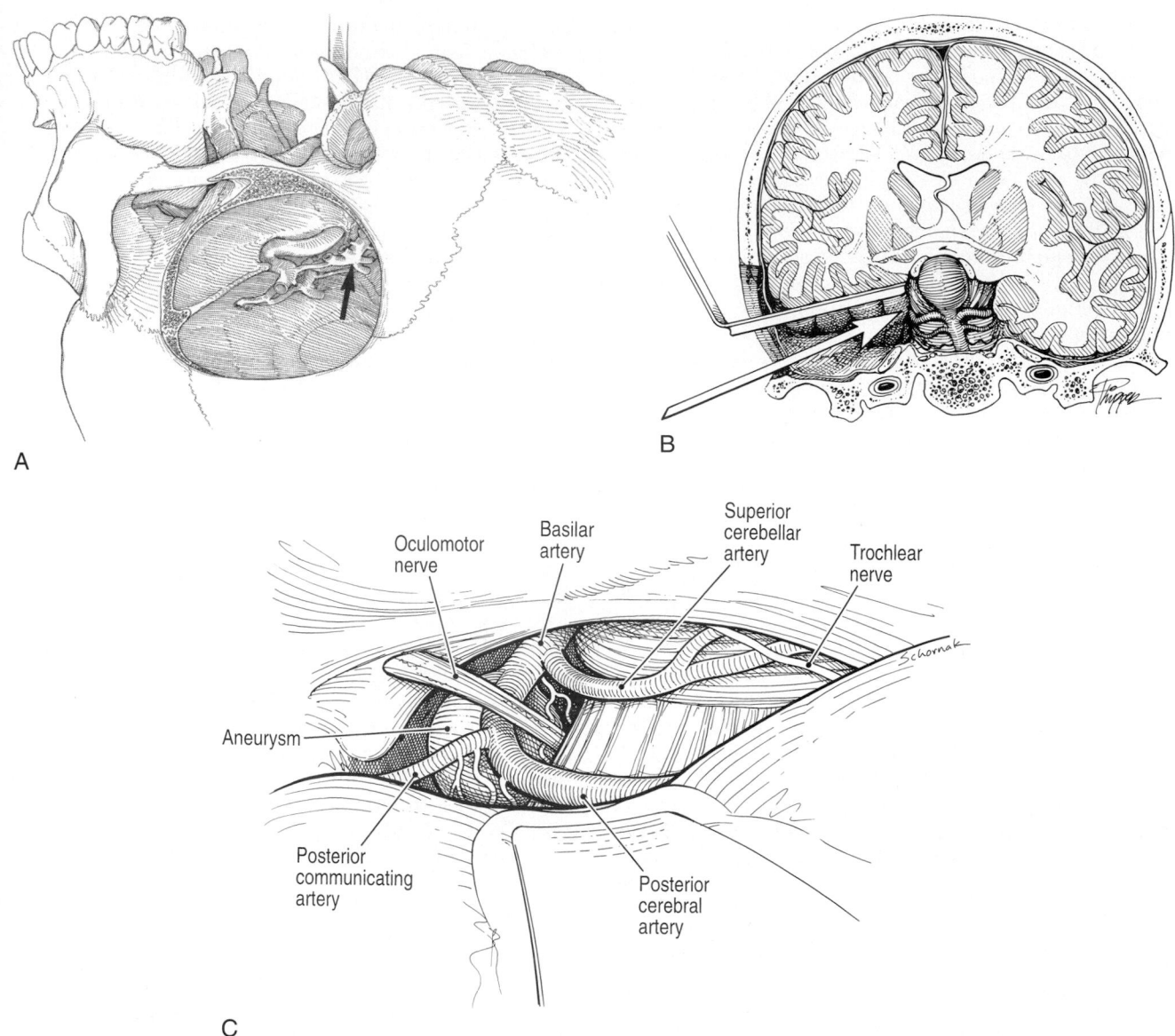

FIGURE 67–12   *Subtemporal exposure. This approach is used for aneurysms of the distal basilar artery, including those arising from the superior cerebellar arteries and the basilar artery tip. A, Lateral view of the skull demonstrates the bony dissection for this approach to the upper basilar artery (arrow). The lateral wall of the temporal bone, along with a portion of the root of the zygoma, has been removed with a high-speed drill. Removal of bone minimizes the extent of temporal lobe retraction needed to expose the basal cisterns. B, Coronal section through the midportion of the temporal fossa illustrates the extent of temporal lobe retraction required for this approach. Because of the potential risks associated with temporal lobe retraction, this approach is usually performed from the non-dominant (right) side. C, The pertinent anatomy seen from a right subtemporal exposure for a basilar tip aneurysm. This approach provides good visualization of the perforating branches extending along the posterior surface of the aneurysm. It is particularly well suited for those aneurysms that angle posteriorly; however, it may be difficult for the surgeon to visualize the contralateral posterior cerebral artery and oculomotor nerve. (Courtesy of the Barrow Neurological Institute.)*

rior cerebral arteries are then followed medially to the basilar apex, and the aneurysm is dissected and clipped.

Pterional–Trans-sylvian Approach. The pterional craniotomy was popularized by Yasargil as an approach to basilar apex aneurysms.[281,284,285,292,293] It is familiar to most neurosurgeons because it is the standard approach used for most anterior circulation aneurysms (see earlier discussion). Compared with the subtemporal trajectory, the pterional trajectory is more anterolateral, providing a better

overall view of arterial and cranial nerve anatomy. However, the posterior perforating arteries are usually obscured by the aneurysm fundus; consequently, the surgeon must manipulate the aneurysm to see the perforators. The more anterior approach also places the ICA in the center of the surgical corridor, making it an obstacle between the surgeon and the basilar apex.

To expose the basilar apex through this approach, the surgeon must split the sylvian fissure, widely open the cisterns around the optic nerve and carotid artery, and gently retract the frontal and temporal lobes (Fig. 67–13). Some temporal bridging veins may have to be divided to mobilize the temporal pole, but this maneuver is usually well tolerated. The posterior communicating artery is followed back through Liliequist's membrane to the posterior cerebral artery, which is then followed medially to the basilar apex (see Fig. 67–13). Opening the choroidal fissure and mobilizing the anterior choroidal artery posteriorly as it courses along the optic tract allow wider separation of the frontal and temporal lobes and provide a better line of sight for aneurysms that ride high above the clivus. The anterior temporal artery can sometimes limit temporal lobe retraction posteriorly, especially when the artery arises proximally on the middle cerebral artery. Dividing this small artery can dramatically enhance exposure and is usually well tolerated.

With the pterional approach, the ICA becomes an obstacle in the operative field and can obscure access to the basilar apex. Three routes around the ICA are available. A medial route runs through the triangle formed by the lateral edge of optic nerve, the medial ICA, and the A_1 segment of the anterior cerebral artery (optic-carotid triangle). A superior route runs through the space between A_1, M_1, and the optic tract. A lateral route runs through the interval between the lateral internal carotid surface and the oculomotor nerve. We generally prefer the lateral route because the optic-carotid triangle is narrow and the superior approach is obscured by small but crucial perforating arteries from the ICA. The lateral route usually provides ample access and can be expanded through further medial mobilization of the ICA if necessary. Some-

times, multiple routes of exposure are needed to dissect different parts of the aneurysm or to pass different instruments.

Orbitozygomatic-Pterional Approach. The orbitozygomatic-pterional approach expands the pterional approach by removing the superior and lateral orbit (Fig. 67–14), thereby creating more space in the operative corridor and providing a more anterior trajectory than the standard pterional approach. This trajectory allows an extended upward view of the basilar apex (see Fig. 67–14).[294–307] For these reasons, it has become our preferred approach for basilar apex aneurysms. The approach requires additional work to remove the orbitozygomatic bone unit and poses additional risks, including frontalis nerve injury, pulsatile enophthalmos, orbital entrapment, diplopia from extraocular muscle or nerve injury, blindness, communication with the frontal sinus that can cause infection or CSF leaks, and greater periorbital bruising. In our opinion, however, the incidence of these complications is sufficiently low that the advantages gained by the increased exposure far outweigh the risks.

The orbitozygomatic approach adds two steps to the pterional approach—soft tissue dissection to expose the orbitozygomatic bone unit and osteotomies to free it. The zygoma and orbital rim are ensheathed in two layers of the temporalis fascia, which are elevated to expose the bone. Exposure can be accomplished by either an interfascial dissection that peels the layers apart or a subfascial dissection that cuts the inner layer as it passes under the zygoma, thereby releasing the fascia. The subfascial dissection is simple, fast, and preferred. It does not disturb the frontalis branch of the facial nerve, which runs

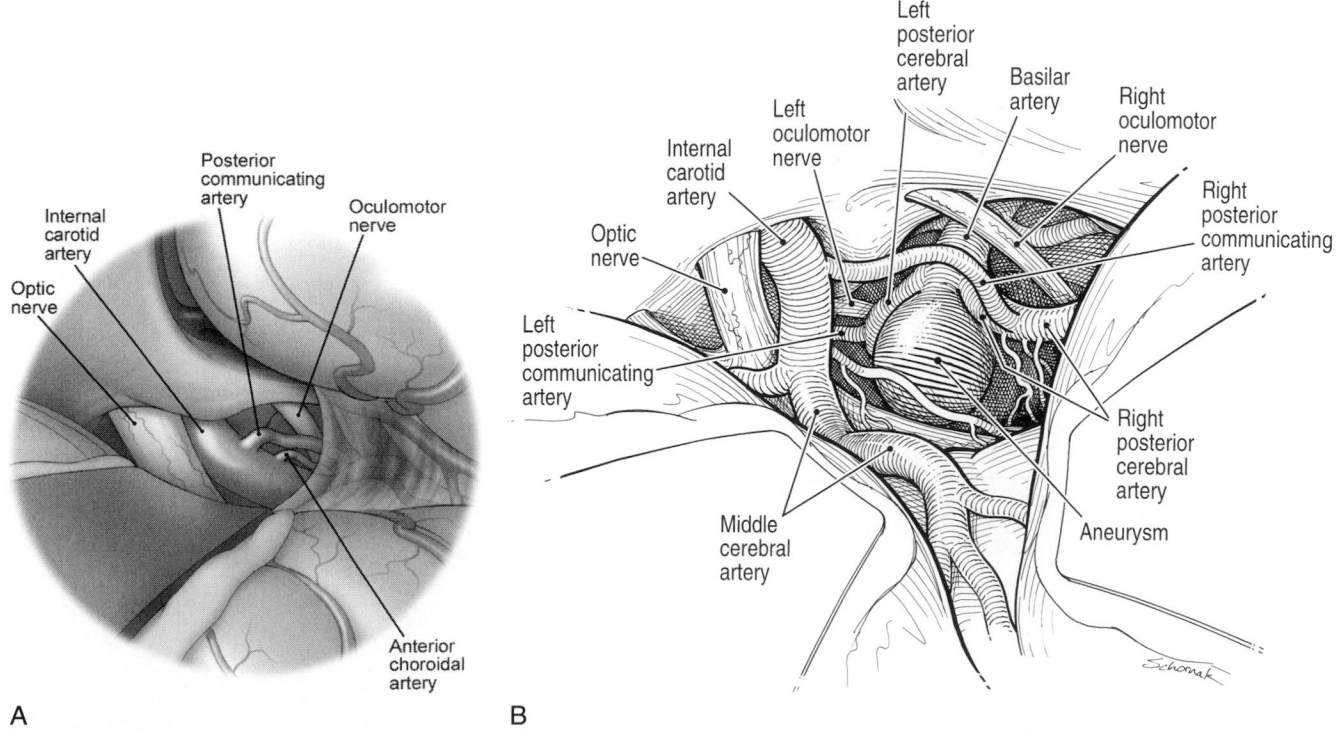

FIGURE 67–13 *A, This intraoperative view shows the microsurgical anatomy of the pterional approach. B, Splitting the sylvian fissure allows the frontal and temporal lobes to be mobilized and the deep anatomy around the basilar apex to be visualized.*

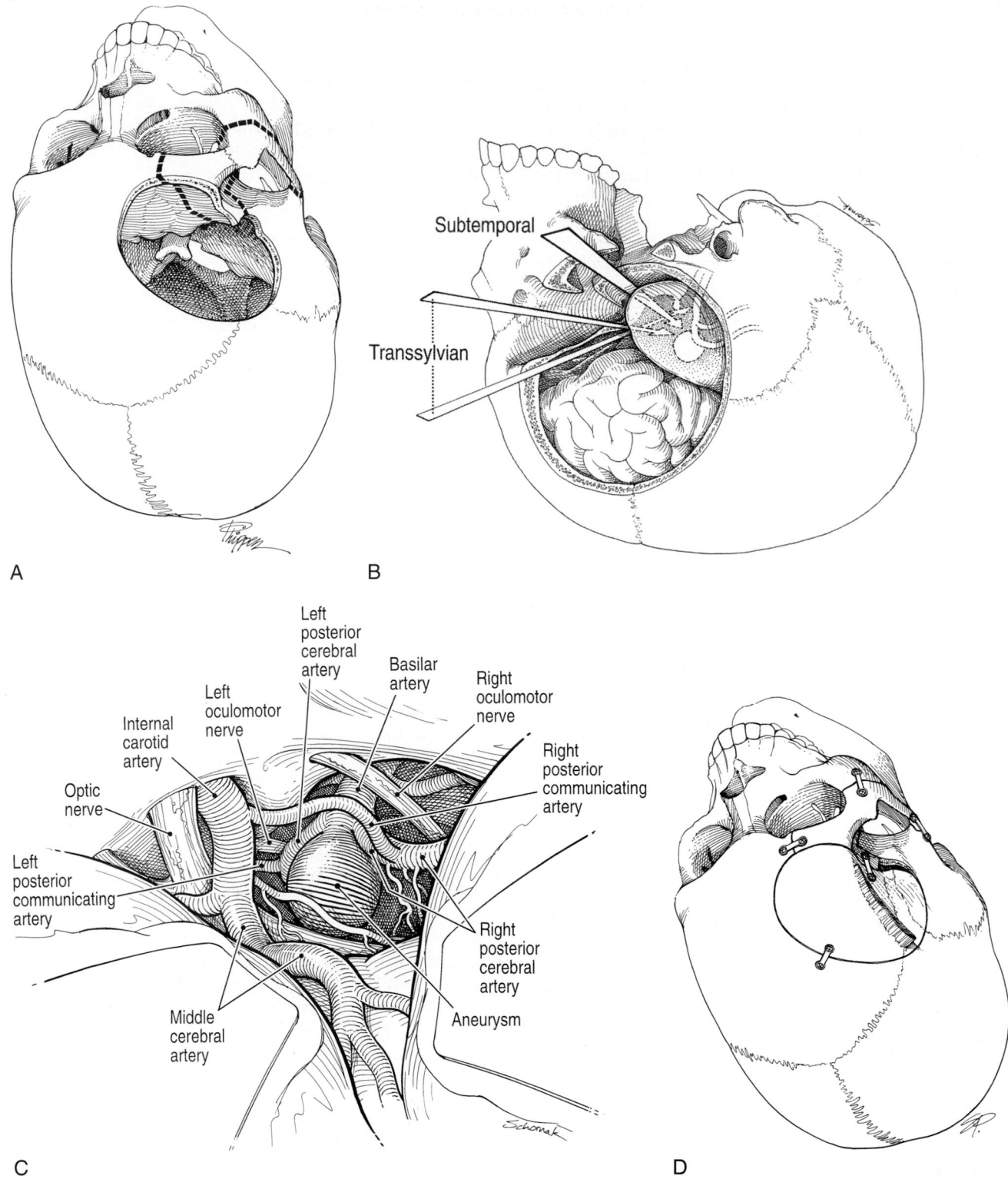

A

B

Subtemporal

Transsylvian

C

Left posterior cerebral artery

Basilar artery

Right oculomotor nerve

Right posterior communicating artery

Left oculomotor nerve

Internal carotid artery

Optic nerve

Left posterior communicating artery

Right posterior cerebral artery

Middle cerebral artery

Aneurysm

D

FIGURE 67–14 *Orbitozygomatic approach. This approach is used for aneurysms of the upper third of the basilar artery. A, The exposure begins with a standard pterional craniotomy. The roof and lateral wall of the orbit along with the zygoma are then removed as one piece by means of the combination of osteotomies (dashed lines) illustrated in this sketch. B, The extensive bony removal provides a wide corridor of exposure with multiple angles of approach to the upper basilar artery and its branches, including trans-sylvian and subtemporal routes (arrows). C, The pertinent anatomy seen from a right orbitozygomatic trans-sylvian approach for a basilar tip aneurysm is illustrated. The sylvian fissure has been widely opened, and dissection extended along the anterior choroidal artery, allowing the anterior tip of the temporal lobe to be retracted laterally. The carotid and middle cerebral arteries are displaced anteriorly to expose the aneurysm. If exposure is limited by the posterior communicating artery, the vessel can be divided between hemostatic clips. This approach allows good visualization of the contralateral posterior cerebral artery and oculomotor nerve. D, Reconstruction and fixation of the orbitozygomatic osteotomy and pterional bone flap with miniplates and screws give an excellent cosmetic result. (Courtesy of the Barrow Neurological Institute.)*

superficial to the outer fascial layer. The periorbita, which is continuous with the outer layer of temporal fascia and keeps the periorbital fat in place, is carefully stripped from the orbit, facilitating the orbital osteotomies. Once the orbitozygomatic unit is exposed, the temporalis muscle is mobilized inferiorly, a frontotemporal craniotomy is made, and the dura of the frontal lobe is elevated from the superior and lateral walls of the orbit down to the superior orbital fissure. Removing the orbit obviates drilling of the pterion.

The orbitozygomatic unit consists of the orbital rim, orbital roof, lateral orbital wall, and zygomatic arch. It is released by a series of five osteotomies (see Fig. 67–14) made with a high-speed reciprocating saw. The first cut is made across the zygomatic root, with care taken to avoid the temporomandibular joint. A fixation plate is placed in the zygoma and registered to improve the cosmetic results after closure. The second cut is made across the zygomatic bone in two parts, first from the inferolateral margin of the zygomatic bone halfway across to the lateral orbital rim, and then from the inferior orbital fissure to the same endpoint. When this osteotomy is made in two cuts, the resulting V in the zygomatic bone keeps the fragment secured into position when replaced. The third cut is along the medial orbital roof, just lateral to the supraorbital notch. The frontal dura and underlying brain must be protected during these cuts. The fourth cut crosses the posterior orbital roof, approximately 2.5 cm posterior to the inner table of frontal bone (to preserve the orbital roof), and finishes laterally in the thick bone of the sphenoid ridge and pterion. The fifth cut crosses the lateral orbital wall, connecting the cut across the orbital roof with the inferior orbital fissure. The orbitozygomatic unit is then removed as a single piece, and additional bone is removed over the orbital apex around the superior orbital fissure with a small rongeur. A dural flap based over the orbit is tented forward with tacking sutures to depress the globe gently and thereby gain a wide exposure of the sylvian region (see Fig. 67–14).

The intradural exposure with the orbitozygomatic approach is the same as that with the pterional approach. The difference is the larger space provided by removal of the bony prominences of the superior and lateral walls of the orbit. The fulcrum of the trajectory drops lower across the orbit, resulting in a higher view above the posterior clinoid process. Opening the choroidal fissure and mobilizing the temporal pole laterally are important maneuvers that widen this view. Occasionally, an anterior temporal artery that originates proximally on the M_1 may tether the temporal lobe, requiring division to allow mobilization of the lobe.

Extended Orbitozygomatic Approach. The differences in cranial exposures for the subtemporal, pterional, and orbitozygomatic approaches create dramatically different trajectories to the basilar apex. Often, the optimal angle for dissecting the aneurysm cannot be predicted from the preoperative angiogram or axial imaging studies. Other factors, such as the course of the ICA, the axis of the aneurysm neck, and the aneurysm's relationship to the bone of the clivus, influence the optimal surgical trajectory and are understood only during surgery. Consequently, an approach that allows a full range of trajectories gives the surgeon flexibility to shift trajectories during the dissection, without interrupting the microsurgery for additional extradural bone resection. The subtemporal, pterional, and orbitozygomatic approaches can be combined through simple extension of the posteroinferior cranial exposure of an orbitozygomatic approach.[305]

The extended orbitozygomatic approach is analogous to the combined subtemporal and pterional approach that has been called the "half-and-half" or "one-and-a-half" approach. All that is required is a slightly larger craniotomy that extends more posteriorly followed by drilling of the inferior margin of this craniotomy flush with the middle fossa floor. During the microdissection of a large aneurysm, an anatomic survey of the basilar apex and dissection of the contralateral arteries and nerves can be performed from an orbitozygomatic angle. Perforators can be separated from the back of the aneurysm, and the clip can be applied from a subtemporal angle. Taking advantage of multiple views within this 90-degree window of exposure can significantly improve the definition of anatomy, rendering aneurysm clipping easier and safer.

Skull Base Exposures. The outer cranial bone work brings the aneurysm within reach, but with variations in basilar artery anatomy, parts of the skull base (e.g., posterior clinoid process, dorsum sella, and clivus) may partially obscure the surgeon's corridor. The ICA, the optic nerve, or the oculomotor nerve can block access to the neck of a basilar aneurysm if the artery lies too high. The tentorium and cavernous sinus can block access to the neck of a basilar aneurysm if the artery lies too low. Ultimately, the success or failure of an operation can be determined by the manner in which these small inner hurdles are handled.

Access to the basilar artery below the superior cerebellar artery is crucial for proximal control of a basilar apex aneurysm. In most cases, this access is available without additional maneuvers. For low-lying aneurysms, however, the posterior clinoid process may block the way. They can be resected to expose the artery and gain proximal control.[308–310] The posterior clinoid process is bordered laterally by the oculomotor nerve and the cavernous sinus and medially by the sella, dorsum, and clivus. When the posterior clinoid process is large or only minimal additional exposure is needed, bony resection can be accomplished without encroachment on the cavernous sinus and clival venous plexus.

An alternative route to the proximal basilar artery is laterally through the tentorium. A pretemporal or subtemporal trajectory that skirts under the oculomotor nerve can offer the exposure needed for proximal control without any cutting of the tentorium. A tacking suture in the tentorium can pull it inferolaterally and can enlarge this corridor. When these maneuvers are inadequate, the tentorium can be cut, providing a wider view into the posterior fossa. An incision in the tentorium that begins medially behind the dural sleeve of cranial nerve (CN) IV protects this nerve and avoids the cavernous sinus (transtentorial-retrocavernous) but may be posterior enough that it can be reached only subtemporally.[311] An incision in the tentorium that begins medially between CN III and CN IV can be reached from a pretemporal trajectory but risks transecting CN IV and entering the cavernous sinus (transtentorial-transcavernous). Most patients tolerate sacrifice of CN IV, and cavernous sinus bleeding can be controlled easily with packing. Although neither transtentorial approach provides an optimal solution, they can be used to increase the exposure needed for proximal control of the basilar artery.

For basilar tip aneurysms that lie even lower in the posterior fossa, a more extensive transclinoidal approach is needed. Two transclinoidal approaches are available, an inferolateral approach through the cavernous sinus (transclinoidal-transcavernous)[308,312,313] and an inferomedial approach through the dorsum and upper clivus outside the cavernous sinus (transclinoidal-extracavernous).[305]

The transclinoidal-transcavernous approach requires anterior clinoidectomy, posterior clinoidectomy, and opening of the cavernous sinus. Anterior clinoidectomy only marginally increases exposure of the basilar artery, but it allows the distal dural ring around the ICA to be opened so the artery can be moved medially, enlarging the opening into and through the cavernous sinus. An incision is made in the roof of the cavernous sinus, or carotid-oculomotor membrane, medial to the oculomotor nerve, and the cavernous sinus is packed to control venous bleeding. Working in the bend of the intracavernous bend of the ICA, the surgeon can drill away the posterior clinoid and lateral upper clivus. An incision in the clival dura then reveals the basilar trunk below the superior cerebellar arteries. This approach creates a deep corridor into the posterior fossa through the cavernous sinus and upper clivus.

The transclinoidal-extracavernous approach aims medially to the medial wall of the cavernous sinus. The posterior clinoid process, dorsum, and upper clivus are drilled away, and the clival venous plexus is cauterized or occluded with pressure. This approach avoids entry into the cavernous sinus. In addition, resection of the anterior clinoid process and dissection of the carotid dural rings are not required. However, this approach may open a medial corridor of exposure that does not parallel the course of the basilar artery, and therefore does not increase exposure. Still, it is an easy method of gaining exposure and can be attempted before the more bloody transcavernous route.

Medial petrosectomy is another skull base maneuver that can augment the standard subtemporal approach. The details of the technique are discussed in the next section as it applies to the extended middle fossa approach. Extradural removal of petrous bone in Kawase's triangle allows inferior retraction of the trigeminal ganglion and incision of the medial tentorium, thereby creating a corridor into the posterior fossa for access to low-lying basilar apex aneurysms that are approached from the subtemporal trajectory.

Surgical Approaches to the Basilar Trunk

Aneurysms of the basilar trunk are best targeted from a lateral trajectory, and the principal obstacles between the surgeon and the aneurysm are the petrous bone and the sigmoid sinus. The sinus is avoided by traversing anterior to it (presigmoid), and the petrous bone is resected to open a surgical corridor. The extent of bone removal varies from a retrolabyrinthine resection to a radical transcochlear petrosectomy. Transpetrosal routes in front of the labyrinth (extended middle fossa approach through Kawase's triangle), which involve removing the medial petrous apex to arrive at the lower basilar trunk through a narrow window, are suited only for small vertebrobasilar aneurysms. More

extensive approaches combine transpetrosal and subtemporal exposures, in which the intervening tentorium is divided to widen the cerebellopontine angle significantly. Transoral approaches, which can access the midbasilar artery, are mentioned for completeness, although we do not use such approaches because they are associated with high rates of CSF leakage, meningitis, and other complications.

Transpetrosal Approaches. Transpetrosal approaches expose the basilar trunk from a lateral trajectory through presigmoid surgical corridors excavated in the petrous bone. These lateral approaches provide good proximal and distal control of the basilar artery but often put the aneurysm dome between the surgeon and the neck of the aneurysm. Although this positioning can be nettlesome, the approach is typically from the same side as the aneurysm. Approaches on the side away from the dome require more complicated clipping techniques and the use of fenestrated clips. From laterally, some cranial nerves are in the way, placing them at risk, and limits operative maneuverability, but this approach is still preferable to the anterior (transoral) route. Lastly, the petrous drilling required for these approaches is usually outside the neurosurgeon's expertise and therefore necessitates a skull base team including neuro-otologists.

Removal of temporal bone is categorized into the following three variations according to the increasing extent of bone resection: (1) retrolabyrinthine, (2) translabyrinthine, and (3) transcochlear (Fig. 67–15). The retrolabyrinthine approach removes temporal bone between the semicircular canals anteriorly and the posterior fossa dura on the posterior aspect of the temporal bone.[314–316] The semicircular canals are skeletonized, but not violated, to enlarge the working space. The translabyrinthine approach removes more bone and, in the process, removes the semicircular canals and sacrifices hearing.[303,315,317–319] Exposure increases anteriorly to the limit of the internal auditory canal, but the facial nerve is left in its bony sheath, thereby protecting the function of the nerve. The transcochlear approach opens the canal of the facial nerve, transposes the nerve posteriorly, and thereby provides access to the cochlea, which is then removed.[303,315,320,321] This approach eliminates the petrous bone as an obstacle almost completely and provides the greatest exposure of the brainstem, clivus, and basilar trunk.

The three types of temporal bone dissections represent a gradual increase in the amount of petrous bone resection, with a corresponding increase in anterior exposure. The price of this larger exposure is a greater sacrifice of hearing and facial nerve function. Preservation of the inner ear with the retrolabyrinthine approach leaves the hearing and facial nerve function intact. Violating the inner ear with the translabyrinthine and transcochlear approaches sacrifices hearing, and facial nerve function is temporarily, and sometimes permanently, affected.

Extended Retrolabyrinthine Approach. With the extended retrolabyrinthine approach, the patient is positioned supine with a shoulder roll to minimize neck rotation, and the head is positioned by means of skull fixation with the midline parallel to the floor and the vertex slightly downward, making the mastoid bone the highest point in the operative field. The incision begins 1 cm anterior to the tragus and 2 cm above the zygoma, curving gently around the ear to the mastoid tip (see Fig. 67–15), and the scalp flap is retracted anteriorly.

The drilling begins with an initial cut along the temporal line, the bony ridge that continues from the superior border of the zygomatic arch posteriorly to the mastoid cortex, marking both the inferior limit of temporalis muscle insertion and the floor of the middle fossa. A second cut is made perpendicularly, running inferiorly to the mastoid tip. A large cutting burr is used to perform a rapid simple mastoidectomy. Bone in the sinodural angle and covering the sigmoid sinus is removed completely to allow identification of the sigmoid sinus, which is the critical anatomic landmark. Posterior retraction of the sinus and presigmoid dura exposes the middle and posterior fossa dura and the sinodural angle between them. The superior petrosal sinus lies deep to the sinodural angle and represents the posterosuperior margin of the petrous bone. Dissection into the mastoid antrum reveals the horizontal semicircular canal, which leads to other anatomic guideposts, including the external genu of CN VII medially and inferiorly, the posterior semicircular canal posteriorly, and the epitympanum and superior semicircular canal anteriorly. The posterior and superior semicircular canals are skeletonized, and drilling is carried as far anteriorly as possible (see Fig. 67–15). Resection of temporal bone above and below the otic capsule exposes the medial dura of the middle fossa floor, the superior petrosal sinus, and the jugular bulb. A large dural surface is thereby exposed that, when opened, allows access to the cerebellopontine angle.

The retrolabyrinthine approach provides excellent exposure of the cerebellopontine angle but by itself rarely results in enough exposure to allow access to aneurysms on the basilar trunk. Other maneuvers are needed if the

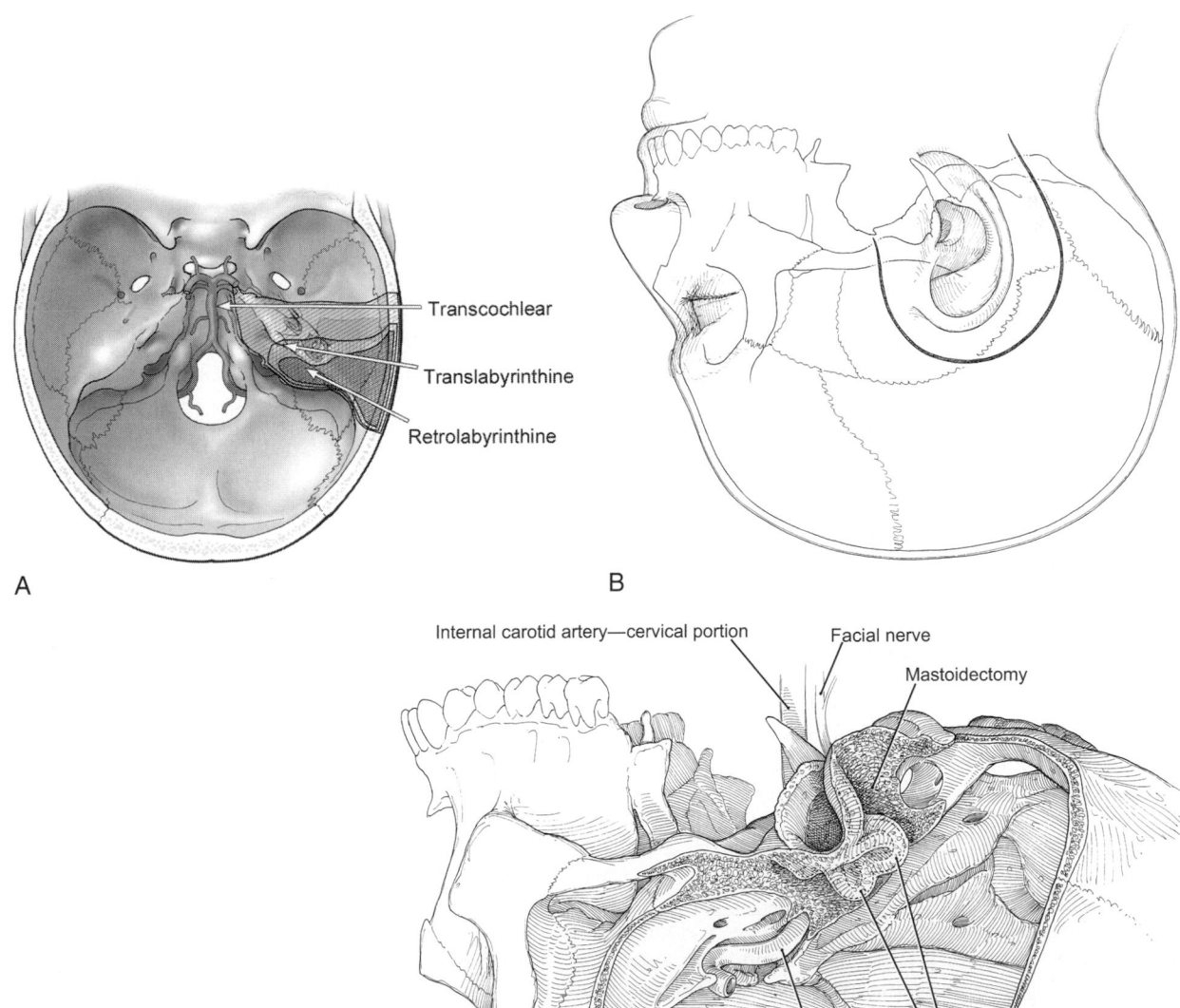

FIGURE 67–15 A, *The three types of presigmoid transpetrosal approaches are illustrated.* B, *The head is positioned laterally and the C-shaped skin incision is the same for all three approaches.* C, *The retrolabyrinthine approach consists of mastoidectomy and removal of temporal bone anteriorly to the posterior semicircular canal.*

Transcochlear

Translabyrinthine

Retrolabyrinthine

A

B

Internal carotid artery—cervical portion

Facial nerve

Mastoidectomy

Posterior and superior semicircular canals

Internal carotid artery—horizontal portion

C

Continued

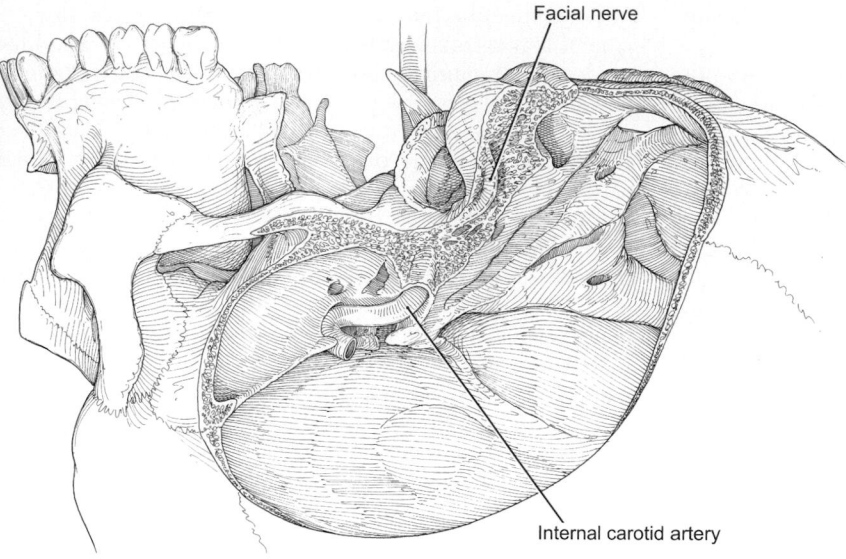

D

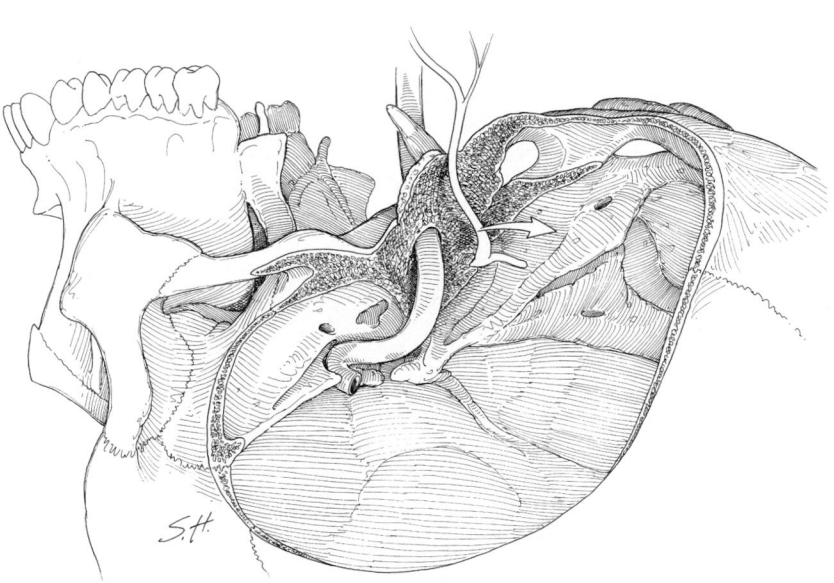

E

FIGURE 67–15, cont'd. D, *The translabyrinthine approach removes the semicircular canals and skeletonizes the internal auditory canal and the descending segment of the facial nerve. E, The transcochlear approach transposes the facial nerve posteriorly to allow complete removal of temporal bone anteriorly to the petrous internal carotid artery.*

petrosectomy is limited to a retrolabyrinthine approach. One such maneuver involves the ligation and division of the sigmoid sinus.[322] A trans-sigmoid dural opening eliminates the constraint of the sigmoid sinus and allows greater posterior retraction of the cerebellum than is possible with an intact sigmoid sinus. Nonetheless, this retrolabyrinthine–trans-sigmoid approach should be used only with smaller aneurysms of the basilar trunk. Another useful modification of the retrolabyrinthine approach is tentoriotomy in conjunction with a subtemporal exposure. This modification constitutes the "combined" approach, which is discussed later.

Translabyrinthine Approach. The translabyrinthine approach is used when more exposure is needed than a simple retrosigmoid approach can provide. The initial part of this approach is the same as the retrolabyrinthine approach, but then all three semicircular canals are drilled away, thereby exposing the posterior half to two thirds of

the internal auditory canal (see Fig. 67–15). The medial walls of the vestibule and the superior semicircular canal ampulla represent the lateral wall of the fundus of the internal auditory canal, and minimal bone removal at this location exposes the canal. The dura lining the internal auditory canal is not opened when this approach is used for aneurysm surgery, but the surgeon keeps the location of CN VII in mind to protect it during the approach. CN VII lies anterosuperiorly in the canal and is separated from the superior vestibular nerve posterosuperiorly by a shelf of bone (Bill's bar). Electrophysiologic monitoring of facial nerve function helps protect the nerve throughout the drilling.

The distal segment of CN VII is skeletonized with a diamond bit along its horizontal (tympanic) segment, external or second genu, and descending (mastoid) segment. The nerve is left in its thinned bony canal to minimize its risk of injury. Additional exposure is gained by removal of petrous bone anteriorly and medially above the internal auditory canal in Kawase's triangle. Inferiorly, the sigmoid sinus is unroofed to the jugular bulb to maximize inferior exposure beneath the internal auditory canal.

The translabyrinthine exposure extends further anteriorly than the retrolabyrinthine approach. The cerebellopontine angle, anterolateral brainstem, and inferior clivus are better seen, but the surgical corridor is still narrow and suitable only for small aneurysms of the basilar trunk unless maneuvers such as division of the sigmoid sinus or tentorium are added.

Transcochlear Approach. A forward extension of the translabyrinthine approach, the transcochlear approach unsheathes and mobilizes CN VII, removes the cochlea, and opens the cerebellopontine angle to expose the anterolateral brain stem, clivus, and basilar trunk. This approach provides the greatest transpetrosal exposure by essentially resecting the entire petrous bone.

The initial procedure is the same as for the translabyrinthine approach, except that the external auditory canal is transected and oversewn in two layers. The facial nerve is skeletonized along its course from its entrance into the internal auditory canal to its exit from the stylomastoid foramen. The facial recess is a tract of air cells bounded medially by the descending segment of the facial nerve, laterally by the chorda tympani, and superiorly by the fossa incudis. Opening the facial recess exposes the middle ear space, the stapes and incus, the promontory of the cochlea, Jacobson's nerve, and the horizontal segment of the facial nerve. The ossicles are removed through this opening into the epitympanum. The chorda tympani is sectioned inferiorly at its origin from the descending portion of the facial nerve, and the facial recess is expanded inferiorly to the hypotympanum and retrofacial area. The greater superficial petrosal nerve is sectioned anteriorly at its origin from the geniculate ganglion. These maneuvers untether the facial nerve so it can be swung posteriorly after being dissected from its bony canal.

The cochlea is then drilled out completely, beginning with the promontory that houses the basal turn of the cochlea. Bone is removed forward to the septum between the basal turn and the petrous ICA. The ICA and internal jugular vein leave the carotid sheath and enter the skull base near each other. The jugulocarotid septum, a ridge of bone that separates the carotid artery as it turns anteriorly from the jugular vein as it turns posteriorly, is removed to expose the jugular bulb completely. The close relationship of CN IX, CN X, and CN XI within the jugular foramen must be kept in mind so that injury these nerves can be avoided. During the extensive drilling of the temporal bone, the dura of the internal auditory canal is kept intact to protect this part of CN VII.

When the drilling is completed, the entire temporal bone is gone (see Fig. 67–15). The superior petrosal sinus, stretching from the sinodural angle laterally to Meckel's cave medially, forms the superior boundary of this exposure. The inferior petrosal sinus and jugular bulb are the inferior border. Bone removal extends medially to the clivus and anteriorly to the ICA and periosteum of the temporomandibular joint. The bone of the carotid canal can be removed superiorly to the middle fossa floor. The transcochlear approach gives the greatest exposure of the

transpetrosal approaches, resulting in a wide triangular corridor that leads directly to the basilar trunk and through which even large aneurysms can be exposed adequately for dissection, proximal and distal control, and clipping. The maneuvers that are added to the retrolabyrinthine and translabyrinthine approaches (i.e., division of the sigmoid sinus or tentorium) are seldom necessary to make the transcochlear approach suitable for basilar trunk aneurysms.

Combined Supratentorial and Infratentorial Approach. When petrous-sparing approaches like the retrolabyrinthine and even the translabyrinthine approaches are used to preserve hearing or facial nerve function, the surgical corridor is limited by residual petrous bone anteriorly, the tentorium superiorly, and the sigmoid sinus posteriorly to an extent that dissection and clipping may still be unsafe for large midbasilar aneurysms. Two maneuvers dramatically enhance exposure after petrosectomy, division of the tentorium and posterior mobilization of the sigmoid sinus.[303,315,321,323,324] The petrosectomy then becomes the cornerstone of a combination approach that relaxes these confining superior and posterior barriers. The two critical additions to the transpetrosal approaches, therefore, are (1) a supratentorial and infratentorial craniotomy that crosses the transverse sinus and (2) a tentoriotomy that permits free communication between the supratentorial and infratentorial compartments. This provides extensive exposure of the medial petrous and clival regions and associated neurovascular structures, with minimal brain retraction.

When the temporal bone drilling is complete, an edge of middle fossa dura above the petrosectomy defect and an edge of posterior fossa dura behind the sigmoid sinus have been exposed. These dural exposures serve as burr holes for a subtemporal-suboccipital craniotomy that crosses the transverse sinus. After the bone flap has been removed, a large dural surface that includes the transverse, sigmoid, and superior petrosal sinuses is visible (Fig. 67–16). Before the dura is opened, the brain is relaxed with hyperventilation, mannitol, and the removal of CSF through a lumbar drain. The first dural incision starts anteriorly over the temporal lobe and curves posteriorly and inferiorly to the superior petrosal sinus below where it enters the sigmoid sinus. A second dural incision starts inferiorly in front of the sigmoid sinus, curving up to the superior petrosal sinus. The superior petrosal sinus is cauterized or clipped and then divided. The surgeon should beware of low-lying veins of Labbé that need to be carefully preserved when opening the dura.

The sigmoid sinus can be sacrificed if the contralateral transverse and sigmoid sinuses are patent and communicate with the ipsilateral transverse and sagittal sinuses through a patent torcular Herophili. For added assurance, sigmoid sinus pressure can be measured before and after test occlusion of the sigmoid sinus to confirm that sinus pressure does not rise more than 10 mm Hg. These measurements are made after the superior petrosal sinus has been divided. When angiographic and hemodynamic criteria are met, the sigmoid sinus can be sacrificed safely. It is divided below its confluence with the superior petrosal sinus. The vein of Labbé consistently and reliably enters the transverse sinus above this junction and therefore drains contralaterally. Division of the sigmoid sinus is rarely necessary, however, because a presigmoid dural opening is usually adequate to expose the tentorium and to mobilize the sigmoid sinus.

When the dural incisions are complete and the superior petrosal sinus is divided, the tentorium is incised medially to the tentorial hiatus, posterior to the tentorial entrance of the trochlear nerve (see Fig. 67–16). This crucial maneuver connects the supratentorial and infratentorial compartments and relaxes neural structures. The posterior

temporal lobe is elevated with care to avoid traction on the vein of Labbé, which is connected to the transverse sinus. The petrous apex, clivus, brainstem, cranial nerves, and vessels of the posterior circulation are now visible, and the surgeon can access an aneurysm by working between cranial nerve bundles.

This approach provides wide exposure along the skull base from the foramen magnum to the dorsum sella with minimal brain retraction. The combined approach works

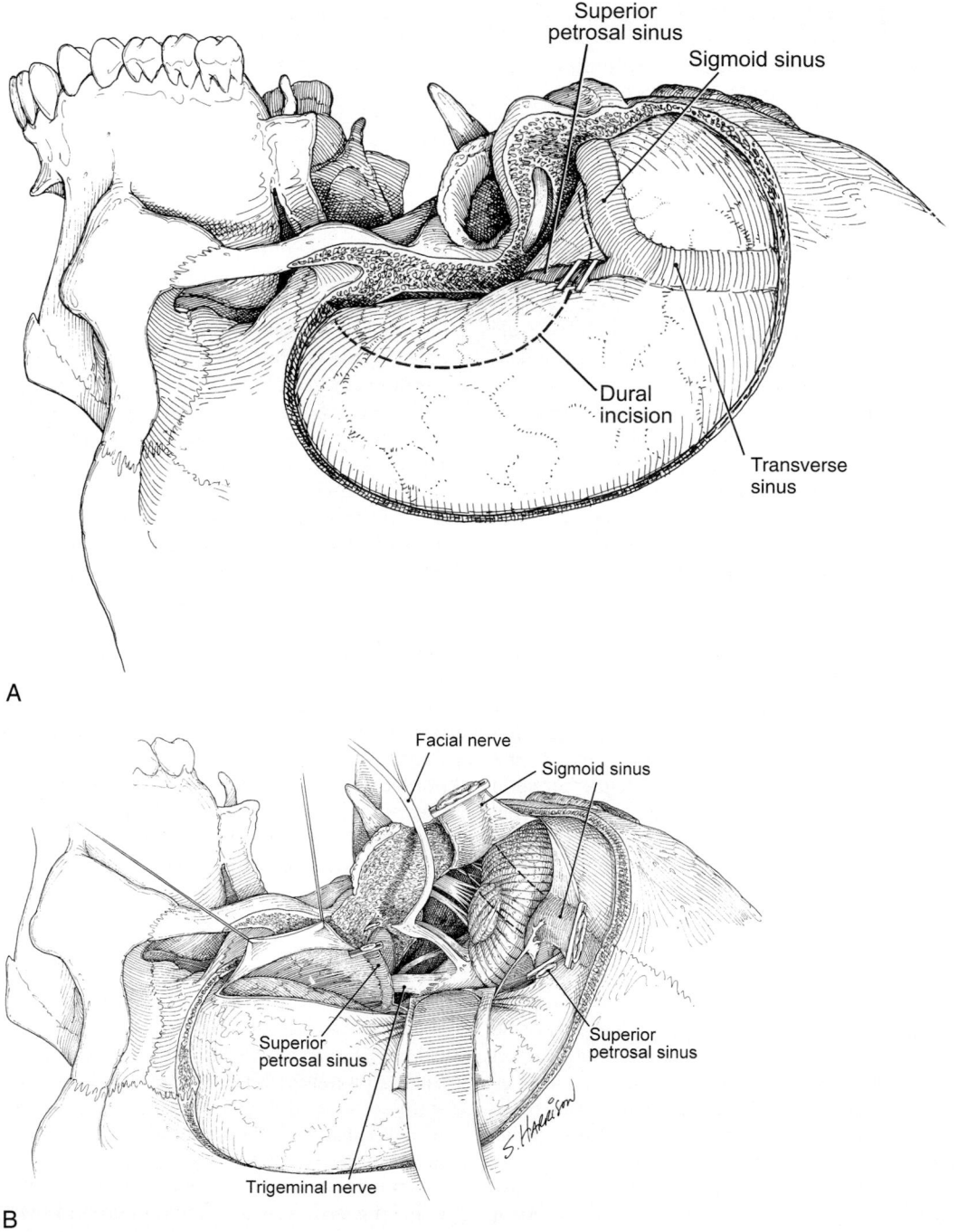

FIGURE 67–16 *The combined supratentorial and infratentorial approach. is a combination of the subtemporal and transpetrosal approaches. A, The approach begins with temporal bone resection, which then serves as a burr hole for a craniotomy that crosses the transverse sinus and exposes temporal lobe and cerebellar dura. A dural incision can then be made across the superior petrosal sinus. B, Division of the tentorium from the transverse-sigmoid junction to the incisura exposes the cranial nerves, brainstem, clivus, and basilar artery.*

with any of the three types of petrosectomy. Typically, it is used with a retrolabyrinthine approach when petrous bone must be conserved and facial nerve function and hearing preserved. The added maneuvers of the combined approach therefore are designed to compensate for less presigmoid exposure.

Extended Middle Fossa Approach. The middle fossa approach was developed to remove small, intracanalicular acoustic neuromas with less than 5 mm of extension into the cerebellopontine angle. This approach provides a direct route to the internal auditory canal, keeps the hearing apparatus intact, and offers a good chance to preserve hearing in patients who have useful hearing preoperatively.[325–327] The approach has been adapted for use with basilar aneurysms not only through skeletonization of the internal auditory canal but also through resection of the medial petrous apex. This approach has several names, including the extended middle fossa approach, Kawase's approach, and the rhomboid approach.[309,310,328] The anterior subtemporal–medial transpetrosal approach is similar, except that the surgeon works intradurally in the middle fossa instead of extradurally.[329] The extended middle fossa approach differs from the other lateral transpetrosal approaches in that the basilar artery is reached from a more anterolateral and superior trajectory in front of the otic capsule and the posterolateral temporal bone is left intact.

Kawase described the extended middle fossa approach to basilar aneurysms, which requires resection of bone in the triangle that bears his name (also called a *quadrangle,* it is actually a complex three-dimensional space).[328] Kawase's triangle is formed by the internal auditory canal posteriorly, the greater superficial petrosal nerve laterally, the lateral margin of the trigeminal nerve and ganglion anteriorly, and the medial edge of the petrous bone medially.[330] The triangle extends inferiorly to the inferior petrosal sinus. Between these neurovascular boundaries are temporal bone and air cells. Resection of Kawase's triangle opens a corridor through which the basilar artery can be reached. The trajectory of this narrow bony corridor and the orientation of the fifth, seventh, and eighth cranial nerve bundles limit the view of the vertebrobasilar junction and provide minimal working space, making the approach impractical for most basilar trunk aneurysms. The approach is described here because it can be used for selected small aneurysms and because the relevant anatomy is important.

The patient is positioned supine with the head fixated as for a subtemporal approach. With a question-mark or horseshoe-shaped incision, the skin and temporalis muscle flaps are reflected anteriorly. A 5 × 5–cm craniotomy is made in the squamosal portion of the temporal bone two-thirds anterior and one-third posterior to the external auditory canal. The inferior edge of the craniotomy is drilled flush to the middle fossa floor. The dura is elevated from the middle fossa floor medially toward the petrous ridge, where a self-retaining retractor is placed with its tip over the lip of the ridge. The middle meningeal artery is followed along the dura to the foramen spinosum, coagulated, and divided. The greater superficial petrosal nerve, which is located approximately 1 cm medially, originates from the geniculate ganglion of the facial nerve and runs superficially along the middle fossa floor in an anteromedial direction. This nerve and the geniculate ganglion are vulnerable

to injury during the dissection. Lateral to the greater superficial petrosal nerve is Glasscock's triangle, through which the petrous ICA can be exposed as it runs horizontally toward the cavernous sinus.

The arcuate eminence is a bony prominence in the middle fossa floor that is almost perpendicular to the petrous ridge and marks the underlying superior semicircular canal. The greater superficial petrosal nerve and arcuate eminence form a 120-degree angle that is bisected by a line paralleling the internal auditory canal. The internal auditory canal can be exposed by drilling along this line medially, where there are no adjacent neurovascular structures. The surgeon removes bone around the porus acusticus and internal auditory canal, working from medial to lateral. The lateral internal auditory canal (fundus) is bounded anteriorly by the cochlea, whose basal turn is particularly vulnerable to entry during drilling in the angle between the greater superficial petrosal nerve and the internal auditory canal. Perforation of the cochlea causes complete loss of hearing. The vestibule and ampulla of the superior semicircular canal are immediately posterior to the fundus. As drilling proceeds laterally, the exposure is narrowed to avoid the cochlea and superior semicircular canal. The dura of the internal auditory canal is exposed laterally to Bill's bar.

The medial petrous apex is removed, with drilling between the borders of Kawase's triangle. The horizontal segment of the petrous ICA is identified laterally in Glasscock's triangle and skeletonized to increase the exposure anteriorly and inferiorly. After drilling is completed, the petrous dural exposure extends from the superior petrosal sinus to the inferior petrosal sinus. The superior petrosal sinus is coagulated and divided just lateral to the trigeminal ganglion. The posterior dura is opened to allow entry into the posterior fossa. The middle fossa dura is incised laterally, and the tentorium is incised medially to the incisura, just behind the entrance of the fourth cranial nerve in its dural canal. The lower basilar artery is then dissected through this opening. The dissection proceeds between CN V and CN VII.

Transoral Approaches. Transoral approaches to basilar trunk aneurysms are used with great reluctance and are mentioned here only for the sake of completeness.[331–335]

The patient is positioned supine. Unless an oral retraction system adequately depresses the tongue and endotracheal tube out of the surgical field, a tracheostomy and gastrostomy are performed. A lumbar subarachnoid drain is also inserted to help divert CSF after surgery, to prevent an oral-CSF fistula. The pharyngeal cavity is prepared with povidone-iodine, and a midline incision is made in the pharyngeal mucosa. After the soft tissues have been elevated and the proper trajectory has been confirmed fluoroscopically, the clivus is drilled to create a rectangular opening in the midline. The clival dura is opened in the midline, and the basilar trunk is exposed. Closure requires packing of the clival defect with abdominal fat and closure of the pharyngeal mucosa in layers. CSF drainage and prophylactic antibiotics are used postoperatively.

Surgical Approaches to the Vertebral Trunk

The third category of surgical approaches targets aneurysms of the intradural vertebral artery. These approaches, which provide posteroinferior trajectories along the axis of the vertebral trunk, are the midline suboccipital approach, the far-lateral approach, and the extended far-lateral approach. The inner exposure of a lateral suboccipital approach is enlarged by resection of the occipital condyle and jugular tubercle and, occasionally, by mobilization of the extradural vertebral artery—all skull base techniques that are the hallmarks of the far-lateral approach. This approach can be combined with a transpetrosal approach in the "combined-combined" approach for even greater exposure of the vertebral and basilar arteries.

Midline Suboccipital Approach. The suboccipital approach, a standard approach to cerebellar lesions and the fourth ventricle, is occasionally used to deal with aneurysms arising from the distal posterior inferior cerebellar artery after it courses around the anterior and lateral medulla.[286,311,336] Bilateral proximal vertebral artery lesions are sometimes best accessed through a midline approach that provides equal access to the two sides. Bypass procedures involving the distal posterior inferior cerebellar artery are also performed through a midline suboccipital approach. The midline approach does not provide good exposure of aneurysms located distally on the vertebral artery or near the usual origin of the posterior inferior cerebellar artery.

The patient is positioned prone with the chin tucked to open the interval between the foramen magnum and posterior arch of C1 (Fig. 67–17). In this position, the surgeon can operate while seated over the patient's head. A midline skin incision is made from above the inion to the spinous process of C4. The superior nuchal line and posterior cervical fascia are exposed approximately 3 cm to each side of midline to enable a Y-cut in the fascia. This kind of fascial incision readily exposes the midline nuchal ligament, allows the posterior cervical musculature to be separated in an avascular plane, and provides fascial cuffs that can be reapproximated to prevent CSF leaks. The paraspinous muscles are swept laterally to expose the occiput, foramen magnum, and posterior elements of C1 and C2. Complete exposure of the C2 spinous process facilitates soft tissue retraction. The dural adhesions around the foramen magnum are released with an angled curette, and a craniotomy can be made, with use of the lip of the foramen magnum as the epidural access point for the drill (see Fig. 67–17). In elderly patients with adherent dura, a suboccipital burr hole with subsequent cuts down to the foramen magnum may help preserve the dura. Additional lateral bone around the foramen magnum is rongeured off to widen the exposure.

The dura is opened in a Y-shaped fashion, with careful control of bleeding from the circular sinus of the foramen magnum. The arachnoid of the cisterna magna is opened, and the cervicomedullary junction is exposed. The vertebral arteries can be identified anterior to the dentate ligaments coursing anteromedially. Dissection in the tonsillomedullary fissure exposes the posterior inferior cerebellar arteries as they run between the cerebellar hemispheres. For more distal exposure, the interhemispheric fissure can be split between the tonsils, and the course of the posterior inferior cerebellar arteries through the cranial loop can be followed.

Far-Lateral Approach. The far-lateral approach is the most common approach to aneurysms of the vertebral

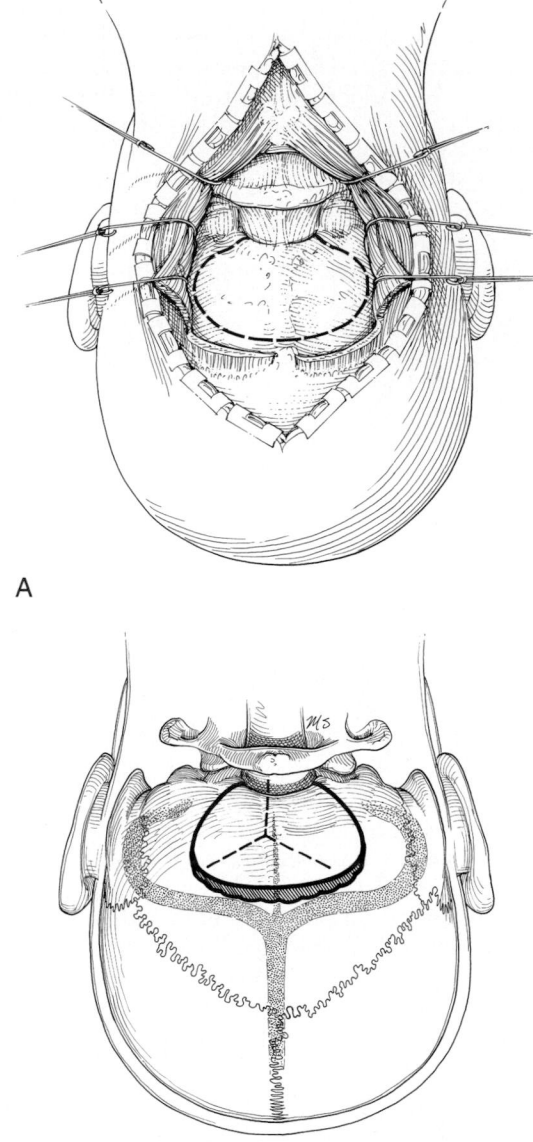

A

B

FIGURE 67–17 *The midline suboccipital approach. A, The patient is positioned prone with the head flexed to open the suboccipital-cervical angle. A midline linear skin incision is used, and the superior nuchal ligament is left as a cuff by which to reattach the muscles at closure. B, The craniotomy extends from the foramen magnum to the torcula and as far laterally as a linear midline incision will allow. The Y-shaped dural incision is shown (dashed line).*

trunk.[303,337–341] Most such aneurysms are unilateral and extend ventrally and medially beyond the region that can be accessed through a midline suboccipital exposure. Therefore, the craniotomy can be limited to one side, and the patient's position can be changed from prone to three-quarter prone. These modifications substantially improve exposure of the vertebral artery by swinging the surgical corridor laterally. The outer cranial exposure is enhanced by the resection of the posterior arch of the first cervical vertebra and resection of the posteroinferior skull base (including the posterolateral foramen magnum, the posterior half of the occipital condyle, and the jugular tubercle). Synonyms for the far-lateral approach include the lateral suboccipital approach, extreme lateral approach, and extreme lateral inferior transcondylar exposure (ELITE).[309] Resection of bone in the angle between the lower medulla and cerebellum creates a surgical corridor along the axis of the vertebral artery through which aneurysms can be exposed with minimal cerebellar retraction.

An important element of the far-lateral approach is the patient's position (Fig. 67–18). A modified park-bench or three-quarter-prone position is used, with the affected side upward. The operating table is extended by placing a 3/4-inch-thick plastic board under the mattress and pulling both the mattress and the board 6 inches beyond the edge of the table. This extender creates a gap between the Mayfield head holder and its attachment to the table, allowing the dependent arm to hang comfortably over the extended end of the table, where it is cradled in a padded sling. Dropping the arm and shoulder down effectively rotates the head into position. This position minimizes brachial plexus compression and improves venous return compared with the full prone position.

The following three maneuvers are essential to position the head optimally: (1) flexion in the anteroposterior plane until the chin is one finger-breadth from the sternum, (2) rotation 45 degrees away from the side of the lesion, and (3) lateral flexion 30 degrees down toward the floor. This position puts the axis of the clivus perpendicular to the floor so the surgeon can look down the axis of the vertebral and basilar arteries and work between the horizontally arrayed cranial nerves. The ipsilateral mastoid process becomes the highest point in the operative field, and the posterior cervical-suboccipital angle is opened wide to increase the operating space. The shoulder facing up may have to be taped to keep the cervical-suboccipital angle free of obstructions.

A hockey-stick incision is made (see Fig. 67–18) beginning in the cervical midline over the C5 spinous process. This incision extends cephalad to the inion, courses laterally along the superior nuchal line to the mastoid bone, and finishes inferiorly at the mastoid tip. The midline nuchal ligament is identified so that the paraspinous musculature can be split in this avascular plane. A cut just below the superior nuchal line detaches the paraspinous muscles, which are then swept inferolaterally to expose the occipital bone and foramen magnum while also leaving behind a cuff for reattachment of the muscle during closure. Mobilization of the paraspinous musculature in this manner provides adequate exposure of the lateral foramen magnum and eliminates the need to dissect or transect these muscles, thereby reducing postoperative pain. Retraction of soft tissue is facilitated by exposure down to and around the C2 spinous process. The vertebral artery courses from the transverse foramen of the lateral mass of C1, through the sulcus arteriosus of the C1 vertebral arch, to its dural entry point; it must be completely but carefully exposed. The lateral epidural venous plexus can cause troublesome bleeding but is easily preserved by blunt dissection.

Bone is removed in three parts as follows: (1) C1 laminotomy, (2) lateral occipital craniotomy, and (3) condylec-tomy (Fig. 67–19). The arch of C1 is removed with the drill; one cut is made just lateral to the sulcus arteriosus, and another across the contralateral arch. Additional atlantal bone can be removed under the vertebral artery lateral to the transverse foramen. A unilateral suboccipital craniotomy is made that extends as far laterally as possible. The rim of the foramen magnum is rongeured to extend the opening medially across the midline and laterally toward the condyle.

Finally, the lateral aspect of the foramen magnum, the posteromedial half of the occipital condyle, and the jugular tubercle are removed with a drill and a diamond bit to minimize injury to adjacent emissary veins. The anterior extent of condylar resection is defined either by the hypoglossal canal, the condylar emissary vein, or removal of bone to expose dura as it begins to curve anteromedially. This bone removal provides a curving slope that is centered on the condyle and completely flat. The dural incision (see Fig. 67–18) curves from the cervical midline across the circular sinus and laterally to the edge of the craniotomy. An inferior cut made laterally under C1 mobilizes the flap further laterally against the margin of the craniotomy. The cisterna magna is opened with use of the operating microscope, and the arachnoid layers are reflected.

The proximal vertebral artery just beyond its point of dural penetration is available for proximal control of the aneurysm. Exposure here keeps temporary clips out of the deeper region near the posterior inferior cerebellar artery and vertebrobasilar junction, and typically requires division of the dentate ligament. The corridor along the vertebral artery is exposed by dissection of the tonsillomedullary fissure and mobilization of the ipsilateral cerebellar tonsil away from the medulla. The vertebral artery is dissected from proximal to distal, but the posterior inferior cerebellar artery is dissected from distal to proximal. These converging lines lead to the posterior inferior cerebellar artery's origin, where most of the aneurysms treated with this approach are located. The surgeon can follow the vertebral artery farther to the vertebrobasilar junction by operating around and through the lower cranial nerves.

The far-lateral approach provides wide exposure of the vertebral trunk and anterolateral brainstem with minimal retraction on the cerebellum. It is the preferred approach to this region and is suitable for most aneurysms located there.

Extended Far-Lateral Approaches. The exposure of the far-lateral approach can be extended superiorly by removal of occipital bone to the junction of the transverse and sigmoid sinuses.[342] This retrosigmoid addition provides access to the cerebellopontine angle and large vertebral artery aneurysms in this region. The trajectories from the far-lateral and retrosigmoid approaches are almost perpendicular; consequently, the retrosigmoid extension does not improve the exposure of the far-lateral approach. It does, however, provide a complementary view of the anatomy, which can help clarify operative strategy.

The approach is identical to the far-lateral technique, but the superolateral edge of the craniotomy is defined by drilling through the mastoid bone to identify the transverse-sigmoid junction. The sigmoid sinus is skeletonized

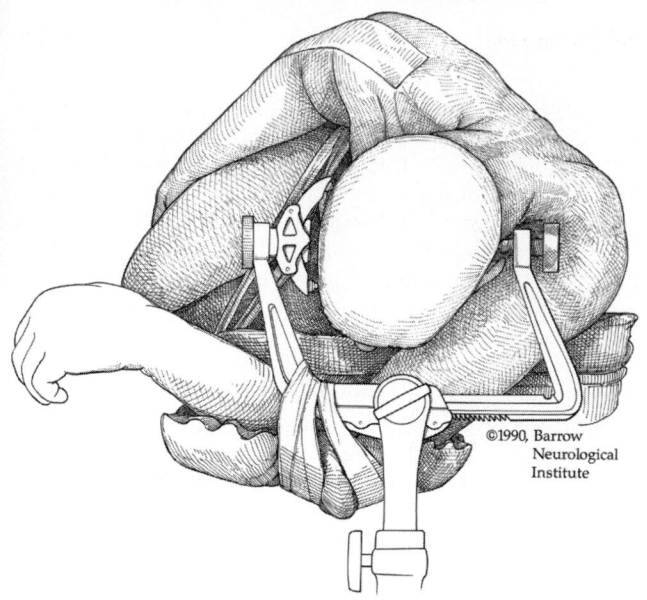

A

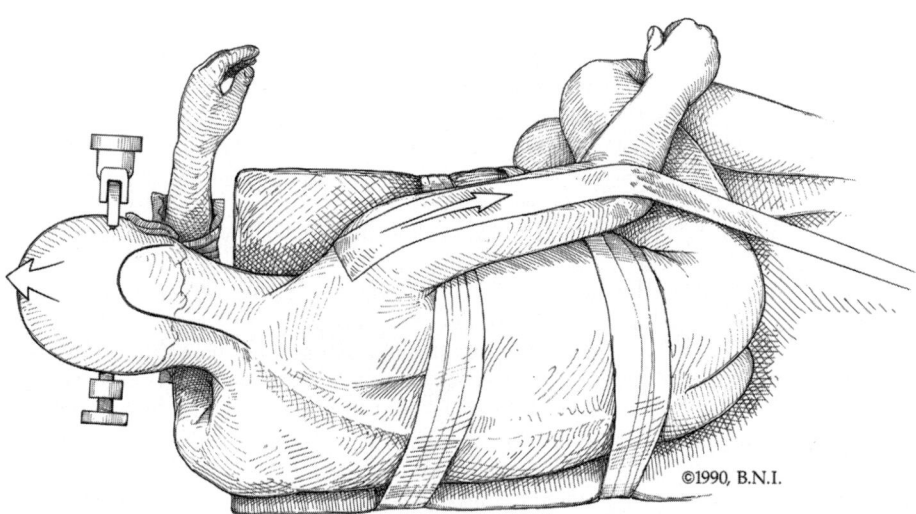

B

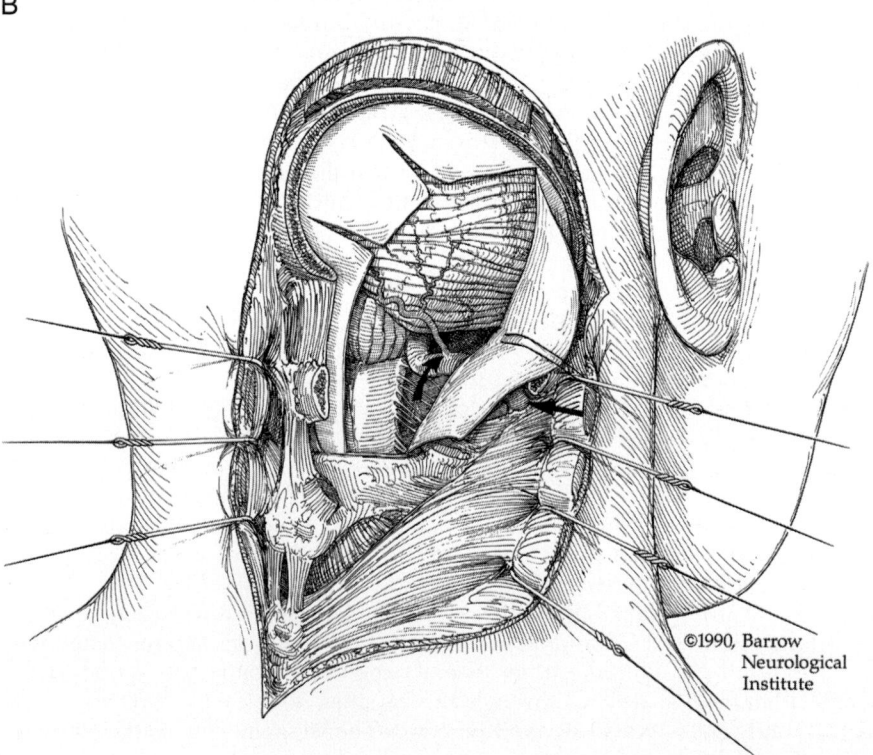

C

FIGURE 67–18 *Approach used for exposure of vertebral artery aneurysms. A, The patient is placed in the park-bench position. Care is taken to ensure proper padding of all pressure points. Note the cradle support for the lower arm. B, Surgeon's view of the operative position. The incision for exposing the right vertebral artery is outlined. C, The surgical exposure has been completed. The posterior arch of the first cervical vertebra has been resected laterally on the right side to the edge of the bony foramen of the vertebral artery (straight arrow). The suboccipital bone dissection has been carried to the sigmoid sinus and the medial edge of occipital condyle. The vertebral artery is visible intradurally as it courses medially to give rise to the origin of the posterior inferior cerebellar artery (curved arrow). (Courtesy of the Barrow Neurological Institute.)*

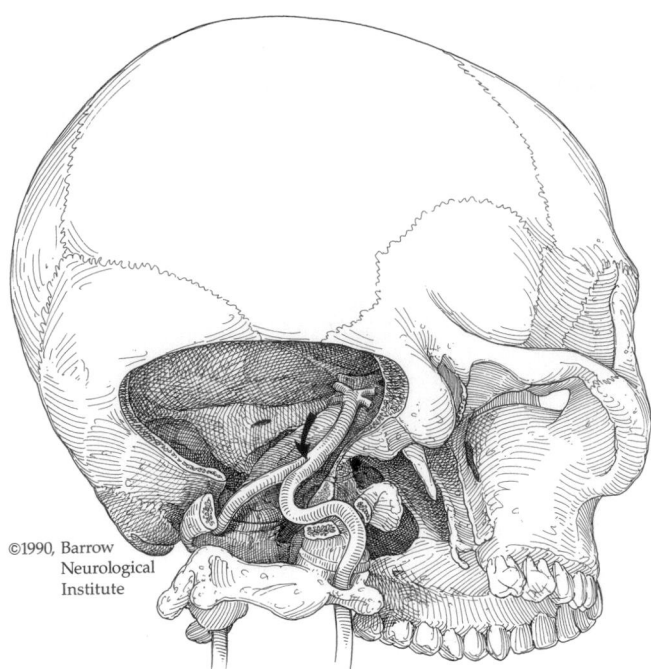

©1990, Barrow
Neurological
Institute

FIGURE 67–19 *Far-lateral suboccipital exposure for visualizing aneurysms arising from the vertebrobasilar junction (arrow). The posterior arch of the first cervical vertebra is resected laterally to completely free the vertebral artery from its bony foramen. The suboccipital bone dissection is carried to the edge of the sigmoid sinus and through the medial third of the occipital condyle. This bony dissection minimizes retraction of the cerebellum and brainstem, which is poorly tolerated. (Courtesy of the Barrow Neurological Institute.)*

down to the jugular bulb. The subsequent far-lateral craniotomy then connects to this exposed dura and the craniotomy flap is enlarged. The dura is opened with a flap based along the sigmoid sinus; when tacked anteriorly, the flap pulls the sinus forward to open the cerebellopontine angle. The standard far-lateral dural flap then connects with this flap.

Far-Lateral Combined Supratentorial and Infratentorial (Combined-Combined) Approach. Occasionally, giant aneurysms involving the vertebrobasilar junction or lower basilar trunk require an exposure that spans almost the entire length of the skull base from the dorsum sellae to the foramen magnum. The far-lateral approach, when used with the combined supratentorial and infratentorial approach, exposes the entire petroclival region.[321,343,344] Such an approach joins the transpetrosal, subtemporal, and far-lateral approaches, overcoming the limitations of a transpetrosal approach or an extended far-lateral approach when used alone. This approach, the most extensive of the combination approaches, is referred to as the "combined-combined" approach.

The patient is placed in the park-bench position (Fig. 67–20) with the head fixated as it would be for the far-lateral approach. The hockey-stick incision is enlarged, beginning anteriorly at the zygoma, coursing superiorly around the ear and toward the inion, and ending inferiorly in the midline at C5 (see Fig. 67–20). A myocutaneous flap

is elevated to expose the lateral temporal bone, mastoid, posterior cranium, and laminae of C1 and C2. A cuff of nuchal fascia is left to reattach the cervical muscles at the end of the procedure.

Bone removal consists of four parts—petrosectomy, C1 laminotomy, craniotomy, and condylectomy. The neurotologist first drills the temporal bone. Rotation of the head can be adjusted during the petrosectomy to bring the head parallel to the floor to facilitate drilling. The arch of C1 is exposed, the vertebral artery is identified, and a C1 laminotomy is performed. The craniotomy cut then connects the midline foramen magnum with the anterior margin of the petrosectomy overlying the inferior temporal lobe, crossing the transverse sinus just lateral to the torcular. A second cut connects the lateral foramen magnum with the posteroinferior margin of the petrosectomy, immediately behind the sigmoid sinus. The underlying dural sinuses are dissected carefully from the bone flap, which is then removed. A large dural surface is exposed (see Fig. 67–20) with the transverse and sigmoid sinuses in the middle. Finally, the lateral aspect of the foramen magnum, posteromedial two thirds of the occipital condyle, and jugular tubercle are removed.

The dura can be opened either in two flaps in front of and behind the sigmoid sinus to preserve it, or in a single flap that sacrifices the sigmoid sinus. The two dural flaps are simply the standard openings for the combined approach plus the standard opening for the far-lateral approach. The flaps create two windows of exposure on either side of the preserved sigmoid sinus. In contrast, sacrificing the sigmoid sinus and crossing it below the sinodural angle joins these two incisions to create a single flap extending from the anterior margin of the craniotomy over the temporal lobe, across the sigmoid sinus, and down to C1 (see Fig. 67–20). When the tentorium is incised to the hiatus, a large unobstructed opening is created that exposes the anterolateral brainstem from the midbrain to the upper cervical spinal cord (see Fig. 67–20). Arachnoid dissection reveals the cranial nerves extending from the optic to the hypoglossal nerves, both vertebral arteries, the posterior inferior cerebellar arteries, the anterior spinal artery, the vertebrobasilar junction, the basilar artery, and the entire length of the clivus. The exposure of this approach is unsurpassed, but it is needed only rarely for unusual giant aneurysms.

Special Considerations

Management of Infectious Intracranial Aneurysms (Mycotic Aneurysms)

Infectious intracranial aneurysms are rare aneurysms that develop from infection in the arterial wall caused by circulating infectious material, often from foci of infection within the endocardium or cardiac valves.[345] They occur primarily as a complication of subacute bacterial endocarditis (SBE) but are also seen in patients with congenital heart disease and prominent right-to-left shunts. Approximately 17% of patients with SBE are reported to have symptoms of cerebral embolization. Clinical and pathologic studies have demonstrated the presence of mycotic aneurysms in approximately 4% of patients with SBE. Infectious emboli lodge in small, distal cerebral

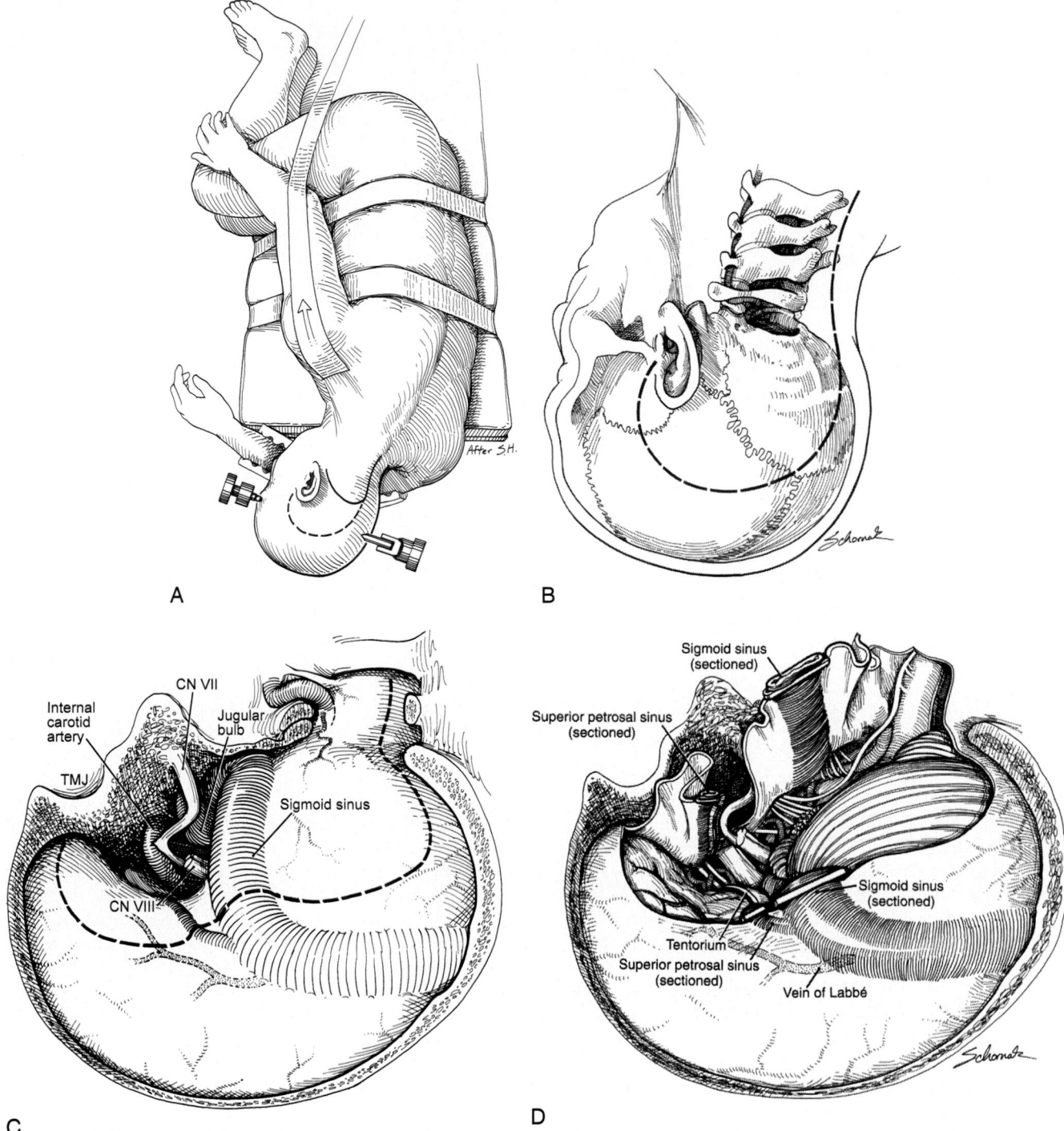

FIGURE 67–20   *The far-lateral combined supratentorial and infratentorial ("combined-combined") approach. A, The park-bench position used for the far-lateral approach is used for this approach. B, Instead of the hockey-stick incision of the far-lateral approach (solid line), the incision is extended anteriorly and superiorly to the zygoma (dashed line). Bony resection includes petrosectomy, condylectomy, C1 laminectomy, and a large suboccipital-temporal craniotomy. C, When this bone exposure is completed, a trans-sigmoid dural incision is made. D, With the dura opened, the vertebrobasilar system is accessible as the surgeon works in between cranial nerve bundles.*

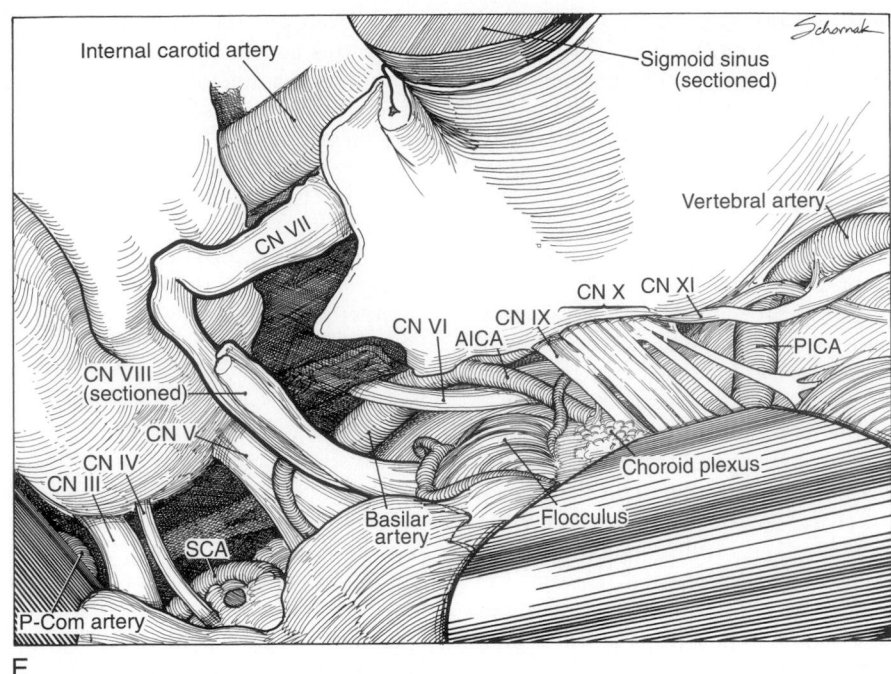

FIGURE 67–20, cont'd. E, *The microsurgical anatomy of basilar artery, its branches, and the cranial nerves is shown. AICA, anterior inferior cerebellar artery; PICA, posterior inferior cerebellar artery; SCA, superior cerebellar artery; P-Com, posterior communicating artery; TMJ, temporomandibular joint.*

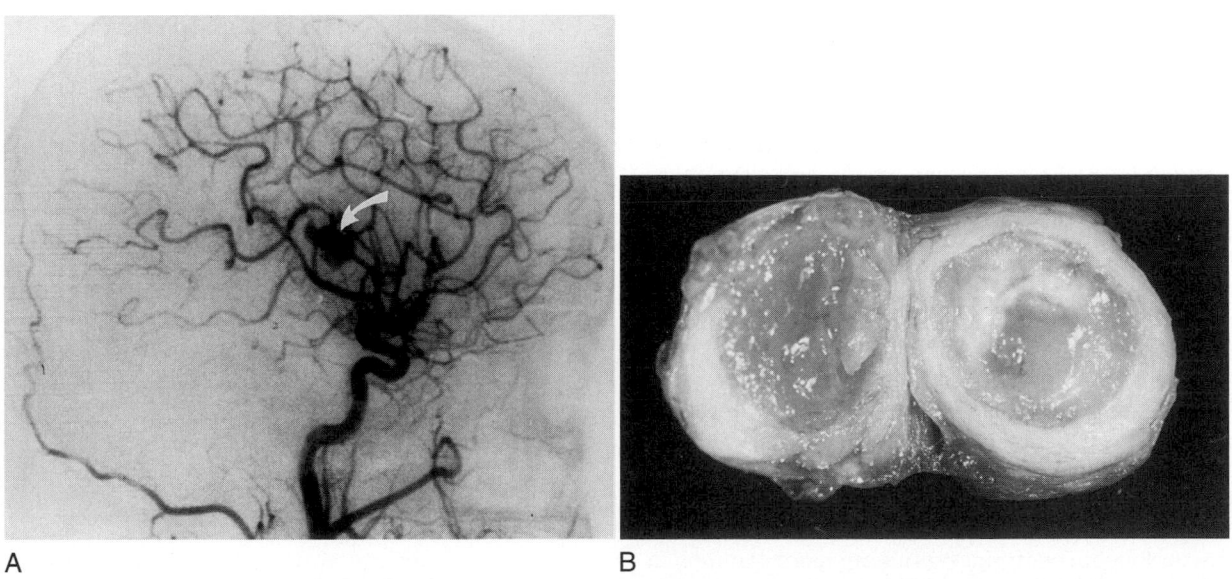

FIGURE 67–21 *Angiographic appearance (A) and gross pathologic appearance (B) of mycotic middle cerebral artery aneurysm (arrow) in a middle-aged man who presented with a history of left hemisphere transient ischemic attacks as well as signs and symptoms of subacute bacterial endocarditis, including dyspnea, fever, chills, and a grade V/VI systolic ejection murmur.*

arteries, occlude flow, and elicit intense inflammation in the adventitia and media, destroying the integrity of the artery wall. Usually, infectious intracranial aneurysms are fusiform and eccentric, without the necks that characterize saccular aneurysms.[346] Unlike congenital aneurysms, which are normally located at the proximal branching points of the circle of Willis, mycotic aneurysms are typically located more peripherally (Fig. 67–21).

Because these aneurysms routinely arise from septic emboli, CT and angiography are required for patients with SBE and focal neurologic findings. In centers with high-resolution MRI, screening for aneurysms with the combination of MRI of the brain and magnetic resonance angiography of the head is a reasonable option; conventional angiography should be used to confirm abnormal findings before treatment.

Patients with unruptured infectious aneurysms should be managed medically with antibiotics and serial angiography.[345] If the aneurysm disappears, or the parent artery spontaneously thromboses, the bleeding risk is eliminated and no further intervention is needed. If the aneurysm remains unchanged but has not ruptured, continued angiographic surveillance is required. If the aneurysm enlarges or changes shape, the destructive process that has caused arterial weakening and aneurysm formation remains active and the bleeding risk is probably high; the patient with such findings should undergo endovascular or open surgical obliteration of the aneurysm, depending on the medical condition of the patient and the eloquence of the brain territory supplied by the parent artery. The patient with a ruptured aneurysm without hematoma and the patient with an aneurysm that does not involve eloquent vascular territory should undergo endovascular obliteration of the aneurysm, with the recognition that the treatment may sacrifice the parent artery. The patient with a ruptured aneurysm and hematoma causing mass effect or increased ICP and the patient with a ruptured aneurysm that involves eloquent vascular territory should undergo open surgical obliteration of the aneurysm, with the hope of preserving or, if needed, reconstructing the parent artery.

Giant, Fusiform, and Dolichoectatic Aneurysms

Giant, fusiform, and dolichoectatic aneurysms are uncommon compared with routine saccular aneurysms and also differ in their clinical presentation and treatment options. Giant aneurysms, defined as more than 25 mm in diameter,[347] constitute 3% to 5% of most aneurysms series, with a female-to-male ratio of about 3:1.[25,45,95,347–349] They most commonly occur in patients 30 to 60 years of age, the same age range as those at risk for aneurysms in general. Fusiform and dolichoectatic aneurysms are even more rare, and most reviews of large autopsy or angiogram series suggest an incidence of less than 0.1%.[50,350,351] Incidence peaks in patients in their late 40s, although patients of all ages have been reported. In most series, giant aneurysms in the anterior circulation outnumber giant aneurysms in the posterior circulation by 2:1.[352,353]

The distribution of fusiform and dolichoectatic aneurysms is more controversial. Drake and Peerless,[354] reviewing their series of 4000 aneurysms treated surgically from 1965 to 1992, found 120 fusiform or dolichoectatic aneurysms; of these, 95 were in the posterior circulation and 25 in the anterior circulation. This finding suggests that fusiform or dolichoectatic aneurysms are more common in the posterior circulation.[351,355–357] However, results of other series indicate that the distribution of these aneurysms between the anterior and posterior circulation may be more equal or may even favor the anterior circulation.[50,350,358–362]

How giant, fusiform, and dolichoectatic aneurysms form is not entirely clear. They have commonly been attributed to atherosclerosis of the intracranial circulation. Dandy[355] first proposed this mechanism, and several subsequent pathology series demonstrated fusiform aneurysms with intimal thickening and hyalinization, lipid-laden phagocytes and cholesterol clefts.[50,351,363,364] Some later studies have noted that intracranial atherosclerosis is a common disorder, but giant, fusiform, and dolichoectatic aneurysms are exceedingly rare in comparison. Giant aneurysms often

have atherosclerotic changes at the neck. Fusiform aneurysms and many dolichoectatic aneurysms, however, are almost completely devoid of atherosclerotic change, although the walls of parent vessels may contain atheromatous plaques.[359,365–368] It is now believed that intracranial atheromas may exacerbate a preexisting structural abnormality but that the plaques themselves are not the inciting factor in formation of these aneurysms.[360,367,369–372] Instead, many of these aneurysms may originate from undiagnosed intracranial arterial dissections.[350,367,369–373]

Exact rates of rupture are hard to determine, but the literature suggests 30% to 80% of giant aneurysms manifest as SAH.[45,283,347,348,354,374,375] The rates of hemorrhage from dolichoectatic and fusiform aneurysms are not as well defined. Many series suggest that the number of patients with fusiform aneurysms manifesting as aneurysmal SAH is lower than that of patients with saccular aneurysms,[350,351,354,359,376] but other series report a rate of rupture similar to that of saccular aneurysms.[377–379] Anson[358] has suggested that the actual rate of hemorrhage may be the same for nonsaccular or dolichoectatic and saccular aneurysms but that fusiform aneurysms are more likely to be diagnosed from symptoms related to compression or ischemia, thereby leading to a lower relative incidence of presentation with SAH.

Giant, fusiform, and dolichoectatic aneurysms commonly cause neurologic signs due to mass effect and ischemia, which may be due to the formation and expansion of thrombus within the aneurysm and detachment of emboli that close off downstream arteries.[305,347,348,352,353,375,380–384] The deficits that result depend on the location of the aneurysm and the afferent and efferent arteries involved. In general, giant and fusiform aneurysms of the anterior circulation are more likely to manifest as episodic speech or motor deficits consistent with transient ischemic attacks or stroke, whereas those of the posterior circulation cause progressive deficits through mass effect. Because the supratentorial compartment can accommodate an enlarging aneurysm, giant, dolichoectatic, and fusiform aneurysms in the anterior circulation do not usually give rise to symptoms from mass effect, although headache and compression of the optic nerves and chiasm or upper cranial nerves due to mass effect from anterior circulation dolichoectatic aneurysms have been reported.[359,385–388] In contrast, aneurysms in the posterior circulation are more likely to cause mass effect within the tight quarters of the posterior fossa and can lead to cranial neuropathies, quadriparesis, ataxia, and respiratory insufficiency.[351,356,359,376,386,389–403] Giant fusiform basilar aneurysms can compress the cerebral aqueduct, the third ventricle, or the foramen of Monro and cause hydrocephalus.[376,404–407] Posterior circulation aneurysms are less likely to manifest ischemic symptoms, but they, too, can shower emboli from intramural thrombus or close off perforating vessels to the brainstem through thrombus expansion. In addition, extreme ectasia of the basilar artery can cause brainstem infarction by stretching and distorting perforating brainstem paramedian branches.[376,408]

High-quality four-vessel cerebral angiography is essential in the preoperative evaluation of patients with giant, fusiform, and dolichoectatic aneurysms, but MRI and CT are also needed (Fig. 67–22). Many of these aneurysms are

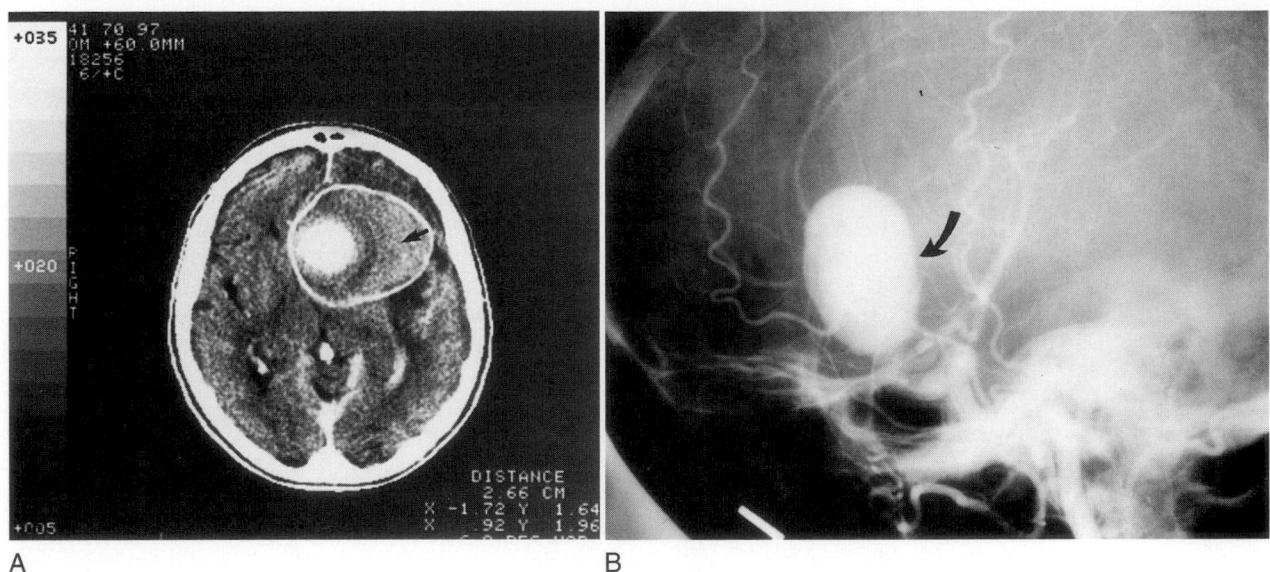

FIGURE 67–22 *A 56-year-old woman presented with dementia and progressive right-sided weakness.* A, *Contrast-enhanced head CT scan demonstrates a large, centrally enhancing mass with a thin rim of contrast bordering the lesion, producing the so-called target sign. This picture is nearly pathognomonic for a partially thrombosed giant aneurysm; the nonenhancing portion of the mass (arrow) represents thrombus within the aneurysm dome.* B, *Lateral view of the left internal carotid artery angiogram in the same patient confirms the diagnosis of a giant internal carotid artery aneurysm (arrow). Note that the size of the aneurysm is grossly underestimated from the angiogram (compare with the CT scan), because only the central portion of the lesion fills with contrast.*

partially thrombosed, and the internal dimensions of the lumen demonstrable by angiography do not accurately reflect the true size of the aneurysm. CT and CT angiography often demonstrate a calcified eggshell border that defines the true diameter of the aneurysm and can also better define an aneurysm's relationship to the bony anatomy of the skull base before surgery. MRI demonstrates a signal void within a patent lumen as well as alternating high-intensity and low-intensity signals on T1-weighted images corresponding to hemosiderin and methemoglobin within the layers of thrombus.[409,410] MRI also allows exquisite delineation of the mass as it relates to the brainstem and cranial nerves. This modality helps define the extent of preoperative brain injury due to intraparenchymal hematoma or ischemia due to hypoperfusion caused by luminal compression or perforator blockade.

The natural history of giant, fusiform, and dolichoectatic aneurysms is dismal because of the high risks of hemorrhage, progressive neurologic deficits from compression, and distal thromboembolism. Mortality rates are almost 70% after 2 years and 85% after 5 years.[28,349,354,365,379,411–413] In contrast, surgical results in many series are better, with good neurologic outcome in 61% to 86% of cases; surgical mortality ranged between 5% and 22% in spite of the technical challenges posed by these aneurysms.[281,283,305,350,352–354,358,414–418] When the surgical results are compared with the natural history of giant, fusiform, and dolichoectatic aneurysms, the imperative for aggressive treatment is clear.

The surgical management of giant intracranial aneurysms must overcome special problems. The necks of these lesions may become so wide that they incorporate the origins of adjacent branches, making direct obliteration by clipping impossible. In other cases, calcification of the neck

or partial thrombosis of the aneurysm makes attempts at clipping extremely hazardous. Finally, the sheer size of these lesions combined with awkward locations may make it impossible to dissect the necks properly. A variety of surgical techniques have been developed to deal with these problems, including ligation or trapping procedures with or without microvascular bypass, partial resection of the aneurysm combined with direct microsurgical repair of the parent vessel, and clipping or direct repair with the use of hypothermic circulatory arrest. The indications and basic principles of these techniques are described later.

Parent Artery Occlusion

Parent artery occlusion is the simplest method to treat giant, fusiform, and dolichoectatic aneurysms. It may involve occlusion of inflow (Hunter's operation), occlusion of outflow, or both (trapping). The goal of surgery is to eliminate, reduce, or reverse flow through the aneurysm.[347,419–422] Complete elimination of flow is ideal, because the risk of rupture or growth of the aneurysm is also eliminated, but this goal typically requires trapping. The length of parent artery occluded by trapping should be minimized, with the points of occlusion immediately proximal and distal to the aneurysm. Trapping can be performed safely if normal branches from the parent artery can be excluded from the trapped segment or if collateral blood flow to distal territories is adequate. The first requirement cannot always be met, particularly along the supraclinoid segment of the ICA, M_1 segment of the middle cerebral artery, and basilar artery where the anterior choroidal artery, lenticulostriate arteries, and brainstem perforating arteries, respectively, may be intimately associated with the aneurysm base. In such cases, it is advisable to limit the parent artery occlusion to only proximal occlusion, which eliminates inflow but still allows collateral flow to perfuse these branches. Assessing the second requirement (adequate collateral blood flow) may require provocative testing (balloon test occlusion; see later).

Proximal parent artery occlusion may not eliminate flow through an aneurysm, but it typically reverses and reduces flow. Retrograde collateral flow through a proximally occluded aneurysm is usually minimal, with enough to supply perforator and branch arteries but with sluggish or stagnant flow in the aneurysm itself. The hemodynamics typically induce thrombus formation, particularly in large and giant aneurysms with preexisting thrombus. Proximal occlusion with thrombosis of a dolichoectatic aneurysm is usually sufficient treatment, because the risk of hemorrhage of such an aneurysm is small. Sometimes the thrombosis induced by proximal occlusion aggravates compressive symptoms, in which case a debulking procedure may be indicated. Distal parent artery occlusion is usually reserved for a large or giant dolichoectatic aneurysm in which exposure of the proximal artery is difficult (e.g., basilar trunk aneurysms) and the aneurysm is thick-walled, thrombus-filled, or both, with low risk of rupture from the arterial pressures that persist within it.

Parent artery occlusions can often be performed endovascularly, with the use of either inflatable balloons or detachable coils. Advantages of endovascular occlusion include minimal invasiveness and easy access to arteries that might require extensive surgery. The disadvantage of such an approach is the need to occlude a wider segment of the normal parent artery with the balloon or coil. These endovascular agents do not provide the discrete "point" occlusion of a surgically placed clip. Some parent arteries, like the posterior inferior cerebellar artery, have critical perforators that cannot be visualized angiographically; they may be better treated with clip occlusion rather than endovascular occlusion.

Cerebral infarction is a major immediate complication of carotid artery occlusion: Approximately 10% to 20% of patients are unable to tolerate carotid artery occlusion.[421,423,424] Numerous techniques, including balloon test occlusion, the measurement of carotid artery stump pressures, EEG monitoring, jugular venous blood sampling, gradual occlusion, and cerebral blood flow measurements, have been proposed to help predict whether a patient can withstand permanent carotid occlusion, but these tests reduce rather than eliminate ischemic complications, because the onset of ischemic deficits may be delayed for hours to days. The majority of these delayed complications after carotid artery occlusion are most likely caused by thromboembolic propagation rather than low flow rates. Clearly, however, there are patients in whom the limited availability of collateral blood supplies markedly raises the risks of neurologic injury after parent artery occlusion. It is also important to remember that parent artery occlusion does not protect the patient completely from the risk of rebleeding. Norlen and Olivecrona[425] reported a 16% incidence of death from recurrent SAH in the 1- to 14-year follow-up of patients undergoing internal or common carotid ligature, or both. In a report of the Cooperative Study, Nishioka[424] reported an 8% rebleeding rate on long-term follow-up in 39 patients who underwent carotid artery occlusion for the treatment of ruptured aneurysms; these patients also had a 16.6% incidence of delayed stroke ipsilateral to the internal carotid ligation.

Direct Clipping

With modern microsurgical techniques, the majority of giant intracranial aneurysms can be directly clipped. Management often requires temporary trapping of the aneurysm. As discussed earlier, temporary vessel occlusion appears to be safe for 10 to 20 minutes if the patient is under deep barbiturate anesthesia with burst suppression of EEG activity. To enhance the collateral blood supply, the patient should be kept normotensive or mildly hypertensive during temporary vessel occlusion.

The first and most important surgical decision in the treatment of giant, fusiform, and dolichoectatic aneurysms is selection of the approach that provides the widest exposure and most direct access to the aneurysm. For these aneurysms in the anterior circulation, the question becomes whether or not an orbitozygomatic osteotomy can enhance the routine pterional exposure enough to justify its use.[302,426,427] The extra space provided by an orbitozygomatic osteotomy is particularly important for giant, fusiform, and dolichoectatic aneurysms in the anterior circulation; maneuvers such as anterior clinoid removal, ICA exposure in Glasscock's triangle, and deep bypass procedures all profit from the additional maneuvering room provided by the orbitozygomatic osteotomy.

For giant, fusiform, and dolichoectatic aneurysms in the posterior circulation, it is best to think of the vertebrobasilar trunk as having five divisions and then to choose the approach according to the portion of the vertebrobasilar trunk involved.[305] Aneurysms in the upper basilar zone (upper two fifths of the basilar artery) are best approached through an extended orbitozygomatic craniotomy; aneurysms in the lower vertebrobasilar zone (lower two fifths of the basilar artery and the intradural segment of the vertebral arteries) are best approached through an extended far-lateral craniotomy; and aneurysms in the basilar midregion (middle fifth of the basilar artery) are best approached through a transpetrosal craniotomy. Aneurysms that span these boundaries may need one of the combination approaches (see earlier discussion of surgical approaches to posterior circulation aneurysms).

Once the surgical approach has been performed and exposure is complete, great care must be taken to ensure that all branches and adjacent vessels have been identified and dissected free before clipping is attempted. For giant aneurysms, temporary clipping of the parent vessel and major branches decreases the risk of rupture during the final stages of dissection and clipping. If preoperative studies demonstrate extensive thrombus within the aneurysm sac or if the aneurysm is difficult to collapse, thrombectomy may be required (Fig. 67–23). This requirement may change the goal of surgery from elimination of the aneurysm to reduction of mass effect. Thrombectomy is particularly useful for giant posterior circulation aneurysms, in which the neurologic effects of brainstem compression are so devastating and the ability to reconstruct the posterior circulation arteries through a narrow surgical corridor is limited. Thrombus is removed piecemeal with cup forceps or an ultrasonic aspirator. An ultrasonic aspirator is especially effective for the delicate

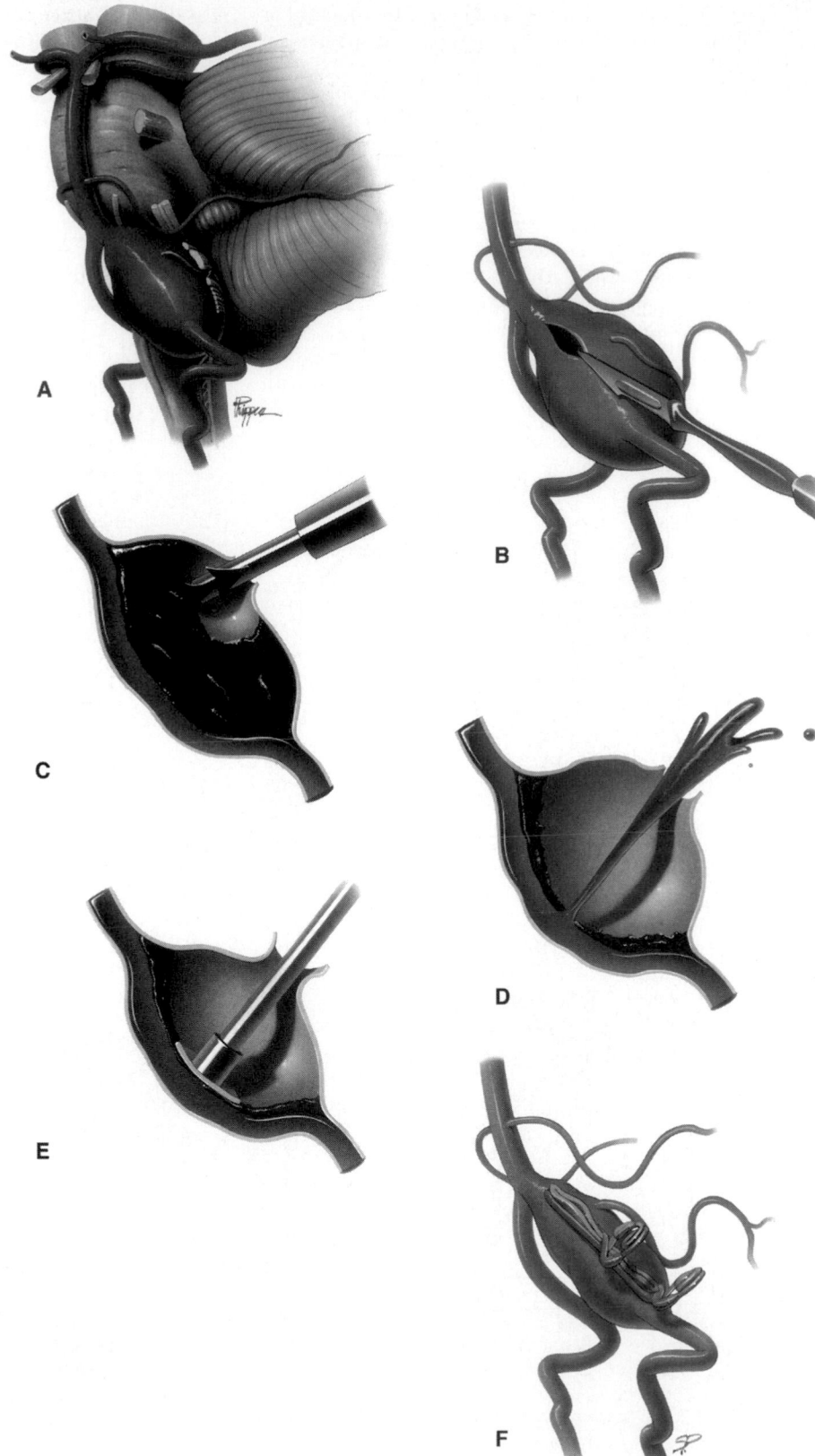

FIGURE 67–23 *Dolichoectatic aneurysms involving the intradural vertebral artery typically produce symptoms from compression of the brainstem and cranial nerves (A). This mass is eliminated by opening the aneurysm with a No. 11 blade (B) and removing thrombus with an ultrasonic aspirator (C). The thrombectomy proceeds until the lumen of the aneurysm is encountered (D). Bleeding is controlled with absorbable knitted fabric (Surgicel) (E), and the walls of the aneurysm are brought together with clips to reconstruct the lumen of the parent artery (F). Note that the thrombectomy eliminates mass effect and generates the redundant vessel wall needed to reconstruct the artery. (Reproduced with permission from Barrow Neurological Institute.)*

removal of hardened thrombus, as it avoids the traction or manipulation of the aneurysm required by piecemeal removal with cup forceps.

Thrombectomy proceeds until either the thrombus has been adequately debulked or the lumen of the aneurysm is encountered, at which point bleeding is controlled with application of a hemostatic agent and gentle pressure. Excavating the thrombus in this manner not only eliminates the mass effect but also generates a redundant aneurysm wall that can be used to reconstruct the artery lumen with clips. All important branch arteries are carefully identified and preserved. It can be difficult to determine whether the reconstructed channel through the aneurysm has a sufficient internal caliber to supply these distal branches, particularly when the aneurysm wall is thickened with atherosclerotic disease or when there is intraluminal

thrombus. Therefore, clips are applied to leave a generous lumen. Intraoperative Doppler to ensure patency of the parent vessel and angiography are useful. Of the techniques discussed for giant, fusiform, and dolichoectatic aneurysms, clip reconstruction is the most elegant because it eliminates the aneurysm and preserves distal flow.

Bypass Procedures

A small number of giant aneurysms, particularly those involving the cavernous portion of the ICA, are best managed with the combination of a trapping procedure with an arterial bypass or venous jump graft.[305,352,353,414,415,418,428,429] A wide variety of bypasses are available for anterior circulation aneurysms, and the choice of bypass depends on the location of the aneurysm and the flow requirements of the distal territory (Fig. 67–24).

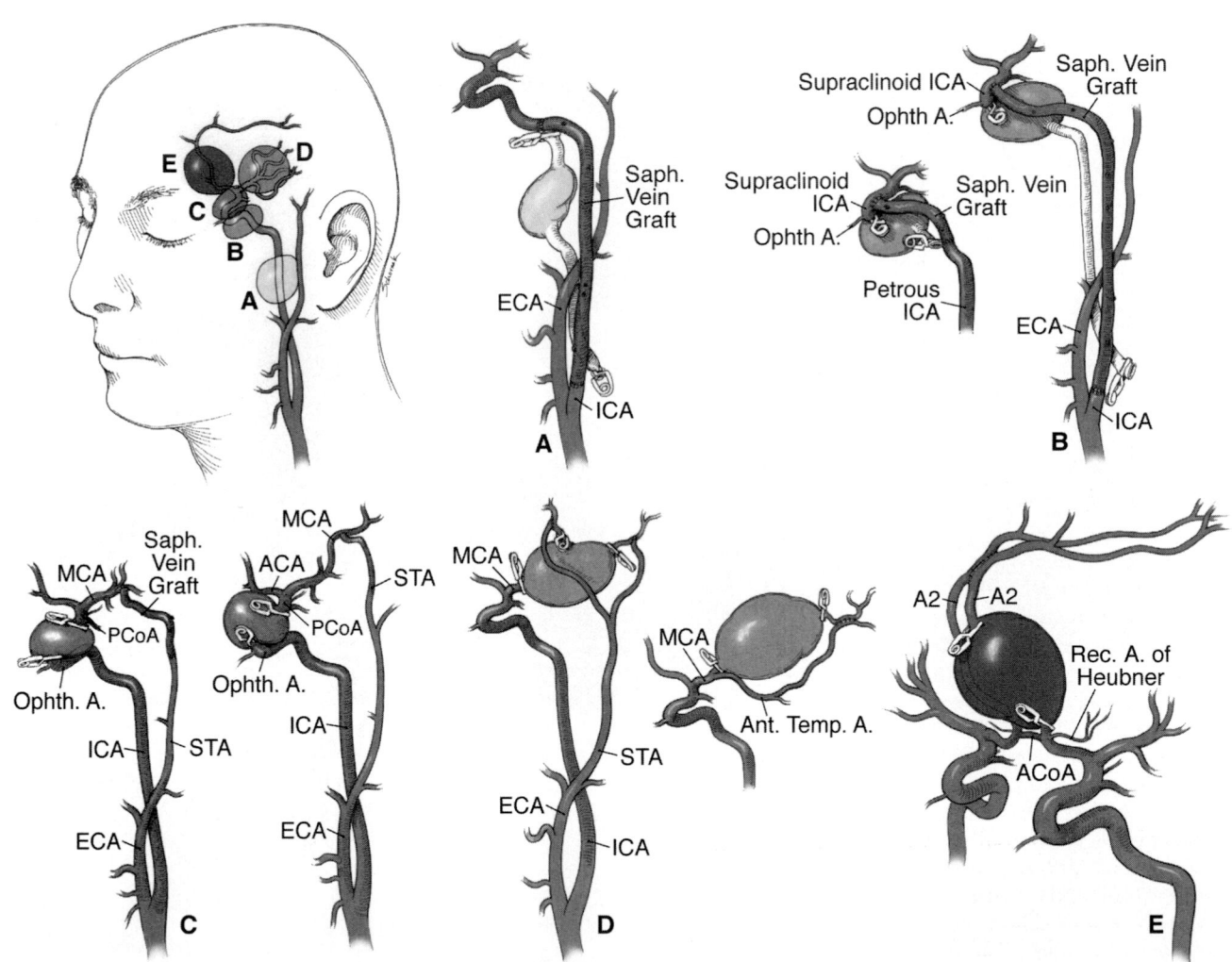

FIGURE 67–24 *Surgical approaches to revascularization of the anterior circulation. Overview showing the anterior circulation and common locations for aneurysms. A, The internal carotid artery (ICA) aneurysm at the skull base is trapped and revascularized with a cervical–petrous carotid artery bypass with a saphenous vein graft. B, The cavernous ICA aneurysm is trapped and revascularized with a petrous–supraclinoid carotid artery bypass with a saphenous vein graft or, alternatively, with a cervical–supraclinoid carotid artery bypass. C, The supraclinoid ICA is trapped and revascularized with a superficial temporal artery–middle cerebral artery (STA-MCA) bypass or, alternatively, with an STA-MCA bypass with a saphenous vein graft. D, The MCA aneurysm is trapped and revascularized with a "double-barrel" STA-MCA bypass or, alternatively, with an anterior temporal artery–MCA in situ bypass. E, The anterior cerebral artery aneurysm is trapped and revascularized with an A$_2$-A$_2$ in situ bypass. ACoA, anterior communicating artery; Ant. Temp. A., anterior temporal artery; ECA, external carotid artery; Ophth. A., ophthalmic artery; PCoA, posterior communicating artery; Rec. A., recurrent artery of Heubner; Saph., saphenous. (Reproduced with permission from Barrow Neurological Institute.)*

Aneurysms located on the carotid artery at the skull base can be trapped proximally in the neck and distally along the petrous carotid artery, and then bypassed by an extradural cervical–petrous carotid artery anastomosis. Intracavernous ICA aneurysms are difficult to expose, and attempts to clip them are complicated by venous bleeding from the sinus and injury of adjacent cranial nerves. Instead, these aneurysms can be trapped after insertion of a saphenous vein bypass that spans from the petrous to the supraclinoid carotid artery, or from the cervical to the supraclinoid carotid artery (Fig. 67–25). The latter bypass is easier, but the former bypass uses a shorter segment with a potentially higher patency rate.

Revascularization after occlusion of the supraclinoid carotid artery can be achieved with a superficial temporal

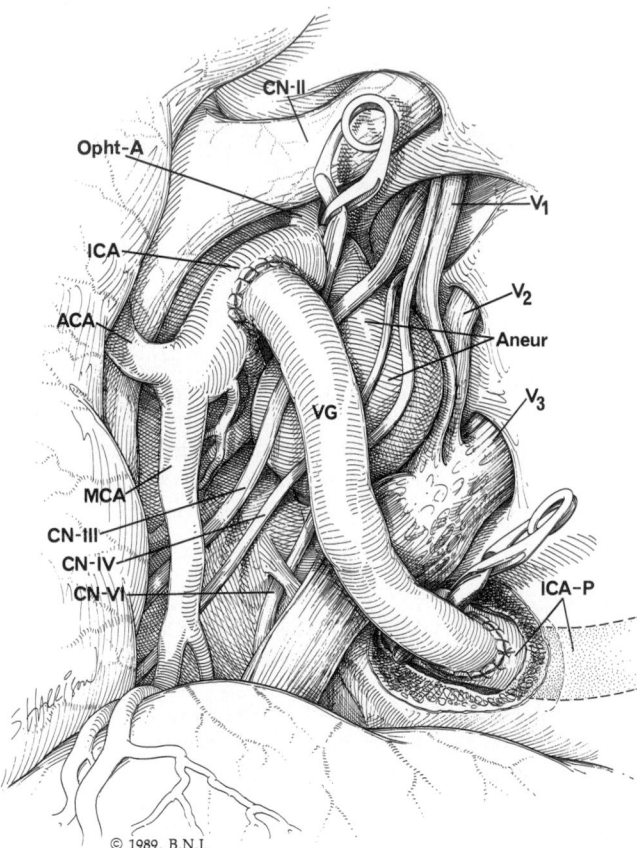

FIGURE 67–25 *Vein graft (VG) from the petrous segment of the internal carotid artery (ICA-P) to the supraclinoid segment of the internal carotid artery (ICA) for the treatment of a giant aneurysm (Aneur) involving the cavernous segment of the internal carotid artery. Note that the aneurysm has been eliminated from the circulation by the placement of proximal and distal clips. For the purpose of illustration, the lateral wall of the cavernous sinus has been removed in this drawing to allow visualization of the course of the third, fourth, and sixth cranial nerves (CN), and the fifth cranial nerve. Other labeled structures are the ophthalmic artery (Opht-A), anterior cerebral artery (ACA), middle cerebral artery (MCA), and the optic nerve (CN-II). (Adapted from Spetzler RF, Fukushima T, Martin N, et al: Petrous carotid-to-intradural carotid saphenous vein graft for intracavernous giant aneurysm, tumor, and occlusive cerebrovascular disease. J Neurosurg 73:496–501, 1990.)*

artery–middle cerebral artery (STA-MCA) bypass. Patients with poor tolerance to balloon temporary occlusion will probably require a high-flow saphenous bypass from the cervical carotid to the middle cerebral artery. An STA-MCA bypass is also used to revascularize the distal middle cerebral artery territory after trapping of aneurysms. A "double-barrel" STA-MCA bypass, which connects both frontal and parietal branches of the superficial temporal artery to different branches of the middle cerebral artery, can further increase the blood flow to this territory or can be used to revascularize both trunks of the middle cerebral artery bifurcation as they exit a trapped aneurysm.

If the superficial temporal artery is damaged during the craniotomy or is too narrow to provide sufficient flow for bypass, an in situ bypass can anastomose the anterior temporal artery side-to-side to a middle cerebral artery branch distal to the aneurysm. Similarly, an uninvolved middle cerebral branch can serve as a donor vessel to an adjacent branch that has been occluded proximally, using either an end-to-side implantation or a side-to-side anastomosis. If an aneurysm involves one of the anterior cerebral arteries distal to the anterior communicating artery, then a side-to-side anastomosis between the involved anterior cerebral artery and its contralateral mate can preserve distal flow through both arteries.

A number of bypasses are available to revascularize parent arteries in the posterior circulation (Fig. 67–26). The upper basilar artery can be revascularized with use of the superficial temporal artery as a donor artery and either the superior cerebellar artery or the posterior cerebral artery as a recipient artery. The superior cerebellar artery is preferred because temporary occlusion is better tolerated by this artery than by the posterior cerebral artery. High-flow saphenous vein grafts can also revascularize the basilar apex when the superficial temporal artery is insufficient, with either the cervical carotid artery or the middle cerebral artery used as the donor artery. If direct access to a basilar artery aneurysm is needed during the same operation as the bypass, a combined supratentorial and infratentorial approach is used, and a bypass from the intradural vertebral artery to the superior cerebellar artery or posterior cerebral artery is performed. Radial artery grafts are often easier to harvest than saphenous vein grafts when a lateral or three-quarter-prone position is used for a posterior fossa craniotomy. Once the bypass is completed, this approach provides direct access to the aneurysm for trapping or proximal occlusion; this access is not usually available when a skull base approach to the basilar apex, such as the orbitozygomatic-pterional approach, is used.

The anterior inferior cerebellar artery and the midbasilar trunk are revascularized with the occipital artery. Rarely is a high-flow bypass needed here, but such bypasses are available. The vertebral artery is readily accessible through the far-lateral approach, making it possible to reconstruct the artery with an interposition graft. The posterior inferior cerebellar artery commonly originates from the base of aneurysms here, and its perforators to the anterior and lateral medulla make preservation of its flow a priority. Fortunately, posterior inferior cerebellar artery can be revascularized with the occipital artery, the contralateral posterior inferior cerebellar artery in a side-to-side bypass, or a graft from the proximal vertebral artery. Reconstitution of flow in

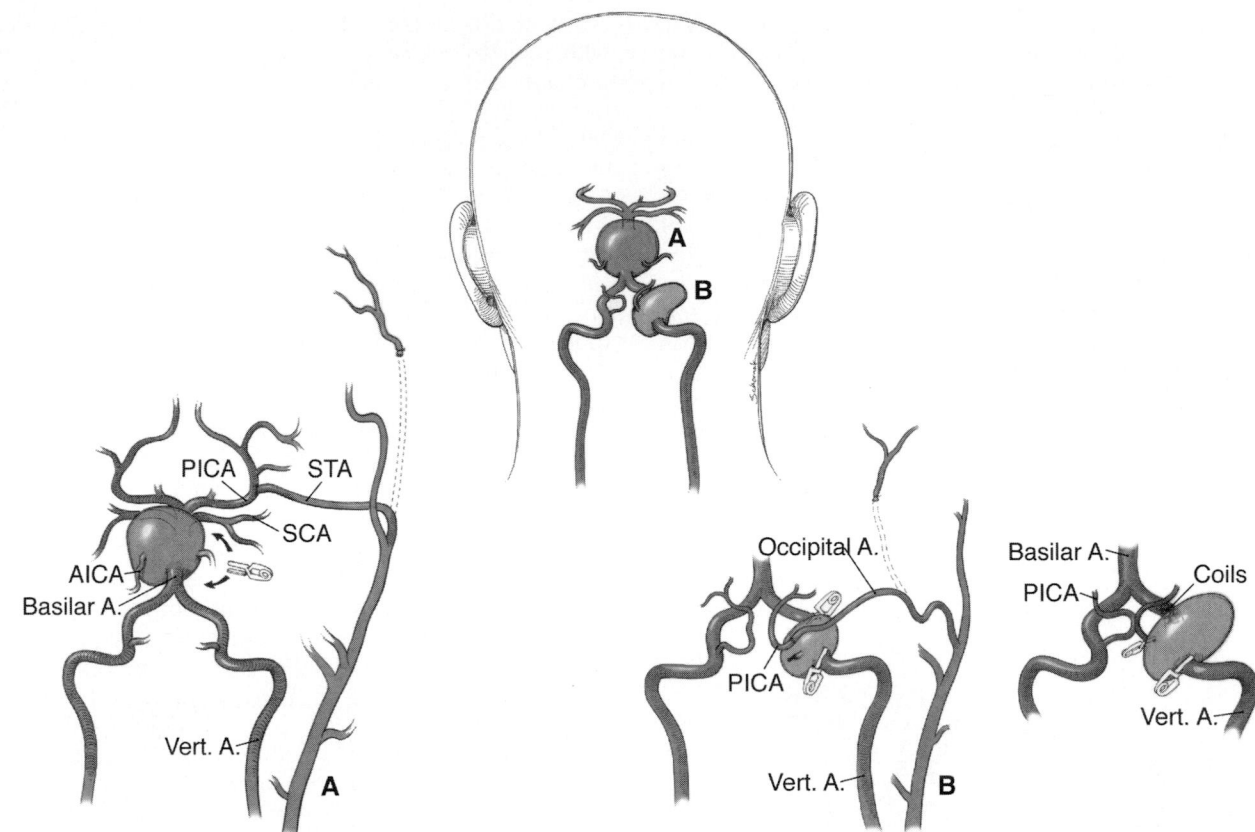

FIGURE 67–26 *Surgical approaches to revascularization of the posterior circulation. Overview showing the posterior circulation and common locations for aneurysm. A, The midbasilar artery is occluded proximal or distal to the aneurysm and revascularized with a superficial temporal artery (STA)–posterior cerebral artery bypass or with an STA–superior cerebellar artery bypass. B, The vertebral artery aneurysm is trapped and revascularized with a posterior inferior communicating artery (PICA)–PICA in situ bypass. Alternatively, an occipital artery–PICA bypass is shown. AICA, anterior inferior cerebellar artery; SCA, superior cerebellar artery; Vert. A., vertebral artery. (Reproduced with permission from Barrow Neurological Institute.)*

the distal posterior inferior cerebellar artery enables this artery to be occluded as it exits the aneurysm, after which retrograde filling from the bypass perfuses the medullary perforators. Furthermore, a patent contralateral vertebral artery that joins with the basilar artery allows the surgeon to occlude the vertebral artery proximal to the aneurysm.

Hypothermic Circulatory Arrest

The surgical management of giant aneurysms of the vertebrobasilar system presents special problems. Because of the awkward location of these lesions, they cannot readily be controlled by temporary clipping of feeding vessels. In addition, these aneurysms are surrounded by numerous small but highly important perforating branches that supply the brainstem and cerebellum. Accurate dissection and clipping of the aneurysm neck with preservation of these perforators are paramount for a good outcome. A useful adjunct for the treatment of these lesions is total circulatory arrest with deep hypothermia. Hypothermic circulatory arrest provides complete vascular control, obviates the use of temporary clips, eliminates the risk of aneurysm rupture, and enhances cerebral protection. Disadvantages include femoral artery and vein cannulation that can injure these vessels, heparinization which increases the risk of hemorrhagic complications, red blood cell and platelet consump-

tion, slowed coagulation parameters owing to hypothermia and hemodilution, risk of ischemic brain injury, and expense.[305,353,430,431] Several groups have reported better results with this technique in the treatment of giant intracranial aneurysms.[402,432–435] We reserve the use of this technique for giant, fusiform, and dolichoectatic aneurysms involving the vertebrobasilar system.

A multispecialty team with good coordination and understanding among its members is essential. The team should include a neurosurgeon, a cardiothoracic surgeon, a pump technician, and an anesthesiologist with experience in both neurologic and cardiovascular surgery. Figure 67–27 illustrates the typical layout of the room and the location of the team members. The aneurysm is exposed through one of the previously described approaches, which is dictated by the aneurysm's location, and the neck is inspected. Occasionally, the neck of the aneurysm is free of perforating branches and can be readily clipped without circulatory arrest. More commonly, the size of the aneurysm blocks the necessary visualization to allow safe clipping. In such cases, further dissection is delayed while the patient is prepared for cardiopulmonary bypass. The femoral vessels are exposed, the patient is fully heparinized, and the femoral artery and vein are cannulated (Fig. 67–28). Extracorporeal circulation is initiated, and

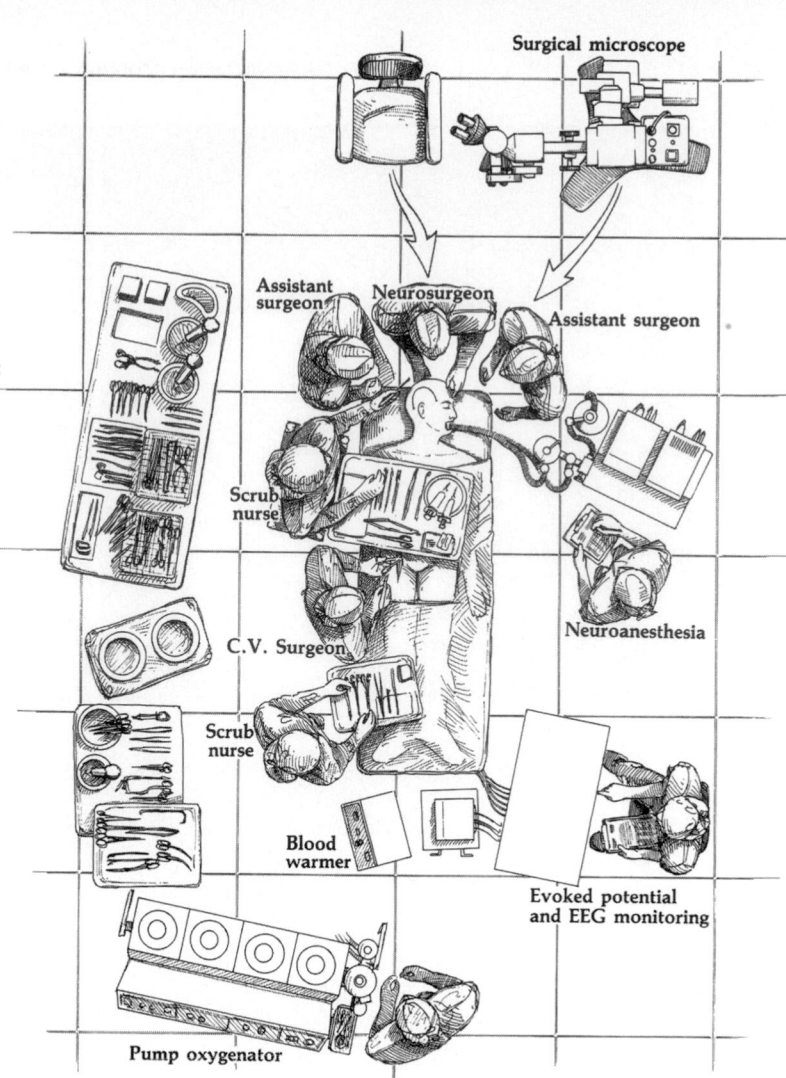

FIGURE 67–27 *Layout of the operating room in neurosurgical cases that involve the use of hypothermic circulatory arrest. (From Blazier CJ, Cavanaugh E, Antonoli L: Surgical treatment of complex cerebrovascular lesions utilizing hypothermia and circulatory arrest: Nursing implications. BNI Q 5:33, 1990.)*

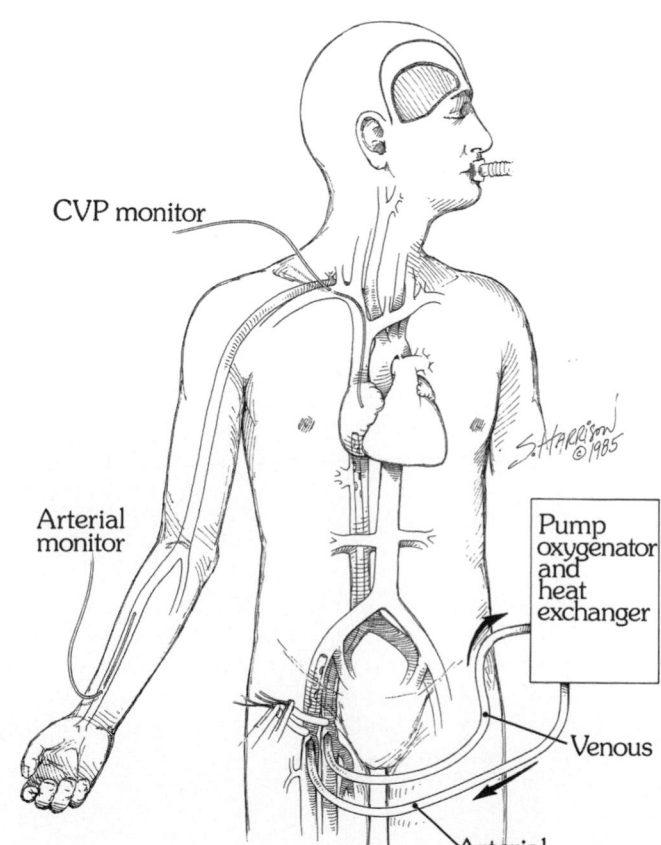

FIGURE 67–28 *Technique used to establish extracorporeal circulation during hypothermic circulatory arrest for intracranial aneurysms. The femoral artery and vein are cannulated in the groin and connected to the pump oxygenator and heat exchanger. This approach allows the cardiovascular and neurosurgical teams to work simultaneously as illustrated in Figure 67–27. CVP, central venous pressure. (From Spetzler RF, Hadley MN, Rigamonti D, et al: Aneurysms of the basilar artery treated with circulatory arrest, hypothermia, and barbiturate cerebral protection. J Neurosurg 68:868, 1988.)*

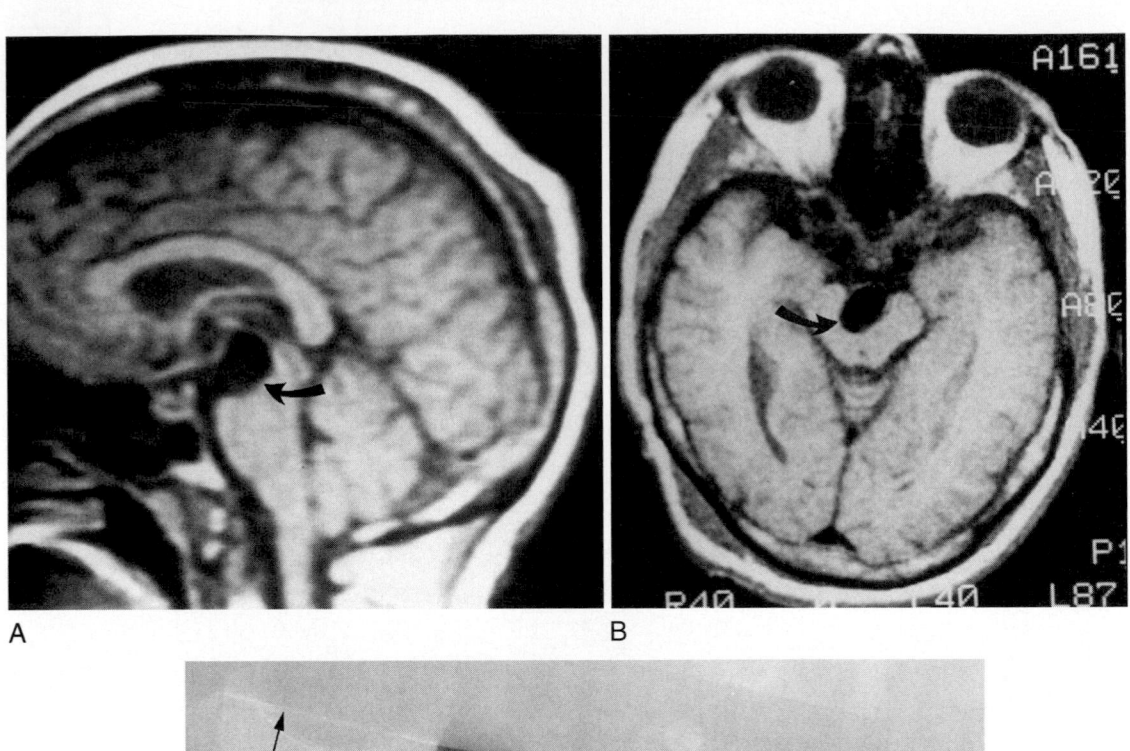

A   B

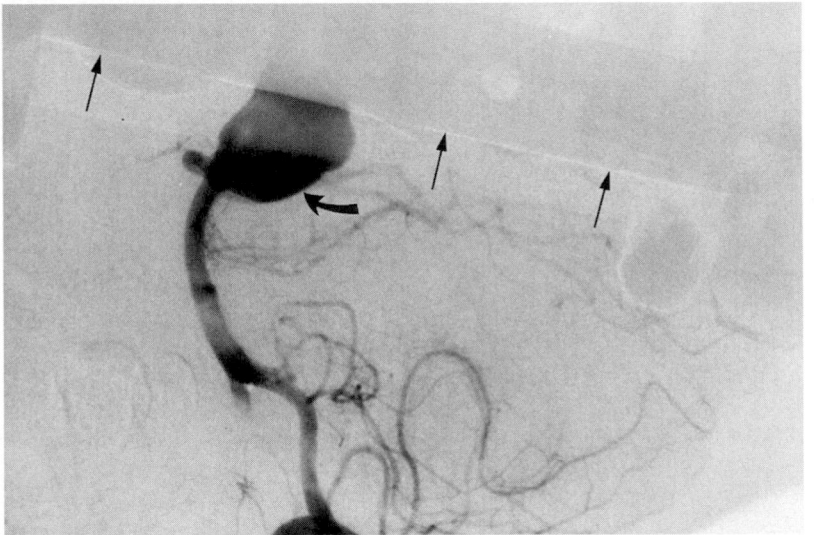

C

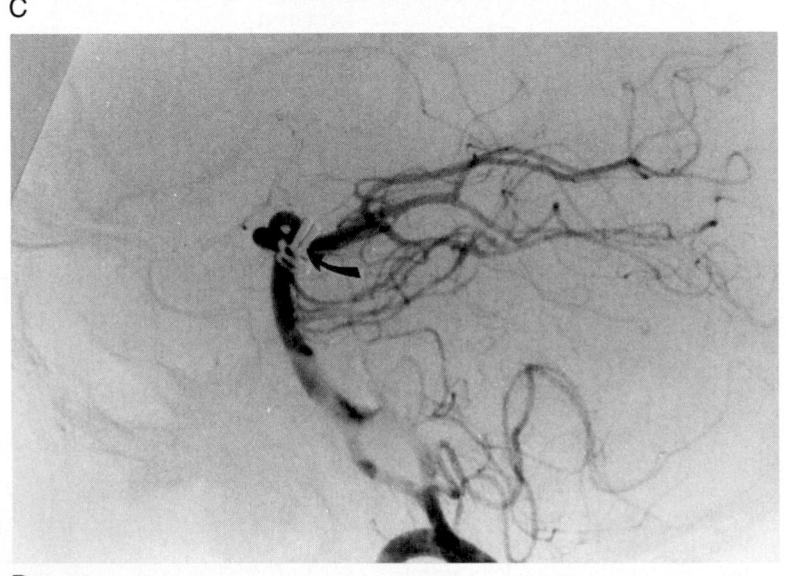

D

FIGURE 67–29 *A 51-year-old woman sustained a cervical spine fracture and mild head trauma in a motor vehicle accident. MRI of the head and neck was performed as part of the initial trauma evaluation. A and B, Sagittal and transverse T1-weighted images revealed a giant, incidental basilar tip aneurysm (arrows). The cervical spine fracture was treated by immobilization of the patient with a halo vest and ring. C, A lateral view of the vertebral artery angiogram confirmed the diagnosis of a giant basilar tip aneurysm (curved arrow). Artifact from the halo ring is apparent (straight arrows). On both the MR images and the angiogram, the aneurysm dome angles up and back, distorting and displacing the brainstem. The cervical spine fracture healed without complication. Four months after her accident, the patient underwent elective clipping of the aneurysm via a subtemporal approach and with the use of hypothermic circulatory arrest. Her recovery was quick and uneventful. D, Lateral view of the postoperative vertebral angiogram shows complete obliteration of the aneurysm with preservation of the parent vessels. A single straight clip is faintly visible across the neck of the aneurysm (arrow).*

the patient is gradually cooled to a core temperature of approximately 15°C. The pump is stopped and the blood is allowed to drain into the bypass pump reservoir, collapsing the aneurysm. Dissection of the aneurysm neck is completed, with care being taken to free all perforating vessels and major branches. If the aneurysm contains extensive thrombosis, it can be opened and partially evacuated to enable clipping of the neck.

After the aneurysm is clipped, the pump is restarted and the patient is gradually rewarmed. The risk of intracerebral hematoma formation is minimized by avoiding any movement of the retractors after the patient has been heparinized and before rewarming and weaning from extracorporeal circulation and the heparin is reversed. In addition, clotting factors and platelets are replenished by transfusion of one to two units of autologous, fresh, whole blood that was removed during the initial exposure of the aneurysm. If necessary, the pump can be primed with one to two units of packed red blood cells to maintain an adequate hemoglobin level.

Using this technique, we have had good results (Fig. 67–29).[431] In the series of patients who have undergone hypothermic circulatory arrest for treatment of lesions at the Barrow Neurological Institute, the surgical morbidity and mortality rates associated with hypothermic circulatory arrest were 13.3% and 8.3%, respectively. At late follow-up, 76% of the patients had good outcomes (Glasgow Outcome Scale scores of 1 and 2), 5% had poor outcomes (Glasgow Outcome Scale scores of 3 and 4), and 18% had died. Patient outcome correlated with preoperative neurologic condition. Preservation of perforating arteries was paramount to achieving a good outcome; duration of circulatory arrest was not. These findings are commensurate with those of other series.[402,430,432,434,436–442]

SUMMARY

Advances in neuroanesthesia, the development of new microsurgical instruments, and the rapid evolution of microvascular techniques have dramatically reduced the operative morbidity and mortality associated with the surgical management of intracranial aneurysms. In patients with acute aneurysmal SAH, early surgical intervention has now virtually eliminated the risk of rebleeding, whereas changes in perioperative management, including the use of hypervolemic-hypertensive therapy and calcium antagonists, have significantly blunted the devastating effect of vasospasm. In patients admitted in good condition, early surgery and aggressive management have reduced morbidity and mortality to as little as 10% to 15%. The management of patients with giant aneurysms of the vertebrobasilar system remains a significant challenge. Hypothermic circulatory arrest provides a useful adjunct for the treatment of these rare lesions, but innovative strategies are needed.

References

1. Symonds CP: Spontaneous subarachnoid hemorrhage. Q J Med 18:93, 1924.
2. Cushing H: Contributions to the clinical studies of intracranial aneurysms. Guys Hosp Rep 73:159, 1923.
3. Moniz E: L'encephalographie artérielle, son importance dans la localisation des tumeurs cérébrales. Rev Neurol 2:72, 1927.
4. Dott NM: Intracranial aneurysms: Cerebral arterioradiography: Surgical treatment. Trans Med Chir Soc Edinburgh 47:219, 1932.
5. Dandy WE: Intracranial aneurysm of internal carotid artery cured by operation. Ann Surg 107:654, 1938.
6. Ljunggren B, Brandt L, Kagstrom E, et al: Results of early operations for ruptured aneurysms. J Neurosurg 54:473, 1981.
7. Ljunggren B, Saveland H, Brandt L: Aneurysmal subarachnoid hemorrhage—historical background from a Scandinavian horizon. Surg Neurol 22:605, 1984.
8. Ljunggren B, Saveland H, Brandt L, et al: Aneurysmal subarachnoid hemorrhage: Total annual outcome in a 1.46 million population. Surg Neurol 22:435, 1984.
9. Inagawa T: Trends in incidence and case fatality rates of aneurysmal subarachnoid hemorrhage in Izumo City, Japan, between 1980–1989 and 1990–1998. Stroke 32:1499, 2001.
10. Inagawa T, Aoki H, Ishikawa S, et al: Aneurysmal subarachnoid hemorrhage in Izumo City and Shimane Prefecture of Japan: Seasonal variation. Hiroshima J Med Sci 37:17, 1988.
11. Linn FH, Rinkel GJ, Algra A, et al: Incidence of subarachnoid hemorrhage: Role of region, year, and rate of computed tomography: A meta-analysis. Stroke 27:625, 1996.
12. Ohno K, Suzuki R, Masaoka H, et al: A review of 102 consecutive patients with intracranial aneurysms in a community hospital in Japan. Acta Neurochir (Wien) 94:23, 1988.
13. Sarti C, Tuomilehto J, Salomaa V, et al: Epidemiology of subarachnoid hemorrhage in Finland from 1983 to 1985. Stroke 22:848, 1991.
14. Broderick JP, Brott T, Tomsick T, et al: The risk of subarachnoid and intracerebral hemorrhages in blacks as compared with whites. N Engl J Med 326:733, 1992.
15. Mayberg MR, Batjer HH, Dacey R, et al: Guidelines for the management of aneurysmal subarachnoid hemorrhage: A statement for healthcare professionals from a special writing group of the Stroke Council, American Heart Association. Stroke 25:2315, 1994.
16. Ingall TJ, Whisnant JP, Wiebers DO, et al: Has there been a decline in subarachnoid hemorrhage mortality? Stroke 20:718, 1989.
17. Haley EC Jr, Kassell NF, Torner JC: The International Cooperative Study on the Timing of Aneurysm Surgery: The North American experience. Stroke 23:205, 1992.

18. Haley EC Jr, Kassell NF, Torner JC: A randomized trial of nicardipine in subarachnoid hemorrhage: Angiographic and transcranial Doppler ultrasound results: A report of the Cooperative Aneurysm Study. J Neurosurg 78:548, 1993.

19. Haley EC Jr, Kassell NF, Torner JC: A randomized controlled trial of high-dose intravenous nicardipine in aneurysmal subarachnoid hemorrhage: A report of the Cooperative Aneurysm Study. J Neurosurg 78:537, 1993.

20. Haley EC Jr, Kassell NF, Torner JC, et al: A randomized trial of two doses of nicardipine in aneurysmal subarachnoid hemorrhage: A report of the Cooperative Aneurysm Study. J Neurosurg 80:788, 1994.

21. Kassell NF, Torner JC, Haley EC Jr, et al: The International Cooperative Study on the Timing of Aneurysm Surgery. Part 1: Overall management results. J Neurosurg 73:18, 1990.

22. Kassell NF, Torner TC: Epidemiology of intracranial aneurysms. Int Anesthesiol Clin 20:13, 1982.

23. Pickard JD, Murray GD, Illingworth R, et al: Effect of oral nimodipine on cerebral infarction and outcome after subarachnoid haemorrhage: British aneurysm nimodipine trial. BMJ 298:636, 1989.

24. Pickard JD, Walker V, Brandt L, et al: Effect of intraventricular haemorrhage and rebleeding following subarachnoid haemorrhage on CSF eicosanoids. Acta Neurochir (Wien) 129:152, 1994.

25. Weir B: Intracranial aneurysms and subarachnoid hemorrhage: An overview. In Wilkins RH, Rengachary SS (eds): Neurosurgery. New York, McGraw-Hill, 1994, p 1308.

26. Jellinger K: Pathology of intracerebral hemorrhage. Zentralbl Neurochir 38:29, 1977.

27. Hassler O: Morphological studies on the large cerebral arteries with reference to etiology of subarachnoid haemorrhage. Acta Psychiatr Scand 154:1, 1961.

28. McCormick WF, Acosta-Rua GJ: The size of intracranial saccular aneurysms: An autopsy study. J Neurosurg 33:422, 1970.

29. Locksley HB: Natural history of subarachnoid hemorrhage, intracranial aneurysms and arteriovenous malformations. J Neurosurg 25:321, 1966.

30. Kassell NF, Torner JC: Aneurysmal rebleeding: A preliminary report from the Cooperative Aneurysm Study. Neurosurgery 13:479, 1983.

31. Kassell NF, Torner JC: The International Cooperative Study on Timing of Aneurysm Surgery—an update. Stroke 15:566, 1984.

32. Kassell NF, Torner JC, Jane JA, et al: The International Cooperative Study on the Timing of Aneurysm Surgery. Part 2: Surgical results. J Neurosurg 73:37, 1990.

33. Burrows PF, Robertson RL, Barnes PD: Angiography and the evaluation of cerebrovascular disease in childhood. Neuroimaging Clin North Am 6:561, 1996.

34. Herman JM, Rekate HL, Spetzler RF: Pediatric intracranial aneurysms: Simple and complex cases. Pediatr Neurosurg 17:66, 1991.

35. Husson RN, Saini R, Lewis LL, et al: Cerebral artery aneurysms in children infected with human immunodeficiency virus. J Pediatr 121:927, 1992.

36. Kanaan I, Lasjaunias P, Coates R: The spectrum of intracranial aneurysms in pediatrics. Minim Invasive Neurosurg 38:1, 1995.

37. Kasahara E, Murayama T, Yamane C: Giant cerebral arterial aneurysm in an infant: Report of a case and review of 42 previous cases in infants with cerebral arterial aneurysm. Acta Paediatr Jpn 38:684, 1996.

38. Koelfen W, Wentz U, Freund M, et al: Magnetic resonance angiography in 140 neuropediatric patients. Pediatr Neurol 12:31, 1995.

39. Norris JS, Wallace MC: Pediatric intracranial aneurysms. Neurosurg Clin North Am 9:557, 1998.

40. Proust F, Toussaint P, Garnieri J, et al: Pediatric cerebral aneurysms. J Neurosurg 94:733, 2001.

41. Roche JL, Choux M, Czorny A, et al: [Intracranial arterial aneurysm in children: A cooperative study: Apropos of 43 cases]. Neurochirurgie 34:243, 1988.

42. Storrs BB, Humphreys RP, Hendrick EB, et al: Intracranial aneurysms in the pediatric age-group. Childs Brain 9:358, 1982.

43. terBrugge KG: Neurointerventional procedures in the pediatric age group. Childs Nerv Syst 15:751, 1999.

44. Yazbak PA, McComb JG, Raffel C: Pediatric traumatic intracranial aneurysms. Pediatr Neurosurg 22:15, 1995.

45. Locksley HB: Natural history of subarachnoid hemorrhage, intracranial aneurysms and arteriovenous malformations: Based on 6368 cases in the cooperative study. J Neurosurg 25:219, 1966.

46. Locksley HB, Sahs AL, Knowler L: Report on the cooperative study of intracranial aneurysms and subarachnoid hemorrhage. Section II: General survey of cases in the central registry and characteristics of the sample population. J Neurosurg 24:922, 1966.

47. Meyer FB, Sundt TM Jr, Fode NC, et al: Cerebral aneurysms in childhood and adolescence. J Neurosurg 70:420, 1989.

48. Ostergaard JR: A long-term follow-up study of juvenile aneurysm patients. Acta Neurochir (Wien) 77:103, 1985.

49. Ostergaard JR, Voldby B: Intracranial arterial aneurysms in children and adolescents. J Neurosurg 58:832, 1983.

50. Housepian EM, Pool JL: A systematic analysis of intracranial aneurysms from the autopsy file of the Presbyterian Hospital, 1914–1956. J Neuropathol Exp Neurol 17:409, 1958.

51. Biller J, Adams HP Jr: Cerebrovascular disorders associated with pregnancy. Am Fam Physician 33:125, 1986.

52. Hunt HB, Schifrin BS, Suzuki K: Ruptured berry aneurysms and pregnancy. Obstet Gynecol 43:827, 1974.

53. Minielly R, Yuzpe AA, Drake CG: Subarachnoid hemorrhage secondary to ruptured cerebral aneurysm in pregnancy. Obstet Gynecol 53:64, 1979.

54. Barno A, Freeman DW: Maternal deaths due to spontaneous subarachnoid hemorrhage. Am J Obstet Gynecol 125:384, 1976.

55. Fliegner JR, Hooper RS, Kloss M: Subarachnoid haemorrhage and pregnancy. J Obstet Gynaecol Br Commonw 76:912, 1969.

56. Giannotta SL, Daniels J, Golde SH, et al: Ruptured intracranial aneurysms during pregnancy: A report of four cases. J Reprod Med 31:139, 1986.

57. Heidrich R, Niedner K: Pregnancy and subarachnoid haemorrhage. Eur Neurol 3:38, 1970.

58. Piotin M, de Souza Filho CB, Kothimbakam R, et al: Endovascular treatment of acutely ruptured intracranial aneurysms in pregnancy. Am J Obstet Gynecol 185:1261, 2001.

59. Robinson JL, Hall CJ, Sedzimir CB: Subarachnoid hemorrhage in pregnancy. J Neurosurg 36:27, 1972.

60. Robinson JL, Hall CS, Sedzimir CB: Arteriovenous malformations, aneurysms, and pregnancy. J Neurosurg 41:63, 1974.

61. Singer JR, Hummelgard AB, Martin EM: Ruptured aneurysm in pregnancy. J Neurosurg Nurs 17:230, 1985.

62. Stoodley MA, Macdonald RL, Weir BK: Pregnancy and intracranial aneurysms. Neurosurg Clin North Am 9:549, 1998.

63. Witlin AG, Friedman SA, Egerman RS, et al: Cerebrovascular disorders complicating pregnancy—beyond eclampsia. Am J Obstet Gynecol 176:1139, 1997.

64. Pool JL: Treatment of intracranial aneurysms during pregnancy. JAMA 192:209, 1965.

65. Barrow DL, Reisner A: Natural history of intracranial aneurysms and vascular malformations. Clin Neurosurg 40:3, 1993.

66. Newton CL, Bell SD: Arteriovenous malformation in the pregnant patient: A case study. J Neurosci Nurs 27:109, 1995.

67. Wilkins RH: Natural history of intracranial vascular malformations: A review. Neurosurgery 16:421, 1985.

68. D'Haese J, Christiaens F, D'Haens J, et al: Combined cesarean section and clipping of a ruptured cerebral aneurysm: A case report. J Neurosurg Anesthesiol 9:341, 1997.

69. Spike J: Brain death, pregnancy, and posthumous motherhood. J Clin Ethics 10:57, 1999.

70. Rhoton AL Jr: Anatomy of saccular aneurysms. Surg Neurol 14:59, 1980.

71. Rhoton AL Jr, Saeki N, Perlmutter D, et al: Microsurgical anatomy of common aneurysm sites. Clin Neurosurg 26:248, 1979.

72. Rhoton AL: Microsurgical anatomy of saccular aneurysms. In Wilkins RH, Rengachary SS (eds): Neurosurgery. New York, McGraw-Hill, 1996, p 2215.

73. Unruptured intracranial aneurysms—risk of rupture and risks of surgical intervention. International Study of Unruptured Intracranial Aneurysms. N Engl J Med 339:1725, 1998.

74. Andrews RJ, Spiegel PK: Intracranial aneurysms: Age, sex, blood pressure, and multiplicity in an unselected series of patients. J Neurosurg 51:27, 1979.

75. Nehls DG, Flom RA, Carter LP, et al: Multiple intracranial aneurysms: Determining the site of rupture. J Neurosurg 63:342, 1985.

76. Ostergaard JR, Hog E: Incidence of multiple intracranial aneurysms: Influence of arterial hypertension and gender. J Neurosurg 63:49, 1985.

77. Cervoni L, Delfini R, Santoro A, et al: Multiple intracranial aneurysms: Surgical treatment and outcome. Acta Neurochir (Wien) 124:66, 1993.

78. Ellamushi HE, Grieve JP, Jager HR, et al: Risk factors for the formation of multiple intracranial aneurysms. J Neurosurg 94:728, 2001.

79. Juvela S: Risk factors for multiple intracranial aneurysms. Stroke 31:392, 2000.

80. Weir B: Unruptured intracranial aneurysms: A review. J Neurosurg 96:3, 2002.

81. Inagawa T: Multiple intracranial aneurysms in elderly patients. Acta Neurochir (Wien) 106:119, 1990.

82. Martelli N, Colli BO, Assirati JA Jr, et al: Surgical treatment of multiple intracranial aneurysms. Arq Neuropsiquiatr 46:107, 1988.

83. Orz Y, Osawa M, Tanaka Y, et al: Surgical outcome for multiple intracranial aneurysms. Acta Neurochir (Wien) 138:411, 1996.

84. Rinne J, Hernesniemi J, Niskanen M, et al: Management outcome for multiple intracranial aneurysms. Neurosurgery 36:31, 1995.

85. Vajda J, Juhasz J, Orosz E, et al: Surgical treatment of multiple intracranial aneurysms. Acta Neurochir (Wien) 82:14, 1986.

86. Hackney DB, Lesnick JE, Zimmerman RA, et al: MR identification of bleeding site in subarachnoid hemorrhage with multiple intracranial aneurysms. J Comput Assist Tomogr 10:878, 1986.

87. Jaskolski DJ, Zawirski M, Jakubowski J: A clinical evaluation of computed tomography in patients with subarachnoid haemorrhage and multiple intracranial aneurysms. Zentralbl Neurochir 50:138, 1989.

88. Stone JL, Crowell RM, Gandhi YN, et al: Multiple intracranial aneurysms: Magnetic resonance imaging for determination of the site of rupture: Report of a case. Neurosurgery 23:97, 1988.

89. Hino A, Fujimoto M, Iwamoto Y, et al: False localization of rupture site in patients with multiple cerebral aneurysms and subarachnoid hemorrhage. Neurosurgery 46:825, 2000.

90. Lee KC, Joo JY, Lee KS: False localization of rupture by computed tomography in bilateral internal carotid artery aneurysms. Surg Neurol 45:435, 1996.

91. Heiskanen O: Risk of bleeding from unruptured aneurysm in cases with multiple intracranial aneurysms. J Neurosurg 55:524, 1981.

92. Solander S, Ulhoa A, Vinuela F, et al: Endovascular treatment of multiple intracranial aneurysms by using Guglielmi detachable coils. J Neurosurg 90:857, 1999.

93. Bonita R, Thomson S: Subarachnoid hemorrhage: Epidemiology, diagnosis, management, and outcome. Stroke 16:591, 1985.

94. Vapalahti M, Ljunggren B, Saveland H, et al: Early aneurysm operation and outcome in two remote Scandinavian populations. J Neurosurg 60:1160, 1984.

95. Weir B: Aneurysms Affecting the Nervous System. Baltimore, Williams & Wilkins, 1987.

96. Jane JA, Winn HR, Richardson AE: The natural history of intracranial aneurysms: Rebleeding rates during the acute and long term period and implication for surgical management. Clin Neurosurg 24:176, 1977.

97. Jane JA, Kassell NF, Torner JC, et al: The natural history of aneurysms and arteriovenous malformations. J Neurosurg 62:321, 1985.

98. Kassell NF, Drake CG: Timing of aneurysm surgery. Neurosurgery 10:514, 1982.

99. Adams HP Jr, Kassell NF, Kongable GA, et al: Intracranial operation within seven days of aneurysmal subarachnoid hemorrhage: Results in 150 patients. Arch Neurol 45:1065, 1988.

100. Aoyagi N, Hayakawa I: Study on early re-rupture of intracranial aneurysms. Acta Neurochir (Wien) 138:12, 1996.

101. Piepgras DG, Khurana VG, Whisnant JP: Ruptured giant intracranial aneurysms. Part II: A retrospective analysis of timing and outcome of surgical treatment. J Neurosurg 88:430, 1998.

102. Vermeij FH, Hasan D, Bijvoet HW, et al: Impact of medical treatment on the outcome of patients after aneurysmal subarachnoid hemorrhage. Stroke 29:924, 1998.

103. Solenski NJ, Haley EC Jr, Kassell NF, et al: Medical complications of aneurysmal subarachnoid hemorrhage: A report of the multicenter, cooperative aneurysm study. Participants of the Multicenter Cooperative Aneurysm Study. Crit Care Med 23:1007, 1995.

104. Adams CB, Fearnside MR, O'Laoire SA: An investigation with serial angiography into the evolution of cerebral arterial spasm following aneurysm surgery. J Neurosurg 49:805, 1978.

105. Adams HP Jr, Jergenson DD, Kassell NF, et al: Pitfalls in the recognition of subarachnoid hemorrhage. JAMA 244:794, 1980.

106. Adams HP Jr: Prevention of brain ischemia after aneurysmal subarachnoid hemorrhage. Neurol Clin 10:251, 1992.

107. Adams HP Jr, Kassell NF, Torner JC, et al: Predicting cerebral ischemia after aneurysmal subarachnoid hemorrhage: Influences of clinical condition, CT results, and antifibrinolytic therapy: A report of the Cooperative Aneurysm Study. Neurology 37:1586, 1987.

108. Allen GS, Ahn HS, Preziosi TJ, et al: Cerebral arterial spasm—a controlled trial of nimodipine in patients with subarachnoid hemorrhage. N Engl J Med 308:619, 1983.

109. Petruk KC, West M, Mohr G, et al: Nimodipine treatment in poor-grade aneurysm patients: Results of a multicenter double-blind placebo-controlled trial. J Neurosurg 68:505, 1988.

110. Philippon J, Grob R, Dagreou F, et al: Prevention of vasospasm in subarachnoid haemorrhage: A controlled study with nimodipine. Acta Neurochir (Wien) 82:110, 1986.

111. Adams HP Jr: Calcium antagonists in the management of patients with aneurysmal subarachnoid hemorrhage: A review. Angiology 41:1010, 1990.

112. Mayberg MR: Cerebral vasospasm. Neurosurg Clin North Am 9:615, 1998.

113. Shibuya M, Suzuki Y, Sugita K, et al: Effect of AT877 on cerebral vasospasm after aneurysmal subarachnoid hemorrhage: Results of a prospective placebo-controlled double-blind trial. J Neurosurg 76:571, 1992.

114. Wijdicks EF, Ropper AH, Hunnicutt EJ, et al: Atrial natriuretic factor and salt wasting after aneurysmal subarachnoid hemorrhage. Stroke 22:1519, 1991.

115. Wijdicks EF, Vermeulen M, Hijdra A, et al: Hyponatremia and cerebral infarction in patients with ruptured intracranial aneurysms: Is fluid restriction harmful? Ann Neurol 17:137, 1985.

116. Brouwers PJ, Wijdicks EF, Hasan D, et al: Serial electrocardiographic recording in aneurysmal subarachnoid hemorrhage. Stroke 20:1162, 1989.

117. Kuroiwa T, Morita H, Tanabe H, et al: Significance of ST segment elevation in electrocardiograms in patients with ruptured cerebral aneurysms. Acta Neurochir (Wien) 133:141, 1995.

118. Mayer SA, LiMandri G, Sherman D, et al: Electrocardiographic markers of abnormal left ventricular wall motion in acute subarachnoid hemorrhage. J Neurosurg 83:889, 1995.

119. Weir B, Disney L, Grace M, et al: Daily trends in white blood cell count and temperature after subarachnoid hemorrhage from aneurysm. Neurosurgery 25:161, 1989.

120. Fisher CM, Kistler JP, Davis JM: Relation of cerebral vasospasm to subarachnoid hemorrhage visualized by computerized tomographic scanning. Neurosurgery 6:1, 1980.

121. Hunt WE, Hess RM: Surgical risk as related to time of intervention in the repair of intracranial aneurysms. J Neurosurg 28:14, 1968.

122. Kistler JP, Crowell RM, Davis KR, et al: The relation of cerebral vasospasm to the extent and location of subarachnoid blood visualized by CT scan: A prospective study. Neurology 33:424, 1983.

123. Teasdale GM, Drake CG, Hunt W, et al: A universal subarachnoid hemorrhage scale: Report of a committee of the World Federation of Neurosurgical Societies. J Neurol Neurosurg Psychiatry 51:1457, 1988.

124. Bailes JE, Spetzler RF, Hadley MN, et al: Management, morbidity and mortality of poor-grade aneurysm patients. J Neurosurg 72:559, 1990.

125. Le Roux PD, Winn HR: Management of the ruptured aneurysm. Neurosurg Clin North Am 9:525, 1998.

126. Le Roux PD, Elliott JP, Newell DW, et al: Predicting outcome in poor-grade patients with subarachnoid hemorrhage: A retrospective review of 159 aggressively managed cases. J Neurosurg 85:39, 1996.

127. Chyatte D, Fode NC, Sundt TM Jr: Early versus late intracranial aneurysm surgery in subarachnoid hemorrhage. J Neurosurg 69:326, 1988.

128. Disney L, Weir B, Petruk K: Effect on management mortality of a deliberate policy of early operation on supratentorial aneurysms. Neurosurgery 20:695, 1987.

129. Ljunggren B, Brandt L: Timing of aneurysm surgery. Clin Neurosurg 33:159, 1986.

130. Suzuki J, Onuma T, Yoshimoto T: Results of early operations on cerebral aneurysms. Surg Neurol 11:407, 1979.

131. Hugenholtz H, Elgie RG: Considerations in early surgery on good-risk patients with ruptured intracranial aneurysms. J Neurosurg 56:180, 1982.

Therapy

132. Saveland H, Ljunggren B, Brandt L, et al: Delayed ischemic deterioration in patients with early aneurysm operation and intravenous nimodipine. Neurosurgery 18:146, 1986.

133. Weir B, Aronyk K: Management mortality and the timing of surgery for supratentorial aneurysm. J Neurosurg 54:146, 1981.

134. Kassell NF, Torner JC: The International Cooperative study on timing of aneurysm surgery. Acta Neurochir (Wien) 63:119, 1982.

135. Auer LM: Acute operation and preventive nimodipine improve outcome in patients with ruptured cerebral aneurysms. Neurosurgery 15:57, 1984.

136. Auer LM: Preventive nimodipine and acute aneurysm surgery: Heading for the control of complications after aneurysmal subarachnoid hemorrhage. Neurochirurgia (Stuttg) 28(Suppl 1):87, 1985.

137. Auer LM, Brandt L, Ebeling U, et al: Nimodipine and early aneurysm operation in good condition SAH patients. Acta Neurochir (Wien) 82:7, 1986.

138. Ljunggren BC, Brandt JL, Saveland HG: Outcome in patients subjected to early aneurysm operation and intravenous nimodipine. Minerva Med 77:1087, 1986.

139. Ljunggren B, Saveland H, Brandt L, et al: Early operation and overall outcome in aneurysmal subarachnoid hemorrhage. J Neurosurg 62:547, 1985.

140. Ohman J, Heiskanen O: Timing of operation for ruptured supratentorial aneurysms: A prospective randomized study. J Neurosurg 70:55, 1989.

141. Saveland H, Brandt L: Which are the major determinants for outcome in aneurysmal subarachnoid hemorrhage? A prospective total management study from a strictly unselected series. Acta Neurol Scand 90:245, 1994.

142. Le Roux PD, Elliot JP, Newell DW, et al: The incidence of surgical complications is similar in good and poor grade patients undergoing repair of ruptured anterior circulation aneurysms: A retrospective review of 355 patients. Neurosurgery 38:887, 1996.

143. Le Roux PD, Elliott JP, Downey L, et al: Improved outcome after rupture of anterior circulation aneurysms: A retrospective 10-year review of 224 good-grade patients. J Neurosurg 83:394, 1995.

144. Batjer HH, Samson DS: Emergent aneurysm surgery without cerebral angiography for the comatose patient. Neurosurgery 28:283, 1991.

145. Brandt L, Sonesson B, Ljunggren B, et al: Ruptured middle cerebral artery aneurysm with intracerebral hemorrhage in younger patients appearing moribund: Emergency operation? Neurosurgery 20:925, 1987.

146. Nowak G, Schwachenwald R, Arnold H: Early management in poor grade aneurysm patients. Acta Neurochir (Wien) 126:33, 1994.

147. Steudel WI, Reif J, Voges M: Modulated surgery in the management of ruptured intracranial aneurysm in poor grade patients. Neurol Res 16:49, 1994.

148. Ausman JI: The New England Journal of Medicine report on unruptured intracranial aneurysms: A critique. Surg Neurol 51:227, 1999.

149. Ausman JI, Roitberg B: A response from the ISUIA: International Study on Unruptured Intracranial Aneurysms. Surg Neurol 52:428, 1999.

150. Bederson JB, Awad IA, Wiebers DO, et al: Recommendations for the management of patients with unruptured intracranial aneurysms: A statement for healthcare professionals from the Stroke Council of the American Heart Association. Circulation 102:2300, 2000.

151. Berenstein A, Flamm ES, Kupersmith MJ: Unruptured intracranial aneurysms. N Engl J Med 340:1439, 1999.

152. Brennan JW, Schwartz ML: Unruptured intracranial aneurysms: Appraisal of the literature and suggested recommendations for surgery, using evidence-based medicine criteria. Neurosurgery 47:1359, 2000.

153. Brett A: Unruptured intracranial aneurysms. N Engl J Med 340:1441, 1999.

154. Broderick JP: Coiling, clipping, or medical management of unruptured intracranial aneurysms: Time to randomize? Ann Neurol 48:5, 2000.

155. Connolly ES Jr, Mohr JP, Solomon RA: Unruptured intracranial aneurysms. N Engl J Med 340:1440, 1999.

156. Caplan LR: Should intracranial aneurysms be treated before they rupture? N Engl J Med 339:1774, 1998.

157. Solomon RA, Fink ME, Pile-Spellman J: Surgical management of unruptured intracranial aneurysms. J Neurosurg 80:440, 1994.

158. Stieg PE, Friedlander R: Unruptured intracranial aneurysms. N Engl J Med 340:1441, 1999.

159. Tsutsumi K, Ueki K, Morita A, et al: Risk of rupture from incidental cerebral aneurysms. J Neurosurg 93:550, 2000.

160. Wiebers DO, Piepgras DG, Brown RD Jr, et al: Unruptured aneurysms. J Neurosurg 96:50, 2002.

161. Winn HR, Jane JA Sr, Taylor J, et al: Prevalence of asymptomatic incidental aneurysms: Review of 4568 arteriograms. J Neurosurg 96:43, 2002.

162. Piepgras DG: Unruptured aneurysms. J Neurosurg 96:63, 2002.

163. Juvela S, Porras M, Poussa K: Natural history of unruptured intracranial aneurysms: Probability of and risk factors for aneurysm rupture. J Neurosurg 93:379, 2000.

164. Wiebers DO: Natural history of unruptured intracranial aneurysms. Operative Techniques in Neurosurgery 3:166, 2000.

165. Piepgras DG, Kassell NF, Torner J: A response from the ISUIA. Surg Neurol 52:428, 1999.

166. Connolly ES Jr, Solomon RA: Management of symptomatic and asymptomatic unruptured aneurysms. Neurosurg Clin North Am 9:509, 1998.

167. Johnston SC, Gress DR, Kahn JG: Which unruptured cerebral aneurysms should be treated? A cost-utility analysis. Neurology 52:1806, 1999.

168. Juvela S: Recommendations for the management of patients with unruptured intracranial aneurysms. Stroke 32:815, 2001.

169. Kobayashi S, Orz Y, George B, et al: Treatment of unruptured cerebral aneurysms. Surg Neurol 51:355, 1999.

170. Mitchell P, Jakubowski J: Risk analysis of treatment of unruptured aneurysms. J Neurol Neurosurg Psychiatry 68:577, 2000.

171. Orz YI, Hongo K, Tanaka Y, et al: Risks of surgery for patients with unruptured intracranial aneurysms. Surg Neurol 53:21, 2000.

172. Raaymakers TW, Rinkel GJ, Limburg M, et al: Mortality and morbidity of surgery for unruptured intracranial aneurysms: A meta-analysis. Stroke 29:1531, 1998.

173. Riina HA, Spetzler RF: Unruptured aneurysms. J Neurosurg 96:61, 2002.

174. Dumont AS, Lanzino G, Kassell NF: Unruptured aneurysms. J Neurosurg 96:52, 2002.

175. Sarner M, Crawford MD: Ruptured intracranial aneurysm: Clinical series. Lancet 2:1251, 1965.

176. Scott BA, Weinstein z, Pulliam MW: Computed tomographic diagnosis of ruptured giant posterior cerebral artery aneurysms. Neurosurgery 22:553, 1988.

177. Naff NJ: Intraventricular hemorrhage in adults. Curr Treat Options Neurol 1:173, 1999.

178. Yoshimoto Y, Wakai S, Satoh A, et al: Intraparenchymal and intrasylvian haematomas secondary to ruptured middle cerebral artery aneurysms: Prognostic factors and therapeutic considerations. Br J Neurosurg 13:18, 1999.

179. Kallmes DF, Lanzino G, Dix JE, et al: Patterns of hemorrhage with ruptured posterior inferior cerebellar artery aneurysms: CT findings in 44 cases. AJR Am J Roentgenol 169:1169, 1997.

180. Ishibashi A, Yokokura Y, Sakamoto M: Acute subdural hematoma without subarachnoid hemorrhage due to ruptured intracranial aneurysm—case report. Neurol Med Chir (Tokyo) 37:533, 1997.

181. Kraus GE, Herman JM, Marciano F, et al: Ruptured giant aneurysm of an occluded middle cerebral artery in a severe-grade patient: Case report. Neurosurgery 36:169, 1995.

182. Barami K, Ko K: Ruptured mycotic aneurysm presenting as an intraparenchymal hemorrhage and nonadjacent acute subdural hematoma: Case report and review of the literature. Surg Neurol 41:290, 1994.

183. Sadato N, Numaguchi Y, Rigamonti D, et al: Bleeding patterns in ruptured posterior fossa aneurysms: A CT study. J Comput Assist Tomogr 15:612, 1991.

184. Adams HP Jr, Kassell NF, Torner JC, et al: CT and clinical correlations in recent aneurysmal subarachnoid hemorrhage: A preliminary report of the Cooperative Aneurysm Study. Neurology 33:981, 1983.

185. Alberico RA, Patel M, Casey S, et al: Evaluation of the circle of Willis with three-dimensional CT angiography in patients with suspected intracranial aneurysms. AJNR Am J Neuroradiol 16:1571, 1995.

186. Alberico RA, Ozsvath R, Casey S, et al: Helical CT angiography for the detection of intracranial aneurysms. AJNR Am J Neuroradiol 17:1002, 1996.

187. Baxter AB, Cohen WA, Maravilla KR: Imaging of intracranial aneurysms and subarachnoid hemorrhage. Neurosurg Clin North Am 9:445, 1998.

188. Gonzalez-Darder JM, Pesudo-Martinez JV, Feliu-Tatay RA: Microsurgical management of cerebral aneurysms based in CT angiography with three-dimensional reconstruction (3D-CTA) and without preoperative cerebral angiography. Acta Neurochir (Wien) 143:673, 2001.

189. Hashimoto H, Iida J, Hironaka Y, et al: Use of spiral computerized tomography angiography in patients with subarachnoid hemorrhage in whom subtraction angiography did not reveal cerebral aneurysms. J Neurosurg 92:278, 2000.

190. Hirai T, Korogi Y, Ono K, et al: Preoperative evaluation of intracranial aneurysms: Usefulness of intraarterial 3D CT angiography and conventional angiography with a combined unit—initial experience. Radiology 220:499, 2001.

191. Lenhart M, Bretschneider T, Gmeinwieser J, et al: Cerebral CT angiography in the diagnosis of acute subarachnoid hemorrhage. Acta Radiol 38:791, 1997.

192. Matsumoto M, Sato M, Nakano M, et al: Three-dimensional computerized tomography angiography-guided surgery of acutely ruptured cerebral aneurysms. J Neurosurg 94:718, 2001.

193. Seruga T, Bunc G, Klein GE: Helical high-resolution volume-rendered 3-dimensional computer tomography angiography in the detection of intracranial aneurysms. J Neuroimaging 11:280, 2001.

194. Tampieri D, Leblanc R, Oleszek J, et al: Three-dimensional computed tomographic angiography of cerebral aneurysms. Neurosurgery 36:749, 1995.

195. Velthuis BK, Rinkel GJ, Ramos LM, et al: Subarachnoid hemorrhage: Aneurysm detection and preoperative evaluation with CT angiography. Radiology 208:423, 1998.

196. Velthuis BK, Van Leeuwen MS, Witkamp TD, et al: Computerized tomography angiography in patients with subarachnoid hemorrhage: From aneurysm detection to treatment without conventional angiography. J Neurosurg 91:761, 1999.

197. Vieco PT: CT angiography of the intracranial circulation. Neuroimaging Clin North Am 8:577, 1998.

198. Young N, Dorsch NW, Kingston RJ, et al: Intracranial aneurysms: Evaluation in 200 patients with spiral CT angiography. Eur Radiol 11:123, 2001.

199. Le Roux PD, Dailey AT, Newell DW, et al: Emergent aneurysm clipping without angiography in the moribund patient with intracerebral hemorrhage: The use of infusion computed tomography scans. Neurosurgery 33:189, 1993.

200. Rinkel GJ, van Gijn J, Wijdicks EF: Subarachnoid hemorrhage without detectable aneurysm: A review of the causes. Stroke 24:1403, 1993.

201. Rinkel GJ, Wijdicks EF, Hasan D, et al: Outcome in patients with subarachnoid haemorrhage and negative angiography according to pattern of haemorrhage on computed tomography. Lancet 338:964, 1991.

202. du Mesnil de Rochemont R, Heindel W, Wesselmann C, et al: Nontraumatic subarachnoid hemorrhage: Value of repeat angiography. Radiology 202:798, 1997.

203. Duong H, Melancon D, Tampieri D, et al: The negative angiogram in subarachnoid haemorrhage. Neuroradiology 38:15, 1996.

204. Rinkel GJ, Wijdicks EF, Vermeulen M, et al: Nonaneurysmal perimesencephalic subarachnoid hemorrhage: CT and MR patterns that differ from aneurysmal rupture. AJNR Am J Neuroradiol 12:829, 1991.

205. Cioffi F, Pasqualin A, Cavazzani P, et al: Subarachnoid haemorrhage of unknown origin: Clinical and tomographical aspects. Acta Neurochir (Wien) 97:31, 1989.

206. Juvela S: Minor leak before rupture of an intracranial aneurysm and subarachnoid hemorrhage of unknown etiology. Neurosurgery 30:7, 1992.

207. Schwartz TH, Solomon RA: Perimesencephalic nonaneurysmal subarachnoid hemorrhage: Review of the literature. Neurosurgery 39:433, 1996.

208. Gomez PA, Lobato RD, Rivas JJ, et al: Subarachnoid haemorrhage of unknown aetiology. Acta Neurochir (Wien) 101:35, 1989.

209. Rinkel GJ, Wijdicks EF, Vermeulen M, et al: The clinical course of perimesencephalic nonaneurysmal subarachnoid hemorrhage. Ann Neurol 29:463, 1991.

210. Hamilton MG, Williams FC: Perioperative management of subarachnoid hemorrhage. In Carter LP, Spetzler R, Hamilton MG (eds): Neurovascular Surgery. New York, McGraw-Hill, 1994, p 603.

211. Dangor AA, Lam AM: Anesthesia for cerebral aneurysm surgery. Neurosurg Clin North Am 9:647, 1998.

212. Torner JC, Kassell NF, Wallace RB, et al: Preoperative prognostic factors for rebleeding and survival in aneurysm patients receiving antifibrinolytic therapy: Report of the Cooperative Aneurysm Study. Neurosurgery 9:506, 1981.

213. Barker FG 2nd, Ogilvy CS: Efficacy of prophylactic nimodipine for delayed ischemic deficit after subarachnoid hemorrhage: A meta-analysis. J Neurosurg 84:405, 1996.

214. McKhann GM 2nd, Le Roux PD: Perioperative and intensive care unit care of patients with aneurysmal subarachnoid hemorrhage. Neurosurg Clin North Am 9:595, 1998.

215. Awad IA, Carter LP, Spetzler RF, et al: Clinical vasospasm after subarachnoid hemorrhage: Response to hypervolemic hemodilution and arterial hypertension. Stroke 18:365, 1987.

216. Kassell NF, Peerless SJ, Durward QJ, et al: Treatment of ischemic deficits from vasospasm with intravascular volume expansion and induced arterial hypertension. Neurosurgery 11:337, 1982.

217. Origitano TC, Wascher TM, Reichman OH, et al: Sustained increased cerebral blood flow with prophylactic hypertensive hypervolemic hemodilution ("triple-H" therapy) after subarachnoid hemorrhage. Neurosurgery 27:729, 1990.

218. Sloan MA, Haley EC Jr, Kassell NF, et al: Sensitivity and specificity of transcranial Doppler ultrasonography in the diagnosis of vasospasm following subarachnoid hemorrhage. Neurology 39:1514, 1989.

219. Harrison MJ: Influence of haematocrit in the cerebral circulation. Cerebrovasc Brain Metab Rev 1:55, 1989.

220. Graff-Radford NR, Torner J, Adams HP Jr, et al: Factors associated with hydrocephalus after subarachnoid hemorrhage: A report of the Cooperative Aneurysm Study. Arch Neurol 46:744, 1989.

221. Kosteljanetz M: CSF dynamics in patients with subarachnoid and/or intraventricular hemorrhage. J Neurosurg 60:940, 1984.

222. Nornes H, Magnaes B: Intracranial pressure in patients with ruptured saccular aneurysm. J Neurosurg 36:537, 1972.

223. Voldby B, Enevoldsen EM: Intracranial pressure changes following aneurysm rupture. Part 1: Clinical and angiographic correlations. J Neurosurg 56:186, 1982.

224. Voldby B, Enevoldsen EM: Intracranial pressure changes following aneurysm rupture. Part 3: Recurrent hemorrhage. J Neurosurg 56:784, 1982.

225. Voldby B, Enevoldsen EM: Intracranial pressure changes following aneurysm rupture. Part 2: Associated cerebrospinal fluid lactacidosis. J Neurosurg 56:197, 1982.

226. Hasan D, Vermeulen M, Wijdicks EF, et al: Management problems in acute hydrocephalus after subarachnoid hemorrhage. Stroke 20:747, 1989.

227. Milhorat TH: Acute hydrocephalus after aneurysmal subarachnoid hemorrhage. Neurosurgery 20:15, 1987.

228. Rajshekhar V, Harbaugh RE: Results of routine ventriculostomy with external ventricular drainage for acute hydrocephalus following subarachnoid haemorrhage. Acta Neurochir (Wien) 115:8, 1992.

229. Mohr G, Ferguson G, Khan M, et al: Intraventricular hemorrhage from ruptured aneurysm: Retrospective analysis of 91 cases. J Neurosurg 58:482, 1983.

230. van Gijn J, Hijdra A, Wijdicks EF, et al: Acute hydrocephalus after aneurysmal subarachnoid hemorrhage. J Neurosurg 63:355, 1985.

230a. Alleyne CH, Hassan M, Azbramski JM: The efficacy and cost of prophylactic versus periprocedural antibiotics in patients with external ventricular drains. Neurosurgery 47:1124–1129, 2000.

231. Lyke KE, Obasanjo OO, Williams MA, et al: Ventriculitis complicating use of intraventricular catheters in adult neurosurgical patients. Clin Infect Dis 33:2028, 2001.

232. Rebuck JA, Murry KR, Rhoney DH, et al: Infection related to intracranial pressure monitors in adults: Analysis of risk factors and antibiotic prophylaxis. J Neurol Neurosurg Psychiatry 69:381, 2000.

233. Hader WJ, Steinbok P: The value of routine cultures of the cerebrospinal fluid in patients with external ventricular drains. Neurosurgery 46:1149, 2000.

234. Holloway KL, Barnes T, Choi S, et al: Ventriculostomy infections: The effect of monitoring duration and catheter exchange in 584 patients. J Neurosurg 85:419, 1996.

235. Diringer M, Ladenson PW, Stern BJ, et al: Plasma atrial natriuretic factor and subarachnoid hemorrhage. Stroke 19:1119, 1988.

236. Hasan D, Wijdicks EF, Vermeulen M: Hyponatremia is associated with cerebral ischemia in patients with aneurysmal subarachnoid hemorrhage. Ann Neurol 27:106, 1990.

237. Wijdicks EF, Vermeulen M, ten Haaf JA, et al: Volume depletion and natriuresis in patients with a ruptured intracranial aneurysm. Ann Neurol 18:211, 1985.

238. Wijdicks EF, Vermeulen M, van Gijn J: Hyponatraemia and volume status in aneurysmal subarachnoid haemorrhage. Acta Neurochir (Wien) Suppl 47:111, 1990.

239. Doczi T, Joo F, Vecsernyes M, et al: Increased concentration of atrial natriuretic factor in the cerebrospinal fluid of patients with aneurysmal subarachnoid hemorrhage and raised intracranial pressure. Neurosurgery 23:16, 1988.

240. Rosenfeld JV, Barnett GH, Sila CA, et al: The effect of subarachnoid hemorrhage on blood and CSF atrial natriuretic factor. J Neurosurg 71:32, 1989.

241. Shimoda M, Yamada S, Yamamoto I, et al: Atrial natriuretic polypeptide in patients with subarachnoid haemorrhage due to aneurysmal rupture: Correlation to hyponatremia. Acta Neurochir (Wien) 97:53, 1989.

242. Mori K, Arai H, Nakajima K, et al: Hemorheological and hemodynamic analysis of hypervolemic hemodilution therapy for cerebral vasospasm after aneurysmal subarachnoid hemorrhage. Stroke 26:1620, 1995.

243. Solomon RA, Fink ME, Lennihan L: Early aneurysm surgery and prophylactic hypervolemic hypertensive therapy for the treatment of aneurysmal subarachnoid hemorrhage. Neurosurgery 23:699, 1988.

244. Hasan D, Vermeulen M, Wijdicks EF, et al: Effect of fluid intake and antihypertensive treatment on cerebral ischemia after subarachnoid hemorrhage. Stroke 20:1511, 1989.

245. Fodstad H: Antifibrinolytic treatment in subarachnoid haemorrhage: Present state. Acta Neurochir (Wien) 63:233, 1982.

246. Kassell NF, Haley EC, Torner JC: Antifibrinolytic therapy in the treatment of aneurysmal subarachnoid hemorrhage. Clin Neurosurg 33:137, 1986.

247. Vermeulen M, Lindsay KW, Murray GD, et al: Antifibrinolytic treatment in subarachnoid hemorrhage. N Engl J Med 311:432, 1984.

248. Pinna G, Pasqualin A, Vivenza C, et al: Rebleeding, ischaemia and hydrocephalus following anti-fibrinolytic treatment for ruptured cerebral aneurysms: A retrospective clinical study. Acta Neurochir (Wien) 93:77, 1988.

249. Dernbach PD, Little JR, Jones SC, et al: Altered cerebral autoregulation and CO2 reactivity after aneurysmal subarachnoid hemorrhage. Neurosurgery 22:822, 1988.

250. Hitchcock ER, Tsementzis SA, Dow AA: Short- and long-term prognosis of patients with a subarachnoid haemorrhage in relation to intra-operative period of hypotension. Acta Neurochir (Wien) 70:235, 1984.

251. Voldby B, Enevoldsen EM, Jensen FT: Regional CBF, intraventricular pressure, and cerebral metabolism in patients with ruptured intracranial aneurysms. J Neurosurg 62:48, 1985.

252. Voldby B, Enevoldsen EM, Jensen FT: Cerebrovascular reactivity in patients with ruptured intracranial aneurysms. J Neurosurg 62:59, 1985.

253. Ishii R: Regional cerebral blood flow in patients with ruptured intracranial aneurysms. J Neurosurg 50:587, 1979.

254. Tenjin H, Hirakawa K, Mizukawa N, et al: Dysautoregulation in patients with ruptured aneurysms: Cerebral blood flow measurements obtained during surgery by a temperature-controlled thermoelectrical method. Neurosurgery 23:705, 1988.

255. Ausman JI, Diaz FG, Malik GM, et al: Management of cerebral aneurysms: Further facts and additional myths. Surg Neurol 32:21, 1989.

256. Ausman JI, Diaz FG, Malik GM, et al: Current management of cerebral aneurysms: Is it based on facts or myths? Surg Neurol 24:625, 1985.

257. Jabre A, Symon L: Temporary vascular occlusion during aneurysm surgery. Surg Neurol 27:47, 1987.

258. Samson D, Batjer HH, Bowman G, et al: A clinical study of the parameters and effects of temporary arterial occlusion in the management of intracranial aneurysms. Neurosurgery 34:22, 1994.

259. McDermott MW, Durity FA, Borozny M, et al: Temporary vessel occlusion and barbiturate protection in cerebral aneurysm surgery. Neurosurgery 25:54, 1989.

260. Mizoi K, Yoshimoto T: Permissible temporary occlusion time in aneurysm surgery as evaluated by evoked potential monitoring. Neurosurgery 33:434, 1993.

261. Ogilvy CS, Carter BS, Kaplan S, et al: Temporary vessel occlusion for aneurysm surgery: Risk factors for stroke in patients protected by induced hypothermia and hypertension and intravenous mannitol administration. J Neurosurg 84:785, 1996.

262. Batjer H, Samson D: Intraoperative aneurysmal rupture: Incidence, outcome, and suggestions for surgical management. Neurosurgery 18:701, 1986.

263. Lavine SD, Masri LS, Levy ML, et al: Temporary occlusion of the middle cerebral artery in intracranial aneurysm surgery: Time limitation and advantage of brain protection. J Neurosurg 87:817, 1997.

264. Branston NM, Hope DT, Symon L: Barbiturates in focal ischemia of primate cortex: Effects on blood flow distribution, evoked potential and extracellular potassium. Stroke 10:647, 1979.

265. Hoff JT, Pitts LH, Spetzler R, et al: Barbiturates for protection from cerebral ischemia in aneurysm surgery. Acta Neurol Scand Suppl 64:158, 1977.

266. Selman WR, Spetzler RF: Therapeutics for focal cerebral ischemia. Neurosurgery 6:446, 1980.

267. Selman WR, Spetzler RF, Anton AH, et al: Management of prolonged therapeutic barbiturate coma. Surg Neurol 15:9, 1981.

268. Selman WR, Spetzler RF, Roessmann UR, et al: Barbiturate-induced coma therapy for focal cerebral ischemia: Effect after temporary and permanent MCA occlusion. J Neurosurg 55:220, 1981.

269. Selman WR, Spetzler RF, Roski RA: Barbiturate resuscitation from focal cerebral ischemia—a review. Resuscitation 9:189, 1981.

270. Selman WR, Spetzler RF, Roski RA, et al: Barbiturate coma in focal cerebral ischemia: Relationship of protection to timing of therapy. J Neurosurg 56:685, 1982.

271. Batjer HH, Kopitnik TA, Giller CA, et al: Surgery for paraclinoidal carotid artery aneurysms. J Neurosurg 80:650, 1994.

272. Cawley CM, Zipfel GJ, Day AL: Surgical treatment of paraclinoid and ophthalmic aneurysms. Neurosurg Clin North Am 9:765, 1998.

273. Day AL: Aneurysms of the ophthalmic segment: A clinical and anatomical analysis. J Neurosurg 72:677, 1990.

274. Day AL: Clinicoanatomic features of supraclinoid aneurysms. Clin Neurosurg 36:256, 1990.

275. Gibo H, Lenkey C, Rhoton AL Jr: Microsurgical anatomy of the supraclinoid portion of the internal carotid artery. J Neurosurg 55:560, 1981.

276. Heros RC, Nelson PB, Ojemann RG, et al: Large and giant paraclinoid aneurysms: Surgical techniques, complications, and results. Neurosurgery 12:153, 1983.

277. Oikawa S, Kyoshima K, Kobayashi S: Surgical anatomy of the juxtadural ring area. J Neurosurg 89:250, 1998.

278. Pikus HJ, Heros RC: Surgical treatment of internal carotid and posterior communicating artery aneurysms. Neurosurg Clin North Am 9:785, 1998.

279. Day AL, Morcos JJ, Revilla F: Management of aneurysms of the anterior circulation. In Youmans JR (ed): Neurological Surgery: A Comprehensive Guide to the Diagnosis and Management of Neurosurgical Problems, 4th ed. Philadelphia, WB Saunders, 1996, p 1272.

280. Ohno K, Monma S, Suzuki R, et al: Saccular aneurysms of the distal anterior cerebral artery. Neurosurgery 27:907, 1990.

281. Yasargil MG: Microneurosurgery. Clinical Considerations, Surgery of Intracranial Aneurysms, and Results. New York, GT Verlag, 1984, vol 2.

282. Yasargil MG, Carter LP: Saccular aneurysms of the distal anterior cerebral artery. J Neurosurg 40:218, 1974.

283. Drake CG: Giant intracranial aneurysms: Experience with surgical treatment in 174 patients. Clin Neurosurg 26:12, 1979.

284. Peerless SJ, Drake CG: Posterior circulation aneurysms. In Rengachary SS (ed): Neurosurgery. New York, McGraw-Hill, 1985, p 1422.

285. Peerless SJ, Drake CG: Management of aneurysms of the posterior circulation. In Youmans JR (ed): Neurological Surgery: A Comprehensive Guide to the Diagnosis and Management of Neurosurgical Problems, 3rd ed. Philadelphia, WB Saunders, 1990, p 1764.

286. Wright DC, Wilson CB: Surgical treatment of basilar aneurysms. Neurosurgery 5:325, 1979.

287. Drake CG: Bleeding aneurysms of the basilar artery: Direct surgical management in four cases. J Neurosurg 26:335, 1961.

288. Drake CG: Surgical treatment of ruptured aneurysms of the basilar artery: Experience with 14 cases. J Neurosurg 23:457, 1965.

289. Drake CG: Further experience with surgical treatment of aneurysm of the basilar artery. J Neurosurg 29:372, 1968.

290. Drake CG: The surgical treatment of aneurysms of the basilar artery. J Neurosurg 29:436, 1968.

291. Drake CG: The treatment of aneurysms of the posterior circulation. Clin Neurosurg 26:96, 1979.

292. Yasargil MG, Fox JL: The microsurgical approach to intracranial aneurysms. Surgical Neurology 3:7, 1975.

293. Yasargil MG, Antic J, Laciga R, et al: Microsurgical pterional approach to aneurysms of the basilar bifurcation. Surg Neurol 6:83, 1976.

294. al-Mefty O: Supraorbital-pterional approach to skull base lesions. Neurosurgery 21:474, 1987.

295. Fujitsu K, Kuwabara T: Zygomatic approach for lesions in the interpeduncular cistern. J Neurosurg 62:340, 1985.

296. Hakuba A, Liu S, Nishimura S: The orbitozygomatic infratemporal approach: A new surgical technique. Surg Neurol 26:271, 1986.

297. Hakuba A, Tanaka K, Suzuki T, et al: A combined orbitozygomatic infratemporal epidural and subdural approach for lesions involving the entire cavernous sinus. J Neurosurg 71:699, 1989.

298. Ikeda K, Yamashita J, Hashimoto M: Orbitozygomatic temporopolar approach for a high basilar tip aneurysm associated with a short intracranial internal carotid artery: A new surgical approach. Neurosurgery 29:105, 1991.

299. Jane JA, Park TS, Pobereskin LH, et al: The supraorbital approach: Technical note. Neurosurgery 11:537, 1982.

300. Lee JP, Tsai MS, Chen YR: Orbitozygmatic infratemporal approach to lateral skull base tumors. Acta Neurol Scand 87:403, 1993.

301. McDermott MW, Durity FA, Rootman J, et al: Combined frontotemporal-orbitozygomatic approach for tumors of the sphenoid wing and orbit. Neurosurgery 26:107, 1990.

302. Sano K: Temporo-polar approach to aneurysms of the basilar artery at and around the distal bifurcation: Technical note. Neurol Res 2:361, 1980.

303. Sekhar LH, Kalia KK, Yonas H, et al: Cranial base approaches to intracranial aneurysms in the subarachnoid space. Neurosurgery 35:472, 1994.

304. Uttley D, Archer DJ, Marsh HT, et al: Improved access to lesions of the central skull base by mobilization of the zygoma: Experience with 54 cases. Neurosurgery 28:99, 1991.

305. Lawton MT, Daspit CP, Spetzler RF: Technical aspect and recent trends in the management of large and giant midbasilar aneurysms. Neurosurgery 41:513, 1997.

306. Zabramski JM, Kiris T, Sankhla SK, et al: Orbitozygomatic craniotomy: Technical note. J Neurosurg 89:336, 1998.

307. al-Mefty O, Anand VK: Zygomatic approach to skull-base lesions. J Neurosurg 73:668, 1990.

308. Dolenc VV: Anatomy and Surgery of the Cavernous Sinus. New York, Springer-Verlag, 1989.

309. Day JD, Fukushima T, Giannotta SL: Cranial base approaches to posterior circulation aneurysms. J Neurosurg 87:544, 1997.

310. Day JD, Fukushima T, Giannotta SL: Microanatomical study of the extradural middle fossa approach to the petroclival and posterior cavernous sinus region: Description of the rhomboid construct. Neurosurgery 34:1009, 1994.

311. Kopitnik TA: Temporary arterial occlusion for giant intracranial aneurysms: Indications and limitations. Tech Neurosurg 4:99, 1998.

312. Nutik SL: Pterional craniotomy via a transcavernous approach for the treatment of low-lying distal basilar artery aneurysms. J Neurosurg 89:921, 1998.

313. Dolenc VV, Skrap M, Sustersic J, et al: A transcavernous-transsellar approach to the basilar tip aneurysms. Br J Neurosurg 1:251, 1987.

314. Brackman DE, Hitselberger WE: Retrolabyrinthine approach: Technique and newer indications. Laryngoscope 88:286, 1978.

315. Sekhar LN, Bucur SD: Cranial base approaches to large and giant aneurysms. Tech Neurosurg 4:133, 1998.

316. Spetzler RF, Hamilton MG, Daspit CP: Petroclival lesions. Clin Neurosurg 41:62, 1994.

317. Morrison AW, King TT: Experiences with a translabyrinthine-transtentorial approach to the cerebello-pontine angle. J Neurosurg 38:382, 1973.

318. House WF: Translabyrinthine approach. In Luetje CM (ed): Acoustic Tumors. Baltimore, University Park, 1979, p 43.

319. Brackmann DE, Green JD: Translabyrinthine approach for acoustic tumor removal. Otolaryngol Clin North Am 25:311, 1992.

320. House WF, Hitselberger WE: The transcochlear approach to the skull base. Arch Otolaryngol 102:334, 1976.

321. Lawton MT, Daspit CP, Spetzler RF: Transpetrosal and combination approaches to skull base lesions. Clin Neurosurg 43:91, 1996.

322. Giannotta SL, Maceri DR: Retrolabyrinthine transsigmoid approach to basilar trunk and vertebrobasilar artery junction aneurysms: Technical note. J Neurosurg 69:461, 1988.

323. Spetzler RF, Daspit CP, Pappas CT: The combined supra- and infratentorial approach for lesions of the petrous and clival regions: Experience with 46 cases. J Neurosurg 76:588, 1992.

324. Hitselberger WE, House WF: A combined approach to the cerebellopontine angle: A suboccipital-petrosal approach. Arch Otolaryngol 84:267, 1966.

325. House W: Surgical exposure of the internal auditory canal and its contents through the middle cranial fossa. Laryngoscope 71:1363, 1961.

326. House WF, Shelton C: Middle fossa approach for acoustic tumor removal. Otolaryngol Clin North Am 25:347, 1992.

327. Brackmann DE, House JR 3rd, Hitselberger WE: Technical modifications to the middle fossa craniotomy approach in removal of acoustic neuromas. Am J Otol 15:614, 1994.

328. Kawase T, Toya S, Shiobara R, et al: Transpetrosal approach for aneurysms of the lower basilar artery. J Neurosurg 63:857, 1985.

329. MacDonald JD, Antonelli P, Day AL: The anterior subtemporal, medial transpetrosal approach to the upper basilar artery and pontomesencephalic junction. Neurosurgery 43:84, 1998.

330. Kawase T, Toya S, Shiobara R, et al: Transpetrosal approach for aneurysms of the lower basilar artery. J Neurosurg 63:857, 1985.

331. Hadley MN, Spetzler RF, Sonntag VK: The transoral approach to the superior cervical spine: A review of 53 cases of extradural cervicomedullary compression. J Neurosurg 71:16, 1989.

332. Menezes AH, van Gilder JC: Transoral-transpharyngeal approach to the anterior craniocervical junction: 10 year experience with 72 patients. J Neurosurg 69:895, 1988.

333. Ogilvy CS, Barker FG 2nd, Joseph MP, et al: Transfacial transclival approach for midline posterior circulation aneurysms. Neurosurgery 39:736, 1996.

334. Crockard HA, Koksel T, Watkin N: Transoral transclival clipping of anterior inferior cerebellar artery aneurysm using new rotating applier: Technical note. J Neurosurg 75:483, 1991.

335. Crockard HA: The transoral approach to the base of the brain and upper cervical cord. Ann R Coll Surg Engl 67:321, 1985.

336. de Oliveira E, Rhoton AL Jr, Peace D: Microsurgical anatomy of the region of the foramen magnum. Surg Neurol 24:293, 1985.

337. Heros RC: Lateral suboccipital approach for vertebral and vertebrobasilar artery lesions. J Neurosurg 64:559, 1986.

338. Spetzler RF, Grahm T: The far-lateral approach to the inferior clivus and the upper cervical region: Technical note. BNI Q 6:35, 1990.

339. Sen CN, Sekhar LN: An extreme lateral approach to the intradural lesions of he cervical spine and foramen magnum. Neurosurgery 27:197, 1990.

340. Wen HT, Rhoton AL, Katsuta T, et al: Microsurgical anatomy of the transcondylar, supracondylar, and paracondylar extensions of the far lateral approach. J Neurosurg 87:555, 1997.

341. George B, Dematons C, Cophigon J: Lateral approach to the anterior portion of the foramen magnum: Application to surgical removal of 14 benign tumors: Technical note. Surg Neurol 29:484, 1988.

342. Tedeschi H, Rhoton AL: Lateral approaches to the petroclival region. Surg Neurol 41:180, 1994.

343. Baldwin HZ, Spetzler RF, Wascher TM, et al: The far lateral-combined supra- and infratentorial approach: Clinical experience. Acta Neurochir (Wien) 134:155, 1995.

344. Baldwin HZ, Miller CG, van Loveren HR, et al: The far lateral/combined supra- and infratentorial approach: A human cadaveric prosection model for routes of access to the petroclival region and ventral brain stem. J Neurosurg 81:60, 1994.

345. Chun JY, Smith W, Halbach VV, et al: Current multimodality management of infectious intracranial aneurysms. Neurosurgery 48:1203, 2001.

346. Molinari GF, Smith L, Goldstein MN, et al: Pathogenesis of cerebral mycotic aneurysms. Neurology 23:325, 1973.

347. Morley TP, Barr HW: Giant intracranial aneurysms: Diagnosis, course, and management. Clin Neurosurg 16:73, 1969.

348. Whittle IR, Dorsch NW, Besser M: Giant intracranial aneurysms: Diagnosis, management, and outcome. Surg Neurol 21:218, 1984.

349. Pia HW, Zierski J: Giant cerebral aneurysms. Neurosurg Rev 5:117, 1982.
350. Anson JA, Lawton MT, Spetzler RF: Characteristics and surgical treatment of dolichoectatic and fusiform aneurysms. J Neurosurg 84:185, 1996.
351. Hayes WT, Bernhardt H, Young JM: Fusiform arteriosclerotic aneurysm of the basilar artery: Five cases including two ruptures. Vasc Surg 1:171, 1967.
352. Lawton MT, Spetzler RF: Surgical management of giant intracranial aneurysms: Experience with 171 patients. Clin Neurosurg 42:245, 1995.
353. Lawton MT, Spetzler RF: Surgical strategies for giant intracranial aneurysms. Neurosurg Clin North Am 9:725, 1998.
354. Drake CG, Peerless SJ: Giant fusiform intracranial aneurysms: Review of 120 patients treated surgically from 1965 to 1992. J Neurosurg 87:141, 1997.
355. Dandy WE: Intracranial Arterial Aneurysms. New York, Hafner, 1944.
356. Resta M, Gentile MA, Di Cuonzo F, et al: Clinical-angiographic correlations in 132 patients with megadolichovertebrobasilar anomaly. Neuroradiology 26:213, 1984.
357. Stehbens WE: Pathology of the Cerebral Blood Vessels. St. Louis, CV Mosby, 1972, p 351.
358. Anson JA: Treatment strategies for intracranial fusiform aneurysms. Neurosurg Clin North Am 9:743, 1998.
359. Little JR, St. Louis P, Weinstein M, et al: Giant fusiform aneurysm of the cerebral arteries. Stroke 12:183, 1981.
360. Yu YL, Moseley IF, Pullicino P, et al: The clinical picture of ectasia of the intracerebral arteries. J Neurol Neurosurg Psychiatry 45:29, 1982.
361. Suzuki S, Takahashi T, Ohkuma H, et al: Management of giant serpentine aneurysms of the middle cerebral artery—review of literature and report of a case successfully treated by STA-MCA anastomosis only. Acta Neurochir 117:23, 1992.
362. Yasargil MG: Microneurosurgery, vol I: Pathological Considerations. New York, Thieme-Stratton, 1984, p 279.
363. Courville CB: Arteriosclerotic aneurysms of the circle of Willis: Some notes on their morphology and pathogenesis. Bull L A Neurol Sci 27:1, 1962.
364. Hulten-Gyllensten IL, Lofstedt S, von Reis G: Observations on generalized arteriectasis. Acta Med Scand 163:125, 1959.
365. Nijensohn DE, Saez RJ, Reagan TJ: Clinical significance of basilar artery aneurysms. Neurology 24:301, 1974.
366. Moffie D: Fusiform aneurysm of intracranial arteries. Psychiatr Neurol Neurochir 71:85, 1968.
367. Sacks JG, Lindenburg R: Dolicho-ectatic intracranial arteries: Symptomatology and pathogenesis of arterial elongation and distention. Johns Hopkins Med J 125:95, 1969.
368. Nakasu Y, Saito A, Handa J: Fusiform aneurysm of the anterior communicating artery. Surg Neurol 21:511, 1984.
369. Greitz T, Lofstedt S: The relationship between the third ventricle and the basilar artery. Acta Radiol 42:85, 1954.
370. Hegedus K: Ectasia of the basilar artery with special reference to possible pathogenesis. Surg Neurol 24:463, 1985.
371. Ley A: Compression of the optic nerve by a fusiform aneurysm of the carotid artery. J Neurol Neurosurg Psychiatry 13:75, 1950.
372. Nakatomi H, Segawa H, Kurata A, et al: Clinicopathological study of intracranial fusiform and dolichoectatic aneurysms: Insight on the mechanism of growth. Stroke 31:896, 2000.
373. Mizutani T, Aruga T: "Dolichoectatic" intracranial vertebrobasilar dissecting aneurysm. Neurosurgery 31:765, 1992.
374. Battaglia R, Pasqualin A, Da Pian R: Italian cooperative study on giant intracranial aneurysms. 1: Study design and clinical data. Acta Neurochir (Wien) Suppl 42:49, 1988.
375. Drake CG: Ligation of the vertebral (unilateral or bilateral) or basilar artery in the treatment of large intracranial aneurysms. J Neurosurg 43:255, 1975.
376. Nishizaki T, Tamaki N, Takeda N, et al: Dolichoectatic basilar artery: A review of 23 cases. Stroke 17:1277, 1986.
377. Aymard A, Fobin YP, Hodes JE, et al: Endovascular occlusion of vertebral arteries in the treatment of unclippable vertebrobasilar aneurysms. J Neurosurgery 74:393, 1991.
378. Gobin YP, Vinuela F, Gurian JH, et al: Treatment of large and giant fusiform intracranial aneurysms with Guglielmi detachable coils. J Neurosurg 84:55, 1996.
379. Shokunbi MT, Vinters HV, Kaufmann JC: Fusiform intracranial aneurysms: Clinicopathologic features. Surg Neurol 29:263, 1988.
380. Bokemeyer C, Frank B, Brandis A, et al: Giant aneurysm causing frontal lobe syndrome. J Neurol 237:47, 1990.
381. Drake CG: Progress in cerebrovascular disease: Management of cerebral aneurysm. Stroke 12:273, 1981.
382. Sonntag VK, Yuan RH, Stein BM: Giant intracranial aneurysms: A review of 13 cases. Surg Neurol 8:81, 1977.
383. Whittle IR, Dorsch NW, Besser M: Spontaneous thrombosis in giant intracranial aneurysms. J Neurol Neurosurg Psychiatry 45:1040, 1982.
384. Lawton MT, Spetzler RF: Surgical strategies for giant intracranial aneurysms. Acta Neurochir (Wien) Suppl 72:141, 1999.
385. Hopkins EW, Poser CM: Posterior cerebral artery ectasia: An unusual cause of ophthalmoplegia. Arch Neurol 29:279, 1973.
386. Moseley IF, Holland IM: Ectasia of the basilar artery: The breadth of the clinical spectrum and the diagnostic value of computed tomography. Neuroradiology 18:83, 1979.
387. Trobe JD, Glaser JS, Quencer RC: Isolated oculomotor paralysis: The product of saccular and fusiform aneurysms of the basilar artery. Arch Ophthalmol 96:1236, 1978.
388. Bloch S, Ronthal M, Danziger J: Visual field defects produced by basilar artery ectasia. Clin Radiol 31:335, 1980.
389. Bollensen E, Buzanoski JH, Prange HW: Brainstem compression by basilar artery anomalies as visualized by MRI. J Neurol 238:49, 1991.
390. Brihaye J, Perier O, Smulders J: Glossopharyngeal neuralgia caused by compression of the nerve by an atheromatous vertebral artery. J Neurosurg 13:299, 1956.
391. Campbell JB, Pearman K, Nahl SS: Basilar artery ectasia: A rare cause of sensorineural deafness. J Laryngol Otol 100:333, 1986.
392. Deeb ZL, Jannetta PJ, Rosenbaum AE, et al: Tortuous vertebrobasilar arteries causing cranial nerve syndromes: Screening by computed tomography. J Comput Assist Tomogr 3:774, 1979.
393. Echivarri HC, Rubino FA, Gupta SR, et al: Fusiform aneurysm of the vertebrobasilar arterial system. Stroke 20:1741, 1989.
394. Frasson F, Ferrari G, Fugazzola C, et al: Megadolichobasilar anomaly causing brainstem syndrome: A case report. Neuroradiology 13:279, 1977.
395. Gibson WP, Wallace D: Basilar artery ectasia (an unusual cause of a cerebello-pontine lesion and hemifacial spasm). J Laryngol Otol 89:721, 1975.
396. Harsh GRT, Wilson CB, Hieshima GB, et al: Magnetic resonance imaging of vertebrobasilar ectasia in tic convulsif: Case report. J Neurosurg 74:999, 1991.
397. Katayama Y, Tsubokawa T, Miyazaki S, et al: Growth of totally thrombosed giant aneurysm within the posterior cranial fossa: Diagnostic and therapeutic considerations. Neuroradiology 33:168, 1991.
398. Kerber CW, Margolis MT, Newton TH: Tortuous vertebrobasilar system: A cause of cranial nerve signs. Neuroradiology 4:74, 1972.
399. Lye RH: Basilar artery ectasia: An unusual cause of trigeminal neuralgia. J Neurol Neurosurg Psychiatry 49:22, 1986.
400. Stark RJ: Supranuclear ophthalmoplegia with basilar artery aneurysms. Surg Neurol 12:447, 1979.
401. Trobe JD, Glaser JS, Quencer RC: Isolated oculomotor paralysis: The product of saccular and fusiform aneurysms of the basilar artery. Arch Ophthalmol 96:1236, 1978.
402. Spetzler RF, Hadley MN, Rigamonti D, et al: Aneurysms of the basilar artery treated with circulatory arrest, hypothermia, and barbiturate cerebral protection. J Neurosurg 68:868, 1988.
403. Boeri R, Passerini A: The megadolichobasilar anomaly. J Neurol Sci 1:475, 1964.
404. Breig A, Ekbom K, Greitz T, et al: Hydrocephalus due to elongated basilar artery: A new clinicoradiological syndrome. Lancet 1:874, 1967.
405. de los Reyes RA, Kantrowitz AB, Boehm FH, et al: Transcallosal, transventricular approach to a basilar apex aneurysm. Neurosurgery 31:597, 1992.
406. Ekbom K, Greitz T, Kalmer M, et al: Cerebrospinal fluid pulsations in occult hydrocephalus due to ectasia of basilar artery. Acta Neurochir (Wien) 20:1, 1969.
407. Rozario RA, Levine HL, Scott RM: Obstructive hydrocephalus secondary to an ectatic basilar artery. Surg Neurol 9:31, 1978.
408. Shirakuni T, Tamaki N, Matsumoto S, et al: Megadolichobasilar anomaly associated with brain stem infarction: A case report. J Comput Tomogr 9:79, 1985.

409. Wascher TM, Spetzler RF: Saccular aneurysms of the basilar bifurcation. In Spetzler RF (ed): Neurovascular Surgery. New York, McGraw-Hill, 1995, p 729.

410. Batjer HH, Kopitnik TA, Purdy PD, et al: Vertebral and PICA aneurysms. In Spetzler RF (ed): Neurovascular Surgery. New York, McGraw-Hill, 1995, p 763.

411. Haddad GF, Haddad FS: Cerebral giant serpentine aneurysm: Case report and review of the literature. Neurosurgery 23:92, 1988.

412. Steinberg GK, Drake CG, Peerless SJ: Deliberate basilar or vertebral artery occlusion in the treatment of intracranial aneurysms: Immediate results and long-term outcome in 201 patients. J Neurosurg 79:161, 1993.

413. Lownie SP, Drake CG, Peerless SJ, et al: Clinical presentation and management of giant anterior communicating artery region aneurysms. J Neurosurg 92:267, 2000.

414. Sundt TM Jr, Piepgras DG, Marsh WR, et al: Saphenous vein bypass grafts for giant aneurysms and intracranial occlusive disease. J Neurosurg 65:439, 1986.

415. Sundt TM Jr, Piepgras DG: Surgical approach to giant intracranial aneurysms: Operative experience with 80 cases. J Neurosurg 51:731, 1979.

416. Hosobuchi Y: Direct surgical treatment of giant intracranial aneurysms. J Neurosurg 51:743, 1979.

417. Ausman JI, Diaz FG, Sadasivan B, et al: Giant intracranial aneurysm surgery: The role of microvascular reconstruction. Surg Neurol 34:8, 1990.

418. Symon L, Vajda J: Surgical experiences with giant intracranial aneurysms. J Neurosurg 61:1009, 1984.

419. Bakay L, Sweet WH: Cervical and intracranial intra-arterial pressures with and without occlusion. Surg Gynecol Obstet 95:67, 1952.

420. Bakay L, Sweet WH: Intra-arterial pressures in the neck and brain: Late changes after carotid closure, acute measurements after vertebral closure. J Neurosurg 10:353, 1953.

421. Tindall GT, Goree JA, Lee JF, et al: Effect of common carotid ligation on size of internal carotid aneurysms and distal intracarotid and retinal artery pressures. J Neurosurg 25:503, 1966.

422. Spetzler RF, Schuster H, Roski RA: Elective extracranial-intracranial arterial bypass in the treatment of inoperable giant aneurysms of the internal carotid artery. J Neurosurg 53:22, 1980.

423. Landolt AM, Millikan CH: Pathogenesis of cerebral infarction secondary to mechanical carotid artery occlusion. Stroke 1:52, 1970.

424. Nishioka H: Results of the treatment of intracranial aneurysms by occlusion of the carotid artery in the neck. J Neurosurg 25:660, 1966.

425. Norlen G, Olivecrona H: The treatment of aneurysms of the circle of Willis. J Neurosurg 10:404–415, 1953.

426. Smith RR, Al-Mefty O, Middleton TH: An orbitocranial approach to complex aneurysms of the anterior circulation. Neurosurgery 24:385, 1989.

427. Origitano TC, Anderson DE, Tarassoli Y, et al: Skull base approaches to complex cerebral aneurysms. Surg Neurol 40:339, 1993.

428. Diaz FG, Ausman JI, Pearce JE: Ischemic complications after combined internal carotid artery occlusion and extracranial-intracranial anastomosis. Neurosurgery 10:563, 1982.

429. Diaz FG, Ohaegbulam S, Dujovny M, et al: Surgical alternatives in the treatment of cavernous sinus aneurysms. J Neurosurg 71:846, 1989.

430. Connolly ES Jr, Solomon RA: Hypothermic cardiac standstill for cerebral aneurysm surgery. Neurosurg Clin North Am 9:681, 1998.

431. Lawton MT, Raudzens PA, Zabramski JM, et al: Hypothermic circulatory arrest in neurovascular surgery: Evolving indications and predictors of patient outcome. Neurosurgery 43:10, 1998.

432. Baumgartner WA, Silverberg GD, Ream AK, et al: Reappraisal of cardiopulmonary bypass with deep hypothermia and circulatory arrest for complex neurosurgical operations. Surgery 94:242, 1983.

433. Drake CG, Barr HWK, Coles JC, et al: The use of extracorporeal circulation and profound hypothermia in the treatment of ruptured aneurysms. J Neurosurg 21:575, 1964.

434. Silverberg GD, Reitz BA, Ream AK: Hypothermia and cardiac arrest in the treatment of giant aneurysms of the cerebral circulation and hemangioblastoma of the medulla. J Neurosurg 55:337, 1981.

435. Uihlein A, MacCarty CS, Michenfelder JD: Deep hypothermia and surgical treatment of intracranial aneurysms: A five-year survey. JAMA 195:639, 1966.

436. Ausman JI, Malik GM, Tomecek FJ, et al: Hypothermic circulatory arrest and the management of giant and large cerebral aneurysms. Surg Neurol 40:289, 1993.

437. Ausman JI, McCormick PW, Stewart M, et al: Cerebral oxygen metabolism during hypothermic circulatory arrest in humans. J Neurosurg 79:810, 1993.

438. Belopavlovic M, Buchthal A: Cerebral function monitoring for assessment of barbiturate therapy under moderate hypothermia in cerebral aneurysm surgery. Acta Anaesthesiol Belg 31(Suppl):93, 1980.

439. Greene KA, Marciano FF, Hamilton MG, et al: Cardiopulmonary bypass, hypothermic circulatory arrest and barbiturate cerebral protection for the treatment of giant vertebrobasilar aneurysms in children. Pediatr Neurosurg 21:124, 1994.

440. Kato Y, Sano H, Zhou J, et al: Deep hypothermia cardiopulmonary bypass and direct surgery of two large aneurysms at the vertebrobasilar junction. Acta Neurochir (Wien) 138:1057, 1996.

441. Silverberg GD: Giant aneurysms: Surgical treatment. Neurol Res 6:57, 1984.

442. Solomon R, Smith CR, Raps EC, et al: Deep hypothermic circulatory arrest for the management of complex anterior and posterior circulation aneurysms. Neurosurgery 29:732, 1991.

443. Spetzler RF, Lee KS: Reconstruction of the temporalis muscle for the pterional craniotomy. Technical note [see comments]. J Neurosurg 73:636, 1990.

444. Blazier CJ, Cavanaugh E, Antonioli L: Surgical treatment of complex cerebrovascular lesions utilizing hypothermia and circulatory arrest: Nursing implications. BNI Q 5:33, 1990.

Chapter Sixty-Eight

Vascular Malformations of the Brain

Andrew T. Parsa and Robert A. Solomon

HISTORICAL PERSPECTIVE

In their comprehensive review of historical developments in the field of the treatment of arteriovenous malformations (AVMs), Yasargil and colleagues[1] give credit to William Hunter for providing many important early concepts. Dr. Hunter's descriptions of extracranial AVMs, documented in his 1762 monograph, formed the basis for testing divergent theories regarding the physiology, pathology, and development of these lesions. Applying Hunter's teleologic framework almost 100 years later, Rokitansky was the first to comprehensively describe angiomas of the intracranial cavity, speculating that they were in fact highly vascular tumors. Later, Virchow and others refined Rokitansky's description to include a rudimentary classification system of telangiectasias and venous, arterial, arteriovenous, and cystic angiomas. Virchow's work is particularly noteworthy because his extensive pathologic studies determined that only a small percentage of angiomas are neoplastic, and that the majority of these represent some type of congenital anomaly. D'Arcy Power described clinical correlation of the pathologic process defined by Virchow and his contemporaries in 1888, as did Steinhil 3 years later. D'Arcy Power's description of a 20-year-old man with right-sided hemiplegia and a left sylvian fissure AVM is an early model for anatomic localization of this disease process.[1]

From the 1890s to the 1930s, as the use of surgery for intracranial mass lesions increased, so did descriptive reports of AVMs. The first well-documented successful excision of an intracranial AVM was performed in 1889. In this case Pean, a French general surgeon, operated on a 15-year-old boy who presented with left-sided seizures and a right-sided frontal-parietal lesion. In 1928, Cushing[2] and Dandy[3] described their individual series of 14 and 15 patients, respectively. In a later 1928 monograph entitled *Tumors Arising from the Blood-vessels of the Brain*, Cushing and Bailey[4] summarized the expert opinions of their era in describing a group of lesions referred to as "angiomatous malformations." These researchers elaborated upon standard principles that form the basis of our treatment strategies today, including surgical ligation of feeding vessels, removal of the nidus, radiation therapy,

and judicious observation. Their remarkably detailed anatomic, pathologic, and surgical primer is a landmark treatise that foreshadowed many of the developments to follow in the 20th century.

No single historical event is more important to the treatment of patients with AVMs than the development of intracerebral angiography. The application of angiography as a diagnostic tool serves as a logical milestone for classifying early experiences. The work of Cushing, Dandy, and Bailey described in the 1920s should be considered distinct from that of pioneers such as Olivecrona, Penfield, Eriksen, and Pilcher, who collectively described through the 1940s the treatment of more than 100 patients with AVMs using preoperative angiograms.[1] The relatively recent development of embolization and the advent of endovascular procedures represent additional treatment milestones. Fundamental developments in neuroimaging, such as computed tomography (CT) and magnetic resonance imaging (MRI), surgical tools such as the operating microscope, and adjuncts such as gamma knife radiosurgery have also optimized outcomes for many patients with AVMs.

Currently, we continue to make diagnostic and therapeutic advances in the treatment of patients with AVMs. Frameless stereotaxis and functional mapping have facilitated lesion localization, and the endovascular field seems to become more refined every year. Despite these technical advances, there currently remains a subpopulation of patients for whom no treatment can be undertaken safely. It is these patients in particular who provide the historical impetus to develop more effective treatment modalities.

There are still no clear answers to many fundamental medical and scientific questions regarding AVMs. Yasargil and colleagues[1] have informed us that there has always been controversy about the pathogenesis, nomenclature, classification, diagnosis, and treatment of AVMs. We would add to these topics the issue of the natural history of these lesions. In the 21st century, the medical staff charged with the care of patients with AVMs face the same questions addressed by early pioneers. Multidisciplinary paradigms of management are being applied as advances in evidence-based medicine raise the possibility of delineating optimal patient care. In this chapter, we detail the clinical and scientific topics that have fostered more effective strategies for the treatment of patients with AVMs. We conclude with a review of eight cases from our institution that exemplify the multidisciplinary approach necessary for obtaining a favorable outcome.

PATHOLOGIC CLASSIFICATION AND RADIOLOGIC CORRELATES

Cushing and Bailey[4] observed, "The fact that brain tissue or traces of it . . . can be demonstrated between the cords of vessel leads us to side with [authors who] favour the view that these lesions are essentially anomalies; and even though they may be capable of growth, they are in no sense comparable to the admittedly neoplastic tumors."

Detailed descriptions of malformations are often confounded by the quality of the operative or postmortem specimen. The propensity for these lesions to bleed as well as the dynamic nature of their growth can obscure pathologic characteristics. Preoperative treatment modalities such as embolization and radiation therapy can also alter the microscopic appearance of malformations. Despite these difficulties, there are fundamental structures that define various malformations. Furthermore, these structural characteristics have a radiologic correlate that can facilitate early diagnosis.

Capillary Telangiectasias

Capillary telangiectasias are composed exclusively of small capillary-type blood vessels that resemble normal capillaries surrounded by normal-appearing parenchyma. They are typically less than 1 cm in diameter and occur most commonly in the pons (Fig. 68–1). These lesions are usually found incidentally at autopsy and rarely have clinical sequelae such as bleeding and thrombosis. Capillary telangiectasias are being recognized with increasing frequency on MRI as new imaging sequences are applied. These lesions enhance with contrast material but are otherwise undetectable on conventional MRI. A typical capillary telangiectasia lacks the hemosiderin rim of cavernous malformations and demonstrates greater susceptibility only on gradient-echo images, probably because of blood oxygen level–dependent contrast.

Capillary telangiectasias are clinically significant because they may represent earlier versions of cavernous malformations. In 1991, Rigamonti and colleagues[5] reviewed the histories of 20 patients with cavernous malformations and analyzed the clinical, radiographic, and surgical-autopsy data associated with these lesions. In some patients, multiple lesions, including cavernous malformations, capillary telangiectasias, and transitional forms between the two, were identified. On the basis of this analysis, these researchers concluded that capillary telangiectasia and cavernous malformations represent two pathologic extremes within the same vascular malformation category, and they proposed grouping them as a single entity. Later, the same group described the juxtaposition of a capillary telangiectasia, cavernous malformation, and developmental venous anomaly in the brainstem of a single patient.[6] Juxtaposition of these three different vascular lesions in the brainstem of an otherwise normal individual suggested that the lesions were related. It is now hypothesized that a developmental event disrupting local capillary-venous structures occurs in capillary telangiectasia, subsequently leading to the formation of cavernous malformations.[6] Capillary telangiectasias can also more rarely occur in association with AVMs.[7]

Cavernous Malformations

Cavernous malformations are composed of cystic vascular spaces lined by a single layer of endothelial cells. These sinusoidal vessels form a compact mass with no intervening neural parenchyma. The lack of neural tissue is a characteristic historically used to distinguish cavernous malformations from capillary telangiectasias. Application of electron microscopy has revealed that endothelial cells within cavernous malformations lack tight junctions.[8]

Upon gross examination, cavernous malformations are well-circumscribed focal areas of reddish purple discoloration up to a few centimeters in size (Fig. 68–2). Hemorrhage results in variable deposition of hemosiderin, reactive gliosis, and focal areas of calcification. The absence of direct arterial input makes it difficult to visualize these lesions on conventional angiography, but their appearance on MRI is very characteristic. Blood of varying ages in and around these lesions gives a stereotypical pattern of heterogeneity (Fig. 68–3).

Venous Malformations

Venous malformations have been described as the most common type of vascular malformation at autopsy.[1] These lesions are composed of anomalous veins separated by normal neural parenchyma. The malformations may be

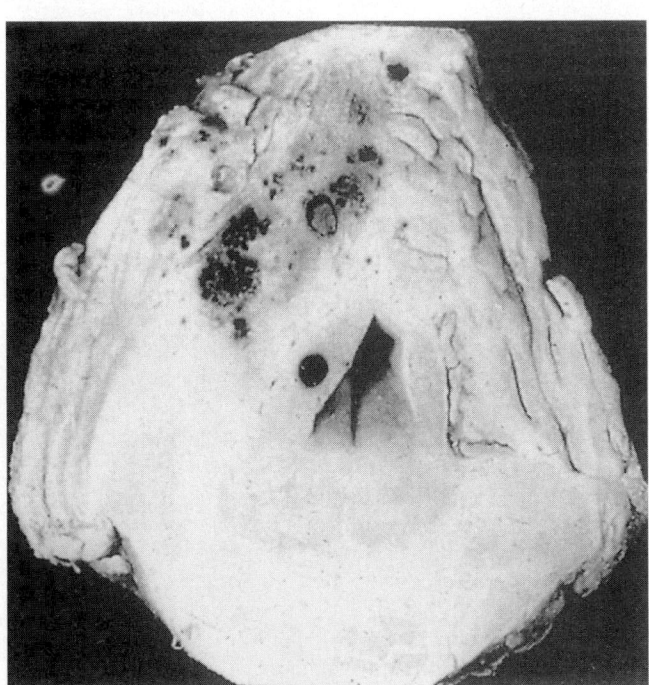

FIGURE 68–1 *Pontine capillary telangiectasia.*

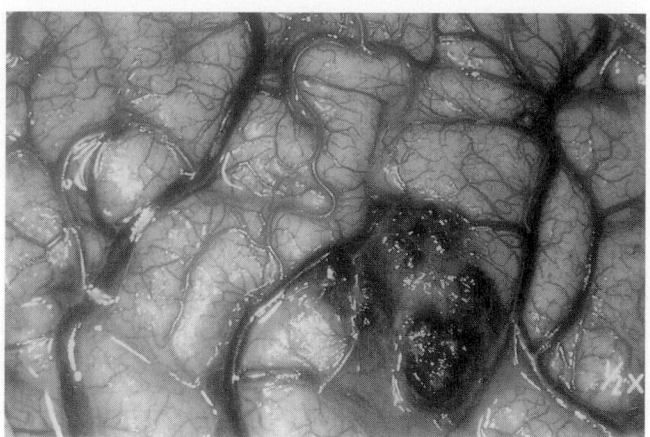

FIGURE 68–2   *Cavernous malformation on the surface of the brain.*

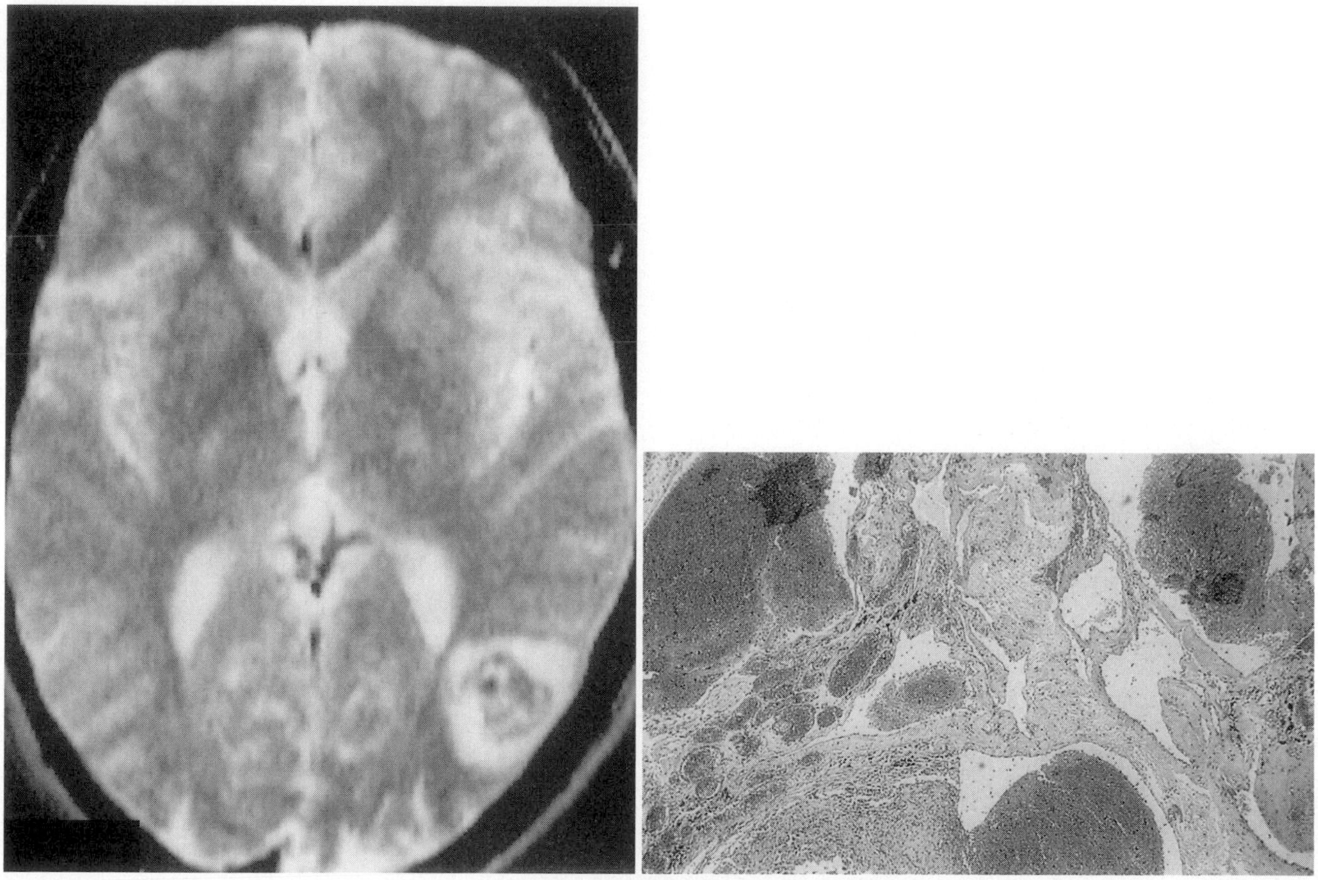

A

B

FIGURE 68–3   *Cavernous malformation showing blood of varying ages.* A, MRI. B, Micrograph.

composed of a single, greatly dilated, tortuous vein or a number of smaller veins coalescing at a single point; they never have direct arterial input. Accordingly, these lesions have a characteristic appearance in the venous phase of an angiogram described as "caput medusae" (Fig. 68–4). Venous malformations can also be visualized as linear signals in unusual locations during contrast-enhanced CT scanning or conventional MRI. From a clinical perspective, these lesions are considered benign, and any hemorrhage associated with a venous malformation is usually secondary to a nearby cavernous malformation.

Arteriovenous Malformations

The essence of the pathology of an AVM is arterial shunting into draining veins without intervening capillaries. Several groups have delineated the nature of structures that facilitate this shunting using conventional histologic methods[9,10] as well as scanning electron microscopy.[11] All three reports described shunting arterioles communicating directly with AVM core vessels. These pathologic hallmarks have distinctive radiographic correlates that span the spectrum of AVM disease. Focal lesions may demonstrate a clear arterial supply of a tight nidus with pathognomonic early draining veins (Fig. 68–5). In contrast, characteristic angiographic features of diffuse lesions included multiple small arterial feeders, small ectatic vessels in the malformation itself, multiple small draining veins, and a diffuse, puddling appearance of the contrast dye.[12]

Most vascular channels within an AVM are venous in morphology, although transitional vessels are quite common. Vascular channels vary in accordance with the spectrum of disease. A tightly compacted nidus without intervening neural parenchyma is characteristic of focal lesions, whereas diffuse lesions contain normal cerebral tissue between abnormal vessels.[12] Regardless of their place in this spectrum of disease, the propensity for AVMs to bleed has a histologic and pathologic correlate. Microscopic areas of hemosiderin deposition and abnormal gliotic parenchyma can be identified even in patients who do not present after an ictal event. These micro-hemorrhages are followed by thrombosis and reparative fibrosis that lead to scar formation and calcification.

Other vascular lesions can be found in association with AVMs, including venous and arterial aneurysms. Venous aneurysms do not typically have a clinicopathologic correlate (Fig. 68–6); however, there are important clinical implications and surgical considerations for the patient with an AVM and an associated arterial aneurysm. These aneurysms have been classified as intranidal, flow-related, or unrelated to the AVM nidus.[13] In a review of 632 patients, Redekop and colleagues[13] found that intranidal aneurysms have a high correlation with hemorrhagic clinical presentation and a risk of bleeding during the follow-up period that considerably exceeds the risk in AVMs without associated aneurysms. Patients with flow-related aneurysms in association with an AVM may present with hemorrhage from either lesion. Aneurysms that arise on distal feeding arteries near the nidus have a high probability of regressing with substantial or curative AVM therapy. In a later analysis of patients with AVMs (240 treated for AVM and 2 for an aneurysm), feeding vessel pedicle aneurysms appeared to occur more frequently in conjunction with infratentorial AVMs.[14]

ARTERIOVENOUS MALFORMATIONS
Embryology

Several aspects of AVM morphologic characteristics resemble the anastomotic plexuses of developing vasculature in the embryo. These similarities have led many investigators to speculate that a fundamental arrest of vascular development is associated with the formation of AVMs.[15] Mullan and colleagues[16] have attempted to correlate several clinical, anatomic, and angiographic features of lesions from patients with AVMs with known events in the development of central nervous system (CNS) vasculature. These investigators hypothesize that AVMs begin in human

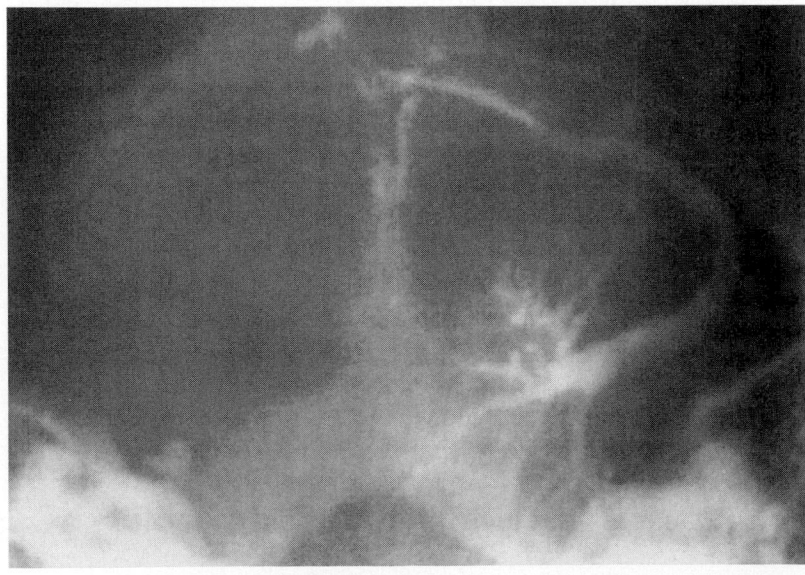

FIGURE 68–4 *Angiographic view of a caput medusae.*

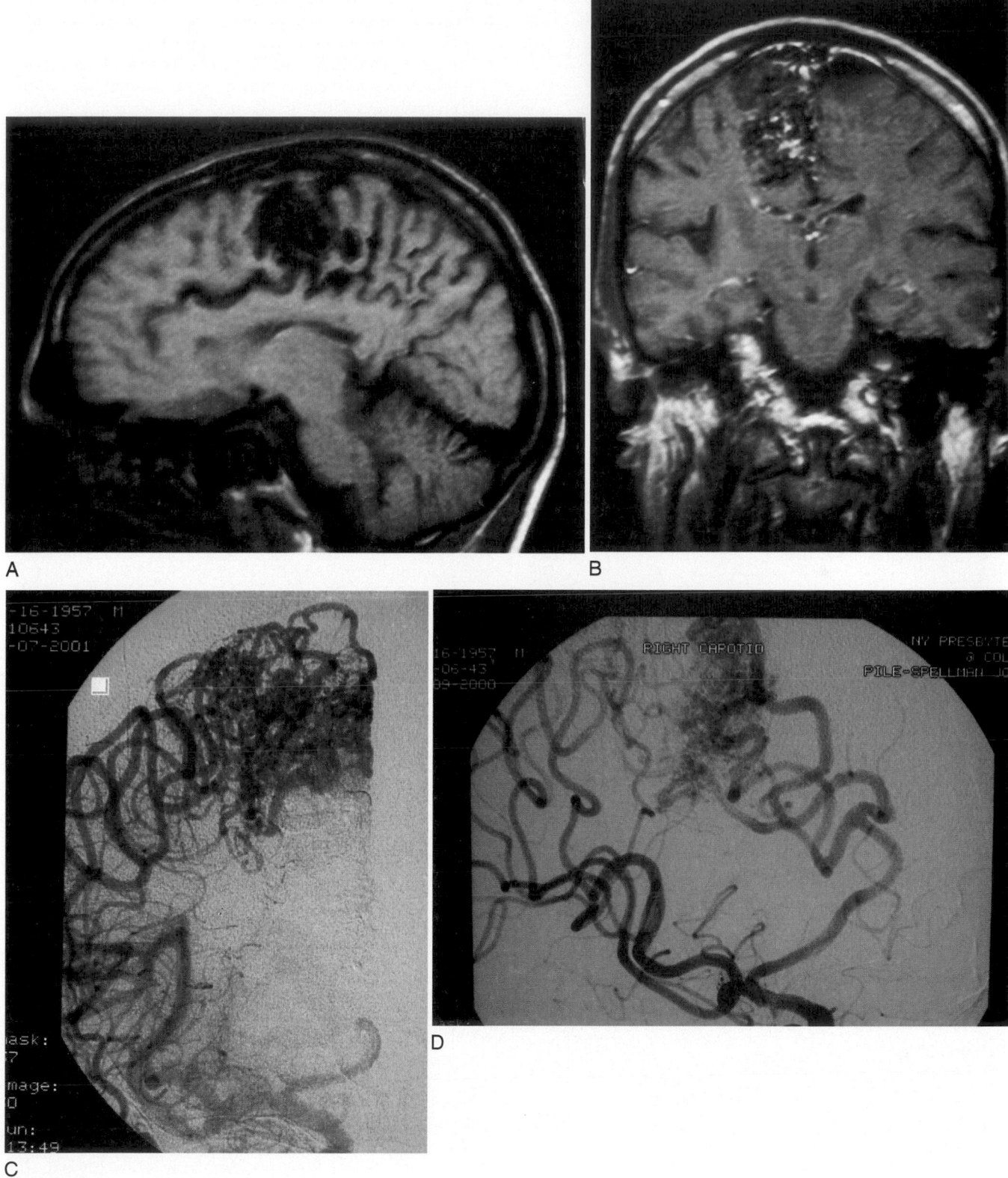

FIGURE 68–5 *Arteriovenous malformation. A and B, MRI. C and D, Preoperative angiograms.*

Continued

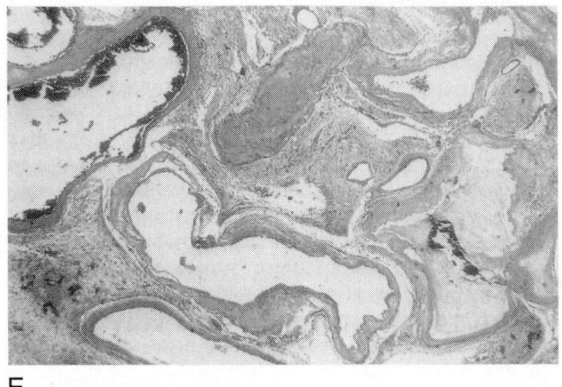

E

FIGURE 68–5, cont'd. E, *Micrograph.*

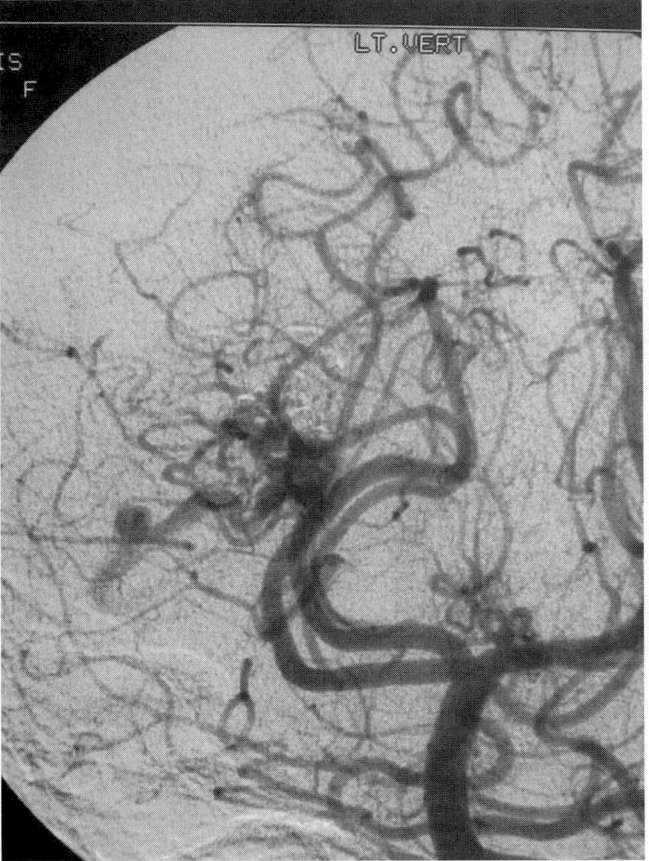

FIGURE 68–6   *Venous aneurysm.*

embryonic development, during the sequential formation and absorption of surface veins; mainly in the 40- to 80-mm length interval. Accordingly, discordance of vein formation and resorption can potentially result in predictable anomalies. Absence of the middle cerebral vein or its failure to communicate with the cavernous sinus in patients with AVMs may correlate with the late embryologic development of that vein or with its even later connection to the cavernous sinus.

Other circumstantial embryologic correlates are the entry of the superior ophthalmic vein into the cavernous sinus through the inferior rather than the superior orbital fissure, the relative infrequency of middle cerebral vein backflow in the presence of an extensive cavernous fistula, and the relative infrequency of hemorrhage in relation to the inferior petrosal fistula.[16] Each of these findings is consistent with a relationship between the anomaly and older venous pathways. The occurrence of hemorrhage in association with a superior petrosal sinus fistula and the failure of the superior petrosal sinus to connect to the cavernous sinus may also have an embryologic correlate.[16] In addition, an insult at the time at which the paired internal cerebral veins fuse into one channel could explain aneurysms of the vein of Galen and absence or deformation of the straight sinus.

This view of Mullan and colleagues,[16] that specific embryologic events are associated with AVMs, is supported by a number of clinical syndromes in children with AVMs.[17–19] These syndromes can range in severity and involvement of other organ systems. Hereditary hemorrhagic telangiectasia (HHT) is an autosomal dominant vascular dysplasia that can involve multiple organs.[19] Visceral involvement includes pulmonary, gastrointestinal, and cerebral AVMs, which have been reported predominantly in adults. Clinical evidence of an embryologic etiology for AVMs also comes from anecdotal case reports that describe as yet unnamed syndromes. An example is the case of a 14-year-old boy with syndactyly of all limbs and an intracranial dural AVM.[20] The coincidence of syndactyly and an AVM in this patient is consistent with a single common intrauterine insult occurring during the second month of gestation. The differentiation of cerebral vessels in utero approximately matches the time frame for normal interdigital tissue regression, at 5 to 7 weeks' gestational age.

Physiology

The physiology of AVMs and surrounding brain can be influenced by many factors, including size, location, associated vascular anomalies, and the presence of hemorrhage. Despite the great variety of attributes found among patients with AVMs, some common principles apply to each of these lesions. In their early review addressing the pathophysiology of cerebral ischemia accompanying AVMs, Spetzler and associates[21] describe several landmark papers that have led to theoretical models of AVMs and facilitated our current understanding. The key components of current models of AVM physiology are the feeding AVM artery, the surrounding brain normally perfused by this artery, and the AV shunt facilitated by the AVM.

A basic theory of AVM physiology has been described by Spetzler and associates[21] to explain the phenomenon of ischemia-related changes in the brain surrounding the AVM. As the AV shunt at the center of the AVM becomes more pronounced, flow preferentially goes toward the shunt (i.e., the path of least resistance), resulting in a reduction of cerebral perfusion pressure in the vascular beds supplied by the feeding artery. This decrease in nutrient flow is directly proportional to the flow rate through the AV shunt, the length of the feeding vessel, and the local venous pressure. In a compensatory response, normal cerebral autoregulation accommodates the reduced blood flow to the surrounding parenchyma by dilating nutrient arterioles. Continuous exposure to low perfusion pressures, however, may result in permanent dilatation of the nutrient arteries and permanent structural changes in the vasculature. Eventually these vascular beds, previously under normal autoregulation, regress into passive networks that are pressure dependent. Autonomic input can no longer dilate vasculature to facilitate increased flow, nor can autonomic input constrict these vessels if the relative pressure into the system suddenly increases. Ischemic changes occur when the capacity for compensatory vasodilation is exceeded by the reduction in nutrient artery flow—which in turn depends on the AV shunt at the core of the AVM.

Applying this model of ischemia, Spetzler and associates[21] have provided a possible explanation for bleeding in areas of brain surrounding a resected AVM. The phenomenon of normal perfusion pressure breakthrough can occur after removal of an AVM and also relates to the loss of autonomic responses in chronically dilated vascular beds. Successful treatment of an AVM is defined as removal of the AV shunt. When an AV shunt is obliterated, the perfusion pressure of surrounding brain can increase from subnormal to normal physiologic values. Under nonpathologic circumstances, the autonomic response to this subtle increase in pressure would be to constrict feeding vessels. However, the chronic dilatation of the vascular beds precludes a normal response, resulting in hemorrhage and edema of the surrounding brain[21] or even of distant areas within the proximal arterial territory supplying the AVM.[22]

The complexity of AVM physiology has become more apparent as tools have been developed to model variable flow rates and perfusion pressures.[23-25] Lo and coworkers[23] have described a biomathematical analysis of hemodynamic alterations in intracranial AVMs based on fluid dynamic formulations of flow rates, cerebral perfusion pressure, intra-AVM pressure gradients, and hemodynamic resistances. Their model demonstrated that (1) vascular steal is inversely proportional to the hemodynamic resistance of the AVM, (2) probability of hemorrhage is related to the distribution of cerebral perfusion pressure across large thin-walled shunts, (3) normal reperfusion pressure after AVM obliteration depends on the resistance of surrounding vasculature to the elevated blood flow, and (4) hyperemic complications after treatment are likely to occur in high-flow AVMs that demonstrate steal. In general, the findings of this mathematical model of AVM physiology reflect the clinical pathophysiology of patients with AVMs.[24]

As techniques evolve for measuring flow rates and pressures in and around AVMs,[26-29] mathematical and computer models of AVM physiology may have more of an impact. Other theories have examined the role of the venous circulation and the relationship to postoperative hyperemic complications. Al-Rodhan and colleagues[30] have proposed that edema and hemorrhage after AVM resection result from venous outflow obstruction; this process leads to passive hyperemia and engorgement of tissues and to stagnant flow in AVM feeding vessels. Schaller and associates[31] and Meyer and colleagues[32] have suggested that postoperative hyperperfusion injury after AVM resection results from the unconstrained arterial inflow into cortical areas rendered ischemic by long-standing preoperative venous hypertension.

No one theory completely explains all the pathophysiologic phenomena that have been observed with cerebral AVMs. Most likely, there is some combination of preoperative steal and postoperative venous occlusion that leads to edema and hemorrhage in a small subset of patients after AVM resection.

Molecular Biology

A Primer in Molecular Biology

The appearance and behavior of a cell, whether normal or abnormal, is due in large part to cellular proteins. The synthesis of a protein and subsequent biologic action of that protein are the endpoints of a series of events (i.e., DNA is transcribed into RNA, which is translated into protein). Genetic mutations occur at the level of genomic DNA and include base-pair changes, deletions, insertions, and inactivation through methylation. Genomic DNA is organized into two sets of chromosomes, each containing specific genes. However, the overwhelming majority of DNA found in the genome does not code for proteins. Instead this noncoding DNA has important regulatory and structural functions. Each gene has a discrete organization that includes genetic sequences designated for transcription into RNA and elements that regulate transcription. Downstream of the transcriptional starting site, the DNA sequence is divided into exons and introns. The final messenger RNA (mRNA) molecule is made up of exons joined together, whereas introns contain intervening sequences that are spliced out during processing. Protein synthesis occurs after mRNA moves from the nucleus into the cytoplasm.

Translation refers to the process that converts the information encoded by nucleic acid sequence into the amino acid sequence constituting a protein. In the flow of genetic information from DNA to protein, RNA is the least stable molecule, with a half-life that can last from seconds to minutes. The relative instability of RNA can make it the rate-limiting molecule in the events that lead up to the synthesis of most proteins. Mutations at the level of DNA are thus carried forward in the form of proteins that are mutated, overexpressed after genetic amplification, or underexpressed after genetic deletion. The process of identifying genetic mutations in an AVM can start with the surgical specimen or with peripheral blood lymphocytes from the patient and family members. Over the last three decades, several techniques have been developed to study DNA, RNA, and protein from freshly obtained or archived specimens. Later technical innovations, such as differential display polymerase chain reaction (PCR) methodology, representational difference analysis, and gene chips are expediting the detection of genetic lesions in vascular malformations.

Genetic Mutations Associated with Vascular Malformations

Two fundamental approaches have been undertaken to identify genetic defects associated with vascular malformations, (1) linkage analysis of patients and family members associated with hereditary disorders and (2) molecular analysis of surgical specimens for defective or missing gene products.

The first of these approaches, linkage analysis, has been applied most successfully in identifying a gene associated with familial cerebral cavernous malformations (CCMs).[33]

Over the course of several years, investigators and clinicians have worked to establish the genetic pattern, location, and identity of genes associated with CCMs. Initially, the recognition of unrelated Hispanic-American families in which CCMs segregated as an autosomal dominant trait established a genetic basis for this disease.[33,34] Linkage analysis subsequently identified locus heterogeneity with disease genes for CCM at chromosomal regions 7q, 7p, and 3q.[35] Efforts that have focused on the 7q locus have identified mutations in the gene Krev Interaction Trapped 1 (*krit1*) in French and Hispanic-American families with CCM.[36-39] The *krit1* gene was originally identified through its interaction with the Ras-family guanosine triphosphatase (GTPase) krev1/rap1a in a two-hybrid screen, inferring a role in GTPase signaling cascades. Collectively, the data from linkage analysis suggests that aberrant Ras signaling pathways may be implicated in the development of cavernous malformations. To date, all mutations of the *krit1* gene result in loss of function; which was recently confirmed in an analysis of four Hispanic-American families with CCM mapping to 7q.[37] In these families, the *krit1* gene revealed a point mutation in exon 6 that predicts the substitution of a premature termination codon for glutamine at codon 248. The search for mutated genes that map to 7p and 3q is ongoing and will be facilitated by progress on the human genome project as well as by investigator consortiums that pool data from multiple families.

The second approach to identifying mutations in genes associated with AVM involves the molecular analysis of surgical specimens for defective or missing gene products. As mentioned previously, hereditary hemorrhagic telangiectasia is an autosomal dominant vascular dysplasia that can involve multiple organs.[19] Most cases of HHT are caused by mutations in the endoglin gene on chromosome 9 (HHT type 1) or the activin receptor–like kinase 1 gene on chromosome 12 (HHT type 2), which leads to telangiectases and AVMs of the skin, mucosa, and viscera. A logical hypothesis generated from these genetic studies is that the genes are missing or mutated in cerebral AVM specimens. However, this hypothesis may in fact be an oversimplification. Bourdeau and colleagues[40] have demonstrated that the endoglin gene product is intact in AVM specimens from patients with HHT type 1. When analyzed by immunostaining and densitometry, normal blood vessels of the brain and vessels adjacent to these AVMs showed a 50% reduction in the ratio of endoglin to PECAM-1 (platelet endothelial cell adhesion molecule-1); this finding suggests that all blood vessels of patients with HHT1 express reduced endoglin in situ and that AVMs are not attributable to a focal loss of endoglin. In the case of HHT1, molecular analysis of intraoperative specimens has demonstrated that the endoglin gene product is intact, providing the impetus to search for alternative genetic mutations.

Epidemiology

Determination of the true epidemiology and natural history of AVMs has been confounded by both the heterogeneity of divergent patient populations and the varying institutional biases toward treatment. Several literature reviews have sought to consolidate relevant retrospective and prospective studies in an effort to provide a consensus view. At our institution, Berman and associates[41] have attempted to determine the incidence and prevalence of AVM by critically reviewing the original sources from which these rates were derived. This group reviewed relevant original literature, including autopsy series, the Cooperative Study of Intracranial Aneurysms and Subarachnoid Hemorrhage, related analyses, and other population-based studies. The results of their analysis showed that many of the prevalence estimates (500 to 600 per 100,000 population) were based on autopsy data, a source that is inherently biased. Other estimates (140 per 100,000 population) originated from an inappropriate analysis of data from the Cooperative Study. The most reliable information came from a population-based study of Olmsted County in Minnesota[42]; however, prevalence data specific to AVMs was not found in that study. Owing to variation in the detection rate of asymptomatic AVMs, Berman and colleagues[41] contend that the most reliable estimate for the occurrence of the disease is the detection rate for symptomatic lesions: 0.94 per 100,000 person-years (95% confidence interval, 0.57–1.30/100,000 person-years). This figure is derived from a single population-based study, but it is supported by a reanalysis of other data sources.[42] The prevalence of detected, active (at-risk) AVM disease is unknown, but it can be inferred from incidence data to be lower than 10.3 per 100,000 population.[41]

In a later review of the literature, Al-Shahi and coworkers[43] concluded that there is very little accurate information about the frequency and clinical course of AVMs because the methods of most studies have been flawed and because AVMs tend to be treated once they are discovered.[43] Consolidation of the relevant literature for AVMs in adults yielded an incidence of AVMs at approximately 1 per 100,000 per year in unselected populations, and a point-prevalence in adults of approximately 18 per 100,000. Further analysis suggested that AVMs (1) account for between 1% and 2% of all strokes, 3% of strokes in young adults, and 9% of subarachnoid hemorrhages and (2) are responsible for 4% of primary intracerebral hemorrhages overall (when not stratified by age) and for up to 33% of primary intracerebral hemorrhages in young adults. With respect to clinical sequelae, Al-Shahi and coworkers[43] concluded that at least 15% of people affected by AVMs are asymptomatic, that about 20% present with seizures, and that for approximately 66%, the dominant mode of presentation is with intracranial hemorrhage. The limited high-quality data available on prognosis suggest that long-term crude annual case fatality is 1% to 1.5%, the crude annual risk of first occurrence of hemorrhage from an unruptured AVM is approximately 2%, but the risk of recurrent hemorrhage may be as high as 18% in the first year, with uncertainty about the risk thereafter. For people with untreated AVMs, the annual risk of development of de novo seizures was determined to be 1%.[43]

One of the few prospective studies on AVMs was published by Ondra and colleagues[44] in 1990. These investigators monitored 166 symptomatic patients with AVMs of the brain who had not undergone surgery. Follow-up data were obtained for 160 (96%) of the original population, with a mean follow-up period of 23.7 years. The rate of major rebleeding was 4.0% per year, and the mortality rate was 1.0% per year. At follow-up review, 23% of the patients were dead from AVM hemorrhage. The combined rate of major morbidity and mortality was 2.7% per year. These annual rates remained essentially constant over the entire period of the study. Most significantly, the investigators concluded that there was no difference in the incidence of rebleeding or death regardless of presentation with or without evidence of hemorrhage. The mean interval between initial presentation and subsequent hemorrhage was found to be 7.7 years.[44] Collectively, many of the questions regarding AVM natural history will remain unanswered until modern-day prospective studies, such as the one just described, are initiated.

Clinical Presentation

Hemorrhage

Intracranial hemorrhage is by far the most common presenting symptom for patients with intracranial vascular malformations. Hemorrhage is the initial symptom related to an AVM for between 50% and 75% of patients.[42,43] The hemorrhages are most often intracerebral because of the location of AVMs within the parenchyma; and they are often accompanied by secondary subarachnoid and intraventricular hemorrhage. Unlike hemorrhages associated with ruptured aneurysms, AVM subarachnoid blood comes from venous channels carrying blood with arterial pressure and is rarely associated with vasospasm. In general, the patient with an AVM bleed survives and improves over time as the intraparenchymal clot resolves. This picture is in stark contrast to that for the patient with a ruptured aneurysm, who has a high risk for rebleeding, vasospasm, or both after the initial hemorrhage.

The clinical sequelae of a hemorrhage depend on the location and extent of intracranial mass effect. Patients with hemorrhage in proximity to functional motor cortex may sustain contralateral hemiparesis or hemiplegia, whereas patients with hemorrhage in clinically silent areas of the brain (i.e., the right frontal lobe) may have no focal deficits. Headaches and seizures may also be associated with intracranial hemorrhage. Recurrent hemorrhages are usually separated by years and sometimes decades. As described previously, the prospective study by Ondra and colleagues[44] suggests a 4% per year risk of major rebleeding.

Seizures

Seizures are the second most common symptom associated with supratentorial intracranial vascular anomalies. Approximately 25% to 50% of all patients with AVMs present with a focal or generalized seizure, without obvious hemorrhage.[43] In general, epilepsy associated with intracranial vascular anomalies can be controlled with effective medical management. Accordingly, the presence of a seizure disorder alone is not sufficient to warrant radical surgical treatment of an AVM or cavernous malformation. Surgical treatment will diminish an associated seizure disorder in some cases; often, however, there is no improvement. The selection of patients for surgical treatment should therefore be based on the risk of future hemorrhage.

Headache

Headaches are a common problem with AVMs but are rarely encountered in other vascular lesions without evidence of hemorrhage.[45,46] A headache disorder similar to classic migraine headaches has been described for patients with AVMs.[47] These headaches are usually unilateral and do not shift from side to side as seen in patients with migraine. However, auras, visual symptomatology, and severe debilitating intermittent headaches have been described in patients with AVMs. Patients with lesions of the occipital lobe are especially prone to development of a migraine-like headache disorder.[46] More generalized headaches related to elevated venous pressures and stretching of venous sinuses and dura have also been reported.[43] These headaches are less dramatic than those seen with occipital lobe AVMs and are rarely of a debilitating nature.

Steal Syndromes

A rare but important symptom associated with AVMs is related to arterial steal phenomenon.[48] This symptom is most relevant to a subgroup of patients who demonstrate progressive neurologic deficits without hemorrhage over many years in conjunction with high-flow AVMs. Although a definitive explanation for this problem is lacking,[49] the deficits that develop are most likely related to the cumulative effect of steal from normal perfusion of the surrounding brain by the AVM. As described previously, the phenomenon of normal perfusion pressure breakthrough may in fact be related to the physiologic environment created by chronic steal syndromes.

Treatment Options and Considerations

Cushing and Bailey[4] advise, "As in most cerebral lesions, however, each case should be considered a law unto itself. There are large aneurysms and small ones; those which are mostly arterial, others mainly venous; some are superficial, others deep, some are in highly important areas of the brain, others in portions largely silent. All of these factors, and finally the patient's wishes in the matter must be weighed."

The choice of treatment for patients should consider risks attendant to each therapeutic option as well as the natural history of the individual patient.[50] Therapeutic alternatives are as follows, either individually or in combination: (1) operative resection or obliteration, (2) endovascular embolization, and (3) radiosurgery. Judicious observation should always be a consideration, especially in patients for whom surgery poses a high risk because of medically related issues, lesion size or location, or vascular anatomy.

In general, venous malformations and capillary telangiectasias do not require therapeutic intervention because of their relatively benign nature. Cavernous malformations are best left untreated when they are found incidentally[51]; however, if they manifest as hemorrhage, surgical resection should be considered.[52,53] Symptomatic cavernous malformations of the supratentorial compartment and spinal cord can often be excised and cured by surgery. Cavernous malformations of the cerebellum can also usually be readily excised when manifesting as hemorrhage. In contrast, cavernous malformations of the brainstem are difficult to treat surgically without incurring significant morbidity.[54] Because the natural history shows the risk of these lesions to be low, only appropriate low-risk surgical procedures should be considered. High-risk surgery to remove deep capsular, basal ganglia, or brainstem malformations requires a clinical prodrome of progressive neurologic decline and multiple hemorrhages.

The most important clinical decision-making with regard to vascular malformations is related to AVM. The age of the patient, the location and size of the AVM, and the vascular configuration are important factors that warrant consideration in the decision about treatment.[50]

Surgical Intervention

Surgical removal of an AVM is the most definitive treatment and offers the patient the best chance of an immediate cure. The presenting symptoms of an AVM are probably the least important factor in deciding whether or not a patient should be subjected to an intracranial operation. The previously described natural history studies clearly demonstrate that even patients who present with nonhemorrhagic seizures and headaches are at significant risk for AVM-associated intracranial bleeding.[44] In general, the risk of surgical intervention cannot be justified in asymptomatic patients older than 55 years. After this age, the risks of surgery are about equal to the risks of allowing the lesions to develop naturally over the projected lifetime of the individual. Location is critical as well. For example, AVMs located in areas such as the brainstem or basal ganglia should be treated surgically only in young patients who present with symptomatic hemorrhage and significant neurologic disability.[55,56] Lesions located in the medial hemisphere also present a high level of operative difficulty compared with other supratentorial lesions.[57] In contrast, malformations that are small, polar in location, and readily accessible can be treated surgically, even in older patients.

The size and vascular configuration of the lesion has formed the basis of a rudimentary classification system described by Spetzler and Martin[58] in 1986. In this system, lesions are graded on the basis of size, pattern of venous drainage, and neurologic eloquence of adjacent brain. All AVMs can be assigned to one of six grades. Grade I malformations are small, superficial, and located in noneloquent cortex; grade V lesions are large, deep, and situated in neurologically critical areas; and grade VI lesions are essentially inoperable. Retrospective and prospective application of this grading scheme to a series of surgically excised AVMs has demonstrated correlation with the incidence of postoperative neurologic complications.[58,59]

The Spetzler-Martin grading scale fails to address many aspects of surgical risks. A very important feature of AVMs that predicts complex surgery and high risk is the presence of deep perforator vessels supplying an AVM. When lenticulostriate vessels, thalamoperforate vessels, or both supply the malformation, critical brain areas must be violated to secure the arterial supply. Similarly, superficial AVMs that have exclusive cortical arterial supply and cortical venous drainage, even lesions that are large and located in eloquent areas of the brain, can be safely excised. Therefore, the decision for or against resection is multifactorial. Ideally, patients should be younger than 50 years and should have small, cortically based lesions that present to the surface with primary cortical arterial supply and cortical venous drainage. Deep malformations, especially those with deep arterial and venous associations, are better treated conservatively or with stereotaxic radiosurgery when appropriate.

Operative Technique

The details of operative approaches to AVM lesions vary significantly according to size, location, and vascular configuration. Several groups have described specific considerations regarding medial hemisphere,[57] basal ganglia,[56,60] posterior fossa,[61–63] and brainstem locations.[55,64,65] The reader is referred to their excellent reviews for technical details on the surgery of lesions in these specific areas. General considerations for operative technique include preoperative evaluation and preparation, intraoperative goals, and postoperative management.

Before surgery, each patient should be thoroughly evaluated for coexisting medical conditions, such as hypertension, that may effect subsequent management. In addition, a complete radiologic assessment should include high-quality angiograms and, when possible, MRI sequences that facilitate localization of the lesion. The patient is prepared for surgery by ensuring adequate blood levels of anticonvulsant drugs. Patients are at a higher risk for seizures after surgical resection, possibly secondary to changes in venous blood flow patterns.[66] Accordingly, it is essential to load patients preoperatively and to ensure maintenance of adequate anticonvulsant drug levels in the immediate postoperative period.

In general, initial intraoperative goals of AVM surgery include lesion localization, exposure of relevant anatomy, and brain relaxation. Localization can be facilitated by correlation of anatomic landmarks with the lesion anatomy or by means of stereotaxis. A wide craniotomy and dural opening is used to expose relevant anatomy. When the dura is opened, it is important to avoid compromise of any dural-based venous drainage of the lesion. Brain relaxation is accomplished by administration of mannitol, appropriate positioning of the patient's head above the heart, hyperventilation, and, occasionally, cerebrospinal fluid (CSF) drainage via a spinal or intraventricular drain.

After adequate exposure, the next surgical goal is to localize the lesion within the surgical field. The arterialized distended veins of an AVM are the best surface landmark and can be correlated with the angiogram to pinpoint the location of arteries that often lie deeper (Fig. 68–7). The bulk of the malformation may flare out under otherwise normal-appearing cortex so that only the tip of the lesion is seen. After exposure of the malformation surface and thorough review of the angiogram, a circumscribing incision is made that avoids normal cortex. Care should be taken during this stage of the operation to avoid disturbing any major draining veins. Smaller vessels may be interrupted, but even with a major deep draining vein, the primary cortical vein should be left intact until much later in the operation. Nutrient arteries are usually found deep in the sulcus. The surgeon cauterizes, clips, and divides them, working circumferentially around the margins of the malformations. Thus, the entire cortical margin and subcortical surface of the malformation are circumscribed, the major veins being avoided while the arterial supply is secured.

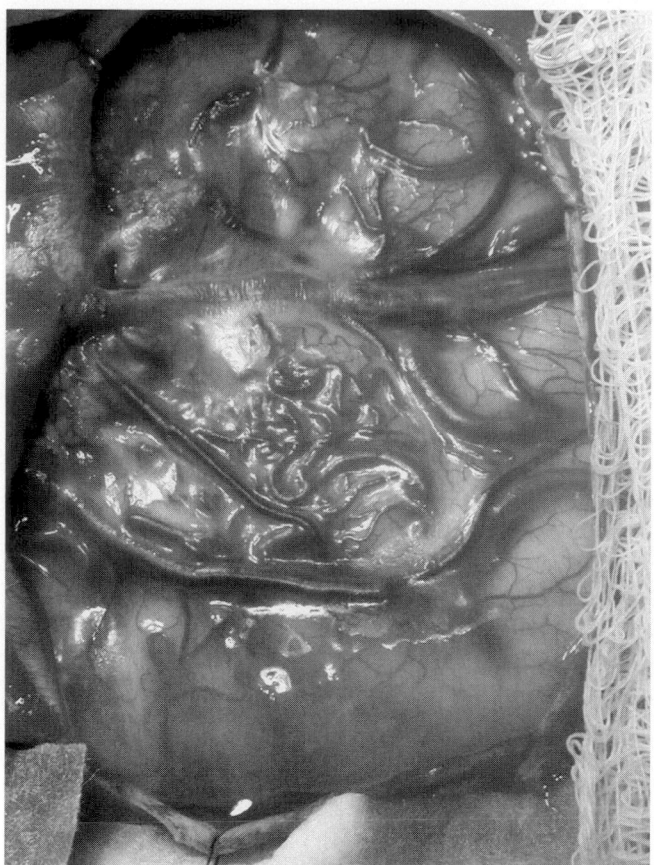

FIGURE 68–7 *Arterialized distended veins of an arteriovenous malformation on the surface of the brain.*

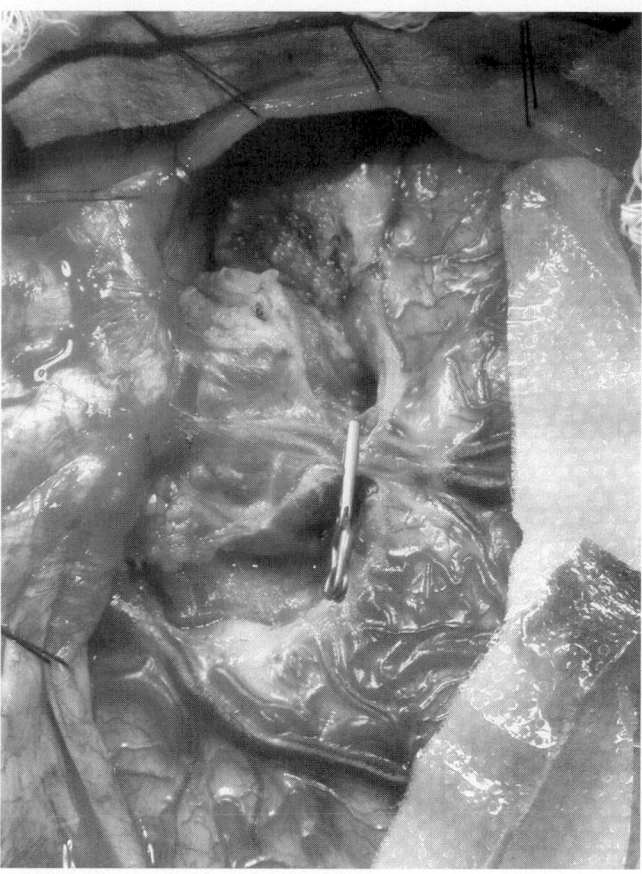

FIGURE 68–8 *Test occlusion of the draining vein in an arteriovenous malformation.*

In general, bipolar cautery is used to secure arterial feeders. Some larger vessels require clipping, and smaller arteries can be cauterized and sectioned primarily. As deeper portions of the malformation are uncovered, a gliotic area surrounding the malformation can be separated from the normal white matter. This separation often affords an excellent plane of dissection that is aided by previous hemorrhages. However, deep areas of the malformation are sometimes supplied by numerous tiny penetrating vessels traversing the white matter, which can be extremely difficult to cauterize. It is these deep portions of the malformation that pose the greatest surgical challenge for hemostasis. Once the lesion has been circumferentially dissected, a test occlusion of the draining vein is undertaken to evaluate the effects of removing the vessel (Fig. 68–8). In addition, the resection cavity should be finally inspected at a systolic blood pressure above the patient's baseline pressure values.

Postoperative Management

After total removal of the AVM, the two most prevalent complications are hemorrhage and seizures.[43] In most cases, clinically significant hemorrhage is the result of residual AVM secondary to incomplete excision. These hemorrhages typically occur within the first 12 to 24 hours postoperatively and are associated with a clinical decline necessitating hematoma evacuation. Other causes of postoperative hemorrhage are insufficient occlusion of major

arterial inputs, venous occlusion, and normal perfusion pressure breakthrough phenomenon.[21] Postoperative maintenance of strict blood pressure parameters is critical, as is formal documentation of complete removal of the AVM by means of a high-quality postoperative angiogram.

We typically procure an angiogram immediately after the operation in a fully equipped angiogram suite (Fig. 68–9). During this immediate postoperative period, the patient is kept intubated and sedated, and the operating room and staff remain available in case residual AVM is found on the angiogram. In most institutions, the quality of the intraoperative angiography is not sufficient to fully evaluate the complex vascular changes often seen after AVM resection. The decision to resect additional cortical and white matter areas that contain abnormal vessels is crucial in terms of potential postoperative deficits. High-quality angiography is required to differentiate dysplastic vessels that will involute spontaneously from dangerous residual AVM.

Seizures may occur postoperatively even if adequate levels of anticonvulsants have been maintained before, during, and after the operation. If a seizure does occur postoperatively, control should be gained as rapidly as possible by means of standard multiple-drug therapy. Once the patient is stabilized in the postictal period, head CT should be performed to document that there is no hematoma. After surgery, 24 hours of monitoring in an intensive care unit (ICU) is sufficient in uncomplicated

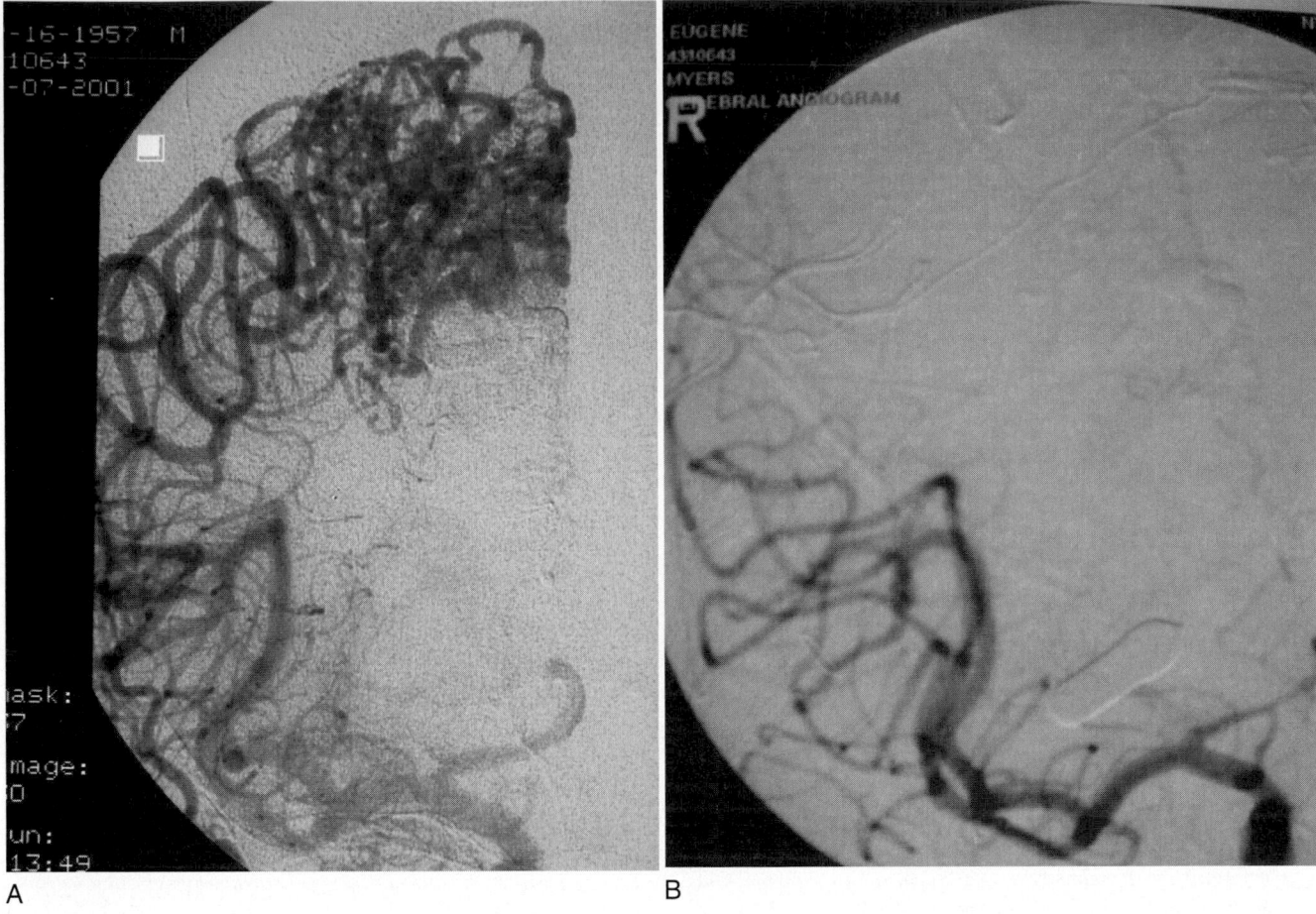

A   B

FIGURE 68–9   *Total removal of an arteriovenous malformation. Preoperative (A) and postoperative (B) angiograms.*

cases. Dexamethasone dosage can then be rapidly tapered off, and patients can begin ambulating. Seizure prophylaxis is generally advisable for approximately 6 months after uncomplicated surgery, but longer periods may be required in patients who have postoperative seizures or a previous (preoperative) history of seizures. In such patients, anticonvulsant medication is continued for at least a year after the last seizure.

Embolization

Endovascular embolization is an important adjunct to the management of patients with AVMs. The technology is rapidly improving with respect to safety and efficacy. In general, the procedure is facilitated by femoral arterial access and fluoroscopic guidance of a catheter into the feeding artery of an AVM. Subsequently, embolic materials such as wire coils, pellets, particulate slurries, and glue are injected in a controlled fashion to occlude the arterial supply of the AVM.[67] Although in rare cases embolization treatment can annihilate an AVM completely, it is almost never appropriate to apply this modality as the sole treatment.[68-71] A partially treated AVM may be more likely to bleed than an untreated AVM; therefore endovascular treatment is not recommended unless it is utilized as part of a multimodality plan geared toward total obliteration of the malformation.

In an optimal scenario, embolization can successfully remove deep feeders to the malformation, greatly decreasing the risk of postoperative hemorrhage and associated morbidity. For a large AVM, the gradual occlusion of flow through the lesion significantly reduces the incidence of arterial and venous circulatory changes that lead to hyperemia and hemorrhage after surgical excision. In some instances, embolization treatment can reduce a large malformation to a small size that may be amenable to radiosurgery.[68] The value of this approach has yet to be proved, because recanalization in treated but not excised AVMs can occur.[72]

The choice to integrate embolization into the treatment plan is actively debated,[73] in part because the risks of embolization may differ according to the experience of the interventional team. Independently assessed data on frequency, severity, and determinants of neurologic deficits after endovascular treatment of AVMs are scarce. At our institution, 233 consecutive patients with AVMs receiving one or more endovascular treatments (for a total of 545 procedures) were analyzed prospectively.[74] The Rankin Scale was used to assess neurologic impairment before and after completion of endovascular therapy. Demographic, clinical, and morphologic predictors of treatment-related neurologic deficits were identified through the use of multivariate logistic regression models. The analysis assessed lesion characteristics such as AVM size, venous drainage pattern, and eloquence of AVM location. Mean follow-up time was 9.6 months (SD [standard deviation], 18.1 months). Two hundred patients (86%) experienced no change in neurologic status after treatment, and 33 patients (14%) showed treatment-related neurologic deficits. Of the latter, 5 patients (2%) had persistent disabling deficits (Rankin score > 2), and 2 (1%) died. Higher patient age, larger number of embolizations, and absence of a pretreatment neurologic deficit were associated with new neurologic deficits. None of the morphologic AVM characteristics tested was found to predict treatment complications. From independent neurologic assessment and prospective data collection, these findings suggest a low rate of disabling treatment complications after endovascular brain AVM treatment in high-volume centers.

Radiosurgery

Cushing and Bailey[4] were among the first to describe radiation therapy for patients with AVMs. Since their initial descriptions, great progress has been made with regard to target resolution and associated reduction in treatment morbidity.[75] The principles of stereotactic radiosurgery are based on delivery of high-energy radiation to a well-defined volume containing the nidus of the malformation. Gradual sclerosis of the blood vessels subsequently occurs, obliterating the AVM over a period of 1 to 2 years.

Radiosurgery was first performed with a device called the gamma knife.[76] However, because this instrument is expensive and depends on high-energy cobalt sources, it is not widely available. Proton beams and linear accelerators have been effectively used for radiosurgery because these high-energy radiation sources are more readily available and can be easily interfaced with standard CT and angiographically directed stereotactic equipment. Depending on several factors, including size and vascular characteristics, obliteration of an AVM seems to take 1 to 2 years after delivery of a therapeutic dose.[77] Regardless of the source utilized, radiosurgery is highly effective for AVMs less than 2.0 cm in largest diameter, but larger malformations are less responsive.[78–80]

With proper dosimetry, the immediate side effects of radiosurgery have been moderate and limited to mild episodes of radiation necrosis.[81] However, the difficulty associated with treating patients with radiosurgery relates to the possibility of post-treatment hemorrhage. Because of the late onset of therapeutic effect, there is a definitive risk for hemorrhage after radiosurgery. The long-term side effects of radiosurgery as well as the risk of bleeding have been studied by a number of different groups.[82–85] In particular, Flickinger and coworkers have been extremely prolific with respect to reporting their collective experience using the gamma knife for the treatment of patients with AVMs. In a series of articles starting in 1995 and continuing to the present, this group has described retrospective data with long-term follow-up on patients treated at their institution as well as patients treated at other collaborative centers.[79,80,86–91] In 1999, a multi-institutional study of 102 patients with AVMs who experienced neurologic sequelae after radiosurgery was described.[86] These patients were derived from a pool of 1255 patients with AVMs treated with radiosurgery. Complications in these 102 patients consisted of evidence of radiation injury to the brain parenchyma in 80 patients (7 also with cranial nerve deficits, 12 also with seizures, and 5 with cyst formation), isolated cranial neuropathies in 12 patients, and only new or worsened seizures in 10 patients. Severity was classified as minimal in 39 patients, mild in 40, disabling in 21, and

fatal in 2. Symptoms resolved completely in 42 patients, for an actuarial resolution rate of 54% ± 7% at 3 years after onset of symptoms after radiotherapy. Multivariate analysis identified significantly greater symptom resolution in patients with no prior history of hemorrhage ($P = 0.01$, 66% vs. 41%), and in patients with symptoms of minimal severity, such as headache or seizure, as the only sequelae of radiosurgery ($P < 0.0001$, 88% vs. 34%). This large study demonstrates that the late sequelae of radiosurgery can manifest in various ways. However, further long-term studies of these problems are needed to take into account symptom severity and prior hemorrhage history. In addition, it will be important to weigh institutional bias toward treatment with respect to its effects on clinical decision-making.

CASE STUDIES

The following eight cases were selected from the senior chapter author's (R.A.S.) experience to exemplify the multimodality treatment necessary to effectively treat AVMs of the brain. Although each case is approached individually, recurrent themes of management warrant general application. In every case, the risk of treatment is weighed against the risk of natural disease progression. In some cases there is no clear-cut answer, underscoring the difficulty of managing these patients in even an optimal, tertiary-care environment. The clinical presentation and description of AVM vascular anatomy is included to provide context for the treatment plan.

Case 1: Arteriovenous Malformation Treated with Embolization and Surgical Excision

A 28-year-old man presenting with a generalized seizure was found upon further evaluation to have a 2.0 × 4.0–cm vascular malformation extending from the surface of the parietal lobe down to the atrium of the left lateral ventricle (Fig. 68–10). The patient recovered to a normal neurologic baseline and was treated with phenytoin for his seizure. He subsequently underwent a series of embolizations over a 1-year period. Arterial flow into the malformation was significantly reduced, as shown in Figure 68–11. A craniotomy and wide dural opening revealed focal abnormalities on the brain surface overlying the malformation (Fig. 68–12), which facilitated localization of the lesion. A circumferential resection was undertaken to carefully remove the lesion en bloc (Fig. 68–13). An immediately postoperative angiogram confirmed complete excision of the malformation, and the patient sustained no postoperative complication. This case illustrates the value of preoperative embolization, as the morbidity associated with removing the lesion shown in Figure 68–11*C* is significantly less than for the lesion shown in Figure 68–11*A* and *B*. In addition, this case illustrates a common mode of presentation (i.e., seizure) and the importance of stabilizing patients with AVMs preoperatively with appropriate anticonvulsant medication.

Case 2: Arteriovenous Malformation Treated Conservatively

A 23-year-old woman presented with a sudden onset of severe headache, nausea, vomiting, and change in mental

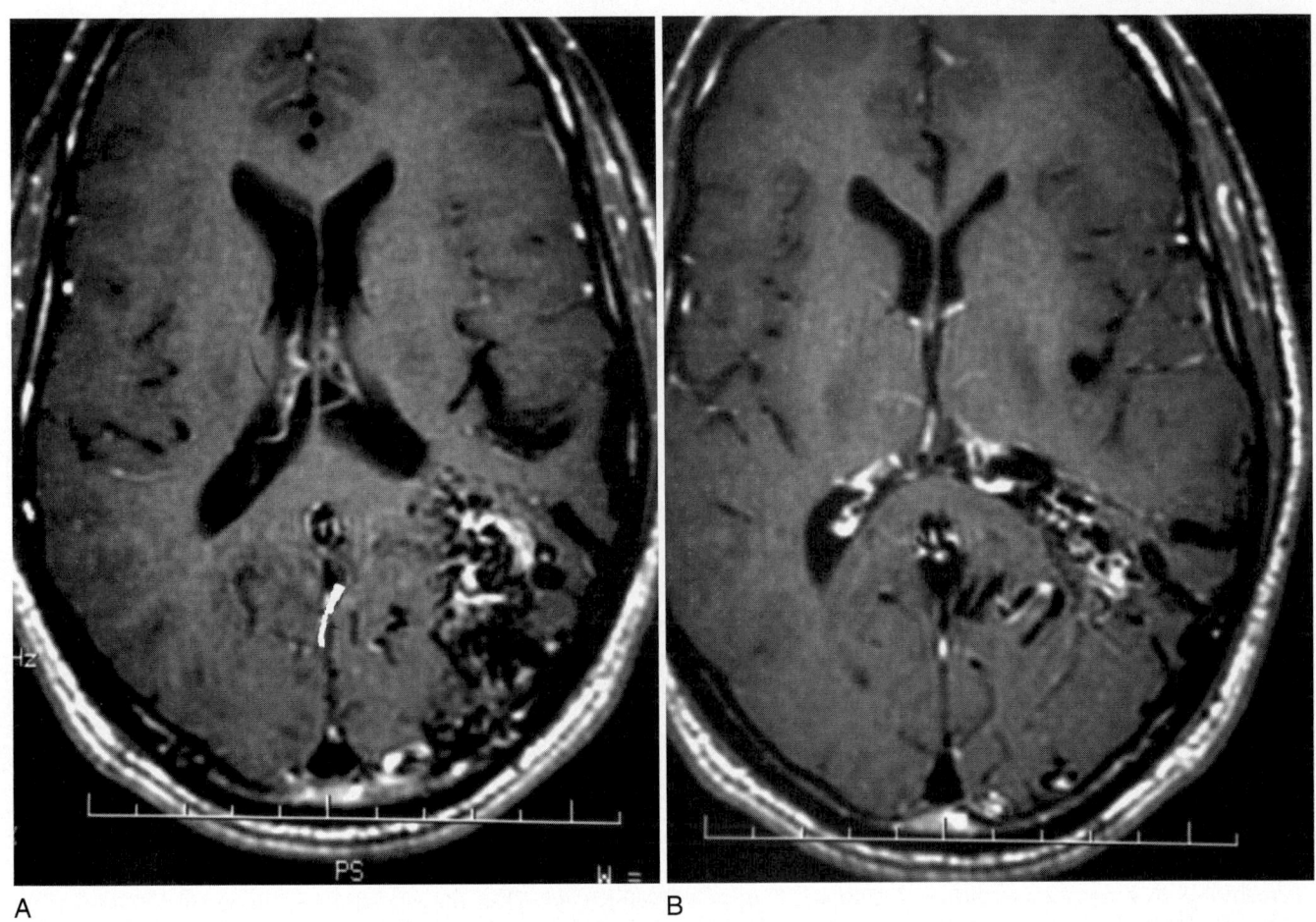

A   B

FIGURE 68–10   A *and* B, *A 28-year-old man with generalized seizure found to have an arteriovenous malformation extending from the surface of the parietal lobe down to the atrium of the left lateral ventricle.*

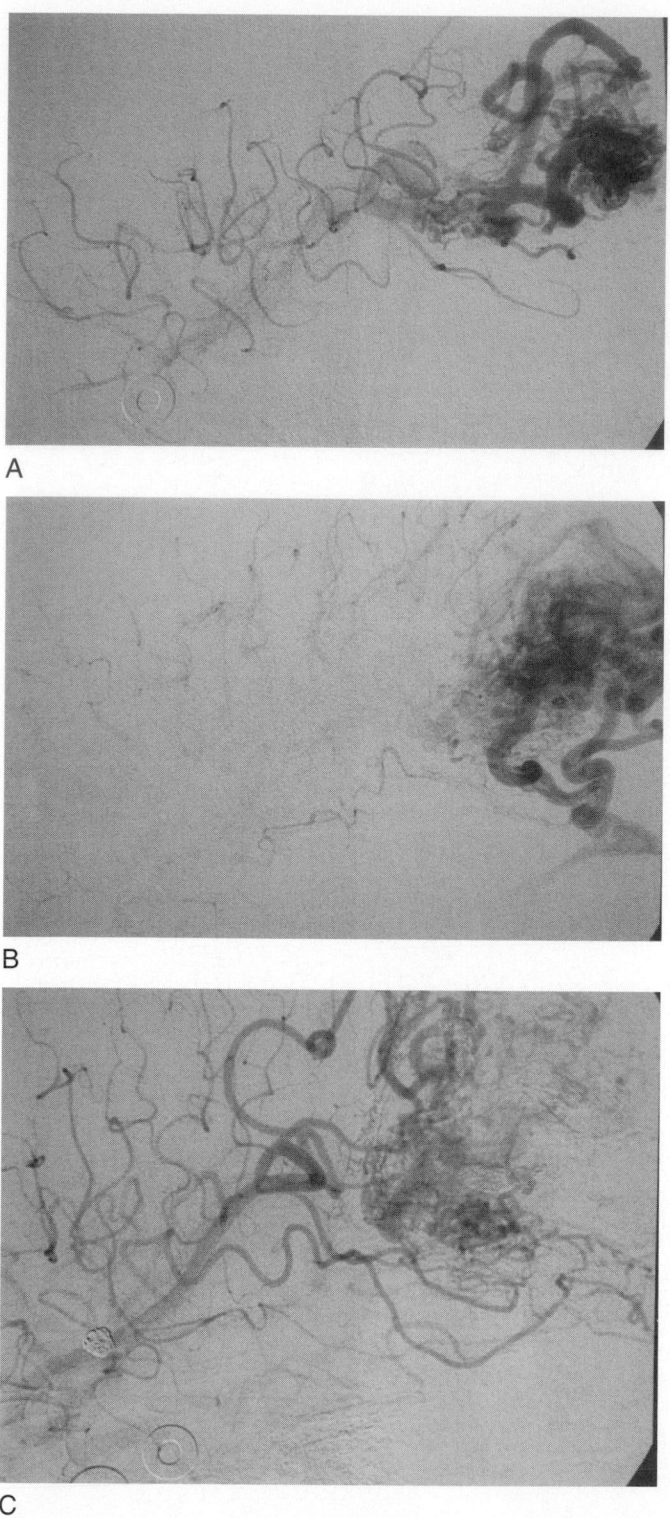

A

B

C

FIGURE 68–11 *Same patient as in Figure 68–10. A, Arterial phase before embolization. B, Venous phase before embolization. C, After embolization.*

Therapy

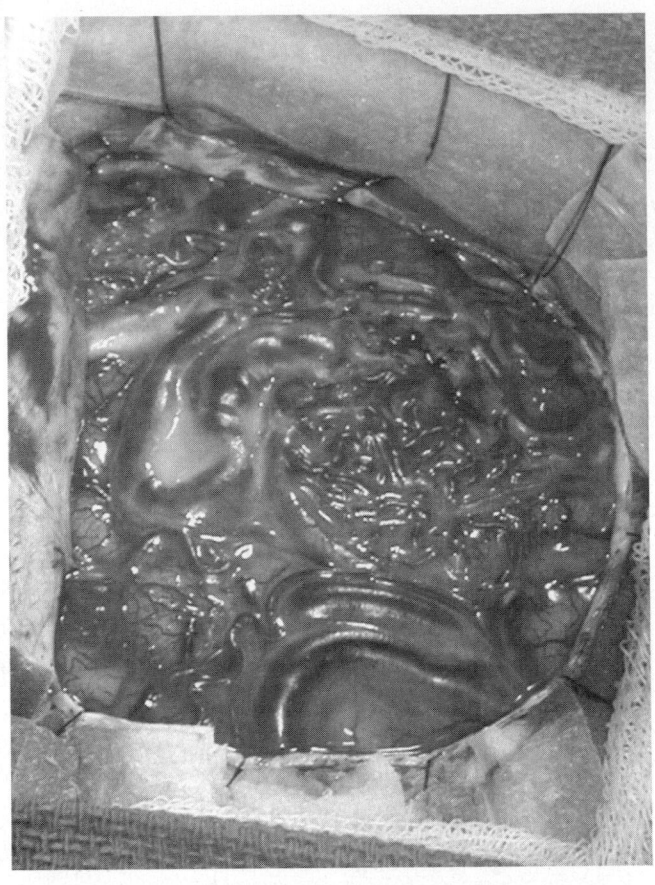

FIGURE 68–12 *Same patient as in Figures 68–10 and 68–11. Focal abnormalities on the brain surface overlying the malformation.*

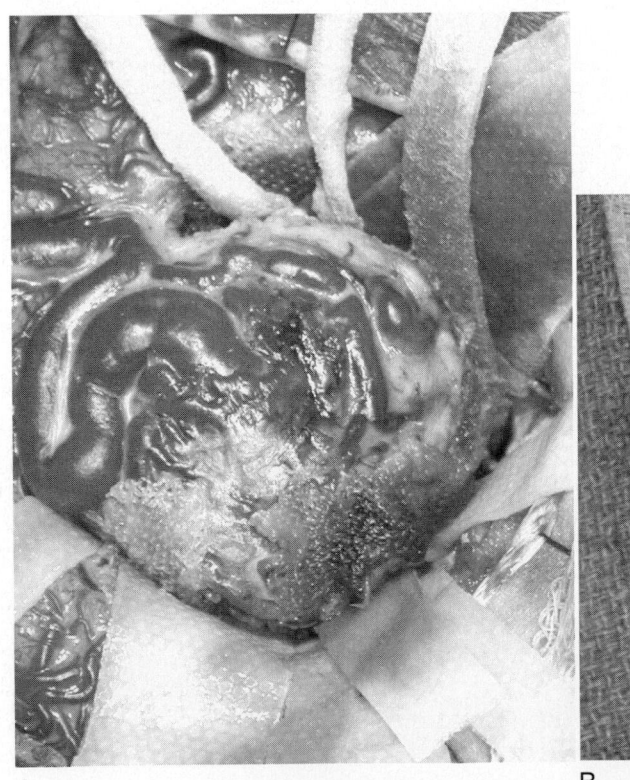

A

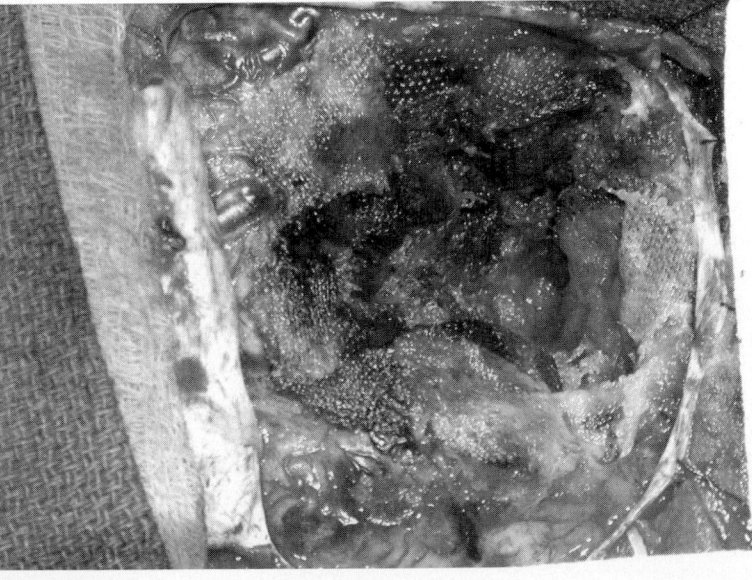

B

FIGURE 68–13 *Same patient as in Figures 68–10 to 68–12. A and B, En bloc surgical resection.*

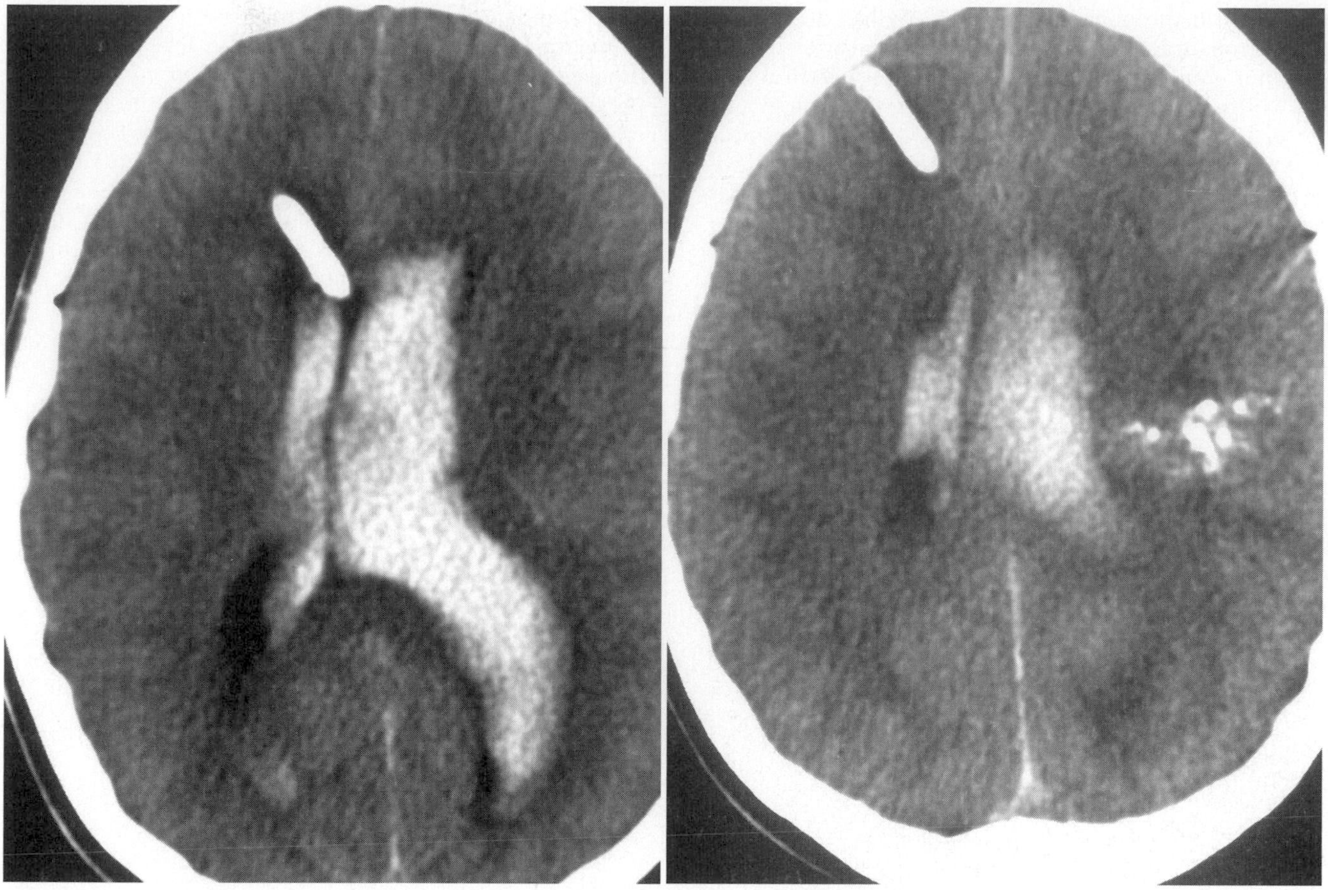

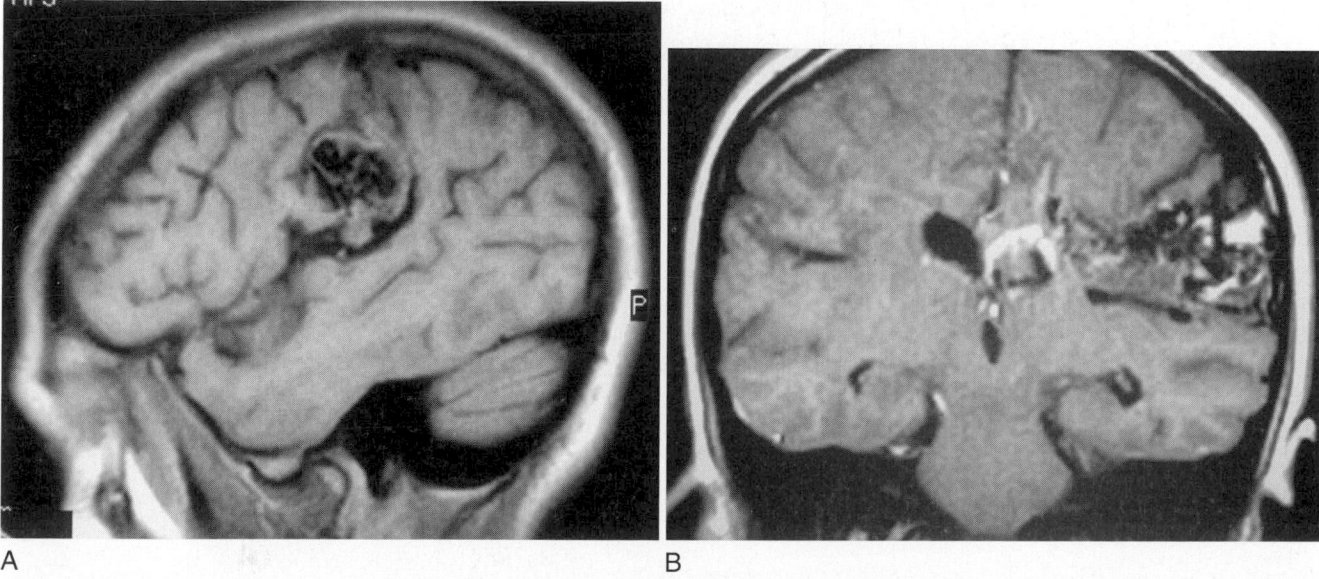

FIGURE 68–14 *A 23-year-old woman with intraventricular hemorrhage. A and B, CT scans.*

status. Head CT at the time of presentation revealed a large intraventricular hemorrhage and calcifications in the left motor region consistent with an AVM (Fig. 68–14). An external ventricular drain was placed on an emergency basis to decompress her ventricles, and after more than 2 weeks in the intensive care unit, she recovered to neurologic baseline with the exception of a subtle balance instability. She did not require permanent CSF diversion. MRI demonstrated a 3.0 × 5.0–cm AVM adjacent to the left motor strip and extending deeply into the ventricle (Fig. 68–15).

FIGURE 68–15 *Same patient as in Figure 68–14. A and B, MRI demonstrating an arteriovenous malformation adjacent to the left motor strip and extending deeply into the ventricle.*

As shown in the angiograms, the AVM has dual arterial supply from branches of the middle cerebral artery and the posterior choroidal vessels of the posterior cerebral arteries, with superficial and deep venous drainage (Fig. 68–16). Although the malformation could be surgically removed after embolization, the morbidity associated with disrupting motor fibers in proximity to the lesion make surgery an unappealing option for this patient.

This case illustrates two important points that come to bear in the management of patients with AVMs. The first point is that in an acute setting, there is little to be gained by attempting emergency decompression of hemorrhage or malformation. The intervention of external ventricular drainage facilitated management of increase in intracranial pressure while affording the medical team the time necessary to procure all the appropriate studies. The second point is that not all AVMs can be treated without incurring significant morbidity. The size of this lesion (i.e., > 3.0 cm) precludes radiosurgery. This AVM's deep perforator supply and deep venous drainage as well as its proximity to the motor strip predict significant risk with endovascular and surgical treatment.

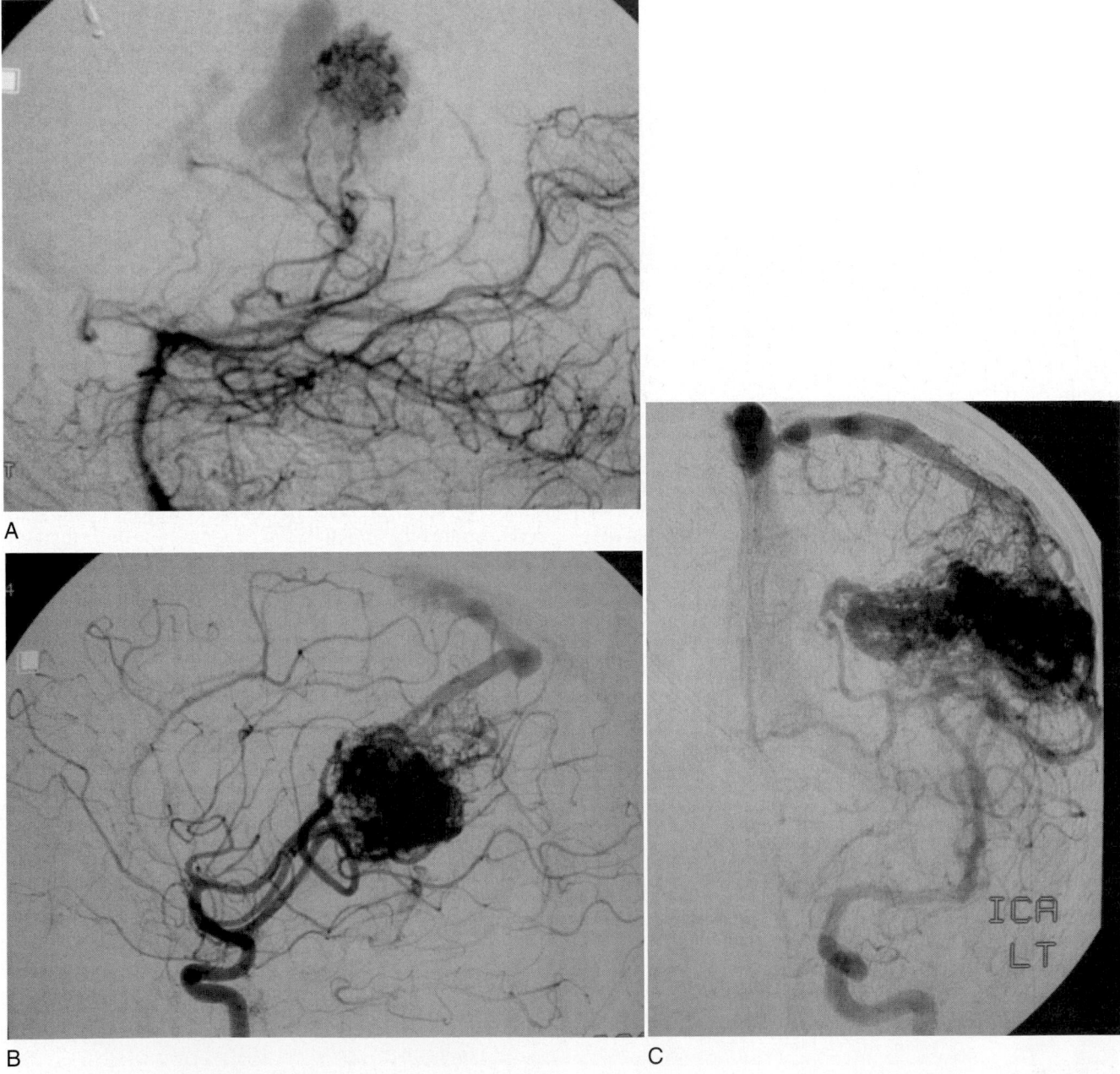

A

B

C

FIGURE 68–16   *Same patient as in Figures 68–14 and 68–15. A to C, Angiograms showing dual arterial supply from branches of the middle cerebral artery and the posterior choroidal vessels of the posterior cerebral arteries, with deep and superficial drainage.*

Case 3: Arteriovenous Malformation Treated with Embolization and Radiosurgery

A 33-year-old woman presented after sustaining a grand mal seizure. Evaluation performed shortly afterward revealed a right posterior temporal AVM that was 3.0 cm in its largest diameter. The AVM was in the inferior temporal gyrus and presented to the surface laterally. Although this lesion was surgically accessible, superselective Wada testing performed during the embolization demonstrated that memory and language functions were heavily localized to the right temporal lobe. Given the inherent risks associated with a surgical procedure in this location, the patient elected to undergo embolization followed by radiosurgery. As shown in Figure 68–17, embolization was performed to reduce arterial inflow, followed by radiosurgery. An angiogram at 3 years' follow-up demonstrates only a small residual component in proximity to the glue cast (Fig. 68–18).

This case illustrates the importance of a multidisciplinary approach and of allowing the patient and physicians to properly evaluate treatment risks. It also demonstrates the value of obtaining follow-up information on treated patients with AVMs. As we begin to accrue these data from multiple centers, a clearer picture will emerge with respect to the efficacy of radiosurgery and the possibility that partial embolization may reduce the cure rate with subsequent stereotactic radiosurgery.

Case 4: Arteriovenous Malformation Treated with Surgery Demonstrating Presence of Postoperative Dysplastic Vessels That Resolve over Time

A 41-year-old woman presented with a sudden, severe headache and blurred vision. Evaluation at that time revealed no subarachnoid hemorrhage. However, the patient was noted to have a right parietal AVM with a large dilated vein (Fig. 68–19). Intraoperatively, the dilated arterialized vein could be appreciated on the surface of the brain and was preserved until the majority of the lesion had

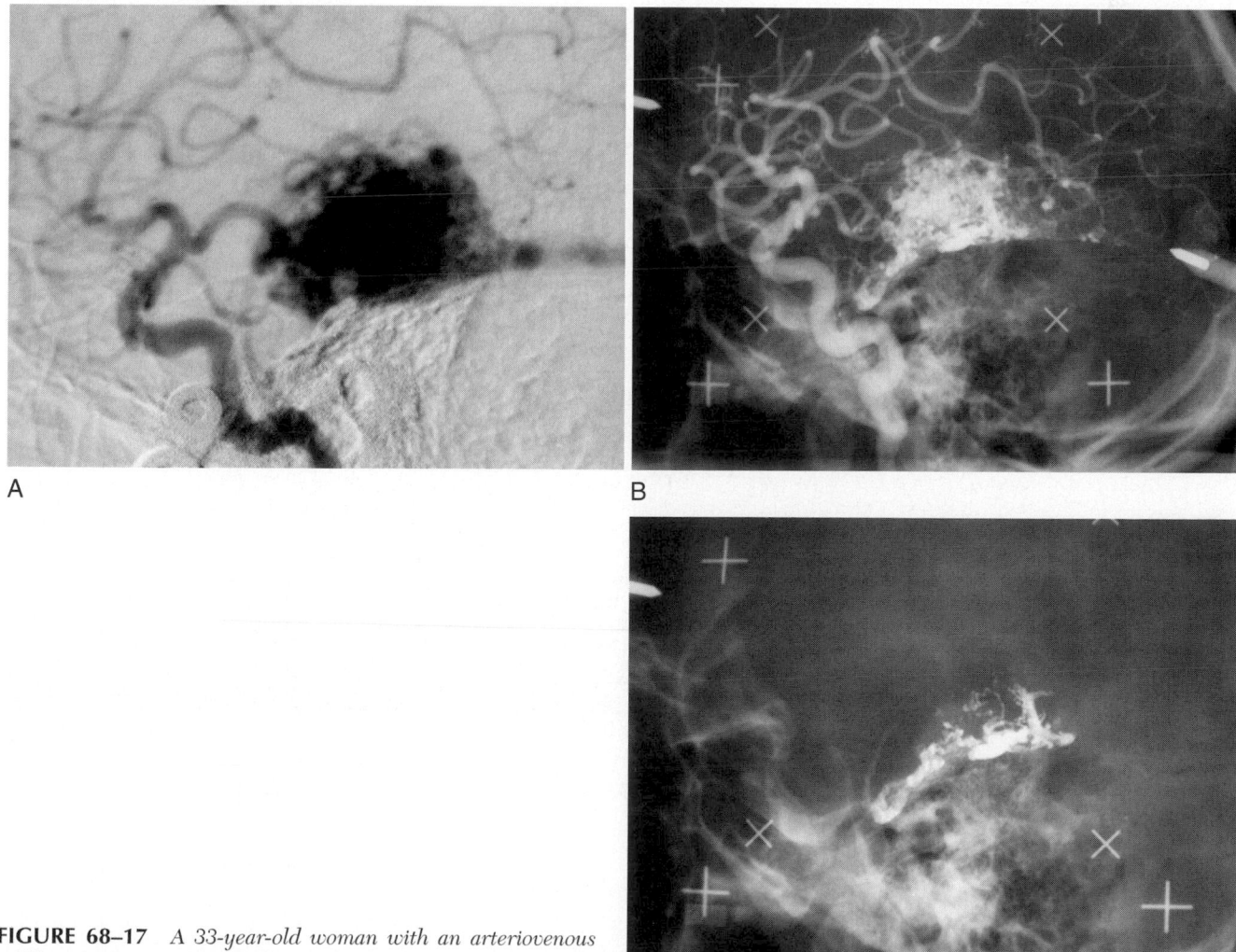

A

B

C

FIGURE 68–17 *A 33-year-old woman with an arteriovenous malformation. A, Preoperative angiogram. B and C, After gamma-knife radiation and embolization.*

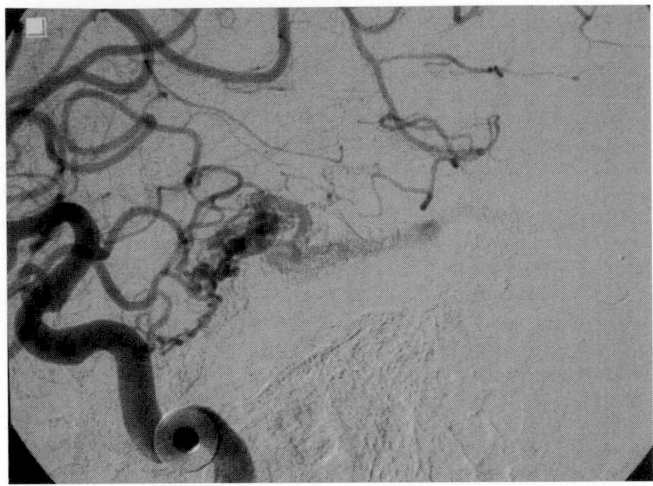

FIGURE 68–18 *Same patient as in Figure 68–17. Three years after treatment, angiogram demonstrates small residual component in proximity to the glue cast.*

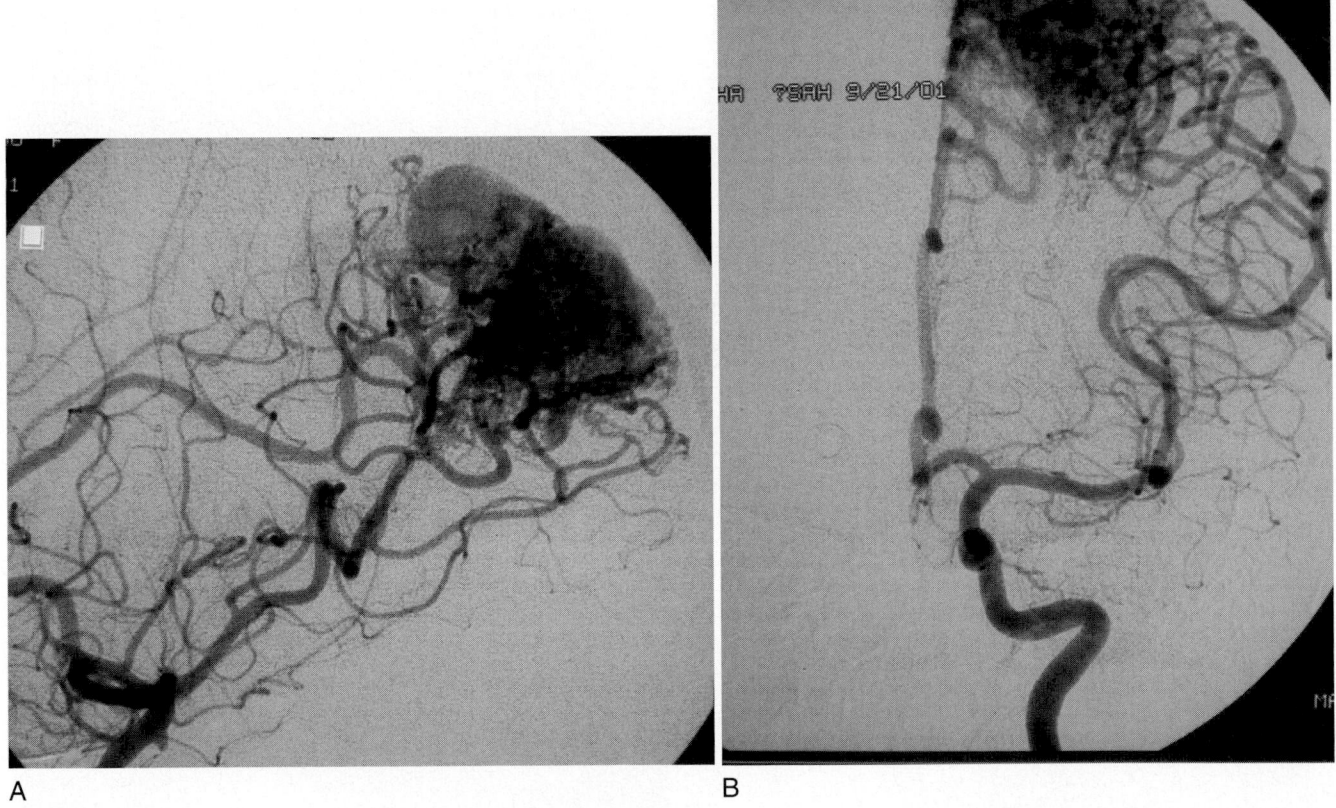

A   B

FIGURE 68–19 *A 41-year-old woman with arteriovenous malformation. Preoperative lateral (A) and anteroposterior (B) angiograms.*

been circumferentially dissected (Fig. 68–20). An immediate postoperative angiogram showed complete resection of the AVM; however, a number of dysplastic vessels were seen that were not associated with an early draining vein (Fig. 68–21). Follow-up angiogram demonstrated resolution of these dysplastic vessels (Fig. 68–22).

This case illustrates the importance of accurately interpreting postoperative angiograms as well as the utility of conservative management in the treatment of dysplastic vessels. Solomon and colleagues[92] have described their experience with abnormal dysplastic vessels discovered after AVM resection in 86 consecutive patients. These patients underwent operations with standard protocol for immediate postoperative angiography while under the same general anesthesia. Angiographic interpretation dictated admission to the intensive care unit or return to the operating room for further resection. In 78 patients, the angiogram revealed complete resection without dysplastic vessels. Two patients were returned to the operating room, one for residual malformation with an early draining vein, and one for resection of residual dysplastic vessels. There was one postoperative hemorrhage in a patient whose postoperative angiogram was falsely negative for residual AVM. Six patients with residual dysplastic vessels mimicking residual AVM, but without an early draining vein, were managed conservatively. Follow-up

angiography demonstrated spontaneous involution of these abnormal vessels in all of these patients, as illustrated by this case.

On the basis of this experience, we believe that residual dysplastic feeding vessels resembling the neovascularity of moyamoya disease, but not associated with an early draining vein, do not represent residual malformation after AVM resection. The abnormal vessels will completely resolve over time and should be followed conservatively.[92] In a follow-up report to this initial description, the predictors and frequency of residual dysplastic vessels on cerebral angiography after AVM surgery were studied in 240 prospectively enrolled surgical patients from the New York AVM Databank.[93] These patients collectively underwent 269 AVM-related surgical procedures, and postoperative brain angiographic findings were classified post hoc as showing (1) persistent dysplastic vessels, (2) a residual AVM, (3) focal hyperemia in the surgical bed, (4) other changes, or (5) normal findings. Univariate and multivariate analysis models were applied to test for an association between residual dysplastic vessels and patient age, patient gender, preoperative AVM size, anatomic AVM location, number of embolization procedures before surgery, and the interval between AVM surgery and the postoperative angiogram. Of the 224 documented postoperative angiograms, 78 (35%) showed dysplastic vessels, 24

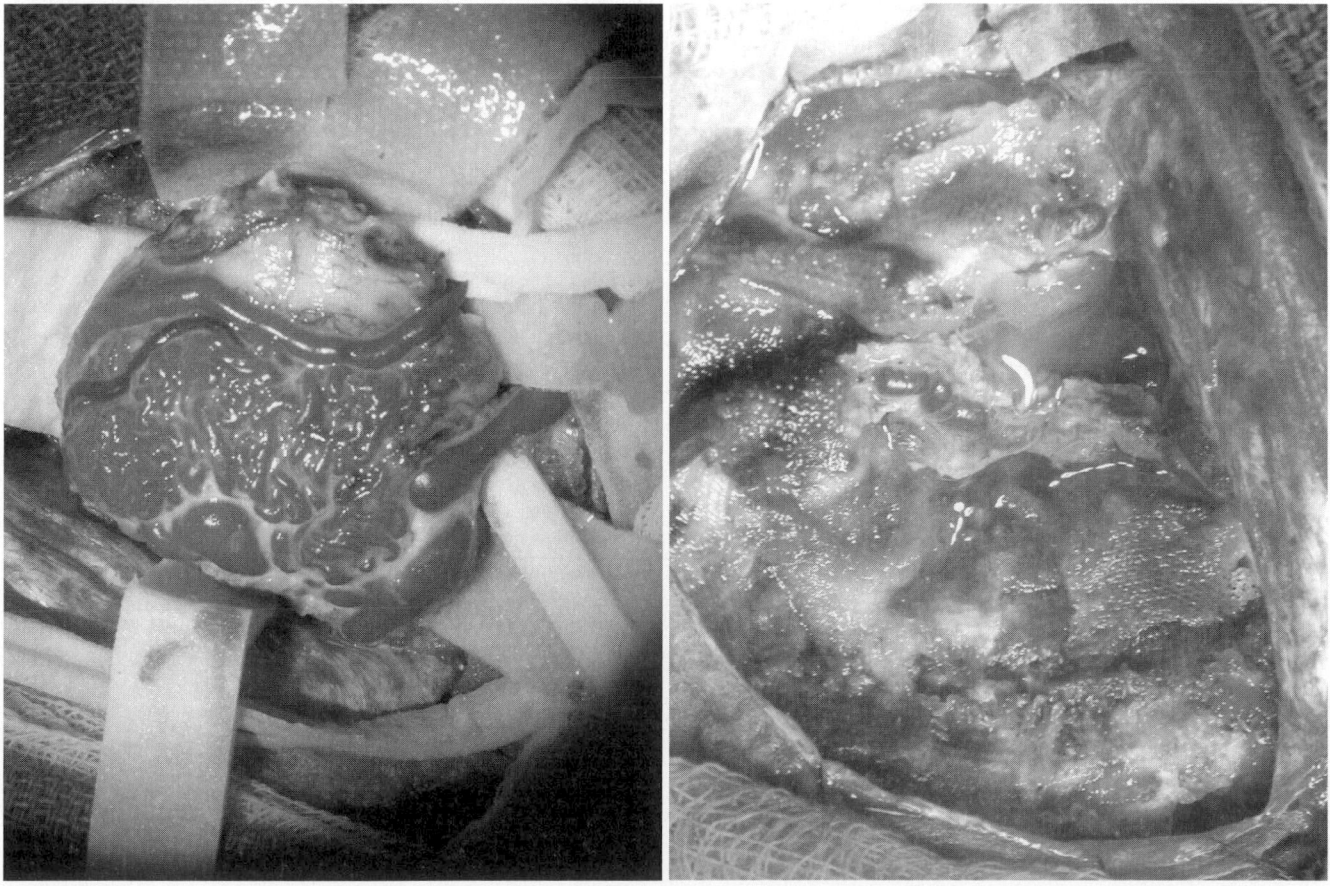

A   B

FIGURE 68–20   *Same patient as in Figure 68–19.* A, *Intraoperative view of dilated arterialized vein.* B, *Post-resection cavity.*

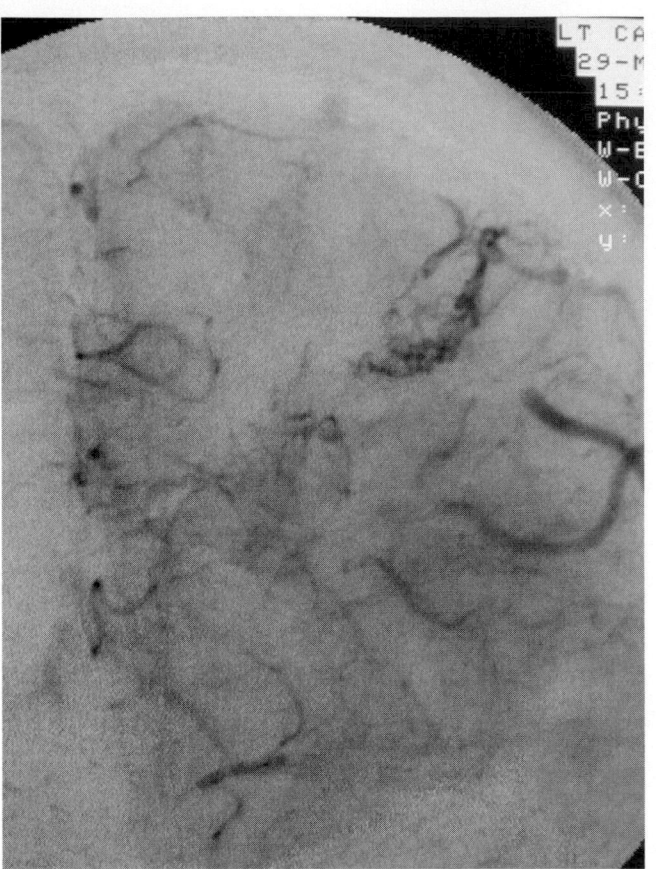

FIGURE 68–21   *Same patient as in Figures 68–19 and 68–20. Immediate postoperative angiogram showing dysplastic vessels not associated with an early draining vein.*

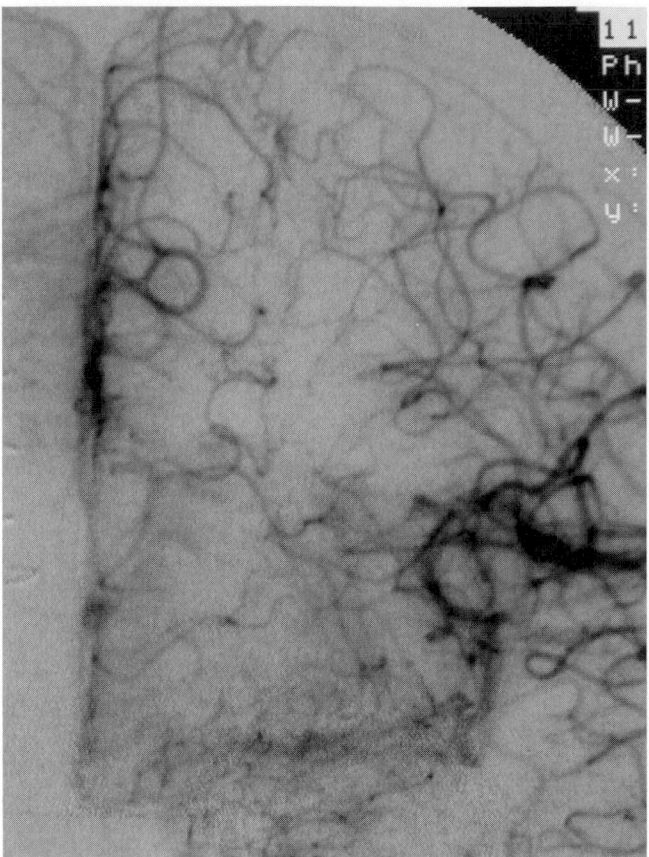

FIGURE 68–22   *Same patient as in Figures 68–19 to 68–21. Follow-up angiogram demonstrating resolution of dysplastic vessels.*

(11%) showed evidence of a residual AVM, 16 (7%) showed focal hyperemia, 6 (2%) revealed other findings, and 100 (45%) were normal. The cases with angiographic evidence of dysplastic vessels were significantly associated with increasing size of the AVM (in millimeter increments; $P = 0.0001$); the mean diameter of AVMs in patients with dysplastic vessels on angiogram after surgery was significantly larger (41 mm, SD ± 14) than in those without residual dysplastic vessels (27 mm, SD ± 13; $P < 0.001$). Symptomatic postoperative intracerebral hemorrhage occurred in 4 patients (1%), in 2 of whom dysplastic vessels were seen on the postoperative angiogram. Collectively, these findings suggest that persistent dysplastic vessels may be found in approximately one third of angiograms after AVM surgery. In addition, preoperative AVM size was found to be an independent predictor for the occurrence of dysplastic vessels on the postoperative angiogram.[93]

Case 5: Dural Arteriovenous Fistula Treated with Embolization

A 68-year-old woman was referred with a 20-year history of left-sided headache radiating to the left side of her scalp and around her left eye. Over the past several years, she underwent multiple MRI evaluations that were inter-

preted as showing no abnormality. More recently, her symptoms progressed to include a pulsatile tinnitus in the left ear. Subsequent evaluation revealed the presence of a dural AV fistula fed primarily from the external carotid branches of the occipital artery and also from the left meningohypophyseal trunk (Fig. 68–23). The fistula was successfully treated with embolization, as shown in Figure 68–24.

This case illustrates a common presentation of dural AV fistulas as well as the utility of embolization in treatment. Although surgical intervention to occlude the fistula is an option for this patient, the future role of surgery in these cases may be reserved for clipping any residual veins that drain intracranially. The presence of intracranial draining veins increases the possibility of intracranial hemorrhage as well as the treatment morbidity.[94,95]

Case 6: Basal Ganglia Arteriovenous Malformation Treated Successfully with Embolization and Radiosurgery

A 33-year-old woman presented with a sudden onset of severe headache and left-sided hemiplegia. Evaluation at that time revealed a large hemorrhage in the right basal ganglia with an associated AVM fed mostly by the lenticulostriate vessels on the right side (Fig. 68–25). It occupied

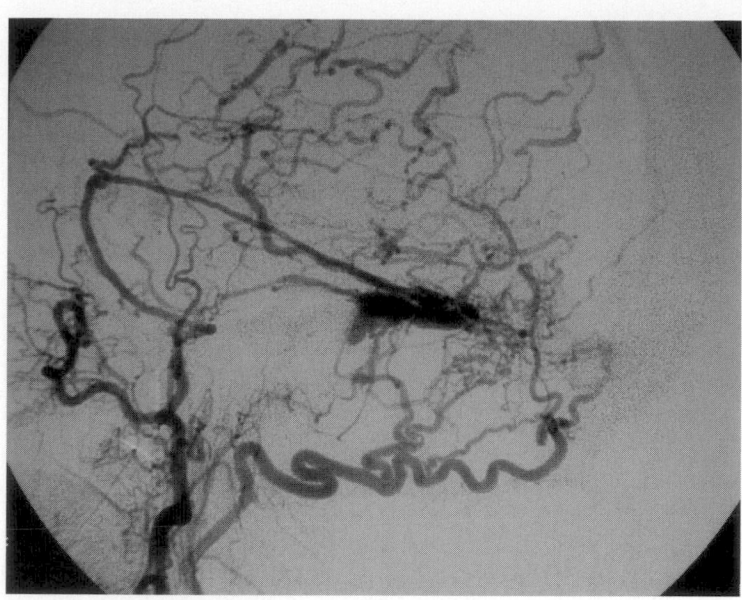

FIGURE 68–23 *Angiogram of a 68-year-old woman with an arteriovenous fistula fed primarily from the external branches of the occipital artery and left meningohypophyseal trunk.*

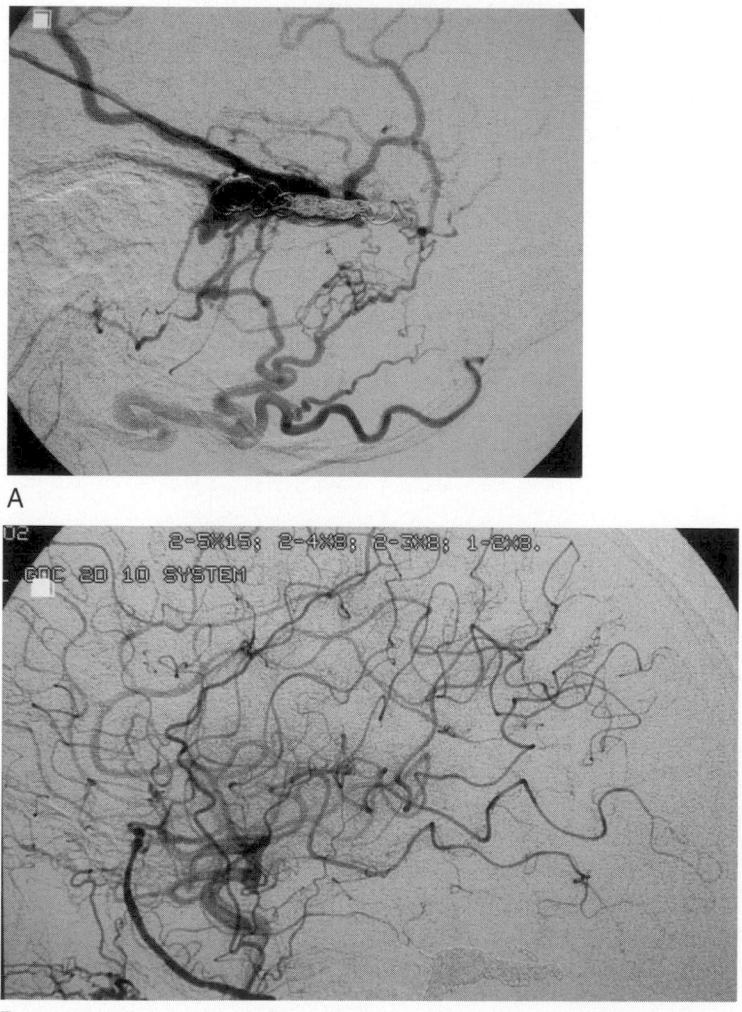

FIGURE 68–24 *Same patient as in Figure 68–23. A, Before treatment. B, Angiogram after successful embolization.*

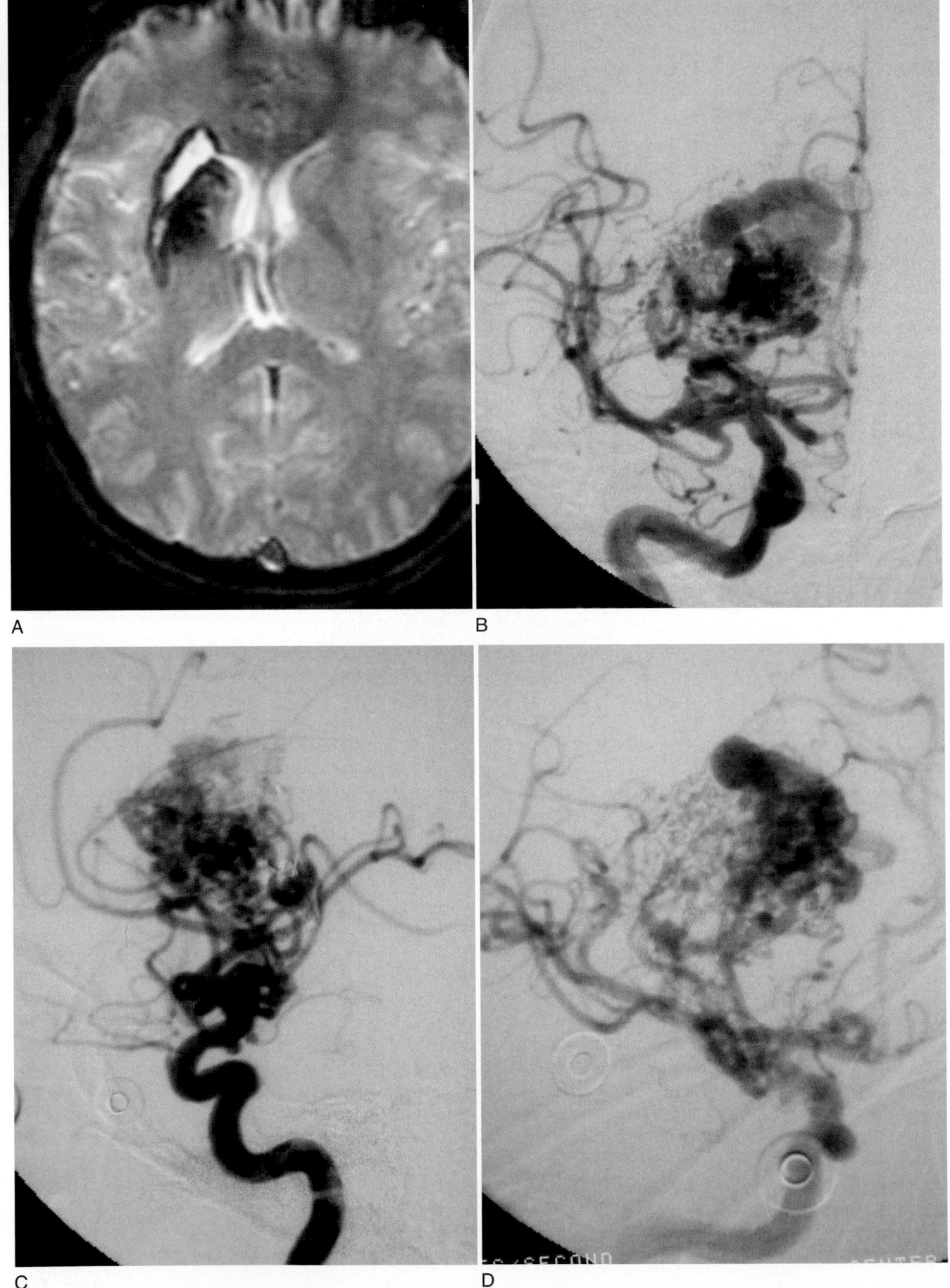

FIGURE 68–25 *A 33-year-old woman with right basal hemorrhage associated with arteriovenous malformation. A, MRI. B to D, Anteroposterior (B), lateral (C), and oblique (D) angiographic views.*

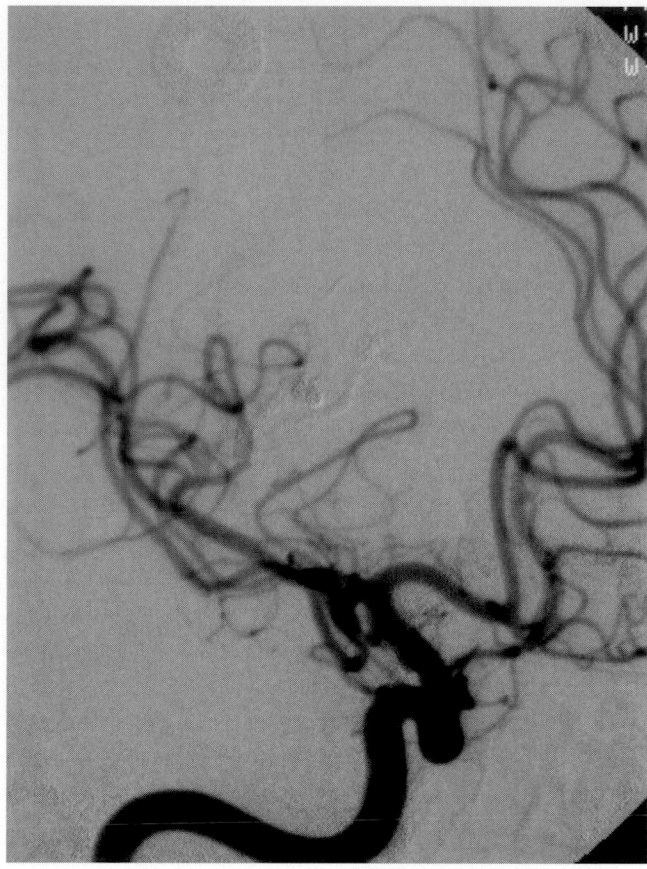

FIGURE 68–26 *Same patient as in Figure 68–25. Postembolization angiogram demonstrating complete obliteration.*

deep basal ganglia structures and drained by a large draining vein that went up the superior sagittal sinus. The patient underwent two stages of embolization and one treatment with radiosurgery. The location of the lesion in proximity to the right thalamus and internal capsule made this a very unfavorable lesion for surgical resection. A follow-up angiogram 3 years after treatment of the AVM with radiosurgery revealed complete obliteration of the lesion (Fig. 68–26). As with case 3, the availability of nonsurgical treatment modalities was critical to optimizing the care of this patient.

Case 7: Arteriovenous Malformation Treated with Embolization and Surgical Resection

A 21-year-old woman presented with a grand mal seizure and no other associated medical problems. MRI performed as part of the evaluation revealed a 3.2-cm AVM located in the anteroinferior aspect of the left temporal lobe (Fig. 68–27). The patient underwent successful staged embolization, which significantly reduced the arterial supply to the AVM (Fig. 68–28). Subsequent surgical resection of the lesion was successful (Fig. 68–29).

Case 8: Cerebellar Arteriovenous Malformation with an Associated Venous Aneurysm

A 28-year-old woman presented to the emergency room with headache, nausea, and vomiting. Head CT revealed a small hemorrhage in the right side of the superior cerebellum. Subsequent MRI and angiogram demonstrated a 2-cm AVM in the superior aspect of the right cerebellar hemisphere with a venous aneurysm and a small hemorrhage or thrombus in the venous aneurysm (Fig. 68–30). The patient underwent staged embolization and surgical resection via a suboccipital craniotomy. A postoperative angiogram showed no residual AVM (Fig. 68–31).

SUMMARY

Great progress in the treatment of patients with vascular malformations has been achieved since Rokitansky's initial description of intracranial AVMs.[1] The prospective analysis of evidence-based clinical outcome data will be critical in accurately determining the long-term effect of many treatment modalities. The advent of endovascular techniques combined with advances in radiosurgery has provided important surgical adjuncts to the treatment of these difficult lesions.

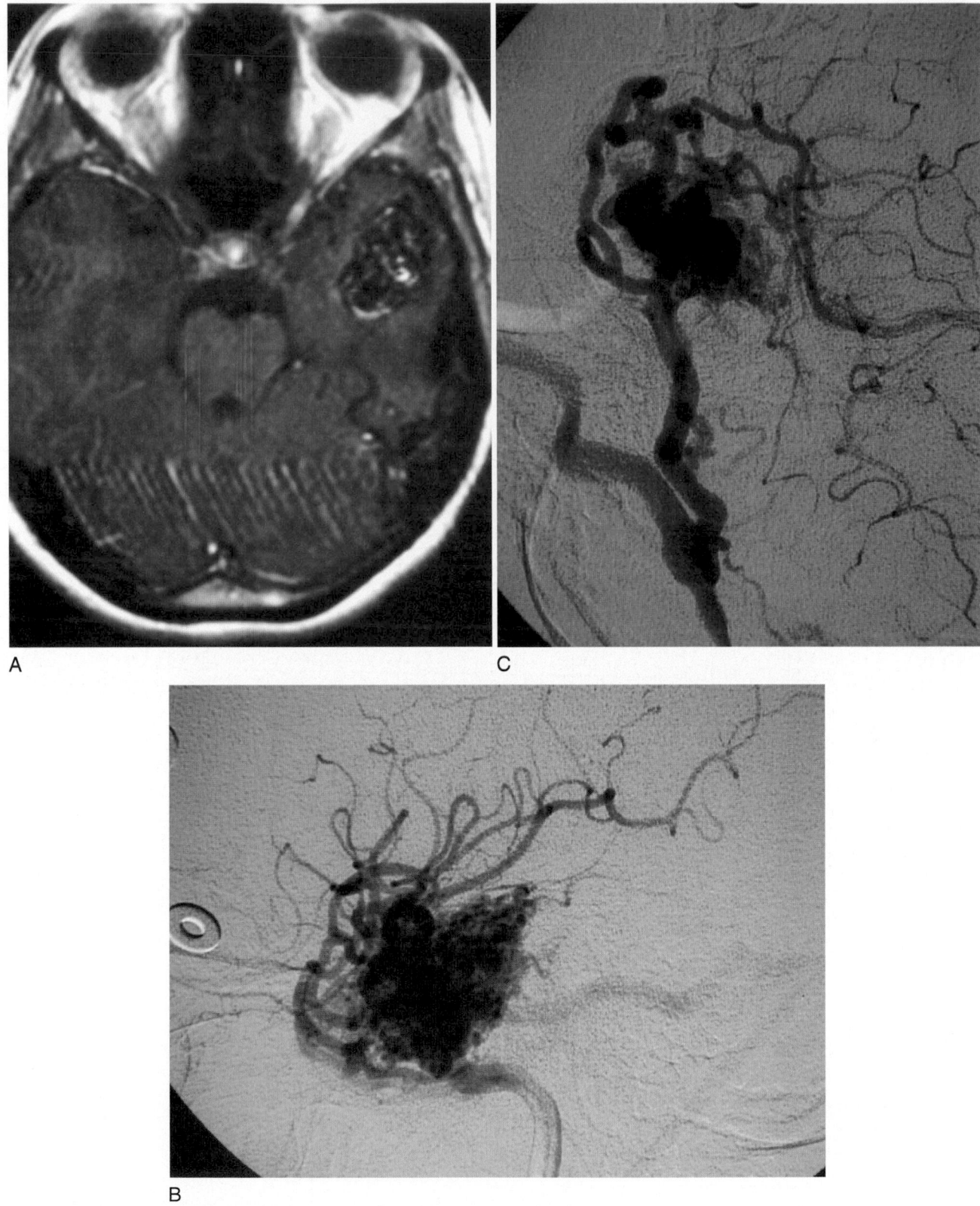

A

C

B

FIGURE 68–27 *A 21-year-old woman with an arteriovenous malformation in the anteroinferior aspect of the left temporal lobe. Preoperative MRI (A) and angiograms (B and C).*

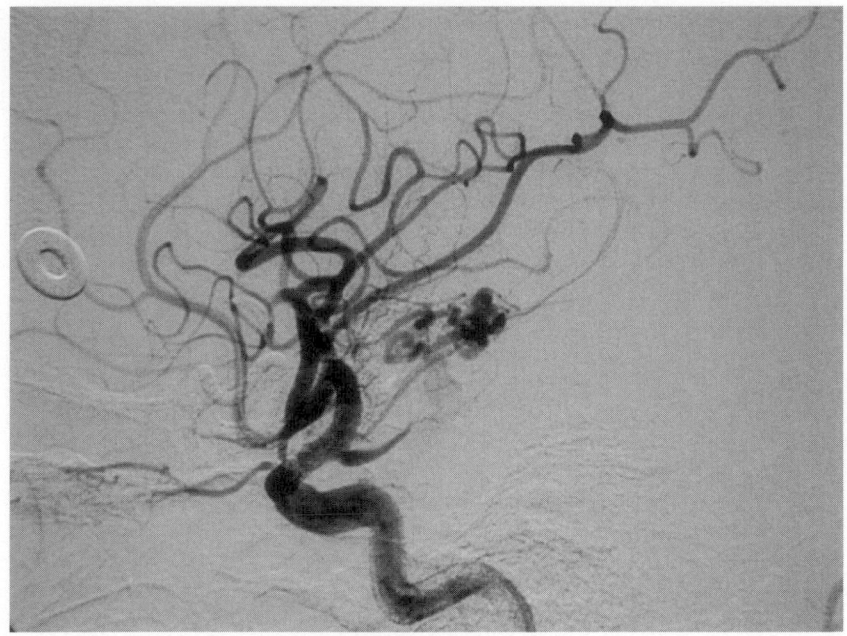

FIGURE 68–28   *Same patient as in Figure 68–27. Postembolization angiogram.*

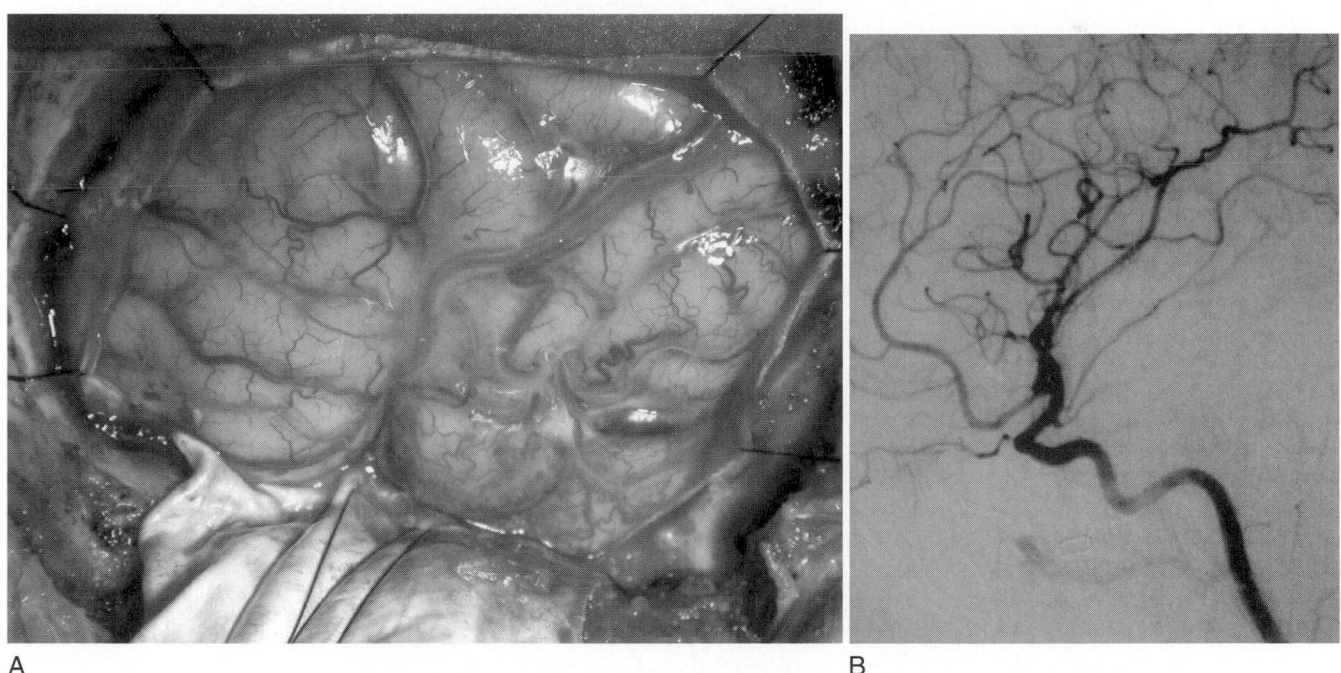

A   B

FIGURE 68–29   *Same patient as in Figures 68–27 and 68–28. A, Intraoperative view of the brain surface. B, Postoperative angiogram.*

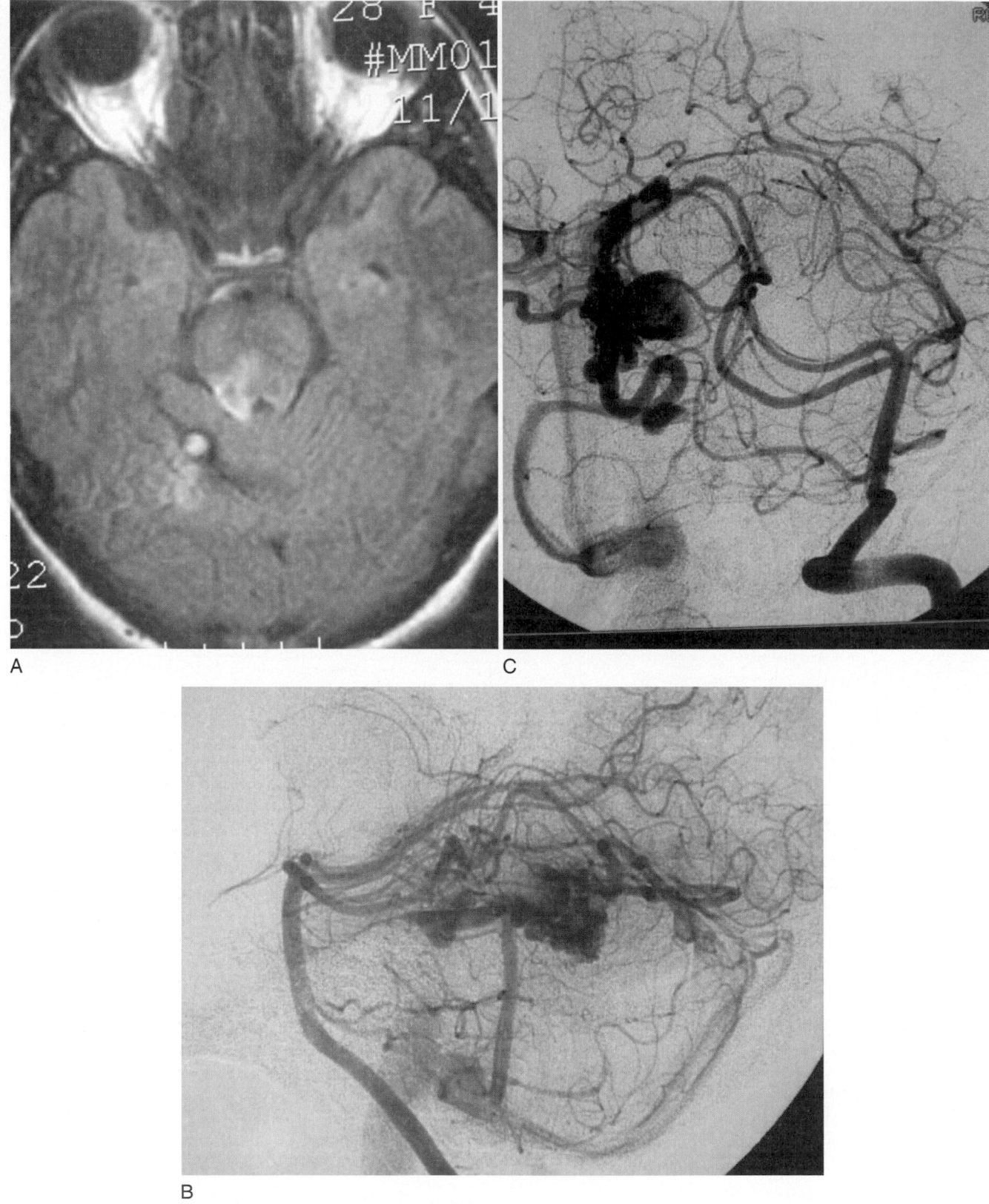

FIGURE 68–30 *A 28-year-old woman with an arteriovenous malformation in the superior aspect of the right cerebellar hemisphere with a venous aneurysm and a small hemorrhage or thrombus in the venous aneurysm. A, Preoperative MRI. B and C, Preoperative angiograms.*

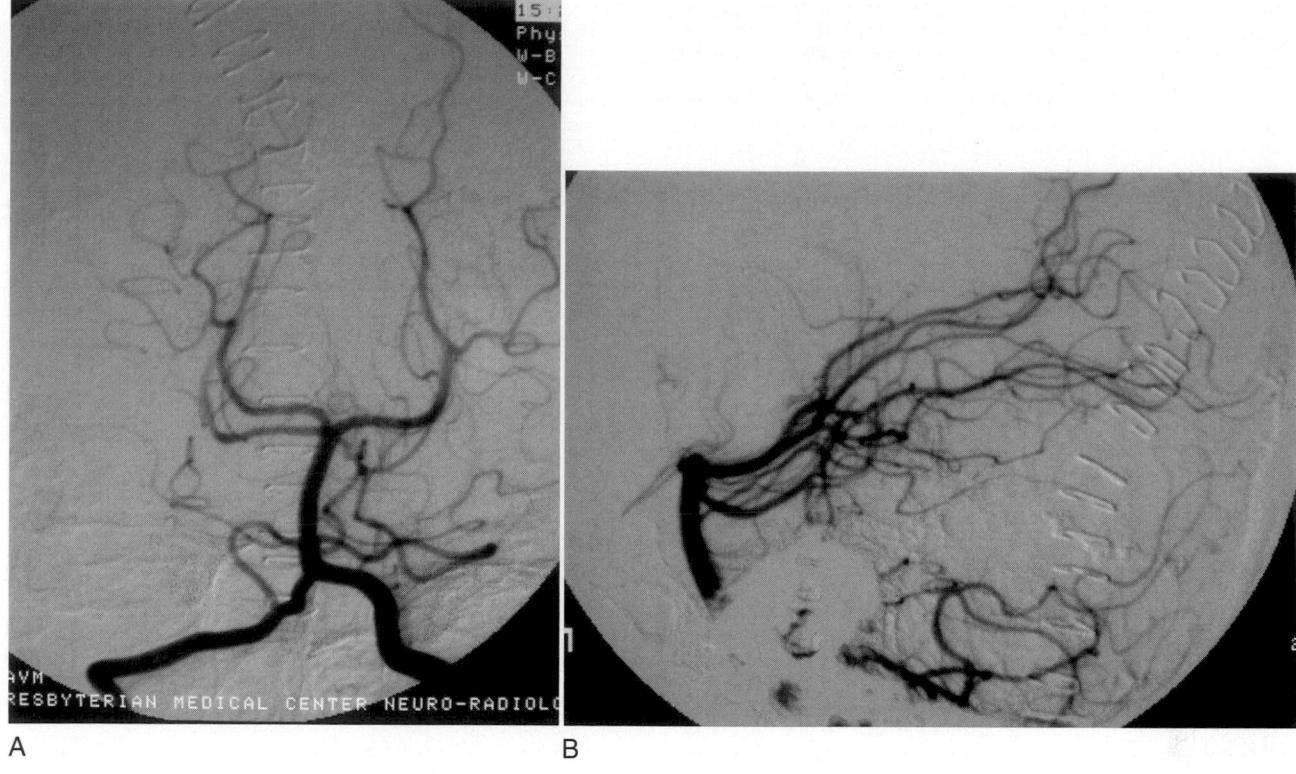

FIGURE 68–31 *Same patient as in Figure 68–30. A and B, Postoperative angiograms showing no residual arteriovenous malformation.*

We look forward to the contributions of clinicians and scientists who have combined efforts to understand the molecular and genetic etiology of these lesions.

References

1. Yasargil M G: Microneurosurgery, Vol 3A. New York, Thieme, 1984.
2. Cushing H: The Harvey Cushing Collection of Books and Manuscripts, Vol 1. New Haven, Yale University Dept of the History of Science and Medicine, 1943.
3. Dandy WE: Selected Writings of Walter Dandy, Vol 1. Springfield, IL, Charles C Thomas, 1957.
4. Cushing H, Bailey P: Tumors Arising from Blood-Vessels of the Brain. Springfield, IL, Charles C Thomas, 1928, p 9.
5. Rigamonti D, Johnson PC, Spetzler RF, et al: Cavernous malformations and capillary telangiectasia: A spectrum within a single pathological entity. Neurosurgery 28:60–64, 1991.
6. Clatterbuck RE, Elmaci I, Rigamonti D: The juxtaposition of a capillary telangiectasia, cavernous malformation, and developmental venous anomaly in the brainstem of a single patient: Case report. Neurosurgery 49:1246–1250, 2001.
7. Awada A, Watson T, Obeid T: Cavernous angioma presenting as pregnancy-related seizures. Epilepsia 38:844–846, 1997.
8. Wong JH, Awad IA, Kim JH: Ultrastructural pathological features of cerebrovascular malformations: A preliminary report. Neurosurgery 46:1454–1459, 2000.
9. Kida Y, Kobayashi T, Tanaka T, et al: Seizure control after radiosurgery on cerebral arteriovenous malformations. J Clin Neurosci 7(Suppl 1):6–9, 2000.
10. Meng JS, Okeda R: Histopathological structure of the pial arteriovenous malformation in adults: Observation by reconstruction of serial sections of four surgical specimens. Acta Neuropathol (Berl) 102:63–68, 2001.
11. Yamada S, Liwnicz B, Lonser RR, Knierim D: Scanning electron microscopy of arteriovenous malformations. Neurol Res 21:541–544, 1999.
12. Chin LS, Raffel C, Gonzalez-Gomez I, et al: Diffuse arteriovenous malformations: A clinical, radiological, and pathological description. Neurosurgery 31:863–868; discussion 868–869, 1992.
13. Redekop G, TerBrugge K, Montanera W, Willinsky R: Arterial aneurysms associated with cerebral arteriovenous malformations: Classification, incidence, and risk of hemorrhage. J Neurosurg 89:539–546, 1998.
14. Westphal M, Grzyska U: Clinical significance of pedicle aneurysms on feeding vessels, especially those located in infratentorial arteriovenous malformations. J Neurosurg 92:995–1001, 2000.
15. Jellinger K: Vascular malformations of the central nervous system: A morphological overview. Neurosurg Rev 9:177–216, 1986.
16. Mullan S, Mojtahedi S, Johnson DL, Macdonald RL: Embryological basis of some aspects of cerebral vascular fistulas and malformations. J Neurosurg 85:1–8, 1996.
17. Kondziolka D, Humphreys RP, Hoffman HJ, et al: Arteriovenous malformations of the brain in children: A forty year experience. Can J Neurol Sci 19:40–45, 1992.
18. Di Rocco C, Tamburrini G, Rollo M: Cerebral arteriovenous malformations in children. Acta Neurochir 142:145–156, 2000.
19. Morgan T, McDonald J, Anderson C, et al: Intracranial hemorrhage in infants and children with hereditary hemorrhagic telangiectasia (Osler-Weber-Rendu syndrome). Pediatrics 109:E12, 2002.
20. Sekhon LH, Morgan MK, Johnston IH: Syndactyly and intracranial arteriovenous malformation: Case report. Br J Neurosurg 8:377–380, 1994.
21. Spetzler RF, Hargraves RW, McCormick PW, et al: Relationship of perfusion pressure and size to risk of hemorrhage from arteriovenous malformations. J Neurosurg 76:918–923, 1992.
22. Solomon RA, Michelsen WJ: Defective cerebrovascular autoregulation in regions proximal to arteriovenous malformations of the brain: A case report and topic review. Neurosurgery 14:78–82, 1984.
23. Lo EH: A haemodynamic analysis of intracranial arteriovenous malformations. Neurol Res 15:51–55, 1993.
24. Kader A, Young WL: The effects of intracranial arteriovenous malformations on cerebral hemodynamics. Neurosurg Clin North Am 7:767–781, 1996.

25. Kailasnath P, Chaloupka JC: Mathematical modeling of AVM physiology using compartmental network analysis: Theoretical considerations and preliminary in vivo validation using a previously developed animal model. Neurol Res 18:361–366, 1996.

26. Kader A, Young WL, Massaro AR, et al: Transcranial Doppler changes during staged surgical resection of cerebral arteriovenous malformations: A report of three cases. Surg Neurol 39:392–398, 1993.

27. Tsuchiya K, Katase S, Yoshino A, Hachiya J: MR digital subtraction angiography of cerebral arteriovenous malformations. AJNR Am J Neuroradiol 21:707–711, 2000.

28. Uggowitzer MM, Kugler C, Riccabona M, et al: Cerebral arteriovenous malformations: Diagnostic value of echo-enhanced transcranial Doppler sonography compared with angiography. AJNR Am J Neuroradiol 20:101–106, 1999.

29. Manchola IF, De Salles AA, Foo TK, et al: Arteriovenous malformation hemodynamics: A transcranial Doppler study. Neurosurgery 33:556–562; discussion 562, 1993.

30. al-Rodhan NR, Sundt TM Jr, Piepgras DG, et al: Occlusive hyperemia: A theory for the hemodynamic complications following resection of intracerebral arteriovenous malformations. J Neurosurg 78:167–175, 1993.

31. Schaller C, Urbach H, Schramm J, Meyer B: Role of venous drainage in cerebral arteriovenous malformation surgery, as related to the development of postoperative hyperperfusion injury. Neurosurg 51:921–927; discussion 927–929, 2002.

32. Meyer B, Urbach H, Schaller C, Schramm J: Is stagnating flow in former feeding arteries an indication of cerebral hypoperfusion after resection of arteriovenous malformations? J Neurosurg 95:36–43, 2001.

33. Gunel M, Awad IA, Finberg K, et al: A founder mutation as a cause of cerebral cavernous malformation in Hispanic Americans. N Engl J Med 334:946–951, 1996.

34. Gunel M, Awad IA, Anson J, Lifton RP: Mapping a gene causing cerebral cavernous malformation to 7q11.2-q21. Proc Natl Acad Sci U S A 92:6620–6624, 1995.

35. Gunel M, Awad IA, Finberg K, et al: Genetic heterogeneity of inherited cerebral cavernous malformation. Neurosurgery 38:1265–1271, 1996.

36. Zhang J, Clatterbuck RE, Rigamonti D, Dietz HC: Cloning of the murine Krit1 cDNA reveals novel mammalian 5′ coding exons. Genomics 70:392–395, 2000.

37. Zhang J, Clatterbuck RE, Rigamonti D, Dietz HC: Mutations in KRIT1 in familial cerebral cavernous malformations. Neurosurgery 46:1272–1277; discussion 1277–1279, 2000.

38. Verlaan DJ, Davenport WJ, Stefan H, et al: Cerebral cavernous malformations: Mutations in Krit1. Neurology 58:853–857, 2002.

39. Notelet L, Chapon F, Khoury S, et al: Familial cavernous malformations in a large French kindred: Mapping of the gene to the CCM1 locus on chromosome 7q. J Neurol Neurosurg Psychiatry 63:40–45, 1997.

40. Bourdeau A, Cymerman U, Paquet ME, et al: Endoglin expression is reduced in normal vessels but still detectable in arteriovenous malformations of patients with hereditary hemorrhagic telangiectasia type 1. Am J Pathol 156:911–923, 2000.

41. Berman MF, Sciacca RR, Pile-Spellman J, et al: The epidemiology of brain arteriovenous malformations. Neurosurgery 47:389–396; discussion 397, 2000.

42. Brown RD Jr, Wiebers DO, Torner JC, O'Fallon WM: Frequency of intracranial hemorrhage as a presenting symptom and subtype analysis: A population-based study of intracranial vascular malformations in Olmsted Country, Minnesota. J Neurosurg 85:29–32, 1996.

43. Al-Shahi R, Warlow C: A systematic review of the frequency and prognosis of arteriovenous malformations of the brain in adults. Brain 124:1900–1926, 2001.

44. Ondra SL, Troupp H, George ED, Schwab K: The natural history of symptomatic arteriovenous malformations of the brain: A 24-year follow-up assessment. J Neurosurg 73:387–391, 1990.

45. Gawel MJ, Willinsky RA, Krajewski A: Reversal of cluster headache side following treatment of arteriovenous malformation. Headache 29:453–454, 1989.

46. Kupersmith MJ, Vargas ME, Yashar A, et al: Occipital arteriovenous malformations: Visual disturbances and presentation. Neurology 46:953–957, 1996.

47. Monteiro JM, Rosas MJ, Correia AP, Vaz AR: Migraine and intracranial vascular malformations. Headache 33:563–565, 1993.

48. Sheth RD, Bodensteiner JB: Progressive neurologic impairment from an arteriovenous malformation vascular steal. Pediatr Neurol 13:352–354, 1995.

49. Mast H, Mohr JP, Osipov A, et al: 'Steal' is an unestablished mechanism for the clinical presentation of cerebral arteriovenous malformations. Stroke 26:1215–1220, 1995.

50. Mattle HP, Schroth G, Seiler RW: Dilemmas in the management of patients with arteriovenous malformations. J Neurol 247:917–928, 2000.

51. Labauge P, Brunereau L, Laberge S, Houtteville JP: Prospective follow-up of 33 asymptomatic patients with familial cerebral cavernous malformations. Neurology 57:1825–1828, 2001.

52. Moriarity JL, Wetzel M, Clatterbuck RE, et al: The natural history of cavernous malformations: A prospective study of 68 patients. Neurosurgery 44:1166–1171; discussion 1172–1163, 1999.

53. Zabramski JM, Wascher TM, Spetzler RF, et al: The natural history of familial cavernous malformations: Results of an ongoing study. J Neurosurg 80:422–432, 1994.

54. Kupersmith MJ, Kalish H, Epstein F, et al: Natural history of brainstem cavernous malformations. Neurosurgery 48:47–53; discussion 53–44, 2001.

55. Solomon RA, Stein BM: Management of arteriovenous malformations of the brain stem. J Neurosurg 64:857–864, 1986.

56. Solomon RA, Stein BM: Interhemispheric approach for the surgical removal of thalamocaudate arteriovenous malformations. J Neurosurg 66:345–351, 1987.

57. Sisti MB, Kader A, Stein BM: Microsurgery for 67 intracranial arteriovenous malformations less than 3 cm in diameter. J Neurosurg 79:653–660, 1993.

58. Spetzler RF, Martin NA: A proposed grading system for arteriovenous malformations. J Neurosurg 65:476–483, 1986.

59. Hamilton MG, Spetzler RF: The prospective application of a grading system for arteriovenous malformations. Neurosurgery 34:2–6; discussion 6–7, 1994.

60. Richling B, Bavinzski G: Arterio-venous malformations of the basal ganglia: Surgical versus endovascular treatment. Acta Neurochir Suppl 53:50–59, 1991.

61. Batjer H, Samson D: Arteriovenous malformations of the posterior fossa: Clinical presentation, diagnostic evaluation, and surgical treatment. J Neurosurg 64:849–856, 1986.

62. Drake CG, Friedman AH, Peerless SJ: Posterior fossa arteriovenous malformations. J Neurosurg 64:1–10, 1986.

63. George B, Celis-Lopez M, Kato T, Lot G: Arteriovenous malformations of the posterior fossa. Acta Neurochir (Wien) 116:119–127, 1992.

64. Sisti MB, Stein BM: Arteriovenous malformations of the brain stem. Neurosurg Clin North Am 4:497–505, 1993.

65. Lawton MT, Hamilton MG, Spetzler RF: Multimodality treatment of deep arteriovenous malformations: Thalamus, basal ganglia, and brain stem. Neurosurgery 37:29–35; discussion 35–26, 1995.

66. Piepgras DG, Sundt TM Jr, Ragoowansi AT, Stevens L: Seizure outcome in patients with surgically treated cerebral arteriovenous malformations. J Neurosurg 78:5–11, 1993.

67. Deveikis JP: Endovascular therapy of intracranial arteriovenous malformations: Materials and techniques. Neuroimaging Clin North Am 8:401–424, 1998.

68. Henkes H, Nahser HC, Berg-Dammer E, et al: Endovascular therapy of brain AVMs prior to radiosurgery. Neurol Res 20:479–492, 1998.

69. Marks MP, Lane B, Steinberg GK, et al: Endovascular treatment of cerebral arteriovenous malformations following radiosurgery. AJNR Am J Neuroradiol 14:297–303; discussion 304–295, 1993.

70. Nakahara I, Taki W, Kikuchi H, et al: Endovascular treatment of aneurysms on the feeding arteries of intracranial arteriovenous malformations. Neuroradiology 41:60–66, 1999.

71. Valavanis A, Yasargil MG: The endovascular treatment of brain arteriovenous malformations. Adv Tech Stand Neurosurg 24:131–214, 1998.

72. Mizutani T, Tanaka H, Aruga T: Total recanalization of a spontaneously thrombosed arteriovenous malformation: Case report. J Neurosurg 82:506–508, 1995.

73. Martin NA, Khanna R, Doberstein C, Bentson J: Therapeutic embolization of arteriovenous malformations: The case for and against. Clin Neurosurg 46:295–318, 2000.

74. Hartmann A, Pile-Spellman J, Stapf C, et al: Risk of endovascular treatment of brain arteriovenous malformations. Stroke 33:1816–1820, 2002.

75. Ogilvy CS: Radiation therapy for arteriovenous malformations: A review. Neurosurgery 26:725–735, 1990.

76. Massager N, Regis J, Kondziolka D, et al: Gamma knife radiosurgery for brainstem arteriovenous malformations: Preliminary results. J Neurosurg 9(Suppl 3):102–103, 2000.

77. Chang JH, Chang JW, Park YG, Chung SS: Factors related to complete occlusion of arteriovenous malformations after gamma knife radiosurgery. J Neurosurg 93(Suppl 3):96–101, 2000.

78. Friedman WA, Bova FJ, Mendenhall WM: Linear accelerator radiosurgery for arteriovenous malformations: The relationship of size to outcome. J Neurosurg 82:180–189, 1995.

79. Flickinger JC, Pollock BE, Kondziolka D, Lunsford LD: A dose-response analysis of arteriovenous malformation obliteration after radiosurgery. Int J Radiat Oncol Biol Phys 36:873–879, 1996.

80. Flickinger JC, Kondziolka D, Maitz AH, Lunsford LD: An analysis of the dose-response for arteriovenous malformation radiosurgery and other factors affecting obliteration. Radiother Oncol 63:347–354, 2002.

81. Werner-Wasik M, Rudoler S, Preston PE, et al: Immediate side effects of stereotactic radiotherapy and radiosurgery. Int J Radiat Oncol Biol Phys 43:299–304, 1999.

82. Voges J, Treuer H, Lehrke R, et al: Risk analysis of LINAC radiosurgery in patients with arteriovenous malformation (AVM). Acta Neurochir Suppl (Wien) 68:118–123, 1997.

83. Voges J, Treuer H, Sturm V, et al: Risk analysis of linear accelerator radiosurgery. Int J Radiat Oncol Biol Phys 36:1055–1063, 1996.

84. Naoi Y, Cho N, Miyauchi T, et al: Usefulness and problems of stereotactic radiosurgery using a linear accelerator. Radiat Med 14:215–219, 1996.

85. Malone S, Raaphorst GP, Gray R, et al: Enhanced in vitro radiosensitivity of skin fibroblasts in two patients developing brain necrosis following AVM radiosurgery: A new risk factor with potential for a predictive assay. Int J Radiat Oncol Biol Phys 47:185–189, 2000.

86. Flickinger JC, Kondziolka D, Lunsford LD, et al: A multi-institutional analysis of complication outcomes after arteriovenous malformation radiosurgery. Int J Radiat Oncol Biol Phys 44:67–74, 1999.

87. Flickinger JC, Kondziolka D, Lunsford LD: Radiosurgery of benign lesions. Semin Radiat Oncol 5:220–224, 1995.

88. Flickinger JC, Kondziolka D, Pollock BE, et al: Complications from arteriovenous malformation radiosurgery: Multivariate analysis and risk modeling. Int J Radiat Oncol Biol Phys 38:485–490, 1997.

89. Flickinger JC, Kondziolka D, Maitz AH, Lunsford LD: Analysis of neurological sequelae from radiosurgery of arteriovenous malformations: How location affects outcome. Int J Radiat Oncol Biol Phys 40:273–278, 1998.

90. Flickinger JC, Kondziolka D, Lunsford LD: Dose selection in stereotactic radiosurgery. Neurosurg Clin North Am 10:271–280, 1999.

91. Flickinger JC, Kondziolka D, Lunsford LD, et al: Development of a model to predict permanent symptomatic postradiosurgery injury for arteriovenous malformation patients. Arteriovenous Malformation Radiosurgery Study Group. Int J Radiat Oncol Biol Phys 46:1143–1148, 2000.

92. Solomon RA, Connolly ES Jr, Prestigiacomo CJ, et al: Management of residual dysplastic vessels after cerebral arteriovenous malformation resection: Implications for postoperative angiography. Neurosurgery 46:1052–1060; discussion 1060–1052, 2000.

93. Stapf C, Connolly ES, Schumacher HC, et al: Dysplastic vessels after surgery for brain arteriovenous malformations. Stroke 33:1053–1056, 2002.

94. Barnwell SL, Halbach VV, Higashida RT, et al: Complex dural arteriovenous fistulas: Results of combined endovascular and neurosurgical treatment in 16 patients. J Neurosurg 71:352–358, 1989.

95. Tomlinson FH, Rufenacht DA, Sundt TM Jr, et al: Arteriovenous fistulas of the brain and the spinal cord. J Neurosurg 79:16–27, 1993.

Chapter Sixty-Nine

Cavernous Malformations and Venous Anomalies: Natural History and Surgical Management

Adetokunbo A. Oyelese, Ian G. Fleetwood, and Gary K. Steinberg

Vascular lesions of the central nervous system (CNS) may be catastrophically lethal in their clinical presentation and symptomatology. Intracranial aneurysms and arteriovenous malformations (AVMs) typically manifest as subarachnoid or intraparenchymal hemorrhage, either of which may result in death or severe neurologic morbidity. The threshold for intervention with these lesions is thus understandably low. Cavernous malformations (CMs) and developmental venous anomalies (DVAs), on the other hand, usually have a less aggressive course; thus, in planning their management, one must consider their natural history.

CAVERNOUS MALFORMATIONS

A considerable amount of knowledge on CMs has been contributed to the medical literature in the last decade. These lesions may be variously described in terms of their radiographic appearance, familial nature, or symptomatic clinical presentation.

Epidemiology and Genetics

Cavernous malformations are vascular lesions characterized by sinusoidal, thin-walled, abnormally enlarged vascular cavities with a single layer of endothelium and the absence of intervening neural parenchyma (Fig. 69–1). Representing 10% to 16% of CNS vascular malformations,[1–3] CMs were previously categorized as angiographically occult vascular malformations (AOVMs), and were considered, like AVMs, to be congenital lesions. It is now clear, however, that they may arise de novo[4–6] or after irradiation.[7–11]

The prevalence of CMs in the general population is difficult to estimate, because not all asymptomatic lesions come to medical attention. The prevalence of CM as based on autopsy series ranges from 0.4% to 0.5%.[2,12,13] Before the advent of magnetic resonance imaging (MRI),

asymptomatic lesions were rarely identified prior to autopsy. However, with the widespread use of MRI, the reported prevalence has ranged from 0.39%[14] to as high as 0.9%.[15] CMs affect males and females equally,[14,16–18] although some groups report a more aggressive clinical course in female patients.[17,19,20] Although patients in all age groups are affected, the lesions are often symptomatic in the second and fourth decades.[14,17,21]

CMs occur in two forms—a nonhereditary (sporadic) form and a familial form inherited in an autosomal dominant pattern.[6,22] It has been suggested that more than half of patients with CMs have the familial variant.[22] Patients with the familial variant are more likely to have multiple lesions, and de novo lesions have been shown to develop in such patients.[4,6,23,24] As many as 84% of patients with the familial CMs[6,20,25–29] and 33% of those with sporadic CMs[14,16,17,30,31] have multiple lesions. One study showed that most sporadic cases with multiple lesions were in fact familial.[24] The development of de novo lesions in the familial form of the disease may explain the observation that the number of lesions increases with age (Fig. 69–2).[4,24]

Characterization of the familial form of CMs in the literature has largely been in Hispanic patients of Mexican descent,[32–35] in Western Europeans,[4,23,24,36] and in people of Chinese descent.[37] French and Icelandic kindreds have also been described.[24,26,38] A mutation on the long arm of chromosome 7 has been identified as accounting for the form of inherited cerebral CM (CCM1) in Hispanic North Americans.[33,39,40] Further genetic analysis of this mutation has shown that a founder effect accounts for most familial cases of CM as well as many apparently sporadic cases within this population, indicating that the mutation was inherited from a common ancestor.[32] Other genetic loci have been identified in non-Hispanic kindreds with familial CM, including mutations on the short arm of chromosome 7 (CCM2) and the long arm of chromosome 3 (CCM3).[35,41] Although messenger RNA (mRNA) coding for the protein KRIT1 has been identified as the

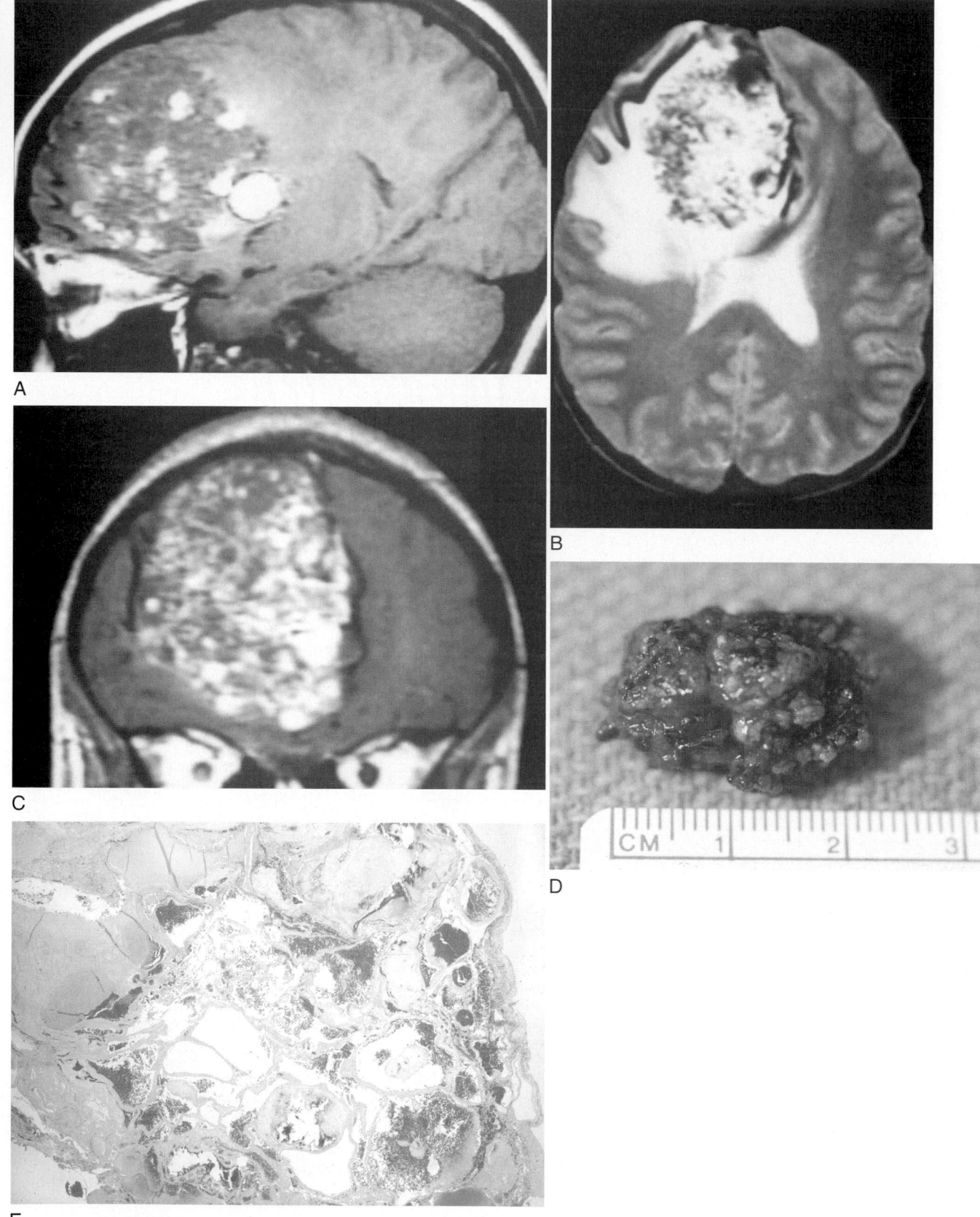

FIGURE 69–1   *Sagittal T1-weighted (A), axial T2-weighted (B) and coronal T1-weighted (C) MR images depicting a large right frontal cavernous malformation (CM) in a patient presenting with headaches. Note the extensive mass effect and edema as well as the characteristic heterogeneous appearance in B. D, Gross resected CM with well-circumscribed, multilobulated, "mulberry-like" appearance in a different patient. E, Histologic examination of the CM shown in D reveals thin-walled, sinusoidal vascular channels with organized thrombus and absence of intervening brain parenchyma on hematoxylin-eosin stain. (A through C courtesy of William Sheridan, MD, Redwood City, CA.)*

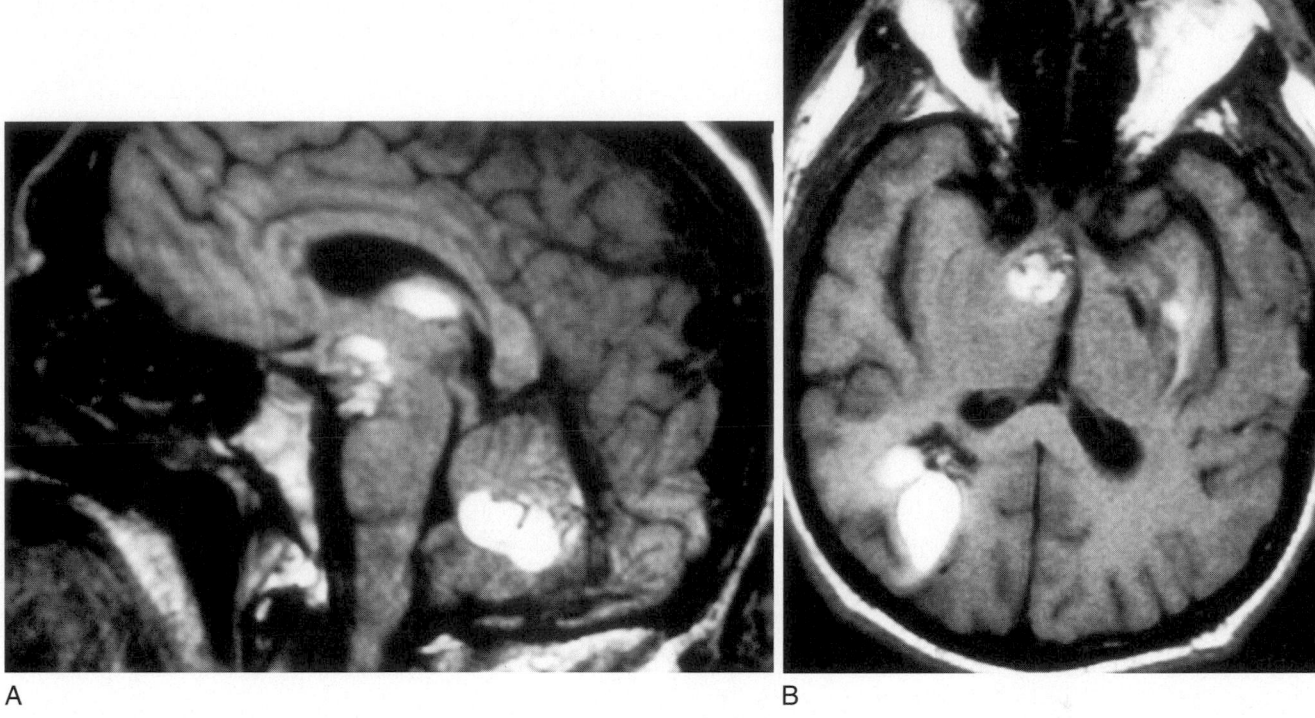

FIGURE 69–2 *Sagittal (A) and axial (B) T1-weighted MRI depicting hypothalamic, thalamic, basal ganglia, temporo-occipital, and cerebellar cavernous malformations in a single patient.*

transcriptional product of the *CCM1* gene,[42–44] no function has been ascribed to this protein, and the etiology of CMs remains unclear.[37] Recent work, however, has begun to establish the differences in molecular biology between CMs and AVMs.[45,46] In all, CMs have been identified in more than 109 families,[47] with onset of symptoms occurring at an earlier age with each subsequent generation—a phenomenon known as *anticipation*.[48,49]

Clinical Presentation

CMs may manifest asymptomatically as incidental lesions, with seizures, or with hemorrhage and mass effect producing a wide range of neurologic symptoms depending on the location of the lesion. Rare cases of CMs manifesting as fatal hemorrhage have been reported.[50] There appears to be a preponderance of supratentorial cerebral lesions compared with thalamic, brainstem, and spinal cord lesions.[1,13,14,17,20,51,52] In their analysis of the literature, Moran and colleagues[53] showed that CMs were distributed above (80%) and below (20%) the tentorium approximately in proportion to the volume of brain tissue in these areas.

Seizures
Perhaps in direct correlation with a supratentorial location, seizures are the most common presenting symptom, occurring in 25% to 55% of cases.[1,6,14,16–18,20,22,52,54,55] Del Curling and associates[14] found the risk of developing seizures to be

1.51% per person-year for 16 subjects. Of this cohort, the risk of seizures was 1.34% per year in subjects with single lesions, and 1.85-fold greater in those with multiple lesions (2.48%). Also, patients with multiple lesions were symptomatic for seizures at an earlier age than those with single lesions (24 ± 8.57 years and 42 ± 3.78 years, respectively). Simple partial seizures were reported in 21% to 31% of patients, complex partial seizures in 6% to 58%, and generalized seizures in 27% to 70%, and some patients experienced multiple seizure types.[21,53,54] Compared with other CNS lesions of similar size and location, CMs appear to be more epileptogenic[21,55] and more frequently associated with medically intractable seizures,[56] particularly when located in the temporal lobe.[21,53]

The underlying cause of seizures in patients with CMs is postulated to be related not only to irritation and compression from repeated hemorrhage but also to exposure of the surrounding brain parenchyma to blood breakdown products, especially hemosiderin and iron.[17,21,22,55,57,58] This theory, however, has not been validated by some clinical studies.[56]

Hemorrhage
Clinically significant hemorrhage is defined as (1) hemorrhage observed on MRI to extend outside the confines of the hemosiderin ring of the CM (extralesional hemorrhage) or (2) hemorrhage that produces neurologic symptoms.[17,21] In contrast, numerous intralesional microhemorrhages may lead to lesion enlargement but have no

clinical sequelae; this latter form of hemorrhage is the hallmark of practically all CMs and accounts for the large number of cases that are asymptomatic despite radiographic evidence of prior hemorrhage. Recurring intralesional hemorrhages also account for the characteristic appearance of CMs on MRI. Clinically symptomatic or significant hemorrhages are less common, occurring in 8% to 37% of lesions[1,14,16,17,19,22,24,26,31,59] and more commonly in female[17,19,59] and pediatric patients.[60,61]

Focal Neurologic Deficits

Acute or progressive focal neurologic deficits represent the third most common presentation of CM. They tend to occur in the setting of intralesional hemorrhage with subsequent enlargement of the CM or in patients in whom extralesional hemorrhage is evident on MRI. Reported frequency in clinical series ranges from about 15% to 45%.* Specific manifestations of the neurologic deficit depend on the location of the CM and occur more commonly in women, in older patients, and with lesions located in the brainstem.[6,17,19,21,24,31,54,59]

Natural History

The natural history of CMs has been the source of much debate in neurological literature (Table 69.1). Earlier reports assumed that these lesions, like AVMs, were present from birth, and therefore, hemorrhage rates were determined on the basis of the lifetime of the individual.[14,16,30] It has now been established that at least in the familial form of the disease, lesions may arise de novo at a rate of 0.4 lesions per patient-year,[4–6,24] thus rendering inaccurate the hemorrhage rates calculated on a lifetime basis. Although it might not be possible to clearly establish the risk of an initial hemorrhage retrospectively, one can more accurately define the risk of rehemorrhage prospectively once an episode has occurred or a lesion has come to clinical attention.

Such prospective analysis has been conducted in a number of studies on patients with sporadic and familial CMs.[6,16,17,20,31,52] Initial hemorrhage rates range from 0.25% to 2.3% per patient-year in retrospective analyses[14,16,30] and from 0.7% to 3.1% per patient-year in prospective analyses.[6,16,17,20,31,52] In a prospective study, Porter and colleagues[31] observed a marked difference in clinical behavior between superficial and deep CMs. Patients with superficial lesions had a negligible rate of clinical deterioration, whereas in those with deep CMs, the annual clinical event rate was 10.6%.[31] However, this finding does not necessarily imply a higher hemorrhage rate for deep lesions. Given the higher density of critical functional tissue in deep locations, smaller hemorrhages in deep structures may cause clinical symptoms more frequently.

Behavior of individual lesions is apparently similar in sporadic and familial CMs.[59] However, the behavior of CMs differs markedly depending on whether the patient is female or whether the lesion is symptomatic, has hemorrhaged previously, or is located within the brainstem.[59,63] In examining the risk of hemorrhages and neurologic events in CMs, one must establish what the expected lesion

behavior is once the CM has come to medical attention, before embarking on an intervention protocol. The hemorrhage or neurologic event rate based on examination of a mixed population of symptomatic and clinically silent lesions has been reported at 0.7%, 2.6%, 4.2%, and 6.5% per patient-year in four separate studies.[6,16,17,31] This rate is lower in clinically silent, nonhemorrhagic lesions (0.39% to 0.6% per patient-year)[16,19,64] than in symptomatic, posthemorrhage lesions (4.5% to about 30% per patient-year).[5,16,19,24,65] In a review of 141 patients presenting with clinically overt hemorrhage and subsequently undergoing treatment with surgery or radiosurgery, Barker and coworkers[65] found that recurrent hemorrhages tend to occur in "clusters" around the initial hemorrhage and to subsequently diminish in frequency with time. This group observed that the recurrent hemorrhage risk decreased from 2% to 1% per month 2.5 years after a hemorrhage, representing a 2.4-fold decline.[65]

The rate of symptomatic hemorrhage or neurologic events has also been found to be higher in female subjects, particularly during pregnancy,[17,21,59,63] despite the fact that there is no gender predilection for prevalence.[14,17,61] Although supratentorial lesions tend to manifest as seizures, brainstem lesions commonly manifest as focal neurologic deficits and generally portend a more morbid prognosis.[5,6,17,19,24,31,59,63] The rehemorrhage rate in brainstem CMs ranges from 5.1% to 30% per patient-year.[5,19,31,66] Porter and colleagues[31] found that the deficits resolved completely in only 37% of patients who had deep lesions and suffered symptomatic hemorrhages.

Finally, Clatterbuck and associates[67] studied punctate CMs (see later section on type IV CMs) and found this subtype to be relatively stable over time, with only a few lesions progressing to a more serious morphology.

Diagnostic Neuroimaging

CMs were formerly classified along with venous anomalies, capillary telangiectasias, and thrombosed AVMs as angiographically occult (or cryptic) vascular malformations because of the inability of angiography to consistently and accurately detect them. This inability stems from the fact that CMs are generally low-flow lesions lacking large feeding arteries or arterialized veins. In some reports, a CM may appear as a capillary blush or an avascular mass on angiography,[58] but the majority of angiographic studies are negative for CMs.

Lesions with calcification, hemorrhage, or a cystic component may be visualized on computed tomography (CT) as hyperdense or heterogeneous lesions with a sensitivity of 70% to 100%.[1,68] However, the specificity of such findings is quite low, because some tumors and other vascular malformations may also have this appearance. The preferred imaging modality for detecting CMs is MRI because of its superior sensitivity and specificity, particularly when gradient-recalled echo (GRE) sequences are employed.[24,37,67] T2-weighted MRI is not 100% sensitive for the diagnosis of CM, because it has at least a 5% false-negative rate[24] and thrombosed AVMs, hematomas, hemorrhagic tumors, and inflammatory lesions of the CNS may occasionally mimic the MRI appearance of CMs.[69] GRE sequences have been shown to be more sensitive in this regard.[24]

---

*See references 1, 6, 14, 17, 20–22, 24, 31, 52, 54, 59, 62.

Table 69.1 Overview of Natural History of Cavernous Malformations

Series (Year)[*]	Findings	Comments
Del Curling et al (1991)[14]	Prevalence = **0.39%** Estimated hemorrhage risk = **0.25%** per person-year Estimated overall risk of seizure development = **1.51%** per person-year (single lesion = 1.34%; multiple lesions = 2.48%)	Retrospective study with rates calculated from birth to initial diagnosis
Robinson et al (1991)[17]	Prevalence = **0.47%** Annualized bleeding rate = **0.7%** Greater risk of overt hemorrhage in females ($P = 0.05$)	Retrospective study with rates calculated over a defined period after diagnosis Includes symptomatic and asymptomatic patients
Zabramski et al (1994)[6]	Incidence of symptomatic hemorrhage = **6.5%** per patient-year or **1.1%** per lesion-year De novo lesions observed in 29% of patients for a rate of 0.4% per patient-year Classification of cavernous malformations into radiographic types I–IV	Prospective study involving 59 members of six families followed with serial MRI for a mean 2.2 years Familial symptomatic and asymptomatic cases
Aiba et al (1995)[19]	Estimated hemorrhage rates for seizure, and incidental groups = **0.39%** per patient-year Estimated hemorrhage rate for hemorrhage group = **22.9%** per patient-year Hemorrhage more common in females <40 yrs old	Retrospective study of 110 treated patients stratified by presentation: hemorrhage (symptomatic), seizure (w/out acute hemorrhage), and incidental diagnosis
Kondziolka et al (1995)[16]	Retrospective annual hemorrhage rate = 1.3% Prospective hemorrhage rate = **2.63%** per year (overall) Prospective hemorrhage rate = 0.6% per year (no prior bleed) Prospective hemorrhage rate = 4.5% per year (prior hemorrhage)	Prospective and retrospective analyses Symptomatic and asymptomatic patients
Porter et al (1997)[31]	Annual event rate = **4.2%** per patient-year Annual symptomatic hemorrhage rate = **1.6%** per patient-year No increase in risk if original presentation was with bleed Infratentorial annual hemorrhage rate = 3.8% per year Supratentorial annual hemorrhage rate = 0.4% per year Deep lesion hemorrhage rate = 4.1% per year (event rate 10.6% per year) Superficial lesion hemorrhage rate = 0% (event rate 0%) No events during pregnancy Deep/infratentorial location most important risk for subsequent events, and rate of complete recovery is only 37%	Combined retrospective and prospective study of 110 patients Differentiates between neurologic events (with or w/out hemorrhage) and hemorrhages (without neurologic symptoms) 88% of patients symptomatic Mean follow-up 46 months
Barker et al (2001)[65]	Temporal clustering of recurrent hemorrhages in early post hemorrhage period Rehemorrhage rate = 2%/month for the first 2.5 years then decreases to <1%/month	Retrospective review of patients with overt hemorrhage to determine whether clustering (change in hazard rate for hemorrhage with time) was a feature of the natural history 141 patients presenting with **clinically overt hemorrhage** with subsequent surgery or stereotactic radiosurgery over an 18-year period

[*]Superscript numbers indicate chapter references.

Zabramski and colleagues[6] have classified CMs into four categories on the basis of the correlation between MRI signal characteristics and pathology. Type I lesions are characterized by a hyperintense core on T1-weighted MRI that corresponds to subacute hemorrhage; a smaller hyperintense core with a surrounding hypointense halo typifies the T2-weighted MRI appearance. Type II lesions contain loculated areas of hemorrhage and thrombosis of varying age surrounded by gliotic, hemosiderin-stained brain parenchyma. It is these lesions that exhibit the characteristic reticulated mixed-signal core and surrounding hypointense rim that is considered pathognomonic for CM on T2-weighted MRI. Type III lesions, which are hypointense on T1- and T2-weighted MRI but particularly so on GRE imaging, represent lesions with chronic resolved hemorrhage. Type IV lesions are well visualized only on GRE imaging, on which they appear as punctuate, hypointense lesions (Fig. 69–3).[6,24,67]

Management of Cavernous Malformations

Indications for Surgery

In considering the management of patients with CMs, the physician must carefully weigh the risks and benefits of various treatment options, such as surgery and radiosurgery, against the natural history of the lesion and

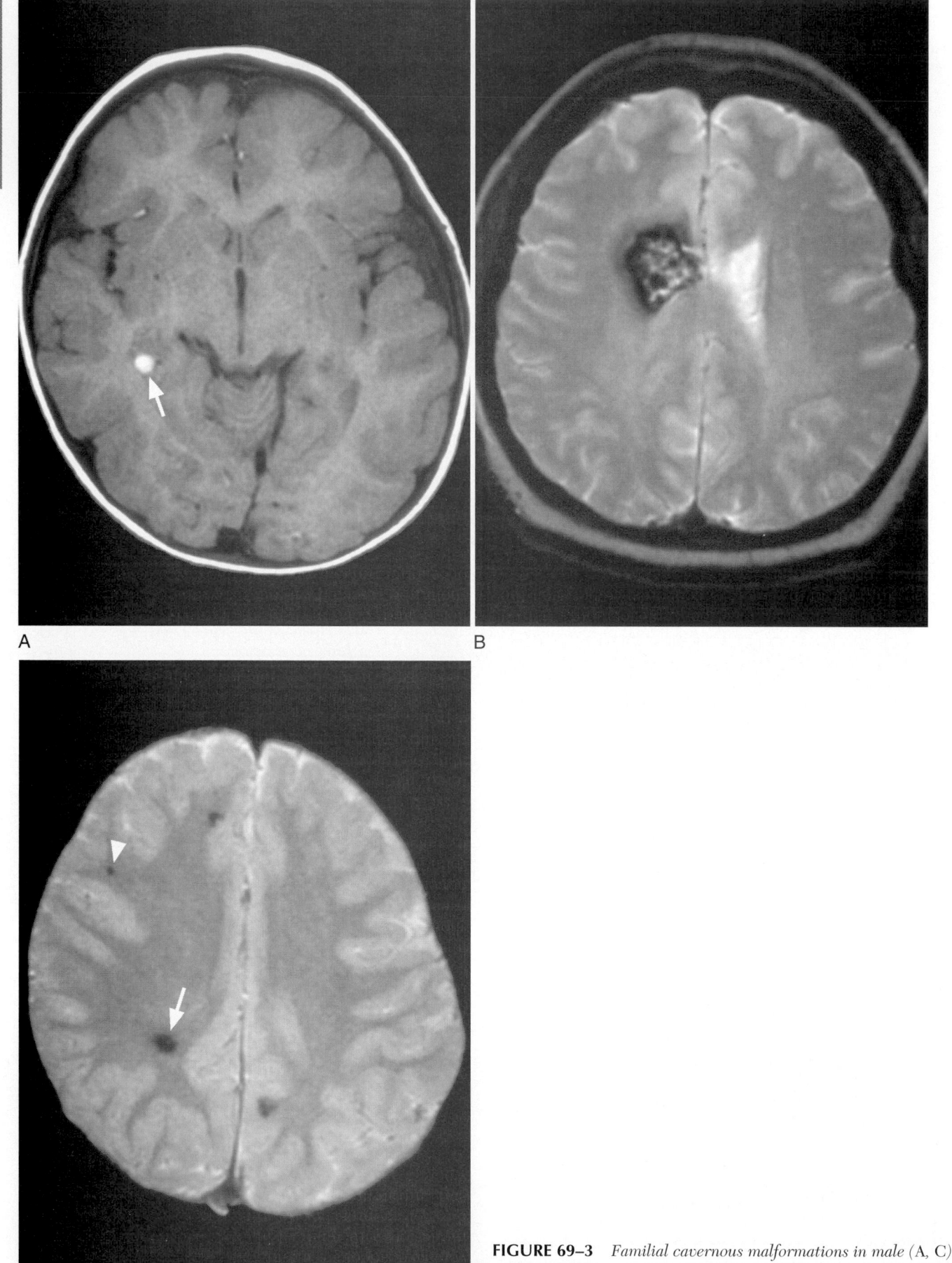

FIGURE 69–3 *Familial cavernous malformations in male* (A, C) *and female* (B) *second-degree relatives of Hispanic descent. Note the presence of type I lesion* (A, arrow), *type II lesion* (B), *and type III* (C, arrow) *and IV* (C, arrowhead) *lesions.*

expectant management. As discussed previously, the natural history or behavior of a lesion may vary according to lesion- and patient-specific traits. CMs tend to be more aggressive in children and females, during pregnancy, and with a brainstem location; this behavior must be factored into the decision-making. Although the indications for treatment of symptomatic lesions remain to be clearly defined, it is currently generally accepted that asymptomatic lesions be observed regardless of location. Intervention is usually considered for three conditions: medically intractable seizures, progressive neurologic deficits (with or without radiographic evidence of new hemorrhage), and recurrent symptomatic hemorrhage.

Asymptomatic and Mildly Symptomatic Accessible Lesions

With the advent of superior diagnostic neuroimaging techniques and subsequent identification of a large number of subjects with asymptomatic sporadic or familial CMs, the role of prophylactic surgical intervention for these lesions has been called into question. Fatal hemorrhage from CMs has been described, but the incidence is low,[50] and therefore the threat of a hemorrhage alone is not typically considered a surgical indication.[14] Even though surgery for accessible lesions carries a low risk of morbidity, it is generally recommended that patients be observed if they present with nonspecific symptoms such as headache. Some groups have suggested resection of such lesions because of the risk of subsequent symptomatic hemorrhage, the psychological burden to the patient, and the cost of serial imaging studies with follow-up.[21] This approach must obviously be considered, however, only after extensive counseling discussions with the patient about the natural history, risks of surgery, and individualized patient factors (Fig. 69–4).

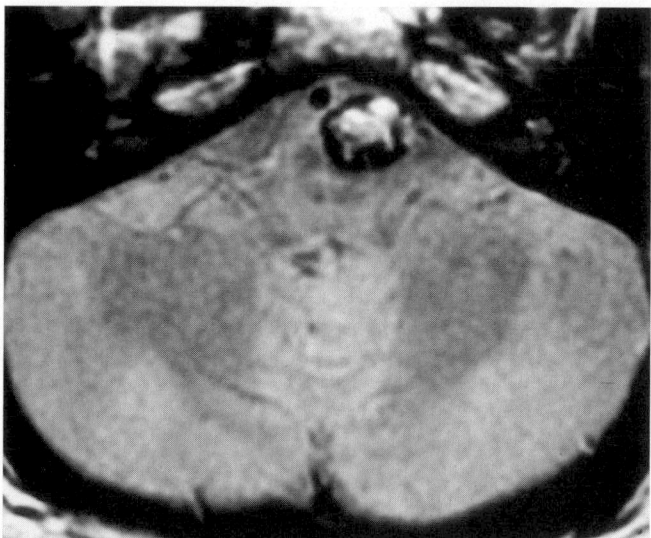

FIGURE 69–4 *Left ventral, pontine cavernous malformation in an asymptomatic 20-year-old patient. The lesion was managed with observation even though it was considered surgically accessible.*

Inaccessible Symptomatic Lesions

Conservative expectant management is also indicated for certain patients with symptomatic but inaccessible lesions (Fig. 69–5A and B). Chang and coworkers[70] developed an elaborate mathematical model that they applied to surgical decision-making in the resection of CMs for hemorrhage. Using calculations of morbidity-free life expectancies, estimated surgical risks, and lesion morbidity, they determined the surgical gain of morbidity-free life-expectancy years for superficial and deep lesions in young and old patients. Their analysis demonstrated that the gain was minimal (0.0 to 1.1 years) for superficial lesions, irrespective of age of patient or eloquence of lesion location. Similar analysis applied to deep lesions yielded the finding of a small gain in patients older than 60 years (1.1 to 3.1 years) and a significant gain (17 to 25 years) in patients younger than 20 years.[70] These researchers thus concluded that the role of surgery for asymptomatic superficial lesions was controversial but that intervention was justified for symptomatic deep lesions, particularly in young patients. This conclusion concurs with natural history studies comparing deep and superficial lesions.[31]

Seizures

Medical therapy is currently the primary treatment modality in the management of patients with CM and epilepsy, but whether surgical or medical treatment is the optimal management for such patients has yet to be determined. The traditional approach is that only the patient with medically intractable epilepsy undergo resection of a CM lesion definitively representing a seizure focus (Fig. 69–6). However, it has been shown that patients with CMs and a more protracted history of seizures have a smaller chance of being seizure free after surgery.[53,71–73] One randomized controlled trial of surgery for temporal lobe epilepsy has determined that surgery was superior to prolonged medical management.[74] In addition to patients with intractable seizures, Giulioni and associates[75] have advocated surgery for CM patients with nonrefractory epilepsy to avoid lesion growth and extension of the epileptogenic region.

Outcome of Surgical Management

Superficial Cavernous Malformations (Cerebral and Cerebellar Lesions)

Surgical resection of supratentorial, hemispheric CMs has been reported extensively in the literature with good outcomes.[61,76–79] Amin-Hanjani and colleagues[77,80] performed a retrospective critical analysis of patients undergoing CM surgery over an 18-year period to determine the risks attributable to surgical management. This cohort included 84 patients with supratentorial hemispheric lesions presenting with seizures (61%), neurologic deficits (18%), and headache (21%) and 8 patients with cerebellar lesions. Complete resection was achieved in all cases, and the outcome was good or excellent in 96.4% of cerebral cases, with a 4.8% permanent morbidity rate. Ninety-six percent of patients with seizures were seizure free postoperatively.[77] For resection of cerebellar lesions, outcome was good or excellent in 87.5% of cases, with no persistent morbidity. Acciarri and coworkers[76] noted a 91% good outcome

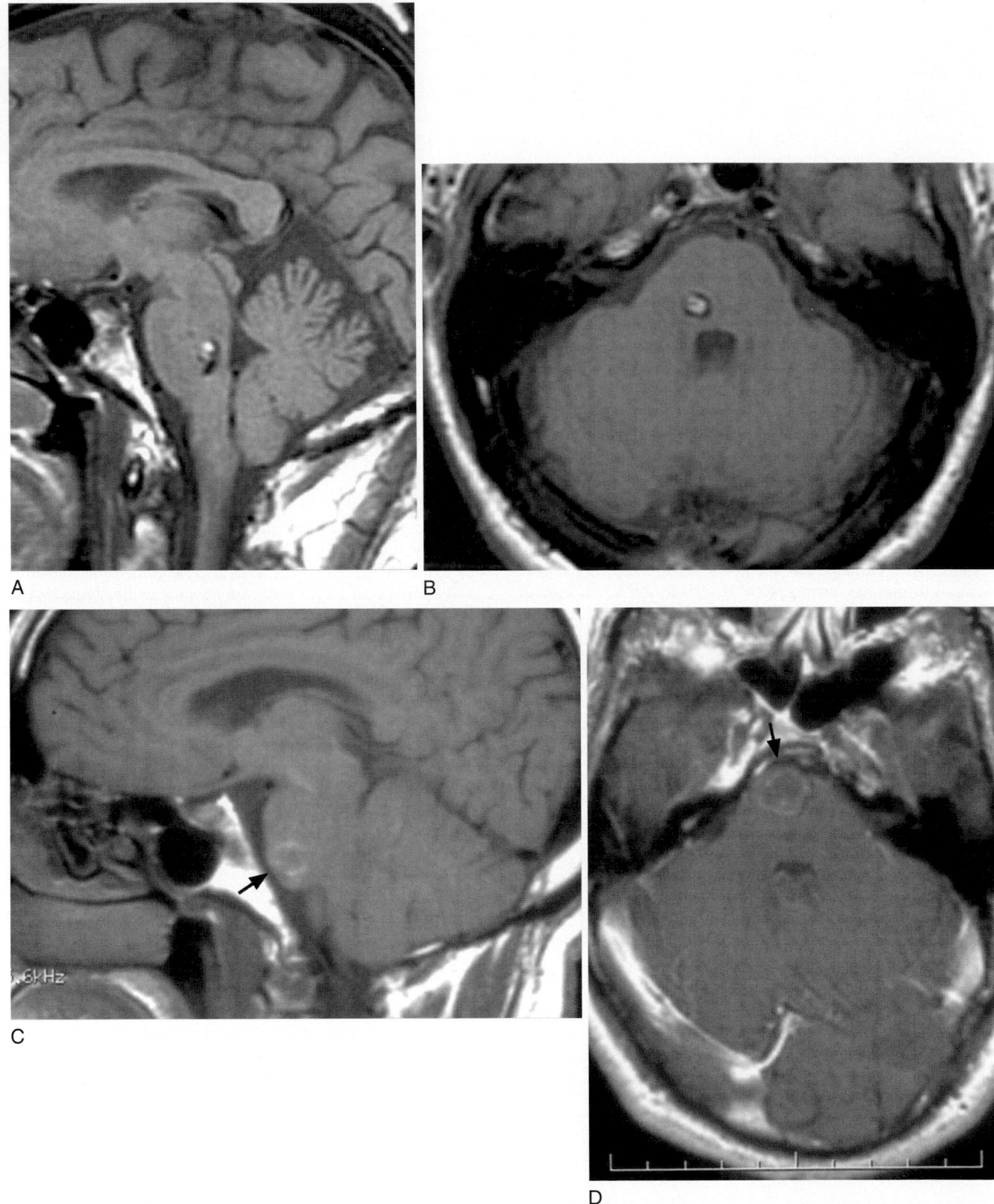

FIGURE 69–5   A *and* B, *Right dorsal pontine cavernous malformation (CM) in a 53-year-old man presenting with numbness and paresthesias. Because the lesion did not abut a pial surface, it was managed by observation only and remained stable with subsequent neuroimaging.* C *and* D, *A right ventral pontomedullary CM in a 59-year-old man who presented clinically with left hemiparesis, facial droop, and dysarthria. The lesion appeared to abut the pial surface* (arrow). *However, at surgery using a far lateral, transcondylar approach, no hemosiderin staining was observed on the brainstem surface. Intraoperative stereotactic localization and electrophysiologic brainstem mapping placed the lesion in the vicinity of the cranial nerves VII and VIII. Therefore, surgical resection was not attempted.*

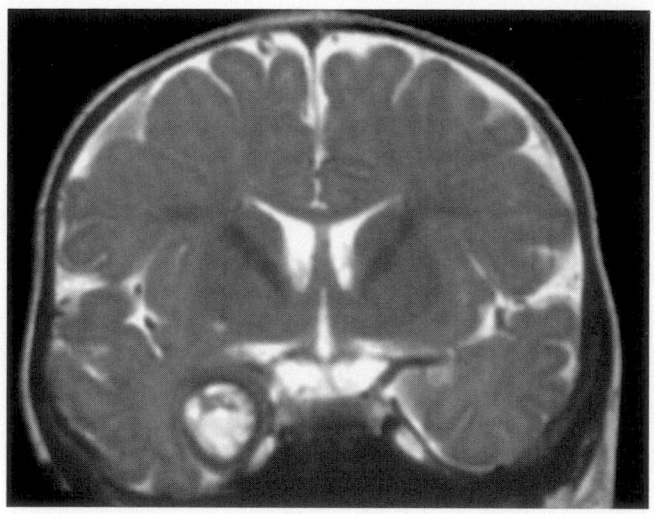

FIGURE 69–6 *Right temporal cavernous malformation (CM) causing intractable seizures in a 7-month-old Hispanic boy with familial CM. The patient has experienced good seizure control after surgical resection of the CM.*

after total resection in 95% of 55 patients with supratentorial lesions; however, 2 of 4 patients with intraventricular lesions died. Similar results have been obtained in smaller series and are summarized in Table 69.2.

Seizures represent the primary presenting symptom of supratentorial CM lesions. Although surgery is indicated for seizures refractory to medications,[55] resection of lesions in patients with single or few medically controlled seizures is emerging as an acceptable indication, given that a longer history of seizures is associated with a less favorable outcome.[53,71–73] Overall results indicate good seizure control after lesionectomy or radical resection of CM for epilepsy.[53,56,71–73,77,81] Zevgaridis and colleagues[73] observed a 95% improvement in seizure control after lesion resection in 77 patients, with 88.3% of patients were seizure free postoperatively. Studies examining whether lesion resection alone (lesionectomy) is equivalent to extensive seizure surgery for control of epilepsy demonstrated that patients with a seizure history shorter than 12 months were treated effectively with lesionectomy. In patients whose seizure history was longer than 12 months or who had experienced more than five seizures, seizure control after lesionectomy

Table 69.2   Overview of Surgical Outcomes for Superficial and Deep Cavernous Malformations

Series (Year)°	Total Number of Patients	Symptoms	Location	Results	Outcome	Complication(s)
Superficial Lesions						
Supratentorial						
Amin-Hanjani and Ogilvy (1999)[77]	84	Seizure, headache, hemorrhage	Not specified	Complete resection: 100%	Excellent/good: 96% Worsened: 4%	None
Chaskis and Brotchi (1998)[78]	16	Not specified	F: 8 T: 6 O: 2	Complete resection: 100%	No recurrent hemorrhage	Not specified
Acciarri et al (1993)[76]	55	Focal deficits Hemorrhage Seizures	F: 20 T: 17 Pa: 10 O: 8	Complete resection: 52 (95%)	Good: 91% Fair: 7% Poor: 2%	Not specified; 2 deaths in patients with intraventricular cavernous malformations
Ojemann et al (1993)[79]	32	Hemorrhage: 20 Seizures: 21 Neuro deficit: 6 Headache: 5	F: 11 T: 10 Pa: 10 O: 1	Complete resection: 100%	Good: 30 Fair: 2 Poor: 0 All patients returned to work	1 patient with new minor deficit
Scott et al (1992)[61]	10	Seizures, deficit, headache	F: 2 T: 2 Pa: 4 Po: 1 O: 1	Complete resection: 100%	No rebleeding in a mean 3.2 years of follow-up	Hemiparesis resolving over 1 year in 1 patient
Infratentorial						
Amin-Hanjani and Ogilvy (1999)[77]	8	Not specified	Cerebellum	Complete resection: 100%	Excellent/good: 87.5%	None
Chaskis and Brotchi (1998)[78]	3	Not specified	Cerebellum	Complete resection: 100%	No recurrent hemorrhage	Not specified

Continued

Therapy

Table 69.2   Overview of Surgical Outcomes for Superficial and Deep Cavernous Malformations—cont'd

Series (Year)*	Total Number of Patients	Symptoms	Location	Results	Outcome	Complication(s)
Acciarri et al (1993)[76]	74	Focal deficits, hemorrhage	CH: 4 V: 1	Complete resection: 80%	Good: 80% Fair: 20%	Death: 2
Ojemann et al (1993)[79]	3	Ataxia	CH	Complete resection: 3	Good: 3	None
Scott et al (1992)[61]	2	Deficit	CH	Complete resection: 2	Good; no rebleeding over 6.5-year mean follow-up	None
Deep Lesions Steinberg et al (2000)[85]	57	Hemorrhage: 100%	Thal: 5 BG: 10 MB: 9 Po: 24 M: 9	Subtotal resection: 7% Total resection: 93%	4.7-yr follow-up: Improved: 52% Unchanged: 43% Worse: 5%	Rebleeding: 4
Chaskis and Brotchi (1998)[78]	18	Not specified	BG, Thal, deep white matter, CC, IV	Subtotal resection: 2	Not specified	Not specified
Bertalanffy et al (1991)[51]	26	Progressive neurologic deficit: 18/16 Seizures: 4/26 Hydrocephalus: 3/26 Rebleed: 1/26	BG: 10 Thal: 2 MB: 5 Po: 8 M: 1	No new deficits: 11/26 Delayed recovery: 7/26 Deterioration: 8/26	Improved: 6/11 Fewer seizures: 4/4	Rebleeding: 2 Long tract injury: 2 Vascular injury: 3 Paradoxical air embolism: 1
Fritschi et al (1994)[82] Literature review	93	All symptomatic Hemorrhage: 88%	MB: 14% MB-P: 12% Po: 62% Po-M: 12% M: 5%	Subtotal resection: 7/93	Complete recovery: 39.8% Minimal disability: 44.1% Moderate disability: 15%	2/7 with subtotal resection had rebleeding within 4.1 years 2/7 residual lesions enlarged
Original patients	29	Focal deficit, seizures, coma Hemorrhage: 76%	MB: 6 Po: 13 Po-M: 6 M: 4	Complete resection: 24	Not specified	Not specified
Porter et al (1999)[5] (includes 26 patients from Fritschi et al, 1994[82])	100	Cranial neuropathies Sensory disturbance Hemiparesis/plegia Ataxia Dysarthia Coma Headache Hydrocephalus Hemorrhage: 97%	MB: 16 MB-P: 15 Po: 39 Po-M: 10 M: 16 Other: 7	Subtotal resection: 1%	Same or better: 87% Worse: 10% Died: 3.5% (one from postoperative hemorrhage) (Mean GOS at 35 months: 4.5)	Permanent or severe morbidity: 12% CN palsies: 7% Weakness: 2% Brachial plexopath: 1% Trach/PEG: 1%
Amin-Hanjani and Ogilvy (1999)[77]	17	Not specified	Not specified	Subtotal resection: 4/17	Excellent/good: 64% Fair: 24% Poor: 12%	Rebleed within three years in 2/4 subtotal resections Permanent complications: 17.6%
Ziyal et al (1999)[87]	9	Hemorrhage: 100% Multiple bleeds: 8/9 Residual deficits: 100%	MB: 2 Po-M: 3 M: 4	Subtotal resection: 2	Excellent/good (GOS 5 or 4): 8/9 Worse (GOS 3): 1/9	Rebled in 1 of 2 with subtotal resection

*Superscript numbers indicate chapter references.
BG, basal ganglia; CC, corpus callosum; CH, cerebellar hemisphere; CN, cranial nerve; F, frontal; GOS, Glasgow Outcome Scale score; IV, intraventricular; M, medulla; MB, midbrain; O, occipital; Pa, parietal; Po, pons; T, temporal; Thal, thalamus; Trach/PEG, tracheostomy/percutaneous gastric feeding tube; V, cerebellar vermis.

alone was less favorable.[71,72] Thus, it appears that more extensive epilepsy surgery should be performed in this latter group of patients.[55]

Deep Cavernous Malformations (Brainstem, Basal Ganglia, and Thalamic Lesions)

CMs within the brainstem, basal ganglia, and thalamus (Fig. 69–7) represent more complex surgical lesions and thus have less favorable operative outcomes.[5,51,60,77,79,82–87] One study noted a 30% recurrent hemorrhage rate in a retrospective analysis of 100 patients.[5] Eighty-six of these patients underwent surgical resection of the lesion, which resulted in neurologic improvement or stability in 87%, deterioration in 10%, a 33% postoperative morbidity that was permanent in 12%, and a surgical mortality of 4%.[5] Pozzati[83] reported on 12 patients with thalamic lesions, of whom 5 were observed, 4 underwent aggressive surgery, and 3 were managed with radiosurgery, ventriculoperitoneal shunt placement, or evacuation of hematoma. The operative mortality was 25% (1/4 patients), and the remaining patients improved or remained the same.

Amin-Hanjani and Ogilvy[77] reported a good or excellent outcome in 64.2% of 14 patients, with a 14.2% rate of persistent disabling morbidity. Our published series involved 56 patients operated on for 57 brainstem, basal ganglia, and thalamic CM lesions at Stanford University Department of Neurosurgery; 42 of the lesions were located in the brainstem and 15 in the basal ganglia or thalamus.[85] In the immediate postoperative period, neurologic status was unchanged in 55% of patients, improved in 16%, and worsened in 29%. At long-term follow-up (>6 months), 43% of patients showed no changed from preoperative neurologic state, 52% had improved, and 5% had worsened.[85] Complete resection was achieved in 93% of lesions with a long-term postoperative morbidity of 5%. Patients in whom the CM had undergone prior stereotactic radiosurgery (SRS) or radiotherapy had a worse outcome. Although there was no perioperative mortality, 2 patients died at 2.5 and 4 years postoperatively; both had undergone prior irradiation. At Stanford, we have now operated on 89 patients with brainstem, basal ganglia, and thalamic CMs (1991 to 2002). The long-term results show 96% of patients with an excellent or good outcome, 2% with a poor outcome, and 2% mortality with 5% permanent surgical morbidity. Outcomes for other surgical series involving resection of deep-seated CMs are listed in Table 69.2.

Surgical Considerations

Preoperative Assessment and Management

A thorough history and physical examination with particular attention to the family history must be obtained. Preoperative neuroimaging studies, preferably MRI with T1-weighted sequences for localization, are required. Angiography is not necessary, although it is sometimes helpful in the identification of a DVA, which can occur in association with a CM (Fig. 69–8). However, DVAs are usually identifiable on contrast-enhanced MRI as well. In patients undergoing resection for seizure control, the evaluation should include electroencephalography (EEG) studies to confirm that there is concordance between the epileptic focus and the CM.

Antibiotics are administered preoperatively and continued for at least 24 hours after surgery. The patient is started on steroid therapy, the dosage of which is rapidly tapered postoperatively in the absence of neurologic complications. After induction of general endotracheal anesthesia (conscious sedation for patients requiring speech mapping) and insertion of a Foley catheter, a lumbar drain may be placed for cerebrospinal fluid drainage, but usually only in patients with lesions of the upper brainstem requiring a subtemporal approach. Intravenous administration of furosemide (10 to 20 mg) and mannitol (0.5 to 1.0 gm/kg) may be considered, with recognition that excessive brain dehydration has the potential to produce relaxation and brain shift, possibly rendering image guidance inaccurate. Anticonvulsants are used selectively in patients who are considered to be at high risk of perioperative seizures or who have prior seizure history. For patients undergoing resection after a hemorrhage, sufficient time should be allowed for stabilization of neurologic symptoms.[88] We prefer to wait about 4 weeks and have found that this delay also provides time for acute hemorrhages to soften or liquefy, facilitating dissection.[85]

Operative Approaches

The surgical approach in the resection of a CM is based on the location of the lesion and the pial surface to which it is closest. The primary goal is to reach the lesion while traversing as little normal brain parenchyma as possible, yet have adequate room for exposure and resection of the lesion with minimal injury to surrounding structures. Surgical approaches in the resection of supratentorial and infratentorial lesions have been described elsewhere[79,84,85,87,89–97] and are summarized in Table 69.3.

Surgical Techniques and Adjuncts

Microsurgical Dissection

Microsurgical resection is performed under high-power magnification with very fine irrigating bipolar coagulation forceps and finely regulated suction. The coagulation is set to low power to limit the spread of current to the surrounding brain. The lesion may be approached through a sulcus or through a small corticotomy in order to avoid injury to the parenchyma. Resection of brainstem lesions should be avoided if they do not present on a pial or ventricular surface (see Fig. 69–5C and D). For lesions in noneloquent brain, total resection of the CM and surrounding hemosiderin rim is the goal. This can be achieved by microsurgical dissection of the gliotic tissue surrounding the lesion to create a cleavage plane. Small blood vessels can be coagulated and divided if they are encountered, although DVAs must be preserved. Larger lesions may be decompressed with suction, microscissors, or the ultrasonic surgical aspirator prior to resection of the capsule.

We define *eloquent brain* as areas with a high density of specialized neurologic function, such as the brainstem, diencephalon, basal ganglia, deep cerebellar nuclei, motorsensory, language, and visual cortices as well as the optic nerve and chiasm. Lesions located in eloquent brain should be resected without dissection of the hemosiderin or gliotic rim surrounding the CM. Associated DVAs

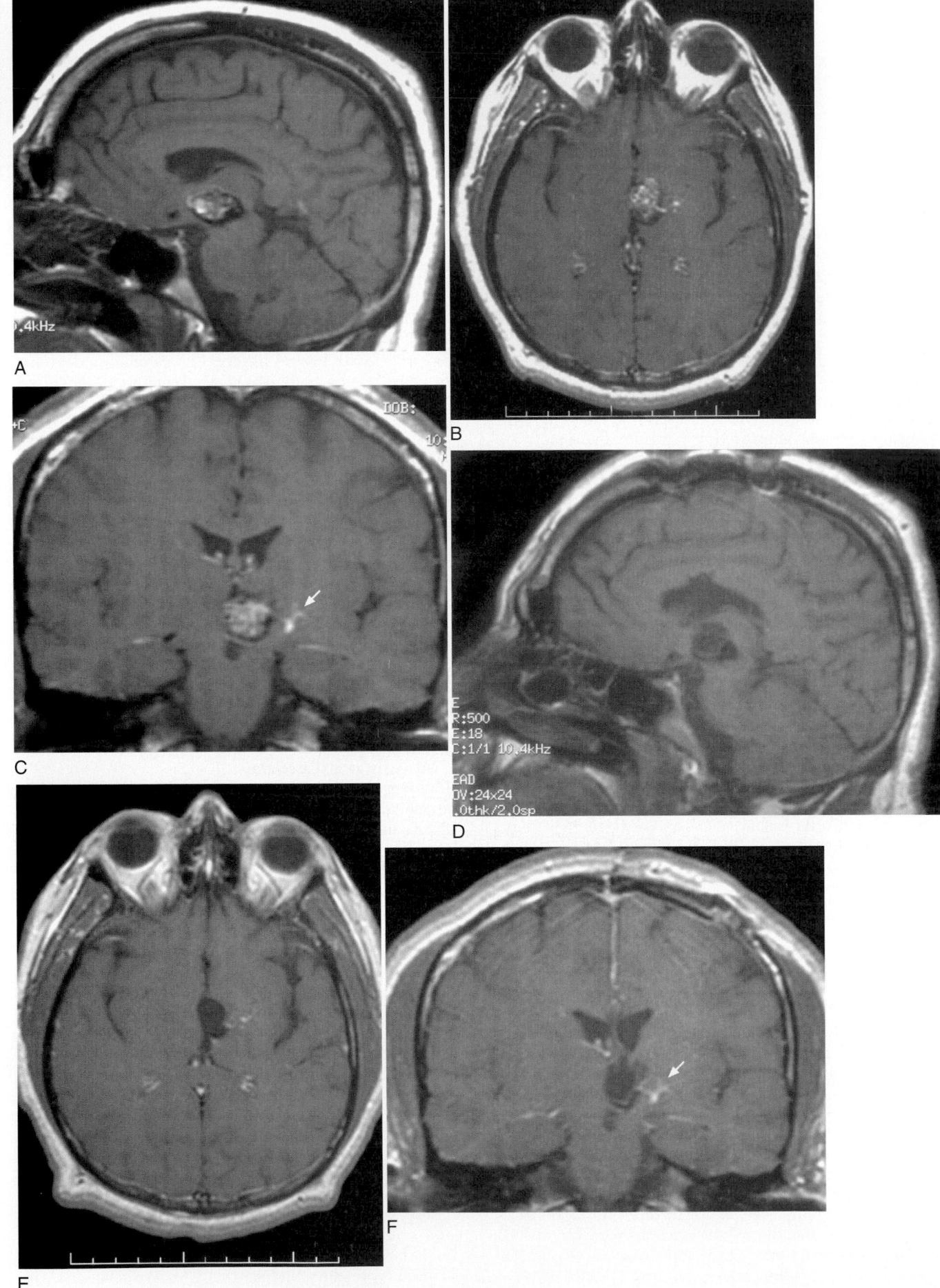

FIGURE 69–7 A *to* C, *Preoperative MRI depicting a hypothalamic cavernous malformation in a 32-year-old man who presented with right-sided hemiparesis and numbness along with dysarthria and cognitive and memory difficulties. After the patient recovered neurologically, the lesion was resected via a left frontal, transcallosal, intraventricular approach, operating through the foramen of Monro and utilizing intraoperative stereotactic navigation.* D *to* F, *Postoperative images. Note an adjacent venous anomaly that was left intact* (arrows, C *and* F).

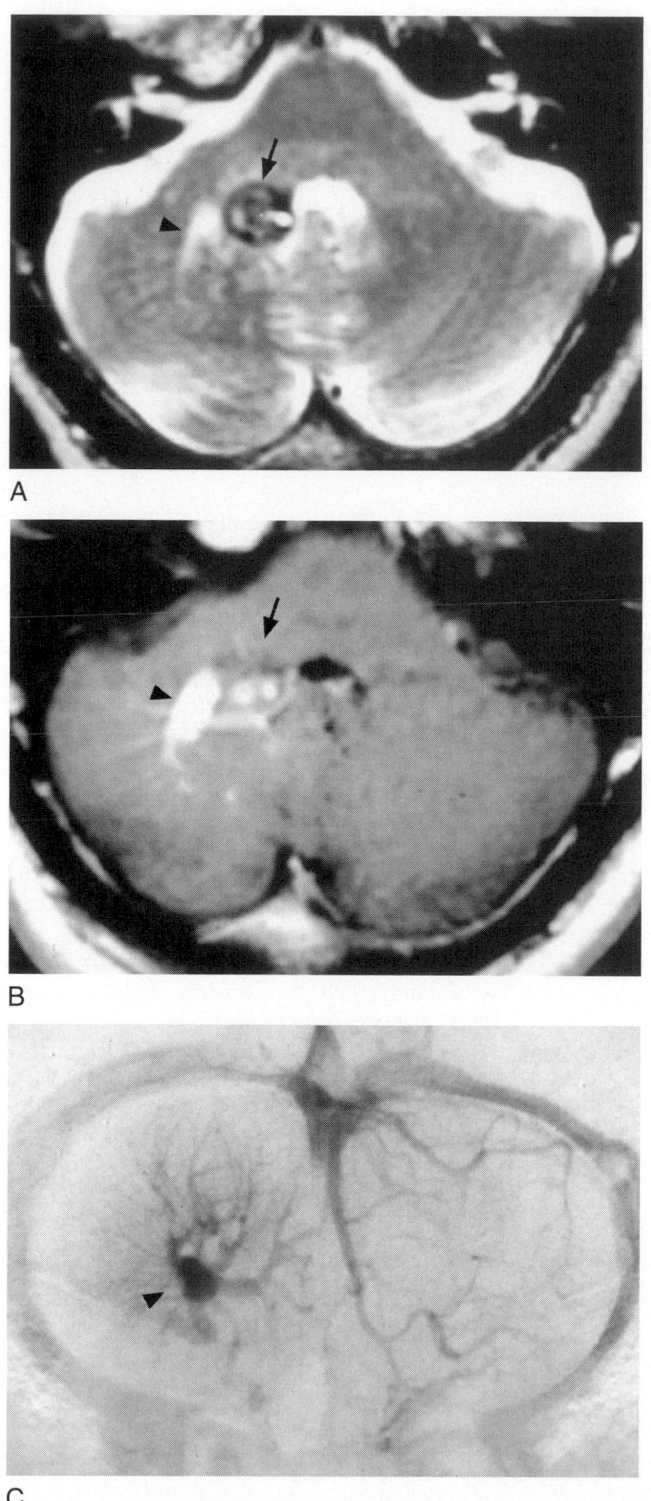

A

B

C

FIGURE 69–8 *Coexistence of a right cerebellar cavernous malformation* (arrow) *with a developmental venous anomaly* (arrowhead) *seen on T2-weighted MRI* (A), *contrast-enhanced T1-weighted MRI* (B), *and angiography* (C).

Table 69.3   Approaches for Resection of Cavernous Malformation Lesions

Lesion Location	Approach	Critical Structures
Supratentorial		
Inferior or lateral frontal	Pterional	
Subfrontal		
Suprachiasmatic		
Medial frontal	Interhemispheric	Anterior corpus callosum, cingulate gyrus, anterior lateral and third ventricles
Anterior and medial temporal lobes	Modified pterional	Amygdala, hippocampus
Posterior temporal	Temporal	
Inferior temporal	Subtemporal	Vein of Labbé
Middle and posterior frontal	Frontal	Rolandic cortex
Medial posterior frontal and parietal	Frontal-parietal	
Posterior parietal	Parietal-occipital	Calcarine cortex
Occipital		
Lateral ventricle (trigone)	Transcortical paramedian	
Thalamus	Interhemispheric, transcallosal	Vein of Galen, internal cerebral veins
Pineal region	Infratentorial supracerebellar	Vein of Galen
Infratentorial		
Inferior medial cerebellar, dorsal medulla	Suboccipital	Cerebellar vermis, medial cerebellar hemispheres, floor of fourth ventricle, dorsal medulla
Superior medial cerebellar, dorsal midbrain (tectum)	Occipital transtentorial, infratentorial/supracerebellar	Superior cerebellar peduncles, vermis, anterior medullary velum, posterior third ventricle, splenium of corpus callosum, quadrigeminal plate, vein of Galen
Anterior and lateral medulla, cervicomedullary junction	Far lateral suboccipital	Vertebral artery, lower cranial nerves, occipital condyle
Ventral and lateral midbrain, pontomesencephalic	Subtemporal/transpetrosal, Pterional-transsylvian	Vein of Labbé, sigmoid sinus, superior petrosal sinus, cranial nerves VII and VIII
Midpons (ventral and lateral)	Combined subtemporal and retromastoid, subtemporal/transpetrosal, combined subtemporal and translabyrinthine	Vein of Labbé, sigmoid sinus, superior petrosal sinus, cranial nerves VII and VIII
Dorsal pons	Suboccipital (± transvermian)	Facial colliculus, hypoglossal trigone, vagal trigone

should be left untouched, because injury to them may result in venous infarction with subsequent devastating consequences. The resection bed is lined with a single layer of strips of absorbable knitted hemostatic fabric (Surgicel; Johnson & Johnson, New Brunswick, NJ), and hemostasis is meticulously maintained.

One of the goals of CM surgery for seizures is to resect the area of hemosiderin staining and gliosis around the lesion, because this material is thought to be epileptogenic. Casazza and associates[56] found, however, that a residual hemosiderin-containing ring, as evidenced by its persistence on postoperative MRI, did not worsen outcome and that conversely, removal of the surrounding hemosiderin-stained tissue did not necessarily improve outcome. Additionally, removal of the glial scar does not appear to offer any added advantage with respect to postoperative seizure control.[73]

Intraoperative Stereotaxy
Intraoperative stereotaxy is a useful adjunct in the localization and resection of lesions located in eloquent areas of the cerebral cortices and brainstem. Currently available frameless stereotaxy systems that utilize an infrared optical tracking system integrated into the operating microscope allow for localization while still achieving submillimeter accuracy. Such systems offer better planning of operative approach, particularly for deep lesions that are not visible on a pial surface (Fig. 69–9). Alternatively, some investigators have used intraoperative ultrasonography for lesion localization, with good results.[77]

Electrophysiologic Monitoring and Mapping
Electrophysiologic monitoring is considered an extremely valuable adjunct in the resection CM lesions located in eloquent areas of the brain and brainstem.[87,98,99] Mapping of motor, sensory, and language cortex should be performed with lesions located in close proximity to these locations. We use bilateral somatosensory evoked potentials (SSEPs), brainstem auditory evoked potentials (BAEPs), and bilateral monitoring of cranial nerve III, V, VII, XI, and XII motor function for deep lesions, particularly those within the brainstem and with approaches involving the fourth ventricle.[98,99]

Hypothermia
We have routinely used mild brain hypothermia by applying a cooling blanket and decreasing core and brain temperature to 33°C in the resection of vascular lesions. Although this modality has not yet been shown to be clinically beneficial in the resection of deep CMs, it is a safe,

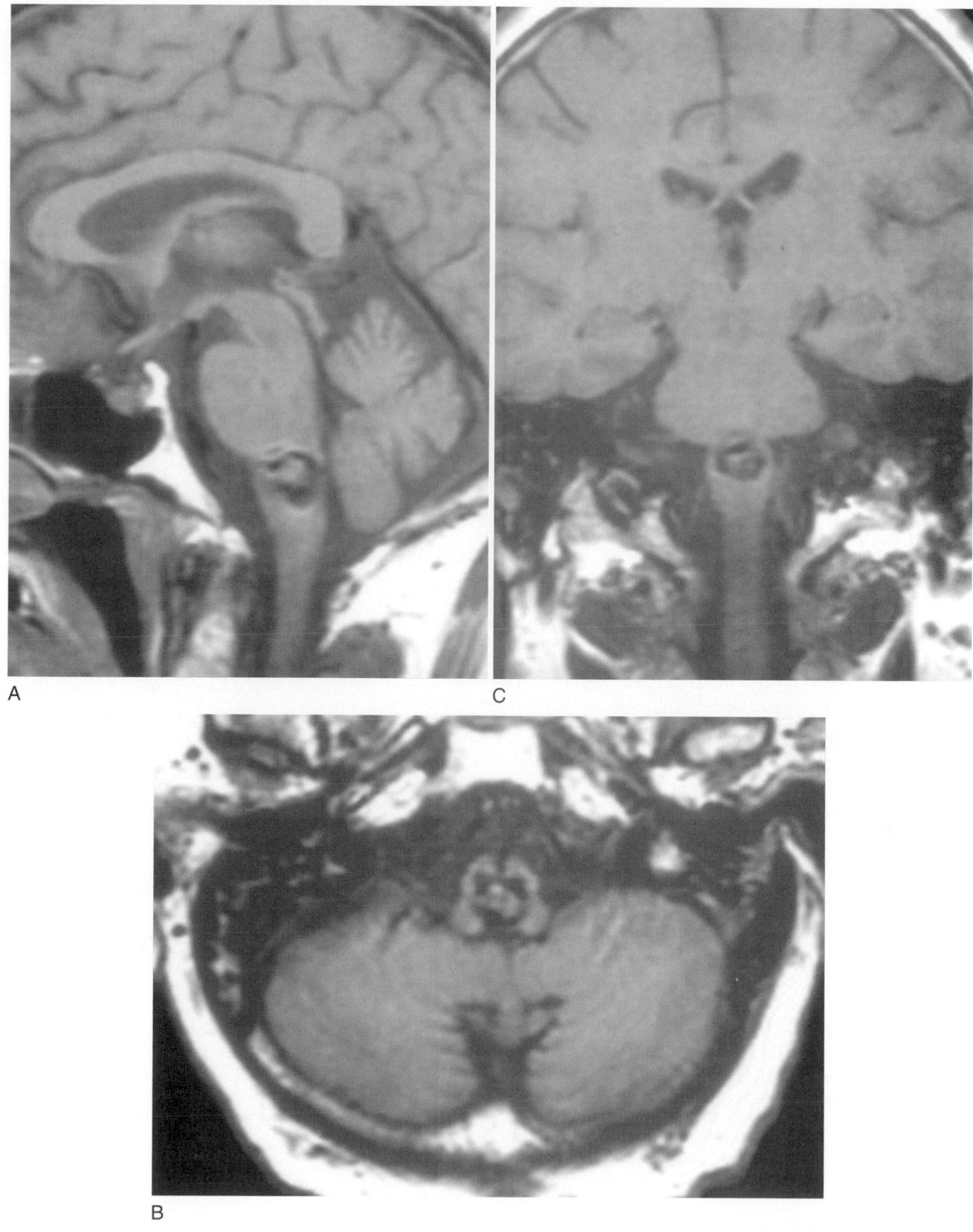

FIGURE 69–9 *A to C, T1-weighted MRI showing a brainstem cavernous malformation (CM) located in the medulla of a 54-year-old man who presented with progressive dysarthria, ataxia, and paresthesias. The lesion was approached suboccipitally through the floor of the fourth ventricle with the use of mild hypothermia and intraoperative electrophysiologic monitoring.*

Continued

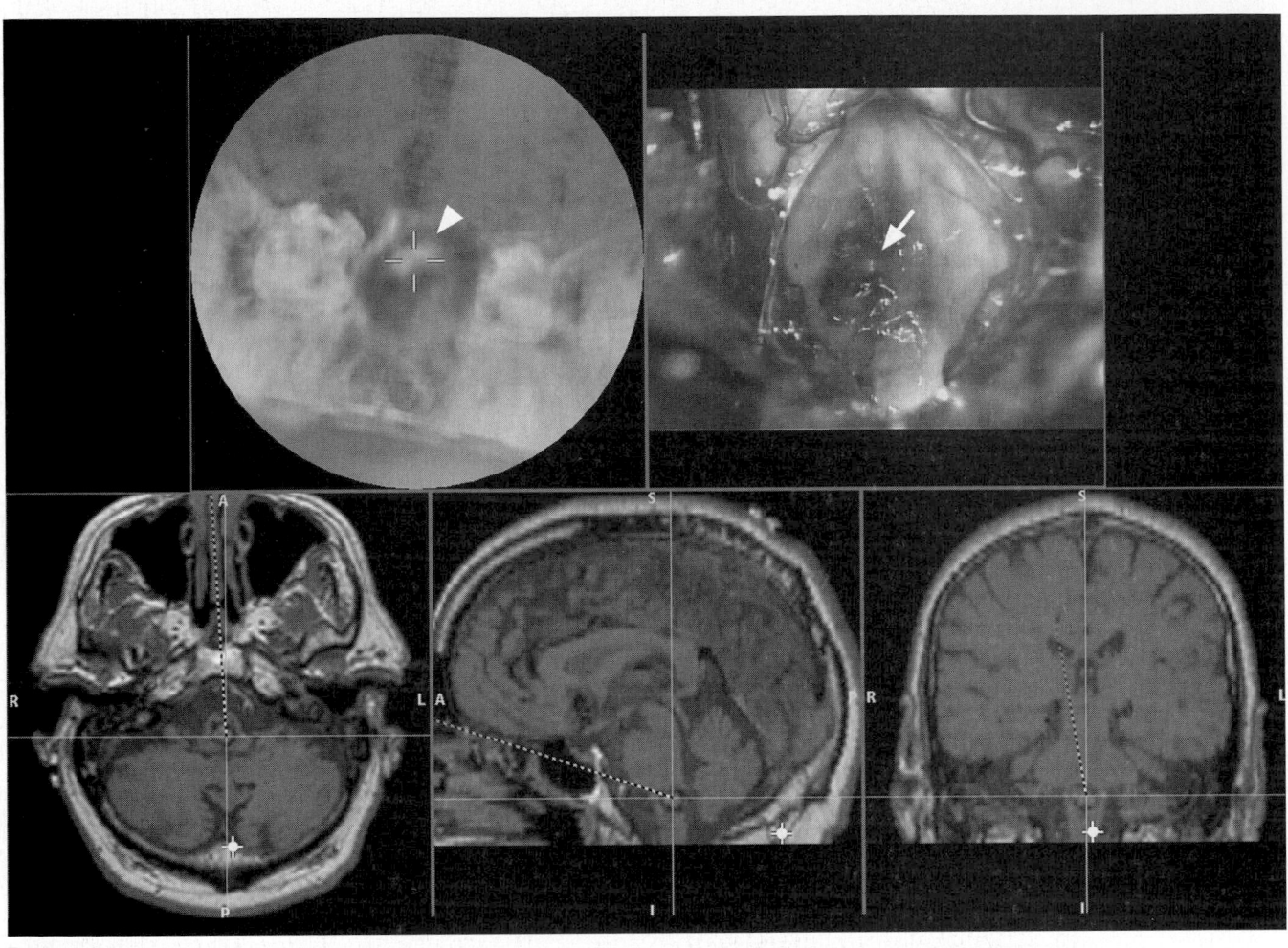

D

FIGURE 69–9, cont'd. D, *Intraoperative stereotactic neuronavigation, utilizing the Cbyon system in this case, allowed for localization of the lesion on axial, sagittal, and coronal MRI planes* (bottom row) *as well as three-dimensional volumetric computer rendering of the CM* (top left, arrowhead) *and overlying bony anatomy, and screen projection of the structures visualized through the microscope* (top right) *with integrated infrared optical tracking* (arrow).

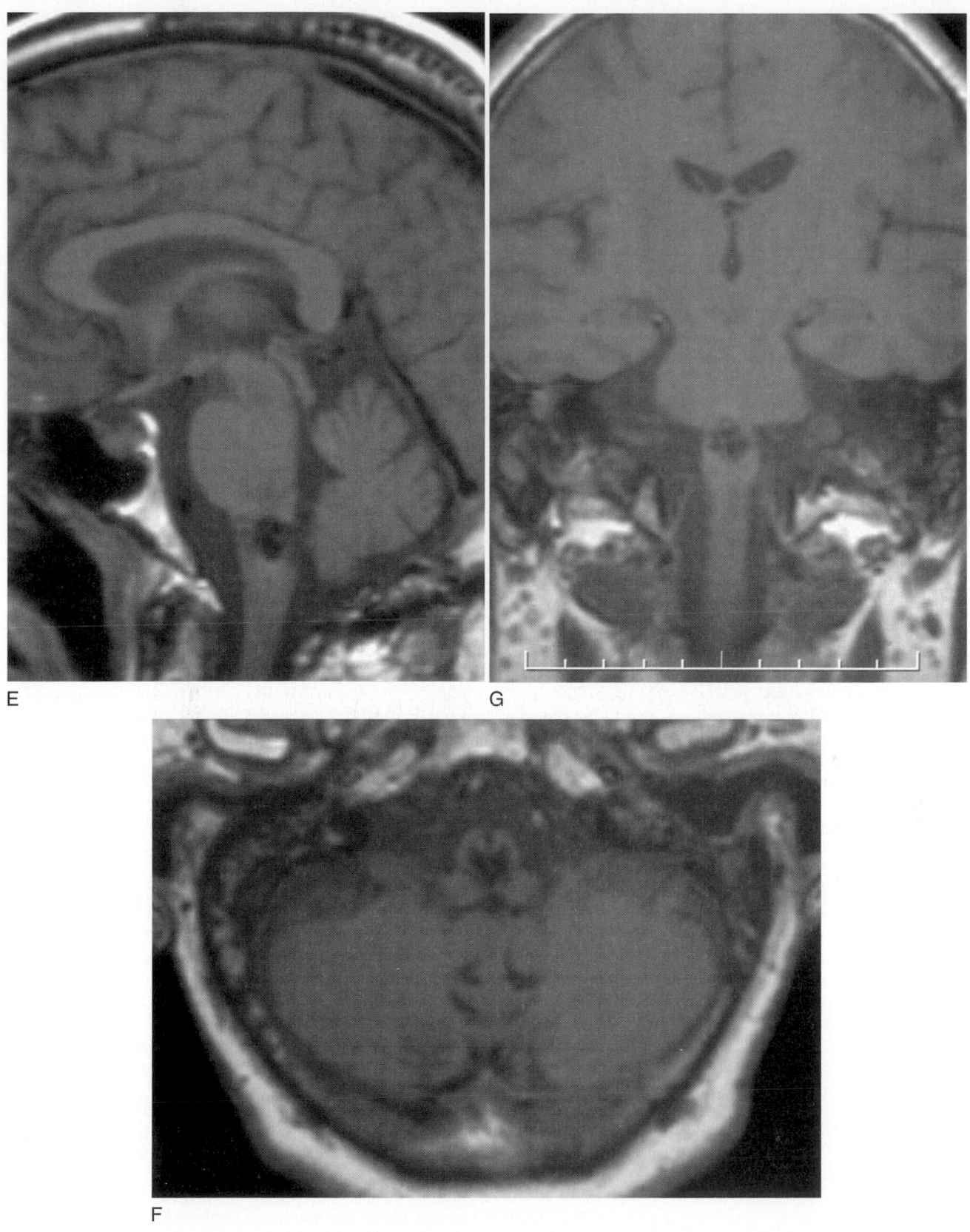

FIGURE 69–9, cont'd. E *to* G, *T1-weighted MRI performed 5 months after surgery show complete resection of the CM.*

feasible intervention that is useful in experimental cerebral ischemia, in global ischemia after cardiac arrest in patients, and possibly after ischemic or traumatic brain injury.[100–103]

Postoperative Care

All patients are observed in the intensive care unit after surgery, with monitoring of airway and mean arterial pressure as well as cardiac and respiratory function. Neurologic function is also closely monitored for signs of deterioration from postoperative hemorrhage, edema, or hydrocephalus. In patients with brainstem lesions, dysfunction of the lower cranial nerves may occur, resulting in breathing or swallowing difficulties that may necessitate placement of a tracheostomy or gastrojejunostomy tube. Steroid therapy is usually maintained postoperatively, with rapid weaning in uncomplicated cases. Administration of antibiotics is continued for 24 hours after surgery. Postoperative CT or MRI is optional. We routinely obtain MRI 2 to 3 months postoperatively to confirm complete resection of the CM.

Complications, Morbidity, and Their Management

Intraoperative and postoperative hemorrhage from inadequate hemostasis after CM resection is rare, partly because the lesion is under very low pressure. However, a potential complication is a subtotal resection with subsequent rehemorrhage. MRI obtained 3 to 6 months postoperatively is useful in confirming complete resection, although not 100% accurate.[85] Management of a residual lesion would depend on its location and the patient's clinical symptomatology.

Neurologic deficits and postoperative morbidity may result from manipulation and resection of lesions in eloquent areas. A percentage of these may result from retraction, manipulation, or perioperative edema and may be transient. A transient internuclear ophthalmoplegia may occur after resection of a midline lesion via a fourth ventricular approach; new or worsening hemiparesis may result from resection of a thalamic or basal ganglia lesion; upper and lower cranial nerve dysfunction and appendicular or gait ataxia may appear after resection of brainstem and cerebellar lesions. Swallowing and respiratory difficulties (Ondine's curse) may result from resection of lesions in the medulla, and their management can be somewhat challenging, often requiring tracheostomy, placement of a feeding tube, or prolonged ventilator dependence. Hydrocephalus may occur from obstruction of the ventricles or cerebral aqueduct by blood and is treated by drainage if symptomatic.

Postoperative wound infection, meningitis, or cerebrospinal fluid leaks may occur, as with other intracranial procedures. The risk of these complications is reduced by meticulous wound and dural closure, proper sterile technique, and administration of perioperative antibiotics.

Radiosurgery

Surgical resection of superficial, accessible CM lesions can be achieved with a low incidence of morbidity and mortality. Resection of lesions that lie deep within the brain represents a much more complex management dilemma. Although the natural history of deep CMs is more ominous than that of superficial lesions in noneloquent brain, the risk of surgical resection is also greater. In patients with progressively symptomatic deep lesions for which surgical extirpation is not an option SRS has been proposed as an alternative treatment modality. Several published reports document experience in the treatment of deep CM with SRS, but few have demonstrated a clear advantage for this intervention. Additionally, SRS has its own attendant morbidity, and our experience suggests that lesions that have been previously treated with SRS are more difficult to resect, with patients demonstrating a poorer outcome.[85]

A caveat in evaluating the efficacy of SRS in the treatment of CMs is that the natural history is still being defined, making it unclear whether the response to SRS is any different from the natural course of the disease. In fact, Barker and colleagues[65] found that the rehemorrhage rate was initially high in the first 2.5 years after a bleed (2% per month) and subsequently decreased (1% per month), a pattern they described as "clustering." Finally, one must consider that technological advances made since the early published results of CM radiosurgery, particularly in frame-based and frameless linear accelerator SRS, may improve overall results.

Karlsson and associates[104] reported a decrease in the hemorrhage rate of CM from 11% to 6% 4 years after treatment with Gamma knife SRS. However, both these rates were higher than that reported without treatment,[16] so the results do not clearly show that SRS influences the natural history of the disease. The clinical outcome in this study was notable for a large number of radiation-induced complications, with resultant neurologic deterioration in 41% of treated patients; 27% required subsequent resection.[104] Chang and coworkers[105] found a reduction in the annual post-SRS hemorrhage rate from 9.4% in the first 36 months to 1.6% thereafter. However, radiation-related complications occurred in 11% of their patients. Additionally, subsequent resection of irradiated CMs found that no lesions were completely thrombosed at a mean of 3.5 years after SRS treatment.[106] Other groups have reported similar findings, suggesting a minimal benefit and a modest complication rate ranging from 16% to 59% with SRS treatment.[107–109]

Tsien and colleagues[110] reported their SRS experience in the treatment of AOVMs primarily thought to consist of CMs that were not amenable to surgical resection because of risk. Although they observed a significant reduction in post-radiosurgery hemorrhage rate, 4 patients experienced radiation-induced side effects. These researchers concluded that although controversial, radiosurgery represents a treatment option for patients with otherwise inaccessible symptomatic CMs.[110]

Kondziolka and associates[111,112] observed an annual rehemorrhage rate of 32% in 47 patients prior to their treatment with SRS. The rehemorrhage rate declined to 8.8% in the first 2 years after SRS, and to 1.1% in the subsequent 4 years. A complication rate of 26% was noted in this series. These findings have held true in an ensuing study, which involved 82 patients and a 5-year follow-up period demonstrating a more than 30-fold reduction in rehemorrhage risk and a 13.4% morbidity.[113] They conclude that there was no observed clustering of hemorrhages, and they accounted for the much higher pretreatment rehemorrhage rate of 33.9% by noting that patients in their cohort had suffered at least two pretreatment hemorrhages and thus represented a higher-risk population. However, given the current morbidity rates, further clarification of the natural history and effect of SRS is required before it can be recommended as an alternative to surgery or conservative management of CMs.

Management of Cavernous Malformations in the Pediatric Population

Although CMs tend to be symptomatic between the second and fourth decades,[11,54] occurrence in the pediatric population has been well documented and children account for about one fourth of all CM patients.[18,21,54,114] Pediatric patients appear to have a bimodal distribution of age at symptomatic presentation, with one peak occurring at less than 3 years and the other at 11 years.[114,115] The literature appears to support a different natural history of CM in the pediatric population, with earlier onset of familial cases[4,24,26] and a tendency for presentation with acute neurologic deficits and overt hemorrhage.[21,114] Along with ruptured AVMs, CMs are the major cause of spontaneous intracerebral hemorrhage in otherwise healthy children.[114] Nonetheless, as in adult patients, the natural history of the disease in children remains yet to be definitively described. Cranial irradiation in children has been implicated as a cause of CM.[10]

CMs in pediatric patients may manifest clinically as focal neurologic deficits, seizures, and hemorrhage, like those in adults, but may also appear as macrocephaly, irritability, and failure to thrive. The evaluation and general principles of management are quite similar to those in adult patients. Appropriate imaging studies are especially important, because CMs in the pediatric population may mimic neoplasms and other lesions.[69,114]

Surgical decision-making is based on appropriate balancing of the symptomatic presentation, known natural history, and the accessibility of the lesion. Frim and Scott[116] have recommended that certain symptomatic lesions in eloquent locations and small asymptomatic single lesions be resected. Asymptomatic multiple lesions and symptomatic deep lesions involve a more complex decision-making, given the associated morbidity.[61,116] Mottolese and coworkers[114] have suggested that surgery is indicated in all cases of acute hemorrhage and neurologic deficit, including deep lesions if they are present on a pial surface.[114] However, they recommend conservative management for deep lesions separated from the pial surface by normal brain. It is crucial to avoid major blood loss in young children, thus excluding certain skull base approaches.[114]

The outcome for seizure control after resection of CMs in children is favorable.[75,116] Giulioni and associates[75] reported 100% seizure control with or without medication in 11 children with CM who were experiencing seizures despite adequate medical therapy. Radiosurgery is not recommended as a treatment modality for CM in the pediatric population, because no data currently exist to support its efficacy.[114,116]

VENOUS MALFORMATIONS

Overview

Developmental venous anomalies (DVAs), also known as venous malformations or angiomas, are congenital vascular malformations of the brain thought to arise from anomalous development of normal venous drainage.[117–123] Although often discovered incidentally on neuroimaging studies, DVAs are the most common intracranial vascular lesions, accounting for up to 63% of such lesions and with a reported overall prevalence of 2.6% in autopsy series.[3] Angiographic studies demonstrate a characteristic caput medusae appearance in the late venous phase with a normal circulation time and absence of venous filling during the arterial phase.[124] On MRI, a DVA may appear as a stellate vascular or contrast-enhanced mass (Fig. 69–10).[125,126] The specific etiology in the generation of these lesions is not completely understood. It has been suggested that venous anomalies represent the anatomically abnormal but physiologically normal venous outflow pathway for a portion of the brain after an intrauterine ischemic event.[127–129]

Natural History

DVAs have often been associated with nonspecific, vague neurologic symptoms, such as headaches, dizziness, and incoordination, as well as more specific signs, such as seizures and hemorrhage.[126] However, this association has not translated into a definitive causality. Headaches are the primary symptom in a majority of patients presenting with DVAs,[123] but the headaches are usually not attributable to the lesion.[130] Similarly, in most patients, there is no clear correlation between seizures and an epileptiform focus corresponding to the region of a DVA.[129–131] DVAs may occur in association with other intracranial vascular malformations,[5,127,132–136] which in turn may be the cause of various neurologic signs and symptoms or hemorrhage, raising the question whether DVAs themselves are a cause of hemorrhage.

The risk of hemorrhage from a DVA is unclear but appears to be low. Garner and associates[131] calculated a retrospective hemorrhage rate of 0.22% in 100 patients. McLaughlin and colleagues,[126] examining the hemorrhage rate of DVAs in 80 patients over a 10-year period, found a retrospective rate of 0.61% per year before clinical presentation and a prospective rate of 0.68% per year after a documented hemorrhage. The actual symptomatic hemorrhage rate was 0.34% per year, and these investigators suggested that hemorrhage associated with a DVA might in fact be from an as yet unrecognized underlying CM.[126] There were no cases of severe neurological morbidity or mortality in either of these studies.

Management

The vast majority of patients with DVAs are asymptomatic or experience nonspecific symptoms such as headaches. Therefore, when patients with DVAs present with seizures, hemorrhage, or neurologic deficits, a careful evaluation for other associated lesions should be performed. The evaluation should include high-field MRI with contrast administration.[123,135] Seizures in patients with DVAs are usually well controlled with anticonvulsant medication alone. The common association of these lesions with other vascular lesions makes it difficult to determine the source of a hemorrhage when one does occur in the vicinity of the DVA. Frequently, the hemorrhage is secondary to a related CM

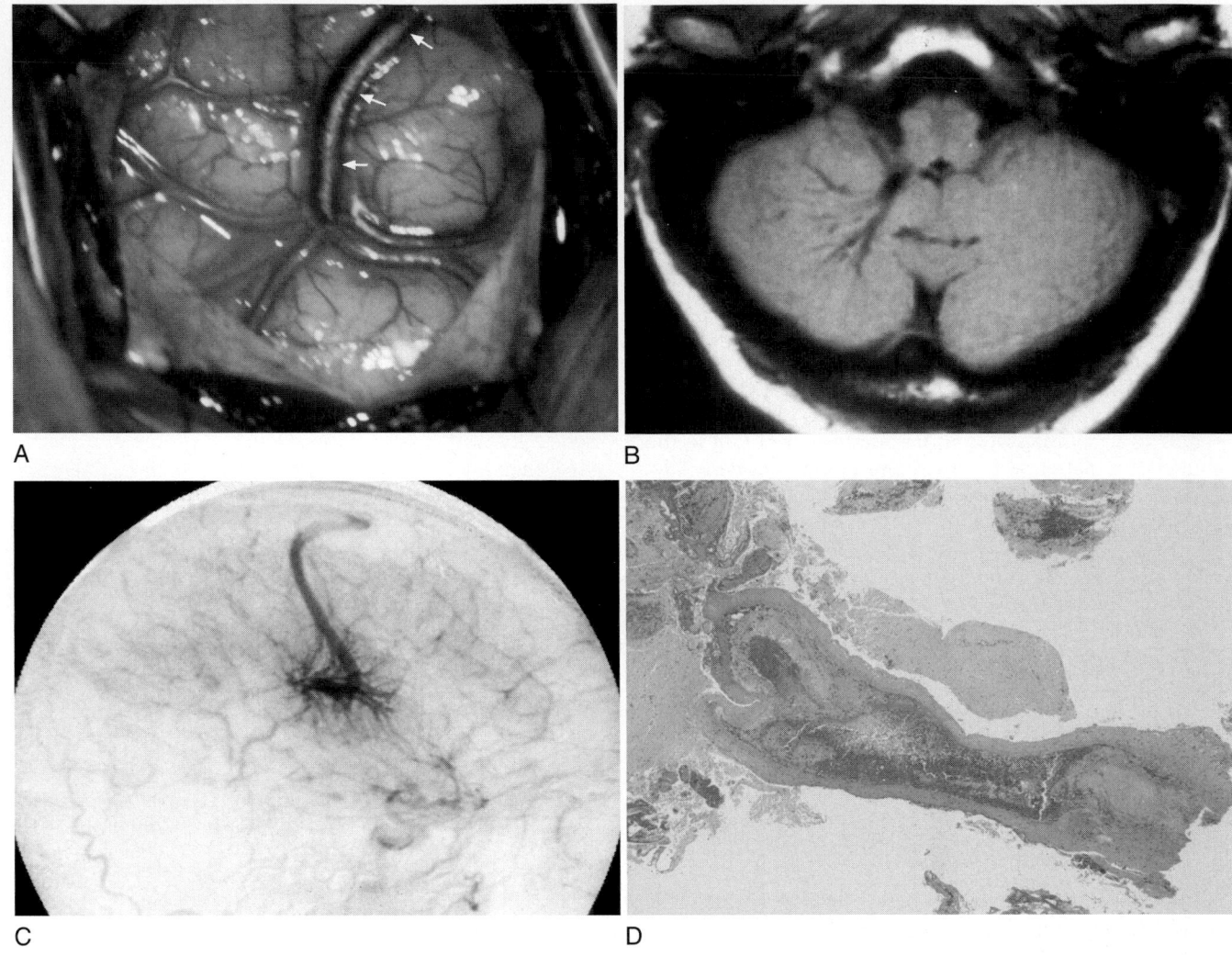

FIGURE 69–10   A, *Intraoperative photograph during resection of a cavernous malformation depicting an adjacent developmental venous anomaly (DVA) on the cortical surface* (arrows). B, *T1-weighted MRI from a different patient shows typical appearance of DVA with caput medusae.* C, *Venous phase angiogram in a different patient showing a DVA.* D, *Pathologic specimen of a DVA demonstrating a large venous channel.*

or other vascular lesion; therefore, in evacuation of the hemorrhage or resection of the associated lesion extreme, caution must be exercised so as not to interfere with the normal or aberrant venous drainage of a DVA.[85] Indeed, fatal and severe neurologic consequences have been reported from venous infarction after surgical obliteration of a DVA.[68,121] Most surgeons recommend a conservative approach to management, with preservation of the DVA at all costs.[85,117,119,131]

SRS has been advocated as an alternative treatment modality for these lesions, under the supposition that a gradual occlusion of venous channels would induce recruitment of collateral drainage and prevent the occurrence of venous infarction.[137] However, incomplete venous obliteration and a high incidence of neurologic morbidity have been observed after SRS of DVAs.[137]

Thus, although DVAs may be associated with mild neurologic symptoms, they are rarely the cause of overt symptomatic hemorrhage or severe neurologic dysfunction. These lesions therefore are rarely symptomatic and never warrant surgical excision. When surgical evacuation of hemorrhage due to an associated vascular lesion is performed, the DVA must be preserved at all costs.

References

1. Giombini S, Morello G: Cavernous angiomas of the brain: Account of fourteen personal cases and review of the literature. Acta Neurochir 40:61–82, 1978.
2. McCormick WF, Hardman JM, Boulter TR: Vascular malformations ("angiomas") of the brain, with special reference to those occurring in the posterior fossa. J Neurosurg 28:241–251, 1968.
3. Sarwar M, McCormick WF: Intracerebral venous angioma: Case report and review. Arch Neurol 35:323–325, 1978.
4. Brunereau L, et al: De novo lesions in familial form of cerebral cavernous malformations: Clinical and MR features in 29 non-Hispanic families. Surg Neurol 53:475–482, discussion 482–483, 2000.
5. Porter RW, et al: Cavernous malformations of the brainstem: Experience with 100 patients. J Neurosurg 90:50–58, 1999.
6. Zabramski JM, et al: The natural history of familial cavernous malformations: Results of an ongoing study. J Neurosurg 80:422–432, 1994.

7. Detwiler PW, et al: De novo formation of a central nervous system cavernous malformation: Implications for predicting risk of hemorrhage. Case report and review of the literature. J Neurosurg 87:629–632, 1997.

8. Detwiler PW, et al: Radiation-induced cavernous malformation. J Neurosurg 89:167–169, 1998.

9. Pozzati E, et al: Occult cerebrovascular malformations after irradiation. Neurosurgery 39:677–682, discussion 682–684, 1996.

10. Larson JJ, et al: Formation of intracerebral cavernous malformations after radiation treatment for central nervous system neoplasia in children. J Neurosurg 88:51–56, 1998.

11. Maraire JN, et al: De novo development of a cavernous malformation of the spinal cord following spinal axis radiation: Case report. J Neurosurg 90(Suppl):234–238, 1999.

12. McCormick WF, Boulter TR: Vascular malformations ("angiomas") of the dura mater. J Neurosurg 25:309–311, 1966.

13. Otten P, et al: [131 cases of cavernous angioma (cavernomas) of the CNS, discovered by retrospective analysis of 24,535 autopsies] [French]. Neurochirurgie 35:82–83, 1989.

14. Del Curling O Jr, et al: An analysis of the natural history of cavernous angiomas. J Neurosurg 75:702–708, 1991.

15. Sage MR, et al: Cavernous haemangiomas (angiomas) of the brain: Clinically significant lesions. Australas Radiol 37:147–155, 1993.

16. Kondziolka D, Lunsford LD, Kestle JR: The natural history of cerebral cavernous malformations. J Neurosurg 83:820–824, 1995.

17. Robinson JR, Awad IA, Little JR: Natural history of the cavernous angioma. J Neurosurg 75:709–714, 1991.

18. Hsu F, Rigamonti D, Huhn SL: Epidemiology of cavernous malformations. In Awad IA, Barrow DL (eds): Cavernous Malformations. Park Ridge, IL, AANS Publications Committee, 1993, pp 13–23.

19. Aiba T, et al: Natural history of intracranial cavernous malformations. J Neurosurg 83:56–59, 1995.

20. Moriarity JL, et al: The natural history of cavernous malformations: A prospective study of 68 patients. Neurosurgery 44:1166–1171, discussion 1172–1173, 1999.

21. Maraire JN, Awad IA: Intracranial cavernous malformations: Lesion behavior and management strategies. Neurosurgery 37:591–605, 1995.

22. Rigamonti D, et al: Cerebral cavernous malformations: Incidence and familial occurrence. N Engl J Med 319:343–347, 1988.

23. Brunereau L, et al: Familial form of intracranial cavernous angioma: MR imaging findings in 51 families. French Society of Neurosurgery. Radiology 214:209–216, 2000.

24. Labauge P, et al: Hereditary cerebral cavernous angiomas: Clinical and genetic features in 57 French families. Societé Francaise de Neurochirurgie. Lancet 352:1892–1897, 1998.

25. Steichen-Gersdorf E, et al: Familial cavernous angiomas of the brain: Observations in a four generation family. Eur J Pediatr 151:861–863, 1992.

26. Hayman LA, et al: Familial cavernous angiomas: Natural history and genetic study over a 5-year period. Am J Med Genet 11:147–160, 1982.

27. Duong H, et al: Multiple intracerebral cavernous angiomas. Can Assoc Radiol J 42:329–334, 1991.

28. Bicknell JM, et al: Familial cavernous angiomas. Arch Neurol 35:746–749, 1978.

29. Dobyns WB, et al: Familial cavernous malformations of the central nervous system and retina. Ann Neurol 21:578–583, 1987.

30. Kim DS, et al: An analysis of the natural history of cavernous malformations. Surg Neurol 48:9–17, discussion 17–18, 1997.

31. Porter P, et al: Cerebral cavernous malformations: Natural history and prognosis after clinical deterioration with or without hemorrhage. J Neurosurg 87:190–197, 1997.

32. Gunel M, et al: A founder mutation as a cause of cerebral cavernous malformation in Hispanic Americans. N Engl J Med 334:946–951, 1996.

33. Gunel M, et al: Mapping a gene causing cerebral cavernous malformation to 7q11.2-q21. Proc Natl Acad Sci U S A 92:6620–6624, 1995.

34. Polymeropoulos MH, et al: Linkage of the locus for cerebral cavernous hemangiomas to human chromosome 7q in four families of Mexican-American descent. Neurology 48:752–757, 1997.

35. Craig HD, et al: Multilocus linkage identifies two new loci for a mendelian form of stroke, cerebral cavernous malformation, at 7p15–13 and 3q25.2–27. Hum Mol Genet 7:1851–1858, 1998.

36. Labauge P, et al: The natural history of familial cerebral cavernomas: A retrospective MRI study of 40 patients. Neuroradiology 42:327–332, 2000.

37. Chen DH, et al: Cerebral cavernous malformation: Novel mutation in a Chinese family and evidence for heterogeneity. J Neurol Sci 196:91–96, 2002.

38. Kidd HA, Cumings JN: Cerebral angiomata in an Icelandic family. Lancet 1:747–748, 1947.

39. Davenport WJ, et al: CCM1 gene mutations in families segregating cerebral cavernous malformations. Neurology 56:540–543, 2001.

40. Dubovsky J, et al: A gene responsible for cavernous malformations of the brain maps to chromosome 7q. Hum Mol Genet 4:453–458, 1995.

41. Gunel M, et al: Genetic heterogeneity of inherited cerebral cavernous malformation. Neurosurgery 38:1265–1271, 1996.

42. Laberge-le Couteulx S, et al: Truncating mutations in CCM1, encoding KRIT1, cause hereditary cavernous angiomas. Nat Genet 23:189–193, 1999.

43. Zhang J, et al: Mutations in KRIT1 in familial cerebral cavernous malformations. Neurosurgery 46:1272–1277, discussion 1277–1279, 2000.

44. Zhang J, et al: Interaction between krit1 and icap1alpha infers perturbation of integrin beta1-mediated angiogenesis in the pathogenesis of cerebral cavernous malformation. Hum Mol Genet 10:2953–2960, 2001.

45. Uranishi R, et al: Further study of CD31 protein and messenger ribonucleic acid expression in human cerebral vascular malformations. Neurosurgery 50:110–115, discussion 115–116, 2002.

46. Uranishi R, et al: Vascular smooth muscle cell differentiation in human cerebral vascular malformations. Neurosurgery 49:671–679, discussion 679–680, 2001.

47. Siegel AM: Familial cavernous angioma: An unknown, known disease. Acta Neurol Scand 98:369–371, 1998.

48. Siegel AM, et al: Anticipation in familial cavernous angioma: A study of 52 families from International Familial Cavernous Angioma Study. IFCAS Group. Lancet 352(9141):1676–1677, 1998.

49. Siegel AM, et al: Anticipation in familial cavernous angioma: Ascertainment bias or genetic cause. Acta Neurol Scand 98:372–376, 1998.

50. Yoshimoto Y, et al: Early fatal rebleeding from a cerebellar cavernous malformation—case report. Neurol Med Chir (Tokyo) 37:343–345, 1997.

51. Bertalanffy H, et al: Microsurgery of deep-seated cavernous angiomas: Report of 26 cases. Acta Neurochir 108:91–99, 1991.

52. Moriarity JL, Clatterbuck RE, Rigamonti D: The natural history of cavernous malformations. Neurosurg Clin North Am 10:411–417, 1999.

53. Moran NF, et al: Supratentorial cavernous haemangiomas and epilepsy: A review of the literature and case series. J Neurol Neurosurg Psychiatry 66:561–568, 1999.

54. Simard JM, et al: Cavernous angioma: A review of 126 collected and 12 new clinical cases. Neurosurgery 18:162–172, 1986.

55. Awad IA, Robinson JR Jr: Cavernous malformations and epilepsy. In Awad IA, Barrow DL (eds): Cavernous Malformations. Park Ridge, IL, AANS Publications Committee, 1993, pp 49–63.

56. Casazza M, et al: Supratentorial cavernous angiomas and epileptic seizures: Preoperative course and postoperative outcome. Neurosurgery 39:26–32, discussion 32–34, 1996.

57. Kraemer DL, Awad IA: Vascular malformations and epilepsy: Clinical considerations and basic mechanisms. Epilepsia 35(Suppl 6):S30–S43, 1994.

58. Rigamonti D, et al: The MRI appearance of cavernous malformations (angiomas). J Neurosurg 67:518–524, 1987.

59. Robinson JR Jr, et al: Factors predisposing to clinical disability in patients with cavernous malformations of the brain. Neurosurgery 32:730–735, discussion 735–736, 1993.

60. Scott RM: Brain stem cavernous angiomas in children. Pediatr Neurosurg 16:281–286, 1990.

61. Scott RM, et al: Cavernous angiomas of the central nervous system in children. J Neurosurg 76:38–46, 1992.

62. Requena I, et al: Cavernomas of the central nervous system: Clinical and neuroimaging manifestations in 47 patients. J Neurol Neurosurg Psychiatry 54:590–594, 1991.

63. Pozzati E, et al: Growth, subsequent bleeding, and de novo appearance of cerebral cavernous angiomas. Neurosurgery 38:662–669, discussion 669–670, 1996.

64. Labauge P, et al: Prospective follow-up of 33 asymptomatic patients with familial cerebral cavernous malformations. Neurology 57:1825–1828, 2001.

65. Barker FG 2nd, et al: Temporal clustering of hemorrhages from untreated cavernous malformations of the central nervous system. Neurosurgery 49:15–24, discussion 24–25, 2001.

66. Kupersmith MJ, et al: Natural history of brainstem cavernous malformations. Neurosurgery 48:47–53, discussion 53–54, 2001.

67. Clatterbuck RE, Elmaci I, Rigamonti D: The nature and fate of punctate (type IV) cavernous malformations. Neurosurgery 49:26–30, discussion 30–32, 2001.

68. Lobato RD, et al: Clinical, radiological, and pathological spectrum of angiographically occult intracranial vascular malformations: Analysis of 21 cases and review of the literature. J Neurosurg 68:518–531, 1988.

69. Steinberg GK, Marks MP: Lesions mimicking cavernous malformations. In Awad IA, Barrow DL (eds): Cavernous Malformations. Park Ridge, IL, AANS Publications Committee, 1993, pp 151–162.

70. Chang HS, et al: Surgical decision-making on cerebral cavernous malformations. J Clin Neurosci 8:416–420, 2001.

71. Cappabianca P, et al: Supratentorial cavernous malformations and epilepsy: Seizure outcome after lesionectomy on a series of 35 patients. Clin Neurol Neurosurg 99:179–183, 1997.

72. Cohen DS, Zubay GP, Goodman RR: Seizure outcome after lesionectomy for cavernous malformations. J Neurosurg 83:237–242, 1995.

73. Zevgaridis D, et al: Seizure control following surgery in supratentorial cavernous malformations: A retrospective study in 77 patients. Acta Neurochir 138:672–677, 1996.

74. Wiebe S, et al: A randomized, controlled trial of surgery for temporal-lobe epilepsy. N Engl J Med 345:311–318, 2001.

75. Giulioni M, et al: Results of surgery in children with cerebral cavernous angiomas causing epilepsy. Br J Neurosurg 9:135–141, 1995.

76. Acciarri N, et al: Intracranial and orbital cavernous angiomas: A review of 74 surgical cases. Br J Neurosurg 7:529–539, 1993.

77. Amin-Hanjani S, Ogilvy CS: Overall surgical results of occult vascular malformations. Neurosurg Clin North Am 10:475–483, 1999.

78. Chaskis C, Brotchi J: The surgical management of cerebral cavernous angiomas. Neurol Res 20:597–606, 1998.

79. Ojemann RG, Crowell RM, Ogilvy CS: Management of cranial and spinal cavernous angiomas (honored guest lecture). Clin Neurosurg 40:98–123, 1993.

80. Amin-Hanjani S, et al: Risks of surgical management for cavernous malformations of the nervous system. Neurosurgery 42:1220–1227, discussion 1227–1228, 1998.

81. Folkersma H, Mooij JJ: Follow-up of 13 patients with surgical treatment of cerebral cavernous malformations: Effect on epilepsy and patient disability. Clin Neurol Neurosurg 103:67–71, 2001.

82. Fritschi JA, et al: Cavernous malformations of the brain stem: A review of 139 cases. Acta Neurochir 130:35–46, 1994.

83. Pozzati E: Thalamic cavernous malformations. Surg Neurol 53:30–39, discussion 39–40, 2000.

84. Samii M, et al: Surgical management of brainstem cavernomas. J Neurosurg 95:825–832, 2001.

85. Steinberg GK, et al: Microsurgical resection of brainstem, thalamic, and basal ganglia angiographically occult vascular malformations. Neurosurgery 46:260–270, discussion 270–271, 2000.

86. Symon L, Jackowski A, Bills D: Surgical treatment of pontomedullary cavernomas. Br J Neurosurg 5:339–347, 1991.

87. Ziyal IM, et al: Surgical management of cavernous malformations of the brain stem. Br J Neurosurg 13:366–375, 1999.

88. Steinberg GK, Vanefsky MA: Management of the patient with an occult vascular malformation. In Hadley MM (ed): Perspectives in Neurological Surgery. St. Louis, Quality Medical, 1994, pp 18–39.

89. Morcos JJ, Heros RC, Frank DE: Microsurgical treatment of infratentorial malformations. Neurosurg Clin North Am 10:441–474, 1999.

90. Ojemann RG, Crowell RM, Ogilvy CS: Cranial and spinal cavernous malformations. In Ojemann RG, Ogilvy CS, Crowell RM (eds): Surgical Management of Neurovascular Disease. Baltimore, Williams & Wilkins, 1995, pp 538–557.

91. Ojemann RG, Ogilvy CS: Microsurgical treatment of supratentorial cavernous malformations. Neurosurg Clin North Am 10:433–440, 1999.

92. Shah MV, Heros RC: Microsurgical treatment of supratentorial lesions. In Awad IA, Barrow DL (eds): Cavernous Malformations.

Park Ridge, IL, AANS Publications Committee, 1993, pp 101–116.

93. Wascher TM, Spetzler RF: Microsurgical treatment of infratentorial lesions. In Awad IA, Barrow DL (eds): Cavernous Malformations. Park Ridge, IL, AANS Publications Committee, 1993, pp 117–132.

94. Reisch R, Bettag M, Perneczky A: Transoral transclival removal of anteriorly placed cavernous malformations of the brainstem. Surg Neurol 56:106–115, discussion 115–116, 2001.

95. Koyama T, et al: Surgery of a cavernous angioma making a tunnel between the fourth ventricle and tubercle. Neurosurg Rev 24:38–40, 2001.

96. Katayama Y, et al: Surgical management of cavernous malformations of the third ventricle. J Neurosurg 80:64–72, 1994.

97. Steinberg GK, Chang SD: Surgical management of angiographically occult vascular malformations of the brainstem, thalamus, and basal ganglia. In SS R (ed): Neurosurgical Operative Color Atlas. Park Ridge, IL, American Association of Neurological Surgeons, 1999, pp 127–133.

98. Chang SD, Lopez JR, Steinberg GK: Intraoperative electrical stimulation for identification of cranial nerve nuclei. Muscle Nerve 22:1538–1543, 1999.

99. Chang SD, Lopez JR, Steinberg GK: The usefulness of electrophysiological monitoring during resection of central nervous system vascular malformations. J Stroke Cerebrovasc Dis 8:412–422, 1999.

100. Marion DW, et al: Treatment of traumatic brain injury with moderate hypothermia. N Engl J Med 336:540–546, 1997.

101. Steinberg GK, Grant G, Yoon EJ: Deliberate hypothermia. In Andrews RJ (ed): Intraoperative Neuroprotection. Baltimore, Williams & Wilkins: 1996, pp 65–84.

102. Mild therapeutic hypothermia to improve the neurologic outcome after cardiac arrest. The Hypothermia After Cardiac Arrest Study Group. N Engl J Med 346:549–556, 2002.

103. Bernard SA, et al: Treatment of comatose survivors of out-of-hospital cardiac arrest with induced hypothermia. N Engl J Med 346:557–563, 2002.

104. Karlsson B, et al: Radiosurgery for cavernous malformations. J Neurosurg 88:293–297, 1998.

105. Chang SD, et al: Stereotactic radiosurgery of angiographically occult vascular malformations: 14-year experience. Neurosurgery 43:213–220, discussion 220–221, 1998.

106. Gewirtz RJ, et al: Pathological changes in surgically resected angiographically occult vascular malformations after radiation. Neurosurgery 42:738–742, discussion 742–743, 1998.

107. Pollock BE, et al: Stereotactic radiosurgery for cavernous malformations. J Neurosurg 93:987–991, 2000.

108. Mitchell P, et al: Stereotactic radiosurgery and the risk of haemorrhage from cavernous malformations. Br J Neurosurg 14:96–100, 2000.

109. Amin-Hanjani S, et al: Stereotactic radiosurgery for cavernous malformations: Kjellberg's experience with proton beam therapy in 98 cases at the Harvard Cyclotron. Neurosurgery 42:1229–1236, discussion 1236–1238, 1998.

110. Tsien C, et al: Stereotactic radiosurgery in the management of angiographically occult vascular malformations. Int J Radiat Oncol Biol Phys 50:133–138, 2001.

111. Kondziolka D, et al: Reduction of hemorrhage risk after stereotactic radiosurgery for cavernous malformations. J Neurosurg 83:825–831, 1995.

112. Maesawa S, Kondziolka D, Lunsford LD: Stereotactic radiosurgery for management of deep brain cavernous malformations. Neurosurg Clin North Am 10:503–511, 1999.

113. Hasegawa T, et al: Long-term results after stereotactic radiosurgery for patients with cavernous malformations. Neurosurgery 50:1190–1198, 2002.

114. Mottolese C, et al: Central nervous system cavernomas in the pediatric age group. Neurosurg Rev 24:55–71, discussion 72–73, 2001.

115. Edwards MSB, Baumgartner JE, Wilson CB: Cavernous and other cryptic vascular malformations in the pediatric age group. In Awad IA, Barrow DL (eds): Cavernous Malformations. Park Ridge, IL, AANS Publications Committee, 1993, pp 163–183.

116. Frim DM, Scott RM: Management of cavernous malformations in the pediatric population. Neurosurg Clin North Am 10:513–518, 1999.

117. Goulao A, et al: Venous anomalies and abnormalities of the posterior fossa. Neuroradiology 31:476–482, 1990.
118. Kondziolka D, Dempsey PK, Lunsford LD: The case for conservative management of venous angiomas. Can J Neurol Sci 18:295–299, 1991.
119. Lasjaunias P, Burrows P, Planet C: Developmental venous anomalies (DVA): The so-called venous angioma. Neurosurg Rev 9:233–242, 1986.
120. Numaguchi Y, et al: Intracranial venous angiomas. Surg Neurol 18:193–202, 1982.
121. Senegor M, Dohrmann GJ, Wollmann RL: Venous angiomas of the posterior fossa should be considered as anomalous venous drainage. Surg Neurol 19:26–32, 1983.
122. Valavanis A, Wellauer J, Yasargil MG: The radiological diagnosis of cerebral venous angioma: Cerebral angiography and computed tomography. Neuroradiology 24:193–199, 1983.
123. Rigamonti D, et al: Cerebral venous malformations. J Neurosurg 73:560–564, 1990.
124. Fierstien SB, Pribram HW, Hieshima G: Angiography and computed tomography in the evaluation of cerebral venous malformations. Neuroradiology 17:137–148, 1979.
125. Rigamonti D, et al: Appearance of venous malformations on magnetic resonance imaging. J Neurosurg 69:535–539, 1988.
126. McLaughlin MR, et al: The prospective natural history of cerebral venous malformations. Neurosurgery 43:195–200, discussion 200–201, 1998.
127. Mullan S, et al: Cerebral venous malformation-arteriovenous malformation transition forms. J Neurosurg 85:9–13, 1996.
128. Mullan S, et al: Embryological basis of some aspects of cerebral vascular fistulas and malformations. J Neurosurg 85:1–8, 1996.
129. Saito Y, Kobayashi N: Cerebral venous angiomas: Clinical evaluation and possible etiology. Radiology 139:87–94, 1981.
130. Topper R, et al: Clinical significance of intracranial developmental venous anomalies. J Neurol Neurosurg Psychiatry 67:234–238, 1999.
131. Garner TB, et al: The natural history of intracranial venous angiomas. J Neurosurg 75:715–722, 1991.
132. Awad I., et al: Mixed vascular malformations of the brain: Clinical and pathogenetic considerations. Neurosurgery 33:179–188, discussion 188, 1993.
133. Robinson JR Jr, et al: Pathological heterogeneity of angiographically occult vascular malformations of the brain. Neurosurgery 33:547–554, discussion 554–555, 1993.
134. Rigamonti D, Spetzler RF: The association of venous and cavernous malformations: Report of four cases and discussion of the pathophysiological, diagnostic, and therapeutic implications. Acta Neurochir 92:100–105, 1988.
135. Abe T, et al: Coexistence of occult vascular malformations and developmental venous anomalies in the central nervous system: MR evaluation. AJNR Am J Neuroradiol 19:51–57, 1998.
136. Pryor J, Setton A, Berenstein A: Venous anomalies and associated lesions. Neurosurg Clin North Am 10:519–525, 1999.
137. Lindquist C, et al: Radiosurgery for venous angiomas. J Neurosurg 78:531–536, 1993.

Chapter Seventy

Dural Arteriovenous Malformations

J. Paul Elliott, Daniel Huddle, and Issam A. Awad

Arteriovenous malformations (AVMs) affecting the central nervous system include a number of pathologic entities, all characterized by abnormal arteriovenous shunting. The cerebral AVMs (CAVMs) consist of a nidus of arteriovenous shunting within brain parenchyma, supplied by the intracranial anterior and posterior circulation and lacking a normal capillary bed. Pial fistulas are characterized by a direct, high-flow shunt from a pial artery to an enlarged vein or varix. The dural AVMs (DAVMs) are composed of arteriovenous shunts within the dural leaflet, typically supplied predominantly by pachymeningeal arteries and located near a major venous sinus.[1]

Historically, the DAVMs have been a confusing entity, in part because of their multiple names and the difficulty of separating their primary abnormality, dural arteriovenous shunting, from other secondary changes. They are distinct from but are often confused with CAVMs. Some investigators believe that DAVMs should be more appropriately named dural arteriovenous shunts, dural arteriovenous fistulas, or dural arteriovenous fistulous malformations.[2]

DAVMs are distinguished from other intracranial vascular lesions by their nidus, which is composed of arteriovenous shunting localized in the leaflets of the dura mater (Fig. 70–1). They are typically localized adjacent to a major dural sinus, and their arterial supply originates from both intradural arteries and pachymeningeal branches of cerebral arteries. Venous drainage occurs through an adjacent dural sinus, other dural and leptomeningeal venous channels, or both. Although their etiology is controversial, DAVMs appear to be acquired lesions.[3] They may remain asymptomatic or may manifest as a wide range of symptoms, including headache, tinnitus, bruit, cranial neuropathy, seizures, dementia, intracranial hypertension, and focal neurologic deficits from venous congestion.[4–8] DAVMs may also cause life-threatening intracranial hemorrhage.[9] Although it remains difficult to prognosticate for a given lesion, the location (anterior cranial fossa or tentorial incisura) and pattern of venous drainage (retrograde leptomeningeal venous drainage) clearly influence clinical presentation.[10–12] Lesions that manifest as hemorrhage are clearly associated with a significantly higher risk for additional morbidity and mortality. Although many unruptured DAVMs are best treated expectantly, some features identify high-risk lesions, which may be definitively treated with an evolving combination of endovascular, radiosurgical, and surgical techniques.

CLINICAL PRESENTATION

DAVMs account for 10% to 15% of cranial vascular malformations. There is a 2:1 female preponderance, with typical presentation at 30 to 50 years of age. Typical locations are in proximity to the major sinuses (50% transverse-sigmoid, 15% cavernous, 10% tentorial, 8% superior sagittal). A few DAVMs manifest early in life and are thus thought to be congenital. They are usually associated with complex congenital anomalies, rare phakomatoses, or a vein of Galen malformation—a special form of DAVM.[1] In these cases, there is often gross malformation of dural sinuses with atresia of venous outflow from a region of dura mater involved in the DAVM. The vast majority of DAVMs manifest later in life and are assumed to be acquired.[13,14] Known or suspected etiologic factors include trauma, infection, vascular disease, and tumor. The most important aspect of these etiologic factors may be a shared propensity for sinus thrombosis with a secondary alteration in venous hemodynamics (restricted outflow and venous hypertension) and development of shunting from preexisting physiologic shunts.

Clinical manifestations of DAVMs are highly variable and are related primarily to the location of the fistula, and both the arterial supply and venous drainage. The manifestations range from minor symptoms to catastrophic intracranial hemorrhage. The vast majority of symptoms can be attributed to the primary or secondary venous manifestations of the DAVM. More benign symptoms such as pain, tinnitus, and bruit are related to arteriovenous shunting and flow in the DAVM. Manifestation of a DAVM may be sudden or slowly progressive. The severity and type of symptoms are determined by venous topography, venous flow pattern, and the capacity of surrounding compensatory venous drainage. The most serious neurologic sequelae of DAVMs are associated with retrograde leptomeningeal venous drainage.[15] Focal neurologic deficits

DURAL AVM

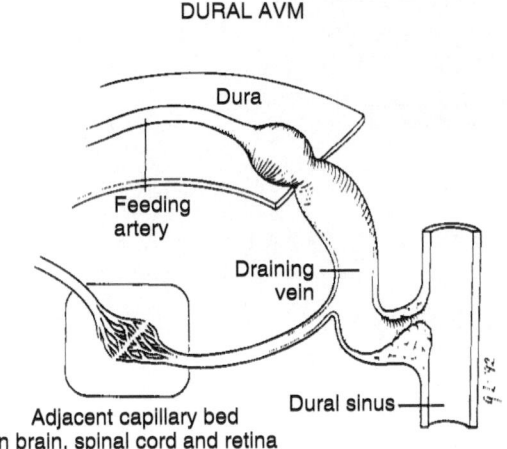

FIGURE 70–1 *Schematic of a dural arteriovenous malformation (AVM). A dural AVM is composed of arteriovenous shunts within the dural leaflet, typically supplied predominantly by pachymeningeal arteries and located near a major venous sinus. Retrograde leptomeningeal venous drainage is associated with a high risk of hemorrhage. (Reprinted with permission of AANS publications.)*

likely result from venous hypertension and intracranial hemorrhage from rupture of arterialized leptomeningeal veins.

There are a wide variety of nonhemorrhagic symptoms.[12,16] Pulsatile tinnitus and other subjective auditory symptoms may occur with or without pain. These symptoms are probably related to high flow through dural vascular channels at the base of the skull. Other painful complaints may be related to orbital congestion or stretching of dural leaflets by engorged vascular channels, or to direct compression of the trigeminal nerve by arterialized venous structures near the petrous apex. Neuro-ophthalmic manifestations of DAVMs include visual and gaze abnormalities caused by venous hypertension as well as orbital or ocular venous hypertension with resulting orbital crowding, venous stasis retinopathy, and glaucoma. Other cranial DAVMs may manifest as symptoms of increased intracranial pressure (ICP) or a poorly defined headache.[7,17] Although the headaches are nonspecific, they do appear to be associated with the dysplastic changes in meningeal vessels, which are often present in DAVMs. There are also a wide spectrum of presenting focal neurologic symptoms, including seizure, hearing loss, cranial nerve palsy, papilledema and other visual symptoms and focal motor-sensory deficits.[18–20]

DAVMs may also alter the hydrodynamics of cerebrospinal fluid (CSF).[6] Dilated venous structures may act as mass lesions, obstructing the CSF circulation and causing hydrocephalus. In other cases, dural venous hypertension may result in decreased absorption of CSF with secondary intracranial hypertension and papilledema. This latter complication appears to be more common in association with high-flow lesions draining into large dural venous sinuses and in the setting of concomitant dural sinus outflow obstruction.

Particular clinical presentations are associated with DAVMs in specific locations.[2,15,16] DAVMs in the region of the transverse or sigmoid sinus, or near the cavernous sinus, often drain into the associated venous sinuses and may cause a variety of clinical manifestations resulting from flow or local venous engorgement. High flow in the region of the transverse-sigmoid sinus junction, for example, often gives rise to pulsatile tinnitus, headache, and bruit. These lesions do not bleed or cause other deficits unless there is associated retrograde leptomeningeal venous drainage. Lesions at the anterior cranial fossa or the tentorial incisura rarely drain into a patent dural venous sinus and are more frequently associated with leptomeningeal venous drainage. They are more likely to cause serious clinical sequelae from venous hypertension and hemorrhage. Hemorrhage has not been reported in the absence of this feature; in all published cases with carefully documented diagnostic findings, hemorrhage from DAVMs is associated with rupture of arterialized venous structures. The prognosis of a first hemorrhage from a DAVM is ominous and is associated with a greater than 30% rate of death or serious disability. Hemorrhage from DAVMs in patients who have undergone anticoagulation has been uniformly fatal.

PATHOPHYSIOLOGY AND LESION EVOLUTION

DAVM is usually acquired.[13,14] It is hypothesized to result from altered angiogenesis within the dura after an inciting event such as trauma, surgery, or chronic infection. Altered angiogenesis is often accompanied by sinus thrombosis. In some cases of documented, angiographically proven dural sinus thrombosis, DAVMs subsequently developed in relationship to the obstructed sinus. Initial microshunts are hypothesized to proliferate in association with the venous hypertension, maturing into clinically significant arteriovenous fistulas. The extent of progression or involution determines the significance of the abnormality. The fistulas may result in hemorrhage or have other focal manifestations, including hemodynamic insufficiency. DAVMs cause decreased regional cerebral blood flow in cortical regions where there is retrograde venous drainage.[21]

The development of DAVMs after trauma and surgery is well known.[22,23] These lesions have also been reported in association with chronic infection, vascular disease, and tumors.[24] Other cases of DAVM have no clear association. They may be identified at anatomic sites distinct from the presumed inciting event. The exact mechanism of development remains unclear. It is hypothesized that development of a DAVM in these diverse settings would probably require a common mechanism as well as a possible anatomic or genetic predisposition.[25,26] Experimental work suggests that the diverse clinical associations of DAVM may be explained by the development of venous obstruction and hypertension with aberrant angiogenesis.[27]

An established DAVM may follow one of several natural courses. Some lesions remain asymptomatic or maintain stable clinical symptoms and angiographic features over many years. Others undergo spontaneous regression, involution, and resolution with stabilization or improvement of neurologic symptoms.[11,28–30] Features that may predispose to such spontaneous involution are not known. DAVMs in the region of the cavernous sinus are particularly prone to this phenomenon, with as many as 40% of reported cases having undergone spontaneous involution. In contrast, some DAVMs may demonstrate increase in size from either arterial or venous enlargement.[1,2,15] Pachymeningeal arterial feeders may be progressively recruited with enlargement of the nidus. The mechanisms behind this progressive recruitment of arterial feeders from numerous sources have not been elucidated. This phenomenon results in hypertrophy of dural arteries and the reappearance of involuted embryonic arteries that may not normally be visible in the adult dura mater.

In some DAVMs, there is also progression of disease on the venous side. Progressive arterialization of the pathologic dural leaflets results in hypertension in adjacent leptomeningeal venous channels; this process may lead to retrograde leptomeningeal venous drainage. Under arterialized pressures, these channels may become tortuous and, eventually, varicose or aneurysmal. Hemorrhage is the unfortunate result. In DAVMs that manifest as intracranial hemorrhage and have retrograde cortical venous drainage, there is a 35% risk of rebleeding within the first 2 weeks.[31]

DIAGNOSIS, CLASSIFICATION, AND INDICATIONS FOR TREATMENT

Diagnosis

Catheter cerebral angiography is the most sensitive and specific diagnostic study for defining DAVMs.[32] In patients with suspected DAVM, the study should include injection of both internal carotid arteries, both vertebral arteries, and both external carotid arteries. In cases of suspected clival or foramen magnum region DAVMs, arch injections may reveal additional ascending muscular or pharyngeal arterial feeders. Imaging should capture the very early arterial phase and continue late into the venous phase. Digital subtraction and magnification techniques and the occasional use of superselective angiography greatly enhance the diagnostic potential of angiography. Cerebral angiography provides the spatial diagnostic detail and dynamic flow information to identify arterial feeders and define the pattern of flow and venous drainage of the DAVM in detail. This information is essential for prognostication and therapeutic decisions.

Other diagnostic tests may reveal indirect evidence of a DAVM. Computed tomography (CT) or magnetic resonance imaging (MRI) is often performed as part of the initial investigation of the patient presenting with neurologic symptoms. These studies may reveal thickening of a region of dura mater, tortuosities of leptomeningeal venous drainage, or secondary changes in brain parenchyma reflective of venous hypertension. Magnetic resonance angiography (MRA) has also been used to detect and follow up DAVMs.[33] To maximize the sensitivity of MRI or MRA, the radiologist should be alerted to the high index of clinical suspicion for the disorder. At present, these adjuvant diagnostic studies are incapable of totally excluding the presence of a DAVM, and they do not define relevant features of the lesion well enough for prognostic and therapeutic decisions to be based on their findings. However, MRI and MRA may be used to screen patients with a low clinical suspicion of a DAVM and to monitor specific features of DAVMs (i.e., development of or enlargement of leptomeningeal venous channels) after baseline correlation with angiography. In the setting of strong clinical suspicion, normal CT or MRI findings should not be used to exclude a DAVM.

Classification

Classification of DAVMs has evolved over time to be useful in guiding therapeutic intervention. Initial attempts were simplistic, emphasizing the anatomic location (e.g., transverse-sigmoid DAVM, cavernous DAVM, sagittal sinus DAVM). These approaches lacked meaningful information in regard to predicting the nature or outcome of the abnormality or treatment options. Subsequent systems incorporated information from diagnostic angiography (Table 70.1).[34–36]

Perhaps one of the most well-recognized classification schemes specific to DAVMs is that developed by Djindjian and colleagues.[34] This system classifies a lesion as one of four types. Type I DAVMs are characterized by normal

Table 70.1   Classification of Dural Arteriovenous Malformations

Type	Djindjian	Cognard	Borden
I	Normal antegrade flow into dural sinus	Normal antegrade flow into dural sinus	Drains directly into venous sinus or meningeal vein
II	Drainage into venous sinus with reflux into adjacent sinus or cortical vein	a. Retrograde flow into sinus b. Retrograde filling of cortical veins only c. Retrograde drainage into sinus and cortical veins	Drains into dural sinus or meningeal veins with retrograde drainage into subarachnoid veins
III	Drainage into cortical veins with retrograde flow	Direct drainage into cortical veins with retrograde flow	Drains into subarachnoid veins without dural sinus or meningeal involvement
IV	Drainage into venous pouch (lake)	Direct drainage into cortical veins with venous ectasia >5 mm and 3× larger than diameter of draining vein	
V		Drainage to spinal perimedullary veins	

antegrade drainage into a venous sinus or meningeal vein; type II lesions drain into a sinus, with reflux into adjacent sinuses or cortical veins; type III DAVMs drain directly into cortical veins with resultant retrograde flow into the cerebral venous compartment; and type IV DAVMs have drainage directly into a venous pouch (venous lake or venous ectasia).

Djindjian and colleagues[34] concluded that type I DAVMs are benign, and that types II through IV have gradually more aggressive characteristics. Since the introduction of the Djindjian classification of DAVMs, other studies have been published in which investigators have attempted to correlate certain features of a DAVM with the likelihood of associated hemorrhage or other specific neurologic complications.[9,12,15,37]

With the advent of more effective endovascular therapeutic techniques, a means of predicting lesion risk and management options emerged. Cognard and associates[35] developed a classification system derived from a modified version of that published by Djindjian's group, defining five types of DAVMs that are based exclusively on the pattern of venous outflow. Type I DAVMs are characterized by normal antegrade flow into the affected dural sinus (Fig. 70–2). Type II lesions are associated with an abnormal direction of venous drainage within the affected dural sinus (Fig. 70–3). The investigators further categorize type II lesions into three subtypes: type IIa, lesions with retrograde flow exclusively into the sinus or sinuses; type IIb, lesions with retrograde venous drainage into the cortical veins only; and type II a + b, lesions with retrograde drainage into both the sinuses and the cortical veins. Type III DAVMs drain directly into a cortical vein or veins without venous ectasia (Fig. 70–4), whereas type IV DAVMs drain into cortical veins with venous ectasia that is greater than 5 mm in diameter and three times larger than the diameter of the draining vein (Fig. 70–5). A type

V DAVM drains into spinal perimedullary veins (Fig. 70–6). Correlation with the clinical data of Cognard and associates[35] yielded the following conclusions: Type I DAVMs are considered benign, and treatment is usually not necessary, except possibly for palliation of symptoms; type IIa lesions are best treated with arterial embolization; type IIb and type IIa + b lesions usually require both transarterial and transvenous embolization for effective obliteration. For type III through V lesions, transarterial and, occasionally, transvenous embolization aimed at complete occlusion of the fistula is necessary and usually must be combined with surgical techniques to eliminate the dangerous cortical venous drainage.

Borden and coworkers[36] have also proposed a classification system emphasizing venous anatomy. This system is appealing in its simplicity, with only three categories. Type I DAVMs drain directly into dural venous sinuses or pachymeningeal veins. Type II lesions drain into dural sinuses or pachymeningeal veins but also have retrograde drainage into subarachnoid (leptomeningeal) veins. Type III DAVMs drain solely into subarachnoid (leptomeningeal) veins and do not have dural sinus or meningeal venous drainage. The validity of both the Cognard and Borden classification systems was confirmed by examination of 102 intracranial DAVMs in 98 patients.[37]

Indications for Treatment

The Borden classification and others emphasize that the primary determinant of a DAVM's prospective aggressive neurologic course is the presence or absence of leptomeningeal venous drainage. This sole feature also primarily determines whether therapeutic interventions, with their associated risks, are justified for these lesions. Because the clinical presentation and natural history of DAVMs are highly variable, treatment should be

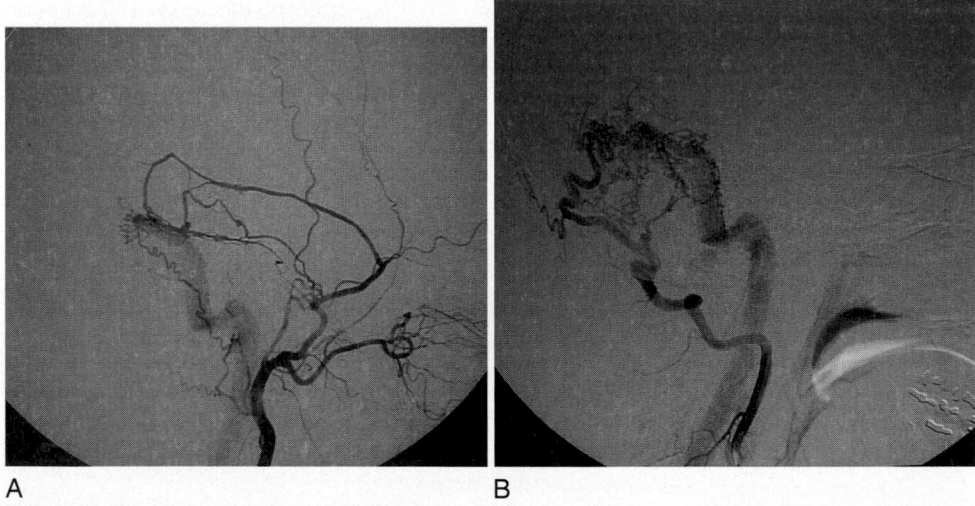

A   B

FIGURE 70–2   *Type I dural arteriovenous malformation in a 35-year-old woman with a new-onset bruit behind the right ear. The patient had experienced head trauma requiring hospitalization 13 years before.* A, *Selective injection of right occipital artery (lateral view). There is arteriovenous shunting via numerous small fistulas from distal arterial branches to the transverse sinus. Venous flow remains antegrade, making this a "benign" lesion.* B, *Selective right external trunk injection (lateral view) showing additional fistulas from middle meningeal and posterior auricular arteries.*

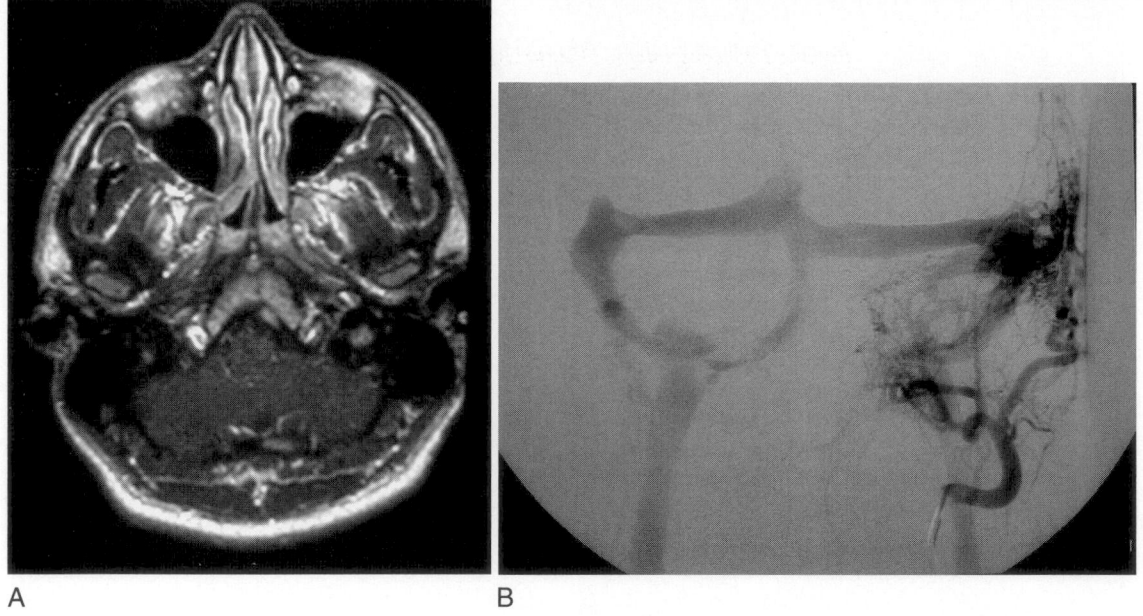

FIGURE 70–3 *Type II dural arteriovenous malformation in a 22-year-old man with a new onset of seizures and no history of head trauma. A, Post–contrast enhancement, T1-weighted axial magnetic resonance image demonstrates increased vascularity along the posteroinferior aspect of the cerebellum. B, Left external carotid injection (frontal view). There is prompt venous opacification during the arterial phase, as well as retrograde filling of the contralateral sinus across the midline. Contribution is primarily from middle meningeal and posterior auricular branches.*

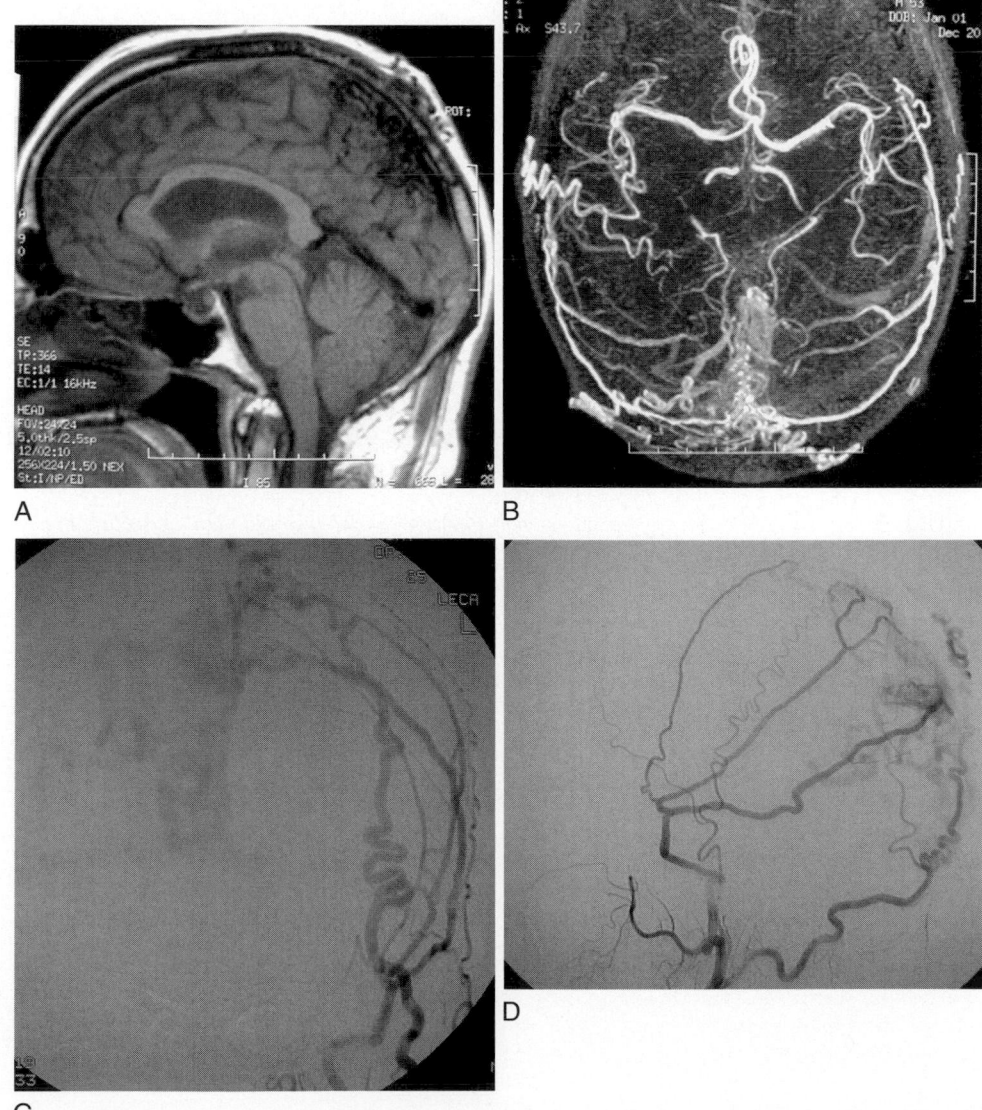

FIGURE 70–4 *Type III dural arteriovenous malformation in a 54-year-old man with new onset of seizure. The patient also noticed a pulsatile mass on his scalp. A, Sagittal T1-weighted, non-contrast magnetic resonance image demonstrates prominent flow voids in the parietal occipital area representing dilated cortical veins. B, Collapsed-view magnetic resonance angiography. Innumerable branches of the external carotid arteries (bilateral) converge near the midline adjacent to the sagittal sinus. Left external frontal (C) and oblique (D) carotid injections. Arteriovenous shunting is noted, with prominent cortical veins to the right of midline and early opacification of the right transverse sinus. Contribution is from superficial temporal, middle meningeal, and occipital arteries.*

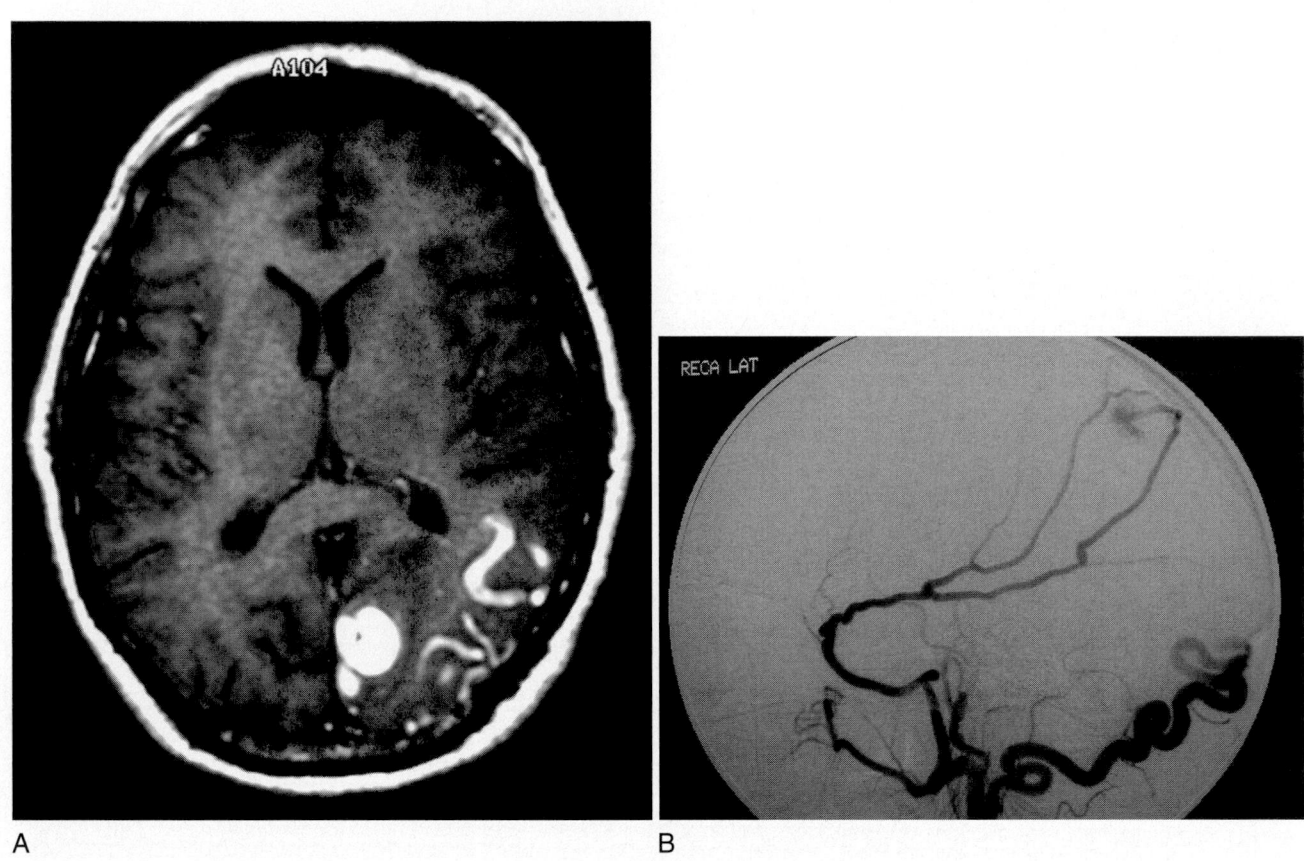

A   B

FIGURE 70–5   *Type IV dural arteriovenous malformation in a 57-year-old man whose family noticed personality changes. The patient described intermittent visual changes. A, Axial T1-weighted magnetic resonance image shows prominent cortical veins. High signal represents slow flow status. Note venous varix (pouch) posteriorly, adjacent to the falx. Right external carotid injection, early (B) and late (C) arterial phase. Markedly dilated middle meningeal and occipital arteries. There is early venous opacification with dilated venous varix.*

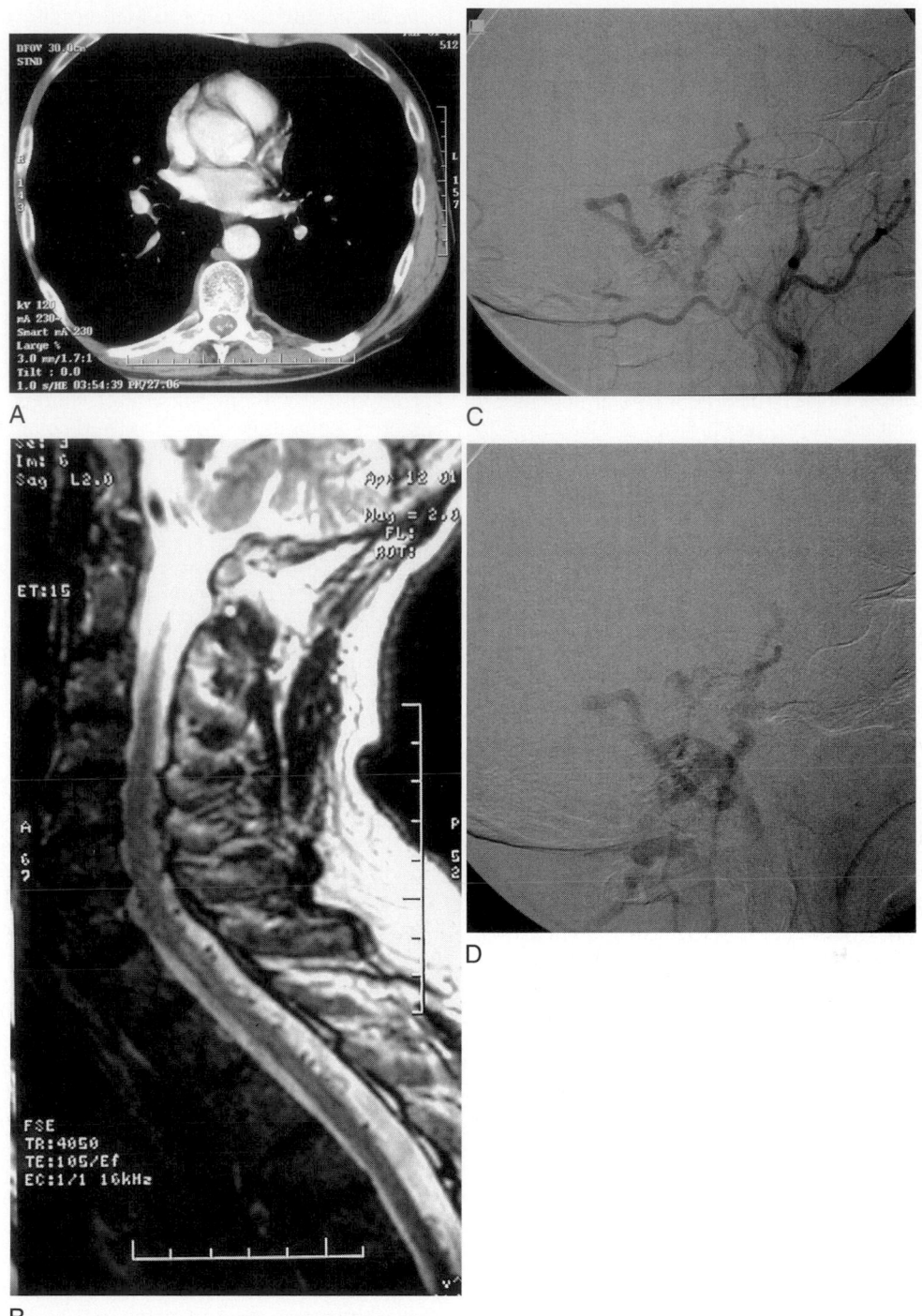

FIGURE 70–6   *Type V dural arteriovenous malformation in a 59-year-old woman with multisystem disease including chronic obstructive pulmonary disease. She had unexplained, progressive difficulty with ambulation. Computed tomography (CT) scanning of the chest was obtained for pulmonary evaluation. A, Post–contrast enhancement CT scan of the chest, axial view. Note the abnormal vascular enhancement within the spinal canal. B, Sagittal T2-weighted magnetic resonance image of the cervical spine. Prominent flow voids are seen dorsal to the spinal cord. These represent prominent venous channels. Left external carotid injection (lateral view), early (C) and delayed (D) images. There is early opacification of venous outflow toward spinal perimedullary veins.*

individualized on the basis of many factors, including patient age and comorbidities, severity of clinical symptoms, predicted risk of rupture, and risk of potential treatment options. In many cases, an expectant approach may be the best option. In other cases, the goal of treatment is most appropriately palliative, often with a goal of limited or partial treatment. Definitive treatment with its associated risks is usually indicated in lesions that have manifested with intracranial hemorrhage or those considered to be high-risk—that is, DAVMs with leptomeningeal venous drainage or variceal or aneurysmal changes in the venous circulation. In a study by Van Dijk and colleagues,[38] patients with these high-risk lesions (Borden types 2 and 3), when given either no treatment or only partial treatment so that persisting cortical venous involvement persisted, suffered a 10% annual mortality and significant additional morbidity.

TREATMENT OPTIONS

Many patients with nonaggressive DAVMs are best treated with only symptomatic palliation, which may consist of reassurance and counseling, biofeedback, and, possibly, jugular massage.[39] The last procedure should be used with caution in the elderly, who might have coexisting carotid disease or may be vulnerable to vasovagal syncope. Patients with dull aching pain or bothersome pulsatile tinnitus may benefit from nonsteroidal anti-inflammatory agents. Carbamazepine may be given for tic-like pain, and short courses of corticosteroids may be particularly effective for retro-orbital discomfort. Patients with DAVMs and tic douloureux should not be treated by percutaneous methods involving puncture of the foramen ovale, which might lead to catastrophic hemorrhage. Once it is decided that a patient with a particular DAVM will benefit from intervention, careful consideration of the available options is required. They include surgery, endovascular treatment, radiosurgery, or a combination of these approaches.

Surgical Technique

The goals of surgical treatment of DAVMs are (1) physical interruption or obliteration of arterialized leptomeningeal venous connections and (2) maximal coagulation or excision of the diseased dura. There is a continuous risk for significant blood loss, particularly early in the procedure, when incomplete surgical exposure may be accompanied by significant bleeding. Beginning with skin infiltration and incision, the operation should proceed a step at a time, with hemostatic control achieved before the next step is taken. This approach is indeed more speedy, more efficient, and safer than a faster procedure, which might require the surgeon to spend time controlling brisk bleeding from many sources. As a rule, no incision should be made unless the surgeon is prepared to control catastrophic bleeding from it. A thorough review of preoperative angiography and judicious use of preoperative embolization help limit the risk of bleeding. Continuous communication with the anesthesia team is critical.

Meticulous attention to hemostasis and microsurgical technique throughout the procedure is imperative.[40] After the abnormal dura is identified, its resection is aided by the irrigating bipolar cautery forceps. The placement of small permanent vascular clips in tandem alternated with dural transection may be useful. Using aneurysm clips to temporarily occlude variceal veins is helpful in determining which veins should be coagulated and sectioned, because occlusion of some veins may significantly affect adjacent cortical venous circulation. It is sometimes possible to identify discrete arteriovenous connections whose occlusion significantly decreases surrounding subarachnoid venous engorgement.

Direct puncture of large varices with intraoperative placement of obliterating coils has been successful.[41] A combination of coils and glue after access has been obtained by craniectomy and direct sinus puncture has also been reported.[42] Resection of the dural sinus can be accomplished without the risk of venous infarction if the resected segment is arterialized and collateral channels are well developed.[43] In some cases, surgical clipping of the draining vein close to the DAVM, with extensive dural coagulation rather than resection, may be preferred.[44] Presigmoid skull base exposures have also been employed, specifically for access to petrosal and sigmoid lesions.[45] Image-guided frameless navigation is useful for flap design and localization of DAVMs or associated cortical venous drainage. Intraoperative angiography helps ensure complete resection in difficult cases.

Endovascular Treatment

Transarterial embolization has been widely used in the treatment of DAVMs.[1,46,47] The use of flow-guided catheter technology and greater experience with particle and glue embolization as well as detachable coils have greatly improved the safety and efficacy of this method.[48-50] However, transarterial embolization rarely succeeds in totally eliminating and curing a DAVM, except in rare instances of limited fistulas with a small number of accessible feeding vessels. More commonly, DAVMs involve a multitude of feeders, which often arise as small twigs from major cerebral arteries that are not amenable to embolization. Transarterial embolization may obliterate the filling of the lesion after one injection, but the DAVM often continues to draw feeders from other sources and reappears on subsequent angiography, possibly in a more ominous configuration. DAVMs that are partially treated with transarterial embolization may later recur and progress to catastrophic hemorrhage.

Transarterial embolization may be effective in palliation of disabling symptoms even when it does not totally "cure" the DAVM. Such a lesion should be monitored as discussed previously. Transarterial embolization also plays an important role in reducing flow through DAVMs before surgical intervention, transvenous obliteration, or radiosurgery.[51-55] This adjunctive, preparatory use of transarterial embolization has greatly enhanced the safety and efficacy of other, more definitive treatment measures.

Symptom palliation may also be accomplished with transarterial embolization of external carotid artery feeders to the DAVM, although such an intervention is not without risk and rarely succeeds in totally eliminating the lesion. Arterial embolization may give a false sense of security that the lesion was "treated," and the DAVM may progress to acquire more aggressive features, including leptomeningeal venous drainage (even in the absence of recurrent symptoms). DAVMs that are observed expectantly or treated palliatively should be monitored closely by means of serial diagnostic studies for the development of leptomeningeal venous drainage, which may occur without a change in clinical symptoms. Noninvasive imaging methods, including MRI and MRA, may be used for interval studies, although these modalities may miss the subtle development of leptomeningeal venous drainage, which may be clinically catastrophic. Depending on the clinical situation and the particular lesion, serial MRI may be performed on a yearly basis, with formal angiography performed every few years, or sooner if symptoms change or if MRI findings suggest new leptomeningeal venous drainage.

Transvenous endovascular obliteration of DAVMs has been used with good results.[54-56] This modality aims at the thrombosis of the venous side of the lesion, often including obliteration of the adjacent dural venous sinus. Occlusion of the venous side of DAVMs is usually well tolerated if the diseased dural sinus is arterialized and does not serve as a site of drainage of cerebrovenous circulation. The diseased dural segment is often associated with harmful retrograde leptomeningeal venous drainage, but these channels are secondarily obliterated with thrombosis of the venous side of DAVMs. This strategy has been used most successfully for the treatment of DAVMs with accessible venous drainage. Transvenous obliteration is particularly effective in the treatment of cavernous sinus DAVMs (access through the inferior petrosal sinus), although these lesions frequently do not require any therapeutic intervention because of their benign clinical symptomatology and tendency for spontaneous regression.

Transvenous obliteration has also been used in cases of transverse-sigmoid sinus DAVMs and may be substantially safer than open surgical approaches to these lesions. However, there may be no accessible transvenous route for many DAVMs, including tentorial incisura DAVMs and

anterior cranial fossa DAVMs, which commonly behave aggressively. Transvenous obliteration may occasionally be performed after open surgical exposure, through puncture of the dural venous sinus or the arterialized venous varix, and the injection of coils or glue.[41] Rarely, transvenous occlusion may result in propagating venous thrombosis or altered hemodynamic patterns with paradoxic clinical deterioration or hemorrhage. Occasionally, a DAVM recurs adjacent to an endovascularly occluded venous sinus; such a development could represent reconstitution of arteriovenous channels within the walls of the occluded sinus or in the organized thrombus within the sinus channel. These cases are amenable to surgical excision of the segment of occluded sinus and disconnection of associated arterialized leptomeningeal veins (Fig. 70–7).

Radiosurgical Treatment

The goal of radiosurgical treatment is sclerosis and obliteration of arteriovenous connections within the diseased dura, which results in secondary thrombosis of the DAVM. Advantages include the noninvasiveness of treatment, which avoids risks associated with invasive procedures. Disadvantages are delayed response to treatment and risk of radiation injury to normal structures in the vicinity of the DAVM.

In a study combining radiosurgery with transarterial embolization, 95% of patients showed symptomatic improvement, and in 87% a cure was demonstrated on angiography performed a median of 12 months after radiosurgery.[57] The complication rate with this treatment strategy was acceptable. Radiosurgery alone was effective when the DAVM was not amenable to embolization, but the time needed for symptomatic improvement was longer. DAVMs of the transverse-sigmoid sinuses treated with a similar strategy yielded a 96% rate of symptom resolution or significant improvement and a total or near-total obliteration at mean angiography 21 months after radiosurgery.[13] There

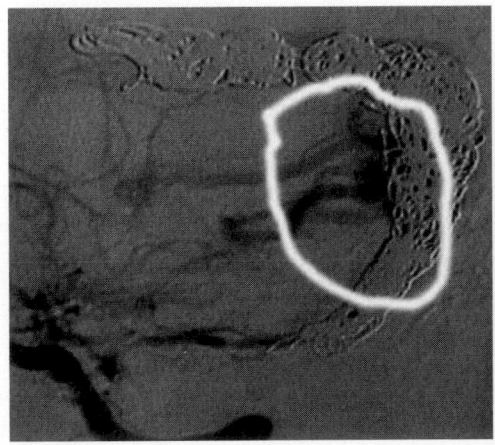
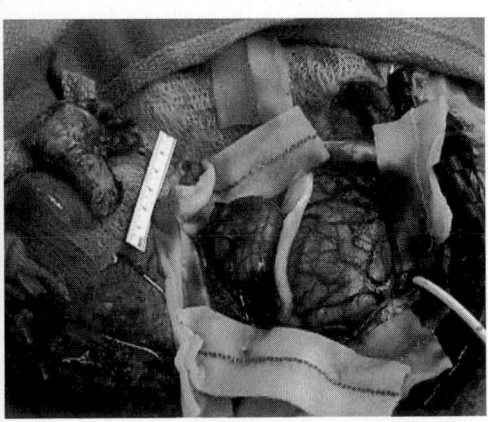

A   B

FIGURE 70–7 *Surgical treatment of recurrent DAVM. A, Angiogram of a 17-year-old boy whose symptoms recurred 2 months after endovascular treatment of a DAVM shows reconstitution of arteriovenous channels within the walls of the previously occluded sinus(white circle). B, Surgical excision of the segment of occluded sinus with disconnection of associated arterialized leptomeningeal veins resulted in cure.*

were no intracerebral hemorrhages or radiation-related complications. Although the ideal treatment parameters and ultimate role of radiosurgery continue to evolve, this method has an established role in the multimodality treatment of DAVMs.

Comprehensive Management Strategy

A DAVM may rarely be discovered on routine imaging studies or on angiograms performed for other indications. Incidental lesions must be carefully assessed for features predisposing to aggressive clinical behavior. Complete angiographic evaluation is indicated in every case of suspected DAVM unless the patient is a poor candidate for therapeutic intervention or refuses invasive diagnostic studies. Lesions should be evaluated specifically for the presence of leptomeningeal venous drainage and for any variceal or aneurysmal changes in the venous circulation. In the absence of these features, the lesion should be observed expectantly. There is no evidence to justify prophylactic treatment of DAVMs that are not associated with leptomeningeal venous drainage. Expectant observation of these lesions should include serial MRI studies for any evidence of development of leptomeningeal venous dilations. Angiographic reexamination of the lesion every few years should be considered, especially for DAVMs at the anterior cranial fossa or the tentorial incisura, which very commonly result in leptomeningeal venous drainage.

Definitive prophylactic treatment should be strongly considered for asymptomatic and incidentally discovered DAVMs that have leptomeningeal venous drainage. The patient should be given the option of open surgical intervention or such alternative radiosurgical or endovascular options as may be appropriate for the lesion's type and location. If treatment does not totally eliminate leptomeningeal venous drainage, either further definitive therapy or very close follow-up of the lesion is indicated. We believe that anticoagulation is contraindicated for DAVMs with leptomeningeal venous drainage.

It appears easiest to justify definitive intervention for DAVMs that have already behaved aggressively. Nevertheless, the morbidity of a first hemorrhage with a DAVM is substantial, and many patients do not survive or do not recover to a condition suitable for therapeutic intervention. Furthermore, little is known about the risk either of subsequent hemorrhage or of the progression of neurologic deficits in this clinical setting. However, there are numerous documented cases of progression of focal neurologic symptoms resulting in death or major disability unless the DAVM is obliterated. We recommend that lesions that have hemorrhaged or that cause focal neurologic symptoms due to parenchymal venous hypertension be considered for definitive treatment. Palliative therapy is not sufficient in this setting.

Lesions that manifest as pain or pulsatile tinnitus are evaluated and treated in the same way as incidental lesions. Nonspecific measures aimed at the symptoms are usually sufficient. Palliative treatment of the DAVM may be considered for the control of symptoms. Rarely is definitive treatment indicated solely for pain or pulsatile tinnitus. We do not believe that the risk of definitive treatment is justified in such DAVMs because they do not exhibit leptomeningeal venous drainage.

Lesions associated with ophthalmoplegia are evaluated on a case-by-case basis. Painful ophthalmoplegia often resolves spontaneously, and many such lesions involute after being subjected to angiography for evaluation. In other cases, ophthalmoplegia may be progressive or associated with retinopathy and visual loss; in such cases, treatment of the associated DAVM is justified. Palliative treatment may be sufficient to stabilize visual symptoms. As in other settings, a radical cure of a DAVM should not be pursued at any risk and is generally not warranted unless the symptoms are truly debilitating or the DAVM is associated with leptomeningeal venous drainage.

The management of DAVMs associated with papilledema and increased intracranial pressure has been discussed previously. In the absence of leptomeningeal venous drainage, the risk of radical treatment of such lesions may not be justified and may or may not achieve subsequent control of intracranial hypertension. Lumboperitoneal shunting or optic nerve sheath decompression may effectively treat the secondary complications of papilledema, and the DAVM can be observed expectantly or treated palliatively or with radiosurgery.

In summary, clinical symptoms other than hemorrhage and neurologic deficits rarely warrant radical treatment of a DAVM, unless the lesion is particularly accessible or is associated with features predisposing to subsequent aggressive clinical behavior. Patient reassurance, symptomatic treatment, or lesion palliation is often sufficient. For DAVMs with features predisposing to an aggressive clinical course, a more definitive treatment strategy should be adopted. It is obvious that the myriad of clinical manifestations of DAVMs and the wide spectrum of possible angiographic and pathophysiologic scenarios call for highly individualized management strategies. Diagnostic investigation should be thorough so as to identify DAVMs with features predisposing to aggressive clinical behavior. Treatment strategies should include a highly individualized choice of modalities from the available armamentarium of symptomatic treatment, lesion palliation, transarterial or transvenous endovascular therapy, open surgical invention, and radiosurgery. For the foreseeable future, the treatment of DAVMs should preferably be entrusted to multidisciplinary teams with expertise in the recognition and management of these lesions, and with experience in a variety of treatment approaches.

Lesions associated with intracranial hypertension and papilledema require special consideration. Palliation or definitive cure of the DAVM frequently (but not always) results in reversal of papilledema and stabilization of visual symptoms. In other instances, the risks of definitive treatment may not be justified. Intracranial hypertension may be treated by lumboperitoneal shunting. Ventriculoperitoneal shunting may not be possible in the patient with small cerebral ventricles and may be dangerous in the setting of arterialized cortical or subependymal veins. Optic nerve sheath decompression has also been used in cases of progressive papilledema and inoperable DAVMs. CSF diversion or optic nerve sheath decompression may be combined with transarterial embolization, radiosurgery, or both in the management of some lesions. Transvenous occlusion is rarely possible in this setting, because it may further compromise intracranial venous outflow.

SUMMARY

Much has been learned about the pathoanatomy, pathophysiology, natural history, and therapeutic options for DAVMs. A better understanding of these lesions has allowed more prompt and precise diagnosis as well as a realistic assessment of features predisposing to an aggressive clinical course. Treatment is guided not only toward the palliation of clinical symptoms but also, and as importantly, toward prevention of future sequelae. The therapeutic armamentarium consists of a number of options with varying risk and effectiveness for individual lesions. Transarterial embolization, transvenous embolization, surgical therapy, and radiosurgery can be used alone or in various combinations as required for individual clinical scenarios.

References

1. Lasjaunias P, Lopez-Ibor L, Abanou A, et al: Radiological anatomy of the vascularization of cranial dural arteriovenous malformations. Anat Clin 6:87–99, 1984.
2. Awad IA, Barrow DL (eds): Dural Arteriovenous Malformations. Park Ridge, IL, American Association of Neurological Surgeons, 1993, pp xi–xii.
3. Lasjaunias P, Berenstein A (eds): Surgical Neuroangiography II: Endovascular Treatment of Cranofacial Lesions. New York, Springer-Verlag, 1987.
4. Aminoff MJ, Kendall BE: Asymptomatic dural vascular anomalies. Br J Radiol 46:662–667, 1973.
5. Fermand M, Reizine D, Melki JP, et al: Long-term follow-up of 43 pure dural arteriovenous fistulas (AVF) of the lateral sinus. Neuroradiology 29:348–353, 1987.
6. Gelwan MJ, Choi IS, Berenstein A, et al: Dural arteriovenous malformations and papilledema. Neurosurgery 22:1079–1084, 1988.
7. Chimowitz MI, Little JR, Awad IA, et al: Intracranial hypertension associated with unruptured cerebral arteriovenous malformations. Ann Neurology 27:474–479,1990.
8. Hurst RW, Bagley LJ, Galetta S, et al: Dementia resulting from dural arteriovenous fistulas: the pathologic findings of venous hypertensive encephalopathy. Am J Neuroradiology 19:1267–1273, 1998.
9. Malik GM, Pearce JE, Ausman JI, et al: Dural arteriovenous malformations and intracranial hemorrhage. Neurosurgery 15:332–339, 1984.
10. Barnwell SL, Malbach VV, Dowd CF, et al: A variant of arteriovenous fistulas within the wall of dural sinuses. J Neurosurg 74:199–204, 1991.
11. Bitoh S, Sakaki S: Spontaneous cure of dural arteriovenous malformation in the posterior fossa. Surg Neurol 12:111–114, 1979.
12. Lasjaunias P, Chiu M, Bruggs KT, et al: Neurological manifestations of intracranial dural arteriovenous malformations. J Neurosurg 64:724–730, 1986.
13. Chardhaury MY, Sachdev VP, Cho SH, et al: Dural arteriovenous malformation of the major venous sinuses: An acquired lesion. Am J Neuroradiol 3:13–19, 1982.
14. Houser OW, Campbell JK, Campbell RJ, et al: Arteriovenous malformation affecting the transverse dural venous sinus: An acquired lesion. Mayo Clin Proc 54:651–661, 1979.
15. Awad IA, Little JR, Akrawi WP, et al: Intracranial dural arteriovenous malformations: Factors predisposing to an aggressive neurologic course. J Neurosurg 72:839–850, 1990.
16. Vinuela F, Fox A, Pelz D, et al: Unusual clinical manifestations of dural arteriovenous malformations. J Neurosurg 64:554–558, 1986.
17. Cognard C, Casasco A, Toevi M, et al: Dural arteriovenous fistulas as a cause of intracranial hypertension due to impairment of cranial venous outflow. J Neurol Neurosurg Psychiatry 65:308–316, 1998.
18. Kim MS, Oh CW, Han DH, et al: Intraosseous dural arteriovenous fistula of the skull base associated with hearing loss. J Neurosurg 96:952–955, 2002.
19. Rizzo M, Bosch EP, Gross CE: Trigeminal sensory neuropathy due to dural external carotid cavernous sinus fistula. Neurology 32:89–91, 1982.
20. Willinsky R, Goyal M, terBrugge K, Montanera W: Tortuous, engorged pial veins in intracranial dural arteriovenous fistulas: Correlations with presentation, location, and MR findings in 122 patients. AJNR Am J Neuroradiol 20:103–136, 1999.
21. Iwama T, Hashimoto N, Takagi Y, et al: Hemodynamic and metabolic disturbances in patients with intracranial dural arteriovenous fistulas: Positron emission tomography evaluation before and after treatment. J Neurosurg 86:806–611, 1997.
22. Ishikawa T, Houkin K, Tokuda K, et al: Development of anterior cranial fossa dural arteriovenous malformation following head trauma: Case Report. J Neurosurg 86:291–293, 1997.
23. Nabors MW, Azzam CJ, Albanna FJ, et al: Delayed postoperative dural arteriovenous malformations: Report of two cases. J Neurosurg 66:768–72, 1987.
24. Yokota M, Tani E, Maeda Y, Yamaura I: Meningioma in sigmoid sinus groove associated with dural arteriovenous malformation: Case report. Neurosurgery 33:316–319, 1993.
25. Singh V, Meyers PM, Halbach VV, et al: Dural arteriovenous fistula associated with prothrombin gene mutation. J Neuroimag 11:319–321, 2001.
26. Yassari R, Jahromi B, Macdonald R: Dural arteriovenous fistula after craniotomy for pilocytic astrocytoma in a patient with protein S deficiency. Surg Neurol 58:59–64, 2002.
27. Lawton MT, Jacobowitz R, Spetzler RF: Redefined role of angiogenesis in the pathogenesis of dural arteriovenous malformations. J Neurosurg 87:267–274, 1997.
28. Magdison MA, Weinberg PE: Spontaneous closure of a dural arteriovenous malformation. Surg Neurol 6:107–110, 1976.
29. Hansen JH, Sogaard I: Spontaneous regression of an extra and intracranial arteriovenous malformation: case report. J Neurosurg 45:338–341, 1976.
30. Olutola PS, Eliam M, Molot M, et al: Spontaneous regression of a dural arteriovenous malformation. Neurosurgery 12:687–690,1983.
31. Duffau H, Lopes M, Janosevic V, et al: Early rebleeding from intracranial dural arteriovenous fistulas: Report of 20 cases and review of the literature. J Neurosurg 90:78–84, 1999.
32. Hu WY, TerBrugge KG: The role of angiography in the evaluation of vascular and neoplastic disease in the external carotid artery circulation. Neuroimag Clin North Am 6:625–644, 1996.
33. Ikawa F, Uozumi T, Kiya K, et al: Diagnosis of carotid-cavernous fistulas with magnetic resonance angiography demonstrating the draining veins utilizing 3-D time-of-flight and 3-D phase contrast techniques. Neurosurg Rev 19:7–12, 1996.
34. Djindjian R, Merland JJ, Theron J (eds): Superselective Arteriography of the External Carotid Artery. New York, Springer-Verlag, 1977, pp 606–628.
35. Cognard C, Gobin YP, Pierot L, et al: Cerebral dural arteriovenous fistulas: Clinical and angiographic correlation with a revised classification of venous drainage. Radiology 194:671–680, 1995.
36. Borden JA, Wu JK, Shucart WA: A proposed classification for spinal and cranial dural arteriovenous fistulous malformations and implications for treatment. J Neurosurg 82:166–179, 1995; erratum appears in J Neurosurg 82:705–706, 1995.
37. Davies MA, terBrugge K, Willinsky R, et al: The validity of classification for the clinical presentation of intracranial dural arteriovenous fistulas. J Neurosurg 85:830–837, 1996.
38. Van Dijk JM, terBrugge KG, Willinsky RA, Wallace MC: Clinical course of cranial dural arteriovenous fistulas with long-term persistent cortical venous reflux. Stroke 33:1233–36, 2002.
39. Halbach VV, Higashida RT, Hieshima GB, et al: Dural fistulas involving the cavernous sinus: Results of treatment in 30 patients. Radiology 163:437–442, 1987.
40. Grisoli F, Vincentelli F, Fuchs S, et al: Surgical treatment of tentorial arteriovenous malformations draining into the subarachnoid space. J Neurosurg 60:1059–1066, 1987.
41. Endo S, Kuwayama N, Takaku A, et al: Direct packing of the isolated sinus in patients with dural arteriovenous fistulas of the transverse-sigmoid sinus. J Neurosurg 88:449–456, 1998.
42. Houdart E, Saint-Maurice JP, Chapot R, et al: Transcranial approach for venous embolization of dural arteriovenous fistulas. J Neurosurg 97:280–286, 2002.

Therapy

43. Sundt TM Jr, Piepgras DG: The surgical approach to arteriovenous malformations of the lateral and sigmoid dural sinuses. J Neurosurg 59:32–39, 1983.

44. Hoh BL, Choudhri TF, Connolly ES Jr, et al: Surgical management of high-grade intracranial dural arteriovenous fistulas: Leptomeningeal venous disruption without nidus excision. Neurosurgery 42:796–804, 1998.

45. Kattner DO, Roth TC, Giannotta SL: Cranial base approaches for the surgical treatment of aggressive posterior fossa dural arteriovenous fistulae with leptomeningeal drainage: Report of four technical cases. Neurosurgery 50:1156–1161, 2002.

46. Hardy RW Jr, Costin JA, Weinstein M, et al: External carotid cavernous fistula treated by transfemoral embolization. Surg Neurol 9:255–256, 1978.

47. Vinuela FV, Debrun GM, Fox AJ, et al: Detachable calibrated-leak balloon for superselective angiography and embolization of dural arteriovenous malformations. J Neurosurg 58:817–823, 1983.

48. Nesbit GM, Barnwell SL: The use of electrolytically detachable coils in treating high-flow arteriovenous fistulas. Am J Neuroradiol 19:1565–69, 1998.

49. Jansen O, Dorfler A, Forsting M, et al: Endovascular therapy of arteriovenous fistulae with electrolytically detachable coils. Neuroradiology 41:951–957, 1999.

50. Liu HM, Huang YC, Wang YH, et al: Transarterial embolisation of complex cavernous sinus dural arteriovenous fistulae with low-concentration cyanoacrylate. Neuroradiology 42:766–770, 2000.

51. Goto K, Sidipratomo P, Ogata N, et al: Combining endovascular and neurosurgical treatments of high-risk dural arteriovenous fistulas in the lateral sinus and the confluence of the sinuses. J Neurosurg 90:289–299, 1999.

52. Collice M, D'Aliberti G, Arena O, et al: Surgical treatment of intracranial dural arteriovenous fistulae: Role of venous drainage. Neurosurgery 47:56–66, 2000.

53. Friedman JA, Pollock BE, Nichols D et al: Results of combined stereotactic radiosurgery and transarterial embolization for dural arteriovenous fistulas of the transverse and sigmoid sinuses. J Neurosurg 94:886–91, 2001.

54. Halbach VV, Higashida RT, Hieshima GB, et al: Transvenous embolization of dural fistulas involving the cavernous sinus. Am J Neuroradiol 10:377–83, 1989.

55. Halbach VV, Higashida RT, Hieshima GB, et al: Transvenous embolization of dural fistulas involving the transverse and sigmoid sinuses. Am J Neuroradiol 10:385–392, 1989.

56. Roy D, Raymond J: The role of transvenous embolization in the treatment of intracranial dural arteriovenous fistulas. Neurosurgery 40:1133–1141, 1997.

57. Pollock BE, Nichols DA, Garrity JA, et al: Stereotactic radiosurgery and particulate embolization for cavernous sinus dural arteriovenous fistulae. Neurosurgery 45:459–466, 1999.

Chapter Seventy-One

Moyamoya Disease: Surgical Aspects

Kazuo Hashi and Masahiko Wanibuchi

In 1957, cases of bilateral occlusion or stenosis of the carotid artery associated with a prominent vascular network at the base of the brain were first noticed in Japan. In 1968, Kudo[1] introduced the condition in the English literature as spontaneous occlusion of the circle of Willis. In 1969, Suzuki and Takaku[2] used the Japanese word *moyamoya*, meaning "hazy" in English, to describe the appearance of the neovascularization. Since then, it has generally been called *moyamoya disease*. In 1976, the Japanese Ministry of Health and Welfare organized an ongoing Research Committee for this condition. However, the cause of the disease remains unknown. There is a possibility that hereditary factors exist, and responsible genes have been reported.[3]

CLINICAL FEATURES

Moyamoya disease is found predominantly in the Japanese and Asian races. It is estimated that approximately 6000 patients were treated in Japan in 1996[4]; that figure is equivalent to a prevalence of approximately 5 cases per 100,000 persons. The incidence of familial occurrence is about 10%.[4] The male-to-female ratio is 1:2.[5] The age of onset shows a bimodal distribution, with a higher peak around 5 years of age and another lower one around 30 to 40 years (Fig. 71–1).[6]

In 2000, the Research Committee proposed the following diagnostic criteria:

1. The diagnosis is made by cerebral angiography and the following findings should be present:
   a. Stenosis or occlusion at the terminal portion of the intracranial carotid artery and/or proximal portions of the anterior and/or middle cerebral arteries.
   b. Abnormal vascular networks in the vicinity of the occlusive or stenotic lesions in the arterial phase.
   c. These findings are present bilaterally.
2. When magnetic resonance imaging (MRI) and magnetic resonance angiography (MRA) clearly show these findings, conventional cerebral angiography may not be required (Fig. 71–2).
3. Similar cerebrovascular conditions associated with the following diseases should be excluded:

a. Atherosclerosis
b. Autoimmune diseases
c. Meningitis
d. Brain tumors
e. Down's syndrome
f. Von Recklinghausen's disease
g. Head injury
h. Irradiation
i. Others

4. Pathologic findings include the following:
   a. Intimal thickening resulting in stenosis or occlusion of the lumen at the terminal portion of carotid arteries on both sides. Sometimes lipid deposits in the thickened intima may be found.
   b. Stenosis or occlusion associated with fibrocellular thickening of the intima, a wavy internal elastic lamina, and an attenuation of the media may be found in the affected vessels.
   c. Numerous small vascular channels (perforators and anastomotic branches) are observed around the circle of Willis.
   d. Reticular conglomerates of small vessels are often seen in the pia mater.

When the three radiologic criteria are met, the diagnosis of moyamoya disease can be made definitively. In pediatric patients, the disease may be diagnosed when the findings are limited to one side or are combined with an apparent stenosis of the terminal portion of the contralateral carotid artery.

Suzuki and Takaku showed the angiographic features of the chronologic progression of the disease and divided the process into six stages, as follows[7]:

Stage 1: Narrowing of the carotid fork. There is a stenosis at the terminal portion of the intracranial carotid arteries with no other findings.
Stage 2: Initiation of the moyamoya changes. Some moyamoya vessels are found at the base in association with stenosis of the carotid arteries and some dilatation of the main intracranial arteries (Fig. 71–3).
Stage 3: Intensification of the moyamoya changes. Moyamoya vessels become more apparent, and the proximal portions of the anterior and middle cere-

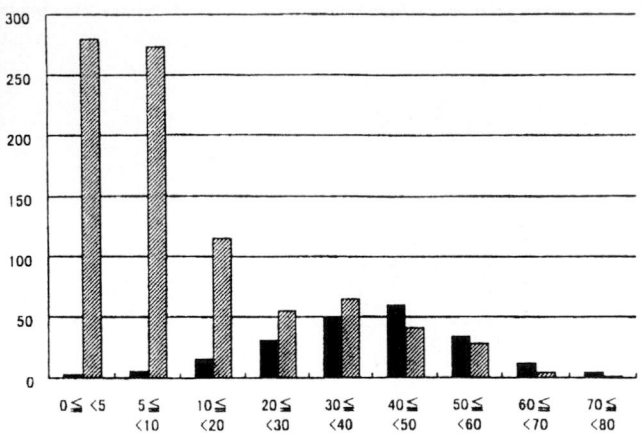

FIGURE 71–1   *Age and clinical pattern of onset of moyamoya disease.* Black bar *indicates cases manifesting as hemorrhage;* gray bar *indicates cases manifesting as symptoms other than hemorrhage. The* abscissa *represents age and the* ordinate *the number of cases. (From Fukuuchi Y, Nogwa S, Yamaguchi K, Dembo T: Follow-up study of registered cases of moyamoya disease in 1999. In Yoshimoto T [ed]: Annual Report 2000 of the Research Committee on Spontaneous Occlusion of the Circle of Willis [Moyamoya Disease]. Tokyo, Ministry of Health, Labor and Welfare, Japan, 2001.)*

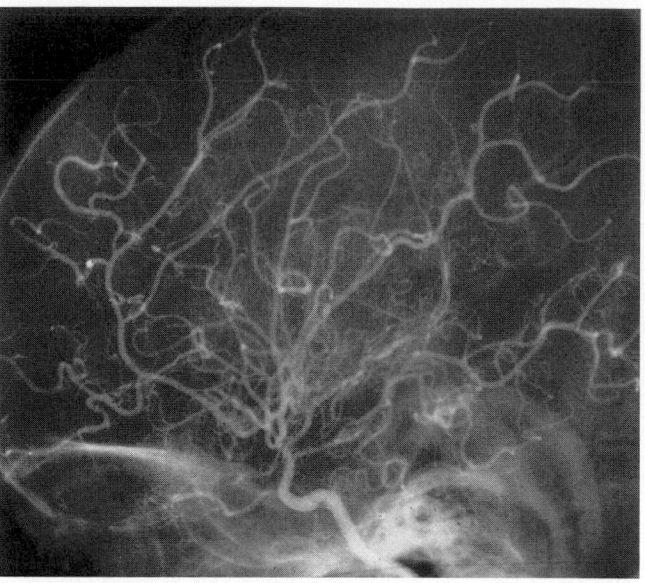

FIGURE 71–3   *Appearance of fine vessels at the base of the brain associated with stenosis of the carotid artery (stage 2 moyamoya disease).*

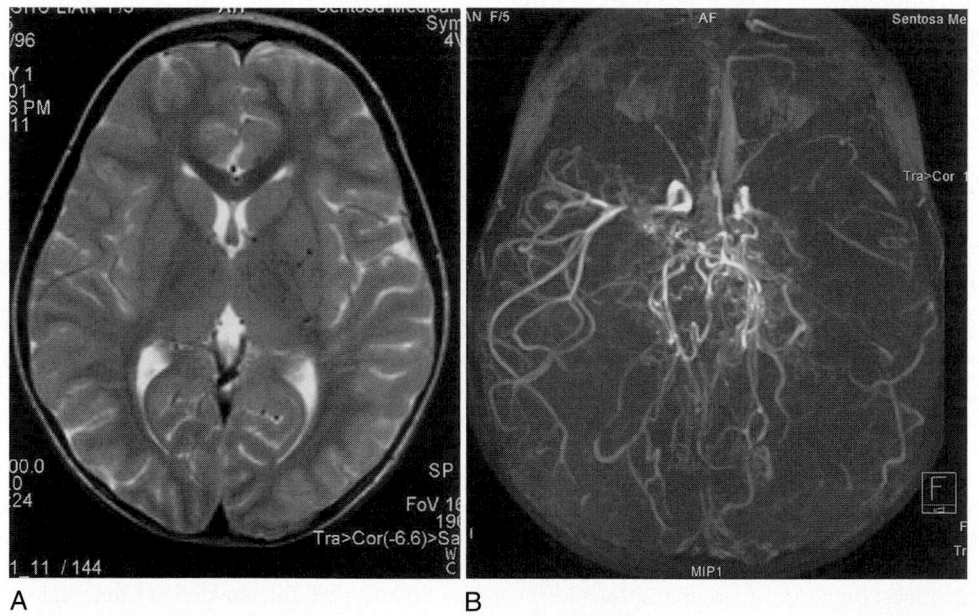

FIGURE 71–2   *MRI and MRA in a 5-month-old girl presenting with a convulsion. A, T2-weighted MRI shows multiple fine flow voids. B, Maximum intensity projection (MIP) image of an axial view of MRA shows fine networks of vessels at the base of the brain.*

bral arteries begin to disappear. Some collateral vessels from the external carotid arterial system may appear (Fig. 71–4).

Stage 4: Minimization of the moyamoya changes. Moyamoya vessels become smaller and finer, and the proximal portions of the anterior and middle cerebral arteries disappear; transdural collateral vessels in the ethmoidal region become prominent (Fig. 71–5).

Stage 5: Reduction of the moyamoya changes. Moyamoya vessels recede and are confined to the terminal portion of the carotid artery; transdural collateral vessels become more prominent (Fig. 71–6).

Stage 6: Disappearance of the moyamoya changes. Moyamoya vessels and intracranial carotid branches disappear, and the vascular supply to the brain becomes completely dependent on the external carotid arterial system.

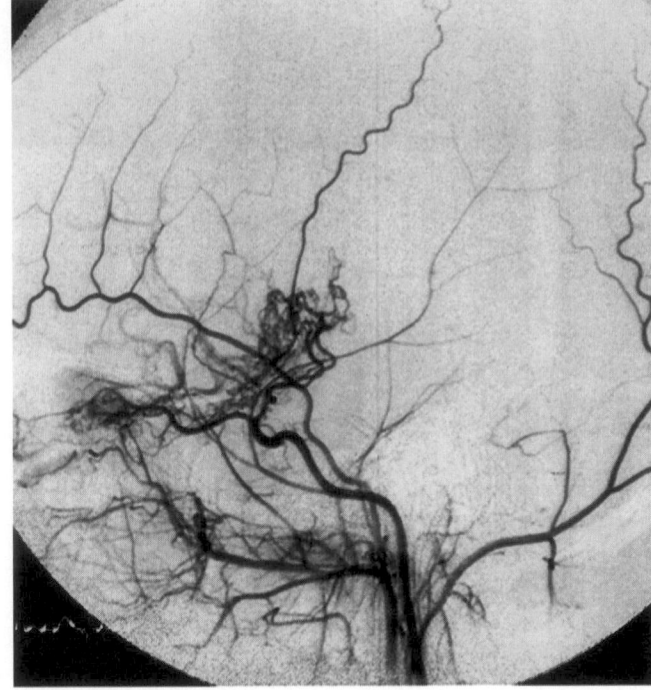

FIGURE 71–6   *Very poor filling of the major cerebral arteries; some moyamoya vessels still at the base (stage 5 moyamoya disease).*

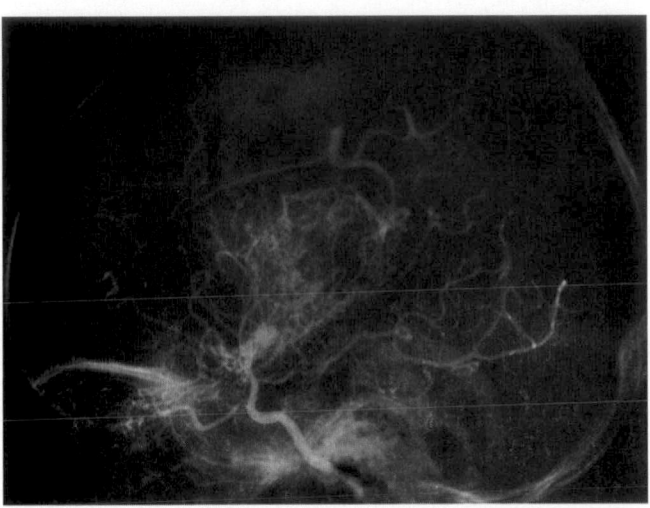

FIGURE 71–4   *Moyamoya vessels are abundant and main trunks of the major cerebral vessels have become more stenotic (stage 3 moyamoya disease).*

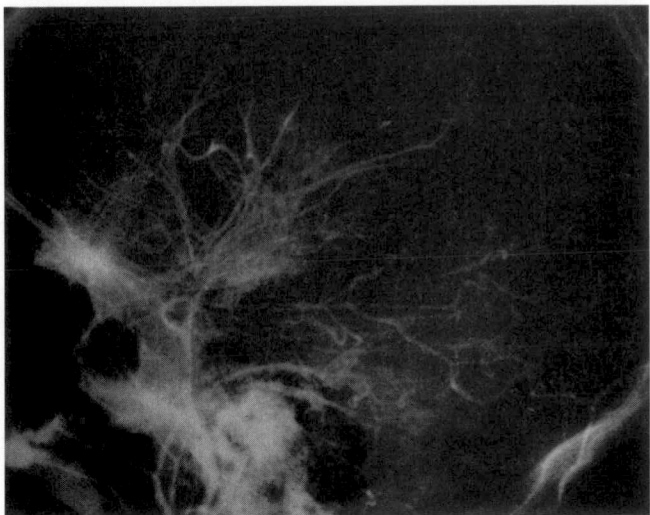

FIGURE 71–5   *Moyamoya vessels have become smaller (stage 4 moyamoya disease).*

The progression is more dynamic in children.[8] It is usual for unilateral involvement in children to progress to bilateral involvement within 1 or 2 years,[9] whereas in adults, unilateral involvement often stays unchanged.

Aneurysms commonly develop at the peripheral portions of cerebral arteries, such as the posterior and anterior choroidal arteries or Heubner's artery, or as pseudoaneurysms within a moyamoya vessel.[10] Most of the major arterial aneurysms are found in the vertebrobasilar system, possibly because of the demand for increased flow in the posterior circulation to compensate for the compromised carotid circulation.

In infants, cerebral ischemia commonly manifests as convulsions. In children, transient ischemic episodes are the most common pattern at onset.[5] Symptoms such as motor, speech, and sensory disturbances, or a combination, alteration of consciousness, involuntary movements, convulsions, or headache may appear suddenly and may have a short duration. Typically, they are provoked by hyperventilation associated with the blowing of a musical instrument or crying. The symptoms may occur repeatedly and sometimes on both sides alternately.

Because the collateral channels may not be adequate to meet the high blood flow demand of the developing brain, the disease is clinically more severe when the onset is earlier. Of patients in whom symptoms begin in the first 2 years of life, approximately 80% experience cerebral infarction and become clinically handicapped with motor or mental deficits (Figs. 71–7 and 71–8).[11] In children, the disease rarely causes death but the process proceeds clinically and radiologically until about the age of 10 years,

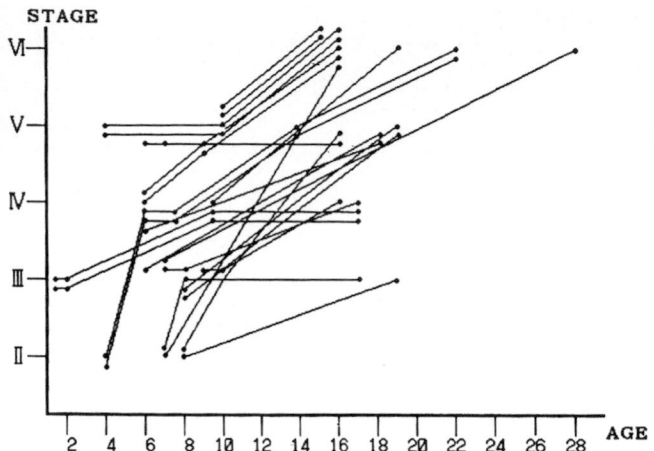

FIGURE 71–7 *Advance in the angiographic stage with increasing age of patients. (From Takahashi A, Fujiwara S, Suzuki Z: Long-term follow-up angiography of moyamoya disease—cases followed up from childhood to adolescence. No Shinkei Geka 14:23–29, 1986.)*

and stabilizes afterwards. However, long-term follow-up studies conducted into adulthood show that the physical or mental condition of the patients is good in less than half of cases.

Electroencephalograms (EEGs) show a peculiar pattern called the "re-buildup phenomenon" in 80% of pediatric cases (Fig. 71– 9).[12] This phenomenon is characterized by the reappearance of slow waves after temporary recovery from the previous buildup or resumption of normal basic rhythm 20 to 60 seconds after cessation of hyperventilation. The mechanism of the re-buildup phenomenon is unknown, but when cerebral ischemia is relieved by external carotid artery–to–internal carotid artery (EC-IC) bypass, the re-buildup phenomenon usually disappears.

More than 50% of cases in adults manifest as intracranial hemorrhage.[3] Hemorrhagic infarction is presumed to be the mechanism, because the hematomas in many cases are in the periventricular tissue, corresponding to the watershed zone between the perforators and the vessels from the cortical surface (Fig. 71–10).[13] In other cases, rupture of an aneurysm may be responsible for the hemorrhagic onset of the disease. Intracranial hemorrhage is the main cause of death or severe neurologic deficit in moyamoya disease. If it is untreated, rebleeding episodes occur with an annual risk of 7%[5] and may occur in the other hemisphere.

SURGICAL TREATMENT

Although antiplatelet agents, vasodilators, and anticonvulsants are usually prescribed, their efficacy is not established.

Since the 1970s, many surgical treatments to increase cerebral perfusion and improve prognosis have been tried. Superficial temporal artery–to–middle cerebral artery (STA-MCA) bypass[14] combined with placement of the tem-

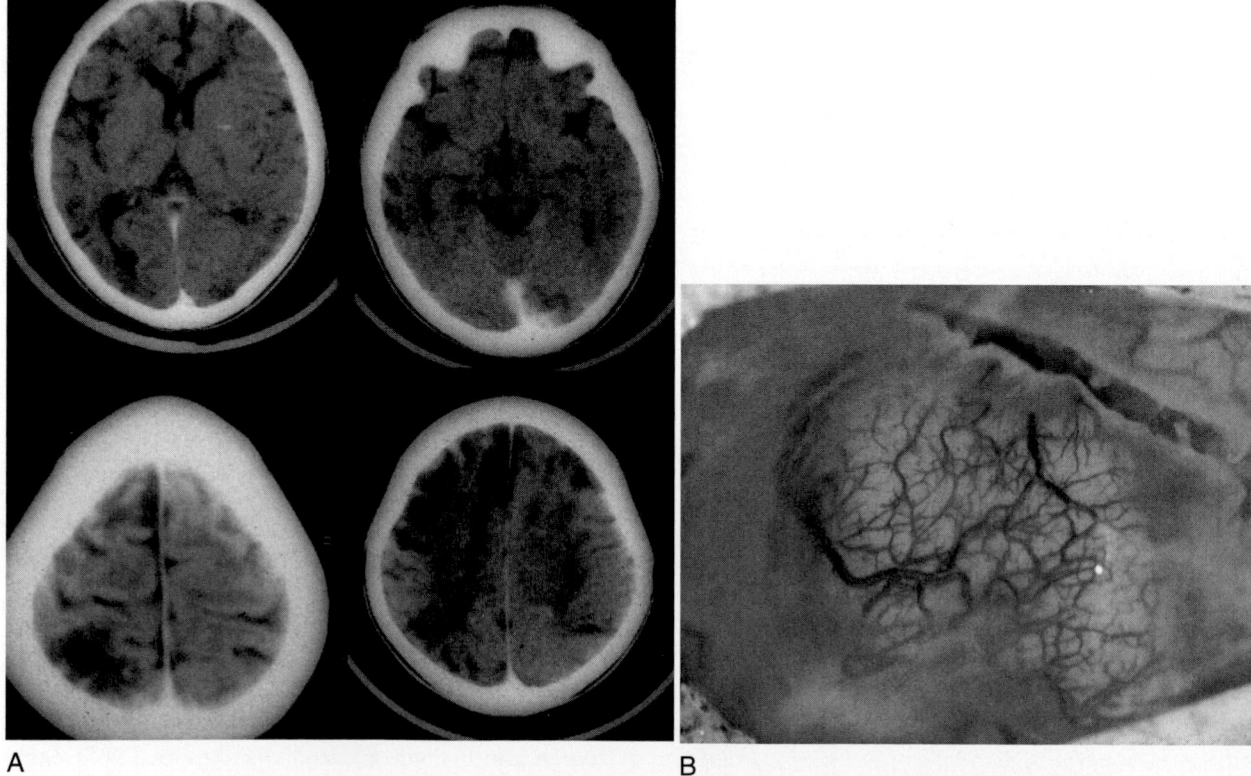

A   B

FIGURE 71–8 A, *Multiple infarctions observed in a 6-year-old patient who had been treated for convulsions that began at age 1 year.* B, *Surface of the brain shows atrophy and many fine, dilated small vessels.*

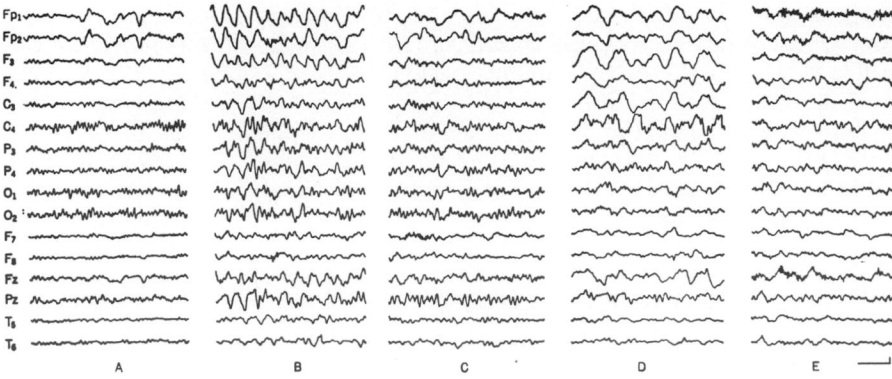

FIGURE 71–9 *Re-buildup phenomenon in electroencephalography in moyamoya disease. A, Resting state; B, during hyperventilation; C, 30 seconds after cessation of hyperventilation; D, 4 minutes after cessation of hyperventilation; E, 7 minutes after cessation of hyperventilation. (From Kodama N, Aoki Y, Hiraga H, et al: Electroencephalographic findings in children with moyamoya disease. Arch Neurol 36:16–19, 1979.)*

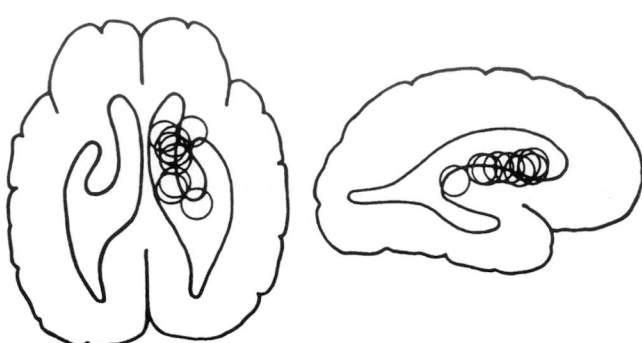

FIGURE 71–10 *Locations of hematomas in cases of hemorrhagic manifestations of moyamoya disease. (From Sasaki T, Sakurai Y, Shimizu Y, et al: Bleeding points in cerebral hemorrhage caused by moyamoya disease in adults: Investigation by CT scan. CT Kenkyu 5:647–655, 1983.)*

poral muscle over the brain surface (encephalomyosynangiosis [EMS])[15] and the placement of the dissected segment of the STA over the brain surface (encephaloduroarteriosynangiosis [EDAS])[16] with various modifications are the principal choices of surgical treatment. Multiple reports attest to the efficacy of these procedures.[17–19]

The advantage of the direct method, STA-MCA bypass combined with EMS, is to achieve an instant revascularization, which can cover a wide area of the brain surface for the subsequent induction of secondary neovascularization. However, the procedure demands a higher level of technical skill because the recipient arteries in children are usually small and fragile. EDAS and its modifications,[20–22] which are indirect methods, are technically easier to perform. They induce secondary neovascularization by placing the dissected strip of STA or middle meningeal artery over the brain surface.

Strict comparison of efficacy between the direct and indirect procedures has never been made. Follow-up results of registered cases in Japan in 1995 showed no remarkable difference in resultant activities of daily living (ADL) for the two methods.[23] However, one report clearly demonstrated the superiority of the direct STA-MCA anastomosis combined with EMS over the indirect method in 16 children with respect to neovascularization and postoperative recovery from ischemic symptoms.[24] The surgical trend has been to choose the direct method initially and to perform the indirect method in cases in which the direct method is technically impossible.

Generally, patients with repeated ischemic episodes and with decreases of regional cerebral blood flow or impairment of vascular reactivity are considered candidates for surgery. The cerebral circulation and metabolism must be evaluated to determine the suitability for operative intervention, usually with single-photon emission computed tomography (SPECT) or positron emission tomography (PET). Reported results show an improvement in circulation and relief of ischemic episodes after surgery.[25] Surgical treatment is strongly recommended for infants or small children because their brains are rapidly developing, even when the sole symptom is a convulsive episode and the decrease in cerebral blood flow is minimal. A decrease in seizure tendency has been reported after surgery.[26]

AIMS OF SURGICAL TREATMENT

At present, it is difficult to improve the circulation in the territory perfused by the anterior cerebral artery. This is a problem because mental disturbances are the major finding in children with early onset of moyamoya disease.[11] Omentum transplantation[27,28] may be the most effective way of improving perfusion over a wide area of frontal and mesial brain, but because of its complexity and invasiveness, this operation is rarely performed. Some investigators have proposed a direct anastomosis between the STA and anterior cerebral arterial branches,[29] the placement of burr holes,[30,31] and dural incision in the frontal region or the insertion of galeal and periosteal strips in the interhemispheric fissure through a small craniotomy to induce neovascularization.[32] The development of some neovascularization was shown by angiography, but the effect of all of these procedures on the prognosis is unknown.

As regards the effect of surgery on patients with hemorrhage, patients who underwent operations were found to do better in ADL and had a lower mortality at follow-up; in particular, the group treated with the direct procedure did better than the group treated with the indirect procedure.[5] Although there is some evidence that STA-MCA bypass was effective in preventing recurrent strokes, including hemorrhage, in adults with a hemorrhagic onset,[33] the preventive effect of surgery on future hemorrhage is not fully established for either direct or indirect procedures. A prospective randomized clinical trial (Japan Adult Moyamoya [JAM] Trial) to investigate this question was started in Japan in 2001.[34]

Direct repair of ruptured saccular aneurysms or some unruptured aneurysms has been performed in a few cases. During such operations, it is vital not to disturb the transdural collateral channels.

OPERATIVE PROCEDURES

STA-MCA Anastomosis Combined with Encephalomyosynangiosis

With the patient supine, the head is turned approximately 60 degrees (Figs. 71–11 and 71–12). A large curvilinear scalp incision is made from the frontal region to the parietal and posterior temporal regions. The scalp flap is turned down, and the STA is dissected. The periosteum is incised along the outer rim of the temporal muscle and is dissected subperiosteally. A large free bone flap is made. The dura is incised and removed to expose the brain surface as widely as possible. The dural defect is later closed with the periosteum attached to the temporal muscle that will be placed later over the brain to cover its surface. The middle meningeal artery is kept patent, so the dural defect is usually created anteriorly and posteriorly to it.

The temporal muscle is dissected in two layers, superficial and deep, and the deep layer is later placed over the brain surface. The STA is cut and is passed through a hole made in the muscle, and an STA-MCA anastomosis is performed with whichever branch of the MCA is chosen by virtue of its size and the location of affected cortex, which

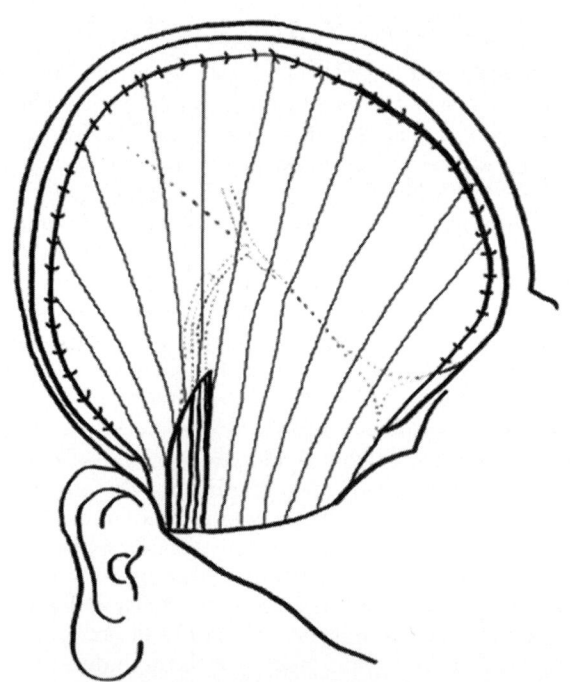

FIGURE 71–11 *Concept of the direct operation consisting of superior temporal artery–to–middle cerebral artery (STA-MCA) anastomosis and encephalomyosynangiosis (EMS).*

is deduced from preoperative symptoms. The arachnoid membrane over the cortex is incised along every exposed sulcus. The brain is covered by the deep layer of the temporal muscle, and the periosteum is sutured to the incised edge of the dura to close the dural defect. The blood supply to the muscle is left undisturbed as much as possible, but meticulous hemostasis should nevertheless be secured. The lower ridge of the bone flap is rongeured to make the passage of the muscle possible. The bone flap is then replaced and fixed. In the presence of a tight brain, it is advisable to fix the bone flap loosely, because hyperventilation should be avoided in moyamoya disease.

The anastomosed STA usually enlarges in the first several weeks postoperatively, but then it gradually becomes smaller and sometimes is seen to be obstructed at follow-up angiography several months later. Numerous fine new vascular networks connect the STA to the branches of MCA (Fig. 71–13). One of the problems of EMS is the bulk of the muscle, which may cause brain compression, although the complication can be avoided by a careful operative procedure. The more serious potential problem of EMS is the induction of epileptic foci by either the formation of scar or action potentials from muscle movements associated with chewing or talking. There are some reports that the incidence of convulsion is higher after EMS.[16,35]

Encephaloduroarteriosynangiosis

The anterior and posterior branches of the STA or the occipital artery can be used as a donor, depending on the site where neovascularization is planned. The head position varies according to the artery used. In principle, the artery is dissected from the surrounding tissue for about 10 cm through a linear incision, with its patency preserved (Fig. 71–14). The underlying attached galea is incised along the course of the artery to make an arterial strip detached from the surrounding tissue.

A small spindle-shaped craniotomy, approximately 2 cm wide and 7 to 8 cm long, is made along the course of the artery, and the dura is incised longitudinally. Care is taken not to cut any large dural artery during this procedure. The strip of artery with galea attached is then placed over the arachnoid membrane along the whole length of the craniotomy, and the galea is sutured in a watertight fashion to the cut edge of the dura. A strip of dura can be removed to ensure that the artery attaches to the brain. The bone flap is replaced and fixed.

The EDAS procedure is simpler than the direct method, and neovascularization occurs within 3 months in many cases, particularly in children. Connections between the placed artery and the middle cerebral arterial branch can be demonstrated (Fig. 71–15).[35,36] The major disadvantages of EDAS are the time lag necessary for neovascularization to develop, the unpredictability of its extent, and the limited brain area covered.

Encephaloduroarteriomyosynangiosis

A modification of EDAS, encephaloduroarteriomyosynangiosis (EDAMS) uses a larger craniotomy with employment of dural strips as an additional source of

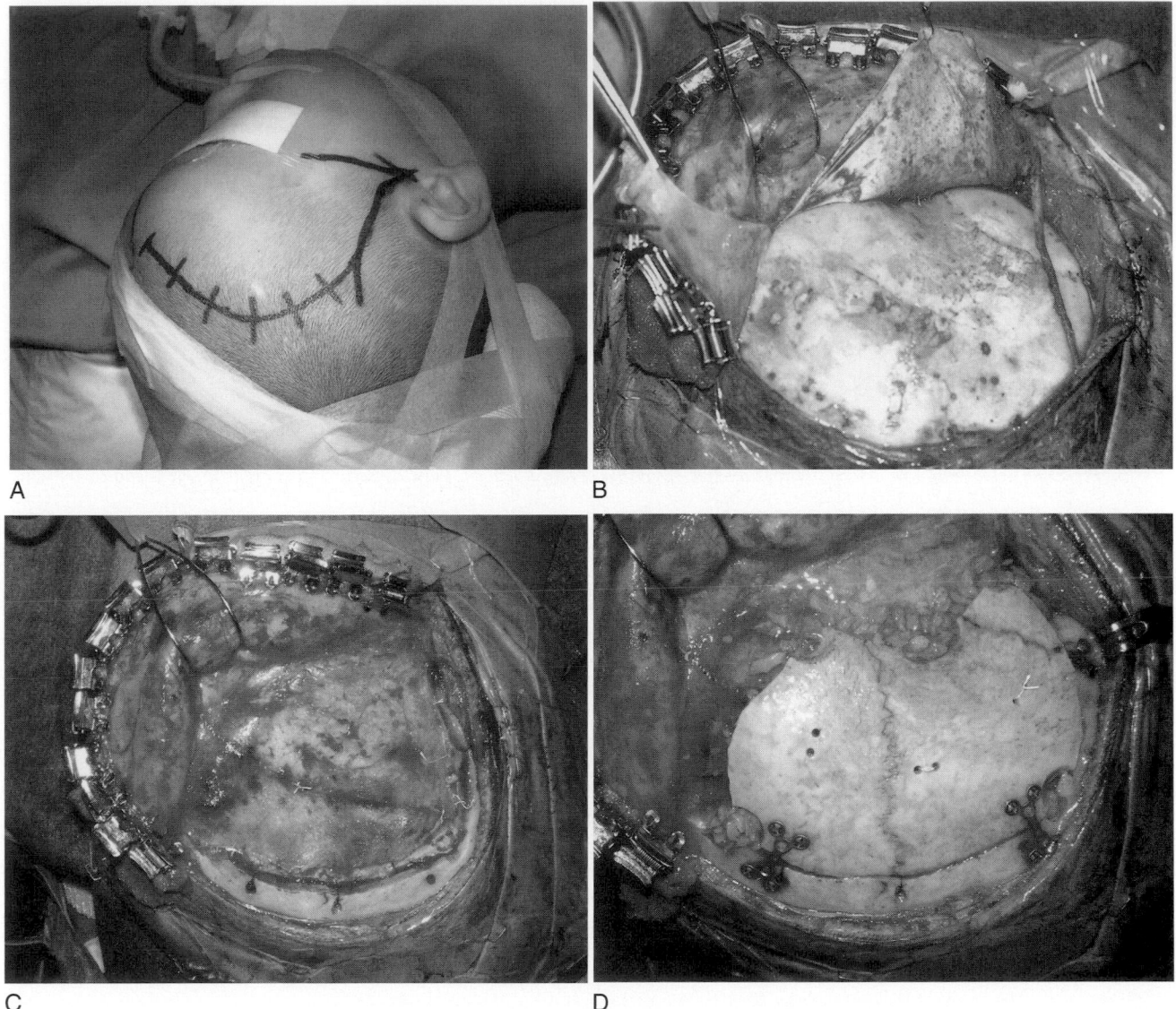

A   B

C   D

FIGURE 71–12 A, *A large craniotomy.* B, *Stripping of the temporal muscle and preparation of the superficial temporal artery for anastomosis.* C, *The brain surface is covered by the temporal muscle after the anastomosis is completed.* D, *The muscle is passed through the space made at the base of the bone flap.*

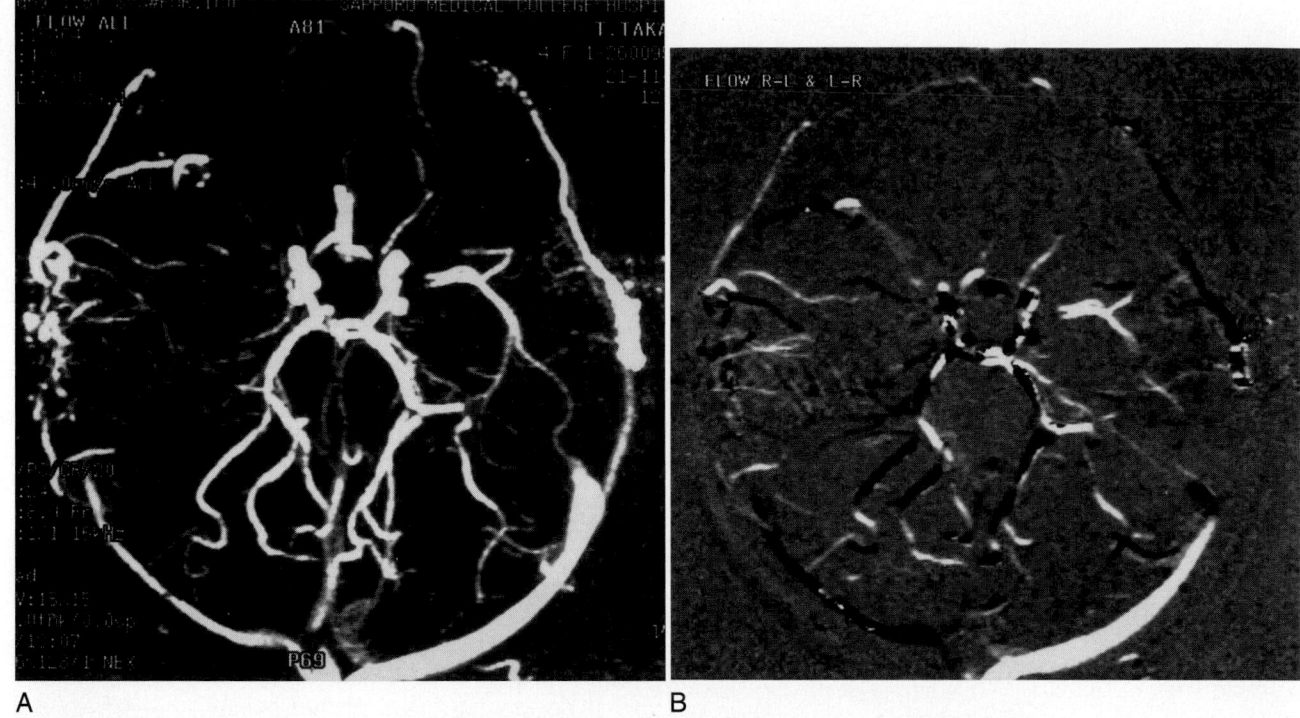

FIGURE 71–13   A, *Magnetic resonance angiogram (MRA) showing neovascularization from the anastomosed superficial temporal artery and the attached muscle 2 years after the operation. B, A phase-resolved MRA for demonstrating the flow direction shows the flow from the superficial temporal artery to the branches of middle cerebral artery. Flow direction from right to left is shown by* white.

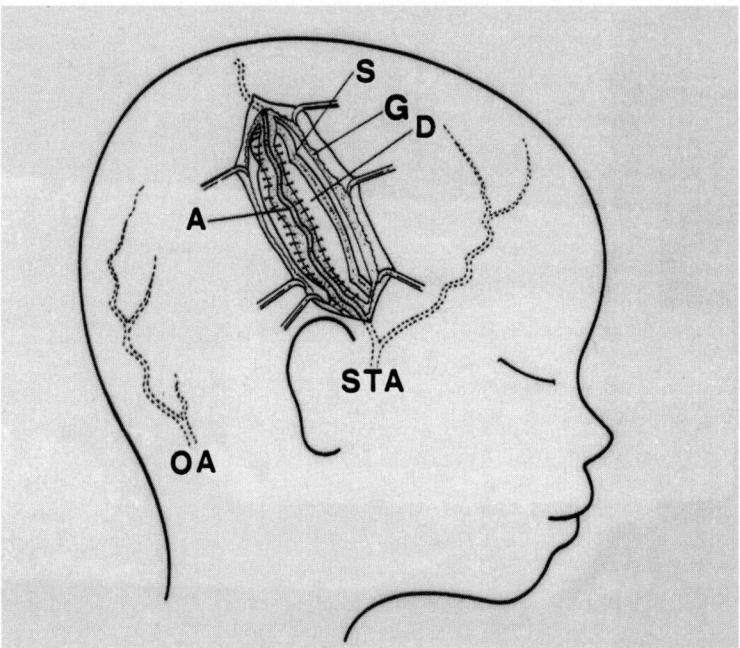

FIGURE 71–14   *Concept of the indirect operation encephaloduroarteriosynangiosis [EDAS]). A, donor scalp artery; D, dura mater; G, galea; OA, occipital artery; S, skull; STA, superficial temporal artery. (From Matsushima Y, Inaba Y: Moyamoya disease in children and its surgical treatment: Introduction of a new surgical procedure and its follow-up angiograms. Childs Brain 11:155, 1984.)*

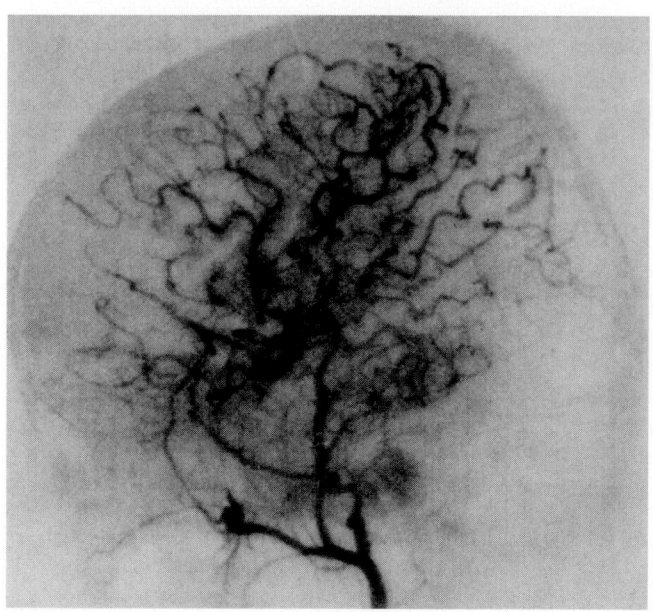

FIGURE 71–15   *Neovascularization observed after encephalo-duroarteriosynangiosis (EDAS). (From Matsushima Y, Inaba Y: Moyamoya disease in children and its surgical treatment: Introduction of a new surgical procedure and its follow-up angiograms. Childs Brain 11:155, 1984.)*

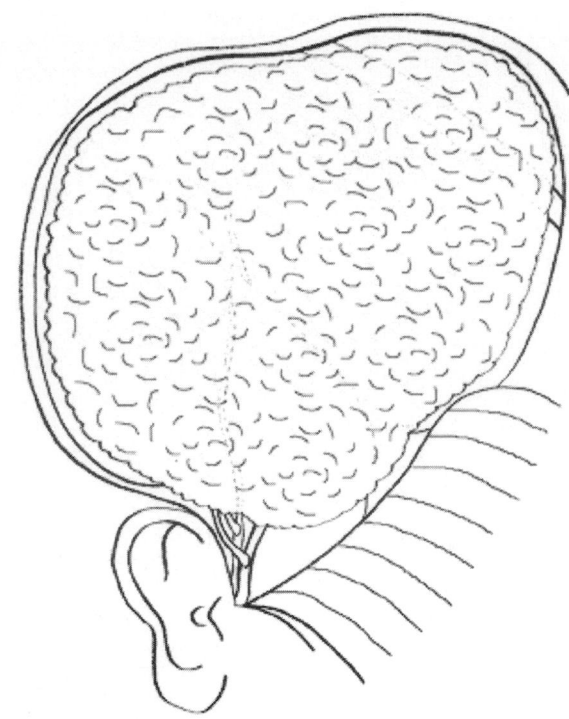

FIGURE 71–16   *Concept of omentum transplantation combined with superficial temporal artery–to–middle cerebral artery (STA-MCA) anastomosis.*

neovascularization, making it a combination of EDAS and EMS. A large frontotemporal craniotomy is made. The STA is stripped away from the scalp with its patency preserved. This STA strip is later placed over the brain, as in EDAS. Two or three linear cuts are made in the dura, and multiple perpendicular cuts are made on each cut edge of the dura to make small, leaflike strips. Branches of the middle meningeal artery are preserved. The arachnoid membrane is incised along the cortical sulci. Then the cut edges of the dura are folded and inserted underneath the dura. The STA is laid on the surface of the brain. The temporal muscle is pulled over the brain surface and loosely sutured to the dura, as in EMS. The bone flap is repositioned and fixed after its lower edge is removed to accommodate the arterial and muscle pedicles.

To enhance neovascularization to the frontal lobe, a small craniotomy at midline of the anterior frontal region may be added in some cases, and through a small dural incision, a galea-periosteal pedicle strip is inserted into the interhemispheric fissure from both sides.[32]

Transplantation of the Omentum

Omental transplantation is a procedure designed to induce prominent neovascularization over a wider area of the brain(Fig. 71–16). It is selected for cases that require such extensive treatment or for which other operations have failed.

A large craniotomy is made; depending on the plan of neovascularization, the craniotomy sometimes includes either frontal lobes or the occipital lobe. The bone flap is made, and the exposed dura is covered with wet gauze until the omentum is ready to be transplanted. The STA and the superficial temporal vein in front of the ear are exposed and prepared for the anastomoses.

The omentum is exposed through a midline laparotomy, and a portion large enough to cover the exposed brain is taken. The surgeon should first confirm that the omental portion is adequately perfused by a vascular loop connected to the large gastroepiploic artery and vein. The gastroepiploic artery of the extirpated omentum is perfused with heparinized blood and saline and is stored wrapped in wet cotton soaked with cooled saline. The abdominal wall is then closed.

The omentum is brought to the craniotomy site, and the gastroepiploic artery and vein are prepared for anastomoses. The gastroepiploic vein is first anastomosed end-to-side to the superficial temporal vein; then the arterial anastomosis is made in the same fashion. Releasing the temporary clips allows confirmation of proper reperfusion of the omentum.

The dura is opened and excised as widely as possible; the arachnoid membrane of the brain surface is incised along the sulci. The omentum is spread over the cortical surface and sutured to the dural edge. The bone flap is loosely fixed if the bulk of omentum is large. If an immediate reperfusion is required, an STA-MCA anastomosis can be performed to an appropriate recipient artery.

The literature on transplantation of the omentum reports induction of good neovascularization over wide areas of the brain (Fig. 71–17), and the prognosis may be better than with other techniques.[28]

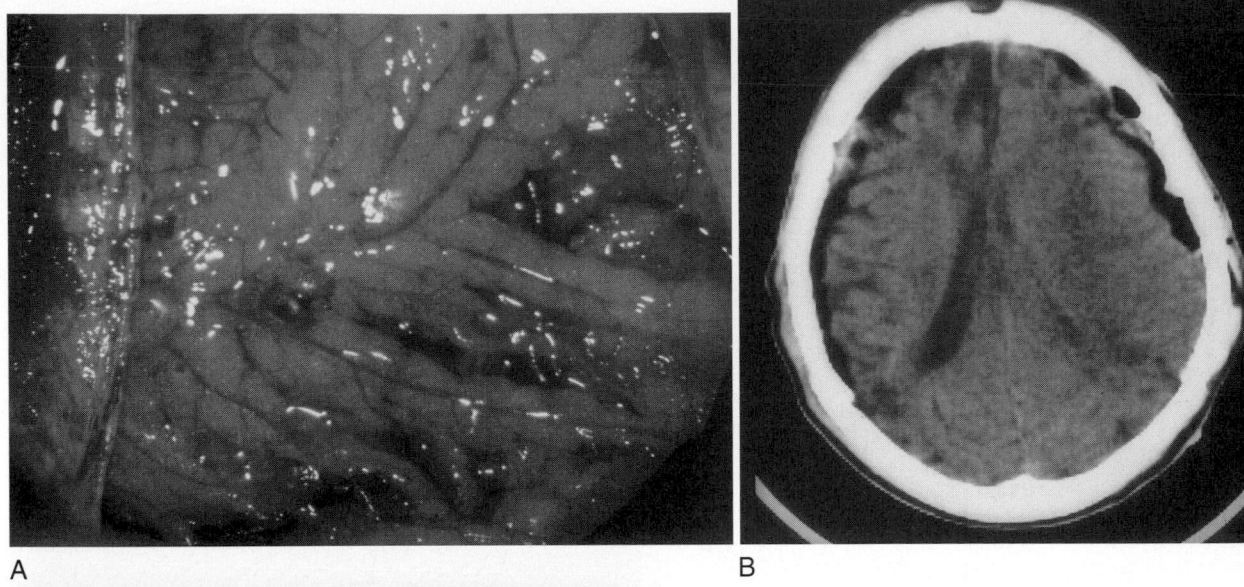

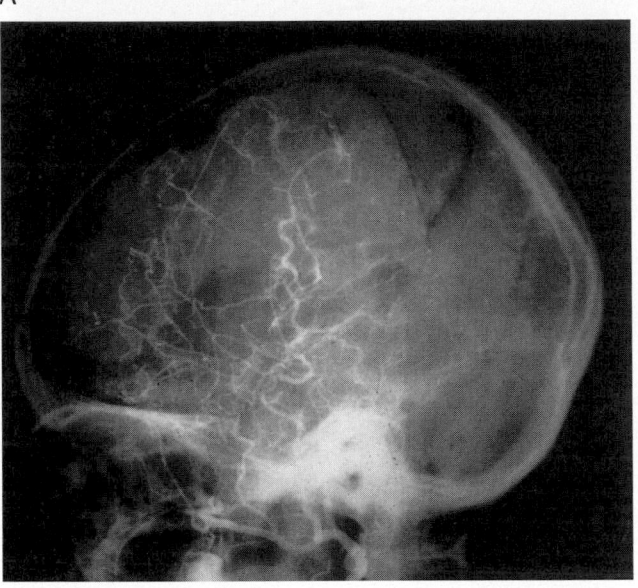

FIGURE 71–17   A, *The brain surface covered by the transplanted omentum.* B, *CT shows omental fat on the brain surface after operation on both sides.* C, *Neovascularization at 1 year after omentum transplantation.*

References

1. Kudo T: Spontaneous occlusion of the circle of Willis: A disease apparently confined to Japanese. Neurology 18:485, 1968.
2. Suzuki J, Takaku A: Cerebrovascular "moyamoya" disease. Disease showing abnormal net-like vessels in base of brain. Arch Neurol 20:288, 1969.
3. Arinami T: Mutation analysis of genes in the moyamoya disease linkage region on chromosome 3p26. In Yoshimoto T (ed): Annual report 2000 of the Research Committee on Spontaneous Occlusion of the Circle of Willis (Moyamoya Disease). Tokyo, Ministry of Health, Labor and Welfare, Japan, 2001, p 61.
4. Fukui M: Current state of study on moyamoya disease in Japan. Surg Neurol 47:138, 1997.
5. Fukuuchi Y, Nogawa S, Yamaguchi K, Dembo T: Follow-up study of registered cases of moyamoya disease in 1999. In Yoshimoto T (ed): Annual Report 2000 of the Research Committee on Spontaneous Occlusion of the Circle of Willis (Moyamoya Disease). Tokyo, Ministry of Health, Labor and Welfare, Japan, 2001, p 7.
6. Yoshimoto T: Guidelines for the diagnosis and the treatment. In Yoshimoto T (ed): Annual Report 2000 of the Research Committee on Spontaneous Occlusion of the Circle of Willis (Moyamoya Disease). Tokyo, Ministry of Health, Labor and Welfare, Japan, 2001, p 73.
7. Suzuki J, Takaku A, Asahi M: Evaluation of a group of disorders showing an abnormal vascular network at the base of the brain with a high incidence among the Japanese. 2 follow-up studies by cerebral angiography. (Japanese) No To Shinkei 18:897, 1966.
8. Takahashi A, Fujiwara S, Suzuki Z: Long-term follow-up angiography of Moyamoya disease: Cases followed up from childhood to adolescence. No Shinkei Geka 14:23–29, 1986.
9. Kawano T, Fukui M, Hashimoto N, et al: Follow-up study of patients with "unilateral" moyamoya disease. Neurol Med Chir (Tokyo) 34:744, 1994.
10. Kawaguchi S, Sakaki T, Morimoto T, et al: Characteristics of intracranial aneurysms associated with moyamoya disease: A review of 111 cases. Acta Neurochir (Wien) 138:1287, 1996.
11. Kurokawa T, Tomita S, Ueda K, et al: Prognosis of occlusive disease of the circle of Willis (moyamoya disease) in children. Pediatr Neurol 1:274, 1985.
12. Kodama N, Aoki Y, Hiraga H, et al: Electroencephalographic findings in children with moyamoya disease. Arch Neurol 36:16–19, 1979.

13. Sasaki T, Sakurai Y, Shimizu Y, et al: Bleeding points in cerebral hemorrhage caused by Moyamoya disease in adults—investigation by CT scan. CT Kenkyu 5:647–655, 1983.
14. Karasawa J, Kikuchi H, Furuse S, et al: Treatment of moyamoya disease with STA-MCA anastomosis. J Neurosurg 49:679, 1978.
15. Karasawa J, Kikuchi H, Furuse S, et al: A surgical treatment of "moyamoya" disease "encephalo-myo-synangiosis." Neurol Med Chir (Tokyo) 17:29, 1977.
16. Matsushima Y, Fukai N, Tanaka K, et al: A new surgical treatment of moyamoya disease in children: A preliminary report. Surg Neurol 15:313, 1981.
17. Kawasawa J, Touho H, Ohnishi H, et al: Long-term follow-up study after extracranial-intracranial bypass surgery for anterior circulation ischemia in childhood moyamoya disease. J Neurosurg 77:84, 1992.
18. Matsushima T, Fukui M, Kitamura K, et al: Encephalo-duro-arterio-synangiosis in children with moyamoya disease. Acta Neurochir (Wien) 104:96, 1990.
19. Isobe M, Kuroda S, Kamiyama H, et al: Cerebral blood flow reactivity to hyperventilation in children with spontaneous occlusion of the circle of Willis (moyamoya disease). No Shinkei Geka 20:399, 1992.
20. Tenjin H, Ueda S: Multiple EDAS (encephalo-duro-arterio-synangiosis): Additional EDAS using the frontal branch of the superficial temporal artery (STA) and the occipital artery for pediatric moyamoya patients in whom EDAS using the parietal branch of STA was insufficient. Childs Nerv Syst 13:220, 1997.
21. Kinugasa K, Mandai S, Kamata I, et al: Surgical treatment of moyamoya disease: Operative technique for encephalo-duro-arterio-myo-synangiosis, its follow-up, clinical results, and angiograms. Neurosurgery 32:527, 1993.
22. Balagura S, Farris WA: Treatment of moyamoya disease by cerebroarteriosynangiosis. Surg Neurol 23:270, 1985.
23. Fukui M, Kawano T: Follow-up study of registered cases in 1995. In Fukui M (ed): Annual Report 1995 of the Research Committee on Spontaneous Occlusion of the Circle of Willis (Moyamoya Disease). Tokyo, Ministry of Health and Welfare, Japan, 1996, p 12.
24. Matsushima T, Inoue T, Suzuki SO, et al: Surgical treatment of moyamoya disease in pediatric patients—comparison between the results of indirect and direct revascularization procedures. Neurosurgery 31:401, 1992.
25. Ikezaki K, Matsushima T, Kuwabara Y, et al: Cerebral circulation and oxygen metabolism in childhood moyamoya disease: A perioperative positron emission tomography study. J Neurosurg 81:843, 1994.
26. Nakase H, Ohnishi H, Touho H, et al: Long-term follow-up study of "epileptic type" moyamoya disease in children. Neurol Med Chir (Tokyo) 33:621, 1993.
27. Karasawa J, Kikuchi H, Kawamura J, et al: Intracranial transplantation of the omentum for cerebrovascular moyamoya disease: A two-year follow-up study. Surg Neurol 14:444, 1980.
28. Ohtaki M, Uede T, Morimoto S, et al: Intellectual functions and regional cerebral haemodynamics after extensive omental transplantation spread over both frontal lobes in childhood moyamoya disease. Acta Neurochir (Wien) 140:1043, 1998.
29. Iwama T, Hashimoto N, Miyake H, et al: Direct revascularization to the anterior cerebral artery territory in patients with moyamoya disease: Report of five cases. Neurosurgery 42:1157, 1998.
30. Kawaguchi T, Fujita S, Hosoda K, et al: Multiple burr-hole operation for adult moyamoya disease. J Neurosurg 84:468, 1996.
31. Endo M, Kawano N, Miyasaka Y, et al: Cranial burr hole for revascularization in moyamoya disease. J Neurosurg 71:180, 1989.
32. Kinugasa K, Mandai S, Tokunaga K, et al: Ribbon encephalo-duro-arterio-myo-synangiosis for moyamoya disease. Surg Neurol 41:455, 1994.
33. Kawaguchi S, Okuno S, Sakaki T: Effect of direct arterial bypass on the prevention of future stroke in patients with the hemorrhagic variety of moyamoya disease. J Neurosurg 93:397, 2000.
34. Miyamoto S: Study on the management of moyamoya disease with hemorrhagic onset. In Yoshimoto T (ed): Annual report 2000 of the Research Committee on Spontaneous Occlusion of the Circle of Willis (Moyamoya Disease). Tokyo, Ministry of Health, Labor and Welfare, Japan, 2001, p 59.
35. Matsushima Y, Inaba Y: Moyamoya disease in children and its surgical treatment: Introduction of a new surgical procedure and its follow-up angiograms. Childs Brain 11:155, 1984.
36. Matsushima Y, Suzuki R, Ohno K, et al: Angiographic revascularization of the brain after encephaloduroarteriosynangiosis: A case report. Neurosurgery 21:928, 1987.

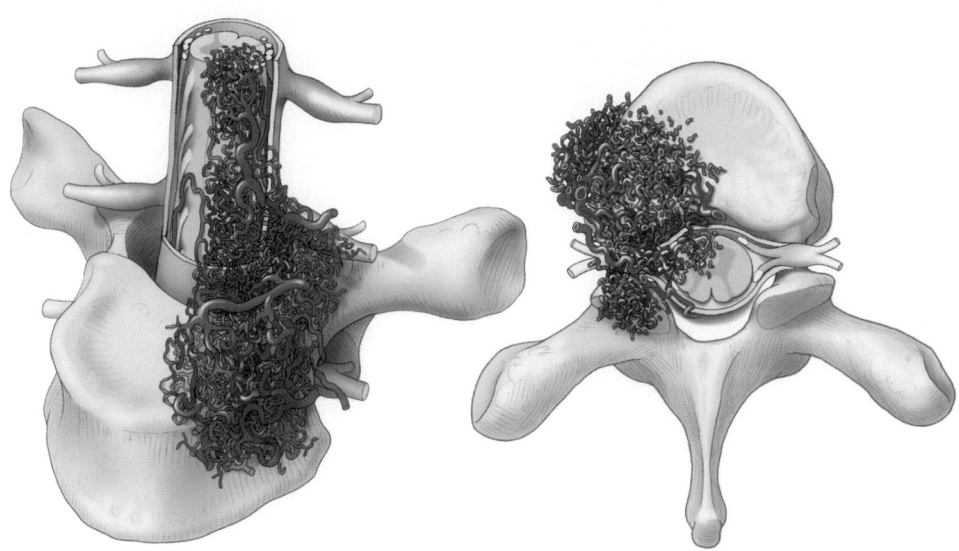

PLATE 72–1 *Intradural-extradural spinal arteriovenous malformation (AVM) is depicted here. Concomitant involvement of adjacent bone and soft tissues is the classic description of this type of AVM. (From Spetzler RF, Detwiler PW, Riina HA, Porter RW: Modified classification of spinal cord lesions. J Neurosurg 96[Suppl]:145–156, 2002.)*

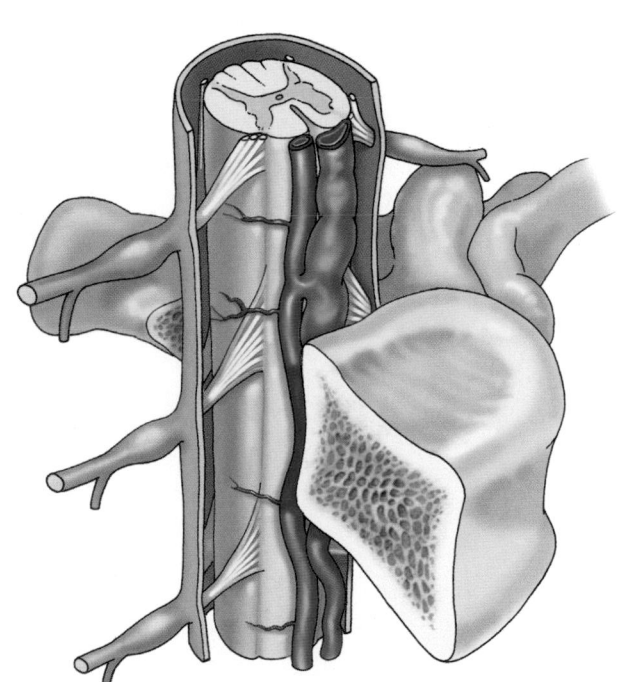

PLATE 72–2 *Drawing of an intradural ventral arteriovenous fistula. The fistula usually arises between the anterior spinal artery and the ventral coronal venous plexus. With permission from Barrow Neurological Institute. (From Spetzler RF, Koos WT [eds] [with contributions from Richling B]: Color Atlas of Microneurosurgery, 2nd ed, Vol III: Cerebral Revascularization, Extracranial Vascular Disease, and Intraspinal Pathology. Stuttgart, George Thieme Verlag, 1999.)297–305, 2001.)*

Chapter Seventy-Two

Spinal Arteriovenous Malformations

Howard A. Riina, G. Michael Lemole, Jr., Louis J. Kim,
and Robert F. Spetzler

Spinal vascular malformations represent a group of complex lesions that often pose both diagnostic and treatment difficulties for neurologists, neurosurgeons, and endovascular surgeons. Advances in imaging modalities and in the design of microcatheters and micro-guidewires combined with improvements in microneurosurgical technique have enhanced our ability to treat these lesions. A multidisciplinary approach to lesions previously thought untreatable can now lead to their complete obliteration. Successful diagnosis and treatment depend on a thorough understanding of the pathophysiology and anatomy of vascular lesions and how they affect the spinal cord. This chapter reviews the diagnosis and treatment of vascular lesions affecting the spinal cord and organizes them into a classification scheme based on the experiences of the senior author (RFS).

Vascular malformations affecting the spinal cord can be divided into three main groups: (1) neoplastic lesions, (2) arteriovenous malformations (AVMs) and arteriovenous fistulas (AVFs), and (3) spinal aneurysms. These three groups form the basis of the modified classification scheme for spinal vascular malformations.[1]

NEOPLASTIC LESIONS AFFECTING THE SPINAL CORD

Neoplastic vascular lesions affecting the spinal cord consist of hemangioblastomas and cavernous malformations. Cavernous malformations are included in this group because they are associated with a known chromosomal derangement, grow exponentially, display familial inheritance, and hence exhibit neoplastic behavioral characteristics.[2–4] Cavernous malformations have also been described as arising de novo in individuals who received irradiation for spinal tumors.[5]

Hemangioblastomas are vascular neoplastic lesions that can affect the spinal cord. They can be so highly vascular that they contain AV shunts and mimic AVMs. In addition to this intense vascularity, the engorged vasculature and often-associated tumor cyst can cause considerable mass effect, leading to spinal cord compression and myelopathy.

Hemangioblastomas are also associated with a chromosomal abnormality and can be observed in a familial inheritance pattern as in the case of von Hippel–Lindau disease.[6]

Both lesions can be diagnosed with conventional magnetic resonance (MRI) with and without gadolinium contrast enhancement. Cavernous malformations and hemangioblastomas have a component that enhances brightly. Cavernous malformations can range from small to large lesions that displace much of the spinal cord parenchyma. Because of their propensity to leak blood products, they are often surrounded by a hemosiderin ring. Combined with their grapelike configuration, this ring often creates a "popcorn"-type appearance on MRI. The hemosiderin ring or halo surrounding the malformation is caused by the imaging characteristics of methemoglobin (Fig. 72–1).[4,7]

The natural history of cavernous malformations is one of bleeding or leaking associated with a period of neurologic decline followed by a period of recovery that never really returns the patient to neurologic normality. In this manner, repeated hemorrhages often cause a significant loss of function over time.

The treatment of cavernous malformations that have bled significantly or repeatedly is microneurosurgical resection. A cavernous malformation that abuts the pial surface or whose hematoma cavity provides a pathway for resection can be managed in this manner. There is no role for radiation therapy in the treatment of cavernous malformations. Furthermore, spinal angiography and embolization also have no role because cavernous malformations are angiographically occult. Cavernous malformations cannot be appreciated on angiography, but the often-associated venous anomaly might be. Care must be exerted at surgery to preserve the developmental venous anomaly, which drains normal tissue. Its loss could result in venous infarction. As many as 20% of patients harbor more than one cavernous malformation and may present after hemorrhage from a second lesion.[8,9]

Hemangioblastomas can commonly be diagnosed with a degree of certainty with the use of MRI. An enhancing mass with a cystic component, spinal syrinx, and surrounding vascular flow voids is highly suspicious for

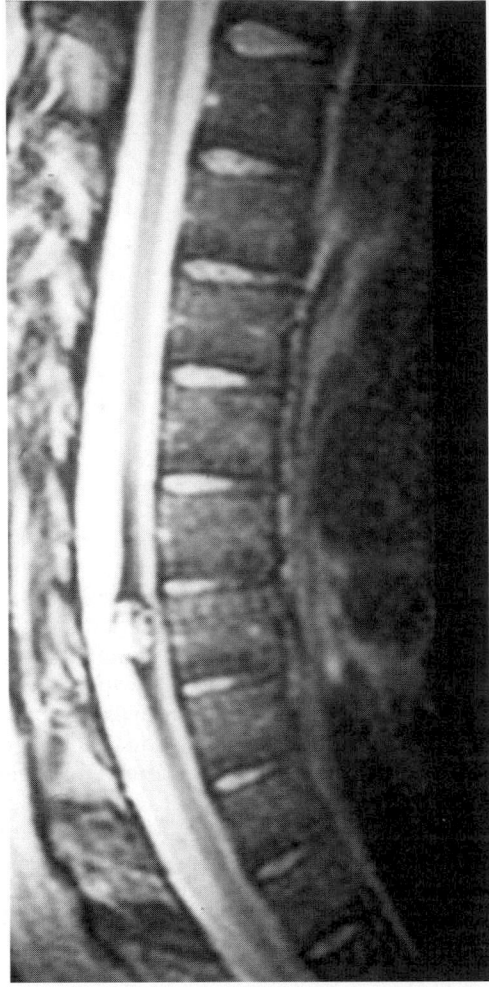

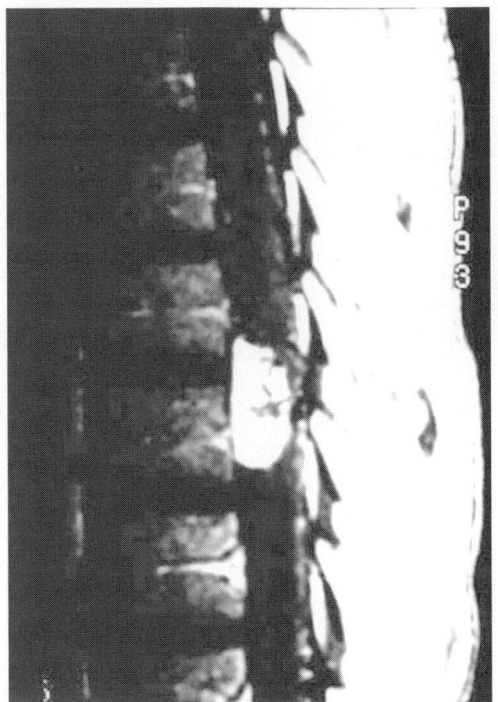

FIGURE 72–2   *Sagittal T1-weighted MR image with gadolinium enhancement demonstrates a homogeneous, brightly enhancing spinal cord hemangioblastoma.*

FIGURE 72–1   *Sagittal T2-weighted MR image of a thoracic intramedullary spinal cord cavernous malformation. Note the significant degree of hemosiderin staining both rostral and caudal to the lesion. The cavernoma itself is heterogeneous in signal characteristics, indicative of prior hemorrhages. These entities usually exhibit minimal or no contrast enhancement and are angiographically occult. (With permission from the Barrow Neurological Institute.)*

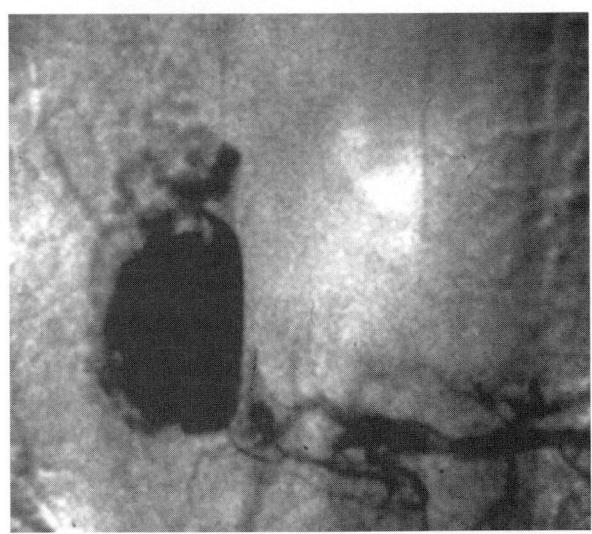

FIGURE 72–3   *Spinal angiogram of the same lesion shown in Figure 72–2 reveals the considerable vascular composition of hemangioblastomas.*

hemangioblastoma (Fig. 72–2).[10–12] Spinal angiography reveals a highly vascular lesion complete with AV shunting mimicking an AVM (Fig. 72–3). If the blood supply to the tumor does not incorporate the anterior spinal artery, preoperative embolization can be performed. Embolization serves to decrease the vascularity of the tumor, facilitating its safe removal. The basis of treatment is therefore microneurosurgical resection after preoperative spinal angiography and preoperative embolization when they can be safely performed.

SPINAL ARTERIOVENOUS LESIONS

Arteriovenous lesions affecting the spinal cord can be divided into AVMs and AVFs.[13] Previous classification schemes have been complicated and confusing. The classification used here is designed to facilitate communication about these lesions and their diagnosis and treatment. AVMs can be either intradural or intradural-extradural. Intradural AVMs are further subdivided into intramedullary, intramedullary-extramedullary, and arteriovenous lesions that affect the conus medullaris. Alternatively, AVFs can be either intradural or extradural; intradural lesions are located either dorsally or ventrally.

Dural-based fistulas have not been observed in the pediatric population.

Intradural-Extradural Arteriovenous Malformations

Intradural-extradural AVMs are vascular malformations that can affect the spinal cord as well as its surrounding tissues. More than a single tissue type is usually affected, and the malformation can include an entire metamere (Plate 72–1). Complete involvement of an entire metamere, including skin, soft tissue, bone, and spinal cord parenchyma, is referred to as *Cobb's syndrome*.[14] Cobb's syndrome represents the full manifestation of the intradural-extradural type of AVM. The old name for these lesions was juvenile or metameric AVMs. As this old name implies, they tend to be more common in children, but they have also been reported in adults.

These highly vascular lesions consist of an extradural component, including part of the vertebral column, surrounding soft tissue, and an intradural component that affects the spinal cord. Spinal angiography delineates the angioarchitecture and clarifies the local vascular anatomy, which must be appreciated before one can proceed with treatment. Therapy consists of a multidisciplinary approach and often begins with endovascular treatment in the form of embolization. Preoperative embolization is usually followed by microneurosurgical resection. Complete obliteration is rare because of extensive tissue involvement.

Intradural Arteriovenous Malformations

Intradural AVMs can be separated into intramedullary lesions, intramedullary-extramedullary lesions, and arteriovenous lesions affecting the conus medullaris.[13] Intramedullary malformations are further subdivided into those with a compact nidus and those with a diffuse nidus.

Intramedullary Lesions

Intramedullary AVMs involve the substance of the spinal cord (Fig. 72–4A). They can be described as being pial, abutting the pial surface, or completely subpial. As mentioned, their nidus can be either diffuse or compact. The type of nidus has significant implications for the success of treatment. Malformations with a focal, compact nidus are more amenable to both embolization and surgical excision (Fig. 72–4B and C). Alternatively, a lesion with a diffuse nidus may be more difficult to embolize safely and effectively. Surgical excision is also more difficult, and repeated operations are often required to achieve successful obliteration. Intramedullary lesions are both high-pressure and high-flow types of malformations. They often become symptomatic from hemorrhage or a compressive myelopathy related to engorged vascular structures. Vascular steal can cause a vascular ischemic myelopathy.

Patients presenting with a spinal cord hemorrhage or myelopathy usually undergo MRI as the initial diagnostic study. Flow voids and dilated vascular structures in addition to any changes seen in the spinal cord itself all suggest a spinal AV-type of malformation. When large enough, these dilated vascular structures can be seen compressing the spinal cord. MRI is followed by spinal angiography, which remains the study of choice for delineating the angioarchitecture of a lesion. This modality allows final diagnosis and suggests a treatment path.

Treatment of an intramedullary AVM can consist of embolization and microneurosurgical resection. Embolization can be performed at the time of spinal angiography to decrease the risk of a second procedure and to facilitate treatment. Surgery then follows embolization within 24 to 48 hours. Postoperative spinal angiography is needed to determine whether complete obliteration has been achieved or residual malformation requires further treatment. Repeat or staged resection is common.

Arteriovenous Malformations Affecting the Conus Medullaris

AVMs affecting the conus medullaris are defined by their predilection for the conus medullaris and cauda equina regions of the spinal cord. We have observed them to extend along the length of the filum terminale. These malformations are characterized by a pattern of complex venous drainage, multiple niduses, and AV shunting through anterior spinal and posterior spinal arterial feeders. The niduses tend to be pial rather than subpial. This location makes them more extramedullary in their behavior.

The patient with AVMs affecting the conus medullaris presents with a complex myeloradiculopathy. The myelopathy is caused by vascular compression of the conus medullaris, but venous hypertension can also contribute to the patient's neurologic deterioration. Involvement of the cauda equina causes radicular symptoms that can dominate the clinical presentation. As with the other vascular malformations of the spine, diagnosis begins with MRI followed by spinal angiography. In select cases, the patient may be a candidate for spinal embolization, which is then followed by microneurosurgical resection. Despite aggressive treatment, these complex lesions tend to recur.

Arteriovenous Fistulas of the Spinal Cord

AVFs are subdivided into intradural and extradural types.[13,15] The intradural fistulas can be further separated into dorsally and ventrally located lesions. Intradural AVFs are the most common type of fistulas described in the literature. They are most commonly observed in the thoracic spine and manifest secondary to venous hypertension (Fig. 72–5A). Spinal angiography shows a low-flow fistula that enters at the level of the nerve root sleeve (Fig. 72–5B). Fistulas with a single feeder are referred to as type A fistulas, and those with multiple feeders are as type B. Venous hypertension due to the AVF fistula causes a clinical picture of myelopathy that can be confused with neurogenic claudication. Most patients experience a continuous and progressive neurologic decline until the fistula is interrupted.

Intradural ventrally located fistulas are subdivided into types A, B, and C (Plate 72–2 and Fig. 72–6). Type A fistulas have slow flow and manifest secondary to venous hypertension, much like the dorsal-type fistulas. Types B and C are characterized by progressively larger shunts and become symptomatic secondary to vascular steal and compression. Diagnosis begins with MRI, which is followed by spinal angiography. For many years, the basis of treatment

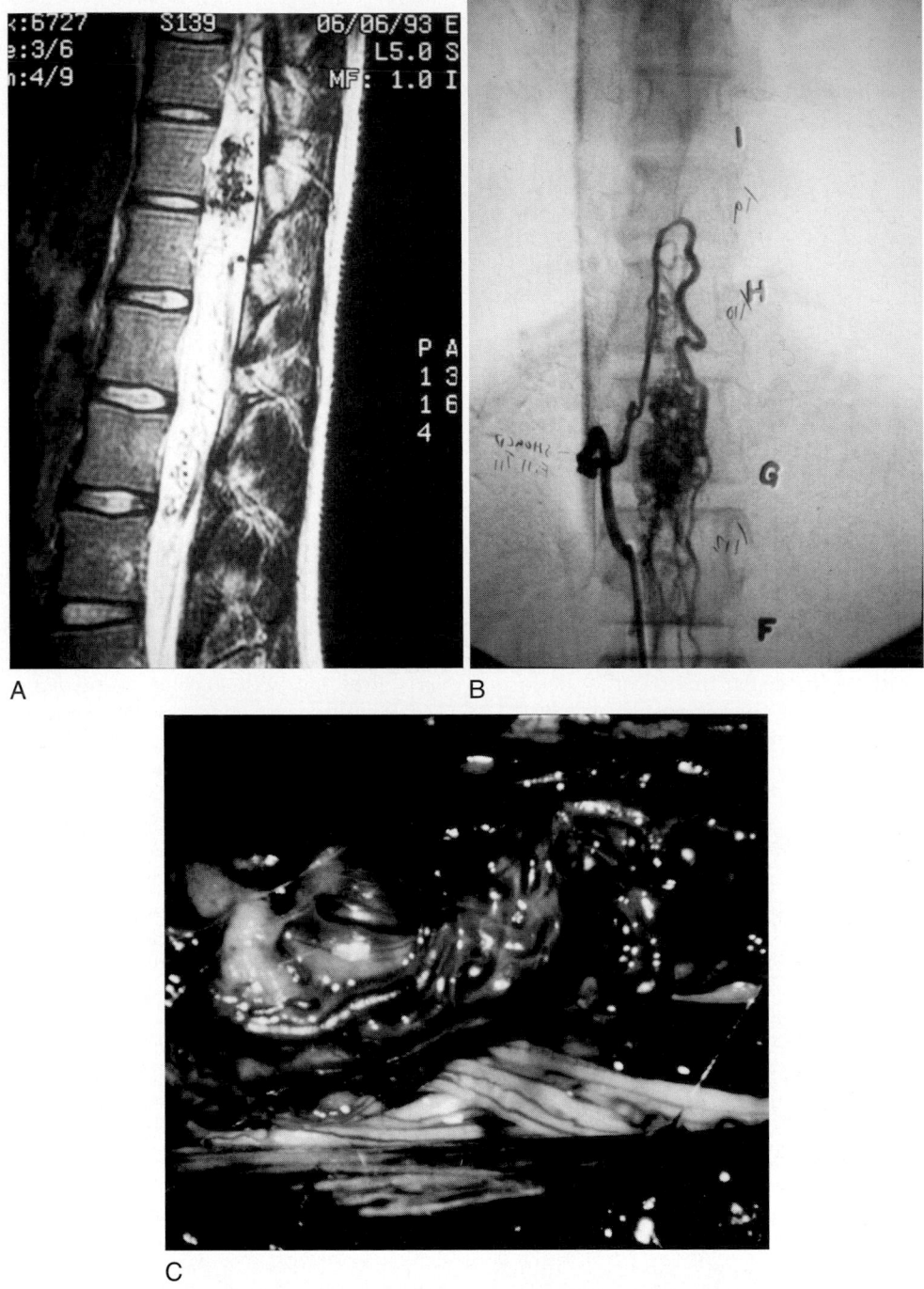

FIGURE 72–4   *A, Sagittal T2-weighted MR image of a compact, intramedullary spinal arteriovenous malformation. Numerous flow voids are evident. B, Spinal angiogram characterizes the complex angioarchitecture of the lesion. C, Intraoperative photograph shows the engorged venous system and large feeding arteries. The potential for vascular steal and spinal cord compression from mass effect is evident. (From Spetzler RF, Koos WT [eds] [with contributions from Richling B]: Color Atlas of Microneurosurgery, 2nd ed, Vol III: Cerebral Revascularization, Extracranial Vascular Disease, and Intraspinal Pathology. Stuttgart, George Thieme Verlag, 1999.)*

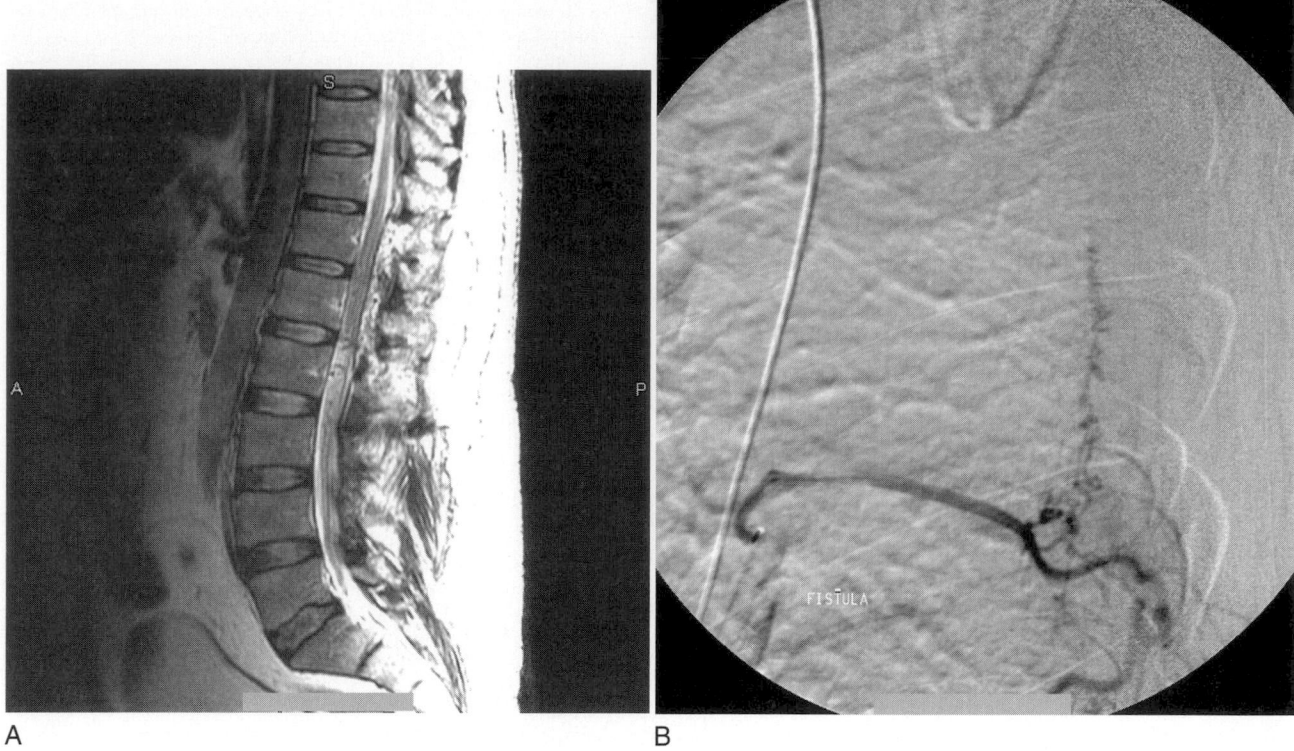

A   B

FIGURE 72–5 A, *MR image of an intradural dorsal arteriovenous fistula (AVF). The flow voids visible reflect the arterialized spinal venous plexus. B, Spinal angiogram of another patient with an intradural dorsal AVF reveals a single fistulous connection from a radicular artery to the venous plexus.*

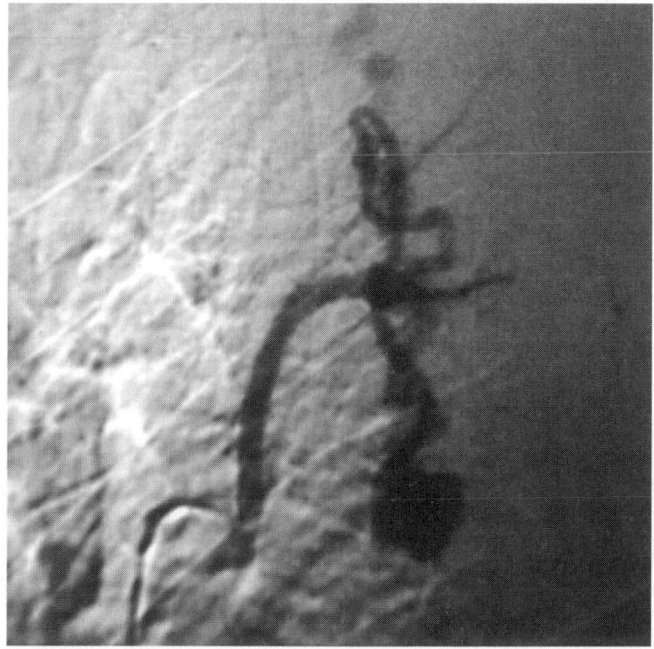

FIGURE 72–6 *Spinal angiogram demonstrates the intradural fistula. (From Spetzler RF, Koos WT [eds] [with contributions from Richling B]: Color Atlas of Microneurosurgery, 2nd ed, Vol III: Cerebral Revascularization, Extracranial Vascular Disease, and Intraspinal Pathology. Stuttgart, George Thieme Verlag, 1999.)*

was microneurosurgical resection alone. Advances in endovascular techniques now allow the endovascular obliteration of select fistulas. Elimination of the fistula leads to an arrest of the patient's neurologic decline, often followed by dramatic neurologic improvement.

SPINAL CORD ANEURYSMS

Aneurysmal lesions affecting the vasculature of the spinal cord are extremely rare. Like aneurysms located in other areas, they develop from a combination of local vessel wall injury and high-flow turbulent states.[16,17] Patients may present with subarachnoid hemorrhage and the onset of radicular symptoms. Diagnosis is confirmed with spinal angiography, and treatment consists of either microneurosurgery or embolization.

DIAGNOSTIC IMAGING

All patients suspected of harboring a spinal vascular malformation should undergo MRI of the spine, both with and without contrast enhancement. Lesions with a significant vascular supply often have dilated vascular structures that can be appreciated on MRI. These serpiginous structures appear as flow voids in and around the spinal cord.[18,19] Mass lesions, such as hemangioblastomas, large cavernous malformations, and large AVMs, can be clearly delineated on MRI.[18–20] Diagnosis can also be made on the basis of MRI alone, but a definitive diagnosis requires spinal angiography. Spinal angiography confirms the diagnosis, defines the angioarchitecture, and often provides an opportunity for spinal embolization either as a preoperative treatment or as definitive therapy. Spinal embolization is part of a pretreatment strategy for hemangioblastomas and many types of AVMs and AVFs. During endovascular procedures, care must be exerted to preserve the anterior spinal artery, injury to which can have catastrophic consequences.

CONCLUSION

Vascular malformations affecting the spinal cord and surrounding tissues are complex lesions that are often difficult to diagnose and treat. Advances in diagnostic imaging, endovascular techniques, and microneurosurgery have made previously unresectable lesions treatable with good outcomes. Despite such advances, these lesions must be treated cautiously to prevent further defects in often neurologically compromised patients. MRI and spinal angiography contribute extensively to our understanding of the vascular anatomy of these lesions and how they relate to the normal neurologic structures of the spinal cord. Only with a thorough understanding of the lesions can surgeons proceed safely with their treatment. Many complex lesions require multiple procedures, often staged, to achieve the desired goals of control and obliteration.

References

1. Spetzler RF, Riina HA, Detwiler PW, et al: Modified classification of spinal cord lesions. J Neurosurg 96(Suppl):145, 2002.
2. Anson JA, Spetzler RF: Surgical resection of intramedullary spinal cord cavernous malformations. J Neurosurg 78:446, 1993.
3. Malis LI: Intramedullary spinal cord tumors. Clin Neurosurg 25:512, 1978.
4. Rutka JT, Brant-Zawadzki M, Wilson CB, et al: Familial cavernous malformations: Diagnostic potential of magnetic resonance imaging. Surg Neurol 29:467, 1988.
5. Maraire JN, Abdulrauf SI, Berger S, et al: De novo development of a cavernous malformation of the spinal cord following spinal axis radiation: Case report. J Neurosurg 90(Suppl):234, 1999.
6. Ismail SM, Cole G: von Hippel-Lindau syndrome with microscopic hemangioblastomas of the spinal nerve roots. J Neurosurg 60:1279, 1984.
7. Furuya K, Sasaki T, Suzuki I, et al: Intramedullary angiographically occult vascular malformations of the spinal cord. Neurosurgery 39:1123, 1996.
8. Cosgrove GR, Bertrand G, Fontaine S, et al: Cavernous angiomas of the spinal cord. J Neurosurg 68:31, 1988.
9. McCormick PC, Michelsen WJ, Post KD, et al: Cavernous malformations of the spinal cord. Neurosurgery 23:459, 1988.
10. Browne TR, Adams RD, Roberson GH: Hemangioblastoma of the spinal cord: Review and report of five cases. Arch Neurol 33:435, 1976.
11. Enomoto H, Shibata T, Ito A, et al: Multiple hemangioblastomas accompanied by syringomyelia in the cerebellum and the spinal cord. Surg Neurol 22:197, 1984.
12. Fox JL, Bashir R, Jinkins JR, et al: Syrinx of the conus medullaris and filum terminale in association with multiple hemangioblastomas. Surg Neurol 24:265, 1985.
13. Anson JA, Spetzler RF: Classification of spinal arteriovenous malformations and implications for treatment. BNI Q 8:2, 1992.
14. Mercer RD, Rothner AD, Cook SA, et al: The Cobb syndrome: Association with hereditary cutaneous hemangiomas. Cleveland Clin Q 45:237, 1978.
15. Gueguen B, Merland JJ, Riche MC, et al: Vascular malformations of the spinal cord: Intrathecal perimedullary arteriovenous fistulas fed by medullary arteries. Neurology 37:969, 1987.
16. Smith BS, Penka CF, Erickson LS, et al: Case report: Subarachnoid hemorrhage due to anterior spinal artery aneurysm. Neurosurgery 18:217, 1986.
17. Vishteh AG, Brown AP, Spetzler RF: Aneurysm of the intradural artery of Adamkiewicz treated with muslin wrapping: Technical case report. Neurosurgery 40:207, 1997.
18. Doppman JL, Di Chiro G, Dwyer AJ, et al: Magnetic resonance imaging of spinal arteriovenous malformations. J Neurosurg 66:830, 1987.
19. Dormont D, Gelbert F, Assouline E, et al: MR imaging of spinal cord arteriovenous malformations at 0.5 T: Study of 34 cases. AJNR Am J Neuroradiol 9:833, 1988.
20. Friedman DP, Flanders AE, Tartaglino LM: Vascular neoplasms and malformations, ischemia, and hemorrhage affecting the spinal cord: MR imaging findings. AJR Am J Roentgenol 162:685, 1994.

Chapter Seventy-Three

Cerebral Vasospasm

R. Loch Macdonald

Clinical reports describing the natural history of patients who in all likelihood had aneurysmal subarachnoid hemorrhage (SAH) and cerebral vasospasm can be found in the literature beginning in the early part of the last century.[1] Ecker and Riemenschneider[2] described, to a skeptical medical community, angiographic arterial narrowing, generally near the site of an aneurysm that had ruptured within 26 days of the angiogram. Since this description 50 years ago, vasospasm has been an important cause of morbidity and mortality in patients who survive the initial SAH. Calcium channel blockers, hemodynamic management, and endovascular therapies for vasospasm have reduced the effect of vasospasm on outcome, although it remains a significant prognostic factor for poor outcome after aneurysmal SAH.

Cerebral vasospasm is defined as reversible narrowing of the intradural subarachnoid arteries that occurs several days after SAH and lasts for days. Other causes of arterial narrowing may mimic cerebral vasospasm, including some that also are a transient constriction of cerebral arteries. The etiology and pathogenesis of vasospasm after SAH, however, are distinct from those of many of the other causes of narrowing of cerebral arteries. *Vasospasm* can refer to the radiologic observation of arterial narrowing (angiographic vasospasm) or to the neurologic deficits attributable to it (symptomatic or clinical vasospasm, delayed cerebral ischemia, or delayed ischemic neurologic deficit).

EPIDEMIOLOGY

Vasospasm can occur after any condition that deposits blood in the subarachnoid space. The arteries that traverse the blood-filled cerebrospinal fluid (CSF) are probably the most affected by vasospasm. Vasospasm occurs after SAH due most commonly to a ruptured aneurysm, which is the most common situation in which there is substantial bleeding into the basal cisterns. However, vasospasm can also develop after rupture of brain vascular malformations, trauma, and hemorrhage associated with surgery in the basal cisterns.[1] Angiographic arterial narrowing has been reported in tuberculous and purulent meningitis, ophthalmoplegic migraine, hypertensive encephalopathy, arteriolar embolization or removal of an embolus from the middle cerebral artery, myelography, electroconvulsive therapy,

and eclampsia as well as in association with unruptured and sometimes unoperated aneurysms. In these conditions not associated with SAH, the time course, etiology, pathology, and pathogenesis of vasospasm probably differ from those of SAH-induced vasospasm.[1]

Vasospasm after SAH begins to appear 3 to 4 days after a single hemorrhage, reaches its maximum incidence and severity between 6 and 8 days, and usually resolves by 12 to 14 days, although it can be seen later.[3] The frequency with which angiographic vasospasm is observed after SAH depends on when angiography is conducted and on other factors that are known to influence the development of vasospasm, chiefly the quantity, density, and persistence of SAH. Severe vasospasm (>50% reduction in arterial diameter) was demonstrated in 23% to 30% of patients receiving placebo in three clinical trials of aneurysmal SAH.[4-6] Dorsch and King,[7] reviewing the world literature published after 1960 for data on angiographic vasospasm, found that angiography performed during the second week after SAH demonstrated vasospasm in 67% of 2738 patients.

Vasospasm produces clinical symptoms and signs chiefly via hemodynamic mechanisms. Whether or not angiographic vasospasm becomes clinically evident therefore depends on (1) the length and severity of the arterial narrowing, (2) other factors that influence cerebral blood flow (CBF), such as blood pressure, intracranial pressure (ICP), blood volume, cardiac output, viscosity, and collateral and anastomotic blood supply, and (3) brain metabolic demand, which is influenced by temperature, seizures, and drugs. In general, symptoms and signs do not develop unless angiography demonstrates a reduction in vessel diameter greater than 50%.

The clinical syndrome due to vasospasm is described as *clinical* or *symptomatic vasospasm* or *delayed ischemic neurologic deficit* or *delayed cerebral ischemia*. The peak day of onset is 8 days after SAH, 1 day later than the peak of angiographic vasospasm. Twenty-eight percent of 3521 patients entered into a cooperative study between 1980 and 1983 had delayed cerebral ischemia.[8] The vast majority were not treated with nimodipine or hemodynamic therapy. A review of 297 publications found delayed ischemic neurologic deficits in 10,445 (32%) of 32,188 patients.[7] Thirty-four percent of 1500 patients in the placebo arms of 5 prospective studies of tirilazad experienced clinical vasospasm.[5,6,9,10]

Symptomatic vasospasm does not progress to infarction in all cases. Development of infarction due to other consequences of SAH makes it difficult to ascertain the risk of infarction specifically from vasospasm. In one study, infarction was observed on computed tomography (CT) scan 3 months after SAH in 51% of patients treated with placebo and in 48% treated with nicardipine.[11] Thirty-one percent of 902 patients entered into a randomized trial within 48 hours of SAH had CT evidence of cerebral infarction by 14 days after SAH.[5]

PATHOLOGY AND PATHOPHYSIOLOGY

Pathology

Vasospastic arteries are constricted or contracted. Platelet aggregates, microthrombi, or both may be present intraluminally. Arterial thrombosis or distal embolization is probably possible, raising the unanswered question whether antiplatelet agents might be of benefit in this condition.[12] The pathologic features are those of arterial contraction, principally constriction of the smooth muscle cells. After 10 to 12 days, as the angiographic phase of vasospasm resolves, arterial fibrosis and proliferation of myointimal cells and extracellular matrix in the tunica intima may be observed.[13]

Vasospasm affects predominantly the large intradural arteries of the circle of Willis. There is no evidence that veins are affected. Vasospasm of small, intraparenchymal arteries has been postulated to occur after SAH, although evidence for this theory comes mainly from controversial positron emission tomography (PET) and CBF studies.[14,15]

SAH is associated with reductions in global CBF and cerebral metabolic rate for oxygen that are more severe with worsening clinical grade. Vasospasm produces a second, additional reduction in CBF in the territories of the vasospastic arteries, and the reductions may be regional, global, or both, depending on the distribution of the vasospasm.[1,16,17] Autoregulation of CBF in response to alterations in cerebral perfusion pressure may be impaired after SAH, even with good clinical grades. The control is not lost in an all-or-none fashion but tends to be progressively impaired with worsening clinical grade and during the time of peak angiographic vasospasm.[16,18] The response of CBF to changes in arterial carbon dioxide is not lost as easily as pressure autoregulation but may be impaired in patients with severe vasospasm.[16]

Pathogenesis

The etiology of vasospasm after SAH is the subarachnoid blood clot itself. Changes in ICP and the tear itself in the aneurysm do not contribute to vasospasm. The most robust predictors of vasospasm are the volume, density, and prolonged presence of subarachnoid blood, usually as observed on CT scan, around the arteries that develop vasospasm (Fig. 73–1).[19–21] Vasospasm can be reproduced experimentally in animals by placement of autologous blood clot next to the cerebral arteries or by injection of adequate amounts of blood into the CSF in the absence of arterial rupture or increased ICP.[1,22,23]

Fractionating the blood placed in the CSF demonstrated repeatedly that erythrocytes are necessary for vasospasm to develop and that hemoglobin within the erythrocytes is an important cause of vasospasm.[24,25] Other components of the erythrocyte and the blood may also contribute. The mechanism by which erythrocyte cytosol and hemoglobin cause vasospasm is uncertain. The key mechanism, however, appears to be a sustained contraction of arterial smooth muscle cells, particularly during the initial peak phase of vasospasm. The ability to reverse vasospasm with selective injection of papaverine into the narrowed arteries suggests that the underlying phenomenon is smooth muscle contraction, although the extent of pharmacologic reversibility decreases with time.[26] The contraction may be due to a variety of interacting pathologic processes, including (1) free radical reactions, (2) alteration in the balance between vasodilator and vasoconstrictor substances normally produced in the arterial wall, such as prostacyclin, nitric oxide, endothelins, and eicosanoids, (3) injury to perivascular nerves, and (4) detrimental effects of the inflammatory reaction induced by SAH.

CLINICAL DIAGNOSIS

Delayed ischemic neurologic deficits due to vasospasm are rare within 3 days of SAH and have their peak incidence of onset 7 to 8 days after SAH (Fig. 73–2). Less than 4% of such deficits occur beyond day 13.[7] Onset can be sudden or insidious and may be preceded or accompanied by increasing headache, neck stiffness, and rising temperature.[27] Classic early signs include confusion, delirium, and progressive decrease in level of consciousness. Focal deficits may supervene acutely or slowly. Fisher and colleagues[27] reported that 75% of deficits could be attributed to spasm of the middle cerebral artery and 25% to spasm of one or both anterior cerebral arteries. There is some relationship to the site of the ruptured aneurysm, because this is the area with the most blood clot in general. Anterior communicating artery aneurysms tend to result in diffuse and bilateral vasospasm (particularly of precommunicating segments of the anterior cerebral arteries), producing changes in consciousness and personality.[28]

FIGURE 73–1   *(On opposite page) A, CT scan on the day of SAH in a 48-year-old man with good clinical grade shows diffuse thick, Fisher grade 3 SAH. Anteroposterior right (B) and left (C) internal carotid angiograms show a small anterior communicating artery aneurysm and no vasospasm. Seven days later, the patient deteriorated clinically; angiograms obtained at this time show severe, diffuse vasospasm of the right (D) and left (E) internal carotid, anterior cerebral, and middle cerebral arteries. The patient was left moderately disabled; a CT scan obtained 3 months later (F) shows bilateral cerebral infarctions in the territories of the middle cerebral arteries.*

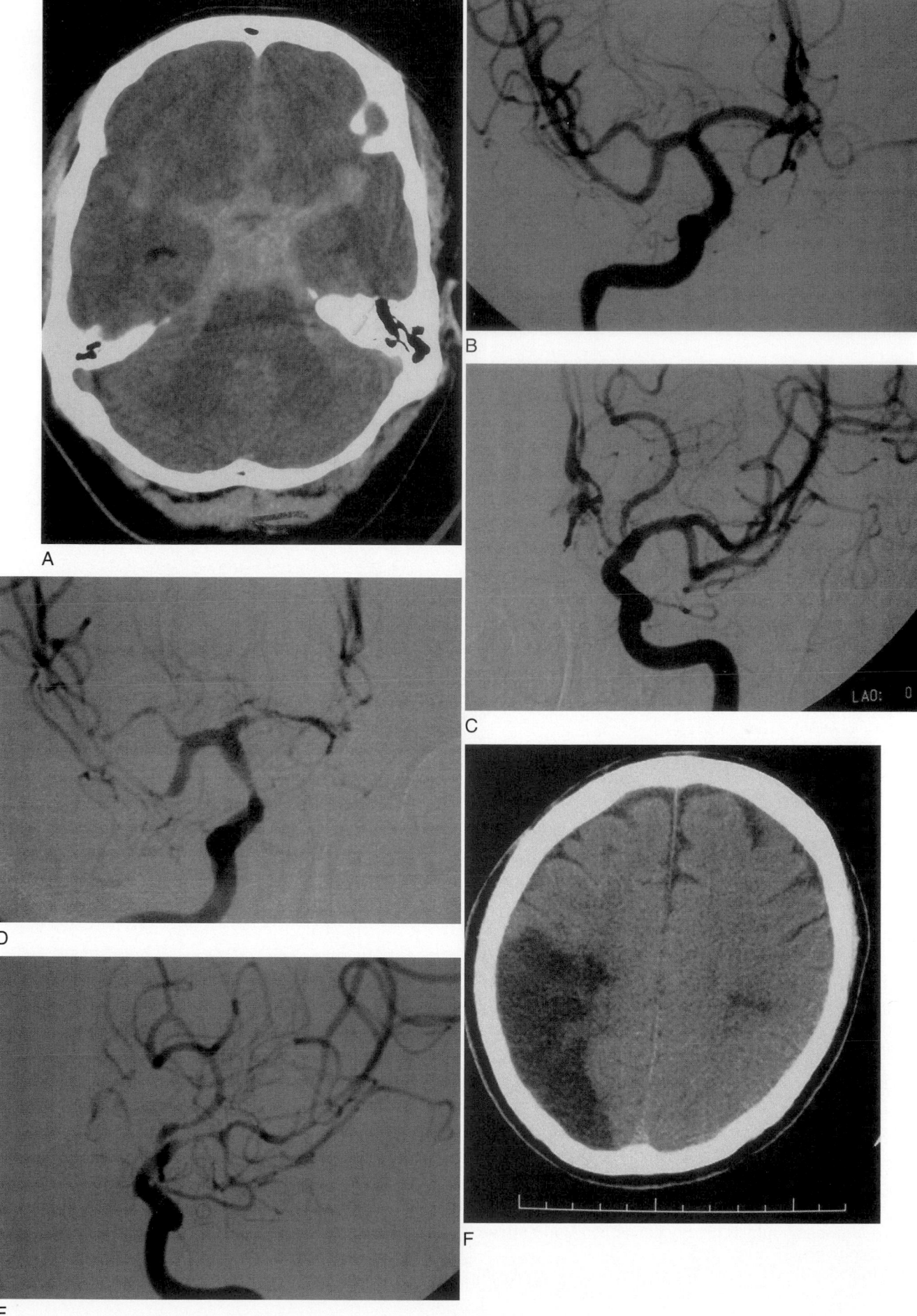

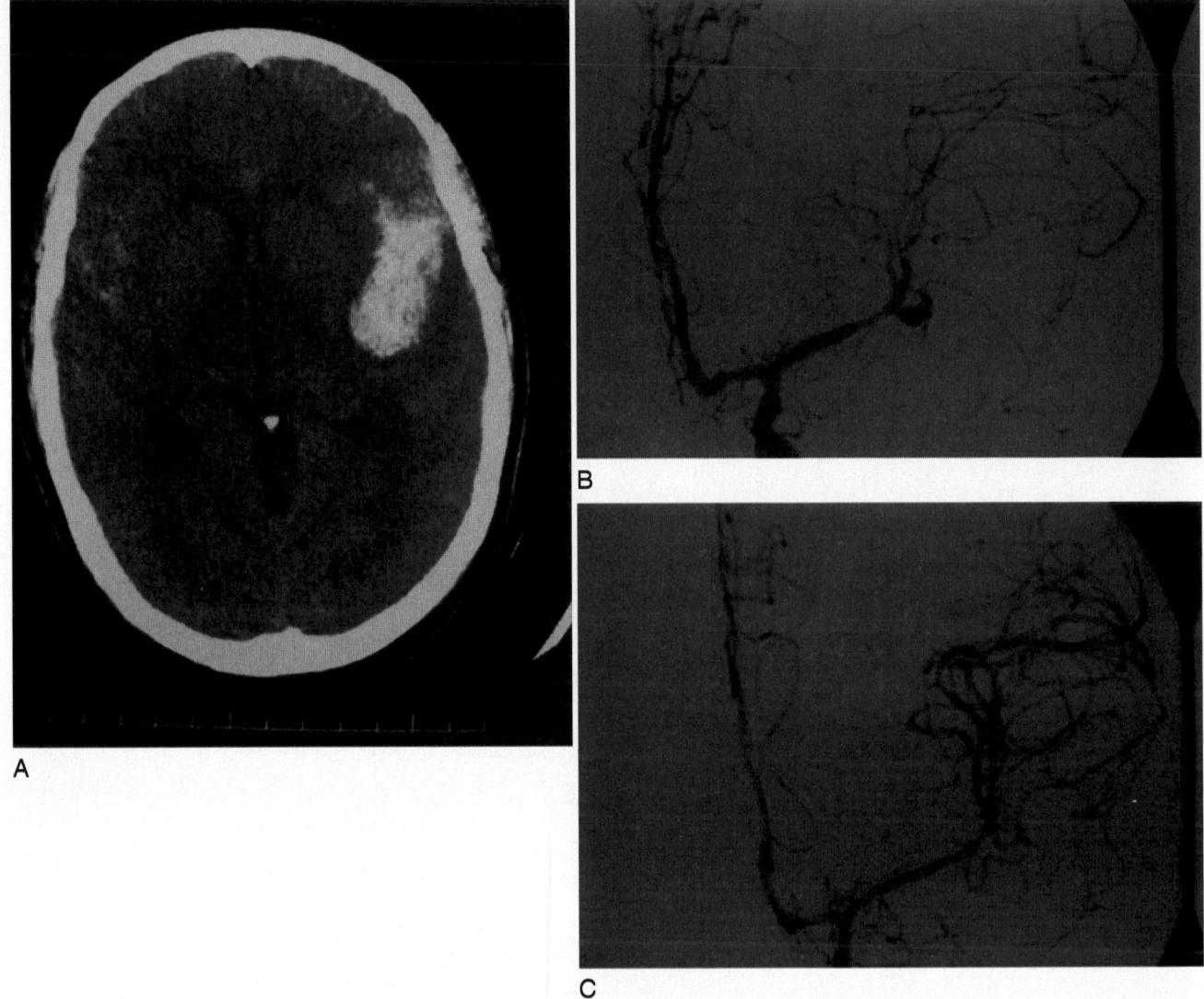

FIGURE 73–2   A, *A 44-year-old woman presented with a ruptured middle cerebral artery aneurysm and had a poor clinical grade. Admission CT scan showed an intracerebral hemorrhage with minimal SAH (Fisher grade 4).* B, *Admission anteroposterior internal carotid angiogram shows narrowing of the middle cerebral artery branches stretched over the hematoma.* C, *The narrowing has resolved 3 days later, during the time of vasospasm; therefore, the narrowing was not due to vasospasm, which would be less likely to develop in a patient with intracerebral hemorrhage. The patient made a good recovery.*

Middle cerebral artery aneurysms may be associated with unilateral vasospasm resulting in focal motor changes, sensory changes, or both, with or without changes in consciousness. Vasospasm after internal carotid aneurysm rupture produces mixed mental and motor changes.

Other conditions enter into the differential diagnosis of vasospasm and may frequently coexist with it (Table 73.1).[29] In general, patients who demonstrate deterioration after SAH during the time of risk of vasospasm undergo neurologic and general examinations, second cranial CT scanning, and blood and radiologic investigations to detect other causes of the deterioration. Transcranial Doppler (TCD) ultrasonography is usually performed, and catheter angiography may be indicated.

Factors identified that predict whether or not vasospasm will develop include the location, volume, density, and persistence of subarachnoid blood as seen on CT scan within 4 to 5 days of SAH. Fisher and colleagues[27] devised a scale for grading the amount of SAH on the initial CT scan obtained within days of SAH. They found that vasospasm was most common in patients with thick clots in the subarachnoid space but was unlikely to occur when no blood was observed or when hemorrhage was exclusively intracerebral or intraventricular (Figs. 73–3 and 73–4, Table 73.2; see Figs. 73–1 and 73–2).[19] The longer the clot persists in the subarachnoid space after SAH and the denser it appears, according to its measure in Hounsfield units on CT scanning, the higher the risk of vasospasm.[1,20,21] This finding is consistent with vasospasm's being a dose-dependent contraction of cerebral arteries in response to hemolyzing erythrocytes in the perivascular subarachnoid space.

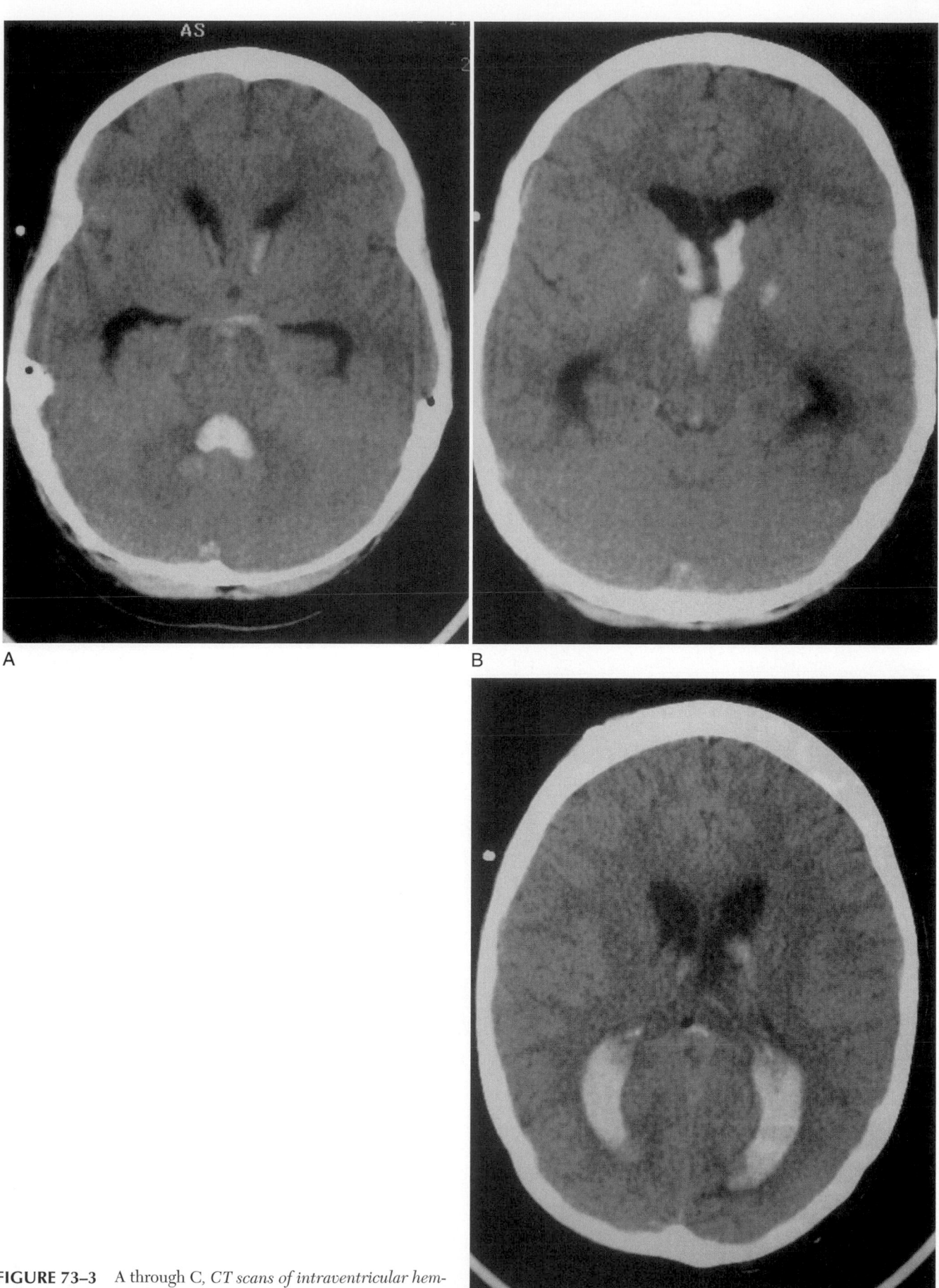

FIGURE 73–3   A through C, CT scans of intraventricular hemorrhage (Fisher grade 4) with minimal SAH from a vertebral artery dissecting aneurysm in a 22-year-old woman.

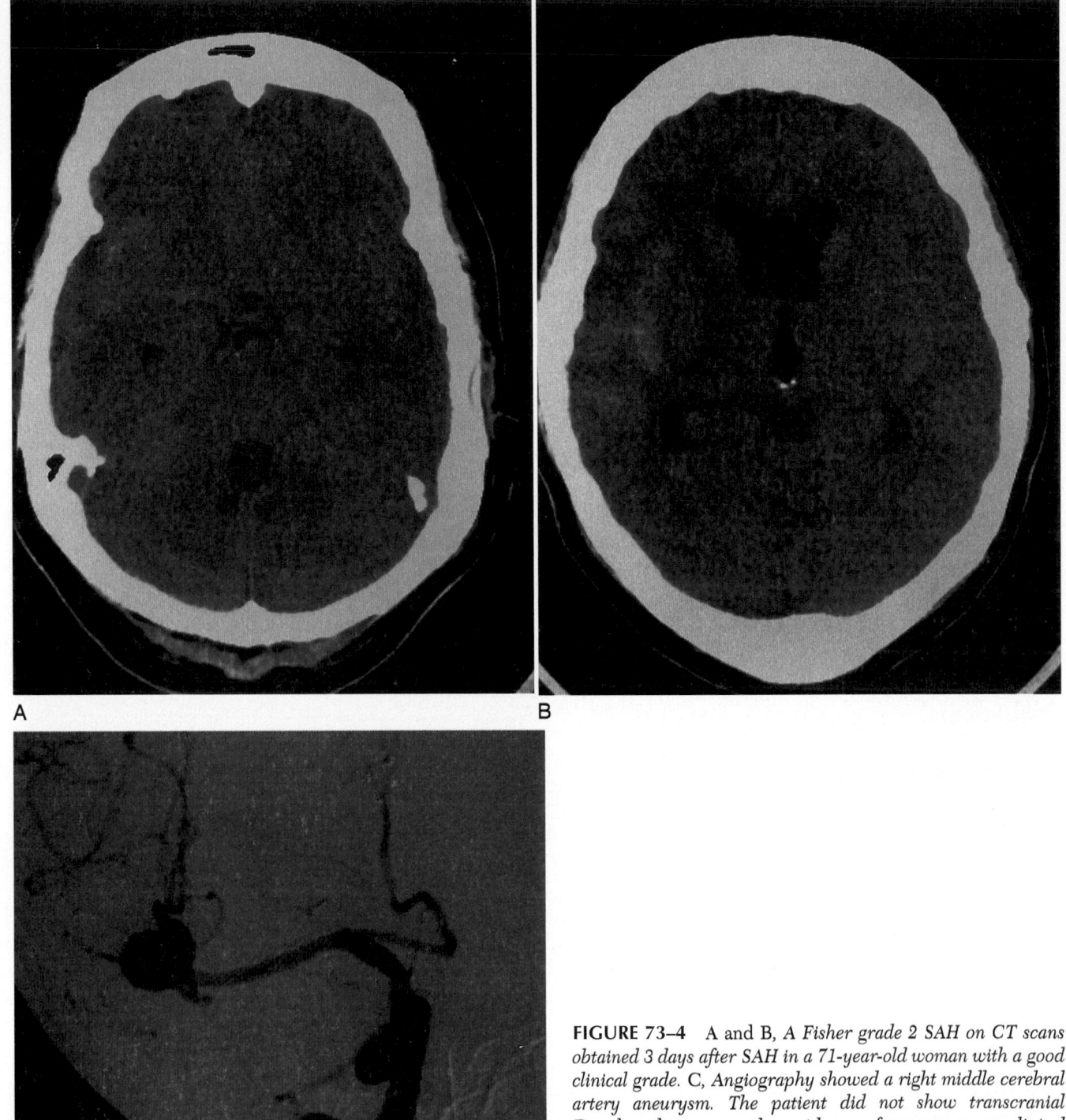

A

B

C

FIGURE 73–4   A and B, *A Fisher grade 2 SAH on CT scans obtained 3 days after SAH in a 71-year-old woman with a good clinical grade. C, Angiography showed a right middle cerebral artery aneurysm. The patient did not show transcranial Doppler ultrasonography evidence of vasospasm or clinical signs of delayed cerebral ischemia.*

Table 73.1 Differential Diagnosis of Delayed Neurologic Deterioration After Subarachnoid Hemorrhage

Metabolic/systemic disorders	Electrolyte disturbances (hyponatremia or hypernatremia)
	Blood gas disturbances (hypoxia, hypercarbia)
	Circulatory disorders (hypotension, arrhythmias)
	Infectious causes (pneumonia, other systemic infections)
	Iatrogenic causes (adverse medication reactions, organ failure)
Neurologic/structural disorders	Rebleeding, intracranial hemorrhage
	Hydrocephalus
	Postoperative complications, intracranial bleeding, subdural hematoma, edema, iatrogenic infarction)
	Meningitis
	Seizures, post-ictal state

Adapted from Peerless SJ: Pre- and postoperative management of cerebral aneurysms. Clin Neurosurg 26:209–231, 1979.

Other factors, such as patient age and gender, have not consistently been shown to predict vasospasm. A prospective observational study on the timing of aneurysm surgery noted an increase in incidence of clinical vasospasm from 27% to 33% when surgery was delayed from days 0 to 3 to days 15 to 32.[30] Other studies have documented a rise in the incidence of ischemic neurologic deficits when surgery is performed during the vasospasm interval (3 or 4 to 14 or so days after SAH).

INVESTIGATIONS

Catheter-based cerebral angiography remains the "gold standard" in the diagnosis of vasospasm. Other causes of arterial narrowing should be distinguished from vasospasm, such as preexisting arterial hypoplasia, atherosclerosis, stretching and displacement of arteries due to mass effect from intracerebral hematoma, diffuse arterial narrowing due to intracranial hypertension, and variations in angiographic technique (see Fig. 73–4). Indications for angiography must be individualized but include neurologic

deterioration attributable to vasospasm without improvement immediately after hemodynamic optimization and patients in whom the diagnosis is uncertain and hemodynamic therapy is difficult or risky, such as the elderly or those with cardiac disease. Catheter angiography carries a 0.5% to 1% risk of stroke.[31]

CT scan is useful for detecting sequelae of SAH, surgery, and vasospasm, such as hemorrhage, hypodense areas, and hydrocephalus. CT angiography has also been used to diagnose vasospasm.[32,33] It carries less risk than catheter angiography but involves administration of contrast medium, which may complicate the conduct of catheter angiography if it is required to diagnose or treat vasospasm. A prospective comparison of helical CT angiography and catheter angiography in 17 patients found that CT angiography was useful for determining whether there was no spasm or severe spasm in proximal arteries but less helpful in detecting distal vasospasm or in differentiating intermediate levels of spasm in the proximal arteries.[32]

Magnetic resonance imaging (MRI) has been used less in patients with SAH, principally because of the time required, the lack of additional information provided that would alter management, and the difficulty in imaging acutely ill patients receiving intensive care. Tamatani and associates[34] examined 125 vasospastic arteries in 32 patients with both catheter angiography and MR angiography (MRA). MRA had a sensitivity of 46% and a specificity of 70%. Motion artifacts and inability to visualize distal vessels were the modality's main limitations.

The main laboratory aid in the diagnosis of vasospasm is TCD ultrasonography. This modality is based on the physics of blood flow, which holds that the velocity of flow through an artery is directly proportional to the volume of flow through the artery and inversely proportional to the square of the diameter of the vessel. Vasospasm is associated with increased TCD ultrasonographic velocities. There can be substantial changes in regional CBF (rCBF) and global CBF after SAH, complicating the diagnosis of vasospasm based solely on TCD ultrasonographic velocity measurements, because velocities decrease as CBF decreases, and vice versa. Aaslid and colleagues[35] presented one of the first comparisons of TCD ultrasonographic and cerebral angiographic findings in patients with SAH. The important findings were that the middle

Table 73.2 Fisher Scale for Grading Subarachnoid Hemorrhage on CT Scan and Relationship to Vasospasm

Grade	Description	Patients with Angiographic Vasospasm	Patients with Clinical Vasospasm	Total Number of Patients
I	No detectable blood	0	0	3
II	Diffuse blood that did not appear dense enough to represent a large, thick homogeneous clot	5	2	14
III	Dense collection of blood that appeared to represent thick clot in the vertical plane (interhemispheric fissure, insular cistern, or ambient cistern) or in the horizontal plane (stem of the sylvian fissure, sylvian cistern, and interpeduncular cistern)	20	19	22
IV	Intracerebral or intraventricular clots but with only diffuse blood or no blood in the basal cisterns	0	0	2

Adapted from Kistler JP, Crowell RM, Davis KR, et al: The relation of cerebral vasospasm to the extent and location of subarachnoid blood visualized by CT scan: A prospective study. Neurology 33:424–436, 1983.

cerebral artery was most readily assessed by TCD ultrasonography and that TCD ultrasonographic findings showed the best correlation with angiographic findings in this vessel. Mean flow velocities in excess of 200 cm/sec were highly suggestive of severe vasospasm, whereas velocities less than 100 cm/sec were rarely associated with significant vasospasm. In general, the sensitivity of the diagnosis of vasospasm based on mean TCD velocities in the range from more than 120 to 150 cm/sec is 50% to 60%, and the specificity exceeds 90%.[1,36]

In addition to false-positive and false-negative results, it may be difficult to predict, as opposed to corroborate, the onset of clinical vasospasm by TCD ultrasonography. Grosset and colleagues[37] studied 121 consecutive patients with SAH and found significantly higher mean flow velocities in patients with clinical vasospasm than in those without (186 ± 6 cm/sec versus 149 ± 5 cm/sec), although the mean flow velocities were not different in the two groups before the development of delayed deficits.[37] The sensitivity of TCD ultrasonographic velocity measurements may be improved by studying daily trends in flow velocities. Increases in velocity of more than 50 cm/sec in 24 hours are suggestive of impending clinical vasospasm.

Another method is to calculate the ratio of middle cerebral artery flow velocity to extracranial internal carotid artery flow velocity (hemispheric or Lindegaard ratio) to compensate for alterations in rCBF.[38] Ratios less than 3 are rare with vasospasm, and ratios higher than 6 are highly suggestive of vasospasm, with intermediate values being less useful. The Lindegaard ratio may differentiate vasospasm from a hyperdynamic state due to hemodynamic therapy or hyperemia. Interpretation of TCD ultrasonographic flow velocities is further hampered by variation in factors that can reduce velocities, such as lower cerebral perfusion pressure, reduced rCBF, and technical factors related to conduct of the examination itself.[39]

The preceding discussion suggests that the noninvasive diagnosis of vasospasm could be improved by measuring CBF. It is well established that rCBF is decreased in the territory of the vasospastic arteries in patients with clinical vasospasm, that measurement of CBF may improve the diagnostic accuracy of noninvasive diagnosis of vasospasm, and that TCD ultrasonographic flow velocities are substantially affected by variations in CBF after SAH.[18,40,41] For example, Clyde and associates[40] retrospectively studied 50 patients with SAH who underwent TCD ultrasonography and xenon CT within 12 hours of each other. Middle cerebral artery CBF values of 31 mL/100 g/min or less corresponded to a peak systolic TCD ultrasonographic velocity of 119 cm/sec, whereas CBF values higher than 31 mL/100 g/min corresponded with a peak velocity of 169 cm/sec, confirming that high flow velocities can be due to increased CBF. Focal neurologic deficits correlated with low CBF in the middle cerebral artery territory on xenon CT, but peak systolic TCD ultrasonographic flow velocities did not.

TREATMENT OF VASOSPASM

General

If vasospasm is caused by persistent subarachnoid clot, removal of this clot should prevent or decrease vasospasm.

When vasospasm is induced by surgical placement of blood clot next to cerebral arteries in nonhuman primates, removal of the clot within 72 hours of placement, either surgically or by administration of intracisternal fibrinolytic drugs, effectively prevents vasospasm. Removal of the clot at a later time reduces the duration and severity of vasospasm; however, the effect is less marked, and the longer the time until clot removal, the longer it takes the effect to manifest.[42-45]

No other preventive strategies for vasospasm have been realized. Management relies on administration of nimodipine and maneuvers to optimize CBF—chiefly, avoidance of various factors, induction of hypertension (hemodynamic therapy), and dilation of spastic arteries by balloon angioplasty, superselective intra-arterial infusion of vasodilators, or both. Another theoretical strategy is neuroprotection.

Clot Removal

Clot removal during aneurysm surgery may reduce the risk of development as well as the severity of vasospasm.[46,47] The effect of clot removal on vasospasm in humans has been variable, probably owing to the difficulty of removing the clot without causing additional brain injury and bleeding. A marked and robust preventive effect of clot lysis with intracisternal tissue plasminogen activator (t-PA) against vasospasm in nonhuman primates[42] stimulated the use of this drug in humans. Prospective observational series described administration of t-PA, either intracisternally at the time of aneurysm surgery or by intracisternal or intraventricular catheter after the surgery.[48-50]

Criteria for treatment with t-PA generally are presentation within 72 hours of SAH and definitive clipping or obliteration of the ruptured vascular lesion. A review of 105 patients meeting these criteria found that the majority had diffuse or localized, thick subarachnoid hematomas and worse clinical grades.[49] Despite this finding, severe and symptomatic vasospasm occurred in only 5% of patients, and mild or moderate arterial narrowing in about 50%. The incidence and severity of vasospasm were lower than in comparable patients described in other studies. For instance, vasospasm developed in 94% of patients with thick SAH in a trial of nimodipine,[51] and in 61%, the vasospasm was severe and diffuse. Good outcome of patients in the t-PA cohort was reported in 76% and death in 7%,[49] compared with a 30% rate of good outcome and a 47% rate of death for the patients in the nimodipine trial of patients with poor-grade disease.[51]

Similar data from prospective, nonrandomized studies are available to support the use of urokinase.[52] A double-blind, placebo-controlled trial of t-PA for prevention of vasospasm randomly assigned 100 patients to receive either a single intracisternal dose of t-PA or placebo after aneurysm clipping.[4] Fifty-seven percent of the treated group made a good recovery at 3 months, compared with 43% of the placebo group. In the subset of patients with thick subarachnoid clot there was a 56% relative risk reduction in severe vasospasm with t-PA. Bleeding complications occurred in 16% of the placebo group and in 19% of the treated group. This study lacked adequate power to demonstrate the efficacy of t-PA, although the trends were all in favor of t-PA, and bleeding complications were not obviously increased with its use.

Hemodynamic Therapy

Hemodynamic therapy involves manipulation of blood pressure, volume, and viscosity and cardiac output in order to optimize CBF. The rationale for induced hypertension seems the soundest compared with the other modalities. SAH and vasospasm may be accompanied by varying degrees of loss of pressure autoregulation. Under these circumstances, elevation of blood pressure may increase CBF, at least in regions of brain that have impaired autoregulation. Early clinical reports documented that patients with delayed ischemic deficits improved when hypertension was induced.[53] No specific randomized studies of induced hypertension for vasospasm have been conducted, and almost all investigators have employed a combination of hypertension and hypervolemia. The use of hypervolemia is based on the observations that patients with SAH are volume-depleted, that infusions of crystalloid, colloid, or both are usually necessary to elevate blood pressure, and that experimental studies suggest that hypervolemia itself may augment CBF.

Complications of induced hypertension and hemodynamic therapy were reported in 24% of patients in six reports.[54] They include rebleeding from the aneurysm if it has not been clipped or coiled, hemorrhagic transformation of infarcts, myocardial ischemia and failure, pulmonary edema, complications of central venous catheterization, and, rarely, hypertensive encephalopathy.[55]

Patients with aneurysmal SAH commonly demonstrate deficits in total circulating blood and red blood cell volumes. More than 3.6 L of fluid per day were necessary to maintain normovolemia for the first 7 days after SAH in one study.[52] At roughly the same time as this fact was being recognized, case series appeared showing improvement in patients with clinical vasospasm after institution of induced hypertension and hypervolemia.[57–60] A review of six reports of vasospasm treatment with hemodynamic therapy found that deficits improved in 68%, resulting in good outcome in 71%; this outcome was judged to be significantly better than the natural history of patients with vasospasm.[54]

The use of induced hypertension with at least the avoidance of hypovolemia as treatment for clinical vasospasm is supported by case series and individual experiences of neurosurgeons. Prophylactic use of these measures, on the other hand, is of less certain value.[7] Origitano and colleagues[61] subjected 43 patients with SAH to aggressive prophylactic hemodynamic therapy using invasive monitoring, vasopressors, and fluids with or without phlebotomy to reduce the hematocrit value to 30%. CBF was elevated in these patients in comparison with historical controls, but the incidence of clinical vasospasm (35%) was not substantially reduced. Lennihan and associates[56] randomly assigned 82 patients to undergo either normovolemia or prophylactic hypervolemia from immediately after SAH through the time of vasospasm. They found that hypervolemia successfully elevated cardiac filling pressures but had no effect on CBF measurements or the incidence of clinical vasospasm.[56] The evidence that elevating intravascular volume above normal increases CBF is controversial, and the beneficial effects of hypervolemia may have been achieved in this study simply through avoidance of hypovolemia or through the simultaneous increase in blood pressure or reduction in hematocrit.[62]

Some investigators have advocated prophylactic or therapeutic hemodilution for vasospasm. A decrease in hematocrit is known to reduce arterial oxygen-carrying capacity and increase CBF. However, whether the increase in CBF is due either to the attempt of regulatory mechanisms to maintain constant oxygen delivery to the brain or to reduced blood viscosity and improved rheologic characteristics remains unresolved. A review of clinical trials of hemodilution for ischemic stroke found evidence of efficacy even when hemodilution was induced within 6 hours of stroke onset.[63]

Pharmacologic Treatments

Nimodipine, a voltage-gated calcium channel antagonist, is administered prophylactically to most patients with aneurysmal SAH on the basis of results of at least 6 randomized placebo-controlled trials (Table 73.3).[51,64–68] Meta-analysis of these studies shows that nimodipine improves the odds of good outcome by 1.86 and reduces the odds of deficit, mortality, or both due to vasospasm and the infarction rate on CT scan by 0.46 to 0.58.[69] These effects were all statistically significant, whereas the slight reduction in overall mortality that occurred in patients treated with nimodipine was not significant. There is no convincing evidence that nimodipine affects angiographic vasospasm, leading to hypotheses that it improves outcome by acting as a neuronal protectant, by improving collateral blood flow, by favorably affecting the rheologic characteristics of blood, or a combination of these actions.

Tirilazad (U74006F) is an antioxidant 21-aminosteroid that is devoid of glucocorticoid side effects. A study of 1023 patients in Europe, Australia, and New Zealand found that treatment with tirilazad 6 mg/kg/day led to statistically significant improvement in good outcome and reduction in death at 3 months.[6] This dose was the dose associated with the highest death rate in an initial study in Canada.[9] A study in North American centers found no significant effect of the same dose, and it was suggested that greater use of anticonvulsants in North America increased drug metabolism, thereby reducing tirilazad's beneficial effects. Two studies of higher tirilazad doses in women did not demonstrate significant improvement in outcome, although the study conducted in Europe, Australia, and New Zealand did find a reduction in symptomatic vasospasm in treated patients.[10,70] The conflicting results of studies, the lack of significant differences between groups in the primary outcome measures in any of the studies, and the absence of consistent effects on angiographic or clinical vasospasm were difficult to explain. The drug has been approved for use in some countries in Europe and Australasia, although it is not in use for this indication in Canada or the United States. Several other antioxidants have been studied in randomized, controlled trials in patients with aneurysmal SAH, but significant effects on outcome were not demonstrated.[71,72]

Other drugs that have been assessed in clinical trials in humans with aneurysmal SAH include the protein kinase inhibitor fasudil (AT877 or HA1077). This drug is widely used in Japan on the basis of results of a randomized trial of 276 patients who underwent aneurysm surgery within 3 days of SAH.[73] Fasudil significantly reduced rates of clinical vasospasm (50% in the placebo group and 35% in the

Table 73.3   Randomized Controlled Trials of Nimodipine Prophylaxis for Subarachnoid Hemorrhage (SAH)

Trial[*]	No. of Patients	Inclusion	Treatment	Outcome
Allen et al (1983)[64]	116	Clinical grades I–II, age 15–80 years, admitted within 96 hours of SAH	0.7 mg/kg orally, then 0.35 mg/kg orally every 4 hours for 21 days Other medical treatment and surgical details not provided	Decreased overall death or severe disability at 21 days No change in overall incidence of clinical vasospasm
Philippon et al (1986)[67]	70	Clinical grades I–III, age 15–65 years, admitted within 72 hours of SAH Patients with hypertension, spasm on initial angiogram, hydrocephalus, and intracerebral hemorrhage excluded	60 mg orally every 4 hours for 21 days Antifibrinolytics used Surgery delayed until after day 3; Excluded if operated before day 3, if vasospasm present on admission angiogram, or if drug could not be started within 72 hours of SAH	Decreased death or severe disability due to vasospasm at 21 days Trend toward decreased incidence of clinical vasospasm
Mee et al (1988)[65]	50	All clinical grades, age 18–65 years, admitted within 96 hours of SAH	200 μg intracisternally at surgery, then 60 mg orally every 4 hours for 21 days No hemodynamic therapy Surgery delayed until a mean of days 9–13	Trend toward more good outcomes at 3 months Significantly reduced 3-month mortality on efficacy analysis only Results potentially confounded by twice as many operative complications in placebo group
Petruk et al (1988)[51]	154	Clinical grades III–V, age >18 years, admitted within 96 hours	60 mg orally every 4 hours for 21 days Hemodynamic treatment allowed Antifibrinolytics used in 20–25% Surgery on day 0–3 in >40%	More good outcomes at 3 months; no difference in mortality Decreased delayed ischemic deficits due to vasospasm alone
Ohman et al (1988)[66]	213	Clinical grades I–III, age 16–70 years, >85% patients admitted within 3 days of SAH, and all by day 10 Patients with intracranial hemorrhage excluded	0.25 μg/kg/min intravenously for 2 hours, then 0.5 μg/kg/min intravenously for 7–10 days, then 60 mg orally every 4 hours until 21 days post-SAH Surgery performed in randomly assigned patient groups on day 0–3, 4–7, or later as part of concurrent trial Antifibrinolytics and hemodynamic therapy not allowed	No overall improvement in outcome at 3 months Subgroup analysis of early surgery group (within 1 week of SAH) showed improved mortality and good outcomes
Pickard et al (1989)[68]	554	All clinical grades, age >18 years, admitted within 96 hours of SAH	60 mg orally every 4 hours for 21 days Other medical treatments unclear Surgery delayed to a mean day of 10–11	Decreased poor outcome (severe disability, vegetative state and death) at 3 months Decreased infarcts Decreased death or disability due to cerebral ischemia

*Superscript numbers indicate chapter references.

fasudil group), moderate to severe angiographic vasospasm (61% for placebo, 38% for fasudil), and cerebral infarcts (50% for placebo, 30% for fasudil). Overall outcome was better in the fasudil group, but the difference did not reach statistical significance.

Shaw and associates[74] compared the endothelin antagonist TAK-044 with placebo in 420 patients treated within 96 hours of SAH. They found no significant differences in outcome or mortality, although there was a trend toward a lower rate of ischemic events in the treated patients (23% for placebo, 21% for TAK-044). Endothelin antagonists are vasodilators, and there were significantly more hypotensive episodes in the treatment group (16% versus 7% for the

placebo group), necessitating greater use of vasopressors in this group. The inability to selectively dilate the cerebral arteries independent of the systemic circulation through administration of intravenous drugs has made hypotension a common and possibly detrimental effect in studies of vasodilator treatment for vasospasm.

Endovascular Treatment

In 1984, Zubkov and colleagues reported the use of balloon angioplasty catheters to dilate 105 vasospastic cerebral arteries in 33 patients after SAH.[75] Even this initial report concluded that balloon angioplasty results in permanent reversal of vasospasm in the treated arteries. Subsequent experience has shown that balloon angioplasty may be indicated in patients with clipped or coiled aneurysms with clinical deterioration from vasospasm despite hemodynamic therapy.[1] A review of reported case series suggests that neurologic improvement occurs in 60% to 80% of treated patients, CBF increases, and TCD ultrasonographic flow velocities diminish in treated arteries. Complications, reported in 5% of cases, include arterial rupture with death and stroke due to arterial occlusion. Because of these risks, balloon angioplasty is generally reserved for patients with neurologic deterioration in whom other treatments for vasospasm have failed and the aneurysm has already been treated by either clipping or coiling. Angioplasty and simultaneous endovascular treatment of the aneurysm with coils might be a reasonable approach; another tactic for patients presenting with vasospasm and an unsecured aneurysm is surgery for clipping and immediately postoperative angioplasty.[76]

Another endovascular treatment is to catheterize the vasospastic artery and infuse papaverine.[77] Vasodilation with this treatment is generally less marked than with balloon angioplasty, and the effect is transient. Vasospasm recurs, as judged from observation of transient clinical improvement or reduction in TCD ultrasonographic flow velocities, and repeated treatments may be necessary. Complications include cerebral infarction, blindness, increased ICP, and neurologic deterioration. As a result, papaverine is generally used only in carefully selected patients with vasospasm inaccessible to treatment with balloon angioplasty in whom the aneurysm is secured and ICP is being directly monitored.[1]

Approach to the Patient with Vasospasm

In general, early aneurysm surgery or coiling is performed, because it effectively prevents rebleeding and facilitates subsequent vasospasm management. Nimodipine treatment is universal, and antifibrinolytics are rarely given. It is important to avoid factors or actions that might reduce CBF or increase brain metabolic demand, such as hyperthermia, hypovolemia, hyponatremia, cardiac arrhythmia, pulmonary congestion, hypoxia, hypercarbia, and raised ICP. Prophylactically induced hypervolemia, hypertension, and hemodilution are not routinely used, although at least 3 L of fluid are administered per day to maintain normovolemia, hypertension is not aggressively treated after aneurysm obliteration, and the hematocrit is not allowed to drop below about 30%.[1,78] It is advisable to maintain normal serum magnesium concentration because low serum magnesium may aggravate cerebral ischemia and vasospasm.[79]

When delayed deterioration occurs, systemic causes are ruled out, and a CT scan is generally obtained to exclude other causes of neurologic compromise (see Table 73.1). The finding of mean TCD ultrasonographic flow velocities greater than 200 cm/sec or less than 120 cm/sec is helpful in ruling vasospasm in or out, respectively, but the ICP and CBF may also have to be considered. Measures are taken to optimize CBF by induction of hypertension and maintenance of fluid volume and cardiac output. Cerebral angiography is usually indicated in patients in whom vasospasm is suspected, who do not show improvement

with the preceding measures, and who may be candidates for endovascular treatment. Angiography may be indicated early in patients who cannot tolerate hemodynamic therapy, to exclude vasospasm as a cause of deterioration and thereby avoid complications or to perform endovascular treatment early.

PROGNOSIS AND OUTCOME FROM VASOSPASM

Vasospasm remains a significant independent adverse factor for outcome in patients with aneurysmal SAH.[8] In the cooperative study on timing of aneurysm surgery, 28% of deaths and 39% of disabilities were attributed to vasospasm; overall, the incidences of death and disability due to vasospasm were 7% and 6%, respectively. Overall outcome at 6 months was death in 26% and complete recovery in 58%. Multivariate analysis of factors predicting poor outcome in this series of 3521 patients included lower level of consciousness on admission, older age, higher admission blood pressure, more SAH on admission CT scan, preexisting medical conditions, posterior circulation aneurysm, vasospasm, and presence of intracerebral or intraventricular hemorrhage. In a review of the world literature, Dorsch and King compared patients with and without vasospasm and found that vasospasm significantly increased mortality from 17% to 31% and reduced the frequency of good outcome from 70% to 44%. A reasonable approximation is that 67% of patients with aneurysmal SAH experience more than mild vasospasm; 33% have delayed ischemia, and 10% die and 10% have permanent neurologic deficits from the delayed ischemia.

Nimodipine and hemodynamic therapy should theoretically reduce death, disability, and cerebral infarction due to vasospasm and, it is hoped, improve outcome. One can compare the data from the surgery timing study that were collected on patients managed in 1980 to 1984,[8] who by and large did not receive these therapies, with the patients entered into the tirilazad studies of a decade or so later.[5,6,10,70] Vasospasm caused death or disability in 17%, the overall outcome was favorable in 69%, and the overall death rate was 16% in the tirilazad studies, compared with 13%, 58%, and 26%, respectively, in the timing study. Outcome seems to have improved, although clearly, major strides still must be made in the prevention and treatment of vasospasm.

References

1. Macdonald RL, Weir B: Cerebral Vasospasm. San Diego, Academic, 2001, p 518.
2. Ecker A, Riemenschneider PA: Arteriographic demonstration of spasm of the intracranial arteries with special reference to saccular arterial aneurysms. J Neurosurg 8:660–667, 1951.
3. Weir B, Grace M, Hansen J, et al: Time course of vasospasm in man. J Neurosurg 48:173–178, 1978.
4. Findlay JM, Kassell NF, Weir BK, et al: A randomized trial of intraoperative, intracisternal tissue plasminogen activator for the prevention of vasospasm. Neurosurgery 37:168–176, 1995.
5. Haley EC Jr, Kassell NF, Apperson-Hansen C, et al: A randomized, double-blind, vehicle-controlled trial of tirilazad mesylate in patients with aneurysmal subarachnoid hemorrhage: A cooperative study in North America. J Neurosurg 86:467–474, 1997.

6. Kassell NF, Haley EC Jr, Apperson-Hansen C, et al: Randomized, double-blind, vehicle-controlled trial of tirilazad mesylate in patients with aneurysmal subarachnoid hemorrhage: A cooperative study in Europe, Australia, and New Zealand. J Neurosurg 84:221–228, 1996.

7. Dorsch NWC, King MT: A review of cerebral vasospasm in aneurysmal subarachnoid hemorrhage. Part 1: Incidence and effects. J Clin Neurosci 1:19–26, 1994.

8. Kassell NF, Torner JC, Haley EC Jr, et al: The International Cooperative Study on the Timing of Aneurysm Surgery. Part 1: Overall management results. J Neurosurg 73:18–36, 1990.

9. Haley EC Jr, Kassell NF, Alves WM, et al: Phase II trial of tirilazad in aneurysmal subarachnoid hemorrhage: A report of the Cooperative Aneurysm Study. J Neurosurg 82:786–790, 1995.

10. Lanzino G, Kassell NF: Double-blind, randomized, vehicle-controlled study of high-dose tirilazad mesylate in women with aneurysmal subarachnoid hemorrhage. Part II: A cooperative study in North America. J Neurosurg 90:1018–1024, 1999.

11. Haley EC Jr, Kassell NF, Torner JC: A randomized controlled trial of high-dose intravenous nicardipine in aneurysmal subarachnoid hemorrhage: A report of the Cooperative Aneurysm Study. J Neurosurg 78:537–547, 1993.

12. Hop JW, Rinkel GJ, Algra A, et al: Randomized pilot trial of postoperative aspirin in subarachnoid hemorrhage. Neurology 54:872–878, 2000.

13. Findlay JM, Weir BK, Gordon P, et al: Safety and efficacy of intrathecal thrombolytic therapy in a primate model of cerebral vasospasm. Neurosurgery 24:491–498, 1989.

14. Grubb RLJ, Raichle ME, Eichling JO, et al: Effects of subarachnoid hemorrhage on cerebral blood volume, blood flow, and oxygen utilization in humans. J Neurosurg 46:446–453, 1977.

15. Yundt KD, Grubb RL Jr, Diringer MN, et al: Autoregulatory vasodilation of parenchymal vessels is impaired during cerebral vasospasm. J Cereb Blood Flow Metab 18:419–424, 1998.

16. Voldby B, Enevoldsen EM, Jensen FT: Cerebrovascular reactivity in patients with ruptured intracranial aneurysms. J Neurosurg 62:59–67, 1985.

17. Yamakami I, Isobe K, Yamaura A, et al: Vasospasm and regional cerebral blood flow (rCBF) in patients with ruptured intracranial aneurysm: Serial rCBF studies with the xenon-133 inhalation method. Neurosurgery 13:394–401, 1983.

18. Touho H, Karasawa J, Ohnishi H, et al: Evaluation of therapeutically induced hypertension in patients with delayed cerebral vasospasm by xenon-enhanced computed tomography. Neurol Med Chir 32:671–678, 1992.

19. Fisher CM, Kistler JP, Davis JM: Relation of cerebral vasospasm to subarachnoid hemorrhage visualized by computerized tomographic scanning. Neurosurgery 6:1–9, 1980.

20. Pasqualin A, Rosta L, Da Pian R, et al: Role of computed tomography in the management of vasospasm after subarachnoid hemorrhage. Neurosurgery 15:344–353, 1984.

21. Suzuki J, Komatsu S, Sato T, et al: Correlation between CT findings and subsequent development of cerebral infarction due to vasospasm in subarachnoid haemorrhage. Acta Neurochir 55:63–70, 1980.

22. Espinosa F, Weir B, Shnitka T, et al: A randomized placebo-controlled double-blind trial of nimodipine after SAH in monkeys. Part 2: Pathological findings. J Neurosurg 60:1176–1185, 1984.

23. Liszczak TM, Varsos VG, Black PM, et al: Cerebral arterial constriction after experimental subarachnoid hemorrhage is associated with blood components within the arterial wall. J Neurosurg 58:18–26, 1983.

24. Mayberg MR, Okada T, Bark DH: The role of hemoglobin in arterial narrowing after subarachnoid hemorrhage. J Neurosurg 72:634–640, 1990.

25. Peterson JW, Kwun BD, Hackett JD, et al: The role of inflammation in experimental cerebral vasospasm. J Neurosurg 72:767–774, 1990.

26. Vorkapic P, Bevan JA, Bevan RD: Longitudinal in vivo and in vitro time-course study of chronic cerebrovasospasm in the rabbit basilar artery. Neurosurg Rev 14:215–219, 1991.

27. Fisher CM, Roberson GH, Ojemann RG: Cerebral vasospasm with ruptured saccular aneurysm—the clinical manifestations. Neurosurgery 1:245–248, 1977.

28. Saito I, Ueda Y, Sano K: Significance of vasospasm in the treatment of ruptured intracranial aneurysms. J Neurosurg 47:412–429, 1977.

29. Peerless SJ: Pre- and postoperative management of cerebral aneurysms. Clin Neurosurg 26:209–231, 1979.

30. Kassell NF, Torner JC, Jane JA, et al: The International Cooperative Study on the Timing of Aneurysm Surgery. Part 2: Surgical results. J Neurosurg 73:37–47, 1990.

31. Leffers AM, Wagner A: Neurologic complications of cerebral angiography: A retrospective study of complication rate and patient risk factors. Acta Radiol 41:204–210, 2000.

32. Anderson GB, Ashforth R, Steinke DE, et al: CT angiography for the detection of cerebral vasospasm in patients with acute subarachnoid hemorrhage. Am J Neuroradiol 21:1011–1015, 2000.

33. Takagi R, Hayashi H, Kobayashi H, et al: Three-dimensional CT angiography of intracranial vasospasm following subarachnoid haemorrhage. Neuroradiology 40:631–635, 1998.

34. Tamatani S, Sasaki O, Takeuchi S, et al: Detection of delayed cerebral vasospasm, after rupture of intracranial aneurysms, by magnetic resonance angiography. Neurosurgery 40:748–753, 1997.

35. Aaslid R, Huber P, Nornes H: Evaluation of cerebrovascular spasm with transcranial Doppler ultrasound. J Neurosurg 60:37–41, 1984.

36. Sloan MA, Haley ECJ, Kassell NF, et al: Sensitivity and specificity of transcranial Doppler ultrasonography in the diagnosis of vasospasm following subarachnoid hemorrhage. Neurology 39:1514–1518, 1989.

37. Grosset DG, Straiton J, McDonald I, et al: Angiographic and Doppler diagnosis of cerebral artery vasospasm following subarachnoid haemorrhage. Br J Neurosurg 7:291–298, 1993.

38. Lindegaard KF, Nornes H, Bakke SJ, et al: Cerebral vasospasm after subarachnoid haemorrhage investigated by means of transcranial Doppler ultrasound. Acta Neurochir (Suppl) 42:81–84, 1988.

39. Klingelhofer J, Dander D, Holzgraefe M, et al: Cerebral vasospasm evaluated by transcranial Doppler ultrasonography at different intracranial pressures. J Neurosurg 75:752–758, 1991.

40. Clyde BL, Resnick DK, Yonas H, et al: The relationship of blood velocity as measured by transcranial doppler ultrasonography to cerebral blood flow as determined by stable xenon computed tomographic studies after aneurysmal subarachnoid hemorrhage. Neurosurgery 38:896–904, 1996.

41. Darby JM, Yonas H, Marks EC, et al: Acute cerebral blood flow response to dopamine-induced hypertension after subarachnoid hemorrhage. J Neurosurg 80:857–864, 1994.

42. Findlay JM, Weir BK, Steinke D, et al: Effect of intrathecal thrombolytic therapy on subarachnoid clot and chronic vasospasm in a primate model of SAH. J Neurosurg 69:723–735, 1988.

43. Handa Y, Weir BK, Nosko M, et al: The effect of timing of clot removal on chronic vasospasm in a primate model. J Neurosurg 67:558–564, 1987.

44. Nosko M, Weir BK, Lunt A, et al: Effect of clot removal at 24 hours on chronic vasospasm after SAH in the primate model. J Neurosurg 66:416–422, 1987.

45. Zhang ZD, Yamini B, Komuro T, et al: Vasospasm in monkeys resolves because of loss of and encasement of subarachnoid blood clot. Stroke 32:1868–1874, 2001.

46. Mizukami M, Kawase T, Usami T, et al: Prevention of vasospasm by early operation with removal of subarachnoid blood. Neurosurgery 10:301–307, 1982.

47. Ohta H, Yasui N, Suzuki A, et al: [Hemorrhagic infarction following vasospasm due to ruptured intracranial aneurysms]. [Japanese]. Neurol Med Chir 22:716–724, 1982.

48. Findlay JM, Weir BK, Kassell NF, et al: Intracisternal recombinant tissue plasminogen activator after aneurysmal subarachnoid hemorrhage. J Neurosurg 75:181–188, 1991.

49. Macdonald RL, Weir BK: Management of vasospasm: Tissue plasminogen activator. In Ratcheson R, Wirth F (eds): Ruptured Cerebral Aneurysms: Perioperative Management. Baltimore, Williams & Wilkins, 1993, pp 168–181.

50. Seifert V, Stolke D, Zimmermann M, et al: Prevention of delayed ischaemic deficits after aneurysmal subarachnoid haemorrhage by intrathecal bolus injection of tissue plasminogen activator (rTPA): A prospective study. Acta Neurochir 128:137–143, 1994.

51. Petruk KC, West M, Mohr G, et al: Nimodipine treatment in poor-grade aneurysm patients: Results of a multicenter double-blind placebo-controlled trial. J Neurosurg 68:505–517, 1988.

52. Sasaki T, Kodama N, Kawakami M, et al: Urokinase cisternal irrigation therapy for prevention of symptomatic vasospasm after aneurysmal subarachnoid hemorrhage: A study of urokinase concentration and the fibrinolytic system. Stroke 31:1256–1262, 2000.

53. Kosnik EJ, Hunt WE: Postoperative hypertension in the management of patients with intracranial arterial aneurysms. J Neurosurg 45:148–154, 1976.

54. Macdonald RL: Cerebral vasospasm. Neurosurg Q 5:73–97, 1995.

55. Amin-Hanjani S, Schwartz RB, Sathi S, et al: Hypertensive encephalopathy as a complication of hyperdynamic therapy for vasospasm: Report of two cases. Neurosurgery 44:1113–1116, 1999.

56. Lennihan L, Mayer SA, Fink ME, et al: Effect of hypervolemic therapy on cerebral blood flow after subarachnoid hemorrhage: A randomized controlled trial. Stroke 31:383–391, 2000.

57. Awad IA, Carter LP, Spetzler RF, et al: Clinical vasospasm after subarachnoid hemorrhage: Response to hypervolemic hemodilution and arterial hypertension. Stroke 18:365–372, 1987.

58. Kassell NF, Peerless SJ, Durward QJ, et al: Treatment of ischemic deficits from vasospasm with intravascular volume expansion and induced arterial hypertension. Neurosurgery 11:337–343, 1982.

59. Muizelaar JP, Becker DP: Induced hypertension for the treatment of cerebral ischemia after subarachnoid hemorrhage: Direct effect on cerebral blood flow. Surg Neurol 25:317–325, 1986.

60. Pritz MB, Giannotta SL, Kindt GW, et al: Treatment of patients with neurological deficits associated with cerebral vasospasm by intravascular volume expansion. Neurosurgery 3:364–368, 1978.

61. Origitano TC, Wascher TM, Reichman OH, et al: Sustained increased cerebral blood flow with prophylactic hypertensive hypervolemic hemodilution ("triple-H" therapy) after subarachnoid hemorrhage. Neurosurgery 27:729–739, 1990.

62. Rosenstein J, Suzuki M, Symon L, et al: Clinical use of a portable bedside cerebral blood flow machine in the management of aneurysmal subarachnoid hemorrhage. Neurosurgery 15:519–525, 1984.

63. Asplund K, Israelsson K, Schampi I: Haemodilution for acute ischaemic stroke. Cochrane Database Syst Rev CD000103, 2000.

64. Allen GS, Ahn HS, Preziosi TJ, et al: Cerebral arterial spasm—a controlled trial of imodipine in patients with subarachnoid hemorrhage. N Engl J Med 308:619–624, 1983.

65. Mee E, Dorrance D, Lowe D, et al: Controlled study of nimodipine in aneurysm patients treated early after subarachnoid hemorrhage. Neurosurgery 22:484–491, 1988.

66. Ohman J, Heiskanen O: Effect of nimodipine on the outcome of patients after aneurysmal subarachnoid hemorrhage and surgery. J Neurosurg 69:683–686, 1988.

67. Philippon J, Grob R, Dagreou F, et al: Prevention of vasospasm in subarachnoid haemorrhage: A controlled study with nimodipine. Acta Neurochir 82:110–114, 1986.

68. Pickard JD, Murray GD, Illingworth R, et al: Effect of oral nimodipine on cerebral infarction and outcome after subarachnoid haemorrhage: British aneurysm nimodipine trial. Br Med J 298:636–642, 1989.

69. Barker FG, Ogilvy CS: Efficacy of prophylactic nimodipine for delayed ischemic deficit after subarachnoid hemorrhage: A meta-analysis. J Neurosurg 84:405–414, 1996.

70. Lanzino G, Kassell NF, Dorsch NW, et al: Double-blind, randomized, vehicle-controlled study of high-dose tirilazad mesylate in women with aneurysmal subarachnoid hemorrhage. Part I: A cooperative study in Europe, Australia, New Zealand, and South Africa. J Neurosurg 90:1011–1017, 1999.

71. Asano T, Takakura K, Sano K, et al: Effects of a hydroxyl radical scavenger on delayed ischemic neurological deficits following aneurysmal subarachnoid hemorrhage: Results of a multicenter, placebo-controlled double-blind trial. J Neurosurg 84:792–803, 1996.

72. Saito I, Asano T, Sano K, et al: Neuroprotective effect of an antioxidant, ebselen, in patients with delayed neurological deficits after aneurysmal subarachnoid hemorrhage. Neurosurgery 42:269–277, 1998.

73. Shibuya M, Suzuki Y, Sugita K, et al: Effect of AT877 on cerebral vasospasm after aneurysmal subarachnoid hemorrhage: Results of a prospective placebo-controlled double-blind trial. J Neurosurg 76:571–577, 1992.

74. Shaw MD, Vermeulen M, Murray GD, et al: Efficacy and safety of the endothelin, receptor antagonist TAK-044 in treating subarachnoid hemorrhage: A report by the Steering Committee on behalf of the UK/Netherlands/Eire TAK-044 Subarachnoid Haemorrhage Study Group. J Neurosurg 93:992–997, 2000.

75. Zubkov YN, Nikiforov BM, Shustin VA: Balloon catheter technique for dilatation of constricted cerebral arteries after aneurysmal SAH. Acta Neurochir 70:65–79, 1984.

76. LeRoux PD, Elliott JP, Grady MS, et al: Anterior circulation aneurysms: Improvement in outcome in good-grade patients 1983–1993. Clin Neurosurg 41:325–333, 1994.

77. Fandino J, Kaku Y, Schuknecht B, et al: Improvement of cerebral oxygenation patterns and metabolic validation of superselective intraarterial infusion of papaverine for the treatment of cerebral vasospasm. J Neurosurg 89:93–100, 1998.

78. Hasan D, Vermeulen M, Wijdicks EFM, et al: Effect of fluid intake and antihypertensive treatment on cerebral ischemia after subarachnoid hemorrhage. Stroke 20:1511–1515, 1989.

79. Veyna RS, Seyfried D, Burke DG, et al: Magnesium sulfate therapy after aneurysmal subarachnoid hemorrhage. J Neurosurg 96:510–514, 2002.

80. Kistler JP, Crowell RM, Davis KR, et al: The relation of cerebral vasospasm to the extent and location of subarachnoid blood visualized by CT scan: A prospective study. Neurology 33:424–436, 1983.

Chapter Seventy-Four

Extracranial-Intracranial Bypass for Cerebral Ischemia

Robert L. Grubb, Jr.

A significant number of atherosclerotic lesions responsible for brain ischemia involve either intracranial arteries or the internal carotid or vertebral arteries at sites inaccessible to extracranial surgical approaches.[1-3] Although many of these atherosclerotic lesions are hemodynamically insignificant and produce ischemic symptoms due to embolization from diseased intima, others can obstruct blood flow to the brain. The development of sophisticated microvascular surgical techniques led to the development of extracranial-intracranial (EC/IC) arterial bypass procedures, which have been applied in an attempt to prevent stroke by improving the hemodynamic status of the circulation distal to a diseased vessel.

The conceptual basis of an EC/IC arterial bypass to increase brain blood flow in patients with symptoms caused by complete carotid artery occlusion was first suggested by Fisher[4] in 1951. The development of these procedures would not have been possible without the pioneering work of Jacobsen and Suarez,[5] who in 1960 described microsurgical techniques that allowed the anastomosis of blood vessels 2 mm in diameter. In 1963, Woringer and Kunlin[6] sutured a saphenous vein graft from the cervical portion of the internal carotid artery (ICA) to its intracranial portion (intracranial ICA). The graft remained patent at the time of the patient's death from coronary artery disease a few days later. Lougheed and colleagues[7] reported a similar procedure in 1971, after which a venous bypass graft remained patent for 9 months. In the 1970s, a patency rate of more than 50% was achieved by Neblett in a series of 22 patients with a cervical carotid artery–to–intracranial ICA saphenous vein graft for carotid occlusion.[8] Yasargil[9] performed an anastomosis between the superficial temporal artery (STA) and the middle cerebral artery (MCA) of a dog in the microsurgical laboratory at the University of Vermont in 1965. This anastomosis and a series of similar anastomoses in dogs remained patent. The first successful STA-MCA bypass procedures in patients were performed independently by Yasargil[9] in Zürich, Switzerland, on October 30, 1967, and Donaghy[8] in Burlington, Vermont, on October 31, 1967. In 1969, Yasargil[10] described in detail the results of 9 patients with cerebrovascular occlusive disease who had undergone successful STA-MCA cortical branch anastomosis.

TECHNIQUES

Various types of EC/IC arterial anastomoses have been performed. These include direct anastomosis of a branch of the external carotid artery (ECA) to a branch of the ICA or vertebrobasilar circulation intracranially, placement of an interposition vein or arterial graft between the extracranial and intracranial circulations, and an indirect anastomosis between ECA branches and the pial circulation of the brain surface. Indirect anastomoses between ECA branches and the brain circulation occur from the gradual development of microvascular collateral channels between a vascularized tissue, usually muscle or omentum, surgically placed on the surface of the brain, and the pial circulation. These procedures are rarely used to treat brain ischemia due to atherosclerotic occlusive disease. They are mainly used to treat progressive ischemia due to moyamoya disease.[11]

EXTRACRANIAL-INTRACRANIAL ARTERIAL BYPASS OF THE INTERNAL CAROTID ARTERY CIRCULATION

The most common EC/IC arterial bypass procedure used in the treatment of cerebral ischemia due to atherosclerotic occlusive disease has been the STA-MCA cortical branch anastomosis (Fig. 74–1). The donor and recipient arteries must be 1 mm or more in diameter. With smaller-diameter arteries, the rate of surgical patency falls sharply. There can be marked dilation of the donor and recipient arteries after this procedure.

The operation is performed by either placing a linear incision over the larger of the frontal or parietal branches of the STA or constructing a large frontotemporal scalp flap that preserves the STA branches.[12-16] With the latter technique, the donor branch of the STA is dissected from the inner surface of the scalp flap. A small craniotomy centered approximately 6 cm above the external auditory canal exposes distal (M_3) segments of the MCA exiting the posterior sylvian fissure. Usually an angular or posterior temporal branch is suitable for the recipient vessel. With the

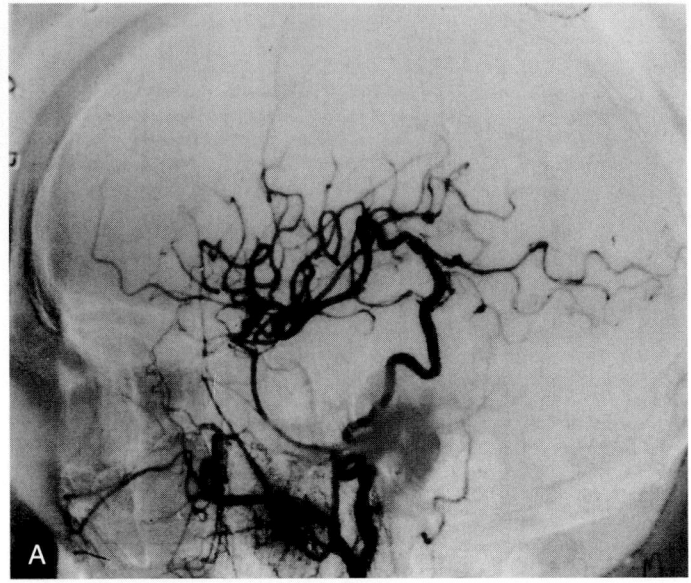

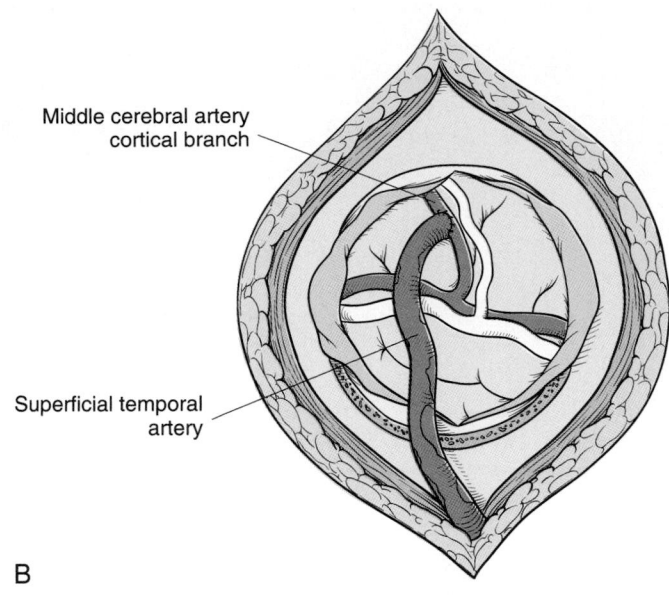

Middle cerebral artery
cortical branch

Superficial temporal
artery

B

FIGURE 74–1   A, *Cerebral angiographic demonstration of successful superior temporal artery-to-middle cerebral artery (STA-MCA) cortical branch anastomosis. B, Diagrammatic representation of STA-MCA cortical branch anastomosis.*

use of microscopic visualization, an end-to-side anastomosis is performed with either interrupted 10-0 monofilament nylon sutures or a combination of interrupted 10-0 nylon and continuous 10-0 polypropylene (Prolene) sutures.[17]

When the STA is not suitable for use as a donor vessel, the occipital artery can be used instead, or a short interposition saphenous vein graft can be placed from the proximal STA to either a cortical (M_3) MCA branch or an M_2 segment branch of the MCA. The latter technique requires two anastomoses, an end-to-end anastomosis proximally and an end-to-side anastomosis distally. Because of the relatively small size of the anastomoses with this procedure, EC-IC arterial bypasses using the STA or occipital artery as a donor vessel can usually be carried out with no more than 30 to 45 minutes of occlusion of the donor and recipient arteries, obviating systemic anticoagulation.

STA-MCA cortical branch anastomosis for symptomatic atherosclerotic occlusive disease of the ICA circulation is the only EC/IC arterial bypass procedure that has been studied with a large randomized trial comparing medical and surgical treatments. In this trial, postoperative patency rates for the bypass were 96%.

When the STA or occipital arteries are not adequate for donor vessels, an interposition graft using the saphenous vein,[7,18,19] radial artery, or a synthetic vascular substitute such as polytetrafluoroethylene (PTFE; Gore-Tex)[20] can be performed, usually between the external or common carotid artery (CCA) and a large, proximal (M_2) branch of the MCA or the intracranial ICA (Fig. 74–2). The innominate, subclavian, and vertebral arteries have also been used as donor arteries. These high-flow bypasses routinely deliver a flow of 75 to 175 mL/min.[19] The procedures are technically more difficult and have a higher rate of complications compared with STA-MCA cortical branch anastomosis.

Venous interposition grafts are usually obtained from the saphenous vein in the lower leg. This vessel commonly

narrows as it approaches the popliteal space, making this portion of the vessel ideal for anastomosis with the intracranial vessel. An incision is made in the neck to expose either the ECA or the subclavian artery. From this incision, the vein is passed subcutaneously, either anterior or posterior to the ear, into a frontotemporal craniotomy that exposes either the intracranial ICA or the anterior sylvian fissure. Usually, a preauricular route is used for passage of the interposition graft if the ICA or an M_2 segment of the MCA is to be used as the recipient vessel. Heparin is then given for systemic anticoagulation. An end-to-side anastomosis of the interposition graft to the donor artery in the neck is then performed, using 6-0 or 7-0 Prolene sutures placed in a continuous fashion. The vein graft is then filled with heparinized saline and temporarily occluded several centimeters proximal to its distal end so as to distend the graft. The vein graft is occluded proximally while an end-to-side anastomosis to the recipient vessel is carried out by means of continuous suturing techniques with 9-0 or 10-0 Prolene. The systemic anticoagulation is then reversed. Long saphenous vein grafts have a lower long-term patency rate than STA-MCA cortical branch anastomoses. The Mayo Clinic reported patency rates of 86% at 1 year, 82% at 5 years, and 73% at 13 years for long saphenous vein bypass grafts to the carotid and vertebrobasilar circulations.[18]

EXTRACRANIAL-INTRACRANIAL ARTERIAL BYPASS OF THE VERTEBROBASILAR CIRCULATION

EC/IC arterial bypass of the vertebrobasilar circulation is technically more difficult to perform than EC-IC arterial bypass of the anterior circulation. Because of the deep sites within the intracranial cavity at which this bypass is performed, very long instruments, which are more difficult

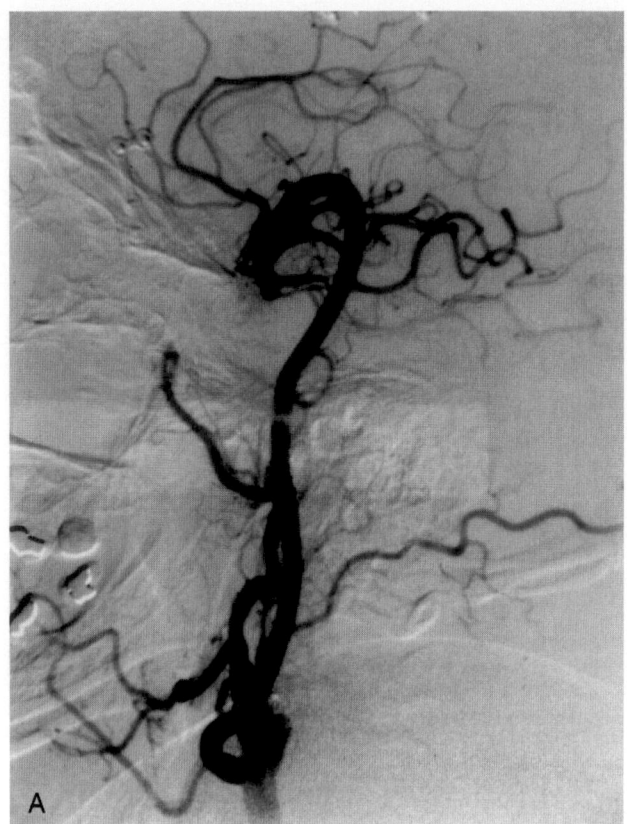

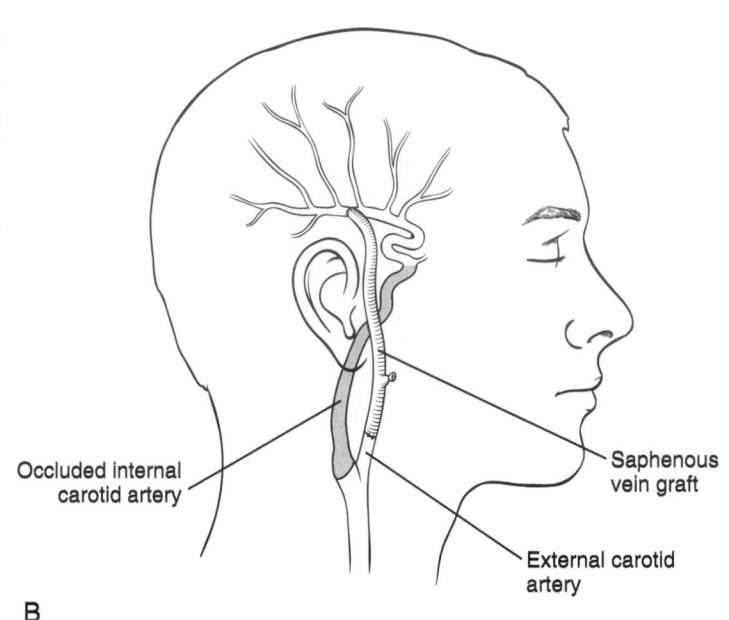

Occluded internal
carotid artery

Saphenous
vein graft

External carotid
artery

A

B

FIGURE 74–2   A, *Cerebral angiographic demonstration of successful saphenous vein interposition graft between the carotid cerebral artery (CCA) and an M_2 segment branch of the middle cerebral artery (MCA). B, Diagrammatic representation of interposition vein graft between the external carotid artery (ECA) and an M_2 segment branch of the MCA.*

to control, are required. The complication rates for EC/IC arterial bypasses of the posterior circulation are higher than those for anterior circulation bypasses.

An occipital artery-to-posterior inferior cerebellar artery (PICA) anastomosis is commonly used for occlusive lesions of the vertebral artery proximal to the origin of the PICA.[21-23] Through a unilateral suboccipital craniotomy, an end-to-side anastomosis is performed, with the tonsillar segment of the PICA, distal to the lateral medullary segment, used as the recipient artery. For occlusive disease of the vertebral arteries distal to the PICA or at the vertebrobasilar junction, the occipital artery is anastomosed to the anterior inferior cerebellar artery (AICA).[24] The operative exposure is nearly the same as that used for an occipital artery–PICA anastomosis. The AICA must be isolated in the cerebellopontine angle at the level of the facial and auditory nerves. The segment of AICA used as a recipient artery must be distal to the origin of brainstem perforating vessels. This anastomosis is extremely difficult to perform because of the small size of AICA and the depth at which sutures must be placed in the anastomosed arteries.

Patients who have stenosis or occlusion of the proximal or middle portion of the basilar artery without collateral flow from the anterior circulation require an EC/IC bypass to the superior cerebellar artery (SCA) or posterior cerebral artery (PCA).[18,19,25,26] Either the STA or a venous interposition graft is used as the donor vessel. A subtemporal craniotomy is performed, and the donor vessel is brought

across the floor of the middle cranial fossa to the lateral aspect of the cerebral peduncle. Systemic anticoagulation is generally not used, because the temporal lobe is retracted during the procedure. An end-to-side anastomosis is performed, with use of either the larger of the rostral and caudal branches of the perimesencephalic portion of the SCA or the P_2 segment of the PCA as the recipient artery. The collateral circulation of the PCA is less extensive than that of the SCA, and a significant risk of performing an anastomosis to the PCA is cortical blindness. An interposition saphenous vein graft from the ECA to the PCA or SCA can achieve early high volume flow, but the incidence of long-term graft failure is higher.

COMPLICATIONS

Major postoperative complications related to EC/IC arterial bypass are most often ischemic or hemorrhagic.[27] Ischemic events may be embolic, secondary to graft occlusion, or hemodynamic in origin.[28-30] Emboli may arise from the donor vessel or an interposition graft, from an anastomotic site, or from a bypassed artery. Focal vasospasm at the site of an arterial anastomosis can occur, leading to ischemia. Hemorrhagic complications can occur secondary to poor suturing techniques, which cause leakage from an anastomosis or from intraparenchymal hemorrhage due to a sudden large increase of blood flow to an area of chronic brain ischemia.[31–33] This latter problem is more common with EC-IC bypass procedures that involve large flow volumes. Postoperative hemorrhagic complications can be reduced by careful blood pressure control after surgery, delay of bypass procedures after recent brain infarction, and avoidance of placement of anastomoses in regions of encephalomalacia.

Other postoperative complications are seizures, cerebral edema, meningitis, subdural hematoma, subdural hygroma, and epidural hematoma. Problems with wound healing, including scalp necrosis and infection, may occur. These problems are more common in patients in whom the STA has been used as a donor artery, leading to devascularization of the scalp. Patients undergoing EC/IC arterial bypass for atherosclerotic occlusive disease also have an increased risk for postoperative cardiac complications, including myocardial infarction.

THE EXTRACRANIAL-INTRACRANIAL ARTERIAL BYPASS TRIAL

In the 1970s EC/IC arterial anastomosis was widely performed for atherosclerotic occlusive disease. An international multicenter randomized trial was conducted between 1977 and 1985 to test the ability of the operation to reduce the rate of subsequent stroke among patients with symptomatic atherosclerotic lesions of the ICA or MCA.[34] Patients who had experienced transient ischemic attacks (TIAs) or minor strokes in the carotid artery distribution within the previous 3 months were eligible for study. The patients were grouped according to the radiologic site of the most distal directly inaccessible lesion, as follows: occlusion of the ICA, stenosis of the ICA at or above the second cervical vertebra, occlusion of the M_1 segment of the MCA, and stenosis of the M_1 segment of the MCA. A total of 1377 patients were entered into the trial, with 714 patients assigned to best medical care (aspirin) and 663 assigned to best medical care with the addition of an STA-MCA cortical branch anastomosis.

The patients were followed for an average of 55.8 months. The 30-day perioperative mortality and morbidity rate was 12.2%. The major stroke rate was 4.5%, and the mortality rate was 1.1%. However, the average delay from randomization to surgery was 9 days, and one third of the perioperative morbidity and mortality occurred in patients before they underwent surgery. During surgery and in the ensuing 30 days, the major stroke rate was 2.5% and the mortality rate was 0.6%. The postoperative bypass patency rate was 96%. Outcome events included stroke, death from stroke, and death from all causes with particular emphasis on stroke occurring in the cerebral hemisphere, which was symptomatic at the time of entry into the trial. The study showed no benefit for surgery. Separate analyses in patients with different angiographic lesions did not identify a subgroup with any benefit from surgery. Secondary survival analyses comparing the medical and surgical groups for major strokes and all deaths, for all strokes and all deaths, and for ipsilateral ischemic strokes demonstrated a similar lack of benefit from surgery. Patients with severe MCA stenosis or persistent ischemic symptoms after ICA occlusion had a substantially worse outcome with surgery.

During the time that this study was being conducted, 2572 other patients, who were not part of the study, underwent EC-IC bypass. This fact led to the suggestion that the patients who had surgery outside the trial were the patients who naturally would have done better with the procedure.[35] However, results reported by 52 centers in the trial that did not operate on patients outside the study were analyzed separately. The patients in these centers, who represented 87% of the subjects enrolled in the study, also had no benefit from the surgical procedure.[36,37]

On the basis of the results of this trial, EC/IC arterial bypass was generally abandoned as a treatment for symptomatic atherosclerotic cerebrovascular disease. The EC-IC bypass trial was also criticized for failing to identify and separately analyze the subgroup of patients with reduction in cerebral perfusion pressure (CPP) in whom surgical revascularization might be more beneficial.[38–40] At the time the trial was conducted, there was no reliable and proven method for identifying a subgroup of patients in whom cerebral hemodynamic factors were of primary pathophysiologic importance. In addition, STA-MCA bypass was criticized for not providing adequate augmentation of blood flow to restore cerebral hemodynamics to normal.

These events led to the development of other surgical revascularization strategies based on the premise that hemodynamic factors are important.[41] The largest subgroup of patients in the EC/IC Arterial Bypass Trial had complete occlusion of the ICA. Prevention of further stroke in patients with complete carotid artery occlusion remains a difficult challenge, because no therapy has been proven effective for preventing subsequent stroke. These patients constitute approximately 15% of patients with carotid territory TIAs or infarction.[42–44] Twelve prospective follow-up studies of angiographically documented symptomatic carotid occlusion of 1261 patients, who were followed for a mean of 45.5 months, found an overall risk of subsequent stroke of 7% per year and a risk of stroke ipsilateral to the occluded carotid artery of 5.9% per year.[45] These risks persist even with the use of platelet-inhibitor drugs and anticoagulants. The relative importance of hemodynamic and embolic factors in these patients remains unclear.[46–51] Such patients may suffer stroke from hemodynamic insufficiency distal to the carotid occlusion or from emboli arising from several sources, including the stump of the occluded ICA in the neck, the tail of the stagnation thrombus that forms distal to the occlusion, and the contralateral carotid artery. Because EC/IC arterial bypass is unlikely to provide protection from embolic stroke, its efficacy in preventing stroke should be greatest in those patients in whom hemodynamic factors are important in the pathogenesis of cerebral infarction.

ASSESSMENT OF CEREBRAL HEMODYNAMICS

The hemodynamic status of the human circulation can be indirectly assessed in vivo with a variety of different imaging techniques. These methods are not interchangeable because they rely on different physiologic mechanisms to infer the presence of hemodynamic compromise. Measurements of cerebral blood flow (CBF) alone are inadequate for this purpose because they cannot distinguish reduction in CBF due to the hemodynamic effects of arterial occlusive disease from compensatory physiologic reductions in CBF caused by the lower metabolic demands of damaged tissue. Thus, it is necessary to rely on indirect assessments based on the compensatory responses made by the brain to progressive reductions in cerebral perfusion pressure (CPP).

When CPP is normal (stage 0 hemodynamic failure), CBF is closely matched to the resting metabolic rate of the tissue. As a consequence of this resting balance between flow and metabolism, the oxygen extraction fraction (OEF) of the brain shows little regional variation. Moderate reductions in CPP have little effect on CBF. Vasodilation of arterioles reduces cerebrovascular resistance, thus maintaining a constant CBF (stage I hemodynamic failure). This phenomenon is known as *cerebrovascular autoregulation*. As a consequence of arteriolar vasodilation, the intravascular cerebral blood volume (CBV) is often elevated, although this finding has been inconsistent. With more severe reductions in CPP (stage II hemodynamic failure), the capacity for compensatory vasodilation is exceeded, and autoregulation fails. CBF begins to decline, but a progressive rise in OEF now maintains cerebral oxygen metabolism and brain function.[49,52,53] This more severe form of cerebral hemodynamic failure has also been called "misery perfusion."[54]

Two basic approaches have been used to assess regional cerebral hemodynamics in humans. The first approach is based on detecting stage I autoregulatory vasodilation by either measuring CBF and CBV or by determining whether there is reduced responsiveness of CBF to a vasodilatory stimulus. A variety of vasodilatory stimuli have been used, including hypercapnia, acetazolamide, and physiologic tasks such as hand movement.[47,49,53,55,56] Normally, each of these vasodilatory stimuli produces a robust increase in CBF. Failure of this augmentation is interpreted as evidence of preexisting autoregulatory vasodilation (stage I hemodynamic failure). The second approach is based on detection of increases in regional OEF (stage II hemodynamic failure).[47,49,53,57,58] Compared with the use of vasodilatory stimuli or CBV measurements, interpretation of increased OEF does not require any inferences about hemodynamic status because it is the direct measurement of a pathophysiologic response.

Measurement of OEF is currently possible only with positron emission tomography (PET). The correlation between the CBF response to vasodilatory agents and increased OEF has been somewhat variable and inconsistent.[59–65] It is not possible at this time to identify a non-PET method of assessing OEF that has sufficient and proven sensitivity and specificity for a substitute method.

CEREBRAL HEMODYNAMICS AND STROKE RISK

Many different methodologies have been used to assess the effect of cerebral hemodynamics on the pathogenesis and treatment of stroke (Table 74.1). In many of these

reports, follow-up information about patients studied with these techniques has been limited and not sufficient to allow definitive conclusions. Stage I hemodynamic compromise was found to be associated with an increased stroke risk in six studies, but three studies did not find an association.

Yonas and coworkers[40] tested cerebrovascular reserve in patients with atherosclerotic occlusive carotid artery disease by means of paired CBF measurements obtained with the stable xenon-CT scanning method, with the cerebral vasodilatory agent acetazolamide given intravenously 20 minutes prior to the second study. Forty-one of the 68 patients in the study had ICA occlusion, and the remainder had greater than 70% carotid artery stenosis. The patients were retrospectively assigned to one of two groups according to the vascular territory found to have the lowest cerebral vasoreactivity and a relatively low baseline CBF. The first group (n = 27) had baseline blood flow values greater than $45 \, \mathrm{mL \cdot 100 \, g^{-1} \cdot min^{-1}}$ or cerebrovascular reserves of 5% or greater. The second group (n = 41) had initial blood flow values less than $45 \, \mathrm{mL \cdot 100 \, g^{-1} \cdot min^{-1}}$ and cerebrovascular reserves of less than 5%. During a mean follow-up of 24 months, there were two contralateral strokes in the first group and eight ipsilateral strokes in the second group (12.6 times greater chance of stroke). None of the 25 patients with ICA occlusion in the first group had an ipsilateral stroke, whereas 5 of 16 patients with ICA occlusion in the second group suffered a subsequent ipsilateral stroke (31% stroke risk). The same investigators subsequently added 27 patients for an analysis of 95 patients with either stenosis of ≤70% or carotid artery occlusion.[66] The patients were classified into two groups on the basis of a paradoxical response to acetazolamide and monitored for a mean of 19.6 months. In the second group, with the more severe impairment of cerebral vasoreactivity, 8 of 38 patients with occlusion of the ICA had a subsequent ipsilateral stroke (21% stroke risk).

In another longitudinal study, Keiser and Widder[67] tested the cerebrovascular reserve capacity in 85 patients with ICA occlusion by means of transcranial Doppler (TCD) ultrasonography. At the time of entry into the study, 46 patients had no symptoms on the side of the ICA occlusion, 13 had presented with TIAs, and 26 had had a minor stroke. MCA blood flow velocity and end-tidal PCO_2 were monitored during steady states of normocapnia, hypercapnia induced by breathing 5% CO_2 in 95% O_2, and hypocapnia produced by voluntary hyperventilation. The patients were prospectively classified into three groups according to the results of the CO_2 reactivity studies and monitored for a mean of 38 months. In the group with normal CO_2 reactivity, 4 of 48 patients had an ipsilateral TIA, but no patient had a stroke. Six of 26 patients with moderate impairment of CO_2 reactivity experienced an ipsilateral ischemic event (3 [12%] strokes, 3 TIAs), and 3 patients a contralateral ischemic event (2 strokes, 1 TIA). In the group with more severe impairment of CO_2 reactivity, 5 of 11 patients (45%) had an ipsilateral stroke, 1 patient had an ipsilateral TIA, and 2 patients had a contralateral hemisphere stroke. There was no significant difference in the risk of subsequent stroke between patients with and patients without a history of neurologic symptoms at the time the ICA occlusion was discovered. This finding is

Table 74.1 Cerebral Hemodynamics and Stroke Risk

Study[°]	Study Design	No. of Patients	Follow-Up (months)	Technique	Cerebral Vasoreactivity (No. of Patients) (Ipsilateral Annual Stroke Risk)[‡]		
					Normal	**Moderate Impairment**	**Severe Impairment**
Powers et al (1989)[75]	Retrospective	30	12	PET	9	21	
				CBV/CBF & OEF	11	0	
Hasegawa et al (1992)[76]	Prospective	51	18.5	SPECT CBF	31	20	
				Acetazolamide test	0	0	
Kleiser and Widder (1992)[67]	Prospective	85[†]	38	Transcranial Doppler Ultrasonography	48	26	11
				CO_2 reactivity	0	7%	24%
Widder et al (1994)[70]	Prospective	86 (111)[†]	1:19 2:31.7	Transcranial Doppler CO_2	2:(48) 1	2:(37) 1%	1:(26) 8%
Yonas et al (1993)[40]	Retrospective	41[†]	24	Xenon-CT CBF	25	16	
				Acetazolamide test	0	16%	
Webster et al (1995)[66]	Retrospective	64°	19.6	Xenon-CT CBF	26	38	
				Acetazolamide test	0	13%	
Yokota et al (1998)[74]	Prospective	105	32.5	SPECT CBF	50	55	
				Acetazolamide test	4%	4%	
Vernieri et al (1999)[71]	Prospective	42[†]	24	Transcranial Doppler Ultrasonography	9	33	
				Breath holding index	0	12%	
Kuroda et al (2001)[73]	Prospective	77	1:18.4 2:43.9 3:48.7	SPECT CBF	3:39	2:27	1:11
				Acetazolamide test	0.6	2%	23.7%
Yamauchi et al (1996)[77]	Prospective	40	12	PET	33		7
				OEF	6%		57%
Yamauchi et al (1999)[78]	Prospective	40	60	PET	33		7
				OEF	3%		11%
Grubb et al (1998)[79]	Prospective	81[†]	31.5	PET	42		39
				OEF	3%		13%

CBF, cerebral blood flow; CBV, cerebral blood volume; OEF, oxygen extraction factor; PET, positron emission tomography; SPECT, single-photon emission computed tomography; xenon-CT, xenon-enhanced computed tomography.

[°]Superscript numbers indicate chapter references.

[†]Only patients with internal carotid artery occlusion.

[‡]Numbers shown in parentheses are numbers of cerebral hemispheres.

puzzling because the prognosis of asymptomatic carotid occlusion is relatively benign.[68,69] The same investigative team later reported on 86 patients with carotid artery occlusion who were monitored for variable periods.[70] A stroke ipsilateral to an occluded ICA occurred in 3 of 26 patients with more severe impairment of CO_2 reactivity, corresponding to an annual stroke rate of 8% (mean follow-up, 19 months). The annual stroke rate in these patients was much lower in this study than in the group of patients previously reported by the same investigators. Only 1 of 37 patients with moderate impairment of CO_2 reactivity and 1 of 48 patients with normal CO_2 reactivity experienced an ipsilateral stroke (mean follow-up, 31.7 months).

Vernieri and colleagues[71] followed 65 patients with occlusion of the carotid artery prospectively for a median follow-up of 24 months; 42 patients were symptomatic (22 with stroke and 20 with TIA), and 23 patients asymptomatic. These researchers studied cerebral hemodynamics with TCD ultrasonography and calculated cerebrovascular reactivity to apnea with the breath-holding index (BHI) in the MCA. Thirty-three of the 42 asymptomatic patients had an abnormal BHI (<0.69). During the follow-up

period, 8 of the 33 symptomatic patients with an abnormal BHI had a stroke ipsilateral to the occluded carotid artery (12.2% annual ipsilateral stroke risk). None of the symptomatic patients with a normal BHI had a subsequent ipsilateral stroke. Twenty of the 23 asymptomatic patients had a normal BHI; only 1 of the 23 patients had a subsequent ipsilateral stroke, and this patient had a normal BHI. All ischemic events occurred between 8 and 25 months in the follow-up period.

In a prospective study, Marekus and Cullinane[72] examined 48 patients who had ICA occlusion with bilateral TCD ultrasonography of the MCAs. The patients either were asymptomatic or had experienced a stroke more than 3 months before they were studied. Cerebrovascular reactivity was tested by having the patients breathe 8% CO_2. During the follow-up period (mean of 1.71 years), there were 5 ipsilateral strokes, 2 ipsilateral TIAs, and 1 stroke and 2 TIAs in other vascular territories. The investigators did not classify the stroke rates according to the presence or absence of impaired reactivity to 8% CO_2. However, they concluded that impaired reactivity to 8% CO_2 was a significant predictor of both ipsilateral stroke and any stroke.

Kuroda and coworkers[73] observed 77 patients with symptomatic occlusion of the ICA or MCA for an average of 42.7 months. The patients had either no or localized cerebral infarction on MRI or CT and no or minimal neurologic deficit. Cerebrovascular reserve capacity was tested with the use of xenon 133 single-photon emission computed tomography (SPECT) to make paired regional CBF (rCBF) measurements, with acetazolamide given intravenously 15 minutes before the second study. The patients were prospectively classified into the following groups: group 1, normal rCBF and normal regional cerebrovascular resistance (rCVR); group 2, normal rCBF and reduced rCVR; group 3, reduced rCBF and reduced rCVR; and group 4, reduced rCBF and normal rCVR. During the follow-up period, 16 strokes occurred, 7 of which were ipsilateral. The annual risks of total and ipsilateral stroke were 35.6% and 23.7%, respectively, in patients with severe cerebral hemodynamic impairment (group 3); 3.85% and 2%, respectively, in patients with moderate cerebral hemodynamic impairment (groups 2 and 4); and 3.8% and 0.6%, respectively, in patients with normal cerebral hemodynamics (group 1).

The largest and methodologically soundest study that did not demonstrate a relationship between stage I impairment of cerebral hemodynamics and the risk of subsequent stroke was a prospective study reported by Yokota and associates.[74] They studied 105 patients who had evidence of ischemic cerebrovascular events, CT findings of minimal infarct, and cerebral angiographic confirmation of unilateral occlusion or severe stenosis (>75% in diameter) of the ICA or proximal MCA. Each patient underwent SPECT study of cerebral perfusion using N-isopropyl-P-[^{123}I-iodoamphetamine] and measurement of cerebrovascular reactivity using acetazolamide. Cerebral vasoreactivity response to acetazolamide was abnormal in 55 patients and normal in 50 patients. The two groups had similar stroke risk factors and vascular lesion sites. The primary endpoint was stroke occurrence. During the follow-up period (mean of 32.5 months), 13 patients experienced a stroke, 11 died, 16 underwent surgical cerebral revascularization procedures (9 EC-IC bypasses and 7 carotid endarterectomies), and 11 were lost to follow-up. There was no significant difference in the rate of subsequent stroke between the two groups. Follow-up SPECT studies with acetazolamide testing showed that cerebrovascular reactivity became normal at an average of 2 years in 11 of 24 patients with initially impaired response to acetazolamide.

A small longitudinal retrospective study monitored 30 medically treated patients with a mixture of cerebrovascular lesions, including carotid artery occlusion and intracranial stenoses, for 1 year.[75] All patients underwent PET measurements of the CBV/CBF ratio and OEF. In 21 patients with increased CBV/CBF ratios distal to a stenotic or occluded artery, no ipsilateral ischemic strokes occurred during follow-up. One of 9 patients with normal cerebral hemodynamics had an ipsilateral ischemic stroke during follow-up. Another small prospective study studied 51 patients for 1.5 years.[76] There was a mixture of asymptomatic and symptomatic carotid artery and intracranial artery stenoses of less than 75% and occlusions in these patients. Each patient underwent a SPECT study of cerebral perfusion using iodine 123 IMP and measurement of cerebrovascular reactivity using acetazolamide. Twenty patients were found to have impaired cerebrovascular reactivity. No patient experienced a stroke during the follow-up period.

A positive association of stage II cerebral hemodynamic compromise and stroke risk has been found by two groups. In these studies, the presence of increased OEF raised the subsequent risk for ipsilateral stroke. A small longitudinal study performed PET measurements of rCBF, rCBV, regional OEF (rOEF), and regional cerebral metabolic rate of oxygen (rCMRO$_2$) in 40 patients with symptomatic occlusion or intracranial stenosis of the ICA or MCA who were treated medically.[77] Six patients had TIAs and 34 patients had minor infarctions. The intervals between the most recent cerebral ischemic event and the PET studies were 1 to 55 months; 17 of the 40 patients were studied 30 to 90 days after their most recent cerebrovascular event. Patients had either normal or increased OEF, based on the absolute mean hemispheric value of OEF in the symptomatic cerebral hemisphere. At 1 year after the PET studies, strokes had occurred in 5 of 7 patients with increased OEF (4 ipsilateral) and in 4 of 33 patients with normal OEF (2 ipsilateral) All the patients experiencing a stroke in the follow-up period had had a minor stroke at entry into the study. In a subsequent study by the same investigators, a 5-year follow-up of these 40 patients was reported.[78] They evaluated increased OEF on the basis of two values, absolute OEF value and ratio of left cerebral hemisphere to right cerebral hemisphere. In the data analysis using absolute values of OEF, ischemic strokes occurred in 5 of 7 patients with increased OEF and 6 of 33 patients with normal OEF. There were 4 ipsilateral ischemic strokes in the group with increased OEF, and 5 in the group with normal OEF. All the strokes in patients with increased OEF occurred within 1 year. When the data were analyzed with the use of OEF asymmetry based on left-to-right cerebral hemisphere OEF ratios, ischemic strokes occurred in 6 of 14 patients with increased OEF and 5 of 26 patients with normal OEF. There were 5 ipsilateral ischemic strokes in patients with increased OEF, and 4 in those with normal OEF.

The strongest evidence of an association of cerebral hemodynamic impairment and stroke was seen in the St. Louis Carotid Occlusion Study.[79] This blinded, prospective study was conducted to test the hypothesis that stage II hemodynamic failure (increased OEF) in the cerebral hemisphere distal to complete carotid artery occlusion was an independent predictor of the subsequent risk of stroke in symptomatic, medically treated patients. The inclusion criterion was (1) occlusion of one or both common or ICAs as demonstrated by contrast-enhanced angiography or MRA in patients with TIAs (including transient monocular blindness) or (2) mild to moderate neurologic deficits (stroke) in the territory of the occluded carotid artery. Patients who had undergone ipsilateral external carotid endarterectomy (CEA) or contralateral CEA before PET were eligible whether or not they had had recurrent symptoms. A patient who underwent subsequent cerebrovascular surgery after the initial PET was dropped from the study at the time of surgery. PET measurements of CBF, CBV, CMRO$_2$, and OEF were carried out. Patients with left-to-right OEF ratios outside the normal range were categorized as having stage II hemodynamic compromise in the hemisphere with higher OEF. These categorizations were made without knowledge of the side of the carotid occlusion or of the clinical course of the patient after the PET study. The primary endpoint was subsequent ischemic stroke. Secondary endpoints were ipsilateral ischemic stroke and death. All living patients were followed for the duration of the study (mean of 31.5 months).

In 81 patients, initial data collection and PET measurements were successful, and they were enrolled in the study. Thirty-nine patients had stage II hemodynamic failure (increased OEF) in one hemisphere, and 42 did not. In all 39 patients with stage II hemodynamic failure, the hemisphere with increased OEF was ipsilateral to the occluded carotid artery. None of the subjects had bilateral carotid occlusion and increased OEF. No significant differences were found between the two groups in baseline risk factors or subsequent medical treatment. Arteriographic confirmation of collateral circulation did not permit distinction between the two groups. Fifteen ischemic strokes occurred, 13 of which were ipsilateral, during follow-up. In the 39 subjects with stage II hemodynamic compromise, 12 total and 11 ipsilateral strokes occurred. In the 42 subjects with normal OEF, there were 3 total and 2 ipsilateral strokes. The annual risk for ipsilateral stroke was 13.3% in patients with increased OEF and 2.7% in patients with normal OEF. Twelve deaths occurred during the follow-up period; 10 were due to non-stroke causes, and 2 resulted from large cerebral infarctions ipsilateral to a symptomatic occluded ICA. Both stroke-related deaths occurred in patients with increased OEF. In the univariate analysis of the relationship between outcome and patient characteristics and subsequent medical treatment, only younger age and stage II hemodynamic failure were significant predictors of both all strokes and ipsilateral ischemic stroke. Both variables remained significant in the multivariate analysis. This study demonstrated that stage II hemodynamic failure (increased OEF) distal to a symptomatic occluded carotid artery is an independent predictor of subsequent ischemic stroke. The study was prospective and blinded and addressed the possible effect of treatment and other risk factors for stroke. The rates of stroke and ipsilateral ischemic stroke in the total group of 81 symptomatic patients were similar to those reported by others, and the risk factor profile was typical for patients with carotid artery disease.[34,45,80]

CEREBRAL HEMODYNAMICS AND EXTRACRANIAL-INTRACRANIAL ARTERIAL BYPASS SURGERY

Multiple studies using PET have demonstrated postoperative improvement of cerebral hemodynamics with STA-MCA bypass surgery.[48,54,81–87] In patients with stage II hemodynamic failure (increased OEF), EC/IC bypass surgery returns hemispheric OEF ratios to normal.[48,82,83,86,87] Improvement in impaired cerebral vasoreactivity to CO_2 or acetazolamide after EC/IC bypass for atherosclerotic occlusive cerebrovascular disease has been reported.[39,56,88–91] In most of these patients, resting rCBF showed little change, although some patients with low

resting rCBF demonstrated improvement in blood flow in the affected cerebral hemisphere after surgery. EC/IC bypass has been recommended for symptomatic patients with appropriate cerebrovascular lesions in whom impaired cerebral vasomotor reactivity to acetazolamide or CO_2 testing is demonstrated.[39,66,92] All of these studies were retrospective analyses of surgical patients. No prospective study of patients with occlusion of the ICA and increased OEF or impaired cerebral vasoreactivity to CO_2 or acetazolamide who were randomly assigned to medical treatment or EC/IC bypass, with other risk factors for stroke controlled, has been reported. Thus, the long-term benefit of using impaired cerebral hemodynamics as a criterion in the selection of patients for EC-IC bypass to prevent stroke remains unproved at this time.

CAROTID OCCLUSION SURGERY STUDY

The results of medical treatment of patients with stage II hemodynamic compromise in the St. Louis Carotid Occlusion Study were poor,[79] being comparable to those reported for medically treated patients with symptomatic severe carotid stenosis.[80] Surgical procedures that improve cerebral hemodynamics, such as EC/IC arterial bypass surgery, would seem to be a logical treatment for these patients. However, in the absence of an empirical trial, it cannot be assumed that the stroke risk in patients who undergo the operation would be equal to that in patients with normal OEF nor that the morbidity and mortality of surgery would be outweighed by any subsequent reduction in stroke risk. The large, multicenter randomized trial of EC/IC bypass surgery conducted from 1977 to 1985 showed no benefit of surgery in preventing subsequent stroke.[34] At the time this trial was conducted, there was no reliable and proven method for identifying a subgroup of patients in whom cerebral hemodynamic factors were of primary pathophysiologic importance. It is now established that such a subgroup can be identified and, furthermore, that they are at high risk for subsequent stroke when treated medically.

On the basis of the findings of the St. Louis Carotid Occlusion Study, a new trial of EC/IC bypass surgery restricted to patients with symptomatic carotid occlusion and stage II cerebral hemodynamic impairment (increased OEF) has been organized.[93] The Carotid Occlusion Surgery Study (COSS), funded by the National Institutes of Health, began patient enrollment in 2002.

References

1. Blaisdell WF, Clauss RH, Galbraith JG, et al: Joint study of extracranial arterial occlusion. IV: A review of surgical considerations. JAMA 209:1889, 1969.
2. Fisher CM, Gore I, Okabe N, et al: Atherosclerosis of the carotid and vertebral arteries—extracranial and intracranial. J Neuropath Exp Neurol 24:455, 1965.
3. Fields WS, North RR, Hass WK, et al: Joint study of extracranial arterial occlusion as a cause of stroke. JAMA 203:955, 1968.
4. Fisher CM: Occlusion of the internal carotid artery. Arch Neurol Psychiatry 65:346, 1951.
5. Jacobsen JH, Suarez E: Microsurgery in anastomosis of small vessels. Surg Forum 11:243, 1960.

6. Woringer E, Kunlin J: Anastomose entré le carotid primitive et la carotide intra-cranienne ou la sylvienne par gréffon selon la technique de la suture suspendue. Neurochirurgie 9:181, 1963.

7. Lougheed WM, Marshall BM, Hunter M, et al: Common carotid to intracranial internal carotid bypass venous graft: Technical note. J Neurosurg 34:114, 1971.

8. Donaghy RMP: History of microneurosurgery. In Wise RJ, Rengachary SS (eds): Neurosurgery. New York, McGraw-Hill, 1985, p 20.

9. Yasargil MG: Experimental small vessel surgery in the dog including patching and grafting of cerebral vessels and the formation of functional extra-intracranial shunts. In Donaghy RMP, Yasargil MG (eds): Micro-Vascular Surgery. Stuttgart, Georg Thieme, 1967, p 87.

10. Yasargil MG: Diagnosis and indications for operations in cerebrovascular occlusive disease. In Yasargil MG (ed): Microsurgery Applied to Neurosurgery. Stuttgart, Georg Thieme, 1969, p 95.

11. Suzuki J, Takaku A: Cerebrovascular "moyamoya" disease: Disease showing abnormal net-like vessels in base of brain. Arch Neurol 20:288, 1969.

12. Yasargil MG: Anastomosis between the superficial temporal artery and a branch of the middle cerebral artery. In Yasargil MG (ed): Microsurgery Applied to Neurosurgery. Stuttgart, Georg Thieme, 1969, p 105.

13. Peerless SJ: Techniques of cerebral revascularization. Clin Neurosurg 23:258, 1976.

14. Ratcheson RA, Grubb RL Jr: Superficial temporal-middle cerebral cortical artery anastomosis. In Smith RR (ed): Stroke and the Extracranial Vessels. New York, Raven Press, 1984, p 255.

15. Reichman OH: Extracranial to intracranial arterial anastomosis. In Youmans JR (ed): Neurological Surgery. Philadelphia, WB Saunders, 1982, p 1584.

16. Tew JM Jr: Techniques of supratentorial cerebral revascularization. Clin Neurosurg 26:330, 1979.

17. Peerless SJ, Gamache FW Jr, Hunter IG: Continuous suture method for microvascular anastomosis: Technical note. Neurosurgery 8:695, 1981.

18. Regli L, Piepgras DG, Hansen KK: Late patency of long saphenous vein bypass grafts to the anterior and posterior cerebral circulation. J Neurosurg 83:806, 1995.

19. Samson DS: Users of extracranial-to-intracranial arterial bypass in current practice. In Tindall GT, Cooper PR, Barrow DH (eds): The Practice of Neurosurgery. Baltimore, Williams & Wilkins, 1996, p 1843.

20. Story JL, Brown WE, Eidelberg E, et al: Cerebral revascularization: Proximal external carotid to distal middle cerebral artery bypass with a synthetic tube graft. Neurosurgery 3:61, 1978.

21. Ausman JI, Chou SN, Lee M, et al: Occipital to cerebellar artery anastomosis for brain stem infarction from vertebrobasilar occlusive disease. Stroke 7:13, 1976.

22. Spetzler RF, Zabramski J: Revascularization of anterior and posterior circulation ischemia. Clin Neurosurg. 29:575, 1982.

23. Sundt TM Jr, Piepgras DG: Occipital to posterior inferior cerebellar artery bypass surgery. J Neurosurg 48:916, 1978.

24. Ausman JI, Diaz FG, los Reyes RA, et al: Anastomosis of occipital artery to anterior inferior cerebellar artery for vertebrobasilar junction stenosis. Surg Neurol 16:99, 1981.

25. Ausman JI, Diaz FG, los Reyes RA, et al: Posterior circulation revascularization: Superficial temporal artery to superior cerebellar artery anastomosis. J Neurosurg 56:766, 1982.

26. Sundt TM Jr, Piepgras DG, Houser OW, et al: Interposition saphenous vein grafts for advanced occlusive disease and large aneurysms in the posterior circulation. J Neurosurg 56:205, 1982.

27. Samson DS, Boone S: Extracranial-intracranial (EC/IC) arterial bypass: Past performance and current concepts. Neurosurgery 3:79, 1978.

28. Heros RC, Scott RM, Kistler JP, et al: Temporary neurological deterioration after extracranial-intracranial bypass. Neurosurgery 15:178, 1984.

29. Khodadad G: Transient postoperative occlusion of the superficial temporal—middle cerebral artery branch anastomosis: Spasm, swelling, or thrombosis. Surg Neurol 3:341, 1975.

30. Reichman OH: Complications of cerebral revascularization. Clin Neurosurg 23:318, 1976.

31. Diaz FG, Pearce J, Ausman JI: Complications of cerebral revascularization with autogenous vein grafts. Neurosurgery 17:271, 1985.

32. Heros RC, Nelson PB: Intracerebral hemorrhage after microsurgical cerebral revascularization. Neurosurgery 6:371, 1980.

33. Sundt TM Jr, Piepgras DG, Marsh WR, et al: Saphenous vein bypass grafts for giant aneurysms and intracranial occlusive disease. J Neurosurg 65:439, 1986.

34. Failure of extracranial-intracranial arterial bypass to reduce the risk of ischemic stroke. Results of an international randomized trial. EC/IC Bypass Study Group. N Engl J Med 313:1192, 1985.

35. Weir B: Extracranial-intracranial bypass surgery. In Webb KMA, Caplan LR, Reis DJ, et al (eds): Primer on Cerebrovascular Diseases. San Diego, Academic Press, 1997, p 578.

36. Barnett HJ, Fox A, Hachinski V, et al: Further conclusions from the extracranial-intracranial bypass trial. Surg Neurol 26:227, 1986.

37. Goldring S, Zervas N, Langfitt T: The Extracranial-Intracranial Bypass Study: A report of the committee appointed by the American Association of Neurological Surgeons to examine the study. N Engl J Med 316:817, 1987.

38. Day AL, Rhoton AL Jr, Little JR: The extracranial-intracranial bypass study. Surg Neurol 26:222, 1986.

39. Schmiedek P, Piepgras A, Leinsinger G, et al: Improvement of cerebrovascular reserve capacity by EC/IC arterial bypass surgery in patients with ICA occlusion and hemodynamic cerebral ischemia. J Neurosurg 81:236, 1994.

40. Yonas H, Smith HA, Durham SR, et al: Increased stroke risk predicted by compromised cerebral blood flow reactivity. J Neurosurg 79:483, 1993.

41. Diaz FG, Ausman JI, Mehta B, et al: Acute cerebral revascularization. J Neurosurg 63:200, 1985.

42. Balow J, Alter M, Resch JA: Cerebral thromboembolism: A clinical appraisal of 100 cases. Neurology 16:559, 1966.

43. Pessin MS, Duncan GW, Mohr JP, et al: Clinical and angiographic features of carotid transient ischemic attacks. N Engl J Med 296:358, 1977.

44. Thiele BL, Young JV, Chikos PM, et al: Correlation of arteriographic findings and symptoms in cerebrovascular disease. Neurology 30:1041, 1980.

45. Hankey GJ, Warlow CP: Prognosis of symptomatic carotid artery occlusion. Cerebrovasc Dis 1:245, 1991.

46. Barnett HJ: Hemodynamic cerebral ischemia: An appeal for systematic data gathering prior to a new EC/IC trial. Stroke 28:1857, 1997.

47. Derdeyn CP, Grubb RL Jr, Powers WJ: Cerebral hemodynamic impairment: Methods of measurement and association with stroke risk. Neurology 53:251, 1999.

48. Grubb RL Jr: Management of the patient with carotid occlusion and a single ischemic event. Clin Neurosurg 33:251, 1986.

49. Grubb RL Jr, Powers WJ: Role of cerebral hemodynamics in ischemic atherosclerotic cerebrovascular disease. Neurosurg Q 3:83, 1993.

50. Grubb RL Jr, Powers WJ: Risks of stroke and current indications for cerebral revascularization in patients with carotid occlusion. Neurosurg Clin N Am 12:473, 2001.

51. Klijn CJ, Kappelle LJ, Tulleken CA, et al: Symptomatic carotid artery occlusion: A reappraisal of hemodynamic factors. Stroke 28:2084, 1997.

52. Gibbs JM, Wise RJ, Leenders KL, et al: Evaluation of cerebral perfusion reserve in patients with carotid-artery occlusion. Lancet 1(8372):310, 1984.

53. Powers WJ: Cerebral hemodynamics in ischemic cerebrovascular disease. Ann Neurol 29:231, 1991.

54. Baron JC, Bousser MG, Rey A, et al: Reversal of focal "misery-perfusion syndrome" by extra-intracranial arterial bypass in hemodynamic cerebral ischemia: A case study with 150 positron emission tomography. Stroke 12:454, 1981.

55. Inao S, Tadokoro M, Nishino M, et al: Neural activation of the brain with hemodynamic insufficiency. J Cereb Blood Flow Metab 18:960, 1998.

56. Kuroda S, Kamiyama H, Abe H, et al: Acetazolamide test in detecting reduced cerebral perfusion reserve and predicting long-term prognosis in patients with internal carotid artery occlusion. Neurosurgery 32:912, 1993.

57. Powers WJ, Grubb RL Jr, Darriet D, et al: Cerebral blood flow and cerebral metabolic rate of oxygen requirements for cerebral function and viability in humans. J Cereb Blood Flow Metab 5:600, 1985.

58. Powers WJ, Press GA, Grubb RL Jr, et al: The effect of hemodynamically significant carotid artery disease on the hemodynamic status of the cerebral circulation. Ann Intern Med 106:27, 1987.

59. Hasegawa Y, Minematsu K, Matsuoka H, et al: CBF responses to acetazolamide and CO_2 for prediction of hemodynamic failure: A PET study. Stroke 28:242, 1997.

60. Hayashida K, Hirose Y, Tanaka Y, et al: Stratification of severity by cerebral blood flow, oxygen metabolism, and acetazolamide reactivity in patients with cerebrovascular disease. In Ishii Y (ed): Recent Advances in Biomedical Imaging. New York, Elsevier Science, 1997, p 113.

61. Herold S, Brozovic M, Gibbs J, et al: Measurement of regional cerebral blood flow, blood volume and oxygen metabolism in patients with sickle cell disease using positron emission tomography. Stroke 17:692, 1986.

62. Hirano T, Minematsu K, Hasegawa Y, et al: Acetazolamide reactivity on ^{123}I-IMP single photon emission computed tomography in patients with major cerebral artery occlusive disease: Correlation with positron emission tomography parameters. J Cereb Blood Flow Metab 14:763, 1994.

63. Kanno I, Uemura K, Higano S, et al: Oxygen extraction fraction at maximally vasodilated tissue in the ischemic brain estimated from the regional CO_2 responsiveness measured by positron emission tomography. J Cereb Blood Flow Metab 8:227, 1988.

64. Nariai T, Suzuki R, Hirakawa K, et al: Vascular reserve in chronic cerebral ischemia measured by the acetazolamide challenge test: Comparison with positron emission tomography. AJNR Am J Neuroradiol 16:563, 1995.

65. Sugimori H, Ibayashi S, Fujii K, et al: Can transcranial Doppler really detect reduced cerebral perfusion states? Stroke 26:2053, 1995.

66. Webster MW, Makaroun MS, Steed DL, et al: Compromised cerebral blood flow reactivity is a predictor of stroke in patients with symptomatic carotid artery occlusive disease. J Vasc Surg 21:338, 1995.

67. Kleiser B, Widder B: Course of carotid artery occlusions with impaired cerebrovascular reactivity. Stroke 23:171, 1992.

68. Bornstein NM, Norris JW: Benign outcome of carotid occlusion. Neurology 39:6, 1989.

69. Powers WJ, Derdeyn CP, Fritsch SM, et al: Benign prognosis of never-symptomatic carotid occlusion. Neurology 54:878, 2000.

70. Widder B, Kleiser B, Krapf H: Course of cerebrovascular reactivity in patients with carotid artery occlusions. Stroke 25:1963, 1994.

71. Vernieri F, Pasqualetti P, Passarelli F, et al: Outcome of carotid artery occlusion is predicted by cerebrovascular reactivity. Stroke 30:593, 1999.

72. Markus H, Cullinane M: Severely impaired cerebrovascular reactivity predicts stroke and TIA risk in patients with carotid artery stenosis and occlusion. Brain 124:457, 2001.

73. Kuroda S, Houkin K, Kamiyama H, et al: Long-term prognosis of medically treated patients with internal carotid or middle cerebral artery occlusion: Can acetazolamide test predict it? Stroke 32:2110, 2001.

74. Yokota C, Hasegawa Y, Minematsu K, et al: Effect of acetazolamide reactivity on long-term outcome in patients with major cerebral artery occlusive diseases. Stroke 29:640, 1998.

75. Powers WJ, Tempel LW, Grubb RL Jr: Influence of cerebral hemodynamics on stroke risk: One-year follow-up of 30 medically treated patients. Ann Neurol 25:325, 1989.

76. Hasegawa Y, Yamaguchi T, Tsuchiya T, et al: Sequential change of hemodynamic reserve in patients with major cerebral artery occlusion or severe stenosis. Neuroradiology 34:15, 1992.

77. Yamauchi H, Fukuyama H, Nagahama Y, et al: Evidence of misery perfusion and risk for recurrent stroke in major cerebral arterial occlusive diseases from PET. J Neurol Neurosurg Psychiatry 61:18, 1996.

78. Yamauchi H, Fukuyama H, Nagahama Y, et al: Significance of increased oxygen extraction fraction in five-year prognosis of major cerebral arterial occlusive diseases. J Nucl Med 40:1992, 1999.

79. Grubb RL Jr, Derdeyn CP, Fritsch SM, et al: Importance of hemodynamic factors in the prognosis of symptomatic carotid occlusion. JAMA 280:1055, 1998.

80. Beneficial effect of carotid endarterectomy in symptomatic patients with high-grade stenosis. North American Symptomatic Carotid Endarterectomy Trial Collaborators. N Engl J Med 325:445, 1991.

81. Baron JC, Rey A, Guillard A: Non-invasive tomographic imaging of cerebral blood flow (CBF) and oxygen extraction fraction (OEF) in superficial temporal artery to middle cerebral artery (STA-MCA) anastomosis. In Meyer JS, Lechner H, Reivich M, et al (eds): Cerebral Vascular Disease. Amsterdam, Excerpta Medica, 1981, p 58.

82. Gibbs JM, Wise RJ, Thomas DJ, et al: Cerebral haemodynamic changes after extracranial-intracranial bypass surgery. J Neurol Neurosurg Psychiatry 50:140, 1987.

83. Iwama T, Hashimoto N, Hayashida K: Cerebral hemodynamic parameters for patients with neurological improvements after extracranial-intracranial arterial bypass surgery: Evaluation using positron emission tomography. Neurosurgery 48:504, 2001.

84. Kawamura S, Sayama I, Yasui N, et al: Haemodynamic and metabolic changes following extra-intracranial bypass surgery. Acta Neurochir 126:135, 1994.

85. Leblanc R, Tyler JL, Mohr G, et al: Hemodynamic and metabolic effects of cerebral revascularization. J Neurosurg 66:529, 1987.

86. Powers WJ, Martin WR, Herscovitch P, et al: Extracranial-intracranial bypass surgery: Hemodynamic and metabolic effects. Neurology 34:1168, 1984.

87. Samson Y, Baron JC, Bousser MG, et al: Effects of extra-intracranial arterial bypass on cerebral blood flow and oxygen metabolism in humans. Stroke 16:609, 1985.

88. Batjer HH, Devous MD Sr, Purdy PD, et al: Improvement in regional cerebral blood flow and cerebral vasoreactivity after extracranial-intracranial arterial bypass. Neurosurgery 22:913, 1988.

89. Bishop CC, Burnand KG, Brown M, et al: Reduced response of cerebral blood flow to hypercapnia: Restoration by extracranial-intracranial bypass. Br J Surg 74:802, 1987.

90. Karnik R, Valentin A, Ammerer HP, et al: Evaluation of vasomotor reactivity by transcranial Doppler and acetazolamide test before and after extracranial-intracranial bypass in patients with internal carotid artery occlusion. Stroke 23:812, 1992.

91. Vorstrup S, Brun B, Lassen NA: Evaluation of the cerebral vasodilatory capacity by the acetazolamide test before EC/IC bypass surgery in patients with occlusion of the internal carotid artery. Stroke 17:1291, 1986.

92. Widder B, Kornhuber HH: Extra-intracranial bypass surgery in carotid artery occlusions: Who benefits? Neurol Psychiat Brain Res 2:126, 1994.

93. Adams HP Jr, Powers WJ, Grubb RL Jr, et al: Preview of a new trial of extracranial-to-intracranial arterial anastomosis: The Carotid Occlusion Surgery Study. Neurosurg Clin N Am 12:613, 2001.

Chapter Seventy-Five

Cerebral Infarction: Surgical Treatment

Bryce Weir

Various surgical approaches have been advocated for the treatment of acute life-threatening cerebral ischemia (Tables 75.1 through 75.6). For those patients in whom early revascularization by thrombolysis is not an option, the removal of a large portion of the skull represents a reasonable therapeutic approach. This decompressive hemicraniectomy has been performed with or without the placement of a dural patch graft. Some surgeons have performed excision of brain that was shown to be infarcted as a type of additional internal decompression. Removal of portions or all of the temporal lobe have sometimes been performed to prevent or treat transtentorial herniation. For an ischemic infarction with an associated region of hematoma, the region has been surgically removed. Ventricular drainage may permit the additional medical treatment of raised intracranial pressure (ICP) and the sampling of cerebrospinal fluid on an ongoing basis. Early revascularization by surgical means has even had its advocates.[1]

Hemicraniectomy permits the expansion of ischemic brain outwards so the likelihood of fatal transtentorial or diencephalic herniation is theoretically diminished. Whether or not the ultimate infarction resulting from ischemia in the middle cerebral artery (MCA) territory is smaller in patients with open skulls than in those with closed skulls is currently not known with certainty. The efficacy of hemicraniectomy has not been established in randomized clinical trials with appropriate controls. General acceptance of this procedure has been impeded by the fear that a reduction in mortality would result in an unacceptable increase in the number of patients with severe impairments.[2]

PATHOLOGY

Shaw and colleagues[3] studied swelling of the brain after cerebral infarction from arterial occlusion in 15 patients who died 18 hours to 3 months after the onset of hemiplegia. Fifty-three percent died less than 4.5 days after onset. Five of these patients died from embolism associated with recent myocardial infarction, 2 after cardiac surgery, 2 as a result of thrombosis of the internal carotid artery (ICA) and MCA associated with atherosclerosis, and 1 from dissection of the aortic arch. From these and other patients, the investigators constructed a series of 69 patients to plot the duration of brain swelling after ischemic infarction in the distribution of the MCA. Swelling was shown to peak in the first few days after the onset of symptoms, with a maximum occurrence around day 4. Transtentorial herniation was specifically recorded in 20 (29%) of the patients dying from ischemic infarction in the MCA territory.[3]

Mayo Clinic investigators reviewed 100 cases for which autopsies showed recent cerebral infarction in the ICA distribution. Transtentorial herniation was the most common cause of death. Thirty-six percent of all the patients and 47% of those with transtentorial herniation died within 48 hours of the onset of cerebral infarction. Sixty-two percent of the deaths due to transtentorial herniation occurred within 3 days, and 81% between days 1 and 4. The majority (68%) of patients with herniation had presented with either altered sensorium or hemiplegia. Altered sensorium alone and hemiplegia alone were relatively poor predictors of subsequent herniation. Fully one third (10/31) of the patients who ultimately died from herniation had neither altered sensorium nor hemiplegia at onset. Other causes of death in this cerebral infarction series were pneumonia (29%), pulmonary embolus (13%), and septicemia (5%).[4]

Of 353 autopsies performed over a decade at Philadelphia General Hospital in patients dying of acute supratentorial infarction, 45 (13%) showed severe brain swelling. Seventy-eight percent of these 45 patients died within 7 days of acute infarction. The rapidly fatal outcome was directly related to brain swelling, transtentorial herniation, brainstem edema, hemorrhage, or a combination of these conditions. Patients who survived longer than a week and died with increased ICP were thought to have sustained further infarctions superimposed upon earlier ones. Complicating visceral diseases were more common in this group and contributed to death in the majority of patients. Of the patients showing severe brain swelling, about two thirds were women. Only 7% of the patients were younger than 50 years; 38% were older than 70 years, and 56% were between 50 and 69 years. For the 45 patients dying with hemispheric swelling, the following findings were noted:

Table 75.1   Potential Surgical Therapy for Acute Cerebral Infarction

Decompressive hemicraniectomy
Durotomy and dural patch
Strokectomy (excision of infarcted brain)
Temporal lobectomy
Hippocampectomy
Removal of associated intracerebral hematoma or hemorrhagic infarct
Ventricular drainage
Early revascularization (extracranial-intracranial bypass)

Table 75.2   Evidence in Favor of Decompressive Hemicraniectomy

- Large numbers of anecdotal case reports and small series suggest that a reduction in mortality can be obtained without an unacceptably high rate of severe disability and complete dependence.
- The benefits appear to be greater in younger, healthier patients who undergo operation before brain edema–induced herniation is established.
- Animal experiments suggest that after occlusion of the middle cerebral artery, the size of infarcts can be reduced by craniectomy and that efficacy relates to the size of the decompression and the promptness with which it is carried out.
- By analogy, cerebellar decompression is generally accepted as efficacious for cerebellar ischemic infarction.

Table 75.3   Capability of Clinical and Imaging Features to Predict Fatal Brain Edema and Herniation in Total Middle Cerebral Artery Territory Ischemia

Reliable predictors	Single-photon emission computed tomography
	Diffusion-weighted and perfusion-weighted magnetic resonance imaging
Less reliable predictors	Routine computed tomography
	T1- and T2-weighted magnetic resonance imaging
	Initial pattern of vessel occlusion on angiography
	Clinical picture

Table 75.4   Potential Benefits of Decompressive Hemicraniectomy for Large Middle Cerebral Artery Infarcts

- Lives may be saved by the reduction of locally raised intracerebral pressure, which aborts brain creep and resultant transtentorial and/or rostral-caudal diencephalic herniation.
- Local reduction in intracerebral pressure may augment the perfusion pressure in the ischemic penumbra thereby decreasing the volume of infarcted tissue which improves neurological outcome

Table 75.5   Potential Adverse Effects of Decompressive Hemicraniectomy for Large Middle Cerebral Artery Infarcts

- A reduction in mortality may result in an increase in the number of severely dependent, depressed patients requiring long-term care.
- The high-intensity care required by this surgical procedure and its expense may negatively affect the availability of care for other patients with a higher potential for recovery.
- Patients are subjected to the usual complications of a major neurosurgical procedure (infection, blood loss, operative site bleeding, venous occlusion, wound dehiscence, cerebrospinal fluid leak, meningitis, complications of general anesthesia).

Table 75.6   Features of the Best Candidates for Decompressive Hemicraniectomy

- Too late for and not previously treated by thrombolysis
- Complete middle cerebral artery (MCA) territory ischemia as a minimum that is destined for infarction
- Young patients who have not yet experienced tentorial herniation
- No prohibitive intercurrent disease
- Personalities/environments/families willing to accept the neurologic deficits from MCA infarction and the risks and expense of surgery

tentorial herniation in 89%, brainstem edema in 80%, foraminal herniation in 76%, brainstem hemorrhage in 60%, falcial herniation in 33%, and secondary necrosis of the hippocampal gyrus in 18%, of the cingulate gyrus in 2%, and of the calcarine sulcus in none. The distribution of infarcts in the 45 cases of severe brain swelling was as follows: MCA, 40%; MCA plus anterior cerebral artery (ACA), 56%; and MCA plus anterior cerebral artery plus posterior cerebral artery (PCA), 4%.[5]

In a series of 845 Japanese patients with stroke reported by Niwa and associates,[6] 61% suffered from brain infarction. The distribution of types of infarction was as follows: atherothrombotic, 31%; cardioembolic, 22%; lacunar, 42%; and other types, 5%.[6]

RELATED OPERATIONS

Decompression for Cerebellar Infarction

Cerebellar infarction is commonly treated by suboccipital craniectomy and decompression with or without excision of infarcted tissue. This procedure is generally performed in patients who deteriorate clinically despite ventriculostomy. Contraindications are far-advanced clinical deterioration, massive brainstem infarction, excessive age, and overwhelming comorbidities. This type of decompressive surgery was accepted earlier and much more readily than cerebral decompressive procedures because neurologic deficits stemming from loss of cerebellar tissue are much easier to accept than overwhelming cognitive and personality deficits.[7-12] The level of consciousness is a powerful predictor of outcome in cerebellar infarction, and the time course is similar to that of cerebral infarction, with deterioration typically occurring between days 2 and 4, principally on the third day. Surgical treatment is not superior to medical treatment in patients who are awake or only drowsy.[10]

Decompression for Traumatic Brain Injury

Decompressive craniectomy has been applied with the use of a variety of surgical techniques for the treatment of uncontrollable ICP after trauma. A review of publications within the last 20 years did not demonstrate a clear benefit. In the personal series reported by Munch and colleagues,[13] 63% of patients undergoing surgical decompression within 4.5 hours of trauma were compared with 37% undergoing decompression later, an average of 56 hours after injury. Patients younger than 50 years who underwent rapid surgical decompression had a significantly better outcome than older patients and patients who underwent later surgical decompression. Craniectomy significantly decreased midline shift and improved visibility of the mesencephalic cisterns. In this group of patients with trauma, a significant decrease in midline shift after craniectomy did not have an observable beneficial effect on outcome. Of potential significance for the use of decompressive hemicraniectomy, the results of this study suggested that the distance of the lower border of the decompressive craniectomy from the temporal cranial base was more important to beneficial effect than the size of the craniectomy.[13]

ANIMAL STUDIES

In 1968, Moody and associates[14] evaluated decompression in a model using gradual inflation of a dural balloon in dogs. All 10 animals in the control group died within 12 hours. Seven of 10 dogs undergoing decompression lived 10 or more days, although none regained consciousness. All the dogs in the decompression group showed hemorrhagic infarcts, necrosis, and edema of the cortex at the decompression site. It is unlikely, however, that the extent of the decompression was sufficient to qualify as a hemicraniectomy.[14] Hatashita and coworkers[15] subjected cats to parietal craniectomy, arterial hypertension induced by aortic balloon catheter placement, or both. These investigators, evaluating the lesions with Evans blue dye extravasation and water content, found that lesions due to arterial hypertension and craniectomy extended further into underlying white matter than those due to hypertension or craniectomy alone. This finding suggests that arterial hypertension should be carefully counteracted in patients who undergo hemicraniectomy.

Forsting and associates[16] induced focal cerebral ischemia in 50 rats using an endovascular occlusion of the MCA technique. Mortality in the untreated group was 35%, whereas none of the animals subjected to decompressive craniectomy died. The average volume of infarction was 161 mm^3 in control animals, 26 mm^3 in animals subjected to craniectomy 1 hour after MCA occlusion, and 59 mm^3 in animals subjected to decompression at 24 hours.

In another study of 182 rats, MCA occlusion was obtained with use of the endovascular technique, followed by reperfusion or craniectomy at 1, 4, or 12 hours.[17] The neurologic score (a graded scale ranging from 0 [no apparent deficits] to 4 [spontaneous contralateral circling]) was 1.8 (better) and infarct volume 79 mm^3 (significantly smaller) in animals undergoing reperfusion at 1 hour. The respective values in the other groups were 3.8 and 225 mm^3 in control animals; 2.8 and 182 mm^3 in those undergoing reperfusion at 4 hours; and 3.7 and 231 mm^3 in those undergoing perfusion at 12 hours. Animals subjected to craniectomy at 1, 4, and 12 hours had better outcomes (neurologic scores of 1.6, 1.9, and 2.6, respectively) and smaller infarcts (96, 109, and 150 mm^3, respectively). These differences were all statistically significant ($P < .05$). Of interest was the finding that the combination of reperfusion and craniectomy was not significantly better than one treatment alone. If one could extrapolate these results to the clinical situation, it would seem that if patients can be treated within 3 hours, the preferred treatment for embolic or thrombotic MCA occlusion would be thrombolysis or mechanical disruption of the obstruction, whereas patients treated after the safe window for thrombolysis would be better candidates for decompressive hemicraniectomy.

NEUROLOGY

Silver and associates[18] reported on a series of 1073 consecutive patients with stroke treated in an intensive care unit, for whom the mortality rate within the first 30 days was 20%. The majority of deaths in the first week were due to transtentorial herniation. Deaths from infarction peaked between the third and sixth days after ictus. Half the deaths in the first week were due to relative immobility (pneumonia, pulmonary embolism, and sepsis), and the rate of deaths from this cause peaked toward the end of the second week. Cardiac deaths occurred throughout the first month and in many patients who had only small functional neurologic deficits.

Chambers and colleagues[19] assessed the factors affecting mortality and quality of life after acute stroke in 1013 patients who were followed for 2 to 8 years. After cerebral infarction, the major determinants of short-term mortality were impaired consciousness, leg weakness, and increasing age. The major determinants of long-term mortality were low levels of activity at hospital discharge, advanced age, male sex, associated heart disease, and hypertension.

All cases of first episodes of brain infarction occurring in Rochester, Minnesota, from 1960 to 1979 were studied by Turney and coworkers.[20] Hemispheric infarction occurred five times more often than brainstem or cerebellar infarction. The magnitude of decline in incidence was the same for each subgroup of infarctions during the 20-year period of the study. The 30-day case-fatality rates of the groups were comparable. Patients with brainstem infarction had better long-term survival and better functional outcome. One third returned to independent living by 1 year, compared with only 22% of survivors of hemispheric infarction. The investigators considered this difference to be the result of residual cognitive and sensory impairments present in survivors of hemispheric infarction. They defined brain infarction as the relatively rapid onset of a focal neurologic deficit arising as the result of a presumed vascular lesion, persisting for 24 hours or longer, and associated with clear cerebrospinal fluid and no evidence of hemorrhage on computed tomography (CT). The average annual incidence rates per 100,000 population fell from 101 at the outset of the study to 55 in the final period (1975 to 1979). Nine percent of patients with cerebral hemispheric infarctions had died by day 7 from ictus. The probability of 30-day survival for patients with hemispheric infarction was 96% for those who were alert on initial presentation but 35% for those who were comatose. At presentation, 803 patients with hemispheric infarction had a 22% incidence of headache and an 80% incidence of motor weakness. Fortyfive percent showed altered consciousness. One-year follow-up in the 505 survivors of hemispheric infarction revealed motor deficits in 57%, cognitive deficits in 34%, and social problems in 12%. Interestingly, 18% of these patients had been dependent (Rankin grade III, IV, or V) before the onset of the episode of infarction that brought them into this study. One year after hemispheric infarction, the distribution by Rankin grade was as follows: grade I, 22%; grade II, 12%; grade III, 17%; and grade IV/V, 13%; 36% of the patients had died. Within 1 week of the onset of hemispheric infarction, cardiac failure occurred in 16%, respiratory infection in 18%, urinary infection in 12%, pulmonary embolus in 1%, and myocardial infarction in 7%.[20]

Widjicks and Diringer[21] studied 42 patients within 24 hours after the onset of MCA occlusion symptoms. Seventy-nine percent of these patients deteriorated. The mortality rate was 27% in the 11 patients younger than 45 years and 91% in the 22 older patients.

In another study, Krieger and associates[22] reviewed data from the placebo arm of a drug trial to identify patients who experienced fatal brain edema. In the 23 patients who died from brain swelling, the minimum baseline National Institutes of Health Stroke Scale (NIHSS) score was 20 in those with left hemispheric infarction and 15 in those with right hemispheric infarction (NIHSS score higher than 22 describes a severe stroke). These investigators then selected 112 subjects from the remaining population who had comparable severe stroke ratings but had not died from brain swelling. The clinical and laboratory characteristics showing the strongest independent association with fatal brain swelling were nausea or vomiting within 24 hours after onset (odds ratio [OR] 5.1) and 12-hour systolic blood pressure 180 mm Hg or higher (OR 4.2). Among radiographic factors, only hypodensity of more than 50% of the MCA territory on the initial CT scan was an independent predictor of fatal swelling (OR 6.1). Krieger and associates[22] concluded that patients with hemispheric infarction are at high risk of subsequent fatal swelling if they have (1) a baseline NIHSS score of either 20 or higher for left hemispheric infarction or 15 or higher for right hemispheric infarction within 6 hours of symptom onset and (2) either nausea or vomiting or CT hypodensity of more than 50% of the MCA territory.

Of 201 patients with large MCA strokes who were identified retrospectively and studied via the case-control method, Kasner and associates[23] found that 47% died of brain swelling, 6% died of nonneurologic causes, and only 47% survived to day 30 after stroke. The odds ratios for predictors of fatal brain edema were as follows: for greater than 50% MCA hypodensity on CT, 6.3; for history of hypertension, 3.0; for history of heart failure, 2.1; for white blood cell (WBC) count per 1000 WBCs/μL, 1.08; and for involvement of vascular territory in addition to the MCA, 3.3. Initial level of consciousness, NIHSS score, early presence of nausea or vomiting, and serum glucose concentration were significantly associated with neurologic deaths in bivariate but not multivariate analysis.[23]

Because most patients with hemispheric infarction survive without decompressive hemicraniectomy, it is obviously very important to restrict this radical therapy to use in patients who are destined to die without it and who have a realistic chance of meaningful quality of life after surgery. The clinical findings by themselves, although important, are an insufficient basis upon which to make this therapeutic decision.

RADICAL NONSURGICAL THERAPY FOR HEMISPHERIC INFARCTION

It does not appear that any nonsurgical therapy or therapeutic combination is likely to be as efficacious as decompressive hemicraniectomy in patients with complete MCA territory infarcts.

Intubation

In a series of 250 patients with acute carotid artery territory ischemic stroke, 8% underwent elective intubation. The procedure was performed a mean of 41 hours after onset of symptoms. Once clinical deterioration began, half the patients needed intubation within an hour. The in-hospital mortality rate was 70%, but only 2 of the patients became independent during follow-up, one of whom underwent hemicraniectomy.[24] ElAd and colleagues[25] found that patients in neurologic intensive care units after cerebral infarction who need mechanical ventilation have an in-hospital mortality of more than 90%. These investigators studied 55 patients with complete MCA territory infarction due to an occlusion of either the distal intracranial carotid artery or the proximal MCA. All patients were assumed to have experienced embolic infarction. The mean Scandinavian Stroke Scale score at admission was 20, and the time course for deterioration varied from 2 to 5 days. Eighty-nine percent of the patients required ventilatory assistance. Seventy-eight percent of the patients died from transtentorial herniation with subsequent brain death. The 22% of patients who survived had a mean Barthel Index of 60 (range 45 to 70).

Complete MCA territory infarction has a very poor prognosis despite intubation. Six percent of the 74 patients with ischemic strokes in the report by Hacke and coworkers[26] required intubation and mechanical ventilation. Signs of brainstem dysfunction predicted a greater likelihood of death, as did male sex. Guujjar and associates[27] report that death, or disability severe enough to necessitate discharge to a nursing facility, occurred in 70% of the 74 mechanically ventilated patients in their series.

Barbiturate Therapy

Schwab and colleagues[28] studied the effect of high-dose barbiturate therapy on ICP and outcome in 60 patients with severe brain edema due to MCA occlusion and hemispheric infarction. In 83%, there was a transient fall in ICP. The investigators concluded that such therapy has no positive effect on neurologic outcome. Only 8% of the patients survived, and 25% of the patients experienced severe side effects from the barbiturate therapy, in addition to arterial hypotension.

Hypothermia

In an uncontrolled study, Schwab and colleagues[29] induced hypothermia to a core temperature of 33° C by means of cold infusion and washings within 14 hours after onset of MCA stroke, and maintained the state for 48 to 72 hours, in 25 patients. Pneumonia developed in 40% of patients, and 44% died. Neurologic outcome, as measured by Scandinavian Stroke Scale score, was 38 (range 28 to 48) at 3 months after stroke. The investigators suggested that this therapy might improve clinical outcome. Induced hypothermia could be carried out as an adjunct to decompressive hemicraniectomy but clearly adds to the potential for iatrogenic injury and demands a high level of resources.

Intracranial Pressure Monitoring

In 12 patients with large infarctions, Ropper and colleagues[30] report that drowsiness was the initial evidence of deterioration and was followed within several hours by pupillary asymmetry, periodic breathing, and the development of contralateral Babinski's sign. Only 4 of their patients survived. An ICP value greater than 15 mm Hg was associated with eventual brain death, and a value less than 15 mm Hg with survival.

Frank[31] measured ICP within 3 hours of onset of deterioration in 19 patients who were deteriorating to stupor because of large hemispheric infarction with edema and in whom other medical complications were ruled out. Stupor began on average about 59 hours after stroke onset, at which time elevation of ICP to more than 15 mm Hg was present in only 26% of the group. The cerebral perfusion pressure was lower than 55 mm Hg in only 11%. Frank[31] concluded that globally elevated ICP is not a common cause of the initial neurologic deterioration from large hemispheric infarction that results in edema.

In a study reported by Schwab and colleagues,[32] epidural probes were used to measure ICP in 48 patients after MCA infarction. The mortality rate was 81%. All the patients who died had ICP higher than 35 mm Hg, and no patient with ICP higher than 35 mm Hg survived.[32] The investigators of this large series of patients undergoing ICP monitoring after MCA infarction concluded that such monitoring may predict clinical outcome but is not helpful in guiding long-term treatment, and they expressed doubt that ICP monitoring had a positive influence on clinical outcome.

Mannitol

Administration of several bolus doses of mannitol may help the occasional patient teetering on the brink of tentorial herniation, but as a sole therapy for complete MCA infarction, this approach is probably of very limited use. Manno

and colleagues[33] used magnetic resonance imaging (MRI) to study the effect of a bolus dose of mannitol on large cerebral infarctions. The therapy led to no change in the measured shift of midline structures. The MCA stroke scale and Glasgow Coma Scale scores improved after mannitol in 29% and 43% of patients, respectively. The pupillary light reflex returned in 29%. The use of a single dose of 1.5 gm/kg of mannitol infused over 10 to 20 minutes did not therefore appear to cause worsening neurologic status at 1 hour. However, it also did not significantly reduce midline shift.[33]

Videen and associates[34] reported that a bolus of mannitol preferentially shrinks noninfarcted brain in patients with acute complete MCA infarctions and CT evidence of midline shift. These researchers performed T1-weighted MRI before and after infusion of a 1.5 gm/kg bolus of mannitol. At 50 to 55 minutes after the baseline scan, the total brain volume had decreased by 8.1 mL. Brain in the noninfarcted hemisphere shrank slightly, (0.8%) and that in the infarcted hemisphere not at all.

Neurochemical Monitoring

Schneweis and coworkers,[35] using microdialysis for neurochemical monitoring of the frontal lobe in patients with large MCA infarction, found increases in concentrations of glutamate and lactate as well as in the lactate-pyruvate ratio. They also observed that ICP rose concurrently, recording levels as high as 124 mm Hg. They suggested that microdialysis might be more predictive of subsequent deterioration than ICP value.[35] Given the current highly invasive nature of neurochemical monitoring and the fact that it monitors only a discrete area of the brain, wide use of this modality is unlikely.

RADIOLOGY

A major problem in the early evaluation of patients after the acute onset of cerebral ischemia is the prediction of the malignant character of the ischemic lesion, which would justify the appropriate early performance of hemicraniectomy. It appears virtually certain that for patients destined to have a malignant course, the earlier the decompression is performed, the less tissue necrosis there will be. On the other hand, the majority of patients who experience acute cerebral ischemia do not have a malignant course and are likely to make recoveries without this prodigious surgical effort.[36]

Computed Tomography

Fifty-three patients who were treated with tissue-type plasminogen activator (t-PA) for acute MCA trunk occlusions were evaluated with CT an average of 2 hours from symptom onset. Parenchymal hypodensity had occurred in 81%, local brain swelling in 38%, and middle cerebral trunk hyperdensity in 47%. A positive predictive value for a fatal clinical outcome was found in 85% of those with hypodensity covering more than 50% of the MCA territory, in 70% of those with local brain swelling, and in 32% of those with hyperdense MCAs. Hypodensity covering more than half of the MCA territory was specific for a fatal outcome in 94% of cases, with a sensitivity of 61%.[32,37]

Kucinski and associates[38] treated 74 patients in whom digital subtraction angiography (DSA) diagnosed acute carotid artery stroke with recombinant tissue-type plasminogen activator (rt-PA) or another fibrinolytic agent. All of the 23% of patients who died had intracranial mass effect and succumbed within a week of stroke onset; also, 53% had initial occlusion of the carotid bifurcation (MCA plus anterior cerebral artery occlusion), but only 29% had (as an initial major early CT sign of ischemia) cortical hypodensity in more than a third of the territory of the MCA.[38]

Von Kummer and colleagues[39] obtained CT scans within 6 hours and then at medians of 1 day and 7 days after onset of ischemic stroke onset in 786 patients. The specificity and positive predictive value of ischemic edema on baseline CT for brain infarcts were 85% and 96%, respectively. The sensitivity and negative predictive values were 64% and 27%, respectively. The patients without early CT findings were less severely affected, had smaller infarcts, had fewer intracranial bleeding events, and had a better clinical outcome at 90 days than patients in whom early CT showed hypoattenuating brain tissue. These investigators concluded that x-ray hypoattenuation on CT scans is highly specific for irreversible ischemic brain damage if it is detected within the first 6 hours.

Single-Photon Emission Computed Tomography

In a study conducted by Hanson and coworkers,[40] patients with hemispheric ischemic stroke were studied with single-photon emission CT (SPECT), which was performed within 6 hours of symptom onset and again at 24 hours. The defect was assessed in semiquantitative manner by means of SPECT using technetium 99m–labeled hexamethylpropyleneamineoxime (99mTc-HMPAO). This agent readily crosses the blood-brain barrier and rapidly localizes in brain tissue in proportion to the blood flow and function at the time of injection. The distribution of activity stabilizes within a few minutes, and there is minimal redistribution for up to 8 hours. Scanning can be performed within 1 to 5 hours after injection. These researchers concluded that there is a strong association between the severity of ischemia on initial SPECT and the long-term outcome as defined by a Barthel Index of 60 or less.

At the time when SPECT findings were clearly abnormal in 13 of the 15 patients in the Hanson study, CT scans showed a suggestive abnormality in only 1. The baseline NIHSS score was not as specific as SPECT in predicting poor outcome in this small series. There was no correlation between the improvement occurring in the NIHSS score and the changes in SPECT findings from initial to later studies. Some patients showed no clinical improvement even though their SPECT findings normalized at 24 hours.[40]

Berrouschot and colleagues[41] performed CT and SPECT using technetium 99m–labeled ethyl-cysteinate-dimer (99mTc-ECD) in 108 patients (37% of their total of 293 admissions for stroke) within 6 hours of the onset of MCA ischemic symptoms. Eleven percent of the patients with MCA ischemia died from infarction. The sensitivity of 99mTc-ECD SPECT for predicting fatal outcome was 82% in both visual and semiquantitative analyses; speci-

ficity was 98% for visual analysis and 99% for semiquantitative analysis. These figures compare very favorably with the sensitivity and specificity of baseline CT studies, which were 36% and 100%, respectively. The sensitivity and specificity values for the Scandinavian Stroke Scale, depressed level of consciousness, and gaze deviation varied between 36% and 86%. These investigators found only the SPECT findings to be independent predictors of malignant MCA infarction or death in a multivariate logistic regression model.[41]

Magnetic Resonance Imaging

Diffusion-weighted imaging (DWI) is based on the modulation of signal intensity caused by water diffusion. The apparent diffusion coefficient (ADC) of water is the quantitative expression of the abnormal water diffusivity in brain parenchyma. Early MRI studies suggested that the presence of a high ADC value and higher than normal T2 value indicated established cellular necrosis.[42] ADC has been found to be consistently and significantly decreased for at least 4 days after stroke onset in large clinical studies of patients with stroke.[43] ADC values are low at less than 1 week after stroke onset and become elevated in later phases.[44]

DWI can rapidly detect acute cerebral ischemic injury as hyperintense signal changes, which reflect a decline in the ADC of water through brain parenchyma, whereas ADC is elevated in the chronic stage because of increased cellular water content. The time course of regional ADC changes in acute human infarction has two stages, a significant reduction lasting for at least 96 hours after stroke onset (58% of controls) and a growing trend for reduction to pseudo-normalization to elevation of values in the subacute and chronic phases of stroke (after 7 days). In a study by Schlaug and associates,[45] 20 patients with acute infarction showed areas of hyperintensity on DWI and concomitant lower ADC values than contralateral normal brain. In sharp distinction, in the studies performed within 6 hours of stroke onset, T2-weighted MRI showed abnormalities in only 1 of the 20 patients.[45]

Perfusion-weighted imaging (PWI), performed after the bolus intravenous injection of gadolinium-containing contrast medium, maps the relative cerebral blood volume. PWI can identify hypoperfused tissue. PWI and DWI can demonstrate cerebral ischemia and ischemic brain injury, respectively, in the first several hours after the onset of symptoms, when proton-density and T2-weighted MRI findings may be normal. In a report by Warach and colleagues,[46] of 19 patients with severely disabling clinical deficits attributable to ischemia in the entire division of the MCA, initial PWI and DWI were more accurate than conventional MRI in predicting occurrence and level of improvement. DWI and PWI correctly predicted outcome category in 89% of cases, whereas conventional MRI did so in only 53%. The superiority of PWI and DWI rose with proximity of study performance to the onset of symptoms. In patients studied within 6 hours, DWI and PWI accurately predicted outcome in 92% of cases; conventional MRI was accurate in only 33%. In none of these cases was the predicted outcome worse than the actual outcome. The presence of a DWI abnormality invariably led to permanent neurologic deficits even when T2-weighted image findings were initially normal.[46]

Standard neurodiagnostic imaging techniques such as CT and T1- and T2-weighted MRI have high false-negative rates when performed on the first day after onset of ischemic symptoms, and negative findings are an unreliable predictor of good outcomes.[43] Lesion volumes determined by DWI in the acute period, however, can predict clinical severity and outcome. DWI can detect ischemic injury within minutes of onset. In 50 patients with acute MCA ischemic lesions, Lovblad and associates[47] found that the volume determined by DWI correlated with the chronic infarct volume as determined by subsequent T2-weighted images. The acute DWI volumes also correlated with clinical severity as measured by NIHSS scores and Barthel Index values. In a study by Beaulieu and coworkers,[48] DWI and PWI performed first within 7 hours of symptom onset detected dynamic changes for the first month after stroke. Ninety-five percent of their patients had increased lesion volume over the first week and then decreases at 1 month. They also found that the mismatch between diffusion and perfusion on the initial scan described lesion growth. The total volume of abnormality on acute DWI and PWI correlated with NIHSS scores.[48]

The ischemic penumbra is a portion of brain with reduced blood supply where there is electrical failure but cellular integrity is maintained. Viable tissue may be found in the ischemic penumbra around an infarction for up to 48 hours after stroke onset. It is a region of low cerebral blood flow (CBF) with relatively preserved or normal cerebral metabolic rates for oxygen and a high oxygen extraction fraction. A decline in the ADC is associated with a decrease in the energy requiring Na^+K^+-ATPase, which permits the identification of the ischemic core as a region of energy failure. Schlaug and colleagues[49] analyzed cases from a stroke database of 25 patients with a mean age of 69 years and a known time of onset of hemispheric ischemic stroke. DWI and PWI studies were performed within 24 hours of onset; follow-up DWI studies performed between 24 and 72 hours after the first studies showed an increase in lesion size. The enlargement of the DWI abnormality between the initial and subsequent studies was 376%. The enlargement of the DWI abnormality occurred within the region of hypoperfusion demonstrated on the initial PWI. The initial PWI regional abnormality was always larger than the initial DWI abnormality. The mean volume of the PWI abnormalities was 97 mL; the mean volume of the DWI abnormalities was 29 mL on the first study and 59 mL on the second. The volume of chronic infarct as shown on T2-weighted MRI was 67 mL; the mean increase of the abnormal chronic T2-weighted MRI volume compared with the initial DWI volume for the entire group was 467%.

The enlargement of the initial diffusion lesion into the oligemic region, as determined by PWI abnormalities, is an operational definition of the ischemic penumbra. CBF probably has to be reduced by more than 20% to cause a significant change in the ADC. The required duration of reduction in CBF or that of other markers that triggers irreversible cell damage and determines the point of no return is unknown. The mean regional ADC within the hyperintense DWI lesion is reduced to approximately 58%

of control values in the acute stage of an infarction. This corresponds to a CBF of 10 to 15 mL/100 g/min. Such studies demonstrate that in the majority of human strokes, there is a mismatch between a smaller diffusion lesion and a larger hypoperfusion lesion. The diffusion lesion grows into the larger and surrounding hypoperfusion region but rarely reaches its size.[49]

In a study reported by Oppenheim and colleagues,[50] 28 patients with MCA infarcts and proven MCA or carotid bifurcation occlusions underwent DWI and MRA within 14 hours of onset of symptoms (median of 5.2 hours). Ten of the patients went on to have malignant MCA infarction. The best predictor of this adverse course was an initial DWI volume greater than 145 cm^3, which achieved 100% sensitivity and 94% specificity. The investigators improved the prediction values to 100% sensitivity and specificity in this series of patients by using a bivariate analysis model that combined DWI volumes and ADC measurements.[50]

SURGERY

In a very early series of "strokectomies," Greenwood[51] described the removal of liquefied necrotic material by suction after infarction, supplemented if necessary by partial frontal and temporal lobectomies. He recommended that surgery be performed before fixation of pupils and deep coma. Of his 9 operated patients, 3 died. In 2 of the 6 survivors, survival disability was rated as moderate; the others were more severely impaired. These cases were not treated by hemicraniectomy. In an early review, Ivamoto and colleagues[52] presented 18 reports of surgical decompression for cerebral infarction. All patients were either hemiplegic or hemiparetic, 78% were in stupor or coma, and 61% had pupillary asymmetry at the time of operation. These researchers also described one of their own patients, a woman who underwent a large craniotomy and subtemporal craniectomy followed by a dural incision in the temporal region with removal of necrotic extruded brain. The patient recovered to the point at which the bone flap could be replaced a month later. She was able to resume some housework and bookkeeping, although she still needed a walker 7 months after the operation.[52]

An influential series appearing in the early 1980s was that of Rengachary and associates,[53] who reported 3 survivors after ipsilateral hemicraniectomy performed for impending death due to uncal herniation. Severe fixed neurologic deficits persisted in 2 patients. These investigators believed that hemicraniectomy was more appropriate for patients with stroke than for those with head injuries, for the following reasons: After trauma, the brain herniates through the cranial defect and tends to become incarcerated outside the skull, leading to the obstruction of venous drainage and contusion of the cortex at the margins. This process is less likely after hemispheric stroke because the brain is already necrotic and the venous drainage is already sluggish or nonexistent. After stroke, the mass effect is strictly unilateral, whereas in traumatic brain swelling it tends to be diffuse. The brainstem is quite viable in patients with stroke unless irreversible changes from herniation have taken place, whereas after trauma, severe acceleration-deceleration injuries have already damaged the brainstem. In patients with head injury, there is a possibility of upward herniation through the tentorium after hemicraniectomy because of posterior fossa swelling. Rengachary and associates[53] suggested that hemicraniectomy after stroke should not be attempted until the patient had received the "full benefits" of nonoperative therapy, including steroids, mannitol, and hyperventilation. Since this paper was written, the futility of such measures in patients with total MCA infarct has been suggested.

Figure 75–1 illustrates the large bone and dural openings required for decompressive craniectomy.

Another encouraging report on decompressive craniectomy was that by Kondziolka and Fazl,[54] published in 1988. They managed five patients with acute supratentorial cerebral infarction that progressed to uncal herniation and impending death from raised ICP and brainstem compression. They performed frontal-temporal craniectomy. All of their patients survived and were walking at follow-up. Two patients actually returned to work. These investigators recommended that craniectomy be performed at the first sign of pupillary dilatation or nonreactivity. Another series of nine cases of hemicraniectomy for cerebral infarction was reported from the University of Virginia in 1990 by Delashaw and coworkers.[55] These patients were an average of 57 years of age and had progressive neurologic deterioration from large right hemispheric cerebral infarction. Mass effect from cerebral edema was diagnosed on the basis of CT scans. One nonneurologic death from lung cancer occurred a month after surgery. At follow-up, which ranged between 5 and 25 months, 89% of the remaining patients were living at home with their families. No patient was fully independent; 38% were "functional" and 63% were "dependent." In half the patients, the Barthel Index at follow-up was less than 60. When asked at follow-up whether they would undergo the procedure again if they had foreknowledge of the outcome, half the patients said unequivocally that they would; three quarters of family members also said that they would agree to their patients' undergoing the procedure.

Using stable xenon-enhanced CT scanning, Kalia and Yonas[56] reported four cases of "strokectomy" in the setting of potentially fatal swelling from massive cerebral infarction. All patients recovered. The patient who did best (only residual upper extremity monoparesis) was 13 years old.

Martins and associates[57] reported on eight patients with ischemic stroke and imminent herniation who underwent surgical decompression with standard temporal lobectomy but without decompressive hemicraniectomy. Six patients survived; in the two who did not, death was attributed to delays in surgical intervention.

Carter and colleagues[58] performed surgical decompression in 14 patients at the Massachusetts General Hospital who presented with right hemispheric infarction and clinical signs of uncal herniation and impending death. Twenty-nine percent underwent surgery within 24 hours of onset, and 43% within 4 days. After the decompression, death from tentorial herniation was prevented in all cases. Eleven patients enjoyed long-term survival; the three deaths were from nonneurologic causes. Eight patients were able to go home and functioned with minimal to moderate assistance, with Barthel Index values greater than 60. Half the patients were able to walk at 1 year after the procedures. The patients averaged 49 years of age, and there was a trend toward better recovery in younger patients. The mean age of patients with Barthel Index values more than 70 was 41 years; that for patients with Barthel Index values less than 70 was 56 years. Twenty-nine percent of the patients became severely depressed. In this series, 64% of patients underwent a temporal lobectomy in addition to the hemicraniectomy, and in 71% of patients, the bone flap was stored within the abdomen. Ten of the 11 surviving patients returned for elective cranioplasty, usually within 2 or 3 months. Of the survivors, 55% said they would go through the hemicraniectomy again knowing what they experienced subsequently, 27% said "Maybe," and 18% answered "Definitely not." The mortality in this series was 3 of 14, and only 1 patient (7%), who was 11 years old, was at home and fully independent at the time of follow-up. In their 1997 report, the investigators reviewed 53 cases of decompressive surgery for stroke and found a mean age of 47 years, with 17% mortality, a 28% rate of poor outcome, and a 55% rate of good outcome.[58] In 24 patients with acute massive cerebral infarction treated by external decompression in Japan, the 2-month outcome after surgery was severe disability in 58%, vegetative state in 8%, and death in 33%.[59]

By 1998, 63 patients enrolled in an open, prospective German trial had undergone hemicraniectomy.[60] Seventy-three percent of the patients survived surgical decompression. Despite complete hemispheric infarction, none of the survivors was completely hemiplegic or completely wheelchair-bound. Interestingly, in the 11 patients with speech-dominant hemispheric infarction, only mild or moderate aphasia was present at 3-month follow-up. The mean Barthel Index value was 65. Patients who underwent surgical decompression within 24 hours of symptom onset

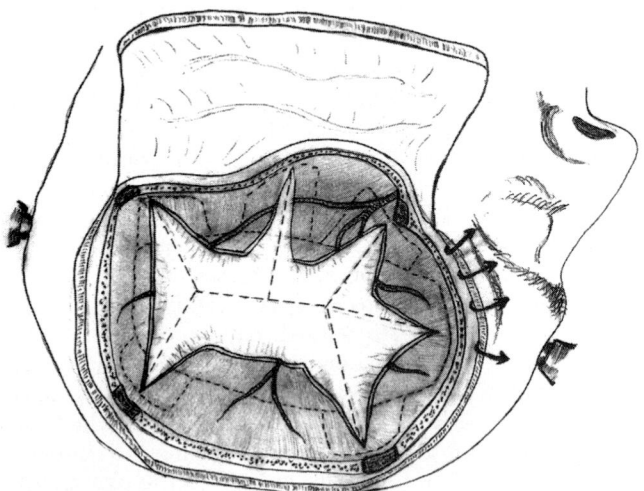

FIGURE 75–1 *The surgeon's "eye view" of the large bone flap removal required in hemicraniectomy and surgical decompression for middle cerebral artery (MCA) territory infarction. Stellate dural incisions permit smooth brain expansion in the territory of the MCA. Areas over the bulged brain are covered with artificial dural substitute. Care should be taken to carry out the decompression over the entire lateral temporal lobe down to the floor of the temporal fossa.*

(mean 21 hours) fared better than those whose surgery was delayed (mean 39 hours). Only 13% of the patients in the early operation group showed signs of herniation preoperatively, compared with 75% in the later operation group. The mortality rate for early surgery was 16%, versus 34% for later surgery. The time in neurosurgery critical care unit was 7.4 days for the early surgery group compared with 13.3 days for the later surgery group. The follow-up Barthel Index value was 69 for the early surgery group, and 63 for the later surgery group.

In the only open, nonrandomized, controlled trial of decompressive hemicraniectomy, conducted by Rieke and associates[61] at the University of Heidelberg over 65 months, 32 patients were prospectively selected for surgical treatment and 21 were treated conservatively. All patients were treated with early full-dose anticoagulation in an effort to prevent re-embolization or the spread of thrombus. This was discontinued 6 hours before and restarted 6 hours after surgery. Nineteen percent of the surgically treated patients had a good outcome, compared with none of the conservatively treated patients. The rate of moderate to severe disability was 47% in patients undergoing surgery, compared with 24% in those treated conservatively. Mortality rates were 34% for surgery and 76% for conservative management. A mean Barthel Index value of 63 was obtained after surgery. One patient had an excellent level of daily activity, 15 required minimal assistance, and 5 were dependent. In the conservatively treated group, all 5 survivors required assistance, with 4 demonstrating a moderately severe handicap. In massive hemispheric stroke victims, surgical decompression can therefore decrease mortality rates to about 1 in 3 with a dependent disability rate of 1 in 4. The surgical technique employed by these investigators was a large decompression with dural patch enlargement. They excluded from the study patients older than 70 years and patients presenting with complete global aphasia, secondary parenchymal hemorrhage, or coma with absence of cortical somatosensory evoked potentials. Initial CT scans in the study subjects showed local swelling and parenchymal hypodensity consistently located in the frontal third of the MCA or in the area of the basal ganglia. No hemorrhagic transformation, midline shift, or loss of mesencephalic cisterns was evident on the initial CT scans. The investigators' review of world literature revealed 79 cases of decompressive surgery for malignant MCA infarctions.

Sixty patients from the an overlapping Heidelberg series were evaluated by serial CT scans before and after craniectomy. The maximum diameter of the hemicraniectomy was determined, and the lesions associated with the surgery were classified as ischemic or hemorrhagic. Parenchymal hemorrhages occurred in 42% of operated cases, and infarction was associated with the hemicraniectomy in 28%. Hemicraniectomy-associated bleeding was related to a higher risk of death. The occurrence of hemicraniectomy-associated bleeding was related to the size of the skull removal, with the frequency of bleeding higher in the smaller hemicraniectomies. Hemicraniectomy-associated hemorrhages were apparently increased in frequency if the skull flap was less than 10 cm in diameter. Doubling the diameter from 6 to 12 cm resulted in an increase in the potential decompressive volume from 9 to 86 mL. The authors recommended keeping the skull flap incision 1 cm lateral to the midline to avoid damaging the bridging veins and possibly causing additional bleeding. They used patches of augmenting dura up to 20 by 3.5 cm.[62] Although cadaveric dura was used in some of the earlier operations, I think it is wiser to use modern substitutes or the patient's own temporal fascia.

In a series reported from Japan, eight patients with an average age of 71.8 years were treated with decompressive craniectomy and were compared with seven historic controls treated conservatively.[63] The mortality rate was 86% in the conservative therapy group and 13% in the surgery group. The surgery group also had a higher functional performance level after treatment.

Demchuk and associates[64] conducted a retrospective case-control study of patients treated at eight institutions over 3 years. The 251 patients had large MCA strokes and were admitted within 48 hours of onset. Forty-three percent died from neurologic causes, 6% died from non-neurologic causes, and 50% survived. Hemicraniectomy was performed in 50 (20%) patients. Hemicraniectomy was performed more commonly in younger patients (average age 50.6 years, versus 67.4 years for conservatively treated patients) who had lower rates of hypertension, diabetes, atrial fibrillation, congestive heart failure, and history of prior stroke. Patients undergoing surgery tended to have more nausea or vomiting in the first 24 hours. They also showed more early ischemic CT changes. The involvement of territories other than the MCA as detected by CT scanning was independently predictive of death in patients undergoing hemicraniectomy (OR 24.9). With data adjusted for baseline differences in age and presence or absence of nausea or vomiting, the 1-month mortality rate after hemicraniectomy was 0.48 compared with conservative treatment. With further adjustments for the baseline NIHSS stroke scale score and CT findings, the odds ratio was even more favorable for hemicraniectomy (0.25 versus conservative treatment).[64]

As a rule, reports of small, personal series or individual cases by neurosurgeons tend to portray a new surgical procedure in an optimistic light. A more sobering account was offered by Holtkamp and colleagues,[65] who reported on 12 patients undergoing hemicraniectomy for MCA infarction. One third died in hospital, and of the 8 survivors, none had a Barthel Index value higher than 60 or a Rankin score less than 4. Of 12 patients concurrently treated by medical means, 10 died, and the 2 survivors had Barthel Index values less than 60 and Rankin scores of 4.[65]

Currently, the literature contains reports of more than 300 decompressive operations for the treatment of acute infarction.[41,50,52–55,57–61,63–77] The quality of the reporting varies widely. Patients who underwent surgery have tended to be younger than patients with ischemic stroke generally. The youngest patient so far was 6 years old.[78] This procedure seems to have a mortality rate of about 1 in 4. In addition, at least 1 in every 4 patients undergoing decompression is severely disabled. If these reports are any indication, the operation is being performed more frequently around the world. Patients in whom the operation is a "success" still must bear the burden of the neurologic deficit resulting from the infarction that necessitated the operation in the first place and must face the hazards of the underlying disease that caused the infarction. It follows that those who are biologically far advanced in age or have significant comorbidities and who do not have a supportive family or social network should not be offered the procedure. The results of current randomized clinical trials will probably refine the indications for the procedure, but individual neurologists and neurosurgeons must still make informed guesses as to the probable outcome for individual patients. Excellent clinical facilities, including "stroke" MRI, ideally should be available to those performing this operation.

References

1. Batjer T, Mickey B, Samson D: Potential roles for early revascularization in patients with acute cerebral ischemia. Neurosurgery 18:283–291, 1986.
2. Auer RN: Hemicraniectomy for ischemic stroke. Can J Neurol Sci 27:269, 2000.
3. Shaw CM, Alvord EC, Berry RG: Swelling of the brain following ischemic infarction with arterial occlusion. Arch Neurol 1:161–176, 1959.
4. Bounds JV, Weibers MD, Whisnant JP, et al: Mechanisms and timing of deaths from cerebral infarction. Stroke 12:474–477, 1981.
5. Ng L, Nimmannitya J: Massive cerebral infarction with severe brain swelling: A clinicopathological study. Stroke 1:158–163, 1970.
6. Niwa J, Kubota T, Chiba M, et al: Acute surgical and endovascular therapy for stroke: Especially patients with brain infarction. No Shinkei Geka 28:499–504, 2000.
7. Andoh T, Sakai N, Yamada H, et al: Cerebellar infarction: Analysis of 33 cases. No Shinkei Geka 18:821–828, 1990.
8. Chen HJ, Lee TC, Wei CP: Treatment of cerebellar infarction by decompressive suboccipital craniectomy. Stroke 23:957–961, 1992.
9. Cioffi FA, Berenini FP, Punzo A, et al: Surgical management of acute cerebellar infarction. Acta Neurochir 74:105–112, 1985.
10. Jauss M, Krieger D, Horning C, et al: Surgical and medical management of patients with massive cerebellar infarctions: Results of the German-Austrian Cerebellar Infarction Study. J Neurol 246:257–264, 1999.
11. Khan M, Polyzoidis KS, Adegbite AB, et al: Massive cerebellar infarction: "Conservative" management. Stroke 14:745–751, 1983.
12. Ogasawara K, Koshu K, Nagamine Y, et al: Surgical decompression for massive cerebellar infarction. No Shinkei Geka 23:43–48, 1995.
13. Munch E, Horn P, Schurer L, et al: Management of severe traumatic brain injury by decompressive craniectomy. Neurosurgery 47:315–323, 2000.
14. Moody RA, Ruamsuke S, Mullan S: An evaluation of decompression in experimental head injury. J Neurosurg 29:586–590, 1968.
15. Hatashita S, Koike J, Sonokawa T, et al: Cerebral edema associated with craniectomy and arterial hypertension. Stroke 16:661–668, 1985.
16. Forsting M, Reith W, Schabitz WR, et al: Decompressive craniectomy for cerebral infarction: An experimental study in rats. Stroke 26:259–264, 1995.
17. Engelhorn T, vonKummer R, Reith W, et al: What is effective in malignant middle cerebral artery infarction: Reperfusion, craniectomy, or both? An experimental study in rats. Stroke 33:617–622, 2002.
18. Silver F, Norris JW, Lewis A, et al: Early mortality following stroke: A prospective review. Stroke 15:492–496, 1984.
19. Chambers BR, Norris JW, Shurvell BL: Prognosis of acute stroke. Neurology 37:221–222, 1987.
20. Turney TM, Garraway WM, Whisnant JP: The natural history of hemispheric and brainstem infarcts in Rochester, Minnesota. Stroke 15:790–794, 1984.
21. Wijdicks E, Diringer MN: Middle cerebral artery territory infarction and early brain swelling: Progression and effect of age on outcome. Mayo Clinic Proc 73:829–836, 1998.
22. Krieger D, Demchuk AM, Kasner SE, et al: Early clinical and radiological predictors of fatal brain swelling in ischemic stroke. Stroke 30:287–292, 1999.
23. Kasner SE, Demchuk AM, Verro P, et al: Predictors of fatal brain edema in massive ischemic stroke [abstract]. Stroke 31:295, 2000.
24. Grotta J, Pasteur W, Khwaja G, et al: Elective intubation for neurologic deterioration after stroke. Neurology 45:640–644, 1995.
25. ElAd B, Bornstein N, Fuchs P, et al: Mechanical ventilation in stroke patients—is it worthwhile? Neurology 47:657–659, 1996.
26. Hacke W, Schwab S, Horn M, et al: "Malignant" middle cerebral artery territory infarction: Clinical course and prognostic signs. Arch Neurol 53:309–315, 1996.
27. Gujjar AR, Deibert E, Manno EM, et al: Mechanical ventilation for ischemic stroke and intracranial hemorrhage: Indications, timing, and outcome. Neurology 51:447–451, 1998.
28. Schwab S, Spranger M, Schwarz S, et al: Barbiturate coma in severe hemispheric stroke: Useful or obsolete? Neurology 48:1608–1613, 1997.
29. Schwab S, Schwarz S, Spranger M, et al: Moderate hypothermia in the treatment of patients with severe middle cerebral artery infarction. Stroke 29:2461–2466, 1998.
30. Ropper AH, Shafran B: Brain edema after stroke: Clinical syndrome and intracranial pressure. Arch Neurol 41:26–29, 1984.
31. Frank J: Large hemispheric infarction, deterioration, and intracranial pressure. Neurology 45:1286–1290, 1995.
32. Schwab S, Schellinger P, Aschoff A, et al: Epidural cerebrospinal fluid pressure measurement and therapy of intracranial hypertension in "malignant" middle cerebral artery infarct. Nervenarzt 67:659–666, 1996.
33. Manno EM, Adams RE, Derdeyn CP, et al: The effects of mannitol on cerebral edema after large hemispheric cerebral infarct. Neurology 52:583–587, 1999.
34. Videen T, Zazulia AR, Manno EM, et al: Mannitol bolus preferentially shrinks non-infarcted brain in patients with ischemic stroke. Neurology 57:2120–2122, 2001.
35. Schneweis S, Grond M, Staub F: Predictive value of neurochemical monitoring in large middle cerebral artery infarction. Stroke 32:1863–1867, 2001.
36. Doerfler A, Engelhorn T, Forsting M: Decompressive craniectomy for early therapy and secondary prevention of cerebral infarction [letter]. Stroke 32:813–814, 2001.
37. vonKummer R, Meyding-Lamade U, Forsting M, et al: Sensitivity and prognostic value of early CT in occlusion of the middle cerebral artery trunk. Am J Neuroradiol 15:9–15, 1994.
38. Kucinski T, Koch C, Grzyska U: The predictive value of early CT and angiography for fatal hemispheric swelling in acute stroke. Am J Neuroradiol 19:839–846, 1998.
39. vonKummer R, Bourquain H, Bastianello S, et al: Early prediction of irreversible brain damage after ischemic stroke at CT. Radiology 219:95–100, 2001.
40. Hanson SK, Grotta J, Rhoades H, et al: Value of single-photon emission-computed tomography in acute stroke therapeutic trials. Stroke 24:1322–1329, 1993.
41. Berrouschot J, Barthel H, vonKummer R: ^{99m}Technetium-ethyl-cysteinate-dimer single-photon emission CT can predict fatal ischemic brain edema. Stroke 29:2556–2562, 1998.
42. Welch KM, Windham J, Knight R, et al: A model to predict the histopathology of human stroke using diffusion and T2 weighted magnetic resonance imaging. Stroke 26:1983–1989, 1995.
43. Warach S, Moseley M, Sorenson M, et al: Time course of diffusion imaging abnormalities in human stroke. Stroke 27:1254–1255, 1996.
44. Lutsep HL, Albers GW, deCrespigny A, et al: Clinical utility of diffusion-weighted magnetic resonance imaging in the assessment of ischemic stroke. Ann Neurol 41:574–580, 1997.
45. Schlaug G, Siewert B, Benfield A, et al: Time course of the apparent diffusion coefficient (ADC) abnormality in human stroke. Neurology 49:113–119, 1997.
46. Warach S, Dashe JF, Edelman RR: Clinical outcome in ischemic stroke predicted by early diffusion-weighted and perfusion magnetic resonance imaging: A preliminary analysis. J Cereb Blood Flow Metab 16:53–59, 1996.
47. Lovblad KO, Baird AE, Schlaug G, et al: Ischemic lesion volumes in acute stroke by diffusion-weighted magnetic resonance imaging correlate with clinical outcome. Ann Neurol 42:164–170, 1997.
48. Beaulieu C, deCrespigny A, Tong DC, et al: Longitudinal magnetic resonance imaging study of perfusion and diffusion in stroke: Evolution of lesion volume and correlation with clinical outcome. Ann Neurol 46:568–578, 1999.
49. Schlaug G, Benfield A, Baird AE: The ischemic penumbra: Operationally defined by diffusion and perfusion MRI. Neurology 53:1528–1537, 1999.

50. Oppenheim C, Samson Y, Manai R, et al: Prediction of malignant middle cerebral artery infarction by diffusion-weighted imaging. Stroke 31:2175–2181, 2000.

51. Greenwood J: Acute brain infarction with high intracranial pressure: Surgical indications. Johns Hopkins Med J 122:254–260, 1968.

52. Ivamoto H, Numoto M, Donaghy MP: Surgical decompression for cerebral and cerebellar infarcts. Stroke 5:365–370, 1974.

53. Rengachary S, Batnitzky S, Morantz R: Craniectomy for acute massive cerebral infarction. Neurosurgery 8:321–328, 1981.

54. Kondziolka D, Fazl M: Functional recovery after decompressive craniectomy for cerebral infarction. Neurosurgery 23:143–147, 1988.

55. Delashaw JB, Broaddus WC, Kassell MD, et al: Treatment of right hemispheric cerebral infarction by hemicraniectomy. Stroke 21:874–881, 1990.

56. Kalia KK, Yonas H: An aggressive approach to massive middle cerebral artery infarction. Arch Neurol 50:1293–1297, 1993.

57. Martins LF, DaCosta V, DaCosta J, et al: Temporal lobectomy in cerebral infarction with mass effect. Arq Neuropsiquiatr 51:118–124, 1993.

58. Carter BS, Ogilvy CS, Candia GJ: One-year outcome after decompression surgery for massive hemispheric infarction. Neurosurgery 40:1168–1175, 1997.

59. Sakai K, Iwahashi K, Terada K: Outcome after external decompression for massive cerebral infarction. Neurol Med Chir (Tokyo) 38:131–135, 1998.

60. Schwab S, Steiner T, Aschoff A, et al: Early hemicraniectomy in patients with complete middle cerebral artery infarction. Stroke 29:1888–1893, 1998.

61. Rieke K, Schwab S, Krieger D, et al: Decompressive surgery in space-occupying hemispheric infarction: Results of an open, prospective trial. Crit Care Med 23:1576–1587, 1995.

62. Wagner S, Schnippering H, Aschoff A, et al: Suboptimum hemicraniectomy as a cause of additional cerebral lesions in patients with malignant infarction of the middle cerebral artery. J Neurosurg 94:693–696, 2001.

63. Kuroki K, Taguchi H, Sumida M, et al: Decompressive craniectomy for massive infarction of middle cerebral artery territory. No Shinkei Geka 29:831–835, 2001.

64. Demchuk AM, Kasner SE, Berrouschot J, et al: Multicenter evaluation of the clinical practice of hemicraniectomy in ischemic stroke [abstract]. Stroke 31:295, 2000.

65. Holtkamp M, Buchheim K, Unterberg A, et al: Hemicraniectomy in elderly patients with space occupying media infarction: Improved

66. Jourdan C, Convert J, Mottolese C, et al: Evaluation of the clinical benefit of decompression hemicraniectomy in intracranial hypertension not controlled by medical treatment. Neurochirurgie 39:304–310, 1993.

67. Koh MS, Goh KY, Tung MY, et al: Is decompressive craniectomy for acute cerebral infarction of any benefit? Surg Neurol 53:225–230, 2000.

68. Kakuk I, Major O, Gubucz I, et al: New methods of intensive therapy in stroke: Hemicraniectomy in patients with complete middle cerebral artery infarction and treatment of intracerebral and intraventricular hemorrhage with urokinase. Ideggyogy Sz 55:118–127, 2002.

69. Young PH, Smith K, Dunn R: Surgical decompression after cerebral hemispheric stroke: Indications and patient selection. South Med J 75:473–475, 1982.

70. Lindegaard KF, Roste GK: Life-saving hemicraniectomy in acute massive brain infarction. Tidsskr Nor Laegeforen 119:4190–4192, 1999.

71. Oro J, Amiridze N, Boyer R: Decompressive craniotomy in medically uncontrollable malignant infarction. Missouri Med 97:17–20, 2000.

72. Sollid S, Kloster R, Ingebrigsten T: Decompression craniectomy: Life-saving treatment in acute cerebral infarction. Tidsskr Nor Laegeforen 119:4199–4210, 1999.

73. Steiger HJ: Outcome of acute supratentorial cerebral infarction in patients under 60. Acta Neurochir 111:73–79, 1991.

74. Tsuruno T, Takeda M, Imaizumi T, et al: Internal decompression with hippocampectomy for massive cerebral infarction. No Shinkei Geka 21:823–827, 1993.

75. Ueno K, Oosato T, Sasaki H, et al: Prophylactic external decompression for massive cerebral infarction. No Shinkei Geka 12:261–267, 1984.

76. vanLeusen HJ, Tans JT, Wurzer JA: Hemicraniectomy for treatment of malignant medial cerebral artery infarctions in 3 patients. Ned Tijdschr Geneeskd 145:639–643, 2001.

77. Walz B, Zimmermann C, Bottger S, et al: Prognosis of patients after hemicraniectomy in malignant middle cerebral artery infarction. J Neurol 249:1183–1190, 2002.

78. Lee MC, Frank JI, Kahana M, et al: Decompressive hemicraniectomy in a 6-year-old male after unilateral hemispheric stroke. Case report and review. Pediatr Neurosurg 38:181–185, 2003.

Therapy

Chapter Seventy-Six

Cerebellar Infarction and Hemorrhage

Kazuhiro Hongo, Junpei Nitta, and Shigeaki Kobayashi

The management of patients with cerebellar infarction and hemorrhage is a complex matter. The pathophysiology and cause of the hemorrhage must be clarified. Surgical indications are determined according to the size and exact location of the hematoma, the extent of brainstem compression as well as the neurologic status. In cases of cerebellar infarction, which vessels are responsible must be established, and hemodynamic status, including collateral circulation, must be ascertained.

ANATOMY OF THE CEREBELLUM

The cerebellum is located in the posterior cranial fossa, which occupies approximately one eighth of the intracranial space. The posterior fossa extends from the tentorial incisura to the foramen magnum and is formed by the occipital, temporal, parietal, and sphenoid bones. If a mass exists in the cerebellum, upward herniation through the tentorial incisura or downward tonsillar herniation through the foramen magnum may occur.

The cerebellum has afferent connections from the spinal cord, vestibular system, reticular formation, pontine nuclei, inferior olive, raphe nuclei, and locus ceruleus, and efferent connections, which terminate in the brainstem and forebrain regions, including the red nuclei and ventrolateral thalamus. Many of the efferent fibers are directly or indirectly related to the descending spinal pathway. The loss of muscular coordination is therefore the most common sign in cerebellar disorders. Besides the cerebellum, the posterior fossa contains such important structures as the brainstem, cranial nerves, basilar and vertebral arteries, and outlets of the ventricular system. The brainstem contains pathways regulating consciousness, vital autonomic functions, motor activities, sensory reception, and body coordination. Consequently, in cases of cerebellar hemorrhage or infarction with mass effect, the symptoms are not limited to cerebellar dysfunction. The ventricular system has its outlets only in the posterior fossa: the foramina of Luschka and Magendie from the fourth ventricle. Therefore, when the fourth ventricle is occluded by the hematoma or cerebellar edema after the ictus, acute obstructive hydrocephalus occurs.

In the cerebellum, there are three major arteries, superior cerebellar artery (SCA), anterior inferior cerebellar artery (AICA), and posterior inferior cerebellar artery (PICA) on each side. The SCA arises near the tip of the basilar artery and passes below the oculomotor and trochlear nerves and above the trigeminal nerve. Then it courses along the cerebellomesencephalic fissure and supplies the superior cerebellar peduncle and the tentorial surface of the cerebellum. Spontaneous cerebellar hemorrhage occurs mostly in the area of the dentate nucleus of the cerebellum, which is usually supplied by the branches of the SCA. The AICA arises from the lower basilar artery and passes above the abducens nerve. It forms a loop at the facial and vestibulocochlear nerves, supplying the middle cerebellar peduncle and the petrosal surface of the cerebellum. The PICA arises from the vertebral artery and courses in close relation to the glossopharyngeal, vagus, accessory, and hypoglossal nerves. It supplies the inferior cerebellar peduncle and the suboccipital surface of the cerebellum. The AICA and PICA sometimes have a common trunk. In such cases, acute occlusion results in a more extensive infarct of the cerebellum.

CEREBELLAR HEMORRHAGE

Clinical Features and Pathophysiology

Spontaneous cerebellar hemorrhage represents approximately 10% of all cases of intracerebral hemorrhage.[1-4] As with the supratentorial intracerebral hemorrhage, cerebellar hemorrhage may be caused by hypertension, amyloid angiopathy, vascular anomalies such as arteriovenous malformations (AVM), and cavernous malformations.

The mortality rate is high because of its location[4,5]; however, the outcome in the survivors with cerebellar hemorrhage is relatively favorable compared with survivors with supratentorial intracerebral hemorrhage. The majority of patients with cerebellar hemorrhage have a history of hypertension. Amyloid angiopathy is also one of the causes of cerebellar hemorrhage in elderly patients. Approximately 5% of patients with cerebellar hemorrhage have an AVM in the cerebellum.[6] Seven percent of intracranial AVMs are located in the posterior fossa, 32% of which are in the cerebellar vermis and 21% in the cerebellar hemispheres.[7]

Although diagnosis of cerebellar hemorrhage is now made easily with computed tomography (CT) scanning and magnetic resonance imaging (MRI), angiography is still an important modality for investigating the cause of hemorrhage. Hypertensive cerebellar hemorrhage usually occurs in the cerebellar hemispheres, especially in the area of the dentate nuclei, and it often results in compression of the brainstem and collapse of the fourth ventricle. Damage to the brainstem is the most important factor for predicting the outcome for a patient, and the existence of acute hydrocephalus is also important in the decision to proceed with emergency surgery.

Indications for Surgery

Taneda and colleagues[8] reported on 75 cases of spontaneous cerebellar hemorrhage, which were classified into three grades according to the deformity of the quadrigeminal cistern seen on CT scans. Disappearance of the cistern predicted a poor prognosis in the patients with cerebellar hemorrhage. Kirollos and associates[9] proposed criteria for decision-making in the management of spontaneous cerebellar hemorrhage based on the deformity of the fourth ventricle on CT scans. The patients with completely obliterated fourth ventricles and Glasgow Coma Scale (GCS) scores lower than 8 at the time of treatment had poor outcomes despite aggressive treatment. Yanaka and coworkers[10] described 31 patients with cerebellar hematoma with GCS scores of 8 or less who underwent hematoma evacuation through the suboccipital craniectomy; eight of those patients had good outcomes. These investigators stressed that the presence of high intensity in the brainstem on postoperative MRI was a predictor of poor prognosis.[10]

Surgical indications depend on neurologic status and CT findings. Deterioration in level of consciousness is a strong indication for emergency surgery. On CT scanning, the larger the hematoma, the greater the degree of deformity of the fourth ventricle or quadrigeminal cistern; progressive hydrocephalus of the supratentorial ventricular system increasingly indicates the necessity for surgery. For hydro-

cephalus associated with a lesser degree of "tightness" of the posterior fossa, some surgeons advocate only ventricular drainage and observation.[9]

Surgical Procedure

After induction of general anesthesia, the patient is placed in the prone position, and the head is fixed in a head frame with the neck slightly flexed. The head is elevated adequately to avoid development of venous hypertension and edema during surgery. Bilateral suboccipital craniectomy is often performed; the extent of the exposure depends on the location and size of the hematoma. A linear skin incision is usually placed between 3 cm above the inion and the spinous process of the C3. When ventricular drainage is required by the presence of obstructive hydrocephalus, a 3-cm-long linear incision is additionally placed at a point 5 cm above the orbitomeatal line and 5 cm posterior to the external auditory meatus, to allow insertion of a ventricular catheter.

We have found that a large question-mark incision is useful to obtain both suboccipital exposure and the ventricular drain site. Additionally, this incision has a cosmetic advantage as the incision is well covered by hair after surgery (Fig. 76–1). Other traditional incisions for this approach are the hockey-stick and horseshoe incisions.

Skin flaps are reflected, and the nuchal fascia and muscles are exposed. The trapezius muscle has an attachment to the medial part of the superior nuchal line, and the sternocleidomastoid muscle has an attachment to the lateral part extending to the mastoid process. An edge of the fascia and muscle is left at the upper incision to facilitate wound closure. The nuchal muscles are split at the midline, and the underlying semispinalis capitis muscle and rectus capitis posterior major and minor muscles are detached from the occipital bone. These muscles are retrogradely dissected from the inferior nuchal line by means of a periosteal elevator or raspatory with minimum cautery, in the same manner as in a frontotemporal craniotomy.[11]

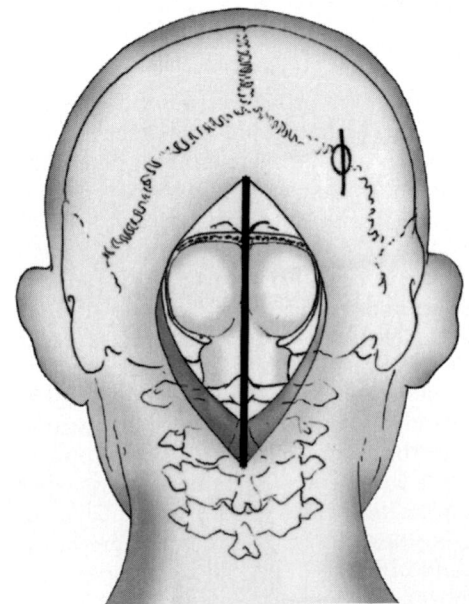
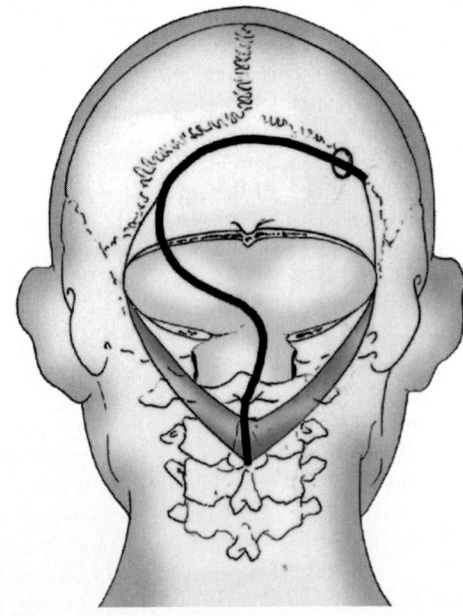

A   B

FIGURE 76–1 *Skin incisions for suboccipital craniectomy and ventricular drainage.* A, *Linear incision.* B, *A large question-mark incision. Note that the question-mark incision provides a large exposure with cosmetic advantages.*

Gentle dissection of these muscles promotes wound healing and prevents postoperative muscle contraction headache. The posterior lamina of C1 is exposed. The myocutaneous flaps are retracted bilaterally with hooks to expose the occipital bone.

Craniectomy is performed with four burr-holes. The craniectomy is widened with a drill and a rongeur laterally and superiorly up to the transverse sinus. The foramen magnum should be opened to secure adequate decompression. After craniectomy, we use ultrasonography to determine the location of the hematoma, and color Doppler ultrasonographic imaging with the color-flow mapping system is helpful when a vascular anomaly has caused a cerebellar hematoma.[12] Prior to the dural opening, a small durotomy is made, and a drainage tube is inserted into the hematoma cavity to evacuate the clots. Then the dura mater is widely opened in a Y shape. The occipital venous sinus is ligated with a silk suture or coagulated and sectioned. The dural flaps are reflected with 3-0 silk sutures. After introduction of the operative microscope, the cerebellar surface is inspected for a vascular anomaly. The corticotomy is extended around the drainage tube, and the hematoma is evacuated with suction. The hematoma is removed from the superficial region to the deeper region. The bleeding points are identified and coagulated. The wall of the hematoma cavity is covered with absorbable knitted fabric (Surgicel) to control oozing.

After adequate removal of the clot, hemostasis should be complete. To confirm hemostasis, the intratracheal pressure is also raised to 30 cm H_2O for 10 seconds (Valsalva maneuver). The hematoma cavity is irrigated with saline solution. A fibrillar collagen (Avitene) may also be used for hemostasis. The dura is closed in a watertight fashion with a continuous suture. In cases requiring further decompression, duraplasty is performed with either artificial dura or a fascia harvested from the parietal region. To prevent venous sinus bleeding, several suspending dural stitches are placed at the edge of the craniectomy. Then the head frame is temporarily loosened and the head is refixed in a neck-extended position to make the nuchal muscles and fascia easier to approximate to the fascia remaining at the superior nuchal line. The muscles are approximated in two layers at the midline, and the skin is sutured. Epidural suction drainage is not recommended, so as to avoid accidental forced drainage of cerebrospinal fluid (CSF).

Postoperative Management

We perform a CT scan in the operating room immediately after surgery, with the general anesthesia maintained.[13] Then the patient is managed in the intensive care unit with monitoring of vital signs. Laboratory data and neurologic signs are important. Auditory brainstem response is monitored when brainstem function is severely impaired. A patient who was comatose, with or without dyspnea preoperatively, is managed with mechanical ventilation and barbiturate therapy. Corticosteroid, mannitol, and a histamine$_2$ blocker are administered intravenously. The systolic blood pressure is maintained at less than 120 mm Hg for 24 hours. A CT scan is taken on the day after surgery to rule out rebleeding and cerebellar edema. Barbiturates are stopped, and the patient is extubated after neurologic status has stabilized and a follow-up CT scan shows improvement in the "tightness" of the posterior fossa. Rehabilitation should start as soon as possible.

Illustrative Case

A 47-year-old man with a history of uncontrolled hypertension had sudden onset of occipital headache and became comatose. On admission, his breathing was ataxic, so he was immediately intubated. A brain CT scan revealed hematoma in both cerebellar hemispheres (Fig. 76–2). The prepontine and quadrigeminal cisterns were obliterated, and the fourth ventricle was completely occluded. The hematoma had ruptured into the fourth ventricle, and the supratentorial ventricular system was dilated. The patient underwent emergency suboccipital decompressive craniectomy with evacuation of the hematoma and ventricular drainage through the occipital horn of the right lateral ventricle. At operation, no vascular anomaly was detected.

Barbiturate therapy was maintained for 2 days after surgery. After weaning from the barbiturate and artificial ventilation, the patient's level of consciousness gradually improved. The postoperative CT scan showed that the posterior fossa had been well decompressed (Fig. 76–3). He had truncal ataxia and bilateral incoordination, but no paresis. He was transferred to another hospital for rehabilitation.

CEREBELLAR INFARCTION

Clinical Features and Pathophysiology

Before the introduction of CT scanning, a correct diagnosis of cerebellar infarction was rarely made during life. With the improvements in CT and MRI, however, diagnosis of cerebellar infarction became easy. Amarenco and colleagues[14] studied the arterial pathology of 88 cerebellar infarcts in 56 patients. Cardiogenic embolism was the cause in 43% of the patients, and atherosclerotic occlusion in 35%. Emboli tend to lodge in the intracranial vertebral artery, resulting in infarction in the PICA territory.

Approximately 13% to 39% of all patients with cerebellar infarction demonstrate mass effect in the posterior fossa.[3,15,16] Large cerebellar infarcts cause edematous changes in the cerebellar hemisphere, resulting in compression of the brainstem whose signs typically start on the third day after the ictus.[17] Initially, an ipsilateral sixth nerve palsy is likely to occur, and facial weakness and Horner's syndrome may be associated. Obstructive hydrocephalus then develops from compression of the fourth ventricle, leading to disturbance of consciousness. The deterioration in consciousness may be rapid. Patients become comatose over several hours once signs of brainstem compression appear.[18] Patients go on to show pinpoint pupils and decerebrate quadriparesis from pontine compression. Ataxic respiration and apnea ultimately occur because of medullary compression from tonsillar herniation, shortly before death.

Indications for Surgery

Patients with small cerebellar infarcts rarely become candidates for surgical treatment. Only in the patient with

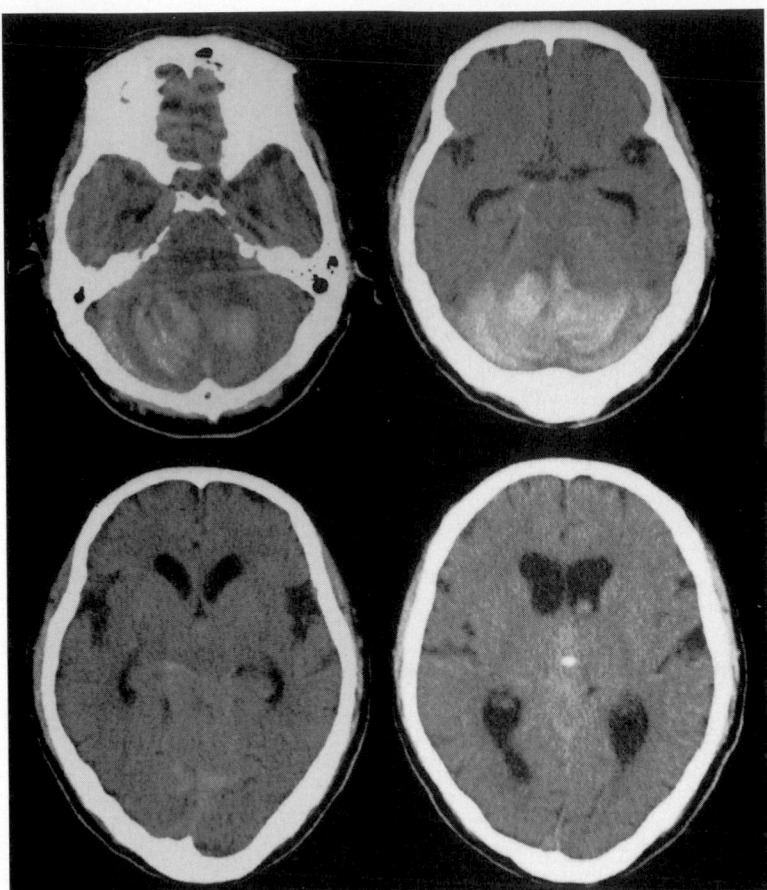

FIGURE 76–2 *CT scans obtained on admission in a 47-year-old man with headache followed by coma. Top left, There is a large cerebellar hematoma in both dentate nuclei with complete obliteration of the fourth ventricle and disappearance of prepontine cistern. Top right, Cerebellar hematoma including the upper vermis with disappearance of the ambient cistern and subarachnoid hemorrhage. Bottom left, Complete obliteration of the quadrigeminal cistern with deformity of the midbrain. Bottom right, Small intraventricular hematomas and dilation of the lateral ventricles.*

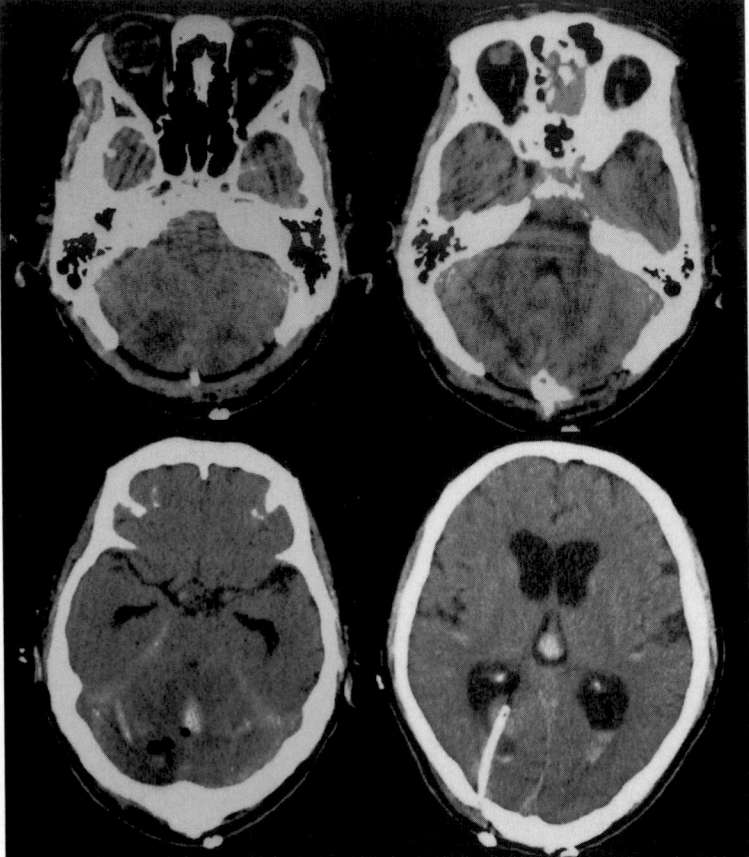

FIGURE 76–3 *CT scans of the same patient as in Fig. 76–2, obtained 24 hours after surgery. Top left, Swollen cerebellum is expanding through the suboccipital craniectomy. Top right, The hematoma has been evacuated, and the fourth ventricle becomes visible. Bottom left, The deformity of the midbrain has improved. Bottom right, A ventricular catheter has been placed in the occipital horn of the right lateral ventricle.*

a rapidly progressing disturbance of consciousness caused by a cerebellar infarction with edematous change is surgical decompression with a large suboccipital craniectomy and dural plasty the treatment of choice. The presence of a hemorrhagic infarction on CT scan does not relate to clinical deterioration,[19] and the finding of vertical displacement of the brainstem on MRI also does not predict deterioration.[3] Detailed and frequent neurologic monitoring is necessary to determine the necessity for surgery.

Some patients who are treated by ventricular drainage alone to relieve an obstructive hydrocephalus have been reported to have good outcomes.[3,20]

Surgical Procedure

Surgical decompression with extensive suboccipital craniectomy and duraplasty is the procedure of choice for massive cerebellar infarction. The craniectomy is essentially the same as that described previously for cerebellar hemorrhage. To achieve effective decompression, the foramen magnum is widely opened, and the craniectomy is extended bilaterally. Laminectomy of C1 is usually added. When an obstructive hydrocephalus is associated, a ventricular catheter into the occipital horn of the lateral ventricle is placed at this stage. If the dura mater is extremely tense, ventricular drainage is not carried out until the dural opening is large enough to avoid upward herniation. The dura mater is incised first near the foramen magnum to drain CSF and then is widely opened. In cases associated with severe edematous change, the grossly necrotic tissue of the cerebellum may be resected for internal decompression. The duraplasty is performed with artificial dura or a piece of fascia harvested from the parietal region.

Illustrative Case

A 52-year-old man with a history of untreated paroxysmal atrial fibrillation presented with a sudden onset of vertigo. He went to a local hospital, where neurologic examinations revealed truncal ataxia and incoordination of the right extremities. A CT scan showed no abnormal findings (Fig. 76–4). He was treated conservatively with the diagnosis of

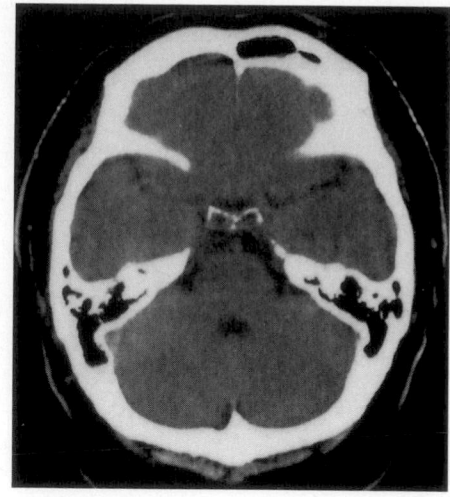

FIGURE 76–4 *CT scan in a 52-year-old man with vertigo, performed just after ictus, shows normal findings.*

right cerebellar infarction. On the following day, a T2-weighted MR image demonstrated a high-intensity area in the territory of the right PICA (Fig. 76–5). Within 3 days after ictus, as he progressively deteriorated, he was transferred to our hospital.

The patient's GCS score was 10. A CT scan taken on admission disclosed a slight high-density area corresponding to the territory of the PICA (Fig. 76–6). The fourth ventricle was compressed, and the supratentorial ventricular system dilated. A diagnosis of hemorrhagic infarction was made. The patient underwent emergency suboccipital decompressive craniectomy with duraplasty and ventricular drainage through the right occipital horn. The patient was treated with barbiturate therapy for 2 days after surgery. The postoperative CT scan showed the posterior fossa well decompressed and a reduction in ventricular size (Fig. 76–7). The patient's level of consciousness completely recovered, and he was discharged with only mild ataxia and right dysmetria. Follow-up MRI performed 3 months after surgery showed a normal brainstem and a slack posterior fossa (Fig. 76–8).

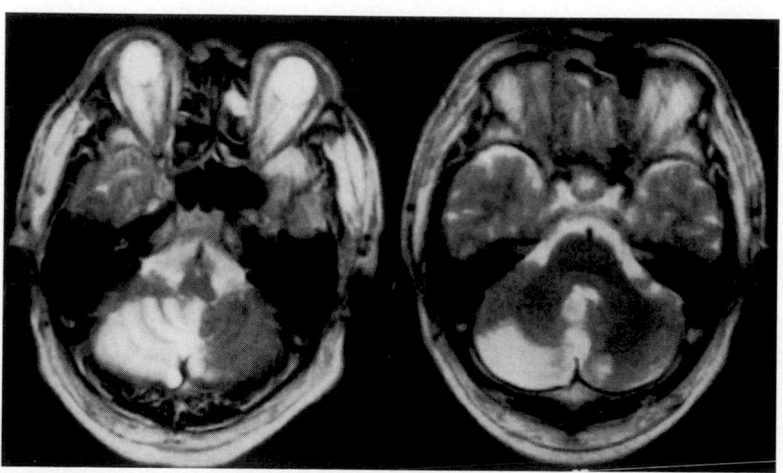

FIGURE 76–5 *T2-weighted MR images (MRI) of the same patient as in Fig. 76–4, performed 24 hours after ictus, showing a high-intensity area in the right posterior inferior cerebellar artery territory.*

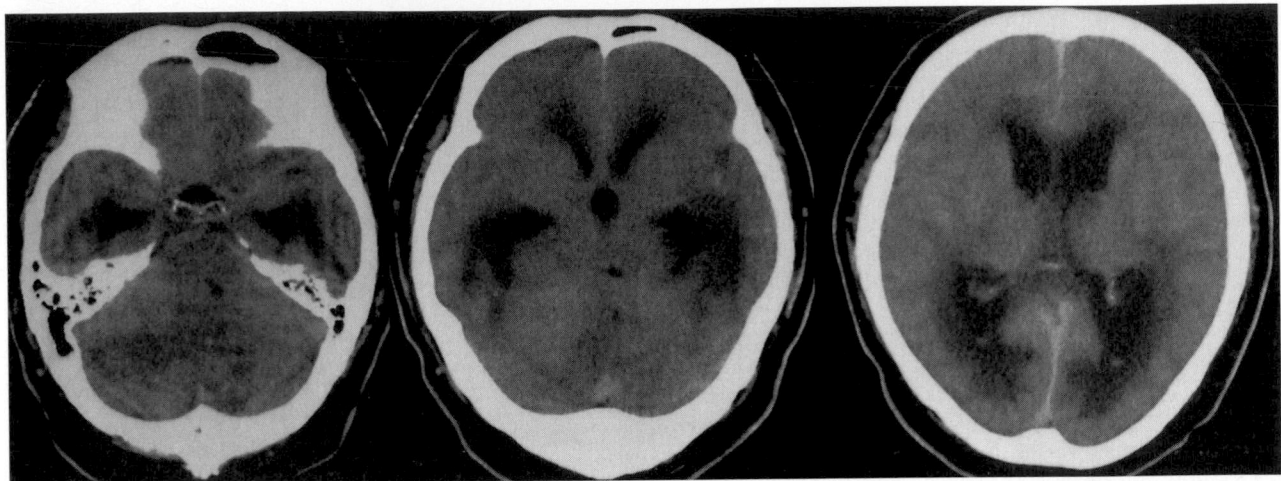

FIGURE 76–6   *CT scans of the same patient as in Fig. 76–4, obtained 3 days after ictus. Left, Fogging effect in the posterior inferior cerebellar artery territory with edema and deformity of the fourth ventricle and marked dilatation of the temporal horn of the lateral ventricles. Middle, Severely compressed quadrigeminal cistern with dilatation of supratentorial ventricular system. Right, Marked ventricular dilatation with disappearance of the sylvian fissures and sulci.*

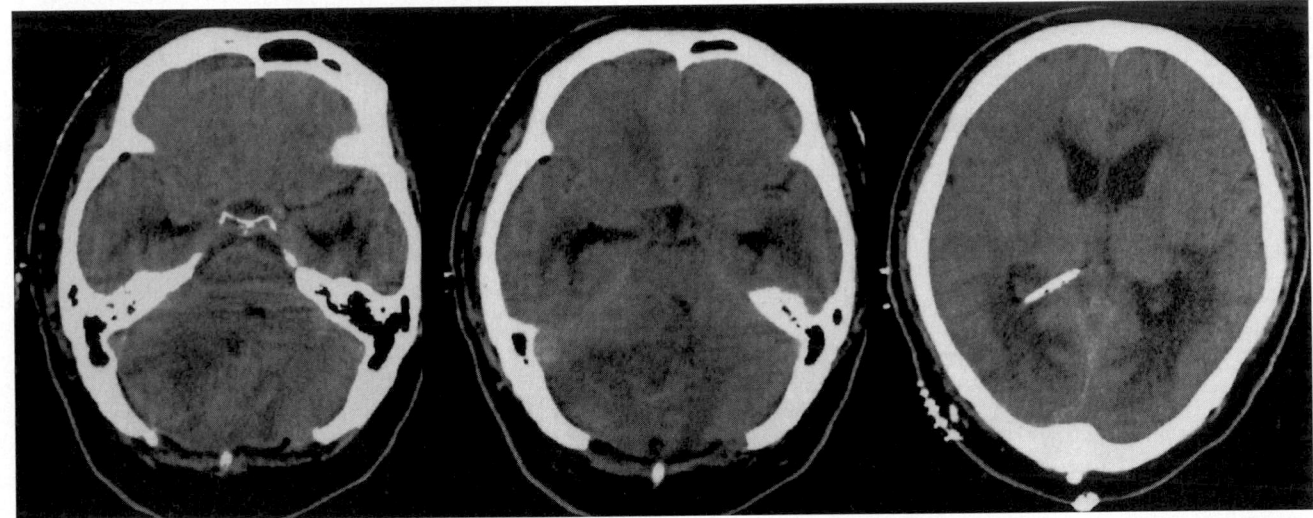

FIGURE 76–7   *CT scans of the same patient as in Fig. 76–4, obtained 24 hours after surgery. Left, The infarcted cerebellum is expanding through the craniectomy and the fourth ventricle deformity. Middle, Marked shrinkage of the temporal horn of the lateral ventricles. Right, A ventricular catheter has been placed in the occipital horn of the right lateral ventricle.*

Vascular Reconstruction

To prevent cerebellar infarction in patients with vertebrobasilar insufficiency, various vascular reconstructions have been carried out. For bilateral occlusion or high-grade stenosis of the distal vertebral artery, various forms of extracranial-intracranial anastomoses have been described, including occipital artery (OA) to PICA, OA-AICA, superficial temporal artery (STA) to SCA, and STA to posterior cerebral artery.[21,22]

OA-PICA anastomosis is the procedure most commonly performed. The patient is positioned prone. An ipsilateral hockey-stick skin incision is made. The attachments of the trapezius and sternocleidomastoid muscles form a tendinous arch, through which the OA and the greater

occipital nerve pass. The OA can be traced between the splenius capitis and semispinalis capitis muscles, and then into the groove of the OA below the mastoid process. The OA is prepared at the time of scalp dissection from the occipital bone. The OA can be harvested from the base of the mastoid process to its most distal part. Unlike the OA between the muscles, the OA in the subcutaneous layer distal to the tendinous arch is tortuous and tightly adherent to the surrounding connective tissue, so dissection of this part takes longer and is tedious. After the OA is dissected, the unilateral suboccipital craniotomy is made. Intradurally, the perimedullary portion of the PICA is identified on the lateral medullary area; then an end-to-side anastomosis of the OA to the perimedullary portion of the PICA is performed.

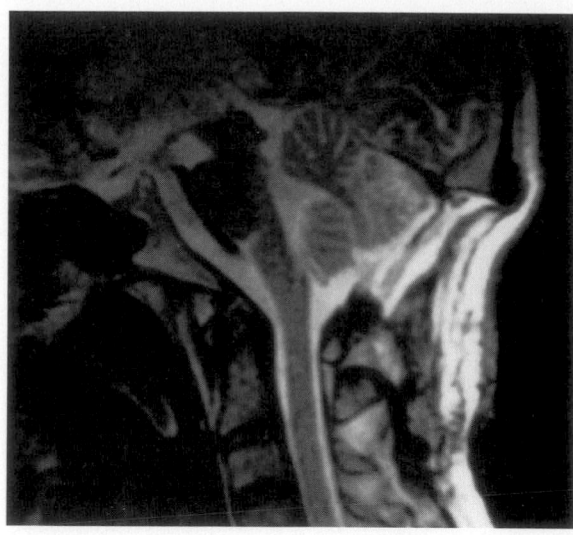

FIGURE 76–8 *Sagittal T2-weighted MR image of the same patient as in Fig. 76–4, obtained 3 months after surgery, shows the posterior fossa slack with no evidence of brainstem injury.*

To prevent cerebellar infarction, the lateral medullary syndrome of one side of the PICA territory, PICA-PICA anastomosis is the procedure of choice. With the patient in the prone position, a midline skin incision is placed. A midline suboccipital craniotomy is performed with the foramen magnum opened. The retrotonsillar segments of the bilateral PICAs course quite close between the bilateral tonsils. A side-to-side anastomosis is performed.

CONCLUSION

The management of cerebellar infarction and hemorrhage is described with focus on the surgical indications and procedures. To achieve the best surgical outcome, the timing of surgery is very important; surgical intervention should be performed without delay when indicated. Perioperative close observation and adequate medical management are important as well.

References

1. Chin D, Carney P: Acute cerebellar hemorrhage with brainstem compression in contrast with benign cerebellar hemorrhage. Surg Neurol 19:406–409, 1983.

2. Heiskanen O: Treatment of spontaneous intracerebral and intra-cerebellar hemorrhages. Stroke 24(Suppl 12):I94–I95, I107–I108.
3. Koh MG, Phan TG, Atkinson JLD, Wijdicks EFM: Neuroimaging in deteriorating patients with cerebellar infarcts and mass effect. Stroke 31:2062–2067, 2000.
4. McKissock W, Richardson A, Walsh L: Spontaneous cerebellar hemorrhage: A study of 34 consecutive cases treated surgically. Brain 83:1–9, 1960.
5. Luparello V, Canavero S: Treatment of hypertensive cerebellar hemorrhage: Surgical or conservative management? Neurosurgery 37:552–553, 1995.
6. Kobayashi S, Sato A, Kageyama Y, et al: Treatment of hypertensive cerebellar hemorrhage: Surgical or conservative management? Neurosurgery 34:246–251, 1994.
7. Drake CG, Friedman AH, Peerless SJ: Posterior fossa arteriovenous malformations. J Neurosurg 64:1–10, 1986.
8. Taneda M, Hayakawa T, Mogami H: Primary cerebellar hemorrhage: Quadrigeminal cistern obliteration on CT scan as a predictor of outcome. J Neurosurg 67:545–552, 1987.
9. Kirollos RW, Tyagi AK, Ross SA, et al: Management of spontaneous cerebellar hematomas: A prospective treatment protocol. Neurosurgery 49:1378–1387, 2001.
10. Yanaka K, Meguro K, Fujita K, et al: Postoperative brainstem high intensity is correlated with poor outcome for patients with spontaneous cerebellar hemorrhage. Neurosurgery 45:1323–1328, 1999.
11. Oikawa S, Mizuno M, Muraoka S, Kobayashi S: Retrograde dissection of the temporalis muscle preventing muscle atrophy for pterional craniotomy. J Neurosurg 84:297–299, 1996.
12. Kitazawa K, Nitta J, Okudera H, Kobayashi S: Color Doppler ultrasound imaging in the emergency management of an intracerebral hamartoma caused by cerebral arteriovenous malformations: Technical case report. Neurosurgery 42:405–407, 1998.
13. Okudera H, Sugita K, Kobayashi S, et al: Clinical experience and utility of a computerized tomographic scanner in the operating room: The operating CT system. Neuroradiology 30:461, 1988.
14. Amarenco P, Hauw JJ, Gautier JC: Arterial pathology in cerebellar infarction. Stroke 21:1299–1305, 1990.
15. Kase CS, Norrving B, Levine SR, et al: Cerebellar infarction: Clinical and anatomic observation in 66 cases. Stroke 24:76–83, 1993.
16. Macdonell RA, Kalnins RM, Donnan GA: Cerebellar infarction: Natural history, prognosis, and pathology. Stroke 18:849–855 1987.
17. Hornig CR, Rust DS, Busse O, et al: Space-occupying cerebellar infarction: Clinical course and prognosis. Stroke 25:372–374, 1994.
18. Heros RC: Cerebellar hemorrhage and infarction. Stroke 13:106–109, 1982.
19. Chaves CJ, Pessin MS, Caplan LR, et al: Cerebellar hemorrhagic infarction. Neurology 46:346–349, 1996.
20. Greenberg J, Skubick D, Shenkin H: Acute hydrocephalus in cerebellar infarct and hemorrhage. Neurology 29:409–413, 1979.
21. Ausman JI, Diaz FG, Vacca DF, Sadasivan B: Superficial temporal and occipital artery bypass pedicles to superior, anterior inferior, and posterior inferior cerebellar arteries for vertebrobasilar insufficiency. J Neurosurg 72:554–558, 1990.
22. Hopkins LN, Budny JL, Spetzler RF: Revascularization of the rostral brain stem. Neurosurgery 10:364–369, 1982.

Chapter Seventy-Seven

Nontraumatic Intracranial Arterial Dissection

Akira Yamaura

TERMINOLOGY

Pathologic studies suggest two categories of nontraumatic intracranial arterial dissections, (1) dissections between the intima and media that cause luminal narrowing or occlusion and (2) dissections between the media and adventitia, or at the media, that cause aneurysmal dilatations.

Cerebral ischemia or infarction may be caused by narrowing of the lumen. The type of dissection associated with external aneurysmal dilatation may rupture into the subarachnoid space, a "true" dissecting aneurysm. These distinctions are seldom absolute. Trauma is an important cause of intracranial arterial dissection, but the posttraumatic condition, including the cerebral circulatory and metabolic environment, produces a clinical picture and necessitates treatment that are largely different from those in the nontraumatic condition.

The internal carotid anterior wall aneurysm was first referred to by the term *internal carotid dorsal aneurysm* by Nakagawa and associates[1] in 1986. In 1996, Sano[2] claimed that *internal carotid anterior or superior aneurysm* would be more accurate. Such an aneurysm often looks like a blood blister, having a very thin wall and a semicircular form, without the neck portion seen in saccular aneurysms, and is easily torn during surgical manipulation. The pathology of this unique lesion is still controversial; Ohkuma and associates[3] found an intramural hematoma in the surgical specimen in one case; in another case, retention of contrast medium in the C2 portion of internal carotid artery on arteriography was associated with a typical dark purple-red lesion at surgery. These findings suggested a dissection of the arterial wall.

Another variety to be briefly discussed in this chapter is dolichoectasia or the megadolichovertebrobasilar anomaly. Mizutani and coworkers[4] reported that magnetic resonance imaging (MRI) disclosed intimal flaps, double lumens, or subacute clot in the false lumens in all four of the dolichoectasias in their series. They suggested that many cases of classic dolichoectasia may be a variety of arterial dissection.

CAUSATIVE FACTORS

Many causative factors have been proposed for arterial dissections. Among them are hypertension, fibromuscular dysplasia, polycystic kidney disease, reticular fiber deficiency, defects in the internal elastic lamina, fibrous or fibroelastic intimal thickening, accumulation of mucoid ground substance, cystic medial degeneration, migraine, moyamoya disease, syphilis, arteritis, atherosclerosis, homocystinuria, and strenuous physical exertion. The presence of a specific causative factor might influence the selection of treatment.

The role of hypertension is not proven in the pathogenesis of arterial dissection, but in the nationwide Japanese study of nontraumatic intracranial arterial dissections, hypertension was found in 47% of hemorrhagic dissections and 43% of nonhemorrhagic dissections.[5] Control of blood pressure is essential in management of patients with subarachnoid hemorrhage (SAH). Before surgery or in patients for whom surgery is not indicated, control of hypertension is the most important and probably the only indicated therapy.

GENERAL ASPECTS AND NATURAL HISTORY

Nontraumatic intracranial arterial dissection was previously and probably still is uncritically accepted as causing only cerebral infarction in otherwise healthy young adults. However, later studies have shown a variety of different clinical pictures, such as SAH, cerebral infarction, and headache not associated with hemorrhage. Understanding the natural history of this unique lesion is important to any decision about treatment modalities. In order to elucidate the general aspects, a nationwide Japanese study was conducted on nontraumatic intracranial arterial dissections from July 1995 to June 1996.[5,6] The inclusion criteria for the study are listed in Table 77.1. Of the 530 neurosurgery training hospitals participating in the study, 208 hospitals encountered such cases during this 1-year period; 350 cases were analyzed.

Table 77.1   Inclusion Criteria of the Japanese Nationwide Study on Nontraumatic Intracranial Arterial Dissection (June 1995–June 1996)

1. Arteriography was mandatory; presence of the following findings:
   a. Tapered narrowing or string sign.
   b. Aneurysmal outpouching.
   c. Intimal flap, contrast medium in a false lumen.
   d. Combination of above findings, such as pearl and string sign.
2. Autopsy confirmed dissection.
3. Head trauma was absent.
4. Patients with magnetic resonance imaging or magnetic resonance angiographic diagnosis but without 1 or 2 were not accepted.

From Yamaura A, Yoshimoto T, Hashimoto N, et al: Nationwide study of nontraumatic intracranial arterial dissection: Clinical features and outcome. Surg Cerebral Stroke 26:79–86, 1998 (Jpn); and Yamaura A, Yoshimoto T, Hashimoto N, et al: Nationwide study of nontraumatic intracranial arterial dissection: Treatment and its results. Surg Cerebral Stroke 26:87–95, 1998 (Jpn).

CLINICAL PICTURE

The data on the clinical picture of intracranial arterial dissections described here are mainly from the nationwide Japanese study.[5,6]

Age

The age distribution showed a peak in patients in their 40s and 50s; none of the patients younger than 30 years experienced bleeding, and in all patients younger than 20 years, the dissection was in the anterior circulation only.

Presentation

The nationwide Japanese study showed that 58% of the patients presented with SAH, 33% with cerebral ischemia from infarction or transient ischemic attack, and 7% with headache not associated with hemorrhage (Table 77.2).

Subarachnoid Hemorrhage

More than 60% of the vertebral artery lesions and approximately 45% of the basilar lesions bled; 40% of the lesions in the anterior circulation bled. SAH has a great influence on the outcome. In addition to the direct effects of the hemorrhage, vasospasm may develop at a remote region. Also, a massive SAH can cause acute hydrocephalus, which may require diversion of cerebrospinal fluid (CSF). Yamaura and colleagues,[7] analyzing 21 patients with ruptured vertebral artery dissections, found visual impairment due to vitreous hemorrhage (Terson's syndrome) in 5 patients (24%). The clinical picture for these patients did not differ from that for patients with SAH due to ruptured saccular aneurysms.

Ischemia or Infarction

Internal bulging of the arterial wall due to dissection between the intima and the media causes narrowing and occlusion of the lumen and ischemia or infarction in the distal region supplied by the affected artery. Some dissec-

Table 77.2   Clinical Picture of Nontraumatic Intracranial Arterial Dissections

Clinical Picture	No. of patients
Subarachnoid hemorrhage	206 (58%)
Brain ischemia (infarction/transient ischemic attack)	118 (33%)
Headache	26 (7%)
Incidental	7 (2%)
Total	357

From Yamaura A, Yoshimoto T, Hashimoto N, et al: Nationwide study of nontraumatic intracranial arterial dissection: Clinical features and outcome. Surg Cerebral Stroke 26:79–86, 1998 (Jpn); and Yamaura A, Yoshimoto T, Hashimoto N, et al: Nationwide study of nontraumatic intracranial arterial dissection: Treatment and its results. Surg Cerebral Stroke 26:87–95, 1998 (Jpn).

tions have a progressive course. Occasionally, however, the stroke proceeds in a stuttering fashion. Also, ischemic complications may arise as a consequence of remote embolization from the dissection site.

Ischemia from a vertebral artery dissection may produce lateral medullary infarction (Wallenberg's syndrome). Okuchi and associates[8] analyzed the cerebral angiograms of 22 patients with Wallenberg's syndrome. The vertebral artery was affected in 15 patients, and the posterior inferior cerebellar artery in 5 patients. Seven (47%) of 15 patients with vertebral artery lesions had dissection (four intracranial and three extracranial).

Hemorrhagic Infarction

Yamashita and colleagues[9] described a 34-year-old man with a posterior inferior cerebellar artery dissecting aneurysm who presented with cerebellar hemorrhagic infarction. This lesion required a decompressive suboccipital craniectomy and internal decompression. Okuno and associates[10] reported on a patient with a dissecting aneurysm who presented with hemorrhagic infarction, visualized on computed tomography (CT) 4 days after presentation. Arteriography showed the "string of pearls" sign in the right A_2 portion of the anterior cerebral artery. The surgical specimen of the affected artery showed dissection in the inner layer of the media.

Mass Effects

A dissecting aneurysm may reach a considerable size and manifest as mass effects. In the series reported by Senter and Sarwar,[11] one patient had pharyngeal and palatal paralysis and nystagmus due to local mass effect. Berger and Wilson[12] reported on six patients, one of whom had a cerebellopontine angle mass causing seventh cranial nerve paralysis. A right vertebral artery dissecting aneurysm of large size in a 56-year-old man was angiographically diagnosed and surgically repaired by Miyazaki and colleagues.[13] Alexander and coworkers[14] reported on a patient with basilar artery dissection that also produced considerable mass effect.

Recurrence

Recurrent clinical events should influence the decision for active treatment and the treatment modality. Yamaura and

Ono[15] reported recurrence in 26 (10%) of their 260 patients. Six (13%) of their 45 patients with anterior circulation lesions and 20 (9%) of their 215 patients with posterior circulation lesions had recurrences. These investigators reported recurrence in 15 (10%) of 147 patients with SAH and 11 (10%) of 113 patients without SAH. There was no apparent difference in frequency of recurrence between the groups with and without SAH. The nationwide Japanese Nationwide study, however, had different results.[5,6] Hemorrhagic lesions rebled in 14% of patients reported in the study, but ischemic lesions recurred in only 4%.

Yamaura and colleagues[7] recorded sudden clinical deterioration in 7 of 21 patients with ruptured intracranial vertebral dissecting aneurysms. Five (24%) had confirmed recurrence of SAH. Rebleeding occurred 3 to 17 days after the first episodes and was less likely thereafter. All 3 patients with ischemia experienced repeated episodes at intervals ranging from 4 days to 8 years and 8 months.

Aoki and Sakai[16] reviewed 60 reported cases of ruptured intracranial vertebral dissection and found that 18 lesions (30%) had rebled. In 8 of the 10 cases for which the interval between the initial bleeding and rebleeding was known, the interval was several hours. This timing of recurrence does not differ from that observed in patients with saccular aneurysms. Yamamoto and coworkers[17] reported an interesting case in which SAH occurred 13 years after the first episode of bleeding from a posterior circulation dissection.

Hemorrhage may occur after an ischemic episode. Takita and associates[18] reported a 33-year-old man who experienced SAH 4 months after an initial brainstem infarction; dissection had extended to the basilar artery from the vertebral artery. Adams and colleagues[19] described a 39-year-old woman who was first seen with pontine infarction and later experienced SAH. They concluded that the initial subintimal dissection had decreased blood flow through penetrating arterioles; subsequent rupture through a thinned adventitia accounted for the SAH. Tsutsumi and coworkers[20] reported a similar case in which the patient presented with lateral medullary infarction and dissection of the vertebral artery. An antiplatelet agent was given, and SAH occurred 2 days later.

The nationwide Japanese study showed that 4 (3%) of 118 patients with ischemic lesions experienced subsequent SAH.[5,6]

RADIOLOGIC DIAGNOSIS

Cerebral angiography remains the most reliable diagnostic modality for arterial dissection; however, erroneous diagnoses have been common, mainly because of the variability of findings, which include the string sign (narrow, tapered lumen), occlusion, proximal or distal dilatation or both, intimal flap, double lumen, retention of contrast medium, or intramural pooling. The sole pathognomonic sign of a dissection is a double lumen (true lumen and intramural false lumen)[21] with intimal flap. However, that combination of findings is rather rare. The false lumen of the dissection would be evident only if the dissection reentered the true lumen distally. Embolic occlusion of the remote branches is commonly seen in vertebral dissections.

The most common error is the misinterpretation of dissection as a ruptured saccular aneurysm of unusual shape, attributed to intraluminal clot and associated with vasospasm of its parent artery.[11,22–24] Such errors in angiographic interpretation could lead to a false judgment regarding the need for surgery.

A specific MRI diagnosis of dissection is possible when parallel dark and bright structures are visualized along the course of the artery. The dark signal represents the patent residual lumen, and the bright signal, intramural clot.[25–27] An intimal flap may be demonstrated by MRI. Subacute or chronic clot in the false lumen is also demonstrable. MRI offers important aid in formulating a plan of interventional radiology and surgery.

Affected Arteries

Another important feature of intracranial arterial dissection is the location of the lesion. More than 80% of dissections arise in the vertebral artery, and 7% in the basilar artery. Only 7% were in the anterior circulation in the nationwide Japanese study.[5,6] This distribution is quite different from that of saccular aneurysms. Most of the surgical procedures for dissections are performed in the posterior fossa.

Multiple Lesions

Multiple dissections are found in 10% of cases. The most common type of multiple dissections consists of lesions in both vertebral arteries. In this situation, it is important to establish which artery was the source of the SAH. Bilateral anterior circulation lesions have also been reported.[15]

Resolution of Dissection

Spontaneous resolution of the dissection is occasionally recognized on "repeat" angiography. Friedman and Drake[23] reported that late angiography showed healing of the dissected artery in two of their patients. One patient showed a complete resolution after 4 years; in the other, only the proximal half of the dissection resolved after 6 months. Berger and Wilson[12] and Shimoji and associates[27] observed similar resolutions. Two of the four patients reported by Pozzati and coworkers[28] also showed spontaneous healing during conservative management.

Yamashita and colleagues[9] reported a PICA dissecting aneurysm that manifested as a sausage-shaped dilatation; arteriography revealed improvement at 146 days and resolution at 258 days.

Persistently Patent False Lumen

Persistently patent false lumen is common. Reentry of the false lumen occurs at the distal portion, after which resistance through the false lumen must diminish remarkably. Such flow through the false lumen may play an important role in the maintenance of a physiologic blood supply. Mizutani and colleagues[29] visualized a persistent double lumen in a middle cerebral artery dissection at 36 months.

They suggested that endothelial formation may have occurred in both the true lumen and the false lumen.

TREATMENT

The optimal treatment of intracranial arterial dissections has not been determined. The first surgical intervention for intracranial dissection took place in 1951, when Poppen[30] operated on a middle cerebral artery dissection.

Surgical Treatment

Indications for Surgery

The indications for surgery remain controversial. Because the dissecting aneurysm cannot be managed by neck clipping in the same way as saccular aneurysms, the choice of surgical treatment is limited to such techniques as proximal occlusion of the parent artery, entrapment of the lesion with[31] or without vascular reconstruction, wrapping, wrapping followed by clipping, and variants of these procedures (Tables 77.3 and 77.4). The remarkable development of endovascular surgery makes it a potentially highly attractive option. The development of appropriate stents has the theoretical advantage of preserving the original lumen while occluding the pathologic dissection.

Dissections in the Posterior Circulation

Dissecting lesions in the posterior circulation are more likely to bleed than those in the anterior circulation. Aoki and Sakai[16] stressed the importance of early operation for ruptured intracranial vertebral dissections, because the acute rebleeding rate in their series was 30%. In my experience, proximal clip occlusion of the parent vertebral artery successfully prevents rebleeding.[7] Some investigators argue that proximal occlusion for dissection is not always safe because rebleeding may still occur postoperatively.[32–34]

Table 77.3 Surgical Treatment of Nontraumatic Intracranial Arterial Dissections: Hemorrhagic Group versus Nonhemorrhagic Group (Single Lesion)

	No. of Procedures		
Procedure	Hemorrhagic Group	Nonhemorrhagic Group	Total
Proximal occlusion	51 (40%)	8 (30%)	59 (38%)
Entrapment	25 (20%)	5 (19%)	30 (19%)
Wrapping/ Coating	13 (10%)	5 (19%)	18 (12%)
Clipping	3 (2%)	2 (7%)	5 (3%)
Other craniotomy	3 (2%)	1 (4%)	4 (3%)
Endovascular surgery	32 (25%)	6 (22%)	38 (25%)
Whole series	127	27	154

From Yamaura A, Yoshimoto T, Hashimoto N, et al: Nationwide study of nontraumatic intracranial arterial dissection: Clinical features and outcome. Surg Cerebral Stroke 26:79–86, 1998 (Jpn), and Yamaura A, Yoshimoto T, Hashimoto N, et al: Nationwide study of nontraumatic intracranial arterial dissection: Treatment and its results. Surg Cerebral Stroke 26:87–95, 1998 (Jpn).

Table 77.4 Surgical Treatment of Nontraumatic Intracranial Arterial Dissections: Anterior Circulation versus Posterior Circulation (Single Lesion)

	No. of Procedures		
Procedure	Anterior Circulation	Posterior Circulation	Total
Proximal occlusion	1 (11%)	54 (39%)	55 (38%)
Entrapment	1 (11%)	29 (21%)	30 (21%)
Wrapping/Coating	5 (56%)	11 (8%)	16 (11%)
Clipping	1 (11%)	4 (3%)	5 (3%)
Other craniotomy	1 (11%)	3 (2%)	4 (3%)
Endovascular surgery	0	36 (26%)	36 (25%)
Whole series	9	137	146

From Yamaura A, Yoshimoto T, Hashimoto N, et al: Nationwide study of nontraumatic intracranial arterial dissection: Clinical features and outcome. Surg Cerebral Stroke 26:79–86, 1998 (Jpn), and Yamaura A, Yoshimoto T, Hashimoto N, et al: Nationwide study of nontraumatic intracranial arterial dissection: Treatment and its results. Surg Cerebral Stroke 26:87–95, 1998 (Jpn).

For patients presenting with ischemia, the number of cases described in the literature is too limited for confident analysis. Pozzati and coworkers[28] recommended angiographic study in neurologically stable patients before surgical intervention is undertaken.

Dissections in the Anterior Circulation

Because dissections of the carotid artery and its branches bleed less often than dissections of the posterior circulation, operations are performed less often. For ruptured dissections, wrapping or some alternative has most commonly been selected in order to keep the lumen patent.

Therapeutic Dilemmas

Yamaura colleagues[7] reported that vertebral dissecting aneurysms are prone to rebleeding within 2 to 3 weeks of the fist episode, after which rebleeding is less likely. Conservative treatment may be justified in selected cases, even if they manifest as hemorrhage. An intimal tear at the entrance of the dissection is commonly found, and on occasion, a second distal tear at the site of reentry of the false lumen, may also be demonstrated. When reentry occurs, the flow of blood can be reestablished through the false lumen. Healing by endothelial lining of the false lumen may result.[35]

Yamaura and colleagues[7] observed during surgery that the affected artery had become whitish gray and firm 4 to 5 weeks after the ictus, probably as a result of organization of the intramural hematoma. This suggests spontaneous healing of the dissection.

Aggressive treatment is based on the significant mortality resulting from rebleeding. Advocates of more conservative therapy point to the possibility of spontaneous resolution. Most procedures require occlusion of the parent artery or true lumen. Surgery is associated with complications, such as lateral medullary infarction, which occurred in 18% of the series reported by Yamaura and associates.[36] In cases of bilateral vertebral dissection, surgical occlusion of one vertebral artery may increase the blood flow through the other artery, with possible adverse effects.

Yamaura and associates[36] retrospectively reviewed a series of 56 consecutive cases of vertebral dissection (42 hemorrhagic and 14 nonhemorrhagic). Among the nonhemorrhagic cases, 11 were treated conservatively; although 2 of these cases showed recurrence at 14 months and 8 years, none of the conservatively treated patients died or had any serious deficits. Conservative therapy appears justified for nonhemorrhagic vertebral dissections.

Of the patients in their series with hemorrhagic vertebral dissections, 29% suffered rebleeding at 0 to 16 days after the ictus. Fourteen cases were not operated upon; 6 patients died, and the other 8 patients did well during a follow-up period of 1 to 15 years (mean 6.6 years). The six fatalities were carefully reviewed; 3 patients might have survived if operation had been performed as soon as possible. Rebleeding occurred on day 0 in the patient who had shown improvement after CSF shunt from an initial classification as Hunt and Kosnik grade 4. The other patients were initially classified as grade 2 and 3, and rebleeding occurred on day 8 in both. If surgery had been performed in all hemorrhagic vertebral dissections as soon as possible, 3 (7%) of 42 patients might have been saved. It is impossible, however, to estimate their quality of life had they survived.

Surgical Techniques

Proximal occlusion and entrapment with or without false lumen obliteration may be performed by endovascular techniques. Takahashi and colleagues[37] stressed the advantages of endovascular occlusion in the treatment of ruptured vertebral dissections. Tsutsumi and coworkers[20] used platinum coils with fiber and Guglielmo detachable coils for intra-aneurysmal embolization and proximal occlusion. Further new endovascular techniques using stents and coils have been developed.[38] In these techniques, the true lumen is kept patent, and the false lumen of the dissection is obliterated by Guglielmo detachable coils through the stent mesh. These techniques may come to play an important role in the treatment of intracranial arterial dissections.

Vertebral artery occlusion is usually safe and successful in producing thrombosis and obliteration of the dissected segment when the dissection involves only the vertebral artery.[23,27] However, the dissection may progress and rebleed even after surgical management.[39]

Su and associates[40] emphasized the importance of monitoring of somatosensory evoked potentials, auditory brain stem responses, and wedge pressure by a balloon occlusion test while preparing for proximal artery occlusion.

Most of the lesions lack a clippable aneurysm neck. However, some surgeons have tried clipping the aneurysmal outpouching with a wrap-and-clip technique or clipping without wrapping. Simple clipping of the outpouching poses a great risk of causing "slipping-out" and rupture or "slipping-in" and luminal occlusion.

In the nationwide Japanese study, 60% of the patients with hemorrhagic dissections underwent surgical treatment, including endovascular surgery, whereas only 18% of those with nonhemorrhagic group were so treated (Table 77.5). More posterior circulation lesions (45%) were treated surgically than anterior circulation lesions (39%) (Table 77.6). The most commonly used technique in both

Table 77.5 Treatment of Nontraumatic Intracranial Arterial Dissections: Hemorrhagic Group versus Nonhemorrhagic Group (Single Lesion)

Treatment	No. of Cases (%)		
	Hemorrhagic Group	Nonhemorrhagic Group	Total
Conservative	80 (38.8%)	124 (82.1%)	204 (57.1%)
Surgical	125 (60.7%)	27 (17.9%)	152 (42.6%)
Not described	1 (0.5%)	0	1 (0.3%)
Whole series	206	151	357

From Yamaura A, Yoshimoto T, Hashimoto N, et al: Nationwide study of nontraumatic intracranial arterial dissection: Clinical features and outcome. Surg Cerebral Stroke 26:79–86, 1998 (Jpn), and Yamaura A, Yoshimoto T, Hashimoto N, et al: Nationwide study of nontraumatic intracranial arterial dissection: Treatment and its results. Surg Cerebral Stroke 26:87–95, 1998 (Jpn).

Table 77.6 Treatment of Nontraumatic Intracranial Arterial Dissections: Anterior Circulation versus Posterior Circulation (Single Lesion)

Treatment	No. of Cases		
	Anterior Circulation	Posterior Circulation	Total
Conservative	14 (60.9%)	165 (55.2%)	179 (55.6%)
Surgical	9 (39.1%)	134 (44.8%)	143 (44.4%)
Whole series	23	299	322

From Yamaura A, Yoshimoto T, Hashimoto N, et al: Nationwide study of nontraumatic intracranial arterial dissection: Clinical features and outcome. Surg Cerebral Stroke 26:79–86, 1998 (Jpn), and Yamaura A, Yoshimoto T, Hashimoto N, et al: Nationwide study of nontraumatic intracranial arterial dissection: Treatment and its results. Surg Cerebral Stroke 26:87–95, 1998 (Jpn).

the hemorrhagic and nonhemorrhagic groups was proximal occlusion of the parent artery at craniotomy. Endovascular techniques were used in 25% of the hemorrhagic cases and 22% of the nonhemorrhagic cases. Wrapping or coating was most commonly used for lesions of the anterior circulation, and proximal occlusion by craniotomy in lesions of the posterior circulation. Endovascular techniques were used only to treat lesions of the posterior circulation.

Given the remarkable advances in endovascular techniques, I believe they are now more widely used.

In comparison with the previous study of mixed series,[15] the nationwide Japanese study showed that more lesions in the anterior circulation than in the posterior circulation were treated surgically.[18] The previous data were as follows: Only 29% of patients with anterior circulation lesions were operated on, compared with 60% of patients with posterior circulation lesions. Operation rates for anterior and posterior circulation lesions were equally high in patients with SAH.

The most commonly employed surgical technique was proximal occlusion of the parent artery, followed by entrapment with or without a bypass, and wrapping. These results were the same in the two studies.

In 1994, Yamaura and Ono[15] found that CSF shunt or drainage was necessary in 32 of 260 cases.

Operative Findings

The most common operative findings were fusiform or tubular dilatations of the affected artery with characteristic discolorations due to intramural hematomas. In the 260 cases reported by Yamaura and Ono,[15] there were 76 observations of discoloration and 81 of fusiform dilatation. The discolorations have been described as black,[24] bluish,[23] bluish black,[23] purple-red,[12,23] brown,[12] and stripes of these colors,[30] depending on the age of the intramural dissection. Yamaura and colleagues[7] pointed out that such characteristic discolorations were recognized only when the operation was performed within 36 days of the hemorrhage. After that time, the affected artery becomes whitish gray and firm, probably because of organization of the intramural hematoma.

Other findings were neovascular patterns and serous fluid beneath the adventitia.[12] Caplan and associates[41] reviewed reported cases of ruptured intracranial vertebral aneurysms. At surgery or necropsy, a bluish or black swelling of the vertebral artery was identified. No obvious stenosis was visible externally. The angiographic narrowing is caused by dissection within the walls of the arteries.

Medical Treatment

There is no established standard for the medical treatment of dissections causing ischemia or infarction. Anticoagulant therapy is potentially helpful for cervical carotid or cervical vertebral dissections, but it is even more controversial for intracranial dissections because of the possibility of SAH.[12] Hochberg and colleagues,[42] for example, reported on a patient whose carotid dissection was treated with heparin because of threatening cerebral infarction and who experienced a cerebral hemorrhage. Other examples of clinical deterioration after anticoagulant therapy have been reported.[43] Tsutsumi and coworkers[20] argued against using antiplatelet therapy and anticoagulant therapy, favoring strict blood pressure control instead. One of their patients presented with lateral medullary infarction, and arteriography showed a dissection of the vertebral artery. Antiplatelet agent was given, and the patient experienced an SAH 2 days after admission.

Caplan and associates[41] reported on a 33-year-old woman with multiple posterior circulation transient ischemic attacks and small strokes in whom lesions of both vertebral arteries were present. Her repeated episodes of ischemia were dramatically controlled by a combination of aspirin and a warfarin analogue. The mechanism of repeated ischemia was considered to be due to intra-arterial emboli of platelet-fibrin-thrombin aggregates.

OUTCOME

Intracranial arterial dissections form a spectrum ranging from benign arteriopathy to a malignant disease resulting in fatal infarction or hemorrhage. In 1984, Berger and Wilson[12] reviewed 36 patients with dissection of the posterior circulation and found that 30 (83%) of them died within a few days to weeks after presentation. Pozzati and coworkers[28] wrote that fatal outcomes tend to be over-reported in comparison with benign ones.

The status at 3 months after ictus of cases in the nationwide Japanese study is shown in Tables 77.7 and 77.8. Outcome is presented in terms of the Glasgow Coma Scale score. In the hemorrhagic group composed of 206 patients, 53% achieved good recovery, 11% were moderately disabled, 6% were severely disabled, 2% were vegetative, and 27% died. The nonhemorrhagic group had a better outcome: 79% had good recoveries, 11% were moderately disabled, 5% were severely disabled, and 3% died. The rate of good recovery was 57% in patients with anterior circulation lesions and 65% in those with posterior circulation lesions (see Table 77.8). More patients with anterior

Table 77.7 Outcome of Nontraumatic Intracranial Arterial Dissections at Latest Contact (3 Months or More After Onset): Hemorrhagic Group versus Nonhemorrhagic Group

Outcome	No. of Cases		
	Hemorrhagic Group	Nonhemorrhagic Group	Total
Good recovery	108 (53%)	119 (79%)	227 (64%)
Moderate disability	22 (11%)	17 (11%)	39 (11%)
Severe disability	13 (6%)	8 (5%)	21 (6%)
Vegetative state	4 (2%)	0	4 (1%)
Death	56 (27%)	5 (3%)	61 (17%)
Not described	3 (1%)	2 (1%)	5 (1%)
Whole series	206	151	357

From Yamaura A, Yoshimoto T, Hashimoto N, et al: Nationwide study of nontraumatic intracranial arterial dissection: Clinical features and outcome. Surg Cerebral Stroke 26:79–86, 1998 (Jpn), and Yamaura A, Yoshimoto T, Hashimoto N, et al: Nationwide study of nontraumatic intracranial arterial dissection: Treatment and its results. Surg Cerebral Stroke 26:87–95, 1998 (Jpn).

Table 77.8 Outcome of Nontraumatic Intracranial Arterial Dissections at Latest Contact (3 Months or More After Onset): Anterior Circulation versus Posterior Circulation

Outcome	No. of Cases		
	Anterior Circulation	Posterior Circulation	Total
Good recovery	13 (57%)	195 (65%)	208 (65%)
Moderate disability	3 (13%)	30 (10%)	33 (10%)
Severe disability	4 (17%)	15 (5%)	19 (6%)
Vegetative state	1 (4%)	3 (1%)	4 (1%)
Death	2 (9%)	51 (17%)	53 (16%)
Not described	0	5 (2%)	5 (2%)
Whole series	23	299	322

From Yamaura A, Yoshimoto T, Hashimoto N, et al: Nationwide study of nontraumatic intracranial arterial dissection: Clinical features and outcome. Surg Cerebral Stroke 26:79–86, 1998 (Jpn), and Yamaura A, Yoshimoto T, Hashimoto N, et al: Nationwide study of nontraumatic intracranial arterial dissection: Treatment and its results. Surg Cerebral Stroke 26:87–95, 1998 (Jpn).

circulation lesions were severely disabled, although the numbers were small.

References

1. Nakagawa F, Kobayashi S, Takemae T, et al: Aneurysm protruding from the dorsal wall of the internal carotid artery. J Neurosurg 65: 303–308, 1986.
2. Sano K: Concerning the nomenclature and classification of internal carotid aneurysms [Japanese with English abstract]. Surg Cereb Stroke 24:333–339, 1996 (Jpn).
3. Ohkuma H, Manabe H, Takahashi T, et al: An etiology of ICA anterior wall aneurysm—with a report of three cases. Surg Cereb Stroke 24:474–480, 1996 (Jpn).
4. Mizutani T, Aruga T: "Dolichoectatic" intracranial vertebrobasilar dissecting aneurysm. Neurosurgery 31:765–773, 1992.
5. Yamaura A, Yoshimoto T, Hashimoto N, et al: Nationwide study of nontraumatic intracranial arterial dissection: Clinical features and outcome. Surg Cereb Stroke 26:79–86, 1998 (Jpn).
6. Yamaura A, Yoshimoto T, Hashimoto N, et al: Nationwide study of nontraumatic intracranial arterial dissection: Treatment and its results. Surg Cereb Stroke 26:87–95, 1998 (Jpn).
7. Yamaura A, Watanabe Y, Saeki N: Dissecting aneurysms of the intracranial vertebral artery. J Neurosurg 72:183–188, 1990.
8. Okuchi K, Watabe Y, Hiramatsu K, et al: Dissecting aneurysm of the vertebral artery as a cause of Wallenberg's syndrome [Japanese with English abstract]. Neurol Surg (Tokyo) 18:721–727, 1990.
9. Yamashita Y, Hayashi S, Saitoh H, et al: Dissecting aneurysm of the posterior inferior cerebellar artery: Study by serial angiography. No Shinkei Geka 29:1057–1062, 2001 (Jpn).
10. Okuno S, Ochiai C, Nagai M: Dissecting aneurysm of the anterior cerebral artery causing hemorrhagic infarction. Surg Neurol 45:25–30, 1996 (Jpn).
11. Senter HJ, Sarwar M: Nontraumatic dissecting aneurysms of the vertebral artery: Case report. J Neurosurg 56:128–130, 1982.
12. Berger MS, Wilson CB: Intracranial dissecting aneurysms of the posterior circulation: Report of six cases and review of the literature. J Neurosurg 61:882–894, 1984.
13. Miyazaki S, Yamaura A, Kamata K, et al: A dissecting aneurysm of the vertebral artery. Surg Neurol 21:171–174, 1984.
14. Alexander CB, Burger PC, Goree JA: Dissecting aneurysms of the basilar artery in 2 patients. Stroke 10:294–299, 1979.
15. Yamaura A, Ono J: Current diagnosis and treatment of intracranial dissecting aneurysms. Neurosurg Q 4:67–81, 1994.
16. Aoki N, Sakai T: Rebleeding from intracranial dissecting aneurysm in the vertebral artery. Stroke 21:1628–1631, 1990.
17. Yamamoto Y, Okada M, Nakamura F: Dissecting aneurysms of vertebrobasilar junction [Japanese with English abstract]. Surg Cerebral Stroke (Tokyo) 19:434–500, 1991.
18. Takita K, Shirato H, Akasaka T, et al: Dissecting aneurysm of the vertebrobasilar artery: A case report and review of previous cases [Japanese with English abstract]. No To Shinkei (Tokyo) 31: 1211–1218, 1979.
19. Adams HP, Aschenbrener CA, Kassell NF, et al: Intracranial hemorrhage produced by spontaneous dissecting intracranial aneurysm. Arch Neurol 39:773–775, 1982.
20. Tsutsumi M, Kawano T, Kawaguchi T, et al: Dissecting aneurysm of the vertebral artery causing subarachnoid hemorrhage after nonhemorrhagic infarction: Case report. Neurol Med Chir (Tokyo) 40:628–631, 2000.
21. Kunze ST, Schiefer W: Angiographic demonstration of a dissecting aneurysm of the middle cerebral artery. Neuroradiology 2:201–206, 1971.
22. Yonas H, Agamarcolis D, Takaoka Y, et al: Dissecting intracranial aneurysms. Surg Neurol 8:407–415, 1977.
23. Friedman AH, Drake CG: Subarachnoid hemorrhage from intracranial dissecting aneurysm. J Neurosurg 60:325–334, 1984.
24. Waga S, Fujimoto K, Morooka Y: Dissecting aneurysm of the vertebral artery. Surg Neurol 10:237–239, 1978.
25. Chen J, Smith R, Keller A, et al: Spontaneous dissection of the vertebral artery: MR findings. J Comput Assist Tomogr 13:326–329, 1989.
26. Hamada J, Sato K, Nagahiro S, et al: Dynamic magnetic resonance appearance of the vertebral dissecting aneurysm: Case report. Neurol Med Chir (Tokyo) 32:698–700, 1992.
27. Shimoji T, Bando K, Nakajima K, et al: Dissecting aneurysm of the vertebral artery: Report of seven cases and angiographic findings. J Neurosurg 61:1038–1046, 1984.
28. Pozzati E, Padovani R, Fabrizi A, et al: Benign arterial dissection of the posterior circulation. J Neurosurg 75:69–72, 1991.
29. Mizutani T: Middle cerebral artery dissecting aneurysm with persistent patent pseudolumen. J Neurosurg 84:267–268, 1996.
30. Poppen JL: Specific treatment of intracranial aneurysms: Experiences with 143 surgically treated patients. J Neurosurg 8:75–102, 1951.
31. Kamiyama H, Nomura M, Abe H, et al: Diagnosis for the intracranial dissecting aneurysms [Japanese with English abstract]. Surg Cereb Stroke 18:50–56, 1990.
32. Yamaura I, Tani E, Yokota M, et al: Endovascular treatment of ruptured dissecting aneurysms aimed at occlusion of the dissected site by using Guglielmi detachable coils. J Neurosurg 90:853–856, 1999.
33. Kitanaka C, Sasaki T, Eguchi T, et al: Intracranial vertebral artery dissections: Clinical, radiological features, and surgical considerations. Neurosurgery 34:620–627, 1994.
34. Ezura M, Takahashi A, Yoshimoto T: Intravascular neurosurgery for ruptured dissecting vertebral artery aneurysms: Angiographical classification and selection of the site of embolization. Surg Cereb Stroke 21:355–360, 1993 (Jpn).
35. Stehbens WE: Dissecting aneurysm of the cerebral arteries. In: Pathology of the Cerebral Blood Vessels. St. Louis, CV Mosby, 1972, pp 440–445.
36. Yamaura A, Ono J, Kubota M: Intracranial dissecting aneurysms—analysis of Japanese and non-Japanese cases. Neurosurgeons 15:54–61, 1996 (Jpn).
37. Takahashi A, Sugawara T, Suga T, et al: Detachable balloon treatment of dissecting vertebral aneurysm in its acute stage of subarachnoid hemorrhage [Japanese with English abstract]. Surg Cereb Stroke (Tokyo) 17:44–48, 1989.
38. Lylyk P, Ceratto R, Hurvitz D, Basso A: Treatment of a vertebral dissecting aneurysm with stents and coils: Technical case report. Neurosurgery 43:385–388, 1998.
39. Irikura K, Miyasaka Y, Ohtaka H, et al: Dissecting aneurysm of the vertebral artery with lateral medullary syndrome: A case report, with special reference to surgical treatment [Japanese with English abstract]. Jpn J Stroke 11:133–139, 1989.
40. Su CC, Watanabe T, Yoshimoto T, et al: Proximal clipping of dissecting intracranial vertebral aneurysm: Effect of balloon Matas' test with neurophysiological monitoring. Acta Neurochir (Wien) 104:59–63, 1990.
41. Caplan LR, Baquis GD, Pessin MS, et al: Dissection of the intracranial vertebral artery. Neurology 38:868–877, 1988.
42. Hochberg FH, Bean C, Fisher CM, et al: Stroke in a 15-year-old girl secondary to terminal carotid dissection. Neurology 25:725–729, 1975.
43. Farrell MA, Gilbert JJ, Kaufmann JCE: Fatal intracranial arterial dissection: Clinical pathological correlation. J Neurol Neurosurg Psychiatry 48:111–121, 1985.

Chapter Seventy-Eight

Interventional Neuroradiologic Therapy

Elad I. Levy, Stanley H. Kim, Bernard R. Bendok, Alan S. Boulos,
Andrew R. Xavier, Abutaher M. Yahia, Adnan I. Qureshi,
Lee R. Guterman, and L. Nelson Hopkins

The treatment of vascular disease has undergone a revolution in the past decade. Previously, open surgical techniques were the only treatment modalities available for vascular disease that resulted in ischemic and hemorrhagic neurologic sequelae. Times have changed. Catheter-based treatment modalities have been developed that rival or surpass open surgical techniques for the treatment of these disease entities.

Cerebral revascularization for the treatment of acute ischemic stroke has become a reality within the past 5 years. Site-specific intra-arterial delivery of thrombolytic agents has enabled recanalization of lesions in the anterior, middle, and posterior cerebral arteries. The application of mechanical techniques to disrupt clot has pushed vessel recanalization rates to 85% as a matter of routine. Hemorrhagic complications still diminish the effectiveness of these techniques, yet a reduction in dosage of thrombolytic agents and greater use of mechanical techniques may drive the clinical utility of these techniques forward. The problem we face is not whether but *how rapidly* recanalization can be achieved—with better education of the public about stroke symptoms ("brain attack") in order to reduce the time to treatment.

Extracranial and intracranial revascularization for atherosclerotic disease has led the vascular revolution for ischemic cerebrovascular disease. Preliminary results suggest that the use of stents for revascularization of the cervical carotid bifurcation will supplant carotid endarterectomy (CEA) in the future. Multiple clinical trials are under way to compare the efficacy of stent placement with that of CEA. These trials will provide level 1 evidence within the next few years. Intracranial atherosclerotic disease is being discovered at an alarming rate by the use of noninvasive imaging techniques like magnetic resonance (MR) and computed tomography (CT) angiography. The application of angioplasty and stent techniques is gaining acceptance. Balloons and stents initially designed for the coronary circulation are being modified for delivery into the tortuous anatomy of the cerebral circulation. As a result, the locations and scope of intracranial lesions that can be treated are increasing. The findings of initial trials have shown high rates of in-stent restenosis, but the use of drug coatings that inhibit fibrous tissue formation within cerebral vessels after manipulation may pave the way for broad application of these techniques for cerebral ischemia.

The treatment and management of cerebrovascular disease changed dramatically in the 1990s. Results of the initial clinical trial of the Guglielmi detachable coil (GDC, Boston Scientific Target, Fremont, CA) in 1990 led the way for a lasting and irreversible change in methods for the treatment of ruptured and unruptured intracranial aneurysms worldwide. At some centers, coil occlusion has become first-line therapy for all aneurysms. Initially, only one platinum coil was available. Today, five companies offer products used for endovascular treatment of intracranial aneurysms. Biologic modification of the platinum coil platform has now been approved by the U.S. Food and Drug Administration (FDA). Coils with polymer and hydrogel modifications may promote complete aneurysm occlusion by inducing scar formation across the aneurysm neck. Intravascular stents have been used to achieve successful reconstruction of the lesion in the parent vessel adjacent to the aneurysm. Liquid polymers have been delivered directly into aneurysms to provide atraumatic methods for complete aneurysm filling. Level 1 evidence indicative of the effectiveness of aneurysm coiling is being amassed from a comparison of endovascular and open surgical techniques. A paradigm shift for the treatment of ruptured and unruptured aneurysms is about to occur.

The treatment of cerebral arteriovenous malformations (AVMs) has benefited from catheter-based technology. Particles and silk, thread, and muscle fragments have been replaced as embolic agents by liquid polymers and sclerosing agents. Advances in catheter technology have enabled access of distal AVM feeding vessels, thereby enabling safer delivery of these substances. New liquid embolic agents show great promise for complete occlusion of AVMs. The ultimate goal of complete, lasting occlusion of the AVM nidus without adjunctive radiosurgery or resection has thus far not been achieved.

In this chapter, we present advances in the use of catheter-based technology for the treatment of cerebrovascular disease and stroke, highlighting new techniques and developments. Although many of the treatment modalities are considered investigational, they represent the current and future treatments for cerebrovascular disease.

CRITICAL CARE

Numerous patients who present with neurologic emergencies are candidates for immediate endovascular rescue. Because both surgical and endovascular approaches may potentially offer patients with acute stroke therapies capable of reversing neurologic deficits, medical optimization in the emergency setting minimizes complications and maximizes the opportunities for success.[1] Emergency endovascular interventions, such as intra-arterial or mechanical thrombolysis, are in their earliest stages of development, and the response to such therapy is highly variable, depending on a number of different factors.[2] In addition to the nature of the underlying neurologic condition, response to endovascular therapy depends on a number of systemic factors, including coagulation status, blood pressure, cardiac function, blood glucose levels, and severity of concomitant medical illnesses. Hence, rapid but careful patient evaluation and selection as well as meticulous periprocedural care are important in ensuring optimal clinical outcome.

Patient Stabilization

As with all life-threatening emergencies, airway protection and evaluation are most important. Some patients require endotracheal intubation before angiography or interventional procedures are performed, either for airway protection or because they cannot cooperate with the study. To ensure patient safety and quality imaging, intubation should be performed by the team member who is most experienced with endotracheal intubations or by an anesthesiologist. The patient must be maximally relaxed with sedatives such as propofol before intubation is attempted, as such agents may confer some neuroprotection in the setting of ischemia and resultant secondary brain injury.[1,3] A short-acting paralytic agent is often used as an adjunct to safe intubation.

After airway stabilization, we keep oxygen saturation at more than 95% during the entire procedure. Immediate chest radiograph, electrocardiogram, and echocardiogram should be sufficient to identify the cause of acute desaturation that is unresponsive to the administration of supplemental oxygen. In the setting of brainstem ischemia and stroke, patients are at an exceptional risk for aspiration because of impaired swallowing due to injury to the nuclei of cranial nerves IX and X. Atelectasis, if suspected, responds well to the use of high positive-end expiratory pressure (PEEP). However, caution should be exercised in patients with acute brain injury, because an elevation of the PEEP can increase intracranial pressure as a result of impaired cerebral venous return. Therefore, careful cardiac and venous pressure monitoring is critical in patients with stroke who are at risk for elevated intracranial

pressure and in whom high PEEP is needed.[4,5] During the acute period and during the intervention, the fraction of inspired oxygen (FiO_2) may be kept at 100%. After the procedure, however, the FiO_2 should be kept below 60% to prevent oxygen toxicity of the bronchial tree.

Focused Differential Diagnosis

Many patients with acute stroke have concomitant coronary artery disease and cardiac dysrhythmias. Clinicians must be cognizant of pulmonary congestion resulting from heart failure, which is another common reason for acute oxygen desaturation. Patients with heart failure may be vulnerable to such complications during long thrombolysis procedures as a result of excessive fluid infusion from the saline flushes through the microcatheters. Pulmonary congestion should be managed with diuretics, fluid restriction, and control of the ventricular rate with an inotropic agent (e.g., dobutamine, dopamine, or norepinephrine). Clinicians must use caution when administering diuretics to or restricting fluids for patients with cerebral ischemic syndromes, because these maneuvers may lower cerebral perfusion pressure and expand the ischemic penumbra. Such critically ill patients benefit from hemodynamic monitoring with placement of a pulmonary artery catheter immediately after the stroke intervention to optimize cardiac output.

A plethora of cerebrovascular emergencies may mimic one another clinically. Presentation in patients with severe neurologic deficits due to ischemic stroke may be similar to that of patients with seizure disorders or intraparenchymal hemorrhages resulting from hypertension, tumors, or AVMs. Immediate attention must be given to normalizing the patient's blood pressure until the diagnosis can be established. A mean arterial pressure of 100 to 130 mm Hg is ideal in the setting of ischemic stroke or for cerebral vasospasm developing after aneurysm coiling. Several investigators caution that although induced hypotension may worsen ischemia, untreated hypertension in acute stroke may lead to swelling, edema, and increased mass effect with a decreased overall functional outcome.[6-8] Hypotensive conditions should be treated with fluid resuscitation; multiple boluses of a combination of colloidal and crystalloid solutions should be tried initially. Inotropic support with norepinephrine should be tried next, unless the patient has baseline bradycardia. In the patient with bradycardia and hypotension, dopamine is the inotropic agent of choice. Dobutamine should be avoided in the setting of hypotensive shock. In the patient about to undergo endovascular intervention, propofol infusion may be an excellent choice for lowering blood pressure, because it can also help sedate the patient and may have some neuroprotective effects.[3,9]

Cardioembolic diseases may be common causes of acute stroke in a select group of patients with atrial fibrillation. In two studies, a cardiac source of emboli was possible in more than half of patients with acute onset of stroke symptoms.[10,11] A heart rate of 60 to 100 beats/min is optimal for providing systemic perfusion without placing excessive strain on the heart. Sinus tachycardia often accompanies cerebral insult and could result from patient confusion and discomfort. Mild sedation with rapid-acting anxiolytics should help to alleviate discomfort. The physician must rule out acute myocardial infarction (MI) by obtaining serial electrocardiograms and cardiac enzyme measurements. In the setting of atrial fibrillation and a rapid ventricular rate, heart rate control can be attempted with intravenous diltiazem and metoprolol first, followed by intravenous amiodarone.

Blood Studies and Imaging

Before sending patients for radiologic imaging, blood samples should be obtained for performance of basic metabolic analysis (electrolytes, urea, creatinine, and glucose), complete hemogram (hematocrit, platelets), and measurement of coagulation parameters (prothrombin time, activated partial thromboplastin time). Even a brief clinical history should address the issue of previous drug intake, particularly the use of antiplatelet agents such as warfarin (as used in patients with atrial fibrillation), clopidogrel, ticlopidine, and aspirin.

Clinicians must be aware of coagulation abnormalities but must use caution in making rapid correction of abnormal coagulation parameters in patients with ischemic syndromes. Blood products such as platelets, fresh frozen plasma, and cryoprecipitate should be available to reverse severe coagulopathies that may result in intracranial hemorrhage (ICH) or may preclude endovascular intervention. We have proceeded with necessary interventions in patients who are receiving heparin for unstable angina. Severe thrombocytopenia is usually a contraindication for interventional procedures. Results of basic metabolic blood analysis are essential before initiation of any intervention or angiographic procedure. Poor renal function may prompt clinicians to use isosmotic contrast agents or gadolinium as an alternative contrast agent.[12] In addition, in the patient with renal dysfunction, use of contrast agents should be reduced as much as possible; and in case of worsening parameters with intractable acidosis, fluid overload, hypertension, or encephalopathy, dialysis is required. Evidence now suggests that the use of fenoldopam, a potent renal vasodilator, may significantly reduce radiocontrast nephropathy.[13]

Once the patient is medically stabilized, rapid diagnosis and assessment of neurologic status are critical for optimal functional outcome. If the diagnosis is not already established, the nature and severity of the underlying neurologic condition should be assessed rapidly. In case of suspected ischemic stroke, a quick neurologic examination should be performed to broadly localize the lesion to either the cerebral hemispheres or the brainstem. The National Institutes of Health Stroke Scale (NIHSS) should be administered by any trained clinician or nurse to every patient with stroke to document initial stroke severity.[14] An urgent non-contrast CT scan of the brain should be performed to exclude evidence of recent hemorrhage and signs of an established infarction. Scans demonstrating hemorrhage or well-demarcated infarction preclude the performance of endovascular procedures involving thrombolysis. Demonstration of a hyperdense middle cerebral artery (MCA) may help localize the occlusion in the patient with acute ischemic stroke and is typically one of the earliest positive CT findings in such patients.[15] CT scans are also examined for evidence of edema, parenchymal shift, and hydrocephalus.

Elective Intubation Before Angiography

Patients with acute neurologic illnesses are often confused and unable to cooperate with clinicians during endovascular procedures. Also, sudden deterioration of patients with acute stroke that occurs during microcatheterization of intracranial vessels may result in catastrophic consequences. We advocate general endotracheal intubation before endovascular procedures are performed for patients with ischemic stroke who have marked deficits. Maximal patient relaxation and comfort are important for the successful completion of the procedure, because clear images with definable lesions are imperative for consideration of all possible therapeutic options; inadequate relaxation may result in significant blood pressure lability or hypertension, raising the patient's risk for hemorrhage. Hence, sedation and intubation with general anesthesia should be used liberally.

APPROACHES FOR VASCULAR ACCESS

As for any procedure, proper patient positioning and access are vital to successful outcome with minimal morbidity. For acute stroke intervention using endovascular techniques, patients are placed supine on the angiography table. Both groins are prepared in usual sterile fashion to provide immediate access to a second puncture site if needed or if the first cannot be successfully accessed. For femoral access, an imaginary line is visualized between the anterior superior region of the iliac spine and the pubic tubercle; a puncture site is localized three finger-breadths below this line. A local anesthetic is then used to infiltrate this area, and a needle is thrust in at a 45-degree angle toward the umbilicus. Some interventionists incise the skin before performing the puncture. The needle may sometimes be used to palpate the bounding pulse of the femoral pulse and redirected to the point where the pulsations are best appreciated.

Once excellent arterial blood return through the puncture needle is visualized, the operator's left hand stabilizes the needle, while a J-shaped wire is inserted through the needle with the right hand. The needle is removed, and a 5F sheath is inserted over the wire and attached to a heparinized saline flush. A diagnostic catheter is inserted through the sheath and advanced into the aortic arch over a hydrophilic guidewire. Diagnostic angiography is performed to elucidate the angiographic anatomy responsible for the patient's neurologic condition.

The femoral artery is an excellent choice for access in the setting of acute stroke interventions for several reasons, including ease of access, familiarity with the approach, and the ability of the vessel to accommodate large sheaths. In some patients, however, femoral access is difficult or is associated with increased morbidity.[16,17] Inasmuch as 10% of the general population, severe peripheral vascular disease, femoral artery occlusion, previous femoral artery bypass graft placement, or morbid obesity precludes successful negotiation of diagnostic or guiding catheters beyond the aortoiliac junction.[16,17] The transradial or transbrachial approach is becoming an alternative to transfemoral access for such patients.

With the advent of smaller delivery apparatus for endovascular thrombolysis, 5F sheaths are needed to allow delivery of the associated balloons, stents, snares, and other devices within the extracranial and intracranial circulation. Cardiologists have long been using the transradial and transbrachial approach for angioplasty and stenting, because the radial artery can accommodate up to an 8F sheath quite well.[18,19] Some investigators have placed 8F sheaths with low rates of complication and permanent occlusion of the radial artery.[20] These large sheaths must be removed immediately after the procedure to minimize the chance of radial artery occlusion. Also, a mixture of heparin (2500-5000 international units/mL), verapamil (2.5 mg), lidocaine (2%, 1 mL), sodium bicarbonate (42 mg), and nitroglycerin (0.2 mg) is infused through the introducer sheath to relieve or prevent vasospasm immediately after insertion of the sheath.

We caution that before the transradial or transbrachial approach is used, adequate collateral circulation of the hand through the ulnar artery must be demonstrated via an Allen test. (The test is performed as follows: After continuous compression of both the radial and ulnar arteries during finger extension, the ulnar artery is released; the time needed to achieve visual capillary refill and at least 92% oxygen saturation at the finger pads are measured).[21] Although several investigators have demonstrated the effectiveness of transradial cerebral angiography and intervention in the elective setting, the transradial approach should be considered in the patient with acute stroke if the transfemoral approach is not feasible.[22-24] Contraindications to the transradial approach include abnormal Allen test result and chronic occlusion of either the ipsilateral subclavian artery or the brachiocephalic trunk (Fig. 78–1).

THROMBOLYSIS OF ACUTE ISCHEMIC STROKE

In 1996, the FDA approved the use of intravenous recombinant tissue plasminogen activator (rt-PA, alteplase) in patients who present within 3 hours of onset of acute ischemic stroke. This approval was based on the positive results of the National Institute of Neurologic Disorders and Stroke (NINDS) study.[25] Currently, intravenous administration of t-PA within the 3-hour time window is the only FDA-approved treatment for acute ischemic stroke. However, two major clinical trials and one prospective observational registry have reported outcomes of death or more than 50% functional dependency at the 3-month follow-up evaluation in patients given this therapy (Table 78.1).[25-27] Moreover, six randomized trials have not demonstrated a significant benefit for intravenous thrombolytic therapy initiated within 3 to 6 hours of stroke onset.[27-32] Multiple randomized trials have evaluated the safety and efficacy of intra-arterial thrombolysis administered 3 to 6 hours after symptom onset.[33,34] In several case series, intra-arterial thrombolysis alone or in combination with mechanical thrombolysis has been reported as an alternative modality for treatment of acute ischemic stroke in a select group of patients.[35-41] A randomized study may be necessary to determine whether thrombolysis with or without mechanical thrombolysis is superior to intravenous thrombolysis for acute ischemic stroke.

The intra-arterial approach to thrombolysis has theoretical advantages. First, angiographic evaluation helps determine whether an occlusion exists and local intra-arterial therapy is necessary. Second, the intra-arterial approach

Table 78.1   **Outcome of Intravenous Alteplase for Acute Ischemic Stroke**

Study*	No. of Patients	% of ICH Symptomatic	% Mortality or Dependency
NINDS[25]	312	6.4	57
ECASS II[27]	81	11.8	58
STARS[26]	389	3.3	57

*Superscript numbers indicate chapter references.
ECASS, European Cooperative Acute Stroke Study; ICH, intracerebral hemorrhage; NINDS, National Institute of Neurological Disorders and Stroke; STARS, Standard Treatment with Alteplase to Reverse Stroke.

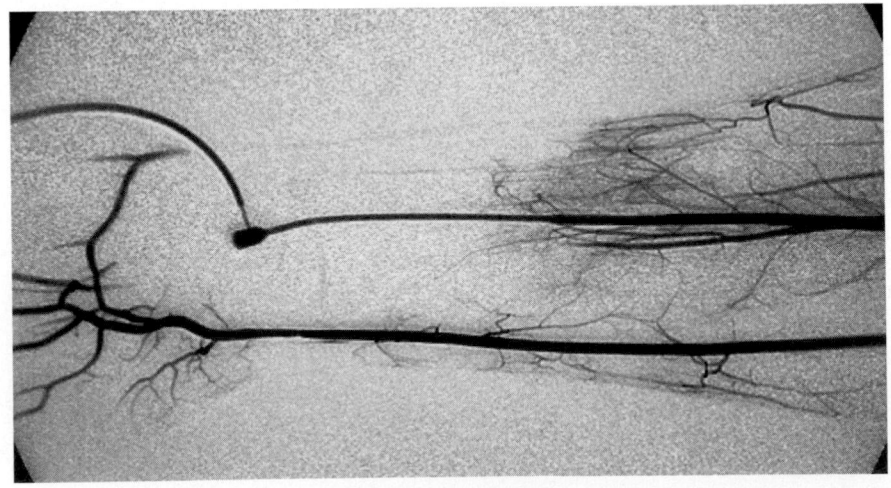

FIGURE 78–1 *Angiogram showing contrast injection through a 5-French sheath in the radial artery. Filling of the radial artery with reflux into the ulnar artery demonstrates excellent collateralization of the hand. (From Levy EI, Boulos AS, Fessler RD, et al: Transradial cerebral angiography: An alternative route. Neurosurgery 51:335–342, 2002.)*

allows delivery of the thrombolytic agent (e.g., t-PA or reteplase) to the site of occlusion without excessive systemic administration (a lesser amount of the drug can actually be used). Third, the endovascular surgeon can titrate the dose of the agent by angiographically visualizing the clot response to lysis. Fourth, when there is a poor response to chemical intra-arterial thrombolysis, angiographic evaluation aids in the selection of methods of mechanical thrombolysis or other endovascular intervention. For example, an acute ischemic stroke from occlusion of the M_1 segment of the MCA may occur in the setting of severe preexisting atherosclerotic stenosis or embolic plaque. Combined use of chemical and mechanical forms of intra-arterial thrombolysis through the use of angioplasty, a stent, or a clot-retrieval device may be required for recanalization (Fig. 78–2). Disadvantages of the intra-arterial approach are time to mobilize the angiography team and obtain vascular access with optimal positioning of the catheter at the occlusion. Additionally, stroke intervention is currently not reimbursed, and thus hospitals are faced with a significant financial burden as a result of device utilization and staffing. With better patient education and earlier recognition of stroke symptoms, the time to treatment can be reduced. Currently, neither the chemical nor the mechanical method of intra-arterial thrombolysis for acute ischemic stroke has been approved by the FDA.

Although chemical and mechanical forms of intra-arterial thrombolysis are promising novel therapies, patients with acute ischemic stroke must still be transported expeditiously to an appropriate facility that can provide acute stroke therapy in a timely fashion. Reducing the time from onset to treatment is paramount, regardless of the type of thrombolytic therapy used. Furthermore, advancements in imaging techniques, such as diffusion-weighted and perfusion-weighted MR imaging (MRI), xenon-enhanced CT (XECT), and CT perfusion scanning, may allow better patient selection for thrombolysis in the future.[42–45] In this section, we review the indications, techniques, and results of intra-arterial thrombolysis reported by major trials as well as from our own experience.

Thrombolytic Agents

A variety of drugs have been used for intravenous or intra-arterial thrombolysis for ischemic stroke in human clinical studies.[46] A summary of thrombolytic agents is given in Table 78.2. All these agents act by converting plasminogen

Table 78.2 Thrombolytic Agents

	Half-life (minutes)	Description
First-generation		
Urokinase	14–20	Serine protease
Streptokinase	18–23	Protein from group C beta-hemolytic streptococci
Second-generation		
Pro-urokinase	20	Proenzyme precursor of urokinase
Alteplase (t-PA)	3–5	Serine protease
Third-generation		
Tenecteplase	17	t-PA mutant
Reteplase	15–18	Deletion mutant of t-PA

t-PA, tissue-type plasminogen activator.

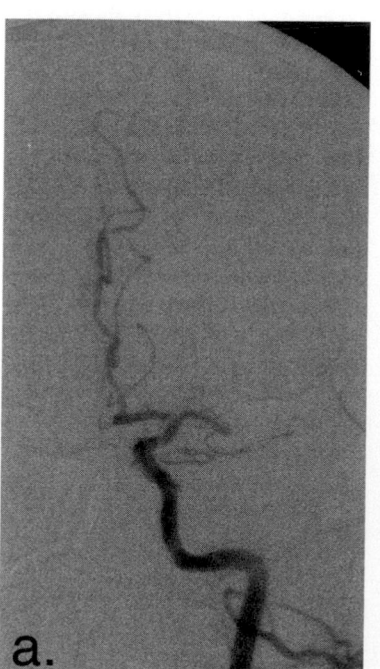
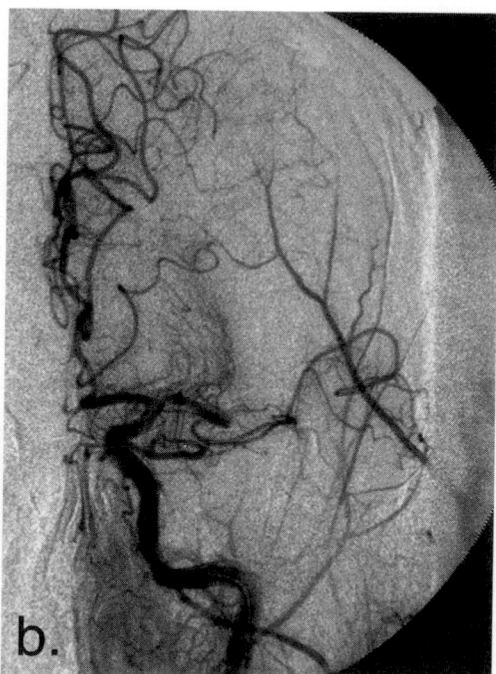
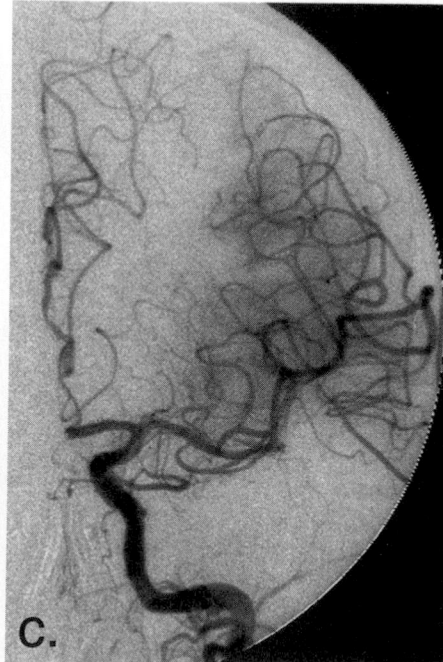

FIGURE 78–2 A, *Cerebral angiogram shows occlusion of the left M_1 segment of the left MCA. B, Persistent occlusion of the M_1 segment of the left MCA after administration of 4 units of reteplase. C, Recanalization of the left MCA after mechanical thrombolysis was performed via a 4-mm snare (Amplatz Goose Neck Microsnare, Microvena, White Bear Lake, MN).*

Table 78.3   Results of Prolyse in Acute Cerebral Thromboembolism (PROACT) Trials I and II

	PROACT I	PROACT II
No. of patients	40	180
CT scan exclusion	ICH, mass effect with midline shift, intracranial tumor, early changes of ischemia	Same as PROACT I, hypodensity or effacement of sulci in more than 1/3 of the MCA territory
Median NIHSS	r-Prourokinase, 17; placebo, 19	r-Prourokinase, 17; placebo, 17
Heparin	All patients received IV heparin; first 16 patients received 100-unit/kg bolus, then 1000-unit/hour infusion during 4 hours; remaining patients received 4000-unit bolus followed by a 500-unit/hour infusion for 4 hours	All patients received 2000-unit heparin bolus IV, then 500-unit/hour infusion for 4 hours
Agent used	6 mg of r-Prourokinase 9 mg over 2 hours	9 mg of r-Prourokinase over 2 hours and heparin
Placebo group	Saline at 30 mL/hour over 2 hours	IV heparin alone
Mechanical thrombolysis	Not permitted	Not permitted

	r-Prourokinase	Placebo	r-Prourokinase	Placebo
% TIMI 2 or 3 recanalization	58	14	66	18
% Symptomatic ICH	15	7	10	2
% Outcome at 90 days				
mRS score 0 to 1	31	21		
mRS score 0 to 2			40	25
% Mortality within 90 days	27	43	25	27

ICH, intracerebral hemorrhage; IV, intravenous; MCA, middle cerebral artery; mRS, modified Rankin Scale; NIHSS, National Institutes of Health Stroke Scale; TIMI, thrombolysis in myocardial infarction.

to plasmin. However, the first-generation thrombolytic agents, such as urokinase (withdrawn from the market) and streptokinase, are not fibrin-specific. Streptokinase is immunogenic and can cause drug resistance, fever, and allergic reactions. The second-generation thrombolytic agents include alteplase (t-PA) and prourokinase (r-ProUK), which are fibrin-selective; high doses of these drugs can lead, however, to lower levels of fibrinogen and plasminogen. Third-generation thrombolytic agents tenecteplase and reteplase are t-PA mutants. They have longer half-lives than alteplase and greater thrombolytic potency.[47] Clinical trials are required to determine the appropriate dosage and identify the candidates for these emerging thrombolytic agents.

Intra-Arterial Thrombolysis Trials

The recanalization efficacy and safety of intra-arterial thrombolysis with recombinant prourokinase has been evaluated in two randomized, multicenter, placebo-controlled trials.[33,34] In the Prolyse in Acute Cerebral Thromboembolism (PROACT) I and II trials, patients with acute ischemic stroke due to MCA occlusion and onset of symptoms within 6 hours underwent intra-arterial thrombolysis with r-prourokinase.[33,34] The results of these trials are summarized in Table 78.3. Recanalization rates are based on the Thrombolysis in Myocardial Infarction (TIMI) grading system (Table 78.4).[48] Recanalization rates (TIMI 2 or 3) were 58% in the r-prourokinase group and 14% in the placebo group in the PROACT I trial. Because of the low number of patients in PROACT I, clinical efficacy of this treatment modality could not be established. However, the safety and recanalization rates observed in PROACT I led to the PROACT II trial. This trial was designed to assess the efficacy of intra-arterial r-prourokinase (9 mg

Table 78.4   Definitions of Perfusion in the Thrombolysis in Myocardial Infarction (TIMI) Trial

Grade	Definition
0 (no perfusion)	There is no antegrade flow beyond the point of occlusion.
1 (penetration without perfusion)	The contrast material passes beyond the area of obstruction but "hangs up" and fails to opacify the entire coronary bed distal to the obstruction for the duration of the cineangiographic filming sequence.
2 (partial perfusion)	The contrast material passes across the obstruction and opacifies the coronary bed distal to the obstruction. However, the rate of entry of contrast material into the vessel distal to the obstruction or its rate of clearance from the distal bed (or both) is perceptibly slower than its entry into or clearance from comparable areas not perfused by the previously occluded vessel (e.g., other coronary artery or the coronary bed proximal to the obstruction).
3 (complete perfusion)	Antegrade flow into the bed distal to the obstruction occurs as promptly as antegrade flow into the bed proximal to obstruction, and clearance of contrast material from the involved bed in the same vessel or the opposite artery.

given over 2 hours, as opposed to 6 mg in PROACT I) as measured by the Modified Rankin Scale (MRS) score of 2 or less at 90 days. For the primary outcome measure of efficacy in PROACT II, 40% of patients receiving r-prourokinase and 25% of those receiving placebo achieved an MRS score of 2 or better at 90 days ($P = .04$).

Recanalization rates (TIMI 2 or 3) were 66% in the r-prourokinase group and 18% in the placebo group in this trial. A 15% absolute increase in favorable outcome was shown with r-prourokinase. For every 7 patients treated with r-prourokinase, 1 would benefit. Despite a higher rate of early symptomatic ICH, intra-arterial r-prourokinase administered within 6 hours of symptom onset in stroke due to MCA occlusion significantly improved clinical outcome.

PROACT II was a landmark trial in that, for the first time in a randomized study, intra-arterial thrombolysis demonstrated clinical efficacy and extended the time window for therapy to 6 hours in a homogeneous group of patients with acute ischemic stroke.[34] This trial was conducted in a standardized fashion in terms of the technique of intra-arterial thrombolysis as well as the agent and the dose used. However, the FDA requested additional data to support the clinical efficacy and safety demonstrated in PROACT II before approving intra-arterial thrombolysis as a standard therapy for patients with acute ischemic stroke. The success of the PROACT II trial was not suffi-cient to gain FDA approval for prourokinase, but the trial has paved the way for additional studies involving intra-arterial thrombolysis (with newer agents) in acute ischemic stroke.

Five studies have evaluated the feasibility, safety, and recanalization rate of a combination of intravenous and intra-arterial thrombolysis in patients with acute ischemic stroke.[49-53] The results are summarized in Table 78.5. The rationale for the combination approach is based on the fact that clinically severe strokes resulting from occlusion of large intracranial vessels respond poorly to intravenous thrombolysis. Combining the two therapies enables patients to receive intravenous therapy during the time required for initiation of intra-arterial thrombolysis, which may be more effective in opening large arteries. Direct comparison of the results of these studies is difficult because of heterogeneity of the study populations, dosages, and types of thrombolytic agents used as well as patient selection criteria. Symptomatic ICH rates within 7 days of treatment range from 6% to 12%. Mortality rates

Table 78.5 Results of Combined Intravenous and Intraarterial Thrombolysis

Study[*]	Study Center	Design	Symptomatic ICH Within 7 Days	Outcome Definition	Outcome	Mortality
EMS Bridging Trial[52]	—	Double-blind randomized placebo-controlled multicenter study comparing safety and feasibility of two treatment strategies	12% (2/17) IV/IA; 6% (1/18) placebo IA	3 months GOS, Barthel index, mRS	No significant differences in outcome between treatment groups	At 90 days: 45% (5/11) in IV/IA; 10% (1/10) in placebo/IA
Emst et al[49]	University of Cincinnati	Retrospective study to assess safety and feasibility of IV t-PA/IA t-PA within 3 hours of symptom onset	6% (1/16)	mRS, follow-up range 2–100 months	44% (7/16) mRS of 0 or 1, 19% (3/16) mRS of 2, 25% (4/16) mRS of 4 or 5	13% (2/16)
Keris et al[51]	Riga, Latvia	Open-label prospective study to assess safety and efficacy of IV t-PA/IA t-PA within 6 hours of symptom onset	None	mRS at 1 month and 12 months good = mRS 0–3; poor = mRS 4–6	67% (8/12) mRS 0–3 at 1 month, 83% (10/12) mRS 0–3 at 12 months	17% at 12 months
Hill et al[50]	University of Calgary, Alberta	Prospective, open-label study to assess safety and feasibility of IV tPA/IA t-PA within 3 hours of symptom onset	None	NIHSS score <3 at 90 days	67% (4/6) NIHSS <3 at 90 days	17% (1/6)
Suarez et al[53]	University Hospitals of Cleveland, Case Western Reserve	Pilot study to assess feasibility of IV t-PA/IA UK or t-PA within 3 hours of symptom onset	10% (2/21) in IV t-PA group only	Barthel index at 90 days: scores of 95 or 100 = good outcome	77% good outcome at 3 months, Barthel index scores >95: 92% (12/13) in IV t-PA/IA UK group, 64% (7/11) in IV t-PA/IV t-PA group, 67% (14/21) in IV t-PA group	16% (7/45)

[*]Superscript numbers indicate chapter references.
EMS, Emergency Management of Stroke; GOS, Glasgow Outcome Scale score; IA, intra-arterial; IV, intravenous; mRS, modified Rankin Scale; NIHSS, National Institutes of Health Stroke Scale; t-PA, recombinant tissue-type plasminogen activator (alteplase); UK, urokinase.

range from 15% to 45%. TIMI 3 recanalization rates range from 19% to 55%.

The Emergency Management of Stroke (EMS) Bridging Trial was designed to assess the safety, feasibility, and recanalization efficacy of this combination approach.[52] However, because of the small sample size (35 patients), the clinical efficacy of this therapy could not be determined from trial results. Suarez and colleagues[53] reported that 78% of patients treated by combination therapy had Barthel index scores higher than 95 at 3 months. Ernst and associates[49] reported MRS scores of 0 or 1 at 2 months' follow-up or later for 44% of patients treated by combination therapy.

On the basis of the results of these initial pilot studies, NINDS funded a Phase II pilot study, the Interventional Management of Stroke (IMS) trial.[54] This trial was an open-label Phase II study designed to provide preliminary results about the safety and efficacy of combination intravenous and intra-arterial t-PA therapies; the therapies were initiated within 3 hours of symptom onset in 80 patients with ischemic stroke and an NIHSS score 10. Patients received 0.6 mg/kg of intravenously administered t-PA over 30 minutes (15% as a bolus), followed by intra-arterially administered t-PA at a dose of up to 22 mg over 2 hours if thrombus is identified on a cerebral angiogram. A preliminary analysis of the study results has shown a 16% rate of mortality at 3 months (compared with 24% in the NINDS placebo group) and a 6% rate of symptomatic ICH (compared with 1% in the NINDS placebo group). TIMI 2 and 3 recanalization rates of 40% and 10%, respectively, were observed. Favorable outcome at 3 months, as defined by an MRS score of 0 or 1, was observed in 30% of patients. Further analysis of the study data is pending.

Qureshi and associates[41] evaluated the safety and efficacy of reteplase (the only third-generation thrombolytic agent available in addition to alteplase for the intra-arterial treatment of acute ischemic stroke) in 16 patients who were poor candidates for intravenous alteplase therapy because (1) the interval from symptom onset to presentation was 3–6 hours or (2) they had severe neurologic deficit on presentation (NIHSS scores ranged from 10 to 26).[41] These investigators used a modified TIMI grading system (Table 78.6) and reported TIMI 3 or 4 (equivalent to the original TIMI grade 3) recanalization rates in 88% of patients. Such a high rate of recanalization was achieved even though 8 of the patients presented with occlusion of either the cervical (n = 4) or intracranial (n = 4) internal carotid artery (ICA). Early neurologic improvement (defined as a decrease of 4 or more points in the NIHSS score at 24 hours) was observed in 44% of patients. Qureshi has developed a new grading scheme to allow more precise location of occlusion in the cerebral vasculature and the existence of collateral circulation, features that are not described by the original and modified TIMI grading schemes.[55] Further studies are needed to evaluate the durability of intra-arterial thrombolysis using reteplase in acute ischemic stroke.

Indications for Intra-arterial Thrombolysis

Inclusion Criteria

On the basis of these major trials and case series, we recommend the following indications and contraindications for intra-arterial thrombolysis in acute ischemic stroke (summarized in Table 78.7).

Patients who present between 3 and 6 hours from the onset of an anterior circulation stroke may be considered for intra-arterial thrombolysis. Through combined efforts of the stroke team, expeditious evaluation, laboratory tests, and imaging studies such as CT, MRI, and cerebral angiography must be completed within 6 hours so that intra-arterial thrombolysis can be initiated. Speed is even more crucial with intra-arterial treatment than with intravenous thrombolysis because of the time needed to prepare for endovascular intervention.

Because of the lack of evidence from randomized clinical trials regarding the efficacy of intra-arterial thrombolysis in the vertebrobasilar artery, we recommend that in patients presenting with posterior circulation stroke, intra-arterial thrombolysis be performed only if treatment can be initiated within 6 hours. There have been anecdotal reports of clinical improvement and successful recanalization of basilar artery occlusion with intra-arterial thrombolysis as long as 24 hours after the onset of stroke symptoms.[2] However, unless diffusion-weighted MRI can be performed to exclude early ischemic changes, we do not recommend performing intra-arterial thrombolysis more than 6 hours from symptom onset. With the development of reliable means of selecting potential candidates on the basis of physiologic rather than chronologic criteria by using advanced imaging systems, it may be possible to determine which patients presenting after the 3- or 6-hour interval may benefit from thrombolysis.

Patients who present with severe neurologic deficits (NIHSS score of 10 or higher) may be considered for intra-arterial thrombolysis. In the Standard Treatment with Alteplase to Reverse Stroke (STARS) study, 389 patients

---

Table 78.6   **Modified Thrombolysis in Myocardial Infarction (TIMI) Grading System**

Grade	Definition
0	No flow
1	Some penetration past the site of occlusion but no flow distal to occlusion
2	Distal perfusion but delayed filling in all vessels
3	Distal perfusion with adequate perfusion in less than half of the distal vessels
4	Distal perfusion with adequate perfusion in more than half of the distal vessels

Table 78.7   **Recommended Indications for Intra-arterial Thrombolysis in Acute Ischemic Stroke**

- Presentation after 3 hours from onset of symptoms with the ability to initiate treatment within 6 hours of onset of symptoms
- Baseline National Institutes of Health Stroke Scale score 10 or higher
- Major surgery within 2 weeks (mechanical and/or chemical thrombolysis may be considered)

who presented within 3 hours of symptom onset underwent intravenous thrombolysis with alteplase.[26] The study showed a 22% decrease in the odds of recovery for every 5-point increase in baseline NIHSS score. Patients in whom the baseline NIHSS score was higher than 10 had a 75% decrease in the odds of recovery. In addition, Tomsick and colleagues[15] reported poor outcomes associated with intravenous thrombolysis administered within 90 minutes of symptoms in patients with NIHSS scores of 10 or higher. We do not mean to imply that an NIHSS score of 10 or higher is a contraindication to intravenous thrombolysis. In fact, in the NINDS study, intravenous thrombolysis resulted in better outcomes than placebo, regardless of the patient's baseline NIHSS score.[25] However, at institutions capable of providing intra-arterial therapy in a timely fashion, this select group of patients may be considered for intra-arterial thrombolysis as an alternative treatment, in view of the poor outcomes observed with intravenous thrombolysis.

Another select group of patients who may be considered for intra-arterial thrombolysis are those who have undergone major surgery within 2 weeks before the onset of stroke symptoms.[56-58] The NINDS trial excluded these patients from intravenous thrombolysis.[25] For these patients, an intra-arterial approach may allow the administration of lower doses of thrombolytic agents needed to achieve recanalization, with or without adjunctive mechanical thrombolysis, than would be required with intravenous thrombolysis. This method may minimize hemorrhagic complications.

Exclusion Criteria

We suggest that the exclusion criteria used in the NINDS study be followed (Table 78.8). In the European Cooperative Acute Stroke Study (ECASS) I, safety and efficacy of thrombolysis with 1.1 mg/kg of body weight of intravenous alteplase were evaluated in patients treated within 6 hours

---

Table 78.8 Recommended Contraindications for Intra-arterial Thrombolysis in Acute Ischemic Stroke

- Failure to initiate treatment within 6 hours from onset of symptoms
- Baseline National Institutes of Health Stroke Scale score <10
- Rapidly improving neurologic status
- Intracranial hemorrhage, parenchymal hypodensity in more than one third of the affected vascular territory, mass effect with midline shift, intracranial tumor (except small meningioma) on CT scanning
- Seizures at onset
- Stroke within previous 6 weeks
- Head trauma within 90 days
- Active or recent hemorrhage within 30 days, known hemorrhagic diathesis
- Baseline international normalized ratios >1.7, activated partial thromboplastin time >1.5 times normal, baseline platelet counts <100,000/μL
- Known sensitivity to contrast agents
- Uncontrolled hypertension, defined as blood pressure >180 mm Hg systolic or ≥100 mm Hg diastolic on three separate occasions at least 10 minutes apart or requiring continuous intravenous therapy

---

of ischemic stroke.[32] However, the enrollment of 17% of the patients (n = 109) was a violation of the study criteria. The most common protocol violation was the inclusion of patients with early signs of infarction within more than one third of the MCA territory on CT. The incidence of ICH was significantly higher in the alteplase group. We recommend strict adherence to this imaging criterion for now, until more clearly defined MRI or other imaging-based selection criteria become available.

Techniques of Chemical Thrombolysis

Before intra-arterial thrombolysis is initiated, heparin is administered because of the risk of thromboembolic complications associated with prolonged microcatheterization of intracranial vessels.[59] In the PROACT I trial, heparin was intravenously infused before selective microcatheterization of the occluded vessel.[33] During the study, however, the dose of intravenous heparin was decreased from a 100-unit/kg bolus, followed by 1000 units administered hourly for 4 hours, to a 2000-unit bolus, followed by 500 units administered hourly for 4 hours; this change led to a lower incidence of ICH. With the initial heparin regimen, the frequency of hemorrhagic transformation within 24 hours was 72.7% in the r-prourokinase group and 20% in the placebo group. After the reduction in the heparin dose, the frequency of ICH at 24 hours decreased to 20% in the r-prourokinase group and to 0 in the placebo group. However, the recanalization rate also decreased, from 81.8% in the high-dose heparin group to 40% in the low-dose heparin group. The PROACT II trial adopted the low-dose heparin regimen used in PROACT I.[34] The use of other antithrombotic or antiplatelet drugs (such as abciximab and reteplase) during the first 24 hours was prohibited by the protocols of these trials. We believe that paying close attention to the activated coagulation time before the initiation of intra-arterial thrombolysis is paramount, because high-dose heparin therapy may augment hemorrhagic complications.

In both PROACT trials, an infusion microcatheter (<3F) was advanced into the proximal third of the MCA thrombus over a microwire.[33,34] If the microcatheter could not be placed in the proximal portion of the thrombus, the catheter was placed just proximal to the thrombus. A superselective angiogram was performed through the microcatheter to document the placement of the microcatheter. Mechanical disruption of the clot was not permitted in these trials. In PROACT II, recombinant r-prourokinase (4.5 mg × 2) or saline placebo was infused at a rate of 30 mL/hr. After 1 hour of r-prourokinase infusion, another angiogram was performed through the microcatheter. If any of the proximal thrombus had dissolved, the endovascular surgeon advanced the microcatheter tip into the proximal portion of any remaining clot in the MCA. For patients in PROACT II, even if complete lysis occurred in the first hour, another 4.5 mg of r-prourokinase was infused into the proximal MCA over the second hour. The final angiogram was performed at 2 hours through the diagnostic catheter in the cervical ICA in both the r-prourokinase and control groups to assess recanalization rates.

We[41] have reported their preliminary experience with intra-arterial reteplase (Retavase, Centocor, Inc., Malvern,

Therapy

PA). The patients were intubated and connected to ventilators before cerebral angiography was performed. Propofol was administered intravenously for sedation. Before selective microcatherization of the occluded vessel, heparin (50 units/kg body weight) was administered intravenously to achieve an activated coagulation time of more than 250 seconds. A 6F guide catheter was placed in the ICA or vertebral artery proximal to the occlusion site. A 2.3F microcatheter was advanced to the occluded vessel in the proximity of the thrombus through the guide catheter over a micro-guidewire. A superselective angiogram was performed via the microcatheter in the occluded vessel to document placement of the microcatheter (Fig. 78–3A). Reteplase was prepared in a 100-mL solution at a concentration of 1 unit of reteplase per 10 mL of sterile normal saline and then infused via the microcatheter at a rate of approximately 1 unit (10 mL) over the course of 10 minutes. Angiograms were performed via the guide catheter after each unit of reteplase was delivered to evaluate the status of recanalization (Fig. 78–3B).

If the technique resulted in recanalization of a large artery occlusion (e.g., basilar artery or cervical ICA) but the thrombus had moved distally to occlude the middle cerebral or posterior cerebral artery, the technique was repeated in the affected distal vessel until recanalization was achieved or the maximum dose of 8 units of reteplase was used (Fig. 78–3C). In contrast to the PROACT trials, we terminated infusion of reteplase before administering the maximum dose if they observed recanalization. Mechanical thrombolysis was performed at the discretion of the endovascular surgeon. Heparin was discontinued at the end of the procedure.

With advancements in the technology of catheters, wires, drugs, and devices for intra-arterial thrombolysis, speedy and improved recanalization is expected in the future. However, the clinical acumen and experience of those who use these tools are very important. Endovascular surgeons not only must be able to identify the potential candidates for intra-arterial thrombolysis but also must know when to stop the procedure and avoid catastrophic consequences. Finally, in the PROACT II trial, there was an average 3-hour delay between patient arrival at a hospital and initiation of intra-arterial thrombolysis.[33] More efficient methods of triage, evaluation, and preparation are needed.

Procedural Complications and Management

The most feared and potentially most life-threatening procedural complication of intra-arterial thrombolysis is ICH. Complications reported in the PROACT I and II trials are summarized in Table 78.9.[33,34] In PROACT I, a total of 105 patients underwent cerebral angiography, but only 46 patients were randomly assigned to receive r-prourokinase or placebo. Seventeen adverse events occurred among 14 of the 105 patients. Procedural complications included transient vasospasm of a catheterized cavernous ICA (n = 1), seizure (n = 1), acute worsening of chronic renal insufficiency due to the radiocontrast agent (n = 1), aspiration pneumonia due to patient's inability to handle oral secretions (n = 1), groin hematoma (n = 10), and worsening of clinical condition (n = 3). Neither trial has reported any incidence of angioneurotic edema, a known complication associated with the intravenous or intra-arterial use of alteplase in ischemic stroke.[50,60,61] Complications of ICH are discussed in the section on post-treatment morbidity.

Management of Bleeding Complications

All hemorrhagic complications in the periprocedural period warrant close evaluation. Potential systemic bleeding associated with the use of heparin and thrombolytic drugs includes gastrointestinal hemorrhage, urinary tract hemorrhage, retroperitoneal hemorrhage, and access site hematoma. These complications may or may not be clinically obvious and require close attention to the results of daily laboratory tests such as hematocrit and hemoglobin levels, partial thromboplastin time, prothrombin time, international normalized ratios (INRs), platelet count, and any additional tests as needed. Frequent examination of the access site during the 24 hours after the procedure and then daily until the day of discharge is important to detect a possible pseudoaneurysm. Retroperitoneal hemorrhage with or without any abdominal symptoms, which can

Table 78.9   Periprocedural Complications in PROACT I and II Trials

	PROACT I		PROACT II	
	r-Prourokinase	**Placebo**	**r-Prourokinase**	**Placebo**
Worsening neurologic symptoms without ICH	Unknown	Unknown	0.8% (1/121)	0
Worsening of chronic renal insufficiency	4% (1/26)	0	Unknown	Unknown
Aspiration pneumonia	4% (1/26)	0	Unknown	Unknown
Anaphylaxis	0	0	0.8% (1/121)	0
Groin hematoma	12% (3/26)	21% (3/14)	7% (9/121)	7% (4/59)
ICH within 24 hours	42% (11/26)	7% (1/14)	35% (38/108)	13% (7/54)
ICH within 10 days	Unknown	Unknown	68% (73/108)	57% (31/54)
ICH within 90 days	50% (13/26)	36% (5/14)	Unknown	Unknown
ICH with neurologic deterioration within 24 hours	15% (4/26)	7% (1/14)	10% (11/108)	2% (1/54)

ICH, intracranial hemorrhage; PROACT, Prolyse in Acute Cerebral Thromboembolism.

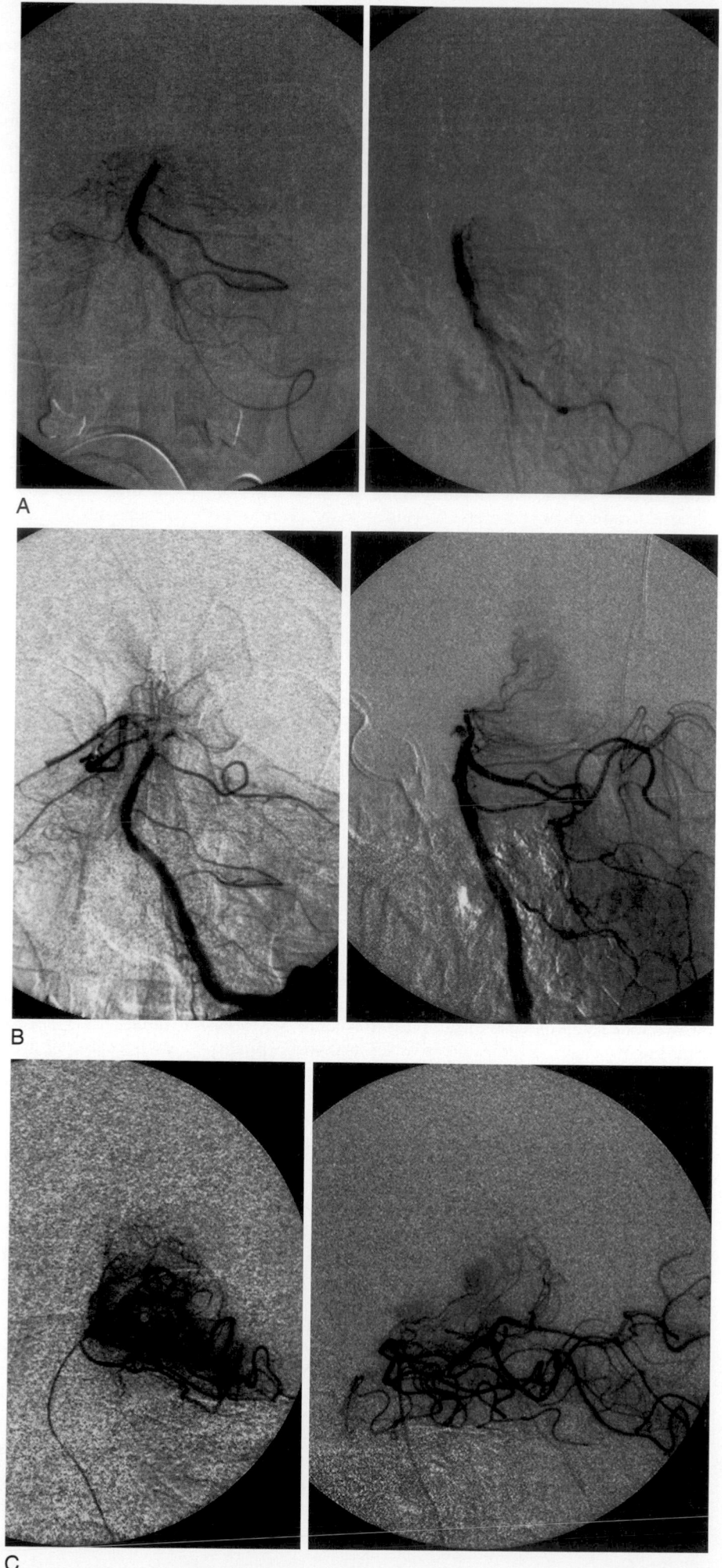

FIGURE 78–3   A, *AP (left) and lateral (right) views of a superselective angiogram via microcatheter show occlusion of the distal BA. B, Left VA angiogram after microcatheter administration of 3.5 units of reteplase directed at the thrombus (AP, left; lateral, right). C, Superselective angiogram via the microcatheter in the left P_1 segment of the posterior cerebral artery (AP, left; lateral, right). BA, basilar artery.*

develop from a complication of a femoral artery puncture or inadequate closure of the puncture site, should be suspected, and an urgent CT scan of the abdomen and pelvis obtained, if there is an unexplained significant or progressive decrease in the patient's hematocrit or hemoglobin level along with signs or symptoms of hemodynamic compromise. An underlying cause of the blood loss or coagulopathy should be evaluated while the necessary blood products (packed red blood cells, cryoprecipitates, fresh frozen plasma, platelets) are administered.

The management of ICH related to intra-arterial thrombolysis requires a multidisciplinary approach. We recommend that patients be intubated and connected to ventilators before the procedure. If ICH is suspected during the procedure because of the extravasation of contrast agent outside the vessel, the thrombolytic drug should be discontinued, and protamine should be administered to reverse the effect of the heparin (1 mg per 100 units of heparin used but not to exceed 50 mg). Coagulation tests should be performed. A cranial CT scan should be obtained immediately. A neurosurgeon should be consulted. A blood transfusion should be considered and administered, especially if a surgical procedure is anticipated. Because of the disruption of the blood-brain barrier, differentiating ICH from contrast enhancement in the affected area is not always easy.[62] Although Hounsfield units can be used to differentiate the two similar-looking signal densities, follow-up cranial CT scan at 24 to 48 hours may show clearance of the contrast material in the absence of ICH.

ICH without significant mass effect, midline shift, uncal herniation, or neurologic deterioration may be managed medically. In the first Global Utilization of Streptokinase and Tissue-plasminogen activator (t-PA) for Occluded Coronary Arteries (GUSTO-I) trial, the incidence of death or disabling stroke with documented hemorrhage was 87%.[63] In this retrospective univariate analysis, surgical evacuation of the hematoma via craniectomy or burr-hole craniotomy was associated with a statistically significant higher survival rate and a trend toward better functional status in patients who experienced ICH after receiving intravenous streptokinase or alteplase for acute MI. Ventriculostomy may be indicated in cases of hydrocephalus or situations for which increased intracranial pressure must be controlled and monitored. We recommend that surgical evacuation be reserved for intracranial hematomas in easily accessible locations in selected patients with progressive neurologic deterioration and substantial mass effect observed on cranial CT scan.

Medical management in the intensive care unit, whether or not surgery is performed, is paramount to improve outcome of patients who have ICH related to intra-arterial thrombolysis. Patients who are lethargic and likely to experience airway compromise should be intubated before angiography is performed. Oxygen saturation level should be kept above 94%. In addition, we recommend keeping systolic blood pressure within the range of 120 to 160 mm Hg and diastolic blood pressure lower than 90 mm Hg within the first 24 hours. The patient's heart rate should be maintained at 60 to 100 beats/min to prevent rate-related cardiac ischemia. Fluid status should be closely observed to avoid dehydration and hypotension as well as fluid overload and cerebral edema. Electrolyte levels should be monitored frequently to prevent arrhythmia. Nutrition should be initiated as soon as possible via a feeding tube for patients who are unable to eat. Patient care in stroke units may reduce secondary complications of stroke and ICH.

Post-Treatment Morbidity and Mortality

ICH is a major risk associated with thrombolytic therapy. The frequency of ICH has been associated with a delay in the initiation of intravenous thrombolysis of 4 to 6 hours or more after stroke onset.[64,65] However, the relationship between ICH and poor outcome, independent of the severity of the initial ischemic event, is not clearly defined. In ECASS II, the higher frequency of severe ICH in the alteplase group (8.1%) than in the placebo group (0.8%) did not result in an overall increase in morbidity and mortality in the alteplase group, as well the rates of favorable outcome were 40% in the treated group and 37% in the placebo group.[27] In the NINDS study, the incidence of symptomatic ICH was 6.4% (20 of 312 patients) in the alteplase group and 0.6% in the placebo group.[25] The mortality rate for patients in the alteplase group who had symptomatic ICH was 45%.

In PROACT I, each of 5 patients found to have hypodensity exceeding 33% of the affected hemisphere on the initial CT scan (ECASS criteria) experienced ICH within 24 hours.[33] In PROACT II, symptomatic ICH occurred only in patients with a baseline NIHSS score of 11 or higher.[34] Symptomatic ICH occurred in 12 of 110 (11%) patients (target population) treated with r-prourokinase and in 2 of 64 (3%) receiving heparin alone. Mortality after symptomatic ICH was 83% (10 of the 12 patients). Blood glucose level exceeding 200 mg/dL at stroke onset was associated with the risk of symptomatic ICH in PROACT II.[66] Severity of stroke, longer time to recanalization, and high glucose levels have been reported as independent predictors of ICH in other series of intra-arterial thrombolysis.[67–70]

In the PROACT I and II trials, the mortality rates at 90 days were 27% and 25% in the r-prourokinase groups and 43% and 27% in the placebo groups, respectively (see Table 78.3).[33,34] In PROACT I, one fatal ICH occurred in each treatment group. Two patients died of cardiac causes, and four patients died of stroke in the r-prourokinase group. In the placebo group, three deaths were related to stroke, and two were cardiac in origin.

In the study conducted by Qureshi and associates,[41] the mortality rate was 56% (9 of 16 patients). All four patients who experienced ICH after thrombolysis died. A higher median NIHSS score of 20 (range 10–26) in this study, compared with a median score of 17 (range 5–27) in PROACT II, may account for the observed differences in the mortality rate. Both PROACT I and PROACT II excluded patients with a baseline NIHSS score exceeding 30. Improved patient selection and an understanding of the mechanisms involved in the development of ICH may reduce the morbidity and mortality associated with intra-arterial thrombolysis.

Mechanical Thrombolysis

During the 1990s, mechanical thrombolysis has evolved as an adjunctive therapy and, potentially, a primary therapy for the treatment of acute ischemic stroke. The main goal of mechanical thrombolysis is to restore cerebral blood flow by removing the obstructive thrombus or disintegrating the thrombus to facilitate activation of the thrombolytic agents. This approach may (1) minimize or obviate the use of thrombolytic agents, thereby reducing the risk of ICH associated with chemical thrombolysis, (2) achieve faster recanalization, and (3) extend the window of intervention beyond 3 to 6 hours.

Devices for mechanical thrombolysis have greatly strengthened the armamentarium of the endovascular surgeon in the treatment of acute ischemic stroke. Also, the use of these devices adds another level of skill and resources to the endovascular surgeon's repertoire. Currently, a variety of devices are being studied, but they are not yet approved by the FDA. Further studies are required to test their safety and efficacy. Here, we briefly review the indications, techniques, and principles of devices that have been used for mechanical thrombolysis in the clinical arena thus far. Rigid guidelines for practice cannot be made at this time, owing to a lack of randomized trials.

Indications for Mechanical Thrombolysis

Mechanical thrombolysis as a primary or the sole therapy for acute ischemic stroke is not recommended at this time, except on a compassionate-use basis. This method of thrombolysis may be indicated for patients in whom standard intra-arterial thrombolysis has failed to achieve recanalization. Lesions in approximately 50% of patients are resistant to intra-arterial chemical thrombolysis.[68,71] This failure of pharmacologic agents in the setting of tenacious clot may be related to site of occlusion, heterogeneous composition of the clot, and underlying atherosclerotic stenosis. Although ranges are wide and variable, lower rates of recanalization are associated with chemical thrombolysis of acute cervical or intracranial ICA occlusions than with distal MCA branch occlusions. In addition, occlusive lesions of the vertebrobasilar artery territory are thought to be more atherothrombotic in nature than MCA occlusions, which may be more embolic.[71,72] As a result, device selection may depend on the occlusion site as well as the vascular disease.

Another indication for mechanical thrombolysis may be in patients for whom the 3-hour window for chemical thrombolysis has passed. Currently, the Mechanical Embolus Removal in Cerebral Ischemia (MERCI) trial is evaluating the safety and recanalization rate of the Concentric Retriever System (Concentric Medical, Mountain View, CA).[73] Inclusion criteria for this trial are (1) diagnosis of acute ischemic stroke, (2) angiographic demonstration of occlusion in the ICA, M_1 segment of the MCA, or basilar artery, (3) contraindications to intravenous t-PA, or (4) presentation of a patient after the 3-hour window in whom treatment can be initiated within 8 hours. Further studies are needed to evaluate the efficacy and therapeutic time window of these mechanical thrombolysis procedures.

Basic Mechanical Thrombolysis Techniques

We have performed mechanical thrombolysis by using snares, angioplasty balloon catheters, microwires, microcatheters, and stents.[38,74] A 6F guide catheter is placed in the ICA or vertebral artery proximal to the lesion. In large vessels such as the ICA, proximal M_1 segment of MCA, and basilar artery, angioplasty was performed with coronary balloons. The diameter of the balloon is undersized in reference to the diameter of the adjacent portion of the occluded vessel. The angioplasty balloon catheters we have used for mechanical thrombolysis are the CrossSail (Guidant, Advanced Cardiovascular Inc, Temecula, CA), OpenSail (Guidant, Advanced Cardiovascular Inc), and NINJA (Cordis Neurovascular, Miami Lakes, FL). In smaller vessels such as the distal MCA (M_2 and M_3) segments, anterior cerebral artery, and posterior cerebral arteries, a microwire, microcatheter, or 4-mm snare (Amplatz Goose-Neck Microsnare, Microvena, White Bear Lake, MN) can be used.

A microwire (0.014 inch) is introduced into a microcatheter (2.3F), and the complex is coaxially advanced through the 6F guide catheter to the site of the occlusion. In smaller vessels, the lesion can be crossed multiple times with a microwire or microcatheter to achieve mechanical disruption of the clot.[75] If a snare is used for mechanical thrombolysis, the lesion is crossed with a microwire and then with the microcatheter. The microwire is exchanged with a snare. We have made multiple passes with a snare through an occluded segment to disrupt the thrombus (Fig. 78–4).

Chopko and coworkers[76] have used a snare for clot retrieval. In this procedure, the snare is gently tightened around the clot, and the microcatheter and guide catheter are withdrawn as a unit. In larger vessels, after the microcatheter is advanced across the lesion, the microwire is exchanged with an exchange wire. The microcatheter is removed, and a balloon catheter is advanced over the exchange wire, facilitating balloon and stent navigation (Fig. 78–5). It is important not to oversize the balloon or the stent so as to avoid dissection or rupture of the affected vessel.

New Devices

Among the new devices for thrombolysis are an ultrasound infusion microcatheter, a laser-driven thrombectomy device, and suction and rheolytic thrombectomy catheters. Preliminary experience with a unique ultrasound infusion microcatheter (EKOS, Bothel, WA) suggests that the technique is safe and yields favorable recanalization rates.[77] In this technique, the catheter is placed within the thrombus and is activated to produce ultrasonic resonance that agitates the thrombus and thereby facilitates the action of the thrombolytic agent.

In animal models of stroke, laser technology using argon and Nd:YAG (neodymium:yttrium-aluminum-garnet) radiation has demonstrated destruction of atheromatous plaque.[78] This technique leads to vaporization of fresh thrombus and plaque without producing significant emboli. However, perforation of the artery wall is a major concern. A pulse-dye laser is unique in that it is tuned to hemoglobin absorption peak. This technique may minimize energy absorption in the vessel wall and allow photoacoustic mechanical disruption of the thrombus. These lasers may be attached to the microcatheter and navigated into the site of occlusion. Further research is under way.

Lutsep and associates[79] reported successful recanalization with suction thrombectomy in three patients with

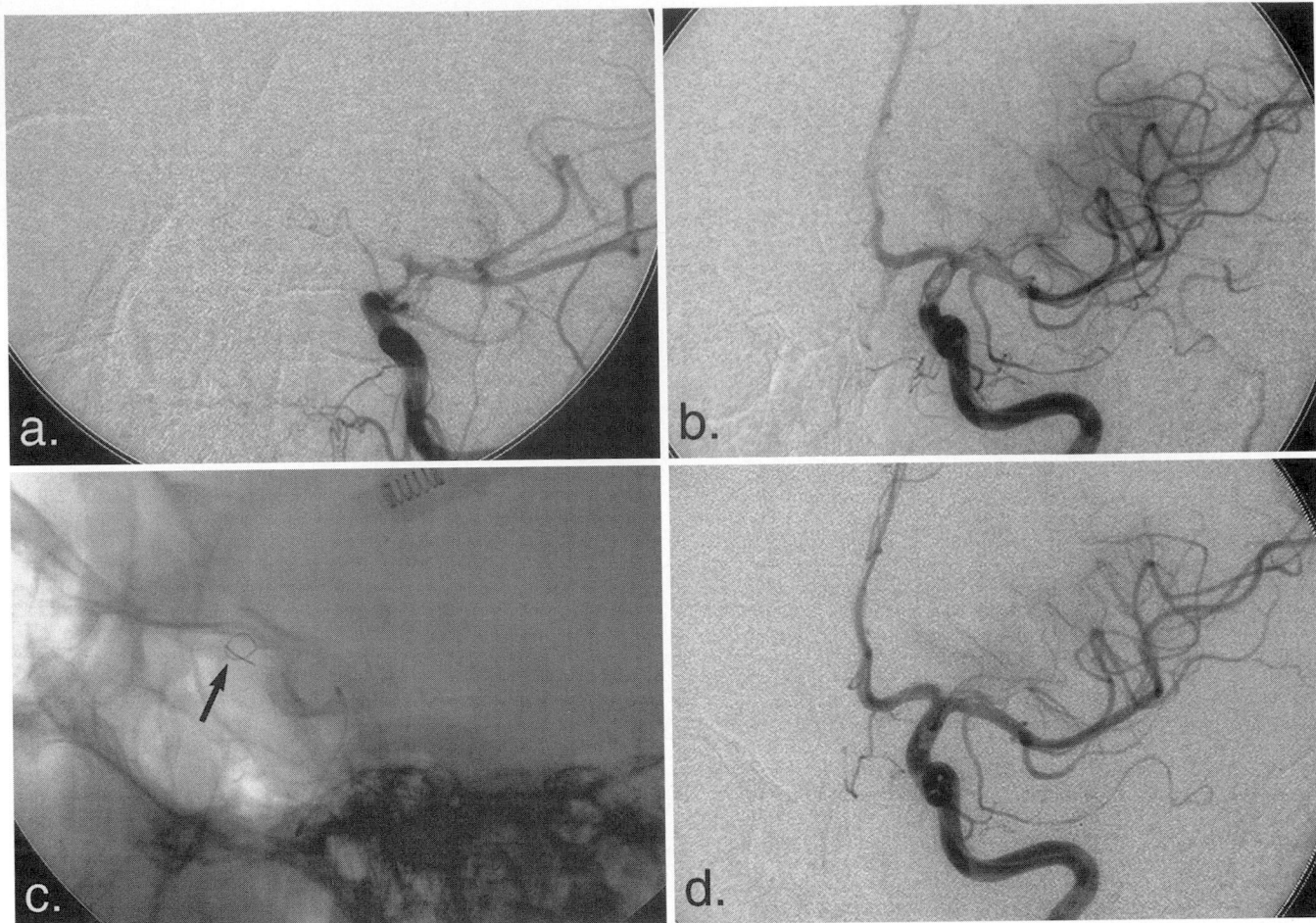

FIGURE 78–4 *A, Left ICA angiogram shows thrombus in the supraclinoid segment of the ICA extending into the left anterior communicating artery (ACA) and MCA. B, Partial resolution of thrombus is observed after infusion of 2 units of reteplase in the supraclinoid segment of the left ICA via the microcatheter. C, A 4-mm snare (Amplatz Goose-Neck Microsnare) is advanced into the thrombus and withdrawn multiple times to disrupt the residual thrombus. D, Near-complete recanalization of the left ACA and MCA was achieved.*

ischemic stroke related to cervical ICA occlusion. In this technique, a 7F guide catheter was navigated over a wire into the proximal third of the thrombus. A 60-mL syringe was used to aspirate the thrombus. The guide catheter was moved in and out of the thrombus several times before slowly being withdrawn to allow for complete removal of the thrombus. This technique may be limited to occlusions in the petrous segment of the ICA.

Another endovascular thrombectomy device is the AngioJet (Possis Medical, Inc., Minneapolis, MN).[80] High-pressure saline jets are directed into the primary evacuation lumen of this thrombectomy catheter to create a hydrodynamic vortex that fragments adjacent thrombus and draws it into the recovery lumen. The use of this device for intracranial thrombectomy is being evaluated in ongoing trials.

Physician and Patient Education

Chemical and mechanical approaches for intra-arterial thrombolysis are promising interventions in acute ischemic stroke. The safety and efficacy of intra-arterial thrombolysis within the 6-hour time window from symptom onset have been demonstrated in major randomized trials as well as case series. Patients with "brain attack" must be expeditiously transferred to institutions with the personnel and resources to provide therapies for the treatment of acute ischemic stroke and must be evaluated to determine their eligibility for such therapies. Time is critical for these patients, regardless of the therapy chosen. Further studies of the efficacy and safety of combination intravenous and intra-arterial therapy must be conducted. Newer fibrinolytic agents and mechanical devices may allow faster recanalization, but the safety of these agents and devices requires further evaluation. The precise role and the limits of newer imaging modalities, such as multimodal MRI, need to be defined to aid in selection of candidates for thrombolysis.

Finally, physicians must assume a pivotal role in educating the public and their colleagues about stroke prevention and treatment locally and nationally. Through the combined efforts of health care professionals, the general

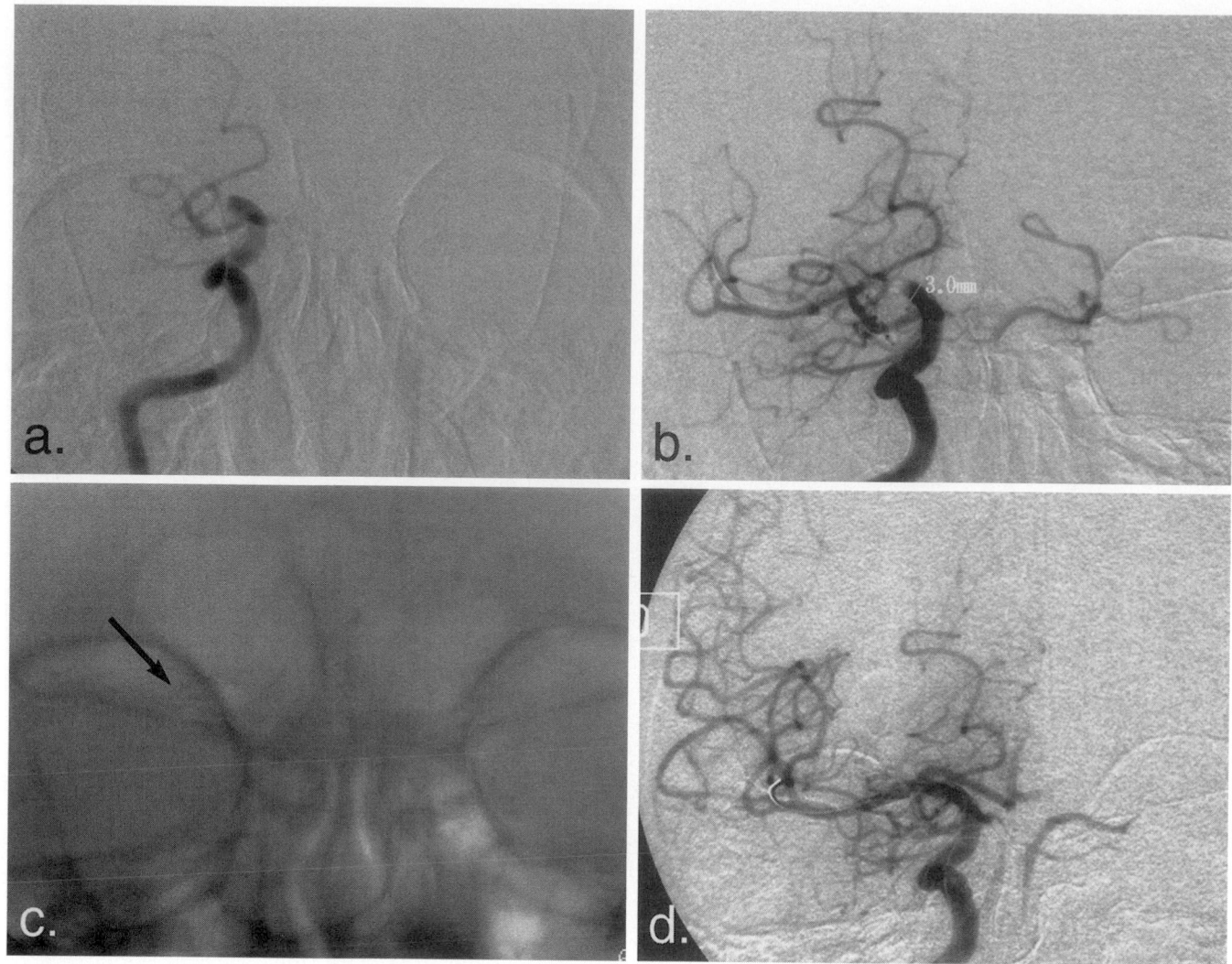

FIGURE 78–5 A, *Right ICA angiogram shows occlusion at the supraclinoid segment of the ICA. B, Right M₁ occlusion persisted despite local infusion of 4 units of reteplase and angioplasty. C, Placement of 2.5-mm × 12-mm S660 stent in the M₁ segment of the MCA. D, Recanalization of right MCA following stent placement.*

public, the American Heart Association, the National Stroke Council, and local and federal governments, management of stroke will improve in the future.

INTRACRANIAL ATHEROSCLEROTIC DISEASE

Intracranial atherosclerotic disease accounts for 8% of all strokes.[81,82] Intracranial atherosclerotic disease is increasingly being discovered with the liberal use of intracranial MR and CT angiography. Both symptomatic and asymptomatic patients are being evaluated more frequently with these noninvasive techniques. The treatment of such lesions has been principally with either antiplatelet (aspirin) or anticoagulant (sodium warfarin) medications. Randomized trials are under way to determine whether aspirin or warfarin is more effective for the treatment of symptomatic intracranial atherosclerotic lesions.[83,84] Because of the

dismal prognosis associated with intracranial atherosclerosis despite medical treatment, alternative treatment options are being explored. Interventional techniques have revolutionized the treatment of coronary atherosclerotic disease and are similarly leading to significant improvements in the treatment of peripheral atherosclerotic disease. Technologic advancements in angioplasty catheters and stents have driven the application of these devices for revascularization of the intracranial circulation. To date, only small patient series have been reported in the literature.

This section consists of a review of the current literature on the natural history of intracranial atherosclerotic disease and the different endoluminal revascularization strategies for the treatment of symptomatic intracranial atherosclerotic lesions. On the basis of this information, laboratory evidence, and our experience, we discuss our revascularization management strategies, including the use of staged stenting procedures. Finally, avoidance and management of complications are mentioned.

Natural History and Medical Management of Intracranial Stenosis

The management of intracranial atherosclerosis remains perplexing. Unlike for atherosclerosis of the extracranial vasculature, only one prospective randomized trial has influenced therapeutic approaches for intracranial disease. The Extracranial-to-Intracranial (EC-IC) Cooperative Bypass Study demonstrated the inefficacy of bypass surgery in preventing recurrence of stroke.[85] This study and other smaller prospective studies have allowed us to define the natural history of intracranial arterial stenosis. In all of these studies, patients were enrolled after the occurrence of a defining neurologic event (transient ischemic attack [TIA] or stroke) referable to the vascular distribution of the intracranial stenotic vessel.

In several studies, including the EC-IC bypass study, a subgroup of patients was treated with aspirin alone. In the bypass study, 714 patients with intracranial ICA or MCA stenosis who received aspirin (1300 mg daily) were observed. The annual stroke rate referable to the stenosis was 7%, with an overall stroke rate of 10%. Craig and associates[86] followed up 58 patients for 2.5 years and discovered a 43% stroke rate and a 15% mortality rate. Marzewski and coworkers[87] followed up 66 patients with distal ICA stenosis and noted a 3.2% annual rate of stroke ipsilateral to the stenosis, with a mortality of 46% over 44 months. Ischemic cerebrovascular disease was responsible for the death of 27% of the patients in these studies.[86,87]

The retrospective arm of the Warfarin-Aspirin Symptomatic Intracranial Disease (WASID) study examined the efficacy of warfarin compared with aspirin for the prevention of major vascular events (stroke, MI, or sudden death).[83] Among 63 patients treated with aspirin, the rate of stroke was 10.4 per 100 patient-years, which correlates well with the rates reported in other studies. Among patients receiving warfarin, however, the stroke rate decreased to 3.6 per 100 patient-years. Three patients had major hemorrhagic complications, in two of whom these were fatal. The rate of hemorrhagic complications for the warfarin-treatment group was 7.8 per 100 patient-years, compared with 1.4 per 100 patient-years for the aspirin treatment group.[83] In summary, the risk of stroke or hemorrhagic event for patients receiving warfarin was 11.4 per 100 patient-years, whereas that for patients receiving aspirin was 11.8 per 100 patient-years.

Adding to the complexity of medication choices are the results of a later trial in Europe, the Stroke Prevention in Reversible Ischemia Trial (SPIRIT). This trial demonstrated a high rate of hemorrhagic complications associated with warfarin therapy in patients who had experienced previous cerebral ischemic events.[88] Moreover, in the Warfarin versus Aspirin in the Secondary Prevention of Stroke Study (WARSS), a randomized controlled study of 2206 patients comparing low-dose anticoagulation (INR 1.4 to 2.8) versus aspirin (325 mg daily) for patients with a non-cardiogenic source of stroke, warfarin was not proven to be more effective than aspirin in preventing stroke recurrence.[84]

In the WASID trial, the occurrence of strokes in vascular territories outside the significant stenosis were nearly eliminated as a result of warfarin therapy.[83] In five of the six patients who had strokes, the strokes occurred in the territory of the compromised vessel. With aspirin, 15 strokes occurred, of which 9 were in the territory of the stenotic artery. Warfarin therapy likely reduces the incidence of stroke outside the territory of the stenotic vessel by reducing the cardioembolic risk of stroke and has been repeatedly shown to significantly reduce the risk of stroke in patients with atrial fibrillation.[89-91] Increasingly, strokes are thought to be caused by a variety of potential cardiac sources in patients without previously identifiable causes. Warfarin, therefore, is probably effective for the prevention of concomitant sources of stroke in the population with potential cardiac sources of thromboemboli and concomitant intracranial atherosclerosis, resulting in the lower stroke rate in these patients than in those treated with aspirin alone.

For patients who experience neurologic symptoms despite antithrombotic treatment, the risk of recurrent events is very high (47.7% over a mean follow-up period of 14.7 months, with a median time to recurrence of 32 days).[92] There is, therefore, some urgency to change the form of treatment once it has failed. In addition, most patients with intracranial disease are more likely to present with a major event (such as a catastrophic stroke) than with a TIA or a minor stroke.[85] This risk of a stroke with potentially irreversible neurologic deficits further complicates medical decision-making as the question arises whether medical management should even be attempted initially.

Asymptomatic Intracranial Atherosclerosis

Intracranial stenosis is a dynamic process whereby repeat angiographic imaging can sometimes reveal dramatically different degrees of arterial blockage. Akins and coworkers[93] presented a retrospective series of serial angiographic studies obtained to study the dynamic morphology of asymptomatic intracranial stenosis. In this series of 21 patients with 45 intracranial stenotic lesions, 40% of the lesions progressed and 20% regressed over a 7-year period. The distal ICA did not seem as predisposed to disease progression as the more distal branches (MCA, anterior cerebral artery, posterior cerebral artery). In 3 patients, regression of the intracranial stenosis was impressive, suggesting that a thrombus was present within the already diseased vessel. In addition, 23% of the patients in this series had strokes during the follow-up period while undergoing different regimens of antithrombotic therapy.

In a later study, significant angiographic improvement of a stenotic vertebrobasilar artery segment was seen after the administration of high-dose atorvastatin, a potent 3-hydroxy-3 methylglutaryl coenzyme A (HMG-CoA) reductase inhibitor, for a 2-week period.[94] This improvement may have occurred from resolution of thrombus, because "statins" promote endogenous fibrinolysis and plaque remodeling.

Pathophysiology of Cerebral Infarction from Arterial Stenosis

There is considerable debate about the mechanism responsible for large vessel stenosis that leads to stroke. Unlike the extracranial carotid artery, in which artery-to-artery embolism is the predominant mechanism, growing evidence in the literature supports a hemodynamic cause for large vessel infarctions. Certainly, a subset of patients has demonstrated a higher rate of stroke recurrence in association with hemodynamic failure.[95–97] More likely, there is an ongoing interaction between the stenosis providing an embolic source and reduced blood flow resulting in diminished ability to clear the emboli. The ischemic events are thus a shift in the balance between embolic load and blood flow.[98] Warfarin is an effective anticoagulant, so the number of emboli generated by an intracranial stenosis may be reduced with its use. Despite warfarin therapy, a significant number of infarctions occurred in the territory of the stenotic vessel in the WARSS and the WASID studies.[83,84] This phenomenon reinforces the supposition that diminished blood flow is the cause of numerous infarctions related to intracranial atherosclerosis. Warfarin is highly effective in treating cardioembolic sources of stroke when blood flow is adequate.

Unlike warfarin, bypass surgery can augment cerebral blood flow and reduce hemodynamic risk of future strokes, but it has little ability to reduce artery-to-artery embolism. The EC-IC bypass study did not demonstrate a reduction in stroke frequency, perhaps because the patient population could not be confined to those with hemodynamic failure.[85] Technology such as positron emission tomography (PET), single-photon emission CT (SPECT), or XECT was unavailable during the study period. Thus, it was difficult to differentiate between TIAs or strokes resulting from emboli and from ischemia. In addition, the EC-IC bypass procedure occasionally precipitates MCA occlusion at the site of the stenotic segment (usually the M_1 segment).[99,100] This thrombosis probably causes perforator occlusion, resulting in deep brain infarction.

In summary, aspirin has demonstrated only mild efficacy for stroke prevention. Warfarin may prove to be more efficacious; despite its use, however, there remains a significant stroke risk to the threatened territory and a possible greater threat of hemorrhagic complication. Endoluminal revascularization, therefore, may have a role in the treatment of both embolic and hemodynamic sources of infarction from the stenotic vessel.

Endoluminal Revascularization: Strategies and Technique

The methods for achieving endoluminal revascularization are primary angioplasty, primary stenting, direct stenting (stenting without immediate balloon predilation), and provisional stenting. In *primary angioplasty*, the operator places an angioplasty balloon to expand the stenotic segment and has no intention of placing a stent. In *primary stenting*, the operator has the intention of placing a stent and may or may not dilate the lesion with an angioplasty balloon before stent placement. If no previous dilation is required, the procedure is called *direct stenting*. *Provisional stenting* refers to stent placement after unsatisfactory luminal recanalization from angioplasty, or stenting as a "bail-out" procedure.

The feasibility and limitations of primary angioplasty were presented in initial patient series.[101–104] The periprocedural risk of stroke or death was 8% to 33%. Later series

have documented a lower incidence of complications, demonstrating a considerable learning curve for these techniques.[105–108] The periprocedural neurologic event rate in these series, which comprised more than 10 patients each, was less than 10%.

The results of these numerous reports are mirrored in the angioplasty series presented by Connors and Wojak.[105] These investigators divided their experience from 1989 to 1998 into three periods. The rate of complications was higher in 17 patients treated during the early and middle periods from 1989 to 1993; complications included dissection in 82%, neurologic events in 6%, and death in 6%. Subsequent to 1993, the rates among 41 patients were dissection in 14%, neurologic events in 8% (of which 4% were TIAs), and death in 2%. Connors and Wojak[105] attribute the improvements to decreasing the balloon diameter to restore the vessel lumen, very slow inflation of the balloon (over 2–5 minutes), and the routine use of glycoprotein IIb/IIIa receptor (GP IIb/IIIa) inhibitors, such as abciximab, during angioplasty. Two hemorrhages (included in the neurologic events rate) occurred during this period. They also avoid crossing a lesion more than once with the angioplasty balloon because that maneuver is likely to raise an intimal flap and cause the vessel to become occluded. One intrinsic advantage of endovascular approaches over surgery is the ability to repeat the angioplasty. A stenotic vessel that has been suboptimally dilated initially can be further dilated on subsequent interventions. Another "pearl" discovered by Connors and Wojak[105] is that the use of shorter angioplasty balloons prevents straightening of the intracranial vessels after balloon inflation, making injury or dissection less likely.

In a single series of clinically symptomatic patients with hemodynamically significant intracranial lesions, Mori and colleagues[107] demonstrated the effectiveness of angioplasty in patients with short (≤5 mm), mildly eccentric or concentric (type A) lesions.[107] In their experience, angioplasty of these lesions resulted in a periprocedural complication rate of 8% (1 stroke in 12). During the 2-year follow-up period, no ipsilateral stroke, neurologic event, or angiographic stenosis occurred; and no bypass surgery or second angioplasty was needed. For angiographic lesions that were longer and more eccentric or chronically occluded, the procedure yielded less effective results. For lesions that were either 5 to 10 mm in length or totally occluded and were less than 3 months old (type B), the success rate was 86%. Angiographic restenosis occurred in 33% of lesions within the 2-year follow-up period. Angioplasty attempts were unsuccessful in 2 of 21 patients. Patients with chronically occluded lesions that were 3 months or older or highly angular or long (>10 mm in length) (type C) fared the worst. Angioplasty was associated with an initial success rate of 33% (3 of 9 patients) and a restenosis rate of 100% at 1 year. These results suggest that angiographic characteristics may help determine feasibility and periprocedural risks of angioplasty. One of 9 patients with type C lesions experienced a stroke from abrupt closure of the stenotic vessel, suggesting that vessels harboring these lesions are extremely tenuous.[107] The cumulative risk of ipsilateral stroke was 12% for type B lesions and 56% for type C lesions. Of note, the natural history of these lesions was not delineated according to lesion type in either the

WASID study or the EC-IC bypass study. Further reports by Mori and colleagues[109,110] suggest that type C and possibly also type B lesions should not be treated by angioplasty alone but rather may benefit from another endovascular technique or from surgery.

Marks and associates[106] reported a periprocedural risk of 5% in their intracranial angioplasty series. Like Connors and Wojak,[105] these investigators undersized the balloon and allowed for residual stenosis. They frequently included anticoagulation (warfarin) therapy in their postprocedural regimen (prescribed for 18 of 23 patients), particularly if there was significant (>50%) residual stenosis or dissection. Two complications occurred during the immediate postprocedural period in this group of 23 patients. A vessel ruptured, resulting in death; and an angioplasty site became occluded by a thrombus. The clot was successfully lysed with intra-arterial tissue plasminogen activator. Two strokes occurred during the follow-up periods of 32 and 37 months. Only one of the strokes involved territory supplied by the treated vessel. This stroke occurred in a vessel with 50% residual stenosis. Including the vessel rupture, the annual rate of stroke in the territory of the previously treated vessel was 3.2%, and the overall rate of stroke during the average 35.4 months of follow-up was 4.8%. This dramatically low frequency of strokes should be acknowledged, because it occurred in patients in whom warfarin therapy was often used in conjunction with revascularization therapy. This combination of therapies may best reduce the risk of strokes from hemodynamic, embolic, and small vessel arteriopathy sources.

Therefore, primary angioplasty provides an effective method of endoluminal revascularization. The intrinsic disadvantages of angioplasty are mirrored in the literature on coronary procedures.[111–113] Coronary angioplasty alone resulted in numerous dissections or vessel recoil that would have been resolved with stent placement. Moreover, there was a low incidence of mortality related to vessel rupture during balloon inflation or hemorrhage associated with reperfusion and use of GP IIb/IIIa inhibitors. Strokes were rare, but ischemic neurologic events occurred either periprocedurally or immediately after angioplasty. The incidence of neurologic events was probably higher in Mori type C lesions. The vessels at greatest risk for restenosis or further strokes were those with residual stenosis, yet the vessels at greatest risk of rupture or dissection were those inflated with a balloon that was the size of the vessel or larger. In follow-up of angioplasty performed for intracranial atherosclerosis, the results appear durable if minimal residual stenosis is apparent. In almost all series reporting delayed neurologic events, the events occurred in patients in whom residual vessel stenosis was seen immediately after completion of the procedure.

The limitations of primary angioplasty prompted investigators to examine the effectiveness of primary stent placement for the treatment of intracranial atherosclerosis. Three series involved at least 10 patients each who underwent intracranial primary stenting for atherosclerotic lesions.[114–116] The first two series report excellent results, with minimal residual stenosis and no neurologic complications.[114,116] Mori and colleagues[116] were unable to deliver a stent in 2 of 12 lesions but were able to successfully perform angioplasty of these lesions. Improvements in trackability and flexibility will make stents easier to deliver. In the series reported by Mori and colleagues,[116] 2 lesions were type C and 8 lesions were type B. One type C lesion could not be accessed for stent delivery, again demonstrating the difficulty in treating this kind of lesion. No restenosis or neurologic events were reported in the early postprocedural period (<4 months). Type B lesions might be best treated with stent placement. Gomez and colleagues[114] successfully placed stents in the basilar or intracranial vertebral arteries in 12 patients. No technical failures or ischemic neurologic events occurred in this series. Three of 12 patients had headaches and 2 had cranial nerve deficits, all of which resolved within 3 months. The cranial nerve deficits were likely related to nerve injury resulting from manipulation of the basilar artery during stent placement.

In the third series reported, Levy and coworkers[115] presented a series of 11 patients with medically refractory vertebrobasilar insufficiency. Primary intracranial stent placement was performed in each case. Technical success was achieved in 9 of 11 patients (82%); four periprocedural complications occurred that resulted in death (mortality rate 36%). In 2 of the remaining 7 patients, intimal hyperplasia developed within or at the end of the stent, and the formation of a pseudoaneurysm was seen at the end of one stent. This series reflects several important findings. Despite routine use of abciximab and heparin, a significant incidence of thromboembolic complications (29%, 2 of 7 surviving patients) resulted from stent placement in the basilar artery. Levy and coworkers[115] mentioned that balloon angioplasty was occasionally performed before stent placement, indicating that most patients in this series were treated with direct stent placement. In addition, intraprocedural rupture was the cause of death in 2 of the 4 patients who died. Vessel rupture occurred in or around the vertebrobasilar junction, where hypoplastic vessels may arise. Because of this anatomical variability, obtaining measurements to select a stent of an appropriate diameter is particularly difficult. In the first two series reported, the stenotic lesions were predilated with an angioplasty balloon before stent placement (primary stent procedure).[114,116]

Ramee and associates[117] have proposed a combined approach for the treatment of symptomatic intracranial stenosis. They used primary angioplasty for revascularization of lesions classified as Mori type A. If the lesion was complex or long, primary stenting was attempted. If the results of primary angioplasty were suboptimal because of dissection or vessel recoil with residual stenosis, a stent was placed. The combined approach yielded an excellent short-term outcome with a 93% success rate and a 53% "unexpected benefit" rate in that 8 of 15 patients had reversal of what was initially thought to be a permanent deficit from a previous stroke. Ten of the 15 patients in this series underwent angioplasty alone. Primary stenting was attempted in 4 patients in whom the lesions were complex and long. Stent placement was unsuccessful in 1 of these patients, who then underwent angioplasty alone, which resulted in 30% residual stenosis. Severe elastic recoil encountered during angioplasty of petrous carotid stenosis in 2 patients necessitated stent deployment to achieve a better initial result (provisional stent placement). This method, described in the coronary literature as provisional stenting, has become popular for coronary revascularization.

Our revascularization management strategies have reflected those depicted in the literature. We used angioplasty alone in our early revascularization experience. We have developed techniques similar to those of Connors and Wojak,[105] in that we typically undersize the vessel and use slow inflation and deflation techniques. One significant difference between our technique and theirs is that we use less compliant coronary balloons that are precisely sized to the vessel for angioplasty procedures. Precise measurements of the stenotic segment and the adjacent parent artery lumen are important to prevent vessel dissection or rupture due to inadvertent oversizing of the angioplasty balloon.

One potential disadvantage associated with the use of less compliant balloons is that the material used to construct the balloon has a higher durometry (i.e., amount of force needed to expand the balloon and, in turn, the amount of force exerted on the parent vessel). As such, more force is required to advance this type of balloon through tortuous vessels. These balloons may be more difficult to navigate into intracranial vessels than more compliant balloons. To facilitate balloon delivery, the shortest balloon length that covers the lesion should be chosen. For short lesions, a 10-mm length balloon would be used. For longer lesions, a 15- or 20-mm balloon can be used. Longer balloons may be more difficult to deliver and may require that the guide wire have firm purchase in the distal vessel. Inflations are kept below 8 atm, and the balloon is slowly inflated and deflated. We typically use coronary exchange length wires that allow us to exchange devices without recrossing the lesion with the wire. Therefore, a suboptimal angioplasty result (because of dissection, vessel recoil, or thrombus) can be treated with either stent placement or second angioplasty with a balloon of a different size.

Anatomically, there are several reasons for different responses of intracranial and coronary vessels to endoluminal revascularization. The high incidence of vessel dissection, rupture, and recoil encountered during intracranial revascularization procedures can be explained by these anatomic differences. The histology and physiology of the intracranial vessels change as these vessels course through the skull base. Once within the skull, they become conduit vessels within a space fixed by the skull with a constant total volume occupied by the brain, cerebrospinal fluid, and blood. Thin-walled subarachnoid vessels transport a large volume of circulating fluid. Cross-sectional histologic specimens of intracranial vessels demonstrate a paucity of vasa vasorum and absence of external elastic membranes. Near absence of the adventitia is noted. The tunica media is composed principally of smooth muscle cells.[118] Such modified vessels are more likely to rupture or dissect during endoluminal revascularization procedures. Moreover, a more robust smooth muscle cell response to angioplasty or stent placement is likely to occur in these vessels, resulting in intimal hyperplasia.

Because of these anatomic differences and the initial results of balloon angioplasty demonstrating a higher incidence of dissection (85%)[105] and rupture (5% to 10%)[105,106] in the intracranial vasculature with the use of coronary techniques (i.e., angioplasty balloons are sized 10% to 20% larger than the reference vessel, and quick inflation and deflation are preferred), alternative methods of revascularization were sought. We use balloons that are clearly smaller in diameter than the parent vessel. For instance, a 1.5- or 2.0-mm balloon will be used in the MCA or basilar artery.

We are increasingly allowing for residual stenosis at the time of the initial intervention (Fig. 78–6). If residual stenosis exists but is not limiting flow (<50%), a staged stent procedure is planned, in which stent placement is performed 6 to 8 weeks after angioplasty. We use this technique because periprocedural risks such as dissection and rupture are minimized by the use of a small-diameter balloon during the initial angioplasty procedure. Residual stenosis portends a higher risk of subsequent symptomatic restenosis or a thromboembolic event; however, in the angioplasty series with the longest follow-up reported in the current literature, most of these thromboembolic events occurred after 6 months (indeed, two strokes occurred at 32 and 37 months after treatment).[106] Therefore, leaving a residual stenosis for 6 to 8 weeks to allow for an intimal response is unlikely to incur a significant neurologic risk. This strategy is particularly useful for complex, long, or recently symptomatic stenoses, for which the risk of periprocedural neurologic complications is highest.[119] If a simple undersized balloon angioplasty is performed first, plaque fracture and injury are less likely to occur. Intimal response that occurs over the ensuing weeks may make subsequent stent placement safer, thereby reducing the chance of dissection, distal embolization, or "snowplowing" (closure of perforating side branches by plaque as the stent or balloon is deployed, as a result of plaque fracture and compression). At our institution, direct stent placement is believed to increase the chances of snowplowing and is therefore no longer used unless the stenosis is in a region without eloquent perforating vessels. Data are needed to evaluate this hypothesis.

We no longer use GP IIb/IIIa inhibitors routinely for intracranial angioplasty and stent placement because of the associated risk of hemorrhage. Connors and Wojak[105] described two hemorrhages in a series of 41 patients. We use abciximab or eptifibatide therapy as a bail-out treatment alternative when thromboembolic complications occur.

Initially, the use of intracranial stents was reserved for cases in which significant vessel recoil or dissection led to the failure of a previous angioplasty procedure. With greater experience, we are learning that certain sites are likely to respond better to stent placement than to angioplasty alone. For instance, angioplasty of a petrous carotid stenosis usually results in significant vessel recoil, so stent placement is necessary.[117,120] This area is also proximal in the vessel tree, allowing more consistent stent placement. Stent delivery, placement, and deployment involve a steep learning curve. Our experience with intracranial stents was preceded by a robust animal experience. We would suggest that these techniques be practiced in models before they are applied clinically.

As mentioned previously, the decision to place a stent should be made on the basis of angioplasty results. Excessive vessel recoil or dissection may mandate stent

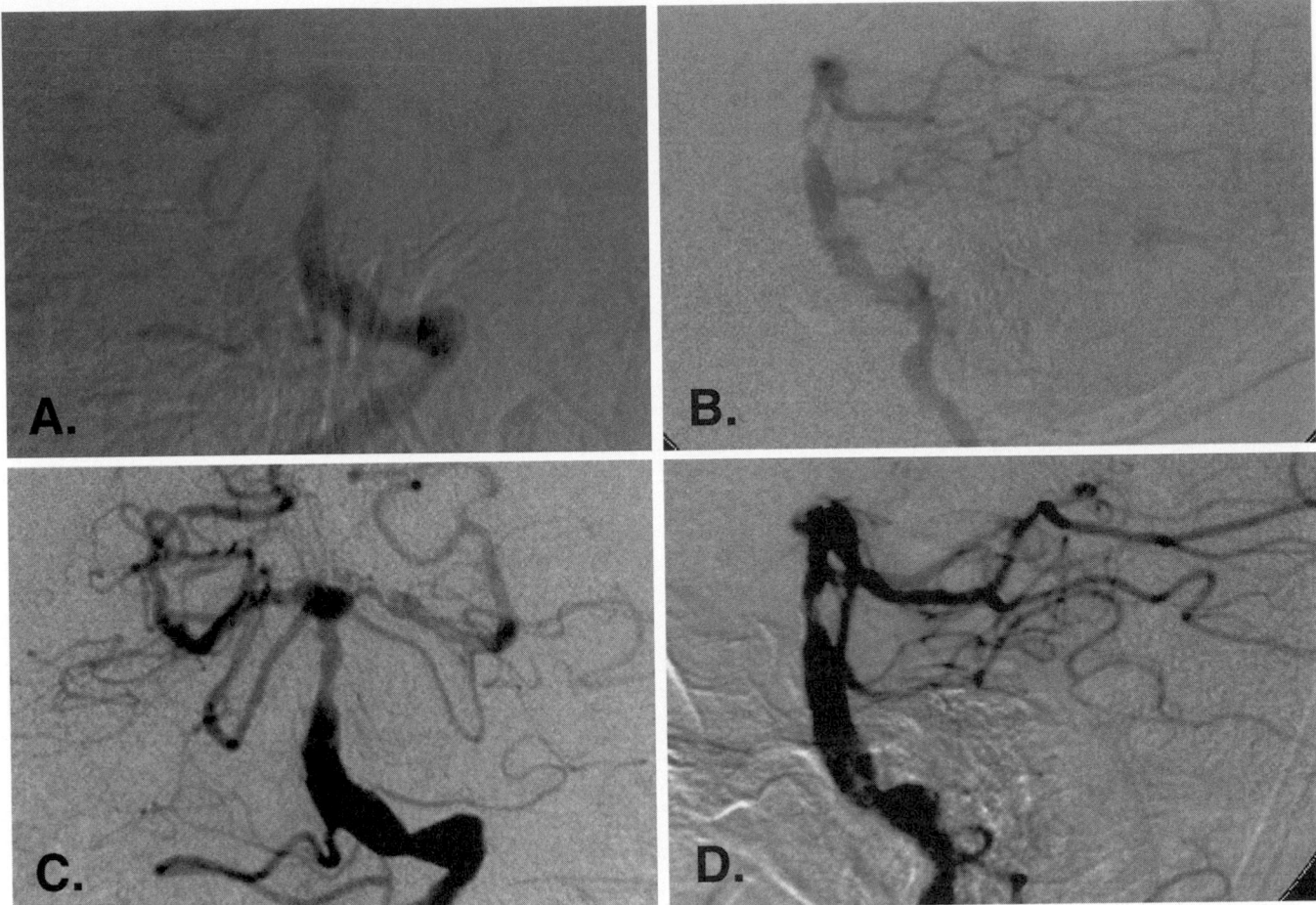

FIGURE 78–6   *AP A, and lateral B, views of an angiogram demonstrating high-grade stenosis of the distal third of the BA with proximal irregularity of the BA. There is a dilatation of the basilar apex involving the origins of the posterior cerebral arteries. AP C, and lateral D, views of the BA following stent-assisted angioplasty of the BA demonstrating residual stenosis but with improved filling of the distal branches and left posterior cerebral artery. Residual stenosis is seen because of the recalcitrant unresponsiveness of the lesion to balloon angioplasty immediately before stenting.*

placement. The stent's diameter should be equal to the normal diameter of the vessel lumen. The stent length should be chosen so that the entire lesion will be covered with an additional 1- to 2-mm overlap onto the healthy vessel on each side. Minimizing the length of the stent is important for navigation of the proximal tortuosity of the skull base. It also may decrease the incidence of intimal hyperplasia.

Stent delivery can be difficult, especially when the radius of curvature of the carotid siphon or vertebral artery near the C1 vertebra is low. It is critical that the guide wire have a firm purchase in the distal vessel. For a stent to be positioned in the supraclinoid carotid artery, the wire should be positioned in the M_2 or M_3 segment of the ipsilateral MCA. For a midbasilar stenosis, the wire should be positioned in the P_2 or P_3 segment of the posterior cerebral artery. During delivery, the position of the distal end of the guide catheter should be carefully monitored. As the stent is negotiated through tight turns in the vasculature, the guide catheter may back out. This movement can result in loss of guide catheter position and distal wire purchase. Extreme caution must be taken in advancing the guide

catheter distally to ensure adequate support for delivery of the stent. On occasion, we place a second wire (V18 Control, Boston Scientific Scimed, Maple Grove, MN) in the guide catheter to improve stability. In later designs, guide catheters are supported by guide sheaths of appropriate length that allow selection of the great vessels arising from the aortic arch. For instance, a Cook shuttle or armored arrow sheath (Cook Inc., Bloomington, IN) is placed 10 to 20 cm proximal to the guide catheter. The guide sheath gives the guide catheter considerable stability, allowing the angioplasty catheter or stent to be advanced through tortuous anatomy.

Once the stent has been advanced across the lesion, careful attention must be paid to positioning. Before deploying the stent, we routinely perform numerous digital subtraction angiographic studies to ensure that the lesion is adequately covered by the stent. Rarely do patients become symptomatic as a result of flow obstruction caused by the stent before deployment. It is advisable to ensure that the stent is positioned properly before deploying it. Deployment should be performed slowly and evenly. The balloon should be expanded fully, and the stent should be embedded into normal vessel proximal and distal to the lesion. Digital subtraction angiography is performed after the procedure to confirm placement, patency, and apposition of the stent to the vessel wall. If post-stent angioplasty is necessary, it can be performed with a slightly larger balloon. If the stent does not adequately cover the lesion, another stent should be placed. Sluggish flow or evidence of thrombus within the stent may require the administration of GP IIb/IIIa inhibitors to prevent acute or subacute thrombosis. Angiograms of the distal vasculature must be carefully examined to ensure that distal embolization has not occurred.

At the conclusion of the procedure, the effect of the heparin is allowed to reverse on its own. The sheath can be left in place and removed when the coagulation cascade has normalized (within 4 to 6 hours), after which pressure can be applied to the groin region to ensure hemostasis. Alternatively, a femoral artery closure device can be used at the conclusion of the procedure. During the periprocedural period, blood pressure is closely monitored and controlled. Clopidogrel, which was administered for the 3 days leading up to the procedure, is continued for 30 days. Aspirin is prescribed for the life of the patient.

We advocate the use of stents for failure of angioplasty. We have begun to also use stent placement routinely in certain sites, such as the petrous carotid artery, and for certain types of lesions. Mori type B and C lesions have a high incidence of restenosis and subsequent neurologic events. For these, we use the aforementioned staged procedure. The initial undersized angioplasty improves cerebral blood flow through the vessel significantly. Then, an intimal response occurs. Six to 8 weeks after the angioplasty, stent placement is performed if significant stenosis remains. When performed in this delayed fashion, the stent procedure may not carry the same thromboembolic risk but does afford the advantage of better early gain (the vessel is opened wider than with angioplasty alone) and a resultant decrease in symptomatic restenosis. On occasion, staged stent placement is not required because the vessel undergoes positive remodeling and the luminal angiographic diameter of the blood vessel improves as a result of the angioplasty alone.

Current Management and Future Directions

The surgeon must understand the natural history of intracranial atherosclerosis well to optimize patient selection for and timing of endoluminal revascularization. Our techniques have evolved such that we perform revascularization in symptomatic patients after angiographic documentation of high-grade intracranial stenosis and blood flow assessment revealing hypoperfusion in the threatened territory. We are increasingly using stent-assisted angioplasty for complex plaques or when initial angioplasty results are suboptimal.

The decision to perform revascularization becomes more difficult when hypoperfusion is not demonstrated on SPECT, PET, or XECT, or a course of treatment with antiplatelet agents has not failed. Patients with these characteristics either could be enrolled in the WASID trial to receive maximal medical therapy or could undergo endoluminal revascularization. Another challenging group consists of asymptomatic patients with MR angiography

evidence of intracranial stenosis. We do not consider these patients for endoluminal revascularization unless radiologic studies show moderate or severe hypoperfusion or lack of reserve in a patient who is to undergo a coronary bypass procedure.

Our techniques for endoluminal revascularization of intracranial stenosis have evolved in accordance with the literature. We use short, undersized angioplasty balloons with slower inflations. Two different antiplatelet agents (clopidogrel and aspirin) are administered for 72 hours before the procedure; GP IIb/IIIa inhibitors may be administered during revascularization of longer, ulcerated lesions. Stent assistance is used as a rescue tactic for dissection or occlusion subsequent to angioplasty. A staged stent procedure is used for complex or difficult stenoses, particularly those in regions of eloquent perforators.[119]

Ongoing advancements in microcatheters, microwires, angioplasty balloons, and intravascular stents have enhanced our ability to successfully treat intracranial atherosclerotic lesions. A role for endoluminal revascularization of these lesions is apparent, particularly in those with concentric, short stenoses. Models for intracranial atherosclerosis and endovascular treatments of these stenoses are necessary to gain insight into the vascular responses after endoluminal device placement. Moreover, the potential use of pharmacologically enhanced stent coatings must be tested with the intracranial vasculature, because these devices may significantly affect the long-term effectiveness of stenting for atherosclerotic disease.

EXTRACRANIAL CAROTID DISEASE: RISK FACTORS AND MANAGEMENT

Identifying the Population for Treatment

Carotid angioplasty and stent placement are becoming increasingly popular interventions for carotid artery disease. It is important for clinicians to become familiar with clinical and radiologic factors that stratify patients to treatment with angioplasty, angioplasty-assisted stenting, or CEA. More importantly, it is imperative that clinicians understand the risk of stroke associated with treatment versus observation alone. As is the case for most other surgical and interventional procedures, minimizing morbidity is achieved by thoughtful analysis of the patient's neurologic condition followed by exquisitely careful patient selection. Treatment for carotid stenosis has undergone rigorous scrutiny involving many multicenter trials for both asymptomatic and symptomatic stenosis. The data obtained from these studies has been used by clinicians to create treatment algorithms. We review some of these trials, specific angiographic data, and technical developments of carotid stenting that may help reduce the risk of stroke for specific cohorts with carotid stenosis.

Among the many trials examining stroke risk after treatment of carotid stenosis, the North American Symptomatic Carotid Endarterectomy Trial (NASCET) attempted to quantify stroke risk after CEA in medically treated patients with symptomatic carotid artery disease.[121] At 30 days from the time of surgery, the incidence of death was 1.1%, that of disabling stroke was 1.8%, and that of nondisabling stroke was 3.7%.[122] Among 26 variables evaluated for stroke risk, the following criteria were found to portend increased risk of stroke: contralateral carotid occlusion, hemispheric TIA, left-sided procedure, ipsilateral ischemic lesion on CT scan, and irregular or ulcerated ipsilateral plaque. Other stroke risk factors were diabetes and elevated diastolic blood pressure.[122] Interestingly, previous cardiac intervention for coronary artery disease was found to reduce the risk of stroke. Results from NASCET demonstrated that patients with 70% or more stenosis had a 17% lower incidence of stroke after CEA than with medical treatment alone.[121] Symptomatic stenosis in the range of 50% to 69% was associated with 5-year rates of ipsilateral stroke of 15.7% among patients treated surgically and 22.2% among those treated medically. No benefit of surgery was found for patients with less than 50% stenosis.[122] We caution that these findings, as well as factors that portend greater stroke risk, were found in a post hoc analysis of the NASCET data set.

In an analysis of patients randomly assigned to undergo CEA in the European Carotid Surgery Trial (ECST), the risk of major ischemic stroke or death after surgery was 7% and did not vary substantially with severity of stenosis.[123] Conversely, the risk of major ischemic stroke ipsilateral to the unoperated symptomatic carotid artery did increase with severity of stenosis, most notably with stenosis of 70% to 80%. For patients with more than 80% stenosis, the Kaplan-Meier estimate of the frequency of a major stroke or death at 3 years was 26.5% for the medical treatment group and 14.9% for the surgery group, an absolute benefit from surgery of 11.6%. It is important to note that measurements of 80% stenosis in the ECST corresponded to approximately 60% stenosis in the NASCET.[122]

Treatment of carotid stenosis in asymptomatic patients has been extensively studied. Of the 721 asymptomatic patients with 60% or more carotid stenosis who underwent CEA in the Asymptomatic Carotid Atherosclerosis Study (ACAS), 1 patient died and 10 others had strokes within 30 days (1.5%).[124,125] The estimated 5-year risk of ipsilateral stroke was 11% for the medical group and 5.1% for the surgical group. Risk factors for stroke included diabetes mellitus, contralateral siphon stenosis, radiation-induced stenosis, previous history of stroke, more than 60% contralateral stenosis, and length of external carotid artery plaque.[126] Use of local or regional anesthesia was associated with a higher risk of TIA and MI.[126] In another analysis of asymptomatic patients with carotid stenosis, the combined incidence of ipsilateral neurologic events was 8.0% in the surgical group and 20.6% in the medical group ($P < 0.001$).[127] The incidence of ipsilateral stroke alone was 9.4% in the medical group and 4.7% in the surgical group.

Increased Operative Stroke and Morbidity Risk

Many factors (mentioned previously) are prognostic for a higher perioperative risk of stroke for patients undergoing CEA. Some of these same risk factors pertain to endoluminal carotid revascularization. Of these, pseudo-occlusion, also known as "slim" sign or "string" sign (angiographic indication of near-complete occlusion of the carotid artery) suggests an increased risk. According to a post hoc analysis of the NASCET data, 106 patients with

near-complete occlusion of the carotid artery were subdivided into those with (n = 29) and those without (n = 77) a string-like lumen. Of patients with near-complete occlusion treated with surgery, 6% had perioperative strokes, as in the group of patients with 70% to 94% stenosis. Only one of the medically treated patients (1.7%) with near-complete occlusion had a stroke within the first month. These data suggest that CEA is not needed on an emergency basis for patients with such lesions and that it does not indicate higher stroke rates for this population than for patients with 70% to 94% stenosis.[128]

Intracranial or extracranial stenoses (such as those found with extracranial tandem lesions) raise the risk of stroke for medically treated patients with carotid stenosis but do not raise the perioperative risk.[129] Although the results from ACAS suggest that contralateral intracranial carotid stenoses increase surgical morbidity, the presence of intracranial stenosis did not raise the surgical risk for a similar subset of patients in the NASCET.

One hundred and fifteen (8.1%) patients enrolled in NASCET had 142 medical complications.[130] The complications were MI and other cardiac disorders (8.1%), respiratory complications (0.8%), transient confusion (0.4%), and other complications (0.7%). Five patients died from these perioperative complications. These results suggest that patients with significant medical comorbidities may be better managed with stent placement than with CEA.

The question arises whether it is possible to identify high-risk patients in need of carotid revascularization who may benefit from angioplasty-assisted stenting and thereby avoid the surgical morbidity of CEA. What is clear are the risk factors that increase the incidence of stroke and the morbidity of surgery after CEA, but more evidence is needed to demonstrate whether stent placement significantly decreases the periprocedural morbidity in this subset of patients. Prospective multicenter trials are currently under way to evaluate the effectiveness of carotid stenting in high-risk patients. Some evidence exists that there is a similar morbidity rate but an overall lower cost and shorter hospital stay after stenting compared with CEA. In one study of nonrandomized groups with similar patient populations, major ipsilateral stroke and death occurred more frequently in the surgical group (2.9%) than in the stent group (0), but the difference was not significant.[131] The stent group also had a significantly shorter hospital stay. In a multicenter registry of 5210 endovascular carotid stent procedures involving 4757 patients, technical success was achieved in 98.4%.[132] TIAs occurred at a rate of 2.82%, with a minor stroke rate of 2.72%. A major stroke rate of 1.49% and a mortality rate of 0.86% were observed. Restenosis rates of carotid stenting were 1.99% and 3.46% at 6 and 12 months, respectively. Roubin and colleagues[133,134] reported their experience of more than 500 carotid stent procedures in a group of asymptomatic and symptomatic patients. There were a 0.6% rate of fatal stroke and a 1% rate of death from causes other than stroke during the 30-day periprocedural period. The major stroke rate was 1%, and the minor stroke rate was 4.8%. Over the 5-year study period, the periprocedural stroke rate improved from 7.1% to 3.1%.

Patient selection and timing of carotid stenting may minimize stroke risk. Recent radiographic evidence of a large infarction or a hemorrhage should delay elective carotid stenting for at least 6 weeks. Bovine or tortuous arches with ostial stenoses, inability to tolerate even temporary anticoagulation, severely tortuous carotid arteries, and poor routes of peripheral access (due to severe peripheral vascular disease) are vascular characteristics that may make CEA a more desirable option. Conversely, patients who have restenosis after a previous endarterectomy, contralateral carotid occlusion, a carotid bifurcation at the level of C2 or higher, dissecting lesions, or severe coronary artery disease, or have undergone radiation therapy to the neck may be more likely to derive greater benefit from stenting. In a study by Lopes and associates,[135] the rate of stroke after stenting and delayed coronary artery bypass surgery was 11%. This stroke rate was lower than that for CEA and coronary bypass surgery performed either simultaneously or sequentially.[136]

In a study of symptomatic and asymptomatic patients with carotid restenosis, treated by stenting, the overall 30-day stroke and death rate was 3.7%.[137] The minor stroke rate was 1.7%, and the major nonfatal stroke rate was 0.8%. The 3-year stroke-free rate was 96%. Another advantage of an endovascular approach in the setting of postsurgical restenosis is the lower incidence of cranial nerve palsies, which can be as high as 10% after CEA for restenosis.[138]

In a cohort of 62 high-risk patients with risk factors such as previous CEA, age greater than 80 years, previous neck irradiation, coronary artery disease, and significant contralateral carotid artery disease, carotid stents were successfully implanted (69 procedures in 62 patients).[139] The major postprocedural complications were two minor strokes (2.9%), one major stroke (1.5%), and one fatal major stroke (1.5%).

As previously mentioned, several multicenter clinical trials are currently under way to investigate the efficacy of carotid stenting (with distal protection) compared with CEA, a time-tested procedure (Table 78.10).

Technical Advances

As carotid artery stenting continues to evolve, technology has become increasingly available to minimize stroke risk. Perhaps the most promising of the technological advances are distal protection with small, retrievable filters or balloons and techniques involving flow reversal. Examples are the PercuSurge Balloon (PercuSurge GuardWire, Medtronic AVE, Santa Rosa, CA), EPI Filterwire (Boston Scientific Embolic Protection Inc, Santa Clara, CA) (Fig. 78–7), and ACCUNET Embolic Protection System (Guidant, Indianapolis, IN).

Table 78.10 Summary of Carotid Stent Trials

Study (Manufacturer or Sponsor)	Design	Clinical Characteristics and Percentage of Stenosis	Stent	Distal Protection Device
ARCHER (Guidant)	Prospective single-arm registry	High-risk Asymptomatic, >80% Symptomatic, >50%	Acculink	Accunet
BEACH (Boston Scientific)	Prospective single-arm registry	High risk Asymptomatic, >80% Symptomatic, >50%	Monorail Wallstent	EPI Filterwire
CABERNET (Boston Scientific and EndoTex)	Prospective single-arm registry	High-risk Asymptomatic, >60% Symptomatic, >50%	NexStent	EPI Filterwire
CARESS (NIH) (excludes CREST patients)	Prospective double-arm registry; physician chooses treatment— 2:1 CEA:CAAS	Asymptomatic, >75% Symptomatic, >50%	Physician's choice	Physician's choice
CREST (NIH, Guidant)	Randomized trial	Symptomatic, >50% stenosis	Acculink	Accunet
MAVEriC (Medtronic AVE)	Prospective single-arm registry	High risk Asymptomatic, >80% Symptomatic, >50%	Maverick	PercuSurge
SAPPHIRE (Cordis)	Prospective registry alongside a randomized trial	High risk (age >80 yrs alone qualifies) Asymptomatic, >80% Symptomatic, >50%	Precise	Angioguard

ARCHER, Acculink for Revascularization of Carotids in High-Risk Patients; BEACH, Boston Scientific EPI: A Carotid Stent for High-Risk Surgical Patients; CAAS, carotid artery angioplasty and stenting; CABERNET, Carotid Artery Revascularization using Boston Scientific EPI Filterwire and EndoTex Stent; CARESS, Carotid Revascularization with Endarterectomy or Stenting Systems; CEA, carotid endarterectomy; CREST, Carotid Revascularization Endarterectomy vs. Stent Trial; MAVEriC, Evaluation of the Medtronic AVE Self-expanding Carotid Stent System with Distal Protection in the Treatment of Carotid Stenosis; NIH, National Institutes of Health; SAPPHIRE, Stenting and Angioplasty with Protection in Patients at High Risk for Endarterectomy.

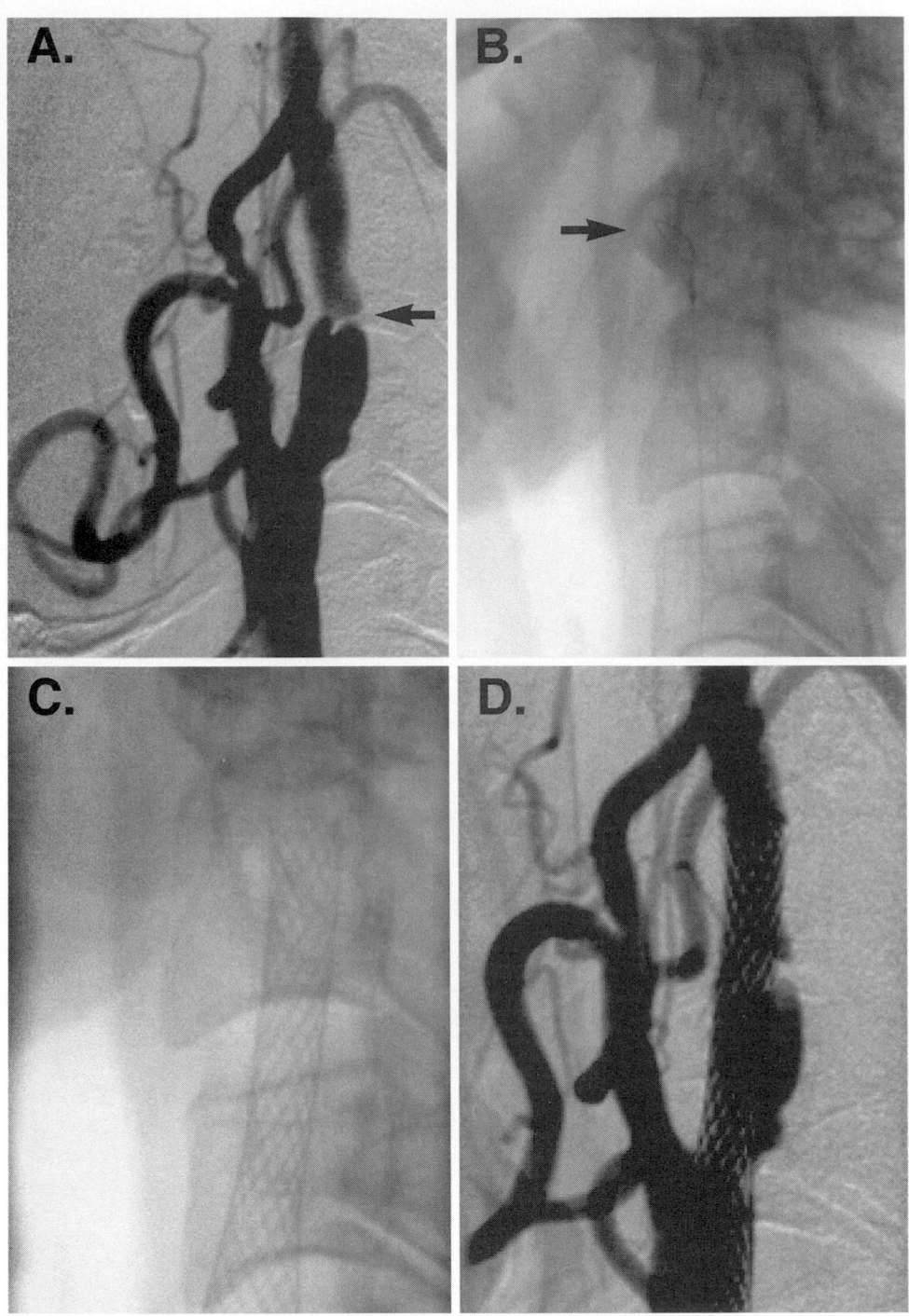

FIGURE 78–7 A, *Lateral angiogram demonstrating focal, ulcerated stenosis of the ICA at the distal portion of the carotid bulb. B and C, Unsubstracted lateral views demonstrating the EPI Filterwire (Boston Scientific Embolic Protection Inc, Santa Clara, CA) in the ICA at the level of C1 (B), and the carotid stent following post-deployment dilatation (C). D, Lateral view demonstrating successful revascularization of the ICA.*

Although the periprocedural incidence of neurologic events is 5% to 9%, the incidence of embolic debris during carotid angioplasty and stent placement is substantially higher at 80% to 90%.[132–134,140–147] The routine use of distal protection devices (available only for patients enrolled in clinical trials in which these devices are being evaluated; see Table 78.10) has demonstrated a 0 to 2% reduction in stroke rates. The protection device should be in place before stent deployment, as this approach has been shown to result in capture of the largest amount of embolic debris (versus at the time when the lesion is predilated and crossed with a wire).[140–143,146,148–150] Clearly, some patients have high-grade stenoses that preclude the passage of high-profile distal protection devices before predilation with an angioplasty balloon. In a review of 14 studies in which stents were placed to treat carotid artery stenosis, 73 (8.8%) of 834 patients had thromboembolic complications, 26 of which were TIAs and 47 (5.6%) were strokes, thereby demonstrating the clinical need for distal protection to prevent emboli.[59] As protection devices decrease in size, there will be fewer lesions that will produce the passage of these devices prior to predilation.

Several centers have described their techniques for carotid stent placement. It is often said that good judgment comes from experience and experience from poor judgment. On the basis of experience from more than 700 carotid artery stenting procedures, our group developed some techniques that maximize procedural success while minimizing morbidity. The following technical points focus on stenting in the setting of irregular or complex anatomy, thus describing techniques that may avoid pitfalls that lead to common complications.

Tortuous aortic arches often pose significant challenges for maneuvering stents into the cervical carotid circulation. Without proper stabilization of the stent delivery device, interventionists often lose position of the catheter and wire, potentially resulting in vessel injury. Techniques for straightening significant tortuosity or stabilizing guide catheters in bovine or wide arches include the use of "vascular scaffolding." Difficult arches can be navigated by temporarily docking a guide sheath in the aortic arch and placing a stabilizing wire in the distal external carotid artery. The guide sheath and obturator are then advanced over this construct, proximal to the carotid artery lesion. A stabilizing, or "buddy," wire may be left in place in the external carotid artery while crossing the stenosis with a 0.014-inch wire in the internal carotid lesion.

Difficulty often arises in the setting of absence or disease of external carotid arteries. In this setting, the insertion of a 6F sidewinder catheter (100 cm or longer) into the common carotid artery may provide sufficient support for subsequent advancement of the guide sheath over the catheter without wire assistance. As a last resort, or in the setting of tandem lesions involving the ostium of the common carotid artery, the guide sheath may be left in the aortic arch, and a stent can be navigated over a wire. Another situation for which stenting from the arch is an option is when the guide catheter has induced flow arrest, which can result from excessive straightening of tortuous anatomy.

ACUTE CAROTID OCCLUSION

Treatment of acute ICA occlusion has been reviewed previously by Meyer and colleagues.[151] Although most of the patients in this review did not experience good neurologic recovery initially after emergency CEA, 26.5% of patients had normal neurologic findings and 11.8% had minimal deficit at follow-up evaluations. Although this series reported a mortality rate of 21%, a mortality rate of 42% was reported in a joint study involving a series of 50 patients who underwent CEA for acute carotid occlusion.[152]

Endovascular therapy is an emerging technique for the treatment of symptomatic, acute occlusion of the ICA (rates of recanalization and hemorrhage are discussed elsewhere in this chapter). Uno and associates[153] have reported promising results with the use of a combination of surgical and endovascular techniques to recanalize acutely occluded carotid arteries. Our group has used microcatheter techniques for opening acute carotid occlusions. After identification of the occlusion by diagnostic angiography, intra-arterial thrombolytic agents (such as reteplase)

may be given. If this therapy fails to completely recanalize the vessel, a microwire may be used to cross the occlusion. Often, the occlusion is tenacious, and a microwire does not have enough stiffness to be navigated through the clot. In this situation, an exchange-length 0.035-inch wire is used to cross the thrombotic occlusion. One must be careful because often there is an underlying severe stenosis (caused by atherosclerosis) that led to the acute thrombotic occlusion. Contrast material should be injected liberally in an attempt to identify the parent vessel lumen distal to the occlusion once a microcatheter has successfully been negotiated distal to this occlusion.[39]

The presence of intracranial tandem embolic occlusions portends a poor outcome for treatment of cervical carotid occlusion with CEA. However, one group reported improvement in four patients with concomitant occlusions after cervical and intracranial intra-arterial thrombolysis with urokinase infusion and mechanical clot disruption.[39] More thrombolytic agent may be infused into the thrombus if diagnostic angiography shows clot burden surrounding the catheter. Once the catheter has traversed the thrombus and is in the true lumen of the parent vessel (distal to the thrombus), mechanical thrombolysis may be used. At this point, the 0.035-inch wire is exchanged for a 0.014-inch wire, and measurements are obtained to determine the caliber of the parent vessel lumen. Unlike in coronary revascularization, one should not liberally oversize the balloons used for carotid revascularization. Techniques used to revascularize acutely occluded cervical carotid arteries include stent-assisted angioplasty of the carotid artery and angioplasty alone in the region of the thrombus.

Once the cervical carotid artery has been successfully opened, careful superselective angiography of the intracranial vasculature, ipsilateral to the lesion, must be completed. Full attention must be paid to the second- and third-order branches of the middle cerebral and anterior cerebral arteries, because branch occlusions may have resulted from distal vessel embolization. Most patients undergoing the procedure are treated after the induction of general anesthesia, so careful evaluation of the angiographic images is crucial to appreciation of subtle occlusion resulting from cervical carotid emboli.

ENDOVASCULAR MANAGEMENT OF DISSECTIONS

Traumatic Carotid Dissections

Dissection of the cervical and intracranial arteries occurs after disruption of the intima and media of the vessel wall. Such disruption typically results in hemorrhage into the vessel wall and subsequent reduction in the true lumen diameter of the native vessel, in turn potentially occluding the vessel.[154] Although several disorders of collagen and vessel wall composition produce a higher incidence of vessel dissection, one of the most common causes of vessel dissection is craniocervical traumatic injury. In a series of 2000 traumatic head injuries, the incidence of carotid injury was 0.5%.[155] Given the incidence of more than 1.5 million traumatic head injuries annually, there is likely a substantial patient population with traumatic arterial lesions potentially resulting in stroke.[156] The incidence of carotid dissection has been reported to be 2.6 per 100,000 persons.[157] Dissections have been reported to be responsible for 20% of strokes in patients younger than 30 years,[158] with neurologic mortality ranging from 20% to 40% and morbidity as high as 80%.[156] It is interesting to note that traumatic lesions to the carotid artery are often missed, because less than half of the patients have cutaneous manifestations and often, a plethora of other severe injuries complicate the diagnosis.[159]

Patients with acute dissection typically present with symptoms related to ischemia or thromboembolic complications. Carotid dissections may cause visual scotoma, contralateral hemiparesis and hypesthesia, or aphasia (with left hemispheric events). Additionally, a Horner's syndrome (miosis, ptosis, and anhidrosis) may occur ipsilateral to the dissection as a result of damage to the sympathetic nerve fibers. Often a partial Horner's syndrome, without anhidrosis, is appreciated because the dissection occurs distal to the common carotid artery bifurcation, usually at the C2–C3 vertebral level.[160] Although patients with dissections typically follow a benign course if the presenting symptoms are localized to headache or neck pain, 15% may progress to severe morbidity or death.[160] Vertebrobasilar artery dissections, which may accompany traumatic carotid dissections, often result in temporary loss of consciousness, cranial nerve palsies, vertigo, or bilateral motor-sensory dysfunction.

Endovascular Treatment of Dissections

Before endovascular techniques were routinely used for the treatment of arterial dissections, medical and surgical modalities were employed to treat symptomatic patients. Medical management involved anticoagulation therapy with warfarin, and surgical options were reserved for patients who had persistent neurologic problems despite anticoagulation therapy. These surgical approaches clearly depended on the sequelae of the dissection. For ischemic symptoms referable to severe residual arterial stenosis resulting from a healed dissection, EC-IC bypass surgery was performed to augment blood flow to a hypoperfused region. Bypass grafting in conjunction with vessel sacrifice was a treatment option in the setting of persistent emboli from dissecting aneurysms.[161,162] In a review of 96 patients, 86% of the patients managed without surgery did poorly versus 53% of patients in the surgical group.[163]

As carotid artery stenting has become increasingly popular, use of this technology has been investigated for the treatment of symptomatic carotid and vertebral artery dissections. Liu and coworkers[164] report performing stent placement for symptomatic artery dissections in seven patients; all seven patients remained symptom free during the follow-up period (average, 3.5 years). Malek and associates[154] described similar findings in a cohort of 10 patients with carotid dissection. Interestingly, this group was able to use multiple overlapping stents to recanalize acute vessel occlusions or "string signs" resulting from severe dissections.

Endovascular salvage procedures have been described for iatrogenic intracranial and extracranial dissections. The frequency of these lesions is likely to rise as more clinicians routinely practice intracranial interventional techniques.

In a review of more than 3000 neurointerventional and diagnostic procedures involving the intracranial circulation, Cloft and colleagues[165] noted iatrogenic dissections in 0.4% of this cohort. These investigators found that the clinical course was benign for most patients with iatrogenic dissections of the carotid artery. On the contrary, another group found that dissections of the intracranial vertebral artery may result in significant neurologic morbidity such as Wallenberg's syndrome, isolated lower cranial neuropathy, Horner's syndrome, and hemisensory dysfunction.[166] In a paper by Dorros and associates,[167] intracranial carotid angioplasty was performed for a flow-limiting petrous carotid artery stenosis. After the angioplasty, the patient was noted to have a dissection that was treated with emergency deployment of a coronary stent. The patient remained asymptomatic without the need for warfarin therapy.

Dissecting aneurysms of the intracranial anterior and posterior circulation are associated with a high rate of recurrent hemorrhage and subsequent neurologic morbidity (Fig. 78–8). The reason for this poor prognosis is probably that these aneurysms occur after acute disruption of the integrity of the vessel wall, often resulting in a false aneurysm (recanalized thrombus). The incidence of vertebral artery dissecting aneurysms is difficult to determine, but some groups have reported rates from 20% to 40%.[168,169] In a report by Kurata and associates,[168] coil embolization was used to occlude dissecting aneurysms of vertebral arteries that had hemorrhaged. The patients treated had no further hemorrhages and good outcomes.

It is important to note that before a dissecting aneurysm of the intracranial vertebral artery is treated, balloon test occlusion is necessary to determine whether the patient can tolerate potential sacrifice of the parent vessel. Additionally, the location of the dissection in relation to the posterior inferior cerebellar artery must be noted, as must the caliber of the contralateral vertebral artery and the posterior communicating arteries and the presence of any vertebral origin disease. Often, anatomic constraints such as hypoplastic contralateral vertebral arteries and absence or small size of posterior communicating arteries may prevent vessel sacrifice of the dominant vertebral artery for treatment of a dissection. Thus, alternative interventions must be found for patients who continue to have symptoms referable to the dissecting vertebral artery aneurysm (usually from thromboembolic debris released from the pseudoaneurysm).

An emerging technology for the treatment of dissecting aneurysms (also discussed in the section on aneurysms) is the use of low-porosity stents (Fig. 78–9). Stents reconstitute the parent vessel lumen, divert the jet of blood away from the inflow zone, and attempt to reestablish laminar flow in the direction of the parent vessel.[170-175] Horowitz and colleagues[176] described the use of stents for the treatment of cervical and extracranial pseudoaneurysms. Our group has treated dissecting aneurysms in four patients with intravascular stents. Although excellent radiographic obliteration of the aneurysm was observed in two cases, the technique has some limitations. In one case, stent thrombosis and subsequent brainstem infarction developed nearly 3 months after treatment in a noncompliant patient with a history of cocaine abuse (Fig. 78–10).[177] We believe that the combination of not adhering to an antiplatelet

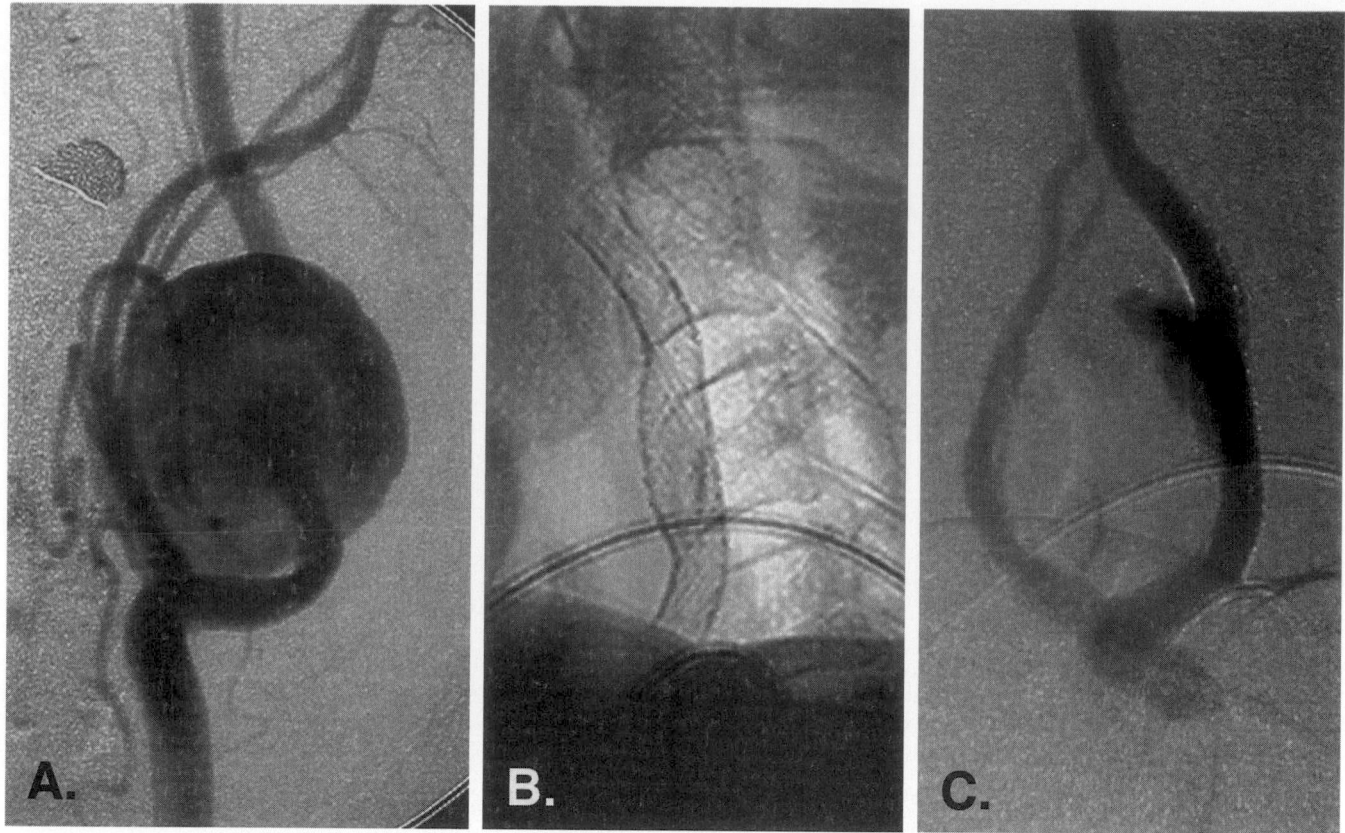

FIGURE 78–8 A, *Angiogram of the carotid artery demonstrating a giant dissecting aneurysm of the cervical ICA. B, Fluoroscopic view showing the carotid stent following successful deployment. C, Angiogram demonstrating immediate resolution of the aneurysm with a small amount of contrast outside the stent lumen (filling a small portion of the aneurysm).*

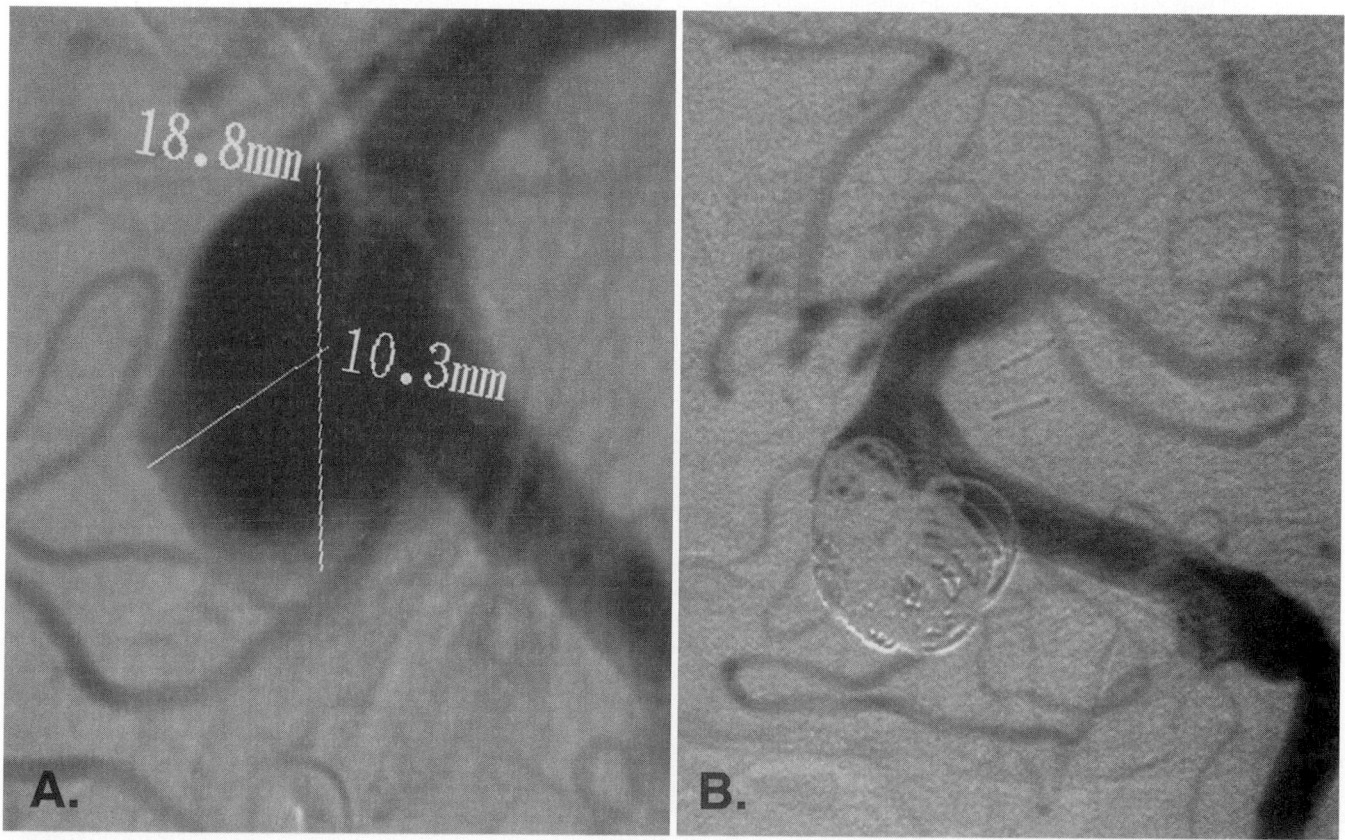

FIGURE 78–9 A, *High-magnification angiography demonstrating a dissection aneurysm of the vertebrobasilar junction. B, Angiogram showing reconstruction of the lumen of the vertebrobasilar junction following stenting and coiling of the aneurysm.*

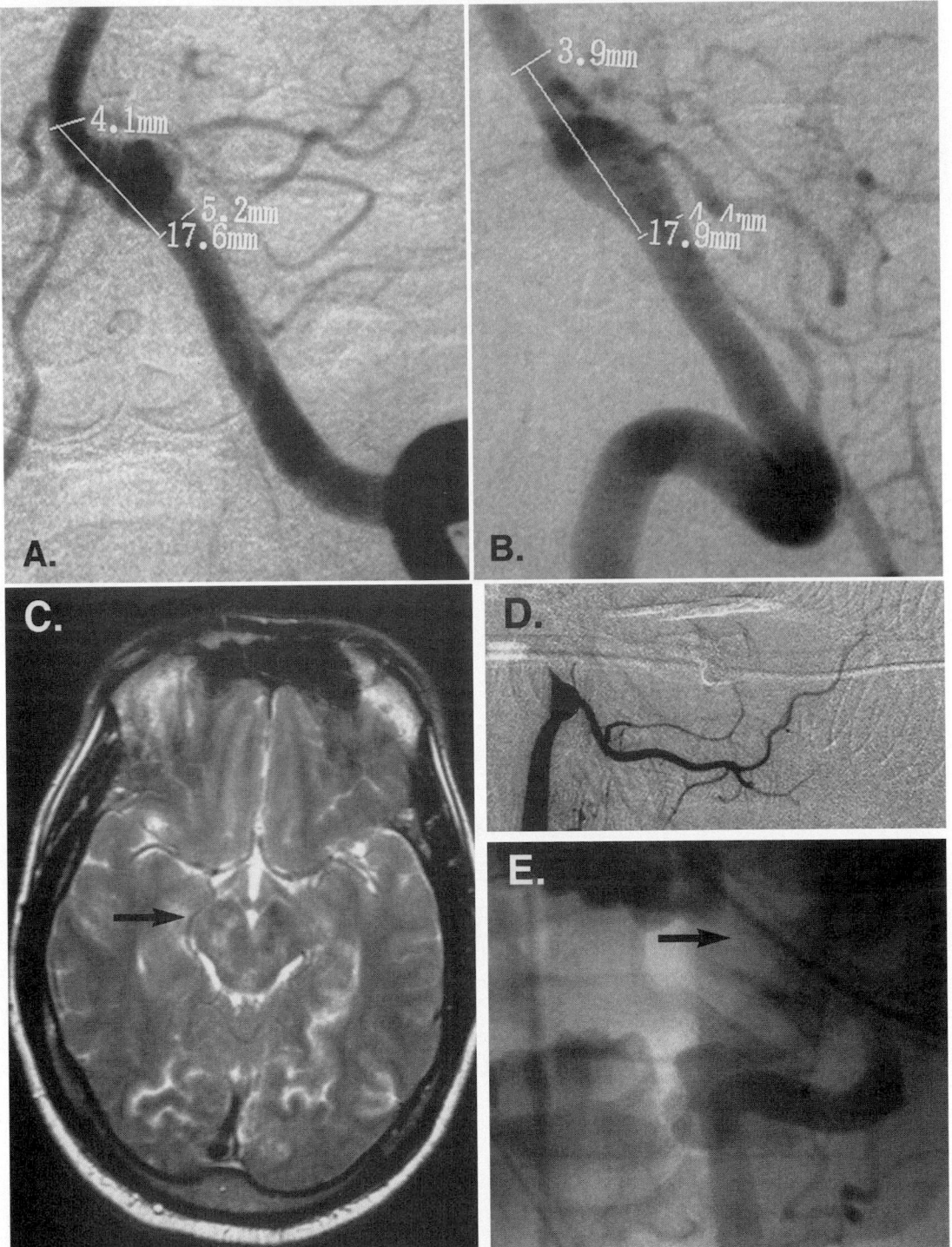

FIGURE 78–10   A, *AP and* B, *lateral views of a digital subtraction angiogram demonstrating a fusiform aneurysm, with measurements indicated along the parent vessel.* C, *Long-TR MR images demonstrating bilateral midbrain infarctions.* D, *Lateral digital subtraction angiogram demonstrating a VA occlusion in the region of a large occipital artery origin proximal to the cranial base.* E, *Unsubtracted angiogram demonstrating stasis and vessel occlusion several centimeters proximal to the stent. (From Levy EI, Boulos AS, Bendok BR, et al: Brainstem infarction following delayed thrombosis of a stented vertebral artery fusiform aneurysm: Case report. Neurosurgery 51:1284–1285, 2002.)*

regimen and ingesting cocaine (a potent platelet aggregator)[178] resulted in delayed onset of stent thrombosis.[177]

Another limitation of current stent technology involves the pliability of low-porosity stents. Low-porosity stents are advantageous in that they significantly reduce the inflow and outflow of blood, a feature that (theoretically) should lead to aneurysm thrombosis. Unfortunately, as porosity declines, the rigidity of the stent increases, lessening the likelihood of successfully navigating the stent through successive tortuosities. One approach to bypassing some of the extracranial vertebral tortuosities involves performing a cut-down on the vertebral artery at the craniocervical junction or at the C1–C2 vertebral level.[179] Once this region of the vertebral artery is adequately exposed, a sheath can be inserted into the vertebral artery. This surgical exposure allows the sheath to be inserted in close proximity to the target lesion, avoiding many tortuosities proximal to the insertion point. Thus, less mechanical energy is translated into the sheath, catheters, and stent delivery apparatus. Additionally, the ability to maneuver the stent may be improved by the mechanical advantage gained by inserting the sheath relatively near the dissection in the intracranial circulation. Meticulous surgical technique is essential to avoid infection, injury to the vertebral artery, iatrogenic dissection during sheath insertion, and loss of sheath position in the vessel. If the patient's anatomy precludes the delivery of a rigid, low-porosity stent, stent-assisted coiling may be used. Although this technique has been described by others for wide-necked or fusiform aneurysms of the posterior circulation, one must be careful when deploying coils in what may be a false lumen.[154,180–182] Techniques for stent-assisted coiling and stenting of the posterior circulation are described later (see aneurysm discussion).

EXTRACRANIAL VERTEBRAL ARTERY STENOSIS

Atherosclerotic occlusive disease of the extracranial vertebral artery, which is present in approximately 25% to 40% of the population, is an important cause of posterior circulation ischemia.[183,184] The V_1 (proximal) segment of the vertebral artery, extending from the origin of the artery at the subclavian artery to the entrance into the transverse vertebral foramen, is the most common site for atherosclerotic occlusive disease in the vertebral artery.[184] These ostial lesions can serve not only as embolic sources but also as flow-limiting stenoses that can produce posterior circulation ischemia. However, the natural history, clinical features, and optimal therapy for atherosclerotic lesions of the extracranial vertebral artery are not clearly defined, for multiple reasons. First, these lesions may not be well visualized by ultrasonography and may require digital subtraction angiography or MR angiography for definitive diagnosis. Second, symptoms of posterior circulation ischemia, such as dizziness and ataxia, may be misinterpreted as nonspecific symptoms, leading to misdiagnosis.[185,186] Third, no prospective randomized trial has been performed to determine which therapy is optimal for symptomatic stenosis of the extracranial vertebral artery. Surgery of these lesions is technically difficult and is associated with significant morbidity and mortality.[187] Medical

therapy, consisting of antiplatelet agents, systemic anticoagulation, avoidance of orthostatic hypotension, and elevation of mean arterial blood pressure, remains empiric. In the last decade, angioplasty with or without stenting has been performed as an alternative treatment for extracranial vertebral artery stenosis.[188–190] In this section, we discuss indications for these procedures along with associated technical features and success and complication rates.

Indications for Vertebral Artery Angioplasty and Stenting

We do not recommend routine performance of vertebral artery angioplasty with or without stenting for asymptomatic patients who have atherosclerotic stenosis of the extracranial vertebral artery. There are situations, however, in which angioplasty or stenting may be indicated for asymptomatic stenosis, such as for stenosis at the vertebral artery origin in a patient with a dominant or single vertebral artery. Further data are needed regarding the natural history of extracranial vertebral artery stenosis as well as the long-term durability of these procedures. Chastain and coworkers[191] reported uncomplicated angioplasty and stenting of extracranial vertebral artery stenosis in 11 asymptomatic patients. These patients were known to have poor intracranial collateral circulation. However, long-term angiographic and clinical follow-up is needed to determine the efficacy of these procedures in this select group of patients.

At this time, we recommend reserving angioplasty with or without stent placement for atherosclerotic extracranial vertebral artery stenosis in the patient whose symptoms do not respond to medical therapy. Angioplasty with or without stenting may be recommended instead of medical therapy for symptomatic patients who have physiologic evidence of hypoperfusion or in whom inadequate intracranial collateral flow is demonstrated by an imaging modality such as PET, SPECT, or XECT. Antiplatelet and anticoagulation therapies may reduce embolic events resulting from vertebral artery stenosis but are unlikely to augment flow distal to these lesions. Wityk and colleagues,[184] reviewing the clinical features and radiographic findings for patients with either occlusion or high-grade stenosis of the V_1 segment who were enrolled in the New England Medical Center Posterior Circulation Registry, found that 16% had TIAs resulting from hemodynamic instability. The advantages of a combination angioplasty and stenting procedure over angioplasty alone include prevention of elastic recoil and of early restenosis.

Technique

The basic principles of preprocedural treatment with antiplatelet medication, intraprocedural heparinization, and guide catheter placement for vertebral angioplasty and stenting are similar to those used for extracranial carotid and peripheral arterial interventions. Although femoral access is used for most cases, brachial or radial access can be used to perform vertebral artery angioplasty and stenting if femoral access is unavailable. Occasionally, the vertebral artery origin is angled to favor delivery of a stent from a brachial or radial approach. The stenotic lesion is typically crossed with a 0.014-inch guidewire and dilated with a slightly undersized, noncompliant balloon (inflated 3–3.5 mm) before stent placement. After angioplasty, a stent is deployed with guidance from the road-mapping function of the angiography unit. Post-stent angioplasty may be performed if residual stenosis is significant. Precise placement of the stent in the ostium of the vertebral artery requires multiple angiographic projections to visualize the ostium as the artery arises posteriorly and superiorly from the subclavian artery (Fig. 78–11). Poor placement of the stent may lead to inadequate coverage of the ostium, resulting in residual ostial stenosis or "watermelon seeding" (forced migration of the stent as a result of asymmetric pressure applied by the vessel onto the stent wall). Alternatively, too much overhang of the stent below the ostium and into the parent lumen may make access into the vertebral artery challenging for post-stent angioplasty.

Selection of the stent depends on the location and anatomy of the vertebral artery stenosis. In general, ostial lesions are prone to elastic recoil after angioplasty. As a result, a stent with adequate radial strength is required to achieve adequate dilation. Hand-mounted Palmaz stents (Johnson & Johnson Interventional Systems, Warren, NJ) and balloon-expandable stents have been used for ostial lesions. Newer flexible coronary stents are available. Lesions in the V_1 or V_2 segment (those located within the transverse foramina at the C1–C6 spinal levels) may be treated with balloon-expandable (Multi-Link Tetra, Guidant Inc, Indianapolis, IN) or self-expanding (Magic Wallstent, Boston Scientific Schneider, Minneapolis, MN) stents. Self-expanding stents should be used with caution for lesions involving the ostium because the exact length and placement of the stent cannot always be predicted. In the future, stents with a special coating (such as heparin, sirolimus, or paclitaxel) to reduce intimal hyperplasia and distal protection devices may play a role in the treatment of vertebral artery origin stenosis. At present, data are insufficient to determine their effectiveness in this setting.

Procedural Complications

Angioplasty and stenting for stenosis of the extracranial vertebral artery are associated with potential complications such as transient arterial spasm, dissection, rupture, occlusion, hemorrhage, stroke, and death, in addition to transient neurologic complications or TIAs. Angioplasty and stenting of the distal vertebral artery may be technically difficult because of the tortuous anatomy, especially in older patients with severe atherosclerotic stenosis. Spasm of the vertebral artery may be relieved by the removal of catheters or the administration of intra-arterial nitroglycerin. A flow-limiting, hemodynamically significant dissection resulting from angioplasty may have to be treated with a stent to avoid permanent occlusion and a potential thromboembolic event. Higashida and coworkers[192] reported an 8.8% occurrence of transient neurologic complications in 34 patients in whom proximal vertebral artery stenosis (>70% stenosis) was treated with angioplasty alone.

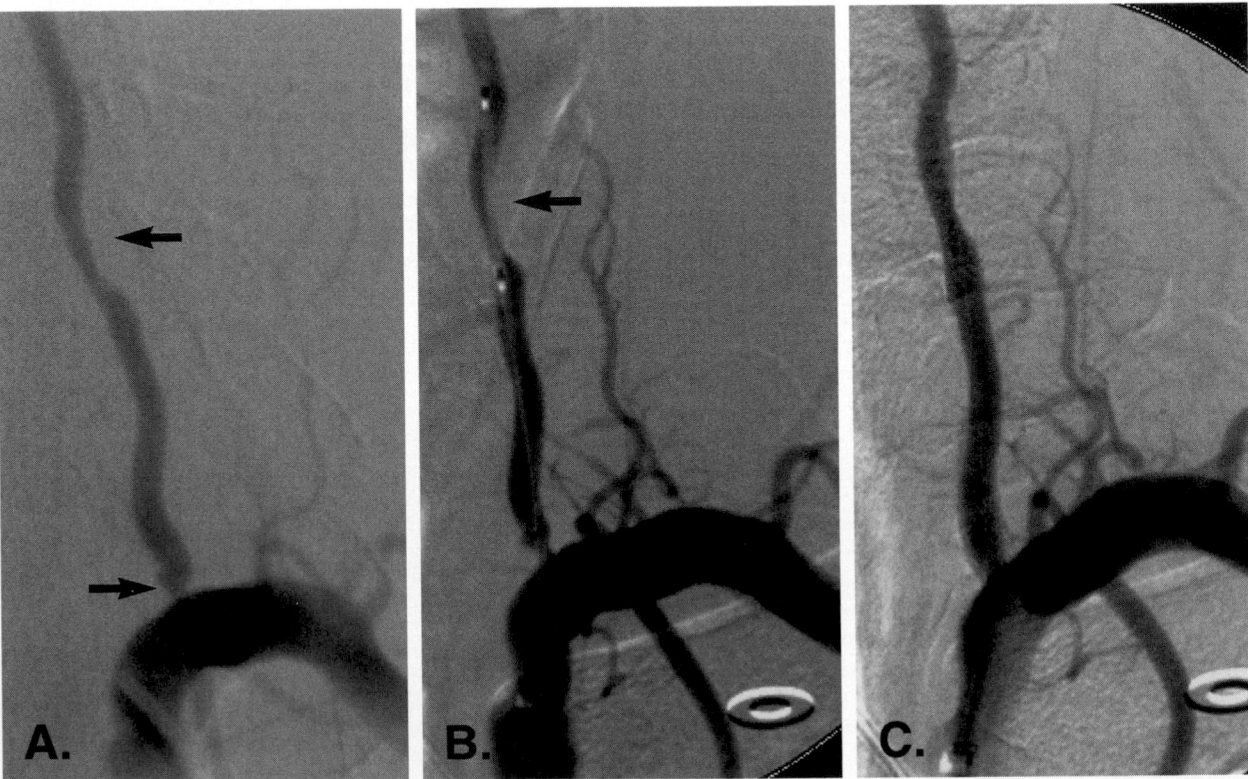

FIGURE 78–11   A, *AP view of the cervical VA demonstrating tandem stenosis at the VA origin and low vertical VA. B, Angiogram showing a stent being placed in the distal lesion. C, Cervical angiogram demonstrating recanalization of the VA origin and tandem stenosis following placement of a stent across each lesion.*

Table 78.11   Results of Vertebral Artery Angioplasty and Stenting for Extracranial Vertebral Artery Stenosis

Series[*]	No. of patients	Procedural Complications (% of Patients)	30-Day Morbidity and Mortality (% of Patients)	Mean Angiographic Follow-up (Months)	Restenosis (% of patients)[†]
Chastain et al (1999)[191†]	50	None	4	25 ± 10	10 (5 of 50 patients) at 6 months
Malek et al (1999)[193]	13	8 (1 of 13 patients) transient ischemic attacks	0	Unknown	Unknown
Piotin et al (2000)[196]	7	None	0	None	0 at mean 15 months
Mukherjee et al (2001)[195]	12	None	0	None	8 (1 of 12 patients) at 7 months
Jenkins et al (2001)[193]	32	3 (1 of 32 patients) transient ischemic attacks	0	None	3 (1 of 32 patients) at 3.5 months

[*]Superscript numbers indicate chapter references.
[†]Restenosis defined as >50% residual luminal stenosis.
[‡]Eleven of 50 patients had asymptomatic extracranial vertebral artery stenosis.

Rates of transient neurologic complications ranging from 3% to 8% have been reported for combination vertebral artery angioplasty and stenting (Table 78.11).[191,193–196] This complication is probably related to a thromboembolic event. Further studies are needed to assess the complications associated with these procedures.

Outcome

Before vertebral artery stenting was introduced, angioplasty alone for symptomatic stenosis of the extracranial vertebral artery was reported as a safe alternative to medical therapy. However, vertebral angioplasty has several limitations. First, an ostial stenosis can be very difficult to dilate adequately with angioplasty alone. In addition to immediate elastic recoil, an 8.8% rate of restenosis (defined as >50% residual luminal stenosis) within 2 to 5 months has been reported.[192] These data have encouraged the use of stents. Mukherjee and associates[195] reported symptomatic restenosis in 1 (8%) of 12 patients who underwent vertebral artery origin angioplasty and stenting. Although most studies report a significant benefit of vertebral angioplasty and stenting in alleviating symptoms of posterior circulation ischemia, the series are small, retrospective, and nonrandomized. Many of these studies lack long-term clinical and angiographic evaluations. More studies are required to evaluate the efficacy of these procedures.

Morbidity and Mortality

In one of the largest series of angioplasty for extracranial vertebral artery stenosis, Higashida and coworkers[192] reported a 5% mortality (2 of 38 patients; 1 death within 30 days). The two deaths were related to angioplasty of stenotic lesions of the vertebral artery located between the C1 and C3 spinal levels. In one case, vessel occlusion leading to stroke resulted in death; in the other, vessel rupture resulted in death several months later. In one of the largest series of combination angioplasty and stenting, Chastain and colleagues[191] reported a 2% rate for both 30-day mortality and morbidity in 50 patients. One patient had

a major stroke during a coronary angiogram 4 days after vertebral artery revascularization. Another patient died of MI 19 days after the procedure. Although these series are small, they suggest that combination angioplasty and stenting of the vertebral artery is associated with low rates of morbidity and mortality and a reduction in the rates of posterior circulation strokes in the setting of medically refractory posterior circulation ischemia.

SUBCLAVIAN STEAL SYNDROME

In 1960, Contorni[197] reported the first angiographic demonstration of retrograde flow in the vertebral artery ipsilateral to a proximal subclavian artery stenosis in a neurologically asymptomatic patient. In 1961, Fisher[198] explained that subclavian artery stenosis or occlusion could result in reduction of blood flow to the arm, reversal of flow to the ipsilateral vertebral artery, and claudication or neurologic deficits of the arm when intracranial or extracranial collateral circulation is inadequate; he named this new vascular disease a "subclavian steal syndrome" (SSS). Since the inception of this term, the clinical significance and natural history of subclavian steal have evolved from those of a disease that is morbid with neurologic symptoms, including vertigo, syncope, ataxia, paresthesia, and motor or visual deficits, to those of a condition that is often asymptomatic.[199–205] Moreover, SSS, which until 1980 was treated surgically even in asymptomatic patients, is now considered for treatment only in patients who have symptoms. This syndrome is reported to occur in approximately 6% of patients who have an asymptomatic cervical bruit.[206] Over the last two decades, noninvasive imaging modalities, such as Doppler ultrasonography, MRI and MR angiography, and XECT have complemented angiography as investigative tools.[207,208] A variety of surgical treatments and complications have been reported for SSS over the past four decades.[209–212] Since Bachman and Kim[213] reported the first successful angioplasty for SSS in 1980, subclavian angioplasty with or without stenting has been performed as an alternative to surgery. In this section, we briefly review the endovascular management of SSS.

Indications

Contrary to earlier beliefs that most patients with SSS have symptoms, the subclavian steal alone is rarely a cause of posterior circulation ischemia.[214] The advancement of noninvasive imaging tools has contributed to better understanding of the natural history of a subclavian steal. Bornstein and Norris[215] reported a 2-year follow-up review of 32 patients with asymptomatic subclavian steal with no cerebrovascular event related to the steal. Moran and associates[216] studied 55 patients with SSS with Doppler ultrasonography over a mean follow-up period of 4.1 years, during which only 7.2% of patients experienced symptoms of vertebrobasilar ischemia. No posterior circulation strokes were reported. However, 18% of the patients had symptoms of anterior circulation ischemia or stroke. Hennerici and colleagues[217] reviewed the medical records of 324 patients in whom subclavian steal was detected on the basis of Doppler ultrasonography and reported symptoms of vertebrobasilar ischemia in only 5% of these patients.[217] The majority of patients (64%) were asymptomatic. The remainder had lateralizing hemispheric symptoms. These studies suggested that SSS might become symptomatic when there is hemodynamic insufficiency in the presence of coexisting severe carotid occlusive disease or inadequate intracranial collateralization. For these reasons, revascularization is not advocated for asymptomatic patients.

Subclavian angioplasty with or without stent placement may be indicated for symptomatic SSS in patients who have comorbid medical conditions that raise the risk of perioperative complications. No prospective, randomized study is available to compare the efficacy of surgical revascularization and endoluminal revascularization for SSS. The advantages of an endovascular approach include the avoidance of the complications of general anesthesia and surgery. The disadvantages of angioplasty with or without stenting include potential dissection, thrombosis, and embolization. The durability of patency after subclavian angioplasty is difficult to interpret because in most series, follow-up angiography has not been performed, the investigators having relied on Doppler ultrasonography. However, long-term patency after subclavian angioplasty alone for stenosis (ranging from 54% to 100% at 2 months to 5 years) appears superior to that for occlusion (<50% at 4 to 88 months of follow-up).[218-222]

In an attempt to improve upon the results of angioplasty, subclavian angioplasty–assisted stenting has been popularized for symptomatic subclavian steal and occlusive disease. Case series have reported minimal rates of complications and high rates of technical success.[223-226] However, functional outcome measures have not been consistently reported. Further studies are needed to evaluate the efficacy and long-term patency of angioplasty with stent placement for symptomatic subclavian steal.

Technique

Innovative techniques, such as insertion of a balloon into the ipsilateral vertebral artery with temporary occlusion of flow and the adjunctive use of thrombolytic agents before subclavian angioplasty and stent placement, have been used since the 1980s. The selection of the periprocedural anticoagulation regimen, anesthesia, vascular access approach, wires, guide catheters, balloons, and stents depends on the patient, the vascular disease, and the endovascular surgeon. We routinely start patients on therapy with 325 mg of aspirin and 75 mg of clopidogrel once daily 3 days before the procedure. A brachial or a femoral artery approach or a combination of the two approaches may be used to perform subclavian angioplasty or stent placement.

Typically, a 6F to 8F sheath (Cook guide sheath, Cook Inc.) is introduced at the femoral or brachial artery access site. Heparin is administered intravenously as a bolus to achieve an activated coagulation time above 250 and up to 300 seconds. Fluoroscopic guidance and road-mapping technique are used throughout the procedure. A 0.035-inch, angled hydrophilic guidewire (Glidewire, Boston Scientific MediTech, Watertown, MA) is inserted into a 5F angled diagnostic catheter (MediTech Boston Scientific). The guidewire-catheter complex is coaxially advanced into the sheath. The stenotic or occluded segment of the subclavian artery is crossed with the guidewire. In the case of balloon angioplasty alone, the angled catheter is removed; then a balloon catheter (diameter ranging from 6 to 10 mm, and length from 3 to 10 cm) is advanced over the guidewire, and angioplasty is performed. The pre-inflation diameter of the balloon should be 1 to 2 mm less than the diameter of the subclavian artery distal to the stenosis or occlusion. Such under-dilation may minimize significant arterial dissection or rupture. If significant (>30%) residual stenosis or occlusion is observed, a second angioplasty may be performed with a slightly larger balloon. Subclavian stenting can be performed at the same sitting if significant stenosis remains after the first or second angioplasty attempt, as long as the residual lumen is large enough to accommodate the stent (Fig. 78–12). In the case of subclavian occlusion, the lesion is crossed with the 0.035-inch guidewire and then the angled catheter; and the guidewire is exchanged for a 0.014- to 0.018-inch wire. Balloon angioplasty, stenting, or both can then be performed over the exchange guidewire.

For subclavian artery stenosis or occlusion near the origin of the vertebral artery, controversy exists as to how close to the vertebral artery origin an angioplasty can be safely performed. Vitek[227] reported no complications with subclavian angioplasty across the vertebral artery origin in 50% of 35 subclavian artery angioplasties but cautioned that angioplasty might be unsafe when the lesion involves the vertebral artery origin.

A variety of balloon-expandable (e.g., Palmaz stent [Johnson & Johnson]) and self-expanding (e.g., Wallstent, Boston Scientific Schneider, Minneapolis, MN) stents are available for subclavian stenting. The selection of the stent depends on the size of the adjacent normal artery and the characteristics (length, calcification) and location of the lesion. A self-expanding stent, such as the Wallstent, may be used for a noncalcified long lesion. However, there are limitations with the Wallstent. The maximal diameter of this stent is 10 mm, which would not be suitable for a subclavian artery with a normal diameter of more than 10 mm. In addition, the length of a fully deployed Wallstent cannot always be accurately predicted. Accuracy is important,

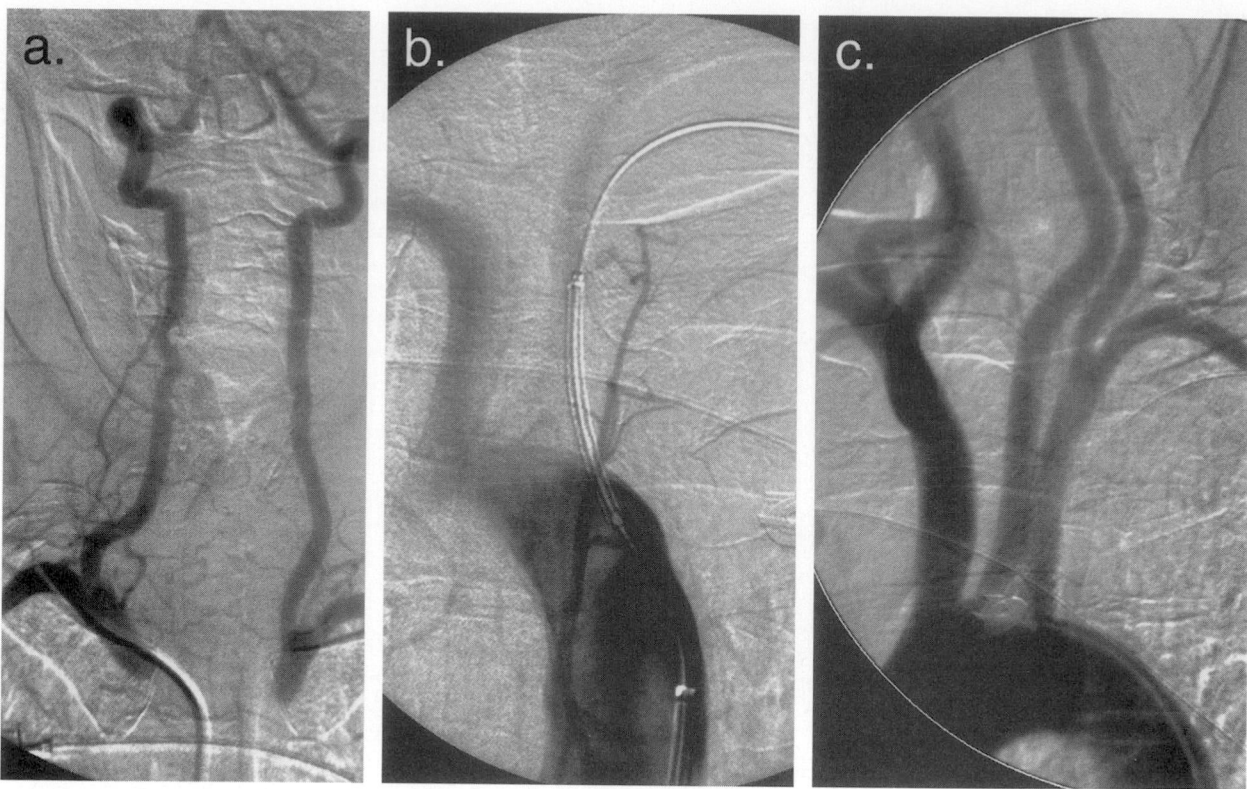

FIGURE 78–12   A, *Right subclavian artery angiography shows retrograde filling of the left vertebral artery (VA) resulting from occlusion of the left subclavian artery proximal to the origin of the left VA. B, Angioplasty is performed over a 0.035-inch glidewire in the left subclavian artery. C, After placement of a 38-mm MEGALINK stent (Guidant Inc.) in the left subclavian artery, angiography reveals anterograde filling of the left VA.*

especially in the ostial lesions off the aortic arch, because a malpositioned stent may protrude into the aortic arch or may completely bypass the ostial lesion. Thus, an ostial lesion may be better treated with a balloon-expandable stent, such as a Palmaz stent, or a self-expanding stent that has more predictable length when deployed, such as the S.M.A.R.T. stent (Cordis Neurovascular, Miami Lakes, FL). Post-stent angioplasty may be performed within the stent if significant residual stenosis remains. Angiography is performed after each angioplasty and stent placement. After the procedure, patients are prescribed 75 mg of clopidogrel daily for 1 month and 325 mg of aspirin for an indefinite period.

Procedural Complications

The main procedural complications associated with subclavian angioplasty and stenting are hematoma, pseudoaneurysm, and thrombosis at the access site; distal arterial emboli; and arterial dissection. The incidence of these complications ranges from 0 to 11.4%.[218–226] Failure to recanalize an occluded subclavian artery is frequently observed with angioplasty alone; early reocclusion rates as high as 13% have been reported.[228] As a result, subclavian artery stenting for the treatment of occlusions has been evaluated at several institutions. Although many series have reported small numbers of cases, initial success rates as high as 100% and asymptomatic and symptomatic

restenosis (>50%) rates of 7% and 3%, respectively, at 1 year have been reported.[218–226]

Morbidity and Mortality

Rodriguez-Lopez and associates[225] reported a 3% incidence of postprocedural TIA in 37 patients after treatment with percutaneous balloon angioplasty and stenting of subclavian artery stenosis.[225] In the occlusion group (15 of 37 patients), no postprocedural cerebrovascular events or deaths occurred. Ringelstein and Zeumer[229] reported that a delay in the reversal of vertebral artery blood flow after percutaneous balloon angioplasty may account for such low rates of neurologic complications. Follow-up ultrasonography in these patients at 9 months showed no restenosis in the occlusion group. Additional studies are needed to determine the long-term morbidity and mortality of subclavian artery stenting for SSS.

SSS is often associated with extracranial atherosclerotic disease. The subclavian steal becomes symptomatic when there is inadequate intracranial collateralization via the circle of Willis. Subclavian angioplasty or stenting is an alternative treatment option for patients with SSS who are at increased risk for surgery because of their medical comorbidities. In cases of subclavian stenosis, percutaneous angioplasty with or without stent placement appears to be safe and feasible. However, for cases of subclavian occlusion or stenosis that are refractory to angioplasty, stenting appears to be a promising method. Further study is needed to evaluate the durability of these procedures.

INTRACRANIAL ANEURYSMS

Epidemiology and Natural History

The epidemiology and natural history of cerebral aneurysms have been the subject of debate.[230] In two autopsy studies, the prevalence of cerebral aneurysms was 2.1%.[231,232] In one of these studies, 1.7% of the aneurysms were ruptured and 0.4% were unruptured.[231] Approximately 30,000 Americans are afflicted with aneurysmal subarachnoid hemorrhage (SAH) yearly.[230] The incidence of SAH has been reported to be between 6 and 16 per 100,000 persons in the United States, with higher numbers reported from Japan and Finland.[230,233–235] Aneurysmal SAH accounts for 25% of cerebrovascular deaths and 8% of all strokes.[236]

In terms of natural history, ruptured and unruptured aneurysms carry significantly different risks. The risk of rupture has also been shown to be a function of aneurysm size and tobacco consumption.[237,238] Although the natural history of ruptured aneurysms has been well defined, there is controversy regarding the natural history of unruptured aneurysms, particularly those less than 10 mm in diameter.[230,237] We refer the reader to recent scholarly reviews of these issues by Weir[230] and by the investigators of the International Study of Unruptured Intracranial Aneurysms.[237]

The most common complication of cerebral aneurysm is SAH.[239] Other complications are cranial nerve deficits, symptoms related to mass effect,[240] and strokes related to emboli released from thrombus within the aneurysm.[241] We briefly review the salient points of each of these consequences.

Subarachnoid Hemorrhage

Modern management of patients with SAH in the critical care unit, along with specialized microsurgical and endovascular expertise, contribute significantly to the prevention of recurrent hemorrhage and stroke after aneurysm rupture. Of paramount concern is the prevention of rehemorrhage because it is associated with a case-fatality rate of 70%.[242] Juvela[243] reported a 22.5% incidence of aneurysm rebleeding within 6 months of the primary hemorrhage in 236 untreated patients. Aneurysm coiling results in a significant reduction in the incidence of rehemorrhage. In the series reported by Vinuela and associates,[244] 97.8% of 403 ruptured aneurysms did not rebleed within 6 months of the primary hemorrhage (rehemorrhage occurred in 9 patients in whom aneurysms were incompletely coiled).

In addition to the morbidity associated with the initial hemorrhage, SAH can result in vasospasm, which can be neurologically detrimental. Reducing the morbidity associated with vasospasm is one of the opportunities to reduce the morbidity and mortality of SAH. Angiography shows vasospasm in 70% of patients with SAH; of these patients, approximately 50% have symptoms.[245] Approximately 20% of symptomatic patients experience stroke or die despite maximal modern therapy.[245] Angiographically evident

vasospasm usually peaks during days 5 to 14 after hemorrhage.[242] Hypertension and hypervolemia have emerged as the first line of therapy for symptomatic vasospasm.[246] Intra-arterial administration of papaverine and balloon angioplasty have been used with some success to treat medically refractory vasospasm.[239] Balloon angioplasty can be used for proximal vessel spasm of the supraclinoid carotid artery, A_1 segment of the ICA, M_1 segment of the MCA, vertebral artery, or basilar artery.[247] Balloon angioplasty can be associated with vessel rupture if not performed carefully with avoidance of overdilation. Improvements in balloon technology may reduce this risk. It has been observed that balloon angioplasty can permanently relieve vasospasm symptoms in 60% to 70% of cases.[247] Papaverine can be used for distal vessel spasm.[248–250] Initial enthusiasm for intra-arterial papaverine has waned over the past several years, however, because it has been observed that the effects of papaverine are short lived.

Mass Effect

In a study by Malisch and coworkers,[240] in which the effect of coiling on symptoms related to the mass effect of aneurysms on cranial nerves was examined, symptoms resolved in 32% of patients and improved in 42%, with no change in 21% and worsening in 5%. It is believed that removing the pulsatility associated with an aneurysm after coiling may be responsible for symptom improvement.[240]

Ischemic Complications

A paucity of data exists with respect to the embolic risk associated with the presence of an aneurysm. Clot can accumulate in the fundus of an aneurysm as a result of flow stasis, particularly in a large aneurysm. In a study by Qureshi and colleagues,[241] complications associated with embolization from the aneurysm fundus occurred in 3.3% of patients presenting with an unruptured aneurysm. In this study, clipping of the aneurysm was associated with a low risk of symptom recurrence. It should be noted that the presence of clot in an aneurysm might be a risk factor for thromboembolic complications during aneurysm coiling.

Results and Technical Advances in Coil Treatment

Although the results of coil treatment of small aneurysms (diameter <12 mm) and aneurysms with small necks (<5 mm) appear to be promising, lesser degrees of success have been observed with aneurysms with larger diameters and wider necks.[251] Technical advances have occurred over the past several years to increase the success rate with coiling of large and wide-necked aneurysms. In the balloon-remodeling technique, which has been championed by Moret and associates,[252] more coils can be packed near the aneurysm neck because a balloon is inflated across the neck during coil placement (Fig. 78–13). The balloon is deflated after each coil is deployed to restore flow temporarily. Stent-assisted coiling appears to be another promising technique for certain wide-necked aneurysms (Fig. 78–14).[253] The stent serves as scaffolding across the aneurysm neck, which holds the coils within the aneurysm

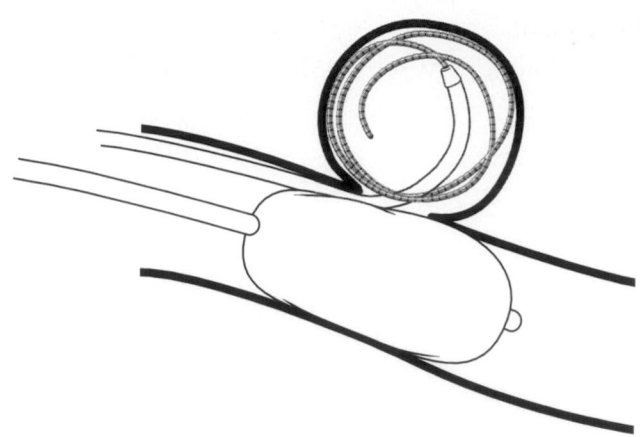

FIGURE 78-13   *Balloon-assisted aneurysm coiling.*

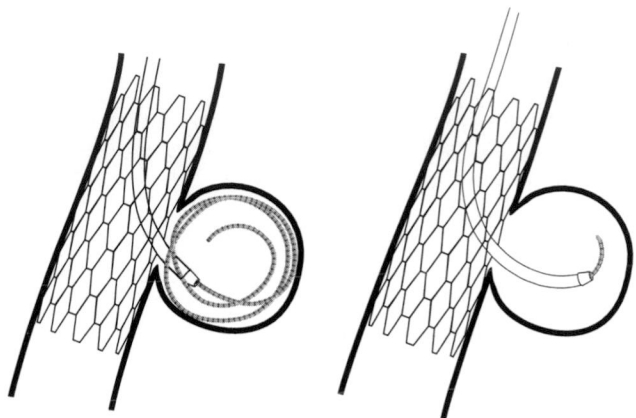

FIGURE 78-14   *Stent-assisted aneurysm coiling.*

sac. Manufacturers have improved coils in an attempt to overcome some of the shortcomings associated with coil technology. Spherical coils (MicruSphere coils, Micrus Corporation, Mountain View, CA) and three-dimensional Guglielmi detachable coils (Boston Scientific Target) appear to allow certain wide-necked aneurysms to be coiled more effectively.

Fusiform Aneurysms

Fusiform aneurysms can lead to mass effect, hemorrhage, or both. The outcomes for patients with fusiform aneurysms remain poor, despite advances in microsurgical and endovascular treatment techniques. The treatment of fusiform aneurysms often requires vessel sacrifice. Over the past several years, we have used stents to treat certain fusiform aneurysms. Stents offer the advantage of maintaining patency of the parent vessel. Preliminary results suggest that stents may play a significant role in the management of this complex disease.[255]

Dissecting Aneurysms

Dissecting aneurysms in patients who present with SAH have a poor natural history.[256] Surgical trapping is often

required to treat these aneurysms because parent vessel reconstruction can be hampered by damage from dissection of the vessel wall.[257] Endovascular occlusion may be an option when sacrifice of the parent vessel can be tolerated.[257] Stents may play a role in treating these rare lesions.

ARTERIOVENOUS MALFORMATIONS

Definition, Pathology, and Epidemiology

An AVM is a congenital lesion that anatomically consists of a collection of abnormal arteries and veins lacking a normal capillary connection. The abnormal arteries form a conglomeration of vessels, which are referred to as the *nidus*. The nidus typically has little to no intervening brain tissue. The lack of a capillary bed causes early venous drainage, venous hypertension, and recruitment of arterial feeders. True arteriovenous shunts are occasionally noted in AVMs. Autopsy data suggest that AVMs occur in 4.3% of the general population.[258] Between 1980 and 1990, the annual incidence of symptomatic AVMs in the Netherlands was 1.1 per 100,000 population.[259]

Aneurysms are the type of vascular lesions most commonly associated with AVMs. According to the literature, this association occurs in 2.7% to 23% of patients.[260,261] The four types of aneurysms observed in conjunction with AVMs are intranidal aneurysms, pedicular aneurysms, proximal aneurysms, and hemodynamically unrelated (Fig. 78-15). Evidence suggests that the first three types of aneurysms occur as a result of the flow dynamics created by the AVM.

Classification

Although multiple classification systems for AVMs have emerged, the Spetzler-Martin grading system has remained the simplest and most practical to use.[262] The system assigns AVMs to grades according to size, eloquence of surrounding brain, and presence or absence of deep venous drainage (Table 78.12). Increased surgical risk

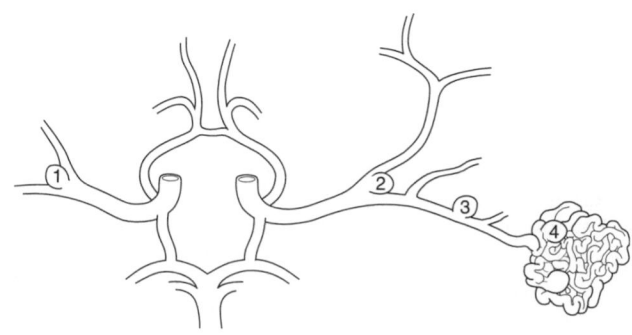

FIGURE 78-15   *The four types of aneurysm associated with AVMs: 1, a hemodynamically unrelated aneurysm; 2, proximal pedicle aneurysm; 3, distal pedicle aneurysm; 4, intranidal aneurysm. (From Bendok BR, Levy EI, Guterman LR, Hopkins LN: Pathophysiology of intracranial aneurysms and arteriovenous malformations and fistula. In Yadav JS [ed]: Textbook of Cerebrovascular Intervention. Philadelphia, Elsevier, in press.)*

Table 78.12   Spetzler-Martin Classification of Arteriovenous Malformations of the Brain*

Feature	Points Awarded
Size	
Small (<3 cm)	1
Medium (3–6 cm)	2
Large (>6 cm)	3
Eloquence of adjacent brain	
Noneloquent	0
Eloquent	1
Pattern of venous drainage	
Superficial only	0
Deep	1

*Grade = [size] + [eloquence] + [venous drainage]; that is [1, 2, or 3] + [0 or 1] + [0 or 1] Adapted from Spetzler RF, Martin NA: A proposed grading system for arteriovenous malformations. *J Neurosurg* 65:478, 1986.

is associated with higher AVM grade. The grading system was initially designed to assess the safety and risk of AVM excision but is used by most practitioners regardless of treatment modality. One study suggests, however, that this grading scheme may not have relevance to modern embolization strategies.[263]

Natural History

AVMs have been associated with seizures, hemorrhage, headaches, and ischemia related to steal (see previous discussion of subclavian steal). In children younger than 2 years, congestive heart failure and hydrocephalus are common presentations. For the purpose of this chapter, we focus on the hemorrhagic and ischemic manifestations of AVMs.

Stroke registries indicate that AVMs are responsible for the symptoms in more than 1% of patients who present with stroke.[264] The risk of AVM hemorrhage is approximately 2% to 3% per year.[258,265-268] Mortality from the first hemorrhage varies from 10% to 30%.[254] An estimated 10% to 20% of survivors have long-term disability.[254,268,269] Kondziolka and associates[270] proposed the following simplified equation to determine the hemorrhage risk in any given patient:

$$\text{Lifetime risk (\%)} = 105 - \text{patient's age (years)}$$

This equation helps put the risk of hemorrhage in perspective when considering patients of varying ages.

The risk of hemorrhage appears to rise during the first year after a hemorrhage. In two studies, the increase was 6%,[267,271] and in one study, 17.8%.[266] Certain radiologic findings appear to be associated with an increased risk of hemorrhage. Among these findings are central venous drainage, intranidal aneurysm, periventricular or intraventricular location, arterial supply via perforators, multiple aneurysms, vertebrobasilar supply, basal ganglia location, single draining vein, impaired venous drainage, and deep venous drainage alone.[254,272,273] Whether a history of AVM hemorrhage portends a higher risk for a second hemorrhage over the long term is controversial.[254,268]

Treatment

The treatment of AVMs has dramatically evolved within the past 30 years as a result of advances in microsurgery, endovascular techniques, and radiation therapy. The current broad treatment categories for AVMs are microsurgery alone, embolization followed by microsurgery, stereotactic irradiation alone, embolization followed by stereotactic irradiation, and embolization alone. For the purpose of this chapter, we focus on the endovascular embolization techniques and strategies used for AVM treatment. Embolization can play a role as a preoperative tool, as a pre–stereotactic irradiation tool, as sole therapy for a cure, as sole therapy for palliation, and to treat associated aneurysms.

Embolization as a Preoperative Tool

Microsurgery has been shown to be a safe and effective treatment for certain AVMs. The long-term protective effects of AVM surgery from hemorrhage risk have been established. In one study by Heros and colleagues,[274] excellent outcomes were achieved by surgery in 98.7% of patients with Spetzler-Martin grade I, II, or III AVMs at a mean follow-up of 3.8 years. Studies and empiric observations have suggested that AVM embolization reduces blood loss and enhances the ease of surgery.[275]

For large AVMs, embolization can achieve the goal of gradually decreasing the volume of the AVM before excision. Although it has never been proven, this strategy is believed to lower the risk of postoperative hemorrhage from normal perfusion pressure breakthrough.[276] According to the normal perfusion pressure breakthrough theory, the increased flow of blood through a large AVM deprives the surrounding brain tissue of adequate blood supply. This deprivation creates a chronic ischemic state and loss of autoregulation. When a large AVM is resected, the surrounding tissue, which was previously ischemic, becomes perfused by a larger blood flow. The lack of autoregulation makes the small vessels vulnerable to hemorrhage. Gradual embolization of these large AVMs is thought to allow the surrounding brain tissue to adjust to gradually increasing amounts of perfusion, hence reducing the risk of hemorrhage after eventual resection of the AVM. Endovascular techniques performed before surgery can also be used to treat an associated aneurysm, particularly if the aneurysm will be difficult to treat during surgical excision.

Embolization Followed by Stereotactic Irradiation

Radiosurgery has emerged as an attractive option for some AVMs, especially those located in surgically prohibitive locations such as the thalamus. Stereotactic technology allows the delivery of radiation precisely and directly to the AVM while limiting exposure of surrounding brain tissue. Radiosurgery results in a 78% to 88% obliteration rate at 3 years for AVMs with diameters equal to or less than 10 mm.[277] Lower obliteration rates and higher complication rates are associated with radiosurgery of larger AVMs. Over the past decade, several centers have reported on the strategy of embolization to reduce large AVMs to sizes amenable to radiosurgery.[278,279] This is an attractive strategy for large AVMs for which surgical excision poses a high risk. Long-term outcomes associated with this type of treatment have not yet been determined, and recanalization remains a concern.[279]

Embolization Alone

Only a small percentage of AVMs can be treated by endovascular techniques alone with current technology.[280] These AVMs are typically small (<3 cm) and have a limited number of arterial feeders (1 or 2).

Embolization for Palliation

Palliative embolization can be used in rare situations to decrease symptoms of large AVMs that are deemed untreatable by other means. Embolization can be used to reduce headaches and reversible neurologic deficits attributable to steal or venous hypertension. Embolization for palliation is only temporary, because the AVM can recur over time as a result of recanalization. No evidence exists that partial embolization of an AVM decreases the long-term risk of hemorrhage.[254]

Embolic Materials

Although a plethora of embolic materials have been reported over the past several decades, N-butyl cyanoacrylate (NBCA) is the agent used most commonly for embolization of cerebral AVMs. NBCA is a liquid adhesive embolic agent that has been found to be relatively safe and effective for this purpose.[275,281] In comparison with other embolic agents, NBCA has superior durability. Onyx Liquid Embolic System (Micro Therapeutics Inc, Irvine, CA) is currently being examined in a national trial as a potential embolic agent for AVMs.

Embolization Tools: Microcatheters and Microwires

Dramatic advances over the past two decades have significantly enhanced the safety and efficacy of AVM embolization. Two types of microcatheters are used to embolize AVMs, over-the-wire catheters and flow-guided catheters. The advantages of using over-the-wire catheters include the ability to precisely navigate the catheter to the target vessel. Disadvantages are the larger size compared with flow-guided catheters, and the need for a wire, which might perforate the fragile vessels near the nidus. Flow-guided catheters are smaller and softer than over-the-wire catheters. They are carried by the high flow toward the nidus. These catheters may be difficult to place in low-flow lesions, however.

The Future of AVM Embolization

Continued refinements in embolic materials, microcatheters, and microwires will likely enhance the ability to safely treat AVMs. Three-dimensional imaging will contribute to an improved understanding of AVM architecture. Moreover, it is possible that transvenous methods will be developed to treat the nidus.

TUMOR EMBOLIZATION

Patients with intracranial neoplasms may present with a variety of neurologic symptoms. These symptoms include cranial nerve palsies, hemiparesis, paresthesias, aphasias, abulia, akinetic mutism, and amnesia, all of which may result from the mass effect of the neoplasm. Paroxysmal onset of symptoms may result from tumor hemorrhage into the tumor bed or into adjacent parenchyma, leading to neurologic deficits.

Most intracranial tumor embolizations have been performed for neoplasms with robust vascular pedicles, such as meningiomas, hemangiopericytomas, and paragangliomas. The earliest reports of tumor embolization surfaced in 1974, when Hekster and colleagues[282] described the use of preoperative tumor embolization to reduce blood loss during subsequent resection. Later reports by others demonstrated the effectiveness of tumor embolization in the reduction of blood loss.[283–287] Intra-arterial therapies for recurrent and malignant brain neoplasms have also been reported.[288–292] Although the results of these studies show promise, especially in that chemotherapeutic agents can be delivered to tumor beds, thus sparing patients many of the systemic toxicities associated with the treatment, larger studies are needed. In a study by Kerber and associates,[293] patients with advanced squamous cell carcinoma of the head and neck were treated with intra-arterial cisplatin at a dose of 150 mg/m² weekly for 4 consecutive weeks. Thiosulfate was given intravenously as an antagonist to counteract systemic toxicity. This method of administering an antitumor drug directly into the lesion while protecting the kidneys and bone marrow from the agent's systemic effects resulted in the control of the carcinoma in more than 90% of the patients who were studied.[293]

Controversy remains regarding preoperative embolization of meningiomas. As modern surgical techniques and tools such as microscopy, electrocautery, and hemostatic agents enable surgeons to resect intracranial tumors with less difficulty, the utility of preoperative embolization of meningiomas is in question. There may be a role for preoperative embolization for patients in whom large tumor vessels and significant vascular blushing are demonstrated by angiography. Most meningiomas, however, are not sufficiently vascular to warrant the risk and expense of preoperative embolization. Most endovascular surgeons agree that the main indications for meningioma embolization are to reduce potential blood loss, to facilitate removal of the tumor (firm, fibrous meningiomas often develop the consistency of fish flesh once they become necrotic from compromised blood supply), and potentially shorten the operative time.

In a study by Bendszus and coworkers,[294,295] 60 patients were prospectively evaluated to determine the utility of preoperative meningioma embolization; 30 patients underwent tumor resection after embolization and the other 30 patients underwent tumor resection alone. The rates of surgical morbidity with permanent neurologic worsening were 16% in the embolization group and 20% in the nonembolization group. One patient (3%) sustained a permanent neurologic deficit caused by the embolization. Thus, the net complication rate in the group treated with preoperative embolization was 19%, which was similar to that of the group treated with surgery alone. The difference between the two groups was the lower intraoperative blood loss in patients in whom tumor embolizations were successful. According to another study, the optimal time for resection of meningiomas after embolization of at least 50% of tumor blood supply is approximately 7 to 9 days, after which tumor necrosis no longer increases.[296] Others have found that tumor necrosis is readily apparent 4 days after embolization and that no revascularization is noted 7 days after embolization.[297] Months after tumor embolization, however, revascularization is readily demonstrated by angiography and MRI.[297] Similar findings of complete tumor necrosis, demonstrated by proton spectroscopy, occur 4 days after meningioma embolization. Within 24 hours, however, lactate levels that are suggestive of necrosis may be appreciated.[298]

Several agents are currently used for tumor embolization. They are polyvinyl alcohol (PVA), absorbable gelatin sponge (Gelfoam), coils, alcohol, and trisacryl gelatin microspheres. The goal of embolization is to saturate the tumor's vascular bed with these agents, not simply to occlude large feeding arteries.[299] Thus, the choice and order of embolic agents used are important in the attempt to first saturate the fine network of vessels that supply the deepest regions of the tumor bed. Gelfoam powder, microspheres, and PVA are available in particle sizes as small as 50 μm and as large as 1 mm. Smaller particles should be used during the initial stages of pedicle emboliza-

tion because they can penetrate and occlude the fine, distal vasculature supplying the tumor bed. As these vessels become saturated with particles, larger particles can be used to embolize more proximal, and therefore larger, vessels supplying the tumor. We caution that smaller particles have an increased risk of penetrating distal branches of normal parenchyma if reflux occurs; larger particles cannot penetrate the tumor bed beyond the more proximal vessels. Some interventionists advocate the use of microspheres during the later stages of tumor embolization, which are less likely to occlude the catheter during slow injections because of their uniform nature (Fig. 78–16).[299]

Bendszus and coworkers[295] compared meningioma embolization using 150- to 300-μm trisacryl gelatin microspheres (n = 30, group 1), 45- to 150-μm PVA particles (n = 15, group 2), and 150- to 250-μm PVA particles (n = 15, group 3); they studied the inflammatory reaction, extent of necrosis, and distal migration (in the vascular tumor bed) of each embolic agent. The microspheres were located more distally in tumor vessels and resulted in less intraoperative blood loss than PVA particles of either size.

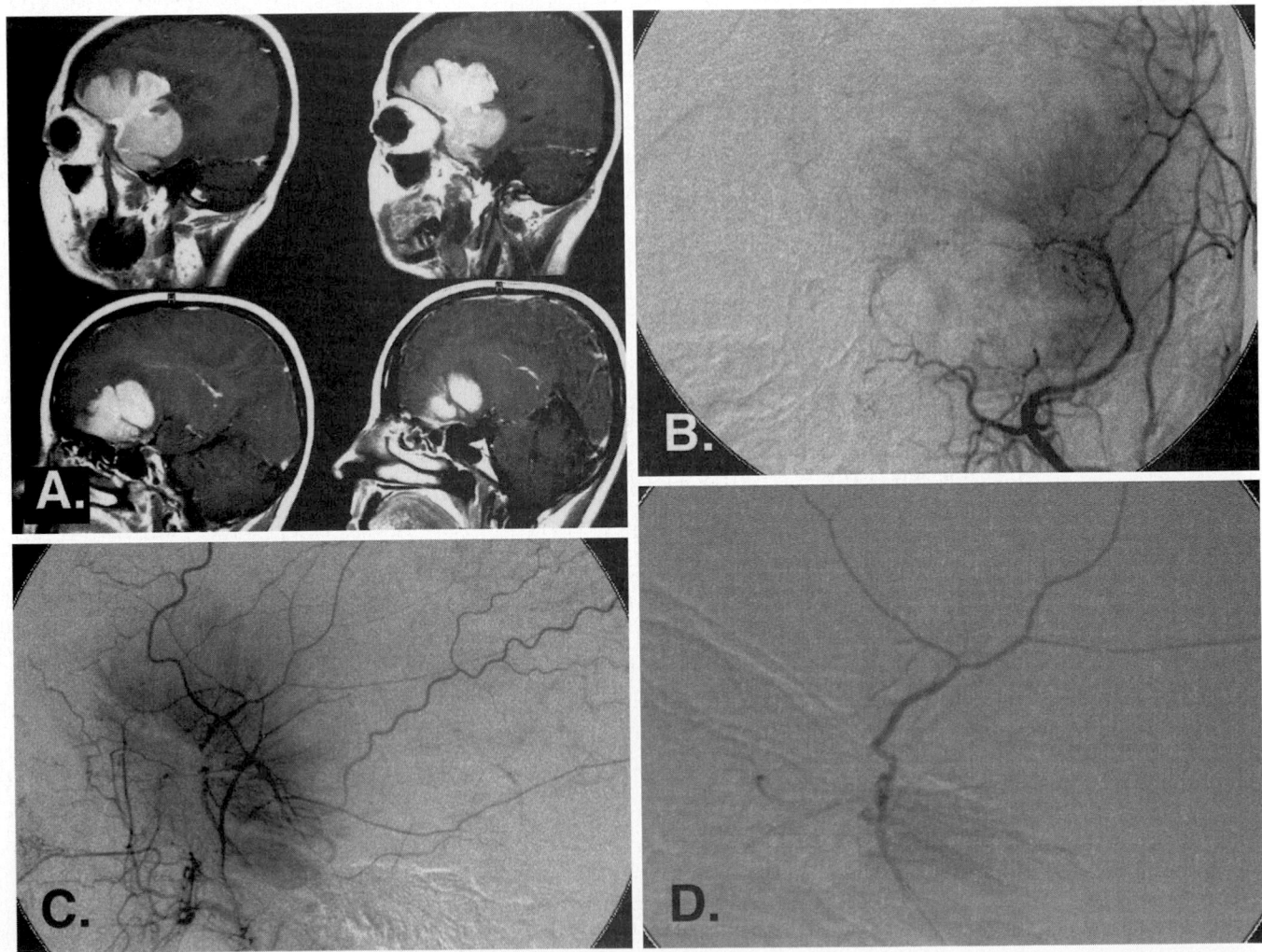

FIGURE 78–16   A, *MR imaging with contrast demonstrating a contrast-enhancing mass consistent with a sphenoid-wing meningioma.* B, *AP and* C, *lateral views showing a significant vascular blush of the tumor bed.* D, *Lateral angiographic view demonstrating near-complete resolution of the tumor blush following embolization with Embosphere microspheres (BioSphere Medical, Rockland, MA).*

Although liquid embolic agents (Fig. 78–17) such as alcohol have been used for tumor embolization, this technique is typically reserved for embolization of distal vessels unreachable by microcatheters. Typically, a balloon is inflated proximal to the microcatheter tip to prevent reflux of the alcohol. Usually, less than 5 mL are needed to attain the desired effects—intimal disruption, inflammation, and tumor necrosis.[299]

With the variety of agents used for embolization of meningiomas, complication rates range from 0 to 9%.[299] An uncommon but potentially devastating neurologic complication is peritumoral or intraluminal hemorrhage from acute changes in the tumor blood supply. Often, a partially embolized tumor may hemorrhage into the tumor capsule or into portions of necrotic tumor.[300] Other complications are the formation of iatrogenic fistulas, such as carotid-cavernous fistulae after vessel perforations.[301] Infarctions to the retina or parenchyma tend to occur when anastomoses between the external and internal carotid arteries are poorly appreciated. Such anastomoses occur between the middle meningeal artery and the ophthalmic artery, between the ascending pharyngeal artery and the vertebral artery, between the occipital artery and the vertebral artery, between the accessory meningeal branches to the inferolateral trunk, and finally through persistent fetal anastomoses. It should be noted that parasagittal or convexity meningiomas may receive bilateral supply from the middle meningeal artery; thus retinal infarctions may occur bilaterally via aberrant anastomoses.[299]

Several techniques are employed by neurointerventionists to avoid some of the aforementioned complications. After careful review of the patient's baseline angiograms, superselective microcatheterization is performed to evaluate the blood supply of the tumor and detect anastomoses

that would be potentially dangerous. Typically, a 6F guide catheter is advanced over a stiff 0.035-inch wire into the appropriate parent artery (external carotid, internal carotid, or vertebral artery) in the cervical region. A microcatheter is then advanced over a steerable microwire into a tumor pedicle, and superselective angiography is performed to visualize any anastomoses with vessels supplying normal tissue. Lidocaine and methohexital are injected into the pedicle, and careful cranial nerve and other neurologic testing is done. Contrast material is mixed with the embolic agent of choice, and the pedicle is then embolized. Using negative road-mapping techniques, the operator may readily see subtle reflux of embolic agent proximal to the catheter tip. At this point, the catheter must be cleared of embolic material with saline. Care must be taken to avoid reflux of embolic material proximal to the catheter tip, which may lead to entry of embolic agents into vessels supplying brain parenchyma or the retina. Additionally, liberal angiography should be done to evaluate the angioarchitecture, because vessels previously "absent" on angiography may become apparent as blood is preferentially shunted through them.[299]

The future of intra-arterial tumor therapy remains exciting, as clinicians try to unite the utility of stereotactic radiosurgery with the potential of endovascular surgery for local delivery of chemotherapeutic agents. The high incidence of metastatic brain neoplasms (approximately 150,000 to 200,000 are newly diagnosed annually), combined with the lack of effective treatments for glioblastoma multiforme, may allow such hybrid therapies to have a significant effect on this current health care dilemma.[302,303] Radiation-sensitizing agents that have affinity for metastatic neoplasms to the brain, such as gadolinium texaphyrin, may be administered intra-arterially at higher doses than intravenous

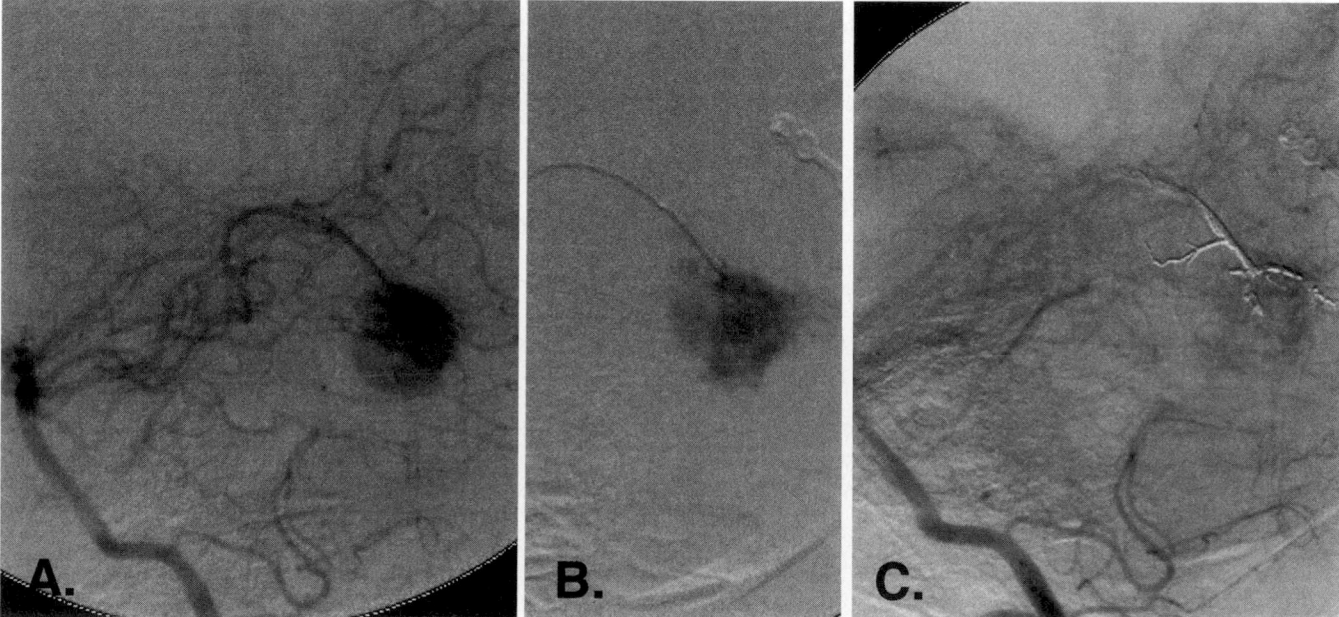

FIGURE 78–17 A, *Lateral angiogram demonstrating vascular tumor blush of a hemangioblastoma following the injection of contrast through the guide catheter. B, Another view following contrast injection through the microcatheter. C, Complete resolution of the tumor blush following infusion of 1 ml of 100% alcohol and NBCA with glacial acetic acid.*

infusion affords, with avoidance of systemic effects.[304,305] After administration of these agents, patients would undergo stereotactic radiosurgery. With the aid of current advances in surface-coating techniques and materials, embolic agents potentially may be coated with antineoplastic agents and then directly injected into the tumor bed.

CONCLUSION

Endovascular neurosurgery is evolving at a frantic pace in which technology often seems far ahead of the clinical strategies for implementing it. Although endovascular technology is still in its infancy, this field holds the promise to provide minimally invasive therapies for cerebrovascular disease resulting in ischemia and stroke. Clearly, clinicians are not yet able to predict the long-term effects of endovascular therapies, such as endoluminal responses to intracranial stent and coil implantations. Nonetheless, short- and middle-term outcomes show promise in that endovascular procedures may obviate the need for craniotomies.

As described in detail in this chapter, endovascular neurosurgeons treat ischemic stroke regularly, whether stroke is the primary problem or a consequence of another primary vascular disorder (such as a ruptured aneurysm resulting in vasospasm). Catheter-based delivery of suspensions or liquid agents, in conjunction with transcatheter mechanical devices (such as balloons, stents, and clot retrieval devices), aimed at targeting the lesion responsible for stroke may improve stroke outcome for a selected patient group. Future applications of transcatheter technology may involve the delivery of growth factors able to reconstitute the vessel lumen across an aneurysm or even of stem cells with the ability to repair and restore parenchyma destroyed by ischemic stroke. Currently, the most significant challenges remain our ability to provide and implement appropriate intra-arterial therapy in a timely manner, educating the public about the various presentations of stroke, and stimulating the imaginations of physicians and industrial scientists.

Acknowledgments

We thank Paul H. Dressel for preparation of the illustrations, the staff at Kaleida Gates Hospital Library for assistance with literature searches and obtaining references, and Debi Zimmer for editorial assistance. The authors have the following financial relationships to disclose: Dr. Bendok, Dr. Boulos, and Dr. Levy receive funding from the AANS/CNS Joint Section on Cerebrovascular Surgery Mullan Neuroendovascular Surgery Award. Dr. Guterman is a Consultant for Guidant Corporation. Dr. Hopkins receives research support from and is a consultant for Boston Scientific, Cordis, Guidant, and Medtronic; in addition, he has a financial interest in Boston Scientific.

References

1. Gibbons KJ, Livingston K: Patient management, complications, and intensive care. Neurosurg Clin North Am 5:555–563, 1994.
2. Levy EI, Firlik AD, Wisniewski S, et al: Factors affecting survival rates for acute vertebrobasilar artery occlusions treated with intra-arterial thrombolytic therapy: A meta-analytical approach. Neurosurgery 45:539–548, 1999.
3. Jevtovic-Todorovic V, Wozniak DF, Powell S, Olney JW: Propofol and sodium thiopental protect against MK-801-induced neuronal necrosis in the posterior cingulate/retrosplenial cortex. Brain Res 913:185–189, 2001.
4. Cooper KR, Boswell PA, Choi SC: Safe use of PEEP in patients with severe head injury. J Neurosurg 63:552–555, 1985.
5. Cotev S, Paul WL, Ruiz BC, et al: Positive end-expiratory pressure (PEEP) and cerebrospinal fluid pressure during normal and elevated intracranial pressure in dogs. Intensive Care Med 7:187–191, 1981.
6. Chamorro A, Vila N, Ascaso C, et al: Blood pressure and functional recovery in acute ischemic stroke. Stroke 29:1850–1853, 1998.
7. Davalos A, Cendra E, Teruel J, et al: Deteriorating ischemic stroke: Risk factors and prognosis. Neurology 40:1865–1869, 1990.
8. Goldstein LB: Should antihypertensive therapies be given to patients with acute ischemic stroke? Drug Safety 22:13–18, 2000.
9. Sagara Y, Hendler S, Khoh-Reiter S, et al: Propofol hemisuccinate protects neuronal cells from oxidative injury. J Neurochem 73:2524–2530, 1999.
10. Hornig CR, Haberbosch W, Lammers C, et al: Specific cardiological evaluation after focal cerebral ischemia. Acta Neurol Scand 93:297–302, 1996.
11. Stirling J, Muramatsu K, Shirai T: Cerebral embolism as a cause of stroke and transient ischemic attack. Echocardiography 13:513–518, 1996.
12. Sancak T, Bilgic S, Sanldilek U: Gadodiamide as an alternative contrast agent in intravenous digital subtraction angiography and interventional procedures of the upper extremity veins. Cardiovasc Intervent Radiol 25:49–52, 2002.
13. Madyoon H, Croushore L, Weaver D, Mathur V: Use of fenoldopam to prevent radiocontrast nephropathy in high-risk patients. Catheter Cardiovasc Interv 53:341–345, 2001.
14. Goldstein LB, Samsa GP: Reliability of the National Institutes of Health Stroke Scale: Extension to non-neurologists in the context of a clinical trial. Stroke 28:307–310, 1997.
15. Tomsick T, Brott T, Barsan W, et al: Prognostic value of the hyperdense middle cerebral artery sign and stroke scale score before ultraearly thrombolytic therapy. AJNR Am J Neuroradiol 17:79–85, 1996.
16. Campeau L: Percutaneous radial artery approach for coronary angiography. Cathet Cardiovasc Diagn 16:3–7, 1989.
17. Spaulding C, Lefevre T, Funck F, et al: Left radial approach for coronary angiography: Results of a prospective study. Cathet Cardiovasc Diagn 39:365–370, 1996.
18. Lotan C, Hasin Y, Mosseri M, et al: Transradial approach for coronary angiography and angioplasty. Am J Cardiol 76:164–167, 1995.
19. Lotan C, Hasin Y, Salmoirago E, et al: The radial artery: An applicable approach to complex coronary angioplasty. J Invasive Cardiol 9:518–522, 1997.
20. Wu SS, Galani RJ, Bahro A, et al: 8 French transradial coronary interventions: Clinical outcome and late effects on the radial artery and hand function. J Invasive Cardiol 12:605–609, 2000.
21. Allen EV: Thromboangiitis obliterans: Methods of diagnosis of chronic occlusive arterial lesions distal to the wrist with illustrative cases. Am J Med Sci 178:237–244, 1929.
22. Levy EI, Boulos AS, Fessler RD, et al: Transradial cerebral angiography: An alternative route. Neurosurgery 51:335–342, 2002.
23. Matsumoto Y, Hokama M, Nagashima H, et al: Transradial approach for selective cerebral angiography: Technical note. Neurol Res 22:605–608, 2000.
24. Matsumoto Y, Hongo K, Toriyama T, et al: Transradial approach for diagnostic selective cerebral angiography: Results of a consecutive series of 166 cases. AJNR Am J Neuroradiol 22:704–708, 2001.
25. Tissue plasminogen activator for acute ischemic stroke. The National Institute of Neurological Disorders and Stroke rt-PA Stroke Study Group. N Engl J Med 333:1581–1587, 1995.
26. Albers GW, Bates VE, Clark WM, et al: Intravenous tissue-type plasminogen activator for treatment of acute stroke: The Standard Treatment with Alteplase to Reverse Stroke (STARS) study. JAMA 283:1145–1150, 2000.
27. Hacke W, Kaste M, Fieschi C, et al: Randomised double-blind placebo-controlled trial of thrombolytic therapy with intravenous alteplase in acute ischaemic stroke (ECASS II). Second European-Australasian Acute Stroke Study Investigators. Lancet 352:1245–1251, 1998.

28. Randomised controlled trial of streptokinase, aspirin, and combination of both in treatment of acute ischaemic stroke. Multicentre Acute Stroke Trial–Italy (MAST-I) Group. Lancet 346:1509–1514, 1995.

29. Thrombolytic therapy with streptokinase in acute ischemic stroke. The Multicenter Acute Stroke Trial–Europe Study Group. N Engl J Med 335:145–150, 1996.

30. Clark WM, Wissman S, Albers GW, et al: Recombinant tissue-type plasminogen activator (alteplase) for ischemic stroke 3 to 5 hours after symptom onset. The ATLANTIS Study: A randomized controlled trial. Alteplase Thrombolysis for Acute Noninterventional Therapy in Ischemic Stroke. JAMA 282:2019–2026, 1999.

31. Donnan GA, Davis SM, Chambers BR, et al: Streptokinase for acute ischemic stroke with relationship to time of administration: Australian Streptokinase (ASK) Trial Study Group. JAMA 276:961–966, 1996.

32. Hacke W, Kaste M, Fieschi C, et al: Intravenous thrombolysis with recombinant tissue plasminogen activator for acute hemispheric stroke. The European Cooperative Acute Stroke Study (ECASS). JAMA 274:1017–1025, 1995.

33. del Zoppo GJ, Higashida RT, Furlan AJ, et al: PROACT: A phase II randomized trial of recombinant pro-urokinase by direct arterial delivery in acute middle cerebral artery stroke. PROACT Investigators. Prolyse in Acute Cerebral Thromboembolism. Stroke 29:4–11, 1998.

34. Furlan A, Higashida R, Wechsler L, et al: Intra-arterial prourokinase for acute ischemic stroke. The PROACT II study: A randomized controlled trial. Prolyse in Acute Cerebral Thromboembolism. JAMA 282:2003–2011, 1999.

35. Eckert B, Koch C, Thomalla G, et al: Acute basilar artery occlusion treated with combined intravenous abciximab and intra-arterial tissue plasminogen activator: Report of 3 cases. Stroke 33:1424–1427, 2002.

36. Endo S, Kuwayama N, Hirashima Y, et al: Results of urgent thrombolysis in patients with major stroke and atherothrombotic occlusion of the cervical internal carotid artery. AJNR Am J Neuroradiol 19:1169–1175, 1998.

37. Jahan R, Duckwiler GR, Kidwell CS, et al: Intraarterial thrombolysis for treatment of acute stroke: Experience in 26 patients with long-term follow-up. AJNR Am J Neuroradiol 20:1291–1299, 1999.

38. Kim SH, Qureshi AI, Suri MFK, et al: Mechanical thrombolysis using balloon angioplasty and snare with low-dose intraarterial reteplase (third-generation thrombolytic) for ischemic stroke: A prospective study (paper 13). J Neurosurg 96:168A, 2002.

39. Nesbit GM, Clark WM, O'Neill OR, Barnwell SL: Intracranial intraarterial thrombolysis facilitated by microcatheter navigation through an occluded cervical internal carotid artery. J Neurosurg 84:387–392, 1996.

40. Qureshi AI, Suri MF, Shatla AA, et al: Intraarterial recombinant tissue plasminogen activator for ischemic stroke: An accelerating dosing regimen. Neurosurgery 47:473–479, 2000.

41. Qureshi AI, Ali Z, Suri MF, et al: Intra-arterial third-generation recombinant tissue plasminogen activator (reteplase) for acute ischemic stroke. Neurosurgery 49:41–50, 2001.

42. Kidwell CS, Saver JL, Mattiello J, et al: Thrombolytic reversal of acute human cerebral ischemic injury shown by diffusion/perfusion magnetic resonance imaging. Ann Neurol 47:462–469, 2000.

43. Kidwell CS, Saver JL, Mattiello J, et al: Diffusion-perfusion MRI characterization of post-recanalization hyperperfusion in humans. Neurology 57:2015–2021, 2001.

44. Kidwell CS, Saver JL, Villablanca JP, et al: Magnetic resonance imaging detection of microbleeds before thrombolysis: An emerging application. Stroke 33:95–98, 2002.

45. Lev MH, Segal AZ, Farkas J, et al: Utility of perfusion-weighted CT imaging in acute middle cerebral artery stroke treated with intra-arterial thrombolysis: Prediction of final infarct volume and clinical outcome. Stroke 32:2021–2028, 2001.

46. Qureshi AI, Ringer AJ, Suri MF, et al: Acute interventions for ischemic stroke: Present status and future directions. J Endovasc Ther 7:423–428, 2000.

47. Davydov L, Cheng JW: Tenecteplase: A review. Clin Ther 23:982–997, 2001.

48. Sheehan FH, Braunwald E, Canner P, et al: The effect of intravenous thrombolytic therapy on left ventricular function: A report on tissue-type plasminogen activator and streptokinase from the Thrombolysis in Myocardial Infarction (TIMI Phase I) trial. Circulation 75:817–829, 1987.

49. Ernst R, Pancioli A, Tomsick T, et al: Combined intravenous and intra-arterial recombinant tissue plasminogen activator in acute ischemic stroke. Stroke 31:2552–2557, 2000.

50. Hill MD, Barber PA, Demchuk AM, et al: Acute intravenous–intra-arterial revascularization therapy for severe ischemic stroke. Stroke 33:279–282, 2002.

51. Keris V, Rudnicka S, Vorona V, et al: Combined intraarterial/intravenous thrombolysis for acute ischemic stroke. AJNR Am J Neuroradiol 22:352–358, 2001.

52. Lewandowski CA, Frankel M, Tomsick TA, et al: Combined intravenous and intra-arterial r-TPA versus intra-arterial therapy of acute ischemic stroke: Emergency Management of Stroke (EMS) Bridging Trial. Stroke 30:2598–2605, 1999.

53. Suarez JI, Zaidat OO, Sunshine JL, et al: Endovascular administration after intravenous infusion of thrombolytic agents for the treatment of patients with acute ischemic strokes. Neurosurgery 50:251–260, 2002.

54. Broderick J: The Interventional Management of Stroke (IMS) Study: Preliminary results. Presented at The 7th International Symposium on Thrombolysis and Acute Stroke Therapy, Lyon, France, May 29–June 1, 2002.

55. Qureshi AI: New grading system for angiographic evaluation of arterial occlusions and recanalization response to intra-arterial thrombolysis in acute ischemic stroke. Neurosurgery 50:1405–1415, 2002.

56. Chalela JA, Katzan I, Liebeskind DS, et al: Safety of intra-arterial thrombolysis in the postoperative period. Stroke 32:1365–1369, 2001.

57. Katzan IL, Masaryk TJ, Furlan AJ, et al: Intra-arterial thrombolysis for perioperative stroke after open heart surgery. Neurology 52:1081–1084, 1999.

58. Moazami N, Smedira NG, McCarthy PM, et al: Safety and efficacy of intraarterial thrombolysis for perioperative stroke after cardiac operation. Ann Thorac Surg 72:1933–1939, 2001.

59. Qureshi AI, Luft AR, Sharma M, et al: Prevention and treatment of thromboembolic and ischemic complications associated with endovascular procedures: Part I: Pathophysiological and pharmacological features. Neurosurgery 46:1344–1359, 2000.

60. Hill MD, Barber PA, Takahashi J, et al: Anaphylactoid reactions and angioedema during alteplase treatment of acute ischemic stroke. CMAJ 162:1281–1284, 2000.

61. Rudolf J, Grond M, Schmulling S, et al: Orolingual angioneurotic edema following therapy of acute ischemic stroke with alteplase. Neurology 55:599–600, 2000.

62. Mericle RA, Lopes DK, Fronckowiak MD, et al: A grading scale to predict outcomes after intra-arterial thrombolysis for stroke complicated by contrast extravasation. Neurosurgery 46:1307–1315, 2000.

63. Mahaffey KW, Granger CB, Sloan MA, et al: Neurosurgical evacuation of intracranial hemorrhage after thrombolytic therapy for acute myocardial infarction: Experience from the GUSTO-I trial. Global Utilization of Streptokinase and Tissue-plasminogen activator (tPA) for Occluded Coronary Arteries. Am Heart J 138:493–499, 1999.

64. Haley EC Jr, Brott TG, Sheppard GL, et al: Pilot randomized trial of tissue plasminogen activator in acute ischemic stroke. The TPA Bridging Study Group. Stroke 24:1000–1004, 1993.

65. Levy DE, Brott TG, Haley EC Jr, et al: Factors related to intracranial hematoma formation in patients receiving tissue-type plasminogen activator for acute ischemic stroke. Stroke 25:291–297, 1994.

66. Kase CS, Furlan AJ, Wechsler LR, et al: Cerebral hemorrhage after intra-arterial thrombolysis for ischemic stroke: The PROACT II trial. Neurology 57:1603–1610, 2001.

67. Kidwell CS, Saver JL, Carneado J, et al: Predictors of hemorrhagic transformation in patients receiving intra-arterial thrombolysis. Stroke 33:717–724, 2002.

68. Suarez JI, Sunshine JL, Tarr R, et al: Predictors of clinical improvement, angiographic recanalization, and intracranial hemorrhage after intra-arterial thrombolysis for acute ischemic stroke. Stroke 30:2094–2100, 1999.

69. Tanne D, Kasner SE, Demchuk AM, et al: Markers of increased risk of intracerebral hemorrhage after intravenous recombinant tissue plasminogen activator therapy for acute ischemic stroke in clinical

practice: The Multicenter rt-PA Stroke Survey. Circulation 105:1679–1685, 2002.

70. Ueda T, Sakaki S, Kumon Y, Ohta S: Multivariable analysis of predictive factors related to outcome at 6 months after intra-arterial thrombolysis for acute ischemic stroke. Stroke 30:2360–2365, 1999.

71. Ringer AJ, Qureshi AI, Fessler RD, et al: Angioplasty of intracranial occlusion resistant to thrombolysis in acute ischemic stroke. Neurosurgery 48:1282–1290, 2001.

72. Ueda T, Sakaki S, Nochide I, et al: Angioplasty after intra-arterial thrombolysis for acute occlusion of intracranial arteries. Stroke 29:2568–2574, 1998.

73. Starkman S, Gobin P, Duckwiler GR, et al: Mechanical Embolus Removal in Cerebral Ischemia (MERCI) Trial. Presented at The 27th International Stroke Conference. San Antonio, TX, The American Stroke Association, February 7–9, 2002.

74. Yahia AM, Qureshi AI, Boulos AS, et al: Balloon-expandable stents for intracranial arterial occlusion in patients with ischemic stroke. Presented at The 7th International Symposium on Thrombolysis and Acute Stroke Therapy, Lyon, France, May 29–June 1, 2002.

75. Barnwell SL, Clark WM, Nguyen TT, et al: Safety and efficacy of delayed intraarterial urokinase therapy with mechanical clot disruption for thromboembolic stroke. AJNR Am J Neuroradiol 15:1817–1822, 1994.

76. Chopko BW, Kerber C, Wong W, Georgy B: Transcatheter snare removal of acute middle cerebral artery thromboembolism: Technical case report. Neurosurgery 46:1529–1531, 2000.

77. Teal PA, Hill MD, Alastair BM: Intra-arterial ultrasound catheter (EKOS) facilitated thrombolysis. Presented at The 7th International Symposium on Thrombolysis and Acute Stroke Therapy. Lyon, France, May 29–June 1, 2002.

78. Watson BD, Prado R, Veloso A, et al: Cerebral blood flow restoration and reperfusion injury after ultraviolet laser-facilitated middle cerebral artery recanalization in rat thrombotic stroke. Stroke 33:428–434, 2002.

79. Lutsep HL, Clark WM, Nesbit GM, et al: Intraarterial suction thrombectomy in acute stroke. AJNR Am J Neuroradiol 23:783–786, 2002.

80. Sharafuddin MJ, Hicks ME, Jenson ML, et al: Rheolytic thrombectomy with use of the AngioJet-F105 catheter: Preclinical evaluation of safety. J Vasc Interv Radiol 8:939–945, 1997.

81. Sacco RL, Kargman DE, Gu Q, Zamanillo MC: Race-ethnicity and determinants of intracranial atherosclerotic cerebral infarction. The Northern Manhattan Stroke Study. Stroke 26:14–20, 1995.

82. Wityk RJ, Lehman D, Klag M, et al: Race and sex differences in the distribution of cerebral atherosclerosis. Stroke 27:1974–1980, 1996.

83. Chimowitz MI, Kokkinos J, Strong J, et al: The Warfarin-Aspirin Symptomatic Intracranial Disease Study. Neurology 45:1488–1493, 1995.

84. Redman AR, Allen LC: Warfarin Versus Aspirin in the Secondary Prevention of Stroke: The WARSS Study. Curr Atheroscler Rep 4:319–325, 2002.

85. The EC-IC bypass study. N Engl J Med 317:1030–1032, 1987.

86. Craig DR, Meguro K, Watridge C, et al: Intracranial internal carotid artery stenosis. Stroke 13:825–828, 1982.

87. Marzewski DJ, Furlan AJ, St Louis P, et al: Intracranial internal carotid artery stenosis: Long-term prognosis. Stroke 13:821–824, 1982.

88. Gorter JW: Major bleeding during anticoagulation after cerebral ischemia: Patterns and risk factors. Stroke Prevention In Reversible Ischemia Trial (SPIRIT). European Atrial Fibrillation Trial (EAFT) study groups. Neurology 53:1319–1327, 1999.

89. Stroke Prevention in Atrial Fibrillation Study: Final results. Circulation 84:527–539, 1991.

90. Risk factors for stroke and efficacy of antithrombotic therapy in atrial fibrillation: Analysis of pooled data from five randomized controlled trials. Arch Intern Med 154:1449–1457, 1994.

91. Petersen P, Boysen G, Godtfredsen J, et al: Placebo-controlled, randomised trial of warfarin and aspirin for prevention of thromboembolic complications in chronic atrial fibrillation. The Copenhagen AFASAK study. Lancet 8631:175–179, 1989.

92. Thijs VN, Albers GW: Symptomatic intracranial atherosclerosis: Outcome of patients who fail antithrombotic therapy. Neurology 55:490–497, 2000.

93. Akins PT, Pilgram TK, Cross DT 3rd, Moran CJ: Natural history of stenosis from intracranial atherosclerosis by serial angiography. Stroke 29:433–438, 1998.

94. Callahan AS 3rd, Berger BL, Beuter MJ, Devlin TG: Possible short-term amelioration of basilar plaque by high-dose atorvastatin: Use of reductase inhibitors for intracranial plaque stabilization. J Neuroimaging 11:202–204, 2001.

95. Ozgur HT, Kent Walsh T, Masaryk A, et al: Correlation of cerebrovascular reserve as measured by acetazolamide-challenged SPECT with angiographic flow patterns and intra- or extracranial arterial stenosis. AJNR Am J Neuroradiol 22:928–936, 2001.

96. Webster MW, Makaroun MS, Steed DL, et al: Compromised cerebral blood flow reactivity is a predictor of stroke in patients with symptomatic carotid artery occlusive disease. J Vasc Surg 21:338–345, 1995.

97. Yonas H, Pindzola RR, Meltzer CC, Sasser H: Qualitative versus quantitative assessment of cerebrovascular reserves. Neurosurgery 42:1005–1012, 1998.

98. Caplan LR, Hennerici M: Impaired clearance of emboli (washout) is an important link between hypoperfusion, embolism, and ischemic stroke. Arch Neurol 55:1475–1482, 1998.

99. Awad IA, Little JR, Furlan AJ: Conversion of an intracranial arterial stenosis to a symptomatic occlusion after EC/IC bypass surgery. Neurosurgery 13:734, 1983.

100. Awad I, Furlan AJ, Little JR: Changes in intracranial stenotic lesions after extracranial-intracranial bypass surgery. J Neurosurg 60:771–776, 1984.

101. Clark WM, Barnwell SL, Nesbit G, et al: Safety and efficacy of percutaneous transluminal angioplasty for intracranial atherosclerotic stenosis. Stroke 26:1200–1204, 1995.

102. Higashida RT, Tsai FY, Halbach VV, et al: Interventional neurovascular techniques in the treatment of stroke state-of-the-art therapy. J Intern Med 237:105–115, 1995.

103. Takis C, Kwan ES, Pessin MS, et al: Intracranial angioplasty: Experience and complications. AJNR Am J Neuroradiol 18:1661–1668, 1997.

104. Terada T, Higashida RT, Halbach VV, et al: Transluminal angioplasty for arteriosclerotic disease of the distal vertebral and basilar arteries. J Neurol Neurosurg Psychiatry 60:377–381, 1996.

105. Connors JJ 3rd, Wojak JC: Percutaneous transluminal angioplasty for intracranial atherosclerotic lesions: Evolution of technique and short-term results. J Neurosurg 91:415–423, 1999.

106. Marks MP, Marcellus M, Norbash AM, et al: Outcome of angioplasty for atherosclerotic intracranial stenosis. Stroke 30:1065–1069, 1999.

107. Mori T, Fukuoka M, Kazita K, Mori K: Follow-up study after intracranial percutaneous transluminal cerebral balloon angioplasty. AJNR Am J Neuroradiol 19:1525–1533, 1998.

108. Nahser HC, Henkes H, Weber W, et al: Intracranial vertebrobasilar stenosis: Angioplasty and follow-up. AJNR Am J Neuroradiol 21:1293–1301, 2000.

109. Mori T, Kazita K, Mori K: Cerebral angioplasty and stenting for intracranial vertebral atherosclerotic stenosis. AJNR Am J Neuroradiol 20:787–789, 1999.

110. Mori T, Mori K, Fukuoka M, et al: Percutaneous transluminal cerebral angioplasty: Serial angiographic follow-up after successful dilatation. Neuroradiology 39:111–116, 1997.

111. George CJ, Baim DS, Brinker JA, et al: One-year follow-up of the Stent Restenosis (STRESS I) Study. Am J Cardiol 81:860–865, 1998.

112. Huang P, Levin T, Kabour A, Feldman T: Acute and late outcome after use of 2.5-mm intracoronary stents in small (< 2.5 mm) coronary arteries. Catheter Cardiovasc Interv 49:121–126, 2000.

113. Morice MC, Bradai R, Lefevre T, et al: Stenting small coronary arteries. J Invasive Cardiol 11:337–340, 1999.

114. Gomez CR, Misra VK, Liu MW, et al: Elective stenting of symptomatic basilar artery stenosis. Stroke 31:95–99, 2000.

115. Levy EI, Horowitz MB, Koebbe CJ, et al: Transluminal stent-assisted angioplasty of the intracranial vertebrobasilar system for medically refractory, posterior circulation ischemia: Early results. Neurosurgery 48:1215–1223, 2001.

116. Mori T, Kazita K, Chokyu K, et al: Short-term arteriographic and clinical outcome after cerebral angioplasty and stenting for intracranial vertebrobasilar and carotid atherosclerotic occlusive disease. AJNR Am J Neuroradiol 21:249–254, 2000.

117. Ramee SR, Dawson R, McKinley KL, et al: Provisional stenting for symptomatic intracranial stenosis using a multidisciplinary approach: Acute results, unexpected benefit, and one-year outcome. Catheter Cardiovasc Interv 52:457–467, 2001.

118. Lang J: Clinical Anatomy of Brainstem Vessels. New Haven, Conn, Miles Pharmaceutical, 1981.

119. Levy EI, Hanel RA, Bendok BR, et al: Staged stent-assisted angioplasty for symptomatic intracranial vertebrobasilar stenosis. J Neurosurg 97:1294–1301, 2002.

120. Fessler RD, Lanzino G, Guterman LR, et al: Improved cerebral perfusion after stenting of a petrous carotid stenosis: Technical case report. Neurosurgery 45:638–642, 1999.

121. Beneficial effect of carotid endarterectomy in symptomatic patients with high-grade carotid stenosis. North American Symptomatic Carotid Endarterectomy Trial Collaborators. N Engl J Med 325:445–453, 1991.

122. Barnett HJ, Taylor DW, Eliasziw M, et al: Benefit of carotid endarterectomy in patients with symptomatic moderate or severe stenosis. North American Symptomatic Carotid Endarterectomy Trial Collaborators. N Engl J Med 339:1415–1425, 1998.

123. Randomised trial of endarterectomy for recently symptomatic carotid stenosis: Final results of the MRC European Carotid Surgery Trial (ECST). Lancet 351:1379–1387, 1998.

124. Study design for randomized prospective trial of carotid endarterectomy for asymptomatic atherosclerosis. The Asymptomatic Carotid Atherosclerosis Study Group. Stroke 20:844–849, 1989.

125. Endarterectomy for asymptomatic carotid artery stenosis. Executive Committee for the Asymptomatic Carotid Atherosclerosis Study. JAMA 273:1421–1428, 1995.

126. Young B, Moore WS, Robertson JT, et al: An analysis of perioperative surgical mortality and morbidity in the asymptomatic carotid atherosclerosis study. ACAS Investigators. Asymptomatic Carotid Atherosclerosis Study. Stroke 27:2216–2224, 1996.

127. Hobson RWI, Weiss DG, Fields WS, et al: Efficacy of carotid endarterectomy for asymptomatic carotid stenosis (Veterans Affairs Cooperative Study Group). N Engl J Med 328:221–227, 1993.

128. Morgenstern LB, Fox AJ, Sharpe BL, et al: The risks and benefits of carotid endarterectomy in patients with near occlusion of the carotid artery. North American Symptomatic Carotid Endarterectomy Trial (NASCET) Group. Neurology 48:911–915, 1997.

129. Kappelle LJ, Eliasziw M, Fox AJ, et al: Importance of intracranial atherosclerotic disease in patients with symptomatic stenosis of the internal carotid artery. The North American Symptomatic Carotid Endarterectomy Trial. Stroke 30:282–286, 1999.

130. Paciaroni M, Eliasziw M, Kappelle LJ, et al: Medical complications associated with carotid endarterectomy. North American Symptomatic Carotid Endarterectomy Trial (NASCET). Stroke 30:1759–1763, 1999.

131. Gray WA, White HJ Jr, Barrett DM, et al: Carotid stenting and endarterectomy: A clinical and cost comparison of revascularization strategies. Stroke 33:1063–1070, 2002.

132. Wholey MH, Wholey M, Mathias K, et al: Global experience in cervical carotid artery stent placement. Catheter Cardiovasc Interv 50:160–167, 2000.

133. Roubin GS, Hobson RW 2nd, White R, et al: CREST and CARESS to evaluate carotid stenting: Time to get to work! J Endovasc Ther 8:107–110, 2001.

134. Roubin GS, New G, Iyer SS, et al: Immediate and late clinical outcomes of carotid artery stenting in patients with symptomatic and asymptomatic carotid artery stenosis: A 5-year prospective analysis. Circulation 103:532–537, 2001.

135. Lopes DK, Mericle RA, Lanzino G, et al: Stent placement for the treatment of occlusive atherosclerotic carotid artery disease in patients with concomitant coronary artery disease. J Neurosurg 96:490–496, 2002.

136. Moore WS, Barnett HJ, Beebe HG, et al: Guidelines for carotid endarterectomy: A multidisciplinary consensus statement from the Ad Hoc Committee, American Heart Association. Circulation 91:566–579, 1995.

137. New G, Roubin GS, Iyer SS, et al: Safety, efficacy, and durability of carotid artery stenting for restenosis following carotid endarterectomy: A multicenter study. J Endovasc Ther 7:345–352, 2000.

138. Hernandez-Vila E, Strickman NE, Skolkin M, et al: Carotid stenting for post-endarterectomy restenosis and radiation-induced occlusive disease. Tex Heart Inst J 27:159–165, 2000.

139. Paniagua D, Howell M, Strickman N, et al: Outcomes following extracranial carotid artery stenting in high-risk patients. J Invasive Cardiol 13:375–381, 2001.

140. Al-Mubarak N, Roubin GS, Vitek JJ, et al: Effect of the distal-balloon protection system on microembolization during carotid stenting. Circulation 104:1999–2002, 2001.

141. Angelini A, Reimers B, Della Barbera M, et al: Cerebral protection during carotid artery stenting: Collection and histopathologic analysis of embolized debris. Stroke 33:456–461, 2002.

142. Ohki T, Roubin GS, Veith FJ, et al: Efficacy of a filter device in the prevention of embolic events during carotid angioplasty and stenting: An ex vivo analysis. J Vasc Surg 30:1034–1044, 1999.

143. Ohki T, Veith FJ: Carotid artery stenting: Utility of cerebral protection devices. J Invasive Cardiol 13:47–55, 2001.

144. Ohki T, Parodi J, Veith FJ, et al: Efficacy of a proximal occlusion catheter with reversal of flow in the prevention of embolic events during carotid artery stenting: An experimental analysis. J Vasc Surg 33:504–509, 2001.

145. Roubin GS: The status of carotid stenting. AJNR Am J Neuroradiol 20:1378–1381, 1999.

146. Vitek JJ, Roubin GS, Al-Mubarek N, et al: Carotid artery stenting: Technical considerations. AJNR Am J Neuroradiol 21:1736–1743, 2000.

147. Wholey MH, Wholey M, Bergeron P, et al: Current global status of carotid artery stent placement. Cathet Cardiovasc Diagn 44:1–6, 1998.

148. Al-Mubarak N, Vitek JJ, Iyer SS, et al: Carotid stenting with distal-balloon protection via the transbrachial approach. J Endovasc Ther 8:571–575, 2001.

149. Al-Mubarak N, Vitek JJ, Iyer S, et al: Embolization via collateral circulation during carotid stenting with the distal balloon protection system. J Endovasc Ther 8:354–357, 2001.

150. Reimers B, Corvaja N, Moshiri S, et al: Cerebral protection with filter devices during carotid artery stenting. Circulation 104:12–15, 2001.

151. Meyer FB, Sundt TM Jr, Piepgras DG, et al: Emergency carotid endarterectomy for patients with acute carotid occlusion and profound neurological deficits. Ann Surg 203:82–89, 1986.

152. Blaisdell WF, Clauss RH, Galbraith JG, et al: Joint study of extracranial arterial occlusion. IV: A review of surgical considerations. JAMA 209:1889–1895, 1969.

153. Uno M, Hamazaki F, Kohno T, et al: Combined therapeutic approach of intra-arterial thrombolysis and carotid endarterectomy in selected patients with acute thrombotic carotid occlusion. J Vasc Surg 34:532–540, 2001.

154. Malek AM, Higashida RT, Phatouros CC, et al: Endovascular management of extracranial carotid artery dissection achieved using stent angioplasty. AJNR Am J Neuroradiol 21:1280–1292, 2000.

155. El Gindi S, Salama M, Tawfik E, et al: A review of 2,000 patients with craniocerebral injuries with regard to intracranial haematomas and other vascular complications. Acta Neurochir 48:237–244, 1979.

156. Burke JP, Marion DW: Cerebral revascularization in trauma and carotid occlusion. Neurosurg Clin North Am 12:595–611, 2001.

157. Schievink WI, Mokri B, Whisnant JP: Internal carotid artery dissection in a community: Rochester, Minnesota, 1987–1992. Stroke 24:1678–1680, 1993.

158. Bogousslavsky J, Regli F: Ischemic stroke in adults younger than 30 years of age: Cause and prognosis. Arch Neurol 44:479–482, 1987.

159. Yamada S, Kindt GW, Youmans JR: Carotid artery occlusion due to nonpenetrating injury. J Trauma 7:333–342, 1967.

160. Guillon B, Levy C, Bousser MG: Internal carotid artery dissection: An update. J Neurol Sci 153:146–158, 1998.

161. Coffin O, Maiza D, Galateau-Salle F, et al: Results of surgical management of internal carotid artery aneurysm by the cervical approach. Ann Vasc Surg 11:482–490, 1997.

162. Treiman GS, Treiman RL, Foran RF, et al: Spontaneous dissection of the internal carotid artery: A nineteen-year clinical experience. J Vasc Surg 24:597–607, 1996.

163. Krajewski LP, Hertzer NR: Blunt carotid artery trauma: Report of two cases and review of the literature. Ann Surg 191:341–346, 1980.

164. Liu AY, Paulsen RD, Marcellus ML, et al: Long-term outcomes after carotid stent placement treatment of carotid artery dissection. Neurosurgery 45:1368–1374, 1999.

165. Cloft HJ, Jensen ME, Kallmes DF, Dion JE: Arterial dissections complicating cerebral angiography and cerebrovascular interventions. AJNR Am J Neuroradiol 21:541–545, 2000.

166. Hosoya T, Watanabe N, Yamaguchi K, et al: Intracranial vertebral artery dissection in Wallenberg syndrome. AJNR Am J Neuroradiol 15:1161–1165, 1994.

167. Dorros G, Cohn JM, Palmer LE: Stent deployment resolves a petrous carotid artery angioplasty dissection. AJNR Am J Neuroradiol 19:392–394, 1998.
168. Kurata A, Ohmomo T, Miyasaka Y, et al: Coil embolization for the treatment of ruptured dissecting vertebral aneurysms. AJNR Am J Neuroradiol 22:11–18, 2001.
169. Yamaura A, Watanabe Y, Saeki N: Dissecting aneurysms of the intracranial vertebral artery. J Neurosurg 72:183–188, 1990.
170. Aenis M, Stancampiano AP, Wakhloo AK, Lieber BB: Modeling of flow in a straight stented and nonstented side wall aneurysm model. J Biomech Eng 119:206–212, 1997.
171. Imbesi SG, Kerber CW: Analysis of slipstream flow in a wide-necked basilar artery aneurysm: Evaluation of potential treatment regimens. AJNR Am J Neuroradiol 22:721–724, 2001.
172. Kerber CW, Heilman CB: Flow in experimental berry aneurysms: Method and model. AJNR Am J Neuroradiol 4:374–377, 1983.
173. Kerber CW, Cromwell LD, Zanetti PH: Experimental carotid aneurysms. Part 2: Endovascular treatment with cyanoacrylate. Neurosurgery 16:13–17, 1985.
174. Kerber CW, Liepsch D: Flow dynamics for radiologists. II: Practical considerations in the live human. AJNR Am J Neuroradiol 15:1076–1086, 1994.
175. Kerber CW, Liepsch D: Flow dynamics for radiologists. I: Basic principles of fluid flow. AJNR Am J Neuroradiol 15:1065–1075, 1994.
176. Horowitz MB, Miller G 3rd, Meyer Y, et al: Use of intravascular stents in the treatment of internal carotid and extracranial vertebral artery pseudoaneurysms. AJNR Am J Neuroradiol 17:693–696, 1996.
177. Levy EI, Boulos AS, Bendok BR, et al: Brainstem infarction after delayed thrombosis of a stented vertebral artery fusiform aneurysm: Case report. Neurosurgery 51:1284–1285, 2002.
178. Heesch CM, Wilhelm CR, Ristich J, et al: Cocaine activates platelets and increases the formation of circulating platelet containing microaggregates in humans. Heart 83:688–695, 2000.
179. Terada T, Nakai E, Tsuura M, et al: Combined surgery and endovascular stenting for basilar artery stenosis refractory to balloon angioplasty: Technical case report. Acta Neurochir 143:511–516, 2001.
180. Horowitz MB, Levy EI, Koebbe CJ, Jungreis CC: Transluminal stent-assisted coil embolization of a vertebral confluence aneurysm: Technique report. Surg Neurol 55:291–296, 2001.
181. Massoud TF, Turjman F, Ji C, et al: Endovascular treatment of fusiform aneurysms with stents and coils: Technical feasibility in a swine model. AJNR Am J Neuroradiol 16:1953–1963, 1995.
182. Phatouros CC, Sasaki TY, Higashida RT, et al: Stent-supported coil embolization: The treatment of fusiform and wide-neck aneurysms and pseudoaneurysms. Neurosurgery 47:107–115, 2000.
183. Phatouros CC, Higashida RT, Malek AM, et al: Endovascular treatment of noncarotid extracranial cerebrovascular disease. Neurosurg Clin North Am 11:331–350, 2000.
184. Wityk RJ, Chang HM, Rosengart A, et al: Proximal extracranial vertebral artery disease in the New England Medical Center Posterior Circulation Registry. Arch Neurol 55:470–478, 1998.
185. Caplan LR, Amarenco P, Rosengart A, et al: Embolism from vertebral artery origin occlusive disease. Neurology 42:1505–1512, 1992.
186. Gomez CR, Cruz-Flores S, Malkoff MD, et al: Isolated vertigo as a manifestation of vertebrobasilar ischemia. Neurology 47:94–97, 1996.
187. Rocha-Singh K: Vertebral artery stenting: Ready for prime time? Catheter Cardiovasc Interv 54:6–7, 2001.
188. Crawley F, Brown MM, Clifton AG: Angioplasty and stenting in the carotid and vertebral arteries. Postgrad Med J 74:7–10, 1998.
189. Drescher P, Katzen BT: Percutaneous treatment of symptomatic vertebral artery stenosis with coronary stents. Catheter Cardiovasc Interv 52:373–377, 2001.
190. Storey GS, Marks MP, Dake M, et al: Vertebral artery stenting following percutaneous transluminal angioplasty: Technical note. J Neurosurg 84:883–887, 1996.
191. Chastain HD 2nd, Campbell MS, Iyer S, et al: Extracranial vertebral artery stent placement: In-hospital and follow-up results. J Neurosurg 91:547–552, 1999.
192. Higashida RT, Tsai FY, Halbach VV, et al: Transluminal angioplasty for atherosclerotic disease of the vertebral and basilar arteries. J Neurosurg 78:192–198, 1993.
193. Jenkins JS, White CJ, Ramee SR, et al: Vertebral artery stenting. Catheter Cardiovasc Interv 54:1–5, 2001.

194. Malek AM, Higashida RT, Phatouros CC, et al: Treatment of posterior circulation ischemia with extracranial percutaneous balloon angioplasty and stent placement. Stroke 30:2073–2085, 1999.
195. Mukherjee D, Roffi M, Kapadia SR, et al: Percutaneous intervention for symptomatic vertebral artery stenosis using coronary stents. J Invasive Cardiol 13:363–366, 2001.
196. Piotin M, Spelle L, Martin JB, et al: Percutaneous transluminal angioplasty and stenting of the proximal vertebral artery for symptomatic stenosis. AJNR Am J Neuroradiol 21:727–731, 2000.
197. Contorni L: Il circolo collaterale vertebro-vertebrale nella obliterazione dell'arterio subclavia all sua origine. Minerva Chir 15:268–271, 1960.
198. Fisher C: A new vascular syndrome: "The subclavian steal" [editorial]. N Engl J Med 265:912–913, 1961.
199. de Bray JM, Zenglein JP, Laroche JP, et al: Effect of subclavian syndrome on the basilar artery. Acta Neurol Scand 90:174–178, 1994.
200. Herring M: The subclavian steal syndrome: A review. Am Surg 43:220–228, 1977.
201. Piccone VA, Leveen HH: The subclavian steal syndrome. Ann Thoracic Surg 9:51–75, 1970.
202. Smith JM, Koury HI, Hafner CD, Welling RE: Subclavian steal syndrome: A review of 59 consecutive cases. J Cardiovasc Surg (Torino) 35:11–14, 1994.
203. Thomassen L, Aarli JA: Subclavian steal phenomenon: Clinical and hemodynamic aspects. Acta Neurol Scand 90:241–244, 1994.
204. Walker PM, Paley D, Harris KA, et al: What determines the symptoms associated with subclavian artery occlusive disease? J Vasc Surg 2:154–157, 1985.
205. Webster MW, Downs L, Yonas H, et al: The effect of arm exercise on regional cerebral blood flow in the subclavian steal syndrome. Am J Surg 168:91–93, 1994.
206. Fields WS, Lemak NA: Joint study of extracranial arterial occlusion. VII: Subclavian steal—a review of 168 cases. JAMA 222:1139–1143, 1972.
207. Ackermann H, Diener HC, Seboldt H, Huth C: Ultrasonographic follow-up of subclavian stenosis and occlusion: Natural history and surgical treatment. Stroke 19:431–435, 1988.
208. Drutman J, Gyorke A, Davis WL, Turski PA: Evaluation of subclavian steal with two-dimensional phase-contrast and two-dimensional time-of-flight MR angiography. AJNR Am J Neuroradiol 15:1642–1645, 1994.
209. AbuRahma AF, Robinson PA, Jennings TG: Carotid-subclavian bypass grafting with polytetrafluoroethylene grafts for symptomatic subclavian artery stenosis or occlusion: A 20-year experience. J Vasc Surg 32:411–419, 2000.
210. Beebe HG, Stark R, Johnson ML, et al: Choices of operation for subclavian-vertebral arterial disease. Am J Surg 139:616–623, 1980.
211. Deriu GP, Milite D, Verlato F, et al: Surgical treatment of atherosclerotic lesions of subclavian artery: Carotid-subclavian bypass versus subclavian-carotid transposition. J Cardiovasc Surg (Torino) 39:729–734, 1998.
212. Owens LV, Tinsley EA Jr, Criado E, et al: Extrathoracic reconstruction of arterial occlusive disease involving the supraaortic trunks. J Vasc Surg 22:217–222, 1995.
213. Bachman DM, Kim RM: Transluminal dilatation for subclavian steal syndrome. AJR Am J Roentgenol 135:995–996, 1980.
214. Taylor CL, Selman WR, Ratcheson RA: Steal affecting the central nervous system. Neurosurgery 50:679–689, 2002.
215. Bornstein NM, Norris JW: Subclavian steal: A harmless haemodynamic phenomenon? Lancet 2(8502):303–305, 1986.
216. Moran KT, Zide RS, Persson AV, Jewell ER: Natural history of subclavian steal syndrome. Am Surg 54:643–644, 1988.
217. Hennerici M, Klemm C, Rautenberg W: The subclavian steal phenomenon: A common vascular disorder with rare neurologic deficits. Neurology 38:669–673, 1988.
218. Farina C, Mingoli A, Schultz RD, et al: Percutaneous transluminal angioplasty versus surgery for subclavian artery occlusive disease. Am J Surg 158:511–514, 1989.
219. Hebrang A, Maskovic J, Tomac B: Percutaneous transluminal angioplasty of the subclavian arteries: Long-term results in 52 patients. AJR Am J Roentgenol 156:1091–1094, 1991.
220. Mathias KD, Luth I, Haarmann P: Percutaneous transluminal angioplasty of proximal subclavian artery occlusions. Cardiovasc Intervent Radiol 16:214–218, 1993.

221. Motarjeme A, Keifer JW, Zuska AJ, Nabawi P: Percutaneous transluminal angioplasty for treatment of subclavian steal. Radiology 155:611–613, 1985.

222. Selby JB Jr, Matsumoto AH, Tegtmeyer CJ, et al: Balloon angioplasty above the aortic arch: Immediate and long-term results. AJR Am J Roentgenol 160:631–635, 1993.

223. Kumar K, Dorros G, Bates MC, et al: Primary stent deployment in occlusive subclavian artery disease. Cathet Cardiovasc Diagn 34:281–285, 1995.

224. Queral LA, Criado FJ: The treatment of focal aortic arch branch lesions with Palmaz stents. J Vasc Surg 23:368–375, 1996.

225. Rodriguez-Lopez JA, Werner A, Martinez R, et al: Stenting for atherosclerotic occlusive disease of the subclavian artery. Ann Vasc Surg 13:254–260, 1999.

226. Sueoka BL: Percutaneous transluminal stent placement to treat subclavian steal syndrome. J Vasc Interv Radiol 7:351–356, 1996.

227. Vitek JJ: Subclavian artery angioplasty and the origin of the vertebral artery. Radiology 170:407–409, 1989.

228. Bogey WM, Demasi RJ, Tripp MD, et al: Percutaneous transluminal angioplasty for subclavian artery stenosis. Am Surg 60:103–106, 1994.

229. Ringelstein EB, Zeumer H: Delayed reversal of vertebral artery blood flow following percutaneous transluminal angioplasty for subclavian steal syndrome. Neuroradiology 26:189–198, 1984.

230. Weir B: Unruptured intracranial aneurysms: A review. J Neurosurg 96:3–42, 2002.

231. de la Monte SM, Moore GW, Monk MA, Hutchins GM: Risk factors for the development and rupture of intracranial berry aneurysms. Am J Med 78:957–964, 1985.

232. Inagawa T, Hirano A: Autopsy study of unruptured incidental intracranial aneurysms. Surg Neurol 34:361–365, 1990.

233. Broderick JP, Brott T, Tomsick T, et al: Intracerebral hemorrhage more than twice as common as subarachnoid hemorrhage. J Neurosurg 78:188–191, 1993.

234. Kiyohara Y, Ueda K, Hasuo Y, et al: Incidence and prognosis of subarachnoid hemorrhage in a Japanese rural community. Stroke 20:1150–1155, 1989.

235. Sarti C, Tuomilehto J, Salomaa V, et al: Epidemiology of subarachnoid hemorrhage in Finland from 1983 to 1985. Stroke 22:848–853, 1991.

236. Mohr JP, Caplan LR, Melski JW, et al: The Harvard Cooperative Stroke Registry: A prospective registry. Neurology 28:754–762, 1978.

237. Unruptured intracranial aneurysms—risk of rupture and risks of surgical intervention. International Study of Unruptured Intracranial Aneurysms Investigators. N Engl J Med 339:1725–1733, 1998.

238. Qureshi AI, Suri MF, Yahia AM, et al: Risk factors for subarachnoid hemorrhage. Neurosurgery 49:607–613, 2001.

239. Bendok BR, Getch CC, Malisch TW, Batjer HH: Treatment of aneurysmal subarachnoid hemorrhage. Semin Neurol 18:521–531, 1998.

240. Malisch TW, Guglielmi G, Vinuela F, et al: Unruptured aneurysms presenting with mass effect symptoms: Response to endosaccular treatment with Guglielmi detachable coils. Part I: Symptoms of cranial nerve dysfunction. J Neurosurg 89:956–961, 1998.

241. Qureshi AI, Mohammad Y, Yahia AM, et al: Ischemic events associated with unruptured intracranial aneurysms: Multicenter clinical study and review of the literature. Neurosurgery 46:282–290, 2000.

242. Mayberg MR, Batjer HH, Dacey R, et al: Guidelines for the management of aneurysmal subarachnoid hemorrhage: A statement for healthcare professionals from a special writing group of the Stroke Council, American Heart Association. Circulation 90:2592–2605, 1994.

243. Juvela S: Rebleeding from ruptured intracranial aneurysms. Surg Neurol 32:323–326, 1989.

244. Vinuela F, Duckwiler G, Mawad M: Guglielmi detachable coil embolization of acute intracranial aneurysm: Perioperative anatomical and clinical outcome in 403 patients. J Neurosurg 86:475–482, 1997.

245. Biller J, Godersky JC, Adams HP Jr: Management of aneurysmal subarachnoid hemorrhage. Stroke 19:1300–1305, 1988.

246. Origitano TC, Reichman OH, Anderson DE: Prophylactic hypervolemia without calcium channel blockers in early aneurysm surgery. Neurosurgery 31:804–806, 1992.

247. Newell DW, Eskridge JM, Mayberg MR, et al: Angioplasty for the treatment of symptomatic vasospasm following subarachnoid hemorrhage. J Neurosurg 71:654–660, 1989.

248. Coskun E: Papaverine and vasospasm. J Neurosurg 96:973–974, 2002.

249. Morgan MK, Jonker B, Finfer S, et al: Aggressive management of aneurysmal subarachnoid haemorrhage based on a papaverine angioplasty protocol. J Clin Neurosci 7:305–308, 2000.

250. Ohkuma H, Ogane K, Tanaka M, Suzuki S: Assessment of cerebral microcirculatory changes during cerebral vasospasm by analyzing cerebral circulation time on DSA images. Acta Neurochir Suppl (Wien) 77:127–130, 2001.

251. Turjman F, Massoud TF, Sayre J, Vinuela F: Predictors of aneurysmal occlusion in the period immediately after endovascular treatment with detachable coils: A multivariate analysis. AJNR Am J Neuroradiol 19:1645–1651, 1998.

252. Moret J, Cognard C, Weill A, et al: Reconstruction technic in the treatment of wide-neck intracranial aneurysms: Long-term angiographic and clinical results. Apropos of 56 cases. J Neuroradiol 24:30–44, 1997.

253. Lanzino G, Wakhloo AK, Fessler RD, et al: Efficacy and current limitations of intravascular stents for intracranial internal carotid, vertebral, and basilar artery aneurysms. J Neurosurg 91:538–546, 1999.

254. Ogilvy CS, Stieg PE, Awad I, et al: AHA Scientific Statement: Recommendations for the management of intracranial arteriovenous malformations: A statement for healthcare professionals from a special writing group of the Stroke Council, American Stroke Association. Stroke 32:1458–1471, 2001.

255. Chiaradio JC, Guzman L, Padilla L, Chiaradio MP: Intravascular graft stent treatment of a ruptured fusiform dissecting aneurysm of the intracranial vertebral artery: Technical case report. Neurosurgery 50:213–216, discussion 216–217, 2002.

256. Berger MS, Wilson CB: Intracranial dissecting aneurysms of the posterior circulation: Report of six cases and review of the literature. J Neurosurg 61:882–894, 1984.

257. Ali MA, Bendok BR, Tawk RG, et al: Trapping and revascularization for a dissecting aneurysm of the proximal posteroinferior cerebellar artery: Technical case report and review of the literature. Neurosurgery 51:258–263, 2002.

258. Michelson W: Natural history and pathophysiology of arteriovenous malformations. Clin Neurosurg 26:307–313, 1978.

259. Jessurun GA, Kamphuis DJ, van der Zande FH, Nossent JC: Cerebral arteriovenous malformations in The Netherlands Antilles: High prevalence of hereditary hemorrhagic telangiectasia-related single and multiple cerebral arteriovenous malformations. Clin Neurol Neurosurg 95:193–198, 1993.

260. Patterson J, McKossoch W: A clinical survey of intracranial angiomas with special reference to their mode of progression and surgical treatment: A report of 110 cases. Brain 79:233–266, 1956.

261. Lasjaunias P, Piske R, Terbrugge K, Willinsky R: Cerebral arteriovenous malformations (C. AVM) and associated arterial aneurysms (AA). Analysis of 101 C. AVM cases, with 37 AA in 23 patients. Acta Neurochir 91:29–36, 1988.

262. Spetzler RF, Martin NA: A proposed grading system for arteriovenous malformations. J Neurosurg 65:476–483, 1986.

263. Hartmann A, Pile-Spellman J, Stapf C, et al: Risk of endovascular treatment of brain arteriovenous malformations. Stroke 33:1816–1820, 2002.

264. Furlan AJ, Whisnant JP, Elveback LR: The decreasing incidence of primary intracerebral hemorrhage: A population study. Ann Neurol 5:367–373, 1979.

265. Brown RD Jr, Wiebers DO, Forbes G, et al: The natural history of unruptured intracranial arteriovenous malformations. J Neurosurg 68:352–357, 1988.

266. Fults D, Kelly DL Jr: Natural history of arteriovenous malformations of the brain: A clinical study. Neurosurgery 15:658–662, 1984.

267. Graf CJ, Perret GE, Torner JC: Bleeding from cerebral arteriovenous malformations as part of their natural history. J Neurosurg 58:331–337, 1983.

268. Ondra SL, Troupp H, George ED, Schwab K: The natural history of symptomatic arteriovenous malformations of the brain: A 24-year follow-up assessment. J Neurosurg 73:387–391, 1990.

269. Hartmann A, Mast H, Mohr JP, et al: Morbidity of intracranial hemorrhage in patients with cerebral arteriovenous malformation. Stroke 29:931–934, 1998.

270. Kondziolka D, McLaughlin MR, Kestle JR: Simple risk predictions for arteriovenous malformation hemorrhage. Neurosurgery 37:851–855, 1995.

271. Forster DM, Steiner L, Hakanson S: Arteriovenous malformations of the brain: A long-term clinical study. J Neurosurg 37:562–570, 1972.

272. Kader A, Young WL, Pile-Spellman J, et al: The influence of hemodynamic and anatomic factors on hemorrhage from cerebral arteriovenous malformations. Neurosurgery 34:801–808, 1994.

273. Miyasaka Y, Yada K, Ohwada T, et al: An analysis of the venous drainage system as a factor in hemorrhage from arteriovenous malformations. J Neurosurg 76:239–243, 1992.

274. Heros RC, Korosue K, Diebold PM: Surgical excision of cerebral arteriovenous malformations: Late results. Neurosurgery 26:570–578, 1990.

275. Jafar JJ, Davis AJ, Berenstein A, et al: The effect of embolization with N-butyl cyanoacrylate prior to surgical resection of cerebral arteriovenous malformations. J Neurosurg 78:60–69, 1993.

276. Spetzler RF, Wilson CB, Weinstein P, et al: Normal perfusion pressure breakthrough theory. Clin Neurosurg 25:651–672, 1978.

277. Pollock BE, Lunsford LD, Flickinger JC, Kondziolka D: The role of embolization in combination with stereotactic radiosurgery in the management of pial and dural arteriovenous malformations. In Connors JJ, Wojak JC (eds): Interventional Neuroradiology. Philadelphia, WB Saunders, 1999, pp 267–275.

278. Fournier D, TerBrugge KG, Willinsky R, et al: Endovascular treatment of intracerebral arteriovenous malformations: Experience in 49 cases. J Neurosurg 75:228–233, 1991.

279. Gobin YP, Laurent A, Merienne L, et al: Treatment of brain arteriovenous malformations by embolization and radiosurgery. J Neurosurg 85:19–28, 1996.

280. Vinuela F, Dion JE, Duckwiler G, et al: Combined endovascular embolization and surgery in the management of cerebral arteriovenous malformations: Experience with 101 cases. J Neurosurg 75:856–864, 1991.

281. Debrun GM, Aletich V, Ausman JI, et al: Embolization of the nidus of brain arteriovenous malformations with n-butyl cyanoacrylate. Neurosurgery 40:112–121, 1997.

282. Hekster RE, Matricali B, Luyendijk W: Presurgical transfemoral catheter embolization to reduce operative blood loss: Technical note. J Neurosurg 41:396–398, 1974.

283. Berenstein A, Russell E: Gelatin sponge in therapeutic neuroradiology: A subject review. Neuroradiology 141:105–112, 1981.

284. Brismar J, Cronqvist S: Therapeutic embolization in the external carotid artery region. Acta Radiol Diagn (Stockh) 19:715–731, 1978.

285. Hieshima GB, Everhart FR, Mehringer CM, et al: Preoperative embolization of meningiomas. Surg Neurol 14:119–127, 1980.

286. Hilal SK, Michelsen JW: Therapeutic percutaneous embolization for extra-axial vascular lesions of the head, neck, and spine. J Neurosurg 43:275–287, 1975.

287. Latchaw RE, Gold LH: Polyvinyl foam embolization of vascular and neoplastic lesions of the head, neck, and spine. Radiology 131:669–679, 1979.

288. Feun LG, Wallace S, Stewart DJ, et al: Intracarotid infusion of cis-diamminedichloroplatinum in the treatment of recurrent malignant brain tumors. Cancer 54:794–799, 1984.

289. Qureshi AI, Suri MF, Khan J, et al: Superselective intra-arterial carboplatin for treatment of intracranial neoplasms: Experience in 100 procedures. J Neurooncol 51:151–158, 2001.

290. Recht L, Fram RJ, Strauss G, et al: Preirradiation chemotherapy of supratentorial malignant primary brain tumors with intracarotid cisplatinum (CDDP) and i.v. BCNU: A phase II trial. Am J Clin Oncol 13:125–131, 1990.

291. Stewart DJ, Grahovac Z, Benoit B, et al: Intracarotid chemotherapy with a combination of 1,3-bis(2-chloroethyl)-1-nitrosourea (BCNU), cis-diaminedichloroplatinum (cisplatin), and 4Ξ-O-demethyl-1-O-(4,6-O-2-thenylidene-β-D-glucopyranosyl)epipodophyllotoxin (VM-26) in the treatment of primary and metastatic brain tumors. Neurosurgery 15:828–833, 1984.

292. Watne K, Hannisdal E, Nome O, et al: Combined intra-arterial and systemic chemotherapy for recurrent malignant brain tumors. Neurosurgery 30:223–227, 1992.

293. Kerber CW, Wong WH, Howell SB, et al: An organ-preserving selective arterial chemotherapy strategy for head and neck cancer. AJNR Am J Neuroradiol 19:935–941, 1998.

294. Bendszus M, Rao G, Burger R, et al: Is there a benefit of preoperative meningioma embolization? Neurosurgery 47:1306–1312, 2000.

295. Bendszus M, Klein R, Burger R, et al: Efficacy of trisacryl gelatin microspheres versus polyvinyl alcohol particles in the preoperative embolization of meningiomas. AJNR Am J Neuroradiol 21:255–261, 2000.

296. Kai Y, Hamada J, Morioka M, et al: Appropriate interval between embolization and surgery in patients with meningioma. AJNR Am J Neuroradiol 23:139–142, 2002.

297. Kuroiwa T, Tanaka H, Ohta T, Tsutsumi A: Preoperative embolization of highly vascular brain tumors: Clinical and histopathological findings. Noshuyo Byori 13:27–36, 1996.

298. Jüngling FD, Wakhloo AK, Hennig J: In vivo proton spectroscopy of meningioma after preoperative embolization. Magn Reson Med 30:155–160, 1993.

299. Horowitz MB, Spiro R, Purdy P, et al: Meningioma embolization. Contemp Neurosurg 23:1–6, 2001.

300. Suyama T, Tamaki N, Fujiwara K, et al: Peritumoral and intratumoral hemorrhage after gelatin sponge embolization of malignant meningioma: Case report. Neurosurgery 21:944–946, 1987.

301. Terada T, Nakai E, Tsumoto T, Itakura T: Iatrogenic arteriovenous fistula of the middle meningeal artery caused during embolization for meningioma—case report. Neurol Med Chir (Tokyo) 37:677–680, 1997.

302. Niranjan A, Lunsford LD, Gobbel GT, et al: Brain tumor radiosurgery: Current status and strategies to enhance the effect of radiosurgery. Brain Tumor Pathol 17:89–96, 2000.

303. Niranjan A, Moriuchi S, Lunsford LD, et al: Effective treatment of experimental glioblastoma by HSV vector-mediated TNFalpha and HSV-tk gene transfer in combination with radiosurgery and ganciclovir administration. Mol Ther 2:114–120, 2000.

304. Radford IR: Gd-Tex Pharmacyclics Inc. Curr Opin Investig Drugs 1:524–528, 2000.

305. Rosenthal DI, Nurenberg P, Becerra CR, et al: A phase I single-dose trial of gadolinium texaphyrin (Gd-Tex), a tumor selective radiation sensitizer detectable by magnetic resonance imaging. Clin Cancer Res 5:739–745, 1999.

Chapter Seventy-Nine

Standards for Surgical Treatment of Cerebrovascular Disease, Circa 2000

Peter D. Le Roux and H. Richard Winn

Stroke is the third leading cause of death in the United States and the leading cause of disability. It is estimated that more than 700,000 strokes occur in the United States each year and there are more than 4.4 million stroke survivors.[1,2] In 1999, the American Heart Association (AHA) estimated the economic burden of stroke in the United States to be $51 billion.[3]

Surgery plays a significant role in stroke management, both in prevention and in treating the acute manifestations of hemorrhagic or ischemic disease. However, even in the best of hands, adverse events and adverse outcomes occur during or after surgery for cerebrovascular disease.[4] Today's cerebrovascular surgeons—unlike their predecessors, who developed many of the procedures and introduced them into clinical use—face stricter standards of legal accountability for adverse events and outcomes, whether or not associated with medical negligence. In a case of medical negligence, it is the purview of the court to determine whether a surgeon's conduct in a particular instance falls below an acceptable "professional standard of care" and, if so, whether that conduct was a cause of the patient's outcome.

One must recognize that an adverse outcome does not imply substandard care. Furthermore, the "standard of care" is often subject to opinion and debate in both medical and legal circles. National attention has also been drawn to variations in the performance of different surgical procedures and different outcomes in different regions.[5] These disparities in the absence of case-mix variations imply better practice in some areas or reflect uncertainty about optimum management or patient selection. These observations and the report from the Institute of Medicine (IOM) on patient safety in hospitals are two of several factors that have increased the interest in the development of evidence-based medicine, best practice guidelines, and standards of care.[6]

In this chapter, we (1) discuss shortcomings in the literature that may limit the establishment of standards; (2) briefly review expected outcomes after some common surgical procedures for cerebrovascular disease, such as those for carotid artery disease, cerebral aneurysms, arteriovenous malformation (AVM), and intracerebral hematoma (ICH), although the reader is referred to the relevant chapters in this text for more comprehensive summaries; (3) examine how patients or third party payers decide "the standard of care"; (4) discuss how and why adverse events occur and how they may be prevented; (5) consider practice guidelines; and (6) examine the definition of "quality" in health care. Our intent is not to establish a "standard of care" but rather to draw attention to the important role that physicians play at the interface between the law and medicine and to highlight the difficulty of establishing a single standard in cerebrovascular surgery.

THE LITERATURE

To establish a standard in cerebrovascular surgery requires literature-based evidence mixed with experience. The IOM's report on medical errors, *To Err Is Human; Building a Safer Health System,*[6] describes a practice consistent with current medical knowledge that incorporates evidence-based medicine as being central to patient safety. The next IOM report, *Crossing the Quality Chasm: A New Health System for the 21st Century,*[7] lists six aims for this new system, including "services based on scientific knowledge." Studies in humans are often confounded by many variables; consequently, every study must be examined for such confounders as well as for study design defects, data quality, and the strength of any statistical conclusions. These concerns are usually addressed by medical journals' peer review processes. However, publication of a study in a prominent peer-reviewed journal does not guarantee that the study results or conclusions are correct.[8]

The validity of a published study can be evaluated with a 13-point scoring system developed by Heyland and colleagues (Table 79.1).[9] In addition, several organizations, including the AHA and the American College of Surgeons (ACS), have classified evidence in medicine according to its quality or level and so base their management recommendations on a grade that reflects consistency and strength of the evidence (Tables 79.1 and 79.2).[10–12] Ideally, standards of care require grade A evidence—that is, validation by large randomized clinical trials (RCTs). Surgical practice, however, has limited high-quality evidence derived from stringent randomized clinical trials, in part because randomization and blinding, which are essential to clinical trials, are difficult to apply in surgery.[13–16] Furthermore, although the performance of a procedure may be randomized, the many technical variations associated with a procedure are more difficult to control for. Many surgeons, therefore, are unconvinced that randomized trials are the only means of defining "best evidence." In addition, it can be misleading to conclude that a particular treatment is not efficacious when a broad case mix is included in a large series.[16a] For example, the Extracranial/Intracranial Bypass Study found no benefit to surgery in stroke prevention. However, this study may have overlooked patients with ongoing hemodynamic compromise; such patients are now the subjects of an ongoing RCT. Finally, to be meaningful, the results of large RCTs, which are frequently conducted at selected, high-performance centers, must be transferred into everyday clinical practice.

In the absence of RCTs, surgeons rely on observational data or data derived from clinical series. One must be cautious when interpreting nonrandomized comparisons of outcome because such studies are frequently subject to selection and institutional biases. For example, there are regional differences in care that can influence outcome not explained by a case mix resulting from referral policies.[14,17–19] Similarly, outcome for the same procedure may vary widely and perhaps independently of patient risk factors or surgical technique, depending on who reports the data (Table 79.3). For example, many surgeons were surprised by the high morbidity and mortality rates observed in the International Study of Unruptured Intracranial Aneurysms (ISUIA),[20] and others have questioned the validity of the International Subarachnoid Aneurysm Trial (ISAT)[21] data because of variances in surgical morbidity that appear to be region dependent. Finally, many studies

Table 79.1   Heyland Criteria for Assessing Methodologic Quality of Published Studies*

Variables	0 Points	1 Points	2 Points
Methods			
Randomization	Not randomized	—	Truly randomized
Blinding	Not blinded	Double blinded	—
Analysis	Other	—	Intention-to-treat
Population			
Patient selection	Selected patients or cannot tell	Consecutive eligible patients	—
Comparability of groups at baseline	No or not sure	Yes	—
Extent of follow-up	<100%	100%	—
Intervention			
Treatment protocol	Poorly described	Reproducibly described	—
Co-intervention	Not described	Described, but not equal or not sure	Well described and all equal
Crossovers	Not described	>10%	<10%

*Adapted from Heyland DK, Cook DJ, King D, et al: Maximizing oxygen delivery in critically ill patients: A methodological appraisal of the evidence. Crit Care Med 24:517–524, 1996.
0, 1, and 2 refer to the points assigned in the scoring system.

Table 79.2   Levels of Evidence and Grades of Recommendation

Levels of evidence
I	Meta-analysis of multiple well-designed, controlled studies; randomized trials with low false-positive (alpha) and low false-negative errors (beta) (i.e., high power)
II	At least one well-designed experimental study; randomized trials with high false-positive (alpha) or high false-negative errors (beta) or both (i.e., low power)
III	Well-designed, quasi-experimental studies, such as nonrandomized, controlled, single-group, preoperative-postoperative comparison, concurrent cohort, time, or matched case-control series
IV	Well-designed, nonexperimental studies, such as nonrandomized historical cohort studies, comparative and correlational descriptive and case studies
V	Case reports and clinical examples

Grades of recommendation
A	Evidence of type I or consistent findings from multiple studies of type II, III, or IV
B	Evidence of type II, III, or IV and generally consistent findings
C	Evidence of type II, III, or IV but inconsistent findings

Adapted from Cook CJ, Guyatt GH, Laupacis A, Sackett DL: Rules of evidence and clinical recommendations on the use of antithrombotic agents. Chest 02(Suppl):305S–311S, 1992; and Sackett DL: Rules of evidence and clinical recommendations on the use of antithrombotic agents. Chest 95(2 Suppl):2S–4S, 1989.

Table 79.3 Outcome After Carotid Artery Surgery Can Be Influenced by Differences in Methodology and Authorship*

Study Type (Number of Studies)	Mortality % (95% CI)	Stroke/Death % (95% CI)
Prospective (19)	1.9 (1.3–2.6)	5.6 (3.9–7.3)
Retrospective (32)	1.5 (1.2–1.8)	5.1 (4.3–5.8)
Neurologist assessor (9)	1.4 (0.2–2.7)	7.7 (5–10.2)
Neurologist author (11)	1.8 (1.2–2.5)	6.4 (4.6–8.1)
Multiple surgeons (26)	1.7 (1.4–1.9)	5.5 (4.8–6.1)
Single surgeon (5)	0.7 (0.4–1.0)	2.3 (1.8–2.7)

*Data from a systematic review of 51 studies published between 1980 and 1996 describing mortality and the risk of stroke and/or death after carotid endarterectomy for symptomatic carotid stenosis.

Adapted from Rothwell PM, Slattery J, Warlow CP: A systematic review of the risks of stroke and death due to endarterectomy for symptomatic carotid stenosis. Stroke 27:260, 1996.

describing management strategies for acute cerebrovascular disorders suffer from methodologic weaknesses, implying that current management for patients with these disorders is based on weak evidence.[22,23]

Despite these limitations, the AHA has attempted to provide practice guidelines for a variety of cerebrovascular disorders, including stroke, carotid endarterectomy (CEA), ICH, unruptured cerebral aneurysms, subarachnoid hemorrhage (SAH), and AVMs.[2,24–28] In the absence of level I or grade A evidence (see Table 79.2), however, these management guidelines represent only literature reviews and consensus statements rather than explicit standards. Nevertheless, this guideline development can be a potent tool for studying deficits in the data. Literature reviews also are provided by the Cochrane Collaboration, an international organization dedicated to organizing and disseminating systematic reviews that assess the success of health care interventions.[29,30] There are, however, very few Cochrane reviews on cerebrovascular surgery.

Attempts to measure quality of medical care have used administrative data, and such information is increasingly being requested by health care networks, payers, and regulatory and accrediting groups to compare health care institutions and individual physicians. Administrative data are readily available, are inexpensive to collect, and may provide insight into characteristics of large patient populations. However, the accuracy and reliability of administrative data in describing diagnoses, surgical procedures, characteristics of individual patients, and adverse outcomes are open to challenge, for multiple reasons. First, these data were never intended to answer a clinical question. Furthermore, hospital administrative data are subject to coding bias, lack important physiologic information, and are ill suited to risk adjustment. Consequently, administrative databases may be inconsistent with important clinical information. For example Best and colleagues[31] compared administrative data with data from the U.S. Department of Veterans Affairs (DVA) National Surgical Quality Improvement Program (NSQIP), which employed trained nurses as data collectors to prospectively gather preoperative patient characteristics and 30-day postoperative outcomes for most major operations in 123 DVA hospitals so as to provide risk-adjusted outcomes. These investigators observed that the sensitivity and positive predictive value of administrative data was poor in comparison with data collected by nurses.[31]

RESULTS OF CEREBROVASCULAR SURGERY

Intracerebral Hemorrhage

Nontraumatic (primary or hypertensive) intracerebral hemorrhage represents less than 15% of all strokes and affects about 45,000 people in the United States each year. Among stroke subtypes, ICH is associated with the highest mortality; only one third of patients are alive 1 year after such an ictus, and among survivors, many are dependent.[2,32] Poor outcome is associated with increased ICH volume, mass effect, and herniation. The AHA established management guidelines for primary ICH in 1999; however, there remains significant controversy about who should be treated, what management is appropriate, and whether surgery is beneficial.[2]

The goals of ICH surgery are to reduce mass effect, to prevent the release of potentially neurotoxic substances from the ICH, and to prevent prolonged contact between the hematoma and normal tissue, which might initiate other pathologic processes. However, the benefit of surgery, particularly for deep basal ganglionic, thalamic, or pontine hemorrhages, is masked by the neural damage sustained during the surgical approach or by the recurrent bleeding once the tamponade effect is lost.

Many nonrandomized clinical series comparing surgery and best medical treatment of ICH have been reported.[2,33] The most consistent finding is significant variability in treatment and outcome. Seven RCTs had been published through early 2003.[32,34–39] The final results of an eighth RCT, STICH, are awaited. Meta-analysis of these 7 trials, including one from the pre–computed tomography (CT) era, performed by the organizers of the STICH trial, demonstrated a trend toward worse outcome after surgery.[40] With exclusion of data from the pre-CT era trial[37], analysis found no difference between surgical and medical treatment. However, a reduction in the likelihood of death and dependency after surgery was observed when data from a Chinese trial[36] were excluded for methodologic reasons. In another meta-analysis of these RCTs as well as three trials of supratentorial hemorrhage involving 249 patients, Hankey and associates[41] observed that 83% of patients who underwent craniotomy were dead or dependent at 6 months. Later small trials have focused on early surgery (median time to surgery about 8 hours); these pilot studies demonstrate the feasibility of early evacuation of ICH but do not demonstrate a clear benefit for surgical evacuation.[33,39,40]

The results of these various randomized trials and clinical series demonstrate that outcome after primary ICH is bad in the vast majority of patients, independent of the treatment provided. The following observations about treatment of ICH can be made:

1. There is significant debate about the initial blood pressure treatment after an ICH. The AHA guidelines

suggest that if the mean arterial pressure is greater than 130 mm Hg, short-acting intravenous drugs should be administered to keep the cerebral perfusion pressure (CPP) above 70 mm Hg.[2]

2. Corticosteroids should be avoided.[42] However, the experience with other medications, such as hypertonic saline and barbiturates, is insufficient for any meaningful conclusions to be made about their use.

3. Aggressive, timely reversal of transtentorial herniation using appropriate hyperventilation, osmotic agents, or surgery may improve outcome.[43]

4. The best surgical results compared to nonsurgical management are seen in patients with a cerebellar ICH for whom the initial Glasgow Coma Scale (GCS) score is less than 14 or in whom the ICH volume is large (≥40 mL).[44] It is therefore common practice for neurosurgeons to evacuate cerebellar ICHs more than 3 cm in diameter. Frequently, when a cerebellar ICH is this size, evacuation is performed independently from the patient's neurologic condition.

5. The role of minimally invasive stereotactic or endoscopic procedures is uncertain, although small feasibility studies suggest that their use may be associated with a trend toward better outcome in certain patients, particularly those with lobar hematomas and those younger than 60 years.[34,39]

Symptomatic Carotid Artery Disease

CEA is the most frequently performed noncardiac vascular procedure. Several large, prospective RCTs have demonstrated that CEA is three times more effective than medical therapy alone in reducing the risk of stroke in patients with symptomatic carotid stenosis between 70% and 99% in severity.[45–50] In addition, the procedure is durable, the risks of disabling ipsilateral ischemic stroke reaching only 4.4% by 10 years.[51] Risk factors for late stroke after carotid surgery include presentation with cerebral symptoms, diabetes, elevated systolic blood pressure, smoking, male sex, increasing age, and less severe preoperative stenosis. Plaque morphology and patch grafting have not been associated with higher risk of late stroke. There were differences in these RCTs, but pooled analysis of data from the three major trials, involving 6092 patients and 35,000 patient-years of follow-up[50] using the same measurements and definitions, provided consistent results.

Surgery is of some benefit for patients with 50% to 69% symptomatic stenosis, and very beneficial for those with greater than 70% symptomatic stenosis but without near-occlusion. However, CEA itself is associated with risks. For example, in the pooled analysis, the overall risk of stroke or death with surgery was 7.1%[50] (Table 79.4), similar to that observed in surgical case series when patients were assessed postoperatively by a neurologist (see Table 79.2).[52] Other complications associated with CEA are myocardial infarction, cranial nerve injuries, wound hematoma, hypertension, hypotension, hyperperfusion syndrome, intracerebral hemorrhage, seizures, and recurrent stenosis (Table 79.5).[49,53] Poorly controlled hypertension raises the risk of postoperative complications, and other risk factors for perioperative stroke have been described in the Sundt classification (Table 79.6).[54,55]

Similarly, the North American Symptomatic Carotid Endarterectomy Trial (NASCET) collaborators observed that a hemispheric rather than a retinal transient ischemic attack (TIA), a left-sided procedure, contralateral carotid occlusion, demonstration of an ipsilateral ischemic lesion on CT, and ulcerated plaque were independent predictors of perioperative stroke or death after carotid surgery.[56] Each of these factors nearly doubled surgical risk and so may be useful in selecting medical therapy in patients for whom surgery offers only marginal benefit.

The most catastrophic event that can occur after CEA is ICH secondary to hyperperfusion. The Mayo Clinic experience in 2362 consecutive CEAs demonstrated that ICH occurred in 0.6% of patients within 2 weeks after surgery.[57] Hemorrhages were large and often fatal (60%) or were associated with poor outcome (25%) in this series. Risk factors for development of ICH after carotid surgery include advanced age, hypertension, presence of high-grade stenosis, poor collateral flow, and angiographic demonstration of slow flow in the middle cerebral artery territory. A final risk factor is reoperation. However, second operations have durable benefits and rates of stroke-free survival similar to those for primary CEA. These variables should be kept in mind when the treating physician considers carotid stenting instead of reoperation (Table 79.7).[58,59]

Guidelines for CEA have been provided by the AHA.[26] The various RCTs have clarified the indications for surgery. However, there is no consensus on how the operation should be performed. Debates continue, for example, over whether local or general anesthesia should be used, whether shunting should be performed all the time, selectively, or never, and whether patching should be applied in all, some, or no cases. Aspirin therapy should be started before surgery in all patients who are to undergo CEA unless there are contraindications; the optimal dose, however, is uncertain.[60] Similarly, patients should be counseled about other risk factors, such as hypertension, cigarette smoking, and hypercholesterolemia. Unstable hypertension is associated with increased perioperative risk, and because unstable blood pressure is observed in more than 70% of patients during the first 24 hours after CEA,[61] patients with perioperative hypertension should be closely monitored after surgery. This monitoring may occur in an intensive care unit (ICU). However, different monitoring standards have been proposed to decrease the procedural cost.[62] There is no reliable data to define an acceptable level or duration of postoperative monitoring, and no RCTs examining the benefit of ICU care after CEA have been conducted. Regardless of whether ICU care is provided, high-risk patients, such as those with preoperative hypertension, should be closely monitored for the first 24 hours after surgery.

These various differences and debates about technique and care notwithstanding, the most important finding of these RCTs is that for the benefit of CEA over medical therapy to be maintained, the procedure should be undertaken only when the surgeon performing the procedure has a low procedure complication rate (e.g., 3%, depending on other risk factors).[63] Consequently, the risks reported in the NASCET and the other RCTs should serve as a guide to best practices. Because minor strokes may often be missed in routine clinical practice outside a

Table 79.4 Risks of Death and Stroke Within 30 Days of Carotid Endarterectomy in Patients Who Underwent Trial Surgery, According to Severity of Symptomatic Carotid Stenosis*

	ECST		NASCET		VA309		Total		P†
	No. Events per No. Patients	% Risk (95% CI)	No. Events per No. Patients	% Risk (95% CI)	No. Events per No. Patients	% Risk (95% CI)	No. Events per No. Patients	% Risk (95% CI)	
Outcome stroke or death									
<50% stenosis	73/1044	6.9% (5.4–8.6)	43/663	6.5% (4.7–8.6)	0/0	—	116/1707	6.7% (5.6–8.0)	.52
50–69% stenosis	37/371	10.0% (6.9–13.1)	30/421	7.1% (4.8–10.0)	2/20	10.0% (1.2–3.2)	69/812	8.4% (6.6–10.5)	.16
≥70% stenosis	17/249	6.8% (4.0–10.7)	14/261	5.4% (3.0–8.8)	5/71	7.0% (2.3–15.7)	36/581	6.2% (4.4–8.5)	.58
Near-occlusion	3/78	3.8% (0.8–10.8)	5/70	7.1% (2.4–15.0)	0/0	—	8/148	5.4% (2.4–10.4)	.48
Total	130/1742	7.5% (6.3–8.8)	92/1415	6.5% (5.3–7.9)	7/91	7.7% (3.1–15.2)	229/3248	7.1% (6.3–8.1)	.30
Outcome death									
<50% stenosis	10/1044	0.9% (0.5–1.7)	7/663	1.1% (0.4–2.2)	0/0	—	17/1707	1.0% (0.6–1.6)	.80
50–69% stenosis	6/371	1.5% (0.6–3.3)	6/421	1.4% (0.5–3.1)	0/20	0% (0–16.8)	12/812	1.4% (0.8–2.5)	.83
≥70% stenosis	1/249	0.4% (0–12.2)	1/261	0.4% (0–2.1)	3/71	4.2% (0.8–1.19)	5/581	0.9% (0.3–2.0)	.97
Near-occlusion	0/78	0% (0–4.6)	1/70	1.4% (0–7.7)	0/0	—	1/148	0.7% (0–3.7)	.29
Total	17/1742	1.0% (0.6–1.6)	15/1415	1.1% (0.6–1.7)	3/91	3.3 (0.7–9.3)	33/3248	1.1% (0.8–1.5)	.86

*Data pooled from the three randomized controlled trials of surgery in symptomatic carotid stenosis.

†Heterogeneity.

CI, confidence interval; ECST, European Carotid Surgery Trial; NASCET, North American Symptomatic Carotid Endarterectomy Trial; VA309, Veterans Affairs Cooperative Studies Program 309.

Adapted from Rothwell PM, Eliasziw M, Gutnikov SA, et al: Analysis of pooled data from the randomised controlled trials of endarterectomy for symptomatic carotid stenosis. Carotid Endarterectomy Trialists' Collaboration. Lancet 361(9352):107, 2003.

Table 79.5   Risks Associated with Carotid Endarterectomy for Symptomatic Carotid Stenosis

Death: 1.1% (90 days)
Stroke risk
    Disabling: 0.9% (90 days)
    Non-disabling stroke: 4.5% (90 days)
    30-day stroke morbidity and mortality: 5.8%
    Risk of ipsilateral stroke at 2-year follow-up: 9%; medical
        treatment alone 26%
    Intracerebral hemorrhage: 0.6%
Nonstroke perioperative complications
    Wound hematoma: 5.5%°
    Cranial nerve palsies: 8.6%
    Myocardial infarct: 1%
    Other cardiovascular complications: 7.1%
    Respiratory complications: 0.4%
Factors associated with increased surgical risk
    Hemispheric transient ischemic attack
    Left carotid endarterectomy
    Contralateral carotid occlusion
    Ipsilateral ischemic lesion on computed tomography
    Irregular or ulcerated plaque
Factors associated with increased medical risk
    Preoperative hypertension
    Angina or myocardial infarct

°In about 1% of patients, reexploration may be necessary, particularly if there is airway compromise.
Data from the North American Symptomatic Carotid Endarterectomy Trial.[49,51,53,56,57]

strictly controlled trial, an audit of operative risk should perhaps be performed by an independent neurologist. Confidential feedback of outcomes data has been demonstrated to lead to changes in management that are associated with improvement in results over time.[64]

Asymptomatic Carotid Stenosis

There is less certainty about the benefit of CEA in unselected patients with asymptomatic carotid disease. Four published RCTs have addressed this question. Results of the Carotid Artery Stenosis with Asymptomatic Narrowing: Operation Versus Aspirin (CASANOVA) study were inconclusive.[65] The Mayo Clinic Asymptomatic Carotid Endarterectomy (MACE) study was stopped because myocardial infarction occurred in 26% of patients in the surgical arm, compared with 9% of patients in the medical arm, who received aspirin.[66] However, surgical patients

did not receive aspirin. The Veterans Affairs Cooperative Study of CEA for patients with asymptomatic carotid artery stenosis demonstrated a significant 38% risk reduction over 2 years for the combined end points of ipsilateral TIA, transient monocular blindness, and stroke.[67] The surgical group had lower rates of fatal stroke (4.7% versus 9.4% for the medical group) and nonfatal stroke (1.2% versus 2.4% per year, respectively). However, this difference was not statistically significant. The largest study, the Asymptomatic Carotid Atherosclerosis Study (ACAS), randomly assigned 1662 patients to either surgery plus medical therapy or medical therapy alone.[50] All patients received aspirin and counseling in risk factor reduction. The study was halted after a median follow-up of 2.7 years (4465 patient-years) because of demonstration of a significant benefit of surgery. The risk of ipsilateral stroke, any perioperative stroke, or death in patients undergoing CEA was estimated at 5% over 5 years; in medically treated patients, the corresponding risk was 11%. Women did not benefit from CEA, and no relationship between surgical outcome and the degree of stenosis was observed.

The results of these various studies have been described in guidelines from the AHA, which can be summarized as follows: CEA may be considered in patients with high-grade asymptomatic carotid stenosis when performed by a surgeon with a procedural morbidity/mortality rate lower than 3% and in patients with life expectancy of at least 5 years. When the procedural complication rate approaches 5%, the benefit of CEA for asymptomatic carotid disease disappears. Some of this risk can be reduced by less reliance on catheter angiography, which in the ACAS was associated with a 1.2% rate of stroke.[32] However, most physicians are not aware of the complication rates of the surgeons to whom they refer patients for CEA.[68]

Cerebral Aneurysms and Subarachnoid Hemorrhage

The majority of cerebral aneurysms remain asymptomatic until aneurysm rupture produces subarachnoid hemorrhage (SAH). Population-based studies demonstrate that aneurysmal SAH occurs in about 10 per 100,000 people each year; this rate may vary by 10-fold among different populations.[17] In patients treated with bed rest alone, a risk of aneurysm rerupture persists indefinitely.[69] Even with treatment, population-based studies suggest that SAH is fatal or disabling in two thirds of those affected.[17,70] In industrialized countries, the 30-day mortality rate is about

Table 79.6   Sundt Classification of Carotid Artery Surgery Risk

Grade	Neurologic Status	Medical Risk[†]	Angiographic Risk[‡]	Morbidity and Mortality (%)
I	Stable	−	−	<1
II	Stable	−	+	1.8
III	Stable	+	±	4.0
IV	Unstable°	±	±	8.5

°Progressive ischemic neurological deficit, infarct <7 days, transient ischemic attack (TIA) <24 hrs, crescendo TIAs.
[†]Angina, myocardial infarct, congestive heart failure, severe hypertension, chronic obstructive pulmonary disease, age >70 yr.
[‡]Occluded opposite ICA, siphon stenosis, plaque extension, high carotid bifurcation, intraluminal thrombosis.
Adapted from Sundt TM, Sordok BA, Whisnart JP: Carotid endarterectomy: Complications and preoperative assessment of risk. Mayo Clin Proc 50:301, 1975.

Table 79.7 Risk of Carotid Endarterectomy or Angioplasty for Carotid Artery Disease*

	Angioplasty	Surgery	OR (95% CI)
Death (%)	0.8	1.2	0.68 (0.43–1.05)
Stroke (%)	7.1	3.3	2.2 (1.62–3.04)
Fatal or disabling stroke (%)	3.2	1.6	2.09 (1.3–3.33)
Stroke or death (%)	3.9	2.2	1.86 (1.22–2.84)

*The risk is calculated from 13 angioplasty studies including 714 patients and 20 surgical studies including 6970 patients.
CI, confidence interval; OR, odds ratio.
Adapted from Golledge J, Mitchell A, Creenhalgh RM, Davies AH: Systematic comparison of the early outcome of angioplasty and endarterectomy for symptomatic carotid artery disease. Stroke 31:1439, 2000.

40%, and by 1 year, about 50% of patients with SAH are dead.[71-76] Among the survivors, approximately 60% remain permanently disabled, often because of cognitive or neuropsychological abnormalities,[17,73,75-78] and only half the survivors who were employed before the hemorrhage return to the same level of work afterwards.[79,80] These outcome results suggest that current SAH management may be inadequate. In part, this state may stem from the heterogeneity and complex pathophysiology of aneurysm rupture.

Practice guidelines for patients with SAH are available.[27] However, there are many different management strategies for SAH, and apparently similar outcomes can occur despite these different strategies. Treatment recommendations for SAH are primarily empirical and derived mainly from observational clinical series that often suffer from methodologic weaknesses—making it difficult to develop a "standard of care."[14,22,23] In addition, the information obtained from the few RCTs that have examined SAH management has many limitations or is applicable only to a small subset of patients (e.g., the ISAT trial), or there is no clear explanation for the benefits observed (e.g., the various nimodipine trials).[81]

Unruptured Aneurysms

Clearly, SAH is a devastating event, so one opportunity to improve outcome is to identify and treat unruptured intracranial aneurysms (UIAs). This would require a clear knowledge of UIA natural history; even with recent studies, however, the natural history remains poorly defined and little understood. For example, data from the ISUIA, which has been severely challenged,[20] suggest that the annual hemorrhage rate for asymptomatic small aneurysms is 0.05%, whereas more recent studies suggest that the rupture rate is 1% to 2% per year,[82-85] consistent with earlier natural history data. It is clear from these various studies that no two UIAs and no two patients are identical. The risk of rupture is greater with larger aneurysms, posterior circulation location, aneurysms associated with AVMs, symptomatic aneurysms, UIAs that are seen on follow-up imaging to have enlarged, and previous SAH from another aneurysm (i.e. multiple aneurysms).[20,86-90] Factors such as cigarette smoking, hypertension, and binge alcohol drinking also may be associated with aneurysm rupture.[88,91-93] Consequently, although UIA treatment guidelines have been published

and extensive decision analysis has been performed, there are no firm standards describing which patient should be treated; instead each patient and each aneurysm should be individually considered for treatment.[25]

What are the results of surgical treatment of UIAs (Tables 79.8 and 79.9)? First, aneurysm surgery is effective; overall more than 90% of surgically treated aneurysms are completely obliterated.[94-99] Failure to occlude an aneurysm is more likely when the aneurysm is large or cerebrovascular atherosclerosis is identified.[97] For example, Solomon and coworkers,[100] treating 202 UIAs surgically, observed complete occlusion in more than 90% of small aneurysms but in only 54% of giant aneurysms. Most of the literature describing UIAs, other than the ISUIA, consists of individual case series. These studies suggest that about 5% of patients die or are disabled after surgical treatment of UIAs.[100-107] In contrast, results of the ISUIA trial, a prospective study involving 1172 patients, suggested that the combined morbidity and mortality may approach 15% at 1 year.[20]

Meta-analyses of surgical series have been performed (see Tables 79.8 and 79.9); most suggest that the combined morbidity and mortality rate is between 3% and 7%. For example, King and associates[108] reviewed 28 clinical series involving 733 patients. Overall, 4.1% of patients were disabled, and 1% died. Later, Raaymakers and colleagues[109] performed a meta-analysis of series published between 1966 and 1996 and involving 2460 patients who underwent surgical repair of UIAs. Surgical morbidity was 10.9%, and surgical mortality 2.6%. The limitations to this meta-analysis, which is a controversial retrospective research tool, are as follows: (1) results are reported primarily by surgeons with an inherent bias, (2) different aneurysm sizes and locations are included, (3) how a UIA was occluded is not always described, (4) postoperative angiography was rarely performed, so the efficacy of surgery is ill-defined, (5) description of outcome measures is often lacking, and (6) cognitive or quality of life assessment was usually absent. These limitations become important in deciding who should be treated and whether surgical or endovascular techniques are more appropriate.

Many variables affect surgical outcome for UIAs. Patient-related factors that increase UIA surgical risk include advanced age, ischemic cerebrovascular disease,

Table 79.8 Summary of Small Published Reviews and Clinical Series Describing Surgical Risk for Unruptured Aneurysms

Study* (reference)	Number of Patients/ Studies	Mortality (95% CI)	Morbidity (95% CI)
Wirth et al (1983)[107]	260/7	0 (0–1)	6.5 (3.9–10.3)
Rosenorn et al (1988)[50]	354/10	0 (0–4)	4 (0–12)
Piepgras (1989)[279]	234/5	0 (0–1.3)	7.3 (4.3–11.4)
Pertuiset et al (1991)[104]	293/10	1 (0.2–3)	2 (0.8–4.4)
King et al (1994)[108]	733/28	1 (0.4–20)	4.1 (2.8–5.8)

*Superscript numbers indicate chapter references.
CI, confidence interval.

Table 79.9   Outcome After Surgical Treatment of Unruptured Intracranial Aneurysms from Large Observational Studies and Meta-Analysis

Study[*]	Type of study	Dates of Data Collection	Number of Patients	Combined Poor Outcome, % (95% CI)	Mortality, % (95% CI)
Raaymakers et al (1998)[109]	Meta-analysis	1966–1996	2460 (61 studies)	10.9 (9.6–12.2)	2.6 (2–3.3)
Johnson et al (1999)[281]	Administrative review	1994–1997	2357	18.5 (16.9–20)	2.3 (1.7–2.9)
Johnson et al (2001)[282]	Administrative review	1990–1998	1699	25 (23.3–27.4)	3.5 (2.6–4.3)
ISUIA, Phases 1 and 2 (2002)[20,283]	Prospective, observational	1992–1998	1916	14%[†]	3.0 (2.2–3.8)

CI, confidence interval; ISUIA, International Study of Unruptured Intracranial Aneurysms.

[†]Includes non-Rankin scale affecting neurocognitive deficiencies.

Adapted from Molyneux A, Le Roux P: Surgical or endovascular treatment of intracranial aneurysms: A comparison of techniques. In Le Roux P, Newell DW, Winn HR (eds): Management of Cerebral Aneurysms. Philadelphia, Elsevier 2004, pp 983–995.

and medical conditions such as diabetes mellitus.[100,107,110,111] Increased aneurysm size, posterior circulation aneurysms, wide aneurysm neck, atherosclerosis, and calcification in the aneurysm neck, among other aneurysm-related variables, are associated with higher risk.[100,107,109,110] A large aneurysm, particularly a giant aneurysm, is probably the most important risk factor for poor surgical outcome, even in expert hands (Table 79.10). For example, Solomon and coworkers[100] observed a favorable outcome in 83% of patients who underwent surgical repair of giant UIAs, whereas 99% of their patients who had UIAs less than 10 mm in diameter experienced good outcomes.

Ruptured Cerebral Aneurysms

Many factors, including patient age, premorbid condition, the time it takes to reach the hospital, clinical grade at admission, amount of SAH on CT, intraventricular hemorrhage (IVH), hydrocephalus, ICH, aneurysm size or location, rebleeding, and vasospasm, can affect outcome after aneurysm rupture. It is thus difficult to apply a single standard of care to all patients and all aneurysms after SAH. Among these many variables, the most important independent factor associated with outcome is the patient's admission clinical status or grade after aneurysm rupture[17,76,112–117];

coma or poor clinical grade has consistently been identified as a predictor of death or poor functional outcome after SAH (Table 79.11). How to manage these very sick patients is uncertain; there is no one successful strategy, and all strategies are derived exclusively from clinical series. These clinical series, however, demonstrate that there is a population of patients with poor clinical grade who can make a meaningful recovery.[113,118–120] This chance of recovery, however, requires an aggressive multidisciplinary approach (Table 79.12). Such management necessitates a large commitment of resources, and in the current era of limited resources, one must ask whether intervention is justified in all patients with poor clinical grade.

The optimal time after aneurysm rupture at which to perform surgical occlusion remains a fundamental question in cerebrovascular surgery. There has been extensive research on the timing of aneurysm surgery. The majority of these studies are large clinical series or describe concurrent cohorts or historical controls.[112,121–128] There is a tendency in these studies for patients undergoing early surgery (within 72 hours of aneurysm rupture) to experience more favorable outcomes. A single randomized study has examined surgical timing after anterior circulation aneurysm rupture in patients with Hunt and Hess clinical

Table 79.10   Outcomes in Surgical Series of Giant Intracranial Aneurysms

Study[*]	No. Patients	Excellent, Good	Fair, Poor	Death
		Outcome (%)		
Kodama & Suzuki (1982)[285]	49	61	16	22
Symon & Vajda (1984)[286]	36	86	6	8
Yasargil (1984)[287]	30	67	23	10
Hosobuchi (1985)[288]	82	84	9	7
Heros (1986)[164]	28	82	7	5
Sundt (1990)[289]	315	80	6	15
Ausman et al (1990)[290]	62	84	11	5
Peerless et al (1990)[291]	305	67	22	11
Lawton & Spetzler (1995)[284]	171	87	8	5

[*]Superscript numbers indicate chapter references.

Adapted from Lawton MT, Spetzler RF: Surgical management of giant intracranial aneurysms: Experience with 171 patients. Clin Neurosurg 42:245,1995.

Table 79.11   The International Cooperative Study on the Timing of Aneurysm Surgery: Admission Level of Consciousness Is Associated with Outcome*

Consciousness Level	Good Recovery (%)	Moderately Disabled (%)	Severely Disabled (%)	Vegetative (%)	Dead (%)	Total (n)
Alert	74.3	7.5	4.1	1.0	13.1	1722
Drowsy	53.5	11.0	6.3	1.7	27.6	1136
Stuporous	30.2	13.8	8.0	4.3	43.7	348
Comatose	11.1	5.4	7.9	3.5	72.1	315
Total	57.6	9.1	5.5	1.8	26.0	3521

*Relationship between admission level of consciousness and outcome: $X^2 = 720.5$; $P < 0.001$.
Modified from Kassell NF, Torner JC, Haley EC Jr: The International Cooperative Study on the Timing of Aneurysm Surgery. I: Overall management results. J Neurosurg 73:18, 1990.

grades I through III.[129] At 3 months, 91.5% of patients undergoing surgery within 72 hours after SAH were independent; the rates were 78.6% for those undergoing surgery between 4 and 7 days, and 80% for those undergoing surgery more than 8 days after SAH.

The international Cooperative Study on the Timing of Aneurysm Surgery (COSTAS)[112,125] was a prospective epidemiologic, but nonrandomized study that gathered information on 3251 patients with SAH in the 1980s. Among patients who were alert at admission, 78% experienced a favorable 6-month outcome when surgery was performed between 0 and 3 days after SAH. Of patients in whom surgery was performed more than 14 days after SAH, 69% experienced a favorable outcome. In separate analysis of 722 patients treated at 27 North American centers, a good recovery was observed in 70.9% of patients undergoing surgery between 0 and 3 days after SAH, but in 62.9% of patients undergoing surgery after 14 days.[123] For each patient with a ruptured aneurysm, several factors influence whether surgery is performed immediately or is delayed; these factors are related to the aneurysm, the hemorrhage, and the patient. Taken together, however, the various data suggest that surgery performed within 3 days of SAH is associated with the best chance of good outcome.

Outcome after SAH has been described in many series dating from before the introduction of the operating microscope to prospective RCTs of drug therapies for SAH performed during the 1990s and RCTs comparing surgery and Guglielmi detachable coils (GDC).[21,112,125,130–133] Although there are some limitations and biases in these larger trials, their results suggest expected outcomes associated with modern SAH treatment (Table 79.13). Results of surgical treatment and medical management are different. However surgical complications such as intraoperative aneurysm rupture, residual aneurysm, major vessel occlusions, cerebral contusion, ICH, wound infection and meningitis may complicate about 20% of cases and are associated with about 10% of the morbidity and mortality after SAH.[9,97,98,112,123–125,134–141] Factors such as inexperience and poor surgical technique may play a role.[4,134,139] However, complications and poor outcome occur with surgery even in the best of hands or when patients are cared for in specialized referral centers. Like the experience with UIAs, surgical complications after SAH are associated primarily with aneurysms' location, increased size, and complex morphology.[75,97,136,141,142,144,145] By contrast,

timing of surgery and clinical status of the patient have little or no impact on the likelihood of surgical complications (Table 79.14).[98,112,121,125,126,128]

How effective is surgery for ruptured aneurysms? When intraoperative or postoperative angiography is routine, residual aneurysms are observed in 5% of cases even if the surgeon believes the clip application is satisfactory.[17,96,98,99,140,146,147] Iatrogenic vessel occlusion occurs in 2% to 5% of patients; half of those affected suffer a disabling stroke.[97,122] These complications are associated primarily with aneurysm-related factors such as increased size, location in the posterior circulation or anterior communicating artery, and presence of atherosclerosis. Among aneurysms with known residua, long-term angiographic follow-up demonstrates growth in 40%, particularly those in which the original residual aneurysm was broad-based.[95] The incidence of rebleeding from these residual aneurysms is estimated to be between 0.5% and 1.9% per year.[95,96,135,148] These data have prompted some researchers to suggest that intraoperative angiography is useful.[146,149] This may be true for some large and complex aneurysms and aneurysms that involve the proximal internal carotid artery. However, intraoperative angiography in general does not provide the high level of visualization obtained in the angiography suite, so it might yield false-positive and false-negative results. The risk of stroke associated with intraoperative or postoperative angiography is very low (<0.4%) in patients with SAH.[97,150] Consequently, intraoperative or postoperative aneurysm imaging should be performed in the vast majority of patients.

Arteriovenous Malformation

Intracranial AVMs are rare. Population-based data are limited but suggest that 1 to 2 people per 100,000 have an AVM.[8,39,142] Because the primary treatment goal for AVMs is elimination of hemorrhage risk, the safety and efficacy of treatment must be measured against the natural history of AVMs. The long-term risk of hemorrhage among people with AVMs and the outcome of this hemorrhage are controversial. A number of potential biases can affect natural history studies—selection bias, treatment intervention bias, inconsistent follow-up, and lack of angiography for all cases. Furthermore, many AVMs are treated when detected.[151] The available data on the natural history of AVMs are level V data (see Table

Table 79.12   Summary of Published Data Describing Overall Management Outcome in Patients with Hunt and Hess Clinical Grade IV or V after SAH

Study[°]	Patients[†]	Age	Management[‡]	Outcome (%)[§] Favorable	Poor	Death
Inamasu et al (2002)[292]	18 (Grade V only)	60.3	Comfort Measures Only	5.5	0	95.5
Hunt & Hess (1968)[293]	47 (17.1%)	NR	Delayed surgery until grade I or II	NR	NR	78.7
Adams et al (1981)[294]	61 (26%)	NR	Delayed surgery; antifibrinolytics	18	24.6	57.4
Testa et al (1985)[295]	80 (36%)	Mean 51.4 yr Range 14–73 yr	Delayed surgery until grade I, II or III; limited ICU care	3.8	8.8	87.4
Freckmann et al (1987)[296]	20 (6.3%)	NR	Delayed surgery unless ICH present; routine CCB, HV	5	20	75
Hijdra et al (1987)[297]	42 (15.9%)	Est[¶] 28% > 60 yr	Delayed surgery until grade I or II; some patients received antifibrinolytics, excluded those >65 yr	5	23	71
Ohno et al (1988)[298]	32 (34.7%)	14 patients >70 yr	Delayed surgery unless ICH present	15.6	15.6	68
Average				9.5	18.4	72.9
Chyatte et al (1988)[121]	80 (32.8%)	NR	Selective early surgery (26%)	25	29	46
Inagawa et al (1988)[299]	157 (24.8%)	44% > 60 yr	Selective early surgery; surgery deferred in 66.8% patients	9.5	15.2	75.2
Petruk et al (1988)[81]	108 (NR)	Est 54 yrs	Multicenter randomized trial of CCB; no standard management	25	21.3	53.7
Sevrain et al (1991)[300]	66 (24.4%)	Mean 47.2 yr Range 20–74 yr	Early surgery except patients with large ICH and abnormal pupils	19.6	12.2	68.2
Medlock et al (1992)[301]	41 (36%)	Mean 53.1 yr	Early surgery; routine HV, no CCB	7	5	88
Miyaoka et al (1993)[127]	370 (22.8%)	NR	Multicenter; selective early surgery (28%)	20.8	15.7	63.5
Average				17.8	16.4	65.8
Bailes et al (1990)[118]	54 (23.3%)	Mean 56 yr	EVD; selective aggressive; routine HV	42.6	7.4	50
Seifert et al (1990)[302]	74 (17.3%)	14 patients > 60 yr	EVD for hydrocephalus; selective aggressive	20.2	12.2	67.4
Nowak et al (1994)[303]	109 (39.4%)	NR	EVD; selective aggressive; routine CCB	21.1	36.7	42.2
Steudel et al (1994)[304]	116 (20.2%)	Est 49.5 yr	EVD for hydrocephalus; selective aggressive	35.3	7.8	56.9
Ungersbock et al (1994)[305]	48 (24.5%)	Mean 53.1 yr Range 31–77 yr	EVD; selective aggressive; routine CCB	21.3	36.2	42.5
Rordorf et al (1997)[120]	118 (NR)	Mean 57.5 yr	EVD: selective aggressive: triple-H and endovascular balloon dilation for vasospasm	31.3	16.1	52.5
Shimoda et al (1999)[306]	191 (50.8%)	Mean 57 yr	EVD, selective aggressive, cisternal drainage, HV, CCB, urokinase for IVH—outcome results for 74 patients selected for treatment	41.8[‖]	28.4[‖]	29.8[‖]
Hutchinson et al (2000)[307]	102 (NR)	Mean 55 yr	EVD for hydrocephalus, IVH, selective aggressive, triple-H	25	8	67
Suzuki et al (2000)[308]	189 (31.3%)	68.4 yr (for selected patients)	EVD, selective aggressive based on 12 hours of ICP control—outcome results for 103 patients selected for treatment	42.7[‖]	20.4[‖]	36.9[‖]
Average[‖]				31.2[‖]	19.2[‖]	50.6[‖]
Le Roux et al (1996)[113]	159 (36.5%)	Median 54 yr	Aggressive surgical management of all patients, routine HV, CCB, selective angioplasty	38.4	18.2	43.4
Kremer et al (1999)[309]	40 (22.3)	Mean 51.5 yr	Endovascular occlusion, triple-H; 23 patients with ICH not included in analysis	40[‖]	20°°°	40°°°

Table 79.12 Summary of Published Data Describing Overall Management Outcome in Patients with Hunt and Hess Clinical Grade IV or V after SAH—cont'd

Study[°]	Patients[†]	Age	Management[‡]	Outcome (%)[§] Favorable	Poor	Death
Groden et al (2001)[310]	41 (NR)	Mean 53.3 yr	Endovascular (n = 20) or surgical (n = 21) occlusion within 5 days, triple-H	29.3	31.7	39
Inamasu et al (2002)[292]	58 (Grade V only)	Mean 62.5 yr	Selective endovascular, if GCS score = 3, no treatment; outcome analysis excludes 17 patients who had surgery or ICH	2.4[°°]	17.1[°°]	80.5[°°]
van Loon et al (2002)[311]	11 (Grade V only)	Mean 48.1 yr	EVD, endovascular occlusion, routine HV, CCB	54.5	27.3	18.2
Average[‖]				31.6[‖°°]	24[‖°°]	44.4[‖°°]

°Superscript numbers indicate chapter references.

†Number of patients presenting with poor clinical grade after aneurysm rupture; percentage of all patients in all clinical grades treated at same institution(s) shown in parentheses.

‡A selective aggressive treatment strategy generally involves the following: (1) resuscitation of all patients with poor clinical grade, although not all patients are intubated and ventilated; (2) craniotomy in patients with ICH, and placement of EVD in other patients; (3) aggressive management, including occlusion of aneurysm within 24 hours in patients demonstrating clinical improvement or if ICP is controlled with EVD or other measures and there is no evidence of brain destruction on head CT; and (4) only comfort measures in other patients.

§Favorable outcome = patient independent, including GOS score indicating good outcome or moderate disability; poor outcome = patient dependent, including GOS score indicating severe disability or vegetative state.

‖The outcome results are limited to only those for patients selected for treatment. In most series, if a selective aggressive treatment strategy is used, nearly 100% of those patients who received only comfort measured died or were severely disabled. On average, therefore, more than 200 patients who presented with clinical grade IV or V are excluded from the outcome analysis. Because these patients inevitably did poorly, the outcome results may over-represent actual favorable outcome.

°°Outcome results do not include patients with aneurysmal ICH.

¶Value estimated from limited data.

CCB, calcium channel antagonist (blocker) therapy; CT, computed tomography; Est, estimate; EVD, external ventricular drainage; GCS, Glasgow Coma Scale; GOS, Glasgow Outcome Scale; HV, hypervolemia; ICH, intracerebral hemorrhage; ICP, intracranial pressure; ICU, intensive care unit; NR, not reported; triple-H, hypervolemia, hemodilution, and hypertension.

Adapted from Le Roux P, Winn HR: Management of the ruptured aneurysm. In Le Roux P, Newell DW, Winn HR (eds): Management of Cerebral Aneurysms. Philadelphia, Elsevier 2004, pp 303–333; and Le Roux P, Winn HR: Intracranial aneurysms and subarachnoid hemorrhage: Management of the poor grade patient. Acta Neurochir Suppl 72:7, 1999.

Table 79.13 Surgical Outcome after Subarachnoid Hemorrhage Reported in Large Observational Studies and Randomized Controlled Trials (RCTs) of Ruptured Aneurysms in Patients with Good Clinical Grade*

Study[†]	Study Type	Data Collection Period	No. of patients with Good Clinical Grade	Proportion "Good" Outcome, % (95% CI)	Mortality in Patients with "Good" Clinical Grade, % (95% CI)
Kassel et al (1990)[112]	Prospective, observational	1983–1986	1882	78.7% (76.7–80.5)	8.3% (7.0–9.6)
Haley et al (1997)[130]	RCT (tirilazad vs. placebo)	1994–1996	696		9.6% (7.5–12)
			886	70% (67–73) all grades	
Koivisto et al (2000)[131]	RCT (coil vs. surgery)	1995–1998	57 all grades	66% (52–78)	16% (7–27) 1 yr
Ogungbo et al (2001)[132]	Prospective observational	1990–1998	1609 (total)	90% (good grade)	6.2% (surgery)
International Subarachnoid Aneurysm Trial (2002)[21]	RCT (coil vs. surgery	1997–2002	1070 (1009 with good grade)	70% (all grades) at 1 year	10.1% (all grades) at 1 year

*Hunt and Hess grade 1, 2, or 3.

†Superscript references indicate chapter references.

Adapted from Molyneux A, Le Roux P: Surgical or endovascular treatment of intracranial aneurysms: A comparison of techniques. In Le Roux P, Newell DW, Winn HR (eds): Management of Cerebral Aneurysms. Philadelphia, Elsevier 2004, pp 983–995.

Table 79.14   Surgical Complications After Surgery for Ruptured Anterior Circulation Aneurysms

Complication	Percentage of Patients with Good clinical Grade (n = 224)	Percentage of Patients with Poor Clinical Grade (n = 131)
New intracerebral hematoma/contusion on computed tomography	2.2	0.8
New intracerebral hematoma, surgery°	4.5	3.8
Aneurysm remnant on postoperative angiogram†	7.1	7.2
Vessel occlusion on postoperative angiogram	7.1	6.3
Wound dehiscence	2.2	0.8
Cerebrospinal fluid leak	1.8	0.8
Meningitis	2.2	2.3
Wound infection	0.4	1.5
Cosmetic	0	1.5

°Intracerebral hematoma requiring surgical evacuation.
†All patients with good clinical grade and 111 patients with poor clinical grade underwent postoperative angiography.
Adapted from Le Roux P, Elliot JP, Newell DW, et al: The incidence of surgical complications is similar in good and poor grade patients undergoing repair of ruptured anterior circulation aneurysms: A retrospective review of 355 patients. Neurosurgery 38:887, 1996.

Table 79.15   Risk of Surgical Treatment of Arteriovenous Malformations

Spetzler-Martin Grade	Surgical Morbidity (%)	Surgical Mortality (%)
1	8	0
2	3	0
3	11	0
4	37	2.4
5	71	4.8

Adapted from Heros RC, Korosue K, Diebold PM: Surgical excision of cerebral arteriovenous malformations: Late results. Neurosurgery 26:570, 1990.

79.2) and indicate an overall initial annual hemorrhage risk between 2% and 3%.[152,154–157] Mortality from the first hemorrhage is between 10% and 30%, and 10% to 20% of survivors have long-term disability,[152,154–159] suggesting a long-term crude annual case-fatality rate of 1% to 1.5% and an annual combined major morbidity and mortality risk of 2.7%.[151,157]

The decision to treat an AVM is complex, and many factors must be considered, such as patient age, treatment risk and success, natural history, and the varied therapies—surgery, stereotactic radiosurgery (SRS), and embolization.[160] The decision how to treat an AVM is limited because there are no level I or II data describing standards of care for AVMs, in large part because of the heterogeneity of these lesions and their relative rarity. Guidelines have been published, but the recommendations are subject to a wide interpretation.[28] There are no RCTs, however, decision analysis that is based on clinical series and retrospective case reports suggest that of all treatments, microsurgery for AVMs offers patients the greatest quality of life, provided that the surgery is associated with less than 7% risk of major neurologic morbidity and mortality.[161] No two AVMs are alike, and surgical risk is defined primarily by AVM morphology or grade. Among the best-known and most popular grading systems is the Spetzler-Martin, which grades AVMs on the basis of size, venous drainage, and functional importance of adjacent brain. The relationship between this grading system and postoperative deficits was described initially from retrospective data,[162] but its validity has been confirmed in a prospective fashion (Tables 79.15 and 79.16).[163]

Surgery for AVMs is generally elective. However, emergency surgery to remove a large, life-threatening ICH may occasionally be necessary. In such a situation, none of the AVM, or at most a limited portion of the AVM, should be removed along with the ICH. The patient then should be allowed to recover, and more information about the AVM obtained through angiography. There are no firm guidelines or standards for perioperative care or that address the value of preoperative embolization, use of the operating microscope, intraoperative angiography, intraoperative mapping, perioperative blood pressure control, or seizure prophylaxis, among other questions.

Reports describing outcome after surgical excision of brain AVMs are based on level V data, most of which have been gathered in a retrospective fashion. Nevertheless, these published clinical series from expert AVM surgeons suggest that 90% to 95% of patients with Spetzler-Martin grade I or II lesions have an excellent or good outcome after surgery (see Table 79.16).[162,164] The rate of excellent or good outcome in grade III lesions is 68.2% for short-term follow-up and 88.6% for long-term follow-up. Such favorable outcomes are also observed in 73% of patients with grade IV AVMs and 57.1% with grade V lesions. In prospective studies, treatment-associated morbidity is observed in 31.2% and 50% of grade IV and grade V lesions, respectively.[163,165] The risk of residual AVM or ICH after AVM surgery is not well described. In a report from the New York AVM Databank involving 240 prospectively enrolled patients who underwent 269 AVM-related surgical procedures, 6% had a residual AVM when a single-step procedure was performed and symptomatic postoperative ICHs were observed in 1%. The risk of residual AVM or dysplastic vessels after surgery is significantly associated with increasing mean diameter of the AVM.[166]

The Role of Multimodality Therapy, Embolization, or Stereotactic Radiosurgery

There are only level V studies in the literature describing multimodality therapy, embolization, and SRS for AVMs, so no specific recommendations for the use of these therapies can be made.[28] However, it does appear that multimodality therapy plays a helpful role in larger lesions (Spetzler-Martin grade III or IV), for which complete obliteration is the goal. All grade V lesions should be managed on an individual basis and with a multidisciplinary approach. Resources to provide multimodality treatment may vary among institutions; however, there is no

Table 79.16 Results of Microsurgical Treatment of Arteriovenous Malformations Less Than 3 cm in Diameter

Study[*]	No. of Patients	Obliteration (%)	Postoperative Hemorrhage	Death	New Permanent Neurologic Deficit (%)	Cases of Major Morbidity (%)	Cases of Minor Morbidity (%)
Spetzler & Martin (1986)[31]	69	100	0	0	NR	1 (1.4)	4 (5.8)
Heros, et al (1990)[312]	91	87	0	0	NR	0 (0)	10 (11)
Sundt et al (1991)[313]	84	100	0	0	2.2	NR	NR
Sisti, et al (1993)[314]	67	94	0	0	1.5	8 (11.9)	24 (35.85)
Hamilton & Spetzler (1994)[113]	71	100	0	0	0	1 (1.4)	8 (11.3)
Schaller & Schramm (1997)[315]	62	98.4	0	0	3.2	NR	NR
Pikus et al (1998)[124]	54	100	0	0	1.9	0 (0)	1 (1.9)

NR, not recorded.
[*]Superscript numbers indicate chapter references.

role for partial treatment of an AVM. Embolization followed by surgery is the cornerstone of multimodality treatment, particularly for larger AVMs.[165,167,168] Numerous clinical studies describe the beneficial effect of preoperative embolization in reducing procedure time and blood loss or in converting high-grade (Spetzler-Martin) lesions to lower-grade lesions which appears to be associated with reduced surgical morbidity and mortality.[165,167,169] No prospective RCTs have been performed to verify this observation, and there are no prospectively controlled studies comparing surgery with and without embolization.

The four basic objectives for AVM embolization are (1) complete AVM occlusion (rare), (2) preparation for surgical excision (including feeding artery aneurysm embolization), (3) reduction in the size before radiosurgery, and (4) palliative flow reduction (rare). Embolization is usually not necessary for small easily accessible AVMs for surgery, being best reserved for deep or relatively inaccessible feeding arteries or for staged preoperative occlusion of large high-flow AVMs to reduce hemodynamic complications.[170] There is no rigorous data to support how AVMs should be embolized. For example, it is unclear whether to use general anesthesia or deep intravenous sedation or what embolization agent is best. Similarly, the use of corticosteroids, anticonvulsants, aspirin, and calcium channel blockers, among other drugs, during embolization procedures has not been rigorously tested.

Only level V data describe the results and efficacy of AVM embolization. Five percent to 10% of cases are

associated with complications, and the rate of death during embolization is about 1% or less (Table 79.17).[165,167,171–173] For example, Gobin and associates[174] observed rates of 5.6% for minor complications, 7.2% for moderate or severe complications, and 1.6% for mortality during the course of embolization in 125 patients. Similarly, Hartmann and colleagues,[169,171] who treated 233 patients with 545 endovascular procedures, observed that 33 patients (14%) showed treatment-related neurologic deficits; 5 (2%) had persistent disabling deficits, and 2 (1%) died. Increasing patient age and number of embolizations but not AVM morphology were associated with increased risk. Complete AVM occlusion is observed in about 10% of patients who undergo embolization (see Table 79.17).[168,170]

SRS is also advocated for selected AVMs. A large number of studies (level IV or V evidence) show that SRS provides satisfactory results for AVM cure (Table 79.18).[175–183] Radiosurgery is most appropriate for patients with small AVMs, particularly those with volumes less than 10 cm^3 or a maximum diameter less than 3 cm, especially when they are located in eloquent brain regions.[175,180,182] Complete AVM obliteration and therefore elimination of the hemorrhage risk is observed in 80% of patients within 2 to 3 years after SRS. Smaller AVMs respond better because more radiation can be delivered safely.[184] Radiosurgery, however, has potential morbidity that corresponds with the time course for AVM obliteration; overall, there is a 5% to 7% risk of treatment-related complications.[180,183,184] In addition, symptomatic patients are

Table 79.17 Results of Embolization of Arteriovenous Malformation

Study[*]	Material	Cases (No.)	Occluded (%)	Minor Deficit (%)	Major Deficit (%)	Mortality (%)
Berenstein (1990)[316]	IBCA	500	17	5	1	1
Wikholm et al (1996)[317]	NBCA, PVA	150	13	32	7	1
Gobin et al (1996)[174]	NBCA	125	11	6	2	0
Debrun et al (1997)[318]	NBCA	54	5	4	2	4
Paulsen et al (1999)[319]	NBCA, PVA	38	3	6	6	0
Song et al (2000)[320]	Silk	230	—	9	4	1

[*]Superscript numbers indicate chapter references.
IBCA, isobutyl-2-cyanocrylate; NBCA, N-butyl cyanoacrylate; PVA, polyvinyl alcohol.

Table 79.18   Results of Stereotactic Radiosurgery for Arteriovenous Malformations

Study°	Cases (No.)	Occluded (%)	Morbidity (%)	Bleeds (%/yr)	Mortality (%)
Steiner et al (1992)[182]	239	81	4	4	5
Friedman et al (1996)[176]	201	—	—	6	1
Flickinger et al (1996)[184]	197	72	—	—	—
Flickinger et al (1997)[321]	307	—	11	—	—
Karlsson et al (1997)[178]	945	87	—	—	—
Sasaki et al (1998)[322]	66	86	7	5	1
Pollack (1999)[323]	97	74	5	5	4

exposed to a 3% to 4% annual hemorrhage risk during the time it takes for the radiation to obliterate the AVM. Moreover, the long-term outcome and risks after radiosurgical treatment are unclear. Tumor induction after irradiation is a recognized risk, and the occurrence of brain tumors after radiation therapy has been described. Excellent results also are obtained from microsurgery of AVMs less than 3 cm in diameter. Although there are no RCTs, comparisons among different case series describing SRS or surgery have led some to suggest that for small, surgically accessible lesions (Spetzler-Martin grade I or II), surgery has fewer risks than radiosurgery and is more likely to provide definitive cure.[28,185]

HOW DO PATIENTS OR THIRD-PARTY PAYERS DECIDE WHERE THEY CAN GET "THE STANDARD OF CARE"?

Many variables affect the outcome of treatment for cerebrovascular disease. Those that are specific to patients or diseases are discussed in the preceding sections as well as the relevant chapters of this book. Other variables associated with outcome, such as socioeconomic status, geographical differences, hospital type, and referral patterns, are beyond the control of the individual physician and are not patient specific.[19,186–188] For example, Whisnant and colleagues[188] found that among patients with SAH treated at the same institution, survival for 30 days after SAH was significantly higher in patients who were referred for treatment from outside the community than in patients from within the community.

Such differences have led patients, insurance companies, corporate purchasers, and policy-makers to use hospital volume as a surrogate indicator of quality and, therefore, of the standard of care, because a growing body of literature has found an association between better outcome and high treatment volume for a wide range of procedures and conditions, including CEA, aneurysm surgery, and SAH.[189–194] These findings have significant clinical, legal, and policy implications. However, the association and the magnitude of the association between volume and outcome are variable. Furthermore, "high volume equals quality or standard of care" is a false premise, because the majority of the studies use administrative data, which is associated with many problems of application to clinical outcomes, as already discussed.[195,196] For example, hospital volume–outcome studies that perform risk adjustment with clinical data are less likely to

observe associations than are studies using administrative data.[192] Second, very few studies examine the processes of care that may be more relevant to outcome than volume alone.

Surgeon volume is another surrogate marker for "standard of care." The two premises for this relationship are "practice makes perfect" and "selective referral." If the former is a valid determinate for quality, it is unclear whether there is a threshold volume. Alternatively, the frequency of performance of a procedure may be important in making a surgeon "perfect."[197] If "selective referral" underlies surgical volume, patients and referring physicians must know outcome results and case mix for a particular surgeon. These data, except for cardiac surgery mortality in some states, are not available and even when they are available, physicians and patients do not base referrals and choices on them.[198,199] Selective referral also implies that patients have a choice about the surgeon who operates on them.

The relationship between individual surgeon volume and outcome has been observed in some[195,200] but not all studies[201,202] examining cerebrovascular surgery, in particular carotid artery surgery. Exactly what constitutes an "adequate" number of CEAs performed for good outcome is not known; some studies suggest five procedures a year is sufficient.[195] Furthermore, some high-volume surgeons have poor outcomes and some low-volume surgeons have good outcomes. Similarly, some high-volume surgeons operate at low-volume institutions. Thus, the relationship of hospital or surgeon volume with, and their relative contribution to, the quality of cerebrovascular surgery is not known.

Public health policies may stem from these observations. Whether they influence the standard of care depends on how well the public understands the complexities in the relationship between volume and outcome, whether risk adjustment is performed, and whether patients can choose their surgeon or hospital. As Rothwell and colleagues[203] suggest after an analysis of surgeon risk in the European Carotid Surgery Trial (ECST), oversimplistic interpretations of crude results may lead to unjustified surgeon criticism and are unlikely to result in improved patient care.

The Leapfrog Group, among other groups, has suggested a policy of selective referral of surgical procedures such as CEA to high-volume hospitals. The implementation of such a policy is controversial, because whether the optimal performance of a surgical procedure depends more on individual surgeons' abilities or on hospital volume alone remains unclear.[200,204,205] In addition, rather than volume alone, several lines of evidence suggest that it is the process of care or organized care that is associated with improved outcome. For example, the relationships between a Level I trauma center and improved outcome and between an organized inpatient multidisciplinary approach to stroke care and better outcome have been described.[206-208] Nursing care and availability of nurses are fundamental to organized health care. There is, however, a shortage of registered nurses (RNs).[209,210] This situation has significant clinical implications, as several studies have demonstrated that there is a significant association between lack of nurses and higher mortality or larger number of adverse events.[211-213] For example, in a cross-sectional analysis of linked data from 10,184 nurses and 232,342 patients in general, orthopaedic, and vascular surgery, Aiken and coworkers[211] observed that for each patient added to the number of patients a nurse cared for, there was a 7% rise in likelihood of a patient dying within 30 days of hospitalization.

MEDICAL ERRORS AND ADVERSE OUTCOME

How Often Do Medical Errors Occur?

Adverse outcomes occur in cerebrovascular surgery even in the best of hands.[4,50] However, an adverse outcome does not imply substandard care. Medical errors may or may not be associated with poor outcome. How often do they occur? The 2000 report from IOM attributes between 44,000 and 98,000 deaths annually to medical error.[6] This conclusion was calculated mathematically from data that is nearly 20 years old. Whether such a relationship is still applicable is not certain. Later studies suggest that medical errors may occur in about one quarter of hospitalized patients[211,214,215] and may contribute to serious consequence, such as death or long-term disability, in 10% to 20%. However, less than 20% of errors are recognized by caregivers,[216] and only 1% to 2% result in legal claims, in large part because errors do not always lead to poor outcome.[214,215] For example, in a prospective observational study that examined adverse events among 1047 patients in three teaching hospitals, Andrews and colleagues[214] observed that 17.7% had at least one serious adverse event, which was usually linked to the seriousness of the illness.

There is limited information on the prevalence of errors or adverse outcomes in neurosurgery. In the National Veterans Administration Surgical Risk Study, a prospective observational study from 44 Veterans Affairs Medical Centers (VAMC) in 83,958 patients undergoing noncardiac surgery, of which 10% was neurosurgery, unadjusted mortality at 30 days was 3.1%; 17% of the patients had one or more major complications, and mean neurosurgical morbidity was 14.2%.[217] Despite the apparent frequency of medical errors and the attention that has been focused on them by the IOM, less than 10% of physicians or patients regard medical errors as one of the largest problems in health care today. Instead, physicians name costs of malpractice insurance and lawsuits and cost of health care, whereas the public names cost of health care and problems with insurance companies and health plans as the major problems facing health care.[215] It is important also to recognize that there is a difference between errors and unexpected outcome. Errors can be an act of omission or commission from individuals or from the system of health care—some but not all errors harm patients. An unexpected or unanticipated outcome is a negative result; it may or may not be associated with a medical error but also may result from biologic variability. Patients undergoing cerebrovascular surgery must be aware of these differences; such awareness, in part, forms the basis of informed consent.

Why Do Medical Errors Occur?

In the IOM's report *To Err Is Human; Building a Safer Health System*,[6] medical errors are largely attributed to system factors rather than to negligent or incompetent individuals.[6] For example, in the Harvard study on which the IOM report was partly based, 1133 patients (3.7%) with disabling injuries caused by medical treatment were identified from 30,195 randomly selected hospital records in New York State.[143,218] Two thirds of those events were considered to have been caused by management errors, most of which were not due to negligence. Forty-eight percent of the adverse events were associated with surgery. However, adverse events during surgery were less likely to be caused by negligence (17%) than nonsurgical errors (37%). The highest proportion of negligence-induced adverse events were associated with diagnostic mishaps, noninvasive therapeutic mishaps (usually error of omission), or were associated with events in the emergency room. In surgery, the highest incidence of adverse events occurs not during the procedure but rather in the subsequent monitoring and daily care.[214] Anesthesia accounts for few adverse events (about 2%), but when anesthesia-related events do occur, they are frequently related to human error.[219] The likelihood of an adverse event is greater with longer hospital stays, with ICU care, or with development of a complication.

There are many reasons why medical errors occur. First, the sheer volume of new information, the National Institutes of Health (NIH) spend $15.6 billion, the pharmaceutical industry $24 billion, and the medical device industry $9 billion on research and development each year. This research generates new knowledge and technologies more rapidly than physicians (even with respect to the research in their medical discipline) or the health care system can absorb. Second, error, including preventable adverse surgical events, may be institution related and may occur more frequently in for-profit, minor teaching, or nonteaching government-owned hospitals than in major teaching hospitals.[220] Third, the incidence of chronic conditions is rising and the population is progressively aging. Fourth, health care remains fragmented and uncoordinated. For example, health care lags far behind other industries in the effective use of state-of-the-art computer systems. Fifth, most errors are intrinsic to the system and result from a multitude or cascade of small errors that can lead to serious errors.[221] For example, administrative decisions can contribute to 10% of medical errors,[214] whereas problems with complex organizational systems, such as not having enough time with patients, health care professional overwork, stress, fatigue, failure of health professionals to work together or communicate as a team, and understaffing of nurses in hospitals are frequently cited as reasons for medical error.[221] Finally, as health care delivery has changed from a fee-for-service, autonomous system to managed care with limited autonomy,[222,223] there has been a significant drop in physician satisfaction[222,224]; this change has been associated with impaired job performance and physician error.[223,225–227]

Can Medical Errors Be Prevented?

The current literature on preventing human error and improving safety is derived mainly from major industrial disasters, airplane accidents, and nuclear explosions.[228] Most reports in medicine describe the problem, but there is limited discussion on how to improve patient safety. Traditionally in medicine, a punitive search has been conducted for an individual culprit. Today, however, there is a better understanding that medical error or substandard care must be approached with a systems method because there is a growing realization that adverse outcomes are rarely due to one large error by one person but instead more commonly result from multiple small system or latent errors. *Latent errors* consist of deficiencies in design, organization, maintenance, training, and management that create conditions in which persons are more likely to make mistakes or that combine, even unexpectedly, to create an adverse outcome.[228] Hence the concept "to err is human."

Surgeons, including cerebrovascular surgeons, tend to practice in an independent and sometimes idiosyncratic fashion. Their actions may be unpredictable or without scientific basis (e.g., choice of suture, whether to place a drain or not, prophylaxis against deep vein thrombosis, and postoperative ambulation).[216,229] In these circumstances, error is inevitable. By contrast, the airline industry has been able to significantly reduce error through a willingness to adopt a system that reduces chances of error stemming from unique practices; that is, they follow strict protocols. Whether protocols can be applied to the many unique aspects of cerebrovascular disease is uncertain. One can put error reduction into perspective, however: If the airline industry were only 99% successful, there would be at least two plane crashes a day at Chicago's O'Hare Airport. By contrast, surgeons and most patients are delighted with a 90% to 95% success rate in surgery. In medicine, anesthesia is perhaps the only specialty that has reduced error through the use of critical-incident analysis, standardization, checklists, changes in training and supervision, and automation of anesthesia machines and alarm systems.[230]

Many organizations, including health care purchasers, insurers, providers and federal and state governments, are attempting to address medical error and standard of care. One such group is the Leapfrog Group a consortium of more than 100 Fortune 500 companies and other health care purchasers that represent more than 35 million employees. This group suggests the following three standards to prevent medical mistakes: (1) use of computerized physician order entry, (2) selection of hospitals with best results or extensive experience for certain high-risk conditions and procedures, and (3) employment of intensivists in ICUs.[231] This last standard, ICU staffing, is particularly appealing because 5 million patients are admitted annually to ICUs, 10% die during hospitalization, and nearly all of those admitted to the ICU suffer a preventable adverse event.[214,232] Furthermore, several studies have demonstrated that increased intensivist staffing in ICUs can improve patient outcomes.[233,234] Other groups, such as the Accreditation Council for Graduate Medical Education (ACGME), have introduced shorter resident work hours to prevent fatigue-induced errors. This change may be only part of the solution, however, because errors have been demonstrated to be associated with discontinuity of care and handoffs that naturally stem from restricted work hours.[235]

Reporting Medical Errors

The IOM report recommended that reporting medical errors, including deaths and serious injuries associated with medical error and also "near misses," may be the best source of data with which to develop systems to raise the "standard of care" and eliminate medical error.[6,7] Consequently many hospitals, professional bodies, and state legislatures, are developing polices and procedures that require error reporting and disclosure. For example, the Joint Commission on Accreditation of Healthcare Organizations (JCAHO) has tied disclosure to accreditation.[236,237] Similarly, the responsibility to disclose adverse outcomes is specifically addressed in the American Medical Association's Code of Ethics and the American College of Physicians' ethics manual.

Health care providers, however, are at present skeptical about error reporting,[238] in part because they believe the data may be misused and may result in punitive action or that such error reporting will encourage malpractice lawsuits. In addition, excessive legislation can be counterproductive. A successful reporting system that can potentially eradicate errors and raise the standard of care should be confidential and nonpunitive and should focus on the system rather than the individual.[215,239] Such a system must be pragmatically integrated with the routine provision of care. Such a system has been available in the airline industry for more than 25 years—the Aviation Safety Reporting System.

The information gained in the analysis of medical errors should be used for a root cause analysis rather than a search for fault.[240] Such an approach will help reduce error, as the JCAHO has recognized,[237] and is consistent with industries that have succeeded in becoming safe (e.g., aviation and nuclear power). Health care, however, is more complex than these industries, and the difficulties are compounded by the current tendency to assign blame for errors, fear of lawsuits, and a focus on individual performance. In addition, the public believes that persons responsible for errors with serious consequences should be sued, fined, and subject to suspension of their professional licenses. These attitudes—shared by legislators and the legal system—are unlikely to change.

Many consumer groups are calling for the National Practitioner Data Bank (NPDB) to be made public. This electronic repository, established by Congress as part of the Health Care Quality Improvement Act of 1986, collects information about adverse license actions, restriction of clinical privileges, and professional society membership as well as data on all payments made on behalf of physicians for liability settlements and judgments. When the NPDB was enacted, the information was to remain confidential. It was not the intent of the NPDB to equate payment with below-standard practice. However, practitioners listed on the NBPB are now regarded in some quarters as practicing below the standard of care. There are many limitations to the NPBD data. For example, there is no threshold of payment, record of physician specialty (variable risk of liability), and liability settlements and judgments rarely note whether the standard of care was violated. In recent years, the number of NPDB-listed physicians has grown by 10% annually, and now includes greater than 20% of U.S. physicians. If making a malpractice payment means practicing below the standard of care, then 20% of U.S. physicians already are practicing below standard.[241]

STANDARDS OF CARE AND PRACTICE GUIDELINES IN CEREBROVASCULAR SURGERY

Standards of Care

The "standards of care" in cerebrovascular surgery are limited. Why? First there are few high-quality data that document the benefits associated with nuances of care or of surgical technique. For example, the CEA RCTs clarify the benefit of CEA but do not "standardize," apart from "safely," how the procedure should be performed. Similarly, there are primarily only empiric data to support whether or not some common medical interventions, such as administration of anticonvulsants after SAH, should be standard. It remains unclear, however, how much data is enough to determine a standard. Second, lawyers dislike "medical standards of care"; they prefer a "standard" only for a particular case but not for all patients. Third, physicians dislike standards because any standard imposed by a third party distorts the doctor-patient relationship and there can be no standard to cover all cases and all aspects of a particular case. If no standard exists for a given procedure, there can be no medical malpractice—it is a priori impossible to contravene a medical standard if it does not exist. External standards, however, are coming in the form of practice guidelines, critical pathways, and utilization reviews, to name a few. The legal system, courts, payers, or legislative bodies cannot and should not set the standard. Instead, for cerebrovascular surgery, organizations such as the American Board of Neurological Surgery (ABNS) and the American Association of Neurological Surgeons (AANS) should, at the very least, establish a database in which members report their experience with any alleged deviations below the standard. Then, when there is an allegation of negligence or substandard care, this database can be used to help describe the spectrum that is associated with "standard of care."

Establishment of a standard may not always safeguard the individual physician in matters of alleged negligence. For example, the courts have found that although custom is relevant in standard of care, "custom should never be conclusive"[242,243]; that is, there are circumstances in which a professional standard may be set aside. This notion has it origins in a landmark case from 1932, *The TJ Hooper*[243] and in the medical context in *Helling v Carey*.[242] In *Hooper*, a tugboat without a radio caused an accident. Even though it was not required or standard for tugboats

to carry radios at the time, the courts turned to "basic reasonableness standard" and set aside the professional standard on the basis of evidence that the standard is unreasonable in light of knowledge and a relatively low cost of other safer practices. In *Helling v Carey*, an ophthalmologist was found guilty of not screening a young woman for glaucoma even though no other ophthalmologists performed such screening nor was it recommended in an authoritative text. This finding implies that an individual medical practitioner can be held to a standard not yet adopted throughout the profession if the courts feel that a standard is lacking. Furthermore, the courts reserve the right to find a whole practice unsound. By contrast, an expert witness held to a standard can accurately describe only what other physicians of comparable training ordinarily do in similar circumstances; he or she cannot find a whole practice unsound.

Practice Guidelines

The IOM defines *practice guidelines* as "systematically developed statements to assist practitioner and patient decisions about appropriate health care for specific clinical circumstances".[244] Practice guidelines, in part, have been considered by some to be synonymous with "standards of care." They are not, however, because in the United States practice guidelines have been stimulated primarily by a desire to reduce economic costs (the economic and societal costs of cerebrovascular disease are well known and staggering). Two primary concerns have fueled practice guideline development, (1) regional differences in performance of procedures, interventions, or surgery and (2) rising health care cost that is associated with reduced payments to hospitals and physicians, as well as greater restriction of physician autonomy.[245,246] Today, hospitals face a diminishing operating margin.[245] Variability in care is known to contribute to cost[246]; consequently, institutions are analyzing delivery of care, searching for ways to address these market pressures. In this situation, it is hoped that practice guidelines can identify appropriate treatment and eliminate the unnecessary "inappropriate care" or variation in care. In short, practice guidelines are more a means to control costs rather than improve patient outcome. For this reason, practice guidelines are important to the government, regulatory bodies, and third party payers. Today, development of such guidelines is no longer only a local or professional responsibility; it is established in federal law and funded by millions of Public Health Service and Medicare dollars.

Practice Guidelines and the Law

The AHA has published practice guidelines or consensus statements describing several aspects of cerebrovascular surgery.[2,24-28] Practice guidelines may have vast legal implications. First, they are germane to the growing body of law and public policy describing forces external to the doctor-patient relationship. This includes large organizations that determine the nature of benefits as well as utilization management, in which the practice guidelines help determine who gets what or what is appropriate care. Second, practice guidelines can be used by credentialing committees and payers to establish standards of care. When used in this manner, however, the guidelines measure physician conformity rather than patient outcome. Third, practice guidelines can be relevant in malpractice. However, adherence to guidelines is not a defense against liability and often may be used against physicians rather than in their defense.[240,247] For example, Hymans and colleagues,[248] who reviewed 259 claims at two insurance companies and a survey from 960 randomly selected malpractice attorneys, observed that practice guidelines were used for inculpatory purposes in more than half the cases, a proportion two- to three-fold greater than for exculpatory purposes. In malpractice, the value of guidelines, particularly when written by expert panels, is that they may reduce liability premiums. The need for surgeon involvement in developing practice guidelines is therefore obvious, because many aspects of cerebrovascular surgery may not lend themselves to definitive statements. Similarly, guidelines cannot cover every conceivable circumstance, and in some situations, the complexity of the problem may prevent development of a guideline. Guidelines thereby become collections of evidence describing good practice.

Desirable features for guidelines include validity, reliability, reproducibility, clinical applicability, clinical flexibility, clarity, and scheduled review.[249] It is also clear that guidelines must reflect the complexity of medical practice and decision-making; if not, they will not be relevant or accepted by the intended audience.[250] Additionally, guidelines need flexibility to allow room for development of the field and for individual physicians to exercise judgment and so protect themselves against the "outlier" (rare and unusual) patient and a wide variety of practice circumstances.

Examination of how practice guidelines affect individual physicians has been limited; studies that have been performed often find that some guidelines are easier to meet than others.[251] This difference is associated, in part, with geographical variation, resources at an institution, and capabilities of other services. For example, Cohen and associates,[252] who evaluated anesthetic outcome in Canada among 27,184 patients at four centers, concluded that "the contribution of anesthesia to perioperative outcomes is uncertain and may be explained by institutional differences which are beyond the control of the anesthetist." The same argument could be made by individual surgeons treating cerebrovascular disease. It is also apparent that guidelines or protocols may not eliminate all surgical error or adverse events. For example, what operating room does not count sponges? Nevertheless sponges still are left in surgical patients, particularly during emergency surgery or when there is an unexpected change in surgery; in other words, there always is an unpredictable element in surgery that may preclude universal application of guidelines.[253] There are other factors, such as the new residency work-hour requirements by which "shift" work can be associated with greater errors[235,254–256] and the critical shortage of nurses that may limit universal application of guidelines in cerebrovascular surgery.[210,211] There is still interest in practice guidelines for individual disease. For example, if risk increases in carotid artery surgery, the surgical benefit is lost. Third party payers and medical managers are therefore interested in guidelines that promote the safety and efficacy of a procedure.

Quality of Care and Its Relationship to Standards of Care

Standards of care and practice guidelines lend themselves to the new health care economy in which the underlying expectation is that physicians and health care organizations will compete on the basis of quality and cost.[257] The means of precisely measuring or defining *quality*, which may in turn delineate a "standard of care," is elusive. Surgeons tend to define *quality* in terms of the results of patient care. The IOM defines it as "the degree to which health services for individuals and populations increase the likelihood of desired health outcomes and are consistent with current professional knowledge."[258] Other definitions, adapted from the science of industrial quality, focus on improving the processes by which care is delivered; *quality* by this light is "a continuous effort by all members of an organization to meet the needs and expectations of patients and other customers."[259] This latter definition is useful in developing standards of care because it (1) emphasizes the value of continuous improvement, (2) suggests that organizational processes of health care provision be studied, and (3) recognizes that patients' evaluations are valid indicators of quality. Process measures (what is done to a patient) may be more sensitive than outcomes measures (what happens to a patient) to determine "quality" care, because adverse outcomes may not occur each time there is an error or omission or when something is done incorrectly.[260] Nonetheless, some critics of process measures argue that if health care dollars are spent on improving the processes of care, health care costs may rise without a corresponding improvement in health.

Performance Measures

The development and application of performance measures is necessary to evaluate "quality" in health care and, in so doing, create standards or perhaps detect substandard practice.[261] Practice guidelines are not performance measures. Guidelines suggest diagnostic or therapeutic interventions for most patients in most circumstances, but the use of guidelines remains at the discretion of the physician. In contrast, *performance measures* are explicit standards of care against which actual clinical care is judged and that imply that physicians are in error if they do not provide care according to the standards. There are two central themes in designing performance measures, (1) demonstration of a link between each intervention and its outcome (harmful or beneficial) and (2) outcomes research, including medical effectiveness, patient functional status, patient satisfaction, and cost effectiveness.[262] For performance measures to be credible, they must demonstrate that differences in outcome will result if the processes of care under the control of the physician or health care system are altered.

Quantifying and improving health care quality and establishing practice guidelines and standards constitute a progressively more important goal in American medicine.[253] For example, the First Scientific Forum on Assessment of Quality of Care and Outcomes Research in Cardiovascular Disease and Stroke was held in 2000.[264] This conference assembled providers, researchers, payers, managed care, industry, and assessors of health care quality to discuss the current state of quality assessment in cardiovascular disease and stroke. It was clear from this conference that quantifying health care quality for stroke is a complicated and demanding process for which public and payer demands exceed current capabilities. The major challenges identified by this forum are as follows:

1. Identification of appropriate patients and patient information, because administrative and retrospective chart reviews have severe limitations. Prospective data collection is ideal but, in the absence of electronic medical records or incorporation of confidential quality measures into routine patient care, may not be feasible.
2. Time sensitivity of assessment and data acquisition. For example, some patients are lost to follow-up, and their characteristics or outcomes may be different from those patients with follow-up data. Some outcomes (e.g., thrombolysis for stroke) can be demonstrated in short-term measures (30 days), whereas the benefits of other interventions, such as CEA, may manifest months or years after discharge. Furthermore, patient care does not end with a patient's discharge from the hospital; many patients recovering from surgery for AVMs or after SAH demonstrate improvement over months after they return home.
3. Risk adjustment is important to ensure that differences in outcome are associated with quality of care and not with underlying patient characteristics. This may be difficult and expensive, and even though there are sophisticated risk adjustment techniques, a great deal of outcome variability remains unexplained. In part this lack of explanation may result from the small sample size associated with some conditions or complications after surgery. It is therefore problematic to try to rank different providers or institutions. Consequently, outcome measurements may be more appropriate for internal quality improvement.

Despite these limitations, many organizations, particularly with the advent of the Internet, publish lists that claim to rank the quality of health care systems and providers. The public regards these lists as a measure of the "standard of care." However, these various rankings often provide contradictory assessments of any given hospital and as yet cannot be relied upon.

Whether quality assurance information can translate into improved outcome remains uncertain, because establishing a relationship between risk-adjusted outcome and quality of care may be difficult.[265] One potential source of difficulty is random variation in low-frequency outcomes. For example, surgical mortality can vary several-fold each year because of chance variation in low-frequency occurrences. There is less variation in operative morbidity because it is more frequent than mortality. However, morbidity is more likely to be influenced by reporting or ascertainment bias. For example, in the National Veterans Administration Surgical Risk Study, risk adjustment had only a modest effect on the rank order of hospitals by rate of postoperative morbidity.[266] The same study showed that quality comparisons between hospitals may be feasible with the use of adjusted, but not unadjusted, mortality rates.[217] Furthermore, mortality rates are so low overall that it is difficult to create models predicting outcome in

individual procedures.[217] Samsa and colleagues[267] used data from the Department of Veterans Affairs NSQIP from different time periods; the correlation between two time periods was low, suggesting that many apparent quality improvement problems may not be as large as they first appear, particularly when based on few complications per facility. Few quality measures have been formally evaluated in stroke and cerebrovascular surgery. There are data showing, however, that an organized approach to stroke care and ICU care may reduce mortality, shorten length of hospital stay, and improve functional outcome.[268,269] These results suggest that the "process of care" rather than the individual practitioner has a greater effect on outcome.

Effect of Medical Education

Although rarely considered, medical school education and residency training may affect standards of care. The number of medical school applications has declined, and surgical residencies have become less attractive during the last several years.[270] The long-standing central tenet of neurosurgical training is to develop good clinical judgment by carefully evaluating each surgical patient and witnessing the progression of disease and the effects of interventions while providing continuity of patient care. This central theme has been eroded by several factors, including same-day admissions, shorter hospital stays, and lack of participation in longer-term outpatient follow-up.[254,271-273] For example, in some programs, residents obtain a history from and perform physical examination in only 10% of the patients on whom they subsequently operate.

Surgical education and the maintenance of a standard of care may be further compromised by the new resident work-hour restrictions required by the ACGME. Proponents of work-hour restrictions cite data demonstrating that fatigue impairs human performance and contend that long work hours cause fatigue and mood changes, which in turn increase medical errors. No studies have been performed that prove that health care personnel fatigue harms patients.[274] Furthermore, malpractice suits alleging that physician fatigue has caused patient harm are surprisingly rare. Early studies examining work-hour restrictions also suggest that they are associated with more complications and longer hospital stays,[275,276] in part because transitions between clinicians and cross-coverage increase the number of preventable adverse events.[235] Instead, "Lack of familiarity with a patient, not fatigue, is the major cause of errors of judgment."[254,277] The limitations on residency work hours may also result in (1) diminished development of accountability and professionalism, the keys to a successful physician-patient relationship (2) interference with educational activities or reduction in contact between residents and attending physicians,[278] (3) reduction in surgical experience, and (4) increased difficulty in recruiting and retaining faculty. All of these unintended secondary consequences of the alteration of work hours in residency training will negatively affect future standards of care for neurosurgical patients.

References

1. American Heart Association: Stroke Statistics. Available online at www.americanheart.org/Heart_and_Stroke_A_Z_Guide/strokes.html/

2. Broderick JP, Adams HP, Barsan W, et al: Guidelines for the management of spontaneous intracerebral hemorrhage: A statement for health care professionals from a special writing group of the Stroke Council, American Heart Association. Stroke 1999;30:905–915

3. American Heart Association: Economic Cost of Cardiovascular Diseases. Available online at www.americanheart.org/statistics/10econom.html (accessed September 2000).

4. Fridriksson S, Saveland H, Jakobsson KE, et al: Intraoperative complications in aneurysm surgery: A prospective national study. J Neurosurg 96:515–522, 2002.

5. Cronenwett J, Birkmeyer J (eds): The Dartmouth Atlas of Vascular Health care. Chicago, AHA Press, 2000.

6. Kohn LT, Corrigan JM, Donaldson MS: To Err Is Human: Building a Safer Health System. Washington, DC, National Academy Press, 2000.

7. Committee on Quality of Health Care in America, Institute of Medicine: Crossing the Quality Chasm: A New Health System for the 21st Century. Washington, DC, National Academy Press, 2001.

8. Relman AS, Angell M: How good is peer review? N Engl J Med 321:827–829, 1989.

9. Heyland DK, Cook DJ, King D, et al: Maximizing oxygen delivery in critically ill patients: A methodologic appraisal of the evidence. Crit Care Med 24:517–524, 1996.

10. Cook DJ, Guyatt GH, Laupacis A, Sackett DC: Rules of evidence and clinical recommendations on the use of antithrombotic agents. Chest 102:305S–311S, 1992.

11. Guyatt GH, Sackett DL, Cook DJ: Users' guide to the medical literature. II: How to use an article about therapy or prevention. A. Are the results of the study valid? JAMA 270:2598–2601, 1993.

12. Sackett DL: Rules of evidence and clinical recommendations on the use of antithrombotic agents. Chest 95(Suppl):2S–4S, 1989.

13. Horton R: Surgical research or comic opera: Questions, but few answers. Lancet 347:984–985, 1996.

14. Le Roux P, Winn HR: Management of cerebral aneurysms: How can current management be improved? Neurosurg Clin 9:421–433, 1998.

15. Malcynski JT, Hoff WS, Reilly PM, et al: Practice management guidelines for trauma patients: Where's the evidence [abstract]? J Trauma 47:1170, 2000.

16. Solomon MJ, McLeod RS: Should we be performing more randomized controlled trials evaluating surgical operations? Surgery 118:459–467, 1995.

16a. The EC/IC Bypass Study Group: Failure of extracranial-intracranial arterial bypass to reduce the risk of ischemic stroke. Results of an international randomized trial. N Engl J Med 313:1191–1200, 1985.

17. Le Roux P, Winn HR: Management of the ruptured aneurysm. In Le Roux P, Newell DW, Winn HR (eds): Management of Cerebral Aneurysms. Philadelphia, Elsevier 2004, pp 303–333.

18. Weir NU, Sandercock PAG, Lewis SC, et al: Variations between countries in outcome after stroke in the International Stroke Trial (IST). IST Collaborative Group. Stroke 32:1370–1377, 2001.

19. Wennberg JE, Freeman JL, Culp WJ: Are hospitalized services rationed in New Haven or over-utilized in Boston. Lancet 8543:1185–1189, 1987.

20. Unruptured intracranial aneurysms: Risks of rupture and risks of surgical intervention. International Study of Unruptured Intracranial Aneurysms Investigators. N Engl J Med 339:1725–1733, 1998.

21. Molyneux A, Kerr R, Stratton I, et al: International subarachnoid aneurysm trial (ISAT) of neurosurgical clipping versus endovascular coiling in 2143 patients with ruptured intracranial aneurysms: A randomized trial. International subarachnoid aneurysm collaborative group. Lancet 360: 267–1274, 2002.

22. van der Schaaf IC, Ruigrok YM, Rinkel GJ, et al: Study design and outcome measures in studies on aneurysmal subarachnoid hemorrhage. Stroke 33:2043–2046, 2002.

23. van Gijn J, Bromberg JEC, Lindsay KW, et al: Definition of initial grading, specific events, and overall outcome in patients with aneurysmal subarachnoid hemorrhage. Stroke 25:1623–1627, 1994.

24. Adams HP Jr, Adams RJ, Brott T, et al: Guidelines for the early management of patients with ischemic stroke: A scientific statement from the Stroke Council of the American Stroke Association. Stroke 34:1056–1083, 2003.

25. Bederson JB, Awad IA, Wiebers D et al: Recommendations for the management of patients with unruptured intracranial aneurysms: A

26. Biller J, Feinberg WM, Castaldo JE, et al: Guidelines for carotid endarterectomy: A Statement for Health care Professionals From a Special Writing Group of the Stroke Council, American Heart Association. Stroke 29:554–562, 1998.

27. Mayberg MR, Batjer HH, Dacey R, et al: Guidelines for the management of aneurysmal subarachnoid hemorrhage: A statement for health care professionals from a special writing group of the Stroke Council, American Heart Association. Stroke 25: 2315–2328, 1994.

28. Ogilvy CS, Stieg PE, Awad I, et al: Recommendations for the management of intracranial arteriovenous malformations. A statement for health care professionals from a special writing group of the Stroke Council, American Stroke Association. Stroke 32:1458–1471, 2001.

29. Cochrane Collaboration. Available at www.cochrane.org; last accessed July 24, 2002.

30. Levin A: The Cochrane Collaboration. Ann Intern Med 135:309–312, 2001.

31. Best WR, Khuri SF, Phelan M, et al: Identifying patient preoperative risk factors and postoperative adverse events in administrative databases: Results from the Department of Veterans Affairs National Surgical Quality Improvement Program. J Am Coll Surg 194:257–266, 2002.

32. Juvela S, Heiskanen O, Poranen A, et al: The treatment of spontaneous intracerebral hemorrhage: A prospective randomized trial of surgical and conservative treatment. J Neurosurg 70:755–758, 1989.

33. Qureshi AI, Tuhrim S, Broderick JP, et al: Spontaneous intracerebral hemorrhage. N Engl J Med 344:1450–1460, 2001.

34. Auer L, Deinsberger W, Niederkorn K, et al: Endoscopic surgery versus medical treatment for spontaneous intracerebral hematoma: A randomized study. J Neurosurg 70:530–553, 1989.

35. Batjer HH, Reisch JS, Allen BC, et al: Failure of surgery to improve outcome in hypertensive putaminal hemorrhage: A prospective randomized trial. Arch Neurol 47:1103–1106, 1990.

36. Chen X, Yang H, Czherig Z: A prospective randomised trial of surgical and conservative treatment of hypertensive intracranial haemorrhage [in Chinese]. Acta Acad Med Shanghai 19:237–240, 1992.

37. McKissock W, Richardson A, Taylor J: Primary intracerebral hemorrhage: A controlled trial of surgical and conservative treatment in 180 unselected cases. Lancet 2:222–226, 1961.

38. Morgenstern LB, Frankowski RF, Shedden P, et al: Surgical Treatment for Intracerebral Hemorrhage (STICH): A single-center, randomized clinical trial. Neurology 51:1359–1363, 1998.

39. Zuccarello M, Brott T, Derex L, et al: Early surgical treatment for supratentorial intracerebral hemorrhage: A randomized feasibility study. Stroke 30:1833–1839, 1999.

40. Fernandes HM, Gregson B, Siddique S, Mendelow AD: Surgery in intracerebral hemorrhage: The uncertainty continues. Stroke 31:2511–2516, 2000.

41. Hankey GJ, Hon C: Surgery for primary intracerebral hemorrhage: Is it safe and effective? A systematic review of case series and randomized trials. Stroke 82:2126–2132, 1997.

42. Poungvarin N, Bhoopat W, Viriyavejakul A, et al: Effects of dexamethasone in primary supratentorial intracerebral hemorrhage. N Engl J Med 316:1229–1233, 1987.

43. Qureshi AI, Geocadin RG, Suarez JI, Ulatowski JA: Long-term outcome after medical reversal of transtentorial herniation in patients with supratentorial mass lesions. Crit Care Med 28:1556–1564, 2000.

44. Kobayashi S, Sato A, Kageyama Y, et al: Treatment of hypertensive cerebellar hemorrhage: Surgical or conservative management? Neurosurgery 32:246–250, 1994.

45. MRC European Carotid Surgery Trial: Interim results for symptomatic patients with severe (70–99%) or with mild (0–29%) carotid stenosis. European Carotid Surgery Trialists' Collaborative Group. Lancet 337:1235–1243, 1991.

46. Randomised trial of endarterectomy for symptomatic carotid stenosis: Final results of MRC European Carotid Surgery Trial (ECST). Lancet 351:1379–1387, 1998.

47. Endarterectomy for asymptomatic carotid artery stenosis. Executive Committee for the Asymptomatic Carotid Atherosclerosis Study. JAMA 273:1421–1428, 1995.

48. Mayberg MR, Wilson SE, Yatsu F, et al: Carotid endarterectomy and prevention of cerebral ischemia in symptomatic carotid steno-

Statement for Health care Professionals from the Stroke Council of the American Heart Association. Stroke 31:2742–2750, 2000.

sis. Veterans Affairs Cooperative Studies Program 309 Trialist Group. JAMA 266:3289–3294, 1991.

49. Beneficial effect of carotid endarterectomy in symptomatic patients with high-grade carotid stenosis. North American Symptomatic Carotid Endarterectomy Trial Collaborators. N Engl J Med 325:445–453, 1991.

50. Rothwell PM, Eliasziw M, Gutnikov SA, et al: Analysis of pooled data from the randomised controlled trials of endarterectomy for symptomatic carotid stenosis. Carotid Endarterectomy Trialists' Collaboration. Lancet 361(9352):107–116, 2003.

51. Cunningham EJ, Bond R, Mehta Z, et al: Long-term durability of carotid endarterectomy for symptomatic stenosis and risk factors for late postoperative stroke. Stroke 33:2658–2663, 2002.

52. Rothwell PM, Slattery J, Warlow CP: A systematic review of the risks of stroke and death due to endarterectomy for symptomatic carotid stenosis. Stroke 27:260–265, 1996.

53. Barnett HJ, Taylor DW, Eliasziw M, et al: Benefit of carotid endarterectomy in patients with symptomatic moderate or severe stenosis. North American Symptomatic Carotid Endarterectomy Trial Collaborators. N Engl J Med 339:1415–1425, 1998.

54. Rothwell PM, Slattery J, Warlow CP: A systematic review of clinical and angiographic predictors of stroke and death due to carotid endarterectomy. BMJ 315:1571–1577, 1997.

55. Sundt TM, Sandok BA, Whisnant JP: Carotid endarterectomy: Complications and preoperative assessment of risk. Mayo Clin Proc 50:301–306, 1975.

56. Ferguson GG, Eliasziw M, Barr HW, et al: The North American Symptomatic Carotid Endarterectomy Trial: Surgical results in 1415 patients. Stroke 30:1751–1758, 1999.

57. Piepgras DG, Morgan MK, Sundt TM Jr, et al: Intracerebral hemorrhage after carotid endarterectomy. J Neurosurg 68:532–536, 1988.

58. AbuRahma AF, Jennings TG, Wulu JT, et al: Redo carotid endarterectomy versus primary carotid endarterectomy. Stroke 32;2787–2792, 2001.

59. Golledge J, Mitchell A, Greenhalgh RM, Davies AH: Systematic comparison of the early outcome of angioplasty and endarterectomy for symptomatic carotid artery disease. Stroke 31:1439–1443, 2000.

60. Taylor D., Barnett HJM, Haynes RB, et al: Low-dose and high-dose acetylsalicylic acid for patients undergoing carotid endarterectomy: A randomized controlled trial. Lancet 353:2179–2184, 1999.

61. Fein JM: Carotid endarterectomy. In Fein JM, Flamm ES (eds): Cerebrovascular Surgery, vol 2. New York, Springer-Verlag, 1985, pp 399–427.

62. Harbaugh KS, Harbaugh RE: Early discharge after carotid endarterectomy. Neurosurgery. 37:219–224, 1995.

63. Fields WS, Maslenikov V, Meyer JS, et al: Joint study of extracranial arterial occlusion. V: Progress report of prognosis following surgery or nonsurgical treatment for transient cerebral ischemic attacks and cervical carotid artery lesions. JAMA 211:1993–2003, 1970.

64. Kresowik TF, Hemann RA, Grund SL, et al: Improving the outcomes of carotid endarterectomy: Results of a statewide quality improvement project. J Vasc Surg 31:918–926, 2000.

65. Carotid surgery versus medical therapy in asymptomatic carotid stenosis. The CASANOVA Study Group. Stroke 22:1229–1235, 1991.

66. Results of a randomized controlled trial of carotid endarterectomy for asymptomatic carotid stenosis. Mayo Asymptomatic Carotid Endarterectomy Study Group. Mayo Clin Proc 67:513–518, 1992.

67. Hobson RW 2nd, Weiss DG, Fields WS, et al: Efficacy of carotid endarterectomy for asymptomatic carotid stenosis: The Veterans Affairs Cooperative Study Group. N Engl J Med 328:221–227, 1993.

68. Goldstein LB, Moore WS, Robertson JT, et al: Complication rates for carotid endarterectomy: A call for action. Stroke 28:889–890, 1997.

69. Winn HR, Richardson AE, Jane JA: The long-term prognosis in untreated cerebral aneurysms. I: The incidence of late hemorrhage in cerebral aneurysm: A 10-year evaluation of 364 patients. Ann Neurol 1:358–370, 1977.

70. King JT Jr: Epidemiology of aneurysmal subarachnoid hemorrhage. Neuroimaging Clin North Am 7:659–668, 1997.

71. Epidemiology of aneurysmal subarachnoid hemorrhage in Australia and New Zealand: Incidence and case fatality from the Australasian Cooperative Research on Subarachnoid Hemorrhage Study (ACROSS). Stroke 31:1843–1850, 2000.

72. Edner G, Kagstrom E, Wallstedt L: Total overall management and surgical outcome after aneurysmal subarachnoid haemorrhage in a defined population. Br J Neurosurg 6:409–420, 1992.

73. Hackett ML, Anderson CS: Health outcomes 1 year after subarachnoid haemorrhage: An international population-based study. Australasian Cooperative Research on Subarachnoid Haemorrhage Study (ACROSS) Group. Neurology 55:658–662, 2000.

74. Ingall T, Asplund K, Mahonen M, Bonita R: A multinational comparison of subarachnoid hemorrhage epidemiology in the WHO MONICA stroke study. Stroke 31:1054–1061, 2000.

75. Ljunggren B, Saveland H, Brandt L: Causes of unfavorable outcome after early aneurysm operation. Neurosurgery 13:629–633, 1983.

76. Longstreth WT Jr, Nelson LM, Koepsell TD, van Belle G: Clinical course of spontaneous subarachnoid hemorrhage: A population-based study in King County, Washington. Neurology 43:712–718, 1993.

77. Romner B, Sonesson B, Ljunggren B, et al: Late magnetic resonance imaging related to neurobehavioral functioning after aneurysmal subarachnoid hemorrhage. Neurosurgery 25:390–397, 1989.

78. Sonesson B, Ljunggren B, Saveland H, Brandt L: Cognition and adjustment after late and early operation for ruptured aneurysm. Neurosurgery 21:279–287, 1987.

79. Buchanan KM, Elias LJ, Goplen GB: Differing perspectives on outcome after subarachnoid hemorrhage: The patient, the relative, the neurosurgeon. Neurosurgery 46:831–838, 2000.

80. Hutter BO, Gilsbach JM, Kreitschmann I: Quality of life and cognitive deficits after subarachnoid haemorrhage. Br J Neurosurg 9:465–475, 1995.

81. Petruk KC, West M, Mohr G, et al: Nimodipine treatment in poor grade aneurysm patients: Results of a multicenter double-blind placebo-controlled trial. J Neurosurg 68:505–517, 1988.

82. Juvela S, Porras M, Poussa K: Natural history of unruptured aneurysms: Probability of and risk factors for aneurysm rupture. J Neurosurg 93:379–387, 2000.

83. Tsutsumi K, Ueki K, Morita A: Risk of rupture from incidental cerebral aneurysms. J Neurosurg 93:550–553, 2000.

84. Winn HR, Jane JA Sr, Taylor J, et al: Prevalence of asymptomatic incidental aneurysms: Review of 4568 arteriograms. J Neurosurg 96:43–49, 2002.

85. Winn HR. Section overview: Unruptured aneurysms. J Neurosurg 96:1–2, 2002.

86. Asari S, Ohmoto T: Natural history and risk factors of unruptured cerebral aneurysms. Clin Neurol Neurosurg 95:205–214, 1993.

87. Brown RD, Wiebers Do, Forbes GS: Unruptured intracranial aneurysms and arteriovenous malformations: Frequency of intracranial hemorrhage and relationship of lesions. J Neurosurg 73:859–863, 1990.

88. Juvela S, Hillbom M, Numminen H, Koskinen P: Cigarette smoking and alcohol consumption as risk factors for aneurysmal subarachnoid hemorrhage. Stroke 24:639–646, 1993.

89. Juvela S, Porras M, Heiskanen O: Natural history of unruptured intracranial aneurysms: A long-term follow-up study. J Neurosurg 79:174–182, 1993.

90. Rinkel GJE, Djibuti M, Algra A, van Gijn J: Prevalence and risk of rupture of intracranial aneurysms: A systematic review. Stroke 29:251–256, 1998.

91. Bonita R: Cigarette smoking, hypertension and the risk of subarachnoid hemorrhage: A population-based case-control study. Stroke 17:831–835, 1986.

92. Longstreth WT Jr, Nelson LM, Koepsell TD, van Belle G: Cigarette smoking, alcohol use, and subarachnoid hemorrhage. Stroke 23:1242–1249, 1992.

93. Teunissen LL, Rinkel GJE, Algra A, van Gijn J: Risk factors for subarachnoid hemorrhage: A systematic review. Stroke 27:544–549, 1996.

94. Acevedo JC, Turjman F, Sindou M: Postoperative angiography in surgery for intracranial aneurysm: Prospective study in consecutive series of 267 operated cases. Neurochirurgie 43:275–284, 1997.

95. David CA, Vishteh G, Spetzler RF, et al: Late angiographic follow-up of surgically treated aneurysms. J Neurosurg 91:396–401, 1999.

96. Feuerberg I, Lindquist C, Lindqvist M: Natural history of postoperative aneurysm rests. J Neurosurg 66:30–34, 1987.

97. Le Roux P, Elliott JP, Eskridge JM, et al: Risks and benefits of diagnostic angiography following aneurysm surgery: A retrospective analysis of 597 studies. Neurosurgery 42:1248–1255, 1998.

98. Le Roux P, Elliott JP, Newell DW, et al: The incidence of surgical complications is similar in good and poor grade patients undergo-

ing repair of ruptured anterior circulation aneurysms: A retrospective review of 355 patients. Neurosurgery 38:887–895, 1996.

99. Rauzzino MJ, Quinn CM, Fischer W: Angiography after aneurysm surgery: Indications for selective angiography. Surg Neurol 49:32–41, 1998.

100. Solomon RA, Fink ME, Pile-Spellman J: Surgical management of unruptured intracranial aneurysms. J Neurosurg 80:440–446, 1994.

101. Deruty R, Gelissou-Guyotat I, Mottolese C, et al: Surgical management of unruptured intracranial aneurysms: Personal experience with 37 cases and discussion of the indications. Acta Neurohir (Wien) 119:35–41, 1992.

102. Eskesen V, Rosenørn J, Schmidt K, et al: Clinical features and outcome in 48 patients with unruptured intracranial saccular aneurysms: A prospective consecutive study. Br J Neurosurg 1:47–52, 1987.

103. Heiskanen O: Risks of surgery for unruptured intracranial aneurysms. J Neurosurg 65:451–453, 1986.

104. Pertuiset B, Mahdy M, Sichez J, et al: Unruptured intracranial saccular aneurysms less than 20 mm in diameter in adults: Surgery in 89 cases. Rev Neurol (Paris) 147:111–120, 1991.

105. Rice BJ, Peerless SJ, Drake CG: Surgical treatment of unruptured aneurysms of the posterior circulation. J Neurosurg 73:165–173, 1990.

106. Rosenorn J, Eskesen V, Schmidt K: Unruptured intracranial aneurysms: An assessment of the annual risk of rupture based on epidemiological and clinical data. Br J Neurosurg 2:369–377, 1988.

107. Wirth FP, Laws ER Jr, Piepgras D, Scott RM: Surgical treatment of intracranial aneurysms. Neurosurgery 12:507–511, 1983.

108. King JT, Berlin JA, Flamm ES: Morbidity and mortality from elective surgery for asymptomatic, unruptured, intracranial aneurysms: A meta-analysis. J Neurosurg 81:837–842, 1994.

109. Raaymakers TW, Rinkel GJ, Limburg M, Algra A: Mortality and morbidity of surgery from unruptured Intracranial aneurysms: A meta-analysis. Stroke 29:1531–1538, 1998.

110. Connolly ES, Solomon RA: Management of symptomatic and asymptomatic unruptured aneurysms. Neurosurg Clin North Am 9:509–524, 1998.

111. Khanna RK, Malik GM, Qureshi N: Predicting outcome following surgical treatment of unruptured intracranial aneurysms: A proposed grading system. J Neurosurg 84:49–54, 1996.

112. Kassell NF, Torner JC, Haley EC Jr, et al: The International Cooperative Study on the Timing of Aneurysm Surgery. Part 1: Overall management results. J Neurosurg 73:18–36, 1990.

113. Le Roux P, Elliott JP, Newell DW, et al: Predicting outcome in poor grade subarachnoid hemorrhage: A retrospective review of 159 aggressively managed patients. J Neurosurg 85:39–49, 1996.

114. Ogden JA, Mee EW, Henning M: A prospective study of impairment of cognition and memory and recovery after subarachnoid hemorrhage. Neurosurgery 33:572–586, 1993.

115. Ogilvy CS, Carter BS: A proposed comprehensive grading system to predict outcome for surgical management of intracranial aneurysms. Neurosurgery 42:959–996, 1998.

116. Roos EJ, Rinkel GJ, Velthuis BK, Algra A: The relation between aneurysm size and outcome in patients with subarachnoid hemorrhage. Neurology 54:2334–2336, 2000.

117. Weir B, Disney L, Karrison T: Sizes of ruptured and unruptured aneurysms in relation to their sites and the ages of patients. J Neurosurg 96:64–70, 2002.

118. Bailes JE, Spetzler F, Hadley MN, Baldwin ME: Management, morbidity and mortality of poor grade aneurysm patients. J Neurosurgery 72:559–566, 1990.

119. Le Roux P, Winn HR: Intracranial aneurysms and subarachnoid hemorrhage: Management of the poor grade patient. Acta Neurochir Suppl 72:7–26, 1999.

120. Rordorf G, Ogilvy CS, Gress DR, et al: Patients in poor neurological condition after subarachnoid hemorrhage: Early management and long-term outcome. Acta Neurochir 13:1143–1151, 1997.

121. Chyatte D, Forde N, Sundt T: Early versus late intracranial aneurysm surgery in subarachnoid hemorrhage. J Neurosurg 69:326–331, 1988.

122. Disney L, Weir B, Petruk K: Effect on management mortality of a deliberate policy of early operation on supratentorial aneurysms. Neurosurgery 20:695–701, 1987.

123. Haley EC Jr, Kassell NF, Torner JC: The International Cooperative Study on the Timing of Aneurysm Surgery: The North American experience. Stroke 23:205–214, 1992.

124. Hernesniemi J, Vapalahti M, Niskanen M, et al: One year outcome in early aneurysm surgery: A 14 year experience. Acta Neurochir (Wien) 122:1–10, 1993.

125. Kassell NF, Torner JC, Jane JA, et al: The International Cooperative Study on the Timing of Aneurysm Surgery. Part 2: Surgical results. J Neurosurg 73:37–47, 1990.

126. Milhorat TH, Krautheim M: Results of early and delayed operations for ruptured intracranial aneurysms in two series of 100 consecutive patients. Surg Neurol 26:123–128, 1986.

127. Miyaoka M, Sato K, Ishii S: A clinical study of the relationship of timing to outcome of surgery for ruptured cerebral aneurysms: A retrospective analysis of 1622 cases. J Neurosurg 79:373–378, 1993.

128. Rosenorn J, Eskesen V, Schmidt K, et al: Clinical features and outcome in 1076 patients with ruptured intracranial saccular aneurysms: A prospective consecutive study. Br J Neurosurg 1:33–46, 1987.

129. Ohman J, Heiskanen O: Timing of operation for ruptured supratentorial aneurysms: A prospective randomized study. J Neurosurg 70:55–60, 1989.

130. Haley EC, Kassels NF, Apperson-Hansen C, et al: A randomised double blind placebo controlled trial of tirilazad mesylate in patients with aneurysmal subarachnoid haemorrhage: A cooperative North American study. J Neurosurg 86:467–474, 1997.

131. Koivisto T, Vanninen R, Hurskainen H, et al: Outcomes of early endovascular versus surgical treatment of ruptured cerebral aneurysms: A prospective randomized study. Stroke 31:2369–2377, 2000.

132. Ogungbo B, Gregson BA, Blackburn A, Mendelow AD: Trends over time in the management of subarachnoid haemorrhage in Newcastle: Review of 1609 patients. Br J Neurosurg 15:388–395, 2001.

133. Vanninen R, Koivisto T, Saari T, et al: Ruptured intracranial aneurysms: Acute endovascular treatment with electrolytically detachable coils—a prospective randomized study. Radiology 211:325–336, 1999.

134. Batjer H, Samson D: Intraoperative aneurysmal rupture: Incidence, outcome, and suggestions for surgical management. Neurosurgery 18:701–707, 1986.

135. Drake CG, Vanderlinden RG: The late consequences of incomplete surgical treatment of cerebral aneurysms. J Neurosurg 27:226–238, 1967.

136. Giannotta SL, Oppenheimer JH, Levy ML, Zelman V: Management of intraoperative rupture of aneurysm without hypotension. Neurosurgery 28:531–536, 1991.

137. Jomin M, Lesoin F, Lozes G: Prognosis with 500 ruptured and operated intracranial arterial aneurysms. Surg Neurol 21:13–18, 1984.

138. Karhunen PJ: Neurosurgical vascular complications associated with aneurysm clips evaluated by postmortem angiography. Forensic Sci Int 51:13–22, 1991.

139. Maurice-Williams R, Kitchen ND: Ruptured intracranial aneurysms: Learning from experience. Br J Neurosurg 8:519–527, 1994.

140. MacDonald RL, Wallace MC, Kestle JR: Role of angiography following aneurysm surgery. J Neurosurg 79:826–832, 1993.

141. Schramm J, Cedzich C: Outcome and management of intraoperative aneurysm rupture. Surg Neurol 40:26–30, 1993.

142. Drake CG, Friedman AH, Peerless SJ: Failed aneurysm surgery: Reoperation in 115 cases. J Neurosurg 61:848–856, 1984.

143. Harvard Medical Practice Study: Patients, Doctors, and Lawyers & Medical Injury, Malpractice Litigation, and Patient Compensation in New York. Cambridge, MA, President and Fellows of Harvard College, 1990.

144. Pasqualin A, Battaglia R, Scienza R, Da Pian R: Italian cooperative study on giant intracranial aneurysms: Results of treatment. Acta Neurochir 42:65–70, 1988.

145. Sundt TM, Whisnant JP: Subarachnoid hemorrhage from intracranial aneurysms: Surgical management and natural history of disease. N Eng J Med 299:116–122, 1978.

146. Tang G, Cawley CM, Dion JE, Barrow DL: Intraoperative angiography during aneurysm surgery: A prospective evaluation of efficacy. J Neurosurg 96:993–999, 2002.

147. Thornton J, Bashir Q, Aletich VA, et al: What percentage of surgically clipped intracranial aneurysms have residual necks? Neurosurgery 46:1294–1300, 2000.

148. Lin T, Fox AT, Drake CG: Regrowth of aneurysm sacs from residual neck following aneurysm clipping. J Neurosurg 70:556–560, 1989.

149. Alexander TD, MacDonald RL, Weir B, Kowalczuk A: Intraoperative angiography in cerebral aneurysm surgery: A prospective study of 100 craniotomies. Neurosurgery 39:10–18, 1996.

150. Cloft HJ, Joseph GJ, Dion JE: Risk of cerebral angiography in patients with subarachnoid hemorrhage, cerebral aneurysm, and arteriovenous malformation: A meta-analysis. Stroke 30:317–210, 1999.

151. Al-Shahi R, Warlow C: A systematic review of the frequency and prognosis of arteriovenous malformations of the brain in adults. Brain 124:1900–1926, 2001.

152. Brown RD, Wiebers DO, Forbes G, et al: The natural history of unruptured intracranial arteriovenous malformations.J Neurosurg. 68:352–357, 1988.

153. Jessurun GA, Kamphuis DJ, van der Zande FH, et al: Cerebral arteriovenous malformations in the Netherland Antilles: High prevalence of hereditary hemorrhagic telangiectasia-related single and multiple cerebral arteriovenous malformations. Clin Neurol Neurosurg 95:193–198, 1993.

154. Crawford PM, West CR, Chadwick DW, et al: Arteriovenous malformations of the brain: The natural history in unoperated patients. J Neurol Neurosurg Psychiatry 49:1–10, 1986.

155. Graf CJ, Perret GE, Torner JC: Bleeding from cerebral arteriovenous malformations as part of their natural history. J Neurosurg 58:331–337, 1983.

156. Mast H, Young WL, Koennecke HC, et al: Risk of spontaneous haemorrhage after diagnosis of cerebral arteriovenous malformation. Lancet 350:1065–1068, 1997.

157. Ondra SL, Troupp H, George ED, et al: The natural history of symptomatic arteriovenous malformations of the brain: A 24 year follow-up assessment. J Neurosurg 73:387–391, 1990.

158. Forster DM, Steiner L, Hakanson S: Arteriovenous malformations of the brain: A long-term clinical study. J Neurosurg 37:562–570, 1972.

159. Hartmann A, Mast H, Mohr JP, et al: Morbidity of intracranial hemorrhage in patients with cerebral arteriovenous malformation. Stroke 29:931–934, 1998.

160. Tew JM, Lewis AI: Management strategies for the treatment of intracranial arteriovenous malformations. Clin Neurosurgery 46: 267–284, 2000.

161. Fisher W: Therapy of AVMs: A decision analysis. Clin Neurosurg 42:294–312, 1995.

162. Spetzler RF, Martin NA: A proposed grading system for arteriovenous malformations. J Neurosurg 65:476–483, 1986.

163. Hamilton MG, Spetzler RF: The prospective application of a grading system for arteriovenous malformations. Neurosurgery 34:2–7, 1994.

164. Heros RC: Management of giant paraclinoid aneurysms. In Kikuchi H, Fukushima T, Watanabe K (eds): Intracranial Aneurysms. Niigata, Japan, Nishimura, 1986, p 273.

165. Spetzler RF, Martin NA, Carter LP, et al: Surgical management of large AVMs by staged embolization and operative excision. J Neurosurg 67:17–28, 1987.

166. Stapf C, Connolly ES, Schumacher HC, et al: Dysplastic vessels after surgery for brain arteriovenous malformations. Stroke 33:1053–1056, 2002.

167. Jafar JJ, Davis AJ, Berenstein A, et al: The effect of embolization with N-butyl cyanoacrylate prior to surgical resection of cerebral arteriovenous malformations. J Neurosurg 78:60–69, 1993.

168. Vinuela F, Dion JE, Duckwiler G, et al: Combined endovascular embolization and surgery in the management of cerebral arteriovenous malformations: Experience with 101 cases. J Neurosurg 75:856–864, 1991.

169. DeMeritt JS, Pile-Spellman J, Mast H, et al: Outcome analysis of preoperative embolization with N-butyl cyanoacrylate in cerebral arteriovenous malformations. AJNR Am J Neuroradiol 16:1801–1807, 1995.

170. Martin NA, Khana R, Doberstein C, Bentson J: Therapeutic embolization of arteriovenous malformations: The case for and against. Clin Neurosurg 46: 295–318, 2000.

171. Hartmann A, Pile-Spellman J, Stapf C, et al: Risk of endovascular treatment of brain arteriovenous malformations. Stroke 33:1816–1820, 2002.

172. Latchaw RE, Madison MT, Larsen DW: Intracranial arteriovenous malformations: Endovascular strategies and methods. In Batjer HH (ed): Cerebrovascular Disease. New York, Lippincott-Raven, 1997, pp 707–725.

173. Purdy PD, Batjer H, Risser RC, et al: Arteriovenous malformations of the brain: Choosing embolic materials to enhance safety and ease of excision. J Neurosurg 77:217–222, 1992.

174. Gobin YP, Laurent A, Schlienger M, et al: Treatment of brain arteriovenous malformations by embolization and radiosugery. J Neurosurg 85:19–28, 1996.

175. Colombo F, Pozza F, Chierego G, et al: Linear accelerator radiosurgery of cerebral arteriovenous malformations: An update. Neurosurgery 34:14–21, 1994.

176. Friedman WA, Blatt DL, Bova FJ, et al: The risk of hemorrhage after radiosurgery for arteriovenous malformations. J Neurosurg 84:912–999, 1996.

177. Friedman WA, Bova FJ, Mendenhall WM: Linear accelerator radiosurgery for arteriovenous malformations: The relationship of size to outcome. J Neurosurg 82:180–189, 1995.

178. Karlsson B, Lax I, Soderman M: Factors influencing the risk for complications following gamma knife radiosurgery of cerebral arteriovenous malformations. Radiother Oncol 43:275–280, 1997.

179. Karlsson B, Lindquist M, Lindquist C: Long-term angiographic outcome of arteriovenous malformations responding incompletely to gamma knife surgery. Radiosurgery 1:188–194, 1996.

180. Lunsford LD, Kondziolka D, Flickinger JC, et al: Stereotactic radiosurgery for arteriovenous malformations of the brain. J Neurosurg 75:512–524, 1991.

181. Pollock BE, Lunsford LD, Kondziolka D, et al: Patient outcomes after stereotactic radiosurgery for "operable" arteriovenous malformations. Neurosurgery 35:1–8, 1994.

182. Steiner L, Lindquist C, Adler JR, et al: Clinical outcome of radiosurgery for cerebral arteriovenous malformations. J Neurosurg. 77:1–8, 1992.

183. Yamamoto Y, Coffey RJ, Nichols DA, Shaw EG: Interim report on the radiosurgical treatment of cerebral arteriovenous malformations: The influence of size, dose, time, and technical factors on obliteration rate. J Neurosurg 83:832–737, 1995.

184. Flickinger JC, Pollock BE, Kondziolka D, et al: A dose-response analysis of arteriovenous malformation obliteration after radiosurgery. Int J Radiat Oncol Biol Phys 36:873–879,1996.

185. Pikus HJ, Beach ML, Harbaugh RE: Microsurgical treatment of arteriovenous malformations: Analysis and comparison with stereotactic radiosurgery. J Neurosurg 88:641–646, 1998.

186. Kapral MK, Wang H, Mamdani M, Tu JV: Effect of socioeconomic status on treatment and mortality after stroke. Stroke 33:268–275, 2002.

187. Lantos JD, Meadow W, Miles SH, et al: Providing and forgoing resuscitative therapy for babies of very low birth weight. J Clin Ethics 3:283–311, 1992.

188. Whisnant JP, Sacco SE, O'Fallon WM, et al: Referral bias in aneurysmal subarachnoid hemorrhage. J Neurosurg. 78:726–732, 1993.

189. Bardach NS, Zhao S, Gress DR, et al: Association between subarachnoid hemorrhage outcomes and number of cases treated at California hospitals. Stroke 33:1851–1856, 2002.

190. Birkmeyer JD, Finlayson EV, Birkmeyer CM: Volume standards for high-risk surgical procedures: Potential benefits of the Leapfrog initiative. Surgery 130:415–422, 2001.

191. Flum DR, Koepsell T, Heagerty P, et al: Outcome analysis of preoperative embolization with N-butyl cyanoacrylate in cerebral arteriovenous malformations. AJNR Am J Neuroradiol 16:1801–1807, 1995.

192. Halm EA, Lee C, Chassin MR: Is volume related to outcome in health care? A systematic review and methodologic critique of the literature. Ann Intern Med 137:511–520, 2002.

193. Perler BA, Dardik A, Burleyson GP, et al: Influence of age and hospital volume on the results of carotid endarterectomy: A statewide analysis of 9918 cases. J Vasc Surg 27:25–33, 1998.

194. Solomon R, Mayer S, Tarmey JJ: Relationship between the volume of craniotomies for cerebral aneurysm performed at New York State Hospitals and in-hospital mortality. Stroke 27:13–17, 1996.

195. Hannan EL, Popp AJ, Tranmer B, et al: Relationship between provider volume and mortality for carotid endarterectomies in New York state. Stroke 29:2292–2297, 1998.

196. Hannan EL, Racz MJ, Jollis JG, et al: Using medicare claims data to assess provider quality for CABG surgery: Does it work well enough? Hlth Serv Res 31:659–678, 1997.

197. Cox CE, Salud CJ, Cantor A, et al: Learning curves for breast cancer sentinel lymph node mapping based on surgical volume analysis. J Am Coll Surg 193;593–600, 2001.

Therapy

198. Schneider EC, Epstein AM: Influence of cardiac surgery performance reports on referral practices and access to care: A survey of cardiovascular specialists. N Engl J Med 335:251–256, 1996.

199. Schneider EC, Epstein AM: Use of public performance reports: A survey of patients undergoing cardiac surgery. JAMA 279:1638–1642, 1998.

200. Cowan J, Justin B, Dimick B, et al: Surgeon volume as an indicator of outcomes after carotid endarterectomy: An effect independent of specialty practice and hospital volume. J Am Coll Surg 195:814–821, 2002.

201. Cebul RD, Snow RJ, Pine R, et al: Indications, outcomes, and provider volumes for carotid endarterectomy. JAMA 279:1282–1287, 1998.

202. O'Neill L, Lanska DJ, Hartz A: Surgeon characteristics associated with mortality and morbidity following carotid endarterectomy. Neurology 55:773–781, 2000.

203. Rothwell PM, Warlow CP: Interpretation of operative risks of individual surgeons. European Carotid Surgery Trialists' Collaborative Group. Lancet 353:2105, 1999.

204. Edwards WH, Morris JA Jr, Jenkins JM, et al: Evaluating quality, cost-effective health care: Vascular database predicted on hospital discharge abstracts. Ann Surg 213:433–439, 1991.

205. Kempczinski RF, Brott TG, Labutta RJ: The influence of surgical specialty and caseload on the results of carotid endarterectomy. J Vasc Surg 3:911–916, 1986.

206. Fabian TC: What's new in trauma and critical care. J Am Coll Surg 192:276–286, 2001.

207. Langhorne P, Duncan P: Does the organization of postacute stroke care really matter? Stroke 32:268–274, 2001.

208. Pasquale MD, Peitzman A, Bednarski J, Wasser T: Outcome analysis of Pennsylvania trauma centers: Factors predictive of non-survival in seriously injured patients [abstract]. J Trauma 47:1168, 2000.

209. American Hospital Association: The hospital workforce: Immediate and future. AHA Trend Watch 3:1–8, 2001.

210. Berliner H, Ginzberg E: Why this hospital nursing shortage is different. JAMA 288:2742–2744, 2002.

211. Aiken, LH, Clarke SP, Sloane DM, et al: Hospital nurse staffing and patient mortality, nurse burnout, and job dissatisfaction. JAMA 288:1987–1993, 2002.

212. Bond CA, Raehl CL, Pitterle ME, et al: Health care professional staffing, hospital characterisitcs and hospital mortality rates. Pharmacotherapy 19:130–138, 1999.

213. Needleman J, Buerhaus PI, Mattke S, et al: Nurse Staffing and Patient Outcomes in Hospitals. Washington, DC, US Department of Health and Human Services, Health Resources and Services Administration, 2001.

214. Andrews LB, Stocking C, Krizek T, et al: An alternative strategy for studying adverse events in medical care. Lancet 349:309–313, 1997.

215. Blendon PJ, DesRoches CM, Brodie M, et al: Patient safety: Views of practicing physicians and the public on medical errors. N Engl J Med 347:1933–1940, 2002.

216. Krizek TJ: Surgical error: Reflections on adverse events. Bull Am Coll Surg 85:18–22, 2000.

217. Khuri SF, Daley J, Henderson W, et al: The National Veterans Administration Surgical Risk Study: Risk adjustment for the comparative assessment of the quality of surgical care. J Am Coll Surg 180:519–531, 1995.

218. Leape LL, Brennan TA, Laird N, et al: The nature of adverse events in hospitalized patients: Results of the Harvard Medical Practice Study II. N Engl J Med 324:377–384, 1991.

219. Williamson JA, Webb RK, Selen A, et al: Human failure: An analysis of 2000 incident reports. The Australian Incident Monitoring Study.Anaesth Intensive Care 21:678–683, 1993.

220. Thomas EJ, Orav EJ, Brennan TA: Hospital ownership and preventable adverse events. J Gen Intern Med 15:211–219, 2000.

221. Reason J: Human error. BMJ 320:768–770, 2000.

222. Murray A, Montgomery JE, Chang H, et al: Doctor discontent: A comparison of physician satisfaction in different delivery system settings, 1986 and 1997. J Gen Intern Med 16:452–459, 2001.

223. Spickard A Jr, Gabbe SG, Christensen JF: Mid-career burnout in generalist and specialist physicians. JAMA 288:1447–1450, 2002.

224. Sullivan P, Buske L: Results for CMA's huge 1998 physician survey point to a dispirited profession. CMAJ 159:525–528, 1998.

225. Crane M: Why burned-out doctors get sued more often. Med Econ 75:210–218, 1998.

226. Firth-Cozens J, Greenhalgh J: Doctors' perceptions of the links between stress and lowered clinical care. Soc Sci Med 44:1017–1022, 1997.

227. Shanafelt TD, Bradley KA, Wipf JE, Back AC: Burnout and self-reported patient care in internal medicine residency programs. Ann Intern Med 136:358–367, 2002.

228. Reason J: Human Error. Cambridge, Cambridge University Press, 1990.

229. Bosk C: Forgive and remember: Managing Medical Failure. Chicago, University of Chicago Press, 1989.

230. Gaba DM, Howard SK, Flanagan B, et al: Assessment of clinical performance during simulated crises using both technical and behavioral ratings. Anesthesiology 89:8–18, 1998.

231. Milstein A, Galvin RS, Delbanco SF, et al: Improving the safety of health care: The leapfrog initiative. Eff Clin Prac 3:313–6, 2000.

232. Lipsett PA, Swoboda SM, Dickerson J, et al: Survival and functional outcome after prolonged intensive care unit stay. Ann Surg 231:262–268, 2000.

233. Carson SS, Stocking C, Podsadecki T, et al: Effects of organizational change in the medical intensive care unit of a teaching hospital: A comparison of 'open' and 'closed' formats. JAMA 276:322–328, 1996.

234. Manthous CA, Amoateng-Adjepong Y, Al-Kharrat T, et al: Effects of a medical intensivist on patient care in a community teaching hospital. Mayo Clin Proc 72:391–399, 1997.

235. Petersen LA, Brennan TA, O'Neil AC, et al: Does housestaff discontinuity of care increase the risk for preventable adverse events? Ann Intern Med 121:866–872, 1994.

236. Joint Commission on Accreditation of Health care Organizations: Comprehensive Accreditation Manual for Hospitals, 2001. Available online at www.jcaho.org/api_frm.html/

237. Joint Commission on Accreditation of Health care Organizations: Revisons to the Joint Commission Standards In Support of Patient Safety and Medical/Health care Error Reduction. Available online at www.jcaho.org/

238. Sexton BJ, Thomas EJ, Helmreich RL: Error, stress, and teamwork in medicine and aviation: Cross sectional surveys. BMJ 320:745–749, 2000.

239. Studdert DM, Brennan TA: No-fault compensation for medical injuries: The prospect for error prevention. JAMA 286:217–223, 2001.

240. Roscoe LA, Krizek TJ: Reporting of medical errors. Bull Am Coll Surg 87:12–17, 2002.

241. Fischer JE: Current status of the National Practitioner Data Bank. Bull Am Coll Surg 86:20–47, 2001.

242. Helling v Carey, 83 Wash2d 514, 519 P2d 9811 (1974).

243. The T. J. Hooper, 60 F 2d 737 (2nd Cir 1932).

244. Field MJ, Lohr KN: Clinical Practice Guidelines: Directions for a New Program. Washington, DC, Institute of Medicine, National Academy Press, 1990.

245. Hospitals' bottom line suffering. OR Manager 16:32, 2000.

246. Reinhardt UE: The economist's model of physician behavior. JAMA 281:462–464, 1999.

247. Felsenthal E: Doctors' own guidelines hurt them in court. Wall Street Journal October 10, 1994, p B1.

248. Hyams AL, Brandenburg JA, Lipsitz SR, et al: Practice guidelines and malpractice litigation: A two-way street. Ann Intern Med 122:450–455, 1995.

249. Salcman M: Practice Guidelines for stroke: Enforceable? Meaningful. In Batjer H (ed): Cerebrovascular Disease. Philadelphia, Lippincott-Raven, 1997, pp 1219–1227.

250. Woolf SH: Manual for Medical Practice Guideline Development: A Draft Protocol for Expert Panels Convened by the Office of the Forum for Quality and Effectiveness in Health Care. Washington, DC, US Government Agency for Health Care Policy and Research, 1990, p 37.

251. Stone SP, Whincup P: Standards for the hospital management of stroke patients. J R Coll Physicians Lond 28:52–58, 1994.

252. Cohen MM, Duncan PG, Pope WD, Biehl D, et al: The Canadian four-centre study of anaesthetic outcomes. II: Can outcomes be used to assess the quality of anaesthesia care? Can J Anaesth 40:79–81, 1993.

253. Gawande AA, Studdert DM, Orav EJ, et al: Patient safety: Risk factors for retained instruments and sponges after surgery. N Engl J Med 348:229–235, 2003.

254. Barden CB, Specht MC, McCarter MD, et al: Effects of limited work hours on surgical training. J Am Coll Surg 195:531–538, 2002.

255. Brennan TA, Hebert LE, Laird NM, et al: Hospital characteristics associated with adverse events and substandard care. JAMA 265:3265–3269, 1991.

256. Petersen LA, Orav EJ, Teich JM, et al: Using a computerized sign-out program to improve continuity of inpatient care and prevent adverse events. Jt Comm J Qual Improv 24:77–87, 1998.

257. Kuttner R: The American health care system: Wall Street and health care. N Engl J Med 340:664–668, 1999.

258. Bodenheimer T: The American health care system: The movement for improved quality in health care. N Engl J Med 340:488–492, 1999.

259. Laffel G, Blumenthal D: The case for using industrial quality management science in health care organizations. JAMA 262:2869–2873, 1989.

260. Rhodes RS: Quality in surgery: From outcomes to process-and back again. Surgery 126:76–77, 1999.

261. Laing RJ: Measuring outcome in neurosurgery. Br J Neurosurg 14:181–184, 2000.

262. Haines SJ: Evidence-based neurosurgery. Neurosurgery 52:36–47, 2003.

263. Chassin MR, Galvin RW: The urgent need to improve health care quality: Institute of Medicine National Roundtable on Health Care Quality. JAMA 280:1000–1005, 1998.

264. Measuring and improving quality of care. A report from the American Heart Association/American College of Cardiology First Scientific Forum on Assessment of Health care Quality in Cardiovascular Disease. Stroke 31:1002–1012, 2000.

265. Donabedian A: The quality of care: How can it be assessed? JAMA 260:1743–1748, 1988.

266. Daley J, Khuri SF, Henderson W, et al: Risk adjustment of the postoperative morbidity rate for the comparative assessment of the quality of surgical care: Results of the National Veterans Affairs Surgical Risk Study. J Am Coll Surg 185:328–340, 1997.

267. Samsa G, Oddone EZ, Horner R, et al: To what extent should quality of care decisions be based on health outcomes data? Application to carotid endarterectomy. Stroke 33:2944–2949, 2002.

268. Hanson CW, Deutschman CS, Anderson HL, et al: Effects of an organized critical care service on outcomes and resource utilization: A cohort study. Crit Care Med 27:270–274, 1999.

269. Indredavik B, Bakke F, Slørdahl SA, et al: Stroke unit treatment improves long-term quality of life: A randomized controlled trial. Stroke 29:895–899, 1998.

270. Association of American Medical Colleges: AAMC Data Book: Statistical Information Related to Medical Schools and Teaching Hospitals. Washington DC, AAMC, 2001.

271. Clark PA: What residents are not learning: Observations in an NICU. Acad Med 76:419–424, 2001.

272. Ludmerer K: Time to Heal. New York, Oxford University Press, 1999.

273. Silen W: Crisis in surgical education. J Am Coll Surg 193;514–515, 2001.

274. Gaba DM, Howard SK: Patient safety: Fatigue among clinicians and the safety of patients. N Engl J Med 347:1249–1255, 2002.

275. Bollschweler E, Krings A, Fuchs KH, et al: Alternative shift models and the quality of patient care. Langenbeck's Arch Surg 386:104–109, 2001.

276. Laine C, Goldman L, Soukup JR, et al: The impact of a regulation restricting medical house staff working hours on the quality of patient care. JAMA 269:374–378, 1993.

277. Statement on Fundamental Characteristics of Surgical Residency Programs (ST-4). The American College of Surgeons. Bull Am Coll Surg 73:22–23, 1988.

278. Kapur N, House A: Working patterns and the quality of training of medical house officers: Evaluating the effect of the 'new deal.' Med Educ 32:432–438, 1998.

279. Piepgras DG: Management of incidental intracranial aneurysms. Clin Neurosurg 35:511–518, 1989.

280. Molyneux A, Le Roux P: Surgical or endovascular treatment of intracranial aneurysms: A comparison of techniques. In Le Roux P, Newell DW, Winn HR (eds): Management of Cerebral Aneurysms. Philadelphia, Elsevier 2004, pp 983–995.

281. Johnson SC, Dudley RA, Gress DR, Ono L: Surgical and endovascular treatment of unruptured intracranial aneurysms at US University Hospitals. Neurology 52:1799–1805, 1999.

282. Johnson SC, Zhaio S, Dudley RA, et al: Treatment of unruptured aneurysms in California. Stroke 32:597–605, 2001.

283. International Study of Unruptured Intracranial Aneurysms (ISUIA) Investigators: ISUIA Phase 2 data. Presented at the 27th International Stroke Conference of the American Stroke Association, San Antonio, TX, February 9, 2002.

284. Lawton MT, Spetzler RF: Surgical management of giant intracranial aneurysms: Experience with 171 patients. Clin Neurosurg 42:245, 1995.

285. Kodama N, Suzuki J: Surgical treatment of giant aneurysms. Neurosurg Rev 5:155, 1982.

286. Symon L, Vajda J: Surgical experiences with giant intracranial aneurysms. J Neurosurg. Dec;61(6):1009–1028, 1984.

287. Yasargil MG: Giant intracranial aneurysms. In Yasargil MG (eds): Microneurosurgery II: Clinical Considerations, Surgery of the Intracranial Aneurysms and Results. New York, Thieme-Stratton, 1984, p 296.

288. Hosobuchi Y: Giant intracranial aneurysms. In Wilkins RH, Rengachary SS (eds): Neurosurgery. New York, McGraw-Hill, 1985, p 1404.

289. Sundt TM Jr: Results of surgical management. In Sundt TM, Jr (ed): Surgical Techniques for Saccular and Giant Intracranial Aneurysms. Baltimore, Williams & Wilkins, 1990, p 19.

290. Ausman JI, Diaz F, Sadasivan B, et al: Giant intracranial aneurysm surgery: The role of microvascular reconstruction. Surg Neurol 34:8, 1990.

291. Peerless SJ, Wallace MC, Drake CG: Giant intracranial aneurysms. In Youmans JR (eds): Neurological Surgery: A Comprehensive Reference Guide to the Diagnosis and Management of Neurological Problems. Philadelphia, WB Saunders, 1990, p 1742.

292. Inamasu J, Nakamura Y, Saito R, et al: Endovascular treatment for poorest-grade subarachnoid hemorrhage in the acute stage: Has the outcome been improved? Neurosurgery 50:1199–206, 2002.

293. Hunt WE, Hess RM: Surgical risk related to time of intervention in the repair of intracranial aneurysms. J Neurosurgery 24:14–19, 1968.

294. Adams HP, Kassel NF, Torner JC, et al: Early management of aneurysmal subarachnoid hemorrhage: A report of the Cooperative Aneurysm Study. J Neurosurg 54:141–145, 1981.

295. Testa C, Andreoli A, Arista A, et al: Overall results in 304 consecutive patients with acute spontaneous subarachnoid hemorrhage. Surg Neurol 24:377–385, 1985.

296. Freckmann N, Noll M, Winkler D, et al: Does the timing of aneurysm surgery neglect the real problems of subarachnoid hemorrhage? Acta Neurochir 89:91–99, 1987.

297. Hijdra A, Braakman R, van Gijn J, et al: Aneurysmal subarachnoid hemorrhage: Complications and outcome in a hospital population. Stroke 18:1061–1067, 1987.

298. Ohno K, Suzuki R, Masaoka H, et al: A review of 102 consecutive patients with intracranial aneurysms in a community hospital in Japan. Acta Neurochir 94:23–27, 1988.

299. Inagawa T, Takahashi M, Aoki H, et al: Aneurysmal subarachnoid hemorrhage in Izumo City and Shimane Prefecture of Japan: Outcome. Stroke 19:176–180, 1988.

300. Sevrain L, Rabenhenoina C, Hattab N, et al: Les anevrismes à expression clinique grave d'emblèe (grades IV et V de Hunt et Hess): Une sèrie de 66 cas. Neurochirurgie 36:287–296, 1990.

301. Medlock MD, Dulebohn SC, Elwood PW: Prophylactic hypervolemia without calcium channel blockers in early aneurysm surgery. Neurosurgery 30:12–16, 1992.

302. Seifert V, Trost HA, Stolke D: Management morbidity and mortality in grade 4 and 5 patients with aneurysmal subarachnoid hemorrhage. Acta Neurochir 103:5–10, 1990.

303. Nowak G, Schwachenwald R, Arnold H: Early management in poor grade aneurysm patients. Acta Neurochir (Wien) 126:33–37, 1994.

304. Steudel WI, Reif J, Voges M: Modulated surgery in the management of ruptured intracranial aneurysm in poor grade patients. Neurol Res 16:49–53, 1994.

305. Ungersbock K, Bocher-Schwarz H, Ulrich P, et al: Aneurysm surgery of patients in poor clinical grade: Indications and experience. Neurol Res 16:31–34, 1994.

306. Shimoda M, Oda S, Shibata M, et al: Results of early surgical evacuation of packed intraventricular hemorrhage from aneurysm rupture in patients with poor-grade subarachnoid hemorrhage. J Neurosurg 91:408–414, 1999.

307. Hutchinson PJ, Power DM, Tripathi P, Kirkpatrick PJ: Outcome from poor grade aneurysmal subarachnoid haemorrhage: Which

poor grade subarachnoid haemorrhage patients benefit from aneurysm clipping? Br J Neurosurg 14:105–109, 2000.

308. Suzuki M, Otawara Y, Doi M, et al: Neurological grades of patients with poor-grade subarachnoid hemorrhage improve after short-term pretreatment. Neurosurgery 47:1098–1105, 2000.

309. Kremer C, Groden C, Hansen HC, et al: Outcome after endovascular treatment of Hunt and Hess Grade IV or V aneurysms: Comparison of anterior versus posterior circulation. Stroke 30:2617–2622, 1999.

310. Groden C, Kremer C, Regelsberger J, et al: Comparison of operative and endovascular treatment of anterior circulation aneurysms in patients in poor grades. Neuroradiology 43:778–783, 2001.

311. van Loon J, Waerzeggers Y, Wilms G, et al: Early endovascular treatment of ruptured cerebral aneurysms in patients in very poor neurological condition. Neurosurgery 50:457–465, 2002.

312. Heros RC, Korosue K, Diebold PM: Surgical excision of cerebral arteriovenous malformations: Late results. Neurosurgery 26:570–578, 1990.

313. Sundt TM, Peipgras DG, Stevens LN: Surgery for supratentorial arteriovenous malformations. Clin Neurosurg 37:49–115, 1991.

314. Sisti MB, Kader A, Stein BM: Microsurgery for 67 intracranial arteriovenous malformations less than 3 cm in diameter. J Neurosurg 79:653–660, 1993.

315. Schaller C, Schramm J: Microsurgical results for small arteriovenous malformations accessible for radiosurgical or embolization treatment. Neurosurgery 40:664–675, 1997.

316. Berenstein A: Cerebral arteriovenous malformations. Am J Neuroradiol 11:220, 1990.

317. Wilkholm G, Lundqvist, Svendsen P: Embolization of cerebral arteriovenous malformations. Part I: Technique, morphology, and complications. Neurosurgery 39:448, 1996.

318. Debrun GM, Aletich V, Ausman JI, et al: Embolization of the nidus of brain arteriovenous malformations with n-butyl cyanoacrylate. Neurosurgery. 40:112–120, 1997.

319. Paulsen RD, Steinberg GK, Norbash AM, et al: Embolization of basal ganglia and thalamic arteriovenous malformations. Neurosurgery 44:991–996, 1999.

320. Song JK, Eskridge JM, Chung EC, et al: Preoperative embolization of cerebral arteriovenous malformations with silk sutures: Analysis and clinical correlation of complications revealed on computerized tomography scanning. J Neurosurg 92:955–960, 2000.

321. Flickinger JC, Kondziolka D, Pollock BE, et al: Complications from arteriovenous malformation radiosurgery: Multivariate analysis and risk modeling. Int J Radiat Oncol Biol Phys 38:485–490, 1997.

322. Sasaki T, Kurita H, Saito I, et al: Arteriovenous malformations in the basal ganglia and thalamus: Management and results in 101 cases. J Neurosurg 88:285, 1998.

323. Pollack B: Stereotactic radiosurgery for arteriovenous malformations. Neurosurg Clin North Am 10:281, 1999.

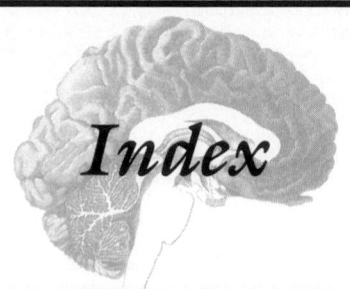

Index

Note: Page numbers followed by the letter f refer to figures, and those followed by t refer to tables. Plate numbers indicate color plates.

Index